The Handbook of
Brain Theory
and Neural Networks

The Handbook of
Brain Theory
and Neural Networks

Second Edition

EDITED BY

Michael A. Arbib

EDITORIAL ADVISORY BOARD

Shun-ichi Amari • John Barnden • Andrew Barto • Ronald Calabrese
Avis Cohen • Joaquín Fuster • Stephen Grossberg • John Hertz
Marc Jeannerod • Mitsuo Kawato • Christof Koch • Wolfgang Maass
James McClelland • Kenneth Miller • Terrence Sejnowski
Noel Sharkey • DeLiang Wang

EDITORIAL ASSISTANT
Prudence H. Arbib

A Bradford Book
THE MIT PRESS
Cambridge, Massachusetts
London, England

This book was set in Times Roman by Impressions Book and Journal Services, Inc., Madison,
Wisconsin, and was printed and bound in the United States of America.

Library of Congress Cataloging-in-Publication Data

The handbook of brain theory and neural networks / edited by Michael A. Arbib;
editorial advisory board, Shun-ichi Amari . . . [et al.]; editorial assistant, Prudence H. Arbib.
    p. cm.
    "A Bradford book."
    Includes bibliographical references and index.
    ISBN 0–262–01197–2
    1. Neural networks (Neurobiology)—Handbooks, manuals, etc.
  2. Neural networks (Computer science)—Handbooks, manuals, etc.
  I. Title: Brain theory and neural networks. II. Arbib, Michael A.
  QP363.3.H36   2002
  612.8′2—dc21   2002038664

Contents

Preface to the Second Edition

Like the first edition, which it replaces, this volume is inspired by two great questions: "How does the brain work?" and "How can we build intelligent machines?" As in the first edition, the heart of the book is a set of close to 300 articles in Part III which cover the whole spectrum of *Brain Theory and Neural Networks*. To help readers orient themselves with respect to this cornucopia, I have written Part I to provide the elementary background on the modeling of both brains and biological and artificial neural networks, and Part II to provide a series of road maps to help readers interested in a particular topic steer through the Part III articles on that topic. More on the motivation and structure of the book can be found in the Preface to the First Edition, which is reproduced after this. I also recommend reading the section "How to Use This Book"—one reader of the first edition who did not do so failed to realize that the articles in Part III were in alphabetical order, or that the Contributors list lets one locate each article written by a given author.

The reader new to the study of *Brain Theory and Neural Networks* will find it wise to read Part I for orientation before jumping into Part III, whereas more experienced readers will find most of Part I familiar. Many readers will simply turn to articles in Part III of particular interest at a given time. However, to help readers who seek a more systematic view of a particular subfield of *Brain Theory and Neural Networks*, Part II provides 22 Road Maps, each providing an essay linking most of the articles on a given topic. (I say "most" because the threshold is subjective for deciding when a particular article has more than a minor mention of the topic in a Road Map.) The Road Maps are organized into 8 groups in Part II as follows:

Grounding Models of Neurons and Networks
    Grounding Models of Neurons
    Grounding Models of Networks
Brain, Behavior, and Cognition
    Neuroethology and Evolution
    Mammalian Brain Regions
    Cognitive Neuroscience
Psychology, Linguistics, and Artificial Intelligence
    Psychology
    Linguistics and Speech Processing
    Artificial Intelligence
Biological Neurons and Networks
    Biological Neurons and Synapses
    Neural Plasticity
    Neural Coding
    Biological Networks
Dynamics and Learning in Artificial Networks
    Dynamic Systems
    Learning in Artificial Networks
    Computability and Complexity
Sensory Systems
    Vision
    Other Sensory Systems
Motor Systems
    Robotics and Control Theory
    Motor Pattern Generators
    Mammalian Motor Control

Applications, Implementations, and Analysis
  Applications
  Implementation and Analysis

The authors of the articles in Part III come from a broad spectrum of disciplines—such as biomedical engineering, cognitive science, computer science, electrical engineering, linguistics, mathematics, physics, neurology, neuroscience, and psychology—and have worked hard to make their articles accessible to readers across the spectrum. The utility of each article is enhanced by cross-references to other articles within the body of the article, and lists at the end of the article referring the reader to road maps, background material, and related reading.

To get some idea of how radically the new edition differs from the old, note that the new edition has 285 articles in Part III, as against the 266 articles of the first edition. Of the articles that appeared in the first edition, only 9 are reprinted unchanged. Some 135 have been updated (or even completely rewritten) by their original authors, and more than 30 have been written anew by new authors. In addition, there are over 100 articles on new topics. The primary shift of emphasis from the first edition has been to drastically reduce the number of articles on applications of artificial neural networks (from astronomy to steelmaking) and to greatly increase the coverage of models of fundamental neurobiology and neural network approaches to language, and to add the new papers which are now listed in the Road Maps on Cognitive Neuroscience, Neural Coding, and Other Sensory Systems (i.e., other than Vision, for which coverage has also been increased). Certainly, a number of the articles in the first edition remain worthy of reading in themselves, but the aim has been to make the new edition a self-contained introduction to brain theory and neural networks in all its current breadth and richness.

The new edition not only appears in print but also has its own web site.

Acknowledgments

My foremost acknowledgment is again to Prue Arbib, who served as Editorial Assistant during the long and arduous process of eliciting and assembling the many, many contributions to Part III. I thank the members of the Editorial Advisory Board, who helped update the list of articles from the first edition and focus the search for authors, and I thank these authors not only for their contributions to Part III but also for suggesting further topics and authors for the *Handbook*, in an ever-widening circle as work advanced on this new edition. I also owe a great debt to the hundreds of reviewers who so constructively contributed to the final polishing of the articles that now appear in Part III. Finally, I thank the staff of P. M. Gordon Associates and of The MIT Press for once again meeting the high standards of copy editing and book production that contributed so much to the success of the first edition.

Michael A. Arbib
Los Angeles and La Jolla
October 2002

Preface to the First Edition

This volume is inspired by two great questions: "How does the brain work?" and "How can we build intelligent machines?" It provides no simple, single answer to either question because no single answer, simple or otherwise, exists. However, in hundreds of articles it charts the immense progress made in recent years in answering many related, but far more specific, questions.

The term *neural networks* has been used for a century or more to describe the networks of biological neurons that constitute the nervous systems of animals, whether invertebrates or vertebrates. Since the 1940s, and especially since the 1980s, the term has been used for a technology of parallel computation in which the computing elements are "artificial neurons" loosely modeled on simple properties of biological neurons, usually with some adaptive capability to change the strengths of connections between the neurons.

Brain theory is centered on "computational neuroscience," the use of computational techniques to model biological neural networks, but also includes attempts to understand the brain and its function through a variety of theoretical constructs and computer analogies. In fact, as the following pages reveal, much of brain theory is not about neural networks per se, but focuses on structural and functional "networks" whose units are in scales both coarser and finer than that of the neuron. Computer scientists, engineers, and physicists have analyzed and applied artificial neural networks inspired by the adaptive, parallel computing style of the brain, but this *Handbook* will also sample non-neural approaches to the design and analysis of "intelligent" machines. In between the biologists and the technologists are the connectionists. They use artificial neural networks in psychology and linguistics and make related contributions to artificial intelligence, using neuron-like unites which interact "in the style of the brain" at a more abstract level than that of individual biological neurons.

Many texts have described limited aspects of one subfield or another of brain theory and neural networks, but no truly comprehensive overview is available. The aim of this *Handbook* is to fill that gap, presenting the entire range of the following topics: detailed models of single neurons; analysis of a wide variety of neurobiological systems; "connectionist" studies; mathematical analyses of abstract neural networks; and technological applications of adaptive, artificial neural networks and related methodologies. The excitement, and the frustration, of these topics is that they span such a broad range of disciplines, including mathematics, statistical physics and chemistry, neurology and neurobiology, and computer science and electrical engineering, as well as cognitive psychology, artificial intelligence, and philosophy. Much effort, therefore, has gone into making the book accessible to readers with varied backgrounds (an undergraduate education in one of the above areas, for example, or the frequent reading of related articles at the level of the *Scientific American*) while still providing a clear view of much of the recent specialized research.

The heart of the book comes in Part III, in which the breadth of brain theory and neural networks is sampled in 266 articles, presented in alphabetical order by title. Each article meets the following requirements:

1. It is authoritative within its own subfield, yet accessible to students and experts in a wide range of other fields.
2. It is comprehensive, yet short enough that its concepts can be acquired in a single sitting.
3. It includes a list of references, limited to 15, to give the reader a well-defined and selective list of places to go to initiate further study.
4. It is as self-contained as possible, while providing cross-references to allow readers to explore particular issues of related interest.

Despite the fourth requirement, some articles are more self-contained than others. Some articles can be read with almost no prior knowledge; some can be read with a rather general knowledge of a few key concepts; others require fairly detailed understanding of material covered in other articles. For example, many articles on applications will make sense only if one understands the "backpropagation" technique for training artificial neural networks; and a number of studies of neuronal function will make sense only if one has at least some idea of the Hodgkin-Huxley equation. Whenever appropriate, therefore, the articles include advice on background articles.

Parts I and II of the book provide a more general approach to helping readers orient themselves. Part I: Background presents a perspective on the "landscape" of brain theory and neural networks, including an exposition of the key concepts for viewing neural networks as dynamic, adaptive systems. Part II: Road Maps then provides an entrée into the many articles of Part III, with "road maps" for 23 different themes. The "Meta-Map," which introduces Part II, groups these themes under eight general headings which, in and of themselves, give some sense of the sweep of the *Handbook*:

Connectionism: Psychology, Linguistics, and Artificial Intelligence
Dynamics, Self-Organization, and Cooperativity
Learning in Artificial Neural Networks
Applications and Implementations
Biological Neurons and Networks
Sensory Systems
Plasticity in Development and Learning
Motor Control

A more detailed view of the structure of the book is provided in the introductory section "How to Use this Book." The aim is to ensure that readers will not only turn to the book to get good brief reviews of topics in their own specialty, but also will find many invitations to browse widely—finding parallels amongst different subfields, or simply enjoying the discovery of interesting topics far from familiar territory.

Acknowledgments

My foremost acknowledgment is to Prue Arbib, who served as Editorial Assistant during the long and arduous process of eliciting and assembling the many, many contributions to Part III; we both thank Paulina Tagle for her help with our work. The initial plan for the book was drawn up in 1991, and it benefited from the advice of a number of friends, especially George Adelman, who shared his experience as Editor of the *Encyclopedia of Neuroscience*. Refinement of the plan and the choice of publishers occupied the first few months of 1992, and I thank Fiona Stevens of The MIT Press for her support of the project from that time onward.

As can be imagined, the plan for a book like this has developed through a time-consuming process of constraint satisfaction. The first steps were to draw up a list of about 20 topic areas (similar to, but not identical with, the 23 areas surveyed in Part II), to populate these areas with a preliminary list of over 100 articles and possible authors, and to recruit the first members of the Editorial Advisory Board to help expand the list of articles and focus on the search for authors. A very satisfying number of authors invited in the first round accepted my invitation, and many of these added their voices to the Editorial Advisory Board in suggesting further topics and authors for the *Handbook*.

I was delighted, stimulated, and informed as I read the first drafts of the articles; but I have also been grateful for the fine spirit of cooperation with which the authors have responded to editorial comments and reviews. The resulting articles not only are authoritative and accessible in themselves, but also have been revised to match the overall style of the *Handbook* and to meet the needs of a broad readership. With this I express my sincere thanks to the editorial advisors, the authors, and the hundreds of reviewers who so constructively contributed to the final polishing of the articles that now appear in Part III; to Doug Gordon and the copy editors and typesetters who transformed the diverse styles of the manuscripts into the style of the *Handbook;* and to the graduate students who helped so much with the proofreading.

Finally, I want to record a debt that did not reach my conscious awareness until well into the editing of this book. It is to Hiram Haydn, who for many years was editor of *The American Scholar*, which is published for general circulation by Phi Beta Kappa. In 1971 or so, Phi Beta Kappa conducted a competition to find authors to receive grants for books to be written, if memory serves aright, for the Bicentennial of the United States. I submitted an entry. Although I was not successful, Mr. Haydn, who had been a member of the jury, wrote to express his appreciation of that entry, and to invite me to write an article for the *Scholar*. What stays in my mind from the ensuing correspondence was the sympathetic way in which he helped me articulate the connections that were at best implicit in my draft, and find the right voice in which to "speak" with the readers of a publication so different from the usual scientific journal. I now realize that it is his example I have tried to follow as I have worked with these hundreds of authors in the quest to see the subject of brain theory and neural networks whole, and to share it with readers of diverse interests and backgrounds.

Michael A. Arbib
Los Angeles and La Jolla
January 1995

How to Use This Book

More than 90% of this book is taken up by Part III, which, in 285 separately authored articles, covers a vast range of topics in brain theory and neural networks, from language to motor control, and from the neurochemistry to the statistical mechanics of memory. Each article has been made as self-contained as possible, but the very breadth of topics means that few readers will be expert in a majority of them. To help the reader new to certain areas of the *Handbook*, I have prepared Part I: Background and Part II: Road Maps. The next few pages describe these aids to comprehension, as well as offering more information on the structure of articles in Part III.

Part I: Background: The Elements of Brain Theory and Neural Networks

Part I provides background material for readers new to computational neuroscience or theoretical approaches to neural networks considered as dynamic, adaptive systems. Section I.1, "Introducing the Neuron," conveys the basic properties of neurons and introduces several basic neural models. Section I.2, "Levels and Styles of Analysis," explains the interdisciplinary nexus in which the present study of brain theory and neural networks is located, with historical roots in cybernetics and with current work going back and forth between brain theory, artificial intelligence, and cognitive psychology. We also review the different levels of analysis involved, with schemas providing the functional units intermediate between an overall task and neural networks. Finally, Section I.3, "Dynamics and Adaptation in Neural Networks," provides a tutorial on the concepts essential for understanding neural networks as dynamic, adaptive systems. We close by stressing that the full understanding of the brain and the improved design of intelligent machines will require not only improvements in the learning methods presented in Section I.3, but also fuller understanding of architectures based on networks of networks, with initial structures well constrained for the task at hand.

Part II: Road Maps: A Guided Tour of Brain Theory and Neural Networks

The reader who wants to survey a major theme of brain theory and neural networks, rather than seeking articles in Part III one at a time, will find in Part II a set of 22 road maps that, among them, place every article in Part III in a thematic perspective. Section II.1 presents a Meta-Map, which briefly surveys all these themes, grouping them under eight general headings:

Grounding Models of Neurons and Networks
  Grounding Models of Neurons
  Grounding Models of Networks
Brain, Behavior, and Cognition
  Neuroethology and Evolution
  Mammalian Brain Regions
  Cognitive Neuroscience
Psychology, Linguistics, and Artificial Intelligence
  Psychology
  Linguistics and Speech Processing
  Artificial Intelligence
Biological Neurons and Networks
  Biological Neurons and Synapses
  Neural Plasticity
  Neural Coding
  Biological Networks

Dynamics and Learning in Artificial Networks
   Dynamic Systems
   Learning in Artificial Networks
   Computability and Complexity
Sensory Systems
   Vision
   Other Sensory Systems
Motor Systems
   Robotics and Control Theory
   Motor Pattern Generators
   Mammalian Motor Control
Applications, Implementations, and Analysis
   Applications
   Implementation and Analysis

This ordering of the themes has no special significance. It is simply one way to approach the richness of the *Handbook*, making it easy for you to identify one or two key road maps of special interest. By the same token, the order of articles in each of the 22 road maps that follow the Meta-Map is one among many such orderings. Each road map starts with an alphabetical listing of the articles most relevant to the current theme. The road map itself will provide suggestions for *interesting* traversals of articles, but this need not imply that an article provides *necessary* background for the articles it precedes.

Part III: Articles

Part III comprises 285 articles. These articles are arranged in alphabetical order, both to make it easier to find a specific topic (although a Subject Index is provided as well, and the alphabetical list of Contributors on page 1241 lists all the articles to which each author has contributed) and because a given article may be relevant to more than one of the themes of Part II, a fact that would be hidden were the article to be relegated to a specific section devoted to a single theme. Most of these articles assume some prior familiarity with neural networks, whether biological or artificial, and so the reader new to neural networks is encouraged to master the material in Part I before tackling Part III.

Most articles in Part III have the following structure: The introduction provides a non-technical overview of the material covered in the whole article, while the final section provides a discussion of key points, open questions, and linkages with other areas of brain theory and neural networks. The intervening sections may be more or less technical, depending on the nature of the topic, but the first and last sections should give most readers a basic appreciation of the topic, irrespective of such technicalities. The bibliography for each article contains about 15 references. People who find their favorite papers omitted from the list should blame my editorial decision, not the author's judgment. The style I chose for the *Handbook* was *not* to provide exhaustive coverage of research papers for the expert. Rather, references are there primarily to help readers who look for an *introduction* to the literature on the given topic, including background material, relevant review articles, and original research citations. In addition to formal references to the literature, each article contains numerous cross-references to other articles in the *Handbook*. These may occur either in the body of the article in the form THE TITLE OF THE ARTICLE IN SMALL CAPS, or at the end of the article, designated as "**Related Reading**." In addition to suggestions for related reading, the reader will find, just prior to the list of references in each article, a mention of the **road map(s)** in which the article is discussed, as well as **background** material, when the article is more advanced.

In summary, turn directly to Part III when you need information on a specific topic. Read sections of Part I to gain a general perspective on the basic concepts of brain theory and neural networks. For an overview of some theme, read the Meta-Map in Part II to choose road maps in Part II; read a road map to choose articles in Part III. A road map can also be used as an explicit guide for systematic study of the area under review. Then continue your exploration through further use of road maps, by following cross-references in Part III, by looking up terms of interest in the index, or simply by letting serendipity take its course as you browse through Part III at random.

Part I: Background

The Elements of Brain Theory
and Neural Networks

Michael A. Arbib

How to Use Part I

Part I provides background material, summarizing a set of concepts established for the formal study of neurons and neural networks by 1986. As such, it is designed to hold few, if any, surprises for readers with a fair background in computational neuroscience or theoretical approaches to neural networks considered as dynamic, adaptive systems. Rather, Part I is designed for the many readers—be they neuroscience experimentalists, psychologists, philosophers, or technologists—who are sufficiently new to *brain theory and neural networks* that they can benefit from a compact overview of basic concepts prior to reading the road maps of Part II and the articles in Part III. Of course, much of what is covered in Part I is also covered at some length in the articles in Part III, and cross-references will steer the reader to these articles for alternative expositions and reviews of current research. In this exposition, as throughout the *Handbook*, we will move back and forth between *computational neuroscience*, where the emphasis is on modeling biological neurons, and *neural computing*, where the emphasis shifts back and forth between biological models and artificial neural networks based loosely on abstractions from biology, but driven more by technological utility than by biological considerations.

Section I.1, "Introducing the Neuron," conveys the basic properties of neurons, receptors, and effectors, and then introduces several simple neural models, including the discrete-time McCulloch-Pitts model and the continuous-time leaky integrator model. References to Part III alert the reader to more detailed properties of neurons which are essential for the neuroscientist and provide interesting hints about future design features for the technologist.

Section I.2, "Levels and Styles of Analysis," is designed to give the reader a feel for the interdisciplinary nexus in which the present study of brain theory and neural networks is located. The selection begins with a historical fragment which traces our federation of disciplines back to their roots in cybernetics, the study of control and communication in animals and machines. We look at the way in which the research addresses brains, machines, and minds, going back and forth between brain theory, artificial intelligence, and cognitive psychology. We then review the different levels of analysis involved, whether we study brains or intelligent machines, and the use of schemas to provide intermediate functional units that bridge the gap between an overall task and the neural networks which implement it.

Section I.3, "Dynamics and Adaptation in Neural Networks," provides a tutorial on the concepts essential for understanding neural networks as dynamic, adaptive systems. It introduces the basic dynamic systems concepts of stability, limit cycles, and chaos, and relates Hopfield nets to attractors and optimization. It then introduces a number of basic concepts concerning adaptation in neural nets, with discussions of pattern recognition, associative memory, Hebbian plasticity and network self-organization, perceptrons, network complexity, gradient descent and credit assignment, and backpropagation. This section, and with it Part I, closes with a cautionary note. The basic learning rules and adaptive architectures of neural networks have already illuminated a number of biological issues and led to useful technological applications. However, these networks must have their initial structure well constrained (whether by evolution or technological design) to yield approximate solutions to the system's tasks—solutions that can then be efficiently and efficaciously shaped by experience. Moreover, the full understanding of the brain and the improved design of intelligent machines will require not only improvements in these learning methods and their initialization, but also a fuller understanding of architectures based on networks of networks. Cross-references to articles in Part III will set the reader on the path to this fuller understanding. Because Part I focuses on the basic concepts established for the formal study of neurons and neural networks by 1986, it differs hardly at all from Part I of the first edition of the *Handbook*. By contrast, Part II, which provides the road maps that guide readers through the radically updated Part III, has been completely rewritten for the present edition to reflect the latest research results.

I.1. Introducing the Neuron

We introduce the *neuron*. The dangerous word in the preceding sentence is *the*. In biology, there are radically different types of neurons in the human brain, and endless variations in neuron types of other species. In brain theory, the complexities of real neurons are abstracted in many ways to aid in understanding different aspects of neural network development, learning, or function. In *neural computing* (technology based on networks of "neuron-like" units), the artificial neurons are designed as variations on the abstractions of brain theory and are implemented in software, or VLSI or other media. There is no such thing as a "typical" neuron, yet this section will nonetheless present examples and models which provide a starting point, an essential set of key concepts, for the appreciation of the many variations on the theme of neurons and neural networks presented in Part III.

An analogy to the problem we face here might be to define *vehicle* for a handbook of transportation. A vehicle could be a car, a train, a plane, a rowboat, or a forklift truck. It might or might not carry people. The people could be crew or passengers, and so on. The problem would be to give a few key examples of form (such as car versus plane) and function (to carry people or goods, by land, air, or sea, etc.). Moreover, we would find interesting examples of co-evolution: for example, modern highway systems would not have been created without the pressure of increasing car traffic; most features of cars are adapted to the existence of sealed roads, and some features (e.g., cruise control) are specifically adapted to good freeway conditions. Following a similar procedure, Part III offers diverse examples of neural form and function in both biology and technology.

Here, we start with the observation that a brain is made up of a network of cells called neurons, coupled to receptors and effectors. Neurons are intimately connected with glial cells, which provide support functions for neural networks. New empirical data show the importance of glia in regeneration of neural networks after damage and in maintaining the neurochemical milieu during normal operation. However, such data have had very little impact on neural modeling and so will not be considered further here. The input to the network of neurons is provided by *receptors*, which continually monitor changes in the external and internal environment. Cells called *motor neurons* (or *motoneurons*), governed by the activity of the neural network, control the movement of muscles and the secretion of glands. In between, an intricate network of neurons (a few hundred neurons in some simple creatures, hundreds of billions in a human brain) continually combines the signals from the receptors with signals encoding past experience to barrage the motor neurons with signals that will yield adaptive interactions with the environment. In animals with backbones (vertebrates, including mammals in general and humans in particular), this network is called the *central nervous system* (CNS), and the brain constitutes the most headward part of this system, linked to the receptors and effectors of the body via the spinal cord. Invertebrate nervous systems (neural networks) provide astounding variations on the vertebrate theme, thanks to eons of divergent evolution. Thus, while the human brain may be the source of rich analogies for technologists in search of "artificial intelligence," both invertebrates and vertebrates provide endless ideas for technologists designing neural networks for sensory processing, robot control, and a host of other applications. (A few of the relevant examples may be found in the Part II road maps, **Vision, Robotics and Control Theory, Motor Pattern Generators,** and **Neuroethology and Evolution**.)

The brain provides far more than a simple stimulus-response chain from receptors to effectors (although there are such reflex paths). Rather, the vast network of neurons is interconnected in loops and tangled skeins so that signals entering the net from the receptors interact there with the billions of signals already traversing the system, not only to yield the signals that control the effectors but also to modify the very properties of the network itself, so that future behavior will reflect prior experience.

The Diversity of Receptors

Rod and cone receptors in the eyes respond to light, hair cells in the ears respond to pressure, and other cells in the tongue and the mouth respond to subtle traces of chemicals. In addition to touch receptors, there are receptors in the skin that are responsive to movement or to temperature, or that signal painful stimuli. These external senses may be divided into two classes: (1) the proximity senses, such as touch and taste, which sense objects in contact with the body surface, and (2) the distance senses, such as vision and hearing, which let us sense objects distant from the body. Olfaction is somewhere in between, using chemical signals "right under our noses" to sense nonproximate objects. Moreover, even the proximate senses can yield information about nonproximate objects, as when we feel the wind or the heat of a fire. More generally, much of our appreciation of the world around us rests on the unconscious fusion of data from diverse sensory systems.

The appropriate activity of the effectors must depend on comparing where the system should be—the current target of an ongoing movement—with where it is now. Thus, in addition to the

external receptors, there are receptors that monitor the activity of muscles, tendons, and joints to provide a continual source of feedback about the tensions and lengths of muscles and the angles of the joints, as well as their velocities. The vestibular system in the head monitors gravity and accelerations. Here, the receptors are hair cells monitoring fluid motion. There are also receptors to monitor the chemical level of the bloodstream and the state of the heart and the intestines. Cells in the liver monitor glucose, while others in the kidney check water balance. Receptors in the *hypothalamus*, itself a part of the brain, also check the balance of water and sugar. The hypothalamus then integrates these diverse messages to direct behavior or other organs to restore the balance. If we stimulate the hypothalamus, an animal may drink copious quantities of water or eat enormous quantities of food, even though it is already well supplied; the brain has received a signal that water or food is lacking, and so it instructs the animal accordingly, irrespective of whatever contradictory signals may be coming from a distended stomach.

Basic Properties of Neurons

To understand the processes that intervene between receptors and effectors, we must have a closer look at "the" neuron. As already emphasized, *there is no such thing as a typical neuron.* However, we will summarize properties shared by many neurons. The "basic neuron" shown in Figure 1 is abstracted from a motor neuron of mammalian spinal cord. From the *soma* (cell body) protrudes a number of ramifying branches called *dendrites*; the soma and dendrites constitute the input surface of the neuron. There also extrudes from the cell body, at a point called the *axon hillock* (abutting the initial segment), a long fiber called the *axon*, whose branches form the *axonal arborization*. The tips of the branches of the axon, called *nerve terminals* or *boutons*, impinge on other neurons or on effectors. The locus of interaction between a bouton and the cell on which it impinges is called a *synapse*, and we say that the cell with the bouton *synapses upon* the cell with which the connection is made. In fact, axonal branches of some neurons can have many varicosities, corresponding to synapses, along their length, not just at the end of the branch.

We can imagine the flow of information as shown by the arrows in Figure 1. Although "conduction" can go in either direction on the axon, most synapses tend to "communicate" activity to the dendrites or soma of the cell they synapse upon, whence activity passes to the axon hillock and then down the axon to the terminal arbo-

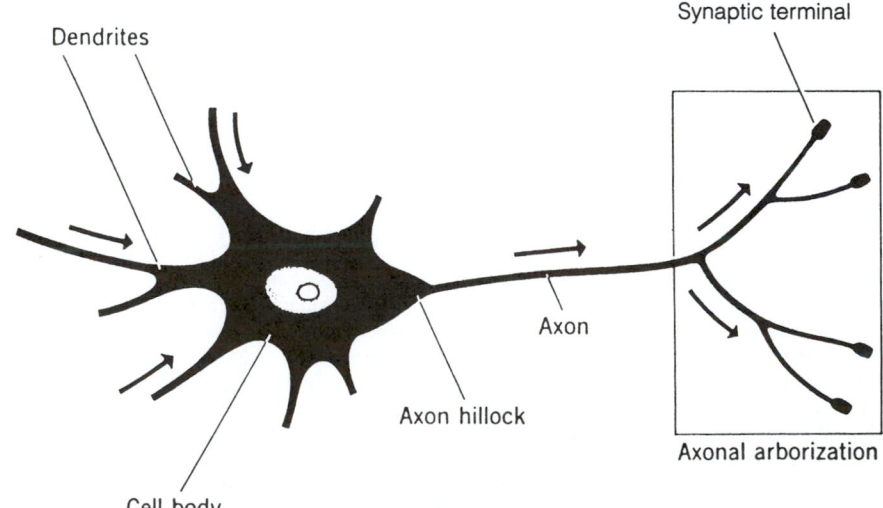

Figure 1. A "basic neuron" abstracted from a motor neuron of mammalian spinal cord. The dendrites and soma (cell body) constitute the major part of the input surface of the neuron. The axon is the "output line." The tips of the branches of the axon form synapses upon other neurons or upon effectors (although synapses may occur along the branches of an axon as well as at the ends). (From Arbib, M. A., 1989, *The Metaphorical Brain 2: Neural Networks and Beyond,* New York: Wiley-Interscience, p. 52. Reproduced with permissions. Copyright © 1989 by John Wiley & Sons, Inc.)

rization. The axon can be very long indeed. For instance, the cell body of a neuron that controls the big toe lies in the spinal cord and thus has an axon that runs the complete length of the leg. We may contrast the immense length of the axon of such a neuron with the very small size of many of the neurons in our heads. For example, amacrine cells in the retina have branchings that cannot appropriately be labeled dendrites or axons, for they are short and may well communicate activity in either direction to serve as local modulators of the surrounding network. In fact, the propagation of signals in the "counter-direction" on dendrites away from the soma has in recent years been seen to play an important role in neuronal function, but this feature is not included in the account of the "basic neuron" given here (see DENDRITIC PROCESSING—titles in SMALL CAPS refer to articles in Part III).

To understand more about neuronal "communication," we emphasize that the cell is enclosed by a membrane, across which there is a difference in electrical charge. If we change this potential difference between the inside and outside, the change can propagate in much the same passive way that heat is conducted down a rod of metal: a normal change in potential difference across the cell membrane can propagate in a passive way so that the change occurs later, and becomes smaller, the farther away we move from the site of the original change. This passive propagation is governed by the *cable equation*

$$\frac{\partial V}{\partial t} = \frac{\partial^2 V}{\partial x^2}$$

If the starting voltage at a point on the axon is V_0, and no further conditions are imposed, the potential will decay exponentially, having value $V_{(x)} = V_0 e^{-x}$ at distance x from the starting point, where the length unit, the *length constant*, is the distance in which the potential changes by a factor of $1/e$. This length unit will differ from axon to axon. For "short" cells (such as the rods, cones, and bipolar cells of the retina), passive propagation suffices to signal a potential change from one end to the other; but if the axon is long, this mechanism is completely inadequate, since changes at one end will decay almost completely before reaching the other end. Fortunately, most nerve cells have the further property that if the change in potential difference is large enough (we say it exceeds a *threshold*), then in a cylindrical configuration such as the axon, a pulse can be generated that will actively propagate at full amplitude instead of fading passively.

If propagation of various potential differences on the dendrites and soma of a neuron yields a potential difference across the membrane at the axon hillock which exceeds a certain threshold, then a regenerative process is started: the electrical change at one place is enough to trigger this process at the next place, yielding a *spike* or *action potential*, an undiminishing pulse of potential difference propagating down the axon. After an impulse has propagated along the length of the axon, there is a short *refractory period* during which a new impulse cannot be propagated along the axon.

The propagation of action potentials is now very well understood. Briefly, the change in membrane potential is mediated by the flow of ions, especially sodium and potassium, across the membrane. Hodgkin and Huxley (1952) showed that the *conductance* of the membrane to sodium and potassium ions—the ease with which they flow across the membrane—depends on the transmembrane voltage. They developed elegant equations describing the voltage and time dependence of the sodium and potassium conductances. These equations (see the article AXONAL MODELING in Part III) have given us great insight into cellular function. Much mathematical research has gone into studying Hodgkin-Huxley-like equations, showing, for example, that neurons can support rhythmic pulse generation even without input (see OSCILLATORY AND BURSTING PROPERTIES OF NEURONS), and explicating trig-

gered long-distance propagation. Hodgkin and Huxley used curve fitting from experimental data to determine the terms for conductance change in their model. Subsequently, much research has probed the structure of complex molecules that form *channels* which selectively allow the passage of specific ions through the membrane (see ION CHANNELS: KEYS TO NEURONAL SPECIALIZATION). This research has demonstrated how channel properties not only account for the terms in the Hodgkin-Huxley equation, but also underlie more complex dynamics which may allow even small patches of neural membrane to act like complex computing elements. At present, most artificial neurons used in applications are very simple indeed, and much future technology will exploit these "subneural subtleties."

An impulse traveling along the axon from the axon hillock triggers new impulses in each of its branches (or *collaterals*), which in turn trigger impulses in their even finer branches. Vertebrate axons come in two varieties, myelinated and unmyelinated. The myelinated fibers are wrapped in a sheath of *myelin* (Schwann cells in the periphery, oligodendrocytes in the CNS—these are glial cells, and their role in axonal conduction is the primary role of glia considered in neural modeling to date). The small gaps between successive segments of the myelin sheath are called *nodes of Ranvier*. Instead of the somewhat slow active propagation down an unmyelinated fiber, the nerve impulse in a myelinated fiber jumps from node to node, thus speeding passage and reducing energy requirements (see AXONAL MODELING).

Surprisingly, at most synapses, the direct cause of the change in potential of the postsynaptic membrane is not electrical but chemical. When an impulse arrives at the presynaptic terminal, it causes the release of *transmitter* molecules (which have been stored in the bouton in little packets called vesicles) through the presynaptic membrane. The transmitter then diffuses across the very small *synaptic cleft* to the other side, where it binds on receptors on the postsynaptic membrane to change the conductance of the postsynaptic cell. The effect of the "classical" transmitters (later we shall talk of other kinds, the neuromodulators) is of two basic kinds: either *excitatory*, tending to move the potential difference across the postsynaptic membrane in the direction of the threshold (*depolarizing* the membrane), or *inhibitory*, tending to move the polarity away from the threshold (*hyperpolarizing* the membrane). There are some exceptional cell appositions that are so large or have such tight coupling (the so-called gap junctions) that the impulse affects the postsynaptic membrane without chemical mediation (see NEOCORTEX: CHEMICAL AND ELECTRICAL SYNAPSES).

Most neural modeling to date focuses on the excitatory and inhibitory interactions that occur on a fast time scale (a millisecond, more or less), and most biological (as distinct from technological) models assume that all synapses *from* a neuron have the same "sign." However, neurons may also secrete transmitters that modulate the function of a circuit on some quite extended time scale. Modeling that takes account of this *neuromodulation* (see SYNAPTIC INTERACTIONS and NEUROMODULATION IN INVERTEBRATE NERVOUS SYSTEMS) will become increasingly important in the future, since it allows cells to change their function, enabling a neural network to switch dramatically its overall mode of activity.

The excitatory or inhibitory effect of the transmitter released when an impulse arrives at a bouton generally causes a subthreshold change in the postsynaptic membrane. Nonetheless, the cooperative effect of many such subthreshold changes may yield a potential change at the axon hillock that exceeds threshold, and if this occurs at a time when the axon has passed the refractory period of its previous firing, then a new impulse will be fired down the axon.

Synapses can differ in shape, size, form, and effectiveness. The geometrical relationships between the different synapses impinging on the cell determine what patterns of synaptic activation will yield the appropriate temporal relationships to excite the cell (see

DENDRITIC PROCESSING). A highly simplified example (Figure 2) shows how the properties of nervous tissue just presented would indeed allow a simple neuron, by its very dendritic geometry, to compute some useful function (cf. Rall, 1964, p. 90). Consider a neuron with four dendrites, each receiving a single synapse from a visual receptor, so arranged that synapses A, B, C, and D (from left to right) are at increasing distances from the axon hillock. (This is not meant to be a model of a neuron in the retina of an actual organism; rather, it is designed to make vivid the potential richness of single neuron computations.) We assume that each receptor re-

acts to the passage of a spot of light above its surface by yielding a generator potential which yields, in the postsynaptic membrane, the same time course of depolarization. This time course is propagated passively, and the farther it is propagated, the later and the lower is its peak. If four inputs reached A, B, C, and D simultaneously, their effect may be less than the threshold required to trigger a spike there. However, if an input reaches D before one reaches C, and so on, in such a way that the peaks of the four resultant time courses at the axon hillock coincide, the total effect could well exceed threshold. This, then, is a cell that, although very

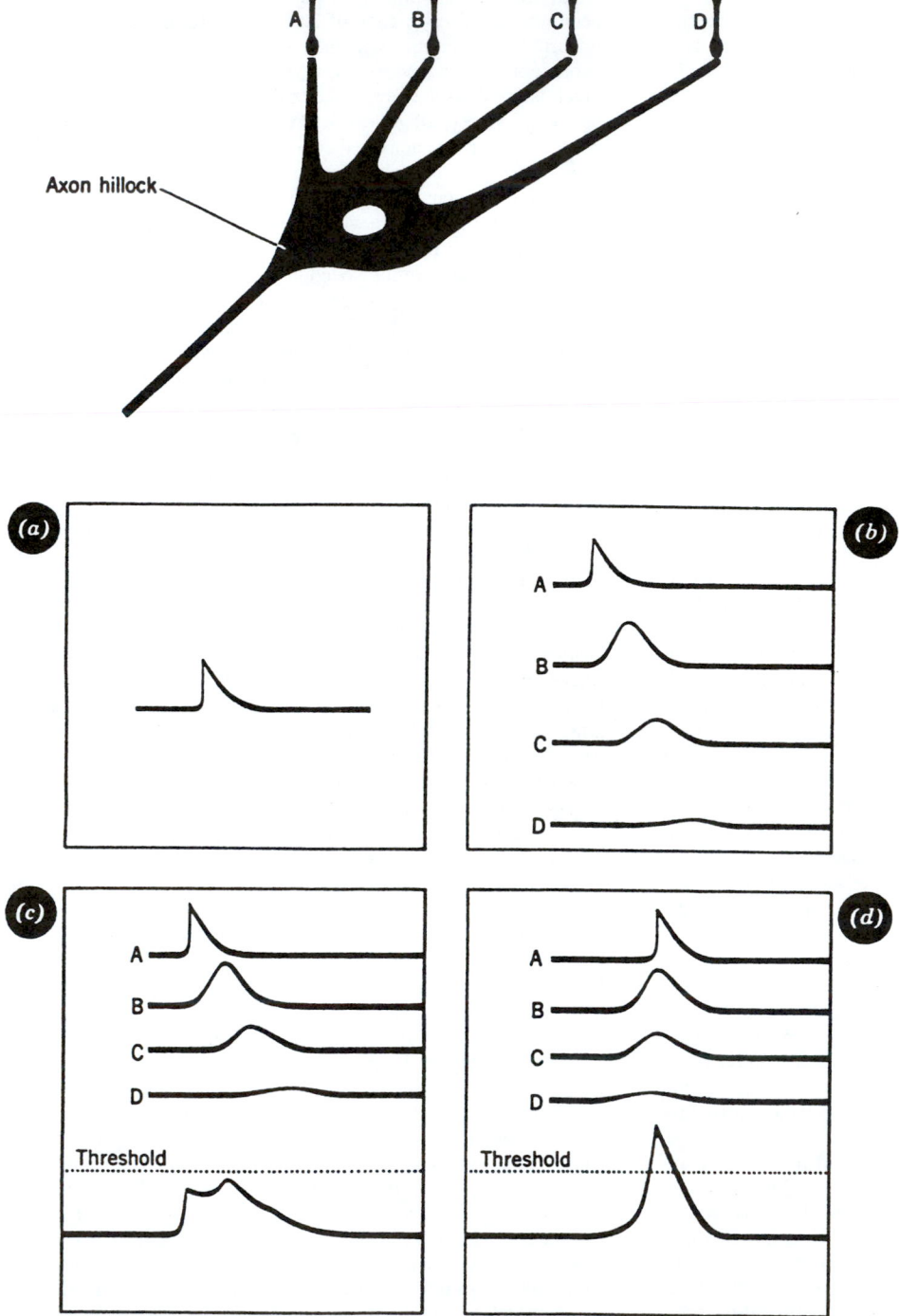

Figure 2. An example, conceived by Wilfrid Rall, of the subtleties that can be revealed by neural modeling when dendritic properties (in this case, length-dependent conduction time) are taken into account. As shown in Part *C*, the effect of simultaneously activating all inputs may be subthreshold, yet the cell may respond when inputs traverse the cell from right to left (*D*). (From Arbib, M. A., 1989, *The Metaphorical Brain 2: Neural Networks and Beyond*, New York: Wiley-Interscience, p. 60. Reproduced with permission. Copyright © 1989 by John Wiley & Sons, Inc.)

simple, can detect direction of motion across its input. It responds only if the spot of light is moving from right to left, and if the velocity of that motion falls within certain limits. Our cell will not respond to a stationary object, or one moving from left to right, because the asymmetry of placement of the dendrites on the cell body yields a preference for one direction of motion over others (for a more realistic account of biological mechanisms, see DIREC-TIONAL SELECTIVITY). This simple example illustrates that the *form* (i.e., the geometry) of the cell can have a great impact on the *function* of the cell, and we thus speak of *form-function* relations. When we note that neurons in the human brain may have 10,000 or more synapses upon them, we can understand that the range of functions of single neurons is indeed immense.

Receptors and Effectors

On the "input side," receptors share with neurons the property of generating potentials, which are transmitted to various synapses upon neurons. However, the input surface of a receptor does not receive synapses from other neurons, but can transduce environmental energy into changes in membrane potential, which may then propagate either actively or passively. (Visual receptors do not generate spikes; touch receptors in the body and limbs use spike trains to send their message to the spinal cord.) For instance, the rods and cones of the eye contain various pigments that react chemically to light in different frequency bands, and these chemical reactions, in turn, lead to local potential changes, called generator potentials, in the membrane. If the light falling on an array of rods and cones is appropriately patterned, then their potential changes will induce interneuron changes to, in turn, fire certain ganglion cells (retinal output neurons whose axons course toward the brain). Properties of the light pattern will thus be signaled farther into the nervous system as trains of impulses (see RETINA).

At the receptors, increasing the intensity of stimulation will increase the generator potential. If we go to the first level of neurons that generate pulses, the axons "reset" each time they fire a pulse and then have to get back to a state where the threshold and the input potential meet. The higher the generator potential, the shorter the time until they meet again, and thus the higher the frequency of the pulse. Thus, at the "input" it is a useful first approximation to say that intensity or quantity of stimulation is coded in terms of pulse frequency (more stimulus ≈ more spikes), whereas the quality or type of stimulus is coded by different lines carrying signals from different types of receptors. As we leave the periphery and move toward more "computational" cells, we no longer have such simple relationships, but rather interactions of inhibitory cells and excitatory cells, with each inhibitory input moving a cell away from, and each excitatory input moving it toward, threshold.

To discuss the "output side," we must first note that a muscle is made up of many thousands of muscle fibers. The motor neurons that control the muscle fibers lie in the spinal cord or the brainstem, whence their axons may have to travel vast distances (by neuronal standards) before synapsing upon the muscle fibers. The smallest functional entity on the output side is thus the *motor unit*, which consists of a motor neuron cell body, its axon, and the group of muscle fibers the axon influences.

A muscle fiber is like a neuron to the extent that it receives its input via a synapse from a motor neuron. However, the response of the muscle fiber to the spread of depolarization is to contract. Thus, the motor neurons which synapse upon the muscle fibers can determine, by the pattern of their impulses, the extent to which the whole muscle comprised of those fibers contracts, and can thus control movement. (Similar remarks apply to those cells that secrete various chemicals into the bloodstream or gut, or those that secrete sweat or tears.)

Synaptic activation at the *motor end-plate* (i.e., the synapse of a motor neuron upon a muscle fiber) yields a brief "twitch" of the muscle fiber. A low repetition rate of action potentials arriving at a motor end-plate causes a train of twitches, in each of which the mechanical response lasts longer than the action potential stimulus. As the frequency of excitation increases, a second action potential will arrive while the mechanical effect of the prior stimulus still persists. This causes a mechanical summation or fusion of contractions. Up to a point, the degree of summation increases as the stimulus interval becomes shorter, although the summation effect decreases as the interval between the stimuli approaches the refractory period of the muscle, and maximum tension occurs. This limiting response is called a *tetanus*. To increase the tension exerted by a muscle, it is then necessary to recruit more and more fibers to contract. For more delicate motions, such as those involving the fingers of primates, each motor neuron may control only a few muscle fibers. In other locations, such as the shoulder, one motor neuron alone may control thousands of muscle fibers. As descending signals in the spinal cord command a muscle to contract more and more, they do this by causing motor neurons with larger and larger thresholds to start firing. The result is that fairly small fibers are brought in first, and then larger and larger fibers are recruited. The result, known as Henneman's Size Principle, is that at any stage, the increment of activation obtained by recruiting the next group of motor units involves about the same percentage of extra force being applied, aiding smoothness of movement (see MOTO-NEURON RECRUITMENT).

Since there is no command that a neuron may send to a muscle fiber that will cause it to lengthen—all the neuron can do is stop sending it commands to contract—the muscles of an animal are usually arranged in pairs. The contraction of one member of the pair will then act around a pivot to cause the expansion of the other member of the pair. Thus, one set of muscles *extends* the elbow joint, while another set *flexes* the elbow joint. To extend the elbow joint, we do not signal the *flexors* to lengthen, we just stop signaling them to contract, and then they will be automatically lengthened as the *extensor* muscles contract. For convenience, we often label one set of muscles as the "prime mover" or *agonist*, and the opposing set as the *antagonist*. However, in such joints as the shoulder, which are not limited to one degree of freedom, many muscles, rather than an agonist-antagonist pair, participate. Most real movements involve many joints. For example, the wrist must be fixed, holding the hand in a position bent backward with respect to the forearm, for the hand to grip with its maximum power. *Synergists* are muscles that act together with the main muscles involved. A large group of muscles work together when one raises something with one's finger. If more force is required, wrist muscles may also be called in; if still more force is required, arm muscles may be used. In any case, muscles all over the body are involved in maintaining posture.

Neural Models

Before presenting more realistic models of the neuron (see PERSPECTIVE ON NEURON MODEL COMPLEXITY; SINGLE-CELL MODELS), we focus on the work of McCulloch and Pitts (1943), which combined neurophysiology and mathematical logic, using the all-or-none property of neuron firing to model the neuron as a binary discrete-time element. They showed how excitation, inhibition, and threshold might be used to construct a wide variety of "neurons." It was the first model to tie the study of neural nets squarely to the idea of computation in its modern sense. The basic idea is to divide time into units comparable to a refractory period so that, in each time period, at most one spike can be generated at the axon hillock of a given neuron. The McCulloch-Pitts neuron (Figure 3A) thus operates on a discrete-time scale, $t = 0, 1, 2, 3, \ldots$, where the

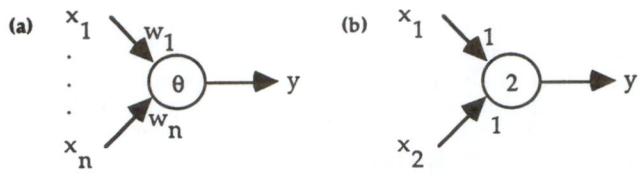

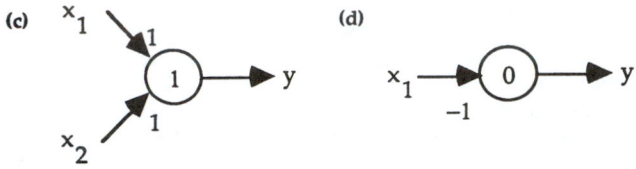

Figure 3. *a*, A McCulloch-Pitts neuron operating on a discrete-time scale. Each input has an attached weight w_i, and the neuron has a threshold θ. The neuron "fires" at time $t + 1$ just in case the weighted values of its inputs at time t is at least θ. *b*, Settings of weights and threshold for neurons that function as an AND gate (i.e., the output fires if x_1 and x_2 both fire). *c*, An OR gate (the output fires if x_1 or x_2, or both fire). *d*, A NOT gate (the output fires if x_1 does NOT fire).

time unit is (in biology) on the order of a millisecond. We write $y(t) = 1$ if a spike does appear at time t, and $y(t) = 0$ if not. Each connection, or *synapse*, from the output of one neuron to the input of another has an attached *weight*. Let w_i be the weight on the *i*th connection onto a given neuron. We call the synapse *excitatory* if $w_i > 0$, and *inhibitory* if $w_i < 0$. We also associate a *threshold* θ with each neuron, and assume exactly one unit of delay in the effect of *all* presynaptic inputs on the cell's output, so that a neuron "fires" (i.e., has value 1 on its output line) at time $t + 1$ if the weighted value of its inputs at time t is at least θ. Formally, if at time t the value of the *i*th input is $x_i(t)$ and the output one time step later is $y(t + 1)$, then

$$y(t + 1) = 1 \quad \text{if and only if} \quad \sum_i w_i x_i(t) \geq \theta$$

Parts *b* through *d* of Figure 3 show how weights and threshold can be set to yield neurons that realize the logical functions AND, OR, and NOT. As a result, McCulloch-Pitts neurons are sufficient to build networks that can function as the control circuitry for a computer carrying out computations of arbitrary complexity; this discovery played a crucial role in the development of automata theory and in the study of learning machines. Although the McCulloch-Pitts neuron no longer plays an active part in *computational neuroscience*, it is still widely used in *neural computing*, especially when it is generalized so that the input and output values can lie anywhere in the range [0, 1] and the function $f(\Sigma_i w_i x_i(t))$, which yields $y(t + 1)$, is a continuously varying function rather than a step function. However, it is one thing to define model neurons with sufficient logical power to subserve any discrete computation; it is quite another to understand how the neurons in actual brains perform their tasks. More generally, the problem is to select just which units to model, and to decide how such units are to be represented. Thus, when we turn from neural computing to computational neuroscience, we must turn to more realistic models of neurons. On the other hand, we may say that neural computing cannot reach its full power without applying new mechanisms based on current and future study of biological neural networks (see the road map **Biological Neurons and Synapses**).

Modern brain theory no longer uses the binary model of the neuron, but instead uses continuous-time models that either rep-

resent the variation in average firing rate of the neuron or actually capture the time course of membrane potentials. It is only through such correlates of measurable brain activity that brain models can really feed back to biological experiments. Such models also require the brain theorist to know a great deal of detailed anatomy and physiology as well as behavioral data. Hodgkin and Huxley (1952) have shown us how much can be learned from analysis of membrane properties about the propagation of electrical activity along the axon; Rall (1964; cf. Figure 2) was a leader in showing that the study of membrane properties in a variety of connected "compartments" of membrane in dendrite, soma, and axon can help us understand small neural circuits, as in the OLFACTORY BULB (q.v.) or for DENDRITIC PROCESSING (q.v.). Nonetheless, in many cases, the complexity of compartmental analysis makes it more insightful to use a more lumped representation of the individual neuron if we are to assemble the model neurons to analyze large networks. A computer simulation of the response of a whole brain region which analyzed each component at the finest level of detail available would be too large to run on even a network of computers. In addition to the importance of detailed models of single neurons in themselves, such studies can also be used to fine-tune more economical models of neurons, which can then serve as the units in models of large networks, whether to model systems in the brain or to design artificial neural networks which exploit subtle neural capabilities.

We may determine units in the brain *physiologically*, e.g., by electrical recording, and *anatomically*, e.g., by staining. In many regions of the brain, we have an excellent correlation between physiological and anatomical units; that is, we know which anatomical entity yields which physiological response. Unfortunately, this is not always the case. We may have data on the electrophysiological correlates of animal behavior, and anatomical data as well, yet not know which specific cell, defined anatomically, yields an observed electrophysiological response. Another problem that we confront in modeling is that we have both too much and too little anatomical detail: too much in that there are many synapses that we cannot put into our model without overloading our capabilities for either mathematical analysis or computer simulation, and too little in that we often do not know which details of synaptology may determine the most important modes of behavior of a particular region of the brain. Judicious choices from available data, and judicious hypotheses concerning missing data, must thus be made in setting up a model, leading to the design of experiments whose results may either confirm these hypotheses or lead to their modification. An important point of good modeling methodology is thus to set up simulations in such a way that we can use different connectivity on different simulations, both to test alternative hypotheses and to respond to new data as they become available.

The simplest "realistic" model consonant with the above material is the *leaky integrator* model. Although some biological neurons communicate by the passive propagation (cable equation) of membrane potential down their (necessarily short) axons, most communicate by the active propagation of "spikes." The generation and propagation of such spikes has been described in detail by the Hodgkin-Huxley equations. However, the leaky integrator model omits such details. It is a continuous-time model based on using the *firing rate* (e.g., the number of spikes traversing the axon in the most recent 20 ms) as a continuously varying *output* measure of the cell's activity, in which the *internal state* of the neuron is described by a single variable, the membrane potential at the spike initiation zone. The firing rate is approximated by a simple, sigmoid function of the membrane potential. That is, we introduce a function σ of the membrane potential m such that $\sigma(m)$ increases from 0 to some maximum value as m increases from $-\infty$ to $+\infty$ (e.g., the sigmoidal function $k/[1 + \exp(-m/\theta)]$, increasing from 0 to its maximum k). Then the firing rate $M(t)$ of the cell is given by the equation:

$$M(t) = \sigma(m(t))$$

The time evolution of the cell's membrane potential is given by a differential equation. Consider first the simple equation

$$\tau \frac{dm(t)}{dt} = -m(t) + h \qquad (1)$$

We say that $m(t)$ is in an *equilibrium* if it does not change under the dynamics described by the differential equation. However, $dm(t)/dt = 0$ if and only if $m(t) = h$, so that h is the *unique* equilibrium of Equation 1. To get more information, we now integrate Equation 1 to get

$$m(t) = e^{-t/\tau}m(0) + (1 - e^{-t/\tau})h$$

which tends to the *resting level h* with *time constant τ* with increasing t so long as τ is positive. We now add synaptic inputs to obtain

$$\tau \frac{dm(t)}{dt} = -m(t) + \sum_i w_i X_i(t) + h \qquad (2)$$

where $X_i(t)$ is the firing rate at the ith input. Thus, an excitatory input ($w_i > 0$) will be such that increasing it will increase $dm(t)/dt$, while an inhibitory input ($w_i < 0$) will have the opposite effect. A neuron described by Equation 2 is called a *leaky integrator neuron*. This is because the equation

$$\tau \frac{dm(t)}{dt} = \sum_i w_i X_i(t) \qquad (3)$$

would simply integrate the inputs with scaling constant τ,

$$m(T) = m(0) + \frac{1}{\tau} \int_0^T \sum_i w_i X_i(t)dt \qquad (4)$$

but the $-m(t)$ term in Equation 3 opposes this integration by a "leakage" of the potential $m(t)$ as it tries to return to its input-free equilibrium h.

It should be noted that, even at this simple level of modeling, there are alternative models. In the foregoing model, we have used subtractive inhibition. But there are inhibitory synapses which seem better described by *shunting* inhibition which, applied at a given point on a dendrite, serves to divide, rather than subtract from, the potential change passively propagating from more distal synapses. Again, the "lumped frequency" model cannot model the relative timing effects crucial to our motion detector example (see Figure 2). These might be approximated by introducing appropriate delay terms

$$\tau \frac{dm(t)}{dt} = -m(t) + \sum_i w_i X_i(t - t_i) + h$$

Another class of neuron models—spiking neurons, including integrate-and-fire neurons—are intermediate in complexity between leaky integrator models in which the output is the average firing rate (see RATE CODING AND SIGNAL PROCESSING) and detailed biophysical models in which the fine details of action potential generation are modeled using the Hodgkin-Huxley equation. In these intermediate models, the output is a spike whose timing is continuously variable as a result of cellular interactions, but the spike is represented simply by its time of occurrence, with no internal structure. For example, one may track the continuous variable (4), then generate a spike each time this quantity reaches threshold, while simultaneously resetting the integral to some baseline value (see INTEGRATE-AND-FIRE NEURONS AND NETWORKS).

Such models include the ability to transmit information very rapidly through small temporal differences between the spikes sent out by different neurons (see SPIKING NEURONS, COMPUTATION WITH).

All this reinforces the observation that there is no modeling approach that is automatically appropriate. Rather, we seek to find the simplest model adequate to address the complexity of a given range of problems. The articles in Part III of the *Handbook* will provide many examples of the diversity of neural models appropriate to different tasks.

More Detailed Properties of Neurons

In Section I.3, the only details we will add to the neuron models just presented will be various, relatively simple, rules of synaptic plasticity. This level of detail (though with many variations) will suffice for a fair range of models of biological neural networks, and for a range of current work on artificial neural networks (ANNs). The road map **Biological Neurons and Synapses** in Part II surveys a set of articles that demonstrate that biological neurons are vastly more complex than the present models suggest. Other road maps show the special structures revealed in "special-purpose" neural circuitry in different species of animals. Table 1 lists some of the relevant articles on such circuits, together with the specific animal types on which the studies were based. The point is that much is to be learned from features specific to many different types of nervous systems, as well as from studies in humans, monkeys, cats, and rats that focus on commonalities with the human nervous system.

An appreciation of this complexity is necessary for the computational neuroscientist wishing to address the increasingly detailed database of experimental neuroscience, but it should also prove important for the technologist looking ahead to the incorporation of new capabilities into the next generation of ANNs. Nonetheless, much can be accomplished with simple models, as we shall see in Section I.3.

Table 1. A Sampling of Articles Showing the Lessons to be Learned from the Study of Nervous Systems Very Different from Those of Humans

Crustacean Stomatogastric System	Crabs and lobsters
Development of Retinotectal Maps	Frogs
Echolocation: Cochleotopic and Computational Maps	Bats
Electrolocation	Electric fish
Half-Center Oscillators Underlying Rhythmic Movements	Various
Invertebrate Models of Learning	*Aplysia* and *Hermissenda*
Locomotion, Invertebrate	Various insects
Locust Flight: Components and Mechanisms in the Motor	Locusts
Motor Primitives	Frogs
Neuromodulation in Invertebrate Nervous Systems	Various
Oscillatory and Bursting Properties of Neurons	Various
Scratch Reflex	Turtles
Sound Localization and Binaural Processing	Owls
Spinal Cord of Lamprey: Generation of Locomotor Patterns	Lampreys
Visual Course Control in Flies	Flies
Visuomotor Coordination in Frog and Toad	Frogs and toads
Visuomotor Coordination in Salamander	Salamanders

I.2. Levels and Styles of Analysis

Many articles in this book show the benefits of interplay between biology and technology. Nonetheless, it is essential to distinguish between studying the brain and building an effective technology for intelligent systems and computation, and to distinguish among the various levels of investigation that exist (from the molecular to the system level) in these related, but by no means identical, disciplines. The present section provides a fuller sense of the disciplines that come together in brain theory and neural networks, and of the different levels of analysis involved in the study of complex biological and technological systems.

A Historical Fragment

Perhaps the simplest history of brain theory and neural networks would restrict itself to just three items: studies by McCulloch and Pitts (1943), Hebb (1949), and Rosenblatt (1958). These publications introduced the first model of neural networks as "computing machines," the basic model of network self-organization, and the model of "learning with a teacher," respectively. (Section I.3 provides a semitechnical introduction to this work and a key set of currently central ideas that build upon it.) The present historical fragment is designed to take us up to 1948, the year preceding the publication of Hebb's book, to reveal our present federation of disciplines as the current incarnation of what emerged in the 1940s and is aptly summed up in the title of the book, *Cybernetics: Or Control and Communication in the Animal and the Machine* (Wiener, 1948). But whereas Wiener's view of cybernetics was dominated by concepts of control and communication, our subject is dominated by notions of parallel and distributed computation, with special attention to learning in neural networks. On the other hand, notions of information and statistical mechanics championed by Wiener have reemerged as a strong strand in the study of neural networks today (see, e.g., the articles FEATURE ANALYSIS and STATISTICAL MECHANICS OF NEURAL NETWORKS in Part III). The articles in Part III will make abundantly clear how far we have come since 1948, and also how many problems remain. My intent in the present "fragment" is to enrich the reader's understanding of current contributions by using a selective historical tour to place them in context.

Noting that the Greek word *cybernetics* (κυβερνετεσ) means the helmsman of a ship (cf. the Latin word *gubernator*, which gives us the word "governor" in English), Wiener (1948) used the term for a subject in which feedback played a central role. Feedback is the process whereby, e.g., the helmsman notes the "error," the extent to which he is off course, and "feeds it back" to decide which way to move the rudder. We can see the importance of this concept in endowing automata ("self-moving" machines) with flexible behavior. Two hundred years earlier, in *L'Homme machine*, La Mettrie had suggested that such automata as the mechanical duck and flute player of Vaucanson indicated the possibility of one day building a mechanical man that could talk. While these clockwork automata were capable of surprisingly complex behavior, they lacked a crucial aspect of animal behavior, let alone human intelligence: they were unable to adapt to changing circumstances. In the following century, machines were built that could automatically counter disturbances to restore desired performance. Perhaps the best-known example of this is Watt's governor for the steam engine, which would let off excess steam if the velocity of the engine became too great. This development led to Maxwell's (1868) paper, "On Governors," which laid the basis for both the theory of negative feedback and the study of system stability (both of which are discussed in Section I.3). Negative feedback was feedback in which the error (in Watt's case, the amount by which actual velocity ex-

ceeded desired velocity) was used to counteract the error; stability occurred if this feedback was apportioned to reduce the error toward zero. Bernard (1878) brought these notions back to biology with his study of what Cannon (1939) would later dub *homeostasis*, observing that physiological processes often form circular chains of cause and effect that could counteract disturbances in such variables as body temperature, blood pressure, and glucose level in the blood. In fact, following publication of Wiener's 1948 book, the Josiah Macy, Jr., Foundation conferences, in which many of the pioneers of cybernetics were involved, became referred to as the Cybernetics Group, with the proceedings entitled *Cybernetics: Circular Causal and Feedback Mechanisms in Biological and Social Systems,* (see Heims, 1991, for a history of the conferences and their participants).

The nineteenth century also saw major developments in the understanding of the brain. At an overall anatomical level, a major achievement was the understanding of localization in the cerebral cortex (see Young, 1970, for a history). Magendie and Bell had discovered that the dorsal roots of the spinal cord were sensory, carrying information from receptors in the body, while the ventral roots (on the belly side) were motor, carrying commands to the muscles. Fritsch and Hitzig, and then Ferrier, extended this principle to the brain proper, showing that the rear of the brain contains the primary receiving areas for vision, hearing, and touch, while the motor cortex is located in front of the central fissure. All this understanding of localization in the cerebral cortex led to the nineteenth century neurological doctrine, perhaps best exemplified in Lichtheim's (1885) development of the insights of Broca and Wernicke into brain mechanisms of language, which viewed different mental "faculties" as being localized in different regions of the brain. Thus, neurological deficits were to be explained as much in terms of lesions of the connections linking two such regions as in terms of lesions to the regions themselves. We may also note a major precursor of the connectionism of this volume, where the connections are those between neuron-like units rather than anatomical regions: the associationist psychology of Alexander Bain (1868), who represented associations of ideas by the strengths of connections between "neurons" representing those ideas.

Around 1900, two major steps were taken in revealing the finer details of the brain. In Spain, Santiago Ramón y Cajal (e.g., 1906) gave us exquisite anatomical studies of many regions of the brain, revealing the particular structure of each as a network of neurons. In England, the physiological studies of Charles Sherrington (1906) on reflex behavior provided the basic physiological understanding of synapses, the junction points between the neurons. Somewhat later, in Russia, Ivan Pavlov (1927), extending associationist psychology and building on the Russian studies of reflexes by Sechenov in the 1860s, established the basic facts on the modifiability of reflexes by conditioning (see Fearing, 1930, for a historical review).

A very different setting of the scene for cybernetics came from work in mathematical logic in the 1930s. Kurt Gödel published his famous *Incompleteness Theorem* in 1931 (see Arbib, 1987, for a proof as well as a debunking of the claim that Gödel's theorem sets limits on machine intelligence). The "formalist" program initiated by David Hilbert, which sought to place all mathematical truth within a single formal system, had reached its fullest expression in the *Principia Mathematica* of Whitehead and Russell. But Gödel showed that, if one used the approach offered in *Principia Mathematica* to set up consistent axioms for arithmetic and prove theorems by logical deduction from them, the theory *must* be incomplete, no matter which axioms ("knowledge base") one started with—there would be true statements of arithmetic that could not be deduced from the axioms.

Following Gödel's 1931 study, many mathematical logicians sought to formalize the notion of an effective procedure, of what could *and could not* be done by explicitly following an algorithm or set of rules. Kleene (1936) developed the theory of partial recursive functions; Turing (1936) developed his machines; Church (1941) developed the lambda calculus, the forerunner of McCarthy's list processing language, LISP, a one-time favorite of artificial intelligence (AI) workers; while Emil Post (1943) introduced systems for rewriting strings of symbols, of which Chomsky's early formalizations of grammars in 1959 were a special case. Fortunately, these methods proved to be equivalent. Whatever could be computed by one of these methods could be computed by any other method if it were equipped with a suitable "program." It thus came to be believed (Church's thesis) that if a function could be computed by any machine at all, it could be computed by each one of these methods.

Turing (1936) helped chart the limits of the computable with his notion of what is now called a *Turing machine*, a device that followed a fixed, finite set of instructions to read, write, and move upon a finite but indefinitely extendible tape, each square of which bore a symbol from some finite alphabet. As one of the ingredients of Church's thesis, Turing offered a "psychology of the computable," making plausible the claim that any effectively definable computation, that is, anything that a human could do in the way of symbolic manipulation by following a finite and completely explicit set of rules, could be carried out by such a machine equipped with a suitable program. Turing also provided the most famous example of a noncomputable problem, "the unsolvability of the Halting Problem." Let p be the numerical code for a Turing machine program, and let x be the code for the initial contents of a Turing machine's tape. Then the halting function $h(p, x) = 1$ if Turing machine p will eventually halt if started with data x; otherwise it is 0. Turing showed that there was no "computer program" that could compute h.

And so we come to 1943, the key year for bringing together the notions of control mechanism and intelligent automata.

In "A Logical Calculus of the Ideas Immanent in Nervous Activity," McCulloch and Pitts (1943) united the studies of neurophysiology and mathematical logic. Their formal model of the neuron as a threshold logic unit (see Section I.1) built on the neuron doctrine of Ramón y Cajal and the excitatory and inhibitory synapses of Sherrington, using notation from the mathematical logic of Whitehead, Russell, and Carnap. McCulloch and Pitts provided the "physiology of the computable" by showing that the control box of any Turing machine, the essential formalization of symbolic computation, could be implemented by a network (with loops) of their formal neurons. The ideas of McCulloch and Pitts influenced John von Neumann and his colleagues when they defined the basic architecture of stored program computing. Thus, as electronic computers were built toward the end of World War II, it was understood that whatever they could do could be done by a network of neurons.

Craik's (1943) book, *The Nature of Explanation*, viewed the nervous system "as a calculating machine capable of modeling or paralleling external events," suggesting that the process of forming an "internal model" that paralleled the world is the basic feature of thought and explanation. In the same year, Rosenblueth, Wiener, and Bigelow published "Behavior, Purpose and Teleology." Engineers had noted that if feedback used in controlling the rudder of a ship were too brusque, the rudder would overshoot, compensatory feedback would yield a larger overshoot in the opposite direction, and so on and so on as the system wildly oscillated. Wiener and Bigelow asked Rosenblueth whether there was any corresponding pathological condition in humans and were given the example of intention tremor associated with an injured cerebellum. This evi-

dence for feedback within the human nervous system (see MOTOR CONTROL, BIOLOGICAL AND THEORETICAL) led the three scientists to advocate that neurophysiology move beyond the Sherringtonian view of the CNS as a reflex device adjusting itself in response to sensory inputs. Rather, setting reference values for feedback systems could provide the basis for analysis of the brain as a purposive system explicable only in terms of circular processes, that is, from nervous system to muscles to the external world and back again via receptors.

Such studies laid the basis for the emergence of cybernetics, which in turn gave birth to a number of distinct new disciplines, such as AI, biological control theory, cognitive psychology, and neural modeling, which each went their separate ways in the 1970s. The next subsection introduces a number of these disciplines and the relations between them; this analysis will continue in many articles in Part III of the *Handbook*.

Brains, Machines, and Minds

Brains. Brain theory comprises many different theories as to how the structures of the brain can subserve such diverse functions as perception, memory, control of movement, and higher mental function. As such, it includes both attempts to extend notions of computing, as well as applications of modern electronic computers to explore the performance of complex models. An example of the former is the study of *cooperative computation* between different structures in the brain which seeks to offer a new paradigm for computing that transcends classical notions associated with serial execution of symbolic programs. For the latter, *computational neuroscience* makes systematic use of mathematical analysis and computer simulation to provide ever better models of the structure and function of living brains, building on earlier work in both neural modeling and biological control theory.

Machines. Artificial intelligence studies how computers may be programmed to yield "intelligent" behavior without necessarily attempting to provide a correlation between structures in the program and structures in the brain. *Robotics* is related to AI but emphasizes the flexible control of machines (robots) which have receptors (e.g., television cameras) and effectors (e.g., wheels, legs, arms, grippers) that allow them to interact with the world.

Brain theory has spawned a companion field of *neural computing*, which involves the design of machines with circuitry inspired by, but which need not faithfully emulate, the neural networks of brains. Many technologists usurp the term "neural networks" for this latter field, but we will use it as an umbrella term which may, depending on context, describe biological nervous systems, models thereof, and the artificial networks which (sometimes at great remove) they inspire. When the emphasis is on "higher mental functions," neural computing may be seen as a new branch of AI (see the road map **Artificial Intelligence** in Part II), but it also contributes to robotics (especially to those robot designs inspired by analysis of animal behavior), and to a wide range of technologies, including those based on image analysis, signal processing, and control (see the road map **Applications**).

For the latter work, many people emphasize adaptive neural networks which, without specific programming, can adjust their connections through self-organization or to meet specifications given by some teacher. There are also significant contributions to the systematic design, rather than emergence through learning, of neural networks, especially for applications in low-level vision (such as stereopsis, optic flow, and shape-from-shading). However, complex problems cannot, in general, be solved by the tuning or the design of a single unstructured network. For example, robot control may integrate a variety of low-level vision networks with a set of competing and cooperating networks for motor control and its planning. Brain theory and neural computing thus have to address the analysis and design, respectively, of networks of networks (see, e.g., HYBRID CONNECTIONIST/SYMBOLIC SYSTEMS and MODULAR AND HIERARCHICAL LEARNING SYSTEMS).

Minds. Here, I want to distinguish the brain from the mind (the realm of the "mental"). In great part, brain theory seeks to analyze how the brain guides the behaving organism in its interactions with the dynamic world around it, but much of the control of such interactions is not mental, and much of what is mental is subsymbolic and/or unconscious (see PHILOSOPHICAL ISSUES IN BRAIN THEORY AND CONNECTIONISM and CONSCIOUSNESS, NEURAL MODELS OF). Without offering a precise definition of "mental," let me just say that many people can agree on examples of mental activity (perceiving a visual scene, reading, thinking, etc.) even if they take the diametrically opposite philosophical positions of dualism (mind and brain are separate) or monism (mind is a function of brain). They would then agree that some mental activity (e.g., contemplation) need not result in overt "interactions with the dynamic real world," and that much of the brain's activity (e.g., controlling normal breathing) is not mental. Face recognition seems to be a mental activity that we do not carry out through symbol manipulation. Indeed, even psychologists who reject Freud's particular psychosexual theories accept his notion that much of our mental behavior is shaped by unconscious forces (for an assessment of Freud and an account of consciousness, see Arbib and Hesse, 1986).

Cognitive psychology attempts to explain the mind in terms of "information processing" (a notion which is continuing to change). It thus occupies a middle ground between brain theory and AI in which the model must explain psychological data (e.g., what tasks are hard for humans, people's ability at memorization, the development of the child, patterns of human errors, etc.) but in which the units of the model need not correspond to actual brain structures. In the 1960s and 1970s, the majority of cognitive psychologists formulated their theories in terms of information theory and/or symbol manipulation, while theories of biological organization were ignored. However, workers in both AI and cognitive psychology now pay increasing attention to the cooperative computation paradigm. The term *connectionism* has come to be used for studies that model human thought and behavior in terms of parallel distributed networks of neuron-like units, with learning mediated by changes in strength of the connections between these elements (see COGNITIVE MODELING: PSYCHOLOGY AND CONNECTIONISM).

The study of brain theory and neural networks thus has a twofold aim: (1) to enhance our understanding of human thought and the neural basis of human and animal behavior (brain theory), and (2) to learn new strategies for building "intelligent" machines or adaptive robots (neural computing). In either case, we seek organizational principles that will help us understand how neurons (whether biological or artificial) can work together to yield complex patterns of behavior. *Brain theory* requires empirical data to shape and constrain modeling, but in return provides concepts and hypotheses to shape and constrain experimentation. In *neural computing*, the criterion for success is the design of a machine that can perform a task cheaply, reliably, and effectively, even if, in the process of making the best use of available (e.g., silicon) technology, the final design departs radically from the biological neural network that inspired it. It will be important in reading this *Handbook*, then, to be clear as to whether a particular study is an exercise in brain theory/computational neuroscience or in AI/neural computing. What will not be in doubt is that the influence of these subjects works both ways: not only can brain mechanisms inspire new technology, but new technologies provide metaphors to drive new theories of brain function. To this it must be added that most workers in ANNs know little of brain function, and relatively few neuroscientists have a deep understanding of brain theory or know much

of neural computing beyond the basic ideas of Hebbian plasticity and, perhaps, backpropagation (see Section I.3). However, the level of interchange has increased since the first edition of this *Handbook* appeared, and this new edition is designed to further increase the flow of information between these scientific communities.

Levels of Analysis

Whether the emphasis is on humans, animals, or machines, it becomes clear that we can seek insight at many different levels of analysis; from large information processing blocks down to the finest details of molecular structure. Much of psychology and linguistics looks at human behavior "from the outside," whether studying overall competence or attending to details of performance. Neuropsychology relates behavior to the interaction of various brain regions. Neurophysiology studies the activity of neurons, both to understand the intrinsic properties of the neurons and to help understand their role in the subsystems dissected out by the neuropsychologist, such as networks for pattern recognition or for visuomotor coordination. Molecular and cell biology and biophysics correlate the structure and connectivity of the membranes and subcellular systems which constitute cells with the way these cells transform incoming patterns or subserve memory by changing function with repeated interactions.

These differing levels make it possible to focus individual research studies, but they are ill-defined, and a scientist who works on any one level needs to make occasional forays, both downward to find mechanisms for the functions studied, and upward to understand what role the studied function can play in the overall scheme of things. *Top-down* modeling starts from some overall behavior and explains it in terms of the interaction of high-level functional units, while *bottom-up* modeling starts from the interaction of individual neurons (or even smaller units) to explain network properties. It requires a judicious blend of the two to connect the clear overview of crucial questions to the hard data of neuroscience or, in the case of neural engineering, to the details of implementation. Most successful modeling will be purely bottom-up or top-down only in its initial stages, if at all—constraints on an initial top-down model will be given, for example, by the data on regional localization offered by the neurologist, or the circuit-cell-synapse studies of much current neuroscience.

We must now distinguish the brain's computation from connectionist computation "in the *style* of the brain." If a connectionist model succeeds in describing some psychological input/output behavior, it may become an important hypothesis that its internal structure is "real" (see RECURRENT NETWORKS: NEUROPHYSIOLOGICAL MODELING). In general, however, much additional work will be required to find and assimilate neurophysiological data to provide brain models in which the neurons are not mere formal units but actually represent biological neurons in the brain.

Much study of the brain is guided by evolutionary and comparative studies of animal behavior and brain function (cf. EVOLUTION OF THE ANCESTRAL VERTEBRATE BRAIN and related articles in the road map **Neuroethology and Evolution**). The information about the function of the human brain that is gained in the neurological clinic or during neurosurgery can thus be supplemented by humane experimentation on animals. (However, as evidenced by Table 1 of Section I.1, we can learn a great deal by studying the *differences*, as well as the similarities, between the brains of different species.) We learn by stimulating, recording from, or excising portions of an animal's brain and seeing how the animal's behavior changes. We may then compare such results with observations using such techniques as positron emission tomography (PET) or functional magnetic resonance imaging (fMRI) of the relative activity of different parts of the human brain during different tasks (see IMAGING THE GRAMMATICAL BRAIN, IMAGING THE MOTOR

BRAIN, and IMAGING THE VISUAL BRAIN). The grand aim of *cognitive neuroscience* (as neuropsychology has now become; see the **Cognitive Neuroscience** road map) is to use clinical data and brain imaging to form a high-level view of the involvement of various brain regions in human cognition, using single-cell activity recorded from animals engaged in analogous behaviors to suggest the neural networks underlying this involvement (see SYNTHETIC FUNCTIONAL BRAIN MAPPING). The catch, of course, is that the "analogous behaviors" of animals are not very analogous at all when it comes to such symbolic activities as language and reasoning. In Part III, we will see that "higher mental functions" tend to be modeled more in connectionist terms constrained (if at all) by psychological or psycholinguistic data (cf. the Part II road maps **Psychology** and **Linguistics and Speech Processing**), while the greatest successes in seeking the neural underpinnings of human behavior have come in areas such as vision, memory, and motor control, where we can make neural network models of animal analogues of human capabilities (cf. the road maps **Vision**, **Other Sensory Systems**, **Neural Plasticity**, **Biological Networks**, **Motor Pattern Generators**, and **Mammalian Motor Control**).

We also learn from the attempt to reproduce various aspects of human behavior in a robot, even though human action, memory, learning, and perception are far richer than those of any machine yet built or likely to be built in the near future (see BIOLOGICALLY INSPIRED ROBOTICS). Thus, when we suggest that the brain can be thought of in some ways as a (highly distributed) computer, we are not trying to reduce humans to the level of extant machines, but rather to understand ways in which machines give us insight into human attributes. This type of study has been referred to as *cybernetics*, extending the concept of Norbert Wiener, who, as we have seen, defined the subject as "the study of control and communication in man and machine."

To the extent that they address "higher mental function," the studies presented in this *Handbook* suggest that there is no single "thing" called *intelligence*, but rather a plexus of properties that, taken one at a time, may be little cause for admiration, but any sizable collection of which will yield behavior that we would label as intelligent. Turing (1950) argued that we would certainly regard a machine as intelligent if it could pass the following test: An experimenter sits in a room with two teletypes by which she conducts a "conversation" with two systems. One is a human, the other is a machine, but the experimenter is not told which is which. If, after asking many questions, she is likely to have much doubt about which is human and which is machine, we should, says Turing, concede intelligence to the machine. However, unless one dogmatically insists that being intelligent entails behaving in a human way, it is "harder" for a machine to pass this *Turing test* than to be intelligent. For instance, whereas a computer can answer problems in arithmetic quickly and correctly, a much more complex program would be required to ensure that it answered as slowly and erratically as a human. Turing's aim was not to find a necessary set of conditions to ensure intelligence, but rather to devise a test which, if passed by a machine, would convince most skeptics that the machine had intelligence.

Schema Theory

The analysis of complex systems, whether they subserve natural or artificial intelligence, requires a coarser grain of analysis to complement that of neural networks. To make sense of the brain, we often divide it into functional systems—such as the motor system, the visual system, and so on—as well as into structural subsystems—from the spinal cord and the hippocampus to the various subdivisions of the prefrontal cortex. Similarly, in distributed AI (see MULTIAGENT SYSTEMS), the solution of a task may be distributed over a complex set of interacting *agents*, each with their

dedicated processors for handling the information available to them locally. Thus, both neuroscience and artificial intelligence require a language for expressing the distribution of function across units intermediate between overall function and the final units of analysis (e.g., neurons or simple instructions).

Since the "units of thought" or the subfunctions of a complex behavior may be quite high-level compared to the fine-grain computation of the myriad neurons in the human brain, SCHEMA THEORY (q.v.; see also Arbib, 1981; Arbib, Érdi, and Szentágothai, 1998, chap. 3) complements connectionism by providing a bridging language between functional description and neural networks. It is based on a theory of the concurrent activity of interacting functional units called *schemas*. Perceptual schemas are those used for perceptual analysis, while motor schemas are those which provide the control systems that can be coordinated to effect a wide variety of movement. Other schemas compete and cooperate to meld action, internal state, and perception in an ongoing action-perception cycle.

Figure 4*A* represents brain theory, while Figure 4*B* offers a similar but distinct picture for distributed AI. We may model the brain either functionally, analyzing some behavior in terms of interacting schemas, or structurally, through the interaction of anatomically defined units, such as brain regions (cf. the examples in the road map **Mammalian Brain Regions**) or substructures of these regions, such as layers or columns. In brain theory, we ultimately seek an explanation in terms of neural networks, since the neuron may be considered the basic unit of function as well as of structure, and much further work in computational neuroscience seeks to explain the complex functionality of real neurons in terms of "subneural" units, such as membrane compartments, channels, spines, and synapses. What makes the story more subtle is that, in general, a functional analysis proceeding "top-down" from some overall behavior need not map directly into a "bottom-up" analysis proceeding upward from the neural circuitry (brain theory) or basic set of processors (distributed AI), and that several iterations from the "middle out" may be required to bring the structural and functional accounts into consonance. Brain theory may then seek to replace an initially plausible schema analysis with one whose schemas may be constituted by an assemblage of schemas which can each be embodied in one structure (without denying that a given brain region may support the activity of multiple schemas). The schemas that serve as the functional units in our initial hypotheses about the decomposition of some overall function may well differ from the more refined hypotheses which provide an account of structural correlates as well. On the other hand, distributed AI may adopt any schema analysis that is technologically effective, and the schemas may be implemented in whatever medium is appropriate, whether as conventional computer programs, ANNs, or special-purpose devices. These different approaches then rest on effective design of VLSI "chips" or other computing materials (cf. the road map **Implementation and Analysis**).

For brain theory, the top-level schemas must be "large" enough to allow an analysis of behavior at or near the psychological level, yet also be subject to successive decomposition down to a level that may, in certain cases, be implemented in specific neural networks. We again distinguish a schema as a *functional* unit from a neural network as a *structural* unit. A given schema may be distributed across several neural networks; a given neural network may be involved in the implementation of several different schemas. The same will be true for relating connectionist units to single biological neurons. If there is to be a fuller rapprochement between connectionism and neuropsychology, it will be important to use a vocabulary (or context) that allows one to make the necessary distinctions between connectionist and biological neurons.

A top-down analysis (decomposing a function) may suggest that a certain schema is embedded in a certain part of the brain; we can then marshal the available data from anatomy and neurophysiology

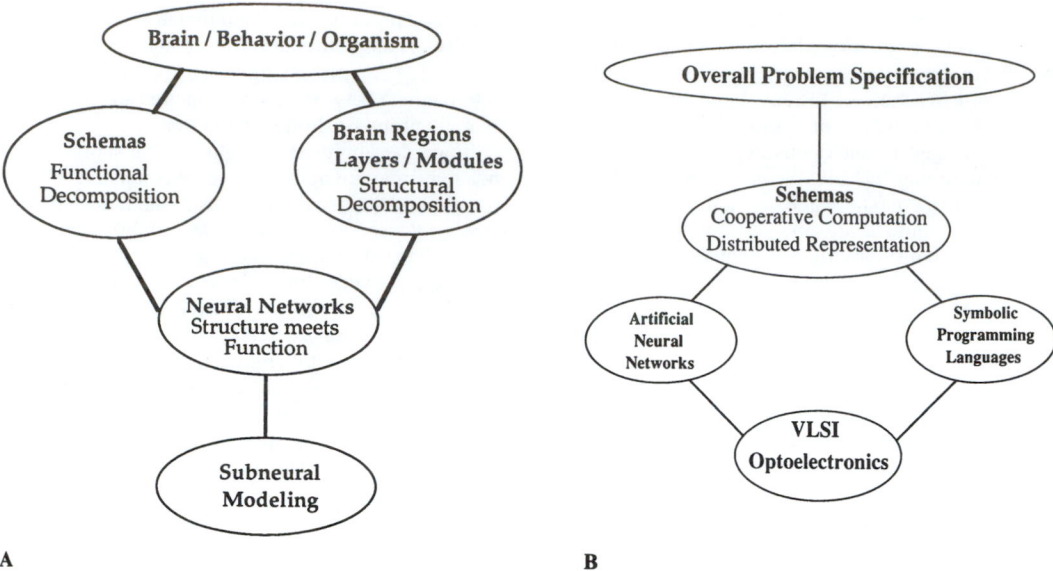

Figure 4. Views of level of analysis of brain and behavior (*A*) and a distributed technological system (*B*), highlighting the role of schemas as an intermediate level of functional analysis in each case.

to assess whether the circuitry can, indeed, subserve an instance of that schema. It often happens that the empirical data are inadequate. We then make hypotheses for experimental confirmation. Alternatively, bottom-up analysis of a brain region (assembling its constituents) may suggest that it subserves a different schema from that originally hypothesized, and we must then conduct a new top-down analysis in the light of these newfound constraints.

To illuminate the notion of experimental insight modifying an initial top-down analysis, we consider an example from *Rana computatrix*, a set of models of visuomotor coordination in the frog and toad (cf. Visuomotor Coordination in Frog and Toad). Frogs and toads snap at small moving objects and jump away from large ones (to oversimplify somewhat). Thus, a simple schema-model of the frog brain might simply postulate four schemas: two perceptual schemas (processes for recognizing objects or situations) and two motor schemas (processes for controlling some structured behavior). One perceptual schema would recognize small moving objects and activate a motor schema for approaching the prey; the other would recognize large moving objects and activate a motor schema for avoiding the predator. Lesion experiments can put such a model to the test if it is enhanced by hypotheses on the localization of each schema in the brain. It was thought that the tectum (a key visual region in the animal's midbrain) was the locus for recognizing small moving objects, while the pretectum (a region just in front of the tectum) was the locus for recognizing large moving objects. Based on these localization hypotheses, the model described would predict that an animal with a lesioned pretectum would be unresponsive to large objects, but would respond normally to small objects. However, the facts are quite different. A pretectum-lesioned toad will approach moving objects, both large and small, and does not exhibit avoidance behavior. This has led to a new schema model in which a perceptual schema to recognize large moving objects is still localized in the pretectum, but the tectum now contains a perceptual schema for *all* moving objects. We then add that activity of the pretectal schema not only triggers the avoidance motor schema but also inhibits approach. This new schema model still yields the normal behavior to large and small moving objects, but also fits the lesion data, since removal of the pretectum removes inhibition, meaning that the ani-

mal will now approach any moving object (Ewert and von Seelen, 1974).

We have thus seen how schemas may be used to provide falsifiable models of the brain, using lesion experiments to test schema models of behavior, and leading to new functional models that better match the structure of the brain. Note again that, in different species, the map from function to brain structure may be different, while in distributed AI the constraints are not those of analysis but rather those of design—namely, for a given function and a given set of processors, a schema decomposition must be found that will map most efficiently onto a network of processors of a certain kind.

While the brain may be considered a network of interacting "boxes" (anatomically distinguishable structures), there is no reason to expect each such box to mediate a single function that is well-defined from a behavioral standpoint. We have just seen that the frog tectum is implicated in both approach and (when modulated by pretectum) avoidance behavior. The language of schemas lets us express hypotheses about the various functions that the brain performs without assuming localization of any one function in any one region, but also allows us to express the way in which many regions participate in a given function, or a given region participates in many functions.

The style of *cooperative computation* (see Cooperative Phenomena) exhibited in both schema theory and connectionism is far removed from serial computation and the symbol-based ideas that have dominated conventional AI. As we shall see in example after example in Part III, the brain has many specialized areas, each with a partial representation of the world. It is only through the interaction of these regions that the unity of behavior of the animal emerges, and the human is no different in this regard. The representation of the world is *the pattern of relationships between all its partial representations*. Much work in AI contributes to schema theory, even when it does not use this term. For example, Brooks (1986) builds robot controllers using layers made up of asynchronous modules that can be considered to be a version of schemas (see Reactive Robotic Systems). This work shares with schema theory, with its mediation of action through a network of schemas, the point that no single, central, logical representation of the world needs link perception and action. It is also useful to view cooperative computation as a social phenomenon. A schema is a self-contained computing agent (object) with the ability to communicate with other agents, and whose function is specified by some behavior. Whereas schema theory was motivated in great part by the study of interacting brain regions (other influences are reviewed in SCHEMA THEORY), much early work in distributed AI was motivated by a social analogy in which the schemas were thought of as "agents" analogous to people interacting in a social setting to compete or cooperate in solving some overall problem, a theme elaborated on by Minsky (1985) and whose current status is reviewed in MULTIAGENT SYSTEMS.

I.3. Dynamics and Adaptation in Neural Networks

Section I.1 introduced a number of key concepts from the biological study of neurons, stressing the diversity of neurons both within the human CNS and across species. It presented several simple models of neurons, noting that computational neuroscience has gone on to produce more subtle and complicated neuronal models, while neural computing tends to use simple neurons augmented by "learning rules" for changing connection strengths on the basis of "experience." The purpose of this section is to introduce two key approaches that dominate the modern study of neural networks: (1) the study of neural networks as dynamic systems (developed more fully in the road map **Dynamic Systems**), and (2) the study of neural networks as adaptive systems (see **Learning in Artificial Networks**). To make this section essentially self-contained, we start by recalling the definitions of the McCulloch-Pitts and leaky integrator neurons from Section I.1, but we do this in the context of a general, semiformal, introduction to dynamic systems.

Dynamic Systems

We motivate the notion of dynamic systems by considering how to abstract the interaction of an organism (or a machine) with its environment. The organism will be influenced by aspects of the current environment—the *inputs* to the organism—while the activity of the environment will be responsive in turn to aspects of the current activity of the organism, the *outputs* of the organism. The inputs and outputs that actually enter into a *theory* of the organism (or machine) are a small sampling of the flux of its interactions with the rest of the universe. There is essentially no limit to how many variables one could include in the analysis; a crucial task in any theory building is to pick the "right" variables.

Depending on the context, we will use the word *system* to denote either the physical reality (which we cannot know in its entirety) or the abstraction with which we approximate it. Inputs and outputs do not constitute a complete description of a system. We cannot predict how someone will answer a question unless we know her state of knowledge; nor can we tell how a computer will process its data unless we know the instructions controlling its computation. In short, we must include a description of the *internal state* of the system which determines what it will extract from its current stimulation in determining its current actions and modifying its internal state. Our abstraction of any real system contains five elements:

1. The set of *inputs*: those variables of the environment which we believe will affect the system behavior of interest to us.
2. The set of *outputs*: those variables of the system which we choose to observe, or which we believe will significantly affect the environment.
3. The set of *states*: those internal variables of the system (which may or may not also be output variables) which determine the relationship between input and output. Essentially, the state of a system is the system's "internal residue of the past": when we know the state of a system, no further information about the past behavior of the system will enable us to refine predictions of the way in which future inputs and outputs of the system will be related.
4. The *state-transition function*: that function which determines how the state will change when the system obtains various inputs.
5. The *output function*: that function which determines what output the system will yield with a given input when in a given state.

Any system in which the state-transition function and output function uniquely determine the new state and output from a specification of the initial state and subsequent inputs is called a *deterministic* system. If, no matter how carefully we specify subsequent inputs to a system, we cannot specify exactly what will be the subsequent states and outputs, we say the system is *probabilistic* or *stochastic*. A stochastic treatment may be worthwhile, either because we are analyzing systems, which are "inescapably" stochastic (e.g., at the quantum level), or because we are analyzing macroscopic systems, which lend themselves to a stochastic description by ignoring "fine details" of microscopic variables. For example, it is usually more reasonable to describe a coin in terms of a 0.5 probability of coming up heads than to measure the initial placement of the coin on the finger and the thrust of the thumb in sufficient detail to determine whether the coin will come up heads or tails.

Continuous-Time Systems

In Newtonian mechanics, the state of the system comprises the positions of its components, which are directly observable, and their velocities, which can be estimated from the observed trajectory over a period of time. Time is continuous (i.e., characterized by the set $\mathbb{R}$ of real numbers), and the way in which the state changes is described by a differential equation: classical mechanics provides the basic example of *continuous-time* systems in which the present state and input determine *the rate at which the state changes*. This requires that the input, output, and state spaces be continuous spaces in which such continuous changes can occur. Consider the simple example of a point mass undergoing rectilinear motion. At any time, its position $y(t)$ is the observable output of the system, and the force $u(t)$ acting upon it is the input applied to the system. Newton's third law says that the force applied to the system equals the mass times the acceleration $\ddot{y}(t) = mu(t)$, where the acceleration $\ddot{y}(t)$ is the second derivative of $y(t)$. According to Newton's laws, the state of the system is given by the position and velocity of the particle. We call the position-velocity pair, at any time, the *instantaneous state* $q(t)$ of the system. In fact, the earlier equation gives us enough information to deduce the rate of change $dq(t)/dt$ of this state. Using standard matrix formalism, we thus have

$$\frac{d}{dt}\begin{bmatrix} y(t) \\ \dot{y}(t) \end{bmatrix} = \begin{bmatrix} \dot{y}(t) \\ \ddot{y}(t) \end{bmatrix} = \begin{bmatrix} \dot{y}(t) \\ mu(t) \end{bmatrix} = \begin{bmatrix} 0 & 1 \\ 0 & 0 \end{bmatrix}\begin{bmatrix} y(t) \\ \dot{y}(t) \end{bmatrix} + \begin{bmatrix} 0 \\ m \end{bmatrix}u(t)$$

while

$$y(t) = \begin{bmatrix} 1 \\ 0 \end{bmatrix}q(t)$$

This is an example of a *linear* system in which the rate of change of state depends linearly on the present state and input, and the present output depends linearly on the present state. That is, there are matrices F, G, and H such that

$$\frac{dq(t)}{dt} = Fq(t) + Gu(t); \; y(t) = Hq(t)$$

More generally, a physical system can be expressed by a pair of equations:

$$\frac{dq(t)}{dt} = f(q(t), u(t))$$

$$y(t) = g(q(t))$$

The first expresses the rate of change $dq(t)/dt$ of the state as a function of both the state $q(t)$ and the input or control vector $u(t)$ applied at any time t; the second reads the output from the current state.

We now present the definition of a *leaky integrator neuron* as a continuous-time system. The internal state of the neuron is its membrane potential, $m(t)$, and its output is the firing rate, $M(t)$. The *state transition function* of the cell is expressed as

$$\tau \frac{dm(t)}{dt} = -m(t) + \sum_i w_i X_i(t) + h \qquad (1)$$

while the *output function* of the cell is given by the equation

$$M(t) = \sigma(m(t)) \qquad (2)$$

Thus, if there are m inputs $X_i(t)$, $i = 1, \ldots, m$, then the *input space* of the neuron is $\mathbb{R}^m$, with current value $(X_1(t), \ldots, X_m(t))$, while the *state* and *output* spaces of the neuron both equal $\mathbb{R}$, with current values $m(t)$ and $M(t)$, respectively.

Let us now briefly (and semiformally) see how a neural network comprised of leaky integrator neurons can also be seen as a continuous-time system in this sense. As typified in Figure 5, we characterize a neural network by selecting N neurons (each with specified input weights and resting potential) and by taking the axon of each neuron, which may be split into several branches

carrying identical output signals, and either connecting each line to a unique input of another neuron or feeding it outside the net to provide one of the K network output lines. Then every input to a given neuron must be connected either to an output of another neuron or to one of the (possibly split) L input lines of the network. Thus the input set $X = \mathbb{R}^L$, the state set $Q = \mathbb{R}^N$, and the output set $Y = \mathbb{R}^K$. If the ith output line comes from the jth neuron, then the *output function* is determined by the fact that the ith component of the output at time t is the firing rate $M_j(t) = \sigma_j(M_j(t))$ of the jth neuron at time t. The state transition function for the neural network follows from the state transition functions of each of the N neurons

$$\tau \frac{dm_i(t)}{dt} = -m_i(t) + \sum_j w_{ij} X_{ij}(t) + h_i \qquad (3)$$

as soon as we specify whether $X_{ij}(t)$ is the output $M_k(t)$ of the kth neuron or the value $x_l(t)$ currently being applied on the lth input line of the overall network.

Discrete-Time Systems

In contrast to continuous-time systems, which *must* have continuous state spaces on which the differential equations for the state transition function can be defined, *discrete-time* systems may have either continuous or discrete state spaces. (A *discrete* state space is just a set with no specific metric or topological structure.) For example, a McCulloch-Pitts neuron is considered to operate on a discrete-time scale, $t = 0, 1, 2, 3, \ldots$, and has connection weights w_i and threshold θ. If at time t the value of the ith input is $x_i(t)$, then the output one time step later, $y(t + 1)$, equals 1 if and only if $\sum_i w_i x_i(t) \geq \theta$. If there are m inputs $(x_1(t), \ldots, x_m(t))$, then, since inputs and outputs are binary, such a neuron has input set $= \{0, 1\}^m$, state set $=$ output set $\{0, 1\}$ (we treat the current state and output as being identical). On the other hand, the important learning scheme known as backpropagation (defined later) is based on neurons which operate on discrete time, but with both input and output taking continuous values in some range, say $[0, 1]$.

In computer science, an *automaton* is a discrete-time system with discrete input, output, and state spaces. Formally, we describe an automaton by the sets X, Y, and Q of inputs, outputs, and states, respectively, together with the *next-state function* δ: $Q \times X \rightarrow Q$ and the *output function* β: $Q \rightarrow Y$. If the automaton is in state q and receives input x at time t, then its next state will be $\delta(q, x)$ and its next output will be $\beta(q)$. It should be clear that a McCulloch-Pitts neural network (i.e., a network like that shown in Figure 5, but a discrete-time network with each neuron a McCulloch-Pitts neuron) functions like a finite automaton, as each neuron changes state synchronously on each tick of the time scale $t = 0, 1, 2, 3, \ldots$. Conversely, it can be shown (see Arbib, 1987; the result was essentially, though inscrutably, due to McCulloch and Pitts, 1943) that any finite automaton can be simulated by a suitable McCulloch-Pitts neural network.

Stability, Limit Cycles, and Chaos

With the previous discussion, we now have more than enough material to understand the crucial dynamic systems concept of *stability* and the related concepts of limit cycles and chaos (see COMPUTING WITH ATTRACTORS and CHAOS IN NEURAL SYSTEMS). We want to know what happens to an "unperturbed" system, i.e., one for which the input is held constant (possibly with some specific "null input," usually denoted by 0, the "zero" input in X). An *equilibrium* is a state q in which the system can stay at rest, i.e., such that $\delta(q, 0) = q$ (discrete time) or $dq/dt = f(q, 0) = 0$ (continuous time). The study of stability is concerned with the issue of whether or not this rest point will be maintained in the face of slight disturbances. To see the variety of equilibria, we use the image of a sticky ball

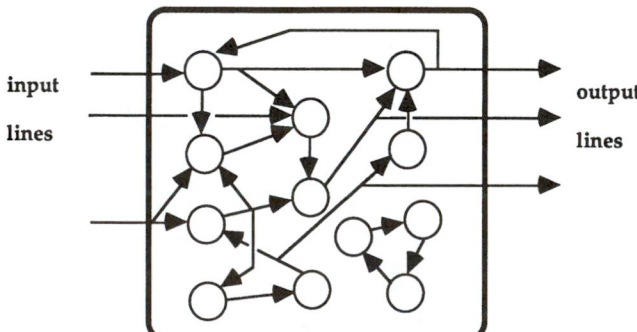

Figure 5. A neural network viewed as a system. The input at time t is the pattern of firing on the input lines, the output is the pattern of firing on the output lines; and the internal state is the vector of firing rates of all the neurons of the network.

input

lines

output

lines

rolling on the "hillside" of Figure 6. We say that point A on the "hillside" in this diagram is an *unstable equilibrium* because a slight displacement from A will tend to increase over time. Point B is in a region of *neutral equilibrium* because slight displacements will tend not to change further, while C is a point of *stable equilibrium*, since small displacements will tend to decrease over time. Note the word "small": in a nonlinear system like that of Figure 6, a large displacement can move the ball from the *basin of attraction* of C (the set of states whose dynamics tends toward C) to another one. Clearly, the ball will not tend to return to C after a massive displacement that moves the ball to the far side of A's hilltop.

Many nonlinear systems have another interesting property: they may exhibit *limit cycles*. These are closed trajectories in the state space, and thus may be thought of as "dynamic equilibria." If the state of a system follows a limit cycle, we may also say it oscillates or exhibits periodic behavior. A limit cycle is *stable* if a small displacement will be reduced as the trajectory of the system comes closer and closer to the original limit cycle. By contrast, a limit cycle is *unstable* if such excursions do not die out. Research in nonlinear systems has also revealed what are called *strange attractors*. These are attractors which, unlike simple limit cycles, describe such complex paths through the state space that, although the system is deterministic, a path that approaches the strange attractor gives every appearance of being random. The point here is that very small differences in initial state may be amplified with the passage of time, so that differences that at first are not even noticeable will yield, in due course, states that are very different indeed. Such a trajectory has become the accepted mathematical model of *chaos*, and it is used to describe a number of physical phenomena, such as the onset of turbulence in a weather system, as well as a number of phenomena in biological systems (see CHAOS IN BIOLOGICAL SYSTEMS; CHAOS IN NEURAL SYSTEMS).

Hopfield Nets

Many authors have treated neural networks as dynamical systems, employing notions of equilibrium, stability, and so on, to classify their performance (see, e.g., Grossberg, 1967; Amari and Arbib, 1977; see also COMPUTING WITH ATTRACTORS). However, it was a paper by John Hopfield (1982) that was the catalyst in attracting the attention of many physicists to this field of study. In a McCulloch-Pitts network, every neuron processes its inputs to determine a new output at each time step. By contrast, a *Hopfield net* is a net of such units with (1) *symmetric* weights ($w_{ij} = w_{ji}$) and no self-connections ($w_{ii} = 0$), and (2) asynchronous updating. For instance, let s_i denote the state (0 or 1) of the ith unit. At each time

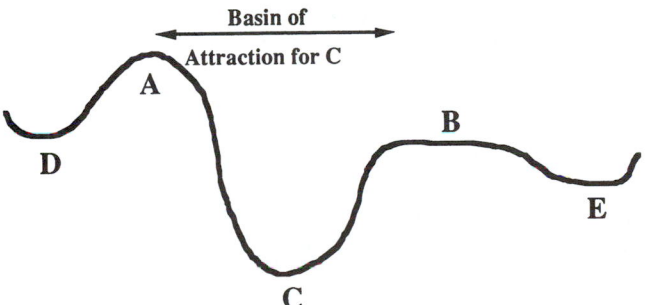

Figure 6. An energy landscape: For a ball rolling on the "hillside," point A is an *unstable equilibrium*, point B lies in a region of *neutral equilibrium*, and point C is a point of *stable equilibrium*. Point C is called an attractor: the basin of attraction of C comprises all states whose dynamics tend toward C.

step, pick just one unit at random. If unit i is chosen, s_i takes the value 1 if and only if $\Sigma w_{ij}s_j \geq \theta_i$. Otherwise s_i is set to 0. Note that this is an *autonomous* (input-free) network: there are no inputs (although instead of considering θ_i as a threshold we may consider $-\theta_i$ as a constant input, also known as a bias).

Hopfield defined a measure called the *energy* for such a net (see ENERGY FUNCTIONALS FOR NEURAL NETWORKS)

$$E = -\tfrac{1}{2} \sum_{ij} s_i s_j w_{ij} + \sum_i s_i \theta_i \qquad (1)$$

This is not the physical energy of the neural net but a mathematical quantity that, in some ways, does for neural dynamics what the potential energy does for Newtonian mechanics. In general, a mechanical system moves to a state of lower potential energy just as, in Figure 6, the ball tends to move downhill. Hopfield showed that his symmetrical networks with asynchronous updating had a similar property.

For example, if we pick a unit and the foregoing firing rule does not change its s_i, it will not change E. However, if s_i initially equals 0, and $\Sigma w_{ij}s_j \geq \theta_i$, then s_i goes from 0 to 1 with all other s_j constant, and the "energy gap," or change in E, is given by

$$\begin{aligned}
\Delta E &= -\tfrac{1}{2} \sum_j (w_{ij}s_j + w_{ji}s_j) + \theta_i \\
&= -\sum_j w_{ij}s_j + \theta_i, \text{ by symmetry} \\
&\leq 0 \text{ since } \sum_j w_{ij}s_j \geq \theta_i
\end{aligned}$$

Similarly, if s_i initially equals 1, and $\Sigma w_{ij}s_j < \theta_i$, then s_i goes from 1 to 0 with all other s_j constant, and the energy gap is given by

$$\Delta E = \sum w_{ij}s_j - \theta_i < 0$$

In other words, with every asynchronous updating, we have $\Delta E \leq 0$. Hence the dynamics of the net tends to move E toward a minimum. We stress that there may be different such states—they are *local* minima, just as, in Figure 6, both D and E are local minima (each of them is lower than any "nearby" state) but not global minima (since C is lower than either of them). Global minimization is not guaranteed.

The expression just presented for ΔE depends on the symmetry condition, $w_{ij} = w_{ji}$, for without this condition, the expression would instead be $\Delta E = -(\tfrac{1}{2})\Sigma_j(w_{ij}s_j + w_{ji}s_j) + \theta_i$ and in this case, Hopfield's updating rule need not yield a passage to energy minimum, but might instead yield a limit cycle, which could be useful in, e.g., controlling rhythmic behavior (see, e.g., RESPIRATORY RHYTHM GENERATION). In a control problem, a link w_{ij} might express the likelihood that the action represented by i would precede that represented by j, in which case $w_{ij} = w_{ji}$ is normally inappropriate.

The condition of *asynchronous* update is crucial, too. If we consider the simple "flip-flop" with $w_{12} = w_{21} = 1$ and $\theta_1 = \theta_2 = 0.5$, then the McCulloch-Pitts network will *oscillate* between the states (0, 1) and (1, 0) or will sit in the states (0, 0) or (1, 1); in other words, there is no guarantee that it will converge to an equilibrium. However, with $E = -(\tfrac{1}{2})\Sigma_{ij}s_i s_j w_{ij} + \Sigma_i s_i \theta_i$, we have $E(0, 0) = 0$, $E(0, 1) = E(1, 0) = 0.5$, and $E(1, 1) = 0$, and the Hopfield network will *converge* to the global minimum at either (0, 0) or (1, 1).

Hopfield also aroused much interest because he showed how a number of optimization problems could be "solved" using neural networks. (The quotes around "solved" acknowledge the fact that the state to which a neural network converges may represent a local, rather than a global, optimum of the corresponding optimization problem.) Such networks were similar to the "constraint satisfaction" networks that had already been studied in the computer vision community. (In most vision algorithms—see, e.g., STEREO CORRESPONDENCE—constraints can be formulated in terms of symmetric weights, so that $w_{ij} = w_{ji}$ is appropriate.) The aim, given a "constraint satisfaction" problem, is to so choose weights for a neural network so that the energy E for that network is a measure of the overall constraint violation. A famous example is the Traveling Salesman Problem (TSP): There are n cities, with a road of length l_{ij} joining city i to city j. The salesman wishes to find a way to visit the cities that is optimal in two ways: each city is visited only once, and the total route is as short as possible. We express this as a constraint satisfaction network in the following way: Let the activity of neuron N_{ij} express the decision to go straight from city i to city j. The cost of this move is simply l_{ij}, and so the total "transportation cost" is $\Sigma_{ij} l_{ij} N_{ij}$. It is somewhat more challenging to express the cost of violating the "visit a city only once" criterion, but we can reexpress it by saying that, for city j, there is one and only one city i from which j is directly approached. Thus, $\Sigma_j (\Sigma_i N_{ij} - 1)^2 = 0$ just in case this constraint is satisfied; a non-zero value measures the extent to which this constraint is violated. This can then be mapped into the setting of weights and thresholds for a Hopfield network. Hopfield and Tank (1986) constructed chips for this network which do indeed settle very quickly to a local minimum of E. Unfortunately, there is no guarantee that this minimum is globally optimal. The article OPTIMIZATION, NEURAL presents this and a number of other neurally based approaches to optimization. The article SIMULATED ANNEALING AND BOLTZMANN MACHINES shows how noise may be added to "shake" a system out of a local minimum and let it settle into a global minimum. (Consider, for example, shaking that is strong enough to shake the ball from D to A, and thus into the basin of attraction of C, in Figure 6, but not strong enough to shake the ball back from C toward D.)

Adaptation in Dynamic Systems

In the previous discussion of neural networks as dynamic systems, the dynamics (i.e., the state transition function) has been fixed. However, just as humans and animals learn from experience, so do many important applications of ANNs depend on the ability of these networks to adapt to the task at hand by, e.g., changing the values of the synaptic weights to improve performance. We now introduce the general notion of an adaptive system as background to some of the most influential "learning rules" used in adaptive neural networks. The key motivation for using learning networks is that it may be too hard to program explicitly the behavior that one sees in a black box, but one may be able to drive a network by the actual input/output behavior of that box, or by some description of its trajectories, to cause it to adapt itself into a network which approximates that given behavior. However, as we will

stress at the end of this section, a learning algorithm may not solve a problem within a reasonable period of time unless the initial structure of the network is suitable.

Adaptive Control

A key problem of technology is to control a complex system so that it behaves in some desired way, whether getting a space probe on course to Mars or a steel mill to produce high-quality steel. A common situation that complicates this *control problem* is that the controlled system may not be known accurately; it may even change its character somewhat with time. For example, as fuel is depleted, the mass and moments of inertia of the probe may change in unpredicted ways. The *adaptation problem* involves determining, on the basis of interaction with a given system, an appropriate "model" of the system which the controller can use in solving the control problem.

Suppose we have available an *identification procedure* which can find an adequate parametric representation of the controlled system (see IDENTIFICATION AND CONTROL). Then, rather than build a controller specifically designed to control this one system, we may instead build a general-purpose controller which can accommodate to any reasonable set of parameters. The controller then uses the parameters which the identification procedure provides as the best estimate of the controlled system's parameters at that time. If the identification procedure can make accurate estimates of the system's parameters as quickly as they actually change, the controller will be able to act efficiently despite fluctuations in controlled system dynamics. The controller, when coupled to an identification procedure, is an *adaptive controller*; that is, it adapts its control strategy to changes in the dynamics of the controlled system. However, the use of an explicit identification procedure is only one way of building an adaptive controller. Adaptive neural nets may be used to build adaptive procedures which may directly modify the parameters in some control rule, or identify the system *inverse* so that desired outputs can be automatically transformed into the inputs that will achieve them. (See SENSORIMOTOR LEARNING for the distinction between forward and inverse models.)

Pattern Recognition

In the setup shown in Figure 7, the *preprocessor* extracts from the environment a set of "confidence levels" for various input features (see FEATURE ANALYSIS), with the result represented by a vector of d real numbers. In this formalization, any pattern x is represented by a point $(x_1, x_2, \ldots, x_d)$ in a d-dimensional Euclidean space $\mathbb{R}^d$ called the *pattern space*. The pattern recognizer then takes the pattern and produces a response that may have one of K distinct values where there are K categories into which the patterns must be sorted; points in $\mathbb{R}^d$ are thus grouped into at least K different sets (see CONCEPT LEARNING and PATTERN RECOGNITION). However, a

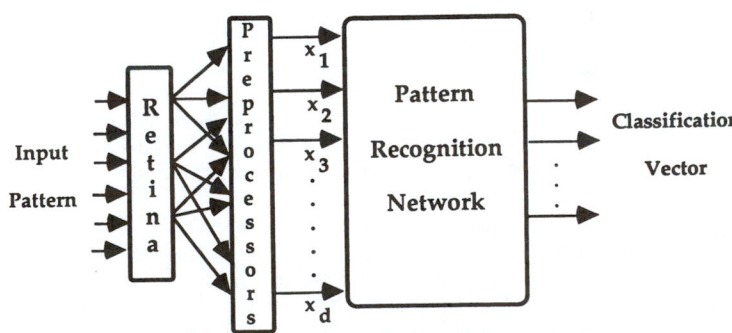

Figure 7. One strategy in pattern recognition is to precede the adaptive neural network by a fixed layer of "preprocessors" or "feature extractors" which replace the image by a finite vector for further processing. In other approaches, the functions defined by the early layers of the network may themselves be subject to training.

category might be represented in more than one region of $\mathbb{R}^d$. To take an example from visual pattern recognition (although the theory of pattern recognition networks applies to any classification of $\mathbb{R}^d$), a and A are members of the category of the first letter of the English alphabet, but they would be found in different connected regions of a pattern space. In such cases, it may be necessary to establish a hierarchical system involving a separate apparatus to recognize each subset, and a further system that recognizes that the subsets all belong to the same set (a related idea was originally developed by Selfridge, 1959; for adaptive versions, see MODULAR AND HIERARCHICAL LEARNING SYSTEMS). Here we avoid this problem by concentrating on the case in which the decision space is divided into exactly two connected regions.

We call a function f: $\mathbb{R}^d \rightarrow \mathbb{R}$ a *discriminant function* if the equation $f(x) = 0$ gives the *decision surface* separating two regions of a pattern space. A basic problem of pattern recognition is the specification of such a function. It is virtually impossible for humans to "read out" the function they use (not to mention *how* they use it) to classify patterns. Thus, a common strategy in pattern recognition is to provide a classification machine with an adjustable function and to "train" it with a set of patterns of known classification that are typical of those with which the machine must ultimately work. The function may be linear, quadratic, polynomial, or even more subtle yet, depending on the complexity and shape of the pattern space and the necessary discriminations. The experimenter chooses a class of functions with parameters which, it is hoped, will, with proper adjustment, yield a function that will successfully classify any given pattern. For example, the experimenter may decide to use a linear function of the form

$$f(x) = w_1 x_1 + w_2 x_2 + \ldots + w_d x_d + w_{d+1}$$

(i.e., a McCulloch-Pitts neuron!) in a two-category pattern classifier. The equation $f(x) = 0$ gives a hyperplane as the decision surface, and training involves adjusting the coefficients (w_1, w_2, $\ldots$, w_d, w_{d+1}) so that the decision surface produces an acceptable separation of the two classes. We say that two categories are *linearly separable* if an acceptable setting of such linear weights exists. Thus, pattern recognition poses (at least) the following challenges to neural networks:

(a) Find a "good" set of preprocessors. Competitive learning based on Hebbian plasticity (see COMPETITIVE LEARNING, as well as the following text) provides one way of finding such features by extracting statistically significant patterns from a set of input patterns. For example, if such a network were exposed to many, but only, letters of the Roman alphabet, then it would find that certain line segments and loops occurred repeatedly, even if there were no teacher to tell it how to classify the patterns.

(b) Given a set of preprocessors and a set of patterns which have already been classified, adjust the connections of a neural network so that it acts as an effective pattern recognizer. That is, its response to a preprocessed pattern should usually agree well with the classification provided by a teacher.

(c) Of course, if the neural network has multiple layers with adaptable synaptic weights, then the early layers can be thought of as preprocessors for the later layers, and we have a case of supervised, rather than Hebbian, formation of these "feature detectors"—emphasizing features which are not only statistically significant elements of the input patterns but which also serve to distinguish usefully to which class a pattern belongs.

Associative Memory

In pattern recognition, we associate a pattern with a "label" or "category." Alternatively, an associative memory takes some "key" as input and returns some "associated recollection" as output (see ASSOCIATIVE NETWORKS). For example, given the sound of a word,

we may wish to recall its spelling. Given a misspelled word, we may wish to recall the correctly spelled word of which it is most plausibly a "degraded image." There are two major approaches to the use of neural networks as associative memories:

In *nonrecurrent* neural networks, there are no loops (i.e., we cannot start at any neuron and "follow the arrows" to get back to that neuron). We use such a network by fixing the pattern of inputs as the key, and holding them steady. Since the absence of loops ensures that the input pattern uniquely determines the output pattern (after the new inputs have time to propagate their effects through the network), this uniquely determined output pattern is the recollection associated with the key.

In *recurrent* networks, the presence of loops implies that the input alone may not determine the output of the net, since this will also depend on the initial state of the network. Thus, recurrent networks are often used as associative memories in the following way. The inputs are only used transiently to establish the initial state of the neural network. After that, the network operates autonomously (i.e., uninfluenced by any inputs). If and when it reaches an equilibrium state, that state is read out as the recollection associated with the key.

In either case, the problem is to set the weights of the neural network so that it associates keys as accurately as possible with the appropriate recollections.

Learning Rules

Most learning rules in current models of "lumped neurons" (i.e., those that exclude detailed analysis of the fine structure of the neuron or the neurochemistry of neural plasticity) take the form of schemes for adjusting the synaptic weights, the "ws." The two classic learning schemes for McCulloch-Pitts-type formal neurons are due to Hebb (see HEBBIAN SYNAPTIC PLASTICITY) and Rosenblatt (the perceptron, see PERCEPTRONS, ADALINES, AND BACKPROPAGATION), and we now introduce these in turn.

Hebbian Plasticity and Network Self-Organization

In Hebb's (1949) learning scheme (see HEBBIAN SYNAPTIC PLASTICITY), the connection between two neurons is strengthened if both neurons fire at the same time. The simplest example of such a rule is to increase w_{ij} by the following amount:

$$\Delta w_{ij} = k y_i x_j$$

where synapse w_{ij} connects a presynaptic neuron with firing rate x_j to a postsynaptic neuron with firing rate y_i. The trouble with the original Hebb model is that every synapse will eventually get stronger and stronger until they all saturate, thus destroying any selectivity of association. Von der Malsburg's (1973) solution was to normalize the synapses impinging on a given neuron. To accomplish this, one must first compute the Hebbian "update" $\Delta w_{ij} = k x_i y_j$ and then divide this by the total putative synaptic weights to get the final result which replaces w_i by

$$\frac{w_{ij} + \Delta w_{ij}}{\sum_k (w_{kj} + \Delta w_{kj})}$$

where the summation k extends over all inputs to the neuron. This new rule not only increases the strengths of those synapses with inputs strongly correlated with the cell's activity, but also decreases the synaptic strengths of other connections in which such correlations did not arise.

Von der Malsburg was motivated by the pattern recognition problem and was concerned with how individual cells in his network might come to be tuned so as to respond to one particular input "feature" rather than another (see OCULAR DOMINANCE AND ORIENTATION COLUMNS for background as well as a review of more recent approaches). This exposed another problem with Hebb's rule: a lot of nearby cells may, just by chance, all have initial random connectivity which makes them easily persuadable by the same stimulus; alternatively, the same pattern might occur many times before a new pattern is experienced by the network. In either case, many cells would become tuned to the same feature, with not enough cells left to learn important and distinctive features. To solve this, von der Malsburg introduced *lateral inhibition* into his model. In this connectivity pattern, activity in any one cell is distributed laterally to reduce (partially inhibit) the activity of nearby cells. This ensures that if one cell—call it A—were especially active, its connections to nearby cells would make them less active, and so make them less likely to learn, by Hebbian synaptic adjustment, those features that most excite A.

In summary, then, when the Hebbian rule is augmented by a normalization rule, it tends to "sharpen" a neuron's predisposition "without a teacher," getting its firing to become better and better correlated with a cluster of stimulus patterns. This performance is improved when there is some competition between neurons so that if one neuron becomes adept at responding to a pattern, it inhibits other neurons from doing so (COMPETITIVE LEARNING). Thus, the final set of input weights to the neuron depends both on the initial setting of the weights and on the pattern of clustering of the set of stimuli to which it is exposed (see DATA CLUSTERING AND LEARNING). Other "post-Hebbian" rules, motivated both by technological efficiency and by recent biological findings, are discussed in several articles in Part III, including HEBBIAN LEARNING AND NEURONAL REGULATION and POST-HEBBIAN LEARNING ALGORITHMS.

In the adaptive architecture just described, the inputs are initially randomly connected to the cells of the processing layer. As a result, none of these cells is particularly good at pattern recognition. However, by sheer statistical fluctuation of the synaptic connections, one will be slightly better at responding to a particular pattern than others are; it will thus slightly strengthen those synapses which allow it to fire for that pattern and, through lateral inhibition, this will make it harder for cells initially less well tuned for that pattern to become tuned to it. Thus, without any teacher, this network automatically organizes itself so that each cell becomes tuned for an important cluster of information in the sensory inflow. This is a basic example of the kind of phenomenon treated in SELF-ORGANIZATION AND THE BRAIN.

Perceptrons

Perceptrons are neural nets that change with "experience," using an *error-correction rule* designed to change the weights of each response unit when it makes erroneous responses to stimuli that are presented to the network. We refer to the judge of what is correct as the "teacher," although this may be another neural network, or some environmental input, rather than a signal supplied by a human teacher in the usual schoolroom sense. Consider the case in which a set **R** of input lines feeds a Pitts-McCulloch neural network whose neurons are called *associator units* and which in turn provide the input to a single McCulloch-Pitts neuron (called the *output unit* of the perceptron) with adjustable weights ($w_1, \ldots, w_d$) and threshold θ. (In the case of visual pattern recognition, we think of **R** as a rectangular "retina" onto which patterns may be projected.) A *simple perceptron* is one in which the associator units are not interconnected, *which means that it has no short-term memory*. (If such connections are present, the perceptron is called *cross-coupled*. A cross-coupled perceptron may have multiple layers and loops back from an "earlier" to a "later" layer.) If the associator units feed the pattern $x = (x_1, \ldots, x_d)$ to the output unit, then the response of that unit will be to provide the pattern discrimination

with discriminant function $f(x) = w_1 x_1 + \ldots + w_d x_d - \theta$. In other words, the simple perceptron can only compute a *linearly separable* function of the pattern as provided by the associator units. The question asked by Rosenblatt (1958) and answered by many others since (cf. Nilsson, 1965) was, "Given a simple perceptron (i.e., only the synaptic weights of the output unit are adjustable), can we 'train' it to recognize a given linearly separable set of patterns by adjusting the 'weights' on various interconnections on the basis of feedback on whether or not the network classifies a pattern correctly?" The answer was "Yes: if the patterns are linearly separable, then there is a learning scheme which will eventually yield a satisfactory setting of the weights." The best-known perceptron learning rule strengthens an active synapse if the efferent neuron fails to fire when it should have fired, and weakens an active synapse if the neuron fires when it should not have done so:

$$\Delta w_{ij} = k(Y_i - y_i)x_j$$

As before, synapse w_{ij} connects a presynaptic neuron with firing rate x_j to a postsynaptic neuron with firing rate y_i, but now Y_i is the "correct" output supplied by the "teacher." (This is similar to the Widrow-Hoff [1960] least mean squares model of adaptive control; see PERCEPTRONS, ADALINES, AND BACKPROPAGATION.) Notice that the rule does change the response to x_j "in the right direction." If the output is correct, $Y_i = y_i$ and there is no change, $\Delta w_j = 0$. If the output is too small, then $Y_i - y_i > 0$, and the change in w_j will add $\Delta w_j x_j = k(Y_i - y_i)x_j x_j > 0$ to the output unit's response to ($x_1, \ldots, x_d$). Similarly, if the output is too large, then $Y_i - y_i < 0$, Δw_j will add $k(Y_i - y_i)x_j x_j < 0$ to the output unit's response. Thus, there is a sense in which the new setting $w' = w + \Delta w$ classifies the input pattern x "more nearly correctly" than w does. Unfortunately, in classifying x "more correctly" we run the risk of classifying another pattern "less correctly." However, the *perceptron convergence theorem* (see Arbib, 1987, pp. 66–69, for a proof) shows that Rosenblatt's procedure does not yield an endless seesaw, but will eventually converge to a correct set of weights if one exists, albeit perhaps after many iterations through the set of trial patterns.

Network Complexity

The perceptron convergence theorem states that, if a linear separation exists, the perceptron error-correction scheme will find it. Minsky and Papert (1969) revivified the study of perceptrons (although some AI workers thought they had killed it!) by responding to such results with questions like, "Your scheme works when a weighting scheme exists, but *when* does there exist such a setting of the weights?" More generally, "Given a pattern-recognition problem, how much of the retina must each associator unit 'see' if the network is to do its job?" Minsky and Papert studied when it was possible for a McCulloch-Pitts neuron (no matter how trained) to combine information in a single preprocessing layer to perform a given pattern recognition task, such as recognizing whether a pattern X of 1s on the retina (the other retinal units having output 0) is *connected*, that is, whether a path can be drawn from any 1 of X to another without going through any 0s. Another question was to determine whether X is of *odd parity*, i.e., whether X contains an odd number of 1s. The question is, "How many inputs are required for the preprocessing units of a simple perceptron to successfully implement f?" We can get away with using a single element, computing an arbitrary Boolean function, and connecting it to all the units of the retina. So the question that really interests us is whether we can get away with a response unit connected to proprocessors, each of which receives inputs from a limited set of retinal units to make a global decision by synthesizing an array of local views.

We convey the flavor of Minsky and Papert's approach by the example of XOR, the simple Boolean operation of addition modulo

2, also known as the exclusive-or. If we imagine the square with vertices $(0, 0)$, $(0, 1)$, $(1, 1)$, and $(1, 0)$ in the Cartesian plane, with (x_1, x_2) being labeled by $x_1 \oplus x_2$, we have 0s at one diagonally opposite pair of vertices and 1s at the other diagonally opposite pair of vertices. It is clear that there is no way of interposing a straight line such that the 1s lie on one side and the 0s lie on the other side. However, we shall prove it mathematically to gain insight into the techniques used by Minsky and Papert.

Consider the claim that we wish to prove wrong: that there actually exists a neuron with threshold θ and weights α and β such that $x_1 \oplus x_2 = 1$ if and only if $\alpha x_1 + \beta x_2 \geq \theta$. The crucial point is to note that the function of addition modulo 2 is symmetric; therefore, we must also have $x_1 \oplus x_2 = 1$ if and only if $\beta x_1 + \alpha x_2 \geq \theta$, and, so, adding together the two terms, we have $x_1 \oplus x_2 = 1$ if and only if $(1/2)(\alpha + \beta)(x_1 + x_2) \geq \theta$. Writing $(1/2)(\alpha + \beta)$ as γ, we see that we have reduced three putative parameters α, β, and θ to just two, namely γ and θ.

We now set $t = x_1 + x_2$ and look at the polynomial $\gamma t - \theta$. It is a degree 1 polynomial, but note: at $t = 0$, $\gamma t - \theta$ must be less than zero ($0 \oplus 0 = 0$); at $t = 1$, it is greater than or equal to zero ($0 \oplus 1 = 1 \oplus 0 = 1$); and at $t = 2$, it is again less than zero ($1 \oplus 1 = 0$). This is a contradiction—a polynomial of degree 1 cannot change sign from positive to negative more than once. We conclude that there is no such polynomial, and thus that there is no threshold element which will add modulo 2.

We now understand a general method used again and again by Minsky and Papert: start with a pattern-classification problem. Observe that certain symmetries leave it invariant. For instance, for the parity problem (is the number of active elements even or odd?), which includes the case of addition modulo 2 when the retina has only two units, any permutation of the points of the retina would leave the classification unchanged. Use this to reduce the number of parameters describing the circuit. Then lump items together to get a polynomial and examine actual patterns to put a lower bound on the degree of the polynomial, fixing things so that this degree bounds the number of inputs to the response unit of a simple perceptron.

Minsky and Papert provide many interesting theorems (for the proof of an illustrative sample, see Arbib, 1987, pp. 82–84). As just one example, we may note that they prove that the parity function requires preprocessors big enough to scan the whole retina if the preprocessors can only be followed by a single McCulloch-Pitts neuron. By contrast, to tell whether the number of active retinal inputs reaches a certain threshold only requires two inputs per neuron in the first layer. (For other complexity results, see the articles listed in the road map **Computability and Complexity**.)

Gradient Descent and Credit Assignment

The implication of the results on "network complexity" is clear: if we limit the complexity of the units in a neural network, then in general we will need many layers, rather than a single layer, if the network is to have any chance of being trained to realize many "interesting" functions. This conclusion motivates the study of training rules for multilayer perceptrons, of which the most widely used is *backpropagation*. Before describing this method, we first discuss two general notions of which it is an important exemplar: *gradient descent* and *credit assignment*.

In discussing Hopfield networks, we introduced the metaphor of an "energy landscape" (see Figure 6). The asynchronous updates move the state of the network (the vector of neural activity levels) "downhill," tending toward a local energy minimum. Our task now is to realize that the metaphor works again on a far more abstract level when we consider learning. In learning, the dynamic variable is not the network state, but rather the vector of synaptic weights (or whatever other set of network parameters is adjusted by the

learning rules). We now conduct *gradient descent in weight space*. At each step, the weights are adjusted in such a way as to improve the performance of the network. (As in the case of the simple perceptron, the improvement is a "local" one based on the current situation. It is, in this case, a matter for computer simulation to prove that the cumulative effect of these small changes is a network which solves the overall problem.)

But how do we recognize which "direction" in weight space is "downhill"? Suppose success is achieved by a complex mechanism after operating over a considerable period of time (for example, when a chess-playing program wins a game). To what particular decisions made by what particular components should the success be attributed? And, if failure results, what decisions deserve blame? This is closely related to the problem known as the "mesa" or "plateau" problem (Minsky, 1961). The performance evaluation function available to a learning system may consist of large level regions in which gradient descent degenerates to exhaustive search, so that only a few of the situations obtainable by the learning system and its environment are known to be desirable, and these situations may occur rarely.

One aspect of this problem, then, is the *temporal* credit assignment problem. The utility of making a certain action may depend on the sequence of actions of which it is a part, and an indication of improved performance may not occur until the entire sequence has been completed. This problem was attacked successfully in Samuel's (1959) learning program for playing checkers. The idea is to interpret predictions of future reward as rewarding events themselves. In other words, neutral stimulus events can themselves become reinforcing if they regularly occur before events that are intrinsically reinforcing. Such *temporal difference learning* (see REINFORCEMENT LEARNING) is like a process of erosion: the original uninformative mesa, where only a few sink holes allow gradient descent to a local minimum, is slowly replaced by broader valleys in which gradient descent may successfully proceed from many different places on the landscape.

Another aspect of credit assignment concerns structural factors. In the simple perceptron, only the weights to the output units are to be adjusted. This architecture can only support maps which are linearly separable as based on the patterns presented by the preprocessors, and we have seen that many interesting problems require preprocessing units of undue complexity to achieve linear separability. We thus need multiple layers of preprocessors, and, since one may not know a priori the appropriate set of preprocessors for a given problem, these units should be trainable too. This raises the question, "How does a neuron deeply embedded within a network 'know' what aspect of the outcome of an overall action was 'its fault'?" This is the *structural* credit assignment problem. In the next section, we shall study the most widely used solution to this problem, called *backpropagation*, which propagates back to a hidden unit some measure of its responsibility.

Backpropagation is an "adaptive architecture": it is not just a local rule for synaptic adjustment; it also takes into account the position of a neuron in the network to indicate how the neuron's weights are to change. (In this sense, we may see the use of lateral inhibition to improve Hebbian learning as the first example of an adaptive architecture in these pages.) This adaptive architecture is an example of "neurally inspired" modeling, not modeling of actual brain structures; and there is no evidence that backpropagation represents actual brain mechanisms.

Backpropagation

The task of backpropagation is to train a *multilayer* (feedforward) *perceptron* (or MLP), a loop-free network which has its units arranged in layers, with a unit providing input only to units in the next layer of the sequence. The first layer comprises fixed input units; there may then be several layers of trainable "hidden units" carrying an internal representation, and finally, there is the layer of output units, also trainable. (A simple perceptron then corresponds to the case in which we view the input units as fixed associator units, i.e., they deliver a preprocessed, rather than a "raw," pattern which connect directly to the output units without any hidden units in between.) For what follows, it is crucial that each unit *not* be binary: it has both input and output taking continuous values in some range, say [0, 1]. The response is a sigmoidal function of the weighted sum. Thus, if a unit has inputs x_k with corresponding weights w_{ik}, the output x_i is given by $x_i = f_i(\Sigma w_{ik}x_k)$, where f_i is a sigmoidal function, say

$$f_i(x) = \frac{1}{1 + e^{-(x + \theta_i)}}$$

with θ_i being a bias or threshold for the unit.

The environment only evaluates the output units. We are given a training set of input patterns p and corresponding desired target patterns t^p for the output units. With o^p the actual output pattern elicited by input p, the aim is to adjust the weights in the network to minimize the error

$$E = \sum_{\text{patterns } p} \sum_{\text{output neurons } k} (t_k^p - o_k^p)^2$$

Rumelhart, Hinton, and Williams (1986) were among those who devised a formula for propagating back the gradient of this evaluation from a unit to its inputs. This process can continue by backpropagation through the entire net. The scheme seems to avoid many false minima. At each trial, we fix the input pattern p and consider the corresponding "restricted error"

$$E = \sum_k (t_k - o_k)^2$$

where k ranges over designated "output units." The net has many units interconnected by weights w_{ij}. The learning rule is to change w_{ij} so as to reduce E by *gradient descent*:

$$\Delta w_{ij} = -\frac{\partial E}{\partial w_{ij}} = 2 \sum_k (t_k - o_k) \frac{\partial o_k}{\partial w_{ij}}$$

Consider a net divided into $m + 1$ layers, with nets in layer $g + 1$ receiving all their inputs from layer g; with layer 0 comprising the input units; and layer m comprising the output units. If i is an output unit (remember, w_{ij} connects from j to i) then the only nonzero term in the last equation has $k = i$. Now $o_k = \Sigma w_{il}o_l$ where $w_{il} \neq 0$ only for o_1 which are outputs from the previous layer. We thus have

$$\Delta w_{ij} = 2(t_i - o_i) \frac{\partial f_i\left(\sum w_{il}o_{m1}\right)}{\partial w_{ij}} = 2(t_i - o_i)f_i'o_j$$

where f_i' is the derivative of the activation function evaluated at the activation level $in_i = \Sigma w_{il}o_l$ to unit i. Thus Δw_{ij} for an output unit i is proportional to $\delta_i o_j$, where $\delta_i = (t_i - o_i)f_i'$.

Next, suppose that i is a hidden unit whose output drives only output units:

$$\Delta w_{ij} = 2 \sum_k (t_k - o_k) \frac{\partial f_k\left(\sum w_{kl}o_l\right)}{\partial w_{ij}}$$

However, the only o_l that depends on w_{ij} is o_i, and so

$$\frac{\partial f_k\left(\sum w_{kl}o_l\right)}{\partial w_{ij}} = \frac{\partial f_k\left(\sum w_{kl}o_l\right)}{\partial o_i} \frac{\partial o_i}{\partial w_{ij}} = [f_k'w_{ki}] \cdot [f_i'o_j]$$

so that $\Delta w_{ij} = 2\Sigma_k(t_k - o_k)[f_k'w_{ki}] \cdot [f_i'o_j]$.

Recalling that $\delta_k = (t_k - o_k)f_k'$ for an output unit k, we may rewrite this as

$$\Delta w_{ij} = 2\left(\sum_k \delta_k w_{ki}\right)f_i'o_j$$

Thus, Δw_{ij} is proportional to $\delta_i o_j$, with $\delta_i = (\Sigma_k \delta_k w_{ki})f_i'$, where k runs over all units which receive unit i's output. More generally, we can prove the following, by induction on how many layers back we must go to reach a unit:

Proposition. Consider a layered loop-free net with error $E = \Sigma_k(t_k - o_k)^2$, where k ranges over designated "output units," and let the weights w_{ij} be changed according to the gradient descent rule

$$\Delta w_{ij} = -\partial E/\partial w_{ij} = 2 \sum_k (t_k - o_k) \frac{\partial o_k}{\partial w_{ij}}$$

Then the weights may be changed inductively, working back from the output units, by the rule

$$\Delta w_{ij} \text{ is proportional to } \delta_i o_j$$

where:

Basis Step: $\delta_i = (t_i - o_i)f_i'$ for an output unit.

Induction Step: If i is a hidden unit, and if δ_k is known for all units that receive unit i's output, then $\delta_i = (\Sigma_k\delta_k w_{ki})f_i'$, where k runs over all units which receive unit i's output.

Thus the "error signal" δ_i *propagates* back layer by layer from the output units. In $\Sigma_k\delta_k w_{ki}$, unit i receives error propagated back from a unit k to the extent to which i affects k. For output units, this is essentially the *delta rule* given by Widrow and Hoff (1960) (see Perceptrons, Adalines, and Backpropagation).

The theorem just presented tells us how to compute Δw_{ij} for gradient descent. It does not guarantee that the above step-size is appropriate to reach the minimum, nor does it guarantee that the minimum, if reached, is global. The backpropagation rule defined by this proposition is, thus, a heuristic rule, not one guaranteed to find a global minimum, but is still perhaps the most diversely used adaptive architecture. Many other approaches to learning, including some which are "neural-like" in at best a statistical sense, rather than being embedded in adaptive neural networks, may be found in the road map **Learning in Artificial Networks** (not just neural networks).

A Cautionary Note

The previous subsections have introduced a number of techniques that can be used to make neural networks more adaptive. In a typical training scenario, we are given a network **N** which, in response to the presentation of any x from some set of input patterns, will eventually settle down to produce a corresponding y from the set Y of the network's output patterns. A training set is then a sequence of pairs (x_k, y_k) from $X \times Y$, $1 \leq k \leq n$. The foregoing results say that, in many cases (and the bounds are not yet well defined), if we train the net with repeated presentations of the various (x_k, y_k), it will converge to a set of connections which cause N to compute a function $f: X \rightarrow Y$ with the property that, over the set of k's from 1 to n, the $f(x_k)$ "correlate fairly well" with the y_k. Of course, there are many other functions $g: X \rightarrow Y$ such that the $g(x_k)$ "correlate fairly well" with the y_k, and they may differ wildly on those "tests" x in X that do not equal an x_k in the training set. The view that one may simply present a trainable net with a few examples of solved problems, and it will then adjust its connections to be able to solve all problems of a given class, glosses over three main issues:

(a) *Complexity*: Is the network complex enough to encode a solution method?

(b) *Practicality*: Can the net achieve such a solution within a feasible period of time? and

(c) *Efficacy*: How do we guarantee that the generalization achieved by the machine matches our conception of a useful solution?

Part III provides many "snapshots" of the research underway to develop answers to these problems (for the "state of play" see, for example, LEARNING AND GENERALIZATION: THEORETICAL BOUNDS; PAC LEARNING AND NEURAL NETWORKS; and VAPNIK-CHERVONENKIS DIMENSION OF NEURAL NETWORKS). Nonetheless, it is clear that these training techniques will work best when training is based on an adaptive architecture and an initial set of weights appropriate to the given problem. Future work on the neurally inspired design of intelligent systems will involve many domain-specific techniques for system design, such as those exemplified in the road maps **Vision** and **Robotics and Control Theory**, as well as general advances in adaptive architectures.

Envoi

With this, our tour of some of those basic landmarks of *Brain Theory and Neural Networks* established by 1986 is complete. I now invite each reader to follow the suggestions of the section "How to Use this Book" of the *Handbook* to begin exploring the riches of Part III, possibly with the guidance of a number of the road maps in Part II.

Acknowledgments. All of Part I is a lightly edited version of Part I as it appeared in the first edition of the *Handbook*. Section I.1 is based in large part on material contained in Section 2.3 of Arbib (1989), while Section I.3 is based on Sections 3.4 and 8.2.

References

Amari, S., and Arbib, M. A., 1977, Competition and cooperation in neural nets, in *Systems Neuroscience* (J. Metzler, Ed.), New York: Academic Press, pp. 119–165.

Arbib, M. A., 1981, Perceptual structures and distributed motor control, in *Handbook of Physiology—The Nervous System*, vol. II, *Motor Control* (V. B. Brooks, Ed.), Bethesda, MD: American Physiological Society, pp. 1449–1480.

Arbib, M. A., 1987, *Brains, Machines, and Mathematics*, 2nd ed., New York: Springer-Verlag.

Arbib, M. A., 1989, *The Metaphorical Brain 2: Neural Networks and Beyond*, New York: Wiley-Interscience.

Arbib, M. A., Érdi, P., and Szentágothai, J., 1998, *Neural Organization: Structure, Function, and Dynamics*, Cambridge, MA: MIT Press.

Arbib, M. A., and Hesse, M. B., 1986, *The Construction of Reality*, New York: Cambridge University Press.

Bain, A., 1868, *The Senses and the Intellect*, 3rd ed.

Bernard, C., 1878, *Leçons sur les phénomènes de la Vie*.

Brooks, R. A., 1986, A robust layered control system for a mobile robot, *IEEE Robot. Automat.*, RA-2:14–23.

Cannon, W. B., 1939, *The Wisdom of the Body*, New York: Norton.

Chomsky, N., 1959, On certain formal properties of grammars, *Inform. Control*, 2:137–167.

Church, A., 1941, *The Calculi of Lambda-Conversion*, Annals of Mathematics Studies 6, Princeton, NJ: Princeton University Press.

Craik, K. J. W., 1943, *The Nature of Explanation*, New York: Cambridge University Press.

Ewert, J.-P., and von Seelen, W., 1974, Neurobiologie and System-Theorie eines visuellen Muster-Erkennungsmechanismus bei Kroten, *Kybernetik*, 14:167–183.

Fearing, F., 1930, *Reflex Action*, Baltimore: Williams and Wilkins.

Gödel, K., 1931, Uber formal unentscheidbare Sätze der *Principia Mathematica* und verwandter Systeme: I, *Monats. Math. Phys.*, 38:173–198.

Grossberg, S., 1967, Nonlinear difference-differential equations in prediction and learning theory, *Proc. Natl. Acad. Sci. USA*, 58:1329–1334.

Hebb, D. O., 1949, *The Organization of Behavior*, New York: Wiley.

Heims, S. J., 1991, *The Cybernetics Group*, Cambridge, MA: MIT Press.

Hodgkin, A. L., and Huxley, A. F., 1952, A quantitative description of membrane current and its application to conduction and excitation in nerve, *J. Physiol. Lond.*, 117:500–544.

Hopfield, J., 1982, Neural networks and physical systems with emergent collective computational properties, *Proc. Natl. Acad. Sci. USA*, 79:2554–2558.

Hopfield, J. J., and Tank, D. W., 1986, Neural computation of decisions in optimization problems, *Biol. Cybern.*, 52:141–152.

Kleene, S. C., 1936, General recursive functions of natural numbers, *Math. Ann.*, 112:727–742.

La Mettrie, J., 1953, *Man a Machine* (trans. by G. Bussey from the French original of 1748), La Salle, IL: Open Court.

Lichtheim, L., 1885, On aphasia, *Brain*, 7:433–484.

Maxwell, J. C., 1868, On governors, *Proc. R. Soc. Lond.*, 16:270–283.

McCulloch, W. S., and Pitts, W. H., 1943, A logical calculus of the ideas immanent in nervous activity, *Bull. Math. Biophys.*, 5:115–133.

Minsky, M. L., 1961, Steps toward artificial intelligence, *Proc. IRE*, 49:8–30.

Minsky, M. L., 1985, *The Society of Mind*, New York: Simon and Schuster.

Minsky, M. L., and Papert, S., 1969, *Perceptrons: An Essay in Computational Geometry*, Cambridge, MA: MIT Press.

Nilsson, N., 1965, *Learning Machines*, New York: McGraw–Hill.

Pavlov, I. P., 1927, *Conditioned Reflexes: An Investigation of the Physiological Activity of the Cerebral Cortex* (translated from the Russian by G. V. Anrep), New York: Oxford University Press.

Post, E. L., 1943, Formal reductions of the general combinatorial decision problem, *Am. J. Math.*, 65:197–268.

Rall, W., 1964, Theoretical significance of dendritic trees for neuronal input–output relations, in *Neural Theory and Modeling* (R. Reiss, Ed.), Stanford, CA: Stanford University Press, pp. 73–97.

Ramón y Cajal, S., 1906, The structure and connexion of neurons, reprinted in *Nobel Lectures: Physiology or Medicine, 1901–1921*, New York: Elsevier, 1967, pp. 220–253.

Rosenblatt, F., 1958, The perceptron: A probabilistic model for information storage and organization in the brain, *Psychol. Rev.*, 65:386–408.

Rosenblueth, A., Wiener, N., and Bigelow, J., 1943, Behavior, purpose and teleology, *Philos. Sci.*, 10:18–24.

Rumelhart, D. E., Hinton, G. E., and Williams, R. J., 1986, Learning internal representations by error propagation, in *Parallel Distributed Processing: Explorations in the Microstructure of Cognition*, vol. 1 (D. Rumelhart and J. McClelland, Eds.), Cambridge, MA: MIT Press/Bradford Books, pp. 318–362.

Samuel, A. L., 1959, Some studies in machine learning using the game of checkers, *IBM J. Res. Dev.*, 3:210–229.

Selfridge, O. G., 1959, Pandemonium: A paradigm for learning, in *Mechanisation of Thought Processes*, London: Her Majesty's Stationery Office, pp. 511–531.

Sherrington, C., 1906, *The Integrative Action of the Nervous System*, New York: Oxford University Press.

Turing, A. M., 1936, On computable numbers with an application to the *Entscheidungsproblem, Proc. Lond. Math. Soc.* (Series 2), 42:230–265.

Turing, A. M., 1950, Computing machinery and intelligence, *Mind*, 59:433–460.

von der Malsburg, C., 1973, Self-organization of orientation-sensitive cells in the striate cortex, *Kybernetik*, 14:85–100.

Widrow, B., and Hoff, M. E., Jr., 1960, Adaptive switching circuits, in *1960 IRE WESCON Convention Record*, vol. 4, pp. 96–104.

Wiener, N., 1948, *Cybernetics: Or Control and Communication in the Animal and the Machine*, New York: Technology Press and Wiley (2nd ed., Cambridge, MA: MIT Press, 1961).

Young, R. M., 1970, *Mind, Brain and Adaptation in the Nineteenth Century: Cerebral Localization and Its Biological Context from Gall to Ferrier*, New York: Oxford University Press.

Part II: Road Maps

A Guided Tour of Brain Theory and Neural Networks

Michael A. Arbib

How to Use Part II

Part II provides a guided tour of our subject in the form of 22 **road maps**, each of which provides an overview of a single theme in brain theory and neural networks and offers a précis of Part III articles related to that theme. The road maps are grouped under eight general headings:

Grounding Models of Neurons and Networks
Brain, Behavior, and Cognition
Psychology, Linguistics, and Artificial Intelligence
Biological Neurons and Networks
Dynamics and Learning in Artificial Networks
Sensory Systems
Motor Systems
Applications, Implementations, and Analysis

Part II starts with the **meta-map** (Section II.1), which is designed to give some sense of the diversity yet interconnectedness of the themes taken up in this *Handbook* by quickly surveying the 22 different road maps. We then offer eight sections, one for each of the above headings, that comprise the 22 road maps. In the road maps, we depart from the convention used elsewhere in this text whereby titles in capitals and small capitals are used for cross-references to all other articles. In the road maps, we reserve capitals and SMALL CAPITALS for articles on the tour, and we use titles in quotation marks to refer to related articles that are not primary to the current road map. We will use **boldface** type to refer to road maps and other major sections in Part II.

Every article in Part III occurs in at least one road map, and a few articles appear in two or even three road maps. Clearly, certain articles unequivocally have a place in a given road map, but as I considered articles that were less central to a given theme, my decisions on which articles to include became somewhat arbitrary. Thus, I invite you to read each road map to get a good overview of the main themes of each road map, and then continue your exploration by browsing Part III and using the articles listed under Related Reading and the index of the *Handbook* to add your own personal extensions to each map.

II.1. The Meta-Map

There is no one best path for the study of brain theory and neural networks, and you should use the meta-map simply to get a broad overview that will help you choose a path that is pleasing, or useful, to you.

Grounding Models of Neurons and Networks

Grounding Models of Neurons
Grounding Models of Networks

The articles surveyed in these two road maps can be viewed as continuing the work of Part I, providing the reader with a basic understanding of the models of both biological and artificial neurons and neural networks that are developed in the 285 articles in Part III. The road maps will help each reader decide which of these articles provide necessary background for their own reading of the *Handbook*.

Brain, Behavior, and Cognition

Neuroethology and Evolution
Mammalian Brain Regions
Cognitive Neuroscience

The road map **Neuroethology and Evolution** places the following road map, **Mammalian Brain Regions**, in a dual perspective. First, by reviewing work on modeling neural mechanisms of the behavior of a variety of nonmammalian animals, it helps us understand the wealth of subtle neural computations available in other species, enriching our study of nervous systems that are closer to that of humans. When we focus on ethology (animal behavior), we often study the integration of perception and action, thus providing a useful complement to the many articles that focus on a subsystem in relative isolation. Second, by offering a number of articles on both biological and artificial evolution, we take the first steps in understanding the ways in which different neural architectures may emerge across many generations. Turning to the mammalian brain, we first look at **Mammalian Brain Regions**. We will also study the role of these brain regions in other road maps as we analyze such functions as vision, memory, and motor control. We shall see that every such function involves the "cooperative computation" of a multiplicity of brain regions. However, **Mammalian Brain Regions** reviews those articles that focus on a single brain region and give some sense of how we model its contribution to key neural functions. The road map **Cognitive Neuroscience** then pays special attention to a range of human cognitive functions, including perception, action, memory, and language, with emphasis on the range of data now available from imaging of the active human brain and the challenges these data provide for modeling.

Psychology, Linguistics, and Artificial Intelligence

Psychology
Linguistics and Speech Processing
Artificial Intelligence

Our next three road maps–**Psychology, Linguistics and Speech Processing**, and **Artificial Intelligence**—are focused more on the effort to understand human psychology than on the need to understand the details of neurobiology. For example, the articles on **Psychology** may overlap those on **Cognitive Neuroscience**, but overall the emphasis shifts to "connectionist" models in which the "neurons" rarely correspond to the actual biological neurons of the human brain (the underlying structure). Rather, the driving idea is that the functioning of the human mind (the functional expression of the brain's activity) is best explored through a parallel, adaptive processing methodology in which large populations of elements are simultaneously active, pass messages back and forth between each other, and can change the strength of their connections as they do so. This is in contrast to the serial computing methodology, which is based on the computing paradigm that was dominant from the 1940s through the 1970s and that now is complemented in mainstream computer science by work in grid-based computing, embedded systems, and teams of intelligent agents.

In short, connectionist approaches to psychology and linguistics use "neurons" that are more like the artificial neurons used to build new applications for parallel processing than they are like the real neurons of the living brain.

In dividing this introduction to connectionism into three themes, I have first distinguished those aspects of connectionist psychology that relate to perception, memory, emotion, and other aspects of cognition in general from those specifically involved in connectionist linguistics before turning to artificial intelligence. The road map **Psychology** also contains articles that address philosophical issues in brain theory and connectionism, including the notion of consciousness, as well as articles that approach psychology from a developmental perspective. The road map **Linguistics and Speech Processing** presents connectionist models of human language performance as well as approaches (some more neural than others) to technologies for speech processing. The central idea in connectionist linguistics is that rich linguistic representations can emerge from the interaction of a relatively simple learning device and a structured linguistic environment, rather than requiring the details of grammar to be innate, captured in a genetically determined universal grammar. The road map **Artificial Intelligence** presents articles whose themes are similar to those in **Psychology** in what they explain, but are part of artificial intelligence (AI) because the attempt is to get a machine to exhibit some intelligent-like behavior, without necessarily meeting the constraints imposed by experimental psychology or psycholinguistics. "Classical" symbolic AI is contrasted with a number of methods in addition to the primary concentration on neural network approaches. The point is that, whereas brain theory seeks to know "how the brain does it," AI must weigh the value of artificial neural networks (ANNs) as a powerful technology for parallel, adaptive computation against that of other technologies on the basis of efficacy in solving practical problems on available hardware. The reader will, of course, find a number of models that are of equal interest to psychologists and to AI researchers.

The articles gathered in these three road maps will not exhaust the scope of their subject matter, for at least two reasons. First, in addition to connectionist models of psychological phenomena, there are many biological models that embody genuine progress in relating the phenomena to known parts of the brain, perhaps even grounding a phenomenon in the behavior of identifiable classes of biological neurons. Second, while **Artificial Intelligence** will focus on broad thematic issues, a number of these also appear in applying neural networks in computer vision, speech recognition, and elsewhere using techniques elaborated in articles of the road map **Learning in Artificial Networks**.

Biological Neurons and Networks

Biological Neurons and Synapses
Neural Plasticity
Neural Coding
Biological Networks

The next four road maps, **Biological Neurons and Synapses**, **Neural Plasticity**, **Neural Coding**, and **Biological Networks**, are ones that, for many readers, may provide the appropriate entry point for the book as a whole, namely, an understanding of neural networks from a biological point of view. The road map **Biological Neurons and Synapses** gives us some sense of how sophisticated real biological neurons are, with each patch of membrane being itself a subtle electrochemical structure. An appreciation of this complexity is necessary for the computational neuroscientist wishing to address the increasingly detailed database of experimental neuroscience on how signals can be propagated, and how individual neurons interact with each other. But such complexity may also provide an eye opener for the technologist planning to incorporate new capabilities into the next generation of ANNs. The road map **Neural Plasticity** then charts from a biological point of view a variety

of specific mechanisms at the level of synapses, or even finer-grained molecular structures, which enable the changes in the strength of connections that underlie both learning and development. A number of such mechanisms have already implied a variety of learning rules for ANNs (see **Learning in Artificial Networks**), but they also include mechanisms that have not seen technological use. This road map includes articles that analyze mechanisms that underlie both development and regeneration of neural networks and learning in biological systems. However, I again stress to the reader that one may approach the road maps, and the articles in Part III of this *Handbook*, in many different orders, so that some readers may prefer to study the articles described in the road map **Learning in Artificial Networks** before or instead of studying those on neurobiological learning mechanisms.

Two more road maps round out our study of **Biological Neurons and Networks**. The simplest models of neurons either operate on a discrete-time scale or measure neural output by the continuous variation in firing rate. The road map **Neural Coding** examines the virtues of other alternatives, looking at both the possible gains in information that may follow from exploiting the exact timing of spikes (action potentials) as they travel along axonal branches from one neuron to many others, and the way in which signals that may be hard to discern from the firing of a single neuron may be reliably encoded by the activity of a whole population of neurons. We then turn to articles that chart a number of the basic architectures whereby biological neurons are combined into **Biological Networks**—although clearly, this is a topic expanded upon in many articles in Part III which are not explicitly presented in this road map.

Dynamics and Learning in Artificial Networks

Dynamic Systems
Learning in Artificial Networks
Computability and Complexity

The next three road maps—**Dynamic Systems**, **Learning in Artificial Networks**, and **Computability and Complexity**—provide a broad perspective on the dynamics of neural networks considered as general information processing structures rather than as models of a particular biological or psychological phenomenon or as solutions to specific technological problems. Our study of **Dynamic Systems** is grounded in studying the dynamics of a neural network with fixed inputs: does it settle down to an equilibrium state, and to what extent can that state be seen as the solution of some problem of optimization? Under what circumstances will the network exhibit a dynamic pattern of oscillatory behavior (a limit cycle), and under what circumstances will it undergo chaotic behavior (traversing what is known as a strange attractor)? This theme is expanded by the study of cooperative phenomena. In a gas or a magnet, we do not know the behavior of any single atom with precision, but we can infer the overall "cooperative" behavior—the pressure, volume, and temperature of a gas, or the overall magnetization of a magnet—through statistical methods, methods which even extend to the analyses of such dramatic phase transitions as that of a piece of iron from an unmagnetized lump to a magnet, or of a liquid to a gas. So, too, can statistical methods provide insight into the large-scale properties of neural nets, abstracting away from the detailed function of individual neurons, when our interest is in statistical patterns of behavior rather than the fine details of information processing. This leads us to the study of self-organization in neural networks, in which we ask for ways in which the interaction between elements in a neural network can lead to the spontaneous expression of pattern; whether this pattern is constituted by the pattern of activity of the individual neurons or by the pattern of synaptic connections which records earlier experience.

With this question of earlier experience, we have fully made the transition to the study of learning, and we turn to the road map which focuses on **Learning in Artificial Networks**, complementing the road map **Neural Plasticity**. (This replaces two road maps from the first edition–Learning in Artificial Neural Networks, Deterministic, and Learning in Artificial Neural Networks, Statistical—for two reasons: (1) the use of statistical methods in the study of learning in ANNs is so pervasive that the attempt to distinguish deterministic and statistical approaches to learning is not useful, and (2) the statistical analysis of learning in ANNs has spawned a variety of statistical methods that are less closely linked to neurobiological inspiration, and we wish these, too, to be included in our road map.) The study of **Computability and Complexity** then provides a rapprochement between neural networks and a number of ideas developed within the mainstream of computer science, especially those arising from the study of complexity of computational structures. Indeed, it takes us back to the very foundations of the theory of neural networks, in which the study of McCulloch-Pitts neurons built on earlier work on computability to inspire the later development of automata theory.

Sensory Systems

Vision
Other Sensory Systems

Vision has been the most widely studied of all sensory systems, both in brain theory and in applications and analysis of ANNs, and thus has a special road map of its own. **Other Sensory Systems**, treated at less length in the next road map, include audition, touch, and pain, as well a number of fascinating special systems such as electrolocation in electric fish and echolocation in bats.

Motor Systems

Robotics and Control Theory
Motor Pattern Generators
Mammalian Motor Control

The next set of road maps—**Robotics and Control Theory**, **Motor Pattern Generators**, and **Mammalian Motor Control**—addresses the control of movement by neural networks. In the study of **Robotics and Control Theory**, the adaptive properties of neural networks play a special role, enabling a control system, through experience, to become better and better suited to solve a given repertoire of control problems, guiding a system through a desired trajectory, whether through the use of feedback or feedforward. These general control strategies are exemplified in a number of different approaches to robot control. The articles in the road map **Motor Pattern Generators** focus on subconscious functions, such as breathing or locomotion, in vertebrates and on a wide variety of pattern-generating activity in invertebrates. The reader may wish to turn back to the road map **Neuroethology and Evolution** for other studies in animal behavior (neuroethology) which show how sensory input, especially visual input, and motor behavior are integrated in a cycle of action and perception. **Mammalian Motor Control** places increased emphasis on the interaction between neural control and the kinematics or dynamics of limbs and eyes, and also looks at various forms of motor-related learning. In showing how the goals of movement can be achieved by a neural network through the time course of activity of motors or muscles, this road map overlaps some of the issues taken up in the more applications-oriented road map, **Robotics and Control Theory**. Much of the material on biological motor control is of general relevance, but the road map also includes articles on primate motor control that examine a variety of movements of the eyes, head, arm, and hand which are studied in a variety of mammals but are most fully expressed in primates and humans. Of course, as many readers will be prepared to notice by now, **Mammalian Motor Control** will, for some readers, be an excellent starting place for their study, since, by showing how visual and motor systems are integrated in a number of primate and human behaviors, it motivates the study of the specific neural network mechanisms required to achieve these behaviors.

Applications, Implementations, and Analysis

Applications
Implementation and Analysis

We then turn to a small set of **Applications** of neural networks, which include signal processing, speech recognition, and visual processing (but exclude the broader set of applications to astronomy, speech recognition, high-energy physics, steel making, telecommunications, etc., of the first edition, since *The Handbook of Neural Computation* [Oxford University Press, 1996] now provides a large set of articles on ANN applications). Since a neural network cannot be applied unless it is implemented, whether in software or hardware, we close with the road map **Implementation and Analysis**. The implementation methodologies include simulation on a general-purpose computer, emulation on specially designed neurocomputers, and implementation in a device built with electronic or photonic materials. As for analysis, we present articles in the nascent field of neuroinformatics which combines database methodology, visualization, modeling, and data analysis in an attempt to master the explosive growth of neuroscience data. (In Europe, the term *neuroinformatics* is used to encompass the full range of computational approaches to brain theory and neural networks. In the United States, some people use *neuroinformatics* to refer solely to the use of databases in neuroscience. Here we focus on the middle ground, where the analysis of data and the construction of models are brought together.)

II.2. Grounding Models of Neurons and Networks

The first two road maps expand the exposition of Part I by presenting basic models of neurons and networks that provide the building blocks for many of the articles in Part III.

Grounding Models of Neurons

Axonal Modeling
Dendritic Processing

Hebbian Synaptic Plasticity
Perceptrons, Adalines, and Backpropagation
Perspective on Neuron Model Complexity
Reinforcement Learning
Single-Cell Models
Spiking Neurons, Computation with

This road map introduces classes of neuron models of increasing complexity and attention to detail. The point is that much can be learned even at high degrees of abstraction, while other phenomena can be understood only by attention to subtle details of neuronal function. The reader of this *Handbook* will find many articles exploring biological phenomena and technological applications at different levels of complexity. The implicit questions will always be, "Do all the details matter?" and "Is the model oversimplified?" The answers will depend both on the phenomena under question and on the current subtlety of experimental investigations. After introducing articles that present neuron models across the range of model complexity, the road map concludes with a brief look at the most widely analyzed forms of synaptic plasticity.

Classes of neuron models can be defined by how they treat the train of action potentials issued by a neuron (see the road map **Neural Coding**). Many models assume that information is carried in the average rate of pulses over a time much longer than a typical pulse width, with the occurrence times of particular pulses simply treated as jitter on an averaged analog signal. A neural model in such a theory might be a mathematical function which produces a real-valued output from its many real-valued inputs; that function could be linear or nonlinear, static or adaptive, and might be instantiated in analog silicon circuits or in digital software. Examples given of such models in SINGLE-CELL MODELS are the McCulloch-Pitts model, the perceptron model, Hopfield neurons, and polynomial neurons. However, some models assume that each single neural pulse carries reliable, precisely timed information. A neural model in such a theory fires only upon the exact coincidence of several input pulses, and quickly "forgets" when it last fired, so that it is always ready to fire upon another coincidence. The simplest such models are the integrate-and-fire models. The article concludes by briefly introducing the Hodgkin-Huxley model of squid axon, based on painstaking analysis (without benefit of electronic computers) of data from the squid giant axon, and then introduces modified single-point models, compartmental models, and computation with both passive dendrites and active dendrites. SPIKING NEURONS, COMPUTATION WITH provides more detail on those neuron models of intermediate complexity in which the output is a spike whose timing is continuously variable as a result of cellular interactions, providing a model of biological neurons that offers more details than firing rate models but without the details of biophysical models. The virtues of such models include the ability to transmit information very quickly through small temporal differences between the spikes sent out by different neurons. Information theory can be used to quantify how much more information about a stimulus can be extracted from spike trains if the precise timing is taken into account. Moreover, computing with spiking neurons may prove of benefit for technology.

AXONAL MODELING is centered on the Hodgkin and Huxley model, arguably the most successful model in all of computational neuroscience. The article shows how the Hodgkin-Huxley equations extend the cable equation to describe the ionic mechanisms underlying the initiation and propagation of action potentials. The vast majority of contemporary biophysical models use a mathematical formalism similar to that introduced by Hodgkin and Huxley, even though their model of the continuous, deterministic, and macroscopic permeability changes of the membrane was achieved without any knowledge of the underlying all-or-none, stochastic, and microscopic ionic channels. The article also describes the differences between myelinated and nonmyelinated axons; and briefly discusses the possible role of heavily branched axonal trees in information processing.

PERSPECTIVE ON NEURON MODEL COMPLEXITY then shows how this type of modeling might be extended to the whole cell. The key point is that one neuron with detailed modeling of dendrites (especially with nonuniform distributions of synapses and ion channels) can perform tasks that would require a network of many simple binary units to duplicate. The point is not to choose the most

complex model of a neuron but rather to seek an intermediate level of complexity which preserves the most significant distinctions between different "compartments" of the neuron (soma, various portions of the dendritic tree, etc.). The challenge is to demonstrate a useful computation or discrimination that can be accomplished with a particular choice of compartments in a neuron model, and then show that this useful capacity is lost when a coarser decomposition of the neuron is used. DENDRITIC PROCESSING especially emphasizes developments in compartmental modeling of dendrites, arguing that we are in the midst of a "dendritic revolution" that has yielded a much more fascinating picture of the electrical behavior and chemical properties of dendrites than one could have imagined only a few years ago. The dendritic membrane hosts a variety of nonlinear voltage-gated ion channels that endow dendrites with potentially powerful computing capabilities. Moreover, the classic view of dendrites as carrying information unidirectionally, from synapses to the soma, has been transformed: dendrites of many central neurons also carry information in the "backward" direction, via active propagation of the action potentials from the axon to the dendrites. These "reversed" signals can trigger plastic changes in the dendritic input synapses. Moreover, it is now known that the fine morphology as well as the electrical properties of dendrites change dynamically, in an activity-dependent manner.

If the most successful model in all of computational neuroscience is the Hodgkin-Huxley model, then the second most successful is Hebb's model of "unsupervised" synaptic plasticity. The former was based on rigorous analysis of empirical data; the latter was initially the result of theoretical speculation on how synapses might behave if assemblies of cells were to work together to store and reconstitute thoughts and associations. HEBBIAN SYNAPTIC PLASTICITY notes that predictions derived from Hebb's postulate can be generalized for different levels of integration (synaptic efficacy, functional coupling, adaptive change in behavior) by simply adjusting the variables derived from various measures of neural activity and the time-scale over which it operates. The article addresses five major issues: Should the definition of "Hebbian" plasticity refer to a simple positive correlational rule of learning, or are there biological justifications for including additional "pseudo-Hebbian" terms (such as synaptic depression due to disuse or competition) in a generalized phenomenological algorithm? What are the spatiotemporal constraints (e.g., input specificity, temporal associativity) that characterize the induction process? Do the predictions of Hebbian-based algorithms account for most forms of activity-dependent dynamics in synaptic transmission throughout phylogenesis? On which time-scales (perception, learning, epigenesis) and at which stage of development of the organism (embryonic, "critical" postnatal developmental periods, adulthood) are activity-dependent changes in functional links predicted by Hebb's rule? Are there examples of correlation-based plasticity that contradict the predictions of Hebb's postulate (termed anti-Hebbian modifications)? The article thus frames many important issues to be developed in the articles of the road map **Neural Plasticity** but that are also implicit, for example, in articles reviewed in the road maps **Psychology** and **Linguistics and Speech Processing**, in which Hebbian (and other) learning rules are used for "formal neurons" that are psychological abstractions rather than representation of real neurobiological neurons or even biological neuron pools. Two other articles serve to introduce the basic learning rules that have been most central in both biological analysis and connectionist modeling. Supervised learning adjusts the weights in an attempt to respond to explicit error signals provided by a "teacher," which may be external, or another network in the same "brain." This model was introduced in the perceptron model, which is reviewed in PERCEPTRONS, ADALINES, AND BACKPROPAGATION (of which more details in the next road map, **Grounding Models of Networks**). On the other hand, REINFORCEMENT LEARNING (of which more details in the road map **Learning in Artificial Networks**) shows how networks can improve their performance when given general reinforcement ("that was good," "that was bad") by a critic, rather than the explicit error information offered by a teacher.

Grounding Models of Networks

ASSOCIATIVE NETWORKS
COMPUTING WITH ATTRACTORS
PERCEPTRONS, ADALINES, AND BACKPROPAGATION
RADIAL BASIS FUNCTION NETWORKS
SELF-ORGANIZING FEATURE MAPS
SPIKING NEURONS, COMPUTATION WITH

The mechanisms and implications of association—the linkage of information with other information—have a long history in psychology and philosophy. ASSOCIATIVE NETWORKS discusses association as realized in neural networks as well as association in the more traditional senses. Many neural networks are designed as pattern associators, which link an input pattern with the "correct" output pattern. Learning rules are designed to construct useful linkages between input and output patterns whether in feedforward neural network architectures or in a network whose units are recurrently interconnected. Special attention is given to the critical importance of data representation at all levels of network operation. PERCEPTRONS, ADALINES, AND BACKPROPAGATION introduces the perceptron rule and the LMS (least-mean-squares) algorithm for training feedforward networks with multiple adaptive elements, where each element can be seen as an adaptive linear combiner of its inputs followed by a nonlinearity which produces the output. It then presents the major extension provided by the backpropagation algorithm for training multilayer neural networks—which can be viewed as dividing the input space into regions bounded by hyperplanes, one for the thresholded output of each neuron of the output layer—and shows how this technique has been used to attack problems requiring neural networks with high degrees of nonlinearity and precision.

COMPUTING WITH ATTRACTORS shows how neural networks (often seen now as operating in continuous time) may be viewed as dynamic systems (a theme developed in great detail by the articles of the road map **Dynamic Systems**). This article describes how to compute with networks with feedback, with the input of a computation being set as an initial state for the system and the result read off a suitably chosen set of units when the network has "settled down." The state a dynamical system settles into is called an *attractor*, so this paradigm is called *computing with attractors*. It is possible to settle down into an equilibrium state, or into periodic or even chaotic patterns of activity. (An interesting possibility, not considered in this article, is to perform computations based on the transient approach to the attractor, rather than on the basis of the attractor alone.) The Hopfield model for associative memory is used as the key example, showing its dynamic behavior as well as how the connections necessary to embed desired patterns can be

learned and how the paradigm can be extended to time-dependent attractors.

SELF-ORGANIZING FEATURE MAPS (SOFMs) introduces a famous version of competitive learning based on a layer of adaptive "neurons" that gradually develops into an array of feature detectors. The learning method is an augmented Hebbian method in which learning by the element most responsive to an input pattern is "shared" with its neighbors. The result is that the resulting "compressed image" of the (usually higher-dimensional) input space forms a "topographic map" in which distance relationships in the input space (expressing, e.g., pattern similarities) are approximately preserved as distance relationships between corresponding excitation sites in the map, while clusters of similar input patterns tend to become mapped to areas in the neural layer whose size varies in proportion to the frequency of the occurrence of their patterns. From a statistical point of view, the SOFM provides a nonlinear generalization of principal component analysis.

SPIKING NEURONS, COMPUTATION WITH discusses both the use of spiking neurons as a useful approximation to biological neurons and the study of networks of spiking neurons as a formal model of computation for which the assumptions need not be biological (see also "Integrate-and-Fire Neurons and Networks"). If the spiking neurons are not subject to significant amounts of noise, then one can carry out computations in networks of spiking neurons where every spike matters, and some finite network of spiking neurons can simulate a universal Turing machine. Spiking neurons can also be used as computational units that function like radial basis functions in the temporal domain. Another code uses the order of firing of different neurons as the relevant signal conveyed by these neurons. Firing rates of neurons in the cortex are relatively low, making it hard for the postsynaptic neuron to "read" the firing rate of a presynaptic neuron. However, networks of spiking neurons can carry out complex analog computations if the inputs of the computation are presented in terms of a space rate or population code.

The last article in this road map gives an example of the utility of studying networks in which the response properties of the individual units are designed not as abstractions from biological neurons, but rather because their response functions have mathematically desirable properties. A multilayer perceptron can be viewed as dividing the input space into regions bounded by hyperplanes, one for the thresholded output of each neuron of the output layer. RADIAL BASIS FUNCTION NETWORKS describes an alternative approach to decomposition of a pattern space into regions, describing the clusters of data points in the space as if they were generated according to an underlying probability density function. Thus the perceptron method concentrates on class boundaries, while the radial basis function approach focuses on regions where the data density is highest, constructing global approximations to functions using combinations of basis functions centered around weight vectors. The article shows that this approach not only has a range of useful theoretical properties but also is practically useful, having been applied efficiently to problems in discrimination, time-series prediction, and feature extraction.

II.3. Brain, Behavior, and Cognition

Neuroethology and Evolution

COMMAND NEURONS AND COMMAND SYSTEMS
CRUSTACEAN STOMATOGASTRIC SYSTEM
ECHOLOCATION: COCHLEOTOPIC AND COMPUTATIONAL MAPS
ELECTROLOCATION

EVOLUTION AND LEARNING IN NEURAL NETWORKS
EVOLUTION OF ARTIFICIAL NEURAL NETWORKS
EVOLUTION OF GENETIC NETWORKS
EVOLUTION OF THE ANCESTRAL VERTEBRATE BRAIN
HIPPOCAMPUS: SPATIAL MODELS

Many readers will come to the *Handbook* with one of two main motivations: to understand the human brain, or to explore the potential of ANNs as a technology for adaptive, parallel computation. The present road map emphasizes a third motivation: to study neural mechanisms in creatures very different from humans and their mammalian cousins—for the intrinsic interest of discovering the diverse neural architectures that abound in nature, for the suggestions these provide for future technology, and for the novel perspective on human brain mechanisms offered by seeking to place them in an evolutionary perspective.

Ethology is the study of animal behavior, in which our concern is with the circumstances under which a particular motor pattern will be deployed as an appropriate part of the animal's activity. Neuroethology, then, is the study of neural mechanisms underlying animal behavior. The emphasis is thus on an integrative, systems approach to the neuroscience of the animal being studied, as distinct from a reductionist approach to, for example, the neurochemistry of synaptic plasticity. Of course, a major aim of this *Handbook* is to create a context in which the reader can see both approaches to the study of nervous systems and ponder how best to integrate them. In particular, the reader will find many examples of the neuroethology of mammalian systems in a wide variety of other road maps, such as **Cognitive Neuroscience**, **Vision**, **Other Sensory Systems**, and **Mammalian Motor Control**. However, the present road map is designed to guide the reader to articles on a number of fascinating nonmammalian systems—as well as a few "exotic" mammalian systems—as a basis for a brief introduction of the evolutionary approach to biological and artificial neural networks.

NEUROETHOLOGY, COMPUTATIONAL suggests that *computational* neuroethology applies not only to animals but also to nonbiological autonomous agents, such as some types of robots and simulated embodied agents operating in virtual worlds (see also "Embodied Cognition"). The key element is the use of sophisticated computer-based simulation and visualization tools to study the neural control of behavior within the context of "agents" that are both embodied and situated within an environment. Other examples include specific neuroethological modeling directed toward specific animals (the computational frog *Rana computatrix* and the computational cockroach *Periplaneta computatrix*) and their implications for the rebirth of ideas first introduced by Grey Walter in his 1950s design of *Machina speculatrix* and later developed in the book *Vehicles* by Valentino Braitenberg.

If a certain interneuron is stimulated electrically in the brain of a marine slug, the animal then displays a species-specific escape swimming behavior, although no predator is present. If in a toad a certain portion of the optic tectum is stimulated in this manner, snapping behavior is triggered, although no prey is present. In both cases, a stimulus produces a rapid ballistic response. Such command functions provide the sensorimotor interface between sensory

pattern recognition and localization, on the one side, and motor pattern generation on the other. COMMAND NEURONS AND COMMAND SYSTEMS analyzes the extent to which a motor pattern generator (MPG) may be activated alone or in concert with others through perceptual stimuli mediated by a single "command neuron" (as in the marine slug) or by more diffuse "command systems" (as in the toad). Three articles then focus specifically on visuomotor coordination. VISUAL COURSE CONTROL IN FLIES explains the mechanisms underlying the extraction of retinal motion patterns in the fly, and their transformation into the appropriate motor activity. Rotatory large-field motion can signal unintended deviations from the fly's course and initiate a compensatory turn; image expansion can signal that the animal approaches an obstacle and initiates a landing or avoidance response; and discontinuities in the retinal motion field indicate nearby stationary or moving objects. Since many of the cells responsible for motion extraction are large and individually identifiable, the fly is quite amenable to an analysis of sensory processing. Similarly, the small number of muscles and motor neurons used to generate flight maneuvers facilitates studies of motor output. VISUOMOTOR COORDINATION IN SALAMANDER shows how low-level mechanisms add up to produce complicated behaviors, such as the devious approach of salamanders to their prey. Coarse coding models demonstrate how the location of an object may be encoded with high accuracy using only a few neurons with large, overlapping receptive fields. (This fits with the fact that the brains of salamanders are anatomically the simplest among vertebrates, containing only about 1 million neurons—frogs have up to 10 times and humans 10 million times as many neurons.) The models have been extended to the case where several objects are presented to the animal by linking a segmentation network and a winner-take-all-like object selection network to the coarse coding network in a biologically plausible way. Compensation of background movement, selection of an object, saccade generation, and approach and snapping behavior in salamanders have also been modeled successfully, in line with behavioral and neurobiological findings. Again, VISUOMOTOR COORDINATION IN FROG AND TOAD stresses that visuomotor integration implies a complex transformation of sensory data, since the same locus of retinal activation might release behavior directed toward the stimulus (as in prey catching) or toward another part of the visual field (as in predator avoidance). The article also shows how the efficacy of visual stimuli to release a response is determined by many factors, including the stimulus situation, the motivational state of the organism itself, and previous experience with the stimulus (learning and conditioning), and the physical condition of the animal's CNS (e.g., brain lesions). In addition, other types of sensory signals can modulate frogs' and toads' response to certain moving visual stimuli. For example, the efficacy of a visual stimulus may be greatly enhanced by the presence of prey odor.

MOTOR PRIMITIVES and SCRATCH REFLEX are two of the articles on nonmammalian animal behaviors that are described more fully in the road map **Motor Pattern Generators**. These articles examine the behavior elicited in frogs and turtles, respectively, by an irritant applied to the animal's skin. The former article examines the extent to which motor behaviors can be built up through a combination of a small set of basic elements; the latter emphasizes how the form of the scratch reflex changes dramatically, depending on the locus of the irritant. Other articles in the road map **Motor Pattern Generators** describe mechanisms underlying a variety of forms of locomotion (swimming, walking, flying).

SOUND LOCALIZATION AND BINAURAL PROCESSING uses data from owls, which are exquisitely skillful in using auditory signals to locate their prey, even in the dark, to anchor models which explain how information from the two ears is brought together to localize the source of a sound. The article focuses on the use of interaural time difference (ITD) as one way to estimate the azimuthal angle of a sound source. It describes one biological model (ITD detection in the barn owl's brainstem) and two psychological models. The underlying idea is that the brain attempts to match the sounds in the two ears by shifting one sound relative to the other, with the shift that produces the best match assumed to be the one that just balances the "real" ITD.

ECHOLOCATION: COCHLEOTOPIC AND COMPUTATIONAL MAPS explores the highly specialized auditory system used by mustached bats to analyze the return signals from the biosonar pulses they emit for orientation and for hunting flying insects. Each biosonar pulse consists of a long constant-frequency (CF) component followed by a short frequency-modulated (FM) component. The CF components constitute an ideal signal for target detection and the measurement of target velocity (relative motion in a radial direction and wing beats of insects), whereas the short FM components are suited for ranging, localizing, and characterizing a target. The article shows how different parameters of echoes received by the bat carry different types of information about a target and how these may be structured in computational maps via parallel-hierarchical processing of different types of biosonar signals. These maps guide the bat's behavior. ELECTROLOCATION discusses another "exotic" sensory system related to behavior, this time the electrosensory systems of weakly electric fish. Animals with active electrosensory systems generate an electrical field around their body by means of an electrical organ located in the trunk and tail, and measure this field via electroreceptors embedded in the skin. Distortions of the electrical field due to animate or inanimate targets in the environment or signals generated by other fish provide inputs to the system, and several distinct behaviors can be linked to patterns of electrosensory input. The article focuses on progress in understanding electrolocation behavior and on the neural implementation of an adaptive filter that attenuates the effects of the fish's own movements.

We now turn to motor systems. CRUSTACEAN STOMATOGASTRIC SYSTEM shows that work on the rhythmic motor patterns of the four areas of the crustacean stomach, the esophagus, cardiac sac, gastric mill, and pylorus, has identified four widely applicable properties. First, rhythmicity in these highly distributed networks depends on both network synaptic connectivity and slow active neuronal membrane properties. Second, modulatory influences can induce individual networks to produce multiple outputs, "switch" neurons between networks, or fuse individual networks into single larger networks. Third, modulatory neuron terminals receive network synaptic input. Modulatory inputs can be sculpted by network feedback and become integral parts of the networks they modulate. Fourth, network synaptic strengths can vary as a function of pattern cycle period and duty cycle.

The lamprey is a very primitive form of fish whose spinal cord supports a traveling wave of activity that yields the swimming movements of the animal's body, yet also persists ("fictive swimming") when the spinal cord is isolated from the body and kept alive in a dish. SPINAL CORD OF LAMPREY: GENERATION OF LOCOMOTOR PATTERNS reviews the data which ground a circuit diagram for the spinal cord circuitry, then shows how the lamprey locomotor network has been simulated. There are a number of neuromodulators present in the lamprey spinal cord that alter the output of the locomotor network. These substances, such as serotonin, dopamine, and tachykinins, offer good opportunities to test our knowledge of the locomotor system by combining the cellular and synaptic actions of the modulators into detailed network models. However, models that do not depend on details of individual cells have also proved useful in advancing our understanding of lamprey locomotion such as the control of turning. Other models probe the nature of the coupling among the rhythm generators, explaining how it may be that the speed of the head-to-tail propagation of the rhythmic activity down the spinal cord can vary with the speed of

swimming even though conduction delays in axons are fixed. LOCUST FLIGHT: COMPONENTS AND MECHANISMS IN THE MOTOR stresses that locust flight motor patterns are generated by an interactive mixture of the intrinsic properties of flight neurons, the operation of complex circuits, and phase-specific proprioceptive input. These mechanisms are subject to the concentrations of circulating neuromodulators and are also modulated according to the demands of a constantly changing sensory environment to produce adaptive behaviors. The system is flexible and able to operate despite severe ablations, and then to recover from these lesions. SENSORIMOTOR INTERACTIONS AND CENTRAL PATTERN GENERATORS analyzes basic properties of the biological systems performing sensorimotor integration. The article discusses both the impact of sensory information on central pattern generators and the less well-understood influence of motor systems on sensory activity. Interaction between motor and sensory systems is pervasive, from the first steps of sensory detection to the highest levels of processing. While there is no doubt that cortical systems contribute to sensorimotor integration, the article questions the view that motor cortex sends commands to a passively responsive spinal cord. Motor commands are only acted upon as spinal circuits integrate their intrinsic activity with all incoming information.

Turning to evolution, we find two classes of articles. We first look at those which focus on simulated evolution in ANNs, with emphasis on the role of evolution as an alternative learning mechanism to fit network parameters to yield a network better adapted to a given task. We then turn to articles more closely related to comparative and evolutionary neurobiology.

When neural networks are studied in the broader biological context of artificial life (i.e., the attempt to synthesize lifelike phenomena within computers and other artificial media), they are sometimes characterized by genotypes and viewed as members of evolving populations of networks in which genotypes are inherited from parents to offspring. EVOLUTION OF ARTIFICIAL NEURAL NETWORKS shows how ANNs can be evolved by using evolutionary algorithms (also known as genetic algorithms). An initial population of different artificial genotypes, each encoding the free parameters (e.g., the connection strengths and/or the architecture of the network and/or the learning rules) of a corresponding neural network, is created randomly. (An important challenge for future research is to study models in which the genotypes are more "biological" in nature, and less closely tied to direct description of the phenotype.) The population of networks is evaluated in order to determine the performance (fitness) of each individual network. The fittest networks are allowed to reproduce by generating copies of their genotypes, with the addition of changes introduced by genetic operators such as mutations (i.e., the random change of a few genes that are selected randomly) or crossover (i.e., the combination of parts of the genotype derived from two reproducing networks). This process is repeated for a number of generations until a network that satisfies the performance criterion set by the experimenter is obtained. LOCOMOTION, VERTEBRATE shows that the combination of neural models with biomechanical models has an important role to play in addressing the evolutionary challenge of seeing what modifications may have occurred in the locomotor circuits between the generation of traveling waves for swimming (the most ancestral vertebrates were close to the lamprey), the generation of standing waves for walking, and the generation of multiple gaits for quadruped locomotion, and on to biped locomotion. One example uses "genetic algorithms" to model the transition from a lamprey-like spinal cord that supports traveling waves to a salamander-like spinal cord that supports both traveling waves for swimming and "standing waves" for terrestrial locomotion, and then shows how vision may modulate spinal activity to yield locomotion toward a goal (see also VISUOMOTOR COORDINATION IN SALAMANDER).

EVOLUTION AND LEARNING IN NEURAL NETWORKS then extends the analysis of ANN evolution to networks that are able to adapt to the environment as a result of some form of lifetime learning. Where evolution is capable of capturing relatively slow environmental changes that might encompass several generations, learning allows an individual to adapt to environmental changes that are unpredictable at the generational level. Moreover, while evolution operates on the genotype, learning affects the phenotype, and phenotypic changes cannot directly modify the genotype. The article shows how ANNs subjected both to an evolutionary and a lifetime learning process have been studied to look at the advantages, in terms of performance, of combining two different adaptation techniques and also to help understand the role of the interaction between learning and evolution in natural organisms. Continuing this theme, LANGUAGE EVOLUTION AND CHANGE offers another style of "connectionist evolution," placing a number of connectionist models of basic forms of language processing in an evolutionary perspective. In some cases, connectionist networks are used as simulated agents to study how social transmission via learning may give rise to the evolution of structured communication systems. In other cases, the specific properties of neural network learning are enlisted to help illuminate the constraints and processes that may have been involved in the evolution of language. The article surveys this connectionist research, starting from the emergence of early syntax, to the role of social interaction and constraints on network learning in the subsequent evolution of language, to linguistic change within existing languages.

With this we turn to the study of evolution in the sense of natural selection in biological systems, building on the insights of Charles Darwin. Since brains do not leave fossils, evolutionary work is more at the level of comparative neurobiology, looking at the nervous systems of currently extant species, then trying to build a "family tree" of possible ancestors. The idea is that we may gain deeper insights into the brains of animals of a given species if we can compare them with the brains of other species, make plausible inferences about the brain structure of their common ancestor, and then seek to relate differences between the current brains and the putative ancestral brains by relating these changes to the possible evolutionary pressures that caused each species to adapt to a specific range of environments. EVOLUTION OF THE ANCESTRAL VERTEBRATE BRAIN notes that efforts to understand how the evolving brain has adapted to specific environmental constraints are complicated because there are always several ways to implement a certain function within existing connections using molecular and cellular mechanisms. In any case, adult diversity is viewed as the outcome of divergent genetic developmental mechanisms. Thus, study of adult structures is aided by placing adult structures within their developmental history as structured by the genes that guide such development. The article introduces a possible prototype of the ancestral vertebrate brain, followed by a scenario for mechanisms that may have diversified the ancestral vertebrate brain. Evolution of the brainstem oculomotor system is used as a focal case study.

The study of gene expression patterns is playing an increasingly important role in the empirical study of brains and neurons, and the pace of innovation in this area has greatly accelerated with the publication of two maps of the human genome as well as genome maps for more and more other species. As of 2002, however, the impact of "genomic neuroscience" on computational neuroscience is still small. To help readers think about the promise of increasing this impact, we not only have the discussion in EVOLUTION OF THE ANCESTRAL VERTEBRATE BRAIN of how during development the CNS becomes polarized and then subdivides into compartments, each characterized by specific pattern of gene expression, but also a companion article, EVOLUTION OF GENETIC NETWORKS, which outlines some of the computational problems in modeling genetic

networks that can direct the establishment of a diversity of neuronal networks in the brain. Since neuronal networks are composed of a wide variety of different cell types, the final fate or end-stage of each cell type represents the outcome of a dynamic amalgamation of gene networks. Genetic networks not only determine the cell fate acquisition from the original stem cell, they also govern contact formation between the cell populations of a given neuronal network. There are intriguing parallels between the establishment and functioning of genetic networks with those of neuronal networks, which can range from simple (on-off switch) to complex. To give some sense of the complexity of organismic development, the article outlines how intracellular as well as cell-cell interactions modify the complexity of gene interactions involved in genetic networks to achieve an altered status of cell function and, ultimately, the connection alterations in the formation of neuronal networks.

OLFACTORY CORTEX describes how, during phylogeny, the paleocortex and archicortex develop in extent and complexity but retain their three-layered character, whereas neocortex emerges in mammals as a five- to six-layered structure. It stresses the evolutionary significance of the olfactory cortex and includes an account for brain theorists interested in principles of cortical organization of the early appearance of the olfactory cortex in phylogeny. Certainly, the cerebral cortex is a distinctive evolutionary feature of the mammalian brain (which does not mean that it is "better" than structures in other genera to which it may be more or less related), and the next articles give two perspectives on its structure. "Grasping Movements: Visuomotor Transformations" presents the interactions of visual areas of parietal cortex with the F5 area of premotor cortex in the monkey brain in serving the visual control of hand movements. The companion article, LANGUAGE EVOLUTION: THE MIRROR SYSTEM HYPOTHESIS, starts from the observations that monkey F5 contains a special set of "mirror neurons" active not only when the monkey performs a specific grasp, but also when the monkey sees others perform a similar task; that F5 is homologous to human Broca's area, an area of cortex usually thought of as related to speech production; but that Broca's area also seems to contain a mirror system for grasping. These facts are used to ground a new theory of the evolution of the human brain mechanisms that support language. It adds a neurological "missing link" to the long-held view that imitation and communication based on hand signs may have preceded the emergence of human mechanisms for extensive vocal communication. With this example to hand, the reader is invited to look through the book for articles that study specific brain mechanisms or specific behaviors in a number of species more or less related to the human. The challenge then is to chart what aspects are common to human brains and the brains more generally of primates, mammals, or even vertebrates; and then, having done so, to see what, if any, distinctive properties human brain and behavior possess. One can then seek an evolutionary account which illuminates these human capacities. For example, it is well known that the human hippocampus is crucial for the creation of episodic memories, our memories of episodes located in specific contexts of space and time (though these memories are eventually consolidated outside hippocampus). On the other hand, HIPPOCAMPUS: SPATIAL MODELS emphasizes the role of the hippocampus and related brain regions in building a map of spatial relations in the rat's world. To what extent can we come to better understand human episodic memory by looking for the generalization from a spatial graph of the environment to one whose nodes are linked in both space and time?

Mammalian Brain Regions

AUDITORY CORTEX
AUDITORY PERIPHERY AND COCHLEAR NUCLEUS
BASAL GANGLIA

This road map introduces the conceptual analysis and neural network modeling of a variety of regions of the mammalian brain. The fact that these regions recur in many articles not listed above emphasizes complementary ways of exploring the mammalian brain in a *top-down* fashion, starting either from the gross anatomy (what does this region of the brain do? the approach of this road map) or from some function (sensory, perceptual, memory, motor control, etc., as in other road maps). These top-down approaches may be contrasted with *bottom-up* approaches, which may start from neurons and seek to infer properties of circuits, or may start from biophysics and neurochemistry and seek to infer properties of neurons (as in much of the road map **Biological Neurons and Synapses**). It must be stressed that whole books can be, and have been, written on each of the brain regions discussed below. The aim of each article is to get the reader started by seeing how a selection of biological data can be addressed by models that seek to illuminate them. In some cases (especially near the sensory or motor periphery), the function of a region is clear, and there is little question as to which phenomena the brain theorist is to explain. But in more central regions, what the experimentalist observes may vary wildly with the questions that are asked, and what the modeler has to work with is more like a Rorschach blot than a well-defined picture.

NEUROANATOMY IN A COMPUTATIONAL PERSPECTIVE notes that a vertebrate brain contains so many neurons, and each neuron has so many connections, that the task of neuroanatomy is not so much to study all the connections in detail, but rather to reveal the typical structural properties of a particular part of the brain, which then provide clues to understanding its various functions. Large brains have comparatively more cortical white matter (i.e., regions containing only axons) than small brains. Moreover, distant elements in a large brain may not be able to collaborate efficiently because of the transmission delays from one point to the other. The way out of this problem may be a higher degree of functional specialization of cortical regions in larger brains. The article provides many data on cortical structure (my favorite is that there are 4 kilometers of axons in each cubic millimeter of mouse cortex) and argues that the data fit Hebb's theory of cell assemblies in that precisely predetermined connections are not required since, as a result of learning, the patterns of interactions between neurons will be different for each brain. What is crucial, however, is an initial connectivity sufficiently rich to allow as many constellations of neuronal activity as possible to be detected and "learned" in the connections.

Many of the articles in this road map are associated with sensory systems: vision, body sense (the somatosensory system), hearing (the auditory system), and smell (the olfactory system). Several articles then discuss brain regions more associated with motor control, learning, and cognition. Five articles take us through the visual system. We start with the RETINA, the outpost of the brain that contains both light-sensitive receptors and several layers of neurons that "preprocess" these responses. Instead of simply coding light intensity, the retina transforms visual signals in a multitude of ways to code properties of the visual world, such as contrast, color, and motion. The article develops a conceptual theory to explain how the structure of the retina is related to its function of coding visual signals. One hypothesis is that much of the retina's signal coding and structural detail is derived from the need to optimally amplify the signal and eliminate noise. But retinal circuitry is diverse. The exact details are probably related to the ecological niche occupied by the organism. In mammals, the retinal output branches into two pathways, the collicular pathway and the geniculostriate pathway. The destination of the former is the midbrain region known as the superior colliculus. COLLICULAR VISUOMOTOR TRANSFORMATIONS FOR GAZE CONTROL charts the role of this brain region in controlling saccades, rapid eye movements that bring visual targets onto the fovea. Even this basic activity involves the cooperation of many brain regions; conversely, the function of the superior colliculus is not restricted to eye movements ("Visuomotor Coordination in Frog and Toad" charts the role of the tectum, which is homologous to the superior colliculus, in approach and avoidance behavior). By virtue of its topographical organization, the superior colliculus has become a key area for experimental and modeling approaches to the question of how sensory signals can be transformed into goal-directed movements. Moreover, the activity in the superior colliculus during saccades to auditory and somatosensory targets conforms to the same motor map, suggesting that considerable sensorimotor remapping must take place.

In mammals, the geniculostriate pathway travels from retina via a specialized region of thalamus called the lateral geniculate nucleus to the primary visual cortex, which is also called the striate cortex because of its somewhat striated appearance. The thalamus has many divisions, not only those involved with sensory pathways, but also those involved in loops linking the cortex to other brain regions like the cerebellum and basal ganglia. The thalamus is the gateway through which all sensory inputs, except olfaction, are relayed to the cortex. THALAMUS shows that the thalamus can effectively control the flow of information to the cortex: during waking, it may subserve attention, selectively enhancing certain inputs to the cortex and attenuating others; during slow-wave sleep, the firing mode of thalamic cells changes, effectively closing the gateway and diminishing the influence of external stimuli on the cortex. Massive feedback from the cortex to the thalamus suggests that the entire thalamo-cortico-thalamic loop plays a role in sustaining and synchronizing cortical activity. Furthermore, certain thalamic nuclei appear to constitute an integral part of the signal flow between different cortical areas. The article reviews the anatomical and neurophysiological data and concludes with a brief discussion of models of the role of thalamus in thalamocortical interactions (see also "Adaptive Resonance Theory" and "Sleep Oscillations"), arguing that the organization of the projections to and from the thalamus is essential to understanding thalamic function.

VISUAL CORTEX: ANATOMICAL STRUCTURE AND MODELS OF FUNCTION reviews features of the microcircuitry of the primary visual cortex, area V1, and physiological properties of cells in its different laminae. It then outlines several hypotheses as to how the anatomical structure and connections might serve the functional organization of the region. For example, a connectionist model of layer IVc of V1 demonstrated that the gradient of change in properties of the layer could indeed be replicated using dendritic overlap through the lower two-thirds of the IVc layer. However, it was insufficient to explain the continuous and sharply increasing field size and contrast sensitivity observable near the top of the layer. However, this discrepancy led to new experiments and related changes in the model which resulted in a good replication of the actual physiological data and required only feedforward excitation. The article continues by analyzing the anatomical substrates for orientation specificity and for surround modulation of visual responses, and concludes by discussing the origins of patterned anatomical connections. VISUAL SCENE PERCEPTION moves beyond V1 to chart the bifurcation of V1 output in monkeys and humans into a pathway that ascends to the parietal cortex (the dorsal "where/how" system involved in object location and setting of parameters for action) and a pathway that descends to inferotemporal cortex (the ventral "what" system involved in object recognition) (see also "Dissociations Between Visual Processing Modes").

SOMATOSENSORY SYSTEM argues that the tactile stimulus representation changes from an original form (more or less isomorphic to the stimulus itself) to a completely distributed form (underlying perception) in a series of partial transformations in successive subcortical and cortical networks. At the level of primary somatosensory cortex, the neural image of the stimulus is sensitive to shape and temporal features of peripheral stimuli, rather than simply reflecting the overall intensity of local stimulation. The processing of somatosensory information is seen as modular on two different scales: macrocolumnar in terms of "segregates" such as the cortical barrels seen in rodent somatosensory cortex, each of which receives its principal input from one of the facial whiskers; and minicolumnar, with each minicolumn in a segregate receiving afferent connections from a unique subset of the thalamic neurons projecting to that segregate. The article argues that the causal factors involved in body/object interactions are represented by the pyramidal cells of somatosensory cortical areas in such a way that their ascending, lateral, and feedback connections develop an internal working model of mechanical interactions of the body with the outside world. Such an internal model can endow the somatosensory cortex with powerful interpretive and predictive capabilities that are crucial for haptic perception (i.e., tactile perception of proximal surroundings) and for control of object manipulation.

The auditory system is introduced in two articles. AUDITORY PERIPHERY AND COCHLEAR NUCLEUS spells out how the auditory periphery transforms a very high information rate acoustic stimulus into a series of lower information rate auditory nerve firings, with the incoming acoustic information split across hundreds of nerve fibers to avoid loss of information. The transformation involves complex mechanical-to-electrical transformations. The cochlear nucleus continues this process of parallelization by creating multiple representations of the original acoustic stimulus, with each representation presumably emphasizing different acoustic features that are fed to other brainstem structures, such as the superior olivary complex, the nuclei of the lateral lemniscus, and the inferior colliculus. These parallel pathways are believed to be specialized for the processing of different auditory features used for sound source classification and localization. From the inferior colliculus, auditory information is passed via the medial geniculate body in the thalamus to the auditory cortex. AUDITORY CORTEX stresses the crucial role that auditory cortex plays in the perception and localization of complex sounds. Although recent studies have expanded our knowledge of the neuroanatomical structure, the subdivisions, and the connectivities of all central auditory stages, relatively little is known about the functional organization of the central auditory system. Nevertheless, a few auditory tasks have been broadly accepted as vital for all mammals, such as sound localization, timbre recognition, and pitch perception. The article discusses a few of the functional and stimulus feature maps that have been found or postulated, and relates them to the more intuitive and better understood case of the echolocating bats (cf. "Echolocation: Cochleotopic and Computational Maps").

The olfactory system is distinctive in that paths from periphery to cortex do not travel via a thalamic nucleus. The olfactory pathway begins with the olfactory receptor neurons in the nose, which project their axons to the olfactory bulb. The function of the olfactory bulb is to perform the initial stages of sensory processing of the olfactory signals before sending this information to the olfactory cortex. The study of the olfactory system offers prime examples of seeking a "basic circuit" that defines the irreducible minimum of neural components necessary for a model of the functions carried out by a region. OLFACTORY BULB offers examples of information processing without impulses and of output functions of dendrites (dendrodendritic synapses). The olfactory cortex is defined as the region of the cerebral cortex that receives direct connections from the olfactory bulb and is subdivided into several areas that are distinct in terms of details of cell types, lamination, and sites of output to the rest of the brain. The main area involved in olfactory perception is the piriform (also called prepyriform) cortex, which projects to the mediodorsal thalamus, which in turn projects to the frontal neocortex. This is often regarded as the main olfactory cortex, and is the subject of the article OLFACTORY CORTEX. Olfactory cortex is the earliest cortical region to differentiate in the evolution of the vertebrate forebrain and is the only region within the forebrain to receive direct sensory input. Models of olfactory cortex emphasize the importance of cortical dynamics, including the interactions of intrinsic excitatory and inhibitory circuits and the role of oscillatory potentials in the computations performed by the cortex.

We now introduce motor cortex, then turn to three systems related to motor control and to visuomotor coordination in mammals (cf. the road map **Mammalian Motor Control**): cortical areas involved in grasping, the basal ganglia, and cerebellum. MOTOR CORTEX: CODING AND DECODING OF DIRECTIONAL OPERATIONS spells out the relation between the direction of reaching and changes in neuronal activity that have been established for several brain areas, including the motor cortex. The cells involved each have a broad tuning function, the peak of which is viewed as the "preferred" direction of the cell. A movement in a particular direction will engage a whole population of cells. It is found that the weighted vector sum of their neuronal preferences is a "population vector" which points in (close to) the direction of the movement for discrete movements in 2D and 3D space. GRASPING MOVEMENTS: VISUOMOTOR TRANSFORMATIONS shows the tight coupling between (specific subregions of) parietal and premotor cortex in controlling grasping. The AIP region of inferior parietal lobe appears to play a fundamental role in extracting intrinsic visual properties ("affordances") from the object for organizing grasping movements. The extracted visual information is then sent to the F5 region of premotor cortex, there activating neurons that code grip types congruent to the size, shape, and orientation of the object. In addition to visually activated neurons in AIP, there are AIP cells whose activity is linked to motor activity, possibly reflecting corollary discharges sent by F5 back to the parietal cortex. (For the possible relation of grasping to language, and the homology between F5 and Broca's area, see "Language Evolution: The Mirror System Hypothesis.")

The basal ganglia include the striatum, the globus pallidus, the substantia nigra, and the subthalamic nucleus. BASAL GANGLIA stresses that all of these structures are functionally subdivided into skeletomotor, oculomotor, associative, and limbic territories. The basal ganglia can be viewed as a family of loops, each taking its origin from a particular set of functionally related cortical fields, passing through the functionally corresponding portions of the basal ganglia, and returning to parts of those same cortical fields by way of specific zones in the dorsal thalamus. The article reviews models of the basal ganglia that attempt to incorporate appropriate anatomical or physiological data, but not those that use only generic neural network architectures. Some models work at a comparatively low level of detail (membrane properties of individual neurons and microanatomical features) and restrict themselves to a single component of the basal ganglia nucleus; others work at the system level with the basal ganglia as a whole and with their interactions with related structures (e.g., thalamus and cortex). Since dopamine neurons discharge in relation to conditions involving the probability and imminence of behavioral reinforcement, dopamine neurons have been seen as playing a role in striatal information processing analogous to that of an "adaptive critic" in connectionist networks (cf. "Reinforcement Learning" and "Dopamine, Roles of").

The division of function between cerebellum and basal ganglia remains controversial. One view is that the basal ganglia play a role in determining when to initiate one phase of movement or another, and that the cerebellum adjusts the metrics of movement, tuning different movements and coordinating them into a graceful whole. CEREBELLUM AND MOTOR CONTROL reviews a number of models for cerebellar mechanisms underlying the learning of motor skills. Cerebellum can be decomposed into cerebellar nuclei and a cerebellar cortex. The only output cells of the cerebellar cortex are the Purkinje cells, and their only effect is to provide varying levels of inhibition on the cerebellar nuclei. Each Purkinje cell receives two types of input—a single climbing fiber, and many tens of thousands of parallel fibers. The most influential model of cerebellar cortex has been the Marr-Albus model of the formation of associative memories between particular patterns on parallel fiber inputs and Purkinje cell outputs, with the climbing fiber acting as "training signal." Later models place more emphasis on the relation between the cortex and nuclei, and on the way in which the subregions of this coupled cerebellar system can adapt and coordinate the activity of specific motor pattern generators. The plasticity of the cerebellum is approached from a different direction in CEREBELLUM AND CONDITIONING. Many experiments indicate that the cerebellum is involved in learning and performance of classically conditioned reflexes. The article reviews a number of models of the role of cerebellum in rabbit eye blink conditioning, providing a useful complement to models of the role of cerebellum in motor control.

The hippocampus has been implicated in a variety of memory functions, both as working memory and as basis for long-term memory. It was also the site for the discovery of long-term potentiation (LTP) in synapses (see "Hebbian Synaptic Plasticity"). Structurally, hippocampus is the simplest form of cortex. It contains one projection cell type, whose cell bodies are confined to a single layer, and receives inputs from all sensory systems and association areas. HIPPOCAMPUS: SPATIAL MODELS builds on the finding that single-unit recordings in freely moving rats have revealed "place cells" in subfields of the hippocampus whose firing is restricted to small portions of the rat's environment (the corresponding "place fields"). These data underlie the seminal idea of the hippocampus as a spatial map (cf. "Cognitive Maps"). The article reviews the data and describes some models of hippocampal place cells and of their role in circuits controlling the rat's navigation through its environment. HIPPOCAMPAL RHYTHM GENERATION provides data and models on theta and other rhythms as well as epileptic discharges, and also introduces the key cell types of the hippocampus and a number of interconnections between the hippocampus that seem to play a key role in the generation of these patterns of activity.

Finally, we turn to prefrontal cortex, the association cortex of the frontal lobes. It is one of the cortical regions to develop last and most in the course of both primate evolution and individual ontogeny. PREFRONTAL CORTEX IN TEMPORAL ORGANIZATION OF ACTION suggests that the late morphological development of this cortex in both cases is related to its support of higher cognitive functions involving the capacity to execute novel and complex ac-

tions, which reaches its maximum in the adult human brain. The lateral region of prefrontal cortex is involved in the representation and temporal organization of sequential behavior. This article emphasizes the physiological functions of the lateral prefrontal cortex in the temporal organization of behavior. Temporal integration of sensory and motor information, through active short-term memory (working memory) and prospective set, supports the goal-directed performance of the perception-action cycle. This role extends to the temporal organization of higher cognitive operations, including, in the human, language and reasoning.

Cognitive Neuroscience

Cognitive neuroscience has been boosted tremendously in the last decade by the rapid development and increasing use of techniques to image the active human brain. The road map thus starts with several articles on ways of observing activity in the human brain and then examines various human cognitive functions.

The organization of large masses of neurons into synchronized waves of activity lies at the basis of phenomena such as the electroencephalogram (EEG) and evoked potentials, as well as the magnetoencephalogram (MEG). The EEG consists of the electrical activity of relatively large neuronal populations that can be recorded from the scalp, while the MEG can be recorded using very sensitive transducers arranged around the head. EEG AND MEG ANALYSIS reviews methods of quantitative analysis that have been applied to extract information from these signals, providing an indispensable tool for sleep and epilepsy research. Epilepsy is a neurological disorder characterized by the occurrence of seizures, sudden changes in neuronal activity that interfere with the normal functioning of neuronal networks, resulting in disturbances of sensory or motor activity and of the flow of consciousness. During an epileptic seizure, the neuronal network exhibits typical oscillations that usually propagate throughout the brain, involving progressively more brain systems. These oscillations are revealed in the EEG (see also "Hippocampal Rhythm Generation"). In general, the same brain sources account for the EEG and the MEG, with the reservation that the MEG reflects magnetic fields perpendicular to the skull that are caused by tangential current dipolar fields, whereas the EEG/MEG reflects both radial and tangential fields. This property can be used advantageously to disentangle radial sources lying in the convexity of cortical gyri from tangential sources lying in the sulci.

EVENT-RELATED POTENTIALS shows how cortical event-related potentials (ERPs) arise from synchronous interactions among large numbers of participating neurons. These include dense local inter-actions involving excitatory pyramidal neurons and inhibitory interneurons, as well as long-range interactions mediated by axonal pathways in the white matter. Depending on the types of interaction that occur in a specific behavioral condition, cortical networks may display different states of synchrony, causing their ERPs to oscillate in different frequency bands, designated delta (0–4 Hz), theta (5–8 Hz), alpha (9–12 Hz), beta (13–30 Hz), and gamma (31–100 Hz). Depending on the location and size of the recording and reference electrodes, recorded cortical field potentials integrate neural activity over a range of spatial scales: from the intracortical local field potential (LFP) to the intracranial electrocorticogram (ECoG) to the extracranial electroencephalogram (EEG). ERP studies have shown that local cortical area networks are able to synchronize and desynchronize their activity rapidly with changes in cognitive state. When incorporated into ANNs, the result could be a metastable large-scale neural network design that recruits and excludes subnetworks according to their ability to reach consensual local patterns, with the ability to implement behavioral schemas and adapt to changing environmental conditions.

Positron emission tomography (PET) and functional magnetic resonance imaging (fMRI) provide means for seeing which brain regions are significantly more active in one task rather than another. Functional neuroimaging is generally used to make inferences about functional anatomy on the basis of evoked patterns of cortical activity. Functional anatomy involves an understanding of what each part of the brain does, and how different brain systems interact to support various sensorimotor and cognitive functions. Large-scale organization can be inferred from techniques that image the hemodynamic and metabolic sequelae of evoked neuronal responses. PET measures regional cerebral blood flow (rCBF) and fMRI measures oxygenation changes. Their spatial resolution is on the order of a few millimeters. Because PET uses radiotracers, its temporal resolution is limited to a minute or more by the half-life of the tracers employed. However, fMRI is limited only by the biophysical time constants of hemodynamic responses themselves (a few seconds).

STATISTICAL PARAMETRIC MAPPING OF CORTICAL ACTIVITY PATTERNS considers the neurobiological motivations for different designs and analyses of functional brain imaging studies, noting that the principles of *functional specialization* and *integration* serve as the motivation for most analyses. Statistical parametric mapping (SPM) is used to identify functionally specialized brain regions that respond selectively to experimental cognitive or sensorimotor changes, irrespective of changes elsewhere. SPM is a voxel-based approach (a voxel is a volume element of a 3D image) employing standard inferential statistics. SPM is a *mass-univariate* approach, in the sense that each data sequence, from every voxel, is treated as a univariate response. The massive numbers of voxels are analyzed in parallel, and dependencies among them are dealt with using random field theory (see "Markov Random Field Models in Image Processing").

One approach to systems-level neural modeling aims at determining the network of brain regions mediating a specific cognitive task. This means finding the nodes of the network (i.e., the brain regions), and determining the task-dependent functional strengths of their interregional anatomical linkages. COVARIANCE STRUCTURAL EQUATION MODELING describes techniques applied to the correlations between PET- or fMRI-determined regional brain activities. These correlations are viewed as "functional connectivities." They thus vary from task to task, as different patterns of excitation and inhibition are routed through the anatomical connections of these regions. Examples of questions that can be answered using this approach are: (1) As one learns a task, do the functional links between specific brain regions change their values? (2) In cases of similar performance, are the same brain networks

being used by normals and patients? The method is illustrated with studies of object and spatial vision showing cross-talk between the dorsal and ventral streams (see "Visual Scene Perception"), which implies that they need not be functionally independent. The article stresses the concept of a *neural context*, where the functional relevance of a particular region is determined by its interactions with other areas. Because the pattern of interactions with other connected areas differs from task to task, the resulting cognitive operations may vary within a single region as it engages in different tasks.

SYNTHETIC FUNCTIONAL BRAIN MAPPING analyzes ways in which models of neural networks grounded in primate neurophysiology can be used as the basis for predictions of the results of human brain imaging. This is crucial for furthering our understanding of the neural basis of behavior. Covariance structural equation modeling helps identify the nodes of the region-by-region network corresponding to a cognitive task, especially when there is little or no nonhuman data available (e.g., most language tasks). Synthetic functional brain mapping uses primate data to form hypotheses about the neural mechanisms whereby cognitive tasks are implemented in humans, with PET and fMRI data providing constraints on the possible ways in which these neural systems function. This is illustrated in relation to the mechanisms underlying saccadic eye movements and working memory.

The next three articles focus on what we are learning about vision, motor activity, and language from functional brain imaging. IMAGING THE VISUAL BRAIN addresses functional brain imaging of visual processes, with emphasis on limits in spatial and temporal resolution; constraints on subject participation; and trade-offs in experimental design. The articles focuses on retinotopy, visual motion perception, visual object representation, and voluntary modulation of attention and visual imagery, emphasizing some of the areas where modeling and brain theory might be testable using current imaging tools. IMAGING THE MOTOR BRAIN shows that the behavioral form and context of a movement are important determinants of functional activity within cortical motor areas and the cerebellum, stressing that functional imaging of the human motor system requires one to study the interaction of neurological and cognitive processes with the biomechanical characteristics of the effectors. Multiple neural systems must interact to successfully perform motor tasks, encode relevant information for motor learning, and update behavioral performance in real time. The article discusses how evidence from functional imaging studies provides insight into motor automaticity as well as the role of internal models in movement. The article also discusses novel mathematical techniques that extend the scope of functional imaging experimentation.

IMAGING THE GRAMMATICAL BRAIN reviews brain imaging results that support the author's view that linguistic rules are neurally real and form a constitutive element of the human language faculty. The focus is on linguistic combinations at the sentence level; but an analysis of cerebral representation of phonological units and of word meaning in its isolated and compositional aspects is provided as background. The study of brain mechanisms supporting language is further advanced in NEUROLINGUISTICS. Neurolinguistics began as the study of the language deficits occurring after brain injuries, and is rooted in the conceptual model of Broca's aphasia, Wernicke's aphasia, and other aphasic syndromes established over a hundred years ago. The article presents data and analyses for between-stage information flow, dynamics of within-stage processing, unitary representations and activation, and processing by constraint satisfaction. (For more background on these two articles, see the road map **Linguistics and Speech Processing**.)

PREFRONTAL CORTEX IN TEMPORAL ORGANIZATION OF ACTION emphasizes the physiological functions of the lateral prefrontal cortex in the temporal organization of behavior, highlighting active short-term memory (working memory) and prospective set. The two cooperate toward temporally integrating sensory and motor information by mediating cross-temporal contingencies of behavior (see also "Competitive Queuing for Planning and Serial Performance"). This temporal integration supports the goal-directed performance of the perception-action cycle. It is a role that extends to the temporal organization of higher cognitive operations, including language and reasoning in humans. CORTICAL MEMORY stresses that some components of memory are localized in discrete domains of cortex, while others are more widely distributed. It outlines a view of network memory in the neocortex that is supported by empirical evidence from neuropsychology, behavioral neurophysiology, and neuroimaging. Its essential features are the acquisition of memory by the formation and expansion of networks of neocortical neurons through changes in synaptic transmission; and the hierarchical organization of memory networks, with a hierarchy of networks in posterior cortex for perceptual memory and another in frontal cortex for executive memory. SEQUENCE LEARNING characterizes behavioral sequences in terms of their serial, temporal, and abstract structure, and analyzes the associated neural processing systems (see also "Temporal Pattern Processing"). Temporal structure is defined in terms of the durations of elements (and the possible pauses that separate them), and intuitively corresponds to the familiar notion of rhythm. Abstract structure is defined in terms of generative rules that describe relations between repeating elements within a sequence. Thus, the two sequences A-B-C-B-A-C and D-E-F-E-D-F are both generated from the same abstract structure 123-213. The article focuses on how the different dimensions of sequence structure can be encoded in neural systems, citing behavioral studies in different patient and control groups and related simulation studies. A recurrent network for manipulating abstract structural relations is implemented in a distributed network that potentially includes the perisylvian cortex in and around Broca's area. It is argued that both transfer of sequence knowledge between domains and abstract rule representation are likely to be neurophysiological realities.

Complementing sequence learning is the study of imitation, the ability to recognize and reproduce others' actions. Imitation is also related to fundamental capabilities for social cognition such as the recognition of conspecifics, the attribution of others' intentions, and the ability to deceive and to manipulate others' states of mind. IMITATION bridges between biology and engineering, reviewing the cognitive and neural processes behind the different forms of imitation seen in animals and showing how studies of biological processes influence the design of robot controllers and computational algorithms. Theoretical models have been proposed to, e.g., distinguish between purely associative imitation (low-level) and sequential imitation (high-level). It is argued that modeling of imitation will lead to a better understanding of the neural mechanisms at the basis of social cognition and will offer new perspectives on the evolution of animal abilities for social representation (see "Language Evolution: The Mirror System Hypothesis" for more on evolution and imitation).

EMOTIONAL CIRCUITS stresses the distinction between emotional experiences and the underlying processes that lead to emotional experiences. (See also "Motivation" for a discussion of the motivated or goal-directed behaviors that are often accompanied by emotion or affect.) The article is grounded in studies of how the brain detects and evaluates emotional stimuli and how, on the basis of such evaluations, appropriate responses are produced, treating emotion as a function that allows the organism to respond in an adaptive manner to challenges in the environment rather than being inextricably compounded with the subjective experience of emotion. The amygdala is shown to play a major role in the evaluation process. It is argued that fearful stimuli follow two main routes. The fast route involves the thalamo-amygdala pathway and responds best to simple stimulus features, while the slow route involves the thalamo-cortical-amygdala pathway and carries more complex features (such as context). The expression of fear is mediated by the outputs of the amygdala to brainstem and hypothalamus, while the experience of fear involves the prefrontal cortex.

One cerebral hemisphere may perform better than the other for such diverse tasks as language, handedness, visuospatial processing, emotion and its facial expression, olfaction, and attention. Behavioral lateralization has not only been demonstrated in people, but also in rodents, birds, primates, and other animals in areas such as vocalization and motor preferences. Many anatomical, biochemical, and physiological asymmetries exist in the brain, but it is generally unclear which, if any, of these asymmetries actually contribute to hemispheric specialization. Pathways such as the corpus callosum connecting the hemispheres appear to mediate both excitatory and longer-term inhibitory interactions between the hemispheres. HEMISPHERIC INTERACTIONS AND SPECIALIZATION first considers models of hemispheric interactions that do not incorporate hemispheric differences, and conversely, models examining the effects of hemispheric differences that do not incorporate hemispheric interactions. It then looks in more detail at recent studies demonstrating how both hemispheric interactions and differences influence the emergence of lateralization in models where lateralization is not initially present.

As we already saw in, e.g., NEUROLINGUISTICS, cognitive neuropsychology uses neurological data on the performance of brain-damaged patients to constrain models of normal cognitive function. LESIONED NETWORKS AS MODELS OF NEUROPSYCHOLOGICAL DEFICITS surveys how connectionist techniques have been employed to model the operation and interaction of "modules" inferred from the neurological data. The advantage over "box-and-arrow" models is that removing neurons or connections in connectionist models leads to natural analogues of real brain damage. Moreover, such models let one explore the possibility that processing is actually more distributed and interactive than the older models implied. The article discusses the effects of simulated lesioning on various models, constructed either as feedforward networks or as attractor networks, paying special attention to the misleading artifacts that may arise when large brains are modeled by small ANNs. Continuing with this theme, NEUROPSYCHOLOGICAL IMPAIRMENTS cautions that the inferences that link a neuropsychological impairment to a particular theory in cognitive neuroscience are not as direct as one might at first assume. The brain is a distributed and highly interactive system, such that local damage to one part can unleash new modes of functioning in the remaining parts of the system. The article emphasizes neural network models of cognition and the brain that provide a framework for reasoning about the effects of local lesions in distributed, interactive systems. In many cases a model's behavior after lesioning is somewhat counterintuitive and so can lead to very different interpretations regarding the nature of the normal system. A model of neglect dyslexia shows how an impairment in a prelexical attentional process could nevertheless show a lexicality effect. Prosopagnosia is an impairment of face recognition that can occur relatively independently of impairments in object recognition. The behavior of some prosopagnosic patients seems to suggest that that recognition and awareness depend on dissociable and distinct brain systems. However, a model of covert face recognition demonstrates how dissociation may occur without separate systems. NEUROLOGICAL AND PSYCHIATRIC DISORDERS shows how neural modeling may be harnessed to investigate the pathogenesis and potential treatment of brain disorders by studying the relation between the "microscopic" pathological alterations of the underlying neural networks and the "macroscopic" functional and behavioral disease manifestations that characterize the network's function. The article reviews computational studies of the neurological disorders of Alzheimer's disease, Parkinson's disease, and stroke, and the psychiatric disorders of schizophrenia and affective disorders.

II.4. Psychology, Linguistics, and Artificial Intelligence

Psychology

Much classical psychology was grounded in notions of association—of ideas, or of stimulus and response—which were well developed in the philosophy of Hume, but with roots going back as far as Aristotle. ASSOCIATIVE NETWORKS shows how these old ideas gain new power because neural networks can provide mechanisms for the formation of associations that automatically yield many further properties. One of these is that neural networks will in many cases have similar responses to similar inputs, a property that is exploited in the study of ANALOGY-BASED REASONING AND METAPHOR. Analogy and metaphor have been characterized as comparison processes that permit one domain to be seen in terms of another. Indeed, many of the advantages suggested for connectionist models—representation completion, similarity-based generalization, graceful degradation, and learning—also apply to analogy, yet analogical processing poses significant challenges for connectionist models. Analogy and metaphor involve structured pattern matching, structured pattern completion, and a focus on common *relational structure* rather than on common object descriptions. The article analyzes current connectionist models of analogy and metaphor in terms of representations and associated processes, not in terms of brain function. Challenges for future research include building analogical models that can preserve structural relations over incrementally extended analogies and that can be used as components of a broader cognitive system such as one that would perform problem solving. Indeed, people continually deal with composite structures whether they result from aggregation of symbols in a natural language into syllables, words, and sentences or aggregation of visual features into contour and regions, objects, and complete scenes. COMPOSITIONALITY IN NEURAL SYSTEMS addresses the question of what sort of neural dynamics allows composite structures to emerge, with the grouping and binding of parts into interpretable wholes. To this day it is still disputed whether ANNs are capable of adequately handling compositional data, and if so, which type of network is most suitable. Basic results have been obtained with simple recurrent networks, but some researchers argue that more complicated dynamics (see, e.g., "Synchronization, Binding and Expectancy") or dynamics similar to classical symbolic processing mechanisms are necessary for successful modeling of compositionality. In a related vein, SYSTEMATICITY OF GENERALIZATIONS IN CONNECTIONIST NETWORKS presents the current "state of play" for Fodor and Pylyshyn's critique of connectionist architecture. They claimed that human cog-

nitive abilities "come in clumps" (i.e., the abilities are systematically related), and that this systematic relationship does not hold in connectionist networks. The present article examines claims and counterclaims concerning the idea that learning in connectionist architectures can engender systematicity, with special attention paid to studies based on simple recurrent networks (SRNs) and recursive auto-associative memory (RAAM). The conclusion is that, for now, evidence for systematicity in such simple networks is rather limited. (One may ponder the fact that animal brains are vastly more complex than a single SRN or RAAM.)

The "units of thought" afforded by connectionist "neurons" are quite high level compared to the fine-grain computation of the myriad neurons in the human brain, and their properties may hence be closer to those of entire neural networks than to single biological neurons. Moreover, future connectionist accounts of cognition will certainly involve the coordination of connectionist modules (see, e.g., "Hybrid Connectionist/Symbolic Systems"). SCHEMA THEORY complements neuroscience's well-established terminology for levels of structural analysis (brain region, neuron, synapse) with a functional vocabulary, a framework for analysis of behavior with no necessary commitment to hypotheses on the localization of each schema (unit of functional analysis), but which can be linked to a structural analysis whenever appropriate. The article focuses on two issues: structuring perceptual and motor schemas to provide an action-oriented account of behavior and cognition (as relevant to the roboticist as the ethologist), and how schemas describing animal behavior may be mapped to interacting regions of the brain. Schema-based modeling becomes part of neuroscience when constrained by data provided by, e.g., human brain mapping, studies of the effects of brain lesions, or neurophysiology. The resulting model may constitute an adequate explanation in itself or may provide the framework for modeling at the level of neural networks or below. Such a neural schema theory provides a functional/structural decomposition, in strong contrast to models that employ learning rules to train a single neural network to respond as specified by some training set.

Connectionism can apply many different types of ANN techniques to explain psychological phenomena, and the article COGNITIVE MODELING: PSYCHOLOGY AND CONNECTIONISM places a sample of these in perspective. The general idea is that much of psychology is better understood in terms of parallel networks of adaptive units than in terms of serial symbol processing, and that connectionism gains much of its power from using very simple units with explicit learning rules. The article points out that connectionist models of cognition can be used both to model cognitive processes and to simulate the performance of tasks and that, unlike many traditional computational models, they are not explicitly programmed by the investigator. However, important aspects of the performance of a connectionist net are controlled by the researcher, so that the achievement of a good fit to the psychological data depends both on the way in which analogs to the data are derived and on the results of "extensional programming," such as decisions about the selection and presentation of training data. The article also notes the work of "cognitive connectionists," whose computational experiments have demonstrated the ability of connectionist representations to provide a promisingly different account of important characteristics of cognition (compositionality and systematicity), previously assumed to be the exclusive province of the classical symbolic tradition. PHILOSOPHICAL ISSUES IN BRAIN THEORY AND CONNECTIONISM asks the following questions: (1) Do neural systems exploit classical compositional and systematic representations, distributed representations, or no representations at all? (2) How do results emerging from neuroscience help constrain cognitive scientific models? (3) In what ways might embodiment, action, and dynamics matter for understanding the mind and the brain? There is a growing emphasis on the computational economies afforded by real-world action and the way larger structures (of agents and artifacts) both scaffold and transform the shape of individual reason. However, rather than seeing representations as opposed to interactive dynamics, the article advocates a broader vision of the inner representational resources themselves, stressing the benefits of converging influences from robotics, systems-level neuroscience, cognitive psychology, evolutionary theory, AI, and philosophical analysis. This philosophical theme is further developed in CONSCIOUSNESS, NEURAL MODELS OF, which reviews the basic ways in which consciousness has been defined, relevant neuropsychological data, and preliminary progress in neural modeling. Among the characteristics needed for consciousness are temporal duration, attentional focus, binding, bodily inputs, salience, past experience, and inner perspective. Brain imaging, as well as insights into single-cell activity and the effects of brain deficits, is leading to a clearer picture of the neural correlates of consciousness. The article presents a specific attention control model of the emergence of awareness in which experience of the prereflective self is identified with the corollary discharge of the attention movement control signal. This signal is posited to reside briefly in its buffer until the arrival of the associated attended input activation at its own buffer. The article concludes by reviewing other neural models of consciousness.

Much of the early work on ANNs was inspired by the problem of "Pattern Recognition" (q.v.). CONCEPT LEARNING provides a general introduction to recent work, placing such ideas in a psychological perspective. Concepts are mental representations of kinds of objects, events, or ideas. The article focuses on learning mental representations of new concepts from experience and how mental representations of concepts are used to make categorization decisions and other kinds of judgments. The article reviews five types of concept learning models: rule models, prototype models, exemplar models, mixed models, and neuroscientific models. The mechanisms discussed briefly here are developed at greater length in many articles in the road map **Learning in Artificial Networks**. The psychology of concept learning receives special application in the study of FACE RECOGNITION: PSYCHOLOGY AND CONNECTIONISM, which relates connectionist approaches to face recognition to psychological theories for the subtasks of representing faces and retrieving them from memory, comparing human and model performance along these dimensions.

Many of the concepts of connectionist psychology are strongly related to work in behaviorism, but neural networks provide a stronger "internal structure" than stimulus-response probabilities. Connectionist research has enriched a number of concepts that seemed "anticognitive" by embedding them in mechanisms, namely, neural nets, which can both support internal states and yield stimulus-response pairs as part of a general input-output map. This is shown in CONDITIONING. During conditioning, animals modify their behavior as a consequence of their experience of the contingencies between environmental events. This article presents formal theories and neural network models that have been proposed to describe classical and operant conditioning. During *classical conditioning*, animals change their behavior as a result of the contingencies between the conditioned stimulus (CS) and the unconditioned stimulus (US). Contingencies may vary from very simple to extremely complex ones. For example, in Pavlov's proverbial experiment, dogs were exposed to the sound of a bell (CS) followed by food (US). At the beginning of training, animals salivated (generated an unconditioned response, UR) only when the US was presented. With an increasing number of CS-US pairings, CS presentations elicited a conditioned response (CR). The article discusses variations in the effectiveness of the CS, the US, and the CS and

US together, as well as attentional models. During *operant* (or *instrumental*) *conditioning*, animals change their behavior as a result of a triple contingency between its responses (R), discriminative stimuli (SD), and the reinforcer (US). Animals are exposed to the US in a relatively close temporal relationship with the SD and R. As in "Reinforcement Learning" (q.v.), during operant conditioning animals learn by trial and error from feedback that evaluates their behavior but does not indicate the correct behavior. The article discusses positive reinforcement and negative reinforcement. Such ideas are further developed in COGNITIVE MAPS. Tolman introduced the notion of a *cognitive map* to explain animals' capacity for place learning, latent learning, detours, and shortcuts. In some models, Tolman's vicarious trial-and-error behavior has been regarded as reflecting the animal's comparison of different expectancies: at choice points, animals make a decision after sampling the intensity of the activation elicited by the various alternative paths. Other models still use Tolman's stimulus-approach view and assume that animals approach the place with the strongest appetitive activation, thereby performing a gradient ascent toward the goal. In addition to storing the representation of the environment in the terms of the contiguity between places, cognitive maps can store information about differences in height and the type of terrain between adjacent places, contain a priori knowledge of the space to be explored, distinguish between roads taken and those not taken, and keep track of which places have been examined. Neural networks with more than two layers can also be used to represent both the contiguity between places and the relative position of those places. Hierarchical cognitive maps can represent the environment at multiple levels. In contrast to their nonhierarchical counterparts, hierarchical maps can plan navigation in large environment, use a smaller number of connections in their networks, and have shorter decision times.

Learning in neural nets can be either supervised or unsupervised, and supervision can be in terms of a specific error signal or some general reinforcement. However, in real animals, these signals seem to have some "heat" to them, which brings us to the issues of motivation and emotion. Motivated or goal-directed behaviors are sets of motor actions that direct an animal toward a particular goal object. Interaction with the goal either promotes the survival of an individual or maintains the species. Motivated behaviors include sleep/wake, ingestive, reproductive, thermoregulatory, and aggressive/defensive behaviors (see also "Pain Networks"). They are often accompanied by emotion or affect. Given the difficulty of defining the terms *drive*, *instinct*, and *motivation* with respect to the neural substrates of behavior, MOTIVATION adopts a neural systems approach that discusses what and how particular parts of the brain contribute to the expression of behaviors that have a motivated character. The approach is based on Hullian incentive models of motivation, where the probability of a particular behavior depends on the integration of information from systems that control circadian timing and regulate arousal state, inputs derived from interosensory information that encode internal state (e.g., hydration state, plasma glucose, leptin, etc.), modulatory hormonal inputs such as gonadal steroids that mediate sexual behavior, and inputs derived from classic sensory modalities. EMOTIONAL CIRCUITS analyzes the nature of emotion, emphasizing its role in behavior rather than the subjective feelings that accompany human emotions, then examines the role of brain structures such as the amygdala, the interaction of body and cognitive states, and the status of neural modeling. The expression of fear is seen as mediated by the outputs of the amygdala to lower brain centers (brainstem, hypothalamus), while the experience of fear involves the prefrontal cortex.

Finally, we turn to development, a theme of special concern in connectionist linguistics (see the next road map). COGNITIVE DEVELOPMENT reviews connectionist models of the origins of knowledge, the mechanisms of change, and the task-dependent nature of developing knowledge across a variety of domains. In each case, the models provided explicit instantiations and controlled tests of specific theories of development, and allowed the exploration of complex, emergent phenomena. However, most connectionist models are "fed" their input patterns regardless of what they output, whereas even very young children shape their environments based on how they behave. Moreover, most connectionist models are designed for and tested on a single task within a single domain, whereas children face a multitude of tasks across a range of domains each day. Capturing such features of development will require future models to take in a variety of types of information and learn how to perform successfully across a number of tasks. DE-VELOPMENTAL DISORDERS uses the comparison of different abnormal phenotypes to explore further the modeling of the developing mind/brain. The article reviews recent examples of connectionist models of developmental disorders. Autism is a developmental disorder characterized primarily by deficits in social interaction, communication, and imagination, but also by a range of secondary deficits. One hypothesis suggests that these structural deficits are consistent with too few neurons in some brain areas, such as the cerebellum, and too many neurons in other areas, such as the amygdala and hippocampus. This grounds a simple connectionist model trained on categorization tasks linking such differences in neuro-computational constraints to some of the secondary deficits found in autism. Other models relate disordered feature maps or hidden unit numbers to higher-level cognitive deficits that characterize autism. Developmental dyslexia has been modeled by changing parameters in models of the normal processes of reading. Another model captures some features of specific language impairment, specifically the difficulty of affected patients in learning rule-based inflectional morphology in verbs, using an attractor network mapping between semantic codes and phonological codes. The article also reports new empirical findings on Williams syndrome patients which reveal a deficit in generalizing knowledge of inflectional patterns to novel forms. Alterations in the initial computational constraints of a connectionist model of past tense development are shown to account for some of the patterns seen in such data, demonstrating how different computational constraints interact in the process of development. Connectionist models thus provide a powerful tool with which to investigate the role of initial computational constraints in determining the trajectory of both typical and atypical development, ensuring that selective deficits in developmental disorders are seen in terms of the outcome of the developmental process itself.

Linguistics and Speech Processing

CONSTITUENCY AND RECURSION IN LANGUAGE
CONVOLUTIONAL NETWORKS FOR IMAGES, SPEECH, AND TIME
    SERIES
HIDDEN MARKOV MODELS
IMAGING THE GRAMMATICAL BRAIN
LANGUAGE ACQUISITION
LANGUAGE EVOLUTION AND CHANGE
LANGUAGE EVOLUTION: THE MIRROR SYSTEM HYPOTHESIS
LANGUAGE PROCESSING
MOTOR THEORIES OF PERCEPTION
NEUROLINGUISTICS
OPTIMALITY THEORY IN LINGUISTICS
PAST TENSE LEARNING
READING
SPEECH PROCESSING: PSYCHOLINGUISTICS
SPEECH PRODUCTION
SPEECH RECOGNITION TECHNOLOGY

The traditional grounding of linguistics is in grammar, a systematic set of rules for structuring the sentences of a particular language.

Much modern work in linguistics has been dominated by the ideas of Noam Chomsky, who placed the notion of grammar in a mathematical framework. His ideas have gone through successive stages in which the formulation of grammars has changed radically. However, two themes have remained stable in the "generative linguistics" that has grown from his work:

- There is a *universal grammar* which defines what makes a language human, and each human language has a grammar that is simply a parametric variation of the universal grammar.
- Language is too complicated for a child to learn from scratch; instead a child has universal grammar as an innate mental capacity. When the child hears example sentences of a language, they set parameters in the universal grammar so that the child can then acquire the grammar of the particular language.

Connectionist linguistics attacks this reasoning on two fronts:

- It says that language processing is better understood in terms of connectionist processing, which, as a performance model (i.e., a model of behavior, as distinct from a competence model, which gives a static representation of a body of knowledge), can give an account of errors as well as regularities in language use.
- It notes that connectionism has powerful learning tools that Chomsky has chosen to ignore. With those tools, connectionism can model how children could acquire language on the basis of far less specific mental structures than those posited in universal grammar.

LANGUAGE PROCESSING reviews many application of connectionist modeling. Despite the insights gained into syntactic structure across languages, the formal study of language has revealed relatively little about learning and development. Thus, as we shall see later in this road map, the connectionist program for understanding language has concentrated on the process of *change*, exploring topics such as language development, language breakdown, the dynamics of representation in complex systems which themselves may be receiving changing input, and even the evolution of language. The article briefly reviews models of lexical processing (reading single words, recognizing spoken words, and word production) as well as higher-level processing. It concludes that there has been important progress in many areas of connectionist-based research into language processing, and this modeling influences both psychological and neuropsychological experimentation and observation. However, it concedes that the major debates on top-down feedback, on the capacity of connectionist models to capture the productivity and systematicity of human language, and on the degree of modularity in language processing remain to be settled.

CONSTITUENCY AND RECURSION IN LANGUAGE then provides more detail on connectionist approaches to syntax. Words group together to form coherent building blocks, *constituents*, within a sentence, so that "The girl liked a boy" decomposes into "the girl" and "liked a boy," forming a subject noun phrase (NP) and a verb phrase (VP), respectively. In linguistics, grammar rules such as Sentence S → NP VP determine how constituents can be put together to form sentences. To capture the full generativity of human language, *recursion* needs to be introduced into the grammar. For example, if we add the rules NP → (det) N(PP) (noun with optional determiner and prepositional phrase) and PP → Preposition NP, then the rules are recursive, because in this case, NP can invoke rules that eventually call for another instance of NP. This article discusses how constituency and recursion may fit into a connectionist framework, and the possible implications this may have for linguistics and psycholinguistics.

LANGUAGE ACQUISITION presents models used by developmental connectionists to support the claim that rich linguistic representations can emerge from the interaction of a relatively simple learning device and a structured linguistic environment. The article reviews connectionist models of lexical development, inflectional morphology, and syntax acquisition, stressing that these models use similar learning algorithms to solve diverse linguistic problems. PAST TENSE LEARNING then presents issues in word morphology as a backdrop for a detailed discussion of the prime debate between a rule-based and a connectionist account of language processing, over the forming of regular and irregular past tenses of verbs in English. The dual mechanism model—use the general rule "add-*ed*" unless an irregular past tense is found in a table of exceptions—was opposed by the view that all past tenses, even for regular verbs, are formed by a connectionist network. The article concludes that most researchers now agree that the mental processing of irregular inflections is not rule governed but rather works much like a connectionist network. Certainly, rules provide an intuitively appealing explanation for regular behavior. Indeed, people are clearly able to consciously identify regularities and describe them with explicit rules that can then be deliberately followed, but this does not imply that a neural encoding of these rules, rather than a connectionist network which yields rule-like behavior, is the better account of "mental reality." The matter is subtle because the brain is composed of neurons. Thus the issue is not "Does the brain's language processing use neural networks?" but whether or not the activity of those networks is best described as explicitly encoding a set of rules.

READING covers connectionist models of reading and associated processes, including the reading disorder known as dyslexia. Where a skilled reader can recognize many thousands of printed words, each in a fraction of a second, with no noticeable effort, a dyslexic child may need great effort to recognize a printed word as a particular word. Most connectionist networks for reading are models of word recognition. However, word recognition is more than an analytic letter-by-letter process that translates spelling into phonology, and so the synthetic-analytic debate provides the organizing theme for this article. The authors argue that, rather than see modeling word recognition as a distinct, separable component of reading, it may be better to investigate more integrative, nonlinear iterative network models. However, SPEECH PROCESSING: PSYCHOLINGUISTICS reviews attempts to capture psycholinguistic data using connectionist models, with the primary focus on speech segmentation and word recognition. This article analyzes how far the problem of segmenting speech into words occurs independently of word recognition; considers the interplay of connectionist models of word recognition with empirical research and theory; and assesses the gap that remains between psycholinguistic studies of speech processing and modeling of the human brain. Although data from neuropsychology and functional imaging are becoming increasingly important (see IMAGING THE GRAMMATICAL BRAIN and NEUROLINGUISTICS), the main empirical constraints on psycholinguistic models are derived from laboratory studies of human language processing that are unrelated to neural data. The article suggests that connectionist modeling helps bridge the gulf between psycholinguistics and neuroscience by employing computational models that embody at least some of the computational principles of the brain.

IMAGING THE GRAMMATICAL BRAIN notes that there is little agreement on the best way to analyze language. Contrary to the connectionist approach (see, e.g., PAST TENSE LEARNING), the author sees inventories of combinatorial rules, and stores of complex objects of several types over which these rules operate, as being at the core of language. The "language faculty," in this view, inheres in a cerebrally represented knowledge base (rule system) and in algorithms that instantiate it. It is divided into levels for the identification and segmentation of speech sounds (universal phonetics), a system that enables the concatenation of phonetic units into se-

quences (phonology), then into words (morphology, where word structure is computed), sentences (syntax), and meaning (lexical and compositional semantics). The article reviews results emanating from brain imaging that support the neural reality of linguistic rules as a constitutive element of the human language faculty. The focus is on linguistic combinations at the sentence level, but an analysis of cerebral representation of phonological units and of word meaning in its isolated and compositional aspects is provided as background. The study of brain mechanisms supporting language is further advanced in NEUROLINGUISTICS. Neurolinguistics began as the study of the language deficits occurring after brain injuries and is rooted in the conceptual model of Broca's aphasia, Wernicke's aphasia, and other aphasic syndromes established over a hundred years ago. However, thanks to recent research, critical details are now seen differently, and finer details have been added. Speech and language are now recognized as the products of interacting dynamic systems, with major implications for modeling normal and abnormal performance and for understanding their neural substrates. The article analyzes between-stage information flow, dynamics of within-stage processing, unitary representations and activation, and processing by constraint satisfaction. How the cognitive elements (nodes) of psychological theorizing correspond to actual neuronal activity is not known for certain. However, the article suggests that the attractor states that can occur in recurrent networks are viable candidates for behaving as nodes. Indeed, many modeling efforts in neurolinguistics have been concerned with the consequences of relatively large-scale assumptions about stages and connections (see "Lesioned Networks as Models of Neuropsychological Deficits").

On the output side, SPEECH PRODUCTION focuses on work in motor control, dynamical systems and neural networks, and linguistics that is critical to understanding the functional architecture and characteristics of the speech production system. The central point is that spoken word forms are not unstructured wholes but rather are composed from a limited inventory of phonological units that have no independent meaning but that can be (relatively freely) combined and organized in the construction of word forms. The production of speech by the lips, tongue, vocal folds, velum, and respiratory system can thus be understood as arising from choreographed linguistic action units. However, when phonological units are made manifest in word and sentence production, their spatiotemporal realization by the articulatory system, and consequent acoustic character presented to the auditory system, is highly variable and context dependent. The speech production system is sometimes viewed as having two components, one (traditionally referred to as phonology) concerned with categorical and linguistically contrastive information, and the other concerned with gradient, noncontrastive information (traditionally referred to as phonetics). However, current work in connectionist and dynamical systems models blurs this dichotomy. MOTOR THEORIES OF PERCEPTION reviews reasons why speech scientists have doubted the claim that the speech motor system participates in speech perception and then argues against such doubts, showing that the theory accrues credibility when it is set in the larger context of investigations of perception, action, and their coupling. The mirror neurons in primates (see LANGUAGE EVOLUTION: THE MIRROR SYSTEM HYPOTHESIS) are seen as providing an existence proof of neuronal perceptuomotor couplings. The article further argues that, although the motor theory of speech perception was motivated by requirements of speaking and listening, real-world functional perception-action coupling is central to the "design" of animals more generally.

We have already contrasted connectionism with rule-based frameworks that account for linguistic patterns through the sequential application of transformations to lexical entries. OPTIMALITY THEORY IN LINGUISTICS introduces optimality theory (OT) as a framework for linguistic analysis that has largely supplanted rule-based frameworks within phonology; it has also been applied to syntax and semantics, though not as widely. Generation of utterances in OT involves two functions, *Gen* and *Eval*. *Gen* takes an input and returns a (possibly infinite) set of output candidates. Some candidates might be identical to the input, others modified somewhat, others unrecognizable. *Eval* chooses the candidate that best satisfies a set of ranked constraints; this optimal candidate becomes the output. The constraints can conflict, so the constraints' ranking, which differs from language to language, determines the outcome. One language might eliminate consonant clusters by deleting consonants; another might retain all input consonants. OT was partly inspired by neural networks, employing as it does the ideas of optimization, parallel evaluation, competition, and soft, conflicting constraints. OT can be implemented in a neural network with constraints that are implemented as connection weights. The network implements a Lyapunov function that maximizes "harmony" ($\Sigma_{ij}a_iw_{ij}a_j$: the sum, for all pairs i, j of neurons, of the product of the neurons' activations and their connection weight). Hierarchically structured representations (e.g., consonants and vowels grouped into syllables) can be represented as matrices of neurons, where each matrix is the tensor product of a vector for a linguistic unit and a vector for its position in the hierarchy.

An approach to language that emphasizes the learning processes of each new speaker rather than the existence of a set of immutable rules shared by all humans seems well equipped to approach the issue of how a language changes from generation to generation. Computational modeling has been used to test competing theories about specific aspects of language evolution under controlled circumstances. Connectionist networks have been used as simulated agents to study how social transmission via learning may give rise to the evolution of structured communication systems. In other cases, properties of neural network learning are enlisted to help illuminate the constraints and processes that may have been involved in the evolution of language. LANGUAGE EVOLUTION AND CHANGE surveys this connectionist research, starting from the emergence of early syntax and continuing on to the role of social interaction and constraints on network learning in subsequent evolution of language. It also discusses linguistic change within existing languages, showing how the inherent generalization ability of neural networks makes certain errors in language transmission from one generation to the next more likely than others. (However, such models say more about the simplification of grammars than about how language complexity arises in the first place.) Where this article stresses computational efficacy of various models proposed for the emergence of features characteristic of current human languages, LANGUAGE EVOLUTION: THE MIRROR SYSTEM HYPOTHESIS focuses on brain mechanisms shared by humans with other primates, and seeks to explain how these generic mechanisms might have become specialized during hominid evolution to support language. It is argued that imitation and pantomime provide a crucial bridging capability between general primate capabilities for action recognition and the language readiness of the human brain.

At present, the state of play may be summarized as follows: generative linguistics has shown how to provide grammatical rules that explain many subtle sentence constructions of English and many other languages, revealing commonalities and differences between languages, with the differences in some cases being reduced to very elegant and compact formulations in terms of general rules with parametric variations. However, in offering the notion of universal grammar as the substrate for language acquisition, generative linguistics ignores issues of learning that must, in any case, be faced in explaining how children acquire the large and idiosyncratic vocabulary of their native tongue. Connectionist linguistics, on the other hand, has made great strides in bringing learning to the center, not only showing how specific language skills (e.g., use of the past

tense) may be acquired, but also providing insight into psycholinguistics, the study of language behavior. However, connectionist linguistics still faces two major hurdles: it lacks the systematic overview of language provided by generative linguistics, and little progress has been made in developing a neurolinguistic theory of the contributions of specific brain regions to language capabilities. It is one thing to train an ANN to yield a convincing model of performance on the past tense; it is quite another to offer an account of how this skill interfaces with all the other aspects of language, and what neural substrates are necessary for their acquisition by the human child.

The remaining articles look at speech processing from a technological perspective rather than in relation to human psycholinguistic data. SPEECH RECOGNITION TECHNOLOGY introduces the way computer systems that transcribe speech waveforms into words rely on digital signal processing and statistical modeling methods to analyze and model the speech signal. Although commercial technology is typically not based on connectionist methods, neural network processing is commonly seen as a promising alternative to some of the current algorithms, and the article focuses on speech recognizers that process large-vocabulary continuous speech and that use multilayer feedforward neural networks. Traditional speech recognition systems follow a hierarchical architecture. A grammar specifies the sentences allowed by the application. (Alternatively, for very large vocabulary systems, a statistical language model may be used to define the probabilities of various word sequences in the domain of application.) Each word allowed by the grammar is listed in a dictionary that specifies its possible pronunciations in terms of sequences of phonemes which are further decomposed into smaller units whose acoustic realizations are represented by statistical acoustic models. When a speech waveform is input to a recognizer, it is first processed by a front-end unit that extracts a sequence of observations, or "features," from the raw signal. This sequence of observations is then decoded into the sequence of speech units whose acoustic models best fit the observations and that respect the constraints imposed by the dictionary and language model. Hidden Markov models (HMMs) have been an essential part of the toolkit for continuous speech recognition, as well as other complex temporal pattern recognition problems such as cursive (handwritten) text recognition, time-series prediction, and biological sequence analysis. HIDDEN MARKOV MODELS describes the use of deterministic and stochastic finite state automata for sequence processing, with special attention to HMMs as tools for the processing of complex piecewise stationary sequences. It also describes a few applications of ANNs to further improve these methods. HMMs allow complex learning problems to be solved by assuming that the sequential pattern can be decomposed into piecewise stationary segments, with each stationary segment parameterized in terms of a stochastic function. The HMM is called "hidden" because there is an underlying stochastic process (i.e., the sequence of states) that is not directly observable but that nonetheless affects the observed sequence of events. CONVOLUTIONAL NETWORKS FOR IMAGES, SPEECH, AND TIME SERIES shows how shift invariance is obtained in convolutional networks by forcing the replication of weight configurations across space. This takes the topology of the input into account, enabling such networks to force the extraction of local features by restricting the receptive fields of hidden units to be local, and enforcing a built-in invariance with respect to translations, or local distortions of the inputs.

Artificial Intelligence

ARTIFICIAL INTELLIGENCE AND NEURAL NETWORKS
BAYESIAN NETWORKS
COMPETITIVE QUEUING FOR PLANNING AND SERIAL
   PERFORMANCE

In the 1950s, the precursors of today's fields of artificial intelligence and neural networks were still subsumed under the general heading of *cybernetics*. Much of the work in the 1960s sought to distance artificial intelligence (AI) from its cybernetic roots, emphasizing models of, e.g., logical inference, game playing, and problem solving that were based on explicit symbolic representations manipulated by serial computer programs. However, work in computer vision and in robotics (discussed in the road maps **Vision** and **Robotics and Control Theory**, respectively) showed that this distinction was never entirely convincing, since these were areas of AI that made use of parallel computation and numerical transformations. For a while, a case could be made that the use of parallelism might be appropriate for peripheral sensing and motor control but not for the "central" processes involved in "real" intelligence. However, work from at least the mid-1970s onward has made this fallback position untenable. For example, in the HEARSAY system, speech understanding was achieved not by serial manipulation of symbolic structures but by the action (implicitly distributed, though in the 1970s still implemented on a serial computer) of knowledge sources (what we would now call "agents") to update numerical confidence levels of multiple hypotheses distributed across a set of "levels" in a data structure known as a blackboard. MULTIAGENT SYSTEMS introduces the methodology that has grown out of such beginnings. What constitutes an "individual" can be highly subjective: an individual to one researcher can, to another, be a complex distributed system comprised of finer-grained agents. Research in brain theory has dealt with different levels, from neurons to brain regions to humans whereas AI work in multi-agent systems has focused on coarse-grained levels of individuality and interaction, where the goal is to draw upon sociological, political, and economic insights. The article is designed to survey enough of this work on multi-agent systems to foster comparisons between the ANN, brain theory, and multi-agent approaches. A crucial notion is that agents either have or learn models of the agents with which they interact. These models allow agents to avoid dealing with malicious or broken agents. Agents may even build nested models of the other agents that include an agent's models of other agents, and so on. By using their models of each other, the agents loosely organize themselves into self-reinforcing communities of trust, avoiding unproductive future interactions with other agents. In another branch of AI, work on *expert systems*—information systems that represent expert knowledge for a particular problem area as a set of rules, and that perform inferences when new data are entered—provided an important application success in which numerical confidence values played a role, but with the emphasis still on manipulation of hypotheses through the serial application of explicit rules. As shown in DECISION SUPPORT SYSTEMS AND EXPERT SYSTEMS, we now see many cases in which the application of separate rules is replaced by transformations effected in parallel by (trainable) neural networks. A *decision system* is either a decision support system or an expert system in the classic AI sense. The article reviews results on connectionist-based decision systems. In particular, trainable knowledge-based neural networks can be used to accumulate both knowledge (rules) and data, building adaptive decision systems with incremental, on-line learning.

As the general overview article ARTIFICIAL INTELLIGENCE AND NEURAL NETWORKS makes clear, there are many problems for which the (not necessarily serial) manipulation of symbolic structures can still outperform connectionist approaches, at least with today's software running on today's hardware. Nonetheless, if we define AI by the range of problems it is to solve—or the "packets of intelligence" it is to implement—then it is no longer useful to define it in opposition to connectionism. In general, the technologist facing a specific problem should choose between, or should combine, connectionist and symbolic approaches on the basis of efficacy, not ideology. On occasion, for rhetorical purposes, authors will use the term AI for a serial symbolic methodology distinct from connectionism. However, we will generally use it in an extended sense of a technology that seeks to realize aspects of intelligence in machines by whatever methods work best. The term *symbolic AI* will then be used for the "classical" approach. The article examines the relative merits of symbolic AI systems and neural networks, and ways of attempting to bridge between the two. In brain theory, everything, whether symbolic or not, is, in the final analysis, implemented in a neural network. But even here, an analysis of the brain will often best be conducted in terms of interacting subsystems that are not all fully explicated in neural network terms. SCHEMA THEORY complements neuroscience's well-established terminology for levels of structural analysis (brain region, neuron, synapse) with a framework for analysis of behavior with no necessary commitment to hypotheses on the localization of each schema (unit of functional analysis), but which can be linked to a structural analysis whenever appropriate. The article focuses on two issues: structuring perceptual and motor schemas to provide an action-oriented account of behavior and cognition (as relevant to the roboticist as the ethologist), and how schemas describing animal behavior may be mapped to interacting regions of the brain. Schema-based modeling becomes part of neuroscience when constrained by data provided by, e.g., human brain mapping, studies of the effects of brain lesions, or neurophysiology. The resulting model may constitute an adequate explanation in itself or may provide the framework for modeling at the level of neural networks or below. Such a neural schema theory provides a functional/structural decomposition, in strong contrast to models that employ learning rules to train a single, otherwise undifferentiated, neural network to respond as specified by some training set. HYBRID CONNECTIONIST/SYMBOLIC SYSTEMS reviews work on hybrid systems that integrate neural (ANN) and symbolic processes. Cognitive processes are not homogeneous, and so some are best captured by symbolic models and others by connectionist models. Correspondingly, from a technological viewpoint, AI systems for practical applications can benefit greatly from a proper combination of different techniques combining, e.g., symbolic models (for capturing explicit knowledge) and connectionist models (for capturing implicit knowledge).

Use of the term *systematicity* in relation to connectionist networks originated with Fodor and Pylyshyn's critique of connectionist architecture. They claimed that human cognitive abilities are systematically related in a way that does not hold in connectionist networks, unlike formal systems akin to propositional logic. SYSTEMATICITY OF GENERALIZATIONS IN CONNECTIONIST NETWORKS starts by noting that this critique made no reference to learning-based generalization, and then proceeds to examine claims and counterclaims concerning the claim that learning in connectionist architectures can engender systematicity. Special attention is paid to studies based on simple recurrent networks (SRNs) and recursive auto-associative memory (RAAM). The article suggests that, for now, evidence for systematicity in such simple networks is rather limited. Perhaps this is not so surprising, given that there is little evidence of systematicity in most animals, and animal brains are vastly more complex than SRNs or RAAMs. Compare "Language Evolution: The Mirror System Hypothesis" for a discussion of how evolution may have shaped the human brain to extend capabilities shared with other species to yield novel human cognitive abilities.

The notion of representation plays a central role in AI. As discussed in SEMANTIC NETWORKS, one classic form of representation in AI is the *semantic network*, in which nodes represent concepts and links represent relations between them. Semantic networks were originally developed for couching "semantic" information, either in the psychologist's sense of static information about concepts or in the semanticist's sense of the meanings of natural language sentences. However, they are also used as a general knowledge representation tool. The more elaborate types of semantic networks are similar in their representational abilities to sophisticated forms of symbolic logic. The article discusses various ways of implementing or emulating semantic networks in neural networks, and of forming hybrid semantic network-neural network systems. STRUCTURED CONNECTIONIST MODELS emphasizes those neural networks in which the translation from symbolic to neural is fairly direct: nodes become "neurons," but now processing is done by neural interactions rather than by an "inference engine" acting on a passive representation. At the other extreme, certain neural networks (connectionist, rather than biological) may transform input "questions" to output "answers" via the distributed activity of neurons whose firing conditions have no direct relationship to the concepts that might normally arise in a logical analysis of the problem (cf. "Past Tense Learning"). In the fully distributed version of the latter approach, each "item" (concept or mental object) is represented as a pattern of activity distributed over a common pool of nodes. However, if "John" and "Mary," for example, are represented as patterns of activity over the entire network such that each node in the network has a specific value in the patterns for "John" and "Mary," respectively, then how can the network represent "John" and "Mary" at the same time? To address such problems, the structured approach often employs small clusters of nodes that act as "focal" nodes for concepts and provide access to more elaborate structures that make up the detailed encoding of concepts (cf. "Localized Versus Distributed Representations"). The discussion of these varying styles of representation is continued in CONNECTIONIST AND SYMBOLIC REPRESENTATIONS. In symbolic representations, the heart of mathematics and many models of cognition, symbols are meaningless entities to which arbitrary significance may be assigned. Composing ordered tuples from symbols and other tuples allows us to create an infinitude of complex structures from a finite set of tokens and combination rules. Inference in the symbolic framework is founded on structural comparison and rule-governed manipulation of these objects. However, AI makes extensive use of nondeductive reasoning methods. Symbolists have moved to more complex formalizations of cognitive processes, using heuristic and unsound inference rules. Connectionists explore a radical alternative: that cognitive processes are mere epiphenomena of a completely different type of underlying system, whose operations can never be adequately formalized in symbolic language. The article examines representation and processing issues in the connectionist move from classical discrete, set-theoretic semantics to a continuous, statistical, vector-based semantics.

In symbolic AI, two concepts can be linked by providing a pointer between them. In a neural net, the problem of "binding" the two patterns of activity that represent the concepts is a more subtle one, and several models address the use of rapidly changing synaptic strengths to provide temporary "assemblages" of currently related data. This theme is developed not only in STRUCTURED CONNECTIONIST MODELS, but also in the articles COMPOSITIONALITY IN NEURAL SYSTEMS (how can inferences about a structure be based on the way it is composed of various elements?), and "Object Structure, Visual Processing" (combining visual elements of an object into a recognizable whole). DYNAMIC LINK ARCHITECTURE, the basic methodology, views the brain's data structure as a graph composed of nodes connected by links. Both units and links bear activity variables changing on the rapid time scale of fractions of a second. The nodes play the role of symbolic elements. The intensity of activity measures the degree to which a node is active in a given time interval, signifying the degree to which the meaning of the node is alive in the mind of the animal, while correlations of activity between nodes quantify the degree to which the signal of one node is related to that of others. The strength of links can change on two time scales, represented by two variables called temporary weight and permanent weight. The permanent weight corresponds to the usual synaptic weight, can change on the slow time scale of learning, and represents permanent memory. The temporary weight can change on the same time scale as the node activity—it is what makes the link dynamic. On this view, dynamic links constitute the glue by which higher data structures are built up from more elementary ones.

Complementing the theme of representation in symbolic AI has been that of planning, going from (representations of) the current state and some desired state to a sequence of operations that will transform the former to the latter. COMPETITIVE QUEUING FOR PLANNING AND SERIAL PERFORMANCE presents neural network studies based on two assumptions: that more than one plan representation can be simultaneously active in a planning layer, and that which plan to enact next is chosen as the most active plan representation by a competition in a second neural layer. Once a plan wins the competition and is used to initiate a response, its representation is deleted from the field of competitors in the planning layer, and the competition is re-run. This iteration allows the two-layer network to transform an initial activity distribution across plan representations into a serial performance. Such models provide a very different basis for control of serial behavior than that given by recurrent neural networks. The article suggests that such a system was probably an ancient invention in the evolution of animals yet may still serve as a viable core for the highest levels of planning and skilled sequencing exhibited by humans.

The final articles in this road map are not on neural nets per se, but instead provide related methods that add to the array of techniques extending AI beyond the serial, rule-based approach. BAYESIAN NETWORKS provides an explicit method for following chains of probabilistic inference such as those appropriate to expert systems, extending Bayes's rule for updating probabilities in the light of new evidence. The nodes in a Bayesian network represent propositional variables of interest and the links represent informational or causal dependencies among the variables. The dependencies are quantified by conditional probabilities for each node given its parents in the network. The network supports the computation of the probabilities of any subset of variables given evidence about any other subset, and the reasoning processes can operate on Bayesian networks by propagating information in any direction. GRAPHICAL MODELS: PROBABILISTIC INFERENCE introduces the graphical models framework, which has made it possible to understand the relationships among a wide variety of network-based approaches to computation, and in particular to understand many neural network algorithms and architectures as instances of a broader probabilistic methodology. Graphical models use graphs to represent and manipulate joint probability distributions. The graph underlying a graphical model may be directed, in which case the model is often referred to as a belief network or a Bayesian network, or the graph may be undirected, in which case the model is generally referred to as a Markov random field. The articles GRAPHICAL MODELS: STRUCTURE LEARNING and GRAPHICAL MODELS: PARAMETER LEARNING present learning algorithms that build on these inference algorithms and allow parameters and structures to be estimated from data. (A fuller précis of the three articles on graphical models can be found in the road map **Learning in Artificial Networks**.) Finally, MEMORY-BASED REASONING applies massively parallel computing to answer questions about a new situation by searching for data on the most similar stored instances. Memory-based reasoning (MBR) refers to a family of nearest-neighbor-like methods for making decisions or classifications. Where nearest-neighbor methods generally use a simple overlap distance metric, MBR uses variants of the value distance metric.

MBR and neural nets form decision surfaces differently, and so will perform differently. MBR can become arbitrarily accurate if large numbers of cases are available, and if these cases are well behaved and properly categorized, whereas neural nets cannot respond well to isolated cases but tend to be good at smooth extrapolation. For each article reviewed in this paragraph, the reader may ponder whether these methods are alternatives to connectionist AI, or whether they can contribute to the emergence of a technologically efficacious hybrid. As stated before, where brain theory seeks to know "how the brain does it," AI must weigh the value of ANNs as a powerful technology for parallel, adaptive computation against that of other technologies on the basis of efficacy in solving practical problems on available hardware.

II.5. Biological Neurons and Networks

Biological Neurons and Synapses

ACTIVITY-DEPENDENT REGULATION OF NEURONAL
  CONDUCTANCES
AXONAL MODELING
BIOPHYSICAL MECHANISMS IN NEURONAL MODELING
BIOPHYSICAL MOSAIC OF THE NEURON
DENDRITIC PROCESSING
DENDRITIC SPINES
DIFFUSION MODELS OF NEURON ACTIVITY
ION CHANNELS: KEYS TO NEURONAL SPECIALIZATION
NEOCORTEX: BASIC NEURON TYPES
NEOCORTEX: CHEMICAL AND ELECTRICAL SYNAPSES
OSCILLATORY AND BURSTING PROPERTIES OF NEURONS
PERSPECTIVE ON NEURON MODEL COMPLEXITY
SINGLE-CELL MODELS
SYNAPTIC INTERACTIONS
SYNAPTIC NOISE AND CHAOS IN VERTEBRATE NEURONS
SYNAPTIC TRANSMISSION
TEMPORAL DYNAMICS OF BIOLOGICAL SYNAPSES

Nearly all the articles in the road maps **Psychology, Linguistics and Speech Processing**, and **Artificial Intelligence** discuss networks made of very simple neurons describable by a single internal variable, either binary or real-valued (the "membrane potential") and that communicate with other neurons by a simple (generally nonlinear) function of that variable, sometimes referred to as the firing rate. Incoming signals are usually summed linearly via "synaptic weights," and these weights in turn may be adjusted by simple learning rules, such as the Hebbian rule, the perceptron rule, or a reinforcement learning rule. Such simplifications remain valuable both for technological application of ANNs and for approximate models of large biological networks. Nonetheless, biological neurons are vastly more complex than these single-compartment models suggest. An appreciation of this complexity is necessary for the computational neuroscientist wishing to address the increasingly detailed database of experimental neuroscience. It is also important for the technologist looking ahead to the incorporation of new capabilities into the next generation of ANNs.

The neocortex is functionally parcellated into vertical columns (~0.5 mm in diameter) traversing all six layers. These columns have no obvious anatomical boundaries, and the topographic mapping of afferent and efferent pathways probably determines their locations and dimensions as well as their functions. NEOCORTEX: BASIC NEURON TYPES shows that these apparently stereotypical microcircuits are composed of a daunting variety of precisely and intricately interconnected neurons and argues that this neuronal diversification may provide a foundation for maximizing the computational abilities of the neocortex. All anatomical cell types can display multiple discharge patterns and molecular expression profiles. Different cell types are synaptically interconnected according to complex organizational principles to form intricate stereotypical microcircuits. The article challenges neural network modelers to incorporate and account for this cellular diversity and the role of different cells in the computational capability of cortical microcircuits. NEOCORTEX: CHEMICAL AND ELECTRICAL SYNAPSES summarizes the diverse functional properties of synapses in neocortex. These synapses tend to be small, but their structure and biochemistry are complex. Both chemical and electrical synapses exist in neocortex. *Chemical synapses* are the "usual synapses" of neural network models, and are far more abundant. They use a chemical neurotransmitter that is packaged presynaptically into vesicles, released in quantized (vesicle-multiple) amounts, and binds to postsynaptic receptors that either open an ion channel directly (voltage-dependent ion channels) or modulate the channel through an intracellular molecule that links the activated receptor to the opening or closing of the channel. The latter molecule is called a "second messenger," to contrast it with the case in which the transmitter itself provides a "primary message" that acts directly on the channel, in this case called "ligand-gated." Second-messenger-based synaptic interaction occurs on a slower time scale than ligand-gated interaction and is called *neuromodulation*, since it may modulate the behavior of the postsynaptic neuron over a time scale of seconds or minutes rather than milliseconds (cf. "Neuromodulation in Invertebrate Nervous Systems" and "Neuromodulation in Mammalian Nervous Systems"). The essential element of an *electrical synapse* is a protein called a connexin; 12 connexins form a single intercytoplasmic ion channel, and a cluster of such channels constitutes a gap junction. Electrical synapses provide a direct pathway that allows ionic current or small organic molecules to flow from the cytoplasm of one cell to that of another. Short-term dynamics allow synapses to serve as temporal filters of neural activity. Long-term synaptic plasticity provides specific, localized substrates for various forms of memory. Modulation of synaptic function by neurotransmitters (see "Neuromodulation in Mammalian Nervous Systems") provides a mechanism for globally altering the properties of a neural circuit during changes of behavioral state. Each of these functions has diverse forms that vary between synapses, depending on their site within the cortical circuit (and elsewhere in the brain).

PERSPECTIVE ON NEURON MODEL COMPLEXITY discusses the wide range of model complexity, from very simple to rather complex neuron models. Which model to choose depends, in each case, on the context, such as how much information we already have about the neurons under consideration and what questions we wish to answer. The use of more realistic neuron models when seeking functional insights into biological nervous systems does not mean choosing the most complex model, at least in the sense of including all known anatomical and physiological details. Rather, the key is to preserve the most significant distinctions between regions (soma, proximal dendritic, distal dendritic, etc.), using "compartmental modeling," whereby one compartment represents each functionally distinct region. SINGLE-CELL MODELS starts by reviewing the "simple" models of Part I (the McCulloch-Pitts, perceptron, and Hopfield models) and the slightly more complex polynomial neuron. It then turns to more realistic biophysical models, most of which are explored in further detail in this road map. These include the Hodgkin-Huxley model of squid axon, integrate-and-fire models, modified single-point models, cable and compartmental models, and models of synaptic conductances.

Before turning to a detailed analysis of mechanisms of neuronal function, we first consider an article that offers a high-level view of the neuron, but this time a stochastic one. Most nerve cells encode their output as a series of action potentials, or spikes, that originate at or close to the cell body and propagate down the axon at constant velocity and amplitude. DIFFUSION MODELS OF NEURON ACTIVITY studies the membrane potential of a single neuron as engaged in a stochastic process that will eventually bring it to the threshold for spike initiation. This leads to the first-passage-time problem, inferring the distribution of neuronal spiking based on the "first passage" of the membrane potential from its resting value to threshold. In addition to using stochastic differential equations, the article shows how the Wiener and Ornstein-Uhlenbeck neuronal models can be obtained as the limit of a Markov process with discrete state spaces. Besides these models, characterized by additive noise terms appearing in the corresponding stochastic differential equations, the article also reviews diffusion models with multiplicative noise, showing that these can be used not only for the description of steady-state firing under constant stimulation, but also for effects of periodic stimulation.

Now for the details of neuronal function. The ionic mechanisms underlying the initiation and propagation of action potentials were elucidated in the squid giant axon by a number of workers, most notably Hodgkin and Huxley. Variations on the Hodgkin-Huxley equation underlie the vast majority of contemporary biophysical models. AXONAL MODELING describes this model and its assumptions, introduces the two classes of axons (myelinated and non-myelinated) found in most animals, and concludes by briefly commenting on the possible functions of axonal branching in information processing. The Hodgkin-Huxley equation was brilliantly inferred from detailed experiments on conduction of nerve impulses. Much research since then has revealed that the basis for these equations is provided by "channels," structures built from a few macromolecules and embedded in the neuron which, in a voltage-dependent way, can selectively allow different ions to pass through the cell membrane to change the neuron's membrane potential. Similarly, channels (also known in this case as receptors) in the postsynaptic membrane can respond to neurotransmitters, chemicals released from the presynaptic membrane, to change the neuron's local membrane potential in response to presynaptic input. These changes, local to the synapse, must propagate down the dendrites and across the cell body to help determine whether or not the axon will "pass threshold" and generate an action potential. ION CHANNELS: KEYS TO NEURONAL SPECIALIZATION notes that channels not only produce action potentials but can set a particular firing pattern, latency, rhythm, or oscillation for the firing of these spikes. Each neuronal class is endowed with a different set of channels, and the diversity of channels between different types of neurons explains the functional classes of neurons found in the brain. Some

neurons fire spontaneously, some show adaptation, some fire in bursts, and so on. Therefore, a channel-based cellular physiology is relevant to questions about the role of different brain regions in overall function.

Biophysically detailed compartmental models of single neurons typically aim to quantitatively reproduce membrane voltages and currents in response to some sort of "synaptic" input. We may think of them as "Hodgkin-Huxley-Rall" models, based on the hypothesis of the neuron as a dynamical system of nonlinear membrane channels distributed over an electrotonic cable skeleton. Such models can incorporate as much biophysical detail as desired (or practical), but in general, all include some explicit assortment of voltage-dependent and transmitter-gated (synaptic) membrane channels. BIOPHYSICAL MECHANISMS IN NEURONAL MODELING first presents general issues regarding model formulations and data interpretation. It then describes the modeling of various features of Hodgkin-Huxley-Rall models, including Hodgkin-Huxley and Markov kinetic descriptions of voltage- and second-messenger-dependent ion channels as well as methods for describing intracellular calcium dynamics and the associated buffer systems and membrane pumps. The models for each of these mechanisms are at an intermediate level of biophysical detail, appropriate for describing macroscopic variables (e.g., membrane currents, ionic concentrations) on the scale of the entire cell or anatomical compartments thereof. Similar models of synaptic mechanisms are covered in SYNAPTIC INTERACTIONS, which provides kinetic models of how synaptic currents arise from ion channels whose opening and closing are controlled (gated) directly or indirectly by the release of neurotransmitter. The article compares several models of synaptic interaction, focusing on simple models based on the kinetics of postsynaptic receptors, and shows how these models capture the time courses of postsynaptic currents of several types of synaptic responses, as well as synaptic summation, saturation, and desensitization.

The membrane potential of central neurons undergoes synaptic noise, fluctuations that depend on both the summed firing of action potentials by neurons presynaptic to the investigated cell and the spontaneous release of transmitter. SYNAPTIC NOISE AND CHAOS IN VERTEBRATE NEURONS argues that, despite its random appearance, synaptic noise may be a true signal associated with neural coding, possibly a chaotic one. In addition to reviewing tools for detecting chaotic behavior, the article pays special attention to Mauthner cells, a pair of identified neurons in the hindbrain of teleost fishes. When the fish is subjected to an unexpected stimulus, one of the cells triggers an escape reaction. Their excitability is controlled by powerful inhibitory presynaptic interneurons that continuously generate an intense synaptic noise. While it is still an open question whether this synaptic noise exhibits deterministic chaos or is truly random, it is worth stressing that the "noise" has adaptive value for the fish: the variability along output pathways introduces uncertainty in the expression of the reflex, and therefore enhances the fish's success in evading predators.

TEMPORAL DYNAMICS OF BIOLOGICAL SYNAPSES complements the many studies of synaptic plasticity in the *Handbook* that focus on long-term changes in synaptic strength by showing how synaptic function can be profoundly influenced by activity over time scales of milliseconds to seconds. Synapses that exhibit such short-term plasticity are powerful computational elements that can have profound impact on cortical circuits (cf. "Dynamic Link Architecture"). Short-term plasticity includes both synaptic depression and a number of components of short-term enhancement (facilitation, augmentation, and posttetanic potentiation) acting over increasingly longer periods of time. Synaptic facilitation appears to result from enhanced transmitter release due to elevated presynaptic calcium levels, while depression is believed to result, in part, from depletion of a readily releasable pool of vesicles. Depression appears to be a particularly prominent feature of transmission at excitatory synapses onto pyramidal cells. In addition to having complex short-term dynamics, synapses are stochastic, and it is argued that constructive roles for unreliable transmission become apparent when short-term plasticity is considered in connection with stochastic transmission, with synapses acting as stochastic temporal filters of their presynaptic spike trains. Indeed, SYNAPTIC TRANSMISSION is concerned with the uncertainties introduced by noise and their relation to synaptic plasticity. The probability that a single activated synapse will release neurotransmitter has a broad distribution, well fitted by a gamma function, with a mean near 0.3. The dynamic regulation of synaptic strength depends on a complicated set of mechanisms that record the history of synaptic use over many time scales, and serve to filter the incoming spike train in a way that reflects the past use of the synapse. The article provides equations which describe how synaptic use determines the number of vesicles available for release, and for the release probability in turn.

OSCILLATORY AND BURSTING PROPERTIES OF NEURONS offers a dynamic systems analysis of the linkage between a fascinating variety of endogenous oscillations (neuronal rhythms) and appropriate sets of channels. However, membrane potential oscillations with apparently similar characteristics can be generated by different ionic mechanisms, and a given cell type may display several different firing patterns under different neuromodulatory conditions. Here, membrane dynamics are described by coupled differential equations, the behavior modes by attractors (cf. "Computing with Attractors"), and the transitions between modes by bifurcations. The rest state is represented by a time-independent steady state, and repetitive firing is represented by a limit cycle. ("Silicon Neurons" shows how such differential equations can be directly mapped into an electronic circuit built using analog VLSI, to allow real-time exploration of the behavior of quite realistic neural models.)

Roughly a dozen different types of ion channels contribute to the membrane conductance of a typical neuron. ACTIVITY-DEPENDENT REGULATION OF NEURONAL CONDUCTANCES takes as its starting point the fact that the electrical characteristics of a neuron depend on the number of channels of each type active within the membrane and on how these channels are distributed over the surface of the cell. A complex array of biochemical processes controls the number and distribution of ion channels by constructing and transporting channels, modulating their properties, and inserting them into and removing them from the neuron's membrane. The point to note here is that channels are small groupings of large molecules, and they are assembled on the basis of genetic instructions in the cell nucleus. Thus, changing which genes are active (i.e., regulating gene expression) can change the set of channels in a cell, and thus the characteristics of the cell. In fact, electrical activity in the cell can affect a range of processes, from activity-induced gene expression to activity-dependent modulation of assembled ion channels. Channel synthesis, insertion, and modulation are much slower than the usual voltage- and ligand-dependent processes that open and close channels. Thus, consideration of activity-dependent regulation of conductances introduces a dynamics acting on a new, slower time scale into neuronal modeling, a feedback mechanism linking a neuron's electrical characteristics to its activity. A similar theme is developed in BIOPHYSICAL MOSAIC OF THE NEURON, which is structured around the metaphor of the mosaic neuron. A mosaic is a collection of discrete parts, each with unique properties, that are fitted together in such a way that an image emerges from the whole in a nonobvious way. Similarly, the neuronal membrane is packed with a diversity of receptors and ion channels and other proteins with a recognizable distribution. In addition, the cytoplasm is not just water with ions, but a mosaic of interacting molecular systems that can directly affect the functional properties of membrane proteins. The argument is that, just as a

mosaic painting provokes perception of a complete image out of a maze of individually diversified tiles, so a given neuron performs a well-defined computational role that depends not only on the network of cells in which it is embedded, but also to a large extent on the dynamic distribution of macromolecules throughout the cell.

DENDRITIC PROCESSING focuses on dendrites as electrical input-output devices that operate on a time scale range of several to a few hundred milliseconds. (See "Dendritic Learning" for modeling of the plasticity of dendritic function and the assertion that the concept of "overall connection strength between two neurons" is ill-defined, since it is the distribution of synapses in relation to dendritic geometry that proves crucial.) The input to a dendrite consists of temporal patterns of synaptic inputs spatially distributed over the dendritic surface, whereas the output is (except, for example, in the case of dendrodendritic interactions) an ionic current delivered to the soma for transformation there, via a threshold mechanism, to a train of action potentials at the axon. The article discusses how the morphology, electrical properties, and synaptic inputs of dendrites interact to perform their input-output operation. It uses cable theory and compartmental modeling to model the spread of electric current in dendritic trees. The variety of excitable (voltage-gated) channels that are found in many types of dendrites enrich the computational capabilities of neurons, with interaction proceeding in both directions, away from and toward the soma. Computer modeling methods for neurons offer numerical methods for solving the equations describing branched cables. DENDRITIC SPINES are short appendages found on the dendrites of many different cell types. They are composed of a bulbous "head" connected to the dendrite by a thin "stem." An excitatory synapse is usually found on the spine head, and some spines also have a second, usually inhibitory, synapse located on or near the spine stem. Models in which the spine is represented as a passive electrical circuit show that the large resistance of a thin spine stem can attenuate a synaptic input delivered to the spine head. Other models address calcium diffusion and plasticity in spines. Current research focuses on the hypothesis that the spine stem provides a diffusional resistance that allows calcium to become concentrated in the spine head and calcium-dependent reactions to be localized to the synapse. This could be very important for plasticity changes, such as those that occur with long-term potentiation.

Neural Plasticity

AXONAL PATH FINDING
CEREBELLUM AND CONDITIONING
CEREBELLUM AND MOTOR CONTROL
CEREBELLUM: NEURAL PLASTICITY
CONDITIONING
DENDRITIC LEARNING
DEVELOPMENT OF RETINOTECTAL MAPS
DYNAMIC LINK ARCHITECTURE
HABITUATION
HEBBIAN LEARNING AND NEURONAL REGULATION
HEBBIAN SYNAPTIC PLASTICITY
INFORMATION THEORY AND VISUAL PLASTICITY
INVERTEBRATE MODELS OF LEARNING: *APLYSIA* AND
   HERMISSENDA
NMDA RECEPTORS: SYNAPTIC, CELLULAR, AND NETWORK
   MODELS
OCULAR DOMINANCE AND ORIENTATION COLUMNS
POST-HEBBIAN LEARNING ALGORITHMS
SHORT-TERM MEMORY
SOMATOTOPY: PLASTICITY OF SENSORY MAPS
TEMPORAL DYNAMICS OF BIOLOGICAL SYNAPSES

Most studies of learning in ANNs involve a variety of learning rules, inspired in great part by the psychological hypotheses of

Hebb and Rosenblatt (cf. Section I.3) about ways in which synaptic connections may change their strength as a result of experience. In recent years, much progress has been made in tracing the processes that underlie the plasticity of synapses of biological neurons. The present road map samples this research together with related modeling. Although the emphasis will be on synaptic plasticity, several articles stress the role of axonal growth in forming new connections, and the road map closes with an article suggesting that changes in location of synapses may be just as important as changes in synaptic strength.

Hebb's idea was that a synapse (what we would now call a Hebbian synapse) strengthens when the presynaptic and postsynaptic elements tend to be coactive. The plausibility of this hypothesis has been enhanced by the neurophysiological discovery of a synaptic phenomenon in the hippocampus known as long-term potentiation (LTP), which is induced by a Hebbian mechanism. Hebb's postulate has received various modifications to address, e.g., the saturation problem.

HEBBIAN SYNAPTIC PLASTICITY shows that a variety of experimental networks ranging from the abdominal ganglion in the invertebrate *Aplysia* to visual cortex and the CA1 region of hippocampus offer converging validation of Hebb's postulate on strengthening synapses by (more or less) coincident presynaptic and postsynaptic activity. In these networks, similar algorithms of potentiation can be implemented using different cascades of second messengers triggered by activation of synaptic and/or voltage-dependent conductances. Most cellular data supporting Hebb's predictions have been derived from electrophysiological measurements of composite postsynaptic potentials or synaptic currents, or of short-latency peaks in cross-correlograms, which cannot always be interpreted simply at the synaptic level. The basic conclusion of these experiments is that covariance between pre- and postsynaptic activity upregulates and downregulates the "effective" connectivity between pairs of functionally coupled cells. The article thus suggests that what changes according to a correlational rule is not so much the efficacy of transmission at a given synapse, but rather a more general coupling term mixing the influence of polysynaptic excitatory and inhibitory circuits linking the two cells, modulated by the diffuse network background activation. Replacing this composite interaction by a single coupling term defines an ideal Hebbian synapse.

The crucial role played in the CA1 form of LTP by channels called NMDA receptors in the synapses is further explained in NMDA RECEPTORS: SYNAPTIC, CELLULAR, AND NETWORK MODELS. NMDA receptors are subtypes of receptors for the excitatory neurotransmitter glutamate and are involved in diverse physiological as well as pathological processes. They mediate a relatively "slow" excitatory postsynaptic potential, and act as coincidence detectors of presynaptic and postsynaptic activity. The interactions between the slow NMDA-mediated and fast AMPA-mediated currents provide the basis for a range of dynamic properties that contribute to diverse neuronal processes. NMDA receptors have attracted much interest in neuroscience because of their role in learning and memory. Their ability to act as coincidence detectors make them an ideal molecular device for producing Hebbian synapses. The article reviews data related to the biological characteristics of NMDA receptors and models that have been used to describe their function in isolated membrane patches, in neurons, and in complex circuits.

A classic problem with Hebb's original rule is that it only strengthens synapses. But this means that all synapses would eventually saturate, depriving the cell of its pattern separation ability. A number of biologically inspired responses to this problem are described in the next two articles. HEBBIAN LEARNING AND NEURONAL REGULATION stresses that, for both computational and biological reasons, Hebbian plasticity will involve many synapses of the same neuron. Biologically, synaptic interactions are inevitable as synapses compete for the finite resources of a single neuron. Computationally, neuron-specific modifications of synaptic efficacies are required in order to obtain efficient learning, or to faithfully model biological systems. Hence neuronal regulation, a process modulating all synapses of a postsynaptic neuron, is a general phenomenon that complements Hebbian learning. The article shows that neuronal regulation may answer important questions, such as: What bounds the positive feedback loop of Hebbian learning and guarantees some normalization of the synaptic efficacies of a neuron? How can a neuron acquire specificity to particular inputs without being prewired? How can memories be maintained throughout life while synapses suffer degradation due to metabolic turnover? In unsupervised learning, neuronal regulation allows for competition between the various synapses on a neuron and leads to normalization of their synaptic efficacies. In supervised learning, neuronal regulation improves the capacity of associative memory models and can be used to guarantee the maintenance of biological memory systems. Our basic tour of Hebbian learning concludes with POST-HEBBIAN LEARNING ALGORITHMS. This article starts by observing that Hebb's original postulate was a verbally described phenomenological rule, without specification of detailed mechanisms. Subsequent work has shown the computational usefulness of many variations of the original learning rule. This article presents background material on conditioning, neural development, and physiologically realistic cellular-level learning phenomena as a prelude to a review of several families of rules providing computational implementations of Hebbian-inspired rules.

CEREBELLUM AND MOTOR CONTROL reviews a number of models for cerebellar mechanisms underlying the learning of motor skills. Cerebellum can be decomposed into cerebellar nuclei and a cerebellar cortex. The only output cells of the cerebellar cortex are the Purkinje cells, and their only effect is to provide varying levels of inhibition on the cerebellar nuclei. Each Purkinje cell receives two types of input: a single climbing fiber, and many tens of thousands of parallel fibers. The most influential model of cerebellar cortex has been the Marr-Albus model of the formation of associative memories between particular patterns on parallel fiber inputs and Purkinje cell outputs, with the climbing fiber acting as "training signal." Later models place more emphasis on the relation between the cortex and nuclei, and on the way in which the subregions of this coupled cerebellar system can adapt and coordinate the activity of specific motor pattern generators. The plasticity of the cerebellum is approached from a different direction in CEREBELLUM AND CONDITIONING. Many experiments indicate that the cerebellum is involved in learning and performance of classically conditioned reflexes; the present article reviews a number of models of the role of cerebellum in rabbit eyelid conditioning. (A more general perspective on conditioning is given in CONDITIONING and described more fully in the road map **Psychology**, which describes several formal theories and neural network models for classical and operant conditioning.) Inspired by the Marr-Albus hypothesis, neurophysiological research eventually showed that coincidence of climbing fiber and parallel fiber activity on a Purkinje cell led to long-term depression (LTD) of the synapse from parallel fiber to Purkinje cell. CEREBELLUM: NEURAL PLASTICITY offers readers an exhaustive overview of the data on the neurochemical mechanisms underlying this form of plasticity. The authors conclude that the timing conditions for LTD induction may account for the temporal specificity of cerebellar motor learning, and suggest that an important future development in the field will be to study developmental aspects of LTD in relation to acquisition of motor skills. However, the article cites only one model of LTD. It is clear that there are immense challenges to neural modelers in exploring the implications of the plethora of neurochemical interactions swirling about this single class of synaptic plasticity and, by implication, the variety of different mechanisms expressed elsewhere in the nervous system.

There is now strong evidence for a process of short-term memory (STM) involved in performing tasks requiring temporary storage and manipulation of information to guide appropriate actions. SHORT-TERM MEMORY addresses three issues: What are the different types of STM traces? How do intrinsic and synaptic mechanisms contribute to the formation of STM traces? How do STM traces translate into long-term memory representation of temporal sequences? The stress is on the computational mechanisms underlying these processes, with the suggestion that these mechanisms may well underlie a wide variety of seemingly different biological processes. The article examines both the short-term preservation of patterns of neural firing in a circuit and ways in which short-term maintained activity may be transferred into long-term memory traces.

There is no hard and fast line between the cellular mechanisms underlying the development of the nervous system and those involved in learning. Nonetheless, the former emphasizes the questions of how one part of the brain comes to be connected to another and how overall patterns of connectivity are formed, while the latter tends to regard the connections as in place, and asks how their strengths can be modified to improve the network's performance. Studies of regeneration—the reforming of connections after damage to neurons or cell tracts—are thus associated more with developmental mechanisms than with learning per se. Another significant area of research that complements development is that of aging, but there is still too little work relating aging to neural modeling.

Study of the regeneration of retinotopic eye-brain maps in frogs (i.e., neighboring points in the frog retina map, in a one-to-many fashion, to neighboring points in the optic tectum) has been one of the most fruitful areas for theory-experiment interaction in neuroscience. Following optic nerve section, optic nerve fibers tended to regenerate connections with those target neurons to which they were connected before surgery, even after eye rotation. This suggests that each cell in both retina and tectum has a unique chemical marker signaling 2D location, and that retinal axons seek out tectal cells with the same positional information. However, in experiments in which lesions were made in goldfish retina or tectum, it was found that topographic maps regenerated in conformance with whatever new boundary conditions were created by the lesions; e.g., the remaining half of a retina would eventually connect in a retinotopic way to the whole of the tectum, rather than just to the half to which it was originally connected. Although there is wide variation between species in the degree of order existing in the optic nerve, it is almost always the case that the final map in the tectum is ordered to a greater extent than is the optic nerve. Theory and experiment paint a subtle view in which genetics sets a framework for development, but the final pattern of connections depends both on boundary conditions and on patterns of cellular activity. This view is now paradigmatic for our understanding of how patterns of neural connectivity are determined. The development of such maps appears to proceed in two stages: the first involves axon guidance independent of neural activity; the second involves the refinement of initially crude patterns of connections by processes dependent on neural activity. AXONAL PATH FINDING focuses on the former events, while DEVELOPMENT OF RETINOTECTAL MAPS discusses the latter. Understanding the molecular basis of retinotectal map formation has been transformed since the appearance of the first edition of the *Handbook* by discoveries centering on ephrins and the corresponding Eph receptors. The Eph/ephrins come in two families, Λ and B, with the Λ family important for mapping along the rostral-caudal axis of the tectum, while the B family may be important for mapping along the dorsal-ventral axis. Most models of development of retinotectal maps take synaptic strengths as their primary variable between arrays of retinal and tectal locations, with initial synaptic strengths then updated according to rules that depend in various ways on correlated activity, competition for tectal space, molecular gradients, and fiber-fiber interactions. However, actual movement or branching of axons to find their correct targets is rarely considered. Thus, future computational models of retinotectal map formation should take into account data on Eph receptors and ephrin ligands, data on the guidance of retinal axons that enter the tectum by ectopic routes, and the results of retinal and tectal ablation and transplantation experiments. Up to now, the great majority of theoretical work in the neural network tradition has focused on changes in synaptic strengths within a fixed connectional architecture, but how axons chart their initial path toward the correct target structure has generally not been addressed. AXONAL PATH FINDING reviews recent experimental work addressing how retinal ganglion cell axons find the optic disk, how they then exit the retina, why they grow toward the optic chiasm, why some then cross at the midline while others do not, and so on—a body of knowledge that now has the potential to be framed and interpreted in terms of theoretical models. Whereas work in neural networks has usually focused on processes such as synaptic plasticity that are dependent on neural activity, models for axon guidance must generally be phrased in terms of activity-independent mechanisms, particularly guidance by molecular gradients. Many fundamental questions remain unresolved, for which theoretical models have the potential to make an important contribution. What is the minimum gradient steepness detectable by a growth cone, and how does this vary with the properties of the receptor-ligand interaction and the internal state of the growth cone? How is a graded difference in receptor binding internally converted into a signal for directed movement? And, how do axons integrate multiple cues?

OCULAR DOMINANCE AND ORIENTATION COLUMNS studies two issues that go beyond basic map formation to provide further insight into activity-dependent development. When cells in layer IVc of visual cortex are tested to see which eye drives them more strongly, it is found that ocular dominance takes the form of a zebra-stripe-like pattern of alternating dominance. Model and experiment support the view that the stripes are not genetically specified but instead form through network self-organization. Another classic example is the formation of orientation specificity. A number of models are reviewed in light of current data, both theoretical analysis based on the idea that leading eigenvectors dominate (cf. "Pattern Formation, Biological" and "Pattern Formation, Neural") and computer simulations.

TEMPORAL DYNAMICS OF BIOLOGICAL SYNAPSES complements the many studies of synaptic plasticity in the *Handbook* that focus on long-term changes in synaptic strength by showing the importance of fast synaptic changes over time scales of milliseconds to seconds. Short-term plasticity includes both synaptic depression and a number of components of short-term enhancement (facilitation, augmentation, and posttetanic potentiation) acting over increasingly longer periods of time. In addition to having complex short-term dynamics, synapses are stochastic (see "Synaptic Transmission"), and it is argued that constructive roles for unreliable transmission become apparent when short-term plasticity is considered in connection with stochastic transmission, with synapses acting as stochastic temporal filters of their presynaptic spike trains. DYNAMIC LINK ARCHITECTURE develops the theme of fast synaptic changes at the level of network function, viewing the brain's data structure as a graph composed of nodes connected by links whose strength can change on two time scales, represented by two variables called temporary weight and permanent weight. The permanent weight corresponds to the usual synaptic weight, can change on the slow time scale of learning, and represents permanent memory. The temporary weight can change on the same time scale as the node activity, providing the dynamic links that, according to this model, constitute the glue by which higher data structures are built up from more elementary ones.

INFORMATION THEORY AND VISUAL PLASTICITY demonstrates some features of information theory that are relevant to the relaying of information in cortex and presents cases in which information theory led people to seek methods for Gaussianizing the input distribution and, in other cases, to seek learning goals for non-Gaussian distributions. The MDL principle (see "Minimum Description Length Analysis") was presented as a learning goal which takes into account the complexity of the decoding network. In particular, the article connects entropy-based methods, projection pursuit, and extraction of simple cells in visual cortex.

As can be seen from the above, neural network models of development and regeneration have been dominated by studies of the visual system. The next article, however, takes us to the somatosensory system. Research in the past decade has demonstrated plastic changes at all levels of the adult somatosensory system in a wide range of mammalian species. Changes in the relative levels of sensory stimulation as a result of experience or injury produce modifications in sensory maps. SOMATOTOPY: PLASTICITY OF SENSORY MAPS discusses which features of somatotopic maps change and under what conditions, the mechanisms that may account for these changes, and the functional consequences of sensory map changes.

Just as the giant squid axon provided invaluable insights into the active properties of neural membrane summarized in the Hodgkin-Huxley equation, so have invertebrates provided many insights into other basic mechanisms (see "Neuromodulation in Invertebrate Nervous Systems" and "Crustacean Stomatogastric System" for two examples). INVERTEBRATE MODELS OF LEARNING: *APLYSIA* AND *HERMISSENDA* does the same for basic learning mechanisms. A ganglion (localized neural network) of these invertebrates can control a variety of different behaviors, yet a given behavior such as a withdrawal response may be mediated by 100 neurons or less. Moreover, many neurons are relatively large and can be uniquely identified, functional properties of an individual cell can be related to a specific behavior, and changes in cellular properties during learning can be related to specific changes in behavior. Biophysical and molecular events underlying the changes in cellular properties can then be determined and mathematically modeled. The present article illustrates this with studies of two gastropod mollusks: associative and nonassociative modifications of defensive siphon and tail withdrawal reflexes in *Aplysia* and associative learning in *Hermissenda*.

HABITUATION describes one of the simplest forms of learning, the progressive decrement in a behavioral response with repeated presentations of the eliciting stimulus, and reveals the complexity in this apparent simplicity. This article reviews the fundamental characteristics of habituation and describes experimental preparations in which the neural basis of habituation has been examined as well as attempts to model habituation. Experimental studies have identified at least two important neural mechanisms of habituation, homosynaptic depression within the reflex circuit and extrinsic descending modulatory input. A number of systems are put forward as good candidates for future modeling. Habituation of defensive reflexes was among the first types of learning explained successfully at the cellular level. Habituation in the crayfish tail-flip reflex, due to both afferent depression as well as descending inhibition, offers the opportunity to analyze the interaction and cooperativity of mechanisms intrinsic and extrinsic to the reflex circuit. The nematode *C. elegans* offers the possibility of a genetic analysis of habituation.

As shown in "Dendritic Processing," dendrites are highly complex structures, both anatomically and physiologically, and are the principal substrates for information processing within the neuron. DENDRITIC LEARNING assesses the consequences of axodendritic

structural plasticity for learning and memory, countering the view that neural plasticity is limited to the strengthening and weakening of existing synaptic connections. In particular, the article supports the view that long-term storage may involve the correlation-based sorting of synaptic contacts onto the many separate dendrites of a target neuron. In the models offered in this article, the output of the cell represents the sum of a moderately large set of separately thresholded dendritic subunits, so that a single neuron as modeled here is equivalent to a conventional ANN built from two layers of point neurons. As a result, the concept of "overall connection strength between two neurons" is no longer well defined, for it is the distribution of synapses in relation to dendritic geometry that proves crucial.

Neural Coding

In the McCulloch-Pitts neuron, the output is binary, generated on a discrete-time scale; at the other extreme, the Hodgkin-Huxley equations can create a dazzling array of patterns of axonal activity in which the shape as well as the timing of each spike is continuously variable. In between, we have models such as the leaky integrator model, in which only the rate of firing of a cell is significant, while in the spiking neuron model the timing but not the shape of spikes is continuously variable. This raises the question of how sensory inputs and motor outputs, let alone "thoughts" and other less mental intervening variables, are coded in neural activity. In answering this question, we must not only seek to understand the significance of the firing pattern of an individual neuron but also probe how variables may be encoded in patterns of firing distributed across a whole population of neurons.

Retinotopic feature maps are the norm near the visual periphery and up into the early stages of the visual cortex. Here, the firing of a cell peaks for stimuli that fall on a specific patch of the retina and also for a specific feature. Perhaps the most famous example of this is provided by the simple cells discovered in visual cortex by Hubel and Wiesel, which are edge-sensitive cells tuned both for the retinal position and orientation of the edge. In such studies, the cell is characterized by its firing rate during presentation of the stimulus. Similar results are seen for other feature types (see "Feature Analysis") and other sensory systems. The issue of how other information may be coded by activity in the nervous systems of animals is addressed in a number of articles. LOCALIZED VERSUS DISTRIBUTED REPRESENTATIONS asks whether the final neural encoding of visual recognition of one's grandmother, say, involves neurons that respond selectively to "grandmother"—so-called "grandmother cells"—or whether the sight of grandmother is never made explicit at the single neuron level, with the representation instead distributed across a large number of neurons, none of which responds selectively to "grandmother" alone. Few neuroscientists argue that individual neurons might explicitly represent particular objects, but many connectionists have used localist representations to model phenomena that include word and letter perception, although they generally insist that the units in their models are not real neurons. The article examines neurophysiological evidence that both distributed and local coding are used in high-order visual areas and then goes "against the stream" by forwarding computational reasons for preferring representations that are more localist in some parts of the brain, before examining how work on temporal coding schemes has changed the nature of the local versus distributed debate. SPARSE CODING IN THE PRIMATE CORTEX marshals theoretical reasons and experimental evidence suggesting that the brain adopts a compromise between distributed and local representations that is often referred to as *sparse coding*. This thesis is illustrated with data on object recognition and face recognition in inferotemporal cortex (the "what" pathway) in monkey.

Perhaps the best-known example of motor coding is that described in MOTOR CORTEX: CODING AND DECODING OF DIRECTIONAL OPERATIONS for the relation between the direction of reaching and changes in neuronal activity that have been established for several brain areas, including the motor cortex. The cells involved each have a broad tuning function the peak of which is considered to be the "preferred" direction of the cell. A movement in a particular direction will engage a whole population of cells. It is found that, during discrete movements in 2D and 3D space, the weighted vector sum of these neuronal preferences is a "population vector" which points in (close to) the direction of the movement. Such examples underlie the more general analysis given in POPULATION CODES. Population codes are computationally appealing both because the overlap among the neurons' tuning curves allows precise encoding of values that fall between the peaks of two adjacent tuning curves and because many cortical functions, such as sensorimotor transformations, can be easily modeled with population codes. The article focuses on decoding, or reading out, population codes. Neuronal responses are noisy, leading to the need for good estimators for the encoded variables. The article reviews the various estimators that have been proposed, and considers their neuronal implementations. Moreover, there are cases where it is reasonable to assume that population activity codes for more than just a single value, and could even code for a whole probability distribution. The goal of decoding is then to recover an estimate of this probability distribution.

INTEGRATE-AND-FIRE NEURONS AND NETWORKS shows how these models offer potential principles of coding and dynamics. At the single neuron level, it is shown that coherent input is more efficient than incoherent spikes in driving a postsynaptic neuron. Questions discussed for homogeneous populations include conditions under which it is possible, in the absence of an external stimulus, to stabilize a population of spiking neurons at a reasonable level of spontaneous activity, and the relation of frequency of collective oscillations to neuronal parameters, and how rapidly population activity responds to changes in the input. An extension to mixed excitatory/inhibitory populations as found in the cortex is also discussed. SYNCHRONIZATION, BINDING AND EXPECTANCY argues that the "binding" of cells that correspond to features of a given visual object may exploit another dimension of cellular firing, namely, the phase at which a cell fires within some overall rhythm of firing. The article presents data consistent with the proposal that the synchronization of responses on a time scale of milliseconds provides an efficient mechanism for response selection and binding of population responses. Synchronization also increases the saliency of responses because it allows for effective spatial summation in the population of neurons receiving convergent input from synchronized input cells. SYNFIRE CHAINS were introduced to account for the appearance of precise firing sequences with long interspike delays, dealing with the ways in which such chains might be generated, activity propagation along the chain, how synfire chains can be used to compute, and how they might be detected in electrophysiological recordings. A synfire chain is composed of many pools (or layers) of neurons connected in a feedforward fashion. In a random network with moderate connectivity, many synfire chains can be found by chance, but such ran-

dom synfire chains may not function reproducibly unless the synaptic connections are strengthened by some appropriate learning rule. A given neuron can participate in more than one synfire chain. The extent to which such repeated membership can take place without compromising reproducibility is known as the *memory capacity* of synfire chains. Synfire chains may be considered a special case of the "cell assembly" suggested by Hebb. However, in Hebb's concepts the cell assembly was a network with multiple feedback connections, whereas the synfire chain is a feedforward net. This allows for much faster computations by synfire chains. While noting that there have also been criticisms of the theory, the article argues that classical anatomy and physiology of the cortex sustain the idea that activity may be organized in synfire chains and that one can create compositional systems from synfire chains.

RATE CODING AND SIGNAL PROCESSING investigates ways in which the sequence of spike occurrence times may encode the information that a neuron communicates to its targets. Spike trains are often quite variable under seemingly identical stimulation conditions. Does this variability carry information about the stimulus? The term *rate coding* is applied in situations where the precise timing of spikes is thought not to play a significant role in carrying sensory information. The article analyzes the sensory information conveyed by two types of rate codes, mean firing rate codes and instantaneous firing rate codes, by adapting classical methods of statistical signal processing to the analysis of neuronal spike trains. While focusing on various examples of rate coding, such as that of neurons of weakly electric fish sensitive to electrical field amplitude, the article also notes cases in which spike timing plays a crucial role.

Recent years have seen an increasing number of quantitative studies of neuronal coding based on Shannon's information theory, in which the "information" or "entropy" of a message is a purely statistical measure based on the probability of the message within an ensemble: the less likely the message is to occur, the greater its information content. SENSORY CODING AND INFORMATION TRANSMISSION reviews two recent approaches to measuring transmitted information. The first is based on direct estimation of the spike train entropies in terms of which transmitted information is defined; the second is based on an expansion to second order in the length of the spike trains. The meaning of any signal that we receive from our environment is modulated by the context within which it appears. ADAPTIVE SPIKE CODING explores the analysis of "context" as the statistical ensemble in which the signal is embedded. Interpreting a message requires both registering the signal itself and knowing something about this statistical ensemble. The relevant temporal or spatial ensemble depends on the task. Information theoretically, representations that appropriately take into account the statistical properties of the incoming signal are more efficient (see OPTIMAL SENSORY ENCODING and "Information Theory and Visual Plasticity"). The article focuses on neural adaptation, reversible change in the response properties of neurons on short time scales. Since the first observations of adaptation in spiking neurons, it had been suggested that adaptation serves a useful function for information processing, preventing a neuron from continuing to transmit redundant information, viewing both the filtering and the threshold function of a neuron as adaptive functions of the input that may implement the goal of increasing information transmission. Issues include adaptation to the stimulus distribution, with the information about the ensemble read off from the statistics of spike time differences; the separation of different time scales in adaptation; and adaptation of receptive fields. The article also explores the role of calcium and of channel dynamics in providing adaptation mechanisms.

OPTIMAL SENSORY ENCODING focuses on the visual system, seeking to understand what type of data encoding for signals passing from retina to cerebral cortex could reduce the data rate without significant information loss, exploiting the fact that nearby image pixels tend to convey similar signals and thus carry redundant information. One strategy is to transform the original redundant signal (e.g., in photoreceptors) to nonredundant signals in the retinal ganglion cells or cortical neurons, as in the Infomax proposal. The article presents different coding schemes with different advantages. The retinal code has the advantage of small and identical receptive field (RF) shapes, involving shorter neural wiring and easier specifications. The cortical multiscale code is preferred when invariance is needed for objects moving in depth. Again, whereas the Infomax principle applies well to explain the RFs of the more numerous class of retinal ganglion cells, the P cells in monkeys or X cells in cats, another class of ganglion cells, M cells in monkeys or Y cells in cats, have RFs that are relatively larger, color unselective, and tuned to higher temporal frequencies. These M cells do not extract the maximum information possible (Infomax) about the input but can serve to extract the information as quickly as possible. It is argued that information theory is more likely to find its application in the early stages of the sensory processing, before information is selected or discriminated for any specific cognitive task, and that optimal sensory coding in later stages of sensory pathways will depend on cognitive tasks that require applications of alternative theories.

Biological Networks

CORTICAL HEBBIAN MODULES
CORTICAL POPULATION DYNAMICS AND PSYCHOPHYSICS
DOPAMINE, ROLES OF
HIPPOCAMPAL RHYTHM GENERATION
INTEGRATE-AND-FIRE NEURONS AND NETWORKS
LAYERED COMPUTATION IN NEURAL NETWORKS
NEUROMODULATION IN INVERTEBRATE NERVOUS SYSTEMS
NEUROMODULATION IN MAMMALIAN NERVOUS SYSTEMS
RECURRENT NETWORKS: NEUROPHYSIOLOGICAL MODELING
SLEEP OSCILLATIONS
TEMPORAL INTEGRATION IN RECURRENT MICROCIRCUITS

We turn now to studies of biological neural networks, a study complemented by articles in the road map **Mammalian Brain Regions** and in other road maps on sensory systems, memory, and motor control.

CORTICAL HEBBIAN MODULES models the activity seen in cortical networks during the delay period following the presentation of the stimulus in a delay match-to-sample or delay eye-movement task. The rates observed are in the range of about 10–20 spikes/s, with the subset of neurons that sustain elevated rates being selective of the sample stimulus and concentrated in localized columns in associative cortex. The article shows how to model these selective activity distributions through the autonomous local dynamics in the column. The model presents neural elements and synaptic structures that can reproduce the observed neuronal spike dynamics; showing how Hebbian synaptic dynamics can give rise, in a process of training, to a synaptic structure in the local module capable of sustaining selective activity during the delay period. The mathematical framework for the analysis is provided by the mean field theory of statistical mechanics.

LAYERED COMPUTTION IN NEURAL NETWORKS abstracts from the biology to present a general framework for modeling computations performed in layered structures (which occur in many parts of the vertebrate and invertebrate brain, including the optic tectum, the avian visual wulst, and the cephalopod optic lobe, as well as the mammalian cerebral cortex). A general formalism is presented for the connectivity between layers and the dynamics of typical units of each layer. Information processing capabilities of neural layers include filter operations; lateral cooperativity and competition that can be used in, e.g., stereo vision and winner-take-all;

topographic mapping that underlies the allocation of cortical neurons to different parts of the visual field (fovea/periphery), or the processing of optic flow patterns; and feature maps and population coding, which may be applied both to sensory systems and to "motor fields" of neurons so that the flow of activity in motor areas can predict initiated movements. In a related vein, CORTICAL POPULATION DYNAMICS AND PSYCHOPHYSICS describes cortical population dynamics in the form of structurally simple differential equations for the neurons' firing activities, using a model class introduced by Wilson and Cowan. The Wilson-Cowan model is powerful enough to reproduce a variety of cortical phenomena and captures the dynamics of neuronal populations seen in a variety of experiments, yet simple enough to allow for analytical treatment that yields an understanding of the mechanisms leading to the observed behavior. The model is applied here to explain dynamical properties of the primate visual system on different levels, reaching from single neuron properties like selectivity for the orientation of a stimulus up to higher cognitive functions related to the binding and processing of stimulus features in psychophysical discrimination experiments.

HIPPOCAMPAL RHYTHM GENERATION notes that global brain states in both normal and pathological situations may be associated with spontaneous rhythmic activities of large populations of neurons. This article presents data and models on the main such states associated with the hippocampus: the two main normally occurring states—the theta rhythm with the associated gamma oscillation, and the irregular sharp waves (SPW) with the associated high-frequency (ripple) oscillation—and a pathological brain state associated with epileptic seizures. Several different modeling strategies are compared in studying rhythmicity in the hippocampal CA3 region.

SLEEP OSCILLATIONS analyzes cortical and thalamic networks at multiple levels, from molecules to single neurons to large neuronal assemblies, with techniques ranging from intracellular recordings to computer simulations, to illuminate the generation, modulation, and function of brain oscillations. Sleep is characterized by synchronized events in billions of synaptically coupled neurons in thalamocortical systems. The early stage of quiescent sleep is associated with EEG spindle waves, which occur at a frequency of 7 to 14 Hz; as sleep deepens, waves with slower frequencies appear on the EEG. The other sleep state, associated with rapid eye movements (REM sleep) and dreaming, is characterized by abolition of low-frequency oscillations and an increase in cellular excitability, very much like wakefulness, although motor output is markedly inhibited. Activation of a series of neuromodulatory transmitter systems during arousal blocks low-frequency oscillations, induces fast rhythms, and allows the brain to recover full responsiveness.

It is a truism that similarity of input-output behavior is no guarantee of similarity of internal function in two neural networks. In particular, a recurrent neural network trained by backpropagation to mimic some biological function may have little internal resemblance to the neural networks responsible for that function in the living brain. Nonetheless, RECURRENT NETWORKS: NEUROPHYSIOLOGICAL MODELING demonstrates that dynamic recurrent network models (see "Recurrent Networks: Learning Algorithms" for the formal background) can provide useful tools to help systems neurophysiologists understand the neural mechanisms mediating behavior. Biological experiments typically involve bits of the system; neural network models provide a method of generating working models of the complete system. Confidence in such models is increased if they not only simulate dynamic sensorimotor behavior but also incorporate anatomically appropriate connectivity. The utility of such models is illustrated in the analysis of four types of biological function: oscillating networks, primate target tracking, short-term memory tasks, and the construction of neural integrators.

As is evident in the road map **Biological Neurons and Synapses**, not all neurons are alike: they show a rich variety of conductances that endow them with different functional properties. These properties and hence the collective activity of interacting groups of neurons are not fixed, but are instead subject to modulation. The term *neuromodulation* usually refers to the effect of neurochemicals such as acetylcholine, dopamine, norepinephrine, and serotonin, and other substances, including neuropeptides. By contrast with the rapid transmission of information through the nervous system by excitatory and inhibitory synaptic potentials, neuromodulators primarily activate receptor proteins, which do not contain an ion channel (metabotropic receptors). These receptors in turn activate enzymes, which change the internal concentration of substances called second messengers. Second messengers cause slower and longer-lasting changes in the physiological properties of neurons, resulting in changes in the processing characteristics of the neural circuit. NEUROMODULATION IN INVERTEBRATE NERVOUS SYSTEMS stresses that the sensory information an animal needs depends on a number of factors, including its activity patterns and motivational state. The modulation of the sensitivities of many sensory receptors is shown for a stretch receptor in crustaceans. Modulators can activate, terminate, or modify rhythmic pattern-generating networks. One example of such "polymorphism" is that neuromodulation can reconfigure the same network to produce either escape swimming or reflexive withdrawal in the nudibranch mollusk *Tritonia*. Mechanisms and sites of neuromodulation include alteration of intrinsic properties of neurons, alteration of synaptic efficacy by neuromodulators, and modulation of neuromuscular junctions and muscles. All this makes clear the subtlety of neuronal function that must be addressed by computational neuroscience and that may inspire the design of a new generation of artificial neurons. Turning to the mammalian brain, we find that the anatomical distribution of fibers releasing neuromodulatory substances in the brain is usually very diffuse, with the activity of a small number of neuromodulatory neurons influencing the functional properties of broad regions of the brain. NEUROMODULATION IN MAMMALIAN NERVOUS SYSTEMS starts by summarizing physiological effects of neuromodulation, including effects on resting membrane potential of pyramidal cells and interneurons, spike frequency adaptation, synaptic transmission, and long-term potentiation. It is stressed that the effect of a neurochemical is receptor dependent: a single neuromodulator such as serotonin can have dramatically different effects on different neurons, depending on the type of receptor it activates. Indeed, a chemical may function as a neurotransmitter for one receptor and as a neuromodulator for another. The second half of the article reviews neural network models that help us understand how neuromodulatory effects that appear small at the single neuron level may have a significant effect on dynamical properties when distributed throughout a network. The article reviews several different models of the function of modulatory influences in neural circuits, including noradrenergic modulation of attentional processes (strangely, noradrenergic neurons are those sensitive to norepinephrine), dopaminergic modulation (by dopamine) of working memory, cholinergic modulation (by acetylcholine) of input versus internal processing, and modulation of oscillatory dynamics in cortex and thalamus. DOPAMINE, ROLES OF then focuses specifically on roles of dopamine in both neuromodulation and in synaptic plasticity. Dopamine is a neuromodulator that originates from small groups of neurons in the ventral tegmental area, the substantia nigra, and in the diencephalon. Dopaminergic projections are in general very diffuse and reach large portions of the brain. The time scales of dopamine actions are diverse, from a few hundred milliseconds to several hours. The article focuses on the mesencephalic dopamine centers because they are the most studied, and because they are thought to be involved in diseases such as Tourette's syndrome, schizophrenia, Parkinson's disease, Huntington's disease, drug addiction, and depression. These centers are also involved in such normal brain functions as working memory, reinforcement learning, and attention. The article discusses the biophysical effects of dopamine, how dopamine levels influence working memory, the ways in which dopamine responses resemble the reward prediction signal of the temporal difference model of reinforcement learning, and the role of dopamine in allocation of attention.

INTEGRATE-AND-FIRE NEURONS AND NETWORKS presents relatively simple models that take account of the fact that most biological neurons communicate by action potentials, or spikes (see also "Spiking Neurons, Computation with"). In contrast to the standard neuron model used in ANNs, integrate-and-fire neurons do not rely on a temporal average over the pulses. Instead, the pulsed nature of the neuronal signal is taken into account and considered as potentially relevant for coding and information processing. However, integrate-and-fire models do not explicitly describe the form of an action potential. Integrate-and-fire and similar spiking neuron models are phenomenological descriptions on an intermediate level of detail. Compared to other single-cell models, they allow coding principles to be discussed in a transparent manner. Moreover, the dynamics in networks of integrate-and-fire neurons can be analyzed mathematically, and large systems with thousands of neurons can be simulated rather efficiently.

TEMPORAL INTEGRATION IN RECURRENT MICROCIRCUITS hypothesizes that the ability of neural computation in behaving organisms to produce a response at any time that depends appropriately on earlier sensory inputs and internal states rests on a common principle by which neural microcircuits operate in different cortical areas and species. The article argues that, while tapped delay lines, finite state machines, and attractor neural networks are suitable for modeling specific tasks, they appear to be incompatible with results from neuroanatomy (highly recurrent diverse circuitry) and neurophysiology (fast transient dynamics of firing activity with few attractor states). The authors thus view the transient dynamics of neural microcircuits as the main carrier of information about past inputs, from which specific information needed for a variety of different tasks can be read out in parallel and at any time by different readout neurons. This approach leads to computer models of generic recurrent circuits of integrate-and-fire neurons for tasks that require temporal integration of inputs and, it is argued, provides a new conceptual framework for the experimental investigation of neural microcircuits and larger neural systems.

II.6. Dynamics and Learning in Artificial Networks

Dynamic Systems

Much interest in ANNs has been based on the use of trainable feedforward networks as universal approximators for functions f: $X \rightarrow Y$ from the input space X to the output space Y. However, their provenance was more general. The founding paper of Pitts and McCulloch established the result that, by the mid-1950s, could be rephrased as saying that any finite automaton could be simulated by a network of McCulloch-Pitts neurons. A *finite automaton* is a discrete-time dynamic system; that is, on some suitable time scale, it specifies the next state $q(t + 1)$ as a function $\delta(q(t), x(t))$ of the current state and input (for articles related to automata and theory of computation, see the road map **Computability and Complexity**). But a neuron can be modeled as a continuous-time system (as in a leaky integrator neuron with the membrane potential as the state variable). A network of continuous-time neurons can then be considered as a continuous-time system with the rate of change of the state (which could, for example, be a vector whose elements are the membrane potentials of the individual neurons) defined as a function $\dot{q}(t) = f(q(t), x(t))$ of the current state and input. When the input is held constant, the network (whether discrete- or continuous-time) may be analyzed by dynamical systems theory. COMPUTING WITH ATTRACTORS shows some of the benefits of such an approach. In particular, a net with internal loops may go to equilibrium (providing a state from which the answer to some problem may be read out), enter a limit cycle (undergoing repetitive oscillations which are useful in control of movement, and in other situations in which a "clock cycle" is of value), or exhibit chaotic behavior (acting in an apparently random way, even though it is deterministic). In particular, the article builds on the notion of a Hopfield network. Hopfield contributed much to the resurgence of interest in neural networks in the 1980s by associating an "energy function" with a network, showing that if only one neuron changed state at a time, a symmetrically connected net would settle to a local minimum of the energy, and that many optimization problems could be mapped to energy functions for symmetric neural nets. ENERGY FUNCTIONALS FOR NEURAL NETWORKS uses the notion of Lyapunov function from the dynamical study of ordinary differential equations to show how the definition of energy function and the conditions for convergence to a local minimum can be broadened considerably. (Of course, a network undergoing limit cycles or chaos will not have an energy function that is minimized in this sense.) OPTIMIZATION, NEURAL shows that this property can be exploited to solve combinatorial optimization problems that require a more or less exhaustive search to achieve exact solutions, with a computational effort growing exponentially or worse with system size. The article shows that ANN methods can provide heuristic methods that yield reasonably good approximate solutions. Recurrent network methods based on deterministic annealing use an interpolating continuous (analog) space, allowing for shortcuts to good solutions (compare "Simulated Annealing and Boltzmann Machines"). The key to the approach offered here is the technique of mean-field approximation from statistical mechanics. While early neural optimizations were confined to problems encodable with a quadratic energy in terms of a set of binary variables, in the past decade the method has been extended to deal with more general problem types, both in terms of variable types and energy

functions, and has evolved to a general-purpose heuristic for combinatorial optimization.

DYNAMICS AND BIFURCATION IN NEURAL NETS notes that the powerful qualitative and geometric tools of dynamical systems theory are most useful when the behavior of interest is stationary in the sense that the inputs are at most time or space periodic. It then shows how to analyze what kind of behavior we can expect over the long run for a given neural network. In ANNs, the final state may represent the recognition of an input pattern, the segmentation of an image, or any number of machine computations. The stationary states of biological neural networks may correspond to cognitive decisions (e.g., binding via synchronous oscillations) or to pathological behavior such as seizures and hallucinations. Another important issue that is addressed by dynamical systems theory is how the qualitative dynamics depends on parameters. The qualitative change of a dynamical system as a parameter is changed is the subject of bifurcation theory, which studies the appearance and disappearance of branches of solutions to a given set of equations as some parameters vary. This article shows how to use these techniques to understand how the behavior of neural nets depends on both the parameters and the initial states of the network. PHASE-PLANE ANALYSIS OF NEURAL NETS complements the study of bifurcations with a technique for studying the qualitative behavior of small systems of interacting neural networks whose neurons are, essentially, leaky integrator neurons. A complete analysis of such networks is impossible but when there are at most two variables involved, a fairly complete description can be given. The article introduces this qualitative theory of differential equations in the plane, analyzing two-neuron networks that consist of two excitatory cells, two inhibitory cells, or an excitatory and inhibitory cell. While planar systems may seem to be a rather extreme simplification, it is argued that in some local cortical circuits we can view the simple planar system as representing a population of coupled excitatory and inhibitory neurons. Computational methods are a very powerful adjunct to this type of analysis. The article concludes with comments on numerical methods and software.

CANONICAL NEURAL MODELS starts from the observation that various models of the same neural structure could produce different results. It thus shows how to derive results that can be observed in a class or a family of models. To exemplify the utility of considering families of neural models instead of a single model, the article shows how to reduce an entire family of Hodgkin-Huxley-type models to a *canonical model*. A model is canonical for a family if there is a continuous change of variables that transforms any other model from the family into this one. As an example, a canonical phase model is presented for a family of weakly coupled oscillators. The change of variables does not have to invertible, so the canonical model is usually lower-dimensional, simple, and tractable, and yet retains many important features of the family. For example, if the canonical model has multiple attractors, then each member of the family has multiple attractors.

Chaotic phenomena, in which a deterministic law generates complicated, nonperiodic, and unpredictable behavior, exist in many real-world systems and mathematical models. Chaos has many intriguing characteristics, such as sensitive dependence on initial conditions. CHAOS IN BIOLOGICAL SYSTEMS provides a view of the appearance of this phenomenon of "deterministic randomness" in a variety of models of physical and biological systems. Features used in assessing time series for chaotic behavior include the power spectrum, dimension, Lyapunov exponent, and Poincaré map. Examples are given from ion channels through cellular activity to complex networks, and "dynamical disease" is characterized by qualitative changes in dynamics in biological control systems. However, the high dimensions of biological systems and the environmental fluctuations that lead to nonstationarity make convincing demonstration of chaos in vivo (as opposed to computer models) a difficult matter. CHAOS IN NEURAL SYSTEMS looks at chaos in the dynamics of axons, neurons, and networks. An open issue is to understand the significance, if any, of observed fluctuations that appear chaotic. Does a neuron function well despite fluctuations in the timing between spikes, or are the irregularities essential to its task? And if the irregularities are essential to the task, is there any reason to expect that deterministic (chaotic) irregularities would be better than random ones? The vexing question of whether chaos adds functionality to neural networks is still open (see also "Synaptic Noise and Chaos in Vertebrate Neurons"). STOCHASTIC RESONANCE is a nonlinear phenomenon whereby the addition of a random process, or "noise," to a weak incoming signal can enhance the probability that it will be detected by a system. Information about the signal transmitted through the system is also enhanced. The information content or detectability of the signal is degraded for noise intensities that are either smaller or larger than some optimal value. Stochastic resonance has been demonstrated at several levels in biology, from ion channels in cell membranes to animal and human cognition, perception, and, ultimately, behavior.

PATTERN FORMATION, BIOLOGICAL presents a general methodology, based on analysis of the largest eigenvalue, for tracing the asymptotic behavior of a dynamical system, and applies it to the problem of biological pattern formation. Turing originally considered the problem of how animal coat patterns develop. He suggested that chemical markers in the skin comprise a system of diffusion-coupled chemical reactions among substances called morphogens. Turing showed that in a two-component reaction-diffusion system, a state of uniform chemical concentration can undergo a diffusion-driven instability, leading to the formation of a spatially inhomogeneous state. In population biology, patchiness in population densities is the norm rather than the exception. In developmental biology, groups of previously identical cells follow different developmental pathways, depending on their position, to yield the rich spectrum of mammalian coat patterns and the patterns found in fishes, reptiles, mollusks, and butterflies. The article closes with a mechanical model of the process of angiogenesis (genesis of the blood supply) and network formation of endothelial cells in the extracellular matrix, as well as a new approach for predicting brain tumor growth. PATTERN FORMATION, NEURAL shows that the Turing mechanism for spontaneous pattern formation plays an important role in studying two key questions on the large-scale functional and anatomical structure of cortex: How did the structure develop? What forms of spontaneous and stimulus-driven neural dynamics are generated by such a cortical structure? In the neural context, interactions are mediated not by molecular diffusion but by long-range axonal connections. This neural version of the Turing instability has been applied to many problems concerning the dynamics and development of cortex. In the former case, pattern formation occurs in neural activity; in the latter it occurs in synaptic weights. In most cases there exists some underlying symmetry in the model that plays a crucial role in the selection and stability of the resulting patterns.

Complementing this theme of pattern formation, SELF-ORGANIZATION AND THE BRAIN contrasts the algorithmic division of labor between programmer and computer in most current man-made computers with the view of the brain as a dynamical system in which ordered structures arise by processes of self-organization. It argues that, whereas the theory of self-organization has so far focused on the establishment of static structures, the nervous system is concerned with the generation of purposeful, nested processes evolving in time. However, if a self-organizing system is to create the appropriate patterns, quite a few control parameters in a system must all be put in the right ballpark. The article argues that, in view of the variability of the physiological state of the nervous system, evolution must have developed general mechanisms to actively and autonomously regulate its systems such as to produce interesting self-organized processes and states. The process of brain organization is seen as a cascade of steps, each one taking place within the boundary conditions established by the previous one, but the theory of such cascades is still nonexistent, posing massive challenges for future research. COOPERATIVE PHENOMENA offers a related perspective, developing what has been a major theme in physics for the last century: statistical mechanics, which shows how, for example, to average out the individual variations in position and velocity of the myriad molecules in a gas to understand the relationship between pressure, volume, and temperature, or to see how variations in temperature can yield dramatic phase transitions, such as from ice to water or from water to steam. The article places these ideas in a general setting, stressing the notion of an *order parameter* (such as temperature in the previous example) that describes the macroscopic order of the system and whose variation can yield qualitative changes in system behavior. Unlike a control parameter, which is a quantity imposed on the system from the outside, an order parameter is established by the system itself via self-organization. The argument is mainly presented at a general level, but the article concludes by briefly examining cooperative phenomena in neuroscience, including pattern formation (see also PATTERN FORMATION, BIOLOGICAL), EEG, MEG, movement coordination, and hallucinations (see also PATTERN FORMATION, NEURAL).

STATISTICAL MECHANICS OF NEURAL NETWORKS introduces the reader to some of the basic methods of statistical mechanics and shows that they can be applied to systems made up of large numbers of (formal) neurons. Statistical mechanics has studied magnets as lattices with an atomic magnet (modeled as, e.g., a spin that can be up or down) at each lattice point, and this has led to the statistical analysis of neural networks as "spin glasses," where firing and nonfiring correspond to "spin up" and "spin down," respectively. It has also led to the study of "Markov Random Field Models in Image Processing," in which the initial information at each lattice site represents some local features of the raw image, while the final state allows one to read off a processed image.

COLLECTIVE BEHAVIOR OF COUPLED OSCILLATORS explains the use of phase models (here, the phase is the phase of an oscillation, not the type of phase whose transition is studied in statistical mechanics) to help understand how temporal coherence arises over populations of densely interconnected oscillators, even when their frequencies are randomly distributed. The phase oscillator model for neural populations exemplifies the idea that certain aspects of brain functions seem largely independent of the neurophysiological details of the individual neurons while trying to recover phase information, i.e., the kind of information encoded in the form of specific temporal structures of the sequence of neuronal spikings. The article reviews the collective behavior of coupled oscillators using the phase model and assuming all-to-all type interconnections. Despite this simplification, a great variety of collective behaviors is exhibited. Special attention is given to the onset and persistence of collective oscillation in frequency-distributed systems, splitting of the population into a few subgroups (clustering), and the more complex collective behavior called slow switching. Collections of oscillators that send signals to one another can phase lock, with many patterns of phase differences. CHAINS OF OSCILLATORS IN MOTOR AND SENSORY SYSTEMS discusses a set of examples that illustrate how those phases emerge from the oscillator interactions. Much of the work was motivated by spatiotemporal patterns in networks of neurons that govern undulatory locomotion. The original experimental preparation to which this work was applied is the lamprey central pattern generator (CPG) for locomotion, but the mathematics is considerably more general. The article discusses several motor systems, then turns to the procerebral lobe of *Limax*, the common garden slug, to illustrate chains of oscillators in a sensory system. Since the details of the oscillators often are not known and difficult to obtain, the object of the mathematics is to find the consequences of what is known, and to generate sharper questions to motivate further experimentation.

AMPLIFICATION, ATTENUATION, AND INTEGRATION focuses on the computational role of the recurrent connections in networks of leaky integrator neurons. Setting the transfer function $f(u)$ to be simply u in the network equations yields a linear network that can be completely analyzed using the tools of linear systems theory. The article describes the properties of linear networks and gives some examples of their application to neural modeling. In this framework, it is shown how recurrent synaptic connectivity can either attenuate or speed up responses; both effects can occur simultaneously in the same network. Besides amplification and attenuation, a linear network can also carry out temporal integration, in the sense of Newtonian calculus, when the strength of feedback is precisely tuned for an eigenmode, so that its gain and time constant diverge to infinity. Finally, it is noted that the linear computations of amplification, attenuation, and integration can be ascribed to a number of brain areas.

WINNER-TAKE-ALL NETWORKS presents a number of designs for neural networks that solve the following problem: given a number of networks, each of which provides as output some "confidence measure," find in a distributed manner the network whose output is strongest. Two important variants of winner-take-all are k-winner-take-all, where the k largest inputs are identified, and softmax, which consists of assigning each input a weight so that all weights sum to 1 and the largest input receives the biggest weight. The article first describes softmax and shows how winner-take-all can be derived as a limiting case; it then describes how they can both be derived from probabilistic, or energy function, formulations; and it closes with a discussion of VLSI and biological mechanisms. "Modular and Hierarchical Learning Systems" addresses a somewhat related topic: Given a complex problem, find a set of networks, each of which provides an approximate solution in some region of the state space, together with a gating network that can combine these approximations to yield a globally satisfactory solution (i.e., blend the "good" solutions rather than extract the "best" solution).

DYNAMICS OF ASSOCIATION AND RECALL uses dynamical studies to analyze the pattern recall process and its relation with the choice of initial state, the properties of stored patterns, noise level, and network architecture. For large networks and in global recall processes, the strategy is to derive dynamical laws at a *macroscopic* level (i.e., dependent on many neuron states). The challenge is to find the smallest set of macroscopic quantities which will obey closed deterministic equations in the limit of an infinitely large network. The article focuses on simple Hopfield-type models, but closes with a discussion of some variations and generalizations.

SHORT-TERM MEMORY asks: What are the different types of STM traces? How do intrinsic and synaptic mechanisms contribute to the formation of STM traces? How do STM traces translate into long-term memory representation of temporal sequences? The stress is on computational mechanisms underlying these processes with the suggestion that these mechanisms may well underlie a wide variety of seemingly different biological processes. The article examines both the short-term preservation of patterns of neural firing in a circuit and ways in which short-term maintained activity may be transferred into long-term memory traces.

Learning in Artificial Networks

ADAPTIVE RESONANCE THEORY
ASSOCIATIVE NETWORKS
BACKPROPAGATION: GENERAL PRINCIPLES
BAYESIAN METHODS AND NEURAL NETWORKS
BAYESIAN NETWORKS
COMPETITIVE LEARNING
CONVOLUTIONAL NETWORKS FOR IMAGES, SPEECH, AND TIME SERIES
DATA CLUSTERING AND LEARNING
DYNAMICS OF ASSOCIATION AND RECALL
ENSEMBLE LEARNING
EVOLUTION AND LEARNING IN NEURAL NETWORKS
EVOLUTION OF ARTIFICIAL NEURAL NETWORKS
GAUSSIAN PROCESSES
GENERALIZATION AND REGULARIZATION IN NONLINEAR LEARNING SYSTEMS
GRAPHICAL MODELS: PARAMETER LEARNING
GRAPHICAL MODELS: PROBABILISTIC INFERENCE
GRAPHICAL MODELS: STRUCTURE LEARNING
HELMHOLTZ MACHINES AND SLEEP-WAKE LEARNING
HIDDEN MARKOV MODELS
INDEPENDENT COMPONENT ANALYSIS
LEARNING AND GENERALIZATION: THEORETICAL BOUNDS
LEARNING NETWORK TOPOLOGY
LEARNING AND STATISTICAL INFERENCE
LEARNING VECTOR QUANTIZATION
MINIMUM DESCRIPTION LENGTH ANALYSIS
MODEL VALIDATION
MODULAR AND HIERARCHICAL LEARNING SYSTEMS
NEOCOGNITRON: A MODEL FOR VISUAL PATTERN RECOGNITION
NEUROMANIFOLDS AND INFORMATION GEOMETRY
PATTERN RECOGNITION
PERCEPTRONS, ADALINES, AND BACKPROPAGATION
PRINCIPAL COMPONENT ANALYSIS
RADIAL BASIS FUNCTION NETWORKS
RECURRENT NETWORKS: LEARNING ALGORITHMS
REINFORCEMENT LEARNING
SELF-ORGANIZING FEATURE MAPS
SIMULATED ANNEALING AND BOLTZMANN MACHINES
STATISTICAL MECHANICS OF GENERALIZATION
STATISTICAL MECHANICS OF ON-LINE LEARNING AND GENERALIZATION
STOCHASTIC APPROXIMATION AND EFFICIENT LEARNING
SUPPORT VECTOR MACHINES
TEMPORAL PATTERN PROCESSING
TEMPORAL SEQUENCES: LEARNING AND GLOBAL ANALYSIS
UNIVERSAL APPROXIMATORS
UNSUPERVISED LEARNING WITH GLOBAL OBJECTIVE FUNCTIONS
YING-YANG LEARNING

The majority of articles in this road map deal with learning in artificial neural networks. Nonetheless, the road map is titled "Learning in Artificial Networks" to emphasize the inclusion of a body of research on statistical inference and learning that can be seen either as generalizing neural networks or as analyzing other forms of networks, such as Bayesian networks and graphical models.

The fundamental difference between a system that learns and one that merely memorizes is that the learning system generalizes to unseen examples. Much of our concern is with supervised learning, getting a network to behave in a way that successfully approximates some specified pattern of behavior or input-output relationship. In particular, much emphasis has been placed on feedforward networks which have no loops, so that the output of the net depends on its input alone, since there is then no internal state defined by reverberating activity. The most direct form of this is a synaptic matrix, a one-layer neural network for which input lines directly drive the output neurons and a "supervised Hebbian" rule sets synapses so that the network will exhibit specified input-output pairs in its response repertoire. This is addressed in Asso-

CIATIVE NETWORKS, which notes the problems that arise if the input patterns (the "keys" for associations) are not orthogonal vectors. Association also extends to recurrent networks, but in such systems of "dynamic memories" (e.g., Hopfield networks) there are no external inputs as such. Rather the "input" is the initial state of the network, and the "output" is the "attractor" or equilibrium state to which the network then settles. For neurons whose output is a sigmoid function of the linear combination of their inputs, the memory capacity of the associative memory is approximately $0.15n$, where n is the number of neurons in the net. Unfortunately, such an "attractor network" memory model has many spurious memories, i.e., equilibria other than the memorized patterns, and there is no way to decide whether a recalled pattern was memorized or not. DYNAMICS OF ASSOCIATION AND RECALL (see the road map **Dynamic Systems** for more details) shows how to move away from microscopic equations at the level of individual neurons to derive dynamical laws at a macroscopic level that characterize association and recall in Hopfield-type networks (with some discussion of variations and generalizations).

Historically, the earliest forms of supervised learning involved changing synaptic weights to oppose the error in a neuron with a binary output (the perceptron error-correction rule), or to minimize the sum of squares of errors of output neurons in a network with real-valued outputs (the Widrow-Hoff rule). This work is charted in PERCEPTRONS, ADALINES, AND BACKPROPAGATION, which also charts the extension of these classic ideas to multilayered networks. In multilayered networks, there is the *structural credit assignment problem*: When an error is made at the output of a network, how is credit (or blame) to be assigned to neurons deep within the network? One of the most popular techniques is called backpropagation, whereby the error of output units is propagated back to yield estimates of how much a given "hidden unit" contributed to the output error. These estimates are used in the adjustment of synaptic weights to these units within the network. BACKPROPAGATION: GENERAL PRINCIPLES places this idea in a broader framework by providing an overview of contributions that enrich our understanding of the pros and cons (such as "plateaus") of this adaptive architecture. It also assesses the biological plausibility of backpropagation.

The underlying theoretical grounding is that, given any function $f: X \rightarrow Y$ for which X and Y are codable as input and output patterns of a neural network, then, as shown in UNIVERSAL APPROXIMATORS, f can be approximated arbitrarily well by a feedforward network with one layer of hidden units. The catch, of course, is that many, many hidden units may be required for a close fit. It is thus often treated as an empirical question whether there exists a sufficiently good approximation achievable in principle by a network of a given size—an approximation that a given learning rule may or may not find (it may, for example, get stuck in a local optimum rather than a global one). Gradient descent methods have also been extended to adapt the synaptic weights of recurrent networks. The backpropagation algorithm for feedforward networks has been successfully applied to a wide range of problems, but what can be implemented by a feedforward network is just a static mapping of the input vectors. However, to model dynamical functions of brains or machines, one must use a system capable of storing internal states and implementing complex dynamics. RECURRENT NETWORKS: LEARNING ALGORITHMS presents, then, learning algorithms for recurrent neural networks that have feedback connections and time delays. In a recurrent network, the state of the system can be encoded in the activity pattern of the units, and a wide variety of dynamical behaviors can be programmed by the connection weights. A popular subclass of recurrent networks consists of those with symmetric connection weights. In this case, the network dynamics is guaranteed to converge to a minimum of some "energy" function (see "Energy Functionals for Neural Networks" and "Computing with Attractors"). However, steady-state solutions are only a limited portion of the capabilities of recurrent networks. For example, they can transform an input sequence into a distinct output sequence, and they can serve as a nonlinear filter, a nonlinear controller, or a finite-state machine. This article reviews the learning algorithms for training recurrent networks, with the main focus on supervised learning algorithms. (See "Recurrent Networks: Neurophysiological Modeling" for the use of such networks in modeling biological neural circuitry.)

One useful perspective for supervised learning views learning as hill-climbing in weight space, so that each "experience" adjusts the synaptic weights of the network to climb (or descend) a metaphorical hill for which "height" at a particular point in "weight space" corresponds to some measure of the performance of the network (or the organism or robot of which it is a part). When the aim is to minimize this measure, the learning process is then an example of what mathematicians call *gradient descent*. The term *reinforcement* comes from studies of animal learning in experimental psychology, where it refers to the occurrence of an event, in the proper relation to a response, that tends to increase the probability that the response will occur again in the same situation. REINFORCEMENT LEARNING describes a form of "semisupervised" learning where the network is not provided with an explicit form of error at each time step but rather receives only generalized reinforcement ("you're doing well"; "that was bad!"), which yields little immediate indication of how any neuron should change its behavior. Moreover, the reinforcement is intermittent, thus raising the temporal credit assignment problem (see also "Reinforcement Learning in Motor Control"): How is an action at one time to be credited for positive reinforcement at a later time? The solution is to build an "adaptive critic" that learns to evaluate actions of the network on the basis of how often they occur on a path leading to positive or negative reinforcement. Methods for this assessment of future expected reinforcement include temporal difference (TD) learning and Q-learning (see "Q-Learning for Robots"). Current reinforcement learning research includes parameterized function approximation methods; understanding how exploratory behavior is best introduced and controlled; learning under conditions in which the environment state cannot be fully observed; introducing various forms of abstraction such as temporally extended actions and hierarchy; and relating computational reinforcement learning theories to brain reward mechanisms (see "Dopamine, Roles of").

The task par excellence for supervised learning is pattern recognition—the problem of classifying objects, often represented as vectors or as strings of symbols, into categories. Historically, the field of pattern recognition started with early efforts in neural networks (see PERCEPTRONS, ADALINES, AND BACKPROPAGATION). While neural networks played a less central role in pattern recognition for some years, recent progress has made them the method of choice for many applications. As PATTERN RECOGNITION demonstrates, properly designed multilayer networks can learn complex mappings in high-dimensional spaces without requiring complicated hand-crafted feature extractors. To rely more on learning, and less on detailed engineering of feature extractors, it is crucial to tailor the network architecture to the task, incorporating prior knowledge to be able to learn complex tasks without requiring excessively large networks and training sets. ENSEMBLE LEARNING describes algorithms that, rather than finding one best hypothesis to explain the data, construct a set (sometimes called a committee or ensemble) of hypotheses and then have those hypotheses vote to classify new patterns. Ensemble methods are often much more accurate than any single hypothesis. For example, the representational problem arises when the hypothesis space does not contain any hypotheses that are good approximations to the true decision function f. In some cases, a weighted sum of hypotheses expands the space of functions that can be represented. Hence, by taking a weighted vote of hypotheses, the learning algorithm may be able to form a more accurate approximation to *f*. The bulk of research into ensemble methods has focused on constructing ensembles of decision trees. The article introduces the techniques of bagging and boosting, among others, and analyzes their relative merits under different conditions.

Many specific architectures have been developed to solve particular types of learning problem. ADAPTIVE RESONANCE THEORY (ART) bases learning on internal expectations. A pattern matching process compares an external input with the internal memory of various coded patterns. ART matching leads either to a *resonant* state, which persists long enough to permit learning, or to a parallel memory search. If the search ends at an established code, the memory representation may either remain the same or incorporate new information from matched portions of the current input. When the external world fails to match an ART network's expectations or predictions, a search process selects a new category, representing a new hypothesis about what is important in the present environment.

The neocognitron (see NEOCOGNITRON: A MODEL FOR VISUAL PATTERN RECOGNITION) was developed as a neural network model for visual pattern recognition that addresses the specific question, "How can a pattern be recognized despite variations in size and position?" by using a multilayer architecture in which local features are replicated in many different scales and locations. More generally, as shown in CONVOLUTIONAL NETWORKS FOR IMAGES, SPEECH, AND TIME SERIES, shift invariance in convolutional networks is obtained by forcing the replication of weight configurations across space. Moreover, the topology of the input is taken into account, enabling such networks to force the extraction of local features by restricting the receptive fields of hidden units to be local, and enforcing a built-in invariance with respect to translations, or local distortions of the inputs. The idea of connecting units to local receptive fields on the input goes back to the perceptron in the early 1960s, and was almost simultaneous with Hubel and Wiesel's discovery of locally sensitive, orientation-selective neurons in the cat's visual system.

Just as a polynomial of too high a degree is not useful for curve fitting, a network that is too large will fail to generalize well, and will require longer training times. Smaller networks, with fewer free parameters, enforce a smoothness constraint on the function found. For best performance, it is therefore desirable to find the smallest network that will "fit" the training data. To create a neural network, a designer typically fixes a network topology and uses training data to tune its parameters such as connection weights. The designer, however, often does not have enough knowledge to specify the ideal topology. It is thus desirable to learn the topology from training data as well. LEARNING NETWORK TOPOLOGY reviews algorithms that adjust network topology, adding neurons and removing neurons during the learning process, to arrive at a network appropriate to a given task. For topology learning, a bias is added to prefer smaller models. It is often found that this bias produces a neural network that has better generalization and is more interpretable. This framework is applied to learning the topologies of both feedforward neural networks and BAYESIAN NETWORKS. In Bayesian networks, all the nodes of the network are given and set, and one searches for a topology by adding or deleting links.

Many articles in the *Handbook* emphasize situations where, e.g., learning from examples is stochastic in the sense that examples are randomly generated and the network behavior is thus to be analyzed from a statistical point of view. Statistical estimation identifies the mechanism underlying stochastic phenomena. LEARNING AND STATISTICAL INFERENCE studies learning by using such statistical notions as Fisher information, Bayesian loss, and sequential estimation, as well as the Expectation-Maximization (EM) algorithm for estimating hidden variables. Nonlinear neurodynamics, learning,

and self-organization are seen as adding new concepts to statistical science. The article examines the dynamical behaviors of a learning network under a general loss criterion. The behavior of learning curves is related to neural network complexity to elucidate the discrepancy between training and generalization errors. This perspective is further developed in NEUROMANIFOLDS AND INFORMATION GEOMETRY. A neural network is specified by its architecture and a number of parameters such as synaptic weights and thresholds. Any neural network of this architecture is specified by a point in the parameter space. Learning takes place in the parameter space and a learning process is represented by a trajectory. The article presents the approach of information geometry which sees the geometrical structure of the parameter space as given by a Riemannian manifold. The article shows how dynamical behaviors of neural learning on these "neuromanifolds" are related to the underlying geometrical structures, using multilayer perceptrons and Boltzmann machines as examples.

GENERALIZATION AND REGULARIZATION IN NONLINEAR LEARNING SYSTEMS sets forth the essential relationship between multivariate function estimation in a statistical context and supervised machine learning. Given a training set consisting of (input, output) pairs (x_i, y_i), the task is to construct a map that generalizes well in that, given a new value of *x*, the map will provide a reasonable prediction for the hitherto unobserved output associated with this *x*. Regularization simplifies the problem by applying constraints to the construction of the map that reduce the generalization error (see also "Probabilistic Regularization Methods for Low-Level Vision"). Ideally, these constraints embody a priori information concerning the true relationship between input and output, though various ad hoc constraints have sometimes been shown to work well in practice. Feedforward neural nets, radial basis functions, and various forms of splines all provide regularized or regularizable methods for estimating "smooth" functions of several variables from a given training set. Which method to use depends on the particular nature of the underlying but unknown "truth," the nature of any prior information that might be available about this "truth," the nature of any noise in the data, the ability of the experimenter to choose the various smoothing or regularization parameters well, and so on.

MODULAR AND HIERARCHICAL LEARNING SYSTEMS solves a complex learning problem by dividing it into a set of subproblems. In the context of supervised learning, modular architectures arise when the data can be described by a collection of functions, each of which works well over a relatively local region of the input space, allocating different modules to different regions of the space. The challenge is that, in general, the learner is not provided with prior knowledge of the partitioning of the input space. To solve this, a "gating network" can learn which module to "listen to" in different situations. The learning algorithms described here solve the credit assignment problem by computing a set of posterior probabilities that can be thought of as estimating the utility of different modules in different parts of the input space. An EM algorithm (cf. LEARNING AND STATISTICAL INFERENCE), an alternative to gradient methods, can be derived for estimating the parameters of both the modular system and its extension to hierarchical architectures. The latter arise when we assume that the data are well described by a multiresolution model in which regions are divided recursively into subregions.

BAYESIAN METHODS AND NEURAL NETWORKS shows how to apply Bayes's rule for the use of probabilities to quantify inferences about hypotheses from given data. The idea is to take the predictions $p(d|h_i)$ made by alternative models h_i about data *d*, and the prior probabilities of the models $p(h_i)$, and obtain the posterior probabilities $p(h_i|d)$ of the models given the data, using Bayes's rule in the form $p(h_i|d) = p(d|h_i)p(h_i)/p(d)$. To apply this to neural networks, regard a supervised neural network as a nonlinear parameterized mapping from an input x to an output $y = y(x; w)$, which depends continuously on the "weights" parameter w. The idea is to choose w from a weight space with some given probability distribution $p(w)$ so as to maximize the likelihood of the nets yielding the given set of (input, output) observations. The Bayesian framework deals with uncertainty in a natural, consistent manner by combining prior beliefs about which models are appropriate with how likely each model would be to have generated the data. This results in an elegant, general framework for fitting models to data that, however, may be compromised by computational difficulties in carrying out the ideal procedure. There are many approximate Bayesian implementations, using methods such as sampling, perturbation techniques, and variational methods. In the case of models linear in their parameters, Bayesian neural networks are closely related to GAUSSIAN PROCESSES (q.v.), where many of the computational difficulties of dealing with more general stochastic nonlinear systems can be avoided. Traditionally, neural networks are graphical representations of functions in which the computations at each node are deterministic. By contrast, networks in which nodes represent stochastic variables are called graphical models (see BAYESIAN NETWORKS and GRAPHICAL MODELS: PROBABILISTIC INFERENCE).

RADIAL BASIS FUNCTION NETWORKS applies Bayesian methods to the case where the approximation to the given $y = y(x; w)$ is based on a network using combinations of "radial basis" functions, each of which is "centered" around a weight vector w, so that the response to input x depends on some measure of "distance" of x from w, rather than on the dot product $w \cdot x = \Sigma_i w_i x_i$ as in many formal neurons. The distribution of the w's may be determined by some form of clustering (see DATA CLUSTERING AND LEARNING). Further learning adjusts the connection strengths to a neuron whose outputs give an estimate of, e.g., the posterior probability $p(c|x)$ that class c is present given the observation (network input) x. However, it is easier to model other related aspects of the data, such as the unconditional distribution of the data $p(x)$ and the likelihood of the data, $p(x|c)$, and then recreate the posterior from these quantities according to Bayes's rule, $p(c_i|x) = p(c_i)p(x|c_i)/p(x)$.

GAUSSIAN PROCESSES continues the Bayesian approach to neural network learning, placing a prior probability distribution over possible functions and then letting the observed data "sculpt" this prior into a posterior using the available data. One can place a prior distribution $P(w)$ on the weights w of a neural network to induce a prior over functions $P(y(x;w))$ but the computations required to make predictions are not easy, owing to nonlinearities in the system. A Gaussian process, defined by a mean function and covariance matrix, can prove useful as a way of specifying a prior directly over function space—it is often simpler to do this than to work with priors over parameters. Gaussian processes are probably the simplest kind of function space prior that one can consider, being a generalization of finite-dimensional Gaussian distributions over vectors. A Gaussian process is defined by a mean function (which we shall usually take to be identically zero), and a covariance function $C(x, x')$ which indicates how correlated the value of the function y is at x and x'. This function encodes our assumptions about the problem (e.g., that the function is smooth and continuous) and will influence the quality of the predictions. The article shows how to use Gaussian processes for classification problems, and describes how data can be used to adapt the covariance function to the given prediction problem.

MINIMUM DESCRIPTION LENGTH ANALYSIS shows how ideas relating to minimum description length (MDL) have been applied to neural networks, emphasizing the direct relationship between MDL and Bayesian model selection methods. The classic MDL approach defined the information in a binary string to be the length of the shortest program with which a general-purpose computer could generate the string. The Bayes bridge is obtained by replacing the Bayesian goal of inferring the "most likely" model M from a set

of observations by minimizing the length of an encoded message which describe M as well as the data D expressed in term of M. MDL and Bayesian methods both formalize Occam's razor in that a complex network is preferred only if its predictions are sufficiently more accurate.

UNSUPERVISED LEARNING WITH GLOBAL OBJECTIVE FUNCTIONS makes the point that even unsupervised learning involves an *implicit* training signal based on the network's ability to predict its own input, or on some more general measure of the quality of its internal representation. The main problem in unsupervised learning research is then seen as the formulation of a performance measure or cost function for the learning to generate this internal supervisory signal. The cost function is also known as an objective function, since it sets the objective for the learning process. The article reviews three types of unsupervised neural network learning procedures: information-preserving algorithms, density estimation techniques, and invariance-based learning procedures. The first method is based on the preservation of mutual information $I_{x;y} = H(x) - H(x|y)$ between the input vector x and output vector y, where $H(x)$ is the entropy of random variable x and $H(x|y)$ is the entropy of the conditional distribution of x given y. The second approach is to assume a priori a class of models that constrains the general form of the probability density function and then to search for the particular model parameters defining the density function (or mixture of density functions) most likely to have generated the observed data (cf. the earlier discussion of Bayesian methods). Finally, invariance-based learning extracts higher-order features and builds more abstract representations. Once again, the approach is to make constraining assumptions about the structure that is being sought, and to build these constraints into the network's architecture and/or objective function to develop more efficient, specialized learning procedures.

The Bayesian articles stress the "global" statistical idea of "find the weights which, according to given probability distributions maximize some expectation" as distinct from the deterministic idea of adjusting the weights at each time step to provide a local increment in performance on the current input. However, gradient descent provides an important tool for finding the weight settings which decrease some stochastic expectation of error, too. STOCHASTIC APPROXIMATION AND EFFICIENT LEARNING shows that gradient descent has a long tradition in the literature of stochastic approximation. Any stochastic process that can be interpreted as minimizing a cost function based on noisy gradient measurements in a sequential, recursive manner may be considered to be a stochastic approximation. "Sequential" means that each estimate of the location of a minimum is used to make a new observation, which in turn immediately leads to a new estimate; "recursive" means that the estimates depend on past gradient measurements only through a fixed number of scalar statistics. Such on-line algorithms are useful because they enjoy significant performance advantages for large-scale learning problems. The article describes their properties using stochastic approximation theory as a very broad framework, and provides a brief overview of newer insights obtained using information geometry (see NEUROMANIFOLDS AND INFORMATION GEOMETRY) and replica calculations (see STATISTICAL MECHANICS OF ON-LINE LEARNING AND GENERALIZATION).

In order to understand the performance of learning machines, and to gain insight that helps to design better ones, it is helpful to have theoretical bounds on the generalization ability of the machines. The determination of such bounds is the subject of LEARNING AND GENERALIZATION: THEORETICAL BOUNDS. Here it is necessary to formalize the learning problem and turn the question of how well a machine generalizes into a mathematical question. The article adopts the formalization used in statistical learning theory, which is shown to include both pattern recognition and function learning. The road map **Computability and Complexity** gives more information on this and related articles, such as "PAC Learning and Neural Networks" and "Vapnik-Chervonenkis Dimension of Neural Networks," which offer bounds on the performance of learning methods. SUPPORT VECTOR MACHINES addresses the (binary) pattern recognition problem of learning theory: given two classes of objects, to assign a new object to one of the two classes. Trying to find the best classifier involves notions of similarity in the set X of inputs. Support vector machines (SVMs) build a decision function as a kernel expansion corresponding to a separating hyperplane in a feature space. SVMs rest on methods for the selection of the patterns on which the kernels are centered and in the choice of weights that are placed on the individual kernels in the decision function. SVMs and other kernel methods have a number of advantages compared to classical neural network approaches, such as the absence of spurious local minima in the optimization procedure, the need to tune only a few parameters, and modularity in the design. Kernel methods connect similarity measures, nonlinearities, and data representations in linear spaces where simple geometric algorithms are performed.

The passage of the "energy" of a Hopfield network to a local minimum can be construed as a means for solving an optimization problem. The catch is the word "local" in local minimum—the solution may be the best in the neighborhood, yet far better solutions may be located elsewhere. One resolution of this is described in SIMULATED ANNEALING AND BOLTZMANN MACHINES. At the expense of great increases in time to convergence, simulated annealing escapes local minima by adding noise, which is then gradually reduced ("lowering the temperature"). The initially high temperature (i.e., noise level) stops the system from getting trapped in "high valleys" of the energy landscape, the lowering of temperature allows optimization to occur in the "deepest valley" once it has been found. The Boltzmann machine then applies this method to design a class of neural networks. These machines use stochastic computing elements to extend discrete Hopfield networks in two ways: they replace the deterministic, asynchronous dynamics of Hopfield networks with a randomized local search dynamics, and they replace the Hebbian learning rule with a more powerful stochastic learning algorithm.

Turning from neural networks to another form of network structure, BAYESIAN NETWORKS (as distinct from BAYESIAN METHODS AND NEURAL NETWORKS) provides an explicit method for following chains of probabilistic inference such as those appropriate to expert systems, extending the Bayes's rule for updating probabilities in the light of new evidence. The nodes in a Bayesian network represent propositional variables of interest and the links represent informational or causal dependencies among the variables. The dependencies are quantified by conditional probabilities for each node, given its parents in the network. The network supports the computation of the probabilities of any subset of variables, given evidence about any other subset, and the reasoning processes can operate on Bayesian networks by propagating information in any direction. HELMHOLTZ MACHINES AND SLEEP-WAKE LEARNING starts by observing that since unsupervised learning is largely concerned with finding structure among sets of input patterns, it is important to take advantage of cases in which the input patterns are generated in a systematic way, thus forming a manifold that has many fewer dimensions than the space of all possible activation patterns. The Helmholtz machine is an analysis-by-synthesis model. The key idea is to have an imperfect generative model train a better analysis or recognition model, and an imperfect recognition model train a better generative model. The generative model for the Helmholtz machine is a structured belief network (i.e., Bayesian network) that is viewed as a model for hierarchical top-down connections in the cortex. New inputs are analyzed in an approximate fashion using a second structured belief network (called the recognition model), which is viewed as a model for the standard, bottom-up connections in cortex. The generative and recognition models are learned from data in two phases. In the *wake phase*, the recognition model is used to estimate the underlying generators for a particular input pattern, and then the generative model is altered so that those generators are more likely to have produced the input that is actually observed. In the *sleep phase*, the generative model fantasizes inputs by choosing particular generators stochastically, and then the recognition model is altered so that it is more likely to report those particular generators if the fantasized input were actually to be observed. YING-YANG LEARNING further develops this notion of simultaneously building up two pathways, a bottom-up pathway for encoding a pattern in the observation space into its representation in a representation space, and a top-down pathway for decoding or reconstructing a pattern from an inner representation back to a pattern in the observation space. The theory of Bayesian Ying-Yang harmony learning formulates the two-pathway approach in a general statistical framework, modeling the two pathways via two complementary Bayesian representations of the joint distribution on the observation space and representation space. The article shows how a number of major learning problems and methods can be seen as special cases of this unified perspective. Moreover, the ability of Ying-Yang learning for regularization and model selection is placed in an information-theoretic perspective.

GRAPHICAL MODELS: PROBABILISTIC INFERENCE introduces a generalization of Bayesian networks. The graphical models framework provides a clean mathematical formalism that has made it possible to understand the relationships among a wide variety of network-based approaches to computation, and in particular to understand many neural network algorithms and architectures as instances of a broader probabilistic methodology. Graphical models use graphs to represent and manipulate joint probability distributions. The graph underlying a graphical model may be directed, in which case the model is often referred to as a belief network or a Bayesian network, or the graph may be undirected, in which case the model is generally referred to as a Markov random field. A graphical model has both a structural component, encoded by the pattern of edges in the graph, and a parametric component, encoded by numerical "potentials" associated with sets of edges in the graph. General inference algorithms allow statistical quantities (such as likelihoods and conditional probabilities) and information-theoretic quantities (such as mutual information and conditional entropies) to be computed efficiently. The article closes by noting that many neural network architectures are special cases of the general graphical model formalism, both representationally and algorithmically. Special cases of graphical models include essentially all models of unsupervised learning, as well as Boltzmann machines, mixtures of experts, and radial basis function networks, while many other neural networks, including the classical multilayer perceptron, can be profitably analyzed from the viewpoint of graphical models. The next two articles present learning algorithms that build on these inference algorithms and allow parameters and structures to be estimated from data. GRAPHICAL MODELS: PARAMETER LEARNING discusses the learning of parameters for a fixed graphical model. As noted, each node in the graph represents a random variable, while the edges in the graph represent the qualitative dependencies between the variables; the absence of an edge between two nodes means that any statistical dependency between these two variables is mediated via some other variable or set of variables. The quantitative dependencies between variables that are connected via edges are specified via parameterized conditional distributions, or more generally nonnegative "potential functions." The pattern of edges is the structure of the graph, while the parameters of the potential functions are parameters of the graph. The present article assumes that the structure of the graph is given, and shows how to then learn the parameters of the graph from data. GRAPHICAL MODELS: STRUCTURE LEARNING turns to the simultaneous learning of parameters and structure. Real-world applications of such learning abound, the example presented being an analysis of data regarding factors that influence the intention of high school students to attend college. For simplicity, the article focuses on directed-acyclic graphical models, but the basic principles thus defined can be applied more generally. The Bayesian approach is emphasized, and then several common non-Bayesian approaches are mentioned briefly.

COMPETITIVE LEARNING is a form of unsupervised learning in which each input pattern comes, through learning, to be associated with the activity of one or at most a few neurons, leading to sparse representations of data that are easy to decode. Competitive learning algorithms employ some sort of competition between neurons in the same layer via lateral connections. This competition limits the set of neurons to be affected in a given learning trial. Hard competition allows the final activity of only one neuron, the strongest one to start with, whereas in soft competition the activity of the lateral neurons does not necessarily drive all but one to zero. One form of competitive learning algorithm can be described as an application of a successful single-neuron learning algorithm in a network with lateral connections between adjacent neurons. The lateral connections are needed so that each neuron can be inhibited from adapting to a feature of the data already captured by other neurons. A second family of algorithms uses the competition between neurons for improving, sharpening, or even forming the features extracted from the data by each single neuron. DATA CLUSTERING AND LEARNING emphasizes the related idea of data clustering, discovering, and emphasizing structure that is hidden in a data set (e.g., the pronounced similarity of groups of data vectors) in an unsupervised fashion. There is a delicate trade-off: not to superimpose too much structure, and yet not to overlook structure. The choice of data representation predetermines what kind of cluster structures can be discovered in the data. Formulating the search for clusters as an optimization problem then supports validation of clustering results by checking that the cluster structures found in a data set vary little from one data set to a second data set generated by the same data source. The two tasks of clustering, density estimation and data compression, are tightly related by the fact that the correct identification of the probability model of the source yields the best code for data compression. PRINCIPAL COMPONENT ANALYSIS shows how, in data compression applications like image or speech coding, a distribution of input vectors may be economically encoded, with small expected values of the distortions, in terms of eigenvectors of the largest eigenvalues of the correlation matrix that describes the distribution of these patterns (these eigenvectors are the "principal components"). However, it is usually not possible to find the eigenvectors on-line. The ideal solution is then replaced by a neural network learning rule embodying a constrained optimization problem that converges to the solution given by the principal components. INDEPENDENT COMPONENT ANALYSIS (ICA) is a linear transform of multivariate data designed to make components of the resulting random vector as statistically independent (factorial) as possible. In signal processing it is used to attack the problem of the blind separation of sources, for example of audio signals that have been mixed together by an unknown process (the "cocktail party effect"). In the area of neural networks and brain theory, it is an example of an information-theoretic unsupervised learning algorithm. When an ICA network is trained on an ensemble of natural images, it learns localized-oriented receptive fields qualitatively similar to those found in area V1 of mammalian visual cortex. ICA has been used to decompose multivariate brain data into components that help us understand task-related spatial and temporal brain dynamics. Thus the same neural network algorithm is being used both as an explanation of brain properties and as a method of probing the brain. Where principal component analysis (PCA) uses second-order statistics (the covariance matrix) to remove correlations between the elements of a vector, ICA uses statistics of all orders. PCA attempts to decorrelate the outputs, while ICA attempts to make the outputs statistically independent. The most widely used adaptive, on-line method for ICA is also the most "neural-network-like" and is the one described in the body of this article.

SELF-ORGANIZING FEATURE MAPS introduces the self-organizing feature map (SOFM or SOM; also known as a Kohonen map), a nonlinear method by which features can be obtained with an unsupervised learning process. It is based on a layer of adaptive "neurons" that gradually develops into an array of feature detectors. The linking of input signals to response locations in the map can be viewed as a nonlinear projection from a signal or input space to the (usually) 2D map layer. The learning method is an augmented Hebbian method in which learning by the element most responsive to an input pattern is "shared" with its neighbors. The result is that the resulting "compressed image" of the (usually higher-dimensional) input space has the property of a topographic map that reflects important metric and statistical properties of the input signal distribution: distance relationships in the input space (expressing, e.g., pattern similarities) are approximately preserved as distance relationships between corresponding excitation sites in the map, and clusters of similar input patterns tend to become mapped to areas of the neural array whose size varies in proportion to the frequency of the occurrence of their patterns. This resembles in many ways the structure of topographic feature maps found in many brain areas, for which the SOFM offers a neural model that bridges the gap between microscopic adaptation rules postulated at the single neuron or synapse level and the formation of experimentally better accessible, macroscopic patterns of feature selectivity in neural layers. From a statistical point of view, the SOFM provides a nonlinear generalization of principal component analysis and has proved valuable in many application contexts.

In order to give a quantitative answer to the question of how well the trained network will be able to classify an input that it has not seen before, it is common to assume that all inputs, both from the training set and the test set, are produced independently and at random. Clearly, the generalization error depends on the specific algorithm that was used during the training, and its calculation requires knowledge of the network weights generated by the learning process. In general, these weights will be complicated functions of the examples, and an explicit form will not be available in most cases. The methods of statistical mechanics provide an approach to this problem, which often enables an exact calculation of learning curves in the limit of a very large network. In the statistical mechanics approach one studies the ensemble of all networks that implement the same set of input/output examples to a given accuracy. In this way the typical generalization behavior of a neural network (in contrast to the worst or optimal behavior) can be described. We thus turn to two articles that apply the methods introduced in the article "Statistical Mechanics of Neural Networks": STATISTICAL MECHANICS OF ON-LINE LEARNING AND GENERALIZATION emphasizes on-line learning in which training examples are dealt with one at a time, while STATISTICAL MECHANICS OF GENERALIZATION emphasizes off-line or memory-based methods, where learning is guided by the minimization of a cost function as averaged over the whole training set. From a statistical physics point of view, the distinction is between systems that can be thought of as being in a state of thermal equilibrium (off-line ≈ on-equilibrium) and away-from-equilibrium situations where the network is not allowed to extract all possible information from a set of examples (on-line ≈ off-equilibrium). While on-line learning is an intrinsically stochastic process, the restriction to large networks, together with assumptions about the statistical properties of the inputs, permits a concise description of the dynamics in terms of coupled ordinary differential equations. These deterministic equations govern the average evolution of quantities that completely define the macroscopic state of the ANN. The average is taken with respect to the data, which is straightforward if the presented examples are statistically independent. The probability that the network will make a mistake on the new input defines its generalization error for a given training set. Its average over many realizations of the training set, as a function of the number of examples, gives the so-called learning curve. Calculation of the learning curve requires knowledge of the network weights generated by the learning process, for which an explicit form will not be available in most cases. The methods of statistical mechanics provide an approach to this problem, in many cases yielding an exact calculation of learning curves in the "thermodynamic limit" of a very large network in which the network size increases in proportion to the number of training examples, while the statistical or information-theoretic approach is applicable to the learning curve of a medium-size network (cf. LEARNING AND STATISTICAL INFERENCE).

MODEL VALIDATION shows how the data analyst tries to infer a "model" that summarizes functional dependencies that may be observed in a given set of empirical data. A good model fit should reproduce the behavior of the studied system in the parameter range to be explained by the model study. Model complexity has to be controlled to avoid both missing essential features of the system (underfitting) and adapting to irrelevant fluctuations in the data (overfitting). Model validation provides the crucial step in modeling between model synthesis and analysis, assessing how appropriate the model is to gain insight into the real-world system. Model validation can make use of bounds of the VC type (cf. "Vapnik-Chervonenkis Dimension of Neural Networks"), which usually contain a complexity term that accounts for the flexibility of the hypothesis class and a fitting term that measures the contraction of measure due to the large number of samples. It is shown how these terms can be controlled either by numerical methods like cross-validation and bootstrap or by analytical techniques from computational learning theory. The trade-off between model complexity and goodness of fit and its relation to the computational complexity of learning remains a deep challenge for research.

HIDDEN MARKOV MODELS describes the use of deterministic and stochastic finite state automata for sequence processing, with special attention to hidden Markov models as tools for the processing of complex piecewise stationary sequences. It also describes a few applications of ANNs to further improve these methods. HMMs allow complex sequential learning problems to be solved by assuming that the sequential pattern can be decomposed into piecewise stationary segments, with each stationary segment parameterized in terms of a stochastic function. The HMM is called "hidden" because there is an underlying stochastic process (i.e., the sequence of states) that is not observable but that affects the observed sequence of events.

TEMPORAL PATTERN PROCESSING notes that time is embodied in a temporal pattern in two different ways: the temporal order among the components of a sequence and the temporal duration of the elements (see also "Sequence Learning"). A sequence is defined as *complex* if it contains repetitions of the same subsequence, and otherwise is *simple*. For the generation of complex sequences, the correct successor can be determined only by knowing components prior to the current one. We refer to the prior subsequence required to determine the current component as the *context* of the component. Temporal processing requires that a neural network have a capacity of short-term memory (STM) in order to maintain a component for some time. Time warping is challenging because we would like to have invariance over limited warping, but dramatic change in relative duration must be recognized differently. Another fundamental ability of human information processing is chunking, which, in the context of temporal processing, means that frequently encountered and meaningful subsequences organize into chunks

that form basic units for further chunking at a higher level. TEMPORAL SEQUENCES: LEARNING AND GLOBAL ANALYSIS studies how elementary pattern sequences may be represented in neural structures at a low architectural and computational cost, seeking to understand mechanisms to memorize spatiotemporal associations in a robust fashion within model neural networks. The article focuses on formal neural networks where the interplay between neural and synaptic dynamics and, in particular, the role of transmission delays can be analyzed using methods from nonlinear dynamics and statistical mechanics. Among the questions studied are how to train a network so that its limit cycles will resemble taught sequences. Such simplified systems are necessarily caricatures of biological structures yet suggest aspects that are important for more elaborate approaches to real neural systems.

EVOLUTION OF ARTIFICIAL NEURAL NETWORKS adds another temporal dimension to the biological process of adaptation, namely, that of evolution. Rather than adapt the weights of a single network to solve a problem in the network's "lifetime," the evolutionary approach applies the methodology of genetic algorithms to evolve a population of neural networks over several generations so that the population becomes better and better suited to some computational ecology. EVOLUTION AND LEARNING IN NEURAL NETWORKS extends this selection of networks on the basis of the result of their adaptation to the environment through lifetime learning. The article shows how studies of ANNs that are subjected both to an evolutionary and a lifetime learning process have been conducted to look at the advantages, in terms of performance, of combining two different adaptation techniques or to help understand the role of the interaction between learning and evolution in natural organisms.

Computability and Complexity

ANALOG NEURAL NETS: COMPUTATIONAL POWER
LEARNING AND GENERALIZATION: THEORETICAL BOUNDS
NEURAL AUTOMATA AND ANALOG COMPUTATIONAL COMPLEXITY
PAC LEARNING AND NEURAL NETWORKS
UNIVERSAL APPROXIMATORS
VAPNIK-CHERVONENKIS DIMENSION OF NEURAL NETWORKS

The 1930s saw the definition of an abstract notion of computability when it was discovered that the set of functions on the natural numbers, $f: \mathbb{N} \to \mathbb{N}$, computable by a Turing machine (an abstraction from following a finite set of rules to calculate on a finite but extendible tape, each square of which could hold one of a fixed set of symbols), lambda functions (which later came to be better known as functions computable by programs written in LISP), and general recursive functions (a class of functions obtained from very simple numerical functions by repeated application of composition, minimization, etc.), were identical. As general-purpose electronic computers were developed and used in the 1940s and 1950s, it was firmly established that these *computable functions* were precisely the functions that could be computed by such computers with suitable programs, provided there were no limitations on computer memory or computation time. This set the stage for the development of complexity theory in the 1960s and beyond: to chart the different subsets of the computable functions that would be obtained when restrictions were placed on computing resources.

Many classification or pattern recognition tasks can be formulated as mappings between subsets of multidimensional vector spaces by using a suitable coding of inputs and outputs, and many types of feedforward networks are *universal* in the sense that, given enough adjustable synaptic weights, they can approximate any mapping between subsets of Euclidean spaces. UNIVERSAL APPROXIMATORS surveys recent developments in the mathematical theory of feedforward networks and includes proofs of the universal approximation capabilities of perceptron and radial basis function networks with general activation and radial functions, and provides estimates of rates of approximation. The article also characterizes sets of multivariable functions that can be approximated without the "curse of dimensionality," which is an exponentially fast scaling of the number of parameters with the number of variables.

NEURAL AUTOMATA AND ANALOG COMPUTATIONAL COMPLEXITY explores what happens when the discrete operations of conventional automata theory are replaced by a computing model in which operations on real numbers are treated as basic. Whereas classical automata describe digital machines, neural models frequently require a framework of analog computation defined on a continuous phase space, with a dynamics characterized by the existence of real constants that influence the macroscopic behavior of the system. Moreover, unlike the flow in digital computation, analog models do not include local discontinuities. Neural networks with real weights are more powerful than traditional models of computation in that they can compute more functions within given time bounds. However, the practicality of an approach based on infinite precision real operations remains to be seen. Nonetheless, the new attention to real numbers has renewed complexity theory and introduced many open problems in computational learning theory and neural network theory. The article thus pays special attention to analog computation in the presence of noise. ANALOG NEURAL NETS: COMPUTATIONAL POWER then analyzes the exact and approximate representational power of feedforward and recurrent neural nets with synchronous update, with a brief discussion of networks of spiking neurons and their relation to sigmoidal nets. Learning complexity increases with increasing representational power of the underlying neural model and care has to be exercised to strike a balance between representational power on the one hand and learning complexity on the other. However, the emphasis of the article is on representational power, i.e., on what can be represented with networks using a given set of activation functions, rather than on learning complexity. Splines (i.e., piecewise polynomial functions) have turned out to be powerful approximators, and they are used here as the benchmark class of activation functions. Much attention is given to studying the properties that a class of activation functions needs to reach the approximation power of splines.

PAC LEARNING AND NEURAL NETWORKS discusses the "probably approximately correct" (PAC) learning paradigm as it applies to ANNs. Roughly speaking, if a large enough sample of randomly drawn training examples is presented, then it should be likely that, after learning, the neural network will classify most other randomly drawn examples correctly. The PAC model formalizes the terms "likely" and "most." The two main issues in PAC learning theory are how many training examples should be presented, and whether learning can be achieved using a fast algorithm. These are known, respectively, as the *sample complexity* and *computational complexity* problems. PAC learning makes use of the Vapnik-Chervonenkis dimension (VC-dimension) as a combinatorial parameter that measures the "expressive power" of a family of functions. This parameter is described more fully in VAPNIK-CHERVONENKIS DIMENSION OF NEURAL NETWORKS. Bounds for the VC-dimension of a neural net **N** provide estimates for the number of random examples that are needed to train **N** so that it has good generalization properties (i.e., so that the error of **N** on new examples from the same distribution is very small, with probability very close to 1). Typically, the VC-dimension for a class of networks grows polynomially (in many cases, between linearly and quadratically) with the number of adjustable parameters of the neural network. In particular, if the number of training examples is large compared to the VC-dimension, the network's performance on training data is a reliable indication of its future performance on subsequent data. The bounds on training set size tend to be large, since they provide generalization guarantees simultaneously for any probability distribution on the examples and for any learning algorithm that minimizes disagreement on the training examples. Tighter bounds are available for some special distributions and specific training algorithms. This theme is further developed in LEARNING AND GENERALIZATION: THEORETICAL BOUNDS in relation to three learning problems: pattern recognition, regression estimation, and density estimation. Because of the looseness of its bounds as well as the difficulty of evaluating them, VC theory was until recently largely neglected by practitioners. This has changed markedly with the development of support vector machines. Using nonlinear similarity measures, referred to as kernels, one can reduce a large class of learning algorithms to linear algorithms in an associated feature space. For the linear algorithms, a VC analysis can be carried out, identifying precisely the factors that need to be controlled to achieve high generalization ability in a variety of learning tasks. "Support Vector Machines" casts these factors into a convex optimization framework, leading to efficient and mathematically well-founded algorithms that have been shown to produce state-of-the-art results on a large variety of problems.

II.7. Sensory Systems

Vision

The topic of **Vision** has provided one of the most fertile fields of investigation both for brain theorists and for technologists constructing ANNs. Six articles in the road map **Mammalian Brain Regions**—RETINA, COLLICULAR VISUOMOTOR TRANSFORMATIONS FOR GAZE CONTROL, "Thalamus," VISUAL CORTEX: ANATOMICAL STRUCTURE AND MODELS OF FUNCTION, and VISUAL SCENE PERCEPTION—introduce various brain regions associated with vision. It is important to emphasize the role of "active vision" in gaining information relevant for animals and robots considered as real-time perception-action systems. This is a theme that is further developed in the road maps **Neuroethology and Evolution** and **Mammalian Motor Control**. Nonetheless, many articles in the present road map will analyze vision as the process of discovering from images what is present in the world: we may see active vision as more like the mode of vision employed by the "where/ how" system described in VISUAL SCENE PERCEPTION, whereas "passive" vision may be closer to the role of the "what" pathway. DISSOCIATIONS BETWEEN VISUAL PROCESSING MODES explores the notion that the visual system has two kinds of jobs to do. One is to support visual cognition, the other is to drive visually guided behavior. Qualitative information about location may be adequate for cognition, but the sensorimotor function needs quantitative egocentrically calibrated spatial information to guide motor acts. The article reviews evidence from neurophysiology, neurological analysis of patients, and psychophysics that the two systems should be modeled as separate maps of visual space rather than as a single visual representation with two readouts. Moreover, spatial information can flow from the cognitive to the sensorimotor representation, but not in the other direction.

However, even "passive" vision is not so passive, since attentional mechanisms are constantly moving the eyes to foveate on items of particular relevance to the current interests of the organism. COLLICULAR VISUOMOTOR TRANSFORMATIONS FOR GAZE CONTROL reviews the role of the superior colliculus in the control of gaze shifts (combined eye-head movements) and its possible involvement in the control of eye movements in 3D space (direction and depth). During attentive fixation, the "Vestibulo-Ocular Reflex" (VOR) and slow vergence maintain binocular foveal fixation to correct for body movements. When the task requires inspection of an eccentric stimulus, a complex synergy of coordinated movements comes into play. Such refixations typically involve a rapid combined eye-head movement (saccadic gaze shift) and often require binocular adjustment in depth (vergence). By virtue of its topographical organization, the superior colliculus has become a key area for experimental and modeling approaches to the question of how sensory signals can be transformed into goal-directed movements. Interestingly, the superior colliculus is not driven by visual input alone. Auditory and somatosensory cues are transformed to register with the visual map in the colliculus for the control of saccades. SENSOR FUSION picks up this theme of ways in which sensory information can be brought together in the brains of diverse

animals (snakes, cats, monkeys, and humans) and surveys biologically inspired technological implementations (such as the use of infrared to enhance vision). PURSUIT EYE MOVEMENTS takes us from saccadic "jumps" to those smooth eye movements involved in following a moving target. Current models of pursuit include "image motion" models, "target velocity" models, and models that address the role of prediction in pursuit. These models make no explicit reference to the neural structures that might be responsible, but the article analyzes the neural pathways for pursuit, stressing the importance of both visual areas of the cerebral cortex and oculomotor regions of the cerebellum.

The RETINA, the outpost of the brain that contains both light-sensitive receptors and several layers of neurons that "preprocess" these responses, transforms visual signals in a multitude of ways to code properties of the visual world such as contrast, color, and motion. The article suggests that much of the retina's signal coding and structural detail is derived from the need to optimally amplify the signal and eliminate noise. But retinal circuitry is diverse. The exact details are probably related to the ecological niche occupied by the organism. In mammals, the retinal output branches into two pathways, the collicular pathway and the geniculostriate pathway. The destination of the former is the midbrain region known as the superior colliculus, discussed above. VISUAL CORTEX: ANATOMICAL STRUCTURE AND MODELS OF FUNCTION reviews features of the microcircuitry of the target of the geniculostriate pathway, the primary visual cortex (area V1), and discusses the physiological properties of cells in its different laminae. It then outlines several hypotheses as to how the anatomical structure and connections might serve the functional organization of the region. For example, a connectionist model of layer IVc of V1 demonstrated that the gradient of change in properties of the layer could indeed be replicated using dendritic overlap through the lower two-thirds of the IVc layer. However, it was insufficient to explain the continuous and sharply increasing field size and contrast sensitivity observable near the top of the layer. The article shows how this discrepancy led to new experiments and related changes in the model which resulted in a good replication of the actual physiological data and required only feedforward excitation. The article goes on to analyze the anatomical substrates for orientation specificity and for surround modulation of visual responses, and concludes by discussing the origins of patterned anatomical connections. OCULAR DOMINANCE AND ORIENTATION COLUMNS discusses further properties of cells in layer IVc of V1. When these cells are tested to see which eye drives them more strongly, it is found that ocular dominance takes the form of a zebra-stripe-like pattern of alternating dominance. Within this high-level organization are "hypercolumns" devoted to a particular retinotopic region of visual space, each hypercolumn being further refined into columns whose cells are best responsive to edges of the same specific orientation. The article also presents models for how these structures might form through self-organization during development. The article reviews data on the orientation specificity of cells of V1 and their columnar organization, and offers models for the way in which development may yield such features of cortical structure. GABOR WAVELETS AND STATISTICAL PATTERN RECOGNITION shows how the response properties of many cells in primary visual cortex may be better described by what are called "Gabor wavelets" than as simple edge detectors. Each Gabor wavelet responds best to patterns of a given spatial frequency and orientation within a given neighborhood. The article relates this notion to both biology and technology. The detection of edge information from within a visual scene is an essential component of visual processing. This processing is believed to be initiated in the primary visual cortex, where individual neurons are known to act as feature detectors of the orientation of edges within the visual scene. Individual neurons can have an *orientation preference* (which states that neuron's preferred orientation of the angle of edges) and *orientation selectivity* (which measures the neuron's sensitivity as a detector of orientation). ORIENTATION SELECTIVITY focuses on mechanisms of orientation selectivity in the visual cortex, arguing that the orientation preference of each neuron and the orderly orientation preference map in cortex are likely to be consequences of a pattern of feedforward convergence. However, the selectivity observed in steady-state and orientation dynamics experiments cannot be achieved by a purely feedforward model. Corticocortical inhibition is a crucial ingredient in the emergence of orientation selectivity in the visual cortex, while the relative importance of corticocortical excitation in enhancing orientation selectivity is still under investigation but appears to be more significant for the function of complex cells than for simple cells in V1. Moving beyond the orientation features of primary visual cortex, INFORMATION THEORY AND VISUAL PLASTICITY demonstrates some aspects of information theory that are relevant to relaying information in cortex and connects entropy-based methods, projection pursuit, and extraction of simple cells in visual cortex. FEATURE ANALYSIS offers a more general view of the characterization of visual features based on the redundancy of the visual signal and the transformation of the signal as it passes along the visual pathway. Describing a particular cell as an "*x* detector" implies that the cell responds when and only when that particular feature is present (e.g., an edge detector responds only in the presence of an edge), but the article argues that describing cells in the early visual system as "detectors" of any type of feature is misleading. Features are useful for describing natural images because the latter have massive informational redundancy. Image space itself is too vast to search directly. Feature analysis depends on the proposition that the search for particular objects can be concentrated in a subspace of image space, the feature space. Localized receptive fields in primary visual cortex provide the primitive basis set for the feature space of vision. These form the basis for the elaboration of neurons responding selectively to geometrical features in area TE of the inferotemporal cortex (IT), and these in turn from the basis for object recognition in different but overlapping areas of IT.

Given that cells in the early stages of the visual system, at least, provide a distributed (more or less retinotopic) set of "features" (in some suitably general sense, given the above caution, of patterns that yield the best response rather than patterns that yield the only response), the issue arises of how those features that correspond to a single object in the visual scene are bound together. CONTOUR AND SURFACE PERCEPTION introduces parallel interacting subsystems that follow complementary processing strategies. Boundary formation proceeds by spatially linking oriented contrast measures along smooth contour patterns, while perceptual surface attributes, such as lightness or texture, are derived from local ratio measures of image contrast of regions lying within contours. Mechanisms of both subsystems mutually interact to resolve initial ambiguities and to generate coherent representations of surface layout. Representations of intrinsic scene characteristics are constrained in terms of the consistency of the set of solutions, which often involve smoothness assumptions for correlated feature estimates. These consistency constraints are typically based on the laws of physical image generation. The article reviews fundamental approaches to computation of intrinsic scene characteristics and various neural models of boundary and surface computation. Each model involves lateral propagation of signals to interpolate and smooth sparse estimates.

ADAPTIVE RESONANCE THEORY (ART) bases learning on internal expectations. A pattern matching process (both for visual patterns and in other domains) compares an external input with the internal memory code for various patterns. ART matching leads either to a *resonant* state, which persists long enough to permit learning, or to a parallel memory search. If the search ends at an established code, the memory representation may either remain the same or incorporate new information from matched portions of the current input. When the external world fails to match an ART network's expectations or predictions, a search process selects a new category, representing a new hypothesis about what is important in the present environment. LAMINAR CORTICAL ARCHITECTURE IN VISUAL PERCEPTION uses the LAMINART model (an extension of ART) to propose functional roles for cortical layers in visual perception. Neocortex has an intricate design that exhibits a characteristic organization into six distinct cortical layers, but few models have addressed the functional utility of the laminar organization itself in the control of behavior. LAMINART integrates data about visual perception and neuroscience for such processes as preattentive grouping and attention. It is suggested that the functional roles for cortical layers proposed here—binding together distributed cortical data through a combination of bottom-up adaptive filtering and horizontal associations, and modulating it with top-down attention—generalize, with appropriate specializations, to other forms of sensory and cognitive processing.

CORTICAL POPULATION DYNAMICS AND PSYCHOPHYSICS models cortical population dynamics to explain dynamical properties of the primate visual system on different levels, reaching from single neuron properties like selectivity for the orientation of a stimulus up to higher cognitive functions related to the binding and processing of stimulus features in psychophysical discrimination experiments. On the other hand, SYNCHRONIZATION, BINDING AND EXPECTANCY argues that the "binding" of cells that correspond to a given visual object may exploit another dimension of cellular firing, namely, the phase at which a cell fires within some overall rhythm of firing. The article presents data consistent with the proposal that the synchronization of responses on a time scale of milliseconds provides an efficient mechanism for response selection and binding of population responses. Synchronization also increases the saliency of responses because it allows for effective spatial summation in the population of neurons receiving convergent input from synchronized input cells. VISUAL SCENE SEGMENTATION tackles the segmentation of a visual scene into a set of coherent patterns corresponding to objects. Objects appear in a natural scene as the grouping of similar sensory features and the segregation of dissimilar ones. Studies in visual perception, in particular *Gestalt* psychology, have uncovered a number of principles for perceptual organization, such as proximity, similarity, connectedness, and relatedness in memory. Scene segmentation requires neural networks to address the binding problem. The temporal correlation approach is to encode the binding by the correlation of temporal activities of feature-detecting cells. A special form of temporal correlation is *oscillatory correlation*, where the basic units are neural oscillators. The article first reviews non-oscillatory approaches in scene segmentation, and then turns to oscillatory approaches. The temporal correlation approach is further developed in DYNAMIC LINK ARCHITECTURE, which views the brain's data structure as a graph composed of nodes connected by links, where both units and links bear activity variables changing on the rapid time scale of fractions of a second. The nodes play the role of symbolic elements. Dynamic links constitute the glue by which higher data structures are built up from more elementary ones.

Beyond the basic issue of how the visual scene is segmented (how visual elements are grouped) into possibly meaningful wholes lies the question of determining for a region so determined its color, motion, distance, shape, etc. These issues are addressed in the next set of articles. COLOR PERCEPTION stresses that color is not a local property inferred from the wavelength of light hitting a patch of retina but is a property of regions of space that depends both on the light they reflect and on the surrounding context. Our visual system "recreates" the world in the form of boundaries that contain surfaces, and color perception involves the perception of aspects of these surfaces. Matching surfaces with the same reflectance properties in different parts of the visual scene or under different illuminants are the two problems of color constancy. In addition, wavelength signals can be used in the course of perceiving form or motion independent of their role in the subjective experience of color. DIRECTIONAL SELECTIVITY first reviews models of retinal direction selectivity (which contributes to oculomotor responses rather than motion perception). Older models depend on the way in which amacrine and other cells of the retina are connected to the ganglion cells, the retinal output cells. A newer model is based on the directionality of synaptic interactions on the dendrites of amacrine cells, involving a spatial asymmetry in the inputs and outputs of a dendrodendritic synapse, and its shunting inhibition. It is argued that development of this latter mechanism might involve Hebbian processes driven by spontaneous activity and light. Cortical directional selectivity (which does contribute to motion perception as well as the control of eye movements) involves many cortical regions. Directionally sensitive cells in primary visual cortex (V1) project to middle temporal cortex (MT) where directional selectivity becomes more complex, MT cells typically having larger receptive fields. From MT, the motion pathway projects to middle superior temporal cortex. Cortical directional selectivity has been modeled in three manners: as a spatially asymmetric excitatory drive followed by multiplication or squaring, via a spatially asymmetric nonlinear inhibitory drive, and through a spatially asymmetric linear inhibitory drive followed by positive feedback. This selectivity might involve Hebbian processes driven by spontaneous activity and binocular interactions. The issues in this article have some overlap with those presented in MOTION PERCEPTION: ELEMENTARY MECHANISMS, which emphasizes measurement of the direction and speed of movement of features in the 2D image linking successive views to infer *optic flow*, which is the pattern of image velocities that is projected onto the retina. The article discusses the cortical correlates of these various representations. MOTION PERCEPTION: NAVIGATION shows how, when an observer moves through the world, the optic flow can inform him about his own motion through space and about the 3D structure and motion of objects in the scene. This information is essential for tasks such as the visual guidance of locomotion through the environment and the manipulation and recognition of objects. This article focuses on the recovery of observer motion from optic flow. It includes strategies for detecting moving objects and avoiding collisions, discusses how optic flow may be used to control actions, and describes the neural mechanisms underlying heading perception. GLOBAL VISUAL PATTERN EXTRACTION continues the study of neural mechanisms which mediate between the extraction of local edge and contour information by orientation-selective simple cells in primary visual cortex (V1) and the high levels of cortical form vision in inferior temporal cortex (IT), where many neurons are sensitive to complex global patterns, including objects and faces. The ventral form vision pathway includes at least areas V1, V2, V4, TEO, and TE (the highest level of IT), raising the question of what processes occur at these intervening stages to transform local V1 orientation information into global pattern representations. Essentially the same question may be posed in cortical motion processing along the dorsal pathway comprising V1, V2, MT, MST, and higher parietal areas. V1 neurons extract only local motion vectors perpendicular to moving edge segments, while MST neurons are sensitive to complex optic flow patterns, including expansion. This article suggests answers to these analogous questions about transitions from local to global processing in both motion and form vision by focusing on intermediate levels of these two pathways, mainly V4 and MST.

PERCEPTION OF THREE-DIMENSIONAL STRUCTURE reviews various computational models for inferring an object's 3D structure from different types of optical information, such as shading, texture, motion, and stereo, and examines how the performance of these models compares with the capabilities and limitations of human observers in judging different aspects of 3D structure under varying viewing conditions. In particular, stereoscopic vision exploits the fact that points in a 3D scene will in general project to different positions in the images formed in the left and right eyes. The differences in these positions are termed *disparities*. The stereo *correspondence problem* is to identify which points in a pair of stereo images correspond to a single point in 3D space. Solving this problem allows the stereo pair to be mapped into a single representation, called a disparity map, that makes explicit the disparities of various points common to both images, thus revealing the distance of various visual elements from the observer. Depth perception is then completed by determining depth values for all points in the images. STEREO CORRESPONDENCE notes that various constraints have been used to help determine which features on the two eyes should be matched in inferring depth. These include compatibility of matching primitives, cohesivity, uniqueness, figural continuity, and the ordering constraint. Various neural network stereo correspondence algorithms are then reviewed, and the problems of surface discontinuities and uncorrelated points, and of transparency, are addressed. The article also reviews neurophysiological studies of disparity mechanisms.

A more abstract approach to the correspondence problem, from the perspective of computer vision rather than psychology or neurophysiology, is offered in TENSOR VOTING AND VISUAL SEGMENTATION. In 3D, as we have seen, surfaces are inferred from binocular images by obtaining depth hypotheses for points and/or edges. In image sequence analysis, the estimation of motion and shape starts with local measurements of feature correspondences, which gives noisy data for the subsequent computation of scene information. Hence, any salient structure estimator must be able to handle the presence of multiple structures and their interaction in the presence of noisy data. This article analyzes approaches to address early to midlevel vision problems, emphasizing the tensor voting methodology for the robust inference of multiple salient structures such as junctions, curves, regions, and surfaces from any combination of points, curve elements, and surface patch element inputs in 2D and 3D. The article describes two regularization formalisms, one that imposes certain physical constraints so that the search space can be constrained and algorithmically tractable, and another using a Bayesian formalism to transform an ill-posed problem into one of functional optimization.

PROBABILISTIC REGULARIZATION METHODS FOR LOW-LEVEL VISION offers regularization theory (cf. "Generalization and Regularization in Nonlinear Learning Systems") as a general mathematical framework to deal with the fact that the problem of inferring 3D structure from 2D images is *ill-posed*: there are many spatial configurations compatible with a given 2D image or set (motion sequence, stereo pair, etc.) of images. The issue then becomes to find which spatial configuration is most probable. We have already seen a number of constraints associated with stereo vision. Deterministic regularization theory defines a "cost function," which combines a measure of how close a spatial configuration comes to yielding the given image (set) with a measure of the extent to which the configuration violates the constraints, and then seeks that configuration which minimizes this cost. The present article emphasizes a more general probabilistic approach in which the "actual" field f and the observed field g are considered as realizations of random fields, with the reconstruction of f understood as an estimation problem. MARKOV RANDOM FIELD MODELS IN IMAGE PROCESSING views the task of image modeling as being one of finding an adequate representation of the intensity distribution of a given image. What is adequate often depends on the task at hand. The general properties of the local spatiotemporal structure of images or image sequences are characterized by a Markov random field (MRF) in which the probability distribution for the image intensity and a further set of other attributes (edges, texture, and region labels) at a particular location are conditioned on values in a neighborhood of pixels (picture elements or image points). The observed quantities are usually noisy, blurred images. The article presents five steps of MRF image modeling within a Bayesian estimation/inference paradigm, and provides a number of examples. Particular attention is paid to maximum a posteriori (MAP) estimates. MRF image models have proved versatile enough to be applied to image and texture synthesis, image restoration, flow field segmentation, and surface reconstruction.

KALMAN FILTERING: NEURAL IMPLICATIONS introduces Kalman filtering, which, under linear and Gaussian conditions, produces a recursive estimate of the hidden state of a dynamic system, i.e., one that is updated with each subsequent (noisy) measurement of the observed system. The article shows how Kalman filtering provides insight into visual recognition and the role of the cerebellum in motor control. In particular, it presents a hierarchically organized neural network for visual recognition, with each intermediate level of the hierarchy receiving two kinds of information: bottom-up information from the preceding level, and top-down information from the higher level. For its implementation, the model uses a multiscale estimation algorithm that may be viewed as a hierarchical form of the extended Kalman filter that is used to simultaneously learn the feedforward, feedback, and prediction parameters of the model on the basis of visual experiences in a dynamic environment. The resulting adaptive process involves a fast dynamic state-estimation process that allows the dynamic model to anticipate incoming stimuli, as well as a slow Hebbian learning process that provides for synaptic weight adjustments in the model.

IMAGING THE VISUAL BRAIN addresses functional brain imaging of visual processes, with emphasis on limits in spatial and temporal resolution, constraints on subject participation, and trade-offs in experimental design. The articles focuses on retinotopy, visual motion perception and visual object representation, and voluntary modulation of attention and visual imagery, emphasizing some of the areas where modeling and brain theory might be testable using current imaging tools. VISUAL ATTENTION offers data and hypotheses for cortical mechanisms to overtly and covertly shift attention (i.e., with and without eye movements). Attention guides where to look next based on both bottom-up (image-based) and top-down (task-dependent) cues—and indeed, the anatomy of the visual system includes extensive feedback connections from later stages and horizontal connections within each layer. Vision appears to rely on sophisticated interactions between coarse, massively parallel, full-field preattentive analysis systems and the more detailed, circumscribed, and sequential attentional analysis system. The articles focus on the brain area involved in visual attention and then analyzes a variety of relevant mechanisms. Yet, having stressed the way in which we normally take a number of shifts of attention to fully take in the details of a visual scene, it is intriguing to learn how much can be absorbed in a single fixation. FAST VISUAL PROCESSING notes that much information can be extracted from briefly glimpsed scenes, even at presentation rates of around 10 frames/s, a technique known as rapid sequential visual presentation (RSVP). Since interspike intervals for neurons are seldom shorter than 5 ms, the underlying algorithms should involve no more than about 20 sequential, though massively parallel, steps. There is an important distinction in neural computation between feedforward processing models and those with recurrent connections that allow feedback and iterative processing. Pure feedforward models (e.g., multilayer perceptrons, MLPs) can operate very quickly in parallel hardware. The article argues that even in systems that use extensive recurrent connections, the fastest behavioral responses may essentially depend on a single feedforward processing wave. It looks at how detailed measurements of processing speed can be combined with

anatomical and physiological constraints to constrain models of how the brain performs such computations.

There is a vast literature on pattern recognition in neural networks (see, for example, "Pattern Recognition" and "Concept Learning"). Here we discuss articles on face recognition and object recognition. The recognition of other individuals, and in particular the recognition of faces, is a major prerequisite for human social interaction and indeed has been shown to employ specific brain mechanisms. The ability to recognize people from their faces is part of a spectrum of related skills that include face segmentation (i.e., finding faces in a scene or image) and estimation of the pose, direction of gaze, and the person's emotional state. FACE RECOGNITION: NEUROPHYSIOLOGY AND NEURAL TECHNOLOGY starts with a review of relevant neurophysiology. Brain injury can lead to prosopagnosia, the loss of ability to recognize individual faces, while leaving intact the ability to recognize general objects. Single-unit recordings in the IT cortex of macaque monkeys have revealed neurons with a high responsiveness to the presence of a face, an individual, or the expression on the face, and neural models for face recognition are reviewed in relation to such data. The article then focuses on computational theories that are inspired by neural ideas (see DYNAMIC LINK ARCHITECTURE; GABOR WAVELETS AND STATISTICAL PATTERN RECOGNITION) but that find their justification in the construction of successful computer systems for the recognition of human faces even when the gallery of possible faces is very large indeed. FACE RECOGNITION: PSYCHOLOGY AND CONNECTIONISM provides a brief history of connectionist approaches to face recognition and surveys the broad range of tasks to which these models have been applied. The article relates the models to psychological theories for the subtasks of representing faces and retrieving them from memory, comparing human and model performance along these dimensions.

OBJECT RECOGNITION focuses on models of viewpoint-invariant object recognition that are constrained by psychological data on human object recognition. It present three main approaches to object recognition—invariant based, model based, and appearance based—and analyzes the strengths of each of these in a framework of decision complexity, noting the trade-off between representations that emphasize invariance and those designed for discriminability. The analysis shows that it is unlikely for a single form of representation to satisfy all kinds of object recognition tasks a human or other visual animal may encounter. The article thus argues that a key ingredient in a comprehensive brain theory for object recognition is a computational framework that allows on-demand selection or adaptation of representations based on the current task and proposes a simple "first past the post" scheme (a temporal winner-take-all scheme) for self-selecting the most appropriate level of abstraction, given a finite set of available representations along a visual processing pathway.

OBJECT STRUCTURE, VISUAL PROCESSING emphasizes structure-processing tasks that call for separate treatment of various fragments of the visual stimulus, each of which spans only a fraction of the visual extent of the object or scene under consideration. Examples of structural tasks include recognition of part-part similarities, and identifying a region in an object toward which an action can be directed. After discussing object form processing in computer vision and relevant neurophysiological data on primate vision, the article focuses on two neuromorphic models of visual structure processing. The JIM model implements a recognition-by-components scenario based on geons ("geometrical elements," which are generalized cylinders formed by moving a cross-section along a possibly curved axis). The Chorus of Fragments model exploits both the "what" and the "where" streams of visual cortex to recognize fragments no matter what their position, but then uses their approximate spatial relationships to see whether they together form cues for the recognition of an object. In particular, then, it avoids the binding problem of explicitly linking neural activity related to a specific object as a prerequisite to analysis of that object's characteristics. (By contrast, SYNCHRONIZATION, BINDING AND EXPECTANCY argues that the brain does solve the binding problem, and does so by synchronization of neural firing for those neurons related to a single object.)

OBJECT RECOGNITION, NEUROPHYSIOLOGY reviews some theoretical approaches to object recognition in the context of mainly neurophysiological evidence. It also considers briefly the analysis of visual scenes. Scene analysis is relevant to object recognition because scenes may themselves be recognized initially at a holistic, object-like level, providing a context or "gist" that influences the speed and accuracy of recognition of the constituent objects. The article proposes that object recognition is based on a distributed, view-based representation in which objects are recognized on the basis of multiple, 2D-feature-selective neurons. Specialist cells appear to play a role in associating such feature combinations into certain nontrivial image transformations, coding for a certain percentage of all stimuli in a largely view-invariant manner. The article offers evidence that a convergent hierarchy is used to build invariant representations over several stages, and that at each stage lateral competitive processes are at work between the neurons. It is argued that the association of views of objects observed over the course of time could play a key role in building up object representations. The review focuses mainly on the "what" stream of IT cortex, seen as the center of object recognition. VISUAL SCENE PERCEPTION also brings in the "where/how" stream of parietal cortex as it analyzes how mechanisms that integrate schemas for recognition of different objects into the perception of some overall scene may be linked to the distributed planning of action. It also presents recent neurophysiology suggesting how the context of a natural scene may modify the response properties of neurons responsive to visual features. The article compares three approaches—the slide-box metaphor, short-term memory in the VISIONS system, and the visuospatial scratchpad—for creating a theory of how the visual perception of objects may be integrated with the perception of spatial layout. The first two stress a schema-theoretic approach, while the latter is strongly tied to visual neurophysiology and modeling in terms of quasi-neural attractor networks. The aim is to open the way to future research that will embed the study of visual scene perception in an action-oriented integration of IT and parietal visual systems.

Other Sensory Systems

AUDITORY CORTEX
AUDITORY PERIPHERY AND COCHLEAR NUCLEUS
AUDITORY SCENE ANALYSIS
ECHOLOCATION: COCHLEOTOPIC AND COMPUTATIONAL MAPS
ELECTROLOCATION
OLFACTORY BULB
OLFACTORY CORTEX
PAIN NETWORKS
PROSTHETICS, SENSORY SYSTEMS
SENSOR FUSION
SOMATOSENSORY SYSTEM
SOMATOTOPY: PLASTICITY OF SENSORY MAPS
SOUND LOCALIZATION AND BINAURAL PROCESSING

Here we analyze sensory systems other than vision—e.g., touch, audition, and pain. Moreover, when one sense cannot provide all the necessary information, complementary observations may be provided by another sense. For example, touch complements vision in placing a peg in a hole when the effector occludes the agent's view. Also, senses may offer competing observations, such as the competition between vision and the vestibular system in maintain-

ing balance (and its occasional side effect of seasickness). Another type of interplay between the senses is the use of information extracted by one sense to focus the attention of another sense, coordinating the two, as in audition cueing vision. SENSOR FUSION explores a number of ways sensory information is brought together in the brains of diverse animals (snakes, cats, monkeys, humans) and surveys biologically inspired technological implementations (such as the use of infrared to enhance vision). (See also "Collicular Visuomotor Transformations for Gaze Control" for an important example of sensor fusion—the transformation of auditory and somatosensory cues into a visual map for the control of rapid eye movements.)

The road map **Mammalian Brain Regions** introduced a number of regions linked to sensory systems other than vision, but we will now meet a number of related and additional topics as well. SOMATOSENSORY SYSTEM shows how the somatosensory system changes the tactile stimulus representation from a form more or less isomorphic to the stimulus to a completely distributed form in a series of partial transformations in successive subcortical and cortical networks. It further argues that the causal factors involved in body/object interactions are explicitly represented by an internal model in the pyramidal cells of somatosensory cortex that is crucial for haptic perception of proximal surroundings and for control of object manipulation. Somatotopy, a dominant feature of subdivisions of the somatosensory system, is defined by a topographic representation, or map, in the brain of sensory receptors on the body surface. SOMATOTOPY: PLASTICITY OF SENSORY MAPS shows that these orderly representations of cutaneous receptors in the spinal cord, lower brainstem, thalamus, and neocortex represent both the peripheral distribution of receptors and dynamic aspects of brain function. The article reviews evidence for somatosensory plasticity involving cortical reorganization after peripheral injury and as a result of training. The article analyzes the features of somatotopic maps that change, the contribution of subcortical changes to cortical plasticity, the mechanisms involved, and the functional consequences of sensory map changes. An important issue is the relation between the plasticity of the sensory and motor systems.

PAIN NETWORKS adds a new dimension to bodily sensation. The pain system encodes information on the intensity, location, and dynamics of tissue-threatening stimuli but differs from other sensory systems in its "emotional-motivational" factors (see also "Motivation"). In the pain system, these factors strongly modulate the relation between stimulus and felt response. At one extreme is allodynia, a state in which the slightest touch with a cotton wisp is agonizing. People display wide individual and trial-to-trial variability in the amount of pain reported following administration of calibrated noxious stimuli; pain sensation is subject to ongoing modulation by a complex of extrinsic (stimulus-generated) and intrinsic (CNS-generated) state variables. The article spells out how these act in the CNS as well as the periphery.

AUDITORY PERIPHERY AND COCHLEAR NUCLEUS spells out how the auditory periphery parcels out acoustic stimulus across hundreds of nerve fibers, and how the cochlear nucleus continues this process by creating multiple representations of the original acoustic stimulus. The article emphasizes monaural signal processing, whereas SOUND LOCALIZATION AND BINAURAL PROCESSING shows how information from the two ears is brought together. The article focuses on the use of interaural time difference (ITD) as one way to estimate the azimuthal angle of a sound source. It describes one biological model (ITD detection in the barn owl's brainstem) and two psychological models. The underlying idea is that the brain attempts to match the sounds in the two ears by shifting one sound relative to the other, with the shift that produces the best match assumed to be the one that just balances the "real" ITD. AUDITORY CORTEX stresses the crucial role that auditory cortex plays in the perception and localization of complex sounds, examining auditory tasks vital for all mammals, such as sound localization, timbre recognition, and pitch perception. AUDITORY SCENE ANALYSIS discusses how the auditory system parses the acoustic mixture that reaches the ears of an animal to segregate a targeted sound source from the background of other sounds. The first stage, segmentation, decomposes the acoustic mixture into its constituent components. In the second stage, acoustic components that are likely to have arisen from the same environmental event are grouped, forming a perceptual representation (stream) that describes a single sound source. At the physiological level, segmentation corresponds (at least in part) to peripheral auditory processing, which performs a frequency analysis of the acoustic input, whereas the physiological substrate of auditory grouping is much less well understood. The article focuses on models that are at least physiologically plausible, while noting that other models of auditory scene analysis adopt a more abstract information processing perspective.

ECHOLOCATION: COCHLEOTOPIC AND COMPUTATIONAL MAPS provides us with a more detailed understanding of the auditory system in a very special class of mammals, the bats. Mustached bats emit echolocation (ultrasonic) pulses for navigation and for hunting flying insects. On the basis of the echo, prey must be detected and distinguished from the background clutter of vegetation, characterized as appropriate for consumption, and localized in space for orientation and prey capture. The bats emit ultrasonic pulses that consist of a long constant-frequency component followed by a short frequency-modulated component. Each pulse-echo combination provides a discrete sample of the continuously changing auditory scene. The auditory network contains two key design features: neurons that are sensitive to combinations of pulse and echo components, and computational maps that represent systematic changes in echo parameters to extract the relevant information.

Electrolocation is another sense that helps the animal locate itself in its world, but this time the animals are electric fishes rather than bats, and the signals are electrical rather than auditory. ELECTROLOCATION relates its topic to the general issue of mechanisms that facilitate the processing of relevant signals while rejecting noise, and of attentional processes that select which stimuli are to be attended to. Weakly electric fish generate an electrical field around their body and measure this field via electroreceptors embedded in the skin to "electrolocate" animate or inanimate targets in the environment. The article emphasizes a widespread but poorly understood characteristic of sensory processing circuits, namely, the presence of massive descending or feedback connections by which higher centers presumably modulate the operation of lower centers. Not only are response gain and receptive field

organization controlled by these descending connections, but there are adaptive filtering mechanisms that can reject stimuli that otherwise might mask critical functions. This use of stored sensory expectations for the cancellation or perhaps the identification of specific input patterns may yield insights into diverse neural circuits, including the cochlear nuclei and the cerebellum, in other species.

Two articles introduce data and models for the olfactory system (see also the road map **Mammalian Brain Regions**). OLFACTORY BULB describes the special circuitry involved in basic preprocessing, while OLFACTORY CORTEX presents a dynamical systems analysis of further olfactory processing. The olfactory bulb receives input from the sensory neurons in the olfactory epithelium and sends its outputs to the olfactory cortex, among other brain regions. The bulb was one of the first regions of the brain for which compartmental models of neurons were constructed, which led to some of the first computational models of functional microcircuits. OLFACTORY BULB gives an overview of olfactory bulb cells and circuits, current ideas about the computational functions of the bulb, and modeling studies to investigate these functions. The olfactory cortex is defined as the region of the cerebral cortex that receives direct connections from the olfactory bulb. It is the earliest cortical region to differentiate in the evolution of the vertebrate forebrain and the only region within the forebrain to receive direct sensory input. Moreover, the olfactory cortex has the simplest organization among the main types of cerebral cortex. OLFACTORY CORTEX thus views it as a model for understanding basic principles underlying cortical organization.

Finally, a very different view of sensory systems is provided by PROSTHETICS, SENSORY SYSTEMS, which discusses how information collected by electronic sensors may be delivered directly to the nervous system by electrical stimulation. After assessing the amenability of all sensory modalities (hearing, vision, touch, proprioception, balance, smell, and taste), the article focuses on auditory and visual prostheses. The great success story has been with cochlear implants. Here the article reviews improved temporospatial representations of speech sounds, combined electrical and acoustic stimulation in patients with residual hearing, and psychophysical correlates of performance variability. Since a prosthesis does not necessarily match natural neural encoding of a stimulus, the success of the prosthesis depends in part on the plasticity of the human brain as it remaps to accommodate this new class of signals. For example, the success of cochlear implants rests in part on the ability of auditory cortex to remap itself in a similar fashion to the remapping of somatosensory cortex described in SOMATOTOPY: PLASTICITY OF SENSORY MAPS.

II.8. Motor Systems

Robotics and Control Theory

ARM AND HAND MOVEMENT CONTROL
BIOLOGICALLY INSPIRED ROBOTICS
IDENTIFICATION AND CONTROL
MOTOR CONTROL, BIOLOGICAL AND THEORETICAL
POTENTIAL FIELDS AND NEURAL NETWORKS
Q-LEARNING FOR ROBOTS
REACTIVE ROBOTIC SYSTEMS
REINFORCEMENT LEARNING IN MOTOR CONTROL
ROBOT ARM CONTROL
ROBOT LEARNING

ROBOT NAVIGATION
SENSORIMOTOR LEARNING

As noted in the "Historical Fragment" section of Part I, the interchange between biology and technology that characterizes the study of neural networks is an outgrowth of work in *cybernetics* in the 1940s. One of the keys to cybernetics was control (the other was communication of the kind studied in information theory). It is thus appropriate that control theory should have become a major application area for neural networks as well as being a key concept of brain theory. The objective of control is to influence the behavior of a dynamical system in some desired fashion. The latter includes maintaining the outputs of systems at constant values (regulation) or forcing them to follow prescribed time functions (tracking). Maintaining the altitude of an aircraft or the glucose level in the blood at constant values are examples of regulation; controlling a rocket to follow a given trajectory is an example of tracking. MOTOR CONTROL, BIOLOGICAL AND THEORETICAL sets forth the basic cybernetic concepts. A motor control system acts by sending motor commands to a controlled object, often referred to as "the plant," which in turn acts on the local environment. The plant or the environment has one or more variables which the controller attempts to regulate. If the controller bases its actions on signals which are not affected by the plant output, it is said to be a feedforward controller. If the controller bases its actions on a comparison between desired behavior and the controlled variables, it is a feedback controller. "Motor Pattern Generation" provides a related perspective (see the road map **Motor Pattern Generators**).

The major advantage of negative feedback control, in which the controller seeks constantly to cancel the feedback error, is that it is a very simple, robust strategy that operates well without exact knowledge of the controlled object, and despite internal or external disturbances. The advantage of feedforward control is that it can, in the ideal case, give perfect performance with no error between the reference and the controlled variable. The main disadvantages are the practical difficulties in developing an accurate controller, and the lack of corrections for unexpected disturbances. IDENTIFICATION AND CONTROL explores the major strategy for developing an accurate controller, namely to "identify" the plant as belonging to (or more precisely, being well approximated by) a system obtained from a general family of systems by setting a key set of parameters (e.g., the coefficients in the matrices of a linear system). By coupling a controller to an identification procedure, one obtains an adaptive controller that can handle an unknown plant even if its dynamics are (slowly) changing. In both biology and many technological applications, nonlinearities and uncertainties play a major role, and linear approximations are not satisfactory. The article presents research using neural networks to handle these nonlinearities and examines the theoretical assumptions that have to be made when such networks are used as identifiers and controllers.

REINFORCEMENT LEARNING IN MOTOR CONTROL recalls the general theory introduced in "Reinforcement Learning" and proceeds to note its utility in motor control. Many motor skills are attained in the absence of explicit feedback about muscle contractions or joint angles. In contrast to supervised learning, such learning depends on "reinforcement" (or evaluative feedback; it need not involve pleasure or pain), which tells the learner whether or not, and possibly by how much, its behavior has improved, or provides an indication of success or failure. Instead of trying to match a standard of correctness, a reinforcement learning system tries to maximize the goodness of behavior as indicated by evaluative feedback. To do this, it has to actively try alternatives, compare the resulting evaluations, and use some kind of selection mechanism to guide behavior toward the better alternatives. Q-LEARNING FOR ROBOTS applies reinforcement learning techniques to robot control. Q-learning does not require a model of the robot-world interaction, and it uses learning examples in the form of triplets (situation, action, Q-value), where the Q-value is the *utility* of executing the action in the situation. Q-learning involves three different functions, *evaluation, memorization,* and *updating*. Heuristically adapted Q-learning has proved successful in applications such as obstacle avoidance, wall following, go-to-the-nest, etc., using neural-based implementations such as multilayer perceptrons trained with backpropagation, or self-organizing maps.

SENSORIMOTOR LEARNING explains how neural nets can acquire "models" of some desired sensorimotor transformation. A *forward model* is a representation of the transformation from motor commands to movements, in other words, a model of the controlled

object. An *inverse model* is a representation of the transformation from desired movements to motor commands, and so can be used as the controller for the controlled object. The managing of multiple models, each with their own range of applicability in given tasks, is given special attention. ROBOT LEARNING focuses on learning robot control, the process of acquiring a sensorimotor control strategy for a particular movement task and movement system. The article offers a formal framework within which to discuss robot learning in terms of the different methods that have been suggested for the learning of control policies, such as learning the control policy directly, learning the control policy in a modular way, indirect learning of control policies, imitation learning, and learning of motor control components. The article also reviews specific function approximation problems in robot learning, including neural network approaches. ROBOT ARM CONTROL addresses related issues concerning the availability of precise mappings from physical space or sensor space to joint space or motor space. Robot arm controllers are usually hierarchically structured from the lowest level of servomotors to the highest levels of trajectory generation and task supervision. In each case an actual motion is made to follow as closely as possible a commanded motion through the use of feedback. The difference lies in the coordinate systems used at each level. At least four coordinate spaces can be distinguished: the task space (used to specify tasks, possibly in terms of sensor readings), the workspace (6D Cartesian coordinates defining a position and orientation of the end-effector), the joint space (intrinsic coordinates determining a robot configuration), and the actuator space (in which actual motions are commanded). Correlational procedures carry out feature discovery or clustering and are often used to represent a given state space in a compact and topology-preserving manner, using procedures such as those described in "Self-Organizing Feature Maps." Error-minimization procedures require explicit data on input-output pairs; their goal is to build a mapping from inputs to outputs that generalizes adequately using, e.g., the least-mean-squares (LMS) rule and backpropagation. In between both extremes lie procedures that use reinforcement learning to build a mapping that maximizes reward. ARM AND HAND MOVEMENT CONTROL discusses some of the most prominent regularities of arm and hand control, and examines computational and neural network models designed to explain them. The analysis reveals an interesting competition between explanations sought on the neural, biomechanical, perceptual, and computational levels that has created its share of controversy. Whereas some topics, such as internal model control, have gained solid grounding, the importance of the dynamic properties of the musculoskeletal system in facilitating motor control, the role of real-time perceptual modulation of motor control, and the balance between dynamical systems models versus optimal control-based models are still seen as offering many open questions.

BIOLOGICALLY INSPIRED ROBOTICS describes how modern robotics may learn from the way organisms are constructed biologically and how this creates adaptive behaviors. (I cannot resist noting here the acronym introduced by R. I. Damper, R. L. B. French, and T. W. Scutt, 2000, ARBIB: An Autonomous Robot Based on Inspiration from Biology, *Robotics and Autonomous Systems*, 31:247–274.) Research on autonomous robots based on inspiration from biology ranges from modeling animal sensors in hardware to guiding robots in target environments to investigating the interaction between neural learning and evolution in a variety of robot tasks. After reviewing the historical roots of the subject, the article provides a general introduction to biologically inspired robotics, with special emphasis on the ideas that the robot is situated in the world and that many complex behaviors are emergent properties of the collective effects of linking a variety of simple behaviors. REACTIVE ROBOTIC SYSTEMS provides a conceptual framework for robotics that is rooted in "Schema Theory" (q.v.) rather than symbolic AI. Here, robot behavior is controlled by the activation of a collection of low-level primitive behaviors (schemas), and complex behavior emerges through the interaction of these schemas and the complexities of the environment in which the robot finds itself. This work was inspired in part by studies of animal behavior (see, e.g., "Neuroethology, Computational" and related articles discussed in the road maps on **Motor Pattern Generators** and **Neuroethology and Evolution**). However, the article not only shows the power of reactive robots in many applications, it also notes the utility of hybrid systems capable of using deliberative reasoning as well as reactive execution (which fits with an evolutionary view of the human brain in which reactive systems handle many functions but can be overruled or orchestrated by, e.g., the deliberative activities of prefrontal cortex).

ROBOT NAVIGATION examines how to get a mobile robot to move to its destination efficiently (e.g., along short trajectories) and safely (i.e., without colliding). If a target location is either visible or identified by a landmark (or sequence of landmarks), a simple stimulus-response strategy can be adopted. However, if targets are not visible, the robot needs a model (or map) of the environment encoding the spatial relationships between its present and desired locations. Sensor uncertainty, together with the inaccuracy of the robot's actuators and the unpredictability of real environments, makes the design of mobile robot controllers a difficult task. It has thus proved desirable to endow robots with learning capabilities in order to acquire autonomously their control system and to adapt their behavior to never experienced situations. The article thus reviews neural approaches to localization, map building, and navigation. More specifically, POTENTIAL FIELDS AND NEURAL NETWORKS examines biological findings on the use of potential fields (which represent, e.g., the force field that drives the motor output of an animal or part of an animal, such as a limb) to characterize the control and learning of motor primitives. The notion of potential fields has also been used to model externally induced constraints as well as internally constructed sensorimotor maps for robot motion control. A robot can reach a stable configuration in its environment by following the negative gradient of its potential field. In this case, the configurations reached will be locally stable but may not be optimal with respect to some behavioral criterion. This deficit can be overcome either by incorporating a global motion planner or by using a harmonic function that does not contain any local minima. The article further indicates how potential field–based motion control can benefit from the use of ANN-based learning. There are links here to the more biological concerns of the articles "Cognitive Maps," "Hippocampus: Spatial Models," and "Motor Primitives."

Motor Pattern Generators

MOTOR PATTERN GENERATION provides an overview of the basic building blocks of behavior (see "Motor Control, Biological and Theoretical" for more general background) to be expanded upon in many of the following articles. The emphasis is on rhythmic behaviors (such as flight or locomotion), but a variety of "one-off" motor patterns (as typified in a frog snapping at its prey) are also studied. The crucial notion is that a central pattern generator (CPG), an autonomous neural circuit, can yield a good "sketch" of a movement, but that the full motor pattern generator (MPG) augments the CPG with sensory input which can adjust the motor pattern to changing circumstances (e.g., the pattern of locomotion varies when going uphill rather than on level terrain, or when the animal carries a heavy load). SENSORIMOTOR INTERACTIONS AND CENTRAL PATTERN GENERATORS discusses both the impact of sensory information on CPGs and the influence of motor systems on sensory activity. It stresses that interaction between motor and sensory systems is pervasive, from the first steps of sensory detection to the highest levels of processing, emphasizing that descending motor commands are only acted upon by spinal circuits when these circuits integrate their intrinsic activity with all incoming information.

COMMAND NEURONS AND COMMAND SYSTEMS analyzes the extent to which an MPG may be activated alone or in concert with others through perceptual stimuli mediated by a single "command neuron" or by more diffuse "command systems." Command functions provide the sensorimotor interface between sensory pattern recognition and localization, on the one side, and motor pattern generation on the other. For example, if a certain interneuron is stimulated electrically in the brain of a marine slug, the animal then displays a species-specific escape swimming behavior, although no predator is present. If in a toad a certain brain area of the optic tectum is stimulated in this manner, snapping behavior is triggered, although no prey is present. In both cases, a stimulus produces a rapid ballistic response.

MOTOR PRIMITIVES and SCRATCH REFLEX look at two behaviors (the former studied in frogs, the latter primarily in turtles) elicited by an irritant applied to the animal's skin. In each case, the position at which the limb is aimed varies with the position of the irritant; there is somatotopic (i.e., based on place on the body) control of the reflex. In both frog and turtle, and thus more generally, spinal cord neural networks can by themselves generate complex sensorimotor transformations even when disconnected from supraspinal structures. Moreover, each reflex has different "modes." To understand this, just think of scratching your lower back. As the scratch site moves higher, the positioning of the limb changes continuously with the position of the irritant until the irritant moves up so much that you make a discontinuous switch to the "over-the-shoulder" mode of back-scratching. The mode changes in these two articles may be compared to the GAIT TRANSITIONS (q.v.), discussed below. In any case, we see here two important issues: how is an appropriate pattern of action chosen, and how is the chosen pattern parameterized on the basis of sensory input? MOTOR PRIMITIVES advances the idea that CPGs construct spinal motor acts by recruiting a few motor primitives from a set encoded in the spinal cord. The best evidence comes from examination of wiping movements and microstimulation of frog spinal cord, where movements are constructed as a sequencing and combination of a collection of force-field motor primitives or fundamental elements. "Visuomotor Coordination in Frog and Toad" discusses how the frog's motor acts may be assembled on the basis of visual input.

With this, we switch to articles in which the emphasis is on rhythmic behavior, with rather little concern for the spatial structure of the movement (for example, the discussion of locomotion will focus on coordinating the rhythms of the legs when the animal progresses straight ahead, rather than on how these rhythms are modified when the animal traverses uneven terrain or turns to avoid an obstacle). CRUSTACEAN STOMATOGASTRIC SYSTEM analyzes specific circuits of identified neurons controlling the chewing (by teeth inside the stomach) behavior of crustaceans. Of particular interest is the finding that neuropeptides (see "Neuromodulation in Invertebrate Nervous Systems") can change the properties of cells and the strengths of connections so that, e.g., a cell can become a pacemaker or a previously ineffective connection can come to exert a strong influence, and with this a network can dramatically change its overall behavior. Thus, the change of "mode" may be under the control of an explicit chemical "switch" of underlying cellular properties. Of course, in some systems, different input patterns of excitation and inhibition may enable a given circuit to act in one of several modes; while in other cases the change of mode may involve the transfer of control from one neural circuit to another. LOCOMOTION, INVERTEBRATE focuses on invertebrate locomotion systems for which quantitative modeling has been done, reviewing computer models of swimming, flying, crawling, and walking, paying special attention to the interaction of neural networks with the biomechanical systems they control. The article also reviews the use of biologically inspired locomotion controllers in robotics, stressing their distributed nature, their robustness, and their computational efficiency. Conversely, robots can serve as an important new modeling methodology for testing biological hypotheses. LOCUST FLIGHT: COMPONENTS AND MECHANISMS IN THE MOTOR narrows the focus to one specific invertebrate motor system. The article emphasizes the interactions of the intrinsic properties of flight neurons, the operation of complex circuits, and phase-specific proprioceptive input, all subject to the concentrations of circulating neuromodulators. Locust flight can adapt to the demands of a constantly changing sensory environment, and the flight system is flexible and able to operate despite severe ablations and then to recover from these lesions.

HALF-CENTER OSCILLATORS UNDERLYING RHYTHMIC MOVEMENTS looks at a set of minimal circuits for generating rhythmic behavior, starting with the half-center oscillator model first proposed to account for the observation that spinal cats (i.e., cats in which connections between brain and spinal cord had been severed) could produce stepping movements even when all sensory feedback from the animal's motion was eliminated. The article shows the utility of models of this type in analyzing rhythms in invertebrates as well as vertebrates—the pelagic mollusk *Clione*, tadpoles, and lampreys—in terms of the intrinsic membrane properties of the component neurons interacting with reciprocal inhibition to initiate and sustain oscillation in these networks. SPINAL CORD OF LAMPREY: GENERATION OF LOCOMOTOR PATTERNS marks an important transition: from seeing how one network can oscillate to seeing how the oscillation of a series of networks can be coordinated. Experiments show that neural circuitry in isolated pieces of the spinal cord of lamprey (a jawless, primitive type of fish) can exhibit oscillations, and when these pieces constitute an intact spinal cord, they all oscillate with the same frequency but form a "traveling wave" with a phase relationship that in the complete fish would yield a wave of bending progressing down the fish from head to tail to yield the coordinated "wiggling" that yields swimming. The article reviews the interaction between experimentation and modeling stimulated by such findings. RESPIRATORY RHYTHM GENERATION presents several alternative models of breathing and evaluates them against mammalian data. These data point to the importance both of endogenous bursting neurons and of network interactions in generating the basic rhythm. In most models, rhythmogenesis is either pacemaker or network driven. The article reviews the data and these models, and then points the way to future models that clarify the integration of endogenous bursting with network interactions. LOCOMOTION, VERTEBRATE shows how neural networks in the spinal cord generate the basic rhythmic patterns necessary for vertebrate locomotion, while higher control centers interact with the spinal circuits for posture control and accurate limb movements, and by sending higher-level commands such as stop and go signals, speed, and heading of motion. In mammals, evolution of the CPGs has been accompanied by important modifications of the descending pathways under the requirements of complex posture control and accurate limb movements, although the extent of the respective changes remains unknown. Computer models that combine neural models with biomechanical models are seen as having an important role to play in studying these issues. One example uses "genetic algorithms" to model the transition from a lamprey-like spinal cord that supports traveling waves to a salamander-like spinal cord that supports both traveling waves for swimming and "standing waves" for terrestrial locomotion, and shows how vision may modulate spinal activity to yield locomotion toward a goal (see also "Visuomotor Coordination in Salamander").

CHAINS OF OSCILLATORS IN MOTOR AND SENSORY SYSTEMS abstracts from the specific circuitry to show how oscillators and their coupling can be characterized in a way that allows the proof of mathematical theorems about patterns of coordination. CPGs are discussed not only for the spinal cord of lamprey, but also for the crayfish swimmeret system and the leech network of swimming. In the context of locomotion, each oscillator is likely to be a local subnetwork of neurons that produces rhythmic patterns of membrane potentials. Since the details of the oscillators often are not known and are difficult to obtain, the object of the mathematics is to find the consequences of what is known, and to generate sharper questions to motivate further experimentation. GAIT TRANSITIONS also studies its topic (e.g., the transition from walking to running) from the abstract perspective of dynamical systems.

Mammalian Motor Control

ACTION MONITORING AND FORWARD CONTROL OF MOVEMENTS
ARM AND HAND MOVEMENT CONTROL
BASAL GANGLIA
CEREBELLUM AND MOTOR CONTROL
COLLICULAR VISUOMOTOR TRANSFORMATIONS FOR GAZE
    CONTROL
EQUILIBRIUM POINT HYPOTHESIS
EYE-HAND COORDINATION IN REACHING MOVEMENTS
GEOMETRICAL PRINCIPLES IN MOTOR CONTROL
GRASPING MOVEMENTS: VISUOMOTOR TRANSFORMATIONS
HIPPOCAMPUS: SPATIAL MODELS
IMAGING THE MOTOR BRAIN
LIMB GEOMETRY, NEURAL CONTROL
MOTOR CONTROL, BIOLOGICAL AND THEORETICAL
MOTOR CORTEX: CODING AND DECODING OF DIRECTIONAL
    OPERATIONS
MOTONEURON RECRUITMENT
MUSCLE MODELS
OPTIMIZATION PRINCIPLES IN MOTOR CONTROL
PROSTHETICS, MOTOR CONTROL
PURSUIT EYE MOVEMENTS
REACHING MOVEMENTS: IMPLICATIONS FOR COMPUTATIONAL
    MODELS
REINFORCEMENT LEARNING IN MOTOR CONTROL
RODENT HEAD DIRECTION SYSTEM
SENSORIMOTOR LEARNING
VESTIBULO-OCULAR REFLEX

Muscle transduces chemical energy into force and motion, thereby providing power to move the skeleton. Because of the intricacies of muscle microstructure and architecture, no comprehensive models are yet able to predict muscle performance completely. MUSCLE MODELS reviews three classes of models each fulfilling a more narrowly defined objective, ranging from attempts to understand the molecular level (cross-bridge models) through lumped parameter mechanical models to input-output models of whole muscle behavior that can be used as part of a broader study of basic musculoskeletal biomechanics or issues of neural control. A motor neuron together with the muscle fibers that it innervates constitutes a motor unit, and each muscle is a composite structure whose force-generating components, the motor units, are typically heterogeneous. Such aggregates can produce much larger forces than a single motor unit. MOTONEURON RECRUITMENT shows how the motor units can be recruited in the service of reflexes, voluntary movement, and posture. The article considers mechanisms that compensate for muscle fatigue and yielding, models the possible role of Renshaw cells in linearization or equalization of motor neuron pool responses, and considers the possible role of cerebellum in control of motor neuron gain, as well as the roles of motor cortex in motor neuron recruitment.

PROSTHETICS, MOTOR CONTROL deals with the use of electrical stimulation to alter the function of motor systems, either directly or indirectly. The article presents three clinical applications. Therapeutic electrical stimulation is electrically produced exercise in which the beneficial effect occurs primarily off-line as a result of trophic effects on muscles and perhaps the CNS. Neuromodulatory stimulation is preprogrammed stimulation that directly triggers or modulates a function without ongoing control or feedback from the patient, and functional electrical stimulation (FES) provides precisely controlled muscle contractions that produce specific movements required by the patient to perform a task. The article also describes subsystems for muscle stimulation, sensory feedback, sensorimotor regulation, control systems, and command signals, most of which are under development to improve on-line control of FES.

MOTOR CONTROL, BIOLOGICAL AND THEORETICAL sets forth the basic cybernetic concepts. A motor control system acts by sending motor commands to a controlled object, often referred to as "the plant," which in turn acts on the local environment. The plant or the environment has one or more variables that the controller attempts to regulate. If the controller bases its actions on signals that are not affected by the plant output, it is said to be a feedforward controller. The full understanding of movement must rest on a full analysis of the integration of neural networks with the biomechanics of the skeletomuscular system. Nonetheless, much has been learned about limb control from a more abstract viewpoint, as the next four articles show. Optimization theory has become an important aid to discovering organizing principles that guide the generation of goal-directed motor behavior, specifying the results of the underlying neural computations without requiring specific details of the way those computations are carried out. OPTIMIZATION PRINCIPLES IN MOTOR CONTROL concedes that not all motor behaviors are necessarily optimal but argues that attempts to identify optimization principles can yield a useful taxonomy of motor behavior. The hypothesis is that in performing a motor task, the brain produces coordinated actions that minimize some measure of performance (such as effort, smoothness, etc.). The article reviews several studies in which such ideas were examined in the context of planar upper limb movements, comparing the purely kinematic minimum jerk model with the more dynamics-based minimum torque change model. Bur how does one go from a kinematic description of the movement of the hand to the pattern of muscle control that yields it? There are still many competing hypotheses. One approach seeks to find control systems that yield optimal trajectories in the absence of disturbances. Another starts from the observation that a muscle is like a controlled-length spring: set its length, and it will naturally return to the equilibrium length that was set. The EQUILIBRIUM POINT HYPOTHESIS builds on this a systems-level description of how the nervous system controls the

muscles so that a stable posture is maintained or a movement is produced. In this framework, the controller is composed of muscles and the spinal-based reflexes, and the plant is the skeletal system. The controller defines a force field that is meant to capture the mechanical behavior of the muscles and the effect of spinal reflexes. The equilibrium point hypothesis views motion as a gradual postural transition, and it is suggested that for the case of multijoint arm movements, one can predict the hand's motion if the supraspinal system smoothly shifts the equilibrium point from the start point to a target location. GEOMETRICAL PRINCIPLES IN MOTOR CONTROL considers a different transition, that from the spatial representation of a motor goal to a set of appropriate neuromuscular commands, which is in many respects similar to a coordinate transformation. (A word of caution: The matter is subtle because the brain rarely has neurons whose firing encodes a single coordinate. Consider, for example, retinotopic coding as distinct from the specific use of (x, y) or (r, θ) coordinates. Thus the issue is whether the activity in certain networks is better described as encoding one representation than another, such as those related to the eye rather than those related to the shoulder.) The article describes three types of coordinate system—end-point coordinates, generalized coordinates, and actuator coordinates—each representing a particular "point of view" on motor behavior, then examines the geometrical rules that govern the transformations between these classes of coordinates. It shows how a proper representation of dynamics may greatly simplify the transformation of motor planning into action. LIMB GEOMETRY, NEURAL CONTROL offers another perspective, starting from a discussion of the role of extrinsic and intrinsic coordinates when a human makes a movement. Multijointed coordination complicates the problem of motor control. Consider the case of arm movements. The activation of an elbow flexor will always contribute a flexor torque at the elbow, but the resulting elbow movement can be flexion, extension, or no motion at all, depending on the actively produced torque at the shoulder. Although in principle a coordinated motor action could be planned muscle by muscle, a more parsimonious solution is to plan more global goals at higher levels of organization and let the lower-level controllers specify the implementation details. The article reviews issues related to the kinematic aspects of limb geometry control for arm movements and for posture and gait.

Fast, coordinated movements depend on the nervous system being able to use copies of motor control signals (the corollary discharge) to compute expectations of how the body will move, rather than always waiting for sensory feedback to signal the current state of the body. ACTION MONITORING AND FORWARD CONTROL OF MOVEMENTS spells out three functions of corollary discharge. The stability of visual perception during eye movements was one of the first physiological applications proposed for an internal comparison between a movement and its sensory outcome. Second, goal-directed behavior implies that the action should continue until the goal has been satisfied, so that motor representations must involve not only forward mechanisms for steering the action but also mechanisms for monitoring its course and checking its completion. Third, similar processes have been postulated for actions aimed at complex and relatively long-term goals, for comparing the representation of the intended action to the actual action and compensating for possible mismatch between the two. Clearly, the effective use of corollary discharge rests on the brain having learned the relation between current state, motor command, and the movement that ensues. SENSORIMOTOR LEARNING explains how neural nets can acquire forward and inverse "models" of some desired sensorimotor transformation. The managing of multiple models, each with its own range of applicability in given tasks, is given special attention. The relevance of such models to the role of cerebellum (CEREBELLUM AND MOTOR CONTROL) is briefly noted, as is the idea that these models may act by controlling lower-level "Motor

Primitives" (q.v.). REINFORCEMENT LEARNING IN MOTOR CON-
TROL, which presents general learning strategies based on adaptive
neural networks, is treated further in the road map **Robotics and
Control Theory**.

With this background, we turn to articles primarily concerned
with visually controlled behaviors for which neurophysiological
data are available from the mammalian (and in many cases the
monkey) brain, as well as behavioral and, in some cases, imaging
data for humans. The road map takes us from basic unconscious
behaviors to those involving skilled action. The vestibulo-ocular
reflex (VOR) serves to stabilize the retinal image by producing eye
rotations that counterbalance head rotations. Vestibular nuclei neurons are much more than a simple relay; their functions include
multimodality integration, temporal signal processing, and adaptive plasticity. VESTIBULO-OCULAR REFLEX reviews the empirical
data, as well as control-theoretic and neural network models for
the neural circuits that mediate the VOR. These perform diverse
computations that include oculomotor command integration, temporal signal processing, temporal pattern generation, and experience-dependent plasticity.

COLLICULAR VISUOMOTOR TRANSFORMATIONS FOR GAZE CON-
TROL analyzes the role of superior colliculus in the control of the
rapid movement, called a saccade, of the eyes toward a target. The
article touches on afferent and efferent mapping, target selection,
visuomotor transformations in motor error maps, remapping models, and coding of dynamic motor error. The theme of remapping
is pursued in DYNAMIC REMAPPING, which distinguishes "one-
shot" remapping (updating the internal representation in one operation to compensate for an entire movement) from a continuous
remapping process based on the integration of a velocity signal or
the relaxation of a recurrent network. In both cases, the problem
amounts to moving a hill of activity in neuronal maps. The article
uses data on arm movements as well as saccades. Models can be
constrained by considering deficits that accompany localized lesions in humans. These data not only provide valuable insights into
the nature of remappings but they might also help bridge the gap
between behavior and single-cell responses. PURSUIT EYE MOVE-
MENTS takes us from saccadic "jumps" to those smooth eye movements involved in following a moving target. Current models of
pursuit vary in their organization and in the features of pursuit that
they are designed to reproduce. Three main types of model are
"image motion" models, "target velocity" models, and models that
address the role of prediction in pursuit. However, these models
make no explicit reference to the neural structures that might be
responsible. The article thus analyzes the neural pathways for pursuit, stressing the importance of both visual areas of the cerebral
cortex and oculomotor regions of the cerebellum, to set goals for
future modeling.

IMAGING THE MOTOR BRAIN shows that the behavioral form and
context of a movement are important determinants of functional
activity within cortical motor areas and the cerebellum, stressing
that functional imaging of the human motor system requires one to
study the interaction of neurological and cognitive processes with
the biomechanical characteristics of the limb. Neuroimaging shows
that multiple neural systems and their functional interactions are
needed to successfully perform motor tasks, encode relevant information for motor learning, and update behavioral performance in
real time. The article discusses how evidence from functional imaging studies provides insight into motor automaticity as well as
the role of internal models in movement.

Two articles explore the way in which the rat charts the spatial
structure of its environment, using both "landmark cues" and a
sense of its head orientation with respect to some key aspects of
its environment. HIPPOCAMPUS: SPATIAL MODELS starts with the
finding that single-unit recordings in freely moving rats have revealed "place cells" in fields CA3 and CA1 of the hippocampus,

so called because their firing is restricted to small portions of the
rat's environment (the corresponding place fields), but the firing
properties of place cells change when the rat is placed in a new
environment. The article focuses on data and models for the role
of place cell firing in the rat's navigation (see "Cognitive Maps"
for a less neurophysiological approach to the same general issues).
RODENT HEAD DIRECTION SYSTEM focuses on head direction cells
in a number of brain areas that fire maximally when the rat's head
is pointed in a specific preferred direction, with a gradual falloff in
firing as the heading departs from that direction. Head direction is
not a simple reflection of sensory stimuli since, for example, the
neural coding can be updated when the animal turns in the dark.
The authors analyze such phenomena using attractor networks.

The next six articles are concerned with reaching and grasping.
MOTOR CORTEX: CODING AND DECODING OF DIRECTIONAL
OPERATIONS spells out the relation between the direction of reaching and changes in neuronal activity that have been established for
several brain areas, including the motor cortex. The cells involved
each have a broad tuning function, the peak of which denotes the
"preferred" direction of the cell. A movement in a particular direction will engage a whole population of cells. It is found that the
weighted vector sum of these neuronal preferences is a "population
vector" that points in (close to) the direction of the movement for
discrete movements in 2D and 3D space. Further observations link
this population encoding to speed of movement as well as to preparation for movement. The present article addresses the question
of how movement variables are encoded in the motor cortex and
how this information could be used to drive a simulated actuator
that mimics the primate arm. ARM AND HAND MOVEMENT CON-
TROL discusses some of the most prominent regularities of arm and
hand control, and examines computational and neural network
models designed to explain them. The analysis reveals the controversies engendered by competition between explanations sought on
different levels—neural, biomechanical, perceptual, or computational. Although some topics, such as internal model control, have
gained solid grounding, the importance of the dynamic properties
of the musculoskeletal system in facilitating motor control, the role
of real-time perceptual modulation of motor control, and the balance between dynamical systems models versus optimal control-
based models are still seen as offering many open questions.
REACHING MOVEMENTS: IMPLICATIONS FOR COMPUTATIONAL
MODELS reviews a number of issues that are emerging from neurophysiological studies of motor control and stresses their implications for development of future models. Data on movement planning, trajectory generation, temporal features of cortical activity,
and overlapping polymodal gradients are used to set challenges for
computational models that will meet the demands of both functional competence and biological plausibility.

EYE-HAND COORDINATION IN REACHING MOVEMENTS focuses
on possible mechanisms responsible for visually guiding the hand
toward a point within the prehension space. Reaching at a visual
target requires transformation of visual information about target
position into a frame of reference suitable for the planning of hand
movement. Accurate encoding of target location requires concomitant foveal and extraretinal signals. The most popular hypothesis
to explain how trajectories are planned is that the trajectory is specified as a vector in the arm's joint space, with joint angle variations
controlled in a synergic way (temporal coupling). The motor command initially sent to the arm is based on an extrafoveal visual
signal; at the end of the ocular saccade, the updated visual signal
is used to adjust the ongoing trajectory. Because of consistent delays in sensorimotor loops, the rapid path corrections observed during reaching movements cannot be attributed to sensory information only but must rely on a "forward model" of arm dynamics. In
any case, where this article focuses on how the hand is brought to
a target, GRASPING MOVEMENTS: VISUOMOTOR TRANSFORMA-

TIONS emphasizes the neural mechanisms that control the shaping of the hand itself to grasp an object, noting the crucial preshaping of the hand during reaching prior to grasping the object. The analysis emphasizes the cooperative computation of visual mechanisms in parietal cortex with motor mechanisms in premotor cortex to integrate sensing and corollary discharge throughout the movement.

CEREBELLUM AND MOTOR CONTROL reviews a number of models of the role of the cerebellum in building "internal models" to improve motor skills. The article asserts that motor control and learning in the brain employ a modsular approach in which multiple controllers coexist, with each controller suitable for one or a small set of contexts. The basic idea is that, to select the appropriate controller or controllers at each moment, each of the multiple inverse models is augmented with a forward model that determines the responsibility each controller should assume during movement. This view is exemplified in the MOSAIC (MOdular Selection And Identification Control) model. Recent human brain imaging studies have started to accumulate evidence supporting multiple internal models of tools in the cerebellum. (One caveat: The article stresses the idea that the cerebellum provides complete motor controllers; other authors emphasize the idea that the cerebellum provides a corrective side path that learns how best to augment controllers located elsewhere in the brain.) Finally, BASAL GANGLIA reviews the structure of this system in terms of multiple loops, with special emphasis on those involved in skeletomotor and oculomotor functions. It also reviews the role of dopamine in motor learning and the mechanisms underlying Parkinson's disease.

II.9. Applications, Implementations, and Analysis

Applications

BRAIN-COMPUTER INTERFACES
DECISION SUPPORT SYSTEMS AND EXPERT SYSTEMS
FILTERING, ADAPTIVE
FORECASTING
KALMAN FILTERING: NEURAL IMPLICATIONS
PROSTHETICS, MOTOR CONTROL
PROSTHETICS, NEURAL
PROSTHETICS, SENSORY SYSTEMS

The road map **Robotics and Control Theory** presents a number of applications of neural networks. Here we offer a representative (but by no means exhaustive) set of other applications, a list that can be augmented by the study of many other road maps. Examples include a variety of topics in vision and speech processing (see the road maps **Vision** and **Linguistics and Speech Processing**, respectively). As noted in the Preface, the discussion of applications of ANNs in areas from astronomy to steel making was a feature of the first edition of the *Handbook* that is not reproduced in the second edition.

Several articles review the various contributions of adaptive neural networks to signal processing. FILTERING, ADAPTIVE notes that adaptive filtering has found widespread use in noise canceling and noise reduction, channel equalization, cochannel signal separation, system identification, pattern recognition, fetal heart monitoring, and array processing. The parameters of an adaptive filter are adjusted to "learn" or track signal and system variations according to a task-specific performance criterion. The field of adaptive filtering was derived from work on neural networks and adaptive pattern recognition. An adaptive filter can be viewed as a signal combiner consisting of a set of adjustable weights (or coefficients represented by a polynomial) and an algorithm (learning rule) that updates these weights using the filter input and output, as well as other available signals. The filter may include internal signal feedback, whereby delayed versions of the output are used to generate the current output, and it may contain some nonlinear components. The single-layer perceptron is a well-known type of adaptive filter that has a binary output nonlinearity (see "Perceptrons, Adalines, and Backpropagation"). The article focuses on the most widely used adaptive filter architecture and describes in some detail two representative adaptive algorithms: the least-mean-square algorithm and the constant modulus algorithm. KALMAN FILTERING: NEURAL IMPLICATIONS then introduces Kalman filtering, a powerful idea rooted in modern control theory and adaptive signal processing. Under linear and Gaussian conditions, the Kalman filter produces a recursive estimate of the hidden state of a dynamic system, i.e., one that is updated with each subsequent (noisy) measurement of the observed system, with the estimate being optimum in the mean-square-error sense. The Kalman filter provides an indispensable tool for the design of automatic tracking and guidance systems, and an enabling technology for the design of recurrent multilayer perceptrons that can simulate any finite-state machine. In the context of neurobiology, Kalman filtering provides insights into visual recognition and motor control. Related applications are discussed in FORECASTING. Neural nets, mostly of the standard backpropagation type, have been used with great success in many forecasting applications. This article looks at the use of neural nets for forecasting with particular attention to understanding when they perform better or worse than other technologies, showing how the success of neural networks in forecasting depends significantly on the characteristics of the process being forecast.

A decision support system is an information system that helps humans make a decision on a given problem, under given circumstances and constraints. Expert systems are information systems that contain expert knowledge for a particular problem area and perform inferences when new data are entered that may be partial or inexact. They provide a solution that is expected to be similar to the solution provided by experts in the field. DECISION SUPPORT SYSTEMS AND EXPERT SYSTEMS uses the collective term *decision system* to refer to either a decision support system or an expert system. The article discusses how neural networks can be employed in a decision system. Such systems help humans in their decision process and so should be comprehensible by humans. The article reviews results of connectionist-based decision systems. In particular, trainable knowledge-based neural networks can be used to accumulate both knowledge (rules) and data, building adaptive decision systems with incremental, on-line learning. (For further developments related to the construction of expert systems, see "Bayesian Networks" and the three articles on "Graphical Models.")

BRAIN-COMPUTER INTERFACES discusses the use of on-line analysis of brainwaves to derive information about a subject's mental state as a basis for driving some external action, such as selecting a letter from a virtual keyboard or moving a robotics device, providing an alternative communication and control channel that does not depend on the brain's normal output pathway of peripheral nerves and muscles, which may be nonfunctional in some patients. The brainwave signals may be evoked potentials generated in response to external stimuli or components associated with spontaneous mental activity. Targets for current research include the extraction of local components of brain activity with fast dynamics that subjects can consciously control. The article reviews the challenge of developing classifiers that work while the subject operates a brain-actuated application, with ANNs providing robust approaches to on-line learning. These studies are complemented by a range of articles on prosthetics. PROSTHETICS, NEURAL provides an overview of the physical components that tend to be common to all neural prosthetic systems. It emphasizes the biophysical factors that constrain the sophistication of those interfaces. Electroneural interfaces for both stimulation of and recording from neural tissue are analyzed in terms of biophysics and electrochemistry. It is also shown how the design of practical neural prostheses must address the systems hardware issues of power and data management and packaging. PROSTHETICS, SENSORY SYSTEMS focuses on sensory prostheses, in which information is collected by electronic sensors and delivered directly to the nervous system by electrical stimulation of pathways in or leading to the parts of the brain that normally process a given sensory modality. After assessing the amenability of all sensory modalities (hearing, vision, touch, proprioception, balance, smell, and taste) the article focuses on auditory and visual prostheses. The great success story has been with cochlear implants. Here the article reviews improved temporospatial representations of speech sounds, combined electrical and acoustic stimulation in patients with residual hearing, and psychophysical correlates of performance variability. Visual prostheses are still in their early days, with no general agreement on the most promising site to apply electrical stimulation to the visual pathways. The article reviews the cortical approach and the retinal approach. Finally, it is noted that since a prosthesis does not necessarily match natural neural encoding of a stimulus, the success of the prosthesis depends in part on the plasticity of the human brain as it remaps to accommodate this new class of signals. PROSTHETICS, MOTOR CONTROL deals with the subset of neural prosthetic interfaces that employ electrical stimulation to alter the function of motor systems, either directly or indirectly. The article presents three clinical applications. Therapeutic electrical stimulation is electrically produced exercise in which the beneficial effect occurs primarily off-line as a result of trophic effects on muscles and perhaps the CNS; neuromodulatory stimulation is preprogrammed stimulation that directly triggers or modulates a function without ongoing control or feedback from the patient; and functional electrical stimulation (FES) provides precisely controlled muscle contractions that produce specific movements required by the patient to perform a task. The article describes subsystems for muscle stimulation, sensory feedback, sensorimotor regulation, control systems, and command signals, most of which are under development to improve on-line control of FES. Electrical stimulation of the nervous system is also being used to treat other disorders, including spinal cord stimulation to control pain and basal ganglia stimulation to control parkinsonian dyskinesias.

To close this road map, we note the importance of using special-purpose VLSI chips to gain the full efficiency of artificial neural network in various applications. Such chips are among the methods for implementation of neural networks discussed in the next road map, **Implementation and Analysis**.

Implementation and Analysis

ANALOG VLSI IMPLEMENTATIONS OF NEURAL NETWORKS
BIOPHYSICAL MECHANISMS IN NEURONAL MODELING
BRAIN SIGNAL ANALYSIS
DATABASES FOR NEUROSCIENCE
DIGITAL VLSI FOR NEURAL NETWORKS
GENESIS SIMULATION SYSTEM
NEUROINFORMATICS

NEUROMORPHIC VLSI CIRCUITS AND SYSTEMS
NEURON SIMULATION ENVIRONMENT
NEUROSIMULATION: TOOLS AND RESOURCES
NSL NEURAL SIMULATION LANGUAGE
PHOTONIC IMPLEMENTATIONS OF NEUROBIOLOGICALLY INSPIRED NETWORKS
PROGRAMMABLE NEUROCOMPUTING SYSTEMS
SILICON NEURONS
STATISTICAL PARAMETRIC MAPPING OF CORTICAL ACTIVITY PATTERNS

Briefly, a neural network (whether an artificial neural network for technological application or a simulation of a biological neural network in computational neuroscience) can be implemented in three main ways: by programming a general-purpose electronic computer, by programming an electronic computer designed for neural net implementation, or by building a special-purpose device to emulate a particular network or parametric family of networks. We discuss these three approaches in turn, and then review a number of articles describing tools and methods for the analysis of brain signals and related activity.

NEUROSIMULATION: TOOLS AND RESOURCES reviews neurosimulators, i.e., programs designed to reduce the time and effort required to build models of neurons and neural networks. A neurosimulator requires, at the very least, a highly developed interface, a scalable design (e.g., through parallel hardware), and extendibility with new neural network paradigms. The review includes programs for modeling networks of biological neurons as well as programs for kinetic modeling of intracellular signaling cascades and regulatory genetic networks but does not cover connectionist simulators. It provides a general picture of the capabilities of several neurosimulators, highlighting some of the best features of the various programs, and also describes ongoing efforts to increase compatibility among the various programs. Compatibility allows models built with one neurosimulator to be independently evaluated and extended by investigators using different programs, thereby reducing duplication of effort, and also allows models describing different levels of complexity (molecular, cellular, network) to be related to one another. The next three articles present some of the methods necessary for efficient simulation of detailed models of single neurons (see, e.g., the articles "Axonal Modeling" and "Dendritic Processing" in the **Biological Neurons and Synapses** road map). BIOPHYSICAL MECHANISMS IN NEURONAL MODELING is a primer on biophysically detailed compartmental models of single neurons (see the road map **Biological Neurons and Synapses** for a fuller précis), but contributes to the topic of neurosimulators by illustrating examples of model definitions using the Surf-Hippo Neuron Simulation System, providing a minimal syntax that facilitates model documentation and analysis. GENESIS SIMULATION SYSTEM describes GENESIS (GEneral NEural SImulation System), which was developed to support "structurally realistic" simulations, computer-based implementations of models designed to capture the anatomical structure and physiological characteristics of the neural system of interest. GENESIS has been widely used for single-cell "compartmental" modeling but is also used for large network models, using libraries of ion channels and complete cell models, respectively. NEURON is a neurosimulator that was first developed for simulating empirically based models of biological neurons with extended geometry and biophysical mechanisms that are spatially nonuniform and kinetically complex. This functionality has been enhanced to include extracellular fields, linear circuits to emulate the effects of nonideal instrumentation, models of artificial (integrate-and-fire) neurons, and networks that can involve any combination of artificial and biological neuron models. NEURON SIMULATION ENVIRONMENT shows how these capabilities have been implemented so as to achieve computational efficiency while maintaining conceptual clarity, i.e., the knowledge that what has been instantiated in the computer model is an accurate representation of the user's conceptual model. Where NEURON has been primarily used for detailed modeling of single neurons, NSL NEURAL SIMULATION LANGUAGE provides methods for simulating very large networks of relatively simple (artificial or biological simulation) neurons. NSL (pronounced "Nissl") models focus on modularity, a well-known software development strategy in dealing with large and complex systems. Full understanding of a system is gained both by simulating modules in isolation and by designing computer experiments that follow the dynamics of the interactions between the various modules. An NSL model can be described either by direct programming in NSLM, the NSL (compiled) Modeling language, or by using the Schematic Capture System (SCS), a visual programming interface to NSLM supporting the description of module assemblages. "Phase-Plane Analysis of Neural Nets" introduces the qualitative theory of differential equations in the plane for analyzing neural networks. Computational methods are a very powerful adjunct to this type of analysis. The article concludes with comments on numerical methods and software. Between them, the articles reviewed in this paragraph make clear the challenge of providing multilevel neurosimulation environments in which one can move effortlessly between the levels of schemas (functional decomposition of an overall behavior), large neural networks, detailed models of single neurons, and neurochemical models of synaptic plasticity. To be fully effective, such an environment will also need visualization tools, and the ability to access a database to provide experimental results for comparison with model-based predictions.

The next two articles address the *digital*, parallel implementation of neural networks. DIGITAL VLSI FOR NEURAL NETWORKS starts by looking at the differences between digital and analog design techniques, with a focus on analyzing cost-performance trade-offs in flexibility (Amdahl's Law), and then considers the use of standard VLSI processors in parallel configurations for ANN emulation. The Adaptive Solutions CNAPS custom digital ANN processor is then discussed to convey a sense of some of the issues involved in designing digital structures for ANN emulation. Although this chip is no longer produced, it is still being used and provides a good vehicle for understanding the trade-offs inherent in emulating neural structures digitally. Finally, the article looks at field programmable gate array (FPGA) technology as a promising vehicle for digital implementation of ANNs. PROGRAMMABLE NEUROCOMPUTING SYSTEMS emphasizes that the design of specialized digital neurocomputers has exploited three items common to many neural (ANN) algorithms to improve cost/performance: the limited numeric precision required; the inherently high data parallelism, where the same operation is performed across large arrays of data; and communication patterns restricted enough to allow broadcast buses or unidirectional rings to support parallel execution of many common neural network algorithms. However, in the future, the work of commercial design teams to incorporate multimedia-style kernels into the workloads they consider during the design of new microprocessors will have as a by-product the ability to dramatically improve performance for ANN algorithms. This suggests that in the future there will be greatly reduced interest in special-purpose neurocomputers but much attention to software strategies to optimize ANN performance on commercially available microprocessors.

However, the above three assumptions are not so useful in the implementation of detailed "compartmental" models of neurons. Here, attention has been paid to the design of highly special-purpose *analog* VLSI circuits. Digital VLSI assigns a different circuit to each bit of information that is to be stored and processed. Each circuit is driven to the limit so that it settles into a 0-state or a 1-state, passing through a linear voltage-current regime to get

from one saturation state to the other. Thus, if a synaptic weight is to be stored with eight-bit precision in digital VLSI, it requires eight such circuits. By contrast, the linear regime of a single circuit element on a VLSI chip can store data with about three bits of precision with far less "real estate" on the chip, and with far less power loss. The price, of course, is that precision cannot be guaranteed on the same scale as for digital circuits, but in many neural net applications, analog precision is more than adequate. ANALOG VLSI IMPLEMENTATIONS OF NEURAL NETWORKS provides an overview of the implementation of circuitry in analog VLSI, and then summarizes a number of technological implementations of such analog chips for ANNs. The article introduces the difference between the constraints imposed by the biological and silicon media and emphasizes that letting the silicon medium constrain the design of a system results in more efficient methods of computation. Special emphasis is given to five properties of a silicon synapse that are essential for building large-scale adaptive analog VLSI synaptic arrays. This article focuses on building neural network integrated circuits (IC), and especially on building connectionist neural network models. SILICON NEURONS takes the same implementation methodology into the realm of computational neuroscience. Biological neural networks are difficult to model because they are composed of large numbers of nonlinear elements and have a wide range of time constants. Simulation on a general-purpose digital computer slows dramatically as the number and coupling of elements increase. By contrast, silicon neurons operate in real time, and the speed of the network is independent of the number of neurons or their coupling. On the other hand, high connectivity still poses problems in 2D chip layouts, and the design of special-purpose hardware is a significant investment, particularly if it is analog hardware, since analog VLSI still lacks a general set of easy-to-use design tools. In any case, NEUROMORPHIC VLSI CIRCUITS AND SYSTEMS charts the virtues of using analog VLSI to build "neuromorphic" chips, i.e., chips whose design is based on the structure of actual biological neural networks. Biological systems excel at sensory perception, motor control, and sensorimotor coordination by sustaining high computational throughput with minimal energy consumption. Neuromorphic VLSI systems employ distributed and parallel representations and computation akin to those found in their biological counterparts. The high levels of system integration offered in VLSI technology make it attractive for the implementation of highly complex artificial neuronal systems, even though the physics of the liquid-crystalline state of biological structures is different from the physics of the solid-state silicon technologies. The article provides a basic foundation in device physics and presents a set of specific circuits that implement certain essential functions that exemplify the breadth possible within this design paradigm. However, VLSI-based neural networks have difficulty in scaling up or interconnecting multiple neural chips to incorporate large numbers of neuron units in highly interconnected architectures without significantly increasing the computational time. This motivates the use of optical interconnections. The success of optic fibers as media for telecommunications has been complemented by the use of holograms and spatial light modulators as mechanisms for storing and processing information via patterns of light (photonics) rather than patterns of electrons (electronics). The current state of photonic approaches to neural network implementation is charted in PHOTONIC IMPLEMENTATIONS OF NEUROBIOLOGICALLY INSPIRED NETWORKS, which provides a perspective on the use of holography as a technique for building adaptive connection matrices for ANNs, as well as earlier discussions of holography as a metaphor for the working of associative memory in actual brains. In photonic implementation of neurobiologically inspired networks, optical (free-space or through-substrate) techniques enable an increase in the number of neuron units and the interconnection complexity by using the off-chip (third) dimension. This merging of optical and photonic devices with electronic circuitry provides additional features such as parallel weight implementation, adaptation, and modular scalability.

The remaining articles provide a number of perspectives on the analysis of data on the brain.

BRAIN SIGNAL ANALYSIS reviews applications of ANNs to brain signal analysis, including analysis of the EEG and MEG, the electromyogram (EMG), and computed tomographic (CT) images and magnetic resonance (MR) brain images, and to series of functional MR brain images (fMRI). Since most medical signals usually are not produced by variations in a single variable or factor, many medical problems, particularly those involving decision making, must involve a multifactorial decision process. In these cases, changing one variable at a time to find the best solution may never reach the desired objective, whereas multifactorial ANN approaches may be more successful. The review is organized according to the nature of brain signals to be analyzed and the role that ANNs play in the applications.

STATISTICAL PARAMETRIC MAPPING OF CORTICAL ACTIVITY PATTERNS describes the construction of statistical maps to test hypotheses about regionally specific effects like "activations" during brain imaging studies. Statistical parametric maps (SPMs) are image processes with voxel values that are, under the null hypothesis, distributed according to a known probability density function (usually Student's T or F distributions), analyzing each and every voxel using any standard (univariate) statistical test. The resulting statistical parameters are assembled into an image, the SPM. SPM{T} refers to an SPM comprising T statistics; similarly, SPM{F} denotes an SPM of F statistics. SPMs are interpreted as spatially extended statistical processes by referring to the probabilistic behavior of stationary Gaussian fields. Unlikely excursions of the SPM are interpreted as regionally specific effects, attributable to the sensorimotor or cognitive process that has been manipulated experimentally.

NEUROINFORMATICS presents an integrated view of neuroinformatics that combines tools for the storage and analysis of neuroscience data with the use of computational models in structuring masses of such data. In Europe, *neuroinformatics* is a term used to encompass the full range of computational approaches to brain theory and neural networks. In the United States, some people use the term neuroinformatics solely to refer to databases in neuroscience. Taking the perspective of the *Handbook*, this article sees the key challenge for neuroinformatics to be to integrate insights from synthetic data obtained from running a model with data obtained empirically from studying the animal or human brain. The problem is that the data, and thus the models, of neuroscience are so diverse. Neuroscience integrates anatomy, behavior, physiology, and chemistry, and studies levels from molecules to compartments and neurons up to biological neural networks and on to the behavior of organisms. The article thus presents an architecture for a federation of databases of empirical neuroscientific data in which results from diverse laboratories can be integrated. It further advocates a cumulative approach to modeling in neuroscience that facilitates the reusability (with appropriate changes) of modules within current neural models, with the pattern of re-use fully documented and tightly constrained by the linkage with this federation of databases. DATABASES FOR NEUROSCIENCE then focuses on the issues in constructing such databases. In order to be able to integrate such diverse sources, the various communities within the neurosciences must begin to develop standards for their community's data. Neuroscientists use many different and incompatible data formats that do not allow for the free exchange of data, and the article stresses the need for standards for the description of the actual data (i.e., a formalized description of the metadata), possibly using extensible markup language (XML) technologies. (On a related theme, NEUROSIMULATION: TOOLS AND RESOURCES examines two of the enabling neurosimulation technologies that will allow modelers to compare and modify models, verify one another's simulations, and extend models with their own tools.) One possible solution to integrating data from sources with heterogeneous data and representation is to extend the conventional wrapper-mediator architecture with domain-specific knowledge. The article concludes with analysis of a specific database of brain images (the fMRI Data Center) and a comprehensive table of neuroscience databases constructed to date.

Part III: Articles

Action Monitoring and Forward Control of Movements

Marc Jeannerod

Introduction

Monitoring its own output is thought to be a basic principle of functioning of the nervous system. This idea, inherited from the cybernetic era, and still operational now, is based on the notion of a comparison of the actual output of the system with the expected, or desired, output. In the domain of motor control, for example, it is assumed that each time the motor centers generate an outflow signal for producing a movement, a "copy" of this command (the "efference copy") is retained. The reafferent inflow signals generated by the movement (e.g., visual, proprioceptive) are compared with the copy. If a mismatch between the two types of signals is recorded, new commands are generated until the actual outcome of the movement corresponds to the desired movement. This comparison cannot be made, however, until the reafferent signals and the efference copy have been rendered compatible with one another. Proprioceptive signals, in principle, should be directly compatible with motor output (they arise from the same muscles and joints that are activated during the movement). Visual signals, by contrast, are generated in a set of coordinates quite different from those of motor output. Thus, a common set of coordinates must be computed to make the comparison useful.

The efference copy can only measure the performance error when the action comes to execution. In order to give this mechanism a predictive role in anticipating the effects of an action, one must assume the existence of a more complex "internal model" of that action. Such a model should be able to simulate the action generation process without waiting for the sensory reafference, or even without performing it. According to Wolpert, Ghahramani, and Jordan (1995), a combination of two processes is required: "The first process uses the current state estimate and motor command to predict the next state by simulating the movement dynamics with a forward model. The second process uses a model of the sensory output process to predict the sensory feedback from the current state estimate. The sensory error—the difference between actual and predicted sensory feedback—is used to correct the state estimate resulting from the forward model" (p. 1881). Several possible applications for this mechanism are reviewed in the following discussion.

Stability of Visual Perception and Target Localization

The stability of visual perception during eye movements was one of the first physiological applications proposed for an internal comparison between a movement and its sensory outcome. When one moves one's eyes across the visual field, objects tend to appear stationary in spite of their displacement on the retina; if, however, the same displacement is produced by an external agent (e.g., by gently pressing against the eye at the external canthus), objects no longer appear stationary. To account for this phenomenon, it has been conjectured that the command signals to the eye muscles are effective in remapping the visual scene and canceling out the visual displacement. In the absence of this signal, the visual displacement becomes visible. Sperry (1950) coined the term of "corollary discharge" (CD) for the centrally arising discharge that reaches the visual centers as a corollary of any command generated by the motor centers. In this way, the visual centers can distinguish the retinal displacement related to a self-generated movement from that produced by a moving scene. Visual changes produced by a movement of the eye are normally "canceled" by a CD of a corresponding size and direction. If, however, the CD is absent or does not

correspond to the visual changes (e.g., when the eye is pressed), these changes are not canceled and are read by the visual system as having their origin in the external world. The combination of the retinal signals and the extraretinal command signals (CD) thus produces a perceived stability of the visual world (Jeannerod, Kennedy, and Magnin, 1979). Signals arising from eye muscle proprioceptors also contribute to visual stability during eye movements (see Gauthier, Nommay, and Vercher, 1990). A CD type of regulation should in principle be more advantageous, however, because of its timing: a discharge propagating directly from the motor to the visual centers should be available to the visual system earlier than discharges arising from the periphery.

The same logic used for perceptual visual stability can also apply to egocentric localization of visual targets. The retinal position of a target cannot in itself be sufficient for its localization in space because, as the eyes move in the head, and the head moves on the trunk, several different retinal positions correspond to the same spatial locus. The spatial location of the target must therefore be reconstructed by combining eye/head position signals with the position of the target on the retina. The relationships between the retinal error signal (the position of the target on the retina) and the eye position signal were first formalized by Robinson (1975). In this influential model, the efference copy from eye position is derived from the output of a neural integrator that maintains the eye at a given position during fixation. It is this signal of actual eye position that is combined with retinal error to provide other motor systems (e.g., the arm) with the target location information. Eye movements are not generated on the basis of retinal error. Instead, the driving signal for the eye to reach the desired eye position relative to the head is the eye motor error signal. This signal is obtained by "subtracting" the actual change in eye position in orbit from the desired position. The movement stops when the motor error equals zero.

Guitton (1992) was able to directly demonstrate the dynamic nature of this process, by showing that output neurons from the superior colliculus—the tectoreticular (TR) neurons—code the change in eye motor error during the movement. Before the movement takes place, a TR neuron with a preferred vector corresponding to the desired eye position will be activated and will drive the eye movement generator. As the movement progresses and motor error is reduced, other TR neurons coding for smaller vectors will be activated until the error is zero. At this point, a TR neuron coding for a zero vector will be activated and fixation will be maintained. Guitton postulates that an internal representation of change in gaze position is generated and compared with the desired gaze position to yield instantaneous gaze motor error. If one assumes that this error is the parameter represented topographically on the collicular map, one can conceive how this signal will activate the proper sequence of TR neurons. Hence Guitton's hypothesis of a moving "hill" of activity shifting across the collicular map, from the caudal part where large vectors are encoded to the rostral part where fixation vectors are encoded. There are some difficulties with this model, however, notably with the timing of discharges in the superior colliculus which, in order to be suitable for coding motor error, should precede those of the eye movement generator.

Representation of Goals of Movements

Goal-directed behavior implies that the action should continue until the goal has been satisfied. Motor representations must therefore involve not only forward mechanisms for steering and directing the action, but also mechanisms for monitoring its course and for checking its completion. This error correction mechanism implies a short-term storage of outflow information processed at each level of action generation. Because reafferent signals during execution of a movement are normally delayed with respect to the command signal, the comparison mechanism must look ahead in time and produce an estimate of the movement velocity corresponding to the command. The image of this estimated velocity is used for computing the actual position of the limb with respect to the target (Hoff and Arbib, 1992). It is only because the current state of the action is monitored on-line (rather than after the movement terminates), that corrections can be applied without delay as soon as the deviation of the current trajectory from the desired trajectory is detected. A subtle mechanism postulated by Miles and Evarts (1979) for the regulation of movements could be useful here. They pointed out that the discharge of muscle spindles in the agonist muscle during a movement (due to the co-activation of the gamma motoneurons) exactly fulfills the criterion for an efference copy that propagates "upward" and is an exact copy of the motor input sent to the alpha motoneurons. This signal could well be used for on-line comparison with incoming signals resulting from the limb movement.

It has been proposed that the information stored in the comparison process should encode, not joint rotations or kinematic parameters, but final configurations (of the body, of the moving segments, etc.) as they should arise at the end of the action. In other words, the goal of the action, rather than the action itself, would be represented in the internal model of the action. This hypothetical mechanism is supported by experimental arguments. Desmurget et al. (1995) recorded reach and grasp movements directed at a handle that had to be grasped with a power grip. When the orientation of the handle was suddenly changed at the onset of a movement, the arm smoothly shifted from the optimal configuration initially planned to reach the object to another optimal configuration corresponding to the object in its new orientation. The shift was achieved by simultaneous changes at several joints (shoulder abduction, wrist rotation), so that the final grasp was effected in the correct position. In this case the comparison between the desired and the actual arm position could be effected dynamically through a process similar to that which has been proposed to solve the problem of coordinate transformation during goal-directed movements. The position of an object in space is initially coded in extrinsic (e.g., visual) coordinates. In order to be matched by the moving limb, however, this position must be transferred into an intrinsic coordinate frame. If the position of the object in extrinsic coordinates and the position of the extremity of the limb in intrinsic coordinates coincide (that is, if these positions correspond to the same point in the two systems of coordinates), the action should logically be considered as terminated (see Carrozzo and Lacquaniti, 1994).

In addition to matching the movement trajectory to the representation of the intended movement, this mechanism has also other potential functions for the control of movements. The comparison between corollary and incoming signals might be used to produce a correspondence between the motor command and the amount of muscular contraction, even if the muscular plant is not linear. Other nonlinearities may also arise from interaction of the moving limb with external forces, especially if it is loaded (for a review, see Weiss and Jeannerod, 1998). This mapping problem, which is a critical factor for producing accurate limb movements, is less important for eye movements, where interactions with the external force field are minimal and where the load of the moving segment is constant. In this case, the pattern of command issued by the eye movement generator should unequivocally reflect the final desired position of the eye, that is, the position where the retinal error is zero.

Action Monitoring

At a still higher level, that of actions aimed at complex and relatively long-term goals, similar processes have been postulated for comparing the representation of the intended action to the actual action and compensating for possible mismatch between the two. Several studies, using brain imaging techniques, have focused on identifying neural structures that would fulfill the requirements for a comparison mechanism or an error detecting device. Carter et al. (1998) studied the activity of the anterior cingulate gyrus, a region lying on the medial cortical surface of the frontal lobe, in a letter detection task designed to increase error rates and manipulate response competition. Activity was found to increase during erroneous responses, but also during correct responses in conditions of high levels of response competition. They concluded that the anterior cingular gyrus detects conditions under which errors are likely to occur, rather than errors themselves. This result suggests that action-monitoring mechanisms anticipate the occurrence of errors, by using internal models of the effects of the action on the world. In other words, the sensory consequences of an action are evaluated before they occur, even in conditions in which the action may not be executed. This mechanism can also become a powerful means of determining whether a sensory event is produced by our own action or by an external agent (and ultimately, if an action is self-produced or not). Blakemore, Rees, and Frith (1998) compared brain activity during the processing of externally produced tones and the processing of tones resulting from self-produced movements. They found an increase in the right inferior temporal lobe activity when the tones were externally produced, suggesting that this area would be inhibited by the volitional system in the self-produced condition. This result raises interesting questions about the possible consequences of a dysfunction of such a system. Increased activity in the primary auditory areas in the temporal lobe has been observed during auditory hallucinations in psychotic patients (Dierks et al., 1999). Hence, it is possibility that a defective self-monitoring system would produce false attribution of one's own speech to an external source.

Road Map: Mammalian Motor Control
Related Reading: Collicular Visuomotor Transformations for Gaze Control; Consciousness, Neural Models of; Eye-Hand Coordination in Reaching Movements; Schema Theory; Sensorimotor Learning

References

Blakemore, S. J., Rees, G., and Frith, C. D., 1998, How do we predict the consequences of our actions? A functional imaging study, *Neuropsychologia*, 36:521–529. ◆

Carrozzo, M., and Lacquaniti, F., 1994, A hybrid frame of reference for visuomanual coordination, *Neuroreport*, 5:453–456.

Carter, C. S., Braver, T. S., Barch, D. M., Botwinick, M. M., Noll, D., and Cohen, J. D., 1998, Anterior cingulate cortex, error detection and the online monitoring of performance, *Science*, 280:747–749. ◆

Desmurget, M., Prablanc, C., Rossetti, Y., Arzi, M., Paulignan, Y., Urquizar, C., and Mignot, J. C., 1995, Postural and synergic control for three-dimensional movements of reaching and grasping, *J. Neurophysiol.*, 74:905–910.

Dierks, T., Linden, D. E. J., Jandl, M., Formisano, E., Goebel, R., Lanferman, H., and Singer, W., 1999, Activation of Heschl's gyrus during auditory hallucinations, *Neuron*, 22:615–621.

Gauthier, G. M., Nommay, D., and Vercher, J. L., 1990, The role of ocular muscle proprioception in visual localization of targets, *Science*, 249:58–61.

Guitton, D., 1992, Control of eye-head coordination during orienting gaze shifts, *Trends Neurosci.*, 15:174–179.

Hoff, B., and Arbib, M. A., 1992, A model of the effects of speed, accuracy and perturbation on visually guided reaching, in *Control of Arm Move-*

ment in Space (R. Caminiti, P. B. Johnson, and Y. Burnod, Eds.), *Experimental Brain Research,* Series 22, pp. 285–306. ◆

Jeannerod, M., Kennedy, H., and Magnin, M., 1979, Corollary discharge: Its possible implications in visual and oculomotor interactions, *Neuropsychologia,* 17:241–258.

Miles, F., and Evarts, E. V., 1979, Concepts of motor organization, *Annu. Rev. Psychol.,* 30:327–362.

Robinson, D. A., 1975, Oculomotor control signals, in *Basic Mechanisms*

of Ocular Motility and Their Clinical Implications (G. Lennerstrand and P. Bach-y-Rita, Eds.), Oxford, UK: Pergamon, pp. 337–374.

Sperry, R. W., 1950, Neural basis of the spontaneous optokinetic response produced by visual inversion, *J. Comp. Physiol. Psychol.,* 43:482–489.

Weiss, P., and Jeannerod, M., 1998, Getting a grasp on coordination, *News in Physiologoical Science,* 13:70–75.

Wolpert, D. M., Ghahramani, Z., and Jordan, M. I., 1995, An internal model for sensorimotor integration, *Science,* 269:1880–1882. ◆

Activity-Dependent Regulation of Neuronal Conductances

Larry F. Abbott and Eve Marder

Introduction

An enormous amount of both theoretical and experimental work has focused on the implications of activity-dependent synaptic plasticity for development, learning, and memory. Less attention has been paid to the fact that the intrinsic characteristics of individual neurons change during development (Spitzer and Ribera, 1998) and can be modified by activity (Franklin, Fickbohm, and Willard, 1992; Desai, Rutherford, and Turrigiano, 1999), yet these too play a vital role in shaping network function.

The electrical characteristics of a neuron depend on the numbers of channels of various types that are active within the cell membrane and on how these channels are distributed over the surface of the cell. The conventional approach to developing a conductance-based model is to attempt to measure all the ionic currents expressed by a neuron, describe them with Hodgkin-Huxley equations, and finally assemble the neuron model (Koch and Segev, 1998). This approach is based on the assumptions that individual neurons of a given class have the same ionic currents expressed at the same levels and that a neuron expresses the same currents whenever it is sampled under a specified set of experimental conditions. However, these assumptions appear to be contradicted by experimental evidence (see, e.g., Liu et al., 1998). In addition, it is rarely possible to make all of the measurements needed to construct a conductance-based model in this manner. Most neurons have many types of ion channels with complex spatial distributions. It is unlikely that all these currents and their spatial distributions can be measured. As a result, conventional conductance-based models depend on considerable hand-tuning of parameters. Each attempt to make neurons more biologically realistic is accompanied by a worsening of this problem. Hand-tuning a detailed, multicompartment, conductance-based model can be extremely time consuming and frustrating.

Neurons accomplish the feat of expressing appropriate numbers of ion channels in the relevant locations without running months of computer simulations. This suggests that a set of parameter adjustment mechanisms may allow neurons to self-tune their conductance densities to produce specific electrophysiological properties. A number of attempts have been made at incorporating such mechanisms into conductance-based neuron models (Bell, 1992; LeMasson, Marder, and Abbott, 1993; Siegel, Marder, and Abbott, 1994; Liu et al., 1998; Golowasch et al., 1999; Stemmler and Koch, 1999). Self-tuning activity-dependent models provide an alternative approach to modeling neurons and networks. This class of models does not assume that neurons necessarily have the same conductance densities over time, nor that individual neurons of a well-defined class are identical. Rather, they depend on simple negative feedback mechanisms to develop and maintain sets of conductances that produce particular firing patterns and response characteristics. In these models, a second-messenger system, which may involve Ca^{2+} influx and a variety of Ca^{2+} sensors, guides the expression of the membrane conductances in a self-regulating manner.

Results

A Model Neuron with Self-Regulating Conductances

Self-regulating models are constructed by specifying a set of activity sensors and the rules by which they modify conductance densities. Experimental work indicates that the intracellular Ca^{2+} concentration is a good indicator of neuronal activity. Intracellular Ca^{2+} concentrations become elevated in response to activity and fall during inactive periods (Ross, 1989). Many Ca^{2+}-dependent cellular processes, controlled by a variety of Ca^{2+} sensors that monitor Ca^{2+} entry through different ion channels, can affect channel densities (Bito, Deisseroth, and Tsien, 1997; Barish, 1998; Finkbeiner and Greenberg, 1998). The intracellular Ca^{2+} concentration itself, or sensors of inward Ca^{2+} currents, can thus be used as feedback elements that monitor activity and change conductances. In general, when the neuron's activity is high, the activity-dependent rules decrease excitability, and when activity is low, they increase excitability by modifying appropriate conductances.

A model neuron constructed on these principles can start with almost any initial conductance densities and self-assemble a set of maximal conductances that produce particular intrinsic characteristics and patterns of activity. An example of a model spontaneously developing a set of maximal conductances that produces bursting behavior, starting from an initially silent state, is shown in Figure 1 (Liu et al., 1998). This illustrates but one example of the many ways that the model can generate bursting activity. Virtually any initial state leads ultimately to bursting, but, interestingly, the sets of conductances constructed by the model differ from trial to trial, although the final pattern of bursting is always similar to that shown in Figure 1. Thus, there is a non-unique map between maximal conductances and activity. The final set of conductances depends on initial conditions and is variable, even though the pattern of activity produced by the model is not.

A Model Network with Self-Regulating Conductances

Circuits of self-regulating neurons can self-assemble into functional circuits. This can be illustrated using a simplified model of the pyloric circuit of the crab stomatogastric ganglion (STG). The pyloric rhythm of the STG consists of alternating bursts of activity in several neurons, including the lateral pyloric (LP) and pyloric

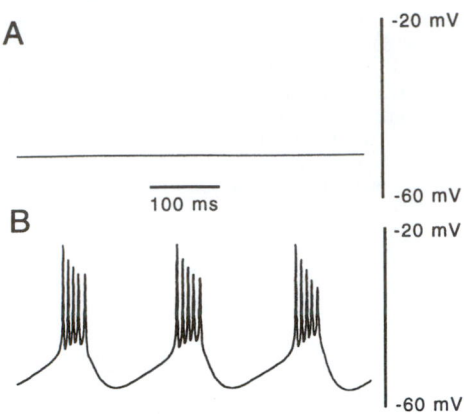

Figure 1. Self-assembly of a bursting model neuron (*B*) starting from different initial conditions (*A*). *A* and *B* represent the voltage traces at the beginning and end of the self-tuning process. (Adapted from Liu et al., 1998).

(PY) neurons, and the anterior burst (AB)/pyloric dilator (PD) pacemaker unit. The model shown in Figure 2 is a three-neuron circuit with individual neurons and synaptic connections similar to those of the LP and PY neurons and the AB/PD unit of the STG. Each model neuron consists of two compartments and has maximal conductances that are regulated by activity as described in the previous section.

When isolated from each other, the individual AB/PD, LP, and PY neurons of the model, like the neuron model shown in Figure 1, self-assemble their conductances. A novel feature of the circuit model is apparent when a realistic pattern of fixed synaptic connections is established between the model cells. In this case, the

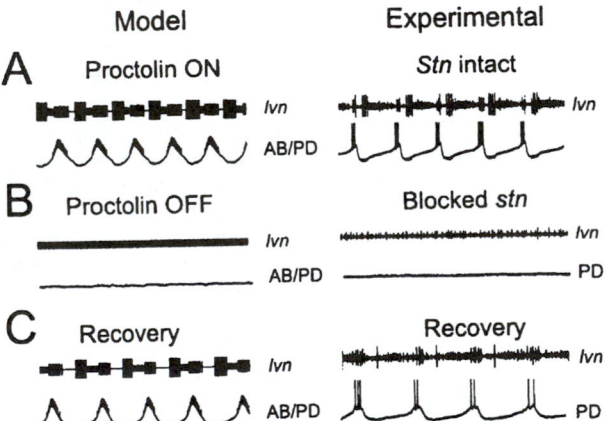

Figure 2. Comparison of a network model and experimental data. *A*, Control conditions in the model (left) and experiment (right). There is a triphasic motor pattern, revealed in the extracellular lvn recording. Intracellular PD recordings are also shown. In the model, the AB/PD and LP neurons contain a proctolin current. In the experiment, the modulatory inputs in the *stn* were left intact. *B*, Immediately after the modulatory inputs are removed, rhythmic activity is lost. Modulatory inputs are removed in the model by setting the proctolin current to zero. In the experiment, impulse activity in the *stn* was blocked to prevent the release of the neuromodulators. *C*, Activity eventually resumes. In the model, the activity-dependent sensors in each cell respond to the change in activity seen in *B*, and slowly modify the conductances of each of the model neurons, resulting in the recovery of rhythmic network activity, as occurred in the experimental case. (Adapted from Golowasch et al., 1999.)

entire network self-assembles to generate a pattern of activity similar to the triphasic rhythm recorded in the intact STG, and it can do so from any initial configuration of the maximal conductances of the three neurons (Golowasch et al., 1999). Interestingly, the intrinsic maximal conductances and responses properties of the individual model neurons are different if they self-assemble as a coupled circuit rather than in isolation. When assembled in a circuit, each of the model neurons ends up similar to its biological counterpart when acutely isolated, and the entire network generates realistic rhythmic activity. Thus, a cell-autonomous, activity-dependent regulatory rule is sufficient to self-assemble an entire circuit, at least in this example. It is not necessary to use any sensor that monitors the output of the whole circuit. Rather, each neuron takes care of its own activity, and the resultant circuit is tuned as a consequence of each cell's independent self-adjustment.

Comparison with Data from STG Organ Culture

Generation of the pyloric rhythm normally requires the presence of neuromodulatory substances released from axon terminals of the stomatogastric nerve (*stn*). If the *stn* is cut or blocked, rhythmic activity slows considerably or ceases. However, if the preparation is maintained over a period of days without *stn* modulatory input, rhythmic activity eventually resumes (Golowasch et al., 1999). Thus, it appears that prolonged removal of modulatory input alters the configuration of the pyloric circuit, allowing it to operate independently of the modulators that it normally requires.

The right side of Figure 2 shows the basic experimental result. Before blockade of the *stn*, the preparation shown on the right side of Figure 2*A* displayed a robust pyloric rhythm. Immediately following blockade of action potential conduction along the *stn*, the rhythm completely terminated (Figure 2*B*, right). However, when the block was maintained for approximately 24 hours, rhythmic pyloric activity resumed (Figure 2*C*, right). This recovery may be due, at least in part, to changes in the intrinsic properties of the neurons of the STG induced by the shift in activity following *stn* blockade, which allows the pyloric network to operate in the absence of neuromodulatory input.

This hypothesis can be studied, using the model discussed in the previous section, by including a proctolin conductance to simulate the effects of neuromodulators released by *stn* axons. The peptide proctolin is only one of many substances released from axon terminals of the *stn*, but it is a particularly potent modulator of the pyloric network. Figure 2 compares the behavior of the model with experimental results. Initially, the activity of the model network with the proctolin current included (Figure 2*A*, left) was similar to the pyloric activity of the experimental preparation with the *stn* intact (Figure 2*A*, right). To simulate the effects of blocking the *stn*, the proctolin conductance in the LP and AB/PD neurons was set to zero (Figure 2*B*, left). This immediately terminated the rhythmic activity of the model network, duplicating the effect of blocking the *stn* in the real preparation (Figure 2*B*, right). The suppression of the rhythm following the elimination of the proctolin conductance caused the activity-dependent conductance regulation mechanisms to modify the maximal conductances of the model neurons. This resulted in restoration of the pyloric rhythm in the model network after elimination of the proctolin conductance (Figure 2*C*, left), matching the natural resumption of the rhythm (Figure 2*C*, right).

It is important to stress that although the pyloric rhythms in Figures 2*A* and 2*C* look similar, they are produced by quite different cellular mechanisms. In Figure 2*A*, the existence of the rhythm depends on the presence of the modulatory proctolin current, while in Figure 2*C* the rhythms are produced in the absence of the modulator.

Discussion

The homeostatic regulation of neuronal circuits is an essential element in their development and maintenance as functioning systems. This is often ignored in the construction of neural networks, because fixed parameters are adjusted and used to control network function. Biological systems do not have the luxury of using fixed constants, because of the continual recycling of the proteins from which they are built. As a consequence, biological networks are typically more robust than artificial networks, and they are self-assembling. The work described here is an attempt to incorporate these features into neural network models.

The model studies described have revealed several interesting consequences of activity-dependent regulation of conductances: (1) Conductance regulation stabilizes a model neuron against activity shifts caused by extracellular perturbations. (2) Intrinsic properties of model neurons are modified by sustained shifts in activity. (3) The regulation scheme described here, applied as a local regulator of channel density in a multicompartment model, can produce a realistic spatial distribution of conductances. (4) Regulation of the activity of individual neurons in a network may, in some case, be sufficient for the development and maintenance of a network pattern requiring coordination across neurons.

One of the most significant messages provided by models of conductance regulation is that the same mechanisms that develop and maintain membrane conductances are likely to modify these conductances in response to long-lasting changes in the activity of the neuron. Furthermore, different neurons, or the same neuron at different times, may exhibit similar characteristics and activity while expressing membrane conductances at quite different levels. These observations make it apparent that neuron models must be much more flexible and dynamic than has conventionally been the case.

Road Map: Biological Neurons and Synapses
Background: Ion Channels: Keys to Neuronal Specialization
Related Reading: Biophysical Mosaic of the Neuron

References

Barish, M. E., 1998, Intracellular calcium regulation of channel and receptor expression in the plasmalemma: Potential sites of sensitivity along the pathways linking transcription, translation, and insertion, *J. Neurobiol.*, 37:146–157.

Bell, A. J., 1992, Self-organization in real neurons: Anti-Hebb in "channel space," in *Advances in Neural Information Processing Systems* (J. Moody, S. Hanson, and R. Lippmann), Eds., San Mateo, Morgan Kaufmann, pp. 59–66.

Bito, H., Deisseroth, K., and Tsien, R. W., 1997, Ca^{2+}-dependent regulation in neuronal gene expression, *Curr. Opin. Neurobiol.*, 7:419–429.

Desai, N. S., Rutherford, L. C., and Turrigiano, G. G., 1999, Plasticity in the intrinsic excitability of cortical pyramidal neurons, *Nature Neurosci.*, 2:515–520.

Finkbeiner, S., and Greenberg, M. E., 1998, Ca^{2+} channel-regulated neuronal gene expression, *J. Neurobiol.*, 37:171–189. ◆

Franklin, J. L., Fickbohm, D. J., and Willard, A. L., 1992, Long-term regulation of neuronal calcium currents by prolonged changes of membrane potential, *J. Neurosci.*, 12:1726–1735.

Golowasch, J., Casey, M., Abbott, L. F., and Marder, E., 1999, Network stability from activity-dependent regulation of neuronal conductances, *Neural Computat.*, 11:1079–1096.

Koch, C., and Segev, I., 1998, *Methods in Neuronal Modeling*, Cambridge, MA: MIT Press. ◆

LeMasson, G., Marder, E., and Abbott, L. F., 1993, Activity-dependent regulation of conductances in model neurons, *Science*, 259:1915–1917.

Liu, Z., Golowasch, J., Marder, E., and Abbott, L. F., 1998, A model neuron with activity-dependent conductances regulated by multiple calcium sensors, *J. Neurosci.*, 18:2309–2320.

Ross, W. N., 1989, Changes in intracellular calcium during neuron activity, *Annu. Rev. Physiol.*, 51:491–506. ◆

Siegel, M., Marder, E., and Abbott, L. F., 1994, Activity-dependent current distributions in model neurons, *Proc. Natl. Acad. Sci. USA*, 91:11308–11312.

Spitzer, N. C., and Ribera, A. B., 1998, Development of electrical excitability in embryonic neurons: Mechanisms and roles, *J. Neurobiol.*, 37:190–197. ◆

Stemmler, M., and Koch, C., 1999, How voltage-dependent conductances can adapt to maximize the information encoded by neuronal firing rate, *Nature Neurosci.*, 2:521–527.

Adaptive Resonance Theory

Gail A. Carpenter and Stephen Grossberg

Introduction

Principles derived from an analysis of experimental literatures in vision, speech, cortical development, and reinforcement learning, including attentional blocking and cognitive-emotional interactions, led to the introduction of adaptive resonance as a theory of human cognitive information processing (Grossberg, 1976a, 1976b). The theory has evolved as a series of real-time neural network models that perform unsupervised and supervised learning, pattern recognition, and prediction (Levine, 2000; Duda, Hart, and Stork, 2001). Models of unsupervised learning include ART 1 (Carpenter and Grossberg, 1987) for binary input patterns and fuzzy ART (Carpenter, Grossberg, and Rosen, 1991) for analog input patterns. ARTMAP models (Carpenter et al., 1992) combine two unsupervised modules to carry out supervised learning. Many variations of the basic supervised and unsupervised networks have since been adapted for technological applications and biological analyses.

Match-Based Learning, Error-Based Learning, and Stable Fast Learning

A central feature of all ART systems is a pattern matching process that compares an external input with the internal memory of an active code. ART matching leads either to a *resonant* state, which persists long enough to permit learning, or to a parallel memory search. If the search ends at an established code, the memory representation may either remain the same or incorporate new information from matched portions of the current input. If the search ends at a new code, the memory representation learns the current input. This *match-based learning* process is the foundation of ART code stability. Match-based learning allows memories to change only when input from the external world is close enough to internal expectations, or when something completely new occurs. This feature makes ART systems well suited to problems that require on-line learning of large and evolving databases.

Match-based learning is complementary to *error-based learning*, which responds to a mismatch by changing memories so as to reduce the difference between a target output and an actual output, rather than by searching for a better match. Error-based learning is naturally suited to problems such as adaptive control and the learning of sensorimotor maps, which require ongoing adaptation to present statistics. Neural networks that employ error-based learning include backpropagation and other multilayer perceptrons (MLPs) (Duda et al., 2001; see BACKPROPAGATION: GENERAL PRINCIPLES).

Many ART applications use *fast learning*, whereby adaptive weights converge to equilibrium in response to each input pattern. Fast learning enables a system to adapt quickly to inputs that occur rarely but that may require immediate accurate recall. Remembering details of an exciting movie is a typical example of learning on one trial. Fast learning creates memories that depend on the order of input presentation. Many ART applications exploit this feature to improve accuracy by voting across several trained networks, with voters providing a measure of *confidence* in each prediction.

Coding, Matching, and Expectation

Figure 1 illustrates a typical ART search cycle. To begin, an input pattern **I** registers itself as a short-term memory activity pattern **x** across a field of nodes F_1 (Figure 1A). Converging and diverging pathways from F_1 to a coding field F_2, each weighted by an adaptive long-term memory trace, transform **x** into a net signal vector **T**. Internal competitive dynamics at F_2 further transform **T**, generating a compressed code **y**, or *content-addressable memory*. With

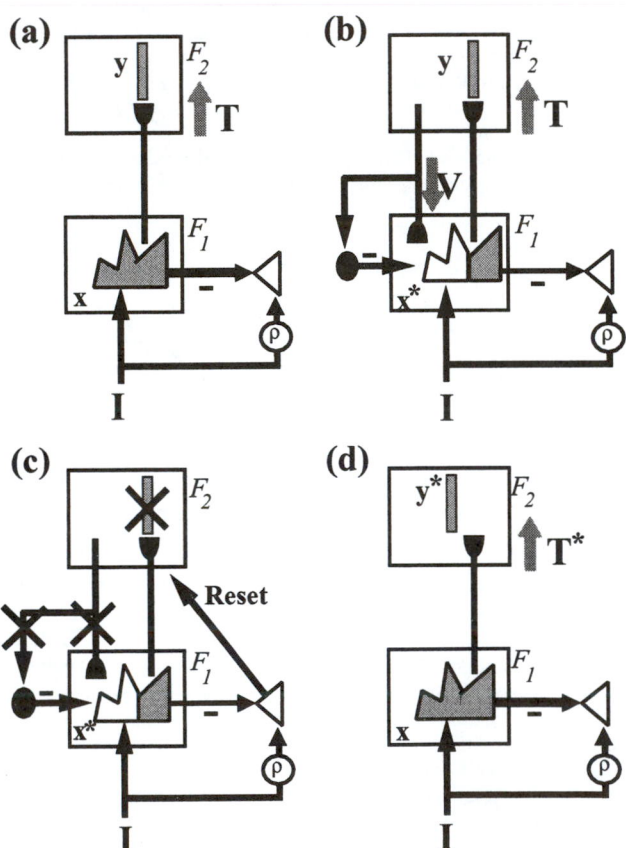

Figure 1. An ART search cycle imposes a matching criterion, defined by a dimensionless vigilance parameter ρ, on the degree of match between a bottom-up input **I** and the top-down expectation **V** previously learned by the F_2 code **y** chosen by **I**. See text for discussion of *A* through *D* sequence.

strong competition, activation is concentrated at the F_2 node that receives the maximal $F_1 \rightarrow F_2$ signal; in this *winner-take-all* mode, only one code component remains positive (see WINNER-TAKE-ALL NETWORKS).

Before learning can change memories, ART treats the chosen code as a *hypothesis*, which it tests by matching the *top-down expectation* of **y** against the input that selected it (Figure 1B). Parallel specific and nonspecific feedback from F_2 implements matching as a real-time locally defined network computation. Nodes at F_1 receive both learned excitatory signals and unlearned inhibitory signals from F_2. These complementary signals act to suppress those portions of the pattern **I** of bottom-up inputs that are not matched by the pattern **V** of top-down expectations. The residual activity **x*** represents a pattern of *critical features* in the current input with respect to the chosen code **y**. If **y** has never been active before, **x*** = **x** = **I**, and F_1 registers a perfect match.

Attention, Search, Resonance, and Learning

If the matched pattern **x*** is close enough to the input **I**, then the memory trace of the active F_2 code converges toward **x***. The property of encoding an *attentional focus* of critical features is key to code stability. This learning strategy differentiates ART networks from MLPs, which typically encode the current input rather than a matched pattern, and hence employ slow learning across many input trials to avoid catastrophic forgetting.

ART memory search begins when the network determines that the bottom-up input **I** is too novel or unexpected with respect to the active code to satisfy a matching criterion. The search process resets the F_2 code **y** before an erroneous association to **x*** can form (Figure 1C). After reset, medium-term memory within the $F_1 \rightarrow F_2$ pathways (Carpenter and Grossberg, 1990) biases the network against the previously chosen node, so that a new code y^* may be chosen and tested (Figure 1D).

The ART matching criterion is determined by a parameter ρ called *vigilance*, which specifies the minimum fraction of the input that must remain in the matched pattern in order for resonance to occur. Low vigilance allows broad generalization, coarse categories, and abstract memories. High vigilance leads to narrow generalization, fine categories, and detailed memories. At maximal vigilance, category learning reduces to exemplar learning. While vigilance is a free parameter in unsupervised ART networks, in supervised networks vigilance becomes an internally controlled variable that triggers a search after rising in response to a predictive error. Because vigilance then varies across learning trials, the memories of a single ARTMAP system typically exhibit a range of degrees of refinement. By varying vigilance, a single system can recognize both abstract categories, such as faces and dogs, and individual examples of these categories.

Supervised Learning and Prediction

An ARTMAP system includes a pair of ART modules, ART_a and ART_b (Figure 2). During supervised learning, ART_a receives a stream of patterns $\{a^{(n)}\}$ and ART_b receives a stream of patterns $\{b^{(n)}\}$, where $b^{(n)}$ is the correct prediction given $a^{(n)}$. An associative learning network and a vigilance controller link these modules to make the ARTMAP system operate in real time, creating the minimal number of ART_a recognition categories, or *hidden units*, needed to meet accuracy criteria. A minimax learning rule enables ARTMAP to learn quickly, efficiently, and accurately as it conjointly minimizes predictive error and maximizes code compression in an on-line setting. A *baseline vigilance* parameter $\bar{\rho}_a$ sets the minimum matching criterion, with smaller $\bar{\rho}_a$ allowing broader categories to form. At the start of a training trial, $\rho_a = \bar{\rho}_a$. A predictive failure at ART_b increases ρ_a just enough to trigger a search, through a feedback control mechanism called *match tracking*. A

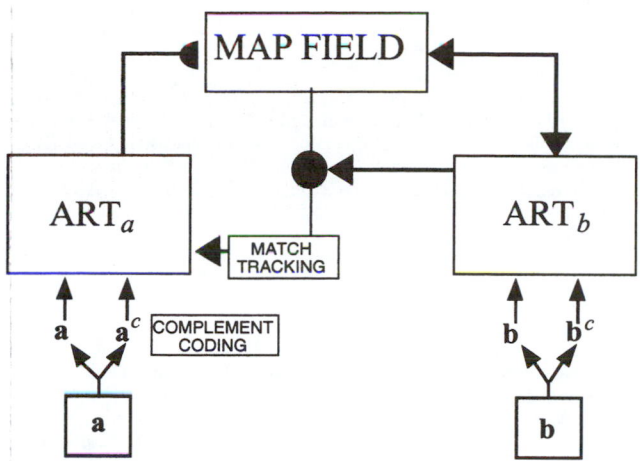

Figure 2. The general ARTMAP network for supervised learning includes two ART modules. For classification tasks, the ART_b module may be simplified.

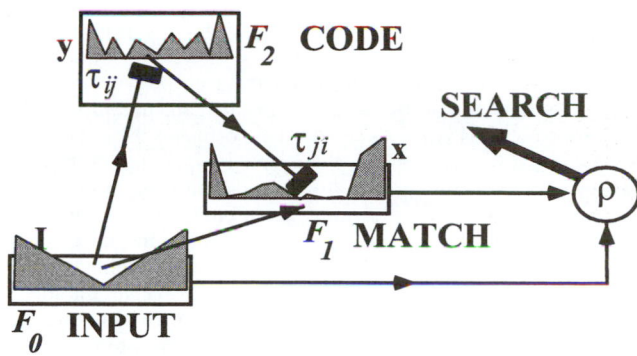

Figure 3. A distributed ART (dART) architecture retains the stability of WTA ART networks but allows the F_2 code to be distributed across arbitrarily many nodes.

newly active code focuses attention on a different cluster of input features, and checks whether these features are better able to predict the correct outcome. Match tracking allows ARTMAP to learn a prediction for a rare event embedded in a cloud of similar frequent events that make a different prediction.

ARTMAP employs a preprocessing step, called *complement coding*, which, by normalizing input patterns, solves a potential category proliferation problem (Carpenter et al., 1991). Complement coding doubles the number of input components, presenting to the network both the original feature vector and its complement. In neurobiological terms, complement coding uses both on-cells and off-cells to represent an input pattern. The corresponding on-cell portion of a weight vector encodes features that are consistently present in category exemplars, while the off-cell portion encodes features that are consistently absent. Small weights in complementary portions of a category representation encode as uninformative those features that are sometimes present and sometimes absent.

Distributed Coding

Winner-take-all activation in ART networks supports stable coding but causes category proliferation when noisy inputs are trained with fast learning. In contrast, distributed McCulloch-Pitts activation in MLPs promotes noise tolerance but causes catastrophic forgetting with fast learning (see LOCALIZED VERSUS DISTRIBUTED REPRESENTATIONS). *Distributed ART* (dART) models are designed to bridge these two worlds: distributed activation enhances noise tolerance, while new system dynamics retain the stable learning capabilities of winner-take-all ART systems (Carpenter, 1997). These networks automatically apportion learned changes according to the degree of activation of each coding node, which permits fast as well as slow distributed learning without catastrophic forgetting.

New learning laws and rules of synaptic transmission in the reconfigured dART network (Figure 3) sidestep computational problems that occur when distributed coding is imposed on the architecture of a traditional ART network (Figure 1). The critical design element that allows dART to solve the catastrophic forgetting problem of fast distributed learning is the *dynamic weight*. This quantity equals the rectified difference between coding node activation and an *adaptive threshold*, thereby combining short-term and long-term memory in the network's fundamental computational unit.

Thresholds τ_{ij} in paths projecting directly from an input field F_0 to a coding field F_2 obey a *distributed instar* (dInstar) learning law,

which reduces to an instar law when coding is winner-take-all. Rather than adaptive gain, learning in the $F_0 \rightarrow F_2$ paths resembles the *redistribution of synaptic efficacy* (RSE) observed by Markram and Tsodyks (1996) at neocortical synapses. In these experiments, pairing enhances the strength, or efficacy, of synaptic transmission for low-frequency test inputs, but fails to enhance, and can even depress, synaptic efficacy for high-frequency test inputs. In the dART learning system, RSE is precisely the computational dynamic needed to support real-time stable distributed coding.

Thresholds τ_{ji} in paths projecting from the coding field F_2 to a matching field F_1 obey a distributed outstar (dOutstar) law, which realizes a principle of atrophy due to disuse to learn the network's expectations with respect to the distributed coding field activation pattern. As in winner-take-all ART systems, dART compares top-down expectation with the bottom-up input at the matching field, and quickly searches for a new code if the match fails to meet the vigilance criterion.

Discussion: Applications, Rules, and Biological Substrates

ART and dART systems are part of a growing family of self-organizing network models that feature attentional feedback and stable code learning. Areas of technological application include industrial design and manufacturing, the control of mobile robots, face recognition, remote sensing land cover classification, target recognition, medical diagnosis, electrocardiogram analysis, signature verification, tool failure monitoring, chemical analysis, circuit design, protein/DNA analysis, three-dimensional visual object recognition, musical analysis, and seismic, sonar, and radar recognition (e.g., Caudell et al., 1994; Griffith and Todd, 1999; Fay et al., 2001). A book by Serrano-Gotarredona, Linares-Barranco, and Andreou (1998) discusses the implementation of ART systems as VLSI microchips. Applications exploit the ability of ART systems to learn to classify large databases in a stable fashion, to calibrate confidence in a classification, and to focus attention on those featural groupings that the system deems to be important based on experience. ART memories also translate to a transparent set of IF-THEN rules that characterize the decision-making process and may be used for feature selection.

ART principles have further helped explain parametric behavioral and brain data in the areas of visual perception, object recognition, auditory source identification, variable-rate speech and word recognition, and adaptive sensorimotor control (e.g., Levine, 2000; Page, 2000). One area of recent progress concerns how the neocortex is organized into layers, clarifying how ART design principles are found in neocortical circuits (see LAMINAR CORTICAL ARCHITECTURE IN VISUAL PERCEPTION).

Pollen (1999) resolves various past and current views of cortical function by placing them in a framework he calls *adaptive resonance theories*. This unifying perspective postulates resonant feedback loops as the substrate of phenomenal experience. Adaptive resonance offers a core module for the representation of hypothesized processes underlying learning, attention, search, recognition, and prediction. At the model's field of coding neurons, the continuous stream of information pauses for a moment, holding a fixed activation pattern long enough for memories to change. Intrafield competitive loops fixing the moment are broken by active reset, which flexibly segments the flow of experience according to the demands of perception and environmental feedback. As Pollen (1999, pp. 15–16) suggests, "[I]t may be the consensus of neuronal activity across ascending and descending pathways linking multiple cortical areas that in anatomical sequence subserves phenomenal visual experience and object recognition and that may underlie the normal unity of conscious experience."

Road Maps: Learning in Artificial Networks; Vision
Related Reading: Competitive Learning; Helmholtz Machines and Sleep-Wake Learning; Laminar Cortical Architecture in Visual Perception

References

Carpenter, G. A., 1997, Distributed learning, recognition, and prediction by ART and ARTMAP neural networks, *Neural Netw.*, 10:1473–1494.

Carpenter, G. A., and Grossberg, S., 1987, A massively parallel architecture for a self-organizing neural pattern recognition machine, *Computer Vision Graphics Image Process.*, 37:54–115.

Carpenter, G. A., and Grossberg, S., 1990, ART 3: Hierarchical search using chemical transmitters in self-organizing pattern recognition architectures, *Neural Networks*, 3:129–152.

Carpenter, G. A., Grossberg, S., Markuzon, N., Reynolds, J. H., and Rosen, D. B., 1992, Fuzzy ARTMAP: A neural network architecture for incremental supervised learning of analog multidimensional maps, *IEEE Trans. Neural Netw.*, 3:698–713.

Carpenter, G. A., Grossberg, S., and Rosen, D. B., 1991, Fuzzy ART: Fast stable learning and categorization of analog patterns by an adaptive resonance system, *Neural Netw.*, 4:759–771.

Caudell, T. P., Smith, S. D. G., Escobedo, R., and Anderson, M., 1994, NIRS: Large scale ART-1 neural architectures for engineering design retrieval, *Neural Netw.*, 7:1339–1350.

Duda, R. O., Hart, P. E., and Stork, D. G., 2001, *Pattern Classification*, 2nd ed., New York: Wiley, section 10.11.2. ◆

Fay, D. A., Verly, J. G., Braun, M. I., Frost, C., Racamato, J. P., and Waxman, A. M., 2001, Fusion of multi-sensor passive and active 3D imagery, in *Proc. SPIE Enhanced Synthet. Vision*, vol. 4363.

Griffith, N., and Todd, P. M., Ed., 1999, *Musical Networks: Parallel Distributed Perception and Performance*, Cambridge, MA: MIT Press.

Grossberg, S., 1976a, Adaptive pattern classification and universal recoding: I. Parallel development and coding of neural feature detectors, *Biol. Cybern.*, 23:121–134.

Grossberg, S., 1976b, Adaptive pattern classification and universal recoding: II. Feedback, expectation, olfaction, and illusions, *Biol. Cybern.*, 23:187–202.

Levine, D. S., 2000, *Introduction to Neural and Cognitive Modeling*, Mahwah, New Jersey: Erlbaum, chap 6. ◆

Markram, H., and Tsodyks, M., 1996, Redistribution of synaptic efficacy between neocortical pyramidal neurons, *Nature*, 382:807–810.

Page, M., 2000, Connectionist modelling in psychology: A localist manifesto, *Behav. Brain Sci.*, 23:443–512.

Pollen, D. A., 1999, On the neural correlates of visual perception, *Cereb. Cortex*, 9:4–19.

Serrano-Gotarredona, T., Linares-Barranco, B., and Andreou, A. G., 1998, *Adaptive Resonance Theory Microchips: Circuit Design Techniques*, Boston: Kluwer Academic.

Adaptive Spike Coding

Adrienne Fairhall and William Bialek

Introduction

The meaning of any signal that we receive from our environment is modulated by the context within which it appears. Our interpretation of color, a spoken phoneme, or a patch of luminance depends critically on its context. Although "context" may be a rather abstract notion, it is often reasonable to understand the term as meaning the statistical ensemble in which the signal is embedded. Interpreting a message requires both registering the signal itself and knowing something about this statistical ensemble. The relevant temporal or spatial ensemble depends on the task. The context may be highly local; we interpret appropriately gradations of light and dark in a scene where local brightness typically varies over orders of magnitude (see FEATURE ANALYSIS). For tasks such as decision making, the relevant statistics may reflect complex descriptions of the world accumulated over long periods.

Neural representations at every level of information processing should be similarly modulated by context. Information theoretically, this has measurable advantages: representations that appropriately take into account the statistical properties of the incoming signal are more efficient. Since the 1950s it has been suggested that efficiency is a design principle of the nervous system, allowing neurons to transmit more useful information with their limited dynamic range (see OPTIMAL SENSORY ENCODING). Thus, one expects that learning the context and implementing this knowledge through coding strategy is inherent in the formation of representations.

Such adjustments occur over a wide range of time scales. Through the genetic code, species adapt to environmental changes over many generations. In a single individual, learning, implemented through neural plasticity, continues throughout life in response to experience of the world; perceptual learning is stored even at low levels of neural information processing (see SOMATOTOPY: PLASTICITY OF SENSORY MAPS). In the article, we discuss even more rapid changes: neural adaptation, which we take to mean reversible change in the response properties of neurons on short time scales.

Since Adrian's first observations of adaptation in spiking neurons, it has been suggested that adaptation serves a useful function for information processing, preventing a neuron from continuing to transmit redundant information and increasing its responsiveness to new stimuli. Within the simplified picture of a neuron as a combination of linear filtering followed by a threshold, or a decision rule for spiking, either or both of the two components—the filter and the threshold function—may be adaptive functions of the input, and both may implement the goal of increasing information transmission. We will discuss both of these possibilities.

Neurons in every sensory modality have been shown to have adaptive properties, and the mechanisms governing various types of adaptation have been at least partially explored (Torre et al.,

1995). Here we will discuss adaptation as the simplest form of learning and memory. We describe recent experiments that explicitly aim to link the phenomenology of adaptive spike coding to its functional relevance, in particular to improved information transmission. A common feature of adaptation is the existence of multiple time scales. In examining mechanisms, we concentrate on recent work suggesting that the long time scales retaining short-term memory can be generated through single-cell properties.

Adaptive Coding

Adaptation of neural firing rate to stationary stimuli has been seen in all modalities of the primary sensory system. In the visual system, photoreceptors adapt to light level, and retinal ganglion cells show rapid contrast gain control. The trade-offs and information processing gains due to adaptation in insect eyes, relevant also for the vertebrate retina, are discussed in Laughlin (1989). Mechanoreceptors in the somatosensory system have been classified into four main types of cells, three of which are distinguished by the time scales of their adaptation (rapidly and slowly adapting), and these time scales in part determine the cells' function: slowly adapting cells are implicated in the perception of spatial form and texture, while the experience of flutter and of motion is mediated by rapidly adapting cells (Johnson, 2001). Thus, the dynamics of adaptation can determine a neuron's functional role.

Adaptation is not limited to primary receptors. In visual cortex, V1 neurons show contrast adaptation, which is thought to occur entirely at the level of cortex. The motion aftereffect, a familiar phenomenon whereby following exposure to motion in one direction, the visual field appears to move in the opposite direction, is thought to be due to adaptation of direction-sensitive neurons in visual cortex.

Adaptation to a Distribution

Understanding the significance of adaptation for information processing requires going beyond fixed stimuli. Recently, studies have focused on adaptation to the stimulus *distribution*. This approach is necessary to characterize coding information theoretically: the evaluation of a coding strategy requires considering the entire ensemble of inputs and outputs. In Smirnakis et al. (1997), retinal ganglion cells were stimulated with dynamic movies of flickering light intensity where the mean light level was fixed but the variance was switched periodically from one value to another. The spike rate of the neurons showed typical adaptive behavior (Figure 1): following an increase in variance, the firing rate increased initially, but gradually returned to a considerably lower level; a decrease in variance led to a sudden dip in firing rate, with eventual recovery.

The experiments of Smirnakis et al. (1997) consider only firing rate. However, the timing of single spikes can convey a great deal of information about the stimulus. In the visual system of the fly, in particular the motion-sensitive identified neuron H1 in the fly's lobula plate, much is understood about single-spike coding, providing an excellent opportunity to study the effects of adaptation in detail.

H1 responds to a simple stimulus, wide-field horizontal motion. The neuron is characterized by its input/output relation $P(\text{spike}|s)$, or the probability of a spike given the projection s of the dynamic stimulus onto a relevant feature, determined by reverse correlation.

When the system has reached steady state through exposure to a zero-mean, white noise velocity stimulus with a given variance σ^2, its input/output relation is measured. The resulting curves, measured for a range of values of the variance, are shown in Figure 2. Clearly, the input/output relation is not a fixed property of the system but adapts to the distribution of inputs. Indeed, it does so in such a way that the stimulus appears to be measured in units of its

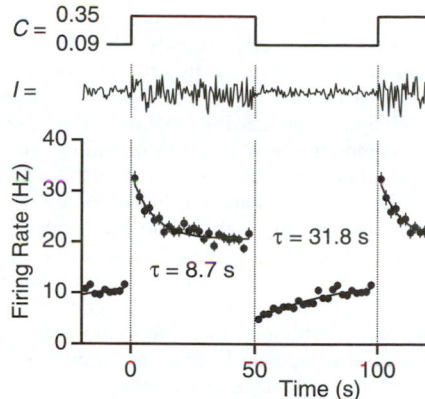

Figure 1. Firing rate of rabbit retinal ganglion cells in response to a flicker stimulus where the variance of the light intensity I switches periodically in time. (From Smirnakis S. M., et al., 1997, Adaptation of retinal processing to image contrast and spatial scale, *Nature*, 386: 69–73. Copyright 1997, Macmillan Publishers Ltd.; reprinted with permission.)

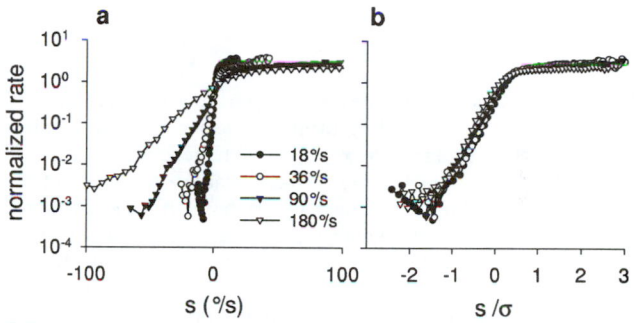

Figure 2. (a) A set of input/output relations relating the probability of spiking to the velocity stimulus, measured for stationary white noise stimuli with different variances. (b) The curves differ only by a scale factor as is shown by normalizing the stimulus by its standard deviation. In this case the curves coincide. (From Brenner, N., Bialek, W., and de Ruyter van Steveninck, R. R., 2001, Adaptive rescaling maximizes information transmission, *Neuron*, 26:695–702. Copyright 2000, Elsevier Science, reprinted with permission.)

standard deviation; when the curves are replotted with the stimulus normalized by its RMS value, they superimpose. Thus, a scale factor λ multiplying the stimulus, and thereby matching the dynamic range of the response to the distribution of the inputs, is a degree of freedom for the system. The value of λ chosen by the system achieves a maximum of information transmission (Brenner, Bialek, and de Ruyter van Steveninck, 2000).

This is a simple form of learning: the system gauges the standard deviation of the signal and modifies its response properties to adjust its dynamic range to the range of inputs. The adjustment must take some time, as the new distribution must be sampled from examples. This sets fundamental physical and statistical limits for the system's estimate of the current variance. We can examine the time scale for learning (Fairhall et al., 2001) by, as in the retina experiments described earlier, switching periodically between two distributions. The firing rate shows the same pattern of adaptation as was seen in the experiments of Smirnakis et al. (1997), but this pattern need not correspond to the time scale for adjustment of the input/output relation. Indeed, it was found that the scale factor of the input/output relations, measured dynamically, adjusts much more rapidly than the relaxation time of the rate—on the order of 100 ms, compared with several seconds. This short time scale is consistent with the limits imposed by estimates of noise from the photoreceptors. One can verify that the dynamic adaptation of the input/output relation maintains information transmission through the system by computing how much information one can extract from the spikes about the stimulus (see SENSORY CODING AND INFORMATION TRANSMISSION and Fairhall et al., 2001). The information rate recovers on comparably short time scales.

For the decoder, a potential drawback of adaptive coding is *ambiguity*: it is necessary to know the context in order to interpret the signal correctly. Thus, information about the context must be conveyed independently. Although this information might be carried by other neurons in the network, here the information about the ensemble is carried simultaneously by the same spike train: it can be read off, either through the rate (taking into account the delays due to the slow relaxation) or, more accurately, through the variance dependence of the statistics of *spike time differences* (Fairhall et al., 2001). Thus, for the code of H1, spikes carry multiple meanings: in absolute timing, as precise markers of single stimulus events, and in relative timing, as indicators of the stimulus ensemble.

Multiple Time Scales

The slow relaxation of the rate appears to be related to a commonly observed property of adapting primary sensory neurons: a power law decay of the firing rate r, $r \sim t^{-\alpha}$. More generally, in the case just presented, the rate is close to the *fractional derivative* of the logarithm of the stimulus variance. For each frequency ω, fractional differentiation shifts the frequency component by a constant phase, and scales each component by ω^α, where α is a power less than 1. Some of the properties of a fractional differentiator are illustrated in Figure 3. Several examples of a power law decay of the rate following a step change in stimulus amplitude were collected by Thorson and Biederman-Thorson (1974; Figure 4) and more have since been observed; examples include various invertebrate mechanoreceptors and photoreceptors, mammalian carotid sinus baroreceptors, and cat retinal ganglion cells.

We have noted a separation of time scales in the adaptation of the input/output relation compared with the rate. This type of adaptation on its own signals the existence of many time scales. Power-law scaling implies the lack of a typical time scale or the presence of multiple time scales. Fractional differentiation is nonlocal; the response at time t_0 is affected by times $t \ll t_0$. This is a linear "memory" mechanism.

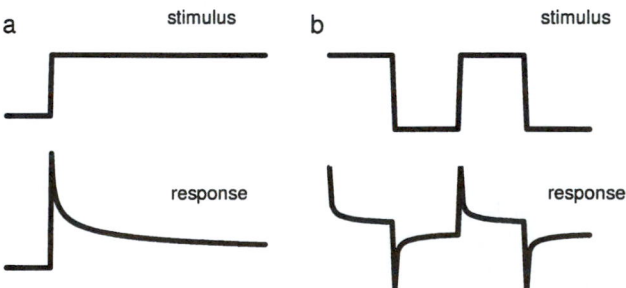

Figure 3. Illustration of some properties of a fractional differentiator with exponent $\alpha = 0.3$. (a) A step function stimulus leads to a power law decaying rate. In a log-log plot the curve would appear as a straight line with slope $-\alpha$. (b) A square wave leads to a similar adaptation curve as shown in Figure 1.

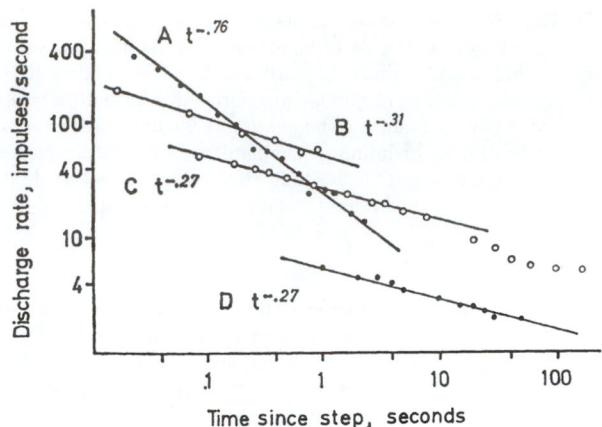

Figure 4. Four curves showing power law adaptation in response to a step increase in stimulus in four different receptors: cockroach leg mechanoreceptor, in response to distortion of the tactile spine on the femur (curve A); slit sensillum on the leg of the hunting spider in response to 1,200 Hz sound (curve B); slowly adapting stretch receptor of the crayfish (curve C); and increase of response over light-adapted level of *Limulus* lateral-eye eccentric cell to an increase in light intensity (curve D). (Examples from Thorson, J., and Biedermann-Thorson, M., 1974, Distributed relaxation processes in a sensory adaptation, *Science*, 183:161–172. Copyright 1974, American Association for the Advancement of Science; reprinted with permission.)

Such adaptation is particularly interesting both because it is so prevalent and because it may have an important role in optimizing information transmission. Fractional-differentiation-like behavior is observed in fly photoreceptors, and in that case, the exponent of the fractional differentiator appears to be matched to the spectrum of natural stimuli (van Hateren and Snippe, 2001). Thus the effect of the transformation is to whiten the spectrum of natural signals. Because many natural stimuli have power-law characteristics, it is intriguing to speculate that fractional differentiation at the sensory periphery may be a general neural mechanism for whitening input statistics.

Mechanisms

Adaptation requires retaining memory of activity over extended time scales. These long time scales can arise from a number of sources. Intracellular calcium concentration has been identified as playing an important role in information processing, acting as a slowly changing "integrator" of activity. Other forms of adaptation, particularly the power-law-like behavior discussed in the previous section, are also likely to be a property of single cells rather than of the network. Recent biophysical studies show that membrane dynamics can have long time scales that retain memory of the history of stimulation/activity over hundreds of seconds (Marom, 1998). This could be brought about either by the modification of intrinsic properties or by intrinsic properties that have built-in long time scales through *state-dependent inactivation* (Turrigiano, Marder, and Abbott, 1996; Marom, 1998).

Calcium as an Integrator of Activity

Each spike introduces a roughly constant amount of calcium into the cell through voltage-dependent Ca^{2+} channels. The Ca^{2+} concentration then decays slowly. Thus, $[Ca^{2+}]$ can be modeled as a leaky integrator of activity, with a decay time scale of ca. 100 ms. This calcium signal can allow activity-dependent regulation of subsequent neural activity through the modification of conductances (see Activity-Dependent Regulation of Neuronal Conductances).

Recent evidence indicates that single-cell properties may contribute to contrast adaptation in cortex (Sanchez-Vives, Nowak, and McCormick, 2000). Previous work has shown that contrast adaptation is associated with hyperpolarization of the membrane potential in cat area 17 neurons. By stimulating the neurons directly with injected current, effects similar to contrast adaptation are seen (though less dramatically than to real visual input). This suggests that these effects can be induced through the modulation of intrinsic cell properties; the activation of Ca^{2+}- and Na^+-dependent potassium conductances is indicated.

State-Dependent Channel Dynamics

In some cases the relevant dynamics may be due to the complex behavior of the channels themselves. Recently it has become clear that the dynamics of inactivation provide the membrane with the possibility for extended history dependence (Marom, 1998).

A simplified picture of the gating of voltage-gated ion channels is a three-state scheme:

$$C \Leftrightarrow O \Leftrightarrow I \qquad (1)$$

where channels can be either closed (C), open (O), or inactivated (I). Generally, the transition between closed and open is voltage-dependent and rapid, on the order of the duration of an action potential. The transition between open and inactivated, on the other hand, is voltage-independent and can have very long time scale dynamics. Intriguingly, studies in vitro show that some sodium channel types have inactivation rates that scale with the duration of the input (Marom, 1998), providing time scales of up to several minutes. The precise mechanism underlying this large variety of time scales is not yet well understood; it is hypothesized that the system cascades through a multiplicity of inactivation states. Earlier theoretical work has shown that the coupling of many states leads to a scaling relation between the duration of activity and the rate of recovery from inactivation.

In a step closer to a realistic preparation, the dynamic clamp was applied to cultured stomatogastric ganglion neurons to add an effective slowly inactivating potassium current (Turrigiano et al., 1996). As had been observed previously, this produced long delays to firing during depolarization, and an increase in excitability with a time scale much longer than the duration of the input. Further, the slow channel dynamics produced a long-lasting effect on the firing properties of the neuron.

In vivo, the contribution of slowly inactivating sodium channels to power-law-like adaptation has been suggested. Mechanosensory neurons in the cockroach femoral tactile spine have been shown to display power-law adaptation. From intracellular measurements, Basarsky and French (1991) found that the spike rate adaptation is due to cumulative slowing of the recovery of the membrane potential between spikes. Previous work had demonstrated that calcium channel blockers or blockers of Ca^{2+}-activated K^+ channels did not reduce adaptation, while modifying sodium channel inactivation did.

These mechanisms might be seen as primitives for short-term "learning and memory."

Modeling

Historically, attempts to model adaptation have considered the process to involve a dynamic threshold. More recently, modeling approaches have taken a functional perspective on the outcome of adaptation and have proposed algorithms whereby the conductances may adjust to provide the cell with desirable properties, such

as approximately constant activity (see Activity-Dependent Regulation of Neuronal Conductances). Closer to our earlier discussion, Stemmler and Koch (1999) derive a learning rule for conductances that maximizes the mutual information between input and output, where the output is taken to be the neuron's firing rate. The learning rule adjusts conductances at every new presentation of the stimulus, subject to biologically plausible constraints. Under this learning rule, a realistic conductance-based model neuron was indeed able to learn a changing distribution and adjust its firing statistics accordingly. The time scales treated were orders of magnitude longer than those observed experimentally in Fairhall et al. (2001) and predicted theoretically from statistical considerations. Experimental evidence is still required to determine whether such a model is realistic.

As noted, many adaptation processes in sensory receptors follow a power-law relaxation. Assuming that most elementary processes involve a single time scale, with exponential dynamics, Thorson and Biederman-Thorson (1974) proposed that power laws may arise from a superposition of many elementary processes with a wide range of time scales. From the definition of the gamma function,

$$t^{-\alpha} = \frac{1}{\Gamma(\alpha)} \int_0^\infty dr \; r^{\alpha-1} e^{-rt} \qquad (2)$$

a power law may be generated by a weighted sum of exponentials with a range of time scales. This distribution was considered to be generated through geometric factors, such as the inhomogeneous distribution of elements within the receptor.

This model has met with some skepticism because of the requirements both for a continuous distribution of time scales and for these to be present in the appropriate proportions. It has been noted that power-law-like behavior results from much less stringent conditions: the superposition of only a few exponentials can produce a power law over the decade or two normally available to experiment. However, recent experimental advances, outlined in the previous section, may provide a better underpinning for the derivation of power-law adaptation from membrane mechanisms.

Adaptation of Receptive Fields

As noted in the Introduction, a neuron can be modeled as a combination of feature extraction (linear filtering) and a nonlinear decision function (or threshold). Although we have discussed the effects of adaptation on the nonlinear decision function, adaptation can also affect the feature that causes the neuron to spike: the receptive field can depend on the ensemble of inputs. Although this result had been frequently observed in work on invertebrate vision, recent experiments demonstrate analogous results for cortical receptive fields. Sceniak et al. (1999) show that the extent of spatial summation implemented by neurons in V1 depends adaptively on contrast; this has parallels in the adaptation of filters in retina (Laughlin, 1989). Theunissen, Sen, and Doupe (2000) found that the spatiotemporal receptive fields of neurons in auditory cortex showed a strong dependence on the stimulus ensemble. This is a natural consequence of neural nonlinearity, but such a dependence is also necessary for optimal information processing.

Discussion

The ubiquity of adaptation throughout the nervous system should be proof of its fundamental importance. Although the phenomenology of adaptation, particularly to constant stimuli, has been extensively explored, recent experimental and theoretical approaches have made contact with the principles of information theory in order to evaluate adaptive coding. For fly motion-sensitive neurons, it was found that the coding strategy of the system adapts rapidly and continuously to track dynamic changes in the statistics of the stimulus.

We have discussed a variety of mechanisms that may implement adaptive coding at the level of single cells. Although it is likely that systems will implement such important behavior at many levels, it is appealing that the simplest elements of neural computation have the power to carry out dynamic aspects of information processing.

Road Map: Neural Coding
Related Reading: Population Codes; Sensory Coding and Information Transmission

References

Basarsky, T., and French, A., 1991, Intracellular measurements from a rapidly adapting sensory neuron, *J. Neurophysiol.*, 65:49–56.

Brenner, N., Bialek, W., and de Ruyter van Steveninck, R., 2000, Adaptive rescaling maximizes information transmission, *Neuron*, 26:695–702.

Fairhall, A. L., Lewen, G., Bialek, W., and de Ruyter van Steveninck, R. R., 2001, Efficiency and ambiguity in an adaptive neural code, *Nature*, 412:787–792.

Johnson, K. O., 2001, The roles and functions of cutaneous mechanoreceptors, *Curr. Opin. Neurobiol.*, 11:455–61. ◆

Laughlin, S. B., 1989, The role of sensory adaptation in the retina, *J. Exp. Biol.*, 146:39–62. ◆

Marom, S., 1998, Slow changes in the availability of voltage-gated ion channels: Effects on the dynamics of excitable membranes, *J. Membr. Biol.*, 161:105–113. ◆

Sanchez-Vives, M., Nowak, L., and McCormick, D., 2000, Membrane mechanisms underlying contrast adaptation in cat area 17 in vivo, *J. Neurosci.*, 20:4267–4285.

Sceniak, M. P., Ringach, D. L., Hawken, M. J., and Shapley, R., 1999, Contrast's effect on spatial summation by macaque V1 neurons, *Nature Neurosci.*, 2:733–739.

Smirnakis, S. M., Berry, M. J., Warland, D. K., Bialek, W., and Meister, M., 1997, Adaptation of retinal processing to image contrast and spatial scale, *Nature*, 386:69–73.

Stemmler, M., and Koch, C., 1999, How voltage-dependent conductances can adapt to maximize the information encoded by neuronal firing rate, *Nature Neurosci.*, 2:521–527.

Theunissen, F., Sen, K., and Doupe, A., 2000, Spectral-temporal receptive fields of nonlinear auditory neurons obtained using natural sounds, *J. Neurosci.*, 20:2315–2331.

Thorson, J., and Biederman-Thorson, M., 1974, Distributed relaxation processes in a sensory adaptation, *Science*, 183: 161–172. ◆

Torre, V., Ashmore, J. F., Lamb, T. D., and Menini, A., 1995, Transduction and adaptation in sensory receptor cells, *J. Neurosci.*, 15:7757–7763. ◆

Turrigiano, G., Marder, E., and Abbott, L., 1996, Cellular short-term memory from a slow potassium conductance, *J. Neurophysiol.*, 75:963–968.

van Hateren, J. H., and Snippe, H. P., 2001, Information theoretical evaluation of parametric models of gain control in blowfly photoreceptor cells, *Vision Res.*, 41:1851–1865.

Amplification, Attenuation, and Integration

H. Sebastian Seung

Introduction

Differential equations such as

$$\tau \dot{x}_i + x_i = f\left(\sum_j W_{ij} x_j + b_i\right) \tag{1}$$

have long been used to model networks of interacting neurons (Ermentrout, 1998; PHASE-PLANE ANALYSIS OF NEURAL NETS). The activity of neuron i is represented by a single dynamical variable x_i, and its input-output characteristics by a single transfer function f. There are more biophysically realistic descriptions of neural networks that include many dynamical variables per neuron, in order to explicitly model dendritic integration, action potential generation, and synaptic transmission. Nevertheless, simplified models like that in Equation 1 have been useful for understanding how the computational properties of neural networks are related to their synaptic organization.

The parameter W_{ij} in Equation 1 represents the strength of the synapse from neuron j to i. These synapses are termed *recurrent*, as they connect to other neurons in the same network. Feedforward synaptic input from outside the network is implicit in the bias b_i. The feedforward synapses could be made explicit by writing $b_i = b_i^0 + \Sigma_a V_{ia} z_a$, where z_a are input neuron activities, V_{ia} the strengths of the feedforward synapses, and b_i^0 any intrinsic tendency of neuron i to be active. But the feedforward connections will be left implicit in the following, so as to focus on the computational role of the recurrent connections.

Accordingly, the biases b_i in Equation 1 will be regarded as the inputs to the network, while the activities x_i are the outputs. If there were no recurrent synapses ($W_{ij} = 0$ for all i and j), then each neuron i would respond by low-pass filtering the signal $f(b_i)$ with time constant τ. When there are recurrent synapses, a general char-

acterization of the response properties of a network is difficult, but the situation is greatly simplified when nonlinearity is neglected. Putting the transfer function $f(u) = u$ in Equation 1 yields the linear network

$$\tau \dot{x}_i + x_i = \sum_j W_{ij} x_j + b_i \tag{2}$$

which can be completely analyzed using the tools of linear systems theory. The modest goal of this article is to describe some properties of linear networks and give examples of their application to neural modeling.

In particular, the focus is on the role of recurrent synaptic connectivity. Provided that they do not lead to instability, the recurrent connections alter both the gain and speed of response to feedforward input. Either they amplify and slow down responses to feedforward input, or they attenuate and speed up responses. Both effects can occur simultaneously in the same network, as can be seen by mathematically transforming the network of interacting neurons into a set of noninteracting eigenmodes. The effect of the recurrent synapses generally varies from mode to mode.

Besides amplification and attenuation, a linear network can also carry out the operation of temporal integration, in the sense of Newtonian calculus. This happens when the strength of feedback is precisely tuned for an eigenmode, so that its gain and time constant diverge to infinity.

Admittedly, the neglect of nonlinearity is a step away from biological realism. Nevertheless, linear models are important because they give insight into the local behavior of nonlinear networks, which can often be linearly approximated in the vicinity of fixed points. And the linear computations of amplification, attenuation, and integration have been ascribed to a number of brain areas.

Autapse

The simplest example of a recurrent synapse is a single neuron with a synapse onto itself, or *autapse*, in the terminology of neurophysiology. For this case, the dynamics (Equation 2) takes the form

$$\tau \dot{x} + x = Wx + b \qquad (3)$$

The autapse has strength W and is said to be excitatory if $W > 0$ and inhibitory if $W < 0$. The example is not meant to be a realistic model of a biological autapse; it is only a simple illustration of some of the effects of recurrent synaptic connections. The parameter W will also be called the strength of *feedback*, in the terminology of engineering. Without feedback ($W = 0$), the neuron acts as a low-pass filter of input b with time constant τ. When the effect of feedback is considered, the first distinction that has to be made is between the unstable $W > 1$ and the stable $W < 1$ cases. (Discussion of the borderline $W = 1$ case is postponed until later.)

If $W > 1$, the autapse is unstable, as can be seen by solving Equation 3 for input b that is constant in time. The solution diverges exponentially to infinity, because the feedback is so strong that it leads to runaway instability. Note that in a more realistic model, the growth of this runaway instability would eventually be limited by nonlinearity, but in the idealized linear model (Equation 3), divergence to infinity is possible.

If $W < 1$, the autapse is stable, and the dynamics (Equation 3) can be rewritten in the form

$$\frac{\tau}{1 - W} \dot{x} + x = \frac{b}{1 - W} \qquad (4)$$

From this formula can be read two numbers that characterize the autapse: the steady-state gain, and the time constant of response. The gain is operationally defined by holding the input constant and allowing the output to relax to the steady-state value $x_\infty = b/(1 - W)$. Then the steady-state gain, defined as the ratio of output x_∞ to input b, is $1/(1 - W)$. By this definition, the gain is exactly unity in the case of no feedback ($W = 0$). Positive ($W > 0$) and negative ($W < 0$) feedback have different effects. Positive feedback amplifies, boosting the gain to a value greater than 1. Negative feedback attenuates, making the gain less than 1.

Positive and negative feedback also have opposite effects on the speed of response. The time constant of the exponential relaxation to the steady state is $\tau/(1 - W)$. In the case of no feedback, this is equal to the fundamental time constant τ. But positive feedback lengthens the time constant, while negative feedback shortens it. This means that there is a trade-off between amplification and speed, sometimes known as the gain-bandwidth trade-off. Intuitively speaking, the trade-off arises because feedback amplification requires that the signal circulate in the feedback loop, so that more amplification requires more time.

In summary, a feedback loop containing a perfectly linear element behaves in a simple way. Positive feedback ($W > 0$) amplifies and slows down response, assuming that it doesn't lead to instability. Negative feedback ($W < 0$) attenuates and speeds up response.

The idea of amplification by positive feedback has been prominent in a number of models of primary visual cortex (Douglas et al., 1995). Neurons in layer 4 receive both feedforward drive from the thalamus and recurrent input from other cortical neurons. It has been proposed that the recurrent interactions amplify the responses to feedforward input. To test this idea, Ferster and colleagues recorded from layer 4 neurons. They inactivated corticocortical inputs both by cooling (Ferster, Chung, and Wheat, 1996) and electrical stimulation (Chung and Ferster, 1998). In both cases, they measured a two- or threefold reduction in the amplitude of cortical

responses to visual stimulation, which was interpreted as a loss of amplification by positive feedback.

The above discussion omitted the special case of $W = 1$, which is the borderline between stability and instability. For $W \neq 1$, there was exactly one steady state, which was either stable or unstable, depending on whether W was less than or greater than 1. In contrast, if $W = 1$, there is not a unique steady state. The number of steady states depends on b. There are infinitely many if $b = 0$, and none at all if $b \neq 0$. To understand the case of non-zero b, it is helpful to return to Equation 3, which reduces to $\tau \dot{x} = b$. In other words, the response x is the time integral of b. Therefore, a linear autapse can act as an integrator, if the strength of feedback is precisely tuned (Seung et al., 2000). Variants of this idea have been used to model neural integrators, brain areas that integrate their inputs in the sense of Newtonian calculus (Robinson, 1989).

Mutually Inhibitory Pair

While the autapse illustrates the gain-bandwidth trade-off in feedback amplification, it involves only a single neuron, and cannot capture genuine population behaviors. A more interesting example consists of two linear neurons with mutual inhibition:

$$\tau \dot{x}_1 + x_1 = -\beta x_2 + b_1 \qquad (5)$$

$$\tau \dot{x}_2 + x_2 = -\beta x_1 + b_2 \qquad (6)$$

The parameter β is assumed to be positive, so that the interaction is inhibitory. This dynamics is more complex than Equation 3 because it involves two differential equations that are coupled to each other. Luckily, it turns out that the equations can be decoupled by adding and subtracting them.

Adding the two equations yields an equation for the common mode $x_c = x_1 + x_2$,

$$\tau \frac{d}{dt}(x_1 + x_2) + (x_1 + x_2) = -\beta(x_1 + x_2) + (b_1 + b_2) \qquad (7)$$

Comparison with Equation 3 reveals that the common mode behaves like an autapse with negative feedback. Therefore the common mode attenuates its input $b_1 + b_2$ with steady-state gain $1/(1 + \beta)$ and time constant $\tau/(1 + \beta)$.

Similarly, subtracting the two equations yields an equation for the differential mode $x_d = x_1 - x_2$,

$$\tau \frac{d}{dt}(x_1 - x_2) + (x_1 - x_2) = \beta(x_1 - x_2) + (b_1 - b_2) \qquad (8)$$

The differential mode behaves like an autapse with positive feedback. If $\beta > 1$, the differential mode is unstable. If $\beta < 1$, then the differential mode amplifies its input $b_1 - b_2$ with steady-state gain $1/(1 - \beta)$ and time constant $\tau/(1 - \beta)$.

To recapitulate, transforming from (x_1, x_2) to (x_c, x_d) formally decoupled the mutually inhibitory pair of neurons into two "virtual" autapses. Note that the transformation is reversible, as x_1 and x_2 can be reconstructed from the common and differential modes, e.g., $x_1 = (x_c + x_d)/2$.

A striking aspect of this example is that mutual inhibition has completely opposite effects on the common and differential modes. For the common mode, inhibition mediates negative feedback, which leads to attenuation. But inhibition mediates positive feedback for the differential mode, which leads to amplification.

The general lesson to be drawn is that no direct correspondence exists between the sign of synaptic connections and the sign of feedback. This is because a synapse is local, belonging to just two neurons. In contrast, feedback strength is global, belonging to a distributed mode of the network. As will be described below, the feedback strength is given in general by the eigenvalues of the synaptic weight matrix W. The autapse is a special exception for which the sign of the synaptic connection directly corresponds to the sign of feedback, but this does not hold true in general.

The idea that inhibition between neurons can amplify differences has been used to explain the fact that visual systems are more sensitive to relative luminance, or contrast, than to absolute luminance. For example, the *Limulus* retina consists of visual receptors that are topographically organized in a two-dimensional network and interact via lateral inhibition. Measurements of retinal output reveal enhancement of luminance differences, a fact that has been successfully explained using network models that are generalizations of the mutually inhibitory pair considered here (Hartline and Ratliff, 1972).

The special case $\beta = 1$ is also of interest. It is the borderline of stability for the differential mode. If $b_1 - b_2$ is zero, then the differential mode $x_1 - x_2$ is constant in time, according to Equation 8, while the common mode $x_1 + x_2$ converges exponentially to the value $(b_1 + b_2)/2$. This is a simple example of a *line attractor*, a line of fixed points to which all trajectories are attracted (Seung, 1996). More complex nonlinear network models with approximate line attractors have been used to model the phenomenon of persistent neural activity (Seung, 1996; Zhang, 1996).

Note that having a continuous set of fixed points is an unusual situation, requiring the precise tuning of the inhibitory strength β and the differential input $b_1 - b_2$. When $b_1 - b_2$ is non-zero, then it is integrated by the differential mode. In this case, inhibitory interactions yield an integrator, in contrast to the autapse, which requires excitatory feedback to integrate. Robinson et al. proposed that lateral inhibition is the mechanism of the oculomotor neural integrator, which converts vestibular and other velocity-coded inputs into eye position outputs (Cannon, Robinson, and Shamma, 1983).

General Network

For a general network of N neurons, the effects of feedback can be understood via eigensystem analysis. It is convenient to rewrite the dynamics in Equation 2 in matrix-vector form as

$$\tau \frac{d}{dt} x + x = Wx + b \tag{9}$$

where x and b are vectors and W is the synaptic weight matrix.

Suppose that the weight matrix can be factorized as $W = S\Lambda S^{-1}$, where Λ is a real diagonal matrix and S is a real invertible matrix. A sufficient condition for a real diagonalization is that the weight matrix W be symmetric, but this is not a necessary condition. The diagonal entries of Λ are the eigenvalues of W. The columns of S are the right eigenvectors of W, and the rows of S^{-1} are the left eigenvectors.

Recall that transforming to the common and differential modes simplified the dynamics of the mutually inhibitory pair. The analogue here is to change from x and b to

$$\tilde{x} = S^{-1}x, \qquad \tilde{b} = S^{-1}b$$

These vectors can be used to express x and b as linear combinations of the right eigenvectors, $x = S\tilde{x}$ and $b = S\tilde{b}$.

The transformation of Equation 9 is effected by multiplying with S^{-1},

$$\tau \frac{d}{dt} \tilde{x} + \tilde{x} = S^{-1}Wx + \tilde{b} \tag{10}$$

$$= S^{-1}WS\tilde{x} + \tilde{b} \tag{11}$$

$$= \Lambda \tilde{x} + \tilde{b} \tag{12}$$

Writing out the last expression component by component yields

$$\tau \frac{d}{dt} \tilde{x}_a + \tilde{x}_a = \lambda_a \tilde{x}_a + \tilde{b}_a$$

where λ_a is the ath diagonal element of Λ, or equivalently the ath eigenvalue of W. This is a great simplification: the network (Equation 9) of N interacting neurons has been transformed into N non-interacting "virtual" autapses. Each autapse has feedback with strength given by the eigenvalues λ_a. Assuming that the eigenvalues are less than or equal to 1, each autapse can perform the operations of amplification, attenuation, or integration.

Discussion

In this article, some effects of recurrent synaptic connectivity on linear networks were characterized. The autapse example demonstrated that there is a gain-bandwidth trade-off in amplification and attenuation by feedback, and the possibility of integration when feedback is precisely tuned. The mutually inhibitory pair illustrated the decoupling of an interacting network into "virtual" autapses, and also illustrated that the sign of feedback is not directly related to the sign of synaptic connections. Such a decoupling is generally possible for any synaptic weight matrix W that is diagonalizable with all real eigenvalues.

More generally, the eigenvalues (and eigenvectors) are complex numbers. When an eigenvalue of W has a non-zero imaginary part, the corresponding eigenmode exhibits oscillatory behavior. Accordingly, linear analyses have been used to explain the existence of oscillations in some neural network models (Li and Hopfield, 1989).

It is natural to ask whether the concepts introduced above have any relevance for *nonlinear* neural networks. A simple way of modeling nonlinearity is to introduce a threshold for activation by choosing $f(x) = \max\{x, 0\}$ for the transfer function in Equation 1. Because the resulting dynamics are piecewise linear, eigenvalues and eigenvectors are still essential for mathematical analysis (Hadeler and Kuhn, 1987; Hahnloser et al., 2000), but the threshold nonlinearity leads to a richer variety of dynamical behaviors. A full discussion of threshold linear networks is beyond the scope of this article, but let us briefly reconsider the example of a mutually inhibitory pair of neurons presented with inputs that are constant in time. For linear neurons, the mutual inhibition caused differences in input to be amplified in the steady-state response. If the neurons are instead threshold linear, *winner-take-all* behavior can result for some choices of model parameters. Then only a single neuron is active at steady state, no matter how small the difference in inputs may be (Amari and Arbib, 1977). As in the purely linear case, the difference in steady-state outputs is greater than the difference in inputs. However, this behavior cannot be explained in terms of a simple linear amplification. For a more detailed explanation, see WINNER-TAKE-ALL NETWORKS.

Road Map: Dynamic Systems
Background: I.3. Dynamics and Adaptation in Neural Networks
Related Reading: Pattern Formation, Neural; Winner-Take-All Networks

References

Amari, S., and Arbib, M. A., 1977, Competition and cooperation in neural nets, in *Systems Neuroscience* (J. Metzler, Ed.), New York: Academic Press, pp. 119–165. ◆
Cannon, S. C., Robinson, D. A., and Shamma, S. 1983, A proposed neural network for the integrator of the oculomotor system, *Biol. Cybern.*, 49:127–136.
Chung, S., and Ferster, D., 1998, Strength and orientation tuning of the thalamic input to simple cells revealed by electrically evoked cortical suppression, *Neuron*, 20:1177–1189.

Douglas, R. J., Koch, C., Mahowald, M., Martin, K. A. C., and Suarez, H. H., 1995, Recurrent excitation in neocortical circuits, *Science*, 269:981–985.

Ermentrout, B., 1998, Neural networks as spatio-temporal pattern-forming systems, *Rep. Prog. Phys.*, 61:353–430. ◆

Ferster, D., Chung, S., and Wheat, H., 1996, Orientation selectivity of thalamic input to simple cells of cat visual cortex, *Nature*, 380(6571):249–252.

Hadeler, K. P., and Kuhn, D., 1987, Stationary states of the Hartline-Ratliff model, *Biol. Cybern.*, 56:411–417.

Hahnloser, R. H., Sarpeshkar, R., Mahowald, M. A., Douglas, R. J., and Seung, H. S., 2000, Digital selection and analogue amplification coexist in a cortex-inspired silicon circuit, *Nature*, 405(6789):947–951.

Hartline, H. K., and Ratliff, F., 1972, Inhibitory interaction in the retina of *Limulus*, in *Handbook of Sensory Physiology: Physiology of Photore-ceptor Organs* (M. G. F. Fuortes, Ed.), Berlin: Springer-Verlag, pp. 382–447.

Li, Z., and Hopfield, J. J., 1989, Modeling the olfactory bulb and its neural oscillatory processings, *Biol. Cybern.*, 61:379–392.

Robinson, D. A., 1989, Integrating with neurons, *Annu. Rev. Neurosci.*, 12:33–45.

Seung, H. S., 1996, How the brain keeps the eyes still, *Proc. Natl. Acad. Sci. USA*, 93:13339–13344.

Seung, H. S., Lee, D. D., Reis, B. Y., and Tank, D. W., 2000, The autapse: A simple illustration of short-term analog memory storage by tuned synaptic feedback, *J. Comput. Neurosci.*, 9:171–185. ◆

Zhang, K., 1996, Representation of spatial orientation by the intrinsic dynamics of the head-direction cell ensemble: A theory, *J. Neurosci.*, 16:2112–2126.

Analog Neural Networks, Computational Power

Bhaskar DasGupta and Georg Schnitger

Introduction

The last two decades have seen a surge in theoretical techniques to design and analyze the performance of neural nets as well as novel applications of neural nets to various applied areas. Theoretical studies on the computational capabilities of neural nets have provided valuable insights into the mechanisms of these models.

In subsequent discussion, we distinguish between feedforward neural nets and recurrent neural nets. The architecture of a feedforward net $\mathcal{N}$ is described by an interconnection graph and the activation functions of $\mathcal{N}$. A node (processor or neuron) v of $\mathcal{N}$ computes a function

$$\gamma_v \left(\sum_{i=1}^{k} a_{v_i,v} u_{v_i} + b_v \right) \tag{1}$$

of its inputs $u_{v_1}, \ldots, u_{v_k}$. These inputs are either external (i.e., representing the input data) or internal (i.e., representing the outputs of the immediate predecessors of v). The coefficients $a_{v_i,v}$ (respectively b_v) in Equation 1 are the *weights* (respectively *threshold*) of node v, and the function γ_v is the *activation function* of v. No cycles are allowed in the interconnection graph, and the output of designated nodes provides the output of the network. A recurrent neural net, on the other hand, allows cycles, thereby providing potentially higher computational capabilities. The *state* u_v of node v in a recurrent net is updated over time according to

$$u_v(t + 1) = \gamma_v \left(\sum_{i=1}^{k} a_{v_i,v} u_{v_i}(t) + b_v \right) \tag{2}$$

In this article, we emphasize the exact and approximate representational power of feedforward and recurrent neural nets. This line of research can be traced back to Kolmogorov (1957), who essentially proved the first existential result on the (exact) representation capabilities of neural nets (cf. UNIVERSAL APPROXIMATORS). The need to work with "well-behaved" activation functions, however, enforces approximative representations of target functions, and the question of the approximation power (with limited resources) becomes fundamental.

The representation power of neural nets has immediate consequences for learning, since we cannot learn (approximately) what we cannot represent (approximately). On the other hand, the complexity of learning increases with increasing representational power of the underlying neural model, and care must be exercised to strike a balance between representational power, on the one hand, and learning complexity, on the other. The emphasis of this article is on representational power, i.e., what can be represented with networks using a given set of activation functions, rather than on learning complexity.

In this article, we discuss only a small subset of the literature on this topic. After introducing the basic notation, we discuss the representational power of feedforward and recurrent neural nets. There follows a brief discussion of networks of spiking neurons and their relation to sigmoidal nets, with a summary statement.

Models and Basic Definitions

In this section we present the notation and basic definitions used in subsequent sections. For real-valued functions we measure the approximation quality of function f by function g (over a domain $D \subseteq \mathbb{R}^n$) by the Chebychev norm,

$$\|f - g\|_D = \sup\{|f(x) - g(x)| : x \in D\}$$

(the subscript D will be omitted when clear from the context). To emphasize the selection of activation functions, we introduce the concept of Γ-nets for a class Γ of real-valued activation functions. A Γ-net $\mathcal{N}$ assigns only functions in Γ to nodes. We assume that each function in Γ is defined on some subset of $\mathbb{R}$, and require that Γ contain the identity function by default (thus allowing weighted additions as node outputs). Finally, we restrict our attention to Γ-nets with a single output node.

The *depth* of a feedforward net $\mathcal{N}$ is the length of the longest path of the (acyclic) interconnection graph of $\mathcal{N}$, and the *size* of $\mathcal{N}$ is the number of nodes. The *hidden nodes* are all nodes excluding all input nodes and the output node.

The class of important activation functions is rather large and includes, among others, the binary threshold function

$$\mathcal{H}(x) = \begin{cases} 0 & \text{if } x \leq 0, \\ 1 & \text{if } x > 0, \end{cases}$$

the cosine squasher, the Gaussian, the standard sigmoid $\sigma(x) = 1/(1 + e^{-x})$, the hyperbolic tangent, (generalized) radial basis functions, polynomials and trigonometric polynomials, splines, and rational functions.

Care must be exercised when using a neural net with continuous activation functions to compute a Boolean-valued function, since in general, the output node computes a real number. A standard output convention in this case is as follows (see Maass, 1994):

Definition 1. A Γ-net $\mathcal{N}$ computes a Boolean function $F: \mathbb{R}^n \to \{0, 1\}$ with separation $\varepsilon > 0$ if there is some $t \in \mathbb{R}$ such that for any input $x \in \mathbb{R}^n$, the output node of $\mathcal{N}$ computes a value that is at least $t + \varepsilon$ if $F(x) = 1$, and at most $t - \varepsilon$ otherwise.

Recurrent neural nets, unlike their feedforward counterparts, allow loops in their interconnection graph. Certainly *asynchronous* recurrent nets are an important neural model, but we assume in Equation 2 that all nodes update *synchronously* at each time step. Typically, besides internal and external data lines, some of the inputs and outputs are validation lines, indicating if there is any input or output present at the time.

Computational Power of Feedforward Nets

The simple perceptron as a feedforward neural net with one layer has only limited computational abilities. For instance, if we restrict ourselves to one-node simple perceptrons and assume monotone, but otherwise arbitrary, activation functions, then the XOR function $\text{XOR}(x_1, x_2) = x_1 \oplus x_2$ cannot be computed.

On the other hand, if we choose the binary threshold function $\mathcal{H}$ as activation function, then the learning problem for simple perceptrons is efficiently solvable by linear programming. This positive result is also extendable to a large class of activation functions, including the standard sigmoid. But simple perceptrons should not be underestimated, since the problem of approximately minimizing the missclassification ratio (when the target function is not representable as a simple perceptron) has been shown to be (probably) intractable (Arora et al., 1997).

However, the power of feedforward nets increases significantly when networks of more layers are considered. In fact, a result of Kolmogorov (refuting Hilbert's 13th problem for continuous functions), when translated into neural net terminology, shows that any continuous function can be computed *exactly* by a feedforward net of depth 3.

Theorem 1 (Kolmogorov, 1957). Let n be a natural number. Then there are continuous functions $h_1, \ldots, h_{2n+1} : [0, 1] \to \mathbb{R}$ such that any continuous function $f: [0, 1]^n \to \mathbb{R}$ can be represented as

$$f(x) = \sum_{j=1}^{2n+1} g\left(\sum_{i=1}^{n} \alpha_i h_j(x_i)\right)$$

where the function g as well as the weights $\alpha_1, \ldots, \alpha_n$ depend on f.

But, unfortunately, the function g depends on the function to be represented. Moreover, the functions h_j are nondifferentiable and hence cannot be used by current learning algorithms. For further discussion, we refer the reader to Poggio and Girosi (1989).

However, if we only allow everywhere differentiable activation functions (such as the standard sigmoid), then we can only represent everywhere differentiable target functions. Thus, one has to relax the requirement of exact representation, and demand only that the approximation error (in an appropriate norm) is small. Applying the Stone-Weierstrass theorem one obtains, for instance, (trigonometric) polynomials as universal approximators, and hence we get neural nets with one hidden layer as universal approximators.

Cybenko (1989) considers activation functions from the class of continuous *discriminatory* functions. This class contains, for instance, *sigmoidal* functions, i.e., continuous functions σ satisfying

$$\sigma(t) \to \begin{cases} 1 & \text{as } t \to +\infty \\ 0 & \text{as } t \to -\infty \end{cases}$$

Theorem 2. Let σ be a continuous discriminatory function and let $f: [0, 1]^n \to \mathbb{R}$ be a continuous target function. Then, for every $\varepsilon > 0$ and for sufficiently large N (where N depends on the target function f and ε), there exist weights α_{ij}, w_j and thresholds β_j, such that $\|f - g\| < \varepsilon$, where $g = \sum_{j=1}^{N} w_j \cdot \sigma(\sum_{i=1}^{n} \alpha_{ij} \cdot x_i + \beta_j)$.

In particular, one hidden layer suffices to approximate any continuous function by sigmoidal nets within arbitrarily small error. Further results along this line are shown by Hornik; Stinchcombe and White; Funahashi, Moore, and Poggio; and Poggio and Girosi, to mention just a few. Whereas most arguments in the above-mentioned results are nonconstructive, Carroll and Dickinson describe a method using Radon transforms to approximate a given L_2 function to within a given mean square error.

Barron (1993) discusses the approximation quality achievable by sigmoidal nets of small size. In particular, let $B_r^n(0)$ denote the n-dimensional ball with radius r around 0 and let $f : B_r^n(0) \to \mathbb{R}$ be the target function. Assume that F is the magnitude distribution of the Fourier transform of f.

Theorem 3 (Barron, 1993). Let σ be any sigmoidal function. Then for every probability measure μ and for every N there exist weights α_{ij}, w_j and thresholds β_j, such that

$$\int_{B_r^n(0)} \left(f(x) - \sum_{j=1}^{N} w_j \cdot \sigma\left(\sum_{i=1}^{n} \alpha_{ij} \cdot x_i + \beta_j\right)\right)^2 \mu(dx)$$
$$\leq \frac{(2\int r \cdot |w| \cdot F(dw))^2}{N}$$

Set $C_f = \int r \cdot |w| \cdot F(dw)$, and the approximation error achievable by sigmoidal nets of size N is bounded by $(2 \cdot C_f)^2/N$. However, C_f may depend superpolynomially on n, and the curse of dimensionality may strike. As an aside, the best achievable squared error for linear combinations of N *basis functions* will be at least $\Omega(C_f / n \cdot N^{1/n})$ for certain functions f (Barron, 1993), and hence neural networks are superior to conventional approximation methods from this point of view.

The results just enumerated show that depth-2 feedforward nets are universal approximators. This dramatically increased computing power, however, has a rather negative consequence. Kharitonov (1993) showed that under certain cryptographic assumptions, no efficient learning algorithm will be able to predict the input-output behavior of binary threshold nets with a fixed number of layers. This result holds even when experimentation is allowed, that is, when the learning algorithm is allowed to submit inputs for classification.

In the next section, we compare important activation functions in terms of their approximation power, when resources such as depth and size are limited. The following section discusses networks of spiking neurons. Lower size bounds for sigmoidal nets are mentioned when we compare networks of spiking neurons and sigmoidal nets.

Efficient Approximation by Feedforward Nets

Our discussion will be informal, and we refer the reader to DasGupta and Schnitger (1993) for details. Our goal is to compare activation functions in terms of the size and depth required to obtain tight approximations. Another resource of interest is the *Lipschitz bound* of the net, which is a measure of the numerical stability of the circuit. Informally speaking, for a net $\mathcal{N}$ to have Lipschitz-bound L, we first demand that all weights and thresholds of $\mathcal{N}$ be bounded in absolute value by L. Moreover, we require that each activation function of $\mathcal{N}$ have (the conventional) Lipschitz-bound L on the inputs it receives. Finally, the actually received inputs have to be bounded away from regions with higher Lipschitz bounds.

We formalize the notion of having *essentially the same approximation power*.

Definition 2. Let Γ_1 and Γ_2 be classes of activation functions.

(a) We say that Γ_2 simulates Γ_1 (denoted by $\Gamma_1 \leq \Gamma_2$) if and only if there is a constant $k \geq 1$ such that for all Γ_1-nets C_2 of size at most s, depth at most d, and Lipschitz bound 2^s, there is a Γ_2-circuit C_1 of size at most $(s + 1)^k$, depth at most $k \cdot (d + 1)$, and Lipschitz bound $2^{(s+1)^k}$, such that

$$\|C_1 - C_2\|_{[-1,1]^n} \leq 2^{-s}$$

(b) We say that Γ_1 and Γ_2 are equivalent if and only if $\Gamma_1 \leq \Gamma_2$ and $\Gamma_2 \leq \Gamma_1$.

In other words, when simulating classes of gate functions, we allow depth to increase by a constant factor size and the logarithm of the Lipschitz bound to increase polynomially. The relatively large Lipschitz bounds should not come as a surprise, since the negative exponential error 2^{-s} requires correspondingly large weights in the simulating circuit.

Splines (i.e., piecewise polynomial functions) have turned out to be powerful approximators, and they are our benchmark class of activation functions; in particular, we assume that a spline net of size s has as its activation functions splines of degree at most s with at most one knot. Which properties does a class Γ of activation functions need to reach the approximation power of splines? The activation functions should be able to approximate polynomials as well as the binary threshold $\mathcal{H}$ with few layers and relatively few nodes.

Tightly approximating polynomials is not difficult as long as there is at least one "sufficiently smooth" nontrivial function $\gamma \in \Gamma$. The crucial problem is to obtain a tight approximation of $\mathcal{H}$. It turns out that γ-nets achieve tight approximations of $\mathcal{H}$ whenever

$$|\gamma(x) - \gamma(x + \varepsilon)| = O(\varepsilon/x^2)$$

$$\text{for } x \geq 1, \quad \varepsilon \geq 0 \quad \text{and} \quad \left|\int_1^\infty \gamma(u^2)du\right| \neq 0$$

Let us call a function with these two properties *strongly sigmoidal*. (We are actually demanding too much, since it suffices to tightly approximate a strongly sigmoidal function γ by small Γ-nets with few layers.) Let us call a class Γ *powerful* if there is at least one "sufficiently smooth" nontrivial function in Γ and if a strongly sigmoidal function can be approximated as demanded above.

Examples of powerful singleton classes include, for instance, $1/x$ as a prime example, and more generally any rational function that is not a polynomial, $\exp(x)$ (since $\exp(-x)$ is strongly sigmoidal) and $\ln(x)$ (since $\ln(x + 1) - \ln(x)$ is strongly sigmoidal), any power x^α provided α is not a natural number, and the standard sigmoid as well as the Gaussian $\exp(-x^2)$.

Theorem 4.

(a) Assume that Γ is powerful. Then splines $\leq \Gamma$.
(b) The following classes of activation function have equivalent approximation power: splines (of degree s for nets of size s), any rational function that is not a polynomial, any power x^α (provided α is not a natural number), the logarithm (for any base), $\exp(x)$, and the Gaussian $\exp(-x^2)$.

Notably missing from the list of equivalent activation functions are polynomials, trigonometric polynomials, and the binary threshold function $\mathcal{H}$ (or, more generally, low-degree splines). Low-

degree splines turn out to be properly weaker. The same applies to polynomials, even if we allow any polynomial of degree s an activation function for nets of size s. Finally, sine nets cannot be simulated (as defined in Definition 2), for instance by nets of standard sigmoids, and we conjecture that the reverse is also true, namely, that nets of standard sigmoids cannot be simulated efficiently by sine nets.

What happens if we relax the required approximation quality from 2^{-s} to s^{-d}, when simulating nets of depth d and size s? Linear splines and the standard sigmoid are still not equivalent, but the situation changes completely if we *count* the number of inputs when determining size and if we restrict the Lipschitz bound of the target function to be at most s^{-d}. With this modification an even larger class of important functions, including linear splines, polynomials, and the sine function, turn out to be equivalent with the standard sigmoid.

The situation for Boolean input and output is somewhat comparable. Maass, Schnitger, and Sontag, and subsequently DasGupta and Schnitger constructed Boolean functions that are computed by sigmoidal nets of constant size (i.e., independent of the number of input bits), whereas $\mathcal{H}$-nets of constant size do not suffice. (See Maass, 1994, for a more detailed discussion.) However, Maass (1993) showed that spline nets of constant degree, constant depth, and polynomial size (in the number of input bits) can be simulated by $\mathcal{H}$-nets of constant depth and polynomial size. This simulation holds without any restriction on the weights used by the spline net.

Thus, analog computation does help for discrete problems, but apparently by not too much. For a thorough discussion of discrete neural computation, see Siu, Roychowdhury, and Kailath (1994).

Sigmoidal Nets and Nets of Spiking Neurons

A formal model of networks of spiking neurons is defined in Maass (1997); see SPIKING NEURONS, COMPUTATION WITH. The architecture is described by a directed graph $G = (V, E)$, with V as the set of nodes and E as the set of edges. We interpret nodes as neurons and edges as synapses, and assign to each neuron v a threshold function $\Theta_v : \mathbb{R}^+ \to \mathbb{R}^+$. ($\mathbb{R}^+$ denotes the set of nonnegative reals.) The value of $\Theta_v(t - t')$ measures the "reluctance" (or the threshold to be exceeded) of neuron v to fire at time t ($t > t'$), assuming that v has fired at time t'. This reluctance can be overcome only if the potential $P_v(t)$ of neuron v at time t is at least correspondingly as large.

The potential of v at time t depends on the recent firing history of the presynaptic neurons (or the immediate predecessors) u of v. In particular, if the synapse between neurons u and v has the efficacy (or weight) w_{uv}, if $\varepsilon_{uv}(t - s)$ is the response to the firing of neuron u at time s ($s < t$) and if the presynaptic neuron u has fired previously for the times in the set $Fire_u^t$, then the potential at time t is defined as

$$P_v(t) = \sum_{(u,v) \in E} \sum_{s \in Fire_u^t} w_{uv} \cdot \varepsilon_{uv}(t - s) \qquad (3)$$

Two models, namely deterministic (respectively noisy) nets of spiking neurons, are distinguished. The deterministic version assumes that neuron v fires whenever its potentials $P_v(t)$ reach $\Theta_v(t - t')$ (with most recent firing t'), whereas the more realistic noisy version assumes that the firing probability increases with increasing difference $P_v(t) - \Theta_v(t - t)$.

Thus we can complete the definition of the formal model, assuming that a response function $\varepsilon_{uv} : \mathbb{R}^+ \to \mathbb{R}$ as well as the weight w_{uv} is assigned to the synapse between u and v. The model computes by transforming a spike train of inputs into a spike train of outputs. For instance assuming temporal coding with constants T and c, the output of a designated neuron with firing times $T + c \cdot t_1, \ldots, T + c \cdot \Sigma_{i=1}^k t_i, \ldots$ is defined as $t_1, \ldots, t_i, \ldots, \Sigma_{i=1}^k t_i, \ldots$.

The power of spiking neurons shows for the example of the element distinctness function ED_n with real inputs $x_1, \ldots, x_n$, where

$$ED_n(x) = \begin{cases} 1 & \text{if } x_i = x_j \text{ for some } i \neq j, \\ 0 & \text{if } |x_i - x_j| \geq 1 \text{ for all } i \neq j, \\ \text{arbitrary} & \text{otherwise.} \end{cases}$$

We assume that the inputs $x_1, \ldots, x_n$ are represented by n input trains of single spikes. Now it is easy to choose a simple threshold function as well as simple (and indeed identical) response functions such that even a single spiking neuron with unit weights is capable of computing ED_n. On the other hand, any sigmoidal net computing ED_n requires at least $(n - 4)/2 - 1$ hidden units (Maass, 1997). This result is also the strongest lower size bound for sigmoidal nets computing a specific function; the argument builds on techniques from Sontag (1997).

Certainly this one-neuron computation requires time, because of the temporal input coding, but the same applies to sigmoidal networks, since, from the point of neurobiology, the x_i's will be obtained after sampling the firing rate of their input neurons.

Nets of spiking neurons are capable of simulating $\mathcal{H}$-nets with at most the same size, and hence are properly stronger than $\mathcal{H}$-nets and at least in some cases stronger than sigmoidal nets. Thus, careful timing is an advantage that synchronized models cannot overcome.

Computational Power of Recurrent Nets

The computational power of recurrent nets is investigated in Siegelmann and Sontag (1994, 1995). (See also Siegelmann, 1998, for a thorough discussion of recurrent nets and analog computation in general.) Recurrent nets include feedforward nets, and thus the results for feedforward nets apply to recurrent nets as well. But recurrent nets gain considerably more computational power with increasing computation time. In the following discussion, for the sake of concreteness, we assume that the piecewise linear function

$$\pi(x) = \begin{cases} 0 & \text{if } x \leq 0 \\ x & \text{if } 0 \leq x \leq 1 \\ 1 & \text{if } x \geq 1 \end{cases}$$

is chosen as the activation function. We concentrate on binary input and assume that the input is provided one bit at a time.

First of all, if weights and thresholds are integers, then each node computes a bit. Recurrent nets with integer weights thus turn out to be equivalent to finite automata, and they recognize exactly the class of regular language over the binary alphabet $\{0, 1\}$.

The computational power increases considerably for rational weights and thresholds. For instance, a "rational" recurrent net is, up to a polynomial time computation, equivalent to a Turing machine. In particular, a network that simulates a universal Turing machine does exist, and one could refer to such a network as "universal" in the Turing sense. It is important to note that the number of nodes in the simulating recurrent net is fixed (i.e., *does not grow* with increasing input length).

Irrational weights provide a further boost in computation power. If the net is allowed exponential computation time, then arbitrary Boolean functions (including noncomputable functions) are recognizable. However, if only polynomial computation time is allowed, then nets have less power and recognize exactly the languages computable by polynomial-size Boolean circuits.

Discussion

We have discussed the computing power of neural nets, including universal approximation results for feedforward and recurrent neural networks as well as efficient approximation by feedforward nets with various activation functions. We emphasize that this survey is far from complete. For instance, we omitted important topics such as the VAPNIK-CHERVONENKIS DIMENSION OF NEURAL NETWORKS (q.v.) and the complexity of discrete neural computation.

Important open questions relate to proving better upper and lower bounds for sigmoidal nets computing (or approximating) specific functions, and achieving a better understanding of size and depth trade-offs for important function classes. Other neural models, such as networks of spiking neurons, significantly change the computing power, and the questions we have identified apply to these models as well.

Road Map: Computability and Complexity
Background: I.3. Dynamics and Learning in Neural Networks
Related Reading: Neural Automata and Analog Computational Complexity; PAC Learning and Neural Networks; Universal Approximators

References

Arora, S., Babai, L., Stern, J., and Sweedyk, Z., 1997, The hardness of approximate optima in lattices, codes and systems of linear equations, *J. Comput. Syst. Sci.*, 54:317–331.

Barron, A. R., 1993, Universal approximation bounds for superpositions of a sigmoidal function, *IEEE Trans. Inform. Theory*, 39:930–945.

Cybenko, G., 1989, Approximation by superposition of a sigmoidal function, *Math. Control Signals Syst.*, 2:303–314.

DasGupta B., and Schnitger, G., 1993, *The Power of Approximating: A Comparison of Activation Functions*, NIPS 5, 615–622. Available: http://www.cs.uic.edu/~dasgupta/resume/publ/papers/approx.ps.Z

Kharitonov, M., 1993, Cryptographic hardness of distribution specific learning, in *Proceedings of the 25th ACM Symposium on the Theory of Computing*, pp. 372–381.

Kolmogorov, A. N., 1957, On the representation of continuous functions of several variables by superposition of continuous functions of one variable and addition, *Dokl. Akad. Nauk USSR*, 114:953–956.

Maass, W., 1993, Bounds for the computational power and learning complexity of analog neural nets, in *Proceedings of the 25th Annual ACM Symposium on the Theory of Computing*, pp. 335–344.

Maass, W., 1994, Sigmoids and Boolean threshold circuits, in *Theoretical Advances in Neural Computation and Learning* (V. P. Roychowdhury, K. Y. Siu, and A. Orlitsky, Eds.), Boston: Kluwer, pp. 127–151.

Maass, W., 1997, Networks of spiking neurons: The third generation of neural network models, *Neural Netw.*, 10:1659–1671.

Poggio, T., and Girosi, F., 1989, A theory of networks for approximation and learning, *Artif. Intell. Memorandum*, No. 1140.

Siegelmann, H. T., 1998, *Neural Networks and Analog Computation: Beyond the Turing Limit*, Boston: Birkhäuser. ◆

Siegelmann, H. T., and Sontag, E. D., 1994, Analog computation, neural networks, and circuits, *Theoret. Comput. Sci.*, 131:331–360.

Siegelmann, H. T., and Sontag, E. D., 1995, On the computational power of neural nets, *J. Comput.*, 50:132–150.

Siu, K.-Y., Roychowdhury, V. P., and Kailath, T., 1994, *Discrete Neural Computation: A Theoretical Foundation*, Englewood Cliffs, NJ: Prentice Hall. ◆

Sontag, E. D., 1997, Shattering all sets of k points in general position requires $(k - 1)/2$ parameters, *Neural Computat.*, 9:337–348.

Analog VLSI Implementations of Neural Networks

Paul Hasler and Jeff Dugger

Introduction

The primary goal of analog implementations of neural networks is to incorporate some level of realistic biological modeling of adaptive systems into engineering systems built in silicon. We cannot simply duplicate biological models in silicon media because the constraints imposed by the biological media and the silicon media are not identical. Approaches that have been successful begin with the constraints that the silicon medium imposes on the learning system. Therefore, letting the silicon medium constrain the design of a system results in more efficient methods of computation.

We will focus our attention on issues concerning building neural network integrated circuits (ICs), and in particular on building connectionist neural network models. Connectionist neural networks, loosely based on biological computation and learning, can be useful for biological modeling if the limitations are understood. These neural systems are typically built as mappings of mathematical models into analog silicon hardware either by using standard building blocks (i.e., Gilbert multipliers: Mead, 1989) or by taking advantage of device physics (Hasler et al., 1995). This approach, related to investigations of adaptation and learning in neurobiological systems, provides the minimum necessary model of synaptic interaction between neurons, even for biological models. Neuromorphic (Mead, 1989, see also NEUROMORPHIC VLSI CIRCUITS AND SYSTEMS) and connectionist approaches develop adaptive systems from different levels of neural inspiration, and therefore lead to different levels of model complexity. Adding dendritic interactions and precise models of biological learning (e.g., LTP) to the connectionist model yields more biological realism. Implementations of fuzzy systems typically follow a similar approach to implementations of neural networks. The related field of cellular neural networks (CNNs), started by Chua, is particularly concerned with the circuit techniques used to build locally connected two-dimensional (2D) meshes of neuron processors (Chua, 1998), but the architecture design is fundamentally different and imposes different constraints on implementation.

Neural Network Basics Focused on Implementation Issues

Figure 1 shows the basic feedforward structure typically used in neural network implementations. Most approaches focus on feedforward structures, since feedback systems and networks with time dynamics (e.g., time delays) are straightforward extensions for silicon implementation, although the algorithm design is considerably more difficult. In this model, we encode a neuron's activity as an analog quantity based on the mean spiking rate in a given time window. One can build linear or nonlinear filters at the input to the sigmoid function. Typically, a low-pass filter is built or modeled, since that will naturally occur for a given implementation or will set a desired convergence to an attractor (i.e., recurrent networks). This model is excellent for describing neurobiology if only mean-firing-rate behavior with minimal dendritic interactions is considered.

A basic model synapse (either digital or analog) must be able to store a weight, multiply its input with the stored weight, and adapt that weight based on a function of the input and a fed-back error signal. We model feedforward computation mathematically as

$$y_i = w_{ij}x_j \rightarrow \mathbf{y} = \mathbf{W}\mathbf{x} \tag{1}$$

where x_j is the jth input ($\mathbf{x}$ is a vector of inputs), y_i is the ith output ($\mathbf{y}$ is a vector of outputs), and w_{ij} is the stored weight at position (i,j) ($\mathbf{W}$ is a matrix of weights). The result of this output is passed through a nonlinear function

$$z_i = \tanh(a(y_i - \theta_i)) \tag{2}$$

where we designate z_i as the result of the computation, a is a gain factor, and θ_j is a variable threshold value. Other nonlinear functions, like radial basis functions (see RADIAL BASIS FUNCTION NETWORKS), are also often used, which would typically modify the

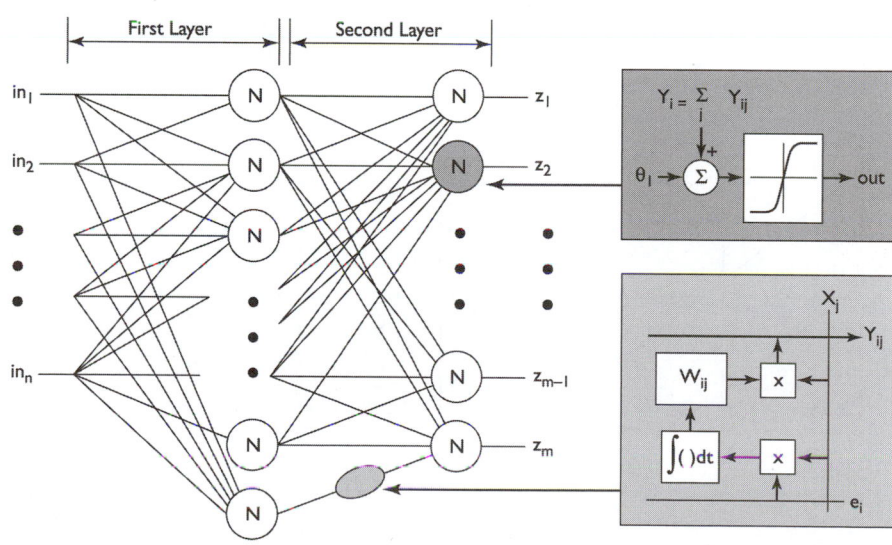

Figure 1. Classic picture of a two-layer neural network from the perspective of implementating these networks in hardware. The neural networks are layers of simple processors, called neurons, that are interconnected through weighting elements, called synapses. The neurons aggregate the incoming inputs (including a threshold or offset) and are applied through a tanh(·) nonlinearity. The synapse elements, which in general are far more numerous than the neuron elements, must multiply the incoming signal by an internally stored value, called the weight, and must adapt this weight according to a particular learning rule. Learning rules implemented in silicon are typically functions of correlations of signals passing through each synapse processor.

Wx computation. We model the weight adaptation mathematically as

$$\tau \frac{d\mathbf{W}}{dt} = f(\mathbf{W}, \mathbf{xe}^T) \tag{3}$$

where **e** is a vector of error signals that is fed back along various rows. We call this an outer-product learning rule, or a *local* learning rule, because of the $\mathbf{xe}^T$ computation. The outer-product learning rule is dependent on the choice of $f(\mathbf{W}, \mathbf{xe}^T)$ and the choice of the error signal.

Several learning algorithms have been proposed that conform to this functional form; representative examples can be found elsewhere in the *Handbook*. Learning algorithms usually divide into two categories, supervised and unsupervised. *Supervised algorithms* adapt the weights based on the input signals and a supervisory signal to train the network to produce an appropriate response. In many supervised algorithms (see PERCEPTRONS, ADALINES, AND BACKPROPAGATION) this weight change is a time average of the product of the input and some fed-back error signal ($\mathbf{e} = \mathbf{y} - \hat{\mathbf{y}}$, where $\hat{\mathbf{y}}$ is the target signal). *Unsupervised algorithms* adapt the weights based only on the input and output signals, and in general the weights are a function of the input statistics. Although these learning algorithms result in very different results, both weight-update rules are similar from an implementation viewpoint. Most unsupervised algorithms are based on Hebbian learning algorithms, which correspond to neurobiological evidence of learning (see HEBBIAN SYNAPTIC PLASTICITY). For a Hebbian synapse, the weight change is a time average of the product of the input and output activity ($\mathbf{e} = \mathbf{y}$).

Neural Network Implementations: Architecture Issues

Before considering circuit implementations of neurons and synapses, we first frame the overall architecture issues involved in implementing neural networks. In most implementations, a single layer of synapses is built as mesh architectures connected to a column of neuron processors (Figure 2). Because silicon ICs are 2D, mesh architectures work optimally with 2D routing constraints.

Feedforward Computation

Figure 2*A* shows the typical mesh implementation of feedforward computation for a single-layer architecture. A mesh of processors is an optimal communication architecture for interconnect limited systems, which is the case for small synapse elements. Currents are preferred for outputs, because the summation typically required for most connectionist models is easily performed on a single wire, and voltages are preferred for inputs because they are easy to broadcast. Local processing is defined as interaction between *physically close* elements, voltage broadcast along global lines (inputs), or current/charge summation along a wire (outputs). As a result, each synapse has only to compute the local computation: $\mathbf{W}_{ij}\mathbf{x}_j$. Because the synapses store a weight value, the picture in Figure 2*A* resembles an analog memory that allows a full matrix-vector multiplication in the equivalent of one memory column access. This approach, called analog computing arrays, is defined and its implication for signal processing is described elsewhere (Kucic et al., 2001). Figure 2*B* shows how to modify a mesh architecture when considering *m*-nearest-neighbor connections. Other sparse

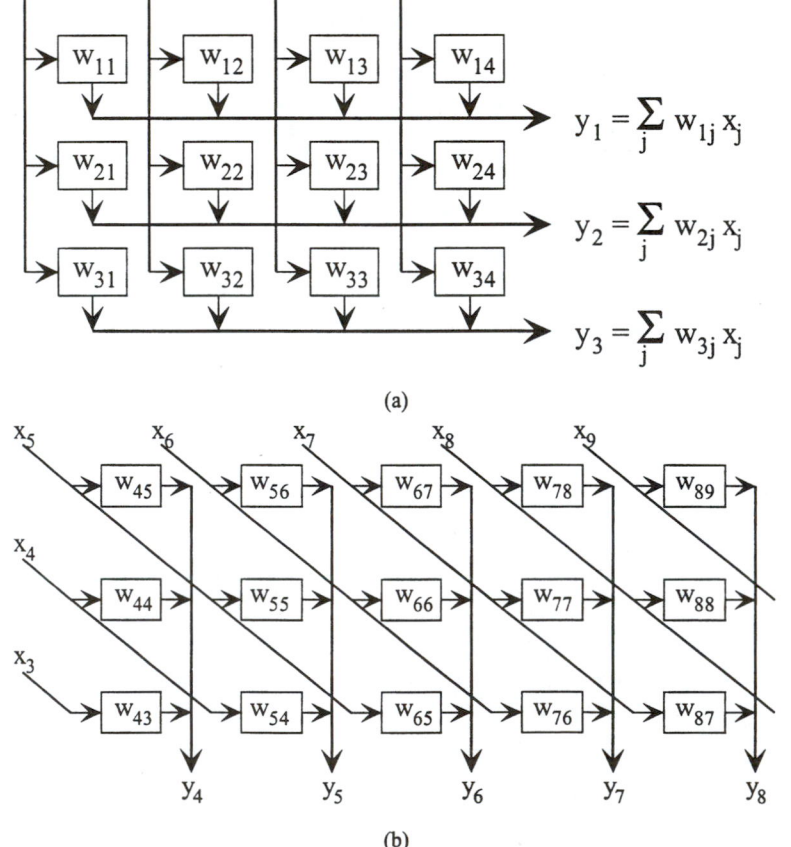

Figure 2. Typical architectures for neural network implementations. Although the routing looks complicated in Figure 1, it can easily be implemented in a mesh architecture. *A*, Diagram of the classic mesh architecture, typically used for fully connected architectures. *B*, Diagram of a mesh processor architecture optimized for nearest-neighbor computations.

encodings require digital communication and processing to handle the addressing schemes (i.e., address translation tables) and additional complexity (i.e., multiplexing scheme to access the inputs of each synapse).

To implement a neuron, we need a function that can compute a tanh(·) function. Fortunately, this function occurs in many IC circuits using either BJT or MOSFET (subthreshold or above-threshold) devices, such as the differential transistor pair (Mead, 1989). Since we only need a column of neuron circuits, they do not have the same area constraints that are imposed on synapse elements. Dynamics (e.g., low-pass filtering) are usually achieved by adding additional capacitance. Often one needs a current to perform voltage conversion between the summed synapse outputs and tanh(·) output, as well as at the output of a differential transistor pair. This conversion often can be nonlinear, or it may have to be nonlinear to interface with later processing stages.

Adaptive Neural Network Architectures

Synapses require both feedforward and adaptation computations; therefore, architectural constraints imposed by the learning algorithm are an essential consideration for any neural network. Only learning algorithms that scale to large numbers of inputs and outputs are practical. A single-layer architecture with a local supervised or unsupervised rule of the form of Equation 3 only requires communicating the *error* signal along each row (Figure 3). The complexity of the synapse computation will depend on the particular learning rule. Many complicated algorithms, such as the generalized Hebbian algorithm (GHA) (Hasler and Akers, 1992) and INDEPENDENT COMPONENT ANALYSIS (ICA) (q.v.), require additional matrix-vector multiplications, but can be developed into a mesh architecture. Algorithms requiring matrix-matrix multiplications are difficult in standard IC technologies.

For multilayer algorithms, the architecture gets more complicated, particularly for supervised algorithms such as multilayer backpropagation. To extend the basic silicon synapse to a backpropagating synapse, we need an additional function: we need an output current that is the product of the fed-back error signal (drain voltage) and stored weight. We show this architecture in Figure 4A. This additional function results in two issues, one concerning the signal-to-noise ratio of the resulting error signal and the other concerning the overall synapse size. The effect of these small error signals, even without the resolution issues, is a slow learning rate.

The neural network literature is replete with possible alternative approaches, but we will base our proposed research on the Helm-

holtz machine concept (see HELMHOLTZ MACHINES AND SLEEP-WAKE LEARNING). Our primary reason for using this approach rests on our desire to use single-layer networks as primitives for building larger networks, as well as the fact that this reciprocal adaptive single-layer network architecture is seen in various models of sensory neurosystems, such as the pathways from retina to LGN to V1 or some of the pathways between the cochlea and auditory cortex (A1). Figure 4B considers a two-layer network implementation of a backpropagation-like learning rule using this Helmholtz block. In this case, we double the number of layers, and therefore double the effective synapse size; for a backpropagation algorithm, we require the same number of floating-gate multipliers, but with significant additional implementation costs that greatly increase the synapse complexity. This approach seems more IC-friendly for the development of adaptive multilayer algorithms than backpropagation approaches, although its digital implementation is nominally equivalent to backpropagation approaches. This approach directly expands to multiple layers and could be used in limited reconfigurable networks because we are building networks with single adaptive layers. Starting with the single-layer network as the basic building block simplifies the abstraction toward system development.

Resulting Synapse Design Criteria

Because the synapse is the critical element of any neural network implementation, we state five properties of a silicon synapse that are essential for building large-scale adaptive analog VLSI synaptic arrays (Hasler et al., 1995):

1. The synapse must store a weight permanently in the absence of learning.
2. The synapse must compute an output current as the product of its input signal and its synaptic weight.
3. The synapse must modify its weight at least using outer-product learning rules.
4. The synapse must consume minimal silicon area, thereby maximizing the number of synapses in a given area.
5. The synapse must dissipate a minimal amount of power; therefore, the synaptic array is not power constrained.

Achieving all five requirements requires a detailed discussion of the circuits used to implement a synapse, which is the subject of the next section.

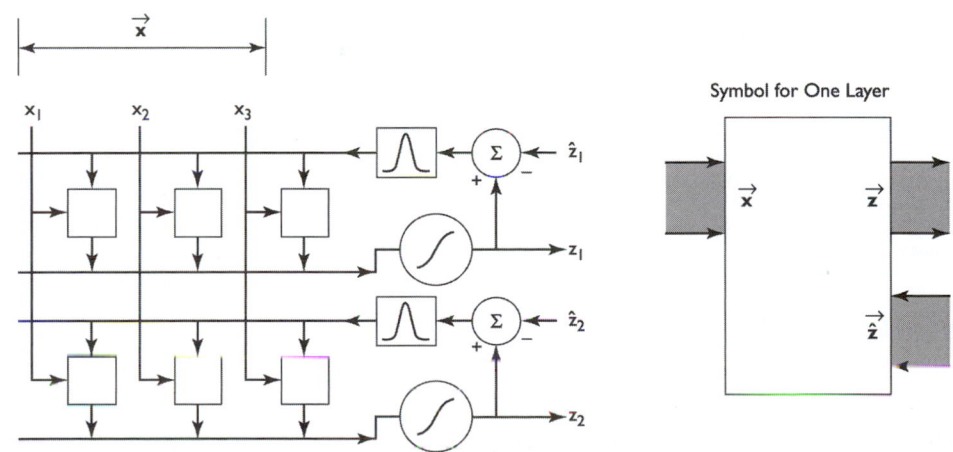

Figure 3. Learning in a single layer. We can build either supervised algorithms (LMS is explicitly shown) or unsupervised one-layer networks in this architecture. For a one-layer supervised case, $\hat{z}$ is the desired or target output signal vector, where $e_j = z_j - \hat{z}_j$. Further, one might apply a nonlinear function to the resulting error signal; in LMS, one applies a nonlinear function to counteract the effect of the sigmoid in the feedforward path. Many unsupervised rules, like Hebbian or Oja rules, can be formulated as $\hat{z} = f(z)$. One can schematically represent this network from its terminals, x, z, and $\hat{z}$, as shown from its block diagram. Finally, the nonlinear (sigmoid) elements typically convert current to voltage.

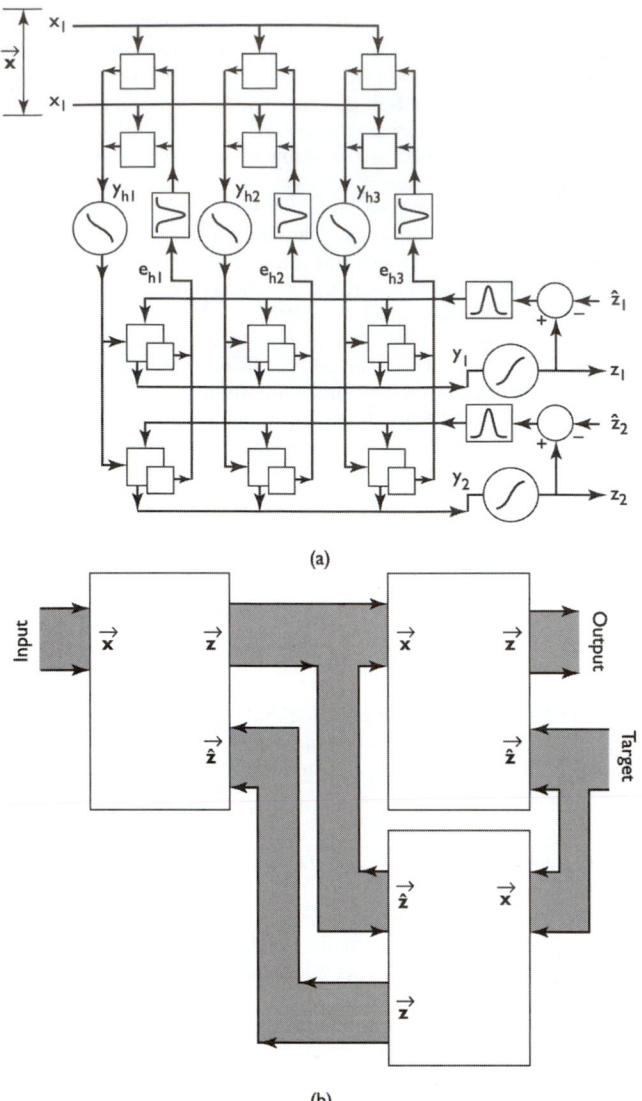

(a)

(b)

Figure 4. Possible architectures for adaptive multilayer neural networks. A, Implementation for backpropagation networks. There are many forms and modifications, but from an implementation viewpoint, these approaches can be modified toward this architecture. This approach significantly increases synapse size, because one typically requires the complexity of two synapses for weight feedback. Further, this approach limits some circuit approaches to building dense synapses. The output from the hidden layer, or layer 1, is $\mathbf{y}_h$ and the error signal given to the hidden layer is $\mathbf{e}_h$. The synapses in the second layer must also output a current proportional to the product of error * stored weight; the sum of these currents along a column is the error for the next layer. As a result, the synapses on the second layer must be more complex. B, Implementation using Helmholtz machine concepts. This approach requires twice as many synapses for all but the first layer, which yields the same complexity as the backpropagation approaches. This approach will converge to the same steady states and requires only a modular tiling of single-layer networks; its reciprocal feedback has a similar feel to communication between layers of cortical neurons.

Neural Network Implementation: Synapse Circuits

Early Research in Synapse Design

Several neural networks have been built in analog silicon hardware. Several good recent implementation techniques can be found in

Cauwenberghs and Bayoumi (1999); here we present an overview. From the architecture discussions, we require a synapse block where an input voltage should modulate an output current, which is summed along a line; therefore, most implementations employ a variable resistance or transconductance element. As a result, a primary issue in synapse circuit designs is developing dense multiplier circuits, because multiplication of an input by a weight is fundamental to every synapse. Earlier approaches for implementating the feedforward synapse computation included fixed resistances (which were among the earliest implementations), switched-capacitor implementations (Tsividis and Satyanarayana, 1987), Gilbert multiplier cells (Mead, 1989), and linearized conductance elements (Dupuie and Ismail, 1990; Cauwenberghs, Neugebaur, and Yariv, 1991; Hasler and Akers, 1992). Intel's ETANN chip was the first commercially available neural network IC that used floating gates for weight storage (Holler et al., 1989). One of the most successful implementations of a large-scale adaptive neural system was the Heuralt-Juetten algorithm, but it required a great deal of circuit complexity (Cohen and Andreou, 1992). Other researchers have implemented unsupervised learning and backpropagation algorithms, with mixed success (Furman, White, and Abidi, 1988; Hasler and Akers, 1992). Successful analog implementations of connectionist networks have included algorithmic modifications that facilitate implementation in silicon. The history of this field has shown that the success of an implementation is strongly correlated with the degree to which the algorithm is adapted to the silicon medium.

Synapses in previous silicon implementations have required large circuit complexity because they have typically been constructed using traditional circuit building blocks to realize memory, computation, and adaptation functions separately, rather than taking advantage of device physics to combine these functions in a compact circuit element. Not only does large circuit complexity consume tremendous circuit area and power, but the chance of a network operating correctly decreases exponentially with cell size.

The most difficult problem to overcome when building efficient adaptive circuits is the effect of p-n junction leakage currents (Hasler et al., 1995; Hasler and Minch, 2002). First, since many implementations dynamically store their weight parameters on a capacitor, these junction leakage currents typically limit the hold time, on the order of seconds; therefore, weight storage often becomes a critical concern in many of these applications. Several on-chip refreshing schemes have been proposed and built (Hasler and Akers, 1992) and are currently finding applications in various ICs (Cauwenberghs and Bayoumi, 1999). Second, since real-time learning often requires time constants from 10 ms to days, junction leakage currents limit the use of capacitor storage techniques, unless prohibitively large capacitor areas are used. Weight update schemes based on weight perturbation methods, i.e., where the error signal is based on random known changes in the weights, can often work in these constraints if some form of dynamic refreshing scheme is used (Cauwenberghs and Bayoumi, 1999). Often, junction leakage is too large for many adaptive system problems.

Single-Transistor Learning Synapses

Current research into analog neural network ICs pursues two directions. The first direction is based on refreshable DRAM elements with adaptation using weight perturbation techniques (Cauwenberghs and Bayoumi, 1999). The second direction is based on a wide range of techniques using floating-gate synapses. Floating gates have seen use in neural networks as storage elements (Holler et al., 1989), which eliminates the long-term weight storage issues but still results in fairly complex synapse circuits. Here, we briefly describe the potential of using floating-gate synapses.

The single-transistor learning synapse (STLS), or transistor synapse, makes use of device physics and constraints inherent to the

Figure 5. Layout, cross-section, and circuit diagram of the floating-gate pFET in a standard double-poly n-well MOSIS process. The cross-section corresponds to the horizonatal line slicing through the layout view. The pFET transistor is the standard pFET transistor in the n-well process. The gate input capacitively couples to the floating gate by either a poly-poly capacitor, a diffused linear capacitor, or a MOS capacitor, as seen in the circuit diagram (not explicitly shown in the other figures). We add floating-gate charge by electron tunneling, and we remove floating-gate charge by hot-electron injection. The tunneling junctions used by the single-transistor synapses is a region of gate oxide between the polysilicon floating gate and n-well (a MOS capacitor). Between V_{tun} and the floating gate is our symbol for a tunneling junction, a capacitor with an added arrow designating the charge flow.

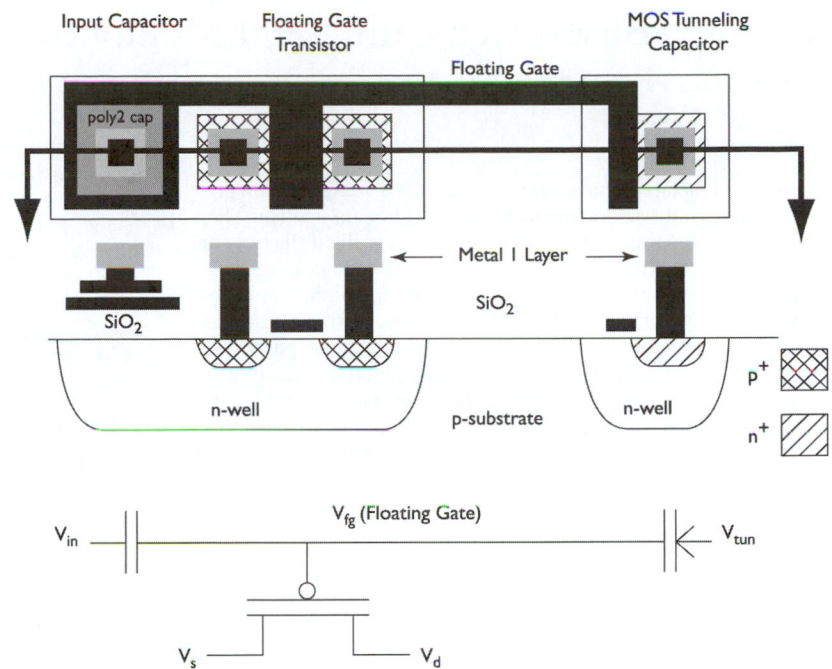

silicon medium to realize learning and adaptation functions, rather than direct implementation of learning rules using traditional circuit building blocks (Hasler et al., 1995). This technology is rooted in floating-gate circuits (Hasler and Lande, 2001; Hasler and Minch, 2002) in which multiple features of a floating-gate transistor are used, not just the nonvolatile storage (Figure 5). These elements utilize physical characteristics of the silicon medium, such as electron tunneling and hot-electron injection, which traditionally have posed problems for engineers. The starting point for this technology is a floating-gate transistor (Hasler et al., 1995; Kucic et al., 2001) operating with subthreshold currents and configured to simultaneously store permanently the weight charge, compute an output current that is the product of the input signal and the synaptic weight, and modify its weight charge based on many outer-product learning rules. This approach meets all five requirements for a silicon synapse. These weights can be automatically programmed, which enables setting fixed weights, setting initial bias conditions, and employing weight perturbation learning rules (Kucic et al., 2001). Further, by setting the appropriate boundary circuits for the synapse array, we can get a wide range of learning rules by continuously enabling our *programming mechanisms* during computation (Kucic et al., 2001). One form of the learning rules looks like

$$\tau \frac{dw_{i,j}}{dt} = \eta E[x_i e_j] - w_{i,j} \qquad (4)$$

where τ is the adaptation time constant and η is the strength of the correlating term.

Road Map: Implementation and Analysis
Related Reading: Digital VLSI for Neural Networks; Photonic Implementations of Neurobiologically Inspired Networks; Silicon Neurons

References

Chua, L. O., 1998, *A Paradigm for Complexity*, vol. 31, in World Scientific Series on Nonlinear Science, Series A, Singapore: World Scientific Publishing.

Cauwenberghs, G., and Bayoumi, M. A., Eds., 1999, *Learning in Silicon*, Boston: Kluwer Academic.

Cauwenberghs, G., Neugebaur, C., and Yariv, A., 1991, An adaptive CMOS matrix vector multiplier for large scale analog hardware neural network applications, in *Proceedings of the International Joint Conference on Neural Networks*, vol. 1, pp. 507–512.

Cohen, M., and Andreou, A. G., 1992, Current-mode subthreshold MOS implementation of the Herault-Jutten autoadaptive network, *IEEE Trans. Solid State Circuits*, 27:714–727.

Dupuie, S. T., and Ismail, M., 1990, High frequency CMOS transconductors, in *Analogue IC Design: The Current-Mode Approach* (C. Toumazou, F. J. Lidgey, and D. G. Haigh, Eds.), London: Peter Peregrinus, pp. 181–238.

Furman, B., White, J., and Abidi, A. A., 1988, CMOS analog IC implementing the backpropagation algorithm, in *Abstracts of the First Annual INNS Meeting*, vol. 1, p. 381.

Hasler, P., and Akers, L., 1992, Circuit implementation of a trainable neural network using the generalized Hebbian algorithm with supervised techniques, in *Proceedings of the International Joint Conference on Neural Networks*, vol. 1, Baltimore, pp. 1565–1568. ◆

Hasler, P., Diorio, C., Minch, B. A., and Mead, C., 1995, Single transistor learning synapses, in *Advances in Neural Information Processing Systems 7*, Cambridge, MA: MIT Press, pp. 817–824.

Hasler, P., and Lande, T. S., Eds., 2001, *Floating-Gate Circuits* (special issue), *IEEE Trans. Circuits Syst II*, 48(1).

Hasler, P., and Minch, B. A., 2002, *Floating-Gate Devices, Circuits, and Systems*, New York: IEEE Press.

Holler, M., Tam., S., Castro, H., and Benson, R., 1989, An electrically trainable artificial neural network with 1024 "floating gate" synapses, in *Proceedings of the International Joint Conference on Neural Networks*, vol. 2, Washington, D.C., pp. 191–196. ◆

Kucic, M., Low, A.-C., Hasler, P., and Neff, J., 2001, A programmable continuous-time floating-gate Fourier process, *IEEE Trans. Circuits and Systems II*, 48:90–99.

Mead, C., 1989, *Analog VSLI and Neural Systems*, Reading, MA: Addison-Wesley. ◆

Tsividis, Y., and Satyanarayana, S., 1987, Analogue circuits for variable synapse electronic neural networks, *Electron. Lett.*, 24(2):1313–1314.

Analogy-Based Reasoning and Metaphor

Dedre Gentner and Arthur B. Markman

Introduction

Analogy and metaphor have been characterized as comparison processes that permit one domain to be seen in terms of another. They are important to connectionism for two reasons. First, there is an affinity at the descriptive level: many of the advantages suggested for connectionist models—representation completion, similarity-based generalization, graceful degradation, and learning—also apply to analogy (Barnden, 1994). Second, analogical processing poses significant challenges for connectionist models. Analogy involves the comparison of *systems of relations* between items in a domain. To model analogy requires representations that include internal relations. Many connectionist models have concentrated instead on statistical learning of correlational patterns over featural or dimensional representations.

Tenets of Analogy and Metaphor

Analogy derives from the perception of relational commonalities between domains that are dissimilar on the surface. These correspondences often suggest new inferences about the target domain. Analogy has been widely studied in humans. In the past decade, psychological research on analogy has converged on a set of benchmark phenomena against which models of analogy can be measured. These eight benchmarks, shown in Table 1, can be organized according to four processing principles. Analogy and metaphor involve (1) structured pattern matching; (2) structured pattern completion, (3) a focus on common relational structure rather than on common object descriptions, and (4) flexibility in that (a) the same domain may yield different interpretations in different comparisons, and (b) a single comparison may yield multiple distinct interpretations. Any model of analogy must account for these phenomena.

We begin by reviewing the principles and benchmarks, and then discuss current connectionist models of analogy and metaphor. Our discussion takes place at Marr's *computational and algorithmic*

Table 1. Eight Benchmark Phenomena of Analogy

1. Relational Similarity	Analogies involve relational commonalities; object commonalities are optional.
2. Structured Pattern Matching	Analogical mapping involves one-to-one correspondence and parallel connectivity.
3. Systematicity	In interpreting analogy, connected systems of relations are preferred over sets of isolated relations.
4. Candidate Inferences	Analogical inferences are generated via structural completion.
5. Alignable Differences	Differences that are connected to the commonalities of a pair are rendered more salient by a comparison.
6. Flexibility (1): Interactive Interpretation	Analogy interpretation depends on both terms. The same term yields different interpretations in different comparisons.
7. Flexibility (2): Multiple Interpretation	Analogy allows multiple interpretations of a single comparison.
8. Cross-mapping	People typically perceive both interpretations of a cross-mapping and prefer the relational interpretation.

levels, at which cognition is explained in terms of representations and associated processes. We will not evaluate the models in terms of brain function, partly because the neural basis is not yet understood, but also because we believe a computational model must first justify itself as a cognitive account. We will focus mainly on analogy, which has been well studied at the processing level. Much of what we know about analogy can be applied to metaphor as well. Later, we will explore ways in which analogy and metaphor may differ.

Structured Pattern Matching

The defining characteristic of analogy and many metaphors is the alignment of relational structure. Alignment involves finding *structurally consistent matches* (those observing parallel connectivity and one-to-one correspondence). *Parallel connectivity* requires that matching relations have matching arguments; *one-to-one correspondence* limits any element in one representation to at most one matching element in the other representation (Gentner and Markman, 1997; Holyoak and Thagard, 1995). For example, in the analogy "The atom is like the solar system," the nucleus in the atom (the *target*) corresponds to the sun in the solar system (the *base*) and the electrons to the planets, because they play similar roles in a common relational structure: e.g., **revolve** (sun, planets) and **revolve** (nucleus, electron). The sun is not matched to both the nucleus and the electron, as that violates one-to-one correspondence. Another characteristic of analogy is *relational focus*: objects correspond by virtue of playing like roles and need not be similar (e.g., the nucleus need not be hot).

There is considerable evidence that people can align two situations, preserving connected systems of commonalities and making the appropriate lower-order substitutions. For example, Clement and Gentner (1991) showed people analogous stories and asked them to state which of two assertions shared by base and target was most important to the match. Subjects chose the assertion connected to matching causal antecedents. More generally, people's correspondences are based both on the goodness of the local match and on its connection to a larger matching system (Markman and Gentner, 1993). This finding demonstrates the systematicity principle: Analogies seek *connected systems of matching relations* rather than isolated relational matches.

When making comparisons, it often occurs that nonidentical items are matched by virtue of playing a common role in the matching system. These corresponding but nonidentical elements give rise to *alignable differences*, and have been shown to be salient outputs of the comparison process (Gentner and Markman, 1997). In contrast, aspects of one situation that have no correspondence in the other, called *nonalignable differences*, are not salient outputs of comparison. For example, when comparing the atom to the solar system, the fact that atoms have electrons and solar systems have planets is an alignable difference. The fact that solar systems have asteroids, while atoms have nothing that corresponds to asteroids, is a nonalignable difference.

Structured Pattern Completion

Analogical reasoning also involves the mapping of inferences from one domain to another. Thus, a partial representation of the target is completed based on its structural similarity to the base. For example, Clement and Gentner (1991) extended the findings described earlier by deleting some key matching facts from the target story and asking subjects to make a new prediction about the target based on the analogy with the base story. Consistent with the previous result, subjects mapped just those predicates that were causally connected to other matching predicates.

Flexibility: Interactive Interpretation

Analogy and metaphor are flexible in important ways. Indeed, Barnden (1994) suggests that analogy and metaphor may reconcile connectionism's flexibility with symbolic AI's structure-sensitivity. One way that analogy and metaphor are flexible is that the interpretations are interactions between the two terms. The same item can take part in many comparisons, with different aspects of the representation participating in each comparison.

For example, Spellman and Holyoak (1992) compared politicians' analogies for the Gulf War. Some likened it to World War II, implying that the United States was acting to stop a tyrant, whereas others likened it to Vietnam, implying that the United States had embroiled itself in a potentially endless conflict between two other opponents. Comparisons with different bases highlighted different features of the target. Flexibility is also evident when the same base term is combined with different targets. For example, the metaphor "A lake is a mirror" highlights that a lake has a flat reflective surface, whereas "Meditation is a mirror" highlights the self-examination aspect of meditation.

Flexibility: Multiple Interpretations of the Same Comparison

A more striking kind of flexibility is that a single base-target comparison can give rise to multiple distinct interpretations. For a comparison like "Cameras are like tape recorders," people can readily provide an object-level interpretation ("Both are small mechanical devices") or a relational interpretation ("Both record events for later display"). Interestingly, children tend to prefer the former and adults the latter.

Despite this flexibility, people generally maintain structural consistency within an interpretation. In one study, Spellman and Holyoak (1992) asked subjects to map the Gulf War onto World War II (WWII). They asked "If Saddam Hussein corresponds to Hitler, who does George Bush correspond to?" Some subjects chose Franklin Delano Roosevelt, whereas others chose Winston Churchill. The key finding was that, when asked to make a further mapping for the United States in 1991, subjects chose structurally consistent correspondences. Those who mapped Bush to Roosevelt usually mapped the US-1991 to the US-during-WWII, and those who mapped Bush to Churchill mapped the US-1991 to Britain-during-WWII.

An extreme case of conflicting interpretations is *cross-mapping*, in which the object similarities suggest different correspondences than do the relational similarities. For example, in the comparison between "Spot bit Fido" and "Fido bit Rover," Fido is cross-mapped. When presented with cross-mapped comparisons, people can compute both alignments. Research suggests that adding higher-order relational commonalities increases people's preference for the relational alignment, whereas increasing the richness of the local object match increases people's preference for the object match. For example, people are more likely to select the relational correspondence in Figure 1B than in Figure 1A. This example also illustrates that the analogical processes we describe can apply to perceptual as well as conceptual materials. The ability to compute relational interpretations (even for the cross-mappings) is central to human analogizing across a wide range of domains.

This flexibility and the ability to process cross-mappings have significant implications for the comparison process, because they

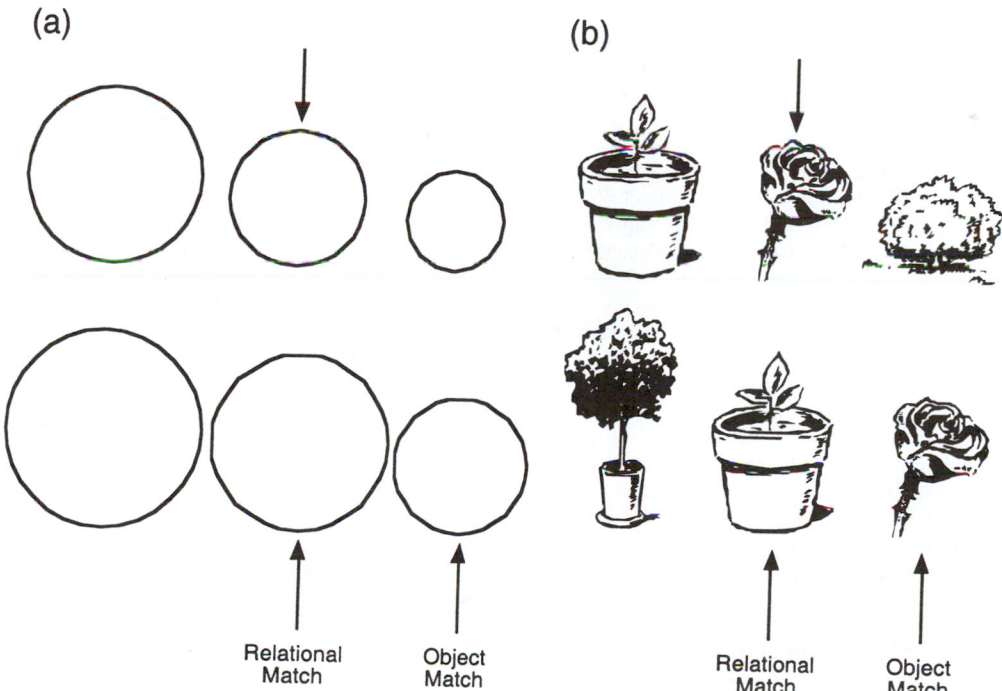

Figure 1. Sets of object triads containing a cross-mapping. A cross-mapping occurs when two similar objects play different roles in a matching relational system. In this case, the similar objects have different relative sizes. (A) shows a sparse pair of objects that are likely to have few distinguishing attributes, whereas (B) shows a rich pair of objects that are likely to have many distinguishing attributes.

mean that simulations cannot simply be trained to generate a particular kind of interpretation. Rather, the comparison process must be able to determine both object matches and structural matches and to attend selectively to one or the other.

Connectionism and Analogical Mapping

As the preceding review makes clear, a central aspect of analogical reasoning and metaphor is alignment and mapping between structured representations. Symbolic models—e.g., Falkenhainer, Forbus, and Gentner's (1989) structure-mapping engine (SME)—have been able to pass the eight benchmarks in Table 1. Advances in connectionist models of analogy and metaphor have come with the development of techniques for representing structure (e.g., Hinton, 1991; STRUCTURED CONNECTIONIST MODELS). The best-developed models to date have been models of analogy rather than models of metaphor, and so we will focus on the analogy models here. We will discuss differences between analogy and metaphor in the following section.

An early connectionist model of analogy was ACME (Holyoak and Thagard, 1989). This model was a localist constraint-satisfaction network in which the nodes represented possible correspondences between elements in the base and target. Nodes were created using the constraint of semantic matching via a table that determined which predicates were seen as semantically similar. Nodes were connected in accordance with structural consistency, with nodes for consistent matches getting excitatory links and nodes for inconsistent matches getting inhibitory links. Finally, a pragmatic constraint was added by activating nodes related to goals and correspondences known in advance. After this activation was set up, the network was allowed to settle, and the most active nodes (above some threshold) determined the correspondences between base and target found by the system. The interpretation found by ACME need not maintain structural consistency, which can lead to problems in making inferences. Hummel, Burns, and Holyoak (1994) point out that the implementation of the pragmatic constraint often causes the important node(s) to map to everything in the other analog. Finally, because ACME settles on a single interpretation of an analogy, its solution to cross-mappings merges the object and relational interpretations.

A model of analogy has also been developed using *tensor product representations* (Smolensky, 1990). In a tensor product, two vectors $\mathbf{X}$ and $\mathbf{Y}$ are bound by taking the outer product of these vectors, $\mathbf{YX}^T$. The outer product normally forms a matrix, but a vector can be constructed from this matrix by concatenating its columns. Given $\mathbf{X}$ and $\mathbf{YX}^T$, the vector $\mathbf{Y}$ can be obtained as $\mathbf{YX}^T\mathbf{X}$ if $\mathbf{X}$ is a unit vector. Variable bindings can thus be captured by using one vector to represent a predicate and the other to represent its argument.

Tensor products have been used in a distributed connectionist model—STAR—that performs a:b::c:d analogies (Halford et al., 1994). STAR represents binary relations ($\mathbf{R}(a, b)$) using tensor products of rank 3 (which are like the binary tensor products just described except that three vectors are bound together). In this model, long-term memory consists of a matrix of tensor products corresponding to various relations the system knows about. To process an analogy, the model takes the a and b terms and probes long-term memory to find a relation between them. It then takes this relation and the c term of the analogy and finds a fourth term that shares that relation with the c term. This model uses a distributed connectionist representation to perform a one-relation analogical reasoning task. Thus, STAR performs analogy through retrieval of known relations. STAR cannot generate multiple distinct interpretations of a comparison. If the system knows many different items that could be the answer to the analogy, the output vector is a combination of them all. Finally, this model does not make use of higher-order relational structure to constrain its matches.

Perhaps the most complete connectionist model of analogy is Hummel and Holyoak's (1997) LISA, which operates over structured representations by using temporal synchrony in unit firing to encode relations. The connections between relations and their arguments are maintained by having individual units, which represent concepts, fire in phase with units that represent particular relational bindings (STRUCTURED CONNECTIONIST MODELS). For example, to represent **kiss** (John, Mary) nodes for kiss, John and *agent* fire in phase. Nodes for kiss, Mary and *patient* also fire in phase (but out of phase with those for John and *agent*). Furthermore, each node representing a concept is connected to a distributed representation designed to capture the meaning of that concept. The semantic similarity of any two concepts is just the dot product of the vectors in the distributed representations of those concepts. Finally, higher-order relations are represented in LISA by chunking relations that are arguments to higher-order relations into a single node.

Mapping takes place in LISA by selecting one domain (either the base or the target) as a driver. A role-argument binding is activated in the driver, and activation flows from the active nodes to the distributed semantic representation, and from the semantic nodes to localist concept nodes in the other domain. LISA has a limited-capacity working memory of 4–6 nodes. This working memory holds onto the correspondences from a small number of previous firings, thus allowing some influence of higher-order relational structure. If the role bindings for a higher-order relation are fired followed by the role bindings for the relational arguments of that higher order relation, then the correspondences suggested by the higher order relation can influence the mapping given to its argument. Trainable connections between nodes in the base and target are updated only after a certain number of firing cycles (depending on the size of working memory). LISA has been tested on a number of analogy problems. It tends to make relational mappings for analogies, and generally finds structurally consistent correspondences. The model selects either the relational mapping or the object mapping for a cross-mapping. On any given run, LISA arrives at only one interpretation; however if the order in which nodes in the driver are activated is varied, the system can find different interpretations on different runs. Finally, because the model can use complex representations, it can use different aspects of the representation of a domain in different comparisons involving that domain.

LISA is the only extant model of analogical mapping to include an explicit working memory constraint. At present, two major questions remain. First, the order in which statements are activated in the driver—a crucial determinant of the outcome of a match—is currently decided by the modeler. Second, the model has not been tested on large representations of the base and target. Thus, it is not clear how it will perform on these representations.

How Metaphor Differs from Analogy

The previous section focused on connectionist models of analogy. There has been little work on connectionist models of metaphor. To some degree, models of analogy could be extended to metaphor. In this section, we discuss some differences between analogy and metaphor that are relevant for developing a connectionist model of metaphor.

Metaphors are nonliteral assertions of likeness. They may be phrased as comparisons, in *simile* form ("A cloud is like a sponge") or as class inclusions, in *metaphor* form ("A cloud is a sponge"). When a novel metaphor is being processed, the two domains in the metaphor are compared using the same process that is applied to analogy. Unlike analogy, however, metaphors need not focus exclusively on relations. For example, the example above could be interpreted as a cloud that is fluffy, which would focus on an attribute of sponges that clouds also possess. This metaphor can also be given a relational interpretation. For example, it might be interpreted to mean that both clouds and sponges soak up water and give it back later. Typically, adults (but not children) prefer relational interpretations of metaphors to attribute interpretations.

There are three key ways in which metaphors differ from analogies. First, whereas analogies tend to have explanatory-predictive functions, metaphors may have expressive purposes and may affect the mood of the piece in which they are embedded. Thus, the primary impact of a metaphor might come in the emotions that it brings out rather than on the information in the comparison that is promoted. Second, not all metaphors are necessarily processed as comparisons. Glucksberg and his colleagues (e.g., Glucksberg and Keysar, 1990) suggest that metaphors might be processed as class inclusion statements rather than as comparisons. While there is debate as to exactly when metaphors are processed as comparisons or as class inclusion statements, some evidence suggests that novel metaphors and similes (e.g., "Some cults are termites") are processed by alignment and mapping, whereas conventional metaphors (e.g., "Some people are sheep") may be processed by accessing a stored metaphorical word sense. Finally, there are often systems of related metaphors in a language (Lakoff and Johnson, 1980). For example, English has a system of metaphors in which anger is described as heated fluid in a container (e.g., "Mary was boiling mad. The pressure built up in her until she finally exploded with rage."). These metaphorical systems might reflect a large-scale mapping between a base and target domain.

One model of system metaphors has been developed by Narayanan (1999). This model uses a localist connectionist system to handle extended metaphors such as the anger as heated fluid example above. In this system, the connection between a base and target domain is assumed to be established by convention, so there is no mapping mechanism for constructing new correspondences. Instead, the model focuses on how understanding a physical base domain can aid the comprehension of an abstract target. The model has a detailed localist network representation of the base domain in which actions can be simulated as transitions through the network. After simulating a possible outcome in the physical domain, the established mapping to the target domain is used by passing activation from the base to corresponding nodes in a belief network representing the target. In this way, metaphorical inferences can be drawn from base to target. These inferences are confined to existing correspondences between the domains; there is no mechanism for establishing new correspondences. A variety of constraints on metaphor interpretation such as the intent of the speaker can be incorporated into the model by treating them as additional sources of activation.

It may be possible to extend connectionist models of analogy to metaphor. Connectionist models may be well suited to capturing emotional aspects of metaphor. Associations between emotions and words (and word sounds) are unlikely to be mediated by strictly symbolic and rule-based processes. Thus, the kinds of soft constraints that are easily implemented in connectionist models might be particularly well suited to understanding this aspect of metaphor comprehension.

Discussion

Analogical and metaphor processing rely heavily on structurally governed correspondences between the two domains. This leads to

the eight benchmarks summarized in Table 1 that pose a challenge for any model of analogy. Connectionist models that address these phenomena have focused on techniques for representing and processing structured representations. LISA, which uses structured representations and structure-sensitive processing, accounts for many of the phenomena in Table 1, although some additional specification and testing of the model is still required.

Some challenges for future research include (1) building analogical models that can preserve structural relations over incrementally extended analogies such as are used in reasoning, (2) developing models that can be used as components of a broader cognitive system such as one that would perform problem solving, and (3) developing models that can handle novel and conventional metaphors.

Road Map: Psychology
Related Reading: Associative Networks; Compositionality in Neural Systems; Concept Learning; Systematicity of Generalizations in Connectionist Networks

References

Barnden, J. A., 1994, On the connectionist implementation of analogy and working memory matching, in *Advances in Connectionist and Neural Computation Theory, Vol 3: Analogy, Metaphor, and Reminding* (K. J. Holyoak and J. A. Barnden, Eds.), Norwood, NJ: Ablex Publishing Company, pp. 327–374. ◆

Clement, C. A., and Gentner, D., 1991, Systematicity as a selection constraint in analogical mapping, *Cognitive Sci.*, 15:89–132.

Falkenhainer, B., Forbus, K. D., and Gentner, D., 1989, The structure-mapping engine: An algorithm and examples, *Artificial Intelligence*, 41:1–63.

Gentner, D., and Markman, A. B., 1997, Structural alignment in analogy and similarity, *Am. Psychol.*, 52(1):45–56. ◆

Glucksberg, S., and Keysar, B., 1990, Understanding metaphorical comparisons: Beyond similarity, *Psychol. Rev.*, 97(1):3–18.

Halford, G. S., Wilson, W. H., Guo, J., Wiles, J., and Stewart, J. E. M., 1994, Connectionist implications for processing capacity limitations in analogies, in *Advances in Connectionist and Neural Computation Theory, Vol. 2: Analogical Connections* (K. J. Holyoak and J. Barnden, Eds.), Norwood, NJ: Ablex, pp. 363–415.

Hinton, G. E., Ed., 1991, *Connectionist Symbol Processing*, Cambridge, MA: MIT Press.

Holyoak, K. J., and Thagard, P., 1989, Analogical mapping by constraint satisfaction, *Cognit. Sci.*, 13(3):295–355.

Holyoak, K. J., and Thagard, P., 1995, *Mental Leaps: Analogy in Creative Thought*, Cambridge, MA: MIT Press. ◆

Hummel, J. E., Burns, B., and Holyoak, K. J., 1994, Analogical mapping by dynamic binding: Preliminary investigations, in *Advances in Connectionist and Neural Computation Theory: Vol. 2: Analogical Connections* (K. J. Holyoak and J. A. Barnden, Eds.), Norwood, NJ: Ablex.

Hummel, J. E., and Holyoak, K. J., 1997, Distributed representations of structure: A theory of analogical access and mapping, *Psychol. Rev.*, 104(3):427–466.

Lakoff, G., and Johnson, M., 1980, *Metaphors We Live By*, Chicago, IL: The University of Chicago Press.

Markman, A. B., and Gentner, D., 1993, Structural alignment during similarity comparisons, *Cognitive Psychology*, 25(4):431–467.

Narayanan, S., 1999, Moving right along: A computational model of metaphoric reasoning about events, in *The Proceedings of AAAI-99*, Orlando, FL: AAAI.

Smolensky, P., 1990, Tensor product variable binding and the representation of symbolic structures in connectionist systems, *Artificial Intelligence*, 48:159–216.

Spellman, B. A., and Holyoak, K. J., 1992, If Saddam is Hitler then who is George Bush? Analogical mapping between systems of social roles, *J. Personality Soc. Psychol.*, 62(6):913–933.

Arm and Hand Movement Control

Stefan Schaal

Introduction

The control of arm and hand movements in human and nonhuman primates has fascinated researchers in psychology, neuroscience, robotics, and numerous related areas. To the uninitiated observer, movement appears effortless. It is only when trying to duplicate such skills with artificial systems or when examining the underlying neural substrate that one discovers a surprising complexity that, so far, has prevented us from understanding the biological implementation, how to repair neural damage, and how to create human-like robots with a human level of movement skills.

Research directed toward understanding motor control can be approached on different levels of abstraction. For example, such research may entail examining the biochemical mechanisms of neuronal firing, the representational power of single neurons and populations of neurons, neuroanatomical pathways, the biomechanics of the musculoskeletal system, the computational principles of biological feedback control and learning, or the interaction of perception and action. No matter which level of inquiry is chosen, however, ultimately we need to solve the "reverse engineering" problem of how the properties of each level correlate with the characteristics of skillful behavior. Motor control of the arm and hand is an excellent example of the difficulties that arise in the reverse engineering problem. Behavioral research has discovered a variety of regularities in this movement domain, but it is hard to determine on which level they arise. Moreover, most of these regularities were examined in isolated arm or hand movement studies, whereas coordination of the arm and hand is a coupled process in which hand and arm movement influence each other. In this article, we discuss some of the most prominent regularities of arm and hand control and consider where these regularities come from, with a particular focus on computational and neural network models. It will become apparent that an interesting competition exists among explanations sought on the neural, biomechanical, perceptual, or computational level. These competing explanations have created a large amount of controversy in the research community over the years.

Behavioral Phenomena of Arm and Hand Control

Most movement skills can be achieved in an infinite number of ways. For instance, during reaching for an object, an arbitrary hand path can be taken between starting point and end point, and the path can be traversed at arbitrary speed profiles. Moreover, because of the excess of the number of degrees of freedom in primate movement systems, there is an infinite number of ways for realizing a chosen hand path through postural configurations (see ROBOT ARM CONTROL). On the biomechanical level there is even more redundancy, because there are many more muscles than degrees of freedom in the human body, and the redundancy increases on the neuronal level. Thus, it is extremely unlikely that two different individuals would use similar movement strategies to accomplish the same movement goal. Surprisingly, however, behavioral research did find a large number of regularities, not just across individuals of a given species but also across different species (see, e.g., Flash and Sejnowski, 2001). These regularities or invariants have become central to understanding perceptuomotor control, as they seem to indicate some fundamental organizational principles in the central nervous system (CNS).

Bell-Shaped Velocity Profiles and Curvature in Reaching Movements

About 20 years ago, Morasso (see OPTIMIZATION PRINCIPLES IN MOTOR CONTROL) discovered that in point-to-point reaching

movements in humans, the hand path in Cartesian (external) space was approximately straight and the tangential velocity trajectory along the path could be characterized by a symmetric bell shape, a result that was duplicated in monkeys. In contrast, velocity profiles in joint space and muscle space were much more complex. These findings gave rise to the hypothesis that point-to-point reaching movements are planned in external coordinates and not in internal ones. Later, more detailed examinations of reaching movements revealed that, although *approximately* straight, reaching movement showed a characteristic amount of curvature as a function of where in the workspace the starting point and end point of the movement were chosen. Also, the symmetry of the velocity profile varies systematically as a function of movement speed (e.g., Bullock and Grossberg, 1988). These behavioral phenomena gave rise to a variety of models to explain them.

Initial computational models of reaching focused on accounting for the bell-shaped velocity profile of hand movement, employing principles of optimal control based on a kinematic optimization criterion for movement planning that favors smooth acceleration profiles of the hand (see OPTIMIZATION PRINCIPLES IN MOTOR CONTROL). As this theory would produce perfectly straight-line movements in Cartesian space and perfectly symmetric bell-shaped velocity profiles, the observed violation of these features in behavioral expression was explained by assuming that these movement plans were executed imperfectly by an equilibrium point controller (see EQUILIBRIUM POINT HYPOTHESIS). Thus, the behavioral features of point-to-point movements were attributed to perfect motor planning and imperfect motor execution.

An alternative viewpoint was suggested by Kawato and coworkers (see OPTIMIZATION PRINCIPLES IN MOTOR CONTROL and EQUILIBRIUM POINT HYPOTHESIS). Their line of research emphasizes that the CNS takes the dynamical properties of the musculoskeletal system into account and plans trajectories that minimize "wear and tear" in the actuators, expressed as a minimum torque-change or minimum motor-command-change optimization criterion. According to this overall view, the behavioral features of arm and hand control are an intentional outcome of an underlying computational principle that employs models of the entire movement system and its environment.

Recently, Harris and Wolpert (see OPTIMIZATION PRINCIPLES IN MOTOR CONTROL) suggested that the features of arm and hand movement could also be due to the noise characteristics of neural firing, i.e., the decreasing signal-to-noise ratio of motor neurons with increasing firing frequency. Thus, the neuronal level together with the behavioral goal of accurate reaching was held responsible for behavioral characteristics.

Several other suggestions were made to account for features of arm and hand control. Perceptual distortion could potentially contribute to the curvature features in reaching, and dynamical properties of feedback loops in motor planning could generate asymmetries of bell-shaped velocity profiles (Bullock and Grossberg, 1988). Moreover, imperfection of motor learning (see SENSORIMOTOR LEARNING) and delays in the control system could equally play into explaining behavior.

Movement Segmentation

For efficient motor learning, it seems mandatory that movement systems plan on a higher level of abstraction than individual motor commands, as otherwise the search space for exploration during learning would become too large to find appropriate actions for a new movement task (see ROBOT LEARNING). Movement primitives (see MOTOR PRIMITIVES), also called units of action, basis behaviors, or gestures (see SPEECH PRODUCTION), could offer such an abstraction. Pattern generators in invertebrates and vertebrates (see MOTOR PATTERN GENERATION) and the few different behavioral modes of oculomotor control (e.g., VOR, OKR, smooth pursuit, saccades, vergence) can be seen as examples of such movement primitives. For arm and hand control, however, whether some form of units of actions exist is a topic of ongoing research (Sternad and Schaal, 1999). Finding behavioral evidence for movement segmentation could thus provide some insight into the existence of movement primitives.

Since the 1980s, kinematic features of hand trajectories have been used as one major indicator to investigate movement segmentation. From the number of modes of the tangential velocity profile of the hand in linear and curvilinear drawing movements, it was concluded that arm movements may generally be created based on discrete strokes between start points, via points, and end points, and that these strokes are piecewise planar in three-dimensional movement (for a review, see Sternad and Schaal, 1999). From these and subsequent studies, stroke-based movement generation and piecewise planarity of the hand movement in Cartesian space became one of the main hypotheses for movement segmentation (Flash and Sejnowski, 2001).

Recent work (Sternad and Schaal, 1999), however, reinterpreted these indicators of movement segmentation partially as an artifact, in particular for rhythmic movement, that, surprisingly, was also assumed to be segmented into planar stokes. Human and robot experiments demonstrated that features of apparent movement segmentation could also arise from principles of trajectory formation that use oscillatory movement primitives in joint space. When such oscillations are transformed by the nonlinear direct kinematics of an arm (see ROBOT ARM CONTROL) into hand movement, complex kinematic features of hand trajectories can arise that are not due to movement segmentation. Sternad and Schaal (1999) therefore suggested that movement primitives may be better sought in terms of dynamic systems theory, looking for dynamical regimes like point and limit cycle attractors and using perturbation experiments to find principles of segmenting movements into these basic regimes.

The 2/3 Power Law

Another related behavioral feature of primate hand movements trajectories, the 2/3 power law, was discovered by Lacquaniti et al. (in Flash and Sejnowski, 2001). In rhythmic drawing movements, the authors noted a power law relationship with proportionality constant k between the angular velocity $a(t)$ of the hand and the curvature of the trajectory path $c(t)$:

$$a(t) = kc(t)^{2/3} \tag{1}$$

There is no physical necessity for movement systems to satisfy this relation between kinematic (i.e., velocity) and geometric (i.e., curvature) properties of hand movements. Since the power law has been reproduced in numerous behavioral experiments (Viviani and Flash, 1995, in Flash and Sejnowski, 2001) and even in population code activity in motor cortices (Schwartz and Moran, 1999, in Flash and Sejnowski, 2001), it may reflect an important principle of movement generation in the CNS.

The origins of the power law, however, remain controversial. Schaal and Sternad (2001) reported strong violations of the power law in large-scale drawing patterns and, in accordance with other studies, interpreted it as an epiphenomenon of smooth movement generation (Flash and Sejnowski, 2001). Nevertheless, the power law remains an interesting descriptive feature of regularities of human motor control and has proved to be useful even in model-

ing the perception of movement (see MOTOR THEORIES OF PERCEPTION).

The Speed-Accuracy Trade-off

In rapid reaching for a target, the movement time MT of reaching the target was empirically found to depend on the distance A of the start point of movement from the target and the target width W—equivalent to the required accuracy of reaching—in a logarithmic relationship: $MT = a + b \log2(2A/W)$, where a and b are proportionality constants in this so-called Fitts' law or speed-accuracy trade-off. Since Fitts' law is a robust phenomenon of human arm and hand movement, many computational models used it as a way to verify their validity. Unfortunately, Fitts' law has been modeled in many different ways, including models from dynamic system theory, noise properties of neuronal firing, and computational constraints in movement planning (for a review, see Mottet and Bootsma, 2001; Bullock and Grossberg, 1988). Thus, it seems that the constraints provided by Fitts' law are too nonspecific to give clear hints as to the organization of the nervous system. Nevertheless, the empirical phenomenon of Fitts' law remains a behavioral landmark.

Resolution of Redundancy

As mentioned earlier, during reaching for a target in external space, the excess number of degrees of freedom in the human body's kinematic structure usually allows an infinite number of postures for each hand position attained during the reaching trajectory. An active area of research in motor control is thus concerned with how redundancy is resolved, whether there is within- or across-subject consistency of the resolution of redundancy, and whether it is possible to deduce constraints on motor planning and execution from the resolution of redundancy.

Early studies by Cruse et al. (in Bullock, Grossberg, and Guenther, 1993) demonstrated that redundancy resolution was well described by a multiterm optimization criterion that primarily tries to keep joint angular position as far as possible away from the extreme positions of each joint and also minimizes some physiological cost. According to this explanation, when a reaching movement is initiated in a rather unnatural posture, the movement slowly converges to the optimal posture on the way to the goal, rather than achieving optimality immediately. This strategy resembles the method of resolved motion rate control in control theory, suggested as a neural network model of human motor planning by Bullock et al. (1993). Grea, Desmurget, and Prablanc (2000) observed similar behavior in reaching and grasping movements. Noting that the final posture at a grasp target was highly repeatable even if the target changed its position and orientation during the course of the reaching movement, the authors concluded that the CNS plans the final *joint space* position for reaching and grasping, not just the final hand position. However, the optimization methods proposed by Bullock et al. (1993) could result in similar behavior, without the CNS explicitly planning the final joint space posture. An elegant alternative view to optimization methods is suggested in GEOMETRICAL PRINCIPLES IN MOTOR CONTROL (q.v.), where motor control and planning based on force fields is emphasized. It is evident more work will be needed before a final conclusion can be reached on the issue of redundancy resolution.

Reaching and Grasping

The coordination of reaching and grasping offers at least three important windows onto motor control. First, reaching and grasping require a resolution of redundancy, as outlined in the previous section. However, small changes in target orientation can lead to the need for drastic changes in arm and hand posture at the target, such that movement planning requires carefully chosen strategies for successful control. Second, reaching and grasping are two separate motor behaviors that may or not be executed independently of each other. This issue allows researchers to examine the superposition and sequencing of movement primitives. Third, grasping has a more interesting perceptual component than reaching, since appropriate grasp points, grasping strategies, and grasping forces need to be selected as a function of target shape, size, and weight. The principles of perceptuomotor coordination can thus be examined in well-controlled experiments, including the grasping of objects that induce visual illusions.

Among the key features of reaching and grasping are the following: (1) a fast initial arm movement to bring the hand close to the target, (2) a slow approach movement when the hand is near the target, and (3) a preshaping phase of the hand with initial progressive opening of the grip, followed by closure of the grip until the object size is matched and the object is finally grasped (Jeannerod et al., 1995; Arbib and Hoff, 1993, in Jeannerod et al., 1995). Although early models of reaching and grasping assumed independence of these different phases and simply executed them in a programmatic way, behavioral perturbation studies that changed the target size, orientation, or distance revealed a coupling between the phases (for a review, see Jeannerod et al., 1995), such that, e.g., the preshaping partially reversed when the target distance was suddenly increased. Using optimization principles, Hoff and Arbib (in Jeannerod et al., 1995) developed a model of these interactions by structuring the reach-and-grasp system in appropriate perceptual and motor schemas (see SCHEMA THEORY), including abstraction of the multifingered hand in terms of two or more virtual fingers to simultaneously model different grip types (e.g., precision grip, power grip) and their opposition spaces for contact selection. This model can also be mapped onto the known functional cortical anatomy in primates. Grip force selection and the anticipation of object properties has been studied by a number of authors (e.g., Flanagan and Beltzner, 2000), who generally agree that the CNS seems to use internal models to adjust grip force. From studies of the resolution of redundancy, it was concluded that the entire arm posture at the target seems to be planned in advance (Grea et al., 2000), but this result may need differentiation as outlined in the previous section. In general, there seems to be a consensus that behavioral features of reaching and grasping are carefully planned by the CNS and are not accidental.

Motor Learning

Because of continuous change in body size and biomechanical properties throughout development, the ability to learn motor control is of fundamental importance in biological movement systems. Moreover, when it comes to arm and hand control, primates show an unusual flexibility in devising new motor skills to solve novel tasks. Learning must therefore play a pivotal role in computational models of motor control.

One of the most visible research impacts of motor learning was the controversy between equilibrium point control (see EQUILIBRIUM POINT HYPOTHESIS) and internal model control (see SENSORIMOTOR LEARNING and CEREBELLUM AND MOTOR CONTROL). Proponents of equilibrium point control believed that the learning of internal models is too complicated to be plausible for biological information processing, while proponents of internal model control accumulated evidence that various, in particular fast, movement behaviors cannot be accounted for by equilibrium point control. At present, there seems to be an increasing consensus that internal model control is a viable concept for biological motor learning, and that the equilibrium point control strategy in its original and appealing simplicity is not tenable. Behavioral learning experiments

that were created in the wake of the equilibrium point control discussion sparked a new branch of research on motor learning (see SENSORIMOTOR LEARNING and GEOMETRICAL PRINCIPLES IN MOTOR CONTROL). Adaptation to virtual force fields, to altered perceptual environments, or to virtual objects are among the main behavioral paradigms to investigate motor learning, with the goal of better understanding the time course, representations, control circuits, retention, and functional anatomy of motor learning (see SENSORIMOTOR LEARNING).

Interlimb Coordination

In robotics, the control of two limbs can be accomplished as if the two systems were completely independent, thus reducing the control problem to that of controlling two robots instead of one. In biological motor control, such independence does not exist, and a rich area of behavioral investigation examines the computational principles and constraints that arise from the coordination of multiple limbs. In arm and hand control, the approach of dynamic pattern formation (e.g., Kelso, 1995) has been a prominent methodology to account for interlimb coordination. In this approach, motor control in general and interlimb coordination in particular are viewed as an assembly of the required degrees of freedom of the motor system into a task-oriented attractor landscape (Saltzman and Kelso, 1987, in Kelso, 1995). Interlimb coordination is thus conceived of as the result of coupling terms in nonlinear differential equations. An important question thus arises as to what kind of equations model the control of movement, and what kind of variables cause the coupling. A variety of models of movement generation with nonlinear dynamics approaches were suggested, based on differential equations, that either generate movement plans (Kelso, 1995; Sternad, Dean, and Schaal, 2000) or directly generate forces. The origin of coupling between limbs, however, remains an issue of controversy. Possible sources could be perceptual, proprioceptive, purely planning-based, interaction force–based, a preference for homologous muscle activation, or neural crosstalk. By demonstrating that the orientation of limbs in external space can explain a certain class of interlimb coordination, recent behavioral results (Mechsner et al., 2001) emphasized that perceptual coupling may be much more dominant than previously suspected. In general, however, there seems to be a strong need for detailed computational modeling to elucidate the computational and neuronal principles of interlimb coordination.

Intralimb Coordination

Investigations of intralimb coordination seek to uncover the specific principles by which individual segments of a limb move relative to one another. Models of arm and hand control that are based on optimal control (see OPTIMIZATION PRINCIPLES IN MOTOR CONTROL) or optimal resolution of redundancy automatically solve the intralimb coordination problem by means of their optimization framework; any kind of special behavioral features would be considered accidental. However, some research has considered whether some special rules of information processing by the CNS can be deduced from the regularities of intralimb coordination. For reaching movements, the simple mechanism of joint interpolation can account for a large set of behavioral features when the onset times of the movements in individual degrees of freedom are staggered, an older observation that has been confirmed in more recent work (Desmurget et al., 1995). For rhythmic movement, it is of interest to know how the oscillations in individual degrees of freedom remain phase-locked to each other, and whether there are preferred phase-locked modes (Schaal et al., 2000). As in interlimb coordination, models of nonlinear differential equations seem the most suitable for capturing the effects of rhythmic intralimb dynamics.

Perception-Action Coupling

Most of the behavioral studies outlined in the previous sections were primarily concerned with specific aspects of *motor control* and less with issues of *perceptuomotor control*. However, the interaction of perception and action reveals many constraints on the nervous system. In the behavioral literature, there is a large body of research that examines particular perceptuomotor skills, such as the rhythmic coordination of arm movement during the juggling of objects or the interaction of external forces and limb dynamics to generate movement (e.g., Sternad, Duarte, et al., 2000). This interesting topic cannot be discussed in detail here.

Discussion

Behavioral phenomena of arm and hand movement have sparked a rich variety of computational models on various levels of abstraction. Although some topics, such as internal model control, have gained solid ground in recent years (Flash and Sejnowski, 2001), many other issues remain controversial and deserve more detailed and computational investigations. Perhaps the most interesting topics for future research are the importance of the dynamic properties of the musculoskeletal system in facilitating motor control, the role of real-time perceptual modulation of motor control, and dynamic systems models versus optimal control-based models.

Road Maps: Mammalian Motor Control; Robotics and Control Theory
Related Reading: Eye-Hand Coordination in Reaching Movements; Grasping Movements: Visuomotor Transformations; Limb Geometry, Neural Control; Robot Arm Control; Sensorimotor Learning

References

Bullock, D., and Grossberg, S., 1988, Neural dynamics of planned arm movements: Emergent invariants and speed-accuracy properties during trajectory formation, *Psychol. Rev.,* 95:49–90. ◆

Bullock, D., Grossberg, S., and Guenther, F. H., 1993, A self-organizing neural model of motor equivalent reaching and tool use by a multijoint arm, *J. Cogn. Neurosci.,* 5:408–435.

Desmurget, M., Prablanc, C., Rossetti, Y., Arzi, M., Paulignan, Y., Urquizar, C., and Mignot, J. C., 1995, Postural and synergic control for three-dimensional movements of reaching and grasping, *J. Neurophysiol.,* 74:905–910.

Flanagan, J. R., and Beltzner, M. A., 2000, Independence of perceptual and sensorimotor predictions in the size-weight illusion, *Nature Neurosci.,* 3:737–741.

Flash, T., and Sejnowski, T., 2001, Computational approaches to motor control, *Curr. Opin. Neurobiol.,* 11:655–662. ◆

Grea, H., Desmurget, M., and Prablanc, C., 2000, Postural invariance in three-dimensional reaching and grasping movements, *Exp. Brain Res.,* 134:155–162.

Jeannerod, M., Arbib, M. A., Rizzolatti, G., and Sakata, H., 1995, Grasping objects: The cortical mechanisms of visuomotor transformation, *Trends Neurosci.,* 18:314–320. ◆

Kelso, J. A. S., 1995, *Dynamic Patterns: The Self-Organization of Brain and Behavior,* Cambridge, MA: MIT Press.

Mechsner, F., Kerzel, D., Knoblich, G., and Prinz, W., 2001, Perceptual basis of bimanual coordination, *Nature,* 414:69–73.

Mottet, D., and Bootsma, R. J., 2001, The dynamics of rhythmical aiming in 2D task space: Relation between geometry and kinematics under examination, *Hum. Movement Sci.,* 20:213–241.

Schaal, S., and Sternad, D., 2001, Origins and violations of the 2/3 power law in rhythmic 3D movements, *Exp. Brain Res.,* 136:60–72. ◆

Schaal, S., Sternad, D., Dean, W., Kotoska, S., Osu, R., and Kawato, M., 2000, Reciprocal excitation between biological and robotic research, in *Sensor Fusion and Decentralized Control in Robotic Systems III, Proceedings of the SPIE,* Boston, MA: SPIE.

Sternad, D., Dean, W. J., and Schaal, S., 2000, Interaction of rhythmic and discrete pattern generators in single joint movements, *Hum. Movement Sci.,* 19:627–665.

Sternad, D., Duarte, M., Katsumata, H., and Schaal, S., 2000, Dynamics of a bouncing ball in human performance, *Phys. Rev. E,* 63:1–8.

Sternad, D., and Schaal, D., 1999, Segmentation of endpoint trajectories does not imply segmented control, *Exp. Brain Res.,* 124:118–136.

Artificial Intelligence and Neural Networks

John A. Barnden and Marcin Chady

Introduction

This article surveys the distinctions between symbolic artificial intelligence (AI) systems and neural networks (NNs), their relative advantages, and ways of attempting to bridge the gap between the two.

For this review we can take AI to consist of the development, analysis, and simulation of computationally detailed, efficient systems for performing complex tasks, where the tasks are broadly defined, involve considerable flexibility and variety, and are typically similar to aspects of human cognition or perception. These broad tasks include natural language understanding and generation; expert problem solving; common-sense reasoning; visual scene analysis; action planning; and learning.

There is nothing in this description of AI that prevents the computational systems from being neural networks. Nevertheless, it is fair to say that the bulk of AI can be called "traditional" or "symbolic" AI, relying on computation over symbolic structures (e.g., logic formulae). The rest of the review will therefore discuss relationships between symbolic AI and NNs.

Relative Advantages

Advantages of Neural Networks

One of the main benefits claimed for NNs is graceful degradation, especially when they are of the distributed variety (LOCALIZED VERSUS DISTRIBUTED REPRESENTATIONS). A computational system is said to exhibit graceful degradation when it can tolerate significant corruption of its input or internal workings. The toleration consists of the system's continuing to perform usefully, though not necessarily perfectly. In NNs, input imperfection is typically a matter of corruption of individual input activation vectors. Internal corruption usually takes the form of deletions of nodes or links or corruptions of the link weights.

Symbolic AI systems, on the other hand, tend not to degrade gracefully. Consider a simple rule-based system. A small corruption of an input data structure is likely to make it fail to match the precise form expected by the rules that would otherwise have applied, so that they totally fail to be enabled. Equally, other rules might erroneously be enabled. Similarly, even minor damage to a rule can have very large effects on how the system operates.

As a special case of graceful degradation, NNs sometimes exhibit *error correction*, whereby an erroneous or corrupted pattern on an input bank of units leads to a corrected version of the pattern appearing in the network, enabling the network to proceed as if the correct version had been provided. Related to this type of error correction is *pattern completion*, whereby an incomplete pattern is filled out to become a more complete pattern somewhere in the network.

Also related to graceful degradation is *automatic similarity-based generalization*, in which previously unseen inputs that are sufficiently similar to training inputs lead naturally to behavior that is usefully similar to (or captures central tendencies in) the behavior elicited by the training inputs. There is a sense in which similarity of representations induces similarity of processing more readily than it does in symbolic AI: there is, by and large, a higher degree of naturally achievable continuity in the mapping from inputs to outputs. In addition, previously unseen blends of different representations will naturally tend to lead to processing that is a blend of the processing that would have arisen from the different representations that have been blended together. Such behavior is possible in symbolic AI but specific system-design effort is needed to achieve it.

Importantly, NNs can *learn* generalizations or category prototypes by exposure to instances, through fairly straightforward, uniform weight modification procedures. These generalizations or prototypes come to be implicit in the adjusted weights. Although learning is intensively studied in symbolic AI, and some learning paradigms in symbolic AI involve adjustment of numerical parameters akin to NN weights, symbolic processing does not provide any specific support to these paradigms. The paradigms could therefore be said to arise less easily and naturally out of symbolic processing than out of NN activity.

The preceding properties of NNs have found their application in *content-based access* (or *associative access*) to long-term memory (see ASSOCIATIVE NETWORKS). This can take two different forms. First, let us assume, as usual, that a neural net's long-term memory is its set of weights. The manipulation of an input vector by the network can be thought of as the bringing to bear of particular content-relevant long-term memories on that vector. Second, in any NN that learns a map from particular inputs to particular outputs, an output can be thought of as a particular long-term memory recalled directly on the basis of the content of the input. Content-based access is not as easily provided in symbolic systems implemented in conventional computers, although it can be obtained to some useful degree by sophisticated indexing schemes (see Bonissone et al. in Barnden and Holyoak, 1994), associative computer memories, or hashing (see Touretzky in Hinton, 1991, for discussion).

NNs can have *emergent rule-like behavior*. Such behavior can be described, approximately at least, as the result of following symbolic rules, even though the system does not contain representations of explicit rules (see Elman, 1991). Emergent rule-like behavior is a central issue in the application of neural networks to high-level cognitive tasks.

More generally, NNs tend to be more sensitive to *subtle contextual effects* than symbolic AI systems are, because multiple sources of information can more easily be brought to bear in a gracefully interacting and parallel way. This property of NNs facilitates *soft constraint satisfaction*. That is, it is possible to arrange for some hypotheses to compete and cooperate with each other, gradually influencing each other's levels of confidence until a stable set of hypotheses is found. Each hypothesis is represented by a node or group of nodes in the neural network, and the constraints are encoded by links joining those nodes or groups. The constraint-satisfaction is soft because no individual constraint needs to be satisfied absolutely. By contrast, although many symbolic AI sys-

tems are designed to do constraint satisfaction, the symbolic framework provides no special support for it, particularly when the constraints are soft.

Finally, NNs are an inherently parallel model of computation whose parallelism is straightforwardly realizable in a physical substrate.

Advantages of Symbolic AI Systems

The symbolic framework is better than NNs at encoding and manipulating the *complex, dynamic structures* of information that appear to be needed in cognition. These structures can, for instance, be interpretations of natural language utterances, descriptions of complex scenes, complex plans of action, or conclusions drawn from other information. The encodings of such structures, whether these encodings are symbolic or otherwise, need to have the following important properties. (See also Shastri in Barnden and Pollack, 1991.)

1. The encodings must often be highly temporary—for instance, encodings of interpretations of natural language sentences and encodings of intermediate conclusions during reasoning need to be rapidly created, modified, and discarded. Although activation patterns in NNs are temporary, temporariness is challenging for NNs when it is combined with properties 2–6.
2. The encoding technique must allow the encoded structures to combine information items (e.g., word senses) that have never been combined before, or never been combined in quite the same way, in the experience of the system.
3. The encodings must allow the encoded information to have widely varying structural complexity. Natural language sentence interpretations provide illustrations of this point.
4. In particular, the encoded structures can be multiply nested. In the sentence "John believes that Peter's angry behavior toward Mary caused her to write him a strongly worded letter," the anger description is nested within a causation description that is nested within a belief report.
5. A given type of information can appear at different levels of nesting. A system might have to represent a sitting *room* that has a wall that bears a picture that itself depicts a dining *room*. As another illustration, a *belief* might be about a hope that is about a *belief*.
6. A given type of information may also have to be multiply instantiated in other ways, as when, for instance, there are three love relationships that need to be simultaneously represented.

Turning to manipulations, cognitive systems must exhibit strong properties of *systematicity* of processing—each information structure J that one cares to mention has an extremely large class of variants that must be able to be subjected to the same sort of processing as J is; and the class of variants is far too large to imagine that each variant is processed by a separate piece of neural network or a separate symbolic module. So, we must have symbolic AI systems and NNs capable of very flexible and general processing. (See also SYSTEMATICITY OF GENERALIZATIONS IN CONNECTIONIST NETWORKS.)

The *variable-binding* problem for neural networks is one manifestation of the need for systematicity of processing. Suppose one wishes a neural network to make inferences that obey the following rule: X is jealous of Z whenever X loves Y, Y loves Z, and X, Y, and Z are distinct people. In this statement of the rule, the variables X, Y, and Z can be replaced by any suitable people-descriptions, such as "Joe Bloggs' father's boss." The systematicity issue in this example is that of avoiding having replication of machinery for all the different possible combinations of values for these variables. (Each such combination is a J in the terms of the previous paragraph.) This issue can also be thought of as the variable binding problem for the example, even if a neural network dealing with it does not have any explicit representation of the rule or the variables in it. In the special case in which a neural network implements the rule as a subnetwork and has particular units, subnetworks, or activation patterns that play the role of the three variables, the variable binding problem, in a narrower sense now, is the problem of how the network is to be able to "bind" such a unit, subnetwork, or activation pattern to a particular value at any given moment, and how the binding is to be used in processing.

Cognitive systems must also exhibit a high degree of *structure-sensitivity* in their processing. Pieces of information that have complex structure must be processed in ways that are heavily dependent on their structure as such, not (just) on the nature of constituents taken individually. For example, consider the operation of inferring from "not both *A* and *B*" that "not *A* or not *B*." The operation is independent of what *A* and *B* are—it is only the "not both . . . and . . ." structure that is important.

These features of information structure encodings and manipulations combine to distinguish the types of information that neural networks for reasoning, natural language understanding, etc. must deal with from the types of information that typical neural networks cater for. Traditional NN techniques were originally developed largely for specific "low level" applications, such as restricted forms of pattern recognition, or for limited forms of pattern association. Because of the resulting continuing limitations in most applications of NNs, it has been sufficient for NNs to adhere, by and large, to the following restrictions (although almost every restriction is violated by some NN subparadigm). These restrictions cause difficulty in trying to apply NNs to natural language understanding, common-sense reasoning, and the like.

1. There is typically no dynamic, rapid creation and destruction of nodes and links. Therefore, temporary information cannot be encoded in temporary network topology changes. (Some of this effect can, however, be obtained by techniques such as dynamic links described in DYNAMIC LINK ARCHITECTURE (q.v.), or by higher-order units, whose activation is sensitive to weighted sums of products of input values, rather than just to weighted sums of input values.)
2. Links in NNs are not differentiated by labeling, unlike the links in symbolic structures such as SEMANTIC NETWORKS (q.v.). Therefore, in an NN, information that could otherwise be put into link labels has to be encoded somehow in activation values, weights, extra links, or other features of network topology, adding significantly to the cumbersomeness of the net and its processing. (See Barnden and Srinivas, 1991, for more discussion.)
3. The resolution of NN activation values is generally not fine enough to allow them individually to encode complex symbolic structures. Most typically, activation values merely encode confidence levels of some sort.
4. Pointers are usually not allowed. That is, activation values or patterns are not allowed to act as names or addresses of parts of the network itself.
5. Stored programs are not allowed. That is, activation values or patterns cannot act as instructions (names of internal computational actions).

Further Comparative Remarks

The advantages claimed here for NNs are not clearcut. For instance, there are types of AI systems that readily exhibit forms of graceful degradation, pattern completion, and similarity-based generalization. In particular, as Barnden in Barnden and Holyoak (1994) argues in detail and other researchers have noted, these benefits are natural properties of suitably designed symbolic analogy-based reasoning systems (see ANALOGY-BASED REASONING AND METAPHOR and also MEMORY-BASED REASONING).

Just as NNs support some types of learning more readily than symbolic AI systems do, the converse holds as well. Symbolic AI systems, by virtue of their ability to handle complex temporary information structures, are in a better position to perform various types of rapid learning, proceeding in large steps rather than lengthy, gradual weight modification. For instance, a symbolic AI system is in a good position to reason about why some plan of action failed, and thus quickly and greatly amend relevant parts of its knowledge base or planning strategies. Also, the ability of neural networks to learn generalizations is often hindered by elaborate, extensive training regimes. It is true that in some learning regimes, such as some forms of Hebbian learning, final weights are calculated in a direct way from single presentations of training items. But more typically, the number of training-item presentations one needs to make to the network runs to tens or hundreds of thousands before useful results can be obtained.

NNs are good at allowing hypotheses to be held with varying degrees of confidence, the degrees being realized as activation levels. However, it is commonplace also in symbolic AI to have numerical degrees of confidence. These appear in DECISION SUPPORT SYSTEMS AND EXPERT SYSTEMS (q.v.) and elsewhere. However, the normal properties of activation spread and activation combination in NNs support confidence levels in a natural way. In symbolic AI systems the computations have to be specially and explicitly designed.

The contrasts between neural networks and symbolic AI that were presented earlier are clouded by the fact that NNs can be *implementational*. Implementational NNs are exact implementations of symbol processing schemes of the sort used in traditional symbolic AI systems. That is, network-unit activations (and/or link weights, possibly) can be regarded as exactly encoding symbolic representations as used in traditional AI systems—such as logic formulas, frames, schemas, or pieces of semantic network—and changes in network state can be regarded as exactly encoding traditional symbolic manipulation steps—such as traversal, concatenation, and rearrangement of structures—that are used in traditional AI for directly effecting reasoning, planning, natural language understanding, etc. See, for example, Barnden's and Shastri's chapters in Barnden and Pollack (1991) and Lange and Wharton's chapter in Barnden and Holyoak (1994).

The *non*implementational style includes NNs that can be usefully viewed as *approximately* manipulating traditional symbolic objects in traditional ways. However, the nearer an NN is to being implementational, the more it runs the danger of inheriting the disadvantages of symbolic AI, such as the tendency to lack graceful degradation.

Bridging the Gap

The discrepancy in the relative advantages of (nonimplementational) NNs and symbolic AI systems has been the focus of much attention during the last decade or so (see, e.g., Barnden and Pollack, 1991; Browne and Sun, 2001; Hinton, 1991; Jagota et al., 1999; McGarry, Wermter, and McIntyre, 1999). We shall review here some representative attempts to tackle the problem.

A common approach to extending conventional types of NN processing to handle complex dynamic structures is to use *reduced representations*, also known as *compressed encodings*. See, e.g., Hinton, Pollack, and St. John's chapter and McClelland's chapter in Hinton (1991), as well as Elman (1991). A reduced representation is a single activation vector that is created from the several activation vectors that encode the constituents of the structure in such a way that the resulting vector is of roughly the same size as each of the constituents' vectors. For example, the constituents could be words, and a sequence of word encodings could represent a sentence. The reduced representation is then a roughly word-sized vector for the whole sentence.

One architecture used to produce reduced representations of sequences of items is a Simple Recurrent Network (SRN). An SRN is typically a three-layer network in which the input to the middle layer consists of an item in the sequence together with the previous activation pattern in the middle layer itself. As a result of back-propagation training, the encodings produced in the middle layer are compressed vectors representing the current input *in the context of* the history of items presented to the network so far. SRNs have been successfully used, for instance, for predicting the category of the next word in a sentence being inputed (Elman, 1991).

A more general-purpose architecture for producing recurrent compressed encodings is Pollack's Recursive Auto-Associative Memory (RAAM) (see Pollack in Hinton, 1991). The input and output layers are divided up into segments that hold constituent encodings. The net is trained to map sequences of constituent encodings to themselves. The activation pattern that appears on the hidden layer of the trained network in response to a particular sequence of constituent encodings on the input layer is the compressed encoding for the sequence. (And a compressed encoding can be decoded by placing it in the hidden layer: a close approximation, hopefully, to the sequence of constituent encodings appears on the output layer.) Also, during training, a hidden layer pattern can be copied into any of the segments in the input and output layer, leading to the ability of the network to handle recursive structures some of whose constituents are themselves sequences of constituents. An example of such a structure is the sentence "John knows that Sally is clever," thought of as having the sentence "Sally is clever" as a constituent.

There are some indications that compressed encodings can support *holistic* structure-sensitive processing by means of conventional NN techniques such as feedforward association networks (see, e.g., Chalmers, 1990; Pollack in Hinton, 1991). The processing is holistic in that the encodings are not uncompressed into the individual activation vectors that encode their notional constituents. For example, Chalmers successfully trained a three-layer backpropagation network to transform compressed encodings of active English sentences into compressed encodings of their passive counterparts. The hidden layer had the same size as the input and output layers (the size of a compressed encoding) and the net operated in one pass of activation, so that it cannot have been working by first decoding the input compressed encodings into the corresponding sequence of constituent encodings.

However, in-depth analysis of RAAM-like systems (Kolen, 1994) reveals that the computation depends on very fine tuning of synaptic weights and highly precise activation levels. The implication is that holistic computation based on RAAM-generated encodings is sensitive to noise, which is a significant drawback given that graceful degradation is a major argument for using neural networks. An additional complication associated with all of the aforementioned techniques of generating reduced representations is the lengthy process of weight training.

These problems are avoided in a related approach of which a central example is the Holographic Reduced Representation (HRR) technique of Plate (1995). See also Rachkovskij and Kussul (2001). HRRs use predefined combination operations (circular convolutions) to produce compressed encodings. No training is required and both encoding as well as decoding are performed in a single step. What is more important, though, is that these transformations offer a more comprehensive account of systematicity. Given a sufficiently large size of code vectors, not only can HRRs recursively bind any number of elements, but also, using simple vector addition, multiple bindings can be combined further to form collections of predicates. Such collections retain superficial and structural sim-

ilarity of structures, so that decoding is not necessary to estimate an item's relevance for certain types of computation. If necessary, any one predicate can be readily extracted using inverse operations, although not without some loss of information due to the nature of circular convolution and vector addition. The operations introduce some degree of noise, which is further amplified by the decoding transformation. However, it can be rectified using an auto-associative memory to recover the original elements. Using this approach, Plate (1995) shows how HRRs can be used to represent sequences and more complex structures, and how to achieve chunking and variable binding.

In a different approach to bridging the gap, Barnden in Barnden and Holyoak (1994) capitalizes on the comment made previously that symbolic analogy-based reasoning possesses many of the main advantages of nonimplementational NNs. The claim is that an implementational NN that implements a symbolic analogy-based reasoning system inherits those advantages, as well as the symbolic AI advantage with respect to complex dynamic information structures.

The preceding approaches assume that it is worthwhile to develop gap-bridging systems that are neural networks in their entirety, rather than developing systems that are some combination of NN machinery with symbolic AI machinery (where the latter is given no NN realization). The latter, hybrid, strategy is a popular approach to bridging the gap (McGarry et al., 1999). The simpler types of hybridization occur in systems that have largely separate neural and symbolic modules (see, e.g., Hendler in Barnden and Pollack, 1991). But more intimate hybridizations have been developed, for instance, in networks where an individual node or link can act partially like those in neural networks and partially like those in symbolic networks.

Although the more implementational an NN is the more it risks inheriting disadvantages of symbolic AI, it may still be that some of the implementational NN techniques could be adapted for use in gap-bridging systems that escape those disadvantages. Therefore, we will now look at some of the techniques.

A crucial aspect of implementational NNs is the way in which they allow representational items to be rapidly and temporarily combined so as to form encodings of temporary complex information structures. One form of this *dynamic combination* (or *temporary association*) issue is the variable binding problem, and a closely related form is the role binding problem. The variable binding problem was described previously. The role binding problem is concerned with giving specific values to the roles (slots) in predicates, frames, schemas, and the like.

An immediately obvious, and somewhat natural, approach to dynamic combination is to combine network nodes or assemblies by adding new links or giving non-zero weights to existing zero-weight links. However, this method is highly cumbersome because network structure is not data that is directly manipulable by the network itself. Another rather similar approach is to facilitate existing (non-zero-weight) connection paths, between nodes/assemblies that are to be combined, by activating intermediate nodes on the paths. These nodes are called binding nodes. Since the dynamic combination structure is now encoded in the activation levels of binding nodes, the net can more easily analyze that structure. However, the processing is still cumbersome (Barnden and Srinivas, 1991).

A distinctly different approach is to deem nodes/assemblies to be bound together when they fire in synchrony (see STRUCTURED CONNECTIONIST MODELS, COMPOSITIONALITY IN NEURAL SYSTEMS, and DYNAMIC LINK ARCHITECTURE). See in particular Shastri in Barnden and Pollack (1991), and Henderson and Lane (1998). The method is an important special case of the more general notion of binding nodes together by giving them similar spatiotemporal activation patterns. This is the pattern-similarity association technique: see Barnden and Srinivas (1991) and Barnden in Barnden and Pollack (1991).

Distinctly different again is the use of positional encodings of dynamic combinations. In the more developed forms of this idea (see Barnden in Barnden and Pollack, 1991), activation patterns are dynamically combined by being put into suitable relative positions with respect to each other, much as bit-strings in computer memory can be put into contiguous memory locations to form records.

A somewhat pointer-like technique has been implemented: see Lange and Wharton in Barnden and Holyoak (1994). Different parts of the network are capable of emitting activation patterns that are thought of as their "signatures." Other parts can then temporarily hold signatures and thereby point, in a sense, to the parts that possess the signatures.

One noteworthy way of achieving temporary association is the use of auto-associative memories with rapid Hebbian learning, as in van der Velde (1995). Van der Velde demonstrates how multiple elements can be stored in a single network while preserving their ordering. Each element in the sequence refers to the next and previous ones by unique pointers that constitute part of the memory trace in an auto-associative module. Using this approach, van der Velde builds a conventional stack-based generator of center-embedded sentences. Despite its implementational architecture, this model manages to retain the graceful-degradation property of nonimplementational NNs. Hebbian association was also used by Hadley et al. (2001) to achieve a strong from of systematicity.

Finally, Smolensky in Hinton (1991) proposed an abstract but influential binding and structure-representation approach based on tensors. Some realizations of this approach involve binding nodes, but the approach can be seen to subsume other concrete techniques as well.

Discussion

One theme of this review has been that the relative advantages of symbolic AI and NNs are less clear-cut than is usually implied. In particular, although NNs have been successful for some purposes and can have advantages such as graceful degradation, most NN research has not addressed the complex information processing issues routinely tackled in symbolic AI research. The latter field has contributed much more, for instance, to the study of how natural language discourse can be understood and common-sense reasoning performed. Nevertheless, pursuing nonsymbolic approaches to the problems is beneficial for as long as the symbolic approaches fail to provide all the answers.

Some of the open questions in the area of this review are: Is it actually necessary to go beyond symbolic AI in order to account for complex cognition? If it is, should symbolic AI be dispensed with entirely, or is some amount of complex symbol-processing unavoidable? How can reasoning, natural language understanding, etc. be effected by neural networks without just implementing conventional symbol processing? How can different styles of system, e.g., implementational and nonimplementational neural networks, or neural networks and non-neural systems, be gracefully combined into hybrid systems?

Road Map: Artificial Intelligence
Related Reading: Compositionality in Neural Systems; Connectionist and Symbolic Representations; Hybrid Connectionist/Symbolic Systems; Multiagent Systems; Philosophical Issues in Brain Theory and Connectionism; Structured Connectionist Models; Systematicity of Generalizations in Connectionist Networks

References

Barnden, J. A., and Holyoak, K. J. (Eds.), 1994, *Advances in Connectionist and Neural Computation Theory, Vol. 3: Analogy, Metaphor and Reminding*, Norwood, NJ: Ablex Publishing Corp.

Barnden, J. A., and Pollack, J. B. (Eds), 1991, *Advances in Connectionist and Neural Computation Theory, Vol. 1: High Level Connectionist Models*, Norwood, NJ: Ablex Publishing Corp. ◆

Barnden, J. A., and Srinivas, K., 1991, Encoding techniques for complex information structures in connectionist systems, *Connection Science*, 3:263–309.

Browne, A., and Sun, R., 2001, Connectionist inference models, *Neural Networks*, 14:1331–1355. ◆

Chalmers, D. J., 1990, Syntactic transformations on distributed representations, *Connection Science*, 2:53–62.

Elman, J. L., 1991, Distributed representations, simple recurrent networks, and grammatical structure, *Machine Learning*, 7:195–225.

Hadley, R. F., Rotaru-Varga, A., Arnold, D. V., and Cardei, V. C., 2001, Syntactic systematicity arising from semantic predictions in a Hebbian-competitive network, *Connection Science*, 13:73–94. ◆

Henderson, J., and Lane, P., 1998, A connectionist architecture for learning to parse, in *Proceedings of COLING-ACL* (Montreal, Canada, 1998), pp. 531–537.

Hinton, G. E. (Ed.), 1991, *Connectionist Symbol Processing*, Cambridge, MA: MIT Press.

Jagota, A., Plate, T., Shastri, L., and Sun, R. (Eds.), 1999, Connectionist symbol processing: Dead or alive?, *Neural Computing Surveys*, 2:1–40. ◆

Kolen, J. F., 1994, Fool's gold: Extracting finite state machines from recurrent network dynamics, in *Advances in Neural Information Processing Systems, Vol. 6* (J. D. Cowan, G. Tesauro, and J. Alspector, Eds.), San Mateo, CA: Morgan Kaufmann, pp. 501–508.

McGarry, K., Wermter, S., and MacIntyre, J., 1999, Hybrid neural systems: From simple coupling to fully integrated neural networks, *Neural Computing Surveys*, 2:62–93.

Plate, T. A., 1995, Holographic reduced representations, *IEEE Transactions on Neural Networks*, 6:623–641.

Rachkovskij, D. A., and Kussul, E. M., 2001, Binding and normalization of binary sparse distributed representations by context-dependent thinning, *Neural Computation*, 13:411–452.

van der Velde, F., 1995, Symbol manipulation with neural networks: Production of a context-free language using a modifiable working memory, *Connection Science*, 7:247–280.

Associative Networks

James A. Anderson

Introduction

The operation of *association* involves the linkage of information with other information. Although the basic idea is simple, association gives rise to a particular form of computation, powerful and idiosyncratic. The mechanisms and implications of association have a long history in psychology and philosophy. Association is also the most natural form of neural network computation. This article will discuss association as realized in neural networks as well as association in the more traditional senses.

Neural networks are often justified as abstractions of the architecture of the nervous system. They are composed of a number of computing units, roughly modeled on neurons, joined together by connections that are roughly modeled on the synapses connecting real neurons together. The basic computational entity in a neural network is related to the pattern of activity shown by the units in a group of many units.

Because of the use of activity patterns—mathematized as state vectors—as computational primitives, the most common neural network architectures are pattern transformers which take an input pattern and transform it into an output pattern by way of system dynamics and a set of connections with appropriate weights. In a very general sense, therefore, neural networks are frequently designed as *pattern associators*, which link an input pattern with the "correct" output pattern. Learning rules are designed to construct accurate linkages. The most common feedforward neural network architectures realize this linkage by way of connections between layers of units (Figure 1). There may be a single set of modifiable connections between input and output (Figure 1*B*), or multiple layers of connections (Figure 1*C*). Another common architecture is realized by a single layer of units where the units in the layer are recurrently interconnected (Figure 1*A*).

One common design goal of a feedforward associator (Figures 1*B* and 1*C*) is to realize what Kohonen (1977) has labeled *heteroassociation*, that is, to link input and output patterns that need have no relation to each other. Another possibility is to realize what Kohonen has called *autoassociation*, where the input and output patterns are identical. Recurrent networks (Figure 1*A*) are well suited to autoassociation.

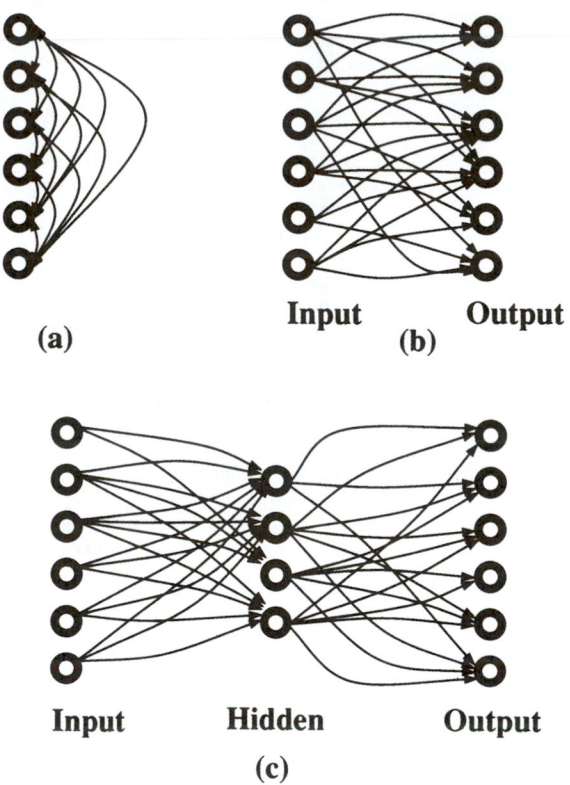

Figure 1. Three common basic neural network architectures. *A*, A set of units connects recurrently to itself by way of modifiable connections. (The connections are drawn as reciprocal.) *B*, A feedforward network in which an input pattern is transformed to an output pattern by way of a layer of modifiable connections. *C*, A more general feedforward network. An input layer projects to an intermediate layer of units. The intermediate layer is often called a *hidden layer* because it may not be accessible from outside the network. The hidden layer then projects to the output units.

Because the input and output patterns must correspond to information about the real world, the *data representation* is of critical importance at all levels of network operation. For example, simple pattern recognizers are often realized by neural networks as a special form of pattern associator by assuming a particular output representation, one where a single active output unit corresponds to the category of the input. Different categories correspond to different active output units. This highly localized representation is sometimes called a *grandmother cell* representation, because it implies that only when one particular unit is active is "grandmother" being represented. The alternative representation is called a *distributed representation*, where representation of a concept like "grandmother" may contain many active units. Choice of representation makes a major difference in how networks are used and how well they work, and is usually more important than the exact choice of network architecture and learning rule. A common situation in engineering applications of neural networks is to have a distributed representation at the input of the network and a grandmother cell representation at the output. In the vertebrate nervous system there is little evidence for this output representation; essentially all normal motor acts involve the coordinated discharge of large groups of neurons. Distributed activity patterns are associated with distributed patterns from one end of most biological networks to the other in vertebrates (but see LOCALIZED VERSUS DISTRIBUTED REPRESENTATIONS), though there are some examples of extreme selectivity in invertebrates. The degree of distribution is a matter for experimental investigation.

Neural Network Associators

Let us give an example of how easily neural network learning rules and architectures give rise to associative behavior. Consider the two-layer network diagrammed in Figure 1*B*. Consider a situation where a pattern of activity, a state vector f, is present at the input set of units and another pattern, state vector g, is shown by the output set of units.

We want to link two patterns so that when f is presented to the input of the network, g will be generated at the output. In this two-layer network (two layers of units, one layer of connections), we will assume that the connections initially are zero and we want to change them to make the association between patterns f and g. We will also assume that all connection strengths are potentially changeable and the set of connection strengths forms a *connection matrix* (or *synaptic matrix*) which we will call W, for "weights."

We have to propose a learning rule, but we also have to make some additional assumptions about the entire system. For example, virtually all artificial neural network learning assumes that the network is learning discrete pairs of patterns, that is, learning takes place only occasionally, when the time is ripe. One could speculate that learning in animals is a dangerous operation—after all, the nervous system is being rewired—and is kept under tight control. Primates are unusual in the degree of learned flexibility their nervous system allows. There is physiological evidence that amount of learning is controlled by diffuse biochemical processes. Dangerous and striking events, causing a biochemical upheaval, give rise to what have been called "flashbulb memories" where everything, including totally irrelevant detail, is learned. ("Where were you when John F. Kennedy was assassinated?" is practically guaranteed to involve a flashbulb memory in those old enough to remember it. September 11, 2001, provides a modern example.) Presumably this corresponds to an undiscriminating "learn" command. In terms of modeling, these observations mean that the decision to learn is decoupled from the act of learning.

Let us assume that we have an input pattern and an output pattern and we wish to associate them for good and sufficient reasons. We assume that we can impress pattern f on the input set of units and pattern g on the output set of units. By far the most common network learning rule used is one or another variant of what is called the "Hebb synapse," described in Hebb (1949). Perhaps the most quoted sentence in the neural network literature is from Hebb: "When an axon of cell A is near enough to excite a cell B and repeatedly or persistently takes part in firing it, some growth process or metabolic change takes place in one or both cells, such that A's efficiency as one of the cells firing B, is increased." (Hebb, 1949:62). The essence of the Hebb synapse is that there has to be a *conjunction* of activity on the two sides of the connection.

There is good physiological evidence for the existence of some form of Hebb synapse in parts of the mammalian central nervous system (see HEBBIAN SYNAPTIC PLASTICITY). However, there are a number of "technical" problems involved in mathematically describing the resulting system. The original formulation by Hebb was concerned with coincident excitation. Nothing was said about coincident inhibition or about coincident excitation and inhibition. Also, the exact function determining strength of modification was not given, and, in fact, is not known. A common assumption in *artificial* network theory is to assume some version of what is called the *generalized Hebb rule* or the *outer product rule*. This states that the change in strength of a connection during learning is given by the *product* of activities on the two sides of the connection, that is, if W_{ij} is the strength of the connection, then the change in strength ΔW_{ij} is proportional to the product, $f_j g_i$, where f_j is the activity of the jth input unit and g_i is the activity of the ith output unit. This convenient expression may have only a weak relationship to physiological reality.

Given the generalized Hebb rule, if we have only a single pair of vectors to associate, the results can be written compactly as

$$W = \eta g f^{\mathrm{T}}$$

where η is a learning constant and W is the connection (or weight) matrix.

By making an additional assumption about the properties of the individual neural elements, this rule leads almost immediately to a simple pattern associator called the *linear associator*. Suppose the elementary computing units are linear, so that the output is given by the inner product between input activity and connection strengths. Then the output pattern is given by the matrix product of an input pattern f and the connection matrix W; that is, the output of the network is Wf. Because we know what W is—it was constructed by the generalized Hebb rule—we can compute the output pattern,

$$(\text{output pattern}) = Wf = \eta g f^{\mathrm{T}} f = (\text{constant})g$$

since $f^{\mathrm{T}} f$ is a constant, the squared length of f. The output pattern is a constant multiple of g and, except for length, we have reconstructed the learned associate of f, that is, g.

Suppose we have a whole set of associations $\{f^i \rightarrow g^i\}$ that we want to teach the network. (Superscripts stand for individual pattern vectors.) If we assume that the overall strength of a connection is the algebraic sum of its past history (an unsupported assumption), then we have the weight matrix W given by

$$W = \sum_i \eta g^i f^{i\mathrm{T}}$$

Notice that in the special case where the input patterns $\{f^i\}$ are orthogonal, that is, $f^i f^j = 0$ if $i \neq j$,

$$Wf^i = (\text{constant})g^i$$

because the contributions to the output pattern from the other terms forming W are identically zero since they involve the inner product $[f_i, f_j] = f_i^{\mathrm{T}} f_j$. This model, and in fact most simple network models, make the prediction that outer product associators will work best and most reliably with representations where different input associations are as orthogonal as possible. For this reason, some cortical

models in the neuroscience literature have explicitly discussed aspects of cortical processing in terms of orthogonalization. The most complete reference for the linear associator and related models is Kohonen (1977, 1984).

It is possible to change almost any assumption and still have an associator. *Hebb learning rules of virtually any kind give rise to associative systems.* As only one example, the nonlinear Hebbian associator proposed by Willshaw, Buneman, and Longuet-Higgins (1969) used binary connections—with strengths either one or zero—and the resulting system still worked nicely as a pattern associator.

Supervised Networks

The outer product associator is less accurate with nonorthogonal patterns. However, observed distortions and human performance are sometimes remarkably similar. (See Anderson, 1995, chap. 11, for a model of "concept formation" that emerges when correlated inputs are stored in the linear associator.)

Most designers of artificial networks prefer networks to produce accurate reproductions of learned associations rather than interesting distortions. (This seemingly natural assumption is not necessarily a good one.) *Supervised* network algorithms can perform more accurate association. Examples of such algorithms would include the Widrow-Hoff (LMS) algorithm, the perceptron, backpropagation, and many others. The basic mechanism employed is *error correction*. Suppose we have an initial training set of patterns to be learned. This means we know what the output patterns are for a number of input patterns. We take an input from the training set and let the network generate an output pattern. We then compare the desired output pattern and the actual output pattern in some way. This process generates an *error signal*. The network is then modified using a learning rule so as to *reduce* the error signal.

The most commonly used error signal is based on the distance between the actual and desired output; however, other error signals can be more desirable. For example, one could incorporate a term penalizing large numbers of connections or large values of connection strength. The network learning problem reduces to a minimization problem where the space formed by the connection strengths (*weight space*) is searched to find the point where error is reduced to as low a value as possible. This process requires the use of control structures that can be complex; for example, there is assumed to be an omniscient *supervisor* who compares desired and actual network output and computes the error term as well as implements the mechanisms to change connection strengths appropriately. The structure of these algorithm is designed to produce good pattern association whether or not this is the aim of the network architects. (See PERCEPTRONS, ADALINES, AND BACKPROPAGATION.)

Autoassociative Models

We have described association as pattern linkage. However, there are alternative descriptions in the neural network literature. For example, in the first sentence of the second chapter of their textbook, *Introduction to the Theory of Neural Computation*, Hertz, Krogh, and Palmer (1991) write, "Associative memory is the 'fruit fly' or 'Bohr atom' problem of the field" (p. 11). Their definition of association is: "Store a set of patterns $\zeta \ldots$ in such a way that when presented with a new pattern ζ_i, the network responds by producing whichever one of the stored patterns most closely resembles ζ_i" (p. 11). This is not, however, a description of association but of a *content addressable memory* where input of partial or noisy information is used to retrieve the correct stored information. The source of this limited view of association lies in the ability of autoassociative systems to reconstruct missing or noisy parts of learned patterns.

Consider the autoassociative version of the linear associator. Suppose we learn one pattern, f, of length 1, with learning constant $\eta = 1$. Then

$$W = ff^T \quad \text{and} \quad Wf = f$$

Suppose we take vector f, with n elements, and set to zero some of the elements, forming a new vector, f'. Let us make a second vector, f'', from only the elements that were set to zero in f'. Then $f' + f'' = f$ and $f' f''^T = 0$. If f' is input to the autoassociator,

$$Wf' = (f' + f'')(f' + f'')f'^T = (\text{constant})f$$

where the constant is related to the length of f'. In operation, by putting a part of f, f', into the network, we retrieve all of f, bar a constant. This behavior is often referred to as the *reconstructive* or *holographic* property of neural networks. Of course, more subtle problems arise when W stores multiple vectors. Anyway, this type of memory is associative because if, for example, the state vector was meaningfully partitioned, then f' is associatively linked to f'' and vice versa in the sense that input of one pattern will produce the other. This kind of associator produces intrinsically bidirectional links (i.e., $f' \rightarrow f''$ and $f'' \rightarrow f'$), unlike feedforward heteroassociators ($f \rightarrow g$).

Some nonlinear "attractor" neural networks with dynamics that minimize energy functions develop their associative abilities largely from their autoassociative architecture. The best-known examples of this kind of associator are Hopfield networks and parallel feedback networks such as the BSB (Brain State in a Box) model (Anderson, 1995, chap. 15). For a general review of attractor networks, see Amit (1989) and COMPUTING WITH ATTRACTORS. Multilayer autoassociators are also possible. The multilayer *encoder networks*, which require the output pattern to be as accurate a reconstruction as possible of the input pattern, also have this form. Many autoassociative networks have close ties to known statistical techniques such as PRINCIPAL COMPONENT ANALYSIS.

A related associative attractor model, called a *bidirectional associative memory*, or BAM (Kosko, 1988), is a nonlinear dynamical system with a reciprocal feedback structure. It assumes two layers of units, as well as pairs of associations to be learned, as in a heteroassociator. There are connections from both input to output and output to input. Given f and g patterns to be learned, assumed to be binary vectors, we can form both a forward and a backward connection matrix. If f is input, then g will be given as the output; g at the output will give rise to f at the input because of the backward connections. Suppose the input is not exactly what was learned. After a few passes back and forth through the system, it can be shown that the network will stabilize, in the noise-free case, to the learned f and g.

Psychological Association

We have shown how neural networks easily form associators of many different kinds. We will now discuss a little of the history of association in psychology to show how associators form a style of computation with considerable power as well as severe limitations.

The major outlines of one way to use an associative computer can be found clearly expressed in Aristotle in the fourth century B.C. Aristotle made two important claims about memory structure: First, the elementary unit of memory is a *sense image*, that is, a sensory-based set of information. Second, links between these elementary memories serve as the basis for higher-level cognition. An English translation by Richard Sorabji (1969) used the term *memory* for the elementary memory unit and *recollection* for reasoning by associations between elementary units. Aristotle discussed at length how one "computes" with memorized sense images. The word *recollection* was used in the translation to denote this process: "Acts of recollection happen because one change is of a nature to occur after another." That is, Aristotle proposed a linkage mechanism between memories. He suggested several ways that linkage could occur: by temporal succession or by "something similar, or opposite, or neighboring." This list of the mechanisms for the formation of associations is approximately what would be given today by psychologists.

Recollection in Aristotle's sense was computation. It was a dynamic and flexible process: "[R]ecollecting is, as it were, a sort of reasoning." Aristotle argued that properly directed recollection is capable of discovering new truths, using memorized sense images as the raw material and learning to traverse new paths through memory (Figure 2).

A practical problem with such an associative net is branching, that is, what to do if there is more than one link leaving an elementary memory. Aristotle was aware of this problem: "[I]t is possible to move to more than one point from the same starting point." A general solution to the branching problem requires a nonlinear mechanism to select one or the other branch.

The most influential psychologists in the twentieth century were the behaviorists, in particular B. F. Skinner, the Harvard psychologist whose ideas about reinforcement learning unfortunately dominated much of the theoretical discussion in psychology for several decades. This school held that learning formed an associative link between a stimulus and a specific response. The link could be strengthened by positive reinforcement (to a first approximation, something useful or pleasant, or the cessation of something unpleasant) or weakened by negative reinforcement (either absence of something pleasant or something actively unpleasant) when the response followed the stimulus. A number of careful experiments showed that there were accurate quantitative "laws of learning" that were followed by animals in some simple situations.

It was debatable whether this view of association is useful in more complex situations. From the beginning, human behavior has seemed to humans to be far richer than stimulus-response ($S \rightarrow R$) association. In the 1950s Skinner wrote a book attempting to explain language behavior using associative rules. In a famous book review, Chomsky (1957) pointed out that simple $S \rightarrow R$ association cannot do some kinds of linguistic computation. The argument used

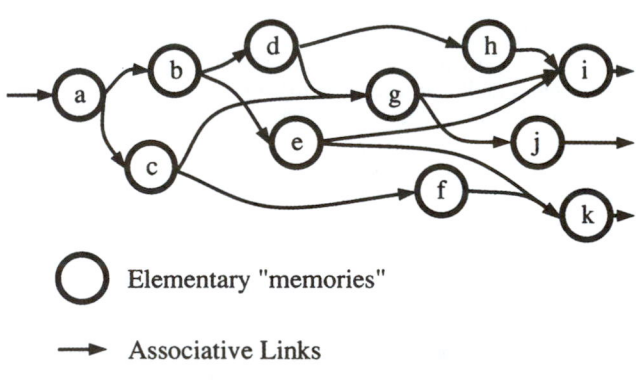

Possible Paths: abdhi, acgi, abei, ...

Figure 2. A simple model of associative computation. Elementary memories ("sense images," according to Aristotle) are associatively linked (arrows) to other sense images. Branches are possible, and they present some difficulties. There are many possible paths through the network. Forming and traversing links between elementary memories is the basis of mental computation.

was that Skinner was proposing a well-defined computing machine with his associative model and that this computing machine was not powerful enough to do the computations we know language users perform. The simple $S \rightarrow R$ models of Skinner had about as much computing power as the simplest heteroassociative neural networks, which no one claimed were general-purpose computers. However, supervised network learning algorithms applied without insight may produce systems with only this degree of overall computational power.

"Connectionist" Models

Much modern work using association assumes that the entities linked, and the links themselves, can have complex internal structure. Flexible systems capable of complex reasoning can be produced by using labeled links: for example, a robin IS-A bird, an IS-A link, or "Fred is the father of Herb," meaning that there is an associative link between Fred and Herb and that the link carries the relationship "Father-of." Complex and sophisticated computational models, *semantic neworks*, can be built from these pieces.

In the 1980s, many of those interested in semantic network models started working with neural networks. The term *connectionism* was often used to indicate the application of neural networks to high-level cognition. Recently there have been many attempts to apply networks to reasoning, to complex concept structures, and, in particular, to language understanding. A heated but illuminating debate arose from an early connectionist paper by Rumelhart and McClelland (1986) that used a neural network to simulate the way young children learn past tenses of verbs. Past tense learning had always been considered to be a good example of the application and misapplication of a specific rule, suggesting symbolic processing. Rumelhart and McClelland's neural network acted as if it were using rules, but the rule-like behavior was the result of generalizing from examples and learning specific cases (see PAST TENSE LEARNING). Perhaps because this model was such a direct attack on the existence of rules in language, a vigorous counterattack developed. As one example, a long paper by Pinker and Prince (1988) finished its abstract with the sentence, "We conclude that connectionists' claims about the dispensability of rules in explanations in the psychology of language must be rejected, and that, on the contrary, the linguistic and developmental facts provide good evidence for such rules" (p. 74). The vigor of the attack is perhaps due in part to the authors' feeling that the connectionists had violated the "central dogma of modern cognitive science, namely that intelligence is the result of processing symbolic expressions" (Pinker and Prince, p. 74). Many other cognitive scientists feel that the "central dogma" is actually more like a central, and open, question.

Less well known outside psychology are several associative neural network models that were constructed to explain the fine structure of experimental data in more traditional areas of psychology such as verbal learning. An interesting example of such a model is the TODAM model of Murdock (see CLASSICAL LEARNING THEORY AND NEURAL NETWORKS in the first edition). TODAM and variants blur the distinction between the network and the representation. In the associative networks we have discussed, there are two formally distinct entities, state vectors and connection matrices. In the TODAM class of models, the association is stored with the items themselves and is therefore the same type of entity. TODAM makes a number of testable qualitative predictions about a wide range of data from the classical verbal learning literature. Recently, models assuming networks composed of large numbers of local networks (a "network of networks") suggest that networks like TODAM might be realizable with neural networks.

Discussion and Open Questions

An often proclaimed virtue of neural networks is their ability to generalize effectively and to do computation based on similarity. Having learned example associations from a training set, the network can then generate correct answers to new examples. Many have pointed out the formal similarity of neural networks to approximation and interpolation as studied in numerical analysis. A properly designed neural network can act as a useful adaptive interpolator with good, even optimal, generalization around the region of the learned examples. However, it is not easy for neural networks to make good generalizations other than by approximation and interpolation. On this basis, Fodor and Pylyshyn (1988) made some telling arguments against the promiscuous application of connectionism to cognition (see SYSTEMATICITY OF GENERALIZATIONS IN CONNECTIONIST NETWORKS). The essential criticism they made is one that an engineer would be happy to make: Associative neural networks are such an inefficient way to compute that it would be foolish to build a cognitive system like that. Neural networks do not generalize well outside of a restricted definition based on mathematical interpolation, they cannot reason effectively, and they cannot extrapolate in any meaningful sense. These criticisms are part of a battle involving the limitations of association that has been going on for centuries. Fodor and Pylyshyn commented, "It's an instructive paradox that the current attempt to be thoroughly modern and 'take the brain seriously' should lead to a psychology not readily distinguishable from the worst of Hume and Berkeley" (p. 64).

Fodor and Pylyshyn contrasted neural network associators with what they call the classical view of mental operation. In essence, this view postulates "a language of thought"; that is, "mental representations have *a combinatorial syntax and semantics*" (p. 12). The classical view is dominant in virtually all branches of traditional artificial intelligence and linguistics. The power of the digital computer arises in part from the fact that it is designed to be an extreme example of this organization: a programming language operating on data is the prototype of the classical view.

Suppose we have a sentence of the form *A and B* that we hold is true. An example Fodor and Pylyshyn used is *John went to the store and Mary went to the store*. The truth of this sentence logically entails the truth of *Mary went to the store*. This conclusion arises from the rules of logic and of grammar. It is not easy for an associative neural network to handle this problem. Such a network could easily learn that *John went to the store and Mary went to the store* is associated with *Mary went to the store*. But the power of the classical approach arises from the fact that every sentence of this form gives rise to the same result. Given the huge number of possible sentences, *it makes practical sense* to assume that some kind of logical syntax exists. It would be hard to figure out how language could function without some global rule-like operations, however implemented.

The ability to understand and answer sentences or phrases that are new to the listener is hard to explain purely with association. To give one example (see MENTAL ARITHMETIC USING NEURAL NETWORKS in the first edition), consider number comparisons such as "Is 7 bigger than 5?" There are nearly 100 such single-digit comparisons, nearly 10,000 two-digit comparisons, and so on. Children cannot possibly learn them as individual cases.

If there is a qualitative difference between human and animal cognition, it lies right here. There have been attempts to build neural networks that realize parts of the classical account, with indifferent success (see Hinton, 1991). Is it possible to build a neural network based largely on natural associators that can reproduce the kind of rule-governed behavior—even in limited domains—that does in fact seem to be part of human cognition? A neural network with this ability would allow for much more powerful and useful generalization than current networks provide. It may not be easy to find this solution. There are many animals with complex nervous systems capable of associative learning, but only our own species, one out of millions of species, is really effective at using these powerful extensions to association.

[Reprinted from the First Edition]

Road Maps: Grounding Models of Networks; Learning in Artificial Networks
Background: I.3. Dynamics and Adaptation in Neural Networks
Related Reading: Artificial Intelligence and Neural Networks; Computing with Attractors

References

Amit, D. J., 1989, *Modelling Brain Function: The World of Attractor Neural Networks*, Cambridge, Engl.: Cambridge University Press.

Anderson, J. A., 1995, *Introduction to Neural Networks*, Cambridge, MA: MIT Press. ◆

Anderson, J. R., 1983, *The Architecture of Cognition*, Cambridge, MA: Harvard University Press.

Chomsky, N., 1957, A review of Skinner's *Verbal Behavior, Language*, 35:26–58.

Fodor, J. A., and Pylyshyn, Z. W., 1988, Connectionism and cognitive architecture: A critical analysis, in *Connections and Symbols* (S. Pinker and J. Mehler, Eds.), Cambridge, MA: MIT Press.

Hebb, D. O., 1949, *The Organization of Behavior*, New York: Wiley.

Hertz, J., Krogh, A., and Palmer, R. G., 1991, *Introduction to the Theory of Neural Computation*, Redwood City, CA: Addison-Wesley. ◆

Hinton, G. E., 1991, *Connectionist Symbol Processing*, Cambridge, MA: MIT Press. ◆

Kohonen, T., 1977, *Associative Memory: A System Theoretic Approach*, Berlin: Springer-Verlag. ◆

Kohonen, T., 1984, *Self-Organization and Associative Memory*, Berlin: Springer-Verlag. ◆

Kosko, B., 1988, Bidirectional associative memories, *IEEE Trans. Sys., Man Cybern.*, 18:49–60.

Pinker, S., and Prince, A., 1988, On language and connectionism: Analysis of a parallel distributed processing model of language acquisition, in *Connections and Symbols* (S. Pinker and J. Mehler, Eds.), Cambridge, MA: MIT Press.

Rumelhart, D. E., and McClelland, J. L., 1986, On learning the past tenses of English verbs, in *Parallel Distributed Processing: Explorations in the Microstructure of Cognition* (D. E. Rumelhart, J. L. McClelland, and PDP Research Group, Eds.), vol. 2, *Psychological and Biological Models*, Cambridge, MA: MIT Press.

Sorabji, R., 1969, *Aristotle on Memory*, Providence, RI: Brown University Press.

Willshaw, D. J., Buneman, O. P., and Longuet-Higgins, H. C., 1969, Nonholographic associative memory, *Nature*, 222:960–962.

Auditory Cortex

Shihab A. Shamma

Introduction

The auditory cortex plays a critical role in the perception and localization of complex sounds. It is the last station in a long chain of processing centers that begins with the cochlea of the inner ear and passes through the cochlear nuclei (CN), the superior olivary complex (SOC), the lateral lemniscus, the inferior colliculus (IC), and the medial geniculate body (MGB) (Figure 1). Recent studies have expanded our knowledge of the neuroanatomical structure, the subdivisions, and the connectivities of all central auditory stages (Winer, 1992). However, apart from the midbrain cochlear and binaural SOC nuclei, relatively little is known about the functional organization of the central auditory system, especially compared to the visual and motor systems. Consequently, modeling cortical auditory networks is complicated by uncertainty about exactly what the cortical machinery is trying to accomplish.

One exception to this state of affairs is the highly specialized echolocating bat, in which these uncertainties are much relieved by the existence of a stereotypical behavioral repertoire that is closely linked to the animal's acoustic environment (see ECHOLOCATION: COCHLEOTOPIC AND COMPUTATIONAL MAPS). This has made it possible to construct a functional map of the auditory cortex, which

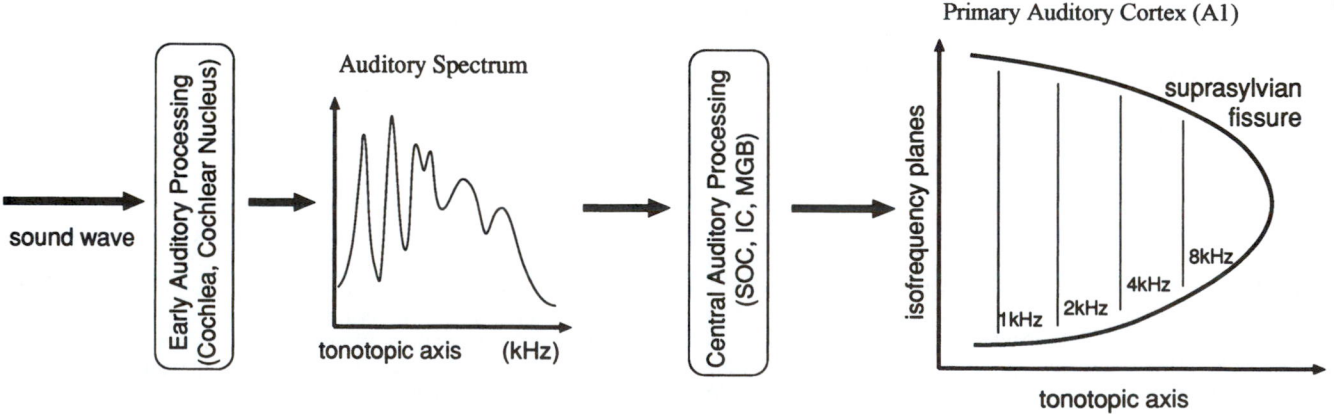

Figure 1. Schematic representation of the multiple stages of processing in the mammalian auditory pathway. Sound is analyzed in the cochlea, and an estimate of the acoustic spectrum (an auditory spectrum) is known to be extracted at the cochlear nucleus (Blackburn and Sachs, 1990). The tonotopic organization of the cochlea is preserved all the way up to the cortex, where it has a two-dimensional layout. The isofrequency plane encodes perhaps other features of the stimulus.

revealed the specific acoustic features extracted and represented in the cortex. In turn, these cortical maps have acted as a guide to discovering the organization and nature of the transformations occurring in lower auditory centers such as the MGB, IC, and SOC. Thus, it has become meaningful in these species to investigate and model cortical and other central auditory neural networks.

In other mammals, it is more difficult to isolate an auditory behavior and its associated stimulus features with comparable specificity. Nevertheless, a few tasks have been broadly accepted as vital for all species, such as sound localization, timbre recognition, and pitch perception. For each, evidence of various functional and stimulus feature maps has been found or postulated, a significant number of them in the last few years. In this review, we elaborate on a few examples of such maps and relate them to the more intuitive and better understood case of the echolocating bats. In each example, our goal is to determine how and whether models of the underlying neural networks can further our understanding of the auditory cortex.

Parcellization and Neuroanatomy of the Auditory Cortex

The layout and neural structure of the auditory cortex is in many respects similar to that of other sensory cortices (Winer, 1992). For instance, based on cytoarchitectonic criteria and patterns of connectivity, it is subdivided into a primary auditory field (AI) and several other surrounding fields, e.g., the anterior auditory field (A) and the secondary auditory cortex (AII). The number and specific arrangement of surrounding fields vary among different species, reflecting presumably the complexity of the animal's acoustic environment. The AI, and possibly other fields, is further subdivided into smaller regions, serving perhaps different functional roles, such as echo delay and amplitude measurements in the bat (see ECHOLOCATION: COCHLEOTOPIC AND COMPUTATIONAL MAPS).

The anatomical parcellization of the auditory cortex into different fields is mirrored by physiologically based divisions. Most important is the systematic frequency organization in different fields, or so-called tonotopic maps. For example, AI cells are spatially ordered based on the tone frequency to which they best respond, i.e., their best frequency (BF). They also respond vigorously to the onset of a tone and exhibit little evidence of adaptation to its repeated presentations. In other fields, cells may be less frequency selective, may respond more adaptively, or may be totally unresponsive to single tones, preferring more spectrally or temporally complex stimuli. A sudden change in these response patterns or in the gradual spatial order of the tonotopic map is usually taken to signify a border between different fields. In the cat, which has the most extensively mapped auditory cortex, four well-ordered tonotopic fields have been described, together with many other less precise secondary areas (Clarey, Barone, and Imig, 1992).

Timbre: Models for the Encoding of Spectral Profiles

Recognizing and classifying environmental sounds is critical for the survival and propagation of many animals. Although a multitude of cues are responsible, the single most important one is the shape of the so-called spectral envelope (or the spectral profile) of the sound. It is largely this cue that allows us to distinguish between speech vowels or between different instruments playing the same note. The spectral profile emerges early in the auditory system as the sound is analyzed into different frequency bands, in effect distributing its energy across the tonotopic axis (the auditory sensory epithelium) (Figure 1). As far as the central auditory system is concerned, the spectral profile is a one-dimensional (1D) pattern of activation analogous to the two-dimensional (2D) distribution of light intensity on the retina.

An important organizational feature of the central auditory system is the expansion of the 1D tonotopic axis of the cochlea into a 2D sheet, with each frequency represented by an entire sheet of cells (Figure 1). An immediate question thus arises as to the functional purpose of this expansion and the nature of the acoustic features that might be mapped along these isofrequency planes. For example, one might conjecture that the amplitude or the local shape of the spectrum is explicitly represented along this new dimension.

In general, there are two ways in which the spectral profile can be encoded in the central auditory system. The first is *absolute*, that is, the spectral profile is encoded in terms of the absolute intensity of sound at each frequency. Such an encoding would in effect combine both the shape information and the overall level. The second way is *relative*, in which the spectral profile shape is encoded separately from the overall loudness of the stimulus. Examples of each of these two hypotheses are discussed next.

The Best-Intensity Model

The first hypothesis is motivated primarily by the strongly nonmonotonic responses as a function of stimulus intensity observed in many cortical and other central auditory cells (Clarey et al., 1992). In a sense, one can view such a cell's response as being selective to (or encoding) a particular intensity. Consequently, a population of such cells, tuned to different frequencies and intensities, can provide an explicit representation of the spectral profile by their spatial pattern of activity (Figure 2). This scheme is not a true transformation of the spectral features represented, but rather is strictly a change in the means of the representation. The most compelling example of such a representation is that in the DSCF area of AI in the mustache bat. However, an extension of this hypothesis to multicomponent stimuli (as depicted in Figure 2) has not been demonstrated in any species.

The Multiresolution Analysis Model

The second hypothesis, in which the relative shape of the spectrum is encoded, is supported by physiological experiments in cat and

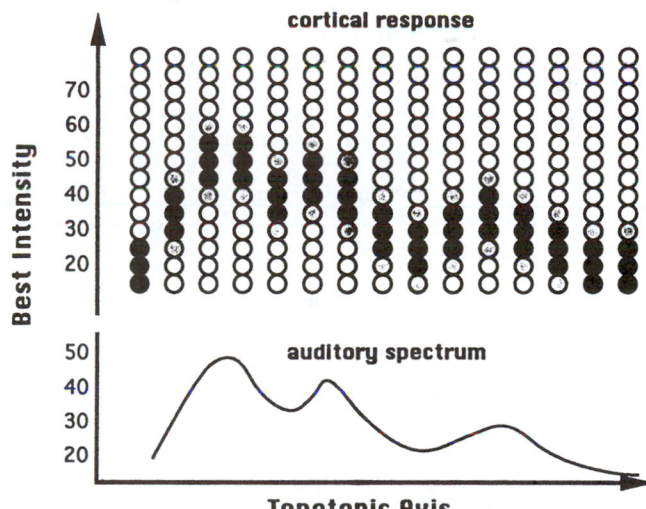

Figure 2. Schematic diagram of the way in which the spectral profile (lower plot) can be encoded by arrays of nonmonotonic cells (circles) tuned to different BFs (along the tonotopic axis) and best intensifies (BIs). The black circles signify strongly activated cells, whereas the white circles indicate weakly activated cells. Thus, a peak in the input pattern located at a given BF and at an intensity of 40 dB would best activate cells with the same BF and BI

ferret AI, coupled with psychoacoustical studies in human subjects. The data reveal a substantial transformation of the way the spectral profile is represented centrally. Specifically, besides the tontopic axis, two features of the response areas of AI neurons (the analogue of the receptive fields in the visual system) are found to be topographically mapped across the isofrequency planes. They are the bandwidth and symmetry of the response areas, depicted schematically in Figure 3A as the *scale* and *symmetry* axes, respectively. In addition, auditory cortical units exhibit systematic response patterns to dynamic spectra that give rise to complex and varied spectrotemporal response areas, as depicted in Figure 3B. These response properties are discussed in greater detail below.

Changes in response area bandwidths. Cell response areas, i.e., the excitatory and inhibitory responses they exhibit to a tone of various frequencies and intensities, change their bandwidth in orderly fashion along the isofrequency planes (Mendelson and Schreiner, 1990). Near the center of AI, cells are narrowly tuned. Toward the edges, they become more broadly tuned. This orderly progression occurs at least twice, and it correlates with several other response parameters such as increasing response thresholds toward the edges.

An intuitively appealing implication of this finding is that response areas of different bandwidths are selective to spectral profiles of different widths. Thus, broad spectral profiles (e.g., broad peaks or gross trends, such as spectral tilts due to preemphasis) would best drive cells with wide response areas. Similarly, narrower spectral profiles (e.g., sharp peaks or edges, or fine details of the spectral profile) would best be represented in the responses of cells with more compact response areas. In effect, having a range of response areas at different widths allows us to encode the spectral profile at different scales or levels of detail (resolution). From a mathematical perspective, this is basically equivalent to analyzing the spectral profile into different scales or "bands," much like performing a Fourier transform of the profile, hence representing it as a weighted sum of elementary sinusoidal spectra (usually known as *ripples*; Shamma, Versnel, and Kowalski, 1995). Coarser scales then correspond to the "low-frequency" ripples, while finer scales correspond to the "high-frequency" ripples.

Changes in response area asymmetry. Response areas exhibit systematic changes in the symmetry of their inhibitory response areas. For instance, cells in the center of AI have sharply tuned excitatory responses around a BF, flanked by symmetric inhibitory response areas. Toward the edges, the inhibitory response areas become significantly more asymmetric, with inhibition dominated by either higher or lower than BF frequencies. This trend is repeated at least twice across the length of the isofrequency plane.

It is intuitively clear that response areas with different symmetries would respond best to input profiles that match their symmetry. For instance, an odd-symmetric response area would respond best if the input profile had the same local odd-symmetry and worst if it had the opposite odd-symmetry. As such, one can state that a range of response areas of different symmetries (symmetry axis in Figure 3A) is capable of encoding the shape of a local region in the profile. From an opposite perspective, it can be shown mathematically that the local symmetry of a pattern can be changed by manipulating only the phase of its Fourier transform (Wang and Shamma, 1995). Therefore, the axis of response area asymmetries in effect is able to encode the phase of the profile transform, thus providing a complementary description to that of the magnitude along the scale axis described above.

Dynamics of cortical responses to spectral profile changes. Auditory cortical units also exhibit systematic and selective responses to dynamic spectra. Specifically, when stimulated by com-

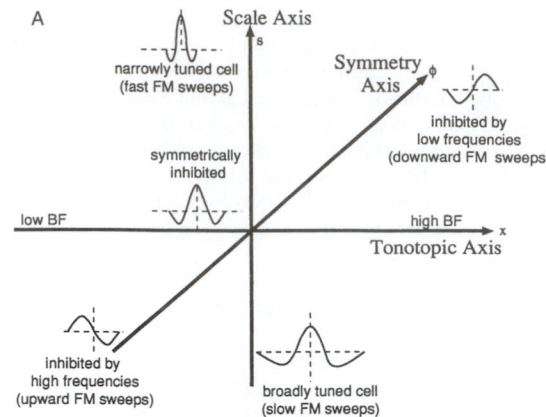

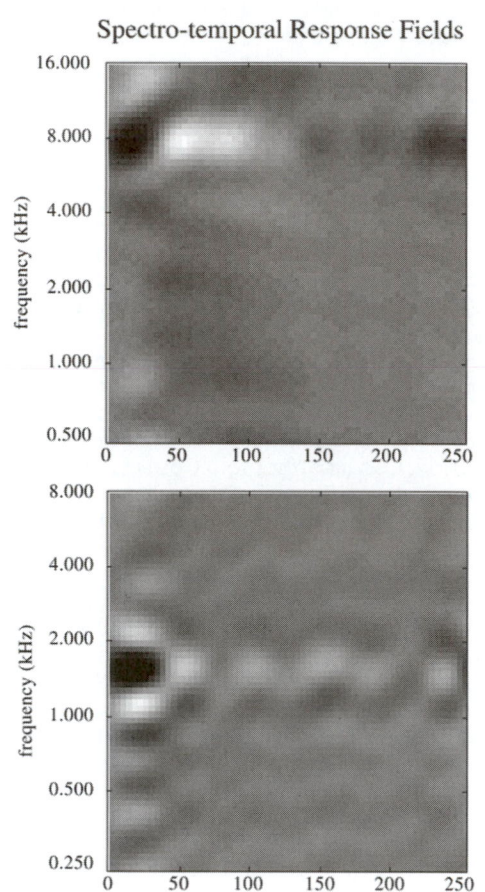

Figure 3. *A*, Schematic diagram of the three representational axes thought to exist in AI: the tonotopic (BF) axis, the scale (or bandwidth) axis, and the symmetry axis. *B*, Examples of spectrotemporal response fields measured from two auditory cortical units of the ferret. In each panel, the strength of the response is represented by the darkness of the display, with black indicating excitatory areas and white indicating regions of suppressed activity. Note that the excitatory central region defines the BF of the unit. Such STRFs exhibit a variety of bandwidths, asymmetry of inhibition relative to the BF, directional selectivity, and temporal dynamics. For instance, the unit in the top panel has significantly slower dynamics and much more asymmetric inhibition about the BF than the unit in the bottom panel. (From Simon, J. Z., Depireux, D. A., and Shamma, S. A., 1998, Representation of complex spectra in auditory cortex, in *Psychophysical and Physiological Advances in Hearing: Proceedings of the 11th International Symposium on Hearing* (A. R. Palmer, A. Ress, A. Q. Summerfield, and R. Meddis Eds.), London: Whurr, 1998, pp. 513–520. Reprinted with permission.)

plex sounds with rippled spectra like those described above, cortical units display preference not only to ripple density and phase, but also to the velocity at which the ripple is drifted past the BF of the cell. Unit selectivities span a wide range of best ripple velocities, from about 20 cycles/s (Hz), down to as low as 1–2 Hz (Kowalski, Depireux, and Shamma, 1996). In addition, auditory cortical units usually exhibit a range of directional sensitivities to upward- and downward-moving ripples.

This directional selectivity is probably directly linked to responses to frequency-modulated (FM) tones, a subject that has been the focus of extensive neural network modeling. These stimuli are important because they mimic the dynamic aspects of many natural vocalizations, as in speech consonant-vowel combinations or the trills of many birds and other animal sounds. The effects of manipulating two specific parameters of the FM sweep, its direction and rate, have been well studied. In several species and at almost all central auditory stages, cells can be found that are selectively sensitive to the FM direction and rate. Most studies have confirmed a qualitative theory in which directional selectivity arises from an asymmetric pattern of inhibition in the response area of the cell

(Wang and Shamma, 1995), whereas rate sensitivity is correlated to the bandwidth of the response area (Heil, Langner, and Scheich, 1992).

The full spectrotemporal response fields. All of above mentioned response area features are integrated into a unified spectrotemporal response area (or field) as illustrated in Figure 3B (deCharms, Blake, and Merzenich, 1998). The full spectrotemporal response field (STRF) summarizes all the response selectivities of a unit by the relative locations, widths, duration, and orientation of its excitatory and inhibitory fields. The overall picture that emerges from these findings is that AI decomposes the auditory spectrum into a multidimensional representation with multiple resolutions along both spectral and temporal dimensions, as illustrated in Figure 4. This spectrotemporal decomposition essentially segregates diverse perceptual features into different streams, e.g., fast, spectrally broad sounds (consonants) from the relatively slow, voiced vowels and the finely resolved harmonics (pitch cues) (Wang and Shamma, 1995). This kind of multiscale analysis is closely analogous to the well-studied organization of receptive fields in the primary visual

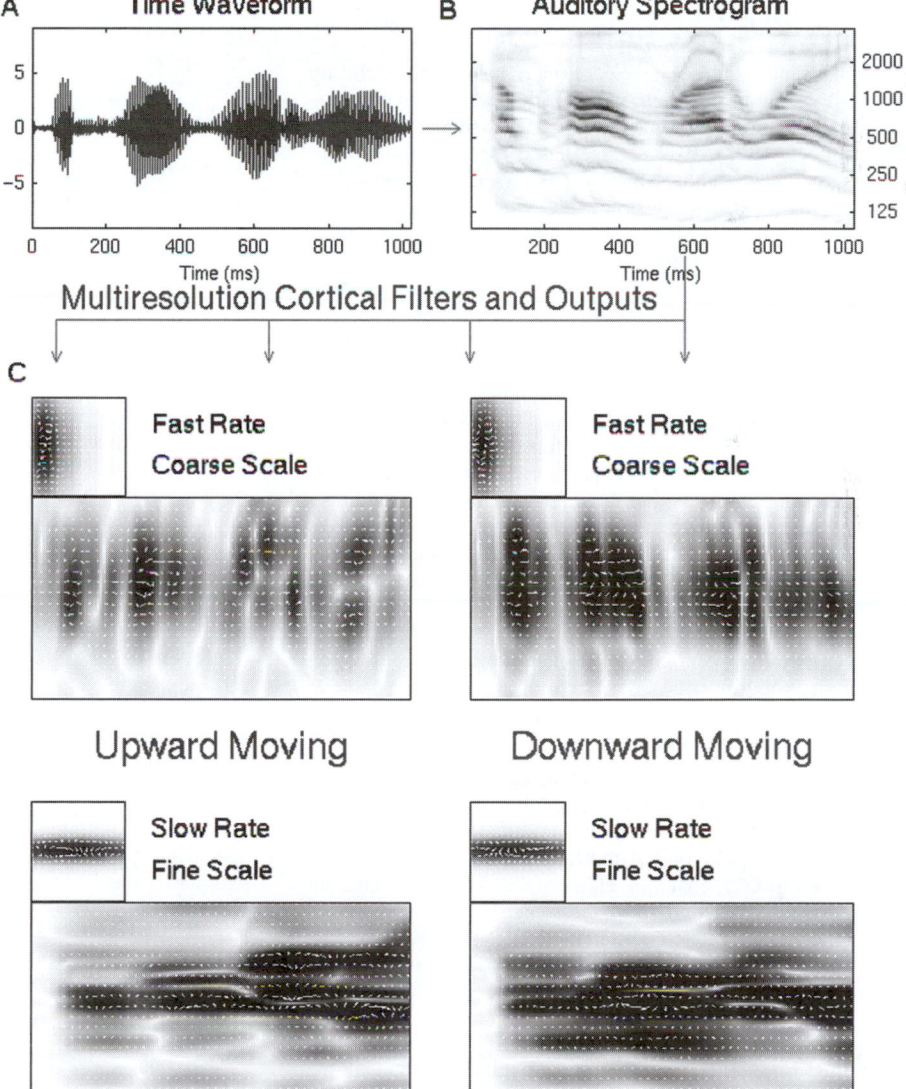

Figure 4. Schematic of the cortical representation of complex dynamic sound spectra. *A,* The time waveform of the acoustic signal /Come home right away/. *B,* The time-frequency representation of the signal (or the auditory spectogram) generated in the early stages of the auditory system. The y-axis represents the logarithmic frequency axis of the cochlea (or the tonotopic axis, as depicted in Figure 1). *C,* Cortical multiscale analysis of the auditory spectrogram along the spectral and temporal dimensions. Each panel represents the activity of a population of cortical cells with the (idealized model) STRF shown in the inset above it. Arrow direction represent the phase of the response; the strength of the response is indicated by the darkness of the display, as in Figure 3B. The two top panels are for broadly tuned but relatively fast STRFs that are selective to motion in opposite directions. The bottom panels are for narrowly tuned and relatively slow units. Different features of the spectrogram are emphasized in different panels. For instance, harmonics (pitch cues) are seen in the lower (fine-scale) panels, whereas onsets due to different consonants are seen only in the upper (fast-rate) panels.

cortex (De-Valois and De-Volois, 1990), and may reflect a general principle of analysis of sensory patterns in all other sensoricortical areas.

Models of Pitch Representation in the Central Auditory System

A sound complex consisting of several harmonics is heard with a strong pitch at the fundamental frequency of the harmonic series, even if there is no energy at all at that frequency. This percept has been variously called the missing fundamental, virtual pitch, or residue pitch. A large number of psychoacoustical experiments have been carried out to elucidate the nature of this percept and its relationship to the physical parameters of the stimulus. Basically, all models fall into one of two camps. In the first camp, the pitch is extracted explicitly from the harmonic spectral pattern. This can be accomplished in a variety of ways, such as by finding the best match between the input pattern and various harmonic templates assumed to be stored in the brain (Goldstein, 1973). In the second camp, the pitch is extracted from the periodicities in the time-waveform of responses in the auditory pathway, which can be estimated, for example, by computing their autocorrelation functions. In this kind of model, some form of organized delay lines are assumed to exist so that the computations can be done, much like those that seem to exist in the FM-FM area of the mustached bat.

In all pitch models, however, the extracted pitch is assumed to be finally represented as a *spatial* map in higher auditory centers. This is because many studies have confirmed that neural synchrony to the repetitive features of a stimulus, be it the waveform of a tone or its AM modulations, becomes progressively worse toward the cortex (Langner, 1992). It is a remarkable aspect of pitch that, despite its fundamental and ubiquitous role in auditory perception, only a few reports exist of physiological evidence of spatial pitch maps, and none has been independently confirmed. One source is NMR scans of the primary auditory cortex in human subjects. The other source of evidence is multiunit mappings in various central auditory structures (Schreiner and Langner, 1988).

Of course, the difficulty of finding spatial pitch maps in the auditory cortex may be due to the fact that it does not exist. This possibility is counterintuitive, given the results of ablation studies showing that bilateral cortical lesions in the auditory cortex severely impair the perception of pitch of complex sounds but do not affect the fine discrimination of frequency and intensity of simple tones. Another possibility is that the maps sought are not at all as straightforward as we imagine. For example, harmonic complexes may evoke stereotypical patterns that are distributed over large areas in the auditory cortex, and not localized, as the simple notion of a pitch map implies (Wang and Shamma, 1995). Finally, it is also possible that AI simply functions as one stage that projects sufficient temporal or spectral cues for later cortical stages to extract the pitch explicitly.

Models of Sound Localization

It has been recognized for many years that the auditory cortex (and especially the AI) is involved in sound localization. Detailed physiological studies further confirmed that AI cells are rather sensitive to all kinds of manipulations of the binaural stimulus (Clarey et al., 1992). For instance, changing either of the two most important binaural cues, the interaural level difference (ILD) or interaural time difference (ITD), causes substantial changes in their firing rate patterns. This sensitivity to interaural cues has its origins early in the auditory pathway, at the SOC, where the first convergence of binaural inputs occurs. However, despite this diversity, two elements typical of a functional organization of AI have been lacking. The first missing element is a significant transformation of the single-unit responses. For example, if ILD-sensitive cells are to

encode the location of a sound source based on this cue, they ought to become uniformly more stable with overall sound intensity. This, however, does not seem to be the case (Semple and Kitzes, 1993). The second element lacking is a topographical distribution of the responses with respect to these cues or to a more complex combination of features (e.g., a map of acoustic space derived from ILD and ITD cues, as in the barn owl) (Sullivan and Konishi, 1986).

A map of auditory space has indeed been found in the superior colliculus of several mammals. No such map, however, has yet been detected in AI or other cortical fields despite intensive efforts (Clarey et al., 1992). What has been found, however, is a topographic order of certain binaural responses along the isofrequency planes of AI. Specifically, cells excited equally well by sounds from both ears (called EE cells) and others inhibited by ipsilateral sounds (called EI cells) are found clustered in alternating bands that parallel the tonotopic axis. One possible functional model that utilizes such maps assumes that EI cells are tuned to particular ILDs, and hence encode the location of a sound source based on this cue. EE cells, in contrast, would encode the absolute level of the sound. However, there is little evidence to support this hypothesis in the sense that neither EE nor EI cells are particularly stable encoders of specific ILD or absolute sound levels. An alternative hypothesis recently proposed is that these cells encode the absolute levels of the stimulus at each ear, rather than the difference and average binaural levels, as previously postulated (Semple and Kitzes, 1993). Finally, it has also been proposed that AI units encode the spatial location of a stimulus through unique patterns of temporal firing, ones that can be discerned using more elaborate pattern recognition neural networks (Middlebrooks et al., 1994).

Discussion

The study of central auditory function has reached a sufficiently advanced stage to allow meaningful quantitative and neuronal network models to be formulated. In most mammals, these models are still systemic in nature, with a primary focus on understanding the overall functional organization of the cortex and other central auditory structures. In the bat and other specialized animals, the models are somewhat more detailed, addressing specific neuronal mechanisms, such as the coincidences and the delay lines of the FM-FM areas. The auditory system, with its multitude of diverse functions and its combination of temporal and spatial processes, should thus prove to be a valuable window into the brain and an effective vehicle for understanding the brain's underlying mechanisms.

Road Maps: Mammalian Brain Regions; Other Sensory Systems
Related Reading: Auditory Periphery and Cochlear Nucleus; Auditory Scene Analysis; Echolocation: Cochleotopic and Computational Maps; Sound Localization and Binaural Processing

References

Blackburn, C. C., and Sachs, M. B., 1990, The representations of the steady-state vowel sound phoneme e in the discharge patterns of cat antero-ventral cochlear nucleus neurons, *J. Neurophysiol.*, 63(5):1191–1212.

Clarey, J., Barone, P., and Imig, T., 1992, Physiology of thalamus and cortex, in *The Mammalian Auditory Pathway: Neurophysiology* (R. Fay, D. Webster, and A. Popper, Eds.), New York: Springer-Verlag, pp. 232–334.

deCharms, R. C., Blake, D. T., and Merzenich, M. M., 1998, Optimizing sound features for cortical neurons, *Science*, 280:1439. ◆

De-Valois, R., and De-Valois, K., 1990, *Spatial Vision*, New York: Oxford University Press.

Goldstein, J., 1973, An optimum processor theory for the central formation of pitch of complex tones, *J. Acoust. Soc. Am.*, 54:1496–1516.

Heil, P., Langner, G., and Scheich, H., 1992, Processing of FM stimuli in the chick auditory cortex analogue: Evidence of topographic representations and possible mechanisms of rate and directional sensitivity, *J. Comp. Physiol. A*, 171:583–600.

Kowalski, N., Depireux, D., and Shamma, S., 1996, Analysis of dynamic spectra in ferret primary auditory cortex: Characteristics of single unit responses to moving ripple spectra, *J. Neurophysiol.*, 76:3503–3523.

Langner, G., 1992, Periodicity coding in the auditory system, *Hearing Res.*, 6:115–142.

Mendelson, J., and Schreiner, C., 1990, Functional topography of cat primary auditory cortex: Distribution of integrated excitation, *J. Neurophysiol.*, 64:1442–1459.

Middlebrooks, J. C., Clock, A. E., Xu, L., and Green, D. M., 1994, A panoramic code for sound location by cortical neurons, *Science*, 264:842–844.

Schreiner, C., and Langner, G., 1988, Periodicity coding in the inferior colliculus of the cat: 2. Topographical organization, *J. Neurophysiol.*, 60:1823–1840.

Semple, M., and Kitzes, L., 1993, Binaural processing of sound pressure level in cat primary auditory cortex: Evidence for a representation based

on absolute levels rather than level differences, *J. Neurophysiol.*, 69:449–461.

Shamma, S., Versnel, H., and Kowalski, N., 1995, Ripple analysis in the ferret primary auditory cortex: 1. Response characteristics of single units to sinusoidally rippled spectra, *J. Aud. Neurosci.*, 1:233–254.

Sullivan, W., and Konishi, M., 1986, Neural map of interaural phase difference in the owl's brainstem, *Proc Natl Acad. Sci. USA*, 83:8400–8404.

Winer, J., 1992, The functional architecture of the medial geniculate body and primary auditory cortex, in *The Mammalian Auditory Pathway: Neuroanatomy* (D. Webster, A. Popper, and R. Fay, Eds.), New York: Springer-Verlag, pp. 232–334.

Wang, K., and Shamma, S., 1995, Representation of spectral profiles in primary auditory cortex, *IEEE Trans. Speech Audio Process.*, 3:382–395.

Auditory Periphery and Cochlear Nucleus

David C. Mountain

Introduction

The auditory periphery transforms a very high information rate acoustic signal into a group of lower information rate neural signals. This process of parallelization is essential because the potential information rate in the acoustic stimulus is on the order of 0.5 megabits per second, and yet typical auditory nerve (AN) fibers have maximum sustained firing rates of 200 per second. The cochlear nucleus (CN) continues the process of parallelization by creating multiple representations of the original acoustic stimulus, with each representation emphasizing different acoustic features.

The major ascending auditory pathways are summarized in Figure 1. Sound is collected by the external ear (pinna) and passes through the ear canal to the eardrum (tympanic membrane), where it excites the middle ear. The middle ear couples the acoustic energy to the fluids of the cochlea, where transduction takes place. The sensory cells of the cochlea (hair cells) convert the mechanical signal to an electrical signal, which is then encoded by the fibers of the auditory nerve and transmitted to the CN in the brainstem. Within the CN, parallel information streams are created that feed other brainstem structures such as the superior olivary complex (SOC), the nuclei of the lateral lemniscus (NLL), and the inferior colliculus (IC). These parallel pathways are believed to be specialized for the processing of different auditory features that are used for sound source classification and localization. From the IC, auditory information is passed on to the medial geniculate body (MGB) in the thalamus, and from there to the auditory cortex.

External Ear

The head and pinna modify the magnitude and phase of the acoustic signal reaching the tympanic membrane in such a way as to provide important cues for sound source localization (Shaw in Gilkey and Anderson, 1997). The transfer function relating tympanic membrane pressure to pressure in the free field is called the head-related transfer function (HRTF) and changes with sound source elevation and azimuth.

Three major mechanisms contribute to the creation of the HRTF. The distance between the ears in most mammals is sufficient to create significant interaural time delays (ITDs) for sound sources off to the side of the head, and the head is large enough to create interaural level differences (ILDs) for frequencies where the wavelength is comparable or smaller than the head. For higher frequencies (above 5 kHz in humans), multiple resonant modes in the pinna add further complexity. These modes are preferentially excited by

sound waves from some directions but not others, resulting in an HRTF with peaks and valleys that change with sound source direction.

Middle Ear and Cochlear Mechanics

The middle ear consists of the tympanic membrane, the three middle-ear bones (ossicles), and the Eustachian tube. The primary function of the middle ear is to match the low acoustic impedance of air to the high acoustic input impedance of the cochlea. The middle-ear transfer function (ratio of intracochlear pressure to ear canal pressure) is high-pass in nature (Rosowski in Hawkins et al.,

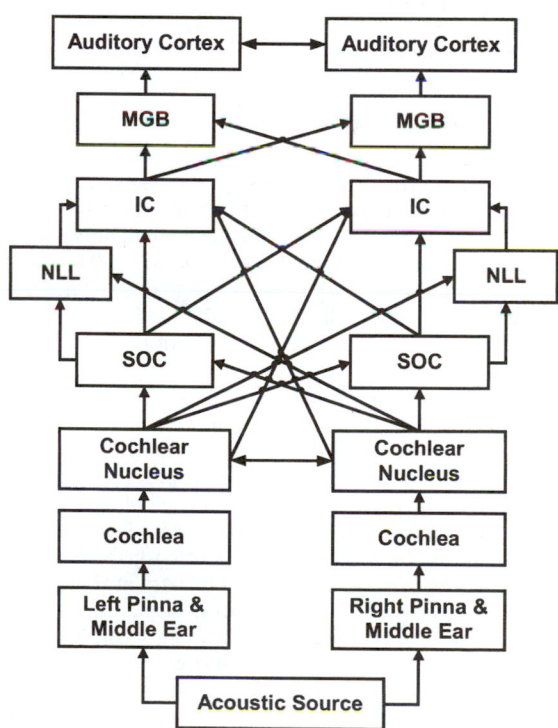

Figure 1. The major ascending auditory pathways. See text for explanation of abbreviations.

1996) and plays a major role in determining the audiogram for a given species.

The cochlea consists of a spiral-shaped, fluid-filled tube embedded in the temporal bone (Slepecky in Dallos, Popper, and Fay, 1996). It is separated into three longitudinal compartments by two membranes: the basilar membrane (BM) and Reissner's membrane. From a hydromechanical and physiological point of view, the BM is the more important of the two. It supports the organ of Corti, which contains the sensory hair cells. Pressure changes in the cochlear fluids produced by the middle ear excite a mechanical traveling wave that propagates along the BM. The traveling wave magnitude peaks at a location that depends on stimulus frequency: high frequencies peak near the base and low frequencies peak near the apex.

Direct measurements of BM motion demonstrate that, at low sound levels, the response can be highly tuned, with each cochlear location only responding to a narrow range of frequencies (Hubbard and Mountain in Hawkins et al., 1996). BM tuning decreases at high sound levels and appears to involve the presence of a group of sensory cells, the outer hair cells (OHCs). All hair cells respond to mechanical stimuli with voltage changes, but in the case of the OHCs, voltage changes result in cell length changes (Holley in Dallos et al., 1996). These voltage-dependent length changes appear to be mediated by voltage-sensitive transmembrane proteins. This novel form of electromotility is piezoelectric in nature, allowing the length changes to achieve very high velocities.

Many hydromechanical models have been proposed to explain these findings (Hubbard and Mountain in Hawkins et al., 1996; de Boer in Dallos et al., 1996), but these hydromechanical models are computationally intense. As a result, it is common practice to represent cochlear mechanics with a bank of digital bandpass filters that capture the salient features of the mechanical frequency response (Hubbard and Mountain in Hawkins et al., 1996). Filters of this type reproduce the magnitude of the cochlear frequency response reasonably well, but they cannot reproduce the changes in cochlear tuning that occur with changes in stimulus level. In order to replicate the nonlinear features of cochlear mechanics in filterbank models, some authors have used filters with parameters that change with stimulus level (cf. Zhang et al., 2001).

Inner Hair Cells

The inner hair cells (IHCs) are the receptor cells that provide most of the input to the auditory nerve. Although much progress has been made in measuring basilar membrane motion, little direct data exist to explain how this motion gets coupled to the IHC hair bundle. Comparisons of IHC receptor potentials to inferred BM motion have led to the hypothesis that hair-bundle motion is a high-pass filtered version (cutoff frequency ~400 Hz) of BM motion. Alternatively, Mountain and Cody (1999) have proposed a model in which the OHCs, through their electromotility, displace the IHC hair bundles more directly, perhaps via movements of the tectorial membrane, rather than via enhanced BM motion.

The mechanical-to-electrical transduction process in hair cells is extremely sensitive, resulting in receptor potentials on the order of 1 mV for hair-bundle displacements of 1 nm. This transduction process is believed to be the result of tension-gated channels located in the hair bundle (Mountain and Hubbard in Hawkins et al., 1996). The relationship between stereocilia displacement x and the mechanically induced conductance change $G(x)$ is most commonly modeled using a first-order Boltzmann model (Mountain and Hubbard in Hawkins et al., 1996).

Although IHCs also contain voltage-dependent conductances (Kros in Dallos et al., 1996), most models include only the mechanically sensitive conductance coupled to a linear leakage resistance and a linear membrane capacitance. The RC nature of the membrane acts as a low-pass filter with a cutoff frequency of around 1 kHz. The effect of this filter is to produce an IHC response that follows the fine structure of the stimulus waveform at low frequencies, while at high frequencies it follows the signal envelope (Mountain and Hubbard in Hawkins et al., 1996).

If a linear filter bank is used to represent cochlear mechanics, then it is often desirable to use a rectification function that includes considerable compression to accommodate the large dynamic range of many acoustic signals. Since the D.C. receptor potentials of IHCs measured using best-frequency tones appear to grow as a logarithmic function of sound pressure, a combination of a half-wave rectifier followed by a logarithmic compressor provides a reasonable model (Mountain and Hubbard in Hawkins et al., 1996).

Auditory Nerve

AN fibers, the cell bodies of which are located in the SG, are divided into two classes, depending on their morphology. Each IHC synapses with 10 to 30 type I AN (AN-I) fibers (Ryugo in Webster, Popper, and Fay, 1992). In most mammals, AN-I fibers synapse only with a single IHC. In contrast, type II fibers (AN-II), which innervate the OHCs, synapse with multiple hair cells. AN-I fibers exhibit spontaneous activity in the absence of sound, and they are often segregated into low (LSR), medium (MSR), and high (HSR) spontaneous rate categories. The pattern of this spontaneous activity is random and is usually modeled as a Poisson or dead-time modified Poisson process. Spontaneous rate tends to correlate with threshold, with HSR fibers being the most sensitive to sound stimuli.

The average firing rate of AN fibers in response to sustained tones is tuned, mimicking the responses at the BM. The peristimulus time histogram (PSTH) exhibits an initial rapid increase, followed by adaptation (Figure 2) to a lower steady-state rate (Ruggero in Popper and Fay, 1992). The steady-state response has only

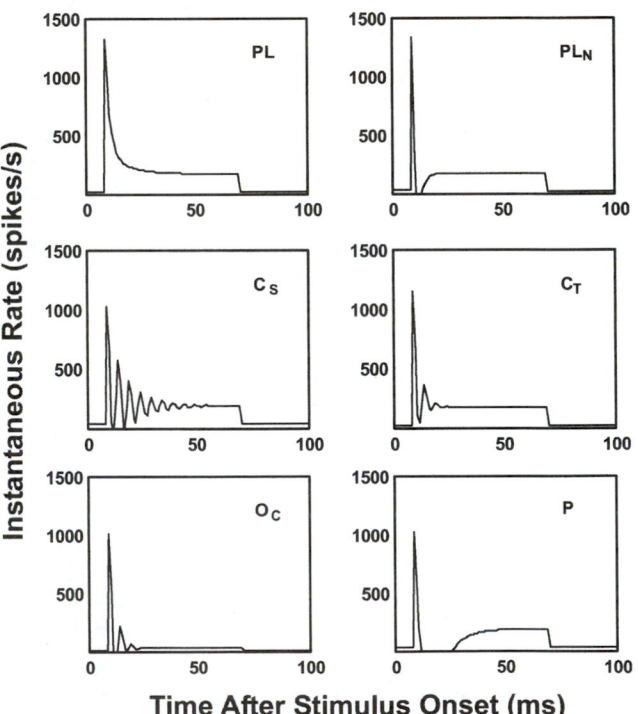

Figure 2. Typical auditory nerve and cochlear nucleus peristimulus time histograms. See text for explanation of abbreviations.

a limited dynamic range, typically saturating at sound levels of approximately 20 dB above the fiber's threshold. There are three components to the adaptation. The fastest component, rapid adaptation, has a time constant of a few milliseconds and creates an onset response with a large dynamic range. The second component, short-term adaptation, has a time constant of a few tens of milliseconds. It creates a slower component immediately after the onset response that has a smaller dynamic range, similar to that of the steady-state response. The third component of adaptation operates on a time scale of seconds and is not included in most auditory models.

On a finer time scale, the instantaneous firing rate (IFR) of AN fibers can be modulated on a cycle-by-cycle basis by the acoustic stimulus (phase locking) up to about 4 kHz (Ruggero in Popper and Fay, 1992). The fast dynamics of the AN IFR, coupled with only modest frequency resolution, suggests that we should think of the AN representation as that of a spectrogram that has been optimized more for temporal resolution than for spectral resolution. This excellent temporal resolution plays an important role in sound-source localization, which relies heavily on cues from interaural time delays.

Scant biophysical data are available for the IHC synapse, but since adaptation is not observed in the IHC receptor potentials, adaptation must be taking place in the IHC-AN synapse. The adaptation processes are most commonly assumed to be the result of synaptic vesicle depletion. Synaptic vesicles are typically divided into two or more pools. One of these pools represents vesicles that are docked at the active zones and is often referred to as the releasable pool or the immediate pool. Additional vesicles, which are located near the release sites but appear to be tethered to the cytoskeleton, are not available for immediate release (Mountain and Hubbard in Hawkins et al., 1996).

Cochlear Nucleus Anatomy

The two CN are the first and only brainstem structures to receive input from the AN. The CN can be anatomically subdivided into several subdivisions, each of which appears to perform a different physiological function. The major subdivisions are the ventral cochlear nucleus (VCN), which is further divided into anteroventral (AVCN) and posteroventral (PVCN) subdivisions, and the DC nucleus (DCN). Fibers of the AN travel through the core of the cochlear spiral and enter the AVCN, where they branch. The ascending branch innervates the AVCN and the descending branch travels through the PVCN and enters the DCN. The ventral regions are surrounded by the marginal shell, which is made up of the small-cell cap (SCC) and the granule-cell layer (GCL). Within a subdivision, the low-frequency fibers project to more ventral regions and the high-frequency fibers project to more dorsal regions. This orderly arrangement of characteristic frequencies is referred to as a *tonotopic projection*.

Cochlear Nucleus Response Types

The most commonly used physiological classification scheme in the CN is based on the PSTH. These histograms are derived by averaging the responses to short tone bursts presented at the cell's characteristic frequency (Rhode and Greenberg in Popper and Fay, 1992). Figure 2 illustrates six of the most common PSTH types found in the CN. The primary-like (PL) PSTHs are similar to the PSTHs recorded from AN fibers. The primary-like with notch (PL$_N$) response type is similar to the PL type but with better synchrony to the stimulus onset, followed by a transient dip in response due to refractory effects. The chopper-cell PSTHs exhibit periodically modulated activity at the beginning of the histogram, which is the result of the regular firing pattern of these cells becoming

synchronized to the stimulus onset. This chopping effect can either be sustained (C$_S$) or transient (C$_T$). The onset cell PSTHs all have large responses to the stimulus onset, followed by reduced or nonexistent activity during the remainder of the stimulus. The onset chopper (O$_C$) PSTH exhibits a transient chopping response after the onset, whereas the O$_L$ type (not shown) shows little or no response after the onset response. Other PSTH types include the pauser (P) and build-up (B) types. The P-type PSTH is characterized by an onset response followed by a period of no activity, which is then followed by a slow build-up of activity. The B-type (not shown) is similar to the P-type but lacks the initial onset response. The different PSTH types are believed to be the result, in part, of differences in intrinsic membrane properties and different degrees of AN fiber convergence and synaptic effectiveness.

Cochlear Nucleus Neural Circuits

Octopus Cells

Octopus cells are located in the PVCN and are characterized by long, thick primary dendrites that usually arise from one side of the cell body and give the cell the appearance of an octopus. The dendrites of octopus cells are oriented perpendicular to the path of incoming AN fibers (Oertel et al., 2000) which means that they receive input from a range of characteristic frequencies. The lower CF fibers synapse on the soma and the higher CF fibers synapse on the dendrites. Octopus cells generally exhibit onset (O$_L$) responses (Rhode and Greenberg in Popper and Fay, 1992) and appear to be more sensitive to broadband stimuli than AN fibers (Oertel et al., 2000). Functionally, octopus cells appear to act as coincidence detectors that detect synchronous events across AN fibers and may form part of networks involving other subthalamic nuclei devoted to processing temporal features such as duration, periodicity, and echo delay. The octopus cells project to contralateral VNLL terminating in calyx endings (Schwartz in Webster et al., 1992). The secure nature of these terminals reinforces the notion that octopus cells play a role in temporal processing. VNLL is primarily a monaural nucleus (Irvine in Popper and Fay, 1992) that provides inhibitory input to the IC (Schwartz in Webster et al, 1992). The octopus cells also provide diffuse innervation to periolivary areas of the SOC (Schwartz in Webster et al., 1992).

Stellate Cells

The stellate cells (SCs) of the VCN are hypothesized to be part of a system that uses a rate code to represent the acoustic spectrum (Rhode and Greenberg in Popper and Fay, 1992). Stellate cells have dendrites that extend away from the soma in all directions and often divide to form secondary and tertiary dendrites. The SCs can be divided into two classes, based on the path taken by their axons. The T-stellate cells project out of the CN by way of the trapezoid body (hence the name T), and the D-stellate cells are interneurons with axons that follow a descending path (hence the name D) on their way to the DCN and contralateral CN. The dendrites of T-stellate cells (also called planar cells) end in tufts and are generally aligned with the isofrequency plane created by the path of AN fibers, whereas those of D-stellate cells (also called radiate cells) extend radially across the isofrequency planes and branch sparingly. Both T- and D-stellate cells have terminal collaterals in the multipolar cell region of the PVCN and in the DCN (Oertel et al., 1990; Doucet and Ryugo, 1997).

D-stellate cells exhibit O$_C$ responses (Figure 2), have a large dynamic range (80 dB or more), and, as would be expected from their dendritic morphology, are more broadly tuned than AN fibers. In contrast, T-stellate cells exhibit C$_T$ responses (Figure 2) and have frequency tuning characteristics similar to those of AN fibers. Stellate cells have a more regular firing pattern than AN fibers and do not preserve timing information as well as the AN fibers do (Rhode and Greenberg in Popper and Fay, 1992).

The basic stellate-cell circuit is illustrated in Figure 3A. The D-stellate cells receive excitatory input from AN-I fibers with a range of CFs and inhibitory input that is believed to come from Golgi cells, which in turn appear to receive their input from AN-II fibers (Ferragamo, Golding, and Oertel, 1998). Golgi cells are small inhibitory interneurons located in the marginal shell with dendrites that branch extensively near the cell body (Cant in Webster et al., 1992). The Golgi cell axons branch even more extensively, forming a plexus with thousands of endings in nearby regions. In contrast to the D-stellate cells, the T-stellate cells receive excitatory input from AN-I fibers with a narrow range of CFs, and they receive inhibitory input from D-stellate cells as well as from vertical cells located in the deep DCN (Ferragamo et al., 1998). The DCN vertical cells receive excitatory input from AN-I fibers with a narrow range of CFs and are strongly inhibited by the more broadly tuned D-stellate cells. The T-stellate cells are the output neurons of this circuit; their axons project to the IC.

Bushy Cells

The major cell types of the AVCN are the spherical bushy cells (SBCs) and the globular bushy cells (GBCs). The term *bushy cell* refers to their appearance, with short primary dendrites that originate from one hemisphere of the cell body and give rise to a profusion of thin, shrub-like appendages. SBCs are believed to play an important role in sound localization and are specialized to preserve timing information. The basic SBC circuit is shown in Figure 3B. SBCs receive their excitatory input from AN-I fibers tuned to a narrow range of frequencies, and in most respects SBCs have response properties, such as their primary-like PSTHs (Figure 2), that are very similar to those of AN fibers. The AN fibers that synapse on the SBC cell body give rise to very large synaptic end-

ings known as the endbulbs of Held (Cant in Webster et al., 1992). These very secure synapses, in combination with a low-threshold potassium conductance in the SBCs, enhance phase locking to the acoustic stimulus (presumably through a coincidence mechanism) to be even more precise than that found in the AN. SBCs receive inhibitory input from vertical cells in the DCN. This inhibitory input is delayed with respect to the excitatory input from the AN and not as effective as the excitatory input, but it may play a role in echo suppression (Rhode and Greenberg in Popper and Fay, 1992).

SBCs project to the ipsilateral and contralateral medial superior olive (MSO), where timing differences (ITD) between the two ears are processed, and the ipsilateral lateral superior olive (LSO), where amplitude differences (ILD) are processed (Oliver in Webster et al., 1992). SBCs project as well to more central nuclei such as the contralateral ventral nucleus of the lateral lemniscus (VNLL) (Oertel and Wickesberg in Oertel, Fay, and Popper, 2002).

The innervation pattern of the GBC is similar to that of the SBC (Figure 3B) and forms a second part of the ILD pathway. They tend to have dendritic fields that are somewhat larger than SBCs and are preferentially contacted by HSR fibers. GBCs, like SBCs, receive extensive input from AN-I fibers on their cell bodies, but these synapses are smaller than the endbulb type found on SBCs. GBCs have response properties similar to those of AN fibers with PL_N PSTHs (Figure 2B), but with a higher degree of synchronization to the acoustic input (Yin in Oertel et al., 2002).

SBCs project primarily to the contralateral SOC, specifically the medial nucleus of the trapezoid body (MNTB), which provides inhibitory input to the LSO (Oliver and Huerta in Webster et al., 1992). The SBC axonal endings terminate in a calyx surrounding the cell bodies of the principal cells of the MNTB. This synaptic specialization suggests that timing is important in the ILD pathway as well as in the ITD pathway. Other projections of the GBCs include the ipsilateral lateral nucleus of the trapezoid body (LNTB), the contralateral VNLL, and periolivary nuclei on both sides (Yin in Oertel et al., 2002).

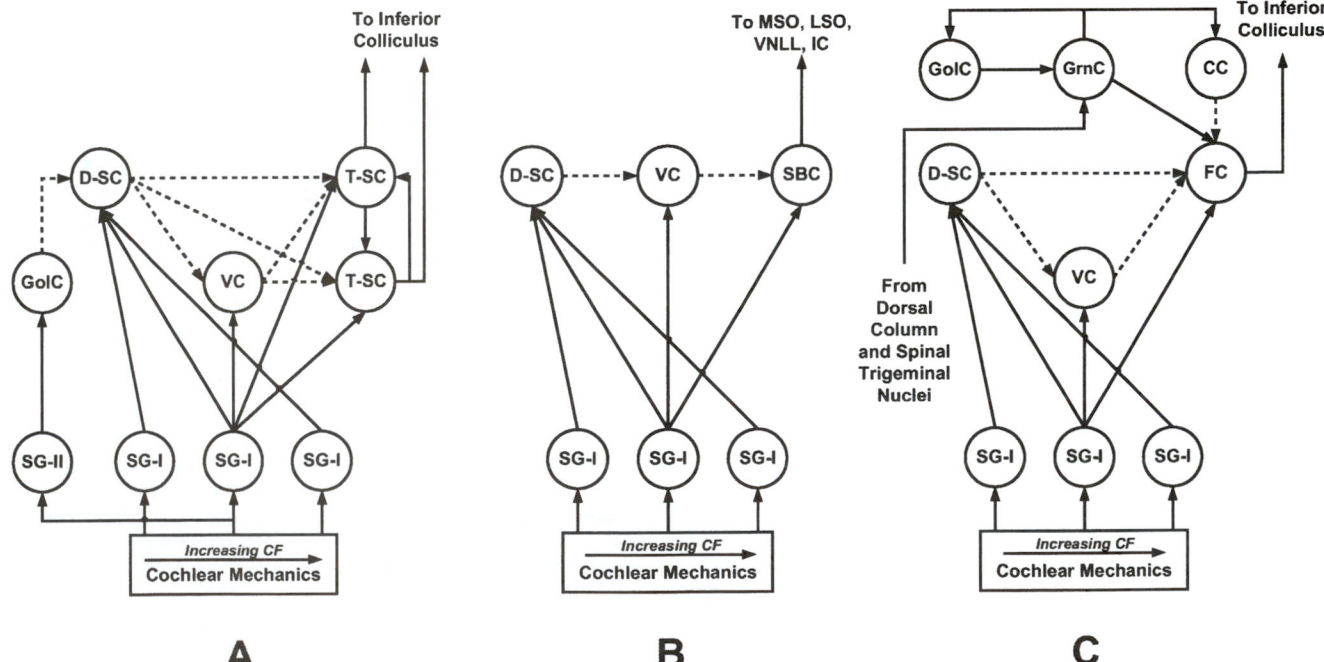

Figure 3. Examples of neural circuits in the cochlear nucleus. Excitatory connections are indicted by solid lines and inhibitory connections are indicated by broken lines. *A*, The stellate cell circuit. *B*, The sperical bushy cell circuit. *C*, The fusiform circuit. See text for explanation of abbreviations.

Fusiform and Giant Cells

The DCN is believed to be involved in processing spectral cues that are important for sound source location, especially source elevation. Cats with lesions to the DCN output pathways exhibit significant deficits in their ability to orient to sources at different locations (Young and Davis in Oertel et al., 2002). The DCN is usually subdivided into three layers, a superficial or molecular layer, an intermediate layer called the granular or fusiform cell layer, and a polymorphic or deep layer. The principal cells of the DCN are the fusiform cells (from which the fusiform cell layer gets its name) and the giant cells located in the deep layer. The apical dendrites of fusiform cells (also called pyramidal cells) are highly branched and extend up into the molecular layer, while the less highly branched basal dendrites extend down into the deep layer. The dendritic morphology of the giant cells is more diverse, ranging from elongate to radiate (Cant in Webster et al., 1992). Beneath the fusiform cells are a group of cells called vertical cells. These cells have their dendritic and axonal arbors confined to an isofrequency lamina. There are two groups of vertical cells. The more superficial group gives rise to only a local axon, the deeper group gives rise to axons that project to the VCN (Rhode, 1999).

The fusiform cell circuit is shown in Figure 3C. The basal dendrites of fusiform cells receive excitatory input from AN-I fibers with a limited range of CFs, a narrow-band inhibitory input from the vertical cells of the DCN, and a wide-band inhibitory input from the D-stellate cells of the VCN. The inhibitory input from the vertical cells is quite strong, and as a result, fusiform cells respond poorly or not at all to pure tones. They respond well to broadband stimuli except when there is a spectral notch at the characteristic frequency, in which case these cells are strongly inhibited (Rhode and Greenberg in Popper and Fay, 1992). As a result of these properties, fusiform cell models create a spectral representation that accentuates spectral notches (Hancock and Voigt, 1999), which are important features of the HRTF for determining sound source elevation. The fusiform cells also receive excitatory input on their apical dendrites from the granule cells, which in turn receive input from the dorsal column and spinal trigeminal nuclei of the somatosensory system. This somatosensory input appears to modify DCN response properties based on head and pinna position (Kanold and Young, 2001).

The giant cell circuit (not shown) is similar to the fusiform cell circuit except that the giant cells do not receive direct input from granule cells and AN input to the giant cells spans a large range of characteristic frequencies. Fusiform and giant cells project to the contralateral ICC and also project to the contralateral DNLL, which provides inhibitory input to both ICs (Oliver and Huerta in Webster et al., 1992).

Discussion

Significant progress has been made in understanding the anatomy and physiology of the subthalamic auditory pathways, but many questions remain. For example, the experimental data suggest that OHCs contribute to the tuned response of the BM and IHCs, but how OHCs perform their function is not well understood. Much of the basic circuitry of the CN has been worked out, but it is not clear how many subpopulations exist for each of the basic cell types described in this article. And perhaps the greatest question of all is, how is information in the parallel pathways leaving the CN reintegrated into a unified percept by higher centers? To answer these questions, future research will need to take an integrated approach, with computational models being used to aid the design and interpretation of anatomical and physiological experiments. These models will need to incorporate the major features of individual cell types as well as the interactions between cell types at different levels of the auditory system. Efforts to create suitable large-scale models have begun (cf. Hawkins et al., 1996), but much remains to be done.

Road Maps: Mammalian Brain Regions; Other Sensory Systems
Related Reading: Auditory Cortex; Auditory Scene Analysis; Echolocation: Cochleotopic and Computational Maps; Sound Localization and Binaural Processing; Thalamus

References

Dallos, P., Popper, A. N., and Fay, R.-R., 1996, *The Springer Handbook of Auditory Research*, vol. 8, *The Cochlea*, New York: Springer-Verlag. ◆

Doucet, J. R., and Ryugo, D. K., 1997, Projections from the ventral cochlear nucleus to the dorsal cochlear nucleus in rats, *J. Comp. Neurol.*, 385:245–264.

Ferragamo, M. J., Golding, N. L., and Oertel, D., 1998, Synaptic inputs to stellate cells in the ventral cochlear nucleus, *J. Neurophysiol.*, 79:51–63.

Gilkey, R. H., and Anderson, T. R., 1997, *Binaural and Spatial Hearing in Real and Virtual Environments*, Mahwah, NJ: Erlbaum.

Hancock, K. E., and Voigt, H. F., 1999, Wideband inhibition of dorsal cochlear nucleus type IV units in cat: A computational mode, *Ann. Biomed. Eng.*, 27:73–87.

Hawkins, H. L., McMullen, T. A., Popper, A. N., and Fay, R.-R., 1996, *The Springer Handbook of Auditory Research*, vol. 6, *Auditory Computation*, New York: Springer-Verlag. ◆

Kanold, P. O., and Young, E. D., 2001, Proprioceptive information from the pinna provides somatosensory input to cat dorsal cochlear nucleus, *J. Neurosci.*, 21:7848–7858.

Mountain, D. C., and Cody, A. R., 1999, Multiple modes of inner hair cell stimulation, *Hear. Res.*, 132:1–14.

Oertel, D., Bal, R., Gardner, S. M., Smith, P. H., and Joris, P. X., 2000, Detection of synchrony in the activity of auditory nerve fibers by octopus cells of the mammalian cochlear nucleus, *Proc. Natl. Acad. Sci. USA*, 97:11773–11779.

Oertel, D., Fay, R. R., and Popper, A. N., 2002, *The Springer Handbook of Auditory Research, vol. 15, Integrative Functions in the Mammalian Auditory Pathway*, New York: Springer-Verlag. ◆

Oertel, D., Wu, S. H., Garb, M. W., and Dizack, C., 1990, Morphology and physiology of cells in slice preparations of the posteroventral cochlear nucleus of mice, *J. Comp. Neurol.*, 295:136–154.

Popper, A. N., and Fay, R.-R., 1992, *The Springer Handbook of Auditory Research*, vol. 2, *The Mammalian Auditory Pathway: Neurophysiology*, New York: Springer-Verlag. ◆

Rhode, W. S., 1999, Vertical cell responses to sound in cat dorsal cochlear nucleus, *J. Neurophys.*, 82:1019–1032.

Webster, D. B., Popper, A. N., and Fay, R.-R., 1992, *The Springer Handbook of Auditory Research*, vol. 1, *The Mammalian Auditory Pathway: Neuroanatomy*, New York: Springer-Verlag.

Zhang, X., Heinz, M. G., Bruce, I. C., and Carney, L. H., 2001, A phenomenological model for the responses of auditory-nerve fibers: I. Nonlinear tuning with compression and suppression, *J. Acoust. Soc. Am.*, 109:648–670.

Auditory Scene Analysis

Guy J. Brown

Introduction

We usually listen in environments that contain many simultaneously active sound sources. The auditory system must therefore parse the acoustic mixture that reaches our ears to segregate a target sound source from the background of other sounds. Bregman (1990) describes this process as *auditory scene analysis* (ASA) and suggests that it takes place in two conceptual stages. The first stage, *segmentation*, decomposes the acoustic mixture into its constituent components. In the second stage, acoustic components that are likely to have arisen from the same environmental event are *grouped*, forming a perceptual representation (*stream*) that describes a single sound source. Streams are subjected to higher-level processing, such as language understanding.

Bregman's account makes a distinction between *schema-driven* and *primitive* mechanisms of grouping. Schema-driven grouping applies learned knowledge of sound sources such as speech in a top-down manner (in this regard, the term "schema" refers to a recurring pattern in the acoustic environment). Primitive mechanisms operate on the acoustic signal in a bottom-up fashion and are well described by Gestalt heuristics such as proximity and common fate (see CONTOUR AND SURFACE PERCEPTION). Primitive organization is both *simultaneous* and *sequential*. Simultaneous grouping operates on concurrent sounds, using principles such as similarity of fundamental frequency. Sequential grouping combines acoustic events over time, according to heuristics such as temporal proximity and frequency proximity.

At the physiological level, segmentation corresponds (at least in part) to peripheral auditory processing, which performs a frequency analysis of the acoustic input. To a first approximation, this frequency analysis can be modeled by a bank of band-pass filters with overlapping passbands, in which each channel simulates the filtering characteristics of one location on the basilar membrane (see AUDITORY PERIPHERY AND COCHLEAR NUCLEUS). From the output of each filter, a simulation of the auditory nerve response can be obtained by rectification and compression or from a detailed model of inner hair cell function. In contrast, the physiological substrate of auditory grouping is much less well understood (Feng and Ratnam, 2000). As a result, models of ASA tend to be functional in approach. In the current review, we focus on models that are at least physiologically plausible; however, it should be noted that there is also a substantial literature that has addressed computational modeling of ASA from a more abstract information-processing perspective (e.g., Rosenthal and Okuno, 1998).

Models of Sequential Grouping

Sequential grouping can be demonstrated by playing listeners a repeating sequence of two alternating tones with different frequencies (ABAB . . .). When the sequence is played rapidly or when the frequency separation between the tones is large, the sequence is heard to split into separate streams (A-A- . . . and B-B- . . .). This phenomenon is known as *auditory streaming* (Bregman, 1990). Listeners are able to direct their attention to only one of the streams, which appears to be subjectively louder than the other. Auditory streaming may therefore be regarded as an example of figure-ground separation.

Auditory streaming may be viewed as a consequence of sequential grouping heuristics that allocate tones to streams depending on their proximity in time and frequency. Several modeling studies have demonstrated that such principles can be implemented by relatively low-level physiological mechanisms. For example, Beauvois

and Meddis (1996) describe a model of auditory streaming that has its basis in mechanisms of peripheral auditory function. The model utilizes two pathways: one in which auditory nerve activity is smoothed by temporal integration and an "excitation-level" path that adds a cumulative random element to the output of the temporal integration path. Firing activity is considered in three auditory filter channels: one at the frequency of each tone and one in between them. The channel with the highest activity in the excitation-level pathway is selected as the dominant "foreground" percept; the remaining channels are attenuated and become the "background." This simple model quantitatively matches auditory streaming phenomena, such as the effect of rate of presentation and frequency separation. Furthermore, the inclusion of a random element in the model (which is assumed to originate from the stochastic nature of auditory nerve firing patterns) explains how spontaneous shifts of attention can occur.

McCabe and Denham (1997) have extended the Beauvois and Meddis model by applying similar principles within a two-layer neural architecture. In their model, "foreground" and "background" neural arrays are connected by reciprocal inhibitory connections, which ensure that activity appearing in one array does not appear in the other (Figure 1). Their network is sensitive to frequency proximity because the strength of inhibitory feedback is related to the frequency difference between acoustic components. Additionally, each layer receives a recurrent inhibitory feedback related to the reciprocal of its own activity. As a result, previous activity in the network tends to suppress differences in subsequent stimuli. This mechanism may be viewed as a neural implementation of Bregman's (1990) "old plus new heuristic," which states that the auditory system prefers to interpret a current sound as a continuation of a previous sound unless there is strong evidence to the contrary. The inclusion of this heuristic within McCabe and Denham's model allows it to explain the effect of background organization on the perceptual foreground.

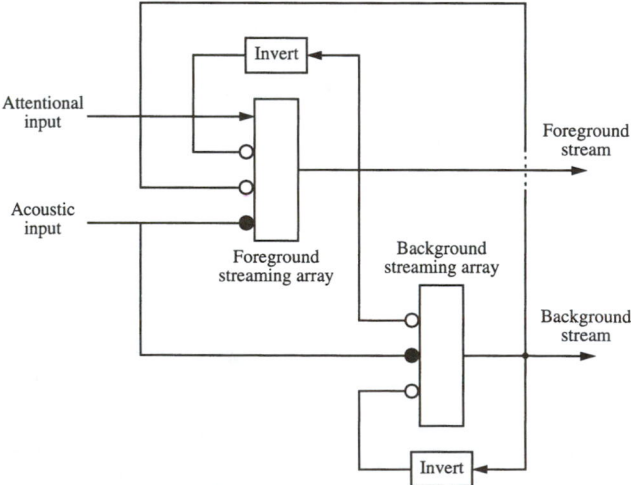

Figure 1. McCabe and Denham's model of auditory stream segregation. Foreground and background streams are encoded by separate neural arrays, which have reciprocal inhibitory connections. Each layer also receives recurrent inhibition. Solid circles indicate excitatory connections; open circles indicate inhibitory connections. (Modified from McCabe and Denham (1997).)

A more central explanation for auditory streaming is given by Todd (1996), who suggests that mechanisms of rhythm perception and stream segregation are underlain by cortical maps of periodicity-sensitive cells. In his model, periodicity detection leads to a spatial representation of the temporal pattern of the stimulus in terms of its amplitude modulation (AM) spectrum. Acoustic events whose AM spectra are highly correlated (as judged by a neural cross-correlation mechanism) are perceptually grouped, whereas events with uncorrelated AM spectra are segregated. Todd's model is able to qualitatively replicate the dependence of auditory streaming on tone frequency and temporal proximity.

The models of Todd (1996) and McCabe and Denham (1997) suggest that the auditory responses associated with different streams are encoded spatially in neural arrays. An alternative is that auditory streams are encoded temporally. For example, Wang (1996) suggests a principle of *oscillatory correlation*, which is a development of von der Malsburg's temporal correlation theory (von der Malsburg and Schneider, 1986). In Wang's scheme, neural oscillators alternate rapidly between relatively stable states of activity (the active phase) and inactivity (the silent phase). Oscillators that encode features of the same stream are synchronized (phase locked with zero phase lag) and are desynchronized from oscillators that represent different streams.

Wang has implemented the oscillatory correlation principle in a model of auditory streaming, in which oscillators are arranged within a two-dimensional time-frequency network. The time axis of the network is assumed to be constructed by a systematic arrangement of neural delay lines. Each oscillator is connected to others in its neighborhood with excitatory connections whose strength diminishes with increasing distance in time and frequency. In addition, every oscillator sends excitation to a global inhibitor, which feeds back inhibition to each oscillator in the network. Oscillators that are close in time and frequency tend to synchronize because the excitatory connections between them are strong. However, groups of oscillators that do not receive mutually supportive excitation tend to desynchronize because of the action of the global inhibitor. As the network dynamics evolve, the combined effects of local excitation and global inhibition cause streams of synchronized oscillators to form. The model qualitatively reproduces a number of auditory streaming phenomena. However, the oscillatory dynamics proceed rapidly, so Wang's network is not able to account for the gradual buildup of the auditory streaming effect over time.

Models of Simultaneous Grouping

Simultaneous grouping mechanisms exploit differences in the characteristics of concurrent sounds in order to perceptually segregate them. For example, the ability of listeners to identify two simultaneously presented vowels ("double vowels") can be improved by introducing a difference in fundamental frequency (F0) between the vowels (Bregman, 1990). Apparently, simultaneous grouping mechanisms are able to segregate the acoustic components related to each F0 and hence retrieve the spectra of the two vowels.

Meddis and Hewitt (1992) describe a model of double-vowel identification based on the *correlogram*, a model of auditory pitch analysis. A correlogram is formed by computing a running autocorrelation at the output of each auditory filter channel, giving a two-dimensional representation in which frequency and time lag are represented on orthogonal axes. Meddis and Hewitt suggest that the correlogram could be computed neurally by using a system of delay lines and coincidence detectors. The F0 of one of the vowels is identified from the correlogram, and channels whose response is dominated by that F0 are removed, thus allowing a clearer view of the second vowel. This mechanism fails to separate the vowels when they both have the same F0 and successfully predicts that

vowel identification performance improves when a difference in F0 is introduced.

The Meddis and Hewitt model is based on a strategy of "exclusive allocation" (Bregman, 1990); all of the energy in a single auditory filter channel is allocated to one vowel or the other. However, this need not be the case. De Cheveigné (1997) describes an approach that uses a "neural cancellation filter" to partition the energy in each channel between vowel percepts. In his scheme, a correlogram is computed, and the fundamental period of one of the vowels is identified. This period is canceled in each channel by a neural comb filter, which is implemented by a neuron with a delayed inhibitory input. This mechanism removes firing activity with a periodicity equal to the inhibitory delay. An advantage of de Cheveigné's approach is that it predicts an increase in listeners' performance with increasing difference in F0 for vowels that are weak in comparison to a harmonic background. The Meddis and Hewitt model is unable to reproduce this result because its exclusive allocation scheme tends to remove the evidence for a weak vowel when the stronger vowel is canceled.

Brown and Wang (1997) have described a neural oscillator model of vowel segregation, which is essentially an implementation of Meddis and Hewitt's (1992) scheme within an oscillatory correlation framework. In their model, each channel of the correlogram is associated with a neural oscillator. Oscillators corresponding to channels that are dominated by the same F0 become synchronized and are desynchronized from channels that are dominated by a different F0. When there is no difference in F0 between the two vowels, a single group of synchronized oscillators forms. However, when a difference in F0 is introduced, the two vowels are segregated according to their F0s, and the channels making up each vowel are encoded as separate groups of synchronized oscillators.

Von der Malsburg and Schneider (1986) describe a related model of simultaneous grouping based on temporal correlation of neural responses. Their scheme employs a neural architecture in which each member of a fully connected network of excitatory cells (E-cells) receives an input from one auditory filter channel. In addition, E-cells receive inhibition from a common inhibitory cell (H-cell). E-cells that receive simultaneous inputs tend to become synchronized by the excitatory links between them and tend to become desynchronized from other cells owing to the influence of inhibition from the H-cell. The network therefore displays a sensitivity to the common onset of acoustic components and may be regarded as implementing a Gestalt principle of common fate (Bregman, 1990).

The Role of Temporal Continuity

With the exception of that of Wang (1996), relatively few modeling studies have demonstrated the integration of simultaneous and sequential grouping principles within the same computational framework. However, several studies have shown how a complex time-frequency mixture can be organized using simultaneous grouping principles and temporal continuity constraints.

Grossberg (1999) describes a multistage model of ASA that implements grouping by common F0 and good continuation. The first stage of his model builds redundant spectral representations of the acoustic input in a "spectral stream" layer. Each stream is represented by a separate neural array. These representations are filtered by neural "harmonic sieves," which connect a node in a "pitch stream" layer with spectral regions near to the harmonics of the corresponding pitch value. Pitch representations compete across streams to select a winner, and the winning pitch node sends top-down signals via harmonic connections to the spectral stream layer. According to an adaptive resonance theory (ART) matching rule, frequency components in the spectral stream that are consistent with the top-down signal are selected, and others are suppressed (see ADAPTIVE RESONANCE THEORY). Selected components reactivate their pitch node, and further top-down signals are produced. In this way, a resonance develops that binds together the frequency components constituting a sound source and its corresponding pitch.

Grossberg's model is able to account for simple simultaneous grouping phenomena, such as the perceptual fusion of components with the same F0. His model also reproduces the auditory continuity illusion (Bregman, 1990), in which a pure tone is heard to continue through a brief interrupting noise, even though the tone is not physically present during the noise burst. It is able to do so because a resonance develops for the tone that is maintained during the noise burst. The ART matching rule then selects the tone from the noise, and competitive interactions cause the tone and residual noise to be allocated to different streams.

Wang and Brown (1999) describe a neural oscillator model whose two-layer architecture echoes the two conceptual stages of ASA. The first (segmentation) layer consists of a two-dimensional time-frequency grid of oscillators with a global inhibitor (Figure 2). In this layer, excitatory connections are formed between auditory filter channels that have a similar temporal response. As a result, segments form in the time-frequency plane and thus correspond to harmonics and formants. The global inhibitor ensures that each segment desynchronizes from the others; the first layer therefore embodies the segmentation stage of ASA, in which the acoustic signal is split into its constituent elements. The second layer receives an input from the first layer. Also, segments in the second layer are connected by excitatory links if they represent time-frequency regions that are dominated by the same F0. As a result, synchronized groups of segments emerge in the second layer, each of which corresponds to a stream with harmonically related components.

Models of Schema-Driven Grouping

Liu, Yamaguchi, and Shimizu (1994) describe a neural oscillator model of vowel recognition that may be regarded as an implementation of schema-driven grouping. The model consists of an input layer and three layers of oscillators labeled A, B, and C, which are likened to regions of the auditory cortex. The A ("feature extraction") layer identifies local peaks in the acoustic spectrum and en-

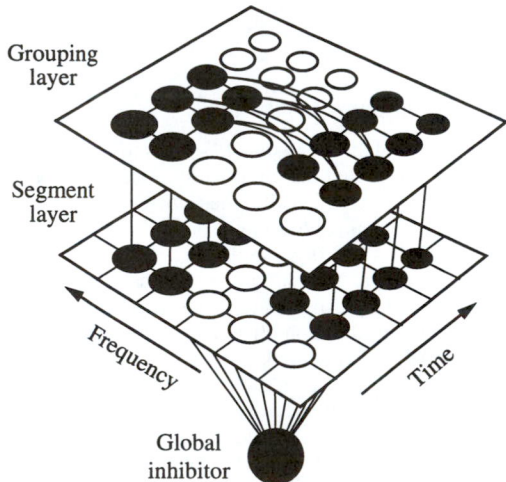

Figure 2. The two-layer neural oscillator model of Wang and Brown (1999). In the first layer, segments are formed that correspond to harmonics and formants. The second layer groups segments according to their fundamental frequency (F0); those with the same F0 form a stream in which all oscillators are synchronized and are desynchronized from other streams. (Modified from Wang and Brown (1999).)

codes them as separate groups of oscillations, which are assumed to correspond to vowel formants. The B ("feature linking") layer acts as a simple associative memory, in which hardwired connections encode the relationship between formant frequencies for different vowels. Associative interactions between the B layer, together with top-down and bottom-up interactions between the A and B layers, lead to the activation of a vowel in terms of a global pattern of synchronized oscillations. The C ("evaluation") layer assesses the synchronization in each formant region and outputs a vowel category. Top-down reinforcement from the B center confers robustness in noise; it is demonstrated that the model is able to recognize vowels robustly in the presence of multispeaker babble.

Discussion

The modeling studies reviewed here propose a neurobiological basis for the principles of auditory organization expounded in Bregman's account of ASA. Clearly, the models differ in their level of explanation, ranging from peripheral (Beauvois and Meddis, 1996) to cortical (Todd, 1996). Without exception, their approach is functional; currently, there is insufficient knowledge about the physiological mechanisms of ASA to attempt a detailed physiological model. It is likely that future research in this field will see a closer synergy between computational modeling studies and neurophysiological investigation.

Various strategies have been proposed for the neural encoding of auditory streams. Beauvois and Meddis (1996) stress that the perceptual separation of sounds need not imply a physical separation of their corresponding representations; in their model, auditory filter channels belonging to a nonattended stream are simply attenuated. This contrasts with the approaches described by Grossberg (1999) and McCabe and Denham (1997), in which different auditory streams are encoded by separate neural arrays. A further approach is to encode streams temporally in the responses of synchronized neural firing patterns (von der Malsburg and Schneider, 1986; Wang, 1996). Although all of these approaches are plausible, none are currently supported by strong neurophysiological evidence.

Many models of ASA require systematic time delays longer than those currently known to exist in the auditory system. Models of double-vowel separation based on the correlogram require delays of the order of 20 ms (Meddis and Hewitt, 1992; de Cheveigné, 1997). Similarly, it is questionable whether the system of delay lines employed in Wang's (1996) neural oscillator model is physiologically realizable. The temporal correlation architecture of von der Malsburg and Schneider (1986) does not suffer from this difficulty, since their network does not have an explicit time axis. However, the explanatory power of their model is weak in comparison to Wang's model, because temporal and frequency relationships between acoustic inputs are not preserved.

Generally speaking, the role of auditory attention has been neglected in computer models of ASA. In auditory streaming, a listener's attention can shift randomly between organizations or may be consciously directed to the high or low tones. The model of Beauvois and Meddis (1996) accounts for the former but not the latter. Similarly, McCabe and Denham's model includes an attentional input (Figure 1), but it is not utilized in their simulations. Wang (1996) suggests that in a neural oscillator framework, attention is paid to a stream when its constituent oscillators reach their active phases; attention therefore alternates quickly among the streams in turn. However, such a scheme does not explain how listeners are able to direct their attention to a particular stream over a sustained period of time.

Also, few models have attempted to model the interaction between top-down and bottom-up grouping mechanisms. In principle, the mechanism of recurrent neural connections described by Liu et al. (1994) could form the basis for such a model. Similarly, Grossberg's (1999) ART scheme could form the basis for a grouping mechanism in which bottom-up features interact with top-down information about the characteristics of sound sources.

The motivation for most of the studies reviewed here is to gain insight into the mechanisms of ASA through computational modeling. However, computer sound separation devices have many real-world applications, such as in hearing prostheses and as preprocessors for robust automatic speech recognition in noise. For example, Wang and Brown (1999) have applied their model to the separation of voiced speech from interfering sounds, with some success. Because they are founded on neurobiological principles, such approaches to sound separation may offer performance advantages over other techniques, such as blind statistical methods.

Road Map: Other Sensory Systems
Related Reading: Auditory Periphery and Cochlear Nucleus; Contour and Surface Perception; Dynamic Link Architecture; Echolocation: Cochleotopic and Computational Maps

References

Beauvois, M. W., and Meddis, R., 1996, Computer simulation of auditory stream segregation in alternating-tone sequences, *J. Acoust. Soc. Am.*, 99:2270–2280.

Bregman, A. S., 1990, *Auditory Scene Analysis*, Cambridge, MA: MIT Press. ◆

Brown, G. J., and Wang, D., 1997, Modelling the perceptual segregation

of double vowels with a network of neural oscillators, *Neural Networks*, 10:1547–1558.

de Cheveigné, A., 1997, Concurrent vowel identification: III. A neural model of harmonic interference cancellation, *J. Acoust. Soc. Am.*, 101:2857–2865.

Feng, A. S., and Ratnam, R., 2000, Neural basis of hearing in real-world situations, *Annu. Rev. Psychol.*, 51:699–725. ◆

Grossberg, S., 1999, Pitch-based streaming in auditory perception, in *Musical Networks: Parallel Distributed Perception and Performance* (N. Griffith and P. Todd, Eds.), Cambridge, MA: MIT Press, pp. 117–140.

Liu, F., Yamaguchi, Y., and Shimizu, H., 1994, Flexible vowel recognition by the generation of dynamic coherence in oscillator neural networks: Speaker-independent vowel recognition, *Biol. Cybern.*, 71:105–114.

McCabe, S. L., and Denham, M. J., 1997, A model of auditory streaming, *J. Acoust. Soc. Am.*, 101:1611–1621.

Meddis, R., and Hewitt, M. J., 1992, Modelling the identification of concurrent vowels with different fundamental frequencies, *J. Acoust. Soc. Am.*, 91:233–245.

Rosenthal, D., and Okuno, H. G. (Eds.), 1998, *Computational Auditory Scene Analysis*, Mahwah, NJ: Lawrence Erlbaum Associates. ◆

Todd, N., 1996, An auditory cortical theory of primitive auditory grouping, *Network: Comput. Neural Syst.*, 7:349–356.

von der Malsburg, C., and Schneider, W., 1986, A neural cocktail-party processor, *Biol. Cybern.*, 54:29–40.

Wang, D., 1996, Primitive auditory segregation based on oscillatory correlation, *Cogn. Sci.*, 20:409–456. ◆

Wang, D., and Brown, G. J., 1999, Separation of speech from interfering sounds based on oscillatory correlation, *IEEE Trans. Neural Networks*, 10:684–697.

Axonal Modeling

Christof Koch and Öjvind Bernander

Introduction

Axons are highly specialized "wires" that conduct the neuron's output signal to target cells—in the case of cortical pyramidal cells up to 10,000 other cortical neurons. As such they are highly specialized, with a relatively stereotypical behavior. Most authors agree that their role in signaling is largely limited to making sure that whatever pulse train is put into one end of the axon is rapidly and faithfully propagated to the other end. This is in contrast to the complexity of electrical events occurring at the cell body and in the dendritic tree, where the information from thousands of synapses is integrated.

Despite the uniformity of electrical behavior, there is great morphological variability that largely reflects a trade-off between propagation speed and packing density. Axonal size varies over four orders of magnitude: diameters range from 0.2-μm fibers in the mammalian central nervous system to 1 mm in squid; lengths range from a few hundred microns to over a meter for motor neurons (Kandel, Schwartz, and Jessell, 2000). Some axons are bound only by the thin cellular membrane, while others are wrapped in multiple sheaths of myelin. An example of an axonal arbor is shown in Figure 1.

The majority of nerve cells encode their output as a series of brief voltage pulses. These pulses, also referred to as *action potentials* or *spikes*, originate at or close to the cell body of nerve cells and propagate down the axon at constant amplitude. Their shape is relatively constant across species and types of neurons. Common to all is the rapid upstroke (depolarization) of the membrane above 0 mV and the subsequent, somewhat slower, downstroke (repolarization) toward the resting potential and slightly beyond to more hyperpolarized potentials. At normal temperatures, the entire sequence occurs within less than 1 ms. A minority of cell types are axonless and appear to use graded voltage as output, such as cells

in the early part of the retina or interneurons in invertebrates (Roberts and Bush, 1981). Action potentials are such a dominant feature of the nervous system that for a considerable period of time it was widely held—and still is in parts of the neural network community—that all neuronal computations involve only these all-or-none events. This belief provided much of the impetus behind the neural network models originating in the late 1930s and early 1940s (see SINGLE-CELL MODELS).

The ionic mechanisms underlying the initiation and propagation of action potentials were elucidated in the squid giant axon by a number of workers, most notably Hodgkin and Huxley (1952). Today, with the widespread availability of cheap and almost unlimited computational power, it is very difficult to imagine the difficulty that Hodgkin and Huxley faced 50 years ago. Not only did they have to derive a proper mathematical formalism based on incomplete data, they also had to solve a nonlinear partial differential equation, the cable equation, using a very primitive hand calculator.

For this work they shared, together with Eccles, the 1963 Nobel prize in physiology and medicine (for a historical overview, see Hodgkin, 1976). Their model has played a paradigmatic role in biophysics; indeed, the vast majority of contemporary biophysical models use essentially the same mathematical formalism Hodgkin and Huxley introduced 50 years ago. This is all the more surprising because the kinetic description of the continuous, deterministic, and macroscopic membrane permeability changes within the framework of the Hodgkin-Huxley model was achieved without any knowledge of the underlying all-or-none, stochastic, and microscopic ionic channels.

Given its importance, we will describe the Hodgkin-Huxley model and its assumptions in some detail in the following section. We then introduce the two classes of axons found in most animals, myelinated and nonmyelinated, and describe their differences. Ax-

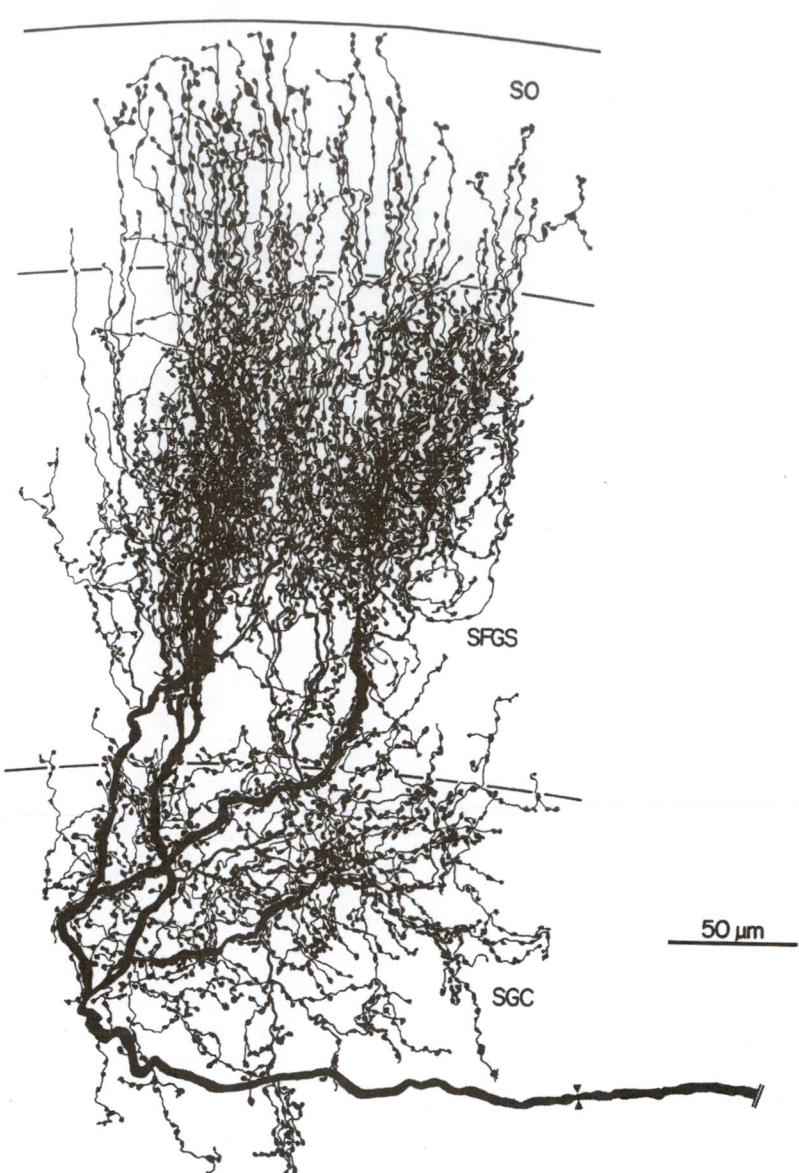

SO

SFGS

50 µm

SGC

Figure 1. Axonal terminations. An axon from nucleus isthmi terminating in turtle tectum was labeled with horseradish peroxidase and reconstructed from a series of parallel sections. The thick parent trunk (3 µm) is wrapped in myelin and shows a node of Ranvier (triangles). The thin (<1 µm) branches are nonmyelinated and are home to approximately 3,600 synaptic boutons (bulbous thickenings), where contact is made onto other cells. The boutons vary greatly in size but average about 1.5 µm in diameter. (From Sereno, M. I., and Ulinski, P. S., 1987, Caudal topographic nucleus isthmi and the rostral nontopographic nucleus isthmi in the turtle, *Pseudemys scripta, J. Comp. Neurol.*, 261:319–346. Copyright © 1987 by Wiley-Liss. Reprinted by permission of John Wiley & Sons, Inc.)

ons possess heavily branched axonal trees. We conclude the overview by briefly alluding to additional complications that arise when attempting to understand the role and function of axonal trees in information processing. For a useful book on the biophysics of dendrites and axons and their computational function, see Koch (1999). For a monograph on the axon in health and disease, see Waxman, Kocsis, and Stys (1995).

The Hodgkin-Huxley Model of Action Potential Generation

Electrical current in nerve cells is carried by the flow of ions through membrane proteins called *channels*. The concentration of sodium ions is high in the extracellular fluid and low in the intracellular axoplasm. This *concentration gradient* gives rise to a tendency for sodium ions to flow into the cell. At some membrane potential, termed the *reversal potential*, the effect of the concentration gradient will be canceled by the *electrical gradient*, and so the net flow of sodium ions will be zero at that point. The channel

transitions into its closed state by virtue of a conformational state in the underlying molecular structure. In the model, this is described by a change in the m variable. A similar situation holds for potassium ions flowing through separate potassium-selective channels, except that the concentration gradient is reversed.

In the squid giant axon, the membrane potential is determined by three conductances: a voltage-independent (passive) leak conductance, g_l, a voltage-dependent (active) sodium conductance, g_{Na}, and an active potassium conductance, g_K. The equivalent circuit used to model the membrane is shown in Figure 2. The conductances are in series with batteries, the values of which correspond to the respective reversal potentials of the ionic currents, E_l, E_{Na}, and E_K. The outside is connected to ground under the assumption that the resistivity of the external medium is negligible.

The time course of an action potential is illustrated in Figure 3. In this simulation of a membrane patch, a brief current pulse initiates an action potential. Before stimulation, the membrane voltage is at rest, $V_m = -65$ mV. At this potential, g_{Na} and g_K are almost fully inactivated. g_K is still much larger than g_{Na}, and the membrane

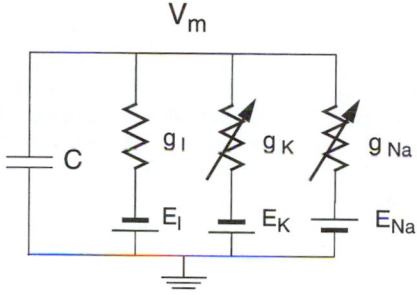

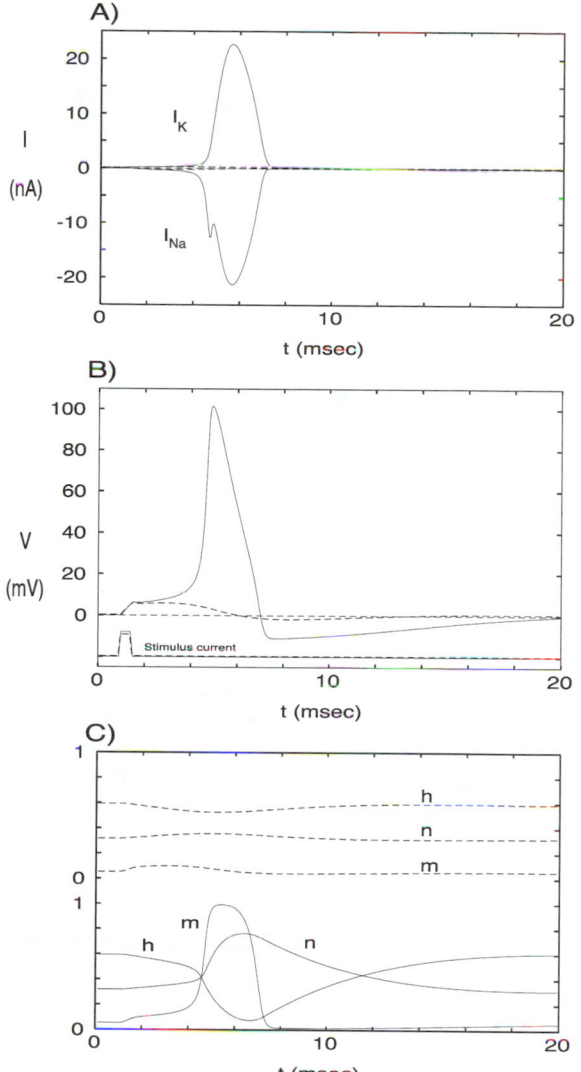

Figure 2. Schematic of ionic channel and neuronal membrane: Equivalent circuit of axonal membrane. The Hodgkin-Huxley model of squid axon incorporates a capacitance and three conductances. Two of the conductances are voltage dependent (active), g_{Na} and g_K, while the third is a passive "leak" conductance, g_l. The maximal conductances are 120, 36, and 0.3 ms/cm^2, respectively. Each conductance is in series with a battery that defines the *reversal potential* for each conductance type. The values are $E_{Na} = 50$, $E_K = -77$, and $E_l = -54.3$ mV. See text for the voltage dependences of g_{Na} and g_K. The top rail corresponds to the axoplasm (inside) of the axon, while the bottom rail, grounded, is the external medium. When a *membrane action potential* or *space clamp* is modeled, only one compartment is used, as shown, and the spatial structure of the membrane is ignored. When *propagating action potentials* are modeled, the specific resistivity of the axoplasm, $R_a = 34.5$ Ωcm, cannot be ignored. R_a is then modeled as a series of resistors connecting identical compartments that correspond to different spatial locations along the axon. The membrane capacitance is 1 μm F/cm^2.

is dominated by the leak current and the residual potassium current. The applied current slowly depolarizes the membrane by charging up the capacitance. As V_m approaches threshold ($V_t \sim -50$ mV), sodium channels begin to open up, allowing for the influx of Na$^+$ ions, which further depolarizes the membrane. About 1 ms later, two events occur to bring the voltage back toward and somewhat beyond the resting value: the sodium conductance inactivates, that is, the sodium channels slowly close again, and potassium channels open up, causing an outward current to flow. This outward current forces the membrane potential below the resting value of -65 mV (hyperpolarization), but the K$^+$ conductance too eventually deactivates, allowing g_l to pull V_m back to rest.

Mathematical Formulation

The equation describing the circuit in Figure 2 is:

$$C \frac{dV_m}{dt} = g_l(E_l - V_m) + g_{Na}(E_{Na} - V_m) + g_K(E_K - V_m) \quad (1)$$

While g_l is constant, g_{Na} and g_K are time and voltage dependent:

$$g_{Na} = \bar{G}_{Na} \cdot m(t)^3 h(t)$$
$$g_K = \bar{G}_K \cdot n(t)^4$$

where the constants $\bar{G}_{Na}$ and $\bar{G}_K$ are the maximal conductances and the time and voltage dependence reside in the so-called *gating variables*, described by the state variables m, h, and n. These fictitious variables follow first-order kinetics, relaxing exponentially toward a steady-state value x_∞ with a time constant τ_x:

$$\frac{dm}{dt} = \frac{m_\infty(V_m) - m}{\tau_m(V_m)}$$
$$\frac{dh}{dt} = \frac{h_\infty(V_m) - h}{\tau_h(V_m)}$$
$$\frac{dn}{dt} = \frac{n_\infty(V_m) - n}{\tau_n(V_m)}$$

Figure 3. Action potential. Computed action potential in response to a 0.5-ms current pulse of 0.4-nA amplitude (solid lines) compared to a subthreshold response following a 0.35-nA current pulse (dashed lines). *A*, Time course of the two ionic currents. Note their large sizes compared to the stimulating current. *B*, Membrane potential in response to sub- and suprathreshold stimuli. The injected current charges up the membrane capacity (with an effective membrane time constant $\tau = 0.85$ ms), enabling sufficient I_{Na} to be recruited to outweigh the increase in I_K (due to the increase in driving potential). The smaller current pulse fails to trigger an action potential, but causes a depolarization followed by a small hyperpolarization due to activation of I_K. *C*, Dynamics of the gating variables. Sodium activation m changes much more rapidly than either h or n. The long time course of potassium activation n explains why the membrane potential takes 12 ms after the potential has first dipped below the resting potential to return to baseline level. (From Koch, C., 1999, *Biophysics of Computation*, Cambridge, MA: MIT Press, p. 150.)

The steady-state activations (m_∞, h_∞, and n_∞) have a sigmoidal dependence on voltage. The *activation* variables m and n have the asymptotes $\lim_{V_m \to -\infty} m_\infty, n_\infty = 0$, $\lim_{V_m \to \infty} m_\infty, n_\infty = 1$, while the reverse holds for the *inactivation* variable h. That is, for very negative voltages, the m and n variables shut off current flow through both channel types, while at very positive potentials, the h particle shuts off the sodium current. The time "constants" (τ_m, τ_h, and τ_n)

are not constant with respect to voltage but rather have a roughly bell-shaped dependence, with peaks in the −80 to −40 mV range. The x_∞ and τ_x values were the ones actually measured by Hodgkin and Huxley using a series of voltage clamp steps. Instead of fitting these curves directly with mathematical functions, which would be sufficient for simulation purposes, they chose to express x_∞ and τ_x in terms of the variables α_x and β_x:

$$x_\infty = \frac{\alpha_x}{\alpha_x + \beta_x}$$

$$\tau_x = \frac{1}{\alpha_x + \beta_x}$$

where α_x and β_x depend on V_m as follows:

$$\alpha_m = \frac{0.1(V_m - 40)}{e^{(V_m - 40)/10} - 1} \qquad \beta_m = 4e^{(V_m - 65)/18}$$

$$\alpha_h = 0.07e^{(V_m - 65)/20} \qquad \beta_h = \frac{1}{e^{(V_m - 35)/10} + 1}$$

$$\alpha_n = \frac{0.01(V_m - 55)}{e^{(V_m - 55)/10} - 1} \qquad \beta_n = 0.125e^{(V_m - 65)/80}$$

Note that the dimensions of τ_x, α_x, and β_x are all in units of 1/s, while n_x is a pure number.

These rate constants assume a temperature of 6.3°C. At higher temperatures, they should be multiplied by a factor of around 3 per 10°C. The functional forms were chosen by Hodgkin and Huxley for two reasons. First, they were among the simplest that fit the data, and second, they resemble the equations that govern the movement of a charged particle in a constant field.

There is no direct way to map this set of equations in a simple manner onto the known molecular correlates of ionic channels, except that many voltage-dependent ionic channels possess four identical subunits, close or identical to the exponent of the activation variable that determines the momentary conductance. How the molecular structure and physical chemistry of these membrane pores explain the high throughput (up to 10^8 ions per second) and selectivity (the potassium channel is at least 10,000 times more permeant to K^+ than to Na^+ ions) has been revealed in stunning detail for potassium channels by atomic-resolution pictures of them (Doyle et al., 1998).

Conceptually, $x_\infty(V_m)$ can be thought of as the probability that an x particle will be in the open state at potential V_m. Each particle follows a two-state Markov model, where α_x is the rate constant from the closed to the open state and β_x is the rate constant from the open to the closed state. The time courses of the three variables are graphed in Figure 3.

This mathematical formalism was laid down in 1952. Since then, most models of voltage-dependent conductances—not only in axons, but also in cell bodies, and dendrites—have used the same formalism, with only minor modifications (Koch and Segev, 1998).

The macroscopic Hodgkin-Huxley equations are both continuous and deterministic, yet the underlying microscopic ionic channels are binary and stochastic. That is, a correct biophysical formulation of the dynamics of the membrane potential needs to take into account the well-known probabilistic behavior of these ionic channels. However, given the large number of channels involved in axonal spike initiation and propagation, it is usually appropriate to approximate the system using the deterministic Hodgkin-Huxley equations. This is not to say, however, that for thin fibers with very high input impedances, a small number of channels, and close to the threshold, stochastic variation in channel behavior might not have large-scale effects on the timing of action potentials (Schneidman, Freedman, and Segev, 1998; Koch, 1999).

Action Potential Propagation

Equation 1 describes a patch of membrane with no spatial extent. This corresponds to the original experiments, in which the axon was "space-clamped": a long electrode was inserted into the axon along its axis, removing any spatial dependence. In response to stimulation, the whole membrane would fire simultaneously as a single isopotential unit. More commonly, one end of the axon is stimulated and an action potential propagates to the other end. The equation that governs extended structures is the cable equation:

$$C\frac{\partial V_m}{\partial t} = \frac{d}{R_a}\frac{\partial^2 V_m}{\partial x^2} + g_l(E_l - V_m)$$
$$+ g_{Na}(E_{Na} - V_m) + g_K(E_K - V_m) \qquad (2)$$

where d is the axon diameter, C is the membrane capacity, and R_a is the intracellular resistivity. The equation rests on the assumption of radial symmetry, i.e., radial current flow can be neglected, leaving only one spatial dimension, the distance x along the cable, in addition to t. If the last two (active) terms are dropped from the right-hand side, we are left with the classical cable equation for passive cables (see DENDRITIC PROCESSING). Associated with that equation is the *space constant* $\lambda = 1/\sqrt{g_l R_a}$, which is the distance across which the membrane potential decays a factor e in an infinite cable under steady-state conditions.

Figure 4 shows the result of a simulation of a 100-cm-long axon of diameter $d = 1$ mm. One end was stimulated with a brief current pulse and the voltage was graphed for five positions along the axon. The form of the action potential is very similar to that in Figure 3; furthermore, the action potential is self-similar as it propagates, showing no signs of dispersion.

The total delay from one end to the other is about 5 ms, giving an average velocity of about 20 m/s. By assuming a constant conduction velocity—that is, by postulating the existence of a wave, $V_m(x, t) = V_m(x - vt)$—Equation 2 shows that the velocity is proportional to the square root of axon diameter: $v \propto \sqrt{d}$ (Rushton, 1951). Indeed, in a truly remarkable test of their model, Hodgkin and Huxley estimated the velocity to be 18.8 m/s, a value within 10% of the experimental value of 21.2 m/s. This is surprisingly

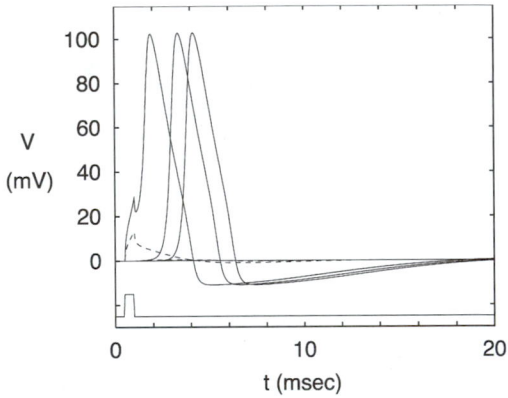

Figure 4. A propagating action potential. Solution to the complete Hodgkin-Huxley model for a long piece of squid axon for a brief suprathreshold current pulse. This pulse generates an action potential that travels down the cable and is shown here at the origin as well as 2 and 3 cm away from the stimulating electrode (solid lines). Note that the shape of the action potential remains invariant due to the nonlinear membrane. If the amplitude of the current pulse is halved, only a local depolarization is generated (dashed curve), which depolarizes the membrane 2 cm away by a mere 0.5 mV (not shown). This illustrates the dramatic difference between active and passive voltage propagation. (From Koch, C., 1999, *Biophysics of Computation*, Cambridge, MA: MIT Press, p. 162.)

accurate, considering that the model was derived from a space-clamped axon. This represents one of the rare instances in which a neurobiological model has made a successful quantitative prediction. The square root relationship had been discovered experimentally in the squid in the late 1930s.

Myelinated and Nonmyelinated Fibers

The principle of action potential generation and propagation appears to be very similar across neuronal types and species. One important evolutionary invention is that of myelination in the vertebrate phylum. Myelin sheaths are white fatty extensions of Schwann cells or neuroglial cells that are wrapped in many layers around axons. Myelin is a major component of the *white matter* of the brain, as opposed to the gray matter of neocortex, which has a high concentration of cell bodies and dendrites. The myelin sheaths extend for up to 1–2 mm along the axon (the *internodes*) and are separated by the *nodes of Ranvier*, which are only a few micrometers long. The internodal distance appears to be approximately linear in fiber diameter.

Myelin insulates the axon from the surrounding medium, increasing the membrane resistance and decreasing the capacitance. This reduces the electrotonic length of the axon for both DC and AC signals, making the cable electrically shorter, thereby significantly increasing the propagation speed. While a 1-mm nonmyelinated axon in the squid has an associated propagation speed of only about 20 m/s (Hodgkin and Huxley, 1952), a myelinated 20-μm vertebrate axon can reach over 100 m/s. For a nonmyelinated axon to reach that velocity, it would have to be an inch thick! This reduction in axon diameter allows for a much higher packing density while conserving speed.

It has been shown both experimentally and theoretically that the velocity of propagation is linear or slightly sublinear in the fiber diameter for myelinated axons. Figure 5 compares the spike propagation velocity for myelinated and nonmyelinated axons for small diameters. The myelinated axons overtake nonmyelinated ones already in the submicrometer range.

As opposed to their uniform distribution in nonmyelinated nerve, the voltage-gated channels in myelinated nerve are highly segregated between node and internode (Hille, 1992). The nodal membrane has a high concentration of fast sodium channels (between 700 and 2,000 per μm^2) and voltage-independent leak channels. The internodal membrane has a low concentration of potassium and leak channels and is virtually devoid of sodium channels. Here, the repolarization of the membrane following the initial phase of the spike is via the leak channels and sodium inactivation. This low density of channels in the internodal membrane, which makes up the more than 99% of the axonal membrane, reduces the average current density across the membrane, resulting in great savings in metabolic energy. Most of the activity occurs at the nodes of Ranvier, while the propagation along the internodes is chiefly passive.

In summary, myelin provides three advantages: propagation speed and packing density are both dramatically increased, while power consumption is decreased.

The Axonal Tree

Some axons branch profusely in the vicinity of the cell body. Others send off one or a few branches that course through the body for up to a meter before branching. Others extend for a few millimeters, giving rise to axonal arbors at regular intervals. The axon often arises at the "axon hillock," a somatic bulge opposite from the trunk of the dendritic tree, though other arrangements are possible, such as the axon's emanating from the dendrite rather than the soma.

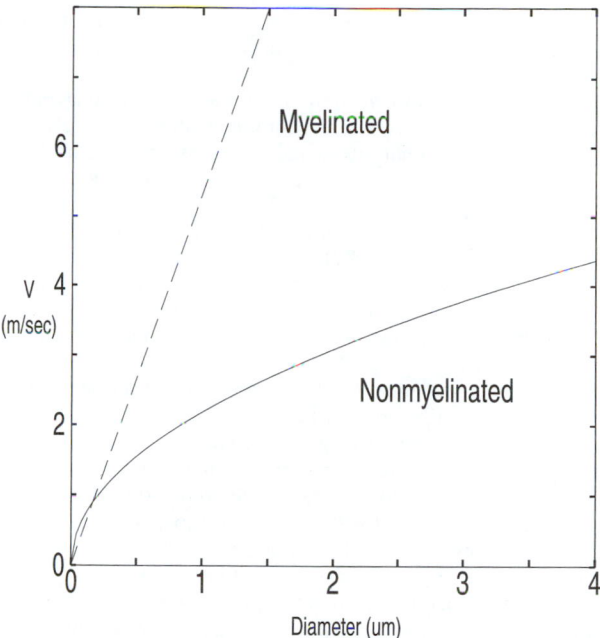

Figure 5. Spike propagation velocity and axonal diameter. The propagation velocity has a square root dependence on diameter for nonmyelinated axons. For myelinated axons, the dependence is linear or slightly sublinear. Myelination increases velocity for axons as thin as 0.2 μm, which are among the smallest found in the brain. (Adapted from Waxman and Bennett, 1972.)

Figure 1 shows an example of a terminal arbor in turtle tectum from a cell originating in nucleus isthmi. This particular axon has a 3-μm myelinated parent trunk and initial daughter branches. These give rise to hundreds of thin, highly varicosed daughter branches that lack myelin. The varicosities are usually the location of synaptic boutons, a local thickening where action potentials trigger the release of neurotransmitter, which in turn induces a conductance change in the postsynaptic target neuron. Boutons of some neurons may receive synaptic input that can inhibit this signal transmission, a process known as presynaptic inhibition. The 3,600 boutons on this arbor average 1.5 μm in diameter, though the size is highly variable, with a few boutons being as large as 7 μm.

The propagation speed along an unbranched axon depends on the diameter, as discussed earlier. In addition, a delay might be introduced at branch points, at varicosities at presynaptic terminals, and at locations where the diameter changes abruptly (Manor, Koch, and Segev, 1991). The delay may be negative (a speed-up), depending on the geometrical aspects, in particular the diameter of the parent branch in relation to that of the daughter branches. In a simulation of a 3.5-mm-long branched terminal axonal tree, Manor et al. found that the total axonal delay from the cell body to the synaptic terminals ranged from about 3 ms to 6 ms. Most of this delay (67%–78%) arose from the properties of unbranched, uniform cables; 16%–26% resulted from branch point delays, and 6%–7% from the presence of varicosities. In theory, the delay at a single branch point may be as large as 2 ms or more, if the temperature is low and the impedance mismatch is large. If the mismatch is too large, however, *branch point failure* may occur, a condition in which the action potential fails to propagate beyond the branch point. The concept of branch point filtering has been put forth by Chung, Raymond, and Lettvin (1970): the branch point may constitute a point of control where selective transmission occurs, allowing the axonal tree to distribute action potentials only to a subset of nerve terminals. Experimentally, little is known concerning the amplitude of temporal dispersion of action potentials due to axonal branching.

While the axonal propagation delay may seem an unavoidable fact of life that slows down neural communication, it may also have important computational advantages. For instance, sound localization (see SOUND LOCALIZATION AND BINAURAL PROCESSING) in the barn owl depends on interaural time differences as small as a tenth of a millisecond and is apparently obtained by using the axon as a delay line (Konishi, 1992), and several models of brain function depend critically on the exact timing of inputs from different sources. Although delays may be imposed by the dendritic trees at the input end of the neuron, the axons are also important candidates for this function.

Debanne and colleagues (1997) discovered that action potentials can be selectively filtered at or beyond axonal branch points via a fast-inactivating A-type of potassium conductance. When a cell is hyperpolarized, a depolarizing step within 10–20 ms that would normally trigger an action potential fails to do so in hippocampal cell bodies. The reason for this selective block is a G_A-like K^+ conductance present somewhere along the axon. If de-inactivated by long-lasting hyperpolarization, it filters out single isolated spikes. It could thereby act to enhance the signal-to-noise ratio of neuronal firing. To what extent this is a general mechanism or an exception to the rule that axons faithfully transmit action potentials from their site of initiation close to the cell body to their postsynaptic target structures remains to be seen.

Over the past several decades, the formalism introduced by Hodgkin and Huxley in 1952—voltage- and time-dependent activation and inactivation variables that determine the current value of the various membrane conductances—has become the de facto standard for modeling an amazing variety of phenomena, including adaptation, calcium-dependent conductances, plateau potentials, first- and second-order inactivation, oscillatory discharges, and several varieties of bursting.

Road Maps: Biological Neurons and Synapses; Grounding Models of Neurons
Related Reading: Activity-Dependent Regulation of Neuronal Conductances; Ion Channels: Keys to Neuronal Specialization; Oscillatory and Bursting Properties of Neurons

References

Chung, S. H., Raymond, S. A., and Lettvin, J. Y., 1970, Multiple meaning in single visual units, *Brain Behav. Evol.*, 3:72–101.

Debanne, D., Guérineau, N. C., Gähwiler, B. H., and Thompson, S. M., 1997, Action-potential propagation gated by an axonal I_A-like K^+ conductance in hippocampus, *Nature*, 389:286–289.

Doyle, D. A., Cabral, J. M., Pfuetzner, R. A., Kuo, A., Gulbis, J. M., Cohen, S. L., Chait, B. T., and MacKinnon, R., 1998, The structure of the potassium channel: Molecular basis of K^+ conduction and selectivity, *Science*, 280:69–77.

Hille, B., 1992, *Ionic Channels of Excitable Membranes*, 2nd ed., Sunderland, MA: Sinauer. ◆

Hodgkin, A. L., 1976, Chance and design in electrophysiology: An informal account of certain experiments on nerve carried out between 1934 and 1952, *J. Physiol.*, 263:1–21.

Hodgkin, A. L., and Huxley, A. F., 1952, A quantitative description of membrane current and its application to conduction and excitation in nerve, *J. Physiol.*, 117:500–544.

Kandel, E. R., Schwartz, J. H., and Jessell, T. M., Eds., 2000, *Principles of Neural Science*, 4th ed., New York: McGraw-Hill.

Koch, C., 1999, *Biophysics of Computation*, Cambridge, MA: MIT Press. ◆

Koch, C., and Segev, I., Eds., 1998, *Methods in Neuronal Modeling*, 2nd ed., Cambridge, MA: MIT Press.

Konishi, M., 1992, The neural algorithm for sound localization in the owl, *Harvey Lect.*, 86:47–64.

Manor, Y., Koch, C., and Segev, I., 1991, Effect of geometrical irregularities on propagation delay in axonal trees, *Biophys. J.*, 60:1424–1437.

Roberts, A., and Bush, B. M. H., Eds., 1981, *Neurones without Impulses: Their Significance for Vertebrates*, Cambridge, Engl.: Cambridge University Press. ◆

Rushton, W. A. H., 1951, A theory of the effects of fibre size in medullated nerve, *J. Physiol.*, 115:101–122.

Schneidman, E., Freedman, B., and Segev, I., 1998, Ionic channel stochasticity may be critical in determining the reliability and precision of spike timing, *Neural Computat.*, 10:1679–1704.

Sereno, M. I., and Ulinski, P. S., 1987, Caudal topographic nucleus isthmi and the rostral nontopographic nucleus isthmi in the turtle, *Pseudemys scripta, J. Comp. Neurol.*, 261:319–346.

Waxman, S. G., and Bennett, M. V. L., 1972, Relative conduction velocities of small myelinated and non-myelinated fibers in the central nervous system, *Nature*, 238:217–219.

Waxman, S. G., Kocsis, J. D., and Stys, P. K., Eds., 1995, *The Axon: Structure, Function and Pathophysiology*, New York: Oxford University Press. ◆

Axonal Path Finding

Geoffrey J. Goodhill

Introduction

Many stages are involved in constructing a biological nervous system. Following the migration of neurons to their proper locations and their phenotypic specification, the initial pattern of connections forms between different regions (Sanes, Reh, and Harris, 2000). Making the right connections is crucial for proper function, and often requires axons to navigate over long distances with great precision (Tessier-Lavigne and Goodman, 1996). Until recently, relatively little was known about this process experimentally; however, the past decade has seen a dramatic increase in knowledge (at least qualitatively) concerning the molecules and mechanisms involved (Mueller, 1999). These insights are now being applied to understanding how axons can be made to regenerate to appropriate

targets after injury to the adult nervous system, such as spinal cord injury.

Until now, the bulk of theoretical work in the neural network tradition has focused on changes in synaptic strengths within a fixed connectional architecture. Although local sprouting within the target has sometimes been considered (as has "sculpting," based on the assumption that when synaptic strengths go to zero, the physical connection is lost), how axons chart their initial path toward the correct target structure has generally not been addressed. An example is the mapping from the eye to more central targets in the brain. Abundant theoretical models address how topographic maps form once axons reach the tectum or visual cortex (see DEVELOPMENT OF RETINOTECTAL MAPS; SELF-ORGANIZING FEATURE MAPS; and OCULAR DOMINANCE AND ORIENTATION COLUMNS), but no theoretical work specifically addresses how retinal ganglion cell axons find the optic disc, how they then exit the retina, why they grow toward the optic chiasm, why some then cross at the midline while others do not, and so on. In recent years important insight into such issues has been gained through innovative experimental work, creating a body of knowledge that now has the potential to be framed and interpreted in terms of theoretical models. A crucial point is that, whereas work in neural networks has usually focused on processes such as synaptic plasticity that are dependent on neural activity, models for axon guidance must generally be phrased in terms of activity-independent mechanisms, particularly guidance by molecular gradients. In this article we first review some of the important experimental data regarding axon guidance, and then discuss some of the theoretical concepts that are relevant to this area.

Experimental Data

Several basic types of mechanisms have been identified to guide axons. (For more detailed discussions of the data summarized in this section, see Tessier-Lavigne and Goodman, 1996; Mueller, 1999; and Song and Poo, 2001.) First, axons can be channeled in particular directions by boundaries of permissive or inhibitory molecules. For instance, a "railroad track" of a permissive molecule may lock an axon into a particular trajectory, or a "wall" of an inhibitory molecule may keep it away from an undesired region. Second, axons can be pushed or pulled by "vector" signals in the form of molecular gradients. These gradients are often established by diffusion of a soluble molecule away from the target region. Third, the path to a distant target may be broken into several short segments, each involving a different type of cue, thus simplifying the problem of long-range guidance. Fourth, once one "pioneering" axon has reached the target, it is often the case that following axons simply fasciculate with (stick to) the pioneering axon. In each of these cases the molecules involved may be substrate-bound (expressed on cell membranes or bound to cells or to the extracellular space) or diffusible (diffusing through the extracellular space).

In the last few years the number of molecules specifically implicated in axon guidance has jumped from virtually none to around 100, most of them previously unknown. (Note that we distinguish between *guidance factors* and *growth factors*: the latter category, which includes the neurotrophins, are often essential for axons to extend, but so far have mostly not been shown to play an active role in axon guidance in vivo.) Guidance factors can be organized into several main families based on their molecular structure, including the netrins, semaphorins, slits, and ephrins. There is an astonishing amount of evolutionary conservation in these families. Homologous molecules perform analogous guidance functions in animals ranging from nematodes to flies to mammals, indicating that the basic molecular tools for wiring a nervous system were established hundreds of millions of years ago. Molecules involved in axon guidance are also often involved in the analogous chemotactic event of cell migration, and recent findings even suggest some commonality with the signal transduction mechanisms important for chemotaxis of leukocytes. Although it was originally thought that the different types of guidance mechanisms might be segregated between different families of molecules, it is now clear that this is not the case. For instance, the same molecule can be attractive in one context but repulsive in another, or it may normally be substrate-bound but have a soluble fragment that can diffuse.

Guidance signals for axons are detected and transduced by the growth cone, a dynamic and motile structure at the tip of the developing axon. This consists of a central region surrounded by web-like veils called lamellipodia, and long, finger-like protrusions called filopodia (Figure 1A). Receptors expressed on the surface of the growth cone can bind molecules of the families mentioned above. The resulting signals are then converted by complex internal transduction pathways into differential rates of actin polymerization in different parts of the growth cone so as to move it forward, left, or right. Dissection of the signaling networks responsible for converting a graded difference in receptor binding into directed movement is currently a very active area of research. One intriguing finding is that the concentration of cAMP within the growth cone

A   **B**

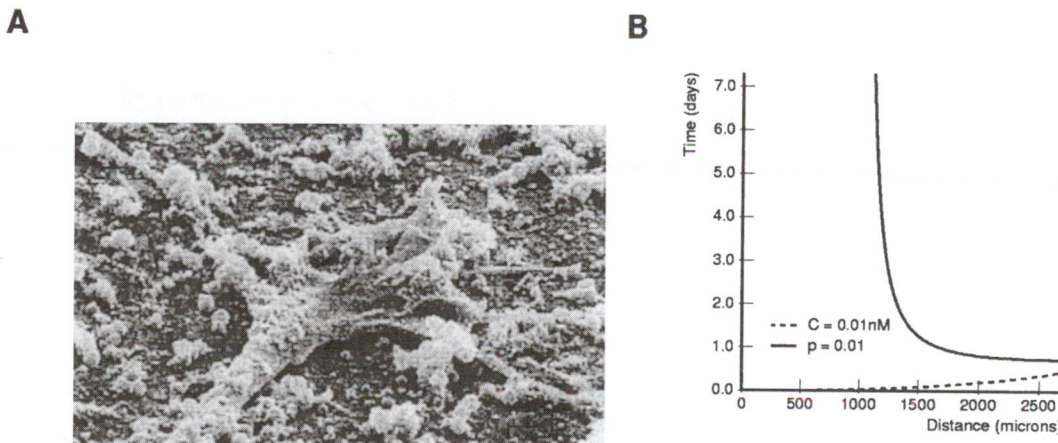

Figure 1. *A*, Electron micrograph of a growth cone at the end of an axon (here the growth cone is resting on a surface irregularly covered with coated beads). The long finger-like protrusions are filopodia. Growth cones are typically about 0.01 mm across. (From Rosentreter, S. M., Davenport, R. W., Löschinger, J. Huf, J., Jung, J., and Bonhoeffer, F., 1998, Response of retinal ganglion cell axons to striped linear gradients of repellent guidance molecules, *J. Neurobiol.*, 37:541–562. © 1998, John Wiley & Sons, Inc. Reprinted with permission.) *B*, Interaction of constraints for guidance by a target-derived diffusible factor. The graph shows, at each distance, the time at which two constraints are satisfied: the low concentration limit, where not enough receptors are bound for a gradient signal to be detected (assumed to be $K_D/100$, with $K_D = 1$ nM), and the fractional change constraint (assumed to be $\Delta C/C = 1\%$). The region between the two curves in each graph is where guidance is possible. The guidance limit imposed by the fractional change constraint once the gradient has stabilized is 1 mm. However, guidance range is extended at earlier times, when the fractional change constraint has yet to take full effect.

helps determine how the growth cone responds to a gradient cue: if the cAMP level is above a certain threshold, the growth cone is attracted; if the cAMP level is below that threshold, the growth cone is repelled.

Theoretical Models

Gradient Detection

Several different areas of theoretical development are relevant to the emerging picture of axon guidance. The general topic of chemotaxis has inspired a large body of theoretical analysis. However, most work has focused on bacteria and leukocytes, and it remains to be established how relevant these models are to axon guidance. Perhaps most important in this category are theories describing the fundamental physical limits on the minimum steepness of gradients detectable by *any* small sensing device. The key hypothesis, first rigorously formulated by Berg and Purcell (1977), is that gradient detection is limited by inherent statistical fluctuations in receptor binding. They calculated the statistical noise in a concentration measurement ΔC_{noise} by a small sensing device that arises from inevitable stochastic variations in the number of receptors bound at any instant. The fractional root mean square error in the measurement of a concentration difference between two spatially or temporally separated points is then $\sqrt{2}\Delta C_{\text{noise}}/C$, where C is the average concentration at the sensing device. For a true gradient to be detected, it must be steep enough so that the actual concentration difference between the two points, ΔC_{grad}, is such that $\Delta C_{\text{grad}} > \sqrt{2}\Delta C_{\text{noise}}$. $\Delta C_{\text{noise}}/C$ can be calculated from first principles using various simplifying assumptions. This approach has been applied to growth cones by Goodhill and Urbach (1999), who derived estimates for the minimum gradient steepness detectable by an axon for a diffusible gradient of order 1% and for a substrate-bound gradient of order 10%. The difference arises because of the lower encounter rate between receptor and ligand molecules for a bound versus a diffusible gradient. Goodhill and Urbach (1999) also showed that the movement of filopodia does not significantly increase the encounter rate, which suggests that filopodia increase gradient sensitivity only by increasing the effective size of the growth cone. However, this approach assumes that the receptor-ligand reaction is diffusion-limited, which may not be the case for the molecules involved in axon guidance. Theoretical work following Berg and Purcell (1977), while still generally founded on the basic assumption that gradient detection is limited by the signal-to-noise ratio, has attempted to relax this and some other assumptions, but these models have not yet been specifically applied to growth cones.

Growth Cones

Theoretical models have been proposed to account for filopodial dynamics. Based on experimentally determined distributions for parameters such as rates of filopodial initiation, extension, and retraction, filopodial length, and angular orientation, Buettner and colleagues (e.g., Buettner, 1995) have developed simulation models describing filopodial structure as a function of time, and growth cone trajectories both during normal growth and when a target is encountered. Goodhill and Urbach (1999) presented a model of growth cone trajectories based on the assumption that each filopodium makes a noisy (in Berg and Purcell's sense) estimate of the concentration in the direction it is pointing, that more filopodia are generated in the direction of higher concentration, and that each filopodium exerts a pull on the growth cone. Other models have proposed hypotheses about how actin and microtubule dynamics lead to filopodia formation, though these models have yet to fully engage with what is known about these processes experimentally.

Another theoretically interesting aspect of growth cones is the signaling events that convert a small difference in receptor binding into a large directed movement. Meinhardt (1999) and others have proposed reaction-diffusion-type models in which a small inhomogeneity in an initially uniform system is amplified via the interaction of a short-range activator with a longer-range inhibitor. However, to return the system to a uniform state so that the directional preference of the growth cone can change with time, a second type of reaction with a longer time constant is invoked, and direct experimental evidence for such processes in growth cones is currently lacking. Tranquillo and Lauffenburger (1987), in the context of leukocyte chemotaxis, simulated and analyzed a model in which two pools of receptors (one on each side of the cell) communicated information about the degree of binding via a single intracellular messenger. This model was quite successful at accounting for various aspects of leukocyte movement, and subsequent versions by Tranquillo and colleagues have examined more complex assumptions regarding the internal signaling dynamics. Bacterial chemotaxis has been extensively studied from the perspective of signal transduction, and theoretical models have been effective at explaining the large amount now known experimentally about this system. A major focus of such models has been to explain the process by which bacteria adapt to background levels of ligand so that they can detect small changes in concentration over many orders of magnitude of absolute concentration. Although such analyses of signaling mechanisms in other chemotacting systems have the potential to be applied to growth cones, it is unclear how similar these systems really are. More generally there is increasing interest in mathematical modeling of the signal transduction pathways underlying cell behavior as a whole, although again, there is little application as yet of these theoretical ideas to axon guidance.

Diffusible Gradients and Optimal Gradients

An important class of gradients for guiding axons both in vivo and in vitro consists of gradients established by diffusion. Hentschel and van Ooyen (1999) investigated a possible role for diffusion in controlling axon fasciculation. They considered a population of axons being guided by a target-derived diffusible factor, and hypothesized that in addition, each axon releases a diffusible attractant that pulls it toward the other axons, hence leading to fasciculation as they grow together toward the target. To account for defasciculation at the target, they hypothesized that each axon also releases a repulsive factor for other axons at a rate dependent on the concentration of the target-derived factor. As the axons approach the target, this repulsive force overcomes the attractive force, leading to defasciculation.

Another approach is to analyze the gradient shapes expected from diffusion processes in particular situations and how these constrain the spatiotemporal domains in which guidance is possible (see Goodhill, 1998, for a review). Goodhill considered a source releasing a diffusible factor at a constant rate into an infinite, spatially uniform three-dimensional volume, a problem for which there is a closed-form solution. As long as the gradient is not too steep, the fractional change in concentration $\Delta C/C$ across the growth cone width a is $\Delta C/C = (\partial C/\partial r)(a/C)$, and can be straightforwardly calculated. It has the perhaps surprising characteristic that, for fixed r, $\Delta C/C$ *decreases* with t. That is, the largest fractional change at any distance occurs immediately after the source starts releasing factor. For large t, $\Delta C/C$ asymptotes at a/r. Thus: (1) At small times after the start of production the factor is very unevenly distributed. The concentration C falls quickly to almost zero moving away from the source, the gradient is steep, and the percentage change across the growth cone $\Delta C/C$ is everywhere large. (2) As time passes, the factor becomes more evenly distributed. C everywhere increases, but $\Delta C/C$ everywhere decreases. (3) For large times, C tends to an inverse variation with the distance from the source r, while $\Delta C/C$ tends to a/r independent of all other parameters. The equation for $\Delta C/C$ can be compared with the size of the smallest gradient the growth cone can detect to yield the regions of parameter space found in which guidance is possible (Figure 1B). Based on data for leukocyte chemotaxis it was assumed that gradient detection occurs when $\Delta C/C \geq p$ and $C \geq C_{\min}$, where p is a threshold assumed independent of C. The positions and times for which the gradient calculated above satisfies these criteria were examined, given appropriate estimates for the relevant parameters. For large times (a few days) after the start of factor production, the maximum range is independent of the diffusion constant and is about 1 mm. This value fits well with both in vitro and in vivo observations. At earlier times, however, the factor is more unevenly distributed, being more concentrated around the source. This makes the fractional change larger than at later times, increasing the range over which guidance can occur. Depending on the parameters, the model predicts that guidance may be possible at distances of several millimeters before the distribution of factor equilibrates. It is conceivable that such a mechanism might be utilized in vivo to extend guidance range beyond the 1 mm limit imposed once the gradient has stabilized.

Similarly, one may inquire as to the optimal gradient shape, in the sense of the shape that guides an axon over the largest possible distance. Assuming the minimal fractional change is constant (not dependent on absolute concentration), the optimal shape is clearly exponential; the maximum guidance distance turns out to be about 1 cm (Goodhill, 1998). It is conceivable that substrate-bound gradients could achieve this shape, and in fact the size of the chick tectum at the time retinotectal maps are forming is about 1 cm. Assuming instead that the minimal fractional change varies with concentration, as predicted by Berg and Purcell, and also assuming a high concentration limit, the order of magnitude of the result remains at 1 cm (Goodhill and Urbach, 1999). More generally, this type of analysis raises the issue of overall scaling between different species. A guidance mechanism (e.g., target-derived diffusible gradient) that works for a small animal will not work in a large animal if the anatomy is simply scaled up. In general, the scale and structure of the anatomy of, say, the elephant nervous system at the time at which long-range navigation occurs are not known in sufficient detail to allow proper comparison with the same features in, say, the rat.

Retinotectal Maps

The most well-developed area of axon guidance modeling concerns the formation of topographic maps in the optic tectum (reviewed in Goodhill and Richards, 1999). The hypothesis of chemospecificity, that graded distributions of molecules are somehow matched to graded distributions of complementary molecules in the tectum so as to form a topographic map, was first proposed qualitatively by Sperry (1963). Although a great deal of experimental work ensued to investigate how such gradients may actually operate, matched gradients of receptors in the retina and ligands in the tectum were discovered only in the mid-1990s. These receptors/ligands are of the Eph/ephrin family, which currently are under intense experimental investigation. Theoretical modeling started in the 1970s (e.g., Willshaw and von der Malsburg, 1979), and early models were based directly on molecular gradients. A key finding was that some kind of normalization is essential to prevent all axons

from targeting the same part of tectum. Although modeling based on gradients has continued (e.g., Gierer, 1987), the focus of most modeling work changed to activity-dependent processes. Here only synaptic strength changes within a fixed architecture are generally considered, rather than the earlier stage of how axons traverse large expanses of the tectum. Data and models in this area are discussed in greater detail in DEVELOPMENT OF RETINOTECTAL MAPS (q.v.).

Discussion

Current experimental work in axon guidance is dominated by techniques and hypotheses at the molecular level. The data are also rapidly evolving, with new molecules and mechanisms important for guidance being discovered at a very fast rate. However, many fundamental questions remain unresolved, and theoretical models have the potential to make an important contribution to answering these questions. What is the minimum gradient steepness detectable by a growth cone, and how does this vary with the properties of the receptor-ligand interaction and the internal state of the growth cone? How is a graded difference in receptor binding internally converted into a signal for directed movement? How do axons integrate multiple cues? And, perhaps most relevant to human health, how can regenerating axons be encouraged to grow toward and reconnect with appropriate targets after injury?

Road Map: Neural Plasticity
Related Reading: Development of Retinotectal Maps

References

Berg, H. C., and Purcell, E. M., 1977, Physics of chemoreception, *Biophys. J.*, 20:193–219.

Buettner, H. M., 1995, Computer simulation of nerve growth cone filopodial dynamics for visualization and analysis. *Cell Motil. Cytoskelet.*, 32:187–204.

Gierer, A., 1987, Directional cues for growing axons forming the retinotectal projection, *Development*, 101:479–489.

Goodhill, G. J., 1998, Mathematical guidance for axons, *Trends Neurosci.*, 21:226–231. ◆

Goodhill, G. J., and Richards, L. J., 1999, Retinotectal maps: Molecules, models, and misplaced data, *Trends Neurosci.*, 22:529–534.

Goodhill, G. J., and Urbach, J. S., 1999, Theoretical analysis of gradient detection by growth cones, *J. Neurobiol.*, 41:230–241.

Hentschel, H. G. E., and van Ooyen, A., 1999, Models of axon guidance and bundling during development, *Proc. R. Soc. Lond. B*, 266:2231–2238.

Meinhardt, H., 1999, Orientation of chemotactic cells and growth cones: Models and mechanisms, *J. Cell Sci.*, 112:2867–2874.

Mueller, B. K., 1999, Growth cone guidance: First steps towards a deeper understanding. *Annu. Rev. Neurosci.*, 22:351–388. ◆

Sanes, D. H., Reh, T. A., and Harris, W. A., 2000, *Development of the Nervous System*, San Diego, CA: Academic Press.

Song, H., and Poo, M-M., 2001, The cell biology of neuronal navigation, *Nature Cell. Biol.*, 3:E81–E88.

Sperry, R. W., 1963, Chemoaffinity in the orderly growth of nerve fiber patterns and connections, *Proc. Natl. Acad. Sci. USA*, 50:703–710.

Tessier-Lavigne, M., and Goodman, C. S., 1996, The molecular biology of axon guidance, *Science*, 274:1123–1133. ◆

Tranquillo, R. T., and Lauffenburger, D. A., 1987, Stochastic model of leukocyte chemosensory movement, *J. Math. Biol.*, 25:229–262.

Willshaw, D. J., and von der Malsburg, C., 1979, A marker induction mechanism for the establishment of ordered neural mappings: Its application to the retinotectal problem, *Philos. Trans. R. Soc. B*, 287:203–243.

Backpropagation: General Principles

Michael A. Arbib

Introduction

Perceptrons are neural nets that use an *error-correction* rule to change the weights of each unit that makes erroneous responses to stimuli that are presented to the network. As already explained in PERCEPTRONS, ADALINES, AND BACKPROPAGATION (q.v.) and Section I.3: "Dynamics and Adaptation in Neural Networks," *backpropagation* is a family of methods for training a *multilayer perceptron*, a loop-free network that has its units arranged in layers, with each unit providing input only to units in the next layer of the sequence. The first layer comprises input units; there may then be several layers of trainable "hidden units" carrying an internal representation, and finally there is the layer of output units, also with trainable synaptic weights.

Rumelhart, Hinton, and Williams (1986) is the most influential paper on the error backpropagation method, providing a formula (see the Proposition below) for propagating back the gradient of error evaluation from a unit to the units that provide its inputs. Since the formulas involve derivatives, the input and output of each unit must take continuous values in some range, here taken to be [0, 1]. The response is a sigmoidal function of the weighted sum. Werbos (1995) provides a historical perspective on precursors of their paper. As a specific example of such a precursor, LEARNING AND STATISTICAL INFERENCE (q.v.) presents a general stochastic descent on-line learning procedure (Amari, 1967), which, when applied to the multilayer perceptron, yields the error backpropagation method.

Proposition. Consider a layered loop-free net with error $E = \Sigma_k(t_k - o_k)^2$, where k ranges over designated output units, and let the weights w_{ij} be changed according to the gradient descent rule

$$\Delta w_{ij} = -\frac{\partial E}{\partial w_{ij}} = 2 \sum_k (t_k - o_k) \frac{\partial o_k}{\partial w_{ij}}$$

Then the weights may be changed inductively, working back from the output units, by the rule Δw_{ij} is proportional to $\delta_i o_j$, where

Basis Step: $\delta_i = (t_i - o_i)f'_i$ for an output unit.

Induction Step: If i is a hidden unit, and if δ_k is known for all units that receive unit i's output, then $\delta_i = (\Sigma_k \delta_k w_{ki})f'_i$, where k runs over all units that receive unit i's output. $\square$

Thus the "error signal" δ_i *propagates* back layer by layer from the output units. In $\Sigma_k \delta_k w_{ki}$, unit i receives error propagated back from a unit k to the extent to which i affects k.

The above proposition tells us how to compute Δw_{ij} for the *online* backpropagation algorithm that adjusts the weights in response to each single input pattern, using the "local error" of the network with its current weight settings for that input. It does not guarantee that the above step size is appropriate to reach the minimum, nor does it guarantee that the minimum, if reached, is global. The backpropagation rule defined by this proposition is, thus, a heuristic rule, not one guaranteed to find a global minimum. The *batch* version of the algorithm cycles through a complete training set of input-output pairs $(x_1, y_1), (x_2, y_2), \ldots, (x_N, y_N)$, with gradient descent applied to the cumulative error of each cycle, until no further changes are required.

As the index to this *Handbook* attests, backpropagation has been perhaps the most diversely used adaptive architecture, especially in technological applications. The purpose of this article is neither to introduce the basics of backpropagation (again, see PERCEPTRONS, ADALINES, AND BACKPROPAGATION and Section I.3: Dy-

namics and Adaptation in Neural Networks) nor to survey its applications (see SPEECH RECOGNITION TECHNOLOGY for one example of a careful analysis of the pros and cons of using multilayer perceptrons), but instead to place backpropagation in a broader context by providing a road map for a number of contributions elsewhere in the *Handbook* that enrich our basic understanding of this adaptive architecture. The article also assesses the biological plausibility of backpropagation.

Auto-Encoding

A basic application for backpropagation networks has been to find compressed representations. In this case, a network with one hidden layer is trained to become an *auto-encoder* or *auto-associator* by learning the identity function: making the desired states of the N output units identical to the states of the N input units for each input-output pair in the training sample. Data compression is achieved by making the number of hidden units $M < N$. Moreover, the features discovered by the hidden units may be useful for processing tasks, such as classification of the input patterns. However, as shown in UNSUPERVISED LEARNING WITH GLOBAL OBEJCTIVE FUNCTIONS, it may not be possible to relate the activities of individual hidden units to specific features that may be found by other means to characterize complicated input patterns. One way to constrain the hidden unit representation is to add extra penalty terms to the error function. For example, a penalty term on hidden unit activations can be chosen that causes these units to represent high-dimensional data as localized bumps of activity in a lower-dimensional constraint surface. This encourages the hidden units to form a map-like representation that best characterizes the input. Other penalty terms lead to other encodings, such as sparse or combinatorial representations (see MINIMUM DESCRIPTION LENGTH ANALYSIS).

RAAM networks (Pollack, 1990) are three-layer backpropagation networks whose input and output layers are each divided into regions. The network is trained to "auto-associate," i.e., to reproduce a given pattern of input on the output layer. The purpose of this training is to permit condensed, distributed encodings of K-tuples of information (i.e., the subpatterns presented to the K regions of the input layer) to be developed on the hidden layer. Once such a distributed encoding has been developed for a given K-tuple of information, that encoding may later be presented as input to a single region of the input layer, while the remaining input regions receive similarly derived distributed encodings, so that the network then develops codes for K-tuples of information. The network may then be trained to auto-associate on this more complex set of input information. Iterating the procedure yields codes for K-tuples of K-tuples, and so on, thus making possible condensed distributed encodings for entire tree structures in the RAAM's hidden layer. SYSTEMATICITY OF GENERALIZATIONS IN CONNECTIONIST NETWORKS (q.v.) discusses the implications of such techniques for the ability, or otherwise, of connectionist models to capture human abilities for symbol processing.

Stochasticity and Plateaus

STOCHASTIC APPROXIMATION AND EFFICIENT LEARNING (q.v.) notes that both on-line and batch backpropagation seek a weight vector w that minimizes the error function, but stresses the statistical notion that inputs must follow some probability distribution so that what we really seek to minimize is the error as averaged over all examples. But should we average over the few examples available in the training set, or over all the complete probability distribution "given by Nature"? The first average is named *empirical risk* and measures only the training set performance. The second average is called the *expected risk* and measures the much more interesting generalization performance (Vapnik, 1998). The *Handbook* introduces a stochastic gradient descent algorithm in which each iteration consists of picking a single random example and updating the weight vector *w* accordingly. This stochastic gradient descent does not need to remember which examples were visited during the previous iterations, making this algorithm suitable for the on-line adaptation of deployed systems. In such a situation, the stochastic gradient descent directly optimizes the expected risk, since the examples are randomly drawn from the "ground truth" distribution. The stochastic gradient descent can also pick examples from a finite training set. This procedure optimizes the empirical risk. The number of iterations is usually larger than the size of the training set. The examples are therefore presented multiple times to the network.

LEARNING AND STATISTICAL INFERENCE (q.v.) offers a general method, called *Fisher efficiency*, of assessing the success of an estimator relating input and output patterns. It then notes that, although backpropagation learning has been used widely, it is not Fisher efficient. Moreover, the method may converge to one of the local minima of the error landscape, which might be different from the global minimum. Intriguingly, convergence may be drastically slow because of "plateaus." The error decreases quickly at the beginning of learning, but its rate of decrease becomes extremely slow. After surprisingly many steps, the error again decreases rapidly. This is understood as showing that weights are trapped in a "plateau" that is not a local minimum but nonetheless provides a region of weight space that learning takes very long to escape from.

Saad and Solla (1995) used statistical mechanics to show that plateaus exist because of the "symmetry" in the hidden units: the output and hence the error measure is invariant under permutations of hidden units in the multilayer perceptron. Whereas this property leads to phase transitions in equilibrium batch training (see STATISTICAL MECHANICS OF GENERALIZATION), the effect in on-line training is that the system approaches a symmetric state from generic initial conditions. STATISTICAL MECHANICS OF ON-LINE LEARNING AND GENERALIZATION (q.v.) discusses how the properties of such plateaus can be investigated in detail by linearizing the dynamics close to the fixed point (Biehl, Riegler, and Wöhler, 1996). Figure 1 in STATISTICAL MECHANICS OF ON-LINE LEARNING AND GENERALIZATION (q.v.) provides a simple example of the breaking of permutation symmetry during learning, showing a typical learning curve in which the learning process is dominated by a pronounced plateau state in which hardly any progress is made while the number of examples increases. Only after an extended period of time does the system leave the plateau and approach its asymptotic state exponentially fast. In the case displayed in the figure, the system is very close to a perfectly symmetric configuration.

There are various acceleration methods for the backpropagation learning rule, but they cannot eliminate plateaus. NEUROMANIFOLDS AND INFORMATION GEOMETRY (q.v.) shows that the natural gradient method (Amari, 1998), based on the Riemannian structure of a neuromanifold, not only eliminates plateaus but is Fisher efficient.

Recurrent Neural Networks

A feedforward network is just a static mapping of input vectors to output vectors, whereas our brain is a high-dimensional nonlinear dynamical system, replete with loops. This provides one motivation (another is technological) for the study of learning algorithms for recurrent neural networks, which have feedback connections and

time delays. In a recurrent network, the state of the system can be encoded in the activity pattern of the units, and a wide variety of dynamical behaviors can be encoded by the connection weights. Network dynamics that converge to a minimum of an "energy" function (see COMPUTING WITH ATTRACTORS) have proved important for associative memory tasks and optimization networks. However, steady-state solutions (fixed-point attractors) are only a limited portion of the capabilities of recurrent networks. A recurrent network can serve as a sequence recognition system or as a sequential pattern generator. RECURRENT NETWORKS: LEARNING ALGORITHMS (q.v.) reviews the learning algorithms for training recurrent networks, focusing on supervised learning algorithms for recurrent networks, with only a brief overview of reinforcement and unsupervised learning algorithms.

Recurrent neural networks use the additional degree of freedom provided by a priori unlimited processing time in order to map the information appropriately. For example, simple recurrent networks (SRNs; Elman, 1990) augments the three-layer backpropagation network with a supplementary context layer of the same size as the hidden layer. Reciprocal links between the hidden layer and the context layer create a loop enabling any activation pattern currently present on the hidden layer to be merged with the activation pattern currently present in the context layer, and vice versa. An extension of the backpropagation algorithm trains these connections as well. Essentially, the activity in the context and hidden layers may be seen as an internal state, so that training serves to update both the definition of a "next-state function" as well as the reading of the output from the internal state in such a way as to enable the system to better and better approximate a training set, which now consists of pairs of input and output sequences, rather than one-shot input vectors and output vectors CONSTITUENCY AND RECURSION IN LANGUAGE (q.v.) exemplifies the use of SRNs in connectionist linguistics.

Other Perspectives

To create a neural network, a designer typically fixes a network topology and uses training data to tune its parameters, such as connection weights. The designer, however, often does not have enough knowledge to specify the ideal topology. In the case of a multilayer perceptron, the only free parameter in "topology space" is the number of hidden units. Too few hidden units and the current task is unlearnable; too many units and the network learns the noise as well as the task relationships. It is thus desirable to learn the topology from training data as well. LEARNING NETWORK TOPOLOGY (q.v.) looks at learning as a search in the space of topologies as well as in weight space. In particular, it provides a general measure of the "goodness" of a topology and some search strategies over the space of topologies to find the best one. This framework is applied to learning the topologies of both feedforward neural networks and Bayesian belief nets (see BAYESIAN NETWORKS).

A basic strategy to avoid false minima is Boltzmann learning (see SIMULATED ANNEALING AND BOLTZMANN MACHINES). Here the units respond in stochastic fashion to their inputs. The degree of "stochasticity" is controlled by a parameter T. As $T \to -\infty$, the unit becomes deterministic; as $T \to \infty$, the unit becomes very noisy. T is often referred to as "temperature," as part of the comparison of large neural networks with the systems treated by statistical mechanics (see STATISTICAL MECHANICS OF NEURAL NETWORKS). Convergence to the global optimum is aided by starting at high T and gradually lowering it—this is the process of "simulated annealing"—with the intuition being that the initial high noise "bumps the system out of the high valleys" of the error landscape, while the eventual low noise allows it to settle in the "low valleys."

MODULAR AND HIERARCHICAL LEARNING SYSTEMS (q.v.) replaces the training of a single network by the training of a set of networks that forms a "mixture of experts," the idea being that each network will become expert at processing inputs from a region of the input space, while a gating network will learn which experts to rely on for processing a given input. As an alternative to gradient methods, Jordan and Jacobs (1994) developed an Expectation-Maximization (EM) algorithm (McLachlan and Krishnan, 1997, give a general treatment of the EM algorithm) that is particularly useful for models in which the expert networks and gating networks have simple parametric forms. Each iteration of the algorithm consists of two phases: (1) a recursive propagation upward and downward in the tree of modules to compute posterior probabilities (the "E step"), and (2) solution of a set of local weighted maximum likelihood problems at the nonterminals and terminals of the tree (the "M step"). Jordan and Jacobs (1994) tested this algorithm on a nonlinear system identification problem (the forward dynamics of a 4-degrees-of-freedom robot arm) and reported that it converged nearly two orders of magnitude faster than backpropagation in a comparable multilayer perceptron network.

GRAPHICAL MODELS: PROBABILISTIC INFERENCE (q.v.) tells us that many neural network architectures are special cases of the general graphical model formalism that the article presents. Special cases of graphical models include essentially all of the models developed under the rubric of "unsupervised learning," as well as Boltzmann machines, mixtures of experts, and radial basis function networks. It is argued that many other neural networks, including the classical multilayer perceptron of the present article, can be analyzed profitably from the point of view of graphical models.

Biological Considerations

REINFORCEMENT LEARNING IN MOTOR CONTROL (q.v.) notes the importance of supervised learning in motor control, but stresses that reinforcement learning (in which positive reinforcement signals success on a task and increasing negative reinforcement gives a measure of increasingly poor performance, but where no explicit error signal for the network's output units is available) is more plausible in many situations involving motor learning; and, indeed, DOPAMINE, ROLES OF (q.v.) shows that certain reinforcement learning methods seem to fit well with the action of dopamine in the brain.

However, RECURRENT NETWORKS: NEUROPHYSIOLOGICAL MODELING (q.v.) argues for the utility of backpropagation as a tool for studying actual networks in the brain. The argument here is that backpropagation provides a means for the computational neuroscientist to adjust the parameters within a given neural network architecture to see whether there is indeed a parameter setting (whose robustness can then be studied) that yields a given type of behavior. The article presents backpropagation not as a model for biological learning, simply as an effective method of obtaining a solution. Biologically plausible learning algorithms will also find similar solutions, but usually take longer. For example, Mazzoni, Andersen, and Jordan (1991) argued that reinforcement learning gave a more biologically plausible learning rule than backpropagation in their study of a network model of cortical area 7a.

But what is the evidence that backpropagation is biologically implausible? HEBBIAN SYNAPTIC PLASTICITY (q.v.) makes a *partial* case for biological plausibility. While conceding that there is no evidence that the backpropagation formula represents actual brain mechanisms, it summarizes new evidence suggesting that activity in one neuron may affect presynaptic neurons, and even neurons presynaptic to those. One might call this *qualitative backpropagation* to stress that the evidence says nothing about the quantitative plausibility of the generalized delta rule. The ability to patch (make local electrode recordings and current injections) at different distances from the soma of a biological neuron has suggested that action potentials propagate back from the soma into the dendrites as well as in the "conventional" direction, from dendrites

to soma (see DENDRITIC PROCESSING). HEBBIAN SYNAPTIC PLASTICITY (q.v.) discusses three distinct mechanisms by which back-propagating spikes can be seen as the "binding signal" emitted by the soma to modify differentially synapses that are active within a precise temporal window. Moreover, the study of identified neurons and synapses in low-density hippocampal cultures has revealed extensive but selective spread of both long-term potentiation (LTP) and long-term depression (LTD) from the site of induction to other synapses in the network (see Bi and Poo, 2001, for a review). LTD induced at synapses between two glutamatergic neurons can spread to other synapses made by divergent outputs of the same presynaptic neuron, to synapses made by other convergent inputs on the same postsynaptic cell, and can even spread in a retrograde direction to depress synapses afferent to the presynaptic neuron (the evidence for qualitative backpropagation). In contrast, LTP can exhibit only lateral spread and backpropagation to the synapses associated with the presynaptic neuron.

Discussion

Backpropagation has provided an effective and widely used architecture for the training of artificial neural networks. We recalled the generalized delta rule for multilayer perceptrons, illustrated its utility with two examples of auto-encoder networks, and showed how the methodology could be extended to recurrent networks. However, statistical analysis showed that backpropagation has problems—a particular example being the likelihood of backpropagation training of multilayer perceptrons getting trapped in plateaus—as well as advantages. We thus provided pointers to stochastic descent methods that avoided these pitfalls, as well as noting extensions of, and alternatives to, backpropagation that can usefully be added to the repertoire of those who train artificial neural networks.

As for biology, we saw that backpropagation may serve as a computational tool to estimate the parameters of a particular biological network even though it does not model the actual learning processes within that network. On the other hand, evidence of "spike backpropagation" provides inspiration for a family of subtle new learning rules that allow the activity of a neuron to affect the neurons presynaptic to its input neurons, but this offers no direct support for the specific formulas of the generalized delta rule. Finally, it should be noted that the modeling and theory summarized in this article are based on neurons with sigmoid outputs. Such units are useful both in artificial neural networks and in connectionist modeling. They can also be considered biological models if their real-valued output is seen to represent a moving-window mean of spiking frequency of the biological neurons (see RATE CODING AND SIGNAL PROCESSING). However, there are cases in which it seems that a better fit to the biology can be obtained if the local temporal structure of spikes in the output of each neuron is taken into account (SPIKING NEURONS, COMPUTATION WITH). This suggests the importance of seeking to define learning rules that do take detailed spike placement, rather than local firing rates, into account. The data reviewed in HEBBIAN SYNAPTIC PLASTICITY (q.v.) may lead brain modelers in the right direction but, unfortunately, no efficient learning algorithm for networks of spiking neurons, whether biological or not, has yet gained wide acceptance.

Road Map: Learning in Artificial Networks
Background: I.3. Dynamics and Adaptation in Neural Networks; Perceptrons, Adalines, and Backpropagation
Related Reading: Computing with Attractors; Hebbian Synaptic Plasticity; Learning and Statistical Inference; Recurrent Networks: Learning Algorithms; Statistical Mechanics of On-Line Learning and Generalization; Stochastic Approximation and Efficient Learning

References

Amari, S., 1967, Theory of adaptive pattern classifiers, *IEEE Trans. Elec. Comp.*, EC-16:299–307.

Amari, S., 1998, Natural gradient works efficiently in learning, *Neural Computat.*, 10:251–276.

Biehl, M., Riegler, P., and Wöhler, C., 1996, Transient dynamics of on-line learning in two-layered neural networks, *J. Phys. A*, 29:4769.

Bi, G., and Poo, M., 2001, Synaptic modification by correlated activity: Hebb's postulate revisited, *Annu. Rev. Neurosci.*, 24:139–166. ◆

Elman, J. L., 1990, Finding structure in time, *Cogn. Sci.*, 14:179–212. ◆

Jordan, M. I., and Jacobs, R. A., 1994, Hierarchical mixtures of experts and the EM algorithm, *Neural Computat.*, 6:181–214.

Mazzoni, P., Andersen, R. A., and Jordan, M. I., 1991, A more biologically plausible learning rule than backpropagation applied to a network model of cortical area 7a, *Cereb. Cortex*, 1:293–307.

McLachlan, G. J., and Krishnan, T., 1997, *The EM Algorithm and Extensions*, New York: Wiley-Interscience.

Pollack, J. B., 1990, Recursive distributed representations, *Artif. Intell.*, 46:77–105.

Rumelhart, D. E., Hinton, G. E., and Williams, R. J., 1986, Learning internal representations by error propagation, in *Parallel Distributed Processing: Explorations in the Microstructure of Cognition*, vol. 1, *Foundations*, (D. E. Rumelhart, J. L. McClelland, and PDP Research Group, Eds.), Cambridge, MA: MIT Press, pp. 318–362. ◆

Saad, D., and Solla, S. A., 1995, On-line learning in soft committee machines, *Phys. Rev. E*, 52:4225–4243.

Vapnik, V. N., 1998, *Statistical Learning Theory*, New York: Wiley.

Werbos, P., 1995, Backpropagation: Basics and new developments, in *The Handbook of Brain Theory and Neural Networks* (M. A. Arbib, Ed.), Cambridge, MA: MIT Press, pp. 134–139. ◆

Basal Ganglia

Tony J. Prescott, Kevin Gurney, and Peter Redgrave

Introduction

Lying on either side of the forebrain/midbrain boundary, at the hub of the mammalian brain, the basal ganglia are a group of highly interconnected brain structures with a critical influence over movement and cognition. The importance of these nuclei for a cluster of human brain disorders, including Parkinson's disease, Hunting-ton's disease, and schizophrenia, has produced a century or more of strong clinical interest, and a prodigious volume of neurobiological research. Given the wealth of relevant data, and a pressing need for a better functional understanding of these structures, the basal ganglia provide one of the most exciting prospects for computational modeling of brain function.

This article will begin by summarizing aspects of the functional architecture of the mammalian basal ganglia and will then describe the computational approaches that have been developed over the course of the past decade (see also Houk, Davis, and Beiser, 1995; Wickens, 1997; Gillies and Arbuthnott, 2000). An important task for an appraisal of computational models is to provide a framework for comparing pieces of work that can differ radically in their breadth of focus, level of analysis, computational premises, and methodology, and whose relative merits can consequently be difficult to ascertain (I.2. Levels and Styles of Analysis). Here, we first distinguish between models that attempt to incorporate appropriate biological data (anatomical and/or physiological) and those that attempt an explanation of function using generic neural network architectures. This review will discuss only those models that incorporate known neurobiological constraints and will consider some of the implications for these models of recent biological data. The models can be divided in two main categories: (1) those that work at a comparatively low level of detail (membrane properties of individual neurons and micro-anatomical features) and that restrict themselves to a single component of the basal ganglia nucleus; and (2) those that deal at the "system level" with the basal ganglia as a whole and/or with their interactions with related structures (e.g., thalamus and cortex). In this article we will also seek to classify system level models in terms of the primary computational role that is being addressed by the neural substrate.

The neuromodulator dopamine is known to play a vital role in regulating basal ganglia processing and also in mediating learning within the basal ganglia. Although some of the likely regulatory functions of dopamine will be considered in this article, a fuller discussion of this topic, including hypotheses and models concerned with the role of dopamine in learning from reinforcement, are the subject of a separate article (DOPAMINE, ROLES OF).

Key Architectural Features

There have been many excellent summaries of the functional anatomy of the basal ganglia (e.g., Mink, 1996; Smith et al., 1998), the following therefore focuses on those aspects most relevant to understanding the models discussed in this article.

The principle structures of the rodent basal ganglia (Figure 1) are the striatum (consisting of the caudate, the putamen, and the ventral striatum), the subthalamic nucleus (STN), the globus pallidus (GP), the substantia nigra (SN), and the entopeduncular nucleus (EP) (homologous to the globus pallidus internal segment in primates). These structures are massively interconnected and form a functional subsystem within the wider brain architecture. There is a growing consensus that the basal ganglia nuclei can be regionally subdivided on the basis of their topographically organized connectivity with each other and with cortical and thalamic regions. Current views of information processing within the basal ganglia are heavily influenced by this suggestion of multiple parallel loops or channels.

The principle input components of the basal ganglia are the striatum and the STN. Afferent connections to both of these structures originate from virtually the entire brain, including cerebral cortex, many parts of the brainstem (via the thalamus), and the limbic system. Input connections provide phasic (intermittent) excitatory input.

The main output nuclei of the basal ganglia are the substantia nigra pars reticulata (SNr) and the entopeduncular nucleus (EP). Output structures provide extensively branched efferents to the thalamus (which project back to the cerebral cortex), and to pre-motor areas of the midbrain and brainstem. Most output projections are normally (tonically) active and inhibitory.

To make sense of the intrinsic connectivity of the basal ganglia it is important to recognize that the main projection neurons from the striatum (medium spiny cells) form two widely distributed populations differentiated by their efferent connectivity and neurochemistry.

One population comprises neurons with mainly D1-type dopamine receptors and projects to the output nuclei (SNr and EP). In the prevailing informal model of the basal ganglia (Albin, Young, and Penney, 1989) this projection constitutes the so-called *direct*

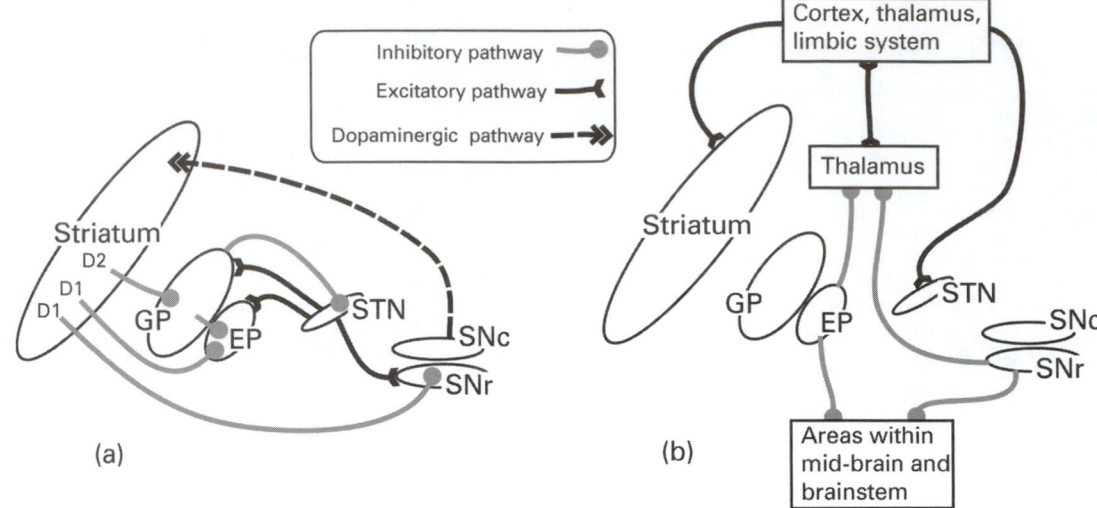

Figure 1. Basal ganglia anatomy of the rat: *A*. Internal pathways. *B*. External pathways. Excitatory and inhibitory pathways are denoted by solid and gray lines, respectively; not all connections are shown. See text for key to abbreviations.

pathway to the output nuclei (see Figure 2A). Efferent activity from these neurons suppresses the tonic inhibitory firing in the output structures, which in turn *disinhibits* targets in the thalamus and brainstem.

A second population of striatal output neurons has predominantly D2-type dopamine receptors. This group projects primarily to the globus pallidus (GP) whose tonic inhibitory outputs are directed both to the output nuclei (SNr and EP) and to the STN. The inhibitory projection from D2 striatal neurons constitutes the first leg of an *indirect pathway* to the output nuclei. Since this pathway has two inhibitory links (Striatum-GP, GP-STN), followed by an excitatory one (STN-EP/SNr), the net effect of striatal activity is

to activate output nuclei, which increases inhibitory control of the thalamus and brainstem.

The main source of dopamine innervation to the striatum is the substantia nigra pars compacta (SNc). Interestingly, the D1 and D2 striatal populations respond differently to dopaminergic transmission, activation of D1 receptors having a predominantly excitatory effect while D2 receptor activation appears to be mainly inhibitory. This arrangement seems to provide dopaminergic control of a "push/pull" mechanism subserved by the direct (inhibitory) and indirect (net excitatory) basal ganglia pathways. Importantly, a key input to the SNc is from striatal areas known as striosomes (areas that project to EP/SNr are known as matri-

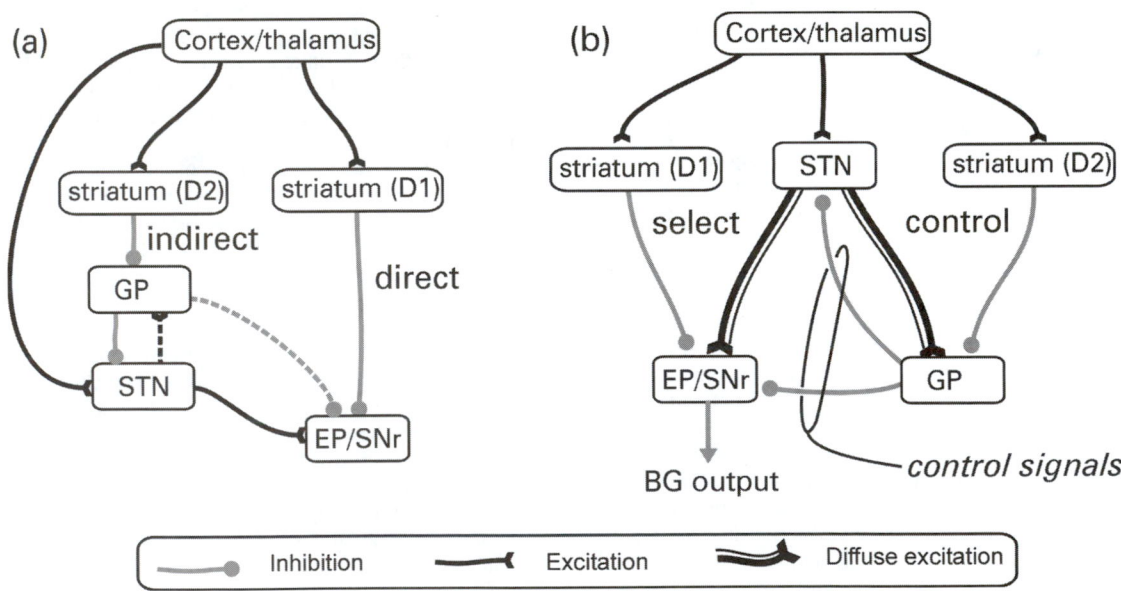

Figure 2. Functional interpretations of the basal ganglia: (a) *Informal* models stress the "direct" and "indirect" pathways and leave the functional consequences of their interactions ill-defined. Other pathways (indicated by dotted lines) have received less emphasis. (b) An alternative interpretation arising from *computational* modeling by Gurney et al. (2001) specifies specific functional roles for the various intrinsic basal ganglia connections summarized by the concept of "selection" and "control" pathways. See text for further explanation.

somes), thus the striatum is a major player in modulating its own dopaminergic input.

Although the preceding description focuses on pathways originating from the striatum, the STN, though much smaller in size, is increasingly recognized as a second important input structure within the basal ganglia functional architecture (see Mink, 1996). STN's excitatory outputs project to both the output nuclei (SNr and EP) and to the intermediary structure GP.

Recent anatomical data by Wu, Richard, and Parent (2000) has suggested that the "direct pathway" is actually branched with a significant output going to GP. Other new data shows the existence of additional inhibitory projections from GP to EP/SNr implying a multiplicity of indirect pathways (Smith et al., 1998). The proliferation of intrinsic basal ganglia circuitry in recent literature has highlighted the need for: (1) a radical reinterpretation of basal ganglia functional anatomy; and (2) an increasingly important role for computational modeling in interpreting the functional properties of the multiple interconnections and loops within the basal ganglia.

Low-Level Models of Individual Basal Ganglia Nuclei

In contrast to the diverse nature of the brain regions projecting to the mammalian striatum, its internal organization appears surprisingly homogeneous. This finding offers hope that an understanding of striatal functioning in one local area could generalize across much of the entire structure. At any given moment the majority of striatal cells are in an inactive "down state," and can only be triggered into an active "up state" (in which they can fire action potentials) by a significant amount of coincident input. Since each neuron has a wide dendritic fan-in (with up to 30,000 synapses), but only a few synapses with any single source neuron, it must receive coincident signals from a large population of inputs to become active (see Wilson in Houk et al., 1995). This organization suggests that striatal spiny neurons may act as "context-specific filters," each one configured to match a specific pattern of activity distributed across multiple loci in one or more brain areas (Mink, 1996).

Recent studies have provided evidence for local inhibition within the striatum mediated either via local interneurones or by reciprocal inhibitory networks among the output cells themselves (see Oorschot et al. in Nicholson and Faull, 2002). Wickens and colleagues (see Wickens, 1997) have investigated the dynamics of such local neighborhoods of striatal neurons using network models. Under varying assumptions of topology and size, they concluded that reciprocal inhibition will usually lead to a network dynamic of competition, that is, the most active neurons will tend to suppress activity in their less active neighbors. This research also examined the effects of simulated dopamine inputs, showing that under circumstances of low dopamine, the dynamic of the network changes from competition to coactivation (where activity is uniformly distributed within the local population of neurons), a pattern that could provide a model for the muscular rigidity seen in dopamine-deficient Parkinson's patients. Using another variant of this model, Wickens explored the implications of dendritic asymmetries based on those observed in the early stages of Huntington's disease. Simulation of asymmetric interconnectivity generated slow traveling waves of activity (where normal symmetric configurations produce stationary activity patterns), suggesting that a similar abnormal network dynamic may underlie the sudden involuntary movements seen in Huntington's patients.

Apart from the striatum, relatively little attention has been given to modeling intrinsic processing within basal ganglia nuclei. One interesting exception is the work by Gillies and Willshaw (see Gillies and Arbuthnott, 2000) on a model of the STN. Having incorporated key physiological and anatomical properties, they showed that the widespread excitatory interconnectivity between STN neurons allows focused input to produce a widely distributed pulse of excitation to SNR and EP. Given that the output of the basal ganglia is largely inhibitory, phasic STN activity could serve to break established patterns of activity in basal ganglia targets thereby acting as a form of interrupt or "reset" mechanism.

The preceding models have as their starting point a wealth of low-level biological constraints with the rationale that the resulting model behavior must approximate observed biological data. Nevertheless, since the phenomena discussed are related to the ability to resolve localized competitions (in striatum) and to interrupt ongoing behaviors (STN), we would argue that these models may be thought of as addressing components of the overall computational problem of action selection (see further discussion later in this article).

System Level Models of Basal Ganglia Circuits and External Functional Loops

Most of the effort so far directed at basal ganglia modeling has been concerned with simulating interactions between the various basal ganglia structures, and between the basal ganglia and other key brain regions such as cortex, thalamus, and brainstem. A comparatively high level of abstraction is usually adopted in this work, in which components of the basal ganglia are decomposed into functional units (e.g., multiple parallel channels). Most work to date has focused on a number of related computational hypotheses—that the basal ganglia function to (1) regulate the degree of action gating, (2) select between competing actions, (3) sustain working memory representations, and (4) store and enact sequences of behavior. These ideas will be the main focus of the remaining discussion.

Action Gating

A key function of the striatum is to provide intermittent, focused inhibition (via the "direct pathway") within output structures that otherwise maintain inhibitory control over motor/cognitive systems throughout the brain. This architecture strongly suggests that a core function of the basal ganglia is to gate the activity of these target systems via the mechanism of disinhibition. Many basal ganglia models employ selective gating, however, that of Contreras-Vidal and Stelmach (1995) is particularly interesting as it explores gating operations in both normal and dysfunctional model variants. These authors coupled a simulation of basal ganglia intrinsic circuitry to a neural network that computed arm movements. Excitatory striatal input resulted in a smoothly varying signal to thalamic targets that provided the "Go" signal for the motor command, and also set its overall velocity. The time taken to execute movements decreased with increasing basal ganglia input thereby matching the results of striatal microstimulation studies. A "dopamine depleted" version of the model exhibited akinesia and bradykinesia similar to that observed in Parkinson's disease.

Selecting Between Competing Actions

The proposal that the basal ganglia act to resolve action selection competitions is based on a growing consensus that a key function of these structures is to arbitrate between sensorimotor systems competing for access to the final common motor path. A computational hypothesis developed from this idea relies on the premise that afferent signals to the striatum encode the salience of "requests for access" to the motor system (Redgrave, Prescott, and Gurney, 1999). Multiple selection mechanisms embedded in the basal ganglia could resolve conflict between competitors and provide clean and rapid switching between winners. First, the up/down states of the striatal neurones may act as a first pass filter to exclude weakly supported "requests." Second, local inhibition within the striatum could selectively enhance the activity of the most salient channels.

Third, the combination of focused inhibition from striatum with diffuse (divergent) excitation from STN could operate as a feedforward, off-center/on-surround network across the basal ganglia as a whole (see Mink, 1996). Last, local reciprocal inhibition within the output nuclei could sharpen up the final selections.

Using the action selection hypothesis as an organizing principle, Gurney, Prescott, and Redgrave (2001) have proposed a reinterpretation of basal ganglia functional anatomy in which the direct/indirect classification is replaced by a new functional grouping based on *selection* and *control* circuits (Figure 2B). Specifically, the focused D1 inhibitory pathway from striatum to EP/SNr (originally the "direct pathway"), together with a *diffuse* excitatory pathway from STN to EP/SNr, form a primary feedforward *selection* circuit. A second group of intrinsic connections centered on the GP acts as a *control* circuit to regulate the performance of the main selection mechanism. Analytical and simulation studies of this model suggest two likely functional roles for this control circuit. First, the inhibition of STN by GP constitutes a negative feedback path that automatically scales the excitatory output of the STN with the number of channels. Second, GP inhibition of EP/SNr forms part of a mechanism that supports dopaminergic regulation of selection. Specifically, increased dopamine in these circuits promotes "promiscuous" selection in which channels are more easily disinhibited, while reduced dopamine results in a "stiffer" competition in which there are fewer winners and higher levels of general target inhibition. The adequacy of this model has been tested by embedding it in the control architecture of a mobile robot equipped with a small repertoire of animal-like behaviors (see Prescott, Gurney et al. in Nicholson and Faull, 2002). This work confirmed that the simulated basal ganglia can provide effective action selection in a real-world context requiring appropriate and timely behavioral switching. The robot model also provided an insight into the emergent consequences of abnormal dopamine modulation of action selection. For instance, and reminiscent of some motor symptoms of Parkinson's disease, reduced dopamine was found to cause failures to select appropriate behavior or to complete behaviors once selected.

An earlier model of the basal ganglia proposed by Berns and Sejnowski (1995) shared the "action selection" premise of Gurney et al., but emphasized possible timing differences between the direct and indirect pathways in a model that included just the feedforward intrinsic basal ganglia connections. An interesting feature of this model is that it incorporated a version of the dopamine hypothesis for reinforcement learning (DOPAMINE, ROLES OF) as a means for adaptively tuning the selection mechanism.

Sustaining Working Memory Representations

The relationship between basal ganglia and cortex is characterized by relatively segregated parallel loops, in which cortical projections to the striatum are channeled through basal ganglia outputs to the thalamus and then back to their cortical areas of origin. The thalamic nuclei in this circuit also have reciprocal, net-excitatory, connections to their cortical targets. This architecture suggests a pattern of cortical-thalamic activity which, once initiated by disinhibitory signals from the basal ganglia, could be sustained indefinitely. Several authors have proposed that this circuit could act as a working memory store (see Houk et al., 1995). An example of this is provided by Arbib and Dominey's model of basal ganglia control of the primate saccadic eye movement system (see article in Houk et al., 1995). These authors modeled an experimental task in which a monkey is required to make a saccade to a remembered target location. They simulated circuits in which cortical cells in the frontal eye fields were activated by the target, which, in turn, excited a population of striatal neurons specialized for delayed saccades. The basal ganglia loops involving these cells disinhibited their thalamic

targets so that the target location was maintained in the cortico-thalamic circuits until the saccade was made.

In our view, the selection and maintenance of specific working memory items can be viewed as an extension of action selection by the basal ganglia to the domain of cognition (selecting from a range of potential cognitive representations those which are to be sustained as working memory). It is interesting to speculate that deficits in this system may underlie the disorders of thought associated with schizophrenia, attention-deficit disorder, and obsessive-compulsive disorder.

Sequence Processing

A plausible use for the working memory mechanism outlined previously would be to link successful selections during the development of behavioral/cognitive sequences. This idea has therefore become a central theme in a number of basal ganglia models. According to Beiser and Houk (1998), sequence encoding can be viewed as the task of translating a temporal ordering into a spatial pattern of neural activity. They propose that the initial item in a sequence selects the basal ganglia loop whose striatal neurons are most attuned to that context. When this channel is disinhibited, the item then becomes encoded as a self-sustaining pattern of cortico-thalamic activity. Later sequence elements are recorded in an identical way, except that, as each new item is added, the cortical activity triggered by its predecessors becomes part of its context (thereby implicitly encoding its position in the temporal order). Rather than recording sequences as spatially distributed patterns, Fukai (1999) has suggested a form of cortical short-term memory for sequences that uses patterns of fast (gamma) and slow (theta) oscillatory activity. Reciprocal inhibition between striatal neurons would allow the basal ganglia to select the first item in such a sequence, while other striatal neurons (and their corresponding basal ganglia outputs) would be recruited to maintain the selection of that item for as long as required. Finally, an excitatory burst from STN terminates the movement and signals the transition to the next item in the sequence. Although differing considerably in detail, these two models share the premise that the basal ganglia is specialized to "unpack" a cortical representation of sequential behavior by selectively gating each of the component movements. Sequence learning is another important theme in basal ganglia modeling. For instance, Dominey, Arbib, and Joseph (1995) have extended their model of delayed saccade control (described previously) to include a mechanism for associative and SEQUENCE LEARNING (q.v.) based, again, on the hypothesis that dopamine provides a reinforcement learning signal.

Discussion

The preceding summary demonstrates that basal ganglia modeling is still at the stage of exploring the space of alternative hypotheses, seeking to operationalize theoretical proposals while trying to match known neurobiological constraints. As a result, there is now a candidate set of "global" basal ganglia functions whose computational requirements we are beginning to understand. It remains to be seen to what extent proposed functions are mutually exclusive and to what extent one may be subsumed within another (for instance, action gating can be viewed as an essential component of action selection). Similar considerations apply when appraising models directed at different levels of basal ganglia function. For example, lower-level models of the striatum or STN may, in the future, be imported as fully functional components into higher-level models. However, some system level models are clearly in direct competition with each other as they ascribe different functional roles to local pathways and nuclei. We anticipate that models based on correct computational assumptions will find it comparatively easy to incorporate new biological constraints, which in most cases will improve their accuracy. In contrast, models making mistaken functional assignments will find it increasingly difficult to incorporate additional biological data while maintaining their functionality. Future work will therefore require ever-closer links between neurobiologists and modelers to refine the models, to formulate questions based on function, and to test the interesting and unforeseen predictions that can emerge from modeling studies.

Road Maps: Mammalian Brain Regions; Mammalian Motor Control
Related Reading: Action Monitoring and Forward Control of Movements; Arm and Hand Movement Control; Dopamine, Roles of; Motor Control, Biological and Theoretical; Reinforcement Learning in Motor Control

References

Albin, R. L., Young, A. B., and Penney, J. B., 1989, The functional anatomy of basal ganglia disorders, *Trends Neurosci.*, 12(10):366–375.

Beiser, D. G., and Houk, J. C., 1998, Model of cortical-basal ganglionic processing: Encoding the serial order of sensory events, *J. Neurophysiol.*, 79(6):3168–3188.

Berns, G. S., and Sejnowski, T. J., 1995, How the basal ganglia make decisions, in *The Neurobiology of Decision Making* (A. Damasio, H. Damasio, and Y. Christen, Eds.), Berlin: Springer-Verlag, pp. 101–113.

Contreras-Vidal, J. L., and Stelmach, G. E., 1995, A neural model of basal ganglia-thalamocortical relations in normal and Parkinsonian movement, *Biol. Cybernetics*, 73(5):467–476.

Dominey, P., Arbib, M., and Joseph, J.-P., 1995, A model of corticostriatal plasticity for learning oculomotor associations and sequences, *J. Cognit. Neurosci.*, 7(3):311–336.

Fukai, T., 1999, Sequence generation in arbitrary temporal patterns from theta-nested gamma oscillations: A model of the basal ganglia-thalamocortical loops, *Neural Networks*, 12(7–8):975–987.

Gillies, A., and Arbuthnott, G., 2000, Computational models of the basal ganglia, *Movement Disorders*, 15(5):762–770. ◆

Gurney, K., Prescott, T. J., and Redgrave, P., 2001, A computational model of action selection in the basal ganglia. I, II, *Biological Cybernetics*, 84(6):401–423.

Houk, J. C., Davis, J. L., and Beiser, D. G., 1995, *Models of Information Processing in the Basal Ganglia*, Cambridge, MA: MIT Press. ◆

Mink, J. W., 1996, The basal ganglia: Focused selection and inhibition of competing motor programs, *Progr. Neurobiol.*, 50(4):381–425. ◆

Nicholson, L. F. B., and Faull, R. L. M., 2002, *Basal Ganglia VII*, New York: Plenum Press.

Redgrave, P., Prescott, T., and Gurney, K., 1999, The basal ganglia: A vertebrate solution to the selection problem? *Neuroscience*, 89:1009–1023.

Smith, Y., Bevan, M. D., Shink, E., and Bolam, J. P., 1998, Microcircuitry of the direct and indirect pathways of the basal ganglia, *Neuroscience*, 86:353–387. ◆

Wickens, J., 1997, Basal ganglia: Structure and computations. *Network-Computation in Neural Systems*, 8(4):R77–R109. ◆

Wu, Y., Richard, S., and Parent, A., 2000, The organization of the striatal output system: a single-cell juxtacellular labeling study in the rat, *Neurosci. Res.*, 38:49–62.

Bayesian Methods and Neural Networks

David Barber

Introduction

An attractive feature of artificial neural networks is their ability to model highly complex, nonlinear relationships in data. However, choosing an appropriate neural network model for data is compounded by the difficulty of assessing the network's complexity. Since we are rarely certain about either our data measurements or model beliefs, a natural framework is to use probabilities to account for these uncertainties. How can we combine our data observations with these modeling uncertainties in a consistent and meaningful manner? The Bayesian approach provides a consistent framework for formulating a response to these difficulties, and is noteworthy for its conceptual elegance (Box and Tiao, 1973; Berger, 1985; MacKay, 1992). The fundamental probabilistic relationship required for inference is the celebrated Bayes rule, which, for general events A, B, C, is

$$p(A|B, C) = \frac{p(B|A, C)p(A|C)}{p(B|C)} \qquad (1)$$

It is convenient to think of different levels of uncertainty in formulating a model. At the lowest level, we may assume that we have the correct model but are uncertain as to the parameter settings θ for this model. This assumption details how observed data are generated, $p(\text{data}|\theta, \text{model})$. The task of inference at this level is to calculate the posterior distribution of the model parameter. Using Bayes's rule, this is

$$p(\theta|\text{data}, \text{model}) = \frac{p(\text{data}|\theta, \text{model})\,p(\theta|\text{model})}{p(\text{data}|\text{model})} \qquad (2)$$

Thus, if we wish to infer model parameters from data, we need two assumptions: (1) how the observed data are generated under the assumed model, or the *likelihood* $p(\text{data}|\theta, \text{model})$, and (2) beliefs about which parameter values are appropriate before the data

have been observed, or the *prior* $p(\theta|\text{model})$. (The denominator in Equation 2 is the normalizing constant for the posterior and plays a role in uncertainty at the higher model level.) That these two assumptions are required is an inescapable consequence of Bayes's rule, and forces the Bayesian to lay bare all necessary assumptions underlying the model.

Coin Tossing Example

Let θ be the probability that a coin will land heads up. An experiment yields the data, $D = \{h, h, t, h, t, h, \ldots\}$, which contains H heads and T tails in $H + T$ flips of the coin. What can we infer about θ from these data? Assuming that each coin is flipped independently, the likelihood of the observed data is

$$p(D|\theta, \text{model}) = \theta^H (1 - \theta)^T \qquad (3)$$

A standard approach in the statistical sciences is to estimate θ by maximizing the likelihood, $\theta^{ML} = \arg\max_\theta p(D|\theta, \text{model})$. This approach is non-Bayesian, since it does not require the specification of a prior. Consequently, theories that deal with uncertainty in ML estimators are primarily concerned with the data likelihood, and not directly with posterior parameter uncertainty (see LEARNING AND GENERALIZATION: THEORETICAL BOUNDS). In the Bayesian approach, however, we need to be explicit about our prior beliefs $p(\theta|\text{model})$. These are updated by the observed data to yield the posterior distribution

$$p(\theta|D, \text{model}) \propto \theta^H (1 - \theta)^T p(\theta|\text{model}) \qquad (4)$$

The Bayesian approach is more flexible than the maximum likelihood approach since it allows (indeed, *instructs*) the user to calculate the effect that the data have in modifying prior assumptions about which parameter values are appropriate. For example, if we believe that the coin is heavily biased, we may express this using the prior distribution in Figure 1A. The likelihood as a function of θ is plotted in Figure 1B for data containing 13 tails and 12 heads. The resulting posterior (Figure 1C) is bimodal, but less extreme than the prior. It is often convenient to summarize the posterior by either the maximum a posteriori (MAP) value or the mean, $\bar{\theta} = \int \theta p(\theta|D)d\theta$. Such a summary is not strictly required by the Bayesian framework, and the best choice of how to summarize the posterior depends on other loss criteria (Berger, 1985).

Model Comparison and Hierarchical Models

The preceding discussion showed how we can use the Bayesian framework to assess which parameters of a model are a posteriori appropriate, given the data at hand. We can carry out a similar procedure at a higher, model level to asses which models are more appropriate fits to the data. In general, the model posterior is given by

$$p(M|D) = \underbrace{p(D|M)}_{\text{Model likelihood}} \underbrace{p(M)}_{\text{Model prior}} /p(D) \tag{5}$$

If the model is parameterized by some unknown variable θ, we need to integrate this out to calculate the model likelihood

$$p(D|M) = \int p(D|\theta, M)p(\theta|M)d\theta \tag{6}$$

Comparing two competing model hypotheses, M_1 and M_2, is straightforward:

$$\frac{p(M_1|D)}{p(M_2|D)} = \underbrace{\frac{p(D|M_1)}{p(D|M_2)}}_{\text{Bayes factor}} \frac{p(M_1)}{(M_2)} \tag{7}$$

In the coin example, we can use this to compare the biased coin hypothesis (model M_1 with prior given in Figure 1A) with a less unbiased hypothesis formed by using a Gaussian prior $p(\theta|M_2)$ with mean 0.5 and variance 0.1^2 (model M_2). This gives a Bayes factor $p(D|M_1)/p(D|M_2) \approx 0.00018$. If we have no prior preference for either model M_1 or M_2, the data more strongly favor model M_2, as

intuition would suggest. If we desired, we could continue in this way, forming a hierarchy of models, each less constrained than the submodels it contains.

Bayesian Regression

Neural networks are often applied to a regression in which we wish to infer an unknown input-output mapping on the basis of observed data $D = \{(\mathbf{x}^\mu, t^\mu), \mu = 1, \ldots P\}$, where $(\mathbf{x}^\mu, t^\mu)$ represents an input-output pair. For example, fit a function to the data in Figure 2A. Since there is the possibility that each observed output t^μ has been corrupted by noise, we would like to recover the underlying clean input-output function. We assume that each (clean) output is generated from the model $f(\mathbf{x}; \mathbf{w})$, where the parameters $\mathbf{w}$ of the function f are unknown, and that the observed outputs t^μ are generated by the addition of noise η to the clean model output,

$$t = f(\mathbf{x}; \mathbf{w}) + \eta \tag{8}$$

If the noise is Gaussian distributed, $\eta \sim N(0, \sigma^2)$, the model M generates an output t for input $\mathbf{x}$ with probability

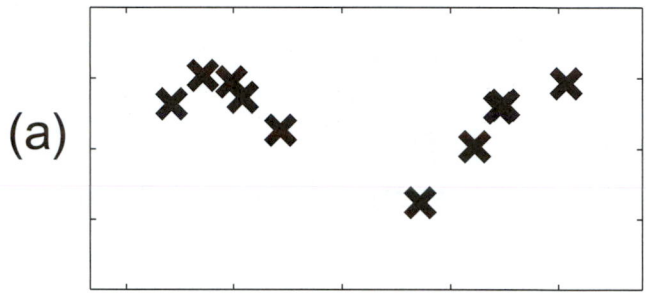

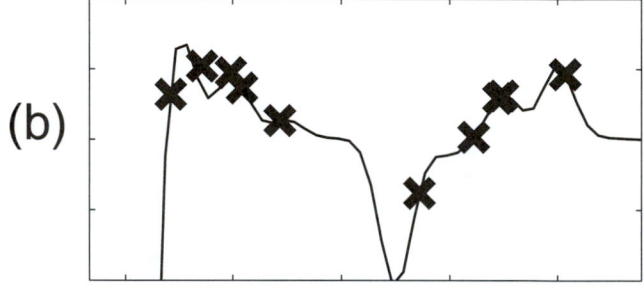

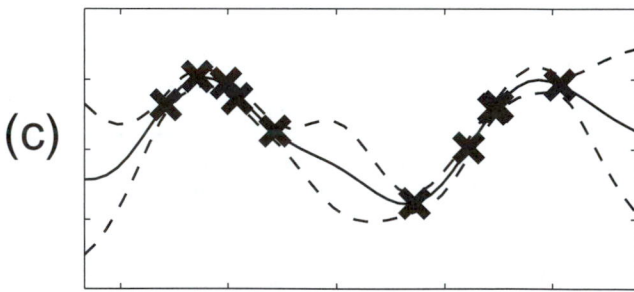

Figure 2. Along the horizontal axis we plot the input x and along the vertical axis the output t. A, The raw input-output training data. B, Prediction using regularized training and fixed hyperparameters. C, Prediction with error bars, using ML-II optimized hyperparameters.

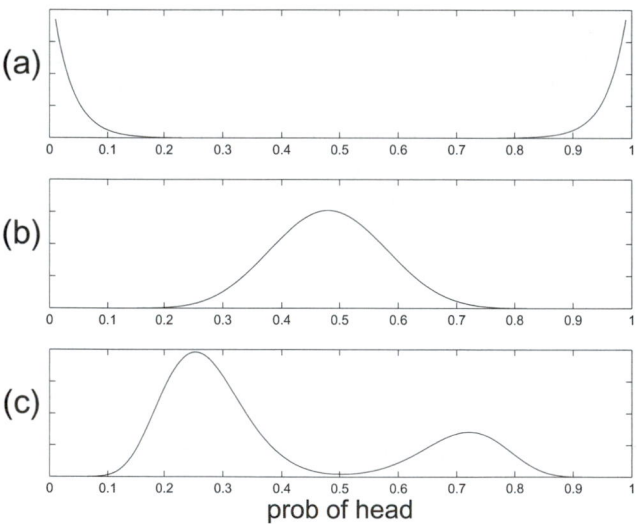

Figure 1. Coin tossing. A, The prior: this indicates our belief that the coin is heavily biased. B, The likelihood after 13 tails and 12 heads are recorded, $\theta^{ML} = 0.48$. C, The posterior: the data have moderated the strong prior beliefs, resulting in a posterior less certain that the coin is biased. $\theta^{MAP} = 0.25$, $\bar{\theta} = 0.39$.

$$p(t|\mathbf{w}, \mathbf{x}, M) = \exp\left\{-\frac{1}{2\sigma^2}(t - f(\mathbf{x}; \mathbf{w}))^2\right\} \bigg/ \sqrt{2\pi\sigma^2} \quad (9)$$

If we assume that each data input-output pair is generated identically and independently from the others, the data likelihood is

$$p(D|\mathbf{w}, M) = \prod_{\mu=1}^{P} p(t^\mu|\mathbf{w}, \mathbf{x}^\mu, M) \quad (10)$$

(Strictly speaking, we should write $p(t^1, \ldots, t^P|\mathbf{w}, \mathbf{x}^1, \ldots, \mathbf{x}^P, M)$ on the left-hand side of Equation 10. However, since we assume that the training inputs are fixed and non-noisy, it is convenient and conventional to write $p(D|\mathbf{w}, M)$.) The posterior distribution $p(\mathbf{w}|D, M) \propto p(D|\mathbf{w}, M)p(\mathbf{w}|M)$ is

$$\log p(\mathbf{w}|D, M) = -\frac{\beta}{2}\sum_\mu (t^\mu - f(\mathbf{x}^\mu; \mathbf{w}))^2$$
$$+ \log p(\mathbf{w}|M) + \frac{P}{2}\log\beta + const. \quad (11)$$

where $\beta = 1/\sigma^2$. Note the similarity between Equation 11 and the sum square regularized training error used in standard approaches to training neural networks (see GENERALIZATION AND REGULARIZATION IN NONLINEAR LEARNING SYSTEMS and Bishop, 1995). In the Bayesian framework, we can motivate the choice of a sum square error measure as equivalent to the assumption of additive Gaussian noise. Typically, we wish to encourage smoother functions so that the phenomenon of overfitting is avoided. One approach to solving this problem is to use a regularizer penalty term to the training error. In the Bayesian framework, we use a prior to achieve a similar effect. In principle, however, the Bayesian should make use of the full posterior distribution, not just a single weight value. In standard neural network training, it is good practice to use committees of networks, rather than relying on the prediction of a single network (Bishop, 1995). In the Bayesian framework, the posterior automatically specifies a committee (indeed, a distribution) of networks, and the importance attached to each committee member's prediction is simply the posterior probability of that network's weight.

Radial Basis Functions and Generalized Linear Models

Generalized linear models have the form

$$f(x; w) = \sum_i w_i \phi_i(\mathbf{x}) \equiv \mathbf{w}^T \Phi(\mathbf{x}) \quad (12)$$

Such models have a linear parameter dependence, but nevertheless represent a nonlinear input-output mapping if the basis functions $\phi(\mathbf{x})$, $i = 1, \ldots, k$ are nonlinear. Radial basis functions (see RADIAL BASIS FUNCTION NETWORKS) are an example of such a network (Bishop, 1995). A popular choice is to use Gaussian basis functions $\phi_i(\mathbf{x}) = \exp(-(\mathbf{x} - \mu^i)^2/(2\lambda^2))$. In this discussion, we will assume that the centers μ^i are fixed, but that the width of the basis functions λ is a hyperparameter that can be adapted. Since the output is linearly dependent on $\mathbf{w}$, we can discourage extreme output values by penalizing large weight values. A sensible weight prior is thus

$$\log p(\mathbf{w}|\alpha) = -\frac{\alpha}{2}\mathbf{w}^T\mathbf{w} + \frac{k}{2}\log\alpha + const. \quad (13)$$

Under the Gaussian noise assumption, the posterior distribution is

$$\log p(\mathbf{w}|\Gamma, D) = -\frac{\beta}{2}\sum_{\mu=1}^{P}(t^\mu - \mathbf{w}^T\Phi(x))^2$$
$$- \frac{\alpha}{2}\mathbf{w}^T\mathbf{w} + const. \quad (14)$$

where Γ represents the hyperparameter set $\{\alpha, \beta, \lambda\}$. (We drop the fixed model dependency wherever convenient.) The weight posterior is therefore a Gaussian, $p(\mathbf{w}|\Gamma, D) = N(\bar{\mathbf{w}}, \mathbf{S})$, where

$$\mathbf{S} = \left(\alpha\mathbf{I} + \beta\sum_{\mu=1}^{P}\Phi(\mathbf{x}^\mu)\Phi^T(\mathbf{x}^\mu)\right)^{-1}$$
$$\bar{\mathbf{w}} = \beta\mathbf{S}\sum_{\mu=1}^{P} t^\mu\Phi(\mathbf{x}^\mu) \quad (15)$$

The mean predictor is straightforward to calculate: $\bar{f}(\mathbf{x}) \equiv \int f(\mathbf{x}; \mathbf{w})p(\mathbf{w}|D, \Gamma)d\mathbf{w} = \bar{\mathbf{w}}^T\Phi(\mathbf{x})$. Similarly, error bars are straightforward, $var(f(\mathbf{x})) = \Phi(\mathbf{x})^T\mathbf{S}\Phi(\mathbf{x})$ (predictive standard errors are given by $\sqrt{var(f) + \sigma_2}$). In Figure 2B, we show the mean prediction on the data in Figure 2A using 15 Gaussian basis functions with width $\lambda = 0.03$ spread out evenly over the input space. We set the other hyperparameters to be $\beta = 100$ and $\alpha = 1$. The prediction severely overfits the data, a result of poor choice of hyperparameters.

Determining Hyperparameters: ML-II

How would the mean predictor be calculated if we were to include the hyperparameters Γ as part of a hierarchical model? Formally, this becomes

$$\bar{f}(\mathbf{x}) = \int f(\mathbf{x}; \mathbf{w})p(\mathbf{w}, \Gamma|D)d\mathbf{w}d\Gamma$$
$$= \int \left\{\int f(\mathbf{x}; \mathbf{w})p(\mathbf{w}|\Gamma, D)d\mathbf{w}\right\}p(\Gamma|D)d\Gamma \quad (16)$$

The term in curly brackets is the mean predictor for fixed hyperparameters. We therefore weigh each mean predictor by the posterior probability of the hyperparameter $p(\Gamma|D)$. Equation 16 shows how to combine different models in an ensemble—each model prediction is weighted by the posterior probability of the model. There are other non-Bayesian approaches to model combinations in which the determination of the combination coefficients is motivated heuristically (see ENSEMBLE LEARNING).

Provided the hyperparameters are well determined by the data, we may instead approximate the above hyperparameter integral by finding the MAP hyperparameters $\Gamma^* = \arg\max_\Gamma p(\Gamma|D)$. Since $p(\Gamma|D) = p(D|\Gamma)p(\Gamma)/p(D)$, if the prior belief about the hyperparameters is weak ($p(\Gamma) \approx const.$), we can estimate the optimal hyperparameters by optimizing the hyperparameter likelihood

$$p(D|\Gamma) = \int p(D|\Gamma, \mathbf{w})p(\mathbf{w}|\Gamma)d\mathbf{w} \quad (17)$$

This approach to setting hyperparameters is called ML-II (Berger, 1985; Bishop, 1995) and assumes that we can calculate the integral in Equation 17. In the case of GLMs, this involves only Gaussian integration, giving

$$2\log p(D|\Gamma) = -\beta\sum_{\mu=1}^{P}(t^\mu)^2 + \mathbf{d}^T\mathbf{S}^{-1}\mathbf{d} - \log|\mathbf{S}|$$
$$+ k\log\alpha + P\log\beta + const. \quad (18)$$

where $\mathbf{d} = \beta\Sigma_\mu\Phi(\mathbf{x}^\mu)t^\mu$. Using the hyperparameters α, β, λ that optimize the above expression gives the results in Figure 2C, where we plot both the mean predictions and standard predictive error bars. This solution is more acceptable than the previous one in which the hyperparameters were not optimized, and demonstrates that overfitting is avoided automatically. A non-Bayesian approach to model fitting based on minimizing a regularized training error would typically use a procedure such as cross-validation to determine the regularization parameters (hyperparameters). Such approaches require the use of validation data (Bishop, 1995). An advantage of the Bayesian approach is that hyperparameters can be set without the need for validation data, and thus all the data can be used directly for training.

Relation to Gaussian Processes

The use of GLMs can be difficult in cases where the input dimension is high, since the number of basis functions required to cover the input space fairly well grows exponentially with the input dimension—the so-called *curse of dimensionality* (Bishop, 1995). If we specify n points of interest $\mathbf{x}^i$, $i \in 1, \ldots n$ in the input space, the GLM specifies an n-dimensional Gaussian distribution on the function values $f_1, \ldots, f_n$ with mean $\bar{f}_i = \bar{\mathbf{w}}^T \Phi(\mathbf{x}^i)$ and covariance matrix with elements $c_{ij} = c(\mathbf{x}^i, \mathbf{x}^j) = \Phi(\mathbf{x}^i)^T \Sigma \Phi(\mathbf{x}^j)$ (see GAUSSIAN PROCESSES). The idea behind a GP is that we can free ourselves from the restriction of choosing a covariance function $c(\mathbf{x}^i, \mathbf{x}^j)$ of the form provided by the GLM prior; any valid covariance function can be used instead. Similarly, we are free to choose the mean function $\bar{f}_i = m(\mathbf{x}^i)$. A common choice for the covariance function is $c(\mathbf{x}^i, \mathbf{x}^j) = \exp(-|\mathbf{x}^i - \mathbf{x}^j|^2)$. The motivation is that the function space distribution will have the property that for inputs $\mathbf{x}^i$ and $\mathbf{x}^j$, which are close together, the outputs $f(\mathbf{x}^i)$ and $f(\mathbf{x}^j)$ will be highly correlated, ensuring smoothness. This is one way of avoiding the curse of dimensionality, since the matrix dimensions depend on the number of training points, and not on the number of basis functions used. However, for problems with a large number of training points, computational difficulties can arise, and approximations again need to be considered.

Multilayer Perceptrons

Consider the case of a single hidden layer neural network

$$f(\mathbf{x}; \mathbf{w}) = \sum_{i=1}^{H} v_i g(\mathbf{x}^T \mathbf{u}^i + b_i) \tag{19}$$

where $g(x)$ is a nonlinear sigmoidal transfer function, for example $g(x) = 1/(1 + \exp(-x))$. The set of all weights (parameters), including input-hidden weights $\mathbf{u}^i$, biases b_i, and hidden-output weights v_i, is represented by the vector $\mathbf{w}$. If the weights are small, the network function f will be smooth, since only the near linear regime of the transfer function g will be accessed. An appropriate prior to control complexity is therefore

$$\log p(\mathbf{w}|\alpha) = -\frac{\alpha}{2} \mathbf{w}^T \mathbf{w} + \frac{k}{2} \log \alpha + const. \tag{20}$$

where $k = dim(\mathbf{w})$. For the moment, we will assume that we know the value of the parameter α. This gives the weight posterior as

$$\log p(\mathbf{w}|\alpha, \beta, D) = -\frac{\beta}{2} \sum_{\mu=1}^{P} (t^\mu - f(\mathbf{x}^\mu; \mathbf{w}))^2$$
$$- \frac{\alpha}{2} \mathbf{w}^T \mathbf{w} + const. \tag{21}$$

where $\beta = 1/\sigma^2$. In Figure 3 we show the result of using a six-hidden-unit network to fit the training data in Figure 3. With $\alpha = 0.1$ and $\beta = 1,000$, we drew a number of weight vectors $\mathbf{w}^l$, $l = 1, \ldots, 15$, from the weight posterior $p(\mathbf{w}|D)$, Equation 21 and considered the corresponding functions $f(\mathbf{x}; \mathbf{w}^l)$. The mean and standard error bars calculated from these samples are plotted in Figure 3. How these samples are obtained is discussed later. Note how the error bars automatically increase in regions of low data density.

Monte Carlo Sampling

In general, the posterior distribution $p(\mathbf{w}|\Gamma, D)$ is non-Gaussian, and the integration required over the weight space to find, for example, the mean predictor

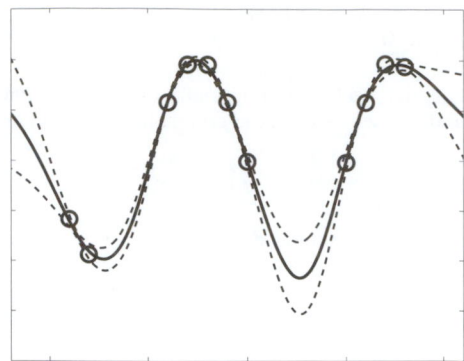

Figure 3. The raw input-output training data, with mean Bayesian MLP predictions (solid curve) and standard error bars (dashed curves). Note how the error bars increase away from the data.

$$\bar{f}(\mathbf{x}) = \int f(\mathbf{x}; \mathbf{w}) p(\mathbf{w}|\Gamma, D) d\mathbf{w} \tag{22}$$

is difficult. An approximate solution is provided by Monte Carlo sampling (Bishop, 1995; Neal, 1996):

$$\int f(\mathbf{x}; \mathbf{w}) p(\mathbf{w}|\Gamma, D) d\mathbf{w} \approx \frac{1}{L} \sum_{i=1}^{L} f(\mathbf{x}; \mathbf{w}^i) \tag{23}$$

where the sample weights $\mathbf{w}^i$ are drawn from the posterior distribution. In principle, this procedure is exact in the limit $L \to \infty$. The great difficulty, however, is in constructing a finite, representative set of samples $\{\mathbf{w}_i\}$, and it is easy to remain trapped in unrepresentative parts of the posterior distribution (Neal, 1996).

Consider the problem of drawing samples from a general distribution $p(\mathbf{x}) \propto \psi(\mathbf{x})$ (Figure 4). Let $\mathbf{x}^{old}$ be a sample point from $p(\mathbf{x})$. We propose a new sample point $\mathbf{x}^{new} = \mathbf{x}^{old} + \eta$ where each element η_i is sampled from a zero-mean Gaussian distribution with variance τ^2. We accept $\mathbf{x}^{new}$ if $\psi(\mathbf{x}^{new}) > \psi(\mathbf{x}^{old})$, since the new candidate sample point is more likely than the old sample point. However, this does not constitute a valid sampling scheme since we only accept increasingly likely points, targeting therefore only the modes of the distribution. To correct for this, we accept a less likely candidate with probability $\psi(\mathbf{x}^{new})/\psi(\mathbf{x}^{old})$. This valid sampling scheme is called the Metropolis method and forms the basis for many generalizations (Neal, 1993, 1996).

In high dimensions, Metropolis sampling can be inefficient, since it is unlikely that testing a new point a long way from the current sample point will result in a more likely point (if you stand on a mountain and jump, it is more likely that you will end up at a point lower than at your current point). Thus, only very small

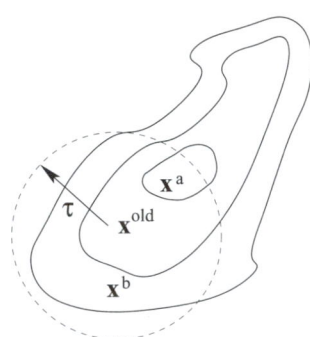

Figure 4. Metropolis Sampling from $p(\mathbf{x}) \propto \psi(\mathbf{x})$. Let $\mathbf{x}^{old}$ be a sample from the distribution $p(\mathbf{x})$. We propose a new candidate $\mathbf{x}^{new}$ by sampling from a Gaussian around $\mathbf{x}^{old}$ with width τ. More likely candidates such as $\mathbf{x}^a$ are accepted. Less likely candidates such as $\mathbf{x}^b$ are accepted with probability $\psi(\mathbf{x}^b)/\psi(\mathbf{x}^{old})$.

jumps will be accepted in high-dimensional spaces, and many samples are required to form a good representation of the distribution. The hybrid Monte Carlo scheme attempts to improve sampling efficiency and allow larger jumps by exploiting gradient information about the distribution and has been successfully employed in Bayesian neural networks (Neal, 1996).

Laplace's Method

Although sampling techniques can be attractive, convergence to a representative set of samples is difficult to assess and can be very slow. Laplace's method is a perturbation technique motivated by the fact that as the number P of training data points is increased, the posterior distribution typically approaches a Gaussian (Walker, 1969) whose variance goes to zero in the limit $P \to \infty$ (we leave aside here the issues of inherent network symmetries). In order to calculate this Gaussian approximation, we consider the posterior distribution, Equation 21:

$$p(\mathbf{w}|D, \Gamma) \propto \exp(-\phi(\mathbf{w})) \tag{24}$$

and expand ϕ around a mode of the distribution, $\mathbf{w}_* = \arg\min \phi(\mathbf{w})$,

$$\phi(\mathbf{w}) \approx \phi(\mathbf{w}_*) + \tfrac{1}{2}(\mathbf{w} - \mathbf{w}_*)^T \mathbf{H}(\mathbf{w} - \mathbf{w}_*) \tag{25}$$

where

$$\mathbf{H} = \nabla\nabla\phi(\mathbf{w})|_{w_*} \tag{26}$$

is the local Hessian matrix. This local expansion defines a Gaussian approximation

$$p(\mathbf{w}|D, \Gamma) \approx \frac{|\mathbf{H}|^{1/2}}{(2\pi)^{k/2}} \exp\{\tfrac{1}{2}(\mathbf{w} - \mathbf{w}_*)^T \mathbf{H}(\mathbf{w} - \mathbf{w}_*)\} \tag{27}$$

The expected value of $f(\mathbf{x}; \mathbf{w})$ as required in Equation 22 can be evaluated by making a further local linearization of the function $f(\cdot, \mathbf{w})$ around the point w_*. In a practical implementation, a standard nonlinear optimization algorithm such as conjugate gradients is used to find a mode w_* of the log posterior distribution (Bishop, 1995).

Determining Hyperparameters

So far we have assumed that the hyperparameters of the MLP are fixed. In a fully Bayesian treatment we would define prior distributions of the hyperparameters, and then integrate them out. Since exact integration is analytically intractable, we can use ML-II to estimate specific values for the hyperparameters by maximizing the marginal likelihood $P(D|\Gamma)$ (Equation 17) with respect to Γ. Using MLPs, the integrand in Equation 17 is non-Gaussian and $p(D|\Gamma)$ needs to be approximated. This can be achieved using Laplace's method by locally expanding the integral to second order in the weights. This leads to simple reestimation formulas for the hyperparameters expressed in terms of the eigenvalue/eigenvector decomposition of the Hessian matrix. This treatment of hyperparameters is called the *evidence* framework (MacKay, 1995) and involves alternating the optimization of $\mathbf{w}$ (mode finding) for fixed hyperparameters with reestimation of the hyperparameters by reevaluating the Hessian matrix for the new value of $\mathbf{w}$. The various approximations involved in this approach improve as the number of data points $P \to \infty$. However, for a finite data set it can be difficult to assess the accuracy of the method. One obvious limitation is that it only takes account of the behavior of the posterior distribution at the mode.

The KL Variational Approach

The Kullback Leibler divergence is a measure of the difference between two probability distributions $p(\mathbf{x})$ and $q(\mathbf{x})$ (Cover and Thomas, 1991)

$$KL(q, p) = \int \{q(\mathbf{x}) \log q(\mathbf{x}) - q(\mathbf{x}) \log p(\mathbf{x})\} d\mathbf{x} \tag{28}$$

This has the advantageous properties $KL \geq 0$ and $KL = 0$ if and only if $p \equiv q$. Consider the KL divergence

$$KL(q(\mathbf{w}), p(\mathbf{w}|\Gamma, D)) \geq 0 \tag{29}$$

Finding the best distribution $q(\mathbf{w})$ in a restricted set of possible distributions by minimizing $KL(q, p)$ gives the best estimate (in the KL sense) to the posterior distribution. From Equation 29 we immediately have the bound

$$\log p(D|\Gamma) \geq \int -q(\mathbf{w}) \log q(\mathbf{w}) d\mathbf{w}$$
$$+ \int q(\mathbf{w}) \log p(D|\Gamma, \mathbf{w}) p(\mathbf{w}) d\mathbf{w} \tag{30}$$

We can make use of this lower bound to carry out an approximate ML-II hyperparameter optimization by the following two-step procedure: First fix the hyperparameters Γ and optimize the bound, Equation 30, with respect to $q(\mathbf{w})$. Then, for fixed $q(\mathbf{w})$, optimize the bound with respect to Γ. This scheme is a generalization of the Expectation-Maximization procedure (see Neal and Hinton in Jordan, 1998) and is also called *ensemble learning* (Barber and Bishop, 1997).

Bayesian Pruning

To this point we discussed the idea of using a prior that encourages smoothness of the input-output mapping. Insofar as neural networks are nonlinear functions of a linear combination of inputs, it is reasonable to use a prior that encourages small weights, $p(\mathbf{w}) \propto \exp(-\mathbf{w}^T \mathbf{A} \mathbf{w}/2)$. Typically, only diagonal matrices $\mathbf{A}$ are considered. We can group weights into clusters containing one or more weights and associate with each cluster c a common hyperparameter α_c. The Bayesian approach results in a posterior distribution over these hyperparameters α_c. Alternatively, we can optimize the hyperparameters using ML-II. If the posterior distribution favors large α_c values, then effectively the weight cluster c is not contributing to the network and may be pruned. A useful choice of clustering is to group all the weights from a single input x_i into the hidden units (note that these weights are different from the weights that fan in to a hidden node). If the hyperparameter α_i (after ML-II optimization) associated with the weights fanning out from input x_i is large, the contribution of input x_i is negligible and can be excluded. This is called *automatic relevance determination* (MacKay, 1995).

The Relevance Vector Machine

In the discussion regarding GLMs, $f(\mathbf{x}) = \Sigma_i w_i \phi_i(\mathbf{x})$, we fixed the centers of the basis functions ϕ_i. Similarly, in the relevance vector machine we use fixed basis functions (Tipping, 2001). By associating with each weight w_i a regularizing prior $p(w_i) \propto \exp(-\alpha_i w_i^2/2)$, we can perform ML-II to optimize the hyperparameters α_i. After optimization, typically many of the α_i will become very large, effectively removing the basis function ϕ_i from the model. This pruning procedure often results in a much sparser representation of the data in terms of only the "relevant" basis functions; this scheme is therefore particularly useful for compression. This sparseness effect is similar, although not equivalent, to the support vector machine (see SUPPORT VECTOR MACHINES), in which training points are effectively removed if they do not affect the prediction of the model.

Classification

The previously described methods can be applied to classification, usually with only minor modification. For convenience, we consider here only problems with two classes. The data set is $D = \{(\mathbf{x}^\mu, t^\mu), \mu = 1, \ldots, P\}$, where $t^\mu \in \{0, 1\}$. In a probabilistic framework, we use the output of the network $f(\mathbf{x}; \mathbf{w})$ to represent the probability that the input is in class 1. In this case, the likelihood is

$$p(D|\mathbf{w}) = \prod_{\mu=1}^{P} f(\mathbf{x}^\mu; \mathbf{w})^{t^\mu} (1 - f(\mathbf{x}^\mu; \mathbf{w}))^{1-t^\mu} \qquad (31)$$

For example, we could take $f(\mathbf{x}) = g(\mathbf{w}^T\mathbf{x})$, where $g(x) = 1/(1 + \exp(-x))$ (Bishop, 1995). In the Bayesian approach, we need to specify a prior belief about the weights. As before, a sensible choice is $p(\mathbf{w}) \propto \exp(-\alpha\mathbf{w}^T\mathbf{w}/2)$, since smaller weights will give less certain predictions. This results in a posterior distribution $p(\mathbf{w}|D) \propto p(D|\mathbf{w})p(\mathbf{w})$. For a novel input $\mathbf{x}$ the probability that it belongs to class 1 is

$$p(t = 1|\mathbf{x}, D) = \int p(t = 1|\mathbf{x}, \mathbf{w})p(\mathbf{w}|D)d\mathbf{w}$$
$$= \int g(\mathbf{w}^T\mathbf{x})p(\mathbf{w}|D)d\mathbf{w} \qquad (32)$$

Consider, for example, fitting the data in Figure 5A. The posterior distribution is given in Figure 5D. The decision boundary ($p(t = 1|\mathbf{x}, \mathbf{w}, D) = 0.5$) for the MAP solution is given in Figure 5B along with the 0.1 and 0.9 decision contours. Another decision boundary associated with the posterior weights $\mathbf{w}^A$ is plotted in Figure 5B. Because the decision boundaries are linear, the predictions of these single networks away from the data remain overly confident. The Bayesian prediction, Equation 32, is plotted in Figure 5C and has decision boundaries that properly account for the uncertainty in the predictions away from the training data.

Since the final integrand in Equation 32 depends only on the weight vector through the "activation" $a = \mathbf{w}^T\mathbf{x}$, we need only know the distribution of this one-dimensional quantity. A reasonable assumption is that the activation will be Gaussian distributed $p(a) = N(\bar{a}, \text{var}(a))$, and the resulting one-dimensional integration $p(t = 1|\mathbf{x}, D) = \int g(a)p(a)da$ can be efficiently performed using quadrature. The statistics of the activation are

$$\bar{a} = \bar{\mathbf{w}}^T\mathbf{x}, \quad \text{var}(a) = \mathbf{x}^T\Sigma\mathbf{x} \qquad (33)$$

where $\bar{\mathbf{w}}$ and Σ are the mean and covariance of the weight posterior $p(\mathbf{w}|D)$. It is convenient to approximate these statistics using Laplace's method.

Discussion

The Bayesian framework deals with uncertainty in a natural, consistent manner by combining prior beliefs about which models are

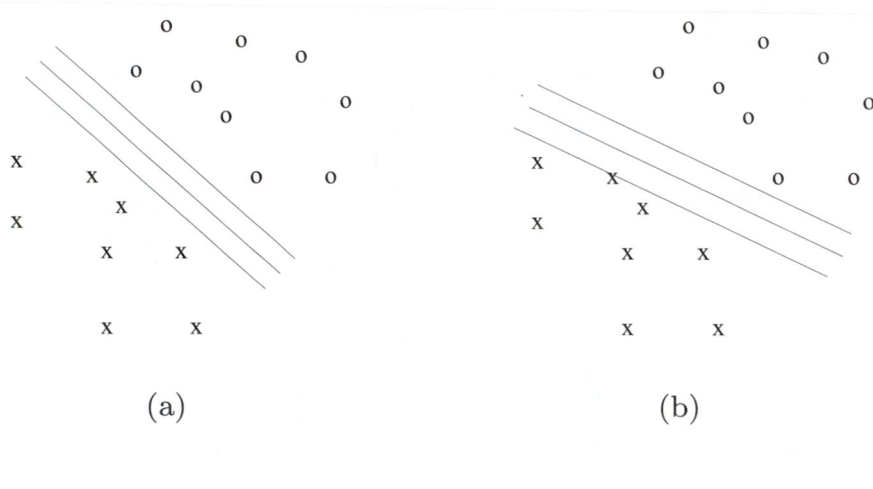

(a)

(b)

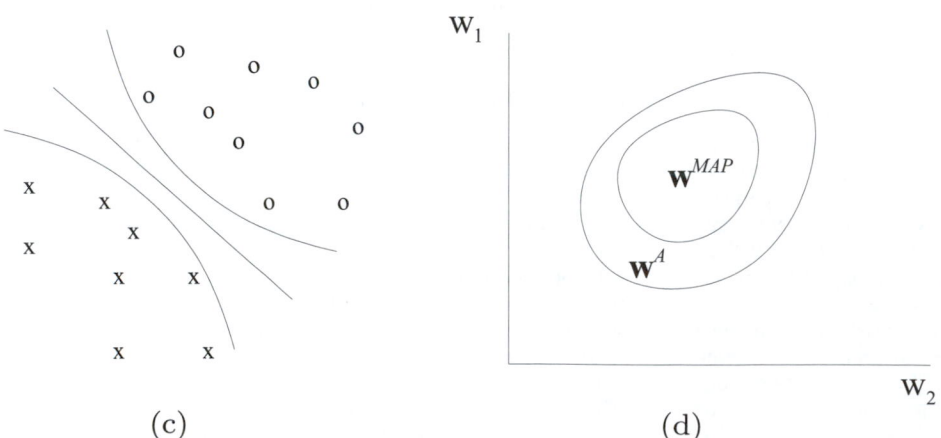

(c)

(d)

Figure 5. *A*, The decision boundary and 0.1, 0.9 decision contours for the most likely predictor $\mathbf{w}^{MAP}$. *B*, The predictions for $\mathbf{w}^A$. *C*, The posterior averaged predictors. *D*, The weight posterior distribution.

appropriate with how likely each model would be to have generated the data. This results in an elegant, general framework for fitting models to data, which, however, may be compromised by computational difficulties in carrying out the ideal procedure. There are many approximate Bayesian implementations, using methods such as sampling, perturbation techniques, and variational methods. Often these enable the successful approximate realization of practical Bayesian schemes. An attractive, built-in effect of the Bayesian approach is an automatic procedure for combining predictions from several different models, the combination strength of a model being given by the posterior likelihood of the model. In the case of models linear in their parameters, Bayesian neural networks are closely related to Gaussian processes, and many of the computational difficulties of dealing with more general stochastic nonlinear systems can be avoided.

Bayesian methods are readily extendable to other areas, in particular density estimation, and the benefits of dealing with uncertainty are again to be found (see Bishop in Jordan, 1998). Traditionally, neural networks are graphical representations of functions, in which the computations at each node are deterministic. In the classification discussion, however, the final output represents a stochastic variable. We can consider such stochastic variables elsewhere in the network, and the sigmoid belief network is an early example of a stochastic network (Neal, 1992). There is a major conceptual difference between such models and conventional neural networks. Networks in which nodes represent stochastic variables are called graphical models (see BAYESIAN NETWORKS) and are graphical representations of *distributions* (GRAPHICAL MODELS: PROBABILISTIC INFERENCE). Such models evolve naturally from the desire of incorporating uncertainty and nonlinearity in networked systems.

Road Map: Learning in Artificial Networks
Related Reading: Bayesian Networks; Gaussian Processes; Graphical Models: Probabilistic Inference; Support Vector Machines

References

Barber, D., and Bishop, C., 1997, Ensemble learning in Bayesian neural networks, in *Neural Networks and Machine Learning* (C. Bishop, Ed.), NATO ASI Series, New York: Springer-Verlag.

Berger, J. O., 1985, *Statistical Decision Theory and Bayesian Analysis*, 2nd ed., New York: Springer-Verlag. ◆

Bishop, C. M., 1995, *Neural Networks for Pattern Recognition*, Oxford, Engl.: Oxford University Press. ◆

Box, G., and Tiao, G., 1973, *Bayesian Inference in Statistical Analysis*, Reading, MA: Addison-Wesley.

Cover, M., and Thomas, J., 1991, *Elements of Information Theory*, New York: Wiley.

Jordan, M., Ed., 1998, *Learning in Graphical Models*, Cambridge, MA: MIT Press.

MacKay, D. J. C., 1992, Bayesian interpolation, *Neural Computat.*, 4(3): 415–447.

MacKay, D. J. C., 1995, Probable networks and plausible predictions: A review of practical Bayesian methods for supervised neural networks, *Netw. Computat. Neural Syst.*, 6(3). ◆

Neal, R. M., 1992, Connectionist learning of belief networks, *Artif. Intell.*, 56:71–113.

Neal, R. M., 1993, *Probabilistic Inference Using Markov Chain Monte Carlo Methods*, Technical Report CRG-TR-93-1, Department of Computer Science, University of Toronto, Toronto, Canada.

Neal, R. M., 1996, *Bayesian Learning for Neural Networks*, Lecture Notes in Statistics 118, New York: Springer-Verlag.

Tipping, M. E., 2001, Sparse Bayesian learning and the relevance vector machine, *J. Machine Learn. Res.*, no. 1, 211–244. ◆

Walker, A. M., 1969, On the asymptotic behaviour of posterior distributions, *J. R. Statist. Soc. B*, 31:80–88.

Bayesian Networks

Judea Pearl and Stuart Russell

Introduction

Probabilistic models based on directed acyclic graphs have a long and rich tradition, beginning with work by the geneticist Sewall Wright in the 1920s. Variants have appeared in many fields. Within statistics, such models are known as *directed graphical models*; within cognitive science and artificial intelligence (AI), they are known as *Bayesian networks*. The name honors the Reverend Thomas Bayes (1702–1761), whose rule for updating probabilities in light of new evidence is the foundation of the approach. The initial development of Bayesian networks in the late 1970s was motivated by the need to model the top-down (semantic) and bottom-up (perceptual) combination of evidence in reading. The capability for bidirectional inferences, combined with a rigorous probabilistic foundation, led to the rapid emergence of Bayesian networks as the method of choice for uncertain reasoning in AI and expert systems, replacing earlier, ad hoc rule-based schemes (Pearl, 1988; Shafer and Pearl, 1990; Jensen, 1996).

The nodes in a Bayesian network represent propositional variables of interest (e.g., the temperature of a device, the sex of a patient, a feature of an object, the occurrence of an event) and the links represent informational or causal dependencies among the variables. The dependencies are quantified by conditional probabilities for each node, given its parents in the network. The network supports the computation of the probabilities of any subset of variables given evidence about any other subset.

Figure 1 illustrates a simple yet typical Bayesian network. It describes the causal relationships among five variables: the season of the year (X_1), whether it's raining or not (X_2), whether the sprinkler is on or off (X_3), whether the pavement is wet or dry (X_4), and whether the pavement is slippery or not (X_5). Here, the absence of a direct link between X_1 and X_5, for example, captures our understanding that there is no direct influence of season on slipperiness;

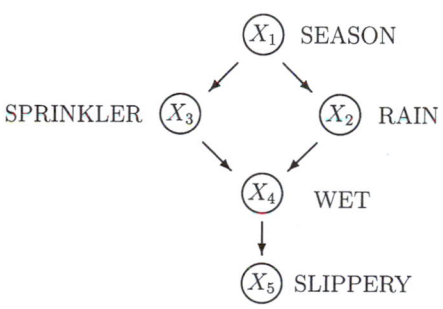

Figure 1. A Bayesian network representing causal influences among five variables. Each arc indicates a causal influence of the "parent" node on the "child" node.

the influence is mediated by the wetness of the pavement. (If freezing is a possibility, then a direct link could be added.)

Perhaps the most important aspect of Bayesian networks is that *they are direct representations of the world, not of reasoning processes.* The arrows in the diagram represent real causal connections and not the flow of information during reasoning (as in rule-based systems and neural networks). Reasoning processes can operate on Bayesian networks by propagating information in any direction. For example, if the sprinkler is on, then the pavement is probably wet (prediction); if someone slips on the pavement, that also provides evidence that it is wet (abduction, or reasoning to a probable cause). On the other hand, if we see that the pavement is wet, that makes it more likely that the sprinkler is on or that it is raining (abduction); but if we then observe that the sprinkler is on, that reduces the likelihood that it is raining (explaining away). It is this last form of reasoning, explaining away, that is especially difficult to model in rule-based systems and neural networks in any natural way, because it seems to require the propagation of information in two directions.

Probabilistic Semantics

Any complete probabilistic model of a domain must, either explicitly or implicitly, represent the *joint distribution*—the probability of every possible event as defined by the values of all the variables. There are exponentially many such events, yet Bayesian networks achieve compactness by factoring the joint distribution into local, conditional distributions for each variable given its parents. If x_i denotes some value of the variable X_i and pa_i denotes some set of values for X_i's parents, then $P(x_i \mid pa_i)$ denotes this conditional distribution. For example, $P(x_4 \mid x_2, x_3)$ is the probability of wetness given the values of sprinkler and rain. The *global semantics* of Bayesian networks specifies that the full joint distribution is given by the product

$$P(x_1, \ldots, x_n) = \prod_i P(x_i \mid pa_i) \qquad (1)$$

In our example network, we have

$$P(x_1, x_2, x_3, x_4, x_5)$$
$$= P(x_1)P(x_2 \mid x_1)P(x_3 \mid x_1)P(x_4 \mid x_2, x_3)P(x_5 \mid x_4) \qquad (2)$$

Provided that the number of parents of each node is bounded, it is easy to see that the number of parameters required grows only linearly with the size of the network, whereas the joint distribution itself grows exponentially. Further savings can be achieved using compact parametric representations, such as noisy-OR models, decision trees, or neural networks, for the conditional distributions. For example, in *sigmoid* networks (see Jordan, 1999), the conditional distribution associated with each variable is represented as a sigmoid function of a linear combination of the parent variables; in this way, the number of parameters required is proportional to, rather than exponential in, the number of parents.

There is also an entirely equivalent *local semantics* that asserts that each variable is independent of its nondescendants in the network given its parents. For example, the parents of X_4 in Figure 1 are X_2 and X_3, and they render X_4 independent of the remaining nondescendant, X_1. That is,

$$P(x_4 \mid x_1, x_2, x_3) = P(x_4 \mid x_2, x_3)$$

The collection of independence assertions formed in this way suffices to derive the global assertion in Equation 1, and vice versa. The local semantics is most useful in *constructing* Bayesian networks, because selecting as parents *all* the direct causes of a given variable invariably satisfies the local conditional independence conditions (Pearl, 2000, p. 30). The global semantics leads directly to a variety of algorithms for reasoning.

Evidential Reasoning

From the product specification in Equation 1, one can express the probability of any desired proposition in terms of the conditional probabilities specified in the network. For example, the probability that the sprinkler is on, given that the pavement is slippery, is

$$P(X_3 = on \mid X_5 = true) = \frac{P(X_3 = on, X_5 = true)}{P(X_5 = true)}$$
$$= \frac{\sum_{x_1, x_2, x_4} P(x_1, x_2, X_3 = on, x_4, X_5 = true)}{\sum_{x_1, x_2, x_3, x_4} P(x_1, x_2, x_3, x_4, X_5 = true)}$$
$$= \frac{\sum_{x_1, x_2, x_4} P(x_1)P(x_2 \mid x_1)P(X_3 = on \mid x_1)P(x_4 \mid x_2, X_3 = on)P(X_5 = true \mid x_4)}{\sum_{x_1, x_2, x_3, x_4} P(x_1)P(x_2 \mid x_1)P(x_3 \mid x_1)P(x_4 \mid x_2, x_3)P(X_5 = true \mid x_4)}$$

These expressions can often be simplified in ways that reflect the structure of the network itself. The first algorithms proposed for probabilistic calculations in Bayesian networks used a local, distributed message-passing architecture, typical of many cognitive activities (Kim and Pearl, 1983). Initially this approach was limited to tree-structured networks, but it was later extended to general networks in Lauritzen and Spiegelhalter's (1988) method of join-tree propagation. A number of other exact methods have been developed and can be found in recent textbooks (Jensen, 1996; Jordan, 1999).

It is easy to show that reasoning in Bayesian networks subsumes the satisfiability problem in propositional logic and, hence, is NP-hard. Monte Carlo simulation methods can be used for approximate inference (Pearl, 1988), giving gradually improving estimates as sampling proceeds. (These methods use local message propagation on the original network structure, unlike join-tree methods.) Alternatively, variational methods provide bounds on the true probability (Jordan, 1999).

Uncertainty over Time

Entities that live in a changing environment must keep track of variables whose values change over time. Dynamic Bayesian networks, or DBNs, capture this process by representing multiple copies of the state variables, one for each time step (Dean and Kanazawa, 1989). A set of variables $\mathbf{X}_t$ denotes the world state at time t and a set of sensor variables $\mathbf{E}_t$ denotes the observations available at time t. The *sensor model* $P(\mathbf{E}_t \mid \mathbf{X}_t)$ is encoded in the conditional probability distributions for the observable variables, given the state variables. The *transition model* $P(\mathbf{X}_{t+1} \mid \mathbf{X}_t)$ relates the state at time t to the state at time $t + 1$. Keeping track of the world, known as *filtering*, means computing the current probability distribution over world states given all past observations, i.e., $P(\mathbf{X}_t \mid \mathbf{E}_1, \ldots, \mathbf{E}_t)$. Dynamic Bayesian networks include as special cases other temporal probability models, such as hidden Markov models (DBNs with a single discrete state variable) and Kalman filters (DBNs with continuous state and sensor variables and linear Gaussian transition and sensor models). For the general case, exact filtering is intractable, and a variety of approximation algorithms have been developed. The most popular and flexible of these is the family of *particle filtering* algorithms (see Doucet, de Freitas, and Gordan, 2001).

Learning in Bayesian Networks

The conditional probabilities $P(x_i \mid pa_i)$ can be updated continuously from observational data using gradient-based or Expectation-Maximization (EM) methods that use just local information derived from inference (Binder et al., 1997; Jordan, 1999), in much the same way as weights are adjusted in neural networks. It is also possible to learn the structure of the network, using methods that trade off network complexity against degree of fit to the data (Friedman, 1998). As a substrate for learning, Bayesian networks have the advantage that it is relatively easy to encode prior knowledge in network form, either by fixing portions of the structure or by using prior distributions over the network parameters. Such prior knowledge can allow a system to learn accurate models from much less data than are required by *tabula rasa* approaches.

Causal Networks

Most probabilistic models, including general Bayesian networks, describe a distribution over possible observed events, as in Equation 1, but say nothing about what will happen if a certain *intervention* occurs. For example, what if I *turn the sprinkler on*? What effect does that have on the season, or on the connection between wetness and slipperiness? A *causal network*, intuitively speaking, is a Bayesian network with the added property that the parents of each node are its direct causes, as in Figure 1. In such a network, the result of an intervention is obvious: the sprinkler node is set to $X_3 = on$, and the causal link between the season X_1 and the sprinkler X_3 is removed. All other causal links and conditional probabilities remain intact, so the new model is

$$P(x_1, x_2, x_3, x_4, x_5) =$$
$$P(x_1)P(x_2 \mid x_1)P(x_4 \mid x_2, X_3 = on)P(x_5 \mid x_4)$$

Notice that this differs from *observing* that $X_3 = on$, which would result in a new model that included the term $P(X_3 = on|x_1)$. This mirrors the difference between seeing and doing: after observing that the sprinkler is on, we wish to infer that the season is dry, that it probably did not rain, and so on; an arbitrary decision to turn the sprinkler on should not result in any such beliefs.

Causal networks are more properly defined, then, as Bayesian networks in which the correct probability model after intervening to fix any node's value is given simply by deleting links from the node's parents. For example, *fire → smoke* is a causal network, whereas *smoke → fire* is not, even though both networks are equally capable of representing any joint distribution on the two variables. Causal networks model the environment as a collection of stable component mechanisms. These mechanisms may be reconfigured locally by interventions, with correspondingly local changes in the model. This, in turn, allows causal networks to be used very naturally for prediction by an agent that is considering various courses of action (Pearl, 2000).

Functional Bayesian Networks

The networks discussed so far are capable of supporting reasoning about evidence and about actions. Additional refinement is necessary in order to process *counterfactual* information. For example, the probability that "the pavement would not have been slippery had the sprinkler been OFF, given that the sprinkler is in fact ON and that the pavement is in fact slippery" cannot be computed from the information provided in Figure 1 and Equation 1. Such counterfactual probabilities require a specification in the form of functional networks, where each conditional probability $P(x_i|pa_i)$ is replaced by a functional relationship $x_i = f_i(pa_i, \epsilon_i)$, where ϵ_i is a stochastic (unobserved) error term. When the functions f_i and the distributions of ϵ_i are known, all counterfactual statements can be assigned unique probabilities, using evidence propagation in a structure called a "twin network." When only partial knowledge about the functional form of f_i is available, bounds can be computed on the probabilities of counterfactual sentences (Pearl, 2000).

Causal Discovery

One of the most exciting prospects in recent years has been the possibility of using Bayesian networks to discover causal structures

in raw statistical data (Pearl, 2000)—a task previously considered impossible without controlled experiments. Consider, for example, the following *intransitive* pattern of dependencies among three events: A and B are dependent, B and C are dependent, yet A and C are independent. If you ask a person to supply an example of three such events, the example would invariably portray A and C as two independent causes and B as their common effect, namely, $A \rightarrow B \leftarrow C$. (For instance, A and C could be the outcomes of tossing two fair coins, and B could represent a bell that rings whenever either coin comes up heads.) Fitting this dependence pattern with a scenario in which B is the cause and A and C are the effects is mathematically feasible but very unnatural, because it must entail fine tuning of the probabilities involved; the desired dependence pattern will be destroyed as soon as the probabilities undergo a slight change.

Such thought experiments tell us that certain patterns of dependency, which are totally void of temporal information, are conceptually characteristic of certain causal directionalities and not others. When put together systematically, such patterns can be used to infer causal structures from raw data and to guarantee that any alternative structure compatible with the data must be less stable than the one(s) inferred; namely, slight fluctuations in parameters will render that structure incompatible with the data.

Plain Beliefs

In mundane decision making, beliefs are revised not by adjusting numerical probabilities but by tentatively accepting some sentences as "true for all practical purposes." Such sentences, called *plain beliefs*, exhibit both logical and probabilistic character. As in classical logic, they are propositional and deductively closed; as in probability, they are subject to retraction and can be held with varying degrees of strength. Bayesian networks can be adopted to model the dynamics of plain beliefs by replacing ordinary probabilities with nonstandard probabilities, that is, probabilities that are infinitesimally close to either zero or one (Goldszmidt and Pearl, 1996).

Discussion

Bayesian networks may be viewed as normative cognitive models of propositional reasoning under uncertainty. They handle noise and partial information using local, distributed algorithms for inference and learning. Unlike feedforward neural networks, they facilitate local representations in which nodes correspond to propositions of interest. Recent experiments suggest that they accurately capture the causal inferences made by both children and adults (Tenenbaum and Griffiths, 2001). Moreover, they capture patterns of reasoning, such as explaining away, that are not easily handled by any competing computational model. They appear to have many of the advantages of both the "symbolic" and the "subsymbolic" approaches to cognitive modeling, and are now an essential part of the foundations of computational neuroscience (Jordan and Sejnowski, 2001).

Two major questions arise when we postulate Bayesian networks as potential models of actual human cognition. First, does an architecture resembling that of Bayesian networks exist anywhere in the human brain? At the time of writing, no specific work has been done to design neurally plausible models that implement the required functionality, although no obvious obstacles exist. Second, how could Bayesian networks, which are purely propositional in their expressive power, handle the kinds of reasoning about individuals, relations, properties, and universals that pervade human thought? One plausible answer is that Bayesian networks containing propositions relevant to the current context are constantly being assembled, as needed, from a more permanent store of knowledge. For example, the network in Figure 1 may be assembled to help explain why this particular pavement is slippery right now, and to decide whether this can be prevented. The background store of knowledge includes general models of pavements, sprinklers, slipping, rain, and so on; these must be accessed and supplied with instance data to construct the specific Bayesian network structure. The store of background knowledge must utilize some representation that combines the expressive power of first-order logical languages (such as semantic networks) with the ability to handle uncertain information. Substantial progress has been made on constructing systems of this kind (Koller and Pfeffer, 1998), but as yet no overall cognitive architecture has been proposed.

Road Maps: Artificial Intelligence; Learning in Artificial Networks
Related Reading: Bayesian Methods and Neural Networks; Decision Support Systems and Expert Systems; Graphical Models: Probabilistic Inference

References

Binder, J., Koller, D., Russell, S., and Kanazawa, K., 1997, Adaptive probabilitic networks with hidden variables, *Machine Learn.*, 29:213–244.

Dean, T., and Kanazawa, K., 1989, A model for reasoning about persistence and causation, *Computat. Intell.*, 5:142–150.

Doucet, A., de Freitas, J., and Gordon, N., 2001, *Sequential Monte Carlo Methods in Practice*, Berlin: Springer-Verlag.

Friedman, N., 1998, The Bayesian structural EM algorithm, in *Uncertainty in Artificial Intelligence: Proceedings of the Fourteenth Conference*

(G. F. Cooper and S. Moral, Eds.), San Mateo, CA: Morgan Kaufmann, pp. 129–138.

Goldszmidt, M., and Pearl, J., 1996, Qualitative probabilities for default reasoning, belief revision, and causal modeling, *Artif. Intell.*, 84:57–112.

Jensen, F. V., 1996, *An Introduction to Bayesian Networks*, New York: Springer-Verlag. ◆

Jordan, M. I., Ed., 1999, *Learning in Graphical Models*, Cambridge, MA: MIT Press. ◆

Jordan, M. I., and Sejnowski, T. J., Eds., 2001, *Graphical Models: Foundations of Neural Computation*, Cambridge, MA: MIT Press.

Kim, J. H., and Pearl, J., 1983, A computational model for combined causal and diagnostic reasoning in inference systems, in *Proceedings of the Eighth International Joint Conference on Artificial Intelligence (IJCAI-83)*, San Mateo, CA: Morgan Kaufmann, pp. 190–193.

Koller, D., and Pfeffer, A., 1998, Probabilistic frame-based systems, in *Proceedings of the Fifteenth National Conference on Artificial Intelligence (AAAI-98)*, Menlo Park, CA: AAAI Press, pp. 580–587.

Lauritzen, S. L., and Spiegelhalter, D. J., 1988, Local computations with probabilities on graphical structures and their application to expert systems (with discussion), *J. R. Statist. Soc.*, series B, 50:157–224.

Pearl, J., 1988, *Probabilistic Reasoning in Intelligent Systems*, San Mateo, CA: Morgan Kaufmann. ◆

Pearl, J., 2000, *Causality: Models, Reasoning, and Inference*, New York: Cambridge University Press. ◆

Shafer, G., and Pearl, J., Eds., 1990, *Readings in Uncertain Reasoning*, San Mateo, CA: Morgan Kaufmann.

Tenenbaum, J. B., and Griffiths, T. L., 2001, Structure learning in human causal induction, in *Advances in Neural Information Processing Systems 13*, Cambridge, MA: MIT Press.

Biologically Inspired Robotics

Noel E. Sharkey

Introduction

At the beginning of the twenty-first century, living organisms have still not been successfully replicated by machines. Computers are much faster at number crunching than humans and can even beat the greatest at chess, and other machines can perform routine physical tasks faster than us and with a precision that we cannot approach. However, animals exhibit such remarkable capacities for flexible adaptation to novel circumstances that roboticists can only gaze in wonder. It is thus an important goal of modern robotics to learn from the way organisms are constructed biologically, and how this creates adaptive behaviors.

Biologically inspired robotics, also known as biomimetic robotics or biorobotics, refers to robotics research in which the life sciences, including biology, psychology, ethology, neuroscience, and evolutionary theory, play a key role in motivating the research. It is necessarily broad because the field is just beginning to emerge as a unified discipline, and so it still has fuzzy boundaries. Biorobotics research ranges from modeling animal sensors in hardware for guiding robots in target environments to investigating the interaction between neural learning and evolution in a variety of robot tasks. There are, however, common themes that will be explored here.

In the following sections, some of the major issues in biorobotics research and the aims of this approach are examined. First we briefly consider the historical roots of the core ideas. The seminal work of Grey Walter (1953) sets the scene and introduces some of the key elements of biologically inspired robotics. The re-introduction and development of the ideas in the 1980s occurred with Braitenberg's *synthetic psychology* and Brook's *behavior-based* robotics. In summarizing the breadth of the current work, we attempt a threefold classification of biologically inspired robotics.

The Roots of Biologically Inspired Robotics

The roots of biologically inspired robotics date back to the early twentieth century, when Hammond constructed a heliotrope based on the biologist Loeb's tropism theory of animal behavior. Loeb proposed that animals are attracted and repelled by stimuli in the environment in a way similar to the phototropic responses of plants. Although Hammond's heliotrope did not model an animal, its mechanized movement toward light was sufficient to satisfy Loeb that his theory has physical plausibility (cf. Sharkey and Ziemke in Ziemke and Sharkey, 1998, pp. 361–392, for an account).

There were a number of robot learning studies during the first half of the twentieth century, before the birth of artificial intelligence (AI). However, the prototypical biorobotics work was conducted by Grey Walter (1953). He went far beyond Hammond in testing the mechanistic plausibility of animal tropism. His aim was to create a self-sustaining artificial life form that could adapt. This required the development of a robot that could seek out a source to recharge its batteries on demand.

Grey Walter used electromechanical robots equipped with two input "receptors": a photo-electric cell for sensitivity to light, and an electrical contact as a touch receptor. The controller, between sensors and motors, was a small artificial nervous system built from miniature valves, relays, condensers, batteries, and small electric motors—no computer. There was a hutch where a robot could drive in to have the battery automatically recharged.

Behavior resulted from the interaction of the internal states of the robot (battery level) and the intensity of light sources, as well as other environmental factors such as obstacles. When the battery levels were high, the robot was repelled by the bright light of the hutch and attracted by the moderate light in the room, where it "explored." With low battery levels, the robot was attracted to the bright light of the hutch for an automatic recharge. In this way Grey Walter demonstrated that mechanical tropism could work as a means of exploration and maintaining energy.

Grey Walter (1953) also investigated adaptation and showed how a simple learning mechanism could extend the behavior of a robot using the conditioned reflex analog (CORA) with a microphone for auditory input.

Biorobotics more or less died when Grey Walter moved on to other research in the 1950s. With the rise of AI and computing, the focus was on providing robots with human-inspired perception and cognition. The new robots had a series of modules, such as visual processing, planning, and reasoning, through which sensory information passed serially. Typically, a decision-making module controlled the output to the actuators. This was in contrast to the more direct control approach of Grey Walter, in which the only mediation between sensing and moving was provided by an artificial neural net consisting of two hardware neurons. Another difference was that whereas AI robotics focused on human cognition, Grey Walter focused on the question of how seemingly complex animal-like behavior could arise from simple mechanisms such as tropisms and reflexes.

Today the term *taxis* is used instead of tropism to refer to the movement of an animal directed by a stimulus, either negatively or positively. Examples of such stimulus-directed activity include chemotaxis (chemical taxis), geotaxis (gravity), phototaxis (light), and phonotaxis (auditory). Although Grey Walter worked only on individual taxes, biologists at the time (e.g., Fraenkel and Gunn; cf. Sharkey and Ziemke in Ziemke and Sharkey, 1998, pp. 361–392) proposed that the behavior of many organisms could be explained by a combination of taxes working together and in opposition. They cited Fraenkel's study of the coastal slug, *Littorina neritoides*. *Littorina* combines positive and negative phototaxis with negative geotaxis to feed and survive. Subsequently, combinations of taxes have been used as powerful explanations of many animal behaviors, from bacteria feeding to insect pheromone trailing to fish breeding and feeding.

These ideas began to emerge in a new wave of robotics during the 1980s as a result of two major influences. First, the neuroanatomist Valentino Braitenberg showed how a number of complex behaviors could emerge from a combination of very simple neural networks encoding different taxes (Braitenberg, 1984). Second, Rodney Brooks's development of subsumption architecture allowed autonomous control by a combination of taxes, and drove home the effectiveness of behavior-based robotics. His major papers from this period are reprinted in Brooks (1999). In this style of robotics, each behavior-producing module, such as *avoid obstacles* or *move toward light*, is encoded as a separate program module such that each is directly under the control of environmental circumstances rather than a central controller. For example, when there is light on the sensors, the *move toward light* module will be active until the light is occluded by an obstacle, at which point the *avoid obstacles* module takes over.

Current Directions in Biorobotics

A large emerging body of research in robotics is making the connection between sensing and moving simple, and the relationship between robot and world tightly coupled. It was the dramatic increase in robotics research, riding on the back of the new behavior-based approach, that enabled biologically inspired robotics to flourish. Since the behavior-based approach grew directly from ideas in the life sciences, it was only natural that once the tools and techniques of the approach had been developed, they would be turned back to work on the source of inspiration.

In this article, biorobotics is divided into three main classes. Although these classes are mutually supportive and their paths often cross, the distinctions between them are nonetheless useful.

- The *generalized* approach follows from the lineage of ideas that inspired Grey Walter to use robots to investigate and extend general mechanistic theories of animal behavior and adaptation. This includes research using neural network adaptation through learning and/or evolutionary methods (see REACTIVE ROBOTIC SYSTEMS).

- The *specific* approach uses methods from the generalized approach to investigate specific species or organisms. The research can range from studies of the physical plausibility of a simple neural explanation for some target behavior pattern to the physical modeling of a particular animal or some of its senses. Models can be evaluated by observing the target behavior of the robot interacting with the environment through sensing and moving. One of the main goals of specific biorobotics is to develop new methods for scientific modeling.

- The *theoretical* division is a mixed bag that provides an examination of the implications of the research for a number of disciplines. The issues range widely, from discussions of robot embodiment to the nature of life. Although all biorobotics has a theoretical component, the theoretical approach is distinct in not requiring empirical work.

The idea was to include only work that at least touched base with the life sciences with respect to the type of controllers and the method of adaptation used. Each of the classes is dealt with in more depth in the following three subsections.

Generalized Biorobotics

The research impetus is to use broad notions derived from the life sciences for robot control. Many of these notions are in the form of implicit assumptions, such as deriving complex behavior from the simplest possible mechanisms or using the ideas of taxis or tropism for automated control. In this sense, Grey Walter's research was prototypical generalized biorobotics. His work on classical conditioning with the CORA architecture also foresaw the modern focus on adaptive techniques in robotics. The biological currency in the generalized biorobotics community mostly consists of abstract models of neural network learning, animal learning, or evolutionary processes, or a mixture. In the next two subsections, the main trends will be discussed.

Evolution. Evolutionary methods have been used for many applications since the 1950s when the first Genetic Algorithm (GA; see EVOLUTION OF ARTIFICIAL NEURAL NETWORKS) was developed by Friedman for his master's thesis on evolving control circuits for autonomous robots. These methods are particularly useful for constraining search in very large search spaces. However, from the perspective of biorobotics, the most important reason for employing evolutionary methods is that they are abstractly related to the Darwinian principle of natural selection and may be seen as analogous to real evolutionary theory; i.e., there is a fitness function to decide how fit a particular program is in the context of the problem it is to solve, and there are mutation and crossover to operate on the computer equivalent of gene strings. Given the intended relationship between the behavior of biorobots and natural biological behavior, the development of an *evolutionary robotics* is a very important step.

A fairly typical example of evolutionary methods for single robots is Nolfi's garbage collector (in Sharkey, 1997, pp. 187–198). The connection weights were evolved to control a miniature robot equipped with distance sensors and a gripper. The task was to "clean" an arena by picking up objects and dropping them off outside. To do this, the robot had to move around the arena, avoid obstacles, locate an object, pick it up, move toward the walls, and release the object outside the arena. After 1,000 generations, robot controllers were evolved that performed the cleaning task to a high degree of accuracy.

Most evolutionary robotics research relies on using a fixed neural network architecture on which the weights are evolved. Another interesting approach is to let the evolutionary method decide on the type of connectivity between the units in the net; i.e., the pattern of connectivity is "genetically" represented (see Husbands et al. in Ziemke and Sharkey, 1998, pp. 185–210).

An important reasearch area in biorobotics is concerned with how the environment and other species co-evolve with a given organism, resulting in an *evolutionary arms race*. This issue has been taken up in the simple form of evolving two competing robot controllers at the same time. For example, Floreano and Nolfi (1997) co-evolved the controllers for predator and prey behavior for two different "species" as part of each other's environment. One of the main problems was that in one generation the predators would win but in the next generation the prey would win because a counterstrategy was evolved. This instability has been overcome by introducing neural network learning during the lifetime of the individuals. In this way the predators were able to adapt to the new evolved strategies of the prey.

The approach of combining the two adaptive techniques of evolutionary methods and neural network learning is proving to be a very effective adaptation technique that has a naturalistic flavor. Much of the research on combining has focused on how learning can help guide evolution—the *Baldwin effect*. The idea is that if the genotype of an individual is close to an optimal combination of genes, learning can allow that individual to increase its suitability for its environment, thereby increasing its probability of survival and reproduction. This could lead to a larger "basin" of fitness around optimal genotypes, channeling evolution toward optimal solutions (see Nolfi and Floreano, 1999, for a review).

Learning. One of the most widely used learning techniques in biorobotics is reinforcement or reward learning (RL) (see, e.g., Krose, 1995). RL has been studied psychologically since the beginning of the twentieth century. An advantage of RL techniques in robotics is that the learner needs only occasional reinforcement. RL is therefore unlike supervised learning, which requires a trainer to provide the learner with an exact target action in every time step, suited for use in unknown environments or tasks (but see Sharkey, 1998, on the use of innate controllers for training supervised learning).

More recently there has been a move toward using the *operant conditioning* techniques developed in the 1940s for studies of animal learning. Operant conditioning involves the shaping of pregiven behaviors. In particular, animals can be trained to produce an experimenter-required behavior when they are rewarded for successive approximations to that behavior. For example, to begin training a rat to press a bar for food, rewards are given for any reaching movement. Then successive approximations to the goal are rewarded until the target behavior is observed. In robotics, this has also been called behavior editing by Dorigo and Colombetti (1998), who have conducted most of the experimental work on this technique. An extension of this work to include incremental shaping is discussed by Urzelai et al. (in Zimke and Sharkey, 1998, pp. 341–360).

In a realistic approach, Saksida et al. (in Sharkey, 1997, pp. 231–249) successfully used operant conditioning to modify the interaction between behaviors that had been preprogrammed into a robot. This departure from using reinforcement learning as a trial-and-error approach to modify existing behaviors is a step toward real animal training. Furthermore, unlike most RL work, the training was conducted by a human trainer rather than a programmed reinforcer. Initially, the robot has three categories of objects: a bright orange jacket, green and pink plastic dog toys, and blue plastic recycling bins. One of its innate behaviors was to approach the plastic dog toys and pick them up. Successful (fast) shaping was shown for a number of new behaviors, including *Follow the Trainer, Recycling,* and *Playing Fetch.*

Specific Biorobotics

One of the attractions of robotics is that there is strong potential for testing the relationship between a model and some hypothesized behavioral consequences in the physical world. When Hammond built his heliotrope in the early twentieth century to test Loebian theory, it was essentially the physical plausibility of the theory that was under scrutiny. This was generalized biorobotics in that the hypotheses were about all animals. One of the goals of specific biorobotics is to extend such physical testing to test specific hypotheses about specific species. The motivation is that mathematical specification and computer simulation provide only a weak test of a model in that the inputs are typically chosen by the researcher and the outputs are designed to be interpretable as data points or graphs. The central idea of specific biorobotics is to test the model by situating the robot in a physical environment that provides the main features of the world of the target species.

There are a number of dangers with this approach, and a number of wrinkles will have to be ironed out before such modeling reaches maturity as a test methodology in biology and psychology. For example, with complex neural networks such as brains, it is not always possible to isolate a mechanism and test its behavioral consequences. Although robotics can offer a window on the possible behaviors resulting from particular models, a model cannot generally be used directly as a robot controller; a number of "gaps" between the sensors, the model, and motor output have to be filled in. This can be advantageous in forcing the theorist to extend the theoretical mechanisms, but care must be taken to ensure that mechanisms outside the theoretical framework do not play a causal role in the robot behavior.

Robotic modeling of living systems has taken a number of different forms, from behavioral modeling (see, e.g., Webb in Gaussier, 1996, pp. 117–134, on cricket phonotaxis; Grasso et al. in Chang and Guadiano, 2000, pp. 115–131 on lobster chemotaxis) to neuroscientific modeling (e.g., Burgess et al. in Ziemke and Sharkey, 1998, pp. 291–300, and Recce et al. in Sharkey, 1997, pp. 393–406, on the rat hippocampus; van der Smagt in Ziemke and Sharkey, 1998, pp. 301–320, on the human cerebellum for arm control) to modeling animal sensing (e.g., Lambrinos et al. in Chang and Guadiano, 2000, pp. 39–64, on ant solar compass sensing; Blanchard et al. in Chang and Guadiano, 2000, pp. 17–38, on locust sensing of approach; Rucci in Chang and Guadiano, 2000, pp. 181–193, on localization of auditory and visual structures in the barn owl) to biomechanics (e.g., Delcomyn and Nelson in Chang and Guadiano, 2000, pp. 5–15, and Quinn and Ritzman in Ziemke and Sharkey, 1998, pp. 239–254, on hexapod walking in the cockroach).

One of the most successful attempts at behavioral modeling has been the work of Webb and her associates (e.g., Webb in Gaussier, 1996, on mate selection in the female cricket). A wheeled robot was used to physically model a female cricket locating a conspecific male by following its calls. The robot was equipped with an auditory system capable of selectively localizing the sound of a male cricket stridulating (rubbing its wings together rapidly to produce a sound that attracts potential mates).

A similar approach has been taken by Lambrinos et al. (in Chang and Gaudiano, 2000, pp. 39–64) for modeling the sensors of the desert ant *Cataglyphus*, which maintains its heading across a largely featureless desert using polarized light sensing. Lambrinos et al. built special-purpose polarized light sensors based on what is known about the neural mechanisms of polarization that the honey bee *Apis mellifera*, the field cricket *Gyrllus campestris*, and the desert ant *Cataglyphus bicolor* use to determine the position of the sun. The sensors were mounted on a wheeled robot and used to test different models of how *Cataglyphus* maintains its heading with polarized light. The research has been successfully conducted on a mobile robot in the ant's natural habitat with a homing performance similar to that of the ant.

As in Webb's work, the "ant robot" was used to model only a small part of the whole process of finding the direction to the nest. It did not, for example, accommodate the movement of the sun across the sky during the day (although this information was used to make corrections to the data). The sun moves relative to Earth at an average of 15° per hour (this figure varies greatly according to the time of day). In the early part of the twentieth century, this fact was used to show that ants both memorized the position of the sun and compensated for its movement. When the ants are imprisoned in a dark box for 2½ hours and released, they deviate from their original bearing by approximately the same number of degrees as the sun moved during their imprisonment. These findings reveal that *Cataglyphus* keeps track of the azimuth during the day and uses this information in maintaining a course.

Another important aspect of robotics used for modeling concerns legged locomotion. This leads to a two-way interaction between model testing and engineering. A number of researchers have turned to insect locomotion as a way to find a type of gait for a legged robot. Quinn and Ritzmann (in Ziemke and Sharkey, 1998, pp. 239–254) have designed and built a hexapod robot based on detailed neurobiological and kinematic observations of the locomotion of the death's head cockroach, *Blaberus discoidalis*. As a result, the robot's kinematics are remarkably similar to those of the real cockroach, and issues addressed in controlling the artificial cockroach have actually lead to new understanding of its natural counterpart.

Moving onto the mammalian nervous system, Burgess, Donnett, and O'Keefe (in Ziemke and Sharkey, 1998, pp. 291–300) used a miniature mobile robot equipped with a camera to test a neuronal model of how internal and external sensory information contribute to the firing of place cells in the rat hippocampus, and how these cells contribute to rat navigation behavior. They tested hypotheses based on their earlier neurophysiological work on the rat hippocampus using single-cell recording techniques. The robot experiments showed that the information provided by the robot's onboard video, odometry, and proximity sensors was sufficient to allow reasonably accurate return to an unmarked goal location. Similar robot modeling work has also been carried out by Recce et al. (in Sharkey, 1997, pp. 393–406) using the hippocampus as a method of absolute localization.

Research in specific biorobotics is gathering momentum as robot and sensing technology continues to improve. There are still many modeling issues to be worked out in conjunction with biology. The next step would be to get the morphology of robots to more accurately model the bodies and movement of the target species and to work continuously toward the goal of modeling whole animals, rather than installing patches to cover the missing bits. Like computational modeling, great care must be taken to ensure that the patches do not have a causal role in the target behavior.

Theoretical Biorobotics

Theoretical biorobotics is the most abstract level of biologically inspired robotics. Essentially, theoretical biorobotics is an all-encompassing category for work that does not involve implementation on a robot but rather addresses metaquestions about robotics. Although wide-ranging, the main theoretical focus of biologically inspired robotics concerns biological and psychological issues. Many of these issues draw on detailed philosophical reasoning. Here we will confine ourselves to setting out some of the main points and referencing more detailed works in the literature.

A strong impetus for the new wave in biologically inspired robotics was the way it differed from traditional AI. Rodney Brooks, one of the prime movers in the mid-1980s, was concerned with the inadequacy of the prevailing methods used in AI for robotics (see, e.g., Brooks, 1999). Based mainly on the cognitivist conception of human intelligence, the sensory input to robots went through a number of strategic stages such as perception, planning, and reasoning before each move. All of the information was presented to a central controller, which decided how to act. This slowed performance to a single small move about every 15 minutes.

Rejecting cognitivism, theoretical biorobotics views intelligence as *embodied* in the machine and in its interactions with the world in which it is situated. Extreme cognitivists hold that mind is essentially a computer program, a language of thought, that could be run on any machine capable of running it. Mind is simply linked to the machine running it and the external world through transducers. Extreme biroboticists might claim that mind is inseparable from the individual machine and the more encompassing environmental machine of which the individual machine is a part. That is, the robot is *situated* in the world and is an *embodied* or *physically grounded* intelligence.

Varela, Thompson, and Rosch (1991) provide an insightful discussion of the details of embodiment in robots and its relation to life and mind. These authors are primarily interested in how living systems are embodied and how they are situated in their interactions with the world. Their purpose is to urge cognitive science to reject the vacuity of ungrounded thought. However, Sharkey and Ziemke (in Ziemke and Sharkey, 1998), while going along with some of the account by Varela et al. of living systems, argue for a weak embodiment in robotics, i.e., that robots can be used to *model* embodiment without themselves being embodied (see Philosophical Issues in Brain Theory and Connectionism).

Another idea that has received considerable attention is that of *emergence* or *emergent behavior*. This is the notion that we can get something for nothing (or very little). One analogy is that from a collection of many molecules of water a cloud emerges that is greater than the sum of the parts. Perhaps a better example is the emergence of collective behavior in insects when each insect carries out very simple behaviors. For example, it is argued that the extraordinary structures that termites build in the desert emerge from very simple behaviors. Clark (1997) provides an in-depth discussion of emergent behavior and describes the two rules required by the termites: "If not carrying anything and you bump into a wood chip, pick it up"; and "If carrying a wood chip and you bump into another one, put it down." The resultant piling behavior emerges from the interplay between simple rules and the constraints of the environment.

The idea, then, is that coherent behavior emerges from a collection of simple taxes working together at the same time. This was an outright rejection of the notion of a central controller for action that was prevalent in AI. The idea in AI was to provide the robot with a model of the world, whereas one of the favorite slogans of the new roboticists is "the world is its own model." Nonetheless, Sharkey and Ziemke (2001) caution that even the taxes are emergent in the sense that they are in the eye of the beholder; i.e., they are distal descriptions of behavior.

One of the healthiest signs in the field is that some mainstream biologists and psychologists have begun to write about the relationship between specific biological findings and robotics. Navigation, for example, is an important topic in both biology and robotics, and biologists (e.g., Collett in Ziemke and Sharkey, 1998, pp. 255–270; Etienne in Ziemke and Sharkey, 1998, pp. 271–290; Franz and Mallot in Chang and Guadiano, 2000, pp. 133–153) have discussed the relation between different aspects of navigation from an insect and mammalian perspective. Moreover, psychologists are beginning to take robot studies using animal learning techniques seriously enough to write detailed discussions of the relationship between the natural and the metallic (e.g., Savage in Ziemke and Sharkey, 1998, pp. 321–340).

Conclusions

The field of biologically inspired robotics has been classified into the three separate subfields of generalized, specific, and theoretical. General and theoretical biorobotics has a long but patchy history that is now a considerable and growing field. Specific biorobotics has gradually emerged from the other two and is fast making headway toward the goal of accurately modeling specific animal species. With the ever-increasing improvements in materials, sensors, and computing equipment, we can look forward to many exciting new developments over the coming decade and the transfer of the findings into engineering.

Road Map: Robotics and Control Theory
Related Reading: Arm and Hand Movement Control; Neuroethology, Computational; Potential Fields and Neural Networks; Reactive Robotic Systems

References

Braitenberg, V., 1984, *Vehicles: Experiments in Synthetic Psychology*, Cambridge, MA: MIT Press. ◆
Brooks, R., 1999, *Cambrian Intelligence: The Early History of the New AI*, Cambridge, MA: MIT Press.
Chang, C., and Gaudiano, P., Eds., 2000, *Biomimetic Robotics, Robot. Auton. Syst.*, 31(1–2):1–218 (special issue).
Clark, A., 1997, *Being There: Putting Brain, Body and World Together Again*, Cambridge, MA: MIT Press.
Dorigo, M., and Colombetti, M., 1998, *Robot Shaping: An Experiment in Behavior Engineering*, Cambridge, MA: MIT Press.
Floreano, D., and Nolfi, S., 1997, Adaptive behaviour in competing co-evolving species, in *Proceedings of the Fourth European Conference on Artificial Life* (P. Husbands and I. Harvey, Eds.), Cambridge, MA: MIT Press.
Gaussier, P., Ed., 1996, *Moving the Frontiers Between Robotics and Biology, Robot. Auton. Syst.*, 16:107–362 (special issue).
Grey Walter, W., 1953, *The Living Brain*, New York: Norton. ◆
Krose, B., Ed., 1995, Special issue on reinforcement learning and robotics. *Robot. Auton. Syst.*, 15:233–340.
Nolfi, S., and Floreano, D., 1999, Learning and evolution, *Auton. Robots*, 7:89–113.
Sharkey, N., Ed., 1997, *Robot Learning: The New Wave, Robot. Auton. Syst.*, 22(3–4):135–274 (special issue). ◆
Sharkey, N., 1998, Learning from innate behaviors: A quantitative evaluation of neural network controllers, *Auton. Robots*, 5:317–334.
Sharkey, N., and Ziemke, T., 2001, Mechanistic vs. phenomenal embodiment: Can robot embodiment lead to strong AI? *Cognit. Syst. Res.*, 2:251–262.
Varela, F., Thompson, E., and Rosch, E., 1991, *The Embodied Mind: Cognitive Science and Human Experience*, Cambridge, MA: MIT Press.
Ziemke, T., and Sharkey, N., Eds., 1998, *Biorobotics, Connect. Sci.*, 10(3–4):161–360 (special issue).

Biophysical Mechanisms in Neuronal Modeling

Lyle J. Graham

Introduction

Models of single neurons span a wide range, with more or less fidelity to biological facts (see PERSPECTIVE ON NEURON MODEL COMPLEXITY; SINGLE-CELL MODELS; MECHANISMS IN NEURONAL MODELING). So-called biophysically detailed compartmental models of single neurons typically aim to quantitatively reproduce membrane voltages and currents in response to some sort of "synaptic" input. We may think of them as Hodgkin-Huxley-Rall models, based on the hypothesis of the neuron as a dynamical system of nonlinear membrane channels (e.g., conductances described by Hodgkin-Huxley kinetics; see ION CHANNELS: KEYS TO NEURONAL SPECIALIZATION; AXONAL MODELING) distributed over an electrotonic cable skeleton (e.g., as described by Rall dendritic cable theory; see DENDRITIC PROCESSING).

Such models can incorporate as much biophysical detail as desired (or practical), but, in general, all include some explicit assortment of voltage-dependent and transmitter-gated (synaptic) membrane channels. Many Hodgkin-Huxley-Rall models also include some system for describing intracellular Ca^{2+} dynamics, for example, to account for the gating of Ca^{2+}-dependent K^+ channels. Modeling these dynamics involves not only Ca^{2+} channels but often associated buffer systems and membrane pumps as well.

This article summarizes the application of the more common mathematical models of these basic biophysical mechanisms (Borg-Graham, 1999; Koch, 1999). The models for each of these mechanisms are at an intermediate level of biophysical detail, appropriate for describing macroscopic variables (e.g., membrane currents, ionic concentrations) on the scale of the entire cell or anatomical compartments thereof.

First, we will discuss general issues regarding model formulations, and data interpretation for contructing models of biophysical mechanisms. We will then describe models for nonlinear channel properties, including Hodgkin-Huxley and Markov kinetic descriptions of voltage and second-messenger-dependent ion channels. Similar models aimed particularly for synaptic mechanisms are covered in SYNAPTIC INTERACTIONS. We will then discuss concentration systems, including models of membrane pumps and concentration buffers. Finally, examples of model definitions are illustrated using the Surf-Hippo Neuron Simulation System (Graham, 2002), pointing out an essential and minimal syntax that facilitates model documentation and analysis.

General Issues for Constructing Biophysical Models

Phenomenological and Mechanistic Models

A first consideration in choosing a mathematical model for a given cellular mechanism is whether the model is intended only to capture an empirical relationship between an independent variable (the input or signal) and a dependent variable (the output or response), or whether the model represents an explicit mechanistic hypothesis. Phenomenological models may be instantiated by a function with few (e.g., a low-dimensional polynomial fit) or many (e.g., look-up table) degrees of freedom, depending on the nature of the problem.

Of course, a mechanistic model can also have few or many parameters, but explanatory power tends to dimish with the number of parameters. The mechanistic and phenomenological model alternatives are not mutually exclusive, since the former may incorporate the latter, and in some ways the distinction between them is rather ad hoc.

Static (Instantaneous) and Dynamic (Kinetic) Models

Another basic consideration is whether the relation between signal and response is instantaneous on the time scale relevant to the entire system at hand. In some cases an instantaneous mechanism may permit analysis by exploiting separation of variables, for example assuming instantaneous activation for Na^+ currents relative to K^+ currents during spiking (see OSCILLATORY AND BURSTING PROPERTIES OF NEURONS). For cellular models that are solved by explicit integration over time, however, instantaneous relationships between state variables can introduce troublesome numerical instabilities unless there are intervening kinetics with slow time constants (relative to the time scale of the integration) that serve to "decouple" element dynamics at the faster time scale.

Deterministic and Stochastic Models

A stochastic component, or "noise," in experimental measures is ubiquitous, for example, in the trial-to-trial variability of spike responses to deterministic stimuli, or in membrane voltage or membrane current fluctuations (especially in vivo). There is accumulating experimental and theoretical evidence that noise places an important constraint on information processing under some conditions while conversely serving a useful computational role in others.

Some system noise can be traced to the inherent stochasticity of molecular kinetics at the cellular level, and there is increasing interest in analyzing single-neuron models that explicitly consider this contribution. For example, simulations with stochastic Hodgkin-Huxley-type channel models can show functional dynamics that would be completely missed by deterministic models. A deterministic approximation should be valid when the number of channels is very large, the usual assumption, but the actual number in a local region of the neuron membrane may be rather low, considering both realistic estimates of channel densities and, especially, the small number of open channels near spike threshold (Schneidman, Freedman, and Segev, 1998).

The Experimenter's Model Versus the Theorist's Model

Every model is based on some empirical data set, but an often overlooked point is how the theorist's model relates to, or rather is constrained by, that of the experimentalist. It may be a bit surprising to discover there is such a thing as an experimentalist's model (which is not the same thing as an *experimental* model). However, in reality, experimental data are never arbitrary but reflect the experimenter's explicit or implicit notion of either the necessary and sufficient parameters of a phenomenon, the functionally relevant mappings between signal and response, what is experimentally tractable (no one is able to do his or her "dream" experiment!), or some combination of all three. The first issue, in particular, is essentially equivalent to assuming some hypothetical model, but importantly, the associated experiments are not normally designed for *testing* that hypothesis (since it is taken as an a priori). Examples include electrophysiological reports on whole-cell current kinetics, which usually focus on voltage-dependent activation and inactivation characteristics according to the classical model of Hodgkin and Huxley (described below). However, this paradigm, while practical, may miss crucial functional characteristics, basically by

not sufficiently characterizing certain important dynamical trajectories. We shall return to this point later in discussing Markov channel models.

Channel Models

Membrane channels underlie both intrinsic neuronal excitablility and the direct postsynaptic action of synaptic transmission. The channel current I, assuming some permeant ion X, may be expressed as the product of a conduction term $f(V, \Delta[X])$ and a gating term $h(V, t, \ldots)$:

$$I = f(V, \Delta[X])h(V, t, \ldots)$$

where V is the membrane voltage, t is time, and $\Delta[X]$ represents the concentration gradient of X across the cell membrane. The ellipsis in the argument of $h()$ stands for the various ligand-dependent processes, for example, Ca^{2+} dependence or the action of synaptic neurotransmitters.

Ohmic and Permeation Conduction Models

The two common models of the conduction term $f()$ are the ohmic model (thermodynamic equilibrium conduction) and the constant-field permeation model (nonequilibrium conduction). In the ohmic model, current is proportional to the difference of the membrane voltage and the reversal potential for I:

$$f(V, \Delta[X]) = \bar{g}_X(V - E_X)$$

where $\bar{g}_X$ is the maximum conductance. The reversal potential E_X for the ion X is given by the Nernst equation:

$$E_X = \frac{-RT}{zF} \text{Log} \frac{[X]_{out}}{[X]_{in}}$$

where R is the gas constant, F is Faraday's constant, and T is temperature in degrees Kelvin. $[X]_{in}$ and $[X]_{out}$ are the intracellular and extracellular concentrations, and z is the valence of the permeant ion X. For more than one permeant ion (all with the same valence) and under some assumptions, the similar Goldman-Hodgkin-Katz voltage equation (e.g., Hille, 2002) may be used. Note that if the effect of channel current on $[X]$ is considered (see section on concentration integration), then the ohmic $f()$ is in fact implicitly nonlinear.

As the conducting ion moves farther from equilibrium (specifically the case for Ca^{2+}), the ohmic model becomes less accurate. A widely used nonequilibrium model is the constant field model, described by the Goldman-Hodgkin-Katz current equation. In this equation (Jack, Noble, and Tsien, 1983; Hille, 2002), the nonlinearity of permeation is explicit:

$$f(V, \Delta[X]) = \bar{p}_X \frac{Vz^2F^2}{RT} \frac{[X]_{in} - [X]_{out} \exp(-zFV/RT)}{1 - \exp(-zFV/RT)}$$

where $\bar{p}_X$ is the permeability (*not* the conductance) of the channel (typically in cm^3/s). Note that at membrane potentials far from the reversal point (e.g., < -20 mV for Ca^{2+} channels) the Goldman-Hodgkin-Katz current equation becomes linear, and thus the ohmic model may suffice if the model voltages are appropriately bounded.

Channel Gating à la Hodgkin and Huxley: Independent Voltage-Dependent Gating Particles

Hodgkin and Huxley (1952) described channel gating as an interaction between independent two-state (open and closed) elements or "particles," all of which must be in the open state for channel conduction (see ION CHANNELS: KEYS TO NEURONAL SPECIALIZATION; AXONAL MODELING). The state dynamics of each particle are described with first-order kinetics:

$$x_C \underset{}{\overset{\alpha(V),\beta(V)}{\rightleftharpoons}} x_O \qquad (1)$$

where x_C and x_O represent the closed and open states of gating particle x, respectively. $\alpha(V)$ and $\beta(V)$ are the forward and backward rate constants of the particle as a function of voltage, respectively.

An Extended Hodgkin and Huxley Model

While Hodgkin and Huxley hypothesized that the steady-state behavior of each particle fit a Boltzmann distribution, their underlying rate equations were essentially ad hoc fits to the experimental data. Although taken as a canonical form by countless cell models, one consequence is that there is not an obvious relationship between the equations' parameters and the more "observable" steady-state, $x_\infty(V)$, and time-constant, $\tau_x(V)$, functions associated with Equation 1.

The Hodgkin-Huxley model can be recast in more explicit form by considering parameters of a single-barrier kinetic model for each particle (Jack et al., 1983; Borg-Graham, 1991, 1999). In its basic form this formulation has five parameters for each particle, compared to six parameters in the Hodgkin-Huxley model. Nevertheless, this formulation may be readily fitted to the original Hodgkin-Huxley equations of squid axon I_{Na} and I_K; the error is comparable to the error between the original equations and the data to which they were fit (cf. Figures 4, 7, and 9 in Hodgkin and Huxley, 1952).

We first derive the expressions the forward, $\alpha'_x(V)$, and backward, $\beta'_x(V)$, rate constants of the single-barrier transition. The parameter z (dimensionless) is the *effective* valence of the gating particle: when positive (negative), the particle opens (closes) with depolarization; thus it is an "activation" ("inactivation") particle. The effective valence is the product of the actual valence of the particle and the proportion of the membrane thickness that the particle moves through during state transitions. γ (dimensionless, between 0 and 1) is the asymmetry of the gating particle voltage sensor within the membrane (symmetric when $\gamma = 0.5$). K is the leading rate coefficient of both $\alpha'_x(V)$ and $\beta'_x(V)$. This term can be described in terms of Eyring rate theory, but here we just take K as a constant. $V_{1/2}$ is the voltage for which $\alpha'_x(V)$ and $\beta'_x(V)$ are equal. The final equations for $\alpha'_x(V)$ and $\beta'_x(V)$ are then:

$$\alpha'_x(V) = K \exp\left(\frac{z\gamma(V - V_{1/2})F}{RT}\right)$$

$$\beta'_x(V) = K \exp\left(\frac{-z(1 - \gamma)(V - V_{1/2})F}{RT}\right)$$

An additional parameter, τ_0 (*not* the passive membrane time constant), is crucial for fitting the expressions to the original Hodgkin-Huxley equations. τ_0 represents a rate-limiting step in the state transition, for example, "drag" on the particle conformation change (similar considerations have been explored for other, more general, kinetic schemes; e.g., Patlak, 1991), and may be incorporated directly into the expression for the time constant $\tau_x(V)$. $x_\infty(V)$, however, is not affected by τ_0:

$$\tau_x(V) = \frac{1}{\alpha'_x(V) + \beta'_x(V)} + \tau_0$$

$$x_\infty(V) = \frac{\alpha'_x(V)}{\alpha'_x(V) + \beta'_x(V)}$$

Two additional parameters, α_0 and β_0, may be considered in some cases, although they are not necessary in reproducing the original Hodgkin-Huxley equations. These parameters are voltage-independent forward and backward rate constants, respectively, of parallel state transitions. If considered, these transitions will change the final forms of $\tau_x(V)$ and $x_\infty(V)$.

The parameters of this form have clear relationships to the corresponding $x_\infty(V)$ and $\tau_x(V)$ functions. Thus, the $V_{1/2}$ parameter gives the midpoint and z sets the steepness of the $x_\infty(V)$ sigmoid. The symmetry parameter γ determines the skew of $\tau_x(V)$: $\gamma = 0.5$ gives a symmetric bell-shaped curve for $\tau_x(V)$, which otherwise bends to one side or the other as γ approaches 0 or 1. z sets the width of $\tau_x(V)$, unless γ is equal to either 0 or 1, in which case $\tau_x(V)$ becomes sigmoidal and thus z sets the steepness as for $x_\infty(V)$.

With this scheme a particle with a voltage-independent rate constant can be represented by setting $1/K \ll \tau_0$ (and $\alpha_0 = \beta_0 = 0$), thus making τ_0 the effective time constant. Likewise, both the time constant and steady state become voltage independent by setting $K = 0$ and choosing the appropriate α_0 and β_0.

Determining the Number of Particles in Hodgkin-Huxley Models

The Hodgkin-Huxley paradigm includes the possibility of multiple gating particles of a given type associated with a given channel. Some experimental papers report fitting integer powers of hypothetical gating particles to the observed kinetics, but more typically steady-state activation or inactivation data are simply the observed macroscopic behavior (that is, reflecting the steady state of the ensemble of particles). Thus, gating particle powers for channel models can often be considered as a free parameter.

Gating particle powers greater than 1 have several kinetic consequences, including a sigmoidal "delayed" time course of activation (Hodgkin and Huxley, 1952), a more rapid approach to 0 in the steady-state characteristic as a function of voltage, and a shift in either the peak (when $0 < \gamma < 1$) or inflection point (when $\gamma = 0$ or 1) of $\tau_x(V)$ in the direction of voltage for which $x_\infty(V)$ tends to 0.

Channel Gating as Dynamical Systems à la Markov Models

The independence and simplicity of the Hodgkin-Huxley gating particle models have at least two advantages: model kinetics can be predicted in an intuitive way, and their numerical evaluation is efficient (Hines, 1984). In addition, as mentioned, electrophysiological measures of whole-cell currents are often guided by this model. The two-state gating model can also be readily adapted to include factors such as intracellular $[Ca^{2+}]$, by using the appropriate functions for α and β (see below).

On the other hand, the independence of the two-state Hodgkin-Huxley particles constrains the equivalent state space description (e.g., allowed state transitions) given by the more general Markovian model (see SYNAPTIC INTERACTIONS). General Markov kinetic models are standard for detailed biophysical analysis of single-channel kinetics, but there have been relatively few applications in the neural modeling literature. One practical limitation is that Markov models are often much more computationally expensive than the Hodgkin-Huxley model. Nevertheless, the richer dynamics of Markov models may prove necessary for capturing functional properties of some channel types, including subthreshold steady-state Na^+ channel rectification (Figure 4), delay of activation for Na^+ and K^+ currents, and the coupling between opening of K^+ channels by Ca^{2+} entering during the action potential and subsequent inactivation (Borg-Graham, 1999).

Although the Markovian framework puts no restrictions on the functions that define state transitions (other than the no-memory condition), the form presented above of the $\alpha(V)$ and $\beta(V)$ functions for the extended Hodgkin-Huxley model is convenient and very general. Another form is the following squeezed exponential formula for the transition rate $\alpha_{ij}(V)$ from state i to state j:

$$\alpha_{ij}(V) = \left(\tau_{min} + \left((\tau_{max} - \tau_{min})^{-1} + \exp\left(\frac{(V - V_{1/2})}{k}\right)\right)^{-1}\right)^{-1}$$

$$(2)$$

where the inverse of τ_{min} (analogous to τ_0 in the extended Hodgkin-Huxley model) and τ_{max} put upper and lower bounds, respectively, on the rate constant $\alpha_{ij}(V)$. Note that there is an implicit coefficient of the exponential term of 1/ms (same units as either $1/\tau_{min}$ or $1/\tau_{max}$) in this equation.

Ca^{2+}-Dependent Gating

Neural models have used a variety of explicit relationships between the concentration of some second messenger and the activation state of the target mechanism. Here we consider a range of examples that have been used to describe Ca^{2+}-dependent K^+ channels.

A simple instantaneous model for Ca^{2+}-dependent gating is given by a static rectified power function of concentration with some threshold θ_{Ca}, reminiscent of firing rate models:

$$w = K \times \sigma([Ca^{2+}]^n - \theta_{Ca})$$

where $\sigma(x) = 0$ for $x < 0$, and $\sigma(x) = x$ otherwise, for the gating variable w.

A simple kinetic model for Ca^{2+}-dependent gating can be described by the following reaction. Assume that w_C and w_O represents the closed and open probabilities, respectively, of a Ca^{2+}-dependent gating particle w with forward and backward rate constants α and β, respectively:

$$w_C + nCa^{2+} \overset{\alpha,\beta}{\rightleftharpoons} w_O$$

Note that the open state w_O is bound to n Ca^{2+} ions. One can also imagine a similar but reverse reaction for the description of Ca^{2+}-dependent inactivation, as has been reported for some Ca^{2+} channels. In the more general Markovian framework, w_C and w_O refer to two adjacent states out of the entire state space. This scheme assumes that binding with Ca^{2+} ions is cooperative: either all binding sites are occupied or none are. We may also consider a τ_0 parameter as in the extended Hodgkin-Huxley model. If we assume that the binding of Ca^{2+} in this reaction does not appreciably change $[Ca^{2+}]$, then the steady-state value for w, w_∞, and the time constant for the kinetics, τ_w, are given by:

$$w_\infty = \frac{\alpha}{\alpha + \beta[Ca^{2+}]_{in}^{-n}}$$

$$\tau_w = \frac{1}{\alpha[Ca^{2+}]_{in}^n + \beta} + \tau_0$$

An important distinction is whether or not a Ca^{2+}-dependent channel is also dependent on voltage. For example, in recordings of the large-conductance Ca^{2+}-dependent K^+ (BK) channel, Barrett, Magleby, and Pallotta (1982) found an approximate third-power relationship between channel open times and $[Ca^{2+}]$ that was strongly facilitated by depolarization. At a membrane voltage of 10 mV, channels became open with a $[Ca^{2+}]$ threshold of about 1 μM.

If the dependences are separable, it may be convenient to consider a product of voltage-only and Ca^{2+}-only gating terms, for example according to the formulations presented earlier. Otherwise, a single gating "particle" must take into account both voltage and Ca^{2+}. A direct voltage dependence of the simple kinetic scheme above can be added in a number of ways, for example by adding a voltage-dependent term to the forward rate constant, now defined as $\alpha(V, [Ca^{2+}]_{in})$:

$$\alpha(V, [Ca^{2+}]_{in}) = \alpha_V(V) \times \alpha[Ca^{2+}]_{in}^n$$

where, e.g., $\alpha_V(V)$ is the squeezed exponential function of voltage in Equation 2, such that the forward reaction speeds up with depolarization.

Moczydlowski and Latorre (1983) proposed a detailed Markovian kinetic scheme for the Ca^{2+}- and voltage-dependent gating of the BK channel, which has been interpreted in several neuron models. The essential dynamics are captured by a two-state scheme as in Equation 1, with rate constants dependent on both voltage and Ca^{2+}, thus:

$$\beta(V, [Ca^{2+}]_{in}) = \beta_0\left(1 + \frac{k_1(V)}{[Ca^{2+}]_{in}}\right)^{-1}$$

$$\alpha(V, [Ca^{2+}]_{in}) = \alpha_0\left(1 + \frac{[Ca^{2+}]_{in}}{k_4(V)}\right)^{-1}$$

where

$$k_i(V) = k_i(0) \times \exp\left(\frac{-V\delta_i FZ}{RT}\right)$$

Ionic Concentration Dynamics

An inevitable consequence of channel currents is that the concentrations on either side of the membrane will change as a function of electrical activity. In addition to the negative feedback on channel currents already mentioned (as a result of a reduction in driving force), such changes can have a variety of other functional consequences. These include the activation of intracellular or extracellular receptors, the most important being those that underlie the myriad Ca^{2+}-dependent pathways (including the Ca^{2+}-dependent channel gating just described). We may also consider the role of the membrane pumps, which tend to maintain ionic gradients (see MECHANISMS IN NEURONAL MODELING), and of the intracellular buffer systems. In the following discussion we emphasize Ca^{2+} dynamics, but similar considerations are relevant for other ions.

Concentration Integrators

Most neuron models that consider concentration changes rely on some partition of the extracellular and intracellular space into a set of well-mixed compartments (e.g., "shells"), with or without an "inifinite" compartment with a fixed concentration. Simple diffusion is normally assumed between compartments, according to the geometry of the partitioning and assumptions about the diffusion coefficient for the free ion, D. Compartments adjacent to the cell membrane also take into account ion flow across the membrane, e.g., due to channels and pumps. The physical partitioning into compartments depends on the question being addressed, with the simplest system being a single intracellular compartment (extracellular concentration being assumed constant).

Any model of $[Ca^{2+}]$ must take into account not only the influx of Ca^{2+} but also some mechanism for the removal of Ca^{2+}. The simplest method is to include a steady-state term in the differential equation(s) describing $[Ca^{2+}]$. In the general case this value is associated with a second parameter corresponding to the time constant for concentration decay.

Membrane Pump Models

More explicit models of ion removal includes mechanisms, such as membrane-bound pumps, that transport Ca^{2+}, K^+, Na^+, and other ions against their respective concentration gradients. A general pump model may be described with a Michaelis-Menton mechanism, assuming no appreciable change in the extracellular $[Ca^{2+}]$:

$$J_{Ca^{2+}} = V_{max} \frac{[Ca^{2+}]_{in}}{K_d + [Ca^{2+}]_{in}} - J_{leak}$$

where $J_{Ca^{2+}}$ is the removal rate of Ca^{2+} per unit area, V_{max} is the maximum flux rate per unit area, and K_d is the half-maximal $[Ca^{2+}]_{in}$. J_{leak} compensates for the resting pump rate and is typically adjusted so that there is no net pump current at rest, given some resting activation of Ca^{2+} channels.

For example, the spine model by Zador, Koch, and Brown (1990) included two Ca^{2+} pumps with Michaelis-Menton kinetics: one high-affinity, low-capacity, corresponding to a Ca ATPase-driven mechanism, and the other low-affinity, high-capacity, corresponding to a Ca^{2+}/Na^+ exchange mechanism (see also Koch, 1999). These pumps were treated as separate currents in the $[Ca^{2+}]$ differential equation. Other models have incorporated a pump that binds to intra- and extracellular Ca^{2+} with various rate constants. These reactions are then solved simultaneously with another binding reaction between $[Ca^{2+}]_{in}$ and a buffer.

Buffer Models

Endogenous intracellular Ca^{2+} buffers have a strong effect on free intracellular $[Ca^{2+}]_{in}$. Cell models that consider Ca^{2+} dynamics have incorporated buffer mechanisms of varying complexities, including solving the dynamical equations for the buffer-Ca^{2+} reaction during the course of the simulation. Note that in some models an explicit (instantaneous) buffer mechanism is replaced by adjusting Ca^{2+} sensitivities of Ca^{2+}-dependent mechanisms, such as Ca^{2+}-dependent K^+ channels.

A simple way to treat intracellular buffering of Ca^{2+} is to assume a nonsaturated buffer (i.e. $[Bu] \gg [Ca^{2+}]_{in}$, where $[Bu]$ is the concentration of buffer binding sites) with instantaneous kinetics. The key parameter, β_{Bu}, in this mechanism equals the ratio of the concentration of bound Ca^{2+} and free Ca^{2+}:

```
(CHANNEL-TYPE-DEF
 `(NA-HH
   (GBAR-DENSITY . 1200)  ; pS/um2
   (E-REV . 50)           ; mV
   (V-PARTICLES . ((M-HH 3) (H-HH 1)))))

(PARTICLE-TYPE-DEF
 `(M-HH
   (CLASS . :HH)
   (ALPHA . (LAMBDA (VOLTAGE)
              (/ (* -0.1 (- VOLTAGE -40))
                 (1- (EXP (/ (- VOLTAGE -40) -10))))))
   (BETA . (LAMBDA (VOLTAGE)
             (* 4 (EXP (/ (- VOLTAGE -65) -18))))))))
```

Figure 1. The Surf-Hippo definitions of the classical Hodgkin-Huxley model of the squid axon Na^+ channel and the associated M-activation gating particle. The plethora of parentheses may seem daunting; however, all formatting (including indentation) is done automatically by Lisp-savvy editors (such as Emacs). The last line in the CHANNEL-TYPE-DEF form specifies three M-HH and one H-HH gating particles. Surf-Hippo model definitions allow concise inclusion of arbitrary functions, in this case for the ALPHA and BETA rate constants (refer to equations of the Hodgkin-Huxley Na^+ channel in AXONAL MODELING, q.v.) in the PARTICLE-TYPE-DEF form. The LAMBDA symbol denotes the beginning of a function definition. In the context of gating particle definitions, Surf-Hippo assumes only that the rate functions take a single VOLTAGE argument (in millivolts), and return a rate value (in ms^{-1}). Comments are indicated with a semicolon. Expression precedence is unambiguous with the prefix notation of Lisp. The first element of each (parenthesized) list defines the operation applied to the rest of the list, and in nested lists everything is evaluated from the inside out: e.g., (+ A (* B C) D) is $A + BC + D$.

$$\beta_{Bu} = \frac{[Ca^{2+}]_{in}^{bound}}{[Ca^{2+}]_{in}^{free}}$$

and thus is a function of $[Bu]$. This mechanism implies that the *measured* $[Ca^{2+}]_{in}$ is equal to the total $[Ca^{2+}]_{in}$ divided by (β_{Bu} + 1). For nondiffusional models of $[Ca^{2+}]_{in}$ (e.g., where there is one Ca^{2+} compartment per electrical compartment), this is the only role of the instantaneous buffer. For multiple-compartment systems, the effective diffusion constant D' applied to the difference in $[Ca^{2+}]$ between compartments must also be adjusted to take into account the instantaneous buffer, by setting D' equal to $D/(\beta_{Bu} + 1)$. A variation on this scheme would be to assume that β_{Bu} is a function of each compartment. In this case the diffusion equation between compartments would reference the original D, with the concentration difference between any two compartments determined by the difference of the total concentrations, weighted by the appropriate β_{Bu}s.

Practical Aspects of Coding Biophysical Models

The translation of experimental data on some biophysical mechanism into simulator code, within the framework of a given mathematical model, and the reverse process (which is a necessary step in formulating experimental predictions from a model) have received little attention. However, these steps have many practical aspects, not the least of which is that as models become more and more complex, the opportunity for errors becomes more and more serious. For this reason it is useful to consider model *syntax* (see NEUROSIMULATION: TOOLS AND RESOURCES; GENESIS SIMULATION SYSTEM; NEURON SIMULATION ENVIRONMENT; NSL NEURAL SIMULATION LANGUAGE).

In most situations, it is desirable that a simulator program act essentially as a "black box," so that model analysis concerns only the input (some collection of model definition files) and the output (numerical data, usually time sequences). Thus, when composing the model definition, one should ideally be able to focus on the model algorithms and their parameters, rather than on their implementation. Model syntax should therefore allow the expression of mathematical (and symbolic, if appropriate) relationships in as close to a "natural" syntax as possible. In other words, one should be able to simply "write down the equations" defining the model. Certainly a practical consequence of such a syntax is that the learning curve for the simulator is reduced, but more important over the long term is simply that if model definitions are easier to read, they are also easier to verify, document, and change.

To illustrate these ideas, here we present examples of biophysical model definitions taken from the Surf-Hippo Neuron Simulation System (Graham, 2002). This system is written in Lisp, an important point, since the system exploits many advantages of this truly high-level language that are well known to the AI community (at the same time having a numerical performance on par with languages such as C). In particular, Lisp supports an emphasis on more

```
(PARTICLE-TYPE-DEF
 `(M-HH-FIT
   (CLASS . :HH-EXT)
   (VALENCE . 2.7)
   (GAMMA . 0.4)
   (BASE-RATE . 1.2)  ; 1/ms
   (V-HALF . -40)     ; mV
   (TAU-0 . 0.07)))   ; ms
```

Figure 2. The Surf-Hippo definition for the extended Hodgkin-Huxley model for the M-activation particle type of the squid axon Na^+ channel.

```
(PARTICLE-TYPE-DEF
 `(NA-X-HPC
   (CLASS . :MARKOV)
   (STATES . (O I C1 C2))
   (OPEN-STATES . (O)
   (STATE-TRANSITIONS .
    ((O   I   3)
     (O   C1  (SQUEEZED-EXPONENTIAL VOLTAGE :V-HALF -51 :K -2 :TAU-MIN 1/3))
     (C1  O   (SQUEEZED-EXPONENTIAL VOLTAGE :V-HALF -42 :K  1 :TAU-MIN 1/3))
     (O   C2  (SQUEEZED-EXPONENTIAL VOLTAGE :V-HALF -57 :K -2 :TAU-MIN 1/3))
     (C2  O   (SQUEEZED-EXPONENTIAL VOLTAGE :V-HALF -51 :K  1 :TAU-MIN 1/3))
     (I   C1  (SQUEEZED-EXPONENTIAL VOLTAGE :V-HALF -53 :K -1 :TAU-MAX 100 :TAU-MIN 1))
     (C1  C2  (SQUEEZED-EXPONENTIAL VOLTAGE :V-HALF -60 :K -1 :TAU-MAX 100 :TAU-MIN 1)))))))
```

Figure 3. The Surf-Hippo definition of a Markovian gating particle for a hippocampal pyramidal cell Na$^+$ channel model (Borg-Graham, 1999). Transition rates between states, in ms^{-1}, are defined with either constants (for example, 3 ms^{-1} for the transition from state O to state I) or functions of voltage (as indicated by the "dummy" variable VOLTAGE). The SQUEEZED-EXPONENTIAL function (Equation 2) is built into Surf-Hippo (when :TAU-MAX is not specified, then the minimum rate is 0).

declarative descriptions (emphasizing *what* kind of model is desired), rather than imperative ones (emphasizing *how* to construct a model). Thus, model syntax in Surf-Hippo is designed to minimize the actual code for mechanism specification: correspondingly, these examples illustrate the necessary and sufficient parameters for each mechanism, avoiding "overhead" code that would be simulator specific. Surf-Hippo also includes automatic generation of mechanism definition code, for example, allowing capture of the "state" of a given mechanism model that has been modified on-line during automatic or manual parameter exploration. This capability, which is facilitated by both the minimal requirements for model specification and the relative ease with which Lisp programs may be able to write Lisp code, is important for avoiding errors when documenting model results.

Figure 1 illustrates the definitions of the classical Hodgkin-Huxley model of the squid axon Na$^+$ channel and the associated M-activation gating particle, showing in particular how arbitrary functions are represented. Once the basic syntax of Lisp is grasped, the human readability of this format is enhanced because it includes only the essential kinetic parameters. As a comparison, the equivalent source code in similar simulation systems such as GENESIS and NEURON is about two to three times larger.

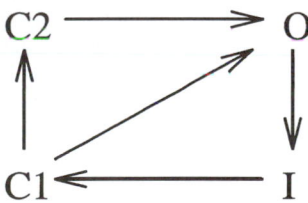

Figure 4. State diagram of a hypothetical Markov gating model used for I_{Na} in a model of hippocampal pyramidal cells (Borg-Graham, 1999). From the single inactivated state I, the two closed states C_i are reached with increasing hyperpolarization. The $C_i \rightarrow O$ transitions implement in effect distinct thresholds, occuring at progressively lower potentials with increasing i. Likewise, the $I \rightarrow C_1$ and $C_1 \rightarrow C_2$ transitions occur at voltages hyperpolarized to the associated $C_1 \rightarrow O$ and $C_2 \rightarrow O$ transitions, respectively, somewhat like a rachet mechanism. The $O \rightarrow I$ transition is voltage independent. The arrows denote the dominant transitions during spike depolarization/repolarization. One important aspect of this model is that the inactivation state is reached only after channel opening, as reported from studies of single Na$^+$ channels (Patlak, 1991; Hille, 1992). Such coupling contradicts the central assumption of independent activation and inactivation kinetics in the Hodgkin-Huxley model.

Several parameterized models of biophysical mechanisms are included in Surf-Hippo, including those discussed in this article. For example, Figure 2 shows the definition for the extended Hodgkin-Huxley model of the Na$^+$ channel M-gating particle. Markov models for particle gating are also readily represented in this system. As an example, Figure 3 illustrates the definition of a Markovian gating particle for a hippocampal pyramidal cell Na$^+$ channel model (Borg-Graham, 1999); the state diagram is shown in Figure 4.

Discussion

Biophysical details are likely to be crucial for understanding neural computation (see MECHANISMS IN NEURONAL MODELING). This process entails an informed trade-off between incorporating every known experimental nuance of a given cellular mechanism and the practical application of abstractions and simplifications that capture essential dynamic relationships between biological molecules and various neuronal signals. In this article we have presented some of the more commonly used mathematical descriptions for these relationships. We note in closing that an increasingly important (and unavoidable) problem with complicated neural models that rely on these sorts of mechanisms is the lack of formal or analytic verification. This situation calls for alternative methods, in particular the cross-validation of numerical results using several tools of similar capability (e.g., NEURON, GENESIS, Surf-Hippo). Practical aspects of coding biophysical models, such as the minimal model syntax discussed here, should facilitate such efforts.

Road Map: Biological Neurons and Synapses
Related Reading: Activity-Dependent Regulation of Neuronal Conductances; Axonal Modeling; GENESIS Simulation System; Ion Channels: Keys to Neuronal Specialization; NEURON Simulation Environment; Neurosimulation: Tools and Resources; NSL Neural Simulation Language; Oscillatory and Bursting Properties of Neurons; Perspective on Neuron Model Complexity; Single-Cell Models; Synaptic Interactions

References

Barrett, J. N., Magleby, K. L., and Pallotta, B. S., 1982, Properties of single calcium-activated potassium channels in cultured rat muscle, *J. Physiol.*, 331:211–230.
Borg-Graham, L., 1991, Modelling the non-linear conductances of excitable membranes, in *Cellular Neurobiology: A Practical Approach* (J. Chad and H. Wheal, Eds.), New York: IRL/Oxford University Press, chap. 13.

Borg-Graham, L., 1999, Interpretations of data and mechanisms for hippocampal pyramidal cell models, *Cereb. Cortex*, 13:19–138. ◆

Graham, L., 2002, The Surf-Hippo Neuron Simulation System, available: http://www.cnrs-gif.fr/iaf/iaf9/surf-hippo.html, v3.0.

Hille, B., 2002, *Ionic Channels of Excitable Membranes*, 3rd ed., Sunderland, MA: Sinauer. ◆

Hines, M., 1984, Efficient computation of branched nerve equations, *Int. J. Biomed. Comput.*, 15:69–76.

Hodgkin, A. L., and Huxley, A. F., 1952, A quantitative description of membrane current and its application to conduction and excitation in nerve, *J. Physiol.*, 117:500–544.

Jack, J. J. B., Noble, D., and Tsien, R. W., 1983, *Electric Current Flow in Excitable Cells*, Oxford, Engl.: Clarendon Press. ◆

Koch, C., 1999, *The Biophysics of Computation: Information Processing in Single Neurons*, Oxford, Engl.: Oxford University Press. ◆

Moczydlowski, E., and Latorre, R., 1983, Gating kinetics of Ca^{2+}-activated K^+ channels from rat muscle incorporated into planar lipid bilayers, *J. Gen. Physiol.*, 82:511–542.

Patlak, J., 1991, Molecular kinetics of voltage-dependent Na^+ channels, *Physiol. Rev.*, 71:1047–1080.

Schneidman, E., Freedman, B., and Segev, I., 1998, Ion-channel stochasticity may be critical in determining the reliability and precision of spike timing, *Neural Computat.*, 10:1679–1703.

Zador, A., Koch, C., and Brown, T. H., 1990, Biophysical model of a Hebbian synapse, *Proc. Natl. Acad. Sci. USA*, 87:6718–6722.

Biophysical Mosaic of the Neuron

Lyle J. Graham and Raymond T. Kado

Introduction

In this article we broadly review the biophysical mechanisms of neurons that are likely to be relevant to computational function (Table 1). These mechanisms operate within the complex three-dimensional anatomy of the single neuron and are manifested by electrical and chemical interactions between ions on either side of the cell membrane and the diverse proteins and other molecules

Table 1. Neuronal Biophysical Mechanisms Relevant to Computational Function

Ion channels
  Control by intrinsic signals (membrane voltage, intracellular molecules)
  Control by extrinsic signals (extracellular molecules, e.g., released from presynaptic terminals)
Receptors
  Ionotropic: Direct control of ion channels
  Metabotropic: Indirect control of ion channels and other internal systems
  External binding sites (synaptic and pancrinic)
  Internal binding sites associated with neuronal and organelle membranes
  Control of internal biochemical systems
Enzymes (kinases and phosphatases, which determine the state of most proteins; others)
Gap junctions
Pumps, transporters, exchangers (electrogenic and nonelectrogenic)
Organelles
  Ca^{2+} sequestering and release (endoplasmic recticulum, mitochondria)
  Protein synthesis and metabolism
  Maintenance and modulation of three-dimensional structure (spines, dendritic morphology)
  Transmitter sequestering and release (synaptic vesicles)
Cytoplasmic biochemical systems
  Transmitter synthesis and degradation
  G proteins: Initiate second messenger release after receptor activation
  Second messengers: Diffusible molecules linking various stages of internal biochemical systems
  Effectors: Targets of second messengers, including channels and enzymes (kinases, phosphatases)
Three-dimensional structure
  Macroscopic anatomy (soma, dendritic and axonal trees)
  Microscopic anatomy (spines, synaptic junctions, variations in dendritic or axonal dimensions)
  "Electrotonic" anatomy (modulated by state of local membrane)
  Geometrical synaptic and channel distribution
  Functional synaptic localization (e.g., retinotopic, tonotropic)
  Computational synaptic localization (e.g., on-the-path interactions, coincidence detection)

embedded in the membrane and within the cytoplasm (Figure 1). The signals mediating these interactions may be defined by the voltage across the cell membrane or by concentrations of specific molecules in specific conformational or metabolic states. The first case relies on the voltage sensitivity of various membrane proteins; the second relies on a vast multitude of receptor proteins that link the functional state of neuronal proteins with the external or internal concentrations of ions and molecules.

It may be noted that none of these cellular mechanisms is unique to neurons. For example, essentially all the mechanisms discussed in this article may be relevant when considering a possible computational role of the neuroglia network (Laming et al., 2000). By the same token, neurons (and glial cells) include the essential mosaic of biochemical systems found in all cells required for metabolism, reproduction, growth, and repair. The complexity is daunting. Here we focus on the better-known elements most clearly linked to the reception, processing, and transmission of neuronally represented information. It may seem that there are so many such elements, and an even larger number of unknown relationships, that it would not be possible for a theory to take all of the actual dynamic behaviors into consideration. Nevertheless, it also seems likely that an oversimplification of these interactions—for example, in the extreme case by describing single neuron function as an abstracted trigger device—may put fundamental limits to the explanatory and predictive power of any neural model. The challenge remains, then, to develop a description of single neuron function that can serve as the foundation for a practical yet sufficient neural theory.

We start with a metaphor, the mosaic neuron. A *mosaic* is a collection of discrete parts, each with unique properties, fitted together in such a way that an image emerges from the whole in a nonobvious way. Similarly, the neuronal membrane is packed with a diversity of receptors and ion channels and other proteins with a recognizable distribution. In addition, the cytoplasm is not just water with ions, but a mosaic of interacting molecular systems that can directly affect the functional properties of membrane proteins. Whether for the developing or for the mature neuron, this mosaic is not stationary. To begin with, neuronal proteins are constantly recycled, as is the case for all cells. Furthermore, on both long and short time scales, most mechanistic theories for learning and memory implicate physical changes in various cellular constituents. On time scales of seconds or less, different signaling systems impinging on the neuron from the network or present in the cytoplasm can modify the properties of the mosaic elements, and in some cases their distribution within the cell (see ACTIVITY-DEPENDENT REGULATION OF NEURONAL CONDUCTANCES). Thus, just as a mo-

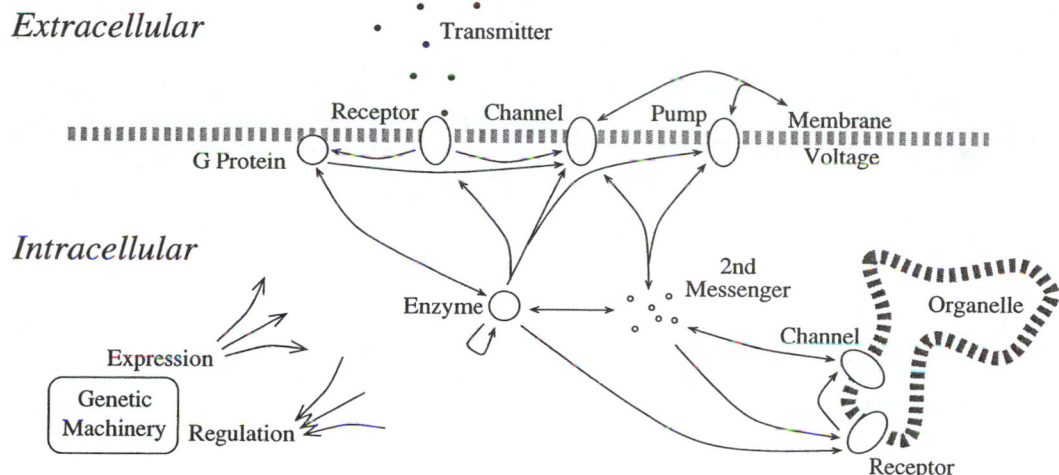

Figure 1. Sketch of the molecular circuit underlying the neuron's biophysical mosaic. This caricature outlines the many interrelated control paths among the molecular elements that determine the functional properties of the neuron. For example, activation of an ionotropic synapse starts with the binding of extracellular transmitter to the membrane receptor, which then directly turns on an associated ion channel. Alternatively, activation of a metabotropic synapse is initiated by transmitter binding to a receptor, which then activates a G protein, which turns on an enzyme, which raises the concentration of a second messenger, which, finally, activates a target ion channel. Many control pathways are immediately bidirectional: current through an ion channel changes the membrane voltage, which in turn can control the gating of that same channel. Some elements can even control themselves, for example autophosphorylating enzymes.

saic painting provokes perception of a complete image out of a maze of individually diversified tiles, current thinking holds that a given neuron performs a well-defined computational role that depends not only on the network of cells in which it is embedded but also to a large extent on the dynamic distribution of macromolecules throughout the cell.

The Minimal Essential Model and the Biophysical Mosaic

It remains an open question as to what constitutes a minimal neuron model for reproducing functional neuronal computation (Meunier and Segev, 2000; see also CANONICAL NEURAL MODELS). This is in part because to date, only a handful of neuron circuit models come close to predicting known experimental data in any nontrivial way. The question of finding a minimal model is hardly an academic one, as can be appreciated by reviewing the dimensionality of the mosaic neuron (Table 2).

Whatever the minimal essential model turns out to be, a detailed knowledge of neuronal biophysics is most likely necessary for understanding the system behavior (even if this understanding is not sufficient). The clearest evidence for this point of view comes from psychopharmacology: although we lack a clear understanding of the mechanisms, we know that adding certain chemicals to the brain parenchyma can qualitatively alter cognitive behavior. We know that the direct action of psychotropic drugs is probably to change one or more biophysical properties at the microscopic cellular level, such as blocking an ion channel, altering the binding kinetics of a receptor, modulating a biochemical pathway, and so on, rather than acting at a more macroscropic systems level, such as cleanly disconnecting a circumscribed subcircuit from the entire network. We know that physical access to the brain is necessary for this action (preventing a drug from crossing the blood-brain barrier eliminates its effect), and we also know, in many cases, that some neurons have highly specific membrane receptors for a given psychotropic molecule that are often localized in very restricted areas at the level of brain substructures and even at the single-cell level. Often there is direct evidence of a drug's effect in electro-physiological measurements of single cells, when a change in intrinsic response properties or synaptic dynamics is seen after a given chemical is added to the fluid bathing the nervous tissue.

The Mosaic's Tiles

We will now review the major proteins that compose the neuron mosaic and discuss some basic implications of their diversity and complexity. These macromolecules include ion channels, receptors (described along with the molecules that activate them), enzymes, gap junctions, pumps, exchangers, and transporters. Note that these classifications can sometimes overlap. For example, an ionotopic receptor is a protein multimer that includes both a receptor part and a channel part.

Several texts may be consulted for more detail on these mechanisms (Johnston and Wu, 1995; Weiss, 1996; Koch and Segev, 1998; Fain, 1999; Hille, 2002). In particular, the textbook by Koch (1999) provides an explicit foundation for the computation/algorithm/implementation trinity that is fundamental for understanding brain function.

Ion Channels

Ion channels are membrane-spanning proteins that, owing to their conformational states which allow the passage of ionic current, are the primary basis for the dynamical electrical behavior of neurons (see ION CHANNELS: KEYS TO NEURONAL SPECIALIZATION). The permeability of the conducting states and the kinetics governing state transitions (generally referred to as channel gating) can be affected by a variety of factors, principally the membrane voltage and the intra- and extracellular concentrations of the permeable ions and other specific molecules. Sensitivity to extracellular molecules is generally mediated by either direct action on the channel or various receptor proteins (e.g., in response to neurotransmitters), as discussed below. Molecules that affect channel gating from the inside include second messengers. The kinetic relationship between membrane voltage, the concentration of neurotransmitters, second messengers, and a channel's conductance state can be quite complex, a point we return to later.

Table 2. Quantitative Summary of the Neuron's Biophysical Mosaic Relevant to Computational Function

Spatial scales (voltage and concentration transients): <1 to thousands of microns
Temporal scales
   Kinetics of gating, binding, and diffusion: <1 ms to seconds
   Gene expression: days to years?
Anatomy
   Tens to hundreds of dendritic and axonal branches
   Models of electrotonic structure can require thousands of compartments
Synapses and channels
   Thousands of pre- and postsynaptic sites
   Five major categories of charge carriers: Na^+, K^+, Ca^{2+}, Cl^-, other (e.g., "cationic," proton, etc.)
   Tens of types for each category, several of which may be expressed in a single neuron
Receptors and associated agonists (neurotransmitters, second messengers, etc.)
   Approximately 30 major types, several of which may be expressed in a single neuron
   Possibly tens of identified subtypes for some major receptor types

A brute force map of a single neuron would be very large indeed. For example, compartmental models of the dendritic tree can require hundreds or thousands of coordinates, corresponding to spatial scales relevant for representing gradients of membrane voltage or of the concentration of intracellular molecules. A given neuron may have thousands of synaptic inputs, each associated with one of several types of receptors, and the cell membrane can include tens of types of ion channels. Furthermore, the different synaptic receptor and channel types are typically scattered inhomogeneously over the neuron. It is also important to consider the stationarity of the map. For computations over hundreds of milliseconds or less, the map may properly be thought to be static, but at longer time scales it may be necessary to consider a dynamic layout of the mosaic. For another *carte du monde* of computational cellular mechanisms and their spatial and temporal scales, see Figure 21.2 in Koch, 1999.

Since channels are the most direct mechanism determining the basic firing properties of the cell (e.g., regular adapting, bursting, fast spiking), and since channels are subject to functional modulation on a variety of time scales, it is not surprising that a given neuron can exhibit more than one "stereotypical" firing behavior, depending on the conditions (see NEOCORTEX: BASIC NEURON TYPES).

Receptors and Their Agonists and Antagonists: Neurotransmitters, Neuromodulators, Neurohormones, and Second Messengers

Receptors are membrane proteins whose functional action is triggered by the reversible binding of specific molecules called ligands (Cooper, Bloom, and Roth, 1996; see NMDA RECEPTORS: SYNAPTIC, CELLULAR, AND NETWORK MODELS). A given molecule may be a ligand for more than one kind of receptor, with very different or even opposite functional effects; likewise, a given receptor may be able to be activated by more than one endogenous (or artificial, that is, experimental or pharmaceutical) ligand. A ligand that tends to upregulate the functional activity of a receptor protein is called an agonist for that receptor. Conversely, antagonists are molecules that inhibit the activity of a receptor.

There are two basic types of receptors, ionotropic and metabotropic. Ionotropic receptors are directly associated with an ion channel whose gating is controlled by the presence of the receptor agonist. The action of metabotropic receptors is more complex: upon binding to an agonist, these receptors activate a G protein (so named because their action involves the conversion between guan-

osine diphosphate and guanosine triphosphate), which may directly control channel gating or may initiate a biochemical cascade mediated by second messengers. The end point of this "chain reaction" can be, for example, the opening of a channel, or the phosphorylation of a receptor by the activation of a kinase.

Agonists are properly called neurotransmitters when released by the presynaptic terminal of an axon (or possibly a dendrite) arising from another neuron (see NEOCORTEX: CHEMICAL AND ELECTRICAL SYNAPSES). Extracellular agonists also include neuromodulators and neurohormones, with the latter distributed through the vasculature as well as the perineuronal space (see NEUROMODULATION IN MAMMALIAN NERVOUS SYSTEMS and NEUROMODULATION IN INVERTEBRATE NERVOUS SYSTEMS). From a functional viewpoint, the main difference between these agonists and neurotransmitters is that neurotransmitters generally mediate synaptic communication between two specific pre- and postsynaptic cells, whereas the release of a neuromodulator or neurohormone into the extracellular space mediates *pancrinic* transmission, affecting a local region of tissue rather than a single postsynaptic site. Another, somewhat arbitrary, difference is that neuromodulators and neurohormones tend not to overtly excite or inhibit their targets, but rather shape the response of a neuron to classical synaptic transmitters in various and subtle ways (Kaczmarek and Levitan, 1987). Note that a given molecule can be assigned more than one of these roles (e.g., neurotransmitter versus neuromodulator), depending on the cell type or region in the nervous system.

Intracellular second messengers are called such because their concentration is often subsequent to the message delivered by neurotransmitters (e.g., after activation of a metabotopic receptor). Second messengers may have direct actions or, as mentioned, may participate in more complicated reaction schemes. Depending on the complexity of the reaction, the functional action of second messengers can be quite delayed and last for minutes if not longer. In addition, the more complicated the biochemical cascade, the more opportunities there are for interactions with modulatory pathways.

The most well-known second messenger is the Ca^{2+} ion, which modulates various membrane channels and biochemical cascades, including many neurotransmitter release systems, and whose intracellular concentration is mediated by a variety of Ca^{2+}-permeable channels, pumps, buffers, and intracellular stores (involving as well the extensive endoplasmic recticulum network, which may support regenerative intracellular Ca^{2+} waves [Berridge, 1998]).

There is a vast array of receptor types, some of which are associated with classical point-to-point synaptic transmission, others that mediate pancrinic transmission, and still others that function as links along intracellar pathways. Presynaptic membrane may also express extracellular receptors whose agonist is either the transmitter released by the same terminal (and thus implementing an immediate feedback loop) or another substance, which then may modulate the presynaptic terminal properties. A given neuron may express many different types of receptors in response to the signaling molecules released from other cells, normally in a nonuniform distribution over its surface. In contrast, the number of neuroactive compounds that a single neuron releases itself is usually one, probably (according to current knowledge) at most two or three.

Enzymes

Among the wide variety of enzymes distributed in the neuron's cytoplasm, the most important types for signal processing include kinases and phosphatases, as well as those involved in the metabolism of signaling molecules (e.g., synthases and lipases). The kinases and phosphatases respectively phosphorylate (add a phosphate group) and dephosphorylate specific target proteins, as a result modifying the functional properties of the target. This is the most common mechanism of regulating the activity of neuronal proteins, for example, by altering the responsiveness of a receptor to an agonist, or the voltage dependency or conductance of an ion channel.

Gap Junctions

Gap junctions are membrane proteins that form a direct electrical path between two neurons, essentially as a nonlinear, nonselective ion channel (see NEOCORTEX: CHEMICAL AND ELECTRICAL SYNAPSES). Thus, on the one hand, these connections are like conventional synapses in that they mediate information flow from cell to cell, but on the other hand, they are quite unlike conventional synapses in that this flow is (more or less) reciprocal and instantaneous. As with essentially all the other neuronal elements, gap junctions can be functionally modulated, typically by Ca^{2+} or other second messengers.

Pumps, Exchangers, and Transporters

Pumps, exchangers, and transporters are membrane proteins responsible for the active maintenance of concentration gradients of different ions and molecules crucial for neural signal processing, and thus are able to modify the membrane potential, either directly or indirectly.

For example, the enzyme Na/K ATPase maintains the characteristic Na^+ and K^+ gradients across all cell membranes; related proteins include the calcium and proton pumps. The action of these pumps depends on the hydrolysis of adenosine triphosphate (ATP) to adenosine diphosphate (ADP), and thus they are tightly coupled to the metabolic machinery of the neuron. Since these cations directly or indirectly contribute to the membrane potential, and since the kinetics of the pump can be modulated, a pump can set the neuron's long-term electrical behavior.

In addition to driving channel currents, the Na^+ and K^+ gradients across the cell membrane also provide the energy for exchangers and transporters. Exchanger proteins move ions such as Ca^{2+} and protons out of the neuron, against their gradients, in exchange for Na^+ moving down its gradient. The exchangers react faster than pumps and thus provide early protection against excessive accumulation of various ions. Transporter proteins move molecules such as glutamate and GABA (respectively the principal excitatory and inhibitory neurotransmitters in the central nervous system) back into the neuron (and into surrounding glia as well) after being released into the extracellular space during synaptic transmission.

The activity of some of these proteins is electrogenic. For example, the Na/K pump cycles two K^+ ions in for three Na^+ ions out, and therefore directly generates a net outward current that can cause a hyperpolarization of many millivolts, depending on conditions. Although not always inherently electrogenic, there is an indirect link between the activity of exchangers and transporters and the membrane potential. Since they are driven by the inward movement of Na^+, an increase in exchanger or transporter activity leads to an increase in the cytoplasmic concentration of Na^+, which will then be countered by increased Na/K ATPase activity and its attendent electrogenic effect.

Implications of Neuronal Macromolecule Diversity and Complexity

Channels, receptors, pumps, enzymes, and so on are comprised of one or several individual proteins, called subunits, each of which is coded by a specific gene. For any given type of channel (etc.) there may be many variations of the complete ensemble, or *multimer*, as one subunit substitutes for another, which often imparts different peculiarities to the functional properties of the multimeric

protein (binding sites, effect on kinetics, etc.—in fact, the same sort of properties that may be affected by protein phosphorylation). Thus, a particular Ca^{2+} channel type, for example, may have ten or so identified variants or subtypes (with the strong likelihood that more remain to be discovered). There are as yet but few demonstrations, either by explicit functional studies or by model prediction, that these differences between subtypes are relevant for neural computation. Nevertheless, correlations are increasingly being found between particular disease states and subtle functional alterations of cellular elements, or, in the opposite sense, functional (e.g., behavioral) expressions of genetic manipulation (e.g., knockout) protocols. Thus, the reality of subtype diversity suggests an important limitation for models that employ a single stereotypical kinetic model of a given type of neural protein.

Subunit substitution in a receptor, channel, or other neural protein can, among other things, determine different endogenous modulatory agonists or antagonists. Since there are many candidates for pancrinic pathways at most neurons, this mechanism is important for understanding circuitry dynamics in the intact brain. This functional diversity also has extremely important implications for clinical pharmacology: different subunits can also impart sensitivities to different exogenous compounds, allowing the eventual possibility of targeting very specific synapses or other cellular elements with the appropriately chosen (or designed) drug.

Individual proteins are comprised of contorted chains of thousands of amino acids. This fundamental complexity allows for, in principle, several mechanisms by which a protein may be influenced by its local environment. Thus, there may be an important location dependence of the functional properties of a particular kind of protein, reflecting subtle variations in the protein's microenvironment. For the same reason, it is not surprising that the behavior of a channel, for example, may be modified by the membrane voltage or by binding with a signaling molecule. In this context, we may note that quantitative experimental measurements of a given channel or receptor type in different cell types are inevitably different, beyond what would be expected from experimental variability. Sometimes such differences are seen even between different locations of a single cell type (in particular somatic versus dendritic). Thus, there are at least two possible explanations for such differences: they may be intrinsic to the neural protein under investigation (i.e., a difference in subunit composition), or they may reflect how different local environments, specific to different cell types or location within a single cell, can influence the protein's behavior.

Neuron Models and the Biophysical Mosaic

We now return to the question of neuron models and how they might relate to cellular details. In the most general sense, a single neuron provides a dynamic mapping from a spatiotemporal pattern of pulsed inputs impinging on its dendrites and soma, into a single sequence of output spikes at the axon hillock, which may then be further altered by distinct mechanisms in the axonal tree and presynaptic boutons. Overall, the neuron models employed by theorists describe the time-varying three-dimensional biophysical mosaic underlying this complex signal processing to varying degrees (see PERSPECTIVE ON NEURON MODEL COMPLEXITY and SINGLE-CELL MODELS).

At the simplest level, an extreme abstract model might be a point integrator whose output is passed through a static sigmoid transfer function, where the scalar output is analogous to the firing rate of a spiking neuron. Here the biophysical basis is essentially limited to the resistive nature of the neuron membrane and the spike threshold. As a next step, the basic temporal characteristics of neuronal function may be represented by a leaky integrate-and-fire model that captures the resistive-capacitive nature of the neuron membrane and the action potential–based point process communication between neurons (see INTEGRATE-AND-FIRE NEURONS AND NETWORKS). Among other things, this scheme allows for encoding by both firing rate and higher-order statistics of spike trains, as well as a more tractable analysis of generalized stochastic mechanisms (see ADAPTIVE SPIKE CODING, RATE CODING AND SIGNAL PROCESSING, and SENSORY CODING AND INFORMATION TRANSMISSION).

A more explicit description of biophysical mechanisms might start with the characteristics of membrane channels and dendritic cables (see DENDRITIC PROCESSING). For example, a single neuron model may include transmitter-gated synaptic conductance inputs distributed on a linear (or "passive") cable tree topology, with conductance-based (i.e., voltage-dependent channels) spike generation at a central somatic node. An anatomically based dendritic cable structure provides an explicit basis for synaptic weights via different coupling impedances to the soma, as well as cable-dependent (e.g., "on-the-path") nonlinear synaptic interactions. Simple channel models can capture basic spike firing properties such as absolute and relative refractory period, adaptation, or non-zero minimum firing rates.

A model with increased biophysical realism could include voltage-dependent membrane properties distributed throughout the cell (Stuart, Spruston, and Häusser, 1999; see DENDRITIC PROCESSING). Intrinsic and synaptic mechanisms can be modeled with less or more sophisticated kinetic descriptions, either deterministic or stochastic (see BIOPHYSICAL MECHANISMS IN NEURONAL MODELING; TEMPORAL DYNAMICS OF BIOLOGICAL SYNAPSES, SYNAPTIC INTERACTIONS; and SYNAPTIC NOISE AND CHAOS IN VERTEBRATE NEURONS). Further details of functional properties may require descriptions of the microphysiology of extra- and intracellular systems, and thus explicit modeling of biochemical dynamics, including Ca^{2+} diffusion, buffering, sequestration, and release; protein conformations; and enzyme activation/inactivation. Finally, the most faithful cellular model would require a four-dimensional construct whose biophysical properties vary with both space and time, in particular depending on past activity, or "experience" (see HEBBIAN SYNAPTIC PLASTICITY).

State Variables and Functional Compartments of the Mosaic Neuron

The many cellular elements we have described suggest a similar number of variables that characterize the functional state of a neuron as a signal processing device, each of which may be thought of as representing information. The most classical variable, of course, is the membrane voltage, which defines the immediate integration of synaptic input onto the dendritic tree and soma and, eventually, the action potential output of the cell. However, it may be argued that for predicting spike output, the first derivative of the membrane voltage may be nearly as important as the actual value of the voltage, a behavior that is easily predicted by Hodgkin-Huxley-type models (see AXONAL MODELING; BIOPHYSICAL MECHANISMS IN NEURONAL MODELING; and ION CHANNELS: KEYS TO NEURONAL SPECIALIZATION). Other variables that may be important include the concentration of ions and various neuroactive molecules (e.g., transmitters and second messengers) both inside and outside the cell, and the metabolic or conformational state of various membrane and intracellular proteins. Finally, it may be useful to consider structural or anatomical parameters of the single neuron as functional state variables, such as number and distribution of spines or postsynaptic sites.

All of these state variables are determined by complex relationships between the cellular constituents. For example, the membrane voltage at any given point in the neuron is determined by the spatial distribution of electrically conducting membrane channels and their reversal potentials, the membrane capacitance, and the electrical coupling to the rest of the cell as determined by the three-dimensional branching cable structure and cytoplasmic resistivity. In turn, the ion concentration gradients that underlie channel reversal potentials are determined by an interplay between the currents through the appropriate channels (which tend to reduce the gradients) and membrane pumps, exchangers, transporters, and intracellular buffer and sequestering systems (which in general tend to maintain the gradients). Finally, in some cases ions passing through a given membrane channel can subsequently bind with and then modulate the conduction state of either the same or possibly other types of channels. Clearly, feedback pathways are the rule rather than the exception in the mosaic's interactions (see Figure 1).

The state variables of a neuron can be associated with a variety of functional compartments, with spatial scales that range from less than a micron to the entire cell. These compartments may correspond to the spatial gradients of voltage (e.g., as determined by dendritic cable properties) or second messenger concentration (e.g., determined by diffusion constant and geometry of the intracellular space), or to the localization of a given biochemical pathway, or to an explicit subcellular structure (e.g., a dendritic spine, an organelle, the cell nucleus). In summary, for most state variables the neuron is far from a classical "well-mixed" system. Rather, an extreme internal heterogeneity is usually the case: a single cell thus becomes a cell of cells.

Emergent State Properties of Intracellular Chemical Systems

Recent work has demonstrated the possibility of various stable arrangements between the concentrations of certain intracellular molecules or the metabolic states of certain proteins, all of which in turn can participate in various biochemical pathways, including those regulating membrane properties and plasticity (Weng, Bhalla, and Iyengar, 1999). From an information processing viewpoint, these combinations can be thought of as essentially distinct states that partially define the functional input-output properties of the neuron. It has also been proposed that changes in cellular properties on even longer time scales may be due to self-stabilizing conformational states of proteins such as CAM kinase II or others. Of course, any mechanism underlying a long-lasting modification of the neuronal transfer function is a candidate for the molecular basis of memory (see INVERTEBRATE MODELS OF LEARNING: APLYSIA AND HERMISSENDA).

Discussion: How Much Biophysics Needs to Be Known for a Compelling Brain Theory?

Where does the complexity of the mosaic neuron leave us in terms of formulating a theory for the brain? In particular, how detailed does a model of the neuron have to be, and how does the power of current methods compare with the computational complexity inherent at various levels of biophysical description? These open questions have a very practical importance, since there are few opportunities for formal analyses of these nonlinear dynamical systems. Furthermore, the increasing experimental knowledge of neuronal cellular mechanisms is daunting. The details seem to have an almost fractal quality; no matter what level is being examined, underneath any given mechanism there is another Pandora's box of parameters waiting to be described. Today, so many biophysical properties are known to be present in the neuron membrane that the biggest risk is to choose to include only those that will give the model the properties desired. This leads to a model that is unlikely to fail, and therefore unlikely to teach us anything that we did not know before.

The brute force strategy is to construct a bottom-up, biophysically detailed cell model in order to cover as much as possible the high-order interactions between various mechanisms. Once the map has been laid out, sufficiently rich deterministic or stochastic kinetic equations for the membrane elements and intracellular dynamics may then be assigned. Such maps can be evaluated, at least in principle, since all known biophysical mechanisms can be described by nonlinear partial differential equations, and thus are amenable to standard numerical integration techniques.

However, it may appear that at some point there will be too many equations with too many free parameters for practical evaluation or, more important, for true *understanding*. (On the other hand, the rapid evolution of computing power suggests that the threshold for "impractical" is hard to define.) An optimistic view is that once a sufficiently elaborate biophysical cellular model is constructed, its behavior may be well enough understood so that a more abstract model that captures the functional essentials with considerably less computational expense may be derived. But until there are some formal criteria for establishing what exactly "essential" means, this process will inevitably be an iterative one, moving back and forth between an analysis of detailed cell models in isolation and in nontrivial networks (limited most probably by the available tools) and an analysis of more abstract neural networks. The fundamental challenge to theorists, then, is to go beyond this sort of "reverse engineering" approach and develop a method that is at once commensurate with the complexity of the brain, yet can produce a bona fide theory whose detail avoids that of the actual biological reality.

Road Map: Biological Neurons and Synapses
Related Reading: Activity-Dependent Regulation of Neuronal Conductances; Adaptive Spike Coding; Axonal Modeling; Dendritic Processing; Hebbian Synaptic Plasticity; Ion Channels: Keys to Neuronal Specialization; Neocortex: Chemical and Electrical Synapses; NMDA Receptors: Synaptic, Cellular, and Network Models; Rate Coding and Signal Processing; Synaptic Interactions; Synaptic Noise and Chaos in Vertebrate Neurons; Temporal Dynamics of Biological Synapses

References

Berridge, M. J., 1998, Neuronal calcium signaling, *Neuron*, 21:13–26.
Borg-Graham, L., 1999, Interpretations of data and mechanisms for hippocampal pyramidal cell models, *Cereb. Cortex*, 13:19–138. ◆
Cooper, J. R., Bloom, F. E., and Roth, R. H., 1996, *The Biochemical Basis of Neuropharmacology*, 7th ed., Oxford, Engl.: Oxford University Press. ◆
Fain, G. L., 1999, *Molecular and Cellular Physiology of Neurons*, Cambridge, MA: Harvard University Press. ◆
Hille, B., 2002, *Ionic Channels of Excitable Membranes*, 3rd ed., Sunderland, MA: Sinauer. ◆
Johnston, D., and Wu, S. M.-S., 1995, *Foundations of Cellular Neurophysiology*, Cambridge, MA: MIT Press. ◆
Kaczmarek, L. K., and Levitan, I. B., Eds., 1987, *Neuromodulation: The Biochemical Control of Neuronal Excitability*, Oxford, Engl.: Oxford University Press.
Koch, C., 1999, *The Biophysics of Computation: Information Processing in Single Neurons*, Oxford, Engl.: Oxford University Press. ◆
Koch, C., and Segev, I., Ed., 1998, *Methods in Neuronal Modeling*, 2nd ed., Cambridge, MA: MIT Press. ◆
Laming, P. R., Kimelberg, H., Robinson, S., Salm, A., Hawrylak, N., Müller, C., Roots, B., and Ng, K., 2000, Neuronal-glial interactions and behaviour, *Neurosci. Biobehav. Rev.*, 24:295–340.
Meunier, C., and Segev, I., 2000, Neurons as physical objects: Structure, dynamics and function, in *Handbook of Biological Physics* (F. Moss and Gielen S., Eds.), New York: Elsevier.
Stuart, G., Spruston, N., and Häusser, M., Eds., 1999, *Dendrites*, Oxford, Engl.: Oxford University Press. ◆
Weiss, T. F., 1996, *Cellular Biophysics* (2 vol.), Cambridge, MA: MIT Press. ◆
Weng, G., Bhalla, U. S., and Iyengar, R., 1999, Complexity in biological signaling systems, *Science*, 284:92–96.

Brain Signal Analysis

Jeng-Ren Duann, Tzyy-Ping Jung, and Scott Makeig

Introduction

Artificial neural networks (ANNs) have now been applied to a wide variety of real-world problems in many fields of application. The attractive and flexible characteristics of ANNs, such as their parallel operation, learning by example, associative memory, multifactorial optimization, and extensibility, make them well suited to the analysis of biological and medical signals. In this study, we review applications of ANNs to brain signal analysis, for instance, for analysis of the electroencephalogram (EEG) and magnetoencephalogram (MEG) or electromyogram (EMG), and as applied to computed tomographic (CT) images and magnetic resonance (MR) brain images, and to series of functional MR brain images (i.e., fMRI).

Most ANNs are implemented as sets of nonlinear summing elements interconnected by weighted links, forming a highly simplified model of brain connectivity. The basic operation of such artificial neurons is to pass a weighted sum of their inputs through a nonlinear hard-limiting or soft "squashing" function. To form an ANN, these basic calculating elements (artificial neurons) are most often arranged in interconnected layers. Some neurons, usually those in the layer farthest from the input, are designated as output neurons. The initial weight values of the interconnections are usually assigned randomly.

The operation of most ANNs proceeds in two stages. Rules used in the first stage, training (or learning), can be categorized as supervised, unsupervised, or reinforced. During training, the weight values for each interconnection in the network are adjusted either to minimize the error between desired and computed outputs (supervised learning) or to maximize differences (or minimize similarities) between the output categories (unsupervised or competitive learning). In reinforced learning, an input-output mapping is learned during continued interaction with the environment so as to maximize a scalar index of performance (Haykin, 1999). The second stage is recall, in which the ANN generates output for the problem the ANN is designed to solve, based on new input data without (or sometimes with) further training signals.

Because of their multifactorial character, ANNs have proved suitable for practical use in many medical applications. Because most medical signals of interest usually are not produced by variations in a single variable or factor, many medical problems, particularly those involving decision making, must involve a multifactorial decision process. In these cases, changing one variable at a time to find the best solution may never reach the desired objective (Dayhoff and DeLeo, 2001), whereas multifactorial ANN approaches may be more successful. In this article, we review recent applications of ANNs to brain signal processing, organized according to the nature of brain signals to be analyzed and the role that ANNs play in the applications.

Roles of ANNs in Brain Signal Processing

To date, ANNs have been applied to brain data for the following purposes:

- *Feature extraction, classification, and pattern recognition.* ANNs in this application serve mainly as nonlinear classifiers. The inputs are preprocessed so as to form a feature space. ANNs are used to categorize the collected data into distinct classes. In other cases, inputs are not subjected to preprocessing but are given directly to an ANN to extract features of interest from the data.
- *Adaptive filtering and control.* In this application, ANNs operate within closed-loop systems to process changing inputs, adapting their weights "on the fly" to filter out unwanted parts of the input (adaptive filtering), or mapping their outputs to parameters used in on-line control (adaptive control).
- *Linear or nonlinear mapping.* In this application, ANNs are used to transform inputs to outputs of a desired form. For example, an ANN might remap its rectangular input data coordinates to circular or more general coordinate systems.
- *Modeling.* ANNs can be thought of as function generators that generate an output data series based on a learned function or data model. ANNs with two layers of trainable weights have proved capable of approximating any nonlinear function.
- *Signal separation and deconvolution.* In this application, ANNs separate their input signals into the weighted sum or convolution of a number of underlying sources using assumptions about the nature of the sources or of their interrelationships (e.g., their independence).
- *Texture analysis and image segmentation.* Image texture analysis is becoming increasingly important in image segmentation, recognition, and understanding. ANNs are being used to learn spatial or spatial-frequency texture features and, accordingly, to categorize images or to separate an image into subimages (image segmentation).
- *Edge detection.* In an image, an edge or boundary between two objects can be mapped to a dark band between two lighter areas (objects). By using the properties of intensity discontinuity, ANNs can be trained to recognize these dark bands as edges, or can learn to draw such edges based on contrast and other information.

Application Areas

In this section, we describe some applications of ANNs to brain signals by means of examples involving neurobiological time series and brain images. Neurobiological signals of clinical interest recorded noninvasively from humans include electroencephalographic (EEG), magnetoencephalographic (MEG), and electromyographic (EMG) data. Research in brain imaging includes the analysis of structural brain images, mainly focused on the extraction of three-dimensional (3D) structural information, from various kinds of brain images (e.g., magnetic resonance images, or MRIs), as well as the analysis of functional brain imaging series that mainly reveal changes in the brain state during cognitive tasks using medical imaging techniques (e.g., functional MRI, or fMRI, and positron emission tomography, or PET). These examples by no means cover all the applications in the field.

Neurobiological Signals

EEG and MEG. EEG provides a noninvasive measure of brain electrical activity recorded as changes in the potential difference between two points on the scalp. MEG is the magnetic counterpart of EEG. In accordance with the assumption that the ongoing EEG can be altered by stimulus or event to form respectively the event-related potential (ERP) or the evoked potential (EP), these changes, though tiny, can be recorded through the scalp. It is possible for researchers to apply pattern recognition algorithms to search for the differences in brain status while the brain is performing different tasks. Thus, Peters, Pfurtscheller, and Flyvbjerg (2001) applied an autoregressive model to four-channel EEG potentials to obtain features that were used to train an ANN using a backpropagation algorithm to differentiate the subject's intention to move the left or right index finger or right foot. They suggested that the framework might be useful for designing a direct brain-computer interface. In the study of Zhang et al. (2001), ANNs were trained to determine the stage of anesthesia based on features extracted from the middle-latency auditory-evoked potential (MLAEP) plus other physiological parameters. By combining power spectral estimation, principal component analysis (PCA), and ANNs, Jung et al. (1997) demonstrated that continuous, accurate, noninvasive, and near real-time estimation of an operator's global level of alertness is feasible using EEG measures recorded from as few as two scalp sites. The results of their ANN-based estimation compared favorably with results obtained using a linear regression model applied to the same PCA-reduced EEG power spectral data.

Sun and Sclabassi (2000) employed an ANN as a linear mapping device to transform the EEG topography obtained from a forward solution in a simple spherical model to a more realistic spheroidal model whose forward solution was difficult to compute directly. In that study, a backpropagation learning algorithm was used to train an ANN to convert spatial locations between spherical and spheroid models. Instead of computing the infinite sums of the Legendre functions required in the asymmetric spheroidal model, the calculations were carried out in the spherical model and then converted by the ANN to the more realistic model for display and evaluation.

Recently, ANNs have made a substantial contribution to the analysis of EEG/MEG by separating the problem of EEG/MEG source identification from that of source localization, a mathematically underdetermined problem: any scalp potential distribution can be produced by a limitless number of potential distributions within the head. Because of volume conduction through cerebrospinal fluid, skull, and scalp, EEG and MEG data collected from any point on the scalp may include activity arising in multiple locally synchronous but relatively independent neural processes within a large brain volume. This has made it difficult to relate EEG measurements to underlying brain processes and to localize the sources of EEG and MEG signals. Progress has been made by several groups in separating and identifying the distinct brain sources from their mixtures in scalp EEG or MEG recordings, assuming only their temporal independence and spatial stationarity (Makeig et al., 1997; Jung et al., 2001), using a class of independent component analysis (ICA) or blind source separation algorithms.

Muscle and movement signals. From recordings of muscle stretching (mainly the EMG), it is possible to predict the intent of subjects to perform actions such as hand or finger movements, or to judge the disability of a specific bundle of muscle cells. For example, Khalil and Duchene (2000) used wavelet coefficients obtained from uterine EMG to train ANNs to separate the inputs into four labeled categories: uterine contractions, fetal movements, Alvarez waves, and long-duration low-frequency band waves. They reported that the system was useful for maintaining preterm births. On the other hand, Stites and Abbas (2000) used an ANN as a pattern shaper to refine the output patterns of a functional neuromuscular stimulation system that served as a pattern generator of control signals for cyclic movements to help the paraplegic patient stand using functional neuromuscular stimulation.

Brain Images

Structural images. In structural brain image analysis, ANNs may play roles in image segmentation, image labeling, or edge detection. Image segmentation is the first and probably the most important step in digital image processing. Segmentation may be a labeling problem in which the goal is to assign, to each voxel in a gray-level image, a unique label that represents its belonging to an anatomical structure. The results of image segmentation can be used for image understanding and recognition, 3D reconstruction, visualization, and measurements, including brain volume changes in developmental brain diseases such as Alzheimer's disease and autism. The rapid pace of development of medical imaging devices such as MRI and computed tomography permits a better understanding of anatomical brain structure without, prior to, or even during neurosurgery. However, the results are highly dependent on the quality of the image segmentation processes.

Here we give some examples using ANNs in image segmentation: Dawant et al. (1991) presented a backpropagation neural network approach to the automatic characterization of brain tissues from multimodal MR images. The ability of a three-layer backpropagation neural network to perform segmentation based on a set of MR images (T1-weighted, T2-weighted, and proton density-weighted) acquired from a patient was studied. The results were compared with those obtained using a maximum likelihood classifier. Dawant et al. found no significant difference in the results obtained by the two methods, although the backpropagation neural network gave cleaner segmentation images. Using the same analysis strategy, Reddick et al. (1997) first trained a self-organizing map (SOM) on multimodal MR brain images to efficiently extract and convert the 3D inputs (from T1-, T2- and proton density-weighted images) into a feature space and utilized a backpropagation neural network to separate them into classes of white matter, gray matter, and cerebrospinal fluid. Their work demonstrated high intraclass correlation between the automated segmentation and classification of tissues and standard radiologist identification, as well as high intrasubject reproducibility.

Functional images. Today, not only are medical imaging devices able to provide impressive spatial resolution and details of the fine structure of the human brain, they can also reveal changes in brain status in awake subjects who are performing a task or even daydreaming, by measuring ongoing metabolic changes, including cerebral blood flow, cerebral blood volume (by PET), and blood oxygenation level–dependent signal levels (by fMRI). We will give some examples, mainly from fMRI analysis.

Functional brain imaging emerged in the early 1990s, based on the observation that increases in local neuronal activity are followed by local changes in oxygen concentration. Changing the amount of oxygen carried by hemoglobin changes the degree to which hemoglobin disturbs a magnetic field, as a result of which in vivo changes in blood oxygenation could be detected by MRI (Ogawa et al., 1992). The subsequent changes in the MRI signal became known as the blood oxygenation level–dependent or BOLD signal. This technique was soon applied to normal humans during functional brain activation (the subjects performed cognitive tasks), giving birth to the rapid growing field of fMRI.

Theoretically, the fMRI BOLD signal from a given brain voxel can be interpreted as a linear combination of different sources with distinguishable time courses and spatial distributions, including use-dependent hemodynamic changes, blood, or CSF flows, plus subject movement and machine artifacts. Recently, ANNs (especially those using ICA), applied to fMRI data, have proved to be a powerful method for detecting and separating task-related activations with either known or unanticipated time courses (McKeown et al., 1998) that could not be detected using standard hypothesis-driven analyses. Duann et al. (2002) have given further details of applying ICA to the fMRI BOLD signal. They showed that the hemodynamic response to even widely spaced stimulus presentations may be dependent on the trial, site, stimulus, and subject. Thus, the standard regression–based method of applying a fixed hemodynamic response model to find stimulus- or task-related BOLD activations needs to be reconsidered.

Discussion

The use of ANNs as classifiers currently dominates their applications in the field of brain signal analysis. This includes classification of brain or related signals as exhibiting normal or abnormal features or processes. Not surprisingly, published studies report promising results.

If the measurements can be modeled as an additive mixture of different sources, including task-related signals and artifacts, applying blind source separation prior to the further processing, visualization, or interpretation may better reveal the underlying physical phenomena (such as different brain processes), which in the raw data could be contaminated or overwhelmed by other processes of no interest.

A survey of relevant papers shows that the most popular architecture for ANNs is the multilayer perceptron (MLP). The MLP architecture is both simple and straightforward to implement and use. In MLPs, information flows in one direction except during training, when error terms are backpropagated. Backpropagation updates network weights in a supervised manner. Although it cannot guarantee a globally minimal solution, backpropagation at least arrives at a local minimum through gradient descent. Various techniques have been derived in an attempt to avoid overfitting to a local minimum. Once the network weights have been learned and fixed, feedforward networks can be implemented in hardware and made to run in real time. All of these characteristics make the backpropagation algorithm most popular in biomedical applications.

In some applications, target outputs may not be available or may be too expensive to acquire. In these cases, unsupervised learning algorithms may be used. Among unsupervised learning algorithms, self-organizing maps (SOMs) are the most popular for biomedical applications. During training, SOMs attempt to assign their input patterns to different output regions. Often SOMs may converge after only few learning cycles.

Application Issues

Although most published papers have concluded that ANNs are appropriate for their domain of interest, many issues still have to be resolved before ANNs can be claimed to be the general method of choice. Unfortunately, most published studies have not gone beyond demonstrating application to a very limited amount of data. As with any type of method, ANNs have their limitations that should be carefully considered:

- Every study should provide a rationale for the data chosen as input. For example, ANN-based computer-aided diagnostic systems may give misleading results if the ANNs are not given adequately representative features and sufficient naturally occurring data variations in their training data. With ANNs, any input may yield some sort of output, correct and useful or not ("garbage in, garbage out"). Therefore, the keys to success of ANN applications are not only to pick an appropriate architecture or learning algorithm, but also to choose the right data and data features to train the network.

- Although methods of applying ANNs to biomedical signals have already shown great promise, great care must be taken to examine the results obtained. The issue of trust in the outputs of ANNs always deserves informed as well as statistical consideration. Since medical diagnosis is nearly always a multifactorial and multidisciplinary problem, medical experts should always evaluate network outputs in light of other direct or indirect convergent evidence before making final decisions affecting the health of patients.

- Before practical implementation is planned, ANN methods should be compared to more direct ways of obtaining the same answers, as these might sometimes prove more accurate or cost effective.

Model Mining

Since the first wave of popularization of backpropagation networks nearly two decades ago, an ever greater number and variety of ANN models have been devised to tackle an ever greater variety of problems. The overall insight that ANNs both embody and exemplify is perhaps that our human intelligence is multifactorial and highly adaptable to using whatever forms of information are available to us. In this spirit, we suggest that researchers always attempt to interpret the physiological meaning both of the features of their input data and of the data models that their trained ANNs represent. Too often ANNs have been treated like black boxes. We believe it is time to open the black boxes and interpret what is happening inside them. Such interpretations might even yield new insights into the nature of the biomedical signals, or suggest new or more efficient ways to look at the input data. It is also possible that the ANN models and methods might suggest more efficient methods to collect input data. Such "model mining" might even prove to be the most rewarding result of applying ANNs. Researchers who simply recount classification accuracy may ignore nuggets of novel information about brain processes hidden in the ANN models that they and the data have jointly constructed.

Road Map: Implementation and Analysis
Related Reading: EEG and MEG Analysis; Muscle Models; Neuroinformatics; Statistical Parametric Mapping of Cortical Activity Patterns

References

Dawant, B. M., Ozkan, M., Zijdenbos, A., and Margolin, R., 1991, A computer environment for 2D and 3D quantitation of MR images using neural networks, *Magn. Reson. Imaging*, 20:64–65.

Dayhoff, J. E., and DeLeo, J. M., 2001, Artificial neural networks: Opening the black box, *Cancer*, 91:1615–1635. ◆

Duann, J. R., Jung, T. P., Kuo, W. J., Yeh, T. C., Makeig, S., Hsieh, J. C., and Sejnowski, T. J., 2002, Single-trial variability in event-related BOLD signals, *NeuroImage*, 15:823–835. ◆

Haykin, S., 1999, *Neural Network: A Comprehensive Foundation*, Englewood Cliffs, NJ: Prentice Hall. ◆

Jung, T.-P., Makeig, S., Stensmo, M., and Sejnowski, T. J., 1997, Estimating alertness from the EEG power spectrum, *IEEE Trans. Biomed. Eng.*, 44:60–69.

Jung, T.-P., Makeig, S., McKeown, M. J., Bell, A. J., Lee, T.-W. and Sejnowski, T. J., 2001, Imaging brain dynamics using independent component analysis, *Proc. IEEE*, 89:1107–1122. ◆

Khalil, M., and Duchene, J., 2000, Uterine EMG analysis, a dynamic approach for change detection and classification, *IEEE Trans. Biomed. Eng.*, 47:748–756.

Makeig, S., Jung, T.-P., Bell, A. J., Ghahremani, D., and Sejnowski, T. J., 1997, Blind separation of auditory event-related brain responses into independent components, *Proc. Natl. Acad. Sci. USA*, 94:10979–10984. ◆

McKeown, M. J., Jung, T.-P., Makeig, S., Brown, G. G., Kindermann, S. S., Lee, T.-W., and Sejnowski, T. J., 1998, Spatially independent activity patterns in functional MRI data during the Stroop color-naming task, *Proc. Natl. Acad. Sci. USA*, 95:803–810. ◆

Ogawa, S., Tank, D., Menon, R., Ellermann, J., Kim, S., Merkle, H., and Ugurbil, K., 1992, Intrinsic signal changes accompanying sensory stimulation: Functional brain mapping with magnetic resonance imaging, *Proc. Natl. Acad. Sci. USA*, 89:5951–5959. ◆

Peters, B. O., Pfurtscheller, G., and Flyvbjerg, H., 2001, Automatic differentiation of multichannel EEG signals, *IEEE Trans. Biomed. Eng.*, 48:111–116.

Reddick, W. E., Glass, J. O., Cook, E. N., Elkin, T. D., and Deaton R. J., 1997, Automated segmentation and classification of multispectral magnetic resonance images of brain using artificial neural networks, *IEEE Trans. Med. Imaging*, 16:911–918.

Stites, E. C., and Abbas, J. J., 2000, Sensitivity and versatility of an adaptive system for controlling cyclic movements using functional neuromuscular stimulation, *IEEE Trans. Biomed. Eng.*, 47:1287–1292. ◆

Sun, M., and Sclabassi, R. J., 2000, The forward EEG solution can be computed using artificial neural networks, *IEEE Trans. Biomed. Eng.*, 47:1044–1050. ◆

Zhang, X.-S., Roy, R. J., Schwender, D., and Daunderer, M., 2001, Discrimination of anesthetic states using mid-latency auditory evoked potential and artificial neural networks, *Ann. Biomed. Eng.*, 29:446–453.

Brain-Computer Interfaces

José del R. Millán

Introduction

There is a growing interest in the use of physiological signals for communication and operation of devices for the severely motor disabled as well as for able-bodied people. Over the last decade evidence has accumulated to show the potential of analyzing brainwaves on-line to derive information about the subject's mental state that is then mapped into some external action such as selecting a letter from a virtual keyboard or moving a robotics device. A *brain-computer interface (BCI)* is an alternative communication and control channel that does not depend on the brain's normal output pathway of peripheral nerves and muscles (Wolpaw et al., 2000).

Most BCI systems use electroencephalogram signals (EEG and MEG ANALYSIS) measured from scalp electrodes that do not require invasive procedures. Although scalp EEG is a simple way to record brainwaves, it does not provide detailed information on the activity of single neurons (or small clusters of neurons) that could be recorded by implanted electrodes in the cortex (PROSTHETICS, NEURAL). Such a direct measurement of brain activity may, in principle, enable faster recognition of mental states and even more complex interactions.

A BCI may monitor a variety of brainwave phenomena. Some groups exploit evoked potentials generated in response to external stimuli (see Wolpaw et al., 2000, for a review). Evoked potentials are, in principle, easy to pick up but are constrained by the fact that the subject must be synchronized to the external machinery. A more natural and practical alternative is to rely on components associated with spontaneous mental activity. Such spontaneous components range from slow cortical potentials of the EEG (e.g., Birbaumer et al., 1999), to variations of EEG rhythms (e.g., Wolpaw and McFarland, 1994; Kalcher et al., 1996; Anderson, 1997;

Roberts and Penny, 2000; Millán et al., 2002b), to the direct activity of neurons in the cortex (e.g., Kennedy et al., 2000; Wessberg et al., 2000).

Direct Brain-Computer Interfaces

Direct BCIs involve invasive procedures to implant electrodes in the brain (PROSTHETICS, NEURAL). Apart from ethical concerns, a major difficulty is to obtain reliable long-term recordings of neural activity. Recent advances have made it possible to develop direct BCIs with animals and even human beings.

Kennedy and colleagues (2000) have implanted a special electrode into the motor cortex of several paralyzed patients. These electrodes contain a neurotrophic factor that induces growth of neural tissue within the hollow electrode tip. With training, patients learn to control the firing rates of the multiple recorded neurons to some extent. One of them is able to drive a cursor and write messages.

Wessberg et al. (2000) have recorded the activity of ensembles of neurons with microwire arrays implanted in multiple cortical regions involved in motor control, as monkeys performed arm movements. From these signals they have obtained accurate real-time predictions of arm trajectories and have been able to reproduce the trajectories with a robot arm. Although these experiments do not describe an actual BCI, they support the feasibility of controlling complex prosthetic limbs directly by brain activity. In addition, earlier work by Nicolelis and colleagues showed that neural predictors can be derived for rats implanted with the same kind of microelectrodes (see Nicolelis, 2001, for details and reference). The rats were trained to press a bar to move a simple device delivering water, and later learned to operate this device through neural activity only.

For a more detailed analysis and prospects of this area, see Nicolelis (2001).

Noninvasive Brain-Computer Interfaces

Noninvasive BCIs are based on the analysis of EEG phenomena associated with various aspects of brain function. Thus, Birbaumer et al. (1999) measure slow cortical potentials (SCP) over the vertex (top of the scalp). SCP are shifts in the depolarization level of the upper cortical dendrites and indicate the overall preparatory excitation level of a cortical network. Other groups look at local variations of EEG rhythms. The most commonly used rhythms are related to the imagination of movements and are recorded from the central region of the scalp overlying the sensorimotor cortex. In this respect, there exist two main paradigms. Pfurtscheller's team works with event-related desynchronization (ERD, EEG and MEG ANALYSIS) computed at fixed time intervals after the subject is commanded to imagine specific movements of the limbs (Kalcher et al., 1996; Obermaier, Müller, and Pfurtscheller, 2001). Alternatively, Wolpaw and co-workers analyze continuous changes in the amplitudes of the μ (8–12 Hz) or β (13–28 Hz) rhythms (Wolpaw and McFarland, 1994). Finally, in addition to motor-related rhythms, Anderson (1997) and Millán et al. (2002b) also analyze continuous variations of EEG rhythms, but not only over the sensorimotor cortex and in specific frequency bands. The reason is that a number of neurocognitive studies have found that different mental tasks—such as imagination of movements, arithmetic operations, or language—activate local cortical areas to different extents. The insights gathered from these studies guide the placement of electrodes to obtain more relevant signals for the different tasks to be recognized. In this latter case, rather than looking for predefined EEG phenomena as in the previous paradigms, the approach aims at discovering EEG patterns embedded in the continuous EEG signal associated with different mental states.

Most of the existing BCIs are based on synchronous experimental protocols in which the subject must follow a fixed repetitive scheme to switch from one mental task to the next (Wolpaw and McFarland, 1994; Kalcher et al., 1996; Wolpaw and McFarland, 1994; Birbaumer et al., 1999; Obermaier et al., 2001). A trial consists of two parts. A first cue warns the subject to get ready and, after a fixed period of several seconds, a second cue tells the subject to undertake the desired mental task for a predefined time. The EEG phenomena to be recognized are time locked to the last cue and the BCI responds with the average decision over the second period of time. In these synchronous BCI systems, the shortest trial lengths that have been reported are 4 s (Birbaumer et al., 1999) and 5 s (Obermaier et al., 2001). This relatively long time is necessary because the EEG phenomena of interest, either SCP or ERD, need some seconds to recover. On the contrary, other BCIs rely on more flexible asynchronous protocols where the subject makes self-paced decisions on when to stop doing a mental task and start immediately the next one (Roberts and Penny, 2000; Millán et al., 2002b). In this second case, the time of response of the BCI goes from 0.5 s (Millán et al., 2002b) to several seconds (Roberts and Penny, 2000).

EEG signals are characterized by a poor signal-to-noise ratio and spatial resolution. Their quality is greatly improved by means of a Surface Laplacian (SL) derivation, which requires a large number of electrodes (normally 64–128). The SL estimate yields new potentials that represent better the cortical activity originated in radial sources immediately below the electrodes (for details see McFarland et al., 1997; Babiloni et al., 2001; and references therein). The superiority of SL-transformed signals over raw potentials for the operation of a BCI has been demonstrated in different studies (e.g., McFarland et al., 1997). Although significant progress has been obtained (and will still continue) with studies using a high number of EEG electrodes (from 26 to 128), today's practical BCI systems should have a few electrodes (no more than 10) to allow their operation by laypersons, as the procedure of electrode positioning is time consuming and critical. Most groups have developed BCI prototypes with a limited number of electrodes that, however, do not benefit from SL transformations. On the contrary, Babiloni et al. (2001) and Millán et al. (2002b) compute SL derivations from a few electrodes, using global and local methods, respectively.

Wolpaw and McFarland (1994) as well as Birbaumer et al. (1999) have demonstrated that some subjects can learn to control their brain activity through appropriate, but lengthy, training in order to generate fixed EEG patterns that the BCI transforms into external actions. In both cases the subject is trained over several months to modify the amplitude of either the SCP or μ rhythm, respectively. A few other groups follow machine learning approaches to train the classifier embedded in the BCI. These techniques range from linear classifiers (Babiloni et al., 2001; Obermaier et al., 2001), to compact multi-layer perceptrons and Bayesian neural networks (Anderson, 1997; Roberts and Penny, 2000), to variations of LVQ (Kalcher et al., 1996), to local neural classifiers (Millán, 2002; Millán et al., 2002b). Most of these works deal with the recognition of just two mental tasks (Roberts and Penny, 2000; Babiloni et al., 2001; Obermaier et al., 2001), or report classification errors bigger than 15% for three or more tasks (Kalcher et al., 1996; Anderson, 1997). An exception is Millán's approach that achieves error rates below 5% for three mental tasks, but correct recognition is 70% (Millán, 2002; Millán et al., 2002b). Obermaier et al. (2001) reports on a single disabled person who, after several months of training, has reached a performance level close to 100%. It is also worth noting that some of the subjects who follow Wolpaw's approach are able to control their μ rhythm amplitude at four different levels. These classification rates, together with the number of recognizable tasks and duration of the trials, yield bit rates from approximately 0.15 to 2.0.

Some approaches are based on a mutual learning process in which the user and the brain interface are coupled together and adapt to each other (Roberts and Penny, 2000; Obermaier et al., 2001; Millán, 2002; Millán et al., 2002b). This should accelerate the training time. Thus, Millán's approach has allowed subjects to achieve good performances in just a few hours of training (Millán, 2002; Millán et al., 2002b). Analysis of learned EEG patterns confirms that for a subject to operate a personal BCI satisfactorily, the BCI must fit the individual features of the user (Millán et al., 2002a).

Another important concern in BCI is the incorporation of rejection criteria to avoid making risky decisions for uncertain samples. This is extremely important from a practical point of view. Roberts and Penny (2000) apply Bayesian techniques for this purpose, while Millán et al. (2002b) use a confidence probability threshold. In this latter case, more than ten subjects have experimented with their BCI (Millán, 2002; Millán et al., 2002b). Most of them were trained for a few consecutive days (from three to five). Training time was moderate, around half an hour daily. Experimental results show that, at the end of training, the correct recognition rates were 70% (or higher) for three mental tasks. This figure is more than twice random classification. This modest rate is largely compensated by two properties: wrong responses were below 5% (in many cases even below 2%) and decisions were made every half-second. Some other subjects have undertaken consecutive training sessions (from four to seven) in a single day. None of these subjects had previous experience with BCIs and, in less than two hours, all of them reached the same excellent performance as noted previously. It is worth noting that one of the subjects was a physically impaired person suffering from spinal muscular atrophy.

Brain-Actuated Applications

These different BCI systems are being used to operate a number of brain-actuated applications that augment people's communication capabilities, provide new forms of education and entertainment, and also enable the operation of physical devices. There exist virtual keyboards for selecting letters from a computer screen and writing a message (Birbaumer et al., 1999; Obermaier et al., 2001; Millán, 2002). Using these three different approaches, subjects can write a letter every 2 minutes, every 1 minute, and every 22 seconds, respectively. Wolpaw's group has also its own virtual keyboard (Wolpaw, personal communication). A patient who has been implanted with Kennedy and colleagues' special electrode has achieved a spelling rate of about three letters per minute using a combination of neural and EMG signals (Kennedy et al., 2000).

On the other hand, it is also possible to make a brain-controlled hand orthosis open and close (see references in Wolpaw et al., 2000; Obermaier et al., 2001) and even guide in a continuous manner a motorized wheelchair with on-board sensory capabilities (Millán, 2002). In this latter case, the key idea is that users' mental states are associated with high-level commands that the wheelchair executes autonomously (ROBOT NAVIGATION). Another critical aspect for the control of the wheelchair is that subjects can issue high-level commands at any moment, as the operation of the BCI is self-paced and does not require waiting for specific events.

Finally, Millán (2002) illustrates the operation of a simple computer game, but other educational software could have been selected instead.

Discussion

Despite recent advancements, BCI is a field still in its infancy and several issues must be addressed to improve the speed and performance of BCI. One of them is the exploration of local components of brain activity with fast dynamics that subjects can consciously

control. For this we will need increased knowledge of the brain (where and how cognitive and motor decisions are made) as well as the application of more powerful digital signal processing (DSP) methods than those commonly used currently. In addition, extraction of more relevant features, by means of these DSP methods, together with the use of more appropriate classifiers, will improve BCI performance in terms of classification rates and the number of recognizable mental tasks. It may be possible to apply recurrent neural networks to exploit temporal dynamics of brain activity. However, a main limitation in scaling up the number of recognizable mental tasks is the quality—signal-to-noise ratio (SNR)—and resolution of the measured brain signals. This is especially true in the case of EEG-based BCIs, in which the SNR is very poor and we cannot get detailed information on the activity of small cortical areas unless we use a large number of electrodes (64, 128, or more). It is thus crucial to develop better electrodes that are also easy to position, thereby enabling the use of a large number of electrodes even by laypersons. Finally, another key concern is to keep the BCI constantly tuned to its owner. This requirement arises because, as subjects gain experience, they develop new capabilities and change their EEG patterns. In addition, brain activity changes from one session (with which data the classifier is trained) to the next (where the classifier is applied). The challenge here is to adapt the classifier on-line while the subject operates a brain-actuated application, even if the subject's intention is not known until later. In this respect, local neural networks are better suited for on-line learning (STATISTICAL MECHANICS OF ON-LINE LEARNING AND GENERALIZATION) than other methods, due to their robustness against catastrophic interference. This list of topics is not exhaustive, but space limits prevent further discussion (see Wolpaw et al., 2000, for additional details on these and other issues).

Although the immediate application of BCI is to help physically impaired people, its potentials are extensive. Ultimately, they may lead to the development of truly adaptive interactive systems that, on the one hand, augment human capabilities by giving the brain the possibility to develop new skills and, on the other hand, make computer systems fit the pace and individual features of their owners. Most probably, people will use BCI in combination with other sensory interaction modalities (e.g., speech, gestures) and physiological signals (e.g., electromyogram, skin conductivity). Such a multimodal interface will yield a higher bit rate of communication with better reliability than would occur if only brainwaves were utilized. On the other hand, the incorporation of other interaction modalities highlights a critical issue in BCI, namely the importance of filtering out from the recorded brain signals non-CNS artifacts originated by movements of different parts of the body. INDEPENDENT COMPONENT ANALYSIS (q.v.) is a method of detecting and removing such artifacts.

Road Map: Applications
Related Reading: Event-Related Potentials; Kalman Filtering: Neural Implications; Prosthetics, Motor Control; Prosthetics, Sensory Systems

References

Anderson, C. W., 1997, Effects of variations in neural network topology and output averaging on the discrimination of mental tasks from spontaneous EEG, *J. Intell. Syst.*, 7:165–190.
Babiloni, F., Cincotti, F., Bianchi, L., Pirri, G., Millán, J. del R., Mouriño, J., Sallinari, S., and Marciani, M. B., 2001, Recognition of imagined hand movements with low resolution surface Laplacian and linear classifiers, *Med. Eng. & Physics*, 23:323–328.
Birbaumer, N., Ghanayim, N., Hinterberger, T., Iversen, I., Kotchoubey, B., Kübler, A., Perelmouter, J., Taub, E., and Flor, H., 1999, A spelling device for the paralysed, *Nature*, 398:297–298.
Kalcher, J., Flotzinger, D., Neuper, C., Gölly, S., and Pfurtscheller, G., 1996, Graz brain-computer interface II, *Med. Biol. Eng. Comput.*, 34:382–388.

Kennedy, P. R., Bakay, R. A. E., Moore, M. M., Adams, K., and Goldwaithe, J., 2000, Direct control of a computer from the human central nervous system, *IEEE Trans. Rehab. Eng.*, 8:198–202.

McFarland, D. J., McCane, L. M., David, S. V., and Wolpaw, J. R., 1997, Spatial filter selection for EEG-based communication, *Electroenceph. Clin. Neurophysiol.*, 103:386–394.

Millán, J. del R., 2002, Adaptive brain interfaces, *Comm. of the ACM*, to appear. ◆

Millán, J. del R., Franzé, M., Mouriño, J., Cincotti, F., and Babiloni, F., 2002a, Relevant EEG features for the classification of spontaneous motor-related tasks, *Biol. Cybern.*, 86:89–95.

Millán, J. del R., Mouriño, J., Franzé, M., Cincotti, F., Varsta, M., Heikkonen, J., and Babiloni, F., 2002b, A local neural classifier for the recognition of EEG patterns associated to mental tasks, *IEEE Trans. on Neural Networks*, 11:678–686.

Nicolelis, M. A. L., 2001, Actions from thoughts, *Nature*, 409:403–407. ◆

Obermaier, B., Müller, G., and Pfurtscheller, G., 2001, "Virtual Keyboard" controlled by spontaneous EEG activity, in *Proceedings of the International Conference on Artificial Neural Networks*, Heidelberg: Springer-Verlag.

Roberts, S. J., and Penny, W. D., 2000, Real-time brain-computer interfacing: A preliminary study using Bayesian learning, *Med. Biol. Eng. Computing*, 38:56–61.

Wessberg, J., Stambaugh, C. R., Kralik, J. D., Beck, P. D., Laubach, M., Chapin, J. K., Kim, J., Biggs, S. J., Srinivassan, M. A., and Nicolelis, M. A. L., 2000, Real-time prediction of hand trajectory by ensembles of cortical neurons in primates, *Nature*, 408:361–365.

Wolpaw, J. R., and McFarland, D. J., 1994, Multichannel EEG-based brain-computer communication, *Electroenceph. Clin. Neurophysiol.*, 90:444–449.

Wolpaw, J. R., Birbaumer, N., Heetderks, W. J., McFarland, D. J., Peckham, P. H., Schalk, G., Donehin, E., Quatrano, L. A., Robinson, C. J., and Vaughan, T. M., 2000, Brain-computer interface technology: A review of the first international meeting, *IEEE Trans. on Rehab. Eng.*, 8:164–173. Special Section on Brain-Computer Interfaces. ◆

Canonical Neural Models

Frank Hoppensteadt and Eugene M. Izhikevich

Introduction

Mathematical modeling is a powerful tool for studying the fundamental principles of information processing in the brain. Unfortunately, mathematical analysis of a certain neural model could be of limited value, because the results might depend on the particulars of that model: various models of the same neural structure could produce different results. For example, if an investigator obtains results with a Hodgkin-Huxley-type model (see AXONAL MODELING) and then augments the model by adding more parameters and variables to take into account more neurophysiological data, would similar results emerge? A reasonable way to circumvent this problem is to derive results that are largely independent of the model and that can be observed in a class or a family of models.

Having understood the importance of considering families of neural models instead of a single model, we carry out this task by reducing an entire family of Hodgkin-Huxley-type models to a canonical model (for precise definitions, see Section 4.1 in Hoppensteadt and Izhikevich, 1997). Briefly, a model is *canonical* for a family if there is a continuous change of variables that transforms any other model from the family into this one, as we illustrate in Figure 1. For example, the entire family of weakly coupled oscillators of the form in Equation 1 can be converted into the canonical phase model described by Equation 6, where H_{ij} depend on the particulars of the functions f_i and g_{ij}. The change of variables does not have to be invertible, so the canonical model is usually lower dimensional, simple, and tractable. Yet it retains many important features of the family. For example, if the canonical model has multiple attractors, then each member of the family has multiple attractors.

The major advantage to considering canonical models is that one can study universal neurocomputational properties that are shared by all members of the family, since all such members can be put into the canonical form by a continuous change of variables. Moreover, an investigator need not actually present such a change of variables explicitly, so that derivation of canonical models is possible even when the family is so broad that most of its members are given implicitly, e.g., in the abstract form of Equation 1. For example, the canonical phase model in Equation 6 reveals universal computational abilities (e.g., oscillatory associative memory) that are shared by all oscillatory systems, regardless of the nature of

each oscillator or the particulars of the equations that describe it. Thus, the canonical model approach provides a rigorous way to obtain results when only partial information about neuron dynamics is known. Many examples are given subsequently in this article.

The process of deriving canonical neural models is more an art than a science, because a general algorithm for doing so is not known. However, much success has been achieved when we consider weakly connected networks of neurons whose activity is near a bifurcation, a situation that often occurs when the membrane potential is near the threshold value (see DYNAMICS AND BIFURCATION IN NEURAL NETS and PHASE-PLANE ANALYSIS OF NEURAL NETS). We review such bifurcations and corresponding canonical

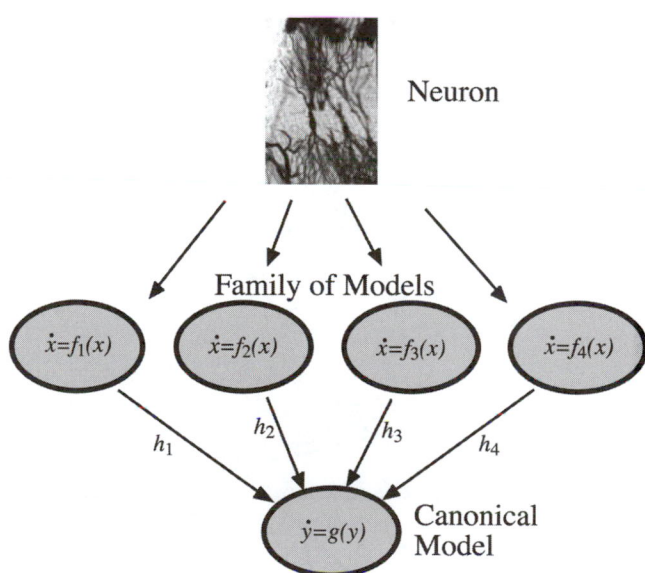

Figure 1. Dynamical system $\dot{y} = g(y)$ is a canonical model for the family $\{f_1, f_2, f_3, f_4\}$ of neural models $\dot{x} = f(x)$ because each such model can be transformed into the form $\dot{y} = g(y)$ by the continuous change of variables h_i.

models. Their rigorous derivation and detailed analysis can be found in Hoppensteadt and Izhikevich (1997).

Weakly Connected Neural Networks

The assumption of weak neuronal connections is based on the observation that the typical size of a postsynaptic potential is less than 1 mV, which is small in comparison with the mean size necessary to discharge a cell (around 20 mV) or the average size of the action potential (around 100 mV) (for a detailed review of relevant electrophysiological data, see Hoppensteadt and Izhikevich, 1997, chap. 1). From the mathematical point of view, this results in neural models of "weakly connected" form

$$\dot{x}_i = f(x_i, \lambda_i) + \varepsilon \sum_{j=1}^{n} g_{ij}(x_i, x_j, \varepsilon) \qquad (1)$$

where each vector $x_i \in \mathbb{R}^m$ describes membrane potential, gating variables, and other electrophysiological variables of the ith neuron (see ION CHANNELS: KEYS TO NEURONAL SPECIALIZATION). Each vector $\lambda_i \in \mathbb{R}^l$ denotes various biophysical parameters of the neuron. The function f describes the neuron's dynamics, and the functions g_{ij} describe connections between the neurons. The dimensionless parameter $\varepsilon \ll 1$ is small, reflecting the strength of connections between neurons.

Bistability and Hysteresis

Bistable and hysteretic dynamics are ubiquitous in neural models, and they may play important roles in biological neurons. The cusp bifurcation depicted in Figure 2 is one of the simplest bifurcations leading to such dynamics. For example, the sigmoidal neuron

$$\dot{x} = -x + aS(x), \quad S(x) = 1/(1 + e^{-x})$$

is at a cusp bifurcation point $x = 0.5$ when $a = 4$. It is bistable when $a > 4$. If each neuron in the weakly connected network described by Equation 1 is near a supercritical cusp bifurcation, then the entire network can be transformed into the canonical form (Hoppensteadt and Izhikevich, 1997)

$$y_i' = r_i - y_i^3 + \sum_{j=1}^{n} s_{ij} y_j \qquad (2)$$

where each scalar $y_i \in \mathbb{R}$ describes rescaled dynamics of the ith neuron. Particulars of the functions f and g_{ij} and the value of the

parameters λ_i do not affect the form of the canonical model. They only affect the parameters r_i and s_{ij}. Thus, by studying the canonical model in Equation 2 one can gain some insight into the neurocomputational behavior of any neural model near a cusp bifurcation, whether it is a simple sigmoidal neuron or a biophysically detailed conductance-based (Hodgkin-Huxley-type) neuron.

The canonical model in Equation 2 is quite simple: each equation has only one nonlinear term, namely, y_i^3, and two internal parameters, r_i and s_{ii}. Still, the Cohen-Grossberg-Hopfield convergence theorem applies, which means that the canonical model has the same neurocomputational properties as the standard Hopfield network (see COMPUTING WITH ATTRACTORS).

Theorem 1 (Cohen-Grossberg-Hopfield Convergence Theorem)

If the connection matrix $S = (s_{ij})$ is symmetric, then the canonical neural network of Equation 2 is a gradient system.

One can easily check that

$$E(y) = -\sum_{i=1}^{n} (r_i y_i - \tfrac{1}{4} y_i^4) - \tfrac{1}{2} \sum_{i,j=1}^{n} s_{ij} y_i y_j$$

is a potential function for Equation 2 in the sense that $y_i' = -\partial E/\partial y_i$ (see also ENERGY FUNCTIONALS FOR NEURAL NETWORKS).

Small-Amplitude Oscillations

Many biophysically detailed neural models can exhibit small-amplitude (damped) oscillations of the membrane potential, especially when the system is near transition from rest state to periodic activity. In the simplest case this corresponds to the supercritical

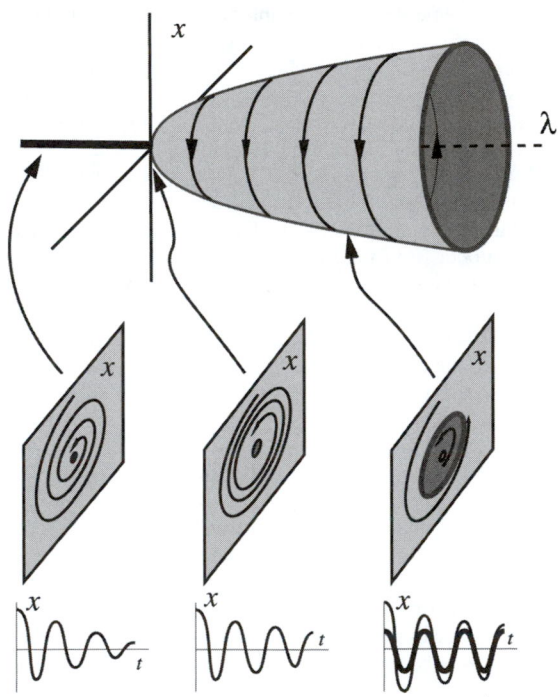

Figure 3. Supercritical Andronov-Hopf bifurcation in $\dot{x} = f(x, \lambda)$. On the left, the rest state is stable. In the middle, the rest state is losing stability, giving birth to a stable limit cycle corresponding to periodic activity. On the right, the system exhibits periodic activity.

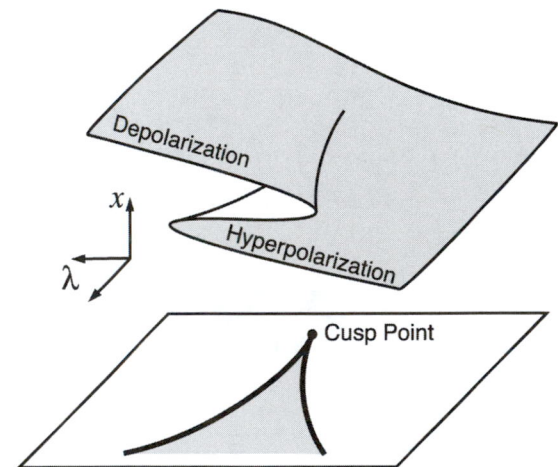

Figure 2. Cusp surface.

Andronov-Hopf bifurcation in Figure 3. Many weakly connected networks (in the form of Equation 1) of such neurons can be transformed into the canonical model

$$z_i' = (r_i + i\omega_i)z_i - z_i|z_i|^2 + \sum_{j=1}^{n} c_{ij}z_j \qquad (3)$$

by a continuous change of variables (Aronson, Ermentrout, and Kopell, 1990). Here $i = \sqrt{-1}$, and each complex variable $z_i \in \mathbb{C}$ describes oscillatory activity of the ith neuron. Again, particulars of the form of the functions f and g_{ij} in Equation 1 affect only the values of the parameters r_i and ω_i and the complex-valued synaptic coefficients $c_{ij} \in \mathbb{C}$.

Even though the canonical model in Equation 3 exhibits oscillatory dynamics, one can still prove the following analogue of the Cohen-Grossberg convergence theorem, which implies that the canonical model in Equation 3 has oscillatory associative memory; that is, it can memorize and retrieve complex oscillatory patterns (Hoppensteadt and Izhikevich, 1996) (Figure 4).

Theorem 2 (Synchronization Theorem for Oscillatory Neural Networks)

If in the canonical neural network in Equation 3 all neurons have equal frequencies $\omega_1 = \ldots = \omega_n$ and the connection matrix $C = (c_{ij})$ is self-adjoint, i.e.,

$$c_{ij} = \bar{c}_{ji} \quad \text{for all } i \text{ and } j \qquad (4)$$

then the network always converges to an oscillatory phase-locked pattern; that is, the neurons oscillate with equal frequencies and constant, but not necessarily identical, phases. There could be many such phase-locked patterns corresponding to many memorized images.

The proof follows from the existence of an orbital energy function

$$E(z) = -\sum_{i=1}^{n} (r_i|z_i|^2 - \tfrac{1}{2} |z_i|^4) - \sum_{i,j=1}^{n} c_{ij}\bar{z}_i z_j$$

for Equation 3 (see ENERGY FUNCTIONALS FOR NEURAL NETWORKS).

The self-adjoint synaptic matrix arises naturally when one considers complex Hebbian learning rules (Hoppensteadt and Izhikevich, 1996):

$$c_{ij} = \frac{1}{n} \sum_{s=1}^{k} \xi_i^s \bar{\xi}_j^k \qquad (5)$$

where each vector $\xi^s = (\xi_1^s, \ldots, \xi_n^s) \in \mathbb{C}^n$ denotes a pattern of phase relations between neurons to be memorized (see also HEBBIAN SYNAPTIC PLASTICITY). Notice that the problem of negative (mirror) images does not arise in oscillatory neural networks, since both ξ^k and $-\xi^k$ result in the same phase relations.

The key difference between the Hopfield-Grossberg network and the oscillatory network (Equation 3) is that memorized images correspond to equilibrium (point) attractors in the former and to limit cycle attractors in the latter. Pattern recognition by an oscillatory neural network involves convergence to the corresponding limit cycle attractor, which results in synchronization of the network activity with an appropriate phase relation between neurons, as in Figure 4 (see also COMPUTING WITH ATTRACTORS).

Large Amplitude Oscillations

Suppose that neurons in the weakly connected network described by Equation 1 exhibit periodic spiking (Figure 5; see also CHAINS OF OSCILLATORS IN MOTOR AND SENSORY SYSTEMS, COLLECTIVE BEHAVIOR OF COUPLED OSCILLATORS, and PHASE-PLANE ANALYSIS OF NEURAL NETS). If they have nearly equal frequencies, then the network can be transformed into the phase canonical model

$$\varphi_i' = \omega_i + \sum_{j=1}^{n} H_{ij}(\varphi_j - \varphi_i) \qquad (6)$$

where each $\varphi_i \in \mathbb{S}^1$ is a one-dimensional (angle) variable that describes the phase of the ith oscillator along the limit cycle attractor corresponding to its periodic spiking (see Figure 5), and each H_{ij} is a function that depends on f and g_{ij} that can be explicitly computed using Malkin's theorem (Theorem 9.2 in Hoppensteadt and Izhikevich, 1997).

The phase canonical model (Equation 6) describes frequency locking, phase locking, and synchronization properties of the original system in Equation 1. Therefore, to understand these and other nonlinear phenomena that might take place in oscillating neural

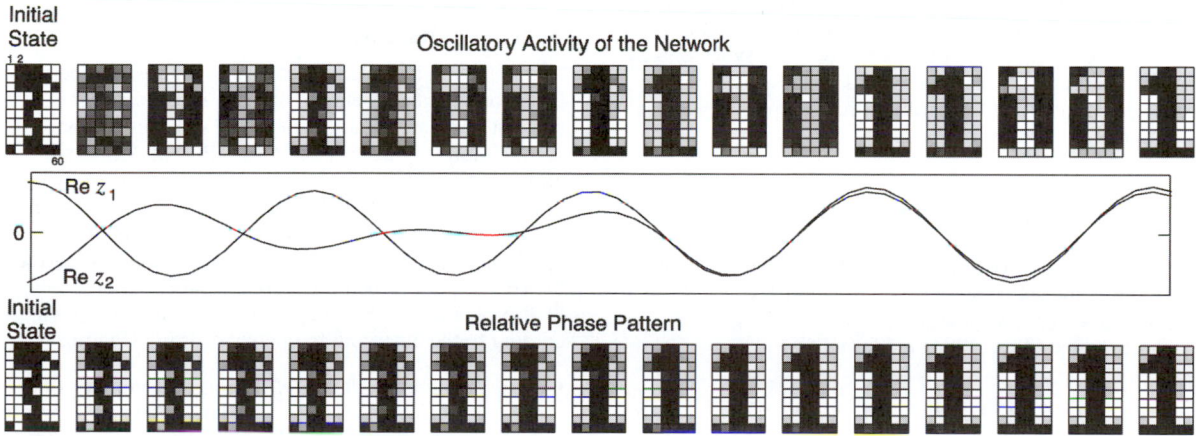

Figure 4. Pattern recognition via phase locking by the oscillatory canonical model (Equation 3). Complex Hebbian learning rule (5) was used to memorize patterns "1," "2," and "3." When the distorted pattern "1" is presented as an initial state, the neurons synchronize with the phase relations corresponding to the memorized pattern "1."

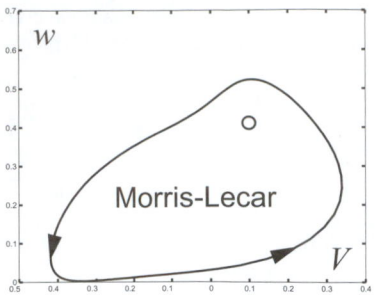

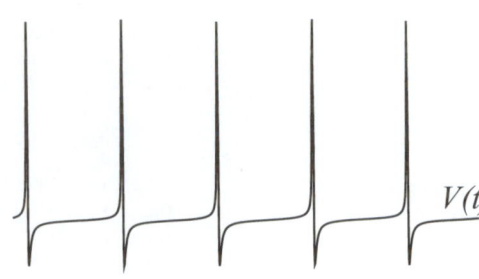

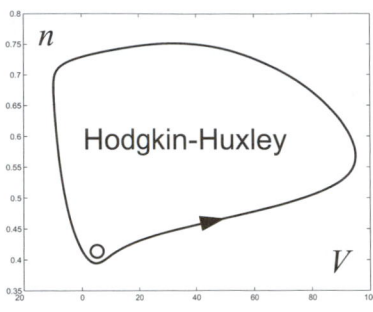

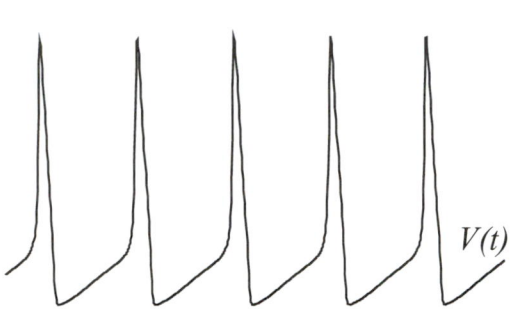

Figure 5. Examples of large-amplitude limit cycle attractors corresponding to periodic spiking in two biophysically detailed neural models, Morris and Lecar (1981) and Hodgkin and Huxley (1952).

networks, it usually suffices to consider the phase model. In particular, one can glimpse the universal computational abilities that are shared by all oscillatory systems, regardless of the nature of each oscillator or the particulars of the equations that describe it. Indeed, one can prove the following analogue of Theorem 2.

Theorem 3 (Synchronization Theorem for Oscillatory Neural Networks)

If all oscillators in Equation 6 have equal frequencies, i.e., $\omega_1 = \ldots = \omega_n$, and the connection functions H_{ij} have pairwise odd form, i.e.,

$$H_{ij}(-\psi) = -H_{ji}(\psi) \qquad (7)$$

for all i and j, then the canonical phase model in Equation 6 converges to a phase-locked pattern $\varphi_i(t) \to \omega_1 t + \phi_i$ for all i, so the neurons oscillate with equal frequencies (ω_1) and constant phase relations ($\varphi_i(t) - \varphi_j(t) = \phi_i - \phi_j$). In this sense the network dynamic is synchronized. There could be many stable synchronized patterns corresponding to many memorized images.

The proof is based on the observation that the phase canonical model in Equation 6 has the energy function

$$E(\varphi) = \frac{1}{2} \sum_{i,j=1}^{n} R_{ij}(\varphi_j - \varphi_i)$$

where R_{ij} is the antiderivative of H_{ij}; that is, $R'_{ij} = H_{ij}$ (see Theorem 9.15 in Hoppensteadt and Izhikevich, 1997, and ENERGY FUNCTIONALS FOR NEURAL NETWORKS).

For example, Kuramoto's (1984) model

$$\varphi'_i = \omega_i + \sum_{j=1}^{n} s_{ij} \sin (\varphi_j + \psi_{ij} - \varphi_i) \qquad (8)$$

has such an oscillatory associative memory when $\omega_1 = \ldots = \omega_n$:

$$s_{ij} = s_{ji} \quad \text{and} \quad \psi_{ij} = -\psi_{ji}$$

for all i and j. If we denote $c_{ij} = s_{ij} e^{i\psi_{ij}}$, then these conditions have the form shown by Equation 4. The energy function for Kuramoto's model is

$$E(\varphi) = -\frac{1}{2} \sum_{i,j=1}^{n} s_{ij} \cos (\varphi_j + \psi_{ij} - \varphi_i)$$

There are various estimates of the storage capacity of the network, as discussed by Vicente, Arenas, and Bonilla (1996). In particular, those authors found a time scale during which oscillatory networks can have better performance than Cohen-Grossberg-Hopfield-type attractor neural networks.

Since neither the form of the functions f and g_{ij} nor the dimension of each oscillator in Equation 1 were specified, one could take the above result to the extreme and claim that *anything that can oscillate can also be used for computing*, as for associative pattern recognition, etc. The only problem is how to couple the oscillators so that Equation 7 is satisfied.

Neural Excitability

An interesting intermediate case between rest and periodic spiking behavior is when a neural system is *excitable*; that is, it is at rest, but can generate a large-amplitude spike in response to a small perturbation (Figure 6) (see PHASE-PLANE ANALYSIS OF NEURAL NETS and OSCILLATORY AND BURSTING PROPERTIES OF NEURONS). A simple but useful criterion for classifying neural excitability was suggested by Hodgkin (1948), who stimulated cells by applying currents of various strengths. When the current is weak the cell is quiet. When the current is strong enough, the cell starts to fire repeatedly. He suggested the following classification according to the emerging frequency of firing (Figure 7):

- *Class 1 neural excitability*: Action potentials can be generated with arbitrarily low frequency. The frequency increases as the applied current is increased.
- *Class 2 neural excitability*: Action potentials are generated in a certain frequency band that is relatively insensitive to changes in the strength of the applied current.

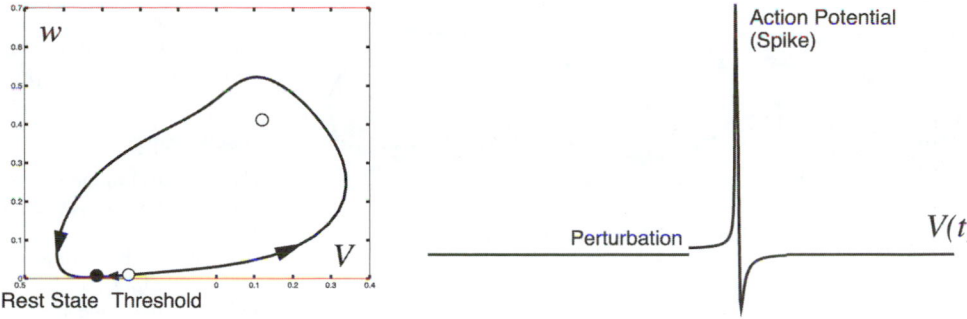

Figure 6. Neural excitability in Morris and Lecar (1981) neuron having fast Ca^{2+} and slow K^+ voltage-gated currents. The rest state (solid circle) is stable, but small perturbations can push the voltage beyond the threshold (open circle), thereby causing a large-amplitude excursion, or action potential. The voltage variable changes slowly near the rest states but fast during the generation of action potentials.

Their class of excitability influences neurocomputational properties of cells (see review in Izhikevich, 2000). For example, class 1 neural systems have a well-defined threshold manifold for their state variables, beyond which they generate a large-amplitude spike. They generate an all-or-none response, and they act as *integrators*, meaning that the higher the frequency of the incoming pulses, the sooner they fire. In contrast, class 2 neural systems may not have a threshold manifold. They could generate spikes of arbitrary intermediate amplitude, and they could act as *resonators*. That is, they respond to certain resonant frequencies of the incoming pulses. Increasing the incoming frequency may delay or even terminate their response.

A canonical model for class 1 excitable systems is described in the next section. The canonical model for class 2 systems has yet to be found.

Class 1 Excitable Systems

Class 1 excitable systems are understood relatively well (Rinzel and Ermentrout, 1989; Ermentrout, 1996; Hoppensteadt and Izhi-

kevich, 1997; Izhikevich, 2000). The transition from rest to periodic spiking in such systems occurs via a saddle node on invariant circle bifurcation, as shown in Figure 8 (see also DYNAMICS AND BIFURCATION IN NEURAL NETS and OSCILLATORY AND BURSTING PROPERTIES OF NEURONS). A weakly connected network of such neurons can be transformed into a canonical model, which can be approximated by

$$\vartheta_i' = 1 - \cos \vartheta_i + (1 + \cos \vartheta_i)\left(r_i + \sum_{j=1}^{n} s_{ij}\delta(\vartheta_j - \pi)\right) \quad (9)$$

where $\vartheta_i \in \mathbb{S}^1$ is the phase of the ith neuron along the limit cycle corresponding to the spiking solution. Again, particulars of the functions f and g_{ij} in Equation 1 do not affect the form of the canonical model in Equation 9, but only affect the values of the parameters r_i and s_{ij}, which can be computed explicitly (Hoppensteadt and Izhikevich, 1997, chap. 8). Notice that the canonical model in Equation 9 is pulse coupled, whereas the original weakly coupled network in Equation 1 is not. The qualitative reason for pulse coupling is that the voltage changes are extremely slow most

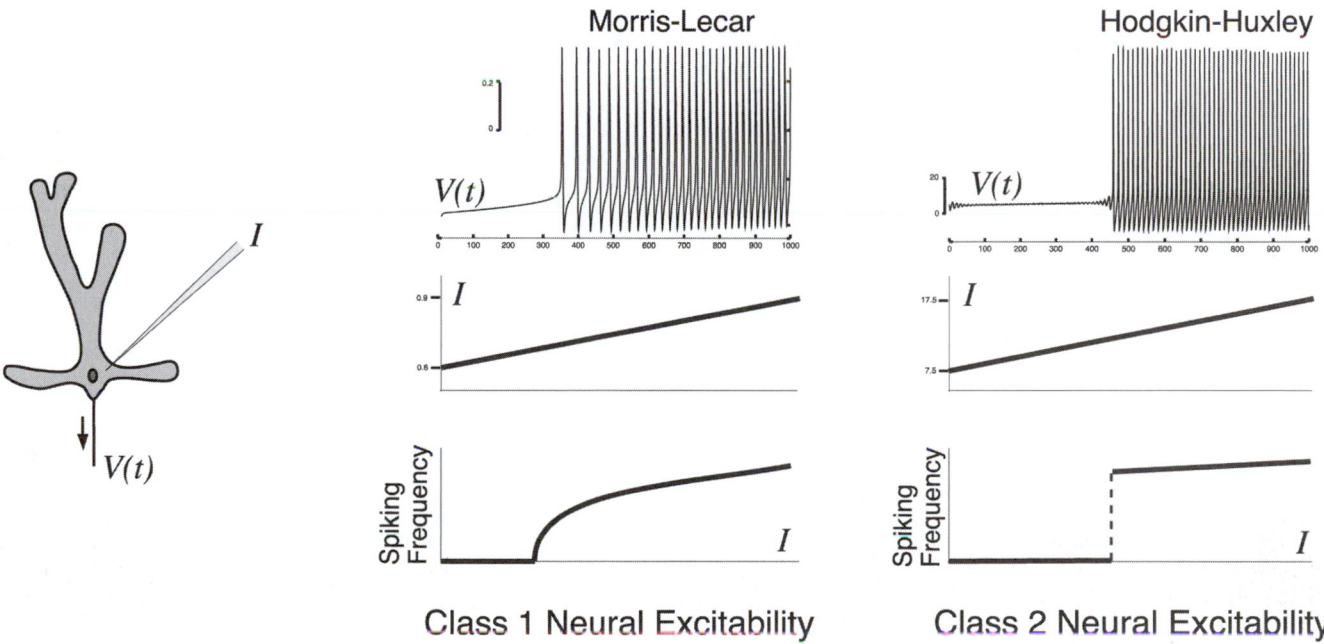

Figure 7. Transition from rest to repetitive spiking in two biophysical models when the strength of applied current, I, increases. The neural excitability is classified according to the frequency of emerging spiking.

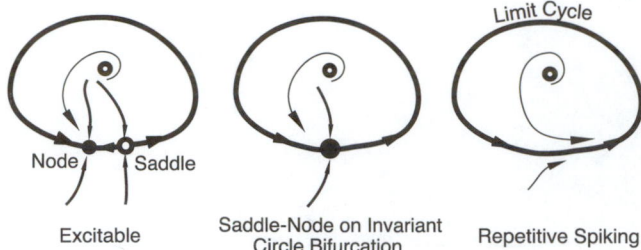

Figure 8. Class 1 neural excitability via saddle node on invariant circle bifurcation: The threshold state (saddle) approaches the rest state (node), they coalesce and annihilate each other leaving only limit cycle attractor. The oscillation on the attractor has two time scales: slow transition through the "ghost" of the saddle-node bifurcation and fast rotation along the rest of the limit cycle.

of the time because of the proximity to the rest state, but they are relatively instantaneous during the generation of an action potential. Hence the duration of coupling looks infinitesimal on the slow time scale.

The neuron is quiescent when $r_i < 0$ (Figure 8, left) and fires periodically when $r_i > 0$ (Figure 8, right). It fires a spike exactly when ϑ_i crosses the value π, which results in a step-like increase in the phases of other neurons. Hence, the canonical model in Equation 9 is a *pulse coupled neural network* (Izhikevich, 1999). It has many important physiological features, including absolute and relative refractory periods (Figure 9). Indeed, the effect of every incoming pulse depends on the internal state of the neuron, since it is multiplied by the function $(1 + \cos\vartheta_i)$. The effect is maximal when the neuron is near rest, since $(1 + \cos\vartheta_i) \approx 2$ when $\vartheta_i \approx 0$. It is minimal when the neuron is generating a spike, since $(1 + \cos\vartheta_i) \approx 0$ when $\vartheta_i \approx \pi$.

A canonical model for *slowly* connected class 1 excitable neurons with spike frequency adaptation has the form (Izhikevich, 2000):

$$\vartheta_i' = 1 - \cos\vartheta_i + (1 + \cos\vartheta_i)\left(r_i + \sum_{j=1}^{n} s_{ij}w_j\right)$$

$$w_i' = \delta(\vartheta_i - \pi) - \eta w_i$$

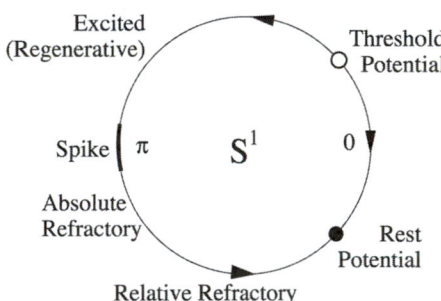

Figure 9. Diagram of the canonical model in Equation 9 for class 1 neural excitability. (From Hoppensteadt and Izhikevich, 1997.)

where w_i describes slow synaptic processes. The term $s_{ii}w_i$ denotes not a self-synapse but a slow spike frequency adaptation ($s_{ii} < 0$) or facilitation ($s_{ii} > 0$) process.

Discussion

The canonical model approach to computational neuroscience provides a rigorous way to derive simple yet accurate models that describe single-cell or network dynamics (see SINGLE-CELL MODELS). Such a derivation is possible even when no assumptions are made regarding the detailed form of equations describing neural activity. Indeed, we specify neither f nor g_{ij} in Equation 1. The only assumptions we make are those concerning the dynamics of each neuron—whether it is quiescent, excitable, periodic spiking, and so on. Nevertheless, any such neural system can be transformed into a canonical model by a piecewise continuous change of variables.

The derivation of canonical models can be a daunting mathematical task. However, once found, the canonical models provide invaluable information about universal neurocomputational properties shared by a large family of neural systems. For example, studying the canonical model in Equation 9 sheds light on the behavior of *all* class 1 excitable systems and their networks, regardless of the details of equations describing their dynamics.

Road Map: Dynamic Systems
Background: Dynamics and Bifurcation in Neural Nets; Phase-Plane Analysis of Neural Nets
Related Reading: Axonal Modeling; Chains of Oscillators in Motor and Sensory Systems; Collective Behavior of Coupled Oscillators; Computing with Attractors; Cooperative Phenomena; Energy Functionals for Neural Networks; Pattern Formation, Neural

References

Aronson, D. G., Ermentrout, G. B., and Kopell, N., 1990, Amplitude response of coupled oscillators, *Physica D*, 41:403–449.

Ermentrout, G. B., 1996, Type I membranes, phase resetting curves, and synchrony, *Neural Computat.*, 8:979–1001. ◆

Hodgkin, A. L., 1948, The local electric changes associated with repetitive action in a non-medulated axon, *J. Physiol.*, 107:165–181.

Hodgkin, A. L., and Huxley, A. F., 1952, A quantitative description of membrane current and application to conduction and excitation in nerve, *J. Physiol.*, 117:500–544.

Hoppensteadt, F. C., and Izhikevich, E. M., 1996, Synaptic organizations and dynamical properties of weakly connected neural oscillators: II. Learning of phase information, *Biol. Cybern.*, 75:129–135. ◆

Hoppensteadt, F. C., and Izhikevich, E. M., 1997, *Weakly Connected Neural Networks*, New York: Springer-Verlag.

Izhikevich, E. M., 1999, Class 1 neural excitability, conventional synapses, weakly connected networks, and mathematical foundations of pulse-coupled models, *IEEE Trans. Neural Netw.*, 10:499–507

Izhikevich, E. M., 2000, Neural excitability, spiking, and bursting, *Int. J. Bifurcat. Chaos*, 10:1171–1266. ◆

Kuramoto, Y., 1984, *Chemical Oscillations, Waves, and Turbulence*, New York: Springer-Verlag.

Morris, C., and Lecar, H., 1981, Voltage oscillations in the barnacle giant muscle fiber, *Biophys. J.*, 35:193–213.

Rinzel, J., and Ermentrout, G. B., 1989, Analysis of neural excitability and oscillations, in *Methods in Neuronal Modeling* (C. Koch and I. Segev, Eds.), Cambridge, MA: MIT Press. ◆

Vicente, C. J., Arenas, A., and Bonilla, L. L., 1996, On the short-term dynamics of networks of Hebbian coupled oscillators, *J. Phys. A*, L9–L16.

Cerebellum and Conditioning

Jeffrey S. Grethe and Richard F. Thompson

Introduction

For many years, psychologists and neurobiologists have been searching for the substrates underlying learning and memory. Aristotle hypothesized that learning involved the association of ideas with one another. Pavlov (1927, cited in Gormezano, Kehoe, and Marshall, 1983) combined the concepts of learning and association with the production of reflexes (see CONDITIONING). Classical conditioning (CC) has been extremely useful in examining the substrates underlying learning and memory. The standard CC paradigm (Figure 1) consists of pairing a neutral stimulus, the conditioned stimulus (CS), with an aversive stimulus, the unconditioned stimulus (US). At the beginning of training, the only response to the stimuli is the unconditioned response (UR) to the US. Over repeated pairings of the stimuli, an association is formed between the CS and US, resulting in the performance of a conditioned response (a response that resembles the UR).

By varying stimulus parameters, a large number of behavioral-conditioning phenomena can be observed (Gormezano et al., 1983). Eye-blink conditioning can occur with a CS-US interstimulus interval (ISI) ranging from 100 ms to well over 1 s. The rate of learning and asymptotic response level are optimal at an ISI of about 250 ms. After 100–200 training trials at the optimal ISI, rabbits give CRs on more than 90% of trials. The CR onset initially develops near the US onset, gradually begins earlier in the trial over the course of training, and generally peaks near the US onset (Figure 1). More complex conditioning phenomena can also be observed (see CONDITIONING).

Cerebellar Substrates of Classical Eye-Blink Conditioning

Current evidence from extensive anatomical, lesion, and physiological studies argues very strongly that the essential memory trace for the classically conditioned nictitating membrane response is formed and stored in the cerebellum (Thompson et al., 1997). This research has identified much of the network subserving classical conditioning (Figure 2). Information regarding the US is transmit-

ted by the dorsal accessory olive to the cerebellum through the climbing fibers. Stimulation of the dorsal accessory olive, in place of a corneal airpuff, has been shown to be an effective US. If the dorsal accessory olive is lesioned before paired presentations of the CS and US, learning of the conditioned response is prevented. In addition, the interpositus provides inhibitory feedback to the inferior olive, and over the course of learning, the inhibitory feedback increases, thereby decreasing the output of the inferior olive. This evidence points to the olivary climbing fiber system as being the essential reinforcing pathway that transmits an error signal to the cerebellum. Information regarding the CS is transmitted to the cerebellum from the pontine nuclei by the mossy fibers. Stimulation of the pontine nuclei or mossy fibers has been shown to be an effective CS. The CR pathway consists of the anterior interpositus nucleus, magnocellular red nucleus, and finally the accessory abducens nucleus and the facial (seventh) nucleus. This circuit points to the cerebellum as the site of convergence where associative learning may take place. Experimental evidence supports this view, since lesions of the cerebellum, including the critical regions of the interpositus nucleus, completely abolish the conditioned response without affecting the UR.

One of the first theories to detail how associative memories could be formed in the cerebellum was proposed by Albus (1971). The most striking aspect of this model was that the parallel fiber synapses on Purkinje cells were modifiable. This theory of parallel fiber–Purkinje cell plasticity now has considerable experimental support. In addition, Albus predicted the occurrence of long-term depression at this synapse (see CEREBELLUM: NEURAL PLASTICITY). Furthermore, Albus predicted that climbing fiber spikes are the US and that mossy fiber activity patterns are the CS, predictions that are now supported by the conditioning literature. However, this theory does not account for the temporal dynamics of the CR. One of the more interesting features of classical conditioning is that of the well-timed response. Over the course of training, the timing of the response to the CS becomes more precise (i.e., the CR predicts the onset of the US). Most models of the cerebellum and its involvement in the classically conditioned eye-blink response focus on the production of this well-timed CR.

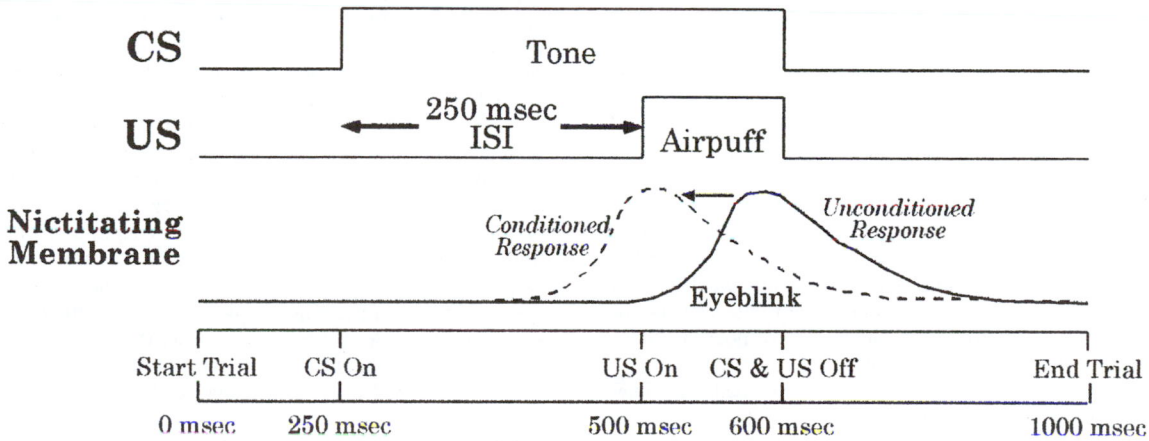

Figure 1. Standard delay conditioning paradigm. The CS is a 350-ms tone and the US is a 100-ms airpuff directed at the cornea. Early in training, the animal responds to the airpuff (UR). Over time, the animal learns to associate the tone with the airpuff, and produces a defensive blink that coincides with the airpuff (CR).

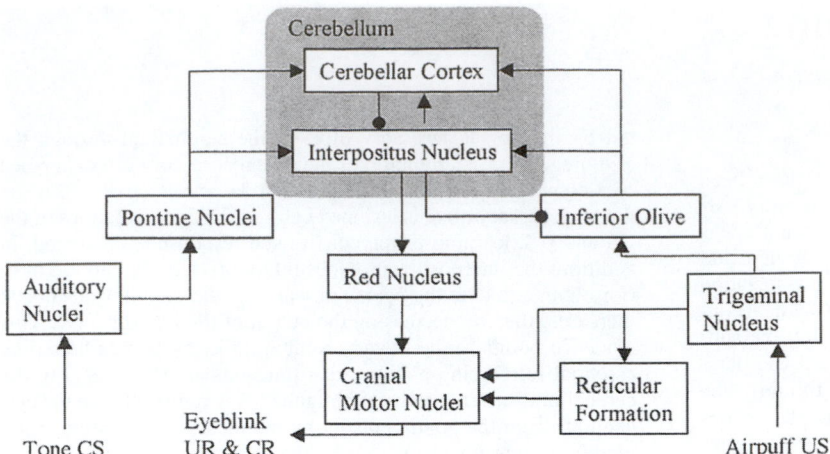

Figure 2. Essential circuitry for the classically conditioned nictitating membrane response.

Modeling the Role of the Cerebellum in Classical Conditioning

One of the first theories as to how the cerebellum could control movement timing was proposed by Braitenberg (1961). He suggested that parallel fibers could act as tapped delay lines, with the conduction time of the parallel fibers yielding movement timing. However, this theory cannot account for movements with time scales on the order of hundreds of milliseconds; it can only account for delays on the order of a few milliseconds. Many current models, however, still rely on this notion.

Moore, Desmond, and Berthier (1989) constructed a model of the cerebellum based on an earlier adaptive network model. In order to temporally associate the CS and US, the CS inputs are not discrete events but rather stimulus traces that persist for some time after the CS is gone (see CONDITIONING). Learning is then allowed to occur when the CS trace and the US coincide. In the cerebellar implementation the adaptive unit is the Purkinje cell, whereas the Golgi cell learns to gate an image of the CR from the brainstem to the Purkinje cell. Purkinje and Golgi cell plasticity, combined with the model's tapped delay lines, yields anticipatory CRs for delay and trace conditioning at all ISIs. The learning rules follow the form of Rescorla and Wagner's (1972) model and thus account for the same stimulus context effect. One problem with this model is that the tapped delay lines must be on the order of hundreds of milliseconds, and no physiologically plausible mechanism has been suggested for this. Another problem is the existence of the CR image: the model does not include learning of this hypothesized image. Moore et al. have hypothesized that this image is located around the trigeminal nucleus. Learning-induced models of the CR are present in the region bordering the trigeminal; however, evidence has shown that this model is relayed to the trigeminal from the interpositus via the red nucleus. It is interesting to note that a cerebellar implementation of the Sutton and Barto tapped delay model (Moore and Choi, 1997) also requires feedback from extracerebellar structures. In order to properly determine the difference between the predicted reinforcement and actual reinforcement, the model uses an efference copy of the conditioned response from the red nucleus and spinal trigeminal nucleus.

Jaffe (1990) proposed a model that moved the tapped delay lines from the network and placed them at the level of the neuron. The model proposed that single interpositus neurons can generate the full range of delays for CRs by adjusting their input weights and exploiting the phenomenon of delayed inhibitory rebound. The most significant problem with this model is that the interpositus cell must be quiescent at CS onset and cannot fire through the delay period. However, most neurons in the interpositus are spontaneously active, and it seems unlikely that a few neurons silent during the delay could account for the production of the CR.

Fiala, Grossberg, and Bullock (1996) also developed a neuron-centered tapped delay line model of the metabotropic glutamate receptor (mGluR) second-messenger system (see CEREBELLUM: NEURAL PLASTICITY), which is responsible for the well-timed CR. Temporal correlation between the CS (parallel fiber–induced mGluR response) and US causes a phosphorylation of AMPA receptors and calcium-dependent potassium channels. Phosphorylation of the calcium-dependent potassium channels results in a reduction in Purkinje cell firing during the CS-US interval. This model is very interesting in that it explores possible biochemical mechanisms for production of the well-timed response. However, for this model to produce responses across the full range of timing, the variety in the density of mGluR receptors on dendritic spines must be highly variable, which may not be physiologically plausible.

In addition to tapped delay line models, researchers began investigating how dynamical network processes within the cerebellum could yield precise timing. Buonomano and Mauk (1994) developed a semirealistic population model of the cerebellar cortex. The CS activates a subset of mossy fibers, which in turn excites a population of granule cells. Both the mossy fibers and the granule cells excite a population of Golgi cells. The resulting Golgi inhibition of the granule cells produces a varying pattern of granule cell activity over time in which different subsets of granule cells are active at different times. Learning of the CR would occur through weakening of the parallel fiber synapses that were active around the occurrence of the US. An extension of this model (Mauk and Donegan, 1997) includes two sites of plasticity within the cerebellum, the cerebellar cortex and interpositus nucleus. More important, the model showed that long-term depression of the parallel fiber–Purkinje cell synapses, coupled with recurrent projections between the interpositus and inferior olive, produces a stable learning system. The most pressing problem with these models is extreme sensitivity to noise. If there is a substantial amount of noise in the network or if the input pattern varies during the CS, the Purkinje cell timing would be disrupted due to the changes in the granule cell activity pattern.

Bartha (1992) developed a network simulation of the cerebellum and associated circuitry that stressed the input and output representation of the cerebellum. The input representation was constrained by known properties of the mossy fibers and the output representation was modeled through detailed information on the CR pathway and oculomotor plant. The cerebellar model consists of two populations of granule cells, one responsive to the tone CS and one unresponsive. The Golgi cell's inhibitory influence on the tone-unresponsive granule cells is to produce a variety of firing patterns so that the granule cells display differing periods of depression. The Purkinje cell then selects the granule cells (through long-term depression) that display the proper time interval of depression to produce a properly timed eye-blink. With realistic single-neuron parameters, the model is able to reproduce many aspects of CR timing and form. One concern with the model lies with the Golgi cells. For the Golgi cell to be able to produce the proper spectrum of delays for short ISIs, the time constant of the Golgi cells' influence on the granule cells must fall within the 100 ms to 250 ms range, which can be considered physiological. However, to produce properly timed blinks of longer latencies, the time constant of this inhibitory effect must be considerably longer, which does not seem physiologically plausible.

Grethe (2000) developed a model that focuses on the cerebellar microcomplex as a Hebbian cell assembly (a highly interconnected group of neurons that forms a reverberatory circuit that can sustain activity). Each microcomplex contains a set of Purkinje cells and their related nuclear neurons. The cerebellar cortex receives mossy fiber input from both pontine nuclei and recurrent projections from the interpositus nucleus. This basic architecture allows the recurrent excitation in the excitatory interpositus cells to be modulated by the Purkinje cells in the cerebellar cortex. The architecture of the model tries to preserve the topographic projections between the cerebellar cortex and the deep nuclei as well as the beam-like organization of Purkinje cells receiving input from the parallel fibers. Local reverberations in the cerebellum, between the cerebellar cortex and deep nuclei, are responsible for the response topography and timing. Long-term depression at the parallel fiber–Purkinje cell synapse is responsible for the precise timing of the response. The reverberations are controlled by the anatomical connectivity, the bistability of Purkinje neurons, and the process of synaptic fatigue. One interesting aspect of the model is the effect of stimulation intensity on the response timing of the assembly. Since the timing of the model is inherently dependent on the recurrent projections, this timing process can be sped up by increasing the stimulation intensity of the CS, which has been found experimentally.

Gluck and associates (2001) developed a connectionist-level model of classical eye-blink conditioning incorporating basic features of the essential cerebellar circuitry, based on the Rescorla-Wagner model, a most successful trial-level behavioral formulation of classical conditioning. The Rescorla-Wagner model assumes that the change in association between a neutral CS and a response-evoking US is a function of the difference between the US and an animal's *expectation* of the US, given all CSs present in the trial. Because the discrepancy, or "error," between the animal's expectations and what actually occurs drives learning in this theory, the theory is referred to as an "error-correcting" learning procedure.

Thirty years after its publication, the Rescorla-Wagner model stills stands as the most influential and powerful model in psychology for describing and predicting animal learning behavior in conditioning studies. Moreover, its influence has extended far beyond animal conditioning. The model's basic error correction principle has been rediscovered within cognitive psychology and cognitive neuroscience in the form of connectionist network models, many of which rely on the same principle. In addition, the most commonly used connectionist learning procedure, back propagation (see PERCEPTRONS, ADALINES, AND BACKPROPAGATION), along with its simpler predecessor, the delta rule (see CONDITIONING), both are generalizations of the Rescorla-Wagner model.

Although the Gluck et al. model does not attempt to model neuronal processes, it includes two key features of cerebellar circuitry:

positive feedback via the pontine nuclei and negative feedback via inhibition of the inferior olive. This rather simple connectionist model successfully predicts a wide range of behavioral phenomena of classical conditioning, including, in particular, adaptive timing of the CR and blocking. In the model, adaptive timing depends on positive feedback; if this feedback is blocked, adaptive timing no longer occurs. The model circuitry predicts that inhibition of the inferior olive-climbing fiber input system is necessary for the behavioral phenomenon of blocking. This prediction was empirically verified by Kim, Krupa, and Thompson (1998), who showed that blocking interpositus-evoked GABA inhibition of the inferior olive during compound-stimulus training completely prevented behavioral blocking.

Discussion

Currently, no model accounts for all the data on cerebellar neurobiology and conditioning. However, models of conditioning that take into account the neurobiology of the cerebellum can pose questions that researchers may be able to examine. For example, in order to experimentally test some of the network models presented, single-unit recordings from the granule would be necessary. These recordings are difficult because granule cells are small and closely spaced. Moreover, it would be difficult to obtain these recordings while the task is being performed. The predictions from several of the models regarding granule cells are all different:

- Buonomano and Mauk predict that a subset of granule cells will exhibit nonperiodic activity.
- Bartha predicts that the subset of granule cells will primarily show depressions in activity at all conditionable intervals after the presentation of a CS.
- Grethe predicts that activation of the granule cells in the cell assembly should occur in a wave-like fashion as the cell assembly's reverberating activity increases.

The future will bring new experiments that test these and future models, which in turn will lead to further experiments and models.

Road Map: Mammalian Brain Regions
Related Reading: Cerebellum and Motor Control; Cerebellum: Neural Plasticity; Conditioning

References

Albus, J. S., 1971, A theory of cerebellar function, *Math. Biosci.*, 10:25–61.

Bartha, G. T., 1992, A computer model of oculomotor and neural contributions to conditioned blink timing, Ph.D. diss., University of Southern California.

Braitenberg, V., 1961, Functional interpretation of cerebellar histology, *Nature*, 190:539–540.

Buonomano, D. V., and Mauk, M. D., 1994, Neural network model of the cerebellum: Temporal discrimination and the timing of motor responses, *Neural Computat.*, 6:38–55.

Fiala, J. C., Grossberg, S., and Bullock, D., 1996, Metabotropic glutamate receptor activation in cerebellar Purkinje cells as substrate for adaptive timing of the classically conditioned eye-blink response, *J. Neurosci.*, 16:3760–3774.

Gluck, M. A., Allen, M. T., Myers, C. E., and Thompson, R. F., 2001, Cerebellar substrates for error-correction in motor conditioning, *Neurobiol. Learn. Mem.*, 76:314–341.

Gormezano, I., Kehoe, E. J., and Marshall, B. S., 1983, Twenty years of classical conditioning research with the rabbit, *Prog. Psychobiol. Physiol. Psychol.*, 10:197–275. ◆

Grethe, J. S., 2000, Neuroinformatics and the cerebellum: Towards an understanding of the cerebellar microzone and its contribution to the well-timed classically conditioned eyeblink response, Ph.D. diss., University of Southern California.

Jaffe, S., 1990, A neuronal model for variable latency response, in *Analysis and Modeling of Neural Systems* (F. H. Eeckman, Ed.), Boston: Kluwer, pp. 405–410.

Kim, J., Krupa, D., and Thompson, R. F., 1998, Inhibitory cerebello-olivary projections and blocking effect in classical conditioning, *Science*, 27:570–573.

Mauk, M. D., and Donegan, N. H., 1997, A model of pavlovian eyelid conditioning based on the synaptic organization of the cerebellum, *Learn. Mem.*, 4:130–158.

Moore, J. W., and Choi, J-S., 1997, The TD model of classical conditioning: Response topography and brain implementation, in *Neural-Network Models of Cognition* (J. Donahoe and V. Dorsel, Eds.), North-Holland: Elsevier, pp. 387–405.

Moore, J. W., Desmond, J. E., and Berthier, N. E., 1989, Adaptively timed conditioned responses and the cerebellum: A neural network approach, *Biol. Cybern.*, 62:17–28.

Rescorla, R. A., and Wagner, A. R. A., 1972, A theory of pavlovian conditioning: Variations in the effectiveness of reinforcement and nonreinforcement, in *Classical Conditioning: II. Current Research and Theory* (A. H. Black and W. F. Prokasy, Eds.), New York: Appleton-Century-Crofts.

Thompson, R. F., Bao, S., Berg, M. S., Chen, L., Cipriano, B. D., Grethe, J. S., Kim, J. J., Thompson, J. K., Tracy, J., and Krupa, D. J., 1997, Associative learning, in *The Cerebellum and Cognition* (J. Schmahmann, Ed.), *Int. Rev. Neurobiol.*, 41:151–189 (special issue). ◆

Cerebellum and Motor Control

Mitsuo Kawato

Introduction

Fast, smooth, and coordinated movements cannot be achieved by basic feedback control alone because delays associated with feedback loops are long (about 200 ms for visual feedback and 100 ms for somatosensory feedback) and feedback gains are low. Additionally, feedback controllers such as the commonly used PID (proportional, integral, and derivative) controllers do not incorporate predictive dynamic or kinematic knowledge of controlled objects or environments. Two major feedforward control schemes have been proposed: the equilibrium point control hypothesis and the inverse dynamics model hypothesis (see EQUILIBRIUM POINT HYPOTHESIS and MOTOR CONTROL, BIOLOGICAL AND THEORETICAL). Some versions of the former scheme advocate that the central nervous system (CNS) can avoid inverse dynamics computation by relying on the spring-like properties of muscles and reflex loops. For this mechanism to work efficiently, the mechanical and neural feedback gains, which can be measured as mechanical stiffness in perturbation experiments, must be quite high. The low stiffness of the arm, which was measured during visually guided point-to-point multijoint movements (Gomi and Kawato, 1996), suggests the necessity of inverse dynamics models in these well-practiced and relaxed movements. The internal models in the brain must be acquired through motor learning in order to accommodate the changes that occur with the growth of controlled objects such as hands, legs, and torso, as well as the unpredictable variability of the external world.

Where in the brain are internal models of the motor apparatus likely to be stored? First, the locus should exhibit a remarkable adaptive capability, which is essential for acquisition and continuous update of internal models of the motor apparatus. A number of physiological studies have suggested important functional roles of the cerebellum in motor learning and remarkable synaptic plasticity in the cerebellar cortex (Ito, 1984, 2001). Second, the biological objects of motor control by the brain, such as the arms, speech articulators, and the torso, possess many degrees of freedom and complicated nonlinear dynamics. Correspondingly, neural internal models should receive a broad range of sensory inputs and possess a capacity high enough to approximate complex dynamics. Extensive sensory signals carried by mossy fiber inputs and an enormous number of granule cells in the cerebellar cortex seem to fulfill these prerequisites for internal models. (See Figure 1 for cerebellar circuitry and its connection to the cerebellar nucleus in the case of the lateral cerebellum.) Finally, the cerebellar symptoms usually classified as the "triad" of hypotonia, hypermetria, and intention tremor could be understood as degraded performance when control is forced to rely solely on primitive feedback control after internal models are destroyed or cannot be updated. This is because precise, fast, coordinated movements can be executed if accurate internal models of the motor apparatus can be utilized during trajectory planning, coordinate transformation, and motor control, while primitive feedback controllers with long feedback delays and small gains can attain only poor performance in these computations and usually lead to oscillatory instability for forced fast movements.

Miall et al. (1993) grouped into classes many theories regarding the role of the cerebellum (such as coordination, studied by Flourens; comparators, studied by Holmes; gain controllers; associative learning). The most complete class of theories, these authors suggested, comprises theories in which the cerebellum forms an internal model of the motor system; such theories can encompass all the alternative theories, while fitting many of the known facts of cerebellar organization. These theories require that the cerebellum be an adaptive system capable of learning and of updating a model as the behavior of the motor system changes. They also require that the cerebellum store relevant parameters of the motor system, as these parameters form part of the description of the motor system behavior. Another requirement is timing capabilities: the motor system is dynamic, so a useful model will also need dynamic (i.e., time-dependent) behavior. How might internal models be acquired in the cerebellum through motor learning?

Marr-Albus Model and Synaptic Plasticity

Purkinje cells are the only output neurons from the cerebellar cortex. They receive two major synaptic inputs, from parallel fibers and from climbing fibers (Figure 1). Waveforms of neuronal spikes generated by the two kinds of synaptic inputs are different and can be discriminated even on extracellular recordings: simple spikes are triggered by parallel fibers and complex spikes are triggered by climbing fibers. Modularity is the basic design principle in the cerebellum. In the spinocerebellum, somototopic fractured maps have been identified for parallel fiber inputs to the cerebellar cortex. Furthermore, microzones as long as several centimeters along the longitudinal axis of the cerebellar folia and as wide as 0.2 mm have been identified for climbing fiber inputs (Ito, 1984).

Marr (1969) and Albus (1971) proposed a detailed model of the cerebellum, according to which the cerebellum can form associative memories between particular patterns on parallel fiber inputs and Purkinje cell outputs. The basic idea is that the parallel fiber–Purkinje cell synapses can be modified by input from the climbing

Figure 1. Schematic diagram of a neural circuit for voluntary movement learning control by a cerebrocerebellar communication loop (see Ito, 1984, for details). Although the lateral part of the cerebellum hemisphere is shown and the input and output of other cerebellar regions are vastly different, the neural circuit of the cerebellar cortex is rather the same and uniform. It must be emphasized that only one climbing fiber makes contact with a single Purkinje cell, whereas parallel fibers make 200,000 synapses on a single Purkinje cell. The number of granule cells, the origin of parallel fibers, is about 10^{11}. CF, climbing fiber; BC, basket cell; GO, Golgi cell; GR, granule cell; MF, Mossy fiber; PC, Purkinje cell; PF, parallel fiber; ST, stellate cell; DE, dentate nucleus; IO, inferior olivary nucleus; PN, pontine nuclei; RNp, parvocellular red nucleus; VL, ventrolateral nucleus of the thalamus.

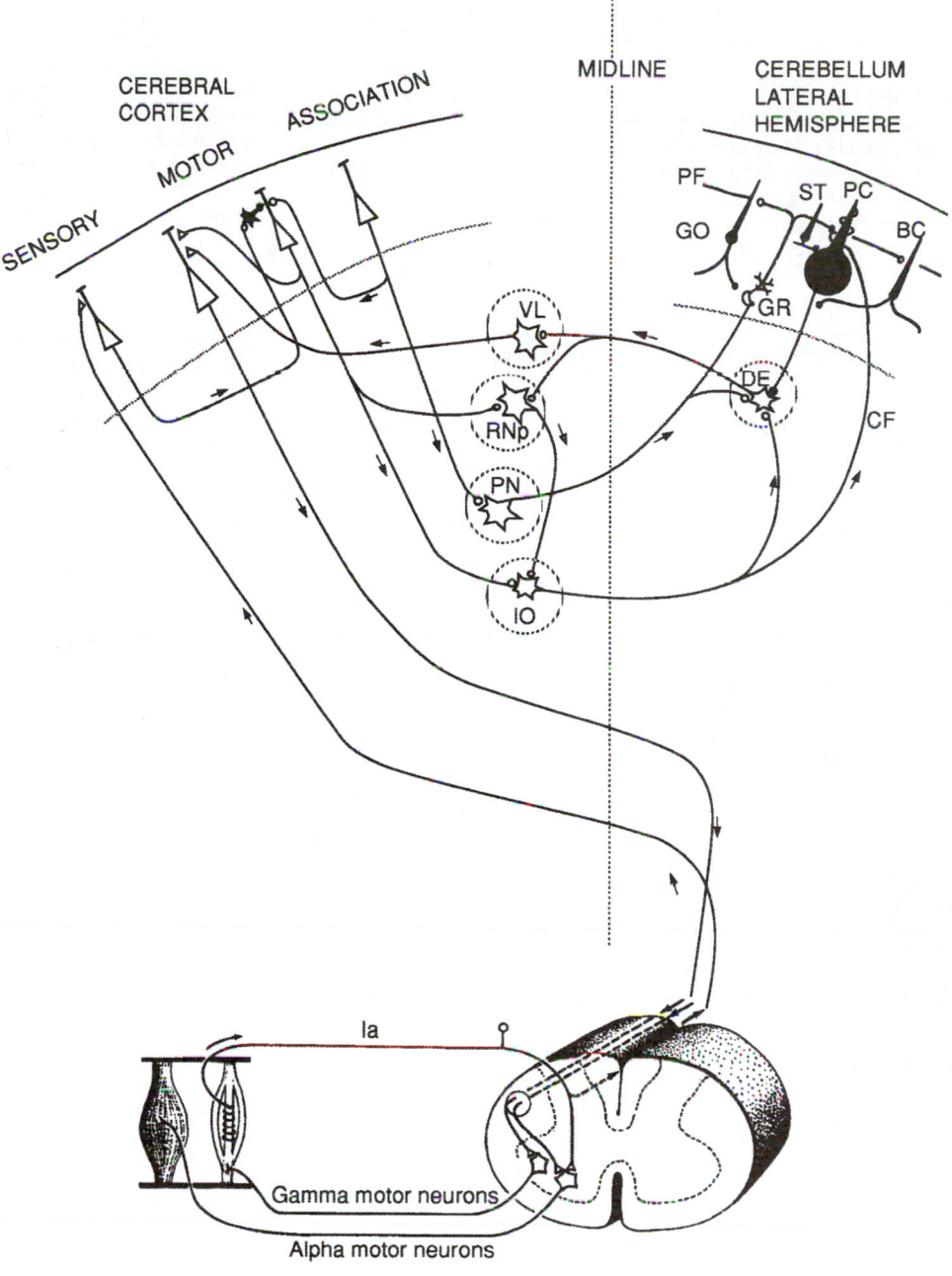

fibers. In the perceptron models, the efficacy of a parallel fiber–Purkinje cell synapse is assumed to change when there exists a parallel fiber and climbing fiber input conjunction. The presence of the putative heterosynaptic plasticity of Purkinje cells was demonstrated as a long-term depression (LTD) (Ito, 2001).

The original Marr-Albus model did not take into account the dynamic and temporal characteristics of sensorimotor integration and was inappropriate in proposing simple associative memories for motor control problems. More satisfactory dynamic modeling in cerebellar learning was started by Fujita (1982). An associative LTD found in Purkinje cells can be modeled as the following heterosynaptic plasticity rule (Fujita, 1982): the rate of change of the synaptic efficacy of a single parallel fiber synapse is proportional to the negative product of the firing rate of that synapse's input and the increment of the climbing fiber firing rate from its spontaneous level:

$$\tau dw_i/dt = -x_i(F - F_{\text{spont}}) \tag{1}$$

where τ is the time constant, w_i is the synaptic weight of the ith parallel fiber–Purkinje cell synapse, x_i is the firing frequency of the ith parallel fiber–Purkinje cell synapse, F is the firing frequency of the climbing fiber input, and F_{spont} is its spontaneous level. This single rule reproduces both the LTD and the long-term potentiation (LTP) found in Purkinje cells. When the climbing fiber and the parallel fiber are stimulated simultaneously, the parallel fiber synaptic efficacy decreases. In contrast, the parallel fiber synaptic efficacy increases when only the parallel fiber is stimulated (that is, when the climbing fiber firing frequency is lower than its spontaneous level). From a computational viewpoint, if the Purkinje cell output is the linear weighted summation of the parallel fiber inputs, Equation 1 can be regarded as the steepest descent of the error function defined as the square of the second factor. That is, this equation could provide a supervised learning rule if and only if the climbing fiber firing rate encodes an error signal.

Although early-day cerebellar models (Marr, 1969; Albus, 1971) were epoch-making in proposing Purkinje cell plasticity as a basis of cerebellar learning at the hardware level, they were not satisfactory at the representational and computational theory levels. What is actually learned and stored in the cerebellum? What neural representations are used in inputs and outputs of the Purkinje cells? Recent models and experimental efforts point to answers entirely different from those suggested by the early-day models.

Models of Limb Motor Control in the Cerebellum

Boylls (1975) proposed that the spatiotemporal neural firing patterns formed by the excitatory loop due to the cerebellar reverberating circuit and the inhibitory loop via the Purkinje cells are computationally beneficial for the generation of rhythmic interlimb coordination patterns in locomotion. In Boylls's theory, the purpose of cerebellar computation is to create synergically meaningful excitation profiles on a cerebellar nucleus, whose profiles are subsequently transmitted via an "output nucleus" to spinal levels. Boylls's model was later extended by Houk and Barto (1992) to accommodate motor learning in the cerebellum as an adjustable pattern generator (APG) model of the cerebellum. Temporal patterns of movement are acquired through motor learning, based on the LTD of Purkinje cells in combination with the reverberating circuit. Artificial neural network models with recurrent connections that can learn and generate arm trajectories were the computational bases of their model. The learning scheme proposed is mathematically based on associative reward-penalty learning (see REINFORCEMENT LEARNING IN MOTOR CONTROL). One of its attractive features is that a temporal movement pattern is selected and generated, which is impossible with a simple internal forward or inverse model. Correspondingly, however, learning is more difficult.

Cerebellar Feedback-Error-Learning Model

Internal models can be largely classified into forward models and inverse models (see SENSORIMOTOR LEARNING). Forward models predict the sensory consequences of movements from an efference copy of issued motor commands. Inverse models compute necessary feedforward motor commands from desired movement information. Both kinds of internal models are assumed to be located in the cerebellum (Kawato, 1999). However, the evidence for the forward models is much more circumstantial than is the evidence for the inverse models (see MOTOR CONTROL, BIOLOGICAL AND THEORETICAL). Learning forward models are generally much easier than inverse models because actual sensory feedback can be utilized as a teaching signal in the supervised learning equation (Equation 1), except for the difficulty associated with the delay in sensory feedback. Miall et al. (1993) proposed that the cerebellum forms two types of forward internal models. One model is a forward model of the motor apparatus. The second is a forward model of the transport time delays in the control loop (due to receptor and effector delays, axonal conductance, and cognitive processing delays). The second model delays the copy of prediction made by the first model so that it can be compared in temporal registration with actual sensory feedback from the movement. The second model resolves the difficulty of a temporal mismatch between the sensory signal delayed by the feedback loop and the output calculated by forward internal models.

Acquiring an inverse dynamics model through motor learning is computationally difficult because the necessary teaching signal for the desired motor command, which is the output of the inverse dynamics model, is not available. Several computational learning schemes to resolve this difficulty have been proposed (see SENSORIMOTOR LEARNING). Kawato and colleagues (Kawato, 1999) proposed a cerebellar feedback-error-learning model (CBFELM; Figure 2), which turned out to be the most biologically plausible of the various proposals as a model of the cerebellum. In this model, simple spikes (SS) represent feedforward motor commands and the parallel fiber inputs represent the desired trajectory as well as the sensory feedback of the current status of the controlled object. A microzone of the cerebellar cortex constitutes (part of) an inverse model of a specific controlled object such as an eye or an arm. Most important climbing fiber inputs are assumed to carry a copy of the feedback motor commands generated by a crude feedback control circuit. Thus, the complex spikes (CS) of Purkinje cells activated by climbing fiber inputs are predicted to be sensory error signals already expressed in motor command coordinates. The supervised learning equation (Equation 1) allows an interpretation that a crude feedback controller could generate approximation to the necessary error signal in motor commands. Stability and convergence of the CBFELM have been proved mathematically in the recent control theory literature.

Experimental Supports for the Cerebellar Feedback-Error-Learning Model

The CBFELM model was directly supported by neurophysiological studies in the ventral paraflocculus (VPFL) of monkey cerebellum

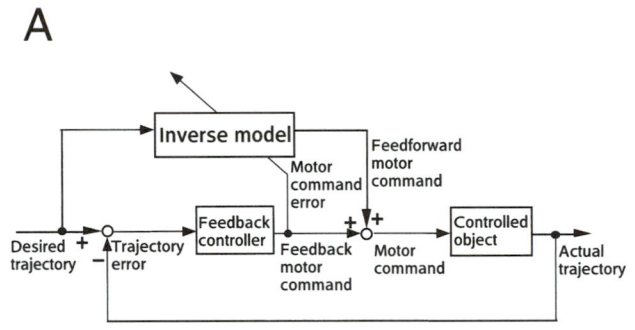

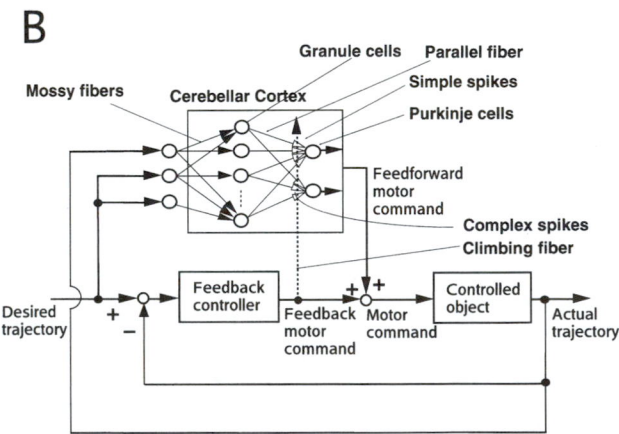

Figure 2. *A*, The general feedback-error-learning model. *B*, The cerebellar feedback-error-learning model (CBFELM) (Kawato, 1999). The "controlled object" is a physical entity that needs to be controlled by the CNS, such as the eyes, hands, legs, or torso.

during ocular following responses (OFRs) (Shidara et al., 1993; Kawato, 1999; Yamamoto et al., 2002). OFRs are tracking movements of the eyes evoked by movements in a visual scene and are thought to be important for the visual stabilization of gaze. The phylogenetically older, crude feedback circuit of the CBFELM is comprised of the retina, the accessory optic system (AOS), and the brainstem. The phylogenetically newer, more sophisticated feedforward pathway and the inverse dynamics model of the CBFELM correspond to the cerebral and cerebellar cortical pathway and the cerebellum, respectively.

During OFRs, the temporal waveforms of SS firing frequency of VPFL Purkinje cells show complicated patterns. However, they (Figure 3, thin curve) were quite accurately reconstructed by using an inverse dynamics representation of the eye movement (Figure 3, thick curve; Shidara et al., 1993). The model fit was good for the majority of the neurons studied under a wide range of visual stimulus conditions. The same inverse dynamics analysis of firing frequency was applied to neurons in the area MST and dorsolateral pontine nucleus (DLPN), which provide visual mossy fiber inputs to the VPFL. In this area neural firing patterns were not well reconstructed. Taken together, these data suggest that the VPFL is the major site of the inverse dynamics model of the eye for OFRs.

The CBFELM model assumes that motor commands, which are conveyed by SS, are directly modified and acquired through synaptic plasticity by motor command errors, which are conveyed by climbing fiber inputs. For this to work, the motor commands and climbing fiber inputs must have comparable temporal and spatial characteristics, but the ultra-low discharge rates of the latter (1–2 spikes/s) would appear to rule this out. This apparently discrete and intermittent nature of climbing fiber inputs once suggested a reinforcement learning type of theory of cerebellar learning. However, if thousands of trials were averaged to compute firing frequencies of the climbing fiber inputs, the firing rates actually conveyed very accurate and reliable temporal waveforms of motor command error (Figure 3Cb). Because the LTD is a rather slow process of several tens of minutes of time constants, the averaging over many trials can actually be conducted by the LTD dynamics itself. Consequently, the firing probability of climbing fiber inputs aligned with the stimulus motion onset had high-frequency temporal dynamics matching those of the dynamic command signals. Thus, the most critical assumption of the CBFELM model was satisfied.

The preferred directions of MST and DLPN neurons were evenly distributed over 360 degrees. Thus, the visual coordinates for OFRs are uniformly distributed over all possible directions. On the other hand, the spatial coordinates of the extraocular muscles lie in either the horizontal or vertical directions, and are entirely different from the visual coordinates. The preferred directions of Purkinje cell SS were either downward or ipsilateral, and at the site of each recording, electrical stimulation of a Purkinje cell elicited eye movement toward the preferred direction of the SS of that Purkinje cell. This observation indicates that the SS coordinate framework is already that of the motor commands. Thus, at the parallel fiber–Purkinje cell synapse, a drastic visuomotor coordinate transformation occurs. Hence, the neural representation dramatically changes from population coding in MST and DLPN to firing rate coding of Purkinje cells at the parallel fiber–Purkinje cell synapse. What is the origin of this drastic transformation? According to the CBFELM model, the CS and eventually the AOS are the source of this motor command spatial framework. The preferred directions of pretectum neurons are upward, and those of nucleus of optic tract neurons are contralateral, and they are propagated to the inferior olive neurons and the CS of Purkinje cells. Yamamoto et al. (2002) reproduced all these experimental findings of Purkinje cell firing

characteristics during OFRs based on CBFELM, thus providing quite strong evidence for the theory.

Although direct and rigorous support of the CBFELM model was limited to a small portion of the cerebellum and to only several types of eye movements (OFR, VOR, OKR, smooth pursuit), because the neural circuit of different parts of the cerebellum is uniform and LTD is ubiquitous, we believe that the computational principle and the neural architecture demonstrated are common to all parts of the cerebellum. Recent physiological and brain imaging experiments provided further support of the CBFELM model in visually guided arm reaching movements (Kitazawa, Kimura, and Yin, 1998) and in the learning of a new tool (Imamizu et al., 2000).

Discussion

Humans can manipulate a vast number of tools, and exhibit an almost infinite number of behaviors in different environments. Given this multitude of contexts for sensorimotor control, there are two qualitatively distinct strategies to motor control and learning. The first is to use a single controller that uses all the contextual information in an attempt to produce an appropriate control signal. However, such a controller would have to be enormously complex to allow for all possible scenarios. If this controller were unable to encapsulate all the contexts, it would need to adapt every time the context of the movement changed before it could produce appropriate motor commands. This would produce transient but possibly large performance errors. Alternatively, a modular approach could be used in which multiple controllers coexist, with each controller suitable for one or a small set of contexts. Depending on the current context, only those appropriate controllers should be active to generate the motor command.

The modular approach has several computational advantages over the nonmodular approach. First, by using multiple inverse models, each of which might capture the motor commands necessary when interacting with a particular object or within a particular environment, we could achieve an efficient coding of the world. In other words, the large set of environmental conditions in which we are required to generate movement requires multiple behaviors or sets of motor commands, each embodied within a module. Second, the use of a modular system allows individual modules to adapt through motor learning, without affecting the motor behaviors already learned by other modules. Third, many situations that we encounter are derived from combinations of previously experienced contexts, such as novel conjoints of manipulated objects and environments. By modulating the contribution to the final motor command of the outputs of the inverse modules, an enormous repertoire of behaviors can be generated. With as few as 32 inverse models, in which the output of each model either contributes or does not contribute to the final motor command, we have 2^{10} behaviors—sufficient for a new behavior for every second of one's life. Therefore, multiple internal models can be regarded conceptually as *motor primitives*, which are the building blocks used to construct intricate motor behaviors with enormous vocabulary (see MOTOR PRIMITIVES).

Based on the benefits of a modular approach and the experimental evidence for modularity in observed behaviors, Wolpert and Kawato (1988) have proposed that the problem of motor learning and control is best solved using multiple controllers—that is, inverse models. At any given time, one or a subset of these inverse models will contribute to the final motor command (Figure 4 gives the details of the model). However, if there are multiple controllers, then there must also be some scheme to select the appropriate controller or controllers at each moment in time. The basic idea is that multiple inverse models exist to

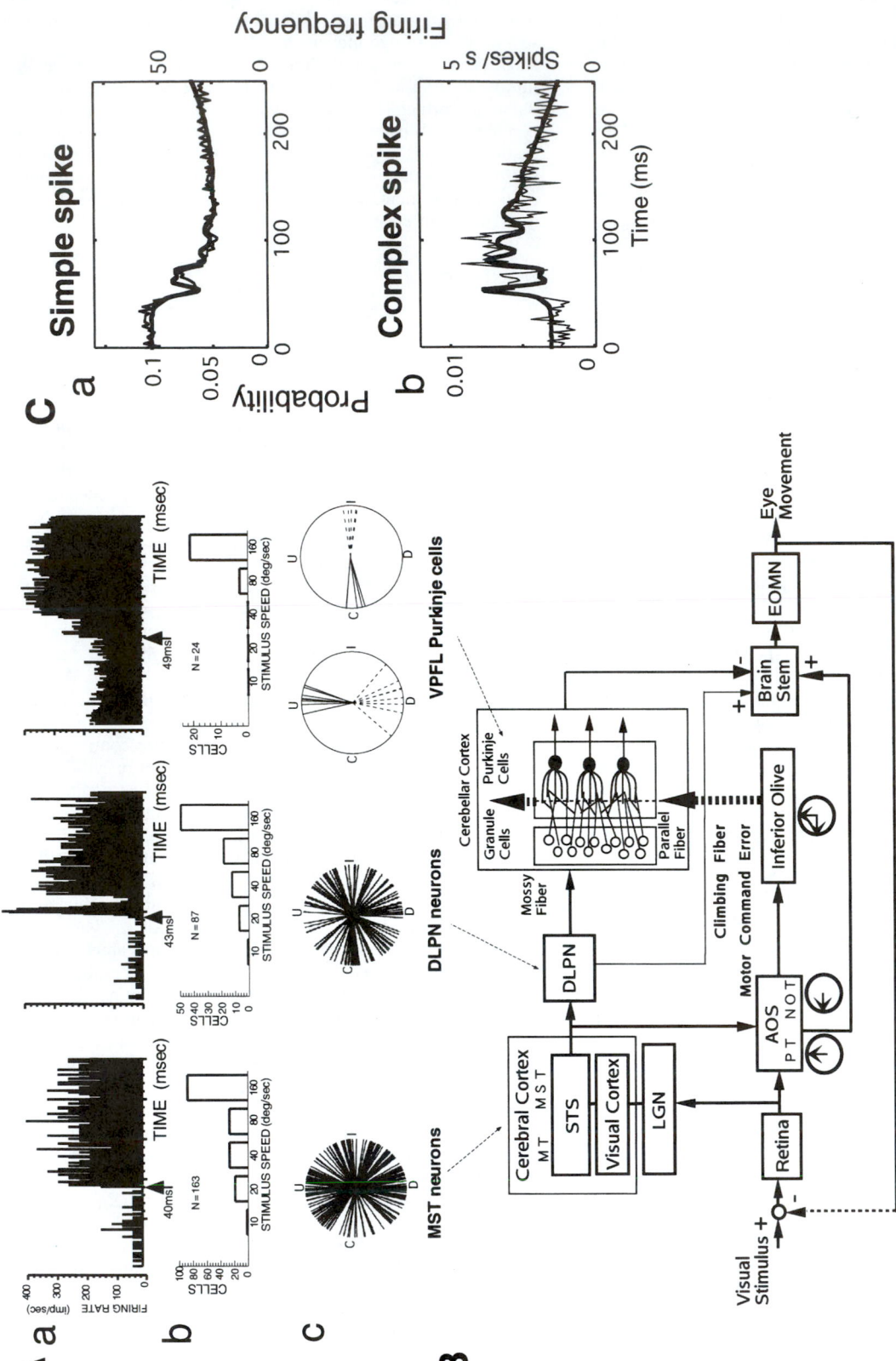

Figure 3. Change of neural codes and learning of inverse dynamics model in the cerebellum for ocular following responses (OFRs) (see Yamamoto et al., 2002, for a model reproduction of this experimental data). A, The firing characteristics of MST, DLPN, and VPFL neurons. B, A schematic neural circuit for OFR. C, The temporal firing patterns of VPFL Purkinje cells in upward eye movements induced by upward visual motion. In A, the left, middle, and right columns are for MST, DLPN, and VPFL neurons. In a, post-stimulus-time histograms of the firing rates of a typical neuron in each of the three areas are shown. The origin of time is the onset of visual stimulus motion. In b, histograms of a number of cells within a given range of the optimum stimulus speeds are shown. In c, polar plots of optimum stimulus directions are shown. U, C, D, and I indicate upward, contralateral, downward, and ipsilateral, respectively. VPFL Purkinje cells were classified into two groups, vertical cells and horizontal cells, based on simple spike (dotted line) and complex spike (solid line) optimum directions. The upper part shows the corticocortical (the cerebral cortex to the cerebellar cortex) pathway, which corresponds to the feedforward arc of the feedback-error-learning model. The lower part shows the phylogenetically older feedback pathway containing the accessory optic system, which corresponds to a crude feedback controller in the feedback-error-learning scheme. C, Temporal firing patterns of nine Purkinje cells accumulated (thin curves) and their reconstruction based on an inverse-dynamics model (bold curves). The model predicts that the temporal firing patterns of simple spikes (a) and complex spikes (b) should be mirror images of each other, and this was confirmed experimentally. MST, medial superior temporal area; DLPN, dorsolateral pontine nucleus; VPFL, ventral paraflocculus; AOS, accessory optic system; PT, pretectum; NOT, nucleus of optic tract; MT, middle temporal area; STS, superior temporal sulcus; LGN, lateral geniculate nucleus; EOMN, extraocular motor neurons.

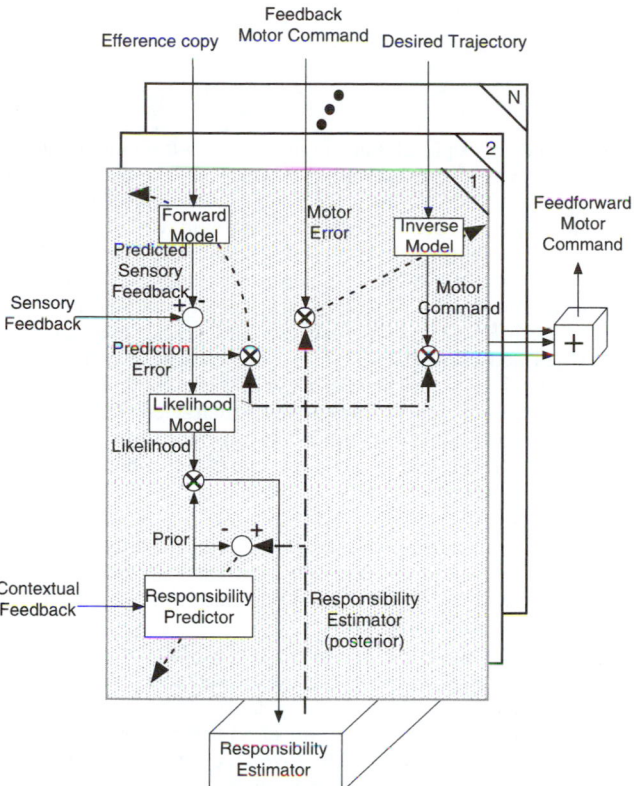

Figure 4. A schematic of the MOSAIC model (Wolpert and Kawato, 1998). *N*-paired modules are shown as stacked sheets (the dotted lines represent training signals and three-signal multiplication). The details of the first module are shown. Interactions between modules take place through the responsibility estimator. Each module consists of three interacting parts. The first two, the forward model and the responsibility predictor, are used to determine the responsibility of the module. This responsibility signal reflects the degree to which the module captures the current context and should, therefore, participate in control.

control the system, and each is augmented with a forward model that determines the responsibility each controller should assume during movement. This responsibility signal reflects, at any given time, the degree to which each pair of forward and inverse models should be responsible for controlling the current behavior. Within each module, the inverse and forward internal models are tightly coupled during their acquisition, through motor learning. This ensures that the forward models learn to divide up experience so that at least one forward model can predict the consequence of actions performed in any given context. By coupling the learning of the forward and inverse models, the inverse models learn to provide appropriate control commands in contexts in which their paired forward model produces accurate predictions. The model was once called the multiple paired forward and inverse models, but it was later renamed MOSAIC (MOdular Selection And Identification Control). MOSAIC is a version of the mixture-of-experts architecture (see MODULAR AND HIERARCHICAL LEARNING SYSTEMS).

Recent human brain imaging studies have started to accumulate evidence supporting multiple internal models of tools in the cerebellum (Imamizu et al., 2000, and successive studies). Other imaging studies suggest forward models in the cerebellum as well as inverse models. Each modular internal model in MOSAIC could have good anatomical correspondence with microzones. MOSAIC is capable of learning to produce appropriate motor commands in a variety of contexts and can switch rapidly between controllers as the context changes. These features are important for a full model of motor control and motor learning, as it is clear that the human motor system is capable of very flexible, modular adaptation. Furthermore, MOSAIC has the potential to explain many human cognitive capabilities such as thinking, communication, and language. This point is intriguing, since the cerebellum was shown to be involved in these uniquely human cognitive activities.

Road Maps: Mammalian Brain Regions; Mammalian Motor Control; Neural Plasticity
Background: Motor Control, Biological and Theoretical
Related Reading: Cerebellum and Conditioning; Imaging the Grammatical Brain; Sensorimotor Learning

References

Albus, J. S., 1971, A theory of cerebellar functions, *Math. Biosci.*, 10:25–61.

Boylls, C. C., 1975, *A Theory of Cerebellar Function with Applications to Locomotion: I. The Physiological Role of Climbing Fiber Inputs in Anterior Lobe Operation*, COINS Technical Report, Amherst: University of Massachusetts, Computer and Information Science.

Fujita, M., 1982, Adaptive filter model of the cerebellum, *Biol. Cybern.*, 45:195–206.

Gomi, H., and Kawato, M., 1996, Equilibrium-point control hypothesis examined by measured arm stiffness during multi-joint movement, *Science*, 272:117–120.

Houk, J. C., and Barto, A. G., 1992, Distributed sensorimotor learning, in *Tutorial in Motor Behavior II* (G. E. Stelmach and J. Requin, Eds.), Amsterdam: Elsevier, pp. 71–100.

Imamizu, H., Miyauchi, S., Tamada, T. Sasaki, Y., Takino, R., Puetz, B., Yoshioka, T., and Kawato, M., 2000, Human cerebellar activity reflecting an acquired internal model of a new tool, *Nature*, 403:192–195. ◆

Ito, M., 1984, *The Cerebellum and Neural Control*, New York: Raven Press.

Ito, M., 2001, Long-term depression: Characterization, signal transduction, and functional roles, *Physiol. Rev.*, 81:1143–1195. ◆

Kawato, M., 1999, Internal models for motor control and trajectory planning, *Curr. Opin. Neurobiol.*, 9:718–727. ◆

Kitazawa, S., Kimura, T., and Yin, P., 1998, Cerebellar complex spikes encode both destinations and errors in arm movements, *Nature*, 392:494–497.

Marr, D., 1969, A theory of cerebellar cortex, *J. Physiol.*, 202:437–470.

Miall, R. C., Weir, D. J., Wolpert, D. M., and Stein, J. F., 1993, Is the cerebellum a Smith predictor? *J. Motor Behav.*, 25:203–216.

Shidara, M., Kawano, K., Gomi, H., and Kawato, M., 1993, Inverse dynamics model eye movement control by Purkinje cells in the cerebellum, *Nature*, 365:50–52.

Wolpert, D., and Kawato, M., 1998, Multiple paired forward and inverse models for motor control, *Neural Netw.*, 11:1317–1329. ◆

Yamamoto, K., Kobayashi, Y., Takemura, A., Kawano, K., and Kawato, M., 2002, Computational studies on acquisition and adaptation of ocular following responses based on cerebellar synaptic plasticity, *J. Neurophysiol.*, 87:1554–1571. ◆

Cerebellum: Neural Plasticity

Hervž Daniel and Francis Crepel

Introduction

The participation of the cerebellum in motor learning was postulated by Brindley as early as 1964 and then formalized by Marr and Albus (see CEREBELLUM AND MOTOR CONTROL for details) around 1970. Purkinje cells (PCs) are the only output neurons of the cerebellar cortex. Each PC receives two excitatory synaptic inputs displaying distinct characteristics. The first and most powerful one-to-one synaptic input corresponds to climbing fibers (CFs) that originate from neurons in the contralateral inferior olive and make multiple synapses on primary and secondary dendrites of PCs. The second, weaker excitatory input corresponds to parallel fibers (PFs) that originate from cerebellar granule cells; 80,000 PFs converge onto tertiary dendrites of each PC, where each PF makes few synapses. PFs and CFs are likely to use the excitatory amino acid glutamate (Glu) as a neurotransmitter.

Given the dual arrangement of these excitatory synaptic inputs and taking into account current models of memory, it has been proposed that during motor learning, the gain of synaptic transmission at PF-PC synapses changes if and only if these synapses are repetitively activated at low rates in conjunction with CF impinging on the same PC. In this scheme, the CF acts as an external teacher to instruct PF-PC synapses to change their gain to adapt the cerebellar cortex output to the motor command (see CEREBELLUM AND MOTOR CONTROL). Thus, Marr's theory of motor learning predicts that repeated coincident activation of CFs and PFs leads to a long-term potentiation (LTP) of the PF synaptic inputs. However, Albus proposed instead that a long-term depression (LTD) occurs rather than LTP at PF-PC synapses during motor learning, to avoid saturation of neuronal networks.

The first experimental support in favor of this theory was provided by Ito and co-workers in a series of in vivo experiments on rabbits (Ito, Sakurai, and Tongroach, 1982). They demonstrated that LTD is associative, since only concomitant stimulation of PFs at low frequency (1–4 Hz) and of the CF impinging on the same PC leads to LTD of synaptic transmission at PF-PC synapses. In contrast, activation either of the CF or of PFs alone has no long-term effect. In addition, this long-term change in synaptic strength is restricted to PF-PC synapses activated in conjunction with CFs and is thus considered to be input specific. This is a crucial point for deciphering the mechanisms involved in motor learning (Ito et al., 1982). With the experimental advantages of in vitro brain slices and culture preparations, more recent studies have elucidated, at least in part, the complex processes of glutamate receptor activation and subsequent second-messenger cascades controlling the induction and the expression of this form of synaptic plasticity. The present article presents a detailed review of the findings of many experimentalists. Since space does not allow a comprehensive bibliography, the reader is referred to Daniel, Levenes, and Crepel (1998) and Daniel et al. (1999) for a full bibliography and citation of these many researchers.

Glutamatergic Receptors Involved in LTD Induction

We first examine the components in Figure 1. In marked contrast to most other neurons in the brain, PCs in the mature brain do not bear functional *N*-methyl-D-aspartate (NMDA) ionotropic receptors (see NMDA RECEPTORS: SYNAPTIC, CELLULAR, AND NETWORK MODELS). As such, fast excitatory synaptic transmission at PF-PC synapses is entirely mediated by non-NMDA ionotropic receptors, mostly of the AMPA type. These synapses also possess type-1α metabotropic glutamatergic receptors (mGluR1) coupled to phospholipase C, the activation of which leads to the production of inositol 1,4,5-triphosphate (IP$_3$) and of diacylglycerol (DAG, a protein kinase C (PKC) activator). There is now wide agreement that LTD induction of PF-mediated synaptic responses in PCs in acute slices and of Glu-induced currents in cultured PCs requires the activation of these two receptor groups. In cultured PCs, evidence for AMPA receptor participation in LTD has been provided by Linden and co-workers (1991). They have shown that iontophoretic application of quisqualate (an agonist of both mGluRs and AMPA receptors) induces LTD of quisqualate-mediated excitatory currents when combined with PC depolarization sufficient to produce Ca^{2+} entry through voltage-gated Ca^{2+} channels (VGCCs). This LTD is blocked by bath application of CNQX (a selective antagonist of AMPA receptors) during the pairing protocol (Linden et al., 1991). Likewise, using acute slices, other workers demonstrated that application of CNQX during a classical pairing protocol (PC depolarization/PF stimulation) prevents induction of LTD of PF-EPSCs but not its expression.

Concerning mGluRs, it was shown that application of mGluR1-inactivating antibodies or of the mGluR antagonist MCPG completely blocks LTD induction, while LTD induced by a classical pairing protocol is significantly impaired in knockout (KO) mice lacking functional mGluR1s. Moreover, LTD in mGluR1-null mutant mice can be rescued either by bypassing the disrupted mGluR1s with direct pharmacological activation of downstream intracellular cascades (activation of IP3 signal transduction pathway by photolytic release of IP3) (Daniel et al., 1999) or by transfecting

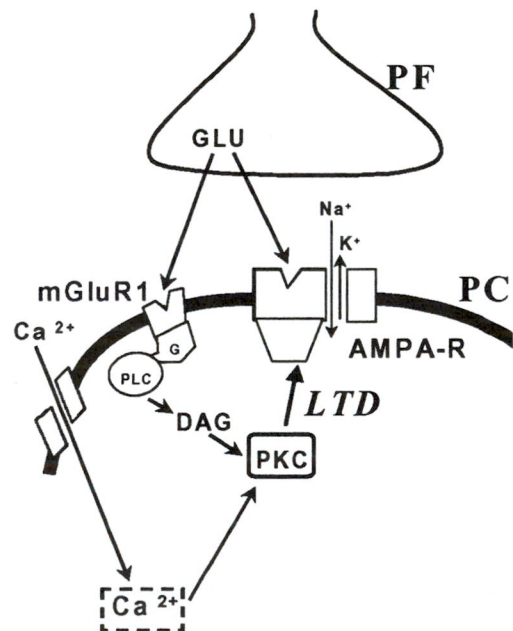

Figure 1. Schematic diagram of signal transduction processes involving the glutamatergic receptors proposed to participate in LTD induction: AMPA receptor (AMPA-R), and G (G)-protein-coupled-type 1-metabotropic glutamate receptor (mGluR1), which is positively coupled to phospholipase C (PLC) and can therefore lead to the production of 1,2-diacylglycerol (DAG), a protein kinase C (PKC) activator. Other abbreviations: GLU: Glutamate, PC: Purkinje cell, PF: parallel fiber.

functional mGluR1s in these KO mice under the control of the PC-specific L7 promoter (Ichise et al., 2000). Thus, these studies demonstrate the key role of mGluR1 in PCs for LTD induction, as they rule out the possibility that impairment of LTD in mGluR1 KO mice is due to some indirect developmental defects.

Involvement of Increases in Intracellular Ca²⁺ in LTD Induction

The crucial role of increases in Ca^{2+} resulting from VGCC activation for LTD induction was initially demonstrated in acute slices maintained in vitro with induction of LTD of PF-mediated synaptic responses by concomitant stimulation of PFs and CF impinging on the same PC prevented when PC intracellular free Ca^{2+} is buffered by 1,2-*bis*(2-aminophenoxy)ethane-N,N,N',N'-tetra-acetic acid (EGTA). The involvement of Ca^{2+} increases following VGCC activation in LTD induction was also evidenced in this same preparation, where LTD of PF-mediated responses was consistently induced by pairing these synaptic responses with direct depolarization of PCs sufficient to produce Ca^{2+} entry through VGCCs, thus mimicking activation of CFs. Likewise, as shown by Crepel and Krupa (1988) in acute slices and by Linden et al. (1991) in cultured PCs, LTD of responses elicited in PCs by iontophoretic application of Glu in their dendritic fields is also induced when these responses are combined with membrane depolarization, giving rise to Ca^{2+} spike firing. Finally, in patch-clamped PCs in acute slices, combining recordings of synaptic currents with fluorometric measurements of intracellular Ca^{2+} concentration directly demonstrates that PF stimulation paired with depolarization-induced Ca^{2+} transients is sufficient to induce LTD (see Figure 2).

In addition to Ca^{2+} entry through VGCCs, it was hypothesized that the cascade of events leading to LTD in PCs may involve Ca^{2+} release from IP3- or ryanodine-sensitive internal stores (Daniel et

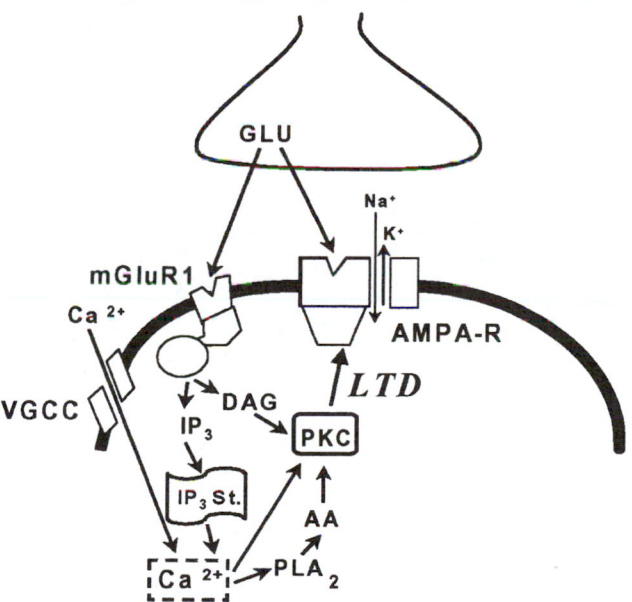

Figure 2. Schematic diagram of signal transduction processes proposed to participate in LTD induction involving increase in intracellular calcium, resulting from voltage-gated calcium channel (VGCC) activation and/or from calcium release from Inositol-1,4,5-trisphosphate (IP3)-internal stores (IP3 St), and involving the full PKC activation which requires in addition to the intracellular cascade leading to DAG production, the activation of the calcium-dependent enzyme phospholipase A₂ (PLA₂) leading to arachidonic acid (AA) production. Other abbreviations as in Figure 1.

al., 1998). However, in acute slices, the extent to which this process is involved seems to depend crucially on experimental conditions. Two groups have shown that both inhibition of Ca^{2+} release from IP3-sensitive stores with heparin (an antagonist of IP3 receptors) or with a specific antibody against IP3-receptor type 1 block LTD induced by a classical pairing protocol. Likewise, slices prepared from mice with a disrupted IP3-receptor type 1 gene, which is predominantly expressed in PCs, lack LTD induced by the same pairing protocol. Finally, and as mentioned before, the impairment of LTD induced by a classical pairing protocol in mGluR1-deficient PCs is pharmacologically rescued by photolysis of a caged IP3-compound. Along the same line, LTD can be rescued in transgenic mice with defective IP3-mediated Ca^{2+} signaling in spines, by local photolysis of a caged Ca^{2+} compound. Taken together, these data seem to establish that Ca^{2+} release from internal stores are critical for LTD induction in slices, at least in certain experimental conditions, but they do not reveal the precise mechanisms of their involvement in more physiological conditions. Indeed, synaptically driven Ca^{2+} mobilization from internal stores by PF stimulation has been now detected in PC spines and dendritic microdomains with confocal microscopy as well as with the use of two-photons laser scanning microscopy.

The problem of the participation of Ca^{2+} release from internal stores in LTD induction has been recently elucidated in an elegant series of experiments using two-photon laser scanning microscopy. In particular, it has been shown that with conjunctive activation of CF and of small number of PFs, both Ca^{2+} signals and LTD are confined to the activated synapses and require Ca^{2+} release from IP3-sensitive stores. In contrast, with co-activation of CF and of a large number of PFs, Ca^{2+} signals spread to dendritic shafts, and LTD induced in these conditions is now entirely mediated by VGCC-dependent Ca^{2+} entry. These results may reconcile previous conflicting findings regarding the involvement of Ca^{2+} release from internal stores in LTD induction in acute slices. Indeed, depletion of internal Ca^{2+} stores with thapsigargin blocks induction of LTD of PF-EPSPs induced by PC depolarization/bath application of mGluR agonist (1S-3R ACPD) without PF stimulation but does not prevent the induction of LTD by a classical pairing protocol (PC depolarization/PF stimulation).

In cultured PCs, the results are also puzzling, since certain studies have reported that inhibition of Ca^{2+} release from ryanodine or IP3-sensitive internal Ca^{2+} stores blocks LTD induced by Glu/depolarization conjunctive stimulation. In contrast, others have shown that LTD induction appears to be independent from Ca^{2+} release from IP3-sensitive stores. Thus, the potential involvement of Ca^{2+} release from internal stores in LTD induction in these reduced preparations is unclear, especially in the light of a recent study demonstrating that Ca^{2+} release from internal stores in PCs maintained in culture is impaired (Womack, Walker, and Khodakhah, 2000).

Second Messengers and LTD Induction: Cascades Involving PKC Activation and Nitric Oxide (NO)-cGMP-Dependent Protein Kinase (PKG) Activation

PKC Pathway

We now examine other aspects of the pathway shown in Figure 2. It is now well accepted that the second-messenger cascades following rises in internal Ca^{2+} involve PKC activation. Since PKCγ is abundantly expressed in PCs (Daniel et al., 1998) and mGluR1 activation also results in DAG production (see above), it was tempting to postulate that the cascade of events leading to LTD involves the activation of PKC by Ca^{2+} entry through VGCCs and DAG produced by mGluR activation following Glu release from PFs (Crepel and Krupa, 1988). Indeed, studies by Crepel and Krupa

(1988) in acute slices and later studies in cultures showed that direct activation of PKC by phorbol esters induces LTD of the responsiveness of PCs to exogenously applied Glu or quisqualate, whereas inactive analogs are without effect. Moreover, studies in acute cerebellar slices have shown that the potent protein kinase inhibitor polymixin B or the selective PKC inhibitory peptide PKC[19-36] abolishes LTD induction by conventional pairing protocols (PC depolarization/PF stimulation). Likewise, PKC[19-36] also blocks LTD induction by Glu/depolarization conjunction in cultured PCs. Moreover, in this reduced preparation, full activation of PKC is required to induce LTD and involves activation of the calcium-dependent enzyme phosphoplipase A$_2$(PLA$_2$) leading to arachidonic acid (AA) production, in addition to the intracellular cascade leading to DAG production. Such an involvement of PLA$_2$ in LTD induction was also evidenced more recently in acute slices by Reynolds and Hartell (2001). Finally, the crucial role of PKC activation in the cellular mechanisms leading to LTD induction was recently supported by the introduction of an additional player in the game, that is, the corticotropin-releasing factor that is contained in CFs and is critical for LTD induction in cerebellar slices, probably acting by enhancing activation of PKC.

However, and surprisingly enough, mice with null mutation in protein kinase Cγ exhibit apparently normal cerebellar LTD and this LTD is still abolished by specific PKC inhibitors. These puzzling results suggest that compensatory processes involving other subtypes of PKC are activated in these mutants to sustain LTD or, as was recently proposed, PKCα and/or PKCβ_1 but not PKCγ are involved in LTD induction (Hirono et al., 2001). More straightforward results were obtained by using transgenic mice selectively expressing the pseudosubstrate PKC inhibitor, PKC[19-31] in PC, since no LTD could be produced in these cells either in cultures or (Goossens et al., 2001) in acute slices. Thus, altogether, there is now a wide agreement that induction of cerebellar LTD requires PKC activation in in vitro brain slices and in culture preparations.

NO-cGMP-PKG Pathway

Further mechanisms are summarized in Figure 3. Inhibition of postsynaptic protein phosphatase activity through a cascade involving nitric oxide (NO), cGMP production, and cGMP-dependent protein kinase (PKG) activation is also required for LTD induction. In neurons, increases in intracellular Ca^{2+} can induce the formation of NO from arginine, by activating calmodulin-dependent NO-synthase (NO-S). As early as 1990, it was shown, in acute slices, that LTD of PF-mediated EPSPs induced by a conventional pairing protocol is prevented by bath application of NO-S inhibitors and furthermore that this blocking effect is reversed by addition of an excess of arginine in the bath. In the same year, it was shown that, again in acute slices, bath application of NO-S inhibitor prevents enduring desensitization of AMPA receptors of PCs resulting from successive exposures of slices to quisqualate. Moreover, it was shown later on that an LTD-like phenomenon can be induced by bath application of NO donors or by dialyzing such NO donors in the recorded cell through the recording patch pipette. However, neuronal nitric oxide synthase (nNO-S) has not been identified in PCs, even following RT-PCR analysis of mRNAs directly harvested from these neurons during patch-clamp experiments. In contrast, nNO-S is highly expressed in neighboring elements such as PFs and basket cells. Further studies, with NO-sensitive electrodes inserted into the molecular layer of cerebellar slices, have shown that protocols that are known to induce LTD lead to NO release, most probably originating from PFs. Finally, it has been shown that photolytic release of NO and Ca^{2+} inside PCs could replace the conjunctive PF stimulation and depolarization, respectively, required for LTD induction, suggesting that NO release is sufficient to replace PF stimulation. If this finding underlines the potential

role of NO in LTD induction, it is somewhat puzzling, as it contradicts previous experiments demonstrating that activation of AMPA receptors and of mGluRs are necessary for LTD induction (see the previous section). This apparent discrepancy could be due to the use of the photolytic release of NO, which is a powerful pharmacological tool but may exaggerate the participation of this NO pathway in LTD induction, which otherwise might be much less prominent in physiological conditions. Nevertheless, taken together, data obtained in acute slices are entirely consistent with a role for NO in LTD induction in PCs.

The target for NO is likely to be the soluble enzyme guanylate cyclase (sGC), which is abundantly expressed in PCs. Indeed, it is now indirectly established (by measurements of cGMP-dependent activation of phosphodiesterases) that NO, either pharmacologically applied or endogenously released following electrical stimulation of the molecular layer, triggers cGMP production in Purkinje cells (Hartell et al., 2001). Numerous studies have examined the potential role of cGMP on LTD induction. A long-lasting depression of PF-mediated responses is induced by direct dialysis of cGMP into the recorded PCs through the recording patch-pipette or by bath application of 8-bromo-cGMP (a membrane-permeative cGMP analog). In addition, this cGMP-induced LTD-like phenomenon partially occludes subsequent induction of LTD by classical pairing protocols. Moreover, LTD induced by a classical pairing protocol is totally inhibited by intracellular injection of the selective and potent inhibitor of sGC, 1H-(1,2,4)oxadiazolo(4,3-a)quinoxalin-1-one (ODQ), confirming that the sGC of PCs is the target of NO.

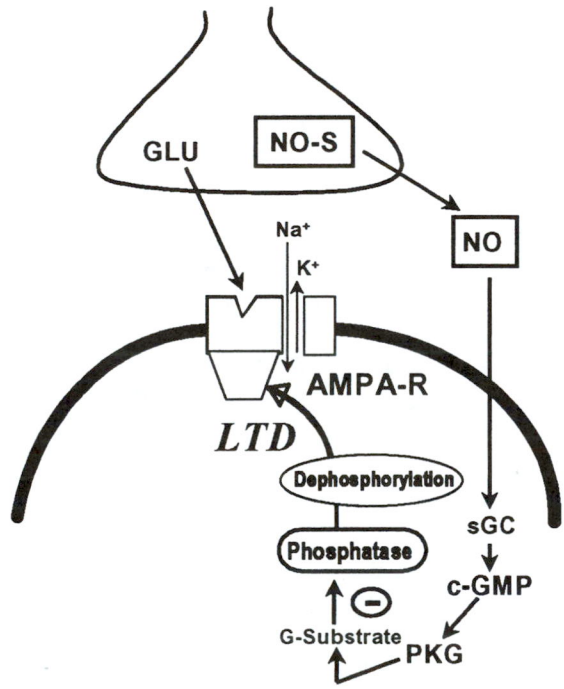

Figure 3. Schematic diagram of signal transduction processes involving the NO-cGMP-PKG pathway proposed to participate in LTD induction: Nitric oxide (NO), produced by NO-synthase (NO-S), activates synthesis of cyclic guanosine monophosphate (cGMP) by the catalytic action of the soluble guanylate cyclase (sGC); cGMP production in turn activates Protein kinase G (PKG), a cGMP-dependent protein kinase, thereby allowing phosphorylation of its specific endogenous "G-substrate," which is, in the phosphorylated state, a powerful inhibitor of protein phosphatase. Other abbreviations as in Figure 1.

In keeping with these findings, Ito and Karachot suggested in 1992 that cGMP production would in turn activate a cGMP-dependent protein kinase (PKG), thereby allowing phosphorylation of its specific endogenous G-substrate, which is, in the phoshorylated state, a powerful inhibitor of protein phosphatases. In keeping with such a hypothesis, it has been shown that selective inhibition of PKG blocks LTD induced by co-activation of PFs and CFs or LTD induced by PF stimulation paired with PC depolarization (Reynolds and Hartell, 2001). In addition, it has been reported that bath application of the protein phosphatase inhibitor calyculin A induces LTD in acute slices.

All these experiments support the view that the NO-cGMP-PKG pathway participates in cellular events leading to LTD. Because of its ability to diffuse over large distances, the role of NO in LTD cannot be to bring synapse specificity for this change in synaptic strength. Rather, this compound might allow recruitment of additional synapses into the pool of those exhibiting LTD following co-activation of PFs and CFs, thus increasing the signal-to-noise ratio of this process.

While the involvement of NO-cGMP signaling in LTD induction in cerebellar slices is now firmly established, the induction of LTD of glutamate-evoked currents in cultured PCs is unaffected by treatments that stimulate or inhibit this signaling pathway. This discrepancy might be due to the fact that in reduced preparations, putative NO donors such as PFs and basket cells are more scarcely represented. Alternatively, it is also conceivable that mechanisms of LTD induction are different in neurons grown in dissociated cultures versus those in acute brain slices from young adult animals.

Changes in the Functional Characteristics of Postsynaptic AMPA Receptors During LTD Expression

In early in vivo experiments, Ito and co-workers showed that co-activation of PCs by CF stimulation and iontophoretic Glu application into their dendritic fields induced a long-lasting decrease in their responsiveness to this agonist (Ito et al., 1982). This result led Ito to propose that induction of LTD might ultimately lead to a long-term desensitization of PC postsynaptic ionotropic Glu receptors. Consistent with this view, experimental evidence based on the use of the coefficient of variation (CV) applied to PF-EPSCs suggests that LTD of PF-EPSCs, induced either by a classical pairing protocol or by bath application of NO donors in acute slices, is entirely expressed at a postsynaptic level. Moreover, a true modification of Glu receptor properties during LTD expression has been also suggested in acute slices. Indeed, it has been shown that aniracetam, a compound that is known to markedly reduce desensitization of AMPA receptors, has a larger potentiating effect on PF-EPSCs after induction of LTD than before, which suggests that LTD involves a true desenzitization of postsynaptic AMPA receptors at PF-PC synapse. These results support the view that this change in long-term synaptic efficacy involves a genuine change in the functional characteristics of postsynaptic AMPA receptors.

Redistribution of AMPA Receptors and LTD Expression

In addition to functional modifications of AMPA receptors, recent studies have shown that trafficking of these receptors could play a crucial role in the expression of LTD (see Xia et al., 2000). Indeed, LTD expression in cultured PCs is associated with a rapid endocytotic-dependent decrease in the number of GluR2-containing synaptic AMPA receptors. This internalization requires clathrin-complex-mediated endocytosis, since peptides that inter-

fere with this complex block LTD. Additionally, this process depends on the intracellular carboxy-terminal domain of AMPA receptor subunit GluR2(/3), which has been identified as a likely candidate region to interact with proteins of the postsynaptic density, allowing their intracellular anchoring. These latest studies have made substantial advance toward a molecular understanding of LTD expression by establishing a potential link between the internalization of AMPA receptors and PKC activation (see above). Indeed, phosphorylation of Ser 880 in the C-terminal domain of GluR2(/3) by pharmacological PKC activation is accompanied by a reduction in the binding affinity of this subunit to an anchoring protein of the postsynaptic density termed "glutamate receptor interacting protein" (GRIP) (Figure 4), thereby leading to significant disruption of postsynaptic GluR2 clusters (Matsuda et al., 2000). In addition, treatments that disrupt the interaction between the carboxy-terminal of GluR2(/3) and PICK1 (another protein component of the postsynaptic density interacting with protein kinase C) (Figure 4) strongly attenuated both LTD induced by glutamate/depolarization pairing and a LTD-like phenomenon produced by exogenous application of PKC-activating phorbol ester (Xia et al., 2000). Taken together, these findings demonstrate that expression

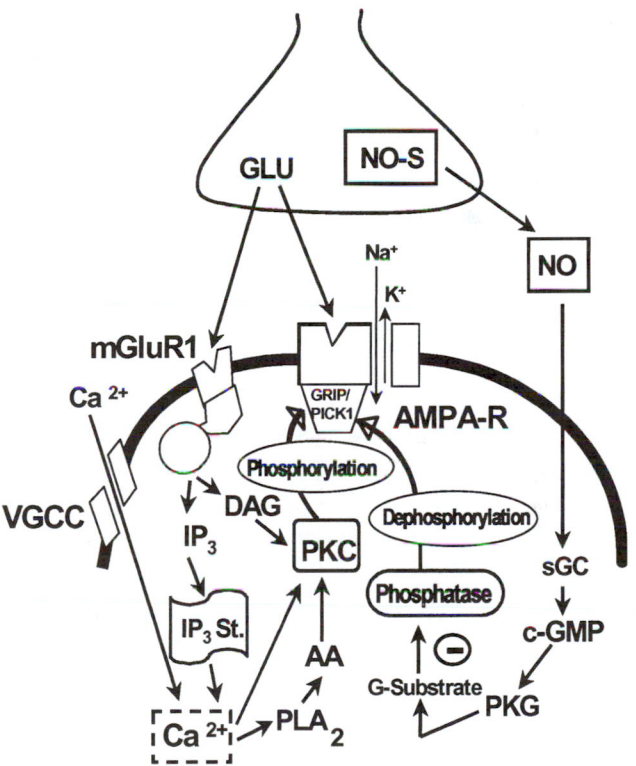

Figure 4. General schematic diagram of signal transduction processes leading to the phosphorylation and internalization of AMPA receptors, proposed to participate in LTD induction (glutamate receptor interacting protein (GRIP) and protein interacting with protein kinase C (PICK1) are proteins of the postsynaptic density interacting with AMPA receptors). Other abbreviations as in previous figures (Abbreviations: AA: arachidonic acid, AMPA-R: AMPA receptor, cGMP: cyclic guanosine monophosphate, DAG: 1,2-diacylglycerol, G: G protein, GLU: glutamate, GRIP: glutamate receptor interacting protein, IP$_3$: inositol-1,4,5-trisphosphate, IP$_3$ St.: inositol-1,4,5-trisphosphate internal Ca^{2+} stores, mGluR1: type-1 metabotropic glutamate receptor, NO: nitric oxide, NOS: nitric oxide synthase, PC: Purkinje cell, PF: parallel fiber, PICK1: protein interacting with C-kinase 1, PKC: protein kinase C, PKG: protein kinase G, PLA$_2$: phospholipase A$_2$, PLC: phospholipase C, sGC: soluble guanylate cyclase.)

of cerebellar LTD requires PKC-regulated interaction between the carboxy terminal of GluR2(/3) and specific proteins of the postsynaptic density. Ultimately, internalization and/or changes in the properties of AMPA receptors could then create a disturbance in the postsynaptic density, which might in turn initiate a cascade of events that leads to a reorganization of the dendritic cellular cytoskeleton, thereby creating a permanent imprint of LTD.

Transcription Factors, Protein Synthesis, and LTD Expression

Recent findings have demonstrated that the mechanisms involved in the maintenance phase of LTD (which may underlie long-term memory) include the expression of transcription factors and require protein synthesis in addition to modifications of AMPA receptor properties and/or changes in their distribution. The experimental protocols that are known to induce LTD trigger expression of the immediate-early genes c-Fos and Jun-B, suggesting that the expression of these genes may help to establish cerebellar long-term depression. Moreover, translational inhibitors that were perfused immediately after the induction protocol abolished LTD of glutamate responsiveness in cultured PCs only after a delay of 45 minutes, suggesting that postsynaptic protein synthesis is specifically involved in the establishment of the late phase of LTD. However, Karachot et al. (2001) have reported more recently that translational inhibitors entirely abolish the LTD induced by conjunctive stimulation of PFs and CF in acute slices, including its early phase, even if this early phase is less sensitive to these inhibitors.

Discussion

After two decades of research, the understanding of the cellular and molecular mechanisms pathways underlying LTD has made rapid progress. Although part of the signal transduction pathways remains obscure, the stable phosphorylation of AMPA receptors appears to play a key step for expressing LTD (Figure 4). Thus, taking into account the experimental data available so far, Kuroda and coworkers have recently established a very interesting computational model that links kinetics of phosphorylation of AMPA receptors with different phases of LTD expression (Kuroda, Schweighofer, and Kawato, 2001).

Despite remaining uncertainties in the current understanding of the cellular and molecular mechanisms underlying the induction and expression of LTD, this associative and input specific form of synaptic plasticity has been proposed as the cellular basis for error-driven learning and memory in the motor system (see MOTOR CONTROL, BIOLOGICAL AND THEORETICAL). In particular, recent in vivo experiments point toward a role of LTD in the adaptation of the vestibulo-ocular reflex (VOR). This conclusion has been strengthened by the observations that selective expression of PKC inhibitors in PCs not only blocks cerebellar LTD without affecting PC excitability in alert transgenic mice, but also is accompanied by a lack of VOR adaptation in these animals (Goossens et al., 2001). Such a correlation between impairment of LTD and deficiency of associative learning of eyeblink conditioning has also been consistently found in other types of transgenic mice, such as mice that are deficient in mGluR1 (Aiba et al., 1994, in Daniel et al., 1998) or GFAP (Shibuki et al., 1996, in Daniel et al., 1998). Thus, there is now a growing consensus to support the notion that the associative nature of LTD makes it an attractive candidate for the cellular substrate underlying motor learning in the cerebellum. Moreover, the timing conditions for LTD induction may account for the temporal specificity of cerebellar motor learning. In this respect, an important future development in the field will be to study developmental aspects of LTD in relation to acquisition of motor skills.

Road Map: Neural Plasticity
Related Reading: Cerebellum and Conditioning; Cerebellum and Motor Control; NMDA Receptors: Synaptic, Cellular, and Network Models

References

Crepel, F., and Krupa, M., 1988, Activation of protein kinase C induces a long-term depression of glutamate sensitivity of cerebellar Purkinje cells: An in vitro study, *Brain Res.*, 458:397–401. ◆

Daniel, H., Levenes, C., and Crepel, F., 1998, Cellular mechanisms of cerebellar LTD, *Trends Neurosci.*, 21:401–407.

Daniel, H., Levenes, C., Fagni, L., Conquet, F., Bockaert, J., and Crepel, F., 1999, Inositol-1,4,5-trisphosphate-mediated rescue of cerebellar long-term depression in subtype 1 metabotropic glutamate receptor mutant mouse, *Neuroscience*, 92:1–6. ◆

Goossens, J., Daniel, H., Rancillac, A., van der Steen, J., Oberdick, J., Crepel, F., De Zeeuw, C. I., and Frens, M. A., 2001, Expression of protein kinase C inhibitor blocks cerebellar long-term depression without affecting Purkinje cell excitability in alert mice, *J. Neurosci.*, 21:5813–5823.

Hartell, N. A., Furuya, S., Jacoby, S., and Okada, D., 2001, Intercellular action of nitric oxide increases cGMP in cerebellar Purkinje cells, *NeuroReport*, 12:25–28.

Hirono, M., Sugiyama, T., Kishimoto, Y., Sakai, I., Miyazawa, T., Kishio, M., Inoue, H., Nakao, K., Ikeda, M., Kawahara, S., Kirino, Y., Katsuki, M., Horie, H., Ishikawa, Y., and Yoshioka, T., 2001, Phospholipase Cβ4 and protein kinase Cα and/or protein kinase CβI are involved in the induction of long term depression in cerebellar Purkinje cells, *J. Biol. Chem.*, 276:45236–45242.

Ichise, T., Kano, M., Hashimoto, K., Yanagihara, D., Nakao, K., Shigemoto, R., Katsuki, M., and Aiba, A., 2000, mGluR1 in cerebellar Purkinje cells essential for long-term depression, synapse elimination, and motor coordination, *Science*, 288:1832–1835.

Ito, M., Sakurai, M., and Tongroach, P., 1982, Climbing fiber induced depression of both mossy fiber responsiveness and glutamate sensitivity of cerebellar Purkinje cells, *J. Physiol.*, 324:113–134. ◆

Karachot, L., Shirai, Y., Vigot, R., Yamamori, T., and Ito, M., 2001, Induction of long-term depression in cerebellar Purkinje cells requires a rapidly turned over protein, *J. Neurophysiol.*, 86:280–289.

Kuroda, S., Schweighofer, N., and Kawato, M., 2001, Exploration of signal transduction pathways in cerebellar long-term depression by kinetic simulation, *J. Neurosci.*, 21:5693–5702.

Linden, D. J., Dickinson, M. H., Smeyne, M., and Connor, J. A., 1991, A long-term depression of AMPA currents in cultured cerebellar Purkinje neurons, *Neuron*, 7:81–89. ◆

Matsuda, S., Launey, T., Mikawa, S., and Hirai, H., 2000, Disruption of AMPA receptor GluR2 clusters following long-term depression induction in cerebellar Purkinje neurons, *EMBO J.*, 19:2765–2774.

Reynolds, T., and Hartell, N. A., 2001, Roles for nitric oxide and arachidonic acid in the induction of heterosynaptic cerebellar LTD, *NeuroReport*, 12:133–136.

Womack, M. D., Walker, J. W., and Khodakhah, K., 2000, Impaired calcium release in cerebellar Purkinje neurons maintained in culture, *J. Gen. Physiol.*, 115:339–346.

Xia, J., Chung, H. J., Wihler, C., Huganir, R .L., and Linden, D. J., 2000, Cerebellar long-term depression requires PKC-regulated interactions between GluR2/3 and PDZ domain-containing proteins, *Neuron*, 28:499–510.

Chains of Oscillators in Motor and Sensory Systems

Nancy Kopell and G. Bard Ermentrout

Introduction

Collections of oscillators that send signals to one another can phase-lock with many patterns of phase differences. This article discusses a set of examples that illustrate how those phases emerge from the oscillator interactions. Much of the work was motivated by spatiotemporal patterns in networks of neurons that govern undulatory locomotion. The original experimental preparation to which this work was applied is the lamprey central pattern generator (CPG) for locomotion (see SPINAL CORD OF LAMPREY: GENERATION OF LOCOMOTOR PATTERNS). However, the mathematics is considerably more general, and can be used to gain insight into other systems. In addition to the lamprey CPG, we will briefly discuss related pattern generators in the crayfish swimmeret system (Skinner, Kopell, and Mulloney, 1997) and the leech network of swimming (Friesen and Pearce, 1993), as well as waves of activity in other oscillatory neural tissue (Kleinfeld et al., 1994). For relationships to other patterns in the nervous system, see SYNCHRONIZATION, BINDING AND EXPECTANCY; OLFACTORY BULB; and OLFACTORY CORTEX.

Though much has been written about chains of oscillators in the context of physical problems, very little of that literature is relevant to chains of biological oscillators. Much of the the physics literature depends on the existence of certain conserved quantities that are irrelevant in a biological setting. Biological oscillators have other structure that is important to the behavior of collections of such oscillators. For example, unlike models of mechanical oscillators, models of biological oscillators have stable limit cycles (see PHASE-PLANE ANALYSIS OF NEURAL NETS). In the context of locomotion, each "oscillator" is likely to be a local subnetwork of neurons that produces rhythmic patterns of membrane potentials. Since the details of the oscillators often are not known and difficult to obtain, the object of the mathematics is to find the consequences of what is known, and to generate sharper questions to motivate further experimentation.

Physical Models and Phase Models

Each of the examples we describe below can be considered, roughly, as an array of oscillators. In the absence of knowledge of details, it is desirable to keep the oscillator description as general as possible. Thus, we assume only that the local network can be described by some (possibly high-dimensional) system of ordinary differential equations having a stable limit cycle, with no concern for the mechanistic origin of that oscillation.

In general, the behavior of interacting oscillators can be arbitrarily complex (Guckenheimer and Holmes, 1983, chap. 6). However, in some circumstances, the network behaves like a much more simply described collection of units. For example, suppose that the coupling is (sufficiently) weak. Then the collection of oscillators acts as if there were a well-defined "phase" to each oscillator, and the signals between the oscillators become dependent only on the differences of the phases (Kopell, 1987). The form of the equations is then

$$\theta_j' = \omega_j + \sum H_{jk}(\theta_k - \theta_j) \qquad (1)$$

Here θ_j is the phase of the jth oscillator and ω_j is its frequency when uncoupled. The interaction functions $H_{jk}(\phi)$ measure how much the jth oscillator is sped up or slowed down by the interaction with the kth oscillator; they can be computed from the original, more complicated equations by averaging the effects of the coupling terms over a cycle, and depend on the properties of the oscillators as well as the coupling (Guckenheimer and Holmes, 1983, chap. 4). There are also other computational ways of producing (at least the relevant parts of) the coupling functions, including a method that can in principle be done in the absence of explicit knowledge of the equations (see SPINAL CORD OF LAMPREY: GENERATION OF LOCOMOTOR PATTERNS).

The existence of this reduction procedure allows us to come back to questions about how details of the oscillators or the coupling can affect the network behavior via their effects on the functions H_{jk}. The simple description in Equation 1 can also be valid in some circumstances relevant to CPGs in which the coupling is strong. For example, if each oscillator is itself a composite of cells and emits coupling signals several times per cycle, the system can behave like the averaged one (see Cohen et al., 1992, for reference).

Mechanisms for the Production of Traveling Waves

We now consider arrays of oscillators, of which nearest-neighbor coupled chains are the simplest example. When the above reduction is valid, the equations have the form

$$\theta_j' = \omega_j + H_A(\theta_{j+1} - \theta_j) + H_D(\theta_{j-1} - \theta_j) \qquad (2)$$

Here H_A and H_D are the functions that represent the coupling in the ascending and descending directions of the chain. There are at least two different mechanisms that can produce waves in Equation 2. One of these relies on differences in natural frequency along the chain and the other on properties of the coupling.

The first mechanism is easy to illustrate, using the simple choice of coupling functions $H_A(\phi) = H_D(\phi) = \sin(\phi)$, where ϕ denotes the relevant phase difference. Such functions arise from the reduction procedure when the differential equations producing the oscillations have, for example, odd symmetry and the interaction is via the standard mathematical description of diffusion between compartments (Ermentrout and Kopell, 1984). In this case, if the natural frequencies are all equal, the synchronous solution ($\theta_j = \theta_k$ for all j, k) is the stable output of the chain. If the frequencies are not all the same, however, other behavior is produced. For example, a gradient in frequencies produces a traveling wave of activity from the oscillator with the highest frequency to the one with the lowest (Cohen, Holmes, and Rand, 1982), but not one with constant phase lags (i.e., independent of position along the chain).

Waves induced by frequency differences are important in the electrical activity produced by smooth muscle of the intestines, where there is a linear gradient in the uncoupled frequencies (Ermentrout and Kopell, 1984). They are also known to exist in the leech CPG for swimming (Friesen and Pearce, 1993) and appear to be the mechanism underlying waves in *Limax* (Ermentrout, Flores, and Gelperin, 1998). There is no evidence for such a gradient in the lamprey or crustacean swimmeret system.

A variation on the frequency gradient idea has an oscillator at one or both ends of the chain with a different frequency than the ones in the middle. Even with symmetric coupling such as $H_A(\phi) = H_D(\phi) = \sin(\phi)$, there can be waves of activity. In this case, the waves can have constant phase lags.

Another mechanism that produces traveling waves in chains of locally coupled oscillators relies on the properties of the coupling, allowing the frequencies to be identical. The essential property for H_A or H_D is that, if there is one-way coupling using either of these functions, the oscillators would lock with a non-zero phase difference. A simple example of such a coupling function is $H_A(\phi) =$

$\alpha\sin\phi + \beta\cos\phi$, with $\beta \neq 0$, while $H_B(\phi) = 0$. We note that for almost all kinds of coupling between two oscillators (in particular for models of chemical synapses), $H(0) \neq 0$. An important special exception is the mathematical description of simple diffusion across a membrane, which is a standard model of electrical synapses.

To understand how this mechanism works, consider a chain of oscillators coupled only in one direction, e.g., the ascending direction. Then the equations take the form

$$\theta'_j = \omega + H_A(\phi_j); \; j \neq N$$
$$\theta'_N = \omega \qquad\qquad (3)$$

where $\phi_j = \theta_{j+1} - \theta_j$. The hypothesis about H_A implies that $H_A(0) \neq 0$, i.e., that the zero ϕ_0 of H_A satisfies $\phi_0 \neq 0$. Since all equations with $j \neq N$ are the same, we get equal phase lags $\phi_j = \phi_0$. This corresponds to a wave traveling at constant speed determined by ϕ_0. The direction of the wave depends on the sign of ϕ_0; if $\phi_0 > 0$, the wave travels in the ascending direction; if $\phi_0 < 0$, the wave travels in the opposite direction. Thus, the direction of the coupling does not determine the direction of the wave.

If the coupling is in both directions, and/or if the frequencies are not uniform, the outcome can still be calculated (Kopell and Ermentrout, 1986). We will say more about this later in the context of particular applications. One of the applications (to *Limax*) uses a generalization of the ideas of coupling-induced waves. In that example, there is a gradient of coupling strength, so the equations have the form

$$\theta'_j = \omega_j + s_j H_A(\theta_{j+1} - \theta_j) + s_j H_D(\theta_{j-1} - \theta_j) \qquad (4)$$

Here s_j denotes the strength of the connections to the jth cell; a gradient in coupling strength corresponds to the s_j changing monotonically with j.

The Lamprey Central Pattern Generator for Swimming

This CPG is described in more detail in SPINAL CORD OF LAMPREY: GENERATION OF LOCOMOTOR PATTERNS (q.v.). The most striking aspect of the lamprey CPG for undulatory locomotion is the linear geometry of the network. That is, the network can be portrayed crudely as a chain of oscillators (Cohen et al., 1982). The linear geometry provides important constraints on the behavior of the network, making it possible to use the theory described above. It is also important that the number of oscillators associated with the circuit be fairly large: there are approximately 100 segments, and small numbers (at least two) of isolated segments are known to be able to oscillate. The general theory in (Kopell and Ermentrout, 1986) is addressed to understanding the behavior of such long chains of oscillators; as we will see in the section on crayfish, CPGs that correspond to small numbers of oscillators must have a different construction in order to have a similar behavior. Although long fibers are known to exist in the lamprey cord, we consider first only local coupling; this was remarkably successful in explaining the behavior of the spinal cord. For references to the long fibers, see Cohen et al. (1982).

The first issue to be addressed about this preparation is the mechanism for producing the traveling wave that is observed in the spinal cord (see SPINAL CORD OF LAMPREY: GENERATION OF LOCOMOTOR PATTERNS). This wave has a constant speed (i.e., the phase lag between adjacent oscillators is independent of position along the chain). For the large class of equations for which the representation in Equation 2 is valid, the general theory of Kopell and Ermentrout (1986) tells us what properties of the oscillators and coupling are necessary to produce this constant speed wave.

In general, if there are frequency differences among the oscillators, the wave speed is not constant along the chain. (This can be mitigated by creating coupling that connects each oscillators to multiple neighbors; see Cohen et al., 1992.) Thus, frequency gradients do not provide the basis for waves in the lamprey. Chains with differences in frequency for the first and last oscillators do produce constant speed waves. However, small sections from any portion of the isolated lamprey cord produce local phase differences identical to the differences produced in the whole cord, invalidating the hypothesis that the ends of the cord are intrinsically different from the rest.

The edges of a piece of cord *are* different, not because of their intrinsic properties but because of their placement, and this can produce waves driven by edge effects. We saw in the previous section that one-way coupling provides constant speed waves if the uncoupled frequencies of the oscillators are equal; in that mechanism, the relevant edge is the oscillator that gets no input.

The theory of Kopell and Ermentrout (1986) proves the surprising fact that, even with two-way coupling, a long but finite chain in general behaves like one with only one-way coupling. (For this, the coupling must be asymmetric.) That is, for the purpose of determining the phase lags between any two points on the chain, one of the two directions of coupling is dominant over the other; the output is almost as if the other coupling were silent. The phase lags among the oscillators are affected by the nondominant coupling only near one end of the chain, where there is a "boundary layer" of phase lags different from those in the rest of the chain. (This occurs only for long chains; when the chain is short, as in the swimmeret system discussed later, the boundary layer can be most of the chain.) This dominance can be understood from a linearized version of the equations (see SPINAL CORD OF LAMPREY: GENERATION OF LOCOMOTOR PATTERNS); however, the linearized equations do not reproduce other effects elicited by experimental perturbations. An important result of the theory is that the lags depend only on the coupling functions; changes in the frequency uniformly along the chain do not change the expression of phase lags.

Three sets of experiments have been done with the isolated lamprey spinal cord to test the ideas described above. Theory based on Kopell and Ermentrout (1986) and other mathematical work was used in each case to predict an effect that should be seen only if one direction of the coupling was dominant, and to determine the dominant direction. In one of these experiments, a small motor was attached to one end of an otherwise pinned-down cord and used to wag the cord periodically at measured frequencies; the predicted effect concerned the range of frequencies over which the cord could be entrained by the forcing at either end of the cord. In another set of experiments, the local frequency of the intrinsic circuits was manipulated to be different in different parts of the cord; the mathematics makes predictions about changes in phase lags due to the frequency perturbations. The third set of experiments concerned the existence of "boundary layers" in phase lags at one end of the chain. In each case, the predicted effect was found, and the data revealed that the dominant direction of coupling is caudal to rostral (ascending), though the wave itself is descending.

For more information on the the experiments and interpretation, see SPINAL CORD OF LAMPREY: GENERATION OF LOCOMOTOR PATTERNS and Cohen et al. (1992) and the references therein; the Cohen article has the references to the mathematical work. We note that if the edge effects needed to create the waves are produced by changing the frequencies of the first and last oscillators in a chain that would otherwise display synchrony, the mathematics says that the consequences of the experimental perturbation would not be as observed.

The central question that motivated the lamprey work concerned the constancy of the phase lags as swimming speed is increased. In vivo, the swimming speed of an animal is proportional to the frequency of the local oscillators of the spinal cord. In the isolated spinal cord, the frequency can be manipulated directly; changing the oscillatory frequency uniformly does not change the phase lags along the cord. The theory described above provides a first step toward explaining this constancy; it says that changing the frequencies uniformly along the cord should not change the phase lags, provided that the zero of the dominant coupling does not change. In the lamprey spinal cord, changes of frequency may be achieved in ways that also change the coupling. Thus, the theory raises the sharper question of how the local network is constructed so that the excitation that increases the frequency leaves unchanged the relevant zero crossing.

Swimmeret Systems of Crayfish

The swimmeret system of crayfish is another example of modular control of motor behavior via oscillatory components. The swimmerets are four paired, jointed limbs in the abdomen of the animal that move rhythmically to propel the animal through the water. Each swimmeret is controlled by a local oscillatory neural circuit in a ganglion containing motor neurons that innervate the swimmeret and interneurons that produce the rhythm (Skinner and Mulloney, 1998).

During a bout of swimming, the circuits all oscillate with the same frequency and maintain a constant phase relationship. The left and right sides are synchronized and there is approximately a quarter-cycle phase difference between neighboring circuits, with a posterior circuit leading its anterior neighbor. Thus, the chain of circuits produces a traveling wave whose direction is opposite to that of the lamprey. As in the lamprey, the wave produced has a wavelength approximately that of the body length, and the phase lag between adjacent segments is the same between any pair of segments. Other parallels with the lamprey swimming CPG are (1) there is no evidence for frequency differences between uncoupled local circuits, and (2) pharmacologically induced uniform changes in frequency of the circuits do not affect the phase lags.

In the swimmeret system, intersegmental coordination between the local circuits is accomplished by interneurons projecting to neighboring circuits. The details of connectivity and how the rhythms are produced are not known. Thus, as in the lamprey investigation, it is useful to consider the network behavior from a more abstract point of view, to understand what constraints on the bidirectional connectivity and local oscillators are necessary to reproduce key experimental observations. Based on recordings from isolated ganglia bathed in nicotinic agonists to produce swim-like patterns, some observations are as follows: (1) when anterior or posterior ganglia are selectively excited, a significant change in phase lag occurs at the excitation boundary, and (2) the frequency of the swimmeret pattern increases with an increase in the number of ganglia excited.

A model having the same form as Equation 2 can reproduce the basic findings about normal phases and perturbations in phase and frequency due to experimental perturbations (see Skinner and Mulloney, 1998, for references). However, in order for this to be so, there are critical differences from the lamprey work in assumptions about the coupling. For the lamprey, the length of the chain of oscillators allows one direction of coupling to dominate; the other direction makes its presence known (at least with respect to the phase lags) only in a small boundary layer. For a short chain (four oscillators), both directions of coupling contribute significantly, and must be coordinated in order for the phase lags to be appropriate. The mathematical theory suggests that the two coupling directions must be constructed so that each, by itself, would produce the appropriate lag of 90 degrees. Since the lags are measured in a fixed direction (e.g., $(j + 1)$-st to jth ganglion), this requires a zero crossing for the ascending coupling to be 90 degrees, and that for the descending coupling to be -90 degrees. That is, the coupling in the two directions must be asymmetric in a very particular way. If they have the same strength and that asymmetry, all the experimental observations follow Skinner et al. (1997).

The Leech Central Pattern Generator for Swimming

The 21 segmental ganglia of the leech are responsible for producing the traveling wave that enables the animal to swim. A small number of neurons in each ganglion have been identified as responsible for producing the rhythms. These can be crudely divided into three groups according to the phase in the cycle when they fire: (1) $-10°$ to 70°, (2) 130° to 180°, and (3) 220° to 260°. Most of the interactions are inhibitory, and the three groups essentially divide the cycle into 120° subgroups. The fact that the coupling signals occur at different phases in the cycle motivated the idea of temporal averaging that was used to create the phase models described in the preceding sections for the lamprey circuits.

In the leech, the coupling appears to be important in the creation of the oscillations: an isolated ganglion is able to produce a crude oscillatory rhythm, but the rhythm is much more regular in the intact chain. The coupling within the leech CPG has many long-range connections. While the lamprey also has such connections, the success of the simple nearest-neighbor models in explaining many of the details of the lamprey swim pattern suggests that the long-range connections are not as important as they are in the leech. The length of the coupling is important in the formation of the phase lags for the leech CPG; unlike the lamprey CPG, the intersegmental phase lags are smaller for the intact cord than for pieces of the cord. This can be understood from mathematical work showing that coupling to multiple neighbors in general decreases the phase lag (see Cohen et al., 1992, for a reference).

In this CPG, there is a systematic gradient in the intrinsic frequency of each of the ganglia; the gradient is opposite the direction of the wave, which is rostrocaudal. The general mathematical theory in Kopell and Ermentrout (1986) shows that there can be waves in locally coupled chains with both frequency gradients and asymmetric coupling. However, the theory does not address the effects of the significant conduction delays in the leech cord, or the effects of coupling that might extend for a large fraction of the cord. Thus, the creation of the phase lags is less understood in the leech than in the other two examples presented above.

The Procerebral Lobe of *Limax*

Waves in the nervous system occur not only in locomotor activities but in sensory processing as well. A well-studied example occurs in the procerebral (PC) lobe of the *Limax*, or common garden slug, that is responsible for the olfactory processing of the slug. The PC lobe can be isolated from the animal along with the sensory apparatus. Under resting conditions, optical imaging of the lobe reveals a regular slow oscillatory wave that travels from the distal region of the lobe to the basal region (Kleinfeld et al., 1994). The frequency is about a half a cycle per second and the velocity is about 250 μm per second. The lobe itself is about 500 μm, so that, as in the lamprey, at any given point in time, there is only one wave on the lobe. When the animal is exposed to a novel odor, the oscillations quickly synchronize for several cycles and then return to the traveling waves. The reasons for the waves and the synchronization are not known, although it is believed that they may be crucial in odor learning and recognition. Blocking the oscillations impairs the animal's ability to be conditioned to odor stimuli.

In a recent paper, Ermentrout, Flores, and Gelperin (1998) developed a minimal model for the oscillations and waves in the lobe under a variety of experimental conditions. As in the lamprey work, the intent was to suggest a general model that was not dependent on biophysical details that are not known for the PC lobe. Since the lobe consists of many coupled intrinsically oscillating cells, modeling it as a network of coupled oscillators is natural.

The lobe consists of two layers, the cell layer and the neuropil. The source of the waves appears to be intrinsically oscillatory bursting cells in the cell layer. There are many interneurons that send processes into the neuropil and are likely important in the maintenance of the wave and the switch to synchrony. The double layer of cells is an important part of the anatomical structure to be retained in the model. One layer represents the locally connected bursting neurons and the other represents the diffusely coupled interneurons. Interneuron connections, believed to be an important part of the odor associative memory, are globally coupled, while the bursting neurons are coupled locally. Each layer consists of an $N \times m$ array of oscillators, with N representing the apical-basal axis (the direction of wave propagation) and m representing the axis parallel to the wave fronts. Each bursting cell influences only the interneuron in its immediate neighborhood, while each interneuron influences every bursting cell. The interneuron coupling is very weak during the resting state; the odor stimulus induces greater activity in the interneurons, which is modeled by an increase in their coupling strength.

In the PC lobe, the mechanism for wave production was hypothesized by Ermentrout et al. (1998) to be a gradient in the coupling strength, with the neurons in the basal end having stronger coupling than the neurons in the apical end. The reason for this choice is that the basal end is thicker and broader than the apical end, so that there could be more neurons involved in the rhythm at the thicker end. The interaction function for each layer was

$$H(\phi) = C + K \sin(\phi - \xi) \tag{5}$$

with slightly different values of C and K for the two layers. The layer with the locally connected bursting neurons is responsible for producing the waves, while the other layer has connections that collapse the wave to synchrony when there is an odor stimulant. Considering a slice in the direction of the waves, the relevant form of the full set of equations for the layer of oscillators is given by Equation 4.

As in the simpler Equation 2, without a gradient in coupling strengths, there is a dominant direction of coupling that determines the phase lags. The major role of the gradient is to determine which coupling direction is dominant. (It is the one with coupling from the larger strengths to the weaker ones if the ascending and descending coupling is the same.) In particular, the coupling strengths do not change the phase lags. This can be deduced from the general equations in Kopell and Ermentrout (1990), and can be seen easily from equations for one-way coupling, as in Equation 3, with coupling strengths included.

An interesting feature of a model in which the dominance is determined by coupling gradients is that it mimics one feature of a frequency gradient while still producing constant speed waves: If a chain of oscillators has a frequency gradient, splitting the chain at some point produces two smaller chains having different locked frequencies; this is also true if the chain has a gradient in coupling strengths. This feature is seen in the *Limax* preparation.

Long-Range Coupling

The theory discussed in the previous sections deals only with local coupling (nearest neighbor and multiple neighbor, but still short compared to the length of the chain). There have been few studies so far on the effects of long-range coupling (see Cohen et al., 1992, for some references). One of these (Ermentrout and Kopell, 1994a) was motivated by trying to understand why the wavelength of the traveling wave in lamprey (and other anguiliform species that swim by undulation) is approximately one body length. Although the theory discussed above provides a framework for understanding how the wavelength can stay constant when the swimming speed changes, it does not provide any clues to why that wavelength should be related to the body length.

Ermentrout and Kopell showed that long coupling between the ends and an interior region, adjusted so that the coupling produces antiphase between the oscillators directly coupled, can create trav-

eling waves that have the correct wavelength. With the same architecture, but changes in the relative strengths of the ends-to-middle coupling versus middle-to-ends coupling, a new, stable pattern can emerge: the chain displays a standing wave, characteristic of the spinal cord of amphibia during a trotting gait. Thus, this architecture is a substrate for both swimming movements (traveling wave) and trotting movements in an amphibian (Ermentrout and Kopell, 1994a). The long fibers cannot be essential to the production of the phase lags in adult lamprey, since the waves form in small portions of the animal. It is possible that a mechanism involving long fibers is responsible for creating the appropriate phase lags in young animals, and that learning mechanisms then enable this information to be encoded in local synapses, which can then work without global connectivity (Ermentrout and Kopell, 1994b).

Phase Oscillators and Relaxation Oscillators

Equation 1 is derived from a physical description of oscillators and their interactions by a reduction procedure described in a previous section. When the reduction procedure is not valid, the emergent behavior of the collection of oscillators can be very different from that of the chains described in the preceding sections.

One such situation in which the reduction procedure is not generally valid involves relaxation oscillators coupled using models of excitatory chemical synapses (see PHASE-PLANE ANALYSIS OF NEURAL NETS). Such oscillators have critical differences in the mechanisms by which the phase lags are determined. For interactions mimicking fast chemical synapses, Somers and Kopell (1995) described a coupling scheme they called fast threshold modulation, or FTM. In that mathematical description, at sufficiently high or low voltages of the presynaptic cell, the synaptic conductance saturates, so that the postsynaptic cell receives a current that is (on the high or low branch) independent of the trajectory of the presynaptic cell. Thus, the postsynaptic cell is essentially uncoupled from the presynaptic one, but has its voltage equation (and so its effective threshold for firing) changed during the input.

The different mechanisms lead to some important contrasts in properties. One is that variations in frequency or in inputs among relaxation oscillators coupled by FTM need not lead to phase differences among the oscillators, as occurs for Equation 2 (Somers and Kopell, 1995). This provides a potential mechanism to be used in constructing a network whose phase lags are well regulated even if the frequencies are not. A second difference concerns speed of locking: long chains of oscillators of the form of Equation 2 can take many, many cycles to approach the locked solution, with the time increasing with the length of the chain. By contrast, a long chain of relaxation oscillators can lock within a couple of cycles (Somers and Kopell, 1995).

It is difficult to obtain traveling waves in a chain of such oscillators; the usual outcome is approximate synchrony unless the coupling is very weak (in which case the averaging procedure is relevant). Indeed, changes in gating of synapses or voltage range of the presynaptic cell can change the mechanism of the interaction from that of phase oscillator-like behavior to that of FTM, changing waves into almost synchronous cell assemblies. Thus, a generalized signal in the network that changes, e.g., the threshold or sharpness of the synapses can provide a stimulus-induced change in mechanism, and hence of emergent behavior (Somers and Kopell, 1995). We saw in the *Limax* example how a stimulus produced change from waves to synchrony; this provides another kind of mechanism for such a change.

In a recent paper, Izhikevich (2000) has shown that it is possible to derive coupled-phase models derived from relaxation oscillators. The corresponding interaction functions, $H(\phi)$, have a discontinuity at the origin. This implies that a reciprocally coupled pair will synchronize even if there is a difference in the intrinsic frequencies. Thus, in theory one can connect fast-threshold modulation with phase models and obtain the properties of the former by using the easily analyzed formalism of the latter.

Chains of relaxation oscillators have also featured in models of a single dendrite of the basal ganglia dopaminergic neuron. Based on the experiments and models of Wilson and Callaway, Medvedev and Kopell modeled the compartments of the dendrite as a chain of coupled relaxation oscillators. (For a reference to the work of Wilson and Callaway, see Medvedev and Kopell, 2001.) The aim of the work was to understand the origin of long transients in frequency observed in slice preparations and biophysical models. The model was able to explain how the electrical coupling between the compartments can produce a spiking rate decreasing over many cycles; this decrease is analogous to spike frequency adaptation, but does not use any unusual currents normally associated with adaptation.

More complicated local circuits, with several different elements within a local circuit, may have some features of each type. The properties of such composite oscillators were studied in the context of the swimmeret CPG system (Skinner and Mulloney, 1998). In that system, the theory using averaged coupling is successful in understanding phase lags in normal and perturbed settings. A model based on the biophysical underpinnings of the component cells allows one to address finer questions relating to control of burst durations and frequency.

Road Maps: Dynamic Systems; Motor Pattern Generators
Related Reading: Collective Behavior of Coupled Oscillators; Half-Center Oscillators Underlying Rhythmic Movements; Spinal Cord of Lamprey: Generation of Locomotor Patterns

References

Cohen, A., Ermentrout, G. B., Kiemel, T., Kopell, N., Sigvardt, K., and Williams, T., 1992, Modelling of intersegmental coordination in the lamprey central pattern generator for locomotion, *Trends Neurosci.,* 15:434–438. ◆

Cohen, A. H., Holmes, P. J., and Rand, R. H., 1982, The nature of the coupling between segmental oscillators of the lamprey spinal generator for locomotion: A mathematical model, *J. Math. Biol.,* 13:345–369.

Ermentrout, G. B., Flores, J., and Gelperin, A., 1998, Minimal model of oscillations and waves in the *Limax* olfactory lobe with tests of the model's predictive power, *J. Neurophysiol.,* 79:2677–2689.

Ermentrout, G. B., and Kopell, N., 1984, Frequency plateaus in a chain of weakly coupled oscillators: I, *SIAM J. Math. Anal.,* 15:215–237.

Ermentrout, G. B., and Kopell, N., 1994a, Inhibition-produced patterning in chains of coupled nonlinear oscillators, *SIAM J. Appl. Math.,* 54:478–507.

Ermentrout, G. B., and Kopell, N., 1994b, Learning of phase-lags in coupled neural oscillators, *Neural Computat.,* 6:225–241.

Friesen, W. O., and Pearce, R. A., 1993, Mechanisms of intersegmental coordination in leech locomotion, *Semin. Neurosci.,* 5:41–47. ◆

Guckenheimer, J., and Holmes, P., 1983, *Nonlinear Oscillations, Dynamical Systems and Bifurcations of Vector Fields,* New York: Springer-Verlag. ◆

Izhikevich, E., 2000, Phase equations for relaxation oscillators, *SIAM J. Appl. Math.,* 60:1789–1805.

Kleinfeld, D., Delaney, K. R., Fee, M. S., Flores, J. A., Tank, D. W., and Gelperin, A., 1994, Dynamics of propagating waves in the olfactory network of a terrestrial mollusk: An electrical and optical study, *J. Neurophysiol.,* 72:1402–1419.

Kopell, N., 1987, Toward a theory of modeling central pattern generators, in *Neural Control of Rhythmic Movements in Vertebrates* (A. H. Cohen, S. Grillner, and S. Rossignol, Eds.), New York: Wiley, pp. 369–413. ◆

Kopell, N., and Ermentrout, G. B., 1986, Symmetry and phaselocking in chains of weakly coupled oscillators, *Commun. Pure Appl. Math.* 39:623–660.

Kopell, N., and Ermentrout, G. B., 1990, Phase transitions and other phenomena in chains of coupled oscillators, *SIAM J. Appl. Math.,* 50:1014–1052.

Medvedev, G., and Kopell, N., 2001, Synchronization and transient dynamics in chains of FitzHugh-Nagumo oscillators with strong electrical coupling, *SIAM J. Appl. Math.,* 61:1762–1801.

Skinner, F., and Mulloney, B., 1998, Intersegmental coordination of limb movements during locomotion: Mathematical models predict circuits that drive swimmeret beating, *J. Neurosci.,* 18:3831–3842.

Somers, D., and Kopell, N., 1995, Waves and synchrony in networks of oscillators of relaxation and non-relaxation type, *Physica D,* 88:1–14.

Skinner, F., Kopell, N., and Mulloney, B., 1997, How does the crayfish swimmeret system work: Insights from nearest neighborcoupled models, *J. Comp. Neurosci.,* 4:151–160.

Chaos in Biological Systems

Leon Glass

Introduction

Chaotic dynamics, i.e., *aperiodic dynamics in deterministic systems displaying sensitivity to initial conditions,* has emerged from a relatively obscure topic of mathematics to an area that is of great current interest among scientists as well as the general public. The important characteristics of chaos are the apparent irregularity of time traces and the divergence of the trajectories over time (starting from two nearby initial conditions) in a system that is deterministic. Although the rhythm is irregular, the underlying deterministic equations can lead to structure in the dynamics (Figure 1).

Deterministic chaotic dynamics is different in principle from what is commonly known as random dynamics. In random dynamics, prediction is intrinsically impossible, except in a statistical sense. A natural system believed to be random is the radioactive decay of isotopes, leading to random time intervals between decay events.

Chaotic dynamics is now well-documented in a variety of different mathematical models, physical systems, and biological systems (Cvitanovic, 1989). Introductions to chaotic dynamics suitable for biology include Glass and Mackey (1988), Kaplan and Glass (1995), Strogatz (1994), and Liebovitch (1998). Research in biology has extended from studies of dynamics in well-controlled model systems to analysis of spontaneous dynamics in organisms. Although all agree that spontaneous activity is very complicated, reflecting the interactions of the intrinsic physiological control mechanisms with the fluctuating environment, the extent to which concepts developed in simpler chaotic systems can be applied is controversial. The word *chaos* has been used with so many different nuances of meaning and operational definitions that the original technical meaning (i.e., the highlighted phrase in the opening sentence of this article) can no longer be assumed. However, in this article, I will stick to this original technical definition of chaos.

Identifying Chaos

Chaos in Deterministic Systems

In a deterministic system there is a definite equation governing the dynamics. Biological systems have been modeled by difference

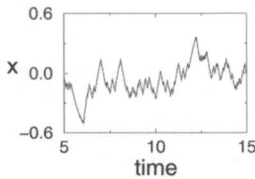

Figure 1. Dynamics from a deterministic high-dimensional differential equation representing a highly interconnected gene or neural network. The extremely irregular dynamics reflect deterministic chaos rather than random noise, but it would be difficult to develop criteria to determine this without huge amounts of data. The network is of the sort discussed in Mestl et al. (1997) with 32 model "neurons," each of which has 15 randomly chosen inputs. The graph shows the values of one of those variables as a function of time.

equations, differential equations, delay-differential equations, and partial differential equations that display chaotic dynamics. As long as one is dealing with deterministic equations, the signature of deterministic chaos is clear. It is easy to numerically integrate the equations starting from two nearby initial conditions and to watch the evolution. Chaotic systems display aperiodic dynamics with the same statistical properties (such as density histograms) for both trajectories. In addition, the trajectories should diverge but remain in a bounded region. Many equations also show characteristic bifurcations (changes in qualitative dynamics) as parameters change that are representative of well-studied routes to chaos. Perhaps the best known of these, the "period doubling route to chaos," has been found in a variety of simple equations and experimental systems. As a parameter of an equation changes, the period of an oscillation undergoes successive doublings. For example, if the period of an oscillation was initially 1 s, as a parameter changed the period would have doubled to 2 s, then as the parameter changed a bit more the period would have doubled to 4 s, and so forth. However, the parameter range over which each successively doubled period persists decreases geometrically, so that in practice it is very difficult to observe experimentally more than two or three of the successive doublings. The period doublings lead eventually to chaotic dynamics, which arise after a parameter crosses a threshold (Cvitanovic, 1989).

When dealing with dynamics in experimental systems or in natural systems, it is much more problematic to figure out the dynamic origins of complicated rhythms that are not periodic. Such rhythms will usually arise from the interaction between a deterministic system and random noise, and it is difficult to dissect out the relative effects of the determinism and the noise (Ruelle, 1994). Since there is no clear operational definition for chaos in experimental data, analyses generally focus on other properties of time series that can be defined operationally. However, if chaos has property C, and a time series has a property C, it does not follow that the time series is chaotic. Several books and web sites deal with time-series analysis methods and their pitfalls (Ott, Sauer, and Yorke, 1994; Abarbanel, 1996; Kantz and Schreiber, 1997; Goldberger et al., 2000).

I now summarize many features that are assessed in analyses of time series.

Power spectrum. The power spectrum of a time series can be easily determined using fast Fourier transform algorithms. However, since one can always construct random models that have the same power spectrum as a deterministic model, the power spectrum is not a good measure for defining chaos.

Dimension. Grassberger and Procaccia (1983) defined the correlation dimension of a set of points embedded in d dimensions. The set of points could be generated in a variety of ways, including

discrete time processes (e.g., time intervals between neural spikes or outputs of a difference equation) or continuous processes (e.g., recording from an electroencephalogram or a continuous differential equation). Call r the distance away from a given point. The point correlation function, $C_i(r)$ is proportional to the number of points lying within a radius r of a point i. The spatial correlation function, $C(r)$, is an average of the $C_i(r)$ over all points. Then the correlation dimension is v, if $C(r) = kr^v$ for small values of r. For random points distributed in d dimensions, $C(r) = kr^d$, so that the dimension is an integer equal to the dimension of the space in which points are distributed. Thus a line has dimension 1, a plane has dimension 2, and so forth. However, some sets of points, called *fractals*, have a fractional dimension. Some workers take a fractional correlation dimension as a definition for deterministic chaos, since many chaotic dynamical systems have attractors with a fractional dimension. However, there are many pitfalls associated with determining the dimension, and not all chaotic systems have a fractional dimension. Consequently, a fractional correlation dimension cannot be accepted as a definition for chaos.

Lyapunov exponent. The Lyapunov exponent measures the rate at which trajectories diverge. A negative Lyapunov exponent indicates convergence of trajectories and a positive Lyapunov exponent indicates divergence of trajectories. Therefore, for a time series a positive Lyapunov exponent is a necessary condition for chaotic dynamics. However, the numerical algorithms for determination of the Lyapunov exponent may yield a positive exponent for periodic oscillations with large first derivatives, or in noisy systems. Therefore, a positive Lyapunov exponent found using numerical methods from naturally occurring data cannot be taken as a definition for chaos.

Poincaré map. Certain difference equations display period doubling bifurcations and chaos. An example is the quadratic map in which the value of a variable at one time is a quadratic function of the value at the previous time. The period doubling route to chaos is observed as the height of the quadratic function is increased. Some experimental data can be plotted so that the value of a variable at one time is plotted as a function of its value at the preceding time. For example, given a sequence of interspike intervals, it is possible to plot one interspike interval as a function of the preceding interval. If data plotted in this fashion clearly fall on a one-dimensional curve that is known to give chaotic dynamics, then this is good evidence for chaotic dynamics in the data. However, most biological examples in which data are plotted in this fashion do not give such clear-cut results, but rather give clouds of points.

Determinism and prediction. Since chaotic dynamics are generated by deterministic equations, in chaotic systems it should be possible either to demonstrate determinism or to predict dynamics that will occur in the proximate future. Several methods have been developed to try to make predictions based on past dynamics without necessarily knowing the equations of motion. A confounding factor of prediction tests is that random inputs to linear and nonlinear systems lead to correlations for short times that enable prediction even though the system is not deterministic and hence not chaotic. Random signals in which there are brief randomly inserted segments, all of which have the same waveform, would also be expected to show short-term predictability, but the underlying signal would not be chaotic.

Surrogate data. None of the above measures can be simply applied to determine if a given data set displays deterministic chaos. Consequently, several people have advocated generating "surrogate" data sets that have similar statistical properties to a given data set but are generated from a random process (Kantz and Schreiber, 1997). For example, it is a simple matter to generate a random time series that has an identical power spectrum to a given time series. Statistical analyses are then carried out using the time series under investigation and surrogates. The results of the analysis of the surrogate data are compared with the analysis of the original data. The origins of significant differences are then analyzed. They may be due to deterministic chaos, although other hypotheses, such as failure to capture some important aspect in the surrogate data set, need to be entertained. Application of this technique has led to the recognition that many earlier claims for deterministic chaos were in error.

Chaos at Subcellular and Cellular Levels

Carefully controlled experiments, in which it is possible to generate large amounts of high-quality data while varying critical control parameters, have demonstrated chaotic dynamics in chemical, electronic, and hydrodynamic systems (Cvitanovic, 1989). Observations of chaotic dynamics in biological systems are more problematic. I will briefly review some of the areas in which there have been claims for chaotic dynamics.

Subcellular Dynamics: Ion Channels

The basis for neural activity lies in the changes of conductance of specialized protein molecules called ion channels that allow ions to pass between the intracellular and the extracellular medium. For example, action potentials of nerve cells are usually associated with the opening of sodium ion channels. Classical intracellular electrophysiological techniques record the average activity over the thousands of ion channels present on a single nerve cell. Macroscopic ionic models describe this average activity and its dependence on the membrane voltage. An important technological advance, called the patch clamp, enabled researchers to measure directly the conductance of a single ion channel during its open state. Experimental recording of a single ion channel typically shows a complex switching behavior in which the channel makes transitions between open and closed states in a seemingly random manner. Most researchers believe that this switching is random and have developed appropriate theoretical descriptions. However, deterministic chaotic models may show the same statistical features as the random models (Liebovitch, 1998). At the current time, new information about the structural properties of ion channels is accumulating, and this should yield new insights into the molecular basis of the conformational changes that underlie the channel activity. Independent of the outcome of that endeavor, the observation that subcellular ion channel events are following a random (or perhaps chaotic) dynamics raises a conceptual problem: Why is it possible to study cellular or supercellular processes using deterministic ionic models? Presumably, the thousands of channels in a single cell, and the millions and billions in collections of cells, enable an averaging, so that macroscopic equations are valid, with fluctuations being small.

Cellular Activity in Single Cells

The electrical activity of single cells can be easily measured using intracellular or extracellular microelectrodes, either in vitro or in vivo. The activity can be measured during spontaneous activity or in response to manipulation of environmental parameters. In my opinion, the most convincing demonstrations of chaotic dynamics in biological systems have been carried out in this scale of preparation. Periodic stimulation of oscillatory or excitable biological systems, such as nerve or cardiac tissue, has identified chaotic dynamics over restricted ranges of stimulation parameters (Glass and Mackey, 1988). Over other stimulation ranges there are regular rhythms in which there are repeating sequences of stimuli and action potentials. This work is placed on a firm footing by extensive theoretical analyses and numerical simulation mathematical mod-

els. Depending on the stimulation parameters, the theoretical models display periodic behavior or deterministic chaos in agreement with experimental observations. Moreover, in the chaotic region, plotting the stimulus phase as a function of the preceding stimulus phase to generate the Poincaré map can give a plot that is similar to the quadratic map (Glass and Mackey, 1988), further supporting the identification of chaos. However, there is no clear functional role for chaos at a cellular level.

Complex Dynamics in Biological Networks

Chaos in Complex Networks

One of the outstanding characteristics of biological systems is that they are characterized by complex networks of interacting elements. Thus, schematic diagrams of biological systems controlling metabolism, hormone secretion, gene activation, hormone secretion, motor activity, and heart rate are notable for being incredibly complex, with multiple feedbacks. Mathematical models developed for complex biological networks often demonstrate chaotic dynamics (Arbib, Érdi, and Szentágothai, 1997; Goldbeter, 1997; Mestl, Bagley, and Glass, 1997; Glass and Mackey, 1988; Sreenivasan, Pradhan, and Rapp, 1999). However, because there are no well-established operational tests for chaos, analyses that claim chaos in experimental or clinical data are often subject to alternative interpretations. Thus, the extent to which data such as heart rate variability or electroencephalographic data reflect deterministic chaos has been hotly debated. In recent years, there have been suggestions that many biological time series that had previously been called chaotic are not chaotic but may be better described using other adjectives ($1/f$ long-range scaling, fractal, multifractal). However, these terms do not have clear implications with regard to the underlying mechanisms. Independent of the detailed mechanisms of fluctuations, a variety of studies have suggested implications for the study of health and disease.

Chaos and Health

Although early studies of biological control networks often emphasized that they served to maintain homeostasis—a relatively constant internal environment—there is now increasing recognition that normal, healthy individuals can be expected to show complex fluctuations in important physiological functions (Goldberger, 1996). Many diseases can be characterized by qualitative changes in dynamics in biological control systems. Since these changes may be associated with bifurcations in appropriate mathematical models of the physiological systems, Mackey and I proposed the term "dynamical disease" to capture the dynamic aspects of disease (Glass and Mackey, 1988).

There are many examples of altered physiological dynamics associated with disease. Diminished heart rate variability is associated with a higher risk of sudden cardiac death. However, since patients do not die from reduced heart rate variability, it is important to clarify the underlying mechanisms. One hypothesis is that impaired cardiac function leads to increased sympathetic nervous activity associated with elevated levels of circulating chemicals (catecholamines). This in turn will increase the heart rate and lead to less variability. Further, since circulating catecholamines are pro-arrhythmic, there can be an increased risk of arrhythmia. In addition, patients with impaired heart function are also more likely to be taking drugs that blunt fluctuations in heart rate, or may even have implanted artificial pacemakers that might lead to a more regular rhythm. Clinical studies that associate higher risk for sudden cardiac death with decreased heart rate variability do not always address these potentially confounding factors. Independent of the mechanism, since low heart rate variability is associated with a higher risk for sudden cardiac death, the analysis of heart rate variability in the clinic has practical utility.

In a similar vein, in neurology, there have been claims that time-series analysis techniques can be useful in predicting the occurrence of an epileptic episode (Schiff, 1998). These types of claims are often hard to validate, since the data sets and the analysis algorithms often are not readily available. However, the recently established Research Resource for Complex Physiologic Signals (Goldberger et al., 2000) may provide an important avenue for publishing both data sets and data analysis packages.

Another practical direction is to apply to biological systems (Moss and Gielen, 2000) methods that can successfully control chaotic dynamics in mathematical models and in physical systems (Ott et al., 1994). Control methods have been applied to control comparatively simple rhythms associated with deterministic dynamics in model experimental systems. However, in cases in which the rhythms are more complex and not definitely associated with deterministic dynamics, further research is needed to validate the utility of chaos control methods.

Discussion

Theoretical studies have demonstrated chaotic dynamics in mathematical models of biological systems ranging from the subcellular level to the organismal level. The most convincing experimental observations of chaotic dynamics in biological systems are associated with the response of biological systems in vitro to periodic stimulation of comparatively well-defined cells or assemblies of cells. The high dimensions of biological systems, the fluctuating environment (leading to nonstationarity), and the subtleties of the numerical methods are factors that make convincing demonstration of chaos in vivo a difficult matter. Therefore, although it might not be surprising that clear demonstrations of deterministic chaos in biology are rare, it is surprising that exaggerated claims founded on weak experimental evidence have been widely accepted without sufficient critical analysis.

Insofar as real biological systems (as opposed to computer models of these systems) are exposed to random thermal and other fluctuations and are composed of large numbers of interacting elements (i.e., they are high-dimensional), it is not easy to decide the appropriate class of theoretical model for a given system. Another difficult issue is to understand the biological significance, if any, of the observed fluctuations. Consider complex fluctuations in the timing between spikes of a neuron: does the neuron function well despite these irregularities, or are the irregularities essential to its task? And if the irregularities are essential for the task, is there any reason to expect that deterministically chaotic irregularities would be better than random ones? Although there have been several interesting speculations about an association of chaos with health and a possible role for chaos in information processing (for a summary, see Arbib et al., 1997), convincing demonstrations of the function of chaos are not yet available. Probably what drives many in brain theory is to understand the neural correlates of the human mind: higher cognitive function, originality, and free will. Humans be-

have neither in a random manner nor in a totally predictable manner. Although it seems inevitable that the mathematical concept of chaos will help us interpret the human brain, definite results pointing in that direction are still meager.

Road Map: Dynamic Systems
Background: I.3. Dynamics and Adaptation in Neural Networks
Related Reading: Chaos in Neural Systems; Stochastic Resonance; Synaptic Noise and Chaos in Vertebrate Neurons

References

Arbib, M. A., Érdi, P., and Szentágothai, J., 1997, *Neural Organization: Structure, Function, and Dynamics*, Cambridge, MA: MIT Press, Sect. 4.3.
Abarbanel, H. D. I., 1996, *Analysis of Observed Chaotic Data*, Berlin: Springer-Verlag. ◆
Cvitanovic, P., Ed., 1989, *Universality in Chaos*, 2nd ed., Bristol: Adam Hilger.
Glass, L., and Mackey, M. C., 1988, *From Clocks to Chaos: The Rhythms of Life*, Princeton, NJ: Princeton University Press. ◆
Goldberger, A. L., 1996, Non-linear dynamics for clinicians: Chaos theory, fractals, and complexity at the bedside, *The Lancet*, 347:1312–1314.
Goldberger, A. L., Amaral, L. A. N., Glass, L., Hausdorff, J. M., Ivanov, P. C., Mark, R. G., Mietus, J. E., Moody, G. B., Peng, C.-K., and Stanley, H. E., 2000, PhysioBank, PhysioTools, and PhysioNet: Components of a New Research Resource for Complex Physiologic Signals, *Circulation*, 101:e215–e220. [*Circulation* electronic pages; http://circ.ahajournals.org/cgi/content/full/101/23/e215]. See also http://www.physionet.org for online data collections.
Goldbeter, A., 1997, *Biochemical Oscillations and Cellular Rhythms: The Molecular Bases of Periodic and Chaotic Behaviour*, Cambridge, Engl.: Cambridge University Press.
Grassberger, I., and Procaccia, I., 1983, Measuring the strangeness of strange attractors, *Physica D*, 9:189–208.
Kantz, H., and Schreiber, T., 1997, *Nonlinear Time Series Analysis*, Cambridge, Engl.: Cambridge University Press. Software available at: http://www.mpipks-dresden.mpg.de/tisean. ◆
Kaplan, D., and Glass, L., 1995, *Understanding Nonlinear Dynamics*, New York: Springer-Verlag. ◆
Liebovitch, L. S., 1998, *Fractals and Chaos Simplified for the Life Sciences*, New York: Oxford University Press. ◆
Ott, E., Sauer, T., and Yorke, J. A., Eds., 1994, *Coping with Chaos*, New York: Wiley.
Mestl, T., Bagley, R. J., and Glass, L., 1997, Common chaos in arbitrarily complex feedback networks, *Phys. Rev. Lett.*, 79:653–656.
Moss, F., and Gielen, S., Eds., 2000, *Handbook of Biological Physics*, vol. 4, *Neuro-informatics, Neural Modelling*, Amsterdam: Elsevier, chaps. 6 and 7.
Ruelle, D., 1994, *Physics Today*, 47:24–30.
Schiff, S. J., 1998, Forecasting brain storms, *Nature Med.*, 4:1117–1118.
Sreenivasan, R., Pradhan, N., and Rapp, P. E., Eds., 1999, *Nonlinear Dynamics and Brain Functioning*, Nova Science Publishers.
Strogatz, S. H., 1994, *Nonlinear Dynamics and Chaos: With Applications in Physics, Biology, Chemistry, and Engineering (Studies in Nonlinearity)*, Cambridge, MA: Perseus. ◆

Chaos in Neural Systems

Kazuyuki Aihara

Introduction

From the viewpoint of dynamical systems theory, biological neurons and neural networks can be understood as nonlinear dynamical systems. Therefore, research on neural systems is a combination of brain science and nonlinear science.

The progress of nonlinear science in the twentieth century deepened our understanding of interesting dynamical phenomena called

deterministic chaos, or simply chaos, although the research history of chaos can be traced back at least to Poincaré's work on the three-body problem in celestial mechanics 100 years ago. Chaotic phenomena, in which a deterministic law generates complicated, non-periodic, and unpredictable behavior, exist in many real-world systems and mathematical models. Chaos has many intriguing characteristics, such as a sensitive dependence on initial conditions, or the so-called butterfly effect (i.e., the influence of a small perturbation in the initial condition diverges with time), and fractal geometrical structure (i.e., chaotic behavior is represented by a strange attractor with a noninteger dimension in the state space) (Ott, Sauer, and Yorke, 1994; see also CHAOS IN BIOLOGICAL SYSTEMS; DYNAMICS AND BIFURCATION IN NEURAL NETS).

In this article, the nonlinear behavior of neural systems is considered with respect to deterministic chaos. Although many of the neural systems that have been studied so far for neural computation have simple dynamics that converge into a steady state corresponding to an equilibrium point or a limit cycle, neural systems with chaotic dynamics produce much more dynamical behavior that may be functional from the viewpoint of information processing (see also COMPUTING WITH ATTRACTORS).

Neurodynamics and Chaos

The nonlinear dynamics of a single neuron can naturally generate deterministic chaos under some conditions. For example, nerve membranes of squid giant axons respond to periodic forcing, such as sinusoidal and periodic pulse stimulation, not only periodically but also chaotically, depending on parameter values of the frequency and the strength of the force and states of nerve membranes (Aihara, 2002). Figure 1 demonstrates a chaotic response observed experimentally in squid giant axon. Chaotic and various other neuronal responses, which provide possible mechanisms of synaptic coding, are also observed in biological neurons stimulated through synapses (Segundo et al., 1998; see also SYNAPTIC NOISE AND CHAOS IN VERTEBRATE NEURONS). Thus, the behavior of a single neuron is essentially very dynamical, although some computational aspects of excitable neurodynamics can be reduced to static and logical calculations typically modeled by the McCulloch-Pitts neuron. Furthermore, chaotic dynamics in neural systems may also be discussed both in the more microscopic level of ion channels and in the mesoscopic and more macroscopic levels of neural networks (Elbert et al., 1994; Freeman, 2000; see also CHAOS IN BIOLOGICAL SYSTEMS).

Although chaotic behavior appears extremely irregular and complicated, it differs entirely from stochastic randomness because chaos is generated according to a definite deterministic rule. This deterministic dynamics enables control, short-term prediction, and change through bifurcation of chaotic behavior. On the other hand, because real neural systems operate in noisy environments, it is an important and delicate problem to clarify the effects of noise on chaotic neurodynamics (Freeman, 2000; Kaneko and Tsuda, 2000; Tsuda, 2001).

Models of Chaotic Neural Networks

Can deterministic chaos in neural systems play a useful role? Biologically based answers to this question are few (Glass, 2001; see also CHAOS IN BIOLOGICAL SYSTEMS), but possible functions of chaos have been explored using theoretical models of chaotic neural networks.

Various models of neurons and neural networks with chaotic dynamics, in both discrete time and continuous time, have been proposed (Aihara, Takabe, and Toyoda, 1990; Lewis and Glass, 1992; Nara et al., 1995; van Vreeswijk and Sompolinsky, 1996; Rabinovich and Abarbanel, 1998; Freeman, 2000; Kaneko and Tsuda, 2000; Tsuda, 2001). For example, chaos in nerve membranes can be well described by continuous-time nerve equations like the Hodgkin-Huxley and FitzHugh-Nagumo equations (Aihara, 2002). It is an important research subject to extend such biologically realistic neuronal models by considering difference of excitability types (see CANONICAL NEURAL MODELS) and input effects through both chemical and electrical synapses (see NEOCORTEX: CHEMICAL AND ELECTRICAL SYNAPSES; TEMPORAL DYNAMICS OF BIOLOGICAL SYNAPSES).

On the other hand, simpler neuron models are desirable for elucidating possible principles of information processing with chaotic dynamics in large-scale neural networks both mathematically and numerically. For this purpose, a simple discrete-time model of chaotic neural networks has been proposed in which the neuronal elements qualitatively reproduce chaotic responses experimentally observed in squid giant axons (Aihara et al., 1990; Aihara, 2002). This model, based on the earlier Caianiello's neuronic equations and the Nagumo-Sato model with refractoriness, considers spatiotemporal external inputs from outside the network, spatiotemporal feedback inputs through mutual interactions among constituent neurons in the network, and refractory effects as a general discrete-

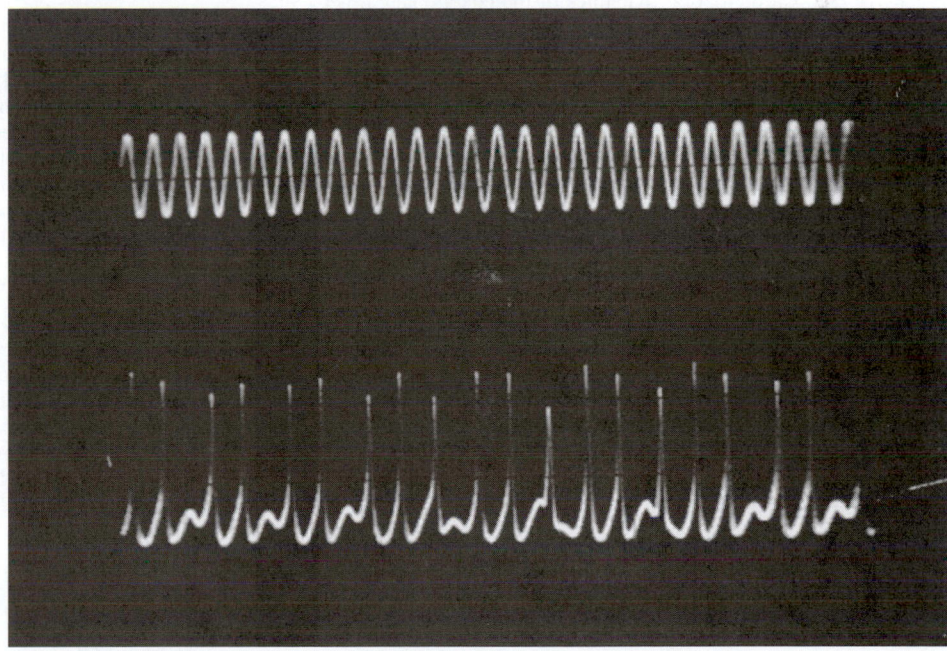

Figure 1. An example of chaotic response (below) of squid giant axon in a state of self-sustained oscillation to stimulation of a sinusoidal current (above).

time model of neural networks composed of neurons with their own chaotic dynamics (Aihara et al., 1990; Adachi and Aihara, 1997; Aihara, 2002). In fact, by adjusting the values of parameters, the model of chaotic neural networks can include many conventional discrete-time neuron models, such as the McCulloch-Pitts neurons with the Heaviside output function, analog neurons with the logistic output function used in backpropagation neural networks, and the Nagumo-Sato neurons with response characteristics of complete devil's staircases. Thus, with the model of chaotic neural networks, chaotic dynamics can be introduced into conventional discrete-time neural networks to explore possible functions and computational roles of spatiotemporal chaos in neural information processing by comparing the performance of the chaotic neural networks with that of the conventional neural networks in the common framework.

There is another approach to modeling chaos in neural systems. Rather than connecting chaotic neuronal elements, network dynamics can produce chaos by devising interactions through feedback connections among simpler neuronal elements, as follows: piecewise linear models (Lewis and Glass, 1992), balanced excitation and inhibition with sparsely connected strong synapses (van Vreeswijk and Sompolinsky, 1996), reduction of asymmetric connectivity storing cyclic memories by a pseudo-inverse method (Nara et al., 1995), coupled mesoscopic oscillators with different delayed feedback loops (Freeman, 2000), and two recurrent neural networks with excitatory and inhibitory feedback connections and stochastic renewal of dynamics representing synaptic noise (Kaneko and Tsuda, 2000; Tsuda, 2001).

Possible Functions of Spatiotemporal Chaos in Neural Networks

Several aspects of useful computational dynamics with spatiotemporal chaos in neural systems are reviewed with the model of chaotic neural networks below. Since each constituent element of the chaotic neural network model has its own chaotic dynamics, the spatiotemporal dynamics of the whole network is fundamentally very rich, complicated, flexible, and dependent on the coupling of chaotic neuronal elements. The adjustment of chaotic dynamics in elemental neurons by constraining architecture, interactions among neurons, and other parameters in the model leads to functional harnessing of the spatiotemporal dynamics of the chaotic neural networks (Aihara et al., 1990; Rabinovich and Abarbanel, 1998; Kaneko and Tsuda, 2000).

Dynamical Association

Associative memory is one of the most popular applications of neural networks (see ASSOCIATIVE NETWORKS; COMPUTING WITH ATTRACTORS; DYNAMICS OF ASSOCIATION AND RECALL; STATISTICAL MECHANICS OF NEURAL NETWORKS). As an example, we can consider the nonlinear dynamics of autoassociative memory networks composed of 100 chaotic neurons, where the synaptic weights are determined by the correlation matrix of four stored patterns: "cross," "triangle," "wave," and "star" (Adachi and Aihara, 1997).

Figure 2A shows spatiotemporal patterns generated by the associative dynamics of the chaotic neural network. In a recalling process in the conventional autoassociative memory network, the network state quickly converges from a perturbed stored pattern to the exact stored pattern, which is an asymptotically stable fixed point of the network dynamics. The network state of the chaotic neural network, on the other hand, displays itinerant behavior among stored patterns, as shown in Figure 2A, if the network parameters are appropriately adjusted so that the refractoriness is strong enough to escape from any fixed points except the totally

quiescent state at which all neurons are resting. The pattern at $t = 1$ in Figure 2A is very close to the stored pattern of "wave." If the network were the conventional autoassociative memory, it would keep this pattern of "wave" forever after $t = 1$. However, the chaotic network continues recalling different stored patterns and their reversed patterns successively, intermittently, nonperiodically, and unpredictably; e.g., the patterns at $t = 23$ and $t = 80$ in Figure 2A are very close to the pattern "cross" and the reversed pattern of "triangle," respectively. It should be noted that this dynamical association process is different from cyclic memory, in which the order of recalled patterns is predictably periodic, as designed by synaptic connections.

Moreover, external inputs to neurons corresponding to a stored pattern can attract the spatiotemporally chaotic dynamics near the stored pattern for a while but not eternally, as shown in Figure 2B, where external inputs corresponding to the stored pattern "triangle" are applied to the chaotic neural network of Figure 2A. Actually, chaotic dynamics is effective for achieving a quick response to changing external inputs (van Vreeswijk and Sompolinsky, 1996; Rabinovich and Abarbanel, 1998).

The spatiotemporal dynamics of Figure 2A can be interpreted as either searching stored patterns or generating spatiotemporal patterns composed of static patterns memorized by synaptic weights. This dynamic may be related to a nonlinear phenomenon called *chaotic itinerancy*, widely observed in different nonlinear models of cortical neural networks, globally coupled maps, and optical turbulence (Kaneko and Tsuda, 2000; Tsuda, 2001). Recurrent neural networks composed of McCulloch-Pitts types of neurons display similar dynamics with chaotic association when reducing asymmetric connectivity storing cyclic memories (Nara et al., 1995).

Related to this kind of memory dynamics, Freeman and colleagues proposed, on the basis of their physiological experiments on the olfactory neural system, an intriguing hypothesis: Chaotic neural activities play functional roles in a global and unstructured basal state with the capability of rapid and unbiased access to learned patterns evoked by trained odors and a catchbasin state classifying and learning unknown patterns evoked by novel or unfamiliar odors (Freeman, 2000).

Dynamical Optimization

The spatiotemporal searching dynamics demonstrated in Figure 2A also can be applied as a new kind of heuristic method to combinatorial optimization problems, especially the *NP*-hard problems that are quite important in many industrial and engineering applications. In the field of neural computation, gradient descent neurodynamics with a computational energy function has been applied to combinatorial optimization problems like the traveling salesman problems (TSP) (see OPTIMIZATION, NEURAL). Although this dynamical method for combinatorial optimization is an interesting heuristic technique, its naive applications would usually suffer from the so-called local minimum problem.

Since the spatiotemporal dynamics of the chaotic neural networks can easily escape from local minimum states, the performance of the chaotic neural networks for *NP*-hard problems is expected to be better than that of the conventional neural networks with simple gradient descent dynamics. This method utilizes chaotic fluctuation rather than stochastic fluctuation for combinatorial optimization. We can theoretically guarantee the global searching capability of the chaotic neural networks under some sufficient conditions for fully developed chaotic dynamics (Aihara, 2002). However, it is speculated that efficient searching is achieved when the chaotic dynamics generates an appropriate strange attractor with fractal structure, which may be a zero measure with respect to the Lebesque measure of the whole state space but includes globally

Figure 2. Associative dynamics of a chaotic neural network with four stored patterns. The network is composed of 100 chaotic neurons with refractoriness (Adachi and Aihara, 1997). *A*, Spatiotemporally chaotic patterns of the chaotic neural network. The output pattern of 100 constituent neurons is displayed in the form of a 10 × 10 matrix with black and white squares showing firing and quiescent neurons, respectively. *B*, Response of the chaotic neural network to the stimulation corresponding to the stored pattern "triangle."

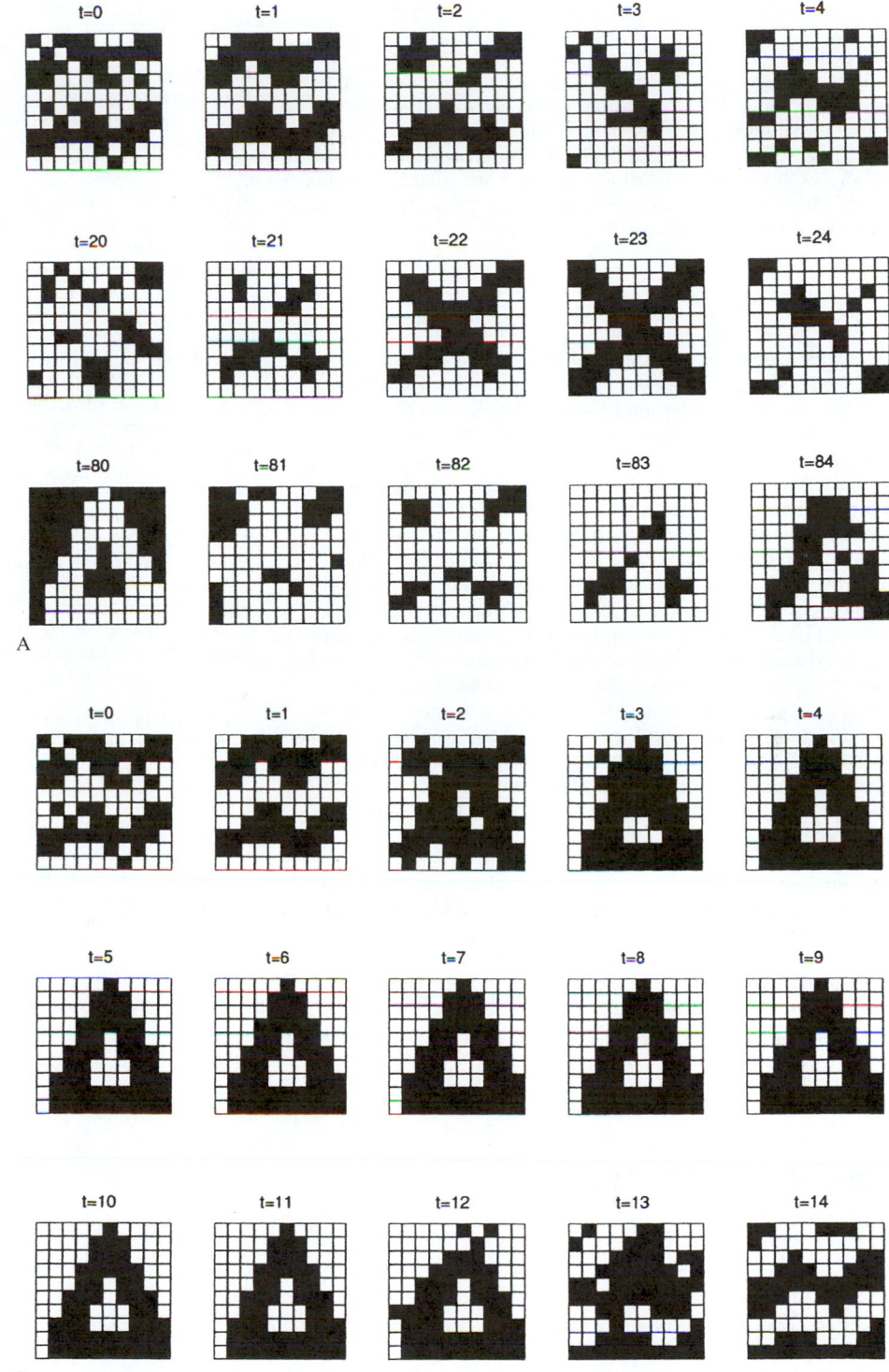

optimal or near-optimal solutions. The optimization efficiency can be further improved by introducing chaotic simulated annealing with changing network bifurcation parameter values ranging from fully chaotic states to fixed points and by combining chaotic neurodynamics with effective heuristic methods like the 2-opt algorithm and the tabu search algorithm (Aihara, 2002).

Cantor Coding

Tsuda and colleagues (Tsuda, 2001) proposed a chaos-driven contracting system, a simple example of which is a chaotic neural network with three neurons in which an unstable chaotic neuron drives a contracting system composed of a stable excitatory neuron and a stable inhibitory neuron. In this network, information of a symbolic sequence generated by the forcing chaotic neuron is encoded on a Cantor-like set in the state space of the contracting subsystem. Because the system can be extended to a more general architecture composed of a recurrent neural system with chaotic itinerant dynamics and a contracting neural network stimulated by the former network, similar phenomena are expected to be experimentally observed at CA3 and CA1 in the hippocampus and at the olfactory bulb and the prepyriform cortex in the olfactory neural system. These neural networks may ultimately be involved in the formation of episodic memory (Tsuda, 2001).

Discussion

The chaotic neural networks and the possible computational dynamics with dynamical association, combinatorial optimization, and Cantor coding have been reviewed as simple examples of neural systems with chaotic dynamics. Although theoretical and experimental studies on chaos in neural systems further suggest other possible roles of chaotic neurodynamics in relation to higher functions of the brain, such as adaptation, perception, episodic memory, learning, awareness, intentionality, and thought (Freeman, 2000; Tsuda, 2001), it is still an important open question to experimentally prove or disprove the existence of these functions of chaos in real biological systems (Glass, 2001; see CHAOS IN BIOLOGICAL SYSTEMS). It is certain, however, that real nerve membranes have chaotic dynamics, while many artificial neuronal models are based upon oversimplified threshold dynamics. The chaotic dynamics in the level of single neurons may be the key to emergence of organized functions in biological neural networks (Rabinovich and Abarbanel, 1998). Thus, it is an important future problem to examine in detail dynamical cell assemblies and possible spatiotemporal coding (Fujii et al., 1996) in neural networks composed of chaotic neurons.

Neural systems with chaotic spatiotemporal dynamics, on the other hand, can be attractive models for analog neurocomputing (see also ANALOG NEURAL NETS: COMPUTATIONAL POWER; NEURAL AUTOMATA AND ANALOG COMPUTATIONAL COMPLEXITY; SPIKING NEURONS, COMPUTION WITH) because chaotic dynamics can read out the complexity of a real number with time due to instability and nonlinearity. In fact, analog IC chips of chaotic neural networks have already been implemented as a new kind of analog computing circuits for practical applications of spatiotemporal chaos in the fields of engineering (Aihara, 2002).

Road Map: Dynamic Systems
Background: Computing with Attractors
Related Reading: Chaos in Biological Systems; Synaptic Noise and Chaos in Vertebrate Neurons

References

Adachi, M., and Aihara, K., 1997, Associative dynamics in a chaotic neural network, *Neural Networks*, 10:83–98.

Aihara, K., 2002, Chaos engineering and its application to parallel distributed processing with chaotic neural networks, *Proc. IEEE*, 90(5): 919–930. ◆

Aihara, K., Takabe, T., and Toyoda, M., 1990, Chaotic neural networks, *Phys. Lett. A.*, 144:333–340.

Elbert, T., Ray, W. J., Kowalik, Z. J., Skinner, J. E., Graf, K. E., and Birbaumer, N., 1994, Chaos and physiology: Deterministic chaos in excitable cell assemblies, *Physiol. Rev.*, 74:1–47. ◆

Freeman, W. J., 2000, *Neurodynamics: An Exploration in Mesoscopic Brain Dynamics*, London: Springer-Verlag. ◆

Fujii, H., Ito, H., Aihara, K., Ichinose, N., and Tsukada, M., 1996, Dynamical cell assembly hypothesis: Theoretical possibility of spatio-temporal coding in the cortex, *Neural Networks*, 9:1303–1350. ◆

Glass, L., 2001, Synchronization and rhythmic processes in physiology, *Nature*, 410:277–284. ◆

Kaneko, K., and Tsuda, I., 2000, *Complex Systems: Chaos and Beyond*, Berlin: Springer-Verlag. ◆

Lewis, J. E., and Glass, L., 1992, Nonlinear dynamics and symbolic dynamics of neural networks, *Neural Computat.*, 4:621–642.

Nara, S., Davis, P., Kawachi, M., and Totsuji, H., 1995, Chaotic memory dynamics in a recurrent neural network with cycle memories embedded by pseudo-inverse method, *Int. J. Bifurc. Chaos*, 5:1205–1212.

Ott, E., Sauer, T., and Yorke, J. A. (Eds.), 1994, *Coping with Chaos: Analysis of Chaotic Data and the Exploitation of Chaotic Systems*, New York: Wiley. ◆

Rabinovich, M. I., and Abarbanel, H. D. I., 1998, The role of chaos in neural systems, *Neuroscience*, 87:5–14.

Segundo, J. P., Sugihara, G., Dixon, P., Stiber, M., and Bersier, L. F., 1998, The spike trains of inhibited pacemaker neurons seen through the magnifying glass of nonlinear analyses, *Neuroscience*, 87:741–766.

Tsuda, I., 2001, Towards an interpretation of dynamic neural activity in terms of chaotic dynamical systems, *Behav. Brain Sci.*, 24:575–628. ◆

van Vreeswijk, C., and Sompolinsky, H., 1996, Chaos in neuronal networks with balanced excitatory and inhibitory activity, *Science*, 274:1724–1726.

Cognitive Development

Yuko Munakata

Introduction

Two classic questions in the study of cognitive development are:

1. *Where does our knowledge come from?* Questions about origins (whether of knowledge, life, the universe, etc.) form the basis for some of the most interesting, challenging, and hotly debated issues in science and popular culture. In regard to the origins of knowledge, the debate has taken the form of nature versus nurture, and more recently of specifying the interactions between them.
2. *How does change occur?* This question builds on the question of origins. A complete developmental account must specify not only the beginnings (of knowledge, life, the universe, etc.), but also the mechanisms that govern change in the system. The

question of change is one of the most important yet relatively unanswered questions in the study of cognitive development. How do we progress, for example, from not speaking a word to communicating with short phrases to participating in lengthy, complex conversations?

Answering these two classic questions requires the ability to assess what is known at different points in development. For example, what do newborns, older infants, and toddlers know about the permanence of objects in the world? Specifying the time course of development of such knowledge could shed light on questions about the origins of this knowledge and how change occurs. Toward this end, researchers have developed a variety of clever techniques to assess knowledge in children of all ages, even preverbal infants. However, children sometimes provide conflicting impressions of what they know across this variety of techniques, raising another important question:

3. *Why does what children know depend so much on how they are tested*? That is, why is children's knowledge so task dependent? Why do children pass one measure of knowledge with flying colors, while simultaneously failing another measure meant to tap the same knowledge? For example, infants as young as 3.5 months seem to understand the permanence of objects, as assessed by their looking times at events with occluded objects (Baillargeon, 1995). However, infants fail to understand object permanence for many more months, as assessed by whether or not they search for toys that are presented and then hidden.

Resolving these discrepancies in what children seem to know is critical for understanding the origins of knowledge and how change occurs.

Connectionist models have provided a useful tool for exploring these three fundamental questions, as well as many other facets of cognitive development (McClelland and Plunkett, 1995; Elman et al., 1996). Such models provide a useful complement to behavioral studies in general (O'Reilly and Munakata, 2000), and particularly in the study of development. This article describes contributions from connectionist models in exploring the origins of knowledge, mechanisms of change, and the task-dependent nature of children's knowledge. These models span the domains of perception, memory, language, problem solving, and rule use.

Origins of Knowledge

The debate about origins has played out in the domain of infants' perception of the world—whether they experience a "blooming, buzzing confusion," as William James claimed, or come equipped to make sense of objects moving around them. Young infants appear sensitive to the continuity of object motion, the fact that objects move only on connected paths, never jumping from one place to another without traveling a path in between. For example, infants as young as 2.5 months look longer at events in which objects appear to move discontinuously than at events in which the objects move continuously (Spelke et al., 1992). Such longer looking times suggest that infants find the discontinuous events unnatural, and so possess some understanding of object continuity. What are the origins of such knowledge?

An understanding of object continuity may be part of our innate core knowledge (Spelke et al., 1992). However, the label of "innate" leaves many questions unanswered about the origins of knowledge. For example, how do infants come to understand object continuity, and what are the mechanisms underlying such understanding?

These questions were explored in a connectionist model initially developed to explore imprinting behavior in chicks, and object recognition more generally (O'Reilly and Johnson, 2002). The model viewed a simplified environment in which objects moved continuously. Based on this experience, the model developed receptive field representations of objects that encoded continuous locations in space, thereby demonstrating a sensitivity to object continuity.

What were the origins of the model's sensitivity to object continuity? First, the network had recurrent excitatory connections and lateral inhibitory connections in the hidden layers that allowed active units to remain active; specifically, active units continued to send activation to themselves via the recurrent excitatory connections, and they prevented other competing units from becoming active via the lateral inhibitory connections. Thus, when the network viewed an object, certain hidden units became active, and they tended to stay active even as the object moved around in the

input. As a result, the network represented the different input patterns associated with a moving object as the same object on the hidden layer. Second, the network learned according to a Hebbian learning rule, which led the model to associate this hidden unit pattern of activity with the object in different locations in the input. As a result, whenever the object appeared in any of these locations, the network came to activate the same hidden units, or the same object representation. In this way, with exposure to events in the world that conformed to the principle of continuity, the model developed receptive field representations of objects that encoded continuous locations in space, and so learned to "recognize" objects that moved continuously in its environment. Thus, the model provided a precise specification of the potential origins of knowledge about object continuity: a system with recurrent excitatory and lateral inhibitory connections and a Hebbian learning rule, and an environment with objects that move continuously.

One might describe this model in terms of an innate predisposition to understand the continuity of objects, given that the network was structured "from birth" with recurrent excitatory and lateral inhibitory connections and a Hebbian learning rule; all it needed was the typical experience of viewing objects moving continuously in its environment. However, again, it is not clear what benefits would be conferred by calling the developmental timecourse of the model innate. In contrast, the benefits of the model should be clear in providing an explicit, mechanistic account of the potential origins of sensitivity to object continuity.

Mechanisms of Change

Most connectionist models, including the object continuity model, address some aspect of change. Networks change as activations are propagated through them, connection weights adjust during learning, and new forms emerge from the complex interactions of elements in the networks (as with the development of representations of object continuity). Here, we focus on models exploring two important issues regarding developmental changes: critical periods and stages.

Critical Periods

Humans mature at a slower rate than any other species. Counterintuitively, this slow rate of development may provide the perfect biological environment (and a critical period) for mastering complex domains such as language. A connectionist model was developed to explore such critical periods in language learning (Elman, 1993). The model "heard" sentences of varying degrees of complexity, with the goal of predicting what word would come next at each point in a sentence. From this experience, the model learned to hold on to words it had heard recently in order to predict what might come next, allowing it to abstract the grammatical structure of the language. The model could thus correctly predict grammatically appropriate words within a sentence, even in complex sentences such as "Dogs see boys who cats who Mary feeds chase." The model displayed a critical period, in that "young" networks were able to master the language input, while "older" networks were unable to.

Why did this model display a critical period? The young and older networks differed only in their working memory spans, or how many words they could keep in mind. Although children of different ages differ in many more ways, this single manipulation in the model allowed the potential contribution of working memory to be isolated and evaluated. The young network could keep only three or four words in mind, because its working memory was cleared after every three or four words that were heard; this span was increased gradually as the network aged. In contrast, for the older network, no such clearing of working memory ever occurred, so it could keep more words in mind from the start of learning. Intuitively, one might have expected the older network to be more capable of learning. Instead, by being able to keep more in mind, the older network got bogged down in all of the information it was processing, and was unable to abstract the key kernels (of grammatical category, number, and verb argument type) for understanding the structure of its language. (Imagine trying to learn grammar by studying complex sentences like the "dogs" example above—there is quite a bit to get lost in!) In contrast, by being able to keep only a few words in mind, the young network was better able to focus on these key kernels. (Imagine trying to learn grammar by studying simple portions of complex sentences like the "dogs" example above, e.g., "Dogs see boys"—much less to get lost in.) After abstracting these key kernels, the young network was then able to build on this grammatical knowledge to process more complex sentences as its working memory span increased. Elman (1993) referred to this advantage of limited capacity as "the importance of starting small."

The model thus instantiated an explicit, mechanistic account for the potential causes of critical periods in language learning, leading to the conclusion of the importance of starting small. The conclusions from the simulations are bolstered by similar conclusions from the detailed analyses of behavioral results, and the conclusions from the behavioral results are bolstered by the working implementation in a connectionist model of the somewhat counterintuitive theory.

Stages

Children appear to pass through qualitatively different stages in solving certain tasks. For example, in the balance-scale task, children view a scale with weights on each side at particular distances from the fulcrum, and they must decide which arm of the scale will fall when supports underneath the scale are released. Children initially answer these problems randomly, using no apparent rule about the physical properties of weight and distance to guide their decisions. They next attend only to the amount of weight on each side of the fulcrum (rule I), then include the distance of weights from the fulcrum if weights are equal on each side of the fulcrum (rule II), and eventually attend to both weight and distance information regardless of whether weights are equal on each side (rule III) (Siegler, 1976).

A connectionist model of the balance-scale task (McClelland, 1995) demonstrated how such stage-like progressions can result from small, successive adjustments to connection weights. The model received balance scale problems as patterns of activity corresponding to weight and distance information, and simulated children's performance of progressing from no-rule behavior to rule I, rule II, and rule III behavior.

Why did the model display stage-like behavior? Using error-driven learning, the network's initially random weights were slowly modified with each experience to reduce the discrepancies between the network's predictions about balance scale problems and the actual outcomes. For some time the network's answers were random, because the connections from input to hidden layer and from hidden layer to output layer were not yet meaningful. The network then began to develop representations of weight in its hidden layer. In one simulation, the earlier sensitivity to weight over distance arose because the network received greater exposure to problems where weight predicted the balance-scale outcome (reflecting the possibility that children have more experience with the effects of variations in weight than with the effects of variation in distance). In subsequent simulations, the earlier sensitivity to weight arose with equal exposure to the two cues, owing to the weight cue (a single piece of information) being more simple than the distance cue, which requires computing the relation between

two pieces of information. As the hidden layer representations of weight became more fully formed, such that units were becoming more distinct in their activation patterns, units could be more readily credited for their contribution to the network's correct performance, or blamed for their contribution to the network's errors. The connections from the hidden units to the output units (and from the input units to the hidden units) could then be adjusted appropriately to improve the network's performance, producing a stage-like transition from random answers to rule I answers based on weight.

Sensitivity to the distance cue followed this same pattern of gradual development of hidden unit representations, facilitating credit and blame assignment and the adjustment of connections, leading to a stage-like transition to rules II and III. In this way, incremental weight adjustments in neural networks can result in small representational changes that then support relatively fast learning, producing stage-like behavior.

Task-Dependent Behavior

Children's task-dependent behavior provides a challenge to stage theories, and to developmental theories more generally as discussed earlier. If children are in a given stage or have mastered a particular construct, why do they simultaneously pass and fail different measures of this knowledge? This section focuses on models that explore task-dependent behavior in two domains: memory for hidden objects (often studied under the rubric of a concept of object permanence) and perseveration (the repetition of behaviors that no longer make sense).

Object Permanence

Infants show an incredible range of task-dependent behaviors in their memory for hidden objects. One of the most salient is their failure to search for hidden objects for months after demonstrating sensitivity to hidden objects in their looking times (specifically, looking longer at impossible than at possible events with objects that become occluded; Baillargeon, 1995). Competing interpretations of such task-dependent behaviors have fueled controversies surrounding the origins of knowledge and the mechanisms of change in this domain.

A connectionist model demonstrated how object permanence knowledge could develop without being prespecified, and how such knowledge could lead to success in one task but not another (Munakata et al., 1997). The model viewed a simplified environment in which objects conformed to the principle of object permanence (e.g., disappearing from view behind occluders and reappearing after the occluders were removed). Based on this experience, in the absence of any explicit signal that hidden objects continued to exist, the model became sensitive to the permanence of objects, continuing to represent objects even after they were hidden.

What were the origins of the model's knowledge of object permanence? As in the object recognition model described above, the object permanence model had recurrent excitatory connections that allowed active units to remain active. Like the language learning and balance scale models, the object permanence model also had a goal of predicting what would happen in its environment. Through error-driven learning, the network adjusted its weights if its predictions were incorrect, for example, if the network predicted that an occluded object would not reappear when the occluder was removed, and then the object did in fact reappear. So, when an object moved out of view, the network gradually learned to use its recurrent connections to maintain a representation of the object, allowing the network to accurately predict its environment (and the reappearance of such hidden objects).

Why was the model's knowledge of object permanence task dependent? The network's memory for hidden objects was graded in nature, gradually becoming more like the network's representations of visible objects. The network's perceptual prediction system could use weak memories of occluded objects to expect their reappearance, whereas the network's reaching system, with a delayed and slowed time course of development, could not use these weak memories of occluded objects to reach. This early inability to reach to occluded objects was not due simply to deficits in the reaching system, because this system was able to reach for visible objects (for which the network quickly developed strong representations). Thus, the strength of the graded representations was critical to the task-dependent behavior of the network. Moreover, the strengthening of the networks' memories alone was sufficient to allow the system to progress from initially reaching only for visible objects to then reaching for occluded objects as well. In this way, memory development may be critical to infants' increasing abilities to demonstrate sensitivity to hidden objects across a range of tasks.

Thus, with exposure to events that conformed to the principle of object permanence, the model provided an explicit, mechanistic account of the potential origins of our sensitivity to the permanence of objects, and of the task-dependent nature of infant knowledge in this domain.

Perseveration

Task-dependent behaviors may be most compelling when infants and children *perseverate*, repeating prepotent or habitual behaviors when they no longer make sense. In these cases, participants pass and fail different measures of the same knowledge in a single testing paradigm, at the same moment or very close in time. For example, as soon as infants will search for a toy that is presented and then hidden, they search perseveratively, continuing to reach back to old hiding locations after watching as the toy is hidden in a new location (Diamond, 1985). However, even as infants reach perseveratively, they occasionally gaze at the correct hiding location. Similarly, after 3-year-olds correctly sort cards according to one set of rules (e.g., with blue cards going into one pile and red cards going into another pile), most perseverate in sorting by this rule even after the rules have changed (e.g., to sort the cards by their shape rather than their color) (Zelazo, Frye, and Rapus, 1996). However, the children can correctly answer questions about the new rule they should be using, such as where trucks should go in the shape game. Thus, even as infants and children perseverate with their previous responses, they sometimes seem to indicate through other measures that they have some awareness of the correct response.

Connectionist models have been used to explore the mechanisms that lead to perseveration, support improvements with development, and yield task-dependent behaviors (Munakata, Morton, and Stedron, in press). These models simulate all of these aspects of performance based on a competition between "active" and "latent" memory traces. In the connectionist framework, active traces take the form of sustained activations of network processing units, and latent traces take the form of changes to connection weights between units. Latent traces build as a network repeats a behavior (e.g., searching in one hiding location, or sorting according to one rule), biasing the network to repeat that behavior. These latent traces are thought to be subserved by posterior cortical areas, and to develop quite early in life. The ability to maintain active traces of currently relevant information (e.g., a new hiding location or rule) appears to depend on gradual developments in the prefrontal cortex. The strength of these active traces is manipulated in the models in terms of the strength of recurrent connections within a layer, which allow active units to maintain their activity. Networks perseverate when latent traces for previously relevant information

are stronger than active memory traces for current information. Improvements in active memory abilities allow networks to overcome their prior biases when the task changes. Thus, perseveration may be understood in terms of neural specializations for different types of representations, which develop at different rates and compete with one another (see O'Reilly and Munakata, 2000, for further discussion of neural/computational trade-offs and their behavioral consequences).

Why do the models show task-dependent perseveration? As in the object permanence model, the strengthening of active representations is not an all-or-nothing process; these representations are graded in nature. The models can use weak active representations for certain tasks but not for others. For example, a network can use a weak active representation of a new card sorting rule to answer questions about the rule ("Where do trucks go in the shape game?"), because there is no competition from latent representations (e.g., to sort by color) in this task. No conflict needs to be resolved to answer this question, so weak representations suffice. In contrast, the network cannot use such weak representations to sort cards correctly. The inherent conflict in the sorting task (e.g., a card is both red and a truck) requires the active representation of the new rule to be strong enough to overcome the latent bias toward the old rule.

Similarly, a network can use weak memories for a toy's current hiding location for some tasks (gazing at the correct location) but not for others (reaching to the correct location). In this case, the gazing system updates more frequently than the reaching system (reflecting the general difference between these systems in infants, as well as in how often infants are allowed to use them in the typical toy-hiding task). Networks can thus gaze successfully with relatively weak memories, because they can update their gaze to the proper location frequently, thereby countering perseverative tendencies. In contrast, networks require stronger memories to reach to the correct location, because longer delays pass before they update their reaching, by which time they have become more susceptible to perseverative biases.

Discussion

Connectionist models have thus addressed several key issues in the study of cognitive development—the origins of knowledge, the mechanisms of change, and the task-dependent nature of developing knowledge—across a variety of domains (see also LANGUAGE ACQUISITION; PAST TENSE LEARNING; and DEVELOPMENTAL DISORDERS). In each case, the models provided explicit instantiations and controlled tests of specific theories of development, and allowed the exploration of complex, emergent phenomena. As a result, these models have provided insight into how sophisticated object-processing mechanisms might develop in the first months of life, why we might have critical periods for learning language, how some problem-solving skills can progress in stages, and how we can simultaneously pass and fail different measures of memory and rule use.

Many challenges remain, however, for connectionist models to provide more complete accounts of cognitive development. Two important areas for advancement are the following:

1. *Models that shape their environments.* Most connectionist models are "fed" their inputs, activity pattern after activity pattern, regardless of what they output. For example, language learning models hear sentence after sentence, no matter how poorly the models do in their comprehension. Similarly, models see the same objects in their environments regardless of how they behave toward the objects. Quite in contrast, even very young children shape their environments based on how they behave. For example, infants who reach for objects receive different

sensory information about the objects than infants who simply gaze at the objects. Children who show more advanced language skills may shape the ways in which caregivers speak to them. Capturing these important aspects of development requires models that shape their environments, such that their behaviors influence their subsequent inputs (e.g., Schlesinger and Parisi, 2001).

2. *Models that are more all-purpose.* Most connectionist models are designed for and tested on a single task within a single domain, such as the balance-scale task or the task of searching for hidden objects. A single model sees only this single task during the course of its development. Again, quite in contrast, children face a multitude of tasks across a range of domains each day. Capturing this important aspect of processing requires models that take in a variety of types of information and determine how to appropriately process them to perform successfully across a number of tasks (Karmiloff-Smith, 1992).

These kinds of developments in modeling, together with further explorations of the origins of knowledge, mechanisms of change, and task-dependent behaviors, should help to advance our understanding of fundamental issues in cognitive development.

Road Map: Psychology
Related Reading: Concept Learning; Developmental Disorders; Language Acquisition

References

Baillargeon, R., 1995, Physical reasoning in infancy, in *The Cognitive Neurosciences* (M. Gazzaniga, Ed.), Cambridge, MA: MIT Press.

Diamond, A., 1985, Development of the ability to use recall to guide action, as indicated by infants' performance on A$\bar{B}$, *Child Dev.*, 56:868–883.

Elman, J. L., 1993, Learning and development in neural networks: The importance of starting small, *Cognition*, 48:71–99.

Elman, J. L., Bates, E. A., Johnson, M. H., Karmiloff-Smith, A., Parisi, D., and Plunkett, K., 1996, *Rethinking Innateness: A Connectionist Perspective on Development*, Cambridge, MA: MIT Press. ◆

Karmiloff-Smith, A., 1992, *Beyond Modularity: A Developmental Perspective on Cognitive Science*, Cambridge, MA: MIT Press. ◆

McClelland, J. L., 1995, A connectionist perspective on knowledge and development, *Developing Cognitive Competence: New Approaches to Process Modeling* (T. J. Simon and G. S. Halford, Eds.), Hillsdale, NJ: Erlbaum, pp. 157–204. ◆

McClelland, J. L., and Plunkett, K., 1995, Cognitive development, in *The Handbook of Brain Theory and Neural Networks*, 1st ed. (M. A. Arbib, Ed.), Cambridge, MA: MIT Press, pp. 193–197.

Munakata, Y., McClelland, J. L., Johnson, M. H., and Siegler, R., 1997, Rethinking infant knowledge: Toward an adaptive process account of successes and failures in object permanence tasks, *Psychol. Rev.*, 104:686–713.

Munakata, Y., Morton, J. B., and Stedron, J. M., in press, The role of prefrontal cortex in perseveration: Developmental and computational explorations, in *Connectionist Models of Development* (P. Quinlan, Ed.), East Sussex: Psychology Press. ◆

O'Reilly, R. C., and Johnson, M. H., 2002, Object recognition and sensitive periods: A computational analysis of visual imprinting, in *Brain Development and Cognition: A Reader*, 2nd ed. (M. H. Johnson, Y. Munakata, and R. O. Gilmore, Eds.), Oxford, Engl.: Blackwell, pp. 392–413.

O'Reilly, R. C., and Munakata, Y., 2000, *Computational Explorations in Cognitive Neuroscience: Understanding the Mind by Simulating the Brain*, Cambridge, MA: MIT Press. ◆

Schlesinger, M., and Parisi, D., 2001, The agent-based approach: A new direction for computational models of development, *Dev. Rev.*, 21:121–146.

Siegler, R., 1976, Three aspects of cognitive development, *Cognit. Psychol.*, 8:481–520.

Spelke, E., Breinlinger, K., Macomber, J., and Jacobson, K., 1992, Origins of knowledge, *Psychol. Rev.*, 99:605–632.

Zelazo, P. D., Frye, D., and Rapus, T., 1996, An age-related dissociation between knowing rules and using them, *Cognit. Dev.*, 11:37–63.

Cognitive Maps

Nestor A. Schmajuk and Horatiu Voicu

Introduction

According to Tolman (1932), animals acquire the *expectancy* that the performance of response R1 in a situation S1 will be followed by a change to situation S2 (S1-R1-S2 expectancy). Tolman hypothesized that a large number of local expectancies can be combined, through inferences, into a *cognitive map*. Tolman proposed that place learning, latent learning, detours, and shortcuts illustrate animals' capacity for reasoning by generating inferences. In place learning, animals learn to approach a given spatial location from multiple initial positions, independently of any specific set of responses. In latent learning, animals are exposed to a maze without being rewarded at the goal box (Figure 1). When a reward is later presented, animals demonstrate knowledge of the spatial arrangement of the maze, which remains "latent" until reward is introduced. Detour problems are those in which animals have to take an alternative, longer path to the goal. Shortcuts are those problems in which animals can take an alternative, shorter path to the goal.

When seeking reward in a maze, organisms compare the expectancies evoked by alternative paths. For Tolman, *vicarious trial-and-error behavior*, i.e., the active scanning of alternative pathways at choice points, reflects the animal's generation and comparison of different expectancies. At choice points, animals sample different stimuli before making a decision. For example, a rat often looks back and forth between alternative stimuli before approaching one or the other. According to Tolman's *stimulus-approach* view, organisms learn that a particular stimulus situation is appetitive, and therefore it is approached. It has been suggested that, in the presence of numerous intra- and extramaze cues, animals typically learn to approach a set of stimuli associated with reward and to avoid a set of stimuli associated with punishment. However, in a totally uniform environment, animals learn to make the correct responses that lead to the goal.

Maze Learning

Deutsch (1960) presented a formal description of cognitive mapping that incorporates many of Tolman's cognitive concepts. Deutsch assumed that when an animal explores a given environment, it learns that stimuli follow one another in a given sequence. Internal representations of the stimuli are linked together in the order the stimuli are encountered by the animal. Deutsch suggested that a given drive activates its goal representation, which in turn activates the linked representations of stimuli connected to it. When the animal is placed in the maze, it searches for stimuli stimulated by the goal representation. When a stimulus activated by the goal

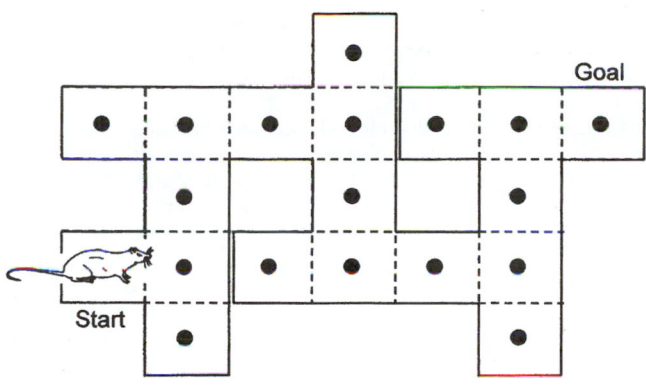

Figure 1. Latent learning. Schematic top view of a multiple T-maze. Places used in Figure 3 are represented by squares in broken lines, with the centers indicated by solid circles.

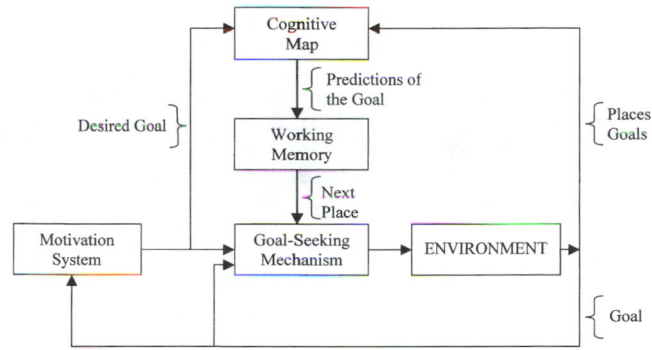

Figure 2. The model. Interactions between the motivation system, cognitive map, working memory, goal-seeking mechanism, and environment. (After Voicu and Schmajuk, 2001a.)

is perceived, the activation of lower stimuli in the chain is cut off, and behavior is controlled by the stimulus that is closer to the goal. Deutsch's theory can account for latent learning in the following terms. When animals are exposed to the maze without being rewarded at the goal box, they learn about the connections between different places in the maze. When a reward is subsequently presented, activation of the goal representation activates the representations of the stimuli connected to it.

Milner (1960) proposed a system capable of building a Tolmanian spatial map and of using it to control the animal's movements in a spatial environment. The model has nodes that are active only when a particular response (R_i) has been made in a particular location (S_j). The output of these nodes can be associated with nodes representing the location (S_k) that results from making response R_i at location S_j. When the organism is placed in location S_j, random responses are generated. When response R_i appears, the node with inputs S_j and R_i is active and, in turn, activates the node representing S_k. If S_k is associated to an appetitive stimulus, it activates a mechanism that holds R_i in the response generator, and location S_k can be reached. Some views of hippocampal function (e.g., McNaughton, 1989) suggest that S_j-R_i-S_k associations would be stored in the hippocampus (see HIPPOCAMPUS: SPATIAL MODELS).

Lieblich and Arbib (1982) addressed the question of how animals build a cognitive model of the world. Lieblich and Arbib posited that spatial representations take the form of a directed graph in which nodes represent *recognizable situations* in the world. In Lieblich and Arbib's scheme, a node represents not only a place, but also the motivational state of the animal. Consequently, a place in the world might be represented by more than one node if the animal has been there under different motivational states. Lieblich and Arbib postulated that each node in the world graph is labeled with *learned* vectors, **R**, that reflect the drive-reduction properties for multiple motivations of the place represented by that node. Based on the value of **R**, the animal moves to the node most likely to reduce its present drive. More recently, Guazelli et al., (1998), following O'Keefe and Nadel's (1978) notions, integrated the world graph model, used for map-based navigation, with a "behavioral orientation" model, used for route navigation, in order to explain experimental data in normal and fornix-lesioned rats.

Hampson (1990) analyzed maze navigation in terms of a model that combines stimulus-response and stimulus-stimulus mechanisms into a system capable of assembling action sequences in order to reach a final goal.

Schmajuk and Thieme (1992) presented a real-time, biologically plausible neural network approach to purposive behavior and cog-

nitive mapping. This biologically plausible theory includes (1) an action system, consisting of a goal-seeking mechanism with goals set by (2) a motivation system; (3) a cognitive system, in which a neural network implements a cognitive map; and (4) a working memory, where the readings of the cognitive map are temporarily stored (Figure 2).

The goal-seeking mechanism in the action system changes from exploratory behavior to approach behavior when either (1) the goal is found or (2) one place in the cognitive map generates a prediction of the goal that is stronger than the predictions generated by all other alternative places.

The cognitive map is a *topological map* that represents the adjacency, but not distances or directions, between places, as well as the associations between places and goals. Figure 3 shows a heteroassociative network (Kohonen, 1977) capable, through recurrent connections, of cognitive mapping. The network includes three types of inputs: current places, neighboring places, and goals. Cur-

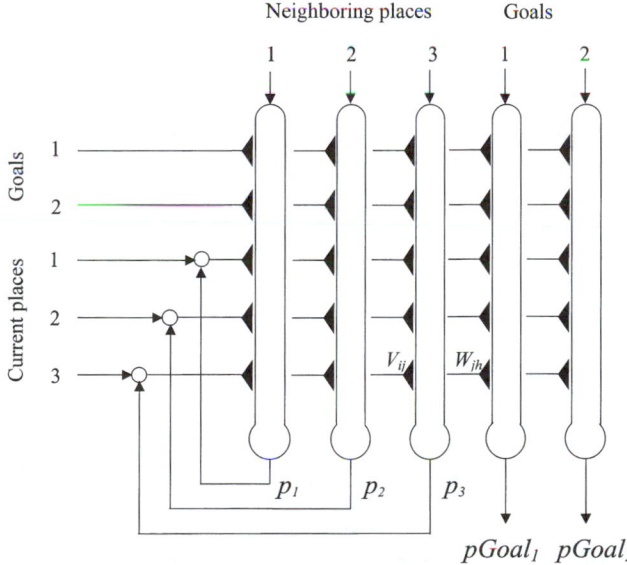

Figure 3. Cognitive Map. The prediction of neighboring place j, p; is fed back into the neuron representing place j as a current place. V_{ij}: association between place i and place j. W_{hi}: association between goal h and place i W_{ih}: association between place i and goal h g_h: activation of goal h. Arrows denote fixed excitatory connections; triangles denote variable excitatory connections. (After Voicu and Schmajuk, 2001a.)

rent places and neighboring places are defined by a system that determines the position of the animal in space. Goals represent a feature (e.g., food, unexamined places) that, under the appropriate motivation (e.g., hunger, exploration), the agent wants to approach.

Associations between place i and place j, $V_{i,j}$, are the elementary internal learned representations of the links in the external world. These associations are stored in modifiable synapses, indicated by triangles in Figure 3. Whereas a positive $V_{i,j}$ association means that place j can be accessed from place i, a positive $V_{j,i}$ association means that place i can be accessed from place j. In both cases, $V_{i,j} = V_{j,i} = 0$ mean that each place cannot be accessed from the other. At the beginning of the exploration, all adjacent places are assumed to be linked in the cognitive map (all $V_{i,j} = 1$). As the agent explores the environment, connections $V_{i,j}$ are modified in order to reflect the real environment. "Trodden" links between places are represented by stronger connections ($V_{i,j} = V_{j,i} > 1$) than unexplored links.

At the beginning of the exploration, each place is designated as "unexamined," $W_{j,\text{GOAL}h} = W_{\text{GOAL}h,j} = 1$. When place j can be accessed and occupied by the agent, it changes its status to "examined," $W_{j,\text{GOAL}h} = W_{\text{GOAL}h,j} = 0$, meaning that it is no longer a goal for exploration. When place j, adjacent to place i currently occupied by the agent, can be examined, place j also changes its status to examined, $W_{j,\text{GOAL}h} = W_{\text{GOAL}h,j} = 0$, even if it cannot be entered.

The cognitive map combines multiple associations $V_{i,j}$ to infer spatially remote locations. This is achieved by recurrently reinjecting the signal representing neighboring place j (as predicted by place i according to $V_{i,j}$) into the representation of current place j. Current place j now predicts neighboring place k according to $V_{j,k}$, and the signal representing neighboring place k is reinjected into the representation of current place k. At each reinjection, the signal representing a neighboring place is attenuated, for instance, in half. The process is halted when the representation of the remote position is eventually activated.

The network successfully describes how rats demonstrate latent learning, detour behavior, and place learning. In order to ascertain the power of the network in problem solving, Schmajuk and Thieme (1992) applied the network to the Tower of Hanoi task. Simulations show that the network takes a few trials to solve the problem in the minimum number of movements.

Schmajuk, Thieme, and Blair (1993) incorporated a route system to the network described by Schmajuk and Thieme (1992). Whereas the cognitive map stores associations between places and reward, the route system establishes associations between cues and reward. Both systems compete with each other to establish associations with the reward, with the cognitive system generally overshadowing the route system. In agreement with O'Keefe and Nadel (1978), after hippocampal lesions (see HIPPOCAMPUS: SPATIAL MODELS), animals navigate through mazes by making use of the route system.

Recently, Voicu and Schmajuk (2001a, 2001b) introduced some modifications to the Schmajuk and Thieme (1992) model. First, whereas the early model assumed no a priori knowledge of the space to be explored, the modified model assumes a representation of the environment as a set of potentially connected and unexamined locations, each approximately the size of the footprint of the agent. Second, instead of random exploratory behavior, the model assumes that a curiosity drive guides the animal to examine all unvisited places. Third, whereas in the original model the decision of what place to move to next was based on a comparison of the predictions of the goal when each of the alternative places is briefly entered, in the new model this decision is based on a comparison of the activation of each of the alternative places when the goal is activated. This approach is similar to that described by Deutsch (1960) and subsequently used by Mataric (1991) and Reid and

Staddon (1998). Fourth, the model differentiates between links that connect places but have not been traversed by the agent, and those that have. These links are part of what is referred to as "trodden path."

In addition to latent learning, detour behavior, and place learning, the new model (1) performs a thorough and efficient exploration of the environment, (2) describes shortcuts, and (3) generates novel predictions for a case in which animals have to circumvent an obstacle placed on their path to the goal and then either retake their usual route (detour) or advance directly to the goal (shortcut).

As mentioned above, in order to plan the shortest path between any two places, the model presented by Voicu and Schmajuk (2001a, 2001b) spreads activation between the representations of the goal and the current location of the animal. The resulting activities are stored in working memory. However, two problems might arise when navigating in a large environment. One, the capacity of working memory might be too small to store the activity of all intermediate places. Two, the attenuation suffered by the spreading activation is too large to reach the representation of the location of the animal. These potential problems call for the use of a hierarchical cognitive map (Voicu and Schmajuk, 2002).

In the hierarchical map, the environment is represented at multiple levels. At the highest level, the environment is divided in a number of regions equal to the size of working memory. The size of the working memory is such that the activation spreading through it can reach and activate the most remote spatial representations. At the lowest level, the environment is divided in parts equal in size to that of the footprint of the organism. Between the highest and the lowest level, each part of the previous level is divided in a number of parts equal to the size of the working memory. Path planning starts at the level that contains the points between which navigation is desired and ends at the lowest level, at which motion is produced.

According to the hierarchical cognitive model, and in agreement with experimental data, when information about the relationship between two places that belong to two different regions (e.g., Seattle and Montreal) is lacking, humans wrongly rely on the relation between the regions where those places are located (e.g., United States and Canada). Also in agreement with experimental results, the hierarchical cognitive model suggests that spatial memory is organized in a hierarchical fashion even when objects are uniformly distributed in space. Finally, experimental results suggest that hierarchical spatial representations support semantic priming, a result that the hierarchical model can explain in terms of one item activating the representation of a second one in the cognitive map, and therefore decreasing the response time to the second item.

Discussion

In the last decades, Tolman's (1932) ideas about cognitive maps have been refined and given mechanistic embodiments. In recent models (e.g., Voicu and Schmajuk, 2001a), Tolman's vicarious trial-and-error behavior has been regarded as reflecting the animal's comparison, but not the generation, of different expectancies. Expectancies are generated by activating the representation of the location of the goal with the motivation system. That activation is subsequently spread over the cognitive map until the representation of the location of the agent becomes active. At choice points, animals make a decision after sampling the intensity of the activation elicited by the different alternative paths. Several models (Mataric, 1991; Reid and Staddon, 1998; Voicu and Schmajuk, 2001a) still use Tolman's stimulus-approach view and assume that animals approach the place with the strongest appetitive activation, thereby performing a gradient ascent toward the goal.

Interestingly, Tolman (1932, p. 177) suggested that the relations between initial and goal positions can be represented by a directed graph, and called this graph a means-end field. Current artificial intelligence theories describe problem solving as the process of finding a path from an initial to a desired state through a directed graph (see COMPETITIVE QUEUING FOR PLANNING AND SERIAL PERFORMANCE).

In addition to storing the representation of the environment in terms of the contiguity between places (Schmajuk and Thieme, 1992), cognitive maps can store information about differences in height and in the type of terrain between adjacent places, contain a priori knowledge of the space to be explored (Reid and Staddon, 1998; Voicu and Schmajuk, 2001a), distinguish between roads taken and those not taken (Voicu and Schmajuk, 2002), and keep track of which places have been examined.

Schmajuk et al. (1993) used Kohonen's (1977) two-layer associative network to mechanistically implement the cognitive map. Networks with more than two layers can also be used to represent not only the contiguity between places, but also the relative position of those places.

Recently, Voicu and Schmajuk (2001b) introduced the idea of hierarchical cognitive maps in which the environment is represented at multiple levels. At each level, the environment is divided into a number of parts equal to the size of working memory. In contrast to their nonhierarchical counterparts, hierarchical maps can plan navigation in large environments, use a smaller number of connections in their networks, and have shorter decision times.

Road Map: Psychology
Related Reading: Hippocampus: Spatial Models; Potential Fields and Neural Networks

References

Deutsch, J. A., 1960, *The Structural Basis of Behavior*, Cambridge, Engl.: Cambridge University Press.

Guazelli, A., Corbacho, F. J., Bota, M., and Arbib, M. A., 1998, Affordances, motivations, and the world graph theory, *Adapt. Behav.*, 6:435–471.

Hampson, S. E., 1990, *Connectionistic Problem Solving*, Boston: Birkhauser.

Kohonen, T., 1977, *Associative Memory*, Berlin: Springer-Verlag.

Lieblich, I., and Arbib, M. A., 1982, Multiple representations of space underlying behavior, *Behav. Brain Sci.*, 5:627–659. ◆

Mataric, M. J., 1991, Navigating with a rat brain: A neurobiologically-inspired model of robot spatial representation, in *From Animals to Animats 1*, Cambridge, MA: MIT Press, pp. 169–175.

McNaughton, B. L., 1989, Neuronal mechanisms for spatial computation and information storage, *Neural Connections and Mental Computations* in (L. Nadel, L. Cooper, P. Culicover, and R. Harnish, Eds.), New York: Academic Press.

Milner, P. M., 1960, *Physiological Psychology*, New York: Holt, Rinehart, and Winston.

O'Keefe, J., and Nadel, L., 1978, *The Hippocampus as a Cognitive Map*, Oxford, Engl.: Clarendon Press.

Reid, A. K., and Staddon, J. E. R., 1998, A dynamic route finder for the cognitive map, *Psychol. Rev.*, 105:585–601.

Schmajuk, N. A., and Thieme, A. D., 1992, Purposive behavior and cognitive mapping: An adaptive neural network, *Biol. Cybern.*, 67:165–174. ◆

Schmajuk, N. A., Thieme, A. D., and Blair, H. T., 1993, Maps, routes, and the hippocampus: A neural network approach, *Hippocampus*, 3:387–400.

Tolman, E. C., 1932, Cognitive maps in rats and men, *Psychol. Rev.*, 55:189–208. ◆

Voicu, H., and Schmajuk, N. A., 2001a, Three-dimensional cognitive mapping with a neural network, *Robot. Auton. Syst.*, 35:21–35

Voicu, H., and Schmajuk, N. A., 2001b, Hierarchical cognitive maps, presented at the Fifth International Conference on Cognitive and Neural Systems, Boston, MA, May 29.

Voicu H., and Schmajuk, N. A., 2002, Exploration, navigation and cognitive mapping, *Adapt. Behav.*, 8:207–223.

Cognitive Modeling: Psychology and Connectionism

Amanda J. C. Sharkey and Noel E. Sharkey

Introduction

Connectionism has had a major impact on psychology and cognitive modeling. In the next section we consider this influence, identifying four typical features of connectionist models of cognition:

1. They can be used both to model cognitive processes and to simulate the performance of tasks.
2. Data analogues can be derived from the models in such a way as to provide a good fit to data from cognitive psychology experiments.
3. Unlike traditional computational models, connectionist models are not explicitly programmed by the investigator.
4. They encourage the development of new accounts of empirical data.

Having identified these features, we point out that although the connectionist stance has some real benefits, it would be unwise to assume that it has been fully developed. There are aspects of it that still need to be understood and clarified. For instance, establishing equivalences between the performance of a net and the tasks it simulates involves a number of assumptions. At the same time, important aspects of the performance of a connectionist net are controlled by the researcher, by means of *extensional programming*. In particular, decisions are made about the selection and presentation of training data. This means that the achievement of a good fit to the psychological data depends both on the way in which analogues to the data are derived and on the results of extensional programming. Nonetheless, a major advantage of a connectionist approach to the modeling of psychological processes is that it has encouraged the development of new accounts of old data in a number of domains.

We subsequently consider the potential of connectionist computation for the development of a new theory of cognition. Rather than modeling the details of psychology experiments, the research efforts of a new breed of "cognitive connectionists" have been directed toward computational experiments. These experiments have demonstrated the ability of connectionist representations to provide a viable and different account of important characteristics of cognition (compositionality and systematicity), previously assumed to be the exclusive province of the classical symbolic tradition. Although connectionism has only an abstract relationship to neural processing, the promise here is that the use of brain-style computation will enable steps to be taken toward a unified account of how a mind emerges from a brain. Of course, it is not yet known whether connectionism will ultimately be able to account for all aspects of cognition. We discuss the likelihood that a more complete connectionist account of cognition will almost certainly involve the coordination of connectionist modules, and we point to the beginning of a debate over the extent to which such coordination requires a classical architecture or could be accomplished in a purely connectionist manner.

Models of Cognition

In 1986, a two-volume edited work by McClelland and Rumelhart presented a number of connectionist models of different aspects of cognition that had been *trained* by exposure to samples of the required tasks. This work was indebted to earlier pioneering neural network research related to cognitive processing and memory (e.g., Anderson, 1972), but it was these two volumes that set the agenda for connectionist cognitive modelers and offered a methodology that has become the standard. Connectionist cognitive models are now legion. The domains that have been simulated include, in memory, retrieval and category formation; in language, phoneme recognition, word recognition, speech perception, acquired dyslexia, and language acquisition; and in vision, edge detection and object and shape recognition.

In this article we have chosen to discuss only supervised learning techniques, as these techniques have been most commonly used in connectionist cognitive modeling. In the simplest case of supervised learning, a net consists of a set of input units, a layer of hidden units, and a set of output units, each layer being connected to the next via modifiable weights. This is a feedforward net. When the net is trained on a set of input-output pairs, the weights are adjusted via a learning algorithm (e.g., backpropagation) until the required output is produced in response to each input in the training set. When tested on a set of previously unseen inputs, the net will, to a greater or lesser extent, display an ability to generalize, that is, to go beyond the data it was trained on, and to produce an appropriate response to some of the test inputs. The ability of the net to generalize depends on the similarity between the function extracted as a result of the original training and the function that underlies the test set. If the training set was sufficiently representative of the required function, generalization results are likely to be good. Where the inputs and outputs of such a net are given an interpretation relevant to the performance of a cognitive task, the net may be seen as a model of that task.

In addition to their basic architecture and mode of operation, it is also possible to identify four typical features of connectionist models of cognition that, in combination, account for much of the popularity of the approach they exemplify: (1) They can be used both to model mental processes and to *simulate* the actual behavior involved. (2) They can provide a "good fit" to the data from psychology experiments. (3) The model, and its fit to the data, is achieved without explicit programming, or "handwiring." (4) They often provide new accounts of the data. We discuss each of these features in turn.

The first two features, namely, the way in which connectionist nets can both provide a model of a cognitive process and simulate a related task, and their ability to provide a good fit to the empirical data, combine some of the characteristics of two earlier routes to modeling. One of these routes, taken by the cognitive psychology community, involved building models that could account for the results from psychology experiments with human subjects but did not incorporate simulations of experimental tasks. The second route, followed by the artificial intelligence (AI) community, was to build computer models that actually performed the task in ways that resembled human performance, without regard to detailed psychological evidence. The connectionist approach, as described here, provides the benefits both of simulating the performance of

human tasks and, at the same time of fitting the data from psychological investigations.

As an example of the latter, consider Seidenberg and McClelland's (1989) model of word pronunciation. This model simulates a number of experimental behaviors, including pronunciation of novel items, differences in performance on lexical decision and naming tasks, and ease of pronunciation in relation to variables such as frequency of occurrence, orthographic redundancy, and orthographic-phonological regularity. At the same time, the model is generally accepted as providing a good fit to the experimental data. This is achieved by deriving an analogue to the data from the performance of the model. In the case of Seidenberg and McClelland's account of lexical decisions, the comparison with lexical decision data is accomplished by computing an "orthographic error score," based on the sum of squares of the differences between the feedback pattern computed by the network and the actual input to the orthographic units. Here a low error score is equated with a fast reaction time. Others have assumed different data analogues. For example, Plaut et al., (1996) present an attractor network that accounts for latency data in time to settle on a response.

The third typical feature of connectionist models of cognition is that the model and its fit to the data are achieved without explicit handwiring. This feature can be favorably contrasted to the symbolic programming methodology employed in AI, where the model must be programmed step by step, leaving room for ad hoc modifications and kludges.

The fourth feature, perhaps the most scientifically exciting, is the possibility of providing a novel explanation of the data. In their model of word pronunciation, Seidenberg and McClelland (1989) showed that their network provided an integrated (single mechanism) account of data on both regular and exception words; by contrast, the old cognitive modeling conventions had forced an explanation in terms of a dual route. A criticism of the Seidenberg-McClelland model was that it failed to provide an account of the reading of nonwords. However, a more recent formulation of the model (Plaut et al., 1996) shows that a single mechanism is able to provide an account of the basic patterns of word and nonword reading within a single mechanism. (See Christiansen, Conway, and Curtin, 2000, for a more recent example of a connectionist model that exhibits rule-like behavior from a single mechanism.)

On first consideration, the four features discussed above seem to provide support in favor of a connectionist approach to cognitive modeling, as opposed to the approaches taken in the two preceding routes to cognition, by AI and cognitive modelers. When the result has been the development of new, and simpler, accounts of the data, there are obvious benefits. The connectionist approach would also seem to be preferable to more symbolic approaches inasmuch as it makes it possible both to simulate the tasks and to provide a good fit to the data, and to do this without having to program these abilities in hand. However, we must tread warily here in claiming a clear distinction between the connectionist approach and those that preceded it.

Let us first reexamine the idea that connectionist network models are not explicitly programmed by hand. Although this statement is strictly true, a number of decisions that affect the subsequent performance of the model still have to be made by the researcher. The following factors, for example, both govern the creation of a model and are in the hands of the researcher: (1) the architecture of the net and its initial structure, (2) the learning technique, (3) the learning parameters (e.g., the learning rate), (4) the input and output representations, and (5) the training sample. The term *extensional programming* can be used to refer to the manipulation of these factors. By means of extensional programming, the clever experimenter can determine the ultimate form of a model and hence its performance in terms of any data set.

Control of the content and presentation of the training sample is an important aspect of extensional programming. Its potential influence on the performance of a connectionist model can be illustrated by considering some of the criticisms of McClelland and Rumelhart's past tense model (see PAST TENSE LEARNING). Their model is said to mirror several aspects of human learning of verb endings. However, Pinker and Prince (1988) pointed out that the experimenters had unrealistically tailored the environment to produce the required results and that the results were an artifact of the training data. More specifically, the results indicated a U-shaped curve in the rate of acquisition, as occurs with children, but, Pinker and Prince argued, this curve occurred only because the net was exposed to the verbs in an unrealistically structured order. These criticisms have largely been answered by further research, but the point remains. Selection of the input, and control of the way that it is presented to the net, affect what the net learns. A similar argument can be made about the selection of input representations. Plaut et al. (1996), in their model of normal and impaired word reading, explicitly discuss the role of their chosen input representation in achieving their results, claiming that is the change in input representation from the earlier Seidenberg and McClelland model that accounts for an improved ability to handle nonword data.

If the performance of a connectionist net is determined by its extensional programming, this means that there are a number of parameters that can be altered until a good data fit is achieved. Moreover, accepting that a good fit to the data has been achieved requires accepting a number of other assumptions about the way that the relevant tasks have been simulated, the consequent way that analogues to the data have been derived from the performance of the model, and so on. Thus, when a model is said to explain the empirical data from lexical decision tasks, the model does not actually perform a lexical decision task as humans do, outputing a yes when the input is a word and a no when it is not. An equivalence must be drawn between the task as it is performed by humans and the actual input-output relationships encoded by the net. In fact, the actual task in question is rarely performed by the model. What is performed is often something that approximates the task and is assumed to capture its essential characteristics. Thus, in a model of word pronunciation, the output of the model does not take the form of spoken words but rather a set of phonological features. Here the approximation is fairly straightforward, but in other cases the relationship is less obvious. Ratcliff (1990), for instance, equates the phenomenon of "recognition memory" with that of auto-association, assuming that the ability of a net to reproduce its inputs as outputs corresponds to the human ability to recognize inputs that have been seen before.

From the foregoing discussion it is apparent that some of the advantages of connectionist models of cognition are not entirely straightforward. Nonetheless, their potential for developing new accounts that go beyond the data is an important justification for their employment. Much of the excitement in the psychology community has been about their ability to handle apparently rule-governed phenomena without any explicit rules, and in particular to account for the processing of regular and exceptional material. For example, learning to produce the appropriate past tense form of verbs was always considered a rule-governed phenomenon until McClelland and Rumelhart (1986) showed that the behaviors could be trained in a model that did not contain any explicit rules. The different style of computation afforded by connectionism has also been the focus of much debate. The issue being debated is the extent to which connectionism is able to support the operations required of a theory of mind, namely, structure-sensitive operations. This debate is examined in the next section.

An Emerging Theory of Cognition

The past two decades saw considerable discussion about whether or not the new connectionism actually constituted a paradigm shift.

Whatever the eventual outcome of this discussion may be, it is clear that the adoption of connectionist modeling techniques has led to changes. One such change has been the emergence of a new breed of cognitive modelers who are concerned to explore the implications of connectionist computation for a new theory of cognition, with the ultimate aim of providing an account of the way in which a mind emerges from a nervous system. The methodology employed by these "cognitive connectionists" represents a move away from the detailed modeling of cognitive psychology experiments toward more abstract computational experimentation. This should broaden the scope of their investigations, for although there are benefits to models that provide a new explanation of a wide spectrum of data, the maintenance of a close relationship between model and data can limit investigations to previously identified questions from an older paradigm.

The promise of a new connectionist theory of cognition is that it will further our understanding of the relationship between brain and mind. However, this does not necessarily mean that such a theory will incorporate details of neural processing. It is important to make a clear distinction between the use of *brain-style* computation and neuropsychological modeling. Although connectionist models are sometimes described as being "neurally inspired," their relationship to neural processing is delicate and tenuous. In a model of cognitive processes, it is unlikely that the computation performed corresponds to what goes on at the neural level. Indeed, it has been suggested (Edelman, 1987) that it may take units on the order of several thousand neurons to encode stimulus categories of significance to animals. Clearly, when the inputs to a net are entities like noun phrases or disease symptoms or even the phonological representations of words, the inputs cannot be equated with neural inputs but must represent substantially preprocessed stimuli. In fact, there are few cases in which actual facts about the nervous system are used to constrain the architecture and design of a model. It is, of course, important to build computational models of real brain circuits in all of their glorious detail. But if one is concerned with cognition rather than with the details of neural processes, an appropriate research strategy is to use broader brush strokes, relying on computational abstractions.

In support of a movement away from the details of neurophysiology and away from psychology experiments, we can cite an example of progress from the history of connectionism itself. Arguably, it was two major simplifying assumptions made by McCulloch and Pitts that enabled them to develop their theoretical analyses without getting bogged down in the physical and chemical complexity of the nervous system. Their first simplification was based on the observation that neural communication is thresholded, and thus the spike activation potential is all or none: it either fires or does not fire. Thus, the neuron could be conceived of as a binary computing device. The second simplification was to view synapses as numerical weightings between simple binary computing elements. This meant that computation proceeded by summing the weighted inputs to an element and using the binary threshold as an output function (see Sharkey and Sharkey, 1994, for historical details). The position of the cognitive connectionist described here is therefore that we can best proceed by being constrained by simplifying but principled assumptions about neural computation and cognition.

Nonetheless, if the use of connectionist computation, as opposed to symbolic computation, is to lead to the development of a new theory of cognition, connectionist computation must first be shown to be capable, in principle, of supporting higher mental processes, and to do so in a novel manner; mere implementation of symbolic architectures will not do. The question of whether or not connectionism is capable of supporting a cognitive architecture has mainly been addressed in the context of discussions about the novelty and value of connectionist representation. This question is considered below. (See also STRUCTURED CONNECTIONIST MODELS; CONNECTIONIST AND SYMBOLIC REPRESENTATIONS; COMPOSITIONALITY IN NEURAL SYSTEMS.)

One of the properties of uniquely connectionist representations, as identified by N. E. Sharkey (1997), is that they are distributed and nonsymbolic. Proponents of the classical symbolic tradition have claimed that such representations are in principle incapable of supporting a cognitive architecture, because in order to account for the systematic nature of human thought, representations must be able to support structure-sensitive processes, and this requires compositional representations. The assumption is that there is only one kind of compositionality, namely, the concatenative compositionality of symbolic strings. This permits structure-sensitive operations, because in their mode of combination, the constituents of complex expressions are tokened whenever the complex expression is tokened. For example, in order to develop an expression from a sentence like "John kissed Mary," arbitrary symbols representing the constituents JOHN, KISSED, and MARY are combined in a contextually independent concatenation to produce the propositional representation KISS (JOHN, MARY). Whenever this latter complex expression is tokened, its constituents, KISS, MARY, and JOHN, are also tokened. This makes the manipulation of the representations by a mechanism sensitive to the syntactic structure resulting from concatenative compositionality relatively easy.

Distributed representations, on the other hand, do not exhibit this kind of compositionality. Instead, cognitive connectionists have identified an alternative form of compositionality, one that has been described as merely functional, nonconcatenative compositionality (see COMPOSITIONALITY IN NEURAL SYSTEMS). Distributed representations combine tokens without those tokens appearing in the complex expression, since the tokens of the input constituents are destroyed in their combination. The point is that such representations can still be shown to be *functionally* compositional, because there exist general and reliable procedures for combining constituents into complex expressions and for decomposing those expressions back into the constituents. It is possible, for example, to encode simple syntactic trees in terms of connectionist distributed representations, and to decode them back into the same syntactic trees (Pollack, 1990). Thus the constituents of the tree have been combined into a form of representation that is nonconcatenative but that preserves the necessary information.

A considerable and growing body of research has shown that not only are distributed representations compositional, they can also enable *systematic* structure-sensitive operations. Chalmers (1990), for example, found that it was possible to use connectionist nets to transform distributed representations for active sentences into distributed representations for passive sentences. Thus, distributed representations allow at least a limited form of systematicity without emergence onto the symbol surface. Moreover, this is not just an example of old wine in new bottles, a mere implementation of the classical account. These uniquely connectionist representations operate in a different manner.

N. E. Sharkey (1997) describes seven major properties of uniquely connectionist representations. In addition to properties that overlap with those we identified earlier in this article, he identifies a further property of uniquely connectionist representations: namely, they are reusable, or portable, for other tasks. This property has been demonstrated in a number of cognitive tasks, such as Chalmers' (1990) active-passive transformations, and more recently in a control task. N. E. Sharkey (1997) reports the development of a disembodied arm control system in which the connectionist representations that had been developed as a result of training a net to output transformationally invariant position classes were reused as input to a net trained to direct a mobile robotic arm to pick up objects.

There is ongoing debate over the extent to which connectionism is capable of supporting a new style of cognitive architecture. The arguments in favor stress the capability of connectionist representations for both compositionality and systematicity, that the representations are reusable for other tasks, and that they accomplish these properties by different means than those of classical symbolic representations. Opponents stress the problems connectionists have in dealing with structured representations and expressing relationships between variables, and our ability to immediately follow a linguistically expressed rule (see Marcus, 2001). However, it should be noted that although it can be argued that connectionist representations can support structure-sensitive operations, or that connectionist nets can process regular and exception material within a single mechanism, it does not necessarily follow that the connectionists assume that the brain should be modeled as a unitary mechanism. There are a number of reasons for assuming that connectionist modeling of more complex cognitive functions will require some degree of modularization. For instance, there is the observed difficulty of training a net to perform two unrelated tasks at the same time, and concomitantly the advantages often observed in terms of performance when a task is modularized (A. J. C. Sharkey, 1999).

It seems likely that future connectionist research will have to attend to issues of modularity and the control and coordination of distinct connectionist modules. This research area is receiving increasing attention in the field of behavior-based robotics (see REACTIVE ROBOTIC SYSTEMS; BIOLOGICALLY INSPIRED ROBOTICS), where the challenge is not only to coordinate modules but also to provide an account of the way in which distinct modules, and the representations they employ, emerge in the first place (N. E. Sharkey, 1998). A related classical versus connectionist debate may also surface here, regarding the extent to which the coordination of modules requires a classical architecture (Hadley, 1999) or can be achieved without resource to a central executive (N. E. Sharkey, 1998).

Discussion

This article began by outlining the main characteristics of connectionist models of cognition. Two of the main apparent advantages of connectionist models are (1) their ability to both model and simulate empirical data, and (2) their ability to do so without being explicitly programmed. These features segregate connectionist models from the earlier models of cognitive psychologists, who modeled the data without simulating the tasks involved, and from AI models, which are explicitly programmed and which simulate behavior without regard to the details of psychological evidence. On further reflection, however, the distinction between connectionist models and earlier approaches becomes less clear. Obtaining a good fit to the data relies on a number of assumptions and is not, as is sometimes supposed, achieved without experimental intervention. The researcher must make a number of decisions that determine the performance of the model. We introduced the term extensional programming to refer to these decisions, which include the selection of the training set and its manner of presentation. Nonetheless, even if there are some aspects of connectionist models that bear further consideration, it is still the case that the novel style of computation they embody often encourages the development of new accounts of previously investigated data.

Subsequently we considered the ability of connectionism to support a new theory of cognition. Cognitive connectionists, are more concerned to exploit the implications of connectionist computation than to provide detailed models of psychological data. An important issue for the cognitive connectionist is the notion of connectionist representation. It has been claimed that connectionist representations are in principle incapable of supporting an account of higher mental processes. To counter this claim, computational experiments have been conducted with the aim of demonstrating that connectionist representations have a complex internal structure, capable of fulfilling the requirements for a cognitive architecture.

Connectionist representations have been shown to be capable of much of the systematicity and compositionality required of them by their critics. They do not merely implement symbolic computation but operate in a novel manner. Whether it will be possible to provide a connectionist account of all aspects of cognition remains to be seen. An important issue to be addressed is that of modularity, in particular the extent to which the coordination of distinct modules implies a classical architecture or can be accomplished in a uniquely connectionist manner.

Road Map: Psychology
Related Reading: Artificial Intelligence and Neural Networks; Philosophical Issues in Brain Theory and Connectionism; Systematicity of Generalizations in Connectionist Networks

References

Anderson, J. A., 1972, A simple neural network generating an interactive memory, *Math. Biosci.*, 8:137–160.

Chalmers, D. J., 1990, Syntactic transformations on distributed representations, *Connect. Sci.*, 2:53–62.

Christiansen, M., Conway, C. M., and Curtin, S., 2000, A connectionist single mechanism account of rule-like behaviour in infancy, in *Proceedings of the 22nd Annual Conference of the Cognitive Science Society*, Mahwah, NJ: Erlbaum, pp. 83–88.

Edelman, G. M., 1987, *Neural Darwinism*, New York: Basic Books.

Hadley, R. F., 1999, Connectionism and novel combinations of skills: Implications for cognitive architecture, *Minds Machines*, 9:197–221.

Marcus, G. F., 2001, *The Algebraic Mind: Integrating Connectionism and Cognitive Science*, Cambridge, MA: MIT Press. ◆

McClelland, J. L., Rumelhart, D. E., and PDP Research Group, Eds., 1986, *Parallel Distributed Processing: Explorations in the Microstructure of Cognition* (2 vols.), Cambridge, MA: MIT Press.

Pinker, S., and Prince, A., 1988, On language and connectionism: Analysis of a parallel distributed processing model of language acquisition, in *Connections and Symbols* (S. Pinker and J. Mehler, Eds.), Cambridge, MA: Bradford/MIT Press, pp. 73–194.

Plaut, D. C., McClelland, J. L., Seidenberg, M. S., and Patterson, K., 1996, Understanding normal and impaired word reading: Computational principles in quasi-regular domains, *Psychol. Rev.*, 103:56–115.

Pollack, J., 1990, Recursive distributed representations, *Artif. Intell.*, 46:77–105.

Ratcliff, R., 1990, Connectionist models of recognition memory: Constraints imposed by learning and forgetting functions, *Psychol. Rev.*, 96:523–568.

Seidenberg, M. S., and McClelland, J. L., 1989, A distributed, developmental model of visual word recognition and naming, *Psychol. Rev.*, 96:523–568.

Sharkey, A. J. C., 1999, Multi-net systems, in *Combining Artificial Neural Nets: Ensemble and Modular Multi-Net Systems* (A. J. C. Sharkey, Ed.), New York: Springer-Verlag, pp. 1–30. ◆

Sharkey, N. E., 1997, Artificial neural networks for coordination and control: The portability of experiential representations, *Robot. Auton. Syst.*, 22:345–359.

Sharkey, N. E., 1998, Learning from innate behaviours: A quantitative evaluation of neural network controllers, *Machine Learn.*, 31:115–139.

Sharkey, N. E., and Sharkey, A. J. C., 1994, Emergent cognition, in *Handbook of Neuropsychology*, vol. 9, *Computational Modeling of Cognition* (J. Hendler, Ed.), Amsterdam: Elsevier. ◆

Collective Behavior of Coupled Phase Oscillators

Yoshiki Kuramoto

Introduction

Certain aspects of brain functions seem largely independent of the neurophysiological details of the individual neurons and their interconnections. The phase oscillator model for neural populations, like other neural network models, relies on this anticipation, still trying to recover the *phase information* that has been ignored by conventional models using all-or-none threshold elements. Here, phase information means the kind of information encoded in the form of specific temporal structures of the sequence of neuronal spikings that the real brain should make full use of. In this article, we present a brief survey of the collective behavior of coupled oscillators using the phase model and assuming all-to-all type interconnections. With these mathematical simplications, a number of definite results can be obtained. Because such a model could be too idealistic for practical purposes, we will not try to interpret the types of behavior obtained as relevent to specific brain activities.

Within the above restrictions on the model, the variety in collective behavior exhibited is still great. We will particularly be concerned in this article with the onset and persistence of *collective oscillation* in frequency-distributed systems; splitting of the population into a few subgroups, called *clustering*; and the more complex collective behavior called *slow switching*. It turns out that knowing the type of phase coupling between an interacting pair of oscillators is helpful for interpreting the resulting collective behavior. In the final section, a few remarks are provided on the limitations of the present model.

Phase Model

By suitably defining the phase ϕ (mod 2π) on the limit-cycle orbit of a given oscillator, its free motion can always be described by $\dot{\phi} = \omega$. When weak coupling is introduced between a pair of identical oscillators 1 and 2, each described by $\dot{\phi}_{1,2} = \omega$, phase reduction theory (Kuramoto, 1984) tells that these equations are modified as

$$\dot{\phi}_1 = \omega + \Gamma_{12}(\phi_1 - \phi_2) \tag{1}$$

combined with the similar equation for oscillator 2, where the coupling functions $\Gamma_{ij}(x)$ are 2π-periodic. What is important here is that the coupling depends only on the phase difference. Whenever necessary, $\Gamma_{ij}(x)$ can be computed numerically from knowledge of the original dynamical system model for the coupled oscillators.

The above argument can easily be generalized to systems of slightly nonidentical oscillators by replacing ω with $\omega + \delta\omega_{1,2} \equiv \omega_{1,2}$. Thus, a general network of N similar oscillators with pairwise coupling reduces to

$$\dot{\phi}_i = \omega_i + \sum_{j=1}^{N} \Gamma_{ij}(\phi_i - \phi_j) \tag{2}$$

This model, possibly with generalizations by including systematic and/or random forcing terms, provides a canonical model for oscillator networks.

Whether or not the weak coupling assumption is valid, the phase model has also been used as a convenient phenomenological model for the study of visual processing, motor control, and other life processes (Cohen, Holmes, and Rand, 1982; Ermentrout and Kopell, 1984; Sompolinsky et al., 1991).

Types of Phase Coupling

Phase coupling functions can be classified into a few basic types, and they lead to qualitatively different dynamics of a coupled pair. Assuming that the coupling is symmetric, or $\Gamma_{12}(x) = \Gamma_{21}(x) \equiv \Gamma(x)$, we obtain the equation for the phase difference $\psi \equiv \phi_1 - \phi_2$ in the form

$$\dot{\psi} = \Delta\omega + \Gamma_a(\psi) \tag{3}$$

where $\Delta\omega = \omega_1 - \omega_2$ and $\Gamma_a(\psi)$ is twice the antisymmetric part of $\Gamma(\psi)$, i.e., $\Gamma_a = \Gamma(\psi) - \Gamma(-\psi)$. Note that $\Gamma_a(x)$ satisfies $\Gamma_a(0) = \Gamma_a(\pm\pi) = 0$. When the oscillators are identical ($\Delta\omega = 0$), there are three typical situations (Figure 1). For type A coupling, $\Gamma_a'(0) < 0$ and $\Gamma_a'(\pm\pi) > 0$, so that the phase-synchronized state $\psi = 0$ is stable, while the antiphase state $\psi = \pm\pi$ is unstable. This form of coupling is called *in-phase type*. For type B coupling, in contrast, we have $\Gamma_a'(0) > 0$ and $\Gamma_a'(\pm\pi) < 0$, so that the coupling is called *antiphase type*. For type C coupling, both the in-phase and antiphase states are unstable, while the phase difference is locked at some intermediate value. We will call this *out-of-phase type* coupling. More complicated situations are possible where multiple values of ψ become stable.

When the oscillators are nonidentical, each $\dot{\psi}$ versus ψ curve in Figure 1 will be shifted upward or downward, so that the stable

value of ψ also changes. Clearly, outside a certain range of $\Delta\omega$, no fixed point can exist. Then the oscillators fail to synchronize, and the system as a whole exhibits quasi-periodic motion with two independent frequencies, their difference being given by the long-time average of $\dot{\psi}$. Numerical computation of Γ_a for some neural oscillator models in a self-oscillatory regime assuming diffusive or pulsatile coupling suggests that any of these three types of coupling is possible in real neural systems. It is remarkable that type C coupling can be obtained for self-oscillatory Hodgkin-Huxley neurons with excitatory synaptic coupling (Hansel, Mato, and Meunier, 1993a).

Neural oscillators are often modeled with the so-called leaky integrate-and-fire (LIF) neurons. In order to see the connection of this model to the phase model (Kuramoto, 1990), let a LIF neuron be described with variable u ($0 \le u \le 2\pi$), and identify the states $u = 0$ and 2π just as we did for the phase variable. The intrinsic dynamics of this neuron is such that u is monotone increasing with t, so that when u reaches the level $u = 2\pi$, it is immediately reset to the zero value. This instant is interpreted as the time of firing. Specifically, u is supposed to obey the equation

$$\dot{u} = a - u \tag{4}$$

Obviously, the neuron repeats firing if $a > 2\pi$, while it is non-oscillatory but only excitable when $a < 2\pi$. As for coupling with another LIF neuron, the usual assumption is that u changes by a small amount ε each time $t_n (n = 1, 2, \ldots)$ the second neuron fires. The coupling is excitatory if $\varepsilon > 0$ and inhibitory otherwise. This dynamical rule is conveniently represented by the term $\varepsilon\Sigma_n\delta(t - t_n)$ added to the right-hand side of Equation 4.

In the self-oscillatory regime ($a > 2\pi$), the natural frequency is given by $\omega = 2\pi/|\ln(1 - 2\pi/a)|$. It can be shown that the network of self-oscillatory LIF neurons with weak coupling is equivalent to that of phase oscillators given by the form of Equation 2 with the coupling function $\Gamma(\psi) = \varepsilon\omega a^{-1}\exp(\psi/\omega)$ ($0 \le \psi < 2\pi$). Note that $\Gamma(\psi)$ has a discontinuity at $\psi = 0$. It is easy to check that for positive (negative) ε, the in-phase (antiphase) state gives a unique and strongly stable state.

Throughout the subsequent sections, the coupling will be assumed to be pairwise and symmetric, belonging to either A, B, or C type.

Collective Oscillation

The collective behavior of coupled phase oscillators differs drastically for different coupling types. If the coupling is of the in-phase type and the oscillators are identical, then the whole assembly is in perfect phase synchrony, behaving as a single giant oscillator.

Many examples of collective oscillations in living and nonliving systems are known (Pikovsky, Rosenblum, and Kurths, 2001). With respect to sensory processing in the brain, in particular, collective synchronization may play a crucial role in the linking of sensory inputs across multiple receptive fields (Gray & Singer, 1998; Malsburg and Schneider, 1986). There are some studies on the last topic using the phase oscillator model (Sompolinsky et al., 1991).

Collective oscillations, if functionally relevant at all, should persist robustly against random perturbations from various sources, as would be unavoidable in the real world. How such robustness is guaranteed can theoretically be explained by using our phase model with all-to-all coupling. For a short history of this small branch of nonlinear science, see the review article by Strogatz (2000). The simplest model for this problem is given by

$$\dot{\phi}_i = \omega_i + \frac{1}{N}\sum_{j=1}^{N}\Gamma(\phi_i - \phi_j) \tag{5}$$

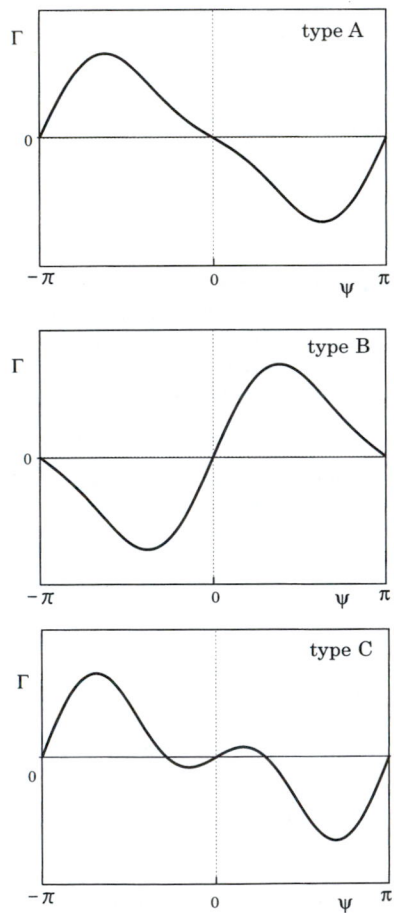

Figure 1. Three types of phase coupling functions.

Here the randomness is assumed in the natural frequencies ω_i with distribution $g(\omega)$, which is unimodal and symmetric about $\omega = \Omega$. For the simplest coupling function $\Gamma(x) = -K \sin x$, and in the limit of the population size N going to infinity, an exact solution with phase-transition-like behavior is available in a rather simple form. Macroscopic oscillation amplitude can be measured by the complex *order parameter* $w = N^{-1}\Sigma_{j=1}^{N}e^{i\phi_j}$. Analysis shows that the order parameter behaves like $w = \sigma \exp(i\Omega t)$, where σ satisfies the transcendental equation

$$\sigma = K\sigma \int_{-\pi/2}^{\pi/2} dx g(\Omega + K\sigma \sin x) \cos x e^{ix} \equiv S(\sigma) \quad (6)$$

$S(\sigma)$ is an S-shaped odd function saturating to 1 as $\sigma \to \infty$. Therefore, besides the trivial solution $\sigma = 0$, which always exists, a nontrivial solution appears when K exceeds a critical value given by $K_c = 2/(\pi g(\Omega))$ at which $S'(0) = 1$. It is remarkable that the period Ω of the macroscopic oscillation becomes infinitely precise as $N \to \infty$.

There are also studies for more general coupling functions. A noticeable result of such studies is that the order parameter for K slightly larger than K_c behaves like $\sigma \propto (K - K_c)^\beta$ with the exponent $\beta = 1$ rather than the classical value $\frac{1}{2}$, insofar as the coupling function is not completely free from the second harmonic component.

As the origin of randomness, the distribution in natural frequency may be replaced with external noise. When the noise is additive, white Gaussian, and drives the oscillators individually, the collective dynamics can also be studied analytically by means of a Fokker-Planck equation for the number density $\rho(\phi, t)$. Similar phase-transition-like behavior with $\beta = \frac{1}{2}$ is then obtained. Such a stochastic population model with the extension of including external stimuli, and with particular emphasis on its phase-resetting characteristics, was extensively studied by Tass (1999) with a view to medical applications such as the analysis of magnetoencephalography/electroencephalography data and deep brain stimulation techniques used in Parkinsonian patients.

Clustering and Complex Collective Behavior

We now consider the population dynamics of Equation 5 for the out-of-phase type coupling. The oscillators are assumed to be identical. Actually, owing to the desynchronizing nature of the coupling, the effects of randomness would be of secondary importance in causing complex collective behavior. Since perfect coherence is impossible, we want to find out what types of collective behavior can arise. The extreme opposite of perfect coherence is perfect *incoherence*, for which the phase distribution $\rho(\phi)$ is uniform. Such ρ certainly exists as a particular solution of the problem. However, analysis shows that its stability is guaranteed only for a special form of the coupling function. Thus, what occurs generically seems to be something intermediate between perfect coherence and perfect incoherence. Numerical study shows that most commonly, the whole population splits into two-point clusters, each in perfect phase synchrony, their phase difference preserving a constant value. Such collective behavior is obtained for the coupling function

$$\Gamma(\psi) = -\sin \psi + a \sin 2\psi \quad (7)$$

and illustrated in Figure 2 in comparison with the case of perfect coherence. The size proportion of the clusters, $p : 1 - p$, is not unique and depends on initial conditions; there is a certain range of p in which such two-cluster states remain stable. On a macroscopic level, the transition from one-cluster state to two-cluster state may appear as *rhythm splitting*, such as is often reported in the literature on circadian oscillations.

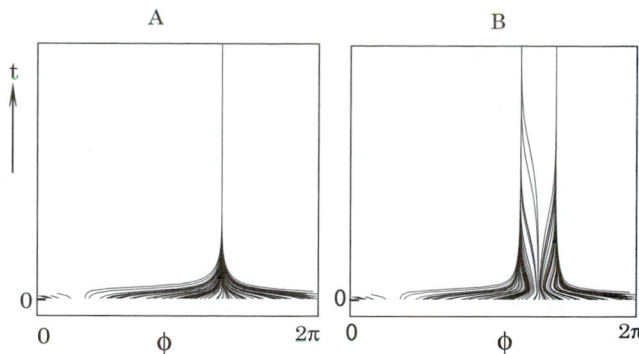

Figure 2. Formation of phase-synchronized clusters in a co-moving frame of reference for which ϕ remains constant for steady oscillation. A coupling function (Equation 7) with $\alpha = 0$ and random initial conditions are assumed. For $a = 0.4$ (A), the whole assembly converges to a single point cluster, while for $a = 0.7$ (B) it splits into two subpopulations, each in perfect phase synchrony.

The two clusters rigidly rotating in the phase space may become unstable for any p. When this happens, one or the other cluster may further split into multiple clusters, or otherwise a peculiar behavior called *slow switching* may occur (Hansel, Mato, and Meunier, 1993b). The latter phenomenon can be described as follows. For most periods, the system stays practically in a two-cluster state even if it is unstable. However, one of the clusters eventually becomes unable to maintain its internal phase synchrony, and starts to dissolve. This is followed by a short period of strong disorder. The entire system then relaxes to another two-cluster state, i.e., the state obtained by a constant phase shift of the original two-cluster state. Since the last state is also unstable, the same process repeats indefinitely, but with longer and longer time scales. The peculiar dynamics here is interpreted as resulting from the formation of an attracting heteroclinic loop connecting the first and second two-cluster states mentioned above. In the presence of weak randomness, in the form of either external noise or inhomogeneity, the switchings occur nearly periodically, with the period prolonged as the randomness is decreased.

Discussion

A few remarks should be about the two simplifying assumptions we have worked with. They are first, the weak coupling assumption, which enabled the phase description, and second, the all-to-all coupling. The first assumption has two implications. First, it implies that the oscillators practically keep staying on their intrinsic limit-cycle orbit when perturbed by the other oscillators. This allows us to ignore all degrees of freedoms other than the phases. Second, the time scale associated with the coupling is so long (much longer than the period of oscillation) that the effect of coupling can be time-averaged over one cycle of oscillation. This results in the coupling function depending only on the phase difference, thus fascilitating the mathematical analysis greatly. Assuming the weakness in coupling in the first sense seems neurobiologically quite reasonable (Hoppensteadt and Izhikevich, 1997). However, the second condition seems more restrictive. For instance, whenever neural oscillators establish mutual synchronization only within a few interspike intervals, this condition must certainly be violated.

Regarding the connectivity of neural oscillators, all-to-all coupling is apparently an extreme idealization. Local coupling represents another idealization. Actual coupling must be something in between, but the studies on coupled oscillator networks with general nonlocal coupling are still few. A neurobiologically plausible form of coupling often employed is characterized by short-range excitation and long-range inhibition. For this specific coupling type, and using relaxation oscillators, Terman and Wang (1995) studied the collective dynamics of the network in an attempt to lay a physical foundation for the oscillatory correlation theory of feature binding.

Road Map: Dynamic Systems
Related Reading: Chains of Oscillators in Motor and Sensory Systems; Synchronization, Binding and Expectancy; Visual Scene Segmentation

References

Cohen, A. H., Holmes, P. J., and Rand, R. H., 1982, The nature of the coupling between segmental oscillators of the lamprey spinal generator for locomotion: A mathematical model, *J. Math. Biol.*, 13:345–369.

Ermentrout, B., and Kopell, N., 1984, Frequency plateaus in a chain of weakly coupled oscillators, *SIAM J. Math. Anal.*, 15:215–237.

Gray, C. M., and Singer, W., 1989, Stimulus-specific neuronal oscillations in orientation columns of cat visual cortex, *Proc. Natl. Acad. Sci. USA*, 86:1698–1702.

Hansel, D., Mato, G., and Meunier, C., 1993a, Phase dynamics for weakly coupled Hodgkin-Huxley neurons, *Europhys. Lett.*, 23:367–372.

Hansel, D., Mato, G., and Meunier, C., 1993b, Clustering and slow switching in globally coupled phase oscillators, *Phys. Rev. E.*, 48:3470–3477.

Hoppensteadt, F. C., and Izhikevich, E. M., 1997, *Weakly Connected Neural Networks*, New York: Springer-Verlag.

Kuramoto, Y., 1984, *Chemical Oscillations, Waves, and Turbulence*, Berlin: Springer-Verlag. ◆

Kuramoto, Y., 1990, Collective synchronization of pulse-coupled oscillators and excitable units, *Physica D*, 50:15–30.

Malsburg, C. von der, and Schneider, W., 1986, A neural cocktail-party processor, *Biol. Cybern.*, 54:29–40.

Pikovsky, A., Rosenblum, M., and Kurths, J., 2001, *Synchronization: A Universal Concept in Nonlinear Science*, Cambridge, Engl.: Cambridge University Press. ◆

Sompolinsky, H., et al., 1991, Cooperative dynamics in visual processing, *Phys. Rev. A.*, 43:6990–7011.

Strogatz, S. H., 2000, From Kuramoto to Crawford: exploring the onset of synchronization in populations of coupled oscillators, *Physica D*, 143:1–20.

Tass, P. A., 1999, *Phase Resetting in Medicine and Biology*, Berlin: Springer-Verlag.

Terman, D., and Wang, D., 1995, Global competition and local cooperation in a network of neural oscillators, *Physica D*, 81:148–176.

Collicular Visuomotor Transformations for Gaze Control

J. A. M. Van Gisbergen and A. J. Van Opstal

Introduction

Neurophysiological studies on oculomotor control started in the early 1970s with descriptions of firing patterns at the motoneuron and the premotor level. Meanwhile, a wealth of information has become available on signal processing in the midbrain superior colliculus (SC) and at cortical levels. This article examines recent developments concerning the role of the SC in the control of gaze shifts (combined eye-head movements) and its possible involvement in the control of eye movements in 3D space (direction and depth). New experimental paradigms, putting fewer behavioral constraints on the eye and head motor systems, have led to novel views on the nature of collicular signals.

In classifying modes of oculomotor behavior, it appears useful to make a distinction between two behavioral states that alternate continuously in daily life. During attentive fixation the vestibulo-ocular reflex (VOR) and slow vergence maintain binocular foveal fixation to correct for body movements. When the task requires inspection of an eccentric stimulus, a complex synergy of coordinated movements comes into play. Such refixations typically involve a rapid combined eye-head movement (saccadic gaze shift) and often require binocular adjustment in depth (vergence). It is thought that the system responsible for rapid eye-head movements is actively suppressed during fixation, so that a gating signal (WHEN signal) is required which enables it to respond to the signals that specify the amplitude and the direction of movement (WHERE signals). There is evidence that large gaze shifts involve concurrent suppression of the VOR, which would otherwise counteract the system's effectiveness. As discussed later in this article, there is good reason to think that the SC is involved in this cyclic alternation between gaze holding and gaze shifting. This article will review related theoretical concepts, together with the underlying experimental data. For a broader orientation, see Scudder, Kaneko, and Fuchs (2002), and Wurtz (1996).

Fixation cells (FIX) in the rostral pole of the SC are active during attentive fixation and pause during large saccades (see Wurtz, 1996,

for review). In the caudal zone, the pattern of activity is just the opposite. A group of saccade-related cells (SAC) becomes active prior and during the saccade and has low levels of activity during active fixation. A similar antagonistic pattern of activity, functionally reminiscent of the rostral-caudal distinction in the SC, characterizes omnipause neurons and saccadic burst cells in the brainstem. These cells pause and burst during saccades; it is thought that they are driven by FIX and SAC cells, respectively. The brainstem pause cells, and burst cells have mutual inhibition and it has recently been suggested that this is also the case for FIX and SAC cells in the SC (Munoz and Istvan, 1998). In the visual system, target position is topographically coded. At the level of burst cells and motoneurons, saccade size is coded temporally by the number of spikes in the burst or the instantaneous firing rate. This transition from spatial to temporal coding is a classical problem in the study of the saccadic system in which the SC is thought to play a key role. Early studies of SAC cells suggested that the SC contains a topographical map specifying desired saccade displacement. These recordings showed that each SAC neuron is recruited only for a limited range of saccade amplitudes and directions, denoted as its movement field. As one moves from the fixation zone to the caudal border, the movement field of local SAC neurons becomes larger and more eccentric. Since saccade direction is coded along the perpendicular dimension, the colliculus can be considered as a map of saccade amplitude and direction that is organized in polar coordinates. By virtue of its topographical organization, the SC has become a key area for experimental and modeling approaches to the question of how sensory signals can be transformed into goal-directed movements. It has become clear that the SC activity during saccades to auditory and somatosensory targets conforms to the same motor map, suggesting that considerable sensorimotor remapping must take place (for references and further explanation see Dynamic Remapping).

An early electrical stimulation study by Robinson showed for the first time that the SC motor map is highly nonhomogeneous:

relatively more space is devoted to the representation of small saccades. Based on these results, the collicular motor representation in the monkey has been modeled by a complex-logarithmic mapping function (Van Gisbergen, Van Opstal, and Tax, 1987). This description characterizes the relation between retinal target location and the site of maximum SAC cell activity (afferent mapping) as well as the inverse relation between the locus of movement cell activity and the resulting saccade vector (efferent mapping). In the model, the population activity resembles a Gaussian function centered on the point defined by the afferent mapping. This activity profile is translation-invariant so that the number of active cells is assumed constant, independent of saccade size. Such a topographical representation may generate goal-directed saccades if each cell has fixed connections with the horizontal and vertical burst cells downstream, allowing it to generate a small movement vector, proportional to its firing rate, into the direction of the retinal location to which it is connected by the afferent mapping.

Several recent developments have called for extensions of the model. For example, microstimulation in the SC (Van Opstal, Van Gisbergen, and Smit, 1990) has revealed that the eye displacement, encoded by a given site, can be systematically modified by the stimulation parameters. Furthermore, it now seems clear that the SC is involved with rapid gaze movements rather than being a purely saccadic eye-movement control center. Finally, there is increasing evidence that the SC is also involved in directing the eyes in depth. These latter two developments will now be discussed.

Role of the Superior Colliculus in the Control of Gaze Shifts

That activity in the colliculus can generate gaze movements has become clear from electrical stimulation studies in a number of species. The possibility that the monkey SC may code desired gaze displacement has been investigated at the single unit level by Freedman and Sparks (1997). Their approach was to compare the activity of movement cells in trials in which either the gaze displacement vector, the eye displacement vector, or the head displacement vector was constant while the other two vectors varied widely. The conclusion from this work is that a gaze displacement signal is derived from the locus of activity in the SC motor map, which is subsequently decomposed into separate eye and head displacement signals downstream from the colliculus (see Figure 1). The work of Cullen and Guitton (1997) suggests that this separation is not yet evident at the level of premotor burst cells (see discussion later in this article).

Less is known about the extent to which the WHEN systems for eye and head are coupled. If omnipause cells would govern both subsystems, one would expect the onset latencies of eye and head movements to be strongly coupled. Although microstimulation in cat SC seems to support this notion, experiments in primates reveal a considerable degree of independence, arguing against a single shared WHEN system.

Struck by the similarities between eye and head contributions to natural gaze shifts in the cat, Guitton, Munoz, and Galiana (1990) have suggested the possibility that eye and head are driven by a common signal. However, experiments in humans where eye and head had nonaligned starting positions before the gaze movement started (Goossens and Van Opstal, 1997) revealed that their movements may have different directions, incompatible with a common input signal. This led them to propose a model in which eye and head are driven by signals expressed in oculocentric and craniocentric coordinates, respectively, which are nevertheless derived from a common collicular gaze displacement command. One feature of the model is that the driving signals for both the eyes and the head depend on absolute eye position (see Figure 1). The need for such an arrangement has also become apparent from electrical

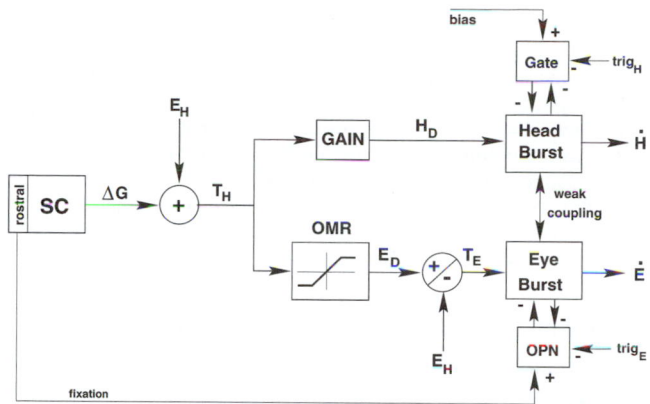

Figure 1. Primate gaze control model. As explained in the text, the collicular gaze displacement command, ΔG, cannot be used to drive eyes and head directly. The scheme proposes that it is first transformed into a desired craniocentric position, T_H, by adding current eye position, E_H. A scaled version of this signal (H_D, desired head position) controls the head movement generator and accounts for the finding that the head-movement gain is typically less than one. The craniocentric signal is also passed through a neural saturation element (OMR) to prevent the oculomotor system from running against the limits of its motor range. Dynamic eye motor error, T_E, which drives the oculomotor burst generator, is then obtained by subtracting current eye position from the clipped T_H signal, E_D (dynamic desired eye position). The model also proposes a weak excitatory coupling between the two motor systems (Galiana and Guitton, 1992; Goossens and Van Opstal, 1997). This coupling accounts for the differences in eye and head contributions to the gaze shift, as well as for the modulation of head movement trajectories by eye position. The gating mechanisms for the eye (OPN) and head burst generators (Gate) each have their own trigger and bias signals. Internal feedback loops that are assumed to control the eye and head burst generators to ensure that the eye reaches the target, as well as the role of the vestibular system, have been omitted for clarity (after Goossens and Van Opstal, 1997).

stimulation studies in the superior colliculus of the head-free monkey (Freedman, Stanford, and Sparks, 1996).

Activity of Burst Cells During Gaze Shifts

Earlier discussions of the role to be assigned to the SC in models of the oculomotor system have generally taken for granted that the role of short-lead burst neurons (BN) was already well established. These cells were thought to carry a saccadic velocity signal. However, since the underlying evidence was based on studies in head-fixed animals, it cannot be excluded that the activity of these cells may in fact be related to gaze velocity. The main reason for considering this possibility is that the colliculus, their major source of input, is now thought to specify a desired gaze shift (see previous discussion).

Cullen and Guitton (1997) have made a thorough study of saccadic burst cells to find out whether their activity during head-free gaze shifts might be gaze rather than eye-related. To investigate this question, they fitted the discharge patterns of BNs during head-free gaze shifts, $B(t)$, with a descriptive model of the form: $B(t) = a + b.\dot{E} + c.\dot{H}$ where a is a bias term, $\dot{E}$ represents instantaneous eye velocity, $\dot{H}$ is current head velocity, and b and c are coefficients. This formulation provides a framework for unambiguous definitions of gaze-related versus eye-related coding and yields numbers allowing each cell to be placed along the continuum between these two extremes.

If a cell is to code gaze velocity, it should not matter by which combination of eye and head velocity the gaze-velocity signal was created. In such an idealized cell, coefficients b and c would have identical values. In a pure eye velocity cell, coefficient c would be zero. Remarkably, the tacit assumption in the literature that burst cells are pure eye velocity cells, which seemed to make sense because these neurons have direct connections with oculomotoneurons, was not confirmed. Most cells had a head-velocity contribution in addition to the expected eye-velocity term. On the other hand, the cells were not straightforward gaze cells either because the weights are generally not equal ($c < b$) so that, in fact, their behavior is a compromise between eye related and gaze related.

Control of Refixations in Direction and Depth

Delineation of the Problem

Most refixations made in daily life involve both a change in direction and in depth. It has long been held that these movements are made by largely independent subsystems, the saccadic and the vergence system, which were conceived of as binocular controllers. The striking contrast between the quite slow movements in pure vergence and the rapidity of saccades tended to support the idea that these systems are quite different in nature. Early modeling studies have further emphasized the notion of distinct systems with unique properties. It was recognized early on that saccades are much too fast to allow the benefit of direct sensory feedback to guide the movement on a moment to moment basis. By contrast, it has often been proposed that pure vergence movements are slow enough to be under direct visual feedback. These distinctions, based on the extreme cases of pure vergence and pure saccades, become much less clear in the more common situation where both systems act together as occurs during refixations in 3D visual space. The finding that, in such cases, vergence shows a very clear velocity enhancement during the saccade has led to the proposal that perhaps saccades may be disconjugate (unequal in the two eyes). It should be noted that, for the portion of the vergence response that is executed as part of a fast movement, the role of direct sensory feedback must be extremely limited.

Since the saccadic and the vergence subsystems typically operate in joint fashion, we must ask how this coordination comes about. Some provision is necessary to ensure that the saccadic system and the vergence system will move to the same target when there are several alternatives. Chaturvedi and Van Gisbergen (1998) performed behavioral experiments in humans instructed to make binocular refixations to a green target in 3D space and to ignore a red distracter at another location. In short-latency responses, errors (to the red stimulus) and compromising responses (in between) were not uncommon but it appeared that the two systems always worked in unison, strongly suggesting that there must be a common central target selection system operating on 3D stimulus location information.

Possible Role of SC in Coding Refixations in 3D Space

Recent evidence suggests that the SC, which receives depth information from parietal cortex, may be directly involved in saccade-vergence coordination. Chaturvedi and Van Gisbergen (1999) applied electrical stimulation in the caudal SC when the monkey was just preparing or executing the 3D refixation to a visual target. Electrical stimulation alone produced a saccade without an overt vergence component. Stimulation in midflight, just after the monkey had started his visually guided movement, caused a compromise saccade and a marked reduction of the fast vergence component. The vergence perturbation was not simply an epiphenomenon of a change in saccade duration and was comparable in strength to the saccadic disturbance. The vergence effect cannot be understood from classical models proposing that the SC

specifies only the movement in the frontal plane, leaving the depth movement coding to some other area (see above). Instead, Chaturvedi and Van Gisbergen (1999) proposed that the population of cells at any SC locus shares the same direction movement vector, like in the old 2D-coding schemes, but suggest that there is also a depth movement component. The latter is different from cell to cell so that the entire depth dimension along the locally represented direction in space is covered (see Figure 2). With such an extended scheme it is understandable, in principle, why electrical stimulation in isolation may cause only a pure saccadic movement, without any overt sign of vergence. In this situation, the local cells with different depth tuning will be excited indiscriminately, thereby causing a zero vergence displacement command which can counteract the visually induced vergence signal. By contrast, the saccadic signal will still emerge during such local artificial intervention by virtue of the topographical organization of the motor map, which represents the desired horizontal and vertical components spatially on a much courser scale.

Coding of Eye Movements by Burst Cells

At this point it is interesting to consider how fast eye movements in 3D are coded at the premotor level. It was thought until very recently that burst cells in the reticular formation coded saccades binocularly by providing a conjugate velocity signal. From a systematic study based on eye movements in 3D space, Zhou and King (1998) concluded that most cells code eye velocity for either one or the other eye, irrespective of the depth component involved. This means that the total population contains a 3D code, including both directional and depth components, and that the old idea that they

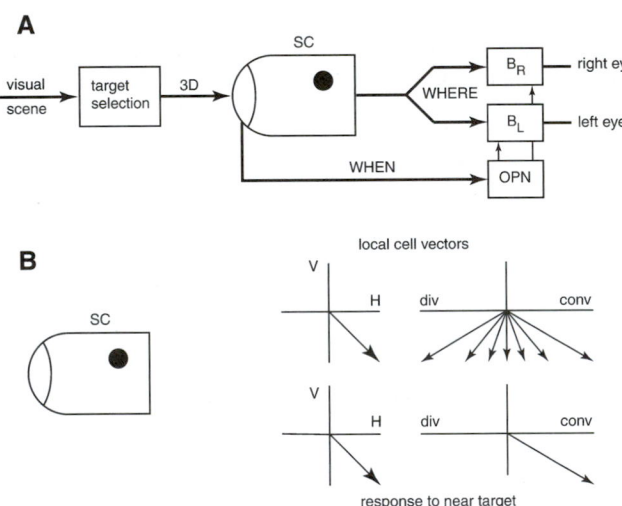

Figure 2. Possible role of SC in control of rapid eye movements in direction and depth. *A*, Based on evidence discussed in the text, the scheme proposes that the SC receives 3D information about the location of the selected target and emits a 3D WHERE signal to activate the populations of right eye and left eye burst cells in the brainstem (Zhou and King, 1998). The initiation system (WHEN) is embodied by the rostral zone in the SC and omnipause cells in the brainstem (OPN). The locus of the active zone in the SC determines the change in fixation in the frontal plane but has no topographic organization for depth coding. *B*, Proposal on how activity in the SC may code direction and depth. All the cells in the active zone code for an oblique downward movement but the cells differ in their depth coding directions as shown in the upper-right panel. For a near target in the locally represented direction of the visual field, the population will yield the direction vector shown at bottom left and the net convergence movement shown in the bottom-right panel.

code only conjugate saccades must be abandoned. It is tempting to suggest that the 3D coding at the level of the burst cells may be a further elaboration of the proposed 3D coding in the SC, which is known to be a major source of input signals for these neurons.

Discussion

Decomposition of SC Signals for Eye and Head

As explained in the previous section, it is now thought that the deep layers of the SC specify a desired gaze displacement, which typically involves movement of both the eyes and the head (Guitton et al., 1990; Freedman et al., 1996; Freedman and Sparks, 1997). However, accumulating evidence indicates that this signal cannot be used directly to drive eyes and head. First, the desired gaze shift may encode a movement well beyond the oculomotor range. For example, suppose a SC site that specifies a 40° rightward gaze displacement is active. When the eyes are looking 20° to the left, the entire movement could be covered by the oculomotor system alone. However, when the eyes start from a position 20° to the right, part of the gaze shift has to be made by the head so that the relative contributions of the eyes and the head to the total gaze shift will (in part) be determined by the initial position of the eyes in the orbit. Second, experiments have shown that the movement directions of eyes and head can be quite different when their initial starting positions are unaligned. Both motor systems appear to move in the direction of the spatial target position. Multiple regression of human data has shown that the direction of head movement is best described by the head motor-error vector (rather than by gaze error). In contrast, the eye-in-head displacement is best described in terms of an eye motor-error signal (Goossens and Van Opstal, 1997). Third, in primates the difference in movement onset of eyes and head varies considerably from trial to trial (see previous discussion). This variability is largely explained by the relative contributions of the two motor systems to the gaze shift: the larger the planned head movement, the earlier it starts (Freedman et al., 1996; Goossens and Van Opstal, 1997). These relative contributions are not fully determined by initial eye position, since stimulus modality is also an important factor: auditory gaze shifts tend to have larger (and thus earlier) head movements (Goossens and Van Opstal, 1997). Finally, the movement trajectories of the head are influenced by eye position, which suggests a subtle coupling between the two motor systems. The simplified scheme in Figure 1 incorporates these different aspects, and highlights the transformations that are required between the SC and the two motor systems.

Binocular Versus Monocular Control of Eye Movements

The question of how the brain coordinates binocular eye movements has been debated already in the previous century, long before any neurophysiological evidence was available. One view, known as the principle of equal innervation, advocates that there are two binocular control systems that affect both eyes. The conjugate system moves both eyes equally and in the same direction. The disconjugate system in this scheme moves both eyes equally in opposite directions, to generate vergence movements. In this way, all binocular eye movements can be described mathematically as the linear sum of a conjugate and a disconjugate movement command, but it is not known whether this is also a valid description of how the real system operates.

The alternative idea is that each eye is controlled separately (monocular control systems). Quite unexpectedly, a recent study by Zhou and King (1998) has yielded evidence for the latter scheme at the level of burst cells. That the situation is not simple is indicated by the even more surprising finding by Zhou and King that

motoneurons in the abducens nucleus often carry binocular signals. This is counterintuitive since, at first glance, it would seem hard to think of a more likely candidate for monocular eye movement coding than the oculomotorneuron level. The finding of monocular coding in premotor burst celld raises interesting questions for the organization at more central levels. If the SC indeed contains a 3D code for rapid eye movements, as discussed above, the question to be faced is how the functional projections of its cells may be organized. Sylvestre, Galiana, and Cullen (2002) have recently proposed a model featuring a shared vergence/saccade controller in the SC, which can yield monocular burst cells without requiring an exceedingly complex wiring diagram.

Is the SC an Open-Loop Controller?

The two schemes in this chapter suggest that the SC provides a motor command to downstream platforms in open-loop fashion. There is general agreement that vision is much too slow to provide feedback during saccadic refixations. In other words, if ongoing platform movements are to affect current SC activity, the only possibility is to use internal (or local) feedback. Currently, there is no clear evidence for the idea that the SC has access to fast moment-to-moment local feedback about saccade execution. There are signs of a limited degree of local feedback but its precise role remains to be determined. For an extensive review on experimental and theoretical work in this vast and highly controversial field we refer to Scudder et al. (2002).

Road Maps: Mammalian Brain Regions; Mammalian Motor Control; Vision

Related Reading: Dynamic Remapping; Pursuit Eye Movements; Vestibulo-Ocular Reflex

References

Chaturvedi, V., and Van Gisbergen, J. A. M., 1998, Shared target selection for combined version-vergence eye movements, *J. Neurophysiol.*, 80:849–862.

Chaturvedi, V., and Van Gisbergen, J. A. M., 1999, Perturbation of combined saccade-vergence movements by microstimulation in monkey superior colliculus, *J. Neurophysiol.*, 81:2279–2296.

Cullen, K. E., and Guitton, D., 1997, Analysis of primate IBN spike trains using system identification techniques. II. Relationship to gaze, eye, and head movement dynamics during head-free gaze shifts, *J. Neurophysiol.*, 78:3283–3306.

Freedman, E. G., Stanford, T. R., and Sparks, D. L., 1996, Combined eye-head gaze shifts produced by electrical stimulation of the superior colliculus in rhesus monkeys, *J. Neurophysiol.*, 76:927–952.

Freedman, E. G., and Sparks, D. L., 1997, Activity of cells in the deeper layers of the superior colliculus of the rhesus monkey: Evidence for a gaze displacement command, *J. Neurophysiol.*, 78:1669–1690.

Galiana, H. L., and Guitton, D., 1992, Central organization and modeling of eye-head coordination during orienting gaze shifts, *Ann. NY Acad. Sci.*, 656:452–471.

Goossens, H. H. L. M., and Van Opstal, A. J., 1997, Human eye-head coordination in two dimensions under different sensorimotor conditions, *Exp. Brain Res.*, 114:542–560.

Guitton, D., Munoz, D. P., and Galiana, H. L., 1990, Gaze control in the cat: Studies and modeling of the coupling between orienting eye and head movements in different behavioral tasks, *J. Neurophysiol.*, 64:509–531.

Munoz, D. P., and Istvan, P. J., 1998, Lateral inhibitory interactions in the intermediate layers of the monkey superior colliculus, *J. Neurophysiol.*, 79:1193–1209.

Scudder, C. A., Kaneko, C. R. S., and Fuchs, A. F., 2002, The brainstem burst generator for saccadic eye movements, *Exp. Brain Res.*, 142:439–462. ◆

Sylvestre, P. A., Galiana, H. L., and Cullen, K. E., 2002, Conjugate and vergence oscillations during saccades and gaze shifts: Implications for integrated control of binocular movement, *J. Neurophysiol*, 87:257–272.

Van Gisbergen, J. A. M., Van Opstal, A. J., and Tax, A. A. M., 1987, Collicular ensemble coding of saccades based on vector summation, *Neuroscience*, 21:541–555.

Van Opstal, A. J., Van Gisbergen, J. A. M., and Smit, A. C., 1990, Com- parison of saccades evoked by visual stimulation and collicular electrical stimulation in the alert money, *Exp. Brain Res.*, 79:299–312.

Wurtz, R. H., 1996, Vision for the control of movement, *Invest. Opthalmol. Vis. Sci.*, 37:2131–2145.

Zhou, W., and King, W. M., 1998, Premotor commands encode monocular eye movements, *Nature*, 393:692–695.

Color Perception

Robert Kentridge, Charles Heywood, and Jules Davidoff

Introduction

Color is the name we assign to the experience elicited by an attribute of a surface, namely, its spectral reflectance. Color sensations have a reliable, though complex, relationship to the spectral composition of light received by the eyes. The visual system tackles a series of computational problems in the course of processing wavelength. Variation in the wavelength of light is isolated from variation in its intensity. The spectral reflectance properties of surfaces are isolated from the effects of the spectral composition of light illuminating them (matching surfaces with the same reflectance properties in different parts of the visual scene or under different illuminants are the two problems of color constancy). Finally, the resulting continuous color space is partitioned into discrete color categories. In addition, it will become clear that wavelength signals can be used in the course of perceiving form or motion, independent of their role in the subjective experience of color.

Wavelength-Dependent Differences Within the Visual System

Color percepts derive from light that varies in both wavelength and intensity. A single type of photoreceptor in the eye responds with differing efficiency to light over a wide range of wavelengths. Consequently, a visual system in which there is only a single type of photoreceptor inevitably confounds wavelength and intensity. A visual system containing photoreceptors that differ in their spectral response can, in principle, disambiguate wavelength and intensity by comparing the responses of different types of receptors.

Receptors

Wavelength-selective processing can be traced from differentially wavelength-sensitive cone types in the retina to the lateral geniculate nucleus (LGN) and then on to striate cortex and extrastriate areas beyond it. There are three cone types in the human retina, with peak sensitivities at 560 nm, 530 nm, and 430 nm and referred to as L, M, and S (long-, medium-, and short-wavelength-sensitive) cones, respectively. In some people one or more of these cone types are missing; hence, color sensations that would normally be perceived as distinct are confused, and the individuals are "color-blind." The functions relating the sensitivities of these cone types to the wavelength of stimulating light can be inferred by comparing the wavelength sensitivities of color-blind and normal observers or by examining the effects of adaptation to light of one wavelength on sensitivity to light of other wavelengths. Figure 1 shows the relative absorption efficiencies of the three cone types and the typical pattern of behavioral sensitivity to intensity modulation.

The output of cones provides information about an object's state, for example, allowing ripe and unripe fruit to be discriminated. The peak sensitivities of photoreceptors appear exquisitely matched to maximize the discriminability of the foliage or fruits that form the

diets of a number of species of primates (Sumner and Mollon, 2000). Studies of the genetic coding of cone pigments indicate that human trichromacy evolved from ancestral dichromacy through the division of a single long-wavelength-sensitive pigment into distinct L and M pigments (Bowmaker, 1998).

The Combination of Receptor Signals in the M, P, and K Channels

Three anatomically distinct cell types in the retina combine cone signals in distinct ways (Dacey, 2000). In all cases, the response has a "center-surround" organization. A set of cones from one part of the visual field influences the cell in one way, while a set of cones from the surrounding area influences it in a different way. Parasol cells receive input from L and M, but not S, cones. Inputs from L and M cones are summed in both the center and surround fields of parasol cells (Figure 2A). Parasol cells cannot convey information about wavelength independent of intensity. They project to the magnocellular layer of the LGN, which in turn projects to layers 4Cα and 4B of primary visual cortex (V1). This pathway, and its onward projections, is known as the M-channel. The M-channel contributes to the perception of luminance and motion but does not convey wavelength-coded signals.

Midget ganglion cells have color-opponent receptive fields. This center-surround organization sharpens the effective wavelength selectivity of the ganglion cell, helping to unconfound wavelength and intensity variation. Consider first a nonopponent cell, sensitive to medium wavelength light. This cell will produce the same re-

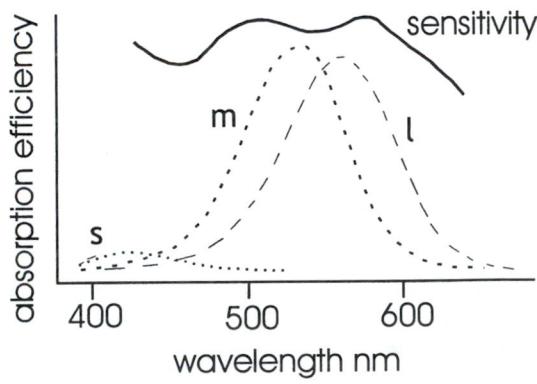

Figure 1. The relative absorption efficiencies of short-, medium-, and long-wavelength cone types, labeled s, m, and l, are shown as dotted, short-dashed, and long-dashed lines, respectively. The solid line shows sensitivity to increments in luminance for lights of different wavelengths. The sensitivity decreases falling between the peaks of the cone absorption spectra are known as Sloan-Crawford notches.

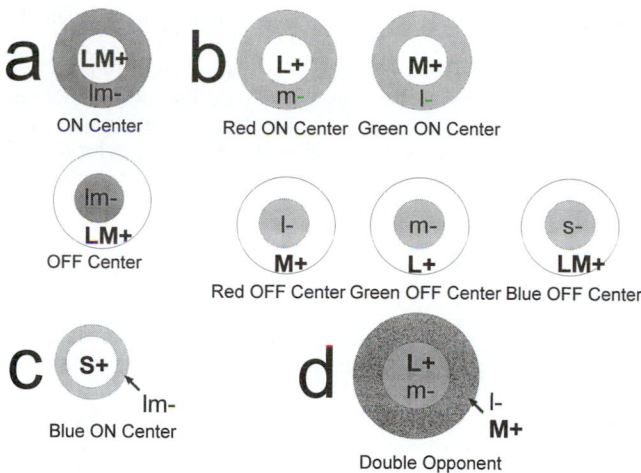

Figure 2. Schematic representations of receptive field organization of cells in (*A*) the M-channel, (*B*) the P-channel, and (*C*) the K-channel. (*D*) An example of receptive field organization of a cortical double-opponent cell.

sponse to a given intensity of medium wavelength light, or a stronger intensity of longer wavelength light. Although its peak sensitivity is to medium rather than longer wavelength light, because sensitivity only reduces gradually as wavelength deviates from the peak, the longer wavelength light still produces a response. Now consider the responses of an opponent cell excited by medium wavelength light in the center of its field and inhibited by long wavelength light in the surround to different intensities and wavelengths of light falling on its entire receptive field. Medium wavelength light produces excitation in the center and no inhibition in the surround; there is a net increase in the cell's firing rate. Higher intensities of medium wavelength light elicit stronger net responses. A slightly longer wavelength produces some excitation in the center field of the ganglion cell but also a small inhibitory response in the surround. These roughly balance, and so the firing rate of the cell is largely unaffected by the stimulus. The same situation applies to a high-intensity stimulus; again, central excitation is balanced by surround inhibition. This ganglion cell is therefore capable of conveying information solely about the intensity of medium wavelength light.

The vast majority of foveal midget ganglion cells are driven by L or by M cones in the center of their receptive field; these centers can be either excitatory or inhibitory. Away from the fovea, midget ganglion cells lose their spectral opponency, as more than one cone type drives both the center and surround. There appears to be little input from S cones to midget ganglion cells, just as there are very few S cones in the retina. About 2%–3% of parafoveal midget ganglion cells have S-OFF central receptive fields with an ON surround driven by both L and M inputs (Figure 2*B*). There are no S-ON center midget ganglion cells.

Small bistratified ganglion cells receive inputs from all three cone types; however, their central field always appears to be driven by an excitatory input from S cones, while their surround combines inhibitory L and M inputs. The bipolar cells that convey signals from cones to the central field receive inputs only from S cones and are driven by multiple cells, unlike the bipolar cells that drive the central fields of midget ganglion cells, which receive inputs from single cones. The result is that, although these cells do show clear spatial and spectral opponency, the size of the central field (100 μm standard deviation) is much larger than that found in midget ganglion cells (25 μm) (Figure 2*C*). The surround fields of small bistratified cells are smaller than those of midget ganglion

cells (140 μm and 205 μm, respectively), so these cells show relatively weak spatial opponency. One additional consequence of the S-cone specificity of the small bistratified cells is that the S-ON center, LM-OFF surround organization extends into the peripheral visual field, whereas midget ganglion cells lose spectral opponency beyond the parafovea. There are no S cones in the central 0.3 degrees of the visual field, so foveal vision is effectively color-blind to color variation mediated by S cones.

Midget ganglion cells project to the parvocellular layer of the LGN, and thence to layer 4Cβ of V1. This pathway, and its onward projections, is known as the P-channel. The P-channel conveys information about long and medium wavelengths and fine detail. It has been suggested that small bistratified ganglion cells conveying short wavelength information also contribute to the P-channel. However, it is now widely believed that small bistratified cells drive a distinct class of geniculate cells. The P-channel does contribute to motion perception; however, its contribution is weaker than that of the M-channel and nonveridical—the speed of perceived motion depends on the chromatic contrast of the stimulus.

Small bistratified ganglion cells form the start of the K-channel (Hendry and Reid, 2000). They project to koniocellular neurons in the LGN, distinguished from magno and parvo cells on the basis of their cell membrane chemistry. These cells mainly form layers intercalated between the parvo- and magnocellular layers, but some K-cells are also found in the parvocellular layer, with a smaller number being found in the magnocellular layer. K-cells project not only to layer 1 of V1, but also directly to V2. There is a particularly rich innervation of V2 by K-cells with foveal receptive fields. K-cells' receptive fields are large (at least as large as those of cells in the magnocellular layer) and often have irregular shapes. K-cells convey information contributing to color sensations, depending on contrasts of the output of S cones to combinations of M and L cone outputs; they may also contribute to motion perception.

The position summarized above remains controversial and has been challenged on a number of counts. In particular, it has been argued that the K-channel alone conveys chromatic signals (including L versus M information), while the P-channel is dedicated to fine spatial vision (Calkins and Sterling, 1999).

Primary Visual Cortex

The M, P, and K pathways project to groups of cells within V1 that can be distinguished on the basis of cytochrome oxidase reactivity (Livingstone and Hubel, 1984). K and P, but not M, pathways innervate cytochrome oxidase–stained regions known as blobs. P and M, but not K, pathways innervate the remaining regions, known as interblobs. There is recent evidence that cells show different specificities for wavelength processing in V1 (Conway, 2001; Johnson, Hawken, and Shapley, 2001). The cells discussed earlier in this article had a "single-opponent" organization. They can convey information about the intensities of light of particular wavelengths while being relatively uninfluenced by other wavelengths. They cannot, however, convey information about wavelength contrast. This requires "double-opponent" cells in which a central receptive field excited by one wavelength and inhibited by another is surrounded by a field in which the same two wavelengths have the opposite actions (Figure 1*D*). Double-opponent organization allows a cell to convey a consistent response to the boundary between two surfaces, regardless of the light illuminating them. If the illuminant changes, for example lengthening in wavelength, then longer wavelength light will be reflected from both sides of the boundary. Consider a double-opponent cell whose central receptive field is excited by long wavelengths and inhibited by medium wavelengths and whose surrounding field is inhibited by long wavelengths and excited by medium wavelengths. Imagine that the cell's receptive fields fall on a boundary between a pair of surfaces, one of which is good and one poor at reflecting long wavelength light, so that the good reflector falls in the cell's central field. The net result will be excitation—that ratio of long to medium wavelength light is high in the central field and low in the surround. When the light illuminating both sides of the boundary lengthens in wavelength, the L/M ratios in both the excitatory center and the inhibitory surround will increase. The response of the cell is therefore largely unaffected by a change in illuminant. Obviously, such cells perform the preliminary computation necessary for color constancy. Of course, their responses only indicate spatially local changes in surface reflectance. To recover absolute reflectances throughout a scene, then, one also needs to estimate the response likely to be elicited by some fixed "anchoring" color in that scene and then to integrate local border contrasts from that anchoring point (see, e.g., Gilchrist et al., 1999, for similar arguments with respect to lightness perception). Until recently, evidence for the existence of double-opponent cells was controversial; however, recent findings indicate that such cells occur in V1 and, moreover, are sensitive to the orientation of chromatic (wavelength-dependent) borders as well as to the contrast of cone ratios across them.

Extrastriate Cortex

The clinical condition of cerebral achromatopsia, in which patients lose the ability to perceive color not as a result of retinal abnormalities but rather as a consequence of brain damage, provides strong evidence that brain areas specialized for color perception exist beyond striate cortex. The identification of these areas is, however, wreathed in controversy. The damaged areas include extrastriate cortex in the vicinity of the fusiform and lingual gyri. Neuroimaging studies have also shown increases in cerebral blood flow (implying increased brain activity) in these areas when normal subjects observed colored scenes. Zeki et al. (1991) therefore suggested that there was a specific color center in human extrastriate cortex. Early studies in which the responses from single neurons in monkeys were recorded in response to visual stimuli suggested that the color center might correspond to cortical area V4. A number of problems arose with this interpretation. The selectivity of the response of neurons to particular characteristics of stimuli differs only in degree between brain areas. Some neurons in nearly all visual areas respond selectively to wavelength; the proportion in V4 is not comparatively large. In addition, damage to area V4 in monkeys did not cause deficits in discriminations based on wavelength, although deficits were induced by damage to areas anterior to V4 (Heywood and Cowey, 1998). These findings appeared consistent with neuroimaging studies in humans identifying a color-selective area anterior to V4, christened V8 (Hadjikhani et al., 1998). Whether V8 really corresponds to the anterior areas that, when damaged, caused deficits for wavelength discrimination in monkeys remains controversial.

Wavelength Information Contributes to More Than Color Perception

The fact that our visual system can disambiguate wavelength and intensity makes it possible to ignore variations or sharp changes in intensity caused by shadows. One role of a wavelength-selective visual system is therefore segmentation of the visual scene on the basis of chromatic boundaries. Often chromatic boundaries will provide better cues for segmenting objects from their backgrounds than brightness boundaries—for example, in the dappled sunlight of a forest floor.

The residual abilities found in cerebral achromatopsia indicate that wavelength is exploited in more than one way. Although cerebral achromatopsics deny a phenomenal experience of color and cannot discriminate between stimuli differing only in wavelength, they can effortlessly perceive boundaries between areas differing only in wavelength (Heywood, Kentridge, and Cowey, 1998). Their ability to use wavelength information to perceive form or motion, but not to perceive color, suggests that these functions may have distinct anatomical bases. Destruction of the putative color center, be it V4 or V8, disrupts the perception and experience of color, but not other functional uses of wavelength.

Discussion

Some of the earliest insights into the coding of color derived from work on color mixing. Following his discovery of the composition of white light, Newton developed the concept of the color circle, an arrangement of light sources around the periphery of a circle in which the mixture of any pair of diametrically opposite lights would produce white. Despite the color circle showing a continuum of light sources, Newton identified five primary colors (red, yellow, green, blue, and a violet-purple). However, attempts were soon made to discover how few colors were required in order to produce all other colors by mixing. Although there was some disagreement about which colors were primary, it was apparent to most investigators that three were sufficient. This culminated in the Young-Helmholtz trichromatic theory of color vision. Young believed that the primaries were red, green, and violet.

The fact that we require three primary colors in order to produce the full range of colored sensations reflects the fact that we have photoreceptors sensitive to three distinct wavelength distributions. The consequence is that any combination of lights that produces the same amount of activation in the three receptor types will produce the same response in the visual system and the same perception of color. There are, therefore, a large number of colors that are potential primaries.

Other features of color perception suggest an alternative to the trichromatic theory. In particular, there are limits to our abilities to see pairs of colors tinting one another. People perceive bluish reds and yellowish reds, but never greenish reds; they perceive reddish yellows and greenish yellows, but never bluish yellows. These opponent color pairings, red-green and blue-yellow, are also apparent in afterimages, color shadows, and color contrast. Observations such as these led Hering in 1905 to suggest a four-color opponent-process theory of color vision.

Both these theories assumed that the similarities between color sensations are completely determined by the outputs of the wavelength-dependent neurons in the visual system. For example, it is tempting to believe that opponent processes operating in V1 are the direct precursors of our space of colors. They have been taken as the sources of four primary colors (red, green, yellow, and blue) that are irreducible to other colors, and each contains one sensation that is pure (unique) in that it contains no trace of any other primary. However, the outputs of the cells in V1 would not produce these unique colors even if there were agreement as to what they might be (Saunders and van Brakel, 1997; Webster et al., 2000). Nor would the categories of color arise from variation in discrimination across the visible spectrum. The wavelengths at which there are minima in threshold do not correspond to the boundaries between primary colors. Controversially, it has been argued from cross-lingual evidence that color categories are determined by the speaker's color terms. The neurophysiology produces a given percept, but the assignment of that percept to a color category is a matter of agreement among observers.

Road Map: Vision
Related Reading: Contour and Surface Perception; Retina

References

Bowmaker, J. K., 1998, Evolution of color vision in vertebrates, *Eye*, 12:541–547.

Calkins, D. J., and Sterling, P., 1999, Evidence that circuits for spatial and color vision segregate at the first retinal synapse, *Neuron*, 24:313–321.

Conway, B. R., 2001, Spatial structure of cone inputs to color cells in alert macaque primary visual cortex (V-1), *J. Neurosci.*, 21:2768–2783.

Dacey, D. M., 2000, Parallel pathways for spectral coding in primate retina, *Annu. Rev. Neurosci.*, 23:743–775. ◆

Gilchrist, A., Kossyfidis, C., Bonato, F., Agostini, T., Cataliotti, J., Li, X. J., Spehar, B., Annan, V., and Economou, E., 1999, An anchoring theory of lightness perception, *Psychol. Rev.*, 106:795–834.

Hadjikhani, N., Liu, A. K., Dale, A. M., Cavanagh, P., and Tootell, R. B. H., 1998, Retinotopy and color sensitivity in human visual cortical area V8, *Nature Neurosci.*, 1:235–241.

Hendry, S. H. C., and Reid, R. C., 2000, The koniocellular pathway in primate vision, *Annu. Rev. Neurosci.*, 23:127–153. ◆

Heywood, C. A., and Cowey, A., 1998, With color in mind, *Nature Neurosci.*, 1:171–173.

Heywood, C. A., Kentridge, R. W., and Cowey, A., 1998, Cortical color blindness is not "blindsight for color," *Consciousness Cognit.*, 7:410–423.

Johnson, E. N., Hawken, M. J., and Shapley, R., 2001, The spatial transformation of color in the primary visual cortex of the macaque monkey, *Nature Neurosci.*, 4:409–416.

Livingstone, M. S., and Hubel, D. H., 1984, Anatomy and physiology of a color system in the primate visual cortex, *J. Neurosci.*, 4:309–356.

Saunders, B. A. C., and Van Brakel, J., 1997, Are there non-trivial constraints on colour categorization? *Behav. Brain Sci.*, 20:167–228. ◆

Sumner, P., and Mollon, J. D., 2000, Catarrhine photopigments are optimized for detecting targets against a foliage background, *J. Exp. Biol.*, 203:1963–1986.

Webster, M. A., Miyahara, E., Malkoc, G., and Raker, V. E., 2000, Variations in normal color vision: II. Unique hues, *J. Opt. Soc. Am.*, 17:1545–1555.

Zeki, S., Watson, J. D. G., Lueck, C. J., Friston, K. J., Kennard, C., and Frackowiak, R. S. J., 1991, A direct demonstration of functional specialization in human visual-cortex, *J. Neurosci.*, 11:641–649.

Command Neurons and Command Systems

Jorg-Peter Ewert

Introduction

If a certain interneuron is stimulated electrically in the brain of a marine slug, the animal then displays a species-specific escape swimming behavior, although no predator is present. If a certain brain area of the optic tectum of a toad is stimulated in this manner, snapping behavior is triggered, although no prey is present. In both cases, a commanding trigger, which in the natural situation is associated with adequate predator or prey signals, activates an appropriate motor program. We address the notion "command" to a stimulus which elicits a rapid ballistic response. The transformation involves sensory pattern recognition and localization on the one side and motor pattern generation on the other; command functions provide the sensorimotor interface (Kupfermann and Weiss, 1978). This interface translates a specific pattern of sensory input mediated by sensory neurons (SN) into an appropriate spatiotemporal pattern of activity in premotor and motor neurons. The latter coordinate the corresponding action pattern, which, in various animal groups and depending on the task, may be rather stereotyped (fixed action pattern) or may leave room for variability (modal action pattern). This correspondence can be innate, modified innate, or acquired, strategy related. Commands are motivated. Once an action pattern is commanded, it tends to carry on to completion, although there may be cases in which a command is "countermanded." How does the sensorimotor interface operate?

Before we tackle this question in depth, a few comments on pattern generation are in order (see MOTOR PATTERN GENERATION). In the present context, a motor pattern generator (MPG) is defined as an internuncial network that, in response to a commanding input, coordinates appropriate muscle contractions. The network is activated if and only if a specific (combination of) input occurs. An intrinsic pattern of neuronal connectivity in the network ensures the generation of a consistent spatiotemporal distribution of excitation and inhibition, often involving oscillatory circuits. The output of the network, mediated by premotor neurons, has privileged access to the requisite motor neuronal pools. Proprioceptive and internal feedback—or feedback from components of the motor network to the command neuron(s)—can play a role in the coordination and maintenance of a motor pattern (e.g., Jing and

Gillette, 2000). Hence, command neurons can be involved to carry timing information for the MPG. Recurrent feedback from the motor system to the command and from the command to the sensory afferents may terminate the command and may also prevent sensory input during the animal's movement.

There are cases in which a short-term command *triggers* the corresponding MPG whose activity outlasts the command activity. In other cases, a sustained (tonic) command is necessary to drive the MPG. The efficacy of a triggering or a driving command depends on the requirements under which an action pattern is released: (1) locus of the stimulus, (2) presence of adequate stimulus features, (3) behavioral state (dominance), (4) motivation (variable on a relatively long time scale), attention, and arousal (variable in the short-term), (5) gating input, and (6) evaluation of the stimulus in connection with prior experience. The first two listed concern aspects of the releasing stimulus; the latter four refer to modulatory functions.

Sensorimotor interfaces with command functions occupy an important topic in neuroethology, the science of the neurobiological fundamentals of behavior (e.g., see Carew, 2000). Neuroethology contributes a valuable perspective to neuroscience of which the present article presents one component.

The Command Neuron Concept

The question as to whether a sensorimotor command can be mediated by a command neuron (CN),

$$\text{sign stimulus} \rightarrow \text{SN} \rightarrow \textbf{CN} \rightarrow \text{MPG} \rightarrow \text{behavior pattern}$$

was and occasionally still is controversial (Kupfermann and Weiss, 1978; Eaton, Lee, and Foreman, 2001). After a definition by Kupfermann and Weiss (1978), a command neuron (CN) is an interneuron whose excitation is both necessary (n) and sufficient (s) to activate the corresponding MPG. Test criteria of this n&s condition include (1) the recording of the activity from the putative CN during the presentation of a stimulus signal in registration with the corresponding action pattern (link between stimulus and motor activity), (2) electrical stimulation of the putative CN with demonstration that this action pattern is executed (s-criterion), and (3) removal of the putative CN and demonstration that this action pattern is no longer elicited by the stimulus signal (n-criterion).

The best candidates for this approach are among the identified CNs of various invertebrates, such as the pair of lateral giant fibers in crayfish that, in response to mechanical stimulation, trigger the fast tail flip escape reaction. For the function of the lateral giant, the term "command" was first introduced by C.A.G. Wiersma and K. Ikeda (for a review, see Edwards, Heitler, and Krasne, 1999). Among vertebrates, there is the reticulospinal Mauthner cell of teleost fish, which, in response to certain acoustic-vibratory stimulation, commands the fast C-shaped body bend escape reaction, called "C-start" (Eaton et al., 2001). The C-start is triggered by a spike in one of the bilateral pair of Mauthner cells.

However, in such cases in which identified putative CNs activate corresponding MPGs, it was not trivial to evaluate the n&s condition. Eaton and co-workers performed a scholarly structured examination on the Mauthner cell (see Eaton et al., 2001). Surprisingly, it turned out that the n-criterion was not fulfilled clearly; after both Mauthner cells in the goldfish were lesioned, the C-start escape reaction could still be elicited by acoustic sign stimuli—however, at a longer latency. This suggests that appropriate auditory receptive "backup" systems, which are normally inhibited by Mauthner cell activation, commanded the C-start. Interestingly, also the s-criterion was not fulfilled unequivocally, because electrical stimulation of the Mauthner cell did not trigger the complete C-start. This suggests that for the full C-start pattern, the activity in other, parallel descending reticulospinal cells is required, too.

Is the CN concept restricted to very few cases, or is it even obsolete? Regarding unknown network interactions (serial, parallel, convergence, divergence, feedforward, and lateral inhibition), the n&s condition may be too rigorous in many cases. Depending on a sensorimotor function, we therefore envision a spectrum of possibilities by which command functions can be executed. The idea behind the revisited command concept (cf. Eaton et al., 2001) is furthermore fruitful both in the neurophysiological analysis of behavior (e.g., Ewert, 1997; Edwards et al., 1999) and in perceptual robotics (e.g., Lukashin, Amirikian, and Georgopolous, 1996; REACTIVE ROBOTIC SYSTEMS).

Experiments to test the n&s condition of particular neurons for triggering behavioral acts are a historical fact that is part of the research record on these types of systems. However, this should not distract us from the complex results that emerge from the experiments done to test this paradigm or from the complex ways in which these cells really function.

Command (Releasing) Systems

Plastic ballistic behavior elicited by distributed networks is triggered by populations of command-like interneurons that form a command system (CS) (Kupfermann and Weiss, 1978). Such a CS consists of collectively operating neurons, each of which is called a command element (CE) or command-like neuron. For just one CE of a CS, the n&s condition cannot be fulfilled. For example, if the CEs of a CS are connected to the MPG like a logical AND-gate, in this case a CE fulfills the n-criterion but not the s-criterion; if the CEs of a CS are connected to the MPG like a logical OR-gate, in that case a CE fulfills the s-criterion but not the n-criterion. However, when the CEs of a CS are treated as a unit, the CS will meet the n&s condition in both cases. We learn that the CS notion has a much broader applicability than the CN notion. In fact, the pair of identified bilateral cerebral interneurons of the type cc5 in the marine snail Aplysia works conjointly as a two-neuron CS that fulfills the n&s condition for the bilateral pedal arterial-shortening component of defensive head withdrawal behavior (Xin, Weiss, and Kupfermann, 1996).

In Mauthner cell-initiated escape behavior, the current concept suggests that the C-start is elicited by a CS consisting of at least two groups of command-like reticulospinal neurons (CEs). One group, in which the Mauthner cell participates, controls the agonist muscular contraction; another group controls the antagonist contraction that, depending on the direction of the acoustic stimulus, precisely shapes the trajectory for certain C-start escape angles (Eaton et al., 2001). If we ask how the two parts of the CS control trajectory, it appears, for example, that the agonist and antagonist CEs can vary their respective output magnitudes and timing patterns to regulate the escape trajectory. This example introduces more sophisticated CSs and relates to the question whether a "backup" system really exists. Since it is difficult to explain how a backup system could evolve, it is a simpler interpretation to recognize the parallel nature of the CS. The role of the parallel output may be to produce variable trajectory angles. A consequence of its organization is that it is "robust" such that if one element (e.g., a Mauthner cell) does not participate, the behavior still can occur. But it could well be that an organism that is missing one Mauthner cell may not be able to accurately control its trajectory.

The concept of a command-releasing system (CRS) is suggested for functions requiring a more complex perception of the sensory input (Ewert, 1997). Different types of electrically uncoupled CEs (a population of each) cooperatively trigger an MPG. Each type of CE evaluates a certain aspect of the releasing stimulus signal, such as features or feature combinations and their location in space, respectively; we call this a *sensorimotor code*. The concept of coded commands stresses that firing of various types of efferent neurons (CEs) in a certain combination (CRS) characterizes an object in space and selects the appropriate goal-directed action pattern (MPG). In amphibians, such cells with different visual response properties project their axons from the optic tectum (T-type neurons) or thalamic/pretectal nuclei (TH-type neurons) to the bulbar/spinal motor systems via discrete tecto-bulbarspinal and pretectobulbar/spinal pathways (Figure 1). The hypothesis illustrated in Figure 1 suggests the following:

- The code {**T4, X, T5.2**} says: "an object is moving anywhere in the visual field [T4]" and "the object occurs at a certain position in the visual field x-y coordinates [X]" and "the object has prey features [T5.2]" → *orient!*
- The code {**T1.3, T3, T5.2**} says: "an object is moving in the frontal binocular field of vision at a narrow distance [T1.3]" and "the small object is approaching [T3]" and "the object has prey features [T5.2]" → *snap!*
- The code {**TH6, T6**} says: "a large object is moving in the dorsal visual field [T6]" and "the large object is approaching [TH6]" → *duck!*

After the hypothesis, in such a multifunctional network, on one hand, the same goal can be reached by differently combined CRS whose CEs may be distributed in different brain structures; on the other hand, certain CEs can be shared by different CRSs for different goals. Evidence of such multifunctional properties, for example, is provided for *Aplysia* by Xin et al. (1996): The type cc5 neuron contributes to different aspects of behavior, such as defensive head withdrawal, tentacular withdrawal, feeding, and locomotion. For some (aspects of) behaviors, the neuron probably acts as CE; for other aspects or components of behavior, however, the same interneuron may participate in a distributed circuit where it is neither necessary nor sufficient.

Also, Mauthner cells participate in behaviors other than escape, such as prey capture. The story of Mauthner cell function may be even more complex. In the electric fish *Gymnotus carapo*, auditory activation of Mauthner cell leads, by its connections to medullary pacemaker neurons of the electric organ, to an abrupt and pro-

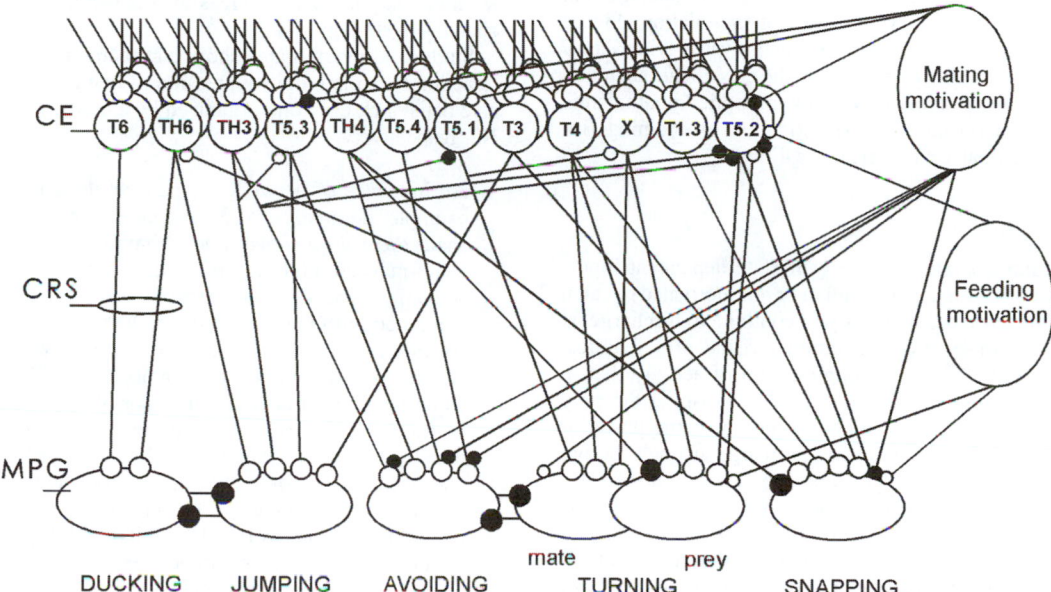

Neuronal properties

T6 monocular dorsal large receptive field, sensitive to moving large objects

TH6 monocular wide receptive field, sensitive to approaching big objects

TH3*,T5.3* monocular receptive fields of 30-50° diameter, sensitive to moving large objects

TH4* receptive field encompassing the visual field of one or both eyes, sensitive to moving large objects

T5.4* monocular receptive field of about 35° diameter, sensitive to moving big compact objects

T5.1* monocular receptive fields of 20-30°, sensitive to moving objects of small or intermediate size

T3* nasal monocular receptive field of 20-30°, sensitive to approaching objects

T4* receptive field encompassing the visual field of one or both eyes, sensitivity like T5.1 or T5.2

X hypothetic tegmental neurons computing retinal topography and body segment orientation

T1.3* nasal binocular receptive field of 15-30°, responsive to objects moving at narrow distance

T5.2* monocular receptive field of 20-30°, sensitive to small objects with preference to
   objects elongated in the direction of their movement

Figure 1. Concept of sensorimotor codes implemented by command-releasing systems (CRSs) in common toads. Different subsets of functionally identified types of visual thalamic/pretectal (TH) and tectal (T) neurons as command elements (CE) contribute to commanding and parameterizing motor patterns of feeding (prey orienting, snapping), escape (ducking, jumping, avoidance turning), and orienting by the male toad toward the female in the mating season. For example, *T5.1* neurons respond sensitively to prey objects, whereas *T5.2* neurons display prey-selective properties with respect to configurational visual cues; *T6, TH6, TH4,* and *T5.4* neurons respond best to various aspects of predator stimuli. Breeding motivation and hunger state deliver different modulatory influences. Each circle represents a set of neurons, each oval stands for a motor-pattern-generating circuit (MPG) with access to motor neuronal pools. The open dots refer to excitatory inluences, and the solid dots to inhibitory influences; the CE level obtains sensory inputs, for example, from retinal ganglion cells and interneurons. The asterisk indicates that the projective character of the neuron (command element) is evidenced by means of the antidromic stimulation/recording method. (Modified from Ewert, 1997.)

longed increase in the rate of discharges of the electric organ. This probably enhances the electrolocative sampling of the environment during Mauthner cell mediated escape or prey-catching behavior (Curti et al., 1999).

Properties of Commands

With respect to requirements 1 through 6 listed in the introduction, the properties of a command can be manyfold. We select three aspects.

Localization

Certain CEs of a CRS monitor the stimulus in space to select and direct the behavior in relation to the target. Visual space, the *x-y-z*

position of an object, are translated into appropriate motor space. In mammals, the superior colliculus is involved in visual orientation of the eye, head, and trunk. Information about the position of these movable segments must be integrated in the topographic correspondence between sensory input and motor output. For example, the sensory map in the collicular superficial layers is transformed into a motor map in the deep layers, in which a vector from an initial eye position to a goal eye position is represented. Hypotheses concerning gaze, eye, and head displacement commands are discussed by Freedman and Sparks (1997).

Information on visual depth can be obtained in various ways, such as by binocular vision or motion parallax. Such information is necessary not only to select appropriate behavior, but also to estimate the real size of the target.

Feature Analysis

Certain CEs of a CRS are involved in the feature analysis of the sensory signal. For example, the toad's visual system selects between prey and nonprey through an analysis of the moving object in terms of configurational features, namely, the dimensions of an object parallel versus perpendicular to its direction of movement. A bug or a millipede is thus not recognized explicitly; rather, they are implicit in the prey schema determined by an object-features-relating algorithm (Ewert, 1997). The discharge rate of toad's prey-selective *T5.2* neurons in response to a moving object is correlated with the probability that the configuration of this object fits the prey schema. These neurons, as CEs, obviously display predictive responses, since they show a strong premotor buildup of activity before the animal orients toward prey, but they are silent before or during a spontaneous head movement. In the response properties of *T5.2* neurons, certain kinds of interactions of distributed tectal (T) and thalamic/pretectal (TH) neuronal populations are expressed. This feature analyzing T/TH filter system is integrated in a macronetwork that allows various kinds of modulation (Figure 2), for example, with respect to response gating (involving basal/ganglionic nuclei) or to raising or lowering the classification threshold depending on motivation (involving preoptic/hypothalamic structures) or to generalization or specification by learning (involving the hippocampal ventral medial pallium).

Motivation and Attention

A command cannot operate effectively if state-dependent inputs are not appropriate. If a toad is inattentive or not motivated to catch prey, the prey-selective *T5.2* neurons will continue to discharge, at a lower rate, in response to configurational visual prey features; however, they do not show the strong buildup of activity that in prey-responsive animals precedes and predicts grasping the prey with the tongue. Comparably, neurons of area 5 of the posterior parietal association cortex in monkeys discharge strongly before the animal performs a ballistic grasping movement with its arm toward a rewarding banana. In keeping with the proposal by Mountcastle and co-workers, these "arm projection neurons" function in a broad sense as a command system for the motivated exploration of extrapersonal space (for a complementary point of view, see GRASPING MOVEMENTS: VISUOMOTOR TRANSFORMATIONS). However, if the monkey was satiated, the banana did not elicit the predictive buildup of activity in these neurons required to elicit grasping. So whether or not the s-criterion is met depends on the behavioral state. This illustrates again one of the problems with rigidly designating neuronal function according to the n&s paradigm: Whether the cell is either n or s for a behavior depends on the conditions.

In crickets, the efficacy of the calling-song commanding interneuron, too, depends on the behavioral state (Hedwig, 2000). In silent animals that were previously singing, experimentally evoked commands by this interneuron triggered the song according to the s-criterion. In the resting state, however, experimentally evoked commands by the interneuron elicited an incomplete calling song, so the interneuron failed to meet the s-criterion.

Behavioral Choice

Behavioral dominances exist, and these may depend, for example, on the season due to hormonal influences. In summertime, the toad's predator-avoiding behavior overrides prey-catching behavior if appropriate visual releasers are present simultaneously, whereas the male toad's mate-approaching behavior to an adequate stimulus is absent. In spring during the mating season, mate-approaching behavior dominates predator-avoiding behavior, whereas prey-catching behavior fails to occur. The behavioral choice may result from dual excitatory/inhibitory influences to the toad's tectal or thalamic/pretectal CEs and/or MPGs (cf. Figure 1).

The rat's colliculus superior (SC), too, in response to certain unexpected visual stimuli can initiate rapid ballistic opposite behaviors such as orienting/approaching versus freezing/avoiding. Each type of behavior is commanded by a different set of neurons located in the intermediate or deep SC layers, respectively, that project their axons in discrete phylogenetically old SC-bulbar/spinal pathways (homologous to the tecto-bulbar/spinal pathways in amphibians). Krout et al. (2001) provide anatomic evidence for the hypothesis that the decision in the SC to select one of these behaviors—approach versus avoidance—in an appropriate stimulus situation involves visual projections from SC to (1) thalamo-basal/ganglionic, (2) thalamo-amygdaloid, and (3) thalamocortical circuits. It is suggested that loop 1 is involved in behavioral choice via disinhibitory (gating) and inhibitory (selecting) pathways, and the connections with loop 2 add information related to emotional learning and memory, whereas the connections with loop 3 allow changes in strategy.

Studies in invertebrates show that there are several ways of interaction to explain the suppression of one of two mutually exclusive behaviors, each one organized by a network N1 and a network N2, respectively.

1. An influence of network N1 cancels the command in N2: for example, dominance of escape swimming over feeding in the snail *Pleurobranchaea*; the behavioral switch is caused by swim-induced inhibition of feeding command neurons, that is, activation of feeding interneurons that inhibit the feeding command neurons (Jing and Gillette, 2000).
2. An influence of network N1 suppresses both the command in N2 and the MPG in N2: for example, choice of the body shortening withdrawal behavior in favor of swimming in the leech; in response to mechanical stimuli, body shortening is commanded by a set of interneuronal parallel pathways that inhibit one of the swim command interneurons and an interneuron of the swim MPG (Shaw and Kristan, 1999).
3. An influence of network N1 inhibits the MPG in N2 but not the command in N2: for example, in stridulating crickets, wind-evoked signals that are silencing the calling song do not inhibit the ongoing activity of the interneuron that commands this song but do inhibit the song MPG. This allows immediate singing when the wind wanes (Hedwig, 2000).

CRS and Schema Theory

A command-releasing system (CRS) can be regarded as the neurobiological correlate of Nico Tinbergen's concept of (innate) releasing mechanism (see Ewert, 1997), originally called by Konrad Lorenz "the (innate) releasing schema."

SCHEMA THEORY (q.v.) offers an interdisciplinary science that allows one to treat principles of neuroethology or neural engineering in the same language. In the language of schema theory, the sensorimotor code of a CRS embodies a *perceptual schema* that exists for only one purpose: to determine the conditions for the activation of a specific MPG embodying a *motor schema*. The CRS must also ensure that the resultant movement is directed in relation to the target. A schema and its instantiation usually are coextensive; that is, instantiation of a schema appears to be identifiable with appropriate activity in certain populations of neurons of the brain, whereby each schema may involve several cell types or brain regions, while a given cell type or brain region may be involved in several schemas. The motor schemas of directed appetitive behaviors and consummatory behavior need not occur in a fixed order; rather, each may proceed to completion, followed by perceptual

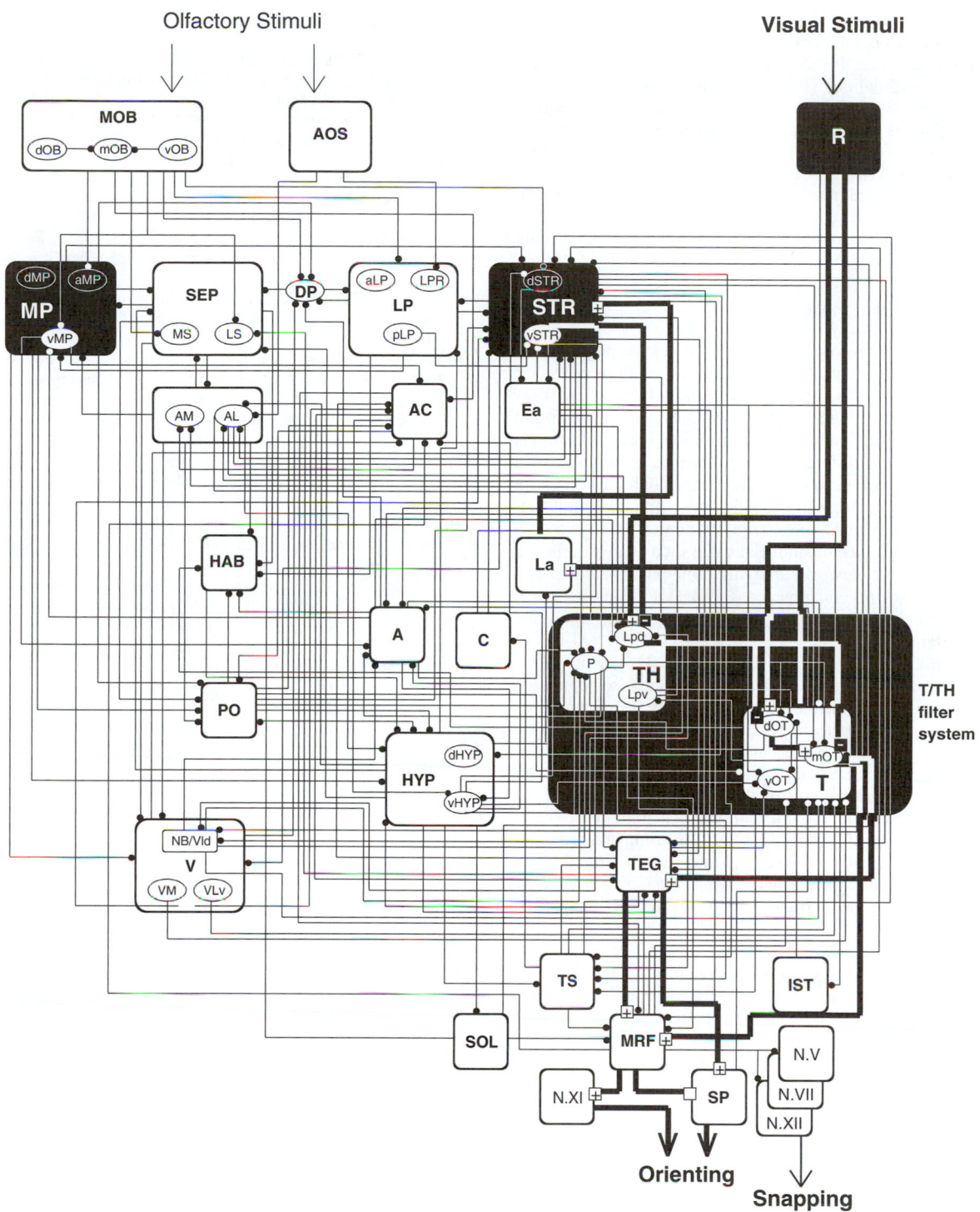

Figure 2. The visual configurational prey schema of common toads results from interactions between retina (R)-fed optic tectal (T) networks and retina-fed thalamic/pretectal (TH) networks. The former network evaluates the dimension of an object parallel to the direction of its movement; the latter evaluates its dimension perpendicular to the direction of movement. Pretectotectal inhibitory influences determine the prey-selective properties of tecto-bulbar/spinal projecting neurons of the type *T5.2* (cf. Figure 1). The T/TH filter system (see the black labeled large area) is integrated in a macronetwork, whose components may influence this system in different ways. For example, the basal ganglionic ventral striatum (vSTR) is involved in gating the orienting response toward prey (cf. thick labeled lines): retinal (R) output is fed both to T and TH (Lpd nucleus); vSTR obtains T-information via the lateral anterior thalamic nucleus (La); a descending striato(vSTR)-pretecto (Lpd)-tectal (T) disinhibitory connection gates the tecto (T)/tegmento (TEG)-bulbar (MRF)/spinal (SP) processing stream. As a result, visual perception (prey recognition) is translated into action (prey-catching orienting). Suggested excitatory and inhibitory influences are indicated by plus and minus signs, respectively. Other, not labeled, loops involving the hippocampal ventral medial pallium (vMP) via anterior thalamic (A), preoptic (PO), and hypothalamic nuclei (HYP) modify the selectivity of the prey schema in the course of nonassociative or associative learning, such as by combining visual and olfactory cues. (For details, see Ewert et al., 2001.)

schemas that will determine which motor schema is to be executed next. Schemas may be linked by so-called *coordinated control programs*. Motor schemas, for example, can take the form of compound motor coordinations (such as a frog's programmed jump-snap-gulp sequence), which make up a set that will proceed to completion without intervening perceptual tests, for example, in such a manner that schema A proceeds to completion, and completion of schema A triggers the initiation of schema B, or that schema A passes a parameter X to schema B. It is also possible that two or more motor schemas are co-activated simultaneously and interact through competition and cooperation to yield a more complicated motor pattern.

Perspectives

Operations between sensory analysis and motor response represented by sensorimotor codes (CRS) are of general importance. Of particular interest are the alternative ways in which different organisms solve similar problems. For example, it was shown that the same algorithm that underlies configurational prey selection is implemented by such different neuronal networks as those of a toad, which is a vertebrate, and a praying mantis, which is an insect (Prete, 1992). This biologically justifies the artificial neural network approach. Cervantes-Pérez (see VISUOMOTOR COORDINATION IN FROG AND TOAD) demonstrates that such an algorithm can be modeled by neural networks applying principles of parallel-distributed processing and convergence. Pavlásek (1997) uses artificial neuronal networks to investigate how the precise timing and structuring of neural commands controlling goal-directed movements can be realized in general. Lukashin et al. (1996) apply a computational paradigm that utilizes the actual impulse population activity of directionally tuned cells recorded from the motor cortex of monkey during the performance of a motor task as command signals to drive an artificial mechanical device: an artificial neuronal network recodes the brain signals into the motor schema of a simulated actuator, a method that is suitable for electronically driven prostheses such as a multijoint artificial limb. This is just one example of the applications of research on command functions in sensorimotor systems for perceptual and reactive robotics (cf. also REACHING MOVEMENTS: IMPLICATIONS FOR COMPUTATIONAL MODELS; REACTIVE ROBOTIC SYSTEMS; and ROBOT ARM CONTROL).

Road Map: Motor Pattern Generators; Neuroethology and Evolution
Related Reading: Motor Pattern Generation; Neuroethology, Computational; Visuomotor Coordination in Frog and Toad

References

Carew, T. J., 2000, *Behavioral Neurobiology: The Cellular Organization of Natural Behavior*, Sunderland, MA: Sinauer. ◆

Curti, S., Falconi, A., Morales, F. R., and Borde, M., 1999, Mauthner cell-initiated electromotor behavior is mediated via NMDA and metabotropic glutaminergic receptors on medullary pacemaker neurons in a Gymnotid fish, *J. Neurosci.*, 19(20):9133–9140.

Eaton, R. C., Lee, R. K. K., and Foreman, M. B., 2001, The Mauthner cell and other identified neurons of the brainstem escape network of fish, *Prog. Neurobiol.*, 63:467–485. ◆

Edwards, D. H., Heitler, W. J,. and Krasne, F. B., 1999, Fifty years of a command neuron: The neurobiology of escape behavior in the crayfish, *Trends Neurosci.*, 22(4):153–161. ◆

Ewert, J.-P., 1997, Neural correlates of key stimulus and releasing mechanism: A case study and two concepts, *Trends Neurosci.*, 20:332–339. ◆

Ewert J.-P., Buxbaum-Conradi, H., Dreisvogt, F., Glagow, M., Merkel-Harff, C., Röttgen, A., Schürg-Pfeiffer, E., and Schwippert, W. W., 2001, Neural modulation of visuomotor functions underlying prey-catching behaviour in anurans: Perception, attention, motor performance, learning, *Comp. Biochem. Physiol. A*, 128:417–461.

Freedman, E. G., and Sparks, D. L., 1997, Activity of cells in the deeper layers of the superior colliculus of the rhesus monkey: Evidence for a gaze displacement command, *J. Neurophysiol.*, 78:1669–1690.

Hedwig, B., 2000, Control of cricket stridulation by a command neuron: Efficacy depends on the behavioral state, *J. Neurophysiol.*, 83(2):712–722.

Jing, J., and Gillette, R., 2000, Escape swim network interneurons have diverse roles in behavioral switching and putative arousal in *Pleurobranchaea*, *J. Neurophysiol.*, 83(3):1346–1355.

Krout, K. E., Loewy, A. D., Westby, G. W. M., and Redgrave, P., 2001, Superior colliculus projections to midline and intralaminar thalamic nuclei of the rat, *J. Comp. Neurol.*, 431:198–216.

Kupfermann, I., and Weiss, K. R., 1978, The command neuron concept, *Behav. Brain Sci.*, 1:3–39. ◆

Lukashin, A. V., Amirikian, B. R., and Georgopoulos, A. P., 1996, A simulated actuator driven by motor cortical signals, *Neuroreport*, 7(15–17):2597–2601.

Pavlásek, J., 1997, Timing of neural commands: A model study with neuronal networks, *Biol. Cybern.*, 77(5):359–365.

Prete, F. R., 1992, Discrimination of visual stimuli representing prey versus non-prey by the praying mantis *Sphodromantis lineola* (Burr.), *Brain Behav. Evol.*, 39:285–288.

Shaw, B. K., and Kristan, W. B., Jr., 1999, Relative roles of the S cell network and parallel interneuronal pathways in the whole-body shortening reflex of the medicinal leech, *J. Neurophysiol.*, 82(3):1114–1123.

Xin, Y., Weiss, K. R., and Kupfermann, I., 1996, An identified interneuron contributes to aspects of six different behaviors in *Aplysia*, *J. Neurophysiol.*, 16(16):5266–5279.

Competitive Learning

Nathan Intrator

Introduction

Competitive learning is described by a family of algorithms that use some sort of competition between lateral neurons during learning and normal activity. In a typical competitive network architecture, neurons in each layer are connected to the next layer, but, in addition, there are lateral connections between neurons in the same layer that cause the competition. Competitive learning includes a wide variety of algorithms performing different tasks, such as encoding, clustering, and classification.

The notion of a limited pool of individually adaptable tuned units is more than a functional abstraction useful for psychological modeling. The reality of a distributed representational substrate whose members compete for a share in the representation of the stimulus has been demonstrated in a variety of electrophysiological studies (Gilbert, 1994). These studies can be divided into two major groups. In the first group, competition among members of a pool of tuned units has been enhanced by the withdrawal of stimulation from some of the units. For instance, the induction of a retinal scotoma leads to invasion of the visual space of affected cells by the receptive fields of other, neighboring cells. An analogous effect, albeit on a much longer time scale, is observed in the somatosensory modality (Merzenich et al., 1988). In comparison, in the second group, the increased prominence of a subpopulation of functional units (whose emergence may in itself be a product of learning) is precipitated merely by the prevalence of the preferred stimuli of those units in the sensory repertoire of the system. For example, in the monkey, this phenomenon has been glimpsed in relation to face representation (Rolls et al., 1989), as well as the representation of general natural and artificial (Logothetis and Scheinberg, 1996) objects.

Overview

In recent years, competitive learning has received considerable attention because of its demonstrated applicability and its biological plausibility. The idea of competition between neurons leads to sparse representations of data that are easy to decode and conserve energy. Current competitive learning algorithms can be distinguished by their learning rule (which is driven by their desired objective function) or by the form and role of the competition during learning. One form of competitive learning algorithms can be described as an application of a successful single neuron learning algorithm in a network with lateral connections between adjacent neurons. The lateral connections are needed so that each neuron can extract a different feature from the data. For example, if one has an algorithm for finding the principal component in a data set, i.e., the first eigenvector of the correlation matrix of the data, then a careful application of this learning rule in a lateral inhibition (competitive) network gives an algorithm that finds the first few principal components of the data (Sanger, 1989). This set of algorithms can be characterized by the fact that if the lateral connections are turned off, then neurons are likely to learn the most easily extracted feature in the data (based on the objective function), or the feature that corresponds to the closest local minimum of the objective function. For example, in a principal components network with no lateral inhibition, all neurons will converge to the first principal component of the data. In such algorithms, it is often sufficient to study the learning rule of a single neuron and deduce from it the performance of the network as a whole.

A second family of algorithms is characterized by the fact that turning off the lateral connections will result in a great loss of ability to extract useful features. Thus, the competition between neurons has an important role in improving, sharpening, or even forming the features extracted from the data by each single neuron. This is an important distinction that suggests that competitive learning may be useful in cases where other forms of learning may have difficulties. One such example is a network that searches for clusters. Clustering is the process of grouping together data points based on some measure of distance. When no inhibition exists between neurons, it is likely that neurons will converge to the mean of the data distribution. This follows from the fact that based on a Hebbian rule, neuronal weights (of radial basis neurons) tend to converge to the center of the distribution in order to maximize correlation of input activity with output activity. An algorithm that looks for tight clusters will probably find those that are occurring with highest probability, or those cluster centers that are closest to the initial weight values. When inhibition is turned on, the cluster centers will move to new locations and will become sharper and more distinct. There is evidence that inhibition plays a similar role in various brain functions such as the creation of orientation columns in visual cortex (Ramoa, Paradiso, and Freeman, 1988) or sharpening receptive fields in sensory cortex (Merzenich et al., 1988).

There are other points of view on competitive learning, in particular, competition over presynaptic versus postsynaptic resources (Willshaw et al., 1997). A more detailed review of these issues can be found in Intrator and Edelman (1997).

Local Competition over Space

Frequently in a classification problem, there are regions in pattern space in which classification is easier, while there are other regions in which classification is not that simple and thus requires a larger (more complex) network. For example, there may be regions in which the different classes are linearly separable and other regions in which the boundary is highly nonlinear. Therefore, one of the key ideas in machine learning and statistical parameter estimation is recursive partitioning of the observation space in order to separate such regions. Motivation comes from the desire to study structure of high dimensional space by searching for homogeneous subregions that present a simpler structure than the original whole input space. Statistical theory suggests that the variance of the estimator, which directly influences generalization performance, is affected by the complexity of the estimator (polynomial degree, number of hidden units, etc.). Thus, performing the estimation with a simpler architecture is likely to improve generalization performance. However, if the network architecture is "too simple," in the sense that the architecture is not rich enough to allow a flexible enough function to fit the data, a large training error is unavoidable.

One solution to this trade-off is to recursively partition the data into several homogeneous regions so that a smaller network will suffice for each region. In this context we shall discuss in the next section the network of competing experts.

In a lateral competition network, a cluster center (the mean of a Gaussian distribution) is associated with a neuronal weight vector, and neurons compete between themselves to add each of the input patterns to their cluster. For a given pattern, the winner, in hard competition, is the neuron with highest probability for that pattern to belong to the Gaussian distribution represented by its center (see WINNER-TAKE-ALL NETWORKS). In soft competition, the cluster centers are organized in such a way that the distance of each data point from each of the cluster centers corresponds to the probability of this point under each of the Gaussian distribution (Jacobs et al., 1991).

If an input $x \in R^n$ is drawn with probability π_i from one of J independent Gaussians (for simplicity, assume that the Gaussians are radially symmetric), its a posteriori probability of belonging to the jth Gaussian is $\pi_j p_j(x)$, for

$$p_j(x) = \frac{1}{M\sigma_j} \exp\left(-\frac{\|x - \mu_j\|^2}{2\sigma_j^2}\right)$$

where $\sigma_j^2 I$ is the covariance matrix of Gaussian j, and M is a normalizing constant. The partial likelihood that measures the probability of the data under the model of input x_k in this model is $L(x_k) = \Sigma_j \pi_j p_j(x_k)$. The partial likelihood of a pattern set $\{x_k\}_{k=1}^K$ is

$$\mathcal{L} = \prod_k L(x_k)$$

assuming K independent patterns. This could be turned into a likelihood if the marginal probabilities are taken into account to convert the partial likelihood into a probability function, but since the marginals do not participate in the optimization, there is no need to do that. Parameter estimation of such a model involves adjusting the centers $\{\mu_j\}$, the covariances $\{\sigma_j^2\}$, and the prior probabilities $\{\pi_j\}$ so as to maximize the likelihood of the model for a given training set. It is mathematically equivalent but more convenient to maximize the log likelihood, since the maximization is then on summation and not multiplication. In a radial basis function network realization of this model, there are J radial basis hidden units and a linear output unit that gives the likelihood function under the conditions of the model.

Assuming for simplicity that σ_j are equal, the hard competition approach for solving this problem would assume that each input can belong to only one cluster center. (Thus, the competition between neurons will lead to only one active neuron at a time), and, therefore, the above definition of $P(x)$ is replaced by

$$P(x) = \max_i \pi_i p_i(x)$$

The analytic solution for cluster centers (under assumptions about radial symmetry and σ_i and π_i being equal) is

$$\mu_i = \frac{\sum_{k \in C_i} x_k}{N_i}$$

where C_i is the set of training patterns that were assigned to belong to the cluster center i and N_i is the number of these patterns. Note that this is not an explicit solution, since C_i depend on all of the μ_ks. A learning rule that converges to this solution is given by

$$\Delta\mu_{ij} = \eta(x_{ki} - \mu_{ij})p_i(x)$$

for the winning cluster i, and no change for the other clusters. This learning rule moves the closest cluster center in the direction of the data points that belong to that cluster, finally forming stable cluster boundaries and converging to the mean of the cluster. During this process, input patterns may "cross" from one cluster to another as a result of the movement of the cluster center. However, the process will converge to a stable solution simply because the mean squared distance of the patterns from their corresponding cluster centers goes down.

The soft competition paradigm assumes that each pattern can belong to any of the clusters. In this case, the solution that maximizes the likelihood of the model is given by

$$\mu_i = \frac{\sum_k p(i|x_k)x_k}{\sum_k p(i|x_k)}$$

where

$$p(i|x_k) = \frac{p_i(x_k)}{\sum_j p_j(x_k)}$$

A learning rule for the soft competition is similar to that for the hard competition. The difference is that each of the cluster centers is modified in the direction of the line connecting the cluster center and pattern x_k in proportion to the probability that it belongs to that cluster. This follows from the formulation of the data as a mixture-of-Gaussians model. The soft competition approach is closely related to k-means clustering (Duda and Hart, 1973).

In practice, this algorithm does not perform well when the number of cluster centers is not known a priori or when the clusters are not radially symmetric. A lateral inhibition network in which each unit is locally pushing other units not to become selective to the region it is normally selective to can alleviate those problems. Kohonen's self-organizing map (SOM) is one of the earlier implementations of such networks (Kohonen, 1984). Its 2D lateral inhibition structure, which is also called learning vector quantization, implements clustering and has been shown to be useful in numerous applications, most recently in the WEBSOM project for text clustering.

The idea of having experts (entire modules), rather than units, compete globally over the whole space is a direct extension of the more local competitive learning approach. It leads to a competitive network and hierarchical mixture of experts (see MODULAR AND HIERARCHICAL LEARNING SYSTEMS).

Competitive Learning and Resource Allocation

Competition over limited resources and the allocation of such resources are important characteristics of learning in biological sys-

tems. How do such systems manage and distribute their resources? It seems plausible to assume that a sophisticated system would choose an allocation strategy in response to the characteristics of the task. Consider, for instance, a situation that involves two consecutive learning tasks. In such a case, one may distinguish between two possibilities: (1) the second task involves the same data as the first one; (2) the second task involves new data (albeit presented in the same sensory modality).

We hypothesize the existence of a low-dimensional internal representation of the data, whose computation incurs a cost in terms of time and effort. It is then clear that in case 1, the system will be better off if it retains the same internal representation in both tasks. In comparison, in case 2, the existing representation may be modified, or a new one may be created. An intriguing glimpse into the approach taken by the brain in such a situation is provided by recent experimental results concerning the representation of extracorporal space in rat hippocampus (Wilson and McNaughton, 1993; see HIPPOCAMPUS: SPATIAL MODELS). In that study of place cells, Wilson and McNaughton used chronic multielectrode implantation techniques that allowed long-term recording of cell activities. They recorded more than a hundred cells from free-moving rats that had been trained so they were familiar with part of a simple maze. In these rats, certain hippocampal cells fired in relation to their place in the maze; when the rats were suddenly exposed to a new place, they underwent a short (about 5 minutes) phase of learning in which cells that were silent in the previous location were recruited to encode the new location. This process is consistent with a possible effective reduction in inhibition of cells that have not been recently active. Such a reduction in inhibition may enable them to modify their response patterns rapidly and to become coherently active in the new location.

Discussion

There are various ways in which one can construct controller networks and they resemble various statistical approaches. One can construct either a wide shallow network, in which input patterns are split only once into one of several experts performing the task, or a deep tree with many splits, so that the regression or classification task is performed only by a bottom (terminating) node of the tree. This approach, known as the CART method, has gained considerable attention with the appearance of the classification and regression trees (Breiman et al., 1984). This method constructs a tree leading to different decisions in different regions of pattern space. A direct extension of competitive learning ideas motivated by the success of the above recursive partitioning methods is the hierarchy-of-experts approach (see MODULAR AND HIERARCHICAL LEARNING SYSTEMS).

There is no doubt about the importance of competition in the formation of neural and artificial networks. Experimental evidence from olfactory cortex suggests the performance of hierarchical clustering by a biological network (Lynch, 1986) and has led to the proposal of a model for hierarchical clustering as well. It uncovered the potential of recursive partitioning in complex pattern encoding and classification. Work by Merznick on motor cortex demonstrates that when inhibition is reduced (through amputation), a cortical region that has been responsive to input from one sensory region very quickly adapts to become sensitive to adjacent sensory regions. Competition between units and between collections of units is crucial for such a process. The exact nature of such competition, as well as the optimal architectures that exploit competition for self-organizing, have yet to be uncovered and are likely to benefit from recent advances in multiple cell recording.

Road Map: Learning in Artificial Networks
Related Reading: Data Clustering and Learning; Self-Organizing Feature Maps; Winner-Take-All Networks

References

Breiman, L., Friedman, J. H., Olshen, R. A., and Stone, C. J., 1984, *Classification and Regression Trees*, Wadsworth Statistics/Probability Series, Belmont, CA: Wadsworth.

Duda, R. O., and Hart, P. E., 1973, *Pattern Classification and Scene Analysis*, New York: Wiley.

Gilbert, C. D., 1994, Neuronal dynamics and perceptual learning, *Curr. Biol.*, 4:627–629.

Intrator, N., and Edelman, S., 1997, Competitive learning in biological and artificial neural computation, *Trends Cognit. Sci.*, 7:268–272. ◆

Jacobs, R. A., Jordan, M. I., Nowlan, S. J., and Hinton, G. E., 1991, Adaptive mixtures of local experts, *Neural Computat.*, 3:79–87.

Kohonen, T., 1984, *Self-Organization and Associative Memory*, Berlin: Springer-Verlag.

Logothetis, N. K., and Scheinberg, D. L., 1996, Visual object recognition, *Annu. Rev. Neurosci.*, 19:577–621.

Lynch, G., 1986, *Synapses, Circuits and the Beginnings of Memory*, Boston: MIT Press. ◆

Merzenich, M. M., Recanzone, G., Jenkins, W. M., Allard, T. T., and Nudo, R. J., 1988, Cortical representation plasticity, in *Neurobiology of Neocortex* (P. Rakic and W. Singer, Eds.), New York: Wiley, pp. 41–68. ◆

Ramoa, A. S., Paradiso, M. A., and Freeman, R. D., 1988, Blockade of intracortical inhibition in kitten striate cortex: Effects on receptive field properties and associated loss of ocular dominance plasticity, *Exp. Brain Res.*, 73:285–296.

Rolls, E. T., Baylis, G. C., Hasselmo, M. E., and Nalwa, V., 1989, The effect of learning on the face selective responses of neurons in the cortex in the superior temporal sulcus of the monkey, *Exp. Brain Res.*, 76:153–164.

Sanger, T. D., 1989, Optimal unsupervised learning in a single-layer linear feedforward neural network, *Neural Netw.*, 2:459–473.

Willshaw, D., Hallam, J., Gingell, S., and Lau, S. L., 1997, Marr's theory of the neocortex as a self-organizing neural network, *Neural Computat.*, 9:911–936. ◆

Wilson, M. A., and McNaughton, B. L., 1993, Dynamics of hippocampal ensemble code for space, *Science*, 261:1055–1058. ◆

Competitive Queuing for Planning and Serial Performance

Daniel Bullock and Bradley J. Rhodes

Introduction

In neural network studies of planning and serial performance, there is a long history of what Hartley and Houghton (1996) called *competitive queuing* (CQ) models (Figure 1). Such models follow naturally from two assumptions: (1) More than one plan representation can be simultaneously active in a planning layer; and (2) The most active plan representation is chosen, in a second neural layer, by a competition run to decide which plan to enact next. In CQ models, activation is the "common currency" used to compare alternative plans, and simple maximum-finding or winner-take-all (WTA) dynamics can be used as the choice mechanism in the choice layer. Once a plan wins the competition and is used to initiate a response, its representation is deleted from the field of competitors in the planning layer, and the competition is run again. This iteration allows the two-layer network to transform an initial activity distribution across plan representations, often called a *primacy gradient*, into a serial performance (Grossberg, 1978).

As a representation of serial order, the primacy gradient across plan representations in a CQ model is a fundamentally parallel representation. For this reason, CQ models provide a much different basis for control of serial behavior than what have come to be called recurrent neural networks (RNNs). An RNN, in this restrictive usage, is a network in which each output is fed back to the input (or other pre-output) stage as a way of helping to create a distinctive context for eliciting the correct next output. In such an RNN, the representation of the learned sequence is itself fundamentally serial, in the sense that the information that specifies the sequence only becomes available as the serial performance unfolds. In contrast, all the information needed to specify a forthcoming sequence is present in the current state of the planning level of a CQ system, although this current state may itself be dynamically evolving. Having such an explicit, parallel, activation-based representation of sequential plans becomes a substantial advantage for many purposes. For example, such representations can be learned and recalled via compressive and expansive coding operations, as noted later in this article.

Although CQ networks are a radically different basis for sequence control than RNNs, CQ networks also use neural signal recurrence, or internal feedback, for various purposes. The deletion signal sent to the planning layer once a plan is chosen for enactment is one example. Moreover, Grossberg (1978) showed how to implement both the planning layer and the choice layer of a CQ model as *recurrent competitive fields* (RCFs), which exhibit approximate normalization of the total activity level distributed across competing sites in a neural layer. These RCFs were interpreted as parts of a working memory system, in which activity distributions are maintained through significant intervals by recurrent self-excitation combined with recurrent inhibition of competitors. Yet simple changes of signal functions can transform a pattern-holding RCF into a WTA RCF, or even an RCF that quickly forgets initial activity differences. Beyond this ready tunability to realize both the pattern-holding and WTA properties of a CQ system, RCFs have two further properties that enhance their suitability as core models of the planning layers within biological CQ systems. If one plan representation is deleted (by zeroing its activity) from a planning layer RCF, then activity automatically redistributes among the remaining plan representations in a way that preserves the rank ordering of preexisting activation levels. This third property is crucial if iterated deletion is not to disrupt the planning layer's parallel representation of the serial order of subsequent plans.

A fourth property is another consequence of RCF normalization in the planning layer. Because total activity is conserved, *more* simultaneously active plans imply *less* activation per plan, including the plan scheduled to be performed first. If the initial activation level of this plan predicts the reaction time (RT) to perform the first planned action (as is the case if the choice layer is a WTA network with a high threshold for generating an output to the response execution system, and the latter system is set to perform as soon as it receives an input) then this variant of a CQ model makes a surprising prediction. The RT to *initiate* performance of a prepared sequence should increase with the number of plans in the prepared sequence. Such a "sequence length effect on RT" is true for humans performing lightly practiced sequences from working

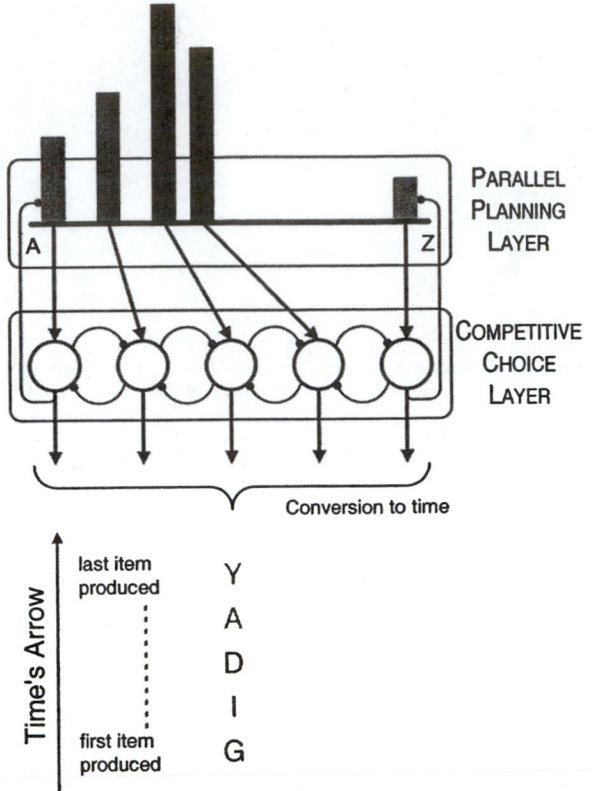

Figure 1. Initial state of a two-layer competitive queuing (CQ) system, prior to production of a five-letter sequence. The sequence that will emerge is shown in the lower part of the figure. Excitatory connections terminate with arrowheads, inhibitory connections with filled circles. The most active plan is selected for execution in the lower, competitive choice, layer by a winner-take-all dynamic whose outcome is wholly determined (in the absence of noise) by the activation gradient (representing the to-be-performed sequence) present in the parallel planning layer. Once a plan representation wins at the competitive layer, a large output signal is sent to initiate execution of the corresponding response (descending arrow) and to delete the plan's representation in the parallel activation layer (ascending path to parallel planning layer). This process iterates until all plans have been enacted and all planning layer activities deleted. The result is sequential plan execution that corresponds to the initial rank ordering (primacy gradient) of plan activation levels in the upper field of the CQ network. Although each competitive layer node would send an inhibitory connection to its correspondent in the parallel planning layer, only two such connections are shown here, to avoid clutter. In this example, which uses recurrent inhibition in the choice layer, each competitive layer node would inhibit all others, but only nearest-neighbor inhibition is actually depicted. (Adapted from Rhodes, 1999, with permission.)

memory (Sternberg et al., 1978; review in Rhodes, 1999). Simulations by Boardman and Bullock (1991) verified these RT properties for a two-layer CQ system coupled to a response generation network. They also showed that the model correctly predicted patterns of inter-item intervals observed in the Sternberg et al. RT task. Bradski et al. (1994, cited in Rhodes, 1999) developed a neural network that could serve as a perceptual preprocessor for a CQ model. In this network, a sequence of perceptual inputs induced an appropriate primacy gradient across plan representations in the planning layer of the CQ circuit.

Applying the CQ Model to Immediate Serial Recall

In the Sternberg et al. (1978) task, subjects were told to repeat short prepared lists as fast as possible following an external signal. This

qualified it as an RT task. A related list-recall task is the immediate serial recall (ISR) task, in which subjects also recall a short list from working memory, but without explicit instruction to initiate or perform recall as fast as possible. This non-RT sequence production task has also been modeled within the CQ framework. To the three core assumptions noted previously (primacy gradient, deletion on enactment, and iterated competitive choice of most-active remaining plan), Page and Norris (1998) added two auxiliary assumptions: that the choice is noisy, and that decay of activity in the planning layer occurs during input to the planning layer and during intervals spent performing items from the list. Error data favor both assumptions, and this extended model was able to address data on errors of serial recall. One kind of error, simple failure to recall, is most probable for list-final plans in long sequences. The extended model explains this as a consequence of their low initial activation level (due to being last in the primacy-gradient-coded sequence), which in turn makes them more susceptible to falling into inactivity due to the decay that can occur during enactment of the prepared sequence. Another feature of error data from ISR studies is that the vast majority of transposition errors (items are recalled, but in incorrect order) are simple exchanges with immediately adjacent items in the planned sequence. Given moderately noisy choice, this likewise follows from the gradient representation, because noise in the choice layer is less likely to illicitly promote a plan by two positions in the activity gradient than by one position.

Brain Substrates of Competitive Queuing

Data that strikingly confirm one of the main physiological predictions of CQ models was recently reported in Chafee et al. (2001). Since the CQ model depends on a working memory to hold a gradient of activations across plan representations prior to and during performance, the model predicts that such a gradient will be observable in the part of the brain responsible for working memory, namely the prefrontal cortex (PFC). Chafee et al. observed three ensembles of prefrontal activities corresponding to three segments of a forthcoming line drawing that a monkey had been trained to produce. The relative strength of activation of the three cellular ensembles predicted the order of the forthcoming segments: the higher the premovement activation, the earlier in the sequence the corresponding segment was produced. Error data were also in accord with predictions of the CQ model.

Another property of some versions of the CQ model is the normalization of total activity in the planning layer. This property predicts that peak frontal cortical activities associated with plan representations will decline as the number of coactive plans increases. Data that confirm this prediction for plan representations' activities were recently reported by Cisek and Kalaska (2002). They found a class of cells in the rostral part of the dorsal premotor cortex (rPMd) that they called "potential response cells." Different subsets of such cells, representing different potential responses, were coactive during a delay period when there was uncertainty regarding which, if any, of one or two alternative responses should be performed. This delay period activity was much more vigorous in each plan representation (cell subset) when there was only one potential response to hold in working memory than when there were two potential responses to hold in working memory.

These data on rPMd and PFC are consistent with representations in a normalized working memory capable of storing a primacy gradient—the planning layer of a CQ system. What part of the brain serves as the choice layer for frontocortical plan representations? One idea that has grown in popularity in recent years is that the striatum, a subcortical structure that encompasses the caudate, putamen, and accumbens nuclei of the basal ganglia, may provide competitive arenas in which cortically represented plans vie for execution. According to the recent model of Brown, Bullock, and Grossberg (2000), the winning plan selectively activates a small subset of spiny projection neurons (SPNs) in the striatum, which receives a massive excitatory input from the cerebral cortex. Via a return pathway that traverses the pallidum and thalamus, this focal striatal activation enables selective activation of output cells in a cortical layer (layer Vb) that is below, and excited by, the layer in which the cortical planning cells are found. One point of current debate regards how the striatum runs its competition to choose the next plan to execute. This debate arises because the striatum contains both feedback inhibition, mediated by SPNs, and feedforward inhibition, mediated by inhibitory interneurons which, like the SPNs, are direct recipients of excitatory input from the cortex. The simulations reported in Brown et al. (2000) were based on recent physiological data indicating that the dominant factor in striatal choice making is feedforward inhibition, not recurrent inhibition. In a situation with many strongly activated competing plans, reliance on feedback inhibition to resolve the competition would require that many cells in the choice field would be transiently active. Therefore a high threshold downstream from the choice field would be necessary to prevent multiple premature response activations. With feedforward competition, none of the choice field's output cells—in the striatal case, the SPNs—need activate until the moment that the competition yields a winner.

Plan Layer Loading by Rapid Parallel Recall from Procedural Long-Term Memory

One of the advantages of CQ models' explicit parallel representation of sequential plans—an advantage unavailable to RNNs as such—is that these distributed representations can be learned and recalled via compressive and expansive coding operations. In the Sternberg task and the ISR task mentioned previously, novel sequence information was provided to the performer. According to the CQ interpretation, performers hold a corresponding parallel representation for a few seconds in working memory (WM) before generating the sequence under the guidance of WM. However, Verwey (1996), among others, showed that a very high number of practice trials with short fixed sequences leads to *disappearance* of the sequence length effect on RT originally discovered by Sternberg et al. (1978). Is this result explicable in terms of a CQ model that uses activity normalization in the planning layer? Rhodes and Bullock (2002) have recently reported successful simulations of several sets of list learning and performance data, using a neural network in which the cerebellum, modeled as a substrate for procedural long-term memory (LTM), learns activation gradients over item nodes and rapidly recalls them into a normalized motor buffer (planning layer), which is a WM for action plans. The recall process is rapid because it entails *parallel loading of sequence chunks* into a WM from LTM. When the procedural LTM of a fixed sequence representation becomes strong enough (due to extensive practice), it causes preselection of the first list item within the CQ subsystem. Such preselection explains the disappearance of the sequence length effect on RT, which Verwey (1996) showed to be a reliable effect if subjects were given high levels of practice. This hybrid cerebellar-CQ model's assumption that the cerebellum can load parallel sequence representations into a frontocortical motor buffer is supported by recent neuroanatomical tracing studies, which have discovered pathways that run from the dentate nuclei of the cerebellum, via the thalamus, to several frontocortical zones, including premotor cortex and the PFC. More generally, the hybrid model illustrates how the CQ model, which focuses on WM dynamics that support sequential performance, can be interfaced with an LTM system that compressively learns and stores, and expansively recalls, oft-used sequences. Such a system is critical for functions that require frequent re-use of subsequences, such as musical performance or language production.

CQ as a General Basis for Serial Behavior

For CQ to qualify as a core model for all sequence planning and control, it must be shown that it is extensible to a full range of human serial performance domains. Given the pervasive involvement of the brain substrate outlined previously, it is reasonable to look for CQ signatures far beyond the types of skill tasks considered thus far. The most highly developed example of human serial behavior, syntactic language production, is a critical test case for the thesis that CQ is general. Another instructive case is sequential control of attentional focus during information pickup from complex scenes.

Is CQ Extensible to Language Production?

It might be thought that the CQ model cannot apply to syntactic language production, because sequencing errors in language production do not usually follow the "immediately adjacent items exchange" pattern found in ISR studies (which typically use nongrammatical item sequences). In most sequencing errors in language production, exchanges respect grammatical constraints, as when a sequencing error transforms the intended "flying saucers" into the spoonerism "sighing flossers." But note: the same example supports the CQ postulate that the initial segments of both words were already coactive in a planning field prior to production of either word. Moreover, it is plausible that the exchange error occurred because noise transiently rendered the plan for "fl" less active than the plan for "s" at the instant that "flying" should have been spoken. In fact, several neural network theorists have used CQ as a core of extended models that have offered explanations of many of the grammar-respecting patterns of sequencing-errors observed in language production (e.g., Dell, Burger, and Svec, 1997; Hartley and Houghton, 1996).

The most sustained treatment of CQ in language generation is that in Ward (1994). Far from simply explaining how the "emergent choice" that operates in CQ models is compatible with grammar-respecting sequencing errors in language production, Ward argues that *only* emergent choice offers a basis for overcoming more traditional language generators' failures to mimic the "flexible incremental generation" (FIG) exhibited in the real-time behavior of human speakers as they compose sentences "on the fly." Ward's FIG model combines CQ principles with principles inspired by *construction grammar* (e.g., Goldberg, 1995) to build a comprehensive connectionist model of grammatical sentence generation. The FIG algorithm is an iterated cycle: (1) Each node of an input conceptualization is a source of activation to "construction" nodes of various types, including words; (2) Activation is allowed to flow freely through the structured network of nodes; (3) When the network settles (or is forced to make an output) the most highly activated word representation is selected and enacted; (4) Any node or nodes of the input conceptualization that are expressed by the enacted word are inhibited, and activation levels are updated to represent the new current state; and (5) Steps 2–4 iterate until the conceptual content of the input has been expressed by the enacted word sequence. For the system to work well, the word plan that has the highest activation must be for a word that will be both syntactically and semantically correct if spoken as the next word in the utterance. This requirement is met, in part, by having the activation level of a word be determined by the product of its semantic and syntactic inputs, not by their sum.

Although much remains to test such models of CQ in the service of language production, initial simulation successes indicate that CQ may provide an ideal foundation for speech and language production models: one that is well grounded in neurobiology, and one that overcomes the inflexibility and other limitations inherent in more traditional, less parallel, theories.

Can CQ Be Considered an Attention Control Mechanism?

To gather information from the visible world around us, we typically, and rapidly, move our attention sequentially from one part of the scene to another. Often such search is purposeful, as when we are attempting to find a particular item or object, such as a familiar face in a crowd. In other cases, the scan sequence can be driven by salient features present in the visible scene. Either way, there must exist some mechanism for determining where to focus attention first, where to move the focus next, and so on. As defined previously, CQ provides a very simple and elegant candidate mechanism. The combination of a "saliency map" with an "inhibition of return" mechanism forms the basic mechanism for controlling attention deployment in contemporary computational models of focal visual attention (e.g., Itti and Koch, 2001). The most salient location in the map has the highest activation and draws the focus of attention to that location, whereupon map activity at that location is inhibited. Consequently, some other location in the map becomes most active—i.e., most salient—and now attracts the attentional focus. This process is another example of CQ. That it applies to attention shifts is no surprise because of the close link between such shifts and saccadic eye movements, sequential control of which has been attributed to interactions between frontal cortex and the basal ganglia (e.g., Brown et al., 2000).

Discussion

The fundamental scenario represented by the CQ model is almost palpable. We seem to be able to feel that two considered plans, or candidate words, begin with nearly equal potency, but that upon further deliberation, one waxes as the other wanes, and the waxing plan is first used to guide performance. Moreover, our capacity to simultaneously consider multiple plans in WM is limited to a small number. This limitation is predicted by the activity normalization property, which itself is needed to preserve the computational function of differences in activation levels. If forced to decide quickly, we feel that we choose the more vivid plan even if the rejected or deferred plan is also vivid and attractive. In the brain's parallel planning system, some common currency must be available for incrementing and decrementing the value of response alternatives, and in biological neural networks the use of excitation and inhibition to achieve these effects leaves activation level as the natural measure of relative priority. This, in combination with a maximum-finding network, creates a CQ system, which is probably an ancient invention in the evolution of animals. Recent computational studies, cited previously, have begun to explore how this ancient system

may still serve as a viable core for the highest levels of planning and skilled sequencing exhibited by humans.

Road Map: Artificial Intelligence
Related Reading: Artificial Intelligence and Neural Networks; Decision Support Systems and Expert Systems; Multiagent Systems; Recurrent Networks: Learning Algorithms; Winner-Take-All Networks

References

Boardman, I., and Bullock, D., 1991, A neural network model of serial order recall from short-term memory, in *Proceedings of the International Joint Conference on Neural Networks* (Seattle) vol. II, Piscataway, NJ: IEEE Service Center, pp. 879–884.

Brown, J., Bullock, D., and Grossberg, S., 2000, How laminar frontal cortex and basal ganglia circuits interact to control planned and reactive saccades, *Boston University Technical Report CAS/CNS-2000-023.*

Chafee, M. V., Averbeck, B. B., Crowe, D. A., and Georgopoulos, A. P., 2001, Motor sequence representation of prefrontal neurons predicts error patterns in drawing, *Abstr. Soc. Neurosci.*, 533.3.

Cisek, P., and Kalaska, J. F., 2002, Simultaneous encoding of multiple potential reach directions in dorsal premotor cortex, *J. Neurophysiol.*, 87:1149–1154.

Dell, G. S., Burger, L. K., and Svec, W. R., 1997, Language production and serial order: A functional analysis and a model, *Psychol. Rev.*, 104:123–147. ◆

Goldberg, A. E., 1995, *Constructions: A Construction Grammar Approach to Argument Structure*, Chicago, IL: U. of Chicago Press.

Grossberg, S., 1978, A theory of human memory: Self-organization and performance of sensory-motor codes, maps, and plans, in *Progress in Theoretical Biology*, vol. 5 (R. Rosen and F. Snell, Eds.), New York, NY: Academic Press, pp. 233–374. ◆

Hartley, T. A., and Houghton, G., 1996, A linguistically constrained model of short-term memory for nonwords, *J. Mem. Lang.*, 35:1–31.

Itti, L., and Koch, C., 2001, Computational modelling of visual attention, *Nature Rev. Neurosci.*, 2:194–203.

Page, M. P. A., and Norris, D., 1998, The primacy model: A new model of immediate serial recall, *Psychol. Rev.*, 105:761–781. ◆

Rhodes, B., 1999, *Learning-Driven Changes in the Temporal Characteristics of Serial Movement Performance: A Model Based on Cortico-Cerebellar Cooperation*, Doctoral Dissertation, Cognitive and Neural Systems Department, Boston University. ◆

Rhodes, B., and Bullock, D., 2002, Neural dynamics of learning and performance of fixed sequences. Latency pattern reorganizations and the N-STREAMS model. *Boston University Technical Report CAS/CNS-02-005.*

Sternberg, S., Monsell, S., Knoll, R. L., and Wright, C. E., 1978, The latency and duration of rapid movement sequences: Comparisons of speech and typewriting, (Reprinted) in *Perception and Production of Fluent Speech* (R.A. Cole, Ed.), 1980, Hillsdale, NJ: Erlbaum, pp. 469–505.

Verwey, W. B., 1996, Buffer loading and chunking in sequential key pressing, *JEP: Human Perception and Performance*, 22:544–562.

Ward, N., 1994, *A Connectionist Language Generator*, Norwood, NJ: Ablex Publishing. ◆

Compositionality in Neural Systems

Barbara Hammer

Introduction

In real life, people deal with composite structures: Written English language is built out of 26 characters (and a few additional symbols) that form syllables, words, sentences, articles, road maps, and finally the *Handbook of Brain Theory*. Spoken language consists of raw acoustic waves at a basic level; at a higher level, it can be decomposed into phonemes that form words, sentences, a poem or a speech. Visual data can be decomposed into pixels with various colors and intensities; alternatively, the raw image data may be represented by features like edges or texture, which are grouped to complex contours, objects, and, finally, a complete scene, such as the image of a grandmother sitting in a chair and knitting. Moreover, not only real-life data are processed as composite objects:

artificial data created by humans or virtual objects also have a composite structure. As examples, web sites consist of single pages with a head and body, links, tabulars, figures, enumerations, and so on. Computer programs decompose into procedures and functions, or objects and methods. Logical formulas and terms are recursive objects built out of symbols for constants, variables, and functions, logical connectives, and quantors.

In respect to neural systems, two questions arise:

1. Artificial neural networks are developed in order to model important aspects of the human brain and to explain how biological neural networks process information. A common characteristic of the way in which data are created, processed, and stored by humans is compositionality. *Which neural dynamics allow composite structures, grouping, and binding to emerge* in such a way that the single parts can be restored rapidly and, at the same time, the whole composite structure can be identified with a single object?

2. Artificial neural networks are a powerful and universal machine learning tool that is used in scientific and industrial applications for data contained in a finite dimensional vector space. Everyday data are composite. *How can we adapt standard neural techniques to composite structures* such that connectionistic methods can be used in everyday applications and combined with other compositional machine learning tools?

These two questions constitute extreme positions in a single problem spectrum: How is information processed in the brain? Since it is unlikely that models that are satisfactory with regard to both efficiency and biological plausibility will become available in the near future, the focus can be on one of two aspects: either one can develop practically applicable and efficiently trainable approaches or one can design biologically plausible and universal systems. Most existing approaches lie somewhere in between, partly because biological systems are indeed very effective, suggesting the universal principle of compositionality and dynamic binding, e.g., in the visual system (Bienenstock, 1996) (see DYNAMIC LINK ARCHITECTURE).

Properties of Compositionality

What are the general properties of composite objects like the sentences "John loves Mary" or "Mary loves that John loves Mary"? The structures are composed of *basic primitives*—here, the words *John, Mary, loves*, and *that*. The primitives are instances of a certain *type*, e.g., a noun or verb. Composite expressions arise if the primitives are combined in specified *relations*. The sentence "John loves Mary" is an instance of a relation of the form subject–predicate–object, where subject and object can be instantiated with a specific noun, for example. Alternatively, these positions may be filled with composite objects, such as "John loves Mary" in the example "Mary loves that John loves Mary." The complexity of recursively generated structures is usually not limited a priori. As an example, we could build the sentences "John loves that Mary loves that John loves Mary," or "Mary loves that John loves that Mary loves that John loves Mary," and so on. Hence, as pointed out in van Gelder (1990), the combination of primitives of certain types within constituency relations yields composite structures of *a priori unlimited complexity and an infinite number of possible combinations*.

The *semantics* of composite objects is determined by the semantics of the simple primitives and their relation in the structure. The primitives alone do not determine the semantics. The sentences "John loves Mary" and "Mary loves John," for example, have identical constituents but different meanings. Moreover, the decomposition of complex objects into simpler parts and their interpretation may depend on the whole structure: the meaning of *her* in the sentence "Mary loves that John loves her" depends on the context of the part "John loves her." Conversely, the same situation

may be described with different composite objects, such as "Mary loves that John loves Mary" or "Mary loves that John loves her." In other words, parts of a structure may be substituted by entirely different representations without affecting the semantics. Hence, the whole structure as well as the involved primitives and their relation should be available for referring the semantics.

Although an unlimited number of combinations of the primitives in constituency relations is possible in principle, commonly only a small number of all possible combinations are used in practice and make sense. Either basic syntactic rules or semantic limitations restrict the variety of possible compositions. "That John loves Mary loves Mary" does not make sense, for example, if the composite structure "that John loves Mary" is used as subject. Restrictions of possible combinations are often context dependent. For example, the sentence "John loves himself" would be preferred to "John loves John" unless the word "John" refers to two different persons.

Humans are capable of understanding and producing composite objects. Moreover, they can deal with new complex structures although they have never seen the specific combination of primitives before. As an example, having read the above sentences concerning John and Mary and the sentence "Mary loves Peter," people would be capable of understanding the sentence "John loves that Mary loves Peter," and they would possibly infer that this sentence is false. People can infer the meaning of partially new structures. They have knowledge about primitives and relations, and additional information such as rules for composition or experience with similar structures. Moreover, compositional structures play an important role if the capability of humans for analogy-based reasoning is investigated (see ANALOGY-BASED REASONING AND METAPHOR).

Appropriate artificial neural systems for use in processing compositional data should take these properties into account. Although they have to deal with an unrestricted amount of partially new and ambiguous data, they can use the sparseness and hierarchical structure of the data for efficient processing.

Neural Systems and Compositionality

Popular neural methods perform pattern recognition, for which classical statistics provides a well-founded theory (see PATTERN RECOGNITION). Standard neural networks are adapted to real vectors contained in a finite dimensional Euclidean real-vector space. Concerning compositional structures, the question arises how to encode and process an arbitrary amount of information with this finite dimensional machinery.

Compared to their biological counterparts, artificial neural networks often neglect the fine temporal structure of spike trains (see OSCILLATORY AND BURSTING PROPERTIES OF NEURONS and ADAPTIVE SPIKE CODING): standard artificial networks process real values or binary values in a well-defined topological order. Real values correlate to the mean spiking frequence of the biological neurons; hence, the local temporal structure and respective correlation of spikes are not taken into account. Binary values might encode single spikes, although the topology allows processing on a discrete or fixed time scale only. Experiments provide evidence that the fine temporal structure may indeed carry important information for encoding complex scenes in biological networks (Engel et al., 1992). However, the precise way in which information is encoded in the respective parts of the brain is not yet understood. Moreover, some effects can possibly already be explained at the abstract level of rate coding (see RATE CODING AND SIGNAL PROCESSING). Hence it is worth considering the whole spectrum of neural architectures capable of dealing with compositionality. Our taxonomy for characterizing the various approaches is based on the connection structure of the neural architectures and on their fundamental dynamical behavior.

A key property of appropriate systems is their capability of processing a priori unlimited information. *Static solutions* with feedforward networks have the advantage that efficient training algorithms are readily available (see BACKPROPAGATION: GENERAL PRINCIPLES). Unfortunately, either their capacity is limited or they need an a priori unlimited amount of neural resources.

Recurrent neural networks use the additional degree of freedom provided by a priori unlimited processing time in order to map the information appropriately. Recurrent networks may be *partially recurrent*, where the processing dynamics are determined by the respective data structure. The restriction to limited recursive data structures allows the immediate generalization of efficient standard learning tools (see RECURRENT NETWORKS: LEARNING ALGORITHMS). Alternatively, the networks may be *fully recurrent*, in which case the dynamics are determined by the respective process. This allows more flexibility, but the processing time cannot be limited a priori, and alternative learning algorithms are necessary (see TEMPORAL SEQUENCES: LEARNING AND GLOBAL ANALYSIS). In particular, continuous-time fully recurrent neural networks can use the fine temporal structure for encoding complex information, such as in networks of spiking neurons (see INTEGRATE-AND-FIRE NEURONS AND NETWORKS). These approaches are biologically plausible and flexible. Unfortunately, no efficient learning algorithm comparable to standard backpropagation for feedforward networks has been established for networks of spiking neurons until today.

Static Approaches

The *grandmother neuron doctrine* assumes that each simple or composite object is represented by the activity of a specific neuron for this object (see LOCALIZED VERSUS DISTRIBUTED REPRESENTATIONS). Neurons for complex objects are hierarchically connected to neurons representing their simple parts, and they only become active if all neurons for their parts become active. Putative "grandmother cells" have been found in the visual system of the macaque monkey, for example (see SPARSE CODING IN THE PRIMATE CORTEX) but the data do not preclude the firing of such cells for a variety of patterns. Some invariance, for example with respect to the specific lighting, may be involved in the hierarchical computation, such that the neuron that encodes our grandmother fires independent of the specific context. Naturally, this approach requires additional neural resources for each new primitive, relation, or composite object, and therefore suffers from combinatorial limitations. Moreover, it is not obvious how entirely new combinations of well-known ingredients could be processed properly, i.e., in such a way that the possibility of analogies and transfer is taken into account. However, the hierarchical feedforward computation makes it possible to identify each neuron with a specific meaning and to use standard neural techniques.

Alternatively, composite objects may be represented in a *distributed manner* via the activation of a group of neurons for the single features (see POPULATION CODES). This reduces the number of necessary neurons, but it is not obvious how invariance and not instantiated or new features are to be integrated. The necessary amount of resources depends on the respective task and cannot be uniformly limited. Moreover, the composition of two objects into a composite object is to be distinguished from the simple superposition of the activation of each; otherwise, the respective decomposition would become ambiguous.

Naturally, both encodings may be combined in *localized distributed representations* of objects that correspond to the firing of neurons at a certain area of the pool. This encoding is suggested by the presence of topology-preserving maps in biological systems where similar stimuli cause neural activities in similar neural regions (see OCULAR DOMINANCE AND ORIENTATION COLUMNS).

Either localized or distributed encoding of composite objects in a vector space of fixed dimension has so far been the standard encoding for practical applications (see LOCALIZED VERSUS DISTRIBUTED REPRESENTATIONS). Hierarchical extraction of relevant features and finally of the respective class is a promising technique that has been successfully applied in various applications, such as the recognition of visual objects or text processing (Riesenhuber and Poggio, 1999; Mel and Fiser, 2000). Given the limits with respect to the number of recognized objects, static approaches suffer from a priori limitations and can only explain parts of biological information processing.

Partially Recurrent Systems

Discrete time partially recurrent neural networks are widely used in time series prediction, speech recognition, and the processing of sequences of real vectors in general (Kremer, 2001) (see CONSTITUENCY AND RECURSION IN LANGUAGE; IDENTIFICATION AND CONTROL). They deal with sequences of real vectors as opposed to simple real vectors and hence are capable of processing very simple composite objects with a priori unlimited informational content. Their dynamics directly mirror the recursive structure of the data: a standard feedforward network encodes in its internal activations the context of the computation, i.e., the first part of a sequence, and recursively maps one entry of the sequence after another to new contexts, depending on its internal state. Since the dynamic is fixed according to the data structure, standard gradient descent techniques can be used for supervised learning of mappings with sequences as inputs or outputs (see RECURRENT NETWORKS: LEARNING ALGORITHMS).

The a priori unlimited information in the data structure changes the learning theoretical properties compared to standard feedforward networks: On the one hand, the power of recurrent networks can be demonstrated by relating them to classical symbolic computing mechanisms, such as Turing machines (Hammer, 2002) (see NEURAL AUTOMATA AND ANALOG COMPUTATIONAL COMPLEXITY). On the other hand, valid generalization can no longer be guaranteed for training set sizes that are both independent of the underlying input distribution and independent of the specific output of the training algorithm (Hammer, 2002) (see PAC LEARNING AND NEURAL NETWORKS; VAPNIK-CHERVONENKIS DIMENSION OF NEURAL NETWORKS).

One can think of the recursive dynamics of simple recurrent networks as a recursive coding of sequences to distributed representations in a finite dimensional vector space. This idea can immediately be generalized to more complex composite objects, provided they have a recursive structure: trees consist of a label and a fixed number of subtrees. Hence, a network that is to encode trees instead of simple sequences can recursively map the root's label and the already computed codes for the subtrees to a code for the entire tree. It can also decode a distributed representation of a tree by computing the root's label and codes for the subtrees, which can be recursively processed further (Frasconi, Gori, and Sperduti, 1997; Hammer, 2002). This mechanism can be found in various STRUCTURED CONNECTIONIST MODELS (q.v.). Note that terms and formulas have a natural representation as tree structures: the single symbols are contained in the respective nodes, and the subformulas or subterms respectively correspond to subtrees. Thus, networks capable of encoding or decoding tree structures constitute a universal mechanism that enables the use of neural techniques in symbolic domains.

Concrete implementations of this basic idea differ in how the respective networks are trained. With the dynamics being determined by the data structure, gradient descent techniques can be used for supervised learning of general mappings, with trees as input or output. Recursive networks are trained directly for the specific learning problem (Frasconi et al., 1997; Hammer, 2002). The recursive autoassociative memory trains only encoding and decoding, such that their composition yields the identity on the data, leading to universal encoding (Frasconi et al., 1997; Sperduti, 1994). Holographic reduced representation uses a fixed transition function that is not trained at all (Plate, 1995). These approaches have been successfully applied in such different areas as chemistry, theorem proving, and language processing (Frasconi et al., 1997; Hammer, 2002). Learning is quite similar to the training of simple recurrent networks as far as practical algorithms as well as theoretical properties like approximation and generalization capability are concerned (Hammer, 2002).

This approach, however, is limited to recursive compositions with a well-defined recursive structure; cyclic structures cannot be processed in this way. Moreover, gaining access to single parts of recursive structures may be time-consuming and subject to noise, depending on the level of recurrence. There exist fundamental mathematical limitations to the possibility of coding infinite tree structures in a finite dimensional vector space: encoding has to be nested or fractal, which means that the Euclidean metric is no longer appropriate for the resulting distributed representations (Hammer, 2002). Thus, various neural methods that are based on the Euclidean metric cannot be used for further processing. Reliable decoding is a difficult task with a lower-bounded complexity (Hammer, 2002) (see VAPNIK-CHERVONENKIS DIMENSION OF NEURAL NETWORKS). Therefore, neural networks with the above dynamics are not appropriate for efficiently decoding a large amount of distributed data.

Fully Recurrent Systems

Fully recurrent neural systems are networks where the neuron's activations evolve in time in a continuous or discrete manner. Commonly, the dynamics can be described by nonlinear difference equations in discrete time or differential equations in continuous time. The main difference from partially recurrent networks is that the processing dynamics and consequently the required computation time are not directly determined by the data structures. Time and complexity of computation and representation of information are a priori unlimited. The systems may use the temporal structure of the neuron's activations for storing important information in specific spatiotemporal activation patterns such as synfire chains, i.e., successive spiking of specified neurons in precise time intervals (see SYNFIRE CHAINS). As proposed by Bienenstock (1996), for example, the synchronous oscillation of different neurons or assemblies may indicate that they represent objects that are bound together (see SYNCHRONIZATION, BINDING AND EXPECTANCY and ADAPTIVE SPIKE CODING). This type of binding could easily be further processed with coincidence detectors. Alternatively, information may be stored in simple localized or distributed patterns of the neuron's activities, as in the static and partially recurrent approaches. Various systems obey a gradient dynamics as an example and converge to a fixed point that contains the important information (see TEMPORAL SEQUENCES: LEARNING AND GLOBAL ANALYSIS).

Concrete implementations differ considerably in their complexity and intention. Several approaches merely demonstrate that important effects such as *oscillation, synchronization*, and *coincidence detection* can be found in experiments on biological neural activities and can be simulated in an artificial, though biologically plausible, environment (see CHAOS IN NEURAL SYSTEMS; COLLECTIVE BEHAVIOR OF COUPLED OSCILLATORS, and CORTICAL POPULATION DYNAMICS AND PSYCHOPHYSICS). Particularly in the context of networks of spiking neurons, methods that allow a mathematical investigation of complex systems have been developed over the last years (see INTEGRATE-AND-FIRE NEURONS AND NETWORKS). First steps in possible training mechanisms use the principles of self-organization and Hebbian learning (see POST-HEBBIAN LEARNING ALGORITHMS). Binding via the temporal structure and synchronous oscillation is a biologically plausible mechanism that is supported by experimental results (Engel et al., 1992). It is not yet obvious how complex recursive and hierarchical structures can be represented in this way, since methods such as iterated period doubling or a superposition of the oscillation, for example, are restricted by the computation accuracy of neurons. Moreover, efficient learning algorithms for practical applications are not yet available.

Other approaches *develop practical tools for concrete tasks* that involve binding mechanisms, such as feature grouping or edge detection in images (see VISUAL SCENE SEGMENTATION). Grouping may be encoded in synchronously oscillating neurons or in the localized activation of specific neurons in a limiting state that minimizes an energy function, such as in the competitive layer model (Wersing, Steil, and Ritter, 2001). Most approaches are based on appropriate excitation of similar neurons and an inhibition of cells with dissimilar activation. Again, only limited possibilities of automatic learning of the connections are available so far.

Finally, recurrent systems for *complex analogical reasoning and symbolic processing* have been proposed (see STRUCTURED CONNECTIONIST MODELS). Popular approaches are LISA, SHRUTI, and INFERNET, which have in common that binding is realized via synchronous oscillation of neurons or pools of neurons (Hummel and Holyoak, 1997; Sougné, 1999; Shastri, 1999). Structures are represented through localized or distributed cell activations. Rules correspond to specific neural connections that allow human-like analogical reasoning and are mostly hand encoded. They are capable of simulating various effects and limitations of human-like reasoning. However, like most fully recurrent approaches, the systems suffer from the lack of universal and efficient training algorithms.

Discussion

Compositionality as a common principle of information processing should find its counterpart in artificial neural systems. Solutions may either enhance static feedforward systems and represent the objects by static activation patterns, or may rely on recursive and adaptive encoding mechanisms in partially recurrent networks, or may use complex dynamics and the fine temporal structure of the neuron's activation for reliable representation. Of course, it is possible to transfer more practical tools and theoretical guarantees from classical network techniques to these systems if they are similar to classical systems. It should be pointed out that it is still disputed whether artificial neural networks are capable of adequately handling compositional data, and if so, which type of network is the most suitable one. Remarkable results have been obtained with simple recurrent networks, although some researchers argue that more complicated dynamics or dynamics similar to classical symbolic processing mechanisms are necessary for successful modeling within the context of compositionality (see CONNECTIONIST AND SYMBOLIC REPRESENTATIONS and Elman (1998) and references therein for a discussion of this subject).

Important directions for future research include the exploration of real neural codes in biological systems. Of particular interest is whether effects such as synchronous activation indeed contain information that is necessary for the representation of relations. Oscillations could constitute a byproduct of information processing that merely enables efficient adaptation in biological systems.

Restrictions on compositionality are another avenue of exploration. In practice, only a small subset of all possible combinations of primitives and relations occurs. Mathematical analysis of structure-processing systems implies usually a worst-case analysis and might indicate, for example, that static approaches are not appropriate for this field. However, neural mechanisms that are not capable of representing arbitrary composite objects in principle might be well suited for restricted, though important, domains.

Road Map: Artificial Intelligence
Related Reading: Analogy-Based Reasoning and Metaphor; Dynamic Link Architecture; Structured Connectionist Models; Systematicity of Generalizations in Connectionist Networks

References

Bienenstock, E., 1996, Composition, in *Brain Theory: Biological Basis and Computational Theory of Vision* (A. Aertsen and V. Braitenberg, Eds.), New York: Elsevier, pp. 269–300. ◆

Elman, J., 1998, Generalization, simple recurrent networks, and the emergence of structure, in *Proceedings of the Twentieth Annual Conference of the Cognitive Science Society* (M. A. Gernsbacher and S. J. Derry, Eds.), Mahwah, NJ: Erlbaum.

Engel, A. K., König, P., Kreiter, A. K., Chilien, T. B., and Singer, W., 1992, Temporal coding in the visual cortex: New vista on integration in the nervous system, *Trends Neurosci.*, 15:218–225.

Frasconi, P., Gori, M., and Sperduti, A., 1997, A general framework for adaptive processing of data sequences, *IEEE Trans. Neural Netw.*, 9:768–786. ◆

Hammer, B., 2002, Recurrent networks for structured data: A unifying approach and its properties, *Cogn. Systems Res.* (in press). ◆

Hummel, J. E., and Holyoak, K. J., 1997, Distributed representation of structure: A theory of analogical access and mapping, *Psychol. Rev.*, 104:427–466.

Kremer, S. C., 2001, Spatio-temporal connectionist networks: A taxonomy and review, *Neural Computat.*, 13:249–306. ◆

Mel, B., and Fiser, J., 2000, Minimizing binding errors using learned conjunctive features. *Neural Computat.*, 12:247–278.

Plate, T., 1995, Holographic reduced representations, *IEEE Trans. Neural Netw.*, 6:623–641.

Riesenhuber, M., and Poggio, T., 1999, Are cortical models really bound by the "binding problem"? *Neuron*, 24:87–93.

Shastri, L., 1999, Advances in SHRUTI: A neurally motivated model of relational knowledge representation and rapid inference using temporal synchrony, *Appl. Intell.*, 11(1):79–108.

Sougné, J. P., 1999, *INFERNET: A neurocomputational model of binding and inference*, PhD thesis, Université de Liège.

Sperduti, A., 1994, Labeling RAAM, *Connect. Sci.*, 6:429–459.

van Gelder, T., 1990, Compositionality: A connectionist variation on a classical theme, *Cognit. Sci.*, 14:355–384. ◆

Wersing, H., Steil, J. J., and Ritter, H., 2001, A competitive layer model for feature binding and sensory segmentation of features, *Neural Computat.*, 13:357–387.

Computing with Attractors

John Hertz

Introduction

This article describes how to compute with networks with feedback that exhibit complex dynamical behavior. In order to compute with any machine, we need to know how data are to be fed into it and how the result of a computation is to be read out. These questions are trivial for layered feedforward networks, but not for networks with feedback. A natural proposal is to wait until the network has "settled down" and then read the answer off a suitably chosen set of units. The state a dynamical system settles into is called an *attractor*, so this paradigm is called computing with attractors.

The term "settling down" is not meant to restrict this picture to cases in which the dynamical state of the network stops changing. This is one kind of attractor, but it is also possible to settle down into periodic or even chaotic patterns of activity, as described below.

It is possible in principle to perform computations based on the transient approach to the attractor, in addition to or instead of on the basis of the attractor alone. However, we will not consider this alternative in this article.

Computing with attractors is appealing because it does not require the person reading the result to observe the entire evolution of the network. Neither need she know when the computation was started or how long it took. All that is required is the identification of the attractor that a given initial condition evolves toward (and a way of recognizing that the network has reached the attractor). Therefore, this survey will begin with a brief description of the kinds of attractors one can meet: fixed points, limit cycles, and strange attractors. We will illustrate the paradigm with a simple example, the Hopfield model for associative memory. We then indicate briefly both how the connections necessary to embed desired patterns can be learned and how the paradigm can be extended to time-dependent attractors. Finally, we examine the possible relevance of attractor computation to the functioning of the brain.

Networks, Attractors, and Stability

We will focus our attention on networks described by systems of differential equations like

$$\tau_i \frac{du_i}{dt} + u_i(t) = \sum_{j \neq i} w_{ij} g[u_j(t)] + h_i(t) \qquad (1)$$

Here $u_i(t)$ is the net input to unit i at time t and $g(\ )$ is a sigmoidal activation function ($g' > 0$), so that $V_i = g(u_i)$ is the activation of unit i. The connection weight to unit i from unit j is denoted w_{ij}, $h_i(t)$ is an external input, and τ_i is a relaxation time.

We can also consider discrete-time systems governed by

$$V_i(t + 1) = g\left[\sum_j w_{ij} V_j(t) + h_i(t)\right] \qquad (2)$$

Here it is understood that all units are updated simultaneously.

These models are deterministic. Noisy networks can be analyzed by the methods of statistical mechanics and are treated extensively elsewhere in this *Handbook* (see, e.g., STATISTICAL MECHANICS OF NEURAL NETWORKS and STATISTICAL MECHANICS OF GENERALIZATION).

Viewing such a network as a computer, data can be read into it in two ways. One is as the $h_i(t)$ on a subset of the units, which we can call input units. The $h_i(t)$ values might be held fixed or varied in time, depending on the problem. This way of loading data is, of course, just carried over directly from the conventional input-output paradigm as we normally apply it to feedforward networks. Alternatively, we can load the data by setting the values of the initial activations $V_i(0)$. For layered feedforward networks this procedure is equivalent to the previous one, but for recurrent nets it is fundamentally different. We can also use both these input mechanisms simultaneously. The first is appropriate when we want to have the output vary with the input (e.g., continuous mapping), while we use the second when we want an output to be insensitive to small changes in the input (e.g., error correction). As the second one is intrinsic to recurrent networks, we will focus most of our attention on it.

The program of such a computer is its connection weights w_{ij}. Some of them may be zero, but the questions we address here are rather trivial unless there is some feedback, i.e., unless our networks are *recurrent*. We will not restrict our attention to symmetric connections; w_{ij} need not equal w_{ji}.

Finding the correct weights to implement a particular computation is a highly complex problem. However, for recurrent networks, we must first understand something about the attractors that represent the results of computations, so we now turn our attention to this problem.

To describe the dynamics of our networks, we make use of a picture in which the activation of each unit in the network is associated with a direction in a multidimensional space, called the *configuration space*. Every point in this space represents a possible state of the network, called the *state vector*, and the motion of this vector represents its evolution in time. For all recurrent networks of interest, there are just three possibilities for the asymptotic state:

1. The state vector comes to rest, i.e., the unit activations stop changing. This is the simplest case to analyze and is called a *fixed point*. Different results of a computation (owing to different input data) are characterized by settling into different fixed points. The region of initial states that settles into a single fixed point is called its *basin of attraction*. Most of the examples of recurrent networks in the literature, such as the Hopfield model and many related ones, compute with fixed points.
2. The state vector settles into a periodic motion, called a *limit cycle*.
3. The state vector moves chaotically, in the sense that two copies of the system that initially have nearly identical states will grow more and more dissimilar as they evolve: the two state vectors diverge from each other. However, the way they diverge is restricted. At any time the two state vectors are actually growing closer together in many directions in the configuration space; the divergence occurs only in some (typically a few) directions. A Poincaré map showing, e.g., the states of some of the units every time the state vector passes through some hyperplane in configuration space will be a fractal object with a dimensionality greater than zero (Schuster, 1989). This kind of attractor is called *strange* (see CHAOS IN BIOLOGICAL SYSTEMS and CHAOS IN NEURAL SYSTEMS).

Which kind of attractor we obtain will depend on the connections in the network and, possibly, the input data. Suitable learning algorithms make it possible to design the desired type. In simple applications, fixed points are naturally easiest to deal with. However, it may sometimes be advantageous to exploit the richer dynamical possibilities available in non-fixed-point attractors. For example, limit cycles allow the timing of the network's response to be controlled.

For all three kinds of attractors, the computation performed is a mapping from an initial condition to a particular attractor. It is evident that the dynamics partitions the configuration space into basins of attraction around the attractors. All initial conditions within a given basin map to the same attractor; that is, they are classified in the same way by the computation.

There are conditions under which the attractors will always be fixed points. For nets described by the continuous dynamics of Equation 1, a sufficient (but not necessary) condition is that the connection weights be symmetric: $w_{ij} = w_{ji}$.

General results about the stability of recurrent nets were proved by Cohen and Grossberg (1983). They showed that for static external input h_i, if the connection matrix w_{ij} is symmetric, the at-

tractors of Equation 1 are always fixed points, even if the activation function is allowed to differ from unit to unit, the $u_i(t)$ on the left-hand side is replaced by a general monotonic function $b_i(u_i)$, and τ_i is a (positive) function of u_i.

The proof illustrates the basic mathematical strategy for proving stability. Suppose we can find some quantity, a nontrivial function of the state variables u_i, which always decreases under the dynamics described in Equation 1 except for special values of u_i at which it does not change. These values are fixed points. For values of u_i near such a point, the system will evolve either toward it (an attractor) or away from it (a repellor). For almost all starting states, the dynamics will end at one of the attractor fixed points. Furthermore, these are the only attractors. If there were a limit cycle, for example, our function would decrease everywhere on a closed curve, which is impossible. Thus, whether such a quantity exists for a given network is very important. A function with this property is called a *Lyapunov function*.

There is indeed such a function for the Cohen-Grossberg extension of the dynamics described in Equation 1:

$$L(\mathbf{u}) = \sum_i \int^{u_i} [b_i(u) - h_i]g_i'(u)du - \tfrac{1}{2}\sum_{ij} w_{ij}g_i(u_i)g_j(u_j) \quad (3)$$

We can show directly that it is a Lyapunov function by computing its time derivative. Making use of the equations of motion and the symmetry of w_{ij}, we find

$$\dot{L} = -\sum_i g_i'(u_i)\tau_i(u_i)\dot{u}_i^2 \le 0 \quad (4)$$

Thus L is always decreasing, except at the fixed points $\dot{u}_i = 0$.

When a Lyapunov function exists, we may think about the dynamics in terms of sliding downhill on a surface in configuration space, the height of which is given by $L(\mathbf{u})$. The motion is not simple gradient descent, since $\dot{u}_i$ is not exactly proportional to $-\partial L/\partial u_i$ (there is an extra factor $g_i'(u_i)\tau_i(u_i)$). Nevertheless, the motion is always downhill, and the bottoms of the valleys correspond to the fixed points.

If we know the form of the Lyapunov function for a particular kind of network, this picture gives us a clue about how to program desired fixed-point attractors: we try to choose the connection weights w_{ij} and biases h_i so that L has minima at these points in configuration space.

To gain a little more insight, we restrict ourselves to the case $b_i(u) = u$ and an activation function $g(u) = \tanh(\beta u)$. Using the activation variables $V_i = g(u_i)$ instead of u_i, we find that we can write L in the form

$$L(\mathbf{V}) = \frac{1}{\beta}\sum_i \int^{V_i} dy \tanh^{-1} y - \sum_i h_i V_i - \tfrac{1}{2}\sum_{ij} w_{ij}V_i V_j \quad (5)$$

For large gain β, the first term is small. It is natural to think of the other two simply as a "potential energy" that the system tries to minimize. The w_{ij} and h_i should thus be chosen so that their sum has minima at or near the desired fixed points. The main effect of the first term is just to prevent the activations from reaching 1 or -1, since its derivatives diverge there.

Sometimes it is simple to construct a potential energy with the desired minima, at least approximately. In other problems, this strategy may be inadequate, and we have to resort to iterative learning algorithms to determine the network parameters.

Limit cycles and strange attractors are harder to handle mathematically. Often, however, it is possible to proceed in some kind of analogy with the fixed-point case.

Associative Memory

The most celebrated application of computing with fixed points is ASSOCIATIVE NETWORKS (q.v.). Here we follow the treatment due to Hopfield (1984) (see also Hertz, Krogh, and Palmer, 1991, chaps. 2 and 3). There is a set of patterns to be stored somehow by the computer. Given as input a pattern that is a corrupted version of one of these, the result of the computation should be the corresponding uncorrupted one.

The strategy for solving this problem is to try to guess a form for the potential energy part of Equation 5 that will have minima at the configurations corresponding to the patterns to be stored. We take patterns $\xi_i^\mu = \pm 1$. The subscript i labels the N elements of the pattern (e.g., pixel values), and the superscript μ labels the p different patterns in the set. The patterns are assumed random and independent for both different i and different μ. (This assumption is artificial for most potential applications, but studying this simple case affords us some insight into how the network works, and we will see how to relax it in the next section.) If we wanted to store just one such pattern ξ_i, a natural choice is just to take the potential energy function proportional to $-(\Sigma_i \xi_i V_i)^2$. The quantity $\Sigma_i \xi_i V_i$ measures the similarity between the pattern and the state of the network. It achieves its maximal value at $+N$, and therefore $-(\Sigma_i \xi_i V_i)^2$ is minimal if and only if every V_i coincides with ξ_i. For more than one pattern we try one such term for each pattern, yielding a total potential energy

$$H = -\frac{1}{2N} \sum_{\mu=1}^{p} \left(\sum_i \xi_i^\mu V_i \right)^2 \tag{6}$$

Multiplying out the square of the sum, we can identify the connection weights in Equation 5 as

$$w_{ij} = \frac{1}{N} \sum_\mu \xi_i^\mu \xi_j^\mu \tag{7}$$

The form of this equation suggests a Hebbian interpretation (see HEBBIAN SYNAPTIC PLASTICITY). For each pattern, there is a contribution to the connection weight proportional to the product of sending (ξ_j^μ) and receiving (ξ_i^μ) unit activities when the network is in the state $V_i = \xi_i^\mu$. This is just the form of synaptic strength proposed by Hebb (1949) as the basis of animal memory, so this is sometimes called a Hebbian storage prescription. This matrix is symmetric and has positive definite eigenvalues, so our earlier results guarantee that the attractors of our network dynamics are fixed points for both continuous and discrete-time dynamics.

The hope is that this will produce a fixed point of the network dynamics at or near each ξ_i^μ. (Because our H is purely quadratic in the V_i, we also expect fixed points near $-\xi_i^\mu$.) We can see how well this works by examining the stationary points of the Lyapunov function described by Equation 5, which are

$$V_i = \tanh \left(\beta \sum_j w_{ij} V_j \right) \tag{8}$$

We would first like to know whether there are solutions of Equation 8 that vary across the units like the individual patterns ξ_i^μ.

The quality of retrieval of a particular stored pattern ξ_i^μ is measured by the quantity $m_\mu = N^{-1} \Sigma_i \xi_i^\mu V_i$. Using Equation 8, with the weight formula of Equation 7, we obtain

$$m_\mu = \frac{1}{N} \sum_i \xi_i^\mu \tanh \left(\beta \sum_v \xi_i^v m_v \right) \tag{9}$$

The kind of solution we are looking for should describe a state of the network that is correlated with only one of the stored patterns, i.e., just one of the $m_\mu \neq 0$. With this restriction, Equation 9 reduces to

$$m = \tanh (\beta m) \tag{10}$$

where m is the value of the one non-zero m_μ. This equation has nontrivial solutions whenever $\beta > 1$. Next we have to inquire

whether these solutions are truly attractors, i.e., whether they are stable. At this point the story gets mathematically involved, so we simply survey the results (Kühn, Bös, and van Hemmen, 1991). Everything here is derived in the limit of a large network, i.e., $N \to \infty$; thus, the tools of statistical mechanics can be brought to bear.

The story is quite simple when p (the number of stored patterns) is a negligible fraction of N, the number of units in the network. Then the nontrivial solutions are globally stable, while the solution $m = 0$ is unstable, whenever $\beta > 1$.

If the gain is high enough, there are other attractors in addition to the ones we have tried to program into the network with the choice of Equation 7. In the simplest of these, the state of the network is equally correlated with three of the ξ_i^μ, say, $\xi_i^{\mu_1}$, $\xi_i^{\mu_2}$, and $\xi_i^{\mu_3}$. These other attractors are thus mixtures of three of our desired attractors. Such solutions exist whenever $\beta > 1$, but they are locally stable only when $\beta > 2.17$. Turning the gain up higher still, combinations of greater numbers of the desired memories also become stable. Thus, by keeping the gain between 1 and 2.17, we can limit the attractor set to the desired states.

When p is of the same order as N, the analysis is more involved. The root of the problem is that the different terms in the weight formula in Equation 7 interfere with each other, even for independent random patterns. (The overlap between two patterns is of order $N^{-1/2}$, but as there are of order N such overlaps, the net effect is of order 1.) This cross-talk has three important effects. First, it induces small mismatches, which grow with increasing $\alpha = p/N$, between the original patterns ξ_i^μ and the attractors. Second, and more dramatically, it destroys the pattern-correlated attractors completely above a critical value of α, α_c. This critical value depends on the gain β, and in the limit $\beta \to \infty$, α_c approaches 0.14. Finally, one finds that whenever the gain exceeds $\beta_s = (1 + 2\sqrt{\alpha})^{-1} \leq 1$ there are infinitely many fixed points, all completely uncorrelated with the patterns ξ_i^μ.

Nevertheless, as long as we are not trying to store too many patterns ($\alpha < \alpha_c$), there will be attractors that are strongly correlated with the patterns. The unwanted other attractors can no longer be completely eliminated by suitable tuning of the gain, but as they are uncorrelated with the patterns, they do not have much effect on the retrieval of a pattern, starting from an initial configuration not too far from the attractor.

Thus, attractor computation works in this system over a wide range of model parameters. It can be shown to be robust with respect to many other variations as well. These include dilution (random removal of connections), asymmetry (making some of the $w_{ij} \neq w_{ji}$), and quantization or clipping of the weight values.

Obviously, both this network and the kind of computation it performs are very simple. It is not directly applicable to problems like scene analysis, where several objects, as well as relationships between them, have to be identified and characterized. It is possible to construct more complex networks, with modular and hierarchical structure, to perform such computations, but space does not permit us to treat them here.

A number of other problems, in particular in optimization theory, have been treated using the same strategy of choosing the connections so that the potential energy has minima in the appropriate places (see OPTIMIZATION, NEURAL). The features we have noted in the associative memory problem appear to be universal. It is possible to obtain the desired attractors (at least approximately), but other, undesired attractors are generally also created. These can be controlled in some degree by suitable adjustment of the gain or other parameters.

Learning

The weight formula in Equation 7 was only an educated guess. It is possible to obtain better weights that reduce the cross-talk and increase α_c by employing systematic learning algorithms.

One of the simplest of these is *Boltzmann learning* (see SIMU-LATED ANNEALING AND BOLTZMANN MACHINES and Hertz et al., 1991, chap. 7). Originally, Boltzmann learning was formulated for stochastic binary units. Here we use a formulation for continuous-valued deterministic units. Suppose, as above, that we want to make an attractor of the configuration in which the unit activations are proportional to pattern ξ_i^μ. Now if we start the network in the configuration $V_i = \xi_i^\mu$, it will settle into some fixed point V_i^μ. The algorithm is to change the weights according to

$$\Delta w_{ij} = \eta(\xi_i^\mu \xi_j^\mu - V_i^\mu V_j^\mu) \qquad (11)$$

The first term is a Hebb-like learning term, like Equation 7, and the second term ensures that learning stops when the fixed point V_i^μ coincides with ξ_i^μ. This is then performed for every pattern and repeated until the attractors converge to the desired locations. It is evident from Equation 11 that the resulting connections will be symmetric if the initial ones are. Boltzmann learning can also be used when there are hidden units. In that case, when i or j is a hidden unit, the patterns ξ_i^μ or ξ_j^μ are simply replaced by the stationary values those units take when the nonhidden units are clamped at the pattern values.

In the stochastic Boltzmann machine algorithm, the degree of stochasticity is controlled by a "temperature" parameter T. It corresponds in our deterministic network of continuous-valued units to the degree of softness in the sigmoidal activation function $g(u)$. (For $g(u) = \tanh \beta u$, the parameter β can be identified with $1/T$.) For both kinds of networks, convergence to the fixed point V_i^μ is aided by starting at high T and gradually lowering it. This procedure goes by the name *simulated annealing*.

The other simple learning rule that can be used to learn particular attractors is the delta rule. When there are no hidden units, its weight updating rule is

$$\Delta w_{ij} = \eta(\xi_i^\mu - V_i^\mu)\xi_j^\mu \qquad (12)$$

As in Equation 11, the role of the second or "unlearning" term in the parentheses is to turn learning off when the desired fixed points are achieved. With hidden units, the delta rule becomes what is known as *backpropagation* (see PERCEPTRONS, ADALINES, AND BACKPROPAGATION). There is insufficient space here to go into the mathematical description of backpropagation in recurrent networks (but see RECURRENT NETWORKS: LEARNING ALGORITHMS). We only remark that it is describable as propagating weight adjustments through the original network with all the directions of the connections reversed (see Hertz et al., 1991, chap. 7).

Nonstationary Attractors

So far, we have worked with networks with first-order dynamics (1 or 2) and a symmetric weight matrix. If we relax either of these conditions, non-fixed-point attractors are possible.

It is possible to extend the Hopfield model described above to store pattern sequences, by including suitable delays into the discrete-time dynamics (2). This problem is treated in detail in TEMPORAL SEQUENCES: LEARNING AND GLOBAL ANALYSIS (q.v.). It can be mapped onto the one with static patterns, and much of the analysis for that model can be carried over to the dynamic case. Recent experimental investigations (Markram et al., 1997; Bi and Poo, 1998) have found synaptic changes that depend in sign on the relative timing of pre- and postsynaptic spikes. Such synaptic dynamics could provide a physiological substrate for sequence learning.

In a purely computational context, iterative learning algorithms can also be brought to bear to stabilize specific desired limit cycles. In particular, the recurrent backpropagation algorithm mentioned above for learning fixed points can be extended rather straightfor-

wardly to learning arbitrary time-dependent patterns (see Hertz et al., 1991, chap. 7).

If networks can learn arbitrary periodic attractors, the obvious next question is whether they can learn strange attractors. The answer to this is also affirmative. The initial work on this problem was done by Lapedes and Farber (1987), who succeeded in teaching a network a strange attractor generated by a nonlinear differential-delay equation known as the Mackey-Glass equation, which was originally introduced in a model of blood production.

Discussion: Attractors in the Brain?

Both local (see MOTOR PATTERN GENERATION) and macroscopic neural activity (as in epilepsy; see EEG and MEG ANALYSIS) can be described in terms of non-fixed-point attractors. However, the most interesting questions about attractors in the brain have to do with their functional roles in processes such as perception, recognition, and memory. For example, are particular attractors associated with the recognition of particular objects? Can the settling of the brain's activity into such an attractor be identified with the recognition process?

It has also been suggested (Skarda and Freeman, 1987) that a strange attractor in which the system hops irregularly between two or more regions of configuration space can provide a model for understanding why the brain does not get trapped forever in a fixed-point or limit-cycle attractor.

There is progress toward more biologically realistic modeling of the neural structures that could carry out the kinds of computations we have been discussing (see CORTICAL HEBBIAN MODULES).

Some interesting evidence in favor of attractor computation comes from modeling by Griniasty, Tsodyks, and Amit (1993) of some experiments in which monkeys learn to identify a set of visual patterns. During training, the patterns are presented in a particular order. After learning, the patterns are presented in random order and multicellular recordings are made in a small region of anterior ventral temporal cortex during the period between stimuli. The spatial pattern of the mean firing rates across the electrode array is found to be stimulus specific. The interesting finding is that although the stimuli are not correlated with each other, the resulting firing patterns are. Strong correlations are found only between pairs of activity patterns evoked by stimuli that were close together in the training sequence.

In the theoretical analysis, the firing rate patterns are identified with attractors of the cortical dynamics. They suppose there are pre- and postsynaptic delays in the learning of the patterns, which leads to new terms proportional to $N^{-1}\Sigma_\mu \xi_i^\mu \xi_j^{\mu \pm 1}$ added to the weight formula of Equation 7. This has the consequence that the attractor corresponding to a particular pattern is correlated with those of nearby patterns in the sequence. The form of this correlation can be calculated and is quite similar to that observed in Miyashita's experiments. This result lends credence to both the idea of attractor computation and the Hebbian learning picture.

Another phenomenon in which attractor networks appear to play an important role is working memory. The basic experimental finding is the following. Macaque monkeys perform a match-to-sample task: in each trial the animal sees a sequence of visual patterns, and it must press a bar when the one shown first is repeated. It thus has to keep a memory of the first stimulus during the intervening ones in the sequence. Some neurons in prefrontal (PF) cortex that are selectively sensitive to the first (sample) pattern exhibit continuing activity, above background level, in the entire delay period up to the re-presentation of that pattern, despite the intervening stimuli. Some neurons in inferior temporal (IT) cortex, which provides input to PF, exhibit similarly persistent "delay activity," but this activity is terminated by the presentation of different, intervening stimuli. Thus, these areas seem to be involved in the temporary storage of memories for visual patterns.

Associative memory networks incorporating important features of cortical circuitry and firing dynamics and exhibiting delay activity for learned attractors were developed by Amit and Brunel (1997). Their approach was developed further and applied to the phenomenology described above by Renart, Parga, and Rolls (2000) and Renart et al. (2001), who modeled IT and PF cortices as a pair of coupled associative memory modules. For appropriate coupling between the modules, the initial stimulus leads to an attractor state, associated with the first pattern, that persists in the PF module, even after the stimulus is changed and the state of the IT module is pushed into another attractor by the new (different) stimulus.

Related work by Compte et al. (2000), focusing on PF cortex alone, models experiments on an oculomotor delayed-response task in which a monkey has to remember the location of a visual cue during a delay period of a few seconds before it makes a behavioral response. Although the details of the two groups' models differ, both reproduce the phenomenology of the experiments quite well, lending support to an interpretation in terms of attractor computation.

It is thus evident that the attractor hypothesis at least provides a useful framework within which to address a number of problems in cortical computation, both theoretically and experimentally. It is too soon to know how widely it will be applicable, but it plays a key role in the current interplay of theory and experiment, as we try to build a coherent mathematical framework for cognitive neuroscience.

Road Maps: Dynamic Systems; Grounding Models of Networks
Related Reading: Dynamics and Bifurcation in Neural Nets; Energy Functionals for Neural Networks

References

Amit, D. J., and Brunel, N., 1997, Model of global spontaneous activity and local structured activity during delay periods in the cerebral cortex, *Cerebral Cortex*, 7:237–252.

Bi, G. Q., and Poo, M. M., 1998, Synaptic modifications in cultured hippocampal neurons: Dependence on spike timing, synaptic strength, and postsynaptic cell type, *J. Neurosci.*, 18:10464–10472.

Compte, A., Brunel, N., Goldman-Rakic, P. S., and Wang, X-J., 2000, Synaptic mechanisms and network dynamics underlying spatial working memory in a cortical network model, *Cerebral Cortex*, 10:910–923.

Cohen, M., and Grossberg, S., 1983, Absolute stability of global pattern formation and parallel memory storage by competitive neural networks, *IEEE Trans. Syst. Man Cybern.*, 13:815–826.

Griniasty, M., Tsodyks, M. V., and Amit, D. J., 1993, Conversion of temporal correlations between stimuli to spatial correlations between attractors, *Neural Computat.*, 5:1–17.

Hebb, D. O., 1949, *The Organization of Behavior*, New York: Wiley. ◆

Hertz, J. A., Krogh, A. S., and Palmer, R. G., 1991, *Introduction to the Theory of Neural Computation*, Redwood City, CA: Addison-Wesley. ◆

Hopfield, J. J., 1984, Neurons with graded responses have collective computational properties like those of two-state neurons, *Proc. Natl. Acad. Sci. USA*, 79:3088–3092.

Kühn, R., Bös, S., and van Hemmen, L., 1991, Statistical mechanics of graded-response neurons, *Phys. Rev. A*, 43:2084–2087.

Lapedes, A., and Farber, R., 1987, Nonlinear Signal Processing Using Neural Networks: Prediction and Signal Modelling, Technical Report LA-UR-87-2662, Los Alamos, NM: Los Alamos National Laboratory.

Markram, H., Lubke, J., Frotscher, M., and Sakmann, B., 1997, Regulation of synaptic efficacy by coincidence of postsynaptic APs and EPSPs, *Science*, 275:213–215.

Renart, A., Moreno, R., de la Rocha, J., Parga, N., and Rolls, E. T., 2001, A model of the IT-PF network in object working memory which includes balanced persistent activity and tuned inhibition, *Neurocomputing*, 38–40:1525–1531.

Renart, A., Parga, N., and Rolls, E. T., 2000, A recurrent model of the interaction between prefrontal and inferotemporal cortex in delay tasks, *Adv. Neural Inform. Proc. Syst.*, 12:171–177.

Skarda, C. A., and Freeman, W. J., 1987, How brains make chaos in order to make sense of the world, *Behav. Brain Sci.*, 10:161–195.

Schuster, H. G., 1989, *Deterministic Chaos*, 2nd ed., Weinheim, Germany: VCH Verlagsgesellschaft. ◆

Concept Learning

Thomas J. Palmeri and David C. Noelle

Introduction

Concepts are mental representations of kinds of objects, events, or ideas. We have concepts because they allow us to see something as a kind of thing rather than just as a unique individual. Concepts allow generalization from past experiences: By treating something as a kind—as an instantiation of some concept—as a member of some category—we can use what we have learned from other examples of that kind. Concepts permit inferences: Deciding predator from prey, edible from inedible, friend from enemy involves concepts. Concepts facilitate communication: Describing something as a kind of thing may obviate the need to provide details of the thing itself. Concepts permit different levels of abstraction: We know the difference between objects and ideas, animals and plants, dogs and cats, and terriers and collies. Concepts bring cognitive economy: What we learn about animals generally can be applied to specific animals without needless replication of that knowledge throughout our conceptual hierarchy. Concepts are fundamental building blocks of human knowledge (see Margolis and Laurence, 1999).

The focus of this article is on learning mental representations of new concepts from experience. We will also address how we use mental representations of concepts to make categorization decisions and other kinds of judgments.

Overview of Concept Learning Models

One goal of model development is to test specific hypotheses regarding the kinds of representations created during learning and the kinds of processes used to act upon those representations to make decisions. In order to develop a formal model of concept learning, a modeler must specify what perceptual information is provided by the sensory system, how that information is represented, how that information is compared with what has been learned about a concept, how this previously learned knowledge is represented in memory, and how decisions are made based on comparing perceptual information with stored conceptual representations (see PATTERN RECOGNITION).

A tacit assumption of many models of concept learning is that the perceptual system extracts information from the environment, passing a perceptual representation on to a conceptual stage of processing, which in turn generates an action. In the parlance of neural networks, the perceptual system provides the inputs to the network, the association weights and activation functions encode the conceptual representations, and decision processes use the outputs to generate a response. Most concept learning models characterize the perceptual system as a dimensionality reduction device (see OBJECT RECOGNITION and OBJECT STRUCTURE, VISUAL PROCESSING). For example, in the case of vision, the input on the retina is an extremely high-dimensional representation, with every photoreceptor effectively encoding an independent dimension of sensation. The perceptual system creates a relatively low-dimensional representation by recoding the retinal input in terms of a smaller number of features or dimensions. These vectors of features or dimensions serve as the inputs to the concept learning network.

The distinction between features and dimensions is fully discussed elsewhere (e.g., Tversky, 1977). The members of a category—the extension of a concept—may be seen as clusters of perceptual vectors in a psychological space. An important type of concept learning entails associating regions in that space with particular category labels.

A *featural representation* in a neural network essentially consists of a vector of input nodes encoding the presence or absence of primitive elements. Similar stimuli share many common features. Dissimilar stimuli correspond to uncorrelated vectors. Often in simulation modeling, feature representations have no direct relationship to the actual stimuli of an experiment, but are instead designed to capture the statistical relationships among stimuli.

A *dimensional representation* is not discrete, but represents information in terms of values along continuously varying psychological dimensions. Similar stimuli have similar values along the dimensions, occupying adjacent locations in psychological space. Often in simulation modeling, dimensional representations may be derived from physical properties of actual stimuli or may be derived from similarity ratings (or other measures of psychological proximity) made by subjects using techniques such as multidimensional scaling (although feature representations can be derived as well).

The core of this article reviews models of how concepts are learned and represented in neural networks. One important distinction between models is whether concepts have LOCALIZED VERSUS DISTRIBUTED REPRESENTATIONS (q.v.). Another is whether conceptual knowledge relies on abstractions, such as rules or prototypes, or relies on specific exemplar knowledge. Most models focus on supervised learning, where trial-by-trial feedback is supplied, but some models address unsupervised learning. Most models focus on how concepts are learned within a category learning paradigm, whereby subjects learn to produce the correct label for each stimulus, but some models address how subjects can learn to infer properties other than the category label. Most models focus on

learning from induction over examples, but some address learning from instruction or from explanation as well.

Concept Learning Models

Rule Models

Early philosophers conjectured that all concepts were decomposable into necessary and sufficient conditions for membership (e.g., Plato in Margolis and Laurence [1999]). A "triangle" is a closed form with three sides, a "bachelor" is an unmarried adult male, and so forth. Conceptual rules are like carefully worded definitions provided to a student. Indeed, a strength of this hypothesis is the apparent alignment of mental representations with self-reports of conceptual knowledge. Generally, to be considered a rule, a concise definition is required—if arbitrarily complex rules are allowed, the rule hypothesis becomes vacuous, because virtually any representation can be characterized by complex rules. Therefore, rule representations typically include just a small set of dimensions—sometimes only a single dimension. Although this may seem overly restrictive, humans frequently exhibit reliance on individual dimensions during concept learning (Nosofsky, Palmeri, and McKinley, 1994).

Simple neural network units may be connected to compute logical functions (see NEURAL AUTOMATA AND ANALOG COMPUTATIONAL COMPLEXITY). A rule involving a threshold along a single dimension is the simplest example, and serves as the basis for rules in some concept learning models (e.g., Ashby et al., 1998; Erickson and Kruschke, 1998). Assuming a dimensional input representation, a single-dimension rule simply involves a learned weighted connection w_{ij} from input node a_i to output unit o_j with learned bias θ_j

$$o_j = \frac{1}{[1 + \exp(-w_{ij}a_i - \theta_j)]} \tag{1}$$

The sigmoidal activation of this unit is proportional to the likelihood of category membership. A network of this kind essentially implements a linear decision boundary in psychological space, with the boundary orthogonal to one of the psychological dimensions, and with the position of the boundary specified by the learned bias θ_j (see Figure 1A).

Prototype Models

Although people often report conceptual knowledge in terms of rules, there are reasons to question rules as the universal basis for conceptual knowledge. Many common concepts are difficult to de-

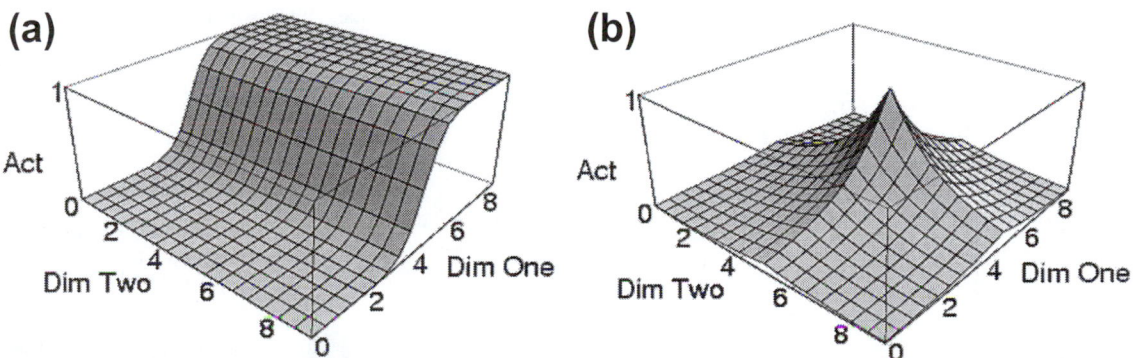

Figure 1. Examples of activation (Act) as a function of location in a two-dimensional psychological space (Dim One × Dim Two) for (a), the logistic sigmoidal function in Equations 1–3 and for (b), the radial-basis function in Equation 4.

fine using rules—Wittgenstein suggested the example of "games" as appearing to defy definition (see Margolis and Laurence, 1999). Instead, concepts seem to possess "family resemblances," with instances bearing many similarities but no characteristics common to all members. Human performance often belies the existence of rules in that some items appear to be "better" members than others in terms of typicality ratings, speed of processing, and inductive power.

Such findings led to an alternative view of conceptual knowledge based on abstract prototypes (see Rosch and also Lakoff in Margolis and Laurence, 1999). A prototype need never be directly experienced, but can be formed by averaging across observed instances. In psychological space, the prototype is the centroid of a cloud of instances. New items are classified according to their relative similarity to learned prototypes, with typicality effects emerging from this process. Learning just two prototypes effectively partitions psychological space into two regions separated by a linear boundary, but this boundary is a fuzzy (probabilistic) one and is unconstrained in terms of its orientation within psychological space.

A simple two-layer prototype model assumes an input layer of features (or dimensions) with learned associations to category output nodes. Each output unit o_j corresponds to a single concept prototype, and the weights w_{ij} from inputs a_i to each o_j reflects the strength of association of particular stimulus features with that concept:

$$o_j = \frac{1}{\left[1 + \exp\left(-\sum_i w_{ij} a_i - \theta_j \right) \right]} \quad (2)$$

The probability $P(j)$ of categorizing a stimulus as a member of category j can simply be given by the relative activation of node j compared to all other nodes. Other more dynamic mechanisms, such as lateral inhibition, can also introduce competition between concepts in WINNER-TAKE-ALL NETWORKS (q.v.).

This simple network learns to associate input stimuli with their corresponding categories. A related approach is to train ASSOCIATIVE NETWORKS (q.v.) to reproduce the features of each training instance as well as the correct category label (e.g., McClelland and Rumelhart, 1985). This pattern completion approach permits the network to not only categorize stimuli, but also to infer other missing features as well. More powerful pattern completion arises when COMPUTING WITH ATTRACTORS (q.v.) such as in the Brain State in a Box model (see ASSOCIATIVE NETWORKS). Recurrent connections between all category label units and all feature units permit the network to encode soft constraints guiding how activation settles over time. In addition to their pattern completion properties, learned basins of attraction in such networks can instantiate nonlinear decision boundaries between categories, potentially creating

a kind of prototype model that incorporates information about both the mean and the variability of a distribution of category exemplars.

Exemplar Models

Simple concept learning networks of the sort just described can learn category structures (a) and (b) depicted in Figure 2—linearly separable categories—but cannot learn category structure (c)—nonlinearly separable categories. This is the classic XOR problem that stymied early developments in neural networks (see PERCEPTRONS, ADALINES, AND BACKPROPAGATION). In contrast, multilayered networks with an input layer, a hidden layer, and an output layer can learn these category structures. Activation of hidden and output nodes is determined by a nonlinear sigmoid function like that shown in Equation 2. Learning takes place via gradient descent on error, with knowledge fully distributed throughout the network connections (see BACKPROPAGATION: GENERAL PRINCIPLES). These "backpropagation networks" are powerful learning devices and, with sufficient hidden nodes, they can acquire concepts of nearly unlimited complexity.

Psychological models of concept learning attempt to model human behavior, with all its errors and apparent inefficiencies. Although backpropagation networks are powerful machine learning devices, they make relatively poor models of human concept learning. For one, backpropagation networks are insensitive to the psychological dimensional structure within the categories. From a statistical standpoint, structure (a) and structure (b) in Figure 2 have equivalent complexity, so backpropagation networks learn both types equally quickly. But people find structure (a) far easier to learn than structure (b) because structure (a) permits attending to a single dimension. Backpropagation networks generally learn linearly separable categories, such as structure (b), far more quickly than nonlinearly separable categories, such as structure (c). By contrast, people find structure (c) easier to learn. More generally, people are not constrained by linear separability, and often exhibit more rapid learning of nonlinearly separable than linearly separable categories. Finally, backpropagation networks suffer from catastrophic forgetting in which new concept learning overwrites previous concept learning. There have been many modifications to simple backpropagation networks to combat this problem. Common to many approaches is the use of semilocalized representations instead of fully distributed representations (see LOCALIZED VERSUS DISTRIBUTED REPRESENTATIONS).

Exemplar-based models assume local representations (see Smith and Medin in Margolis and Laurence, 1999). In contrast to rule and prototype models, concepts are represented extensionally, in terms of specific category instances. A number of variations of exemplar models have been proposed, and a vast set of empirical phenomena is consistent with them (Nosofsky and Kruschke, 1992). Perhaps the best-known neural network exemplar model is ALCOVE (Kruschke, 1992), which is largely derived from the gen-

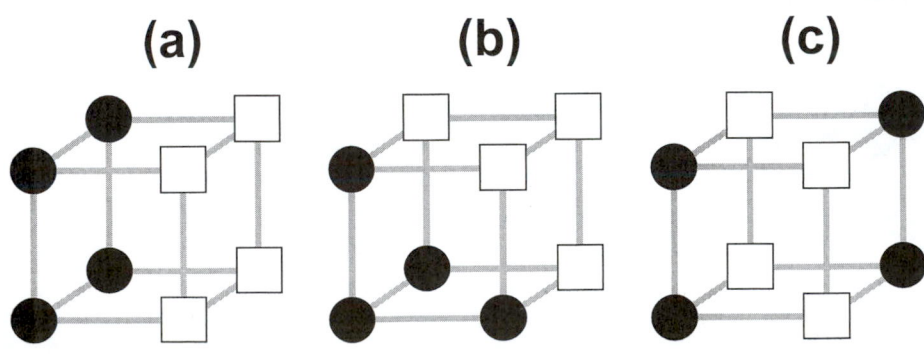

Figure 2. Depictions of three category structures. Individual stimuli are composed of three binary-valued dimensions. The dimensional values of a stimulus are specified by its location in the three-dimensional psychological space. For each structure, black circles represent stimuli in one category and white squares represent stimuli in another category.

eralized context model of categorization (Nosofsky, 1986), but incorporates error-driven learning.

ALCOVE is a three-layered feedforward network in which activation passes from a dimensional input layer, with each dimension scaled by a learned selective attention weight, to an exemplar-based hidden layer, to a category output layer via learned association weights. In contrast to backpropagation networks (compare Figures 1(a) and 1(b)), activation h_j of hidden exemplar node j is based on its similarity to the input stimulus

$$h_j = \exp\left[-c\left(\sum_i \alpha_i |e_{ji} - a_i|^r\right)^{1/r}\right] \quad (3)$$

where a_i is the value of the input stimulus along dimension i, e_{ji} is the value of exemplar j along dimension i, α_i is the learned attention to dimension i, c is a similarity scaling parameter, and r determines the psychological distance metric (see also RADIAL BASIS FUNCTION NETWORKS). When optimally allocated, selective attention weights emphasize differences along diagnostic dimensions and deemphasize differences along nondiagnostic dimensions (Nosofsky, 1986).

ALCOVE also learns to associate exemplars with category outputs. Activation of category output node k is given by

$$o_k = \sum_j w_{kj} h_j \quad (4)$$

where w_{kj} is the learned association weight between exemplar j and output node k. The probability of categorizing the input stimulus as a member of category K is given by

$$P(K) = \frac{\exp(\varphi o_K)}{\sum_k \exp(\varphi o_k)} \quad (5)$$

where φ is a response mapping parameter. Attention weights (α_i) and association weights (w_{kj}) are learned by gradient descent on error.

Although exemplar models like ALCOVE have accounted for a wide variety of fundamental categorization phenomena (Nosofsky and Kruschke, 1992), until recently they have ignored the time-course of making a categorization decision. One avenue of recent theoretical development has addressed the time-course of the accumulation of perceptual evidence used to categorize a stimulus (Lamberts, 2000), modeling how perceptual processes make some information available sooner than others. Another avenue of development has examined the time-course of making categorization decisions. Nosofsky and Palmeri (1997) proposed a stochastic exemplar-retrieval model with a competitive decision process to account for both categorization response probabilities and response times. Although this theoretical development was formalized using mathematical modeling tools, such as a random walk decision process, the dynamics of these stochastic, competitive categorization models could be implemented in various neural network architectures as well.

Mixed Models

Exemplar models have been shown to account for a variety of results, including some that were originally thought to unequivocally indicate rules or prototypes as concept representations. Yet, there seems to be some emerging evidence that people do use abstractions, particularly abstract rules, as concept representations. Clearly, people can be instructed to use rules before they have experienced any examples (Palmeri, 1997; Noelle, Cottrell, and McKinley, 2002). Also, it appears that people may approach the task of learning categories by testing simple categorization rules (e.g., Nosofsky et al., 1994), although people may eventually shift to using exemplars with experience (Johansen and Palmeri, in press). One important focus of current research is developing and testing formal models with mixed representations. At one extreme are models that posit functionally independent rule-based and exemplar-based systems that race to completion (e.g., Palmeri, 1997); exemplar-based representations gain strength with repeated exemplar experience and eventually win the race. Alternatively, rule and exemplar representations may be functionally independent, but the outputs of these systems may compete based on strength of evidence rather than completion time (e.g., Ashby et al., 1998). Erickson and Kruschke (1998) proposed a neural network model (ATRIUM) with separate rule and exemplar representations that compete, with the model learning whether rule-based or exemplar-based information should be used to categorize a particular instance. Finally, other architectures have proposed combinations of rules, exemplars, and perhaps other representations within a single representational medium.

Neuroscientific Models

Neurobiological findings have begun to constrain concept learning models by ruling out mechanisms that resist reasonable neural implementation. Some recent models have included hypotheses concerning how conceptual knowledge is instantiated in the brain.

COVIS is one example of a model grounded in neurophysiology (Ashby et al., 1998). COVIS is a mixed representational model, incorporating implicit decision boundaries and explicit unidimensional rules. The implicit learning system, assumed to reside within the striatum, encodes a category decision boundary (although other representations—such as exemplar-like coarse-coded topological maps of psychological space with regions associated with category labels—also fits within this general framework). Verbal rule processing is assumed to exist in the prefrontal cortex, with the selection of rule-attended dimensions handled by a reinforcement learning process in the anterior cingulate, mediated by projections from the basal ganglia. Given a stimulus, the implicit and rule-based systems compete to provide a category response. This model has been applied to concept learning deficits seen in the very old and the very young, in patients with Parkinson's disease and Huntington's disease, in clinically depressed patients, in individuals with focal brain lesions, and in nonhuman animals.

Other neurally oriented concept learning models have focused on the role of prefrontal cortex in representing and actively maintaining rule-based information during categorization (Noelle et al., 2002; O'Reilly et al., 2002). A distinguishing feature of these models is the use of signals that encode changes in expected future reward (see REINFORCEMENT LEARNING)—emanating from the basal ganglia dopamine system (see DOPAMINE, ROLES OF)—to determine when a useful rule representation has been found and should be gated into a prefrontal working memory system. Like COVIS, these dopamine-gating models incorporate a mixed representation, integrating rules with a kind of procedural knowledge. Unlike COVIS, these models focus on procedural knowledge embedded in multilayer networks, presumably located within the cortex, rather than on a special implicit learning system within the striatum. Rule representations, stored as patterns of activity in a prefrontal attractor network (see COMPUTING WITH ATTRACTORS), do not directly compete with these procedural systems, but rather modulate them through the injection of activity. Models of this kind have provided explanations for frontal lesion data, suggested a coarse topological organization for prefrontal cortex, captured patterns of performance on dynamic classification tasks, explained interference effects in instructed category learning, and illuminated learning deficits in schizophrenia.

Discussion

In this article, we limited our discussion to the kinds of representations and processes that subserve a particular aspect of concept learning, namely learning to categorize. Recent work has investigated other topics, as well, including how people learn to infer properties other than the category label and how learning about categories may influence perceptual processing in a top-down manner (e.g., Schyns, Goldstone, and Thibaut, 1998).

An important focus of current research was outlined in this article: Do people use different kinds of concept representations, how are those representations learned, and is the dominance of particular representations modulated by experience or other task demands? In order to help answer these questions, and in order to develop neurally plausible models of concept learning, some researchers are beginning to incorporate the constraints imposed by various neuroscientific sources of evidence, including studies of patients with focal brain damage, functional imaging and evoked potential studies, and single unit recordings in animals.

Road Map: Psychology
Related Reading: Feature Analysis; Object Recognition; Pattern Recognition

References

Ashby, F. G., Alfonso-Reese, L. A., Turken, A. U., and Waldron, E. M., 1998, A formal neuropsychological theory of multiple systems in category learning, *Psychol. Rev.*, 105:442–481.

Erickson, M. A., and Kruschke, J. K., 1998, Rules and exemplars in category learning, *J. Exp. Psychol.*, 127:107–140.

Johansen, M. K., and Palmeri, T. J., (in press), Are there representational shifts during category learning? *Cognitive Psychology*.

Kruschke, J. K., 1992, ALCOVE: An exemplar-based connectionist model of category learning, *Psychol. Rev.*, 99:22–44.

Lamberts, K., 2000, Information-accumulation theory of speeded categorization, *Psychol. Rev.*, 107:227–260.

Margolis, E., and Laurence, S., 1999, *Concepts: Core Readings*, Cambridge, MA: MIT Press. ◆

McClelland, J. L., and Rumelhart, D. E., 1985, Distributed memory and the representation of general and specific information, *J. Exp. Psychol.*, 114:159–188.

Noelle, D. C., Cottrell, G. W., and McKinley, C. R. M., 2002, Modeling individual differences in the specialization of an explicit rule, Manuscript under review.

Nosofsky, R. M., 1986, Attention, similarity, and the identification-categorization relationship, *J. Exp. Psychol.*, 115:39–57.

Nosofsky, R. M., and Kruschke, J. K., 1992, Investigations of an exemplar-based connectionist model of category learning, in *The Psychology of Learning and Motivation*, vol. 28 (D. L. Medin, Ed.), San Diego, CA: Academic Press, pp. 207–250. ◆

Nosofsky, R. M., and Palmeri, T. J., 1997, An exemplar-based random walk model of speeded classification, *Psychol. Rev.*, 104:266–300.

Nosofsky, R. M., Palmeri, T. J., and McKinley, S. C., 1994, Rule-plus-exception model of classification learning, *Psychol. Rev.*, 101:53–79.

O'Reilly, R. C., Noelle, D. C., Braver, T. S., and Cohen, J. D., 2002, Prefrontal cortex and dynamic categorization tasks: Representational organization and neuromodulatory control, *Cerebral Cortex*, 12:246–257.

Palmeri, T. J., 1997, Exemplar similarity and the development of automaticity, *J. Exp. Psychol.*, 23:324–354.

Schyns, P. G., Goldstone, R. L., and Thibaut, J. P., 1998, The development of features in object concepts, *Behav. Brain Sci.*, 21:1–40. ◆

Tversky, A., 1977, Features of Similarity, *Psychology Review*, 84:327–352.

Conditioning

Nestor A. Schmajuk

Introduction

During conditioning, animals modify their behavior as a consequence of their experience of the contingencies between environmental events. This article delineates several formal theories and neural network models that have been proposed to describe classical and operant conditioning. Other important theories, omitted here owing to space limitations, are described by Schmajuk (1997).

Classical Conditioning

During classical conditioning, animals change their behavior as a result of the contingencies between the conditioned stimulus (CS) and the unconditioned stimulus (US). Contingencies may vary from very simple to extremely complex ones. For example, in Pavlov's famous experiment, dogs were exposed to the sound of a bell, the CS, followed by food, the US. At the beginning of training, animals only generated unconditioned responses (UR), salivation, when the US was presented. With an increasing number of CS-US pairings, CS presentations elicited a conditioned response (CR). In general, a CR is analogous to the UR (dogs salivate in response to the bell), CR onset precedes the US onset (salivation precedes food presentation), and the peak CR amplitude tends to be located around the time of the occurrence of the US. When acquisition is followed by presentations of CS alone, the CR extinguishes.

Different CS-US interstimulus intervals (ISI) may be employed. Conditioning is negligible with short ISIs, increases dramatically at an optimal ISI that depends on the response being conditioned, and gradually decreases with increasing ISIs.

Second-order conditioning consists of a first phase in which CS_1 is paired with the US. In a second phase, CS_1 and CS_2 are paired together in the absence of the US. Finally, when CS_2 is presented alone, it generates a CR. Sensory preconditioning consists of a first phase in which two CSs, CS_1 and CS_2, are paired together in the absence of the US. In a second phase, CS_1 is paired with the US. Finally, when CS_2 is presented alone, it generates a CR.

In latent inhibition, pre-exposure to CS retards the acquisition of CS-US associations. Latent inhibition is characterized by a large number of properties. In blocking, an animal is first conditioned to CS_1, and this training is followed by conditioning to a compound consisting of CS_1 and a second stimulus, CS_2. This procedure results in a weaker conditioning to CS_2 than would be attained if paired separately with the US. In overshadowing, an animal is conditioned to a compound consisting of CS_1 and CS_2. This procedure results in weaker conditioning to each CS than it would achieve if it was independently trained.

In conditioned inhibition, CS_2 acquires inhibitory conditioning following CS_1 reinforced trials interspersed with CS_1-CS_2 nonreinforced trials. In contrast to excitatory conditioning, presentations of CS_2 alone do not extinguish inhibitory conditioning.

In compound conditioning, two or more stimuli are presented together in the presence of the US. In a feature-positive discrimination, animals receive reinforced simultaneous compound presentations (CS_1 overlapping with CS_2) alternated with nonreinforced presentations of CS_2. Animals learn to respond to CS_1 but not to CS_2. In an occasion-setting paradigm, animals receive reinforced serial compound presentations (CS_1 preceding CS_2) alternated with nonreinforced presentations of CS_2. Animals learn to respond to the CS_1-CS_2 compound but not to CS_1 or CS_2. In negative patterning, presentations of a reinforced component (CS_1 or CS_2) are intermixed with nonreinforced compound (CS_1-CS_2) presentations. Negative patterning is attained if the response to the compound is smaller than the sum of the responses to the components. In positive patterning, reinforced compound (CS_1-CS_2) presentations are intermixed with nonreinforced component (CS_1 or CS_2) presentations. Positive patterning is attained if the response to the compound is larger than the sum of the responses to the components.

Associations, Predictions, and Connections

Modern learning theories assume that the association between events CS_i and CS_k, $V_{i,k}$, represents the *prediction* that CS_i will be followed by CS_k. Neural network or connectionist theories frequently assume that the association between CS_i and CS_k is represented by the efficacy of the synapses, $V_{i,k}$, that connect a presynaptic neural population excited by CS_i with a postsynaptic neural population that is excited by CS_k (event k might be another CS or the US). When CS_k is the US, this second population controls the generation of the CR. At the beginning of training, synaptic strength $V_{i,US}$ is small, and therefore, CS_i is incapable of exciting the second neural population and generating a CR. As training progresses, synaptic strengths gradually increase, and CS_i comes to generate a CR.

Although some models of conditioning describe changes in $V_{i,k}$ on a trial-to-trial basis, real-time networks describe the unbroken, continuous temporal dynamics of $V_{i,k}$. In general, real-time neural networks assume that CS_i gives rise to a trace, $\tau_i(t)[d(\tau_i)/dt = K_1(CS_i - \tau_i)]$, in the central nervous system that increases over time to a maximum and then gradually decays to zero. The increment in $V_{i,k}$ is a function of the intensity of the CS_i trace at the time the US is presented.

Changes in synaptic strength $V_{i,k}$ might be described by $\Delta V_{i,k} = f(CS_i)f(CS_k)$, where $f(CS_i)$ represents the presynaptic activity and $f(CS_k)$ the postsynaptic activity. Different $f(CS_i)$ and $f(CS_k)$ functions have been proposed. Learning rules for $V_{i,k}$ either assume variations in the effectiveness of CS_i, $f(CS_i)$, the US, $f(CS_k)$, or both. The following sections describe how different types of models deal with the many experimental results presented before.

Variations in the Effectiveness of the CS: Attentional Models

Attentional theories assume that the formation of CS_i-US associations depend on the magnitude of an internal representation of CS_i, $f(CS_i)$. In neural network terms, attention may be interpreted as the modulation of the CS representation that activates the presynaptic neuronal population involved in associative learning. When focused on a particular CS, selective attention enhances the internal representation of that specific CS.

Mackintosh's (1975) attentional theory suggests that CS_i associability, $f(CS_i)$, increases when CS_i is the best predictor of (the CS most strongly associated with) the US and decreases otherwise. Mackintosh's model describes latent inhibition, overshadowing, and blocking. In contrast to Mackintosh's (1975) view, Pearce and Hall (1980) suggested that $f(CS_i)$ increases when CS_i is a poor predictor of the US, $f(CS_i) = |US - \Sigma_j V_{j,US}CS_j|$, where $\Sigma_j V_{j,US}CS_j$ represents the aggregate prediction of the US computed on all CSs present at a given moment. In addition to latent inhibition, blocking, and overshadowing, the Pearce and Hall model correctly predicts that latent inhibition might be obtained after training with a weak US. According to Grossberg's (1975) neural attentional theory, pairing of CS_i with a US causes both an association of $f(CS_i)$ with the US and an association of the US with $f(CS_i)$. Sensory representations $f(CS_i)$ compete among themselves for a limited-capacity short-term memory activation that is reflected in CS_i-US associations.

Variations in the Effectiveness of the US: Simple and Generalized Delta Rules

A popular rule, proposed independently in psychological (Rescorla and Wagner, 1972) and neural network (see PERCEPTRONS, ADALINES, AND BACKPROPAGATION for the Widrow-Hoff rule) domains, has been termed the delta rule. The delta rule describes changes in the synaptic connections between the two neural populations by way of minimizing the squared value of the difference between the output of the population controlling the CR generation and the US. According to the "simple" delta rule, CS_i-US associations are changed until $f(US) = US - \Sigma_j V_{j,US}CS_j$ is zero. In neural network terms, $f(US)$ can be construed as the modulation of the US signal that activates the postsynaptic neural population involved in associative learning. Rescorla and Wagner showed that the model describes acquisition, extinction, conditioned inhibition, blocking, and overshadowing.

Sutton and Barto (1981) presented a temporally refined version of the Rescorla-Wagner model. In the model, the effectiveness of CS_i is given by the temporal trace $\tau_i = f(CS_i(t)) = Af(CS_i(t)) + BCS_i(t)$, which does not change over trials. The effectiveness of the US changes over trials according to $f(US(t)) = (y(t) - y'(t))$, where the output of the model is $y(t) = f[\Sigma_j V_{j,US}f(CS_j) + f(US)]$, $f(US)$ is the temporal trace of the US, and $y'(t) = Cy'(t) - (1 - C)y(t)$. Computer simulations show that the model correctly describes acquisition, extinction, conditioned inhibition, blocking, overshadowing, primacy effects, and second-order conditioning. In 1990 the authors proposed a new rendering of the Sutton and Barto (1981) model, designated the temporal difference model, in which $f(US) = (US + \gamma y'(t + 1) - y'(t))$. The temporal difference model correctly describes ISI effects, serial-compound conditioning, no extinction of conditioned inhibition, second-order conditioning, and primacy effects.

Kehoe (1988) presented a network that incorporates a hidden-unit layer trained according to a delta rule. In addition to the paradigms described by the Rescorla-Wagner model, the network describes stimulus configuration, learning to learn, savings effects, and positive and negative patterning.

Schmajuk and DiCarlo (1992) introduced a model that, by employing a generalized delta rule (also known as backpropagation; see PERCEPTRONS, ADALINES, AND BACKPROPAGATION) to train a layer of hidden units that configure simple CSs, is able to solve negative and positive patterning. Interestingly, this biologically plausible, real-time rendition of backpropagation differs from the original version in that the error signal that is used to train hidden units, instead of including the derivative of the activation function of the hidden units, simply contains their activation function. Figure 1 shows real-time simulations on trials 1, 4, 8, 12, 16, and 20 in a delay-conditioning paradigm with a 200-ms CS, a 50-ms US, and a 150-ms ISI. As CR amplitude increases over trials, output weights VS_i and VN_j and hidden weights VH_{ij} may increase or decrease.

The network provides correct descriptions of acquisition of delay and trace conditioning, extinction, acquisition-extinction series, blocking, overshadowing, discrimination acquisition and reversal, compound conditioning, feature-positive discrimination, conditioned inhibition, negative patterning, positive patterning, and generalization.

Gluck and Myers (1993) presented a network that also trains a hidden layer through a backpropagation procedure. The authors assume three three-layer networks that work in parallel. The output and hidden layers of one of the networks are trained to associate CS inputs with those same CS inputs and the US. The output layers

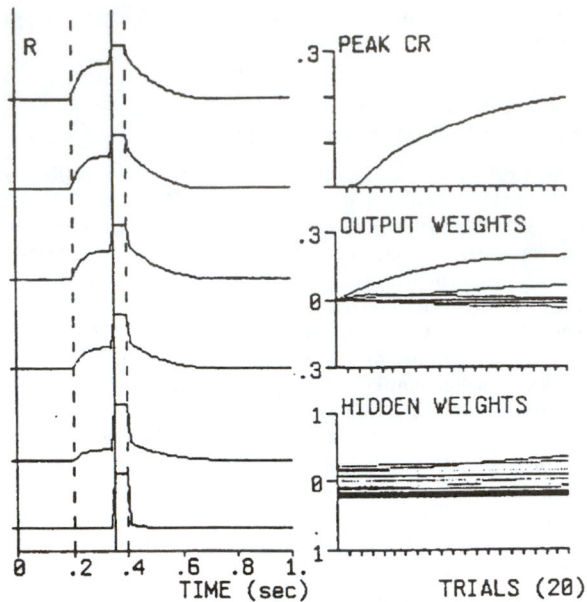

Figure 1. Acquisition of classical conditioning. *Left*, Real-time simulated conditioned and unconditioned response on trials 1, 4, 8, 12, 16, and 20. Vertical dashed lines indicate CS onset and offset. Vertical solid line indicates US onset. Trial 1 is represented at the bottom of the panel. *Right*, Peak CR: Peak CR as a function of trials. Output weights: Average VSs and VNs as a function of trials. Hidden weights: Average VHs as a function of trials. (After Schmajuk and DiCarlo, 1992.)

of the other two networks are also trained by the US, but their hidden units are trained by the hidden units of the first network.

Variations in the Effectiveness of Both the CS and the US

To account for a wider range of classical conditioning paradigms, some theories have combined variations in the effectiveness of both the CS and the US. For example, Wagner (1978) suggested that CS_i-US associations are determined by (1) $f(US) = (US - \Sigma_j V_{j,US} CS_j)$ as in the Rescorla-Wagner model, and (2) $f(CS_i) = (CS_i - V_{i,CX} CX)$, where CX represents the context and V_{iCX} the strength of the CX-CS_i association.

Schmajuk, Lam, and Gray (1996) introduced a theory that assumes that $f(CS_i)$ is modulated by the association of the internal representation of CS_i with the total environmental novelty, z_i. Total environmental novelty is given by $\Sigma_j |\bar{\lambda} - \bar{B}_j|$, that is, the sum of the absolute values of the differences of the average predicted and the average observed event j. Schmajuk et al. (1996) showed that the model correctly describes most of the properties of latent inhibition.

Buhusi and Schmajuk (1996) showed that when combined with the Schmajuk and DiCarlo (1992) model (see Figure 2), the Schmajuk et al. (1996) approach can describe a wide variety of classical conditioning data; see the figure caption for details.

Multiple Representations of the CS: Timing

The fact that the peak CR amplitude tends to be located around the time of the occurrence of the US suggests that animals learn about the temporal relationship between the CS and the US. Grossberg

and Schmajuk (1989) proposed a neural network (called the spectral timing model) that is capable of learning the temporal relationships between the CS and the US. The model consists of three layers of neural elements. A step function, activated by the CS presentation, excites the first layer that contains many elements, each one having a different reaction time. The output of each element in the first layer is a sigmoid function that activates a second layer of habituating transmitter gates. In turn, the output of each transmitter gate activates a $f(CS_i)$ element. Those $f(CS_i)$ elements active at the time of the US presentation become associated with the US in proportion to their activity. All $f(CS_i)$ elements activate their corresponding $V_{i,US}$ weights and are added to generate the CR. During testing, the CR shows a peak at the time when the $f(CS_i)$ elements that have been active simultaneously with the US are active again. The model is able to describe ISI curves with single and multiple USs and a Weber's law for temporal generalization. Grossberg and Schmajuk (1989) showed that the model can explain the effects of increasing CS and US intensity, an inverted U in learning as a function of ISI, multiple timing peaks, effect of increasing US duration, and the effect of drugs on timed motor behavior.

Church and Broadbent (1991) presented a connectionist version of Church's scalar timing theory. The model consists of the following components: (1) a pacemaker that emits pulses, (2) a switch that is opened at the onset of the event to be timed and closed at its offset, (3) a counter that accumulates pulses, (4) a reference memory that accumulates pulses of reinforced times and a working memory that stores the total number of pulses accumulated in a particular trial, and (5) a comparator that compares the values stored in both memories. Values stored in working memory are compared to values stored in reference memory, and if they are similar, a response is produced. Notice that the number of stored pulses increases with the measured time. The model is able to describe timing with single but not with multiple USs and describes a Weber's law for temporal generalization.

Operant Conditioning

During operant (or instrumental) conditioning, animals change their behavior as a result of a triple contingency between its responses (R), discriminative stimuli (S_D), and the reinforcer (US). Animals are exposed to the US in a relatively close temporal relationship with the S_D and R. As they experience the S_D-R-US contingency, animals emit R when S_D is presented.

Four classes of S_D-R-US contingencies are possible: (1) positive reinforcement, in which R is followed by the presence of an appetitive US; (2) punishment, in which R is followed by the presence of an aversive US; (3) omission, in which R is followed by the absence of an appetitive US; and (4) negative reinforcement (escape and avoidance), in which R is followed by the absence of an aversive US. As in reinforcement learning (see REINFORCEMENT LEARNING), during operant conditioning, animals learn by trial and error from feedback that evaluates their behavior but does not indicate the correct behavior.

Positive Reinforcement

Operant conditioning can be obtained with free operant procedures, in which the operant response may occur repeatedly. Free operant paradigms are usually run in a Skinner box. In such a box, rats learn to press a bar (R) or pigeons learn to peck a key (R) to obtain food (US) from a dispenser when a light (S_D) is lit.

Dragoi and Staddon (1999) introduced a model that describes the major properties of free operant conditioning. According to their theory, (1) responses and stimuli become associated with re-

Figure 2. Diagram of a network that incorporates (a) an attentional system and (b) a configural system. In the attentional system, the internal representations of CS_i are modulated by the total environmental novelty, Novelty', computed in the novelty system. In the configural system, the internal representations of simple stimuli XS_i become *configured* with the internal representations of other CSs in hidden units that represent configural stimuli CN_j. In the associative system, both CS_i and CN_i become associated with the ohter CSs and the US. The attentional system permits the description of latent inhibition, and the configural system permits the description of occasion setting. CS_i: conditioned stimulus; ZS_i, YS_i: attentional associations; XS_i: CS_i internal representation; CN_j: configural representation; VS_{ik}: XS_i-CS_k association; VS_{iUS}: XS_i-US association; VN_{ik}: CN_i-CS_k associations; US: unconditioned stimulus; B_k: CS_k aggregate prediction; B_{US}: US aggregate prediction; $\overline{CS}_k$: CS_k average observed value; $\overline{B}_k$: CS_k average predicted value; CR: conditioned response. Arrows represent fixed synapses. Solid circles represent variable synapses. (After Buhusi and Schmajuk, 1996).

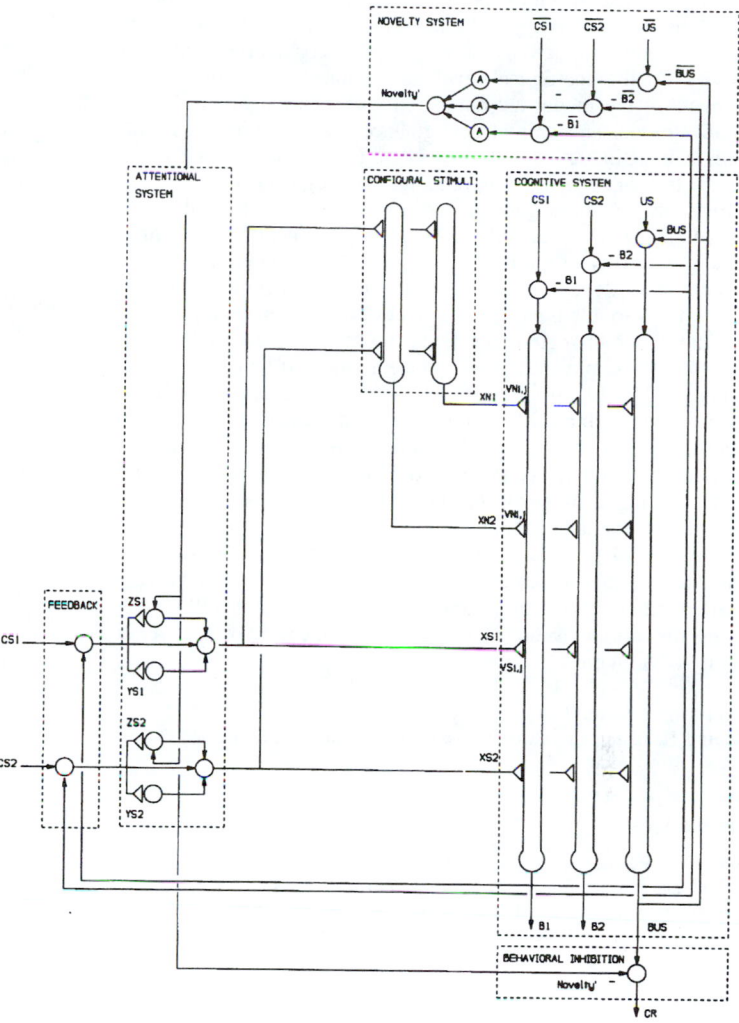

inforcement, (2) response-reinforcement and stimulus-reinforcement associations are combined to generate learning expectancy, and (3) the operant response is controlled by the interaction between expected and experienced events. The model describes qualitative features of operant behavior such as discrimination learning, response selection, contingency effects, effects of reinforcement delay, matching in choice experiments, development of preference, contrast effects, resistance to extinction, spontaneous recovery, regression, serial-reversal learning, and overtraining reversal effect.

Negative Reinforcement

Operant conditioning can also be obtained with discrete trial procedures, in which the operant response occurs only once on a given trial. For instance, discrete-trial avoidance paradigms are usually run in a two-way shuttle box. The shuttle box is a chamber with two compartments separated by a barrier with a door. Each compartment has a metal grid floor that can deliver a shock (US). Lights above the chambers provide warning signals (WS) for the US. The experiment starts with both compartments being illuminated. At time zero, the light above the compartment where the animal is located turns off (WS), and the door separating both compartments opens. If the animal has not crossed to the opposite side after a given time (that may vary between 2 and 40 s), the shock US is

applied. If the animal has crossed to the opposite side before that time, it avoids the US, and the separating door closes behind it. After a constant or an average intertrial interval that varies from 15 s to 4 minutes, the whole sequence restarts.

Schmajuk, Urry, and Zanutto (1998) presented a real-time two-process theory of avoidance that combines elements of classical and operant conditioning. The network incorporates two processes: classical and operant conditioning. Whereas the classical conditioning process controls US-US, WS-US, and R-US associations, the operant conditioning process controls US-R_{escape} and WS-$R_{avoidance}$ associations. Whereas classical conditioning is regulated by a delta rule, $f(US) = US - \Sigma_j V_{j,US} X_j$, where X represents WS, R, or the US, operant conditioning is regulated by a novel algorithm that mirrors the classical conditioning algorithm, $f(US) = - (US - \Sigma_j V_{j,US} X_j)$. Schmajuk et al. (1998) applied the network to the description of escape and avoidance behavior in a shuttle box, running wheel, leg flexion, or lever-pressing paradigms as Sidman avoidance. Schmajuk et al. (1998) demonstrated through computer simulations that the model describes most of the features that characterize avoidance behavior.

Discussion

Theories and neural networks of conditioning can be evaluated at different levels. At the behavioral level, simulated behavioral results are compared with experimental data. At the computational level, simulated activity of the neural elements of the model are compared with the activity of single-neuron or neural population activity. At the anatomical level, interconnections among neural elements in the model are compared with neuroanatomical data. Finally, model and animal performances can be compared after brain lesions, induction and blockade of long-term potentiation, or administration of different psychopharmacological drugs.

Examples of these good matches include the Schmajuk et al. (1996) model, which describes a very large number of conditioning paradigms, many of the behavioral properties of latent inhibition, the activity of dopamine neurons in the nucleus accumbens as coding for the variable novelty, the effect of lesions of the hippocampus and different regions on the accumbens on latent inhibition, the effect of administration of amphetamine and haloperidol also on latent inhibition. Another interesting case is the Sutton and Barto (1990) model, which, when combined with some of the principles used in the Grossberg and Schmajuk (1998) model, describes the activity of dopamine neurons of the ventral tegmental area and substantia nigra in terms of the prediction errors for rewards (Schultz, Dayan, and Montague, 1997).

Good models are characterized by (1) a large percentage of simulation results that match experimental results and (2) a relatively small number of equation parameters. As Schmajuk (1997) explains, the ratio between (1) and (2) gives a measure of the overall quality of a model.

Road Maps: Neural Plasticity; Psychology
Related Reading: Cognitive Maps; Concept Learning; Embodied Cognition; Motivation

References

Buhusi, C. V., and Schmajuk, N. A., 1996, Attention, configuration, and hippocampal function. *Hippocampus, 6*, 621–642. ◆
Church, R. M., and Broadbent, H. A., 1991, A connectionist model of timing, in *Neural Network Models of Conditioning and Action* (M. Commons, S. Grossberg, and J. E. R. Staddon, Eds.), Hillsdale, NJ: Erlbaum, pp. 225–240.
Dragoi, V., and Staddon, J. E. R., 1999, The dynamics of operant conditioning, *Psychol. Rev.*, 106:20–61.
Gluck, M. A., and Myers, C. E., 1993, Hippocampal mediation of stimulus representation: A computational theory, *Hippocampus*, 3:491–516.
Grossberg, S., 1975, A neural model of attention, reinforcement, and discrimination learning, *Int. Rev. Neurobiol.*, 18:263–327.
Grossberg, S., and Schmajuk, N. A., 1989, Neural dynamics of adaptive timing and temporal discrimination during associative learning, *Neural Networks*, 2:79–102.
Kehoe, E. J., 1988, A layered network model of associative learning: Learning to learn and configuration, *Psychol. Rev.*, 95:411–433.
Mackintosh, N. J., 1975, A theory of attention: Variations in the associability of stimuli with reinforcement, *Psychol. Rev.*, 82:276–298.
Pearce, J. M., and Hall, G., 1980, A model for Pavlovian learning: Variations in the effectiveness of conditioned but not of unconditioned stimuli, *Psychol. Rev.*, 87:532–552.
Rescorla, R. A., and Wagner, A. R., 1972, A theory of Pavlovian conditioning: Variation in the effectiveness of reinforcement and nonreinforcement, in *Classical Conditioning II: Theory and Research* (A. H. Black and W. F. Prokasy, Eds.), New York: Appleton-Century-Crofts.
Schmajuk, N. A., 1997, *Animal Learning and Cognition: A Neural Network Approach*. New York: Cambridge University Press. ◆
Schmajuk, N. A., and DiCarlo, J. J., 1992, Stimulus configuration, classical conditioning, and the hippocampus, *Psychol. Rev.*, 99:268–305.
Schmajuk, N. A., Lam, Y. W., and Gray, J. A., 1996, Latent inhibition: A neural network approach, *J. Exp. Psychol. Anim. Behav. Process*, 22: 321–349. ◆
Schmajuk, N. A., Urry, D., and Zanutto, B. S., 1998, The frightening complexity of avoidance: An adaptive neural network, in *Models of Action: Mechanisms of Adaptive Behavior* (C. Wynne and J. E. R. Staddon, Eds.), Hillsdale, NJ: Erlbaum, pp. 201–238.
Schultz, W., Dayan, P., and Montague, P. R., 1997, A neural substrate of prediction and reward, *Science*, 275:1593–1599.
Sutton, R. S., and Barto, A. G., 1981, Toward a modern theory of adaptive networks: Expectation and prediction. *Psychol. Rev.*, 88:135–170.
Wagner, A. R., 1978, Expectancies and the priming of STM, in *Cognitive Processes in Animal Behavior* (S. H. Hulse, H. Fowler, and W. K. Honig, Eds.), Hillsdale, N.J.: Erlbaum, pp. 177–209.

Connectionist and Symbolic Representations

David S. Touretzky

Introduction

In symbolic representations, the heart of mathematics and most models of cognition, symbols are meaningless entities to which arbitrary significances may be assigned (Newell, 1980; Harnad, 1990). Composing ordered tuples from symbols and other tuples allows us to create an infinitude of complex structures from a finite set of tokens and combination rules. Inference in the symbolic framework is founded on structural comparison and rule-governed manipulation of these objects.

Many aspects of language and cognition appear rule-like but, on closer inspection, are not so amenable to axiomatization. A famous example is the production of past tense forms of English verbs (Rumelhart and McClelland, 1986; see PAST TENSE LEARNING). Regular verbs add /t/ or /d/ or /ed/ to derive their past tense phonetic form, depending on the final sound of the stem, e.g., "flipped" versus "fibbed" versus "fitted." People generate regular past tenses of novel forms, such as "bork" to "borked," as if they were "applying the rule." But multiple classes of irregular verbs follow different conventions, e.g., sing/sang, bring/brought, or leave/left. People sometimes apply these patterns to novel forms, as in

"bling"/"blang," or misapply them to stems that follow a different irregular convention ("bring" to "brang" instead of "brought"). There are stages in child language acquisition where the regular suffix is not only misapplied, as in "bring" to "bringed," but sometimes combined with the output of an exception pattern, producing forms such as "broughted." The interactions of regular and exception forms, and the developmental phenomena associated with past tense acquisition, are difficult to formalize. Thus, it seems unlikely that children are constructing explicit past tense *rules* in their heads.

The aim of the formal symbolic approach to understanding is to give a precise account of a domain in the language of that domain, e.g., a theory of grammar expressed in terms of morphemes, words, and phrases, or a theory of vision formulated in terms of pixels, regions, boundaries, etc. Axioms (rules) determine the structures that may be composed and the inferences that may be drawn from them. The approach has had great success in formalizing mathematics, but the hope that language, perception, or other aspects of cognition might succumb to similar treatment has faded.

It is important to note here that rule-based systems are not limited to deductively sound, consistent inferences. Artificial intelligence makes extensive use of nondeductive reasoning methods. For example, case-based reasoning tries to match a problem description against a library of cases for which the solution is already known. Match scores are determined heuristically, in some instances simply by counting the number of shared features. The cases retrieved provide only a best guess at an answer, but this may be sufficient.

The search for sound deductive rules for cognitive domains having long been abandoned, the debate between symbolists and connectionists is over how much of the formalist enterprise should be retained. Symbolists have moved to more complex formalizations of cognitive processes, using heuristic and unsound inference rules. (No one claims humans are sound reasoners. Heuristics have proved very useful, and suitably constrained inference systems might never suffer the consequences of their unsoundness.) Connectionists explore a radical alternative: that cognitive processes are mere epiphenomena of a completely different type of underlying system, whose operations can never be adequately formalized in symbolic language (Smolensky, 1988; see PHILOSOPHICAL ISSUES IN BRAIN THEORY AND CONNECTIONISM).

That connectionist models are implemented on digital computers does not make them symbolic models. The past tense model can be described in terms of nodes and links and activation values, but there is no isomorphism between this description and one phrased in the domain language, i.e., in terms of verb stems and affixes. The relationships between elements at the two levels can only be hinted at. This is what makes the model nonsymbolic.

In summary, connectionism replaces classical discrete, set-theoretic semantics with continuous, statistical, vector-based semantics. In the following sections we examine representation and processing issues from a connectionist perspective.

Feature Vector Representations

If arbitrary symbols are replaced by feature vectors, the similarity of two concepts can be measured by their dot product. This is an attractive alternative to defining explicit axioms for determining, say, whether *chair* should be more similar to *table* than to *couch*. Similar concepts will naturally have similar vector representations, which facilitates generalization in neural networks.

Early models in this vein used hand-constructed feature vectors, often with familiar semantic features such as "human," "animate," "solid," etc. But other types of representations were also used. Rumelhart and McClelland's past tense model represented present tense verb forms with a triplet encoding. The phonemic sequence /stop/ would be encoded in triplet form as $_\#s_t$, $_st_o$, $_to_p$, and $_op_\#$. The encoding used in Rumelhart and McClellands's model was actually a finer-grained representation that used triplets of phonetic features instead of whole phonemes. Words were encoded as 460-element vectors, with each element corresponding to a possible triplet. A network trained on some past tense forms could thus generalize correctly to novel forms.

The advent of backpropagation learning led to the creation of feature vectors by the networks themselves. Hinton's (1990, pp. 47–76) family tree model learned relationships about three generations of people, such as "Victoria is the mother of Colin," "Victoria is the wife of James," and "Penelope is the mother of Victoria." The network took as input a pair such as "Victoria" and "mother," and was trained to activate the output unit for "Colin." A separate unit was used to represent each individual or relationship, but these units projected to small hidden layers that in turn projected to the central hidden layer. After training on 104 tuples defined over 24 persons and 12 relationships, feature vector representations developed in the dedicated person and relationship hidden layers that reflected the similarity structure of the domain. For example, one unit came to be strongly inhibited when coding for people in the third generation. The unit was weakly active for peo-

ple in the middle generation; and strongly active for grandparents, i.e., persons in the first generation.

Connectionist representations have been termed subsymbolic (Smolensky, 1988) because they capture graded, messy, but statistically important aspects of a domain. This idea has also been explored in Latent Semantic Analysis (Foltz, 1996), which derives feature vector representations for words in a large text corpus. First a matrix of occurrence information for each word in each of many contexts is constructed. A context can be a document, a paragraph, or even a sentence. The matrix is then reduced to a lower-dimensional form by singular value decomposition (SVD), similar to Principal Components Analysis. The result is a set of 100–300 dimensional feature vectors, one per word, which are useful for many kinds of text matching and retrieval applications. These features capture information about linguistic relations but do not look anything like the semantic features normally used in linguistic analysis. Once again, dot product can be used to compute similarity.

A problem with fixed feature vector representations is that what should count as similar is often context dependent. Another problem is that while feature vectors are a natural way to represent individual concepts, they are not so convenient for representing relationships among concepts; the latter may have to be generated on the fly during reasoning rather than constructed gradually through gradient descent learning.

Composite Structure

Symbolic models create trees of increasing size to encode structures with more components, but this route is not open to connectionist networks, which use fixed-length vectors (see COMPOSITIONALITY IN NEURAL SYSTEMS). Several solutions have been proposed. Encoder/decoder networks created using backpropagation can map composite objects into points in a vector space. Simple recurrent networks (SRNs; see Elman in Touretzky, 1991) represent sequences this way, and Recurrent Auto-Associative Memories (RAAMs; see Pollack in Hinton, 1990) use a similar approach to represent trees. The problem with this method is that the inductive bias of backpropagation learning does nothing to enforce systematicity in these representations, so novel inputs will not be treated correctly unless the model has been trained on a substantial fraction of the set of all possible structures to be encoded.

An alternative approach employs simple combinatorial operations on vectors to perform composition and extraction operations, thereby enforcing systematicity (see SYSTEMATICITY OF GENERALIZATIONS IN CONNECTIONIST NETWORKS). Plate's (2000) holographic reduced representation is the most promising example. Holographic reduced representations encode frame-like objects where each role and each filler is a vector of several thousand bits. Roles are paired with fillers using a circular convolution operator, which produces a vector result. Multiple role/filler pairings are then combined by vector addition and normalization. *John kissed Mary* might be encoded as *agent* $\otimes$ *john* + *patient* $\otimes$ *mary* + *action* $\otimes$ *kissed*. The vectors encoding composite objects can themselves serve as roles or fillers, providing a limited form of structural recursion. But the primitive vectors, e.g., for *john* and *mary*, must be nearly orthogonal to prevent interference between overly similar patterns, which precludes the use of a meaningful feature vector representation. On the other hand, dot product can still be used to do matching and retrieval, and even to measure analogical similarity (Eliasmith and Thagard, 2001).

Nonlinear Mapping

Certain types of representation support certain types of processing better than others. Most of the inference in connectionist networks takes place via nonlinear mapping of vectors, implemented by one or more weight matrices. Properly constructed, such matrices can simulate the effects of discrete inference rules, combine rules with exceptions, express graded inferences, exploit statistical structure in the domain, and incorporate information from multiple evidence sources. Most important, these mappings can be constructed automatically using learning procedures.

A single layer of weights was sufficient to allow the Rumelhart and McClelland past tense model to capture both the regular past tense rules and various classes of exceptions. More powerful mappings can be achieved with additional layers of weights, and by allowing a network to feed back on itself. In SRNs (Elman in Touretzky, 1991), the hidden layer activity at time t is fed back as an additional input to the network at time $t + 1$ (see CONSTITUENCY AND RECURSION IN LANGUAGE). SRNs process information sequentially and can learn finite-state grammars. But Servan-Schreiber, Cleeremans, and McClelland (in Touretzky, 1991) showed that these networks do more than that: they learn and exploit the statistical structure of the training data. Servan-Schreiber et al. suggest that statistical differences between main and embedded clauses might help a language learner track long-range dependencies generated by recursive grammatical constructs.

The problems with the nonlinear mapping approach are that it requires lots of training data to adequately cover a small domain, and the "rules" are often learned imperfectly, so the network does not always generalize correctly. On the other hand, it provides a way to study complex phenomena without having to formulate rules explicitly. Plaut (1999) showed that lesioning a network that mapped orthographic to phonetic representations (and that also had attractor dynamics) could reproduce many interesting effects observed in word reading and acquired dyslexias (see LESIONED NETWORKS AS MODELS OF NEUROPSYCHOLOGICAL DEFICITS). Some of these effects, such as characteristic mixtures of error types, have proved difficult to explain with symbolic models.

Rohde's connectionist sentence comprehension and production model (CSCP) shows that nonlinear maps can challenge symbolic language models in nontrivial domains (Rohde, 2002). CSCP is a collection of SRNs that learns a substantial fragment of English grammar, including many types of embedded and relative clauses. The model has a 300-word vocabulary and contains both parsing and sentence production components. It required 2 months on a fast workstation to train. Although its performance is not perfect, its coverage is impressive.

Parallel Constraint Satisfaction

Rule-based systems have trouble determining the best interpretation of an ambiguous stimulus because of the difficulty of formulating explicit rules that weigh multiple sources of evidence in a flexible manner. Connectionist networks approach this as a constraint satisfaction problem. Evidence sources impose weak constraints on the stimulus interpretation, and the activity of the network evolves to reflect the collective effect of all these influences.

One of the simplest constraint satisfaction architectures is the interactive activation network, in which constraints are expressed as weighted excitatory or inhibitory links between nodes standing for concepts. Semantically related units have mutually excitatory connections, while units that code for alternative hypotheses inhibit each other. Consider the treatment of *The astronomer married the star* in Waltz and Pollack's (1985) interactive parsing model. There are two word-meaning nodes for *star*, one being "heavenly body" and the other "movie star." There is an excitatory link from astronomer to the heavenly body node because the two are semantically related. Hence, the model predicts that this meaning of star will be primed by "astronomer," and will initially be favored over "movie star." But when *married* is encountered, it imposes a constraint that the subject and object must be human. This ultimately leads to suppression of activity in the heavenly body node, causing movie star to become active.

Neural net constraint satisfaction systems, unlike their symbolic counterparts, are attractor networks (see COMPUTING WITH ATTRACTORS). We can draw on dynamical systems theory to understand their behavior. Most of these networks use "localist" or symbolic rather than "distributed" or vector representations (see LOCALIZED VERSUS DISTRIBUTED REPRESENTATIONS), but their inference mechanism is still nonaxiomatic.

More sophisticated constraint satisfaction can be done with Boltzmann machines, which employ hidden units to express nonlinear interactions among constraints, and simulated annealing search to find the best interpretation of the input. An example of spreading activation and simulated annealing using localist representations is Hofstadter and Mitchell's analogy-making program, CopyCat (Mitchell, 1993). One of the few annealing reasoners developed to date that employs feature vector representations is microKLONE (Derthick in Hinton, 1990), which translated a frame-based semantic network language into a complex structure of nodes and links expressing semantic constraints among slot fillers. microKLONE was able to use these constraints not only to fill in missing information, but also to produce plausible inferences in counterfactual situations.

Discussion

Connectionist representations promise a continuous, statistical, vector-based alternative to rule-based reasoning over discrete symbol structures. Although too abstract to map directly onto neural circuitry, the new conceptual framework has strongly influenced theorizing about the brain.

As yet we have only glimmerings of how connectionist models might surpass the abilities of symbolic reasoners. One suggestion of how they might do this is Hinton's (1990, pp. 47–76) notion of a "reduced description," in which the encoding of a concept like "room" contains abbreviated but directly accessible information about affiliated concepts such as "window," "door," "doorknob," and "keyhole." A reasoner could thus immediately recognize how a room could have a keyhole, rather than having to follow a chain of pointers to reach that concept via "door" and "doorknob." But we have not yet seen a successful implementation of reduced descriptions, much less a mechanism to automatically tailor such descriptions to the requirements of a domain.

The elements discussed in this article—feature vector representations, composite structure, nonlinear maps, and parallel constraint satisfaction—do not yet work well together. Multiple conceptual breakthroughs are likely required before they can be incorporated into a unified connectionist theory of symbol processsing.

Road Map: Artificial Intelligence
Related Reading: Artificial Intelligence and Neural Networks; Compositionality in Neural Systems; Hybrid Connectionist/Symbolic Systems; Systematicity of Generalizations in Connectionist Networks

References

Eliasmith, C., and Thagard, P., 2001, Integrating structure and meaning: A distributed model of analogical mapping, *Cognit. Sci.*, 25:245–286.
Foltz, P. W., 1996, Latent Semantic Analysis for text-based research, *Behav. Res. Meth. Instr. Comput.*, 28:197–202.
Harnad, S., 1990, The symbol grounding problem, *Physica D*, 42:335–346.
Hinton, G. E., Ed., 1990, *Connectionist Symbol Processing, Artif. Intell.*, 46 (special issue). ◆
Mitchell, M., 1993, *Analogy-Making as Perception*, Cambridge, MA: MIT Press.
Newell, A., 1980, Physical symbol systems, *Cognit. Sci.*, 4:135–183.

Plate, T., 2000, Analogy retrieval and processing with distributed vector representations, *Expert Syst. Int. J. Knowledge Engn. Neural Netw.*, 17:29–40. ◆

Plaut, D. C., 1999, Computational modeling of word reading, acquired dyslexia, and remediation, in *Converging Methods in Reading and Dyslexia* (R. Klein and P. A. McMullen, Eds.), Cambridge, MA: MIT Press, pp. 339–397.

Rohde, D. R., 2002, A connectionist model of sentence comprehension and production, Ph.D. diss., Carnegie Mellon University. Available: http://www.cs.cmu.edu/~dr/Thesis.

Rumelhart, D. E., and McClelland, J. L., 1986, On learning the past tense of English verbs, in *Parallel Distributed Processing: Explorations in the Microstructure of Cognition* (J. L. McClelland and D. E. Rumelhart, Eds.), Cambridge, MA: MIT Press, vol. 2, pp. 216–217.

Smolensky, P., 1988, On the proper treatment of connectionism, *Behav. Brain Sci.*, 11:1–74. ◆

Touretzky, D., Ed., 1991, *Connectionist Approaches to Language Learning, Machine Learn.*, 7(2–3):105–252 (special issue).

Waltz, D. L., and Pollack, J. B., 1985, Massively parallel parsing: A strongly interactive model of natural language interpretation, *Cognit. Sci.*, 9:51–74.

Consciousness, Neural Models of

John G. Taylor

Introduction

The construction of neural theories of consciousness faces the difficulty that, by its very nature, consciousness is subtle, and its defining characteristics are still poorly discerned. This leads to uncertainty about what properties create consciousness in the brain and even regarding the location of the sites of consciousness creation, the so-called neural correlates of consciousness (NCC). In order to prevent the NCC from wandering all over the brain, whether in the primary sensory or unimodal associative cortices (Pollen, referred to in Taylor, 2001), or now in the prefrontal cortex (Crick and Koch, 1998), care must be taken in assessing evidence in support of various possible sites of the NCC. New experimental results from brain imaging, as well as further insights into single cell activity and the effects of brain deficits, are now leading to a clearer picture of the NCC (Taylor, 1999, 2001a). This is an important advance, since concentration can now be turned to the nature of the neural representations crucially involved in consciousness. Neural network ideas and explicit models are helping to pin down what these representations consist of and how they function. Thus, progress is slowly being made to understand scientifically this most mysterious of human phenomena: the race for consciousness has started in earnest (Taylor, 1999).

Yet consciousness is not easy to define precisely. In order to make initial progress without spending time in logic chopping, let us follow the article on consciousness in the previous edition of the *Handbook* (Velmans, 1995). The definition given there is initially appropriate for the present purposes:

Consciousness is synonymous with awareness or conscious awareness (sometimes phenomenal awareness). The contents of consciousness encompass all that we are conscious of, aware of or experience.

This distinguishes consciousness from other mental activity; there is much in the mind of which the possessor is not conscious, so that consciousness is a special faculty of the mind. The nature of its function has been vigorously debated (Velmans, 1995), although with no justification of either extreme: consciousness has no purpose, but is solely an epiphenomenon, or alternatively it is the ultimate control system of the mind. Comments supporting the latter view will be given later in this article, as well as further discussion of the validity of the above definition.

If consciousness is difficult to define and its function is hard to discern, at least some features involved with its creation are more generally agreed upon. Characteristics needed for consciousness are as follows:

1. *Temporal duration.* Neural activity is needed to be present for at least 200 ms for awareness to arise. This is supported by the data of Libet and colleagues (1964) and by the duration of activity in buffer working memory sites, suggested by a number of workers as being the sites of creation of consciousness (Taylor, 1999).

2. *Attentional focus.* It is widely supposed that consciousness can only arise of an object at the focus of attention; there is experimental support for this position (Mack and Rock in Wright, 1997). The resulting amplification of the attended input allows it to attain consciousness and also be laid down in long-term memory, for later conscious access.

3. *Binding.* The binding of features, analyzed in separate areas of cortex, to allow recognition and experience of objects, has long been regarded as crucial for the explanation of consciousness. Such binding has been proposed to occur by several means, especially by simultaneous activations, such as by coupled oscillatory modules (Crick and Koch, 1990) or by attentive competitive/amplificatory processing (Triesman in Wright, 1997). There is evidence for both of these being involved in cortical processing.

4. *Bodily inputs.* The availability of such inputs is needed to give a perspective to inputs, following detailed investigations by psychologists (Bermudez, Marcel, and Eilan, 1995).

5. *Salience.* Coded in the limbic system, salience is needed to give a suitable level of importance to a given input, and can arise, for example, from the cingulate cortex, as involving motivational activation, or from other limbic sites.

6. *Past experience.* This gives content to conscious experience, by reactivating previous relevant experience (Taylor, 1999); such memories are especially involved in defining the self.

7. *Inner perspective*: Besides having awareness of an input, we each possess an inner perspective, without which we cannot experience the mental world as belonging to us. The inner perspective is thus that of ownership of our awareness. Without it we would be zombies, having content but no sense of "what it is like to be me" (Nagel, 1974).

Only by a concerted attack on the underlying brain structures involved in the creation of consciousness, and their detailed modelling, can real progress be made. Recent advances on the three counts—the "where," the "what," and the "how" of consciousness—will be described in this article. Several recent experimental results from brain imaging, single-cell data, and brain deficits will be described in the next section. These help in determining a site for the NCC. From these data, the inferior parietal lobes are concluded to be the most appropriate region for the site of consciousness (Taylor, 2001a). In the following section the notion of the central representation will be developed; it contains the crucial contents for consciousness. A general model of attention control, the CODAM model, which incorporates the central representation and is appropriate for simulating the associated emergence of consciousness, is then presented in the next section. Relations to other models are described briefly in the penultimate section, and a short conclusion and discussion of open questions finishes the review.

Experimental Data

The data to be considered are of a variety of sorts: from single cells, lesion effects on behavior, and from brain imaging (especially that using PET and fMRI). The single-cell data involves information on the presence or absence of significant activity observed in an animal under anesthesia. This has little effect on the level of early sensory cortical responses, for example, in V1 and MT or in inferotemporal cortex. We will later consider the important effects of attention on such activity, although this does not change the overall story. There is considerable effect of anesthesia on parietal lobe single-cell responses, which led to great difficulty in measuring from such cells before the advent of the ability to record from awake, behaving monkeys. Thus, occipital and temporal cortices are not sufficient for consciousness, while parietal may be.

As a start to considering lesion effects, we note the singular lack of loss of consciousness due to frontal deficits brought about either by disease or injury, as numerous reports show. For example, there is the famous case of Phineas Gage (described in Taylor, 1999), who had a tamping iron blown through his frontal lobes with considerable loss of frontal cortex but without successive loss of consciousness as he was carried to the local doctor. There is also the case of the young man who was born bereft of most of his frontal lobes (mentioned in Taylor, 2001), but yet, apart from great social problems, lived a normal conscious existence.

One area of brain lesions of particular relevance to the NCC is that of neglect (which can be either of visual inputs or control of actions). Patients usually suffer a loss of the right parietal lobe, and subsequently lose awareness of input from their left hemifield. This loss, for example, is observed in the inability to cross out lines on the left of their field of view. It is now agreed that neglect arises specifically from damage to the inferior parietal lobe (Milner, 1997).

Much is also being discovered by brain imaging about the siting in cortex of buffer working memories. Those for spatial vision are in the right, those for language and temporal estimation in the left, inferior parietal lobes. Extinction, involving loss of awareness of the right-hand object of two similar objects, one on the left, one on the right, is sited separately in the superior parietal lobe (Milner, 1997).

Recent fMRI data indicates that the experience of the motion aftereffect (MAE) most occurs strongly in BA 40 (the supramarginal gyrus), in the inferior parietal lobe. The experimental paradigm to observe this uses motion adaptation to a set of horizontal bars moving vertically downward for 30 s, and then stopping. Subjects exposed to such a display usually experience the MAE for 9 or so s after cessation of the movement of the bars.

Whole-head fMRI measurements during this paradigm (Taylor et al., 2000) showed a network of connected areas, as in Figure 1. This network has a posterior group, involving especially the motion area MT, which was found to be responsive to all forms of motion as well as the MAE. On the other hand, there is a set of anterior modules, shown in Figure 1, which are particularly active both during the MAE period and just after the cessation of oscillatory movement of the bars both up and down (after which there is no MAE experience reported). Finally, there are inferior parietal re-

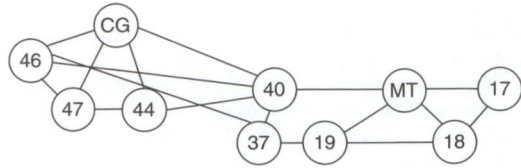

Figure 1. The network of areas active in the brain during the MAE experiment (Schmitz et al., 1998, referred to in Taylor, 2001). The lines joining the various modules denote those for which the correlation coefficient is at least 0.4. MT denotes the middle temporal area, and the other areas are numbered according to Brodmann's numeration.

gions, which demonstrate activity almost solely in response to the MAE period.

All of the inputs required to support the features described in the first section are available, it would seem almost uniquely, for the inferior parietal lobe. Thus, the buffer working memory sites for space and time (and language) have been noted previously as being there, as is a competition for consciousness associated with these sites (Taylor, 1999). Bodily inputs are also available there, as noted from effects of manipulation of the body in neglect, as well as from known neuroanatomy (connections with the vestibular apparatus and the cerebellum are well known). The limbic system is also well connected to the inferior parietal lobe and so is episodic memory.

We conclude that the inferior parietal lobe (IPL) is suitably connected and structured to satisfy all of the criteria A–F in the first section. We will discuss its relevance to criterion G when we consider the CODAM model of a Heution control.

The Central Representation

Evidence from neglect studies and brain imaging on healthy subjects has been presented in this article to implicate the IPL as playing a crucial role in controlling attention and creating awareness. Attention can occur in a range of possible frames of reference: neglect can be observed tied to an object, or to a trunk-centered frame of reference or a variety of other reference frames (Milner, 1997). This implies that the IPL is composed of a set of modules carrying information from the environment as well as modulation by possible body input. Thus, the IPL is eminently suited to carry what is termed the "Central Representation," defined as: "The combined set of multi-modal activations involved in fusing sensory activity, body positions, salience and intentionality for future planning; it involves a competitive process between the various working memory modules it contains to single out one to be conscious and be used for report to other working memory sites for further planning or action" (Taylor, 2001a).

There are several important features of the central representation (CR) that need discussion, in relation to the criteria in the introduction to the article:

1. The CR must have access to sensory input, such as in vision, coded at a high level. Thus, it must have good access to temporal lobe representations, so as to use the categorization built there to guide action.
2. It also must have access to the bodily input needed to guide actions in terms of the intentionality coded in the superior parietal lobe. Such intentionality is coded for various sorts of actions: of the limbs, eyes, head, or fingers. This intentionality must be furnished with the parameters of the objects on which the actions must be taken; thus, cerebellar and vestibular input must also be accessible to the central representation, as it is in the parietal lobes. A neural model of this intentionality has been presented in Fagg and Arbib (1998).

3. Salience of the inputs in the sensory field is an important attribute for the guidance of actions; that arises from limbic input already activated to provide saliencies of inputs from the orbitofrontal cortex by way of the cingulate. This is compounded by activations in the posterior cingulate gyrus, encoded as parts of episodic memory.

4. Several modules in the CR are involved in the IPL; the total activity must undergo an overall competition, possibly aided by thalamonucleus reticularis processing. A simulation of such a model has been given earlier (described in Taylor, 1999). The existence of such competition is supported by attention deficits observed in subjects with pulvinar lesions.

5. Siting the emergence of awareness in the IPL, as the result of the competition ongoing there, is supported by simulation of the data of Libet and colleagues (1964). The original experiment involved the creation of sensory experience (that of a gentle touch on the back of the patient's hand) by direct stimulation of cortex in patients being operated on for movement problems. The simulation (described in Taylor, 1999) used a simplified model of the corticothalamo-nucleus reticularis circuit, and led to the observed dependence of the delay of awareness on the strength of the threshold current for experiencing the touch on the back of the patient's hand.

6. Such a competition has also been suggested (described in Taylor, 1999) as occurring to explain experimental results of subliminal effects on lexical decision response times obtained by Marcel (1980). The experiment involved measurement of the reaction times of subjects to deciding if the first or third of three letter strings were words or not. Subliminal exposure to priming words occurred for the second letter string under one condition, with the presentation of polysemous words such as "palm," on which the lexical decision had to be made to the third word. The prior exposure caused the decision to be speeded up or delayed in characteristic ways according to the semantic relations of the three words to each other; the simulation was able to explain these results by means of a competition assumed to occur on the phonological store, aided and abetted by activations from a semantic memory store.

In conclusion, we site the CR in the IPL as the site for attention and short-term memory processing, with confluence there of information on salience, episodic memory, high level coding of inputs, and information on body state.

An Attention Control Model (CODAM) of the Emergence of Awareness

Attention, the respectable face of consciousness for neuroscience, has received surprisingly short shrift recently from those directly attacking the problem of consciousness. This is in spite of the phenomenon of inattentional blindness, that there is no perception without attention, as noted by Mack and Rock (in Wright, 1997), and the many claims by those working on attention that there is no consciousness of an unattended input. There is now improved understanding of attention arrived at by brain imaging using a range of psychophysical paradigms and ever more careful single-cell experiments. A control view of attention is now accepted, in which signals from outside early cortex modulate inputs so as to allow selection of a desired target input from a set of distracters. We will now develop this view, describing how the Central Representation supports the creation of consciousness by means of a suitable control model.

In such a control model, there are the "plant" components of primary and secondary sensory and motor cortices containing input activations being attended to, an inverse controller in parietal/frontal as source of the attention signal, and a rules module containing the desired state into which attended input should be transformed (there being a prefrontal top-down rules module, and a bottom-up component in superior colliculus). Further components of a so-called forward model (or observer) can also be tentatively identified. This resides as buffer sites in inferior parietal and updating areas in prefrontal, as well as parts involved in monitoring effectiveness of response under the guidance of the rules modules, sited in cingulate cortex. This model (shown in Figure 2) has been simulated for a variety of paradigms (Taylor and Rogers, 2001), being an engineering control formalization of many neural models of attention.

To bring consciousness to the foreground inside the control model of attention, we turn to recent developments in phenomenology to guide us: there are two components of consciousness: "consciousness of" and the pre-reflective self. The pre-reflective self is experienced as the ownership of one's conscious experience and as the basis of all awareness; without it there would be content but no owner of that content.

To incorporate this important component in the attention control model, a very conjectural step was made in Taylor (2000): it was proposed that an observer is present that contains a buffered copy of the controller signal (more properly called a *corollary discharge*, since it is coded in the same manner as attended sensory activation on its buffer). This copy is used to achieve more rapid updating of the movement control signal. Such a copy will not be bound in any attention-based manner to the content of consciousness, since that can only be present on feedback from the plant. The corollary discharge signal will therefore not have any content. It can, however, be identified with the experience of "ownership," that of the about-to-appear amplified input that is being attended to. Such a signal can grant immunity to error through misidentification of the first-

Figure 2. A simple attention movement control model (shown in bold lines), composed of attended cortex (containing activity representing an attended input), an attention movement generator, a rules module (for either top-down or bottom-up control of attention), and a monitor (based on the error between the required attention state and that occurring as determined by a sensory buffer). The additional module and connections (in dotted lines) completes the CODAM model. It involves a buffer to hold the corollary discharge of attention movement. This corollary discharge signal is employed to speed up movement of attention as well as prevent incorrect updating of the sensory buffer until attention has been moved to the correct place (as assessed by the corollary discharge buffer acting as an observer or attention state estimator).

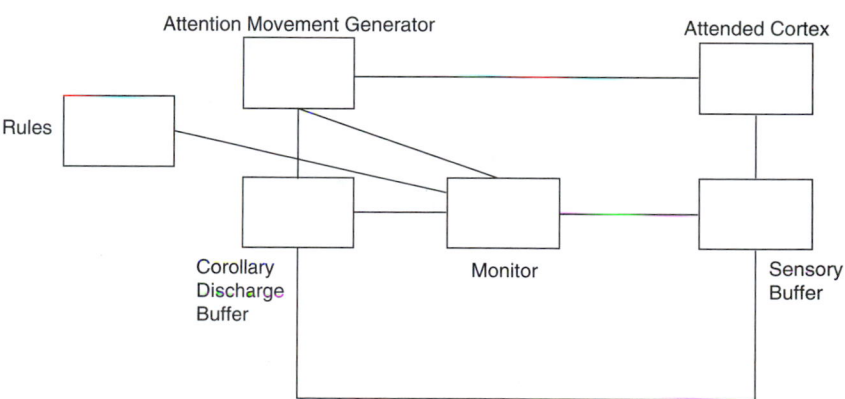

person pronoun. This would follow if the corollary discharge acts only to let onto the buffer what it has been told to by the inverse attention controller. As such, it inhibits all other possible entrants to contentful consciousness. This occurs for the brief period before the attentionally amplified input from sensory cortex arrives. The corollary discharge is then supposed to be inhibited in its turn. Such complex processing is supported by the siting of much of the attention control structures nearby in the parietal lobe, singled out recently as crucial for consciousness to arise. A simple model for such usage of the corollary discharge is shown in Figure 2, involving an additional observe component (shown in dotted lines), beyond the control model used in Taylor and Rogers (2001).

Following many experimental results, we site the attention controller in superior parietal lobe, the prefrontal cortex or superior colliculus, the attended plant in sensory cortices, working memory buffers in inferior parietal lobe, the monitor in the cingulate, and the goals module in the prefrontal cortex.

This approach results in the corollary discharge of attention movement (CODAM) model of consciousness (Taylor, 2000, 2001b):

> Experience of the pre-reflective self is identified with the corollary discharge of the attention movement control signal residing briefly in its buffer until the arrival of the associated attended input activation at its own buffer.

The CODAM model achieves the required unpacking of the Central Representation: its essential constituents are (1) that of a signal of ownership in the corollary discharge buffer (with no content), (2) contents of external inputs represented by activity subsequently stored on the attended input buffer. There is a strict temporal order of activation, with the former briefly activated first, followed by the attended input buffer. More extended duration of the corollary discharge signal is suggested as the source of the meditatory states of samadhi or nirvana: this is attention observing itself (Taylor, 2002). The presence of the pre-reflective self implies that the definition of consciousness given in the introductory section is incomplete; it needs extension by addition of the sentence "Those contents include awareness of consciousness itself, as occurs in the pre-reflective self."

The above model is only presented at the "arrows and boxes" level. Detailed neural implementations of various components are possible:

1. *Temporal duration*: achieved by the neural field recurrence—the bubble model, in which bubbles are temporally extended but spatially localised regions of neural activity with a certain degree of independence from inputs (Taylor, 1999).
2. *Attention focus*: numerous neural models of attention processing in terms of object recognition have been created, such as the feedback amplification system of Mozer and Sitton (referred to in Taylor and Rogers, 2002, and see references therein). A general control framework encompassing such models has been suggested (Taylor, 2000, 2001b). A specific simulation, using competitive processing on the IMC is given in Taylor and Rogers (2001). Global competition across the CR is achieved by the NRT (with simulation described in Taylor, 1999).
3. *Binding*: achieved by attention processing in the models noted above, to which synchronized activity can be added.
4. *Bodily inputs*: the effect of these on attention processing in the parietal lobe has been modeled by modulations using various neural methods.
5. *Salience*: amygdala encoding salience of inputs has been used in models of frontal set shifting (discussed in Taylor, 1999).
6. *Episodic memory*: various hippocampal models have been created, although the manner in which episodic memory is built in cortex is still unclear (see discussion in Taylor, 1999).

There are numerous important questions to be answered before the CODAM model can be accepted as a source of inner experience:

Would it pass the Turing test if it were included in a full neural simulation?
How does the control aspect of attention, regarded as the highest control system in the brain, achieve learning of effective motor responses so as to achieve automaticity?
How is language (and thought) built from this overall framework?
It is hoped that answers to these questions will be forthcoming by subsequent work.

Other Neural Models of Consciousness

Numerous models have been presented in the past to explain consciousness; only neural models will be considered here, and those only briefly.

1. Gray's Hippocampal Predictor model (see Gray et al. in Freeman and Taylor, 1997). This suggests that the hippocampus enables predictions to be made of future experiences, so creating consciousness. Various amnesic subjects, without hippocampus, however, still respond in a conscious manner in conversation, in spite of severe long-term memory deficits.
2. Aleksander's MAGNUS (see Browne et al. in Freeman and Taylor, 1997). This is based on a set of attractors, built by learning in a recurrent net in RAM-based hardware. Activation of an attractor is claimed to be the "artificial consciousness" of the system of the related input. This model has the defect that it involves no "internal experience" associated with attractor activity; it is a useful, if broad, model of the contents of consciousness.
3. Shallice's SAS (see reference in Taylor, 1999). This assumes total control of neural activity by the frontal "supervisory attention system." However, evidence against the NCC being sited in the frontal lobes was given in the section on experimental data. Better consistency with the CODAM model of the previous section can be achieved by extending the supervisory attention system to include parietal sites.
4. Baar's Global Workspace (see Newman et al. in Freeman and Taylor, 1997). This regards consciousness as the gaining of access to a "global workspace" (GW), considered as being on layer 1 of cortex. The GW is an incompletely defined concept, especially since it also does not necessarily have any internal experience. It can be related to the CODAM model by regarding access to the GW as the important process for determining the pre-reflective self. The CODAM model indicates how this access is controlled by suitable buffer activity, as well as determining the temporal nature of activity on ensuing access, when content enters consciousness.
5. Crick and Koch's 40 Hz (1990). That gamma-band oscillations are important for binding and segmenting is now well established (both experimentally in the brain and by computation). However, since such oscillations are observed in anesthetized animals, such activity cannot be regarded as sufficient for consciousness.
6. Pollen's Early model (see reference in Taylor, 2001). This supposes consciousness arises from feedback and relaxation to a fixed point of an attractor dynamics. Yet there is such re-entrance at many levels in the brain, such as between LGN and V1. The activity in LGN is not in consciousness, so indicating that the existence of such feedback is not sufficient for consciousness to be created.
7. Zeki's "local homunculus" (see references in Taylor, 2001a). This proposes that micro-consciousnesses arise in numerous

early cortical areas. However not only does this proliferation of homunculi add to the difficulties of consciousness but is also contradicted by the results presented in the section on experimental data.

8. Edeleman's Reentrant Theory (see reference in Taylor, 1999). This is based on the special use of reentrant circuits, and so suffers from the difficulties of item 6 of this list.

9. Roll's Higher Order Theory (HOT; expanded in Roll's article in Freeman and Taylor, 1997). This uses language to enable higher order thoughts of lower order experienced inputs. The original HOT theory faces the difficulty that it rules out non-reflective consciousness in animals other than humans. Moreover the perspectival nature of experience cannot be incorporated into the HOT model in any obvious manner.

10. Harth's Inner Sketchpad Model (see Harth in Freeman and Taylor, 1997). This is based on the use of the reentry of a global scalar quantity, the degree of overlap between the input and activation, to achieve hill-climbing or attractor relaxation; it has the same defect as that of item 6 of this list, being involved in much dynamical processing in the brain but not just that specifically producing consciousness.

11. The Competitive Relational Mind model (Taylor, 1999). That a competitive process occurs in and between working memory sites for the emergence of consciousness is now becoming clear, but is still insufficient for the production of any perspectival account of awareness at the level of the pre-reflective self (Taylor, 2001b). Further circuitry is needed to build on this approach, as described in the section on the CODAM model.

In spite of the defects pointed out in the above models, they all involve important components in overall brain processing. The CODAM model introduced earlier is to be regarded as an extra component that benefits from the various computational features emphasised in the models of the previous section.

Discussion

Our main conclusions are:

1. The IPL is the essential site in the brain for consciousness.
2. The central representation, based there, gives conscious content (through activity in attended sites bound to the central representation by various mechanisms).
3. A simple control model of the movement of attention, supported by experimental data, can be extended to a mechanism for the creation of consciousness through the CODAM model. This led to a computational understanding of the minimal or pre-reflective self.

The broad range of the review touched on many areas, all of which require considerable further work. If the basic CODAM prin-

ciples are correct—as is so far supported by a range of material (Taylor, 2001b)—it provides a first viable neural approach to understanding human consciousness. It could even lead to the creation of a viable blueprint for machine consciousness. The greatest challenge facing the computational neuroscience community is to create simulations that can properly test the ideas presented here. At the same time, the challenge to neuroscience is to develop experimental proof or disproof of the CODAM model.

Road Map: Psychology
Related Reading: Action Monitoring and Forward Control of Movements; Cognitive Maps; Embodied Cognition; Emotional Circuits; Language Evolution: The Mirror System Hypothesis

References

Bermudez, J. L., Marcel, A. J., and Eilan, N., 1995, *The Body and the Self,* Cambridge, MA: MIT Press.

Crick, F. H. C., and Koch, C., 1990, Towards a neurobiological theory of consciousness, *Sem. Neurosci.,* 2:263–275.

Crick, F. H. C., and Koch, C., 1998, Consciousness and neuroscience, *Cerebral Cortex,* 8:97–107. ◆

Fagg, A. H., and Arbib, M. A., 1998, Modeling parietal-premotor interactions in primate control of grasping, *Neural Networks,* 11:1277–1304. ◆

Freeman, W., and Taylor, J. G., 1997, Neural Networks for Consciousness, Special Issue, *Neural Networks,* 10(7).

Libet, B., Alberts, W. W., Wright, E. W., DeLattre, L. D., Levin, G., and Feinsein, B., 1964, Production of threshold levels of conscious sensation by electrical stimulation of human somatosensory cortex, *J Neurophysiol,* 27:546–578

Marcel, A. J., 1980, Conscious and preconsious recognition on polysemous words: locating the selective effects of prior verbal contexts, in *Attention and Performance VIII* (R. S. Nickerson, Ed.), Hillsdale NJ: Lawrence Erlbaum.

Milner, A. D., 1997, Neglect, extinction and the cortical streams of visual processing, in *Parietal Lobe: Contributions to Orientation in 3D Space* (P. Thier and H.-O. Karnath, Eds.), Heidelberg: Springer, pp. 3–22. ◆

Nagel, T., 1974, What is it like to be a bat? *Philos. Rev.,* 83:434–450. ◆

Taylor, J. G., 1999, *The Race for Consciousness,* Cambridge, MA: MIT Press.

Taylor, J. G., 2000, Attentional movement: The control basis for consciousness, *Neurosci. Abst.,* 30:2231. Abstract No. 839.3.

Taylor, J. G., 2001, The central role of the parietal lobes for consciousness, *Consc. Cognit.,* 10:379–417; 421–424.

Taylor, J. G., 2002, From matter to mind, *J. Consc. Stud.,* 9:3–22.

Taylor, J. G., and Rogers, M., 2002, A control model for the movement of attention, *Neural Networks,* 15:309–326.

Taylor, J. G., Schmitz, N., Ziemons, K., Gross-Ruyken, M.-L., Mueller-Gaertner, H.-W., and Shah, N.-J., 2000, The network of areas involved in the motion after-effect, *NeuroImage,* 11:257–270. ◆

Velmans, M., 1995, Consciousness, theories of, in *The Handbook of Brain Theory and Neural Networks* (M. A. Arbib, Ed.), Cambridge, MA: MIT Press, pp. 247–250.

Wright, R., (Ed.), 1997, Visual attention. Oxford: Oxford University Press.

Constituency and Recursion in Language

Morten H. Christiansen and Nick Chater

Introduction

Upon reflection, most people would agree that the words in a sentence are not merely arranged like beads on a string. Rather, the words group together to form coherent building blocks within a sentence. Consider the sentence, *The girl liked a boy*. Intuitively, the chunks *the girl* and *liked a boy* constitute the basic components

of this sentence (compared to a simple listing of the individual words or alternative groupings, such as *the girl liked* and *a boy*). Linguistically, these chunks comprise the two major *constituents* of a sentence: a subject noun phrase (NP), *the girl*, and a verb phrase (VP), *liked a boy*. Such *phrasal* constituents may contain two types of syntactic elements: other phrasal constituents (e.g., the NP *a boy* in the above VP) or *lexical* constituents (e.g., the determiner *the* and the noun *girl* in the NP *the girl*). Both types of constituent are typically defined *distributionally* using the so-called replacement test: If a novel word or phrase has the same distribution as a word or phrase of a known constituent type—that is if the former can be *replaced* by the latter—then they are the same type of constituent. Thus, the lexical constituents *the* and *a* both belong to the lexical category of determiners because they occur in similar contexts and therefore can replace each other (e.g., *A girl liked the boy*). Likewise, *the girl* and *a boy* belong to the same phrasal category, NP, because they can be swapped around, as in *A boy liked the girl* (note, however, that there may be semantic constraints on constituent replacements. For example, replacing the animate subject NP *the girl* with the inanimate NP *the chair* yields the semantically anomalous sentence, *The chair liked a boy*).

In linguistics, grammar rules and/or principles determine how constituents can be put together to form sentences. For instance, we can use the following phrase structure rules to describe the relationship between the constituents in the example sentences above:

$$S \rightarrow NP\ VP$$
$$NP \rightarrow (det)\ N$$
$$VP \rightarrow V\ (NP)$$

Using these rules we obtain the following relationships between the lexical and phrasal constituents:

$$[_S[_{NP}[_{det} \text{The }][_N \text{ girl }]][_{VP}[_V \text{ liked }][_{NP} [_{det} \text{ a }][_N \text{ boy }]]]]$$

To capture the full generativity of human language, *recursion* needs to be introduced into the grammar. We can incorporate recursion into the above rule set by introducing a new rule that adds a potential prepositional phrase (PP) to the NP:

$$NP \rightarrow (det)N(PP)$$
$$PP \rightarrow prep\ NP$$

These rules are recursive because the expansion of the right-hand sides of each can involve a call to the other. For example, the complex NP *the flowers in the vase* has the simple NP *the vase* recursively embedded within it. This process can be applied arbitrarily often, creating, for instance, the complex NP with three embedded NPs:

$$[_{NP} \text{ the flowers } [_{PP} \text{ in } [_{NP} \text{ the vase}$$
$$[_{PP} \text{ on } [_{NP} \text{ the table}$$
$$[_{PP} \text{ by } [_{NP} \text{ the window}]]]]]]]]$$

Recursive rules can thus generate constructions of arbitrary complexity.

Constituency and recursion are some of the most fundamental concepts in linguistics. As we saw above, both are defined in terms of relations between symbols. Symbolic models of language processing therefore incorporate these properties by fiat. In this article, we discuss how constituency and recursion may fit into a connectionist framework and the possible implications for linguistics and psycholinguistics.

Constituency

Connectionist models of language processing can address constituency in three increasingly radical ways. First, some connectionist models are *implementations* of symbolic language processing models in "neural" hardware. Many early connectionist models of syntax used this approach; an example is Fanty's (1986) network implementation of a context-free grammar. This kind of model contains explicit representations of the constituent structure of a sentence in just the same way as a nonconnectionist implementation

of the same model would. Connectionist implementations of this kind may be important; they have the potential to provide feasibility proofs that traditional symbolic models of language processing are compatible with a "brain-style" computational architecture. But these models add nothing new with respect to the treatment of constituency.

The remaining two classes of connectionist models *learn* to process constituent structure, rather than having this ability hardwired. One approach is to have a network learn from input "tagged" with information about constituent structure. For example, Kim, Srinivas, and Trueswell (2002) train a network to map a combination of orthographic and co-occurrence-based "semantic" information about a word onto a structured representation encoding the minimal syntactic environment for that word. With an input vocabulary consisting of 20,000 words, this model has an impressive coverage and can account for certain results from the psycholinguistic literature concerning ambiguity resolution in sentence processing. But because constituent structure has been "compiled" into the output representations that the network was trained to produce, this kind of model does not offer any fresh insight into how linguistic constituency might operate, based on connectionist principles.

The third class of connectionist models addresses the more ambitious problem of learning the constituent structure of a language from untagged linguistic input. Such models have the potential to develop a new or unexpected notion of constituency, and hence may have substantial implications for theories of constituency in linguistics and psycholinguistics.

To understand how the more radical connectionist models address constituency, we need to frame the problem more generally. We can divide the problem of finding constituent structure in linguistic input into two interrelated parts: segmenting the sentence into chunks that correspond, to some extent, to linguistic constituents, and categorizing these units appropriately. The first problem is an aspect of the general problem of *segmenting* speech into appropriate units (e.g., phonemes, words) and more generally is an aspect of perceptual grouping. The second problem is an aspect of the general problem of classifying linguistic units—for instance, recognizing different classes of phonemes or establishing the parts of speech of individual lexical items. The segmentation and classification problems need not be solved sequentially. Indeed, there may be mutual influence between the decision to segment a particular chunk of language and the decision that it can be classified in a particular way. Nonetheless, it is useful to keep the two aspects of the analysis of constituency conceptually separate.

It is also important to stress the difference between the problem of assigning constituent structure to novel sentences where the language is known and the problem of acquiring the constituent structure of an unknown language. Statistical symbolic parsers are able to make some inroads into the first problem (Charniak, 1993). For highly stylized language input, and given a prestored grammar, they can apply grammatical knowledge to establish one or more possible constituent structures for novel sentences. But symbolic methods are much less advanced in acquiring the constituent structure of language, because this requires solving the hard problem of learning a grammar from a set of sentences generated by that grammar. It is therefore in relation to the acquisition of constituency that connectionist methods, with their well-developed learning methods, have attracted the most interest.

We begin by considering models that focus on the problem of classifying, rather than segmenting, the linguistic input. One connectionist model (Finch and Chater, 1993) learns the part of speech of individual words by clustering words together on the basis of the immediate linguistic contexts in which they occur. The rationale is based on the replacement test mentioned earlier: if two words are observed to occur in highly similar immediate contexts in a corpus, they probably belong to the same syntactic category. Finch and Chater used a single-layer network with Hebbian learning to store co-occurrences between "target" words and their near neighbors. This allowed each target word to be associated with a vector representing the contexts in which it typically occurred. A competitive learning network classified these vectors, thus grouping together words with similar syntactic categories. This method is able to operate over unrestricted natural language, in contrast to most symbolic and connectionist models. From a linguistic perspective, the model slices lexical categories too finely, producing, for example, many word classes that correspond to nouns or verbs. On the other hand, the words within a class tend to be semantically related, which is useful from a cognitive perspective. The same method can be extended to classify sequences of words as NPs, VPs, etc. An initial classification of words is used to recode the input as a sequence of lexical constituents. Then, short sequences of lexical constituents are classified by their context, as before. The resulting groups of "phrases" (e.g., determiner-adjective-noun) are readily interpretable as NPs, and so on, but again, these groupings are too linguistically restrictive (i.e., only a small number of NPs are included in any particular cluster). Moreover, this phrasal level classification has not yet been implemented in a connectionist network.

A different attack on the problem of constituency involves training simple recurrent networks (SRNs) on linguistic input (Elman, 1990). An SRN involves a crucial modification to a feedforward network: the current set of hidden unit values is "copied back" to a set of additional input units, and paired with the *next* input to the network. The current hidden unit values can thus directly affect the next hidden unit values, providing the network with a memory for past inputs. This enables it to tackle sentence processing, where the input is revealed gradually over time rather than being presented at once.

Segmentation into constituents can be achieved in two ways by an SRN trained to *predict* the next input. One way is based on the assumption that predictability is higher within a constituent than across constituent boundaries, and hence that high prediction error indicates a boundary. This method has been advocated as potentially applicable at a range of linguistic levels (Elman, 1990), but in practice it has been successfully applied only on corpora of unrestricted natural language input in finding word boundaries (Cairns et al., 1997). Even here, the prediction strategy is a very partial cue to segmentation. If the network is provided with information about naturally occurring pauses between utterances (or parts of utterances), an alternative method is to assume that constituent boundaries occur where the network has an unusually high expectation of an *utterance boundary*. The rationale is that pauses tend to occur at constituent boundaries, and hence the prediction of a possible utterance boundary suggests that a constituent boundary may have occurred. This approach seems highly applicable to segmenting sentences into phrases, but it, too, has primarily been used for finding word boundaries in real corpora of language, when combined with other cues (Christiansen, Allen, and Seidenberg, 1998).

So far we have considered how SRNs might find constituents. But how well do they classify constituents? At the word level, cluster analysis of hidden unit activations shows that, to some extent, the hidden unit patterns associated with different word classes group naturally into syntactic categories, for SRNs trained on simple artificial grammars (Elman, 1990). These results are important because they show that even though the SRN may not learn to classify constituents explicitly, it is nevertheless able to *use* this information to process constituents appropriately.

Another way of assessing how SRNs have learned constituency is to see if they can generalize to predicting novel sentences of a language. The logic is that to predict successfully, the SRN must exploit linguistic regularities that are defined across constituents, and hence develop a notion of constituency to do so. However,

Hadley (1994) points out that this type of evidence is not compelling if the novel sentences are extremely similar to the network's training sentences. He suggests that, to show substantial evidence for generalization across constituents, the network should be able to handle novel sentences in which words appears in sentence locations where they have not previously occurred (see SYSTEMACITY OF GENERALIZATIONS IN CONNECTIONIST NETWORKS). For example, a novel sentence might involve a particular noun in object position, where it has previously occurred only in subject position. To generalize effectively, the network must presumably develop some abstract category of nouns. Christiansen and Chater (1994) demonstrated that an SRN can show this kind of generalization.

Despite this demonstration, though, connectionist models do not mirror classical constituency precisely. That is, they do not derive rigid classes of words and phrases that are interchangeable across contexts. Rather, they divide words and phrases into clusters without precisely defined boundaries, and they treat words and phrases differently, depending on the linguistic contexts in which they occur. This *context-sensitive* constituency can be viewed either as the undoing of connectionist approaches to language or as their radical contribution.

The potential problem with context-sensitive constituency is the productivity of language. To take Chomsky's famous example, how do we know that the statement *colorless green ideas sleep furiously* is syntactically correct, except by reference to a context-*in*sensitive representation of the relevant word classes? This seems necessary, because each word occurs in a context in which it has rarely been encountered before. But Allen and Seidenberg (1999) argue that this problem may not be fatal for context-sensitive notions of constituency. They trained a network to mutually associate two input sequences, a sequence of word forms and a corresponding sequence of word meanings. The network was able to learn a small artificial language successfully: it was able to regenerate the word forms from the meanings, and vice versa. Allen and Seidenberg then tested whether the network could recreate a sequence of word forms presented to it, by passing information from form to meaning and back. Ungrammatical sentences were recreated less accurately than grammatical sentences, and the network was thus able to distinguish grammatical from ungrammatical sentences. Importantly, this was true for sentences in which words appeared in novel combinations, as specified by Hadley's criterion and as exemplified by Chomsky's famous sentence. Thus, the context sensitivity of connectionist constituency may not rule out the possibility of highly creative and novel use of language, because abstract relations may be encoded at a semantic level as well as at the level of word forms.

If the apparent linguistic limitations of context-sensitive constituency can be overcome, then the potential psychological contribution of this notion is enormous. First, context sensitivity seems to be the norm throughout human classification. Second, much data on sentence processing seem most naturally to be explained by assuming that constituents are represented in a fuzzy and context-bound manner. The resulting opportunities for connectionist modeling of language processing are extremely promising. Thus, connectionist research may provide a more psychologically adequate notion of constituency than is currently available in linguistics.

Recursion

As with constituency, connectionist models have dealt with recursion in three increasingly radical ways. The least radical approach is to hardwire recursion into the network (e.g., as in Fanty's (1986) implementation of phrase structure rules) or to add an external symbolic ("first-in-last-out") stack to the model (e.g., as in Kwasny and Faisal's (1990) deterministic connectionist parser). In both cases, recursive generativity is achieved entirely through standard symbolic means, and although this is a perfectly reasonable approach to recursion, it adds nothing new to symbolic accounts of natural language recursion. The more radical connectionist approaches to recursion aim for networks to *learn* to deal with recursive structure. One approach is to construct a modular system of networks, each of which is trained to acquire different aspects of syntactic processing. For example, Miikkulainen's (1996) system consists of three different networks: one trained to map words onto case-role assignments, another trained to function as a stack, and a third trained to segment the input into constituent-like units. Although the model displays complex recursive abilities, the basis for these abilities and their generalization to novel sentence structures derive from the configuration of the stack network combined with the modular architecture of the system, rather than being discovered by the model. The most radical connectionist approaches to recursion attempt to learn recursive abilities with minimal prior knowledge built into the system. In this type of model, the network is most often required to discover both the constituent structure of the input and how these constituents can be recursively assembled into sentences. As with the similar approach to constituency described in the previous section, such models may provide new insights into the notion of recursion in human language processing.

Before discussing these modeling efforts, we need to assess to what extent recursion is observed in human language behavior. It is useful to distinguish *simple* and *complex* recursion. Simple recursion consists in recursively adding new material to the left (e.g., the adjective phrases (AP) in *the gray cat → the fat gray cat → the ugly fat gray cat*) or the right (e.g., the PPs in *the flowers in the vase → the flowers in the vase on the table → the flowers in the vase on the table by the window*) of existing phrase material. In complex recursion, new material is added in more complicated ways, such as through center-embedding of sentences (*The chef admired the musicians → The chef who the waiter appreciated admired the musicians*). Psycholinguistic evidence shows that people find simple recursion relatively easy to process, whereas complex recursion is almost impossible to process with more than one level of recursion. For instance, the following sentence with two levels of simple (right-branching) recursion, *The busboy offended the waiter who appreciated the chef who admired the musicians*, is much easier to comprehend than the comparable sentence with two levels of complex recursion, *The chef who the waiter who the busboy offended appreciated admired the musicians*. Because recursion is built into the symbolic models, there are no *intrinsic* limitations on how many levels of recursion can be processed. Instead, such models must invoke *extrinsic* constraints to accommodate the human performance asymmetry on simple and complex constructions. The radical connectionist approach models human performance directly without the need for extrinsic performance constraints.

The SRN model developed by Elman (1991) was perhaps the first connectionist attempt to simulate human behavior on recursive constructions. This network was trained on sentences generated by a small context-free grammar incorporating center-embedding and a single kind of right-branching recursive structure. In related work, Christiansen and Chater (1994) trained SRNs on a recursive artificial language incorporating four kinds of right-branching structures, a left-branching structure, and center-embedding. The behavior of these networks was qualitatively comparable with human performance in that the SRN predictions for right-branching structures were more accurate than on sentences of the same length involving center-embedding, and performance degraded appropriately as the depth of center-embedding increased. Weckerly and Elman (1992) further corroborated these results, suggesting that semantic bias (incorporated via co-occurrence restrictions on the verbs) can facilitate network performance in center-embedded constructions, similar to the semantic facilitation effects found in human processing. Using abstract artificial languages, Christiansen

and Chater (1999) showed that the SRN's general pattern of performance is relatively invariant across network size and training corpus, and concluded that the human-like pattern of performance derived from intrinsic constraints inherent to the SRN architecture.

Connectionist models of recursive syntax typically use "toy" fragments of grammar and small vocabularies. Aside from raising concerns over scaling-up, this makes it difficult to provide detailed fits with empirical data. Nonetheless, some attempts have recently been made to fit existing data and derive new empirical predictions from the models. For example, the Christiansen and Chater (1999) SRN model fits grammaticality rating data from several behavioral experiments, including an account of the relative processing difficulty associated with the processing of center-embeddings (with the following relationship between nouns and verbs: $N_1N_2N_3V_3V_2V_1$) versus cross-dependencies (with the following relationship between nouns and verbs: $N_1N_2N_3V_1V_2V_3$). Human data have shown that sentences with two center-embeddings (in German) are significantly harder to process than comparable sentences with two cross-dependencies (in Dutch). The simulation results demonstrated that the SRNs exhibited the same kind of qualitative processing difficulties as humans on these two types of complex recursive constructions.

Just as the radical connectionist approach to constituency deviates from classical constituency, the above approach to recursion deviates from the classical notion of recursion. The radical models of recursion do not acquire "true" recursion because they are unable to process infinitely complex recursive constructions. However, the classical notion of recursion may be ill-suited for capturing human recursive abilities. Indeed, the psycholinguistic data suggest that people's performance may be better construed as being only quasi-recursive. The semantic facilitation of recursive processing, mentioned earlier, further suggests that human recursive performance may be partially context sensitive. For example, the semantically biased sentence, *The bees that the hive that the farmer built housed stung the children*, is easier to comprehend than the neutral sentence, *The chef that the waiter that the busboy offended appreciated admired the musicians*, even though both sentences contain two center-embeddings. This dovetails with the context-sensitive notion of constituency and suggests that context sensitivity may be a more pervasive feature of language processing than is typically assumed by symbolic approaches.

Discussion

This article has outlined several ways in which constituency and recursion may be accommodated within a connectionist framework, ranging from direct implementation of symbolic systems to the acquisition of constituency and recursion from untagged input. We have focused on the radical approach, because this approach has the greatest potential to affect psycholinguistics and linguistic theory. However, much of this research is still preliminary. More work is needed to decide whether the promising but limited initial results can eventually be scaled up to deal with the complexities of real language input, or whether a radical connectionist approach is beset by fundamental limitations. Another challenge is to find ways—theoretically and practically—to interface models that have been proposed at different levels of linguistic analyses, such as models of morphology with models of sentence processing.

Nevertheless, the connectionist models described in this article have already influenced the study of language processing. First, connectionism has helped promote a general change toward replacing "box-and-arrow" diagrams with explicit computational models. Second, connectionism has reinvigorated the interest in computational models of learning, including learning properties, such as recursion and constituent structure, that were previously assumed to be innate. Finally, connectionism has helped increase interest in the statistical aspects of language learning and processing.

Connectionism has thus already had a considerable impact on the psychology of language. But the final extent of this influence depends on the degree to which practical connectionist models can be developed and extended to deal with complex aspects of language processing in a psychologically realistic way. If realistic connectionist models of language processing can be provided, then the possibility of a radical rethinking not just of the nature of language processing, but of the structure of language itself, may be required.

Road Map: Linguistics and Speech Processing
Background: Language Processing
Related Reading: Language Acquisition; Recurrent Networks: Learning Algorithms

References

Allen, J., and Seidenberg, M. S., 1999, The emergence of grammaticality in connectionist networks, in *The Emergence of Language* (B. MacWhinney, Ed.), Mahwah, NJ: Erlbaum, pp. 115–151.

Cairns, P., Shillcock, R. C., Chater, N., and Levy, J., 1997, Bootstrapping word boundaries: A bottom-up corpus-based approach to speech segmentation, *Cogn. Psychol.*, 33:111–153.

Charniak, E., 1993, *Statistical Language Learning*, Cambridge, MA: MIT Press. ◆

Christiansen, M. H., Allen, J., and Seidenberg, M. S., 1998, Learning to segment speech using multiple cues: A connectionist model, *Lang. Cogn. Proc.*, 13:221–268.

Christiansen, M. H., and Chater, N., 1994, Generalization and connectionist language learning, *Mind Lang.*, 9:273–287.

Christiansen, M. H., and Chater, N., 1999, Toward a connectionist model of recursion in human linguistic performance, *Cogn. Sci.*, 23:157–205. ◆

Elman, J. L., 1990, Finding structure in time, *Cogn. Sci.*, 14:179–211. ◆

Elman, J. L., 1991, Distributed representation, simple recurrent networks, and grammatical structure, *Machine Learn.*, 7:195–225.

Fanty, M. A., 1986, Context-free parsing with connectionist networks, in *Neural Networks for Computing* (J. S. Denker, Ed.), New York: American Institute of Physics, pp. 140–145.

Finch, S., and Chater, N., 1993, Learning syntactic categories: A statistical approach, in *Neurodynamics and Psychology* (M. Oaksford and G. D. A. Brown, Eds.), New York: Academic Press, pp. 295–321.

Hadley, R. F., 1994, Systematicity in connectionist language learning. *Mind Lang.*, 9:247–272.

Kim, A. E., Srinivas, B., and Trueswell, J. C., 2002, The convergence of lexicalist perspectives in psycholinguistics and computational linguistics, in *Sentence Processing and the Lexicon: Formal, Computational and Experimental Perspectives* (P. Merlo and S. Stevenson, Eds.), Amsterdam: John Benjamins Publishing, pp. 109–135.

Kwasny, S. C., and Faisal, K. A., 1990, Connectionism and determinism in a syntactic parser, *Connect. Sci.*, 2:63–82.

Miikkulainen, R., 1996, Subsymbolic case-role analysis of sentences with embedded clauses, *Cogn. Sci.*, 20:47–73.

Weckerly, J., and Elman, J. L., 1992, A PDP approach to processing center-embedded sentences, in *Proceedings of the Fourteenth Annual Meeting of the Cognitive Science Society*, Hillsdale, NJ: Erlbaum, pp. 414–419.

Contour and Surface Perception

Heiko Neumann and Ennio Mingolla

Introduction

Accumulating evidence from psychophysics and neurophysiology indicates that the computation of visual object representations is organized into parallel interacting subsystems, or streams, that consist of mechanisms following complementary processing strategies. *Boundary formation* proceeds by spatially linking oriented contrast measures along smooth contour patterns, whereas *perceptual surface* attributes, such as lightness or texture, are derived from local ratio measures of image contrast of regions taken along contours. Mechanisms of both subsystems mutually interact to resolve initial ambiguities and to generate coherent representations of surface layout.

Even when viewing single-gray-level images, people can discern important characteristics of visual scenes, including brightness, reflectance, surface orientation, texture, transparency, and relative depth. It has been proposed that these inferences are based on neural mechanisms that compute distinct and spatially registered representations of such characteristics or features, so-called *intrinsic images*. This approach has been formalized on the basis of statistical inference theory, in which the a posteriori likelihood of estimating several scene characteristics given the available image is optimized. Common to these approaches is the requirement that representations of intrinsic scene characteristics are constrained in order to guarantee the consistency of the set of solutions, which often involve smoothness assumptions for correlated feature estimates. These consistency constraints are typically based on the laws of physical image generation, such as Lambertian surface reflectance properties, and thus the overall process comprises an ideal observer seeking an optimal solution to the problem of inferring physical scene properties from images.

After briefly summarizing fundamental approaches to the computation of intrinsic scene characteristics, we consider an alternative literature of neural models of boundary and surface computation.

Intrinsic Images and the Neural Processing of Surface Layout

Barrow and Tenenbaum (1978) proposed a framework for machine vision based on computation of view-centered families of representations of local estimates of intrinsic scene characteristics, such as illumination, surface reflectance, and orientation. The resulting images are spatially registered with the single achromatic luminance image in which all the attributes are encoded pointwise. In order to regularize the inverse problem of computing several attributes from image data, several constraints, or assumptions, need to be incorporated into the recovery mechanisms. For example, in order to achieve the continuity of homogeneous surface attributes, each intrinsic image incorporates lateral smoothing of values in a discrete grid unless an edge breaks the local continuity. Discontinuities need to be in registration with intensity edges, and the recovered values for attributes need to fulfill the image irradiance equation at each grid point. This approach has been formalized in terms of coupled Markov random field (MRF) models in which the a posteriori probability for scene interpretation given an image, $p(scene|image) \propto \exp(-E/T)$ (E is an energy function that sums the image and prior constraints, T is a temperature term), can be maximized utilizing a stochastic sampling scheme (simulated annealing; see SIMULATED ANNEALING AND BOLTZMANN MACHINES). The MRF formulation allows us to incorporate a line pro-

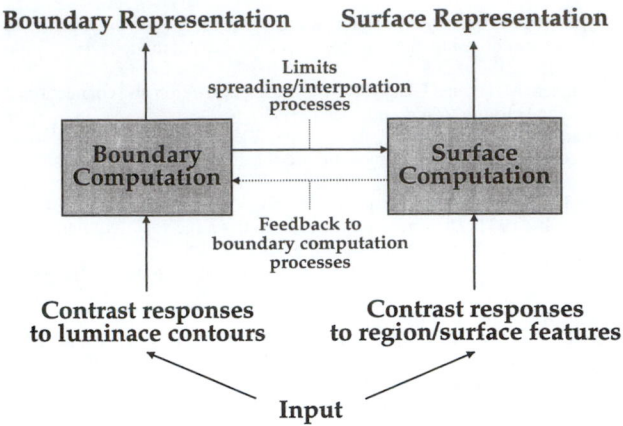

Boundary Representation   **Surface Representation**

Figure 1. Schematic of the macroscopic computational elements for computing boundaries and surfaces. The flow of computation is segregated into parallel but interacting streams to determine boundaries and surface attributes. See text for details.

cess (representing discontinuities) in the form of additional associated energy terms that can break the smoothness within an intrinsic attribute representation at locations where the tension of the recovered surface exceeds certain limits. These interactions correspond to the bidirectional coupling of boundary and surface computation depicted in Figure 1. More recent developments of the MRF approach take into account the computation of perceptual surface attributes, such as transparency (Kersten, 1991).

These approaches share the same basic computational principles: representations of smooth surface characteristics are generated by interpolating sparse data from initial estimates, and an edge map is extracted to depict the discontinuities in one or several attributes. In order to generate mutually consistent maps of intrinsic image characteristics, or attributes, the energy function used in the MRF model must utilize the prior probabilities of image characteristics, which in turn are derived from physical imaging models, e.g., for reflectance or transparency. In that sense the estimation process defines an ideal observer that utilizes knowledge about image formation by trying to invert the optical image generation process. Perceptual findings, however, indicate that, for example, an attribute such as lightness (the perceived surface reflectance) depends on surface size and that the judgment of surface orientation is unreliable over variations in surface curvature or lighting conditions. These observations cannot uniquely be accounted for by the intrinsic image approach, since size effects impose constraints not considered by such local processes as are employed in implementing an inverse optics solution.

In addition, line processes representing physical discontinuities in a surface property are modeled as separate MRFs. In order to be computationally tractable their prior probability structure is formulated over a small local pixel neighborhood only. Empirical observations again suggest that contour processes act over long spatial distances in order to reliably integrate contour fragments to form surface boundaries under variable imaging conditions. In all, these observations motivate the investigation of the neural mechanisms underlying the computation of perceptual boundaries and the subsequent assignment of surface attributes.

Elements of Spatial Long-Range Integration in Boundary Finding

Formal approaches to the Gestalt concept of *good continuation* have garnered increasing attention since Field, Hayes, and Hess

(1993) popularized the notion of an "association field," an elongated spatial zone aligned with oriented contour segments denoting facilitatory perceptual interactions with other segments. This geometry of spatial integration is summarized in the "bipole" icon of Figure 2, a figure-eight-shaped zone that was introduced as a "cooperative cell" unit in a neural network model for grouping by Grossberg and Mingolla (1985). The strength of spatial integration in the presently considered models is always some function of the distances and relative alignments of oriented units, such as contrast edges. Imagine that a contrast pattern occurs along the orientations denoted by the long axes of the dark and light ellipses at locations **x** and **x′**. The influence of the edge at the light ellipse on the representation of the contour strength in the region of the dark ellipse is calculated using the following fundamental quantities: (1) the distance, **r**, between the centers of the two ellipses; (2) the angle, ϑ, between the ray passing through the centers of the two ellipses and the principal axis of the dark ellipse; and (3) the difference in orientation, φ, of the principal axes of the two ellipses.

The bipole shape expresses the region of relatively high coupling strength for the influence of contour segments remote from the central ellipse on a unit whose positional and orientational preferences are denoted by the ellipse at the center. Its shape and connectivity pattern is justified by recent investigations in psychophysics, physiology, and anatomy. For example, the co-occurrence of edge segments in natural scenes have been shown to have a bipole distribution, and cortical cells of similar orientation selectivity in tree shrew are preferentially connected along the axis of their visuotopic alignment to cells of compatible orientational preference (see Neumann and Mingollia, 2001, for details). Thus, the bipole icon for grouping of contour segments, originally suggested on intuitive grounds, is validated by a growing body of empirical data.

The bipole concept can be embedded in a framework in which the pattern of connectivity among relatively tightly coupled neural units is described formally by a *spatial weighting*, or kernel, function, coding the strength of connections between units in a spatial array. Items that are closely spaced are more likely to be grouped than candidates that are located far apart. The underlying neighborhood function often selectively facilitates a sector of a spatial surround to define an anisotropic coupling that is compatible with the feature domain. Elementary features along dimensions such as (tangential) orientation, motion direction, and disparity provide the

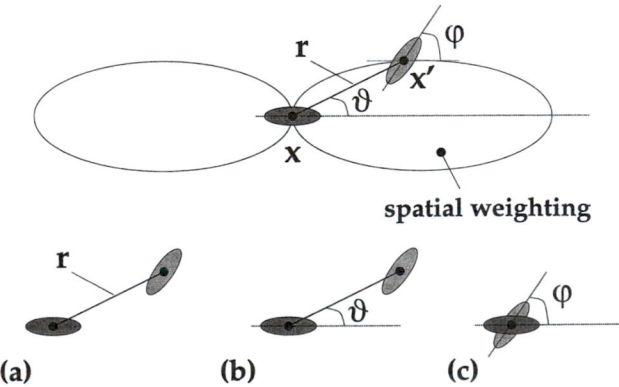

spatial weighting

(a)   **(b)**   **(c)**

Figure 2. *Top*, The "bipole icon" for modeling feature integration in spatial grouping. The quantity to be assessed is the "contribution" of activation in an oriented unit, denoted by the light ellipse, to the activation at the center unit, denoted by the dark ellipse. *Bottom*, The figure-eight shape of a bipole expresses relations among three fundamental quantities: (a) the distance, **r**, between spatial locations, (b) the angle, ϑ, between the virtual line and the target orientation, and (c) the difference in orientation, φ, of the two ellipses.

dimensions of the visual representation space. The feature *relatability* (or *compatibility*) between stimulus items is defined along these dimensions. Herein, the most likely appearance of meaningful structure is encoded to represent "what feature goes with what." In the following treatment we will focus on grouping mechanisms for static form processing and therefore consider only *orientation* as the relevant feature dimension.

The result of integration of items defines the *support* of a localized feature measurement at a given spatial location based on the configuration of other items. Based on the bipole structure of left and right subfields (Figure 2), the support of a target item can be defined as a function

$$\text{support}_{xy,feature} = \{\text{left-input}_{xy,feature}\} \circ \{\text{right-input}_{xy,feature}\} \quad (1)$$

where $\circ$ denotes some operation to define the *combination of subfields*. Subscripts *xy* denote spatial locations in a two-dimensional (2D) retinotopic map, and *feature* identifies the feature dimension involved in the grouping process—in our case, *orientation*. The *activation* of the corresponding target cell results as a function $f(\cdot)$ of the support. The formal description of the mechanisms underlying the computation of activations "left-input" and "right-input," respectively, necessitates the detailed specification of the interaction of activities in grouping.

In most models the connectivity pattern of the relatable features is prespecified, or *programmed*, referring to some measure of geometric entities. These are designed to encode static efficacies between *n*-tuples, e.g., pairs, of feature measurements at given locations optimizing a given functionality. To date, few approaches have investigated the possible *self-organization* of such lateral interactions in a neural architecture. Note that the spatial weighting function and the feature relatability define the components of the net *coupling strength*. This function specifies a metric for the similarity measure in the ⟨*xy, feature*⟩-space and thus defines the distance function of *feature cooperation* for the clustering of a visual pattern in accordance with a relatability measure that underlies the visual interpolation in spatial grouping for object recognition (Kellman and Shipley, 1991). *Input activations* at the different sites are necessary to gather any support. Here, two different types of interactions can be distinguished: (1) a convergent feedforward mechanism is defined when the *bottom-up* input is integrated at the target location, whereas (2) a mechanism of (nonlinear) *lateral* interaction is defined when activity is horizontally integrated within a neural layer.

Taken together, the activation of, say, "left-input" derived from the feature integration process using the bipole mechanism is computed by

$$\text{left-input}_{\mathbf{x}\theta} = \sum_{\mathbf{x}'\phi} \{\text{act}_{\mathbf{x}'\phi} \cdot \text{relate}_{\mathbf{x}\mathbf{x}'\theta\phi} \cdot \text{weight}^L_{\mathbf{x}\mathbf{x}'\theta}\} \quad (2)$$

where "weight" denotes the spatial weighting kernel, "relate" the feature relatability, and "act" the input activations. The "right-input" activity is computed similarly. Here, $\mathbf{x} = (x, y)$ and θ correspond to the location and orientation of the target feature, respectively. Other parameters refer to the specific location ⟨$\mathbf{x}'$, ϕ⟩ in the space-orientation neighborhood (see Figure 2).

Grouping Models and Their Components

The initial processing stages of these models consist of some form of filtering the input luminance image. A (possibly nonlinear) center-surround mechanism (resembling segregated ON and OFF contrast channels at the retina and LGN) computes contrast ratios throughout the image. These outputs drive oriented simple and complex cells, which are often modeled as localized spatial frequency filters, such as Gabor or wavelet kernels. Their output of different orientation fields defines the interface representation for subsequent grouping processes. We focus on those models that (1) have their roots in the explanation of empirical data and (2) were most influential for subsequent scientific developments. A comprehensive treatment can be found in Neumann and Mingolla (2001).

The Boundary Contour System (BCS) has been developed as part of a unified modeling framework called FACADE (Form-And-Color-And-DEpth). As described by Ross, Gossberg, and Mingolla (2000), the BCS consists of a series of boundary detection, competition, and cooperation stages. The general layout of basic processing stages is presented in Figure 3 (left). Long-range boundary cooperation of this scheme (stage 3) accomplishes the grouping of consistent boundaries and the completion of interrupted boundaries. Spatial weighting and relatability, as elements of the support function, in this model are defined as $\text{weight}^{L/R}_{\mathbf{x}\mathbf{x}'\theta} = [\pm\Gamma^{rad}_{\mathbf{x}\mathbf{x}'} \cdot \Gamma^{ang}_{\mathbf{x}\mathbf{x}'\theta}]^+$ (for a scheme separable in polar coordinates; $[\cdot]^+$ denoting half-wave rectification) and $\text{relate}_{\mathbf{x}\mathbf{x}'\theta\phi} = \cos^q(2 \tan^{-1}((y' - y)/(x' - x)) - (\theta + \phi))$ (for a co-circularity constraint; q controlling the angular width of the lobes). The support and activation function is computed employing bipole cells that fire only if both lobes of their integration fields are sufficiently activated. The left/

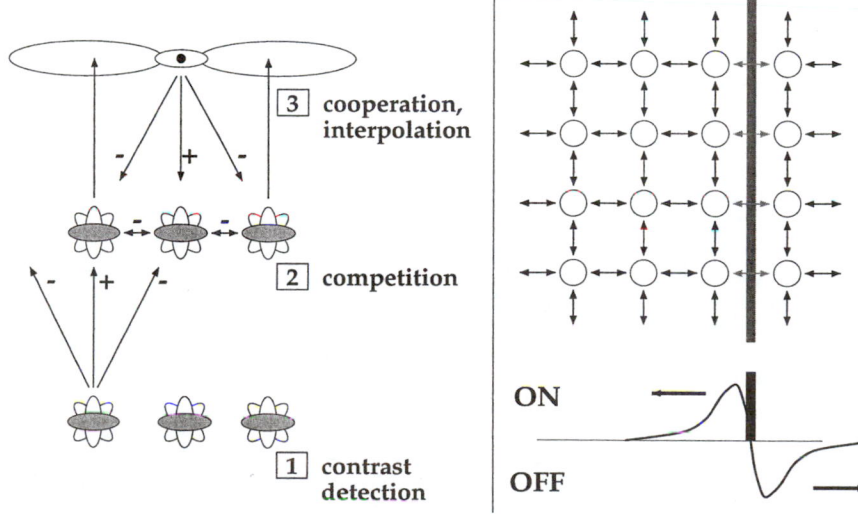

Figure 3. Details of the mechanisms involved in boundary and surface computations. *Left*, The three major stages for *boundary computation* involve contrast detection and competition between responses in space and orientation domain. Resulting responses are integrated over longer distances utilizing oriented bipoles, which lead to on-center/off-surround feedback interaction. *Right*, Lateral interaction for *surface computation* between sites of a regular grid. Local contrast signals measured near boundaries are laterally propagated to fill in regions void of activities. The lateral interaction is controlled by an inhibitory mechanism to reduce or switch off lateral couplings by high boundary activation, as indicated by the light shaded arrows. See text for details.

3 | cooperation, interpolation

2 | competition

1 | contrast detection

ON

OFF

right subfield combination thus realizes a multiplicative, or AND gate, combination of input terms. The cooperative-competitive (CC) feedback loop between stages 1 and 3 (Figure 3, left) acts to complete and enhance spatially and orientationally consistent boundary groupings while inhibiting inconsistent ones, thereby also suppressing noise. This mechanism of long-range completion is also capable of signaling boundaries over gaps in the image, that is, over regions void of any contrast signals, and thus can generate illusory contours for images in which humans perceive them.

Relaxation labeling schemes have been developed as optimization procedures to find consistent interpretations for measurement problems with uncertainty. The computational goal seeks to achieve a consistent labeling assigning graded activations, or probabilities, to a limited set of labels for nodes in a graph representation. For contour integration, the labeling problem can be formulated as one of finding the most likely set of orientations for discrete grid locations corresponding to the graph nodes (a "no-line" label is taken into account to represent the nonresponsiveness of cells at locations that are not boundary elements). Parent and Zucker (1989) determine unambiguous orientation estimates along contours by evaluating consistency constraints based on a measure of compatibility between pairs of orientations. Initial responses are generated by oriented filters (Figure 3, left, stage 1) that were normalized in order to allow filter activations treated as probabilities for assigning orientation labels (stage 2). The individual strengths for orientation measures at a given image location are iteratively updated through the support that is gathered from relatable activities in a spatial neighborhood. Spatial weighting and relatability are defined as $\text{weight}_{\mathbf{xx}'\theta}^{L/R} = P_{\mathbf{xx}'\theta}^{length,L/R} \cdot d(\mathbf{x}, \mathbf{x}')$, where P denotes a predicate to compensate for path length differences on discrete grids and $d(\cdot)$ compensates for differences in interpixel distances, and $\text{relate}_{\mathbf{xx}'\theta\phi} = c_{\mathbf{xx}'\theta\phi} \cdot K_{\mathbf{xx}'\theta\phi}^k \cdot C_{\mathbf{xx}'\theta\phi}^{kk'}$. Here the co-circularity measure c is augmented by two binary predicates to exclude any candidates of incompatible local contour curvature. Input activations in the orientation field are thinned by nonmaximum suppression in order to generate localized representations of contours. The support and activation function is computed by integrating responses from the subfields of the spatial weighting functions (stage 3). Activities are iteratively updated by a nonlinear recurrent competitive/cooperative mechanism.

Contrary to the previous approaches, Heitger et al. (1998) proposed a feedforward scheme of successive filtering for contour grouping that selectively integrates activities from oriented single end-stopped (ES) filters, which respond to, e.g., line ends and corners. The result of such grouping is combined with the representation of oriented contrast responses to generate a final contour map. The core mechanism of grouping again utilizes spatial weighting functions (bipoles) virtually equivalent to those of the BCS (Figure 3, left, stage 3). Two grouping rules are distinguished for corners (para grouping) and line ends (ortho grouping). The responses of ortho and para grouping are linearly interpolated. Different curvature classes are distinguished, similar to the relaxation scheme (see above), by partitioning the bipoles into subfields such that only some of them in the left lobe can cooperate with their counterparts in the right lobe. Left/right lobes are combined in a multiplicative fashion via an AND-gating mechanism, similar to the BCS approach. This makes the grouping scheme selective to complete activations between localized ES features. The elongated bipole lobes are also capable of signaling boundaries over gaps, and thus generate illusory contours. This model does not incorporate any feedback mechanism and must, therefore, employ some stages of postprocessing in order to sharpen the final boundary response.

Based on the previous "core models," other approaches have been developed that elaborate aspects of the general framework. For example, random walks of particles in a discrete lattice of the sampled space-orientation domain have been investigated to determine the paths of spatially relatable items at a given location (x, y, θ) and another point (i, j, ϕ). Particles were initiated at sparse keypoint locations corresponding to localized responses of ES cells. The probability densities in the stochastic completion field represent the strengths—and therefore likelihood—of smooth paths connecting pairs of key points. Another study investigated how V1 horizontal long-range integration could functionally account for the enhancement of texture region boundaries and pop-out effects in visual search. Here, the spatial integration field is subdivided into spatially nonoverlapping parts of excitatory and inhibitory contribution. An elongated bipole integrates activities of cells oriented such that they form smooth interpolations with the target cell at the bipole center. Activities of like orientation from a sector orthogonal to the target cell orientation generate the inhibitory signal. In a similar spirit, a scheme of excitatory long-range integration has been used that consists of two spatial regions: one coaxial bipole with cocircular relatability and one sector that extends orthogonally from the target cell's orientation axis and integrates units oriented parallel to that of the cell. The latter component contributes to a facilitation of simple symmetric shape axes. Each cell inhibits itself based on a threshold of the average input from its immediate neighbors, so that only salient arrangements produce a net output.

Contrast integration for boundary grouping addresses the particularly important question about what the core principles are that underlie the establishing of spatial integration and grouping. Yet there still is an ongoing debate about the role of feedforward and feedback mechanisms involved in spatial grouping and the dominance of their individual contributions in visual processing. Aspects of *temporal coding* principles based on oscillator mechanisms or spiking neurons may play another important role in grouping tasks. Several neurophysiological studies indicate that distributed representations of related scene fragments are linked by temporally correlated, or synchronized, neural activation. The temporal coding hypothesis studied in isolation appears, however, to be incomplete. The temporal establishment of grouping addresses the signaling of binding, but not the "how" or "what" of its computation. The mechanisms of oriented long-range interactions for integration provide the underlying basis for grouping to establish perceptual items related to surface boundaries.

Complementary Mechanisms of Surface Perception

The computation of perceptual surface qualities complements the formation of their boundaries. Image regions that are sufficiently homogeneous in luminance or statistical distribution of contrasts can give rise to the impression of color, texture, brightness, or lightness, also known as achromatic color. How is the generation of smooth representations of surface qualities accomplished? Paradiso and Nakayama (1991) provided compelling psychophysical evidence for a long-hypothesized neural process that propagates local estimates of lightness from boundaries into region interiors. Further psychophysical as well as physiological investigations of temporal properties of brightness and texture filling-in revealed further details of the neural machinery underlying the integration of perceptual surface properties.

Computational models for the generation of perceptual surface quantities generally pursue one of three basic strategies: (1) filtering and rule-based symbolic interpretation, (2) spatial integration via inverse filtering and labeling, or (3) filling-in. In the first scheme, (nonlinear) combinations of filter responses and subsequent rule-based decision operations lead to the final prediction of lightness. The latter two approaches both begin with local luminance ratios estimated along boundaries. Computation of surface qualities proceeds by propagating local estimates into region interiors in order to generate a spatially contiguous representation of homogeneous properties (Figure 3, right). In the spatial integration approach, the lateral propagation is the consequence of an iterative process to invert previous spatial derivative operations labeling region interiors with estimates of quantities derived at region boundaries. Filling-in approaches spread activity in a neural map such that at locations coding region interiors, activation is generated by a spatial diffusion process integrating estimates of local contrasts from remote boundaries.

Spatial filtering approaches utilize initial stages of either isotropic or oriented filters, or both, over multiple bandpass channels of spatial frequency. The filter outputs are scaled nonlinearly by a gain-control mechanism and thresholded, individually interpreted by a set of rules, and finally combined over several scales. In two dimensions this strategy leads to results that depend on the direction of the sequential application of interpretation rules. Authors pursue a simple averaging of results from forward and backward scanning over different orientations (McArthur and Moulden, 1999). Approaches in this category follow a tradition that the input luminance distribution is processed through a sequence of filtering steps during the early stages of the visual system. It is assumed that specific features in the responses directly contribute to observable brightness effects by implicitly propagating local qualities into region interiors as a consequence of applying some interpretation rules.

Spatial integration models attempt to recover object lightness of a surface by utilizing the sequence of processing stages *Filtering/ Differentiation → Boundaries/Thresholding → Integration*. Differentiation and subsequent thresholding operations are intended to detect salient changes in the luminance signal, which in turn trigger the integration from local luminance ratios. Luminance ratios provide the basis to infer surface-related properties that are invariant against gradual illumination changes, thus discounting the illuminant. Furthermore, lightness can be influenced by luminances at regions remote from each other. The Retinex algorithm by Land and McCann (1971) accounts for these observations by integrating contrasts along several pathways of different lengths. The logarithms of luminance ratios at thresholded contrast locations are summed such that, as a net effect, ratios measured between the target region and distant regions are integrated and averaged. A center-surround interaction accounts for this process in an approximate form. Alternative formulations of lightness integration numerically invert the differentiated 2D luminance image. Under certain boundary conditions a unique solution exists that can be computed by numerical techniques (Hurlbert, 1986). Changes in reflectance properties occur locally, thus comprising a high spatial frequency pattern, while inhomogeneous illumination constitutes a phenomenon at low spatial frequencies. Suppression of influences in low spatial frequencies could be achieved by homomorphic filtering in which low-frequency components are reduced or even suppressed and higher frequencies are amplified. Following this idea, approximate approaches for lightness computation utilize multiple spatial frequency channels of center-surround mechanisms based on divisive, or shunting, interactions of different scales.

As a second computational strategy of spatial integration models, *filling-in* approaches proceed by taking local ratios along boundaries and subsequently propagate these measures into the void spaces of bounded regions. Generating a representation of surface quality utilizes the processing stages *Filtering → Boundaries → Filling-in*. The algorithm proposed by Grossberg and Todorović (1988) was the first implementation in two dimensions of the complementary operations of the combined BCS and Feature Contour System (FCS) model of brightness perception that was able to explain a wide variety of phenomena, such as simultaneous contrast and the Craik-O'Brien-Cornsweet illusion. The model was later demonstrated to also account for the temporal properties of brightness filling-in (Paradiso and Nakayama, 1991). Filling-in of local

contrast ratios taken along extended figural boundaries is laterally propagated in a diffusion process. Such a diffusion is controlled by a gradual permeability function Y utilizing a boundary signal such as the one generated by mechanisms of long-range integration (compare Figure 2 and Figure 3, right). This renders filling-in a spatially inhomogeneous diffusion process that generates a maximum likelihood (regularized) solution of a brightness surface given the sparse contrast estimates at the boundaries, where Y is monotonically decreasing to split apart regions of homogeneous surface properties. In the case that the function Y is solely controlled by an auxiliary boundary signal, the function solves a simple gradient descent of finding a dense activity distribution representing surface brightness. In general, Y could also depend on gradients of the filling-in signal itself, such that boundary *and* surface computation become mutually interdependent (dotted arrow in Figure 1) and the overall system becomes nonlinear.

Ross and Pessoa (2000) describe an important extension of previous models by suggesting a context-sensitive weighting of contrast measures prior to a final integration stage. Emphasis is put on a computational mechanism that tags boundaries from contrast detection and grouping to (partially) segment an image into different context domains. The segmentation is triggered by the presence of T-junctions, which are used as seed points to propagate the tagging signal along the roof of the Ts and the adjoining smooth boundary segments, thus generating a map of context boundaries. These boundaries are subsequently used to suppress initial contrast measures along the corresponding contours via a gating mechanism. As a result, the contribution of contrast measures that could lead to erroneous lightness estimates over segmentation boundaries is reduced or even suppressed. This computational mechanism is capable of producing region lightness estimates that account for several effects that have been previously shown to be unexplainable by simple local mechanisms of contrast integration, e.g., White's effect, the Benary cross, and Adelson's folded-card stimuli.

Although not described here, the FACADE model, with which the Ross and Pessoa model has certain parallels, proposes related explanations of the just-mentioned and related lightness effects (Grossberg, 1994). FACADE has also been developed to account for the perception of such phenomena as amodal surface completion, whereby occluded portions of objects are sensed as being present in specific locations behind foreground objects, and more generally the separation of surface regions seen as figures from backgrounds. The development of this and other models (Heitger et al., 1998) that attempt to account for more complex aspects of surface perception than are captured in planar arrays indicates that an exciting new phase of inquiry into surface perception is under way.

Stochastic Formulation of Boundary/Surface Computations

In the tradition of intrinsic image architectures, some approaches formulate the above-outlined boundary and surface computations in a Bayesian framework. For example, Lee (1995) utilized a variant of a nonlinear diffusion mechanism that incorporated piecewise smoothness of filling-in domains that were separated by contour segments denoting breaks in the smooth surface signal. Statistical signals from initial responses of oriented Gabor filters of different frequency selectivity served as filling-in signals. These inputs were subsequently diffused in the space-frequency domain incorporating a spatial modulation by the boundary signal. Mutual interaction between boundary and surface processes were modeled as MRF processes in which Bayesian priors propagated bidirectionally and interacted through local connections in each area. Since this approach focuses on texture region segregation, an explicit modeling of the optical image generation process, as in classical intrinsic image approaches, is not necessary here. This renders the model a Bayesian interpretation of above-mentioned neural processes for surface/boundary extraction.

Discussion

We have seen that the key stages of a common framework of computational models for generating perceptual surface representations utilize separate subsystems for boundary and surface computation. Depending on the modeling framework, different processes of mutual interaction are defined to achieve the goal of generating a coherent representation of object surfaces and their attributes. Modeling the *neural* processes of a perceptual surface layout has focused on the processes of contour completion based on long-range integration based on some variation of the structure of the bipole kernel and a number of additional computational principles in evaluating related activities in feature space. The bipole kernel itself graphically visualizes the oriented fan-like connectivity between sites in a space-orientation feature space.

In comparison with processes of boundary finding, the situation with respect to surface quality perception is considerably less developed, most especially with respect to attributes such as texture perception, which we have not reviewed. All models presented are based on some mechanism to laterally propagate activities to interpolate and smooth sparse estimates. Improved empirical techniques juxtaposed with hypotheses developed by computational modelers offer the hope that coming years will see a convergence in this area, as has already occured in the field of contour completion.

Road Map: Vision
Related Reading: Global Visual Pattern Extraction; Laminar Cortical Architecture in Visual Perception; Perception of Three-Dimensional Structure; Stereo Correspondence

References

Barrow, H. G., and Tenenbaum, J. M., 1978, Recovering intrinsic scene characteristics from images, in *Computer Vision Systems* (A. R. Hanson and E. M. Riseman, Eds.), New York: Academic Press, pp. 3–26.

Field, D. J., Hayes, A., and Hess, R. F., 1993, Contour integration by the human visual system: Evidence for a local "association field," *Vision Res.*, 33:173–193.

Grossberg, S., 1994, 3-D vision and figure-ground separation by visual cortex, *Percept. Psychophys.*, 55:48–120.

Grossberg, S., and Mingolla, E., 1985, Neural dynamics of perceptual grouping: Textures, boundaries, and emergent segmentation, *Percept. Psychophys.*, 38:141–171.

Grossberg, S., and Todorović, D., 1988, Neural dynamics of 1-D and 2-D brightness perception: A unified model of classical and recent phenomena, *Percept. Psychophys.*, 43:723–742.

Heitger, F., von der Heydt, R., Peterhans, E., Rosenthaler, L., and Kübler, O., 1998, Simulation of neural contour mechanisms: Representing anomalous contours, *Image Vision Comput.*, 16:407–421.

Hurlbert, A., 1986, Formal connections between lightness algorithms, *J. Opt. Soc. Am. A*, 3:1684–1693. ◆

Kellman, P. J., and Shipley, T. F., 1991, A theory of visual interpolation in object perception, *Cognit. Psychol.*, 23:141–221. ◆

Kersten, D., 1991, Transparency and the computation of scene attributes, in *Computational Models of Visual Processing* (M. S. Landy and J. A. Movshon, Eds.), Cambridge, MA: MIT Press, pp. 209–228. ◆

Land, E. H., and McCann, J. J., 1971, Lightness and Retinex theory, *J. Opt. Soc. Am.*, 61:1–11.

Lee, T. S., 1995, A Bayesian framework for understanding texture segmentation in the primary visual cortex, *Vision Res.*, 35:2643–2657.

McArthur, J. A., and Moulden, B., 1999, A two-dimensional model of brightness perception based on spatial filtering consistent with retinal processing, *Vision Res.*, 39:1199–219.

Neumann, H., and Mingolla, E., 2001, Computational neural models of spatial integration in perceptual grouping, in *From Fragments to Objects: Grouping and Segmentation in Vision* (T. F. Shipley and P. J. Kellman, Eds.), Amsterdam: Elsevier, pp. 354–400. ◆

Paradiso, M. A., and Nakayama, K., 1991, Brightness perception and filling-in, *Vis. Res.*, 31:1221–1236.

Parent, P., and Zucker, S., 1989, Trace inference, curvature consistency, and curve detection, *IEEE Trans. Pattern Anal. Machine Intell.*, 11:823–839.

Ross, W. D., Grossberg, S., and Mingolla, E., 2000, Visual cortical mechanisms of perceptual grouping: Interacting layers, networks, columns, and maps, *Neural Netw.*, 13:571–588.

Ross, W. D., and Pessoa, L., 2000, Lightness from contrast: A selective integration model, *Percept. Psychophys.*, 62:1160–1181.

Convolutional Networks for Images, Speech, and Time Series

Yann LeCun and Yoshua Bengio

Introduction

The ability of multilayer backpropagation networks to learn complex, high-dimensional, nonlinear mappings from large collections of examples makes them obvious candidates for image recognition or speech recognition tasks (see PATTERN RECOGNITION). In the traditional model of pattern recognition, a hand-designed feature extractor gathers relevant information from the input and eliminates irrelevant variabilities. A trainable classifier then categorizes the resulting feature vectors (or strings of symbols) into classes. In this scheme, standard, fully connected multilayer networks can be used as classifiers. A potentially more interesting scheme is to eliminate the feature extractor, feeding the network "raw" inputs (e.g., normalized images) and relying on learning algorithms to turn the first few layers into an appropriate feature extractor. Although this can be done with an ordinary fully connected feedforward network with some success for tasks such as character recognition, there are problems.

Firstly, typical images, or spectral representations of spoken words, are large, often with several hundred variables. A fully connected first layer with, say a few hundred hidden units would already contain tens of thousands of weights. Overfitting problems may occur if training data are scarce. In addition, the memory requirement for that many weights may rule out certain hardware implementations. But the main deficiency of unstructured nets for image or speech applications is that they have no built-in invariance with respect to translations or local distortions of the inputs. Before being sent to the fixed-size input layer of a neural net, character images, spoken word spectra, or other two-dimensional (2D) or one-dimensional (1D) signals must be approximately size normalized and centered in the input field. Unfortunately, no such preprocessing can be perfect: handwriting is often normalized at the word level, which can cause size, slant, and position variations for individual characters; and words can be spoken at varying speed, pitch, and intonation. This causes variations in the position of distinctive features in input objects. In principle, a fully connected network of sufficient size could learn to produce outputs that are invariant with respect to such variations. However, learning such a task would probably result in multiple units with identical weight patterns positioned at various locations in the input. Learning these weight configurations requires a very large number of training instances to cover the space of possible variations. Conversely, in convolutional networks, shift invariance is automatically obtained by forcing the replication of weight configurations across space.

Secondly, a deficiency of fully connected architectures is that the topology of the input is entirely ignored. The input variables can be presented in any (fixed) order without affecting the outcome of the training. But images, or spectral representations of speech, have a strong 2D local structure, and time series have a strong 1D structure: variables (or pixels) that are spatially or temporally nearby are highly correlated. Local correlations are the reasons for the well-known advantages of extracting and combining *local* features before recognizing spatial or temporal objects. Convolutional networks force the extraction of local features by restricting the receptive fields of hidden units to be local.

Convolutional Networks

Convolutional networks combine three architectural ideas to ensure some degree of shift and distortion invariance: local receptive fields, shared weights (or weight replication), and, sometimes, spatial or temporal subsampling. A typical convolutional network for recognizing characters is shown in Figure 1 (from LeCun et al., 1990). The input plane receives images of characters that are approximately size normalized and centered. Each unit of a layer receives inputs from a set of units located in a small neighborhood in the previous layer. The idea of connecting units to local receptive fields on the input goes back to the perceptron in the early 1960s, and was almost simultaneous with Hubel and Wiesel's discovery of locally sensitive, orientation-selective neurons in the cat's visual system. Local connections have been reused many times in neural models of visual learning (see Mozer, 1991; see also NEOCOGNITRON: A MODEL FOR VISUAL PATTERN RECOGNITION). With local receptive fields, neurons can extract elementary visual features such as oriented edges, end points, or corners (or similar features in speech spectrograms). These features are then combined by the higher layers. As stated earlier, distortions or shifts of the input can cause the position of salient features to vary. In addition, elementary feature detectors that are useful on one part of the image are likely to be useful across the entire image. This knowledge can be applied by forcing a set of units whose receptive fields are located at different places on the image to have identical weight vectors (Rumelhart, Hinton, and Williams, 1986). The outputs of such a set of neurons constitute a *feature map*. At each position, different types of units in different feature maps compute different types of features. A sequential implementation of this, for each feature map, would be to scan the input image with a single neuron that has a local receptive field and to store the states of this neuron at corresponding locations in the feature map. This operation is equivalent to a convolution with a small-size kernel, followed by a squashing function. The process can be performed in parallel by implementing the feature map as a plane of neurons that *share* a single weight vector. Units in a feature map are constrained to perform the same operation on different parts of the image. A convolutional layer is usually composed of several feature maps (with different weight vectors), so that multiple features can be extracted at each location. The first hidden layer in Figure 1 has four feature maps with 5 × 5 receptive fields. Shifting the input of a convolutional layer will shift the output but leave it unchanged otherwise. Once a feature has been detected, its exact location becomes less important, as long as its approximate position relative to other features is preserved. Therefore, each convolutional layer is followed by an additional layer that performs a local averaging and a subsampling, reducing the resolution of the feature map, and reducing the sensitivity of the output to shifts and distortions. The second hidden layer in Figure 1 performs 2 × 2 averaging and subsampling, followed by a trainable coefficient, a trainable bias, and a sigmoid. The trainable coefficient and bias control the effect of the squashing nonlinearity (for example, if the coefficient is small, then the neuron operates in a quasi-linear mode). Successive layers of convolutions and subsampling are typically alternated, resulting in a *bi-pyramid* at each layer, the number of feature maps is increased as the spatial resolution is decreased. Each unit in the third hidden layer in Figure 1 may have input connections from several feature maps in the previous layer. The convolution/subsampling combination, inspired by Hubel and Wiesel's notions of "simple" and "complex" cells, was implemented in the neocognitron model, although no globally supervised learning procedure such as backpropagation was available then.

Since all the weights are learned with backpropagation, convolutional networks can be seen as synthesizing their own feature extractor. The weight-sharing technique has the interesting side effect of reducing the number of free parameters, thereby reducing the "capacity" of the machine and improving its generalization ability (see LeCun, 1989, on weight sharing, and LEARNING AND GENERALIZATION: THEORETICAL BOUNDS for an explanation of capacity and generalization). The network in Figure 1 contains about 100,000 connections, but only about 2,600 free parameters because

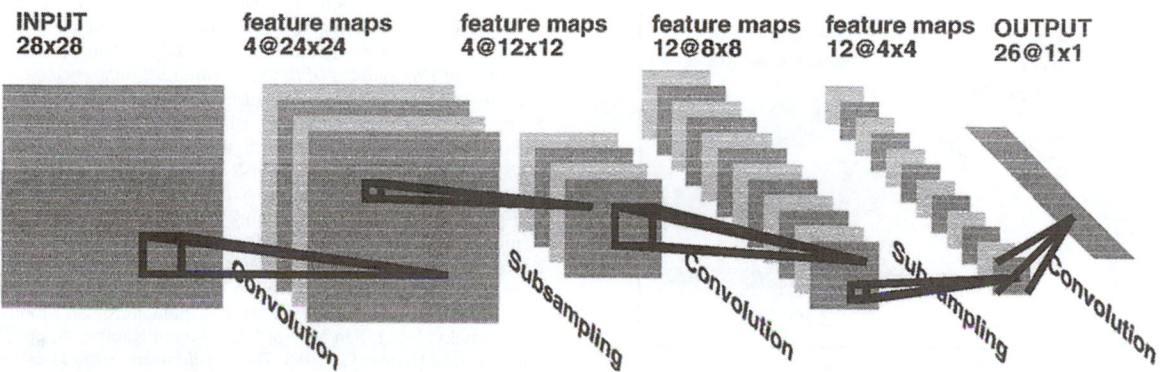

Figure 1. Convolutional neural network for image processing, e.g., handwriting recognition.

of the weight sharing. Such networks compare favorably with other methods on handwritten character recognition tasks (Bottou et al., 1994; see also PATTERN RECOGNITION), and they have been deployed in commercial applications (LeCun et al., 1998).

Fixed-size convolutional networks that share weights along a single temporal dimension are known as time-delay neural networks (TDNNs). TDNNs have been used in phoneme recognition (without subsampling) (Lang and Hinton, 1988; Waibel et al., 1989), spoken word recognition (with subsampling) (Bottou et al., 1990), and on-line handwriting recognition (Guyon et al., 1991).

Variable-Size Convolutional Networks: SDNNs

While characters or short spoken words can be size normalized and fed to a fixed-size network, more complex objects such as written or spoken words and sentences have inherently variable size. One way of handling such a composite object is to segment it heuristically into simpler objects that can be recognized individually (e.g., characters, phonemes). However, reliable segmentation heuristics do not exist for speech or cursive handwriting. A brute force solution is to scan (or replicate) a recognizer at all possible locations across the input. While this can be prohibitively expensive in general, convolutional networks can be scanned or replicated very efficiently over large, variable-size input fields. Consider one instance of a convolutional net and its alter ego at a nearby location. Because of the convolutional nature of the networks, units in the two nets that look at identical locations on the input have identical outputs; therefore their output does not need to be computed twice. In effect, replicating a convolutional network can be done simply by increasing the size of the field over which the convolutions are performed and replicating the output layer, effectively making it a convolutional layer (see Figure 2). An output whose receptive field is centered on an elementary object will produce the class of this object, while an in-between output may be empty or may contain garbage. The outputs can be interpreted as evidence for the categories of objects centered at different positions of the input field. A postprocessor is therefore required to pull out consistent interpretations of the output. Hidden Markov models (HMMs) or other graph-based methods are often used for that purpose (see LeCun et al., 1998; see also HIDDEN MARKOV MODELS, SPEECH RECOGNITION TECHNOLOGY, and PATTERN RECOGNITION). The replicated network and the HMM can be trained simultaneously by backpropagating gradients through the HMM. Globally trained, variable-size TDNN/HMM hybrids have been used for speech recognition (see PATTERN RECOGNITION for a list of references) and on-line handwriting recognition (Schenkel et al., 1993). Two-dimensional

replicated convolutional networks, called *space displacement neural networks* (SDNNs), have been used in combination with HMMs or other elastic matching methods for handwritten word recognition (Keeler, Rumelhart, and Leow, 1991; Bengio, LeCun, and Henderson, 1994). Another interesting application of SDNNs is in object spotting (Wolf and Platt, 1994).

An important advantage of convolutional neural networks is the ease with which they can be implemented in hardware. Specialized analog/digital chips have been designed and used in character recognition and in image preprocessing applications (Boser et al., 1991). Speeds of more than 1,000 characters per second were obtained with a network with around 100,000 connections (shown in Figure 1).

The idea of subsampling can be turned around to construct networks that are similar to TDNNs but can generate sequences from labels. These networks are called reverse TDNNs because they can be viewed as upside-down TDNNs: temporal resolution increases from the input to the output, through alternated oversampling and convolution layers (Simard and LeCun, 1992).

Discussion

Convolutional neural networks are a good example of an idea inspired by biology that resulted in competitive engineering solutions that compare favorably with other methods (Bottou et al., 1994; LeCun et al., 1998). Although applying convolutional nets to image recognition removes the need for a separate hand-crafted feature extractor, normalizing the images for size and orientation (if only approximately) is still required. Shared weights and subsampling bring invariance with respect to small geometric transformations or distortions, but fully invariant recognition is still beyond reach. Radically new architectural ideas, possibly suggested by biology, will be required for a fully neural image or speech recognition system.

Road Maps: Learning in Artificial Networks; Linguistics and Speech Processing
Related Reading: Feature Analysis; Hidden Markov Models; Pattern Recognition; Speech Recognition Technology

References

Bengio, Y., LeCun, Y., and Henderson, D., 1994, Globally trained handwritten word recognizer using spatial representation, space displacement neural networks and hidden Markov models, in *Advances in Neural Information Processing Systems 6* (J. Cowan, G. Tesauro, and J. Alspector, Eds.), San Mateo, CA: Morgan Kaufmann, pp. 937–944.

Boser, B., Sackinger, E., Bromley, J., LeCun, Y., and Jackel, L., 1991, An analog neural network processor with programmable topology, *IEEE J. Solid-State Circuits*, 26:2017–2025.

Bottou, L., Cortes, C., Denker, J., Drucker, H., Guyon, I., Jackel, L., LeCun, Y., Muller, U., Sackinger, E., Simard, P., and Vapnik, V., 1994, Comparison of classifier methods: a case study in handwritten digit recognition, in *Proceedings of the International Conference on Pattern Recognition*, Los Alamitos, CA: IEEE Computer Society Press.

Bottou, L., Fogelman-Soulie, F., Blanchet, P., and Lienard, J. S., 1990, Speaker independent isolated digit recognition: Multilayer perceptrons vs dynamic time warping, *Neural Netw.*, 3:453–465.

Guyon, I., Albrecht, P., Le Cun, Y., Denker, J. S., and Hubbard, W. H., 1991, Design of a neural network character recognizer for a touch terminal, *Pattern Recognit.*, 24:105–119.

Keeler, J., Rumelhart, D., and Leow, W., 1991, Integrated segmentation and recognition of hand-printed numerals, in *Advances in Neural Information Processing Systems 3* (R. P. Lippmann, J. M. Moody, and D. S. Touretzky, Eds.), San Mateo, CA: Morgan Kaufmann, pp. 557–563.

Lang, K., and Hinton, G., 1988, *The Development of the Time-Delay Neural Network Architecture for Speech Recognition*, Technical Report CMU-CS-88-152, Carnegie-Mellon University. Pittsburgh, PA.

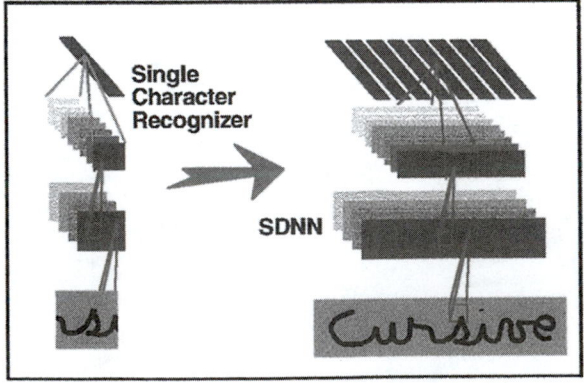

Figure 2. Variable-size replicated convolutional network called a space-displacement neural network (SDNN).

LeCun, Y., 1989, *Generalization and Network Design Strategies*, Technical Report CRG-TR-89-4, Department of Computer Science, University of Toronto.

LeCun, Y., Boser, B., Denker, I., Henderson, D., Howard, R., Hubbard, W., and Jackel, I., 1990, Handwritten Digit Recognition with a Back-Propagation Network, in *Advances in Neural Information Processing Systems 2* (D. Touretzky, Ed.), pages 396–404, Demer 1989. Morgan Kaufmann, San Mateo.

LeCun, Y., Bottou, L., Bengio, Y., and Haffner, P., 1998, Gradient based learning applied to document recognition, *Proc. IEEE*, 86:2278–2324.

Mozer, M., 1991, *The Perception of Multiple Objects: A Connectionist Approach*, Cambridge, MA: MIT Press.

Rumelhart, D., Hinton, G., and Williams, R., 1986, Learning representations by back-propagating errors, *Nature*, 323:533–536.

Schenkel, M., Weissman, H., Guyon, I., Nohl, C., and Henderson, D., 1993, Recognition-based segmentation of on-line hand-printed words, in *Advances in Neural Information Processing Systems 5* (C. Hanson and L. Giles, Eds.), San Mateo, CA: Morgan Kaufmann, pp. 723–730.

Simard, P., and LeCun, Y., 1992, Reverse TDNN: An architecture for trajectory generation, in Moody, J., Hanson, S., and Lipmann, R., editors, *Advances in Neural Information Processing Systems 4* (J. Moody, S. Hanson, and R. P. Lipmann, Eds.), San Mateo, CA: Morgan Kaufmann, pp. 579–588.

Waibel, A., Hanazawa, T., Hinton, G., Shikano, K., and Lang, K., 1989, Phoneme recognition using time-delay neural networks, *IEEE Trans. Acoustics Speech Signal Process.*, 37:328–339.

Wolf, R., and Platt, J., 1994, Postal address block location using a convolutional locator network, in *Advances in Neural Information Processing Systems 6* (J. Cowan, G. Tesauro, and J. Alspector, Eds.), San Mateo, CA: Morgan Kaufmann, pp. 745–752.

Cooperative Phenomena

Hermann P. J. Haken

Introduction

Most objects of scientific study in physics, chemistry, biology, neuroscience, and many other fields are composed of many individual parts that interact with each other. By their interaction, the individual parts may produce cooperative phenomena that are connected with the emergence of new qualities that are not present at the level of the individual subsystems. For instance, the human brain consists of a network of some 100 billion neurons that, through their cooperation, bring about pattern recognition, associative memory, decision making, steering of locomotion, speech, emotions, and so on. Physical systems may serve as model systems or as testing grounds for the development of new concepts and mathematical tools. One important class comprises systems in thermal equilibrium that may undergo a phase transition when the temperature changes. A typical example is water freezing to ice. At the microscopic level, where we are concerned with the motion of individual molecules, molecules above freezing temperature exhibit disordered movement. Below freezing temperature, also called the *critical temperature*, water molecules take their positions in the highly ordered ice crystal. Incidentally, at the macroscopic level, the properties of ice are different from those of water, as is quite evident in the mechanical properties of the two substances. Another example is afforded by ferromagnets. Ferromagnets are composed of many individual elementary magnets that change their orientation randomly but interact to align with each other below a critical temperature, the *Curie temperature*, and may thus produce a macroscopic magnetization typical for ferromagnets. While in metals at a somewhat elevated temperature the electrons move entirely independently of each other, in superconducting metals below a critical temperature the electrons form pairs. At the macroscopic level, the electrical resistance drops to zero, and the metals become superconducting. In both of these cases the macroscopic properties of the system change dramatically when the temperature of the system is changed from the outside and passes through a critical value. Theories that address these phase transitions were originally developed by Landau (cf. Landau and Lifshitz, 1959) and later by K. G. Wilson (1971) and others.

In contrast to biological systems, whose functioning is maintained by a continuous flux of energy or matter through them, the physical systems just described are truly dead. There are, however, physical systems whose spatial, temporal, or spatiotemporal structures are produced and maintained by a continuous influx of energy and/or matter and which may show phase-transition-like phenomena. Thus, they seem suited to act as model systems for biological systems (including the brain), and they may also guide the development of new types of neural nets. Typical examples are provided by lasers, fluids, plasmas, and semiconductors.

Let us consider a solid state laser (Haken, 1983). In a solid matrix, laser-active atoms are embedded that are excited ("pumped") by, for example, light from other lamps. When the excitation level is low, the individual atoms emit their light independently of each other so that microscopically chaotic—i.e., irregular—light waves emerge. If the pump power exceeds a critical value, the properties of the light change dramatically. It is now composed of a single, almost infinitely long wave track that shows only minor fluctuations in phase and amplitude. In the laser, the emission acts of the electrons of the individual atoms have become correlated to produce the collective phenomenon of coherent light. This ordering phenomenon is brought about by the system itself, not by an outside agent interfering with the system, and for this reason this ordering phenomenon is called *self-organization*. The basic mechanism for the emergence of a single coherent light wave is as follows: When a light wave has been emitted from an excited atom, it may hit another excited atom and force that atom to enhance the impinging light wave by the process of stimulated emission (as formulated by Einstein). When a number of atoms are excited, an avalanche of that light wave is generated. Again and again such avalanches are generated, and thus start to compete with each other. The one that has the largest growth rate wins the competition and establishes the laser light wave. Because the energy supply to the system is limited, the light wave eventually saturates. The light wave so established forces the individual electrons of the atoms into its rhythm (synchrony) and thus forces them to support it. In the terminology of synergetics (Haken, 1983), the light wave acts as the *order parameter*. This is a variable that describes the macroscopic order of the system and gives orders to the individual parts of it. In the laser, the order parameter *enslaves* the electrons of the atoms.

When the pump power to the laser is further increased, new effects may appear. For instance, several coherent waves may be produced simultaneously and may lead to specific spatiotemporal intensity distributions; ultrashort regular light pulses may occur; or light may show deterministic chaos. Thus, a single, rather unspecific input variable—namely, the pump power—controls the self-organization of the system, resulting in the production of entirely new temporal or spatiotemporal structures. This input variable is called the *control parameter*. Note the difference between the concepts of order parameter and control parameter: a *control parameter* is a quantity that is imposed on the system from the outside, whereas an *order parameter* is established by the system itself via self-organization.

A variety of similar phenomena related to the formation of spatiotemporal patterns can be observed in fluid layers heated from below or from above, in fluids between two vertical, coaxial, rotating cylinders, and in semiconductors that are driven away from thermal equilibrium. Additional examples of pattern formation can be found in specific chemical reactions. All of these structure-forming processes in nonequilibrium systems are studied in the interdisciplinary field of synergetics, which affords a unified approach to such processes.

Outline of the Mathematical Approach

In order to make visible the profound analogies between the formation of patterns by quite different systems, and to prepare the ground for establishing an important analogy between pattern formation and pattern recognition, we have to adopt a rather abstract level of formulation (Haken, 1983). To describe a system at the microscopic level, we introduce the state vector

$$\mathbf{q} = (q_1, q_2, \ldots, q_n) \tag{1}$$

In the example of a laser, the individual components q_j may stand for the time-dependent field amplitudes used in a decomposition of the electric field strength of the laser light into so-called modes. The modes are typically standing or running sinusoidal waves that fit in between the mirrors of the laser. Further components q_j may stand for the dipole moments of the individual atoms and for the inversion (i.e., degree of excitation) of the atoms. In fluids, q_j denotes the density, the components of the velocity field, and the temperature field. In semiconductors, q_j stands for the densities of electrons, holes, impurity centers, and the electric field. In these cases, the components are both space and time dependent. In models of chemical reactions, q_j may stand for the concentration of a chemical of kind j. In general, the state vector develops in the course of time; this time evolution is described by evolution equations of the form

$$\dot{\mathbf{q}} = \mathbf{N}(\mathbf{q}, \nabla, \alpha) + \mathbf{F}(t), \tag{2}$$

where α represents one or several control parameters. The left-hand side is the temporal derivative of the state vector $\mathbf{q}$, which is determined by the right-hand side of this equation. $\mathbf{N}$ is a nonlinear function of the state vector. The state vector may be subjected to spatial differential operations $\nabla = (\partial/\partial x, \partial/\partial y, \partial/\partial z)$. Finally, $\mathbf{F}$ represents stochastic forces that stem from internal or external fluctuations. In chemical reactions the typical reaction-diffusion equations are of the form

$$\dot{\mathbf{q}} = \mathbf{N}(\mathbf{q}, \alpha) + \mathbf{F}(t) + D\Delta\mathbf{q} \tag{3}$$

where D is a diffusion matrix and $\Delta \cdot \nabla^2$ is the Laplace operator.

Equation 2 in this general form covers an enormous range of phenomena, and at first glance it appears impossible to devise a general method of solution. From the experimental point of view, however, we are often confronted with situations like the following. Below a certain pump power threshold, a laser acts as a lamp without the emission of coherent light. When we slowly increase the pump power, suddenly the laser forms coherent laser light. In

other words, the former state has become unstable and has been replaced by a new state. This suggests the following strategy: We assume that, for a given control parameter value α_0, a solution $\mathbf{q}_0$ of Equation 2 (with $\mathbf{F} \equiv 0$) is known. The general procedure allows us to treat all kinds of $\mathbf{q}_0$ as such a reference state; $\mathbf{q}_0$ may be time-independent (representing a fixed point), time-periodic (representing a limit cycle), time-quasi-periodic (forming a torus), or time-chaotic (forming a chaotic attractor). Common features and differences with respect to bifurcation theory, an important branch of dynamic systems theory, are worth mentioning. Dynamic systems theory also considers bifurcation from a fixed point and from time-periodic solutions; however, it neglects the very important impact of fluctuations as well as dynamical behavior (i.e., relaxation processes), whereas in synergetics these phase-transition effects are included, as is the bifurcation from quasi-periodic and chaotic reference states $\mathbf{q}_0$. Here we explicitly consider the case of a fixed-point $\mathbf{q}_0$. To check the stability of the state $\mathbf{q}_0$ when we change the control parameter, we make the hypothesis that, for α close to α_0, the state $\mathbf{q}_\alpha$ can be written as

$$\mathbf{q}_\alpha = \mathbf{q}_0 + \mathbf{w}(\mathbf{x}, t) \tag{4}$$

where $\mathbf{w}$ is assumed to be a small quantity. We may thus insert Equation 4 into Equation 2. In the resulting equation for $\mathbf{w}$ (still with $\mathbf{F} \equiv 0$), we keep only the linear terms and obtain

$$\dot{\mathbf{w}} = L(\mathbf{q}_0)\mathbf{w} \tag{5}$$

where L is a linear operator. It can be shown quite generally in all the previously mentioned cases of $\mathbf{q}_0$ that the solutions $\mathbf{w}$ can be written in the form

$$\mathbf{w}(\mathbf{x}, t) = \begin{cases} e^{\lambda t}\mathbf{v}_u(\mathbf{x}, t), & Re\lambda \geq 0 \\ e^{\lambda t}\mathbf{v}_S(\mathbf{x}, t), & Re\lambda < 0 \end{cases} \tag{6}$$

where we distinguish between the two sets of modes: *unstable modes*, with $Re\lambda \geq 0$, and *stable modes*, with $Re\lambda < 0$ (Re = real part of). Here, $\mathbf{v}$ depends on t in a way that is weaker than an exponential growth or decay. The λ's are the eigenvalues of Equation 5. Any linear combination of Equation 6 is, of course, again a solution of Equation 5. In what follows, it, however, will be crucial to treat the solutions in Equation 6 individually and to distinguish between those eigenvalues λ whose real part is positive or zero and those whose real part is negative. It is our goal to solve the nonlinear stochastic Equation 2 exactly, i.e., not only in a linear approximation. To this end, we expand the unknown function $\mathbf{q}$ into a superposition of the individual eigenfunctions $\mathbf{v}$ of the linear operator L in Equation 5:

$$\mathbf{q}(\mathbf{x}, t) = \mathbf{q}_0 + \sum_u \xi_u(t)\mathbf{v}_u(\mathbf{x}) + \sum_s \xi_s(t)\mathbf{v}_s(\mathbf{x}) \tag{7}$$

In the mathematical sense, this is a complete superposition representing $\mathbf{q}$ as a function of x. The amplitudes ξ_u and ξ_s are still unknown functions of time. To obtain equations for ξ_u, ξ_s, we insert the expansion of Equation 7 into Equation 2. On the right-hand side of Equation 2 we expand the nonlinear function $\mathbf{N}$ that has become a function of ξ_u and ξ_s into a power series of ξ_u and ξ_s. The terms *linear* in ξ_u or ξ_s read $\xi_u L(\mathbf{q}_0)\mathbf{v}_u$ or $\xi_s L(\mathbf{q}_0)\mathbf{v}_s$, respectively. Because of Equation 5, in the case of a fixed point $\mathbf{q}_0$, we may replace, for instance, $L\mathbf{v}_u$ by $\lambda_u\mathbf{v}_u$.

Keeping these and all higher-order terms and projecting both sides of Equation 2 on the modes $\mathbf{v}$, we obtain the following two sets of equations:

$$\dot{\xi}_u = \lambda_u\xi_u + \hat{N}_u(\xi_u, \xi_s) + \hat{F}_u(t) \tag{8}$$

and

$$\dot{\xi}_s = \lambda_s \xi_S + \hat{N}_s(\xi_u, \xi_s) + \hat{F}_u(t) \tag{9}$$

The first term on the right-hand side of Equations 8 and 9, respectively, stems from the linear part of N, where use was made of the fact that $\mathbf{v}_u$ and $\mathbf{v}_s$ are eigenfunctions of the linear operator L in Equation 5 with the eigenvalues λ that occur on the right-hand side of Equation 6. These equations are entirely equivalent to the former Equation 2. However, provided the inequality

$$|Re\lambda_s| \gg |Re\lambda_u| \tag{10}$$

holds, the *slaving principle* of synergetics (Haken, 1983) can be applied. According to this principle, the mode amplitudes ξ_s are uniquely determined (enslaved) by ξ_u. The possibility of expressing ξ_s by ξ_u can be made plausible in the following fashion: Let us assume that according to Equation 10, the mode amplitudes ξ_s relax much faster than the mode amplitudes ξ_u. Consider Equation 9 with slowly varying ξ_u that act as driving forces on ξ_s. When we neglect transients, ξ_s being driven by ξ_u changes much more slowly than it normally would because of the first term on the right-hand side in Equation 10. In other words, this means that $\dot{\xi}_s$ can be neglected against $\lambda_s \xi_s$, or that $\dot{\xi}_s = 0$. This turns Equation 9 into an algebraic equation that can be solved for ξ_s, expressing ξ_s by ξ_u. This approximation is called *adiabatic approximation*. The slaving principle ensures that this procedure is a first step toward a systematic procedure by which ξ_s can be expressed uniquely and exactly by ξ_u and $\hat{F}_s$:

$$\xi_s(t) = f_s(\xi_u(t), t) \tag{11}$$

The explicit dependence of f_s on t stems from the time dependence of the fluctuating forces, but not of that of the amplitudes ξ_u. In most cases of practical interest, f_s can be approximated by a low-order polynomial in ξ_u.

In practically all cases that have been treated in the literature, the systems are of very high dimension—i.e., they contain very many variables—but the number of unstable mode amplitudes ξ_u is very small. The amplitudes ξ_u are called *order parameters*, whereas the variables ξ_s can be called *enslaved variables*. The order parameter concept allows an enormous reduction in the degrees of freedom. Think of a single-mode laser in which we have one mode and, say, 10^{16} degrees of freedom stemming from the dipole moments and inversions of the individual laser atoms. The order parameter in the single-mode laser is identical with the lasing mode, i.e., a single degree of freedom. Once we have expressed the enslaved modes by means of the order parameters ξ_u via Equation 11, we may insert Equation 11 into Equation 8 and thus find equations for the order parameters alone:

$$\dot{\xi}_u = \lambda_u \xi_u + \hat{N}_u(\xi_u, f_s(\xi_u, t)) + \hat{F}_u(t) \tag{12}$$

In a number of cases, these equations can be put into *universality classes* describing the similar behavior of otherwise quite different systems. The term *universality classes* is chosen in analogy to universality classes in the theory of phase transitions of systems in or close to thermal equilibrium, such as superconductors or ferromagnets, although the classes treated here are of a more general character. In the present context, the term means that Equation 12 can be put into specific general forms (see below). For instance, a single-mode laser, the formation of a roll

pattern in a fluid, or the formation of a stripe pattern in chemical reactions obey the same basic order parameter equation. Such universality classes can be established because of the following facts:

- When we are dealing with a *soft transition* of a system, its order parameters are small, close to the instability point. In analogy to conventional phase transition theory, we call a transition a soft transition if the order parameters change smoothly with the control parameter. This allows us to expand $\hat{N}_u$ into a power series with respect to the order parameters, where we may keep only a few, leading terms.
- Furthermore, we may exploit symmetries. For instance, given a term $\beta \xi_u^2$, if there is an inversion symmetry of the system, it follows that $\beta = 0$. Symmetries lead also in a number of cases to relationships between coefficients.
- Finally, we may invoke so-called normal form theory to simplify the nonlinear functions on the right-hand side of Equation 13.

Some Examples for the Formation of Patterns

We illustrate the procedure just described with a few typical examples encountered in concrete, important cases. In the case of a *single real or complex order parameter*, a typical order parameter equation reads:

$$\dot{\xi}_u = \lambda \xi_u - \beta |\xi_u|^2 \xi_u + F(t) \tag{13}$$

where λ plays the role of a control parameter. The state vector reads

$$\mathbf{q}(\mathbf{x}, t) = \mathbf{q}_0 + \xi_u(t)\mathbf{v}_u(\mathbf{x}) + \sum_s \xi_s(t)\mathbf{v}_s(\mathbf{x}) \tag{14}$$

where the sum over the enslaved modes, s, is in general small, so that the evolving pattern is determined by the second term on the right-hand side, which is called the mode skeleton because it represents the basic features of the evolving pattern. If the system is originally spatially homogeneous, $\mathbf{q}_0$ does not depend on the space coordinate, and $\mathbf{v}_u(\mathbf{x})$ as a solution of Equations 5 and 6 is basically a sine function. If λ is real, a spatial stripe pattern is formed (stripes in chemical reactions, rolls in fluids, current filaments in semiconductors, etc.). If λ is complex, a coherent (and spatially modulated) wave emerges (single-mode laser). The stochastic force F leads to amplitude fluctuations and phase diffusion.

In the case of *two order parameters*, the mode skeleton is determined by

$$\mathbf{q}(\mathbf{x}, t) = \mathbf{q}_0 + \xi_1(t)\mathbf{v}_1(\mathbf{x}) + \xi_2(t)\mathbf{v}_2(\mathbf{x}) \tag{15}$$

Depending on the order parameter Equation 12, modes $\mathbf{v}_u$ may either coexist or compete, with the result that only one remains. In the case of competition, either ξ_1 or ξ_2 vanishes, and a stripe pattern appears. In the case of coexistence, both are nonvanishing, so that the total pattern becomes a superposition of the patterns $\mathbf{v}_1$ and $\mathbf{v}_2$ (square pattern).

A further example for pattern formation in physics is provided by the computer simulation shown in Figure 1, where a liquid in a circular vessel is heated from below. Depending on a prescribed initial state, different stripe patterns may evolve, where in one stripe the fluid is up- and downwelling. In such a case the fluid has the property of an associative memory; i.e., an incomplete set of data (one stripe) is supplemented automatically by the system to a full stripe pattern.

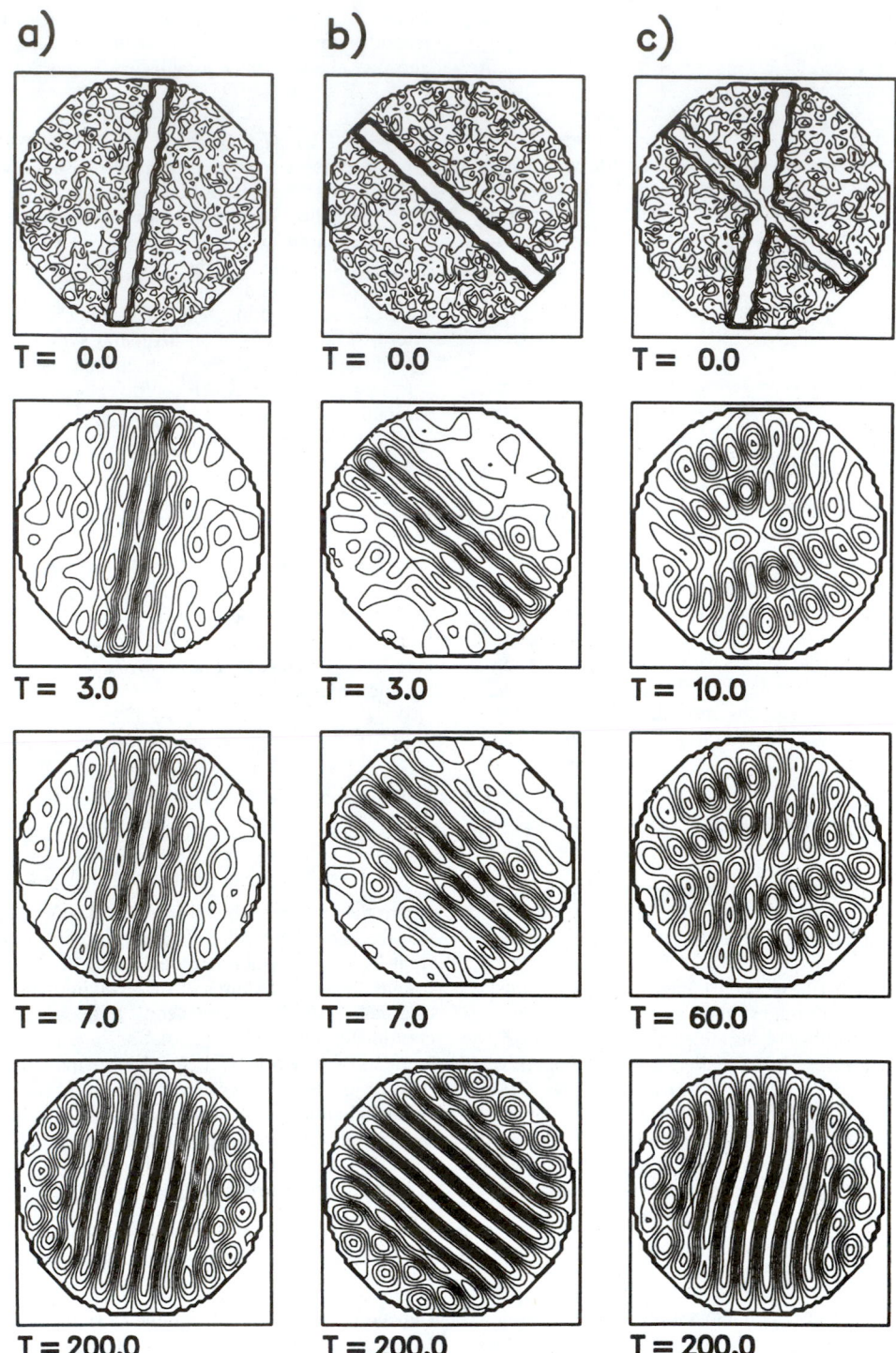

Figure 1. Computer simulation of a fluid heated from below in which initially one upwelling stripe is given. *Left column*, Completion of the single stripe to a full stripe pattern in the course of time. *Middle column*, The same as before, but with a different orientation of the initial stripe. *Right column*, Two initially given upwelling stripes, where one stripe is somewhat stronger than the other one. In the course of time, the originally stronger stripe wins the competition and determines the whole stripe pattern.

Phenomenological and Macroscopic Approaches

In many complex systems, such as biological systems, the basic microscopic evolutions in Equation 2 are not or not fully known.

Nevertheless, in this case also we may capitalize on the results shown earlier under the assumption that a nonequilibrium phase transition happens. This is the case if the macroscopic behavior of the system studied changes qualitatively. In such a case, we may phenomenologically postulate order parameter equations. We may also analyze spatiotemporal patterns by invoking the decomposition formulated in Equation 7 and simple forms of the order parameter equations and using experimental data on evolving or changing spatiotemporal patterns.

Cooperative Phenomena in Neuroscience I

Pattern Recognition

Cooperative phenomena according with the models and interpretations discussed to this point abound in neuroscience. In all of these cases the brain is understood as a self-organizing (synergetic) system. It is possible that important aspects of brain function can be described in terms of order parameters and enslavement.

We have just seen that synergetic systems may act as an associative memory (Kohonen, 1987). This allows us to devise an algorithm (or model) for pattern recognition based on an analogy between pattern formation and pattern recognition (Haken, 1991). In both cases, an incomplete set of data (fluid: a single stripe; pattern recognition: part of a pattern) is completed to a full set of data (fluid: complete stripe pattern; pattern recognition: complete pattern) by means of order parameters and the slaving principle. The algorithm can be formulated as follows: We consider a set of prototype patterns stored in our system. These patterns are represented by vectors $\mathbf{v}^{(k)}$ of a high-dimensional space, where one component $v_i^{(k)}$ corresponds to the gray value or color value of a specific pixel, i, of a pattern labeled by an index k. In the same way we encode a starting or test vector $\mathbf{q}$ (a pattern to be recognized).

By means of these vectors $\mathbf{v}_i^{(k)}$ we construct a dynamics for the test vector $\mathbf{q}$ in the following sense: The test vector $\mathbf{q}$ becomes a time-dependent quantity undergoing a gradient dynamics in a potential field, which may be visualized as a mountainous landscape. This potential field possesses those and only those minima that correspond to the stored prototype pattern vectors $\mathbf{v}^{(k)}$. Note that this approach avoids the well-known difficulty of a number of neural networks, in particular of the Hopfield type (Hopfield, 1982), in which the system can be trapped in spurious minima that do not correspond to any stored patterns (compare the concept of the Boltzmann machine). Here the dynamical system leads to an identification of prototype patterns without the need to introduce simulating annealing, i.e., a statistical pushing of the test vector $\mathbf{q}$ (see SIMULATED ANNEALING AND BOLTZMANN MACHINES).

In Figure 2, the associative property of the dynamical system is shown using three different initial conditions: part of a face, the name of a pattern, and a pattern that is disturbed by noise. In every case there is complete restoration of the original prototype. The dynamics of a "synergetic computer" can be interpreted or realized by means of a parallel network in which each component q_j of $\mathbf{q}$ represents the activity of a model neuron j. By means of the hypothesis

$$\mathbf{q}(t) = \sum_{k'=1}^{M} \xi_{k'}(t)\mathbf{v}^{(k')} + \mathbf{w}(t) \qquad (16)$$

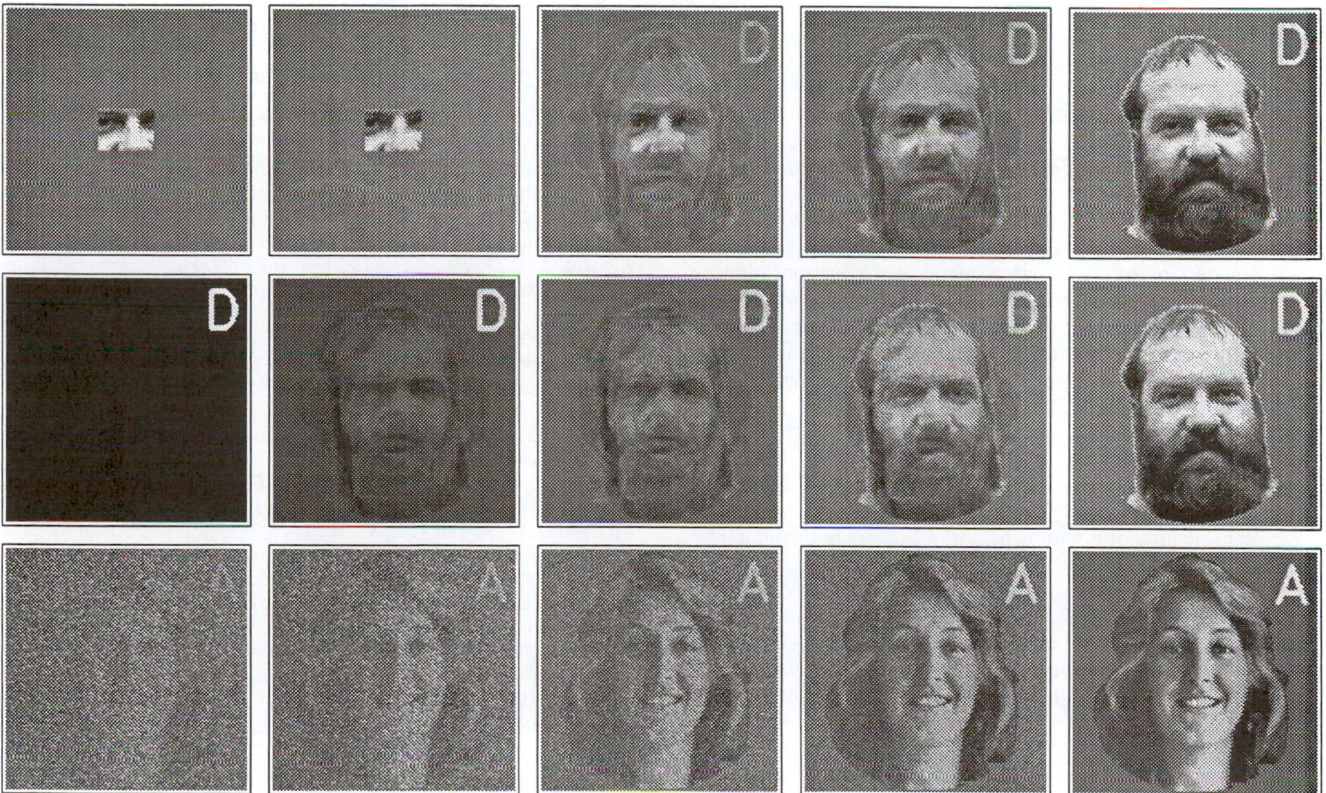

Figure 2. *Upper row,* Restoration of a full face from part of it. *Middle row,* Restoration of a full face from the single letter coding for the name. *Bottom row,* Restoration of a face from an originally noisy face.

where **w** is a residual vector, the dynamics of **q** can be transformed into the order-parameter equations

$$\dot{\xi}_k = \lambda_k \xi_k - B \sum_{k' \neq k}^{M} \xi_{k'}^2 \xi_k - C \sum_{k'=1}^{M} \xi_{k'}^2 \xi_k \qquad (17)$$

The attention parameters λ_k play the role of control parameters and serve to amplify each order parameter, while the second term serves for a discrimination and the last term for a saturation of the order parameters. In this way, an individual order parameter ξ_k is attached to each perceived pattern. The formalism allows one to treat time-dependent attention parameters and the properties of the perception of ambiguous patterns (Haken, 1991, 1996). The formalism can be extended to model stereovision (cf. Haken, 1996).

Thus far we have described a formal model (algorithm) that can be implemented on a serial computer or realized by some parallel devices. But we can go a step farther. The "enslaved" parts are the neurons with their activities, while the order parameters are interpreted as the percepts. In this "synergetics" approach, a connection between the microscopic level, described by the individual parts of a system, and the macroscopic level, described by order parameters, is established. This separation is made possible by a separation of time scales for the reaction of the parts and of the order parameters. Whereas in the brain, the typical time constants of neurons are on the order of milliseconds, those of the brain's macroscopic performance, such as recognition and speech, are on the order of hundreds of milliseconds. At the microscopic level we may mention in particular the neural network model by McCulloch and Pitts (1943), who modeled the individual neurons as two-state elements. A fruitful subsequent step was recognition of the analogy between the McCulloch-Pitts network and spin glasses, which allowed Hopfield (1982) to introduce an energy function for that network, and which gave rise to an avalanche of studies, in particular by theoretical physicists.

Cooperative Phenomena in Neuroscience II

EEG, MEG, Movement Coordination, Hallucinations

An important and very comprehensive model of brain action in terms of neurons (spike rates of action potentials) was established by Wilson and Cowan (1972), who solved their equations numerically. The spatiotemporal patterns found by the authors (for instance, to model hallucinations) can be, at least qualitatively, re-derived in the terms set out in this article. Further evidence for the occurrence of adequate order parameters in brain activities is as follows:

1. The identification of low-dimensional chaos (describable by order parameters) by Babloyantz (1985).
2. The identification of low-dimensional attractors in the olfactory bulb by Freeman (1975).
3. The analysis of petit mal epilepsy, describable by Shilnikov chaos (Friedrich and Uhl, 1992).
4. The MEG analysis of sensorimotor coordination by Kelso (Kelso, Fuchs, and Haken, 1992; see also Haken, 1996). In this work, MEG changes (in both frequency and time domains) in response to auditory and visual stimuli are revealed.

5. The analysis of movement coordination by Haken, Kelso, and Bunz (1985); see also Haken, 1996.

Because in some EEG and MEG measurements, multi-electrode or squid derivations were possible, the spatiotemporal patterns could be determined and, in particular, the basic modes in the sense of a mode decomposition could be identified. In a number of experiments, a surprisingly low number of dominating modes and thus order parameters could be found.

In conclusion, the strategy of searching for order parameters describing brain functions has found some justification, but considerable work remains to be done. Important work about connecting levels of description of cortical and behavioral dynamics in a systematic way has been done by Kelso's group (Kelso, Fuchs, and Jirsa, 1999).

Road Map: Dynamic Systems
Background: Self-Organization and the Brain
Related Reading: EEG and MEG Analysis; Pattern Formation, Biological; Pattern Formation, Neural

References

Babloyantz, A., 1985, Evidence of chaotic dynamics of brain activity during the sleep cycle, in *Dimensions and Entropies in Chaotic Systems* (G. Mayer-Kress, Ed.), Berlin and New York. Springer-Verlag.

Freeman, W., 1975, *Mass Action in the Nervous System: Examination of the Neurophysiological Basis of Adaptive Behavior Through the EEG*, San Diego, CA: Academic Press.

Friedrich, R., and Uhl, C., 1992, Synergetic analysis of human electroencephalograms: Petit-mal epilepsy, in *Evolution of Dynamical Structures in Complex Systems* (R. Friedrich and A. Wunderlin, Eds.), Berlin and New York: Springer-Verlag.

Haken, H., 1983, *Synergetics: An Introduction*, 3rd ed., Berlin and New York: Springer-Verlag. ◆

Haken, H., 1991, *Synergetic Computers and Cognition*, Berlin and New York: Springer-Verlag.

Haken, H., 1996, *Principles of Brain Functioning*, Berlin and New York: Springer-Verlag. ◆

Haken, H., Kelso, J. A. S., and Bunz, H., 1985, A theoretical model of phase transitions in human hand movements, *Biol. Cybern.*, 51:347–356.

Hopfield, J. J., 1982, Neural networks and physical systems with emergent computational abilities, *Proc. Natl. Acad. Sci. USA*, 79:2554–2558.

Kelso, J. A. S., Fuchs, A., and Haken, H., 1992, Phase transitions in the human brain: Spatial mode dynamics, *Int. J. Bifurcat. Chaos*, 2:917–939.

Kelso, J. A. S., Fuchs, A., and Jirsa, V. K., 1999, Traversing scales of brain and behavioral organization, in *Analysis of Neurophysiological Brain Functioning* (C. Uhl, Ed.), Berlin and New York: Springer-Verlag, pp. 73–125. ◆

Kohonen, T., 1987, *Associative Memory and Self-Organization*, 2nd ed., Berlin and New York: Springer-Verlag.

Landau, D., and Lifshitz, I. M., 1959, in *Course of Theoretical Physics*, vol. 5, *Statistical Physics*, London. Pergamon Press.

McCulloch, W. S., and Pitts, W. H., 1943, A logical calculus of the ideas immanent in nervous activity, *Bull. Math. Biophys.*, 5:115–133.

Wilson, H. R., and Cowan, J. D., 1972, Excitatory and inhibitory interactions in localized populations of model neurons, *Biophys. J.*, 12:1–24. ◆

Wilson, K. G., 1971, Renormalization group and critical phenomena: I. Renormalization group and the Kadanoff scaling picture, *Phys. Rev. B*, 4:3174–3183; II. Phase-space cell analysis of critical behavior, *Phys. Rev. B*, 4:3184–3205.

Cortical Hebbian Modules

Daniel J. Amit

Introduction

Before describing model networks of cortical Hebbian modules, we will briefly review some experimental findings. Primates are trained to perform a delay match-to-sample (DMS) task or a delay eye-movement (DEM) task in which a relatively large set of stimuli is presented. The behaving monkey must remember sufficient information about the sample (eliciting) stimulus in order to decide on its behavioral response following the presentation of a second (test) stimulus. The test stimulus is, with equal likelihood, identical to or different from the first stimulus in the DMS task, and a "go" signal in the DEM task. Using single-unit extracellular recordings, neurophysiologists have observed elevated spike rates during the delay period, after the eliciting (sample) stimulus was removed. These elevated spike rates are reproducible and occur in areas such as inferotemporal cortex (IT) and prefrontal cortex, which have been suggested to be part of a working memory system (Fuster, 1995; Goldman-Rakic, 1987). Neurons in rather compact columns have been observed to exhibit stimulus-selective elevated rates that can persist for as long as 30 s, a very long time on the scale of neural time constants. The rates observed are in the range of about 10–20 spikes/s, against a background of spontaneous activity of a few per second. The subset of neurons that sustain elevated rates in the absence of a stimulus is selective of the preceding, first, or sample stimulus. The distribution of rates during the delay among the neurons of the cortical module, or the *delay activity distribution* (DAD), could therefore act as a neural representation and an active memory of the identity of the eliciting stimulus, the representation or memory being transmitted for processing later, when the stimulus is no longer present (Amit, 1995).

The DADs appear to be concentrated in localized columns in associative cortex. The estimate is that this column is about 1 mm^2 in cross-section parallel to the cortical surface. The delay activities corresponding to all the stimuli (as many as 100 in some studies) are constrained to this small module: it contains some 10^5 cells, and 1%–2% of the cells participate in the DAD of a given stimulus (Brunel, 1996); i.e., 1,000–2,000 cells would propagate elevated rates.

The absence of the external stimulus during delay activity leads to the conclusion that the selective activity distributions must be an expression of autonomous local dynamics in the column, whose substrate either forms during the training process or is innate. Some exegesis is needed here. First, the selective delay activity may, of course, be a result of a structure in the afferents arriving at the column under observation. In other words, the particular column may be a mere readout board. However, the absence of the stimulus implies that the structured activity must be maintained somewhere in the brain, and an autonomous mechanism for sustaining a DAD must exist and be formed by learning in the alternative location. We will assume that it is sustained where it is observed. There is some experimental evidence to support such a position.

A second point concerns the assertion that the local structure underlying the delay dynamics could be formed by learning. This statement is supported by the fact that when new stimuli are added to the set after the appearance of DADs, no delay activity is observed for the new stimuli. The alternative situation may describe prefrontal cortex, where DADs appear to be built-in (Goldman-Rakic, 1987).

These observations raise two preliminary issues concerning possible models to account for the computational aspects: (1) the necessary neural elements and synaptic structures that can reproduce

the observed neuronal spike dynamics, and (2) the synaptic dynamics that can give rise, in the process of training, to a synaptic structure in the local module that is capable of sustaining selective DADs. We will concentrate on the first issue and limit ourselves to a few comments about the second.

A successful treatment of the first issue would conclude with a network of neural elements of a given internal dynamics and synaptic matrices that would lead to neurons emitting spikes in spontaneous activity, at low rates, in a very stable way, and, when stimulated by prelearned stimuli, would maintain selective DADs for a large set of eliciting stimuli. For each stimulus, a small fraction of the cells in the module would have elevated rates, and the rest of the cells would maintain spontaneous activity. The spike activities, both spontaneous and structured, would be rather noisy. In other words, there would be large variability in interspike intervals (Softky and Koch, 1992).

At this point we arrive at the second issue: the effect of neuronal activities on synaptic efficacies, which is at the basis of learning. This issue can be broken down into two major parts for further discussion. One part has to do with the feedforward synaptic dynamics, leading to the formation of the module by afferents from preceding cortical areas, the same module for an entire set of different stimuli. The other part has to do with the formation of collateral synapses within the module. The synaptic matrices, which should sustain the various structured activity distributions, must be generated in the process of training via the neuronal activities. If neuronal activities are expressed in terms of spikes, synaptic efficacies must be sensitive to pre- and postsynaptic spikes, in order to affect Hebbian learning, that is, to be potentiated when presynaptic and postsynaptic neurons are simultaneously active and to be depressed when the activities of the two are anticorrelated. There is a tension between the need to learn at least something from every stimulus, so as to accumulate memory, and the need for synaptic stability on long time scales (hours, days, years). Some synapses must change for every stimulus, but the learning process must be immune to spontaneous activity; synapses should not change too easily. Moreover, since neuronal spike dynamics is governed by the emerging synapses, the learning process (synaptic acquisition) may deviate while learning goes on. All of these considerations impose rather severe constraints on both neuronal and synaptic dynamics, over and above the constraints implied by the collective network dynamics (see, e.g., Fusi et al., 2000).

Minimal Elements for a Spiking Network

As a minimal model we take neurons to be of the form described in Equation 1, that is, simple point RC integrators of their afferent currents that emit a spike when the integrated level of depolarization V reaches a threshold θ, followed by an absolute refractory period τ_0 and a resetting of the depolarization to H—an integrate-and-fire (IF) device (see INTEGRATE-AND-FIRE NEURONS AND NETWORKS). Formally, the dynamics of the depolarization is given by

$$\tau \dot{V} = -V + \sum_{i=1}^{C} J_i \tau \sum_k \delta(t_i^k - t) \tag{1}$$

where τ is the integrator's time constant (RC of the equivalent circuit). Effectively, the depolarization $V(t)$ is a sum of unit contributions, each with amplitude J_i, over the interval τ. This simplified form presupposes that the dynamics of the synaptic conductances is much faster than that of the depolarization (for extensions,

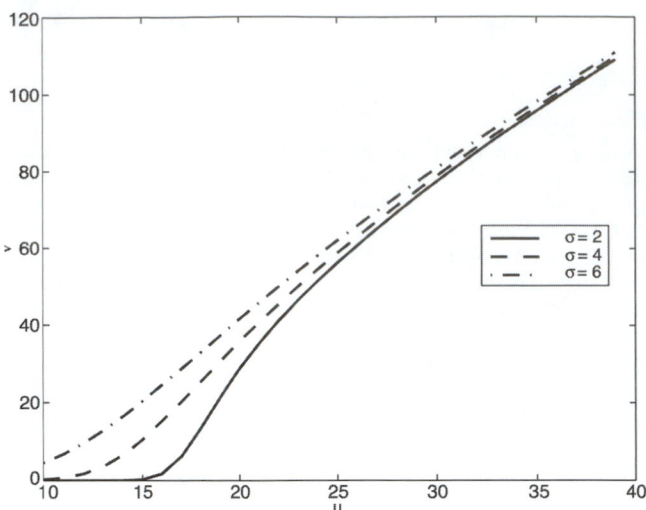

Figure 1. Gain function of integrate-and-fire neuron: rate versus afferent current (μ), for several values of the noise σ, for afferent Gaussian current.

see Brunel and Sergi, 1998). In that case the synaptic efficacies J_i are equivalent to the depolarization provoked by a single afferent spike.

The output spike rate of such a neuron is the inverse of the mean time between two consecutive events in which the depolarization reaches threshold. It is the mean first passage time across the threshold. If the neuron is depolarized by a current of Gaussian distribution, uncorrelated at different times, the output rate can be calculated explicitly (Tuckwell, 1988) by the following:

$$
v_{\text{out}} = \left(\tau_0 + \tau \int_{(H-\mu)/\sigma}^{(\theta-\mu)/\sigma} du \sqrt{\pi} \, \exp(u^2)[1 + \text{erf}(u)] \right)^{-1}
$$
$$
\equiv \Phi(\mu, \sigma) \tag{2}
$$

where τ_0 is the absolute refractory period, μ is the mean of the Gaussian afferents depolarizing the cell per τ, and σ is the corresponding standard deviation (SD).

Note that the response function of this neuron depends not only on the constant part of the afferent current but also on its variance σ, and is an extension of common mean-field results (see, e.g., Amit and Brunel, 1997a). The rate versus the average part of the current (μ) is represented in Figure 1 for several levels of the noise (σ). For low noise, it is zero below a threshold and is convex throughout; with increasing noise a concave region appears, allowing for more than one stable rate. It is the concave part that makes possible the coexistence of spontaneous and selective, elevated spike rate distributions (see, e.g., Fusi and Mattia, 1999; Brunel, 2000).

The assumption of an afferent current of Gaussian distribution is quite useful in cortical conditions. If neurons emit spikes at low rates and receive them via a large number of independent channels (synapses), the total current will be a sum of Poisson processes and hence a Gaussian process. The various assumptions can be verified in microscopic simulations.

The Network

Such minimal elements are put together in a 4:1 ratio of excitatory to inhibitory neuron populations and in large numbers (if not quite as large as the 10^5 of anatomy), in a module that represents a cortical column. A putative assumption for the connectivity pattern would be total randomness, implying that (1) every neuron in the module can synapse on any other neuron; (2) the set of neurons in the local module synapsing on any given cell is chosen at random, constrained only by a mean connectivity given by anatomy (about 10%); (3) synaptic efficacies (excitatory and inhibitory) are random, centered on some plausible mean for each population of synapses; and (4) spike transmission delays are randomly distributed among the synapses (with an average of a couple of milliseconds).

In addition to collateral connections, neurons receive afferents from outside the module (Figure 2). Those afferents may represent a general arousal level or a selective stimulus. The fraction of such synapses is estimated by Braitenberg and Schüz (1991) to be roughly equal to the collateral one. In the absence of structured stimulation, these afferents will be considered uncorrelated, nonselective, and of a fixed spike rate. Stimulation will consist of attributing to the external afferents of a given subset of neurons in the module a higher rate. This leads to higher response rates in that subset of neurons and corresponds to the "visual response" of neurons observed experimentally.

Estimates of J range from 0.05 to 0.5 mV. If one uses an average of 0.2 mV for the excitatory efficacy and a threshold of 20 mV, some 100 simultaneous excitatory synaptic events are required to bring the postsynaptic neuron to threshold.

The above description of neural elements and connectivity of the network can be studied in simulations once the numerical parameters are set. Spike activity in the simulation can be recorded under different conditions, much as would be done in a neurophysiological experiment. One can also record spikes from single or multiple neurons and observe spike rasters, peristimulus histograms (see Figure 4), and cross-correlations of spike emission times prior to learning, in spontaneous activity states. Then, one can impose a synaptic matrix, presumed to have been formed by learning, and observe the same quantities inside and outside of the subset of selective neurons. These are quantities that can also be sampled by electrodes in the cortex of performing animals.

Extended Mean-Field Theory

When the network is in asynchronous activity states, i.e., when neural spike emissions of different neurons are essentially inde-

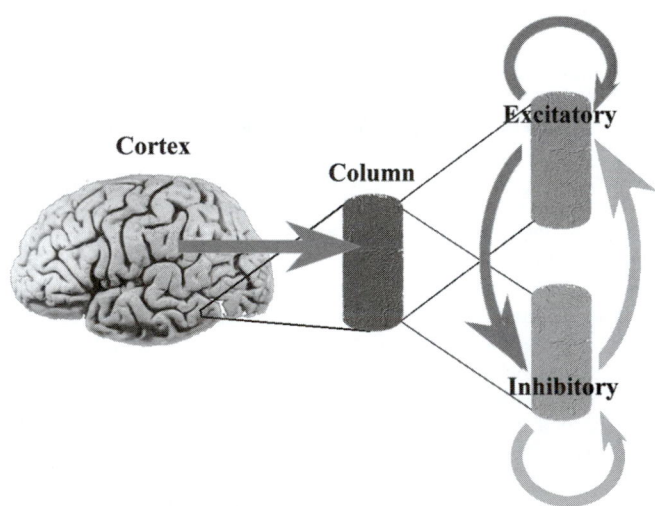

Figure 2. Connectivity scheme. The local network, embedded in the cortex and represented as a column, is divided in two populations of neurons, the excitatory population and the inhibitory population. Neurons in the local network receive collateral connections from excitatory and inhibitory neurons in the same module, as well as from excitatory neurons elsewhere in the cortex.

pendent, there are compact, analytical tools to study a wide variety of properties of large subpopulations of neurons—the collective, computational properties of the network. In other words, if the dynamics of the network leads to large subpopulations within each of which neurons act in a statistically similar way, then the dynamics of the very large network can be described at a level of computational complexity equal to the number of populations that are expected to express different statistical properties. This may appear as a severe restriction. However, one should keep in mind that observable neural phenomena must involve large numbers of neurons acting in essentially the same fashion; otherwise the probability of an electrode detecting a neuron representative of a behavioral correlate would be too low. Similarly, macroscopic probes, as in FMRI or EEG, would not have a large enough signal representing a specific phenomenon. What makes the theory particularly simple is that each neuron (in cortex) receives a very high number of afferents.

The assembly of neurons can be divided into subsets according to neuron types (e.g., excitatory, inhibitory), different sets of afferent synapses (e.g., potentiated or depressed by learning a given stimulus, or not), currently driven by a stimulus or not (e.g., receiving selective external currents), and so on. The network is divided into P subpopulations Π_δ, $\delta = 1, \ldots, P$. Each neuron in population δ is assumed to have the same time constant τ_δ, the same rate v_δ, the same mean number of afferents from population γ—$C_{\delta\gamma}$, and the same mean afferent synaptic efficacy $\langle J_\delta \rangle_\gamma$. The mean afferent current to a neuron in population δ can be written as:

$$\mu_\delta = \tau_\delta \sum_\gamma C_{\delta\gamma} \langle J_\delta \rangle_\gamma v_\gamma(t) + \langle I_{ext,\delta} \rangle \qquad (3)$$

where the sum is over all populations γ. $I_{ext,\delta}$ is the afferent current from outside the module. Here, for simplicity, we assume the rate to be constant for all neurons inside a population (for extensions, see Amit and Brunel, 1997a).

Spike trains are assumed to be Poissonian, so the variance of the input to a neuron in population δ is given as:

$$\sigma_\delta^2 = \tau_\delta \sum_\gamma C_{\delta\gamma} (\text{Var}(J_\delta)_\gamma + \langle J_\delta \rangle_\gamma^2) v_\gamma(t) + \sigma_{ext}^2) \qquad (4)$$

Writing $\text{Var}(J_\delta) = \Delta \langle J_\delta \rangle^2$ (Δ independent of γ) we obtain:

$$\sigma_\delta^2 = (1 + \Delta)\tau_\delta \sum_\gamma C_{\delta\gamma} \langle J \rangle_\gamma^2 v_\gamma(t) + \sigma_{ext}^2 \qquad (5)$$

The afferent currents are converted to output rates via the response function, Equation 2:

$$v_{out,\delta} = \Phi(\mu_\delta, \sigma_\delta) \qquad (6)$$

For a specified network, μ_δ and σ_δ are functions of the set of rates in the different populations. Hence, if we impose the condition that rates on the left-hand side of Equation 6 be equal to the input rates forming the currents, Equations 6 become a set of self-consistent equations, whose number is equal to the number of populations, for the same number of unknowns: the set of stationary rates in the network. A solution of this set of equations provides a set of rates for the populations selected, and an accompanying study of their stability will determine which of the solutions is an attractor—a DAD. The fact that the feedback depends not only on the mean of the current but also on its variance is where mean-field theory is extended.

The importance of mean-field theory goes well beyond its analytic, compact treatment of the behavior of the spiking network. The theory also allows us to identify the *collective variables* characterizing the dynamics of the system, such variables as can be observed experimentally and by other components of a multimodular brain.

Dynamic Mean-Field Theory

In addition to the self-consistent equations given in the preceding sections, a very effective tool for testing the stability of the different stationary states is the dynamic extension of mean-field theory. From the depolarization dynamics of Equation 1 one obtains evolution equations for $\mu[V]$ and $\sigma^2[V]$, which are the asymptotic mean and variance of the depolarization in absence of a threshold (Tuckwell, 1988; Amit and Brunel, 1977b):

$$\tau_\delta \frac{d\mu_\delta[V(t)]}{dt} = -\mu_\delta[V(t)] + \tau_\delta \sum_\gamma A_{\delta,\gamma} v_\gamma + \mu_{\delta,ext}$$

$$\tau_\delta \frac{d\sigma_\delta^2[V(t)]}{dt} = -2\sigma_\delta^2[V(t)] + \tau_\delta \sum_\gamma B_{\delta,\gamma} v_\gamma + \sigma_{\delta,ext}^2 \qquad (7)$$

where $A_{\delta,\gamma}$ and $B_{\delta,\gamma}$ are the coefficients of the rates, as in the sums in Equations 3 and 5. But μ_δ and δ_δ^2, required for the response function that determines the output rate of the neuron, are the means and variances of the afferent currents.

The connection between $(\mu_\delta[V], \sigma_\delta^2[V])$, computed in the dynamic equations, and $(\mu_\delta, \sigma_\delta^2)$ is made in the following manner. In a stationary state, when the left-hand sides of Equations 7 vanish, we have:

$$\mu_\delta[V(t)] = \mu_\delta = \tau_\delta \sum_\gamma A_{\delta,\gamma} Av_\delta + \mu_{\delta,ext}$$

$$2\sigma_\delta^2[V(t)] = \sigma_\delta^2 = \tau_\delta \sum_\gamma A_{\delta,\gamma} Bv_\delta + \sigma_{\delta,ext}^2 \qquad (8)$$

When the temporal variation of the input currents (and hence of the rates) is slow, Equations 8 can also be used away from the stationary state, and we can substitute $\mu_\delta[V(t)]$ and $2\sigma_\delta^2[V(t)]$ for μ_δ and σ_δ^2, respectively, in Equation 2 and obtain a relation between $v_\delta(t)$ and $(\mu_\delta[V(t)], 2\sigma_\delta[V(t)])$. Substituting this relation in Equations 7 gives us a closed set of dynamical equations for $\mu_\delta[V(t)]$ and $\sigma_\delta[V(t)]$, which determines the dynamics of $v_\delta(t)$. A variation in $\mu_\delta[V(t)]$ and $\sigma_\delta[V(t)]$, as given in Equations 7, leads to a shift in the rates, which are then fed back into the dynamical equations.

A set of rates v satisfying Equations 6 and 8 is a stationary point of the dynamics (Equations 7), and vice versa. Thus, solving numerically for the stationary states of Equations 7 is one way of solving Equations 6, with the bonus that such solutions are stable, since they attract.

The Currents

Spontaneous Activity

To proceed, one expresses the mean and variance of the afferent currents in terms of the instantaneous values of the rates in different neural populations that are assumed to behave in a homogeneous way. For example, if the network is expected to sustain only spontaneous activity, one would expect two populations only, a population of excitatory neurons and a population of inhibitory neurons. They would be distinguishable either because the two types of neurons would have different physiological characteristics or because there would be different distributions of synaptic efficacies on the dendrites.

Suppose each neuron receives $C_E(C_i)$ excitatory (inhibitory) synapses on average, whose efficacy has a Gaussian distribution of mean $J_E(J_i)$ and variance $J^2\Delta$ for both. Let the time constants be $\tau_E(\tau_I)$ and their average emission rates be $v_E(v_I)$. Then,

$$\mu_E = \tau_E(C_E J_E v_E - C_i J_i v_I) + \mu_{ext}$$

$$\mu_I = \tau_I(C_E J_E v_E - C_i J_i v_I) + \mu_{ext} \qquad (9)$$

where μ_{ext} is the average afferent, excitatory, nonselective current from outside the module, taken equal for both types of neurons.

The variances of the external currents are σ_{ext}^2. The variances of the total afferent currents are:

$$\sigma_E^2 = \tau_E\left(C_E J_E^2 \nu_E - C_i J_I^2 \nu_I\right) + \sigma_{\text{ext}}^2$$

$$\sigma_I^2 = \tau_I\left(C_E J_E^2 \nu_E - C_I J_I^2 \nu_I\right) + \sigma_{\text{ext}}^2 \qquad (10)$$

When the μs and the σs are introduced in the transduction functions (Equation 2) of the two types of neurons (differing by the integration constants τ_E and τ_I), one obtains two self-consistent equations (like Equation 6) for the average stationary rates in the two populations.

Selective Delay Activity

A richer example is one where learning has taken place and sets of synapses have been modified in response to stimuli presented. Each stimulus presented to the network produces an increase in the spike rates of neurons in a subpopulation of the module; those are the neurons with *visual response*. Mean-field theory is simple if one assumes that no neuron is visually selective to more than one stimulus. Hebbian learning is then expressed by the fact that synapses between neurons responding to a given stimulus have their average efficacy increased, $J_E \rightarrow J_+$, whereas synapses between a neuron responsive to a stimulus and one that is not have their average efficacy depressed, $J_E \rightarrow J_-$.

In this case, the neurons in the module can be divided into four distinct, homogeneous groups: (1) neurons selective to the current stimulus (such as those responding to an image currently presented to a monkey); (2) neurons selective to another stimulus in the set used for training but not activated in the present trial; (3) neurons not responsive to any of the stimuli used (hence with unmodified synapses); and (4) inhibitory neurons. If the number of excitatory (inhibitory) neurons in the module is $N_E(N_i)$, if the number of neurons selective to a stimulus is fN_E, and if the number of stimuli used is p, then the number of neurons in each of the four classes is, respectively, fN_E, $(p-1)fN_E$, $(1-pf)N_E$, and N_i.

In this case one has four self-consistency equations (Equations 3 through 6), or the dynamic version (Equations 7), to find the various stationary activity states of the network following learning, at different stages before, during, and after stimulus presentation, and to study their stability. In the process one constructs the μ's and the σ^2s for each of the populations (eight expressions in all). For example, the mean and variance of the afferent current to neurons in the selective population are

$$\mu_1 = \tau_E C_E[fJ_+\nu_1 + (1-fp)J_-\nu_+ + f(p-1)J_-\nu_-] - C_I J_I \nu_I + \mu_{\text{ext}}$$

$$\sigma_1^2 = \tau_E C_E[fJ_+^2\nu_1 + (1-fp)J_-^2\nu_+ + f(p-1)J_-^2\nu_-] + C_I J_I^2\nu_I + \sigma_{\text{ext}}^2 \qquad (11)$$

in which ν_1, ν_+, ν_-, and ν_I are, respectively, the rates in the four different classes of neuron described above.

Stability and Other Dependence on Parameters

The example of spontaneous activity is very rudimentary, but not without significant lessons (Amit and Brunel, 1997b). The main lesson obtained from mean-field theory is about stability: in the absence of inhibition, spontaneous activity, with spike rates in the range observed, is not possible. Moreover, inhibition must be strong enough to overcome excitation for the collateral part of the afferent currents, even though there are many fewer inhibitory neurons than excitatory ones. Inhibitory neurons can win by possessing either stronger synapses ($J_I > J_E$) or faster internal dynamics ($\tau_I <$

τ_E). In either of these conditions, spikes can be emitted by neurons of the assembly only because of afferents from outside the module.

Another issue that can be studied in detail in this framework is the range of potentiation, following the appearance of selective delay activity, in which spontaneous activity can coexist with the DAD, both of which are observed experimentally and are stable. Which of them manifests itself depends on whether the stimulus presented is familiar or not. The various regimes of stability are presented in the mean-field bifurcation diagram in Figure 3. The two solid curves are the equilibrium rates of spontaneous (flat, low) and persistent delay activity. Below a potentiation of 2.05, only spontaneous activity is stable, at about 3 Hz. For potentiation between 2.05 and 2.3, both are stable, and the dotted curve delineates their corresponding basins of attraction. To the right of 2.3, the stability of spontaneous activity is destroyed, and only the selective delay activity is stable.

Simulations Versus Theory

Generic conclusions require a theory, but the theory must be confronted with simulation of the spiking system that the theory purports to describe. This comparison is quite satisfactory (Amit and Brunel, 1997a), even though the assumption about the absence of correlations in the spike processes reaching a neuron via different afferent channels is not fully justifiable, as has become evident from cross-correlations measured on simultaneously "recorded" cells in the simulation.

An example of a confrontation of theory with simulation is presented in Figure 4. A network of 16,000 excitatory and 4,000 inhibitory neurons is connected as described earlier in this article. The distribution of connectivities and of synaptic efficacies is random. Five groups of 1,600 excitatory neurons each have the average synaptic efficacies connecting them potentiated by a factor of 1.9. Each neuron receives 1,600 excitatory afferents from outside the network, at a rate of $4/\text{s}^{-1}$. The simulation is then launched with an initial random distribution of depolarizations. The neurons start in a spontaneous activity state, as is seen in the figure in the

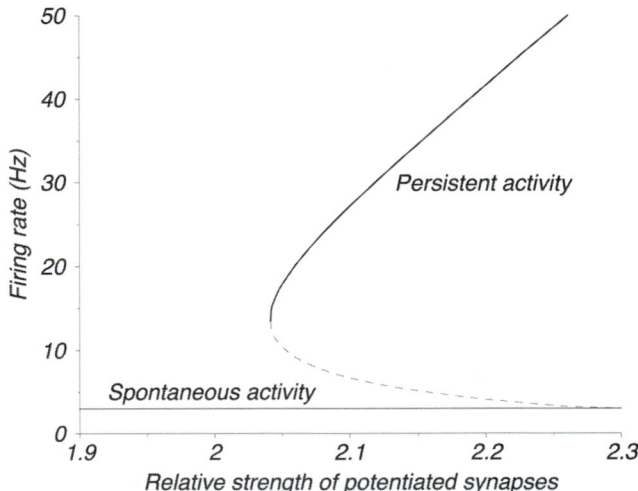

Figure 3. Bifurcation diagram: regions in potentiation-rate plane for stable stationary states of spontaneous activity and selective delay activity. Solid curves denote rates in stable states versus potentiation. Dashed curves indicate a stationary, unstable state, with separating basins of attraction of the two solutions (when both exist). For low potentiation (<2.05), there is only spontaneous activity. For intermediate potentiation (≥2.05, ≤2.3), there are two stable states. With high potentiation (≥2.3), spontaneous activity is unstable (after Brunel, 2000).

Figure 4. Simulations: time evolution of the average emission rate in four neural populations. From the top: an excitatory subpopulation activated by the stimulus (*selective*); excitatory neurons selective to *other stimuli* (grouped together); excitatory neurons nonselective to any stimulus; and the inhibitory population (I). After 1,000 ms of spontaneous activity, a stimulus is presented for 500 ms. When it is removed, the selective subpopulation continues its delay activity at a high rate. Horizontal lines indicate the average rate as given by the dynamic mean-field theory (after Brunel, 2000).

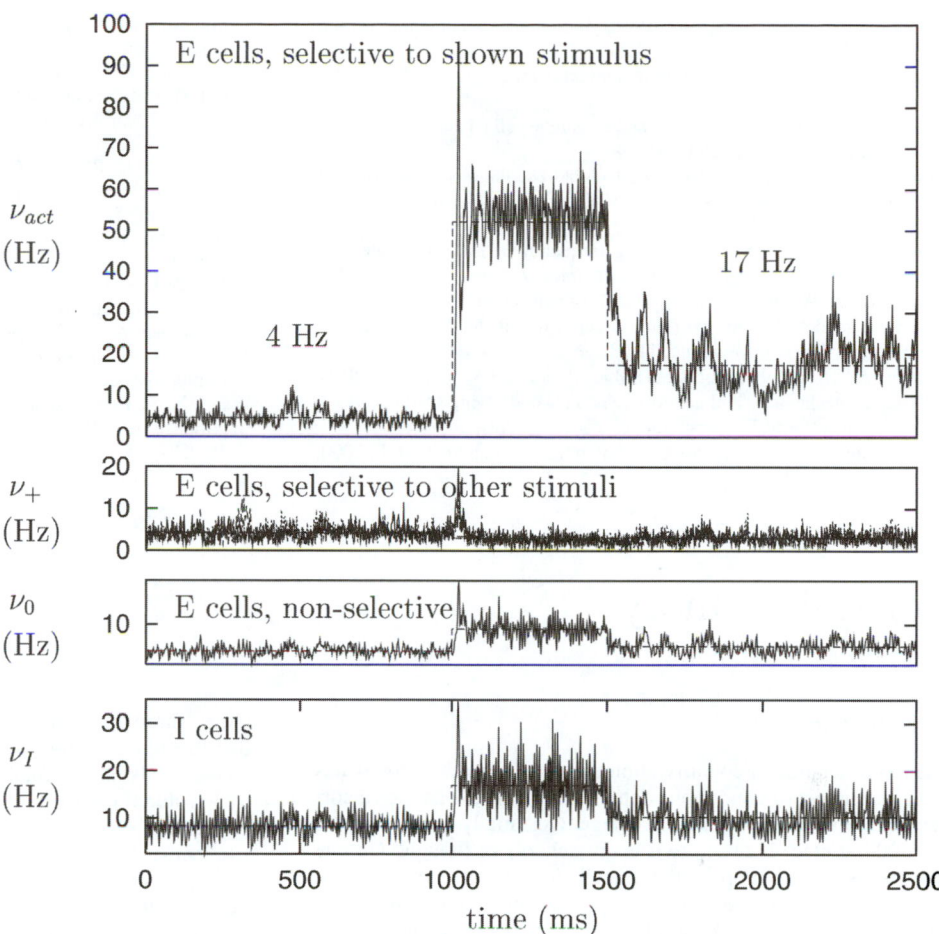

first 1,000 ms. What is plotted is the instantaneous average rate in each population. For the first second, all neurons have low rates. Then a stimulus is presented for 500 ms, by raising the rate of the external afferents to the neurons in one of the populations of selective neurons. The rate in that population rises sharply. Following the removal of the stimulus, one observes 1 s of propagation of a DAD, in which the selective population maintains an elevated rate (lower than under stimulation). The horizontal lines give the mean rate in each population as predicted by mean-field theory.

Discussion

The extended mean-field approach described in this chapter has been applied in richer situations. In particular, it has provided an account of context correlations generated in learning the DMS paradigm with images organized in fixed sequences (Amit, Brunel, and Tsodyks, 1994). Attractor dynamics in localized circuits has also been applied to the gaze fixation problem (Seung, 1996), after having been extended to include line attractors. Recently, such models have been made much more biologically plausible with respect to robustness and realistic rates (Wang, 1999) by the introduction of receptor dynamics, leading to a successful description of working memory immune to distractors (Brunel and Wang, 2001), and to the modeling of spatial working memory (Compte et al., 2000).

Although fruitful, even extended mean-field theory has its limitations. It deals with uniform populations and stationary states, and hence it is insensitive to transmission delays and nonuniform

instabilities. The approach has seen significant extensions capable of satisfactorily handling oscillatory instabilities (Brunel and Hakim, 1999). With the extension of mean-field theory to situations of rich structural complexity, another important step will have been accomplished.

Simulations remain a central tool, functioning as a crucial check on theory. And because the simulation represents an underlying model of the cortical module, the validity of the model as a description of biological reality must often be confronted on levels that theory does not reach, such as simultaneous multicell data, spike emission statistics, and much more.

Road Map: Biological Networks
Background: Hebbian Synaptic Plasticity
Related Reading: Dynamic Remapping; Short-Term Memory; Statistical Mechanics of Neural Networks

References

Amit, D. J., 1995, The Hebbian paradigm reintegrated: Local reverberations as internal representations, *Behav. Brain Sci.*, 18:617. ◆

Amit, D. J., and Brunel, N., 1997a, Dynamics of a recurrent network of spiking neurons before and following learning, *Network*, 8:373. ◆

Amit, D. J., and Brunel, N., 1997b, Model of global spontaneous activity and local structured activity during delay periods in the cerebral cortex, *Cereb. Cortex*, 7:237. ◆

Amit, D. J., Brunel, N., and Tsodyks, M. V., 1994, Correlations of cortical Hebbian reverberations: Experiment versus theory, *J. Neurosci.*, 14:6445.

Braitenberg, V., and Schüz, A., 1991, *Anatomy of the Cortex*, Berlin: Springer-Verlag.

Brunel, N., 1996, Hebbian learning of context in recurrent neural networks, *Neural Computat.*, 8:1677.

Brunel, N., 2000, Persistent activity and the single cell f-I curve in a cortical network model, *Network*, 11:261. ◆

Brunel, N., and Hakim, V., 1999, Fast global oscillations in networks of integrate-and-fire neurons with low firing rates, *Neural Computat.*, 11:1621.

Brunel, N., and Sergi, S., 1998, Firing frequency of leaky integrate-and-fire neurons with synaptic currents dynamics, *J. Theor. Biol.*, 195:87.

Brunel, N., and Wang, X.-J., 2001, Effects of neuromodulation in a cortical network model of object working memory dominated by recurrent inhibition, *J. Comput. Neurosci.*, 11:63. ◆

Compte, A., Brunel, N., Goldman-Rakic, P. S., and Wang, X.-J., 2000, Synaptic mechanisms and network dynamics underlying spatial working memory in a cortical network model, *Cereb. Cortex*, 10:910.

Fusi, S., Annunziato, M., Badoni, D., Salamon, A., and Amit, D. J., 2000, Spike-driven synaptic plasticity: Theory, simulation, VLSI implementation, *Neural Computat.*, 12:2227.

Fusi, S., and Mattia, M., 1999, Collective behavior of networks with linear (VLSI) integrate and fire neurons, *Neural Computat.*, 11:633.

Fuster, J., 1995, *Memory in the Cerebral Cortex*, Cambridge, MA: MIT Press.

Goldman-Rakic, P., 1987, Circuitry of primate prefrontal cortex and regulation of behavior by representational memory, in *Handbook of Physiology*, vol. 5, *The Nervous System* (Editor), chap. 9, Bethesda, MD: American Physiological Society. ◆

Seung, H. S., 1996, How the brain keeps the eye still, *Proc. Natl. Acad. Sci. USA*, 93:13339.

Softky, W. R., and Koch, C., 1992, Cortical cells should spike regularly but do not, *Neural Computat.*, 4:643.

Tuckwell, C. T., 1988, *Introduction to Theoretical Neurobiology*, vol. 2, Cambridge, Engl.: Cambridge University Press.

Wang, X. J., 1999, Synaptic basis of cortical persistent activity: The importance of NMDA receptors to working memory, *J. Neurosci.*, 19:9587. ◆

Cortical Memory

Joaquín M. Fuster

Introduction

The representation of cognitive functions in the cerebral cortex has been the subject of continuous debate since Broca identified a cortical area involved in spoken language. Essentially, the debate has been taking place between two major schools of thought. On one side are those who propose the parcellation of cortex into discrete regions or modules dedicated to special functions, such as language, memory, and perception, or to their specific contents. This is the "localizationist" point of view, which is essentially similar to that of phrenology but legitimized by the scientific method. On the other side of the debate is the "holistic" position, adopted by those who propose the distribution of cognitive functions in wide and overlapping expanses of cortex. As in any theoretical debate, we also find here the eclectics and compromisers, who espouse an intermediate position: some functions or contents are localized and others are distributed. It is increasingly recognized that memory is one such function, with some of its components localized in neuronal networks that are circumscribed to discrete domains of cortex and others widely distributed in networks that extend beyond the boundaries of cortical areas defined by cellular architecture. Thus, the aggregate of experience and knowledge about oneself and the surrounding world would be represented in cortical networks of widely varying size and distribution. This concept does not exclude extracortical structures from memory storage and function or the possibility that, after being acquired in the cortex, some memory is relegated to some of those structures, such as the basal ganglia. Historically, the concept of cortical network memory has two roots. The first is the indirect empirical evidence, gathered by physicians and experimentalists in the past two centuries, that discrete lesions of the cerebral cortex rarely result in deficits of memory or any of its behavioral manifestations, while commonly affecting sensory or motor functions. Karl Lashley (1950) was the first to obtain systematically that kind of indirect evidence by ablations of cortical areas in animals; from their results, he inferred that memory must be widely distributed in the cortex, and further, that dispersed neuronal assemblies could represent the same memories, or *engrams*. The second root of the concept is theoretical. Hayek (1952) was the first to formalize it by postulating large-scale cortical networks (he called them maps) that would represent all the experience obtained through the senses. Subsequently, that concept gained further theoretical support from the fields of artificial intelligence and connectionism. The fundamental idea is that mnemonic information is stored in distributed, net-like patterns of cortical connectivity that are established by experience. In more recent times, neuroscientists have developed several theoretical variants of that idea by adding to it structural and functional constraints and by extending it to other cognitive functions, such as perception.

This article presents in broad outline a model of network memory in the neocortex that is supported by a large body of empirical evidence from neuropsychology, behavioral neurophysiology, and neuroimaging. Its essential features are (1) the acquisition of memory by the formation and expansion of networks of neocortical neurons through changes in synaptic transmission, and (2) the hierarchical organization of memory networks, with a hierarchy of networks in posterior cortex for perceptual memory and another in frontal cortex for executive memory.

Formation of Memory

Toward the end of the nineteenth century, Cajal proposed that memory is essentially formed and stored by changes in the connections between nerve cells. That notion was subsequently expressed by many others, and for many years it remained widely accepted but unproved. It was theoretically formulated in considerable detail by Hebb (1949), and more recently received substantial support by the discovery of two general categories of facts (see Kandel, 1991, for a review): (1) the electrical induction of persistent synaptic changes in cellular assemblies of the hippocampus—a phylogenetically ancient sector of cortex—and (2) the induction of similar changes in the neural circuits of invertebrate animals by behavioral conditioning. Less direct evidence indicates that synaptic plasticity is at the foundation of memory in the cerebral cortex (Fuster, 1999) and the cerebellum (Thompson, 1986). It is now widely accepted that the acquisition of memory consists essentially in the modulation of synaptic transmission, and also, to some extent, in the elimination of synapses.

Hebb (1949), referring to the cortex, postulated that "two cells or systems that are repeatedly active at the same time will tend to become associated, so that activity in one facilitates activity in the other." Thus, temporally coincident inputs would tend to associate the neurons that receive them, by facilitating the synapses between them. This principle, which has been called synchronous convergence (Fuster, 1999), would lead to the formation of the hebbian "cell assembly," a basic neural net of cortical representation in sensory and parasensory cortex. Based on data bearing on the plasticity of responses of visual cortical cells to optic stimuli, Stent (1973) made a strong theoretical argument for the operation of that principle in the neocortex.

Whereas simple sensory memories may be formed and represented in cell assemblies, nets, or modules of sensory and parasensory cortex, the neuropsychologal evidence from humans and animals indicates that the more complex memories of individual experience, as well as abstract knowledge, extend into areas of the cortex of association. Temporally coincident or near-coincident experiences of one or more sense modalities will modulate synaptic contacts between cells in those areas, thus leading to the formation of wider networks that represent assorted items of individual memory and, at higher cortical levels, of knowledge, which is the conceptual or semantic form of memory. The boundaries of those larger networks extend beyond those of any given cytoarchitectonic area, however defined.

The formation of the associative neuronal networks that support and contain memory follows gradients of corticocortical connectivity, which have been most thoroughly investigated in the nonhuman primate (Pandya and Yeterian, 1985). That connectivity departs from primary sensory and motor areas and flows into progressively higher areas of unimodal and multimodal association. The connectivity is reciprocal throughout, such that each connective step, from one area to the next, is reciprocated by fibers running in the opposite direction. Some connections converge and others diverge. Thus, at all levels and between levels, three basic structural features can be recognized in connective networks: convergence, divergence, and feedback or recurrence. In addition, cortical areas of one hemisphere are connected, again reciprocally, with homologous areas of the other hemisphere.

To some extent, the connectivity mediating memory formation follows also maturational gradients, in that it proceeds from area to area following the order in which cortical areas have myelinated in early ontogeny (Fuster, 1997). It also follows gradients of sensory and motor processing. As memories increase in complexity, in terms of the variety and complexity of associated experiences and the sensory inputs that convey them, their networks become progressively wider, and thus span progressively more associative cortical areas of polymodal convergence.

Whereas synaptic modulation and synchronous convergence seem essential features of the process of memory network formation, the process in more general terms is one of self-organization (Kohonen, 1984). The networks and their connective substrate are auto-constituted as the result of the interactions of the organism with its environment. Through these interactions, and mostly by synchronous convergence, new cortical nets are formed and old ones expanded in a dynamic process that persists throughout the life of the organism. In the formation of a memory network, synaptic facilitation is produced not only by the simultaneity of external inputs but also by the simultaneity of these inputs with "inputs" internally generated by the concomitant activation or retrieval of preexisting components of the network. Thus, new memory is formed from old memory.

In recent years, there has been increasing neuropsychological evidence that the hippocampus plays a critical role in the formation of neocortical memory networks (Squire, 1987). It has been established that the hippocampus is reciprocally connected with the cortical areas of association, though not with primary sensory or motor cortex (Amaral, 1987). That connectivity courses through and under the cortex of the peri- and entorhinal region, in the medial and inferior aspects of the temporal lobe. In this manner, reciprocal connections link the hippocampus with the associative cortices of the posterior (postrolandic) regions of the cerebral hemispheres as well as with those of the frontal lobe (prerolandic), notably the prefrontal cortex. The mechanisms by which the hippocampus mediates the formation of memory networks in the neocortex are not known. Possibly, long-term potentiation (LTP) is one of those mechanisms. Further, there is reason to suspect that certain excitatory glutaminergic receptors, notably NMDA receptors, take part in the process. That process would result in protein changes in the membrane of cortical cells, which in turn would strengthen their synapses and thus imprint memories in cortical networks. Inputs from the amygdala, a limbic structure essential for the evaluation of the emotional and motivational significance of sensory information, may also intervene in the process.

Phyletic Memory

The primary sensory and motor cortices lie in the interface between the environment and the cortex of association. Primary sensory cortices provide the inlets of sensory information for the formation of perceptual memory (episodic, semantic, etc.) in posterior cortex of association; primary motor cortex, on the other hand, provides the outlet of frontal association cortex (executive memory) to lower motor structures (e.g., basal ganglia, cerebellum). Thus, primary cortices—ontogenetically the first to myelinate—constitute the cortical gate from sensation to memory, and from memory to action.

It is physiologically plausible to view primary sensory and motor cortices as the foundation of all individual memory, themselves constituting a form of universal memory. These cortices constitute a basic form of memory that I have termed *phyletic memory*. According to this view, phyletic memory is simply the structure of the primary sensory and motor cortex at birth, common to all animals of the same species. Thus, phyletic memory is the most basic of all memories, the memory that the organism has formed through millions of years and countless generations in its interactions with the surrounding world. Those genetically predetermined structures of cortex devoted to the analysis of elementary sensory features and to the integration of the elementary primitives of movement would form the basic template on which all individual memory would grow. In summary, primary cortices can legitimately be called memory, because they retain a form of basic and retrievable information: the memory of the species, the sensory and motor information that the organism has acquired and stored in the course of evolution for survival and procreation. Thus, phyletic memory, the primary sensory and motor cortices, contains already at birth much of the adaptive power of the species. After necessary "rehearsal" in the critical periods of early ontogeny, phyletic memory remains ready for "recall" through a lifetime—ready, that is, to recognize the essential features of the world, and to retrieve and organize the basic patterns of movement for adaptation to the environment. On that foundation of phyletic memory, all the memory of the individual will be developed and hierarchically organized by experience and according to the principles mentioned in the previous section: a hierarchy of perceptual memories will be formed in posterior cortex and a hierarchy of motor memories in frontal cortex.

Perceptual Memory

All memory acquired through the senses qualifies as perceptual memory. This includes a vast fund of individual experience, from the simplest forms of sensory memory to abstract knowledge—in other words, to all that we commonly understand as the memory or knowledge of events, objects, persons, animals, facts, names, and concepts. Perceptual memories, and their cortical substrate, appear hierarchically organized, as the diagram of Figure 1 schematically represents. Such an organization can be inferred from the gradients of cortical connectivity and from neuropsychological evidence, namely, from the study of the psychological effects of cortical lesions. This evidence, however, is somewhat confounded by the variability between subjects and by the profuse relationships of association between the various categories of memory—in other words, by the heterarchy within the hierarchy.

The base of the perceptual hierarchy is sensory phyletic memory, the structure of primary sensory cortices. Immediately above it, in cortex of sensory association, are the memories of the sensory qualities of objects and experiences, unimodal and polymodal. Further up in the hierarchy, in higher associative cortex, memories become more personal and complex, with specific temporal and spatial tags. These memories fall under the category of what is commonly designated declarative memory, the memory of events and experiences. Finally, at the highest levels of the hierarchy, in areas of the temporal and parietal lobes called transmodal (Mesulam, 1998), resides the knowledge of facts, concepts, and names.

At every stage of the hierarchy of perceptual memory, memory networks are essentially made of connections between neuronal aggregates at that stage and by convergence of inputs from below, ultimately from the senses. Thus, at the first associative sensory stage beyond phyletic memory, networks are formed by associations between sensory representations of the same modality to form assemblies or networks of unimodal sensory memory. Above, in polysensory association cortex, and with inputs from unimodal areas, more complex networks of polymodal memory are formed that associate sensory features of multiple origins. Those polymodal networks constitute the substrate for diverse forms of episodic and sematic memory, with wide distribution in higher association areas of posterior cortex. Networks of the transmodal cortex of areas 39 and 40, including cortex of the superior temporal gyrus (Wernicke's area), probably represent the highest forms of conceptual and semantic knowledge. Lesion of these areas induces certain forms of sensory aphasia and agnosia, including the loss of perceptual memory of speech and objects, or object categories.

In general, memory networks expand as they gain in hierarchical level. They fan up from their sensory base as they penetrate progressively higher layers of cortical organization with progressively broader and higher associations. Once established, memories and their networks are linked not only horizontally, within their hierachical layer, but vertically, between layers (symbolized by vertical bidirectional arrows in Figure 1). A low-level sensory network, for

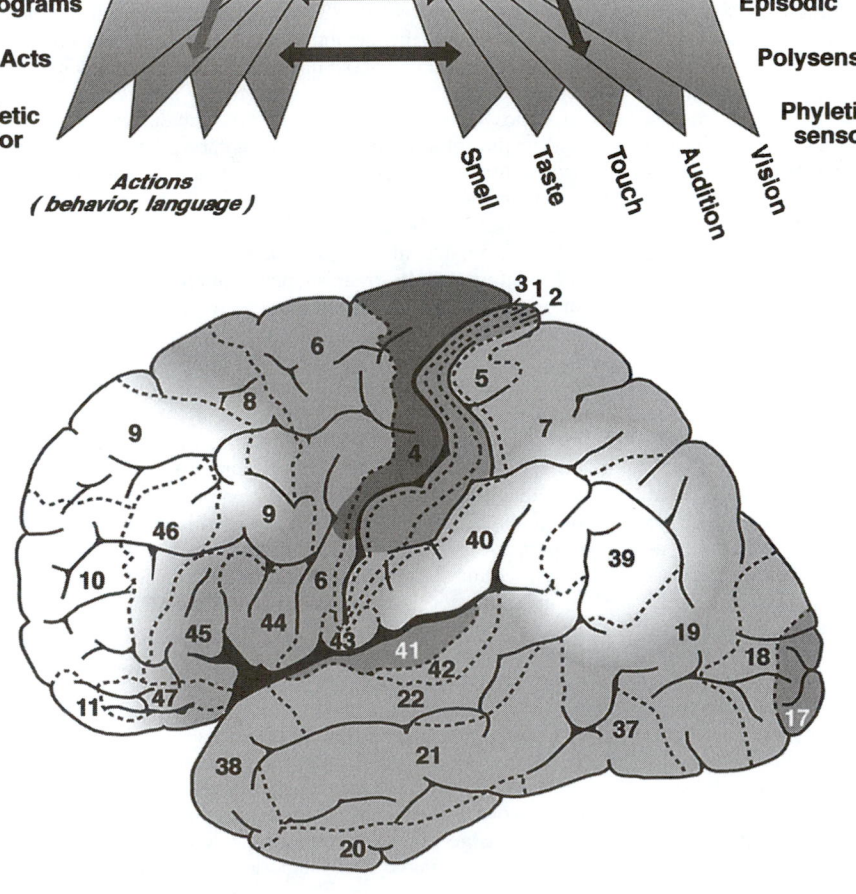

Figure 1. Schematic diagram of the hierarchical organization of memories in accord with the model presented in this article.

example, will establish associations with high-level semantic or conceptual networks. This will result from the co-occurrence of new sensory experiences with the activation of the high-level networks they elicit. In any event, the latter networks will be largely formed by ascending connections from lower levels. Assorted sensory experiences with common attributes will contribute to the formation of conceptual networks at the higher, semantic level. As a consequence of these dynamic interactions, networks of lower and concrete content will be nested within the higher-level conceptual and semantic networks that they have helped establish and that represent the higher and more abstract aspects of perceptual memory. As a consequence of these interactions within and between layers, memory networks profusely share cells and fibers. Conversely, any cortical cell and its connections may be part of many memory networks.

Further, as memory networks gain in hierarchical category, they become not only broader but more resilient, perhaps from increased number and redundancy of associations. Whereas sensory memories are especially vulnerable to discrete local damage (notably the phyletic structure of primary sensory cortices), high-level associative memories are less vulnerable. Since the latter are anchored in multiple sensory experiences, abstract knowledge is less liable to cortical damage than the concrete aspects of declarative memory, such as dates, names, faces, and places. The clinical evidence shows that these concrete elements of memory are especially liable to cortical injury. To some extent, which varies with the individual, these concrete elements of memory are subject to gradual loss as a function of normal aging. On the other hand, it takes a massive cortical lesion for the loss of conceptual perceptual memory to occur, that is, for the loss of what Kurt Goldstein called the "abstract attitude," meaning the utilization of conceptual knowledge in daily life.

Executive Memory

Motor memory, the representation of motor acts and behaviors, is widely distributed throughout the central nervous system. The spinal cord, the brainstem, and the cerebellum constitute the lowest levels of the hierarchy of brain structures harboring motor memories. These structures are the depositories of much of the motor phyletic memory of the organism at birth. This memory is largely innate, stereotypical, and dedicated to the fulfillment of essential drives. Some of it is conditionable and subject to cortical control and modulation.

The highest levels of motor memory, both phyletic and acquired, are supported by the cortex of the frontal lobe (Figure 1). The cortical networks of motor memory are formed essentially in accord with the same principles that guide the formation of perceptual memory, notably synchronous convergence. Here, however, the simultaneously converging signals are of both sensory and motor origin. This includes visual and auditory stimuli that coincide with motor action, or release it by one mechanism or another, and kinesthetic stimuli that accompany the action; in addition, some of the signals are "efferent copies" of the action as it is executed, copies that are provided by recurrent or collateral inputs from the motor system (corollary discharge). Consequently, many motor networks of the frontal cortex are extensions of perceptual networks of posterior cortex. Long corticocortical connections—in the uncinate fasciculus—would provide the functional substrate for those extensions (horizontal arrows in Figure 1).

At the base of the cortical executive or motor hierarchy is the primary motor cortex of the precentral gyrus, the substrate of phyletic motor memory in the neocortex. It supports the representation and execution of elementary motor acts that are defined by the contraction of particular muscles and muscle groups. Hierarchically above primary cortex is the premotor cortex (area 6), which several

lesion and unit studies implicate in the representation of motor acts and programs defined by goal and trajectory (Wiesendanger, 1981; Alexander and Crutcher, 1990). This cortex also participates in the elementary structuring of language. The more complex and novel programs of acquired behavior and language are represented in the prefrontal cortex, which is the highest level of the executive hierarchy. The prefrontal cortex is the cortex of association of the frontal lobe. Both phylogenetically and ontogenetically, it is one of the latest neocortical regions to develop (Fuster, 1997). In the human, it does not reach full maturation until the second decade of life. It receives abundant connections from posterior cortex, limbic formations, and the brainstem.

Neuropsychological studies implicate the prefrontal cortex in the representation of schemas of goal-directed action. Human subjects who have sustained lesions of lateral prefrontal cortex have difficulty remembering and formulating new plans of behavior and structures of language. Monkeys have difficulty learning and executing behavioral tasks that require the sequencing of motor acts, especially if the sequencing contains temporal gaps that have to be bridged by active memory ("working memory"). This kind of behavior is epitomized by the so-called delay tasks (e.g., delayed response, delayed matching). In both the human and nonhuman primate, lesions of the lateral prefrontal cortex impair performance on such tasks. There is some apparent specificity within the lateral prefrontal areas for the kinds of sensory information and motor activity that are processed in those tasks. Regional specificity, however, is secondary to temporal factors. Prefrontal lesions cause deficits in the formation and execution of temporal sequences of behavioral action ("temporal gestalts"), whatever the sensory and motor components of those sequences.

The practice and repeated execution of behavioral sequences seems to lead to the relocation of their representation from prefrontal cortex to lower stages of the motor hierarchy, especially the basal ganglia. Frontal lesions in human subjects induce deficits in the performance of complex voluntary movements without impairing automatic ones. This occurs even if these automatic movements are just as complex and require just as much effort as when they were originally learned. By neuroimaging, it is possible to follow to some degree the migration of executive memories from the prefrontal cortex to other structures of lower hierarchical rank. In the initial stages of the learning of a sequential motor task, certain areas of the dorsolateral prefrontal are activated (Jenkins et al., 1994). As the task becomes routine, parts of the cerebellum and the basal ganglia become more active, and the prefrontal cortex less. Still represented in prefrontal cortex, presumably, are those aspects of the task that are subject to uncertainty or ambiguity. Such is the case with delay tasks, where stimuli and responses contain both uncertainty and ambiguity. This is the reason why the correct performance of these tasks, even after learning, continues to depend on the functional integrity of the prefrontal cortex, and prefrontal cells continue to be involved in that performance.

Retrieval of Memory

Just as the formation of a memory is an associative phenomenon, so is the retrieval of that memory from permanent storage. Both associative phenomena are interdependent. New memory networks are formed by association between co-occurring sensory inputs and between these inputs and older networks that they activate by association. Therefore, new memory is in many respects the expansion of old memory. Whereas individual memories and their networks are expansions of phyletic memory, new individual networks are expansions of old ones. The essential point is that every act of memory formation is accompanied by retrieval of established memory. Retrieval is indispensable for memory formation. That may be the reason why the hippocampus appears to play an important role in both the acquisition and the recall of memory in the neocortex.

Electrophysiological studies in the monkey and neuroimaging in the human indicate that the retrieval of a memory, whether spontaneous or evoked, essentially consists in the activation of the cortical network that represents it (reviewed in Fuster, 1999). The neuronal mechanisms of retrieval are not known but can be presumed to involve the correlated activation of all the neuronal elements of a perceptual network by the sensory or internal (mental) activation of one of its associated components. If the network has executive or motor components, then the activation will extend to an associated executive network of frontal cortex. Above a certain threshold, that activation of an executive network may lead to the execution of action. If the action is sequential and dependent on serial perceptual inputs, then cell prefrontal assemblies will interact with posterior cortical assemblies in the mechanisms of working memory and preparatory set at the foundation of the perception-action cycle (Fuster, 1997; see also PREFRONTAL CORTEX IN TEMPORAL ORGANIZATION OF ACTION). Those mechanisms are still poorly understood. However, it seems increasingly plausible that they include the reverberation of activity in memory networks through recurrent circuits (Zipser et al., 1993).

Discussion

This article presents a general connectionist model of memory. It is proposed that memories consist in, and are represented by, widely distributed and profusely interactive networks of neocortical neurons. Memory networks are formed by modulation of synaptic contacts between concomitantly activated neurons representing discrete features of the external and internal environment. This takes place in the neocortex under the agency of limbic structures, notably the hippocampus. Memory formation is a highly dynamic process closely interdependent with retrieval, and memory networks remain in constant change throughout life, subject to expansion by new associations—and to age-related attrition. Memory networks are hierarchically organized in two broad sectors of neocortex: perceptual memory in posterior (postrolandic) cortex and executive memory in frontal (prerolandic) cortex. At the base of each cortical hierarchy there is a layer of phyletic memory (the structure of primary sensory or motor cortex). Above that layer, in cortex of association, lie the memories of the individual, from the lowest perceptual and motor representations to the highest conceptual representations of perception and action. The semantic and conceptual representations of perception lie in transmodal areas of posterior cortex, whereas the schematic and conceptual representations of action lie in areas of prefrontal cortex. Both are interconnected by long corticocortical fibers, thus forming high-level sensorimotor networks. In the organization of complex behavior, the two sectors of neocortex, posterior and prefrontal, interact dynamically at the summit of the perception-action cycle.

Road Map: Cognitive Neuroscience
Related Reading: Hebbian Synaptic Plasticity; Sequence Learning; Short-Term Memory; Visual Scene Perception

References

Alexander, G. E., and Crutcher, M. D., 1990, Functional architecture of basal ganglia circuits: Neural substrates of parallel processing, *Trends Neurosci.*, 13:266–271.

Amaral, D. G., 1987, Memory: Anatomical organization of candidate brain regions, in *Handbook of Physiology: Nervous System*, vol. V: *Higher Functions of the Brain*, Part 1 (F. Plum Ed.), Bethesda, MD: American Physiological Society, pp. 211–294.

Fuster, J. M., 1997, *The Prefrontal Cortex* (3rd ed.), Philadelphia: Lippincott-Raven.

Fuster, J. M., 1999, *Memory in the Cerebral Cortex*, Cambridge, MA: MIT Press. ◆

Hayek, F. A., 1952, *The Sensory Order*, Chicago: University of Chicago Press.

Hebb, D. O., 1949, *The Organization of Behavior*, New York: Wiley. ◆

Jenkins, I. H., Brooks, D. J., Nixon, P. D., Frackowiak, R. S. J., and Passingham, R. E., 1994, Motor sequence learning: A study with positron emission tomography, *J. Neurosci.*, 14:3775–3790.

Kandel, E. R., 1991, Cellular mechanisms of learning and the biological basis of individuality, in *Principles of Neural Science* (E. R. Kandel, J. H. Schwartz, and T. M. Jessell, Eds.), Norwalk, CT: Appleton and Lange, pp. 1009–1031.

Kohonen, T., 1984, *Self-Organization and Associative Memory*, Berlin: Springer-Verlag. ◆

Lashley, K. S., 1950, In search of the engram, *Symp. Soc. Exp. Biol.*, 4:454–482.

Mesulam, M., 1998, From sensation to cognition, *Brain*, 121:1013–1052. ◆

Pandya, D. N., and Yeterian, E. H., 1985, Architecture and connections of cortical association areas, in *Cerebral Cortex*, vol. 4 (A. Peters and E. G. Jones, Eds.), New York: Plenum Press, pp. 3–61. ◆

Squire, L. R., 1987, *Memory and Brain*, New York: Oxford University Press.

Stent, G. S., 1973, A physiological mechanism for Hebb's postulate of learning, *Proc. Natl. Acad. Sci. USA*, 70:997–1001.

Thompson, R. F., 1986, The neurobiology of learning and memory, *Science*, 233:941–947.

Wiesendanger, M., 1981, Organization of secondary motor areas of cerebral cortex, in *Handbook of Physiology* (S. R. Geiger, Ed.), Bethesda, MD: American Physiological Society, pp. 1121–1147.

Zipser, D., Kehoe, B., Littlewort, G., and Fuster, J., 1993, A spiking network model of short term active memory, *J. Neurosci.*, 13:3406–3420. ◆

Cortical Population Dynamics and Psychophysics

Udo A. Ernst and Christian W. Eurich

Introduction

Visual cortex is one of the most extensively studied regions in the mammalian brain. Over the past decade, much anatomical, physiological, and psychophysical knowledge about its properties has been accumulated experimentally. Considerable effort has been expended on theoretical and computational work to reproduce basic phenomena and to explain their underlying mechanisms.

In this article, we discuss one specific computational approach that has been successfully applied to a variety of problems on different levels of cortical information processing. The approach describes the cortical population dynamics in the form of structurally simple differential equations for the neurons' firing activities. The model class was introduced by Wilson and Cowan (1972, 1973) and is still very popular for, in our opinion, two reasons: first, it is powerful enough to reproduce a variety of cortical phenomena, and it captures the dynamics of neuronal populations seen in numerous experiments; and second, its degree of complexity is still low enough to allow analytical treatment that yields an understanding of the mechanisms leading to the observed behavior.

In the next section, we introduce the model class and discuss some of its basic properties. The following sections show how this model can be applied to explain dynamical properties of the primate visual system on different levels, from single neuron properties like selectivity for the orientation of a stimulus to higher cognitive functions related to the binding and processing of stimulus features in psychophysical discrimination experiments.

The goal of this article is to show that a model that abstracts from biophysical details is often sufficient to identify possible neuronal mechanisms of cortical information processing. The diversity of the examples we mention demonstrates that even a simplifying approach can place seemingly unrelated or even controversial findings in one coherent, unifying framework.

The Wilson-Cowan Model Class

A basic introduction to differential equations in the context of neural systems and the class of models described here can be found in Wilson (1999).

Single Units

The basic unit of the model is a neuronal population. The dynamics of an uncoupled population is described by an ordinary differential equation for its activity $A(t)$, which consists of a decay term and the synaptic input $I(t)$ (τ is a time constant),

$$\tau \frac{dA(t)}{dt} = -A(t) + h(I(t)) \tag{1}$$

The gain function, h, describes the activation of a population dependent on its synaptic input I. Wilson and Cowan (1972) derived this equation from a more general integro-differential equation by applying a temporal filter (*time coarse graining*). Therefore, the resulting Equation 1 is structurally simple, but not exact: one has to bear in mind that temporal variations on a small time scale have been averaged out. In the original publication of Wilson and Cowan, the activity A was identified by the *proportion* of active neurons in a population. For this reason, the gain function h was chosen to be a sigmoid function that saturates at 1 for high input levels (no more than all neurons can be active at a specific time). However, A can equally well be interpreted as the population's firing rate (this will be the case throughout this article). Then h is no longer bound to saturate at 1, and one of the simplest choices is a function that is 0 up to some threshold, and then increases linearly. This piecewise linear function may allow for an analytical treatment by considering appropriate case distinctions. Omitting the saturation regime at high I does not impose serious restrictions, because cortical neurons usually operate within the linear regime of their gain function. Futhermore, diverging network activity in the model will be an indication of an unphysiological parameter regime in which the overall network activity is not dynamically regulated, as it is likely to be in the cortex.

Columns

Cortical nervous tissue contains both excitatory and inhibitory neurons in a dense network. A general model of this network necessarily has to include both cell types, forming one excitatory population (e) and one inhibitory population (i). Each population typically represents some hundreds of single neurons. The populations are mutually connected with weights w_{ee}, w_{ie}, w_{ei}, and w_{ii}. Index pairs like ei are interpreted as a connection originating at the excitatory population and targeting the inhibitory population. We will identify the resulting dynamical system (Wilson and Cowan, 1972) with the concept of a cortical column:

$$\tau_e \frac{dA_e(t)}{dt} = -A_e(t) + h_e(w_{ee}A_e(t) - w_{ie}A_i(t) + I_e(t)) \tag{2}$$

$$\tau_i \frac{dA_i(t)}{dt} = -A_i(t) + h_i(w_{ei}A_e(t) - w_{ii}A_i(t) + I_i(t)) \tag{3}$$

At this point, we would like to note that two very similar model classes exist in the literature. Their dynamics differ in the sense that in the first class, A describes the activation or the firing rate of a population (in this case the nonlinearity in h is applied to the total synaptic input, $\dot{A} = -A + h(wA + I)$), while in the second class, A denotes the membrane potential (in that case h is applied directly to A, $\dot{A} = -A + wh(A) + I$). A reader of the original publications should not be confused, because both variants lead to qualitatively similar results and are often equally well suited to tackle a specific modeling problem.

Layers

A neuronal layer may be described as a multitude of columns arranged in a topographically ordered space. This space may have a varying number of dimensions. For example, some authors have used a one-dimensional chain representing the orientation preference axis; others identify a two-dimensional layer with the surface of the cortical tissue. With $\vec{x}, \vec{x}' \in C$ denoting positions within such a layer, the columns are coupled by appropriately chosen functions $W_{\{ei,ie,ee,ii\}}(\vec{x}, \vec{x}')$ (so-called *lateral couplings*). Mathematically, the neuronal layer is described as a pair of coupled partial differential equations (Wilson and Cowan, 1973):

$$\tau_e \frac{\partial A_e(\vec{x}, t)}{\partial t} = -A_e(\vec{x}, t)$$
$$+ h_e\left(w_{ee} \int_C A_e(\vec{x}', t)W_{ee}(\vec{x}, \vec{x}')d\vec{x}'\right.$$
$$\left. - w_{ie} \int_C A_i(\vec{x}', t)W_{ie}(\vec{x}, \vec{x}')d\vec{x}' + I_e(\vec{x}, t)\right) \tag{4}$$

$$\tau_i \frac{\partial A_i(\vec{x}, t)}{\partial t} = -A_i(\vec{x}, t)$$
$$+ h_i\left(w_{ei} \int_C A_e(\vec{x}', t)W_{ei}(\vec{x}, \vec{x}')d\vec{x}'\right.$$
$$\left. - w_{ii} \int_C A_i(\vec{x}', t)W_{ii}(\vec{x}, \vec{x}')d\vec{x}' + I_i(\vec{x}, t)\right) \tag{5}$$

The inputs $I_{\{e,i\}}$ are typically calculated by integrating a stimulus $S(\vec{x}, t)$ over an *afferent* coupling function $V_{\{e,i\}}(\vec{x}, \vec{x}')$:

$$I_{\{e,i\}}(\vec{x}, t) = \int_R S(\vec{x}', t)V_{\{e,i\}}(\vec{x}, \vec{x}')d\vec{x}' \tag{6}$$

where $\vec{x}, \vec{x}'$ are elements of an input space R. A convenient choice for the lateral as well as the afferent couplings are functions decaying with the distance between two populations, as has been shown in anatomical and physiological studies. Choosing W satisfying $W(\vec{x}, \vec{x}') = W(|\vec{x} - \vec{x}'|)$, the model becomes translationally and rotationally invariant. A commonly used prototype for these kernels is an n-dimensional Gaussian function defined as

$$W_{\{ee,ei,ie,ii\}}(|\vec{x} - \vec{x}'|) = \frac{1}{(\sqrt{2\pi\sigma_{\{e,i\}}^2})^n} \exp\left(-\frac{(\vec{x} - \vec{x}')^2}{2\sigma_{\{e,i\}}^2}\right) \tag{7}$$

The computational advantage of these kernels is that the integration reduces to a multiplication in Fourier space, which speeds up computation time considerably.

For most of this article, we will assume that connections originating from inhibitory populations will be longer than those originating from excitatory populations. Following this scheme, the effective coupling between two columns will have the shape of a Mexican hat (difference of Gaussians). This assumption, which is often made in modeling studies, is questionable insofar as long-ranging patchy excitatory connections exist, at least in the mature primary visual cortex. This may not be a problem, because the layout of primary visual cortex revealed by the structure of the orientation preference map suggests that inhibitory couplings dominate, at least over intermediate distances. Nevertheless, we will also discuss which different or additional phenomena are observed in the presence of long-range axons. For a more detailed introduction to neural layers, see LAYERED COMPUTATION IN NEURAL NETWORKS.

Dynamical Regimes and Orientation Preference

Quasi-linear and Marginally Stable Regimes

With different choices of the system parameters in Equations 4 and 5, almost all model variants exhibit one of two different dynamical behaviors: if the strength of the afferent input dominates over the lateral feedback, a homogeneous and constant input will lead to an activation pattern that is also spatially and temporally constant. This steady state is stable against noise. The parameter regime where this behavior occurs is called the *quasi-linear regime* (upper region in Figure 1). As soon as the inhibitory feedback gets weaker or the excitatory feedback gets stronger, the system enters a second regime, called the *marginally stable regime* (Ben-Yishai, Bar-Or, and Sompolinsky, 1995). Now the steady state is unstable, and even the smallest perturbation leads to the emergence of a pattern of activation clusters commonly called *blobs* (central portion of Figure 1). The mechanism for this type of pattern formation is easy to understand: if the input at one position is slightly increased, this perturbation of the steady state will be amplified by the dominating

excitatory feedback, while the longer-ranging inhibition will suppress the activity in the surround of the emerging blob. For related reading, see WINNER-TAKE-ALL NETWORKS.

Lateral Feedback and Orientation Selectivity

The existence of a marginally stable regime could have consequences for the emergence of orientation selectivity in primary visual cortical neurons. Ben-Yishai et al. (1995) observed that the shape of the blobs remains invariant against different input levels. In a one-dimensional model of a cortical hypercolumn, where $\bar{x} \in C$ is identified with the orientation preference Φ, they demonstrated that the response behavior of neurons to oriented gratings is accurately reproduced: the orientation tuning width remains largely invariant under changes of the stimulus amplitude (contrast). This finding indicates that cortical dynamics may be dominated by lateral feedback rather than by feedforward excitation. A weak afferent orientation bias, such as that emerging from a Hubel-Wiesel arrangement of LGN receptive fields, would then suffice to induce a sharply tuned orientation tuning curve. This idea, with its pros and cons and also the experimental evidence for the origin of orientation tuning, is discussed in detail in ORIENTATION SELECTIVITY (q.v.).

Inhomogeneities and Cortical Maps

Localization of Activation Clusters

In the marginally stable regime, each perturbation lays the seed for the emergence of an activation cluster. This perturbation could be induced by the afferent input, but also by structural inhomogeneities in the model. For example, the lateral coupling function may not be perfectly translationally and rotationally invariant but could be subject to small random jitter. Then, even a homogeneous and constant input would lead to the emergence of activation clusters. Preferentially, these clusters will be located at positions where by

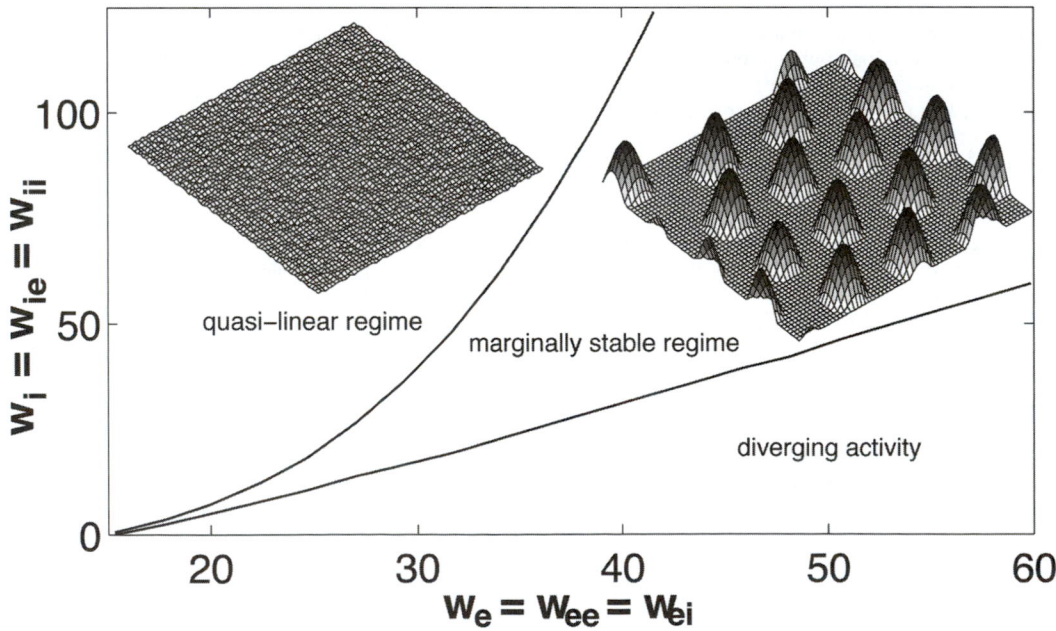

Figure 1. Phase diagram of the spatiotemporal Wilson-Cowan equations (Equations 4 and 5) for a two-dimensional sheet of neurons with threshold-linear h. Three dynamical regimes can be distinguished, depending on the weights w_e and w_i: the quasi-linear and the marginally stable regimes, as described in the text, and a biologically unplausible regime where neural firing rates diverge. Drawings in the quasi-linear and marginally stable regimes show a typical steady-state activity pattern of the excitatory layer for a constant input I plus a small amount of noise.

chance the lateral excitatory feedback is slightly stronger than at other positions nearby. If this jitter comes together with inhomogeneous afferent inputs, both effects will add up, and blobs will choose positions where the afferent input plus the lateral feedback will be largest. Note that in this model, the noise breaks the symmetry of the coupling kernels, and the model will no longer be rotationally and translationally invariant.

Instantaneous Emergence of Cortical Maps

Ernst et al. (2001) simulated a two-dimensional Wilson-Cowan model in which they put a small amount of static noise on the lateral coupling matrix, as can be expected in a biological system, with all its irregularities. They presented moving gratings or bars as stimuli, generating an inhomogeneous afferent input. By recording the model's response to differently oriented gratings (Figure 2A), they found that orientation and direction preference maps naturally emerged when the blobs localized at the spatial inhomogeneities in the model cortex (Figure 2B).

This model has several advantages over other approaches to map development because it reproduces seemingly controversial findings from experimental studies. First, the structure of the maps shows up within milliseconds and does not require any learning. Second, due to the intracortical origin of the map structure seeded by the random jitter of the lateral connections, the feature maps are identical for stimulation of either of the two eyes. Third, the gratings induce an oscillatory movement of the blobs around their preferred positions, which is different for opposite directions of movement. This suggests a new mechanism for directional selectivity of the neuronal response (for a detailed discussion, see DIRECTIONAL SELECTIVITY). And finally, the model reproduces the known relationships between different kinds of feature maps. Taken together, these properties qualify this approach as a model for the initial phase in cortical development where the coarse layout of the maps is determined, which then could get subsequently refined and rearranged by self-organizing mechanisms (see Swindale, 1996, for an extensive review and discussion).

Long-Range Connections and Contour Integration

Up to now, the couplings have been chosen as if there were no long-ranging excitatory connections in the brain. However, those connections exist, and they preferentially link neurons having similar orientation preferences. What dynamical phenomena can one expect if these connections are included?

Long-Range Connections

Several authors employ a connection scheme that locally has the shape of a Mexican hat but extends over that region, sending out additional excitatory connections targeting inhibitory and excitatory populations with a similar orientation preference. The columns in these models have a position (x_1, x_2) within the nervous tissue and an orientation preference Φ; thus, $C \ni \bar{x} = (x_1, x_2, \Phi)$. While the response of the *classical* model without long-range interactions would follow the dynamics described in the previous sections, the addition of long-range connections opens up the possibility that spatially extended stimuli modulate this response. The modulation will depend on the strength, or contrast, and the orientation of the stimuli presented. One important aspect of this excitatory modulation is that the net effect on the column's firing rate depends on activation of the target column, especially in cases where the populations have different thresholds or gains. The reason for this is that long-range input converges onto inhibitory and excitatory target populations; thus, the excitatory target population receives direct excitation and indirect inhibition. The balance between those two sources determines whether the total input inhibits or excites the target population (*differential interaction*).

Nonclassical Receptive Fields

Models with long-range connections have been examined to find an explanation for the so-called nonclassical receptive fields of neurons. Most visual cortical cells have shown dramatic changes in their response to a stimulus within their normal receptive field, when an additional stimulus has been presented outside that region (this additional stimulus alone would elicit no response). Typical phenomena include an increase in the response, if the two stimuli have orthogonal orientations, and a decrease if the stimuli are parallel in orientation (Sillito et al., 1995). The latter modulatory effect may change its sign when the stimuli are presented at a lower luminance level. These findings can largely be explained by population models with long-range interactions; in particular, it is easy to explain the sign change with dynamical properties relying on

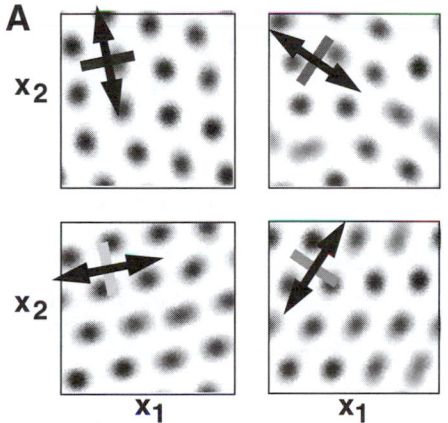
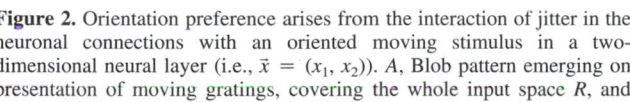
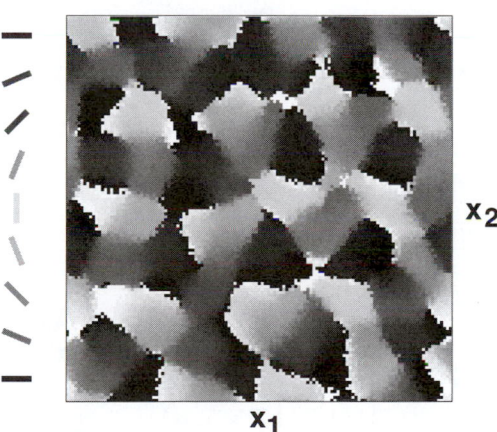

Figure 2. Orientation preference arises from the interaction of jitter in the neuronal connections with an oriented moving stimulus in a two-dimensional neural layer (i.e., $\bar{x} = (x_1, x_2)$). *A*, Blob pattern emerging on presentation of moving gratings, covering the whole input space R, and having different orientations, as shown by the bars. *B*, Vectorial sum of the single-condition blob patterns in *A* for different orientations, coded in scales of gray. The picture strongly resembles orientation maps obtained experimentally with voltage-sensitive dyes. (Adapted from Ernst et al., 2001.)

the differential interaction scheme (see Stetter, Bartsch, and Obermayer, 2000, and references therein). More information on nonclassical receptive fields can be found in VISUAL CORTEX: ANATOMICAL STRUCTURE AND MODELS OF FUNCTION (q.v.).

Association Fields

Another type of cortical coupling function is motivated by *association fields* measured in psychophysical experiments. Association fields quantify how the presentation of a bar at position (x_1, x_2) with orientation Φ will increase or decrease the threshold for detecting a bar at position (x'_1, x'_2) with orientation Φ'. The coupling matrix and model dimension are similar to the models employed in the last paragraph, with one important difference: the coupling function W is chosen according to the association field and therefore is not only orientation selective, but also directionally biased. In other words, two columns best responding to oriented bars being aligned in succession will be connected with a positive weight, while two columns best responding to oriented bars being aligned in parallel will be connected with a negative weight (Figure 3A) or will remain unconnected.

Contour Integration

An aspect of cortical information processing that can be examined and understood in this type of model is the dynamics of contour integration. Contours can be interpreted as a succession of aligned bars; thus, a coupling matrix based on the association field is especially suited to enhance the activity of columns stimulated by elements of the contour, whereas the activity of columns stimulated by distractors becomes suppressed. Li (1999, 2001) has accumulated evidence that contour integration may be explained by this kind of cortical model (Figures 3B and 3C). A close relation of

modeling work and psychophysical experiment shows that the structural simplicity of the Wilson-Cowan model class allows making specific predictions about certain experiments while opening the door to an understanding of the mechanisms at work behind the scenes.

Transient Dynamics and Feature Binding

The modeling approaches discussed so far have focused on the long-term behavior of solutions of Wilson-Cowan type of equations. In particular, steady states of the system and their stability have been associated with phenomena of cortical physiology and psychophysics. In this section, we study the transient dynamics of coupled neural populations and link it to perceptual phenomena in the context of feature binding.

Feature Inheritance and Shine-through

The spatiotemporal behavior of the visual system can be assessed psychophysically through experiments in which stimuli are presented successively for short time intervals. The visual system is thus forced to work at its spatial and temporal limit, resulting in illusions that elucidate cortical mechanisms of signal processing.

Two such illusions have recently been described (Herzog and Koch, 2001; Herzog, Fahle, and Koch, 2001). In the so-called *feature inheritance effect* (Figure 4A), a single vernier—two bars that are slightly displaced—is presented for a brief time (i.e., 10–30 ms, depending on the individual performance of the subject). The vernier is followed by a double grating of five nondisplaced bars that is presented for 300 ms. Psychophysically, subjects are not aware of the vernier but perceive a displaced grating. That is, the vernier is masked by the grating, which inherits the vernier's displacement. The inheritance effect has also been demonstrated for other fea-

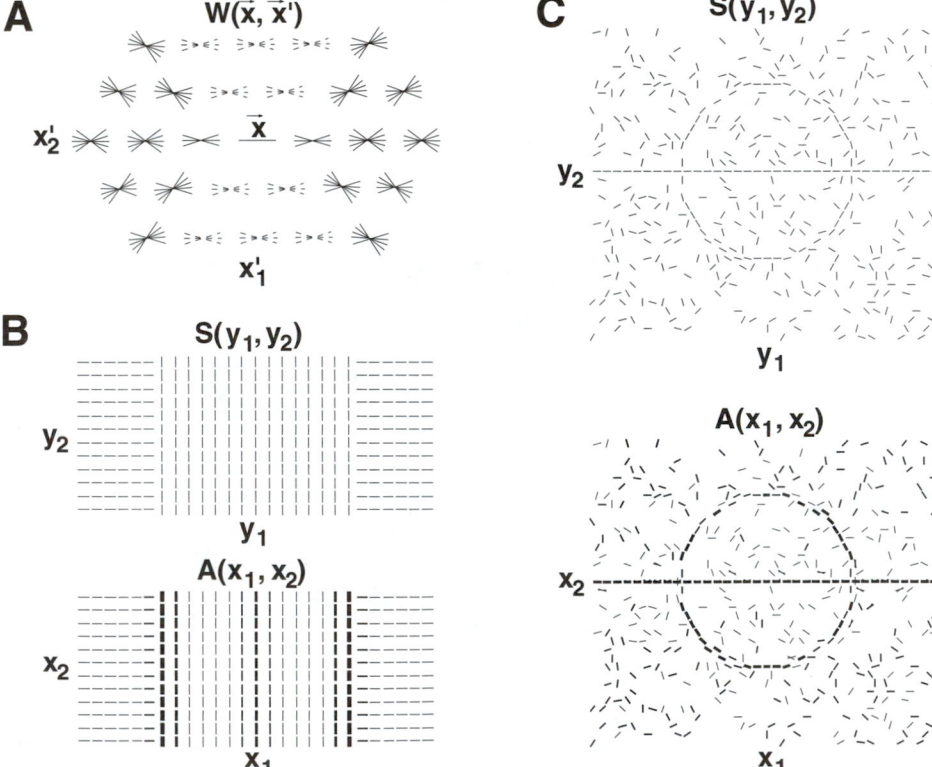

Figure 3. *A*, Coupling scheme W connecting the center column at $\bar{x}$ with the surround columns at $\bar{x}'$ ($\bar{x} = (x_1, x_2, \Phi)$). Excitatory connections are marked with thin bars, inhibitory connections with broken bars. The orientation of the bars denotes the difference in orientation preference of the connected columns. *B* and *C*, Sample stimuli $S(\bar{y})$, $\bar{y} \in R$, and the corresponding activation pattern $A(\bar{x})$, $\bar{x} \in C$. The activation level and the orientation preference of the corresponding column are coded by the thickness and the orientation of the bar, respectively. The connection scheme together with the model's dynamics lead to the enhancement of (orientation) discontinuites (*edge detection, B*) and to an increase in the activity of detectors stimulated by a closed contour (*contour integration, C*). (Adapted from Li, 1999.)

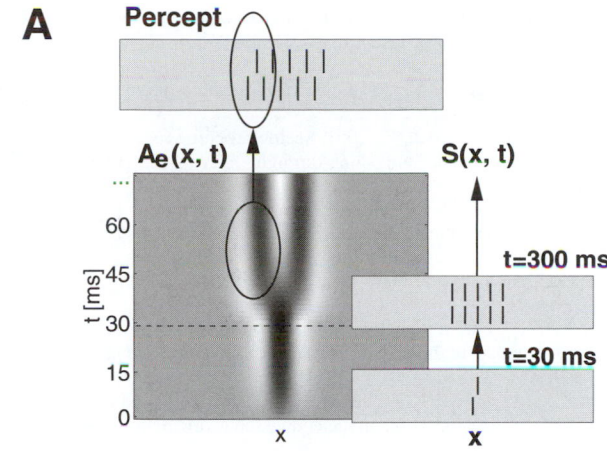

Figure 4. Stimuli, visual percept, and simulation result for the feature inheritance and shine-through effects. In the feature inheritance condition (A), a single vernier is followed by presentation of a grating of five bars (right panels). The percept is a displaced grating (top). The simulation shows the activity of the excitatory population in gray-scale coding. The central peak resulting from the vernier is rapidly suppressed by the edge activity of the grating. In the shine-through condition (B), the vernier is followed by presentation of an elongated grating of 25 bars (right). Perceptually, the vernier looks superimposed on the grating (top). The simulation of the excitatory population reveals that in this case, the central vernier activity persists for a longer time, leading to conscious perception of the shine-through element.

tures, such as orientation and apparent motion (Herzog and Koch, 2001).

Changes in the geometrical arrangement of the grating can modify or even abolish the feature inheritance effect. An example is shown in Figure 4B, where an extended grating of 25 bars follows the presentation of the vernier. In this case, subjects are aware of the vernier, which appears superimposed on the grating (*shine-through effect*).

Vernier Visibility as a Transient Effect

The spatiotemporal version of the Wilson-Cowan equations (Equations 4 and 5) can be used to account for the vernier visibility in the different masking conditions. To elucidate the underlying neural mechanisms, a simple, one-dimensional version without the property of orientation tuning is employed. Consider an excitatory and an inhibitory population of cortical neurons arranged along a one-dimensional axis, $C = \mathbb{R}$. The input space is also taken to be one-dimensional, $R = \mathbb{R}$. For reasons of simplicity, we assume symmetry in the weights ($w_{ee} = w_{ei}$; $w_{ie} = w_{ii}$) and in the interaction kernels ($W_{ee} = W_{ei} \equiv W_e$; $W_{ie} = W_{ii} \equiv W_i$). The latter are modeled as Gaussians (cf. Equation 7). The external input current is identical for both populations, $I_e(x, t) = I_i(x, t) \equiv I(x, t)$, and is given by a convolution of the presented spatiotemporal stimulus intensity $S(x, t)$ with a Mexican hat type of filter $V(x - x')$ whose integral vanishes,

$$V(|x - x'|) = \frac{1}{\sqrt{2\pi\sigma_E^2}} \exp\left(-\frac{(x - x')^2}{2\sigma_E^2}\right)$$
$$- \frac{1}{\sqrt{2\pi\sigma_I^2}} \exp\left(-\frac{(x - x')^2}{2\sigma_I^2}\right)$$

resembling on-off receptive field properties of LGN neurons. The stimulus $S(x, t)$ takes the value 1 if it is part of the vernier or a bar element, and 0 otherwise.

The system parameters—kernel widths, synaptic weights, population time constants, and gain functions—are adjusted considering symmetries and relations in cortical anatomy and physiology.

Numerical results for the feature inheritance and shine-through conditions as described above are given in Figure 4. The gray-

scale-coded activities of the excitatory populations show peaks at the position of the vernier and at the edges of the gratings, whereas almost no activity emerges in the bulk of the gratings. A comparison of the central peaks reveals that in the feature inheritance condition (Figure 4A), the vernier activity decays earlier than in the shine-through condition (Figure 4B). This is due to a strong inhibition by the active neurons representing the nearby edges of the grating. However, in the extended grating comprised of 25 bars, the edges are too far away to exert an influence on the center. The fast suppression of the vernier activity by the small grating shown in Figure 4A leads to a complete masking of the vernier element and a subsequent erroneous binding of its feature, the displacement, to the grating. On the other hand, conditions that allow a longer persistence of the vernier activity, like the one shown in Figure 4B, result in a conscious perception of the vernier and its displacement. Thus, the occurrence of feature inheritance or shine-through is explained by the transient dynamics of a Wilson-Cowan type of model.

The model can be applied to a number of further stimulus conditions and provides quantitative predictions for the visibility of the vernier element with a single set of model parameters. The model is robust with respect to parameter changes, and the overall results are the same no matter whether the dynamical equations are formulated for the population firing rates or the average membrane potentials. In fact, Li was also able to see the described transient behavior in her cortex model (Li, personal communication). The reduced one-dimensional model presented here also yields an analytical access and allows the identification of neural mechanisms responsible for the observed psychophysical effects (Herzog, Ernst, and Eurich; see http://www-neuro.physik.uni-bremen.de/institute/research/vernier.html)

Discussion

The Wilson-Cowan model class yields a description of the behavior of coupled neural populations on a coarse time scale. Versions of the model include purely temporal behavior and spatiotemporal behavior in one and two spatial dimensions, and may incorporate further stimulus features such as the orientation of edges as additional model dimensions. The relatively simple structure of the equations allows an analytical and thorough numerical access to the system dynamics. In recent years the model class has been successfully employed to account for various physiological and psychophysical phenomena of the visual system such as orientation selectivity, cortical map formation, figure-ground segregation, feature binding, and masking effects.

Phenomena outside the visual system are beyond the scope of this article. The same holds for several dynamical aspects of the population equations that have not been addressed; among these are hysteresis phenomena and limit-cycle activity (Wilson and Cowan, 1972). For example, Tsodyks et al. (1997) have modeled oscillatory neural activity in rat hippocampus.

An important extension of the Wilson-Cowan model class is obtained if the simplification of time coarse graining is dropped. The search for appropriate equations describing the behavior of neural populations also on fast time scales and under the consideration of noise is a topic of much current interest. A suggestion that has been put forward in this context is the use of a Fokker-Planck equation; see INTEGRATE-AND-FIRE NEURONS AND NETWORKS and Knight (2000) and references therein for a framework of a variety of such approaches.

Road Map: Neural Coding
Related Reading: Direction Selectivity; Integrate-and-Fire Neurons and Networks; Layered Computation in Neural Networks; Orientation Selectivity; Pattern Formation, Neural; Visual Cortex: Anatomical Structure and Models of Function; Winner-Take-All Networks

References

Ben-Yishai, R., Bar-Or, R., and Sompolinsky, H., 1995, Theory of orientation tuning in visual cortex, *Proc. Natl. Acad. Sci. USA*, 92:3844–3848.

Ernst, U. A., Pawelzik, K. R., Sahar-Pikielny, C., and Tsodyks, M. V., 2001, Intracortical origin of visual maps, *Nature Neurosci.*, 4:431–436.

Herzog, M. H., Fahle, M., and Koch, C., 2001, Spatial aspects of object formation revealed by a new illusion, shine-through, *Vision Res.*, 41:2325–2335.

Herzog, M. H., and Koch, C., 2001, Seeing properties of an invisible object: Feature inheritance and shine-through, *Proc. Natl. Acad. Sci. USA*, 98:4271–4275.

Knight, B. W., 2000, Dynamics of encoding in neural populations: Some general mathematical features, *Neural Computat.*, 12:473–518.

Li, Z., 1999, Visual segmentation by contextual influences via intra-cortical interactions in the primary visual cortex, *Netw. Comput. Neural Syst.*, 10:187–212.

Li, Z., 2001, Computational design and nonlinear dynamics of a recurrent network model of the primary visual cortex, *Neural Computat.*, 13:1749–1780.

Sillito, A. M., Grieve, K. L., Jones, H. E., Cudeiro, J., and Davis, J., 1995, Visual cortical mechanisms detecting focal orientation discontinuities, *Nature*, 378:492–496.

Stetter, M., Bartsch, H., and Obermayer, K., 2000, A mean field model for orientation tuning, contrast saturation and contextual effects in area 17, *Biol. Cybern.*, 82:291–304.

Swindale, N. V., 1996, The development of topography in the visual cortex: A review of models, *Netw. Comput. Neural Syst.*, 7:161–247. ◆

Tsodyks, M. V., Skaggs, W. E., Sejnowski, T. J., and McNaughton, B. L., 1997, Paradoxical effects of external modulation of inhibitory interneurons, *J. Neurosci.*, 17:4382–4388.

Wilson, H. R., 1999, *Spikes, Decisions, and Actions*, Oxford: Oxford University Press. ◆

Wilson, H. R., and Cowan, J. D., 1972, Excitatory and inhibitory interactions in localized populations of model neurons, *Biophys. J.*, 12:1–24.

Wilson, H. R., and Cowan, J. D., 1973, A mathematical theory of the functional dynamics of cortical and thalamic nervous tissue, *Kybernetik*, 13:55–80.

Covariance Structural Equation Modeling for Neurocognitive Networks

Anthony Randal McIntosh

Introduction

Covariance structural equation modeling (CSEM) has proven to be an important analytic tool in functional neuroimaging research. Along with other network analytic methods that are focused on relating the interactions between brain areas with cognition, CSEM can provide important insights into the operation of large-scale neurocognitive systems. This review is divided into three sections. The first outlines the theoretical and technical basis for the examination of large-scale neural systems. The second provides a brief summary of some applications of CSEM to human neuroimaging data collected using either positron emission tomography (PET) or functional magnetic resonance imaging (fMRI). There are several applications of CSEM to studies of normal aging and patient populations that will not be reviewed here (Maguire, Vargha-Khadem, and Mishkin, 2001). The article concludes with some speculation on the utility of network analyses in developing brain theory and how it may be used in conjunction with synthetic neural modeling approaches. For related points on this topic, see SYNTHETIC FUNCTIONAL BRAIN MAPPING.

Theoretical Basis of Network Analysis and the Tools

The driving assumption behind the use of CSEM is that the covariances/correlations of activity are measures of neural interactions. The activity measures may be electromagnetic (e.g., field potentials) or hemodynamic (e.g., cerebral blood flow, oxygen consumption). Neural interactions refer to influences that different elements in the nervous system have on each other via synaptic communication (the term "elements" refers to any constituent of the nervous system, either a single neuron or collections thereof). Activity changes in one neural element usually result from a change in the influence of other connected elements, so focusing only on activity in one area cannot identify the change in afferent influence. Furthermore, it is logically possible for the influences on an element to change without an appreciable change in measured activity. The simplest example would be one in which an afferent influence switches from one source to another without a change in the strength of the influence. Monitoring regional activity alone would miss this shift, but measures of the relation of activity between elements—e.g., the covariance—would not.

Structural Equation Modeling

The foundation for covariance analysis in neuroimaging was laid by Horwitz in a number of papers that looked at regional interrelations in a pairwise manner (Horwitz, Duara, and Rapoport, 1984). Covariance structural equation modeling (CSEM), or path analysis, is a logical extension from this; it uses the anatomical connections between areas in an attempt to characterize the effects between areas, called path coefficients, within a larger functional network (for a complete review, see Bollen, 1989; McIntosh and Gonzalez-Lima, 1994). The covariances among the variables, computed either across subjects within a specific cognitive task or across tasks within a subject, are used to provide weights for the anatomical links in a manner similar to a multiple linear regression.

Covariances used in multivariate analyses can identify the dominant functional and/or effective connections during the performance of a cognitive or behavioral operation. In the context of neuroimaging, *functional connectivity* is a statement that two regions show some non-zero correlation of activity but does not specify how this correlation comes about, while *effective connectivity* is a statement about the direct effect one region has on another, accounting for mutual or intervening influences (Friston, 1994). For the present review, measures of covariances are estimations of functional connectivity while the path coefficients derived from CSEM are estimates of effective connectivity.

In terms of basic equations, consider a four-node network that can be expressed by a series of structural equations (regression equations) as follows:

$$A = \psi_A$$
$$B = wA + \psi_B$$
$$C = vA + yB + \psi_C$$
$$D = xA + zB + \psi_D$$

where w, x, y, and z are parameters to be estimated (the path coefficients) and ψ denotes a residual influence unique to that region. The residual term is best conceived of unique effects on the region that are not part of the network under consideration.

The network can also be expressed as a series of matrices:

$$
\begin{pmatrix} \eta \\ A \\ B \\ C \\ D \end{pmatrix}
=
\begin{pmatrix} \beta \\ 0 & 0 & 0 & 0 \\ w & 0 & 0 & 0 \\ v & y & 0 & 0 \\ x & z & 0 & 0 \end{pmatrix}
*
\begin{pmatrix} \eta \\ A \\ B \\ C \\ D \end{pmatrix}
+
\begin{pmatrix} \psi \\ \psi_A & 0 & 0 & 0 \\ 0 & \psi_B & 0 & 0 \\ 0 & 0 & \psi_C & 0 \\ 0 & 0 & 0 & \psi_D \end{pmatrix}
$$

where η contains the variances of the regions, β contains the path coefficients, and ψ contains the residuals.

Estimates of the path coefficients and residuals are derived from the original interregional covariances. Let the covariance matrix among regions be σ, and let the covariances implied by the estimates for β and ψ be Σ, which is computed by

$$\Sigma = inv(I - \beta)^T * (\psi^T * \psi) * inv(I - \beta)$$

where inv denotes matrix inversion, I is an identity matrix, and T denotes a matrix transpose. Initial estimates for β and ψ are usually done by using a variation of least squares, and then the estimates are improved through iterative fitting to minimize the difference between σ and Σ. There are a number of different iterative search algorithms and fitting functions that have been used in CSEM, which are reviewed by Bollen (1989).

The path coefficients can also be compared statistically between different tasks or groups. This has been the primary application of CSEM to neuroimaging, where the goal is to determine whether the effective connections within the same anatomical network vary depending on cognitive challenge. Some recent extensions have used CSEM to test hypothesized models of effective connections for specific cognitive operations (Bullmore et al., 2000).

Empirical Examples

Dorsal and Ventral Stream Processing in Perceptual Matching

One well-established functional distinction in the brain is between object and spatial visual pathways. The foundation for this dual organization can be traced at least as far back as the 1930s, and one of its strongest expressions to date is in the dorsal and ventral cortical processing streams, described by Ungerleider and Mishkin (1982), which corresponds to object and spatial processing pathways, respectively. A similar duality was identified in humans with the aid of PET (Haxby et al., 1991). In an attempt to characterize the interactions within these cortical pathways, McIntosh et al. (1994) used CSEM to explore cortical interactions that were specific to object and spatial processing.

A match-to-sample task for faces was used to explore object vision. For spatial vision, a match-to-sample task for the location of a dot within a square was used. The results from the right hemisphere analysis are presented in Figure 1 (left hemisphere interactions did not differ between tasks). Path coefficients along the ventral pathway from cortical area 19v extending into the frontal lobe were stronger in the face-matching model, while interactions along the dorsal pathway from area 19d to the frontal lobe were relatively stronger in the location-matching model. Among posterior areas, the differences in path coefficients were mainly in magnitude. Occipitotemporal interactions between area 19v and area 37 were stronger in the face-matching model, while the impact of area 17/18 to 19d and the occipitoparietal influences from area 19d to area 7 were stronger in the location matching model.

The anatomical connections allowed for interactions between the dorsal and ventral pathways with connections from area 37 to area 7 and from area 7 to area 21. The interactions among these areas showed task-dependent differences in magnitude and sign. The functional networks show that while the strongest positive interactions in each model may have preferentially been in one pathway, the parallel pathways were not functioning independently. Strong interactions between parallel pathways have been a consistent finding in all CSEM applications to imaging data. Therefore, while a certain pathway or area may be critical for a particular function, operations in the intact brain involve interactions among many regions.

Spatial Attention

Network interactions that underlie cognitive operations are expressed as a change in the effective connections between parts of the network. As is illustrated above, if visual attention is directed to the features of an object, effective connections among ventral posterior cortical areas tend to be stronger, whereas visual attention directed to the spatial location leads to stronger interactions among dorsal posterior areas. Another way that cognitive operations may express is through the modulation of effective connections between regions. In this case, an area may provide an enabling condition to foster communications between regions. Such an effect was the focus of a model of visuospatial attention by Buchel and Friston (1997).

In this fMRI study, subjects alternated between periods of overt attention for a change to a moving visual dot pattern and periods when they were not attending to the display. Two models were evaluated. The first was a feedforward network from primary visual (V1) to dorsal occipital cortex (V5) to posterior parietal (PP) cortices. In this model, the "attend" condition showed stronger path coefficients than when there was no direct attention to the display. The second model assessed whether prefrontal

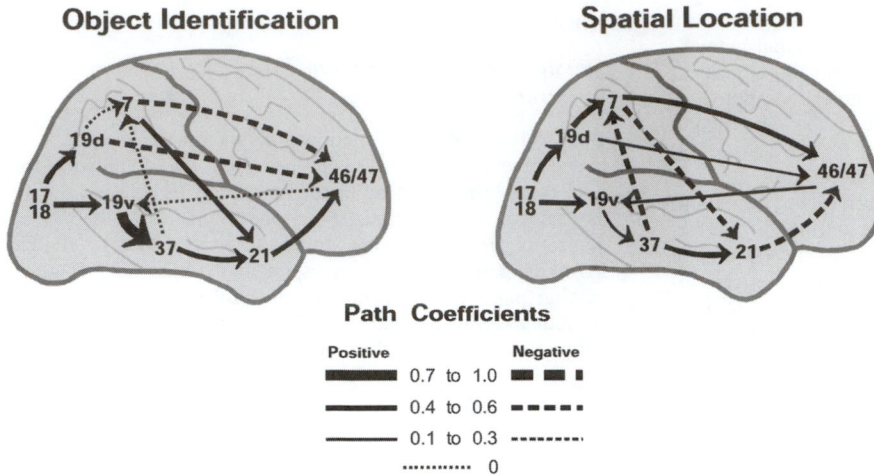

Figure 1. Functional interactions between cortical areas in the right hemisphere for object and spatial vision operations. The numbers on the cortical surface refer to Brodmann areas (d = dorsal, v = ventral). The arrows represent the anatomical connections between areas, and the magnitude of the direct effect from one area to another is proportional to the arrow width for each path.

cortex (PFC) had a modulatory effect in the effective connections between V5 and PP. This model had a direct influence from V5 to PP as well as the interaction term where the effect from V5 to PP depended on PFC (PFCmod). The expectation was that if the attentional effects manifest only on the direct connection from V5 to PP, then the estimate for PFCmod would be zero. The authors demonstrated that the modulatory effect was significant for all subjects. This modulatory effect seemed to vary in an activity-dependent manner in which the relation between V5 and PP was stronger during periods when PFC activity was highest.

This model demonstrated two important points. From the methodological point, it shows how more complex neurobiological effects can be modeled in CSEM. Buchel and Friston modeled a simple interaction term, but that same approach can be used to model true nonlinear effects (Bollen, 1989). From the neurobiological perspective, it demonstrates that cognition can be expressed in the brain either as changes in the direct effect between regions, as a modulatory effect, or in some cases both. What CSEM provides is a quantitative method to examine these possibilities.

Associative Learning

One example of the use of network analysis to test specific hypotheses about regional interactions comes from study of sensory learning (McIntosh, Cabeza, and Lobaugh, 1998). The task had subjects learn an association between a tone and a visual stimulus. Using PET, brain activity was measured in response to the tone across acquisition of the association. The expectation was that as the tone acquired behavioral significance, presentation of the tone would elicit activity in visual areas. Because the activation of visual areas would occur without overt visual stimulation, the second hypothesis was that this activation would be mediated through effects from higher-order cortical areas, likely posterior association or prefrontal cortices. The effective connections between visual cortex and anterior regions were quantified by using CSEM to determine which of these candidates exerted the strongest influence on these visual areas.

Activation of occipital cortex in area 18 to the tone was observed as training proceeded, confirming the first expectation. CSEM of influences on area 18 suggested that two areas in particular seem to exert the dominant influence as the association was learned. Superior temporal cortex (auditory association, area 41/42) and prefrontal cortex near area 10 both changed their ef-

fect on area 18 from suppressive to facilitory as the association was learned.

This study demonstrated learning-related changes in effective connectivity. Although the areas selected for CSEM were related to behavior, it is not clear whether the changes in effective connectivity impacts directly on learning-related performances changes. Buchel, Coull, and Friston (1999) provided a convincing demonstration that changes in effective connectivity related directly to learning. Subjects learned to associate visually presented objects with their location in space. To confirm that the behavioral changes across the experiment related directly to network dynamics, the changes in effective connections between dorsal and ventral processing stream were correlated with subject's learning rate. A robust correlation was found between the learning rate and the change in the influence of posterior parietal cortex (dorsal stream area) on inferotemporal cortex (ventral stream area). This is consistent with the task demands and demonstrates that network dynamics can be directly related to overt changes in behavior.

Awareness and Prefrontal Cortex Interactions

As a follow-up to the simple associative learning study described above, McIntosh and colleagues further investigated the neural interactions subserving cross-modal learning using differential conditioning (McIntosh, Rajah, and Lobaugh, 1999). Two tones were used that had differential relations to the visual stimuli. One tone was a strong predictor of the presentation of a visual stimulus (Tone+), and the other tone was a weak predictor (Tone−). The sample of subjects was divided perfectly in half into those who were aware of the stimulus associations and those who were not. Furthermore, only *aware* subjects learned the differentiation between the tones, while *unaware* subjects showed no behavioral evidence of learning.

The strongest group difference in brain activity elicited by the tones was in left prefrontal cortex (LPFC) near area 9. In aware subjects, LPFC activity showed progressively greater activity to Tone− than Tone+. In unaware subjects, no consistent changes were seen in LPFC or in any of the other regions. At first, these results seem to confirm the prominent role of PFC in monitoring functions and especially its putative role in awareness. However, PFC activation has also been found in tasks in which there was no overt awareness (Berns, Cohen, and Mintun, 1997). It was thus possible that interactions of PFC with other brain regions,

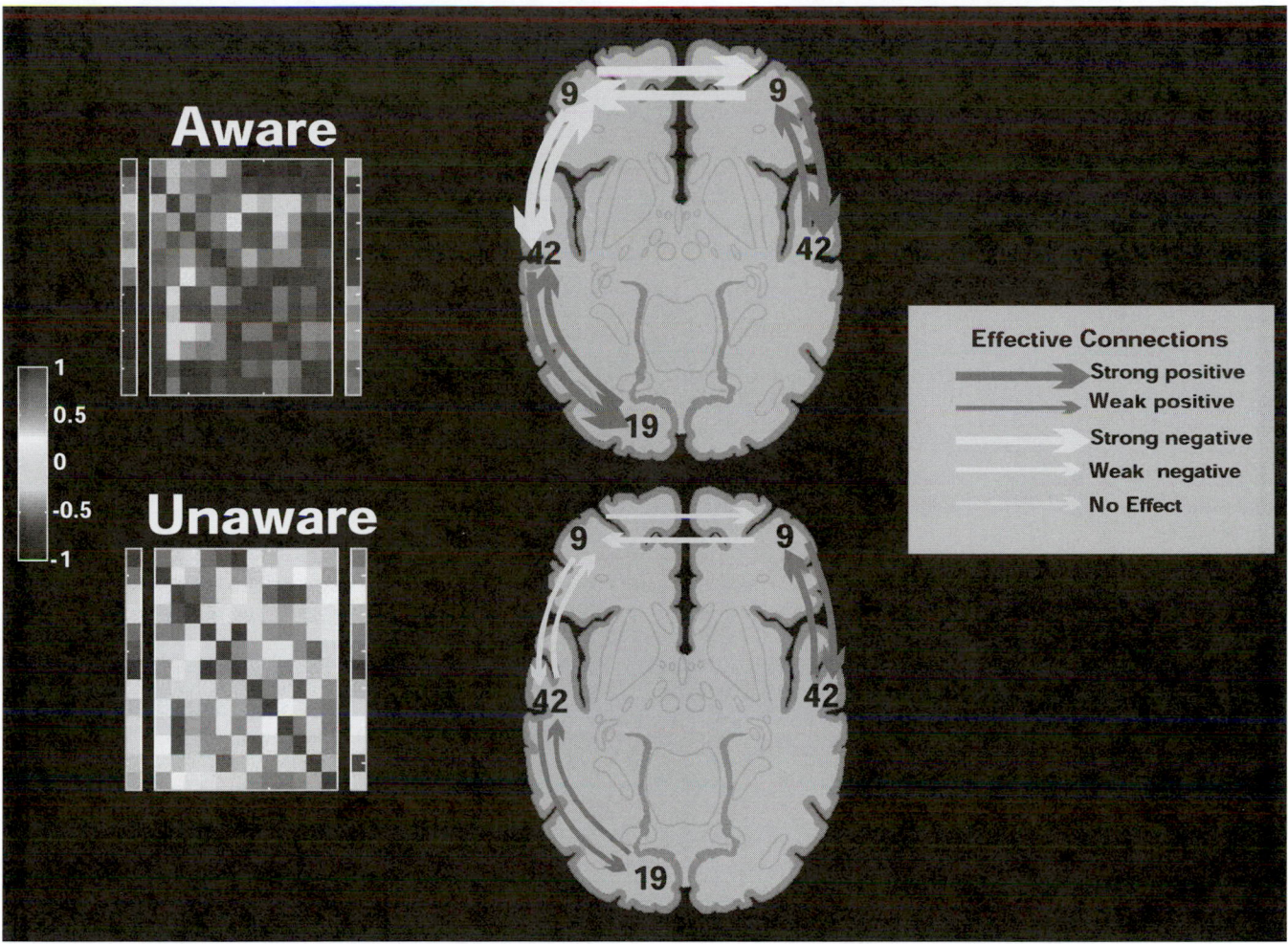

Figure 2. Correlation plots and functional networks from late phases of training in a differential sensory conditioning task. The plots on the left of the figure are pseudo-colored matrices of the correlations of left prefrontal cortex area 9 (first column) with sensory and association cortices, and the correlations of all regions with behavior are shown in the last column of the matrix. The correlation values are represented as color gradations, according to the scale on the far left of the figure. The matrices are symmetric about the major diagonals, which are all ones. The right of the figure shows the functional networks for the two groups. Aware subjects showed strong effective connections involving left prefrontal area 9 and other regions. Conversely, the network for the unaware subjects showed no strong left prefrontal involvement.

present in aware but not in unaware subjects, would better describe the neural system underlying awareness in this task.

When the interactions of LPFC was assessed between the two groups, large differences were found in the strength and pattern of functional connections among several brain areas, including right PFC, bilateral superior temporal cortices (auditory association), occipital cortex, and medial cerebellum. These areas were much more strongly correlated in aware subjects than unaware subjects (Figure 2). To explore some of the network interactions within an anatomical reference, CSEM was applied to a subset of these regions.

As may be expected from the correlation matrices, there were significant differences in the effective connections for aware subjects, including robust interactions involving LPFC. The functional network for unaware subjects differed from that for aware subjects, but there were no significant changes in effective connections across the experiment for the unaware group, and the involvement of LPFC was weak. This confirms that LPFC was not interacting systematically across subjects in the unaware group.

Discussion: Implications for Computational Modeling and Theoretical Efforts

Object and Spatial Vision

Aside from the confirmation of the dorsal/ventral distinction, it was noted that these functionally independent parallel systems could interact during different operations. While there were dominant interactions along dorsal and ventral streams in spatial and object tasks, respectively, there was cross-talk between the two streams, which implies that they need not be functionally independent. The study of Buchel et al. (1999) demonstrates that the interactions between pathways can depend on experience, and the study of Buchel and Friston (1997) suggests mechanisms whereby other cortical areas may modulate the interactions between posterior sensory regions.

Neural Context and Network Operations

A consistent observation in CSEM applications to neuroimaging is that similar areas are engaged in many cognitive functions, and what discriminates these cognitive operations are the pattern of interactions within large-scale networks rather than the involvement of a particular area. This has led to the concept of a *neural context,* in which the functional relevance of a particular region is determined by its interactions with other areas (McIntosh, 1999). Systems-level neuroanatomy shows that brain regions receive projections from many areas and send projections to many others. Neural context emphasizes that the precise pattern of these functionally engaged structural connections defines the translation of brain operations into cognitive operations. Consequently, the same region may show identical levels of activity across many different tasks. Because the pattern of interactions with other connected areas differs, the resulting cognitive operations vary, yet the same region is involved in each task. Stated differently, the neural context within which an area is active embodies the cognitive operation. The implications for computational modeling would be to develop models that can carry out more than one cognitive function through a change in the pattern of interactions among nodes. Thus, the focus would go from trying to model the computations in a single task to deriving a single model configuration that can do multiple tasks.

The relationship between neural modeling and experimental neuroscience continues to mature. The primary utility of modeling comes when they are derived to support specific hypotheses, and serve as frameworks for understanding complex data. Modeling efforts, whether empirically based like CSEM, theoretical, or computational, are all approximations of reality and as such are ultimately false. However, it is not necessarily the model that furthers our knowledge base. Rather, when a model is falsified and subsequently reformulated, scientific progress is made.

Road Map: Cognitive Neuroscience
Related Reading: Imaging the Visual Brain; Object Recognition, Neurophysiology; Schema Theory; Synthetic Functional Brain Mapping

References

Berns, G. S., Cohen, J. D., and Mintun, M. A., 1997, Brain regions responsive to novelty in the absence of awareness, *Science,* 276:1272–1275.

Bollen, K. A., 1989, *Structural Equations with Latent Variables,* New York: Wiley. ◆

Buchel, C., and Friston K., 1997, Modulation of connectivity in visual pathways by attention: Cortical interactions evaluated with structural equation modeling and fMRI, *Cereb. Cortex,* 7:768–778.

Buchel, C., Coull, J. T., and Friston, K. J., 1999, The predictive value of changes in effective connectivity for human learning, *Science,* 283:1538–1541.

Bullmore, E., Horwitz, B., Honey, G., Brammer, M., Williams, S., and Sharma, T., 2000, How good is good enough in path analysis of fMRI data? *Neuroimage,* 11:289–301.

Friston, K. J., 1994, Functional and effective connectivity: A synthesis, *Hum. Brain Mapp.,* 2:56–78.

Haxby, J. V., Grady, C. L., Horwitz, B., Ungerleider, L. G., Mishkin, M., Carson, R. E., Herscovitch, P., Schapiro, M. B., and Rapoport, S. I., 1991, Dissociation of object and spatial visual processing pathways in human extrastriate cortex, *Proc. Natl. Acad. Sci. USA,* 88:1621–1625.

Horwitz, B., Duara, R., and Rapoport, S. I., 1984, Intercorrelations of glucose metabolic rates between brain regions: Application to healthy males in a state of reduced sensory input, *J. Cereb. Blood Flow Metabol.,* 4:484–499.

Maguire, E. A., Vargha-Khadem, F., and Mishkin, M., 2001, The effects of bilateral hippocampal damage on fMRI regional activations and interactions during memory retrieval, *Brain,* 124:1156–1170.

McIntosh, A. R., 1999, Mapping cognition to the brain through neural interactions, *Memory,* 7:523–548.

McIntosh, A. R., and Gonzalez-Lima, F., 1994, Structural equation modeling and its application to network analysis in functional brain imaging, *Hum. Brain Mapp.,* 2:2–22. ◆

McIntosh, A. R., Cabeza, R. E., and Lobaugh, N. J., 1998, Analysis of neural interactions explains the activation of occipital cortex by an auditory stimulus, *J. Neurophysiol.,* 80:2790–2796.

McIntosh, A. R., Rajah, M. N., and Lobaugh, N. J., 1999, Interactions of prefrontal cortex related to awareness in sensory learning, *Science,* 284:1531–1533.

McIntosh, A. R., Grady, C. L., Ungerleider, L. G., Haxby, J. V., Rapoport, S. I., and Horwitz, B., 1994, Network analysis of cortical visual pathways mapped with PET, *J. Neurosci.,* 14:655–666.

Ungerleider, L. G., and Mishkin, M., 1982, Two cortical visual systems, in *Analysis of Visual Behavior* (D. J. Ingle, M. A. Goodale, and R. J. W. Mansfield, Eds.), Cambridge, MA: MIT Press, pp. 549–586.

Crustacean Stomatogastric System

Scott L. Hooper

Introduction

The stomatogastric nervous system (STNS) of decapod crustacea generates the rhythmic motor patterns of the four areas of the crustacean stomach—the esophagus, cardiac sac, gastric mill, and pylorus—and contains some of the best-understood central pattern–generating networks in neurobiology. This work has identified four widely applicable properties of STNS networks. First, rhythmicity in these highly distributed networks depends on both network synaptic connectivity and slow (tens to hundreds of milliseconds), active neuronal membrane properties. Second, modulatory influences can induce individual STNS networks to produce multiple outputs, "switch" neurons between networks, or fuse individual networks into single larger networks. Third, modulatory neuron terminals receive network synaptic input. Modulatory inputs can be sculpted by network feedback, and become integral parts of the networks they modulate. Fourth, network synaptic strengths can vary as a function of pattern cycle period and duty cycle. Similar complex properties are present in many biological neural networks (see ION CHANNELS: KEYS TO NEURONAL SPECIALIZATION; HALF-CENTER OSCILLATORS UNDERLYING RHYTHMIC MOVEMENTS; OSCILLATORY AND BURSTING PROPERTIES OF NEURONS). Introducing such neurons into artificial neural networks may afford significant functional advantages.

Background

Morphology

All known STNS motor neurons and interneurons are monopolar and have inexcitable somata; synaptic contacts and the voltage-dependent channels underlying slow-wave activity are located in neuropil processes. Spike initiation zones are located near the axon and are electrically distant from the cell body (Selverston et al., 1976).

Synapses

Input and output synapses are located side by side on neuropil processes. Neuronal output thus results from local integration in the neuropil instead of the whole-cell integration present in neurons with distinct pre- and postsynaptic regions (Selverston et al., 1976). In the two best-studied STNS networks, the pyloric and gastric networks, synaptic release is a graded (analogue) function of membrane potential (Graubard, Raper, and Hartline, 1983). Multiple transmitters and receptors, each with their own time course, are present in STNS networks. In particular, many STNS synapses induce slow responses with characteristic times as long as 100 ms (Miller, 1987).

Cellular Properties

STNS neurons display a variety of active, long-duration cellular properties. Many show postinhibitory rebound (PIR); i.e., inhibition induces a subsequent, postsynaptic membrane–generated, active depolarization above rest (Selverston et al., 1976). Some are endogenous oscillators—neurons that spontaneously depolarize and hyperpolarize in a rhythmic fashion. Others have "plateau properties." A plateau neuron has, in addition to a stable rest potential, a quasi-stable depolarized plateau membrane potential. Plateau transitions are regenerative; depolarization from rest above a threshold voltage activates voltage-dependent conductances that drive the neuron to the plateau, and small hyperpolarizations from the plateau induce active repolarization to rest (Russell and Hartline, 1978). Plateau properties nonlinearly transform inputs in amplitude and time in that small-amplitude inputs can induce a full transition, and brief inputs (tens of microseconds) induce long-lasting responses (uninhibited plateaus can last for seconds). STNS models suggest that oscillation, plateaus, and PIR are essential for reproducing the dynamic properties of STNS networks (Golowasch et al., 1992; Marder and Selverston, 1992; Nadim et al., 1998).

Neuromodulation

Synaptic strength and cellular properties in STNS networks are altered by modulatory influences. These influences can induce individual neurons to express plateaus or to become endogenous oscillators (Harris-Warrick, Nagy, and Nusbaum, 1992), and dramatically increase the functional repertoire of STNS neurons and networks.

Mechanisms of Central Pattern Generation

The pyloric network is the best-understood STNS network and will be used to illustrate several general principles that underlie rhythmic pattern generation in this and other systems. The pyloric network is a central pattern generator, i.e., it endogenously generates rhythmic patterns without timing cues from the rest of the nervous system. The right portion of Figure 1 shows simultaneous recordings from all six pyloric neuron types. Each cycle consists of a sequence of bursts of action potentials from the pyloric neurons (Figure 1 shows two cycles). Pyloric dilator (PD) motor neuron activity is classically used to define the beginning of the sequence; they and the anterior burster (AB) interneurons fire together. The lateral pyloric (LP) and inferior cardiac (IC) motor neurons fire next, and finally the pyloric (PY) and ventricular dilator (VD) motor neurons fire. The network's synaptic connectivity (Miller, 1987) is shown in Figure 1, left. Small circles represent inhibitory chemical synapses, resistors represent bidirectional electrical coupling,

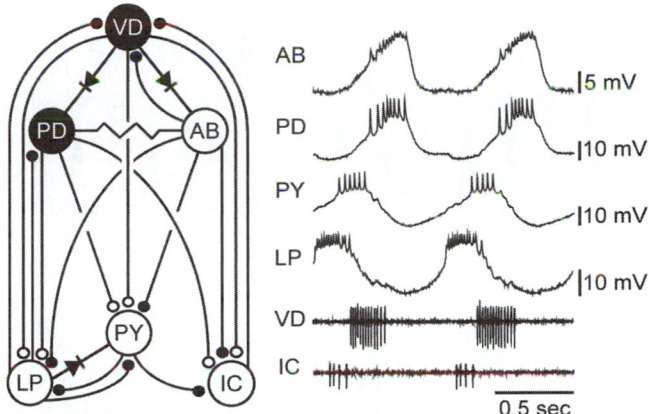

Figure 1. Pyloric network synaptic connectivity (left) and output (right). Small circles represent chemical synapses, resistors represent bidirectional electrical coupling, and the diode represents rectifying electrical coupling. Calibration bar: 20 mV for PD and LP neurons, 10 mV for other neurons.

and the diode represents rectifying electrical coupling (current flows only in the direction of the arrow). The white neurons are glutamatergic and induce rapid, short-lasting inhibition in their followers; the black neurons are cholinergic and induce slow, long-lasting inhibition.

It might be difficult initially to understand how a network dominated by inhibitory synapses is rhythmically active. One solution would be for all network neurons to be endogenous oscillators, and under some circumstances all pyloric neurons can be (Bal, Nagy, and Moulins, 1988). However, the network also produces a slow, but correctly ordered, rhythmic output even in cases in which none of its neurons are endogenous oscillators (Miller, 1987). This rhythmicity arises because the network has multiple locations in which two neurons inhibit each other. Mutual inhibition can lead, in neurons possessing PIR and plateau potentials, to a synaptically based rhythmicity called half-center oscillation. Rhythmicity arises in this synaptic arrangement because the inhibition caused by one neuron's firing induces a delayed PIR, plateau, and firing in the second. The inhibition of the first neuron caused by the second neuron's firing induces in turn a delayed PIR, plateau, and firing in the first neuron, after which the process repeats. This multiplicity of mechanisms makes it difficult to ascribe specific aspects of network function to specific network neurons. Network rhythmicity and pattern instead arise emergently from a combination of neuronal cellular properties and the network's distributed synaptic connectivity.

Nonetheless, a qualitative understanding of pyloric activity can be achieved by considering the cellular properties of the network's neurons and the network's synaptic interconnectivity. The AB neuron is generally the fastest oscillator and drives the PD neurons through their electrical coupling. These neurons inhibit all other pyloric neurons. The LP and IC neurons rebound most quickly after this inhibition and fire next. These neurons inhibit the VD and PY neurons, but eventually the PY neurons rebound and fire. PY neuron firing inhibits the IC and LP neurons and releases the VD neuron from inhibition. The PY and VD neurons are turned off by the next AB/PD neuron burst, and the cycle repeats.

Multifunctional Networks

The pyloric network produces different outputs in response to modulatory inputs (Harris-Warrick et al., 1992). Pyloric network complexity may thus exist to allow construction of many functional

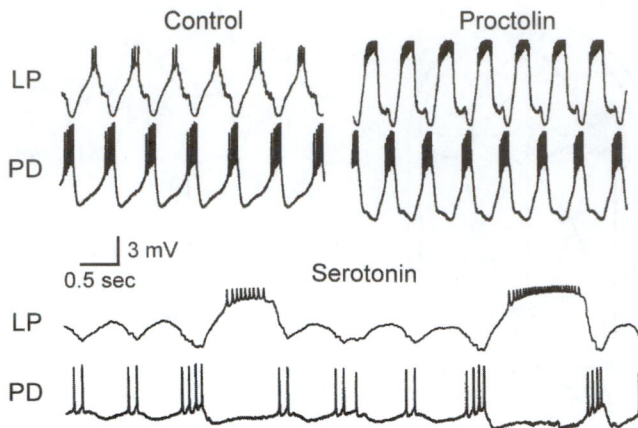

Figure 2. Proctolin (top right panel, 10^{-6}M) and serotonin (bottom panel, 10^{-4}M) induce the pyloric network to produce different motor patterns. (Modified from Marder, E., Hooper, S. L., and Eisen, J. S., 1987, Multiple neurotransmitters provide a mechanism for the production of multiple outputs from a single neuronal circuit, in *Synaptic Function* (G. M. Edelman, W. E. Gall, and M. W. Cowan, Eds.), New York: Wiley, pp. 305–327.)

configurations from a single anatomical network. Figure 2 shows the pyloric outputs induced by the neuromodulators proctolin and serotonin. Proctolin increases LP neuron activity (top trace). Serotonin induces a pattern in which, instead of the LP and PD neurons bursting in alternation, the LP neuron bursts once every two to three PD neuron bursts. Network multifunctionality is not limited to the pyloric network; the gastric mill network also produces multiple outputs. Work in in vivo and semiintact preparations shows that these networks produce multiple outputs in the animal as well, and thus the multiple outputs observed in vitro (and the network switches and fusions noted below) may be behaviorally relevant. Direct evidence for this contention exists in two cases. The first is modulation of the gastric mill rhythm by a cholecystokinin-like hormone whose hemolymph concentration rises after feeding. The second is feedback from stomach proprioceptive neurons that contain acetylcholine and serotonin and that have short-acting, classical (cholinergic) and long-lasting modulatory (serotonergic) effects that would increase pyloric and gastric mill activity (Turrigiano and Heinzel, 1992).

The cellular targets of several modulators are known (Harris-Warrick et al., 1992). This work has two generally relevant results. First, many modulators alter the inherent cellular properties of their target neurons. Second, because directly affected neurons alter the activity of other network neurons, and because these changes modify the responses of directly affected neurons, network activity changes cannot be explained solely by considering the directly affected neurons. Network rearrangements are instead global responses of the entire network, and so not only network rhythmicity but also network modulatory responses are *distributed* functions in these networks.

Neuron Switching and Network Fusion

Until now the four STNS networks have been treated as separate entities. However, the stomach is anatomically compact, adjoining stomach regions are mechanically coupled, and coordination of the motor patterns these networks produce is likely critical for behavior. Considerable internetwork connectivity exists, and network boundaries are variable. These interactions range from simple coordination between networks to cases in which neurons are switched between networks to cases in which networks fuse to form

new networks. Figure 3 shows an example of fusion (Meyrand, Simmers, and Moulins, 1991). The upper panel shows simultaneous recordings, obtained under control conditions, of the VD and PD neurons (pyloric network) and the gastric mill (GM) and lateral posterior gastric (LPG) neurons (gastric mill network). The bottom panel shows the activity of these neurons after discharge of an identified modulatory neuron; the two networks now produce a single conjoint rhythm different from either the pyloric or the gastric rhythm.

The mechanisms underlying network switching and fusion are known in two cases. In one (a switch), the change was due to plateau suppression in the switching neuron (Hooper and Moulins, 1989); in the other (a fusion), it was due to increased strength of an internetwork synaptic connection (Dickinson, Mecsas, and Marder, 1990). Nevertheless, the effects on total network activity again could be understood only by considering the entire network. Long-lasting cellular properties and distributed network architecture thus underlie not only STNS central pattern generation and multifunctionality, but also many aspects of internetwork interaction and restructuring.

Sculpting of Modulatory Input by Network Local Feedback

Many STNS modulatory fibers arise from physically distant cell bodies. The terminals of these fibers receive presynaptic input from, and can serve as integral members of, the networks they modulate. Figure 4 shows one such input, modulatory commissural neuron 1 (MCN1) (Coleman, Meyrand, and Nusbaum, 1995). MCN1 chemically excites the lateral gastric (LG) neuron and interneuron 1 (Int1) of the gastric mill network, and is electrically coupled to the LG neuron (Figure 4A). When MCN1 is active, Int1 fires first, owing to MCN1's fast chemical synapse onto it. Int1 firing inhibits the LG neuron, and this reduces the effectiveness of MCN1's electrical input to the LG neuron (left, Figure 4B). MCN1's slow chemical excitation eventually brings the LG neuron to threshold. LG neuron firing inhibits Int1, presynaptically inhibits

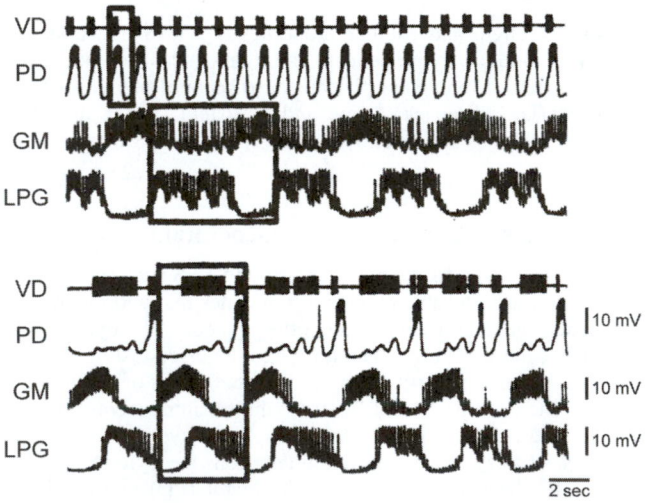

Figure 3. A defined modulatory input fuses networks that are generally distinct (top panel; pyloric, VD, PD neuron traces; gastric mill, GM, LPG neuron traces) into a single network that produces a novel output (bottom panel). (From Meyrand, P., Simmers, J., and Moulins, P., 1991, Construction of a pattern-generating circuit with neurons of different networks, *Nature*, 351:60–63, Figure 3. © 1991, Macmillan Magazines Ltd. Reprinted with permission.)

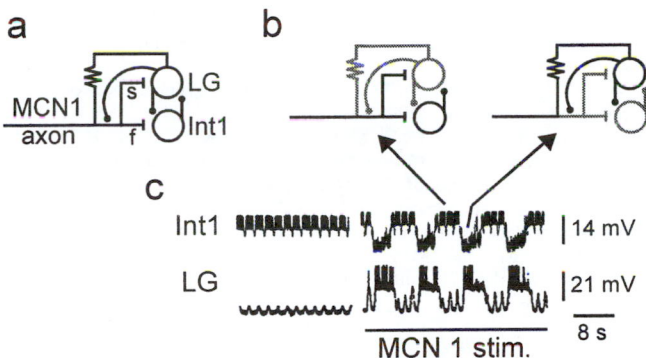

Figure 4. Presynaptic inhibition can sculpt modulator input, and make input terminals integral parts of the networks they modulate. *A,* Synaptic connectivity pattern. MCN1 (a descending modulatory input) makes a fast excitatory synapse onto Int1 and a slow excitatory synapse onto the lateral gastric (LG) neuron. The LG neuron is electrically coupled to, and presynaptically inhibits, the MCN1 axon. The LG neuron and Int1 inhibit each other. *B,* Local feedback rhythmically switches the active mode of MCN1 input. *C,* Tonic MCN1 input (MCN1 active in right panel) activates the gastric mill network. (From Coleman, M. J., Meyrand, P., and Nusbaum, M. P., 1995, A switch between two modes of synaptic transmission mediated by presynaptic inhibition, *Nature,* 378:502–505. © 1995, Macmillan Magazines Ltd. Reprinted with permission.)

MCN1's chemical input to the LG neuron and Int1, and increases the effectiveness of MCN1's electrical input to the LG neuron (right, Figure 4*B*). This electrical input maintains LG neuron activity for a period, but eventually, owing to the lack of MCN1 excitatory chemical input, the LG neuron ceases firing. This removes the LG neuron's presynaptic inhibition of MCN1 input to Int1, Int1 is driven to fire, and the cycle repeats. This switching between different modes of MCN1 input to the gastric mill network, itself driven by gastric activity, continues throughout gastric cycling (Figure 4*C*, right, arrows; the left part shows gastric mill activity before MCN1 activity).

Dependence of Synaptic Strength on Pattern Activity

As noted earlier, modulatory effects cannot be fully understood without considering the entire network. A striking example is the observation that synaptic strength depends on pattern cycle period (Figure 5; Manor et al., 1997). The panels show PD neuron response to rhythmic, square-wave LP neuron depolarizations (recall that pyloric neurons release transmitter as a graded function of membrane potential) at 2.5-s (left) and 0.75-s (right) periods. The PD neuron response is much less at the faster period: Inputs that

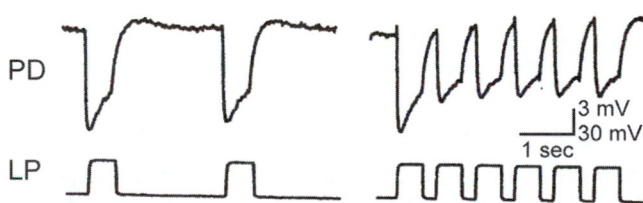

Figure 5. LP to PD neuron synaptic strength varies as a function of LP neuron cycle period. PD neuron postsynaptic response is much less at a 0.75-s LP neuron cycle period (right) than at a 2.5-s period (left). (Modified from Manor, Y., Farzan, N., Abbott, L. F., and Marder, E., 1997, Temporal dynamics of graded synaptic transmission in the lobster stomatogastric ganglion, *J. Neurosci.,* 17:5610–5621.)

alter pattern period can thus alter synaptic strength without directly affecting synaptic transmission. These activity-dependent synaptic strength changes clearly would be fundamentally important in shaping network response to modulation, and provide additional evidence of the interlinking of direct and indirect responses that allow these networks to respond to modulatory input in a global fashion.

Discussion

Work in a well-defined invertebrate nervous system has revealed several cellular and synaptic properties essential for biological function that often are not included in artificial neural networks. Chief among these are the following:

1. Synapses with different characteristic time courses present in the same network.
2. Neurons with long-lasting (tens to hundreds of milliseconds) voltage-dependent conductances that give rise to complex, long-duration cellular characteristics (oscillation, plateaus, PIR).
3. Neuromodulatory inputs that alter synaptic strength and inherent cellular properties.
4. Local feedback that alters neuromodulatory input activity and makes modulatory inputs an integral part of the network they modulate.
5. Network synaptic strengths that depend on network activity (cycle period, duty cycle).

Modeling work shows that many of the functional characteristics (rhythmic pattern production, multiple pattern production, neuron switching, network fusion) of STNS networks require model neurons and networks that incorporate these properties (Golowasch et al., 1992; Marder and Selverston, 1992; Nadim et al., 1998). Including model neurons with similar properties in neural network simulations may enhance artificial neural network capability and deepen understanding of both artificial and biological neural network function.

Road Maps: Motor Pattern Generators; Neuroethology and Evolution
Related Reading: Half-Center Oscillators Underlying Rhythmic Movements; Ion Channels: Keys to Neuronal Specialization; Neuromodulation in Invertebrate Nervous Systems; Oscillatory and Bursting Properties of Neurons; Respiratory Rhythm Generation

References

Bal, T., Nagy, F., and Moulins, M., 1988, The pyloric central pattern generator in crustacea: A set of conditional neuronal oscillators, *J. Comp. Physiol.,* 163:715–727.

Coleman, M. J., Meyrand, P., and Nusbaum, M. P., 1995, A switch between two modes of synaptic transmission mediated by presynaptic inhibition, *Nature,* 378:502–505.

Dickinson, P. S., Mecsas, C., and Marder, E., 1990, Neuropeptide fusion of two motor pattern generator circuits, *Nature,* 344:155–158.

Golowasch, J., Buchholtz, F., Epstein, I. R., and Marder, E., 1992, Contribution of individual ionic currents to activity of a model stomatogastric ganglion neuron, *J. Neurophysiol.,* 67:341–349.

Graubard, K., Raper, J. A., and Hartline, D. K., 1983, Graded synaptic transmission between identified spiking neurons, *J. Neurophysiol.,* 50:508–521.

Harris-Warrick, R. M, Nagy, F., and Nusbaum, M. P., 1992, Neuromodulation of stomatogastric networks by identified neurons and transmitters, in *Dynamic Biological Networks: The Stomatogastric Nervous System* (R. M. Harris-Warrick, E. Marder, A. I. Selverston, and M. Moulins, Eds.), Cambridge, MA: MIT Press, pp. 87–138. ◆

Hooper, S. L., and Moulins, M., 1989, A neuron switches from one network to another by sensory induced changes in its membrane properties, *Science,* 244:1587–1589.

Manor, Y., Farzan, N., Abbott, L. F., and Marder, E., 1997, Temporal dynamics of graded synaptic transmission in the lobster stomatogastric ganglion, *J. Neurosci.*, 17:5610–5621.

Marder, E., and Selverston, A. I., 1992, Modeling the stomatogastric nervous system, in *Dynamic Biological Networks: The Stomatogastric Nervous System* (R. M. Harris-Warrick, E. Marder, A. I. Selverston, and M. Moulins, Eds.), Cambridge, MA: MIT Press, pp. 161–196.

Meyrand, P., Simmers, J., and Moulins, M., 1991, Construction of a pattern-generating circuit with neurons of different networks, *Nature*, 351:60–63.

Miller, J. P., 1987, Pyloric mechanisms, in *The Crustacean Stomatogastric System* (A. I. Selverston and M. Moulins, Eds.), Berlin: Springer-Verlag, pp. 109–136. ◆

Nadim, F., Manor, Y., Nusbaum, M. P., and Marder, E., 1998, Frequency regulation of a slow rhythm by a fast periodic input, *J. Neurosci.*, 18:5053–5067.

Russell, D. F., and Hartline, D. K., 1978, Bursting neural networks: A reexamination, *Science*, 200:453–456.

Selverston, A. I., Russell, D. F., Miller, J. P., and King, D. G., 1976, The stomatogastric nervous system: Structure and function of a small neural network, *Prog. Neurobiol.*, 7:215–290. ◆

Turrigiano, G. G., and Heinzel, H.-G., 1992, Behavioral correlates of stomatogastric network function, in *Dynamic Biological Networks: The Stomatogastric Nervous System* (R. M. Harris-Warrick, E. Marder, A. I. Selverston, and M. Moulins, Eds.), Cambridge, MA: MIT Press, pp. 197–220. ◆

Data Clustering and Learning

Joachim M. Buhmann

Introduction

Intelligent data analysis extracts symbolic information and relations between objects from quantitative or qualitative data. A prominent class of methods are clustering or grouping principles which are designed to discover and extract structures hidden in data sets (Jain and Dubes, 1988). The parameters that represent the clusters are either estimated on the basis of quality criteria or cost functions or, alternatively, they are derived by local search algorithms that are not necessarily following the gradient of a global quality criterion. This approach to inference of structure in data is known as unsupervised learning in the neural computation literature. Clustering as a fundamental pattern recognition problem can be characterized by the following design steps:

1. *Data representation*: What data types represent the objects in the best way to stress relations between the objects, e.g., similarity?
2. *Modeling*: How can we formally characterize interesting and relevant cluster structures in data sets?
3. *Optimization*: How can we efficiently search for cluster structures?
4. *Validation*: How can we validate selected or learned structures?

It is important to note that the data representation issue predetermines what kind of cluster structures can be discovered in the data. Vectorial data, proximity or similarity data, and histogram data are three examples of a wide variety of data types that are analyzed in the clustering literature. On the basis of the data representation, the modeling of clusters defines the notion of groups of clusters in the data and separates desired group structures from unfavorable ones. We consider it mandatory that the modeling step yields a quality measure that is either optimized or approximated during the search for hidden structure in data sets. Formulating the search for clusters as an optimization problem allows us to validate clustering results by large deviation estimates; i.e., robust cluster structures in data should vary little from one data set to a second data set generated by the same data source.

The reader should note that the clustering literature in pattern recognition and applied statistics as well as in communications and information theory pursues two apparently different goals, namely, either (1) *density estimation* or (2) *data compression*. Both goals, however, are tightly related by the fact that the correct identification of the probability model of the source yields the best code for data compression. Mathematically, data compression aims at optimal

partitionings of the data, and stochastic sampling of partitions yields density estimates that are optimized in the maximum entropy sense. This issue is addressed in more detail later in this article.

Data Representations for Clustering

Various data types have been introduced in the pattern recognition literature. Mathematically, we distinguish between the object or design space $\mathcal{O}$ that contains different object configurations $\mathbf{o} \in \mathcal{O}$ and the measurement space $\mathcal{F}$ with measurements $\mathbf{x} \in \mathcal{F}$. Objects might be faces of people, and the corresponding measurements might be intensity or range images. A datum is defined as a relation between a design space $\mathcal{O}$ and a measurement space $\mathcal{F}$. This relation $(\mathbf{o}, \mathbf{x}) \in \mathcal{O} \times \mathcal{F}$ can represent a functional dependence $\mathbf{x} : \mathbf{o} \mapsto \mathbf{x}(\mathbf{o})$ between objects and measurements or a stochastic dependence $\mathbf{P}\{\mathbf{x}|\mathbf{o}\}$. The following categories of data types are most commonly used in data analysis problems:

- *Vectorial data* characterize an object $\mathbf{o}$ by a number of attributes which are combined to a d-dimensional feature vector $\mathbf{x}(\mathbf{o}) \in \mathcal{F} \subset \mathbb{R}^d$.
- *Distributional data* of an object $\mathbf{o}$ are described by an empirical probability distribution or histogram $\mathbf{P}\{\mathbf{x}|\mathbf{o}\}$ over features $\mathbf{x} \in \mathcal{F}$.
- *Proximity data* are characterized by pairwise comparisons between objects according to a proximity measure, e.g., $\mathbf{x}(\mathbf{o}_i) := \{D(\mathbf{o}_i, \mathbf{o}_j) \in \mathbb{R}; 1 \le j \le n\}$. Dissimilarity measures $D(., .)$ often fulfill additional properties, e.g., nonnegativity, vanishing self-dissimilarity, symmetry, and the triangular inequality.

Various polyadic data types such as co-occurrence data (e.g., word bigrams in linguistics, consumer behavior data in economics) or even more complex data types (trigrams) are occasionally considered in the empirical sciences but are not further discussed here.

Modeling Cluster Structure

The goal of clustering is to assign objects with similar properties to the same clusters and dissimilar objects to different clusters. Mathematically, assignments of objects to clusters is represented by an assignment function $m : \mathcal{O} \to \{1, 2, \ldots, k\}$, $\mathbf{o} \mapsto m(\mathbf{o})$. Data clustering pursues the goal to determine a partitioning of object space into subsets $\mathcal{G}_\alpha \equiv \{\mathbf{o} \in \mathcal{O} : m(\mathbf{o}) = \alpha\}$, $1 \le \alpha \le k$. The space of all clustering solutions is the set of all assignment functions $\mathcal{M} = \{m : \mathcal{O} \to \{1, 2, \ldots, k\}\}$. The quality of these partitions is evaluated by an appropriate homogeneity measure for the respective data type. Depending on the clustering goal, either the quality is optimized or the optimum is approximated that might yield a unique solution or a set of approximating solutions. The most commonly used clustering costs are invariant under permutations of the cluster indices. Hierarchical and topological clustering methods impose additional structure on the partitions. These principles are briefly sketched for all three data types.

Central Clustering or Vector Quantization

Clustering n objects that are represented as vectorial data $\mathscr{X} := \{\mathbf{x}_i \in \mathscr{F} : 1 \leq i \leq n\}$ induces a partitioning of the feature space $\mathscr{F} \subset \mathbb{R}^d$. The set of objects is partitioned into clusters in such a way that the average distance from data points to their cluster centers $\mathscr{Y} = \{\mathbf{y}_v \in \mathscr{F} : 1 \leq v \leq k\}$ is minimized. The representation of data $\mathbf{x}_i$ by the centroid $\mathbf{y}_{m(i)}$ induces distortion/quantization costs $D_{i,m(i)}$ due to information loss. The functional form of $D_{i,m(i)}$ depends on the weighting of data distortions, in which quadratic costs $D_{i,m(i)} = \|\mathbf{x}_i - \mathbf{y}_{m(i)}\|^2$ and k-means $\mathbf{y}_\alpha = \sum_{\mathbf{o}_i \in \mathscr{G}_\alpha} \mathbf{x}_i / |\mathscr{G}_\alpha|$ is the most common choice. More general distortion measures like l_p-norms are occasionally considered. The cost function for k-means clustering is defined as

$$H^{cc}(m; \mathscr{X}) = \sum_{i \leq n} \|\mathbf{x}_i - \mathbf{y}_{m(i)}\|^2 \qquad (1)$$

In neural networks, the centroids $\mathbf{y}_{m(i)}$ can be implemented by neural feature detectors that are equipped with radially symmetric receptive fields and a global activity normalization. The size k of the cluster set, i.e., the complexity of the clustering solution, has to be determined a priori or by a problem-dependent complexity measure (Buhmann and Kühnel, 1993). A minimum of the cost function formulated in Equation 1 can be found by varying the assignments $m(i)$, which effectively is a search in a discrete space with exponentially many states. The optimization procedure implicitly yields the cluster means $\{\mathbf{y}_v\}$ by estimating optimized assignments $\{m(i)\}$. A supervised version of central clustering is discussed as LEARNING VECTOR QUANTIZATION (q.v.) in the literature.

Distributional Clustering

Distributional data represent the co-occurrence of objects and features by histograms (Pereira, Tishby, and Lee, 1993). Denote by $\mathscr{D} = \mathbb{O} \times \mathscr{F}$ the data space, i.e., the product space of objects $\mathbf{o} \in \mathbb{O}$ and features $\mathbf{x} \in \mathscr{F}$. In information retrieval, objects might be documents and features might be keywords. The $\mathbf{o} \in \mathbb{O}$ is characterized by an empirical conditional distribution $\hat{\mathbf{P}}\{\mathbf{x}|\mathbf{o}\}$ (histograms); i.e., we count the occurrence of a feature value $\mathbf{x}$ given the object $\mathbf{o}$.

In distribution clustering, objects are grouped according to the similarity of their histograms $\hat{\mathbf{P}}\{\mathbf{x}|\mathbf{o}\}$, with a cluster-specific prototypical distribution of features $\mathbf{P}\{\mathbf{x}|\theta_{m(\mathbf{o})}\}$ that is parametrized by θ_α. The natural distortion measure between two histograms is defined by the Kullback-Leibler divergence (see LEARNING AND STATISTICAL INFERENCE), i.e., $D_{\mathbf{o},m(\mathbf{o})} = \hat{\mathbf{P}}\{\mathbf{o}\}D^{KL}(\hat{\mathbf{P}}\{\mathbf{x}|\mathbf{o}\}\|\mathbf{P}\{\mathbf{x}|\theta_{m(\mathbf{o})}\})$. This idea behind distributional clustering closely resembles k-means clustering when the Euclidian distance is replaced by the KL-divergence. The costs of distributional clustering sum up all distortions of objects, i.e.,

$$H^{hc}(m, \theta; \mathscr{X}) = |\mathbb{O}| \sum_{\mathbf{o} \in \mathbb{O}} \hat{\mathbf{P}}\{\mathbf{o}\}D^{KL}(\hat{\mathbf{P}}\{\mathbf{x}|\mathbf{o}\}\|\mathbf{P}\{\mathbf{x}|\theta_{m(\mathbf{o})}\}) \qquad (2)$$

The costs formulated in Equation 2 define the log-likelihood of a statistical model that explains the data $\mathscr{X}$ by a mixture of data sources: (1) select an object $\mathbf{o} \in \mathbb{O}$ with probability $\mathbf{P}\{\mathbf{o}\}$; (2) choose the cluster α according to the cluster membership of $\alpha =$

$m(\mathbf{o})$; (3) select $\mathbf{x} \in \mathscr{F}$ according to the class-conditional distribution $\mathbf{P}\{\mathbf{x}|\theta_{m(\mathbf{o})}\}$. A very insightful relation to rate distortion theory with side information (Cover and Thomas, 1991) has been described in Tishby, Pereira, and Bialek (1999) and it is called the information bottleneck method.

Pairwise Clustering

Clustering nonmetric data that are characterized by proximity information and not by explicit Euclidean coordinates can be formulated as a graph optimization problem. Given is a graph (v, ε) with weights $\mathscr{D} := \{D_{ij}\}$ on the edges (i, j). The vertices denote the objects to be grouped and the edge weights encode dissimilarity information. Compact clusters are represented by a partition of the vertex set with small dissimilarities between all objects that belong to the same cluster. To simplify the notation, the subset of edges with one vertex in cluster α and one vertex in cluster β is denoted by $\varepsilon_{\alpha\beta} = \{(i, j) \in \varepsilon : \mathbf{o}_i \in \mathscr{G}_\alpha \wedge \mathbf{o}_j \in \mathscr{G}_\beta\}$. A meaningful cost function for pairwise clustering that primarily avoids grouping dissimilar objects into one cluster is defined by

$$H^{pc}(m; \mathscr{D}) = \sum_{v \leq k} \left(|\mathscr{G}_v| \sum_{(i,j) \in \varepsilon_{vv}} \frac{D_{ij}}{|\varepsilon_{vv}|} \right) \qquad (3)$$

Preferred clusters are subsets of objects with minimal average intracluster dissimilarities, weighted by the cluster size $|\mathscr{G}_v|$. This cost function has the remarkable and, for applications, extremely valuable invariance that the assignments do not change if all dissimilarities are changed by the same off-diagonal offset D_0; i.e., arg $\min_m H^{pc}(m; D) = $ arg $\min_m H^{pc}(m; \tilde{D})$, with $\tilde{D} = D_{ij} + D_0(1 - \delta_{ij})$.

An alternative to the pairwise clustering cost function in Equation 3 has been proposed by Shi and Malik (2000) in the context of image segmentation. The clustering criterion

$$H^{nc}(m; \mathscr{D}) = \sum_{v \leq k} \left(\frac{\sum_{(i,j) \in \varepsilon_{vv}} D_{ij}}{\sum_{(i,j) \in \varepsilon : i \in \mathscr{G}_v j \in \mathscr{G}_v} D_{ij}} \right) \qquad (4)$$

weighs the intracluster compactness with the integrated dissimilarities between objects $i \in \mathscr{G}_v \vee j \in \mathscr{G}_v$ in cluster v and all other objects. Good approximate solutions to Equation 4 can be found by spectral graph theory. Originally, this method was developed for similarity data $S_{ij} = \exp(-D_{ij}/\Delta)$ and it was formulated as a minimization of the normalized cut of similarities between two clusters.

A pairwise clustering principle based on local object similarity rather than global cluster compactness has been suggested in Blatt, Wiseman, and Domany (1997) exploiting an analogy to granular magnets. Locality is achieved by the exponential transformation $S_{ij} = \exp(-D_{ij}/\Delta)$, which effectively decouples objects with $D_{ij} \gg \Delta$. The granular magnet concept has been abstracted to the method of typical (multiway) cuts (Gdalyahu, Weinshall, and Werman, 2001), which produces randomized approximations to clustering solutions with small intercluster similarity. The costs for this percolation-type model is given by

$$H^{mc}(m; S) = \sum_{(i,j) \in \varepsilon} S_{ij} - \sum_{v \leq k} \sum_{(i,j) \in \varepsilon_{vv}} S_{ij} = \sum_{v \leq k} \sum_{\substack{\mu \leq k \\ \mu \neq v}} \sum_{(i,j) \in \varepsilon_{vv}} S_{ij} \qquad (5)$$

The identity in Equation 5 relates similarity to neighbors of the same cluster to the combinatorial optimization problem to find a multicut in the graph (v, ε). $H^{mc}(m; S)$ stresses local consistency in clustering, whereas $H^{pc}(m; D)$ emphasizes global compactness of clusters. The granular magnet clustering model generalizes the nearest neighbor linkage method, a popular graph theoretic clustering technique (Duda, Hart, and Stork, 2001).

Topological and Hierarchical Clustering

The four proposed clustering criteria for vectorial, histogram, and proximity data evaluate cluster configurations in a permutation-invariant way. In neurobiology, a topological organization of neurons is often imposed to ensure that nearby neurons process related information in feature space. Respective network structures are known as SELF-ORGANIZING FEATURE MAPS (q.v.). All the introduced clustering principles (Equations 1–5) can be generalized to topology-preserving clustering methods by replacing the unique assignments $\mathbf{o} \mapsto m(\mathbf{o})$ with probabilistic assignments $\mathbf{o} \mapsto \alpha$ with probability $\mathbf{T}_{m(\mathbf{o}),\alpha}$. The cost function for clustering vectorial data translates to

$$H^{\text{som}}(m; \mathcal{X}) = \sum_{i \leq n} \sum_{v \leq k} \mathbf{T}_{m(i),v} \|\mathbf{x}_i - \mathbf{y}_v\|^2 \qquad (6)$$

In case that $\mathbf{T}$ defines a $\tilde{d}$-dimensional neighborhood system, the costs in Equation 6 prefer arrangements of centroids on a $\tilde{d}$-dimensional smooth manifold in the d-dimensional feature space. The additional quantization errors inflicted by the probabilistic assignments are also known in the information theory literature (Cover and Thomas, 1991) as index confusion $v \to \alpha$ due to channel noise. The same principle can be formulated for histogram clustering and for pairwise clustering.

In many application areas a hierarchical partitioning of the object space is favored over unconstraint or topological partitions. The reasons for this preference either are computational, since tree-like structures support rapid data access and efficient algorithmics, or else the data source is hypothesized to be of a tree-like nature. The assignments of objects to clusters have to observe an inclusion principle (Jain and Dubes, 1988) that ensures that subpartitions at a fine level observe the partitions higher up in the tree. It is important to include information of the tree topology in the clustering criterion. Cluster trees resemble decision trees in classification, and they can be naturally implemented in biological brains by layered neural networks.

Optimization

The clustering cost functions can be minimized by various deterministic or stochastic methods from combinatorial and continuous optimization. A widely used class of methods estimates the clustering parameters in an iterative way by first keeping the continuous cluster parameters (centroids, prototype histograms) fixed and optimizing the assignments. In a second step, the continuous parameters are calculated from the new assignments.

The k-Means Algorithm

A well-known algorithm for on-line estimation of prototypes in central clustering is the k-means algorithm (MacQueen, 1967). The k means $\{\mathbf{y}_v : 1 \leq v \leq k\}$ are initialized by the first k data points $\{\mathbf{x}_i : 1 \leq i \leq k\}$. A new data vector $\mathbf{x}_{t+1}$, $t \geq k$ is assigned to the closest mean $\mathbf{y}_\alpha$ according to the nearest neighbor rule

$$m(t + 1) = \arg \min_v \|\mathbf{x}_{t+1} - \mathbf{y}_v\| \qquad (7)$$

with ties being handled appropriately. The new mean vector is adjusted in response to data vector $\mathbf{x}_{t+1}$ according to the learning rule

$$\mathbf{y}_{m(t+1)}^{(t+1)} = \mathbf{y}_{m(t+1)}^{(t)} + \frac{1}{|\mathcal{G}_{m(t+1)}|} (\mathbf{x}_{t+1} - \mathbf{y}_{m(t+1)}^{(t)}) \qquad (8)$$

All other means $\mathbf{y}_v$, $v \neq m(t + 1)$ remain unchanged. The learning rule in Equation 8 adjusts the closest mean $\mathbf{y}_\alpha$ proportional to the deviation $(\mathbf{x}_{t+1} - \mathbf{y}_\alpha^{(t)})$ normalized by the number of data vectors that have already been assigned to this cluster center.

Probabilistic Partitioning Algorithms

The class of stochastic optimization algorithms with SIMULATED ANNEALING AND BOLTZMANN MACHINES (q.v.) as the most prominent techniques plays an eminent role in pattern recognition. The variables of the optimization problem, e.g., the assignments in clustering, are treated as random variables of a stochastic (Markovian) process. The Markov chain Monte Carlo algorithm samples from a set of data partitionings, all of which are considered to be compatible with the data. The size of this set has to be controlled by a cluster validation scheme. Robust clustering methods are derived from the maximum entropy principle, which states that assignments are distributed according to the Gibbs distribution

$$\mathbf{P}(m; \mathcal{X}) = \exp(-(H^{\text{cc}}(m; \mathcal{X}) - F)/T), \qquad (9)$$

$$F = -T \log \sum_{m \in \mathcal{M}} \exp(-H^{\text{cc}}(m; \mathcal{X})/T) \qquad (10)$$

The "computational temperature" T serves as a Lagrange parameter for the expected costs. The free energy F in Equation 10 can be interpreted as a smoothed version of the original cost function H^{cc} (Rose, Gurewitz, and Fox 1990). The cost function H^{cc}, which is linear in the assignments, yields a factorized Gibbs distribution

$$\mathbf{P}(m; \mathcal{X}) = \prod_{i \leq n} \frac{\exp(-D_{i,m(i)}/T)}{\sum_{\mu \leq k} \exp(-D_{i,\mu}/T)} = \prod_{i \leq n} \mathbf{P}_{i,m(i)} \qquad (11)$$

$$\mathbf{P}_{i,v} := \frac{\exp(-D_{i,v}/T)}{\sum_{\mu \leq k} \exp(-D_{i,\mu}/T)}, \quad \forall v \in \{1, \ldots, k\} \qquad (12)$$

$\mathbf{P}_{i,v}$ denote expectation values of assignments. The centroids have to maximize the entropy of the Gibbs distribution, which yields the centroid constraint

$$0 = \sum_{i \leq n} \mathbf{P}_{i,v} \frac{\partial}{\partial \mathbf{y}_v} D_{i,v}, \quad \forall v \in \{1, \ldots, k\} \qquad (13)$$

The Gibbs distribution in Equation 11 can also be interpreted as the complete data likelihood for mixture models with parameters $\mathcal{Y}$. Basically, the Gibbs distribution of the k clusters describes a mixture model with equal priors for each component and equal, isotropic covariances. The assignments $m(i)$ and their expectations $\mathbf{P}_{i,v}$ correspond to the unobservable variables in mixture models and the component densities, respectively. Algorithmically, the centroids and the expected assignments are estimated in an iterative fashion by solving the centroid Equation 13 for fixed expected assignments and, subsequently, inserting the centroids in Equation 12 (Rose et al., 1990; Buhmann and Kühnel, 1993).

The temperature parameter T controls the uncertainty of the clustering problem; i.e., in the limit $T \to 0$, the solution of Equation 12 corresponds to hard clustering with Boolean assignments $\mathbf{P}_{i,v} \in \{0, 1\}$ of a data vector $\mathbf{x}_i$ to the closest cluster center $\mathbf{y}_v$. Large temperature represents the uncertain limit with partial assignments of data vectors to several clusters ($0 \leq \mathbf{P}_{i,v} \leq 1$). The reader should note that the iterative search for solutions of Equations 12 and 13 is guaranteed to yield a local minimum of the costs that, however, could be far from the global minimum.

Gaussian Mixture Models

Natural clusters in data sets are modeled by a mixture of stochastic data sources (McLachlan and Basford, 1988). Each component of this mixture, a data cluster, is described by a univariate probability density that is the stochastic model for an individual cluster. The sum of all component densities forms the probability density of the mixture model

$$P(\mathbf{x}; \Theta) = \sum_{v \leq k} \pi_v p(\mathbf{x}; \theta_v) \qquad (14)$$

Let us assume that the functional form of the probability density $P(\mathbf{x}; \Theta)$ is completely known up to a finite and presumably small number of parameters $\Theta = (\theta_1, \ldots, \theta_k)$. For the most common case of Gaussian mixtures, the parameters $\theta_v = (\mathbf{y}_v, \Sigma_v)$ are the coordinates of the mean vector and the covariance matrix. The a priori probability π_v of the component v, which is assumed to be known, is called the mixing parameter.

Adopting this framework of parametric statistics, the detection of data clusters reduces mathematically to the problem of how to estimate the parameters Θ of the probability density for a given mixture model. A powerful statistical technique for finding mixture parameters is the maximum likelihood method (Duda et al., 2001); i.e., one maximizes the probability of the independently, identically distributed data set $\{\mathbf{x}_i : 1 \leq i \leq n\}$ given a particular mixture model. For analytical purposes it is more convenient to maximize the log-likelihood

$$L(\Theta) = \sum_{i \leq n} \log P(\mathbf{x}_i; \Theta) = \sum_{i \leq n} \log \left(\sum_{v \leq k} p(\mathbf{x}_i; \theta_v)\pi_v \right) \qquad (15)$$

which yields the same maximum likelihood parameters Θ. The straightforward maximization of Equation 15 results in a system of transcendental equations with multiple roots. The ambiguity in the solutions originates from the lack of knowledge of which mixture component v has generated a specific data vector $\mathbf{x}_i$, and therefore which parameter θ_v should be influenced by $\mathbf{x}_i$ in the estimation procedure.

An efficient solution to overcome the computational problem of how to estimate parameters of mixture models with the maximum likelihood method is provided by the Expectation-Maximization (EM) algorithm (Dempster, Laird, and Rubin, 1977). The EM algorithm estimates the unobservable assignments in a first step. The estimates are denoted by $\mathbf{P}_{i,v}$. On the basis of these maximum likelihood estimates $\{\mathbf{P}_{i,v}\}$, the parameters Θ are calculated in a second step. An iteration of these two steps renders the following algorithm for Gaussian mixtures:

- *E-step*: The expectation value of the complete data log-likelihood is calculated conditioned on the observed data $\{\mathbf{x}_i\}$ and the parameter estimates $\hat{\Theta}$. This yields the expected assignments of data to mixture components, i.e.,

$$\mathbf{P}_{i,\alpha}^{(t+1)} = \frac{p(\mathbf{x}_i; \hat{\mathbf{y}}_\alpha^{(t)}, \hat{\Sigma}_\alpha^{(t)})\pi_\alpha}{\sum_{v \leq k} p(\mathbf{x}_i|\hat{\mathbf{y}}_v^{(t)}, \hat{\Sigma}_v^{(t)})\pi_v}$$

$$= \frac{\pi_\alpha |\hat{\Sigma}_\alpha^{(t)}|^{-1/2} \exp(-\frac{1}{2}(\mathbf{x}_i - \hat{\mathbf{y}}_\alpha^{(t)})^T(\hat{\Sigma}_\alpha^{(t)})^{-1}(\mathbf{x}_i - \hat{\mathbf{y}}_\alpha^{(t)}))}{\sum_{v \leq k} \pi_v |\hat{\Sigma}_v^{(t)}|^{-1/2} \exp(-\frac{1}{2}(\mathbf{x}_i - \hat{\mathbf{y}}_v^{(t)})^T(\hat{\Sigma}_v^{(t)})^{-1}(\mathbf{x}_i - \hat{\mathbf{y}}_v^{(t)}))}$$

$$(16)$$

- *M-step*: The likelihood maximization step estimates the mixture parameters, e.g., centers and variances of the Gaussians (Duda et al., 2001, p. 89):

$$\hat{\mathbf{y}}_\alpha^{(t+1)} = \frac{\sum_{i \leq n} \mathbf{P}_{i,\alpha}^{(t+1)} \mathbf{x}_i}{\sum_{i \leq n} \mathbf{P}_{i,\alpha}^{(t+1)}}, \qquad (17)$$

$$\hat{\Sigma}_\alpha^{(t+1)} = \frac{1}{\sum_{i \leq n} \mathbf{P}_{i,\alpha}^{(t+1)}} \sum_{i \leq n} \mathbf{P}_{i,\alpha}^{(t+1)}(\mathbf{x}_i - \hat{\mathbf{y}}_\alpha^{(t+1)})(\mathbf{x}_i - \hat{\mathbf{y}}_\alpha^{(t+1)})^T \qquad (18)$$

Note that Equations 17 and 18 have a unique solution after the expected assignments $\{\mathbf{P}_{i,\alpha}^{(t+1)}\}$ have been estimated. The monotonic increase in the likelihood up to a local maximum guarantees the convergence of the EM algorithm.

Mean Fields for Pairwise Clustering

Minimization of the quadratic cost function formulated in Equation 3 turns out to be algorithmically complicated because of pairwise, potentially conflicting correlations between assignments. The deterministic annealing technique, which produces robust reestimation equations for central clustering in the maximum entropy framework, is not directly applicable to pairwise clustering since there is no analytical technique known to capture correlations between assignments $m(i)$ and $m(j)$ in an exact way. Mean field annealing, however, approximates the intractable Gibbs distribution by the best factorial distribution. The influence of the random variables $m(j), j \neq i$, on $m(i)$ is treated by a mean field that measures the average feedback on $m(i)$. Mathematically, the approximation problem to calculate the Gibbs distribution is replaced by a minimization of the Kullback-Leibler divergence between the approximating factorial distribution and the Gibbs distribution (Hofmann and Buhmann, 1997). A maximum entropy estimate of the mean fields h_{iv} yields the transcendental equations

$$\mathbf{P}_{i,v} = \frac{\exp(-h_{iv}/T)}{\sum_{\mu \leq k} \exp(-h_{i\mu}/T)} \qquad (19)$$

$$h_{iv} = \frac{1}{n\pi_v} \sum_{(i,j) \in \varepsilon} \mathbf{P}_{j,v} \left(D_{ij} - \frac{1}{2n\pi_v} \sum_{(j,r) \in \varepsilon} \mathbf{P}_{r,v} D_{jr} \right) \qquad (20)$$

The variables h_{iv} depend on the given distance matrix D_{ik}, the averaged assignment variables $\{\mathbf{P}_{i,v}\}$, and the cluster weights $\pi_v := \sum_{i \leq n} \mathbf{P}_{i,v}$. Equation 20 suggests an algorithm for learning the optimized cluster assignments that resembles the EM algorithm. In the E-step, the assignments $\{\mathbf{P}_{i,v}\}$ are estimates for given $\{h_{iv}\}$. In the M-step, the $\{h_{iv}\}$ are reestimated on the basis of new assignment estimates. This iterative algorithm converges to a consistent solution of assignments for the pairwise data clustering problem that locally maximizes the entropy.

Cluster Validation

One of the most important problems in data analysis, besides proper modeling, is to test solutions of pattern recognition problems for robustness. The influence of noise in the data on the estimates of cluster centers in central clustering should be minimal in the large data limit. The data analyst, therefore, requests that the clustering solution should be similar if the clustering algorithm partitions a second data set from the same data source. This robustness requirement limits the number of clusters that can be reliably inferred from the data. If too many clusters are supposed to be estimated, then the noise will strongly influence the values of the clustering parameters.

The field of statistical learning theory addresses robustness questions and model complexity issues in the context of supervised learning, in particular for classification and regression. The same trade-off between the complexity of the hypothesis class and the amount of data limits the inference precision in unsupervised learning tasks as data clustering. Theoretical results have to estimate the probability of large deviations between solutions found on two different sample sets. Assume that the cluster solution is quantified by the costs $H(m; \mathscr{X})$ and that we have two data sets, $\mathscr{X}^{(1)}$ and $\mathscr{X}^{(2)}$. The costs $H(m; \mathscr{X})$ might have the combinatorial forms of Equations 1–5, or they could be the log-likelihood (Equation 15) for density estimation. The optimal cluster assignments with respect to the two data sets are $m^{(1)}$ and $m^{(2)}$. A robustness criterion based on large deviation theory should bound from above the probability

$$\mathbf{P}\{H(m^{(1)}; \mathcal{X}^{(2)}) - H(m^{(2)}; \mathcal{X}^{(2)}) > \varepsilon\} \leq \delta \qquad (21)$$

i.e., we require that the optimal solution on the first data set also perform well on a second data set $\mathcal{X}^{(2)}$ with high probability $1 - \delta$. Statistical learning theory relates this deviation to the complexity of the solution space $\mathcal{M}$. Algorithmically, such a complexity control can be implemented by cross-validation, where the algorithm stops to further improve the solution in the optimization process when the costs on the second sample set increase again. This procedure tries to avoid overfitting of model parameters to the data.

Classical strategies to validate clustering solutions are based on Bayesian model selection. The number of modes in mixture model inference can be limited by regularization, e.g., by the minimum description length principle (Duda et al., 2001), which implements the Occam's razor principle for inference (see MINIMUM DESCRIPTION LENGTH ANALYSIS). Alternatives to this criterion are the Bayesian information criterion (BIC), Akaike's information criterion (AIC), or the network information criterion (NIC) (Ripley, 1996), all of which penalize the complexity of the model, e.g., the number of clusters and their cluster parameters. These criteria are asymptotic ($n \to \infty$) in nature.

Discussion

Data clustering as one of the most fundamental information processing procedure to extract symbolic information from subsymbolic data follows the four design steps of pattern recognition: (1) data representation, (2) structure definition, (3) structure optimization, and (4) structure validation. It is still very speculative how these mathematical structures are implemented in biological brains. Neurons with localized receptive fields might provide the neural correlate of centroids in Euclidian feature spaces. Relational data might be represented by neurons that function as comparators. The stochastic dynamics of neurons naturally introduces randomness in the search process for compact cluster structures, and thereby introduces robustness against fluctuations in the data analysis process.

Road Map: Learning in Artificial Networks
Background: Learning Vector Quartization
Related Reading: Principal Component Analysis; Stochastic Approximation and Efficient Learning

References

Blatt, M., Wiseman, S., and Domany, E., 1997, Data clustering using a model granular magnet, *Neural Computat.*, 9:1805–1842.
Buhmann, J., and Kühnel, H., 1993, Vector quantization with complexity costs. *IEEE Trans. Inform. Theory*, 39:1133–1145.
Cover, T. M., and Thomas, J. A., 1991, *Elements of Information Theory*, New York: Wiley. ◆
Dempster, A. P., Laird, N. M., and Rubin, D. B., 1977, Maximum likelihood from incomplete data via the EM algorithm, *J. R. Statist. Soc. Ser. B*, 39:1–38.
Duda, R. O., Hart, P. E., and Stork, D. G., 2001, *Pattern Classification*, New York: Wiley. ◆
Gdalyahu, Y., Weinshall, D., and Werman, M., 2001, Self-organization in vision: Stochastic clustering for image segmentation, perceptual grouping, and image database organization, *IEEE Trans. Pattern Anal. Machine Intell.*, 23:1053–1074.
Hofmann, T., and Buhmann, J. M., 1997, Pairwise data clustering by deterministic annealing, *IEEE Trans. Pattern Anal. Machine Intell.*, 19:1–14.
Jain, A. K., and Dubes, R. C., 1988, *Algorithms for Clustering Data*, Englewood Cliffs, NJ: Prentice Hall. ◆
MacQueen, J., 1967, Some methods for classification and analysis of multivariate observations, in *Proceedings of the 5th Berkeley Symposium on Mathematical Statistics and Probability*, pp. 281–297.
McLachlan, G. J., and Basford, K. E., 1988, *Mixture Models*, New York: Marcel Dekker.
Pereira, F., Tishby, N., and Lee, L., 1993, Distributional clustering of English words, in *Proceedings of the 30th Annual Meeting of the Association for Computational Linguistics*, Columbus, OH, pp. 183–190.
Ripley, B. D., 1996, *Pattern Recognition and Neural Networks*, Cambridge, Engl.: Cambridge University Press.
Rose, K., Gurewitz, E., and Fox, G., 1990, A deterministic annealing approach to clustering, *Pattern Recognit. Lett.*, 11:589–594.
Shi, J., and Malik, J., 2000, Normalized cuts and image segmentation, *IEEE Trans. Pattern Anal. Machine Intell.*, 22:888–905.
Tishby, N., Pereira, F., and Bialek, W., 1999, The information bottleneck method, in *Proceedings of the 37th Allerton Conference on Communication, Control and Computing*, Champaign: University of Illinois Press, pp. 368–377.

Databases for Neuroscience

Jeffrey S. Grethe

Introduction

The advancement of science depends heavily on researchers' ability to share, exchange, and organize large quantities of heterogeneous data in an efficient manner. This is especially true for researchers who are involved in the construction of simulations of the nervous system. Data spanning a wide range of disciplines (e.g., anatomy, physiology, behavior) are needed to conceptualize, design, and validate such simulations. The need for informatics research related to databases is highlighted by the increasingly important role it has played in various scientific communities to help achieve their goals. This is most evident in the molecular biology community (Persidis, 1999; Roos, 2001), where since the beginning of the 1980s, a large collection of specialized data repositories has been constructed. As part of these developments, the National Center for Biotechnology Information (http://www.ncbi.nlm.gov)

was established to develop and maintain public databases and tools for searching and analyzing genomic information. These tools have resulted in incredible scientific advancement within the genomic community, most notably the dissemination of information concerning the human genome (http://www.ncbi.nlm.nih.gov/genome/guide/human/). The success of the Human Genome Project has influenced the application of informatics research to other disciplines, namely, neuroscience.

The amount of neuroscience information being collected is increasing dramatically. This information explosion makes it difficult to search and organize basic research data (Huerta, Koslow, and Leshner, 1993). To that end, the Human Brain Project (http://neuroinformatics.nih.gov) was initiated in September 1993 to provide informatics tools to help manage this data explosion. A main component of the initiative is to provide neuroscientists access to information at all levels of integration through a collection of network-accessible databases. Just as bioinformatics proved to be indispensable for the growth of the molecular biology community, neuroinformatics will become a key component in future neuroscience research. However, the neuroscience community faces some unique challenges.

Neuroscience data are extremely varied and complex. A myriad of structured, textual, graphical, and other information captures experimental results, hypotheses, scientific assumptions, conclusions, formal presentations of theories, and observations. This poses a particularly interesting and important problem for informatics research: to build on state-of-the-art techniques and mechanisms to accommodate the characteristically distinct needs of neuroscience, develop solutions to those problems, and transfer these results to the neuroscience community. Over the last decade, neuroinformatics research has begun to provide mechanisms for the storage of data from varied neuroscientific disciplines (see Table 1 for an overview of database projects). Owing to the great diversity of the databases being developed, we cannot discuss each of these database projects in detail here. Therefore, this article presents and discusses several issues regarding the development of databases for the neuroscience community (for other reviews, see Chicurel, 2000; Kötter, 2001).

Issues in the Development of Neuroscience Databases

Diversity of Neuroscience Data

The interplay of anatomical structure, biochemical processes, and electrical signals gives rise to natural and disease processes. To investigate the underlying mechanisms responsible for these processes, information from varied sources must be integrated. For example, the search for clinical treatments for Parkinson's disease requires information from a wide variety of sources. Information concerning neurotransmitters and receptors, anatomical pathways, neuronal properties, and the information processing that occurs across areas of the basal ganglia must be synthesized and related to clinical, pharmacological, and genetic information. As this example illustrates, neuroscience is an extremely diverse field involving many disciplines. In addition to its diversity, the information of interest to neuroscience researchers is archived throughout the world and stored in a myriad of formats that are accessible through a variety of interfaces and retrieval languages. The data sources can include conventional databases that are accessed through a database query language to web archives accessed by a web browser. Compounding the problem for the neurosciences is that unlike the genomic community, in which data tend to be stored in a few large databases, the neurosciences community will have to be able to access a large, heterogeneous collection of databases.

To be able to integrate such diverse sources, the various communities within the neurosciences must begin to develop standards for their community's data. Currently, in these communities, there exist many different and incompatible data formats that do not allow for the free exchange of data. In addition to needing standards for the raw data themselves, these communities must also develop standards for the description of the actual data (i.e., a formalized description of the meta-data). A possible solution to this problem can be found in the adoption of extensible markup language (XML) technologies. XML (Bosak and Bray, 1999) is a markup language that allows one to describe semistructured representations of information. More specifically, it allows one to annotate data with semantic tags that describe the structure and content of the data. For example, in the modeling community, the Neural Open Markup Language (NeuroML) (Goddard et al., 2001) is being developed to allow researchers to describe models at varying levels of complexity, from cell membranes to large-scale neural networks. In addition

to the ability to exchange data within a community, integration of data from diverse biological disciplines will be needed. In contrast to integration problems found in typical database federations (i.e., different representations of the same information), the neurosciences must be able to integrate data from sources with heterogeneous data and representations. One possible solution for this type of integration has been to extend the conventional wrapper-mediator architecture with domain-specific knowledge (Gupta, Ludäscher, and Martone, 2000).

Data Representation

Data representation is a critical issue for many of the database projects that are currently under way in the neurosciences. One of the first and most central issues in representing data from the brain is the manner in which one describes the fundamental objects of neuroscience. As an example, one need only to look at the classification of brain areas. Currently, there are a number of classification schemes that are not completely compatible. The problem becomes even worse when one considers the difficulty in classifying analogous brain regions across species. How, then, is one supposed to represent location of brain data within a database? Just specifying the textual location might not be sufficient. One partial solution to this problem would be to reference all locations as three-dimensional coordinates within a reference coordinate system (Mazziotta et al., 1995).

The complexity of the experimental paradigms is another critical issue for the representation of neuroscience data. The field of neuroscience is evolving rapidly, and the diversity of these descriptors does not allow one to know a priori what information will need to be stored for future experiments. To address this problem, many database projects stress the importance of an extensible foundation (Nadkarni et al., 1999; Arbib and Grethe, 2001; Gardner et al., 2001) that allows for varying information to be archived in a structured fashion.

User Access

For researchers to be able to navigate and integrate all the information to be provided, user interfaces need to be developed that will give the researcher a seamlessly integrated view of the information concerning a particular topic. These interfaces for neuroscience information would provide a number of novel opportunities that are not available when access is provided only to individual pieces of information. However, the vast amount of information available to researchers over the Internet poses several issues when one attempts to integrate this information. These issues include knowing where the relevant information is located, being able to access that information, integrating and transforming the data into a unified framework, and methods for visualizing the data in an appropriate way.

It is important to realize that the multidisciplinary nature of neuroscience dictates an important additional requirement for these interfaces. Researchers who wish to examine data related to a specific topic will not be experts in every aspect of that topic. For example, a neurochemist studying the kinetics and binding properties of various neurotransmitter receptors might not be aware of the latest clinical information regarding the neurotransmitter in question. Using structured review and summary information as a framework for the presentation of data from varied sources will be imperative when data are to be provided to such a diverse user community.

A Case Study

With support from the National Science Foundation, the National Institutes of Health, and the Keck Foundation, the fMRI Data Cen-

Table 1. Databases Being Developed for the Neurosciences. This table provides a list of databases covering a wide range of subdisciplines within the neurosciences. All databases listed include a brief description, a URL, and a notation as to what forms of data the database is primarily concerned with.

Database	Description	Data
3D Neuron Centered Database **http://www-ncmir.ucsd.edu/NCDB/**	System integrating three-dimensional cellular microscopic data characterizing the realistic locations, surface morphology, and cellular constituents	Cellular, morphology
Brain Image Database (BRAID) **http://braid.rad.jhu.edu/**	Archive of normalized spatial and functional neuroimaging data with an analytical query mechanism	Neuroimaging
BrainInfo **http://braininfo.rprc.washington.edu/**	Helps to identify structures in the brain and provides additional information about these structures	Anatomy
BrainMap **http://ric.uthscsa.edu/projects/brainmap.html**	Database for meta-analysis of author-supplied activations from select human functional brain-mapping literature	Neuroimaging
Brain Models on the Web **http://www-hbp.usc.edu/Projects/bmw.htm**	Database of neural models at the network level, synaptic and kinetic levels, and models that integrate across the levels	Simulation
BrainWeb Simulated Brain Database **http://www.bic.mni.mcgill.ca/brainweb/**	Database of realistic MRI data produced by a simulator to evaluate the performance of various image analysis methods	Neuroimaging
Cell Signaling Networks Database **http://geo.nihs.go.jp/csndb/**	A knowledge base for signaling pathways of human cells	Cellular
CoCoMac **http://www.cocomac.org/**	Database of anatomical connectivity in the macaque	Anatomy
Cortical Neuron Net Database **http://cortex.med.cornell.edu/**	Database of electrophysiological and other information describing cortical neurons	Physiology
Digital Anatomist Project **http://www9.biostr.washington.edu/da.html**	Anatomy information system that is available over the web	Anatomy
European Computerised Human Brain Database **http://fornix.neuro.ki.se/ECHBD/Database/index.html**	Database for relating function to microstructure of the cerebral cortex of humans	Neuroimaging
fMRI Data Center **http://www.fmridc.org**	Publicly accessible repository of peer-reviewed fMRI studies and their underlying data	Neuroimaging
GENESIS Modeler's Workspace **http://www.genesis-sim.org/hbp/**	System to help users create and organize models and interact with other databases and simulation software	Simulation
ICBM **http://www.loni.ucla.edu/ICBM/**	Developing a probabilistic reference system for the human brain	Neuroimaging
Ligand Gated Ion Channel Database **http://www.pasteur.fr/recherche/banques/LGIC/LGIC.html**	Sequence database for neurotransmitter receptors	Sequence
NeuARt **http://www-hbp.usc.edu/Projects/neuart.htm**	Database to retrieve graphical data from a neuroanatomical database	Anatomy
NeuroCore **http://www-hbp.usc.edu/Projects/neurocore.htm**	Database framework for the storage of data from neuroscientific experiments that can be extended to meet a specific lab's requirements	Physiology, chemistry
NeuroGenerator **http://www.neurogenerator.org/**	Database generator for anatomical and functional images of the human brain	Neuroimaging
NeuroScholar **http://chasseur.usc.edu/ns/**	Knowledge management system for literature	Literature
NeuroSys **http://cns.montana.edu/research/neurosys/**	Lightweight peer-to-peer data-sharing system with a database front end	Cellular, physiology
NTSA Workbench **http://soma.npa.uiuc.edu/isnpa/isnpa.html**	Tools for the storage and retrieval of large neuronal time series data sets	Physiology
SenseLab **http://ycmi-hbp.med.yale.edu/senselab/**	Collection of six related databases that focus on information processing in nerve cells of the olfactory system	Anatomy, physiology, sequence, simulation
Surface Management System (SuMS) Database **http://stp.wustl.edu/sums/**	Surface-based database of neuroimaging data intended to aid in cortical surface reconstruction, visualization, and analysis	Neuroimaging
Virtual Neuromorphology Electronic Database **http://www.krasnow.gmu.edu/L-Neuron/database/index.html**	A database for three-dimensional neuronal structures	Morphology, cellular
XANAT **http://stp.wustl.edu/resources/xanat.html**	A graphical anatomical database of neural connectivity	Anatomy

ter (Van Horn et al., 2001) was established in the autumn of 1999 with the objective of creating a mechanism by which members of the neuroscientific community may more easily share functional neuroimaging data. By building a publicly accessible repository of raw data from peer-reviewed studies, the Data Center aims to create a successful environment for the sharing of neuroimaging data in the neurosciences. By increasing the number of scientists who can examine, consider, analyze, and assess the neuroimaging data that have already been collected and published, the center hopes to speed the progress of understanding cognitive processes, the neural substrates that underlie them, and the diseases that affect them. The development of such an archive for neuroimaging data posed certain challenges.

The most critical issue that needed to be addressed in the building of the Data Center was the representation of the data to be archived. In and of itself, raw functional imaging data may not be particularly useful. Proper analysis requires at least knowledge of how the data were acquired. Therefore, in addition to the data sets themselves, the Data Center must store all technical descriptions of the data necessary for someone other than the study's authors to accurately reproduce and interpret the original results. This includes both the information regarding the scanning parameters and the experimental protocols (information and timing of the stimuli) presented to the subject during the collection of the data. The Data Center cannot know a priori all the descriptors required for studies being submitted and therefore relies on an extensible framework for the storage of the data.

The descriptors that are used in describing a neuroimaging experiment constitute one type of meta-data (i.e., data that contain information about the data). These meta-data will allow the data to be organized in a suitable fashion for keyword-based queries. However, it is also important to be able to offer the researcher the ability to query the content of the imaging data directly. Querying the raw functional data directly is not feasible, owing to the amount of imaging data present in the archive (e.g., studies archived at the Data Center can be on the order of hundreds of megabytes to tens of gigabytes). To be able to perform content-based queries on the image data, concise meta-data need to be generated to describe the individual images and time series of images. The meta-data can then be used as a means to quickly find studies of interest based on features derived from the data themselves. Researchers may then further examine these data using more rigorous analysis methods.

Another critical challenge for the Data Center was the protection of human subjects data. This problem is not unique to the Data Center; any database archiving data from human subjects must comply with U.S. government regulations on the protection of such data. To that end, the Data Center makes every reasonable effort to ensure that all data included within the Data Center's archive are anonymized so that data being used by researchers cannot be linked back to the individual subjects who provided it. Neuroimaging data are also unique in that the data themselves can be used as an identifier. It is possible to reconstruct recognizable images of a subject's face from high-resolution structural magnetic resonance data. To that end, all structural data must be stripped (i.e., removal of facial features) before being included in the data archive.

Currently, the Data Center hosts a web site where authors from around the world have been submitting entire, raw data sets from peer-reviewed journals. Visitors to the Data Center's web site may search its holdings via a MEDLINE-inspired query interface. This allows researchers to easily access and search the Data Center's resources without the need to learn a new interface and query language. A researcher who finds data sets of interest can request that they be shipped to him or her on either CD (at no charge) or digital tape. As of July 2002, the Data Center had shipped over 400 data requests to researchers in over 35 countries.

By providing raw neuroimaging data, tools for screening the details of the experimental and scanner protocols, as well as techniques for data discovery and mining, the Data Center will give researchers access to a much larger pool of data than can be found in any single fMRI study. Thus, dynamic analyses across data sets and experiments may be performed, new statistical techniques can be developed, improved techniques for image processing can be investigated, and novel neuroscientific questions may be explored.

Conclusion

Providing scientists access to an ever increasing collection of information in a coherent framework is vital to the future advancement of science. Already in 1985, a National Academy of Sciences report (Morowitz, 1985) suggested that biological research had reached a point at which "new generalizations and higher order biological laws are being approached but may be obscured by the simple mass of data." It is hoped that the continued progress of neuroinformatics in the development of databases and tools for neuroscience will help researchers navigate the masses of data and information that are being generated. In addition to the development of tools for the community, the success of neuroinformatics will depend on how these technologies are accepted by the community at large. The future success of neuroscience databases and neuroinformatics in general will require the neuroscience community to make a paradigm shift similar to those that have already taken place in the molecular biology community.

Road Map: Implementation and Analysis
Related Reading: Neuroinformatics; Neurosimulation: Tools and Resources

References

Arbib, M. A., and Grethe, J. S., 2001, *Computing the Brain: A Guide to Neuroinformatics*, San Diego: Academic Press. ◆

Bosak, J., and Bray, T., 1999, XML and the second generation web, *Scientific American*, 280:89–93. ◆

Chicurel, M., 2000, Databasing the brain, *Nature*, 406:822–825.

Gardner, D., Knuth, K. H., Abato, M., Erde, S. M., White, T., DeBellis, R., and Gardner, E. P., 2001, Common data model for neuroscience data and data model interchange, *J. Am. Med. Inform. Assoc.*, 8:17.

Goddard, N. H., Hucka, M., Howell, F., Cornelis, H., Shankar, K., and Beeman, D., 2001, Towards NeuroML: Model description methods for collaborative modeling in neuroscience, *Philos. Trans. R. Soc. Lond. B Biol. Sci.*, 356:1209–1228.

Gupta, A., Ludäscher, B., and Martone, M. E., 2000, Knowledge-based integration of neuroscience data sources, *12th International Conference on Scientific and Statistical Database Management (SSDBM)*, Berlin, Germany, IEEE Computer Society, July 2000.

Huerta, M. F., Koslow, S. H., and Leshner, A. I., 1993, The human brain project: An international resource, *Trends Neurosci.*, 16:436–438.

Kötter, R., 2001, Neuroscience databases: Tools for exploring brain structure-function relationships, *Philos. Trans. R. Soc. Lond. B Biol. Sci.*, 356:1111–1120. ◆

Mazziotta, J. C., Toga, A. W., Evans, A., Fox, P. T., and Lancaster, J., 1995, A probabilistic atlas of the human brain: Theory and rationale for its development. *NeuroImage* 2:89–101.

Morowitz, H. J., 1985, *Models for Biomedical Research, A New Perspective*, Washington, DC: National Academy Press.

Nadkarni P. M., Marenco, L., Chen, R., Skoufos, E., Shepherd, G., and Miller, P., 1999, Organization of heterogeneous scientific data using the EAV/CR representation. *J. Am. Med. Inform. Assoc.*, 6:478–493.

Persidis, A, 1999, Bioinformatics, *Nat. Biotechnol.*, 17:828–830.

Roos, D. S., 2001, Bioinformatics: Trying to swim in a sea of data. *Science*, 291:1260–1261. ◆

Van Horn, J. D., Grethe, J. S., Kostelec, P., Woodward, J. B., Aslam, J. A., Rus, D., Rockmore, D., and Gazzaniga, M. S., 2001, The fMRIDC: The challenges and rewards of large scale databasing of neuroimaging studies, *Philos. Trans. R. Soc. Lond. B Biol. Sci.*, 356:1323–1339.

Decision Support Systems and Expert Systems

Nikola Kasabov

Introduction

The complexity and the dynamics of many real-world problems, such as decision making and the prediction of economic and financial indexes, decision making in medicine, knowledge discovery in bioinformatics, adaptive intelligent control of industrial processes, on-line decision making based on a large amount of continuous and dynamically changing information on the World Wide Web, and many other problems, impose certain requirements on the information systems, methods, and tools used for this purpose. The information systems and tools must:

- Deal with different types of data and knowledge.
- Adjust incrementally to dynamic changes in the operating environment, accommodating new data and introducing new variables and features as needed without the requirement of redesigning or retraining the whole system. Such adaptation may have to occur in an on-line, real-time mode.
- Update the system's knowledge in a dynamic way.
- Explain in an appropriate way what knowledge is contained in the system, or what knowledge has been learned during the system's operation.

The area of information science and artificial intelligence that is concerned with these issues is called *decision support systems*. A decision support system is an information system that helps humans make a decision about a given problem, under given circumstances and constraints. A decision-making system is a system that makes final decisions and takes actions. Some examples are automated trading systems on the Internet, or systems that grant loans through electronic submissions.

Expert systems belong to the subject area, as they are information systems that contain expert knowledge about a particular problem and perform inference when new data are entered that may be partial or inexact. They provide a solution that is expected to be similar to the solution provided by experts in the field. An expert system usually consists of several parts: (1) a knowledge base, where the expert knowledge resides; (2) a database, where historical and new data are stored; (3) an inference machine, which provides different types of inferences; (4) an efficient interface to users; (5) an explanation module, which provides an explanation of *how* and *why* a certain decision was recommended by the system; and (6) a module that learns and accumulates new knowledge, based on the system's operation and on new incoming data (see Duda and Shortliffe, 1983; Kasabov, 1996).

In the rest of this article we will use the collective term *decision system* to refer to either a decision support system, or a decision-making system, or the most sophisticated among them, the expert system.

Because decision systems deal with different types of data and problem knowledge in different modes (e.g., static versus dynamic data, fixed versus adaptive knowledge, off-line versus on-line mode, and so on), different methods and approaches have been used to build them. These methods include statistical methods (e.g., clustering, principal components analysis, hidden Markov models), mathematical modeling, finite automata, methods used in artificial intelligence (e.g., logic systems, rule-based systems, case-based reasoning, different types of neural networks), and hybrid methods that combine all of the foregoing (Duda and Shortliffe, 1983; Kasabov, 1996).

Decision systems, as presented here, are both human-oriented and human-like systems. The human brain is the ultimate decision system. This article discusses how neural networks, which are vague analogues of the human brain, can be employed in a decision system. We will be concerned with the human-like implementation of decision systems, which is one of their aspects. But the most important aspect of decision systems is their functionality. Because decision systems help humans in the decision process, they should be comprehensible by humans; they should incorporate elements of human-like thinking and human-like information and knowledge processing; and they must be human oriented.

Neural networks and connectionist-based systems have been applied in decision systems as either learning machines or knowledge representation machines, or both. The following listing enumerates some of these applications.

1. Neural networks are used as low-level data-processing and pattern-matching modules, while rule-based modules are used for higher-level decision making (Fu, 1989; Kasabov, 1990). Neural networks are incorporated as part of a production system or of a first-order logic system for decision support.
2. A base consisting of a fixed set of flat rules is incorporated into a connectionist structure with a predefined built-in inference mechanism (Gallant, 1993). No learning is applied.
3. All elements of a production system (e.g., rules, facts, inference machine) are represented in different connectionist modules (Touretzky and Hinton, 1988). No learning is applied on the structure.
4. Trainable knowledge-based neural networks that have fixed structures in terms of number of neurons and connections are used to accommodate both knowledge (rules) and data (Fu, 1989; Towell and Shavlik, 1993; Cloete and Zurada, 2000). Such knowledge-based neural networks are the fuzzy neural networks (Kasabov, 1996).
5. Knowledge-based neural networks that develop (evolve) their structure, their functionality, and their knowledge in time from incoming data, starting from an initial set of knowledge (if such is available), are used for building adaptive, incremental, on-line learning decision systems (Kasabov, 2002).

We will call a decision system that has neural network modules in its structure a *connectionist-based decision system* (CBDS). The following discussion presents different architectures and applications of such systems, starting with the general framework of a CBDS.

General Framework of a Connectionist-Based Decision System

The framework of a CBDS is shown in Figure 1. It consists of the following parts:

- Preprocessing part (e.g., to perform data filtering and feature extraction).
- Neural network part, consisting of neural network modules that are trained on data and incorporate knowledge.
- Higher-level knowledge-based part (e.g., rules for producing final decisions).
- Adaptation part. This part evaluates the system's performance and makes changes to the system's structure and functionality. For example, output error can be used to adjust relevant neural network modules.

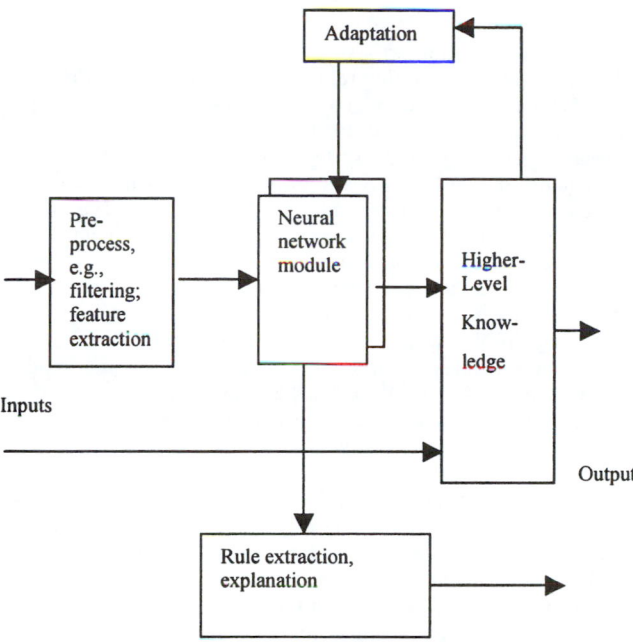

Figure 1. A framework of a connectionist-based decision system (CBDS).

- Rule extraction and explanation part. This part uses both extracted rules from the neural network modules and rules from the decision part to explain *what* the system "knows" about the problem it is designed to solve, and *why* a particular decision for a concrete input vector has been made.

Different types of neural networks (e.g., multiplayer perceptrons, self-organizing maps, radial basis functions, fuzzy neural networks) can be used as part of a CBDS. The most commonly used networks are the knowledge-based neural network.

Knowledge-Based Neural Networks

Knowledge-based neural networks are prestructured neural networks that allow for data and knowledge manipulation, including learning from data, rule insertion, rule extraction, adaptation, and reasoning (Towell and Shavlik, 1993; Cloete and Zurada, 2000; Mitra and Hayshi, 2000). Knowledge-based neural networks have been developed either as a combination of symbolic AI systems and neural networks, or as a combination of fuzzy logic systems and neural networks, or as other hybrid systems.

The knowledge represented in knowledge-based neural networks is mainly in the form of different types of IF-THEN rules. Some of them are listed below:

1. Simple propositional rules (e.g., IF x_1 is A AND/OR x_2 is B, THEN y is C, where A, B, and C are constants, variables, or symbols of true/false type) (Gallant, 1993).
2. Propositional rules with certainty factors (e.g., IF x_1 is A (CF_1) AND x_2 is B (CF_2), THEN y is C (CF_c)) (Fu, 1989; Touretzky and Hinton, 1988).
3. Zadeh-Mamdani fuzzy rules (e.g., IF x_1 is A AND x_2 is B, THEN y is C, where A, B, and C are fuzzy values represented by their membership functions).
4. Takagi-Sugeno fuzzy rules (e.g., IF x_1 is A AND x_2 is B, THEN y is $a.x_1 + b.x_2 + c$, where A, B, and C are fuzzy values and a, b, and c are constants)

5. Rules that have associated degrees of importance and certainty degrees (e.g., IF x_1 is A (DI_1) AND x_2 is B (DI_2), THEN y is C (CF_c), where DI_1 and DI_2 represent the importance of each of the condition elements for the rule output, and the CF_c represents the strength of this rule) (Kasabov, 1996).
6. Rules that represent associations of clusters of data from the problem space (e.g., Rule j: IF [an input vector x is in the input cluster defined by its center (x_1 is A_j, to a membership degree of MD_{1j}, AND x_2 is B_j, to a membership degree of MD_{2j}) and by its radius $R_{j\text{-in}}$], THEN [y is in the output cluster defined by its center (y is C, to a membership degree of MD_c) and by its radius $R_{j\text{-out}}$, with Nex(j) examples represented by this rule] (Kasabov, 2002).
7. Temporal rules (e.g., IF x_1 is present at a time moment t_1 (with a certainty degree and/or importance factor of DI_1) AND x_2 is present at a time moment t_2 (with a certainty degree/importance factor DI_2), THEN y is C (CF_c)).
8. Temporal, recurrent rules (e.g., IF x_1 is A(DI_1) AND x_2 is B(DI_2) AND y at the time moment $(t - k)$ is C, THEN y at a time moment $(t + n)$ is D(CF_c)).

There are several methods for rule extraction from a knowledge-based neural network. Three of them are explained below:

1. Activating a trained knowledge-based neural network on input data and observing the patterns of activation.
2. Rule extraction through analysis of the connections in a trained knowledge-based neural network.
3. Methods that combine 1 and 2.

In terms of applying knowledge-based neural networks to make new inferences, three types of methods can be used:

1. Rules extracted from a knowledge-based neural network are interpreted in another inference machine (e.g., fuzzy inference, production system).
2. The rule-based learning and reasoning modules constitute an integrated connectionist structure, so that reasoning is performed in the connectionist structure.
3. The two options above are combined in one CBDS.

In terms of learning and rule extraction in a knowledge-based neural network, we can differentiate the following cases: (1) offline learning and static rule set extraction: first, learning is performed, and then rules are extracted, which is an one-off process; (2) on-line learning: rules can be extracted at any time during a continuous on-line learning process.

In terms of learning and optimization in a knowledge-based neural network, there are three cases: (1) globally optimized networks: for every new example all the connections change during learning; (2) locally optimized networks: for a new example only few connections change. Local optimization in a knowledge-based neural network would allow for adjusting the network to accommodate new data through tuning a small number of elements, and also for extracting locally meaningful rules. The rules can be tuned as the system works.

(3) Fuzzy neural networks are neural networks that can be interpreted in terms of fuzzy rules; neuro-fuzzy inference systems are fuzzy systems that can be structurally represented in a connectionist way (Kasabov, 1996; Cloete and Zurada, 2000). A review of neuro-fuzzy systems for rule generation has been published by Mitra and Hayashi (2000).

One example of a fuzzy neural network is shown in Figure 2 (Kasabov, 1996, 2002). The architecture consists of five layers of neurons and four layers of connections. The first layer of neurons receives the input information. The second layer calculates the

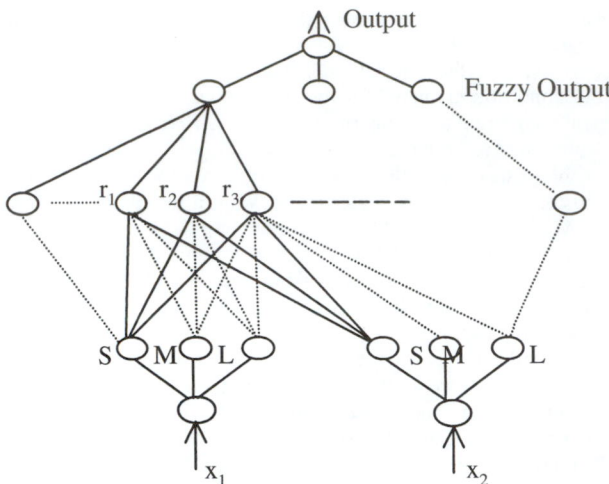

Figure 2. A simple neuro-fuzzy inference system with two inputs, three membership functions, and one output. Rule node r_1 can be represented as a rule: IF x_1 is S and x_2 is S, THEN output is S (certain statistical and linguistic parameters are attached).

fuzzy membership degrees to which the input values belong to predefined fuzzy membership functions, e.g., small, medium, or large. The membership functions can be kept fixed or can change during training. The third layer of neurons represents associations between input and output variables, or fuzzy rules. The fourth layer calculates the degrees to which output membership functions are matched by the input data, and the fifth layer does defuzzification and calculates values for the output variables.

Static Versus Dynamic, Evolving CBDS

A static CBDS is trained on a data set, but it is not continuously updated and adjusted on any new data during its operation. It may be trained regularly on new data plus the previously used data so that the system learns the new data and maintains the previous information as well (the plasticity/stability dilemma). An example is given below.

Example: A CBDS for mortgage approval. A neural network is trained on data for decision making on mortgage approval (the data are also available from the web site http://divcom.otago.ac.nz/infosci/KEL/data). The following attributes are used: Input1: character (0—doubtful; 1—good); Input2: total asset; Input3: equity; Input4: mortgage loan; Input5: budget surplus; Input6: gross income; Input7: debt-servicing ratio; Input8: term of loan; Output: decision (disapprove; approve). In a particular experimental CBDS, neural networks are trained on ten different sets of data, each of them containing both positive (applications are approved) and negative (applications are rejected) examples. Each trained neural net-

work is tested on another data set of positive and negative examples. The generalization error of the neural network is evaluated. Rules are extracted from the trained neural network that explains the decision process. The trained neural network is not incrementally trained on new data and it is used as part of a CBDS.

Dynamic, evolving CBDS systems evolve their structure, their functionality, and their knowledge from incoming data rather than having a predefined structure and a fixed set of rules. They learn and improve continuously over time, as is shown in Figure 3. An example of a set of methods that can be used to build an evolving CBDS is the evolving connectionist systems (ECOS) paradigm (Kasabov, 2002).

Evolving CBDS systems adapt to a changing environment, possibly in real time. They can learn in a "lifelong" learning mode, and they are able to explain what they have learned in terms of rules and other types of knowledge. An evolving CBDS would have a modular, open structure evolving over time. Initially, the neural network can be a mesh of nodes (neurons) with very few connections between them, predefined through prior knowledge or "genetic" information. An initial set of rules can be inserted in this structure. Gradually, through self-organization, the system becomes more and more "wired." The network learns different patterns (exemplars, prototypes) from the training examples. For example, in an ECOS architecture, a node is created and designated to represent an individual example if this example is significantly different from the previous ones (with the level of differentiation established through dynamically changing parameters). In addition to a growing procedure, a pruning procedure is defined. It allows for removing neurons and their corresponding connections that are not actively involved in the functioning of the ECOS, thus making space for new input patterns. Different modes of learning in ECOS are possible, among them are an active learning mode (learning is performed when a stimulus—input pattern—is presented and kept active) and a passive (e.g., sleep) learning mode (learning is performed when there is no input pattern presented at the input of the ECOS).

Adaptive CBDS usually operate as on-line decision systems that make decisions and adjust their knowledge through an incremental, continuous learning from incoming data. Such systems, for example, learn the dynamic changes in a stock index, or adjust their knowledge to include new gene discoveries in Bioinformatics.

Example: On-line financial decision making based on on-line prediction of the MIB30 stock index. Figure 4 shows the use of a neural network for on-line learning and prediction 5 days ahead of the moving average values of the MIB30 stock index (the Milan stock index). Here, an evolving fuzzy neural network (Kasabov, 2002) is used as the neural network. The neural network is trained on-line on consecutive data vectors. Inputs to the neural network are 5-day moving averages of the following variables: DJ(t), DJ(t − 1), MIB30(t), MIB30(t − 1), euro/US\$(t), euro/US\$(t − 1).

At any time of the functioning of the evolving fuzzy neural network, rules can be extracted. The rules represent the current asso-

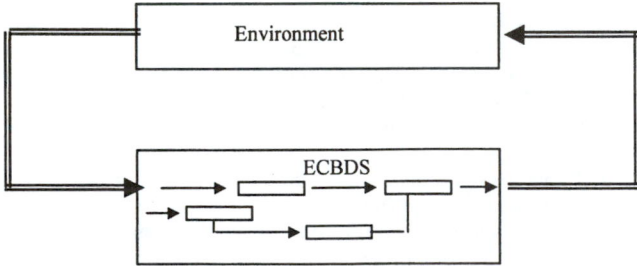

Figure 3. Adaptive, evolving CBDS learn their structure and functionality through interaction with the environment

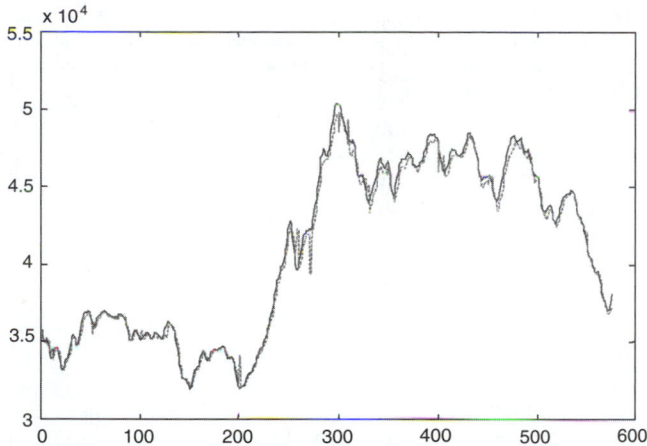

Figure 4. Adaptive CBDS in financial decision making, showing the process of on-line learning and prediction 5 days ahead of the MIB30 index. Chart shows the desired versus the predicted output value for 576 consecutive days.

ciation between the input variables and the output variable, as is illustrated in the rule below:

Rule: IF [DJ(t) is (Medium 0.828) and DJ($t - 1$) is (Medium 0.840) and MIB30(t) is (Low 0.885) and MIB30($t - 1$) is (Low 0.887)] (receptive field = 0.808), THEN MIB30($t + 5$) will be (Low 0.852) (accommodated training examples 182 out of 576).

Connectionist-Based Decision Systems in Economics and Finance

Beltraffi, Margarita, and Terna (1996) describe a variety of CBDS systems in the area of finance and economics. These include CBDS for solving problems such as stock trading, portfolio decision, exchange rate prediction, fraud detection, credit scoring, and many more. Some CBDS systems contain expert rules and make decisions similar to the decisions made by experts, as illustrated in the next example.

Example: A CBDS for simulation and prediction of decisions made by the European Central Bank (ECB) on interest rate intervention (Rizzi et al., 2002). The ECB meets regularly to make a decision on the interest rate for the European Union countries. Modeling this decision-making process is extremely difficult, as it requires both the comprehensive knowledge the ECB members have and fast adaptation to new situations. The system developed by Rizzi et al. (2002) consists of two parts. The first part has several neural networks that use six groups of economic indicators (total of 17 variables) and produces intermediate outputs that include the predicted values for some time series. These values, as well as other economic variables, are fed into a rule-based system that consitutes the second part of the system. The system finally suggests what ECB decisions on the interest rate might be expected at the next three consecutive meetings. Figure 5 shows some test results. The system learns and improves over time after each new datum is entered.

Connectionist-Based Decision Systems in Bioinformatics

Processing a large amount of data, such as in medicine, biochemistry, or molecular biology, and making decisions based on this

information is a task where CBDS systems have been successfully applied. Baldi and Brunak (2001) have demonstrated the application of machine learning techniques, including neural networks, to solving difficult problems, such as DNA promoter recognition, RNA splice junction identification, secondary structure protein prediction, and so on.

Example: CBDS for RNA splice junction identification. Figure 6 shows a simple three-layer perceptron neural network for identifying a biological feature, such as a splice junction from an input RNA sequence. The neural network has 60 inputs, which is the length of the RNA window sequence, five intermediate neurons (nodes), and one output neuron to encode for the feature (1—present, 0—not present). (The data set used for training is available at http://www.ics.uci.edu/~mlearn/MLRepository.html.) The splice junction predicted by the trained neural network from new input data should be further analyzed before a final decision is made.

An on-line training and prediction system for the same problem that is based on an evolving fuzzy neural network is available at http://divcom.otago.ac.nz/infosci/kel/CBIIS/GenIn/. The system can also extract rules, such as the rule shown below:

Rule: IF -----C--C-C-TCC-G--CTC-GT-C--GGTGAGTG--GGC---C---G-GG-C--CC- THEN [Junction Exon-Intron] Receptive field = 0.216. Examples covered by the rule are 26 out of 1,000.

Future Directions for Connectionist-Based Decision Systems

CBDS systems are a fast-growing area. New applications expected to be developed include new techniques for learning, data mining, and knowledge discovery, and practical applications in finance and economics, bioinformatics and life sciences, process control and manufacturing, medicine, and the social sciences.

Road Map: Artificial Intelligence; Applications
Related Reading: Forecasting; Hybrid Connectionist/Symbolic Systems

ECB Intervention	Forecasts of the Expert System		
Date (t)	Date ($t + 1$)	Date ($t + 2$)	Date ($t + 3$)
3 Feb. 2000 0.25	16 Mar. 2000 0.25 (0.25)	27 Apr. 2000 0 (0.25)	8 Jun. 2000 0 (0.50)
16 Mar. 2000 0.25	27 Apr. 2000 0.25 (0.25)	8 Jun. 2000 0.25 (0.50)	31 Aug. 2000 0.25 (0.25)
27 Apr. 2000 0.25	8 Jun. 2000 0.25 (0.5)	31 Aug. 2000 0.25 (0.25)	19 Oct. 2000 0.25 (0.25)
8 Jun. 2000 0.5	31 Aug. 2000 0.25 (0.25)	19 Oct. 2000 0.25 (0.25)	30 Nov. 2000 0.25
31 Aug. 2000 0.25	19 Oct. 2000 0.25 (0.25)	30 Nov. 2000 0.25	18 Jan. 2001 0.25

Figure 5. CBDS in economics: the interest rate decision intervention by the European Central Bank (ECB) at five ECB meetings, versus the calculated ahead intervention by an expert system. After each intervention index decided by the ECB is made available, the expert system adjusts to this decision and then suggests what the ECB decision at three consecutive meetings ahead might be. The real intervention indexes are the numbers in parentheses.

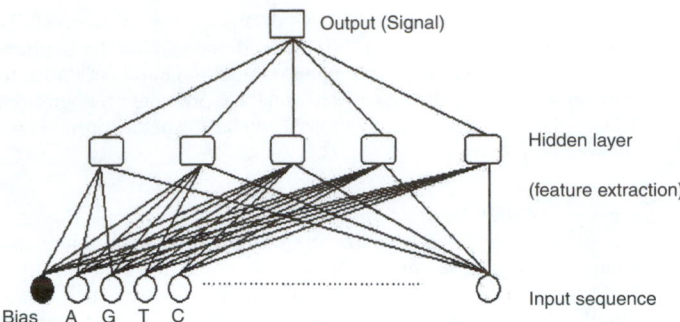

Output (Signal)

Hidden layer

(feature extraction)

Input sequence

Bias   A   G   T   C

Figure 6. CBDS in bioinformatics. A neural network that takes an input vector of 60 nucleotides from an RNA data and evaluates the probability for having exon-intron, or intron-exon splice junction in the middle of the sequence, or no junction at all.

References

Baldi, P., and Brunak, S., 2001, *Bioinformatics: A Machine Learning Approach*, Cambridge, MA: MIT Press. ◆

Beltraffi, A., Margarita, S., and Terna, P., 1996, *Neural Networks for Economics and Financial Modelling*, New York: Interational Thomson Computer Press.

Cloete, I., and Zurada, J., Eds., 2000, *Knowledge-Based Neurocomputing*, Cambridge, MA: MIT Press.

Duda, R. O., and Shortliffe, E. H., 1983, Expert systems research, *Science*, 220:261–268.

Fu, L. M., 1989, Integration of neural heuristics into knowledge-based inference, *Connect. Sci.*, 1:325–340. ◆

Gallant, S. I., 1993, *Neural Network Learning and Expert Systems*, Cambridge, MA: MIT Press. ◆

Kasabov, N. K., 1990, Hybrid connectionist rule-based systems, in *Artificial Intelligence: Methodology, Systems, Applications* (P. Jorrand and V. Sgurev, Eds.), Amsterdam, North-Holland: Elsevier, pp. 227–235.

Kasabov, N., 1996, *Foundations of Neural Networks, Fuzzy Systems and Knowledge Engineering*, Cambridge, MA: MIT Press. ◆

Kasabov, N., 2002, *Evolving Connectionist Systems: Methods and Applications in Bioinformatics, Brain Study and Intelligent Machines*, London: Springer-Verlag.

Mitra, S., and Hayshi, Y., 2000, Neuro-fuzzy rule generation: Survey in soft computing framework, *IEEE Trans. Neural Net.*, 11 No. 3

Rizzi, R., Bazzana, F., Kasabov, N., Fedrizzi, M., and Erzegovesi, L., 2002, A connectionist-based decision support system for modelling the interest rate intervention made by the European Central Bank, *Eur. J. Operat. Res.*, Special Issue on Decision Support Systems.

Sima, J., and Cervenka, J., 2000, Neural knowledge processing in expert systems, in *Knowledge-Based Neurocomputing* (I. Cloete and J. Zurada, Eds.), Cambridge, MA: MIT Press, pp. 419–466.

Towell, G. G., and Shavlik, J. W., 1993, Extracting refined rules from knowledge-based neural networks, *Machine Learn.*, 13:71–101.

Touretzky, D., and Hinton, G., 1988, A distributed connectionist production system, *Cognit. Sci.*, 12:1423–1466.

Dendritic Learning

Bartlett W. Mel

Introduction

In most neurons of the vertebrate central nervous system (CNS), dendritic trees are the primary input surfaces of neurons, receiving thousands to hundreds of thousands of synaptic contacts from other neurons. During development, a period during which the brain is first "wired up," the physical interface between axons and dendrites is extremely dynamic (Cline, 1999), involving large-scale growth, retraction, and remodeling of axonal and dendritic arbors on time scales of minutes to hours. In the adult nervous system, contrary to the connectionist view that neural plasticity is limited to the strengthening and weakening of existing synaptic connections, evidence suggests that physical remodeling of axons and dendrites, including the formation of new synaptic contacts and elimination of existing ones, continues to some degree throughout life (Klintsova and Greenough, 1999). Given that dendrites are highly complex structures both anatomically and physiologically and are the principal substrates for information processing within the neuron itself (Stuart, Spruston, and Häusser, 1999), the question arises as to the consequences of axodendritic structural plasticity for learning and memory. In other words, does experience-dependent remodeling of the physical interface between axons and dendrites have any special role in the long-term storage of information in the brain, beyond that associated with the establishment of the brain's basic neuron-to-neuron wiring diagram?

A critical assumption of most models of learning and development holds that the *neuron* is the appropriate level of granularity for analysis, where the outcome of learning is expressed in terms of changes in the strengths of connections w_{AB} between point neurons *A* and *B* (see HEBBIAN SYNAPTIC PLASTICITY). The enormous physical complexity of individual neurons compels us to consider other types of plasticity, however. For example, activity-dependent rules appear to modulate the density and spatial distribution of the ion channels governing a cell's basic electrical behavior (see ACTIVITY-DEPENDENT REGULATION OF NEURONAL CONDUCTANCES), and can modulate neurite outgrowth and branching (van Ooyen et al., 2002). Both examples involve changes in the neural substrate that are not naturally described in terms of changes in neuron-to-neuron connection strengths.

In this article, we explore the possibility that long-term learning in the mature brain may depend on structural remodeling at the interface between axons and dendrites, a process that continues throughout life. In particular, we cite evidence for the view that long-term storage may involve the correlation-based sorting of synaptic contacts onto the *many separate dendrites* of a target neuron, just as conventional models of neural development typically involve the sorting of synaptic contacts onto the *many separate neurons* of a target population (see DEVELOPMENT OF RETINOTECTAL MAPS; OCULAR DOMINANCE AND ORIENTATION COLUMNS; SELF-ORGANIZING FEATURE MAPS). This shift in granularity is justified by the assumption that individual dendrites, or parts of dendritic trees, act as separately thresholded neuron-like subunits, functionally analogous to the point neurons that populate coarser-grained models of learning and development. We focus on the main projection neurons of cortical tissue, pyramidal cells, although our discussion likely applies to other types of cells as well.

The Neuron as Two-Layer Neural Network

The dendrites of pyramidal cells contain a large number and variety of voltage-dependent channels that profoundly influence their integrative behavior (Häusser, Spruston, and Stuart, 2000). A variety of evidence from intracellular recordings and imaging studies suggests that active spike-like responses can be localized within individual thin branches (Schiller et al., 2000), supporting the idea that individual dendritic branches can act as surrogate "neurons" capable of separately thresholding their synaptic inputs.

Anatomical hints are similarly supportive of such a possibility. If advantages accrue to a cell that maintains multiple integrative subregions within its dendritic tree, one might expect pyramidal cell morphologies to maximize the number of subunits available for independent synaptic processing, subject to practical constraints such as that the cell remain of manageable size, that nonlinear synaptic interactions remain confined to individual subunits, and so on. Pace, Tieman, and Tieman (2000) found that among layer 4 stellate cells of the cat striate cortex, the number of long, thin, terminal sections is nearly constant (around 40) and is independent of the number of primary dendritic branches emanating from the cell body (Figure 1). Given that most of the synapses onto basal dendrites lie on the long, thin, unbranched terminal sections (Elston and Rosa, 1998), the data of Pace et al. suggest a developmental program that tightly regulates the production of mutually isolated dendritic subunits, and then arranges for synapses to be formed primarily there.

What are the implications of this type of morphology for synaptic integration? Cable theory (Koch, 1999) suggests that a dendritic arbor consisting of many thin-branched subtrees radiating outward from a much larger-diameter cell body or dendritic trunk is ideally suited to isolate voltage responses within individual thin branches. Indeed, the possibility that dendritic trees could support complex multisite nonlinear operations, including logic-like operations, has been explored in a number of modeling studies (see Mel, 1999; Segev and London, 2000).

One recent study utilized a simplified model pyramidal cell whose dendrites contained AMPA/NMDA synapses and low concentrations of voltage-dependent Na^+/K^+ channels capable of generating dendritic spikes (Archie and Mel, 2000). When total synaptic drive to the cell was held constant but was distributed in varying spatial patterns to two dendritic branches, the average firing rate of the cell was approximated by a sum-of-squares model. The finding is intriguing in that it suggests a possible connection between the computation carried out within the dendrites and the quadratic "energy" models used to describe several types of visual receptive field properties (Mel, 1999). This study provided the first direct test of the "sum of subunits" model for synaptic integration, in which (1) the thin dendritic branches act like separately thresholded nonlinear subunits and (2) the outputs of the thin branch subunits are summed linearly via the main trunks and cell body prior to global thresholding:

$$y(\mathbf{x}) = g\left(\sum_{i=1}^{m} \alpha_i b\left(\sum_{j=1}^{k} w_{ij}x_{ij}\right)\right) \tag{1}$$

where m is the number of subunits, k is the number of synapses per subunit, w_{ij} is the weight, and x_{ij} is the activity of the jth input to the ith subunit, b is the subunit nonlinearity, α_i is the coupling of the ith subunit to the cell body, and g is a global output nonlinearity. Of interest, Equation 1 also describes the input-output relation of a conventional two-layer neural network.

Structural Plasticity at the Axodendritic Interface

The possibility that neurons contain multiple, separately thresholded dendritic subunits has profound implications for the mechanisms governing the formation and remodeling of the axodendritic interface, and for the physical substrate for long-term information storage in neural tissue. The point may be illustrated from the perspective of axon i in the process of "choosing" which subunit $s \in \{1 \ldots k\}$ to enervate on postsynaptic neuron j during learning or development. The subunit thresholding function b, which generates nonlinear interactions among the set of inputs to each subunit, ensures that i's effectiveness in driving cell j depends not just on its own activity x_i and associated weights w_{ijs}, but also on the activity and weights of the other axons providing input to the same subunits. Thus, given compartmentalized neurons, the "receptive field" of the neuron changes, in general, when any single axon withdraws

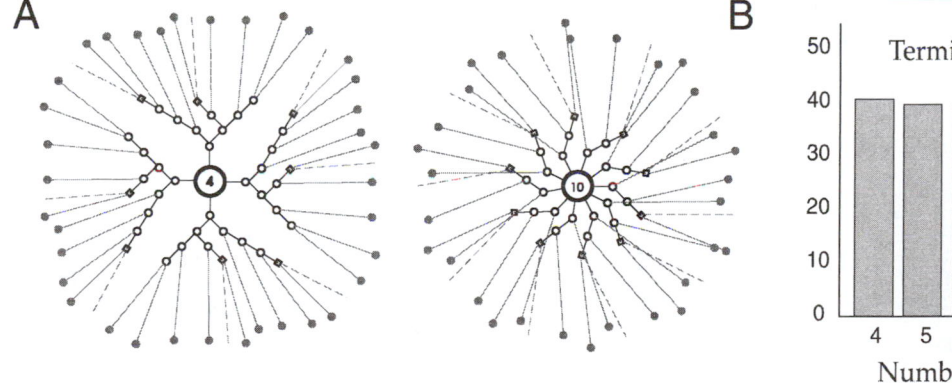
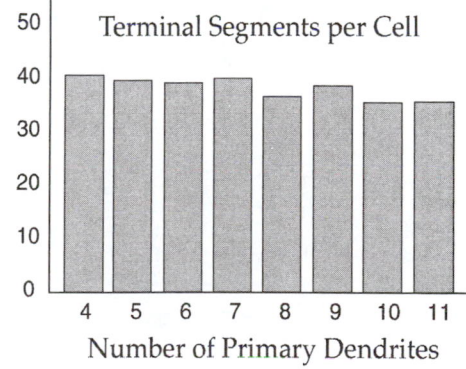
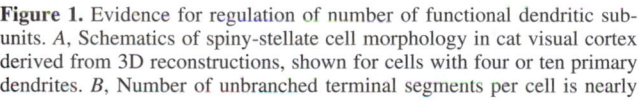

Figure 1. Evidence for regulation of number of functional dendritic subunits. *A*, Schematics of spiny-stellate cell morphology in cat visual cortex derived from 3D reconstructions, shown for cells with four or ten primary dendrites. *B*, Number of unbranched terminal segments per cell is nearly constant (around 40) for cells with widely varying numbers of primary dendrites. (Adapted with permission from Pace, Tieman, and Tieman, 2000.)

a synaptic contact from one subunit and forms a new contact on another, even when the "change of address" involves two branches of the same postsynaptic cell. By contrast, learning models operating at neuron-level granularity, which encode only the overall connection strength between pairs of neurons, lack the parameters needed to represent such changes.

Partnership Combinatorics

The possibility that learning-related mechanisms could orchestrate the correlation-based sorting of synaptic contacts, not just onto whole neurons but a level down, on to specific dendritic subunits, raises the question of whether the physical interface between axons and dendrites in cortical tissue is amenable to this type of fine-scale structural plasticity. The question is important in that, when a neuron contains subunits, its capacity to absorb learned information is closely tied to the *addressing flexibility* of the tissue, that is, the flexibility to establish arbitrary partnerships between presynaptic axons and postsynaptic dendritic subunits (Poirazi and Mel, 2001).

It is now well established that axons, dendrites, and spines are highly dynamic structures, both during development and in the adult brain (Cline, 1999; Klintsova and Greenough, 1999). One model of neural development holds that (1) synapses are initially formed between axons and dendrites in a random, activity-independent fashion, and (2) synapses that are frequently co-activated with their neighbors within the same postsynaptic compartment are structurally stabilized and retained, while those that are poorly correlated with their neighbors are eliminated. If, however, the relevant postsynaptic unit is the individual thin dendrite rather than the whole neuron, then these same neurobiological mechanisms could also drive the separate mapping of like-activated synaptic cohorts onto distinct dendritic subregions.

Although the idea is intriguing, a serious practical difficulty arising from the need to establish on-demand partnerships between arbitrary pairs of axons and dendrites is that of physical proximity, or the lack thereof: it is unreasonable to expect that during the course of learning, particularly in the densely packed neuropil of the mature brain, axons or dendrites should be regularly required to advance and retract over long distances in search of appropriate partnerships.

What physical properties of axons and dendrites might enhance their partnership flexibility, minimizing the need for long-distance travel to form arbitrary pairings between presynaptic axons and dendritic subunits? Axonal and dendritic arborizations are heavily interdigitated within the three-dimensional (3D) volume of the cortical neuropil, an arrangement that maximizes the probability of a close approach between any given axon and any given compartment of a postsynaptic cell. This qualitative observation is illustrated by the montage of an axon and a dendrite shown in Figure 2.

Implications of Dendritic Subunits and Structural Plasticity for Long-Term Memory Storage

We recently set out to quantify the excess trainable storage capacity contained in the selective mapping of synaptic contacts onto dendritic subunits, and to characterize how this excess capacity depends on dendritic geometry (Poirazi and Mel, 2001). We compared the capacity of a subunit containing neuron with m branches (subunits) and k synapses per branch (Equation 1) to that of a point neuron with the same number of synaptic sites but a linear summation rule, that is, with $b(x) = x$ in Equation 1. The two neuron models were thus identical except for the presence or absence of a fixed subunit nonlinearity.

Assuming synaptic contacts of unit weight—although any of the d input lines could form multiple connections to the same or different branches—we derived upper bounds on the capacity of a linear (B_L) versus nonlinear (B_N) cell:

$$B_L = 2 \log_2 \binom{s + d - 1}{s}$$

$$B_N = 2 \log_2 \left(\binom{\binom{k + d - 1}{k} + m - 1}{m} \right) \qquad (2)$$

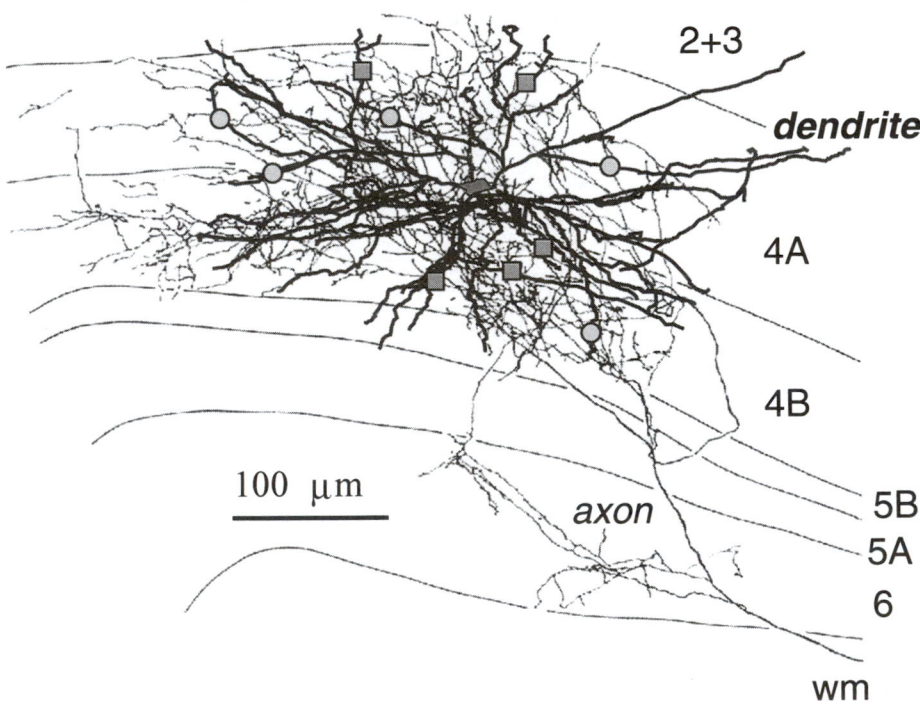

Figure 2. Interdigitated axonal and dendritic trees provide an ideal interface for flexible partnering between a presynaptic axon and the several dozen dendritic subunits of a single postsynaptic neuron. The picture was created by superimposing a dendritic arbor from a cat layer 4 spiny stellate cell (courtesy of Judith Hirsch) on a thalamocortical afferent taken from Freund et al. (1985, *J. Comp. Neurol.*, 242:263). Geometric symbols illustrate locations where minor extensions or retractions could lead to the establishment of new contacts (circles) and the elimination of old contacts (squares) between the axon and dendrite during the course of learning.

The expressions in each case estimate the number of distinct input-output functions that can be expressed by the respective model when assigning $s = m \cdot k$ synaptic contacts with replacement from d distinct input lines. The combinatorial terms take into account the redundancies associated with the two models, that is, the changes in synaptic connectivity that have no effect on the cell's "receptive field"; the logarithm converts the raw function counts into *bits*. B_L and B_N are plotted in Figure 3A for a cell with 10,000 synaptic contacts and three values of d. Capacity is shown on the y-axis for a range of cell geometries represented along the x-axis. The values of B_L are shown on the left and right edges of the plot, since the capacity of a point neuron is equivalent to a subunitized neuron in a degenerate state with either a single branch containing 10,000 synapses or with 10,000 branches containing one synapse each. The peak capacity occurs for cells containing approximately 1,000 subunits of size 10, where the optimal geometry depends little on d over the order-of-magnitude range tested.

The optimal subunit size predicted by Equation 2 ($k = 10$) is considerably smaller than would be expected for a pyramidal cell, whose individual thin terminal branches typically contain hundreds of synapses. This discrepancy could be explained in part by our assumption here that synaptic weights are binary valued; in pilot runs with multivalued weights, the optimal subunit size was pushed to substantially larger values ($k = 25$ for 4-level weights). Furthermore, the assumption that all input axons have ready access to all dendrites is unlikely to hold in neural tissue. Wherever this assumption is violated, pressure would exist to grow longer dendritic subunits, thereby permitting each subunit to gain access to a larger fraction of the "input vector."

Empirical Testing of Memory Capacity

To validate the analytical model, we trained both linear and nonlinear cells on random old/new classification problems using a stochastic gradient descent learning rule (Poirazi and Mel, 2001). Memory capacity was measured for cells with different dendritic geometries by determining the size of the training set that could be internalized with a recognition error rate of 2%. A comparison of analytical versus empirical capacities for both linear and nonlinear cells is shown in Figure 3B. The curves are remarkably similar in form, with peak capacity occurring for cells of similar shape. The optimal nonlinear cell with 10,000 synapses outperformed its size-matched linear counterpart by a factor of 46, learning 27,400 versus 600 patterns at the 2% error criterion. In further experiments with a population of independently trained cells, we found the excess storage capacity available to a structural learning rule could easily approach two orders of magnitude (Poirazi and Mel, 2001).

Discussion

Several types of evidence were cited that call into question the classical "point neuron" as a model for a pyramidal cell or other large dendritic neuron of the CNS. We presented an alternative model supported by physiological, anatomical, and modeling studies, in which the output of the cell represents the sum of a moderately large set of separately thresholded dendritic subunits—a formulation that at a mathematical level is identical to that of a

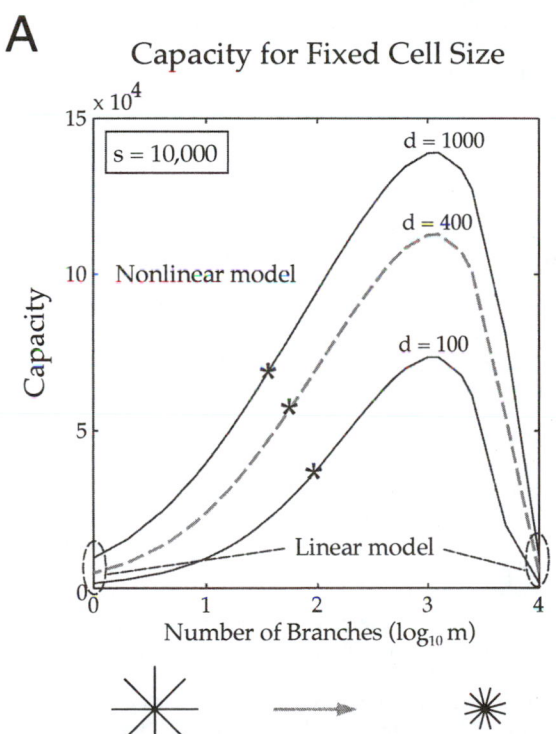

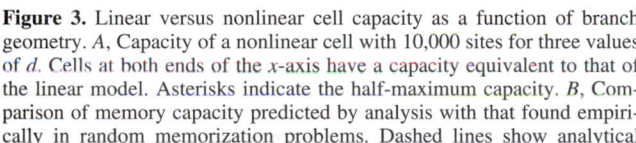

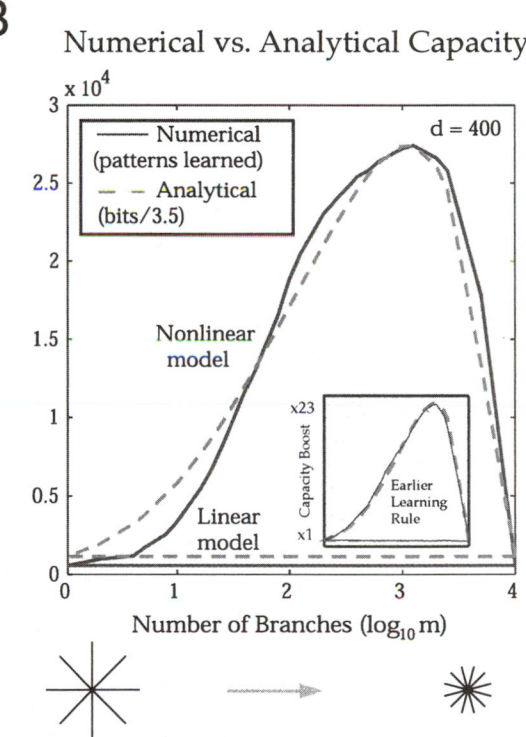

Figure 3. Linear versus nonlinear cell capacity as a function of branch geometry. A, Capacity of a nonlinear cell with 10,000 sites for three values of d. Cells at both ends of the x-axis have a capacity equivalent to that of the linear model. Asterisks indicate the half-maximum capacity. B, Comparison of memory capacity predicted by analysis with that found empirically in random memorization problems. Dashed lines show analytical curves for linear and nonlinear cells (nonlinear capacity curve corresponds to dashed curve in A). Solid curves show capacity measured empirically at 2% error criterion. Analytical curves were scaled down together by a factor of 3.5, to align peak analytical and empirical capacity values for nonlinear model. (Adapted from Poirazi and Mel, 2001.)

conventional artificial neural network built from two layers of point neurons. Multisubunit neurons, if and where they are used in the brain, could help to minimize hardware-associated costs, including brain size, processing delays, error-signal management overhead, and so on.

Although the validity of the subunitized-neuron hypothesis remains to be proved empirically, we have nonetheless explored some of its major consequences for learning and memory. The two main consequences are as follows. First, in a functionally compartmentalized neuron, the formation of new synapses and the elimination of old ones during learning can no longer be viewed simply as a means to increase or decrease the overall connection strength between two neurons, a common interpretation of new synapse or spine formation. Indeed, the concept of "overall connection strength between two neurons" is no longer well-defined, in the sense that the interaction between two neurons can no longer be captured by a single positive or negative coefficient. The granularity has changed: we must now worry about the role of learning-related mechanisms in tuning the connection strengths between a many-fingered presynaptic fiber and the multiple dendritic subunits of a given postsynaptic cell.

Second, from the perspective of learning theory, this change in granularity brings with it a large increase in the number of modifiable parameters available to the neural tissue. And this a not a purely theoretical construct: we have found in simulation studies that these extra parameters translate directly into additional long-term storage capacity, hidden in the fine structure of the axodendritic interface. Interestingly, other sources of "hidden" capacity have been proposed to exist, based on still other kinds of modifiable parameters, including a cell's capacity to discriminate among time-varying signals by varying passive time constant and spike threshold (Zador and Pearlmutter, 1996), or to maximize mutual information between input and output firing rates by varying properties of the resident voltage-dependent ion channels (Stemmler and Koch, 1999). Future experiments will ultimately determine the extent to which these reservoirs of structure-, channel-, or time-based capacity are in fact exploited within the living brain.

Road Map: Neural Plasticity
Related Reading: Dendritic Processing; Development of Retinotectal Maps; Ocular Dominance and Orientation Columns

References

Archie, K. A., and Mel, B. W., 2000, An intradendritic model for computation of binocular disparity, *Nature Neurosci.*, 3:54–63.

Cline, H. T., 1999, Development of dendrites, in *Dendrites* (G. Stuart, N. Spruston, and M. Häusser, Eds.), Oxford, Engl.: Oxford University Press, pp. 35–67. ◆

Elston, G. N., and Rosa, M. G., 1998, Morphological variation of layer III pyramidal neurones in the occipitotemporal pathway of the macaque monkey visual cortex, *Cereb. Cortex*, 8:278–294.

Häusser, M., Spruston, N., and Stuart, G. J., 2000, Diversity and dynamics of dendritic signaling, *Science*, 290:739–744. ◆

Klintsova, A. Y., and Greenough, W. T., 1999, Synaptic plasticity in cortical systems, *Curr. Opin. Neurobiol.*, 9:203–208. ◆

Koch, C., 1999, *Biophysics of Computation*, Oxford, Engl.: Oxford University Press.

Mel, B. W., 1999, Why have dendrites? A computational perspective, in *Dendrites* (G. Stuart, N. spruston, and M. Häussser, Eds.), Oxford, Engl.: Oxford University Press, pp. 271–289. ◆

Pace, C. J., Tieman, D. G., and Tieman, S. B., 2000, Neuronal form: Patterns of dendritic branching in layer 4 stellate cells, *Soc. Neurosci. Abstr.*, 2(794.2):489.

Poirazi, Y., and Mel, B. W., 2001, Impact of active dendrites and structural plasticity on the memory capacity of neural tissue, *Neuron*, 29:779–796.

Schiller, J., Major, G., Koester, H. J., and Schiller, Y., 2000, NMDA spikes in basal dendrites of cortical pyramidal neurons, *Nature*, 404:285–289.

Segev, I., and London, M., 2000, Untangling dendrites with quantitative models, *Science*, 290:744–750. ◆

Stemmler, M., and Koch, C., 1999, How voltage-dependent conductances can adapt to maximize the information encoded by neuronal firing rate, *Nature Neurosci.*, 2:521–527.

Stuart, G., Spruston, N., and Häusser, M., Eds., 1999, *Dendrites*, Oxford, Engl.: Oxford University Press.

van Ooyen, A., Corner, M., Kater, S., and van Pelt, J., 2002, Activity-dependent neurite outgrowth and network development, in *Modeling Neural Development* (A. van Ooyen, Ed.), Cambridge, MA: MIT Press.

Zador, A., and Pearlmutter, B. A., 1996, VC dimension of an integrate-and-fire model neuron, *Neural Computat.*, 8:611–624.

Dendritic Processing

Idan Segev and Michael London

Introduction

We are fortunate to be in the midst of the "dendritic revolution" that emerged when the first edition of the *Handbook* appeared in 1995. For the first time ever, systematic and intimate electrical and optical visits became possible to the dendrites (Figure 1)—the largest component of the mammalian brain in both surface area and volume. These ongoing visits have yielded a much more fascinating picture of the electrical behavior and chemical properties of dendrites than one could have imagined only a few years ago. It is now clear that the dendritic membrane hosts a variety of nonlinear voltage-gated ion channels that endow dendrites with potentially powerful computing capabilities. Our century-old perception of dendrites as electrical devices that carry information unidirectionally, from the many dendritic (input) synapses to the soma and (output) axon, has undergone a dramatic revision. The surprising finding is that dendrites of many central neurons also carry information "backward," via active propagation of action potentials (APs) from the axon to the dendrites. These "backpropagating APs" trigger plastic changes in the dendritic input synapses, and these changes are believed to be the fundamental processes that underlie learning and memory in the brain. Our view of dendrites as static elements has also changed: we now know that the fine morphology as well as the electrical properties of dendrites change dynamically, in an activity-dependent manner. Indeed, one of the major challenges in the years to come is to understand how these changes are correlated with the behavior and learning of the animal.

This article affords a brief introduction to the newly discovered charms of dendrites. For the dendritic-minded reader, several recent reviews are recommended, including the book *Dendrites*, edited by Stuart, Spruston, and Häusser (1999), the quartet of reviews of work on dendrites in *Science* (October 27, 2000), and the review by Euler and Denk (2001).

Dendrites—What Made the Revolution Possible

A combination of several new technologies has made it possible to view dendrites with unprecedented acuity, notably differential-

Figure 1. Dendrites have unique shapes, a feature that is used to characterize neurons into types. In many neuron types, synaptic inputs from a given source are preferentially mapped into a particular region of the dendritic tree. *A*, Cerebellar Purkinje cell of the guinea pig (reconstructed by M. Rapp). *B*, CA1 pyramidal neuron from the rat (reconstructed by B. Claiborne). *C*, Neostriatal spiny neuron from the rat. (Courtesy of C. Wilson.) *D*, Axonless interneurons of the locust (reconstructed by G. Laurent). Typically, synaptic inputs are distributed nonrandomly over the dendritic surface. (*C'* from Wilson, in McKenna, T., Davis, J., and Zornetzer, S. F., Eds., 1992, *Single Neuron Computation*, Boston Academic Press. Reproduced with permission.)

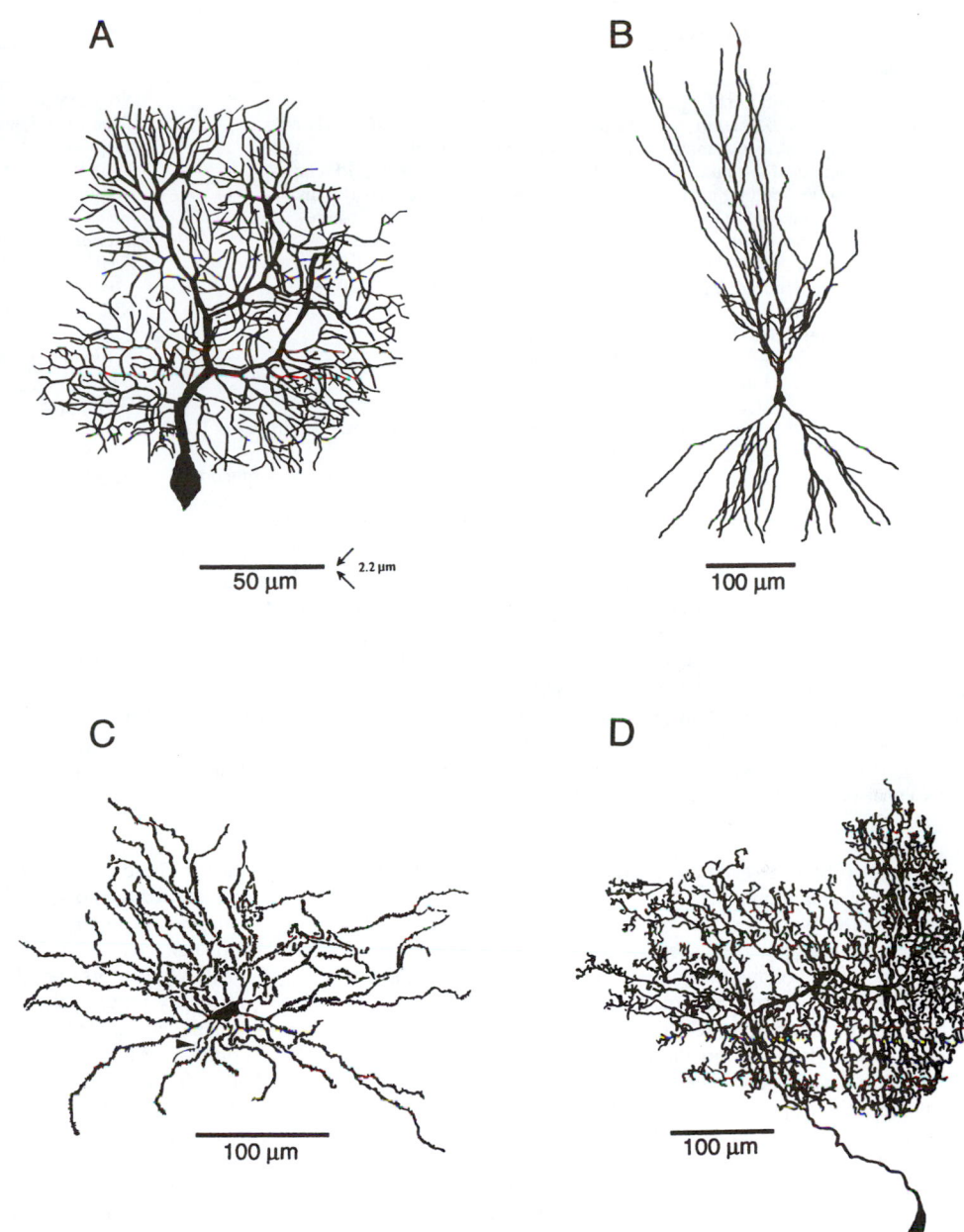

interference contrast (DIC) video microscopy and two-photon microscopy (for a review, see Euler and Denk, 2001). These methods allow researchers to systematically record electrically (using microelectrodes) and optically (using ion-dependent dyes) from identified dendritic locations. Consequently, the effect of a single synaptic input can be monitored in both its dendritic origin and simultaneously in the soma/axon region. Direct measurements of the electrical properties of the dendritic ion channels are now feasible (Johnston et al., 1996; Reyes, 2001); and, with molecular methods (Crick, 1999), specific membrane proteins in dendrites can be marked and manipulated to identify the type and distribution of the various receptors and ion channels in the dendritic membrane. When combined with sophisticated analytic and numerical models, the beginnings of a functional picture emerge from these diverse experimental data. Some of the key experimental and theoretical findings are described below.

Fundamental Facts About Dendrites: Morphological Face, Electrical Character, and Synaptic Inputs

Table 1 summarizes the functionally important facts about dendrites. Because dendrites come in many shapes and sizes, such a summary inevitably presents only a rough range of values. Nonetheless, several important functional conclusions can be drawn from this table.

1. *Morphologically*, dendrites tend to ramify, creating large and complicated trees. Dendrites are thin processes, starting with a diameter of a few micrometers near the soma; the branch diameter typically falls below 1 μm with successive branching, often reaching a distance of 1 mm from the soma. Many (but not all) types of dendrites are studded with abundant tiny branches, or appendages, called dendritic spines. When present,

Table 1. Range of Values for Dendritic Machinery

Morphology	Physiology	Synaptology
Diameter near soma: 1–6 μm	*Passive properties of dendrites*[a]	No. of synapses/neuron: 500–200,000
Diameter at distal tips: 0.3–1 μm	Membrane resistivity (R_m): 1–100K Ωcm^2	Type I (excitatory): 60%–90%[c]; distributed, majority on
Average path length: 0.15–1.5 mm	Axial resistivity (R_i): 70–300 Ωcm	spines
Total dendritic length: 1–10 mm	Membrane capacitance (C_m): 1–2 μF/cm^2	Type II (inhibitory): 10%–40%[c]; near soma, some on
Dendrite area: 2,000–750,000 μm^2	Membrane time constant (τ_m): 1–100 ms	spines
Dendritic trees/neuron: 1–16	Dendrite space constant (λ): 0.2–1 mm	
Dendritic tips/neuron: 10–400	Electrotonic length ($L = x/\lambda$): 0.2–2	*Excitatory synaptic input*[d]
Dend. spines/neuron: 300–200,000	Soma input resistance (R_N): 1–10^3 MΩ	AMPA: g_{peak}: 0.1–0.3 ns; t_{peak}: 0.3–1 ms (may increase
Spine density/1 μm dendrite: 0.5–14	Input resistance at tips (R_T): 10^2–10^3 MΩ	with distance from soma)
Spine length: 0.1–2 μm	Steady-state attenuation factor:	NMDA: g_{peak}: 0.05–0.5 ns; t_{peak}: 5–50 ms
Spine neck diameter: 0.04–0.5 μm	Soma $\rightarrow$ tip: 1.1–2	
Spine head diameter: 0.3–1 μm	Tip $\rightarrow$ soma: 2–15	*Inhibitory synaptic input*[e]
Spine volume: 0.005–0.3 μm^3		GABA$_A$: g_{peak}: 0.4–1 ns; t_{peak}: 0.2–1.2 ms
	Excitable properties of dendrites[b]	GABA$_B$: g_{peak}: 0.1–0.3 ns; t_{peak}: 40–150 ms
	Ca^{2+} channels (L, N, P type)—local dendritic Ca^{2+} AP:	
	Ca^{2+} concentration in spines	
	Na$^+$ channels: Fast activating/inactivating—supports	
	soma $\rightarrow$ dendritic backpropagating AP	
	K$^+$ channels, I$_A$, and mixed current, I$_h$—Increased	
	density with distance from soma—"shock absorbers,"	
	linearization, and temporal normalization.	

[a]The passive properties of dendrites can be strongly modulated by synaptic activity as well as by voltage-gated channels.

[b]Characterization of the voltage-gated ion channels in dendrites (i.e., type, distribution, density, and kinetics) is only beginning to emerge through the use of molecular probes and patch clamp techniques. For reviews, see Koch and Segev (1998, chap. 5) and Reyes (2001).

[c]Based on data from cortical and hippocampal pyramidal neurons.

[d]See, e.g., Stern, P., Edwards, F. A., Sakmann, B., 1992, Fast and slow components of unitary EPSCS on stellate cells elicited by focal stimulation in slices of rat visual-cortex, *J. Physiol. (Lond.)*, 449:247–278.

[e]See, e.g., Otis, T. S., De Koninck, Y., and Mody, I., 1993, Characterization of synaptically elicited GABA$_B$ responses using patch-clamp recordings in rat hippocampal slices, *J. Physiol. (Lond.)*, 463:391–407.

DENDRITIC SPINES (q.v.) are the major postsynaptic targets for *excitatory* synaptic inputs.

2. *Electrically*, dendrites can be characterized by their *passive* properties (the passive "skeleton"), to which the (nonlinear) synaptic- and voltage-dependent ion channels are added. The passive (near resting potential) skeleton can be characterized by the specific membrane resistivity, R_m, of dendrites, which is relatively high (R_m is on the order of 1,000–100,000 Ωcm^2), implying that the dendritic membrane is a good electrical insulator. With a specific capacitance, C_m, of approximately 1 μF/cm^2, the dendritic membrane time constant, τ_m (which sets the range for the time window for the integration of synaptic inputs), is on the order of $\tau_m = R_m C_m = 10$–100 ms. The axial (longitudinal) resistivity of the dendritic cytoplasm, R_i, ranges between 70 and 300 Ωcm, and this, together with the small dimensions of distal arbors, implies a large input resistance (impedance) in the dendrites. The increase in dendritic diameter as one approaches the soma implies a large attenuation factor (on the order of 100) of the peak synaptic potential as it spreads from its origin at the distal dendritic site to the soma (Figure 3A, B).

The *active* properties of dendrites are the outcome of the excitable channels embedded in their membrane. It has been known for years that some types of dendrites, most notably the cerebellar Purkinje cell, can even generate local dendritic AP. More recently, data have indicated that many central neurons can generate dendritic spikes under favorable conditions, and indeed, most of the different types of excitable ion channels in neurons are hosted by the dendrites. Dendrites of different neuron types (e.g., hippocampal CA1, layer V pyramids) bear different combinations of ion channel types, which to a large extent dictate the input-output style of these neurons. A large amount of new information about these ion channels has accumulated in the past few years (see, e.g., Koch and Segev, 1998; Reyes,

2001). These nonlinear ion channels have significant consequences for the computational capabilities of dendrites.

3. *Synaptically*, dendrites of central neurons are covered with synaptically activated (transmitter-gated) receptors. The AMPA and NMDA receptors for glutamate are typically associated with excitatory inputs, whereas GABA$_A$ and GABA$_B$ receptors are typically associated with inhibition. These receptors are not randomly distributed over the dendritic surface (Pettit and Augustine, 2000), and their density can be dynamically modified in an activity-dependent manner. In many, but not all, types of central neurons, the inhibitory-mediated receptors are more proximal than the excitatory synapses (see Shepherd, 1998).

Both the excitatory and the inhibitory synaptic inputs operate in most cases by locally increasing the conductance of the postsynaptic membrane (opening specific ion channels). Therefore, the synaptic input itself perturbs the electrical properties of dendrites, and thus the synaptic input is inherently nonlinear. The time course of the synaptic conductance change may vary by one or two orders of magnitude. The fast excitatory (AMPA) and inhibitory (GABA$_A$) inputs operate on a time scale of a few milliseconds and have a peak conductance on the order of 1 ns; this peak conductance is approximately ten times larger than the slow excitatory (NMDA) and inhibitory (GABA$_B$) inputs, which both act on a time scale of 10–100 ms.

Dendritic Modeling

In two groundbreaking studies, Rall (1959, 1964) established the theoretical foundation that allowed the morphological, electrical, and synaptic properties of dendrites to be linked together in a functionally meaningful framework (see Segev, Rinzel, and Shepherd, 1995). Rall's passive cable theory for dendrites, complemented by his compartment modeling approach, laid the groundwork for a quantitative exploration of the integrative (input-output) function of dendrites.

Passive Cable Theory for Dendrites

Rall described current flow (and the spread of the resultant voltage) in morphologically and physiologically complicated passive dendritic trees using the one-dimensional cable equation

$$\frac{\partial^2 V}{\partial X^2} = \frac{\partial V}{\partial T} + V(X,T) \qquad (1)$$

where V is the voltage across the membrane (interior minus exterior, relative to the resting potential); $X = x/\lambda$, where x is the distance along the core conductor (cm) and the *space constant*, λ, is defined as $\sqrt{r_m/r_i}$; and $T = t/\tau_m$, where the *time constant*, τ_m, is $r_m c_m$. Further, r_m is the membrane resistance for unit length (in Ωcm), c_m is the membrane capacitance per unit length (in F/cm), and r_i is the cytoplasm resistance per unit length (in Ω/cm). A complete derivation of the cable equation can be found in the chapter by Rall (in Koch and Segev, 1998, chap. 2; see also Jack, Noble, and Tsien, 1983, and Perspective on Neuron Model Complexity).

The solution to Equation 1 depends on, in addition to the electrical properties of the membrane and cytoplasm and dimensions of the dendritic tree, the boundary condition at the ends of the segment toward which the current flows. Rall showed that Equation 1 could be solved analytically for passive dendritic trees with arbitrary branching. He modeled the dendritic tree as a collection of short cylindrical segments (Figure 2B), where the tree attached to the end of each segment acts as a sink for the longitudinal current (i.e., a "leaky end").

An example of such a solution for the steady-state case is depicted in Figure 3A and for the transient case in Figure 3B. Several important implications of Figure 3 are discussed later in this article and in Segev and London (2000). Recent extensions of the passive cable theory for dendrites have used the different moments of the transient synaptic potential to explicitly define the notion of input synchrony and propagation delay in dendrites (reviewed in Koch and Segev, 1998, chap. 2). The correspondence between cable theory and the Schrödinger eigenvalue problem for the one-dimensional bounded motion of a particle in quantum mechanics was also used to study the effect of spatially nonuniform membrane conductance on signal transfer in dendrites (see Stuart et al., 1999, chap. 9).

Compartmental Modeling Approach

The compartmental modeling approach complements cable theory by overcoming the assumption that the membrane is passive and that the input is a current source. Mathematically, the compartmental approach is a finite-difference (discrete) approximation to the (nonlinear) cable equation. It replaces the continuous cable equation (Equation 1) with a set, or a matrix, of ordinary differential equations; typically, numerical methods are employed to solve this system (which can include thousands of compartments and thus thousands of equations) for each time step. In the compartmental model, dendritic segments that are electrically short are assumed to be isopotential and are lumped into a single RC (circuit of resistors and capacitors) (either passive or active) membrane compartment (Figure 2C). Compartments are connected to each other via a longitudinal resistivity according to the topology of the tree. Hence, differences in physical properties (e.g., diameter, membrane properties) and differences in potential occur between compartments rather than within them. When the dendritic tree is

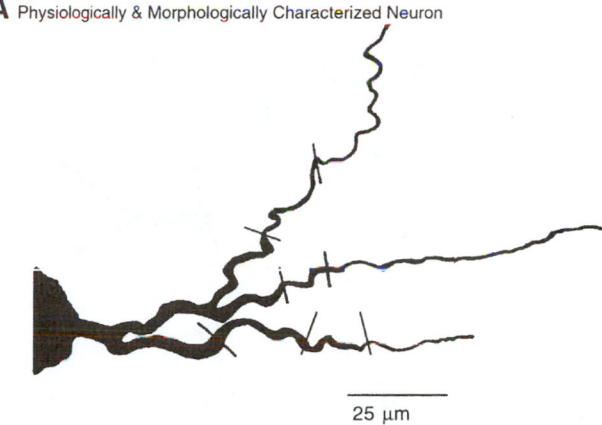

A Physiologically & Morphologically Characterized Neuron

25 μm

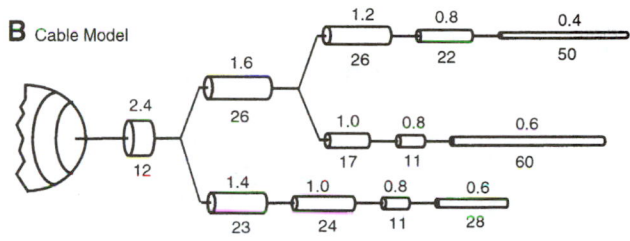

B Cable Model

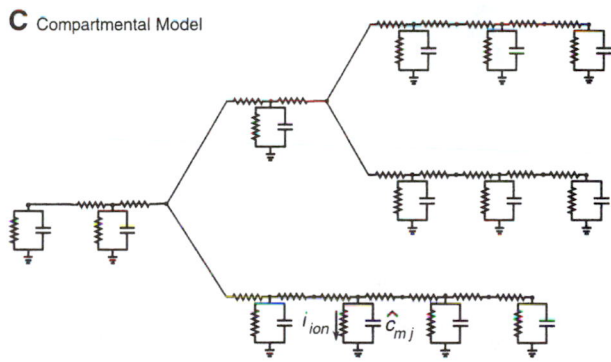

C Compartmental Model

Figure 2. Dendrites (*A*) are modeled either as a set of cylindrical membrane cables (*B*) or as a set of discrete, isopotential RC compartments (*C*). In the cable representation (*B*), the voltage at any point in the tree is computed from Equation 1 and the appropriate boundary conditions are imposed by the tree. In the compartmental representation the tree is discretized into a set of interconnected RC compartments; each is a lumped representation of a sufficiently small dendritic segment. Membrane compartments are connected via axial, cytoplasmic resistances. Here the voltage can be computed at each compartment for any nonlinear input and voltage- and time-dependent membrane properties.

divided into sufficiently small segments (compartments), the solution to the compartmental model converges with that of the continuous cable model. Compartments can represent a patch of membrane with a variety of voltage-gated (excitable) and synaptic (time-varying) channels. Popular public domain computer programs have been developed to simulate compartmental modeling; the most notable are NEURON (NEURON Simulation Environment) and GENESIS (GENESIS Simulation System). A review of the compartmental modeling approach can be found in Koch and Segev (1998, chap. 3).

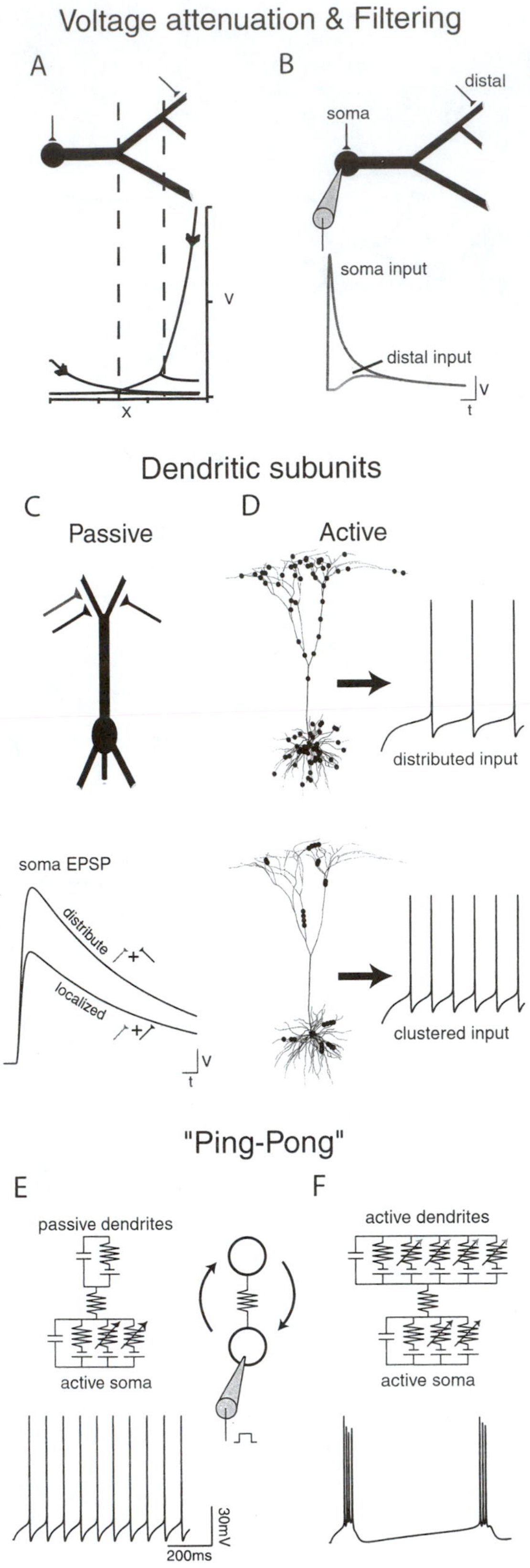

Voltage attenuation & Filtering

Dendritic subunits

"Ping-Pong"

Figure 3. Effects of dendrites on synaptic inputs processing. *Top panel*, Passive dendrites impose voltage attenuation and low-pass filtering on their synaptic inputs. (*A*) Voltage response to a brief current pulse in a simple branched dendritic model (top). Attenuation of voltage peak is plotted for two cases, somatic input and dendritic input. The attenuation is asymmetric and is much steeper in the dendrite-to-soma direction. The voltage response at the input site is much larger for the distal dendritic input (large input impedance). (*B*) Voltage is transient at the soma for somatic input and dendritic input. The filtering effect of the dendrite gives rise to a temporal delay and to an increase in half-width of the distal dendritic input. *Middle panel*, The soma output depends on the degree of synaptic clustering on dendritic subunits. (*C*) In passive dendrites, sublinear summation of synaptic inputs is less pronounced (saturation is reduced) when the inputs are distributed in different dendritic arbors. (*D*) In excitable dendrites, a certain degree of spatial clustering of excitatory synapses (bottom) may result in a significant boosting of the synaptic charge that reaches the soma, because it produces larger local dendritic depolarization that may activate the local excitable channels. As a consequence, the axon fires more vigorously (right). One hundred excitatory synapses were used in both cases: *top*, ten clusters of ten synapses each; *bottom*, 100 clusters of one synapse each. Each synapse was activated 40 times per second for 1 s. *Bottom panel*, Backward-forward "Ping-Pong" interaction between the ion channels in the soma/axon region and the excitable channels in dendrites shapes the output pattern of spikes firing in the axon. Two models of a cortical pyramidal neuron were used, one with passive dendrites (*E*) and the other with excitable dendrites (*F*). For passive dendrites, the axon fires regularly in response to steady soma depolarization, whereas in the model with excitable dendrites, it fires repeated spike bursts. The geometry of the dendritic tree plays a crucial role in this "Ping-Pong" interaction.

Interaction Between Dendrites and Synapses: Main Insights

The theoretical background just outlined and the many results from modeling and experimental studies on dendrites over the last 40 years provide important insights into the input-output properties of dendrites. These properties can be summarized as follows:

Attenuation. Dendritic trees are electrically distributed (rather than isopotential) elements. Consequently, voltage gradients exist over the tree when synaptic inputs are activated locally. In passive dendrites, the voltage tends to attenuate much more severely in the dendrite-to-soma direction (up to a few hundredfold for brief synaptic inputs at distal sites) than in the opposite direction (Figure 3A). This attenuation implies that many (several tens) of excitatory inputs should be activated within the integration time window of about 1 τ_m, in order to build up enough depolarization to reach the threshold for spike firing at the soma and axon. Several experimental as well as theoretical studies (e.g., Reyes, 2001) have proposed that voltage-dependent currents might amplify or "boost" distal synaptic inputs while propagating toward the soma, but it is still an open question to what extent these mechanisms operate in the in vivo situation.

In contrast to the severe attenuation of the voltage *peak amplitude* in passive dendrites, the attenuation of the synaptic charge is relatively small. In many situations the charge is the relevant parameter for determining the firing rate at the axon, and thus, in these cases, the "cost" of placing the synapse at the dendrites rather than at the soma is quite small. Active dendritic currents can boost the synaptic charge, and this boosting is expected to be larger at distal dendritic sites, where the local input resistance (and local depolarization) is large. For example, synapses that are located on excitable dendritic spines (see DENDRITIC SPINES) can trigger regenerative activity that may spread and indirectly activate nearby dendritic regions (a "chain reaction" between active dendritic spines). Synaptic inputs that are mediated by NMDA receptors may implement a similar mechanism for amplification, in which a certain degree of spatial clustering of excitatory inputs is more likely to activate these NMDA receptors and enhance charge transfer to the soma. In this case, the output at the axon depends sensitively on the size and site of the "cluster" (Figure 3D).

Filtering. With passive (RC) properties, dendrites behave like low-pass filters for their synaptic inputs. As a result, synaptic potentials are delayed and become significantly broader as they spread away from the dendritic input site (Figure 3B). The large sink imposed by the tree at distal arbors enhances the decay of local synaptic potentials; smaller enhancement (and thus broader local potentials) is expected at more proximal input sites. The difference in the width of the synaptic potential at different parts of the dendritic tree implies multiple time windows for synaptic integration in the tree. At the soma, the time window for synaptic integration is primarily governed by τ_m, whereas at distal dendritic arbors it may be as short as 0.1 τ_m or less (Koch and Segev, 1998, chap. 2, p. 65). The massive synaptic activity present in vivo greatly affects the apparent membrane conductance and effectively changes the properties of the dendritic filter (Koch and Segev, 1998, chap. 3, p. 125). Extensive background activity can reduce the effective membrane time constant by tenfold. The presence of voltage-activated currents in the dendrites also affects dendritic filtering. Slow currents might turn the dendrites into bandpass filters by suppressing very slow frequencies (Hutcheon and Yarom, 2000). These bandpass filters can be sharpened by the presence of amplifying currents, such as persistent sodium. Other currents might change the apparent capacitance of the filter (Reyes, 2001).

Dendritic inhibition—local veto operation. Inhibitory synapses (which are associated with a conductance change in series with a battery whose value is near the resting potential) are more effective when located on the path between the excitatory input and the "target" region (soma) than when placed distal to the excitatory input. Thus, when strategically placed, inhibitory inputs can specifically veto parts of the dendritic tree and not others (see Rall, 1964; Koch, Poggio, and Torre, 1982; Jack et al., 1983; Segev et al., 1995).

Spatiotemporal integration. Because of dendritic delay, the somatic depolarization that results from activation of excitatory inputs in the dendrites is very sensitive to the temporal sequence of the synaptic activation. It is largest when the synaptic activation starts at distal dendritic sites and progresses proximally. Activation of the same synapses in the reverse order in time will produce smaller somatic depolarization. Thus, the output of neurons with dendrites is inherently *directionally selective* (see PERSPECTIVE ON NEURON MODEL COMPLEXITY).

Gain control. Active dendritic currents (both inward and outward) may serve as a mechanism for synaptic gain control. The membrane potential dynamically controls active conductances in the membrane, which in turn modify the integrative capabilities of the neuron (e.g., its input resistance, electrotonic length); hence the neuron output depends on its state (its membrane potential). Active currents (e.g., outward K^+ current) can act to counterbalance excitatory synaptic inputs (negative feedback) and thus stabilize the input-output characteristics of the neuron. At other voltage regimes, active currents may effectively increase the input resistance and reduce the electrotonic distance between synapses (positive feedback), with the consequence of nonlinearly boosting a specific group of coactive excitatory synapses (Stuart et al., 1999, and references in Segev and London, 2000).

Ping-Pong interactions between synaptic inputs and dendritic spikes. The presence of dendritic spikes (both backpropagating Na^+ spikes as well as local Ca^{2+} spikes) in some neuron types may lead to interesting and nontrivial interactions in the tree. For example, a precise temporal coincidence between the backpropagating Na^+ spike and a distal synaptic input in the apical tree of cortical pyramids may trigger a broad dendritic Ca^{2+} spike that, in turn, leads to a burst of Na^+ spikes at the axon (Reyes, 2001). Thus, a burst of Na^+ spikes in the axon reflects the co-occurrence of input to a basal tree (which generates a backpropagating spike) and an excitatory input to the distal apical tree. Theoretical studies show that slow ion currents in the dendritic tree may interact with the fast spike-generating mechanism at the soma/axon hillock, and this "Ping-Pong" interaction can give rise to many complex spiking patterns in the axon, ranging from regular, high-frequency spiking to spike bursting (Figure 3E; for details, see Koch and Segev, 1998, chap. 5, p. 206).

Computational Function of Dendrites

Different brain areas are specialized in computing specific functions, and each of these areas consists of different types of dendritic structures. Do the unique morphology and electrical properties of the dendrites in a given brain area play a key role in implementing the computational task of this particular piece of brain? Unfortunately, in most cases it is hard to define the specific computational function the neuron executes. Furthermore, we rarely know the nature of the synaptic output that a particular neuron receives while the system computes. Therefore, current theoretical efforts are focusing on exploring the kinds of computations that neurons could potentially implement with their dendrites and synaptic inputs. Several such computations were mentioned earlier; here the major ones are discussed more fully.

Selectivity for Direction of Motion

Because the depolarization in the axon is sensitive to the spatiotemporal order of synaptic activation over the dendritic surface, neurons with dendrites can compute the direction of motion (see Figure 4 and PERSPECTIVE ON NEURON MODEL COMPLEXITY; for details, see Segev et al., 1995; Koch and Segev, 1998). Already at the vertebrate retina some ganglion cells show directional selectivity such that their firing rate is significantly higher when a visual stimulus moves in one direction (preferred direction) rather than the opposite direction (null direction; Figure 4). Whether this computation is implemented postsynaptically by the dendrites of the ganglion cells or is already computed in neurons that are presynaptic to the ganglion cells is still under debate (see Taylor et al., 1999, and Borg-Graham, 2000—references in Euler and Denk, 2001). This debate highlights the need to record from dendrites during the processing of sensory input; recent developments in optical recording from dendrites are likely to provide a direct means of exploring the computational role of dendrites (Single and Borst, 1998; Euler and Denk, 2001)

Indeed, the most direct evidence for dendritic computation comes from work by Single and Borst (1998; see also reviews in Segev and London, 2000, and VISUAL COURSE CONTROL IN FLIES). This study explored the processing of visual information in the fly, in which a population of large interneurons, the tangential cells (TCs), spatially integrates the output signals of many thousands of columnar neurons, each of which is sensitive to a very small part of the visual scene. These TCs are all motion-sensitive: they are excited by motion in one direction and are inhibited by motion in the opposite direction. By combining intracellular recordings and calcium imaging from dendrites in vivo, two major processing steps that are implemented by the TC dendrites were identified. Through the processing of opponent input elements having opposite preferred directions, the directional selectivity of presynaptic neurons is significantly enhanced in the TCs. It was also shown that dendritic filtering helps distinguish a change in contrast due to stimulus motion from changes due to purely local patterns of the stimulus. The result of this integration is a graded depolarization in the axon of the tangential cells; this depolarization represents information about image velocity with high fidelity (Single and Borst, 1998).

Coincidence Detection

Neurons with dendrites can function simultaneously in multiple time windows. Distal arbors act more like coincidence detectors, whereas the soma acts more like an integrator when brief synaptic inputs (i.e., AMPA and $GABA_A$) are involved (Koch and Segev, 1998, chap. 2). Active dendrites provide an additional mechanism for coincidence detection based on local dendritic Na^+ spikes (see SINGLE-CELL MODELS) or on the temporal coincidence between backpropagating Na^+ spikes and local excitatory synaptic input, which gives rise to a broad local dendritic Ca^{2+} spike and a corresponding burst of Na^+ spikes in the axon (see Reyes, 2001, and Figure 4). Ca^{2+} accumulation in dendritic spines can also serve as a detector for coincidence between back propagating Na^+ spikes and excitatory input to the spine (see DENDRITIC SPINES).

The coincidence detector (CD) neurons in the auditory brainstem constitute a special case (Agmon-Snir, Carr, and Rinzel, 1998). These neurons possess bipolar dendrites, each of which receives excitatory synaptic inputs from only one ear. The neuron fires only if the inputs arriving from both ears occur within a very narrow time window (tens of microseconds); this is used by these cells to detect interaural time differences, and therefore the location of the sound source. The problem is how to distinguish a strong input arriving from one ear and an input that arrives simultaneously from both ears. This task cannot be achieved by a neuron that sums its inputs linearly. Agmon-Snir et al. (1998) have shown, using a simplified model of CD neurons, that a strong input arriving at one dendrite (from one ear) cannot drive the cell to fire, because of synaptic saturation, whereas inputs that reach both dendrites summate more linearly with each other at the soma and can trigger an output spike. Thus, segregation of the inputs from each ear to different dendrites, together with the inherent nonlinearity of synaptic summation, improves sound localization.

Feature Extraction, Input Classification, and Logical Operations

Neurons with dendrites can implement a multidimensional classification task where the neurons' output is sensitive to a specific combination of active synapses over the dendritic tree (Stuart et al., 1999, chap. 11). For example, biophysical modeling of cortical pyramidal neurons shows that, with appropriate mapping of synaptic inputs from the lateral geniculate body (LGN) to the dendritic tree, and using local dendritic nonlinearities (mediated via NMDA receptors or excitable channels), these model neurons exhibit several nonlinear features of visual neurons, including phase invariance orientation tuning (a critical feature of complex cells), binocular disparity, and nonlinear boosting of tuning curves (Figure 4).

AND-NOT type of logical operations could be implemented by strategically placed excitatory and inhibitory synaptic inputs over the dendritic tree (Koch et al., 1982, and Figure 4). Because neurons with dendrites can function as many quasi-independent functional subunits, the dendritic tree as a whole can implement a rich repertoire of logical operations. Also, within each of these functional subunits, very localized plastic processes can take place (e.g., on a single dendritic spine; see DENDRITIC SPINES).

Dendritic Learning

Over the past few years, it has become evident that dendrites are not static elements. Rather, there is a continuous change in the morphology of dendritic spines (Segev and London, 2000) and a dynamic change in the distribution of ion channels and synapses on the dendritic surface. Two recent computational studies suggest that these plastic properties of dendrites might play a role in learning. Stemmler and Koch (1999) demonstrated that by changing the distribution of membrane ion channels in a dendritic compartment via a learning rule, the neurons' output can optimize the representation of sensory information. The segregation of ion channels between the dendritic compartment and the soma axon compartment is critical for this mechanism to work. Poirazi and Mel (see DENDRITIC LEARNING) have shown that by spatially reallocating (reshuffling) synapses that are temporally correlated so that they will contact nearby dendritic locations, active dendritic subunits are created whereby the coactivation of synapses within a subunit results in significant synaptic boosting by local nonlinear dendritic mechanisms. This spatial clustering of temporally correlated inputs over the dendritic tree greatly increases the input classification capacity of the neuron.

Discussion

Nature apparently uses dendrites as the basic building blocks for a wide range of nervous systems, from the simplest organism to the most sophisticated one (us?). Dendrites, therefore, need to provide

Computation	Implementation (Biophysical mechanism)	Example
Direction selectivity	1. Dendritic delay + temporal sequence of synaptic activation 2. Asymmetric mapping of inhibition and excitation 3. Integration of many local direction selective detectors	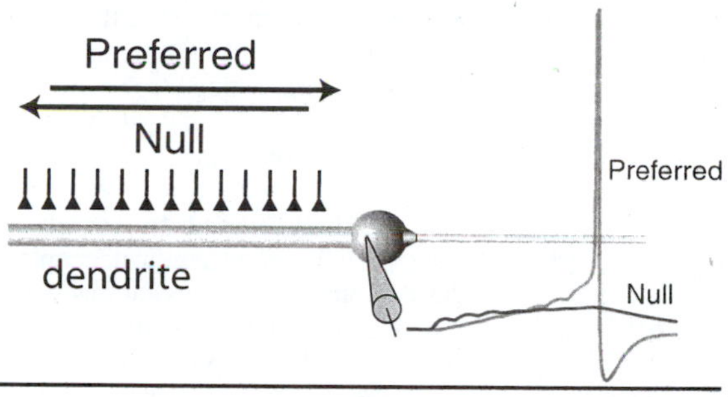
Coincidence detection	1. Backpropagating Na spike + Dendritic Ca spike 2. Input segregation on dendrites + synaptic saturation 3. Backpropagating Na spike + NMDA (Ca in spines) 4. Local dendritic Na spike generated by priciesly timed excitation 5. Short local delays in thin dendrites	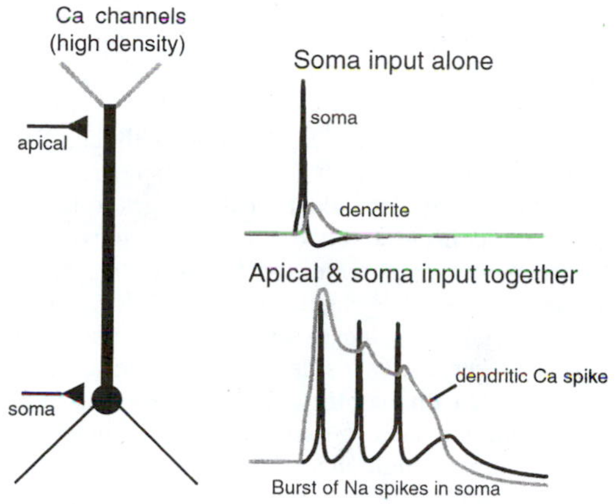
Logical operation	1. "On path" dendritic inhibition + distal excitation (AND-NOT) 2. Local spike in dendritic spines (AND, OR)	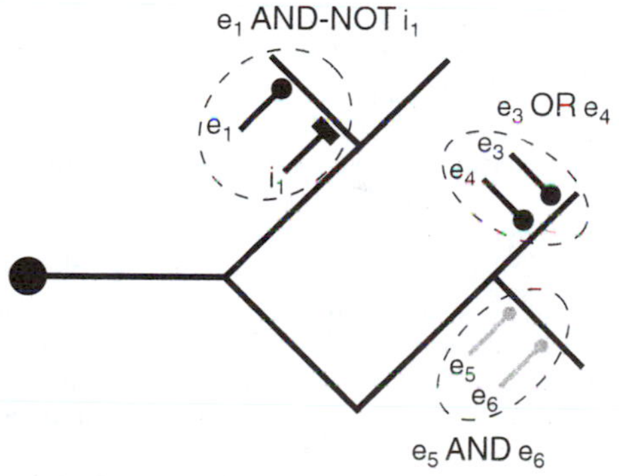
Feature extraction	1. Mapping synaptic inputs to distinct nonlinear dendritic subunits	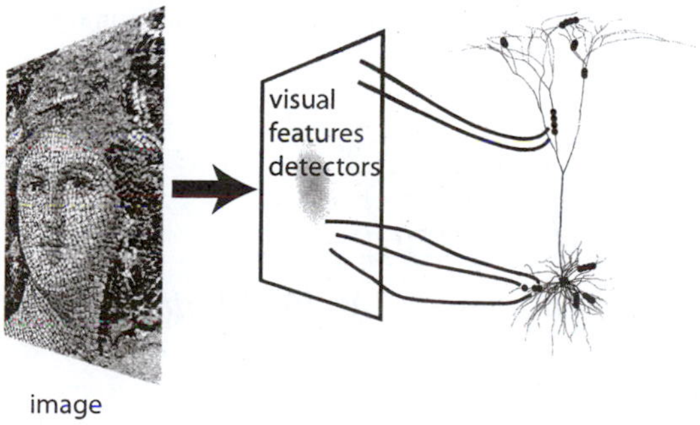

Figure 4. Summary of dendritic computation.

a good solution for the real-life problems that behaving animals must deal with, and the challenge is to explore how the intricacies of dendrites provide such credible solutions. In principle, dendrites could optimize several constraints simultaneously, from the wiring requirements of neural networks to chemical and electrical constraints imposed by the nervous system.

In terms of brain connectivity, dendrites enable the spatial segregation of different types of inputs at different dendritic regions, thus providing a natural means of preserving strong local interactions among specific types of input sources and, at the same time, integrating different input sources onto the same postsynaptic neuron.

The electrical distributed structure of dendrites can give rise to functional subtrees that are partially electrically decoupled from each other. In each of these subtrees, local operations could take place, including local synaptic boosting, local dendritic spiking, local dampening of the backpropagating spike, and so forth. The spatiotemporal (backward-forward) interaction between the different dendritic subtrees could result in a wide range of firing repertoires that would be hard to replicate with spherical (isopotential) neurons. The dendritic tree also behaves like a sink for the excitable channels in the axon; thus it tends to stabilize network activity.

From a chemical perspective, dendrites with their fine diameters and their specialization, such as dendritic spines, allow rapid and very specific activity-dependent local changes to take place in intracellular ion concentrations (e.g., of Ca^{2+} ions). This chemical compartmentalization provides the means for triggering local plastic processes (local "synaptic learning," local morphological changes in dendritic spines). Moreover, the maintenance of ion gradients between the two sides of the dendritic membrane consumes energy. In this context, dendrites may optimize the ratio between membrane area (required for connecting a large number of synapses onto a single neuron) and cell volume, thus reducing energy consumption.

Whether or not dendrites contribute to network computation should be assessed within a wider framework, namely, in terms of the effect of the complexity of the computation executed by a single neuron on the network function. Artificial neural networks typically assume that neurons are simple computational units and that the computation that the nervous system performs emerges as a collective phenomenon. In this framework, the computation at the single neuron level (e.g., orientation selectivity) merely reflects network dynamics. However, as was shown in this article, real neurons can potentially do much more than integrate their input and compare it to a fixed threshold. Moreover, in some cases (mainly in invertebrates), it is clear that single identified neurons actually perform many of the computations required for accomplishing a specific behavioral task.

Thus, the challenge to neural modelers is to better understand whether, and how, the complexity of the single neuron significantly enhances the computational capacity of the network. Once theoretical studies are able to proceed hand in hand with direct measurements obtained from dendrites during actual behavior (and while their nervous system is computing), we will gain a better understanding of the computational role of dendrites. At this point the "dendritic revolution" will come to a close.

Road Map: Biological Neurons and Synapses; Grounding Models of Networks
Background: Single-Cell Models
Related Reading: Dendritic Learning; Dendritic Spines; Perspective on Neuron Model Complexity

References

Agmon-Snir, H., Carr, C. E., and Rinzel, J., 1998, The role of dendrites in auditory coincidence detection, *Nature*, 393:268–272.

Crick, F., 1999, The impact of molecular biology on neuroscience, *Philos. Trans. R. Soc. Lond. B Biol. Sci.*, 354:2021–2025.

Euler, T., and Denk, W., 2001, Dendritic processing, *Curr. Opin. Neurobiol.*, 11:415–422. ◆

Hutcheon, B., and Yarom, Y., 2000, Resonance, oscillation and the intrinsic frequency preferences of neurons, *Trends Neurosci.*, 23:216–222.

Jack, J. J. B., Noble, D., and Tsien, R. W., 1983, *Electrical Current Flow in Excitable Cells*, Oxford, Engl.: Oxford University Press.

Johnston, D., Magee, J. C., Colbert, C. M., and Cristie, B. R., 1996, Active properties of neuronal dendrites, *Annu. Rev. Neurosci.*, 19:165–186.

Koch, C., Poggio, T., and Torre, V., 1982, Retinal ganglion cells: A functional interpretation of dendritic morphology, *Philos. Trans. R. Soc. Lond. B Biol. Sci.*, 298:227–263.

Koch, C., and Segev, I., Eds., 1998, *Methods in Neuronal Modeling: From Ions to Networks*, Cambridge, MA: MIT Press. ◆

Pettit, D. L., and Augustine, G. J., 2000, Distribution of functional glutamate and GABA receptors on hippocampal pyramidal cells and interneurons, *J. Neurophysiol.*, 84:28–38.

Rall, W., 1959, Branching dendritic trees and motoneuron membrane resistivity, *Exp. Neurol.*, 2:503–532.

Rall, W., 1964, Theoretical significance of dendritic trees for neuronal input-output relations, in *Neural Theory and Modeling* (R. F. Reiss, Ed.), Stanford, CA: Stanford University Press.

Reyes, A., 2001, Influence of dendritic conductances on the input-output properties of neurons, *Annu. Rev. Neurosci.*, 24:653–675. ◆

Segev, I., and London, M., 2000, Untangling dendrites with quantitative models, *Science*, 290:744–750. ◆

Segev, I., Rinzel, J., and Shepherd, G., Eds., 1995, *The Theoretical Foundation of Dendritic Function*, Cambridge, MA: MIT Press.

Shepherd, G. M., Ed., 1998, *The Synaptic Organization of the Brain*, New York: Oxford University Press. ◆

Single, S., and Borst, A., 1998, Dendritic integration and its role in computing image velocity, *Science*, 281:1848–1850.

Stemmler, M., and Koch, C., 1999, How voltage-dependent conductances can adapt to maximize the information encoded by neuronal firing rate, *Nat. Neurosci.*, 2:521–527.

Stuart, G., Spruston, N., and Häusser, M., Eds., 1999, *Dendrites*, New York: Oxford University Press. ◆

Dendritic Spines

William R. Holmes and Wilfrid Rall

Introduction

The function of dendritic spines has been debated ever since they were discovered by Ramón y Cajal in 1891. Although it was widely believed that spines were important for intercellular communication, this was not demonstrated until 1959 when Gray, using the electron microscope, showed that synapses are present on spines. Why should synapses exist on spines, rather than on dendrites? What role does spine morphology play in their function? Early theoretical studies of these questions focused on the electrical resistance provided by the thin spine stem and suggested that changes in stem diameter might be important for synaptic plasticity. Later investigations found that if voltage-dependent conductances were present on spines, then spines could increase the computational possibilities of a cell. Recent studies suggest that spines are isolated compartments in which highly localized calcium signals can occur. The amplitude and time course of these calcium signals can initiate localized cascades of biochemical reactions important for synaptic plasticity. (For reviews, see Harris, 1999; Nimchinsky, Sabatini, and Svoboda, 2002; and Sabatini, Maravall, and Svoboda, 2001.)

Spine Morphology

Dendritic spines are short, appendage-like structures found on many different cell types. Spines are composed of a bulbous "head" connected to the dendrite by a thin "neck" or "stem." An excitatory synapse is usually found on the spine head, and some spines also have a second, usually inhibitory, synapse located near or on the spine neck. Spines typically are small in size, but because they occur in densities of 1–2 spines/μm or more, spine membrane area can comprise 40–60% of the total neuron membrane area.

Attempts have been made to classify spines based on their size, shape, and dendritic location. Jones and Powell (1969) categorized spines as sessile (stemless) or pedunculated (having a peduncle, or stem), with sessile spines more common in proximal regions and pedunculated spines in distal regions. Peters and Kaiserman-Abramof (1970) classified spines as (1) stubby, (2) mushroom shaped, or (3) thin or long-thin (Figure 1). Stubby spines were most numerous in proximal regions, long-thin spines dominated distal regions, and mushroom-shaped spines were distributed almost uniformly. These categories are arbitrary since spine shape varies continuously and all types of spines are found in all areas. In some brain regions, it has not been possible to categorize spines in any systematic manner, but categories and a range of dimensions are useful for models.

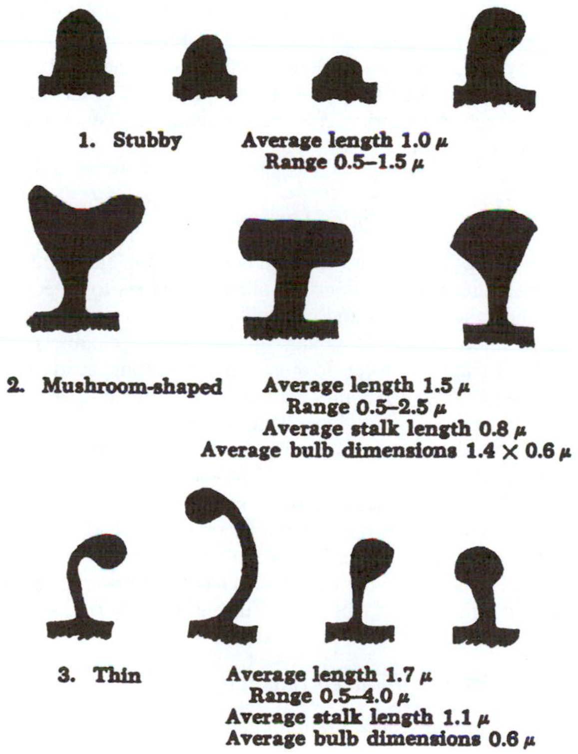

Passive Models of Spine Function

Models in which the spine is represented as a passive electric circuit show that the resistance of a thin spine stem can attenuate a synaptic input delivered to the spine head. This can be seen by considering the circuit pictured in Figure 2.

Assuming a constant synaptic conductance, currents flowing in the spine head can be described by Kirchhoff's law as:

$$V_{SH}/R_{SH} + g_{syn}(V_{SH} - V_{EQ}) + V_{SH}/(R_{SS} + R_{BI}) = 0 \quad (1)$$

where the first term is leakage current across the spine head membrane, the second is the synaptic current, and the third is the flow of current through the spine stem to ground. Because R_{SH} is large, the first term is negligible compared to the other two terms and can be ignored. With this simplification, the steady-state spine head potential is

$$V_{SH} = V_{EQ}/[1 + 1/\{g_{syn}(R_{SS} + R_{BI})\}] \quad (2)$$

Similarly, the currents in the dendrite are described as

$$V_{BI}/R_{BI} + (V_{BI} - V_{SH})/R_{SS} = 0 \quad (3)$$

which can be rearranged as

$$V_{BI} = V_{SH}R_{BI}/(R_{BI} + R_{SS}) \quad (4)$$

Combining Equations 2 and 4, the voltage at the dendrite is

$$V_{BI} = V_{EQ}/[1 + 1/(g_{syn}R_{BI}) + R_{SS}/R_{BI}] \quad (5)$$

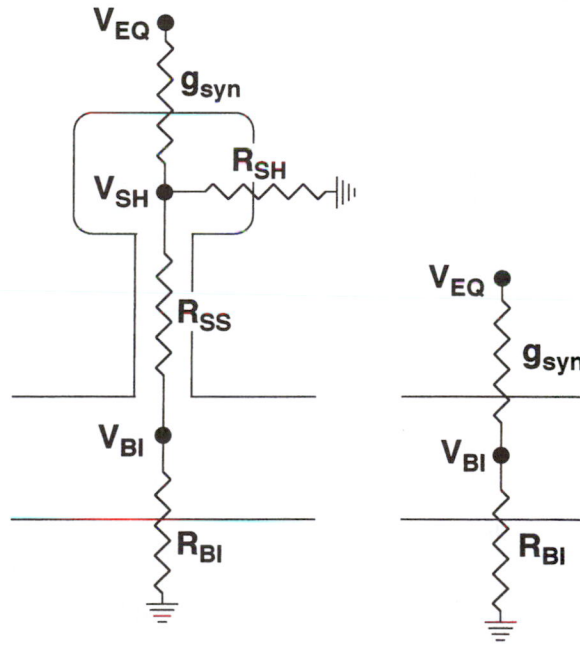

Figure 1. Variety of spine shapes in parietal cortex. (Adapted from Peters and Kaiserman-Abramof, 1970, Table 1. Copyright © 1970 by the Wistar Institute of Anatomy and Biology. Used by permission of John Wiley & Sons, Inc.)

1. **Stubby**   Average length 1.0 μ
Range 0.5–1.5 μ

2. **Mushroom-shaped**   Average length 1.5 μ
Range 0.5–2.5 μ
Average stalk length 0.8 μ
Average bulb dimensions 1.4 × 0.6 μ

3. **Thin**   Average length 1.7 μ
Range 0.5–4.0 μ
Average stalk length 1.1 μ
Average bulb dimensions 0.6 μ

Figure 2. Electrical circuit of a dendritic spine. V_{EQ} is the synaptic reversal potential, V_{SH} is the voltage in the spine head, and V_{BI} is the voltage in the dendrite at the base of the spine. R_{SH} is the spine head resistance, R_{SS} is the spine stem resistance, and R_{BI} is the branch input resistance at the base of the spine. g_{syn} is the synaptic conductance. The corresponding circuit for input on a dendrite is shown on the right.

If, however, the synapse were on the dendrite, Kirchhoff's current law says that

$$g_{syn}(V_{BI} - V_{EQ}) + V_{BI}/R_{BI} = 0 \qquad (6)$$

Rearranging, we have

$$V_{BI} = V_{EQ}/[1 + 1/(g_{syn}R_{BI})] \qquad (7)$$

The only difference between Equations 5 and 7 is the presence of the ratio R_{SS}/R_{BI} in the denominator of Equation 5, and this term accounts for voltage attenuation when the synapse is on the spine instead of the dendrite.

Spines also attenuate synaptic current. The synaptic currents for spine and dendritic inputs can be computed by substituting expressions for V_{SH} and V_{BI} in Equations 2 and 7 in place of V in $g_{syn}(V - V_{EQ})$. The resulting currents are given by the right side of Equations 5 and 7 divided by R_{BI}. The size of the synaptic current entering the spine is attenuated because, for identical g_{syn}, the voltage in the spine head owing to input there is closer to V_{EQ} than the voltage change with a dendritic input.

The R_{SS}/R_{BI} ratio in these equations suggests another possible function for dendritic spines. If a neuron can adjust spine stem morphology (and hence R_{SS}), then spines provide a mechanism to allow synaptic weights to be modified (Rall, 1978). For this mechanism to be important, the value of R_{SS}/R_{BI} should lie between 0.1 and 10 times $1 + 1/(g_{syn}R_{BI})$, because within this range a small change in R_{SS}/R_{BI} can have a significant effect on V_{BI} (see Equation 5). Early experimental estimates of R_{SS}/R_{BI} suggested that it might lie in this effective operating range. This encouraged investigators to look for spine dimension changes in various experimental situations. However, recent estimates of g_{syn}, R_{SS}, and R_{BI} suggest that R_{SS}/R_{BI} may not fall in this range. For example, if $g_{syn} = 0.5$ nS and $R_{BI} = 200$ MΩ, then $1/(g_{syn}R_{BI}) = 10$. This means that R_{SS} should be 220–2,200 MΩ; morphological measurements and imaging experiments indicate, however, that R_{SS} is 5–150 MΩ in many neuron types (Svoboda, Tank, and Denk, 1996). This would seem to rule out the possibility that the function of spines can be explained by changes in passive electrical properties caused by changes in spine dimensions.

Models of Excitable Spines

If voltage-dependent conductances exist on spines, then spines might exist to amplify synaptic inputs. Early theoretical studies showed that postsynaptic potential and charge transfer were five- to ten-fold larger for synaptic input on spines with voltage-dependent conductances than for input to passive spines. Subsequent studies found that interactions among excitable spines could create a number of interesting computational possibilities for information transfer (reviewed in Segev and Rall, 1998). Chain reactions of spine head action potentials, spreading a certain distance proximally and distally, were theoretically possible. Considerable amplification of the initial input could occur even if only a small percentage of spines possessed voltage-dependent channels. Alternatively, subthreshold depolarization could inactive channels and prevent amplification of later inputs.

Although the prediction that spines exist to amplify synaptic input has received some limited experimental support, the level of amplification is likely to be much less than predicted by the models for two reasons. First, the models assume large densities of voltage-dependent ionic channels in spines (~500–1000 channels per spine) while recent estimates place the number of calcium channels in spines at 1–20 (Sabatini and Svoboda, 2000). Second, the models require a large R_{SS} to get the interesting interaction effects. The latest models reduce the required R_{SS} value to 95 MΩ by assuming kinetics for a low threshold calcium action potential in the spine

head, but this value is still at the high end of the 5–150 MΩ range quoted earlier.

Models of Calcium Diffusion in Spines

The theoretical studies described above searched for a function for spines that depended on the electrical resistance of the spine neck. Besides providing an electrical resistance to current flow, the thin spine neck provides a *diffusional* resistance to the flow of ions and molecules. The spine neck, by restricting the flow of materials out of the spine head, might effectively isolate the spine head and provide a localized environment where reactions specific to a particular synapse can occur.

Calcium is a prime candidate for a substance that might be selectively concentrated in the spine head. Calcium is important for a large number of metabolic processes and has been shown to be necessary for the induction of long-term potentiation (LTP), but high concentrations of calcium can lead to cell death. Spines might provide isolated locations where high concentrations of calcium can be attained safely without disrupting other aspects of cell function.

Compartmental models of dendritic spines that included calcium diffusion, buffering, and extrusion tested this idea. The models predicted that calcium influx at the spine head could produce transient spine head calcium concentrations greater than 10 μM, while an equivalent influx at the dendrite would produce only a small concentration change. Spine head calcium concentration changes greater than 10 μM were subsequently observed experimentally.

Large increases in calcium concentration occur because of the small volume of the spine head and because incoming calcium cannot be buffered or pumped out instantaneously. These large transient increases are restricted to the spine head because of the diffusional resistance of the spine neck. The thin spine neck acts as a constriction that slows calcium diffusion. Any calcium that does enter the spine neck is further hindered from diffusing to the dendrite by the presence of calcium buffer and pumps in the spine neck. Calcium that diffuses through the spine neck to the dendrite has little effect on dendritic calcium concentration because of the large dendritic volume.

Spines Allow Coincidence Detection

Amplification of spine head calcium concentration can occur with backpropagating action potentials, allowing spines to detect temporal coincidence of pre- and postsynaptic activity. Although calcium can enter spines via voltage-gated calcium channels or be released from internal stores, in most cells, most spine head calcium enters through NMDA receptor channels. These ligand-gated channels are subject to voltage-dependent magnesium block. Theoretical studies predict a sharp increase in spine head calcium influx when synaptic input occurs slightly before action potential invasion of spines. This occurs because the voltage boost provided by the action potential relieves magnesium block of the NMDA receptor channels. Increases in spine head calcium concentration with coincident pre- and postsynaptic activity has been observed experimentally in a number of labs (e.g., Yuste et al., 1999).

Modeling Calcium-Induced Plasticity in Spines

Spine head calcium concentration changes are important because synaptic plasticity involves cascades of biochemical reactions that are activated or deactivated to different degrees depending on temporal characteristics of the calcium signal. For example, large increases in spine head calcium concentration allow calcium to bind to calmodulin and the calcium-calmodulin complex then activates a number of kinases including calcium-calmodulin-dependent protein kinase II (CaMKII). CaMKII constitutes 20% of the total protein in the postsynaptic density and is thought to play a key role in LTP induction. Recent spine models include predictions of levels of CaMKII activation in the spine head for various input conditions (Holmes, 2000).

The CaMKII pathway is just one of many pathways affected by calcium. Future spine models will study how dozens of different molecules and proteins interact, form signaling complexes, and produce LTP. This is a daunting task, but progress has been made defining network pathways and compiling the necessary rate constants.

Factors Affecting Spine Calcium Dynamics

A number of factors affect the dynamics of the spine head calcium transient. The most important of these are buffer concentration, the magnitude and duration of the calcium current, and spine shape. Buffer concentration and calcium currents in spine heads have been difficult to quantify experimentally, but the range of spine shapes is known for several neuron types. Simulations suggest that spines with fat spine necks are not able to concentrate calcium as quickly or to the same high levels as spines with long-thin necks. Thus, spine shape changes that occur with LTP (Yuste and Bonhoeffer, 2001) are likely to affect the rates and types of calcium-dependent reactions that can occur in a particular spine. During development spines are particularly motile and experimental advances now allow these spine morphology changes to be observed in real time (Matus, 2000). These motility changes can continuously alter calcium decay kinetics in spines.

Discussion

Early theoretical work with passive spine models showed the importance of the electrical spine stem resistance for synaptic transmission and demonstrated how synaptic weights might be modified by changes in this resistance. Later modeling showed that input could be amplified or transformed in a variety of interesting ways if spines have excitable membrane. However, experimental measurements suggest that spine stem *electrical* resistance is too small to play a significant role in electrical signaling in all but a small percentage of spines.

The current hypothesis is that spines, by restricting diffusion of substances away from the synapse, provide a safe, local, and isolated environment in which specific biochemical reactions can occur. In particular, the spine stem provides a *diffusional* resistance that allows calcium to become concentrated in the spine head and

calcium-dependent reactions to be localized to the synapse. This could be very important for plasticity changes, such as those that occur with long-term potentiation. Spine morphology may determine the magnitude of the diffusional resistance and play a role in determining, or restricting, the types of biochemical reactions that can take place at a synapse.

Road Map: Biological Neurons and Synapses
Related Reading: Dendritic Processing; Hebbian Synaptic Plasticity; Ion Channels: Keys to Neuronal Specialization; Neocortex: Chemical and Electrical Synapses

References

Gray, E. G., 1959, Axo-somatic and axo-dendritic synapses of the cerebral cortex: An electron-microscopic study, *J. Anat.*, 93:420–433.
Harris, K. M., 1999, Structure, development, and plasticity of dendritic spines, *Curr. Opin. Neurobiol.*, 9:343–348. ◆
Holmes, W. R., 2000, Models of calmodulin trapping and CaM kinase II activation in a dendritic spine, *J. Computat. Neurosci.*, 8:65–86.
Jones, E. G., and Powell, T. P. S., 1969, Morphological variations in the dendritic spines of the neocortex, *J. Cell. Sci.*, 5:509–529.
Matus, A., 2000, Actin-based plasticity in dendritic spines, *Science*, 290:754–758
Nimchinsky, E. A., Sabatini, B. L., and Svoboda, K., 2002, Structure and function of dendritic spines, *Annu. Rev. Physiol.*, 64:313–353. ◆
Peters, A., and Kaiserman-Abramof, I. R., 1970, The small pyramidal neuron of the rat cerebral cortex: The perikaryon, dendrites and spines, *Am. J. Anat.*, 127:321–356.
Rall, W., 1978, Dendritic spines and synaptic potency, in *Studies in Neurophysiology* (R. Porter, Ed.), New York: Cambridge University Press, pp. 203–209.
Ramón y Cajal, S., 1891. Sur la structure de l'écorce cerebrale de quelques mammiferes, *Cellule*, 7:124–176
Sabatini, B. L., Maravall, M., and Svoboda, K., 2001, Ca^{2+} signaling in dendritic spines, *Curr. Opin. Neurobiol.*, 11:349–356. ◆
Sabatini, B. L., and Svoboda, K., 2000, The number and properties of calcium channels in single dendritic spines determined by optical fluctuation analysis, *Nature*, 408:589–593.
Segev, I., and Rall, W., 1998, Excitable dendrites and spines: Earlier theoretical insights elucidate recent direct observations, *Trends Neurosci.*, 21:453–460. ◆
Svoboda, K., Tank, D. W., and Denk, W., 1996, Direct measurement of coupling between dendritic spines and shafts, *Science*, 272:716–719.
Yuste, R., and Bonhoeffer, T., 2001, Morphological changes in dendritic spines associated with long-term synaptic plasticity, *Annu. Rev. Neurosci.*, 24:1071–1089. ◆
Yuste, R., Majewska, A., Cash, S. S., and Denk, W., 1999, Mechanisms of calcium influx into hippocampal spines: Heterogeneity among spines, coincidence detection by NMDA receptors, and optical quantal analysis, *J. Neurosci.*, 19:1976–1987.

Development of Retinotectal Maps

Geoffrey J. Goodhill

Introduction

A common feature of many axonal projections between different regions of the nervous system is their organization into topographic maps, whereby nearby cells in the input structure project to nearby cells in the output structure. How do such maps form? The best studied example of this phenomenon is the formation of maps from the retina to more central targets. In frogs, fishes, and chicks, the main visual center is the optic tectum. During development, fibers

grow from each retina to the opposite tectum, crossing at the optic chiasm, to form a "retinotopic" map. This map is oriented such that the nasal-temporal and dorsal-ventral axes of each retina map to the caudal-rostral and lateral-medial axes of each tectum, respectively (Figure 1A). In mice, there are topographic projections from the retina to both the superior colliculus (SC) and the lateral geniculate nucleus (LGN). The SC receives connections only from the contralateral eye, as in the retinotectal projection in frogs, fishes, and chicks, whereas the LGN receives in addition a small

	Perturbation	Outcome
a	Normal	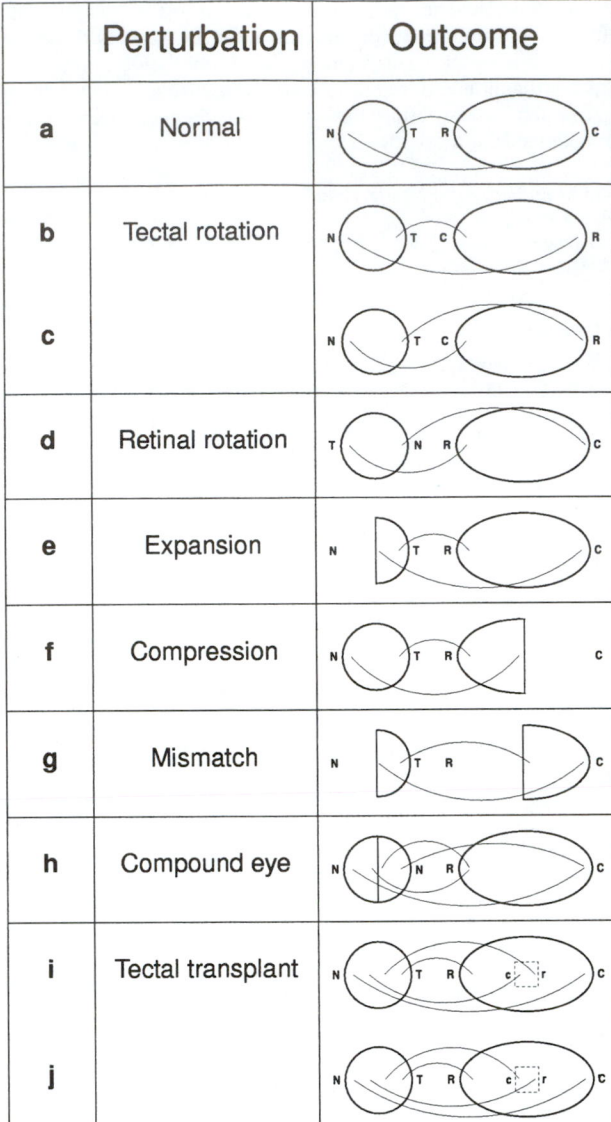
b	Tectal rotation	
c		
d	Retinal rotation	
e	Expansion	
f	Compression	
g	Mismatch	
h	Compound eye	
i	Tectal transplant	
j		

Figure 1. Summary of the outcomes of surgical manipulation experiments in the retinotectal system. The circle represents the retina and the ellipse represents the tectum. N, nasal; T, temporal; R, rostral; C, caudal. See text for more details.

ipsilateral projection. For many purposes, this system can be considered as a sheet of retinal ganglion cells connected to a sheet of tectal/SC/LGN cells by a bundle of ganglion cell fibers. Although there is wide variation among species in the degree of order existing in the optic nerve, it is almost always the case that the final map in the tectum is ordered to a greater extent than is the optic nerve (reviewed in Udin and Fawcett, 1988). The development of such maps appears to proceed in two stages: the first involves axon guidance independent of neural activity, while the second involves the refinement of initially crude patterns of connections by processes dependent on neural activity. This article focuses on the former events (see also AXONAL PATH FINDING); for a discussion of the latter see SELF-ORGANIZING FEATURE MAPS and OCULAR DOMINANCE AND ORIENTATION COLUMNS.

Experimental Data

The Chemospecificity Hypothesis

The main hypothesis driving experimental work in this area has been the idea of "chemospecificity," proposed by Sperry in 1963:

> The establishment and maintenance of synaptic associations [is] conceived to be regulated by highly specific cytochemical affinities that arise systematically among the different types of neurons involved via self-differentiation, induction through terminal contacts, and embryonic gradient effects. . . . [I propose] an orderly cytochemical mapping in terms of two or more gradients of embryonic differentiation that spread across and through each other with their axes roughly perpendicular. These separate gradients successivly superimposed on the retinal and tectal fields and surroundings would stamp each cell with its appropriate latitude and longitude expressed in a kind of chemical code with matching values between the retinal and tectal maps (p. 707).

The most obvious test of this hypothesis is to uncover the molecular identity of these gradients and show that the pattern of these molecules is crucial for proper map formation. However, such a molecular approach has borne fruit only very recently (see below). Instead, much research immediately following Sperry until the 1980s adopted the approach, more rooted in classical embryology, of disrupting the normal development (or, more typically, regeneration) of this system and comparing the outcome with the predictions of Sperry's hypothesis. These experiments are summarized in the next section and in Figure 1. For more detailed discussions, including original references, see Udin and Fawcett (1988), Holt and Harris (1993), and Goodhill and Richards (1999).

Surgical Manipulations

Shifting connections. In fishes and frogs, the retina expands radially during development, while the tectum expands mostly along one dimension. The retinotectal map remains ordered throughout this time, indicating that the retinotectal projection is continually shifting.

Ectopic targeting. Retinal axons entering the tectum via abnormal trajectories can still find their appropriate termination sites.

Rotation. If in *Xenopus* a presumptive tectum is rotated early enough during development, a map is formed that is normal relative to the whole animal (Figure 1*B*), whereas later rotations lead to a rotated map (Figure 1*C*). Initially it was thought that eye rotation could also lead to both a normal outcome if performed early enough and a rotated outcome if performed later. However, more recent experiments have always found rotated maps (Figure 1*D*).

Retinal ablation ("expansion"). The map formed after removal of half of the retina initially covers half the tectum, but then gradually expands to fill the whole tectum (Figure 1*E*). Axon terminal density remains the same. If the optic nerve is then made to regenerate again, an expanded map is immediately formed.

Tectal ablation ("compression"). If half of the tectum is ablated, the regenerated map is compressed into the remaining tectal space (Figure 1*F*). If "mismatched" halves of the retina and tectum are ablated, a topographic map still forms (Figure 1*G*).

Compound eye experiments. When a whole eye is created by fusing together two half-eye rudiments before connections are made, with the two halves being from opposite eyes but of the same type (i.e., nasal, ventral, or temporal), they each map across the whole tectum in the mirror image of each other (Figure 1*H*). When fragments smaller than half a retina are substituted early in development ("pie-slice" eyes), the retinal fragments map appropriately for their original position, although they can also show some degree of reprogramming.

Translocation. If two parts of the tectum are reciprocally translocated, regenerating retinal axons innervate their normal piece of tectum, and also appropriately reverse their order if the tectal fragment is rotated (Figure 1*I*). However, in some cases a map can be formed that ignores the translocation; i.e., the fibers tend to align with fibers in the surrounding tectum, regardless of the orientation of the transplant (Figure 1*J*).

Branching. In frogs and fishes, retinal axons grow to their final termination zones directly. In chicks and rodents, however, retinal axons grow past their final termination zone initially, form axon collaterals along the whole axon shaft (but preferentially in their topographically correct region), and then select their specific topographic termination zone by stabilizing an axon collateral while the distal part of the axon is pruned back.

Direct Evidence for Molecular Gradients

A major breakthrough in the understanding of the molecular basis of retinotectal map formation came in the mid-1990s, with discoveries centering on the erythropoetin-producing hepatocellular (Eph) family of receptor tyrosine kinases and their associated ligands, the ephrins (reviewed in Flanagan and Vanderhaeghen, 1998, and O'Leary, Yates, and McLaughlin, 1999). The Eph/ephrins come in two families, A and B, with promiscuous binding within a family but little affinity between families. It now appears that the A family is important for mapping along the rostral-caudal axis of the tectum, while the B family may be important for mapping along the dorsal-ventral axis.

In chick retina (and on the axons of retinal ganglion cells), Eph A3 is expressed in an increasing nasal to temporal gradient, while Eph A4 and A5 are uniformly expressed (Figure 2). In chick tectum, levels of both ephrin-A2 and ephrin-A5 rise from rostral to caudal, with the latter being restricted to more caudal locations and rising more steeply. In mouse retina, Eph A4 and Eph A5 are expressed, with Eph A4 being expressed uniformly and Eph A5 expressed in an increasing nasal to temporal gradient. In mouse SC, levels of ephrin-A5 rise from rostral to caudal, while levels of ephrin-A2 drop off at both ends of the SC.

A GPI-linked molecule, possibly ephrin-A5, in rostral tectum can preferentially induce branch formation of temporal retinal axons in chicks, and ephrin-A5 has been shown to act as a promotor of axonal branching in the formation of layer-specific circuits in the cortex. Ephrin-A2 and ephrin-A5 are also expressed in the retina in an increasing temporal to nasal gradient, though the functional implications of this phenomenon are still unclear. Several lines of evidence suggest that these receptor-ligand interactions are *repulsive*.

Theoretical Models

The development of retinotectal maps has inspired a large number of theoretical models. Some models have attempted to closely match the large array of data specific to the system in particular species; others have postulated more abstract and generic mechanisms for topographic map formation that can be applied across many systems. This section reviews in historical order some of the models designed to account for the initial activity-independent

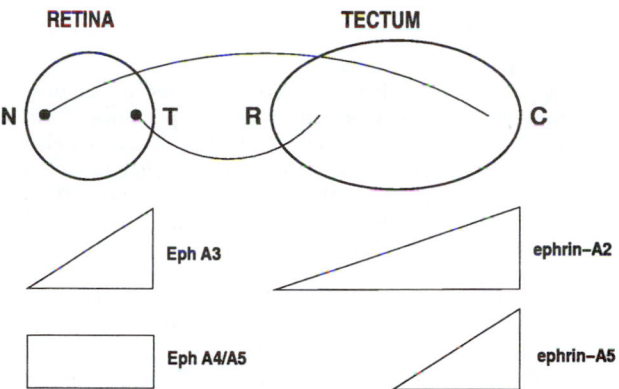

Figure 2. The normal retinotectal mapping and the distribution of Eph receptors and ephrin ligands in the chick. Note that the gradients run in opposite directions. Gradient shapes are not precisely linear. N, nasal; T, temporal; R, rostral; C, caudal.

stage of map formation and specific results, such as expansion, compression, translocation, and rotation of maps.

Prestige and Willshaw's Model

Prestige and Willshaw (1975) were the first to formalize notions of chemospecific matching suggested by Sperry's hypothesis. They distinguished between two forms of chemical matching, which they termed group I and group II (or type I and type II). In group I matching, each presynaptic cell *j* has an affinity for just a small neighborhood of postsynaptic cells, with peak affinity for the cell topographically matching to *j* in the postsynaptic sheet. Although such a rigid scheme can form a map under normal conditions, it cannot account for certain experimental data without invoking the unsatisfactory notion of respecification. In group II matching,

> *all* axons have maximum affinity for making and retaining contacts at one end of the postsynaptic sheet of cells, and progressively less for the cells at greater distances from that end. Similarly, all postsynaptic cells have maximum affinity for axons from one end of the postsynaptic set, and axons remote from this end have correspondingly less likelihood of retaining *any* contact. We may thus talk of *graded affinity* within both pre- and postsynaptic sets . . . (pp. 82–83).

Simulations showed that this mechanism is capable of forming an ordered map if competition is introduced, in the form of normalization. Prestige and Willshaw specified that each presynaptic cell could make only a fixed number of contacts N_{pre} among the postsynaptic cells, and similarly each postsynaptic cell could only support a fixed number of contacts N_{post} from presynaptic cells. This ensures an even spread of connections: without competition for postsynaptic sites, every presynaptic cell would connect only to the highest-affinity end of the postsynaptic set, while without competition for presynaptic sites, every postsynaptic cell would receive connections only from cells at the highest-affinity end of the presynaptic set. However, to explain compression and expansion of retinotectal maps, Prestige and Willshaw found that it was necessary to make the additional assumption ("regulation") that N_{pre} and N_{post} were also altered. For instance, if half the postsynaptic set is removed, then, unless N_{post} is increased, connections will only be made from the highest-affinity end of the presynaptic set.

The Arrow Model

In the "arrow" model of Hope, Hammond, and Gaze (1976), it is assumed that (1) retinal fibers that terminate next to each other in the tectum are able to compare their relative positions of origin, and (2) retinal fibers can identify both rostral-caudal and medial-lateral axes of the tectum (this could be implemented in terms of a polarity gradient of marker along each of these axes). The procedure is then basically the bubblesort algorithm, although a biological implementation for this is not described. Starting from initially random connections in which each retinal fiber contacts one tectal cell, two retinal fibers that terminate next to each other in the tectum are chosen at random. Their retinal positions are compared, and if they are appropriate, the sites of termination of the fibers are exchanged. This simple algorithm is capable of forming topographic maps under normal conditions, and also rotated maps when a piece of the tectal array is rotated. However, it fails to account for the translocated map experiments.

The Tea Trade Model

Willshaw and von der Malsburg (1979) proposed a model based on Sperry's idea that map formation is somehow dependent on induction of molecules from the retina into the tectum. The model is expressed in terms of molecular markers, but markers intrinsic only to the presynaptic sheet. There are no preexisting markers in the postsynaptic sheet: it is assumed that presynaptic markers are transported to the postsynaptic sheet via induction along retinal axons. Several markers exist in the presynaptic sheet, the sources of which are spaced out in the presynaptic sheet at fairly regular intervals. An analogy presented to explain the working of the model was the import of tea from plantations in India to British towns; hence the name "tea trade model."

Initially, markers diffuse in the presynaptic sheet until a stable distribution is set up. It is assumed that each presynaptic axon then induces the vector of markers existing at that point in the presynaptic sheet into the postsynaptic sheet, where the markers diffuse according to the same rule as in the presynaptic sheet. The rate of induction at each synapse is proportional to the strength of that synapse. Synaptic strengths are updated periodically according to the degree of similarity between the vector of markers each fiber carries and the vector of markers already existing at those points it contacts in the postsynaptic sheet. Synaptic updating occurs with a molecular analogue of Hebb's rule: the strength of connection between presynaptic cell i and postsynaptic cell j is increased in proportion to the similarity of their vectors of molecular markers. A slight overall bias in the connection strengths is specified initially in order to provide a global orientation for the map. Synaptic strengths are normalized by division so that each presynaptic cell can only support a certain total strength of connections. This ensures that every presynaptic axon makes contacts in the postsynaptic sheet. Willshaw and von der Malsburg (1979) showed that such a process reaches a stable state and can form appropriate maps under normal conditions, and also correctly predict the outcome of a range of results under abnormal conditions. In particular, some regeneration experiments can be accounted for under this scheme by assuming that when regeneration occurs, the postsynaptic sheet holds a "memory" of the previous pattern of innervation in terms of the previous stable distribution of markers. An algorithm similar to the tea trade model was analyzed mathematically for the one-dimensional case by Häussler and von der Malsburg (1983).

Gierer's Model

Gierer (1983) proposed a model based on the matching of preexisting gradients in retina and tectum as in the chemoaffinity hypothesis. He imagined that mapping is controlled by the concentration of an inhibitory substance $p(x, u)$, where x indicates tectal position and u indicates retinal position. p is produced by a reaction of the graded distribution of a retinal marker present on the tips of retinal axons with a graded distribution of a tectal marker. Axons then grow down the gradient of p to a minimum, stopping when $\partial p/\partial x = 0$.

For this to form a map, it is obviously required that the position of this minimum vary smoothly as a function of retinal origin u; in the simplest case when $x = u$. There is an infinite number of combinations of gradient shapes and reaction rules that accomplish this; Gierer specifically considered exponential gradients. He also suggested a possible mechanism for gradient change in response to surgical manipulations such as retinal or tectal ablation. Reminiscent of the tea trade model, the idea is that

> retinal fibre terminals induce, in the tectum, a slow increase in source (e.g. an enzyme) producing an additional contribution to p, and that the rate of increase is proportional to the local density of retinal fibre terminals. If the sources thus produced persist on the tectum while fibre terminals continuously move to respecified positions of minimal p, this process will eventually smooth out differences in the density of fibre terminals, giving rise to compression or expansion in the dimensions of ablation (p. 84).

The specific trajectories that axons might take to their targets under such a gradient matching scheme were also simulated.

Honda (1998) presented a simpler model in which axons grow to the tectal position where the retinal receptor concentration $R[u]$ times the tectal ligand concentration $L[x]$ equals a constant S, or $R[u]L[x] = S$, where S is the same for all axons. A brief analytical investigation of this type of model can be found in Goodhill and Richards (1999).

Fraser's Model

In a more abstract vein, Fraser (e.g., Fraser and Perkel, 1990) introduced the notion that the state of the system could be described by an "adhesive free energy" G, which depends on how successfully a number of constraints are satisfied. In his model the form of the final mapping is found from minimizing G by simulated annealing. The constraints employed (in order of decreasing weighting in G) are (1) a position-independent adhesion between retinal and tectal cells, (2) a general competition among retinal axons for tectal space, (3) a tendency for neighboring axon terminations in the tectum to stabilize if those axons come from neighboring positions in the retina, (4) a dorsoventral gradient of adhesive specificity in retina and tectum, and (5) an anteroposterior gradient in retina and tectum. Although this model accounts (at least qualitatively) for a large proportion of the experimental literature, a developmental mechanism that could perform such a minimization was not provided.

Cowan's Model

Whitelaw and Cowan (1981) attempted to integrate both marker- and activity-based mechanisms in map formation by combining a gradient of adhesive specificity with activity-dependent synaptic updating. Changes in synaptic strengths are multiplied by the degree of "adhesion" between the corresponding pre- and postsynaptic cells, and both pre- and postsynaptic normalization are employed. The model predicts a range of the experimental literature (including expansion and compression, mismatch, rotation, and compound eye experiments), and also draws attention to experimental evidence contradictory to the induction hypothesis of the tea trade model. More recent additions to this model, for instance a tendency for fibers to stick to their retinal neighbors, have increased the range of data it can account for (see, e.g., Weber et al., 1997).

Discussion

Consideration of the wide variety of data described in the preceding sections—Eph/ephrin gradients, disturbances of normal development and regeneration, and branching—suggests two major limitations of previous models. First, few of them take into account recent discoveries regarding molecular gradients and their role in retinotectal mapping. Second, most of the previous models take synaptic strengths as their primary variable between arrays of retinal and tectal locations. They generally assume each retinal location is initially connected to all tectal locations, or at least to a topographically specific subset. Synaptic strengths are then updated according to rules that depend in various ways on correlated activity, competition for tectal space, molecular gradients, and fiber-fiber interactions. However, these last three effects enter only as terms modulating the development of synaptic strengths. With rare exceptions, actual movement or branching of axons to find their correct targets is not considered. The key experimental results that future computational models of retinotectal map formation should attempt to account for, besides normal map development, include the results of single and multiple knockout experiments of the relevant Eph receptors and ephrin ligands, results of experiments in which Eph/ephrins are misexpressed in retina or tectum, the correct guidance of retinal axons that enter the tectum by ectopic routes, and the results of retinal and tectal ablation and transplantation experiments.

Road Maps: Neural Plasticity; Vision
Related Reading: Axonal Path Finding; Collicular Visuomotor Transformations for Gaze Control; Ocular Dominance and Orientation Columns; Pattern Formation, Neural

References

Flanagan, J. G., and Vanderhaeghen, P., 1998, The ephrins and Eph receptors in neural development, *Annu. Rev. Neurosci.,* 21:309–345. ◆
Fraser, S. E., and Perkel, D. H., 1990, Competitive and positional cues in the patterning of nerve connections, *J. Neurobiol.,* 21:51–72.
Gierer, A., 1983, Model for the retinotectal projection, *Proc. Roy. Soc. Lond. B,* 218:71–93.
Goodhill, G. J., and Richards, L. J., 1999, Retinotectal maps: Molecules, models, and misplaced data, *Trends Neurosci.,* 22:529–534. ◆
Häussler, A. F., and von der Malsburg, C., 1983, Development of retinotopic projections: An analytical treatment, *J. Theor. Neurobiol.,* 2:47–73.
Holt, C. E., and Harris, W. A., 1993, Position, guidance, and mapping in the developing visual system, *J. Neurobiol.,* 24:1400–1422. ◆
Honda, H., 1998, Topographic mapping in the retinotectal projection by means of complementary ligand and receptor gradients: A computer simulation study, *J. Theoret. Biol.,* 192:235–246.
Hope, R. A., Hammond, B. J., and Gaze, R. M., 1976, The arrow model: Retinotectal specificity and map formation in the goldfish visual system, *Proc. R. Soc. Lond. B,* 194:447–466.
O'Leary, D. D. M., Yates, P. A., and McLaughlin, T., 1999, Molecular development of sensory maps: Representing sights and smells in the brain cell, *Cell,* 96:255–269.
Prestige, M. C., and Willshaw, D. J., 1975, On a role for competition in the formation of patterned neural connexions, *Proc. R. Soc. Lond. B,* 190:77–98.
Sperry, R. W., 1963, Chemoaffinity in the orderly growth of nerve fiber patterns and connections, *Proc. Natl. Acad. Sci. USA,* 50:703–710.
Udin, S. B., and Fawcett, J. W., 1988, Formation of topographic maps, *Annu. Rev. Neurosci.,* 11:289–327. ◆
Weber, C., Ritter, H., Cowan, J., and Obermayer, K., 1997, Development and regeneration of the retinotectal map in goldfish: A computational study, *Philos. Trans. R. Soc. Lond. B,* 352:1603–1623.
Whitelaw, V. A., and Cowan, J. D., 1981, Specificity and plasticity of retinotectal connections: A computational model, *J. Neurosci.,* 1:1369–1387.
Willshaw, D. J., and von der Malsburg, C., 1979, A marker induction mechanism for the establishment of ordered neural mappings: Its application to the retinotectal problem, *Philos. Trans. R. Soc. B,* 287:203–243.

Developmental Disorders

Annette Karmiloff-Smith and Michael S. C. Thomas

Introduction

Connectionist models have recently provided a concrete computational platform from which to explore how different initial constraints in the cognitive system can interact with an environment to generate the behaviors we find in normal development (Elman et al., 1996; Thomas and Karmiloff-Smith, 2002a). In this sense, networks embody several principles inherent to Piagetian theory, the major developmental theory of the twentieth century. By extension, these models provide the opportunity to explore how shifts in these initial constraints (or boundary conditions) can result in the emergence of the abnormal behaviors we find in atypical development. Although this field is very new, connectionist models have already been put forward to explain disordered language development in Specific Language Impairment (Hoeffner and McClelland, 1993), Williams syndrome (Thomas and Karmiloff-Smith, 2002b), and developmental dyslexia (Seidenberg and colleagues; see, e.g., Harm and Seidenberg, 1999) and to explain unusual characteristics of perceptual discrimination in autism (Gustafsson, 1997; Cohen, 1998). In this article, we examine the types of initial computational constraints that connectionist modelers typ-ically build in to their models and how variations in these constraints have been proposed as possible accounts of the causes of particular developmental disorders. In particular, we examine the claim that these constraints are candidates for what will constitute innate knowledge. First, however, we need to consider a current debate concerning whether developmental disorders are a useful tool to explore the (possibly innate) structure of the normal cognitive system. We will find that connectionist approaches are much more consistent with one side of this debate than the other.

Developmental Disorders and Modularity

Cognitive neuropsychology assumes that the adult cognitive system has a modular structure, whereby the system can be decomposed into specialized functional components (although whether these components correspond to localized areas of the brain or can be captured by brain-imaging techniques remains an open question). In addition, cognitive neuropsychology assumes that that selective behavioral deficits in adults with brain damage can reveal this modular structure. Developmental disorders can also produce apparently specific deficits in the end state of development. For example, Williams syndrome (WS), a developmental disorder caused by a microdeletion of contiguous genes on one of the alleles of chromosome 7, is characterized by a behavioral profile of relative proficiency in language, face processing, and theory-of-mind (attributing mental states to others) but severe deficits in other skills such as visuospatial processing, number, and problem solving (Karmiloff-Smith, 1998). In hydrocephalus with associated myelomeningocele (a protrusion of the membranes of the brain or spinal cord through a defect in the skull or spinal column), language can be the only area of proficiency. Individuals suffering from Specific Language Impairment (SLI) show the opposite pattern, often apparently performing within the normal range in all domains except language. In autism, even individuals with normal IQs are selectively impaired in tasks that require judging another's mental states (Baron-Cohen, Tager-Flusberg, and Cohen, 1993).

Evidence in many of these disorders of specific high-level deficits at the end of development has encouraged some researchers to view developmental disorders as offering the same theoretical insights into the static structure of the cognitive system that cases of adult brain damage provide. Where such disorders are of a genetic origin, selective developmental deficits are interpreted as revealing innate underpinnings for such structure. For example, Baron-Cohen et al. (1993) have argued that in individuals with autism, an apparent deficit in reasoning about mental states can be explained by the impairment of an innate, dedicated module for such reasoning (the theory-of-mind module). Van der Lely (1997) maintains that selective behavioral deficits in the language performance of children with grammatical SLI can be explained by damage to an underlying, innate module representing syntactic (rule-based) information. Clahsen and Almazan (1998) have proposed that a behavioral deficit in WS language supports the view that while their syntactic skills are "intact," individuals have a deficit to a specific aspect of their (modular) language knowledge: that of accessing information about words that are exceptions to syntactic rules.

However, there are a number of problems with the adult brain damage approach to developmental disorders (Karmiloff-Smith, 1998; Thomas and Karmiloff-Smith, in press). These boil down to the suspicion that such an approach massively underestimates the complexity of the path from gene to behavior. The prevalence of many-to-many, very indirect mappings in the relationship of genes to cognition undermines the claim that direct specific mappings will exist between particular genes and individual high-level cognitive abilities. To the extent that genes are involved in the causal chain of several cognitive domains, it will be less likely that they code anything specific to a single domain. Indeed, direct mappings are unlikely, given that spatial distributions of gene expression in the brain are rarely narrowly confined to subsequent areas of functional specialization in the adult brain and therefore seem unable to code directly for domain-specific developmental outcomes. Even if they could, the idea that behavioral deficits that are identified in the end state of a developmental disorder could reflect the impairment of a single functional module is predicated on the dubious assumption that the rest of the cognitive system could nevertheless develop normally. For this to be true requires either that functional modules develop independently of overall brain growth or that the content of modules is fixed in advance (i.e., the content is innately specified). But neither of these assumptions is likely to be true. With regard to the first, Bishop (1997) has argued persuasively that interactivity rather than independence is the hallmark of early development. With regard to the second, it seems likely that modular structure in the cognitive system and in the brain is an outcome of development rather than a precursor to it and that the neonate brain does not support innate representations with specific content (Elman et al., 1996; Johnson, 1997). A growing number of studies show how both neural localization and neural specialization for

biologically important functions, such as species recognition (Johnson, 1997) and language (Neville, 1991), take place gradually across development.

An alternative to the use of the adult brain damage model is the neuroconstructivist approach (Elman et al., 1996; Karmiloff-Smith, 1998). This approach views developmental disorders in terms of different developmental trajectories, caused by initial differences at a neurocomputational level. Thus, there might be differences in the microcircuitry of the brain or the firing properties of neurons, as opposed to discrete lesions to particular large-scale brain structures or pathways. In this view, development is an interactive process in which the cognitive system self-organizes in response to interactions with a structured environment. Interestingly, this approach suggests that people with developmental disorders may exhibit strengths as well as weaknesses. This prediction is consistent with the superior face recognition skills found in WS and the superior perceptual discrimination abilities found in autism. Neuroconstructivism further suggests that equivalent behavior across normal and abnormal phenotypes may mask different underlying cognitive processes. The notion that an ability is "intact" or "spared" because there is no apparent deficit at the behavioral level employs terminology from the adult brain damage model that may be misleading. To take an example, people with Williams syndrome can display scores on some language and face-processing tasks that are in the normal range. Nevertheless, closer examination suggests that different *cognitive* processes underlie the equivalent *behavioral* scores (Karmiloff-Smith, 1998).

Initial Constraints in Connectionist Models

Current connectionist models of developmental disorders employ alterations to the initial model constraints that, after training, lead to an end state exhibiting behavioral deficits. Connection weights are usually randomized so that the normal network has no specific knowledge prior to training. Thus, it follows that the atypical network has no specific deficit in knowledge prior to training. The behavioral deficits that emerge when these atypical networks are trained are often quite different from the effects of damaging a normal network model after training has been completed. This holds even when the network manipulations are the same in each case (Thomas and Karmiloff-Smith, in press). Thus, current connectionist models are more consistent with the neuroconstructivist approach to developmental disorders than with the adult brain damage approach.

What, then, are the initial constraints that connectionist modelers build into their models of cognitive development? And how do changes to these constraints alter the trajectory of development? In fact, the constraints that connectionist models build in are quite strong ones, and this may come as a surprise to some readers. Connectionist models are often mischaracterized as being unitary, homogeneous, seamless, or undifferentiated domain-general learning devices, whereby the environment is all-powerful in shaping the behavior of the final system. In fact, current connectionist models have a great deal of pre-existing structure built into them prior to any exposure to their training environment. What is general about connectionism are the principles of computation (Seidenberg, 1993). When the general principles of computation are combined with the boundary conditions for a specific domain, the result is a domain-specific model. It is the generality of these principles that gives the connectionist approach its explanatory power. That is, connectionism seeks not just to formulate descriptive generalizations about empirical phenomena, but also to show how they derive from underlying and independently motivated principles (Seidenberg, 1993). However, connectionist models are just as reliant on the constraints of a given domain as they are on the computational principles. Without justified limitations in the design of network models, they become overpowerful data-fitting devices that can at best provide descriptively adequate accounts of cognitive abilities. In short, connectionist models of development do include initial structure but not initial representational content (Elman et al., 1996). The point is that in interacting with a training environment, networks create representational content and become increasingly structured. This additional structure reflects the nature of the training environment.

The structure or boundary conditions that these models build in prior to training typically involve the following:

1. *The initial state of the network, in terms of the number of units, layers, connections, and the pattern of connectivity, collectively known as the network architecture.* The architecture determines the computational power of the network and the type of computations to which the network will be suited. For example, recurrent networks are suited to processing sequential information, whereas associative networks are suited to pattern recognition. The a priori choice of the architecture will have a central role in determining the adequacy of the network in modeling a given domain of cognitive development. A reduction in the number of processing units, or the elimination of internal (hidden) processing units, will restrict the computational power of the network and, depending on the nature of the domain, cause some or all parts of the problem to be learned inadequately. Addition of layers of internal units beyond a single layer tends to delay learning, without a marked increase in effective computational power. Increase of hidden units within a single layer tends to improve performance on the training set but may impair generalization beyond the training set.

2. *The way a particular cognitive problem is presented to the network, in terms of the input and output representations.* For a given domain, the representations determine the nature of the computational problem that the network will face. When the network has to extract a function from the training set (such as a general rule or regularity), the representational scheme will be crucial in determining how transparent or opaque this function is to the network. For instance, if a network is given a training set in a form that masks the relevant similarity between those items in the problem domain that obey a rule, the network will have difficulty in extracting this regularity.

3. *The learning algorithm that the network will use to change its connection weights (and, potentially, its architecture).* Most networks are trained by changing weights to minimize some cost function, such as the difference between the actual output and a target output. The rate at which weights are changed can have an impact on the success of a network in learning a problem. In particular, in complex domains, if weights are changed too quickly, the network may commit too early to a partial solution to the problem and be resistant to change with subsequent training. The learning algorithm is key in determining the plasticity of the network to further learning. Some algorithms allow on-line changes to network architecture depending on how well the network is learning a problem. The way in which the network's computational power is altered on-line will again have a considerable influence on the success of the network in capturing a cognitive ability (see 1 above).

4. *The regime of training that the network will undergo.* After modelers determine the network and the learning rule, they then expose the network to a training set. Often, the network is exposed to the entire training corpus from the start of training. However, in some cases, the network might be trained on an initially limited training set, perhaps based on assumptions about the nature of a child's early learning environment. This initial restriction will affect later training. It may aid learning if the smaller set is representative of the larger set or if it allows the construction of internal representations that will be useful in learning the larger set. On the other hand, it may impair learning if the initial training set contains detail that is irrelevant to the full domain. Alterations in network parameters early in training may have the same effect as restricting the initial training set, as Elman's work on learning syntax with recurrent networks has demonstrated (Elman et al., 1996).

In the connectionist framework, these constraints represent some of the candidates for innateness (although, equally, in principle, any of the constraints could also be experience dependent). Alterations in one or more of these constraints may then lead to the emergence of disordered representations and impaired behavior in a model of atypical development.

We have noted that these models do not support innate representational content in that their weights are initially randomized. However, it is an open question as to whether initial computational constraints (along with sensory input determined by the individual's interaction with the environment) are sufficient to drive development. One possible addition is the postulation of innate attentional predispositions (Elman et al., 1996). In this theory, innate knowledge is built into the subcortical part of brain in the form of a low acuity predisposition to attend certain stimuli. This predisposition then ensures the representation of input that will subsequently drive learning in the more powerful cortical system. For example, such an innate predisposition in face recognition might encourage the newborn infant to attend preferentially to visual stimuli containing a single blob positioned centrally below two blobs (see Johnson, 1997). Innate predispositions provide another candidate factor that might be altered in the start state of the atypical system.

In general, current connectionist models of normal development do not restrict themselves to computational constraints and innate attentional predispositions in their start states, since these models incorporate high-level, domain-specific representations. These models must therefore be seen as a halfway house. In the future they need to be extended to show how their domain-specific representations emerge from some prior process operating over lower-level information (and with its own computational constraints).

We now turn to consider recent examples of connectionist models of developmental disorders.

Recent Models

Autism

Autism is a developmental disorder characterized primarily by a central triad of deficits in social interaction, communication, and imagination but also by a range of secondary deficits. These include a restricted repertoire of interests, an obsessive desire for sameness, excellent rote memory, improved perceptual discrimination, and an impaired ability to form abstractions or generalize knowledge to new situations. Evidence from neuropathological investigations of the brains of affected individuals is suggestive of abnormal wiring patterns in various brain regions, perhaps caused by deficits in neuronal migration during fetal development, curtailment of normal neuronal growth, and/or aberrant development. Cohen (1998) has argued that these structural deficits are consistent with too few neurons in some brain areas, such as the cerebellum, and too many neurons in other areas, such as the amygdala and hippocampus. Cohen has proposed that simple connectionist models trained on categorization tasks can link such differences in neurocomputational constraints to some of the secondary deficits found in autism. In some cases, children with autism have trouble acquiring simple discriminations and attend to a restricted range of stimuli, while in others, children with autism have good discrimination and indeed very good memory but seem to rely on representing too many unique details of stimuli. Cohen showed that simple backpropagation networks with too few hidden units showed a failure to learn classifications tasks, while those with a surfeit of hidden units showed very fast learning, but subsequently generalization became poor, and the network increasingly responded according to particular details of the training set.

In a related proposal, Gustafsson (1997) speculated that the combination of a failure to generalize and heightened perceptual discrimination might be traced to the atypical development of cortical feature maps. In particular, he suggested that higher-than-normal levels of within-layer inhibition in the initial cortical sheet would lead to overly fine-tuned perceptual features, permitting good discrimination but preventing good generalization.

Although Gustafsson did not support this idea with implementations, related work by Oliver et al. (2000) offers an insight into how feature map formation can be developmentally disrupted by changes in the initial properties of a self-organizing connectionist network. Oliver et al. employed a neurobiologically constrained network in which a two-dimensional output layer received information from a single input retina. The network was shown a set of stimuli in the form of bars lying across the input retina. Oliver et al. showed that, using their initial parameter set, the output layer formed a topographic map of the possible inputs: Certain areas of the output layer specialized in responding to each input, and areas representing similar inputs were adjacent to each other in the output layer. Oliver et al. then re-ran the model, disrupting the network in different ways before exposing it to the training stimuli. They varied the threshold of the output units, disrupted the connectivity between the input and the output layers, disrupted the connectivity responsible for lateral inhibition in output layer, and changed the similarity of the input stimuli to each other. These manipulations demonstrated that tiny differences in the initial constraints under which the model developed could have a very significant impact on the outcome of development. The resulting topographic map suffered a range of disruptions, including output units failing to specialize at all or simply turning off, specialization emerging but not in organized areas, and organized areas emerging but without adjacent areas representing similar-looking bars.

Much work remains to be done to develop these proposals exploring the neurocomputational underpinnings of developmental disorders such as autism and, in particular, to relate disordered feature maps or hidden unit numbers to higher-level cognitive deficits such as those in social interaction, communication, and imagination that characterize autism. Nevertheless, such work importantly illustrates a new conception of such disorders in terms of development operating under atypical constraints, rather than in terms of deficits to high-level modules in a static model of the normal adult cognitive system.

Developmental Dyslexia

This disorder has been the focus of much connectionist research, given the success of models in capturing the normal processes of reading. A number of models by Seidenberg and colleagues have sought to change initial constraints in models of reading to simulate either surface dyslexia (in which the subject has difficulty reading words that are exceptions to normal rules of pronunciation), phonological dyslexia (in which the reading of novel words is impaired), or a combination of both. Typically, these models learn mappings between codes representing orthography, phonology, and semantics. Surface dyslexia has been simulated by employing "too few" hidden units in the model or by reducing the learning rate. Phonological dyslexia has been simulated by degrading the phonological representations in some way, for instance, in the type of coding scheme used. For example, Harm and Seidenberg (1999)

pretrained one part of their model to develop appropriate phonological representations prior to learning the reading task. When this "phonological" part of the model was impaired, either by reducing its initial computational power or by limiting the size of the connection weights it could develop, the result was a network exhibiting phonological dyslexia at the end of training on the reading task.

Specific Language Impairment

Hoeffner and McClelland (1993) sought to capture deficits found in the morphosyntax of subjects with SLI, specifically their difficulty in the learning of rule-based inflectional morphology in verbs. Hoeffner and McClelland employed an attractor network mapping between semantic codes and phonological codes. They simulated SLI by changing the initial phonological representations, in line with a hypothesis that SLI may be caused by early perceptual impairments. Specifically, they impaired the network's ability to represent word-final stops and fricatives (including /t/, /d/, and /s/). Although the model they used didn't show an ideal fit to the normal data when unimpaired, it nevertheless captured a number of the key deficits of SLI when trained with impaired representations, particularly a selective difficulty with the formation of regular (+ed) past tenses. In this case, the initial phonological deficit obscured precisely the information that the network required to be able to learn the relevant generalizations about regular past tense formation. However, it should be noted that the perceptual deficit account of SLI remains controversial, and this disorder may well turn out to be heterogeneous, with several different causes.

Williams Syndrome

Recent work in our laboratory has examined underlying deficits in the language of individuals with Williams syndrome (WS). Their language was initially thought to be "spared," but closer examination revealed a number of subtle deficits. It had been reported that individuals with WS show difficulties in forming the past tense of irregular verbs while showing good performance on the regular, rule-based past tense formations (Clahsen and Almazan, 1998). Our recent empirical work suggests that much of this apparently selective deficit is due to an overall delay in language development (young children also find irregular verbs difficult). However, individuals with WS do appear to show a deficit in generalizing knowledge of inflectional patterns to novel forms. These two patterns (selective difficulty with irregular inflections versus reduced levels of generalization) continue to be argued for in the literature on WS language.

Thomas and Karmiloff-Smith (2002b) set out to explore whether alterations to the initial computational constraints of a connectionist model of past tense development could account for either of these patterns of data. The past tense network mapped from verb stem to past tense form in the presence of lexical-semantic information. Various theoretical claims have been made that the WS language system develops under different constraints. These include the proposals that their phonological representations may be atypical and perhaps rely on sensitive auditory processing, that their lexical-semantic representations may show anomalous organization, or that lexical-semantic information about words may be poorly integrated with phonology. To explore the viability of these different accounts to explain the pattern of performance in the past tense task, Thomas and Karmiloff-Smith altered the initial constraints of the network model to implement each type of lower-level deficit.

The results revealed that reduced generalization was consistent with atypical phonological representations (specifically with reduced similarity and redundancy) or interference in integrating lexical-semantic and phonological knowledge. A range of computational constraints caused poorer acquisition of irregular verbs; these verbs are in the minority, and their acquisition can be disrupted under nonoptimal learning conditions. However, attenuated activation from lexical-semantics was able to selectively delay irregular acquisition, offering a link to one of the proposed deficits in WS. Finally, the model demonstrated for the first time precisely how different computational constraints interact in a system in the process of development: The atypical trajectory that is found in WS may arise from the combination of more than one altered constraint.

Further empirical work remains to be carried out to clarify which of the WS patterns is the correct one. However, this modeling work has determined which of the competing accounts are viable within an existing developmental framework and therefore provided a focus for future investigations. Once again, this contrasts with previous theoretical work that construed the WS language system in terms of selective deficits to a static model of the normal adult language system (e.g., Clahsen and Almazan, 1998).

Discussion

Developmental disorders can inform the study of normal development because they provide a broader view of the parameter space within which development takes place. The empiricist argues that the environment specifies a capacity so strongly that systems with a wide variety of initial structures must come to reflect it. The nativist argues that the environment specifies a capacity so poorly that the system must come equipped with pre-existing structure if it is to find the correct solution given the environmental input. The neuroconstructivist argues that the robustness of the cognitive system to changes in its initial setup (as long as we can come to understand precisely what these changes are) will tell us how evolution has placed its bets concerning the capacities that can be trusted to emerge through experience and the capacities that must be given a firmer guiding hand through development. Connectionist models provide a powerful tool with which to investigate the role of initial computational constraints in determining the trajectory of both typical and atypical development. For developmental disorders in which selective deficits in high-level behaviors are reported, the connectionist framework ensures that these deficits are properly seen in terms of the outcome of the developmental process itself.

Road Map: Psychology
Related Reading: Cognitive Development; Language Acquisition; Neurological and Psychiatric Disorders

References

Baron-Cohen, S., Tager-Flusberg, H., and Cohen, D. J., 1993, *Understanding Other Minds: Perspectives from Autism*, Oxford, Engl.: Oxford University Press.

Bishop, D. V. M., 1997, Cognitive neuropsychology and developmental disorders: Uncomfortable bedfellows, *Quarterly Journal of Experimental Psychology*, 50A:899–923.

Clahsen, H., and Almazan, M.,1998, Syntax and morphology in Williams syndrome, *Cognition*, 68:167–198.

Cohen, I. L., 1998, Neural network analysis of learning in autism, in *Neural Networks and Psychopathology* (D. Stein and J. Ludick, Eds.), Cambridge, Engl.: Cambridge University Press, pp. 274–315.

Elman, J. L., Bates, E. A., Johnson, M. H., Karmiloff-Smith, A., Parisi, D., and Plunkett, K., 1996, *Rethinking Innateness: A Connectionist Perspective on Development*, Cambridge, MA: MIT Press. ◆

Gustafsson, L., 1997, Inadequate cortical feature maps: A neural circuit theory of autism, *Biol. Psychiatry*, 42:1138–1147.

Harm, M., and Seidenberg, M. S., 1999, Phonology, reading acquisition, and dyslexia: Insights from connectionist models. *Psychol. Rev.*, 106:491–528.

Hoeffner, J. H., and McClelland, J. L., 1993, Can a perceptual processing deficit explain the impairment of inflectional morphology in developmental dysphasia? A computational investigation, in *Proceedings of the 25th Child Language Research Forum* (E. V. Clark, Ed.), Stanford University, CA: Center for the Study of Language and Information, pp. 38–49.

Johnson, M. H., 1997, *Developmental Cognitive Neuroscience*, Oxford, Engl.: Blackwell. ◆

Karmiloff-Smith, A., 1998, Development itself is the key to understanding developmental disorders, *Trends Cogn. Sci.*, 2:389–398. ◆

Neville, H. J., 1991, Neurobiology of cognitive and language processing: Effects of early experience, in *Brain Maturation and Cognitive Development: Comparative and Cross-Cultural Perspectives. Foundation of Human Behavior* (K. R. Gibson and A. C. Peterson, Eds.), New York: Aldine de Gruyter, pp. 355–380.

Oliver, A., Johnson, M. H., Karmiloff-Smith, A., and Pennington, B., 2000, Deviations in the emergence of representations: A neuroconstructivist framework for analysing developmental disorders, *Dev. Sci.*, 3:1–23.

Seidenberg, M., 1993, Connectionist models and cognitive theory, *Psychol. Sci.*, 4:228–235.

Thomas, M. S. C., and Karmiloff-Smith, A., 2002a, Modeling typical and atypical cognitive development, in *Handbook of Childhood Development* (U. Goswami, Ed.), Oxford, Engl.: Blackwell, pp. 575–599. ◆

Thomas, M. S. C., and Karmiloff-Smith, A., 2002b, Modeling language acquisition in atypical phenotypes. Manuscript submitted for publication.

Thomas, M. S. C., and Karmiloff-Smith, A., in press, Are developmental disorders like cases of adult brain damage? Implications from connectionist modelling. *Behav. Brain Sci.*

Van der Lely, H. K. J., 1997, Language and cognitive development in a grammatical SLI boy: Modularity and innateness, *J. Neurolinguistics*, 10:75–107.

Diffusion Models of Neuron Activity

Luigi M. Ricciardi and Petr Lánský

Introduction

We offer a survey of one-dimensional stochastic diffusion models for the membrane depolarization of a single neuron, with emphasis on the related first-passage-time (FPT) problems, namely, on the determination of the neuronal output. In complex deterministic neuronal models, such as the Hodgkin-Huxley or the Fitzhugh-Nagumo models, the generation of action potentials is automatically included, being itself an essential component of the equations defining and characterizing these models. By contrast, for simple models (usually stochastic, such as those reviewed here), a firing threshold has to be introduced; the generation times of the action potentials are then identified with the instants when the membrane depolarization, which is modeled on the analogy of a particle randomly diffusing in a liquid, equals the firing threshold. Although these times are unique for deterministic models, in the case of stochastic models, and apparently also for many types of real neurons, the time interval that elapses between an action potential and the next one is at least partly random. In the sequel, such a time interval will be viewed as a random variable. The properties of this random variable are mathematically investigated by studying the related FPT problem.

Hereafter, we shall make use of the formalism of stochastic differential equations (SDEs). These equations can be heuristically described as ordinary differential equations in which a rapidly and irregularly fluctuating term (usually involving white noise, in additive or mutiplicative forms) is also present; they are also referred to as to Langevin equations, after the renowned physicist Paul Langévin. To elucidate the nature and the assumptions underlying diffusion models, in a couple of paradigmatic instances we shall sketch how neuronal stochastic diffusion models can be constructed from first principles, that is, without resorting to SDEs. We shall thus indicate how the much-celebrated Wiener and Ornstein-Uhlenbeck (OU) neuronal models stem from simple Markov processes with discrete state spaces after a suitable limiting procedure.

The broad applicability and intuitive appeal of the OU model follow from the circumstance that, if formulated by means of an SDE, up to the stochastic term it coincides with the most common phenomenological deterministic neuronal model, the so-called "leaky integrate-and-fire model." Hence, the OU model represents a natural bridge between deterministic and stochastic modeling of neurons' activity. The success of the Wiener model, which is a special case of the OU model, is instead based on the fact that it is largely solvable in closed form. For this reason, it may serve as a prototype for possible comparisons.

Besides the OU and Wiener models, which are characterized by additive noise terms appearing in the corresponding SDEs, diffusion models with multiplicative noise will also be reviewed. Although neuronal models of the diffusion type are primarily used for the description of steady-state firing under a constant stimulation, some results that are obtained in the case of periodic stimulation will also be mentioned. Irrespective of the type of applied noise, the approach employed here is based on frequency coding presumption.

Stochastic diffusion models are not primarily aimed at direct comparisons with experimental data, being mathematical abstractions of less tractable but more realistic or transparent models. They mainly serve to study the properties of other models by mathematical methods and to produce qualitative predictions, as in the extensive investigations performed on the possibility of stochastic resonance in neurons and neuronal models. For this reason, direct analyses of experimental data by diffusion models are relatively rare. For some references on this matter, see Inoue, Sato, and Ricciardi (1995). More references and expanded commentary can be found in a recent review article (Lánský and Sato, 1999). Additional references and detailed treatment of some models are in Ricciardi (1977) and Tuckwell (1988). For a review on the FPT problem for diffusion processes, see Ricciardi and Sato (1989).

Diffusion Processes and Neuronal Modeling

From a biophysical point of view, neuronal models of single cells reflect the electrical properties of the membrane via electric circuit models that contain energy storage elements. Such circuit models can be described by means of differential equations for the membrane potential. A consistent body of data, recorded from a large variety of different neuronal structures and under different experimental conditions, suggests that the presence of stochastic variables should in general be included in the mathematical models of the neuron's input-output activity, even though the role and influence of these variables are expected to depend on the nature of the specific questions one wishes to answer. Hereafter, we assume that there is a random component, generally denoted as *noise*, embedded in the neuron's input. A second source of noise can be attrib-

uted to the neuron itself, where a random component is added to the incoming input signal. Taking this fact into account, the differential equation describing the neuronal membrane potential then includes a noisy term, and hence becomes itself an SDE whose solution can sometimes be approximated by a diffusion process. In other cases—for instance, when the neuron has very few synaptic inputs near the trigger zone—a Poisson-driven differential equation may be a biologically more appropriate model.

Here we shall assume that the membrane potential between two consecutive neuronal firings (spikes) is represented by a scalar diffusion process $X(t)$. Such a process can be described by the SDE

$$dX(t) = \mu[X(t), t]dt + \sigma[X(t), t]dW(t),$$
$$P\{X(t_0) = x_0\} = 1 \tag{1}$$

where μ and σ are real-valued functions of their arguments satisfying certain regularity conditions, and $W(t)$ is the standard Wiener process. (See Ricciardi, 1977, for an expository discussion of SDEs.) The Wiener process has historically been exploited as the first mathematical model of Brownian motion, namely, the highly irregular and ceaseless motion characterizing all particles immersed in a fluid, irrespective of their nature, that was discovered by Robert Brown as early as 1827. Only in the year 1905 was a mathematical explanation of this mysterious phenomenon provided by Albert Einstein. In the mid-1930s Einstein's theory was refined, completed, and made mathematically more rigorous and general by various physicists and mathematicians, including Norbert Wiener, after whom a fundamental stochastic diffusion process was named. In short, the foundations of a new branch of the theory of stochastic processes were laid, based on a formalism involving equations similar to those describing the time change of the temperature in each point of a metal rod initially heated at one point, or the change of density in each point of a liquid after dropping in it a specified amount of salt. Thus were the "diffusion equations" born.

A stochastic process $W(t)$ is said to be a Wiener process if

(a) $W(0) = 0$.

(b) $W(t)$ has stationary independent increments.

(c) For every $t > 0$, $W(t)$ is normally distributed.

(d) For all $t > 0$, $E[W(t)] = 0$.

These axioms imply $\text{Var}[W(t)] = a^2 t$, where a^2 is a positive parameter, usually representing an empirical characteristic of the process, to be determined by observations. In this paper, we refer to the so-called *standard Wiener process* for which $a = 1$. The reference level for $X(t)$ in Equation 1 is usually taken to be equal to the resting potential. The initial voltage—namely, the reset value instantly attained following a spike—is often assumed to be equal to the resting potential: $X(t_0) = x_0$, where $t_0 \in \mathbb{R}$ denotes the initial time after spike generation.

Because of the simplicity of Equation 1, the process of the action potential generation is not an inherent part of the model, as it is in more complex models, and so the existence of a firing threshold potential $S(t)$—customarily assumed to be a deterministic function of time such that $S(t_0) > x_0$—must be imposed here. The model neuron fires whenever such a threshold potential is reached; then $X(t)$ is instantly reset to its initial value x_0. This situation corresponds to an FPT problem for the associated diffusion process. The interspike intervals are identified with the FPT of $X(t)$ across $S(t)$, namely, with the random variable

$$T = \inf_{t \geq t_0} \{t : X(t) > S(t)\}, \quad X(t_0) = x_0 \tag{2}$$

The importance of interspike intervals is due to the generally accepted hypothesis that the information transferred within the nervous system is usually encoded by the timing of neuronal spikes.

In addition, the reciprocal relationship holding between the firing frequency and the interspike interval naturally leads to the problem of determining the probability density function (pdf) of T, namely, the function $g[S(t), t|x_0, t_0] = \partial_t P\{T \leq t\}$. Particularly when this density cannot be obtained analytically (which is practically the rule) or when it is too difficult to give sufficiently precise estimations of it, the analysis is focused on its statistical moments, and primarily on the mean $E(T)$ and variance $D^2(T)$. The coefficient of variation, $D(T)/E(T)$, is also used, as it is a measure of the relative spread of the distribution and of its deviation from exponentiality. The reciprocal relationship between the firing frequency, on the one hand, and the interspike interval on the other hand suggests plotting the inverse of the value of $E(T)$ versus the intensity of stimulation (reflected by μ) as a stochastic counterpart of the input-output frequency curve.

In the following, we shall restrict our considerations to constant thresholds, and hence we shall set throughout $S(t) = S$, with $S > x_0$. The more realistic models based on time-dependent thresholds, aimed to simulate various aspects of the time varying behavior of the neuron, are mainly used to mimic the relative refractory period, namely, the time change of sensitivity of the neuron to incoming stimuli after a spike has been released. Hence, time-dependent thresholds should be characterized by a very large initial value (possibly infinity), followed by a decay to the constant value S. A realistic example of such a threshold is provided by the function $S(t) = S + S_1 \exp(-t/\gamma)$, where S_1 denotes a very large positive constant and $\gamma > 0$ determines how fast the asymptotic value S is approached.

An alternative description of the process $X(t)$ is obtained via the so-called *diffusion equations approach*. First, one defines the transition pdf of $X(t)$ conditional on $X(t_0) = x_0$:

$$f(x, t|x_0, t_0) = \frac{\partial}{\partial x} P\{X(t) \leq x|X(t_0) = x_0\} \quad (3)$$

It can then be seen that in most cases, f satisfies the Fokker-Planck (FP) equation

$$\frac{\partial f}{\partial t} = -\frac{\partial}{\partial x}[A_1(x, t)f] + \frac{1}{2}\frac{\partial^2}{\partial x^2}[A_2(x, t)f] \quad (4)$$

with initial condition $\lim_{t \downarrow t_0} f(x, t|x_0, t_0) = \delta(x - x_0)$, and the Kolmogorov (K) equation

$$\frac{\partial f}{\partial t_0} + A_1(x_0, t_0)\frac{\partial f}{\partial x_0} + \frac{1}{2}A_2(x_0, t_0)\frac{\partial^2 f}{\partial x_0^2} = 0 \quad (5)$$

with initial condition $\lim_{t_0 \uparrow t} f(x, t|x_0, t_0) = \delta(x_0 - x)$, where δ denotes the Dirac delta function. Here the coefficients $A_1(x, t)$ and $A_2(x, t)$ are the *infinitesimal moments*, or the *drift*, and *infinitesimal variance*, defined as

$$A_i(x, t) := \lim_{\Delta t \downarrow 0} \frac{1}{\Delta t} E\{[X(t + \Delta t) - X(t)]^i|X(t) = x\}$$

$$= \lim_{\Delta t \downarrow 0} \frac{1}{\Delta t}\int (y - x)^i f(y, t + \Delta t|x, t)dy \quad (6)$$

$$(i = 1, 2)$$

It is essential to mention that the quantities $A_1(x, t)$ and $A_2(x, t)$ are related in the following way (Ricciardi, 1977) to the functions μ and σ considered in Equation 1:

$$A_1(x, t) = \mu(x, t) \quad (7)$$

$$A_2(x, t) = \sigma^2(x, t) \quad (8)$$

Equations 1, 4, and 5 characterize the class of diffusion processes. While the description by Equation 1 is more intuitive and suitable for computer simulations, Equations 4 and 5 are suitable

for analytical and numerical treatments of the model. The parameter $A_1(x, t)$ (Equation 7) reflects the strength of the signal impinging on the neuron, while the parameter $A_2(x, t)$ (Equation 8) characterizes the level of noise associated with the signal. If we are interested in modeling the *spontaneous* or *resting* activity of a neuron or its *steady-state* response to a constant stimulus—which is usually required before attempting to model the neuron's response to time-varying stimuli—independence of time can be assumed in Equations 7 and 8. Then, the neuronal output modeld by FPT is a renewal process (intervals between firings are independent and identically distributed random variables), so that without any loss of generality, we can set $t_0 = 0$.

Neuronal Models with Additive Noise

Wiener Process

The year 1964 marks the beginning of the history of neuronal models based on diffusion processes. Indeed, in a much-celebrated article, Gerstein and Mandelbrot (1964) postulated that for a number of experimentally monitored neurons subject to spontaneous activity, the firing pdf could be modeled by the FPT pdf of a Wiener process. Actually, these authors were able to show that, by suitably choosing the parameters of the model, the experimentally recorded interspike interval histograms of many units could be fitted to an excellent degree of approximation by means of the FPT pdf of a diffusion process, characterized by the constant infinitesimal moments

$$A_1(x) = \mu, \quad \mu \in \mathbb{R} \quad (9)$$

$$A_2(x) = \sigma^2, \quad \sigma \in \mathbb{R}^+ \quad (10)$$

As is well known, in this case the transition pdf (Equation 3) is normal, with mean $\mu t + x_0$ and variance $\sigma^2 t$. By means of the methods outlined, for instance, in Ricciardi (1977), one can prove that the FPT pdf of such a process is given by

$$g(S, t|x_0) = \frac{S - x_0}{\sigma\sqrt{2\pi t^3}} \exp\left[-\frac{(S - x_0 - \mu t)^2}{2\sigma^2 t}\right] \quad x_0 < S \quad (11)$$

which in statistical literature is known as the Inverse Gaussian distribution. For $\mu \geq 0$, neuronal firing is a sure event, since the function in Equation 11 is normalized to unity. If one takes $\mu < 0$, the above FPT pdf can be interpreted as the firing pdf conditional on the event "firing occurs." The case $\mu = 0$ is also of interest, since Equation 11 expresses a so-called "stable law." This case provides an interpretation of numerous experimental results indicating that the shapes of histograms are sometimes preserved when the adjacent interspike intervals are summed. Making use of Equation 11, the moments of the density $g(S, t|x_0)$, i.e., the moments of the interspike intervals (that exist for all $\mu > 0$), can be calculated (Ricciardi et al., 1999).

To provide an interpretation of the model based on assumptions formulated in Equations 9 and 10, let us imagine that the neuron's membrane potential undergoes a simple random walk under the effect of excitatory and inhibitory synaptic actions. For simplicity, let us assume that the neuronal dynamics develops on a discrete time scale $0, \tau, 2\tau, \ldots$, with $\tau > 0$ as an arbitrary time unit. Passing to the limit as $\tau \to 0$, it can be shown (Ricciardi, 1977) that the random walk can be made to converge to the diffusion process having drift μ and infinitesimal variance σ^2, in other words, to a Wiener process. This procedure provides the simplest example in which the Wiener model for neuronal activity can be constructed.

The assumptions underlying this model are undoubtedly oversimplified, as some well-known electrophysiological properties of neuronal membrane are not taken into account. Therefore, the Wiener process should be viewed as a statistical descriptor of data rather than as a biologically sound model. However, it must be stressed that the fittings of some experimental data by the FPT pdf (Equation 11) is truly remarkable (see Gerstein and Mandelbrot, 1964).

We should finally point out that if a time-varying threshold is introduced to account for relative refractoriness—which is mainly relevant in high firing rate conditions—the determination of the firing pdf for the Wiener neuronal model cannot be generally accomplished analytically. Hence, ad hoc numerical methods had to be devised.

Ornstein-Uhlenbeck Process

Despite the excellent fitting of some data, the neuronal model based on the Wiener process has been the object of various criticisms, chiefly because it does not include the well-known spontaneous decay of the membrane depolarization. A diffusion model that includes this specific feature is the Ornstein-Uhlenbeck (OU) neuronal model. This is defined as the diffusion process characterized by the following drift

$$A_1(x) = -\frac{x}{\vartheta} + \mu \qquad (12)$$

and by the constant infinitesimal variance given in Equation 10. The new parameter $\vartheta > 0$ in Equation 12 reflects the required decay (the membrane time constant). This model is referred to as the "leaky integrator stochastic neuronal model." Comparing Equations 12 and 9, we see that now the drift is state dependent. However, in the limit as $\vartheta \to \infty$, the moments of Equation 12 are identical to those in Equation 9, meaning that the OU model yields the Wiener (or perfect integrator) model in the limit of an infinitely large time constant. Recalling Equations 1, 7, and 8, we can interpret the OU model as generated by the following SDE:

$$dX(t) = \left[-\frac{X(t)}{\vartheta} + \mu\right]dt + \sigma dW(t), \quad P\{X(t_0) = x_0\} = 1 \qquad (13)$$

where $W(t)$ is the standard Wiener process.

Equation 13 can be taken as defining the OU model. However, such a model can also be obtained from first principles by using the formalism of diffusion equations. To this end, let us initially assume that the neuron is subject to a sequence of excitatory and inhibitory postsynaptic potentials of constant magnitudes $e > 0$ and $i < 0$ occurring in time in accordance with two independent Poisson processes of parameters α_e and α_i, respectively. The membrane potential is thus viewed as a stochastic process $X(t)$ in continuous time with a discrete space consisting of the lattice $x_0 + ki + he$ ($h, k = 0, \pm 1, \ldots$) with the points of discontinuity randomly occurring in time. Again, let x_0 ($x_0 < S$) denote the fixed initial depolarization at which the sample paths start at the fixed initial time $t_0 = 0$. The firing pdf is thus modeled as the pdf of the instants when the sample paths for the first time reach, or cross in the upward direction, the threshold S. In Ricciardi et al. (1999) it is shown that if the input rates are made larger and larger and the postsynaptic potentials are simultaneously made smaller and smaller (with a suitable constraint), the membrane potential "converges" to the diffusion process having infinitesimal moments given by Equations 10 and 12 with $\mu = 0$. The case $\mu \neq 0$ can be obtained by a slightly more complicated model in which multiple Poisson-distributed excitatory and inhibitory inputs impinge on the neuronal membrane. Equation 13, in turn, can be obtained by a limit procedure starting from the differential equation expressing the spontaneous exponential decay of the membrane depolarization after including in it excitatory and inhibitory Poisson-distributed independent input processes.

Solving either the FP equation (Equation 4) or the K equation (Equation 5) with parameters of Equations 10 and 12 under the

appropriate delta-initial conditions, and then setting $t_0 = 0$ (since the process is temporally homogeneous), one obtains (cf. Ricciardi and Sacerdote, 1979):

$$f(x, t|x_0) = [2\pi V(t)]^{-1/2} \exp\left\{-\frac{[x - M(t|x_0)]^2}{V(t)}\right\} \qquad (14)$$

Hence, at each time t the transition pdf (Equation 14) is normal with mean $M(t|x_0) = \mu\vartheta[1 - \exp(-t/\vartheta)] + x_0 \exp(-t/\vartheta)$ and variance $V(t) = \sigma^2\vartheta[1 - \exp(-2t/\vartheta)]/2$.

It must be pointed out that the OU model differs from the Wiener model in several respects. First, an equilibrium regime exists, since in the limit as $t \to \infty$, the pdf (Equation 14) becomes normal with mean $\mu\vartheta$ and variance $\sigma^2\vartheta/2$. Furthermore, attainment of the firing threshold is a sure event, irrespective of the value of μ. However, in contrast to the Wiener model, the FPT problem is in general very complicated, even in the case of constant thresholds.

Two distinct firing regimes can be established for the OU model. In the first one, the asymptotic mean depolarization $\lim_{t\to\infty} M(t|x_0) = \mu\vartheta$ is far above the firing threshold S, and the interspike intervals are relatively regular (deterministic firing). In the second one, it is $\mu\vartheta \ll S$, and firing is caused only by random fluctuations of the depolarization (stochastic or Poissonian firing). The term Poissonian firing is motivated by the circumstance that as the thresholds move farther and farther above the steady-state depolarization $\mu\vartheta$, the firing patterns achieve the characteristics of a Poisson point process.

Equally important to the construction of a model is its verification. Although the Wiener model has often been tested by with experimental data, only relatively recently has the OU model been systematically fitted to interspike histograms (Inoue et al., 1995), owing to the very complicated and cumbersome procedure required for estimating the parameters of the model from interspike intervals data. The available—and as yet unexploited—methods for estimating parameters are based on intracellular recording of the sample paths of $X(t)$ (Lánský, 1983).

The models encountered in the application of diffusion processes to theoretical neuroscience have been predominantly time homogeneous, as reflected in the fact that the functions μ and σ in Equation 1 do not depend on t. Recently, however, an interest in stochastic resonance (a cooperative effect that may arise out of the coupling between deterministic and random dynamics in a nonlinear system) has motivated studies on diffusion neuronal models with time-dependent parameters. As already mentioned, in the OU model two distinct regimes can be identified, deterministic and Poissonian firing. In the first regime, the signal (μ term) is large enough that firing events occur even in the absence of noise. The noise-activated regime corresponds to the situation in which the drift term alone is not sufficient to cause firings, which are instead induced by the noise. The methods of stochastic resonance extend this view mainly to subthreshold periodic signals. Two sources of periodicity can be expected in the signal: either an *endogenous periodicity* or a periodicity of input intensities, the *exogenous periodicity* (Lánský, 1997). Both these instances are included in the following model of the membrane depolarization:

$$dX(t) = \left[-\frac{X(t)}{\vartheta} + \mu + A\cos\omega t\right]dt + \sigma dW,$$
$$P\{X(t_i) = x_0\} = 1, t \geq t_i \qquad (15)$$

where the notation is the same as in Equation 13, $A > 0$ is a constant characterizing the amplitude of the input signal, t_i is the time of the last release of an action potential, and ω is the angular frequency of the driving force modulation ($2\pi/\omega$ is the modulation period). After each firing the membrane potential is instantly reset to its initial value x_0. For exogenous periodicity, the phase of the signal continues after a spike, while in the endogenous case it is always reset, which simplifies the calculations. In the case of endogenous periodicity, the intervals between firing form a renewal process, which quite naturally leads us to consider an FPT problem for the OU process (Equation 13) and a periodic boundary. It is intuitive that by a suitable transformation, an FPT problem for the process modeled by Equation 15 through a constant threshold S can be changed into an FPT problem for a time-independent OU model through a periodic boundary. For exogenous periodicity a different method has to be invoked. In both cases there exists an optimum level σ of noise for which the input frequency ω is best reflected in the output signal (Bulsara et al., 1996; Shimokawa, Pakdaman, and Sato, 1999; Plesser and Geisel, 2001).

It should not pass unnoticed that the deterministic versions of Equations 13 and 15, obtained in the limit $\sigma \to 0$, have long been known in the literature as the Lapicque model, or *leaky integrator* neuronal model (Tuckwell, 1988), presently revived within the context of artificial neural networks.

We conclude this section by pointing out that, especially for experimental purposes, it is sufficient to obtain information only on shape and location of the firing pdf, without finer details. This can be achieved via some of the moments of the firing time. The knowledge of the moments can also, at times, provide some extra valuable information. For example, after a systematic computations of mean and variance of the firing time and of the skewness (a measure of the deviation from symmetry of the firing pdf expressed as the ratio of the third-order central moment to the cube of the standard deviation), for a variety of thresholds and initial states a striking and unsuspected feature of the OU model has emerged: for boundaries of the order of a couple of units or more above the steady-state depolarization $\mu\vartheta$, the variance of the firing time equals the square of its mean value, to an excellent degree of approximation. Moreover, the skewness is equal to 2 to a very high precision. Finally, the goodness of these approximations increases with increasing values of the threshold. When all this information was put together, the conjecture emerged that the firing pdf is susceptible to an excellent exponential approximation for a wide range of thresholds. In addition, these "experimental observations" have led to quantitative results concerning the asymptotic exponential behavior of the FPT pdf not only for the OU process, but also for a wider class of diffusion processes, both for constant and for time-varying boundaries (see Ricciardi et al., 1999, and references therein).

As expected, the convergence to the exponential distribution for increasing thresholds is accompanied by a large increase in the mean firing time. This is in agreement with the finding that for some neurons, the histograms of the recorded interspike intervals are increasingly better fitted by exponential functions as the firing rates decrease.

Neuronal Models with Multiplicative Noise

In order to embody additional physiological features of real neurons, several alternative models have been proposed. It is well known (and as reflected in the Hodgkin-Huxley model), the change in membrane depolarization caused by a synaptic input depends on its current value. Basically, the depolarization of the membrane caused by an excitatory postsynaptic potential decreases linearly with decreasing distance of the membrane potential from the excitatory reversal potential, V_E. In the same manner, the hyperpolarization caused by an inhibitory postsynaptic potential is smaller if the membrane potential is closer to the inhibitory reversal potential, V_I. In this way the depolarization $X(t)$ is confined to the interval (V_I, V_E), whereas in the models presented in the preceeding section it was considered unrestricted. Inequalities $V_I < x_0 < S <$

V_E express obvious conditions relating reversal potentials, initial depolarization, and firing threshold. Although the only diffusion model of linear summation (with exponential decay) of the input signal is the OU process (Equation 13), there is a whole class of diffusion processes that are appropriate if reversal potentials are taken into account. In all these models the drift takes the form

$$A_1(x) = -\frac{x}{\vartheta} + \mu_1(V_E - x) + \mu_2(x - V_I) \qquad (16)$$

where the parameter $\vartheta > 0$ is the membrane time constant, as in Equation 12, and $\mu_1 > 0$, $\mu_2 < 0$ are new parameters reflecting excitation and inhibition, now separately specified, in contrast to the case of Equation 12. Although both moments given by Equations 12 and 16 are linear, the interpretations underlying the two drifts are significantly different. Indeed, in Equation 12 there is a constant "leakage term" ϑ^{-1}, while for the models with reversal potentials the leakage ($\vartheta^{-1} + \mu_1 - \mu_2$) is explicitly input dependent.

The diffusion models that take into account the existence of the reversal potentials always lead to a multiplicative noise effect. This is in agreement with the general notion that an additive noise is generated by events independent of the transmitted message, whereas the multiplicative noise arises inside the processing unit, viz., inside the system. Common forms of infinitesimal variance in models with reversal potentials are the following:

$$A_2(x) = \sigma^2(x - V_I) \qquad (17)$$

$$A_2(x) = \sigma^2(x - V_I)(V_E - x) \qquad (18)$$

$$A_2(x) = \sigma_1^2(x - V_E)^2 + \sigma_2^2(x - V_I)^2 \qquad (19)$$

The first one stresses the importance of the inhibitory reversal potential, which restricts the state space of $X(t)$ from below; the second and third form of the infinitesimal variance attribute equal relevance to both reversal potentials. The main difference between infinitesimal variances in Equations 17 and 18, on the one hand, and Equation 19 on the other lies in the fact that for model 19, the reversal potentials lose their natural role of boundaries of the depolarization (Hanson and Tuckwell, 1983). This fact strongly handicaps model 19. In models characterized by Equations 17 and 18, the behavior at the boundaries V_I and V_E is mathematically rather subtle.

Similarly to the OU model, the statistical moments of T can be calculated for the models defined by Equations 17 and 18. As for the OU process, here also the asymptotic exponentiality holds for low excitation levels. Thus, the only (though very substantial) effect stemming from the models we have considered with reversal potentials consists of the parameter interpretation. From the modeling point of view, the variety of forms identified for the infinitesimal variance and the linear form of the drift are not unexpected. Indeed, these models are meant to reflect, through an "equivalent" noisy ordinary differential equation, the properties, at a single location, of a spatially distributed neuron with noisy inputs, thus corresponding to a stochastic partial differential equation. The linear drift describes the passive electrical circuit properties of the membrane at the trigger zone and the mean effect of the noisy input. The infinitesimal variance, on the other hand, must take into account not only the diversity of spatial configurations for different neurons, but the location and type of synaptic input on that neuron as well. Hence, a variety of forms for this term in the diffusion equation are conceivably appropriate.

It must be emphasized that for neuronal diffusion models originating from SDEs that include either additive or multiplicative noise terms, the FPT problem is in general intractable with analytical tools. However, some efficient procedures have been devised to obtain accurate numerical evaluations of g for the general case of time-varying firing thresholds and for arbitrary diffusion models (not necessarily of the OU type). This is an important target, because to calculate the unknown FPT pdf, one would have to solve Equations 4 or 5 under the appropriate initial delta conditions, and usually, as well, in the presence of complicated boundary conditions when the resulting equations are singular—a very difficult task that rarely leads to analytical solutions. Efficient numerical algorithms are thus especially desirable if one has to deal with time-varying neuronal thresholds. The standard procedure is based on the remark that the FPT pdf $g[S(t), t|x_0, t_0]$ can be proved to be a solution of the following integral equation:

$$f[S(t), t|x_0, t_0] = \int_0^t f[S(t), t|S(\tau), \tau]g[S(\tau), \tau|x_0, t_0]d\tau \quad (20)$$

with $x_0 < S(t_0)$. This is a first-kind Volterra integral equation whose solution is made complicated by the circumstance that the kernel $f[S(t), t|S(\tau), \tau]$ exhibits a singularity of the type $1/\sqrt{t - \tau}$ as $\tau \uparrow t$. Hence, the problem of determining $g[S(t), t|x_0, t_0]$ from Equation 20 via numerical methods is by no means trivial. Furthermore, all classic available algorithms necessitate the use of large computation facilities and sophisticated library programs. As a consequence, they are expensive to run and not suitable for suggesting to the modeler in real time how to identify the various parameters to fit the recorded data.

An entirely different approach that is quite general, although specifically useful for handling neuronal firing problems, was therefore developed. The guiding idea is to prove that the singular Equation 20 can be replaced by a nonsingular second-kind Volterra integral equation for g that possesses an extra degree of freedom, which can be used to remove the singularity of the kernel or, in some instamces, to directly obtain a closed-form expression for $g[S(t), t|x_0, t_0]$. (See Ricciardi et al., 1999, and references therein for a description of the method and of related computational algorithms.)

Discussion

In this article we have outlined a few stochastic models for single neurons' activity based on the theory of diffusion processes. As we have sketched out, prediction of the firing pdf is a difficult problem whose solution can usually be approached only by numerical or simulation procedures. It must be stressed that the neuronal behavior described by diffusion models ultimately implies that for time-constant input, the neuron's output is a renewal process. However, one can conceive models aimed, for instance, at simulating the clustering effect in spike generation. Serial dependence among interspike intervals can be modeled in various ways, for instance by adjusting the reset value after each spike in the OU process. Another possibility consists of the inclusion of some kind of feedback in the model, usually the often experimentally observed *self-inhibition*. A further generalization is achieved by taking into account the spatial properties of a neuron. In the simplest way, this can be done by assuming that the model neuron consists of two compartments: (1) the dendritic compartment, described by a standard diffusion model, and (2) the trigger-zone compartment, including the spontaneous decay of depolarization and the firing mechanism (Lánský and Rodriguez, 1999).

To conclude this bird's-eye view of the topic, we would like to mention an alternative approach to the construction of diffusion models that are able to fit experimental data: reversing the problem. That is, instead of formulating a neuronal model $X(t)$ based on some reasonable assumptions, and then trying to compute the firing pdf as an FPT pdf through a preassigned threshold, one can proceed as follows. First, construct the histogram of the experimentally recorded spike train and try to fit it by a function $g(S, t|x_0)$, with S

and x_0 parameters to be determined by the standard methods. Once this task has been accomplished, ask the following questions: Can $g(S, t|x_0)$ be viewed as the FPT pdf, through the threshold S, of a diffusion process conditioned on $X(0) = x_0$? If the answer is yes, can such a process be uniquely determined? This is, so to speak, the inverse of the FPT problem. Quite surprisingly, a precise answer to this question can be provided, at least in principle (Capocelli and Ricciardi, 1972).

In summary, for modeling purposes we have essentially looked at a neuron as a black box, characterized by an input and an output, for which two distinct problems can be posed: (1) to determine the output for a given input, which has led us to an FPT problem, and (2) to guess the input by analyzing the output, which could be viewed as the *inverse* of an FPT problem. In both cases the class of input functions had to be specified beforehand in order to make these problems mathematically sound. The need for such a specification, in conjunction with a large body of well-known experimental data, has led us to assume that input stimulations and random components are such that the neuron's membrane potential is ultimately modeled by one-dimensional diffusion processes. A sketch of some of the ensuing diffusion models for neurons' activity, and their place in the biological literature, was the object of this article.

Road Map: Biological Neurons and Synapses
Background: Single-Cell Models
Related Reading: Rate Coding and Signal Processing

References

Bulsara, A. R., Elston, T. C., Doering, C. R., Lowen, S. B., and Lindberg, K., 1996, Cooperative behavior in periodically driven noisy integrate-and-fire models of neuronal dynamics, *Phys. Rev. E*, 53:3958–3969.
Capocelli, R. M., and Ricciardi, L. M., 1972, On the inverse of the first passage time probability problem, *J. Appl. Prob.*, 9:270–287.
Gerstein, G. L., and Mandelbrot, B., 1964, Random walk models for the spike activity of a single neuron, *Biophys. J.*, 4:41–68.
Hanson, F. B., and Tuckwell, H. C., 1983, Diffusion approximations for neuronal activity including synaptic reversal potentials, *J. Theor. Neurobiol.*, 2:127–153.
Inoue, J., Sato, S., and Ricciardi, L. M., 1995, On the parameter estimation for diffusion models of single neurons' activities, *Biol. Cybern.* 73:209–221.
Lánský, P., 1983, Inference for diffusion models of neuronal activity, *Math. Biosci.*, 67:247–260. ◆
Lánský, P., 1997, Sources of periodical force in noisy integrate-and-fire models of neuronal dynamics, *Phys. Rev. E*, 55:2040–2044.
Lánský, P., and Rodriguez, R., 1999, Two-compartment stochastic model of a neuron, *Physica D: Nonlinear Phenomena*, 132:267–286.
Lánský, P., and Sato, S., 1999, The stochastic diffusion models of nerve membrane depolarization and interspike interval generation, *J. Periph. Nerv. Syst.*, 4:27–42. ◆
Plesser, H. E., and Geisel, T., 2001, Stochastic resonance in neuron model: Endogenous stimulation revisited, *Phys. Rev. E*, 63:Article 031916 (6 pages).
Ricciardi, L. M., 1977, *Diffusion Processes and Related Topics in Biology, Lecture Notes in Biomathematics*, Berlin: Springer-Verlag. ◆
Ricciardi, L. M., Di Crescenzo, A., Giorno, V., and Nobile, A. G., 1999, Theoretical and algorithmic approaches to first passage time problems, *Math. Japonica*, 50:247–322. ◆
Ricciardi, L. M., and Sacerdote, L., 1979, The Ornstein-Uhlenbeck process as a model for neuronal activity, *Biol. Cybern.*, 35:1–9.
Ricciardi, L. M., and Sato, S., 1989, Diffusion processes and first-passage-time problems, in *Lectures in Applied Mathematics and Informatics* (L. M. Ricciardi, Ed.), Manchester, Engl.: Manchester University Press, pp. 206–285.
Shimokawa, T., Pakdaman, K., and Sato S., 1999, Time-scale matching in the response of a leaky integrate-and-fire neuron model to periodic stimulus with additive noise, *Phys. Rev. E*, 59:3427–3443.
Tuckwell, H. C., 1988, *Introduction to Theoretical Neurobiology*, Cambridge: Engl.: Cambridge University Press. ◆

Digital VLSI for Neural Networks

Dan Hammerstrom

Introduction

The computational overhead required to simulate artificial neural network (ANN) models, whether simplistic or realistically complex, is a key problem in the field because of the computational complexity of these models. Network simulations are required both for research and for commercial products. Most researchers currently perform these simulations on standard computer technology, such as high-end workstations or personal computers. However, as the field progresses, researchers are moving to larger and ever more complex models that challenge even the fastest computers.

A reasonably realistic neural model could approach one million neurons and tens of billions of connections, where a "connection" is a data transfer path between two neurons. In addition to size, the models themselves are becoming more complex as we move from simple inner products to spiking neurons with temporal time course that require a convolution to be performed at each synapse.

For these reasons, there has been much interest in developing custom hardware for ANNs. The inherent parallelism in ANN and connectionist models suggests an opportunity to speed up the simulations. Their simple, low-precision computations also suggest an opportunity to employ simpler and cheaper, low-precision digital hardware implemented by full-custom silicon or by field-programmable gate arrays (FGPAs).

This chapter discusses digital electronic implementations of ANNs. First, we look at the differences between digital and analog design techniques with a focus on performance/cost trade-offs. Second, we consider the use of traditional processors in parallel configurations for ANN emulation. Third, to convey a sense of some of the issues involved in designing digital structures for ANN emulation, a custom digital ANN processor is discussed: the Adaptive Solutions CNAPS. Although this chip is no longer produced, it is still being used. Its simple architecture makes it a good vehicle to understand the trade-offs inherent in emulating neural structures digitally. Fourth, we look briefly at FPGA technology as a promising alternative for digital implementation of ANNs.

Why Digital?

Performance/Cost

One commonly held belief in the ANN research community is that analog computation, in which signals are transmitted and manipulated as strengths, generally voltage or current, is inherently superior to digital computation, in which signals are transmitted and manipulated as serial or parallel streams of 1s and 0s. But in fact, both technologies have advantages and disadvantages. The best choice depends on a variety of factors.

Why is analog appealing? An important reason is that it provides 10–100 times greater computational density than digital computation. *Computational density*—the amount of computation per unit area of silicon—is important because the cost of a chip is generally proportional to its total area. In analog circuitry, complex, nonlinear operations such as multiply, divide, and hyperbolic tangent can be performed by a handful of transistors. Digital circuitry requires hundreds or even thousands of wires and transistors to perform the same operations. Analog computation also performs these operations using far less power per computation than digital computation.

If analog is so good, why are people still building digital chips, and why are most commercial products digital? One important reason is familiarity. People know how to build digital circuits, and

they can do it reliably, no matter the size and complexity of the system. This is partly the legacy of having thousands of digital designers all over the world constantly tweaking and improving design techniques and software. It is also easier to create a digital version of a computation, in which a computer program represents the algorithm, than an analog version, in which the circuit itself represents the algorithm. This is particularly true if you are trying to build a system that is robust and reliable over the wide temperature and voltage ranges needed in commercial products. Analog design is an uncommon capability, and it is becoming less common as people find that they can do more with digital circuitry. For example, digital signal processors now perform most of what was once the domain of analog circuitry. Another advantage of the digital emulation of neural networks is that it significantly eases the integration of the neural network portion of the design with the larger digital system to which it connects.

Flexibility

Another factor working in favor of digital is that analog designs are generally algorithms wired into silicon. Such designs are inflexible. Though there is an interesting class of designs that are programmable analog. Perhaps the most powerful and widely studied is the Cellular Neural Network (Chua and Roska, 2001).

Digital designs can be either hardwired or programmable. Their flexibility is a major benefit, since it allows software control as well as an arbitrary level of precision (low to high and fixed or floating point). The price of this flexibility is reduced performance/cost, but the result is a chip that can solve a larger part of a problem. It also leads to a device that has broader applicability and can track incremental algorithm improvements by changing the software, not by redesigning the circuitry.

The role flexibility plays in system performance/cost can be understood more clearly by examining *Amdahl's law* (Hennessy and Patterson, 1991) that describes the execution time benefits of parallelizing a computation. Briefly, a computing task has portions or *subtasks* that often can be executed in parallel. Other, sequential tasks cannot begin until a previous task has been completed, which forces a sequential ordering of these tasks.

Amdahl's law states that no matter how many processors are available to execute subtasks, the speed of a particular task is roughly proportional to the subtasks that cannot be executed in parallel. In other words, sequential computation dominates as parallelism increases. Amdahl quantifies the relationship as follows:

$$S = 1/(op_s + (op_p/p))$$

where S is the total speed-up, op_s is the number of operations in the serial portion of the computation, op_p is the number of operations in the parallel portion, and p is the number of processors. As p gets large, S approaches $1/op_s$.

For example, suppose we have two chips to choose from. The first can perform 80% of the computation with a $20\times$ speed-up on that 80%. The second can perform only 20% of the computation but executes that 20% with a $1000\times$ total system speed-up. Plugging into the equation, the first chip gives us a total speed up of over $4\times$, while the second—and "faster"—chip has only a $1.25\times$ total system speed-up. A programmable device that accelerates several phases of an application generally offers a much larger benefit than a dedicated device.

Below we discuss FPGAs, which are flexible to the point of allowing the arbitrary configuration of physical digital circuitry.

They are a promising approach to efficiently implementing the inherent parallelism of neural-like structures.

Signal Intercommunication

One difference between silicon and biological networks is that for silicon, internode communication is relatively more expensive than for biological systems. Although several levels of wire interconnect (8–10 today) are available in most silicon processes, each level is restricted to two-dimensional interconnection because wires on the same level cannot pass over or touch one another.

Two-dimensional layout and large expensive wires require us to modify our biologically derived computational models to more closely match the strengths and weaknesses of the implementation technology. To show the need for such modifications, Bailey and Hammerstrom (1988) modeled a hypothetical neural circuit. This circuit, modest by biological standards, had one million "neurons" with one thousand inputs each, or one billion connections total.

The first calculation assumed a direct implementation—that is, one connection per wire. This billion-connection ANN required tens of square meters of silicon for dedicated communication pathways. Since silicon averages tens of dollars per square centimeter, such a system is too costly to be practical. These costs result from a theorem showing that the metal area required by direct communication is proportional to the *cube* of the fan-in or "convergence" at each node.

Their second calculation assumed a multiplexed interconnect structure, one in which several connections shared a metal wire. Wire multiplexing adds complexity at each end. Likewise, an address must be sent with each data packet to identify the sender, and some decoding must be performed on that address. Bailey and Hammerstrom (1988) showed that with the proper communication architecture, a $100\times$ reduction in silicon area over the direct approach was possible with little impact on performance. Since only a few nodes will be active in any given time interval for these large networks, multiplexing interconnect makes even more sense.

Even analog designers of neuromorphic circuitry have recognized the need for multiplexed interconnect. However, analog voltages and currents are difficult to multiplex. One alternative is to represent analog values by using pulses. There are several ways in which pulses can be used to represent information, including pulse rate, phase, and interpulse interval. It is possible for different pulse streams to share a single wire by sending, at the time the pulse occurs, the address of the pulse stream. This approach is called address event representation, or AER (Boahen, 2000). Pulse or "spike" signal representation is also much more neurobiologically plausible.

Digital Neural Networks: Off-the-Shelf Processors

One successful approach to high-speed ANN simulation has been to use arrays of commercial microprocessors. This approach works because desktop machines, thanks to Moore's law, have achieved a tremendous level of performance/cost. Moore's law states that the number of transistors that can be manufactured economically on a single silicon die doubles every 24 months. Moore's law has held constant for roughly 32 doublings, which is truly impressive. There are not many industries that can claim exponential growth over such a long period.

In addition to raw clock speed, another effect of Moore's law is that more transistors are available to dedicate to specialized functionality. Today, the latest microprocessors offer on-board single instruction multiple data (SIMD) parallel coprocessors. For Intel, these coprocessors have evolved from MMx to SSE (Pentium III) and now to SSE2 (Pentium 4) (Intel, 2001). The Motorola/IBM PowerPC has the similar AltiVec system. Although these coprocessors have been designed primarily for basic image processing, video codecs, and graphics, they can also be used to emulate certain ANN models.

A problem these machines have, though, is limited memory bandwidth. Most applications have a fair amount of referencing locality, in which a collection of physically contiguous addresses are referenced multiple times. Reference locality allows the processor to use several layers of cache memory (the Pentium IV has three). However, neural network algorithms typically require that an entire network be accessed for each state update. Since this network can be very large, it generally does not fit in the caches. Consequently, there is a significant slowdown as the processor ends up waiting for data from memory.

Perhaps the best approach is to use a commercial multiprocessor computer that hides the memory bandwidth problems by providing large numbers of processors. For example, the NASA Ames Research Center has several large Silicon Graphics parallel machines (Shan et al., 2000). The largest currently has 1024-processors. These systems use very high-speed interconnects and are able to emulate large, complex neural network structures. Our research group at OGI has simulated simple association networks approaching one million nodes on this machine.

However, such computational power is typically not available to the average researcher. One popular alternative has been to build large computer clusters using relatively inexpensive PCs. Often known as Beowulf clusters (Reschke et al., 1996), these systems connect large numbers of simple processors and are typically built from off-the-shelf hardware (PCs and LAN switches). The software is usually free. Programming is done by using traditional languages and MPI (the message-passing interface) or PVM (parallel virtual machine). Unfortunately, the interprocessor communication tends to be fairly slow relative to the computation, which compromises the total speed-up to some degree. However, they can be fairly efficient if complex models of the neuron are used that require more computation than intercommunication.

As neural network models become larger and more complex, the model connectivity issues become a major factor in the speed of emulation regardless of the hardware platform. Real neural structures demonstrate *sparseness*, that is, a small subset of all possible connections are actually made, and *locality*, that is, there is a higher probability of connections to neurons that are physically near each other. However, ANN models have typically not exhibited significant sparseness or locality, which is another reason for researchers to study more biologically plausible systems so that we can create structures that are computationally robust and have sparse, localized connections.

Digital Neural Networks: Full Custom Processors: CNAPS

Designing specialized architectures that are customized for ANN simulation permits significant improvements in performance/cost, since the processors and their interconnection architecture are optimized for the computations they perform. This section discusses the Adaptive Solutions CNAPS architecture, which was, for a time, a successful commercial product but is no longer produced. It represents the specialized functionality end of the design spectrum of digital chips.

The CNAPS architecture (Hammerstrom, 1995) had multiple processor nodes (PNs) connected in a one-dimensional structure, forming a SIMD array (Figure 1). SIMD architectures have one instruction storage and decode unit and many execution units, simplifying system design and reducing costs. Unlike a PC cluster, each CNAPS PN did not have program storage and sequencing hardware, and each executed the same instruction each clock. Node

Figure 1. CNAPS architecture. This is a single instruction multiple data (SIMD) architecture, in which all processor nodes (PNs) execute the same instruction during each clock. There is a single broadcast data bus that allows efficient one-to-many and many-to-many communication.

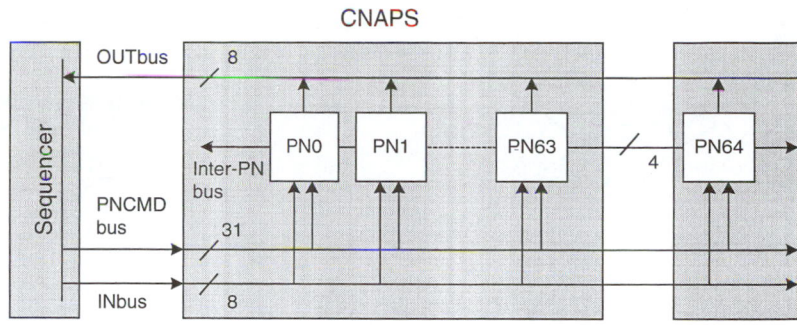

outputs were broadcast from each PN to all the others over a single broadcast bus.

Another major simplification of the CNAPS architecture, which is found in other digital ANN chips, was the use of limited-precision, fixed-point arithmetic. Many researchers have shown that floating point and high precision are unnecessary in ANN simulation (Fahlman and Hoehfeld, 1992). CNAPS supported 1-, 8-, and 16-bit precision in hardware. Consequently, the PNs were smaller and cheaper. This reduced precision was more than adequate for the applications implemented on CNAPS.

The CNAPS architecture had 64 PNs per chip. At the then frequency of 25 MHz, each chip executed at a rate of 1.6 billion connections computed per second. A single chip executed back-propagation learning at a rate of 300 million connection updates per second; each update consists of reading the weight associated with the connection, modifying it, and then writing it back. Each PN (Figure 2) had 4096 bytes of on-chip local memory, used to store synaptic weight data and other local values. Hence, a 64 PN

chip could store up to 256 KB of information. Multiple chips could be combined to create larger, more powerful systems. The general programmability of the device allowed it to execute a large range of functions, including many non-ANN algorithms such as the discrete Fourier transform, nearest neighbor classification, image processing, and dynamic time warping.

Figure 3 shows a simple two layer network mapped to a CNAPS array. The network nodes are labeled CN0–CN7; the processor nodes are labeled PN0–PN3. Multiple network nodes map to a single processor node; in this example, one node from each layer is mapped to a single PN. For feedforward calculation, assume that the outputs of nodes CN0–CN3 have been computed. To compute the inner product of nodes CN4–CN7, the output value of node CN0 is broadcast on the bus to all PNs in the first clock. Each PN then multiplies the CN0 output with the corresponding weight element, which is different for each PN. On the next clock, CN1's output is broadcast, and so on. After four clocks, all 16 products have been computed: $O(n^2)$ connections in $O(n)$ time.

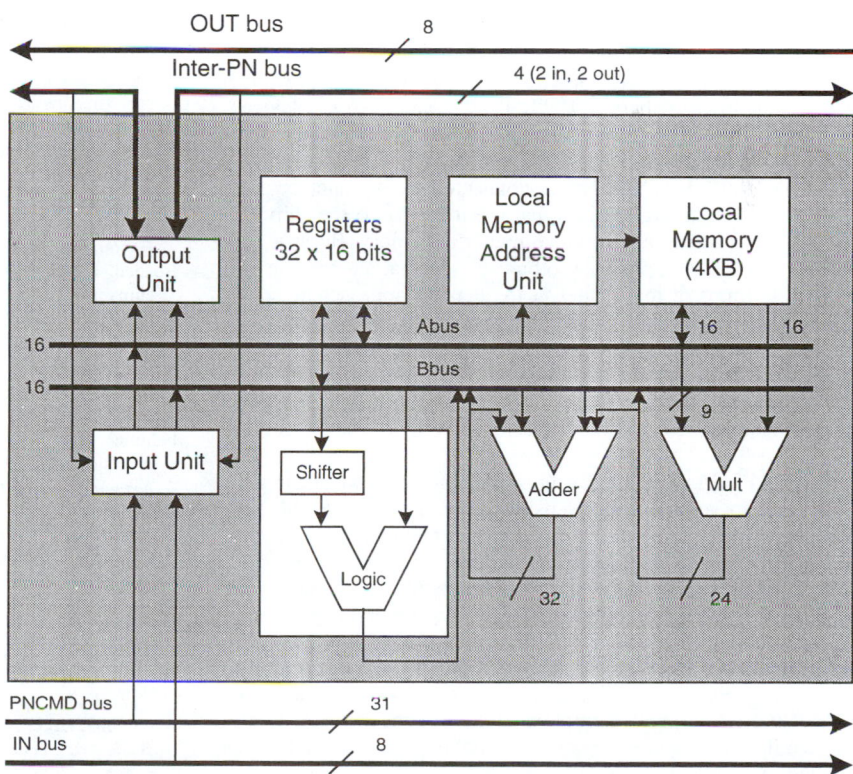

Figure 2. CNAPS PN architecture. A single PN has a multiplier, accumulator, logic/shifter unit, register file, and separate memory address adder. Each PN also has its own memory for storing weights, lookup tables, and other data. Each PN generates its own unique address to memory.

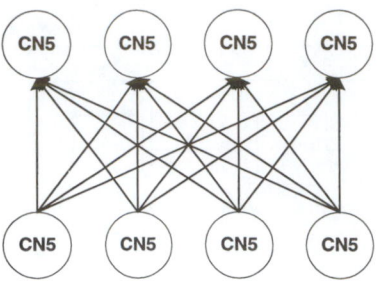

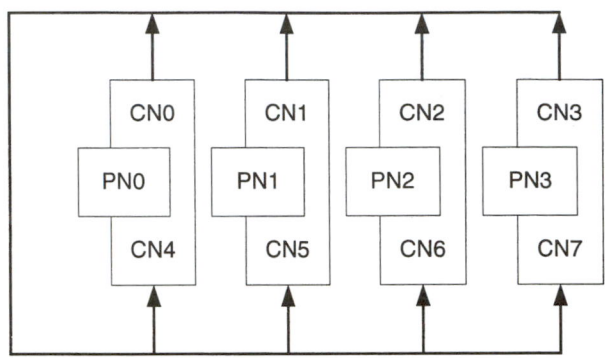

Figure 3. Mapping of a simple two-layer feedforward network to the CNAPS array. When emulating a feedforward network, each layer is spread across the PN array. The neuron outputs of one layer are broadcast sequentially to all PNs while they compute the multiply accumulations for the next layer of neurons.

Digital Neural Networks: Field Programmable Gate Arrays

Perhaps the most promising approach to emulating neural models digitally is the FPGA (Sharma, 1998). Briefly, an FPGA is a device with a large number of generic logic blocks and generic interconnect between those blocks. The functions that the logic blocks implement and how these blocks are connected to one another are determined by configuration bits that are loaded into the chip as one would load a program into a computer's memory. Because of Moore's law, it is now possible to buy FPGAs that are capable of emulating millions of logic gates at frequencies approaching several hundred megahertz. There are very sophisticated design tools that allow logic to be expressed in a high-level hardware description language and then be converted to FPGA configuration bits by an automated synthesis process. These devices can implement large neural structures in parallel (see, for example, Hatano et al., 1999).

Although FPGAs are appearing with larger on-chip memory, they still cannot approach the density of commercial DRAM. So for emulating very large networks, off-chip memory needs to be used to store the various parameters and state information associated with each neuron. However, unlike traditional processors, FPGAs are capable of supporting the access to several high-speed memory structures at once. Consequently, a board with several FPGAs could emulate networks at much higher speeds than a high-speed desktop PC. In addition, the inherent parallelism in each FPGA would allow parallel implementation of the various structures within the neuron, such as sophisticated spike-based computation.

Discussion

It is difficult to predict technology trends, but speculation is always possible. Today, most ANNs are used for pattern recognition. The final stage of most pattern recognition algorithms involves checking a series of classification results to see whether they fit in the larger context of the domain in question. Including this contextual knowledge can be as simple as spell checking, or it can be as complex as accessing high-order rules or schemas that reflect complex syntactical and semantic relationships. Since classification is imperfect, contextual processing, which makes knowledge of such higher-order relationships available to the classification process, is essential to guarantee the accuracy of the final result.

Although the results are still speculative, research (Ambros-Ingerson et al., 1990; Braitenberg and Schüz, 1998) has shown that scaling to large contexts requires networks with relatively sparse interconnect and sparse activation, in which only a few nodes are actively firing at a time. On the basis of research into VLSI connectivity (Bailey, 1993), digital-based systems can handle such networks more efficiently than analog. Therefore, at some point in the processing, the data will probably need to be converted from analog to digital representation. Today, the conversion is done at or just after the input transducer. On the basis of the state of analog technologies, systems of the future will probably take advantage of the computational density of analog VLSI to perform the feature extraction and some preliminary classification at the front end, with conversion to digital form for contextual processing and final classification by "higher-level brain regions."

Road Map: Implementation and Analysis
Related Reading: Analog VLSI Implementation of Neural Networks; Photonic Implementations of Neurobiologically Inspired Networks; Programmable Neurocomputing Systems

References

Ambros-Ingerson, J., Granger, R., et al., 1990, Simulation of paleocortex performs hierarchical clustering, *Science*, 247:1344–1348.

Bailey, J., 1993, A VLSI interconnect strategy for biologically inspired artificial neural networks, Ph.D. thesis, Department of Computer Science/Engineering, Oregon Graduate Institute, Beaverton, OR.

Bailey, J., and Hammerstrom, D., 1988, Why VLSI implementations of associative VLCNs require connection multiplexing, *1988 International Conference on Neural Networks*, San Diego, CA, pp. 173–180.

Boahen, K. A., 2000, Point-to-point connectivity between neuromorphic chips using address events, *IEEE Trans. Circuits and Systems II—Analog and Digital Signal Processing*, 47(5):416–434. ◆

Braitenberg, V., and Schüz, A., 1998, *Cortex: Statistics and Geometry of Neuronal Connectivity*, New York: Springer-Verlag.

Chua, L., and Roska, T., 2001, *Cellular Neural Networks and Visual Computing*, Cambridge, Engl.: Cambridge University Press.

Fahlman, S. E., and Hoehfeld, M., 1992, Learning with limited numerical precision using the cascade-correlation algorithm, *IEEE Trans. Neural Networks*, 3(4):602–611.

Hammerstrom, D., 1995, A digital VLSI architecture for real-world applications, in *An Introduction to Neural and Electronic Networks* (S. F. Zornetzer, J. L. Davis, C. Lau, and T. McKenna, Eds.), San Diego, CA: Academic Press, pp. 335–358. ◆

Hatano, F., et al., 1999, Implementation of cell array neuro-processor by using FPGA, paper presented at IEEE International Joint Conference on Artificial Neural Networks, Washington, DC. ◆

Hennessy, J. L., and Patterson, D. A., 1991, *Computer Architecture: A Quantitative Approach*, Palo Alto, CA: Morgan Kaufmann.

Intel, 2001, *IA-32 Intel Architecture Software Developer's Manual*, vol. 1: *Basic Architecture*, Santa Clara, CA: Intel.

Reschke, C., Sterling, T., et al., 1996, A design study of alternative network topologies for the Beowulf parallel workstation, in *Proceedings of the IEEE International Symposium on High Performance Distributed Computing*, Piscataway, NJ: IEEE.

Shan, H., Singh, J. P., et al., 2000, A comparison of three programming

models for adaptive applications on the Origin2000, in *Proceedings of SC2000*, Dallas, TX.

Sharma, A. K., 1998, *Programmable Logic Handbook: PLDs, CPLDs & FPGAs*, New York: McGraw-Hill Handbooks.

Directional Selectivity

Norberto M. Grzywacz and David K. Merwine

Introduction

Directional selectivity refers to a neuron's ability to produce substantially different responses for stimulus motions of different direction. A directionally selective (DS) cell will fire many spikes in response to object motion in one direction (the preferred direction) while responding weakly, if at all, for motion in the opposite (null) direction. This directional "trigger feature" is often essentially independent of the contrast, contrast polarity, color, shape, or speed of the moving object. Cells displaying directional selectivity are found in the retinas and visual cortices of all the major vertebrate classes. These neurons support a host of visual tasks, ranging from motion perception, image segregation, and deblurring to the control of eye movements. The extraction of direction of motion is so crucial for vision that it is the first motion-related variable encoded in the visual pathway.

It is impossible, however, to determine the direction of a motion using an individual DS neuron. First, because these neurons have relatively small receptive fields, they can only report motion components that are perpendicular to the gradient of illumination. This phenomenon is known as the aperture problem. Second, motions orthogonal to the preferred-null axis will elicit intermediate, ambiguous responses. Moreover, nonmotion parameters, such as contrast, and motion parameters, such as speed, will affect the amplitude of the DS cell's response. However, by comparing over a population of DS cells, the true direction of a motion can be determined. One needs to compare the responses of DS neurons with different preferred directions. Regardless of object contrast or speed, the neuron whose preferred direction is closest to the actual direction of visual motion will have the largest response. Thus, a comparison of responses over a population of DS neurons can disambiguate the veridical motion direction.

Optic Flow

According to physics, the most fundamental variable of motion is velocity, a vector composed of direction and speed. Animals perceive three-dimensional (3D) velocities in the world through the world's two-dimensional (2D) projection onto these animals' retinas. Therefore, the true values of velocity in the world cannot be directly determined using the information from the eyes. A more useful velocity-related variable for the animal is *optic flow*. This is the spatial distribution of velocity vectors that is obtained by projecting the moving 3D world onto the 2D retina. An example of the utility of optic flow analysis occurs when an animal moves forward in a straight line. The resultant optic flow is that of an expansion, and the animal can maintain its heading by keeping the focus of expansion constant (see also MOTION PERCEPTION: NAVIGATION). To find this focus, information about directional selectivity must be combined across the image by "higher" cortical areas. One area that may contribute to this computation is the middle superior temporal cortex (MST), which appears to contain neurons

tuned to expansion and contraction (for a review, see Andersen, 1997).

Mathematically, the most popular definition of optic flow uses the image constraint equation $dE/dt = 0$, where E is the brightness of the image (see Grzywacz, Harris, and Amthor, 1994, for details and references). This equation assumes that brightness varies slowly over time and defines the optic flow $\vec{v}$ as

$$\nabla E \cdot \vec{v} + \frac{\partial E}{\partial t} = 0 \qquad (1)$$

This brightness-related definition is not unique, as nonmotion parameters, such as reflectance, can influence the solutions of the equation. Other definitions emphasize different useful components of the motion. For instance, the directional components alone have proved sufficient for determining heading direction as well as for recovering structure from motion and performing image-segregation tasks.

Speed

Before we embark on a detailed discussion of directional selectivity, we would like to comment briefly on the measurement of speed. This variable is considerably more difficult to measure than direction, as a local determination of speed in the image requires precise spatiotemporal information. In contrast, a measure of direction of motion requires two fairly imprecise positional measurements separated in time. For this reason, the visual system computes local speed with relatively less precision than direction and does so at a later stage of processing.

Computational models have been proposed that use DS signals to obtain local speed (reviewed in Grzywacz et al., 1994). For instance, Grzywacz and Yuille developed such a model by using model DS cells with receptive field profiles based on Gabor functions. They organized these cells in a 3D space whose coordinates were the optimal temporal frequency and the two components of optimal spatial frequency of the cells. They found that any arbitrary translation with constant velocity would yield maximal responses that fell on a plane in this space. Local speed and direction could then be determined by measuring the slant and tilt of this plane. Grzywacz and Yuille proposed a plausible neural architecture for performing this measurement.

Theory of Directional Selectivity

Reichardt, Poggio, and colleagues (Poggio and Reichardt, 1976) described the theoretical requirements for any model of directional selectivity (see also MOTION PERCEPTION, ELEMENTARY MECHANISMS). The first requirement is spatial asymmetry. If a neuron responds better to a motion coming from the left than to a motion coming from the right, then there must be some difference in the inputs from the left and right sides of the cell's receptive field.

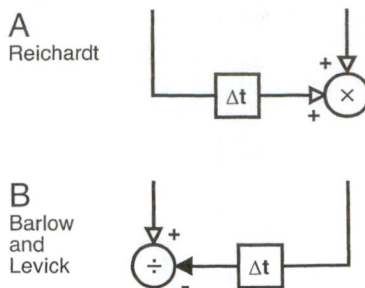

A Reichardt

B Barlow and Levick

Figure 1. Models for directional selectivity. In each case, preferred direction is from left to right. The lines with arrows are inputs to the nonlinear interaction sites (circles). These inputs originate at different spatial locations as indicated by the nonarrow ends of the lines. Boxes with "Δt" symbols indicate that their corresponding lines are slow. Hence, movement going from the slow line to the fast line will generate signals that arrive together at the interaction sites but the opposite movement will not. In the Reichardt model, a multiplication exploits this difference to create directional selectivity. In the Barlow and Levick model, the difference is exploited by an inhibitory (possibly division-like) interaction.

Models for this asymmetry have always included a temporally asymmetric component, that is, some difference in time course between the left- and right-side inputs. However, this need not be the case. For example, the left-side input could "gate" the right-side input (Grzywacz et al., 1994). In this case, the cell will fire only when the motion comes from the left and opens the gate, before reaching the right-side input.

The second requirement for directional selectivity is a nonlinear mechanism. A spatiotemporal asymmetry alone will yield a directional difference in the responses (i.e., differing waveforms, depending on the direction of stimulus motion). However, such an asymmetry alone is not sufficient to produce two different single-number responses for preferred- and null-direction motions, a requirement to decide what the estimated direction of motion is. Poggio and Reichardt's work proves that, without a nonlinear mechanism, any numbers obtained from the waveforms of the responses will be equal for all directions of motion. The nonlinearity can be as simple as a threshold or the gating mechanism mentioned above, but it must be present.

Figure 1A illustrates the simplest model proposed by Reichardt and colleagues for the insect's retinal directional selectivity (RDS). For simplicity, the model uses inputs from only two locations. The proposed spatial asymmetry in this model is temporal. Inputs from the preferred side (the side first encountered by an object moving in the preferred direction, left in the figure) are propagated to the interaction site on a slow time scale compared with those from the null side. The proposed nonlinearity for the interaction is a multiplication. Thus, if an object moves in the preferred direction at an appropriate speed, the slowness of the left-side pathway is compensated for by the earlier arrival time of the stimulus, causing both inputs to arrive at the decision site at the same time, yielding a positive multiplication. For null-direction motions, the inputs will arrive at the decision site separately, and the result of the multiplication will be zero. The multiplicative nonlinearity therefore acts as a coincidence detector.

This multiplicative nonlinearity is one of many quadratic nonlinearity models supported by insect data. Poggio and Reichardt used the Volterra series formulation to examine the predictions common to all quadratic models of directional selectivity. For such a formulation of a smooth, time-invariant, nonlinear interaction between the responses to stimuli in spatial locations $a(z_a)$ and $b(z_b)$, the output is

$$y(t) = h_{0,0} + \sum_{m=1}^{\infty} \sum_{j=0}^{m} h_{j,m-j} *^m z_a^{(j)} z_b^{(m-j)} \qquad (2)$$

where $*^m$ is the mth-order convolution and where $h_{j,m-j}$ are the mth-order kernels of the interaction. The mth-order kernel describes the nonlinear interaction between the responses to stimuli at m different instants in time. A quadratic nonlinearity is one for which if $m \geq 3$, $h_{j,m-j} = 0$. A quadratic nonlinearity thus describes multiplicative interactions between pairs of stimulus responses.

Two predictions of quadratic nonlinearity models are frequency doubling and superposition of nonlinearities. Frequency doubling is the appearance in the Fourier spectrum of the response to moving sinusoidal gratings of energy at a frequency of twice the fundamental but not at frequencies higher than that. In superposition of nonlinearities, the average of the nonlinear response to a grating composed of two sinusoidal gratings of different frequencies (whose ratio is a rational number) is equal to the sum of the responses to the two individual gratings. Both frequency doubling and superposition of nonlinearities can be used to test whether a system computes directional selectivity solely through quadratic nonlinearities.

Retinal Directional Selectivity

Although DS retinal neurons have been described in a number of vertebrates, the vast majority of work has been performed in the rabbit. In this animal, two types of DS cells have been described. The first, the On-Off DS ganglion cell, responds well to moving spots, bars, edges, or gratings of both contrast polarities over a broad range of speeds. Additionally, these cells can detect the direction of motion of long edges for displacements less than the spacing between photoreceptors, hence mediating directional hyperacuity. Four subtypes of On-Off DS cell exist, one each for temporal, nasal, superior, and inferior motions. Each subtype independently tiles the retinal surface and thus can independently sample the visual world. The second DS cell type (the On DS cell) responds only to bright edges and to considerably slower speeds than those preferred by the On-Off type. The On DS cells exist in three subtypes whose preferred directions are aligned with the animal's semicircular canals. These cells have receptive fields whose areas are more than three times larger at any given eccentricity than the On-Off type, and their tiling is correspondingly less dense (Vaney et al., 2001). The On DS type supports optokinetic nystagmus through projections to subcortical areas. As they are infrequently encountered, the mechanisms responsible for these cells' directional selectivity have not been well investigated, and they will not be considered further here.

Spatial Asymmetry

Although a spatial asymmetry is required for generating a DS circuit, no obvious asymmetry exists in the anatomical structure of the On-Off DS cell. The dendritic trees of these ganglion cells have a unique, looping morphology. But there is no relationship between asymmetries in the tree and the cell's preferred direction of motion (Vaney et al., 2001). Therefore, the spatial asymmetry has been conjectured to exist in the connectivity between DS cells and their inputs. No spatially asymmetric connections have been conclusively identified to date. However, two strong candidates exist. First, cross-correlational and anatomical studies of the cholinergic amacrine cell and the On-Off DS cell suggest that the former makes spatially asymmetric connections to the latter. Support for this suggestion comes from the elimination of DS responses to moving gratings by cholinergic antagonists (Grzywacz, Amthor, and Merwine, 1998). Second, asymmetric connections may also exist from some GABAergic amacrine cells to the DS cells. GABA antagonists strongly reduce directional selectivity.

Nonlinearities

In their seminal work on rabbit retinas, Barlow and Levick (1965) performed two-slit apparent-motion experiments on DS cells. They discovered that when two stimuli were presented in null sequence (as if an object were moving in the null direction), then the number of spikes elicited was far less than the sum of the spikes for each stimulus in isolation. From this, they concluded that RDS arises from a nonlinear, *inhibitory* mechanism that "vetoes" responses to null sequences (equivalent to the logical AND-NOT operation). As shown in Figure 1B, their proposed spatial asymmetry has two components. A central component is excitatory and is conducted to the interaction site quickly. A second, inhibitory component is offset to the null side and is conducted with a delay. Thus, an asymmetry exists in both the sign and time course of the two spatially separated components. This asymmetry causes motions in the preferred direction to yield responses, while responses to null-direction motions are vetoed. However, despite Barlow and Levick's proposal, this veto mechanism turns out not to be a perfect veto. Studies reviewed by Grzywacz et al. (1994) show that a better description for the inhibitory interaction is a division-like nonlinearity, as shown in Figure 1B.

Torre and Poggio proposed a biophysical implementation of Barlow and Levick's inhibition (see Grzywacz et al., 1994, for a review). Because RDS can be elicited by motions spanning remarkably short distances almost anywhere within the DS cell's receptive field (Barlow and Levick, 1965), Torre and Poggio suggested that the inhibition acted separately within each branch of the cell's dendritic tree. To constrain the computation spatially, they suggested that the inhibition works through a synapse that causes local changes of membrane conductance (shunting inhibition) and little hyperpolarization. To understand such a synapse, consider a patch of membrane receiving excitatory (g_e) and shunting inhibitory (g_i) synaptic conductances. Setting without loss of generality the resting and inhibitory reversal potentials to zero, the voltage V obeys

$$C \frac{dV(t)}{dt} + (g_e(t) + g_i(t) + g_{\text{leak}})V(t) = g_e(t)E_e + g_{\text{leak}}E_{\text{leak}}$$

(3)

where C is membrane capacitance, g_{leak} is the membrane's leak conductance, and E_e and E_{leak} are reversal potentials of g_e and g_{leak}, respectively. When $g_i \gg g_e$, then V falls toward the following equilibrium value:

$$V(t) \rightarrow \frac{g_e E_e + g_{\text{leak}} E_{\text{leak}}}{g_i}$$

(4)

which is small, because g_i is large. Therefore, this inhibition is division-like rather than subtraction-like. Torre and Poggio argued that a shunting-inhibition mechanism might also be consistent with the insect's quadratic nonlinearity, because, for sufficiently low contrasts, one can ignore the higher-order nonlinearities, as in a Taylor series approximation. However, experimentally a quadratic approximation is not valid for rabbit DS cells, as they fail both the frequency-doubling and superposition-of-nonlinearities tests even at near-threshold contrasts.

Although a shunting-inhibition mechanism can theoretically produce the localized interactions necessary to explain many DS properties, it has not been possible to record intracellularly within dendrites to test this mechanism. Recently, two additional nonlinearities have been proposed that could support dendritically lo-

calized directional selectivity. First, it has been suggested that this nonlinearity could be due to excitatory voltage-dependent conductances at the dendrites. There is evidence of dendritic spikes in rabbit's ganglion cells. Second, it has been proposed that the unusual predominance of NMDA glutamatergic receptors on DS cells may have functional significance. The NMDA channel has a nonlinear behavior, due to channel blockade by magnesium ions at hyperpolarized potentials. Therefore, glutamatergic binding must occur *during depolarization* for the channel to operate. Even weak, null-direction inhibition could cause the NMDA channel to hyperpolarize and close. It could therefore act as the veto site hypothesized by Barlow and Levick (1965). When tested in magnesium-free medium, RDS is severely reduced, suggesting a critical role for NMDA receptors. The NMDA, spiking, and shunting nonlinearities need not be mutually exclusive, and each could play an important role in supporting robust RDS.

Pre- or Postsynaptic Nonlinearities?

In addition to the null-direction inhibition just described, it is known that preferred-direction motions facilitate DS cell responses (Barlow and Levick, 1965). If the spatiotemporal parameters of the stimulus are appropriate, then preferred-direction facilitation can be as strong as null-direction inhibition (reviewed in Grzywacz et al., 1994). Facilitation is believed to come to the DS cell from the cholinergic amacrine cells. A spatial asymmetry has been shown to exist in the input-output relationship of these cells' dendrites. These dendrites receive excitatory inputs along their length, but they release excitatory transmitter (ACh) and may receive inhibitory inputs (through GABA) only at their tips (Figure 2A). If the GABA-inhibition acts in a division-like manner, then each dendrite contains a spatial asymmetry and a nonlinearity, and thus can act as an autonomous DS unit. Hence, it has been proposed that DS signals are at least partially generated presynaptically and flow from the cholinergic dendrites to the DS cell. DS cells would then

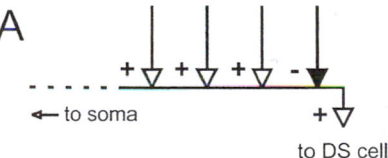

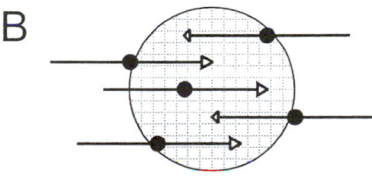

Figure 2. Schemes for presynaptic retinal directional selectivity. *A*, Model of a cholinergic-dendritic DS subunit. The bent line represents a dendrite of the cholinergic amacrine cell making a synapse onto a DS cell. This dendrite receives excitatory inputs throughout its length (open arrows) and inhibitory inputs (filled arrow) near the synaptic ending. Therefore, the output synapse is directionally selective, as the dendrite behaves like a Barlow-and-Levick model (Figure 1B). *B*, Spatial relationship between cholinergic dendrites and the DS cell's receptive field (circle). Arrowhead size indicates synaptic strength, and black discs mark the cholinergic somas. Although all dendrites are directionally selective, the DS cell receives more inputs from the left than from the right. Consequently, its preferred direction is to the right.

preferentially sample from dendrites with the same preferred direction (Figure 2*B*).

There is accumulating evidence, however, that both pre- and postsynaptic asymmetries may be involved in RDS. Complete blockade of cholinergic synapses does not fully eliminate RDS to moving bars (Grzywacz et al., 1998). The residual direction selectivity is GABAergic and appears to be postsynaptic. In turn, GABA blockade not only does not always eliminate RDS, it occasionally reverses its preferred and null directions. Computer simulations of the cholinergic-dendritic RDS can account for these reversals as a result of synaptic saturation (reviewed in Grzywacz et al., 1994). Thus, asymmetric postsynaptic inhibition and asymmetric presynaptic facilitation may act cooperatively to produce robust RDS for a broad range of visual stimuli.

Development

The development of RDS is not well understood. In turtles, RDS emerges late in development, that is, after the establishment of concentric receptive fields, inhibitory surrounds, and orientation selectivity (selectivity to spatial orientation of anisotropic stimuli, such as lines) (Sernagor and Grzywacz, 1995). Evidence suggests that turtle RDS may emerge at the expense of orientationally selective (OS) cells. It has thus been proposed that turtle DS cells are modified OS cells. This late emergence of RDS suggests two hypotheses for its development: (1) it requires light exposure, and/or (2) it requires the late emergence of an inhibitory drive onto the network mediating orientation selectivity.

In rabbits, however, RDS emerges relatively early. The percentage of DS cells and DS cell gap-junctional coupling patterns both appear adult-like within a few days of eye opening. Directionally selective responses have been recorded from rabbit retinas before eye opening. Therefore, some authors have suggested that rabbit RDS is initially generated in the presynaptic cholinergic circuit. The primary excitatory stimulus for this mechanism would be the bursting spontaneous waves of activity known to occur during development (see Sernagor and Grzywacz, 1995, for references on developmental spontaneous activity). In this case, the first challenge for the DS cells would be to connect selectively to cholinergic dendrites of similar orientation. (Recall that the amacrine cell dendrites can each act as a DS subunit.) A Hebbian correlational process that would reinforce statistical biases in the initial contacts from the cholinergic dendrites to proto-DS cells could produce this selectivity. GABAergic null-direction inhibition would then be added to the cell's established directional preference.

Cortical Directional Selectivity

DS cells are found in multiple locations in the cortices of mammals, beginning with simple DS cells in the lateral geniculate nucleus (LGN) input layers of the primary visual cortex (V1). Nearly every simple and complex cell in mammalian V1 has some degree of directional selectivity. However, the strength of directionality varies widely. For example, only about 20% of macaque V1 DS cells achieve preferred-versus-null response ratios greater than 3:1 (De Valois et al., 2000). In comparison, rabbit retinal DS cells typically have preferred-null ratios around 10:1. As with the retinal DS cells, the preferred direction of motion cannot be accounted for by any spatial asymmetries in the dendritic trees of the cortical DS cells. However, unlike retinal DS cells, cortical DS cells are highly selective for the orientation and spatial frequency of the moving stimulus. Moreover, it is often possible to predict the preferred direction of motion for a simple DS cell from its spot-mapped receptive field. This has led to the development of quasilinear models of cortical directional selectivity, which we discuss below.

There is abundant evidence that cortical directional selectivity supports motion perception. Perceptual decisions in motion tasks correlate with the performance of cortical DS neurons (Andersen, 1997). Furthermore, lesions and/or current injections in MT affect motion integration tasks, biasing motion perception in specific and replicable ways (Salzman et al., 1992). In addition to the contribution of cortical DS cells to perception, they probably also assist in the control of eye movements. For instance, neuroanatomical data demonstrate that both MT and MST send large projections to the dorsolateral pons, an area known to be involved in smooth-pursuit eye movements.

Hierarchy

As a first-order approximation, motion is computed hierarchically in the cortex (Andersen, 1997). The hierarchy begins with the simple and complex DS cells in layers IV and VI of cortical area V1, as just described. (In animals phylogenetically close to primates, retinal DS cells project primarily to subcortical centers. Evidence suggests that directional selectivity in the primary visual cortex is computed independently from RDS.) The DS cells in V1 project to the MT cortical area (MT or V5) and to V2, which also projects to MT. Directional selectivity becomes more complex in MT; that is, cells there typically have very large, orientation-independent receptive fields, and many will respond best to the composite motion of a plaid, as opposed to its individual components. From MT, the motion pathway projects to MST, wherein directional selectivity information is further combined to produce neurons sensitive to complex motions, such as rotation, expansion, and contraction (Andersen, 1997).

Psychophysical Models

One class of models for the first stage of cortical directional selectivity is based on human psychophysics and is similar to the Reichardt model in Figure 1*A*. In these models a slow, laterally displaced input and a fast central input are multiplied. As described above, the two signals from these inputs will arrive simultaneously, yielding a response, for only one direction of object motion. Another class, called motion-energy models (Adelson and Bergen, 1985), proposes a distributed spatiotemporal asymmetry and a squaring nonlinearity (Figure 3*A*). The distributed spatial asymmetry occurs because different locations in the receptive field have different impulse responses. This property is known as space-time (S-T) inseparability and is illustrated in Figure 3*B*. For this type of space-time arrangement, it is only for preferred-direction motions that the responses of all areas occur simultaneously. Simple linear summation then results in differential responses to preferred- and null-direction motions, and the squaring nonlinearity converts this directional difference into directional selectivity.

Physiological Models

There is substantial physiological evidence for S-T inseparability in simple DS cells in visual cortex. Figure 3*C* shows an idealized simple-cell receptive field map as would be obtained from reverse-correlation experiments (De Valois et al., 2000). The cell contains on and off subregions with different time courses in different portions of space, resulting in an oriented spatiotemporal receptive field. Assorted variations of linear energy-motion models with static nonlinearities have been proposed that can account for approximately 50%–80% of the response of simple DS cells (Reid, Soodak, and Shapley, 1991; De Valois et al., 2000). However, the correlation between simple-cell S-T profile and direction selectivity varies widely in V1. Cells in layer IVB show very high correlation, those in IVA show only moderate correlation, and those in layer

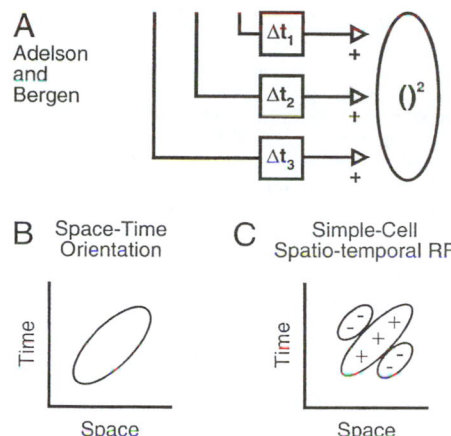

Figure 3. Motion-energy models of cortical directional selectivity. *A*, The Adelson and Bergen model. The symbols here are as in Figure 1, with "( )^2" indicating a squaring operation. *B*, Space-time orientation. If in *A*, $\Delta t_3 < \Delta t_2 < \Delta t_1$, then a plot of the response of the model to stimulation at different positions in space looks like this figure; that is, it is oriented in space-time. Hence, a motion going from left to right will have a positive slope in this plot and cause much response, whereas the opposite motion will not. *C*, Idealized representation of a simple-cell receptive field. The inhibitory flanks help to inhibit motions in the null (nonpreferred) direction (lines with negative slopes).

VI show very low correlation, despite equivalent directional tuning (Murthy et al., 1998). Thus, S-T structure alone cannot fully account for simple DS cell responses. In addition, quasilinear models of simple cells generally overestimate nonpreferred responses and sometimes underestimate preferred responses (Reid et al., 1991). And linear feedforward models also do not predict onset transients, which are commonly observed. Therefore, inhibitory (Reid et al., 1991; Heeger, 1993) or excitatory (Douglas and Martin, 1992) nonlinear feedback interactions between cortical cells have been proposed to account for these discrepancies. It has also been suggested that nonpreferred direction suppression might be due to a cortical inhibitory network devoted to response normalization (Heeger, 1993).

Although it has been accepted for many years that magnocellular cells from the LGN provide the input to the motion system, motion-energy models require inputs to simple DS cells that differ in latency (or temporal phase). Magno cells all have essentially identical response timings and therefore could not provide the range of latencies needed without an intracortical mechanism for creating delays (De Valois et al., 2000). It has been shown that blockade of cortical GABA$_A$ inhibition reduces but does not eliminate S-T inseparability. Thus, intracortical inhibition may contribute to, but cannot be solely responsible for, input latency differences. Humphrey, Saul, and Fiedler (1998) note that about 40% of parvocellular geniculate cells display absolute phase delays and long latencies (lagged cells) relative to the remaining parvo cells (nonlagged cells). Because lagged and nonlagged timing signatures are identifiable in simple-cell receptive fields, these authors attribute S-T inseparability to converging lagged and nonlagged parvo cell inputs with spatially shifted receptive fields. De Valois et al. (2000), however, suggest that the requisite latency differences arise from two classes of nondirectional (preferred-null ratios <3:1) cortical cells, which receive inputs from magno and parvo cells. Both nondirectional types can be found in a single cortical column and have appropriate differences in response waveforms. Additionally, these two nondirectional cell types are often shifted 90° in spatial phase, though centered on the same spatial location. Thus, they have ex-

actly the spatiotemporal profile required to detect direction of motion using a linear energy-motion model.

Complex DS cells are generally found in the upper and lower layers of V1. Unlike most simple DS cells, complex DS cells lack first-order (linear) S-T oriented receptive fields. However, these cells show second-order (quadratic) S-T structure. In other words, it is the interactions between two sequentially stimulated locations in the cell's receptive field that are S-T inseparable. Thus, dynamic nonlinearities have been proposed to account for complex-cell directional selectivity. These nonlinearities would facilitate or inhibit, respectively, the responses to preferred- or null-direction motions. Similarly, S-T separable simple cells have also been shown to display some second-order, that is, nonlinear S-T structure. Because there is evidence for complex-to-simple-cell interactions, it has been proposed that directional selectivity and second-order S-T inseparability in simple cells arise from complex-cell inputs.

Development

At least 5% of the cells in areas V1 and V2 of the kitten are directionally selective at eye opening. Thus, some of the cortical directional selectivity is either genetically coded or epigenetically derived through developmental spontaneous activity. Interestingly, selective biases in the distribution of preferred directions can be produced in kittens by exposing them to stripes moving in a particular direction after eye opening. In addition, one can nearly eliminate cortical directional selectivity by raising animals in an environment that is illuminated only by brief, low-frequency, stroboscopic flashes of light. Under these rearing conditions, only about 10% of V1 cells develop directional selectivity, and their directional selectivity is considerably weaker than normal. Not surprisingly, elimination of S-T inseparability accompanies the loss of directional selectivity (Humphrey et al., 1998). Perceptually, strobe-reared cats require contrasts at least ten times higher than normal to determine the direction of a moving grating. Furthermore, these elevations in contrast threshold can be permanent. No recovery of S-T structure or improvement in contrast threshold was found in two cats that had received 12 years of training following strobe rearing. Thus, it appears that some critical period exists during development during which directional selectivity must be established or it is forever compromised.

Based on the loss of S-T inseparability during strobe rearing, some authors have modeled the development of cortical directional selectivity as due to inputs with different response timings forming connections with a common cortical cell. These connections would self-organize through a Hebbian process that would strengthen the synaptic connections of well-correlated inputs (Humphrey et al., 1998). Strobe rearing would restrict the range of timings that could be associated, and therefore could eliminate cortical directional selectivity.

Discussion

In this article, we have discussed the first step in the perception of motion—the determination of motion direction. This information is encoded by ensembles of directionally selective neurons both in the retina and within multiple visuocortical nuclei. Elucidating the cellular mechanisms subserving directional selectivity has been a major goal of neurobiologists for nearly 40 years.

Road Map: Vision
Related Reading: Feature Analysis; Motion Perception: Elementary Mechanisms; Retina; Visual Cortex: Anatomical Structure and Models of Function

References

Adelson, E. H., and Bergen, J. R., 1985, Spatio-temporal energy models for the perception of motion, *J. Opt. Soc. Am. A*, 2:284–299.

Andersen, R. A., 1997, Neural mechanisms of visual motion perception in primates, *Neuron*, 18:865–872. ◆

Barlow, H. B., and Levick, W. R., 1965, The mechanism of directionally selective units in rabbit's retina, *J. Physiol.*, 178:477–504.

De Valois, R. L., Cottaris, N. P., Mahon, L. E., Elfar, S. D., Wilson, J. A., 2000, Spatial and temporal receptive fields of geniculate and cortical cells and directional selectivity, *Vision Res.*, 40:3685–3702.

Douglas, R. J., and Martin, K. A. C., 1992, Exploring cortical microcircuits: A combined anatomical, physiological, and computational approach, in *Single Neuron Computation* (T. McKenna, J. Davis, and S. F. Zornetzer, Eds.), Orlando, FL: Academic Press, pp. 381–412. ◆

Grzywacz, N. M., Amthor, F. R., and Merwine, D. K., 1998, Necessity of acetylcholine for retinal directionally selective responses to drifting gratings in rabbit, *J. Physiol.*, 512:575–581.

Grzywacz, N. M., Harris, J. M., and Amthor, F. R., 1994, Computational and neural constraints for the measurement of local visual motion, in *Visual Detection of Motion* (A. T. Smith and R. J. Snowden, Eds.), London: Academic Press, pp. 19–50. ◆

Heeger, D. J., 1993, Modeling simple cell direction selectivity with nor-malized, half-squared, linear operators, *J. Neurophysiol.*, 70:1885–1898.

Humphrey, A. L., Saul, A. B., and Fiedler, J. C., 1998, Strobe rearing prevents the convergence of inputs with different response timings onto area 17 simple cells, *J. Neurophysiol.*, 80:3005–3020.

Murthy, A., Humphrey, A. L., Saul, A. B., and Fiedler, J. C., 1998, Laminar differences in the spatiotemporal structure of simple cell receptive fields in cat area 17, *Vision Neurosci.*, 15:239–256.

Poggio, T., and Reichardt, W. T., 1976, Visual control of orientation behaviour in the fly: Part II. Towards the underlying neural interactions, *Q. Rev. Biophys.*, 9:377–438. ◆

Reid, R. C., Soodak, R. E., and Shapley, R. M., 1991, Directional selectivity and spatiotemporal structure of receptive fields of simple cells in cat striate cortex, *J. Neurophysiol.*, 66:505–529.

Salzman, C. D., Murasugi, C. M., Britten, K. H., and Newsome, W. T., 1992, Microstimulation in visual area MT: Effects on direction discrimination performance, *J. Neurosci.*, 12:2331–2355.

Sernagor, E., and Grzywacz, N. M., 1995, Emergence of complex receptive field properties of ganglion cells in the developing turtle retina, *J. Neurophysiol.*, 73:1355–1364.

Vaney, D. I., He, S., Taylor, W. R., and Levick, W. R., 2001, Direction-selective ganglion cells in the retina, *in Motion Vision: Computational, Neural, and Ecological Constraints* (J. M. Zanker and J. Zeil, Eds.), Berlin: Springer-Verlag, pp. 13–56. ◆

Dissociations Between Visual Processing Modes

Bruce Bridgeman

Introduction

The visual system has two kinds of jobs to do. One is to support visual cognition or perception—knowledge about the identities and locations of objects and surfaces in the world. Another, sensori-motor, function is to control visually guided behavior. The two functions require different kinds of visual information.

The cognitive function is concerned with pattern recognition and with the positions of objects relative to one another. Executing this function requires extensive interaction between bottom-up image data and top-down information about objects, faces, etc. Qualitative location information may be adequate for this function; humans are poor at quantitatively estimating distances, directions, etc. if the measures of these abilities are perceptual judgments rather than motor behaviors.

The sensorimotor function, in contrast, needs quantitative ego-centrically calibrated spatial information to guide motor acts. It does not need the minute-of-arc acuity of the cognitive function, however: calibration is more important than resolution. As a result, the brain's sensorimotor representations can be much smaller than those supporting cognition.

It is an empirical question whether these two functions, the cognitive and the sensorimotor, should be modeled as a single visual representation with two readouts or as separate maps of visual space. There is now extensive evidence for two distinct maps or sets of maps of visual space in the brain, one set handling perception and the other supporting visually guided behavior (Figure 1). Evidence comes from physiological recordings from the separate maps, from neurological patients in which one system or the other is damaged, from fMRI and PET scans of humans doing cognitive or sensorimotor tasks, and from psychophysical work in which different spatial values are inserted into the two systems simultaneously.

Some of the earliest evidence for the two-visual-systems distinction came from experiments in hamsters, where lesions of the midbrain's superior colliculus led to the inability to orient appropriately in a T-maze, combined with preserved abilities in pattern discrimination. In other animals, visual cortex lesions disturbed pattern discrimination without interfering with maze orienting (Schneider, 1969). This forebrain-midbrain distinction changed over the course of evolution, as both spatial orientation and pattern recognition became corticalized in primates.

Neurophysiology

The visual pathways begin as a unified system, from the retinas through the lateral geniculate nucleus of the thalamus to the primary visual cortex of the occipital lobe. From here, visual signals are relayed to approximately 27 topographic maps in other visual areas (VISUAL SCENE PERCEPTION). This characteristic of visual systems raises a question: do all of these maps work together in a

Information Flow

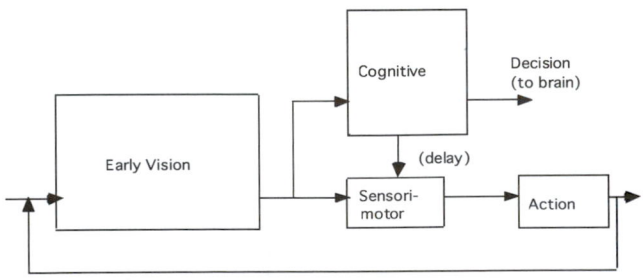

Figure 1. Information flow in cognitive and sensorimotor visual pathways. Visual image input is from the left, and cognitive or motor output to the right.

single visual representation, or are they functionally distinct? If they are distinct, how many functional maps are there and how do they interact?

The evidence reveals that the multiple maps support at least two functionally distinct representations of the visual world. The representations do not always function independently, but communicate with one another in some ways. Each representation uses several of the retinotopic maps; cognitive and sensorimotor representations correspond roughly to pathways into temporal and parietal cortex, respectively (Mishkin, Ungerleider, and Macko, 1983).

The temporal pathway consists of a number of regions in which neurons generally respond to stimuli in larger and larger regions of the visual field, but require increasing amounts of specific features or properties to excite them. This processing pathway culminates in the inferotemporal cortex, which specializes in pattern recognition problems involving choice and discrimination. Neurons in this region typically respond to very large areas of the visual field, usually including the fovea, and their responses are highly modified by visual experience and by the nature of the visual task currently being executed.

The parietal pathway, in contrast, specializes in physical features of the visual world, such as motion and location. One area contains a map of the cortex that specializes in motion of objects, whereas others contain neurons that respond both to characteristics of the visual world and to intended movements (GRASPING MOVEMENTS: VISUOMOTOR TRANSFORMATIONS). The areas serving the sensorimotor functions of vision are only a small part of the parietal lobe; dividing the cognitive and sensorimotor functions into temporal and parietal areas is a convenient first approximation, but several areas anatomically superior to the primary visual cortex (in occipito-parietal regions) are involved in the "temporal" stream. Some areas are involved in both functions.

A key task of the parietal stream is transformation of visual information into motor coordinates. As a first approximation, parietal visual cortex can be divided into five regions: (1) the lateral intraparietal area activated by both saccades and attention; (2) the parietal reach region that is activated by pointing and is also modulated by eye position; (3) the anterior intraparietal area active during visual grasp and also tactile manipulation; (4) the caudal intraparietal sulcus involved in object matching and grasping; and (5) the ventral intraparietal area, responding to visual motion toward the face (Culham and Kanwisher, 2001). Parietal regions are central to attention, eye movements, and orienting.

The spatial function can be further subdivided into two pathways that reflect different modes of spatial coding. Receptive fields of neurons in the lateral intraparietal area are spatially corrected before each rapid eye movement, so that they respond to stimuli that will be in their retinotopic receptive fields (i.e., in retinally based coordinates) following a planned eye movement (Duhamel, Colby, and Goldberg, 1992). The changes in these receptive fields can also be conceived as activity that signals candidates for planned eye movements.

A second coding scheme is seen in parietal area 7a. Neurons in this area provide information sufficient to reconstruct spatial position in head-centered coordinates (Andersen, Essick, and Siegel, 1985). These neurons respond strongly only if the eyes are in a particular position in the orbit and a target occupies a particular retinal location, in a multiplicative interaction. Simulations showed that such a network of cells codes information sufficient to derive spatiotopic output (Zipser and Andersen, 1988). A parallel distributed processing network was trained to respond to targets at particular locations in a visual field. After training, the response properties of the nodes in the model resembled the receptive fields of neurons in area 7a.

Spatial processing may be too basic a function to be limited to the parietal cortex, a relatively high-order structure that is well differentiated only in primates. Some features of the midbrain superior colliculus, such as broad intermodal integration and close connection to oculomotor control, suggest a role in sensorimotor vision (COLLICULAR VISUOMOTOR TRANSFORMATIONS FOR GAZE CONTROL), reflecting the earlier midbrain/forebrain distinction.

Clinical Evidence

Damage to part of the primary visual cortex in human patients results in functional blindness in the affected field—a scotoma. Patients have no visual experience in the scotoma, but when forced to point to targets located there, which they insist they cannot see, they point fairly accurately by using sensorimotor information unavailable to their perception. Visual information coexisting with a lack of visual experience is called blindsight (Weiskrantz et al., 1974); it is an example of visually guided behavior without the experience of perception. It may be made possible by an alternative pathway from the retina to nonstriate visual cortex through the superior colliculus or other subcortical structures. Recent work has shown surprisingly sophisticated processing without awareness, including orientation and color discriminations.

Another example of dissociation of sensoriomotor and cognitive function has been found in a patient with damage to lateral occipital and occipitoparietal cortex (Goodale and Milner, 1992). When asked to match line orientations, the patient could not reliably distinguish horizontal from vertical, though she had no scotoma in which visual experience was altogether absent. Asked to put a card through a slot at varying orientations, however, she oriented the card correctly even as she raised her hand from the start position. There was a dissociation between her inability to perceive object orientation and her ability to direct accurate reaching movements toward objects of varying orientations. Her cognitive representation of space was unavailable, while sensorimotor representation remained intact. The complementary dissociation, with retention of perception accompanied by loss of ability to use visual information to control movements of the limb and hand, is seen clinically under the label of optic ataxia.

Such examples demonstrate separate cognitive and sensorimotor representations, but only in patients with brain damage. When a human suffers brain damage with partial loss of visual function, there is always the possibility that the visual system will reorganize itself, isolating fragments of the machinery that normally function as a unit. The clinical examples, then, leave open the possibility that the system may function differently in intact humans. Any rigorous proof that normal visual function shows the cognitive/sensorimotor distinction must include psychophysical measures in intact humans.

Psychophysics of Space

Some of the earliest evidence for a cognitive/sensorimotor distinction in normal subjects came from studies of rapid (saccadic) eye movements. Subjects are normally unaware of sizable displacements of the visual world if the displacements occur during saccadic eye movements. This implies that information about spatial location is degraded during saccades. There is a seeming paradox to this degradation, however, for people do not become disoriented after saccades, implying that spatial information is maintained. Experimental evidence supports this conclusion. For instance, the eyes can saccade accurately to a target that is flashed (and mislocalized) during an earlier saccade, and hand-eye coordination remains fairly accurate following saccades. How can perceptual information be lost while visually guided behavior is preserved?

To resolve this paradox, it should be noted that the conflicting observations use different response measures. The experiments on perception of displacement during saccades require a symbolic response, such as a nonspatial verbal report or a button press, with an arbitrary spatial relationship to the target. Orienting of the eye or hand, in contrast, requires quantitative spatial information, defined as requiring a 1:1 correspondence between a target position and a motor behavior, such as directing the hand or the eyes to the target. The conflict might be resolved if the two types of measure, which can be labeled as cognitive and sensorimotor, could be combined in a single experiment. If two visual pathways process different kinds of information, spatially oriented motor activities might have access to accurate position information even when that information is unavailable at a cognitive level.

The two conflicting observations (perceptual suppression on one hand and accurate motor behavior on the other) were combined by asking subjects to jab the position of a target that had been displaced and then extinguished (reviewed in Bridgeman, Peery, and Anand, 1997). On some trials the target jump was detected, while on others the jump went undetected due to a simultaneous eye movement (monitored photoelectrically). As one would expect, subjects could point accurately to the position of the now-extinguished target following a detected displacement. Pointing was equally good, however, following an undetected displacement. It appeared that updating information was available to the motor system but not to perception.

This result implied that quantitative control of motor activity was unaffected by the perceptual detectability of target position. One can also interpret the result in terms of signal detection theory as a high response criterion for the report of displacement. The first control for this possibility was a two-alternative forced-choice measure of saccadic suppression of displacement. This criterion-free measure showed an inability to perceive displacements under conditions where pointing was accurate even when the target had been displaced (Bridgeman and Stark, 1979). Information was available to a sensorimotor system controlling pointing, but not to a cognitive system informing visual perception.

Dissociation of cognitive and sensorimotor function has also been demonstrated by giving cognitive and sensorimotor systems opposite signals at the same time. This is a more rigorous way to separate cognitive and sensorimotor systems. A signal was inserted selectively into the cognitive system with stroboscopic induced motion. In this illusion a surrounding frame was displaced, creating the illusion that a target jumps although it remains fixed relative to the subject. We know that induced motion affects the cognitive system, because we experience the effect and subjects can make verbal judgments of it. But the above saccadic suppression experiments (Bridgeman and Stark, 1979) implied that the information used for motor behavior might come from sources unavailable to perception.

In the experiment, a target spot jumped in the same direction as a frame, but not far enough to cancel the induced motion. The spot still appeared to jump in the direction opposite the frame. Saccadic eye movements followed the actual jump direction, even though subjects perceived stroboscopic motion in the opposite direction (Wong and Mack, 1981). If a delay in responding was required, however, eye movements followed the perceptual illusion. This implies that the sensorimotor system has no memory, but must rely on information from the cognitive system when responding to what was previously present rather than what is currently present.

All of these techniques involve motion or displacement, leaving open the possibility that the dissociations are associated in some way with motion systems, rather than with representation of visual location per se. Motion and location may be confounded in some kinds of visual coding schemes. A newer design allows the examination of visual context in a situation where there is no motion

or displacement at any time (Bridgeman et al., 2000). The design is based on the Roelofs effect, a perceptual illusion seen when a static frame is offset to the left or the right of a subject's centerline. Objects that lie within the frame tend to be mislocalized in the direction opposite the offset of the frame. For example, in an otherwise featureless field, a rectangle is presented to the subject's left. Both the rectangle and stimuli within it tend to be localized too far to the right.

A Roelofs effect is seen with a perceptual measure, but subjects point without error. If a delay in responding causes subjects to switch from using sensorimotor information directly to using information imported from the cognitive representation, delaying the response should force them to switch to using cognitive information. By delaying the response cue long enough, all subjects showed a Roelofs effect in both pointing and judging. Thus, this design showed a switch from motor to cognitive information in directing the motor response; the cognitive illusion appears after a delay of about 2 s (Bridgeman et al., 2000; Rossetti, 2000). In the delay case, information flowed from the cognitive system, with the illusion, to the sensorimotor system and thence to behavior. However, the perception of the Roelofs effect shows that accurate sensorimotor information never corrects perception. Thus the arrow from cognitive to sensorimotor in Figure 1 extends in only one direction.

An even longer motor memory is seen for the slopes of hills, where veridical information endures for several minutes despite exaggerated perceptions of the slopes (Creem and Proffitt, 1998). The sensorimotor branch of the system seems to hold spatial information just long enough to direct current motor activity, but no longer. These authors have also shown that the sensorimotor system does not have access to top-down information about the conventional uses of an object. A group of objects is arrayed before a subject with their handles facing away. They will be grasped by their handles if the cognitive system is available to help organize the movement, but if the cognitive system is distracted by another, non-motoric task, the objects will be grasped skillfully but inappropriately by their closest parts. This result raises another issue, the extent of object coding in the sensorimotor system.

Psychophysics of Objects

The cognitive system needs detailed information to identify top-down information about the meanings and uses of objects, while the sensorimotor system needs only information about size, location, and graspability.

Research on object properties has followed several methods. One method is based on the Ebbinghaus illusion, also called the Titchner circles illusion. A circle looks larger if it is surrounded by smaller circles than if it is surrounded by larger circles. Haffenden and Goodale (1998) measured the illusion by asking subjects either to indicate the apparent size of a circle or to pick it up. In both cases neither hand nor target could be seen during the movement. The illusion was larger for the size estimations than for the grasp, indicating that the sensorimotor system was relatively insensitive to the illusion.

A challenge to this line of research came from Franz et al. (2000), who analyzed the Ebbinghaus illusion into two half-illusions: comparing a circle surrounded by larger circles to a circle alone, and comparing a circle surrounded by smaller circles to a circle alone. When the small-circle context and the large-circle context are compared directly, a super-additivity occurs: the illusion is larger than the sum of the two half-illusions. Because grasp necessarily involves a circle alone, the differences between grasp and perception were explained. Goodale has recently clarified this issue by showing that it is the physical distance between the inducing circles and the target circle, not the size of the circles, that influences grasp aperture. Perception, in contrast, is based on the size difference between the inducing circles and the target circle.

Discussion

Information about egocentric spatial location and some object properties is available at a motor level despite cognitive illusions of location. Egocentric localization information is available to the sensorimotor system even while the cognitive system, relying on relative motion and relative position information, holds unreliable information about location. Spatial information can flow from the cognitive to the sensorimotor representation if the sensorimotor information has degraded due to delay, but information cannot flow in the other direction. The two-visual-systems conception applies not only to the localization of objects, but also to their properties.

Road Map: Vision
Related Reading: Object Recognition; Face Recognition: Neurophysiology and Neural Technology; Visual Attention; Visual Scene Perception

References

Andersen, R. M., Essick, G., and Siegel, R., 1985, The encoding of spatial location by posterior parietal neurons, *Science*, 230:456–458.
Bridgeman, B., Gemmer, A., Forsman, T., and Huemer, V., 2000, Processing spatial information in the sensorimotor branch of the visual system, *Vision Research*, 40:3539–3552.
Bridgeman, B., Peery, S., and Anand, S., 1997, Interaction of cognitive and sensorimotor maps of visual space, *Perception and Psychophysics*, 59:456–469.
Bridgeman, B., and Stark, L., 1979, Omnidirectional increase in threshold for image shifts during saccadic eye movements, *Perception and Psychophysics*, 25:241–243.
Creem, S., and Proffitt, D., 1998, Two memories for geographical slant: Separation and interdependence of action and awareness, *Psychonomic Bull. Rev.*, 5:22–36. ◆
Culham, J. C., and Kanwisher, N. G., 2001, Neuroimaging of cognitive functions in human parietal cortex, *Curr. Opin. Neurobiol.*, 2001, 11:157–163
Duhamel, J., Colby, C., and Goldberg, M. E., 1992, The updating of the representation of visual space in parietal cortex by intended eye movements, *Science*, 255:90–92.
Franz, V., Gegenfurtner, K., Bülthoff, H., and Fahle, M., 2000, Grasping visual illusions: No evidence for a dissociation between perception and action, *Psychol. Sci.*, 11:20–25.
Goodale, M. A., and Milner, A. D., 1992, Separate visual pathways for perception and action, *Trends Neurosci.*, 15:20–25. ◆
Haffenden, A. M., and Goodale, M. A., 1998, The effect of pictorial illusion on prehension and perception, *J. Cognit. Neurosci.*, 10:122–136.
Mishkin, M., Ungerleider, L., and Macko, K., 1983, Object vision and spatial vision: Two cortical pathways, *Trends Neurosci.*, 6:414–417. ◆
Rossetti, Y., 2000, Implicit perception in action: Short lived motor representations of space, in *Consciousness and Brain Circuitry* (P. Grossenbacher, Ed.), Amsterdam: John Benjamins Publishers, pp. 131–179.
Schneider, G. E., 1969, Two visual systems, *Science*, 163:895–902.
Weiskrantz, L., Warrington, E., Sanders, M., and Marshall, J., 1974, Visual capacity in the hemianopic field following a restricted occipital ablation, *Brain*, 97:709–728.
Wong, E., and Mack, A., 1981, Saccadic programming and perceived location, *Acta Psychologica*, 48:123–131.
Zipser, J., and Andersen, R. A., 1988, A back-propogation programmed network that simulates response properties of a subset of posterior parietal neurons, *Nature*, 33:679–684.

Dopamine, Roles of

Jean-Marc Fellous and Roland E. Suri

Introduction

Dopamine (DA) is a neuromodulator (see NEUROMODULATION IN INVERTEBRATE NERVOUS SYSTEMS) that originates from small groups of neurons in the mesencephalon [the ventral tegmental area (A10), the substantia nigra (A9) and A8], and the diencephalon (area A13, A14 and A15). Dopaminergic projections are in general very diffuse and reach large portions of the brain. The time scales of dopamine actions are diverse, from a few hundred milliseconds to several hours. This chapter will focus on the mesencephalic dopamine centers because they are the most studied, and because they are thought to be involved in diseases such as Tourette's syndrome, schizophrenia, Parkinson's disease, Huntington's disease, drug addiction, and depression (see Tzschentke, 2001). These centers are also involved in normal brain functions, such as working memory, reinforcement learning, and attention. This chapter briefly summarizes the main roles of dopamine with respect to recent modeling approaches.

Biophysical Effects of Dopamine

The effects of dopamine on membrane currents and synaptic transmission are complex and depend on the nature and distribution of the postsynaptic receptors. At the single-cell level, in the in vitro rat preparation, DA has been found to either increase or decrease the excitability of neurons, through the modulation of specific sets of sodium, potassium, and calcium currents (see Gulledge and Jaffe, 1998, and Nicola, Surmeier, and Malenka, 2000, for reviews). Although the exact nature of the modulation is still debated, it is likely to depend on the opposing contributions of the D1/D5 and D2/D3 family of dopamine receptors that are respectively positively and negatively coupled with adenylate cyclase. Studies in monkey cortical tissue showed that the D1/D5 family of receptor was 20-fold more abundant than the D2/D3 family, and that these receptors were present distally in both pyramidal and nonpyramidal cells (Goldman-Rakic, Muly, and Williams, 2000).

Dopamine modulates excitatory and inhibitory synaptic transmission. Although the nature of neuromodulation of inhibitory transmission is still debated, it appears that in both the cortex and the striatum, D1 receptor activation selectively enhances NMDA but not AMPA synaptic transmission. Because of their voltage dependence, NMDA currents are smaller at rest than in a depolarized state when the postsynaptic cell is firing. Experimental and theoretical evidence suggest that the dopamine enhancement of NMDA currents may be used to induce working memory-like (see later discussion) bistable states in large networks of pyramidal neurons (Lisman, Fellous, and Wang, 1998).

In rats in vivo, stimulation of the ventral tegmental area or local application of dopamine decreases the spontaneous firing of the prefrontal cortex (Thierry et al., 1994), striatum, and nucleus accumbens (Nicola et al., 2000), suggesting that dopamine may be able to control the levels of noise, and hence signal-to-noise ratios.

Given that dopamine modulation strongly depends on the particular distribution of D1/D5 and D2/D3 receptors and on the particular pattern of incoming synaptic transmission, the biophysical effects of dopamine on the intrinsic and synaptic properties is likely to differ from one neuron to the next, raising the intriguing possibility of the existence of several subclasses of neurons that differ mainly by their responses to this neuromodulator.

Dopamine Levels Influence Working Memory

Working memory refers to the ability to hold a few items in mind, with the explicit purpose of working with them to yield a behavior (SHORT-TERM MEMORY). Typically, working memory tasks, such as spatial delayed match-to-sample tasks, consist of the brief presentation of a cue-stimulus (bright dot flashing once) in one of the four quadrants of a screen, followed by a delay period of several seconds, and by a test in which the subject has to respond only if the test stimulus appears the same quadrant as the cue-stimulus. Single-cell studies in monkeys revealed that some prefrontal cortical cells increased their firing rate during the delay period, when the stimulus is no longer present but when the animal has to remember its location in order to later perform the correct action. Both pyramidal cells and interneurons may present this property. The activity of these cells is stimulus dependent, so that only the cells that encode for the spatial location where the cue-stimulus occurred remain active during the delay period.

Local iontophoretic administrations of DA in the prefrontal cortex of monkeys performing a working memory task increase the cells' firing rate during the delay period, without increasing background noise, essentially increasing the signal-to-noise ratio during the task. There is, however, an optimal level of dopamine concentration above and below which working memory becomes impaired. Current theories propose that this effect is due to the enhancement by dopamine of excitatory inputs on pyramidal cells and interneurons. Because DA is more effective in facilitating excitatory transmission on pyramidal cells than on interneurons, intermediate levels of DA improve performance, while higher levels of DA recruit feedforward inhibition and decrease pyramidal cell output, thereby resulting in impairments in the task. Low levels of DA would not be sufficient to induce excitatory facilitation, yielding a poor pyramidal cell output, and hence an impairment (Figure 1 and Goldman-Rakic et al., 2000). There have been a few attempts at modeling the neural substrate of working memory, but very little has yet been done to account for the role of dopamine (Tanaka, 2001).

Dopamine Responses Resemble Reward Prediction Signal of TD Model

A large body of experimental evidence led to the hypothesis that Pavlovian learning depends on the degree of the unpredictability of the reinforcer (Dickinson, 1980). According to this hypothesis, reinforcers become progressively less efficient for behavioral adaptation as their predictability grows during the course of learning. The difference between the actual occurrence and the prediction of the reinforcer is usually referred to as the "error" in the reinforcer prediction. This concept has been used in the temporal-difference model (TD model) of Pavlovian learning (REINFORCEMENT LEARNING IN MOTOR CONTROL). If the reinforcer is a reward, the TD model uses a reward prediction error signal to learn a reward prediction signal. The error signal progressively decreases and shifts to the time of earlier stimuli that predict the reinforcer. The characteristics of the reward prediction signal are comparable to those of anticipatory responses such as salivation in Pavlov's experiment.

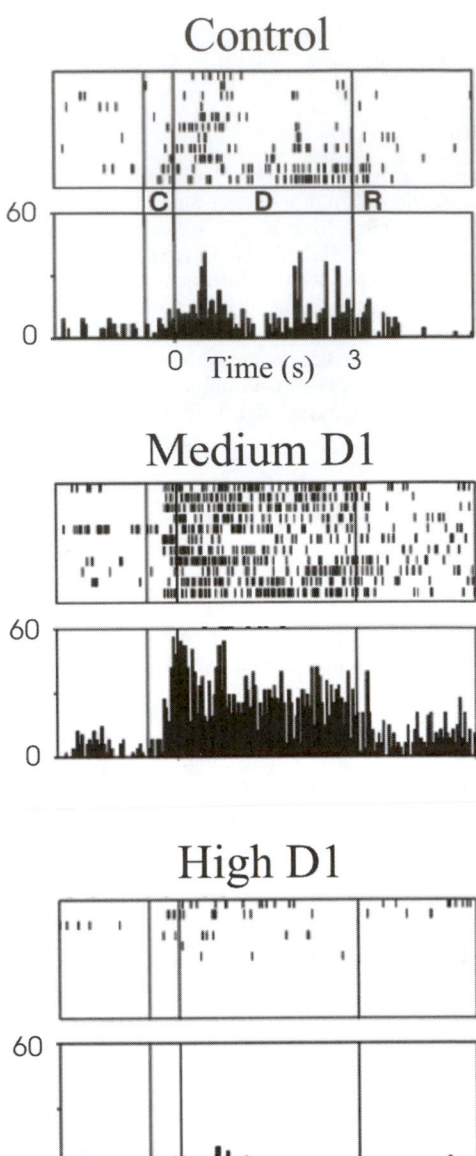

Figure 1. Biphasic effects of dopamine during a working memory task. The task consisted of the brief presentation of a cue (C), a delay of 3 seconds (D), and a response (R). Moderate levels of local application of SCH39166 (25 nA), a D1 receptor agonist, dramatically enhanced the activity of this cell, without significantly increasing its background activity (before cue). Higher levels of SCH39166 (75 nA) decreased the activity of this cell throughout the task. Histogram units are spikes/s. (Figure adapted from Goldman-Rakic, Muly, and Williams, 2000.)

The reward prediction error signal of the TD model remained a purely hypothetical signal until researchers discovered that the activity of midbrain dopamine neurons is strikingly similar to the reward prediction error of the TD model (Figure 2A) (Montague, Dayan, and Sejnowski, 1996; Schultz, 1998). Advances in reinforcement learning theories, as well as evidence for the involvement of dopamine in sensorimotor learning and in cognitive functions, led to the development of the Extended TD model. The reward prediction error signal of the TD model by Suri and Schultz (1999) reproduces dopamine neuron activity in several situations: (1) upon presentation of unpredicted rewards, (2) before, during,

Figure 2. *A*, Prediction error signal of the TD model (left) similar to dopamine neuron activity (right). If a neutral stimulus A is paired with reward, prediction error signal and dopamine activity respond to the reward (before learning). After repeated pairings, the prediction error signal and dopamine activity are already increased by stimulus A and on baseline levels at the time of the reward (after learning). If the stimulus A is conditioned to a reward but is occasionally presented without reward, the prediction error signal and dopamine activity are decreased below baseline levels at the predicted time of reward (omitted reward). *B*, Interactions between cortex, basal ganglia, and midbrain dopamine neurons according to the Actor-Critic models. The limbic areas correspond to the Critic and the sensorimotor areas to the Actor. The striatum is divided into matrisomes (sensorimotor) and striosomes (limbic). Limbic cortical areas project to striosomes, whereas neocortical areas chiefly project to matrisomes. Midbrain dopamine neurons are contacted by medium spiny neurons in striosomes and project to both striatal compartments. They are proposed to influence sensorimotor learning in the matrisomes (instrumental learning) and learning of reward predictions in the striosomes (Pavlovian learning). Striatal matrisomes inhibit the basal ganglia output nuclei Gpi/SNr and can elicit actions due to their projections via thalamic nuclei to motor cortical areas. Several additional functions of this architecture were proposed in Suri, Bargas, and Arbib, 2001. (Figure adapted from Suri and Schultz, 1998.)

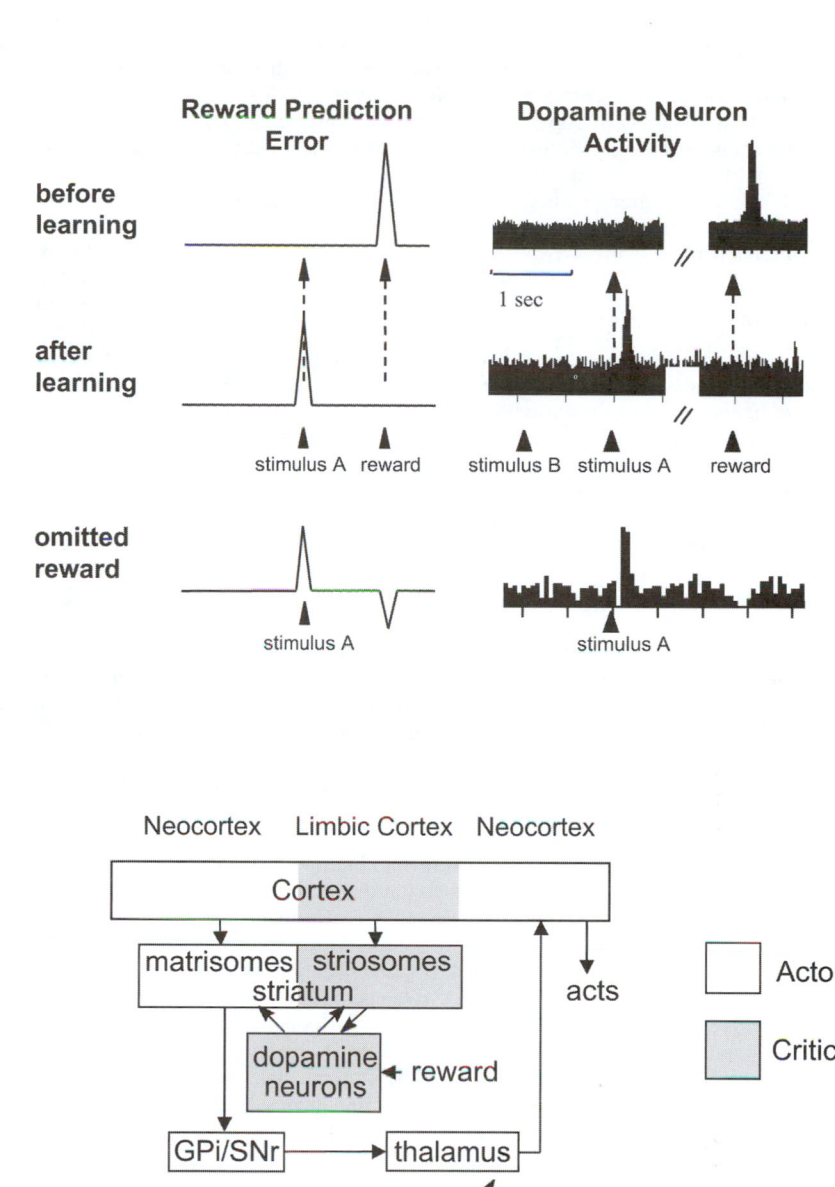

and after learning that a stimulus precedes a reward, (3) when two stimuli precede a reward with fixed time intervals, (4) when the interval between the two stimuli are varied, (5) when a reward is unexpectedly omitted, (6) when a reward is delayed, (7) when a reward occurs earlier than expected, (8) when a reward-predictive stimulus is unexpectedly omitted, (9) when there is a novel, physically salient stimulus that has never been associated with reward (see allocation of attention, discussed later in this chapter), (10) and when a blocking paradigm is used. To reach this close correspondence, three constants of the TD model were tuned to characteristics of dopamine neuron activity (learning rate, decay of eligibility trace, and temporal discount factor), some weights were initialized with positive values to achieve (9), and some ad hoc changes of the TD algorithm were introduced to reproduce (7) (see later discussion).

In Pavlov's experiment, the salivation response of the dog does not influence food delivery. The TD model is a model of Pavlovian

learning and therefore computes predictive signals, corresponding to the salivation response, but does not select optimal actions. In contrast, instrumental learning paradigms, such as learning to press a lever for food delivery, demonstrate that animals are able to learn to perform actions that optimize reward. To model sensorimotor learning in such paradigms, a model component called the Actor is taught by the reward prediction error signal of the TD model. In such architectures, the TD model is also called the Critic. This approach is consistent with animal learning theory and was successfully applied to machine learning studies (REINFORCEMENT LEARNING IN MOTOR CONTROL). Midbrain dopamine neurons project to the striatum and cortex and are characterized by rather uniform responses throughout the whole neuron population. Computational modeling studies with Actor-Critic models show that such a dopamine-like reward prediction error can serve as a powerful teaching signal for learning with delayed reward and for learning of motor sequences (Suri and Schultz, 1999). These models are also consistent with the role of dopamine in drug addiction and electrical self-stimulation (see later discussion). Comparison of the Actor-Critic architecture to biological structures suggests that the Critic may correspond to pathways from limbic cortex via limbic striatum (or striosomes) to dopamine neurons, whereas the Actor may correspond to pathways from neocortex via sensorimotor striatum (or matrisomes) to basal ganglia output nuclei (BASAL GANGLIA) (Figure 2B). Although this standard Actor-Critic model mimics learning of sensorimotor associations or habits, it does not imply that dopamine is involved in anhedonia.

Allocation of Attention

Several lines of evidence suggest that dopamine is also involved in attention processes. Although the firing rates of dopamine neurons can be increased or decreased for aversive stimuli, dopamine concentration in striatal and cortical target areas are often increased (Schultz, 1998). Both findings are not necessarily inconsistent, since small differences in firing rates of dopamine neurons are hard to detect with single neuron recordings, and measurement methods for dopamine concentration usually have less temporal resolution than methods used to measure spiking activity. Furthermore, dopamine concentration is not only influenced by dopamine neuron activity but also by local regulatory processes. Slow changes in cortical or striatal dopamine concentration may signal information completely unrelated to reward. Also, relief following aversive situations may influence dopamine neuron activity as if it were a reward, which would be consistent with opponent processing theories (CONDITIONING). Allocation of attentional resources seems to determine dopamine neuron activity in situations when a reward is delivered earlier than usual. In contrast to any linear model, including the standard TD model, dopamine neuron activity is on baseline levels at the time of the expected reward in this situation. This suggests that delivery of the reward earlier than usual seems to reallocate attentional resources through competitive mechanisms (Suri and Schultz, 1999).

Dopamine neurons respond to a novel, physically salient stimulus even if the stimulus has never been associated with a reward (Schultz, 1998). In contrast to reward-predictive responses, for stimuli of equal physical salience, the increase due to novelty responses seems to be smaller and is followed by a pronounced decrease of neural activity below baseline levels. (Brief and less pronounced decreases of dopamine neuron activity sometimes also occur after a response to a reward.) In contrast to responses to conditioned stimuli, novelty responses extinguish for repeated stimulus presentations. The characteristics of this novelty response are consistent with the TD model if certain associative weights are initialized with positive values instead of using initial values of zero (Suri and Schultz, 1999). Such weights initialization with positive values was proposed in machine learning studies to stimulate exploration of novel actions. Simulation studies demonstrated that such a novelty bonus hardly influences slow movements of more than 100 msec duration because the effects of the two phases in the firing of dopamine neurons cancel out and the movement starts after the biphasic response. However, dopamine novelty responses may stimulate exploration for very brief actions, which may include saccades or allocation of attentional resources (Suri and Schultz, 1999).

Redgrave and collaborators (Redgrave, Prescott, and Gurney, 1999) argued that the latency of dopamine responses is too short to be consistent with the hypothesis that dopamine is a reward prediction signal. Onsets of dopamine novelty responses as well as reward responses seem to occur just before the start of the saccade or during the saccade. The dopamine response will likely occur after the superior colliculus has detected a visual target but prior to the triggering (by collicular neurons) of the saccadic movement required to bring the target to the fovea. If it is assumed that the animal must execute a saccade to a visually presented stimulus before it can adequately assess its predictive value, the latency of dopamine response would be too short to signal reward. We argue against this view. Neural activities in cortical and subcortical areas reflect the anticipated future visual image before a saccade is elicited (Ross et al., 2001). Therefore, the representations of future visual images may influence dopamine neuron activity as if the saccade has already been executed, and thus the dopamine response may start slightly before the saccade. The Extended TD model computes such predictive signals and uses them to select goal-directed actions in a cognitive task (Suri, Bargas, and Arbib, 2001). According to this Actor-Critic model, the interactions between dopamine neuron activities (computed by Critic) and activities that reflect the preparation for intended actions (in Actor) select the actions that maximize reward predictions. The model evaluates the expected values of future actions, without necessarily executing them, in order to select the action with the optimal predicted outcome. The model selects the optimal action from such "action ideas" or "imagined actions." This optimal action is selected by assuming that dopamine neuron activity increases the signal-to-noise-ratio in target neurons. According to this advanced Actor-Critic model, dopamine improves focusing of attention to intended actions and selects actions. Since some neural activities anticipate the retinal images that result in saccades before these saccades are executed (Ross et al., 2001), animals may indeed use such predictive mechanisms for the selection of intentional saccades. Furthermore, similar internal mechanisms may bias intentional switching capabilities of the basal ganglia to facilitate the allocation of behavioral and cognitive processing capacity toward unexpected events (see BASAL GANGLIA and Redgrave et al., 1999). If we assume similar functions of dopamine for short-term memory, this model suggests that dopamine may select the items that should be kept in short-term memory and may also help to sustain their representation over time.

Conclusions

In vitro studies of the biophysical effects of dopamine demonstrate a wide range of dopamine effects on the intrinsic and synaptic properties of individual cells. In vivo studies suggest, however, that the main overall effect of dopamine may be to control noise levels and to selectively enhance the signal-to-noise-ratio of neural processing. This action may behaviorally lead to an improvement of working memory and to better selection of goal-directed actions. The TD model reproduces dopamine neuron activity in many behavioral situations and suggests that dopamine neuron activity codes for an error in reward prediction. This chapter described a TD model that solves cognitive tasks including goal-directed actions (also called planning or intentional actions) and that attempts to reproduce the function of dopamine in attention and preparation processes.

Road Map: Biological Networks
Related Reading: Basal Ganglia; Emotional Circuits; Neuromodulation in Invertebrate Nervous Systems; Neuromodulation in Mammalian Nervous Systems

References

Dickinson, A., 1980, Contemporary animal learning theory, Cambridge, UK: Cambridge University Press.
Goldman-Rakic, P. S., Muly III, E. C., and Williams, G. V., 2000, D(1) receptors in prefrontal cells and circuits, *Brain Res. Rev.*, 31:295–301.
Gulledge, A. T., and Jaffe, D. B., 1998, Dopamine decreases the excitability of layer V pyramidal cells in the rat prefrontal cortex, *J. Neurosci.*, 18:9139–9151.

Lisman, J. E., Fellous, J.-M., and Wang, X.-J., 1998, A role for NMDA-receptor channels in working memory, *Nature Neurosci.*, 1:273–275. ◆

Montague, P. R., Dayan, P., and Sejnowski, T. J., 1996, A framework for mesencephalic dopamine systems based on predictive Hebbian learning, *J. Neurosci.*, 16:1936–1947.

Nicola, S. M., Surmeier, J., and Malenka, R. C., 2000, Dopaminergic modulation of neuronal excitability in the striatum and nucleus accumbens, *Annu. Rev. Neurosci.*, 23:185–215.

Redgrave, P., Prescott, T. J., and Gurney, K., 1999, Is the short-latency dopamine response too short to signal reward error? *Trends Neurosci.*, 22:146–151.

Ross, J., Morrone, M. C., Goldberg, M. E., and Burr, D. C., 2001, Changes in visual perception at the time of saccades, *Trends Neurosci.*, 24:113–121.

Schultz, W., 1998, Predictive reward signal of dopamine neurons, *J. Neurophysiol.*, 80:1–27.

Suri, R. E., and Schultz, W., 1998, Learning of sequential movements by neural network model with dopamine-like reinforcement signal, *Exp. Brain Res.*, 121:350–354.

Suri, R. E., and Schultz, W., 1999, A neural network model with dopamine-like reinforcement signal that learns a spatial delayed response task, *Neurosci.*, 91:871–890. ◆

Suri, R. E., Bargas, J., and Arbib, M. A., 2001, Modeling functions of striatal dopamine modulation in learning and planning, *Neurosci.*, 103:65–85. ◆

Tanaka, S., 2001, Computational approaches to the architecture and operations of the prefrontal cortical circuit for working memory, *Prog. Neuropsychopharmacol. Biol. Psychiat.*, 25:259–281. ◆

Thierry, A. M., Jay, T. M., Pirot, S., Mantz, J., Godbout, R., and Glowinski, J., 1994, Influence of afferent systems on the activity of the rat prefrontal cortex: Electrophysiological and pharmacological characterization, in *Motor and Cognitive Functions of the Prefrontal Cortex* (A. M. J. Thierry, P. S. Goldman-Rakic, and Y. Christen, Eds.), New York: Springer-Verlag. pp. 35–50.

Tzschentke, T. M., 2001, Pharmacology and behavioral pharmacology of the mesocortical dopamine system, *Prog. Neurobiol.*, 63:241–320.

Dynamic Link Architecture

Christoph von der Malsburg

Introduction: The Architecture

The dynamic laws governing the brain's physical elements and their interaction enable it to fall into functionally useful states. The term neural architecture is taken here as referring to the shape of these dynamic laws. This article presents and discusses *dynamic link architecture* (DLA; von der Malsburg, 1981, 1985, 1986). There are various ways in which DLA has been couched in terms of equations (von der Malsburg, 1985; von der Malsburg and Schneider, 1986; von der Malsburg and Bienenstock, 1987; Bienenstock and von der Malsburg, 1987; Wiskott and von der Malsburg, 1996; Zhu and von der Malsburg, 2001). Because DLA has not yet received a canonical mathematical description, it is described here in abstract verbal terms. DLA is a construction site, and this article is an invitation to work at it.

According to DLA, the brain's data structure has the form of graphs composed of nodes (called units) connected by links. The graphs of DLA are dynamic: both units and links bear activity variables changing on the rapid functional time scale of fractions of a second. Graphs form a very versatile data format that is probably able to render the structure of any mental object. A particularly important feature is the ability of graphs to compose more complex data structures from simpler ones, an important requirement for the expression of cognitive structures (see COMPOSITIONALITY IN NEURAL SYSTEMS).

The units of DLA play the role of symbolic elements. This follows the tradition of associating neurons with elementary meaning (the identification of units with neurons is, however, not taken for granted here; see below). Units are endowed with structured signals changing in time. These signals can be evaluated under two aspects, intensity and correlation. Intensity measures the degree to which a unit is active in a given time interval, signifying the degree to which the meaning of the unit is alive in the mind of the animal. Correlations, on the other hand, quantify the degree to which the signal of one unit is related to that of others. The general idea is that identical signal patterns are strongly correlated, whereas statistically independent signal patterns have zero correlation. A correlation can be a binary relation, characterizing two units, or an n-ary relation, to be evaluated for n units at a time.

The strength of links can change on two time scales, represented by two variables called *temporary weight* and *permanent weight*.

The permanent weight corresponds to the usual synaptic weight, can change on the slow time scale of learning, and represents permanent memory. The temporary weight is constrained to the interval between zero and the permanent weight and can change on the same time scale as the unit activity (hence the name dynamic links).

Dynamic links constitute the glue by which higher data structures are built up from more elementary ones. Conversely, the absence of links (temporary or permanent) keeps mental objects separate from each other and prevents their direct interaction. In the simplest case, a link binds a descriptor to an object. For example, a link may bind a unit representing a color to another unit that stands for a specific object. More generally, mental objects are formed by binding together units representing constituent parts. The infinite richness and flexibility of the mind is thus made possible as a combinatorial game. The mental activity of familiar objects (like my grandmother, or a yellow Volkswagen) may be reliably correlated with the activity of specialized units, but these objects still acquire their substance—their imagined visual appearance, and so on—by the dynamical binding of appropriately structured arrays of other units. Units can be part of different functional contexts. They are integrated into a specific one by the activation of appropriate links. Dynamic links are the means by which the brain specializes its circuit diagram to the needs of the particular situation at hand.

Graph Dynamics

Under the influence of signal exchange, graphs and their units and links are subject to dynamic change, constituting a game of network self-organization (see SELF-ORGANIZATION AND THE BRAIN). The dynamic links have a resting strength near the value of the permanent weight. When the units connected by a permanent link become active, there is rapid feedback between the units' signal correlations and the link's strength, with a strong link tending to increase signal correlation and a strong correlation controlling the link to grow in strength toward the maximum set by the permanent weight. This feedback can also lead to a downward spiral, with a weak correlation reducing a link's strength and a weak link losing its grip on signals, which, under the influence of other links, drift apart toward lower correlation. Thus, links between active units tend to be driven toward one of their extreme values, zero or the maximum set by the permanent weight.

Links are subject to divergent and convergent competition: links converging on one unit compete with each other for strength, as do links diverging from one unit. This competition drives graphs to sparsity. Links are also subject to cooperation. Several links carrying correlated signal structure cooperate in imposing that signal structure on a common target unit, helping them all to grow. Because the ultimate cause for all signal structure is random, correlations can only be generated on the basis of common origin of pathways. Thus, cooperation runs between pathways that start at one point and converge to another point. The common origin of converging pathways may, of course, be an event or a pattern in the environment.

Cooperation and competition conspire to favor certain graph structures. These are distinguished by being sparse (that is, activating relatively few of the permanent links in or out of units) and by having a large number of cooperative meshes—arrangements of alternative pathways from one source to one target unit. Beyond these statements, a general characterization of graph attractor states is an open issue. However, there are certain known graph structures that have been shown in simulations to be attractor states and that prove to be very useful (see the section on applications). All of these graph structures may be characterized as "topological graphs": if their units are mapped appropriately into a low-dimensional display space (one- or two-dimensional in the known examples), the links of those graphs all run between units that are neighbors in the display space.

Slow Plasticity

In classical neural architectures, learning is modeled by *synaptic plasticity*, or the change of permanent synaptic weights under the control of neural signals. This general idea is also part of the dynamic link architecture. However, DLA imposes a further refinement in that a permanent weight grows only when the corresponding dynamic link has converged to its maximum strength, which happens only in the context of an organized graph structure. For a permanent link to grow, it is thus not sufficient for the two connected units to have high intensity in the same brain state; in addition, their signals must be correlated and their link must be active. This puts the extra condition on the growth of permanent connection weights that they be validated by indirect evidence, in the form of active indirect pathways between the units connected, and in the form of relative freedom from competition, the two conditions characterizing a well-structured dynamic graph. Thus, only the very few connections that are significant in this sense can grow.

Neural Implementation of Dynamic Links

How can the units, links, and dynamical rules of DLA be identified with known neural structures? This is possible in several ways. It will turn out that to some extent, DLA can be seen as a fair interpretation of known structures, whereas some experimental predictions also flow from it.

Units Are Individual Neurons

At the most fundamental level, units are to be identified with neurons, links with axons and synapses, signals with neural spike trains, and permanent weights with conventional synaptic strengths. Signal intensity is evaluated as firing rate, averaged over intervals of length Δ, whereas the stochastic signal fine structure within that interval is evaluated in terms of correlations with a resolution time τ, two spikes arriving within τ of each other being counted as simultaneous. The smallest reasonable choice for Δ is probably 100 ms or a little less; the smallest choice for τ may be 3 ms, as proposed in von der Malsburg (1981). Neural signals in the cerebral cortex have a very rich stochastic structure on all time scales, much of which is not correlated strongly with external stimuli in neurophysiological experiments (and is usually suppressed by averaging in a post-stimulus time histogram).

A point of contention at the present time is the precision with which nervous tissue can process temporal signal structure. Some authors (e.g., Shadlen and Movshon, 1999) believe that fine temporal structure cannot be transmitted by neurons, and that meaningful signal correlations cannot be extracted. The proposed argument is, however, circular, as it was assumed that neural input signals are random and independent. If this assumption is violated in the brain, the argument falls flat. Indeed, it has been shown (Mainen and Sejnowski, 1995) that spike timing of cortical neurons can be reliable with 1-ms precision if neural input is sufficiently structured, and similarly precise spike timing was found in response to temporally structured visual input seven synaptic generations behind the retina (Bair and Koch, 1995). The latter and other studies would encourage the assumption of a τ of 1 ms. A heated discussion has also sprung up around the status of the interpretation of signal correlations in terms of dynamic binding (SYNCHRONIZATION, BINDING AND EXPECTANCY) as proposed in von der Malsburg (1981; see also Shadlen and Movshon, 1999; Gray, 1999; Singer, 1999; von der Malsburg, 1999, and other articles in the same issue of *Neuron*). At the present time, the issue is the subject of intensive experimental study in many laboratories.

Dynamic links are realized at the single-neuron level as rapid reversible synaptic plasticity (RRP). Starting from a resting value, the temporary weight of a synapse is increased by correlations between the pre- and postsynaptic signals and is decreased if both signals are active in a given time period but are not correlated. The resting weight of a synapse is probably not too far from the maximum set by the permanent weight (so that RRP will manifest itself mainly in the form of rapid weight reduction). The interactions between temporary synaptic strength and signals is such as to constitute a positive feedback loop. Changes in temporary synaptic weights must take place on a fast time scale to be of functional significance, possibly as quickly as within 10 ms. In the prolonged absence of presynaptic or postsynaptic activity, the temporary weight rises or falls back toward its resting value, with a time scale that corresponds to short-term memory (perhaps a few dozen seconds), or it is reset by an active mechanism (for example, in the visual cortex during saccades). Convergent synaptic competition (competition between synapses at the same postsynaptic neuron) could be implemented by the signals arriving on one synapse or one set of synapses spoiling the postsynaptic activity for others. Divergent competition could be implemented with the help of inhibition between the target cells, making it difficult or impossible to synchronize them all with the same presynaptic signal.

The existence of rapid reversible changes in synaptic strength in cortex is a broadly documented experimental fact (see Hempel et al., 2000, for examples and a review of the experimental literature; see also TEMPORAL DYNAMICS OF BIOLOGICAL SYNAPSES). What has not been investigated experimentally in any detail is the dependence of rapid synaptic change on postsynaptic signals, and without such study the type of control postulated in RRP cannot be ascertained. There are many open details that must be determined experimentally. Among them is the identity of the relevant postsynaptic signal (membrane potential, some second messenger, e.g., Ca^{2+}, action potential, or other) and the precise definition of the dynamics of synaptic strength (which could require a delay between the presynaptic and postsynaptic signals, as described for long-term potentiation in Senn, Markram, and Tsodyks, 2001, and experimental work reviewed therein).

As was pointed out, implementation of DLA at the single-neuron level can be realized on a hierarchy of time scales Δ and the concomitant resolution time τ. So far I have discussed the faster end of the hierarchy. If Δ is taken to be a large fraction of a second or longer, we are in the domain of overt attention and the well-studied phenomenon of the mind shifting context sequentially on smaller and larger time scales. There is no doubt that a very important function of attention is keeping topics separate if their simultaneous activation would lead to confusion, and thus to provide temporal binding. A proper understanding of the mechanisms of attention will have to provide an answer to the question of how the focus of attention is formed. Part of the answer will be, of course, that it must unite elements that have something to do with each other (as recorded by the links between them), and not to activate simultaneously what would lead to confusion. The conceptual framework of DLA and its network self-organization are therefore appropriate for the description of attention dynamics.

Multicellular Units

Just as the DLA interpretation of neural dynamics can be applied at different temporal scales, it can also be applied at different spatial scales, either by identifying units with single neurons, as above, or by identifying units with groups of neurons. In this perspective, all individual neurons in a group, called a *multicellular unit* (MCU), are interpreted to have the same meaning. They differ, however, in the synaptic connections they have to neurons in other MCUs. The signal intensity of an MCU is the combined neural activity of all of its neurons. Signal correlations, however, are calculated by paying attention to the distribution of activity in MCUs and determining the combined synaptic weights of all connections between currently active cells in a pair of MCUs. By changing the distribution of activity over its neurons, an MCU can control the connectivity pattern it has to other MCUs. An important example of MCUs is constituted by the hypercolumns in visual cortex. All neurons in a hypercolumn have the same theme, subserving, by definition, one point in visual space. The neurons differ, however, in how they are connected with afferent neurons (which gives them different meaning on a more fine-grained level) and how they are connected to neurons in other hypercolumns.

MCU implementation of DLA differs in important points from the single-neuron implementation. The variables that constitute dynamic links are not temporary synaptic weights but neural spike activity, and correlations are not computed by time-consuming temporal integration over pairs of neural signals but by the instantaneous and parallel evaluation of the signals and connection weights of all active neurons in the MCUs involved. In consequence, with MCUs there is a much greater capacity to express highly structured graphs than in the single-cell implementation. The price for this greater power is much reduced flexibility, because appropriately specialized connectivity patterns within and between MCUs must first be installed.

Implementations of DLA on different temporal and spatial scales are not mutually exclusive and are probably realized concurrently in our brain. The single-cell version is indispensable because of its great flexibility and the absence of any need for specialized preexisting connectivity structures, but it is limited in its capacity to distinguish detailed link structures in limited time. The MCU version is very powerful and may be seen as just an unconventional view of networks in classic architecture, but it requires highly specialized connectivity structures and appropriately tuned activity dynamics.

Applications

The aim of DLA is to serve as a framework for understanding brain functions. Conventional neural network architecture, lacking the

equivalent of dynamic binding, may be a universal medium for realizing individual functions when they are defined ahead of time (such that appropriate combination-coding neurons and connectivity patterns can be defined and binding ambiguities avoided), but in decades of modeling attempts, this architecture has shown itself to be too narrow to go beyond elementary functions. DLA has the full functional repertoire of conventional neural network architecture but goes beyond it in being able to build up structured objects, have them interact in a structured way, or keep them from interfering. The full potential of DLA is far from realized, but some applications have already been modeled, as briefly reviewed in von der Malsburg (1999).

Figure-ground segmentation in visual scenes or other modalities is most naturally modeled by DLA (see VISUAL SCENE SEGMENTATION). So far, most concrete models have employed temporal signal correlations to bind all elements of a figure together and to keep them separate from elements belonging to the ground. For this type of model there is experimental evidence, as reviewed in Gray (1999) and Singer (1999). Also, MCU implementations have been realized in which each unit is subdivided into two subpopulations, one for figure, one for ground, and in a final state all units belonging to the figure restrict their activity to the "figure" neurons, all units in the ground just activate their "ground" neurons.

Many mental objects are met first as sensory arrays of local features. They are most naturally handled, stored, and recognized if the neighborhood relations between features are expressed as bindings and stored and retrieved as dynamic links. This has been realized as *dynamic link matching* for the purpose of invariant visual object recognition (reviewed in von der Malsburg, 1999, and FACE RECOGNITION: NEUROPHYSIOLOGY AND NEURAL TECHNOLOGY). Dynamic link matching, implemented in terms of temporal binding, has rightly been criticized as too slow to account for object recognition in adults. However, a recent implementation employing direct interaction between links (to be implemented with the help of MCUs, for instance) was shown to be very fast, requiring only one or a few iterations (Zhu and von der Malsburg, 2001).

As to the potential of DLA for modeling brain function and cognitive processes, the cited applications are but the tip of the iceberg. Processing and learning the syntactical structure of natural language on the basis of conventional neural architecture has proved very difficult to impossible. The reason is that the flexibility to analyze or to form novel sentences requires dynamic binding. It is particularly important here to realize the general process of instantiation, in which an abstract syntactical structure is applied to a concrete set of elements. Instantiation requires the manipulation of dynamic links between abstract roles and concrete role fillers, and requires the recognition of structural relations between abstract structures and concrete instances. Both of these functions are not part of the repertoire of conventional neural networks.

Road Maps: Artificial Intelligence; Neural Plasticity; Vision
Related Reading: Structured Connectionist Models; Synchronization, Binding and Expectancy; Visual Scene Segmentation

References

Bair, W., and Koch, C., 1995, Precision and reliability of neocortical spike trains in the behaving monkey, in *Computation and Neural Systems* (J. Bower, Ed.), Norwell, MA: Kluwer, pp. 53–58.

Bienenstock, E., and von der Malsburg, C., 1987, A neural network for invariant pattern recognition, *Europhys. Lett.*, 4:121–126.

Gray, C. M., 1999, The temporal correlation hypothesis of visual feature integration: Still alive and well, *Neuron*, 24:31–47.

Hempel, C. M., Hartman, K. H., Wang, X.-J., Turrigiano, G. G., and Nelson, S. B., 2000, Multiple forms of short-term plasticity at excitatory synapses in rat medial prefrontal cortex, *J. Neurophysiol.*, 83:3031–3041.

Mainen, Z. F., and Sejnowski, T. J., 1995, Reliability of spike timing in neocortical neurons, *Science*, 268:1503–1506.

Senn, W., Markram, H., and Tsodyks, M., 2001, An algorithm for modifying neurotransmitter release probability based on pre- and postsynaptic spike timing. *Neural. Computation*, 13:35–67.

Shadlen, M. N., and Movshon, J. A., 1999, Synchrony unbound: A critical evaluation of the temporal binding hypothesis, *Neuron*, 24:67–77.

Singer, W., 1999, Neuronal synchrony: A versatile code for the definition of relations? *Neuron*, 24:49–65.

von der Malsburg, C., 1981, *The Correlation Theory of Brain Function*, MPI Biophysical Chemistry, Internal Report 81–2, reprinted in *Models of Neural Networks II* (E. Domany, J. L. van Hemmen, and K. Schulten, Eds.), Berlin: Springer-Verlag, 1994, chap. 2, pp. 95–119. ◆

von der Malsburg, C., 1985, Nervous structures with dynamical links, *Ber. Bunsenges. Phys. Chem.*, 89:703–710.

von der Malsburg, C., 1986, Am I thinking assemblies? in *Proceedings of the Trieste Meeting on Brain Theory, October 1984* (G. Palm and A. Aertsen, Eds.), Berlin: Springer-Verlag, pp. 161–176.

von der Malsburg, C., 1999, The what and why of binding: The modeler's perspective, *Neuron*, 24:95–104.

von der Malsburg, C., and Bienenstock, E., 1987, A neural network for the retrieval of superimposed connection patterns, *Europhys. Lett.*, 3:1243–1249.

von der Malsburg, C., and Schneider, W., 1986, A neural cocktail-party processor, *Biol. Cybern.*, 54:29–40.

Wiskott, l., and von der Malsburg, C., 1996, Face recognition by dynamic link matching, in *Lateral Interactions in the Cortex: Structure and Function* (J. Sirosh, R. Miikkulainen, and Y. Choe, Eds.), electronic book, available: http://www.cs.utexas.edu/users/nn/web-pubs/htmlbook96/.

Zhu, J., and von der Malsburg, C., 2001, Synapto-synaptic interactions speed up dynamic link matching, presented at the Computational Neuroscience Meeting (CNS*01), San Francisco, CA, June 30–July 5, 2001.

Dynamic Remapping

Alexandre Pouget and Terrence J. Sejnowski

Introduction

The term *dynamic remapping* has been used in many different ways, but one of the clearest formulations of this concept comes from the mental rotation studies by Georgopoulos et al. (1989) (see also MOTOR CORTEX: CODING AND DECODING OF DIRECTIONAL OPERATIONS). In these experiments monkeys were trained to move a joystick in the direction of a visual stimulus or 90° counterclockwise from it. The brightness of the stimulus indicated which movement was required on a particular trial; a dim light corresponded to a 90° movement and a bright light to a direct movement. An analysis of reaction time suggested that, by default, the initial motor command always pointed straight at the target and then continuously rotated if the cue indicated a 90° rotation, an interpretation that was subsequently confirmed by single unit recordings.

The term *remapping* is also commonly used whenever a sensory input in one modality is transformed to a sensory representation in another modality. The best-known example in primates is the remapping of auditory space, from head-centered in the early stages of auditory processing to the retinotopic coordinates used in the superior colliculus (Jay and Sparks, 1987). This type of remapping, equivalent to a change of coordinates, is closely related to sensorimotor transformations. It does not have to be performed over time but could be accomplished by the neuronal circuitry connecting different representations.

This review is divided into three parts. In the first part, we briefly describe the types of cortical representations typically encountered in dynamic remapping. We then summarize the results from several physiological studies where it has been possible to characterize the responses of neurons involved in temporal and spatial remappings. Finally, in the third part, we review modeling efforts to account for these processes.

Neural Representation of Vectors

A saccadic eye movement toward an object in space can be represented as a vector **S** whose components S_x and S_y correspond to the horizontal and vertical displacement of the eyes. Any sensory, or motor, variable can be represented by a similar vector. There are two major ways of representing a vector in a neural population—by a topographic map and by a nontopographic vectorial representation.

The encoding of saccadic eye movements in the superior colliculus is an example of a topographic map representation. A saccade is specified by the activity of a two-dimensional layer of neurons organized as a Euclidean manifold (see COLLICULAR VISUOMOTOR TRANSFORMATIONS FOR GAZE CONTROL). Before a saccade, a bump of activity appears on the map at a location corresponding to the horizontal and vertical displacement of the saccade.

Another example of a vectorial code is the code for the direction of hand movements in the primate motor cortex. Neurons in the primary motor cortex respond maximally for a particular direction of hand movement with a cosine tuning curve around this preferred direction (Georgopoulos et al., 1989). This suggests that each cell encodes the projection of the vector along its preferred direction. [Todorov (2000) questions this interpretation, but the precise identity of the vector being encoded in motor cortex is not critical to the issue of remapping.]

In both cases, the original vector can be recovered from the population activity pattern using statistical estimators. Various examples of such estimators are described in POPULATION CODES.

Neurophysiological Correlates of Remapping

Continuous Remappings

Georgopoulos et al. (1989) studied how the population vector varies over time in the mental rotation experiment described in the introduction. They found that for movement 90° counterclockwise from the target, the vector encoded in M1 initially pointed in the target direction and then continuously rotated 90° counterclockwise, at which point the monkey initiated a hand movement (Figure 1A). This is consistent with the interpretation of the reaction time experiments: The monkey had initially planned to move toward the stimulus, and then updated this command according to the task requirement.

Similar continuous remapping occurs in the postsubiculum of the rat, one of the cortical structures involved in navigation of space. Neurons in the postsubiculum provide an internal compass that encodes the direction of the head with respect to remembered visual landmarks. The neurons have bell-shaped tuning curves around their best direction, similar to the code for hand direction in the primary motor cortex. Electrophysiological recordings have revealed that this vector is continuously updated as the head of the

Figure 1. *A*, Rotation of population vector in the primary motor cortex when the brightness of the target (star) indicates a 90° clockwise movement. (Adapted from Georgopoulos et al., 1989.) *B*, Saccade remapping. The monkey makes a double saccade (S1 and S2) to the remembered positions of T1 and T2. *C*, Post-stimulus-time histograms showing the responses of two cells with receptive fields RF1 and RF2 illustrated in Figure 1*B*. The second cell (RF2) responds only after the first eye movement, encoding the new retinal location of T2, even though it is no longer present on the screen.

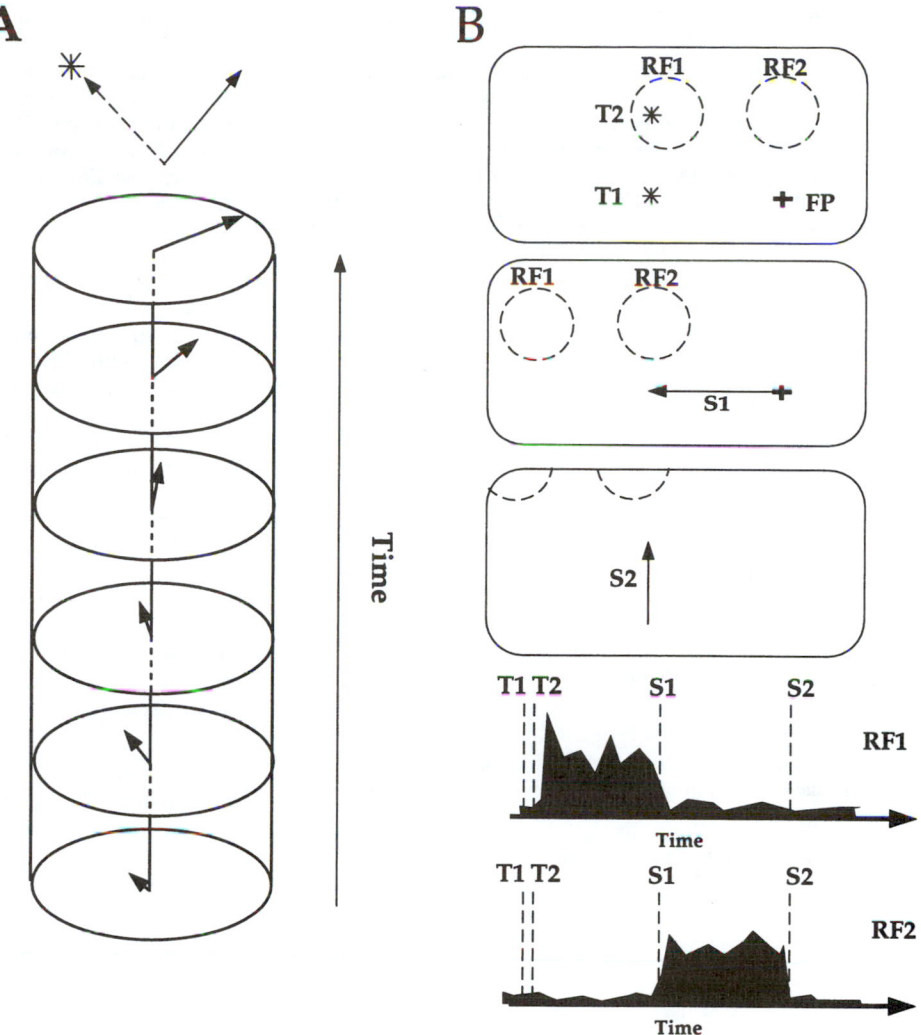

rat moves in space, even in complete darkness, suggesting that vestibular inputs are used for this updating (see RODENT HEAD DIRECTION SYSTEM).

Another example of continuous remappings has been reported in a double saccade task. In these experiments, two targets are briefly flashed in succession on the screen and the monkey makes successive saccades to their remembered locations (Figure 1*B*). Monkeys can perform this task with great accuracy, demonstrating that they do not simply keep a trace of the retinotopic location of the second target, since after the first eye movement this signal no longer corresponds to where the target was in space. Single unit recordings in the superior colliculus, frontal eye field, and parietal cortex have shown that the brain encodes the retinotopic location of the second target before the first saccade occurs. Then while the first eye movement is executed, this information is updated to represent where the second target would appear on the retina after the first saccade (Figure 1*C*; Mays and Sparks, 1980). In certain cases, this update is predictive; i.e., it starts prior to the eye movement (Duhamel, Colby, and Goldberg, 1992).

Graziano, Hu, and Gross (1997) have reported that the same mechanism appears to be at work in the premotor cortex. Bimodal, visuotactile neurons with receptive fields on the face remap the position of remembered visual stimuli after head movements. It is therefore becoming increasingly clear that continuous remappings

are widespread throughout the brain and play a critical role in sensorimotor transformations.

Although all these examples clearly involve vector remappings, it is not entirely clear that the remappings are continuous. Hence, in the Georgopoulos et al. (1989) experiment, the population vector rotation could be a consequence of the simultaneous decay and growth of the initial planned hand direction and the final one, respectively, without ever activating intermediate directions. This is an example of one-shot remapping considered in the next section. Moreover, it is often difficult to determine whether a remapping in one particular area is computed in that area or is simply the reflection of a remapping in an upstream area.

One-Shot Sensory Remapping

In the inferior colliculus and primary auditory cortex, neurons have bell-shaped auditory receptive fields in space whose positions are fixed with respect to the head. In contrast, in the multisensory layer of the superior colliculus, the positions of the auditory receptive fields are fixed in retinotopic coordinates, which implies that the auditory map must be combined with eye position (Jay and Sparks, 1987). Therefore, the auditory space is remapped in visual coordinates, presumably for the purpose of allowing auditory targets to be foveated by saccadic eye movements, a function mediated by the superior colliculus.

A similar transformation has been found in the striatum and the premotor cortex, where some of the cells have visual receptive fields in somatosensory coordinates (skin-centered; Graziano et al., 1997). In all cases, these remappings are thought to reflect an intermediate stage of processing in sensorimotor transformations.

These remappings can be considered as a change of coordinates, which correspond to a translation operation. For example, the auditory remapping in the superior colliculus requires the retinal location of the auditory stimulus, **R**, which, to a first approximation, can be computed by subtracting its head-centered location, **A**, from the current eye position, **E**:

$$\mathbf{R} = \mathbf{A} - \mathbf{E} \qquad (1)$$

Remapping Models

The remappings we have described so far fall into two categories: vector rotation with a vectorial code (e.g., mental rotation) and vector translation within a topographic map (e.g., auditory remapping in the superior colliculus). These transformations are similar, since rotating a vector within a vectorial representation consists of translating a pattern of activity around a circle. Therefore, in both cases the remapping involves translating a bell-shaped pattern of activity across a map. Most models perform this operation either dynamically through time or in one shot through the hidden layer of a feedforward network (Figure 2).

Dynamical Models

Two kinds of mechanisms have been used in models of continuous remapping: the integration of a velocity signal or the relaxation of a recurrent network.

Integrative model for remapping.   In the double saccade paradigm described above, the retinal coordinates of the second target were updated during the first saccade, a process that might involve moving a hill of activity within the parietal cortex. A model by Droulez and Berthoz (1991) shows how this bump of activity could be moved continuously across the map by integrating the eye velocities during the first saccade (Figure 1A). Their model is essentially a *forward* model of motion: Given a velocity signal, it generates the corresponding moving image. Interestingly, the equations are similar to those used for *inverse* models of motion processing. In both cases, the analysis relies on the assumption that the temporal derivative of a moving image is zero. In other words, the overall gray level profile in the image is unchanged; only the positions of the image features change. It is possible to design a recurrent network to implement this constraint (Droulez and Berthoz, 1991), and the resulting network moves arbitrary patterns of activity in response to an instantaneous velocity signal.

Several variations of this idea have been developed. Dominey and Arbib have shown that an approximation of eye velocity, obtained from the eye position modulated neurons found in the parietal cortex is sufficient for this architecture to work (Dominey and Arbib, 1992). Their simulations show patterns of activation very similar to the ones shown in Figure 1B in the part of their model corresponding to the parietal cortex, FEF, and superior colliculus. Zhang (1996) has used line attractor networks to model head direction cells in the postsubiculum of the rat. In this model, the hill is moved by using the velocity signal—in this case a head velocity signal—to temporarily modify the efficacy of the lateral connections.

Recurrent networks.   Mental rotation of a population vector can be reproduced by training a neural network to follow a circular trajectory over time. In this case, the population vector rotates as a consequence of the network dynamics in the absence of any input signals. This approach has been used by Lukashin and Georgopou-

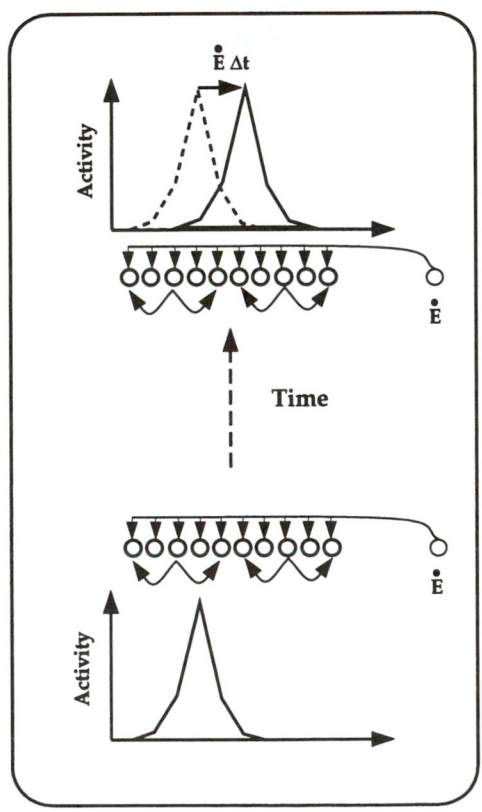
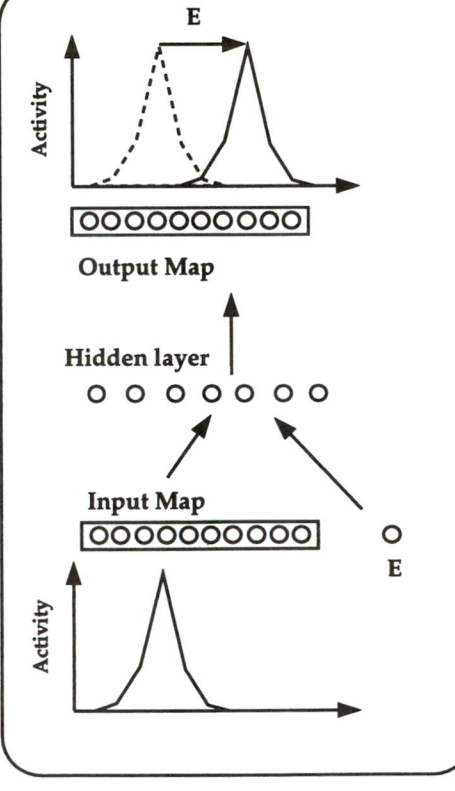

Figure 2. In a map representation, remappings involve moving hills of activity. These hills can be moved continuously in a recurrent network (*A*), or in one shot in a feedforward network (*B*). *A*, The recurrent network dynamically moves the hill of activity according to a velocity signal, $\dot{E}$. As described in the text, there are several ways to achieve this result. Droulez and Berthoz (1991) integrate the eye velocity signals through the lateral connections while Zhang (1996) uses the eye velocity signals to temporally bias the lateral connections. *B*, In feedforward remapping, the hill is moved in one shot by the full amount of the current displacement, *E*, via an intermediate stage of processing in the hidden layer. The weights can be adjusted with a learning algorithm such as backpropagation. Alternatively, one can use basis function units in the hidden layer and train the weights to the output units with a simple learning algorithm such as the delta rule.

los (1994) to model the generation of hand trajectories, but when the trajectory is a circle, mental rotation and a circular hand trajectory are equivalent. Although the model generates a rotating vector, additional mechanisms must be specified to stop the rotation.

Single-Shot Models

Feedforward models have been used for vectorial as well as map representations. They are used whenever the amplitude of the shift is available to the brain beforehand, such as auditory remapping in the superior colliculus in which the shift is directly proportional to the current eye position (Equation 1). In contrast, for mental rotation, the amplitude of the shift is specified by an external stimulus.

Shifter models. As demonstrated by Touretzky, Redish, and Wan (1993), rotation within a vectorial representation can be performed by using a shifter circuit (for more details on shifter circuits, see ROUTING NETWORKS IN VISUAL CORTEX in the First Edition). Their architecture uses N independent circuits, each implementing a rotation through a particular angle. This mechanism is limited in resolution since it rotates only by multiples of $360/N$ degrees. Whether such shifter circuits actually exist in the brain remains to be demonstrated.

Feedforward network models. There are many examples of three-layer networks, and variations thereof, that have been trained or handcrafted to perform sensory remappings. Since these remappings perform vector addition, it might appear unnecessary to deploy a fully nonlinear network for such a task. However, with a map representation, vector addition requires moving a hill of activity in a map as illustrated in Figure 2B, an operation that is highly nonlinear.

Special-purpose nonlinear circuits can be designed to perform this operation (Groh and Sparks, 1992), but more biologically realistic solutions have been found with networks of sigmoidal units trained with backpropagation. Hence, the model of Zipser and Andersen (see GAZE CODING IN THE POSTERIOR PARIETAL CORTEX in the First Edition), which was trained to compute a head-centered map from a retinotopic input, uses hidden units with retinotopic receptive fields modulated by eye position, as in parietal neurons (see also Krommenhoek et al., 1993).

However, backpropagation networks are generally quite difficult to analyze, providing realistic models but little insight into the algorithm used by the network. Pouget and Sejnowski (2001) have explored a way to analyze such networks using the theory of basis functions.

Basis functions. The process of moving a hill of activity in a single shot can be better understood when considered within the larger framework of nonlinear function approximation. For example, consider the feedforward network shown in Figure 2B, applied to a remapping from retinotopic, R_x, to head-centered coordinates, A_x. Because of the map format used in the output later, the responses of the output units are nonlinear in the input variables, namely, the retinal position, R_x, and eye position, E_x.

Therefore, the actual goal of the network is to find an appropriate intermediate representation to approximate this output function. One possibility is to use basis functions of R_x and E_x in the hidden layer (Pouget and Sejnowski, 2001; Salinas and Abbot, 1995).

Perhaps the best-known set of basis functions is the set of cosine and sine functions used in the Fourier transform. Another example is the set of Gaussian or radially symmetric functions with local support (see RADIAL BASIS FUNCTION NETWORKS). A good model

of the response of parietal neurons, which are believed to be involved in remapping, is a set of Gaussian functions of retinal position multiplied by sigmoid functions of eye position. The resulting response function is very similar to that of gain-modulated neurons in the posterior parietal cortex [see GAZE CODING IN THE POSTERIOR PARIETAL CORTEX in the First Edition, and Pouget and Snyder (2000) for a review].

Conclusions

Remappings can be continuous and dynamic or a single shot through several layers of neurons. In both cases, the problem amounts to moving a hill of activity in neuronal maps. Whether some models are better than others is often difficult to establish simply because the neurophysiological data available are relatively sparse. Models can be further constrained by considering deficits that accompany localized lesions in humans (see Pouget and Sejnowski, 2001). These data not only provide valuable insights into the nature of remappings but also might help bridge the gap between behavior and single-cell responses.

Road Map: Vision
Related Reading: Collicular Visuomotor Transformations for Gaze Control; Motion Perception: Elementary Mechanisms; Pursuit Eye Movements; Visual Attention; Visual Scene Perception

References

Dominey, P., and Arbib, M., 1992, A cortico-subcortical model for the generation of spatially accurate sequential saccades, *Cerebral Cortex*, 2:153–175. ◆

Droulez, J., and Berthoz, A., 1991, A neural model of sensoritopic maps with predictive short-term memory properties, *Proc. Natl. Acad. Sci. USA*, 88:9653–9657. ◆

Duhamel, J. R., Colby, C. L., and Goldberg, M. E., 1992, The updating of the representation of visual space in parietal cortex by intended eye movements, *Science*, 255(5040):90–92.

Georgopoulos, A. P., Lurito, J. T., Petrides, M., Schwartz, A. B., and Massey, J. T., 1989, Mental rotation of the neuronal population vector, *Science*, 243:234–236.

Graziano, M., Hu, X., and Gross, C., 1997, Coding the locations of objects in the dark, *Science*, 277:239–241.

Groh, J., and Sparks, D., 1992, Two models for transforming auditory signals from head-centered to eye-centered coordinates, *Biol. Cybernetics*, 67:291–302.

Jay, M. F., and Sparks, D. L., 1987, Sensorimotor integration in the primate superior colliculus: I. Motor convergence, *J. Neurophysiol.*, 57:22–34.

Krommenhoek, K. P., Van Opstal, A. J., Gielen, C. C. A., and Van Gisbergen, J. A. M., 1993, Remapping of neural activity in the motor colliculus: A neural network study, *Vision Res.*, 33:1287–1298.

Mays, L. E., and Sparks, D. L., 1980, Dissociation of visual and saccade-related responses in superior colliculus neurons, *J. Neurophysiol.*, 43:207–232.

Pouget, A., and Sejnowski, T. J., 2001, Simulating a lesion in a basis function model of spatial representations: Comparison with hemineglect, *Psychol. Rev.*, 108:653–673. ◆

Pouget, A., and Snyder, L., 2000, Computational approaches to sensorimotor transformations, *Nature Neurosci.*, 3:1192–1198.

Salinas, E., and Abbot, L., 1995, Transfer of coded information from sensory to motor networks, *J. Neurosci.*, 15:6461–6474. ◆

Todorov, E., 2000, Direct cortical control of muscle activation in voluntary arm movements: A model, *Nature Neurosci.*, 3:391–398.

Touretzky, D., Redish, A., and Wan, H., 1993, Neural representation of space using sinusoidal arrays, *Neural Computation*, 5:869–884.

Zhang, K., 1996, Representation of spatial orientation by the intrinsic dynamics of the head-direction cell ensemble: A theory, *J. Neurosci.*, 16:2112–2126. ◆

Dynamics and Bifurcation in Neural Nets

Bard Ermentrout

Introduction

A *recurrent neural net*, whether it is continuous or discrete in space and time, defines a dynamical system. Thus, it is possible to apply the powerful qualitative and geometric tools of dynamical systems theory to understand the behavior of neural networks. These techniques are most useful when the behavior of interest is stationary in the sense that the inputs are at most time- or space-periodic. Thus, we can ask what kind of behavior we can expect over the long run for a given neural network. Such information is important both in artificial neural networks and biological neural nets. In the former, the final state of the neural network may represent the recognition of an input pattern, the segmentation of an image, or any number of machine computations. The stationary states of biological neural networks may correspond to cognitive decisions (e.g., binding via synchronous oscillations) or to pathological behavior such as seizures and hallucinations.

Another important issue that is addressed by dynamical systems theory is how the qualitative dynamics depends on parameters. The qualitative change in a dynamical system as a parameter is changed is the subject of *bifurcation theory*. The word *bifurcation* is derived from the Greek word for branching; we are concerned with the appearance and disappearance of branches of solutions to a given set of equations as some parameters vary. There are now a large number of very good general books on the mathematical theory behind dynamical systems and bifurcation. In this article we show how to use these techniques to understand the behavior of neural nets. A fundamental problem for both artificial and biologically motivated neural nets is to understand how the solutions depend on the parameters and the initial states of the network.

For excellent introductions to nonlinear dynamics and bifurcation theory, see Ermentrout (1998), Guckenheimer and Holmes (1983), Kuznetsov (1998), and Wiggins (1990).

Some Basic Definitions

A *dynamical system* consists of a phase space, X, a time domain, T, and a function that describes the evolution of the phase space, $\phi(x, t)$. The function ϕ gives the value of an element in the phase space at time t, given that at $t = 0$ it was x. The two main motivating examples are differential equations and maps. In the former case, the time domain is the real line (continuous time); in the latter the time domain is the integers (discrete time). Consider the ordinary differential equation:

$$\frac{dx}{dt} = F(x) \qquad x \in X, t \in R \qquad (1)$$

Then we define $\phi(x_0, t)$ to be the solution to Equation 1 with initial condition x_0. For example, if

$$\frac{dx}{dt} = x \qquad x(0) = x_0$$

then $x(t) = \phi(x_0, t) \equiv x_0 e^t$. (We have restricted our attention to *autonomous* systems in which there is no explicit time dependence.) Consider next the iteration:

$$x(n + 1) = F(x(n)) \qquad x \in X, n \in Z \qquad (2)$$

Then $\phi(x_0, n)$ is defined as the solution to Equation 2 with initial conditions $x = x_0$. For example, if

$$x(n + 1) = 2x(n) \qquad x(0) = x_0$$

then $x(n) = \phi(x_0, n) = x_0 2^n$.

There is nothing that prevents us from considering infinite dimensional dynamical systems such as partial differential equations (see PATTERN FORMATION, BIOLOGICAL) or neural networks distributed in space. The set of states $\Gamma(x_0) = \{ \phi(x_0, t) : t \in T, \phi(x_0, t)$ defined$\}$ is called the *orbit* or *trajectory* through x_0. The orbit is a curve in state space for continuous systems and a sequence of points for discrete systems. If $\Gamma(x_0)$ consists of a single point in phase space, then we say that x_0 is a *fixed point* or *equilibrium* for the system. Fixed points are easily found by solving $F(x_0) = 0$ or $F(x_0) = x_0$ for continuous and discrete dynamical systems, respectively. If $\phi(x_0, t + P) = \phi(x_0, t)$ for some non-zero value P, then the orbit is called *periodic*, with period P. A set S is *invariant* with respect to the dynamical system if $y \in S$ implies that $\phi(y, t) \in S$ for all $t \in T$. Thus, any orbit is an invariant set, as is any fixed point or periodic solution. The partitioning of the state space into orbits is called the *phase portrait* of the dynamical system and is one of the goals of dynamical systems.

Another key question in dynamical systems is the issue of stability. We say that an invariant set S_0 is *stable* if for any y close to S_0, $\phi(y, t)$ stays close to S_0 for all $t \in T$. An invariant set is *asymptotically stable* if for any y near S_0, the distance between $\phi(y, t)$ and S_0 tends to zero as $t \to \infty$. The stability of a fixed point in a discrete or continuous dynamical system is easily determined by studying the eigenvalues of an associated linear operator or matrix. Suppose that x_0 is a fixed point. Let $A = DF(x_0)$ be the matrix obtained by taking the partial derivatives of F with respect to the state variables and evaluating it at the fixed point. The dynamical system obtained by replacing $F(x)$ with Ax is called the *linearized system*. For Equation 1, if all of the eigenvalues of A have strictly negative real parts, then the fixed point is asymptotically stable (and all solutions to the linearized system decay to 0). If any eigenvalue has a positive real part, then the fixed point is unstable. For Equation 2, if all of the eigenvalues of A lie inside the unit circle, then the fixed point is asymptotically stable. If any eigenvalue lies outside the unit circle, then the fixed point is unstable. As long as none of the eigenvalues have zero real part (respectively, lie on the unit circle), we say the fixed point of the differential Equation 1 (respectively map, Equation 2) is *hyperbolic*. Eigenvalues that have negative real parts (lie in the unit circle) are called *stable eigenvalues*, those with positive real parts (lie outside the unit circle) are called *unstable eigenvalues*, and those that have zero real parts (lie on the unit circle) are called *neutral eigenvalues* for the continuous-time (discrete-time) fixed point. The invariant set $W^s(x_0) = \{ y \in X : \phi(y, t) \to x_0$ as $t \to \infty \}$ (respectively $W^u(x_0)\{ y \in X : \phi(y, t) \to x_0$ as $t \to -\infty \}$) is called the *stable manifold* (respectively *unstable manifold*) of the fixed point x_0. The stable (unstable) manifold is just the set of all points that tend to the fixed point as time increases (decreases) to infinity (negative infinity). The dimension of the stable (respectively, unstable) manifold is the number of stable (respectively unstable) eigenvalues of the linearized system. A fixed point that has both unstable and stable eigenvalues is called a *saddle point*. If the fixed point is asymptotically stable, then the stable manifold has the same dimension as the phase space and is then often called the *basin of attraction* for the fixed point. For neutral eigenvalues there is a *center manifold* that is invariant and has the same dimension as the number of neutral eigenvalues. The center manifold is extremely useful and important, as we shall see, since it allows one to study the behavior of high-dimensional systems in a lower-dimensional setting.

So far, the discussion of asymptotic behavior has been restricted to fixed points. A continuous dynamical system can often be re-

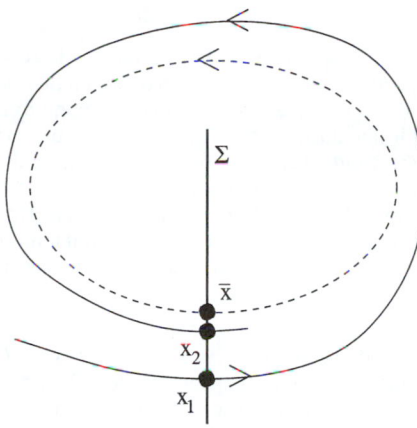

Figure 1. Construction of the Poincaré map for a two-dimensional system.

duced to a discrete one by introducing a *Poincaré map*. Suppose the system has a periodic orbit. A *cross-section* for an *n*-dimensional continuous dynamical system is an $n - 1$-dimensional hypersurface that is orthogonal to the tangent of the periodic orbit (Figure 1). A point on the surface that starts near the periodic orbit will be brought back to the surface at a later time. This produces a locally defined map from the surface back to itself, which is then a discrete dynamical system. From Figure 1, it is clear that a fixed point of the Poincaré map corresponds to a periodic solution of the original system. Thus, we can determine stability, stable, unstable, and center manifolds for periodic solutions just by studying the behavior of a Poincaré map defined in some local neighborhood of it. An isolated periodic solution is called a *limit cycle* and its stability is determined by studying the stability of the fixed point for the associated Poincaré map. A limit cycle solution is hyperbolic if the fixed point of the Poincaré map is hyperbolic.

Invariant sets are not all as simple as periodic solutions and fixed points. In fact, they can be quite complicated. A stable invariant set that has irregular behavior (e.g., it is not a simple curve or point) is called a *strange attractor*. Similarly, the behavior of an invariant set can be quite complex as well. We say that an invariant set is *chaotic* if it displays sensitive dependence on initial conditions; that is, the orbits through two arbitrarily close points on the set diverge from each other exponentially. (For examples of chaotic behavior in neurons, see CHAOS IN NEURAL SYSTEMS; SYNAPTIC NOISE AND CHAOS IN VERTEBRATE NEURONS; and CHAOS IN BIOLOGICAL SYSTEMS).

A dynamical system that has only hyperbolic fixed points and periodic orbits will maintain the same qualitative behavior if the parameters are varied slightly. Thus, qualitative changes are seen when the fixed points and periodic orbits become nonhyperbolic. This happens when eigenvalues cross the critical axis and thus a fixed point loses stability. This is one of the key ideas behind *bifurcation theory*. Roughly, we expect to see qualitative changes as a parameter varies when some of the fixed points or periodic orbits become nonhyperbolic. Bifurcation theory gives us a method of studying arbitrary dynamical systems near these critical values of parameters. The idea is that near a critical parameter value, there will be some neutral eigenvalues. This will imply that there is a nontrivial center manifold and in fact the local dynamics of the full system can be completely understood by studying the dynamics restricted to this center manifold. Bifurcation methods give a recipe for computing the form of the equations on this low-dimensional system. This means that one can study a possibly infinite-dimensional system by looking at the dynamics of a possibly one-dimensional system!

The simplified dynamical systems that one obtains near critical values of the parameters are called *normal forms*. Thus, the understanding of the local behavior of the full system comes from studying the behavior of the relevant normal form.

Local Bifurcations

Local bifurcation theory allows one to study the behavior of discrete and continuous dynamical systems near fixed points. Since the behavior of periodic solutions to continuous systems reduces to the analysis of fixed points of the Poincaré map, local bifurcation of maps enables us to analyze bifurcations of limit cycles in continuous systems.

Continuous-Time Systems

There are two ways in which a fixed point of a continuous-time dynamical system can become nonhyperbolic as a parameter varies: (1) an eigenvalue crosses zero or (2) a pair of complex eigenvalues crosses the imaginary axis. In the case of a zero eigenvalue, this signifies the appearance of new fixed points near the original one. In the most general setting, with no symmetries, a zero eigenvalue implies a *fold* or *turning point* bifurcation. In this bifurcation, the deviation from the fixed point obeys one-dimensional dynamics:

$$r' = ar^2 + c(\mu - \mu^*) \tag{3}$$

where a, c are problem-dependent parameters, $r \in R$, and μ is the parameter that is varied. The fixed points of this simple system (called the normal form) correspond to fixed points of the full system even if it is infinite dimensional. In Figure 2A, steady-state solutions are shown for a, $c > 0$. As μ increases past μ^*, two fixed points, a stable one and an unstable one, coalesce and disappear, leaving no nearby fixed point. (The picture is essentially the same

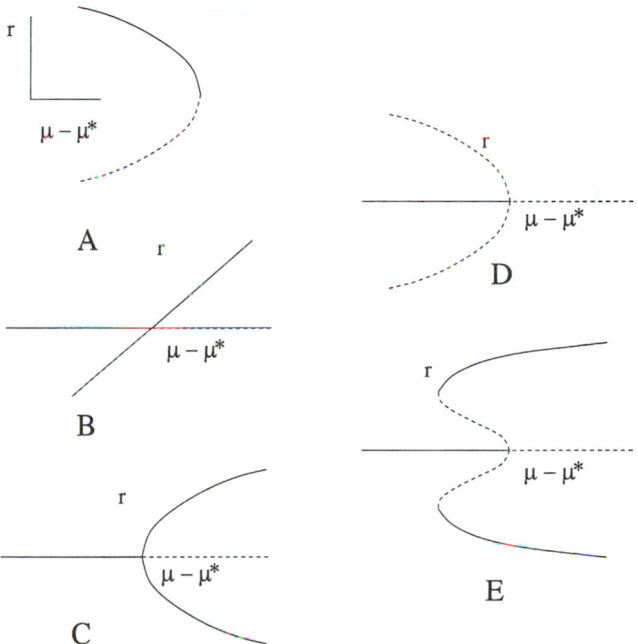

Figure 2. Bifurcation diagrams for fixed points of continuous-time dynamical systems. Solid lines are stable, dashed unstable. *A*, Steady-state solutions for a fold or turning point bifurcation. *B*, A transcritical or exchange-of-stability bifurcation. *C*, A supercritical bifurcation. *D*, A subcritical bifurcation. *E*, Subcritical pitchfork bifurcations turning around at a pair of fold points and restabilizing, leading to bistability.

for other choices of c, a.) In cases with additional symmetry (such as the requirement that there always be at least one fixed point or that the system have some symmetry), there are two additional common normal forms:

$$r' = ar^2 + cr(\mu - \mu^*) \tag{4}$$

$$r' = ar^3 + cr(\mu - \mu^*) \tag{5}$$

Equation 4 leads to the *transcritical* bifurcation shown in Figure 2B. This is also called an *exchange-of-stability* bifurcation since the stability of the two fixed points switches at the point of bifurcation. As in the fold, the signs of a, c are irrelevant to the picture. With additional symmetry, Equation 5 occurs, and this is called the *pitchfork* bifurcation. In this case, the sign of a is important. If $a < 0$, then the bifurcation is *supercritical*, and two new *stable* fixed points arise (Figure 2C). If $a > 0$, then two new *unstable* fixed points occur, and the bifurcation is called *subcritical* (Figure 2D). In many biological and physical systems, subcritical pitchfork bifurcations "turn around" at a pair of fold points and restabilize (as in Figure 2E). This leads to *bistability* between several fixed points and to hysteresis.

Suppose that stability is lost when a pair of complex eigenvalues crosses the imaginary axis. Then the system can undergo what is called a *Hopf* or *Andronov* bifurcation. The dynamics are locally determined by the simple complex differential equation:

$$z' = az^2\bar{z} + cz(\mu - \mu^*) + iwz \quad a, c, z \in C \tag{6}$$

If the real part of a is negative, then a stable periodic orbit will bifurcate from the fixed point with amplitude that is proportional to $\sqrt{\mu - \mu^*}$. The bifurcation is called *supercritical*. If the real part of a is positive, then an *unstable* periodic orbit bifurcates from the fixed point and the bifurcation is called *subcritical*. The bifurcation diagrams look like those of the pitchfork bifurcation (Figures 2C and 2D), where $r = |z|$. As with the pitchfork bifurcation, physical systems that have subcritical Hopf bifurcations often restabilize, as in Figure 2E. Thus, there will be a range of the parameter for which there is a stable limit cycle and a stable fixed point (analogous to Figure 2E.)

Discrete Dynamics

For a discrete dynamical system to undergo a local bifurcation, eigenvalues must cross the unit circle. There are three ways in which this can happen: (1) an eigenvalue is $+1$, (2) an eigenvalue is -1, or (3) a complex pair of eigenvalues lies on the unit circle. The first case, an eigenvalue of 1, is completely analogous to the case of a zero eigenvalue for continuous systems. The third case is similar to the Hopf bifurcation for continuous systems and is called a *Neimark-Sacker* bifurcation. However, the dynamics of the bifurcating solution can be complicated, and all one can conclude is that there is a small invariant circle. The second case, $a - 1$ eigenvalue, is called a *flip* or *period-doubling* bifurcation. The dynamics is determined by the behavior of the simple one-dimensional map:

$$r_{n+1} = -r_n + c(\mu - \mu^*)r_n + ar_n^3 \tag{7}$$

If $a > 0$, then a stable period 2 fixed point appears; that is, every other iterate of the map is the same. If $a < 0$, then an unstable period 2 fixed point occurs. Period-doubling bifurcations are very important, as they often signal the onset of chaotic behavior. Indeed, often a period 2 point itself will become unstable through another period-doubling bifurcation to a period 4 point. This continues as the parameter is changed, and a whole *cascade* of period doublings occurs, terminating in chaotic behavior.

Periodic Orbits in Continuous Systems

Periodic orbits undergo bifurcations similar to those of discrete dynamical systems since their local behavior is reducible to a discrete system. Folds of the Poincaré map correspond to the annihilation of a stable and unstable limit cycle; flips correspond to period doubling of the limit cycle; Neimark-Sacker bifurcations correspond to the appearance of an invariant 2-torus.

In addition to these local bifurcations, there are two common *global* bifurcations in which the period of the orbit tends to infinity. A *heteroclinic* orbit, $\gamma(t)$, is a nonconstant orbit satisfying

$$\lim_{t \to \pm\infty} \gamma(t) = x^\pm$$

where $x^\pm$ are fixed points. If $x^+ = x^-$, we call $\gamma(t)$ a *homoclinic* orbit. In general, one cannot expect to find a homoclinic orbit; rather, as some parameter μ changes, the homoclinic orbit appears at one value of that parameter, μ^* (Figure 3A). Thus, the appearance of a homoclinic is a bifurcation. If the fixed point $x^+ = x^-$ is a hyperbolic saddle, then, as the parameter moves away from criticality, a periodic orbit arises, and the period of this orbit goes to infinity as the homoclinic orbit is approached. The period is given by

$$T_{hom} \sim K \log \frac{1}{|\mu - \mu^*|}$$

If instead of a hyperbolic saddle point, the fixed point is a fold point, then a *saddle node on a limit cycle* occurs (Figure 3B). Limit cycles occur as the parameter is moved from criticality with a period

$$T_{sn} \sim \frac{K}{\sqrt{|\mu - \mu^*|}}$$

Applications to Continuous-Time Neural Nets

So far, we have introduced definitions but not used them in the context of neural networks. Numerous papers have used bifurcation

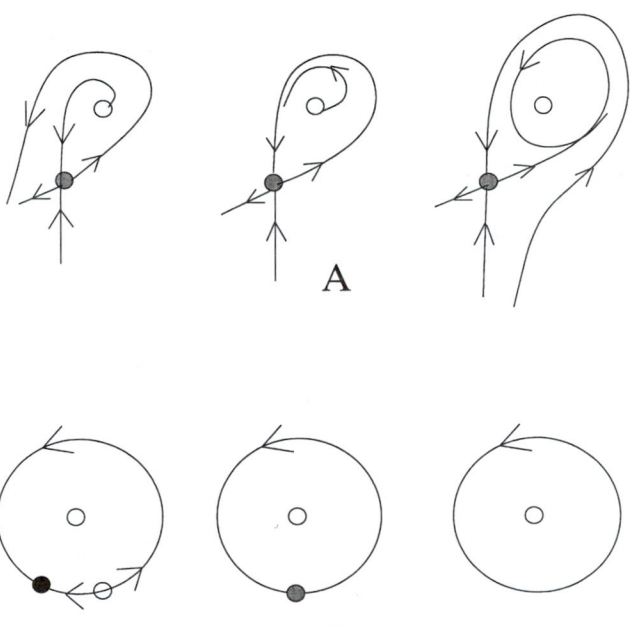

Figure 3. Two distinct types of homoclinic bifurcation. Bifurcation of (A) a homoclinic orbit from a hyperbolic saddle or (B) a saddle node on a limit cycle, leading to periodic orbits.

methods to analyze neural networks (see, e.g., PHASE-PLANE ANALYSIS OF NEURAL NETS; COOPERATIVE PHENOMENA; OSCILLATORY AND BURSTING PROPERTIES OF NEURONS; and PATTERN FORMATION, NEURAL; see also Izhikevich, 2000, for a long and well-illustrated review). The types of neural net models to which the theory has been applied generally have one of the following two forms:

$$\tau_j \frac{du_j}{dt} = -u_j + F_j\left(\sum_k W_{jk}u_k + I_j\right) \qquad (8)$$

$$u_j(n+1) = \mu_j u_j + F_j\left(\sum_k W_{jk}u_k(n) + I_j\right) \qquad (9)$$

The functions F_j are generally monotone and increasing, W_{jk} are the weights, I_j are the inputs, and $1/\tau_j$, $1 - \mu_j$ are decay rates. With proper limits, the sums in Equations 8 and 9 can go to integrals over space in order to represent a continuum model for neural nets. In this case the interaction takes the form

$$\int_\Omega W(x, y)u(y)dy$$

where Ω is the spatial domain, a one- or two-dimensional region in space. The behavior of these models is generally impossible to analyze completely except in certain simple cases. For example, Hopfield (1984) shows that if the weights W_{jk} are symmetric, then all solutions to Equation 8 tend to be fixed points. In the case of one or two dimensions, Equation 8 can be completely analyzed (see Hoppensteadt and Izhikevich, 1997, chap. 2; PHASE-PLANE ANALYSIS OF NEURAL NETS). The discrete system in Equation 9 can be completely characterized only in one dimension.

Local Bifurcations of Fixed Points

To see how bifurcation methods can be used in neural nets, consider a simple continuous neural network with no inputs and satisfying $\tau_j = 1$, $F_j(u) = F(u)$ with $F(0) = 0$, $F'(0) = \mu$, a gain parameter. Thus the trivial state of the network, $u_j = 0$, is a fixed point. To study stability and bifurcation, we linearize about $u_j = 0$ and obtain the matrix

$$M_{jk} = -\delta_{jk} + \mu W_{jk}$$

where δ_{jk} is the Kronecker delta function. If λ is an eigenvalue of W_{jk}, then $-1 + \mu\lambda$ is an eigenvalue for M; thus, if the gain is sufficiently small, the trivial fixed point is stable. If some of the eigenvalues of the weight matrix W have positive real parts, then, for sufficient gain, some of the eigenvalues of M will cross the imaginary axis and the rest state will lose stability. In particular, let λ_0 be the eigenvalue with maximal real part and let Φ_0 be the corresponding eigenvector. Since this is a continuous dynamical system, there are only two cases of interest. Suppose that λ_0 is real. Then if $\mu = \mu^* = 1/\lambda_0$, there will be a zero eigenvalue and a bifurcation to new fixed points. Since 0 is always a fixed point, the bifurcation will be transcritical, or a pitchfork. In any case, the new solution will have a non-zero amplitude and be proportional to Φ_0. This is the essence of pattern formation. The trivial state $u_j = 0$ loses stability and a new state that is coded in the weight matrix bifurcates from rest. Analysis of pattern formation in neural networks (and for that matter, any pattern formation models) all comes down to this calculation (see Murray, 1989). If the weight matrix is symmetric, then the eigenvalues are real and the initial bifurcation from the rest state will always be through a zero eigenvalue. If the weight matrix is non-negative, then the eigenvalue with largest modulus will be real and positive and the first bifurcating mode will be proportional to the principal component of the weight matrix.

Suppose the weight matrix is not symmetric and not all the same sign; that is, there are "inhibitory" and "excitatory" interactions. Then the eigenvalue with maximal real part could be a complex eigenvalue. This means that the first instability is through a Hopf bifurcation and an oscillatory pattern of activities can bifurcate. In situations in which there is symmetry or in which the network has a particular geometry, this type of bifurcation can lead to periodic wave trains. Recently, Hoppensteadt and Izhikevich (1997) proposed a general theory of neural networks that exploits the kind of local analysis that we have only sketched here.

Beyond Local Bifurcations

To go beyond the simple bifurcation analysis described above, it is necessary to turn to numerical methods. There are several numerical packages for the analysis of bifurcations in nonlinear dynamics. AUTO (Doedel et al., 1997) is among the best of them and works on many operating systems. To illustrate the concepts discussed in the previous sections, I present a global numerical diagram for a six-neuron model whose weight matrix was chosen randomly from a uniform distribution with mean 0 and a standard deviation of 0.5. (Note that this particular example was picked because of its rich behavior.) The function $F(x) = \tanh(\mu x)$ was chosen for simplicity. Once the weight matrix is chosen, there is only one parameter, the gain, μ. Figure 4 shows the norm of the solutions that are computed numerically as the gain is increased. The eigenvalues for the weight matrix are approximately -0.83, $0.25 \pm 0.2i$, -0.16, 0.12, -0.47. Thus, for positive gains, there will be a Hopf bifurcation at approximately $\mu = 4$ and a pitchfork bifurcation at approximately $\mu = 8.33$. Both of these branches are shown in the diagram (labeled H1 and P, respectively). The pitchfork is subcritical and undergoes a fold bifurcation (labeled F1) and stabilizes. A subcritical Hopf bifurcation (H3) occurs on this branch,

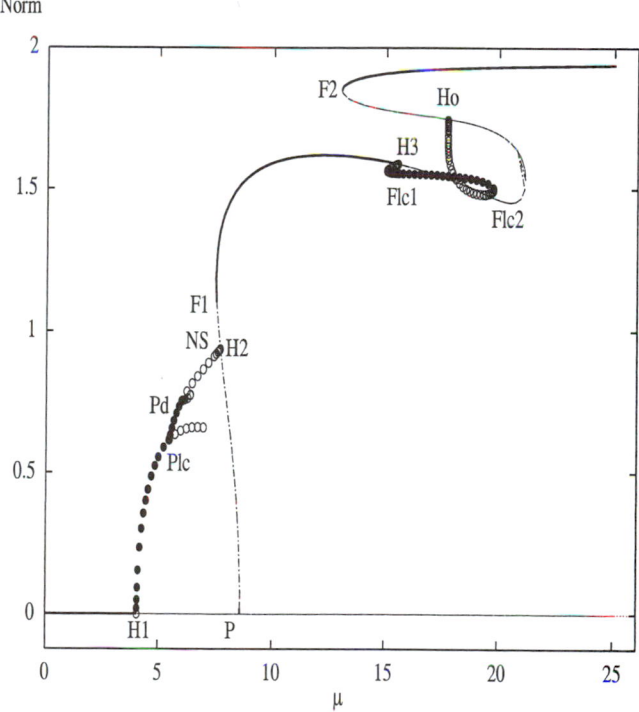

Figure 4. Numerically computed bifurcation diagram for a six-neuron network with random weights chosen between -0.5 and 0.5.

which turns around at the limit-cycle fold bifurcation (Flc1), giving rise to a stable periodic orbit. This orbit turns around again at Flc2, and the resulting unstable limit cycle terminates at a homoclinic bifurcation (Ho). The curve of fixed points turns around at F2, leaving a stable fixed point that persists for all higher values of μ.

The fate of the periodic orbit that arises at H1 is more interesting. This orbit is supercritical and leads to small-amplitude, stable periodic solutions. As μ increases, the periodic orbit (and hence the fixed point to the Poincaré map) loses stability as an eigenvalue crosses $+1$. This results in a pitchfork bifurcation at Plc. The unstable periodic orbit appears to persist for all values of μ beyond the bifurcation point, but never restabilizes. The pitchfork bifurcation of the Poincaré map is supercritical and results in a stable periodic orbit. This orbit becomes unstable at a flip or period-doubling bifurcation (Pd); the branch eventually terminates at a Hopf bifurcation (H2) on the branch of fixed points that bifurcated at P. The periodic branch also undergoes a Neimark-Sacker bifurcation (NS), resulting in an unstable torus. The flip bifurcation is supercritical and leads to a new branch of periodic solutions with twice the period. This branch in turn undergoes a flip bifurcation, and so on, producing a period-doubling cascade. The regimen between $\mu = 5.5$ and $\mu = 7.5$ is very complicated. There are many bifurcations, and the appearance of many stable and unstable periodic orbits as well as chaotic behavior, that are not described on this plot. In order to depict this behavior, we plot the Poincaré map whose cross-section is defined as the hyperplane where $u'_4 = 0$. The u_2 component of this map is shown in Figure 5 as a function of μ. In this diagram, each dot represents an iteration of the Poincaré map, so that for a fixed value of μ, a single dot implies a periodic solution, a pair is a period 2 orbit, and so on. The period-doubling cascades are clear. A period 3 orbit at about $\mu = 6.85$ is seen to undergo a period-doubling cascade as μ is decreased. Chaotic behavior terminates near a saddle point at $\mu \approx 7.57$ and disappears "instantly." This global bifurcation is called a *crisis* by Yorke.

Conclusion

The general behavior of recurrent neural networks as parameters vary remains an open problem. Dynamical systems methods and bifurcation theory provide a general approach to analyzing these interesting systems. Pattern formation, spatiotemporal behavior, and complex dynamics are all aspects of recurrent neural networks that can be understood by these useful mathematical tools. Analytical methods along with the careful use of numerical methods allow one to globally characterize complex biological and artificial neural networks.

Appendix

The neural network used in Figures 3 and 4 has the form:

$$U'_j = -U_j + \tanh\left(\mu \sum_{k=1}^{6} W_{jk}U_k\right)$$

where

$$W = \begin{pmatrix} -0.42473 & 0.243325 & -0.267939 & 0.308063 & -0.0370201 & 0.394969 \\ -0.166832 & 0.474204 & -0.0151443 & 0.476774 & 0.211162 & 0.401305 \\ -0.427914 & 0.370044 & -0.0675567 & 0.276535 & 0.45988 & -0.457168 \\ -0.362131 & 0.033334 & -0.196538 & -0.037606 & -0.125548 & 0.143851 \\ 0.429334 & -0.306886 & 0.402954 & -0.166799 & -0.45518 & -0.0304156 \\ 0.294663 & -0.346348 & -0.138444 & 0.334973 & 0.13884 & -0.364227 \end{pmatrix}$$

Road Map: Dynamic Systems

Related Reading: Chaos in Neural Systems; Computing with Attractors; Oscillatory and Bursting Properties of Neurons; Pattern Formation, Biological; Phase-Plane Analysis of Neural Nets

References

Doedel, E., Champneys, A., Fairgrieve, T., Kuznetsov, Y., Sandstede, B., and Wang, X. J., 1997, AUTO97: Continuation and bifurcation software for ordinary differential equations (with HomCont), Montreal: Computer Science Department, Concordia University available: ftp://ftp.cs.concordia.ca/pub/doedel/auto.

Ermentrout, B., 1998, Neural networks as spatio-temporal pattern-forming systems, *Rep. Prog. Phys.*, 61:353–430. ◆

Guckenheimer, J., and Holmes P. J., 1983, *Nonlinear oscillations, Dynamical Systems, and Bifurcations of Vector Fields.*, Heidelberg: Springer-Verlag.

Hopfield, J., 1984, Neurons with graded response have collective computational properties like those of two-state neurons, *Proc. Natl. Acad. Sci. USA*, 81:3088–3092.

Hoppensteadt, F., and Izhikevich, E., 1997, *Weakly Connected Neural Networks*, New York: Springer-Verlag. ◆

Izhikevich, E. M., 2000, Neural excitability, spiking, and bursting, *Int. J. Bifurcat. Chaos*, 10:1171–1266.

Kuznetsov, Y. A., 1998, *Elements of Applied Bifurcation Theory*, New York: Springer-Verlag. ◆

Murray, J. D., 1989, *Mathematical Biology*, Heidelberg: Springer-Verlag.

Wiggins, S., 1990, *Introduction to Applied Nonlinear Dynamical Systems and Chaos*, New York: Springer-Verlag.

U$_2$

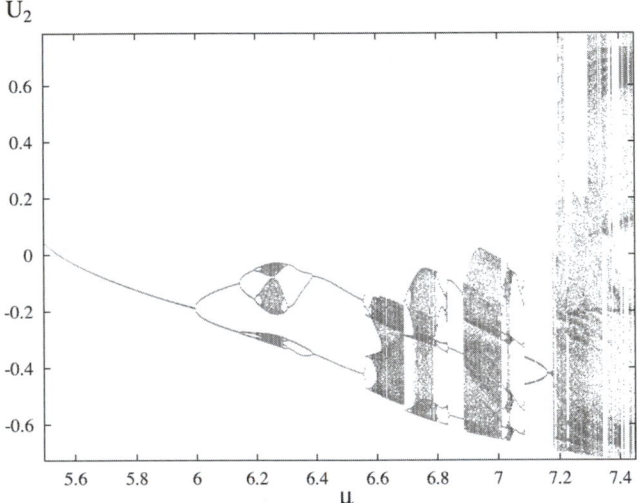

Figure 5. Poincaré map of a region from Figure 3 showing complex dynamics.

Dynamics of Association and Recall

Ton Coolen

Introduction

The concept and relevance of associative memory in neural networks are discussed elsewhere in this *Handbook* (see, e.g., ASSO-CIATIVE NETWORKS, STATISTICAL MECHANICS OF NEURAL NETWORKS, and CORTICAL HEBBIAN MODULES). Associative memory networks are usually (but not always) recurrent, which implies that one cannot simply write down the values of successive neuron states (as with layered networks). The latter must be solved from coupled dynamic equations. Dynamical studies shed light on the pattern recall process and its relation to the choice of initial state, the properties of the stored patterns, the noise level, and the network architecture. In addition, for nonsymmetric networks (where the equilibrium statistics are not known), dynamical techniques are the *only* tools available. Since our interest is usually in large networks and in global recall processes, the common strategy of the theorist is to move away from the *microscopic* equations (i.e., equations at the level of individual neurons) and to derive dynamical laws at a *macroscopic* level (i.e., in terms of quantities that depend on many neuron states). One then faces the following questions:

- Which are the appropriate macroscopic quantities we should attempt to calculate?
- How do we extract the corresponding macroscopic equations from the microscopic ones?

All research in this field basically involves launching or elaborating proposals for dealing with these two issues, which are related in that the "natural" set of macroscopic quantities can be defined as the *smallest* set that will obey *closed deterministic* equations in the limit of an infinitely large network. Since the mid-1970s, many theoretical approaches to recall dynamics have been developed in parallel, while their relations were only understood later. To give an overview of the field I will therefore not always discuss papers in chronological order, but use the benefit of hindsight. In the absence of recent textbooks or reviews that deal with recall dynamics in a satisfactory manner (at least from the viewpoint of what we know today), most of the references will indeed be to research papers. In the interest of transparency, in this article I restrict myself mainly to simple Hopfield-type models, and discuss some variations and generalizations in a final section.

The Core of the Problem

In Hopfield-type models one has N binary neurons, with states $S_i \in \{-1, 1\}$. I will write $S = (S_1, \ldots, S_N)$. The S_i evolve stochastically, driven by postsynaptic potentials (or "local fields") h_i:

$$S_i(t + \Delta) = \text{sgn}[h_i(S(t)) + \eta_i(t)] \qquad h_i(S) = \sum_{j \neq i} J_{ij} S_j \quad (1)$$

The $\eta_i(t)$ are independent random variables, modeling threshold noise. The updates in Equation 1 can be executed in parallel or sequentially. Comparable time units result when choosing $\Delta = 1$ for parallel dynamics and $\Delta = 1/N$ for sequential dynamics. Hopfield networks are equipped with Hebbian-type synapses:

$$J_{ij} = \frac{c_{ij}}{c} \sum_{\mu=1}^{p} \xi_i^\mu \xi_j^\mu \qquad (2)$$

These involve p patterns $\xi^\mu = (\xi_1^\mu, \ldots, \xi_N^\mu) \in \{-1, 1\}^N$. The $c_{ij} \in \{0, 1\}$ specify the network connectivity ($c_{ij} = 1$ if a connection $j \to i$ is present, $c_{ij} = 0$ if not), whereas the factor $c = \langle (1/$

$N) \Sigma_{ij} c_{ij} \rangle$ (the average number of neurons contributing to a local field) ensures that the local fields remain finite as $N \to \infty$. One usually defines also the relative load factor $\alpha = p/c$ (the number of patterns stored per synapse). A fully connected network thus corresponds to $c_{ij} = 1$ for all (i, j) and $c = N$. A so-called randomly extremely diluted network, on the other hand, would have $\lim_{N \to \infty} c^{-1} = 0$ and $\lim_{N \to \infty} c/N = 0$ (i.e., the number of synapses attached to a typical neuron diverges but remains small when compared to the total number of neurons). Theorists often choose to study these two connectivity types because they are found to simplify the analysis of the dynamics (e.g., one need not worry about spatial aspects).

The process of interest is that where, triggered by correlation between the initial state $S(0)$ and a stored pattern ξ^λ, the state vector S evolves toward ξ^λ. If this happens, pattern ξ^λ is said to be recalled. Numerical simulations of a simple fully connected network (with randomly drawn patterns) already clearly illustrate the main features and complications of recall dynamics. Here the correlation between a state vector and the stored patterns is measured by so-called overlaps (or "directional cosines"):

$$m_\mu(S) = \frac{1}{N} \sum_i \xi_i^\mu S_i \qquad (3)$$

For large N we distinguish structural overlaps, where $m_\mu(S) = \mathbb{O}(1)$, from accidental ones, where $m_\mu(S) = \mathbb{O}(N^{-1/2})$ (as for a randomly drawn S). Figure 1 shows the result of measuring the quantities

$$m = m_1(S) \qquad r = \alpha^{-1} \sum_{\mu>1} m_\mu^2(S) \qquad (4)$$

following initial states that are correlated with pattern ξ^1 only. Overlaps with non-nominated patterns are seen to remain $\mathbb{O}(N^{-1/2})$, i.e., $r(t) = \mathbb{O}(1)$. We immediately observe competition between pattern recall ($m \to 1$) and interference of non-nominated patterns ($m \to 0$, with r increasing). The initial overlap (the "cue") needed to trigger recall is found to increase with increasing α (the loading) and increasing T (the noise), until beyond a critical value $\alpha_c(T)$ recall is no longer possible and all trajectories will ultimately lead to the $m = 0$ state (irrespective of the initial state). The competing forces are easily recognized when working out the local fields described by Equation 1, using Equation 2 with $c = N$:

$$h_i(S) = \xi_i^1 m_1(S) + \frac{1}{N} \sum_{\mu>1} \xi_i^\mu \sum_{j \neq i} \xi_j^\mu S_j + \mathbb{O}(N^{-1}) \qquad (5)$$

The first term in Equation 5 drives S toward pattern ξ^1 as soon as $m_1(S) > 0$. The other terms represent interference caused by correlations between the state vector S and non-nominated patterns. One easily shows that for $N \to \infty$, the fluctuations in the values of the recall overlap m must vanish at any time, and that for the present types of initial states and threshold noise, the overlap m will obey

$$m(t + 1) = \int dz \, P_t(z) \, \tanh[\beta(m(t) + z)] \qquad (6)$$

$$P_t(z) = \lim_{N \to \infty} \frac{1}{N} \sum_i \left\langle \delta\left[z - \frac{1}{N} \sum_{\mu>1} \xi_i^1 \xi_i^\mu \sum_{j \neq i} \xi_j^\mu S_j(t)\right] \right\rangle \qquad (7)$$

(with $\beta = T^{-1}$). For general (symmetric) threshold noise distributions, one just substitutes $\tanh[\beta x] \to 2\int_0^x d\eta \, w(\eta)$. Note that Equation 6 can be interpreted as describing the dynamics of the average firing state $m(t) = \langle S(t) \rangle$ of a single "effective neuron" with an effective local field $h(t) = m(t) + z(t)$, where $z(t)$ (distrib-

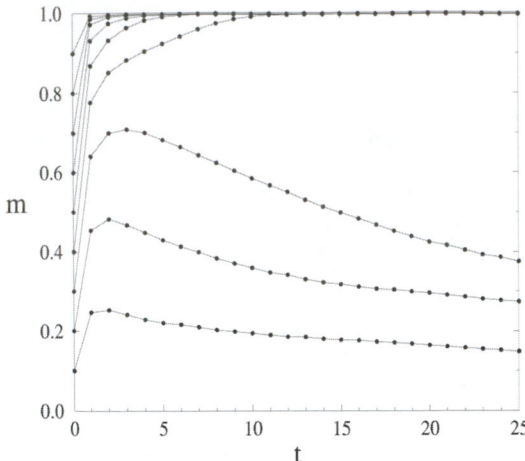

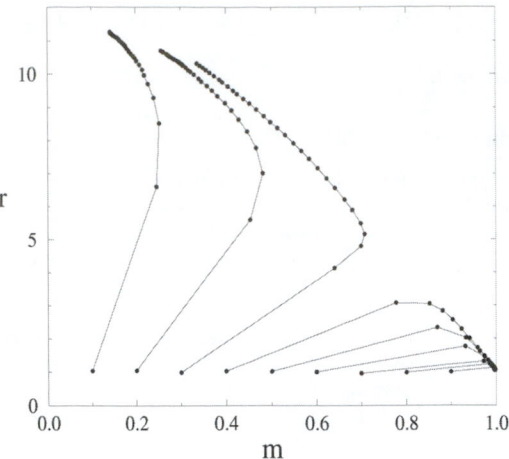

Figure 1. Simulations of a fully connected Hopfield model with $N = 30,000$, threshold noise distribution $w(\eta) = (1/2T)[1 - \tanh^2(\eta/T)]$, $\alpha = T = 0.1$, parallel dynamics, and randomly drawn pattern bits. *Left*, Overlap $m = m_1(S)$ with pattern 1 as functions of time, following initial states $S(0)$ correlated with pattern 1 only, with $m_1(S(0)) \in \{0.1, \ldots, 0.9\}$. *Right*, Corresponding trajectories in the (m, r) plane, where the observable $r = \alpha^{-1}\Sigma_{\mu>1}m_\mu^2(S)$ measures the overlaps with non-nominated patterns.

uted according to $P_t(z)$) acts as an extra contribution to the threshold noise. If all $S_i(0)$ are drawn independently, $\text{Prob}[S_i(0) = \pm\xi_i^1] = (1/2)[1 \pm m(0)]$, the central limit theorem tells us that $P_0(z)$ is Gaussian. One easily derives $\langle z \rangle_0 = 0$ and $\langle z^2 \rangle_0 = \alpha$, so that at $t = 0$, Equation 6 reduces to

$$m(1) = \int \frac{dz}{\sqrt{2\pi}} e^{-(1/2)z^2} \tanh[\beta(m(0) + z\sqrt{\alpha})] \qquad (8)$$

The above ideas, and Equation 8 in particular, go back to Amari (1977). For times $t > 0$, however, the independence of the states S_i need no longer hold. Solving the recall dynamics thus boils down to calculating the (often nontrivial) interference noise distribution $P_t(z)$ in Equation 6 for non-zero times.

Small Numbers of Patterns

The simplest way to avoid trouble is to study situations where the interference noise vanishes in the $N \to \infty$ limit, which happens, for example, in fully connected networks when $\alpha = \lim_{N\to\infty} p/N = 0$ (as with finite p). Equation 6 and its sequential dynamics counterpart now reduce to (with the integrated threshold noise distribution $f[x] = 2\int_0^x d\eta \, w(\eta)$)

$$\text{parallel: } m(t + 1) = f[m(t)]$$

$$\text{sequential: } \frac{d}{dt} m = f[m] - m$$

This situation was exploited by several authors (e.g., Buhmann and Schulten, 1987; Coolen and Ruijgrok, 1988; Riedel, Kühn, and van Hemmen, 1988), who, in view of the simplicity of the finite p regime, were able to consider more complicated choices than Equation 2 for the synapses and arbitrary initial states $S(0)$. If, for instance, we choose the more general form $J_{ij} = (1/N)\Sigma_{\mu\nu=1}^p \xi_i^\mu A_{\mu\nu}\xi_j^\nu$ (with p finite) and if we put $\boldsymbol{m} = (m_1, \ldots, m_p)$, we find the above equations for a single overlap generalizing to coupled equations involving all p overlaps:

$$\text{parallel: } \boldsymbol{m}(t + 1) = \langle \boldsymbol{\xi} f[\boldsymbol{\xi} \cdot \boldsymbol{Am}(t)] \rangle_\xi$$

$$\text{sequential: } \frac{d}{dt} \boldsymbol{m} = \langle \boldsymbol{\xi} f[\boldsymbol{\xi} \cdot \boldsymbol{Am}] \rangle_\xi - \boldsymbol{m}$$

with $\langle g[\boldsymbol{\xi}] \rangle_\xi = 2^{-p}\Sigma_{\xi\in\{-1,1\}^p} g[\boldsymbol{\xi}]$ and $\boldsymbol{A} = \{A_{\mu\nu}\}$. These equations, and more elaborate versions (with, e.g., neuronal transmis-

sion delays) have since been used extensively to study recall properties of models storing static patterns and of models storing pattern sequences (with nonsymmetric J_{ij}). It is even possible to generalize the allowed synapse types further to all matrices of the form $J_{ij} = (1/N)Q[\boldsymbol{\xi}_i; \boldsymbol{\xi}_j]$, with $\boldsymbol{\xi}_i = (\xi_i^1, \ldots, \xi_i^p)$, such as the "clipped Hebbian" synapses $J_{ij} = (1/N)\text{sgn}[\Sigma_\mu \xi_i^\mu \xi_j^\mu]$, by using a different (and larger) set of macroscopic quantities than the p pattern overlaps.

Gaussian Approximations

Let us now return to the nontrivial regime, where $\alpha > 0$ and the interference noise problem must be confronted. As a simple approximation one could just assume that the S_i remain uncorrelated at all times, i.e., $\text{Prob}[S_i(t) = \pm\xi_i^1] = (1/2)[1 \pm m(t)]$ for all $t \geq 0$, such that the argument given earlier for $t = 0$ (leading to a Gaussian interference noise distribution $P(z)$) would hold generally, and where the mapping described by Equation 7 would describe the overlap evolution at all times:

$$m(t + 1) = \int \frac{dz}{\sqrt{2\pi}} e^{-(1/2)z^2} f[m(t) + z\sqrt{\alpha}] \qquad (9)$$

(again with $f[x] = 2\int_0^x d\eta \, w(\eta)$). This equation, however, must be generally incorrect: Figure 1 already shows that, at least for fully connected networks, knowledge of $m(t)$ *only* does not yet permit prediction of $m(t + 1)$. However, for extremely and asymmetrically diluted networks, which are constructed by drawing the synaptic wiring variables c_{ij} in Equation 2 independently at random from $p(c_{ij}) = (c/N)\delta_{c_{ij},1} + (1 - (c/N))\delta_{c_{ij},0}$, with $\lim_{N\to\infty}c/N = 0$ and $c \to \infty$, Equation 8 is indeed found to be correct on finite times (Derrida, Gardner, and Zippelius, 1987). In these networks the time it takes for correlations between neuron states to build up diverges with N, so that correlations are simply not yet noticeable on finite times. For the common choice $f[x] = \tanh[x/T]$ (i.e., $w(\eta) = (1/2T)[1 - \tanh^2(\eta/T)]$), Equation 9 predicts a critical noise level (at $\alpha = 0$) of $T_c = 1$, and a storage capacity (at $T = 0$) of $\alpha_c = 2/\pi \approx 0.637$.

Rather than taking all S_i to be independent, a weaker assumption would be only to assume the interference noise distribution $P_t(z)$ to be a zero-average Gaussian one at any time (with statistically independent noise variables z at different times): $P_t(z) =$

$[\sigma(t)\sqrt{2\pi}]^{-1}e^{-(1/2)z^2/\sigma^2(t)}$. One can then derive (for $N \to \infty$ and fully connected networks) an evolution equation for the width $\sigma(t)$, giving (Amari and Maginu, 1988; Nishimori and Ozeki, 1993):

$$m(t+1) = \int \frac{dz}{\sqrt{2\pi}} e^{-(1/2)z^2} f[m(t) + z\sigma(t)]$$

$$\sigma^2(t+1) = \alpha + 2\alpha m(t+1)m(t)h[m(t),\sigma(t)] + \sigma^2(t)h^2[m(t),\sigma(t)]$$

$$h[m,\sigma] = \int \frac{dz}{\sqrt{2\pi}} e^{-(1/2)z^2} f'[m + z\sigma]$$

These equations describe correctly the qualitative features of recall dynamics, and are found to work quite well when retrieval actually occurs. For nonretrieval trajectories, however, they appear to underestimate the impact of interference noise, and for $f[x] = \tanh[x/T]$, they predict $T_c = 1$ (at $\alpha = 0$) and a storage capacity (at $T = 0$) of $\alpha_c \approx 0.1597$ (whereas this should have been roughly 0.139). A final refinement of the Gaussian approach by Okada (1995) consisted in allowing for correlations between the noise variables z at different times (while still describing them by Gaussian distributions). This then results in a hierarchy of macroscopic equations that improve upon the previous Gaussian theories and even predict the correct stationary state and phase diagrams, but still fail to be correct at intermediate times.

There is a fundamental problem with all Gaussian theories, however sophisticated: apart from special cases, the interference noise distribution is generally *not* of a Gaussian shape. This becomes clear when we follow Nishimori and Ozeki (1993) and return to the simulation experiments of Figure 1 to measure the distribution $P_t(z)$ of Equation 7, resulting in Figure 2. $P_t(z)$ is only (approximately) Gaussian when pattern recall occurs. Hence the successes of Gaussian theories in describing recall trajectories, and their perpetual problems in describing the nonrecall ones.

Exact Results

The only exact procedure known at present is based on a philosophy different from those described so far. Rather than using the probability $p_t(S)$ of finding a microscopic state S at time t in order to calculate the statistics of a macroscopic observable $m(S)$ at time t, one here turns to the probability $\mathrm{Prob}[S(0), \ldots, S(t_m)]$ of finding

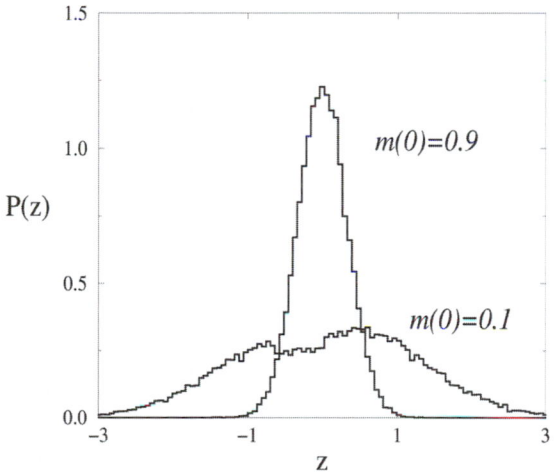

Figure 2. Distributions of interference noise variables $z_i = (1/N)\Sigma_{\mu>1}\xi_i^1\xi_i^\mu\Sigma_{j\neq i}\xi_j^\mu S_j$, as measured in the simulations of Figure 1, at $t = 10$. Unimodal histogram: noise distribution following $m(0) = 0.9$ (leading to recall). Bimodal histogram: noise distribution following $m(0) = 0.1$ (not leading to recall).

a microscopic *path* $S(0) \to S(1) \to \ldots \to S(t_m)$. One also adds time-dependent external sources (similar to injected currents) to the local fields, $h_i(S) \to h_i(S) + \theta_i(t)$, to probe the networks via small perturbations. The statistics of paths are fully captured by the following moment-generating function:

$$Z[\psi] = \langle e^{-i\Sigma_i\Sigma_{t=0}^{t_m}\psi_i(t)S_i(t)} \rangle \quad (10)$$

It generates expectation values of most relevant observable quantities, including those involving neuron states at different times, such as correlation functions $C_{ij}(t, t') = \langle S_i(t)S_j(t')\rangle$ and response functions $G_{ij}(t, t') = \partial\langle S_i(t)\rangle/\partial\theta_j(t')$:

$$\langle S_i(t)\rangle = i\lim_{\psi\to0}\frac{\partial Z[\psi]}{\partial\psi_i(t)} \quad C_{ij}(t, t') = -\lim_{\psi\to0}\frac{\partial^2 Z[\psi]}{\partial\psi_i(t)\partial\psi_j(t')}$$

$$G_{ij}(t, t') = i\lim_{\psi\to0}\frac{\partial^2 Z[\psi]}{\partial\psi_i(t)\partial\theta_j(t')}$$

The idea is next to assume (correctly) that for $N \to \infty$, only the statistical properties of the stored patterns will influence the above macroscopic quantities, so that the generating function $Z[\psi]$ can be averaged over all pattern realizations, i.e., $Z[\psi] \to \overline{Z[\psi]}$. After a certain amount of algebra to evaluate $\overline{Z[\psi]}$ one finds that the recall dynamics can again be described in terms of a single "effective neuron" $S(t)$ with an effective local field. However, this effective local field will generally depend on past states of the neuron and on zero-average but temporally correlated Gaussian noise contributions $\phi(t)$:

$$h(t|\{S\}, \{\phi\}) = m(t) + \theta(t) + \alpha\sum_{t'<t}K(t, t')S(t') + \sqrt{\alpha}\phi(t) \quad (11)$$

The first comprehensive neural network studies along these lines, dealing with fully connected networks, were carried out by Rieger, Schreckenberg, and Zittartz (1988) and Horner et al. (1989), followed by applications to asymmetrically and symmetrically extremely diluted networks (Kree and Zippelius, 1991; Watkin and Sherrington, 1991) (in symmetrically diluted networks the dilution is subject to the constraint $c_{ij} = c_{ji}$ for all (i, j)). More recent applications include sequence processing networks (Düring, Coolen, and Sherrington, 1998), where the overlap m is defined with respect to the "moving" target, i.e., $m(t) = (1/N)\Sigma_i S_i(t)\xi_i^t$. The differences between the results obtained for different models are mainly in the actual form taken by the effective local field in Equation 11, i.e., in the dependence of the "retarded self-interaction" kernel $K = \{K(t, t')\}$ and the covariance matrix $\Phi = \{\Phi(t, t') = \langle\phi(t)\phi(t')\rangle\}$ of the interference-induced Gaussian noise on the macroscopic quantities $C = \{C(s, s') = \lim_{N\to\infty}(1/N)\Sigma_i C_{ii}(s, s')\}$ and $G = \{G(s, s') = \lim_{N\to\infty}(1/N)\Sigma_i G_{ii}(s, s')\}$. For instance:

Model	Synapses J_{ij}	$K(t, t')$	$\langle\phi(t)\phi(t')\rangle$
Fully connected, static patterns	$\frac{1}{N}\sum_{\mu=1}^{\alpha N}\xi_i^\mu\xi_j^\mu$	$(\mathbf{I} - \mathbf{G})^{-1}\mathbf{G}$	$(\mathbf{I} - \mathbf{G})^{-1}\mathbf{C}(\mathbf{I} - \mathbf{G}^\dagger)^{-1}$
Fully connected, pattern sequence	$\frac{1}{N}\sum_{\mu=1}^{\alpha N}\xi_i^{\mu+1}\xi_j^\mu$	0	$\sum_{n\geq0}(\mathbf{G}^\dagger)^n\mathbf{C}\mathbf{G}^n$
Symmetric extremely diluted, static patterns	$\frac{c_{ij}}{c}\sum_{\mu=1}^{\alpha c}\xi_i^\mu\xi_j^\mu$	$\mathbf{G}$	$\mathbf{C}$
Asymmetric extremely diluted, static patterns	$\frac{c_{ij}}{c}\sum_{\mu=1}^{\alpha c}\xi_i^\mu\xi_j^\mu$	0	$\mathbf{C}$

The correlation and response functions are to be solved self-consistently from the following (closed) equations, involving the statistics of the single effective neuron experiencing the field described by Equation 10:

$$C(t, t') = \langle S(t)S(t')\rangle \qquad G(t, t') = \frac{\partial}{\partial\theta(t')} \langle S(t)\rangle \qquad (12)$$

In the case of sequential dynamics the picture is found to be very similar to the one above; instead of discrete time labels $t \in \{0, 1, \ldots, t_m\}$, path summations, and matrices, there one has a real-time variable $t \in [0, t_m]$, path integrals, and integral operators.

It is now clear what happens with Gaussian theories: they can at most produce exact results for asymmetric networks. Any degree of symmetry in the synapses is found to induce, via the kernel $K(t, t')$ a non-zero retarded self-interaction that constitutes a non-Gaussian contribution to the local fields. One also sees that it is not extreme dilution that is responsible for a drastic simplification of the dynamics, but synaptic asymmetry. This is underlined by Figure 3, which shows the phase diagrams of the asymmetrically and the symmetrically extremely diluted Hopfield model (both with $\lim_{N\to\infty} c/N = 0$ and $c \to \infty$), as derived from the above equations. The indirect effect on the dynamics of (even partial) synaptic symmetry is fundamental and can be understood as follows: such (partial) symmetry implies that an excitatory synapse $i \to j$ is more likely to be accompanied by an excitatory synapse $j \to i$ than an inhibitory one; conversely, an inhibitory synapse $i \to j$ is more likely to be accompanied by an inhibitory synapse $j \to i$. In both cases the net effect for an active (inactive) neuron i is an effective self-excitation (self-inhibition); any degree of synaptic symmetry thus acts as a retarded "mirror," which complicates (and slows down) the dynamics.

Non-Gaussian Approximations

Owing to the generally complicated nature of a rigorous treatment of recall dynamics, there is still a market for approximate theories. In view of the non-Gaussian shape of the interference noise distribution, several attempts have been made to construct non-Gaussian

approximations. In all cases the aim is to arrive at a theory involving only macroscopic quantities with a *single* time argument. Henkel and Opper (1990) approximated the theory of a fully connected network with parallel dynamics by replacing the field in Equation 10 with the simpler expression

$$h(t) = m(t) + \theta(t) + d(t)S(t-1) + \sqrt{\alpha}\phi(t)$$

$$\langle \phi(t)\phi(t')\rangle = \sigma^2(t)\delta_{tt'}$$

(with independent zero-average Gaussian fields $\phi(t)$), followed by a self-consistent calculation of $d(t)$ (representing the retarded self-interaction) and of the width $\sigma(t)$ of the distribution of $\phi(t)$. This results in an interference noise distribution $P_t(z)$ (Equation 6), which is the sum of *two* Gaussians, which appears sensible in view of Figure 2, and a nice (but not perfect) agreement with numerical simulations.

A different philosophy was followed by Coolen and Sherrington (1994). Here (as yet exact) equations are derived for the evolution of the macroscopic quantities m and r in Equation 4 (for sequential dynamics), which both involve $P_t(z)$:

$$\frac{d}{dt} m = \int dz\, P_t(z)\, \tanh[\beta(m + z)]$$

$$\frac{d}{dt} r = \frac{1}{\alpha} \int dz\, P_t(z)z\, \tanh[\beta(m + z)] + 1 - r$$

Next one closes these equations *by hand*, using a maximum-entropy (or "Occam's razor") argument: Instead of calculating $P_t(z)$ with the (unknown) distribution $p_t(S)$, it is calculated upon assigning equal probabilities to all states S with $m(S) = m$ and $r(S) = r$, followed by averaging over all realizations of the stored patterns. This results in an explicit (non-Gaussian) expression for the noise distribution in terms of (m, r) only, a theory that is exact for short times and in equilibrium, accurate predictions of the macroscopic flow in the (m, r) plane, but (again) deviations in predicted time dependences at intermediate times. This theory, and its performance, was later improved by applying the same ideas to a derivation of a dynamic equation for the function $P_t(z)$ itself (rather than for m and r only).

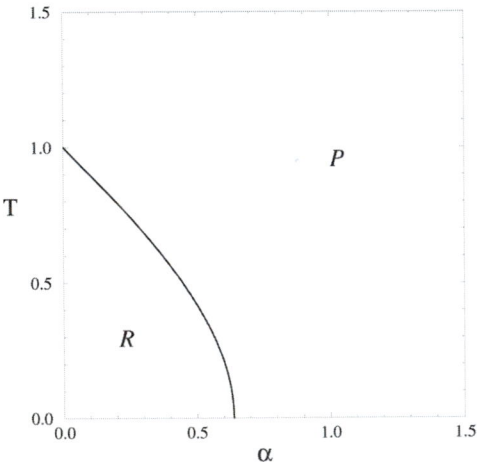

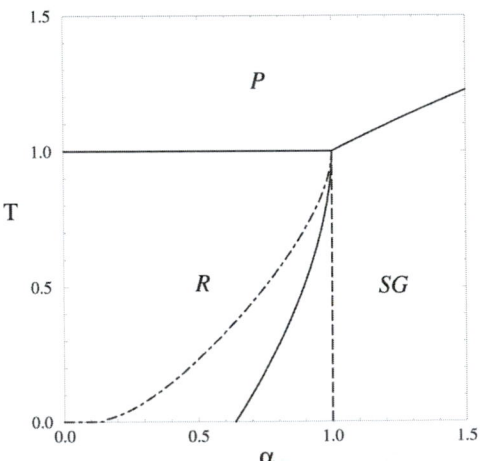

Figure 3. *Left*, Phase diagram of *asymmetrically* extremely diluted networks. Solid line traces continuous transition, separating a paramagnetic (P) region (with pseudo-random motion) from a recall (R) region, reaching the $T = 0$ axis at $\alpha_c = 2/\pi \approx 0.637$. *Right*, Phase diagram of *symmetrically* extremely diluted networks. Solid lines indicate continuous transitions, separating a paramagnetic region from a recall region ($\alpha < 1$) and from a spin-glass region (SG) ($\alpha > 1$) (SG describes the unwanted state where m

$= 0$ and $r > 0$, in the language of Figure 1), and separating the recall region from a spin-glass region (calculated using the so-called replica symmetry assumption). Dashed-dotted line indicates the AT instability (where this assumption breaks down), reaching the $T = 0$ axis at $\alpha_c^{RS} = 2/\pi \approx 0.637$; replica symmetry breaking displaces the solid line to a new (dashed) line, with a new storage capacity $\alpha_c^{RSB} = 1$.

Discussion

In this review I have attempted to explain the various theories that have been developed since the mid-1970s, in often disjunct communities, to understand the dynamics of pattern recall in recurrent neural networks. The methods and ideas described in this review can be, and indeed have been, extended and generalized in many ways. This includes networks with spatial structure, axonal or neuronal delays, nonbinary neurons such as graded-response or integrate-and-fire ones, correlated patterns, networks of coupled oscillators, and so on. Increased biological realism of a model is, as always, paid for by a proportionate reduction in how far one can push the mathematical analysis. However, remarkable progress has been made over the last two decades, with a wave of dynamical studies especially around 1990 (unfortunately, many popular textbooks on neural network theory were written in about 1989, and thus contain very little on recall dynamics), but with new ground being covered up to the present day. Recall dynamics is interesting and relevant in its own right (and a nice challenge for the theorist), yet one can hardly underestimate the importance, especially to those interested in understanding recurrent modules in real nervous tissue, of the other deliverable of dynamical studies: they open up for mathematical analysis the area of recurrent networks with *non-symmetric* (i.e., biologically more realistic) synapses, which is not accessible with the more common equilibrium tools.

Road Maps: Dynamic Systems; Learning in Artificial Networks
Related Reading: Computing with Attractors; Statistical Mechanics of Neural Networks

References

Amari, S. I., 1977, Neural theory of association and concept-formation, *Biol. Cybern.*, 26:175–185. ◆

Amari, S. I., and Maginu, K., 1988, Statistical neurodynamics of associative memory, *Neural Netw.*, 1:63–73.

Buhmann, J., and Schulten, K., 1987, Noise driven temporal association in neural networks, *Europhys. Lett.*, 4:1205–1209.

Coolen, A. C. C., and Ruijgrok, T. W., 1988, Image evolution in Hopfield networks, *Phys. Rev. A*, 38:4253–4255. ◆

Coolen, A. C. C., and Sherrington, D., 1994, Order parameter flow in the fully connected Hopfield model near saturation, *Phys. Rev. E*, 49:1921–1934; *Phys. Rev. E*, 49:5906.

Derrida, B., Gardner, E., and Zippelius, A., 1987, An exactly solvable asymmetric neural network model, *Europhys. Lett.*, 4:167–173.

Düring, A., Coolen, A. C. C., and Sherrington, D., 1998, Phase diagram and storage capacity of sequence processing neural networks, *J. Phys. A Math. Gen.*, 31:8607–8621.

Henkel, R. D., and Opper, M., 1990, Distribution of internal fields and dynamics of neural networks, *Europhys. Lett.*, 11:403–408.

Horner, H., Bormann, D., Frick, M., Kinzelbach, H., and Schmidt, A., 1989, Transients and basins of attraction in neural network models, *Z. Phys. B*, 76:383–398.

Kree, R., and Zippelius, A., 1991, Asymmetrically diluted neural networks, in *Models of Neural Networks* (R. Domany, J. L. van Hemmen, and K. Schulten, Eds.), Berlin: Springer-Verlag, pp. 193–212.

Nishimori, H., and Ozeki, T., 1993, Retrieval dynamics of associative memory of the Hopfield type, *J. Phys. A Math. Gen.*, 26:859–871.

Okada, M., 1995, A hierarchy of macrodynamical equations for associative memory, *Neural Netw.*, 8:833–838.

Riedel, U., Kühn, R., and van Hemmen, J. L., 1988, Temporal sequences and chaos in neural networks, *Phys. Rev. A*, 38:1105–1108.

Rieger, H., Schreckenberg, M., and Zittartz, J., 1988, Glauber dynamics of the Little-Hopfield model, *Z. Phys. B*, 72:523–533.

Watkin, T. L. H., and Sherrington, D., 1991, The parallel dynamics of a dilute symmetric Hebb-rule network, *J. Phys. A Math. Gen.*, 24:5427–5433.

Echolocation: Cochleotopic and Computational Maps

Nobuo Suga

Introduction

The order *Chiroptera* (bats) accounts for one-fifth of mammalian species and has two suborders, Megachiroptera, with 154 species, and Microchiroptera, with about 800 species. All microchiropterans thus far studied echolocate, but only one megachiropteran, the genus *Rousettus*, does. The morphology and ecology of bats are so diverse that echolocation behavior and orientation sounds (biosonar pulses, or simply pulses) are quite different among different species of bats. Accordingly, the auditory system differs among species. Studies in the neuroscience of echolocation have been mainly performed with four different species of microchiropterans: *Pteronotus parnellii* (mustached bat), *Rhinolophus ferrumequinum* (horseshoe bat), *Myotis lucifugus* (little brown bat), and *Eptesicus fuscus* (big brown bat). Among them, the parallel/hierarchical processing of biosonar information was best explored in *Pteronotus*. Thus, the neurophysiology of the auditory system of *Pteronotus* is mainly described in this article.

Properties of Biosonar Signals

For insect capture and orientation, certain microchiropterans emit constant-frequency (CF) and/or frequency-modulated (FM) sounds. The biosonar pulses of *Pteronotus* always consist of a long CF component followed by a short FM component. Since each biosonar pulse contains four harmonics (H_{1-4}), there are potentially eight major components (CF_{1-4} and FM_{1-4} in Figure 1*A*). The second harmonic (H_2) is always predominant, with CF_2 at about 61 kHz and FM_2 sweeping from 61 kHz to about 49 kHz. The CF_2 "resting" frequency differs among individual bats and is sexually dimorphic. In target-directed flight, a CF-FM pulse varies in duration and emission rate, but its spectrum changes little. Target echoes usually overlap with the emitted pulses (Figure 1*B*). *Rhinolophus* also emits CF-FM sounds with H_2 at about 83 kHz. In comparison, *Myotis* and *Eptesicus* emit FM pulses that sweep downward about one octave within a range between 100 and 15 kHz. The properties of FM pulses vary, depending on the species and situations in echolocation. Target echoes usually do not overlap with the emitted pulses (Figure 1*C* and 1*D*).

Different components or parameters of echoes carry different types of target information (Table 1). The long CF component is an ideal signal for target detection and measurement of target relative velocity (2.84 m/s/kHz Doppler shift for a 61-kHz carrier) and the velocity of an insect's wing beat. *Pteronotus* optimizes the acquisition of velocity information by an acoustic behavior called Doppler-shift compensation, by which the frequency of the echo CF_2 is stabilized at approximately 61 kHz. The short FM component is more appropriate for ranging (17.3 cm/ms), localization, and characterization of a target. Since bats emit acoustic pulses at rates of 5–200/s, their auditory system creates stroboscopic acoustic images through enormous parallel processing of pulse-echo pairs in all aspects listed in Table 1.

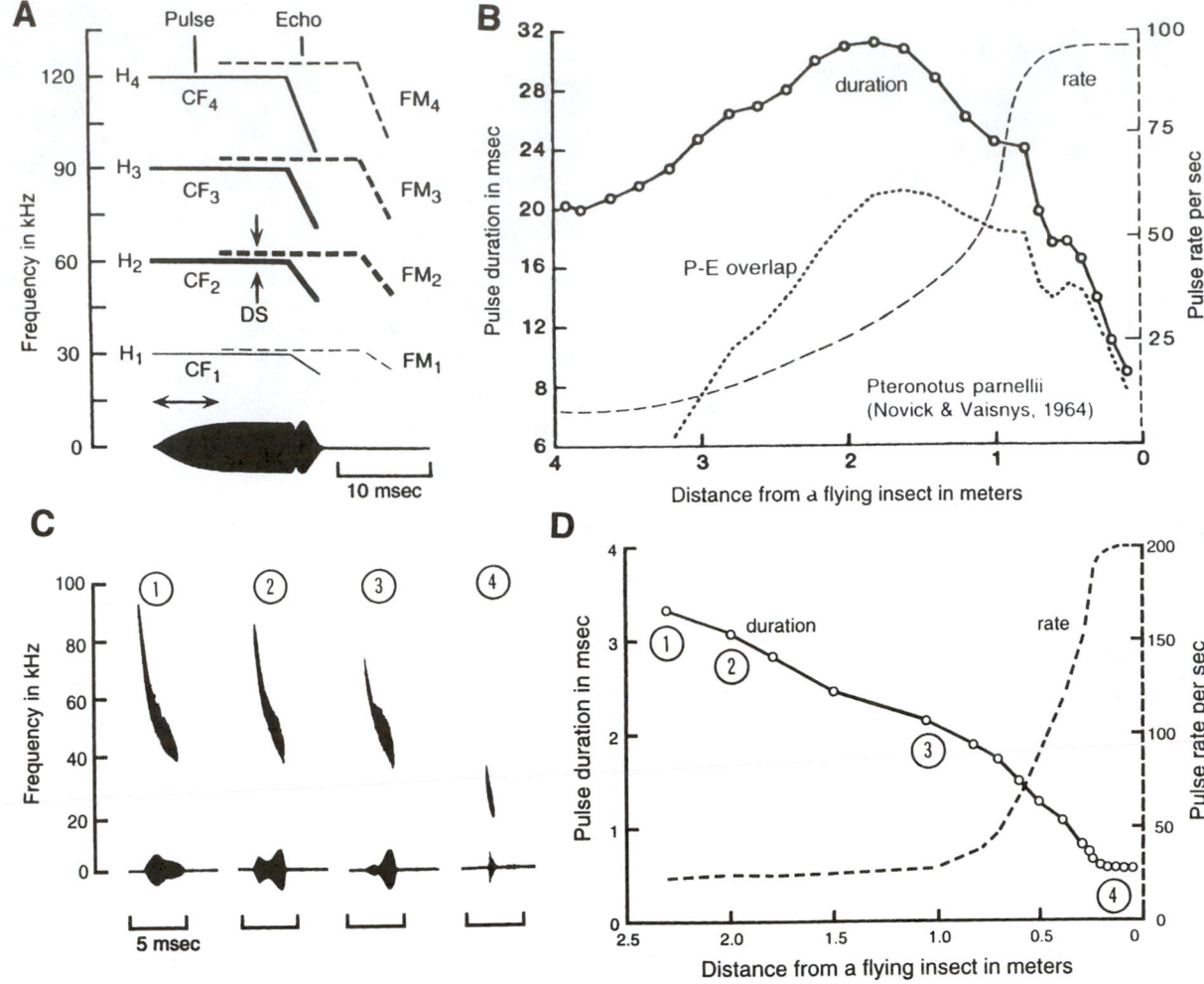

Figure 1. Biosonar "pulses" of the mustached bat, *Pteronotus parnellii* (*A*, *B*) and the little brown bat, *Myotis lucifugus* (*C*, *D*). *A*, The four harmonics (H_{1-4}) of a *Pteronotus* biosonar pulse each consist of a long CF component terminating in a short FM sweep, so that there are eight components, CF_{1-4} and FM_{1-4}. Most of the sound energy is in the second harmonic (H_2), with CF_2 at approximately 61 kHz and FM_2 sweeping from approximately 61 kHz to approximately 49 kHz. As the bat approaches a target, a reflected echo is Doppler-shifted (DS) in frequency, and its delay from the pulse becomes shorter. *B*, During target-directed flight, *Pteronotus* increases the rate of its pulse emissions. The bat initially lengthens the duration of the pulse and then systematically shortens it. Pulse-echo overlap is maximal when the pulses emitted are longest in duration. *C*, *Myotis* emits a short, downward-sweeping FM pulse. *D*, During target-directed flight, *Myotis* increases the rate of pulse emissions, shortens pulse duration as to avoid pulse-echo overlap, and lowers the frequency sweep range of the pulse. Circled numbers 1–4 correspond to those in *C*. (*B* adapted from Novick, A., and Vaisnys, J. R., 1964, Echolocation of flying insects by the bat, Chilonycteris parnellii. *Biol. Bull.*, 127:478–488.)

Table 1. Different acoustic parameters of an echo relative to the biosonar pulse at the ear carry different types of target information

Echo	Target
Doppler shift	Velocity
Steady component	Relative velocity
Periodic component	Insect wingbeat
Amplitude	Subtended angle
Steady component	Relative size
Periodic component	Insect wing beat
Delay	Range
Amplitude + delay	Absolute size
Amplitude spectrum	Fine characteristics
Envelope	Fine characteristics
Binaural cues	Azimuth
Pinna-tragus cue	Elevation

The Auditory System

The gross structure of the auditory system of *Pteronotus* is basically the same as that of other mammals, but it shows a unique functional organization reflecting the properties of its biosonar pulse and echolocation behavior. One of the most striking features is the extremely sharp tuning and the large population of neurons at the auditory periphery for fine frequency analysis of the CF_2 component at approximately 61 kHz. Because of this extremely sharp tuning, they can easily code the small frequency modulation of echoes that would be evoked by the wings of flying insects. The CF_2 processing channel is disproportionately large, from the cochlea through the auditory cortex. The other striking feature of the auditory system of *Pteronotus* is the parallel/hierarchical organization to extract certain types of biosonar information by "combination-sensitive" neurons, as described below.

All the CF and FM components of the biosonar pulse differ in frequency (Figure 1A), and hence they are separately analyzed in the cochlea and are sent in parallel into the brain by different auditory nerve fibers. At the auditory periphery, frequency is represented by the location along the basilar membrane in the cochlea and phase (or stimulus)-locked discharges of auditory nerve fibers. There are no anatomical axes for the representation of stimulus amplitude (intensity) and time (i.e., duration of stimuli and interval between the stimuli). In the central auditory system, divergent/convergent interactions repeatedly take place, and multiple frequency maps and neuronal response properties are formed that differ from those at the periphery. Inhibition (in particular, lateral inhibition), coincidence detectors (AND gates), and multipliers play important roles in the processing of auditory information in the frequency and amplitude domains, whereas delay lines, in addition to the above three, play key roles in time domain processing. For example, the response properties of neurons tuned to echo delays, durations, repetition rates, sequences of sounds, or interaural time differences are created with these four neural mechanisms. The length of delay lines is very short for the processing of interaural time differences, but it can be very long for the processing of other acoustic parameters. Long delay lines are created by inhibition that evokes rebound off-response.

In the CF_{1-3} processing channels, the frequency-tuning curves of peripheral neurons are much sharper than those in other channels. However, they are still triangular in shape, so that the ambiguity in coding frequency by a single neuron is large at high-stimulus amplitudes. All these peripheral neurons respond not only to tone bursts, but also to FM sounds and noise bursts. They are not "combination sensitive." At higher levels, however, many neurons show sharp "level-tolerant" frequency tuning for further analysis of CF signals. A level-tolerant tuning curve has a very narrow bandwidth regardless of stimulus level (amplitude) and plays a role in level-tolerant fine-frequency analysis. Level-tolerant tuning is created by lateral inhibition, which occurs at different levels of the central auditory system (Figure 2). Sharpening of tuning by lateral inhibition is most dramatic in the CF_2 processing channel, and it is practically completed in the medial geniculate body. Inhibition also creates amplitude selectivity, so that some central auditory neurons are tuned not only in frequency but also in amplitude (Figure 2). The CF_2 processing channel mostly projects to the Doppler-shifted CF (DSCF) area of the primary auditory cortex (Figure 3). For the extraction of velocity information from biosonar pulse-echo pairs, the parts of the CF_{1-3} processing channels are integrated in the inferior colliculus (IC), and perhaps in the medial geniculate body (MGB). (It is likely that this integration greatly depends on corticofugal feedback.) As a result, CF/CF combination-sensitive neurons are produced (Figure 4). These neurons project to the CF/CF and DIF areas in the auditory cortex (AC) (Figure 3).

In the FM_{1-4} processing channels, some neurons at higher levels respond selectively to FM sounds because of neural circuits incorporating *disinhibition* and/or *facilitation*. The IC has frequency-versus-latency coordinates. Part of the latency axis is perhaps used as delay lines, as explained later. The parts of the FM_{1-4} processing channels are integrated in the inferior colliculus to create FM-FM neurons, which are tuned to particular echo delays for the extraction of target-distance information from biosonar pulse-echo pairs. The neural mechanisms for creating FM-FM neurons consist of at least

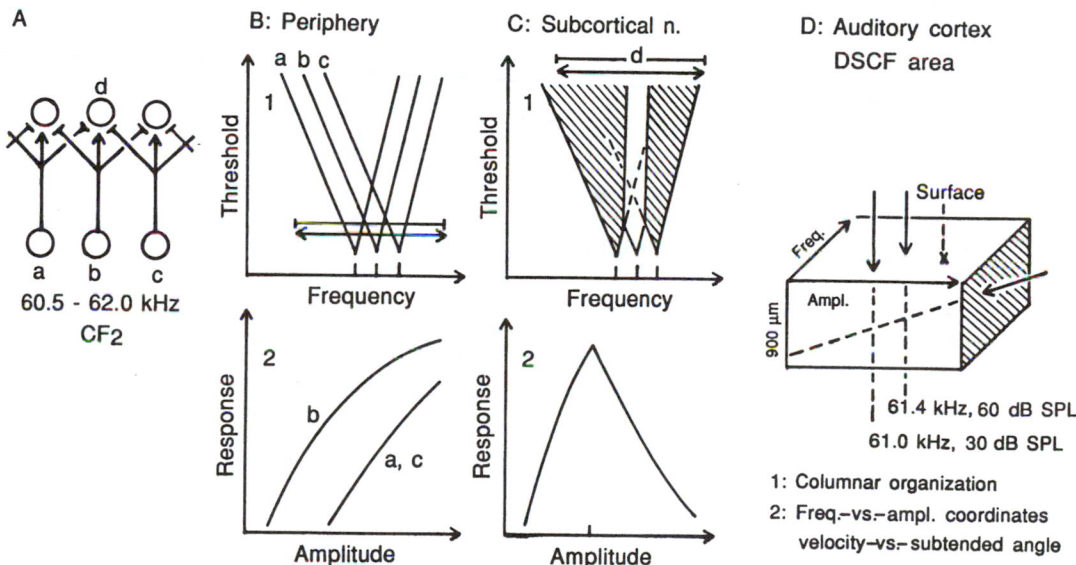

Figure 2. Sharpening of frequency-tuning curves and creation of amplitude tuning by inhibition. *A*, Neural circuit for lateral inhibition. The arrowheads and bar heads represent excitatory and inhibitory synapses, respectively. *B*, Frequency-tuning curves (*B1*) and impulse-count functions (*B2*) of three peripheral neurons: a, b, and c in *A*. The impulse-count functions are measured with a tone burst at a best frequency of neuron b. The double-headed arrow in *B1* indicates that the neurons respond to upward as well as downward-sweeping FM sounds and that the threshold of the response is slightly higher than that to a CF tone at a neuron's best frequency. The horizontal bar in *B1* indicates that these neurons respond to a noise burst and that the threshold of the response is slightly higher than those to the FM sounds. *C*, Subcortical neuron d in *A* has a sharp, level-tolerant frequency-tuning curve sandwiched between inhibitory tuning curves (shaded) as a result of lateral inhibition (*C1*). This subcortical neuron is tuned to a weak tone burst because of the inhibition. The impulse-count function measured with a tone burst at a best frequency of neuron d is highly nonmonotonic (*C2*). The double-headed arrow and horizontal bar in *C1* indicate that neuron d does not respond to FM sounds and noise bursts. *D*, The functional organization of the DSCF area in the auditory cortex. The DSCF area shows columnar organization characterized by a particular combination of best frequency and best amplitude. It has the frequency-versus-amplitude coordinates. (Based on Suga, N., 1994, Processing of auditory information carried by complex species-specific sounds, in *Cognitive Neuroscience* (M. S. Gazzaniga, Ed.), Cambridge, MA: MIT Press, pp. 295–318; Suga and Manabe, 1982.)

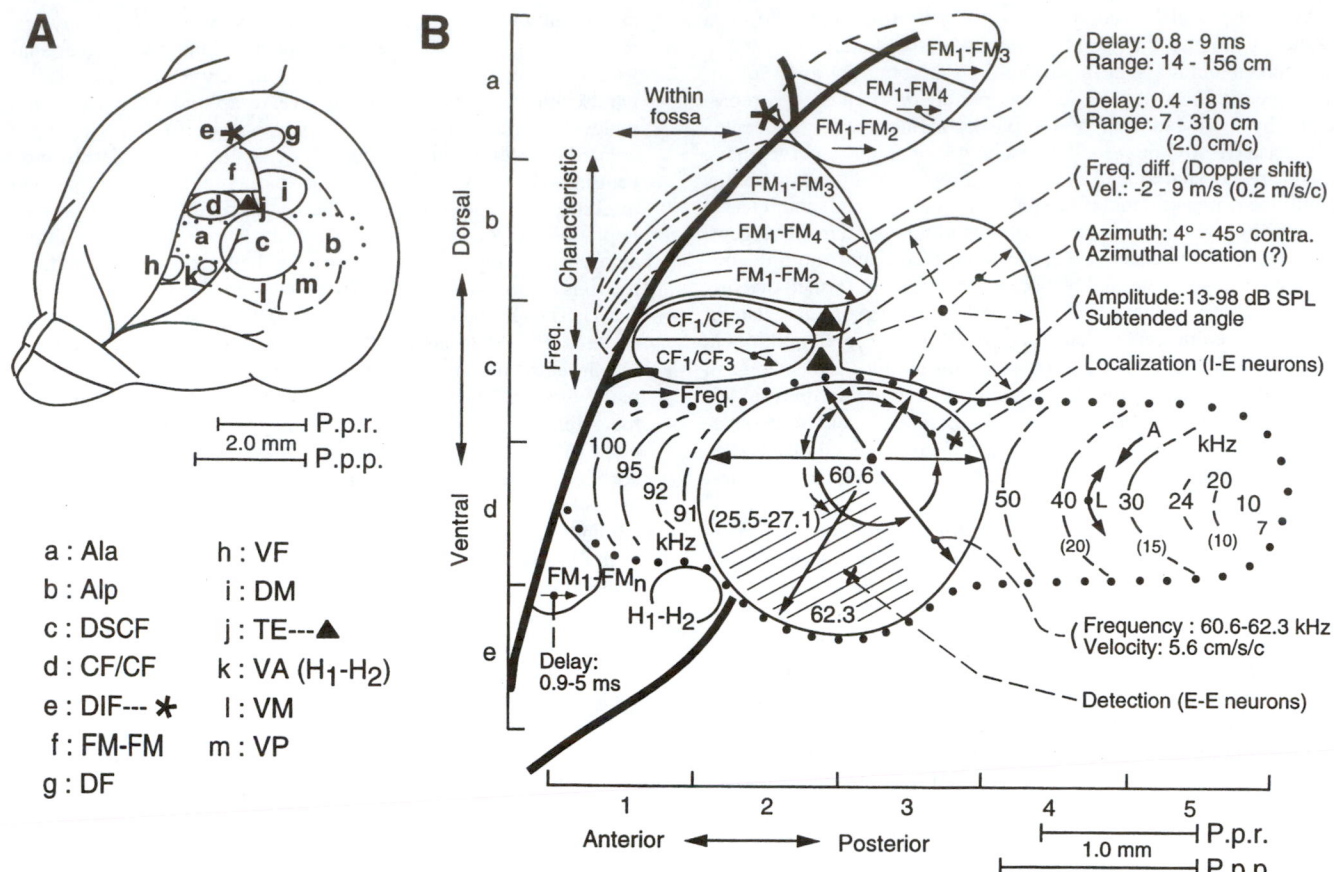

A

a : AIa   h : VF
b : AIp   i : DM
c : DSCF   j : TE---▲
d : CF/CF   k : VA (H$_1$-H$_2$)
e : DIF---✳   l : VM
f : FM-FM   m : VP
g : DF

B

Delay: 0.8 - 9 ms
Range: 14 - 156 cm

Delay: 0.4 -18 ms
Range: 7 - 310 cm
(2.0 cm/c)

Freq. diff. (Doppler shift)
Vel.: -2 - 9 m/s (0.2 m/s/c)

Azimuth: 4° - 45° contra.
Azimuthal location (?)

Amplitude:13-98 dB SPL
Subtended angle

Localization (I-E neurons)

Frequency : 60.6-62.3 kHz
Velocity: 5.6 cm/s/c

Detection (E-E neurons)

Figure 3. The auditory cortex of the mustached bat. *A*, Dorsolateral view of the left cerebral hemisphere and the branches of the median cerebral artery. The long branch is on the fossa. The auditory cortex consists of several areas (a–m), are called AIa, AIp, etc. The functional organization of certain areas has been electrophysiologically explored and is graphically summarized in *B*. *B*, The tonotopic representation of AI (AIa, DSCF, and AIp) and the functional organization of the other areas are indicated by lines and arrows. The DSCF area has axes representing target-velocity information (echo frequency: 60.6–62.3 kHz) or subtended target-angle information (echo amplitude: 13–98 dB SPL). It consists of two subdivisions suited for either target detection (shaded) or target localization (unshaded). These subdivisions are occupied mainly by E-E or I-E binaural neurons. The anterior and posterior halves of the DSCF area are hypothesized to be adapted for processing echoes from either fluttering or stationary targets. Neurons in the DSCF area are sensitive to an FM$_1$-CF$_2$ combination. The FM-FM area consists of three major types of FM-FM neurons (FM$_1$–FM$_2$, FM$_1$–FM$_3$, and FM$_1$–FM$_4$), which form separate clusters. Each cluster has

an axis representing target ranges from 7 to 310 cm (echo delay: 0.4–18 ms). The dorsoventral axis of the FM-FM area probably represents fine target characteristics. The CF/CF area consists of two major types of CF/CF neurons (CF$_1$/CF$_2$ and CF$_1$/CF$_3$), which are also found in separate clusters. Each cluster has two frequency axes and represents a target velocity from −2 to +9 m/s (echo Doppler shift: −0.7 to +3.2 kHz for CF$_2$, and −1.1 to +4.8 kHz for CF$_3$). The DF area consists of the three clusters of FM-FM neurons and has an axis representing target ranges from 7 to 140 cm. The VF area also contains FM-FM neurons and represents target ranges up to 80 cm. The DM area has an axis representing the azimuthal location of the target on the contralateral side in front of the animal. This azimuthal representation is incorporated with tonotopic representation. In the VP area, azimuthal motion-sensitive neurons have been found. The functional organization of the VA and VP areas remains to be studied further. (Adapted from Suga, N., 1994, Processing of auditory information carried by complex species-specific sounds, in *Cognitive Neurosciences* (M. S. Gazzaniga, Ed.), Cambridge, MA: MIT Press, pp. 295–318.)

four physiological components: phasic/constant latency responding neurons, delay lines, coincidence detectors, and amplifiers. An FM sound sequentially stimulates an array of neurons tuned to different frequencies by sweeping across their frequency tuning curves. Phasic/constant latency responders are suited for coding that moment of the stimulus. They code the exact timing of the pulse and its echo, i.e., the echo delay. They are mostly created in the subcollicular nuclei. The other three components are now considered to be in the IC, although part of the delay lines are perhaps created in subcollicular nuclei. Delay lines shift the response to the pulse FM$_1$ in time. A coincidence detector (FM-FM neuron) has two inputs: one input carries activity evoked by the pulse FM$_1$ through a delay line, and the other input carries activity evoked by the echo FM$_n$ without delay lines. An echo always delays acoustically from the

pulse emitted by the bat according to the distance to an echo source. At a coincidence detector whose neural delay is equal to an echo delay, the excitatory response to the echo FM$_n$ arrives at the same time as the delayed excitatory response evoked by the pulse FM$_1$. Then, the coincidence detector shows a strong facilitative response (Figure 5). This facilitation greatly depends on corticofugal feedback.

Collicular FM-FM combination-sensitive neurons produced in this way are tuned to particular echo delays, i.e., target distances. They project to thalamic FM-FM neurons, which show stronger facilitative responses to pulse-echo pairs and sharper delay tuning than the collicular FM-FM neurons. These thalamic FM-FM neurons project to the FM-FM, DF, and VF areas in the AC. The response of these thalamic neurons greatly depends on corticofugal

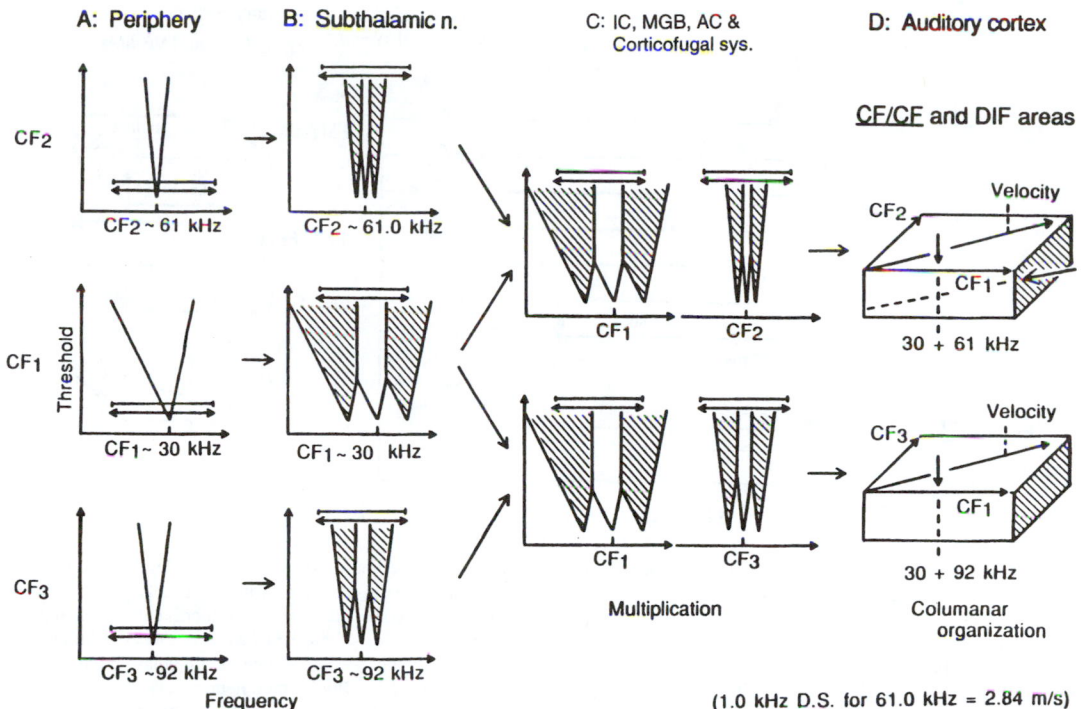

Figure 4. Neural mechanisms for creating frequency-versus-frequency co-ordinates. Triangular frequency-tuning curves of three channels (CF$_{1,2}$ and CF$_3$) at the periphery (*A*) are changed into level-tolerant frequency-tuning curves in the subthalamic auditory nuclei by lateral inhibition (*B*). Then, the CF$_1$ and CF$_2$ or CF$_3$ channels are integrated in the inferior colliculus (IC) and, perhaps, in the medial geniculate body (MGB) to create two types of velocity-tuned, CF/CF combination-sensitive neurons (*C*). These neu-rons project to the CF/CF area in the auditory cortex and form the CF$_1$/CF$_2$ and CF$_1$/CF$_3$ subdivisions. In each subdivision, a cortical minicolumn is characterized by a particular combination of two frequencies. Each subdivision has frequency-versus-frequency coordinates, in which relative velocities of targets are systematically mapped. CF/CF neurons also cluster in the DIF area. (Based on Suga and Tsuzuki, 1985.)

feedback. As a consequence of such parallel-hierarchical processing of complex sounds, there are many functional divisions in the auditory cortex (Figure 3).

Cochleotopic (Frequency) Map in the Auditory Cortex

The central auditory system of *Pteronotus* processes different types of biosonar information and communication calls in a parallel/hierarchical way. As a result, its AC consists of many areas containing different types of combination-sensitive neurons. Therefore, each of these areas has more than one frequency axis. Accordingly, frequency maps based on best frequencies (BFs) of combination-sensitive neurons are much more complex than those based on BFs measured with single-tone stimuli, and indicate the following four important facts. (1) The frequency axes in the AC are not exact copies of the frequency axis along the basilar membrane in the cochlea. Certain portions of the peripheral frequency axis are reduced or enlarged in a cortical frequency axis. (2) Different portions of the peripheral frequency axis are superimposed in parallel or orthogonally across certain cortical areas. (3) An area where the frequency axis can hardly be demonstrated with single-tone stimuli has distinct frequency axes when studied with combination tones. (4) The complex multiple frequency representations in the AC are directly related to the representations of different types of biosonar information.

Computational Maps in the Auditory Cortex

The response properties of certain types of combination-sensitive neurons can be easily related to the processing of particular types of biosonar information, because the CF and FM components of the biosonar signals are suited for the measurements of target velocities and distances, respectively.

Neurons in the DSCF processing area are tuned to particular frequencies and amplitudes of the CF$_2$ component and show a facilitative response to the echo CF$_2$ combined with the pulse CF$_1$ and/or FM$_1$. Most of them are sensitive to periodic frequency modulation. In the DSCF area, individual minicolumns, often called "cortical modules," are characterized by a particular combination of frequency and amplitude. They form frequency-versus-amplitude coordinates for the fine spatiotemporal representation of periodic changes of echoes in frequency and amplitude that would be evoked by insect wing beats (Figure 3*B*). Inactivation of the DSCF area disrupts frequency but not echo-delay discrimination.

Another cortical area (CF/CF) consists of two subdivisions: CF$_1$/CF$_2$ and CF$_1$/CF$_3$ (Figure 3*B*). The responses of CF$_1$/CF$_2$ and CF$_1$/CF$_3$ neurons to an echo CF$_2$ or CF$_3$ are facilitated by the pulse CF$_1$ emitted by the bat when the echo CF$_2$ or CF$_3$ returns from a target with a particular relative velocity and/or with beating wings. Their frequency-tuning curves are extremely sharp. They act as coincidence detectors tuned to particular combinations of CF sounds in the frequency (Doppler shift) domain. Since emitted pulses and Doppler-shifted echoes both vary independently in frequency from each other, the amount of a Doppler shift should be expressed with the frequency-versus-frequency coordinate system. In the CF/CF area, individual minicolumns are characterized by a particular combination of two frequencies. They form the frequency-versus-frequency coordinates by which the relationships between CF$_1$ and CF$_2$ or CF$_3$ (i.e., relative target velocities) are systematically mapped (Figures 3*B* and 4). Some CF/CF neurons are sensitive to

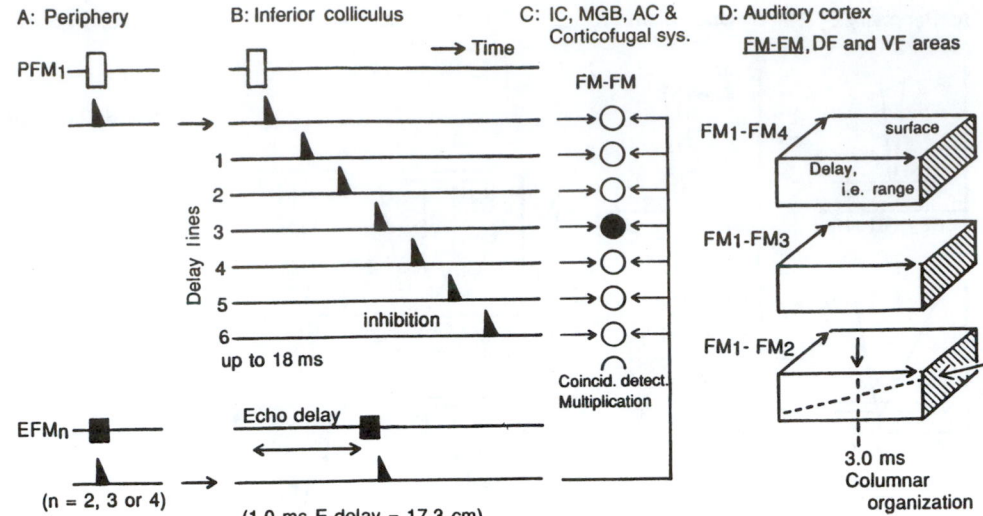

Figure 5. Neural mechanisms for creating delay-tuned neurons and a delay (range) axis. Delay-tuned neurons utilize delay lines (0.4–18 ms long) that are mostly created by inferior collicular neurons tuned to frequencies swept by the FM_1 (top portion of A and B). However, the delay-tuned neurons do not use delay lines created by neurons tuned to frequencies swept by FM_n (n = 2, 3, or 4; bottom portion of A and B). An array of delay-tuned neurons in the inferior colliculus (IC) receives signals from both the FM_1 and FM_n channels (C). In a delay-tuned neuron (filled circle), where an echo FM_n delay from the pulse FM_1 is equal to the neural delay line associated with it, both the signals arrive at the same time. The amount of facilitative ex-

citation of the neuron depends on the degree of coincidence. Three types of thalamic delay-tuned neurons separately project to the FM-FM area of the auditory cortex, forming three subdivisions within the FM-FM area (D). Each subdivision of the FM-FM area shows columnar organization characterized by a particular value of echo delay. It has an echo delay axis, i.e., target-range axis. Delay-tuned neurons also cluster in the DF and VF areas. For simplicity, phasic on-response (onset detector), amplitude tuning, and FM sensitivity are eliminated from the model. (Adapted from Suga, 1990, based on O'Neill and Suga, 1982.)

a combination of three CF signals: CF_1, CF_2, and CF_3. CF/CF neurons are also found in another cortical area (dorsal intrafossa, or DIF) (Figure 3B).

Another specialized area (FM-FM) consists of three subdivisions: FM_1-FM_2, FM_1-FM_3, and FM_1-FM_4 (Figure 3B). The responses of FM-FM neurons to an echo FM_n (n = 2, 3, or 4) are facilitated by the pulse FM_1 emitted by the bat when the echo FM_n returns from a target at a particular distance. They act as coincidence detectors tuned to particular combinations of FM sounds in the time (echo-delay) domain. In the FM-FM area, individual minicolumns are characterized by a particular echo delay. They form an echo-delay (range) map in each subdivision of the FM-FM area (Figures 3B and 5). Some FM-FM neurons are sensitive to a combination of three or even four FM signals. Inactivation of the FM-FM area disrupts delay but not frequency discrimination. FM-FM neurons are clustered not only in the FM-FM area, but also in the dorsal fringe (DF) and ventral fringe (VF) areas, which also have an echo delay map (Figure 3B). It is also important to note that most FM-FM neurons are more sensitive to the combinations of FM sounds than to the combinations of CF tones.

As explained above, velocity and distance information is extracted by combination-sensitive neurons comparing the fundamental of the emitted pulse (CF_1 or FM_1) with the higher harmonics of echo components (CF_n or FM_n). This heteroharmonic sensitivity is one of seven possible mechanisms used to protect the echolocation system from the jamming effect of biosonar pulses produced by conspecifics.

There are many important topics and findings of echolocation that are not described in this short article. One of the important topics to be discussed is sound localization. As in other mammalian and avian species, the bat's auditory system creates binaural neurons tuned to particular interaural time or intensity differences in the subcollicular auditory nuclei and the auditory space map in the

superior colliculus, which is an important nucleus for sensorimotor integration. In this nucleus, some neurons are tuned to a sound source at a combination of a particular azimuth, elevation, and depth. In the AC, however, the auditory space map has not yet been found in any animal, although it has been found that two types of binaural neurons (I-E and E-E) are separately clustered in the DSCF area and that the best azimuth to excite neurons varies systematically along the frequency axis of the AC.

Since the amplitude, velocity, and range maps do not exist in the periphery but are created centrally, these maps are called *computational maps*. The findings made in the AC of the mustached bat and in the visual cortex of the macaque monkey indicate that the auditory and visual systems share an identical principle for processing acoustic or visual scenes: different types of information-bearing elements and parameters are represented/processed in separate cortical areas in parallel. As visual information, auditory information is expressed by spatiotemporal patterns of neural activity in different cortical areas, and cortical neurons contributing to these patterns are quite different from peripheral neurons in response properties. (The cortical areas highly specialized for the processing of biosonar information are also involved in processing communication calls. Each cortical area apparently has multiple functions in auditory information processing.)

Ascending and Descending (Corticofugal) Auditory Systems

Auditory information sent into the brain from the cochlea by the auditory nerve is sent up to the AC in the cerebrum through the brainstem auditory nuclei, the IC in the midbrain, and the MGB in the thalamus. This ascending system is incorporated with the descending (corticofugal) system. In the corticofugal system, neural signals originating from the AC are sent down to the MGB and IC, and then further down to the brainstem auditory nuclei and eventually to the cochlea. The corticofugal system forms feedback loops and plays an important role in adjusting and improving signal processing according to auditory experiences.

Adjustment and Improvement of Cochleotopic and Computational Maps

Corticofugal feedback amplifies excitatory responses to single tones by 1.5 times in the IC and 2.5 times in the MGB, whereas it amplifies facilitative responses to paired sounds by 2.9 times in the IC and 5.6 times in the MGB. Therefore, the auditory responses of subcortical neurons would be very weak without corticofugal feedback. Detailed studies on the corticofugal modulation of subcortical signal processing indicate the following important facts. (1) Neurons in a cortical minicolumn increase the auditory responses of "physiologically matched" subcortical neurons and sharpen, but do not shift, their tuning curves. (2) Neurons in a cortical minicolumn decrease the auditory responses of "physiologically unmatched" subcortical neurons, and sharpen and shift their tuning curves away from the tuning curves of the cortical neurons. (3) As the tuning curves of adjacent neurons along a frequency or echo delay axis overlap each other, the direction of the shift in tuning curve depends on the relative contribution of positive feedback and lateral inhibition. (These cortical functions, mediated by a highly focused positive feedback associated with widespread lateral inhibition, are referred to as *egocentric selection*.) (4) Lateral inhibition spreads only in a given cortical functional area. (5) The effect of egocentric selection is larger on thalamic neurons than on collicular neurons, and is larger on the facilitative responses of combination-sensitive neurons than on the excitatory responses of neurons primarily responding to single tones. (6) Without egocentric selection, the auditory responses of subcortical neurons are significantly weaker than normal. (7) Egocentric selection evoked overrepresentation of a particular value of an acoustic parameter and underrepresentation of adjacent values. In other words, it increases the contrast in neural representation of acoustic signals. (8) Short tone bursts at moderate intensity delivered for 30 minutes can evoke a change (overrepresentation of these tone bursts) in the IC, MGB, and AC. (9) The change becomes larger when the tone bursts become behaviorally relevant. (10) Egocentric selection plays a role in self-organizing the central auditory system according to auditory experiences.

Both the cortical cochleotopic and computational maps are the result not only of divergent and convergent projections in the ascending auditory system, but also of corticofugal feedback. For echolocation, these maps and response properties of central auditory neurons are continuously adjusted and improved by corticofugal feedback according to auditory experience.

Acknowledgments. This work was supported by NIDCD research grant No. DC00175.

Road Map: Other Sensory Systems
Related Reading: Auditory Cortex; Electrolocation; Sound Localization and Binaural Processing

References

Fay, R. R., and Popper, A. N., 1995, *Hearing by Bats*, New York: Springer-Verlag.

Gao, E., and Suga, N., 1998, Experience-dependent corticofugal adjustment of midbrain frequency map in bat auditory system, *Proc. Natl. Acad. Sci. USA*, 95:12663–12670.

Huffman, R. F., and Henson, O. W., Jr., 1990, The descending auditory pathway and acousticomotor systems: Connections with the inferior colliculus, *Brain Res.*, 15:295–232.

Nachtigall, P. E., and Moore, P. W. B., 1988, *Animal Sonar: Process and Performance*, New York: Plenum Press.

Novick, A., and Vaisnys, J. R., 1964, Echolocation of flying insects by the bat, *Chilonycteris, Biol. Bull.*, 127:478–488.

O'Neill, W. E., and Suga, N., 1982, Encoding of target-range information and its representation in the auditory cortex of the mustached bat, *J. Neurosci.*, 2:17–31.

Simmons, J. A., 1989, A view of the world through the bat's ear: The formation of acoustic image in echolocation, *Cognition*, 33:155–199. ◆

Suga, N., 1990, Cortical computational maps for auditory imaging, *Neural Netw.*, 3:3–21.

Suga, N., 1994, Processing of auditory information carried by complex species-specific sounds, in *Cognitive Neurosciences* (M. S. Gazzaniga, Ed.), Cambridge, MA: MIT Press, pp. 295–318. ◆

Suga, N., Gao, E., Zhang, Y., Ma, X., and Olsen, J. F., 2000, The corticofugal system for hearing: Recent progress, *Proc. Natl. Acad. Sci. USA*, 97:11807–11814.

Suga, N., Manabe, T., 1982, Neural basis of amplitude-spectrum representation in auditory cortex of the mustached bat, *J. Neurophysiol.*, 47:225–255.

Suga, N., O'Neill, W. E., Kujirai, K., and Manabe, T., 1983, Specialization of "combination-sensitive," neurons for processing of complex biosonar signals in the auditory cortex of the mustached bat, *J. Neurophysiol.*, 49:573–1626.

Suga, N., and Tsuzuki, K., 1985, Inhibition and level-tolerant frequency tuning in the auditory cortex of the mustached bat, *J. Neurophysiol.*, 53:1109–1145.

Thomas, J., Moss, C., and Vater, M., 1999, *Advances in the Study of Echolocation*, Chicago: University of Chicago Press.

Valentine, D. E., and Moss, C. F., 1997, Spatially selective auditory responses in the superior colliculus of the echolocating bat, *J. Neurosci.*, 17:1720–1733. ◆

Yan, J., and Suga, N., 1996, Corticofugal modulation of time-domain processing of biosonar information in bats, *Science*, 273:1100–1103.

Zhang, Y., Suga, N., and Yan, J., 1997, Corticofugal modulation of frequency processing in bat auditory system, *Nature*, 387:900–903.

EEG and MEG Analysis

Fernando H. Lopes da Silva and Jan Pieter Pijn

Introduction

The electroencephalogram, or EEG, consists of the electrical activity of relatively large neuronal populations that can be recorded from the scalp. Along with the EEG, the magnetic fields generated by these populations can also be recorded as the magnetoencephalogram or MEG using very sensitive transducers. In this article we discuss these two types of activity jointly, since the same methods of analysis apply to both.

Over the course of time, EEG and MEG have became valuable tools in the diagnosis of functional brain disorders, and indispensable in sleep and epilepsy research. The related study of EVENT-RELATED POTENTIALS (q.v.) became essential for studies of brain function in neurology and pathopsychology. This research field received a strong impetus with the development of whole-head MEG systems, since the latter produce data that are less ambiguous in their interpretation. In contrast to EEG, MEG does not need a reference point, and MEG data are more readily modeled in terms of localization of brain sources. These sources of EEG and MEG reflect the dynamics of populations of neurons that have the capacity to work in synchrony. Current understanding emphasizes that synchronous activity in neuronal populations is coupled to the emergence of "local field potentials" (LFPs), which may display oscillations over a wide range of frequencies (Salinas and Sejnowski, 2001).

In general, the same brain sources account for EEG and MEG, with the reservation that the orientation of the active neuronal populations with respect to the cortical surface affects these two modalities differently. MEG signals reflect magnetic fields perpendicular to the skull that are caused by tangential current dipolar fields, whereas EEG signals reflect both radial and tangential fields. This property can be used advantageously to disentangle radial sources lying in the convexity of cortical gyri from tangential sources lying in the sulci.

Over the past few decades, the tools available for functional studies of the brain have been enriched with brain imaging modalities that measure changes in hemodynamics and/or in brain metabolism (e.g., positron emission tomography [PET], functional magnetic resonance imaging [fMRI]). Although these imaging methods have a higher spatial resolution than EEG or MEG, the former have an insurmountable time resolution problem. By contrast, EEG and MEG signals can follow the dynamics of brain activities on a time scale of milliseconds, which corresponds well to the time span for cognitive processing.

A constant preoccupation of EEG research has been to develop techniques to extract information from EEG/MEG signals, recorded at the scalp, that may be relevant for the study of brain functional states and disorders. To this end, a large number of quantitative analytic methods applicable to EEG/MEG have been developed. In general, one can analyze EEG/MEG in time, in space, or both together (spatiotemporal analysis). Recently, the mathematical theory of dynamical nonlinear systems has started to influence the field of brain sciences, in particular by providing a framework that can lead to a better understanding of the dynamics of EEG/MEG signals in relation to brain functions.

In this article we briefly discuss the main aspects of EEG/MEG analysis, considering first, EEG/MEG as a spatiotemporal time series, second, EEG/MEG in terms of the corresponding brain sources, and third, EEG/MEG as a signal that provides information about the state of complex neuronal networks considered as nonlinear dynamical systems (reviewed in Nunez, 1995).

Analysis of EEG/MEG Signals as Spatiotemporal Signals

EEG/MEG signals are complex *spatiotemporal signals*, the statistical properties of which depend on the state of the subject and on external factors. Even when the subject's behavioral state is almost constant, the duration of epochs that have the same statistical properties (i.e., that are *stationary*) is limited. Therefore, EEG/MEG signals present essential *nonstationary* properties. According to the interest of the researcher, emphasis may be placed on analysis of EEG/MEG signals during steady states or on the detection and characterization of transients, such as the paroxysmal patterns that commonly occur in epileptic patients, or alterations of the basic rhythmic activity that occur during changes of the state of alertness (Figure 1). A special type of EEG/MEG transients is formed by event-related, or event-evoked, potentials (see EVENT-RELATED POTENTIALS).

In an analysis of ongoing EEG/MEG activity, it is customary to subdivide EEG/MEG signals into quasi-stationary epochs and to characterize them by a number of statistical parameters, such as probability distributions, correlation functions and frequency, or power spectra. EEG/MEG time series often present a certain degree of *interdependence. Correlation functions* have commonly been used to analyze this property. Here we must distinguish two main questions: the determination of whether within one EEG/MEG signal, a dependency between successive time samples exists, such as in the case of brain rhythmic activity, and the determination of the degree of relationship between two or more EEG/MEG signals. The former can be approached by computing the time average of the product of the signal and a replica of itself shifted by a given time interval—i.e., the *autocorrelation function* (for a more extensive and formal description, see Lopes da Silva, 1999). An important property of the autocorrelation function is that its Fourier transform is the power density spectrum, or simply the *power spectrum*. It gives the distribution of the (squared) amplitude of different frequency components. In general, power spectra represent steady-state variables, but there are also interesting applications to dynamic changes that may reveal how neuronal processes are correlated with specific behaviors. In the latter case, changes in ongoing EEG/MEG activity within given frequency bands, induced by some event (e.g., a sensory stimulus, a cognitive task, or a movement), can be adduced in evidence. Such changes may be characterized by a reduction in EEG/MEG power within a frequency band, usually called event-related desynchronization (ERD), or, in the opposite case, by an increase in power, or event-related synchronization (ERS) (Pfurtscheller and Lopes da Silva, 1999). This form of analysis has been applied to the assessment of cortical areas involved in different behaviors, with interesting results. An example is the planning of specific movements (Figure 2). This example shows that in preparation for a finger movement, the rhythmic activity at 10–12 Hz (i.e., the mu rhythm of the central region) desynchronizes, while a burst of gamma (36–40 Hz) oscillations emerges. The former reflects the focused arousal preparation of the movement, while the latter corresponds to the increase in coupling between clusters of neurons, oscillating within the gamma frequency range, that likely mediates the coordination of the movement. This may be the LFP that corresponds to the neuronal population vector encoding for particular finger movements (Georgopoulos et al., 1999). The postmovement ERS in the beta frequency range probably reflects a reset phenomenon of the dynamical state of the cortical networks engaged in this behavior.

The degree of relationship between two EEG/MEG signals can be estimated using the *cross-correlation function*. Similar to autocorrelation, cross-correlation is the time average of the product of two signals as a function of the time delay between both. The Fourier transform of this function yields the *cross-power spectrum*. The latter is a complex quantity that has magnitude and phase. To quantify the degree of relationship between pairs of EEG/MEG signals as a function of frequency, the magnitude of the cross-power spectrum is usually normalized by dividing it by the value of the autospectra at that frequency of the corresponding signals. This yields a normalized quantity called the *coherence function*. Coherence functions can be used to estimate the degree of the relationship, in the frequency domain, between pairs of EEG/MEG signals.

The counterpart of the coherence function is the *phase function*, which provides information about the time relationship between two signals as a function of frequency. The computation of phase functions has been used to estimate time delays between EEG/MEG signals, in order to obtain evidence for the propagation of EEG/MEG signals in the brain.

As indicated earlier, the correlated activity in neuronal populations (which may display oscillations over a wide range of fre-

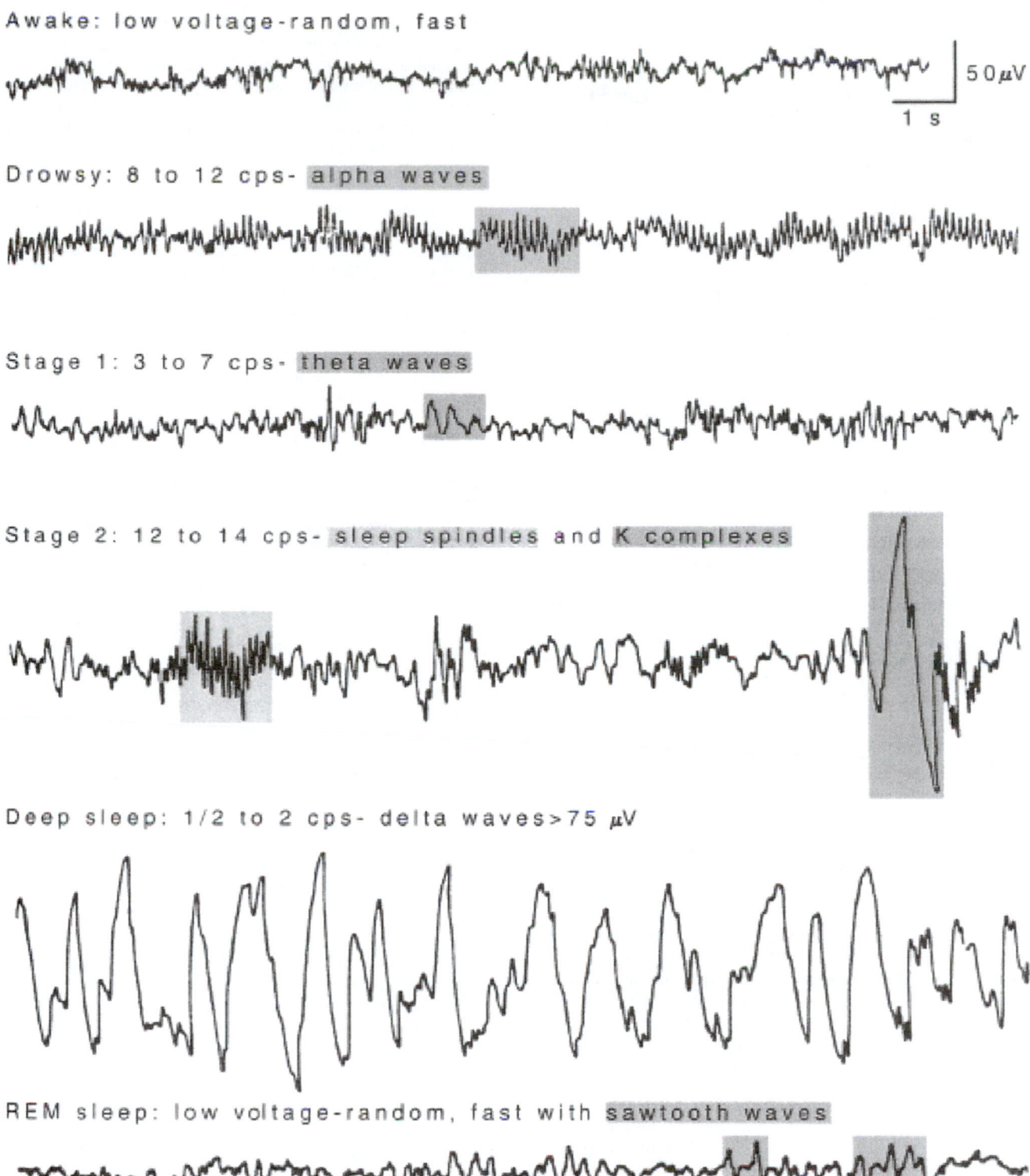

Figure 1. EEG/MEGs recorded during different behavioral stages: awake, drowsy, and sleep stages from superficial sleep (stages 1 and 2) to deep or slow-wave sleep. The last trace shows the EEG during rapid-eye-movement sleep (REM). Note that the awake state is characterized by a mixed pattern, dominated by low-voltage, fast-amplitude (beta/gamma) activities. In the relaxed, drowsy state with the eyes closed, the trace is dominated by oscillations within the alpha frequency range (8–12 Hz). As the subject falls asleep, systematic changes occur: deepening of drowsiness is associated with an increase in slow activitiy, with occasional bursts of 3–7 Hz (theta) waves (shaded area). As sleep deepens, sleep spindles, i.e., bursts of 11 or 12–14 Hz oscillations, and K-complexes (shaded areas), which are evoked responses to afferent stimuli, are the dominant features. During REM sleep the EEG is difficult to distinguish from that of the awake state: it is characterized by low-voltage polyrhythmic activity with occasional "sawtoothed waves" in the 2–6 Hz range (shaded area) that may ocur in conjunction with ocular movements (Modified with permission from Zigmond et al., *Fundamental Neuroscience*, San Diego: Academic Press, 1999.)

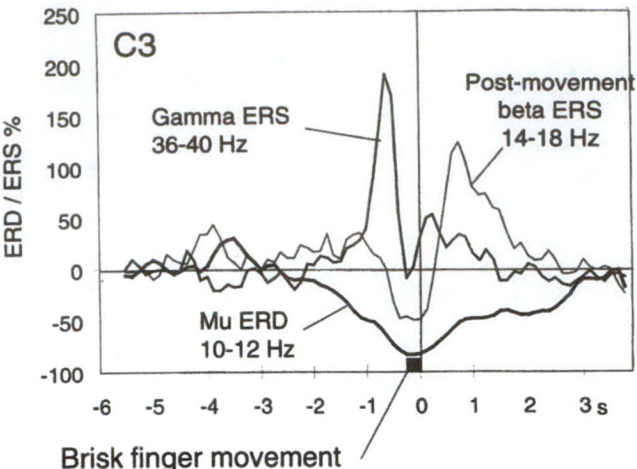

Figure 2. Running power spectra computed for three frequency bands of an EEG recording from electrode site C3, referenced to the left mastoid, and covering the rolandic cortical area, during a brisk right index finger movement. The latter lasted about 240 ms (black bar). The analysis is triggered with respect to movement offset and shows the average of 40 trials. ERD means event-related desynchronization: it consists of a significant power decrease with respect to baseline: ERS indicates the inverse: increase of power or of synchrony. Note that the rhythm in the alpha frequency range (10–12 Hz), called the mu rhythm of the central region, displays ERD starting about 2 s before the movement, while a burst of ERS of gamma frequency components (35–40 Hz) reaches a maximum just before the movement. After movement offset, a rebound ERS in the beta range (14–18 Hz) appears. (Modified with permission from Pfurtscheller, G., and Lopes da Silva, F. H., 1999, Event-related EEG/EMG synchronization and desynchronization: Basic principles, *Clin. Neurophysiol.*, 110:1842–1857.)

quencies as revealed in the EEG and MEG) forms the substrate for a variety of brain functions and associated cognitive processes. Namely transient periods of phase synchrony of oscillating neuronal discharges, particularly in the frequency range of 30–80 Hz (gamma oscillations), appear to act as an integrative mechanism that brings a widely distributed set of neurons together into a coherent ensemble that underlies a cognitive process or the preparation of a movement, as shown in the example of Figure 2. This implies that mechanisms of synchronization at various levels of brain organization, from individual pairs of neurons to LFPs to the much larger scale of EEG and MEG signals recorded from the scalp, are necessary for the coordination of neural activities distributed over distinct brain areas (Varela et al., 2001). Because phase synchrony in EEG/MEG signals must be detected and measured in order to investigate neurocognitive processes, ways of measuring synchrony are of increasing interest. This has led to the development of analytical tools that allow the phase component to be obtained separately from the amplitude component for a given frequency range (Le Van Quyen et al., 2001). With this methodology it was shown, for example, that the scalp EEG/MEG of subjects performing the perceptive task of recognizing human faces induces a long-distance pattern of phase synchronization that represents active coupling of the underlying neural populations. This coupling appears to be necessary for the realization of this cognitive task (Rodriguez et al., 1999).

Estimation of Brain Sources from Scalp EEG/MEG Recordings

A most fundamental aspect of EEG/MEG analysis is to be able to estimate from multiple scalp EEG/MEG recordings the distribution of the corresponding sources within the brain. This implies solving the so-called *inverse problem* of volume conduction theory, i.e., determining the location within the brain tissue of the sources of electrical activity, taking into consideration the properties of both the brain and the conductive media surrounding the brain. This problem has no unique solution: it is not possible to determine a unique current source distribution in a volume conductor from measurements taken at the conductor surface. However, it is possible to solve this problem by putting constraints on the current source distributions, i.e., by defining a specific model of the source. A commonly assumed source model is the equivalent current dipole that represents an active patch of cortex. Therefore, two models are required, one of the source and another one of the volume conductor. Of course, it is necessary to have a sufficient number of measurement points at the scalp in order to obtain a satisfactory solution.

We consider, briefly, the main problems posed by the source and the volume conductor models. The problem of estimating the source is a nonlinear problem that has to be solved iteratively. De Munck (1990) has proposed a general approach that takes into account both the time functions of the activity of the sources and the corresponding spatial properties (positions and orientations). Regarding the volume conductor models, the most commonly used model is a set of concentric spheres that represent, from inside to outside, the brain, the cerebrospinal fluid (in some cases), the skull, and the scalp. However, the head deviates appreciably from a sphere. With the increasing availability of MRI, it is now possible to reconstruct the different head compartments in a more realistic way. This is important, since several simulation studies have shown that deviations from a realistic shape of the head can significantly influence the magnetic fields and the potential distributions (Hämäläinen et al., 1993).

In most applications of EEG/MEG spatial analysis, either in neurology or in psychophysiology, one does not attempt an estimation of the brain sources using the inverse approach, because of the inherent difficulties of this method and the uncertainties of the estimated localizations. Most researchers are satisfied with representing the sets of multiple EEG/MEG signals projected as a map at the surface of the scalp. This is called electric or magnetic *brain mapping*.

EEG/MEG Signals as Expressions of Dynamical Nonlinear Systems

An overview of the basic concepts of nonlinear dynamics can be found in CHAOS IN NEURAL SYSTEMS. Here we briefly state that EEG/MEG signals may correspond to multiple kinds of dynamical states that are characterized by the corresponding attractors, depending on the network's parameters and input conditions. Thus, bifurcations between different modes of dynamics of the same network can take place. This nonlinear dynamical behavior can account for the fact that an epileptic seizure, with a typical paroxysmal EEG/MEG pattern, can emerge suddenly from an apparently normal state characterized by resting EEG/MEG activity.

Quantitative measures for identifying complex nonlinear dynamics have been applied to several kinds of EEG/MEG signals. The *correlation dimension* (D_2) (Grassberger and Procaccia, 1983) has been the most widely used. To interpret estimates of D_2, it is important to use *surrogate* signals (controls) obtained by randomizing the phase of the original EEG/MEG signals. The latter should yield a large D_2 value, since the transformed signal is not distinguishable from Gaussian noise (Theiler, 1990; Pijn et al., 1991). In most cases of ongoing EEG/MEGs, including those recorded during sleep, the difference between the real signals and the surrogate signals is very small, such that the hypothesis that the EEG/MEG signals are generated by a deterministic chaotic process cannot be supported in these cases. However, in the case of EEG/MEG signals recorded during epileptic seizures, the value of D_2 was shown to be much smaller than that of the corresponding surrogate signals. This finding led several groups to explore whether this kind of methodology could be used to unravel changes in EEG/MEG dynamics that may take place *before* an epileptic seizure becomes manifest (Elger and Lehnertz, 1998; Martinerie et al., 1998). Similar results were also obtained from the spatiotemporal evolution of other nonlinear parameters (reviewed by Lehnertz et al., 2001). Taken together, these results indicate that the dynamical properties of the interictal, preictal, ictal, and postictal states are clearly different and have different attractors. This opens the exciting possibility of using these nonlinear analysis methods to predict the occurrence of impending epileptic seizures in clinical practice, and of possibly avoiding their occurrence.

In conclusion, EEG/MEG recordings are complex signals that may provide valuable information about the underlying brain systems, since they have unsurpassed resolution in time, although their spatial resolution is rather limited. Therefore, mapping cortical activity using EEG/MEG signals combined with realistic models of the brain, extracted from MRI scans, may yield new possibilities for functional imaging of dynamical brain states.

Road Map: Cognitive Neuroscience
Related Reading: Brain Signal Analysis; Event-Related Potentials; Hippocampal Rhythm Generation

References

De Munck, J., 1990, The estimation of time-varying dipoles on the basis of evoked potentials, *Electroencephalogrs. Clin. Neurophysiol.*, 77:156–160.

Elger, C. E., and Lehnertz, K., 1998, Seizure prediction by non-linear time series analysis of brain electrical activity, *Eur. J. Neurosci.*, 10:786–789.

Georgopoulos, A. P., Pellizzer, G., Poliakov, A. V., and Schieber, M. H., 1999, Neural coding of finger and wrist movements, *J. Comput. Neurosci.*, 6:279–288.

Grassberger, P., and Procaccia, I., 1983, Measuring the strangeness of strange attractors, *Physica*, 9:183–208.

Hämäläinen, M., Hari, R., Ilmoniemi, R., Knuutila, J., and Lounasmaa, O. V., 1993, Magnetoencephalography: Theory, instrumentation, and applications to noninvasive studies of the working human brain, *Rev. Mod. Phys.*, 65:413–497.

Lehnertz, K., Andrzejak, R. G., Arnhold, J., Kreuz, T., Mormann, F., Rieke, C., Widman, G., and Elger, C. E., 2001, Nonlinear EEG analysis in epilepsy: Its possible use for interictal focus localization, seizure anticipation, and prevention, *J. Clin. Neurophysiol.*, 18:209–222.

Le Van Quyen, M., Foucher, J., Lachaux, J., Rodriguez, E., Lutz, A., Martinerie, J., and Varela, F. J., 2001, Comparison of Hilbert transform and wavelet methods for the analysis of neuronal synchrony, *J. Neurosci. Methods*, 111:83–98.

Lopes da Silva, F. H., 1999, EEG analysis: Theory and practice, in *Electroencephalography: Basic Principles, Clinical Applications and Related Fields* (E. Niedermeyer and F. H. Lopes da Silva, Eds.), 4th ed., Baltimore: Williams and Wilkins, pp. 1135–1163. ◆

Martinerie, J., Adam, C., Le Van Quyen, M., Baulac, M., Clemenceau, S., Renault, B., and Varela, F., 1998, Epileptic seizures can be anticipated by non-linear analysis, *Nature Med.*, 4:1173–1176.

Nunez, P. L., 1995, *Neocortical Dynamics and Human EEG Rhythms*, New York: Oxford University Press. ◆

Pfurtscheller, G., and Lopes da Silva, F. H., 1999, Event-related EEG/MEG synchronization and desynchronization: Basic principles, *Clin. Neurophysiol.*, 110:1842–1857.

Pijn, J. P. M., van Nerveen, J., Noest, A, and Lopes da Silva, F. H., 1991, Chaos or noise in EEG signals: Dependence on state and brain site, *Electroencephalogr. Clin. Neurophysiol.*, 79:371–381.

Rodriguez, E., George N., Lachaux, J. P., Martinerie, J., Renault, B., and Varela, F. J., 1999, Perception's shadow: Long-distance synchronization of human brain activity, *Nature*, 397:430–433.

Salinas, E., and Sejnowski, T. J., 2001, Correlated neuronal activity and the flow of neural information, *Nature Rev. Neurosci.*, 2:539–550. ◆

Theiler, J., 1990, Estimating fractal dimension, *J. Opt. Soc. Am. A*, 7:1055–1073.

Varela, F., Lachaux, J. P., Rodriguez, E., and Martinerie, J., 2001, The brainweb: Phase synchronization and large-scale integration, *Nature Rev. Neurosci.*, 2:229–239.

Electrolocation

Joseph Bastian

Introduction

The electrosensory systems of weakly electric fishes are widely recognized as attractive model systems for studies of the neural bases of behavior. These animals are specialists, relying heavily on information acquired via this unique sensory system, and the importance of electroreception in the animals' life history is reflected in the hypertrophy of brain regions devoted to processing electrosensory information. Animals with active electrosensory systems generate an electric field around their body by means of an electric organ located in the trunk and tail, and measure this field via electroreceptors embedded in the skin. Distortions of the electric field due to animate or inanimate targets in the environment or signals generated by other fishes provide inputs to the system, and several distinct behaviors can be linked to simple patterns of electrosensory input. The ease with which behaviorally relevant stimuli can be identified and simulated, and the wealth of background anatomical and physiological information, are major advantages to studying this system.

Since publication of the first edition of the *Handbook*, advances have been made in understanding the electric organ discharge field of weakly electric fishes and its interaction with targets in the environment (Assad, Rasnow, and Stoddard, 1999). Studies of feeding behavior revealed the motor strategies used during prey capture and have determined detection limits for the system (Nelson and MacIver, 1999). A novel algorithm for determining fish-target distance (depth perception), using information acquired from a single two-dimensional (2D) receptor array, has also been discovered (von der Emde, 1999). Properties of the epidermal electroreceptors have been further defined; numerical models that accurately predict their responses are now available (Nelson, Xu, and Payne, 1997), and analyses of their information-encoding capabilities (see RATE CODING AND SIGNAL PROCESSING) have been completed (Wessel, Koch, and Gabbiani, 1996; Gabbiani and Metzner, 1999). Studies of the primary electrosensory processing region, the electrosensory lateral line lobe (ELL), have revealed how the interaction between ascending sensory information and that descending from higher centers contributes to gain control, receptive field organization, and attentional mechanisms (Berman and Maler, 1999). In addition, these descending inputs participate in an adaptive filtering mechanism, enabling the system to reject predictable patterns of input while preserving sensitivity to novel stimuli (Bastian, 1999; Bell et al., 1997, 1999; Bodznick, Montgomery, and Carey, 1999).

This review focuses on recent progress made in understanding electrolocation behavior, and on the neural implementation of an adaptive filter that attenuates electrosensory stimuli resulting from the fish's own movements. Movement-caused signals can exceed those caused by small prey by more than two orders of magnitude; hence, without a reduction in this "noise," the animal may be unable to detect food efficiently. Reviews of recent progress made in areas ranging from electric fish taxonomy and behavior through the physiology and molecular biology of important neural circuits can be found in Turner, Maler, and Burrows (1999).

Overview of Electroreception

Figure 1*A* illustrates a South American electric fish, *Apteronotus leptorhynchus*. *Apteronotus* produces a quasi-sinusoidal electric organ discharge, or EOD, that ranges in frequency from about 600 to 1,000 Hz, depending on the individual. The bold arrows in Figure 1*A* show the pattern of current flow due to the EOD, which results in a pattern of transdermal potential changes. Electroreceptors specialized to measure the amplitude and timing of this potential are found at high densities within the skin. Objects in the environment having an impedance different from that of the water distort the pattern of EOD current, resulting in a localized change in the transdermal potential or electric image. As the animal moves relative to an object, an EOD amplitude modulation (EOD AM) is produced that is encoded as a change in the firing pattern of electroreceptor afferents (Figure 1*B*). The electroreceptor afferents convey this information to the first processing region in the brain, the ELL. The pyramidal cells (Figure 1*C*) are the principal efferent neurons of the ELL; they receive massive descending or feedback inputs as well as receptor afferent input. Insofar as many of the higher-order neurons providing these feedback signals receive inputs from the pyramidal cells themselves, the ELL is positioned within an electrosensory processing loop, with the result that the functional characteristics of the pyramidal cells are subject to continuous feedback control.

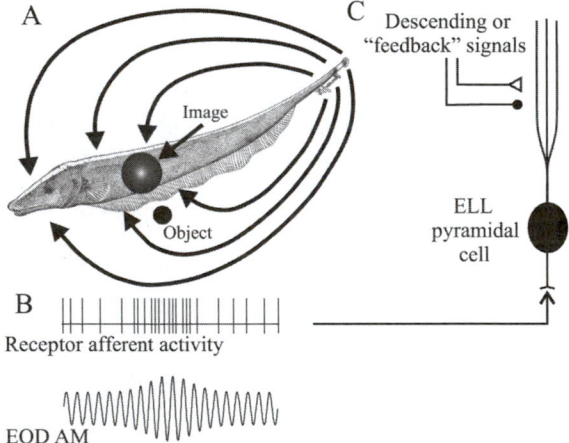

Figure 1. *A*, Pattern of current flow due to the electric organ discharge in *Apteronotus leptorhynchus*. The circle labeled "image" illustrates the pattern of electric organ discharge amplitude modulation (EOD AM) at the animal's body surface as a result of the presence of an object near the fish. *B*, The pattern of EOD AM expected to occur as the animal moves relative to the object, and the resulting change in electroreceptor afferent activity. *C*, Electrosensory lateral line lobe (ELL) pyramidal cell. These "principal cells" of the first-order central electrosensory processing station receive receptor afferent inputs along with feedback signals from higher centers.

Electric Field Measurements and Electrolocation Behavior

Most of the early studies of electrolocation focused on the physiological properties of the receptor afferents and ELL pyramidal cells. Of necessity, these physiological studies used immobilized animals and relatively simple stimulus patterns. Although such studies provided important descriptions of electrosensory system function under well-defined conditions, they were also limited. Natural stimulus patterns such as living prey were not used, and, more important, the animals were not able to engage in normal exploratory behaviors. Recently, high-resolution measurements of the EODs of several species have been completed, and techniques for accurate 3D modeling of the EOD field and various object-caused EOD distortions have become available. These advances have allowed accurate predictions to be made of the spatiotemporal patterns of electrosensory input that occur as a fish encounters targets in its environment. Such studies have also suggested sensory processing algorithms that the animals might use to accomplish critical tasks (Rasnow, 1996; Assad et al., 1999). For example, prey capture based on electrosensory cues requires that the 3D location of the prey relative to the fish be determined. Because the prey or electrolocation target "casts" an electric image on the skin surface (see Figure 1*A*), the 2D position of a target relative to the animal's body surface can be determined from the pattern of activity over the 2D array of electroreceptors. However, estimation of the distance of an object lateral to the fish, or depth perception, is much more difficult. Unlike visual systems, in which depth information can be extracted from paired sensors that view the target from slightly different positions, electrosensory systems probably gauge distance using information from a single receptor array. The peak change in amplitude of the transdermal potential caused by a given object decreases rapidly with increasing lateral distance; hence, this cue could provide information related to target distance. However, the peak amplitude is also a function of object size, resulting in size-distance ambiguities: larger objects at greater distances can generate the same peak potential change as smaller objects closer to the fish. Empirical and modeling studies suggest that distance estimation could be achieved by simultaneous evaluation of multiple image characteristics. It was specifically proposed that measuring the *relative* dimensions of electrical images (e.g., the ratio of electric image width to its peak amplitude) would allow unambiguous distance determination (Rasnow, 1996; Assad et al., 1999).

A series of elegant behavioral experiments demonstrated that another weakly electric fish, *Gnathonemus petersii*, does determine electrolocation target distance using information received over a single 2D receptor array by simultaneously evaluating two electric image characteristics (von der Emde, 1999). Fish were trained to swim through one of two openings in a partition dividing an experimental tank contingent on the relative distances of electrolocation targets positioned behind the openings. Fishes had to choose the opening associated with the object further inside the partition. Not only could the fishes accurately determine the relative distances to identical objects, but, once trained, they could generalize, correctly discriminating relative distance even when objects of different sizes were presented. However, for this species, the maximum slope of the electrical image's spatial profile in combination with peak image amplitude was found to be the best combination of parameters. Von der Emde also found that, at a given distance, spherical objects always produced significantly smaller slopes relative to amplitude than did cubes of the same size. This observation led to the prediction that the animals could be fooled and should misjudge distances when spheres and cubes were compared. This prediction was fulfilled, and the fishes interpreted spherical objects as being farther away than cubes, even when the spheres were as much as 1.5 cm closer to the animal. Such responses to the predicted illusory position of spheres provide compelling evidence in support of the proposed mechanism for distance determination. Furthermore, identification of the sensory processing algorithm used for a given perceptual task provides physiologists with important clues that should greatly facilitate the search for neural correlates of this behavior.

Although it has long been assumed that weakly electric fishes rely heavily on the electrosensory system for prey capture, detailed descriptions of feeding behavior have only recently appeared. Nelson and MacIver (1999) used a video tracking and reconstruction technique to analyze the behavior of two related fishes, *Apteronotus albifrons* and *A. leptorhynchus*, as they fed on small aquatic crustaceans. Stereotyped changes in swimming direction and velocity were found to be associated with prey detection, and, based on the timing of these behavioral landmarks, prey distance at the time of detection was determined. Additionally, given the relationships between electrolocation target size and distance from a fish and the resulting electric image characteristics provided by Rasnow (1996), Nelson and MacIver reconstructed the temporal sequence of electrical images experienced by the fish during prey capture. Finally, given the sequence of electric images as input to a numerical model of electroreceptor afferent responsiveness, Nelson and MacIver arrived at predictions of the spatiotemporal patterns of electroreceptor afferent activity during prey capture. At a typical detection distance of 1 cm, the fishes would experience a peak electric image amplitude of approximately 3 μV, or about 0.3% of the transdermal potential. This translates into a change in receptor afferent firing of about 2.5%, or 7 spikes/s. More recent results also showed that maximum detection distance is dependent on water conductivity, which lends additional support to the idea that the animal's behavior is guided by electrosensory information instead of other cues, such as water turbulence caused by the prey (MacIver, Sharabash, and Nelson, 2001).

These fishes also often change posture during swimming and prey capture; the body is frequently bent into an arc-like posture like that shown in Figure 2. Because the electric organ is located in the trunk and tail, such changes in posture result in large transdermal potential modulations that cause changes in electroreceptor afferent activity 10- to 100-fold greater than changes due to a small prey. These large electrosensory signals resulting from locomotor activity are obviously problematic; they could easily mask small signals due to the presence of prey. However, an adaptive filter operating at the level of the ELL removes the predictable signals related to locomotion while preserving sensitivity to novel signals such as those generated by prey.

Adaptive Plasticity in the Electrosensory Systems

Movements of the trunk and tail of *A. leptorhynchus* through an arc of less than ± 20 degrees, which mimic changes in posture that commonly occur during swimming, cause transdermal potential changes in excess of 100 μV. It has long been recognized that mechanisms must exist that enable the animals to differentiate between such movement-related or reafferent inputs and prey-related signals. Studies in several lower vertebrate species have identified a general mechanism by which reafferent or other predictable and potentially disruptive stimulus patterns can be canceled without compromising sensitivity to relevant stimuli. Importantly, this cancellation process is adaptive; that is, the network mediating the cancellation learns, enabling the system to filter out reafferent inputs that change or evolve over time.

The operation of the ELL pyramidal cell filter is shown diagrammatically in Figure 2. During electrolocation, the fishes often make bending movements of the trunk and tail as they approach and orient to targets (Figure 2A). Consequently, the input to the receptor

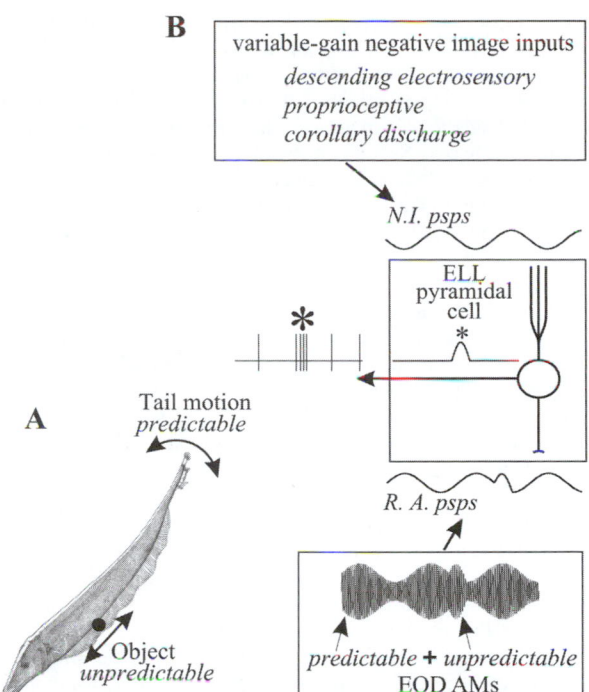

Figure 2. Adaptive filtering by ELL pyramidal cells. *A,* Changes in the fish's posture result in reafferent patterns of afferent input that are *predictable* and can be differentiated from *unpredictable* inputs due to the presence of an object. *B,* ELL pyramidal cells integrate receptor afferent psps (*R.A. psps*) with negative image inputs (*N.I. psps*), with the result that predictable afferent inputs are attenuated while unpredictable inputs are encoded without interference (*).

afferents consists of predictable, often cyclical EOD AMs due to changes in posture as well as unpredictable AMs due to the object. This AM pattern, shown by the lowest waveform in Figure 2*B,* leads to modulation of receptor afferent firing, with the possibility that responses to the cyclical postural changes mask responses to the object. The pattern of receptor afferent synaptic input received by the pyramidal cell is illustrated by the lower waveform, labeled *R.A. psps.* Descending electrosensory, proprioceptive, and corollary discharges of motor commands are received at the pyramidal cell's apical dendrites, and this constellation of excitatory and inhibitory inputs provides a signal that is approximately the inverse of the expected or predictable component of the receptor afferent input. Pyramidal cells sum this negative image input, *N.I. psps,* with the *R.A. psps,* canceling the predictable component of the afference while preserving sensitivity to the unpredictable stimulus (Figure 2*B**).

Very similar mechanisms have been described for four different groups of fishes; elasmobranches, mormyrid weakly electric fish, gymnotid weakly electric fish, and a nonelectric teleost (Bastian, 1999; Bell et al., 1997, 1999; Bodznick et al., 1999). In all cases the neural networks underlying the process are components of the octavolateral system; they process either electroreceptor or normal lateral line inputs and have a cerebellum-like organization. In each case a population of principal cells (e.g., the gymnotid ELL pyramidal cells) receives receptor afferent inputs as well as inputs from large numbers of cerebellar-like parallel fibers. The parallel fibers provide the predictive or negative image inputs. The adaptive characteristic of the cancellation is due to an anti-Hebbian form of synaptic plasticity (see HEBBIAN SYNAPTIC PLASTICITY) at the parallel fiber to principal cell synapse, and a simple set of learning rules can account for the circuit's behavior (reviewed in Bodznick et al., 1999). First, coincident activity of parallel fibers and principal cells leads to a reduction in the strength of active excitatory dendritic synapses. Second, parallel fiber inputs active at times when the postsynaptic cell is inactive lead to increased excitatory synaptic strength. These rules are anti-Hebbian: rather than coincident pre- and postsynaptic activity leading to increased synaptic strength, the opposite occurs. Although these two rules governing plasticity at excitatory synapses are sufficient to account for the adjustment of negative image inputs as described in Figure 2, it is very likely that the strength of inhibitory synapses can also be adjusted, and a complementary pair of rules should govern inhibitory plasticity (Bodznick et al., 1999).

Parallel studies of the cancellation mechanism in these different species have verified that plasticity is associated with parallel fiber to apical dendritic synapses (reviewed in Bastian, 1999; Bell et al., 1999; Bodznick et al., 1999). The plasticity can be blocked by glutamate antagonists applied at these synapses, and it can be evoked by pairing direct electrical stimulation of the parallel fibers with depolarization of the principal cells via intracellular current injection. The depression of excitatory synaptic strength that results is similar to the long-term depression (see CEREBELLUM: NEURAL PLASTICITY) that occurs at cerebellar parallel fiber to Purkinje cell synapses. As in the cerebellum, the depression requires a postsynaptic Ca^{2+} influx; however, unlike in the cerebellum, the depression can be blocked by NMDA receptor antagonists, suggesting that the Ca^{2+} influx may occur via activation of these channels (see NMDA RECEPTORS: SYNAPTIC, CELLULAR, AND NETWORK MODELS). Second-messenger systems operating within the ELL pyramidal cells have also been implicated, and it has been suggested that protein kinase A (PKA) and Ca^{2+}/calmodulin-dependent kinase (CaMK2β) may be involved in pre- and postsynaptic mechanisms underlying the anti-Hebbian plasticity (see Berman and Maler, 1999). Most recently, Han, Grant, and Bell (2000), using an in vitro preparation of the mormyrid ELL, demonstrated that the anti-Hebbian depression at excitatory synapses occurs at the same locus as a nonassociative potentiation. Having both depression and potentiation operative at the same locus has long been recognized as critical to ensuring true reversibility of plastic changes and preventing saturation of potentiation or depression mechanisms. This is the first demonstration of potentiation and depression occurring at the same locus in a cerebellum-like structure.

Discussion

Although electrosensory organisms are highly specialized, they face the same problems and constraints as most other animals do. They must find prey, avoid predators, communicate with conspecifics, and reproduce. Although many of these critical behaviors rely heavily on information acquired via this single sensory system, the properties of the neural circuits involved are likely to reflect general principles operating in many other systems. For example, a widespread but poorly understood characteristic of sensory processing circuits is the presence of massive descending or feedback connections by which higher centers presumably modulate the operation of lower centers. Studies of the ELL of these fishes have shown not only that fundamental properties such as response gain and receptive field organization are controlled by these descending connections, but also that elegant adaptive filtering mechanisms exist that enable the rejection of stimuli that otherwise might mask critical functions. Understanding the cellular mechanisms underlying the synaptic plasticity that forms the basis for this filter should contribute to our understanding of closely related neural circuits such as those found in the cochlear nuclei and the cerebellum. In addition, defining general principles of operation, such as the use of stored sensory expectations for the cancellation or perhaps the identification of specific input patterns, may lead to increased understanding of more diverse neural circuits.

Road Maps: Neuroethology and Evolution; Other Sensory Systems
Related Reading: Auditory Periphery and Cochlear Nucleus; Echolocation: Cochleotopic and Computational Maps; Sound Localization and Binaural Processing

References

Assad, C., Rasnow, B., and Stoddard, P. K., 1999, Electric organ discharges and electric images during electrolocation, *J. Exp. Biol.*, 202:1185–1193.

Bastian, J., 1999, Plasticity of feedback inputs in the apteronotid electrosensory system, *J. Exp. Biol.*, 202:1327–1337. ◆

Bell, C. C., Bodznick, D., Montgomery, J., and Bastian, J., 1997, The generation and subtraction of sensory expectations within cerebellum-like structures, *Brain Behav. Evol.*, 50(suppl. 1):171–178. ◆

Bell, C. C., Han, V. Z., Sugawara, Y., and Grant, K., 1999, Synaptic plasticity in the mormyrid electrosensory lobe, *J. Exp. Biol.*, 202:1339–1347.

Berman, N. J., and Maler, L., 1999, Neural architecture of the electrosensory lateral line lobe: Adaptations for coincidence detection, a sensory searchlight and frequency-dependent adaptive filtering, *J. Exp. Biol.*, 202:1243–1253.

Bodznick, D., Montgomery, J. C., and Carey, M., 1999, Adaptive mechanisms in the elasmobranch hindbrain, *J. Exp. Biol.*, 202:1357–1364. ◆

Gabbiani, F., and Metzner, W., 1999, Encoding and processing of sensory information in neuronal spike trains, *J. Exp. Biol.*, 202:1267–1279. ◆

Han, V. Z., Grant, K., and Bell, C. C., 2000, Reversible associative depression and nonassociative potentiation at a parallel fiber synapse, *Neuron*, 27:611–622.

MacIver, M. A., Sharabash, N. M., and Nelson, M. E., 2001, Prey-capture behavior in gymnotid electric fish: Motion analysis and effects of water conductivity, *J. Exp. Biol.*, 204:543–557.

Nelson, M. E., and MacIver, M. A., 1999, Prey capture in the weakly electric fish *Apteronotus albifrons*: Sensory acquisition strategies and electrosensory consequences, *J. Exp. Biol.*, 202:1195–1203. ◆

Nelson, M. E., Xu, Z., and Payne, J. R., 1997, Characterization and modeling of P-type electrosensory afferent responses to amplitude modulations in a wave-type electric fish, *J. Comp. Physiol. A*, 181:532–544.

Rasnow, B., 1996, The effects of simple objects on the electric field of *Apteronotus leptorhynchus*, *J. Comp. Physiol. A*, 178:397–411.

Turner, R. W., Maler, L., and Burrows, M., 1999, *Electroreception and Electrocommunication*, Cambridge, Engl.: Company of Biologists. ◆

von der Emde, G., 1999, Active electrolocation of objects in weakly electric fish, *J. Exp. Biol.*, 202:1205–1215.

Wessel, R., Koch, C., and Gabbiani, F., 1996, Coding of time-varying electric field amplitude modulations in a wave-type electric fish, *J. Neurophysiol.*, 75:2280–2293.

Embodied Cognition

Olaf Sporns

Introduction

The central tenet of embodied cognition is that cognitive processes emerge from the interactions between neural, bodily, and environmental factors (Varela, Thompson, and Rosch, 1991). Brain, body, and environment are seen as reciprocally and dynamically coupled, with neural and behavioral processes exerting specific effects across the boundaries of brain and body and over different time scales. Clark (1997) has called this complex interplay "continuous reciprocal causation," the coupling of distinct subsystems leading to the emergence of qualitatively new structures. Embodied cognition places strong emphasis on perception-action loops, in which internal and external processes are intricately and cyclically interwoven. The distributed nature of neural, bodily, and environmental interactions has led many authors to deemphasize or, in radical formulations, even abandon some fundamental concepts of cognitive science such as internal representations and the computational nature of mind. They claim that embodied systems generate their cognitive power through real-world interaction, not by manipulating an internal world model, organized in a predominantly sequential (sense-think-act) processing scheme. Whether all internal models (symbolic or neurally based) should be abandoned is a matter of much debate. More balanced theories of embodied cognition would place emphasis on the dynamic coupling between brain and body while allowing for the existence and use of internal models in motor control, planning, and linguistic and symbolic behavior.

Not only has embodied cognition sparked much philosophical and foundational discussion within cognitive science, it has also inspired numerous attempts to build embodied systems as working models of cognitive processes. This article briefly examines embodied models that focus on real-time perception-action coupling, developmental processes, the role of sensorimotor activity in category formation, and value systems. Before we discuss examples of embodied models, we briefly examine some of the underlying design principles.

Design Principles of Embodied Models

While embodied cognitive models show great diversity across different task domains and physical instantiations, most of them fall into distinct classes using different sets of design principles. Roughly, these classes comprise connectionist, dynamic, and neurocomputational (synthetic) models.

Most formal symbolic models rely heavily on computation and representation and do not address neural implementations, learning mechanisms, or the coupling between brain and body. Not surprisingly, embodied cognition eschews such models as appropriate means for implementation. Connectionist models seem more appropriate because they attempt to embed cognitive processes in a neural context. Typical connectionist architectures operate by converting encoded inputs into outputs via intermediate layers, with an emphasis on learning as the search for optimal configurations of synaptic weights. At first glance, however, some basic design principles of connectionist networks appear inconsistent with the philosophy of embodied cognition. Connectionist models employ internal representations in the form of distributed activity patterns that encode higher-order statistical properties of inputs. Motor action is usually not an explicit part of the model and thus rarely contributes to the generation or selection of input patterns. Learning is limited to the optimization of synaptic weights and does not include active exploration or real-world interaction. Although these design principles apply to many classical connectionist architec-

tures (consisting of three layers with hidden units and backpropagation), a number of connectionist approaches have evolved that aim at constructing internal models while taking interactions with the real world into account (see SENSORIMOTOR LEARNING). In addition, numerous connectionist models make explicit reference to neural architectures and dynamics and employ realistic rules of synaptic change. Such neurocomputational models can be embedded in behaving autonomous systems and yield interesting behavior.

A distinct class of models of embodied cognition is based on concepts of dynamical systems theory (Thelen and Smith, 1994; Kelso, 1995). Here the emphasis is less on the mechanistic implementation of neural structures and more on the interplay between the internal dynamics of the agent and the external dynamics of the body and environment. Some central concepts of dynamical systems theory are those of *attractor* and *phase space*. Any point in phase space corresponds to a particular set of values of the system's state variables (which form the dimensions of the space). Over time, the system goes through a trajectory within this phase space, a set of points that are occupied as time progresses. The temporal evolution of the system's trajectory is described by a set of dynamic equations (usually nonlinear differential equations). An attractor is that portion of the state space that the system's trajectory converges upon over time; attractors can be points (stable steady state), limit cycles (periodic states), quasi-periodic, or chaotic. When this formal approach is applied to modeling embodied cognition, cognitive processes (perceiving, planning, deciding, remembering) are described using the language and tools of dynamical systems theory. This has the advantage of unifying the formal treatment of internal and external processes within a common (dynamical) framework. The basic building blocks of dynamical embodied models are state variables, realized as spatially continuous activation fields and usually defined in a behavioral or task-dependent context (e.g., "movement planning field," "decision field"). The temporal evolution of these fields is governed by sets of dynamical equations that ultimately determine behavior.

Another class of models attempts to create autonomous and embodied systems by synthetically assembling such systems from simple components. This approach, also called "synthetic modeling," incorporates explicit mechanisms at all levels and studies their emergent dynamic behavior (Edelman et al., 1992; Pfeifer and Scheier, 1999; Sporns, Almassy, and Edelman, 2000; see also Braitenberg, 1986). In synthetic models, the neural system is defined in terms of a specific physiology and anatomy. When combined with a matching body structure, this approach produces models that often closely resemble particular animal species; examples in the literature include robotic ants, bees, crickets, lobsters, frogs, and primates (see also NEUROETHOLOGY, COMPUTATIONAL). Real and simulated neural systems often attain specific (input- and state-dependent) dynamic states as a result of neuronal interactions. Thus, in synthetic models, large-scale dynamics are the emergent product of low-level components (neurons and connections) and their specific structural and functional properties (e.g., spike dynamics, neuronal morphology, excitatory and inhibitory effects, synaptic plasticity, and connectivity patterns). The synthetic approach allows us to use established principles of computational neuroscience and to relate results obtained with embodied models to the empirical findings of neurobiology. However, the computational expense of simulating realistic neural architectures still places serious limits on the size and complexity of such models, given that they must function in real time as part of a behaving creature.

The emphasis on body structure and environment as causal elements in the emergence of organized behavior requires their explicit inclusion in models of embodied cognition. Although some researchers use simulated environments, more often they use actual robots as physical analogues of real organisms. Robot sensors and effectors are interfaced with a computational model (a neural or dynamic simulation). The robot moves or acts within an environment, either an unconstrained real-world setting (office, lab) or an enclosure containing various kinds of objects. When designing embodied models, it is important to include the relevant physical, dynamic, and kinematic properties of the robot body (Beer et al., 1998), as well as to match the sensorimotor capabilities of the robot and the complexity of its task environment (the principle of "ecological balance"; Pfeifer and Scheier, 1999). Finally, embodied cognitive models must function without human intervention and without the use of supervised learning strategies. A truly autonomous system not only must be embodied, it should also be able to seek out and gather its own sensory inputs ("situatedness") and generate its own experiential and behavioral history. Autonomous systems may exist in a social context. A full account of their behavior and development should include their social interactions and socially mediated processes such as observational or imitation learning.

Real-Time Coupling Between Brain and World

Embodied models of active vision and motor coordination show that several computationally hard problems of information extraction and control are more naturally addressed when the real-time coupling between neural and bodily structures is taken into account. Rather than relying on explicit internal representations or internal world models in computing appropriate outputs, such systems use "the world as its own model."

For example, for many years researchers in machine vision believed that the purpose of vision is to generate an accurate and comprehensive internal representation of the surrounding three-dimensional (3D) world by extracting information from 2D images. According to this view, given an image, the visual system computes a solution, and ultimately issues appropriate motor commands. Movement implements the outcome of perceptual decision making but does not participate in the perceptual process as a source or generator of useful information. About 10 years ago, several authors, among them Dana Ballard and Ruzena Bajcsy (see review in Clark, 1997), proposed an alternative strategy called active or animate vision. According to this approach, vision is best understood in the context of visual behaviors. Organisms use vision to guide motor action in real time, and motor action serves to seek out sources of perceptual information in the environment, for example by orienting sensory surfaces during gaze control. For example, visuomotor behaviors greatly facilitate efficient sampling of sensory environments by autonomous sensorimotor agents. Active vision simplifies several problems of standard machine vision, such as invariant recognition, by using sensorimotor strategies such as foveation to reduce variance across multiple views of the same object. In addition, visual agents can utilize and continually reference objects in the outside world during the generation of behavior instead of relying exclusively on internal models and representations to guide action. Active vision strategies provide only one set of examples of how agent-environment interactions can be exploited in perception; other examples include the use of haptic exploration strategies in active touch.

Another set of examples demonstrating how coupling to the real world can simplify classical control problems comes from embodied models of coordinated movement (see LOCOMOTION, INVERTEBRATE). Several researchers (e.g., Brooks, 1991; Beer et al., 1998) have studied locomotion in insect-like hexapod robots. In these models, walking and other behaviors were not preprogrammed or controlled by a central processor; rather coordination emerged from the interactions between individual leg dynamics, layered control architectures, and the physics of the real world. Real-time coupling to an environment has also been exploited in robotic models of swimming in fish and flying in insects.

Motor Development and the Embodied Perspective

Many theories of human cognitive development primarily rely on the gradual maturation of an internal representation-based processing architecture as an explanatory basis for developmental change. Thelen and Smith (1994) proposed an alternative account focusing on the intimate linkage between brain, body, and environment. These authors claim that, in the course of development, structured action and perception result from dynamic interactions between all these domains, without the necessity for the prior construction of underlying internal representations.

Recently, Thelen and colleagues have investigated the development of Jean Piaget's classic "A-not-B" error in infants. The basic phenomenon involves infants reaching for and retrieving an object from one of two identical containers (labeled A and B) after the object was hidden in full view of the infants. First, the object is repeatedly hidden at and retrieved from location A. If the object is then hidden in container B, the infants, after a brief delay, continue to reach for container A, even though they viewed the object being hidden in B. Numerous contextual effects on the A-not-B task have been demonstrated, including the visual appearance of the containers, timing effects, and infant posture. Several cognitive theories have been proposed to account for the A-not-B error, some suggesting an immature concept of object permanence as the principal cause, others focusing on a dissociation or modular segregation between "knowing" and "acting." Thelen and colleagues (2001) designed a detailed dynamical model to account for the A-not-B error and its context dependency. Important components of the model include a "movement planning field" whose dynamics determine the goal location of the reaching movement. This field receives activation from sensory input fields and from a "memory field" that maintains a memory of recent reaching locations. The A-not-B error emerges dynamically if acute or specific sensory inputs cuing target location B decay (for example, during a brief temporal delay) while inputs from the memory field (with high activity at location A and a slow time course) continue to dominate. Thus, in the model, the A-not-B error is not due to immature or weak internal representations or to a separation between "knowing" and "acting" but is the result of the internal dynamics of the reaching system, specifically the interaction between the effects of memory (long time course) and those of acute sensory inputs (short time course). The model was tested in numerous other contexts and for different sets of task parameters and produced results that were consistent with empirical findings.

A major advance of the dynamical perspective has been to unify processes of neural, bodily, and environmental change within a common dynamical framework. According to this approach, for example, "knowing" and "acting" do not constitute neatly separable modules or domains within the human cognitive architecture. Rather, in the course of human cognitive development, "knowing" and "acting" are intricately coupled and manifest themselves in different contexts of embodied, situated action and individual experience.

Sensorimotor Processes in Category Formation

Perceptual categorization is one of the most fundamental cognitive processes. The formation of new categories is crucial for an organism's ability to continually adapt within a changing and unpredictable environment (Edelman, 1987). A large number of computational and connectionist models of categorization have been proposed (see Pfeifer and Scheier, 1999). The majority of these models work by constructing an optimal mapping between representations of the stimulus (input) and discrete category representations (output). Synaptic weights linking input and output representations are adjusted by using supervised (backpropagation) or unsupervised learning schemes.

Embodied cognition offers a different perspective on category learning. An embodied system is not passively exposed to sensory "data" or to coded feature vectors. Rather, embodied systems exploit movement and interactions with the environment to actively seek out sensory stimulation. In the process, they not only sample but also may generate "good" sensory information, for example by introducing temporal correlations due to bodily movement that help in constructing perceptual invariants. To test this hypothesis, Sporns and colleagues designed an embodied neural model of the development of translation invariance and object selectivity in the primate inferior temporal cortex (Almassy, Edelman, and Sporns, 1998). The model demonstrated that smooth lateral displacement of visual objects due to visual scanning movements are essential for constructing large homogeneous receptive fields of inferior temporal cortical neurons. When such movements were disrupted, translation-invariant and object-selective cells failed to emerge. Even after the initial developmental phase was completed, ongoing synaptic changes within the visual neural maps produced representational experience-dependent plasticity. Groups of neuronal units continued to compete for neural inputs and showed differential increases and decreases reflecting the behavioral history of the model. In another model of category learning, Pfeifer and Scheier (1999) showed that an embodied system can construct sensorimotor categories by generating consistent spatiotemporal correlations across sensor readings while interacting with objects. A simple circling behavior was sufficient to learn the distinction between large and small objects, encountered as a mobile robot navigates its environment.

Both of these models show how embodied systems can actively generate information about objects that is not contained in individual sensor "snapshots." The categorization of objects requires bodily movement and real-world interaction to generate temporally correlated sensory inputs. Correlations can be generated within one sensory modality across time, which may lead to a disambiguation of sensory input through a reduction of the dimensionality of sensory space. In addition, correlations across different sensory channels can be exploited to form cross-modal associations, which are a prerequisite for concept formation. In the context of category and concept formation, embodiment may be viewed as an essential principle that supports the ability of autonomous systems to extract statistical regularities ("knowledge") from an environment. In order to accomplish this function, the temporal dynamics of the nervous system, the morphology of the body (the spatial arrangement and characteristics of its sensors and effectors), and the movement repertoire act together in ways that are not encompassed by pure information-processing approaches.

Value and Embodied Cognition

Embodied cognition requires that neural, bodily, and environmental domains attain dynamically coupled states. Embodied systems need to function coherently within a given environment or task domain. If behavior is to be adaptive, mechanisms must exist by which global functional goals can shape the elementary (neural and bodily) components of the organism, enabling adaptive dynamic states consistently to emerge. In other words, the global performance or adaptiveness of the system must be able to influence its local (internal) structure such that the propensity of the system to behave adaptively is increased. For the system to be truly autonomous, the mechanisms that mold local structure to yield global function must reside wholly within the system itself.

Supervised learning is clearly inconsistent with this requirement. Reinforcement learning (see REINFORCEMENT LEARNING) and in particular temporal difference learning provide a promising set of computational principles, although generally they do not specify the neural mechanisms by which consequences of behavior are sensed by an organism. In mammals, several neuromodulatory systems (including the dopaminergic and noradrenergic systems) are known to project diffusely and widely throughout the cerebral cortex (see DOPAMINE, ROLES OF; NEUROMODULATION IN MAMMALIAN NERVOUS SYSTEMS). They are responsive to salient events in the environment (e.g., reward stimuli) and exert physiological effects on cortical neural activity and plasticity. Sporns and colleagues have implemented such "value systems" in embodied synthetic models (Almassy et al., 1998; Sporns et al., 2000) to study their role in adaptive behavior. Computationally, value acts to gate plasticity during brief episodes of high behavioral saliency. Through synaptic plasticity in sensory afferents to value systems, previously neutral sensory stimuli or modalities can acquire the ability to trigger value and thus become salient to the organism. Sporns et al. (2000) showed how innate and acquired response characteristics can shape the behavioral history of an autonomous robot and provide a neural basis for avoidance and secondary conditioning.

Discussion

Embodied cognition presents a stark contrast to classical views of cognition. The theoretical challenge of embodied cognition has provoked numerous philosophical discussions of core principles of cognition such as representation and the internal world model. It is unclear whether internal models, explicitly symbolic or based on neural representations, should be fully abandoned. Modern neuroscience provides abundant evidence for neural coding in all sensory and motor domains, as well as neural activity underlying internally generated states related to attention, memory, prediction, and planning. Embodied cognition needs to strive for a conceptual synthesis between such internal processes and coupled sensorimotor and behavioral interactions across brain and body. Perhaps it is fair to say that the ultimate success of embodied cognition will depend on whether empirical findings in developmental, cognitive, and neural science buttress its far-reaching theoretical claims and whether implementations of embodied models will compare favorably with those based on other approaches.

In the future we may expect to see a fruitful convergence between the methods and concepts from dynamical systems theory and neuroscience. For example, the large-scale dynamics of an extended network such as the cerebral cortex can be characterized by global interactions between locally specialized (segregated) areas, leading to the emergence of functionally integrated cognitive and perceptual states (Tononi, Edelman, and Sporns, 1998). Thus, in a sense, perceptual and cognitive states are characterized not only by the activity of certain brain regions, but also by their dynamic co- and interactivity. In the future, as we continue to explore the important connection between neural dynamics and cognition (Arbib, Érdi, and Szentágothai, 1998), more advanced synthetic approaches will begin to study neurodynamical processes of increasing complexity within the embodied systems of organisms and robots.

Road Map: Psychology
Related Reading: Neuroethology, Computational; Philosophical Issues in Brain Theory and Connectionism

References

Almassy, N., Edelman, G. M., and Sporns, O., 1998, Behavioral constraints in the development of neuronal properties: A cortical model embedded in a real world device. *Cerebr. Cortex*, 8:346–361.

Arbib, M. A., Érdi, P., and Szentágothai, J., 1998, *Neural Organization: Structure, Function, and Dynamics*, Cambridge, MA: MIT Press.

Beer, R. D., Chiel, H. J., Quinn, R. D., and Ritzmann, R. E., 1998, Biorobotic approaches to the study of motor systems, *Curr. Opin. Neurobiol.*, 8:777–782.

Braitenberg, V., 1986, *Vehicles: Experiments in Synthetic Psychology*, Cambridge, MA: MIT Press.

Brooks, R. A., 1991, New approaches to robotics, *Science*, 253:1227–1232.

Clark, A., 1997, *Being There: Putting Brain, Body and World Together Again*, Cambridge, MA: MIT Press. ◆

Edelman, G. M., 1987, *Neural Darwinism*, New York: Basic Books. ◆

Edelman, G. M., Reeke, G. N., Gall, W. E., Tononi, G., Williams, D., and Sporns, O., 1992, Synthetic neural modeling applied to a real-world artifact, *Proc. Natl. Acad. Sci. USA*, 89:7267–7271.

Kelso, J. A. S., 1995, *Dynamic Patterns*, Cambridge, MA: MIT Press. ◆

Pfeifer, R., and Scheier, C., 1999, *Understanding Intelligence*, Cambridge, MA: MIT Press. ◆

Sporns, O., Almassy, N., and Edelman, G. M., 2000, Plasticity in value systems and its role in adaptive behavior, *Adapt. Behav.*, 8:129–148.

Thelen, E., and Smith, L. B., 1994, *A Dynamic Systems Approach to the Development of Cognition and Action*, Cambridge, MA: MIT Press. ◆

Thelen, E., Schöner, G., Scheier, C., and Smith, L. B., 2001, The dynamics of embodiment: A field theory of infant perseverative reaching, *Brain Behav. Sci.*, 24:1–34.

Tononi, G., Edelman, G. M., and Sporns, O., 1998, Complexity and coherency: Integrating information in the brain, *Trends Cognit. Sci.*, 2:474–484.

Varela, F. J., Thompson, E., and Rosch, E., 1991, *The Embodied Mind*, Cambridge, MA: MIT Press.

Emotional Circuits

Jean-Marc Fellous, Jorge L. Armony, and Joseph E. LeDoux

Introduction

Emotion is clearly an important aspect of the mind; yet it has been largely ignored by the "brain and mind (cognitive) sciences" in modern times. However, there are signs that this is beginning to change. This chapter surveys some issues about the nature of emotion, describes what is known about the neural basis of emotion, and considers some efforts that have been made to develop computer-based models of different aspects of emotion.

What Is Emotion?

The nature of emotion has been debated within psychology for the past century. The formal debate goes back to William James's famous question: Do we run from the bear because we are afraid, or are we afraid because we run? James suggested that we are afraid because we run. Subsequently, the psychological debate over emotion has centered on the question of what gives rise to the subjective states of awareness that we call feelings, or emotional experiences. Theories of emotional experience typically seek to account for how different emotional states come about, and can be grouped into several broad categories: feedback, central, arousal, and cognitive theories (for review, see LeDoux, 1996). Though very different in some ways, each of these theories proposes that emotional experiences are the result of prior emotional processes. Feedback and arousal theories require that the brain detect emotionally significant events and produce responses appropriate to the stimulus; these responses then serve as a signal that determines the content of emotional experience. Central and cognitive appraisal theories, which are in some ways different levels of description of similar processes, assume that emotional experience is based on prior evaluations of situations; these evaluations then determine the content of experience. Interestingly, the evaluative processes that constitute central and appraisal theories are also implicitly necessary for the elicitation of the peripheral responses and arousal states of feedback and arousal theories.

The disparate theories of emotional experience thus all point to a common mechanism—an evaluative system that determines whether a given situation is potentially harmful or beneficial to the individual. Since these evaluations are the precursors to conscious emotional experiences, they must, by definition, be unconscious processes. Such processes are the essence of the ignored half of James's question. That is, we run from a bear because our brain determines that bears are dangerous. Many emotional reactions are likely to be of this type: unconscious information processing of stimulus significance, with the experience of "emotion" (the subjective feeling of fear) coming after the fact.

Although the manner in which conscious experiences emerge from prior processing is poorly understood, progress has nevertheless been made in understanding how brain circuits process emotion. Just as vision researchers have achieved considerable understanding of the neural mechanisms underlying the processing of color while still knowing little about how color experience emerges from color processing (COLOR PERCEPTION), it is possible to study how the brain processes the emotional significance of situations without first solving the problem of how those situations are experienced as conscious content.

The Neural Basis of Emotional Processing

Traditionally, emotion has been ascribed to the brain's limbic system, which is presumed to be an evolutionarily old part of the brain involved in the survival of the individual and species (LeDoux, 2000). Some of the areas usually included in the limbic system are the hippocampal formation, septum, cingulate cortex, anterior thalamus, mammillary bodies, orbital frontal cortex, amygdala, hypothalamus, and certain parts of the basal ganglia. However, the limbic system anatomical concept and the limbic system theory of emotion are both problematic (LeDoux, 2000). The survival of the limbic system theory of emotion is due in large part to the fact that the amygdala, a small region in the temporal lobe, was included in the concept.

The amygdala has been consistently implicated in emotional functions (LeDoux, 1996; Rolls, 1998; Damasio, 1999; various chapters in Aggleton, 2000). Lesions of this region interfere with both positive and negative emotional reactions. Moreover, unit-recording studies show that cells in the amygdala are sensitive to the rewarding and punishing features of stimuli and to the social implications of stimuli. Other limbic areas have been less consistently implicated in emotion, and when they have been implicated, it has been difficult to separate out the contribution of the region to emotion per se as opposed to some of the cognitive prerequisites of emotion. The amygdala therefore serves as an experimentally accessible entry point into the distributed network of brain regions that mediate complex emotional evaluations.

The contribution of the amygdala to emotion results in large part from its anatomical connectivity (reviewed in LeDoux, 2000). The amygdala receives inputs from each of the major sensory systems and from higher-order association areas of the cortex. The sensory inputs arise from both the thalamic and cortical levels. These various inputs allow a variety of levels of information representation (from raw sensory features processed in the thalamus to whole objects processed in sensory cortex to complex scenes or contexts processed in the hippocampus) to impact on the amygdala and thereby activate emotional reactions. Most of these sensory inputs converge in the lateral nucleus of the amygdala, and the higher order information in the basal nucleus (Figure 1). These can be viewed as the sensory and cognitive gateways, respectively, into the amygdala's emotional functions. At the same time, the amygdala sends output projections to a variety of brainstem systems involved in controlling emotional responses, such as species-typical behavioral responses (including facial expressions and whole-body responses such as freezing), autonomic nervous system responses, and endocrine responses. Most of these outputs originate from the central nucleus of the amygdala. Recent anatomical and physiological work has, however, shown that the amygdala consists of several interacting subnuclei that may have specific individual contribution to the overall emotional computation performed (see the following discussion and Figure 1). If the amygdala is consistently found to contribute to the evaluation of the emotional significance of a stimulus, are there systems that control the processing of the amygdala? Recent work suggests that the amygdaloid complex can be modulated by neurochemical systems, such as serotonergic or dopaminergic, that are activated in relation to the overall behavioral state of the organism.

Much of the anatomical circuitry of emotion described previously has been elucidated through studies of fear conditioning, a procedure whereby an emotionally neutral stimulus, such as a tone or light, is associated with an aversive event, such as a mild shock to the foot (LeDoux and Phelps, in Lewis and Haviland-Jones, 2000; Davis, 1998). After such pairings, the tone or light comes to elicit emotional reactions that are characteristically expressed when members of the species in question are threatened. Although there are other procedures for studying emotion, none has been as successfully applied to the problem of identifying stimulus-response connections in emotion. The fear conditioning model is at this point

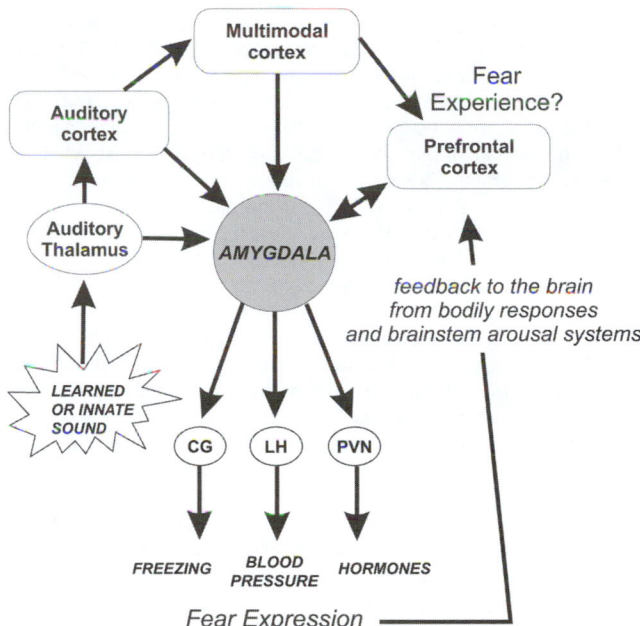

Figure 2. Emotional expression and emotional experience of auditory fear. Fearful stimuli (learned or innate) follow two main routes. The fast route involves the thalamo-amygdala pathway and responds best to simple stimulus features (such as a tone), the slow route involves the thalamo-cortical-amygdala pathway and carries more complex features (such as context). The expression of fear is mediated by the outputs of the amygdala to lower brain centers (brainstem, hypothalamus), while the experience of fear involves the prefrontal cortex circuitry.

particularly attractive since it has laid out pathways from the sensory input stage to the motor output stage of processing, showing how simple stimulus features, stimulus discriminations, and contexts control the expression of behavioral, autonomic, and endocrine responses in threatening situations (Figure 2).

Although many emotional response patterns are hardwired in the brain's circuitry, the particular stimulus conditions that activate these are mostly learned by association through classical conditioning. The amygdala appears to contribute significantly to this aspect of learning and memory and may be a crucial site of synaptic plasticity in emotional learning (LeDoux, 2000). This form of memory is quite different from what has come to be called *declarative memory*, the ability to consciously recall some experience from the past (CORTICAL MEMORY; SHORT-TERM MEMORY). Declarative memory, in contrast to *emotional memory*, crucially requires the hippocampus and related areas of the cortex. When we encounter some stimulus that in the past had aversive consequences, we recall the details of who we were with and where we were and even that it was a bad experience. However, in order to give the declarative memory an emotional flavor, it may be necessary for the stimulus, simultaneously and in parallel, to activate the emotional memory system of the amygdala. It is likely to be this dual activation of memory systems that gives our ongoing declarative memories their emotional coloration. Emotional memories are formed by the amygdala, in the same manner as declarative memories are formed in the hippocampus. The actual site of storage of emotional and declarative memories is still a matter of debate (Cahill et al., 1999), but may involve distant cortical and subcortical areas in addition to the amygdala and hippocampus (LeDoux, 2000).

In the last several years, the basic findings regarding fear conditioning in animals have been confirmed and extended by studies

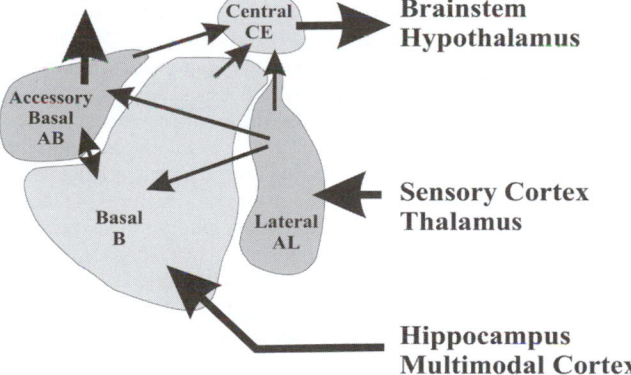

Figure 1. Simplified diagram of the amygdala intrinsic connections. The two main inputs to the amygdala are from the sensory/thalamic structures to AL, providing low level sensory information, and from polymodal and multimodal cortical association areas to B, providing more processed sensory information. The central nucleus receives convergent information from many other amygdaloid nuclei, and generate behavioral outputs (low level motor, autonomic, endocrine responses) that are a reflection of the intrinsic computations performed by the amygdala as a whole. Higher order motor control outputs are generated by the AB. See LeDoux and Pitkanen's chapter and Aggleton's chapter in Aggleton (2000) for more details.

of brain-damaged patients and functional imaging studies. This work has shown that the human amygdala is also involved in fear learning and other emotional processes (for reviews see Damasio, 1999; LeDoux, 2000; and Dolan's chapter in Aggleton, 2000).

At this point, we have mentioned "emotional experience" a number of times, and it may be worth speculating on just what an emotional experience is and how it might emerge. The emotion of fear will be used as an example. All animals, regardless of their stage of evolutionary development, must have the ability to detect and escape from or avoid danger. The widespread distribution of these behaviors in the animal kingdom makes it unlikely that the subjective experience of fear is at the heart of this ability. It may well be the case that subjective, consciously experienced fear is a mental state that occurs when the defense system of the brain (the system that detects threats and organizes appropriate responses) is activated, but only if that brain also has the capacity for consciousness. That is, by this reasoning, fear and other emotions reflect the representation of the activity of neural systems shaped by evolution and the responses they produce as conscious content. If this is true, then it is important that we focus our research efforts on these stimulus-detection and response-organizing systems, as these are the systems that generate the conscious content we call emotions. Although emotional behaviors may be triggered by sensory inputs that bypass or pass through the neocortex, the experience of emotion is likely to involve the cortical representation of the emotional episode. Although our understanding of the cortical representation of emotion episodes (or other conscious experiences) is poor at present, considerable evidence suggests that working memory circuits involving the frontal lobe may play a key role (LeDoux, 2000, and Figure 2). For a different view of the neural basis of emotional experience, see Damasio, 1999.

Computational Models of Emotion

Using computers to understand emotions has always been a challenge. Popular beliefs define computing devices as inherently incapable of exhibiting and experiencing any emotions and, at present, no definite claims have been made that computers may be suitable for such a task. Nevertheless, consistent with the notion put forth in the introduction, computers are used as tools for modeling certain aspects of emotional processing.

Models of Emotional Learning and Memory

As proposed by most central theories, many emotional responses are hardwired in brain circuitry. Nevertheless, in humans and animals, the environmental events that trigger these responses are often learned through experiences in which emotionally neutral stimuli come to be associated with emotionally charged stimuli. One important aspect of emotional processing, therefore, involves the manner in which the brain forms, stores, and uses associations between meaningless and meaningful stimuli.

Grossberg developed models of conditioned affective states based on the notion that conditioned reinforcement involves pairs of antagonistic neural processes, such as fear and relief. The model suggests a mechanism by which neutral events are charged with a reinforcing value (either positive or negative) depending on the previous activity of the model. The simulated neural circuits are suggestive of the role of brain structures involved in the processing of certain emotions, such as the hippocampo-amygdaloid system (described as a zone of convergence of conditioned (CS) and unconditioned (US) stimulus pathways), the septum (described as a zone in which the opposition of the processes is represented), the hypothalamus, the nucleus of the solitary tract, and the reticular formation (described as zones of visceral and somatosensory inputs). These models have been used to explain some aspects of the

dysfunctional behaviors seen in diseases such as schizophrenia (see Grossberg, 2000, for a review).

Armony and co-workers have implemented another connectionist model of emotional learning and memory that, like the previous model, also focuses on zones of convergence of US and CS pathways (Armony et al., 1997). This model is anatomically constrained by the known data of the fear conditioning circuitry. It examines processing in two parallel sensory (CS) transmission pathways to the amygdala from the auditory thalamus and the auditory cortex in a learning situation involving an auditory CS paired with a footshock US. The model is initially trained using a modified Hebb-type learning rule and, under testing conditions, reproduces data related to frequency-specific changes of the receptive fields known to exist in the auditory thalamus and amygdala. The model predicted that lesions of the cortical auditory route would not affect the specificity of the behavioral response to a range of frequencies centered on the training (aversively meaningful) frequency. This prediction has been verified experimentally. Because cortical representations are subject to attentional focus, this modeling study, like the previous one, suggests a close link between the amygdala and the attentional system of the midbrain. A separate connectionist-like model proposed that the amygdala might work in concert with the perirhinal cortex to generate conditioned responses to fear in cases in which the CS-US interval lasts several seconds (Tieu et al., 1999).

Recent anatomical studies coupled to physiological experiments in vivo and in vitro have provided invaluable data that can be used to build biophysically realistic computational models of amygdala circuits. Such models explore the interactions between converging thalamic and cortical inputs onto neurones in the lateral nucleus of the amygdala (Armony and LeDoux, 1997), as well as the role of local feedforward and feedback inhibition in stimulus processing (reviewed in Armony et al., 1997).

Computational Models of Cognitive-Emotion Interactions and Appraisal

Researchers in experimental psychology, artificial intelligence (AI), and cognitive science have long recognized the mutual influences of emotion and cognition. However, these interactions are still not clearly understood. We still do not have adequate theories defining each of these components of human mentation (emotion and cognition), much less a full understanding of how cognition and emotion might relate (EMOTION-COGNITION INTERACTIONS in the First Edition).

As described previously, most theories of emotion recognize the importance of evaluative or appraisal processes. Although there is considerable disagreement as to how these processes should best be viewed, most workers nevertheless see evaluative or appraisal processes as functioning by comparing sensed characteristics of the world to internal goals, standards, and attitude structures, deducing the emotional significance of the stimulus, guiding the expression of emotional behavior and other physiological responses, and influencing other modules pertaining to behavioral decisions.

In principle, it is possible to model appraisal processes using classical symbolic AI techniques (see Picard, 1997, for a review). It is possible, for example, using a vector space approach, to find a plausible mapping between appraisal features (e.g., novelty, urgency, intrinsic pleasantness) and emotion categories (e.g., fear, joy, pride). Relying on a posteriori verbal reports and a predefined set of emotions, one could then derive a limited set of appraisal criteria, sufficient for emotion prediction and differentiation. Other AI approaches, such as decision trees, pattern matching, and production rules (expert systems), are also possible, although each of these methods encounters theoretical difficulties. These types of systems, however, do not generally account for neurophysiological data.

One criticism often made of cognitive models of emotion is related to the complexity of processing involved and to the time they consequently require. From an AI point of view, the criticism has been addressed by introducing reactivity to "classical" cognitive models. Classical AI approaches assume that systems possess a well-defined representation of their environment, state, actions, and goals. In contrast, reactive systems do not make such assumptions; they are mostly based on real-time, incomplete evaluations, their performance being based more on the properties of the evaluative mechanisms than on the quality and quantity of their internal representations (REACTIVE ROBOTIC SYSTEMS).

It is interesting to note that, as we mentioned earlier, appraisal of sensory information might be one of the most prominent functions of the amygdala, placing this structure in a key position to actually perform the mapping of the emotional value of the stimuli. In this view, the relation between amygdala activity and emotion is a computational one (in the broad sense of the term) rather than a subjective one. The existence of multiple pathways to the amygdala from input processing systems of various levels of complexity (see previous discussion) provides a biological resolution to some of the concerns that have been raised about the importance of cognition in driving emotion. The involvement of cognition can be minimal or maximal, depending on the situation.

Models of Facial Expressions of Emotion

Of interest to feedback and arousal theories, the expression of emotion in the face is an important biological aspect of emotion that has significant implications for how emotion is communicated in social situations. Face recognition and analysis of facial expression has only recently been an active field of research in the computer vision community (for review, see Bartlett, 2001). Face analysis can be computationally divided into three subproblems: detecting the face in a scene; identifying the face; and analyzing its expression. At present, each of these tasks uses different features of the face, and different computational approaches. These approaches are based on psychophysical observations and are not yet explicitly based on neurophysiological data. However, a number of neurophysiological studies have been conducted (for review, see Rolls's chapter in Aggleton, 2000). These studies have shown cells selectively responsive to particular faces in areas of the temporal neocortex and in the amygdala. Functional imaging studies of humans have led to similar results (see Dolan's chapter in Aggleton, 2000). Other studies have shown that there might be an influence of facial expressions on the actual neural correlates of the emotional states experienced, through modifications of blood flow characteristics (for review, see Ekman, 1992). Other approaches are more physicomathematical, relying on image processing techniques. These implementations address exclusively the problem of emotional expression (and, possibly, communication of emotions) without relying on any theory of emotional experience (Bartlett, 2001).

Conclusions

It is important to distinguish between emotional experiences and the underlying processes that lead to emotional experiences. One of the stumbling blocks to an adequate scientific approach to emotion has been the focus of the field on constructing theories of the subjective aspects of emotion. Studies of the neural basis of emotion and emotional learning have instead focused on how the brain detects and evaluates emotional stimuli and how, on the basis of such evaluations, emotional responses are produced. The amygdala was found to play a major role in the evaluation process. It is likely that the processing that underlies the expression of emotional responses also underlies emotional experiences, and that progress can be made by treating emotion as a function that allows the organism to respond in an adaptive manner to challenges in the environment rather than to a subjective state. Although computational approaches to subjective experiences of the emotional or nonemotional kind are not likely to be easily achieved, computational approaches to emotional processing are both possible and practical. Although relatively few models currently exist, this situation is likely to change as researchers begin to realize the opportunities that are present in this long-neglected area.

Road Maps: Cognitive Neuroscience; Psychology
Related Reading: Cognitive Maps; Conditioning; Embodied Cognition; Motivation; Pain Networks; Sparse Coding in the Primate Cortex

References

Aggleton, J. P., 2000, *The Amygdala: A Functional Analysis*, 2nd ed., Oxford: Oxford University Press. ◆

Armony, J. L., and LeDoux, J. E., 1997, How the brain processes emotional information, *Ann. NY Acad. Sci.*, 821:259–270. ◆

Armony, J. L., Servan-Schreiber, D., Cohen, J. D., and LeDoux, J. E., 1997, Computational modeling of emotion: Explorations through the anatomy and physiology of fear conditioning, *Trends Cog. Sci.*, 1:28–34.

Bartlett, M., 2001, *Face Image Analysis by Unsupervised Learning*, Boston: Kluwer Academic Publishers.

Cahill, L., Weinberger, N. M., Roozendaal, B., and McGaugh, J. L., 1999, Is the amygdala a locus of "conditioned fear"? Some questions and caveats, *Neuron*, 23:227–228.

Damasio, A., 1999, *The Feeling of What Happens: Body and Emotion in the Making of Consciousness*, New York: Harcourt Brace.

Davis, M., 1998, Anatomic and physiologic substrates of emotion in an animal model, *J. Clin. Neurophysiol.*, 15:378–387.

Ekman, P., 1992, Facial expressions of emotion: New findings, new questions, *Psychol. Sci.*, 3:34–38.

Grossberg, S., 2000, The imbalanced brain: From normal behavior to schizophrenia, *Biol. Psychiat.*, 48:81–98.

LeDoux, J., 1996, *The Emotional Brain*, New York: Simon and Schuster. ◆

LeDoux, J. E., 2000, Emotion circuits in the brain, *Annu. Rev. Neurosci.*, 23:155–184. ◆

Lewis, M., and Haviland-Jones, J. M., 2000, *Handbook of Emotions*, 2nd ed., New York: Guilford Press.

Picard, R. W., 1997, *Affective Computing*: Boston: MIT Press. ◆

Rolls, E. T., 1998, *The Brain and Emotion*, Oxford, UK: Oxford University Press.

Tieu, K. H., Keidel, A. L., McGann, J. P., Faulkner, B., and Brown, T. H., 1999, Perirhinal-amygdala circuit-level computational model of temporal encoding of fear conditioning, *Psychobiology*, 27:1–25.

Energy Functionals for Neural Networks

Eric Goles

Introduction

In this article we survey some of the most common neural network models for which an *energy* can be defined, where an energy is a quantity $E(x(t))$, depending on the current configuration of the network, $x(t)$, that does not increase when the network is updated, i.e., $E(x(t + \tau)) \leq E(x(t))$, and that is constant in steady state. Classically, these quantities appeared in the dynamical study of ordinary differential equations as what is called a Lyapunov function. In fact, the Lyapunov function approach consists in determining a positive quantity that decreases when the differential system approaches the equilibrium points. In such a case, it is possible to study the stability of the solutions (see Grossberg, 1988, and Hirsch, 1989, in the neural networks context). From the physical point of view, the possibility of associating an energy with neural networks arose from the deep analogy between them and the spin-glass magnetic model (Little and Shaw, 1975; Hopfield, 1984; see also OPTIMIZATION, NEURAL). The interest in determining when such quantities exist arises from the fact that their existence allows study of the convergence rate, for specific update modes of the network, to stable or short-period configurations. Moreover, the attractors are local minima of the energy E, so this kind of network can be used to model associative memories (Hopfield, 1982) and hill-climbing optimization strategies.

Energies have been developed for discrete and continuous networks. There are three principal models: discrete transition–discrete time, continuous transition–discrete time, and continuous transition–continuous time. The first model was made famous by Hopfield (1982) for associative memories with Hebb interactions updated asynchronously. It was later extended to sequential and parallel update (Fogelman-Soulié, Goles, and Weisbuch, 1983; Goles, Fogelman-Soulié, and Pellegrin, 1985). The discrete time–continuous function appears in the context of the brain-state-in-a-box model (Golden, 1986). A survey of the energy approach can be found in Goles and Martinez (1990). Finally, the continuous time–continuous transition model has been studied first by Cohen and Grossberg (1983; see COMPUTING WITH ATTRACTORS) and in a particular case by Hopfield (1984). It is important to point out that Hopfield's energy approach was based on a spin-glass analogy of symmetric neural networks. This analogy and some preliminary results were presented in Little (1974) and Little and Shaw (1975).

In this article, we present first the linear argument model for discrete time and continuous transition. We determine, under symmetric assumptions about interconnections, the associated energy. Moreover, we extend the approach to the related class of quasi-symmetric interconnections. In a similar way, we present the discrete time–continuous transition model by taking as a local function a real, bounded, increasing function. It is important to point out that in this case symmetry is also the key hypothesis in determining the energy. Further, we extend the analysis to any increasing function.

For continuous time–continuous transition, we present the general model studied by Grossberg (1988), and we illustrate the energy determination for the particular case developed in Hopfield (1984).

The Binary State–Discrete Time Model

Suppose the neurons take values in a binary set, usually $\{0, 1\}$ or $\{1, 1\}$. We present here the threshold case, i.e., $y_i = 1(\sum_{i=1}^{n} w_{ij}x_j - b_i)$, for $x \in \{0, 1\}^n$ and $1(u) = 1$ iff $u \geq 0$ (0 otherwise).

Throughout this paragraph we will assume, without loss of generality, that for any $x \in \{0, 1\}^n$ and $i \in \{1, \ldots, n\}$, $\sum_{j=1}^{n} w_{ij}x_j - b_i \neq 0$. (Otherwise, it suffices to make a small change in threshold b_i without changing the dynamics; Goles and Martínez, 1990.) The threshold model is the classical one. Other binary models, such as states in the set $\{-1, 1\}$ with the sign transition function, can be reduced to the threshold model, with similar expressions for the energies.

Asynchronous Update

Let us consider the foregoing model with asynchronous update, i.e., the neurons are updated one by one in random order. In this context, we have the following result.

Theorem 1. (Hopfield, 1982; Fogelman-Soulié et al., 1983.) Let $W = (w_{ij})$ be a symmetric $n \times n$ matrix with non-negative diagonal entries (i.e., diag(W) $\geq$ 0). Then the quantity $E(x) = -\frac{1}{2} \sum_{i,j=1}^{n} w_{ij}x_i x_j + \sum_{i=1}^{n} b_i x_i$ is an energy associated with the asynchronous iteration of the network.

Proof. Let $x = (x_1, \ldots, x_n) \in \{0, 1\}^n$ be the current configuration. Suppose we update the kth neuron, obtaining the new configuration $\tilde{x} = (x_1, \ldots, x_{k-1}, \tilde{x}_k, \ldots, x_n)$, where $\tilde{x}_k = 1(\sum_{j=1}^{n} w_{kj}x_j - b_k)$. Let $\Delta_k E = E(\tilde{x}) - E(x)$. Since W is symmetric, we get:

$$\Delta_k E = -(\tilde{x}_k - x_k)\left(\sum_{j=1}^{n} w_{kj}x_j - b_k\right) - \frac{1}{2} w_{kk}(\tilde{x}_k - x_k)^2 \quad (1)$$

By definition of the threshold function, the first term is negative when $\tilde{x}_k \neq x_k$. Since $w_{kk} \geq 0$, we conclude that $\Delta_k E \leq 0$, with $\Delta_k E < 0$ iff $\tilde{x}_k \neq x_k$. □

The first determination of this energy for a particular symmetric threshold model was done by Hopfield (1982) for associative memories and interactions w_{ij} defined by Hebb's rule, i.e., $w_{ij} = \sum_{k=1}^{p} x_i^{(k)}x_j^{(k)}$, $(w_{ij} = 0)$, where $x = \{x^{(1)}, \ldots, x^{(p)}\}$ is the set of prototypes to be memorized. This rule was used before Hopfield in a neural model proposed by Anderson (see ASSOCIATIVE NETWORKS).

As a corollary to the previous theorem, we can state that the only stable states of the network are fixed points, i.e., configurations remaining invariant by the application of the threshold rule. In fact, it suffices to remark that between two successive different configurations, the energy decreases. Furthermore, since the energy is bounded on the set $\{0, 1\}^n$, the network converges in a finite number of steps to a fixed point. We will come back to this aspect in the next section. On the other hand, when diag(W) = 0 (as in Hopfield, 1982), it is easy to verify that the fixed points of the network are local minima of E. In fact, consider a fixed point $x \in \{0, 1\}^n$ and its kth neighborhood in the hypercube, $\tilde{x} = (x_1, \ldots, 1 - x_k, \ldots, x_n)$. Since x is a fixed point and diag(W) = 0, one gets $x_k = 1(\sum_{j \neq k} w_{kj}x_j - b_k)$ and $\Delta_k E = E(\tilde{x}) - E(x) = -(1 - 2x_k)(\sum_{j \neq k} w_{kj}x_j - b_k) > 0$, so x is a local minimum of E. The previous aspect is important for modeling, by hill-climbing neural strategies, some hard combinatorial optimization problems (see OPTIMIZATION, NEURAL)

Periodic Update

Assume now that the neurons are updated one by one in a periodic order: $\{1 \to 2 \to \ldots \to n \to 1\}$. Clearly, this update strategy is a particular case of the asynchronous one, but the periodicity permits us to obtain bounds on the transient time. It is obvious that the network has the same energy, E, as the asynchronous iteration. Given a matrix W and a threshold vector b, we define $\tau(W, b)$ as the maximum number of steps taken by the network, for any initial condition, to reach a stable configuration.

Theorem 2. (Fogelman-Soulié et al., 1983.) Let W be an $n \times n$ symmetric matrix with non-negative diagonal. Then the transient time $\tau(W, b)$ for periodic update is bounded by

$$\tau(W, b) \leq \frac{\|W\|_1 + 2\|b\|_1}{2\left(e + \min_i w_{ij}\right)} \qquad (2)$$

where $e = \min \{|\Sigma_{j=1}^n w_{ij}x_j - b_i| : i \in \{1, \ldots, n\}, x \in \{0, 1\}^n\}$, $\|W\|_1 = \Sigma_{i,j=1}^n |w_{ij}|$, and $\|b\|_1 = \Sigma_{i=1}^n |b_i|$.

Proof. From the proof of Theorem 1, one gets, for any $k \in \{1, \ldots, n\}$, $|\Delta_k E| \geq e + \frac{1}{2} \min_i w_{ii}$. On the other hand, $|E(x)| \leq \frac{1}{2} \Sigma_{i,j=1}^n |w_{ij}| + \Sigma_{i=1}^n |b_i|$. From previous inequalities we obtain the bound directly. $\square$

Better bounds can be obtained with a finer analysis of $|\Delta_k E|$ and $|E(x)|$. See, for instance, Kamp and Hasler (1990) and Goles and Martínez (1990).

Parallel Update

Suppose we update the network synchronously:

$$x_i(t + 1) = 1\left(\sum_{j=1}^n w_{ij}x_j(t) - b_i\right) \quad 1 \leq i \leq n, x(0) \in \{0, 1\}^n \qquad (3)$$

In this context we have the following result.

Theorem 3. (Goles et al., 1985.) Let W be an $n \times n$ symmetric matrix. Then the expression

$$E(t) = -\sum_{i=j=1}^n w_{ij}x_i(t)x_j(t - 1) + \sum_{i=1}^n b_i(x_i(t) + x_i(t - 1))$$

is an energy associated with the parallel update.

Proof. Let $\Delta E = E(t) - E(t - 1)$. Since W is symmetric, one gets

$$\Delta E = -\sum_{i=1}^n (x_i(t) - x_i(t - 2))\left(\sum_{j=1}^n w_{ij}x_j(t - 1) - b_i\right) \quad (4)$$

By definition of the threshold function, $\Delta E \leq 0$ and it is strictly negative when $x(t) \neq x(t - 2)$. $\square$

This energy can also be obtained in the framework of the statistical mechanics model proposed by Little (1974). In fact, the energy $E(t)$ with threshold $b = 0$ is the zero temperature limit of the Hamiltonian: $H(x) = -\beta^{-1}\Sigma_{i=1}^n \log_2 \cosh(\beta n^{-1}\Sigma_{j\neq i}w_{ij}x_i)$, where $\beta = 1/kT$, k being the Boltzmann constant (Peretto, 1984). More information about the physical approach can be found in STATISTICAL MECHANICS OF NEURAL NETWORKS (q.v.).

Corollary 1. For a symmetric matrix W, the parallel iteration converges to fixed points or two-periodic configurations.

Proof. Suppose that $\{x(0), \ldots, x(T - 1), x(T) = x(0)\}$ is a cycle of period T. From Theorem 3 it follows that $E(t)$ is necessarily

constant on the cycle. If $T > 2$, we have $x(0) \neq x(2)$, so $E(2) < E(0)$, which is a contradiction. $\square$

Corollary 2. For a positive-definite matrix W, the parallel update converges to fixed points.

Proof. From Corollary 1 it is enough to prove that there are no two-cycles. Suppose $\{x(0), x(1)\}$ is a two-cycle, i.e., $x(2) = x(0)$. Since W is positive definite, $\alpha = (x(1) - x(0))^T(Wx(1) - x(0)) \geq 0$, with equality only if $x(1) = x(0)$. Further, by Equation 4,

$$\alpha = (x(0) - x(1))^T(Wx(1) - b) - (x(1) - x(0))^T(Wx(0) - b)$$
$$= \Delta_2 E + \Delta_1 E$$

From the proof of Theorem 3, we know that $\Delta_2 E \leq 0$ and $\Delta_1 E \leq 0$, so $\alpha = 0$. Hence, $x(1) = x(0)$, i.e., two-cycles do not exist. $\square$

The application of the foregoing result to associative memory models is straightforward. Consider the Hopfield model with generalized Hebb interconnections on the prototype set $\{x^{(1)}, \ldots, x^{(p)}\} \subseteq \{0, 1\}^n$, with interconnection matrix $W = (1/p)X^TX$, where $X = (x^{(1)}, \ldots, x^{(p)})$. Consider also the projection or pseudo-inverse interconnection model, i.e., $W = (X^TX)^{-1}X^T$. Since in both cases W is positive definite, the parallel updates of previous models converge only to fixed points (Kamp and Hasler, 1990).

From the energy given in Theorem 3, one may determine that the transient time for the parallel update is bounded by $\tau(W, b) \leq (1/e)(\|W\|_1 + 3\|2b - W\bar{1}\|_1 - 2\Sigma_{i=1}^n e_i)$ if $e > 0$ (0 if $e = 0$), where $e = \min\{-E^*(2) - E^*(1): x(0) \neq x(2)\}$, $e_i = \min\{|\Sigma_{j=1}^n w_{ij}u_j - b_i| : u \in \{0, 1\}^n\}$, and $\bar{1} = (1, \ldots, 1)$. Clearly, if all the vectors belong to a two-cycle, then $e = 0$ and $\tau(W, b) = 0$.

It is important to remark that this bound is not necessarily polynomial. In fact, it is possible to build symmetric neural networks of size n with exponential transient time (recall that n neurons corresponds to 2^n states). When the matrix W takes values on the integers, the quantities e_i, e can be controlled and an explicit bound on $\tau(W, b)$ can be given in terms of W, b. Further, there exist symmetric neural networks where the bound is attained. More information about these topics can be found in Goles and Martínez (1990).

Another model that can be studied by using the energy approach is the bidirectional associative memory (BAM) model proposed by Kosko (1988). Roughly, it consists of a two-layer bidirectional network that achieves heteroassociations with a smaller correlation matrix. Given its correlation matrix W and a pair of vectors $(x, y) \in \{0, 1\}^{2n}$, the energy is $E = -x^TWy$ (Wang, Cruz, and Mulligan, 1991).

Energies for Nonsymmetric Models

When the matrix W is no longer symmetric, it is difficult, for general classes of matrices with other nontrivial regularities, to determine energies that ensure convergence to fixed points (in the asynchronous and sequential update) and to fixed points and two-cycles (for the parallel update). That fact is not surprising, since if we permit arbitrary interconnections and enough neurons we can model arbitrary automata (see NEURAL AUTOMATA AND ANALOG COMPUTATIONAL COMPLEXITY).

Furthermore, the dynamics (sequential or parallel) is very dependent on symmetry. In fact, arbitrarily small variations in a symmetric matrix can generate long cycles. A similar situation occurs for the sequential iteration and the non-negativity diagonal hypothesis: a negative diagonal also generates long cycles (Goles and Martínez, 1990). So one may say that the existence of energies relies very much on the hypothesis of symmetric interconnections. Of course, one may find nonsymmetric matrices that accept an energy, but one could not find a nontrivial class, really different from the symmetric one, with the energy property. However, minor variation on symmetry are possible.

One can generalize the foregoing results to the quasi-symmetric class of matrices. We say that a matrix $W = (w_{ij})$ is quasi-symmetric if there exists a positive vector $(u_1, \ldots, u_n)$ such that for any $i, j \in \{1, \ldots, n\}$, $u_i w_{ij} = u_j w_{ji}$. We have the following result.

Theorem 4. (Goles and Martinez, 1990.) Let W be a quasi-symmetric matrix. Then the quantity $E(x) = -\frac{1}{2}\Sigma_{i,j} u_i w_{ij} x_i x_j + \Sigma_{i=1}^n u_i b_i x_i$, is an energy for the asynchronous and sequential update.

The quantity $E(t) = -\frac{1}{2}\Sigma_{i,j=1}^n u_i w_{ij} x_i(t) x_j(t-1) + \Sigma_{i=1}^n u_i b_i(x_i(t) + x_i(t-1))$ is an energy for the parallel update.

The Continuous Transition–Discrete Time Model

Let us now consider a real transition function, $f \colon \mathbb{R} \to \mathbb{R}$, continuous, strictly increasing on an interval $S = (-a, a)$, $f(0) = 0$, and constant outside S, i.e., $f(x) = f(-a)$ for $x \le -a$ and $f(x) = f(a)$ for $x \ge a$. As an example, f could be a truncated "sigmoidal" similar to those used by Hopfield (1984) and classically empolyed in multilayered networks. Another example is the BSB model (Golden, 1986) where f is linear in S. In the previous context, the update function is as follows:

$$y_i = f(\arg_i(x)) \quad 1 \le i \le n, \; x \in S^n \quad (5)$$

where $\arg_i(x) = \Sigma_{j=1}^n w_{ij} x_j - b_i$. For this model and the iterations defined in previous paragraphs we have the following result.

Theorem 5. (Goles and Martínez, 1990.) Suppose W is an $n \times n$ symmetric matrix. Then when $\mathrm{diag}(W) \ge 0$ the asynchronous or periodic update admits the energy

$$E(x) = -\frac{1}{2}\sum_{i,j=1}^n w_{ij} x_i x_j + \sum_{i=1}^n \left(\int_0^{x_i} f^{-1}(s)ds + b_i x_i\right) \quad (6)$$

Furthermore, the quantity

$$E(t) = -\sum_{i,j=1}^n w_{ij} x_i(t) x_j(t-1)$$
$$+ \sum_{i=1}^n \left[\int_0^{x_i(t)} f^{-1}(s)ds + \int_0^{x_i(t-1)} f^{-1}(s)ds\right]$$
$$+ \sum_{i=1}^n b_i(x_i(t) + x_i(t-1)) \quad (7)$$

is an energy associated with the parallel update.

Proof. We first give the proof for the asynchronous (analogous to the periodic) update. Suppose we update the kth neuron, so that $\tilde{x} = (x_1, \ldots, \tilde{x}_k, \ldots, x_n)$, where $\tilde{x}_k = f(\arg_k(x))$. Suppose also that each neuron has been updated at least one time, so $x_k = f(\arg_k(z))$, where $z \in S^n$. Since W is symmetric, one gets

$$\Delta_k E = -(\tilde{x}_k - x_k)\arg_k(x) - \frac{1}{2}w_{kk}(\tilde{x}_k - x_k)^2$$
$$+ \int_0^{\tilde{x}_k} f^{-1}(s)ds - \int_0^{x_k} f^{-1}(s)ds$$

Since $w_{kk} \ge 0$, the quadratic term is clearly negative. For the other two terms, let $u = \arg_k(x)$ and $v = \arg_k(z)$. Then $\Delta_k E = -(f(u) - f(v))u + \int_0^{f(u)} f^{-1}(s)ds - \int_0^{f(v)} f^{-1}(s)ds$.

From the definition of f, we have easily

$$\int_0^{f(\alpha)} f^{-1}(s)ds = \alpha f(\alpha) - \int_0^\alpha f(s)ds \quad (8)$$

so $\Delta_k E = (u - v)f(v) + \int_0^v f(s)ds - \int_0^u f(s)ds$. Since f is an increasing function, one concludes that $\Delta_k E \le 0$. For the parallel update the proof is similar. $\square$

One may also prove that the only finite orbits are fixed points for the asynchronous and periodic update, while fixed points and/or two-cycles are possible for the parallel update.

The generalization to a nonsymmetric interval, and functions such that $f(0) \ne 0$, can be studied in a similar way. A more general approach would suppose that local update functions act in a high-dimensional space. In this framework, by considering $f \colon \mathbb{R}^p \to \mathbb{R}^p$, it has been proved that when f is positive (i.e., $\langle f(x) - f(y), x \rangle \ge 0$ for all $x, y \in \mathbb{R}^p$, where $\langle \, , \rangle$ is a scalar product) the sequential and parallel update for symmetric interconnections admits an energy (Goles, 1985).

Further, if f is a subgradient of a convex function g (i.e., $g(y) \ge g(x) + \langle f(x), y - x \rangle$ for all $x, y \in \mathbb{R}^p$), it can be proved that, under the symmetry hypothesis, the parallel iteration also admits an energy (Goles and Martínez, 1990).

Continuous Transition–Continuous Time Models

Several authors have introduced differential models of neural networks such that the transition function and the time steps are continuous. In this context Cohen and Grossberg (1983) proposed the nonlinear update

$$\frac{dx_i}{dt} = a_i(x_i)\left[b_i(x_i) - \sum_{j=1}^n w_{ij} d_j(x_j)\right] \quad 1 \le i \le n \quad (9)$$

To study the dynamics of Equation 9, the authors assume that $a_i(x) \ge 0$, $d_j'(x) \ge 0$, and the matrix W is symmetric. Then they determine the following energy function:

$$E(x) = -\sum_{i=1}^n \int^{x_i} b_i d_i'(x)dx + \frac{1}{2}\sum_{i,j=1}^n w_{ij} d_i(x_i) d_j(x_j) \quad (10)$$

A particular case of this model was studied by Hopfield (1984):

$$c_i\left(\frac{dy_i}{dt}\right) = \sum_{j=1}^n w_{ij} x_j - \frac{y_i}{R_i} + I_i \quad (11)$$

where $y_i = g_i^{-1}(x_i)$.

Theorem 6. (Hopfield, 1984.) Let W be a symmetric matrix and g_i a sigmoid. Then

$$E(x) = -\frac{1}{2}\sum_{i,j=1}^n w_{ij} x_i x_j + \sum_{i=1}^n \left(\frac{1}{R_i}\right)\int_0^{x_i} g_i^{-1}(s)ds + \sum_{i=1}^n I_i x_i \quad (12)$$

is an energy function associated with Equation 11.

Proof. Since W is symmetric, one gets

$$\frac{dE}{dt} = -\sum_{i=1}^n \frac{dx_i}{dt}\left(\sum_{j=1}^n w_{ij} x_j - \frac{y_i}{R_i} + I_i\right)$$

From Equation 11 we have

$$\frac{dE}{dt} = -\sum_{i=1}^n c_i \frac{dx_i}{dt}\frac{dy_i}{dt} = -\sum_{i=1}^n c_i(g_i^{-1})'(x_i)\left(\frac{dx_i}{dt}\right)^2$$

Since g_i^{-1} is increasing, one concludes that $dE/dt \le 0$. $\square$

Good surveys of differential models of neural networks are provided by Grossberg (1988) and Hirsch (1989).

Discussion

In this article we have reviewed the principal neural models that accept an energy function. In all cases, the existence of such operators depends strongly on regularities of interconnections: symmetry and quasi-symmetry. One may also determine an energy for a class of antisymmetric matrices (Goles and Martínez, 1990), but it seems difficult to find other nontrivial classes of matrices that accept energy functions. In fact, arbitrarily small perturbation of the matrices discussed in this article can induce long cycles in the network dynamics. Necessary and sufficient conditions for the existence of an energy function have been formally studied by Kobuchi (1991) under a plausible decomposition hypothesis of ΔE. But, in practice, the authors recover only the quasi-symmetry class.

Further, some of the results can be extended to high-order networks, i.e., neural networks with polynomial interactions. In this context, under a generalization of the symmetry hypothesis, one may find an energy function for the periodic update (Xu and Tsai, 1990; Kamp and Hasler, 1990).

[Reprinted from the First Edition]

Road Map: Dynamic Systems
Background: I.3. Dynamics and Adaptation in Neural Nets; Computing with Attractors
Related Reading: Dynamics and Bifurcation in Neural Nets

References

Cohen, M., and Grossberg, S., 1983, Absolute stability of global pattern formation and parallel memory storage by competitive neural networks, *IEEE Trans. Syst. Man Cybert.*, SMC-13:815–826.

Fogelman-Soulié, F., Goles, E., and Weisbuch, G., 1983, Transient length in sequential iteration of threshold functions, *Discrete Appl. Math.*, 6:95–98.

Golden, R. M., 1986, The brain-state-in-a-box neural model is a gradient descent algorithm, *J. Math. Psychq.*, 30:73–80.

Goles, E., 1985, Dynamic of positive automata networks, *Theoret. Comput. Sci.*, 41:19–32.

Goles, E., Fogelman-Soulié, F., and Pellegrin, D., 1985, Decreasing energy functions as a tool for studying threshold networks, *Discrete Appl. Math.*, 12:261–277.

Goles, E., and Martínez, S., 1990, *Neural and Automata Networks*, Norwell, MA: Kluwer. ◆

Grossberg, S., 1988, Nonlinear neural networks: Principles, mechanisms, and architectures, *Neural Netw.*, 1:17–61. ◆

Hirsch, M., 1989, Convergent activation dynamics in continuous time networks, *Neural Netw.*, 2:331–349. ◆

Hopfield, J. J., 1982, Neural networks and physical systems with emergent collective computational abilities, *Proc. Natl. Acad. Sci. USA*, 79:2554–2558.

Hopfield, J. J., 1984, Neurons with graded response have collective computational properties like those of two-state neurons, *Proc. Natl. Acad. Sci. USA*, 81:3088–3092.

Kamp, Y., and Hasler, M., 1990, *Réseaux de neurones récursifs pour mémoires associatives*, Lausanne: Presses Polytechniques et Universitaires Romandes. ◆

Kobuchi, Y., 1991, State evaluation functions and Lyapunov functions for neural network, *Neural Netw.*, 4:505–510.

Kosko, B., 1988, Adaptive bidirectional associative memories, *Appl. Opt.*, 26:4947–4960.

Little, W. A., 1974, The existence of persistent states in the brain, *Math. Biosci.*, 19:101–120.

Little, W. A., and Shaw, G. L., 1975, A statistical theory of short and long term memory, *Behav. Biol.*, 14:115.

Peretto, P., 1984, Collective properties of neural networks: A statistical physics approach, *Biol. Cybern.*, 50:51–62.

Wang, Y. F., Cruz, J. B., and Mulligan, J. H., 1991, Guaranteed recall of all training pairs for bidirectional associative memory, *IEEE Trans. Neural Netw.*, 2:559–567.

Xu, X., and Tsai, W. T., 1990, Constructing associative memories using neural networks, *Neural Netw.*, 3:301–309.

Ensemble Learning

Thomas G. Dietterich

Introduction

Learning describes many different activities, ranging from CONCEPT LEARNING (q.v.) to REINFORCEMENT LEARNING (q.v.). The best understood form of statistical learning is known as *supervised learning* (see LEARNING AND STATISTICAL INFERENCE). In this setting, each data point consists of a vector of features (denoted $\mathbf{x}$) and a class label y, and it is assumed that there is some underlying function f such that $y = f(\mathbf{x})$ for each training data point $(\mathbf{x}, y)$. The goal of the learning algorithm is to find a good approximation h to f that can be applied to assign labels to new $\mathbf{x}$ values. The function h is called a *classifier*, because it assigns class labels y to input data points $\mathbf{x}$. Supervised learning can be applied to many problems, including handwriting recognition, medical diagnosis, and part-of-speech tagging in language processing.

Ordinary machine learning algorithms work by searching through a space of possible functions, called *hypotheses*, to find the one function, h, that is the best approximation to the unknown function f. To determine which hypothesis h is best, a learning algorithm can measure how well h matches f on the training data points, and it can also assess how consistent h is with any available prior knowledge about the problem.

As an example, consider the problem of learning to pronounce the letter k in English. Consider the words *desk*, *think*, and *hook*, where the k is pronounced, and the words *back*, *quack*, and *knave*, where the k is silent (in *back* and *quack*, we will suppose that the c is responsible for the k sound). Suppose we define a vector of features that consists of the two letters prior to the k and the two letters that follow the k. Then each of these words can be represented by the following data points:

x_1	x_2	x_3	x_4	y
e	s	–	–	+1
i	n	–	–	+1
o	o	–	–	+1
a	c	–	–	−1
a	c	–	–	−1
–	–	n	a	−1

where $y = +1$ if k is pronounced and -1 if k is silent, and where "_" denotes positions beyond the ends of the word.

One of the most efficient and widely applied learning algorithms searches the hypothesis space consisting of decision trees. Figure 1 shows a decision tree that explains the data points given above. This tree can be used to classify a new data point as follows. Starting at the so-called root (i.e., top) of the tree, we first check whether $x_2 = c$. If so, then we follow the left ("yes") branch to the $y = -1$ "leaf," which predicts that k will be silent. If not, we follow the right ("no") branch to another test: Is $x_3 = n$? If so, we follow

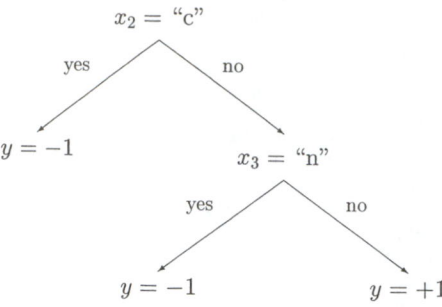

Figure 1. A decision tree for pronouncing the letter k. First, feature x_2 is tested to see if it is the letter c. If not, the feature x_3 is tested to see if it is the letter n. K is pronounced only if x_2 is not c and x_3 is not n.

the left branch to another $y = -1$ leaf. If not, we follow the right branch to the $y = +1$ leaf, where the tree indicates that k should be pronounced.

A decision tree learning algorithm searches the space of such trees by first considering trees that test only one feature (in this case x_2 was chosen) and making an immediate classification. Then they consider expanding the tree by replacing one of the leaves by a test of a second feature (in this case, the right leaf was replaced with a test of x_3). Various heuristics are applied to choose which test to include in each iteration and when to stop growing the tree. For a good discussion of decision trees, see the books by Quinlan (1993) and Breiman et al. (1984).

In addition to decision trees, there are many other representations for hypotheses that have been studied, including PERCEPTRONS, ADALINES, AND BACKPROPAGATION (q.v.), RADIAL BASIS FUNCTION NETWORKS (q.v.), GAUSSIAN PROCESSES (q.v.), graphical models, Helmholtz machines, and SUPPORT VECTOR MACHINES (q.v.). In all cases, these algorithms find one best hypothesis h and output it as the "solution" to the learning problem.

Ensemble learning algorithms take a different approach. Rather than finding one best hypothesis to explain the data, they construct a *set* of hypotheses (sometimes called a *committee* or *ensemble*) and then have those hypotheses "vote" in some fashion to predict the label of new data points. More precisely, an ensemble method constructs a set of hypotheses $\{h_1, \ldots, h_K\}$, chooses a set of weights $\{w_1, \ldots, w_K\}$, and constructs the "voted" classifier $H(\mathbf{x}) = w_1 h_1(\mathbf{x}) + \cdots + w_K h_K(\mathbf{x})$. The classification decision of the combined classifier H is $+1$ if $H(\mathbf{x}) \geq 0$ and -1 otherwise.

Experimental evidence has shown that ensemble methods are often much more accurate than any single hypothesis. Freund and Schapire (1996) showed improved performance on 22 benchmark problems, equal performance on one problem, and worse performance on four problems. These and other studies are summarized in Dietterich (1997).

Why Ensemble Methods Work

Learning algorithms that output only a single hypothesis suffer from three problems that can be partly overcome by ensemble methods: the statistical problem, the computational problem, and the representation problem.

The statistical problem arises when the learning algorithm is searching a space of hypotheses that is too large for the amount of available training data. In such cases, there may be several different hypotheses that all give the same accuracy on the training data, and the learning algorithm must choose one of these to output. There is a risk that the chosen hypothesis will not predict future data points well. A simple vote of all of these equally good classifiers can reduce this risk.

The computational problem arises when the learning algorithm cannot guarantee finding the best hypothesis within the hypothesis space. In neural network and decision tree algorithms, for example, the task of finding the hypothesis that best fits the training data is computationally intractable, so heuristic methods must be employed. These heuristics (such as gradient descent) can get stuck in local minima and hence fail to find the best hypothesis. As with the statistical problem, a weighted combination of several different local minima can reduce the risk of choosing the wrong local minimum to output.

Finally, the representational problem arises when the hypothesis space does not contain any hypotheses that are good approximations to the true function f. In some cases, a weighted sum of hypotheses expands the space of functions that can be represented. Hence, by taking a weighted vote of hypotheses, the learning algorithm may be able to form a more accurate approximation to f.

A learning algorithm that suffers from the statistical problem is said to have high *variance*. An algorithm that exhibits the computational problem is sometimes described as having *computational variance*. And a learning algorithm that suffers from the representational problem is said to have high *bias*. Hence, ensemble methods can reduce both the bias and the variance of learning algorithms. Experimental measurements of bias and variance have confirmed this.

Review of Ensemble Algorithms

Ensemble learning algorithms work by running a base learning algorithm multiple times, and forming a vote out of the resulting hypotheses. There are two main approaches to designing ensemble learning algorithms.

The first approach is to construct each hypothesis independently in such a way that the resulting set of hypotheses is accurate and diverse, that is, each individual hypothesis has a reasonably low error rate for making new predictions and yet the hypotheses disagree with each other in many of their predictions. If such an ensemble of hypotheses can be constructed, it is easy to see that it will be more accurate than any of its component classifiers, because the disagreements will cancel out. Such ensembles can overcome both the statistical and computational problems discussed above.

The second approach to designing ensembles is to construct the hypotheses in a coupled fashion so that the weighted vote of the hypotheses gives a good fit to the data. This approach directly addresses the representational problem discussed above.

We will discuss each of these two approaches in turn.

Methods for Independently Constructing Ensembles

One way to force a learning algorithm to construct multiple hypotheses is to run the algorithm several times and provide it with somewhat different training data in each run. For example, Breiman (1996) introduced the bagging (*bootstrap aggregating*) method, which works as follows. Given a set of m training data points, bagging chooses in each iteration a set of data points of size m by sampling uniformly with replacement from the original data points. This creates a resampled data set in which some data points appear multiple times and other data points do not appear at all. If the learning algorithm is *unstable*—that is, if small changes in the training data lead to large changes in the resulting hypothesis—then bagging will produce a diverse ensemble of hypotheses.

A second way to force diversity is to provide a different subset of the input features in each call to the learning algorithm. For example, in a project to identify volcanoes on Venus, Cherkauer (1996) trained an ensemble of 32 neural networks. The 32 networks were based on eight different subsets of the 119 available input features and four different network sizes. The input feature subsets were selected (by hand) to group together features that were based on different image processing operations (such as principal component analysis and the fast Fourier transform). The resulting ensemble classifier was significantly more accurate than any of the individual neural networks.

A third way to force diversity is to manipulate the output labels of the training data. Dietterich and Bakiri (1995) describe a technique called error-correcting output coding. Suppose that the number of classes, C, is large. Then new learning problems can be constructed by randomly partitioning the C classes into two subsets, A_k and B_k. The input data can then be relabeled so that any of the original classes in set A_k are given the derived label -1 and the original classes in set B_k are given the derived label $+1$. This relabeled data is then given to the learning algorithm, which constructs a classifier h_k. By repeating this process K times (generating different subsets A_k and B_k), an ensemble of K classifiers $h_1, \ldots, h_K$ is obtained.

Now, given a new data point $\mathbf{x}$, how should it be classified? The answer is to have each h_k classify $\mathbf{x}$. If $h_k(\mathbf{x}) = -1$, then each class in A_k receives a vote. If $h_k(\mathbf{x}) = +1$, then each class in B_k receives a vote. After each of the K classifiers has voted, the class with the highest number of votes is selected as the prediction of the ensemble.

An equivalent way of thinking about this method is that each class j is encoded as a K-bit codeword C_j, where bit k is 1 if $j \in B_k$ and 0 otherwise. The kth learned classifier attempts to predict bit k of these codewords (a prediction of -1 is treated as a binary value of 0). When the L classifiers are applied to classify a new point $\mathbf{x}$, their predictions are combined into a K-bit binary string. The ensemble's prediction is the class j whose codeword C_j is closest (measured by the number of bits that agree) to the K-bit output string. Methods for designing good error-correcting codes can be applied to choose the codewords C_j (or, equivalently, subsets A_k and B_k). Dietterich and Bakiri (1995) report that this technique improves the performance of both decision-tree and backpropagation learning algorithms on a variety of difficult classification problems.

A fourth way of generating accurate and diverse ensembles is to inject randomness into the learning algorithm. For example, the backpropagation algorithm can be run many times, starting each time from a different random setting of the weights. Decision tree algorithms can be randomized by adding randomness to the process of choosing which feature and threshold to split on. Dietterich (2000) showed that randomized trees gave significantly improved performance on 14 out of 33 benchmark tasks (and no change on the remaining 19 tasks).

Ho (1998) introduced the random subspace method for growing collections of decision trees ("decision forests"). This method chooses a random subset of the features at each node of the tree, and constrains the tree-growing algorithm to choose its splitting rule from among this subset. She reports improved performance on 16 benchmark data sets. Breiman (2001) combines bagging with the random subspace method to grow random decision forests that give excellent performance.

Methods for Coordinated Construction of Ensembles

In all of the methods described above, each hypothesis h_k in the ensemble is constructed independently of the others by manipulating the inputs, the outputs, or the features, or by injecting randomness. Then an unweighted vote of the hypotheses determines the final classification of a data point.

A contrasting view of an ensemble is that it is an *additive model*, that is, it predicts the class of a new data point by taking a weighted sum of a set of component models. This view suggests developing algorithms that choose the component models and the weights so that the weighted sum fits the data well. In this approach, the choice of one component hypothesis influences the choice of other hy-

potheses and of the weights assigned to them. In statistics, such ensembles are known as *generalized additive models* (Hastie and Tibshirani, 1990).

The Adaboost algorithm, introduced by Freund and Schapire (1996, 1997), is an extremely effective method for constructing an additive model. It works by incrementally adding one hypothesis at a time to an ensemble. Each new hypothesis is constructed by a learning algorithm that seeks to minimize the classification error on a *weighted* training data set. The goal is to construct a weighted sum of hypotheses such that $H(\mathbf{x}_i) = \Sigma_k w_k h_k(\mathbf{x}_i)$ has the same sign as y_i, the correct label of $\mathbf{x}_i$.

The algorithm operates as follows. Let $d_k(\mathbf{x}_i)$ be the weight on data point $\mathbf{x}_i$ during iteration k of the algorithm. Initially, all training data points i are given a weight $d_1(\mathbf{x}_i) = 1/m$, where m is the number of data points. In iteration k, the underlying learning algorithm constructs hypothesis h_k to minimize the weighted training error. The resulting weighted error is $r = \Sigma_i d(\mathbf{x}_i) y_i h_k(\mathbf{x}_i)$, where $h_k(\mathbf{x}_i)$ is the label predicted by hypothesis h_k. The weight assigned to this hypothesis is computed by

$$w_k = \frac{1}{2} \ln\left(\frac{1 + r}{1 - r}\right)$$

To compute the weights for the next iteration, the weight of training data point i is set to

$$d_{k+1}(\mathbf{x}_i) = d_k(\mathbf{x}_i) \frac{\exp(-w_k y_i h_k(\mathbf{x}_i))}{Z_k}$$

where Z_k is chosen to make d_{k+1} sum to 1.

Breiman (1997) showed that this algorithm is a form of gradient optimization in function space with the goal of minimizing the objective function

$$J(H) = \sum_i \exp(-y_i H(\mathbf{x}_i))$$

The quantity $y_i H(\mathbf{x}_i)$ is called the *margin*, because it is the amount by which $\mathbf{x}_i$ is correctly classified. If the margin is positive, then the sign of $H(\mathbf{x}_i)$ agrees with the sign of y_i. Minimizing J causes the margin to be maximized. Friedman, Hastie, and Tibshirani (2000) expand on Breiman's analysis from a statistical perspective.

In most experimental studies (Freund and Schapire, 1996; Bauer and Kohavi, 1999; Dietterich, 2000), Adaboost (and algorithms based on it) gives the best performance on the vast majority of data sets. The primary exception are data sets in which there is a high level of mislabeled training data points. In such cases, Adaboost will put very high weights on the noisy data points and learn very poor classifiers. Current research is focusing on methods for extending Adaboost to work in high noise settings.

The exact reasons for Adaboost's success are not fully understood. One line of explanation is based on the margin analysis developed by Vapnik (1995) and extended by Schapire et al. (1998). This work shows that the error of an ensemble on new data points is bounded by the fraction of training data points for which the margin is less than some quantity $\Theta > 0$ plus a term that grows as

$$\sqrt{\frac{d}{m}} \frac{\log(m/d)}{\Theta}$$

ignoring constant factors and some log terms. In this formula, m is the number of training data points, and d is a measure of the expressive power of the hypothesis space from which the individual classifiers are drawn, known as the VC-dimension. The value of Θ can be chosen to minimize the value of this expression.

Intuitively, this formula says that if the ensemble learning algorithm can achieve a large "margin of safety" on each training data point while using only a weighted sum of simple classifiers, then the resulting voted classifier is likely to be very accurate. Experimentally, Adaboost has been shown to be very effective at increasing the margins on the training data points; this result suggests that Adaboost will make few errors on new data points.

There are three ways in which this analysis has been criticized. First, the bound is not tight, so it may be hiding the real explanation for Adaboost's success. Second, even when Adaboost is applied to large decision trees and neural networks, it is observed to work very well even though these representations have high VC-dimension. Third, it is possible to design algorithms that are more effective than Adaboost at increasing the margin on the training data, but these algorithms exhibit worse performance than Adaboost when applied to classify new data points.

Related Nonensemble Learning Methods

In addition to the ensemble methods described here, there are other nonensemble learning algorithms that are similar. For example, any method for constructing a classifier as a weighted sum of basis functions (see, e.g., RADIAL BASIS FUNCTION NETWORKS) can be viewed as an additive ensemble where each individual basis function forms one of the hypotheses.

Another closely related learning algorithm is the hierarchical mixture-of-experts method (see MODULAR AND HIERARCHICAL LEARNING SYSTEMS). In a hierarchical mixture, individual hypotheses are combined by a gating network that decides, based on the features of the data point, what weights should be employed. This differs from Adaboost and other additive ensembles, where the weights are determined once during training and then held constant thereafter.

Discussion

The majority of research into ensemble methods has focused on constructing ensembles of decision trees. Decision tree learning algorithms are known to suffer from high variance, because they make a cascade of choices (of which variable and value to test at each internal node in the decision tree) such that one incorrect choice has an impact on all subsequent decisions. In addition, because the internal nodes of the tree test only a single variable, this creates axis-parallel rectangular decision regions that can have high bias. Consequently, ensembles of decision tree classifiers perform much better than individual decision trees. Recent experiments suggest that Breiman's combination of bagging and the random subspace method is the method of choice for decision trees: it gives excellent accuracy and works well even when there is substantial noise in the training data.

If the base learning algorithm produces less expressive hypotheses than decision trees, then the Adaboost method is recommended. Many experiments have employed so-called decision stumps, which are decision trees with only one internal node. In order to learn complex functions with decision stumps, it is important to exploit Adaboost's ability to directly construct an additive model. This usually gives better results than bagging and other accuracy/diversity methods. Similar recommendations apply to ensembles constructed using the naive Bayes and Fisher's linear discriminant algorithms. Both of these learn a single linear discrimination rule. The algorithms are very stable, which means that even substantial (random) changes to the training data do not cause the learned discrimination rule to change very much. Hence, methods like bagging that rely on instability do not produce diverse ensembles.

Because the generalization ability of a single feedforward neural network is usually very good, neural networks benefit less from ensemble methods. Adaboost is probably the best method to apply, but favorable results have been obtained just by training several networks from different random starting weight values, and bagging is also quite effective.

For multiclass problems, the error-correcting output coding algorithm can produce good ensembles. However, because the output coding can create difficult two-class learning problems, it is important that the base learner be very expressive. The best experimental results have been obtained with very large decision trees and neural networks. In addition, the base learning algorithm must be sensitive to the encoding of the output values. The nearest neighbor algorithm does not satisfy this constraint, because it merely identifies the training data point $\mathbf{x}_i$ nearest to the new point $\mathbf{x}$ and outputs the corresponding value y_i as the prediction for $h(\mathbf{x})$, regardless of how y_i is encoded. Current research is exploring ways of integrating error-correcting output codes directly into the Adaboost algorithm.

Road Map: Learning in Artificial Networks
Related Reading: Modular and Hierarchical Learning Systems; Radial Basis Function Networks

References

Bauer, E., and Kohavi, R., 1999, An empirical comparison of voting classification algorithms: Bagging, boosting, and variants, *Machine Learn.*, 36:105–139.

Breiman, L., 1996, Bagging predictors, *Machine Learn.*, 24:123–140. ◆

Breiman, L., 1997, *Arcing the Edge*, Technical Report 486, Department of Statistics, University of California, Berkeley. Available: http://citeseer.nj.nec.com/breiman97arcing.html.

Breiman, L., 2001, Random forests, *Machine Learn.*, 45:5–32.

Breiman, L., Friedman, J. H., Olshen, R. A., and Stone, C. J., 1984, *Classification and Regression Trees*, Monterey, CA: Wadsworth and Brooks. ◆

Cherkauer, K. J., 1996, Human expert-level performance on a scientific image analysis task by a system using combined artificial neural networks, in *Working Notes of the AAAI Workshop on Integrating Multiple Learned Models* (P. Chan, Ed.), Menlo Park, CA: AAAI Press, pp. 15–21.

Dietterich, T. G., 2000, An experimental comparison of three methods for constructing ensembles of decision trees: Bagging, boosting, and randomization, *Machine Learn.*, 40:139–158.

Dietterich, T. G., 1997, Machine learning research: Four current directions, *AI Magazine*, 18:97–136. ◆

Dietterich, T. G., and Bakiri, G., 1995, Solving multiclass learning problems via error-correcting output codes, *J. Artif. Intell. Res.*, 2:263–286.

Freund, Y., and Schapire, R. E., 1996, Experiments with a new boosting algorithm, in *Procedings of the 13th International Conference on Machine Learning*, San Francisco: Morgan Kaufmann, pp. 148–156.

Freund, Y., and Schapire, R. E., 1997, A decision-theoretic generalization of on-line learning and an application to boosting, *J. Comput. Syst. Sci.*, 55:119–139.

Friedman, J. H., Hastie, T., and Tibshirani, R., 2000, Additive logistic regression: A statistical view of boosting, *Ann. Statist.*, 28:337–407. ◆

Hastie, T. J., and Tibshirani, R. J., 1990, *Generalized Additive Models*, London: Chapman and Hall. ◆

Ho, T. K., 1998, The random subspace method for constructing decision forests, *IEEE Trans. Pattern Anal. Machine Intell.*, 20:832–844.

Quinlan, J. R., 1993, *C4.5: Programs for Empirical Learning*, San Francisco: Morgan Kaufmann. ◆

Schapire, R. E., Freund, Y., Bartlett, P., and Lee, W. S., 1998, Boosting the margin: A new explanation for the effectiveness of voting methods, *Ann. Statisti.*, 26:1651–1686.

Vapnik, V., 1995, *The Nature of Statistical Learning Theory*, New York: Springer-Verlag.

Equilibrium Point Hypothesis

Reza Shadmehr

Introduction

If one were to take a robot arm and replace each of its motors with a pair of opposing rubber bands, the arm would tend to settle to the same configuration, regardless of where it was released. That configuration is the *equilibrium point* of the system. If we now change the length-tension properties of the rubber bands, such as by changing the resting lengths or stiffnesses, the equilibrium point of the system will change. Our muscles share a property with rubber bands in that the static force they generate depends on length: the greater the length, the greater the force (see MUSCLE MODELS). The activations received by motor neurons, whether from direct descending commands from the brain or from the spinal reflex circuitry, can change the force-length relation for each muscle, resulting in a change in the equilibrium position of the system. When we reach for an object, is the smooth, stable motion a consequence of a simple trajectory of equilibrium points? Are our muscles and the associated spinal reflex circuitry designed in a way that makes control of motion particularly simple for the brain?

If the answer is yes, then it implies that many of the problems inherent to control of a multijoint limb, such as nonlinear state-dependent dynamics, might be simplified by a well-designed low-level control system. In this article I review the evidence regarding this hypothesis.

Mathematical Basis of the Hypothesis

Equilibrium refers to a state of a system in which the forces acting on it are zero. For example, if the dynamics of the system are

$$\dot{q} = h(q, u) \tag{1}$$

where q is the state of the system and $u(t)$ is a control input, then the equilibrium points $q*$ satisfy the following condition:

$$0 = h(q*, u) \text{ for all } t \geq t_0$$

In short, if the system reaches an equilibrium position, it will remain there.

For a mechanical system, the state is an ordered pair $q = \{\theta, \dot{\theta}\}$, where θ and $\dot{\theta}$ are the position and velocity of the system. A change in the state occurs when there are forces acting on it. This can be written in the framework of Equation 1 as

$$\ddot{\theta} = I(\theta)^{-1}(f_c(\dot{\theta}, \theta, u(t)) - f_m(\dot{\theta}, \theta)) \tag{2}$$

where I is the system's inertia, f_c is the external force field imposed on the system due to the controller with control input $u(t)$, and f_m is the force field produced by the motion of the inertial coordinate frames (Coriolis and centripetal) and other forces. It follows that the system is at equilibrium at any state $\{\theta = 0, \dot{\theta} = 0\}$ where the force in the net field $f_c - f_m$ is zero. Any such position $\theta*$ is an equilibrium point for the system.

We call each state where a field has zero force a *null point* of that field. The equilibrium points for the system, however, are a subset of these null points: the equilibrium point exists only at those null points of the force field $f_c - f_m$ where the state has zero velocity.

Let us consider how we could go about controlling the system of Equation 2. Our objective may be to select the input u in such a way that the system follows a desired trajectory $\theta_d(t)$. For this to occur, we might select u at any time t in such a way that if we were at state $\{\theta_d, \dot{\theta}_d\}$, our controller would produce a force $f_c = \hat{f}_m + \hat{I}\ddot{\theta}_d(t)$, where $\hat{x}$ is the controller's estimate of x. Since there may be

uncertainties in the environment, it is a good idea to also have a mechanism to push us toward where we should be if the need arises:

$$f_c = \hat{f}_m + \hat{I}\ddot{\theta}_d - B(\dot{\theta} - \dot{\theta}_d) - K(\theta - \theta_d) \tag{3}$$

where B and K should be positive definite matrices. We can think of the estimates as a feedforward component of the controller and the remainder as the feedback component of the controller. If the estimates were perfect, substitution of Equation 3 into Equation 2 would give:

$$\ddot{e} + c_1\dot{e} + c_2e = 0$$

where $e = \theta - \theta_d$ is the error in tracking our desired trajectory, and c_1 and c_2 are positive definite (because the inertia matrix I is also positive definite for a mechanical system). Therefore, the tracking error would exponentially decline with time and the system would be stable about the desired trajectory.

Equation 3 makes plain the notion that the forces produced by the controller must take into account the system's mass if it is to move the system along the desired trajectory. The estimates are *internal models* that the brain would presumably have to know (see MOTOR CONTROL, BIOLOGICAL AND THEORETICAL for a discussion of how these models might be learned). However, the equilibrium point hypothesis suggests that the feedback system in Equation 3 is designed in a way that largely eliminates the need for the estimates of the dynamics of the limb. In this hypothesis, the muscles and the spinal reflexes function as the feedback system about the desired trajectory, i.e., the stiffness and viscosity of the system. The main question is the extent to which the mechanical behavior of muscles and the reflex system can compensate for the dynamics of the limb.

Biomechanical Behavior at Rest

In a seminal paper by Feldman (1966), it was observed that the spinal control system acting on the elbow joint of the human arm (composed of muscles and the local feedback circuitry) had static characteristics similar to those of a nonlinear spring. When the elbow was displaced from its equilibrium position, muscles produced monotonically increasing force (as measured at the hand):

$$f = a(\exp[b(x(t) - x_\lambda(t))] - 1) \tag{4}$$

where f is muscle force, t is time, $x(t)$ is length of a muscle, and $x_\lambda(t)$ is the threshold length beyond which the muscle will produce force. Feldman's thesis was that the signals sent from the brain to the spinal reflexes and muscles could be interpreted as setting the threshold length $x_\lambda(t)$ for each muscle. Feldman and Orlovsky (1972) later showed that stimulation of a motor center in the brainstem (of cats), resembling what might happen in a voluntary change in the brain's input to the spinal cord, did result in force-length changes in the muscles. These changes appeared as changes in $x_\lambda(t)$ in the above system.

For a constant input $x_\lambda(t)$ in Equation 4, muscle force reflects both the mechanical properties of the isolated muscles (increased production of force when muscle is lengthened) and the effect of local neural feedback (recruitment of more motor neurons if length exceeds a set threshold). There is now independent support for the formulation in Equation 4. Hoffer and Andreassen (1981) measured the rate of change in stiffness with respect to force in muscles of a cat's hindlimb. They found the relation between force and stiffness to be independent of muscle length, and of the form:

$$\frac{df}{dx} = k(1 - \exp[-\alpha f]) \qquad (5)$$

where df/dx is muscle stiffness. Shadmehr and Arbib (1992) noted that the solution to the above differential equation has the form:

$$f = \frac{1}{\alpha} \ln(\exp[\alpha k(x - \lambda)] + 1) \qquad (6)$$

In the above, λ is the constant of integration and depends on the initial conditions for Equation 5. This result demonstrated that an intact muscle reflex system has a static behavior that resembles that of a nonlinear spring with an adjustable threshold.

If a single-joint limb is controlled by a pair of muscles, then setting λ for each muscle sets the equilibrium point of the system and describes a force field about this equilibrium. Hogan (1985) showed that in a multijoint system, this field will be conservative. This means that if the nervous system produces a force field f_c in Equation 3 through setting of threshold lengths for the muscles of the limb, then when $\ddot{\theta}$ and $\dot{\theta}$ are zero, curl of the field f_c should be zero. Mussa-Ivaldi, Hogan, and Bizzi (1985) measured the static component of f_c in humans. The procedure was to have subjects hold on to the handle of a robotic arm. The robot produced force perturbations at various directions and measured the steady-state force response of the subject's arm as a function of position. It was found that the resulting force field was essentially curl-free. Taken together, static behavior of muscles and the spinal control circuitry appeared to be well described as a nonlinear spring with an adjustable threshold length.

Movements as a Shift in Equilibrium Position

When threshold lengths are set for each muscle, the result is a corresponding equilibrium position θ^* for the limb. The major contribution of the equilibrium point hypothesis has been to suggest that motion is generated by the CNS through a gradual transition of equilibrium points along the desired trajectory without an explicit compensation for dynamics. The evidence for this initially came from a simulation study by Flash. She suggested that in the case of human reaching movements in the horizontal plane, it was possible to predict the hand's motion accurately by smoothly shifting the equilibrium point along a straight line from the start point to a target location. Interestingly, she showed that in the simulation, because the controller was not attempting to compensate for the limb's dynamics, the hand's trajectory slightly deviated from a straight line. However, it turns out that the trajectories recorded in human subjects also show similar deviations, matching her simulations. In this model, the controller was composed of a linear spring-dashpot system with adjustable threshold:

$$f_c = K(\theta - \theta^*(t)) + B\dot{\theta}$$

The field had the property that its static behavior about equilibrium was defined by a stiffness matrix K. This matrix was measured about the equilibrium position of a resting arm by Mussa-Ivaldi et al. (1985).

Taking a different approach, Shadmehr, Mussa-Ivaldi, and Bizzi (1993) suggested that if a movement was generated through a gradual shift of the equilibrium position toward the target, then from measurements of the force field about the hand at rest, one should be able to predict the direction and magnitude of forces that should be produced by the muscles during the initiation of the reaching movement (Figure 1). Because the field at rest is not isotropic and depends on the position of the hand, the forces measured during the initiation of a movement should not point toward the target and be position dependent. These movement initiation forces were measured, and it was found that the pattern of forces from measure-

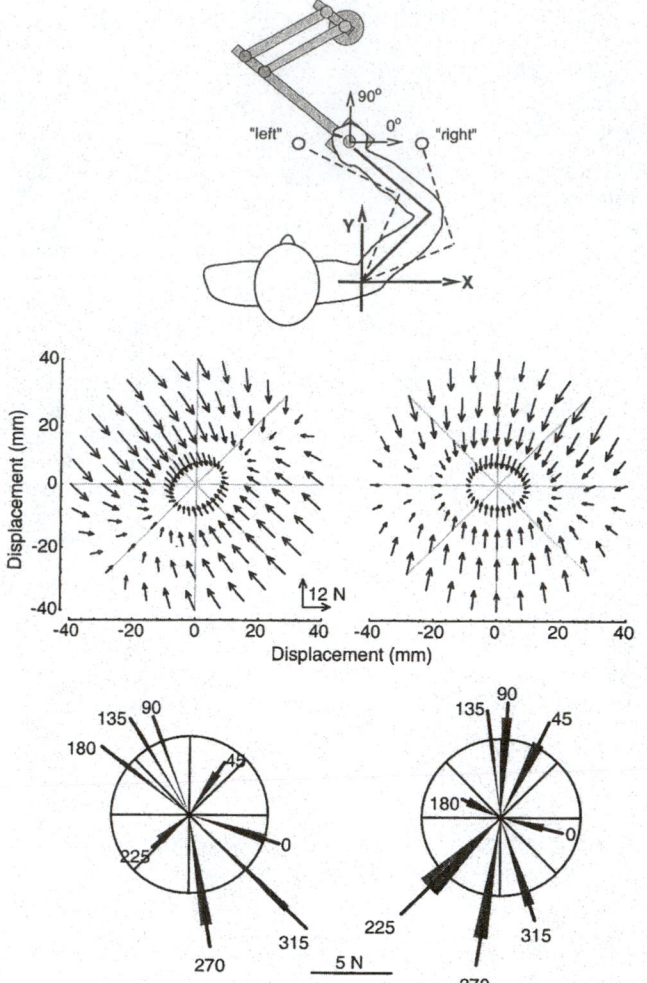

Figure 1. Subject was seated in front of a robotic arm and instructed to hold the handle at either the *right* or *left* configuration. Robot slowly displaced the hand from the origin and measured restoring forces. These forces represent the static component of the force field produced by the muscles, i.e., the postural field. Note the anisotropic shape. Now the subject is told to reach to a target. For randomly selected targets, the robot prevents initiation of the movement (applies a break) and measures the force that the subject is generating in order to make the movement. The magnitude and standard deviations of the movement-related forces are plotted for targets at 0°, 45°, . . . , 315°. The magnitude and direction of movement-related forces are in agreement with the hypothesis that movement is generated through a shift of the equilibrium position of the postural force field toward the target. (From Shadmehr, R., Mussa-Ivaldi, F. A., and Bizzi, R., 1993, Postural force fields of the human arm and their role in generating multijoint movements, *J. Neurosci.*, 13:45–62. Reprinted with permission.)

ments at rest agreed with the measured forces during initiation of movement. In other words, during the start of movements, the equilibrium point of the field had shifted toward the target.

Won and Hogan (1995) went a step further and suggested that during the entire movement, the static component of the field f_c should be similar to that measured when the hand was at rest; i.e., it should converge to an equilibrium position. In their experiment, the hand was displaced from its intended trajectory via a rigid mechanical constraint. It was shown that as the arm was being displaced, it produced forces directed toward the intended trajectory.

The notion of stability about a trajectory (Equation 3) was clearly demonstrated in the data as the controller's output during movement was a force field with an equilibrium point moving roughly along the path connecting the start to the target position.

Dynamics of the Muscle-Reflex System During Movement

Katayama and Kawato (1993) noted that the simulations by Flash used a magnitude of stiffness K that was approximately three times that measured when the arm was at rest. This correctly highlighted the fact that a very stiff system has no need to take into account dynamics of the system in generating its motor output. Although the actual stiffness of the arm was a crucial factor in the simulations, its actual value during movement was unknown, and its estimation had been difficult. Bennett et al. (1992) had found that stiffness during a highly practiced movement was significantly less than that measured when the hand was at rest, while Milner (1993) had found a value that was near the rest levels. It seemed clear that accurate measures of the arm's stiffness during motion were required.

Gomi and Kawato (1996) designed a high-performance robotic manipulandum and measured the arm's stiffness during motion. They found that the stiffness of the arm was near those measured at rest but was temporally modulated about this level during motion. They used measures of local stiffness to estimate the point of convergence of the static component of field f_c by assuming that the static muscle forces were linearly related to distance from equilibrium. Gomi and Kawato concluded that motion of the arm could not be due to a simple shift of the equilibrium point along the desired trajectory. This suggested that ultimately, control of motion required explicit compensation for dynamics of the limb.

The crucial question in the work of Gomi and Kawato (1996) was how to estimate the null point of a force field from local measures of stiffness. Most if not all of the experimental data on intact muscle reflex systems describe only the static behavior, as in Equations 4 and 6. Gomi and Kawato showed that if the dynamic behavior of the muscle reflex system is dominated by its static properties, then it is unlikely that the brain can produce a desired movement via a simple shift of the equilibrium point of the system. But what about the dynamic properties of the muscle reflex system? How do they contribute to control?

Gribble et al. (1998) approached this question by modifying Equation 4 to include the effect of delayed sensory feedback on recruitment of motor neurons, and dependence of muscle force on velocity of contraction and temporal summation of activations. The result was a muscle reflex model that, as before, was controlled via a threshold muscle length, and had a static behavior that remained similar to Equation 4, but was now a complex dynamical system. Remarkably, it was found that if the threshold lengths of the muscles acting on a simulated two-joint arm were shifted along a smooth desired trajectory to the target, the resulting motion was also a smooth trajectory. Furthermore, the local stiffness of the system about the actual trajectory was very similar to that reported by Gomi and Kawato (1996). This suggested that the dynamical behavior of the muscle reflex system was a crucial element in compensating for the arm's dynamic, and that the input to the system might change rather simply from a starting location to a desired end point in order to produce a smooth hand trajectory.

Hodgson and Hogan (2000) performed an elegant experiment that appears to resolve this issue. Rather than estimating a limb's equilibrium position from local stiffness properties and extrapolating to its null point, they perturbed the limb until its equilibrium point was found. Their results (Figure 2) clearly demonstrated that for simple reaching movements, the attractor trajectory was not along the actual trajectory but led it considerably. Therefore, this

demonstrates that while the limb has simple reflex mechanisms that stabilize it in the case of perturbation, the system is not stiff enough that its input can simply ignore dynamics.

Learning and Modulation in Stiffness Properties of the Limb

The motor commands that act on muscles produce not only force but also an attractor that stabilizes the limb about a trajectory. This is a fundamental property that is crucial for control of our movements because there exists a significant delay in tranmission of sensory information from the limbs to our brain. The delay results in multiple levels of feedback: muscles respond with almost no delay with increased force as they are stretched; muscle spindles sense this stretch and activate spinal reflex pathways that enhance this force production with a delay of approximately 30 ms (termed "short-loop" reflexes); the afferent information is conveyed to the thalamus and then to the motor cortex, and the brain responds to the muscle stretch by altering the descending commands, affecting the muscle in approximately 100 ms (termed "long-loop" reflexes). Therefore, the stiffness of the limb and the behavior of the attractor have a time-dependent component. The brain has the ability to modulate the attractor (force response to a displacement) at a time scale of about 100 ms.

Two recent experiments demonstrate that the brain can modulate the long-loop reflexes so as to match the properties of the task. Burdet et al. (2001) asked subjects to make reaching movements while holding a robot that produced a field that was zero along a straight line connecting the start point to end point, but pushed the hand away if the hand strayed from the straight line. Effectively, the hand was traveling along a knife's edge. They demonstrated that the stiffness of the arm increased only along the dimension where the forces were acting (perpendicular to the direction of motion). The results of Wang, Dordevic, and Shadmehr (2001) in subjects who also learned to reach in force fields suggest that this modulation is limited to the long-latency component of the reflex. Therefore, not only do stiffness properties of the limb produce an attractor trajectory that stabilizes the limb during movements, but the brain can also modulate the shape of the restoring forces about the attractor to match the properties of the task.

Summary

Biological muscles are spring-like systems. It was thought that because of their elastic behavior, the CNS might simply describe motor commands in terms of the resting lengths of these springs, effectively producing trajectories in terms of equilibrium points of the system. These commands would ignore the inertial dynamics

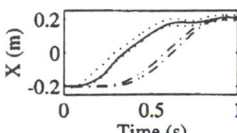 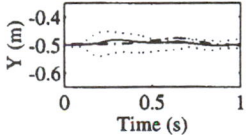

Figure 2. The hand is making a reaching movement while holding a robotic arm. In some cases, the movement is perturbed so that the robot takes the arm along the current estimate of the equilibrium trajectory. The process is repeated until the equilibrium trajectory is found. The bounds for the actual movement are shown by the dash-dot lines. The bounds for the equilibrium trajectory are shown by the dotted lines. The estimate for the equilibrium trajectory is shown by the solid line. Note the large distance by which the equilibrium trajectory leads the actual trajectory. (From Hodgson, A. J., and Hogan, N., 2000, A model-independent definition of attractor behavior applicable to interactive tasks, *IEEE Trans. Syst. Man Cybern.*, 30:105–118. Reprinted with permission.)

of the limb, simplifying the process of control. However, there is now convincing evidence that in programming motor commands to the muscles, the brain does take into account the dynamics of the task (see SENSORIMOTOR LEARNING). The motor commands result in an attractor trajectory that leads the hand in simple reaching movements. It would be expected that both the trajectory of the attractor and the shape of the restoring field about the attractor would change as the dynamics of the task change. Although it is quite possible that biological motor commands can be described in terms of changes in the equilibrium position of the limb, the hypothesis that control of movements by the brain is explicitly performed through this manipulation because it somehow simplifies the process of control appears to be inconsistent with the current data.

Road Maps: Mammalian Motor Control; Dynamic Systems
Related Reading: Arm and Hand Movement Control; Cerebellum and Motor Control; Geometrical Principles in Motor Control; Limb Geometry, Neural Control; Muscle Models; Optimization Principles in Motor Control

References

Bennett, D. J., Hollerbach, J. M., Xu, Y., and Hunter, I. W., 1992, Time varying stiffness of the human elbow joint during cyclic voluntary movement, *Exp. Brain Res.*, 88:433–442.
Burdet, E., Osu, R., Franklin, D. W., Milner, T. E., and Kawato, M., 2001, The central nervous system stabilizes unstable dynamics by learning optimal impedance, *Nature*, 414:446–449.
Feldman, A. G., 1966, Functional tuning of the nervous system with control of movement or maintenance of a steady posture: II. Controllable parameters of the muscles, *Biophysics*, 11:565–578. ◆
Feldman, A. G., and Orlovsky, G. N., 1972, The influence of different descending system on the tonic stretch reflex in the cat, *Exp. Neurol.*, 37:481–494.
Gomi, H., and Kawato, M., 1996, Equilibrium-point control hypothesis examined by measured arm stiffness during multijoint movement, *Science*, 272:117–120. ◆
Gribble, P. L., Ostry, D. J., Sanguineti, V., and LaBoissiere, R., 1998, Are complex control signals required for human arm movement? *J. Neurophysiol.*, 79:1409–1424.
Hodgson, A. J., and Hogan, N., 2000, A model-independent definition of attractor behavior applicable to interactive tasks, *IEEE Trans. Syst. Man Cybern.*, 30:105–118. ◆
Hoffer, J. A., and Andreassen, S., 1981, Regulation of soleus muscle stiffness in premammillary cats: Intrinsic and reflex components, *J. Neurophysiol.*, 45:267–285.
Hogan, N., 1985, The mechanics of multi-joint posture and movement control, *Biol. Cybern.*, 52:315–331.
Katayama, M., and Kawato, M., 1993, Virtual trajectory and stiffness ellipse during multijoint arm movements predicted by neural inverse models, *Biol. Cybern.*, 68:353–362.
Milner, T. E., 1993, Dependence of elbow viscoelastic behavior on speed and loading in voluntary movements, *Exp. Brain Res.*, 93:177–180.
Mussa-Ivaldi, F. A., Hogan, N., and Bizzi, E., 1985, Neural, mechanical, and geometric factors subserving arm posture, *J. Neurosci.*, 5:2732–2743. ◆
Shadmehr, R., and Arbib, M. A., 1992, A mathematical analysis of the force-stiffness characteristics of muscles in control of a single joint system, *Biol. Cybern.*, 66:463–477.
Shadmehr, R., Mussa-Ivaldi, F. A., and Bizzi, E., 1993, Postural force fields of the human arm and their role in generating multi-joint movements, *J. Neurosci.*, 13:45–62.
Wang, T., Dordevic, G. S., and Shadmehr, R., 2001, Learning dynamics of reaching movements results in the modification of arm impedance and long-latency perturbation responses, *Biol. Cybern.*, 85:437–448.
Won, J., and Hogan, N., 1995, Stability properties of human reaching movements, *Exp. Brain Res.*, 107:125–136.

Event-Related Potentials

Steven L. Bressler

Introduction

It is commonly believed that cognition intimately depends on the functioning of the cerebral cortex. Understanding the neural basis of cognition therefore will likely require knowledge of cortical operations at all organizational levels, which may usefully be grouped as microscopic, mesoscopic, and macroscopic. The cellular mechanisms of cortical neurons operate at the microscopic scale and are measured by a host of techniques targeted at that level. Individual cortical neurons contribute to cognitive function, however, by joining in the cooperative actions of neural networks, which operate at the mesoscopic and macroscopic scales. At the microscopic scale, the cooperative fraction of any single neuron's total activity may be exceedingly small, but the cooperative activity of the network exerts effects that are relevant for cognition. The mesoscopic level concerns the cooperative activity of neurons locally in ensembles and area networks, and the macroscopic level concerns the cooperative activity of neurons globally in large-scale networks and entire systems. Thus, many important cortical functions reside in the operations of neural networks and are measured by specialized techniques targeted at the mesoscopic and macroscopic levels.

The event-related potential (ERP) is a neural signal that reflects coordinated neural network activity. The cortical ERP provides a window onto the dynamics of network activity in relation to a variety of different cognitive processes at both mesoscopic and macroscopic levels on a time scale comparable to that of single-neuron activity. Cortical ERPs arise from synchronous interactions among large numbers of participating neurons. These include dense local interactions involving excitatory pyramidal neurons and inhibitory interneurons, as well as long-range interactions mediated by axonal pathways in the white matter. (See NEUROANATOMY IN A COMPUTATIONAL PERSPECTIVE.) Multiple feedback loops involving both excitatory and inhibitory interactions typically cause ERPs to be oscillatory, meaning that they fluctuate within bounds around a central value. Depending on the types of interaction that occur in a specific behavioral condition, cortical networks may display different states of synchrony, causing their ERPs to oscillate in different frequency bands, designated delta (0–4 Hz), theta (5–8 Hz), alpha (9–12 Hz), beta (13–30 Hz), and gamma (31–100 Hz).

The physiological basis of the cortical ERP lies in fields of potential generated by interacting neurons (Lopes da Silva, 1991). Field potentials are largely dendritic in origin, resulting from the summed extracellular currents generated by electromotive forces (EMFs) in the dendrites of synchronously active cortical neurons, primarily pyramidal cells. The EMFs, arising from synaptic activation of postsynaptic ion channels, circulate current in closed loops across the cell membrane and through the intracellular and extracellular spaces. Summed closed-loop currents generated by an ensemble of neighboring neurons flow across the external resistance to form the local ensemble mean field potential (Freeman, 2000).

Depending on the location and size of the recording and reference electrodes, recorded cortical field potentials integrate neural activity over a range of spatial scales: from the intracortical local field potential (LFP) to the intracranial electrocorticogram (ECoG) to the extracranial electroencephalogram (EEG). The LFP (Figure 1) is the most spatially localized signal, integrating the field potential on a submillimeter scale; the ECoG integrates on a submillimeter to millimeter scale; and the EEG integrates over centimeters. The term "field potential" will be used here in reference to the general class of signal subsuming the LFP, ECoG, and EEG. (The intracellular components of the same closed-loop currents that give rise to field potentials are responsible for the closely related magnetic fields, recorded extracranially as the magnetoencephalogram, or MEG.)

A general problem in the investigation of ERPs is that field potential recordings most often contain a combination of potentials, in unknown proportions, from multiple sources. Thus, in addition to the ERP, which is derived from specific networks associated with a behavioral event, the field potential typically also contains potentials derived from the more general field activity of large neural populations. Owing to their fortuitous geometric arrangements and synchronous behavior, these later potentials are mixed with the ERP waveform. Thus, a primary task of all ERP studies is to extract the event-related portion of the recorded field potential. The next section deals with some basic methodology by which this is accomplished for different kinds of ERP.

ERP Varieties and Their Analysis

Whether reflecting mesoscopic or macroscopic activity, the cortical ERP is an electrical signal generated by neuronal networks in relation to a behaviorally significant event. (The corresponding event-related magnetic field has many of the same dynamic and functional properties as the ERP.) Two general classes of ERP are distinguished by whether the relevant event is discrete or continuous. In the case of discrete events, the associated transient ERP is analyzed in short epochs that are time-locked to the event. In the case of continuous events, which usually are periodically modulated sensory stimuli such as a visual flicker, the concurrent steady-state ERP is analyzed in a relatively long time segment.

The traditional approach to the analysis of transient ERPs is to consider the ERP as a characteristic waveform that occurs in relation to the behaviorally significant discrete event. As a simplifying assumption, the ERP waveform is usually treated as if it possesses the same amplitude and phase each time that the event is repeated on multiple trials, although recent analysis shows that

this assumption may not always be valid (Truccolo et al., 2002). Nonetheless, as was discussed above, the recorded single-trial field potential contains contributions from network activity that are both associated (ERP signal) and not associated (noise) with the event. Therefore, averaging of the single-trial field potential time series, time-locked to the event, is commonly employed to extract the ERP from the non-event-related noise. When the relevant event is a sensory stimulus, such phase-locked ERPs are called "evoked." Averaged evoked potentials (Figure 2) are most commonly described in terms of the succession of waveform components that follow stimulus presentation. These components are typically identified according to their polarity (positive or negative) and their time latency following stimulus onset. (Note that the time latency is equivalent to phase in this context.)

Transient ERP waveform components having variable phase may also reliably occur in relation to the repeated event. In this case, time series averaging does not reveal the ERP but instead is destructive, since components of opposite polarity on successive trials tend to be canceled. Non-phase-locked ERPs are referred to as "induced" when they occur following a stimulus and "spontaneous" in the period prior to a stimulus or motor response. This type of ERP may be effectively analyzed by averaging the frequency content of single-trial time series rather than the time series themselves.

Non-phase-locked transient event-related phenomena are detected as frequency-specific changes in the ERP time series. These phenomena may consist of either an event-related increase or decrease of power in one or more of the aforementioned frequency bands. Since the level of ERP power is typically considered to reflect the degree of synchrony within local neuronal populations, a power increase is called event-related synchronization, and a power decrease is called event-related desynchronization (Pfurtscheller and Lopez da Silva, 1999). Frequency analysis has the further advantage of allowing measurement of event-related phase synchronization of ERPs from different cortical sites (Varela et al., 2001). ERP phase synchronization in different frequency ranges has been identified as a fundamental neural correlate of basic sensory and motor processes, as well as higher cognitive processes such as perception and recall of semantic entities. (See SYNCHRONIZATION, BINDING AND EXPECTANCY.)

The study of steady-state ERPs also depends on a variant of frequency analysis. Field potentials recorded during periodically modulated sensory stimulation are narrow-bandpass filtered around the frequency of the driving periodicity to derive the steady-state (periodic) ERPs. Variations in the amplitude and phase of the steady-state ERP are interpreted in terms of driving frequency, spatial location, and behavioral state.

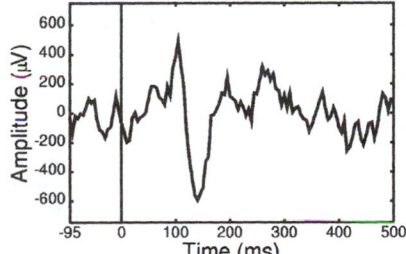

Figure 1. A local field potential (LFP) recorded from the posterior parietal cortex of a macaque monkey in relation to a visual stimulus presented on a display screen for 100 ms, starting at time 0. The LFP was recorded from a chronically implanted bipolar transcortical electrode consisting of 51-μm-diameter Teflon-coated platinum wires with 2.5-mm tip separation.

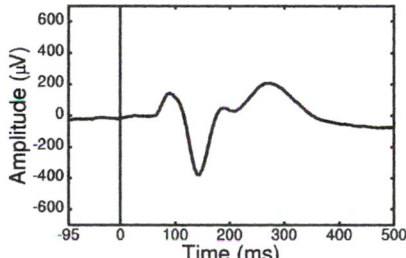

Figure 2. The averaged event-related potential from the same posterior parietal cortex site as in Figure 1, computed from an ensemble of 888 trials. Note the flat prestimulus baseline as compared to the single trial in Figure 1. This illustrates the fact that rhythmic prestimulus activity that is not phase-locked to the stimulus is canceled out by the averaging process.

The Theory of Large-Scale Cortical Networks

Evidence from a variety of sources indicates that neural networks in the cerebral cortex are organized both locally in anatomically segregated areas and on a large scale encompassing multiple distributed areas (Bressler, 2002). Although research on cortical network properties is still in its infancy, a rough depiction of some basic operational features is now possible. Local-area networks process and store information related to specialized sensory, motor, and executive functions, and local synaptic interactions lead to the manifestation of coherent spatial ERP patterns in these specialized informational domains. These interactions also modify the local synaptic matrix with learning. The modified synaptic matrix exerts an essential control on pattern formation in the local-area network by attracting its dynamics to learned (attractor) patterns. In this regard, artificial neural networks that operate according to attractor dynamics bear a resemblance to cortical networks at the local level. (See COMPUTING WITH ATTRACTORS.)

An essential element of overall cortical network function, however, is missing from most artificial network models. Following training on pattern recognition problems, traditional artificial neural networks converge to fixed solutions for a given class of input patterns. Although this behavior has well-known advantages for pattern recognition, it represents an excessive processing rigidity, since these networks lack the ability to adapt to changing external constraints such as are found in real-world situations. Adaptability, in this sense, is a distinguishing feature of normal cortical function.

Theoretical considerations suggest that processing adaptability in the cerebral cortex derives from an essential property of large-scale network dynamics called *metastability*. Cortical metastability refers to a state of dynamic balance among multiply interacting local networks in which the tendency for independent local expression is offset by the tendency for large-scale entrainment (Bressler and Kelso, 2001). The property of metastability permits local networks that are interconnected within the large-scale network architecture of the cortex to coordinate their activities without becoming locked in a fixed pattern of coordination from which they cannot escape.

The ability of local-area networks to form transient coordination relations may represent a basic cortical mechanism for the rapid and flexible association of information from different informational domains. (See ASSOCIATIVE NETWORKS.) It is to be expected that the concurrent coordination of multiple local-area networks imposes conjoint constraints on the spatiotemporal patterning of activity in each local network. The imposition of such constraints may have the important effect of creating associations between activity patterns in different informational domains during the learning process, through the modification of synapses of axons that project from one local network to another. These learned associations would then act during recall on the attractor dynamics of multiple interacting local area networks, causing them to reach a conjunction of consensual patterns that represents an integration of their information. (See COMPUTING WITH ATTRACTORS.)

ERP Evidence for Large-Scale Cortical Network Organization

The theoretical considerations presented in the previous section lead to predictions about the large-scale cortical network organization underlying cognition. One straightforward prediction is that cognitive states should be characterized by unique configurations of interdependent cortical areas in large-scale networks. A confirmation of this prediction is found in the spatial patterning of coactivated cortical areas seen with functional brain imaging techniques such as PET and fMRI. (See COVARIANCE STRUCTURAL EQUATION MODELING.) Like these neuroimaging procedures, ERPs can provide information about the spatial distribution of large-scale network activity underlying a cognitive function. Moreover, because ERPs reflect neurodynamics on a fast time scale (that is inaccessible to current brain imaging technologies), ERPs can also reveal elementary neural subprocesses that subserve that cognitive function. This section uses working memory to illustrate how ERP results can relate large-scale network activity to different subprocesses of a cognitive function.

Working memory consists of several subprocesses for which prominent averaged ERP waveform components have revealed distinct underlying large-scale networks (McEvoy et al., 1998). The mismatch negativity is an early poststimulus ERP component that reflects the maintenance of sensory working memory in the auditory modality. It is elicited by auditory stimuli having physical acoustic properties that deviate from prior (standard) stimuli registered in auditory memory. Occurring between 80 and 200 ms after presentation of deviant auditory stimuli, thus overlapping the N1 and P2 components, the mismatch negativity is isolated by computing the difference wave between averaged ERPs evoked by deviant and standard stimuli. The mismatch negativity is subserved by a large-scale network that includes, in addition to auditory cortical areas, dorsolateral prefrontal cortex, which may serve to control the maintenance of sensory memory in the auditory cortex following one stimulus for comparison with subsequent stimuli (Alain et al., 1998).

A second ERP component, the P3b, occurring roughly 300 ms poststimulus, also results from the comparison of target stimuli with the content of working memory. However, rather than being tuned to the physical characteristics of stimuli, the widely distributed cortical network underlying the P3b is involved in the categorization of stimuli as significant events. Network strength has been found to reflect the degree of consonance resulting from comparison of stimulus attributes with a maintained "expectation" (Kok, 2001).

A third ERP component, related to semantic memory, is the negative-going N400. It occurs between 200 and 500 ms after presentation of a potentially meaningful information-bearing stimulus and varies systematically according to the preexisting context that is established by semantic and long-term memory influences. Specifically, N400 amplitude is reduced as a function of associative, semantic, and repetition priming within or across sensory modalities (Kutas and Federmeier, 2000). Variation of its scalp-recorded topographic distribution with task and stimulus type suggests that the N400 reflects the construction of meaning by cross-modal interactions in a widely distributed neural network. This view is supported by intracranial evidence that the N400 arises from similar waves of activity in multiple brain areas, particularly in the temporal and prefrontal cortices, during the retrieval of information from semantic memory.

Deeper insight into the dynamic organization of large-scale networks underlying working memory comes from studies of the phase synchronization between ERPs from distributed cortical areas. For example, long-range ERP phase synchronization has been reported in the theta frequency range between prefrontal and posterior association areas when subjects retain verbal and spatial items for short periods of time (Sarnthein et al., 1998) and in the beta frequency range between extrastriate areas when they retain visual object representations (Tallon-Baudry et al., 2001). These studies suggest that large-scale cortical network function is based not just on the co-activation of distributed neuronal ensembles, but also on the active coordination of ensemble activity, observable as ERP phase synchronization.

Finally, other ERP types have been used to examine the neural correlates of working memory load. In one investigation, the steady-state visual ERP elicited by a diffuse 13-Hz visual flicker was used to study memory load during the retention period of an object working memory task (Silberstein et al., 2001). The steady-state visual ERP exhibited a load-dependent increase in amplitude at frontal and occipitoparietal sites. By comparison, in a study of event-related synchronization and desynchronization, significant effects of memory load were found in the frontal lobe during a visual sequential letter task (Krause et al., 2000). Event-related synchronization was found at theta frequencies during the initial stages of stimulus processing, whereas event-related desynchronization was observed at alpha frequencies.

Discussion

The cortical ERP reflects the coordinated behavior of large numbers of neurons in relation to a meaningful externally or internally generated event. Single neurons are actively coordinated in the operations of ensembles, local-area networks, and large-scale networks. ERP studies provide a unique avenue of approach to the dynamics of coordination in the cortex at the mesoscopic and macroscopic levels of organization. ERP analysis is an indispensable complement to single-cell neurophysiology and whole-head neuroimaging techniques and can supply a rich source of criteria for neural network modeling efforts.

ERP studies have shown that local cortical area networks are able to synchronize and desynchronize their activity rapidly with changes in cognitive state. These synchronization changes occur between neurons located both within individual local networks and in different local networks. The ability of local area networks to repeatedly reconfigure their activity patterns under constraint of large-scale coordinating influences may allow them to increase the degree of consensus of those local patterns in a short period of time, thereby causing the cortical system as a whole to evolve toward the solution of computational problems. Since it normally operates in a metastable dynamic regime, the cortex is able to balance the coordinated and independent behavior of local networks to maintain the flexibility of this process. When incorporated into artificial neural network designs, a similar computational process could prove useful in avoiding the processing rigidity of many current network models. A metastable large-scale neural network design that recruits and excludes subnetworks according to their ability to reach consensual local patterns has the potential to implement behavioral schema and adapt to changing environmental conditions. Such a system would represent an important advance in machine cognition.

Road Map: Cognitive Neuroscience
Related Reading: Covariance Structural Equation Modeling; EEG and MEG Analysis; Hippocampal Rhythm Generation; Schema Theory; Synchronization, Binding and Expectancy

References

Alain, C., Woods, D. L., and Knight, R. T., 1998, A distributed cortical network for auditory sensory memory in humans, *Brain Res.*, 812:23–37.

Bressler, S. L., 2002, Understanding cognition through large-scale cortical networks, *Curr. Dir. Psychol. Sci.*, 11:58–61.

Bressler, S. L., and Kelso, J. A., 2001, Cortical coordination dynamics and cognition, *Trends Cogn. Sci.*, 5:26–36.

Freeman, W. J., 2000, Mesoscopic neurodynamics: From neuron to brain, *J. Physiol. Paris*, 94:303–322. ◆

Kok, A., 2001, On the utility of P3 amplitude as a measure of processing capacity, *Psychophys.*, 38:557–577.

Krause, C. M., Sillanmaki, L., Koivisto, M., Saarela, C., Haggqvist, A., Laine, M., and Hamalainen, H., 2000, The effects of memory load on event-related EEG desynchronization and synchronization, *Clin. Neurophysiol.*, 111:2071–2078.

Kutas, M., and Federmeier, K. D., 2000, Electrophysiology reveals semantic memory use in language comprehension, *Trends Cogn. Sci.*, 4:463–470.

Lopes da Silva, F., 1991, Neural mechanisms underlying brain waves: From neural membranes to networks, *Electroenceph. Clin. Neurophysiol.*, 79:81–93. ◆

McEvoy, L. K., Smith, M. E., and Gevins, A., 1998, Dynamic cortical networks of verbal and spatial working memory: Effects of memory load and task practice, *Cereb. Cortex*, 8:563–574.

Pfurtscheller, G., and Lopez da Silva, F. H., 1999, Event-related EEG/MEG synchronization and desynchronization: Basic principles, *Clin. Neurophysiol.*, 110:1842–1857.

Sarnthein, J., Petsche, H., Rappelsberger, P., Shaw, G. L., and von Stein, A., 1998, Synchronization between prefrontal and posterior association cortex during human working memory, *Proc. Natl. Acad. Sci. USA*, 95:7092–7096.

Silberstein, R. B., Nunez, Pipingas, A., Harris, P., and Danieli, F., 2001, Steady state visually evoked potential (SSVEP) topography in a graded working memory task, *Int. J. Psychophysiol.*, 42:219–232.

Tallon-Baudry, C., Bertrand, O., and Fischer, C., 2001, Oscillatory synchrony between human extrastriate areas during visual short-term memory maintenance, *J. Neurosci.*, 21:RC177.

Truccolo, W. A., Ding, M., Knuth, K. H., Nakamura, R., and Bressler, A., 2002, Trial-to-trial variability of cortical evoked responses: Implications for the analysis of functional connectivity, *Clin. Neurophysiol.*, 113:206–226.

Varela, F., Lachaux, J. P., Rodriguez, E., and Martinerie, J., 2001, The brainweb: Phase synchronization and large-scale integration, *Nat. Rev. Neurosci.*, 2:229–239. ◆

Evolution and Learning in Neural Networks

Stefano Nolfi

Introduction

Evolution and learning are two forms of adaptation that operate on different time scales. Evolution is capable of capturing relatively slow environmental changes that might encompass several generations. Learning allows an individual to adapt to environmental changes that are unpredictable at the generational level. Moreover, evolution operates on the genotype, but learning affects the phenotype and phenotypic changes cannot directly modify the genotype. Recently, the study of artificial neural networks subjected both to an evolutionary (see EVOLUTION OF ARTIFICIAL NEURAL NETWORKS) and a lifetime learning process has received increasing attention. These studies (see also Nolfi and Floreano, 1999) have been conducted with two different purposes: (1) looking at the advantages, in terms of performance, of combining two different adaptation techniques; (2) understanding the role of the interaction between learning and evolution in natural organisms. The general picture emerging from this body of research suggests that, within an evolutionary perspective, learning has several different adaptive functions:

- It might help and guide evolution by channeling the evolutionary search toward promising directions. For example, learning might significantly speed up the evolutionary search.
- It might supplement evolution by allowing individuals to adapt to environmental changes that cannot be tracked by evolution because they occur during the lifetime of the individual or within few generations.
- It might allow evolution to find more effective solutions and facilitate the ability to scale up to problems that involve large search space.

Learning also has costs. In particular, it might increase the unreliability of evolved individuals (Mayley, 1997). Because learned abilities are also determined by learning experiences, learning individuals might fail to acquire necessary abilities in unfavorable conditions.

How Learning Might Help and Guide Evolution

Hinton and Nowlan (1987) provided a clear and simple demonstration of how learning might influence evolution even if the learned characteristics are not communicated to the genotype. The authors considered a simple case in which (1) the genotype of the evolving individuals consists of 20 genes that encode the architecture of the corresponding neural networks and (2) just a single architecture (i.e., a single combination of gene values) confers added reproductive fitness. Individuals have a genotype with 20 genes that can assume two alternative values (0 or 1). The only combination of genes that provides a fitness value above 0 consists of all 1s. In this extreme case, the probability of finding the good combination of genes is very small, given that the fitness surface looks like a flat area with a spike corresponding to the good combination. Indeed, on such a surface, artificial evolution does not perform better than random search—finding the right combination is akin to discovering a needle in a haystack. The fitness surface metaphor is often used to visualize the search space on an evolutionary algorithm. Any point on the search space corresponds to one of the possible combinations of genetic traits, and the height of each point on the fitness surface corresponds to the fitness of the individual with the corresponding genetic traits.

The addition of learning simplifies the evolutionary search significantly. One simple way to introduce learning is to assume that, in the learning individual, genes can have three alternative values [0, 1, and ?], where question marks indicate modifiable genes whose value is randomly selected within [0, 1], each time step of the individual's lifetime. By comparing learning and nonlearning individuals, one can see that performance increases throughout generations much faster in the former. The addition of learning, in fact, enlarges and smoothes the fitness surface area around the good combination, which can be discovered much more easily in this case by the genetic algorithm. This is because not only the right combination of alleles but also combinations having in part the right alleles and in part unspecified (learnable) alleles might report an average fitness greater than 0. (Fitness increases monotonically with the number of fixed right values because the time needed to find the right combination is inversely proportional, on average, to the number of learnable alleles.) According to Hinton and Nowlan (1987, p. 496), "It is like searching for a needle in a haystack when someone tells you when you are getting close." (On this point, see also BASAL GANGLIA; REINFORCEMENT LEARNING.) A variation of this model has been used to study the interaction between evolution, learning, and culture (Hutchins and Hazlehurst, 1991).

The Hinton-Nowlan model is an extremely simplified case that can be analyzed easily, but it makes several unrealistic assumptions: (1) There is no distinction between genotype and phenotype; (2) learning is modeled as a random process that does not have any directionality; (3) there is no distinction between the learning task (i.e., the learning functions that individuals try to maximize during their lifetimes) and the evolutionary task (i.e., the selection criteria that determine which individuals are allowed to reproduce). Nolfi, Elman, and Parisi (1994) conducted further research that showed how learning and evolution display other forms of mutually beneficial interactions when these limitations are released.

Nolfi et al. (1994) studied the case of artificial neural networks that "live" in a grid world containing food elements. Networks evolve (to become fitter at one task) at the population level and learn (a different task) at the individual level. In particular, individuals are selected on the basis of the number of food elements they are able to collect (evolutionary task) and their capacity to predict the sensory consequences of their motor actions during their lifetime (learning task).

The genotype of the evolving individuals encoded the initial weights of a feedforward neural network which, at each time step, receives sensory information from the environment (the angle and the distance of the nearest food element and the last planned motor action), determines a given motor action selected within four options (move forward, turn left, turn right, or stay still), and predicts the next sensory state (the state of the sensors after the planned action is executed). Sensory information is used both as input and as teaching input for the output units encoding the predicted state of the sensors—the new sensory state is compared with the predicted state, and the difference (error) is used to modify the connection weights through backpropagation. As in the case of the Hinton-Nowlan model, modifications due to learning are not transferred back into the genotype.

The experimental results showed that (1) after a few generations, by learning to predict, individuals increased their performance not only with respect to their ability to predict but also with respect to their ability to find food (i.e., learning produced a positive effect on evolution even if the learning and the evolutionary tasks were different), and (2) the ability to find food increased faster and achieved better results in the case of learning populations than in the case of control experiments in which individuals were not allowed to learn during their lifetime. Further analysis demonstrated that the first observation can be explained by considering that evolution tends to select individuals that are located in regions of the search space where the learning and evolutionary task are dynamically correlated (i.e., where learning-induced changes that produce an increase in performance with respect to the learning task also produce positive effects, on average, with respect to the evolutionary task). And the second observation can be explained by considering that, once learning channels evolution toward solutions in which the learning task and the evolutionary task are dynamically correlated, it allows individuals to recover from deleterious mutations (Nolfi, 1999).

Consider, for example, two individuals, a and b, that are located in two distant locations in weight space but have the same fitness at birth; i.e., the two locations correspond to the same height on the fitness surface (Figure 1). However, individual a is located in a region where the fitness surface and the learning surface are dynamically correlated—a region in which movements that result in an increase in height with respect to the learning surface cause an increase with respect to the fitness surface on average. Individual b, on the other hand, is located in a region where the two surfaces are not dynamically correlated. If individual b moves in weight space, it will go up in the learning surface but not necessarily in the fitness surface. Because of learning, the two individuals will move during their lifetime in a direction that improves their learning performance, i.e., a direction in which their height on the learning surface tends to increase. This implies that individual a, which is located in a dynamically correlated region, will end up with a higher fitness than individual b and will therefore have a better chance to be selected. The final result is that evolution will have a

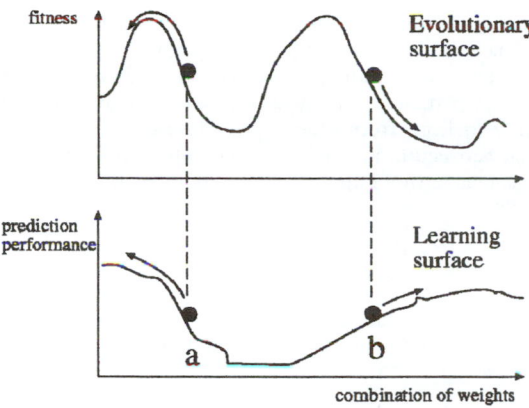

Figure 1. Fitness surface for the evolutionary task and performance surface for the learning task (sensory prediction) for all possible weight matrices. Movements due to learning are represented as arrows.

tendency to progressively select individuals that are located in dynamically correlated regions. In other words, learning forces evolution to select individuals that improve their performance with respect to both the learning and the evolutionary task.

Adapting to Changing Conditions on the Fly

As claimed above, learning might complement evolution by providing a means to master changes that occur too fast to be tracked by the evolutionary process. However, the combination of learning and evolution deeply alters both processes; thus, in individuals that evolve and learn, adaptive characteristics emerge as the result of the interaction between evolutionary and lifetime adaptation and cannot be traced to just one of the two processes.

Nolfi and Parisi (1997) evolved neural controllers for a small mobile robot that was asked to explore an arena (60 × 20 cm) surrounded by walls. The robot was provided with eight infrared sensors that could detect walls up to a distance of about 4 cm and two motors that controlled the two corresponding wheels. The colors of the walls switched from black to white and vice versa each generation because the activity of the infrared sensors is highly affected by the color of the reflecting surface (white walls reflect much more than black walls). Thus, to maximize their exploration behavior, evolved robots should modify their behavior on the fly. In the dark-walled environment, in fact, robots need to move very carefully whenever their sensors are activated; this is because dark walls are detected only when they are very close. In the white-walled environment, robots must begin to avoid walls only when their sensors are strongly activated; this facilitates exploration of the area close to the walls.

Individuals learn during their lifetime by means of self-generated teaching signals. The genotype of the evolving individuals encodes the connection strengths of two neural modules: (1) a teaching module that, each time step, receives the state of the sensors as input and produces a teaching signal as output; (2) an action module that receives the state of the sensors as input and produces motor actions as output. The self-generated teaching signal is used to modify the connection strengths of the action module (for a similar architecture, see Ackley and Littman, 1991). This implies that both the initial behavior produced by the evolving individuals and what the individuals learn are results of the evolutionary process, and neither is determined by the experimenter.

Evolved robots displayed an ability to discriminate between the two types of environments and to modify their behavior accordingly, thereby maximizing their exploration capability. The anal-

ysis of the results revealed that this ability arose from a complex interaction between the evolutionary and learning process. For example, evolved individuals displad an inherited ability to behave so as to enhance the perceived differences between the two environments. This in turns allows the learning process to progressively modify the behavior of the robots so as to adapt to the different environmental conditions.

More generally, this research and that of others has shown that evolution, in the case of individuals able to change during their lifetime as a result of learning, does not tend to directly develop an ability to solve a problem; rather, it tends to develop a predisposition to acquire such ability through learning.

Other experiments conducted by coevolving two competing populations of predator and prey robots (Nolfi and Floreano, 1998) emphasized how lifetime learning might allow evolving individuals to achieve generality, i.e., the ability to produce effective behavior in a variety of circumstances. In these experiments, predators consisted of small mobile robots provided with infrared sensors and a linear camera with a view angle of 36°, which allowed them to detect prey. Prey consisted of mobile robots of the same size; these robots had only infrared sensors, but their maximum available speed was set to twice that of the predators. Each individual was tested against different competitors for ten trials. Predators scored one point for each trial in which they caught prey while prey scored one point for each trial in which they escaped predators.

In this experimental situation, both populations change through the generations as predators and prey face ever-changing, progressively more complex challenges. Interestingly, the authors observed that, in this situation, evolution alone displayed severe limitations; progressively more effective solutions could be developed only by allowing evolving individuals to adapt on the fly through a form of lifetime learning. Indeed, any fixed strategy could master only a limited number of different types of competitors; therefore, only by combining evolution and learning were the authors able to synthesize individuals capable of dealing with competitors adopting qualitatively different strategies. Indeed, by evolving learning individuals, the authors observed the emergence of predators able to detect the current strategy adopted by the prey and to modify their behavior accordingly.

Evolving the Learning Rules

Floreano and Urzelai (2000) conducted a set of experiments in which the genotype of the evolving individuals encoded the learning properties of the neurons of the corresponding neural network. These properties included one of four possible Hebbian learning rules, the learning rate, and the sign of all the incoming synapses of the corresponding neuron. When the genotype is decoded into a neural controller, the connection strengths were set to small random values. After some generations, the genetically specified configuration of learning rules tended to produce changes in the synaptic strengths that allow individuals to acquire the required competencies through lifetime learning. By comparing the results obtained with this method with a control experiment in which the strength of the synapses was directly encoded into the genotype, the authors observed that evolved controllers able to adapt during lifetime can solve certain tasks faster and better than standard nonadaptive controllers. Moreover, they demonstrated that their method scales up well to large neural architectures.

The authors applied this method to evolve neural controllers for mobile robots. Interestingly, the analysis of the synaptic activity of the evolved controllers showed that several synapses did not reach a stable state but kept changing all the time. In particular, synapses continued to change even when the behavior of the robot became rather stable.

Similar advantages have been reported by Husband et al. (1999), who evolved a type of neural network in which neurons, which were distributed over a 2D surface, emitted "gases" that diffused through the network and modulated the transfer function of the neurons in a concentration-dependent fashion, thus providing a form of plasticity.

Finally, the experiments performed by Di Paolo (2000) showed how learning could play the role of a homeostatic process whereby evolved neural networks adapt in order to remain stable in the presence of external perturbations.

Discussion

The interaction between learning and evolution deeply alters both the evolutionary and the learning processes. Evolution in interaction with learning displays dynamics very different from those observed in evolution alone. While in nonlearning individuals the characters that are selected through evolution directly incorporate an ability to produce successful behaviors, in learning individuals they incorporate a predisposition to learn, i.e., a predisposition to acquire necessary abilities through learning. This predisposition to learn may consist of the following:

1. The presence of starting conditions that canalize learning in the right direction. Evolution may select initial weight matrices or network architectures that cause a better and/or a faster learning (Belew, McInerney, and Schraudolph, 1992). This happens either when the learning task and the evolutionary task are the same or when they differ. In the latter case, evolution selects not only individuals that have a predisposition to learn better, but also individuals that, by learning a given task, improve their performance with respect to the evolutionary task.
2. An inherited tendency to behave in such a way that the individual is exposed to the appropriate learning experiences. Evolution tends to select characters that produce initial behaviors that enhance the possibility of learning and/or increase the probability of acquiring adaptive characters through learning. In other words, evolution tends to select individuals whose initial behavior is suitable for learning and not necessarily for solving the evolutionary task.

Similarly, learning within an evolutionary perspective has quite different characteristics from learning studied in isolation, as in "traditional" connectionist research. In individuals that learn but are not subjected to an evolutionary process (e.g., neural networks trained with supervised methods), learning is usually accomplished by ignoring the characters of the individual prior to learning (which are typically generated at random); but in evolving plastic individuals, learning exploits such starting conditions. Moreover, when the learning process itself (i.e., what it is learned during lifetime) is subjected to evolution and not determined in advance, learning does not necessarily tend to incorporate the right solution to the problem; rather, it tends to pull the learning individual in a direction that, given the initial state of the individual, maximizes the chances of adapting to the current environment.

The study of learning within an evolutionary perspective is still in its infancy. But in forthcoming years, it might have an enormous impact on our understanding of how learning and evolution operate in nature. In particular, this type of research might shed light on the ability to learn from others, and more generally on the co-evolution between brain structure and cultural processes such as natural language (for initial explorations of such issue, see Cangelosi, 2001).

Road Maps: Learning in Artificial Networks; Neuroethology and Evolution
Related Reading: Evolution of Artificial Neural Networks; Evolution of Genetic Networks; Language Evolution and Change; Locomotion, Vertebrate

References

Ackley, D. H., and Littman, M. L., 1991, Interaction between learning and evolution, in *Proceedings of the Second Conference on Artificial Life* (C. G. Langton et al., eds.), Reading, MA: Addison-Wesley, pp. 487–509.

Belew, R. K., McInerney, J., and Schraudolph, N. N., 1992, Evolving networks: Using the genetic algorithm with connectionistic learning, in *Proceedings of the Second Conference on Artificial Life* (C.G. Langton et al., Eds.), Reading, MA: Addison-Wesley, pp. 511–548.

Cangelosi, A., 2001, Evolution of communication and language using signals, symbols and words, *IEEE Trans. Evolutionary Computation*, 5(2):93–101.

Di Paolo, E. A., 2000, Homeostatic adaptation to inversion in the visual field and other sensorimotor disruptions, in *From Animals to Animats: Proceedings of the Sixth International Conference on Simulation of Adaptive Behavior* (J.-A. Meyer, A. Berthoz, D. Floreano, H. L. Roitblat, and S. W. Wilson, Eds.), Cambridge, MA: MIT Press, pp. 440–449.

Floreano, D., and Urzelai, J., 2000, Evolutionary robotics with on-line self-organization and behavioral fitness, *Neural Networks*, 13:431–443.

Hinton, G. E., and Nowlan, S. J., 1987, How learning guides evolution, *Complex Systems*, 1:495–502. ◆

Husband, P., Smith, T., Jakobi, N., and O'Schea, M., 1999, Better living through chemistry: Evolving GasNets for robot control, *Connection Science*, 3–4:185–210.

Hutchins, E., and Hazlehurst, B., 1991, Learning in the cultural process, in *Artificial Life II* (C. Langton, C. Taylor, J. D. Farmer, and S. Rasmussen, Eds.), Reading, MA: Addison-Wesley, pp. 689–706.

Mayley, G., 1997, Landscapes, learning costs, and genetic assimilation, *Evolutionary Computation*, 4:213–234.

Nolfi, S., 1999, How learning and evolution interact: The case of a learning task which differs from the evolutionary task, *Adaptive Behavior*, 2:231–236.

Nolfi, S., and Floreano, D., 1998, Co-evolving predator and prey robots: Do "arm races" arise in artificial evolution? *Artificial Life*, 4:311–335.

Nolfi, S., and Floreano, D., 1999, Learning and evolution, *Autonomous Robots*, 1:89–113. ◆

Nolfi, S., and Parisi, D., 1997, Learning to adapt to changing environments in evolving neural networks, *Adaptive Behavior*, 1:75–98.

Nolfi, S., Elman, J. L., and Parisi, D., 1994, Learning and evolution in neural networks, *Adaptive Behavior*, 1:5–28.

Evolution of Artificial Neural Networks

Stefano Nolfi and Domenico Parisi

Introduction

Artificial neural networks may be either computational models of biological nervous systems or computational systems inspired, perhaps loosely, by neurobiology. Natural organisms, however, possess not only nervous systems but also genetic information stored in the nucleus of their cells (genotype). The nervous system is part of the phenotype derived from this genotype through a process called development. The information specified in the genotype determines aspects of the nervous system that are expressed as innate behavioral tendencies and predispositions to learn. When neural networks are viewed in the broader biological context of artificial life (i.e., the attempt to synthesize life-like phenomena within computer and other artificial media), they tend to be accompanied by genotypes and to become members of evolving populations of networks in which genotypes are inherited from parents to offspring (Parisi, 1997).

Artificial neural networks can be evolved by using evolutionary algorithms (Holland, 1975; Koza, 1992). An initial population of different artificial genotypes, each encoding the free parameters (e.g., the connection strengths, the architecture of the network, the learning rules, or some combination thereof) of a corresponding neural network, is created randomly. The population of networks is evaluated in order to determine the performance (fitness) of each individual network. The fittest networks are allowed to reproduce by generating copies of their genotypes with the addition of changes introduced by genetic operators such as mutations (random changes of a few genes that are selected randomly) or crossover (the combination of parts of the genotype derived from two reproducing networks). This process is repeated for a number of generations until a network that satisfies the performance criterion set by the experimenter is obtained (for a review of methodological issues, see Yao, 1993).

The genotype might encode all the free parameters of the corresponding neural network or only the initial values of the parameters and/or other parameters that affect development and learning. In the former case, networks are entirely specified in the genotype and change only phylogenetically as a result of the modifications introduced by genetic operators during reproduction. In the latter case, networks also change ontogenetically (i.e., during the period in which they are evaluated) as a result of both genetic and environmental factors. In this article we review examples of networks that undergo developmental processes such as neural growth. For an analysis of networks that are able to adapt to the environment as a result of a form of lifetime learning see EVOLUTION AND LEARNING IN NEURAL NETWORKS.

Evolution and Development

A cornerstone of biology is the distinction between the inherited genetic code (genotype) and the corresponding organism (phenotype). What is inherited from the parents is the genotype. The phenotype is the complete individual that is formed according to the instructions specified in the genotype.

Evolution is critically dependent on the distinction between genotype and phenotype, and on their relation, i.e., the genotype-to-phenotype mapping. The fitness of an individual, which affects selective reproduction, is based on the phenotype; but what is inherited is the genotype, not the phenotype. Furthermore, while the genotype of an individual is a single entity, the organism is a continuum of different phenotypes taking form during the genotype-to-phenotype mapping process, each derived from the previous one under genetic and environmental influences.

When the genotype-to-phenotype mapping process takes place during an individual's lifetime, we speak of development. In this case, each successive phenotype corresponding to a given stage of development has a distinct fitness. The fitness of a developing individual is a complex function of these developmental phases. Evolution must ensure that all these successive forms are viable and, at the same time, that they comprise a well-formed sequence in which each form leads to the next until a mostly stable (adult) form is reached. This puts various constraints on evolution, but it also offers new means for exploring novelty. Small changes in the developmental rates of different components of the phenotype, for example, can have huge effects on the resulting phenotype. Indeed,

it has been hypothesized that in natural evolution changes affecting regulatory genes that control the rates of development played a more important role than other forms of change such as point mutations (Gould, 1977; see also EVOLUTION OF GENETIC NETWORKS).

Although the role of genotype-to-phenotype mapping and development has been ignored in most experiments involving artificial evolution, awareness of its importance is now increasing. According to Wagner and Altenberg (1996, p. 967), "In evolutionary computer science it was found that the Darwinian process of mutation, recombination and selection is not universally effective in improving complex systems like computer programs or chip designs. For adaptation to occur, these systems must possess *evolvability*, i.e., the ability of random variations to sometimes produce improvement. It was found that evolvability critically depends on the way genetic variation maps onto phenotypic variation, an issue known as the representation problem."

Genetic Encoding

To evolve neural networks one should decide how to encode the network in the genotype in a manner suitable for the application of genetic operators. In most cases, phenotypic characteristics such as synaptic weights are coded in a uniform manner so that the description of an individual at the level of the genotype assumes the form of a string of identical elements (such as binary or floating point numbers). The transformation of the genotype into the phenotypic network is called genotype-to-phenotype mapping.

In direct encoding schemes there is a one-to-one correspondence between genes and the phenotypic characters subjected to the evolutionary process (Yao, 1993). Aside from its biological implausibility (see EVOLUTION OF THE ANCESTRAL VERTEBRATE BRAIN), simple one-to-one mapping has several drawbacks. One problem, for example, is scalability. Since the length of the genotype is proportional to the complexity of the corresponding phenotype, the space to be searched by the evolutionary process increases quadratically with the size of the network (Kitano, 1990).

Another problem of direct encoding schemes is the impossibility of encoding repeated structures (such as network composed of several subnetworks with similar local connectivity) in a compact way. In one-to-one mappings, in fact, elements that are repeated at the level of the phenotype must be repeated at the level of the genotype as well. This affects not only the length of the genotype and the corresponding search space, but also the evolvability of individuals. A full genetic specification of a phenotype with repeated structures, in fact, implies that adaptive changes affecting repeated structures should be independently rediscovered through changes introduced by the genetic operators.

Growing Methods

The genotype-to-phenotype process in nature is not just an abstract mapping of information from genotype to phenotype; it is also a process of physical growth (both in size and in physical structure). Thus, taking inspiration from biology, one may decide to encode in the genotype growing instructions. The phenotype is progressively built by executing the inherited growing instructions.

Nolfi, Miglino, and Parisi (1994) used a growing encoding scheme to evolve the architecture and the connection strengths of neural networks that controlled a small mobile robot. These controllers consisted of a collection of artificial neurons distributed over a 2D space with growing and branching axons (Figure 1, *Top*). Inherited genetic material specified instructions that controlled the axonal growth and the branching process of neurons. During the growth process, when a growing axonal branch of a particular neuron reaches another neuron, a connection is established between the two neurons. The bottom of Figure 1 shows the network re-

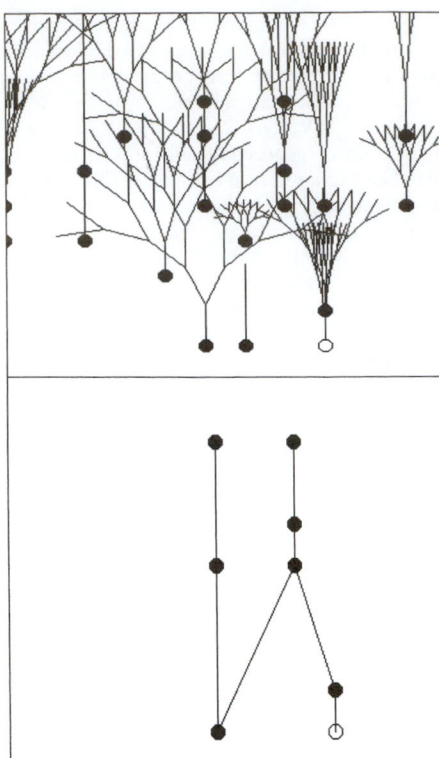

Figure 1. Development of an evolved neural network. *Top*, The growing and branching process of the axons. *Bottom*, The resulting neural network after removal of nonconnecting branches and the elimination of isolated neurons and groups of interconnected neurons.

sulting from this growth process after the elimination of isolated and nonfunctional neurons. Axons grew and branched only if the activation variability of the corresponding neurons was larger than a genetically specified threshold. This simple mechanism is based on the idea that sensory information coming from the environment has a critical role in the maturation of the connectivity of the biological nervous system and, more specifically, that the maturation process is sensitive to the activity of single neurons (Purves, 1994). Therefore, both genetic and environmental factors influenced the developmental process; i.e., the actual sequence of sensory states experienced by the network influenced the process of neural growth.

This method allows the evolutionary process to select neural network topologies that are suited to the task chosen (see LEARNING NETWORK TOPOLOGY). Indeed, analysis of the evolutionary process shows how improvements are due to changes affecting both the neural architecture and the connection weights. Moreover, if some aspects of the task are allowed to vary during the evolutionary process, evolved genotypes display an ability to develop into different final phenotypic structures that are adapted to current conditions.

Cellular Encodings

In natural organisms the development of the nervous system begins with an in-folding of the ectodermic tissue to forms the neural crest. This structure gives rise to the mature nervous system through three phases: the genesis and proliferation of different classes of neurons by cellular duplication and differentiation, the migration of the neurons toward their final destination, and the growth of neurites (axons, dendrites). The growing process described in the previous sec-

tion therefore characterizes very roughly only the last of these phases. A number of attempts inspired by the seminal work of Lindenmayer (1971) have been made to include other aspects of this process in artificial evolutionary experiments.

Cangelosi, Nolfi, and Parisi (1994), for example, extended the model described in the previous section by adding a cell division and migration stage to the already existing stage of axonal growth. The genotype is a collection of rules governing the process of cell division (a single cell is replaced by two daughter cells) and migration (the new cells can move in the 2D space). The genotype-to-phenotype process therefore starts with a single cell which, by undergoing a number of duplication and migration processes, produces a collection of neurons arranged in a 2D space. These neurons grow their axons and establish connections until a neural controller is formed.

Gruau (1994) proposed a genetic encoding scheme for neural networks based on a cellular duplication and differentiation process. The genotype-to-phenotype mapping starts with a single cell that undergoes a number of duplication and transformation processes, ending up in a complete neural network. In this scheme the genotype is a collection of rules governing the process of cell divisions (a single cell is replaced by two daughter cells) and transformations (new connections can be added and the strengths of the connections departing from a cell can be modified). In this model, therefore, connection links are established during the cellular duplication process.

The instructions contained in the genotype are represented as a binary-tree structure as in genetic programming (Koza, 1992). During the genotype-to-phenotype mapping process, the genotype tree is scanned starting from the top node of the tree, then following each ramification. The top node represents the initial cell that undergoes a set of duplication processes to produce the final neural network. Each node of the genotype tree encodes the operations that should be applied to the corresponding cell, and the two subtrees of a node specify the operations that should be applied to the two daughter cells. The neural network is progressively built by following the tree and applying the corresponding duplication instructions. Terminal nodes of the tree (i.e., nodes that have no subtrees) represent terminal cells that will not undergo further duplications. Gruau also considered the case of genotypes formed by many trees where the terminal nodes of a tree may point to other trees. This mechanism allows the genotype-to-phenotype process to produce repeated phenotypic structures (e.g., repeated neural subnetworks) by re-using the same genetic information. Trees that are pointed to more than once, in fact, will be executed more times. This encoding method has two advantages: (1) Compact genotypes can produce complex phenotypic networks; (2) evolution may exploit phenotypes in which repeated substructures are encoded in a single part of the genotype. By evolving neural controllers for a simulated hexapod robot able to walk, the author showed that the problem could be solved only by using a genetic encoding that allows for the possibility of re-using the same genetic information to encode repeated substructures (i.e., similar subnetworks controlling the legs) or by using incremental evolution (i.e., by first evolving oscillator networks to control a single limb, then evolving the coordinating circuitry to yield walking [see also Lewis et al., 1992]).

Discussion

Artificial evolution can be seen as a learning algorithm for training artificial neural networks. From this point of view, one distinctive feature is the limited amount of feedback required. Supervised learning algorithms require immediate and detailed desired answers as feedback. Reinforcement learning algorithms require less—only a judgment of right or wrong, which need not be immediate. Viewed as a learning algorithm, artificial evolution requires still less—only an overall evaluation of the performance of the network over the entire evaluation period. A second distinctive feature is that any parameter of the neural network (e.g., the connection strengths, the network topology, the learning rules, the transfer function of the neurons) can be subjected to the evolutionary process.

Although systematic comparison between artificial evolution and other algorithms has not yet been done, it is reasonable to claim that artificial evolution tend to produce better results when detailed feedback is not available. This is the case, for example, for neural networks that should control mobile robots (Nolfi and Floreano, 2000). In this case, in fact, although the experimenter can provide a general evaluation of how much the behavior of a robot approximates the desired behavior, he or she usually cannot indicate what the robot should do at each time step to produce a desired behavior. Moreover, artificial evolution might prove more effective when certain features of the network (such as the network topology or the transfer functions) that cannot be properly set by hand are crucial. Artificial evolution, in fact, provides a way to co-adapt different types of parameters. Artificial evolution also has drawbacks, such as the time needed to conduct the evolutionary process and the lack of formal criteria for designing effective fitness functions.

The analogy with natural evolution, however, can also be considered more strictly. In this case, the evolutionary process is not seen as an abstract training algorithm but as a process that mimics some of the key aspects of the evolutionary process in nature. From this perspective, neural networks tend to be viewed as a part of a population of artificial organisms that adapt autonomously by interacting with the external environment.

This body of research might contribute to the understanding of natural systems by identifying the key characteristics of natural evolution that make it so successful in producing the extraordinary variety of highly adapted life forms present on the planet. Examples include a better understanding of the role of incremental or staged evolution (i.e., how evolution of animals adapted to one biological niche then provides the basis for further evolution into other niches [Harvey, 1993; Lewis et al., 1992]); the role of competitive coevolution (i.e., how the evolution of two competing populations with coupled fitness may reciprocally drive each other to increasing levels of complexity [Nolfi and Floreano, 2000]); the importance of pre-adaptation (i.e., the possibility of evolving a predisposition to acquire an ability to solve a given problem during lifetime rather than, directly, an ability to solve such a problem [see EVOLUTION AND LEARNING IN NEURAL NETWORKS]).

Road Maps: Learning in Artificial Networks; Neuroethology and Evolution
Related Reading: Evolution and Learning in Neural Networks; Evolution of the Ancestral Vertebrate Brain; Locomotion, Vertebrate

References

Cangelosi, A., Nolfi, S., and Parisi, D., 1994, Cell division and migration in a "genotype" for neural networks, *Network—Computation in Neural Systems*, 5:497–515.

Gould, S. J., 1977, *Ontogeny and Phylogeny*, Cambridge, MA: Harvard University Press.

Gruau, F., 1994, Automatic definition of modular neural networks, *Adaptive Behavior*, 3:151–183.

Harvey, I., 1993, Evolutionary robotics and SAGA: The case for hill crawling and tournament selection, in *Artificial Life 3: Proceedings of the Santa Fe Conference* (C. Langton, Ed.), Reading, MA: Addison-Wesley, pp. 299–326.

Holland, J. J., 1975, *Adaptation in Natural and Artificial Systems*, Ann Arbor, MI: University of Michigan Press.

Kitano, H., 1990, Designing neural networks using genetic algorithms with graph generation system, *Complex Systems*, 4:461–476.

Koza, J. R., 1992, *Genetic Programming: On the Programming of Computers by Means of Natural Selection*, Cambridge, MA: MIT Press.

Lewis, M. A., Fagg, A. H., and Solidum, A., 1992, Genetic programming approach to the construction of a neural network for control of a walking robot, in *Proceedings of the IEEE International Conference on Robotics and Automation*, New York: IEEE Press, pp. 2618–2623.

Lindenmayer, A., 1971, Developmental systems without cellular interactions, their language and grammars, *J. Theor. Biol.*, 30:455–484.

Nolfi, S., and Floreano, D., 2000, *Evolutionary Robotics: The Biology, Intelligence, and Technology of Self-Organizing Machines*, Cambridge, MA: MIT Press/Bradford Books. ◆

Nolfi, S., Miglino, O., and Parisi, D., 1994, Phenotypic plasticity in evolving neural networks, in *Proceedings of the International Conference: From Perception to Action* (D. P. Gaussier and J.-D. Nicoud, Eds.), Los Alamitos, CA: IEEE Press, pp. 146–157.

Parisi, D., 1997, Artificial life and higher level cognition, *Brain Cogn.*, 34:160–184. ◆

Purves, D., 1994, *Neural Activity and the Growth of the Brain*, Cambridge, UK: Cambridge University Press.

Wagner, G. P., and Altenberg, L., 1996, Complex adaptations and the evolution of evolvability, *Evolution*, 50:967–976.

Yao, X., 1993, A review of evolutionary artificial neural networks, *Int. J. Intelligent Systems*, 4:203–222. ◆

Evolution of Genetic Networks

Kirk W. Beisel and Bernd Fritzsch

Introduction

With the completion of an initial draft of the more than 30,000 genes of the human genome we can now establish all the information to make a human from the coded sequences, which are based on a four-nucleotide alphabet. Man has achieved a significant catalog useful for understanding the basis of all evolution through the comparisons of whole genomes ranging from yeast and worms to mice and humans. At present, we can read those four letters and are, to some extent, able to understand words (genes) or phrases (known gene networks). However, most of our current higher level of understanding of the meaning of the DNA sequences and their subsequent organization into gene networks is comparable to an understanding of a poem by Goethe read by a six-year-old. Like the poem, the meta-language of information coding in the human genome needs to be understood above and beyond our current limited insight (Venter et al., 2001). Herein, we offer an outline that specifies some of the computational problems in modeling genetic networks, which can direct the establishment of a diversity of neuronal networks in the brain. Since these neuronal networks are composed of a wide variety of cell types, the final fate or end stage of each cell type represents the outcome of a dynamic amalgamation of gene networks. Genetic networks not only determine the cell fate acquisition from the original stem cell, but also govern the contact formation between the cell populations of a given neuronal network.

In many respects there are numerous intriguing parallels between the establishment and functioning of genetic networks with those of neuronal networks, which can range from simple (on and off switch) to extremely complex (computer logic gate). To appreciate the full complexity of organismic development we outline below how intracellular and cell-cell interactions modify the complexity of gene interactions involved in genetic networks. Such interactions will achieve an altered status of cell function and, ultimately, the connection alterations in the formation of neuronal networks.

Evolving from Operons to Promoters with Enhancers and Suppressors

When Jacob and Monod published their now famous lac operon model of the regulation of the bacterial gene transcription, they initiated what has now become the main problem of developmental biology: unraveling the proximate causes for gene activation and silencing (repression) at the appropriate level. As such, a full understanding of this regulatory process is essential for any higher-level understanding of the information decoding process that unfolds the genome information to form a human being. Simply said, if a muscle cell precursor activates the wrong genetic network, it will form bone around it, like bone cells. The effect of such a developmental "error" would be catastrophic for the organism.

The lac operon (Figure 1) is a gene that consists of two regions. One contains the DNA elements responsible for regulation of gene transcription, and the other encodes for the transcribed protein(s). Regulation of gene transcription to form messenger RNA (mRNA), which is in turn the basis for translating the information coded in the DNA into a protein, is the way the cell regulates the availability of information coded in the genome. The regulatory region is composed of DNA elements, which can be categorized as operator (enhancer/silencer) and promoter sites. Promoters are regions in which RNA transcription is initiated. The operator sites, containing enhancer and silencer elements, are DNA sequences that require proper binding of regulatory proteins to either stimulate or inhibit the promoter region. Initiating transcription requires utilization of regulatory elements within a gene's genomic structure. In the case of the lac operon system, this is achieved by having an operator strand of DNA that initiates gene transcription, controlled by a repressor protein (lacI), which in turn is controlled by an inducer (lactose). The lacI and lactose have specific affinities for each other, such that in the presence of the inducer, the repressor changes its configuration and cannot bind to the operator DNA. This allows transcription of the gene. The product of the gene is an enzyme that metabolizes the inducer (lactose), thus freeing the repressor

(lacI) to block transcription. Once all lactose is metabolized, the repressor binds to the operator, preventing the latter from initiating transcription of an enzyme that is no longer needed. In general terms, both negative (repression) and positive (activation) controlling elements exist for gene transcription.

This basic system of bacterial gene expression regulation has evolved into a much more complicated regulatory process that involves genetic networks rather than single genes. This increase in complexity is further complicated by the evolution of interrupted DNA sequences in multicellular organisms that form exons (parts of the DNA that, when transcribed, are exported from the nucleus and subsequently translated into a protein) and introns (parts of DNA between the exons, which are not translated). This situation does not allow a simple specification of units of information as continuous strands of DNA that specify unique proteins. In general, a single gene specifies each protein, even if this gene is transcribed into a variety of mRNA species through differential splicing of various exons that gives rise to various proteins. It must be recognized that not all genes encode for proteins.

We next have to look at the level of transcription initiation in multicellular organisms, which can have greater complexity compared with that demonstrated by the lac operon. The promoter region requires a basic set of DNA binding proteins to initiate transcription, which is common for all promoter regions. However, for this complex to function, it requires association with one or more specific transcription factors. This transcription factor complex also targets to specific promoter sites. The presence of such transcription factors is therefore essential for the activity mediated by the enhancer and silencer sites on the promoter region of a gene. Such transcription factors regulate the temporal and tissue specific expression of any differentially regulated gene. However, a given enhancer may activate a number of genes, whereas several enhancer sites may be linked to a given promoter region. In addition, the same enhancer may activate transcription of some genes while simultaneously suppressing that of other genes. Most transcription factors can bind to specific DNA sequences, have an activation domain that acts on gene transcription, and also interact with the basic transcription complex as well as other transcription factors. In essence, the promoter region of a gene computes the overall expression of all enhancer/silencer sites that can modify its activity and regulates how much and for how long transcription of a gene occurs. In conclusion, most gene activation/suppression is not on a single gene level, but rather affects multiple genes simultaneously. We propose to use the term *genetic network* for those interactively regulated genes. Essentially, these genetic networks and their complex, spatiotemporally restricted interactions with the DNA provide the basis of the nonlinear relationship of genotype to phenotype.

Modeling Genetic Networks and Their Evolution

In single-celled organisms many of the biochemical pathways represent a hierarchal pathway and as such may represent an intracellular genetic network in its most simplistic form. As organisms evolved, more complex genetic networks formed to control and modify cell-cell interactions and functions. Such networks allowed cells to evolve beyond simple substrate interactions in a continuously active cell and permitted the formation of different cell types, each specialized for specific tasks. Instead of evolving distinct sets of genes for each specific cell type, networks consisting of variable mixes of genetic modules evolved to allow rapid evolution of multiple cell types by rearranging those modules. The establishment of genetic networks was possible only through the evolution of multiple regulatory elements to control gene expression. Once established, a genetic network can be duplicated, then modified to form repeated modules or cassettes.

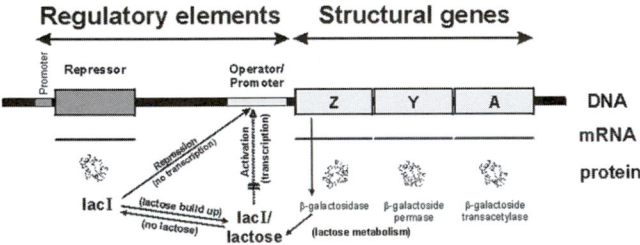

Figure 1. The lac operon model, which shows the regulation of transcription of the Z (β-galactosidase), Y (β-galactoside permase), and A (β-galactoside transacetylase) genes. The promoter regions for the repressor protein and the three structural genes are shown. If no lactose is present, the repressor protein (lacI) will bind with the operator/promoter sites and prevent transcription. If lactose is present, transcript occurs, since lactose binds with lacI and prevents lacI binding with the operator/promoter site. β-Galactosidase will metabolize lactose and thus allows lacI to bind to the promoter to prevent further transcription (negative feedback).

Beyond modularity of genetic networks, developing organisms and the brain also consist of repeated modules. For example, the cerebellum consists of such repetitive modules and has long been viewed as a paradigm for neuronal information processing. Likewise, reiterative development in terms of segmentation and segment transformation has appealed to developmental biologists. This mechanism has allowed us to understand how evolution works by gradually transforming developmental sequences in different segments to generate individuality from commonality. Because of this general interest, we know a great deal of the molecular development of segments and how the basic machinery is altered in various segmented animals as well as how modifiers of development can alter segmental fate (Robert, 2001).

Several models have been developed to theoretically examine genetic networks and how they can impact cellular patterning. Two basic approaches are the standard Boolean network model and the continuous models that approximate neural-like connectionist architectures or biochemical networks of interacting molecules. Salazar-Ciudad and colleagues (Salazar-Ciudad, Newman, and Sole, 2001a; Salazar-Ciudad, Sole, and Newman, 2001b) recently provided a mathematical model for some of those interactions. Building on a previous model to describe the formation of stripes in the fly embryo, Salazar-Ciudad et al. (2001a, b) analyzed properties of various gene networks to form patterns. The basic idea is a reaction-diffusion system that factors in the concentration of a gene product, the interactions of genes (both positive and negative), thresholds of gene responses, and diffusion between cells. Both qualitative and quantitative effects can be mathematically represented so that proximal and distal cell-cell interactions and the resulting effects on the ensuing cellular patterning can be predicted. Salazar-Ciudad et al. (2001a, b) showed that many properties of these larger networks of up to 30 interacting gene products can be broken down into subsets of a genetic network that can form basic patterns such as stripes. Moreover, many of those subsets, called modules, can be combined in various ways to form more complex patterns. Interestingly, this model is close to some models for information processing in neural networks (Salazar-Ciudad et al., 2001a, b).

Building on these properties, they generate two model networks based on the interactions of two diffusible factors that have been identified in setting up segments in insects (Salazar-Ciudad et al., 2001a, 2001b). In one case they assume that one of these diffusible factors increases expression of both factors whereas the other factor inhibits expression of both factors (emergent network). In the second (hierarchic) network, there are no direct or indirect reciprocal relationships between the gene products (Figure 2). Based on these two network properties, they show how either a hierarchic network or an emergent network can represent a realistic model of segmentation. The strength of the emergent network lies in its resilience against change and can result in complex repetitive patterns (three or more stripes). In contrast, the hierarchic network provides a closer relationship between genotype and phenotype and this allows for a more rapid implementation of variation. In addition, hierarchic networks form less complicated repetitive patterns (three or fewer stripes). Moreover, switching between those two networks during developmental steps can provide flexibility in cell fate acquisition and pattern formation. Other patterning processes that lead to the formation of checkerboard patterns can most easily be simulated by employing the lateral inhibition of cell fate assignment provided by the ubiquitous Delta-Notch system of lateral inhibition, again largely simulating network properties well known in computational neurobiology. The genetic networks discussed thus far are essentially suited for simple strings of cells or two-dimensional (2D) sheets of cells and can at best roughly approximate the complexity of three-dimensional organs such as the brain.

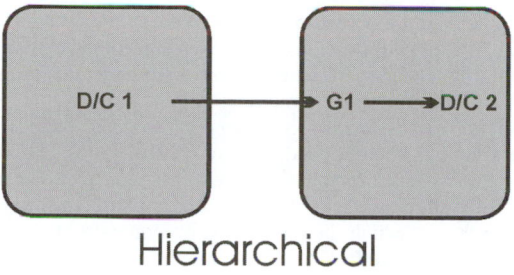

Hierarchical

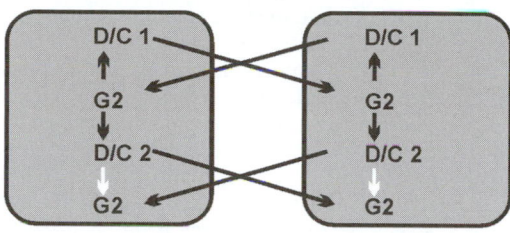

Expansive Emergent

Figure 2. Two interactive modules, which show the interactions between two cells or cell clusters. Diffusible or surface contacting genes (D/C1; D/C2) and nondiffusible gene products (G1; G2) have both activating (black arrows) and inhibiting (white arrows) interactions in the emergent network.

Transcription Factors Belong to a Number of Families

Transcription factors are characterized by a DNA binding domain and by a domain that permits protein-protein interactions to interact with other transcription factors and the transcription activation complex. Many transcription factors can be grouped into larger families depending on certain conserved DNA binding motifs. Perhaps the best-known transcription factors are the homeodomain (Helix-Turn-Helix) proteins, which contain a highly conserved sequence of 60 amino acids. This gene family is present in most eukaryotic organisms and plays a prominent role in controlling the genetic determination of development and implementation of the genetic body plan. Some of the other more famous DNA binding domains are the basic Helix-Loop-Helix (bHLH) domain, the basic Leucine zipper and the Zinc finger domain. Advances in comparative analysis of human, fly, worm, and yeast genomes suggest that, as expected, many transcription factor families have been greatly enlarged in the course of human evolution. For example, while the overall human genome is only about twice as large as the fly genome, and five times as large as the yeast genome, a specific Zinc finger transcription factor family has expanded almost 20 times that of yeast (Venter et al., 2001). Others, like the Forkhead domain, the bHLH domain, and the homeobox domain, have expanded from yeast to humans 10 to 25 times.

In addition to these transcription factors, an expansion of secreted factors that regulate transcription via their specific receptors has played a major role in the evolution of multicellular organisms. Outside of hormones, those secreted factors can be grouped into four families: the Fibroblast Growth Factor (*FGF*) family, the Hedgehog (*Hh*) family, the Wingless (*Wnt*) family, and the Transforming Growth Factor-β (*TGF-b*) superfamily. As is to be expected, these families have been disproportionately enlarged in humans compared to flies (24:1 *FGF*s; 3:1 *Hh*; 18:6 *Wnt*; 29:6

TGF-b). This signifies that expansion of the human genome is not so much a simple duplication of all genes, but rather, an expansion of modulating capacity of gene expression to generate unique contexts in which genes are activated.

A number of researchers consider that some of these contexts involve what has been dubbed "master control genes." Such genes produce transcription factors that, if expressed in areas where they are normally not expressed, can turn those areas into an organ comparable to that in which the normal expression pattern of that gene is apparently involved. A classic example is the *Pax6* gene (reviewed in Pichaud and Desplan, 2002). *Pax6*, together with other genes, is essential for eye formation and forms an interactive gene network. If the mammalian *Pax6* gene is expressed instead of its fly homolog in flies, it can direct fly eye development. Moreover, if it is overexpressed, it can turn areas, like skin at joints, into eye-like structures. It must be noted that eyes form in flies from ectoderm. Thus, only the fly's ectoderm is competent to respond to the enhanced presence of *Pax6*. In analogy to the "grandmother" neuron concept in neurobiology, some people have adopted the view that a single gene can switch on and govern development of an entire organ—in this case, a fly's eye. Most recent research has already modified those initial claims; it has shown that a number of genes [e.g., eyeless1 (*Eya1*) and sine oculis homeobox (*Drosophila*) homolog 3 (*Six3*)], if disrupted by targeted deletion of essential parts of their protein coding regions (knockout), can also cause loss of eyes. Although *Pax6*, *Eya1*, and *Six3* are expressed in a number of organs, they are able to form eyes only if co-expressed in distinct areas. Thus, the genetic context in which a gene is expressed is undeniably important. By changing the context in which a transcription factor is expressed, it can be utilized in a variety of genetic networks and result in the development of a wide range of cell types. This cellular context can also be extended to the spatial and temporal patterning of precursor cells. This is exemplified by the generation of distinct *Drosophila* neuroblast cell lineages, which depend on the timing of the sequential expression of the transcription factors from a common neural precursor (Isshiki et al., 2001).

We have now established that context-dependent gene activation and developmental regulation of dynamically interacting networks of transcription factors are the likely causes for development to take a given pathway. Clearly, if *Pax6* were overexpressed in the endodermal lining of the gut, it would be unable to establish eye formation. The endoderm of the gut is not competent to develop an eye because it lacks the context in which *Pax6* gene activation can govern eye formation. In the following section we explore an example of those networks and their transcriptional regulation.

Cochlea of the Inner Ear: A Paradigm for 2D Developmental Networks Utilizing Boundary Formation

A realistic application of such models would be for the development of an organ with two dimensions conveying crucial structural differences that are functionally meaningful. One such model would be the developmental network that generates the limbs and hands. Here we focus on another, clearly two-dimensionally organized organ—the mammalian cochlea—which converts sound energy into electric signals that convey frequency- and intensity-specific sound information. The mammalian cochlea is a spiral organ in which a functional longitudinal, tonotopic gradient is the basis for frequency-specific sound analysis. The cytoarchitecture of the cochlea is significantly altered across the longitudinal axis, where changes in specific cell types are quite dramatic. The cochlea can also be subdivided radially into the spiral ganglion, organ of Corti (with one row of inner and three rows of outer hair cells), and the lateral wall, which includes the stria vascularis. In essence,

the cochlea represents a 2D organ with concentric and longitudinal differences in cell types. The adult cochlear structure requires at least two concurrent and overlapping developmental networks: one for generating the elongation of the cochlea and another for engendering the radial changes in cell types. In addition, given the existence of functionally distinct rows of single cells (one row of inner hair cells, three rows of outer hair cells), some of the reaction-diffusion models computed by Salazar-Ciudad et al. (2001b), which involve the presence of sharp boundaries, could well apply for cochlear development (Figure 3).

On the molecular side, a number of factors that are crucial for distinct steps in cochlear development have been identified. Several bHLH genes are known to control cell fate determination in the cochlea. The first of these factors to appear in development, *ngn1*, is essential for all sensory neuron formation. *Math1* is essential for all hair cell formation. *Hes1* and *Hes5* are specific for supporting cell formation out of pluripotent supporting cell/hair cell precursors (Zine et al., 2001). Expression of *Math1* drives, through the *Delta/Notch* system for lateral inhibition, the upregulation of *Hes1/5* in supporting cells. Expression of *Hes1/5* is essential to suppress *Math1*; in *Hes1/5* null mutants, some supporting cells assume a hair cell fate, as evidenced by additional hair cell rows (Zine et al., 2001). The exact mechanism(s) for the formation of the spiral ganglion, hair cells, and the supporting cells in their specific topology are still relatively unknown. However, there is evidence for molecular and possibly cellular interactions in assigning distinct cell lines to neuronal and hair cell phenotypes. The mechanisms for upregulation of a specific bHLH gene are tied into those that suppress upregulation of others. Thus, once a cell has upregulated, say, *Math1*, it cannot simultaneously upregulate *Hes1* or *ngn1*. In other words, once upregulated, one of the bHLH factors will activate the genetic network that ultimately leads to the specific cell differentiation.

A gradient exists with respect to the last mitosis of hair cells (first in the apex, last in the base), whereas the process of proliferation and differentiation of spiral ganglion cells starts in the base and finishes in the apex. Interestingly, this apical to basal hair cell proliferation gradient differs from almost all other developmental gradients, which always run from base to apex (e.g., Fariñas et al., 2001). These two complementary developmental genetic networks could be the foundation for the establishment of countergradients of gene expression. The resulting countergradient could lead to a

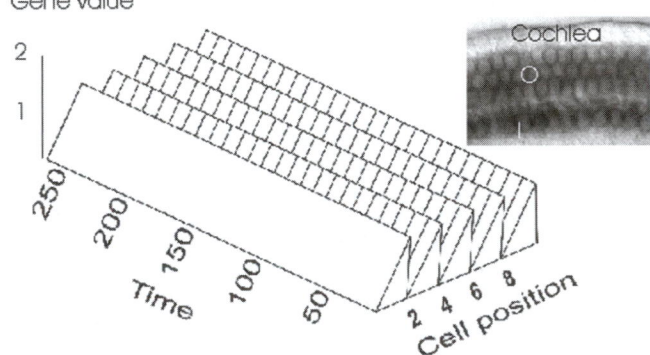

Gene value

Figure 3. The outcome of a simulation using the nonexpansive emergent module is compared to the arrangement of four sensory hair cells in the cochlea (I, one row of inner hair cells; O, three rows of outer hair cells) as revealed by BDNF expression. It is possible that as few as four different genes and their interactions determine the pattern of the hair cell distribution in the cochlea. (Modified from Salazar-Ciudad et al., 2001a, and Fariñas et al., 2001.)

greater disparity of gene expression between the base and apex of the cochlea. A number of regulatory proteins and/or their receptors are expressed in the inner ear during embryonic and postnatal development and could influence the basal to apical longitudinal developmental expression patterns. These are the diffusible factors and their receptors, *BDNF/trkB* and *NT3/trkC, Jag2/Notch,* and *FGF8/FGFR-2(IIIb)* and the transcription factor *GATA3*. For example, in the course of hair cell differentiation the acetylcholine receptor channel $\alpha 9$ gene is upregulated in a basal to apical sweep starting at approximately embryonic day 15.5. In general, ion channel expression patterns in the inner ear follow the general developmental sweep from base to apex first in IHC, then in OHCs. Furthermore, this apparently expansive network may have quantitative effects on downstream gene expression, which could be displayed by differential continuous and discontinuous longitudinal gradients (Beisel et al., 2000).

In many respects, the longitudinal gradient in the cochlea parallels the dorsal-ventral network of bHLH expression in spinal cord and brain. In the brain, a *Mash1* expression domain is ventral to an *ngn* expression domain, which is capped by a *Math1* expression domain. These domains are mutually inhibitory (Gowan et al., 2001) and are directly involved in linking pathways of neurogenesis and regional specification to the formation of distinct functional longitudinal zones (Bermingham et al., 2001). One likely possibility for pattern formation in the cochlea is that the inner ear builds on these developmental regulatory networks. Thus, *ngn1* is expressed in spiral sensory neurons prior to *Math1* expression and inhibits its cellular upregulation, which would specify hair cell formation. Instead of forming longitudinal stripes, as in the brain, the interaction between those genes and the cells carrying them is now forming radially distinct, concentric columns of sensory neurons (more medial, *ngn1* dependent) and hair cells (more lateral, *Math1* dependent). Temporal extension of this interaction by repetitive utilization of this patterning network will result in the longitudinal extension of the cochlea as exemplified in its spiraling growth. Superimposing on this module other developmental modules for finer organization of the existing macropattern will organize the large disparities between the cochlear cell types and the cytoarchitecture.

Beyond these basically 2D models of cellular developmental organization, we next need to investigate 3D pattern formation, which is the real hallmark of brain development.

Realistic Developmental Networks and Their Evolution Involved in the Central Nervous System

The brain can be broken down into longitudinal and transverse compartments. We have already introduced some of the molecular mechanisms for longitudinal functional column formation. Transverse boundaries are in the form of neuromeres, which coincide with specific gene expression domains such as Hox genes. One such transverse boundary has been identified as a major organizing center of molecular and cellular interactions, the midbrain/hindbrain boundary (MHB; Liu and Joyner, 2001). This area is crucial for a number of specific neuronal aspects of the vertebrate brain, notably the cerebellum, the area of the brain that contains the most neurons (Wang and Zoghbi, 2001). This MHB is induced by a negative feedback loop involving two transcription factors, *Otx2* and *Gbx2*, which are expressed in adjacent domains (Figure 4). Absence of *Otx2* reduces the entire forebrain/midbrain formation to the level of the otocyst; absence of *Gbx2* eliminates the MHB and expands the midbrain toward the level of the otic vesicle. Within the expression domain of *Gbx2* an upregulation of *FGF8* occurs, which is inhibited by *Otx2*. But while *FGF8* inhibits *Otx2*, it promotes *Wnt1, Engrailed,* and *Pax2/5* expression. Despite all this information, critical steps in this reasonably complicated in-

teractive network are not yet understood. One obstacle hindering a precise model for the data is that the expression of other genes is eventually lost in a specific knockout (null) mutant (e.g., the *Gbx2* null). The associated genes appear to be upregulated initially in the proper spatiotemporal pattern, suggesting that the underlying patterns specifying the upregulation of these genes are not yet known. However, it is clear that the above outlined genes are essential for the continued expression of the other genes, as indicated in Figure 4.

Previously, we introduced the context dependence of gene expression and its regulation. It is noteworthy that none of the MHB genes, either alone or in combination, can induce formation of a posterior midbrain or a cerebellum in areas such as the caudal hindbrain or the forebrain. This suggests that another set of as yet undiscovered transcription factors must be expressed in the cells of the MHB area to render them competent to respond to the transcription factors outlined above. Those very genes may also be the ones that upregulate the initial expression of *Otx2* and *Gbx2*.

Evolution of the MHB seems to have occurred in steps. An *Otx2* homolog is expressed in the anterior part of the brain vesicle in most chordate species that have been analyzed (Hullond et al., 2000). However, neither spatial nor temporal expressions of all the molecular members necessary to form the mammalian MHB seem to be in place. Specifically, although a homolog of *Wnt1* exists in all chordates, it is not expressed in the typical vertebrate pattern in each chordate (Holland, Holland, and Schubert, 2000). Moreover, the evolution of crucial members of this boundary, such as *FGF8*, is unlikely to be conserved across phyla, as flies have only one *FGF* compared to the 24 *FGFs* known for man (Venter et al., 2001). In addition, formation of the cerebellum and many associated structures further requires the presence of *Math1* (Bermingham et al., 2001). Thus, although certain chordates do have some of the genes that regulate the MHB formation and these genes are expressed in a topologically comparable pattern, even the presence of all those players requires additional implementations of other genes to generate the cellular basis to build a cerebellum. In other words, if fully analyzed, the MHB example may elucidate how an existing expression genetic network implements more genes and expands its regulatory basis to transform midbrain and hindbrain neuronal tissue into a cerebellum.

Discussion

Patterning is an evolving process that can generate new patterns by modifying existing genetic networks (Davidson et al., 2002). Thus, cell fate within those genetic networks can be further modified from existing patterning processes by merging other patterning modules

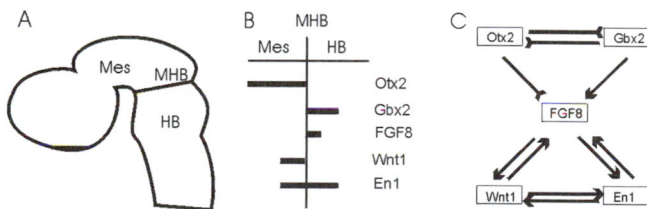

Figure 4. The midbrain/hindbrain boundary (*A*) is one of the best-understood boundaries in brain development. At least five genes (*B*) are interacting to form this boundary in both positive (arrows) and negative interactions (arrow tail; *C*). Each gene is expressed in specific stripes at or across the boundary (*B*). En1, engrailed 1; FGF8, fibroblast growth factor 8; Gbx2, gastrulation brain homeobox 2; Otx2, orthodenticle homolog 2; Wnt1, wingless related MMTV integration site 1. (Adapted from Wang and Zoghbi, 2001, and Liu and Joyner, 2001.)

into an existing genetic network as well as by implementing new downstream players. Currently, the increasing use of knockout (null mutant) mice has greatly facilitated our understanding of genetic networks in development of the central and peripheral neural systems. In many cases these studies demonstrated that knocking out a single gene can affect the expression of hundreds of genes, confirming that genes do not work in isolation. In other null mutants, however, no overt effects are observed, suggesting that biological redundancy may be playing a role. The use of transgenic mice, involving gene dosage or in other cases dominant-negative mutations, may provide additional approaches to elucidate the role of genetic networks in formation and function of neuronal networks. However, these models must be interpreted with caution. Genes, which affect development to yield a variety of CNS deformations, provide limited insights into "how the brain works" because many of these mutations are early lethal and hence cannot be studied. The anticipated extensive use of conditional mutations, in which a gene is deleted in a limited area of the brain only, will likely change this picture dramatically in the near future.

Road Map: Neuroethology and Evolution
Related Reading: Axonal Path Finding; Evolution of Artificial Neural Networks; Evolution of the Ancestral Vertebrate Brain

References

Beisel, K. W., Nelson, N. C., Delimont, D. C., and Fritzsch, B., 2000, Longitudinal gradients of KCNQ4 expression in spiral ganglion and cochlear hair cells correlate with progressive hearing loss in DFNA2, *Brain Res. Mol. Brain Res.*, 82:137–149.

Bermingham, N. A., Hassan, B. A., Wang, V. Y., Fernandez, M., Banfi, S., Bellen, H. J., Fritzsch, B., and Zoghbi, H. Y., 2001, Proprioceptor pathway development is dependent on Math1, *Neuron*, 30:411–422.

Fariñas, I., Jones, K. R., Tessarollo, L., Vigers, A. J., Huang, E., Kirstein, M., de Caprona, D. C., Coppola, V., Backus, C., Reichardt, L. F., and

Fritzsch, B., 2001, Spatial shaping of cochlear innervation by temporally regulated neurotrophin expression, *J. Neurosci.*, 21:6170–6180.

Davidson, E. H., Rast, J. P., Oliveri, P., Ransick, A., Calestani, C., Yuh, C. H., Minokawa, T., Amore, G., Hinman, V., Arenas-Rust, A. G., Pan, Z., Schilstra, M. J., Clarke, P. J., Arnone, M. I., Rowen, L., Cameron, R. A., McClay, D. R., Hood, L., Bolouri, H., 2002, A genomic regulatory network for development, *Science* 295:1669–1678.

Gowan, K., Helms, A. W., Hunsaker, T. L., Collisson, T., Ebert, P. J., Odom, R., and Johnson, J. E., 2001, Crossinhibitory activities of ngn1 and math1 allow specification of distinct dorsal interneurons, *Neuron*, 31:219–232. ◆

Holland, L. Z., Holland, N. N., and Schubert, M., 2000, Developmental expression of AmphiWnt1, an amphioxus gene in the Wnt1/wingless subfamily, *Dev. Genes Evol.*, 210:522–524.

Isshiki, T., Pearson, B., Holbrook, S., and Doe, C. Q., 2001, Drosophila neuroblasts sequentially express transcription factors, which specify the temporal identity of their neuronal progeny, *Cell*, 106:511–521.

Liu, A., and Joyner, A. L., 2001, Early anterior/posterior patterning of the midbrain and cerebellum, *Annu. Rev. Neurosci.*, 24:869–896. ◆

Pichaud, F., Desplan, C., 2002, Pax genes and eye organogenesis, *Curr. Opin. Genet. Dev.* 12:430–434

Robert, J. S., 2001, Interpreting the homeobox: Metaphors of gene action and activation in development and evolution, *Evol. Dev.*, 3:287–295.

Salazar-Ciudad, I., Newman, S. A., and Sole, R. V., 2001a, Phenotypic and dynamical transitions in model genetic networks. I. Emergence of patterns and genotype-phenotype relationships, *Evol. Dev.*, 3:84–94.

Salazar-Ciudad, I., Sole, R. V., and Newman, S. A., 2001b, Phenotypic and dynamical transitions in model genetic networks. II. Application to the evolution of segmentation mechanisms, *Evol. Dev.*, 3:95–103. ◆

Venter, J. C., Adams, M. D., Myers, E. W., et al., 2001, The sequence of the human genome, *Science*, 291:1304–1351. ◆

Wang, V. Y., and Zoghbi, H. Y., 2001, Genetic regulation of cerebellar development, *Nat. Rev. Neurosci.*, 2:484–491.

Zine, A., Aubert, A., Qiu, J., Therianos, S., Guillemot, F., Kageyama, R., and de Ribaupierre, F., 2001, Hes1 and Hes5 activities are required for the normal development of the hair cells in the mammalian inner ear, *J. Neurosci.*, 21:4712–4720.

Evolution of the Ancestral Vertebrate Brain

Bernd Fritzsch

Introduction

Earlier work on the evolution of the vertebrate brain centered on the description and functional analysis of adult brains, with limited attempts to project the origin of various nuclei back to the ventricular surface, thereby generating flat, two-dimensional maps (Nieuwenhuys, ten Donkelaar, and Nicholson, 1997). The remarkable variations in size and shape of parts of the brain were often viewed as evidence of a progressive increase in complexity. The usual implication drawn was that information processing between the sensory input and the motor output became more sophisticated as the number of neurons increased. However, mere size is a tricky issue, as humans and dolphins share both absolute and relative size ratios, but we have no objective way to show which brain is more complex.

In this context it is important to understand that fairly little is known with respect to variations in connections between neurons from topologically comparable areas in different animals. This is unfortunate since altered connections between neurons are crucial functionally relevant aspects of brain variation.

In part this is so because there are always several ways to implement a certain function within existing connections using molecular and cellular mechanisms. These mechanisms are only partly

understood (Koch and Laurent, 1999). It would therefore be naive to work out all connections of every neuron assuming that this alone will help to understand the function of the system in question. Ideally, one would need to have this information and record simultaneously from all neurons involved in a given behavior to unravel the computational properties of even small neuronal networks. Such networks might be those formed by the 302 neurons in the worm *Caenorhabditis elegans*, or the 30 cells of the stomatogastric ganglion. The next best thing is recording from individual neurons under situations of stable behavior, and using these data to simulate a network that can perform the same task using the measured parameters. An excellent example is the fictive swimming in lampreys. Another example is the use of cortical activity to govern robotic movements. For obvious reasons, achieving this in the ancestral vertebrate brain is impossible, and we have to find other ways to gain insights into the origin of the nervous system that evolved into the vertebrate brain.

In this overview I discuss the possible origin of the vertebrate brain, then present a possible ontogenetic way through which the problem of homology/homoplasy may be minimized. In addition, possible mechanisms to diversify the ancestral vertebrate brain are suggested, and data concerning structural changes whose functional implications are as yet unclear are presented

When and How Did the Vertebrate Brain Form?

The origin of the vertebrate brain is tightly coupled to the origin of the vertebrate head, which likely happened around 600 million years ago (Knoll and Carroll, 1999). Next to nothing is known about the central nervous system of these ancestral, bilaterally symmetric animals. We can only assume that it consisted of a simple, dorsally located tube of nerve cells with a barely recognizable specialization of what would become the vertebrate brain at its anterior end.

However, the emerging synthesis of comparative morphology, development, and paleontology offers a new approach to understanding vertebrate brain evolution. Adult diversity is now viewed as the outcome of divergent genetic developmental mechanisms. Thus, resolving brain evolution through comparison of adult structures can be aided by comparative neuroembryology, that is, by comparing adult structures with their specific development and the genes that guide such development. Such comparative embryological data in conjunction with gene expression patterns have aided in clarifying major issues of brain development (Holland and Holland, 1999).

The vertebrate brain forms through invagination of ectoderm (the embryonic "skin") to form a neural tube. During further development the central nervous tissue becomes polarized and then subdivides into compartments, each characterized by a specific pattern of gene expression (Figure 1). It is this latter aspect that may eventually allow us to obtain a map of expression of homologous genes (based on nucleotide sequence identity) to identify topologically comparable and thereby homologous parts of the developing vertebrate brain, irrespective to their structural similarities. Thus far, only rudiments of this map are known, and the relationship of gene expression patterns to the structural evolution of topologically comparable areas is largely unknown (Bermingham et al., 2001). In a few years we will have the molecular delineation of identical subdivisions of the vertebrate brain based on the nested expression of homologous genes. This is a prerequisite to sorting out how identical areas of the brain (defined by their gene expression patterns) have evolved structural differences that serve specific ad-

aptations unique to a specific animal. However, it also appears that molecular identification of major subdivisions of the vertebrate brain, such as forebrain, midbrain, and hindbrain, is possible in all chordates, based on the nested expression of certain homologous genes (Holland and Holland, 1999). Other genes, while conserved in their sequence, appear to have altered their developmental expression patterns in various groups of animals. For example, the left-right asymmetry determination in mice and chickens uses the same molecules but in a different pattern. Moreover, there is ample evidence that developmental genes can be co-opted into novel developmental pathways, either alone or in addition to their original task, (see EVOLUTION OF GENETIC NETWORKS). Moreover, a specific gene can be of conserved importance for forebrain development and evolution but also essential for specific aspects of ear development (Fritzsch, Signore, and Simeone, 2001).

The essence of these findings is that the developmental patterning of the vertebrate brain evolved over 600 million years ago and has been rather stable in many aspects of developmental gene expression. Nevertheless, compartments of the forming brain, once specified in their relative position through conserved gene expression, have diverged to form the unique anatomy of a given species.

The vertebrate head (and brain) evolved in part owing to novel embryonic material, neural crest and placodes, which contribute to all sensory systems of the head. Neural crest is embryonic neuronal material that emerges from the forming neural tube and undergoes extensive migration to form branchial arches, bones, teeth, and peripheral ganglia. Placodes are cake-like epidermal thickenings that contribute sensory neurons to cranial ganglia. Most recently, specific molecules have been identified that are associated with neural crest development. Interestingly, these molecules have also been identified in vertebrate relatives that lack neural crest. This provides molecular evidence that neural crest precursors may exist in the brain and spinal cord of these animals (Corbo et al., 1997). What is important here is that molecular markers may delineate identical populations of neurons that can evolve a novel morphology and function.

The view proposed here is that the evolution of the brain is a sequence of developmental variations leading to modified adult structures. These modified structures serve somewhat different functions that, in turn, are chosen in the process of natural selection (Raff, 1996). Thus the role of mutation in the selection of novel structures and functions is rather indirect (Fritzsch, 1998a). Arguably, the motor system, the common output of the brain, is the best understood part of the brain, as we can clearly define the output in terms of measuring the generated movement and can actually simulate the movement. In addition, we know more about its evolution (Fritzsch, 1998a) and the molecular governance of its compartmentalization (Cordes, 2001) than in any other part of the brain. In the following section I will focus on the evolution of some cranial motor neurons.

Evolution of the Brainstem Oculomotor System

Recent research has shown that developmental selector genes (transcription regulation factors: see EVOLUTION OF GENETIC NETWORKS) play an important role in the differentiating vertebrate brain. These networks appear to form a space map that possibly orchestrates the activation of topologically appropriate structural genes in longitudinal columns and their rostrocaudal subdivisions. Some of these transcription regulators, known as basic helix-loop-helix genes (bHLH genes), may play a role in the dorsoventral patterning of the differentiating brain and spinal cord (Bermingham et al., 2001), while others, known as homeotic genes, play a role in rostrocaudal subdivisions (Cordes, 2001). These genes were identified first in the fruit fly, where they are related, for example, to homeotic transformation (changes in the developmental fate of compartments). Subsequently, homeotic and other selector genes,

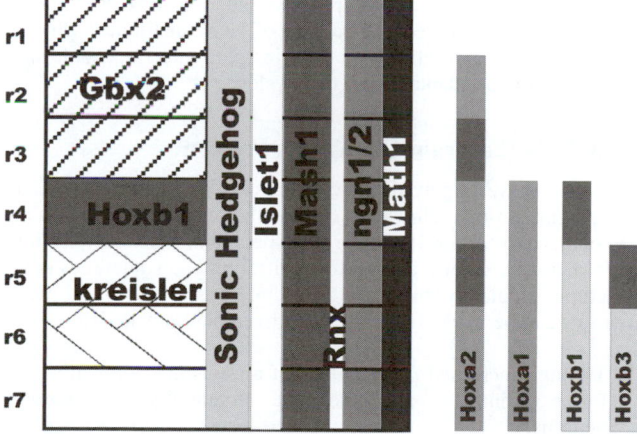

Figure 1. The expression of some longitudinal (Mash1, ngn1/2, Math1, Rnx) and transverse transcription factors (Gbx2, Hoxb1, kreisler) is shown. These expression domains produce an orthogonal grid in which brainstem neuronal phenotypes are uniquely specified. On the left is an idealized flat mounted embryonic day 11 mouse hindbrain. r1–r7 indicate rhombomeres. Note that homeobox genes (Hox) end at different levels with varying expression intensity. Sonic hedgehog defines the floor plate between the two halves of the brain. (Genes and their expression are adapted from Cordes, 2001, and Qian et al., 2001.)

such as bHLH genes were identified in vertebrates, nonvertebrates, and plants. In vertebrates, these genes apparently govern (1) the formation of longitudinal columns of, for example, taste-related nuclei (Qian et al., 2001), and (2) the regionalization of these columns into domains destined to serve a specific cranial nerve (Cordes, 2001). Thus, a developing neuron will undergo activation of a different set from the 30,000+ genes available to differentiate according to its position within this spacemap. This differentiation leads to formation of classes of neurons that will have a characteristic morphology and set of afferents and efferents. However, the detailed connectivity of individual neurons varies as a result of both the regularities and happenstance of development.

The following discussion highlights what is known about the variable organization of a simple system composed of three neuron populations that constitute the vestibulo-ocular pathway, the oculomotor system. The oculomotor system is a unique model because both the input (gravistatic and angular acceleration from the ear) and the output (movement of the eyes) can be quantified and put in the appropriate behavioral context. In its basic pattern, the system has six eye muscles to move the eye and three sets of motor neurons to drive these muscles. A series of bilaterally projecting interneurons (named vestibular nucleus neurons) mediates the input from the ear to the motor neurons. Sensory input from the ear travels via the semicircular canal (for angular acceleration) and two or more gravistatic sensors (for linear acceleration, including earth gravity). Four of the six eye muscles in jawed vertebrates are innervated by the oculomotor motor neurons, but only three out of six eye muscles in lampreys are so innervated (Fritzsch, 1998b). The abducens innervates only one of the six eye muscles (but sometimes an additional muscle, see later discussion) in jawed vertebrates, but it innervates two eye muscles in lampreys (Figure 2). The remaining muscle is innervated by the trochlear motor neurons in all vertebrates. In the ear, jawless vertebrates, such as lampreys, have no horizontal canal, which is one of the major inputs into the oculomotor system of jawed vertebrates that drives compensatory horizontal eye movement.

Thus, the oculomotor system shows two major evolutionary changes in vertebrates: one is related to changes in the eye muscles and their innervation and the other is related to the ear and its additional formation of a semicircular canal. Interestingly, the connections within the brainstem from the inner ear projection to the oculomotor neurons seem to be fairly constant among all vertebrates (Fritzsch, 1998b; Baker, 1998). This common feature apparently provides enough built-in plasticity to accommodate changes on the input and output side without major reorganization of the interconnections.

It is unknown how computation of horizontal acceleration is performed and then transformed into the different coordinates of ocular muscles in lampreys. This vertebrate lacks a horizontal canal but obviously has a functional oculomotor system (Figure 2). If we are to understand the selective advantage (if any) of this reorganization in jawed vertebrates, we have to unravel the structural/functional relationship in this likely primitive pattern of the three-neuron vestibulo-ocular arch in lampreys, then compare this system with the two functionally equivalent vestibulo-ocular systems of jawed vertebrates (Figure 2). Such a comparison could provide exemplary insight into the functional constraints that may accompany the structural transformation of homologous systems. Interestingly, this system has retained its basic function, vestibular governance of eye movement, while at the same time modifying some of its properties.

The major driving force behind this eye muscle reorganization may not have been the need of the system to achieve a different function. Rather, "accidental" developmental changes may have led to a subdivision of eye muscles and their nerves (Fritzsch, 1998b). Alternatively, variation in the inner ear (Fritzsch et al., 2001) may have been the force driving eye muscle reorganization. Once such

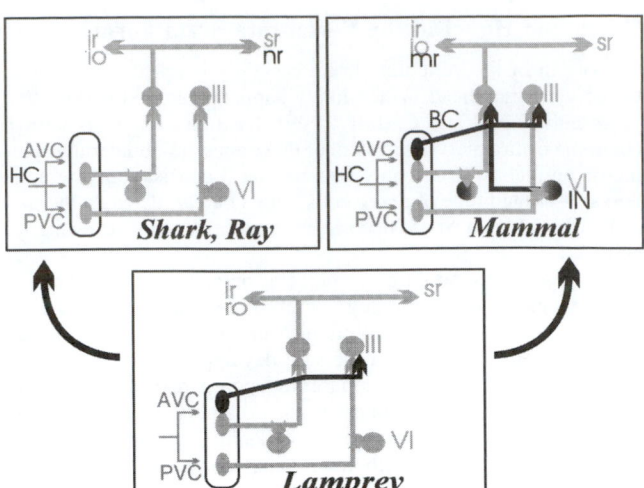

Figure 2. Reorganization of the oculomotor system among vertebrates. Lampreys have three eye muscles (inferior rectus [ir], rostral oblique [ro], and superior rectus [sr]), jawed vertebrates have four eye muscles innervated by cranial nerve III. However, in sharks and rays the nasal rectus (nr) receives a crossed innervation, whereas the functionally equivalent medial rectus (mr) of mammals receives an uncrossed innervation. All vertebrates have a rostral population in the vestibular nuclei that projects uncrossed and a caudal population that projects crossed to oculomotor neurons. Lampreys and mammals have an additional rostral population that projects through the brachium conjunctivum (BC) to the cranial nerve III nucleus. Note that lampreys have no horizontal canal (HC), and that only mammals have internuclear neurons (IN) from cranial nerve VI to III that provide the basis for conjugated horizontal eye movements. This task must be performed differently in lampreys and sharks. AVC, anterior vertical canal; PVC, posterior vertical canal; io. inferior oblique muscle. Dashed line indicates the midline. (Modified from Fritzsch, 1998b.)

changes were in place, the entire oculomotor system implemented the computational alterations generated by this "new" sensory structure into the preexisting connection pattern. This change was nevertheless enough to achieve implementation of horizontal gaze control. Understanding the adaptive implications of these changes would require a detailed comparison of neuroanatomical, physiological, and behavioral data to gain insights into the ecophysiological context of adaptation of this system.

How Does the Brain Change Its Pattern?

Thus far I have largely dealt with factors that keep neuronal development constant. However, despite the overall similarity in the regional subdivisions, it is clear that specific neuronal connections differ between species and perform different and sometimes novel functions. Logically, there are only three possible ways in which neurons can be made available to perform new functions:

1. Through increased proliferation of an existing population that forms redundant and therefore potentially uncommitted neurons.
2. Through loss of an old input and/or target, which frees neurons from their previous functional constraints and allows them to adopt a new commitment, thus adapting their function to changes in the sensory or motor system to which they are linked.
3. Through de novo formation of a novel set of neurons.

The last possibility requires that neurons somehow escape the pattern of gene activation normally mediated through the spatially restricted expression of developmental selector genes (i.e., they were set aside) (Knoll and Carroll, 1999). This could happen in three ways: (1) by alteration of selector gene expression through, for example, upstream changes in regulatory factor gradients that activate these genes, (2) by mutation of selector genes, resulting in changes in the expression pattern and thereby changes in the pattern of activation of downstream genes (see EVOLUTION OF GENETIC NETWORKS), or (3) by mutation of downstream genes to respond differently to selector genes. There is growing evidence that among chordates many selector genes may have a rather stable pattern of expression (Holland and Holland, 1999). Thus, differences in the activation of downstream genes or mutations in downstream genes may be a major mechanism by which nervous system organization is varied.

Increased proliferation and formation of more neurons clearly happened in the evolution of vertebrates, as exemplified by the relatively (brain to body weight) and absolutely larger-sized brains of humans compared to bony fishes. Moreover, specific areas may in some vertebrates become the largest part of the entire brain, while other species may entirely lack these areas. For example, the valvulae cerebelli are unique to bony fishes and can become the largest part of the bony fish brain, much as the forebrain has become the largest part of the human brain (Nieuwenhuys et al., 1997). It is thought that this growth of the valvulae cerebelli is related to the unique electroreceptive sense of these bony fishes, a sense all land vertebrates have lost. In contrast, the growth of the cerebellum in four-legged vertebrates is in part related to the growth of the forebrain (which provides a major input through the pontine nuclei).

This increased proliferation could come about through a simple mutation in genes regulating the proliferation of precursor cells. For example, if four divisions occur in a precursor cell population of ancestors, adding one round of mitosis could double the total number of neurons. Subsequently, some neurons of this initially identical population could develop a different identity. How this new identity could be achieved is still unclear, but one possibility might be that the enlarged population of postmitotic neurons could see a slightly different gradient of selector gene products and could therefore achieve their different phenotypes (Raff, 1996). Thus, neurons were developmentally set aside (Knoll and Carroll, 1999). The differences in function would be obtained by (1) reaching a different target and/or (2) segregation of their perikarya and dendrites (and thus input) through differential migration.

A second possible scenario for the formation of uncommitted neurons may be the loss of either the target or the input. Such a loss would eliminate the constraints normally acting on these neurons and thus would allow them to evolve a new function. A well-known example of this scenario is the evolution of the middle ear ossicles of land vertebrates. There is good comparative and developmental evidence suggesting that these ossicles are derived from former jaw-supporting ossicles. Once their original functional constraint, supporting the jaws, was lost, they underwent a radical change in function.

Experimental reorganization of input changes the function of existing neuronal networks and entire sensory systems. The mechanosensory lateral-line and the electroreceptive system of ampullary organs of fishes and many amphibians is lost in most land vertebrates. Although there is evidence for evolutionary loss of both inputs and targets, it is not yet proven that the neurons freed by such a process from their previous functional constraints are in fact modified to perform a novel, different function. However, it is clear that experimental changes of inputs change the function of existing neuronal networks (Pallas, 2001). Thus, while experimental evidence tends to support the notion of functional changes in existing neuronal networks, there is little evolutionary evidence to support it, and the effect of such a process for brain evolution has not yet been worked out.

From New Neurons to New Functions

Irrespective of how new neurons evolved, they have to achieve new input/output relations to mediate any new function. Clearly, migration of neurons into a new position is a widespread phenomenon in the developing brain. It is widely agreed that neuronal migration correlates with the formation of novel input to this differently positioned subset of neurons. Migration can bring neurons from a dorsal part of the brain to the ventral part, or from one side to the other (Fritzsch, 1998a). One likely scenario is that homologous neurons with comparable function can differ in their position, as occurs in the cases of the laminar nucleus of birds and the medial superior olive in mammals. Both are relay neurons for the auditory pathway, but in birds (and reptiles) they are dorsal, next to the primary auditory nuclei, whereas in mammals they are ventral, near the base of the hindbrain. These differences in position can be reconciled with the assumed homology of these populations by showing that indeed, both nuclei arise dorsally but migrate ventrad in mammals, and that their initial formation is under the control of homologous genes. This change in position of neurons will affect the computation only if the input or output is changed.

In contrast to the well-accepted role of migration in achieving a novel input, how a novel target is reached by the axon is much more controversial. Some ideas have emanated from the undeniable fact of widespread, exuberant projection to different targets during development in birds and mammals. Out of these many targets a single or few targets will be selected by neuronal cell death and axonal pruning. In their ultimate version, such ideas require that no new connections ever form in the brain, arguing that differences are achieved exclusively through the differential loss of connections present in ancestral forms (Ebbesson, 1984). Although appealing, this idea fails to integrate the available data on the development of the peripheral and central nervous system, which show a rather precise selection of pathway choices by a navigating axon with limited developmental "error." Certain molecules have been identified that guide commissural systems in vertebrates and invertebrates alike. Other molecules specify the topology of the retinal projection onto the midbrain. Thus, beyond specifying the identity of topologically restricted populations of neurons, molecules also specify topologically restricted connections within the brain. However, maps generated by different sensors of the world around us form in the brain based on different principles. In the visual system, mapping of the eye onto the midbrain is achieved molecularly by using matching gradients of molecules that provide positional identity of neurons in the retina and target them toward specific areas in the tectum of the midbrain. In contrast, the space map of the hearing system is generated by computing time and intensity differences between both ears into an auditory space map. Thus, there likely will not be a uniform molecular principle for brain map formation in the various sensory modalities. However, the various maps, once established, can be brought into register with each other in certain areas of the brain, such as the roof of the midbrain.

One of the most striking examples of novel pathway selection is the growth of axons from the mammalian cortex to the spinal cord to form the corticospinal tract. The pyramidal neurons are the only cortical neurons in vertebrates that do project to the lumbar spinal cord and thus are considered by most researchers to be a novel tract. Any other interpretation would require the assumption that this tract is ancestral to vertebrates and was lost in all lineages except mammals. Even more compelling evidence for the de novo formation of pathways comes from fiber outgrowth into the periphery. Although these mechanisms were rejected for almost a century, it is now clear that motor neuron axons do not pass through the "ventral roots" of certain chordates. Instead of nerve fibers leaving the spinal cord, muscle fibers project with noncontractile processes to the "ventral roots" of the spinal cord of these small marine animals. One of the major steps in the evolution of the vertebrate brain and spinal cord was then to have motor neurons, which themselves project through the ventral root to reach their target muscles (Fritzsch, 1998a). Although it is still unclear when and how this novel invasion of axons into the periphery happened, those motor neurons had to find a pathway where they had never been before. Moreover, the addition of novel tissue, such as the ear, may have caused redirection of growing fibers.

In the hindbrain of chickens, motor neurons initially form two paramedian strips (Cordes, 2001). Motor neurons within a restricted region project their axons to the facial root to exit the brain (Figure 1). Within the facial nerve some axons reroute to reach the developing ear and function as stato-acoustic efferents. Instead of innervating striated muscle fibers as the facial motor neurons do, they innervate hair cells of the ear (Karis et al., 2001). Moreover, this pathway of efferent fibers to the ear differs among vertebrates. This rerouting within the nerve occurs in chickens and frogs, but not in mammals, where it happens within the brain. In addition, the initially overlapping populations of efferent neurons segregate into different positions within the hindbrain through differential migration.

It is unclear how much the reorganization of the facial motor neurons to the ear to form the stato-acoustic efferents depended on the formation of the ear itself and a concomitant suppression of differentiation of parts of branchial arch–derived muscle fibers. Such losses of target muscles could conceivably have forced a subset of facial motor neurons either to innervate a new target and become the efferents to the ear or to disappear entirely. This highlights but one possibility of how connections within the brain can be changed and the resulting function of the network altered. More detailed connectional data are needed to show how often such changes have happened in the brain.

In conclusion, there is both evidence for ongoing invasion of certain fibers into novel territories and evidence for rather precise pathway selection. This precludes the idea that evolution picked from a completely randomized network. Certain areas, like the forebrain, may in fact benefit from a less constrained development that enables them to form a wider array of initial connections from which only certain connections will be selected in a later developmental step.

Variation in Functionally Relevant Details

Nervous tissue not only undergoes modifications in its long-range connections and formation of new cells, it also shows numerous cellular reorganizations. Such reorganization could manifest as changes in the degree of branching of dendrites, neurotransmitter(s), postsynaptic receptors, and stratification into distinct laminae, or as the absence of these structures in topologically comparable areas of the brain (Nieuwenhuys et al., 1997). For example, the gustatory nuclei in closely related species of bony fishes may be laminated or not. Or the neurons of the cerebellar nuclei, which are all assembled in the white matter in mammals, may become stratified with Purkinje cells into a single cortical layer in bony fishes. What (if any) functional implications these differences in cellular assembly may offer is still unclear, and the variations may represent nothing more than alternative designs to compute the same information. More physiology is needed to distinguish what each network is good for. This is particularly obvious in the stratification of the midbrain tectum of many vertebrates, which apparently can be secondarily reduced without appreciable functional deficits (Nieuwenhuys et al., 1997). Thus, salamanders may have a much less stratified midbrain tectum and yet are fully able to govern the protrusion of their tongue, as accurately as a reptile or a frog, which have a more stratified midbrain. In other words, we may be looking at structural organizations that do little for the underlying function but keep us baffled at how they vary.

Another example is provided by the differences in organization but similarities in function and long-range connections in the forebrain of birds and mammals. Obviously, comparable functions can be accomplished with either a laminar, cortical organization or with a set of interconnected groups of neurons. It has been suggested that "laminar organization of populations is an alternative means of organizing populations of neurons" (Nieuwenhuys et al., 1997). It appears, then, that some of the highly appreciated, laminar networks are but one way in which the brain can implement a specific functional circuit. It is entirely possible that the morphological differences in the forebrain organization of birds and mammals are not driven by their physiology and adaptivity to behavioral tasks but rather reflect alternative developmental strategies that were implemented simply because the outcome is a viable organism.

Discussion

This brief overview has stressed some of the emerging developmental principles presumed to govern the remarkably stable overall pattern of the vertebrate brain throughout its evolution while providing enough room for plasticity in both local interactions as well as long-range connections. The developmental analysis has not yet reached a level that can causally explain how local neuronal assemblies, such as cortical columns, come about during development and how the connections between those neurons are organized to adapt the organism to various tasks.

However, it is proposed that complex interactive genetic networks not only guide overall development but offer room for self-organization of these neuronal assemblies within a set of limitations imposed by the developmental selector genes. Thus, whereas some behavior, such as a reflex, is directly translated from the genes through development into a specific set of connections forming the reflex arc, other connections have enough redundancy to be modified in their response by experience and are able to learn. Evolution not only selects modifications in specific connections that allow for a more adapted response, it also selects neuronal networks that allow for learning and thus adaptation during the life of an organism within the genetic limitations in which the brain and its connections developed.

Looking at the evolution of the brain as the evolution of a system that has both genetically and behaviorally hardwired components and other components that can change their response properties allows us to understand the "adaptiveness" of the brain from a less restricted, more dynamic perspective. Adaptation may be viewed as a compromise between change and development in a system that struggles to stay on top of its changing adaptive landscape (Raff, 1996) by balancing both components in various ways. Clearly, hardwiring a response provides superior response speed but restricts adaptation to change during an organism's lifetime. In contrast, learned responses, while initially slower, allow adaptation over the lifetime of an organism. Modeling such systems must take into account that optimization is constrained by at least these two facts, and thus may never be achieved in any living system to the extent that it can be achieved in artificial systems. Although there have been interesting models of the EVOLUTION OF ARTIFICIAL NEURAL NETWORKS (q.v.), their biological relevance has been somewhat limited by the use of selection on features, such as individual synaptic weighs, that are not necessarily regulated by separate genes in biological nervous systems. Thus, an interesting challenge will be to develop a new generation of models in which evolution occurs within genetically plausible parameters, such as numbers of neurons, variation in long-range output connections, and variation in inputs into the dendrites.

Road Map: Neuroethology and Evolution
Background: Vestibulo-Ocular Reflex
Related Reading: Evolution of Genetic Networks

References

Baker, R., 1998, From genes to behavior in the vestibular system, *Otolaryngol. Head Neck Surg.*, 119:263–275. ◆

Bermingham, N. A., Hassan, B. A., Fernandez, M., Banfi, S., Bellen, H. J., Fritzsch, B., and Zoghbi, H. Y., 2001, Development of the proprioceptor pathway is MATH1-dependent, *Neuron*, 30:411–422.

Corbo, J. C., Erives, A., Di Gregorio, A., Chang, A., and Levine, M., 1997, Dorsoventral patterning of the vertebrate neural tube is conserved in a protochordate, *Development*, 124:2335–2344.

Cordes, S. P., 2001, Molecular genetics of cranial nerve development in mouse, *Nat. Rev. Neurosci.*, 2:611–623. ◆

Ebbesson, S. O. E., 1984, Evolution and ontogeny of neural circuits, *Brain Behav. Sci.*, 7:321–366.

Fritzsch, B., 1998a, Of mice and genes: Evolution of vertebrate brain development, *Brain Behav. Evol.*, 52:207–217. ◆

Fritzsch, B., 1998b, Evolution of the vestibulo-ocular system, *Otolaryngol. Head Neck Surg.*, 119:182–196.

Fritzsch, B., Signore, M., and Simeone, A., 2001, *Otxl* null mutants show partial segregation of sensory epithelia comparable to lamprey ears, *Dev. Genes Evolut.*, 211:388–396.

Holland, L. Z., and Holland, N. D., 1999, Chordate origins of the vertebrate central nervous system, *Curr. Opin. Neurobiol.*, 9:596–602.

Karis, A., Pata, I., van Doorninck, J. H., Grosveld, F., de Zeeuw, C. I., de Caprona, D., and Fritzsch, B., 2001, Transcription factor GATA-3 alters pathway selection of olivocochlear neurons and affects morphogenesis of the ear, *J. Comp. Neurol.*, 429:615–630.

Knoll, A. H., and Carroll, S. B., 1999, Early animal evolution: Emerging views from comparative biology and geology, *Science*, 284:2129–2137. ◆

Koch, C., and Laurent, G., 1999, Complexity and the nervous system, *Science*, 284:96–98.

Nieuwenhuys, R., ten Donkelaar, H. J., and Nicholson, C., 1997, *The central Nervous System of Vertebrates*, Berlin: Springer-Verlag, p. 2200.

Pallas, S. L., 2001, Intrinsic and extrinsic factors that shape neocortical specification, *Trends Neurosci.*, 24:417–423.

Raff, R. A., 1996, *The shape of Life*, Chicago: University of Chicago Press, p. 520.

Qian, Y., Fritzsch, B., Shirasawa, S., Chen, C.-L., and Ma, Q., 2001, Formation of brainstem catecholaminergic neurons and first order relay visceral sensory neurons is dependent on RNX, *Genes Dev.*, 15:2533–2545.

Eye-Hand Coordination in Reaching Movements

Valérie Gaveau, Phillipe Vindras, Claude Prablanc, Denis Pélisson, and Michel Desmurget

Introduction

Despite a century of research, the neural mechanisms involved in eye-hand coordination during reaching movements are still largely unknown. This article addresses this question and describes the mechanisms whereby a visual input is transformed into a motor command. To this end, we consider the different problems that the nervous system has to solve to generate a movement, namely, localizing the target, creating a motor plan, and correcting the ongoing movement if necessary.

Representation of Target Position

Reaching toward a visual target requires transformation of visual information about target position with respect to the line of sight into a frame of reference suitable for the planning of hand movement. This problem is classically decomposed in analytic steps that provide target position information in an eye, head, and ultimately bodily frame of reference. For the sake of clarity, we follow this progression to describe the mechanisms encoding retinal information and extraretinal signals of eye-in-orbit and head-on-trunk positions.

Visual information initially signals the angle separating the target and the line of sight. The reliability of this retinal signal is constrained by the spatial anisotropy of the retina and visual system. Because of the gradient of visual acuity, the encoding of a target location with respect to the line of sight degrades when the stimulus falls in the peripheral visual field. This relative inaccuracy of signals from the peripheral retina can be illustrated by hand-pointing errors observed when the movement is performed while the foveating saccade is prevented. Despite this limitation, it is the peripheral part of the retina that is most often involved in the initial localization of a visual target.

In addition to the retinal signal, the position of the eye in the orbit is necessary to encode the location of the target in a body-centered frame of reference. Paradoxically, without a retinal signal, orbital eye position appears to be only coarsely encoded by extraocular signals. Indeed, when subjects are required to point in dark-ness in the direction of their eyes, the final hand position correlates with eye position, but the scatter is much higher than when the target is a luminous spot (Bock, 1986). Thus, it appears that retinal and extraretinal signals do not simply add but also interact with each other, and that accurate encoding of target location requires concomitant foveal and extraretinal signals. Compatible with this hypothesis are recent studies suggesting that gaze position could influence the encoding of target location for limb motions (Soechting, Engel, and Flanders, 2001).

At the neurophysiological level, the search for interactions between retinal and extraretinal information has stimulated many studies on the neural code of target internal representations. Two different conceptions have emerged: single-unit coding and distributed coding. The single-unit coding concept of integration hypothesizes the existence of individual neurons encoding information about target position, irrespective of eye position. In support of this hypothesis, individual neurons representing symbolic parameters, such as target location in a body-centered reference system, have been described in several studies. For instance, the neuronal activities described by Duhamel et al. (1997) have been shown to encode the position of a visual target respectively in a head-centered frame of reference. This latter coding might hypothetically result from an ultimate stage of coordinate transformation necessary to direct the hand toward a target.

In contrast to the single-unit concept, the distributed coding hypothesis assumes a statistical combination of elementary information about retinal eccentricity and eye position within large neuronal populations. A growing body of evidence of population-based interactions between retinal and extraretinal information supports this concept. Thus, electrophysiological recordings in the parietal cortex of awake monkeys have shown that the activity of the reach-related cells was influenced by eye position information (Batista et al., 1999). With the aid of neural network modeling, Andersen and colleagues (1997) showed that these characteristics of individual neuron discharges are compatible with the existence in the parietal cortex of a distributed code for egocentric target localization.

It may be worth mentioning at this point that the single-unit and distributed concepts are not mutually exclusive. Indeed, symbolic information generated by distributed neuronal populations may ultimately converge at the output level to provide a single-unit representation. For example, the distributed model of Andersen and colleagues yields an output signal of target position relative to the head that is represented at a single-unit level. In addition, a recent electrophysiological study of ventral intraparietal neurons in the monkey showed that the visual response of single units reveals a continuum between head-centered coding and retinotopic coding, leading to the hypothesis that "space may be represented in the cortex both at the population level and at the single cell level" (Duhamel et al., 1997).

How head position signals are integrated with retinal and eye position signals has stimulated less neurophysiological investigation. In 1995, Brotchie et al. reported that the visual response of parietal cortex neurons is modulated by the direction of gaze (integrating both eye and head components). This result suggests that the distributed coding hypothesis of target relative to the head can be generalized to visual target encoding in trunk-centered coordinates. Thus, target-related information in a body reference system seems to be distributed in large neuronal populations.

Planning Movement Trajectory

It is generally admitted that spatiotemporal invariances can give insight into how visually directed movements are planned and controlled by the nervous system. As an example, consider the task of pointing, from a given initial position, toward visual targets distributed within the workspace. In such a situation, two types of regularities can be expected: (1) *extrinsic regularities*, such that the movement displays invariant features in the Cartesian space (e.g., a straight-line path irrespective of the movement direction or amplitude), and (2) *intrinsic regularities*, such that the movement displays invariant features in one of the intrinsic spaces (e.g., a linear relation between joint angle variations). Interestingly, because the relationships between the extrinsic and intrinsic variables are complex and nonlinear, these two potential types of invariances generally cannot occur at the same time. That is, when the hand trajectory is invariant in the extrinsic space, it displays a consistent variability in the intrinsic space, and vice versa.

The task of pointing from a given starting position toward visual targets distributed within the workspace was initially studied by Morasso (1981). Morasso found that joint covariation patterns varied systematically as a function of movement direction, whereas Cartesian hand paths were always roughly straight. Based on this extrinsic stability, he concluded that (1) the hand trajectory in Cartesian space was the primary variable computed during movement planning, and (2) the joint covariation pattern constituted a dependent variable defined secondarily in order to allow the hand to move along the planned trajectory. Futher evidence supporting this view was found in the demonstration that motor planning was a parametric process involving an independent specification of the Cartesian amplitude and Cartesian direction of the upcoming movement (Vindras and Viviani, 1998), as would be expected if these two components were planned separately.

The hypothesis that the hand always follows a straight line path in external space during visually directed reaching has recently been challenged in several studies showing that hand movements can be significantly curved and that the amount of curvature can vary with the movement direction. For instance, Osu et al. (1997) investigated visually directed movements under two conditions: no path instruction (NI), and instruction to move the hand along a straight line (SI). They found that subjects generated much straighter movements in SI than in NI. As indicated by electromyographic activity (EMG), this difference could not be related to an increase in arm stiffness, which suggested that path curvature

was really reflective of the movement planning process. A similar conclusion was reached by Desmurget et al. (1999), who showed, however, that the results reported by Osu et al. were valid only for unconstrained three-dimensional movements. No difference was observed between NI and SI for planar movements. This result might suggest that unconstrained movements, unlike planar movements, are not programmed to follow a straight-line path in the extrinsic space. With respect to this conclusion, several hypotheses have been proposed to explain how unconstrained movements are planned by the central nervous system (CNS). The most popular of these hypotheses suggests that hand trajectory is specified as a vector in the joint space (Flanders, Helms-Tillery, and Soechting, 1992). According to this view, the spatial characteristics of the target are initially converted into a set of arm and forearm orientations. The movement from the starting posture to the target posture is then implemented on the basis of an "angular error vector" whose components represent the difference between the starting and target angles for each joint. During the movement, joint angle variations are not controlled independently, but in a synergic way (temporal coupling). The movement curved path observed in the task space results directly from this temporal coupling.

Eye-Hand Coordination and the Need for On-Line Trajectory Control

For an external observer, the relative coordination of eye, head, and hand during goal-directed reaching appears sequential. When a subject points to a visual target in peripheral space, the eyes move first, followed by the head and ultimately the hand. Because eye movement duration is brief, the gaze generally arrives at the target before or around the time of hand movement onset. Although this sequential organization was initially thought to have a functional foundation, it was subsequently shown to result primarily from inertial factors (Desmurget and Grafton, 2000). Indeed, the EMG discharge is generally synchronized for the eye, head, and arm during fast reaching movements, indicating that the motor command is sent to these different effectors in parallel (the arm moves last simply because it has the greatest inertia). It follows that the motor command initially sent to the arm is based on an extrafoveal visual signal that has been shown to be inaccurate (see first section). At the end of the ocular saccade, which roughly corresponds to the onset of hand movement, the target location can be recomputed on the basis of foveal information. As shown by Prablanc and Martin (1992), this updated visual signal is used by the nervous system to adjust the ongoing trajectory. To demonstrate this point, the authors used a double-step pointing paradigm in which the target location was slightly modified during the course of the ocular saccade when there was saccadic suppression (i.e., the target jump was not perceived consciously by the subject). Results showed that the hand path, which was initially directed to the first target, diverged smoothly toward the second target. Interestingly, corrections were detectable about 110 ms after hand movement onset, showing that hand trajectory was amended very early. As shown by Prablanc and Martin, these corrections were similar whether or not the moving limb was visible to the subject. This suggests that nonvisual feedback loops represent the main process through which extrinsic errors are corrected.

Because of the existence of consistent delays in sensorimotor loops, the rapid path corrections observed during reaching movements cannot be attributed to sensory information only. They can only rely on a "forward model" of the arm dynamics. The idea behind this concept is that the motor system can progressively learn to estimate its own behavior in response to a given command. By integrating information related to the initial movement conditions, the motor outflow, and the sensory inflow, the forward model can determine, and even predict in advance, the probable position and

Figure 1. Forward model of arm dynamics for controlling hand movements. To reach a target, the nervous system has to elaborate a motor plan based on initial conditions (locations of the hand and target). During the execution of the motor command, a forward model of the dynamics of the arm is generated by integration of a copy of motor outflow and sensory inflow. This model then generates an estimation of the movement end-point location. Discrepancies between estimation and target location cause an error signal, which triggers a modulation of the motor command. (From Desmurget, M., and Gafton, S., 2000, Forward modeling allows feedback control for fast reaching movements, *Trends Cognit. Sci.*, 4:423–431. © Elsevier Publishing Co.; reproduced with permission.)

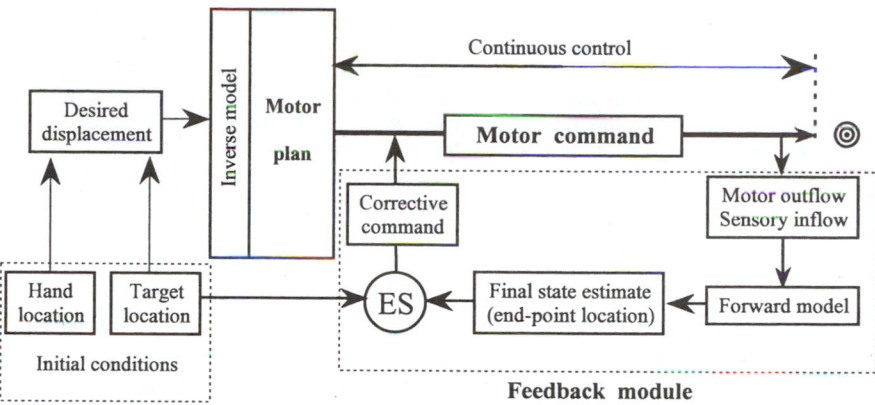

velocity of the effector, thus making feedback strategies possible for fast reaching movements.

This idea was recently operationalized by Desmurget and Grafton (2000), who proposed a simple model through which fast feedback control might be achieved (Figure 1). According to these authors, the forward model of the arm's dynamics generated during a movement is used to predict the movement's end point. By comparing this prediction with the actual target location, the motor system can directly estimate the movement's final accuracy. When a discrepancy is detected between the movement's predicted final location and the target location, an error signal is generated and a corrective command is issued.

The past two decades have been dominated by the hypothesis that reaching movements are primarily under preprogrammed control and that sensory feedback loops exert only a limited influence at the very end of the trajectory. As a consequence, functional investigations have focused primarily on the cerebral structures participating in motor preparation and execution, yielding few insights into the functional anatomy of on-line movement guidance. This latter issue was recently investigated by our group using positron emission tomography (PET) (Desmurget et al., 2001). Seven subjects were required to look at (Eye) or look and point to (EyeArm) visual targets whose location either remained stationary or changed undetectably during the ocular saccade. The latter condition allowed us to increase the amount of correction to be generated during the movement. The functional anatomy of nonvisual feedback loops was identified by comparing the reaching condition involving large corrections (Jump) with the reaching condition involving small corrections (Stationary), after subtracting the activations associated with saccadic movements and hand movement planning [(EyeArm-Jumping minus Eye-Jumping) minus (EyeArm-Stationary minus Eye-Stationary)]. In agreement with earlier observations (Prablanc and Martin, 1992), behavioral recordings indicated that the subjects were both accurate at reaching toward the stationary targets and able to update their movement smoothly and early in response to the target jump. PET difference images showed that these corrections were mediated by a restricted network involving the posterior parietal cortex (PPC), the cerebellum, and the primary motor cortex (M1). As shown in Figure 2, the parietal activation was located in the left intraparietal sulcus, in a region that is generally considered the rostral part of the PPC. The cerebellar activation occurred in the right anterior parasagittal cortex, in a region associated with the production of arm movements. The frontal activation was located in the arm-related area of M1. The contribution of the PPC to movement guidance has recently been confirmed by several studies showing that on-line movement corrections are suppressed when this structure is lesioned or prevented from exerting its function through the application of a transcranial magnetic pulse at the onset of hand movement (Desmurget and Grafton, 2000).

Although the role of the PPC, the cerebellum, and the motor cortex in movement guidance has not been totally elucidated, a general model can be proposed. At a first level, one may suggest that the role of the PPC is to compute a motor error by comparing the target location and the estimated movement end point. This hypothesis is based on two main observations about the PPC, namely, (1) that the PPC has access to a representation of both the target and current hand location through afferent information coming from different sensory modalities and the main motor struc-

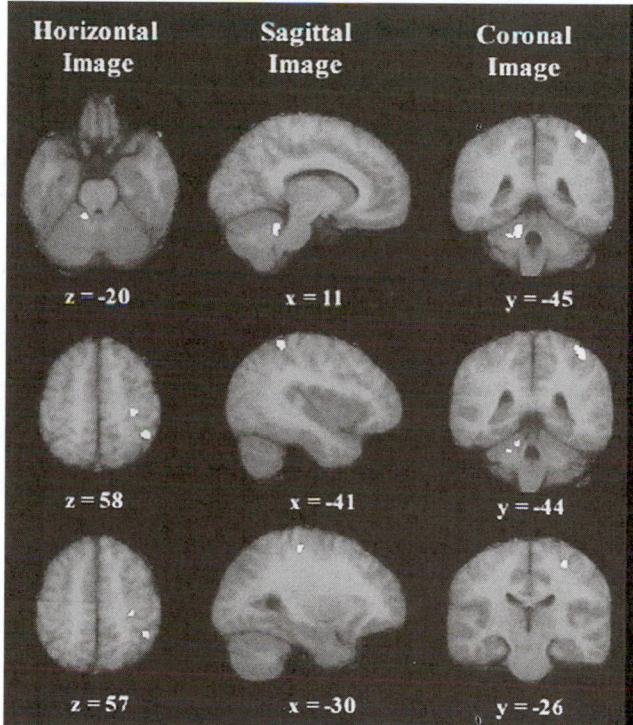

Figure 2. Areas of brain activation superimposed on a mean MRI in Talairach coordinates. On the sagittal images, positive values of *x* designate the hemisphere ipsilateral to the reach arm (right one), and negative values of *x* designate the contralateral hemisphere (left one). Top row is centered on the cerebellar activation site; middle row is centered on the PPC activation site; bottom row is centered on the precentral activation site. (From Desmurget, M., et al., 2001, Functional anatomy of nonvisual feedback loops during reaching: A position emission tomography study, *J. Neurosci.*, 21:2919–2928. © Elsevier Publishing Co.; reproduced with permission.)

tures, and (2) that the PPC is critical for merging the arm- and target-related signals into a common frame of reference (Andersen et al., 1997). Once computed, the motor error needs to be converted into an effective motor command (inverse computation). Converging evidence indicates that this function may be carried out by the cerebellum. In particular, it has been shown that patients with cerebellar lesions are impaired in defining the pattern of muscle activation required to direct the hand along a specific path, and that inverse models are represented within the cerebellum (Wolpert, Miall, and Kawato, 1998). At the extremity of the system, the cerebellar corrective signal might influence the ongoing motor command by modulating the neural signal issued by the primary motor cortex. In agreement with this view, it is known that the primary motor cortex receives substantial input from the cerebellum via the ventrolateral thalamus. Also, it is thought that the motor system is organized in a relative hierarchy such that the primary motor cortex is mainly involved in low-level aspects of motor control. Of course, the previous observations do not imply that other areas are not involved in movement guidance. A role for the basal ganglia, for instance, was proposed in a recent study on patients with Huntington's disease (Smith, Brandt, and Shadmehr, 2000). This role was not, however, confirmed by our group in subsequent work showing that Parkinson's disease patients were able to smoothly and quickly correct ongoing movement in an unconscious double-step study identical to the one used by Prablanc and Martin (1992).

Conclusion

Our knowledge of the neural processes underlying eye-hand coordination has greatly improved over the past two decades. However, our understanding is still far from exhaustive, and many issues remain to be addressed. Current approaches will benefit from the development of independent motor theories within specific experimental and theoretical contexts. Our understanding of the processes whereby a visual input is transformed into a motor command would be greatly improved by comparative studies involving heterogeneous approaches as well as various areas of brain theory and neural networks. The complementary contributions gathered in the *Handbook* are a first step in this promising direction.

Road Map: Mammalian Motor Control
Background: Motor Control, Biological and Theoretical

Related Reading: Collicular Visuomotor Transformations for Gaze Control; Grasping Movements: Visuomotor Transformations; Reaching Movements: Implications for Computational Models

References

Andersen, R. A., Snyder, L. H., Bradley, D. C., and Xing, J., 1997, Multimodal representation of space in the posterior parietal cortex and its use in planning movements, *Annu. Rev. Neurosci.*, 20:303–330. ◆

Batista, A. P., Buneo, C. A., Snyder, L. H., and Andersen, R. A., 1999, Reach plans in eye-centered coordinates, *Science*, 285:257–260.

Bock, O., 1986, Contribution of retinal versus extraretinal signals towards visual localization in goal-directed movements, *Exp. Brain Res.*, 64:476–482.

Brotchie, P. R., Andersen, R. A., Snyder, L. H., and Goodman, S. J., 1995, Head position signals used by parietal neurons to encode locations of visual stimuli, *Nature*, 375:232–235.

Desmurget, M., and Grafton, S., 2000, Forward modeling allows feedback control for fast reaching movements, *Trends Cognit. Sci.*, 4:423–431. ◆

Desmurget, M., Grea, H., Grethe, J. S., Prablanc, C., Alexander, G. E., and Grafton, S. T., 2001, Functional anatomy of nonvisual feedback loops during reaching: A positron emission tomography study, *J. Neurosci.*, 21:2919–2928.

Desmurget, M., Prablanc, C., Jordan, M. I., and Jeannerod, M., 1999, Are reaching movements planned to be straight and invariant in the extrinsic space? *Q. J. Exp. Psychol.*, 52A:981–1020.

Duhamel, J. R., Bremmer, F., BenHamed, S., and Graf, W., 1997, Spatial invariance of visual receptive fields in parietal cortex neurons, *Nature*, 389:845–848.

Flanders, M., Helms-Tillery, S. I., and Soechting, J. F., 1992, Early stages in sensori-motor transformations, *Behav. Brain Sci.*, 15:309–362. ◆

Morasso, P., 1981, Spatial control of arm movements. *Exp. Brain Res.*, 42:223–227.

Osu, R., Uno, Y., Koike, Y., and Kawato, M., 1997, Possible explanations for trajectory curvature in multijoint arm movements, *J. Exp. Psychol. Hum. Percept. Perform.*, 23:890–913.

Prablanc, C., and Martin, O., 1992, Automatic control during hand reaching at undetected two-dimensional target displacements, *J. Neurophysiol.*, 67:455–469. ◆

Smith, M. A., Brandt, J., and Shadmehr, R., 2000, Motor disorder in Huntington's disease begins as a dysfunction in error feedback control, *Nature*, 403:544–549.

Soechting, J. F., Engel, K. C., and Flanders, M., 2001, The Duncker illusion and eye-hand coordination, *J. Neurophysiol.*, 85:843–854.

Vindras, P., and Viviani, P., 1998, Frames of reference and control parameters in visuo-manual pointing. *J. Exp. Psychol. Hum. Percept. Perform.*, 24:569–591.

Wolpert, D. M., Miall, R. C., and Kawato, M., 1998, Internal models in the cerebellum, *Trends Cognit. Sci.*, 2:338–347. ◆

Face Recognition: Neurophysiology and Neural Technology

Rolf P. Würtz

Introduction

The ability to recognize other individuals is a major prerequisite for human social interaction and hence a rather important brain function. The most prominent cue for that recognition is the face. The ability to recognize persons from their faces is part of a spectrum of related skills that includes face segmentation (i.e., finding faces in a scene or image), estimation of the pose, estimating the direction of gaze, and evaluating the person's emotional state. This article focuses on recognition of identity. A more detailed treatment of the other aspects can be found in FACE RECOGNITION: PSYCHOLOGY AND CONNECTIONISM.

Neurophysiology

From neuropsychological studies of patients with brain injuries, it is known that there are subsystems in the brain that are specialized for face processing. Brain injury can lead to loss of the ability to recognize faces, a deficit called *prosopagnosia*, while leaving recognition of general objects intact. The opposite dissociation is reported in Moscovitch, Winocur, and Behrmann (1997), in a patient with intact face recognition together with highly impaired general object recognition. Various stunning perceptual demonstrations show that faces are perceived differently when viewed upside down or as photographic negatives. Those image manipulations make little difference for the perception of general objects but can modify the perception of identity and expression considerably. These findings lead to the assumption that different brain circuits are used for processing general objects and for processing faces, but there is also considerable evidence that not only faces receive special treatment, but all object classes for which there is high expertise (Gauthier, Behrmann, and Tarr, 1999).

Other studies show that patients with prosopagnosia who exhibit no conscious recognition of facial identity still exhibit an unconscious reaction to familiar faces, which is revealed by changes in skin conductance. This mechanism seems to play a major role in the emotional reaction to facial stimuli.

Single-unit recordings of activity in the inferotemporal cortex of macaque monkeys have revealed neurons with a high responsiveness to the presence of a face, an individual, or the expression on a face (see Desimone, 1991, for a review). Although the notion of the optimal stimulus for a cell is very hard to probe experimentally, some of these cells are as close to grandmother cells (see ASSOCIATIVE NETWORKS) as the experimental evidence gets.

In humans, cells that become active when a familiar face is seen have been identified in the inferotemporal gyrus and the fusiform gyrus in both hemispheres. Their clusters do not form anatomically well-defined subregions but are neighbored by modules of different specificity, and their location and extent vary considerably among individuals.

A good account of the current knowledge about face recognition in the human brain is given by Haxby, Hoffman, and Gobbini (2000), whose model refines a cognitive model by Bruce and Young (see Young, 1998, chap. 3) and attaches anatomical locations to its modules. Haxby et al. propose a *core system* for face processing that consists of three interconnected modules. The first, located in the inferotemporal occipital gyrus, is responsible for the early extraction of features relevant for faces. The second, in the superior temporal sulcus, codes for the changeable properties of faces, such as the direction of gaze, lip movement, expression, and the like. Identity as an invariant face property is processed in the lateral fusiform gyrus. This core system communicates with other parts with a need for facial information, such as attention modules, auditory cortex, and emotional centers. The essence of face recognition—to link the visual information to a name and biographical knowledge about particular persons—is carried out in the anterior temporal lobe. These other parts make up the *extended system*.

Computational Theory

As for all cases of object recognition, the main problem to be solved by a face recognition procedure is *invariance*. The same face can produce very different images with changes in position, pose, illumination, expression, partial occlusion, background, and so forth. The task of the recognition system is to generalize over all these variations and capture only the identity.

This sort of invariant recognition is a quotidian property of natural brains but does not come very naturally in current artificial neural network models. Even the simplest case, invariance under translations in the input plane, is difficult to obtain. One major approach starts with the observation that complex cells generalize about small translations of the signal. This can be iterated, and leads to hierarchical networks such as the NEOCOGNITRON: A MODEL FOR VISUAL PATTERN RECOGNITION (q.v.). A huge advantage of such purely feedforward networks is their speed of processing.

Very little is known about how invariant recognition can be learned from examples and generalized to other instances. In an abstract sense, the important long-term goal is to teach a network precisely the invariances required for a given problem domain. This is directly relevant for face recognition, because invariance under expression and slight deformations are very difficult to capture analytically.

If the only invariance required is translation, then template matching (see OBJECT RECOGNITION) can solve the problem rather efficiently. A stored pattern (which we will call "model") is compared to an image by shifting the model across the image and taking the scalar product with appropriate normalization at all possible image locations. The maximum of the resulting matrix can serve as as similarity measure between both images.

In order to extend this method to the more complicated invariances involved in face recognition, the notion of a *correspondence map* is helpful (Figure 1). Correspondence, central to many problems in computer vision, can be defined as follows: *Point pairs from two given images of the same face correspond if they originate from the same point on the physical face.*

Once these correspondences have been established for sufficiently many points, an invariant similarity measure between model and object can be defined as the sum or average over the similarities of local features of all corresponding point pairs. Because the points on the real face are not accessible to either the brain or a computer, these correspondences can only be estimated on the basis of image information. Strictly speaking, correspondences are defined only between images of the same person, but all faces are sufficiently similar in structure that the notion can be extended to correspondence maps between different faces. These maps have many applications beside recognition (see FACE RECOGNITION: PSYCHOLOGY AND CONNECTIONISM).

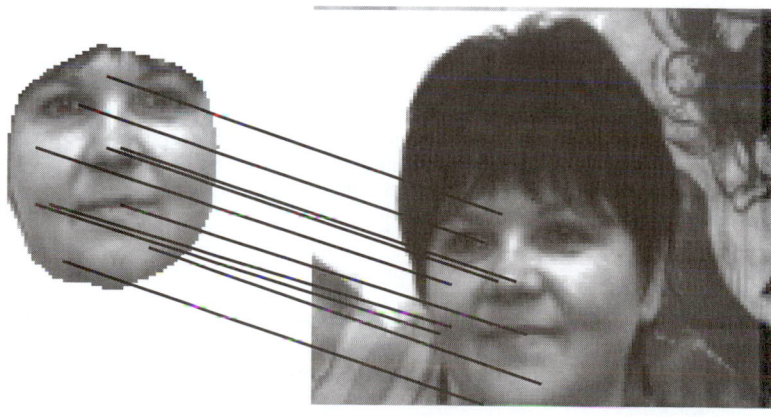

Figure 1. Correspondence maps provide a basis for an invariant similarity measure between two facial images, which can be used for person identification. They also deliver information about pose, size, and expression, and are crucial for animation. Their computation is difficult and rarely perfect. The figure shows selected correspondences obtained with the algorithm from Würtz (1997).

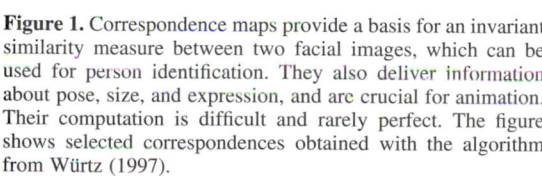

A system to recognize a person out of a collection of known ones can proceed as follows. Correspondence maps are estimated between the given image and all stored models, similarities are calculated on the basis of the correspondence maps, and the model with the highest similarity is picked as the recognized person. A measure for the *reliability* of the recognition can be derived by a simple statistical analysis of the series of all similarity values.

Because correspondence finding is a slow process, the database of known individuals must be organized in such a way that the need for correspondence finding is minimized. Furthermore, it should not be applied to arbitrary images, but some filtering must select image portions that are likely to contain a face for processing and recognition.

Summarizing the computational theory reveals the following building blocks for a successful face recognition system:

1. A representation of the facial images
2. A method of solving the correspondence problem
3. A similarity measure derived from a pair of images and a correspondence map
4. Organization of the database of known individuals
5. Filtering of the visual data (face finding)

For general reviews of face recognition systems, see Grudin (2000) and Chellappa, Wilson, and Sirohey (1995).

Image Representation

Many models for face recognition work directly on image gray values or retinal images. In this case, the correspondence problem becomes particularly difficult, as many points from very different locations share the same pixel value without actually corresponding to each other. A possible remedy consists in combining local patches of pixels. The larger the patch, the more this ambiguity is reduced. On the other hand, the features become more sensitive to distortions and changes in background and thus are of less value for the other required invariances. Patch building may also include linear combinations of pixel values. In this context, *Gabor functions* (see GABOR WAVELETS AND STATISTICAL PATTERN RECOGNITION) as a model of simple and complex cells in V1 have turned out to be a good compromise between locality and robustness and are well-suited for correspondence finding.

The possibility of processing the amplitudes and phases of the Gabor wavelet responses separately is very useful for face processing. Amplitudes (which model the activity of complex cells) vary rather smoothly across the image, and so do the similarities of all image features to a single one. Consequently, they provide smooth similarity landscapes well-suited for matching templates or single feature vectors. The phases, on the other hand, vary as rapidly as dictated by their center frequency and proceed roughly linearly on image paths in the respective direction. Therefore, they can be used to estimate correspondences with subgrid accuracy (Wiskott et al., 1997; Würtz, 1997).

An important alternative for image representation is to use local features that are derived directly from the statistics of facial images. A prominent example is the neural network–based *local feature analysis* (Penev and Atick, 1996), which allows learning local descriptors by minimizing their correlation. This results in a sparse code adapted for the class represented by the training examples.

Correspondence Finding

The representation of a face in terms of local features serves two purposes. First, correspondences must be estimated on the basis of feature similarity, and second, the feature similarities constitute the image similarity. In principle, different features can be used for both purposes.

Because of the ambiguities discussed above, simplifying assumptions must be made about the correspondence maps. A good candidate for such an assumption is *neighborhood preservation*. Consequently, algorithms for correspondence finding usually optimize a combined objective function that favors similarity between local features and smoothness of the correspondence map.

One implementation of this procedure is *elastic graph matching* (EGM) (Lades et al., 1993), in which stored models are represented as graphs vertex-labeled with vectors of local Gabor responses and edge-labeled with a distance constraint. The correspondence problem can be solved by optimizing the similarity between model graph and a (topologically identical) graph in the image in terms of similarity of both edge and vertex labels. This is a high-dimensional optimization problem that is usually simplified by applying a hierarchy of possible graph transformations. It starts with pure translation, later adds scale changes, and finally adds local displacements. In the first steps, Gabor amplitudes are used exclusively, which leads to smooth similarity landscapes and allows separating the different steps.

An alternative method, one that makes use of the pyramidal form of Gabor wavelet transform, is *Gabor pyramid matching* (Würtz, 1997). It starts with standard template matching of the Gabor amplitudes on a sparse grid and low spatial frequency and refines the results using higher spatial frequencies. Thus, neighborhood preservation is not explicitly coded into an objective function but is inherited from the undistorted matching on low frequencies. Very precise correspondences can be obtained by subsequent subgrid estimation using the Gabor phases. This method allows much better background suppression, because the need to know local features for each feature point on all scales is eliminated.

Memory Organization

The importance of memory organization is due to the computational expense of the inevitable correspondence estimation, which should not be carried out separately on all stored models. Consequently, it is necessary to evaluate correspondences *between* the stored models. Adding this idea to EGM results in the so-called *bunch graph* (Wiskott et al., 1997). In that data structure, each vertex is labeled with one local feature vector from each person in the database, and care has to be taken during creation of the bunch graph that these feature vector are indeed taken from corresponding points. In addition to different matching schemes, bunch graphs can be used in two major modes. In one mode, it is assumed that the person to be recognized is indeed in the bunch graph, and is selected according to similarity. Alternatively, the feature most similar to the given image can be selected for each vertex separately, leading to a composition of the face image in terms of the local features of all persons in the bunch graph. Moreover, the vertices can carry additional information, such as sex, beardedness, or a genetic disease of the person they belong to. By majority voting, a decision about that feature for completely unknown persons can be made.

Eigenfaces (Turk and Pentland, 1991) are another technically successful approach to face recognition. Gray-value images of faces are prealigned by an optical flow method and then subjected to PRINCIPAL COMPONENT ANALYSIS (q.v.), which can be interpreted as a neuronal method. It turns out that a few components are sufficient to recognize identity. Recognition proceeds by projecting the image to be classified onto these components and applying a classifier to the resulting low-dimensional vector. Calculating the PC representation from a database of persons is rather time consuming, but projection and classification are very fast. This shows that the major strength of the eigenface method lies in very efficient memory organization.

Neuronal Models

On the technical side, a large variety of neural network models have been applied to the problem of face recognition. They usually start from well-aligned faces with little variation. See Gong et al. (2000) for a good discussion of the application of neural classifiers and an excellent treatment of technical approaches to face recognition.

It is currently not known if there is neuronal machinery in the brain to explicitly estimate correspondences. However, DYNAMIC LINK ARCHITECTURE (q.v.) can be used to solve the correspondence problem, as follows (Lades et al., 1993). Two layers of neurons that represent the image space in model and image, respectively, are fully interconnected by dynamic links. They have an internal wiring that supports moving localized blobs of activity. The development of links is supported by feature similarity and synchronous activation of the connected neurons. The link dynamics then converge to a correspondence mapping. It has been extended by a competition between a multitude of model layers to a full-blown neural face recognition system. This system is sped up by a coarse-to-fine strategy working on the Gabor pyramid. The speedup is due to the possible parallelism between all refinement steps. That system also shows good background invariance, because model and image representation are the same as for pyramid matching.

Face Finding

Having found a correct correspondence map from a stored model into an image in principle implies that segmentation has also been solved. However, applying correspondence-based techniques like bunch graph matching to arbitrary images yields plenty of misclassifications: depending on the parameters, either many faces go undetected or many nonfaces pass as faces.

It seems very difficult to encode the notion of a general face into a program or data structure. Therefore, for *finding* faces in images or video sequences, neural net classifiers are widely used. Typically, a whole set of segmented and roughly normalized face images is used to train a network. Then the network is applied to all points of an image to provide a face/nonface decision. A good review of the facefinding literature can be found in Hjelmås and Low (2000).

Discussion

A correspondence map is a very general model of the variation of appearance of a face. Its estimation is computationally intensive, and the currently known neuronal models that can implement it cannot account for the rapidity of human recognition, even if run on highly parallel hardware like real neurons. The advantage of correspondence maps lies in the fact that much more information, such as the actual position, pose, and expression, can be determined from them.

The quality of technical face recognition systems is difficult to judge. On small data sets (less than 100 individuals), even naive template matching may yield respectable recognition rates. The use of standard databases, which is inevitable for achieving fair comparisons, raises the danger of overadapting the classifiers to the data. To prevent this, the Army Research Laboratory has set up a standard comparison procedure called the FERET test (Philips et al., 2000), in which where the major part of 14,126 images of 1,199 individuals is withheld for independent testing.

With this database, eight competitors underwent a test with the additional information about the (hand-labeled) eye position. Only two competitors, a bunch graph–based system and an eigenface-based system, took the realistic test on the images without any extra information. Both systems performed equally well on the data set with given eye coordinates, and the bunch graph–based system clearly won on the more difficult examples without additional information (Philips et al., 2000). These results underscore the need for very good correspondence estimation for successful face recognition.

Road Map: Vision
Background: Gabor Wavelets and Statistical Pattern Recognition
Related Reading: Dynamic Link Architecture; Face Recognition: Psychology and Connectionism; Object Recognition

References

Chellappa, R., Wilson, C. L., and Sirohey, S., 1995, Human and machine recognition of faces: A survey, *Proc. IEEE*, 83:705–740. ◆

Desimone, R., 1991, Face-selective cells in the temporal cortex of monkeys, *J. Cognit. Neurosci.*, 3:1–8.

Gauthier, I., Behrmann, M., and Tarr, M., 1999, Can face recognition really be dissociated from object recognition? *J. Cognit. Neurosci.*, 11:349–370.

Gong, S., McKenna, S. J., and Psarrou, A., 2000, *Dynamic Vision*, London: Imperial College Press. ◆

Grudin, M. A., 2000, On internal representations in face recognition systems, *Pattern Recogn.*, 33:1161–1177.

Haxby, J. V., Hoffman, E. A., and Gobbini, M. I., 2000, Distributed human neural system for face perception, *Trends Cognit. Sci.*, 4:223–233. ◆

Hjelmås, E., and Low, B. K., 2000, Face detection: A survey, *Comput. Vision Image Understanding*, 83:236–274.

Lades, M., Vorbrüggen, J. C., Buhmann, J., Lange, J., von der Malsburg, C., Würtz, R. P., and Konen, W., 1993, Distortion invariant object recognition in the dynamic link architecture, *IEEE Trans. Comput.*, 42:300–311. ◆

Moscovitch, M., Winocur, G., and Behrmann, M., 1997, What is special about face recognition? Nineteen experiments on a person with visual object agnosia and dyslexia but normal face recognition, *J. Cognit. Neurosci.*, 9:555–604.

Penev, P. S., and Atick, J. J., 1996, Local feature analysis: A general statistical theory for object representation, *Network*, 7:477–500.

Philips, P. J., Moon, H., Rizvi, S. A., and Rauss, P. J., 2000, The FERET evaluation methodology for face-recognition algorithms, *IEEE Trans. Pattern Anal. Machine Intell.*, 22:1090–1104.

Turk, M., and Pentland, A., 1991, Eigenfaces for recognition, *J. Cognit. Neurosci.*, 3:71–86.

Wiskott, L., Fellous, J.-M., Krüger, N., and von der Malsburg, C., 1997, Face recognition by elastic bunch graph matching, *IEEE Trans. Pattern Anal. Machine Intell.*, 19:775–779.

Würtz, R. P., 1997, Object recognition robust under translations, deformations and changes in background, *IEEE Trans. Pattern Anal. Machine Intell.*, 19:769–775. ◆

Young, A., 1998, *Face and Mind*, Oxford, Engl.: Oxford University Press.

Face Recognition: Psychology and Connectionism

Alice J. O'Toole

Introduction

Faces provide humans with rich information about their owners. From a brief glance across a dimly lit room, we can recognize the face of a friend. Faces also provide us with information important for social interaction, including the sex, race, approximate age, and current mood of a person. Humans can extract this information nearly instantaneously from the complex three-dimensional (3D) surface of the head. The skills humans have in perceiving and recognizing faces are even more impressive when we consider the number and diversity of people we must remember as individuals, and the fact that all faces share the same basic set of features (eyes, nose, and mouth), arranged in roughly the same configuration. Quantifying or even specifying the information that makes a face unique is a challenging problem.

Automatic or computer-based approaches to modeling face recognition have a long and relatively successful history among connectionist models of visual recognition. Commercial versions of facial recognition systems are now widely available and have already been employed in a variety of security applications. Although still not at the level of human performance on all tasks, with minimal viewpoint and illumination variation, the performance of these models compares favorably with the performance of humans (see FACE RECOGNITION: NEUROPHYSIOLOGY AND NEURAL TECHNOLOGY).

This article begins with a brief history of connectionist approaches to face recognition. Next, the broad range of tasks to which these models have been applied will be presented. Relating the models to psychological theories is accomplished by breaking the problem into the subtasks of representing faces and retrieving them from memory. Human and model performance can be compared along these dimensions. Finally, the article concludes with an overview of the challenges facing computational models of face processing at the beginning of the twenty-first century.

History and Theoretical Background

Connectionist face recognition models are some of the first successful computational models of a visual recognition task. Perhaps because of the homogeneity of faces as a class of objects, and the utility of recognition within the class of faces, the problem of modeling face recognition has been more tractable than modeling object recognition (see OBJECT RECOGNITION). Early face recognition models date from the beginnings of associative models of memory. In the 1970s, Kohonen (1977) used faces to illustrate the potential of a linear autoassociative network to act as a parallel distributed memory for images. He used simple pixel-based encodings of faces and showed that the model could selectively retrieve memorized faces using partial or occluded memory keys. The work of Kohonen using autoassociative memories with faces provided the cornerstone for most current computational models of face recognition. The autoassociative memory brings together important aspects of the psychology of face recognition and the varied, yet related, computational approaches to the problem.

The key to this connection is that autoassociative memories can be shown to implement PRINCIPAL COMPONENT ANALYSIS (PCA; q.v.), the most common of current connectionist or statistical models of face recognition (cf. Phillips et al., 2000). PCA is a technique for representing a number of correlated variables using a lesser number of uncorrelated or orthogonal variables. Applied to a set of face representations (e.g., images, 3D surfaces), PCA produces a set of orthogonal "feature" axes, known variously as principal components (PCs), eigenvectors, eigenfeatures, or eigenfaces (Turk and Pentland, 1991). These axes are ordered according to the proportion of variance they explain in the set of faces analyzed. A critical property of PCA is that any face in the set of analyzed or "learned" faces can be represented or reconstructed as a weighted combination of PCs. This property is shared by more recent techniques, such as nonnegative matrix factorization, that produce a sparser representation of faces than PCA (Lee and Seung, 1999; see also SPARSE CODING IN THE PRIMATE CORTEX).

From a psychological point of view, it is reasonable to think of PCs as features, and of the weights required for reconstructing a face as its *feature values*. PCA and connectionist-style models have properties reminiscent of human memory for faces. First, the memory is distributed rather than localized. This means that individual face representations interfere with each other in a way that allows for natural confusions between similar faces. Second, at the level of groups of faces, the proportion of variance associated with individual PCs is indicative of the importance of individual features for describing the set of faces. This enables the statistical properties of a particular face-learning history to affect the performance of the model. For example, connectionist models that vary in the racial composition of the training set can simulate the "other-race effect" for human memory (O'Toole et al., 1994). This is the well-known finding that we recognize faces of our own race more accurately than faces of other races.

An important theoretical focus of the last decade has been the integration of connectionist models of face recognition into the *face space theory* of human face processing (Valentine, 1991). Valentine's face space theory posits that human memory for faces can be thought of metaphorically as a multidimensional face space. At the center of the space is the average or "prototype" face. Individual faces are represented as points in the space, with the axes of the space defining the features with which faces are encoded. The distance between any two faces is, therefore, a measure of their similarity.

The face space model accounts for some common psychological findings for face recognition. For example, it is well known that the faces rated by subjects as typical are recognized less accurately than faces rated as distinctive. The face space theory explains this difference based on the probable distribution of faces in the space. Typical faces are close to the average face, where the space is "crowded." Distinctive faces are located in the sparser parts of the space, away from the average. Typical faces, therefore, are more easily confused with other faces than are distinctive faces.

It has become increasingly clear that the majority of connectionist models of face recognition, including those based on PCA, implement a physical version of Valentine's (1991) face space. These physical face spaces provide powerful tools for testing psychological theories about the way humans represent and retrieve faces from memory.

Face-Processing Tasks

Before proceeding, it is worth defining the range of face-processing tasks to which connectionist models have been applied. *Face recognition* involves a judgment about whether or not a face has been learned previously (i.e., is in the model's memory). This is distinct from *face identification*, which requires the retrieval of semantic information about a person whose face has been recognized (i.e., a name, or context or previous encounter). For *face verification*, a face is presented along with identifying information such as a name badge, and the model or machine must affirm or reject the face identification. This task has become increasingly important in recent years with the development of automatic security systems.

In addition to recognizing and identifying the faces of people we know, we must also be able to visually categorize faces along a number of general dimensions, including sex, race, age, and facial expression. Connectionist models have been applied to nearly all of these tasks, with varying levels of success (see O'Toole, Wenger, and Townsend, 2001, for a detailed review of face classification models). Of particular note, recent applications of connectionist models to the task of processing facial expression have become important in the context of human-computer interaction applications. They are also valuable tools for addressing the theoretical issues involved in human perception of emotion. Recent work by two groups have made inroads into the problem using PCA (Calder et al., 2001) and backpropagation models (Dailey, Cottrell, and Adolphs, 2001). Although there is still active debate on the psychological mechanisms involved in the processing of expressions, both models have achieved good performance and offer insight into the human solution to the problem.

Representing Faces

Much of the scientific dialogue associated with connectionist models of face processing over the past 5 to 10 years has focused not on the algorithms, but on the representations to which they are applied. Although the basic models have remained relatively simple, the representations to which they have been applied have evolved quickly and have provided fascinating insights into the complexities of representing the information in faces. As noted, face space models are powerful tools for testing the validity of different underlying representations of faces. The general idea is that the models operate by deriving a face space that is sensitive to the statistical structure of the faces analyzed. However, the way in which these inputs are encoded (e.g., by images, 3D measures, geometrical measures) has a substantial impact on the layout of the face space, and thereby alters the distances between individual faces. This is easy to understand intuitively, as follows. Imagine two faces with highly similar shapes but very different coloring (pigmentation). Representing the faces using images will result in a rather different similarity estimate than representing the faces with 3D surface measures.

The face representations used most commonly in connectionist models of face processing can be divided into three types: (1) raw image codes, (2) partially aligned "pre-morph" codes, and (3) fully corresponded "pre-morph" codes (cf. O'Toole et al., 2001, for additional details).

The first connectionist models represented faces as raw images (Sirovich and Kirby, 1987). Although the faces were spatially scaled and aligned in the image so that the eyes or nose of all faces coincided, this code has the obvious disadvantage of being only minimally tolerant of changes in viewpoint and illumination. Notwithstanding, raw image codes, within these limits, have proved highly effective and accurate at the task of face recognition and have largely remained the standard in state-of-the-art computational models of face recognition (Phillips et al., 2000). Connectionist models based on these codes also provide a reasonable approximation to human judgments about the distinctiveness of a face and human accuracy in recognizing faces (see O'Toole et al., 1994).

More effective ways of aligning faces have been developed based on partially aligned "pre-morph" codes. These codes define a partial correspondence between the features of all faces and help bridge the gap between computational models of face recognition and computer graphics–based face synthesis. Pre-morph codes define a representation that can support a morphable transition between any two faces. Craw and Cameron (1991) first introduced the idea of a pre-morph code for face representation by dividing a face representation into *shape* and *shape-free* encoding. Though not yet exploited to its full potential, this method is valuable to psychologists because it allows independent manipulation of the shape and shape-free components of the face in psychological experiments. Face shape is defined by the spatial positions of a set of facial landmarks (corners of the eyes, mouth, etc.) in an image. Next, a complementary shape-free code of a face is created by morphing (or warping) the face into the average face shape, computed over a large number of faces. The encoding of an individual face, therefore, includes both its shape and shape-free parts. Hancock, Burton, and Bruce (1996) used this separated face code with PCA for modeling human face recognition and found a better fit to human performance than the purely image-based codes used previously.

Dividing the representation of faces in this way enables a separate analysis of the structure of a face and its image-based information, but is costly in terms of the preprocessing required. Successful use of these codes involves locating and marking (often by hand) a relatively large number of facial landmark points that match on all faces. A related representation, inspired by early visual processing, overcomes this problem in an interesting way. This approach characterizes the work of von der Malsburg and his colleagues over the years (see, e.g., Okada et al., 1998, and FACE RECOGNITION: NEUROPHYSIOLOGY AND NEURAL TECHNOLOGY). Okada et al. used banks of Gabor jets—filters with varying orientations and resolutions—to sample face images at multiple locations. The Gabor jets simulate the spatial frequency filtering that occurs in early visual processing in the cortex. Using a dynamic link architecture, face recognition occurs by allowing the relative locations of the Gabor jets to migrate to fit individual faces. In some ways, this implements the partial alignment discussed previously in a biologically plausible way. This model has been shown to support highly accurate face verification and is the basis of commercial identification security systems (see Phillips et al., 2000).

To simulate face synthesis and to implement a face space that is completely continuous (i.e., locations in the space are "possible" faces), however, true correspondences between meaningful facial landmarks are necessary. In recent work using elaborated optic flow algorithms, Blanz and Vetter (1999) have been able to completely automate the feature-matching process to produce "fully corresponded" face representations, using laser scans of human heads. *Fully corresponded* means that the matching process is carried out not only on the landmark points, but on *all* of the sample points. Specifically, Blanz and Vetter aligned the x, y, z and r, g, b sample points for a large number of individuals. From this corresponded representation of the laser scans, they defined a 3D morphable model of faces by analyzing the data with PCA. This model readily fits into the multidimensional face space theory outlined previously, but employs a sophisticated and nearly complete representation of the perceptual information in faces. Psychologists can use this model to precisely manipulate the information in faces. In particular, 3D shape versus 2D reflectance information in faces can be varied selectively. These manipulations have been used to test the contribution of 2D versus 3D information for human face recognition (see O'Toole et al., 2001, for a review of findings).

The morphable model was used to predict high-level face adaptation effects in human perception. Leopold et al. (2001) showed that trajectories can be defined through this space by connecting a face with the average face, and continuing the trajectory to the "other side of the mean" (Figure 1). This defines an "anti-face" or "opposite" to the original face, because it inverts all of the coordinates (feature values) on the PCs. For example, dark faces have light-colored anti-faces, and round, chubby faces have long, skinny anti-faces. Leopold et al. showed that the perception of a face can be facilitated by simply pre-viewing its anti-face for a few seconds.

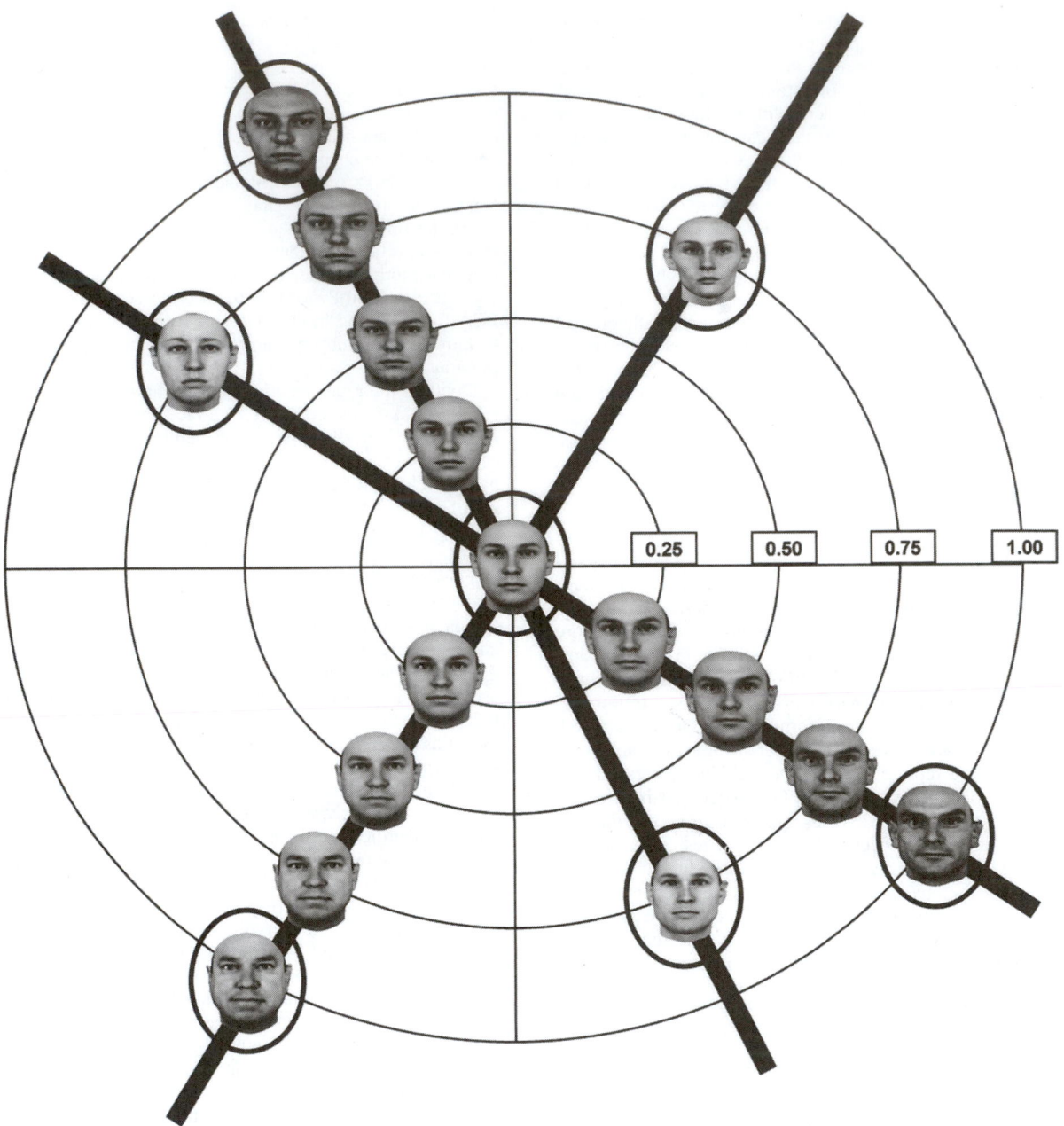

Figure 1. A face space created by the morphable model of Blanz and Vetter (1999) shows the continuous trajectory between a face and the mean or prototype of the face space. Anti-caricatures lie between the face and the prototype. On the other side of the mean is the anti-face, which is an op-posite (i.e., all feature values are reversed) of the original face. (From Leopold, D. A., O'Toole, A. J., Vetter, T., and Blanz, V., 2001, Prototype-referenced shape encoding revealed by high-level aftereffects, *Nature Neurosci.*, 4:89–94. Reprinted with permission.)

This effect has been compared to simpler visual aftereffects, such as the perception of green after viewing red. Trajectories through this complicated face space, therefore, can be used to predict human performance in a rather precise way. Leopold et al. relate these findings to the activity of face-selective cells in inferotemporal cortex, which may encode high-level shape properties of objects.

In summary, face representations have evolved in sophistication and have provided connectionist and statistically based models with better and more precise information about faces. As these representations have improved, so too has the power of the models for simulating aspects of human performance with faces.

Retrieving and Categorizing Faces

In the context of a computational model, face recognition involves a decision about whether or not a face has been learned previously. For the face space framework, this works as follows. The learned faces are points in a multidimensional space. Recognition is implemented by projecting a test face into this space to locate a match. Projection involves the representation of the test face using the features or eigenvectors derived from learned faces. If a good match is found—i.e., if the location of the test face in the space is close to a stored face—then the face should be "recognized." If there is no neighboring face sufficiently close to the test face, the face should be declared "novel." This way of testing face recognition algorithms produces "hit" and "false alarm" data very similar to those acquired in a standard human face recognition experiment.

It is clear that anything that alters the appearance of the face between learning and test time and that is included in the representation (e.g., illumination for a pixel-based code) will affect the accuracy of recognition. This interaction between the model representation and the retrieval process can be used to make predictions about the factors that will determine human accuracy for faces. These predictions can be used to test hypotheses about the kinds of representations employed in the visual system. At present, a variety of algorithms and representations are available. The work of assessing the accord between human and model performance in the context of psychological theories of these processes is under way.

Discussion

Connectionist models of face recognition have a long and distinguished history. Their development has been spurred by the many and varied psychological issues inherent to the perception of human faces, and by a quickly emerging set of industrial applications. These include applications for security systems and biometric analysis of person identification. Connectionist algorithms are available for face recognition, verification, and classification. In the future, we can expect to see systems that track moving people and faces being merged into the better-developed face-processing algorithms discussed here.

Road Maps: Psychology; Vision
Related Reading: Principal Component Analysis; Face Recognition: Neurophysiology and Neural Technology; Object Recognition, Neurophysiology

References

Blanz, V., and Vetter, T., 1999, A morphable model for the synthesis of 3d faces, in *SIGGRAPH'99 Proceedings*, ACM, Computer Society Press, pp. 187–194.

Calder, A. J., Burton, A. M., Miller, P., Young, A. W., and Akamatsu, S., 2001, A principal component analysis of facial expressions, *Vision Res.*, 41:1179–1208.

Craw, I., and Cameron, P., 1991, Parameterising images for recognition and reconstruction, in *Proceedings of the British Machine Vision Conference* (P. Mowforth, Ed.), London: Springer-Verlag, pp. 367–370.

Dailey, M. N., Cottrell, G. W., and Adolphs, R., 2001, A six-unit network is all you need to discover happiness, in *Proceedings of the 22nd Annual Cognitive Science Society Conference*, Mahwah, NJ: Erlbaum.

Hancock, P. J. B., Burton, A. M., and Bruce, V., 1996, Face processing: Human perception and principal components analysis, *Memory Cognit.*, 24:26–40.

Kohonen, T., 1977, *Associative Memory*, New York: Springer-Verlag.

Leopold, D. A., O'Toole, A. J., Vetter, T., and Blanz, V., 2001, Prototype-referenced shape encoding revealed by high-level aftereffects, *Nature Neurosci.*, 4:89–94.

Lee, D. D., and Seung, H. S., 1999, Learning the parts of objects by non-negative matrix factorizations, *Nature*, 401:788–791.

Okada, K., Steffens, J., Maurer, T., Hong, H., Elagin, E., Neven, H., and von der Malsburg, C., 1998, The Bochum/USC face recognition system and how it fared in the FERET Phase III test, in *Face Recognition: From Theory to Applications* (H. Wechsler, P. J. Phillips, V. Bruce, F. Fogelman Soulie, and T. S. Huang, Eds.), Berlin: Springer-Verlag.

O'Toole, A. J., Deffenbacher, K. A., Valentin, D., and Abdi, H., 1994, Structural aspects of face recognition and the other-race effect, *Memory Cognit.*, 22:208–224.

O'Toole, A. J., Wenger, M. J., and Townsend, J. T., 2001, Quantitative models of perceiving and remembering faces: Precedents and possibilities, in *Computational, Geometric, and Process Perspectives on Facial Cognition* (M. J. Wenger and J. T. Townsend, Eds.), Mahwah, NJ: Erlbaum, pp. 1–38. ◆

Phillips, P. J., Moon, H., Rizvi, S., and Rauss, P., 2000, The FERET evaluation method for face recognition algorithms, *IEEE Trans. Pattern Recog. Machine Intell.*, 22:1090–1104. ◆

Sirovich, L., and Kirby, M., 1987, Low dimensional procedure for characterization of human faces, *J. Opt. Soc. Am.*, A4:518–519.

Turk, M., and Pentland, A., 1991, Eigenfaces for recognition, *J. Cognit. Neurosci.*, 3:71–86.

Valentine, T., 1991, A unified account of the effects of distinctiveness, inversion, and race in face recognition, *Q. J. Exp. Psychol.*, 43A:161–204.

Fast Visual Processing

Simon J. Thorpe and Michèle Fabre-Thorpe

Introduction

How long does the visual system take to process an image? Yarbus's pioneering studies of scanning eye movements in the 1960s showed that we typically make about three saccades a second. This finding implies that a few hundred milliseconds is enough for visual analysis and programming the next eye movement. By the 1970s, work by Irv Biederman and Molly Potter had shown that much information can be extracted from briefly glimpsed scenes, even at presentation rates of around 10 frames/s, a technique known as rapid sequential visual presentation (RSVP). In the early 1980s, one of the prime motivations for the development of connectionist and PDP models was Jerry Feldman's "100-step limit." Feldman argued that since many complex cognitive tasks can be performed in about half a second, and since interspike intervals for neurons are seldom shorter than 5 ms, the underlying algorithms should involve no more than about 100 sequential, though massively parallel, steps. These numbers were only ballpark figures and unrelated to any particular task, but Feldman's strategy has recently been taken a step further by measuring processing time on specific high-level visual tasks. In combination with knowledge about underlying anatomy and physiology, such information can provide insights into the processing strategies used by the brain.

There is an important distinction in neural computation between feedforward processing models and those with recurrent connections that allow feedback and iterative processing. Pure feedforward models (e.g., multilayer perceptrons, or MLPs) can operate very quickly in parallel hardware. But many authors, including, for example, Ullman (1996), Rao and Ballard (1999), and Grossberg (2001), have argued that sophisticated visual processing requires the interplay of bottom-up and top-down mechanisms. Such views are supported by the anatomy of the visual system, since neurons at virtually every level are influenced not only by feedforward projections but also by extensive feedback connections from later stages and horizontal connections within each layer. Should one conclude that, because the visual system has recurrent connections, pure feedforward mechanisms have no role to play? Perhaps not, because even in systems that use extensively recurrent connections, the very fastest behavioral responses might essentially depend on a single feedforward processing wave. This article considers how detailed measurements of processing speed can be combined with anatomical and physiological constraints to constrain models of how the brain performs particular computations.

Measuring Processing Speed

The ultimate test for processing speed lies in behavior. If animals can make reliable behavioral responses to specific categories of stimuli with a particular reaction time, there can be no argument about whether the processing has been done. When a fly reacts to displacements of the visual world by changing wing torque 30 ms later, 30 ms is clearly enough for both visual processing and motor execution. Fast behavioral reactions are not limited to insects. For example, tracking eye movements are initiated within 70–80 ms in humans and within around 50 ms in monkeys (Kawano, 1999), and vergence eye movements, required to keep objects within the fixation plane, have latencies of around 85 ms in humans and less than 60 ms in monkeys (Miles, 1997). Such low values probably reflect the relatively simple visual processing needed to detect stimulus movement and the short path lengths in the oculomotor system. How fast could behavioral responses be on tasks that require more sophisticated visual processing?

In 1996, we reported fast behavioral responses on a challenging task for the visual system (Thorpe, Fize, and Marlot, 1996). Presented with color photographs flashed for only 20 ms, subjects had to release a button as quickly as possible if the image contained an animal, and not respond otherwise. Target and nontarget images were extremely varied, with targets including mammals, birds, fish, and insects in their natural environments. Furthermore, no image was shown more than once, which forced subjects to process each image from scratch with minimal contextual help. Despite all these constraints, accuracy was high (around 94%), with mean reaction times (RTs) typically around 400 ms.

While mean RT might be the obvious candidate for measuring processing speed, another useful value is the minimal time needed to complete the task. Using RT distributions, this value can be defined as the first time bin at which correct responses start to significantly outnumber erroneous responses to nontargets. Faster responses occurring with no bias toward targets are presumably anticipations triggered before stimulus categorization was completed. Remarkably, in the animal categorization task, these minimal response times can be less than 250 ms.

It might be thought that images associated with fast responses constitute a subpopulation particularly easy to analyze. However, we found no obvious features that characterize rapidly categorized images (Fabre-Thorpe et al., 2001), implying that, even with highly varied and unpredictable images, the entire processing sequence from photoreceptor to hand movement can be completed in under 250 ms. Remarkably, rhesus monkeys can also perform this task, but their minimal RTs are even faster, around 170–180 ms (Fabre-Thorpe, Richard, and Thorpe, 1998). As in the tracking and vergence eye movement studies mentioned earlier, humans take nearly 50% longer than their monkey cousins to perform a given task.

Such data clearly impose upper limits on the time needed for visual processing. However, they do not directly reveal how long visual processing takes because reaction times also include response execution. How much time should we allow for the motor part of the task? To get at this question, event-related potentials (ERPs) and magnetoencephalography (MEG) recordings can be used to track information processing between stimulus and response. For example, during performance of the animal categorization task, simultaneously recorded ERPs showed that the average response to correct target trials diverged sharply from the average response to correct nontarget trials at about 150 ms post stimulus. This remarkably robust differential ERP response appears specifically related to target detection and occurs well in advance of even the fastest behavioral responses. This value of 150 ms for visual categorization leaves no more than 100 ms for motor execution when behavioral responses occur at around 250 ms.

Processing speed can also be assessed at the level of single neurons by determining the point at which they start to show selectivity for particular visual inputs. By examining the information contained in neuronal responses at different times and in different visual structures, one can follow how processing develops over time. Surprisingly, using response latency to track the time course of visual processing is a relatively recent technique in experimental neuroscience. Nevertheless, by 1989 it was clear that the onset latencies of selective visual responses were a major constraint on models (Thorpe and Imbert, 1989). Face-selective neurons had been described in monkey inferotemporal cortex (IT) with typical onset latencies of around 100 ms. Beyond the visual system as such, neurons in the lateral hypothalamus were known to respond selectively to food after only 150 ms. Although these earlier studies suggested that visual processing could be very fast, they did not specifically determine at which point the neuronal response was fully selective. In 1992 it was demonstrated that even the first 5 ms of the responses in IT neurons could be highly selective to faces (Oram and Perrett, 1992). Since IT neurons can start responding before 100 ms, such data can be used to assign firm limits to the processing time required to reach a certain level of analysis.

Implications for Computational Models

Determining the minimal time required to perform a particular task or computation is not enough to constrain models of the underlying mechanisms without taking into account underlying anatomy and physiology. Even if monkeys can perform an abstract categorization task in as little as 180 ms, this feat would tell us little about the underlying computations if the brain was an unstructured assembly of neurons. However, the underlying anatomical pathways involved are actually quite well known (see VISUAL SCENE PERCEPTION; OBJECT RECOGNITION, NEUROPHYSIOLOGY). Figure 1 illustrates a plausible route involving the various stages in the so-called ventral processing stream that leads to the inferotemporal cortex (V1-V2-V4-PIT-AIT), where neurons selective for complex visual forms are found. But since IT has no direct outputs to the motor system, information has to travel via such areas as prefrontal (PFC), premotor (PMC), and motor cortices (MC) before reaching the spinal cord.

On the basis of this diagram, we can start using neurophysiological data to estimate the processing time available at each step. For example, neurons in V1 can start firing 40 ms after stimulus onset, although 60 ms would be more typical. In IT, the earliest responses start at around 80 ms, with 100 ms being more typical. Given the number of processing steps involved, it would appear that the earliest responses in each area must be produced on the basis of only about 10 ms of activity in the previous stage.

How can such data be used to constrain models of processing? Bear in mind that this 10 ms value includes several components: synaptic transmission, integration of information by postsynaptic cells, spike initiation, and propagation to the next stage. Estimates of conduction velocity for intracortical axons suggest that conduction delays might be considerable. At 1–2 m/s, it would take 15–30 ms simply for information to propagate from V1 to IT (Nowak and Bullier, 1997), a substantial proportion of the 40 ms latency shift between the two areas. Moreover, few if any neurons that receive inputs from the preceding stage project directly to the next stage. In other words, processing in each cortical area almost certainly involves more than one layer of synapses, reducing further the amount of time available at each step. Together, such data imply

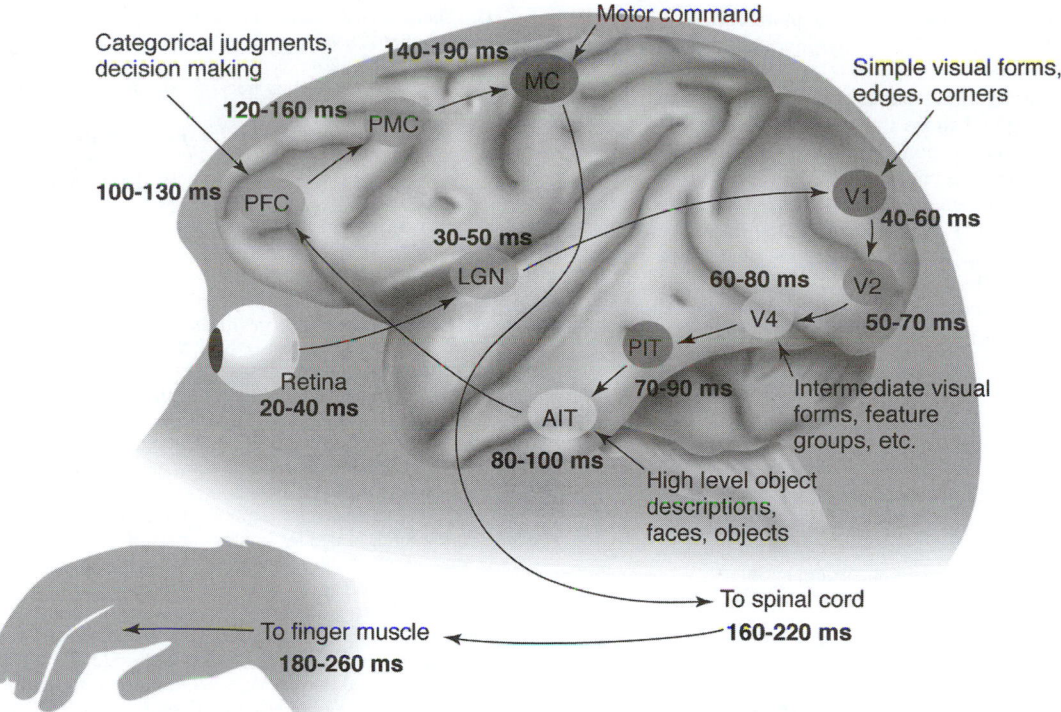

Figure 1. A possible input-output pathway for performing go/no-go visual categorization tasks in monkeys. Information passes from retina to lateral geniculate nucleus (LGN) before arriving in cortical area V1. Further processing occurs in areas V2, V4, and in the posterior and anterior inferotemporal cortex (PIT and AIT) before being relayed to the prefrontal (PFC), premotor (PMC), and motor cortices (MC). Finally, motor neuron activation in the spinal cord triggers hand movement. For each area, the two numbers provide approximate latency values for the earliest responses and for a typical average response. (From Thorpe and Fabre-Thorpe, *Science*, 2001. Reprinted with permission.)

that the earliest responses in any particular area are presumably based on just a few milliseconds of activity in neurons at earlier levels.

This conclusion has some profound implications for cortical computation. First, it implies that, at least in the case of the earliest responses in any particular structure, there will be little time for iterative processing involving recurrent loops at previous stages. Since neurons in areas such as IT have responses that can be selective from the very start, it must presumably be possible to generate such responses on the basis of a pure feedforward pass through the system. This view is also supported by a recent study that analyzed IT responses to sequences of images presented at high rates. As frame rate was progressively increased, response strength dropped, but some neurons were still able to respond selectively at a 72-Hz frame rate, i.e., with images lasting only 14 ms (Keysers et al., 2001). With an onset latency of around 100 ms, it would appear that as many as seven separate images were being processed at the same time in a sequential pipeline, each stage of the visual system effectively processing a different image.

A second major consequence of these temporal constraints concerns the nature of the neural code. It is generally assumed that neurons encode information in their firing rates. Indeed, in the vast majority of artificial neural networks, the spike trains of real neurons are replaced by a single continuous value, often fixed in the range 0 to 1, supposed to represent firing frequency. But how accurately can one determine a firing rate with only a few milliseconds to listen to the output of each neuron? Given that neurons only rarely fire above 100 Hz, very few will generate more than one spike in the time available. This rules out counting several

spikes from the same neuron, or determining the interval between two spikes. Of course, one could measure firing rates across a population of neurons, but this would be an expensive strategy. Yet some alternative coding strategies can operate very efficiently, even with only one spike per neuron. For example, one could use the order in which neurons fire and the fact that the most strongly activated neurons tend to fire first (Thorpe, Delorme, and Van Rullen, 2001). Whatever the solution, it is clear that rapid processing poses a major challenge for computational neuroscience.

Discussion

By combining the detailed time course of visual processing with information about anatomical organization and the characteristics of individual neurons, including their conduction velocities, we can go well beyond the global statements made by Feldman in the early 1980s. Specifically, we have seen that the earliest, highly selective responses of neurons in high-order areas appear to depend almost entirely on a feedforward wave of processing that is so fast that each neuron may well get to fire only one spike. Although this may seem far-fetched, there are simulations showing that simple feedforward networks of neurons that generate only one spike can perform sophisticated tasks that include detecting, localizing, and identifying faces in natural images (Thorpe et al., 2001).

On the other hand, vision cannot be reduced to a feedforward pass. Visual perception is much more complex than simply pressing a button when a particular category of object is present, and there is increasing evidence that this very rapid processing may well be largely unconscious. The formation of a fully segmented, conscious percept may well require far more complex processing than can be achieved in 100–150 ms, involving extensive use of feedback connections. Here again, temporal constraints can help determine the computations that can be performed with only feedforward processing and those that require recurrent mechanisms. For example, neuronal response properties that are not present at the onset of the response but take several tens of milliseconds to develop have recently been reported (Sugase et al., 1999; Lamme and Roelfsema, 2000). This progressive shaping of particular response properties is a hallmark of processing that requires recurrent mechanisms and feedback connections. In such cases, the initial very fast feedforward pass can act as a seeding process that allows subsequent processing to be performed in an intelligent top-down way.

This line of research, in which the details of the time course of visual processing are used to distinguish between different theoretical models of how the brain computes, constitutes a particularly clear example of the way in which experimental and theoretical work in brain theory can complement each other.

Road Map: Vision
Related Reading: Object Recognition, Neurophysiology; Visual Attention; Visual Scene Perception

References

Fabre-Thorpe, M., Delorme, A., Marlot, C., and Thorpe, S., 2001, A limit to the speed of processing in ultra-rapid visual categorization of novel natural scenes, *J. Cognit. Neurosci.*, 13:171–180.

Fabre-Thorpe, M., Richard, G., and Thorpe, S. J., 1998, Rapid categorization of natural images by rhesus monkeys, *NeuroReport*, 9:303–308.

Grossberg, S., 2001, Linking the laminar circuits of visual cortex to visual perception: Development, grouping, and attention, *Neurosci. Biobehav. Rev.*, 25:513–526.

Kawano, K., 1999, Ocular tracking: Behavior and neurophysiology, *Curr. Opin. Neurobiol.*, 9:467–473.

Keysers, C., Xiao, D. K., Foldiak, P., and Perrett, D. I., 2001, The speed of sight, *J. Cognit. Neurosci.*, 13:90–101. ◆

Lamme, V. A. F., and Roelfsema, P. R., 2000, The distinct modes of vision offered by feedforward and recurrent processing, *Trends Neurosci.*, 23:571–579.

Miles, F. A., 1997, Visual stabilization of the eyes in primates, *Curr. Opin. Neurobiol.*, 7:867–871.

Nowak, L. G., and Bullier, J., 1997, The timing of information transfer in the visual system, in *Extrastriate Cortex in Primates* (J. Kaas, K. Rockland, and A. Peters, Eds.), New York: Plenum Press, pp. 205–241. ◆

Oram, M. W., and Perrett, D. I., 1992, Time course of neural responses discriminating different views of the face and head, *J. Neurophysiol.*, 68:70–84.

Rao, R. P., and Ballard, D. H., 1999, Predictive coding in the visual cortex: A functional interpretation of some extra-classical receptive-field effects, *Nature Neurosci.*, 2:79–87.

Sugase, Y., Yamane, S., Ueno, S., and Kawano, K., 1999, Global and fine information coded by single neurons in the temporal visual cortex, *Nature*, 400:869–873.

Thorpe, S., Delorme, A., and Van Rullen, R., 2001, Spike-based strategies for rapid processing, *Neural Netw.*, 14:715–725. ◆

Thorpe, S., Fize, D., and Marlot, C., 1996, Speed of processing in the human visual system, *Nature*, 381:520–522.

Thorpe, S. J., and Imbert, M., 1989, Biological constraints on connectionist models, in *Connectionism in Perspective* (R. Pfeiffer, Z. Schreter, F. Fogelman-Soulié, and L. Steels, Eds.), Amsterdam–North Holland, pp. 63–92.

Ullman, S., 1996, *High-Level Vision: Object Recognition and Visual Cognition*, Cambridge, MA: MIT Press. ◆

Feature Analysis

Michael J. Morgan

Introduction

A popular idea is that natural images can be decomposed into constituent objects, which are in turn composed of features. The space of all possible images is vast, but natural images occupy only a small corner of this space, and images of significant objects such as animals or plants occupy a still smaller region. The visual brain has evolved to analyze only the interesting regions of image space.

A feature description of an image reduces the number of dimensions required to describe the image. An image is a two-dimensional (N by N) array of pointwise (or pixelwise) intensity values. If the number of possible pixel values is p, then the number of possible images is a set $\aleph$, of size pN^2. To distinguish all possible images having N by N pixels, we need a space of N^2 dimensions, which is too large in practice to search for a particular image.

The core idea behind feature analysis is that in real images, objects can be recognized in a space $\Re$ with a much smaller number of dimensions (a smaller dimensionality) than $\aleph$. The space $\Re$ is a *feature space*, and its dimensions are the features. A simple example of a feature space is color space, in which all possible colors can be specified in a three-dimensional space, with axes $L-M$, $L+M-S$ and $L+M+S$, and L, M, and S are the photon catches of the long-, medium-, and short-wavelength receptors, respectively. The reason why a three-dimensional space suffices to distinguish the very much higher-dimensional space of surface reflectance spectra is that there is huge redundancy in natural spectra. The reflectance at a given wavelength is highly correlated with reflectance at nearby wavelengths. We seek similar redundancies in space that will allow dimensional reduction of images.

Features Are Not Necessarily Localized

Note that in this very general framework, there is no implication that features are spatially localized. Features could, for example, be Fourier components. The global Fourier transform has the same dimensionality as the original image and is thus not, according to the present definition, a feature space. But if we throw away Fourier components that are unimportant in distinguishing objects or if we quantize phase, dimensional reduction has been achieved, and we have a feature space. The familiar example of JPEG compression involves a feature space.

To distinguish between spatially localized and nonlocalized features, we shall follow physicists in calling the former *particles* and the latter *waves*. Wavelets (see Olshausen and Field, 1996) are hybrids that are waves within a region of the image but otherwise are particles. Another important distinction is between particles that have place tokens and those that do not. Although all particles have places in the image, it does not follow that these places will be represented by tokens in feature space. It is entirely feasible to describe some images as a set of particles of unknown position. Something like this happens in many descriptions of texture. A very active source of debate in visual psychophysics has been the extent to which the visual system uses place tokens (sometimes called local signs). For example, if the distance between two points *A* and *B* is seen as greater than the distance between two other points *C* and *D*, does this imply that there are place tokens for *A*, *B*, *C*, and *D*, or is some other mechanism involved (Morgan and Watt, 1997)?

The feature concept has proved useful in an impressive variety of different contexts.

Features in Ethology

Lorenz and Tinbergen's concept of the innate releasing mechanism (IRM) with its releasing stimulus foreshadowed much later work in behavior and physiology. The red spot at the base of the herring gull beak, which the young attack to get food from the parent, and the silhouette of the hawk/goose, which elicits fear when moved only in the hawk direction, are classic features that have entered folk psychology.

Features in Physiology

The classic paper "What the Frog's Eye Tells the Frog's Brain" (Lettvin et al., 1959) popularized the idea that special low-level sensory analyzers might exist for the purpose of responding to simple input features, the canonical example being the response of bug-detecting retinal ganglion cells to a small, moving spot. Hubel and Wiesel (1977) described bar and edge detectors in the visual cortex of cat and introduced an influential feature analysis scheme in which hierarchies of mechanisms would combine elementary features into ever increasingly complex objects. The hierarchical scheme, although not without its critics, was supported by the discovery of neurons in inferotemporal cortex (IT) responding selectively to images of complex objects such as a face or hand. Further studies of IT with simpler shapes found a columnar organization of IT with cells having similar response properties organized in repeating columns (Tanaka, 1996) (see Figure 1). The proposal that a ventral pathway leading to IT is responsible for object recognition gains support from lesioning and functional brain-imaging studies, although the idea of a single area for feature analysis is almost certainly too simple (Logothetis and Sheinberg, 1996).

Concept Learning

Most dogs bark and have hair, tails, and ears. But not all dogs bark, and Wittgenstein famously pointed out that some concepts such as

"a game" have no necessary features. Philosophers and animal psychologists met his challenge to the feature concept with the polymorphous concept (Watanabe, Lea, and Dittrich, 1993), an *n*-dimensional feature space in which instances of a concept occupy a subspace without sharp boundaries. Considerable research effort has been devoted to investigating the abilities of animals to learn both natural and artificially polymorphous concepts, a key issue being whether a linear model of feature combination will serve.

Cognitive Psychology

The idea that certain features can be analyzed at a preconscious level has proved fertile. Using the technique of visual search, Treisman (1988) suggested that only certain elementary features, and not their combinations, could serve as preconscious markers (Figure 2). This idea proved especially popular when linked, on rather slender evidence, with the discovery of specialized prestriate cortical areas in monkey devoted to the analysis of color and motion. However, the simple dichotomy between a fast, parallel search for features and a slow, serial search for combinations of features has come to be questioned (see the caption for Figure 2).

Image Compression

The earliest pictures to be sent across the transatlantic telegraph took more than a week to transmit. Engineers soon reduced this time to three hours by encoding the image more economically. Image compression techniques are divided into those that preserve all the information in the original (error-free) and lossy techniques, which try to transmit only the important features (Gonzalez and Woods, 1993). An early pioneer of speeding up telegraph transmission by a lossy feature decomposition was Francis Galton, who proposed a set of features for transmitting face profiles over the telegraph using only four telegraphic "words." Appropriately for the man who invented the fingerprint, he saw this primarily as a forensic aid in sending profiles of wanted criminals around the world. Galton's feature space lays stress on five *cardinal points*. These are the notch between the brow and the nose, the tip of the nose, the notch between the nose and the upper lip, the parting of the lips and the tip of the chin (Figure 3).

The remainder of this review illustrates the concept of feature spaces and describes key issues, some resolved and others not.

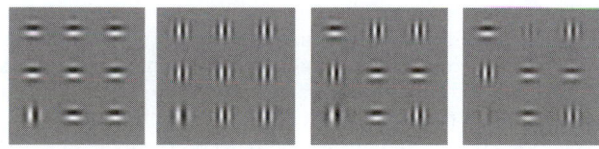

Figure 2. Searching for a single "odd man out" is easy (*A*) when the target has a very different orientation from the background elements or (*B*) when it has a different spatial frequency. Search times do not increase with the number of background elements (parallel search), provided that the orientation difference is sufficiently large. With smaller orientation differences (<10 degrees), search times do increase with the number of background elements, indicating a serial search. It might be thought that orientation and spatial frequency are easy search features because they are represented in primary visual cortex. However, (*C*) the conjunction of a particular spatial frequency and orientation is much harder to find, despite the fact that many V1 neurons are jointly tuned to orientation and frequency. If contrast is randomized (*D*), the search becomes harder still. The most powerful generalization about search is that it becomes harder when the number of different background elements increases. A standard ("back pocket") texture segmentation mechanism that responds to local contrasts in orientation, frequency, contrast, and color can explain most of these findings. (Source: Figures by J. A. Solomon.)

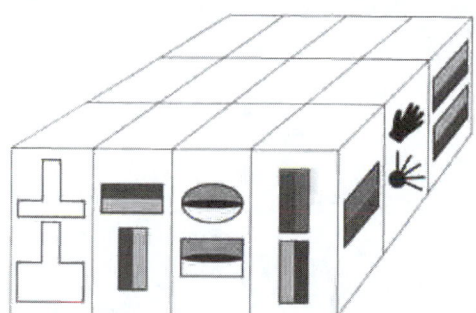

Figure 1. Columnar organization of inferotemporal cortex, based on work of Fujita et al. (see review by Tanaka, 1996). Columns of cells selective for similar complex shapes are interspersed with columns of cells unresponsive to these stimuli but selective to different complex shapes. (Source: Reproduced with permission from Stryker, M. P. (1992), *Nature (Lond.)*, 360:301. Note: In the original, different gray levels are in color, to show color preferences of the cells.)

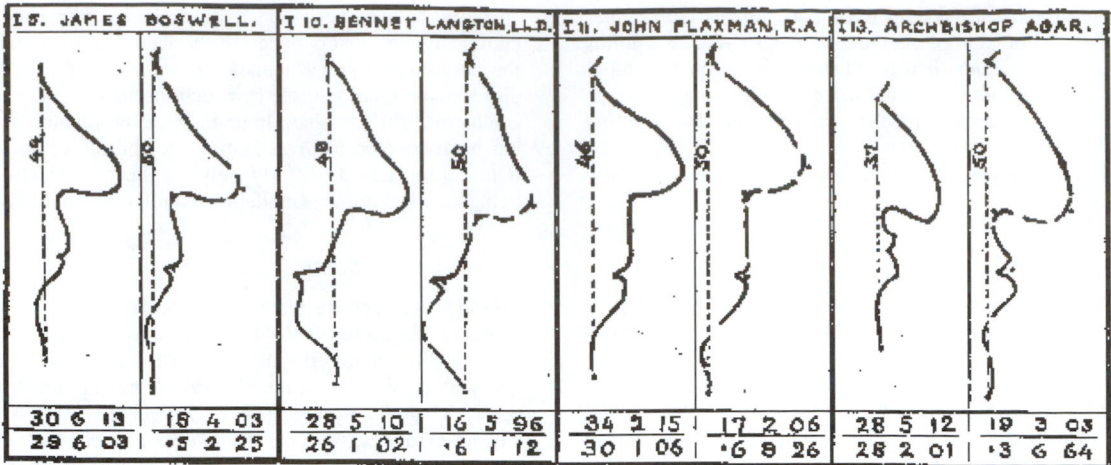

Figure 3. Face profiles described (left member of each pair) and reconstructed (right member of each pair) from 20 telegraphic numbers arranged in five groups of four (bottom). The code uses the relationships between five cardinal points on the profile. Galton was perhaps the first to use the term *cardinal points* to describe a multidimensional feature space for object recognition. (Source: From Galton, F., 1910, *Nature (Lond.)*, March 31, 127–130.)

Principal Component Analysis of Faces

Galton was the first to treat faces as mathematical objects and to add them photographically. The *average face* was held to be especially beautiful, possibly because smallpox scars and other blemishes were removed. Galton also presented the average faces of groups such as rapists, clergymen, and athletes. Any particular face could then be correlated with each average in turn and described by a vector **V**. This vector will tell us the extent of resemblance of that face to the mean rapist, the mean clergyman, the mean athlete, and so on. The average images are a *basis set* for describing all faces. Dimensional reduction has been achieved, as long as the dimension of **V** is less than that of the original image space, N^2. Whether the clergyman-athlete-rapist space is a good one is another matter. It is probably not, because the dimensions are correlated. The aim of most feature analysis, including principal component analysis (PCA), is to ensure that the dimensions of the feature space are uncorrelated, or, in other words, that the axes in the space are *orthogonal*.

The idea behind PCA for faces (or Karhunen-Loeve expansion) is to find a set of features called *eigenvectors* that span the subspace of images in which faces lie (Turk and Pentland, 1991). Each eigenvector has dimensions N^2 and is a linear combination of a set of training faces, each of dimension N by N pixels. Equivalently, each face in the training set is a linear combination of the N^2 eigenvectors. To achieve dimensional reduction, only the most important eigenvectors are chosen as a basis set. These are the vectors that correlate most highly with the members of the training set. The most important, in this sense, is the average image, as defined by Galton.

Since the eigenvectors resemble faces when they are represented as 2D images, they can be called *eigenfaces*. Examples are shown in Figure 4. Once the eigenfaces have been created, each face in the training set can be described by a set of numbers representing its correlation to each of the eigenfaces in turn. If seven eigenfaces are chosen to span the face space, each face will be described by a vector of seven numbers instead of by its pixel values. A huge dimensional reduction has been achieved. The problem of recognizing a face is now a simple one of pattern recognition: finding the vector in memory that it most closely resembles.

PCA has been used for face detection, face recognition, and sex classification. Effective caricatures can be derived by exaggerating the differences of a face from the average. An intriguing experiment by Leopold, O'Toole, and Blanz (2001) suggests that the brain may use a feature space to identify faces. Observers were trained to discriminate "Adam," who was described by a vector in face space, from "Anti-Adam," who had the directly opposite vector. After adapting to Adam for some minutes, observers were more likely to classify the average face (midway between Adam and Anti-Adam) as Anti-Adam than as Adam. The inference is that there exist feature detectors that are tuned in face space and that identification depends on a population code comprising these detectors.

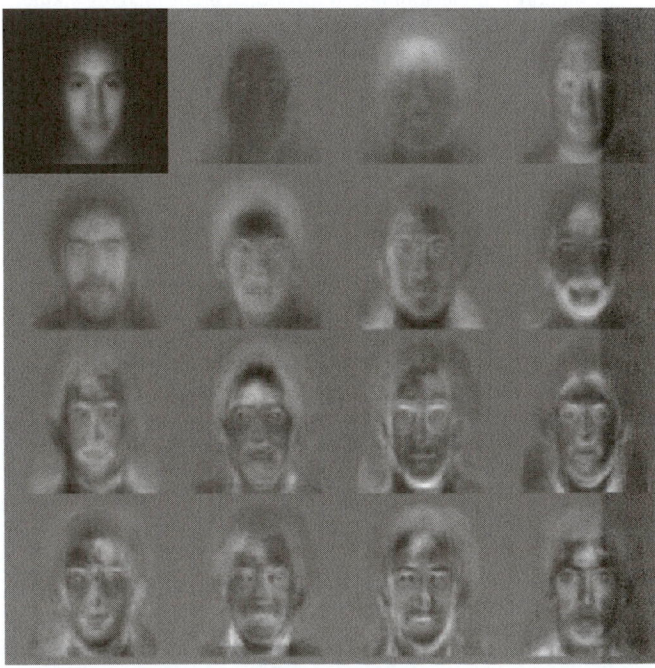

Figure 4. Eigenfaces for face recognition. (Source: Reproduced with permission from the interactive MIT Media Lab Web site: *http://www-white.media.mit.edu/vismod/demos/facerec/basic.html*)

Fourier Freaks and Feature Creatures

In broad terms, we now see that the code for early vision will be cracked when we find the basis set used by the brain for describing the image. One such basis set is the Fourier transform: sinusoids of differing frequency, orientation, and phase are the eigenfunctions of linear systems (Turk and Pentland, 1991). Following the application of certain key ideas in linear systems theory to vision (Robson, 1980), there was much debate about whether feature analysis or Fourier analysis was the preferred vehicle for understanding biological vision. This entertaining but ultimately fruitless debate is now essentially dead and buried. It made sense only when the "Fourier freaks" maintained that objects were recognized exclusively from their global amplitude spectrum. Since no one will now admit to having thought such a thing, it is pointless to provide historical detail.

Contrary to the view that the Fourier amplitude spectrum carries the important information in natural images, it is now recognized that the amplitude spectrum of most images is very similar (Field, 1987). The interesting features of images such as the boundaries of objects are represented in the relative *phases* of Fourier components. An edge or a bar in the image is a place where Fourier components undergo constructive interference. If the global amplitude spectra of two different images such as faces are interchanged, the hybrid images look like the images from which their phase spectra are derived (Figure 5). However, this is true only for the global Fourier transform. If the image is decomposed into a number of overlapping patches and each patch is transformed, it is the amplitude rather than the phase information in the patches that determines the appearance of the image if the patch size is sufficiently small (Figure 5). This is self-evidently true when the patch size is a single pixel, because the transform contains only the DC level and no phase information. But the limit is reached before a single pixel. Further work is needed to determine how the limiting patch size varies in different images and whether it is determined by cycles/image or cycles/degree of visual angle.

The consensus view now is that Fourier analysis in the visual system is limited to a local or *patchwise* Fourier analysis and that this is performed by neurons in V1 with localized, oriented, and spatial-frequency-tuned receptive fields (Robson, 1980). The idea of patchwise spatial frequency analysis fits in well with the architectural division of V1 into *hypercolumns*, each containing a full range of orientations and spatial frequencies, with a scatter of their receptive fields within a region of the image (Hubel and Wiesel, 1977). According to this model, the receptive fields of simple cells in V1 provide a *basis set* for describing local properties of the image, comparable to the wavelet transform in image processing (Olshausen and Field, 1996). Putting this simply, the idea is that an object can be recognized locally in an image by a series of numbers representing its effect on the activity of a population of detectors tuned individually in orientation and spatial frequency. Dimensional reduction is achieved because pointwise intensity values have been discarded and replaced by a more economical code. Just how many types of receptive field are needed to provide a satisfactory basis set for describing natural images is a question of equal interest to psychophysics and image processing.

PCA is far from being the only way to find a suitable basis set for natural images. Receptive fields like those in V1 emerge naturally as a basis set from a learning algorithm that seeks a sparse code for natural images (Olshausen and Field, 1996). The aim of sparse coding is to have each image activate the smallest possible number of members of the basis set. In physiological terms, the aim would be to have as many neurons as possible not activated at all by the image. Using this approach, Olshausen and Field derived a basis set having an impressive similarity to the receptive fields of V1 neurons (Figure 6).

The Primal Sketch

The ability of line drawings to convey shape is very strong evidence that the feature space for object recognition may be of drastically reduced dimensionality, compared to the space of all possible images. Just a few lines drawn on a flat surface can suggest the face of a well-known person or the idea "no skateboarding allowed." Impressed by the effectiveness of cartoons, David Marr (1982) proposed that the earliest stages of vision transform the continuous gray-level image into a neural cartoon, which he called "the primal sketch." Since cartoons emphasize primarily the outlines of shapes, the main objective of the primal sketch is to find *edges* in the image, edges being the loci of points on the 3D object where an object

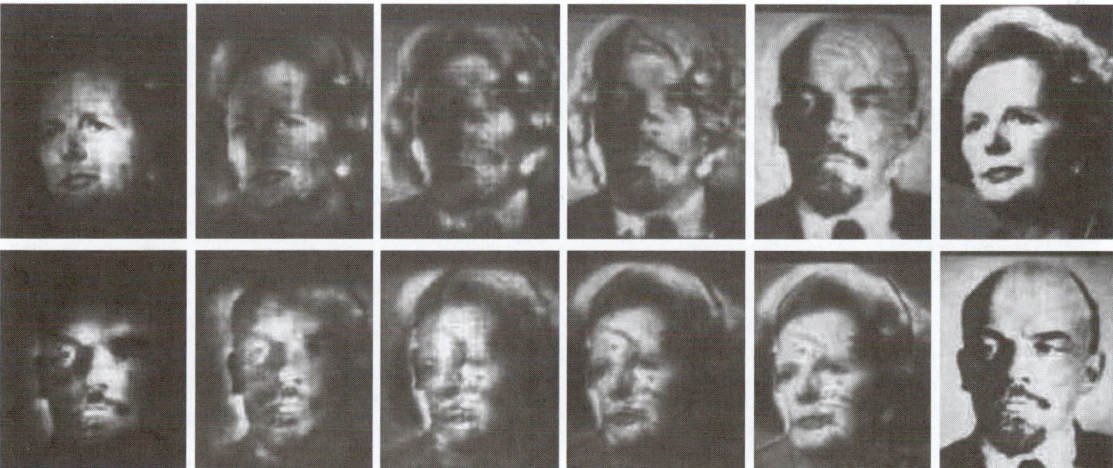

Figure 5. Images of two political theorists (rightmost panels), one of whose ideas have been recently discredited. Each thinker contributes his or her phase from the Fourier transform to each of the images on the left; the amplitude information comes from the other face. The Fourier transform is not global but is rather derived from overlapping patches, the size of which decreases (64, 32, 16, 8, and 4 pixels) from left to right. When the patch size is large, the appearance of the image is dominated by phase information; when it is small, the appearance is dominated by the amplitude of the Fourier components. At intermediate patch sizes, the appearance is composite. (Source: Reproduced with permission from Morgan et al., 1991.)

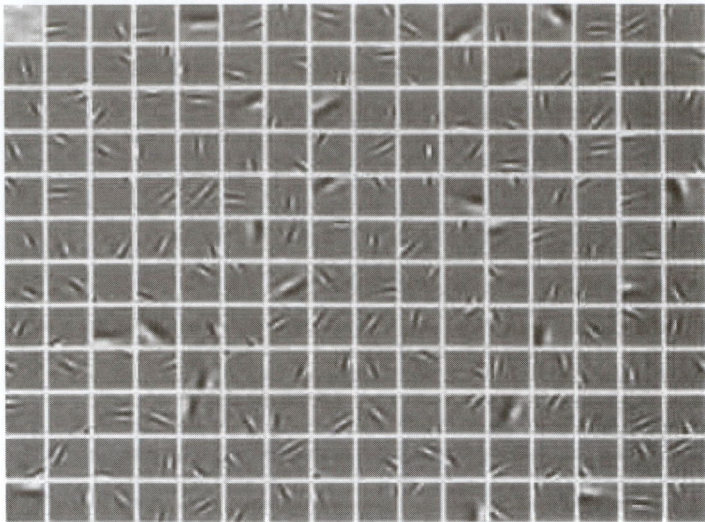

Figure 6. A basis set derived from ten 512 by 512 natural images of the American Northwest by a training algorithm aimed at maximizing the sparseness of the representation. The basis set bears a striking similarity to the receptive fields of V1 neurons, suggesting that they too form an efficient basis set for describing natural images. (Source: Reproduced with permission from Olshausen and Field, 1996.)

occludes itself or objects that are farther away (edge of a cube), or where there is a rapid change in the direction of the tangent plane to the object surface (outline of the nose on a face), or where there is some abrupt change in surface reflectance (boundary of the iris). It is a remarkable fact that much of the edge structure of an object in the image depends on its 3D structure—remarkable because we recognize objects from a variety of viewpoints or from sketches made from a variety of viewpoints.

If we consider an edge such as the outline of the nostril on a face, we shall find in its image a sudden change in luminance, which is not predictable from the gradual changes around it. A discontinuity is conveniently found by a local maximum or minimum in the first spatial derivative of the luminance profile or, equivalently, a *zero-crossing* in the second derivative. Ernst Mach (followed by William McDougall in his quaint "drainage" theory) was the first to conjecture that the visual system uses second derivatives to find features in the luminance profile, his evidence being the appearance of "Mach bands" on the inflection points in luminance ramps. Marr and Hildreth (see Marr, 1982) proposed that the receptive fields of retinal ganglion cells and simple cells in V1 make them nearly ideal second-derivative operators (Laplacians of Gaussians) and that their function is to produce the primal sketch. Different sizes of receptive field produce cartoons at different *spatial scales*, corresponding to the different frequencies in the Fourier transform but agreeing on the position of zero-crossings at the most significant points in the image. This recalls the fact that an edge or a bar in the image is a place where Fourier components undergo constructive interference. The primal sketch neatly uses wavelets to locate edges and turns them into particles.

A wide variety of phenomena have been used to investigate the nature of the "spatial primitives" or features in human vision. These include Mach bands, the Chevreul illusion, the apparent location of bars and edges in gratings and plaids with different spatial frequency components, and edge blur discrimination. Various primitives have been considered, such as zero-crossings, zero-bounded regions, and local energy maxima. Although it is now possible to predict the apparent location of edges and bars in images with a fair degree of accuracy, there is no consensus as yet about the nature or existence of primitives or about the way in which they are combined over spatial scale (Morgan and Watt, 1997).

Summary

Features are useful for describing natural images because the latter have massive informational redundancy. Image space itself is too vast to search directly. Feature analysis depends on the proposition that the search for particular objects can be concentrated in a subspace of image space: *the feature space*. Biologists expect that there will be special sensory mechanisms for searching just the right subspace for a particular task. Ethologists and animal learning theorists concur. Useful hints about likely feature spaces may be obtained from engineers working on image compression. Although in the past feature analysis was contrasted with Fourier analysis, the modern synthesis is that a patchwise Fourier analysis by localized receptive fields in primary visual cortex (V1) provides the primitive basis set for the feature space of vision. These form the basis set for the elaboration of neurons responding selectively to geometrical features in area TE of the inferotemporal cortex, and these in turn from the basis for object recognition in different but overlapping areas of IT.

Road Map: Vision
Related Reading: Gabor Wavelets and Statistical Pattern Recognition; Global Visual Pattern Extraction; Object Recognition, Neurophysiology; Orientation Selectivity

References

Field, D. J., 1987, Relations between the statistics of natural images and the response properties of cortical cells, *J. Opt. Soc. Am. A Opt. Image Sci. Vis.*, 4(12):2379–2394.

Gonzalez, R., and Woods, R., 1993, *Digital Image Processing*, Reading, MA: Addison-Wesley. ◆

Hubel, D. H., and Wiesel, T. N., 1977, Functional architecture of the macaque monkey visual cortex: Ferrier Lecture, *Proc. R. Soc. Lond. B Biol. Sci.*, 198:1–59. ◆

Leopold, D., O'Toole, A. T, and Blanz, V., 2001, Prototype-references shape encoding revealed by high-level aftereffects, *Nature Neurosci.*, 4:89–94.

Lettvin, J. Y., Maturana, R. R., McCulloch, W. S., and Pitts, W. H., 1959, What the frog's eye tells the frog's brain, *Proc. Inst. Rad. Eng.*, 47:1940–1951.

Logothetis, N. K., and Sheinberg, D. L., 1996, Visual object recognition, *Ann. Rev. Neurosci.*, 19:577–621. ◆

Marr, D., 1982, *Vision*, San Francisco: W.H. Freeman. ◆

Morgan, M. J., Ross, J., and Hayes, A., 1991, The relative importance of local phase and local amplitude in patchwise image reconstruction, *Biol. Cybern.*, 65:113–119.

Morgan, M. J., and Watt, R. J., 1997, The combination of filters in early spatial vision: A retrospective analysis of the MIRAGE model, *Perception*, 26:1073–1088. ◆

Olshausen, B., and Field, D, 1996, Emergence of simple-cell receptive field properties by learning a spare code for natural images, *Nature*, 381:607–609.

Robson, J. G., 1980, Neural images: The physiological basis of spatial vision, in *Visual Coding and Adaptability* (C. S. Harris, Ed.), Hillsdale, NJ: Lawrence Erlbaum, pp. 177–214. ◆

Tanaka, K., 1996, Inferotemporal cortex and object vision, *Ann. Rev. Neurosci.*, 19:109–139. ◆

Treisman, A. M., 1988, Features and objects: The 14th Bartlett Memorial Lecture, *Q. J. Exp. Psychol. A*, 40:201–237. ◆

Turk, M., and Pentland, A., 1991, Face recognition using eigenfaces, in *Proceedings of the 1991 IEEE Computer Society Conference on Computer Vision and Pattern Recognition*, Los Alamitos, CA, USA: IEEE Computer Society Press, pp. 586–591.

Watanabe, S., Lea, S., and Dittrich, W., 1993, What can we learn from experiments in pigeon concept formation?, in *Vision, Brain and Behaviour in Birds* (H. Zeigler and H.-J. Bischof, Eds.), Cambridge, MA: MIT Press. ◆

Filtering, Adaptive

John J. Shynk

Introduction

Adaptive filtering is an active area of research that has found widespread use in numerous signal processing and communications applications (Haykin, 2002). These applications include a wide range of important problems, such as noise canceling and noise reduction, channel equalization, co-channel signal separation, system identification, pattern recognition, fetal heart monitoring, and array processing (Ljung and Söderström, 1983; Qureshi, 1985; Giannakis, 1999). Adaptive filters are particularly useful for applications in which the underlying statistics are unknown or nonstationary, which is usually the case in practice (Widrow and Stearns, 1985). The parameters of an adaptive filter are adjusted to "learn" or track signal and system variations according to a performance criterion that is determined by the needs of the specific application.

The field of adaptive filtering was derived partly from work on neural networks and adaptive pattern recognition (Lippmann, 1987; Haykin, 1999). In pattern recognition applications, such as speech recognition and image classification, a neural network can be trained on a wide range of representative input patterns (called the training set). If the training set is sufficiently large, the neural net is capable of successfully classifying new patterns; for example, distorted patterns corrupted by noise will be mapped to the most similar pattern in the training set, as defined by some error criterion. Classification is performed by a threshold or decision device that quantizes the neural net output to one of many different levels representing the various classes.

An adaptive filter can be viewed as a signal combiner consisting of a set of adjustable weights (or coefficients represented by a polynomial) and an algorithm (learning rule) that updates these weights using the filter input and output, as well as other available signals. The filter may include internal signal feedback, whereby delayed versions of the output are used to generate the current output, and it may contain some nonlinear components. The single-layer perceptron is a well-known type of adaptive filter that has a binary output nonlinearity; it is also referred to as *adaline* (for *ada*ptive *lin*ear *neu*ron) (Widrow and Lehr, 1990) (see PERCEPTRONS, ADALINES, AND BACKPROPAGATION). A multilayer perceptron contains many single-layer perceptrons interconnected to form a network that can implement a complex nonlinear system or represent a multidimensional signal pattern (Rumelhart and McClelland, 1986)

It is beyond the scope of this article to cover in depth the different types of adaptive filter configurations and the large number of adaptive algorithms. Instead, we will focus on the most widely used adaptive filter architecture and describe in some detail two representative adaptive algorithms. The least-mean-square (LMS) algorithm (Widrow and Stearns, 1985) computes the coefficients of a tapped delay line (TDL), which is basically a shift register with adjustable coefficients. The constant modulus algorithm (CMA) (Godard, 1980; Treichler and Agee, 1983) also computes the coefficients of a TDL, but, unlike the LMS algorithm, it does not require a training sequence. As we shall see, both algorithms are stochastic-gradient methods that iteratively search for the minimum of well-defined performance (cost) functions. Example CMA performance functions are plotted to reveal their nonquadratic shapes, and computer simulations of the CMA weight trajectories are shown to illustrate the algorithm's learning behavior for an equalization application.

Adaptive Filter Components

An adaptive filter consists of two components: (1) an *adjustable set of weights* that filter or process the input signal and (2) an *adaptive algorithm* that modifies the weights to minimize a performance measure. To be more precise, define the weight vector

$$W(n) \triangleq [w_1(n), w_2(n), \ldots, w_N(n)]^T \tag{1}$$

and the input signal vector

$$X(n) \triangleq [x_1(n), x_2(n), \ldots, x_N(n)]^T \tag{2}$$

where the argument n denotes discrete time and the superscript T is matrix/vector transpose. This particular form of the signal vector contains N distinct inputs and would be appropriate for multidimensional applications such as pattern recognition and array processing. However, there are many signal processing applications involving only one input signal, such as channel equalization, echo cancellation, and system identification. For these cases, the input signal vector would instead be

$$X(n) \triangleq [x(n), x(n-1), \ldots, x(n-N+1)]^T \tag{3}$$

where delayed versions of the input signal $x(n)$ are stored in a shift register or TDL.

The (scalar) filter output is given by the inner product

$$y(n) = W^T(n)X(n) = X^T(n)W(n) \tag{4}$$

It is typically used by the adaptive algorithm in a feedback mechanism that determines how $W(n)$ should be adjusted with each new input vector $X(n)$. In some applications, $y(n)$ is processed by a nonlinear device that yields a decision statistic for an underlying signal contained in the input $X(n)$. For example, in a digital communications application with binary (± 1) transmitted symbols in an additive white Gaussian noise channel (Proakis, 2001), the nonlinearity could be the signum function:

$$\text{sgn}(y(n)) = \begin{cases} +1, & y(n) \geq 0 \\ -1, & y(n) < 0 \end{cases} \qquad (5)$$

where we have arbitrarily assigned $\text{sgn}(0) = +1$. This detector uses the sign of the received signal $y(n)$ to determine the most likely transmitted symbol: $+1$ or -1. The signum function is also used for Rosenblatt's training algorithm (Lippmann, 1987), while a soft nonlinearity such as the hyperbolic tangent is used in the back-propagation algorithm for the multilayer perceptron (Widrow and Lehr, 1990).

The error signal in Figure 1 depends on the application and the performance function; we will provide details of the error in a subsequent section when the adaptive algorithms are discussed. However, at this point we should mention that the error can be generated in (at least) two basic ways. If a training signal $d(n)$ is available (such as in the previously mentioned digital communications application), then the error is a measure of how much $y(n)$ differs from $d(n)$; in this scenario, the training signal is sometimes called the *desired response* in the adaptive filtering literature. For some problems, however, a training signal is not available (also in the digital communications application); in this case, the error is computed in a *blind* manner, which means that it depends only on the adaptive filter input $X(n)$ and output $y(n)$, without any explicit desired-response information.

Applications

Two representative applications of adaptive filtering are described in this section. Many signal processing applications fall into one of these general models. For example, adaptive channel equalization belongs to the field of deconvolution, and some co-channel signal separation techniques utilize an array processing formulation.

Channel Equalization

The configuration for adaptive channel equalization is shown in Figure 2 (Qureshi, 1985). Observe that the adaptive filter is placed in *cascade* with the unknown channel. The goal of the adaptive filter is to mitigate the channel distortion (e.g., multipath propagation) and, in effect, estimate the channel *inverse*. The input of the adaptive filter is obtained from the channel output, which may be corrupted by an additive (Gaussian) noise process $v(n)$. The training signal (desired response) is the transmitted signal $x(n)$. However, since the channel and the adaptive filter each have a finite non-zero delay, it is necessary that the transmitted signal be delayed by an appropriate amount $\Delta > 0$ such that $d(n) = x(n - \Delta)$.

Clearly, since the purpose of any communication system is to transmit information (unknown to the receiver) across the channel,

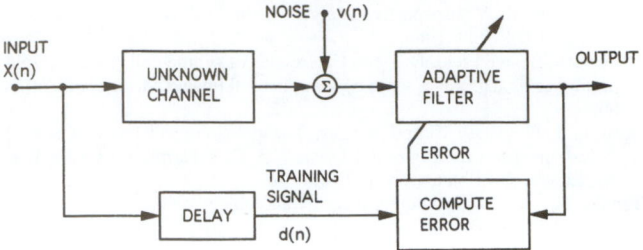

Figure 2. Adaptive channel equalization.

the configuration in Figure 2 for training the adaptive filter is not always feasible. Typically, there is a short training period at the beginning of transmission (start-up) whereby a signal known at the receive end is transmitted and used by the adaptive filter to adjust its weights. When the error rate is sufficiently reduced at the end of training, information can be successfully transmitted across the channel. During this time, the adaptive algorithm stops updating; or, alternatively, a decision-directed or blind adaptive algorithm can be employed that requires knowledge only of certain statistical properties of the transmitted signal (Haykin, 2002).

Co-channel Signal Separation

In cellular communication systems, co-channel interference is becoming an increasingly important issue as the number of subscribers grows (Giannakis, 1999). Co-channel interference is due to frequency reuse, whereby multiple cells operate on the same carrier frequency. To mitigate co-channel interference, it would be desirable to incorporate adaptive antennas that have a directional (beamforming) capability to separate several co-channel signals, thus allowing for greater frequency reuse. In recent years there has been much interest in blind co-channel signal separation algorithms for antenna arrays that can adapt their parameters without using a training signal.

A block diagram of an adaptive array known as the constant modulus (CM) array (Gooch and Lundell, 1986) is shown in Figure 3, where the antenna elements are uniformly spaced and omnidirectional. It consists of two components: (1) a conventional adaptive antenna (beamformer) with weights updated by CMA, and (2) an adaptive signal canceler that removes from the input the co-channel signal captured by the CM array. The weights of the signal canceler are updated by the LMS algorithm using the received array signals as the desired response. A multistage implementation of this architecture, consisting of multiple beamformer/canceler systems in cascade, can be used to separate and recover several co-channel signals (one co-channel signal per stage).

Adaptive Algorithms

In this section, we consider two performance functions: the squared error, which employs a training sequence, and a constant modulus formulation, which yields a blind adaptive algorithm. Both algorithms have the following general form:

$$W(n + 1) = W(n) + \mu[-\nabla(n)] \qquad (6)$$

where $\nabla(n)$ is the *gradient* with respect to $W(n)$ of the corresponding performance function. The positive step size μ controls the transient and steady-state convergence properties of the adaptive weights. The goal of an adaptive algorithm is to adjust $W(n)$ such that it converges to a minimum (stationary point) of the performance function.

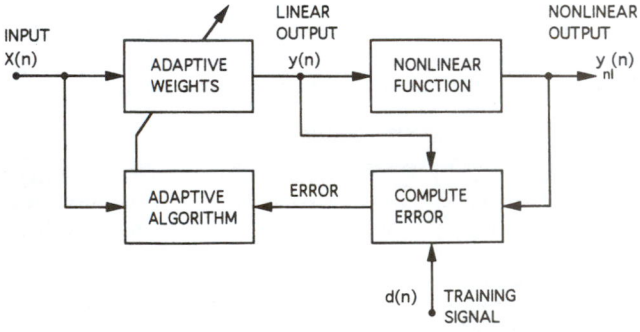

Figure 1. Adaptive filter components.

Figure 3. Co-channel signal separation.

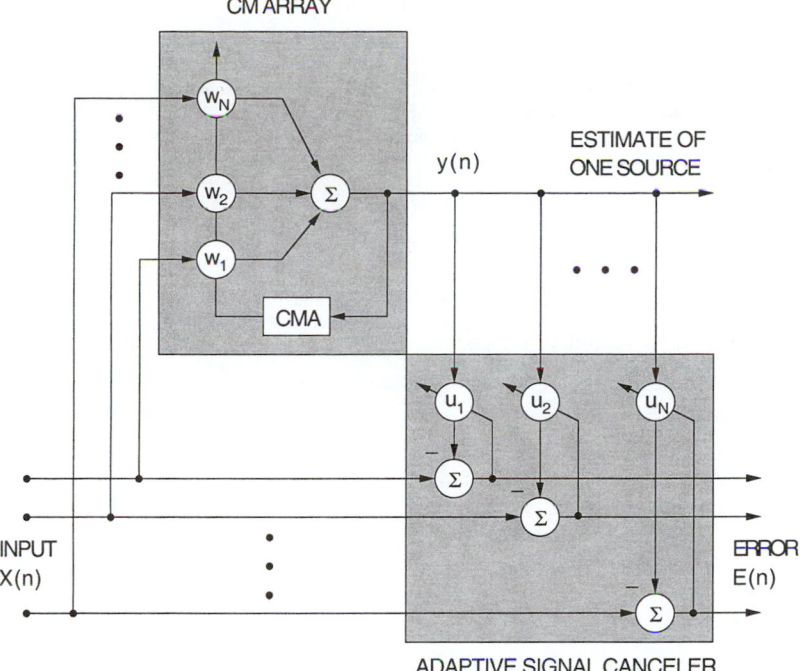

Least-Mean-Square Algorithm

Consider the following performance function:

$$C_{LMS}(n) = e^2(n) \qquad (7)$$

where the error is

$$e(n) = d(n) - y(n) \qquad (8)$$

and $d(n)$ is the training sequence. Note that $C_{LMS}(n)$ is a stochastic variable that fluctuates around the mean square error (MSE), given by

$$\xi_{LMS} = E[e^2(n)] \qquad (9)$$

where $E[\cdot]$ denotes statistical expectation. For this reason, the weight update is referred to as a *stochastic-gradient* algorithm. $C_{LMS}(n)$ can be viewed as a very simple estimate of the ensemble average ξ_{LMS}. (In this article, we interchangeably refer to ξ and its stochastic estimate $C(n)$ as performance functions.) Using Equations 4 and 8, and noting that $\partial(W^T(n)X(n))/\partial W(n) = X(n)$, the gradient of Equation 7 is

$$\nabla_{LMS}(n) = -2X(n)e(n) \qquad (10)$$

resulting in the least-mean-square (LMS) algorithm (Widrow and Stearns, 1985):

$$W(n + 1) = W(n) + 2\mu X(n)e(n) \qquad (11)$$

Thus, with each new set of data $\{X(n), d(n)\}$, the error $e(n)$ is computed and the filter weights are updated in an attempt to learn the underlying signal statistics. The algorithm converges on average (i.e., in the mean) when $E[X(n)e(n)] = \underline{0}$ (the zero vector) which, after substituting $e(n)$, yields the following unique stationary point:

$$W_{LMS} = R^{-1}P \qquad (12)$$

where $R \triangleq E[X(n)X^T(n)]$ and $P \triangleq E[X(n)d(n)]$ are signal correlations (an $N \times N$ matrix and an $N \times 1$ vector, respectively). Observe that the algorithm utilizes the output $y(n)$ before it is pro-

cessed by any subsequent nonlinear device (as illustrated in Figure 1).

Constant Modulus Algorithm

The constant modulus algorithm (CMA) is a blind equalization technique that attempts to restore the constant modulus property of certain communication signals (the binary digital communication signal with values ±1 is such an example). The performance function is a measure of the deviation of the modulus of the equalizer output $y(n)$ from a predetermined constant $r > 0$ according to Treichler and Agee (1983):

$$C_{CMA}(n) = \||y(n)|^p - r^p|^q \qquad (13)$$

where p and q are positive integers, equal to 1 or 2, resulting in four versions of CMA. The scalar r is usually chosen such that the gradient of ξ_{CMA} (the expectation of Equation 13) with respect to the coefficients $W(n)$ is zero when the channel is perfectly equalized. (Note that although $C_{CMA}(n)$ depends on p and q, in order to simplify the notation, we do not indicate this explicitly.)

The gradient of Equation 13 is

$$\nabla_{CMA}(n) = pqX(n)y(n)|y(n)|^{p-2}$$
$$\times (|y(n)|^p - r^p)^{q-1}\text{sgn}[|y(n)|^p - r^p]^q \qquad (14)$$

where $\text{sgn}[\cdot]$ is the signum function previously defined. For convenience, consider the case of $p = q = 2$. Substituting Equation 14 into Equation 6 yields the 2-2 version of CMA:

$$W(n + 1) = W(n) - 4\mu X(n)y(n)(|y(n)|^2 - r^2) \qquad (15)$$

This recursion does not depend on a training sequence; the update is a function only of $X(n)$ and $y(n) = W^T(n)X(n)$. Note that Equation 15 is similar to Equation 11, except that the scalar error $e(n)$ has been replaced by $-2y(n)(|y(n)|^2 - r^2)$.

Unfortunately, since $\xi_{CMA} = E[C_{CMA}(n)]$ is not a quadratic function of $W(n)$ (as is ξ_{LMS}), it is not possible to derive a simple general expression for the stationary point W_{CMA}. In fact, the stationary point is not necessarily unique, and there may be local as well as global minima (the gradient is zero at a local minimum, but a local minimum does not correspond to the overall minimum value of the performance function). However, for the sake of completeness, if we assume that the input $X(n)$ is a Gaussian random vector with zero mean, then it can be shown that the stationary points are given by the following implicit expression (Shynk and Chan, 1993):

$$W_{CMA}^T R W_{CMA} = r^2/3 \qquad (16)$$

Thus, there is an infinity of solutions, all of which achieve the global minimum. Note, however, that this result does not apply in general, because $X(n)$ might be generated by an underlying constant modulus signal (which CMA is designed to handle), in which case $X(n)$ would not be exactly Gaussian.

Convergence Results

In this section, we present some examples of the performance surfaces for CMA, as well as representative trajectories of the CMA weights during adaptation. A *performance surface* is a three-dimensional plot of the performance function versus two of the weight vector components.

CMA Performance Surfaces

Suppose that CMA attempts to equalize a channel with the following transfer function (written using z-transform notation): $C(z) = 1 - 0.6z^{-1} + 0.36\, z^{-2}$. Assume that the transmitted signal is a sequence of binary symbols ± 1 that are independent and equally likely (i.e., Bernoulli with $\Pr(+1) = \Pr(-1) = \frac{1}{2}$). The elements of the corresponding correlation matrix R are $R(1, 1) = R(2, 2) = 1.4896$ and $R(1, 2) = R(2, 1) = -0.8160$. Figure 4A shows the performance surface of a two-weight ($N = 2$) equalizer for the CMA 2-2 performance function. Observe that there are two global minima and two local minima (there is also a local maximum at the origin $W = \underline{0}$). Thus, depending on how the algorithm is initialized, the adaptive weights may converge to any one of these four minima, two of which are not optimal. Similar results are shown in Figure 4B for the CMA 1-1 performance function. In contrast, the performance surface for the LMS algorithm (which uses training) is a paraboloid with a unique global minimum and no local minima (provided R is positive definite) (Widrow and Stearns, 1985).

CMA Weight Trajectories

In adaptive algorithms that employ a gradient update mechanism, such as LMS and CMA, a trade-off exists between the convergence rate and the steady-state value of the MSE (even though the MSE is not the performance function for CMA, it is typically used as a benchmark measure for the performance of a blind algorithm). Both of these properties are controlled by the step size μ, as well as the statistics of the input $X(n)$. When μ is increased, the rate of convergence also increases, but so does the steady-state MSE. Thus, when comparing the convergence behavior of different stochastic-gradient algorithms, it is necessary that the steady-state and transient properties be considered together. For example, the convergence rates of two algorithms can be compared once the step sizes are chosen so that the algorithms achieve the same steady-state MSE.

Figure 5A shows this trade-off for CMA 2-2 for a channel equalization application. These "learning curves" were obtained by averaging the squared error between the equalizer output $y(n)$ and the desired (transmitted) signal $d(n)$ (with an appropriate delay) over ten independent computer runs; the resulting trajectories were then smoothed by a moving average filter. Observe that the steady-state

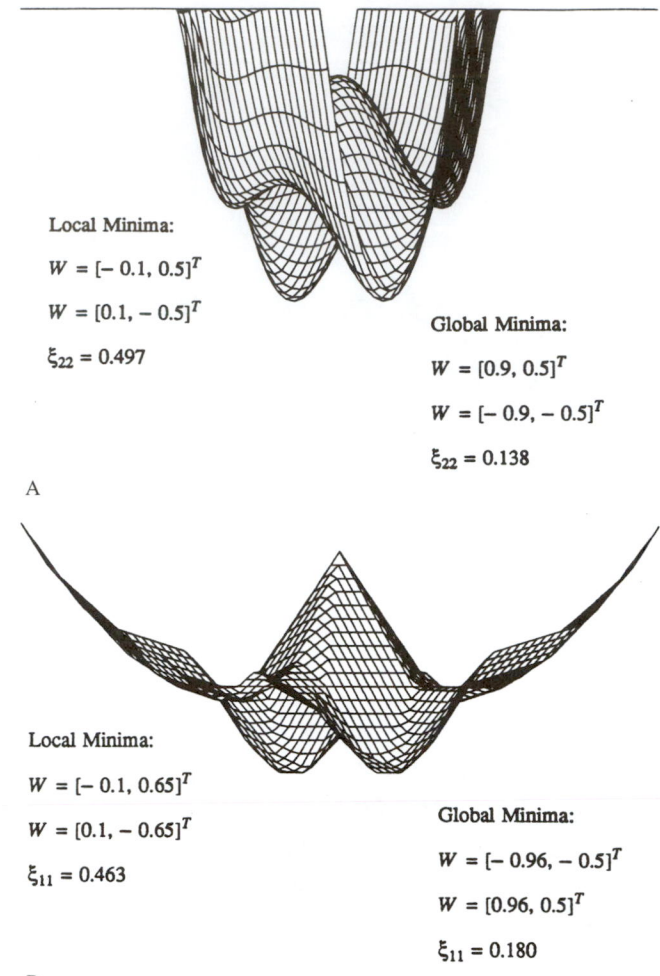

Local Minima:

$W = [-0.1, 0.5]^T$

$W = [0.1, -0.5]^T$

$\xi_{22} = 0.497$

Global Minima:

$W = [0.9, 0.5]^T$

$W = [-0.9, -0.5]^T$

$\xi_{22} = 0.138$

A

Local Minima:

$W = [-0.1, 0.65]^T$

$W = [0.1, -0.65]^T$

$\xi_{11} = 0.463$

Global Minima:

$W = [-0.96, -0.5]^T$

$W = [0.96, 0.5]^T$

$\xi_{11} = 0.180$

B

Figure 4. Performance surfaces ξ_{CMA}. A, CMA 2-2 ($p = q = 2$). B, CMA 1-1 ($p = q = 1$). (From Shynk, J. J., and Chan, C. K., 1993, Performance surfaces of the constant modulus algorithm based on a conditional Gaussian model, *IEEE Trans. Signal Proc.*, 41:1965–1969. © 1993, IEEE. Reprinted with permission.)

MSE and the convergence rate increase with increasing μ. In order to compare algorithms without having to explicitly consider the step size, several simulations can be performed for the algorithms, each simulation with a different value of μ. From this series of simulations, the number of samples required to reach steady state can be determined, along with the steady-state value of the MSE. Using this information, the steady-state MSE can be plotted versus the convergence time for each algorithm. Examples of these "performance curves" for the four versions of CMA are shown in Figure 5B (Shynk et al., 1991). Notice that the performance curve for CMA 1-2 is generally higher than the other curves, indicating that it requires (for this example) more iterations to achieve the same steady-state MSE for a wide range of step size values.

Discussion

Adaptive filters are widely used for a variety of signal processing applications. Although several configurations are possible, the linear combiner shown in Figure 1 is the most common, and the LMS algorithm, which is known to be robust (Haykin, 2002), is the most popular means of adjusting the adaptive weights. There are several

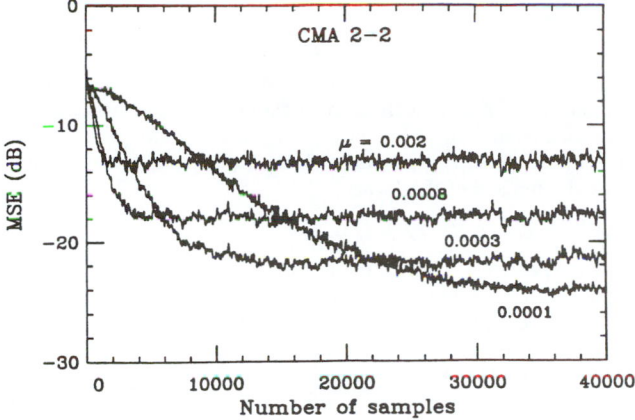

A

B

Figure 5. *A*, CMA learning curves. *B*, CMA performance curves. (From Shynk, J. J., Gooch, R. P., Giridhar, K., and Chan, C. K., 1991, A comparative performance study of several blind equalization algorithms, in *Proceedings of the SPIE Conference on Adaptive Signal Processing.* © 1991, SPIE. Reprinted with permission.)

variations of the LMS algorithm, including those that have less complexity or improved convergence properties. For example, CMA is a blind stochastic-gradient algorithm that can be used instead of the LMS algorithm when an explicit training sequence is not available. The recursive-least-squares (RLS) algorithm is an adaptive algorithm based on the method of least squares that offers faster convergence rates (compared with the LMS algorithm), but at the expense of an increased computational complexity (Haykin, 2002).

The adaptive filter configuration described in this article is the basic component of a multilayer perceptron. These additional layers provide greater nonlinear modeling capabilities, which is usually necessary for complex applications such as speech and image processing. Stochastic-gradient algorithms are typically used to adjust the weights of a multilayer perceptron. They are similar to the adaptive algorithms described in this article, but they have an additional degree of complexity owing to the cascade of layers. One such algorithm, known as the backpropagation algorithm (Rumelhart and McClelland, 1986), has been successfully applied to a number of signal processing problems (Widrow and Lehr, 1990).

Road Map: Applications
Background: Perceptrons, Adalines, and Backpropagation
Related Reading: Forecasting; Kalman Filtering: Neural Implications; Recurrent Networks: Learning Algorithms

References

Giannakis, G. B., Ed., 1999, Highlights of signal processing for communications, *IEEE Signal Proc. Mag.*, 16:14–50. ◆

Godard, D. N., 1980, Self-recovering equalization and carrier tracking in two-dimensional data communication systems, *IEEE Trans. Commun.*, COM-28:1867–1875.

Gooch, R. P., and Lundell, J. D., 1986, The CM array: An adaptive beamformer for constant modulus signals, in *Proceedings of the IEEE International Conference on Acoustics, Speech, and Signal Processing*, New York: IEEE, pp. 2523–2526.

Haykin, S., 1999, *Neural Networks: A Comprehensive Foundation*, Upper Saddle River, NJ: Prentice-Hall. ◆

Haykin, S., 2002, *Adaptive Filter Theory*, 4th ed., Upper Saddle River, NJ: Prentice-Hall. ◆

Lippmann, R. P., 1987, An introduction to computing with neural nets, *IEEE ASSP Mag.*, 4:4–22. ◆

Ljung, L., and Söderström, T., 1983, *Theory and Practice of Recursive Identification*, Cambridge, MA: MIT Press.

Proakis, J. G., 2001, *Digital Communications*, 4th ed., New York: McGraw-Hill. ◆

Qureshi, S. U. H., 1985, Adaptive equalization, *Proc. IEEE*, 73:1349–1387. ◆

Rumelhart, D. E., and McClelland, J. L., Eds., 1986, *Parallel Distributed Processing: Explorations in the Microstructure of Cognition*, Cambridge, MA: MIT Press. ◆

Shynk, J. J., and Chan, C. K., 1993, Performance surfaces of the constant modulus algorithm based on a conditional Gaussian model, *IEEE Trans. Signal Proc.*, 41:1965–1969.

Shynk, J. J., Gooch, R. P., Giridhar, K., and Chan, C. K., 1991, A comparative performance study of several blind equalization algorithms, in *Proceedings of the SPIE Conference on Adaptive Signal Processing*, Bellingham, WA: SPIE, pp. 1565:102–117. ◆

Treichler, J. R., and Agee, B. G., 1983, A new approach to multipath correction of constant modulus signals, *IEEE Trans. Acoust. Speech Signal Proc.*, ASSP-31:459–472.

Widrow, B., and Lehr, M. A., 1990, 30 years of adaptive neural networks: Perceptron, madaline, and backpropagation, *Proc. IEEE*, 78:1415–1441. ◆

Widrow, B., and Stearns, S. D., 1985, *Adaptive Signal Processing*, Englewood Cliffs, NJ: Prentice-Hall. ◆

Forecasting

Lyle H. Ungar

Introduction

Forecasting the future values of sequences of observations is, in many ways, ideally suited for neural networks. Large amounts of

data may be available, and the underlying relationships are often nonlinear and unknown. Neural nets, mostly of the standard backpropagation type (see BACKPROPAGATION: GENERAL PRINCIPLES), have been used with great success in many forecasting applications, including forecasting electricity load, freeway traffic volume, solar cycles, milk yields, tourism demand, grain drying times, ambient air quality, exchange rates, inflation, unemployment, disease epidemics, fish stock levels, sea surface temperatures, sales volumes, flood occurrence in Moravia, and rainfall in Bangladesh. However, in not all of such cases do neural networks outperform conventional ARMA models. This article looks at the use of neural nets for forecasting, with particular attention to understanding when they perform better or worse than other technologies.

The success of neural networks in forecasting depends significantly on the characteristics of the process being forecast. One may want to predict minute-by-minute progress of a chemical reaction, hour-by-hour power usage (load) for an electric power utility, daily weather, monthly prices of products and inventory levels, and quarterly or yearly sales and profits. These problems differ in the quantity and type of information available for forecasting, and hence call for different forecasting techniques. One also needs to choose an appropriate network architecture.

Forecasting problems can be characterized on a number of dimensions: (1) Is a single series of measurements used, as is often done in conventional forecasting, or are multiple related measurements available? (2) Are the data seasonal or not? Monthly or quarterly data such as sales volume or energy use often show strong seasonal variation, while annual data or data measured each second or minute do not. (3) The number of observations and (4) the degree of randomness (signal/noise ratio) of the process also strongly limit the complexity of the model that can be fit. If data are only available annually for the past 10 or 20 years, and if no measurement is available for most of the disturbances, one should not expect to be able to fit a complex model such as a neural network. This is unfortunately the case for many forecasting problems such as those represented in the Makerdakis collection (described below). (5) Finally, for some forecasting problems, one only requires prediction a single time step in the future, while for others, multiple time step forecasts are required. This has implications for the method used to train the neural network.

Before looking at neural networks, we will briefly review conventional forecasting methods. Forecasting has mostly been done using one of two different classes of methods, depending on whether the data are seasonal or not. For monthly data, such as sales or unemployment levels, the seasonal variation is often removed by dividing the series by an index representing the historical seasonal variation. For example, dividing the unemployment rate for each month (perhaps averaged over several years) by the average annual unemployment rate gives an index that indicates monthly variations. This index will have an average value of one. Dividing the actual unemployment rate in a given month by the index for that month gives the seasonally adjusted unemployment rate, which shows overall trends after typical monthly variations are accounted for. A linear or exponential regression (i.e., fitting the data as a linear or exponential function of time), or some form of smoothing such as a moving average, can then be used to make predictions of the deseasonalized unemployment. Actual levels are then forecast by multiplying these base predictions by the index for the month being forecast (Makridakis, Wheelwright, and McGee, 1983).

In contrast, for many complex processes such as chemical plant production, robots, or stock prices, the best prediction of the near future is obtained by using an appropriately weighted combination of recent measurements of the variable being predicted and other correlated variables. The most widely used approach is the Auto-Regressive Moving Average (ARMA) model. For example, to predict the value of a variable y (such as a temperature or a pressure or a stock price) at time $t + 1$ using past values of y and of a second variable z, one would use a linear regression to fit a model of the form

$$y_{t+1} = c_0 + c_1 y_t + c_2 y_{t-1} + c_3 y_{t-2} + \cdots$$
$$+ c_n z_t + c_{n+1} z_{t+1} + \cdots \quad (1)$$

Note that ARMA models differ from the linear regression models mentioned above in that they are functions of previous variables rather than of time.

Neural networks can be used to learn a nonlinear generalization of ARMA models of the form

$$y_{t+1} = f(y_t, y_{t-1}, y_{t-2}, \ldots, z_t, z_{t+1}, \ldots) \quad (2)$$

When the process is nonlinear and sufficient data are available, the neural networks will provide a more accurate model than the linear ARMA model. See Box and Jenkins (1970) for extensive descriptions of conventional ARMA models and the Box-Jenkins modeling approach, which involves picking a model of the form of Equation 1 with some subset of the coefficients set to zero. Later in this article we summarize the results of a number of studies that compare ARMA and neural network models.

Two other modeling methods are also often used by engineers, Kalman filtering and Wiener-Voltera series. Kalman filters (see KALMAN FILTERING: NEURAL IMPLICATIONS) assume a known model structure in which the parameters and their covariance, which is modeled explicitly, may be changing over time. Kalman filters are good for modeling relatively simple but noisy processes, but, unlike neural networks, they do not form nonparametric models that can accurately forecast the behavior of nonlinear systems. Wiener-Voltera series are polynomial expansions fitted to past data. As such, they, like neural nets, can approximate arbitrary functions. However, for models with multiple inputs they require more data than neural networks to obtain an equal level of accuracy.

Using Neural Nets for Forecasting

Neural networks are most often used to fit ARMA-style models of raw time series data from one or more measurements, but they can also be used as a piece of larger forecasting systems, such as in combination with deseasonalizing (i.e., forecasting a time series from which the seasonal component has been removed, as described above). Even for the simpler ARMA-style models, attention to the method is required if one is making forecasts multiple time steps in the future rather than a single time step.

Direct Versus Recurrent Prediction

A simple form of multistep forecasting is direct prediction (Figure 1A), in which a network takes past values as inputs and has separate outputs for predictions one, two, and more time steps in the future. Alternatively, one can train a network to predict one time step in the future and then use the network recursively to make multistep predictions (Figure 1B). Such networks are sometimes called *externally recurrent networks*, in contrast to networks that have internal memory. Direct forecasting networks are easier to build than externally recurrent nets because they do not require unfolding in time (described below), but the predictions are generally less accurate, since they have more parameters that must be fit from the same limited data.

The obvious way to train a network such as is used in Figure 1B is to minimize the error on the one-time-step predictions. Unfortunately, this does not give optimal networks for multistep predictions. To better understand this somewhat confusing point, consider the case of a simple linear ARMA model:

$$y_{t+1} = c_0 + c_1 y_t + c_2 y_{t-1} \quad (3)$$

A two-step-ahead prediction would then take the form

$$y_{t+2} = c_0 + c_1(c_0 + c_1 y_t + c_2 y_{t-1}) + c_2 y_t \quad (4)$$

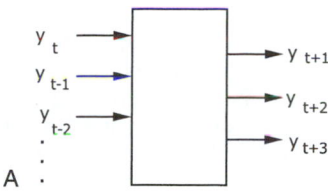

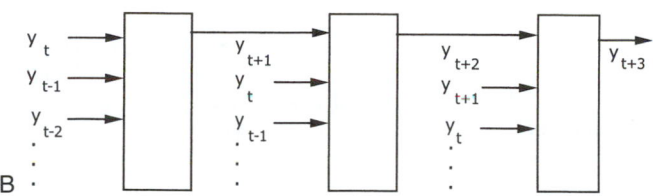

Figure 1. *A*, Direct prediction using a neural network. *B*, Recurrent one-step-ahead prediction using a neural network repeatedly.

Selecting coefficients c_0, c_1, and c_2 to minimize the prediction error for the one-step-ahead error yields a different equation than selecting the same coefficients to minimize the error in the two-step prediction. (Note that the former is a linear regression problem, whereas the latter requires nonlinear regression because the coefficients multiply each other.) More accurate long-range predictions are obtained by training to minimize the multistep prediction error. The solution using backpropagation uses the same unfolding in time or other solution methods as for internally recurrent networks (see RECURRENT NETWORKS: LEARNING ALGORITHMS). This and related issues are covered in detail in books on conventional system identification methods (e.g., Ljung and Torsten, 1983). Much good work has been done using recurrent nets to model time series (e.g., Mozer, 1994).

Combining Neural Networks with Other Methods

There are a number of ways in which neural networks can be combined with data preprocessing techniques, first principles (mechanistic) with partial models of the process being forecast, and with other forecasting techniques. Most commonly, if there is a strong seasonal component to the data, the data may be deseasonalized and the neural net used to forecast the basic trend. It may appear pointless to use a seasonal index when it is well known that neural networks can approximate arbitrary functions, which should include any seasonal variation. Experience indicates that if sufficient data are available, this is true, but that for shorter time series, deseasonalizing gives more accurate forecasts.

Similarly, when modeling complex physical systems, much better forecasts can be obtained with much less data when prior knowledge (e.g., in the form of mass, energy, or kinematic constraints on the variables, or in terms of monotonic relations between measured and forecast variables) is built into the network (Psichogios and Ungar, 1992). In a typical example, the equations governing a fermentation reactor are known except for the growth kinetics of the cells (e.g., yeast) in the reactor. If a neural network is used just to approximate the growth kinetics rather than to model the whole system, models are learned that are more accurate and that extrapolate better to operating regimens where no data are available. Such hybrid or "gray box" methods are popular in science and engineering.

Neural networks can also be used in conjunction with conventional forecasting methods. For example, one can often produce more accurate forecasts by providing several conventional forecasts as input to the neural network. In this case, the network serves partly as a combining method in which the network produces a weighted average of the different forecasts (Foster, Collopy, and Ungar, 1992). Such combining of forecasts is widely practiced in the forecasting community, mostly with relatively arbitrary combining weights.

Assessing Neural Nets for Forecasting

There are several difficulties in assessing forecasting methods. The most serious is that the results of a single forecast tell little about whether the method will be superior for other forecasts. In testing any method, it is important to have a large set of representative time series on which the methods will be tested. An example of such a collection of time series that has been widely used to compare forecasting methods is the Makridakis competition, or M-competition, model (Makridakis et al., 1982). This competition included 1,001 series and evaluated 24 forecasting methods. The series were taken from a variety of organizations in a number of countries and included macroeconomic, microeconomic, industrial, and demographic data such as production levels, net sales, unemployment, spending, GNP, vital statistics, and infectious disease incidence. The series included yearly, quarterly, and monthly series, but no series arising from securities or commodities trading. These time series all involve only a single variable and do not provide correlated variables, which might enhance the predictions.

One must also decide which error criteria to use. The most obvious criterion, and the one that is optimized by standard neural networks, is minimization of the mean squared prediction error. This criterion has the property that a small number of unusual series may have a large effect on the error. In looking at combined errors for different time series, one must, of course, also normalize for the different magnitudes of the series. Thus, forecasters often measure performance by using measures that are more robust to outliers or atypical time series.

Three error measures that have proved particularly robust are the percentage of time a method had a lower absolute error than the "no-change" forecast (or "percent better"), the relative absolute error (or RAE), and the median absolute percent error (or mdAPE). The RAE is calculated as the geometric mean across all series i of

$$\text{RAE}_i = \frac{\sum_{t=1}^{T} |\tilde{x}(t) - x(t)|_i}{\sum_{t=1}^{T} |x(0) - (t)|_i} \tag{5}$$

where $\tilde{x}(t)$ is the forecast and $x(t)$ represents the true value of the series at time t. The RAE represents a comparison over the forecast horizon T for series i of the absolute error of the forecast method, compared to the no-change or random walk forecast. One then calculates a geometric mean over all the series:

$$\text{RAE} = \left[\prod_{i=1}^{n} \text{RAE}_i \right]^{1/n} \tag{6}$$

The median average percent error is defined as the median across all series i of

$$\text{APE}_i = \frac{1}{T} \sum_{t=1}^{T} 100 \frac{|\tilde{x}(t) - x(t)|_i}{|x(t)|_i} \tag{7}$$

Good forecast performance is reflected in higher "percent betters" and lower RAEs and mdAPEs.

In assessing neural networks for forecasting, one must compare the accuracy of the neural networks with that of other statistical tools such as exponential smoothing (for a single time series) or linear ARMA models (for several correlated time series). Surprisingly, many studies fail to compare neural network forecasts with well-made conventional forecasts.

Table 1 lists some applications in which neural networks have been used for forecasting. Almost all of the studies used standard backpropagation networks with less than a dozen inputs and less than a dozen hidden nodes, with the exact architecture being selected by trial and error. Also, most of the studies used data from a single source, and most of the authors evaluated their results on the basis of the mean squared error on out-of-sample forecasts (i.e., error when forecasting data other than that used for building the model). Table 1 does not include any studies using chaotic time series such as from the Mackey-Glass equation, which give little insight into neural network forecasts of realistic data. See Vemuri and Rogers (1994) for a good collection of reprints of a wide variety for neural network forecasting studies, including all studies cited in Table 1 that are not listed in the references. There is also an extensive literature on neural network forecasting for process control (see PROCESS CONTROL in the First Edition). Process control and robotics applications have seen some of the most successful use of neural networks for forecasting, as the processes involved are often sufficiently multivariable and nonlinear to warrant the use of neural networks but sufficiently well characterized and free of noise to allow accurate models to be built.

Dangers in Using Forecasts

Forecasts rely on a number of assumptions. They assume that the system that is modeled remains constant, i.e., that the model that held when the model was built still applies when the forecast is made. If the system structure is evolving over time, techniques from adaptive control may be more appropriate. It is also implicitly assumed when forecasting using neural networks with multiple inputs that the covariance structure of the inputs will remain constant. This presents a major difficulty when modeling systems that have

Table 1. Forecasting Using Neural Nets: Sample Results

Application	Authors	Results	Compared with
Car sales, airline passengers	Tang et al.	NNet better for longer-term forecast; Box-Jenkins better for shorter	Box-Jenkins
Currency exchange rates	Weigend et al.	NNets better	Random guessing
Electric load forecasting	Park et al.	NNet better	Currently used technology (unclear what)
Electrochemical reaction	Hudson et al.	Prediction looks good	—
Flour prices	Chakraborty et al.	NNets better than ARMA	ARMA
Polypropylene sales	Chitra	NNets slightly better than ARMA	ARMA
Stock prices	White	NNets provide no benefit	Random walk
Widely varied (Makridakis collection)	Foster et al.	NNets better on quarterly data, worse on annual data	Many exponential smoothing and deseasonalizing methods

feedback in them, if the feedback structure is variable. For example, consider a house controlled by a thermostat. One will typically find that the heater will be on more often when the house is cold (this is, after all, what the heating system is designed to do). Forecasts of future house temperature can be accurately made using historical temperature measurements. If, however, these forecasts are used as part of the control scheme (the thermostat), then instability often results, since the forecasts fail to account for the new thermostat behavior. Similar situations often occur in economics and marketing, where forecasts can result in new laws being passed or in new prices being charged (and resulting actions by competitors), thus invalidating the original forecast. Unfortunately, there is generally little that one can do other than monitoring forecasts and distrusting them or collecting more data, if the process being forecast changes. (This is true in linear regression as well, where it is impossible to tell which of two highly correlated inputs is responsible for changes in an output, but at least one can easily detect the problem in linear problems by examining the uncertainty on the regression coefficients, whereas it is usually concealed in neural nets.)

Discussion

Neural networks have many demonstrated successes as forecasting tools and a smaller number of documented failures. All the usual warnings about model building apply. In particular, to build a good model, one needs good data. When the data are noisy and occur in short series, neural networks often fail to do better than simple forecasting techniques. For example, the 181 yearly series of the M-competition, which have a mean length of 19 data points on which to base a prediction, do not provide a good basis for complex nonlinear models. Neural networks generally give significant improvements over conventional forecasting methods when applied to monthly data in the M-competition set but not when applied to yearly data (Hill, O'Connor, and Remus, 1996). This is probably due to the high ratio of noise to data in the yearly data.

It may also be the case that the data are truly random or that the key independent variables are not being measured. Research suggests that this is true of the stock market (White, 1988). If this is true, then neural networks will not produce useful market forecasts, although they may help sell forecasting products. Several fund managers claim that they are getting superior predictions using neural networks, but for obvious competitive reasons, they generally do not provide enough information to test the claims. Moody (1998) provides a good discussion of the issues in forecasting the economy.

Neural networks have proved successful in a number of applications such as forecasting prices (Chakraborty et al., 1992), product demand (Chitra, 1993), electric utility loads (Yu, Moghaddamjo, and Chen, 1992), and inventory levels (see Table 1). Such problems are characterized by ample measurements with a relatively high signal-to-noise ratio. In most cases, substantially better performance is obtained by using several related inputs to the network. For example, in forecasting wheat prices in three cities, superior performance was found by using recent wheat prices and measures of the local earning power. Similarly, in forecasting demand for polypropylene production, several macroeconomic variables were fed into the network. On longer, more deterministic time series, such as measuring the progress of a chemical reaction, neural networks have been shown to be a relatively accurate means of forecasting even chaotic series (Hudson et al., 1990; Lapedes and Farber in Vemuri and Rogers, 1994).

All of the applications cited above use standard backpropagation networks, occasionally with some degree of structure built into the network. For example, in the currency exchanges, excess weights were eliminated, while for forecasting wheat prices, past values of prices in three different cities were used to predict the logarithm of flour prices. All have demonstrated better performance than conventional forecasting methods, except when only short time series were available (10 to 30 data points) or when it was unclear if there was an underlying model other than a biased random walk (e.g., stock prices). However, the gains in accuracy over conventional forecasting methods are often relatively small, and overfitting is a common problem. Many companies are now using neural networks for problems such as demand forecasting. When sufficient data are available and care is taken to avoid overfitting, neural networks work well.

Road Map: Applications
Related Reading: Kalman Filtering: Neural Implications; Recurrent Networks: Learning Algorithms

References

Box, G., and Jenkins, G., 1970, *Time Series Analysis: Forecasting and Control*, San Francisco: Holden-Day. ◆

Chakraborty, K., Mehrotra, K., Mohan, C. K., and Ranka, S., 1992, Forecasting the behavior of multivariate time series using neural networks, *Neural Netw.*, 5:961–970. ◆

Chitra, S. P., 1993, Use neural networks for problem solving, *Chem. Eng. Prog.*, April, pp. 44–52. ◆

Foster, B., Collopy, F., and Ungar, L. H., 1992, Neural network forecasting of short noisy time series, *Comput. Chem. Eng.*, 16:293–298. ◆

Hill, T., O'Connor, M., and Remus, W., 1996, Neural network models for time series forecasts, *Manage. Sci.*, 42:1082–1092.

Hudson, J. L., et al., 1990, Nonlinear signal processing and system identification: Applications to time series from electrochemical reactions, *Chem. Eng. Sci.*, 45:2075–2981.

Ljung, L., and Torsten, S., 1983, *Theory and Practice of Recursive Identification*, Cambridge, MA: MIT Press.

Makridakis, S., et al., 1982, The accuracy of extrapolation (time series) methods: Results of a forecasting competition, *J. Forecast.*, 1:111–153.

Makridakis, S., Wheelwright, S., and McGee, V., 1983, *Forecasting: Methods and Applications*, New York: Wiley. ◆

Moody, J., 1998, Forecasting the economy with neural nets: A survey of challenges and solutions, *Lecture Notes Comput. Sci.*, 1524:347–371.

Mozer, M. C., 1994, Neural net architectures for temporal sequence processing, in *Time Series Prediction* (A. S. Weigend and N. A. Gershenfeld, Eds.), Menlo Park, CA: Addison-Wesley, pp. 243–264.

Psichogios, D. C., and Ungar, L. H., 1992, A hybrid neural network: First principles approach to process modeling, *Am. Inst. Chem. Eng. J.*, 38:1499–1512.

Vemuri, V. R., and Rogers, R. D., 1994, *Artificial Neural Networks: Forecasting Time Series*, Los Alamitos, CA: IEEE Computer Society Press. ◆

White, H., 1988, *Economic Prediction Using Neural Networks: The Case of IBM Daily Stock Returns*, in *Proceedings of the IEEE International Conference on Neural Networks*, San Diego, p. II-451.

Yu, D. C., Moghaddamjo, A. R., and Chen, S.-T., 1992, Weather sensitive short-term load forecasting using a nonfully connected artificial neural network., *IEEE Trans. Power Syst.*, 7:1098–1105.

Gabor Wavelets and Statistical Pattern Recognition

John Daugman

Introduction

Starting around 1960, for about three decades investigation into the functioning of the mammalian primary visual cortex was dominated by recordings from single neurons. Using relatively simple stimuli such as oriented bars of light (e.g., Hubel and Wiesel, 1962, 1974), the apparent coding dimensions underlying spatial vision were mapped out by measuring tuning curves of individual neural responses as functions of stimulus parameters. Although methods later moved on, with innovations such as population recordings, noninvasive imaging with photovoltaic dyes, and novel anatomical techniques, the single-unit recording paradigm left a rich legacy of data that lent itself to modeling in engineering terms such as filtering, feature extraction, transform coding, and dimensionality reduction.

In this framework, the key functional concept is that of a neuron's *receptive field*, which specifies that region of two-dimensional (2D) visual space in which image events or structure can influence the neuron's activity. More exactly, the neuron's *receptive field profile* indicates the relative degree to which the cell is excited or inhibited by the distribution of light as a function of its spatial position within the receptive field. Through careful measurements with precisely defined stimuli, the receptive field profile of a *linear* neuron (one obeying proportionality and superposition in its responses to stimuli) reveals how it will respond to *any* pattern and allows the neuron to be analyzed in signal processing terms as a filter. The powerful mathematical tools of linear systems analysis (including Fourier analysis) are the basis of such extrapolations, subject always to the assumption of linearity. More recent findings of adaptive, nonlinear, remote interactions between visual neurons "beyond the classical receptive field" undermine the linear filter perspective and may even call into question the whole notion that a neuron has a stable receptive field profile. Nevertheless, impressive practical results have been achieved in engineering applications of one such model inspired by the classical receptive field data. This article reviews the model that has come to dominate the classical description of cortical simple cells and their inputs to complex cells, and it reviews some successful applications of that scheme within computer vision and statistical pattern recognition.

Receptive Fields and 2D Gabor Wavelets

Typical two-dimensional receptive field profiles of simple cells in the feline visual cortex (Jones and Palmer, 1987) are shown in the top row of Figure 1. There are arguably five major degrees of freedom (i.e., independent forms of variation) spanned by the spatial receptive field structure of such neural populations. These can be regarded as defining the dimensions of the spatial visual code at this cortical level. The first two degrees of freedom are the *location* of a neuron's receptive field, defined by retinotopic coordinates (x, y). The third is the *size* of its receptive field (which can be described using a single scalar diameter, provided we view variation in the field width/length aspect ratio as a secondary population structure). The fourth is the *orientation* of the boundaries separating excitatory and inhibitory regions, as seen in Figures 1 and 3, normally also corresponding to the direction of receptive field elongation. The fifth is the *symmetry*, which may be even or odd, or some linear combination of these two canonical states. (Any function can be decomposed into the sum of an even function plus an odd function, and their relative amplitudes define a continuum that allows this fifth dimension to be regarded as *phase*.)

These degrees of freedom in the spatial visual code also correspond to certain dimensions of the "cortical architecture" (rules of topographic and modular organization), although such structure is

2D Receptive Field Profiles

Fitted 2D Gabor Phasors

Residuals

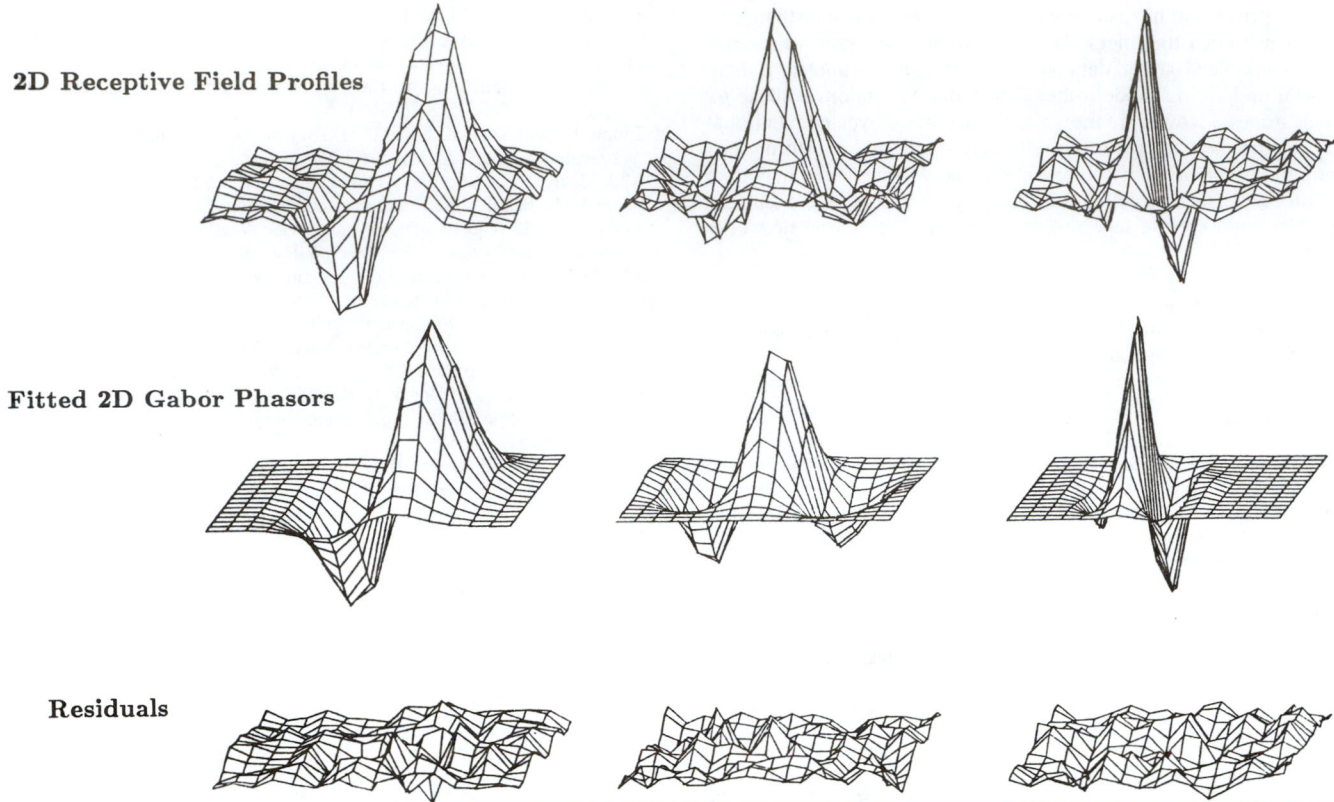

Figure 1. Typical 2D receptive field profiles of simple cells found in cat visual cortex, from measurements by Jones and Palmer (1987). The raw receptive field profiles (top row) are well-described by the 2D Gabor wave- let model (middle row) in 97% of the cells studied, yielding residuals (bot- tom row) that are indistinguishable from random error in chi-squared tests.

less pronounced for some variables than for others. The (x, y) po- sition coordinates of receptive fields in visual space form system- atic (although nonconformal) topographic maps of these two di- mensions across the cortical surface. Third, subpopulations of neurons that share the same orientation preference are grouped to- gether into columns, and successive columns rotate systematically in preferred angle ("sequence regularity"). A similar structure ex- ists for the grouping of cells by the dominant eye from which they receive input, the ocular dominance columns. These rather crystal- line organizational principles were originally documented in sem- inal papers by Hubel and Wiesel (1962, 1974). Of the remaining two degrees of freedom, there is some evidence for pairwise group- ing by quadrature (90°) phase relationship (Pollen and Ronner, 1981), and also some evidence for anatomical grouping by field size, either in different cortical layers or in adjacent columns anal- ogous to those for orientation.

One benefit of identifying the primary degrees of freedom in a spatial image code is that it allows us to characterize the coding strategy in information-theoretic terms. The information-carrying capacity associated with each degree of freedom is a function of the number of individually resolvable states for that dimension. These define a kind of "information budget" that can be allocated in alternative ways among the different available degrees of free- dom. Certain inescapable conflicts arise, however, that limit the extent to which some combinations of information can be simul- taneously resolved. These conflicts take the form of an "uncertainty principle," whose mathematical form (Daugman, 1985) is just a 2D generalization of the one familiar from quantum physics in the famous work of Weyl and Heisenberg. One such conflict, or trade- off, will be intuitively clear from considering the oval receptive

fields in Figure 3. Orientation resolution (the "sharpness" of ori- entation tuning) would be enhanced by making the ovals longer, but this would reduce their resolution for spatial location in that direction. Similarly, increasing the field width by adding more cy- cles of undulation would sharpen the tuning for spatial frequency, but at the cost of lost resolution for spatial location in this direction. The optimal solution for these trade-offs, achieving maximal *con- joint* resolution of image information in both 2D spatial and 2D spectral terms, is the family of complex-valued 2D Gabor wavelets. These were first introduced into vision modeling by Daugman (1980, 1985) as a generalization of the 1D elementary functions, "logons," originally proposed for signal expansions by Gabor (1946).

This family of complex-valued 2D wavelets defining filters with minimal conjoint uncertainty have the following parameterized form in the (x, y) space domain:

$$G(x, y) = e^{-[(x-x_0)^2/\alpha^2 + (y-y_0)^2/\beta^2]}e^{-2\pi i[u_0(x-x_0) + v_0(y-y_0)]} \quad (1)$$

where (x_0, y_0) specify position in the image, (α, β) specify the filter's effective width and length, and (u_0, v_0) specify the filter's modulation wave vector, which can be interpreted in polar coor- dinates as spatial frequency $\omega_0 = \sqrt{u_0^2 + v_0^2}$ and orientation (or direction) $\theta_0 = \arctan(v_0/u_0)$. The real and imaginary parts of this complex filter function describe associated pairs of simple cells in "quadrature phase" (90° phase relation), as were discovered by Pol- len and Ronner (1981). The middle row of Figure 1 shows three examples of the real or imaginary parts of the complex filter of Equation 1, with parameters chosen to fit the experimentally mea- sured receptive field profiles shown in the top row. Neural recordings by Jones and Palmer (1987) confirmed that this family of functions provided good fits to the receptive field profiles of about 97% of the simple cells whose 2D profiles they measured in cat visual cortex. (It should be noted, however, that other investigators have preferred other functions, such as differences of several offset Gaussians, which, having additional fitting parameters, offered better fits to their data.) The top row of Figure 1 illustrates three of the 131 simple-cell 2D receptive field profiles measured by Jones and Palmer. The bottom row shows the residuals obtained by subtracting the best-fitting 2D Gabor wavelet component (middle row) from each measured profile. For nearly all of the cells studied, these residuals were indistinguishable from random error in chi-squared tests. Although alternative analytic forms could be chosen to fit the available 2D receptive field data, there can be no doubt that the 2D Gabor wavelet model specifies an efficient set of coding primitives capturing 2D spatial location, orientation, size (or frequency), and phase (or symmetry) in a natural way.

The 2D Fourier transform $F(u, v)$ of a 2D Gabor wavelet, which reveals its spectral response selectivity in the Fourier plane, has exactly the same functional form as the space-domain function (i.e., it is "self-Fourier"), but with the parameters just interchanged or inverted:

$$F(u, v) = e^{-[(u-u_0)^2\alpha^2 + (v-v_0)^2\beta^2]}e^{2\pi i[x_0(u-u_0) + y_0(v-v_0)]} \quad (2)$$

Thus the 2D Fourier power spectrum $F(u, v)F^*(u, v)$ of a 2D Gabor wavelet is simply a bivariate Gaussian centered on (u_0, v_0). Hence its peak response occurs for an orientation θ_0 and spatial frequency ω_0 as defined earlier, corresponding to the excitatory/inhibitory structure of the receptive field, as one would expect. Some authors have questioned the relevance of the Gabor wavelet property of optimal conjoint resolution in these two domains, or the specialness of the variance metric on which the measure of uncertainty is based. Perhaps the best reply is Aristotle's dictum that "vision is knowing what is where." The extraction of local image structure in terms of oriented undulatory primitives provides information in 2D spectral terms about "what," and the resolution of positional information indicates "where." If we wish to extract visual information simultaneously in terms of both what and where, as Aristotle said, then under the Heisenberg uncertainty principle we cannot do better than to construct our spatial visual code from 2D Gabor wavelets. It would appear that the evolution of the mammalian visual cortex may have been shaped by this criterion and thus converged on the coding primitives that optimize it.

Compact Image Coding and 2D Gabor Transforms

Besides their optimality in terms of the uncertainty relation, 2D Gabor wavelets have many practical properties. They can be used to form a complete and compact image code, as a self-similar 2D wavelet expansion basis, despite their nonorthogonality (Daugman, 1988). Although Gabor wavelets do not technically satisfy the original admissibility conditions for wavelets such as orthogonality and strictly compact support, their practical advantages as coding primitives are not much diminished. For example, they can achieve significant image compression, with appropriate parameterization for wavelet dilations, rotations, and translations. If we take $\Psi(x, y)$ to be a chosen generic 2D Gabor wavelet as specified above in Equation 1, which may be called a "mother wavelet," then we can generate from this one function a complete self-similar family of "daughter wavelets" through the generating operation

$$\Psi_{mpq\theta}(x, y) = 2^{-2m}\Psi(x', y') \quad (3)$$

where the substituted variables (x', y') incorporate dilations of the wavelet in size by octave factors 2^{-m}, translations in position (p, q), and rotations through angle θ:

$$x' = 2^{-m}[x \cos(\theta) + y \sin(\theta)] - p \quad (4)$$

$$y' = 2^{-m}[-x \sin(\theta) + y \cos(\theta)] - q \quad (5)$$

It is noteworthy that as consequences of the similarity, shift, and modulation theorems of 2D Fourier analysis, together with the rotation isomorphism of the 2D Fourier transform, all of these effects of the generating function (Equation 3) applied to a 2D Gabor mother wavelet $\Psi(x, y) = G(x, y)$ in generating the 2D Gabor daughter wavelets $\Psi_{mpq\theta}(x, y)$ will have just corresponding or reciprocal effects on the wavelet's 2D Fourier transform $F(u, v)$ without any other change in functional form (Daugman, 1985). This family of 2D wavelets, and their 2D Fourier transforms, is each closed under the transformation groups of dilations, translations, rotations, and convolutions.

Any image can be represented completely in terms of such a basis of elementary expansion functions. An example of this in a progressive sequence is provided in Figure 2, showing the benchmark "Lena" image reconstructed from increasing numbers of 2D Gabor wavelets. It is interesting that even when only 100 or 500 wavelets are present and distributed across the entire image, already the primary facial features such as the eyes are discernible. Since facial features are essentially just localized undulations, parameterized for scale, position, orientation, and symmetry—that is, the same as the parameterizations of the Gabor wavelets themselves—it is perhaps not surprising that very efficient face codes can be constructed from such wavelets.

An error that occurs frequently in the literature is a confusion between Gabor *projection coefficients* (obtained merely by taking the convolution or inner product of each image region onto a local Gabor wavelet) and Gabor *expansion coefficients* (those needed to reconstruct the image as a linear combination of Gabor wavelets). Because these wavelets are not an orthogonal set (i.e., their mutual inner products are not zero), the expansion coefficients are not the same as the projection coefficients, nor can they easily be obtained from them. For this reason, it is incorrect to refer to the result of image convolutions with Gabor wavelets as a Gabor transform, since the resulting representation is not invertible. One approach for obtaining the Gabor expansion coefficients needed for an invertible image representation (thus defining a true *Gabor transform*) is a relaxation network method introduced in Daugman (1988). The progressive stages of image reconstruction shown in Figure 2 are based on expansion coefficients obtained by that relaxation network.

Interesting issues arise concerning how the "information budget" in a visual code should be allocated. For example, because all Gabor wavelets are indexed by their 2D location, the parameters that specify each wavelet's orientation and spatial frequency can be sequenced much more sparsely than Fourier components in a Fourier transform. Moreover, the necessary density of sampling in orientation and frequency is in a trade-off with the needed density of sampling in position (i.e., how much the wavelets overlap each other). The exact rules for the sampling densities necesssary in these various parameters in order to obtain a *complete* image code are dictated by *frame theory*. Whereas, for example, the 2D Fourier transform must sample the frequency plane along a uniform Cartesian grid, a 2D Gabor transform can sample the frequency plane on just a log-polar grid. This great reduction in sampling density for the higher frequencies is purchased by the wavelet position parameters. Illustrations of self-similar 2D Gabor representations of images, obtained with varying numbers of wavelet orientations (six, four, three, and two orientations in the sampling set), may be

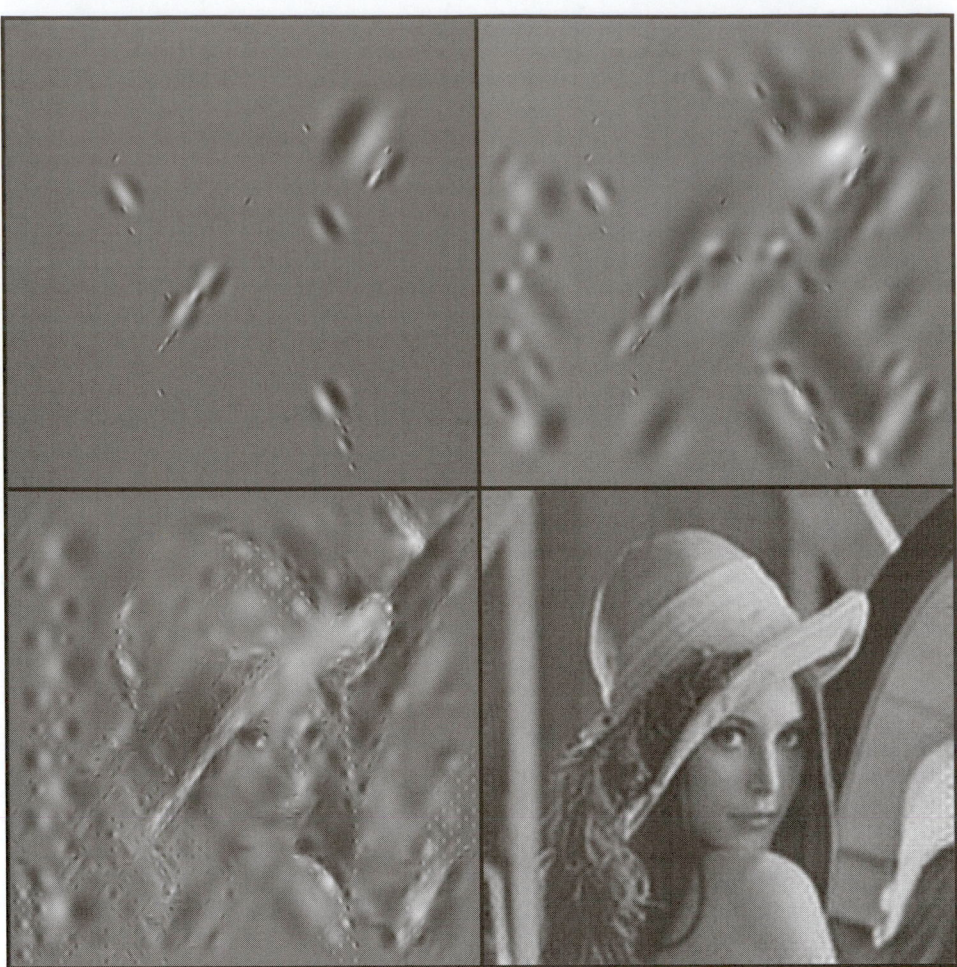

Figure 2. Illustration of the completeness of 2D Gabor wavelets as image coding primitives. The benchmark "Lena" picture is reconstructed by progressive numbers of wavelets in linear combination, of 25, 100, 500, and 10,000. The primary facial features are effectively represented by just a handful of such wavelets. However, because of their nonorthogonality, the wavelets require coefficients that differ from the simple inner product projection of the image onto them.

found in Daugman (1988). These sorts of considerations may be able to answer such longstanding neurobiological questions as "Why are there orientation columns in the cortex, and why is orientation sampled with those bandwidths and intervals? Why do receptive fields overlap this much?" Further neurobiological issues are raised by the fact that the Gabor wavelets are nonorthogonal. The consequences of this include paradoxes in the classical interpretation of what it is that a neuron's receptive field actually enables it to encode about an image. In particular, the classical view that a linear neuron's response (which is determined by the inner product of its receptive field profile with the local image) signifies the "relative presence" of its own structure in the local image region is paradoxical: it implies an incorrect image representation by the ensemble of neurons, given their mutual nonorthogonality.

Facial Analysis and Recognition

Whereas simple cells are regarded as linear filters whose phase sensitivity is clearly determined by their alternating pattern of a few excitatory and inhibitory regions, the so-called "complex" cells that receive input from them have no such phase sensitivity, yet their orientation and spatial frequency tuning are similar to that of simple cells. A natural model therefore supposes that the inputs to complex cells come from quadrature pairs of simple cells, taking the sum of their squared responses, as shown at the top of Figure 3. This nonlinear combination not only achieves a weak kind of

translation invariance (in that the complex cell responds to the stimulus but is indifferent to its phase, or position within the receptive field) but, more important, this arrangement can play a useful role in feature extraction for pattern recognition. This idea is illustrated for the case of a face image in Figure 4 (see the figure caption for a detailed explanation). Since major facial features are essentially localized undulations of a certain scale (frequency) and orientation, it is perhaps not surprising that facial features are easily represented and detected by operations using 2D Gabor wavelets.

This idea has been elaborated further in a number of full face recognition systems based on Gabor wavelets (e.g., Lades et al., 1993). Besides encoding a face by the coefficients of projection of particular regions of the face (centered on fiducial points) onto clusters of multiscale, oriented Gabor wavelets (renamed "jets"), the Lades scheme organizes the data into an elastic graph that can accommodate some distortion. A graph-matching technique searches for matches of the Gabor wavelet projection coefficients while allowing graph distortions corresponding to limited changes in facial expression, perspective angle, and pose. But the approach remains "appearance-based" (i.e., it is a 2D image representation for faces, not a 3D object representation), and as such it is susceptible to changes in perspective geometry and illumination geometry. Such variations in image capture conditions affect the wavelet projection coefficients in a manner for which the graph matching cannot compensate and is not invariant. For similar reasons, all current face recognition algorithms can work only under con-

Quadrature Demodulator Network

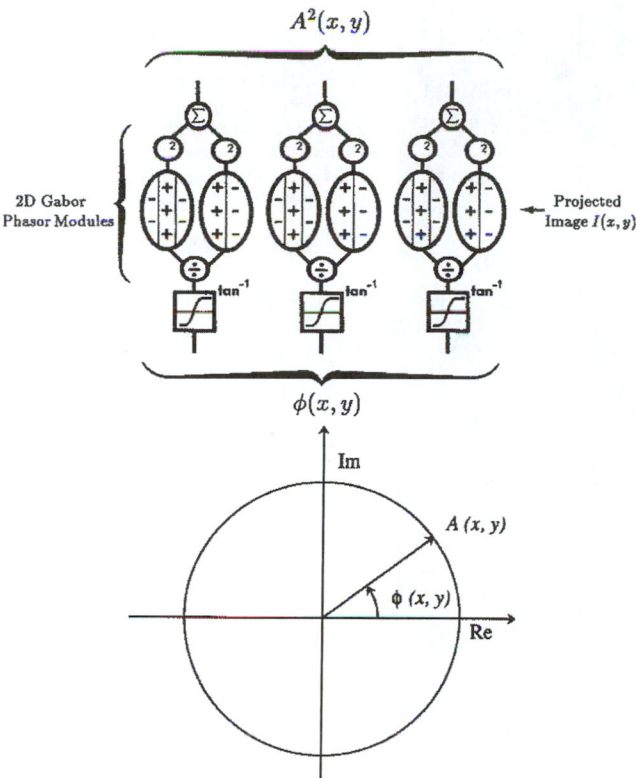

Figure 3. The 2D Gabor wavelet quadrature demodulation network. Even- and odd-symmetric receptive fields, of the kind associated with cortical simple cells, subserve a phasor resolution of information in the complex plane. The sum of the squares of quadrature simple-cell responses extracts an amplitude function $A(x, y)$ or modulus (top of network), while the ratio of their responses resolves the local phase function $\phi(x, y)$ (bottom of network). Such amplitude-and-phase descriptions of image structure can be very useful in computer vision.

strained imaging conditions, with fixed illumination and perspective geometry and relatively fixed expressions. Moreover, in realistic tests, the best systems have error rates approaching 50% when comparing images taken just 1 year apart.

Phase and Amplitude Coding of Texture and Complex Patterns

An important goal of vision is *dimensionality reduction*: creating a succinct and useful representation of image structure having much lower dimension than the raw image itself. In a sense, standard edge detection strategies are examples of this idea, since edge maps can signify object structure, and they clearly have much lower dimension than the raw pixel count. However, many naturally occurring objects, such as faces and bodies, lack the planar or geometrical forms of manufactured objects that generate simple edge maps; instead, they are defined by continuous-tone structure, textures, and undulations, which are not well captured by detecting edges. We saw earlier that facial features are efficiently represented and detected by 2D Gabor wavelets; a similar subspace projection approach using these wavelets was successfully applied by Shustorovich (1994) to the problem of classifying and recognizing handwritten characters. A more general representation for image infor-

mation (Daugman and Downing, 1995) reduces its dimensionality by *decorrelating* it not only in amplitude but also in phase, making use of the intriguing quadrature phase relationship found in the neurobiological recordings from cortical simple cells. As portrayed in Figure 3, the quadrature simple-cell structure not only supports an energy, or modulus, computation emerging from the top of the network as $A^2(x, y)$, but the same paired 2D Gabor receptive fields also support a computation of local phase $\phi(x, y)$, shown emerging from the bottom of the network. The arctangent-like "squashing function" that operates on the ratio of the simple-cell responses is a common feature of many neural network models, but here it serves trigonometrically to resolve a phase angle in the complex plane, as indicated in the phasor diagram at the bottom.

The representation of images in terms of local phase $\phi(x, y)$ and local amplitude $A(x, y)$ is a form of *predictive coding* that takes as its prediction the locally prevalent scale and orientation of image structure, and encodes the full detailed pattern as modulations of that prediction (Daugman and Downing, 1995). This lends itself not only to compact image coding but also to texture segmentation (i.e., the division of an image into regions defined by some local homogeneity of texture). The analysis of texture and its use for image segmentation are important topics in statistical pattern recognition. 2D Gabor wavelets have played dominant roles here, as reviewed in Bovic, Clark, and Geisler (1990) and Navarro, Tabernero, and Cristobal (1996). An alternative approach that explicitly computes Gabor phase rather than just energy for effective texture segmentation is given in du Buf (1990).

Iris Recognition

In this section, we illustrate the principles discussed in this chapter with a practical application that is now coming into wide international use: the automatic visual recognition of persons by their iris patterns. Details about the algorithms that locate an iris and segment it from other tissues, mapping it into a doubly dimensionless coordinate system with invariance for size, translation, and pupil dilation, are given in Daugman (2001). The iris pattern is then demodulated by 2D Gabor wavelets (see Figure 3) in order to extract its *phase sequence* $\phi(x, y)$, with these phase values quantized very coarsely into only the nearest quadrant of the complex plane. This sets two bits of phase information for each wavelet applied in a particular location. An "IrisCode" comprising 2,048 such bits of pattern phase information is then compared against an enrolled database of other IrisCodes in search of a match. These comparisons are performed at the speed of 100,000 IrisCodes per second by the decision network shown in Figure 5. This network transforms the pattern recognition problem into a simple test of statistical independence on the 2D Gabor wavelet phase sequences derived from the patterns.

Results from 9.1 million comparisons between different iris patterns are given in Figure 6, based on images acquired at kiosks in Britain, the United States, Japan, and Korea in public trials of these algorithms over a 3-year period. In these trials, as well as in tests conducted by independent government laboratories (the largest involving 2.73 million iris comparisons), there has never been a single reported false match. The reason is because the 2D Gabor IrisCode extracts about 250 degrees of freedom, whose combinatorics generate binomial distributions with extremely rapidly attenuating tails. Since comparisons of phasor bits are Bernoulli trials whose values of p and q depend on whether a pair of IrisCodes comes from the same or from different eyes, the confidence levels associated with recognition decisions are determined by cumulatives of the binomial probability density of observing a fraction $x = m/N$ "true" exclusive-OR outcomes in N comparisons:

$$f(x) = \frac{N!}{m!(N - m)!} p^m q^{(N-m)} \quad (6)$$

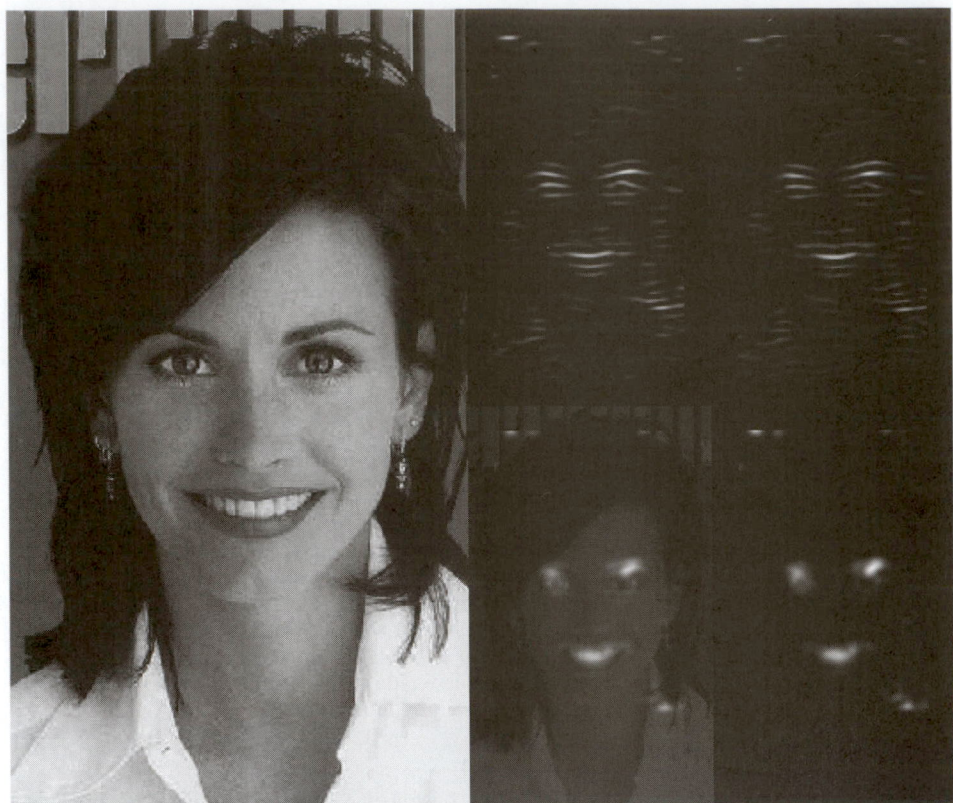

Figure 4. Illustration of facial feature detection by the quadrature demodulator network shown in Figure 3. *Left*, Input image. *Right* (clockwise from top left), the real part of the result of convolution with a 2D Gabor wavelet; the imaginary part from the same convolution (both of these representing the phase-sensitive simple-cell responses); the squared modulus $A^2(x, y)$, representing complex cell response; and this result superimposed on the original (faint) image, illustrating feature detection and localization.

The solid curve in Figure 6 superimposed on the raw data distribution is a plot of the Equation 6 binomial, and it provides a remarkably exact fit. It shows that there is vanishingly small probability that two different iris patterns could agree just by chance in more than about two-thirds of their bits, i.e., produce a fractional Hamming distance smaller than about 0.33. But images acquired

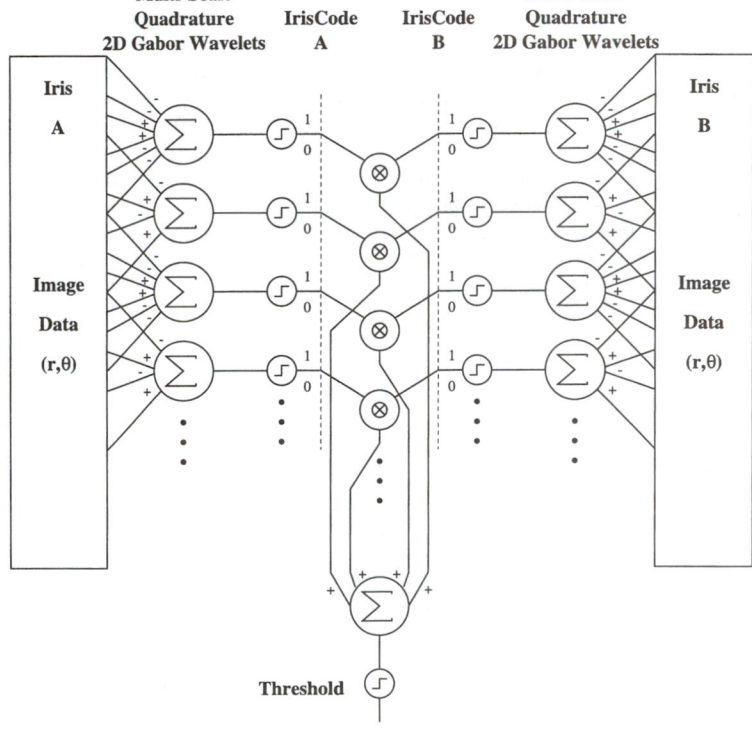

Figure 5. The comparison and recognition network used to make decisions about the identity of iris patterns. In effect, this network transforms the problem of pattern recognition into a test of statistical independence on the iris pattern phase sequences extracted by 2D Gabor wavelet demodulation (Figure 3).

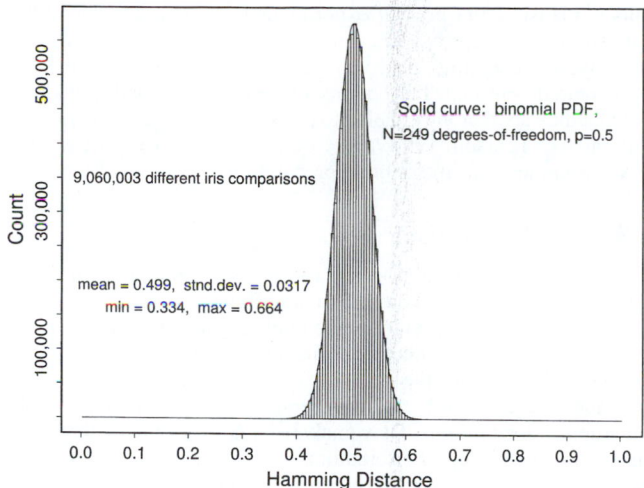

Figure 6. Results of 9.1 million comparisons between human iris patterns. Their Hamming distances are binomially distributed (solid curve, Equation 6). The rapidly decaying tails of such factorial distributions make it almost impossible for two different IrisCodes to disagree by chance in less than about a third of their bits (Hamming distance < 0.33). Thus, the failure of a simple test of statistical independence in this application of 2D Gabor wavelets allows reliable human identification with great tolerance for poor imaging.

from a given iris at different times and under different conditions score Hamming distances well below this, typically in the 0.10–0.15 range. Thus, this complex yet stable textural signature can provide a very accurate basis for automatically recognizing personal identity (in lieu of using PINs, cards, keys, passwords, or documents) for purposes such as border control, building entry, cash machines, computer login, authentication, and security measures in general. All current iris recognition systems installed worldwide use the 2D Gabor wavelet encoding, demodulation, and decision networks described here (Figures 3 and 5). Recent installations of this system include Heathrow Airport, Amsterdam-Schiphol, Washington-Dulles, and Charlotte Airports, for both passenger screening and control of access to restricted areas.

Discussion

The role of 2D Gabor wavelets in the visual sciences began as a model proposed in 1980 for cortical simple-cell 2D receptive field profiles. Today these wavelets are used pervasively in computer vision, image processing, and pattern recognition (for an in-depth review, see Navarro et al., 1996), even though more recent investigations in neuroscience perhaps call into question the very idea that visual neurons even possess stable receptive field profiles. The benefits of performing image coding and analysis using these elementary detectors include the opportunity to describe image structure in terms of local phase and energy, allowing demodulation, which lends itself well to solving pattern recognition problems. Some practical applications now in widespread use include facial and texture analysis, and personal identification by automatic, real-time recognition of iris patterns. These examples illustrate the fruitful interaction that can occur between ideas originating in brain theory and ideas about artificial neural networks.

Road Map: Vision
Related Reading: Face Recognition: Neurophysiology and Neural Technology; Feature Analysis; Orientation Selectivity

References

Bovic, A. C., Clark, M., and Geisler, W. S., 1990, Multi-channel texture analysis using localized spatial filters, *IEEE Trans. Pattern Anal. Machine Intell.*, 12:55–73.
Daugman, J. G., 1980, Two-dimensional spectral analysis of cortical receptive field profiles, *Vision Res.*, 20:847–856.
Daugman, J. G., 1985, Uncertainty relation for resolution in space, spatial frequency, and orientation optimized by two-dimensional visual cortical filters, *J. Opt. Soc. Am. A*, 2:1160–1169. See also: Daugman, J. G., 1993, Quadrature-phase simple-cell pairs are appropriately described in complex analytic form, *J. Opt. Soc. Am. A*, 10:375–377.
Daugman, J. G., 1988, Complete discrete 2D Gabor transforms by neural networks for image analysis and compression, *IEEE Trans. Acoust. Speech Sign. Process.*, 36:1169–1179.
Daugman, J. G., 2001, Statistical richness of visual phase information: Update on recognizing persons by iris patterns, *Int. J. Comput. Vision*, 45:25–38.
Daugman, J. G., and Downing, C. J., 1995, Demodulation, predictive coding, and spatial vision, *J. Opt. Soc. Am. A*, 12:641–660.
du Buf, J. M. H., 1990, Gabor phase in texture discrimination, *Sign. Process.*, 21:221–240.
Gabor, D., 1946, Theory of communication, *J. Inst. Electr. Eng.*, 93:429–457.
Hubel, D. G., and Wiesel, T. N., 1962, Receptive fields, binocular interaction, and functional architecture in the cat's visual cortex, *J. Physiol. (Lond.)*, 160:106–154.
Hubel, D. G., and Wiesel, T. N., 1974, Sequence regularity and geometry of orientation columns in the monkey striate cortex, *J. Comp. Neurol.*, 158:267–293.
Jones, J. P., and Palmer, L. A., 1987, An evaluation of the 2D Gabor filter model of simple receptive fields in cat striate cortex, *J. Neurophysiol.*, 58:1233–1258.
Lades, M., Vorbrüggen, J. C., Buhmann, J., Lange, J., von der Malsburg, C., Würtz, R. P., and Konen, W., 1993, Distortion invariant object recognition in the dynamic link architecture, *IEEE Trans. Comput.*, 42:300–311.
Navarro, R., Tabernero, A., and Cristobal, G., 1996, Image representation with Gabor wavelets and its applications, *Adv. Imaging Electron Phys.*, 97:1–84. ◆
Pollen, D. A., and Ronner, S. F., 1981, Phase relationships between adjacent simple cells in the visual cortex, *Science*, 212:1409–1411.
Shustorovich, A., 1994, A subspace projection approach to feature extraction: The 2D Gabor transform for character recognition, *Neural Netw.*, 7:1295–1301.

Gait Transitions

James J. Collins

Introduction

Legged animals typically employ multiple gaits for terrestrial locomotion. Bipeds, for example, walk, run, and hop, whereas quadrupeds commonly walk, trot, and bound. Animals make transitions between different gaits depending on their speed and the terrain. Experimental studies have demonstrated that animal locomotion is controlled, in part, by a central pattern generator (CPG), which is a network of neurons in the central nervous system (CNS) capable of producing rhythmic output (Shik and Orlovsky, 1976; Grillner, 1981; Pearson, 1993). (The control of locomotion, however, is not purely central; e.g., the output of a locomotor CPG is modulated by feedback from the periphery.) Shik and colleagues, for instance, showed that mesencephalic cats could exhibit a walking gait on a treadmill when the midbrain was electrically stimulated. Moreover, they found that such preparations could switch between different gaits if either the stimulation strength or the treadmill speed was varied.

Although the aforementioned studies established the existence of rhythm-generating networks in the CNS, a vertebrate CPG for legged locomotion remains to be identified or isolated. As a result, little is known about the specific characteristics of the neurons and interconnections making up such systems. Consequently, researchers have resorted to using modeling techniques to gain insight into the possible functional organization of these networks. The most popular approach has involved the analysis of systems of coupled oscillators. Coupled-oscillator models have been used to control the gaits of bipeds (Bay and Hemami, 1987; Taga, Yamaguchi, and Shimizu, 1991), quadrupeds (Stafford and Barnwell, 1985; Schöner, Jiang, and Kelso, 1990; Collins and Stewart, 1993a; Collins and Richmond, 1994), and hexapods (Beer, 1990; Collins and Stewart, 1993b).

The neural mechanisms underlying gait changes are not well understood. A key question in this regard is whether gait transitions involve (1) switching between different CPGs, or (2) bifurcations of activity in a single CPG. In this article, we discuss a number of modeling approaches that have been developed to explore the feasibility of using either one or the other of these mechanisms to generate gait transitions in coupled-oscillator networks.

A Neuromodulatory Approach

As a model for legged-locomotion control, Grillner (1981) proposed that each limb of an animal is governed by a separate CPG, and that interlimb coordination is achieved through the actions of interneurons that couple together these CPGs. Within this scheme, gait transitions are produced by switching between different sets of coordinating interneurons; that is, a locomotor CPG is reconfigured to produce different gaits.

Grillner's proposed strategy has been adopted, in spirit, by several CPG modeling studies. Stafford and Barnwell (1985), for example, used a similar approach in a study of quadrupedal locomotion. They considered a CPG model that was composed of four coupled networks of oscillators. Each network controlled the muscle activities of a limb of a model quadruped. Stafford and Barnwell showed that this model could produce the walk, trot, and bound. In addition, they demonstrated that the walk-to-trot and walk-to-bound transitions could be generated by changing the relative strength of certain interoscillator connections or by eliminating others altogether. (Transitions in the reverse direction, e.g., bound-to-walk, were not reported.) Along similar lines, Bay and Hemami (1987) used a CPG network of four coupled van der Pol oscillators to control the movements of a segmented biped. Each limb of the biped was composed of two links, and each oscillator controlled the movement of a single link. Bipedal walking and hopping were simulated by using the oscillators' output to determine the angular positions of the respective links. Transitions between out-of-phase and in-phase gaits were generated by changing the nature of the interoscillator coupling; for example, the polarities of the network interconnections were reversed to produce the walk-to-hop transition.

This approach is, in principle, physiologically reasonable. For instance, the notion that supraspinal centers may call on functionally distinct sets of coordinating interneurons to generate different

gaits is plausible but not yet experimentally established. In addition, from a different but relevant perspective, it has been shown that rhythm-generating neuronal networks can be modulated—reconfigured—through the actions of neuroamines and peptides, and that they are thereby enabled to produce several different motor patterns (see Pearson, 1993, and CRUSTACEAN STOMATOGASTRIC SYSTEM), at least in invertebrate preparations.

A Synergetic Approach

Synergetics deals with COOPERATIVE PHENOMENA (q.v.) in nonequilibrium systems (Haken, Kelso, and Bunz, 1985). In synergetics, the macroscopic behavior of a complex system is characterized by a small number of collective variables, which in turn govern the qualitative behavior of the system's components.

Schöner et al. (1990) used a synergetic approach in a study of quadrupedal locomotion. They analyzed a network model that was made up of four coupled oscillators. Each oscillator represented a limb of a model quadruped. Three relative phases—the phase differences between the right-front and the left-front, left-hind, and right-hind oscillators, respectively—were used as collective variables to characterize the system's interlimb-coordination patterns. Gait transitions were modeled as nonequilibrium phase transitions, which, in this case, could also be interpreted as bifurcations in a dynamical system (see the next section). Schöner et al. demonstrated that various four-component networks could produce and switch (abruptly or gradually) between different gaits, such as the gallop, trot, and pace, if the coupling terms that operated on the relative phases were varied. Importantly, this work predicted that gait transitions should be accompanied by loss of stability; that is, signs of instability, such as spontaneous gait transitions, should arise near a switching point. Phenomena of this sort have been observed experimentally; the decerebrate cats in the Shik and Orlovsky study, for example, could, near the trot-gallop transition point, switch back and forth spontaneously between the trot and gallop.

This approach is significant in that it relates system parameter changes and stability issues to gait transitions. Its primary weakness, however, is that the physiological relevance of the aforementioned relative-phase coupling terms is unclear. This remains an open issue.

A Group-Theoretic Approach

The traditional approach for modeling a locomotor CPG has been to set up and analyze, either analytically or numerically, the parameter-dependent dynamics of a hypothesized neural circuit. Collins and Stewart (1993a, 1993b), however, approached this problem from the perspective of group theory. Specifically, they considered various networks of symmetrically coupled nonlinear oscillators and examined how the symmetry of the respective systems leads to a general class of phase-locked oscillation patterns. Within this approach, the onset of a given pattern is modeled as a symmetric Hopf bifurcation, and transitions between different patterns are modeled as symmetry-breaking bifurcations of various kinds. In standard Hopf bifurcation, the dynamics of a nonlinear system change as some parameter is varied and a stable steady state becomes unstable, "throwing off" a limit cycle (or periodic solution). At a symmetric analog of a Hopf bifurcation, which is appropriate for symmetric dynamical systems, one or more periodic solutions, usually several, bifurcate. There may also be secondary branches of solutions and other more complicated bifurcations. Successive bifurcations tend to break more and more symmetry; i.e., they lead to states with less and less symmetry. Importantly, the pattern of bifurcations that can occur and the nature of the periodic states that arise through such bifurcations are controlled primarily by the symmetries of the system.

The theory of symmetric Hopf bifurcation thus predicts that symmetric oscillator networks with invariant structure can sustain multiple patterns of rhythmic activity. From the standpoint of CPGs, this prediction challenges the notion that a network's coupling architecture needs to be altered to produce different oscillation patterns. Importantly, the symmetry-breaking analysis is independent of the details of the oscillators' intrinsic dynamics and the interoscillator coupling. (The production of periodic states through symmetric Hopf bifurcation, however, does depend on the variation of some suitable system parameter.) This approach thus provides a framework for distinguishing model-independent features (attributable to symmetry alone) from model-dependent features.

Collins and Stewart used this approach to study the dynamics of symmetric networks of two, four, and six coupled oscillators. These networks were considered as models for bipedal, quadrupedal, and hexapodal locomotor CPGs, respectively. They demonstrated that many of the generic phase-locked oscillation patterns for these models correspond to animal gaits. They also showed that transitions between these gaits could be modeled as symmetry-breaking bifurcations occurring in such systems. These studies led to natural hierarchies of gaits, ordered by symmetry, and to natural sequences of gait bifurcations (Figure 1). This work thus related observed gaits and gait transitions to the organizational structures of the underlying CPGs.

This approach is significant in that it provides a novel mechanism for generating gait transitions in locomotor CPGs. Its primary disadvantage, however, is that its model-independent features cannot provide information about the internal dynamics of individual oscillators. In particular, the stability of the predicted gait patterns and the conditions under which one is selected over another depend on the specific parameters of the model under investigation.

A Hardwired Network Approach

Motivated by the predictions of the above group-theoretic approach, Collins and Richmond (1994) conducted a series of computer experiments with a symmetric, hardwired locomotor CPG model that consisted of four coupled oscillators. They demonstrated that it was possible for such a network to produce multiple phase-locked oscillation patterns that correspond to three quadrupedal gaits: the walk, the trot, and the bound. Transitions between the different gaits were generated by varying the driving signal or by altering internal oscillator parameters. As observed in real animals (Alexander, 1989), transitions between the walk and trot, which were generated by varying the intrinsic frequency of the CPG oscillators and the amplitude of the driving signal, could be either gradual or abrupt, depending on the nature of the parameter variation. Similar parameter changes could also shift the CPG

model from either the walk or the trot into the bound. However, once the CPG model was in bound, it maintained that gait even if the system parameters were returned to their original values for either walk or trot, i.e., there was "total" hysteresis in the network's dynamics. To produce transitions from bound, it was necessary to subject two of the CPG oscillators to an increased driving stimulus before the system parameters were changed to those of the desired gait. (Experimental data that indirectly support such a strategy for generating transitions from bound were provided by Afelt, Blaszczyk, and Dobrzecka, 1983. Specifically, they found that the initiation of the gallop-to-trot transition in dogs was characterized by kinematic changes in a *single pair* of diagonal limbs.) Importantly, the above *in numero* results were obtained without changing the relative strengths or polarities of the system's interconnections; i.e., the network maintained an invariant coupling architecture. Collins and Richmond (1994) also showed that the ability of the hardwired CPG network to produce and switch between multiple gaits was, in essence, a model-independent phenomenon: three different oscillator models—the Stein neuronal model, the van der Pol oscillator, and the FitzHugh-Nagumo model—and two different coupling schemes were incorporated into the network without impeding its ability to produce the three gaits and the aforementioned gait transitions. This general finding was likely attributable to the symmetry of the network, which was maintained in all the numerical experiments.

Earlier, Beer (1990) had designed a hardwired CPG network for controlling hexapodal locomotion (see LOCOMOTION, INVERTEBRATE). In Beer's model, each leg of a model cockroach was controlled by a circuit made up of one pacemaker neuron, two sensory neurons, and three motor neurons. The pacemaker neurons of adjacent leg-controller circuits inhibited one another. If the pacemaker neurons of the network were identical, then the model could generate the tripod gait. To produce metachronal-wave gaits (in which waves of leg movements sweep from the back of the animal to the front), Beer varied the intrinsic frequencies of the pacemaker neurons such that the natural frequency of the back-leg pacemakers was lower than that of the middle-leg pacemakers, which was lower than that of the front-leg pacemakers. With this arrangement, the progression speed of the model cockroach could be changed, and transitions between different gaits could be produced by varying the tonic level of activity of a single command neuron, which was connected to every leg-controller circuit. This model's ability to generate and switch between different gaits was a direct consequence of the interactions between its coupled pacemaker neurons and their respective central and afferent inputs.

A similar model, made up of six coupled unit oscillators, was developed by Taga et al. (1991) to control bipedal locomotion. In this case, each unit oscillator controlled a single joint, i.e., an ankle, knee, or hip, of a multi-link biped. As with Beer's model, the CPG network was driven by a tonic activation signal, and each unit oscillator received feedback about the state of the system's limbs. With this arrangement, the biped's speed could be changed, and abrupt transitions between walking and running could be generated by varying the amplitude of the network's activation signal. Interestingly, these gait transitions exhibited hysteresis; i.e., the walk-to-run transition occurred at a faster progression speed than did the reverse transition. Similar hysteretic behavior has been observed in humans (Alexander, 1989). Taga et al., unfortunately, did not report on the model's ability to switch between out-of-phase gaits (i.e., walking and running) and in-phase gaits (i.e., hopping).

In these studies, gait transitions were produced by varying the CPG's driving signal. From a physiological standpoint, this pattern-switching mechanism is reasonable; e.g., experimental studies have shown that the output of a locomotor CPG can be modified by changes to its descending inputs. Nonetheless, it is important to note that the exact form of the driving signal or signals

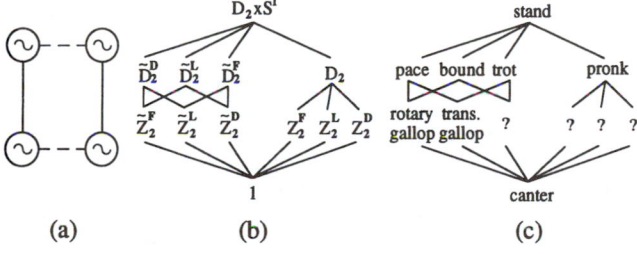

Figure 1. *A*, A rectangularly symmetric network of four coupled oscillators. The solid and dashed lines represent two forms of coupling. *B*, Patterns of symmetry breaking for the network in *A*. The respective group-theoretic symbols are described in Collins and Stewart (1993a). *C*, Quadrupedal gaits corresponding to the patterns in *B*.

acting on a locomotor CPG is unknown. Similarly, it is unclear how externally applied stimulation signals are transmitted to locomotor CPGs. For instance, although the stimulation signal in the Shik and Orlovsky study was amplitude modulated (to produce gait transitions), this does not necessarily mean that the resulting descending signals were also amplitude modulated. In addition, although the results of the Shik study were largely independent of the stimulation frequency, there is evidence that frequency-modulated stimulation signals can affect the output of locomotor CPGs. Lennard and Stein (1977), for example, electrically stimulated the dorsolateral funiculus in spinal and intact turtles and found that an increase in the stimulus frequency resulted in an increased repetition rate of hindlimb swimming movements. Finally, it should be reiterated that it is most likely erroneous to assume (as it has been in several CPG modeling studies) that the net driving signal of a locomotor CPG consists only of descending influences from supraspinal centers. The results from several experimental studies indicate that a CPG "driving" signal may also consist of afferent inputs from peripheral sensory organs (Pearson, 1993).

Discussion

The discussed modeling studies fall into two camps: (1) gait transitions are produced by changing the relative strength or polarity of the interoscillator coupling in a CPG; i.e., "different" CPGs are used to produce different gaits; or (2) gait transitions are generated by changing the CPG's driving signal; i.e., bifurcations in a single CPG are used to generate different gaits. Both of these pattern-switching mechanisms are physiologically plausible, and they each lead to realistic locomotor patterns; e.g., in most of these studies, the stepping frequency or progression speed of the model animal increased when the CPG network switched to "faster" gaits. However, for a consistent theory of gait transitions to emerge, additional experimental data about the functional organization and operation of locomotor CPGs will have to be obtained. In particular, work is needed: (1) to determine whether a locomotor CPG uses functionally distinct sets of coordinating interneurons to produce different motor patterns, (2) to establish the extent to which neuromodulatory mechanisms are employed in vertebrate motor systems, and (3) to clarify the nature of the peripheral and descending inputs that influence the output of a locomotor CPG. Further experimentation is also needed to examine the possible role of bifurcation in gait transitions. In this regard, future investigations should explore the extent of hysteresis in gait transitions and the occurrence of increased instabilities near switching points, as well as consider more extensively the effects of system-parameter variation on gait-transition dynamics.

[Reprinted from the First Edition]

Road Map: Motor Pattern Generators
Background: I.3. Dynamics and Adaptation in Neural Networks
Related Reading: Dynamics and Bifurcation in Neural Nets; Locomotion, Vertebrate; Spinal Cord of Lamprey: Generation of Locomotor Patterns

References

Afelt, Z., Blaszczyk, J., and Dobrzecka, C., 1983, Speed control in animal locomotion: Transitions between symmetrical and nonsymmetrical gaits in the dog, *Acta Neurobiol. Exp.*, 43:235–250.

Alexander, R. McN., 1989, Optimization and gaits in the locomotion of vertebrates, *Phys. Rev.*, 69:1199–1227. ◆

Bay, J. S., and Hemami, H., 1987, Modeling of a neural pattern generator with coupled nonlinear oscillators, *IEEE Trans. Biomed. Eng.*, 34:297–306.

Beer, R. D., 1990, *Intelligence as Adaptive Behavior: An Experiment in Computational Neuroethology*, San Diego: Academic Press.

Collins, J. J., and Richmond, S. A., 1994, Hard-wired central pattern generators for quadrupedal locomotion, *Biol. Cybern.*, 71:375–385.

Collins, J. J., and Stewart, I. N., 1993a, Coupled nonlinear oscillators and the symmetries of animal gaits, *J. Nonlin. Sci.*, 3:349–392. ◆

Collins, J. J., and Stewart, I., 1993b, Hexapodal gaits and coupled nonlinear oscillator models, *Biol. Cybern.*, 68:287–298.

Grillner, S., 1981, Control of locomotion in bipeds, tetrapods and fish, in *The Handbook of Physiology*, section 1: *The Nervous System*, vol. II, *Motor Control* (V. B. Brooks, Ed.), Bethesda, MD: American Physiological Society, pp. 1179–1236.

Haken, H., Kelso, J. A. S., and Bunz, H., 1985, A theoretical model of phase transitions in human hand movements, *Biol. Cybern.*, 51:347–356.

Lennard, P. R., and Stein, P. S. G., 1977, Swimming movements elicited by electrical stimulation of turtle spinal cord: I. Low-spinal and intact preparations, *J. Neurophysiol.*, 40:768–778.

Pearson, K. G., 1993, Common principles of motor control in vertebrates and invertebrates, *Annu. Rev. Neurosci.*, 16:265–297. ◆

Schöner, G., Jiang, W. Y., and Kelso, J. A. S., 1990, A synergetic theory of quadrupedal gaits and gait transitions, *J. Theoret. Biol.*, 142:359–391.

Shik, M. L., and Orlovsky, G. N., 1976, Neurophysiology of locomotor automatism, *Phys. Rev.*, 56:465–501.

Stafford, F. S., and Barnwell, G. M., 1985, Mathematical models of central pattern generators in locomotion: III. Interlimb model for the cat, *J. Motor Behav.*, 17:60–76.

Taga, G., Yamaguchi, Y., and Shimizu, H., 1991, Self-organized control of bipedal locomotion by neural oscillators in unpredictable environment, *Biol. Cybern.*, 65:147–159.

Gaussian Processes

Chris K. I. Williams

Introduction

Much of the work in the field of artificial neural networks concerns the problem of supervised learning. Here we may be interested in regression problems (by which we mean the prediction of some real-valued variable(s)), or classification problems (predicting a class label) given the values of some input variables. Due to factors such as measurement noise, it is necessary to take a statistical view of the learning problem.

Given (possibly noisy) observations of a function at n points, it is necessary to impose extra assumptions about the function if there is to be hope of predicting its value elsewhere. Here we take a Bayesian approach, placing a prior probability distribution over possible functions and then letting the observed data "sculpt" this prior into a posterior using the available data. The Bayesian approach can provide solutions to several problems, such as local optima in weight space, the setting of regularization parameters, overfitting, and model selection (see MacKay, 1992; Neal, 1996; and BAYESIAN METHODS AND NEURAL NETWORKS).

One can place a prior distribution $P(\mathbf{w})$ on the weights $\mathbf{w}$ of a neural network to induce a prior over functions $P(y(\mathbf{x}; \mathbf{w}))$ but the computations required to make predictions are not easy, owing to the nonlinearities in the system, and one needs to resort to analytic approximations or Monte Carlo methods. Gaussian processes are a way of specifying a prior directly over function space; it is often simpler to do this than to work with priors over parameters. Gaussian processes (GPs) are probably the simplest kind of function space prior that one can consider, being a generalization of finite-dimensional Gaussian distributions over vectors.

A finite-dimensional Gaussian distribution is defined by a mean vector and a covariance matrix. A GP is defined by a *mean function* (which we shall usually take to be identically zero), and a *covariance function* $C(\mathbf{x}, \mathbf{x}')$, which indicates how correlated the value of the function y is at $\mathbf{x}$ and $\mathbf{x}'$. This function encodes our assumptions about the problem (for example, that the function is smooth and continuous) and will influence the quality of the predictions.

Gaussian process prediction is illustrated in Figure 1. The upper panel shows a sample of five functions drawn from the prior. The lower panel shows five samples from the posterior after two observations have been made; notice that the posterior is tightly constrained near the observations, but varies more widely further away. Essentially, what has happened is that prior samples not consistent with the observations have been eliminated. The crucial computational point is that it is not necessary to draw samples to make predictions; for regression problems, only linear algebra is required. Below we give more detail on this computation, discuss how to use GPs for classification problems, and describe how data can be used to adapt the covariance function to the given prediction problem.

Further discussion of Gaussian processes is available in Schölkopf and Smola (2001), MacKay (1998), and Williams (1998).

Gaussian Processes

Formal Definition

A stochastic process is a collection of random variables $\{Y(\mathbf{x})|\mathbf{x} \in X\}$ indexed by a set X. In our case X will often be $\mathbb{R}^d$, where d is the number of inputs. The stochastic process is specified by giving the joint probability distribution for every finite subset of variables $Y(\mathbf{x}_1), \ldots, Y(\mathbf{x}_k)$ in a consistent manner. A Gaussian process (GP) is a stochastic process for which any finite set of Y-variables has a joint multivariate Gaussian distribution. A GP is fully specified by its mean function $\mu(\mathbf{x}) = E[Y(\mathbf{x})]$ and its covariance function $C(\mathbf{x}, \mathbf{x}') = E[(Y(\mathbf{x}) - \mu(\mathbf{x}))(Y(\mathbf{x}') - \mu(\mathbf{x}'))]$. For a multidimensional input space, a Gaussian process may also be called a Gaussian random field.

Below we consider Gaussian processes that have $\mu(\mathbf{x}) \equiv 0$. A non-zero $\mu(\mathbf{x})$ can be incorporated into the framework at the expense of a little extra complexity.

Example: Bayesian linear regression. Consider the model $y(x) = \sum_{i=1}^{m} w_i \phi_i(\mathbf{x}) = \mathbf{w}^T \boldsymbol{\phi}(\mathbf{x})$, where $\{\phi_i\}$ is a set of fixed basis functions and $\mathbf{w}$ is a vector of "weights." Let $\mathbf{w}$ have a Gaussian distribution with mean $\mathbf{0}$ and covariance Σ. Then $\mu(\mathbf{x}) = E[y(\mathbf{x})] = E[\mathbf{w}^T]\boldsymbol{\phi}(\mathbf{x}) = 0$ as $E[\mathbf{w}] = \mathbf{0}$. As the mean is zero we have that $C(\mathbf{x}, \mathbf{x}') = \boldsymbol{\phi}^T(\mathbf{x})E[\mathbf{w}\mathbf{w}^T]\boldsymbol{\phi}(\mathbf{x}') = \boldsymbol{\phi}^T(\mathbf{x})\Sigma\phi(\mathbf{x}')$. For example, using basis functions 1 and the components of $\mathbf{x}$ along with $\Sigma = I$ gives $C(\mathbf{x}, \mathbf{x}') = 1 + \mathbf{x}.\mathbf{x}'$.

In the case of a finite dimensional model we can make predictions using calculations in the parameter space (of dimension m), or a GP prediction (which is n-dimensional, where n is the number of data points). For $m < n$ the parameter space method is preferable, but for many useful covariance functions (see, e.g., Equation 1) m is infinite and the GP method is necessary.

Covariance Functions

The only constraint on the covariance function is that it should generate a non-negative definite covariance matrix for any set of points in X. This gives wide scope, and different choices of $C(\mathbf{x}, \mathbf{x}')$ can give rise to such differing priors as straight lines of the form $y = w_0 + w_1 x$ (as discussed above) to the very rough and jagged sample paths associated with a Wiener process (a model for Brownian motion) or an Ornstein-Uhlenbeck process.

One very common form of covariance function is the *stationary* covariance function, where $C(\mathbf{x}, \mathbf{x}')$ is a function of $\mathbf{x} - \mathbf{x}'$. The use of stationary covariance functions is appealing if one would like the predictions to be invariant under shifts of the origin in input space. For example, in one dimension letting $h = x - x'$, the covariance of the Ornstein-Uhlenbeck process is $C_{OU}(h) = v_0 e^{-|h|/\lambda}$, where v_0 sets the overall variance of the process and λ sets a length scale in the input space. Another example of a stationary covariance function is the "squared exponential" covariance function $C_{SE}(h) = v_0 \exp(-h^2/\lambda^2)$ (sometimes called the "Gaussian" covariance function).

One commonly-used covariance function for inputs in $\mathbb{R}^d$ is

$$C(\mathbf{x}, \mathbf{x}') = v_0 \exp\left\{-\sum_{l=1}^{d} \frac{(x_l - x_l')^2}{\lambda_l^2}\right\} \qquad (1)$$

This is simply the product of d squared-exponential covariance functions, but with different length scales on each dimension. The general form of the covariance function expresses the idea that cases with nearby inputs will have highly correlated outputs, and the λ parameters allow a different distance measure for each input dimension. For irrelevant inputs, the corresponding λ_l will become large, and the model will effectively ignore that input. This is closely related to the automatic relevance determination (ARD) idea of MacKay and Neal (Neal, 1996).

The term *kernel function* used in the support vector machines literature is broadly equivalent to the covariance function. Further information on kernel/covariance functions can be found in Schölkopf and Smola (2001, chaps. 4 and 13), MacKay (1998), Williams (1998), and references therein.

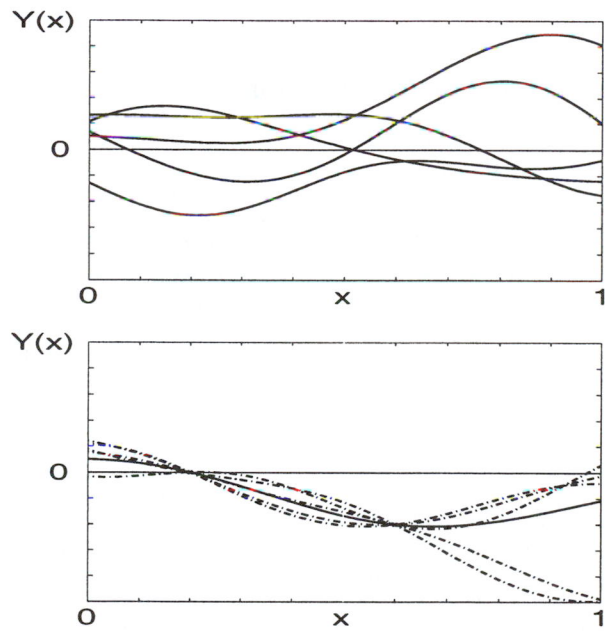

Figure 1. *Top*, Five samples from a Gaussian process prior. *Bottom*, Five samples from the Gaussian process posterior (shown as dot-dash lines) and the posterior mean (solid line), after observing the data points (0.2, 0) and (0.6, −1).

Gaussian Processes for Regression Problems

In the previous section we discussed the properties of Gaussian processes. We now assume that we have input points $\mathbf{x}^n = \mathbf{x}_1, \ldots, \mathbf{x}_n$ and target values $\mathbf{t} = t_1, \ldots, t_n$ and wish to predict the function value y_* corresponding to an input $\mathbf{x}_*$. We assume that the target values t_i are obtained from the corresponding function value y_i by means of additive Gaussian noise, i.e., $t_i = y_i + \varepsilon_i$ for $i = 1, \ldots, n$, where ε_i is an independent zero-mean Gaussian random variable of variance σ_v^2. (The generalization to different variances at each location is straightforward, but notationally a bit more complex.) As the prior is a Gaussian process, the prior distribution over the y_i's is given by $\mathbf{Y} \sim N(\mathbf{0}, K)$, where K is the $n \times n$ covariance matrix with entries $K_{ij} = C(\mathbf{x}_i, \mathbf{x}_j)$. It is then easy to show that the prior distribution over the targets is $N(\mathbf{0}, K + \sigma_v^2 I_n)$ where I_n is the $n \times n$ identity matrix.

To make a prediction for y_* we now need to consider the $n + 1$-dimensional vector, which consists of the n variables in $\mathbf{t}$ with the variable y_* appended, and condition on $\mathbf{t}$ to obtain $P(y_*|\mathbf{t})$. As conditional distributions of jointly Gaussian variables are also Gaussian, it is clear that this distribution will be Gaussian, and our task is to compute the mean $\hat{y}(\mathbf{x}_*)$ and variance $\hat{\sigma}^2(\mathbf{x}_*)$. It turns out that

$$\hat{y}(\mathbf{x}_*) = \mathbf{k}^T(\mathbf{x}_*)(K + \sigma_v^2 I_n)^{-1}\mathbf{t} = \sum_{i=1}^{n} \alpha_i C(\mathbf{x}_i, \mathbf{x}_*) \quad (2)$$

$$\hat{\sigma}^2(\mathbf{x}_*) = C(\mathbf{x}_*, \mathbf{x}_*) - \mathbf{k}^T(\mathbf{x}_*)(K + \sigma_v^2 I_n)^{-1}\mathbf{k}(\mathbf{x}_*) \quad (3)$$

where $\mathbf{k}(\mathbf{x}_*)$ is the $n \times 1$ vector of covariances $(C(\mathbf{x}_1, \mathbf{x}_*), \ldots, C(\mathbf{x}_n, \mathbf{x}_*))^T$, and $\boldsymbol{\alpha} = (K + \sigma_v^2 I_n)^{-1}\mathbf{t}$. Unpacking Equation 2, we see that the prediction function $\hat{y}(\mathbf{x}_*)$ is a linear combination of the kernel functions $C(\mathbf{x}_i, \mathbf{x}_*)$, with coefficients given by the appropriate entries of the vector $\boldsymbol{\alpha}$.

Equations 2 and 3 require the inversion of an $n \times n$ matrix, which is in general an $O(n^3)$ operation. When n is of the order of a few hundred, then this is quite feasible with modern computers. However, once $n \sim O(1000)$, these computations can be quite time-consuming, and much recent research effort has gone into developing approximation methods; see Tresp (2001) for a review. Note that in special cases (notably when the input space is $\mathbb{R}$ and for certain Markovian kernels), the necessary calculations can be carried out in linear time (see Wahba, 1990, for further details).

The use of Gaussian processes for regression problems has been studied extensively by Carl Rasmussen in (Rasmussen, 1996) and in his Ph.D. thesis (available at http://www.cs.utoronto.ca/~carl/). He carried out a careful comparison of the Bayesian treatment of Gaussian process regression with several other state-of-the-art methods on a number of problems and found that its performance is comparable to that of Bayesian neural networks as developed by Neal (1996), and consistently better than the other methods tested.

Adapting the Covariance Function

Given a covariance function, it is straightforward to make predictions for new test points. However, in practical situations we are unlikely to know which covariance function to use. One option is to choose a parametric family of covariance functions (with a parameter vector $\boldsymbol{\theta}$) and then to search for parameters that give good predictions.

Adaptation of $\boldsymbol{\theta}$ is facilitated by the fact that the log likelihood $l = \log P(\mathbf{t}|\boldsymbol{\theta})$ can be calculated analytically as

$$l = -\tfrac{1}{2} \log \det(K + \sigma_v^2 I_n)$$
$$- \tfrac{1}{2} \mathbf{t}^T(K + \sigma_v^2 I_n)^{-1}\mathbf{t} - \frac{n}{2} \log 2\pi \quad (4)$$

This is just the log likelihood of the vector $\mathbf{t}$ under a Gaussian with mean $\mathbf{0}$ and covariance $K + \sigma_v^2 I_n$. The evaluation of the likelihood and its partial derivatives with respect to the parameters takes time $O(n^3)$, unless special structure in the problem can be exploited. Given l and its derivatives with respect to $\boldsymbol{\theta}$, it is straightforward to feed this information to an optimization package in order to obtain a local maximum of the likelihood.

One can also combine $P(\mathbf{t}|\boldsymbol{\theta})$ with a prior $P(\boldsymbol{\theta})$ to yield a Bayesian approach to the problem. Another approach to adapting $\boldsymbol{\theta}$ is to use the cross-validation (CV) or generalized cross-validation (GCV) methods, as discussed in Wahba (1990).

Relationship to Other Methods

Prediction with Gaussian processes is certainly not a very recent topic; the basic theory goes back at least as far as the work of Wiener and Kolmogorov in the 1940s on time series. Gaussian process prediction is also well known in the geostatistics field (see Cressie, 1993), where it is known as "kriging," although this literature naturally has focused mostly on two- and three-dimensional input spaces.

As mentioned above, there is a close relationship between Bayesian approaches and regularization theory. This connection was described in Kimeldorf and Wahba (1970), and further details can be found in Wahba (1990), Poggio and Girosi (1990), and GENERALIZATION AND REGULARIZATION IN NONLINEAR LEARNING SYSTEMS.

When the covariance function $C(\mathbf{x}, \mathbf{x}')$ depends only on $h = |\mathbf{x} - \mathbf{x}'|$, the predictor derived in Equation 2 has the form $\sum_i c_i C(|\mathbf{x} - \mathbf{x}_i|)$ and may be called a *radial basis function* (or RBF) network. This is one derivation of RBFs, which are described in more detail in RADIAL BASIS FUNCTION NETWORKS.

The Gaussian process approach adds a stochastic process view to the regularization viewpoint, giving us "error bars" on the prediction (Equation 3), an expression for $P(\mathbf{t}|\boldsymbol{\theta})$ and its derivatives, and allows us to use the Bayesian machinery for hierarchical models.

Gaussian Processes for Classification Problems

Given training data and an input $\mathbf{x}$, the aim of a classifier is to predict the corresponding class label. This may be done by simply predicting a class label ("hard" classification), or by outputting an estimate of the posterior probabilities for each class $P(k|\mathbf{x})$ ("soft" classification), where $k = 1, \ldots C$ indexes the C classes. Naturally, we require that $0 \leq P(k|\mathbf{x}) \leq 1$ for all k and that $\sum_k P(k|\mathbf{x}) = 1$. A naive application of the regression method for Gaussian processes using, say, targets of 1 when an example of class k is observed and 0 otherwise will not obey these constraints. Soft classification has the advantage that the posterior probability estimates can be used in a principled fashion with loss matrices, rejection thresholds, and so on.

For the two-class classification problem it is only necessary to represent $P(1|\mathbf{x})$, since $P(2|\mathbf{x}) = 1 - P(1|\mathbf{x})$. An easy way to ensure that the estimate $\pi(\mathbf{x})$ of $P(1|\mathbf{x})$ lies in $[0, 1]$ is to obtain it by passing an unbounded value $y(\mathbf{x})$ through an appropriate function that has range $[0, 1]$. A common choice is the logistic function $\sigma(z) = 1/(1 + e^{-z})$ so that $\pi(\mathbf{x}) = \sigma(y(\mathbf{x}))$. The input $y(\mathbf{x})$ to the logistic function will be called the *activation*. In the simplest method of this kind, logistic regression, the activation is simply computed as a linear combination of the inputs, plus a bias, i.e., $y(\mathbf{x}) = \mathbf{w}^T\mathbf{x} + b$. Using a Gaussian process or other flexible methods allows $y(\mathbf{x})$ to be a nonlinear function of the inputs.

For the classification problem with more than two classes, a simple extension of this idea using the "softmax" function gives the predicted probability for class k as

$$\pi(k|\mathbf{x}) = \frac{\exp y_k(\mathbf{x})}{\sum_m \exp y_m(\mathbf{x})} \tag{5}$$

For the rest of this section we shall concentrate on the two-class problem; extension of the methods to the multiclass case is relatively straightforward.

Defining a Gaussian process prior over the activation $y(\mathbf{x})$ automatically induces a prior over $\pi(\mathbf{x})$. To make predictions for a test input $\mathbf{x}_*$ when using fixed parameters in the GP we would like to compute $\hat{\pi}_* = \int \pi_* P(\pi_*|\mathbf{t}, \theta) d\pi_*$, which requires us to find $P(\pi_*|\mathbf{t}) = P(\pi(\mathbf{x}_*)|\mathbf{t})$ for a new input $\mathbf{x}_*$. This can be done by finding the distribution $P(y_*|\mathbf{t})$ (y_* is the activation of π_*) as given by

$$P(y_*|\mathbf{t}) = \int P(y_*|\mathbf{y})P(\mathbf{y}|\mathbf{t})d\mathbf{y} = \frac{1}{P(t)} \int P(y_*|\mathbf{y})P(\mathbf{y})P(\mathbf{t}|\mathbf{y})d\mathbf{y} \tag{6}$$

where $\mathbf{y} = (y_1, \ldots, y_n)$ denotes the activations corresponding to the data points. $P(\pi_*|\mathbf{t})$ can then be found from $P(y_*|\mathbf{t})$ using the appropriate Jacobian to transform the distribution. When $P(\mathbf{t}|\mathbf{y})$ is Gaussian, then the integral in Equation 6 can be computed exactly to yield Equations 2 and 3. However, the usual expression for $P(\mathbf{t}|\mathbf{y}) = \Pi_i P(t_i|y_i)$ and $P(t_i|y_i) = \pi_i$ if $t_i = 1$ and $P(t_i|y_i) = (1 - \pi_i)$ for $t_i = -1$ for classification data (where the t's take on values of 1 or -1) means that the marginalization to obtain $P(y_*|\mathbf{t})$ is no longer analytically tractable. Faced with this problem, we can either use an analytic approximation to the integral in Equation 6 or use Monte Carlo methods to approximate it. These two approaches will be considered in turn.

First, we note that $P(y_*|\mathbf{t})$ is mediated through $P(\mathbf{y}|\mathbf{t})$ and that $P(y_*|\mathbf{y})$ is Gaussian, so that obtaining information about $P(\mathbf{y}|\mathbf{t})$ is the essential step. It is easy to find the maximum of this distribution by optimizing $\log P(\mathbf{y}) + \log P(\mathbf{t}|\mathbf{y})$ with respect to $\mathbf{y}$, e.g., with a Newton-Raphson iteration. It can be shown that the optimization problem is convex. This yields the *maximum a posteriori* estimator $\mathbf{y}^{MAP}$. We could build a classifier based on $\mathbf{y}^{MAP}$ by calculating $y^{MAP}(\mathbf{x}_*)$ as the mean of $P(y_*|\mathbf{y}^{MAP})$. This can then be fed through the logistic function to obtain an approximation to $\hat{\pi}_*$. This MAP solution is the one used in spline-smoothing approaches to classification (Wahba, 1990).

One can also make a Gaussian approximation to $P(\mathbf{y}|\mathbf{t})$ with mean $\mathbf{y}^{MAP}$ and inverse covariance matrix $-\nabla\nabla \log P(\mathbf{y}|\mathbf{t})$. This yields a Laplace approximation to the integral in Equation 6.

Neal (1998) has developed an MCMC method for the Gaussian process classification model. This works by generating samples from $P(\mathbf{y}|\mathbf{t})$ by updating each of the n individual y_i's sequentially using Gibbs sampling. This sampling process can be also be interleaved with sampling for the parameters θ. As with the regression problem, there has been much work on approximation schemes for large data sets; see Tresp (2001) for further details.

Classifiers using splines have been used extensively on a wide variety of problems, see Wahba (1990) and references in GENERALIZATION AND REGULARIZATION IN NONLINEAR LEARNING SYSTEMS. Gaussian process classifiers using MCMC sampling over θ have been described in Williams and Barber (1998).

Relationship to Support Vector Machines

We have seen that the *maximum a posteriori* solution $\mathbf{y}^{MAP}$ is obtained by minimizing $\Psi(\mathbf{y}) = -\log P(\mathbf{y}) - \log P(\mathbf{t}|\mathbf{y})$. This expression can be refined using $-\log P(\mathbf{t}|\mathbf{y}) = -\Sigma_i \log P(t_i|y_i)$ and $-\log P(t_i|y_i) = \log(1 + e^{-t_i y_i})$ to give

$$\Psi(\mathbf{y}) = \tfrac{1}{2} \mathbf{y}^T K^{-1}\mathbf{y} + \sum_i \log(1 + e^{-t_i y_i}) + c \tag{7}$$

where c is a constant independent of $\mathbf{y}$. The criterion optimized by the support vector machine (SVM) learning algorithm (Vapnik, 1995) is very similar, but with $g_{GP}(z) \stackrel{def}{=} \log(1 + e^{-z})$ replaced by $g_{SVM}(z) \stackrel{def}{=} [1 - z]_+$, where $[x]_+ = \max(x, 0)$. These are both monotonically decreasing functions of z, which are linear for $z \to -\infty$. They both decay to zero as $z \to \infty$, but the main difference is that the g_{SVM} takes on the value 0 for $z > 1$, while g_{GP} asymptotes to 0 as $z \to \infty$. The SVM optimization problem is convex, but inequality constraints mean that it is quadratic programming problem.

By replacing g_{GP} with g_{SVM} we obtain $y^{SVM}(\mathbf{x}_*)$ instead of $y^{MAP}(\mathbf{x}_*)$. To make a "hard" ($+1/-1$) prediction, we simply take the predicted class label as $\text{sgn}(y(\mathbf{x}_*))$. This is the SVM classifier. The effect of the flat region of g_{SVM} is to introduce *sparsity* into the prediction of the corresponding $y^{SVM}(\mathbf{x}_*)$, where only those data points with $t_i y_i \leq 1$ contributing; these are known as the support patterns. Note that g_{SVM} is not interpretable as a negative log likelihood as it does not normalize properly. For further discussion, see Wahba (1999) and SUPPORT VECTOR MACHINES.

Discussion

In this article we have seen how Gaussian process priors over functions (which are in general infinite-dimensional objects) can be used in a computationally efficient manner to make predictions.

Methods such as Gaussian processes and support vector machines have come to be known by the umbrella term of *kernel machines* (see Schölkopf and Smola, 2001). The web site http://www.kernel-machines.org/ has extensive links to research publications and software in this area.

One key issue concerning obtaining good performance with kernel methods is the choice of kernel. The squared-exponential kernel is widely used in practice, but it encodes only a general notion of smoothness. For particular problems, incorporation of prior/domain knowledge requires "kernel engineering." A second key issue for kernel methods is developing good approximation algorithms for large data sets.

Road Map: Learning in Artificial Networks
Background: Bayesian Methods and Neural Networks
Related Reading: Generalization and Regularization in Nonlinear Learning Systems; Radial Basis Function Networks; Support Vector Machines

References

Cressie, N. A. C., 1993, *Statistics for Spatial Data*, New York: Wiley.

Kimeldorf, G., and Wahba, G., 1970, A correspondence between Bayesian estimation of stochastic processes and smoothing by splines, *Ann. Math. Statist.*, 41:495–502.

MacKay, D. J. C., 1992, A practical Bayesian framework for backpropagation networks, *Neural Computat.*, 4:448–472.

MacKay, D. J. C., 1998, Introduction to Gaussian processes, in *Neural Networks and Machine Learning* (C. M. Bishop, Ed.), New York: Springer-Verlag. ◆

Neal, R. M., 1996, *Bayesian Learning for Neural Networks*, Lecture Notes in Statistics 118, New York: Springer-Verlag.

Neal, R. M., 1998, Regression and classification using Gaussian process priors (with discussion), in *Bayesian Statistics 6* (J. M. Bernardo et al., Eds.), Oxford, Engl.: Oxford University Press, pp. 475–501.

Poggio, T., and Girosi, F., 1990, Networks for approximation and learning, *Proc. IEEE*, 78:1481–1497.

Rasmussen, C. E., 1996, A practical Monte Carlo implementation of Bayesian learning, in *Advances in Neural Information Processing Systems 8* (D. S. Touretzky, M. Mozer, and M. E. Hasselmo, Eds.), Cambridge, MA: MIT Press, pp. 598–604.

Schölkopf, B., and Smola, A., 2001, *Learning with Kernels*, Cambridge, MA: MIT Press. ◆

Tresp, V., 2001, Scaling kernel-based systems to large data sets, *Data Mining Knowl. Discov.*, 5:197–211.

Vapnik, V. N., 1995, *The Nature of Statistical Learning Theory*, New York: Springer-Verlag.

Wahba, G., 1990, *Spline Models for Observational Data*, SIAM, CBMS-NSF Regional Conference Series in Applied Mathematics. ◆

Wahba, G., 1999, Support vector machines, reproducing kernel Hilbert spaces, and randomized GACV, in *Advances in Kernel Methods* (B. Schölkopf, C. J. C. Burges, and A. J. Smola, Eds.), Cambridge, MA: MIT Press, pp. 69–88.

Williams, C. K. I., 1998, Prediction with Gaussian processes: From linear regression to linear prediction and beyond, in *Learning in Graphical Models* (M. I. Jordan, Ed.), Boston: Kluwer Academic, pp. 599–621. ◆

Williams, C. K. I., and Barber, D., 1998, Bayesian classification with Gaussian processes, *IEEE Trans. Pattern Anal. Machine Intell.*, 20:1342–1351.

Generalization and Regularization in Nonlinear Learning Systems

Grace Wahba

Introduction

In this article we will describe generalization and regularization from the point of view of multivariate function estimation in a statistical context. Multivariate function estimation is not, in principle, distinguishable from supervised machine learning. However, until fairly recently, supervised machine learning and multivariate function estimation had fairly distinct groups of practitioners and little overlap in language, literature, and the kinds of practical problems under study.

In any case, we are given a *training set*, consisting of pairs of input (feature) vectors and associated outputs $\{\mathbf{t}(i), y_i\}$, for n training or example subjects, $i = 1, \ldots, n$. From these data, it is desired to construct a map that *generalizes well*, that is, given a new value of $\mathbf{t}$, the map will provide a reasonable prediction for the unobserved output associated with this $\mathbf{t}$.

Most applications fall into one of two broad categories, which might be called nonparametric regression and classification. In *nonparametric regression,* y may be (any) real number or a vector of r real numbers. The desired algorithm will produce an estimate $\hat{f}(\mathbf{t})$ of the expected value of a (new) y to be associated with a (new) attribute vector $\mathbf{t}$. In the (two-class) *classification* problem, y_i will be an indicator, whether or not the example (subject) came from class $\mathcal{A}$. In some classification applications, the desired algorithm will, given $\mathbf{t}$, return an indicator that predicts whether or not an example with attribute vector $\mathbf{t}$ comes from class $\mathcal{A}$ ("hard") classification. In other applications the desired algorithm will return $p(\mathbf{t})$, an estimate of the *probability* that the example with attribute vector $\mathbf{t}$ is in class $\mathcal{A}$ ("soft" classification). In some applications the feature vector $\mathbf{t}$ of dimension d contains zeros and ones (for example, in a bitmap of handwriting); in others it may contain real numbers representing some physical quantities. Ordered or unordered category indicators are also possible, as in medical demographic studies. *Regularization*, loosely speaking, means that whereas the desired map is constructed to approximately send the observed feature vectors to the observed outputs, constraints are applied to the construction of the map, with the goal of reducing the generalization error (see also PROBABILISTIC REGULARIZATION METHODS FOR LOW-LEVEL VISION). In some applications, these constraints embody a priori information concerning the true relationship between input and output; alternatively, various ad hoc constraints have sometimes worked well in practice. Girosi, Jones, and Poggio (1995) give a wide-ranging review.

Generalization and Regularization in Nonparametric Regression

Single-Input Spline Smoothing

We will use Figure 1 to illustrate the ideas of generalization and regularization in the simplest possible nonparametric regression setup, that is, $d = 1$, $r = 1$, with $\mathbf{t} = t$ any real number in some interval of the real line. The circles (which are identical in each of the three panels of Figure 1) represent $n = 100$ (synthetically generated) input-output pairs $\{t(i), y_i\}$, generated according to the model

$$y_i = f_{TRUE}(t(i)) + \varepsilon_i, \quad i = 1, \ldots, n \qquad (1)$$

where $f_{TRUE}(t) = 4.26(e^{-t} - 4e^{-2t} + 3e^{-3t})$, and the ε_i came from a pseudo-random number generator for normally distributed random variables with mean 0 and standard deviation $\sigma = 0.2$. Given this training data $\{t(i), y_i, i = 1, \ldots, n\}$, the learning problem is to create a map that, if given a new value of t, will predict the response $y(t)$. In this case, the data are noisy, so that even if the new t coincides with some predictor variable $t(i)$ in the training set, merely predicting y as the response y_i is not likely to be satisfactory. Also, this does not yet provide any ability to make predictions when t does not exactly match any predictor values in the training set. It is desired to generate a curve that will allow a reasonable prediction of the response for any t within a reasonable vicinity of the set of training predictors $\{t(i)\}$. The dashed line in each panel of Figure 1 is $f_{TRUE}(t)$; the three solid black lines in the three panels of Figure 1 are three solutions to the variational problem: find f in the (Hilbert) space W_2 of functions with continuous first derivatives and square integrable second derivatives that minimizes

$$\frac{1}{n} \sum_{i=1}^{n} (y_i - f(t(i)))^2 + \lambda \int (f^{(2)}(u))^2 du \qquad (2)$$

for three different values of λ. The parameter λ is known as the *regularization* or *smoothing parameter*. As $\lambda \to \infty$, f_λ tends to the least squares straight line best fitting the data, and as $\lambda \to 0$ the solution tends to that curve in W_2 that minimizes the penalty functional $J(f) = \int (f^{(2)}(u))^2 du$ subject to interpolating the data (provided the $\{t(i)\}$ are distinct). This latter interpolating curve is known as a *cubic interpolating spline*, and minimizers of Equation 2 are known as *smoothing splines*. We remark that, here as well as in the sequel, although a variational problem is being solved in

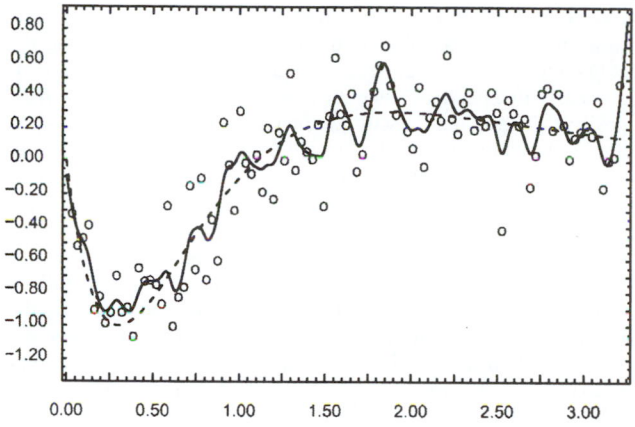

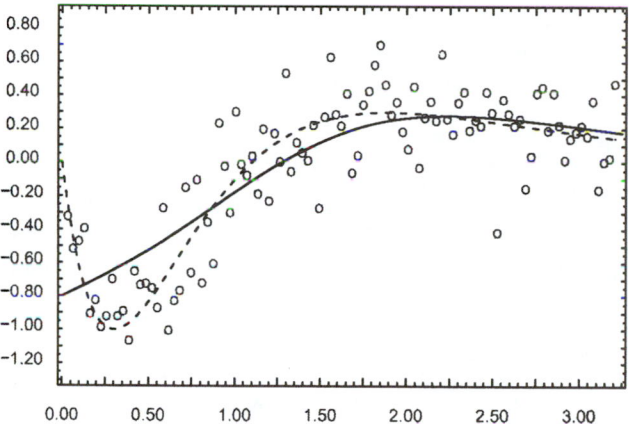

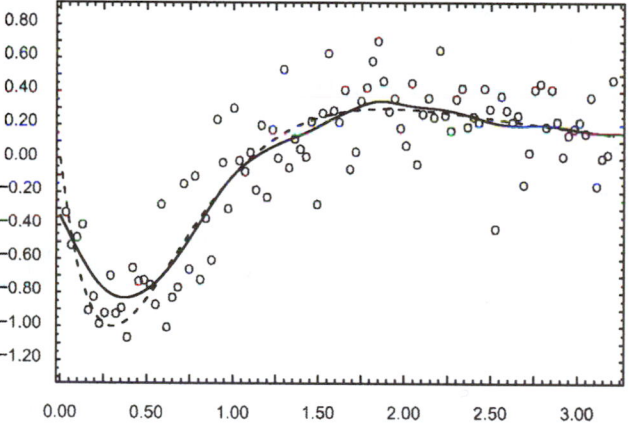

Figure 1. Training data (circles) have been generated by adding noise to $f_{TRUE}(t)$, shown by the dashed curve in each panel. All three panels have the same data. *Top*, Solid curve is fitted spline with λ too small. *Middle*, Solid curve is fitted spline with λ too large. *Bottom*, Solid curve is fitted spline with λ obtained by generalized cross-validation.

be seen that using the wiggly curve in the top panel is not likely to give a good prediction of y, assuming that future predictor-response data are generated by the same mechanism as the training data. In the middle panel, λ has been chosen too large; the curve has been forced to flatten out, and again it can be seen that the heavy line will not give a good prediction of y. In the bottom panel, λ has been chosen by generalized cross-validation (GCV). This is a method that behaves similarly to leaving-out-one in many cases, but with computational and theoretical advantages (see Li, 1986; Wahba, 1990, chap. 4; Girard, 1998). It can be seen that the λ obtained in this way does a good job of choosing the right amount of smoothing to best recover f_{TRUE} of Equation 1. The f_{TRUE} of Equation 1 would provide the best predictor of the response in an expected mean-square-error sense if future data were generated according to Equation 1. The curve in the bottom panel has a reasonable ability to *generalize*, that is, to predict the response given a new value t of the predictor variable, at least if t is not too far from the training predictor set $\{t(i)\}$.

For each positive λ, there exists a unique $\kappa = \kappa(\lambda)$ so that the minimizer f_λ of Equation 2 is also the solution to the problem: Find f in W_2 to minimize

$$L(y, f) = \frac{1}{n} \sum_{i=1}^{n} (y_i - f(t(i))^2 \tag{3}$$

subject to the condition

$$J(f) = \int (f^{(2)}(u))^2 du \le \kappa \tag{4}$$

As λ becomes large, the associated $\kappa(\lambda)$ becomes small, and conversely. In general, the term *regularization* refers to solving some problem involving best fitting, subject to some constraints on the solution. These constraints may be of various forms. When they involve a quadratic penalty involving derivatives, like $J(f)$, the method is commonly referred to as *Tikhonov regularization*. The "tighter" the constraints (i.e., the smaller κ, equivalently the larger λ), the further away the solution f_λ will generally be from the training data; that is, L will be larger. As the constraints get weaker and weaker, ultimately (if there are enough degrees of freedom in the method) the solution will interpolate the data. However, as is clear from Figure 1, a curve that runs through all the data points is *not* a good solution.

A fundamental problem in machine learning with noisy and/or incomplete data is to balance the "tightness" of the constraints with the "goodness of fit" to the data, in such a way as to minimize the generalization error, that is, the ability to predict the unobserved response for new values of t (or $\mathbf{t}$). This trade-off is by now well known as the *bias-variance trade-off*, or, equivalently, the *goodness of fit–model complexity trade-off*. Methods abound in the statistical literature for univariate curve fitting, including Parzen kernel estimates, nearest neighbor estimates, orthogonal series estimates, least squares regression spline estimates, and, recently, wavelet estimates. Each method has one or more regularization parameters, whether they are kernel window widths, number of nearest neighbors included, number of terms in the orthogonal series expansion or regression basis, or factors or thresholds for shrinking or truncating wavelet coefficients, that control this trade-off. (See Ramsay and Silverman, 1997, and references therein.)

Multiple-Input, Single-Hidden-Layer Feedforward Neural Net

A multiple-input, single-hidden-layer feedforward neural net (NN) predictor for the learning problem described in the Introduction is typically of the form

an infinite dimensional Hilbert space, the solution is in an n-dimensional subspace with a known spanning set. (See Wahba, 1990, and references cited there for further information concerning these and other properties of splines, and further references.)

In the top panel of Figure 1 λ has been chosen too small, and the wiggly solid line is attempting to fit the data too closely. It can

$$f_{NN}(\mathbf{t}) = \sigma_0\left(b_o + \sum_{j=1}^{N} w_j \sigma_h(\mathbf{a}_j' \mathbf{t}(i) + b_j)\right) \qquad (5)$$

where the $\mathbf{a}_j$ and $\mathbf{t}$ are d-vectors. The function σ_h is the so-called "activation function" of the hidden layer and σ_0 is the activation function for the output. σ_h is generally a sigmoidal function, for example, $\sigma_h(\tau) = e^\tau/(1 + e^\tau)$, while σ_0 may be linear, sigmoidal or a threshold unit. Here N is the number of hidden units, and the w_j, $\mathbf{a}_j$, and b_j are "learned" from the training data by some appropriate iterative descent algorithm that tries to steer these values toward minimizing some distance measure, typically $L(y, f_{NN}) = (1/n)\sum_{i=1}^{n}(y_i - f_{NN}(\mathbf{t}(i)))^2$. It is clear that if N is sufficiently large and the descent algorithm is run long enough, it should be possible to drive the L as close as one likes to zero. (In practice it is possible to get stuck in local minima.) However, it is also clear intuitively from Figure 1 that driving L all the way to zero is not a desirable thing to do. Regularization in this problem may be done by controlling the size of N, by imposing penalties on the w_j, by stopping the descent algorithm early (that is, by not driving down L as far as it can go), or by various combinations of these strategies. Each will influence how closely f_{NN} will fit the data, how "wiggly" it will be, and how well it will be able to predict unobserved data that are generated by a similar mechanism as the observed data.

Multiple-Input Radial Basis Function and Related Estimates

Radial basis functions are rapidly becoming a popular method for nonparametric regression (see RADIAL BASIS FUNCTION NETWORKS). We first describe a general form of nonparametric regression that will specialize to radial basis functions and other methods of interest. Let $R(\mathbf{s}, \mathbf{t})$ be *any* symmetric, strictly positive definite function on $E^d \times E^d$. Here, *strictly positive definite* means for any $K = 1, 2, \ldots$, the $K \times K$ matrix with j, kth entry $R(\mathbf{s}(j), \mathbf{s}(k))$ is strictly positive definite whenever the $\mathbf{s}(1), \ldots, \mathbf{s}(K)$ are distinct. (A symmetric $K \times K$ matrix M is said to be positive definite if for any K-dimensional column vector $x \neq 0$, $x'Mx$ is greater than or equal to 0, and is said to be strictly positive definite if $x'Mx$ is always strictly greater than 0.) Positive definiteness will play a key role in the discussion below because, among other reasons, any positive definite matrix can be the covariance matrix of a random vector and any positive definite function $R(\mathbf{s}, \mathbf{t})$ can be the covariance function of some stochastic process, $X(\mathbf{t})$. That is, there exists $X(\cdot)$ such that $Cov X(\mathbf{s})X(\mathbf{t}) = R(\mathbf{s}, \mathbf{t})$. Given training data $\{\mathbf{t}(i), y_i\}$, it is always possible in principle to obtain a (regularized) input-output map from this data by letting the model $f_{R,\lambda}$ be of the form

$$f_{R,\lambda}(\mathbf{t}) = \sum_{j=1}^{N} c_j R(\mathbf{t}, \mathbf{s}(j)) \qquad (6)$$

where the $\mathbf{s}(j)$ are $N \leq n$ "centers" that are placed at distinct values of the $\{\mathbf{t}(i)\}$ and $c = (c_1, \ldots, c_N)'$ is chosen to minimize $L(y, f) + \lambda J(f)$. Here

$$L(y, f_{R,\lambda}) = \frac{1}{n} \sum_{i=1}^{n}(y_i - f_{R,\lambda}(\mathbf{t}(i))^2 \qquad (7)$$

and the regularizing penalty $J(\cdot)$ is of the form

$$J(f_{R,\lambda}) = \sum_{j,k=1}^{N} c_j c_k J_{jk} \qquad (8)$$

where J_{kj} are the entries of a non-negative definite quadratic form. The (strict) positive definiteness of R guarantees that

$$L(y, f_{R,\lambda}) + \lambda J(f_{R,\lambda}) \qquad (9)$$

always has a unique minimizer in c, for any non-negative λ. This follows by substituting Equation 6 into Equation 9, and using the fact that the columns of the $n \times N$ matrix with i,j entry $R(\mathbf{t}(i), \mathbf{s}(j))$ are linearly independent since they are just N columns of the $n \times n$ positive definite matrix with i,j entry $R(\mathbf{t}(i), \mathbf{t}(j))$.

Radial basis function estimates are obtained for the special case where $R(\mathbf{s}, \mathbf{t})$ is of the special form

$$R(\mathbf{s}, \mathbf{t}) = r(\|W(\mathbf{s} - \mathbf{t})\|) \qquad (10)$$

where W is some linear transformation on E^d and the norm is Euclidean distance. That is, $R(\mathbf{s}, \mathbf{t})$ depends only on some generalized distance in E_d between $\mathbf{s}$ and $\mathbf{t}$. The regularization—that is, the effecting of the trade-off between goodness of fit to the data and "smoothness" of the solution—is performed by reducing N and/or increasing λ. The choice of W will also affect the "wiggliness" of $f_{R,\lambda}$ in the radial basis function case. Alternatively, a model can be obtained by choosing N small and minimizing $L(y, f)$. In that case, N and W are the smoothing parameters.

In the special case $N = n$, $\mathbf{s}(i) = \mathbf{t}(i)$, the $f_{R,\lambda}$ can (for *any* positive definite R) be shown to be Bayes estimates (see Kimeldorf and Wahba, 1970; Wahba, 1990). Arguments can be given to show that if n is large and $N < n$ is not too small, then they are good approximations to Bayes's estimates (see Wahba, 1990, chap. 7). In the special case $J_{i,j} = R(\mathbf{t}(i), \mathbf{t}(j))$, the Bayes model is easy to describe and we do it here; it is:

$$y_i = X(\mathbf{t}(i)) + \varepsilon_i \qquad (11)$$

with $X(\mathbf{t})$ a zero-mean Gaussian process (see GAUSSIAN PROCESSES) with covariance $EX(\mathbf{s})X(\mathbf{t}) = bR(\mathbf{s}, \mathbf{t})$ and the ε_i independent zero-mean Gaussian random variables with common variance σ^2, and independent of $X(\mathbf{t})$. In this case, the minimizer $f_{R,\lambda}$ of $L(y, f) + \lambda J(f)$, evaluated at $\mathbf{t}$, is the conditional expectation of $X(\mathbf{t})$, given $y_1, \ldots, y_n$, provided that λ is chosen as σ^2/nb. In general, pretending that one has a prior and computing the posterior mean or mode will have a regularizing effect. The preceding discussion extends to symmetric positive definite functions on *arbitrary* domains for $\mathbf{t}$, including those mentioned in the Introduction of this article.

Thin plate splines in d variables (of order m) consist of radial basis functions plus polynomials of total degree less than m in d variables. ($2m - d > 0$ is required for technical reasons.) Letting $\mathbf{t} = (t_1, \ldots, t_d)$, the thin plate splines are minimizers (in an appropriate function space) of

$$\frac{1}{n}\sum_{i=1}^{n}(y_i - f(\mathbf{t}(i))^2 + \lambda \sum_{\alpha_1 + \cdots + \alpha_d = m}\frac{m!}{\alpha_1! \cdots \alpha_d!}\int_{-\infty}^{\infty}\cdots\int_{-\infty}^{\infty}$$
$$\times \left(\frac{\partial^m f}{\partial t_1^{\alpha_1} \cdots \partial t_d^{\alpha_d}}\right)^2 dt_1 \cdots dt_d \qquad (12)$$

Setting $d = 1$, $m = 2$ gives the cubic spline case discussed earlier. Note that there is no penalty on polynomials of total degree less than m; the thin plate splines with a particular choice of λ are Bayes estimates with an improper prior (that is, infinite variance) on the polynomials of total degree less than m (see Wahba, 1990, and references cited therein).

Related variations on regularized estimates include additive smoothing splines, which are of the form

$$f(\mathbf{t}) = \mu + \sum_{\alpha=1}^{d} f_\alpha(t_\alpha) \qquad (13)$$

where μ and the f_α are the solution to a variational problem of the form: Find μ and $f_1, \ldots, f_d$ in a certain function space to minimize

$$\frac{1}{n}\sum_{i=1}^{n}(y_i - f(\mathbf{t}(i))^2 + \sum_{\alpha=1}^{d}\lambda_\alpha J_\alpha(f_\alpha) \qquad (14)$$

The J_α may be of the form of J in Equation 4. Here, there is a *regularization parameter* for each component (see Hastie and Tibshirani, 1990; Wahba, 1990). These additive models generalize to smoothing spline analysis of variance (SS-ANOVA) models. In the SS-ANOVA models, interaction terms of the form $f_{\alpha\beta}(t_\alpha, t_\beta), f_{\alpha\beta\gamma}(t_\alpha, t_\beta, t_\gamma)$, etc., which satisfy side conditions making them uniquely determined, are added to the representation in Equation 13, and corresponding penalty terms with regularization parameters are added in Equation 14. The f_α, etc., may be generalized to themselves, being radial basis functions. Behind these models are positive definite functions that are built up via tensor sums and products of positive definite functions (see Wahba, 1990; Wahba et al., 1995).

Regression spline ANOVA models may be obtained by setting the $f_\alpha, f_{\alpha\beta}$, etc. as linear combinations of a (relatively small) number of basis functions (usually splines). In this case the number of the basis functions is probably the most influential regularization parameter. These and similar methods again all have either explicit or implicit regularization parameters that govern the balance between the complexity of the model and the fit to the data—the bias-variance trade-off.

The usual criterion for the generalization error when the fit involves minimizing the observed residual sum of squares is the expected residual sum of squares for new data, $EL(y_{new}, f_\lambda) \equiv L(f_{TRUE}, f_\lambda) = (1/n)\Sigma_{i=1}^n (f_{TRUE}(\mathbf{t}(i)) - f_\lambda(\mathbf{t}(i)))^2$. Here the y_{new} are new observations at the original $\mathbf{t}(i)$. Leaving out one, leaving out 10%, leaving out a one-third representative sample ("tuning set"), and GCV ("in-sample tuning") are popular methods for choosing the tuning parameters to minimize this criterion. Codes in Splus (smooth.spline()), SAS (tpspline), netlib (entire/gcv directory), Funfits (sreg, tps), R (smooth.Pspline, gss), and elsewhere are available for implementing the univariate spline, thin plate spline, and additive and interaction (ANOVA) splines with GCV to choose single or multiple smoothing parameters. Netlib (http://www.netlib.org/) and Funfits (http://www.cgd.ucar.edu/stats/software.shtml) are freeware. The smooth.Pspline code in R at http://www.r-project.org was used to generate Figure 1.

Generalization and Regularization in Soft Classification

Soft classification is a natural goal in certain kinds of demographic medical studies. For example, suppose a large training set is available from a demographic study, consisting of observations $\{\mathbf{t}(i), y_i\}$, where y_i is an indicator (1 or 0) of the presence or absence of some disease in subject i at the end of the study and $\mathbf{t}(i)$ is a vector of values of risk factors for this subject at the beginning of the study. With this kind of data, it is frequently of interest to make a "soft" classification, that is, to estimate the *probability* $p(\mathbf{t})$ that a new subject with predictor vector $\mathbf{t}$ will contract the disease. A doctor, given this model, may advise new patients which risk factors are important for them to control to reduce the probability of their contracting the disease. A regularized (that is, "smooth") estimate for $p(\mathbf{t})$ is desirable. Regularized estimates can be obtained as follows. First, define

$$f(\mathbf{t}) = \log[p(\mathbf{t})/(1 - p(\mathbf{t}))] \qquad (15)$$

f is known in the statistics literature as the log odds ratio, or logit. Then $p(\mathbf{t})$ is a sigmoidal function of $f(\mathbf{t})$; that is, $p(\mathbf{t}) = e^{f(\mathbf{t})}/(1 + e^{f(\mathbf{t})})$. We will get a regularized estimate for f. $L(y, f)$ of Equation 3 will be replaced by an expression more suitable for 0–1 data, by using the likelihood for these data. To describe the likelihood, note that if y is a random variable with Prob$[y = 1] = p$ and Prob$[y = 0] = (1 - p)$, then the probability density (or likelihood) $P(y, p)$ for y, when p is true, is just $P(y, p) = p^y (1 - p)^{(1 - y)}$. This merely says $P(1, p) = p$ and $P(0, p) = (1 - p)$. Thus, the likelihood for $y_1, \ldots, y_n$ (assuming that the y_i are independent) is

$$P(y_1, \ldots, y_n; p(\mathbf{t}(1)), \ldots, p(\mathbf{t}(n))$$
$$= \prod_{i=1}^n p(\mathbf{t}(i))^{y_i}(1 - p(\mathbf{t}(i)))^{(1 - y_i)} \qquad (16)$$

Substituting f for p in Equation 16 and taking the negative logarithm gives the negative log likelihood $L(y, f)$ in terms of f:

$$-\log P(y_1, \ldots, y_n; f(\mathbf{t}(1)), \ldots, f(\mathbf{t}(n))$$
$$\equiv nL(y, f) = \sum_{i=1}^n [\log(1 + e^{f(\mathbf{t}(i))}) - y_i f(\mathbf{t}(i))] \qquad (17)$$

It is natural for $L(y, f)$ to replace $L(y, f)$ in Equations 3, 7, and 14 when y_i is restricted to 0 or 1, since $L(y, f_{TRUE})$ is (a multiple of) the negative log likelihood for y generated by a model with Gaussian noise, as in Equation 1. A neural net implementation of soft classification would consist of finding $f_{NN}(\mathbf{t}) = \text{logit} p_{NN}(\mathbf{t})$ of the form of Equation 5 to minimize $L(y, f)$ of Equation 17. If N is large enough, then, in principle, f_{NN} may be driven so that $p_{NN}(\mathbf{t}(i))$ is close to 1 if y_i is 1, and is close to 0 if y_i is 0. Again, it is intuitively clear that this is not desirable. As before, a regularized or smooth f_{NN} can be obtained by controlling N, penalizing the w_i, stopping the iterative fitting early, or some combination of these actions.

Penalized likelihood estimates of f are obtained by minimizing $L(y, f) + J_\lambda(f)$, where $J_\lambda(f)$ is a penalty functional corresponding to those in Equations 2, 9, 12, or 14 and its generalizations. A popular definition for the generalization error is the (unobservable) comparative Kullback-Leibler distance of the estimate to the true probability distribution, which can be shown to be given by $EL(y_{new}, f_\lambda) = L(p_{TRUE}, f_\lambda)$. An estimate of λ that minimizes this criterion can be obtained by withholding a representative subset $y_{[left - out]}$ of the training set and choosing λ to minimize $L(y_{[left - out]}, f_\lambda)$. Leaving-out-one estimates are also possible but generally not feasible in this case. Generalized approximate cross-validation (GACV) is a feasible in-sample method of choosing λ; based on a leaving-out-one argument, it has been shown in simulation studies to provide a good estimate of the minimizer of $L(p_{TRUE}; f_\lambda)$ (see Wahba et al., 1999).

Generalization and Regularization in Hard Classification

In the hard classification problem (here we will consider only two classes for simplicity), we are only interested in estimating whether an example with vector $\mathbf{t}$ is in class $\mathcal{A}$ or not. This is the typical situation in, for example, character recognition, voice recognition, and other situations where it is known that the $\mathbf{t}$'s from the two classes being examined are generally well separated. In that case (assuming, for simplicity, that the examples from the two classes are represented in the training set equally as is the future population of interest, and that costs of misclassification are the same for both classes), then the optimum classifier (to minimize the expected cost) would be $\mathcal{A}$ if $p(\mathbf{t})$ is greater than one-half, and not $\mathcal{A}$ otherwise. Equivalently, the same rule can be implemented by examining the sign of the logit $f(\mathbf{t})$. Here we are identifying $\mathcal{A}$ with the 1s, and optimum is with respect to minimizing the expected cost of future misclassification. Unfortunately, in general it is neither desirable nor feasible to estimate the logit f directly by the methods described in the section on soft classification, because in the well-separated case, f takes on values near $\pm\infty$, and solving the penalized likelihood problem of that section is likely to be unstable. Recently, SUPPORT VECTOR MACHINES (q.v.) have been shown to provide an excellent method for classification in this situation (see Burges, 1998).

The support vector machine (SVM) is implemented coding the y_i as ± 1 according as the ith example is in $\mathcal{A}$ or not. Given a positive definite function $R(\mathbf{s}, \mathbf{t})$, we find a function f of the form $f(\mathbf{t}) = b + \sum_{i=1}^{n} c_i R(\mathbf{t}, \mathbf{t}(i))$ by finding b and $c = (c_i, \ldots, c_n)$ to minimize

$$\frac{1}{n} \sum_{i=1}^{n} (1 - y_i f(\mathbf{t}(i))_+ + \lambda \sum_{i,j} c_i c_j R(\mathbf{t}(i), \mathbf{t}(j)) \quad (18)$$

where $(\tau)_+ = \tau$ for $\tau > 0$ and 0 otherwise. Letting f_λ be the minimizer of Equation 18, the classification algorithm is: for a new attribute vector $\mathbf{t}$, assign $\mathcal{A}$ if $f(\mathbf{t}) > 0$ and not $\mathcal{A}$ if $f(\mathbf{t}) < 0$. Lin (1999) has demonstrated the remarkable result that, under general circumstances with appropriately chosen λ, the SVM estimate f_λ tends almost everywhere to either 1 or -1 and is an estimate of $\mathrm{sign} f_{TRUE} \equiv \mathrm{sign}(p_{TRUE} - 1/2)$, which is exactly what is needed to carry out the optimum classification algorithm. It is interesting to note that if the data y_i in the penalized log likelihood estimate were recoded to $y_i = \pm 1$, then the ith term on the right of Equation 17 would become $\log(1 + e^{-y_i f(\mathbf{t}(i))})$, which is bounded below by $(\log 2)(1 - y_i f(\mathbf{t}(i)))_+$. A popular choice for $R(\mathbf{s}, \mathbf{t})$ is $R(\mathbf{s}, \mathbf{t}) = \exp -(1/\sigma^2)\|\mathbf{s} - \mathbf{t}\|^2$, where $\|\cdot\|$ is the Euclidean norm. In this choice of $R(\cdot, \cdot)$ the result may be sensitive to both σ and λ. As before, the λ and σ may be chosen by leaving out a representative subset of the observations and choosing λ and σ to minimize some measure of the generalization error. Here the natural choice for generalization error would be the misclassification rate. A version of GACV for SVMs, again based on a leaving-out-one argument, may be used as an in-sample method for choosing λ and σ (see Wahba, Lin, and Zhang, 2000). The generalization error target for the GACV is $E(1/n)\sum_{i=1}^{n}(1 - y_{i\text{new}} f_\lambda(\mathbf{t}(i)))_+$. However, $(1/2)E(1/n)\sum_{i=1}^{n}(1 - y_{i\text{new}}\mathrm{sign}[f_\lambda(\mathbf{t}(i))])_+$ is the expected misclassification rate, so that to the extent that f_λ resembles $\mathrm{sign} f_\lambda$, this criterion will be appropriate for the generalization error. There is a large literature on the multiclass case, generally involving repeated pairwise or one-versus-many comparisons. A multiclass SVM that deals with all classes simultaneously has recently been developed (Lee, Lin, and Wahba, 2001). This work also demonstrates how to modify the SVM to take into account nonrepresentative training sets and unequal misclassification costs.

Choosing How Much to Regularize

At the time of this writing, it is a matter of lively debate and much research how to choose the various regularization parameters. Leaving out a large fraction of the training sample for this purpose and tuning the regularization parameter(s) to best predict the left-out data (according to whatever criterion of best prediction is adopted) is conceptually simple, defensible, and widely used (this is called out-of-sample tuning). Successively leaving-out-one, successively leaving-out-10%, and the in-sample methods GCV and GACV are all popular. (See also Ye, 1998, who discusses in-sample tuning methods related to GCV in the Gaussian case that allows comparisons across different regularized estimates.) In the normally distributed observational error case, if the standard deviation of the observational error (σ in Equation 1) is known, then unbiased risk estimates become available (see Li, 1986; Wahba, 1990, and references therein). When there is a Bayesian model behind the regularization procedure, then maximum likelihood estimates may be derived (see Wahba, 1985), although in order for these and other Bayesian estimates to do a good job of minimizing the generalization error in practice, it is usually necessary that the priors on which they are based be realistic.

Which Method Is Best?

Feedforward neural nets, radial basis functions, and various forms of splines all provide regularized or regularizable methods for estimating smooth functions of several variables, given a training set

$\{\mathbf{t}(i), y_i\}$. Which approach is best? Unfortunately, there is no single answer to that question, nor is there likely to be one. The answer depends on the particular nature of the underlying but unknown "truth," the nature of any prior information that might be available about this truth, the nature of any noise in the data, the ability of the experimenter to choose the various smoothing or regularization parameters well, the size of the data set, the use to which the answer will be put, and the computational facilities available. From a mathematical point of view, the classes of functions well approximated by neural nets, radial basis functions, and additive and interaction splines (ANOVA splines) are not the same, although all of these methods have the capability of approximating large classes of functions. Of course, if a large enough data set is available, models utilizing all of these approaches can be built, tuned, and compared on data that have been set aside for this purpose. In-sample tuning methods for comparison across different regularized estimates in the hard and soft classification contexts are an area of active research.

Acknowledgments.   This work was supported by NSF grant No. DMS 9704798 and NIH grant No. R01 EY09946.

Road Map: Learning in Artificial Networks
Related Reading: Learning and Statistical Inference; Stochastic Approximation and Efficient Learning

References

Burges, C., 1998, A tutorial on support vector machines for pattern recognition, *Data Mining Knowledge Discovery*, 2:121–167. ◆

Girard, D., 1998, Asymptotic comparison of (partial) cross-validation, GCV and randomized GCV in nonparametric regression, *Ann. Statist.*, 126:315–334.

Girosi, F., Jones, M., and Poggio, T., 1995, Regularization theory and neural networks architectures, *Neural Computat.*, 7:219–269.

Hastie, T., and Tibshirani, R., 1990, *Generalized Additive Models*, New York: Chapman and Hall ◆

Kimeldorf, G., and Wahba, G., 1970, A correspondence between Bayesian estimation of stochastic processes and smoothing by splines, *Ann. Math. Statist.*, 41:495–502.

Lee, Y., Lin, Y., and Wahba, G., 2001, *Multicategory Support Vector Machines*, Technical Report 1043, Madison, WI: University of Wisconsin, Department of Statistics; to appear in *Comput. Sci. Stat.*, 33.

Li, K. C., 1986, Asymptotic optimality of C_L and generalized cross validation in ridge regression with application to spline smoothing, *Ann. Statist.*, 14:1101–1112.

Lin, Y., 1999, *Support Vector Machines and the Bayes rule in Classification*, Technical Report 1014, Madison WI: University of Wisconsin, Department of Statistics, in *Data Mining and Knowledge Discovery*, 6:259–275.

Ramsay, J., and Silverman, B., 1997, *Functional Data Analysis*, New York: Springer-Verlag. ◆

Wahba, G., 1985, A comparison of GCV and GML for choosing the smoothing parameter in the generalized spline smoothing problem, *Ann. Statist.*, 13:1378–1402.

Wahba, G., 1990, *Spline Models for Observational Data*, CBMS-NSF Regional Conference Series in Applied Mathematics, vol. 59, Philadelphia: Society for Industrial and Applied Mathematics. ◆

Wahba, G., Lin, X., Gao, F., Xiang, D., Klein, R., and Klein, B., 1999, The bias-variance tradeoff and the randomized GACV, in *Advances in Information Processing Systems 11* (M. Kearns, S. Solla, and D. Cohn, Eds.), Cambridge, MA: MIT Press, pp. 620–626.

Wahba, G., Lin, Y., and Zhang, H., 2000, Generalized approximate cross validation for support vector machines, in *Advances in Large Margin Classifiers* (A. Smola, P. Bartlett, B. Scholkopf, and D. Schuurmans, Eds.), Cambridge, MA: MIT Press, pp. 297–311.

Wahba, G., Wang, Y., Gu, C., Klein, R., and Klein, B., 1995, Neyman Lecture: Smoothing spline ANOVA for exponential families: With application to the Wisconsin Epidemiological Study of Diabetic Retinopathy, *Ann. Statist.*, 23:1865–1895.

Ye, J., 1998, On measuring and correcting the effects of data mining and model selection, *J. Am. Statist. Assoc.*, 93:120–131.

GENESIS Simulation System

James M. Bower, David Beeman, and Michael Hucka

Introduction

GENESIS (the GEneral NEural SImulation System) was developed as a research tool to provide a standard and flexible means for constructing structurally realistic models of biological neural systems. "Structurally realistic" simulations are computer-based implementations of models whose primary objective is to capture what is known of the anatomical structure and physiological characteristics of the neural system of interest. The GENESIS project is based on the belief that progress in understanding structure-function relationships in the nervous system specifically, or in biology in general, will increasingly require the development and use of structurally realistic models (Bower, 1995). It is our view that only through this type of modeling will general principles of neural or biological function emerge.

There is considerable debate within the computational neuroscience community concerning the appropriate level of modeling. As illustrated in other articles in the *Handbook*, many modeling efforts are currently focused on abstract "general" representations of neural function rather than on detailed, realistic models. However, the history of science clearly indicates that realistic models play an essential role in the development of quantitative understanding of physical systems. For example, philosophers and priests for thousands of years invented "models" to account for the motion of the planets in the night sky. These models, the most famous of which is probably the Ptolemeic system, "replicated the data" and made quantitative predictions. The structure of these planetary models, however, already assumed the general principles on which the universe was organized. It was not until the sixteenth and seventeenth centuries, when Kepler and, later, Newton constructed realistic models of the solar system, that general principles such as universal gravitation emerged. The inverse square law for gravitational attraction fell out of a model that Newton constructed of the moon's movement around Earth; it was not an apple-induced inspiration.

It is our view that neuroscience is not yet ready for its Newton. Instead, we are still in need of Kepler. Viewed most generally, GENESIS is intended to provide a framework for quantifying the physical description of the nervous system in a way that promotes common understanding of its physical structure. At the same time, this physical description also provides the base for simulations intent on understanding fundamental relationships between the structure of the brain and its measurable behavior. Again, looking back at the evolution of planetary science, Kepler's realization that the motion of the planets was elliptical came about as a result of his careful analysis of the detailed positions of the planets obtained by Tycho Brahe. Kepler's development of a mathematical formalism to describe elliptical motion provided a seminal framework for the work of later physicists, including Newton. Similarly, it is our hope and expectation that the formalism being developed within the GENESIS project and other simulation systems such as NEURON (see NEURON SIMULATION ENVIRONMENT) will provide a means for neurobiologists to collaboratively construct a physical description of the nervous system. We believe strongly that general principles of organization, function, and computation will only emerge once this description has been constructed.

GENESIS was designed from the beginning to allow the development of simulations at any level of complexity, from subcellular components and biochemical reactions to whole cells, networks of cells and systems-level models. The earliest GENESIS simulations were biologically realistic large-scale simulations of cortical networks (Wilson and Bower, 1992). The De Schutter and Bower (1994a, 1994b) cerebellar Purkinje cell model is typical of a large, detailed single-cell model, with 4,550 compartments and 8,021 ionic conductances. GENESIS is now being used for large systems-level models of cerebellar pathways (Stricanne, Morissette, and Bower, 1998), and, at the other extreme, is increasingly being used to relate cellular and network properties to biochemical signaling pathways (Bhalla and Iyengar, 1999).

Although GENESIS continues to be widely used for single-cell modeling and for modeling small networks (see, e.g., HALF-CENTER OSCILLATORS UNDERLYING RHYTHMIC MOVEMENTS), we have seen a dramatic increase in the number of publications that report using GENESIS for large network models. We believe that this trend is largely due to the availability of our libraries of ion channels and complete cell models. A description of some notable large-scale network GENESIS simulations (many using parallel computers) that have been published recently can be found at http://www.genesis-sim.org/GENESIS/research/genres.html. This web page also contains links to a list of 170 papers based on research with GENESIS from groups outside of Caltech, and a summary of what various research groups are doing with GENESIS.

GENESIS is implemented in C, using the X Window System, and runs under most varieties of Unix, including Linux. There is also a parallel version of GENESIS (called PGENESIS) that runs on workstation networks, small-scale parallel computers, and large, massively parallel supercomputers. PGENESIS is being used for simulations that must be run many times independently (e.g., parameter searches), and for large-scale models (especially network models with thousands of neurons).

The GENESIS Design Philosophy

The objectives of this project were to reduce redundant software design efforts, establish standards for simulation technology, and provide a common base for the exchange of models and scientific information. The object-oriented nature of the software allows different modelers to easily exchange and reuse whole models or model components. GENESIS also includes a customizable user interface for use by modelers and educators. From the beginning, GENESIS was also designed to serve as an instructional tool, because our involvement in several educational projects had demonstrated that simulations could provide flexible and dynamic learning tools for neuroscience education (Bower and Beeman, 1998).

The design of the GENESIS simulator and interface is based on a building-block approach. Simulations are constructed from modules that receive inputs, perform calculations on them, and then generate outputs. Model neurons are constructed from these basic components, such as compartments (short sections of cellular membrane) and variable conductance ion channels. Compartments are linked to their channels and are then linked together to form multicompartmental neurons of any desired level of complexity. Neurons may be linked together to form neural circuits. This object-oriented approach is central to the generality and flexibility of the system, as it allows modelers to easily exchange and reuse models or model components. In addition, it makes it possible to extend the functionality of GENESIS by adding new commands or simulation components to the simulator, without having to modify the GENESIS base code.

Neural systems are particularly amenable to this object-oriented approach because they typically consist of discrete components interacting in quite stereotyped ways, and because the different simulations tend to use similar neural components, display routines, numerical integration routines, and the like. This modularity means that it is possible to quickly construct a new simulation or to modify an existing simulation by changing modules that are chosen from a library or database of standard simulation components. Individual modules or linked assemblies of modules (such as compartments with channels, entire cells, or networks of cells) can be easily replicated.

Interacting with GENESIS

GENESIS uses a high-level simulation language to construct neurons and their networks. Commands may be issued either interactively to a command prompt, by use of simulation scripts, or through the graphical interface. A particular simulation is set up by writing a sequence of commands in the scripting language that creates the network itself and the graphical interface for a particular simulation. The scripting language and the modules are powerful enough that only a few lines of script are needed to specify a sophisticated simulation. The principal components of the simulation system and the various modes of interacting with GENESIS are shown in Figure 1.

The underlying level of the GENESIS user interface is the Script Language Interpreter (SLI). This is a command interpreter, similar to a Unix system shell, with an extensive set of commands related to building, monitoring, and controlling simulations. GENESIS simulation objects and graphical objects are linked together using the scripting language. The interpreter can read SLI commands either interactively from the keyboard (allowing interactive debugging, inspection, and control of the simulation) or from files containing simulation scripts.

The graphical user interface (GUI) is XODUS, the X-windows Output and Display Utility for Simulations. This provides a higher-level and user-friendly means for developing simulations and monitoring their execution. XODUS consists of a set of graphical objects that are the same as the computational modules from the user's point of view, except that they perform graphical functions. As with the computational modules, XODUS modules can be set up in any manner that the user chooses to display or enter data. Furthermore, the graphical modules can call functions from the script language, so that the full power of the SLI is available through the graphical interface. This makes it possible to interactively change simulation parameters in real time to directly observe the effects of parameter variations. For example, the mouse can be used to plant recording or injection electrodes into a graphical representation of the cell. In addition to provisions for plotting the usual quantities of interest (membrane potentials, channel conductances, and so forth), XODUS has visualization features that permit such choices as using color to display the propagation of action potentials or other variables throughout a multicompartmental model, or to display connections and cell activity in a network model.

The GENESIS simulation engine (see Figure 1) consists of the simulator base code that provides the common control and support routines for the system, including those for input/output and for the numerical solution of the differential equations obeyed by the various neural simulation objects. GENESIS provides a choice of numerical integration methods, including highly accurate and stable implicit methods such as the Crank-Nicholson method (De Schutter and Beeman, 1998).

In addition to receiving commands from the SLI and the GUI, the simulation engine can construct simulations using information from data files and from the precompiled GENESIS object libraries. For example, the GENESIS "cell reader" allows one to build complex model neurons by reading their specifications from a data file instead of from a lengthy series of GENESIS commands delivered to the SLI. Similarly, network connection specifications may be read from a data file with the "fileconnect" command.

The GENESIS object libraries contain the building blocks from which many different simulations can be constructed. These in-

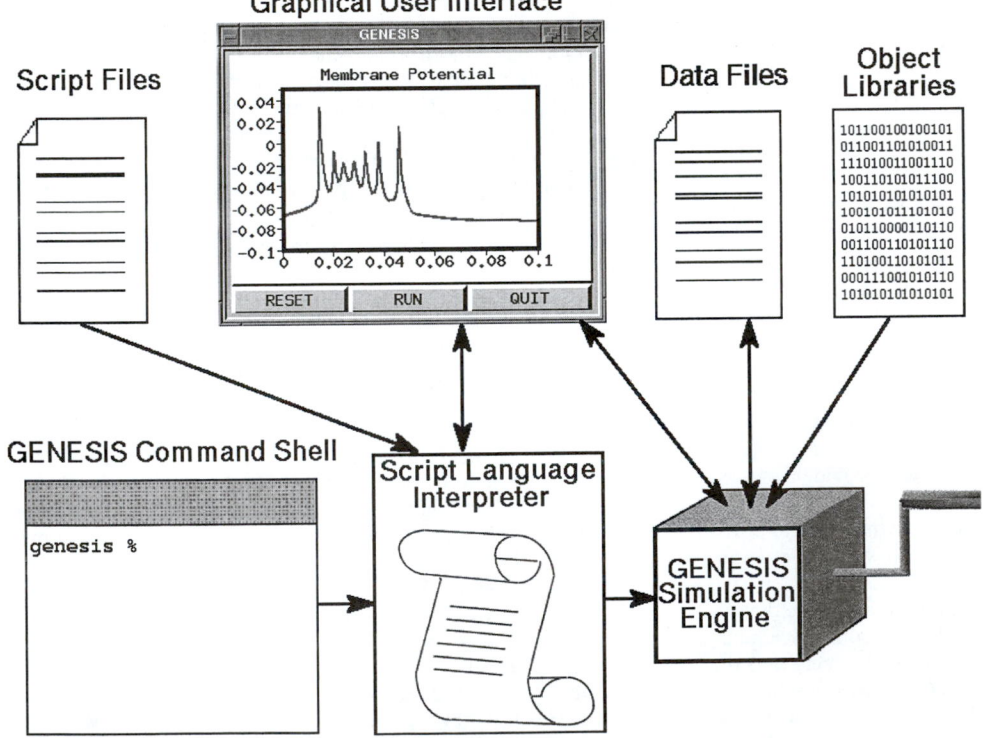

Figure 1. The components of GENESIS and modes of interaction. The Script Language Interpreter processes commands entered through the keyboard, script files, or the graphical user interface, and passes them to the GENESIS simulation engine. The simulation engine also loads compiled object libraries, reads and writes data files, and interacts with the GUI.

clude the spherical and cylindrical compartments from which the physical structure of neurons are constructed, voltage- and/or concentration-activated channels, dendrodendritic channels, and synaptically activated channels with synapses of several types, including Hebbian and facilitating synapses. In addition, there are objects for computing intracellular ionic concentrations from channel currents, for modeling the diffusion of ions within cells, and for allowing ligand gating of ion channels. There are also a number of "device objects" that may be interfaced to the simulation to provide various types of input to the simulation (e.g., pulse and spike generators, voltage clamp circuitry) or measurements (e.g., peristimulus and interspike interval histograms, spike frequency measurements, auto- and cross-correlation histograms).

The kinetics library supports kinetic-level modeling of biochemical pathways. This library currently includes objects for pools (molecular components), *n*-molecular reactions, enzymes, and channels to couple pools of different volume. The parameter search library provides a collection of objects and functions that automate the tedious process of adjusting model parameters to best reproduce experimental measurements carried out on the system being modeled.

GENESIS Script Libraries and Tools

In addition to the object libraries that are compiled into GENESIS, there are a number of libraries that are implemented as simulation scripts. These are available within the GENESIS distribution and in the archives of the GENESIS users group.

The channel library currently contains models for 39 different types of potassium channels (including several types of calcium-dependent channels), 24 types of sodium channels, and 14 types of calcium channels. The available single-cell models include cerebral cortical pyramidal cells, hippocampal pyramidal cells, cerebellar Purkinje cells, mitral, granule, and tufted cells from the olfactory bulb, a hippocampal granule cell model, a thalamic relay cell, and an *Aplysia* R15 bursting pacemaker cell.

GENESIS makes use of the GUI to provide other features to make the simulator more easily usable by people with limited programming experience. A set of kits, implemented as simulation scripts, has been provided to ease the modeling process. Neurokit provides an environment for building, modifying, and testing single-cell models without any programming on the part of the user. Kinetikit is a user-friendly, click-and-drag interface for modeling models of chemical reactions such as occur in biochemical signaling pathways. In addition to defining and running kinetic models, it is intended to facilitate managing kinetic data in these complex models (Bhalla, 1998; Bhalla and Iyengar, 1999).

GENESIS Documentation and Resources

GENESIS comes with extensive documentation. The GENESIS reference manual comes in three forms: a 566-page manual in Postscript format, and corresponding on-line help available either as plain text files viewable within the simulator or as hypertext help, which can be viewed with a web browser.

To complement the reference manual, we have published two editions of *The Book of GENESIS*. The most recent edition (Bower and Beeman, 1998) contains a CD-ROM with the GENESIS distribution, documentation, and files from the users group archives. It is widely used in both research and teaching, and consists of two parts serving complementary needs. Part I is designed to supplement instruction in neurobiology in upper division undergraduate and graduate neuroscience courses and includes chapters on various topics, each written by a known expert, to accompany a particular GENESIS tutorial. These interactive tutorial simulations are user-friendly, with on-line help, and may be used without any prior knowledge of the GENESIS simulator or computer programming. Part II serves as a user's guide to GENESIS, complementing the GENESIS reference manual, by introducing the basic features of GENESIS as well as the process of creating GENESIS simulations, providing a starting point for the development of new simulations. (For further details, please see http://www.genesis-sim.org/GENESIS/bog/bog.html.)

The tutorials mentioned above are included in the GENESIS distribution, along with other tutorials and demonstrations designed to aid new users in building GENESIS simulations. These illustrate the use of advanced GENESIS features, including objects for modeling calcium diffusion; objects for spike analysis, recording, and generation; the use of facilitating and Hebbian synapses; objects for modeling stochastic ion channels; and the parameter search library. Several of the tutorials are based on significant published research simulations, including the piriform cortex model (Wilson and Bower, 1992), the hippocampal pyramidal cell model (Traub et al., 1991), and the detailed cerebellar Purkinje cell model (De Schutter and Bower, 1994a, 1994b). In addition to their educational purpose, these tutorial simulations provide examples of well-constructed GENESIS simulations, and they have been used by others as the basis for the construction of new published research simulations.

Individuals or research groups who make serious use of GENESIS are encouraged to join the GENESIS users group, BABEL. There are currently 347 BABEL memberships, representing approximately 700 users. Members of BABEL are entitled to access the BABEL directories and participate in the e-mail newsgroup. The directories are used as a repository for the latest contributions by GENESIS users and developers. Such contributions include new simulations, libraries of cells and channels, additional simulator components, new documentation and tutorials, bug reports and fixes, and the posting of questions and hints for setting up GENESIS simulations. As the results of GENESIS research simulations are published, many of these simulations are being made available through BABEL.

Use of GENESIS in Education

From its inception, GENESIS has had a strong educational component. We are currently aware of 49 institutions in 11 countries that have used GENESIS in teaching. Many of these institutions use GENESIS in association with *The Book of GENESIS* (Bower and Beeman, 1998).

GENESIS and the tutorials described in the previous sections are now being widely used in graduate and undergraduate instruction. Instructional options include full-semester courses in computational neuroscience or neural modeling, short intensive courses or workshops, course projects, and short units on computational neuroscience within courses on artificial neural nets. An example of the use of GENESIS tutorials as the basis for a short unit on neural modeling is available on the GENESIS web site as an HTML version of two lectures given at the University of Colorado.

GENESIS has also formed the basis for the laboratory section of the Methods in Computational Neuroscience course (1988–1996) at the Marine Biological Laboratory, a course in Mexico City in the summer of 1991, the Crete course in Computational Neuroscience (1996–1998), the EU Advanced Course in Computational Neuroscience (1999–2002), and the Computational Neuroscience course at the National Centre for Biological Sciences in Bangalore (1999–2000).

Discussion

In the many years since the GENESIS project began at Caltech, its development has spread to many other institutions, including the

University of Texas at San Antonio, the University of Antwerp, the National Centre for Biological Studies in Bangalore, the University of Colorado, the Pittsburgh Supercomputer Center, the San Diego Supercomputer Center, and Emory University. In addition, the tools available for GUIs and the decentralization of computational resources as a result of widespread use of the World Wide Web have dramatically changed the environment for computer-based education and research. In a collaborative effort involving many institutions, we are currently redesigning and reimplementing GENESIS in order to modernize the user interface and link the process of modeling with on-line databases of models and model components. Our efforts are taking place in the context of a new software framework called the Modeler's Workspace (Forss et al., 1999; Hucka et al., 2002) and a simulator-independent representation of neural models called NeuroML (Goddard et al., 2001).

Further information about GENESIS and PGENESIS, as well as instructions for downloading and installation, may be obtained from the GENESIS web site, http://www.genesis-sim.org/GENESIS/. Inquiries concerning GENESIS should be addressed to genesis@genesis-sim.org.

Road Map: Implementation and Analysis
Related Reading: Neurosimulation: Tools and Resources

References

Bhalla, U. S., 1998, The network within: Signalling pathways, in *The Book of GENESIS: Exploring Realistic Neural Models with the GEneral NEural SImulation System* (J.M. Bower and D. Beeman, Eds.), 2nd ed., New York: Springer-Verlag, pp. 169–191.

Bhalla, U. S., and Iyengar, R., 1999, Emergent properties of networks of biological signaling pathways, *Science*, 283:381–387.

Bower, J. M., 1995, Reverse engineering the nervous system: An in vivo, in vitro, and in computo approach to understanding the mammalian olfactory system, in *An Introduction to Neural and Electronic Networks*, (S. F. Zornetzer, J. L. Davis, and C. Lau, Eds.), 2nd ed., New York: Academic Press, pp. 3–28. ◆

Bower, J. M., and Beeman, D., 1998, *The Book of GENESIS: Exploring Realistic Neural Models with the GEneral NEural SImulation System*, 2nd ed., New York: Springer-Verlag. ◆

De Schutter, E., and Beeman, D., 1998, Speeding up GENESIS simulations, in *The Book of GENESIS: Exploring Realistic Neural Models with the GEneral NEural SImulation System* (J.M. Bower and D. Beeman, Eds.), 2nd ed., New York: Springer-Verlag, pp. 329–447.

De Schutter, E., and Bower, J. M., 1994a, An active membrane model of the cerebellar Purkinje cell: I. Simulation of current clamps in slice, *J. Neurophysiol.*, 71:375–400.

De Schutter, E., and Bower, J. M., 1994b, An active membrane model of the cerebellar Purkinje cell: II. Simulation of synaptic responses, *J. Neurophysiol.*, 71:401–419.

Forss, J., Beeman, D., Eickler-West, R., and Bower, J. M., 1999, The Modeler's Workspace: A Distributed Digital Library for Neuroscience, *Future Generation Computer Systems*, vol. 16, pp. 111–121. ◆

Goddard, N., Hucka, M., Howell, F., Cornelis, H., Shankar, K., and Beeman, D., 2001, Towards NeuroML: Model description methods for collaborative modelling in neuroscience, *Philos. Trans. R. Soc. Lond. B*, 356:1209–1228. ◆

Hucka, M., Shankar, K., Beeman, D., and Bower, J. M., 2002, The Modeler's Workspace: Making model-based studies of the nervous system more accessible, in *Computational Neuroanatomy: Principles and Methods* (G. Ascoli, Ed.), Totowa, NJ: Humana Press. ◆

Stricanne, B., Morissette, J., and Bower, J. M., 1998, Exploring the sources of cerebellar post-lesion plasticity with a network model of the somatosensory system, *Soc. Neurosci. Abs.*, 23:2364.

Traub, R. D., Wong, R. K. S., Miles, R., and Michelson, H., 1991, A model of a CA3 hippocampal pyramidal neuron incorporating voltage-clamp data on intrinsic conductances, *J. Neurophysiol.*, 66:635–650.

Wilson, M., and Bower, J. M., 1992, Simulating cerebral cortical networks: Oscillations and temporal interactions in a computer simulation of piriform (olfactory) cortex, *J. Neurophysiol.*, 67:981–995.

Geometrical Principles in Motor Control

Ferdinando A. Mussa-Ivaldi

Introduction

The central role played by geometry in the control of motor behaviors was recognized in the early years of the last century by Nikolai Bernstein. Using only the tool of logical reasoning applied to common observations, Bernstein reached the conclusion that "there exist in the higher levels of the CNS projections of space, and not projections of joint and muscles" (Bernstein, 1967). This intuition led others to consider motor planning and execution as separate processes.

The transition from the spatial representation of a motor goal to a set of neuromuscular commands is in many respects similar to a *coordinate transformation*. This analogy is the perspective of this article. We will begin by describing three types of coordinate systems, each one representing a particular point of view on motor behavior. Then, we will examine the geometrical rules that govern the transformations between these classes of coordinates. Finally, we will see how a proper representation of dynamics may greatly simplify the transformation of motor plans into actions.

Coordinate Systems for Motor Control

Endpoint Coordinates

Consider a monkey in the act of reaching for an apple with a wooden stick. The free extremity of the stick is the site at which the monkey interacts with its environment. We call such a site an *endpoint*. The position of the stick is fully determined by six coordinates. This is the smallest set of numbers needed to specify unambiguously the location and orientation of a rigid object in 3D space. The coordinates of the stick can be measured with respect to three orthogonal axes originating, for example, from the monkey's shoulder.

In our example a position in endpoint coordinates is a point

$$r = (x, y, z, \theta_X, \theta_Y, \theta_Z)$$

The coordinates, x, y, and z determine a translation with respect to the orthogonal axes. The angular coordinates, θ_X, θ_Y, and θ_Z, determine an orientation with respect to the same axes. Consistent with this notation, a *force* in endpoint coordinates is a vector with three linear and three angular components:

$$F = (F_X, F_Y, F_Z, \tau_X, \tau_Y, \tau_Z)$$

Generalized Coordinates

A different way of describing the position of the monkey's arm is to provide the set of joint angles that define the orientation of each skeletal segment either with respect to fixed axes in space or with respect to the neighboring segments. Joint angles are a particular instance of *generalized coordinates*. According to the standard definitions of analytical mechanics, generalized coordinates are independent variables that are suitable for describing the dynamics of a system (Goldstein, 1980).

Once a set of generalized coordinates has been defined, one may also define a *generalized force*. For example, if one uses joint angles as generalized coordinates, the corresponding generalized forces are the torques measured at each joint. The dynamics of a mechanical system are described by differential equations relating the generalized coordinates to their first and second time derivatives and to the generalized forces.

In vector notation, the dynamics equations for the skeletal system of the monkey's arm can be written as

$$I(q)\ddot{q} + G(q, \dot{q}) = C(q, \dot{q}, u(t)) \tag{1}$$

where $q = (q_1, q_2, \ldots, q_N)$ is the arm configuration in joint-angle coordinates, $\dot{q}$ and $\ddot{q}$ are, respectively, the first (velocity) and second (acceleration) time derivatives of q, I is an $N \times N$ matrix of inertia (that is configuration dependent) and $G(q, \dot{q})$ is a vector of centripetal and Coriolis torques (Sciavicco and Siciliano, 2000). The whole left-hand side of Equation 1 represents the torque due to the inertial properties of the arm. The term $C(\cdot)$ stands for the net torque generated nonlinearly by the muscles, by the environment (e.g., the gravitational torque), and by other dissipative elements, such as friction. The time-function $u(t)$ is a control vector—for example, a set of neural signals directed to the motoneurons or a representation of a desired limb position at time t (EQUILIBRIUM POINT HYPOTHESIS). Equation 1 may be regarded as a reformulation of Newtons's law: $Ma = F$. The left side represents the passive dynamics associated with limb inertia. The right side is the applied force, which, in this case, is the output of a control process.

Actuator Coordinates

Actuator coordinates afford the most direct representation for the motor output of the central nervous system. A *position* in this coordinate system may be, for example, a collection of muscle lengths, $l = (l_1, l_2, \ldots, l_M)$. Accordingly, a force in the same coordinate system is a collection of muscle tensions, $f = (f_1, f_2, \ldots, f_M)$. The number of actuator coordinates depends on the level of detail of the model of control under consideration. *Unlike generalized coordinates, actuator coordinates do not constitute a system of mechanically independent variables*: one cannot set arbitrary values to l_i without eventually violating some kinematic constraint.

The Workspace and Its Transformations

Both the transformations from generalized coordinates to endpoint coordinates, and from generalized coordinates to actuator coordinates, are, in general, nonlinear mappings. In the case of the monkey's arm, the transformation from joint to hand coordinates is a nonlinear function

$$r = L(q) \tag{2}$$

where r indicates the position of the hand in endpoint coordinates and q is the joint configuration. The transformation from joint to muscle coordinates is another nonlinear mapping

$$l = M(q) \tag{3}$$

We deal briefly with transformations between the different representations of the workspace in the framework of differential geometry. A modern tutorial on this subject can be found in Jose and Saletan (1998).

The Transformation of Vectors and Vector Fields

A function that associates a vector to each point of a multidimensional domain, M, is called a *vector field over M*. For example, one may rearrange the terms of the dynamics in Equation 1 so as to represent the arm's acceleration as a time-varying vector field over the state space described by q and $\dot{q}$:

$$\ddot{q} = I^{-1}(q)[C(q, \dot{q}, u(t)) - G(q, \dot{q})] \tag{5}$$

Another vector field describes the viscoelastic behavior of the arm muscles. This behavior can be measured by stimulating each muscle and recording the resulting tension at different muscle length rates of shortening and times. Then, the collective mechanical output of the skeletomotor system is summarized by a force field in muscle coordinates

$$f = \alpha(l, \dot{l}, t) \tag{5}$$

Vector fields such as those expressed in Equations 4 and 5 determine the way in which a system reacts to its environment on one hand and to its control signals on the other. To investigate the transformation from planning to control of actions, we must understand how such mechanical fields are affected by a change of coordinates.

Let us begin by considering the laws that govern the transformation of a point from a set of coordinates, x, into a new set of coordinates, $\bar{x}$. The coordinate transformation is a nonlinear function

$$\bar{x} = T(x) \tag{6}$$

We assume this function to be continuous and sufficiently differentiable (the existence and continuity of second partial derivatives is enough for most practical purposes.) However, we do not require the existence of an inverse mapping, $x = T^{-1}(\bar{x})$. In many biologically relevant cases the two coordinate systems have different dimensions and the inverse mapping is not defined uniquely or does not exist at all.

Next, consider how a vector field is related to the corresponding vector field in the new coordinate system. Let us begin by considering a field of velocity vectors, $\dot{x} = v(x)$, and apply the chain rule:

$$\dot{\bar{x}} = \frac{d\bar{x}}{dt} = \frac{\partial \bar{x}}{\partial x} \cdot \dot{x}$$

As we are dealing with multivariate functions, the expression $\partial \bar{x}/\partial x$ represents the functional derivative, or *Jacobian* of the transformation T. The Jacobian is a position-dependent matrix, $J(x)$, whose elements are

$$[J(x)]_{i,j} = \frac{\partial \bar{x}_i}{\partial x_j}$$

and the transformation for the velocity vector can be rewritten as

$$\dot{\bar{x}} = J(x) \cdot \dot{x} \tag{7}$$

A vector that changes according to this law is said to be *contravariant*.

Does Equation 7 provide us with a rule for transforming the whole velocity field $v(x)$ into a new field $\bar{v}(\bar{x})$? The answer is generally negative. We may write $\dot{\bar{x}}$ as a function of $\bar{x}$:

$$\dot{x} = J(T^{-1}(\bar{x}))v(T^{-1}(\bar{x})) = \bar{v}(\bar{x})$$

only if the mapping $T(x)$ can be inverted.

If a coordinate transformation cannot be inverted, we know how to transform a contravariant vector *at a given point* but we do not know how to transform a contravariant *field*.

The situation is quite different when dealing with vectors that in a change of coordinates transform like the gradient operator. Again, using the chain rule:

$$\frac{\partial}{\partial x} = \frac{\partial \bar{x}}{\partial x} \cdot \frac{\partial}{\partial \bar{x}}$$

that is,

$$\frac{\partial}{\partial x} = J^T(x) \cdot \frac{\partial}{\partial \bar{x}} \qquad (8)$$

A vector following this type of transformation is said to be *covariant*. Note the dual or reciprocal nature of Equations 7 and 8. An infinitesimal displacement (or a velocity) is transformed by the Jacobian into the new coordinate system. The same Jacobian maps a covariant vector the other way around—from the new to the old coordinate system.

An example of a covariant vector is force, F. The covariance of force derives from the tensor invariance of work and power. *Work and power are indeed true scalar variables whose value is not modified by a change of coordinates*. In the original coordinate system, power is calculated as

$$F^T \dot{x}$$

and in the new coordinate system, as

$$\bar{F}^T \dot{\bar{x}}$$

By equating these two expressions and using Equation 7, we obtain

$$\bar{F}^T J(x)\dot{x} = F^T \dot{x}$$

Hence, the transformation of a force field, $\bar{F}(\bar{x})$, is

$$F(x) = J(x)^T \bar{F}(T(x)) \qquad (9)$$

(compare with Equation 8).

Note that, here, the entire right side has been resolved in terms of x. We reach the important conclusion that unlike contravariant vectors, *covariant vectors transform globally, as fields*. No inverse transformation is required.

Transforming Plans into Action

When we plan a movement such as "trace the shape of a circle with the left hand," we formulate the goal in terms of end point coordinates, without concern for the muscles that participate in the desired behavior. However, once we have decided to trace a circle, our brain must choose which muscles to activate and in which temporal sequence they should be activated. In carrying out this task, our brain must face the challenges associated with *kinematic redundancy*—the imbalance between the number of muscles, joints, and end point coordinates that is typical of any biological system. The issue of kinematic redundancy has attracted considerable attention both in robotics (Mussa-Ivaldi and Hogan, 1991) and in neural modeling (Hinton, 1984; Bullock, Grossberg, and Guenther, 1993).

The purpose of this section is to show how a proper representation of dynamics and of coordinate transformations leads to a simple solution for some problems associated with redundancy. The key for this solution lies in the representation of both the "high level" plans and the "low level" actuator actions as covariant fields of force.

The Transformation of Dynamics

The dynamics of a limb (Equation 1) are expressed as an equilibrium condition between the field of generalized forces, $D(q, \dot{q}, \ddot{q})$, which represent passive elements such as limb inertia and the field of time-varying generalized forces, and $C(q, \dot{q}, t)$, which are generated by the neuromuscular controller:

$$D(q, \dot{q}, \ddot{q}) = C(q, \dot{q}, t) \qquad (10)$$

We formulate the problem of executing a motor plan as the problem of deriving a control field, $C(q, \dot{q}, t)$, that generates a desired end point behavior. *This task is carried out as an approximation problem, after transforming the covariant fields corresponding to the planned behavior and to the neuromuscular mechanics into their corresponding images in generalized coordinates.*

The first step consists of expressing the motor plans as fields of force in endpoint coordinates:

$$F = \pi(r, \dot{r}, t) \qquad (12)$$

For example, a reaching movement of the hand may be planned, as proposed by Flash and Hogan (1985), by specifying a time-varying field whose equilibrium point moves along a smooth trajectory (EQUILIBRIUM POINT HYPOTHESIS). Following a similar approach, the movements of a robotic arm in an obstacle-ridden environment can be efficiently planned by associating a field of repulsive forces to each obstacle and a field of attractive forces to the target location (POTENTIAL FIELDS AND NEURAL NETWORKS).

From our earlier consideration of vector fields, we may conclude that the planned field, $\pi(r, \dot{r}, t)$, has a unique image, $C_\pi(q, \dot{q}, t)$, in configuration space. *This is true regardless of kinematic redundancy*. The only condition for C_π to be defined is that the kinematic transformation from generalized to endpoint coordinates be defined with its first partial derivatives. Operationally, we may construct C_π as a combination of three mappings:

$$C_\pi = l_2 \circ \pi \circ l_1 : (q, \dot{q}, t) \overset{l_1}{\to} (r, \dot{r}, t) \overset{\pi}{\to} F \overset{l_2}{\to} Q$$

The first mapping, l_1, is the direct kinematics transformation ($q \to r$), its Jacobian $(q, \dot{q}, \dot{r})$, and the identity function ($t \to t$). The second mapping is the planned endpoint field, $\pi(r, \dot{r}, t)$. Finally, the third mapping, l_2, is the transformation from endpoint to generalized force, which, again, is provided by the Jacobian of the direct kinematics.

As an example, consider the planning of an endpoint behavior, corresponding to a moving equilibrium position, $r_E(t)$, with linear stiffness and viscosity (that is a linear PD controller in endpoint coordinates):

$$\pi(r, \dot{r}, t) = K(r - r_E(t)) + B\dot{r}$$

The image of this endpoint field in joint coordinates is

$$C_\pi(q, \dot{q}, t) = J^T(q)K(L(q) - r_E(t)) + J^T(q)BJ(q)\dot{q}$$

Note that $r_E(t)$ is a time-varying input function that does not require a measure of the actual hand position. This derivation applies to kinematically redundant limbs, as only the direct transformations, L and J, are required.

On the other end of the planning/execution problem, one must deal with a number of actuators that, in any biological system exceeds the number of generalized coordinates. Microstimulation studies in frogs (Giszter, Mussa-Ivaldi, and Bizzi, 1993) and rats (Tresch and Bizzi, 1999) showed that the focal activation of interneuronal regions within the lumbar spinal cord impose a specific balance of muscle activations. This results in a force field

$$f = \alpha(l, \dot{l}, t) \sum_i \alpha_i \psi_i(l, \dot{l}, t) \qquad (13)$$

This field has a well defined and measurable image in generalized coordinates, $\phi_\alpha(q, \dot{q}, t)$, which can be derived from the combination of three direct transformations:

$$\phi_\alpha = m_2 \circ \alpha \circ m_1 : (q, \dot{q}, t) \xrightarrow{m_1} (l, \dot{l}, t) \xrightarrow{\alpha} f \xrightarrow{m_2} Q$$

The first transformation, m_1, is the actuator kinematics ($M : q \to l$) together with its Jacobian ($q, \dot{q} \to \dot{l}$) and the identity mapping (t). The second transformation is the actuator force field, $\alpha(l, \dot{l}, t)$, and the third transformation, m_2, is again given by the Jacobian of M, $\mu(q) = \partial M(q)/\partial q$.

In generalized coordinates, the force field induced by a synergy of muscles is

$$\phi_\alpha(q, \dot{q}, t) = \sum_i \alpha_i \mu(q)^T \psi_i(M(q), \mu(q)\dot{q}, t)$$

Once again, this derivation of the synergy image in generalized coordinates remains valid for redundant limb because no inverse transformation is involved.

Discussion

Microstimulation studies (Mussa-Ivaldi, Giszter, and Bizzi, 1994) as well as studies of reflex behaviors (Kargo and Giszter, 2000) have demonstrated that multiple muscle synergies can be combined by linear superposition to generate complex behaviors. In particular, Kargo and Giszter found that reflex responses to multiple cutaneous stimuli are accounted for by the linear superposition of the response fields triggered by each stimulus.

The finding of vector summation suggests that under descending supraspinal commands, the fields expressed by the spinal cord may form a broad repertoire:

$$\Gamma = \left\{ C_S(q, \dot{q}, t|c_\alpha) = \sum_\alpha c_\alpha \phi_\alpha(q, \dot{q}, t) \right\} \tag{14}$$

Each element of Γ is generated by the descending commands selecting a group of synergies through the weighting coefficients, c_α. Following this view, the neural control system may approximate a *target field* $C_\pi(q, \dot{q}, t)$ by finding the element of Γ that is closest to the target field. The approximating field may be obtained by least squares methods, that is by determining a set of coefficients, c_α, such that the norm

$$\| C_S(q, \dot{q}, t|c_\alpha) - C_\pi(q, \dot{q}, t) \|^2 \tag{15}$$

is at a minimum.

Field approximation has been directly applied to the generation of a desired trajectory, $q_D(t)$, in generalized coordinates (Mussa-Ivaldi and Bizzi, 2000). In this case, one may attempt to generate the appropriate controller by finding the parameters, c_α, which minimize the difference between passive dynamics and control field in Equation 10 that is by minimizing

$$\| D(q, \dot{q}, \ddot{q}) - C_S(q, \dot{q}, t|c_\alpha) \|^2 \tag{16}$$

along the desired trajectory. Since the parameters, c_α, appear linearly in C_S, this problem has a single global minimum at

$$c_\alpha = \sum_i [\Phi]_{\alpha,i}^{-1} \Lambda_i$$

with

$$\begin{cases} \Phi_{l,m} = \int \phi_l(q_D(t), \dot{q}_D(t), t) \cdot \phi_m(q_D(t), \dot{q}_D(t), t) dt \\ \Lambda_j = \int \phi_j(q_D(t), \dot{q}_D(t), t) \cdot D(q_D(t), \dot{q}_D(t), \ddot{q}(t)) dt \end{cases} \tag{17}$$

The symbol $\cdot$ indicates the ordinary inner product.

The underlying idea of this method is that if the residual force error (16) could be reduced to zero, then the corresponding controller would produce exactly the desired trajectory. If, instead, there is a non-zero residual, then the problem of generating acceptable approximations becomes a problem of local stability: as residual forces may be regarded as a perturbation of the dynamics, one needs to insure that this perturbation does not lead to a motion that diverges from the desired trajectory. A study by Lohmiller and Slotine (1998) showed that the combination of control modules is stable if the modules are "contracting"—a condition germane to exponential stability.

If the modules corresponding to muscle synergies are stable, then the possibility of combining them provide the central nervous system with something equivalent to a movement's representation. The movements of a limb can be considered as "points" in an abstract geometrical space, where the force fields produced by a set of modules play a role equivalent to that of coordinate axes and the selection parameters that generate a particular movement may be regarded as generalized projections of this movement along these axes.

The theoretical view of motor control as a form of function approximation has found support in recent studies of adaptive learning. In a set of elegant experiments, Thoroughman and Shadmehr (2000) have asked subjects to execute movements of the hand against a field of perturbing forces. Subjects learned gradually to compensate these forces, thus recovering the normal kinematics of reaching movements. However, if the forces were suddenly suppressed during "catch trials," subjects showed a transient loss of learning that affected the following movements in variable amounts, depending on the angle between the movement in the catch trial and the following movement. Thorougman and Shadmehr were able to reproduce the process of adaptation as well as the subtle effects of catch trials by assuming that the motor control system composed a representation of the disturbing field as a linear superposition of Gaussian primitives. These primitives encode the force generated in response to a velocity, with a narrow variance parameter (approximately 10 cm/sec). The analysis of motor learning, together with the study of motor primitives in the spinal cord has provided us with a strong support for a theoretical view based on the idea that the central nervous system generate and update a broad spectrum of behaviors by combining elementary building blocks. The mathematical language of force fields and of their transformations is the proper framework for relating this computational mechanism to its observable mechanical effects.

Road Map: Mammalian Motor Control
Related Reading: Equilibrium Point Hypothesis; Eye-Hand Coordination in Reaching Movements; Limb Geometry, Neural Control; Motor Primitives

References

Bernstein, N., 1967, *The Coordination and Regulation of Movement*, Oxford, UK: Pergamon Press.

Bullock, D., Grossberg, S., and Guenther, F. H., 1993, A self-organizing neural model of motor equivalent reaching and tool use by a multijoint arm. *J. Cognit. Neurosci.*, 5:408–435.

Flash, T., and Hogan, N., 1985, The coordination of arm movements: An experimentally confirmed mathematical model, *J. Neurosci.*, 5:1688–1703.

Giszter, S. F., Mussa-Ivaldi, F. A., and Bizzi, E., 1993, Convergent force fields organized in the frog's spinal cord, *J. Neurosci.*, 13:467–491.

Goldstein, H., 1980, *Classical Mechanics*, Reading, MA: Addison-Wesley.

Hinton, G., 1984, Parallel computations for controlling an arm, *J. Motor Behav.*, 16:171–194.

Jose, J. V., and Saletan, E. J., 1998, *Classical Dynamics: A Contemporary Approach*, Cambridge, UK: Cambridge University Press.

Kargo, W. J., and Giszter, S. F., 2000, Rapid correction of aimed movements by summation of force-field primitives, *J. Neurosci.*, 20:409–426.

Lohmiller, W., and Slotine, J,-J. E., 1998, On contraction analysis for nonlinear systems, *Automatica* 34:683–696. ◆

Mussa-Ivaldi, F. A., and Hogan, N., 1991, Integrable solutions of kinematic redundancy via impedance control, *Int. J. Robotics Res.*, 10:481–491.

Mussa-Ivaldi, F. A., Giszter, S. F., and Bizzi, E., 1994, Linear combinations of primitives in vertebrate motor control, *Proc. Natl. Acad. Sci. USA*, 91:7534–7538.

Mussa-Ivaldi, F. A., and Bizzi, E., 2000, Motor learning through the combination of primitives, *Phil. Trans. Roy. Soc. Lond. B*, 355:1755–1769. ◆

Sciavicco, L., and Siciliano, B., 2000, *Modeling and Control of Robot Manipulators*, New York: Springer Verlag.

Thoroughman, K. A., and Shadmehr, R., 2000, Learning of action through adaptive combination of motor primitives, *Nature*, 407:742–747.

Tresch, M. C., and Bizzi, E., 1999, Responses to spinal microstimulation in the chronically spinalized rat and their relationship to spinal systems activated by low threshold cutaneous stimulation, *Exp. Brain Res.*, 129:401–416.

Global Visual Pattern Extraction

Hugh R. Wilson and Frances Wilkinson

Introduction

Decades of research have established that visual pattern recognition begins with the extraction of local edge and contour information by orientation-selective simple cells in primary visual cortex (V1). At the highest levels of cortical form vision in inferior temporal cortex (IT), many neurons are sensitive to complex global patterns, including objects and faces (Desimone, 1991). This raises the key question "What processes occur at intervening stages of the form vision pathway to transform local V1 orientation information into global pattern representations?" It is known that the ventral form vision pathway includes at least areas V1, V2, V4, TEO, and TE (the highest level of IT), so there must be a sequence of transformations. Furthermore, mean receptive field size increases in diameter by roughly a factor of 2.5–2.7 from area to area in this processing hierarchy (Boussaoud, Desimone, and Ungerleider, 1991; Kobatake and Tanaka, 1994). Thus, a mean foveal receptive field diameter of about 0.4° in V1 is transformed into a mean of about 3.0° in V4 and about 15.0°–20.0° in TE. Clearly, such large receptive fields must be combining information from many V1 neurons, but what sorts of combinations actually occur?

Essentially the same question may be posed in cortical motion processing along the dorsal pathway comprising V1, V2, MT, MST, and higher parietal areas. V1 neurons extract only local motion vectors perpendicular to moving edge segments, while MST neurons are sensitive to complex optic flow patterns, including expansion and rotation (Tanaka and Saito, 1989). In the dorsal pathway, receptive field diameter also grows by a factor of 2.5–2.7 from area to area. Thus analogous questions are raised about transitions from local to global processing in both motion and form vision. This article suggests answers to these questions at intermediate levels of these two pathways, primarily V4 and MST.

Global Processes in V4

Although primate V4 was originally believed to be a color vision area, more recent lesion studies have shown that it represents a major intermediate level of the cortical form vision system. Early physiological studies of V4 typically used the bar and grating stimuli that had proved so fruitful in elucidating orientation and spatial frequency selectivity in V1. Such stimuli, however, mainly revealed powerful end inhibition in V4. In a novel approach to V4, Gallant, Braun, and Van Essen (1993) used concentric, radial, and hyperbolic grating stimuli as well as conventional sinusoidal gratings. While many neurons responded well to all stimulus groups, two new groups were found: one responding optimally to concentric gratings and one responding optimally to radial or hyperbolic gratings. Very few neurons responded significantly better to con-

ventional gratings than to the other classes. Using a very different approach, Kobatake and Tanaka (1994) also found that many V4 neurons were selective for concentric, radial, or cross-shaped stimuli.

In an attempt to relate these results to human form vision, it was natural to study Glass patterns, which can convey concentric (Figure 1), radial, and other structures. These patterns are normally generated by randomly placing dot pairs of fixed separation on the pattern such that the orientation defined by the pair is tangent to contours of the desired global pattern (e.g., concentric circles in Figure 1). By randomizing some percentage of the dots, the global structure conveyed by Glass patterns can be degraded. When psychophysical thresholds were measured in this manner, it was discovered that humans are most sensitive to concentric structure, somewhat less sensitive to radial or hyperbolic structure, and least

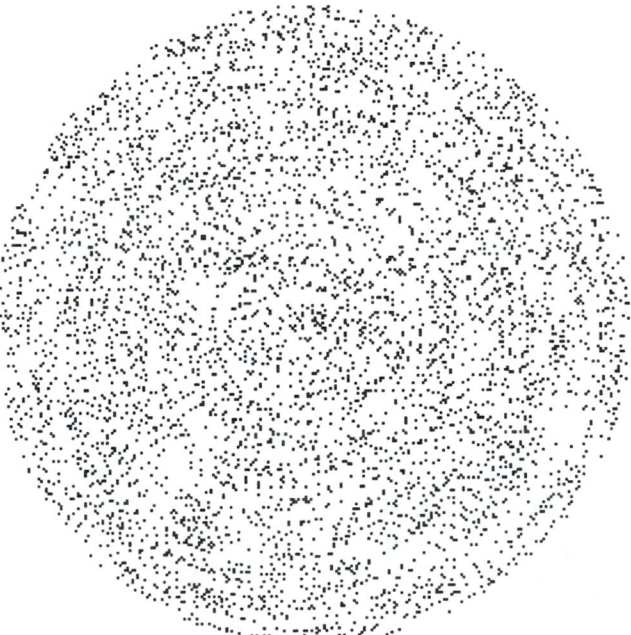

Figure 1. Concentric random dot Glass pattern. The global concentric structure in this pattern is produced by randomly positioning pairs of dots of fixed separation such that the orientation of the pair is locally tangent to a circle (not visible) concentric with the center of the pattern. Radial, hyperbolic, and parallel Glass patterns can be produced analogously.

sensitive to parallel or translational structure (Wilson, Wilkinson, and Asaad, 1997). Further experiments showed that the sensitivity to concentric structure resulted from linear pooling of concentric orientation information within an area estimated to be about 3.0°–4.0° in diameter. Similar results were obtained in experiments with radial Glass patterns (Wilson, 1999b).

The psychophysical data are contrary to what would be expected for V1 but consistent with primate V4 physiology (Gallant et al., 1993; Kobatake and Tanaka, 1994). Accordingly, we asked whether human V4 might also show similar stimulus selectivity. After localizing V1, V4, and the fusiform face area using standard techniques, fMRI responses were measured while viewing concentric, radial, and sinusoidal gratings (Wilkinson et al., 2000). As predicted, the data showed that V1 activation was the same for all three stimulus patterns, while the fMRI signals in V4 were significantly higher for concentric and radial gratings than for sinusoidal gratings (Wilkinson et al., 2000). Interestingly, only concentric gratings and faces produced significant activation of the fusiform face area, suggesting that analysis of concentric structure represents one component of face perception.

Network Model

These data lead to the conclusion that human V4 is selectively sensitive to concentric and radial stimuli (and certainly other configural patterns), as is primate V4. The simple neural network diagrammed in Figure 2 describes a V4 concentric unit model consistent with these data (Wilson et al., 1997; Wilson, 1999b). Three stages make up the model, and these are hypothesized to represent V1, V2, and finally V4 processing. First, the stimulus is processed by oriented filters with properties of V1 simple cells (12 preferred orientations in 15° increments were used). Following this are contrast gain control and full-wave rectification operations for which there is experimental evidence. Next the responses are processed by larger second-stage filters oriented at right angles to their V1 inputs. This combination of filtering, rectification, and orthogonal filtering generates an end-stopped complex cell model that is sensitive to contour curvature (Wilson, 1999b). Finally, V2 responses that are concentric with the center of each V4 receptive field (gray circles) are summed linearly (Σ), and the result is passed through a threshold nonlinearity. An analogous model for V4 radial units has been constructed by simply changing the orientations of the

V1 filters to be parallel to the V2 filters. These V4 models are configural in the sense that they pool all V1 orientations, but each from pattern-specific subregions of the V4 receptive field.

This model offers an explanation for the 2.5- to 2.7-fold increase in receptive field sizes from V1 to V2 and from V2 to V4. The V2 filters must be about this much larger than V1 filters to effectively process curvature, while the V4 receptive fields must sum V2 responses over a diameter around 3.0 times the V2 filter diameter to extract circular or radial structure. Smaller increases in receptive field size from V1 to V4 simply cannot extract the relevant configural information.

The fMRI discovery that concentric gratings activate the fusiform face area is consistent with the hypothesis that V4 concentric units constitute an intermediate stage in face perception. To test this idea, the model in Figure 2 was applied to a variety of faces. For example, model convolution with the transparent face-house image in Figure 3A produced a single peak of activation centered at the black dot (Wilson, Krupa, and Wilkinson, 2000a). Furthermore, the response of this unit was proportional to the mean radius of the head, as indicated by the vertical arrow. This ability of model V4 units to *measure* concentric image structure is produced by the contrast gain control following the V1 filters. This causes the final summation stage Σ to add the number of units active around the pattern circumference, thus producing a signal proportional to radius and independent of contrast over a considerable range (Figure 3B). The model is also capable of encoding aspects of head shape, including axis of elongation and bilateral symmetry, as a sparse population code (Wilson et al., 2000b).

Global Unit Dynamics and Attention

There is considerable evidence that selective attention affects V4 neuron responses, and the evidence suggests that this results from biasing of competitive inhibitory networks (Reynolds, Chelazzi, and Desimone, 1999). Further evidence for such competitive inhibition among V4 concentric units has emerged from analysis of a visual illusion first introduced by Marroquin in 1978 (Wilson et al., 2000a). Marroquin patterns generate percepts of illusory circles appearing and vanishing at multiple locations within the pattern, much like the dynamic fluctuations in binocular rivalry. Psychophysical measurement of the visibility times of illusory circles in

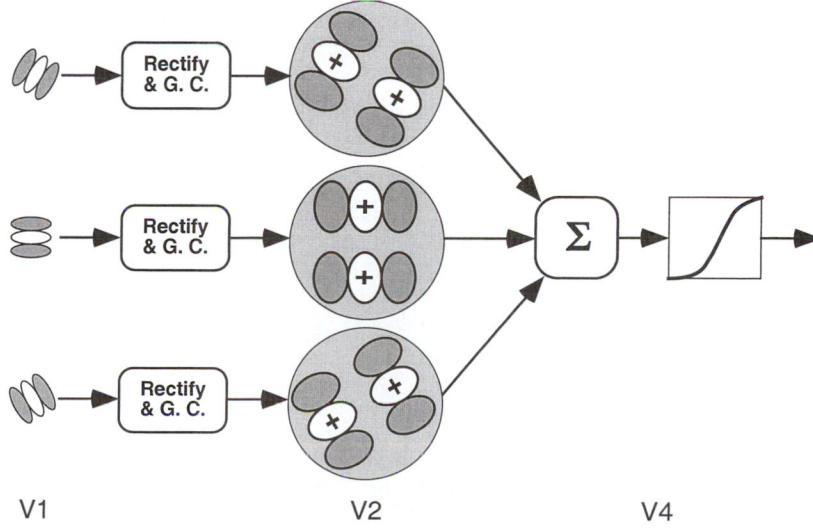

Figure 2. Global pooling model for a V4 concentric unit. Convolving the stimulus with 12 different oriented simple cell filters (only three shown for clarity) having elongated excitatory (white) and inhibitory (gray) zones makes up the V1 stage. This is followed by full-wave rectification and a contrast gain control. V2 processing incorporates filtering by oriented filters that are 2.5–2.7 times the diameter of V1 filters. Finally, responses of concentrically arranged V2 filters are summed (Σ) and passed through a threshold nonlinearity to produce the simulated V4 response. This produces a V4 receptive field size (large gray circles) about 3.0 times that of V2 units, in agreement with cortical physiology.

V1   V2   V4

A

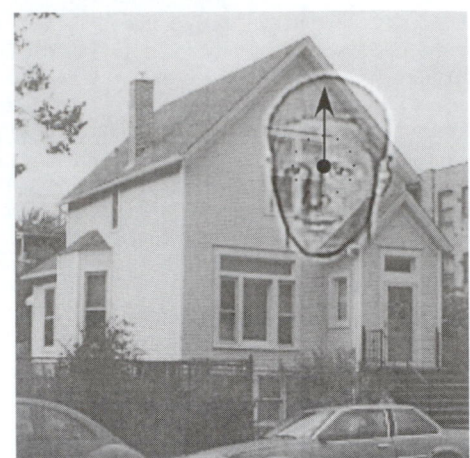

B

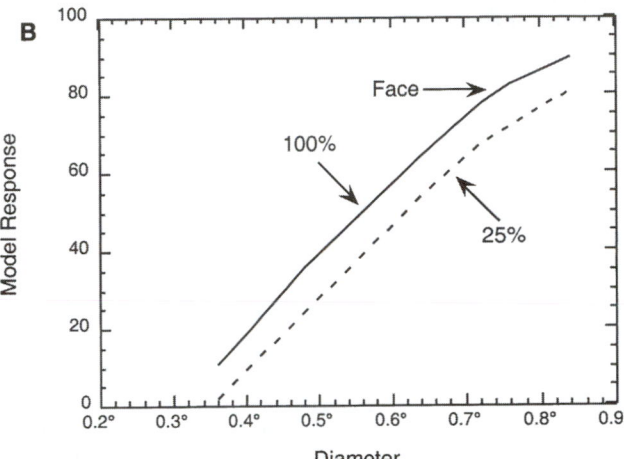

Figure 3. Image processing of a complex scene by the V4 model in Figure 2. *A*, Convolution of the model with a transparent face-house scene produces activation only at the center of the head (black dot), showing that the rectilinear house structure fails to affect model extraction of the ellipsoidal head shape. *B*, Response of maximally active V4 model unit in response to circles of different diameters. Owing to operation of the model contrast gain control, model responses are almost linear functions of diameter over more than a 2:1 size range despite contrast variations from 25% to 100%. The maximum model response to the head in *A* is indicated, and the radius estimated from the graph is plotted as an arrow in *A*.

the Marroquin pattern shows that they typically appear for a mean duration of 2.79 ± 2.75 s and are well described by a gamma distribution (Wilson et al., 2000a).

The V4 concentric unit model was extended to explain data on illusory circle visibility in Marroquin patterns by incorporating nonlinear dynamics and competitive inhibition. Individual neurons were simulated by using Wilson-Cowan-type spike rate equations in which a sigmoid function of postsynaptic potential *P* is approached exponentially in time (Wilson, 1999a):

$$\tau \frac{dE}{dt} = -E + \frac{MP_+^2}{\sigma^2 + P_+^2} \tag{1}$$

where the nonlinearity is a Naka-Rushton function and $P_+ = \max\{P, 0\}$. The maximum spike rate is conventionally $M = 100$, and σ is the semisaturation constant, that is, the value at which the Naka-Rushton function attains the value $M/2$.

Competitive inhibition was introduced by using the recurrent inhibitory spread function $\exp(-R^5/\sigma^5)$, where R is radius between competitors. This network implements a *spatially regional* winner-take-all competition. This means that the most strongly stimulated unit within each mutually inhibitory region will switch on while all others in that region are suppressed by inhibition. As the region is spatially limited, however, there will be multiple regional winners in the network.

Such networks can produce oscillations (rather than approaching a stable equilibrium) only if the regional winners adapt slowly until other winners emerge (Wilson, 1999a). Excitatory neocortical neurons are known to possess ion currents (typically Ca^{2+} mediated K^+ hyperpolarizations) that cause spike frequency adaptation. This reduces excitatory firing rates by a factor of about 3.0 within several hundred milliseconds following stimulus onset. The following equations describe activity in a network with such adaptation (Wilson, 1999a):

$$\tau_E \frac{dE_n}{dt} = -E_n + \frac{100P_+^2}{(10 + H_n)^2 + P_+^2}$$

where

$$P = S_{\text{Marroquin}} - 0.6 \sum_{k \neq n} I_k \exp\left(-\frac{R_{nk}^5}{\sigma^5}\right)$$

$$\tau_I \frac{dI_n}{dt} = -I_n + E_n$$

$$\tau_H \frac{dH_n}{dt} = -H_n + gE_n \tag{2}$$

E_n is the response of an excitatory neuron with a postsynaptic potential P that is the difference between stimulation S derived from the Marroquin pattern minus the spatially weighted inputs from inhibitory neurons I_k, where $n \neq k$, so there is no inhibition of a neuron by the inhibitory neuron it drives. The hyperpolarizing variable H_n produces spike frequency adaptation by increasing the semisaturation constant of the sigmoid nonlinearity in the first equation. Reasonable time constants are $\tau_E = 16$ ms, $\tau_I = 8$ ms, and $\tau_H = 400$ ms, the latter reflecting the much slower rate of spike frequency adaptation.

If Equation 1 is restricted to the case of two mutually inhibitory neurons, one can prove analytically that the system undergoes a Hopf bifurcation to a limit cycle oscillation at a critical value of the hyperpolarizing gain g (Wilson, 1999a). To simulate the illusory oscillating circles of the Marroquin illusion, the equations were extended to a 64×64 neuron array, and input was generated by applying the V4 concentric unit model in Figure 2 to a Marroquin pattern. The resulting model dynamics produced a gamma distribution of visibility durations with mean 2.24 ± 1.93 s (Wilson et al., 2000a), which agrees well with the human data. As Equation 1 represents a totally deterministic network without noise, it might be conjectured that the gamma distribution generated by the network reflects chaotic dynamics. However, the largest Lyapunov exponent was negative, so the dynamics are not chaotic; they apparently represent a very complex, long-period limit cycle.

It is gratifying that model V4 concentric units plus the regional competitive inhibition engendered in Equation 2 can predict an illusion that had remained unexplained for over 20 years. However, the significance of this network probably lies in its relationship to selective attention, which is evident in V4 and is thought to involve biasing of neural competition (Reynolds et al., 1999). Spike frequency adaptation in cortical neurons is controlled by modulatory neurotransmitters (serotonin, dopamine, and histamine), which *reduce* adaptation magnitude. Thus, modulatory transmitters function to tune network parameters, here the hyperpolarizing gain g in Equation 2. Reduction of g for a few excitatory neurons in the network gives them an attentional advantage in subsequent competition. This suggests the hypothesis that biasing in V4 and other cortical areas may result from modulatory control of hyperpolarizing potentials in excitatory cells.

Global Processing in Motion Networks

The V1-V2-MT-MST dorsal motion pathway also shows progressively increasing receptive field size from area to area, with MST receptive fields averaging 50° in diameter (Tanaka and Saito, 1989). As in the ventral form vision pathway, this is indicative of progressively more global processing as information progresses through the hierarchy. Indeed, direction selective neurons in V1 have relatively small receptive fields and respond only to the component of motion perpendicular to local contour orientation. MT neurons pool over a larger visual area, combining V1 and V2 motion vectors over a range of about ±90° to determine the direction of pattern or object motion (Wilson, 1999b). (The restriction of vector pooling to ±90° reflects the ecological constraint that motion vectors in opposite directions cannot result from motion of a single rigid object.) Finally, neurons in MST combine MT responses over broad areas to extract expansion and rotation components of optic flow (Tanaka and Saito, 1989).

Psychophysical evidence that similar motion expansion and rotation units exist in human vision was provided in experiments using a motion analog of Glass patterns (Morrone, Burr, and Vaina, 1995). To generate a percept of rotary motion, for example, a circular patch of random dots is flashed on the screen and followed by a second flashed patch in which each dot is moved a fixed distance around a circular contour from its previous position. If dots are moved outward in the second frame relative to the first, motion expansion is perceived, and so on. Using this approach, Morrone et al. (1995) demonstrated that humans were extremely good at detecting rotary, expanding, and translational motion. Further experiments showed that the visual system globally summed motion vectors directed radially outward in detecting motion expansion. Similarly, clockwise or counterclockwise motion vectors were summed to detect clockwise or counterclockwise rotation, respectively.

These experiments demonstrate global, configural motion summation and are a direct motion analogue of global, configural orientation summation in the detection of concentric and radial Glass patterns (Wilson, 1999b). In consequence, a configural model analogous to the V4 configural model in Figure 2 may be applied to motion. The first stage of a configural motion model would incorporate V1 direction selective Reichardt or motion energy units rather than oriented simple cells. Following rectification, there would be pooling over larger areas to extract local object motions in MT. Finally, there would be configural summation of appropriate MT responses throughout large regions to extract expanding, radial, or translational optic flow.

Discussion

The evidence above indicates that similar global processes in higher cortical areas operate on local V1 orientation responses to extract shape information and on local V1 direction selective responses to detect optic flow patterns. Furthermore, the progressive enlargement of receptive field sizes in moving up either hierarchy is consistent with the requirements of global, configural processing. This leads to the natural question "Just how far do such global summation processes extend in cortical vision?" Certainly, receptive field size continues to increase from V4 to TEO and thence to TE (Boussaoud et al., 1991; Kobatake and Tanaka, 1994). Also, many TE receptive fields have been shown to respond to a complex object such as a face over a range of sizes and locations within visual space (Desimone, 1991). In principle, such size and position

invariance can be generated by obvious extensions of the V4 configural model in Figure 2. Given the evidence for regional competitive inhibition in V4, a larger receptive field sensitive to concentric shape independent of position can be produced by summing V4 concentric unit responses over an area similar to that of the competitive inhibition in Equation 2. Similarly, size invariance can be produced by replicating the V4 model at several different spatial scales, each about an octave apart, allowing regional competition within each scale, and then summing responses across spatial scales in an area beyond V4. Thus, both size and position invariance can be explained by a further stage of global processing with inhibition.

Units that are responsive to global forms such as human and monkey faces have been hypothesized to emerge from configural pooling of appropriate V4 unit responses (Kobatake and Tanaka, 1994). Support for this is provided by the fMRI finding that concentric patterns, which are very effective in activating human V4, are also effective stimuli in the fusiform face area (Wilkinson et al., 2000). Combination of V4 concentric responses with responses of units encoding, for example, the configuration of eyes and nose, could produce face-selective neurons in TE.

Cortical feedback between areas (e.g., V2 to V1, V4 to V2) poses an unsolved problem for models of global pooling, as the models presented here contain no such feedback. Lamme (1995) has shown that V1 responses are enhanced after a 30- to 40-ms latency period if the stimulus is inside an object rather than part of the background, and he has conjectured that this reflects extrastriate feedback. As model V4 concentric units code the location and radius of ellipsoidal regions (see Figure 3), V4 feedback could enhance activity in bounded V1 regions. However, excitatory feedback of this sort, if unchecked, can result in self-organization of network activity into a steady state indicating a hallucination. As hallucinations of circles and faces are common in Charles Bonnet syndrome (Schultz and Melzack, 1993), one can speculate that they result from feedback between cortical areas, including V4. Charles Bonnet syndrome may thus provide a glimpse into the interplay between cortical feedback and global pattern extraction.

Road Map: Vision
Related Reading: Cortical Population Dynamics and Psychophysics; Motion Perception, Elementary Mechanisms; Object Recognition, Neurophysiology

References

Boussaoud, D., Desimone, R., and Ungerleider, L. G., 1991, Visual topography of area TEO in the macaque, *J. Comp. Neurol.*, 306:554–575.

Desimone, R., 1991, Face selective cells in the temporal cortex of monkeys, *J. Cogn. Neurosci.*, 3:1–8. ◆

Gallant, J. L., Braun, J., and Van Essen, D. C., 1993, Selectivity for polar, hyperbolic, and Cartesian gratings in macaque visual cortex, *Science*, 259:100–103.

Kobatake, E., and Tanaka, K., 1994, Neuronal selectivities to complex object features in the ventral visual pathway of the macaque cerebral cortex, *J. Neurophys.*, 71:856–867.

Lamme, V. A. F., 1995, The neurophysiology of figure-ground segregation in primary visual cortex, *J. Neurosci.*, 15:1605–1615.

Morrone, M. C., Burr, D. C., and Vaina, L. M., 1995, Two stages of visual processing for radial and circular motion, *Nature*, 376:507–509.

Reynolds, J. H., Chelazzi, L., and Desimone, R., 1999, Competitive mechanisms subserve attention in macaque areas V2 and V4, *J. Neurosci.*, 19:1736–1753.

Schultz, G., and Melzack, R., 1993, Visual hallucinations and mental state: A study of 14 Charles Bonnet syndrome halluninators, *J. Nerv. Ment. Dis.*, 181:639–643.

Tanaka, K., and Saito, H., 1989, Analysis of motion of the visual field by direction, expansion/contraction, and rotation cells clustered in the dorsal part of the medial superior temporal area of the macaque monkey, *J. Neurophysiol.*, 62:626–641.

Wilkinson, F., James, T. W., Wilson, H. R., Gati, J. S., Menon, R. S., and Goodale, M. A., 2000, An fMRI study of the selective activation of

Graphical Models: Parameter Learning

Zoubin Ghahramani

Introduction

Graphical models combine graph theory and probability theory to provide a general framework for representing models in which a number of variables interact. Graphical models trace their origins to many different fields and have been applied in a wide variety of settings: for example, to develop probabilistic expert systems, to understand neural network models, to infer trait inheritance in genealogies, to model images, to correct errors in digital communication, and to solve complex decision problems. Remarkably, the same formalisms and algorithms can be applied to this wide range of problems.

Each node in the graph represents a random variable (or, more generally, a set of random variables). The pattern of edges in the graph represents the qualitative dependencies between the variables; the absence of an edge between two nodes means that any statistical dependency between these two variables is mediated via some other variable or set of variables. The quantitative dependencies between variables that are connected by edges are specified by means of parameterized conditional distributions, or, more generally, non-negative "potential functions." The pattern of edges and the potential functions together specify a joint probability distribution over all the variables in the graph. We refer to the pattern of edges as the *structure* of the graph, while the parameters of the potential functions are simply called the *parameters* of the graph. In this article, we assume that the structure of the graph is given, and that our goal is to learn the parameters of the graph from data. Solutions to the problem of learning the graph structure from data are given in GRAPHICAL MODELS: STRUCTURE LEARNING (q.v.).

We briefly review some of the notation from GRAPHICAL MODELS: PROBABILISTIC INFERENCE (q.v.) that we will need to cover parameter learning in graphical models. More in-depth treatments of graphical models can be found in Pearl (1988), Heckerman (1996), Jordan (1999), and Cowell et al. (1999).

There are two main varieties of graphical model. *Directed graphical models*, also known as BAYESIAN NETWORKS (q.v.), represent the joint distribution of k random variables $\mathbf{X} = (X_1, \ldots, X_k)$ by a directed acyclic graph in which each node i, representing variable X_i, receives directed edges from its set of parent nodes π_i. The semantics of a directed graphical model are that the joint distribution of $\mathbf{X}$ can be factored into the product of conditional distributions of each variable given its parents. That is, for each setting $\mathbf{x}$ of the variable $\mathbf{X}$,

$$p(\mathbf{x}|\boldsymbol{\theta}) = \prod_{i=1}^{k} p(x_i|\mathbf{x}_{\pi_i}, \boldsymbol{\theta}_i) \tag{1}$$

This factorization formalizes the graphical intuition that X_i depends on its parents $\mathbf{X}_{\pi_i}$. Given its parents, X_i is statistically independent of all other variables that are not descendents of X_i. The set of parameters governing the conditional distribution that relates $\mathbf{X}_{\pi_i}$ to X_i is denoted by $\boldsymbol{\theta}_i$, while the set of all parameters in the graphical model is denoted $\boldsymbol{\theta} = (\boldsymbol{\theta}_1, \ldots, \boldsymbol{\theta}_k)$. Note that 1 is identical to Equation 1 in GRAPHICAL MODELS: PROBABILISTIC INFERENCE (q.v.), except that we have made explicit the dependence of the conditional distributions on the model parameters.

Undirected graphical models represent the joint distribution of a set of variables via a graph with undirected edges. Defining $\mathscr{C}$ to be the set of maximal cliques (i.e., fully connected subgraphs) of this graph, an undirected graphical model corresponds to the statement that the joint distribution of $\mathbf{X}$ can be factored into the product of functions over the variables in each clique:

$$p(\mathbf{x}|\boldsymbol{\theta}) = \frac{1}{Z(\boldsymbol{\theta})} \prod_{C \in C} \psi_C(\mathbf{x}_C|\boldsymbol{\theta}_C) \tag{2}$$

where $\psi_C(\mathbf{x}_C|\boldsymbol{\theta}_C)$ is a potential function assigning a non-negative real number to each configuration $\mathbf{x}_C$ of $\mathbf{X}_C$, and is parameterized by $\boldsymbol{\theta}_C$. An undirected graphical model corresponds to the graphical intuition that dependencies are transmitted via the edges in the graph: each variable is statistically independent of all other variables, given the set of variables it is connected to (i.e., its neighbors). Note again that we have reproduced Equation 2 from GRAPHICAL MODELS: PROBABILISTIC INFERENCE (q.v.), while making explicit the parameters of the potential functions.

The article is organized as follows. We start by concentrating on directed graphical models. In the next section, we discuss the problem of learning maximum likelihood (ML) parameters when all the variables are observed. The following section generalizes this problem to the case in which some of the variables are hidden or missing, and introduces the Expectation-Maximization (EM) algorithm. We then turn to learning parameters of undirected graphical models using both EM and IPF. Finally, we discuss the Bayesian approach, in which a posterior distribution over parameters is inferred from data.

Maximum Likelihood Learning from Complete Data

Assume we are given a data set $\mathbf{d}$ of N independent and identically distributed observations of the settings of all the variables in our directed graphical model $\mathbf{d} = (\mathbf{x}^{(1)}, \ldots, \mathbf{x}^{(N)})$, where $\mathbf{x}^{(n)} = (x_1^{(n)}, \ldots, x_k^{(n)})$. The *likelihood* is a function of the parameters and is proportional to the probability of the observed data:

$$p(\mathbf{d}|\boldsymbol{\theta}) = \prod_{n=1}^{N} p(\mathbf{x}^{(n)}|\boldsymbol{\theta}) \tag{3}$$

We assume that the parameters are unknown and we wish to estimate them from data. We focus on the problem of estimating a single setting of the parameters that maximizes the likelihood formulated in Equation 3. (In contrast, the Bayesian approach to learning described in the last section starts with a prior distribution over the parameters $p(\boldsymbol{\theta})$ that is meant to capture background knowledge we may have about $\boldsymbol{\theta}$, and infers the posterior distribution over parameters given the data $p(\boldsymbol{\theta}|\mathbf{d})$, using Bayes's rule.) Equivalently, we can maximize the log likelihood:

$$\mathscr{L}(\boldsymbol{\theta}) = \log p(\mathbf{d}|\boldsymbol{\theta}) = \sum_{n=1}^{N} \log p(\mathbf{x}^{(n)}|\boldsymbol{\theta}) \tag{4}$$

$$= \sum_{n=1}^{N} \sum_{i=1}^{k} \log p(x_i^{(n)}|\mathbf{x}_{\pi_i}^{(n)}, \boldsymbol{\theta}_i) \tag{5}$$

where the last equality makes use of the factorization (Equation 1) of joint distribution in the directed graphical model. If we assume that the parameters $\boldsymbol{\theta}_i$ governing the conditional probability distribution of X_i given its parents are distinct and functionally independent of the parameters governing the conditional probability distribution of other nodes in the graphical model, then the log likelihood decouples into a sum of local terms involving each node and its parents:

$$\mathscr{L}(\boldsymbol{\theta}) = \sum_{i=1}^{k} \mathscr{L}_i(\boldsymbol{\theta}_i) \tag{6}$$

where $\mathscr{L}_i(\theta_i) = \Sigma_n \log p(x_i^{(n)}|\mathbf{x}_{\pi_i}^{(n)}, \theta_i)$. Each $\mathscr{L}_i$ can be maximized independently as a function of θ_i. For example, if the $\mathbf{X}$ variables are discrete and θ_i is the conditional probability table for x_i given its parents, then the ML estimate of θ_i is simply a normalized table containing counts of each setting of X_i given each setting of its parents in the data set.

Maximum a posteriori (MAP) parameter estimation incorporates prior knowledge about the parameters in the form of a distribution $p(\theta)$. The goal of MAP estimation is to find the parameter setting that maximizes the posterior over parameters, $p(\theta|\mathbf{d})$, which is proportional to the prior times the likelihood. If the prior factorizes over the parameters governing each conditional probability distribution, i.e., $p(\theta) = \Pi_i p(\theta_i)$, then MAP estimates can be found by maximizing

$$\mathscr{L}'(\boldsymbol{\theta}) = \sum_{i=1}^{k} \mathscr{L}_i(\boldsymbol{\theta}_i) + \log p(\boldsymbol{\theta}_i) \qquad (7)$$

The log prior can be seen as a regularizer, which can help reduce overfitting in situations where there are insufficient data for the parameters to be well-determined (see GENERALIZATION AND REGULARIZATION IN NONLINEAR LEARNING SYSTEMS). Although ML estimation is invariant to reparameterization, since the location of the maximum of the likelihood function does not change if you apply a one-to-one transformation $f : \theta \rightarrow \phi$, MAP estimation is not. Indeed, for *any* $\tilde{\theta}$ one can always find a one-to-one mapping such that the MAP estimate of ϕ is $f(\tilde{\theta})$, as long as $p(\theta|\mathbf{d}) > 0$ in a small neighborhood around $\tilde{\theta}$. Thus, care should be taken in the choice of parameterization.

Maximum Likelihood Learning with Hidden Variables

The Expectation-Maximization (EM) Algorithm

Often, the observed data will not include the values of some of the variables in the graphical model. We refer to these variables as missing or hidden variables. With hidden variables, the log likelihood cannot be decomposed as in Equation 6. Rather, we find:

$$\mathscr{L}(\boldsymbol{\theta}) = \log p(\mathbf{x}|\boldsymbol{\theta}) = \log \sum_{\mathbf{y}} p(\mathbf{x}, \mathbf{y}|\boldsymbol{\theta}) \qquad (8)$$

where $\mathbf{x}$ denotes the setting of the observed variables, $\mathbf{y}$ the setting of the hidden variables, and $\Sigma_{\mathbf{y}}$ is the sum (or integral) over $\mathbf{Y}$ required to obtain the marginal probability of the observed data. (For notational convenience, we have dropped the superscript (n) in Equation 8 by evaluating the log likelihood for a single observation.) Maximizing Equation 8 directly is often difficult because the log of the sum can potentially couple all of the parameters of the model. We can simplify the problem of maximizing $\mathscr{L}$ with respect to θ by making use of the following insight. Any distribution $q(\mathbf{Y})$ over the hidden variables defines a *lower bound* on $\mathscr{L}$:

$$\mathscr{L}(\theta) = \log \sum_{\mathbf{y}} p(\mathbf{x}, \mathbf{y}|\boldsymbol{\theta}) = \log \sum_{\mathbf{y}} q(\mathbf{y}) \frac{p(\mathbf{x}, \mathbf{y}|\boldsymbol{\theta})}{q(\mathbf{y})} \qquad (9)$$

$$\geq \sum_{\mathbf{y}} q(\mathbf{y}) \log \frac{p(\mathbf{x}, \mathbf{y}|\boldsymbol{\theta})}{q(\mathbf{y})} \qquad (10)$$

$$= \sum_{\mathbf{y}} q(\mathbf{y}) \log p(\mathbf{x}, \mathbf{y}|\boldsymbol{\theta}) - \sum_{\mathbf{y}} q(\mathbf{y}) \log q(\mathbf{y}) \qquad (11)$$

$$= \mathscr{F}(q, \boldsymbol{\theta}) \qquad (12)$$

where the inequality is known as Jensen's inequality and follows from the fact that the log function is concave. If we define the *energy* of a global configuration $(\mathbf{x}, \mathbf{y})$ to be $-\log p(\mathbf{x}, \mathbf{y}|\theta)$, then some readers may notice that the lower bound $\mathscr{F}(q, \theta) \leq \mathscr{L}(\theta)$ is the negative of a quantity known in statistical physics as the *free energy*: the expected energy under q minus the entropy of q (Neal

and Hinton in Jordan, 1999). The EM algorithm (Dempster, Laird, and Rubin, 1977) alternates between maximizing $\mathscr{F}$ with respect to q and θ, respectively, holding the other fixed. Starting from some initial parameters θ_0, the $\ell + 1$st iteration of the algorithm consists of the following two steps:

$$\textbf{E step:} \quad q_{[\ell+1]} \leftarrow \arg\max_{q} \mathscr{F}(q, \boldsymbol{\theta}_{[\ell]}) \qquad (13)$$

$$\textbf{M step:} \quad \boldsymbol{\theta}_{[\ell+1]} \leftarrow \arg\max_{\theta} \mathscr{F}(q_{[\ell+1]}, \boldsymbol{\theta}) \qquad (14)$$

It is easy to show that the maximum in the E step is obtained by setting $q_{[\ell+1]}(\mathbf{y}) = p(\mathbf{y}|\mathbf{x}, \boldsymbol{\theta}_{[\ell]})$, at which point the bound becomes an equality: $\mathscr{F}(q_{[\ell+1]}, \boldsymbol{\theta}_{[\ell]}) = \mathscr{L}(\boldsymbol{\theta}_{[\ell]})$. This involves inferring the distribution over the hidden variables given the observed variables and the current settings of the parameters, $p(\mathbf{y}|\mathbf{x}, \boldsymbol{\theta}_{[\ell]})$. Algorithms that solve this inference problem are presented in GRAPHICAL MODELS: PROBABILISTIC INFERENCE. These algorithms make use of the structure of the graphical model to compute the quantities of interest efficiently by passing local messages from each node to its neighbors. Exact inference results in the bound being satisfied, but is in general computationally intractable for multiply connected graphical structures. Even these "efficient" message-passing procedures can take exponential time to compute the exact solution in such cases. For such graphs, deterministic and Monte Carlo methods provide a tool for approximating the E step of EM. One deterministic approximation that can be used in intractable models is to increase but not fully maximize the functional with respect to q in the E step. In particular, if q is chosen to be in a tractable family of distributions $\mathfrak{Q}$ (i.e., a family of distributions for which the required expectations can be computed in polynomial time), then maximizing $\mathscr{F}$ over this tractable family

$$\textbf{E step:} \quad q_{[\ell+1]} \leftarrow \arg\max_{q \in \mathfrak{Q}} \mathscr{F}(q, \boldsymbol{\theta}_{[\ell]}) \qquad (15)$$

is called a *variational approximation* to the EM algorithm (Jordan, Ghahramani, Jaakkola, and Saul in Jordan, 1999). This maximizes a lower bound to the likelihood rather than the likelihood itself.

The maximum in the M step is obtained by maximizing the first term in Equation 11, since the entropy of q does not depend on θ:

$$\textbf{M step:} \quad \boldsymbol{\theta}_{[\ell+1]} \leftarrow \arg\max_{\theta} \sum_{\mathbf{y}} p(\mathbf{y}|\mathbf{x}, \boldsymbol{\theta}_{[\ell]}) \log p(\mathbf{y}, \mathbf{x}|\boldsymbol{\theta}) \qquad (16)$$

This is the expression most often associated with the EM algorithm (Dempster et al., 1977), but it obscures the elegant interpretation of EM as coordinate ascent in $\mathscr{F}$. Since $\mathscr{F} = \mathscr{L}$ at the beginning of each M step (following an exact E step), and since the E step does not change θ, we are guaranteed not to decrease the likelihood after each combined EM step.

It is usually not necessary to explicitly evaluate the entire posterior distribution $p(\mathbf{y}|\mathbf{x}, \boldsymbol{\theta}_{[\ell]})$. Since $\log p(\mathbf{x}, \mathbf{y}|\theta)$ contains both hidden and observed variables in the network, it can be factored as before as the sum of log probabilities of each node given its parents (Equation 5). Consequently, the quantities required for the M step are the expected values, under the posterior distribution $p(\mathbf{y}|\mathbf{x}, \boldsymbol{\theta}_{[\ell]})$, of the same quantities (namely the *sufficient statistics*) required for ML estimation in the complete data case.

Consider a directed graphical with discrete variables, some hidden and some observed. Each node is parameterized by a conditional probability table that relates its values to the values of its parents. For example, if node i has two parents, j and k, and each variable can take on L values, then θ_i is an $L \times L \times L$ table, with entries $\theta_{i,rst} = P(X_i = r|X_j = s, X_k = t)$. In the complete data setting where X_i, X_j, X_k are observed, the ML estimate is:

$$\hat{\theta}_{i,rst} = \frac{\#(X_i = r, X_j = s, X_k = t)}{\#(X_j = s, X_k = t)} \qquad (17)$$

where $\#(\cdot)$ denotes the count (frequency) with which the bracketed expression occurs in the data. However, if all three variables were hidden, then one could use the EM algorithm for learning the directed graphical model (Lauritzen, 1995; Russell et al., 1995). The analogous M step for $\theta_{i,rst}$ would be:

$$\hat{\theta}_{i,rst} = \frac{\sum_n P(Y_i = r, Y_j = s, Y_k = t | \mathbf{X} = \mathbf{x}^{(n)})}{\sum_n P(Y_j = s, Y_k = t | \mathbf{X} = \mathbf{x}^{(n)})} \quad (18)$$

The sufficient statistics of the data required to estimate the parameters are the counts of the setting of each node and its parents; no other information in the data is relevant for ML parameter estimation. The *expectation* step of EM computes the expected value of these sufficient statistics.

The EM algorithm provides an intuitive way of dealing with hidden or missing data. The E step "fills in" the hidden variables with the distribution given by the current model. The M step then treats these filled-in values as if they had been observed, and reestimates the model parameters. It is pleasantly surprising that these steps result in a convergent procedure for finding the most likely parameters. Although EM is intuitive and often easy to implement, it is sometimes not the most efficient algorithm for finding ML parameters.

The EM procedure for learning directed graphical models with hidden variables can be applied to a wide variety of well-known models. Of particular note is the special case known as the Baum-Welch algorithm for training hidden markov models (Rabiner 1989; see HIDDEN MARKOV MODELS). In the E step it uses a local message-passing algorithm called the forward-backward algorithm to compute the required expected sufficient statistics. In the M step it uses a parameter reestimation equation based on expected counts, analogous to Equation 18. The EM algorithm can also be used to fit a variety of other models that have been studied in the machine learning, neural networks, statistics, and engineering literatures. These include linear dynamical systems, factor analysis, mixtures of Gaussians, and mixtures of experts (see Roweis and Ghahramani, 1999, for a review). It is straightforward to modify EM so that it maximizes the parameter posterior probability rather than the likelihood.

Parameter Learning in Undirected Graphical Models

When compared to learning the parameters of directed graphical models, undirected graphical models present an additional challenge: the partition function. Even if each clique has distinct and functionally independent parameters, the partition function from Equation 2,

$$Z(\boldsymbol{\theta}) = \sum_{\mathbf{x}} \prod_{C \in \mathcal{C}} \psi_C(\mathbf{x}_C | \boldsymbol{\theta}_C) \quad (19)$$

couples all the parameters together. We examine the effect this coupling has in the context of an undirected graphical model that has had a great deal of impact in the neural networks field: the Boltzmann machine (Ackley, Hinton, and Sejnowski, 1985).

Boltzmann machines are undirected graphical models over a set of k binary variables $S_i \in \{0, 1\}$ (see also SIMULATED ANNEALING AND BOLTZMANN MACHINES). The probability distribution over the variables in a Boltzmann machine is given by

$$P(\mathbf{s}|W) = \frac{1}{Z(W)} \exp \left\{ \frac{1}{2} \sum_{i=1}^{k} \sum_{j \in \text{ne}(i)} W_{ij} s_i s_j \right\}$$

$$= \frac{1}{Z(W)} \prod_{(ij)} \exp \{W_{ij} s_i s_j\} \quad (20)$$

The first equation uses standard notation for Boltzmann machines, where W is the symmetric matrix of weights (i.e., model parame-

ters) and $\text{ne}(i)$ is the set of neighbors of node i in the Boltzmann machine. The second equation writes it as a product of clique potentials, where (ij) denotes the clique consisting of the pair of connected nodes i and j. (Actually, in Boltzmann machines, the maximal cliques in the graph may be very large, although the interactions are all pairwise; because of this pairwise constraint on interactions, we abuse terminology and consider the "cliques" to be the pairs, no matter what the graph connectivity is.)

Assuming that S_i and S_j are observed, taking derivatives of the log probability of the nth data point with respect to W_{ij},

$$\frac{\partial \log P(\mathbf{s}^{(n)}|W)}{\partial W_{ij}} = s_i^{(n)} s_j^{(n)} - \sum_s s_i s_j P(\mathbf{s}|W)$$

$$= \langle s_i s_j \rangle_n^+ - \langle s_i s_j \rangle^- \quad (21)$$

we find that it is the difference between the correlation of S_i and S_j in the data and the correlation of S_i and S_j in the model (the $\langle \cdot \rangle$ notation means expectation). The standard ML gradient descent learning rule for Boltzmann machines therefore tries to make the model match the correlations in the data. The same learning rule applies if there are hidden variables.

The second term arises from the partition function. Note that even for fully observed data, although the first term can be computed directly from the observed data, the second term depends potentially on all the parameters, underlining the fact that the partition function couples the parameters in undirected models. Even for fully observed data, computing the second term is nontrivial; for fully connected Boltzmann machines it is intractable and needs to be approximated.

The IPF Algorithm

Consider the following problem: Given an undirected graphical model, and an initial set of clique potentials, we wish to find the clique potentials closest to the initial potentials that satisfy a certain set of consistent marginals. Closeness of probability distributions in this context is measured using the Kullback-Leibler divergence. The simplest example is a clique of two discrete variables, X_i and X_j, where the clique potential is proportional to the contingency table for the joint probability of these variables $P(X_i, X_j)$, and the marginal constraints are $P(x_i) = \hat{P}(x_i)$ and $P(x_j) = \hat{P}(x_j)$. These constraints could, for example, have come from observing data with these marginals. A very simple and intuitive iterative algorithm for trying to satisfy these constraints is to start from the initial table and satisfy each constraint in turn. For example, if we want to satisfy the marginal on X_i:

$$P_l(x_i, x_j) = P_{l-1}(x_i, x_j) \frac{\hat{P}(x_i)}{P_{l-1}(x_i)} \quad (22)$$

This has to be iterated over X_i and X_j, since satisfying one marginal can change the other marginal. The simple algorithm is known as Iterative Proportional Fitting (IPF), and it can be generalized in several ways (Darroch and Ratcliff, 1972).

More generally, we wish to find a distribution in the form

$$p(\mathbf{x}) = \frac{1}{Z} \prod_c \psi_c(\mathbf{x}_c) \quad (23)$$

that minimizes the Kullback-Leibler divergence to some prior $p_0(\mathbf{x})$ and satisfies a set of constraints (the data) of the form:

$$\sum_{\mathbf{x}} a_r(\mathbf{x}) p(\mathbf{x}) = h_r \quad (24)$$

where r indexes the constraint. If the prior is set to the uniform distribution and the constraints are measured marginal distributions over all the variables in each of the cliques of the graph, then the problem solved by IPF is equivalent to finding the maximum likelihood clique potentials given a complete data set of observations.

IPF can be used to train an ML Boltzmann machine if $\hat{P}(S_i, S_j)$ is given by the data set for all pairs of variables connected in the Boltzmann machine. The procedure is to start from the uniform distribution (i.e., all weights set to 0), then apply IPF steps to each clique potential until all marginals match those in the data. One can generalize this by starting from a nonuniform distribution, which would give a Boltzmann machine with minimum divergence from the starting distribution.

But what if some of the variables in the Boltzmann machine are hidden? Byrne (1992) presents an elegant solution to this problem using ideas from alternating minimization (AM) and information geometry (Csizár and Tusnády, 1984). One step of the alternating minimization computes the distribution over the hidden variables of the Boltzmann machine, given the observed variables. This is the E step of EM, and can also be interpreted within information geometry as finding the probability distribution that satisfies the marginal constraints and is closest to the space of probability distributions defined by the Boltzmann machines. The other step of the minimization starts from $W = 0$ (the maximum entropy distribution for a Boltzmann machine) and uses IPF to find the Boltzmann machine weights that satisfy all the marginals found in the E step, $\hat{P}_{ij} = \langle s_i s_j \rangle^+$. This is the M step of the algorithm; a single M step thus involves an entire IPF optimization. The update rule for each step of the IPF optimization for a particular weight is:

$$W_{ij} \leftarrow W_{ij} + \log\left[\frac{\hat{P}_{ij}}{\langle s_i s_j \rangle^-} \frac{(1 - \langle s_i s_j \rangle^-)}{(1 - \hat{P}_{ij})}\right] \quad (25)$$

This algorithm is conceptually interesting, as it presents an alternative method for fitting Boltzmann machines with ties to IPF and alternating minimization procedures. However, it is impractical for large, multiply connected Boltzmann machines, since computing the exact unclamped correlations $\langle s_i s_j \rangle^-$ can take exponential time.

Although we have presented this EM-IPF algorithm for the case of Boltzmann machines, it is widely applicable to learning many undirected graphical models. In particular, in the E step, marginal distributions over the set of variables in each clique in the graph are computed conditioned on the settings of the observed variables. A propagation algorithm such as the Junction Tree algorithm can be used for this step (see GRAPHICAL MODELS: PROBABILISTIC INFERENCE). In the M step the IPF procedure is run so as to satisfy all the marginals computed in the E step. There also exist Junction-Tree-style propagation algorithms that exploit the structure of the graphical model to solve the IPF problem efficiently (Jiroušek and Přeučil, 1995; Teh and Welling, 2002).

Bayesian Learning of Parameters

A Bayesian approach to learning starts with some a priori knowledge about the model structure—the set of arcs in the Bayesian network—and model parameters. This initial knowledge is represented in the form of a prior probability distribution over model structures and parameters, and is updated using the data to obtain a posterior probability distribution over models and parameters. In this article we will assume that the model structure is given, and we focus on computing the posterior probability distribution over parameters (see GRAPHICAL MODELS: STRUCTURE LEARNING for solutions to the problem of inferring model structure; see also BAYESIAN METHODS AND NEURAL NETWORKS).

For a given model structure $\mathbf{m}$, we can compute the posterior distribution over the parameters:

$$p(\theta|\mathbf{m}, \mathbf{d}) = \frac{p(\mathbf{d}|\theta, \mathbf{m})p(\theta|\mathbf{m})}{p(\mathbf{d}|\mathbf{m})} \quad (26)$$

If the data set is $\mathbf{d} = (\mathbf{x}^{(1)}, \ldots, \mathbf{x}^{(N)})$ and we wish to predict the next observation, $\mathbf{x}^{(N+1)}$, based on our data and model, then the Bayesian prediction

$$p(\mathbf{x}^{(N+1)}|\mathbf{d}, \mathbf{m}) = \int p(\mathbf{x}^{(N+1)}|\theta, \mathbf{m}, \mathbf{d})p(\theta|\mathbf{m}, \mathbf{d})d\theta \quad (27)$$

averages over the uncertainty in the model parameters. This is known as the *predictive distribution* for the model.

In the limit of a large data set, and as long as the prior over the parameters assigns non-zero probability in the region around the ML parameter values, the posterior $p(\theta|\mathbf{m}, \mathbf{d})$ will be sharply peaked around the maxima of the likelihood, and therefore the predictions of a single ML model will be similar to those obtained by Bayesian integration over the parameters.

Often, models are fit with relatively small amounts of data, so asymptotic results are not applicable and the predictions of the ML estimate will differ significantly from those of Bayesian averaging. In such situations it is important to compute or approximate the averaging over parameters in Equation 27. For certain discrete models with Dirichlet distributed priors over the parameters, and for certain linear-Gaussian models, it is possible to compute these integrals exactly. Otherwise, approximations can be used. There are a large number of approximations to the integral over the parameter distribution that have been used in graphical models, including Laplace's approximation, variational approximations, and a variety of MCMC methods (see Neal, 1993, for a review).

Discussion

There are several key insights regarding parameter learning in graphical models. When there are no hidden variables in a directed graphical model, the graph structure determines the statistics of the data needed to learn the parameters: the joint distribution of each variable and its parents in the graph. Parameter estimation can then often occur independently for each node. The presence of hidden variables introduces dependencies between the parameters. However, the EM algorithm transforms the problem so that in each M step the parameters of the graphical model are again uncoupled. The E step of EM "fills in" the hidden variables with the distribution predicted by the model, thereby turning the hidden-data problem into a complete-data problem.

The intuitive appeal of EM has led to its widespread use in models of unsupervised learning where the goal is to learn a generative model of sensory data. The E step corresponds to perception or recognition: inferring the (hidden) state of the world from the sensory data; while the M step corresponds to learning: modifying the model that relates the actual world to the sensory data. It has been suggested that top-down and bottom-up connections in cortex play the roles of generative and recognition models (see HELMHOLTZ MACHINES AND SLEEP-WAKE LEARNING). From a graphical model perspective, the bottom-up recognition model in Helmholtz machines can be thought of as a graph that approximates the distribution of the hidden variables given the observed variables, in much the same way as the variational approximation approximates that same distribution.

Undirected graphical models pose additional challenges. The partition function is usually a function of the parameters, and can introduce dependencies between the parameters even in the case of complete data. The IPF algorithm can be used to fit undirected graphical models from complete data, and an IPF-EM algorithm can be used when there are hidden data as well.

Although ML learning is adequate when there are enough data, in general it is necessary to approximate the average over the parameters. Averaging avoids overfitting; it is hard to see how overfitting can occur when nothing is "fit" to the data. Non-Bayesian methods for avoiding overfitting often also involve averaging, for example, via bootstrap resampling of the data. Even with parameter averaging, predictions can suffer in quality if the assumed structure of the model—the conditional independence relationships—is incorrect. To overcome this, it is necessary to generalize the approach presented in this article to learn the structure of the model as well as the parameters from data. This topic is covered in GRAPHICAL MODELS: STRUCTURE LEARNING (q.v.).

Road Maps: Artificial Intelligence; Learning in Artificial Networks
Background: Bayesian Networks
Related Reading: Graphical Models: Probabilistic Inference; Graphical Models: Structure Learning

References

Ackley, D., Hinton, G., and Sejnowski, T., 1985, A learning algorithm for Boltzmann machines, *Cognit. Sci.,* 9:147–169.

Byrne, W., 1992, Alternating minimization and Boltzmann machine learning, *IEEE Trans. Neural Netw.,* 3:612–620.

Cowell, R. G., Dawid, A. P., Lauritzen, S. L., and Spiegelhalter, D. J., 1999, *Probabilistic Networks and Expert Systems,* New York: Springer-Verlag.

Csizár, I., and Tusnády, G., 1984, Information geometry and alternating minimization procedures, in *Statistics and Decisions,* Supplementary Issue No. 1, (E. J. Dudewicz, D. Plachky, and P. K. Sen, Eds.), Munich: Oldenbourg Verlag, pp. 205–237.

Darroch, J. N., and Ratcliff, D., 1972, Generalized iterative scaling for log-linear models, *Ann. Math. Statist.,* 43:1470–1480.

Dempster, A., Laird, N., and Rubin, D., 1977, Maximum likelihood from incomplete data via the EM algorithm, *J. R. Statist. Soc. B,* 39:1–38.

Heckerman, D., 1996, *A Tutorial on Learning with Bayesian Networks,* Technical Report MSR-TR-95-06, Redmond, WA: Microsoft Research, available: ftp://ftp.research.microsoft.com/pub/tr/TR-95-06.PS. ◆

Jiroušek, R., and Přeučil, S., 1995, On the effective implementation of the iterative proportional fitting procedure, *Computat. Statist. Data Anal.,* 19:177–189.

Jordan, M. I., Ed., 1999, *Learning in Graphical Models,* Cambridge, MA: MIT Press. ◆

Lauritzen, S. L., 1995, The EM algorithm for graphical association models with missing data, *Computat. Statist. Data Anal.,* 19:191–201.

Neal, R. M., 1993, *Probabilistic Inference Using Markov Chain Monte Carlo Methods,* Technical Report CRG-TR-93-1, Department of Computer Science, University of Toronto.

Pearl, J., 1988, *Probabilistic Reasoning in Intelligent Systems: Networks of Plausible Inference,* San Mateo, CA: Morgan Kaufmann. ◆

Rabiner, L. R., 1989, A tutorial on hidden Markov models and selected applications in speech recognition, *Proc. IEEE,* 77:257–286.

Roweis, S. T., and Ghahramani, Z., 1999, A unifying review of linear Gaussian models, *Neural Computat.,* 11:305–345.

Russell, S. J., Binder, J., Koller, D., and Kanazawa, K., 1995, Local learning in probabilistic models with hidden variables, in *Proceedings of an Internation Joint Conference on Artificial Intelligence,* Montreal, Canada: Morgan Kaufmann, pp. 1146–1152.

Teh, Y. W., and Welling, M., 2002, The unified propagation and scaling algorithm, *Adv. Neural Inf. Process. Syst.,* 14:1146–1152.

Graphical Models: Probabilistic Inference

Michael I. Jordan and Yair Weiss

Introduction

A *graphical model* is a type of probabilistic network that has roots in several different research communities, including artificial intelligence (Pearl, 1988), statistics (Lauritzen and Spiegelhalter, 1988), error-control coding (Gallager, 1963), and neural networks. The graphical models framework provides a clean mathematical formalism that has made it possible to understand the relationships among a wide variety of network-based approaches to computation, and in particular to understand many neural network algorithms and architectures as instances of a broader probabilistic methodology.

Graphical models use graphs to represent and manipulate joint probability distributions. The graph underlying a graphical model may be directed, in which case the model is often referred to as a *belief network* or a *Bayesian network* (see BAYESIAN NETWORKS), or the graph may be undirected, in which case the model is generally referred to as a *Markov random field*. A graphical model has both a structural component—encoded by the pattern of edges in the graph—and a parametric component—encoded by numerical "potentials" associated with sets of edges in the graph. The relationship between these components underlies the computational machinery associated with graphical models. In particular, general *inference algorithms* allow statistical quantities (such as likelihoods and conditional probabilities) and information-theoretic quantities (such as mutual information and conditional entropies) to be computed efficiently. These algorithms are the subject of the current article. *Learning algorithms* build on these inference algorithms and allow parameters and structures to be estimated from data (see GRAPHICAL MODELS: PARAMETER LEARNING and GRAPHICAL MODELS: STRUCTURE LEARNING).

Background

Directed and undirected graphical models differ in terms of their Markov properties (the relationship between graph separation and conditional independence) and their parameterization (the relationship between local numerical specifications and global joint probabilities). These differences are important in discussions of the family of joint probability distribution that a particular graph can represent. In the inference problem, however, we generally have a specific fixed joint probability distribution at hand, in which case the differences between directed and undirected graphical models are less important. Indeed, in the current article, we treat these classes of model together and emphasize their commonalities.

Let U denote a set of nodes of a graph (directed or undirected), and let X_i denote the random variable associated with node i, for $i \in U$. Let X_C denote the subset of random variables associated with a subset of nodes C, for any $C \subseteq U$, and let $X = X_U$ denote the collection of random variables associated with the graph.

The family of joint probability distributions associated with a given graph can be parameterized in terms of a product over *potential functions* associated with subsets of nodes in the graph. For directed graphs, the basic subset on which a potential is defined consists of a single node and its parents, and a potential turns out to be (necessarily) the conditional probability of the node given its parents. Thus, for a directed graph, we have the following representation for the joint probability:

$$p(x) = \prod_i p(x_i | x_{\pi_i}) \tag{1}$$

where $p(x_i | x_{\pi_i})$ is the *local conditional probability* associated with node i, and π_i is the set of indices labeling the parents of node i. For undirected graphs, the basic subsets are *cliques* of the graph—

subsets of nodes that are completely connected. For a given clique C, let $\psi_C(x_C)$ denote a general potential function—a function that assigns a positive real number to each configuration x_C. We have

$$p(x) = \frac{1}{Z} \prod_{C \in \mathcal{C}} \psi_C(x_C) \tag{2}$$

where $\mathcal{C}$ is the set of cliques associated with the graph and Z is an explicit normalizing factor, ensuring that $\sum_x p(x) = 1$. (We work with discrete random variables throughout for simplicity.)

Equation 1 can be viewed as a special case of Equation 2. Note in particular that we could have included a normalizing factor Z in Equation 1, but, as is easily verified, it is necessarily equal to 1. Second, note that $p(x_i|x_{\pi_i})$ is a perfectly good example of a potential function, except that the set of nodes that it is defined on—the collection $\{i \cup \pi_i\}$—is not in general a clique (because the parents of a given node are not in general interconnected). Thus, to treat Equation 1 and Equation 2 on an equal footing, we find it convenient to define the so-called *moral graph* $\mathcal{G}^m$ associated with a directed graph $\mathcal{G}$. The moral graph is an undirected graph obtained by connecting all of the parents of each node in $\mathcal{G}$, and removing the arrowheads. On the moral graph, a conditional probability $p(x_i|x_{\pi_i})$ is a potential function, and Equation 1 reduces to a special case of Equation 2.

Probabilistic Inference

Let (E, F) be a partitioning of the indices of the nodes in a graphical model into disjoint subsets such that (X_E, X_F) is a partitioning of the random variables. There are two basic kinds of inference problem that we wish to solve

• *Marginal probabilities*:

$$p(x_E) = \sum_{x_F} p(x_E, x_F)$$

• *Maximum a posteriori (MAP) probabilities*:

$$p^*(x_E) = \max_{x_F} p(x_E, x_F)$$

From these basic computations we can obtain other quantities of interest. In particular, the *conditional probability* $p(x_F|x_E)$ is equal to

$$p(x_F|x_E) = \frac{p(x_E, x_F)}{\sum_{x_F} p(x_E, x_F)}$$

and this is readily computed for any x_F once the denominator is computed—a marginalization computation. Moreover, we often wish to combine conditioning and marginalization, or conditioning, marginalization, and MAP computations. For example, letting (E, F, H) be a partitioning of the node indices, we may wish to compute

$$p(x_F|x_E) = \frac{p(x_E, x_F)}{\sum_{x_F} p(x_E, x_F)} = \frac{\sum_{x_H} p(x_E, x_F, x_H)}{\sum_{x_F} \sum_{x_H} p(x_E, x_F, x_H)}$$

We first perform the marginalization operation in the numerator and then perform a subsequent marginalization to obtain the denominator.

Elimination

In this section we introduce a basic algorithm for inference known as *elimination*. Although elimination applies to arbitrary graphs (as we will see), our focus in this section is on trees.

We proceed via an example. Referring to the tree in Figure 1A, let us calculate the marginal probability $p(x_5)$. We compute this probability by summing the joint probability with respect to $\{x_1, x_2, x_3, x_4\}$. We must pick an order over which to sum, and with some malice aforethought, let us choose the order $(1, 2, 4, 3)$. We have

$$p(x_5) = \sum_{x_3} \sum_{x_4} \sum_{x_2} \sum_{x_1} p(x_1, x_2, x_3, x_4, x_5)$$

$$= \sum_{x_3} \sum_{x_4} \sum_{x_2} \sum_{x_1} p(x_1)p(x_2|x_1)p(x_3|x_2)p(x_4|x_3)p(x_5|x_3)$$

$$= \sum_{x_3} p(x_5|x_3) \sum_{x_4} p(x_4|x_3) \sum_{x_2} p(x_3|x_2) \sum_{x_1} p(x_1)p(x_2|x_1)$$

$$= \sum_{x_3} p(x_5|x_3) \sum_{x_4} p(x_4|x_3) \sum_{x_2} p(x_3|x_2)m_{12}(x_2)$$

where we introduce the notation $m_{ij}(x_j)$ to refer to the intermediate terms that arise in performing the sum. The index i refers to the variable being summed over, and the index j refers to the other variable appearing in the summand (for trees, there will never be more than two variables appearing in any summand). The resulting term is a function of x_j. We continue the derivation:

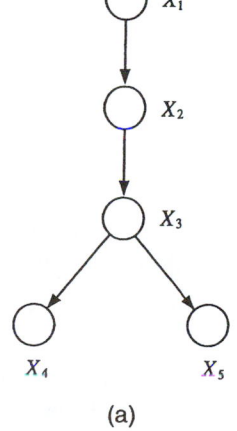

Figure 1. *A*, A directed graphical model. *B*, The intermediate terms that arise during a run of ELIMINATE can be viewed as messages attached to the edges of the moral graph. Here the elimination order was $(1, 2, 4, 3)$. *C*, The set of all messages computed by the sum-product algorithm.

(a)   (b)   (c)

$$p(x_5) = \sum_{x_3} p(x_5|x_3) \sum_{x_4} p(x_4|x_3) \sum_{x_2} p(x_3|x_2)m_{12}(x_2)$$

$$= \sum_{x_3} p(x_5|x_3) \sum_{x_4} p(x_4|x_3)m_{23}(x_3)$$

$$= \sum_{x_3} p(x_5|x_3)m_{23}(x_3) \sum_{x_4} p(x_4|x_3)$$

$$= \sum_{x_3} p(x_5|x_3)m_{23}(x_3)m_{43}(x_3)$$

$$= m_{35}(x_5)$$

The final expression is a function of x_5 only and is the desired marginal probability.

This computation is formally identically in the case of an undirected graph. In particular, an undirected version of the tree in Figure 1A has the parameterization

$$p(x) = \frac{1}{Z}\psi_{12}(x_1, x_2)\psi_{23}(x_2, x_3)\psi_{34}(x_3, x_4)\psi_{35}(x_3, x_5)$$

The first few steps of the computation of $p(x_5)$ are then as follows:

$$p(x_5) = \frac{1}{Z}\sum_{x_3}\psi_{35}(x_3, x_5)\sum_{x_4}\psi_{34}(x_3, x_4)\sum_{x_2}\psi_{23}(x_2, x_3)$$
$$\times \sum_{x_1}\psi_{12}(x_1, x_2)$$

$$= \frac{1}{Z}\sum_{x_3}\psi_{35}(x_3, x_5)\sum_{x_4}\psi_{34}(x_3, x_4)\sum_{x_2}\psi_{23}(x_2, x_3)m_{12}(x_2)$$

and the remainder of the computation proceeds as before.

These algebraic manipulations can be summarized succinctly in terms of a general algorithm that we refer to here as ELIMINATE (Figure 2). The algorithm maintains an "active list" of potentials that, at the outset, represent the joint probability, and at the end represent the desired marginal probability. Nodes are removed from the graph according to an elimination ordering that must be specified. The algorithm applies to both directed and undirected graphs. Also, as we will see shortly, it is in fact a general algorithm, applying not only to trees but to general graphs.

Message-Passing Algorithms

In many problems we wish to obtain more than a single marginal probability. Thus, for example, we may wish to obtain both $p(x_4)$ and $p(x_5)$ in Figure 1A. Although we could compute each marginal with a separate run of ELIMINATE, this fails to exploit the fact that common intermediate terms appear in the different runs. We would like to develop an algebra of intermediate terms that allows them to be reused efficiently.

Suppose in particular that we wish to compute $p(x_4)$ in the example in Figure 1A. Using the elimination order (1, 2, 5, 3), it is easily verified that we generate the terms $m_{12}(x_2)$ and $m_{23}(x_3)$ as before, and also generate new terms $m_{53}(x_3)$ and $m_{34}(x_4)$.

ELIMINATE(G)
    place all potentials $\psi_c(x_C)$ on the active list
    choose an ordering I of the indices F
    for each X_i in I
        find all potentials on the active list that reference X_i
            and remove them from the active list
        define a new potential as the sum (with respect to x_i) of the
            product of these potentials
        place the new potential on the active list
    end
    return the product of the remaining potentials

Figure 2. A simple elimination algorithm for marginalization in graphical models.

As suggested by Figure 1B, the intermediate terms that arise during elimination can be viewed as "messages" attached to edges in the moral graph. Rather than viewing inference as an elimination process, based on a global ordering, we instead view inference in terms of local computation and routing of messages. The key operation of summing a product can be written as follows:

$$m_{ij}(x_j) = \sum_{x_i}\psi_{ij}(x_i, x_j)\prod_{k \in N(i)\backslash j} m_{ki}(x_i) \qquad (3)$$

where $N(i)$ is the set of neighbors of node i. Thus, summing over x_i creates a message $m_{ij}(x_j)$ that is sent to the node j. The reader can verify that each step in our earlier computation of $p(x_5)$ has this form.

A node can send a message to a neighboring node once it has received messages from all of its other neighbors. As in our example, a message arriving at a leaf node is necessarily a marginal probability. In general, the marginal probability at a node is given by the product of all incoming messages:

$$p(x_i) \propto \prod_{k \in N(i)} m_{ki}(x_i) \qquad (4)$$

The pair of equations given by Equations 3 and 4 defines an algorithm known as *sum-product algorithm* or the *belief propagation algorithm*. It is not difficult to prove that this algorithm is correct for trees.

The set of messages needed to compute all of the individual marginal probabilities for the graph in Figure 1A is shown in Figure 1C. Note that a pair of messages is sent along each edge, one message in each direction.

Neural networks also involve message-passing algorithms and local numerical operations. An important difference, however, is that in the neural network setting, each node generally has a single "activation" value that it passes to all of its neighbors. In the sum-product algorithm, on the other hand, individual messages are prepared for each neighbor. Moreover, the message $m_{ij}(x_j)$ from i to j is not included in the product that node j forms in computing a message to send back to node i. The sum-product algorithm avoids double-counting.

Maximum a posteriori (MAP) Probabilities

Referring again to Figure 1A, let us suppose that we wish to compute $p^*(x_5)$, the maximum probability configuration of the variables (X_1, X_2, X_3, X_4), for a given value of X_5. Again choosing a particular ordering of the variables, we compute

$$p^*(x_5) = \max_{x_3}\max_{x_4}\max_{x_2}\max_{x_1} p(x_1)p(x_2|x_1)p(x_3|x_2)p(x_4|x_3)p(x_5|x_3)$$
$$= \max_{x_3} p(x_5|x_3)\max_{x_4} p(x_4|x_3)\max_{x_2} p(x_3|x_2)$$
$$\times \max_{x_1} p(x_1)p(x_2|x_1)$$

and the remaining computation proceeds as before. We see that the algebraic operations involved in performing the MAP computation are isomorphic to those in the earlier marginalization computation. Indeed, both the elimination algorithm and the sum-product algorithm extend immediately to MAP computation; we simply replace "sum" with "max" throughout in both cases. The underlying justification is that "max" commutes with products just as "sum" does.

General Graphs

Our goal in this section is to describe the *junction tree algorithm*, a generalization of the sum-product algorithm that is correct for arbitrary graphs. We derive the junction tree algorithm by returning to the elimination algorithm.

The first point to note is that ELIMINATE is correct for arbitrary graphs—the algorithm simply describes the creation of intermediate terms in a chain of summations that compute a marginal probability. Thus the algorithm is correct, but it is limited to the computation of a single marginal probability.

To show how to generalize the elimination algorithm to allow all individual marginals to be computed, we again proceed by example. Referring to the graph in Figure 3A, suppose that we wish to calculate the conditional probability $p(x_1)$. Let us use the elimination ordering (5, 4, 3, 2). At the first step, in which we sum over x_5, we remove the potentials $\psi_{35}(x_3, x_5)$ and $\psi_{45}(x_4, x_5)$ from the active list and form the sum

$$m_{32}(x_3, x_4) = \sum_{x_5} \psi_{35}(x_3, x_5)\psi_{45}(x_4, x_5)$$

where the intermediate term, which is clearly a function of x_3 and x_4, is denoted $m_{32}(x_3, x_4)$. (We explain the subscripts below.) The elimination of X_5 has created an intermediate term that effectively links X_3 and X_4, variables that were not linked in the original graph. Similarly, at the following step, we eliminate X_4:

$$m_{21}(x_2, x_3) = \sum_{x_4} \psi_{24}(x_2, x_4)m_{32}(x_3, x_4)$$

and obtain a term that links X_2 and X_3, variables that were not linked in the original graph.

A graphical record of the dependencies induced during the run of ELIMINATE is shown in Figure 3B. We could also have created this graph according to a simple graph-theoretic algorithm in which nodes are removed in order from a graph where, when a node is removed, its remaining neighbors are linked. Thus, for example, when node 5 is removed, nodes 3 and 4 are linked. When node 4 is removed, nodes 2 and 3 are linked. Let us refer to this algorithm as GRAPH ELIMINATE.

We can also obtain the desired marginal $p(x_1)$ by working with the "filled-in" graph in Figure 3B from the outset. Noting that the cliques in this graph are $C_1 = \{x_1, x_2, x_3\}$, $C_2 = \{x_2, x_3, x_4\}$, and $C_3 = \{x_3, x_4, x_5\}$, and defining the potentials:

$$\psi_{C_1}(x_1, x_2, x_3) = \psi_{12}(x_1, x_2)\psi_{13}(x_1, x_3)$$
$$\psi_{C_2}(x_2, x_3, x_4) = \psi_{24}(x_2, x_4)$$
$$\psi_{C_3}(x_3, x_4, x_5) = \psi_{35}(x_3, x_5)\psi_{45}(x_4, x_5)$$

we obtain exactly the same product of potentials as before. Thus we have

$$p(x) = \frac{1}{Z}\psi_{12}(x_1, x_2)\psi_{13}(x_1, x_3)\psi_{24}(x_2, x_4)\psi_{35}(x_3, x_5)\psi_{45}(x_4, x_5)$$
$$= \frac{1}{Z}\psi_{C_1}(x_1, x_2, x_3)\psi_{C_2}(x_2, x_3, x_4)\psi_{C_3}(x_3, x_4, x_5)$$

We have essentially transferred the joint probability distribution from Figure 3A to Figure 3B. Moreover, the steps of the elimination algorithm applied to Figure 3B are exactly the same as before, and we obtain the same marginal. An important difference, however, is that in the case of Figure 3B all of the intermediate potentials created during the run of the algorithm are also supported by cliques in the graph.

Graphs created by GRAPH ELIMINATE are known as *triangulated graphs*, and they have a number of special properties. In particular, they allow the creation of a data structure known as a *junction tree* on which a generalized message-passing algorithm can be defined. A junction tree is a tree in which each node is a clique from the original graph. Messages, which correspond to intermediate terms in ELIMINATE, pass between these cliques.

Although a full discussion of the construction of junction trees is beyond the scope of the article, it is worth noting that a junction tree is not just any tree of cliques from a triangulated graph. Rather, it is a maximal spanning tree (of cliques), with weights given by the cardinalities of the intersections between cliques.

Given a triangulated graph, with cliques $C_i \in \mathscr{C}$ and potentials $\psi_{C_i}(x_{C_i})$, and given a corresponding junction tree (which defines links between the cliques), we send the following "message" from clique C_i to clique C_j:

$$m_{ij}(x_{S_{ij}}) = \sum_{C_i \backslash S_{ij}} \psi_{C_i}(x_{C_i}) \prod_{k \in \mathcal{N}(i)\backslash j} m_{ki}(x_{S_{ki}}) \qquad (5)$$

where $S_{ij} = C_i \cap C_j$, and where $\mathcal{N}(i)$ are the neighbors of clique C_i in the junction tree. Moreover, it is possible to prove that we obtain marginal probabilities as products of messages. Thus

$$p(x_{C_i}) \propto \prod_{k \in \mathcal{N}(i)} m_{ki}(x_{S_{ki}}) \qquad (6)$$

is the marginal probability for clique C_i. (Marginals for single nodes can be obtained via further marginalization: i.e., $p(x_i) = \sum_{C\backslash i} p(x_C)$, for $i \in C$.)

The junction tree corresponding to the triangulated graph in Figure 3B is shown in Figure 4, where the corresponding messages are also shown. The reader can verify that the leftward-going messages are identical to the intermediate terms created during the run of ELIMINATE. The junction tree algorithm differs from ELIMINATE, however, in that messages pass in all directions, and the algorithm yields all clique marginals, not merely those corresponding to a single clique.

The sum-product algorithm described earlier in Equations 3 and 4 is a special case of Equations 5 and 6, obtained by noting that the original tree in Figure 1A is already triangulated and has pairs of nodes as cliques. In this case, the "separator sets" S_{ij} are singleton nodes.

Once again, the problem of computing MAP probabilities can be solved with a minor change to the basic algorithm. In particular, the "sum" in Equation 5 is changed to a "max."

There are many variations on exact inference algorithms, but all of them are either special cases of the junction tree algorithm or are close cousins. The basic message from the research literature on exact inference is that the operations of triangulating a graph

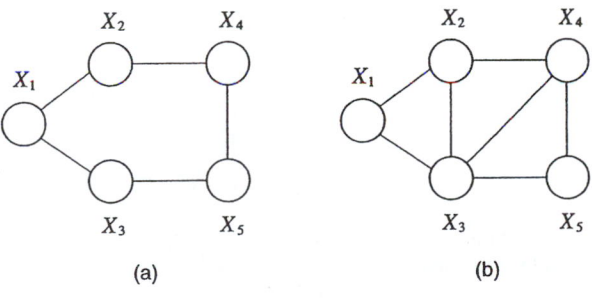

Figure 3. A, An undirected graphical model. B, The same model, with additional edges that reflect the dependencies created by the elimination algorithm.

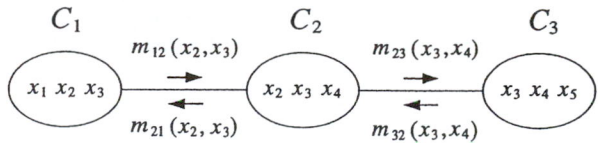

Figure 4. The junction tree corresponding to the triangulated graph in Figure 3B.

and passing messages on the resulting junction tree capture in a succinct way the basic algebraic structure of probabilistic inference.

Cutset Conditioning

In the method of *cutset conditioning*, we identify a "cutset"—defined (in the graphical model literature) as a set of nodes whose removal from the graph yields a tree. For example, in Figure 3*A*, any single node is a cutset. Denoting the indices of the cutset by Q, we loop over all instantiations x_Q, computing the conditional marginals $p(x_i|x_Q)$. The unconditional marginals are then given by $p(x_i) = \Sigma_{x_Q} p(x_i|x_Q) p(x_Q)$.

By considering an augmented graph in which edges are drawn from the nodes in the cutset to all other nodes in the graph, we can view cutset conditioning as a special case of the junction tree algorithm (Shachter, Andersen, and Szolovits, 1994). Note, however, that an implementation of cutset conditioning method involves operating on a single tree at a time, with cliques that are never larger than two nodes. Essentially, cutset conditioning involves implementing the junction tree algorithm in a way that trades time for space.

Computational Complexity

The computational complexity of the junction tree algorithm is a function of the size of the cliques upon which message-passing operations are performed. In particular, summing a clique potential is exponential in the number of nodes in the clique.

The problem of finding the optimal triangulation—the triangulation yielding the smallest maximal clique—turns out to be NP-hard. Clearly, if we had to search over all possible elimination orderings, the search would take exponential time. Triangulation can also be defined in other ways, however, and practical triangulation algorithms need not search over orderings. But the problem is still intractable, and can be a practical computational bottleneck.

An even more serious problem is that in practical graphical models, the original graph may have large cliques, or long loops, and even the optimal triangulation would yield unacceptable complexity. This problem is particularly serious because it arises not during the "compile time" operation of triangulation, but during the "run time" operation of message-passing. Problems in error-control coding and image processing are particularly noteworthy for yielding such graphs, as are discretizations of continuous-time problems and layered graphs of the kinds studied in the neural network field. To address these problems, we turn to the topic of approximate probabilistic inference.

Approximate Inference

The junction tree algorithm focuses on the algebraic structure of probabilistic inference, exploiting the conditional independencies present in a joint probability distribution, as encoded in the pattern of (missing) edges in the graph. There is another form of structure in probability theory, however, that is not exploited in the junction tree framework, and which leads us to hope that successful approximate inference algorithms can be developed. In particular, laws of large numbers and other concentration theorems in probability theory show that sums and products of large numbers of terms can behave in simple, predictable ways, despite the apparent combinatorial complexity of these operations. Approximate algorithms attempt to exploit these numerical aspects of probability theory.

We discuss two large classes of approximate inference algorithms in this section—Monte Carlo algorithms and variational algorithms. Although these classes do not exhaust all of the approximation techniques that have been studied, they capture the most widely used examples.

Monte Carlo Algorithms

Monte Carlo algorithms are based on the fact that while it may not be feasible to compute expectations under $p(x)$, it may be possible to obtain samples from $p(x)$, or from a closely related distribution, such that marginals and other expectations can be approximated using sample-based averages. We discuss three examples of Monte Carlo algorithms that are commonly used in the graphical model setting—Gibbs sampling, the Metropolis-Hastings algorithm, and importance sampling (for a comprehensive presentation of these methods and others, see Andrieu et al., 2003).

Gibbs sampling is an example of a Markov chain Monte Carlo (MCMC) algorithm. In an MCMC algorithm, samples are obtained via a Markov chain whose stationary distribution is the desired $p(x)$. The state of the Markov chain is a set of assignments of values to each of the variables, and, after a suitable "burn-in" period so that the chain approaches its stationary distribution, these states are used as samples.

The Markov chain for the Gibbs sampler is constructed in a straightforward way: (1) at each step one of the variables X_i is selected (at random or according to some fixed sequence), (2) the conditional distribution $p(x_i|x_{U\setminus i})$ is computed, (3) a value x_i is sampled from this distribution, and (4) the sample x_i replaces the previous value of the ith variable.

The implementation of Gibbs sampling thus reduces to the computation of the conditional distributions of individual variables given all of the other variables. For graphical models, these conditionals take the following form:

$$p(x_i|x_{U\setminus i}) = \frac{\prod_{C \in \mathscr{C}} \psi_C(x_C)}{\sum_{x_i} \prod_{C \in \mathscr{C}} \psi_C(x_C)} = \frac{\prod_{C \in \mathscr{C}_i} \psi_C(x_C)}{\sum_{x_i} \prod_{C \in \mathscr{C}_i} \psi_C(x_C)} \qquad (7)$$

where $\mathscr{C}_i$ denotes the set of cliques that contain index i. This set is often much smaller than the set $\mathscr{C}$ of all cliques, and in such cases each step of the Gibbs sampler can be implemented efficiently. Indeed, the conditional of node i depends only on the neighbors of node i in the graph, and thus the computation of the conditionals often takes the form of a simple message-passing algorithm that is reminiscent of the sum-product algorithm.

A simple example of a Gibbs sampler is provided by the *Boltzmann machine*, an undirected graphical model in which the potentials are defined on pairwise cliques. Gibbs sampling is often used for inference in the Boltzmann machine, and the algorithm in Equation 7 takes the form of the classical computation of the logistic function of a weighted sum of the values of neighboring nodes.

When the computation in Equation 7 is overly complex, the *Metropolis-Hastings algorithm* can provide an effective alternative. The Metropolis-Hastings algorithm is an MCMC algorithm that is not based on conditional probabilities and thus does not require normalization. Given the current state x of the algorithm, Metropolis-Hastings chooses a new state $\tilde{x}$ from a "proposal distribution" $q(\tilde{x}|x)$, which often simply involves picking a variable X_i at random and choosing a new value for that variable, again at random. The algorithm then computes the "acceptance probability":

$$\alpha = \min\left(1, \frac{q(x|\tilde{x})}{q(\tilde{x}|x)} \frac{\prod_{C \in \mathscr{C}_i} \psi_C(\tilde{x}_C)}{\prod_{C \in \mathscr{C}_i} \psi_C(x_C)}\right)$$

With probability α the algorithm accepts the proposal and moves to $\tilde{x}$, and with probability $1 - \alpha$ the algorithm remains in state x. For graphical models, this computation also turns out to often take the form of a simple message-passing algorithm.

While Gibbs sampling and Metropolis-Hastings aim at sampling from $p(x)$, *importance sampling* is a Monte Carlo technique for computing expectations in which samples are chosen from a simpler distribution $q(x)$, and these samples are reweighted appropriately. In particular, we approximate the expectation of a function $f(x)$ as follows:

$$
\begin{aligned}
E[f(x)] &= \sum_x p(x)f(x) \\
&= \sum_x q(x)\left(\frac{p(x)}{q(x)} f(x)\right) \\
&\approx \frac{1}{N} \sum_{i=1}^{N} \frac{p(x^{(t)})}{q(x^{(t)})} f(x^{(t)})
\end{aligned}
$$

where the values $x^{(t)}$ are samples from $q(x)$. The choice of $q(x)$ is in the hands of the designer, and the idea is that $q(x)$ should be chosen to be relatively simple to sample from, while reasonably close to $p(x)$ so that the weight $p(x^{(t)})/q(x^{(t)})$ is reasonably large. In the graphical model setting, natural choices of $q(x)$ are often provided by simplifying the graph underlying $p(x)$ in some way, in particular by deleting edges.

The principal advantages of Monte Carlo algorithms are their simplicity of implementation and their generality. Under weak conditions, the algorithms are guaranteed to converge. A problem with the Monte Carlo approach, however, is that convergence times can be long, and it can be difficult to diagnose convergence.

We might hope to be able to improve on Monte Carlo methods in situations in which laws of large numbers are operative. Consider, for example, the case in which a node i has many neighbors, such that the conditional $p(x_i|x_{U\setminus i})$ has a single, sharply determined maximum for most configurations of the neighbors. In this case, it would seem wasteful to continue to sample from this distribution; rather, we would like to be able to compute the maximizing value directly in some way. This way of thinking leads to the variational approach to approximate inference.

Variational Methods

The key to the variational approach lies in converting the probabilistic inference problem into an optimization problem, such that the standard tools of constrained optimization can be exploited. The basic approach has a similar flavor to importance sampling, but instead of choosing a single $q(x)$ a priori, a family of approximating distributions $\{q(x)\}$ is used, and the optimization machinery chooses a particular member from this family.

We begin by showing that the joint probability $p(x)$ can be viewed as the solution to an optimization problem. In particular, define the *energy* of a configuration x by $E(x) = -\log p(x) - \log Z$, and define the *variational free energy* as follows:

$$
\begin{aligned}
F(q) &= \sum_x q(x)E(x) + \sum_x q(x) \log q(x) \\
&= -\sum_x q(x) \log p(x) + \sum_x q(x) \log q(x) - \log Z
\end{aligned}
$$

The variational free energy is equal (up to an additive constant) to the Kullback-Leibler divergence between $q(x)$ and $p(x)$. It is therefore minimized when $q(x) = p(x)$ and attains the value of $-\log Z$ at the minimum. We have thus characterized $p(x)$ variationally.

Minimizing F is as difficult as doing exact inference, and much effort has been invested in finding approximate forms of F that are easier to minimize. Each approximate version of F gives an approximate variational inference algorithm.

For example, the simplest variational algorithm is the *mean field* approximation, in which $\{q(x)\}$ is restricted to the family of factorized distributions: $q(x) = \Pi_i q_i(x_i)$. In this case F simplifies to

$$
\begin{aligned}
F_{MF}(q) = &-\sum_C \sum_{x_C} \log \psi_C(x_C) \prod_{i \in C} q_i(x_i) \\
&+ \sum_i \sum_{x_i} q_i(x_i) \log q_i(x_i)
\end{aligned}
$$

subject to the constraint $\Sigma_{x_i} q_i(x_i) = 1$.

Setting the derivative with respect to $q_i(x_i)$ equal to zero gives

$$
q_i(x_i) = \alpha \exp\left(\sum_{C \in \mathscr{C}_i} \sum_{x_{C\setminus i}} \log \psi_C(x_C) \prod_{j \in C, j \neq i} q_j(x_j)\right) \quad (8)
$$

where α is a normalization constant chosen so that $\Sigma_{x_i} q_i(x_i) = 1$. The sum over cliques C_i is a sum over all cliques that node i belongs to.

Equation 8 defines an approximate inference algorithm. We initialize approximate marginals $q(x_i)$ for all nodes in the graph and then update the approximate marginal at one node based on those at neighboring nodes (note that the right-hand side of Equation 8 depends only on cliques that node i belongs to). This yields a message-passing algorithm that is similar to neural network algorithms; in particular, the value $q(x_i)$ can be viewed as the "activation" of node i.

More elaborate approximations to the free energy give better approximate marginal probabilities. While the mean field free energy depends only on approximate marginals at single nodes, the *Bethe free energy* depends on approximate marginals at single nodes $q_i(x_i)$ as well as on approximate marginals on cliques $q_C(x_C)$:

$$
\begin{aligned}
F_\beta(q) = &\sum_C \sum_{x_C} q_C(x_C) \log \frac{q_C(x_C)}{\psi_c(x_C)} \\
&- \sum_i (d_i - 1) \sum_{x_i} q_i(x_i) \log q_i(x_i)
\end{aligned}
$$

where $d_i - 1$ denotes the number of cliques that node i belongs to.

The approximate clique marginals and the approximate singleton marginals must satisfy a simple marginalization constraint: $\Sigma_{x_{C\setminus i}} q_C(x_C) = q_i(x_i)$. When we add Lagrange multipliers and differentiate the Lagrangian, we obtain a set of fixed point equations. Surprisingly, these equations end up being equivalent to the "sum-product" algorithm for trees in Equation 3. The messages $m_{ij}(x_j)$ are simply exponentiated Lagrange multipliers. Thus the Bethe approximation is equivalent to applying the local message-passing scheme developed for trees to graphs that have loops (see Yedidia, Freeman, and Weiss, 2001). This approach to approximate inference has been very successful in the domain of error-control coding, allowing practical codes based on graphical models to nearly reach the Shannon limit.

Discussion

The unified perspective on inference algorithms that we have presented in this article has arisen through several different historical strands. We briefly summarize these strands here and note some of the linkages with developments in the neural network field.

The elimination algorithm has had a long history. The "peeling" algorithm developed by geneticists is an early example (Cannings, Thompson, and Skolnick, 1978), as are the "decimation" and "transfer matrix" procedures in statistical physics (Itzykson and Drouffe, 1991). For a recent discussion of elimination algorithms, including more efficient algorithms than the simple ELIMINATE algorithm presented here, see Dechter (1999).

Belief propagation has also had a long history. An early version of the sum-product algorithm was studied by Gallager (1963) in the context of error-control codes (see Kschischang, Frey, and Loeliger (2001) for a recent perspective). Well-known special cases of sum-product include the forward-backward algorithm for hidden Markov models (see HIDDEN MARKOV MODELS), and the Kalman filtering/smoothing algorithms for state-space models. A seminal presentation of the sum-product algorithm was provided by Pearl (1988).

The variant of the junction tree algorithm that we have defined is due to Shafer and Shenoy (1990), and has also been called the *generalized distributive law* by Aji and McEliece (2000). A closely related variant known as the *Hugin algorithm* arose from the work of Lauritzen and Spiegelhalter (1988); it is described by Jensen (2001).

Many neural network architectures are special cases of general graphical model formalism, both representationally and algorithmically. Special cases of graphical models include essentially all of the models developed under the rubric of unsupervised learning (see UNSUPERVISED LEARNING WITH GLOBAL OBJECTIVE FUNCTIONS, INDEPENDENT COMPONENT ANALYSIS, and HELMHOLTZ MACHINES AND SLEEP-WAKE LEARNING), as well as Boltzmann machines (see SIMULATED ANNEALING AND BOLTZMANN MACHINES), mixtures of experts (see MODULAR AND HIERARCHICAL LEARNING SYSTEMS), and radial basis function networks (see RADIAL BASIS FUNCTION NETWORKS). Many other neural networks, including the classical multilayer perceptron (see PERCEPTRONS, ADALINES, AND BACKPROPAGATION) can be profitably analyzed from the point of view of graphical models. For more discussion of these links, see the articles in Jordan (1999).

Road Map: Artificial Intelligence; Learning in Artificial Networks
Related Reading: Bayesian Networks; Graphical Models: Parameter Learning; Graphical Models: Structure Learning; Markov Random Field Models in Image Processing

References

Aji, S. M., and McEliece, R. J., 2000, The generalized distributive law, *IEEE Trans. Inform. Theory*, 46:325–343.

Andrieu, C., De Freitas, J., Doucet, A., and Jordan, M. I., 2003, An introduction to MCMC for machine learning, *Machine Learn* (in press). ◆

Cannings, C., Thompson, E. A., and Skolnick, M. H., 1978, Probability functions on complex pedigrees, *Adv. Appl. Probab.*, 10:26–91.

Dechter, R., 1999, Bucket elimination: A unifying framework for probabilistic inference, in *Learning in Graphical Models* (M. I. Jordan, Ed.), Cambridge, MA: MIT Press.

Gallager, R. G., 1963, *Low-Density Parity Check Codes*, Cambridge, MA: MIT Press.

Itzykson, C., and Drouffe, J., 1991, *Statistical Field Theory*, Cambridge, Engl.: Cambridge University Press.

Jensen, F. V., 2001, *Bayesian Networks and Decision Graphs*, New York: Springer-Verlag. ◆

Jordan, M. I., Ed., 1999, *Learning in Graphical Models*, Cambridge, MA: MIT Press. ◆

Jordan, M. I., Ghahramani, Z., Jaakkola, T. S., and Saul, L. K., 1999, An introduction to variational methods for graphical models, *Machine Learn.*, 37:183–233. ◆

Kschischang, F. R., Frey, B. J., and Loeliger, H.-A., 2001, Factor graphs and the sum-product algorithm, *IEEE Trans. Inform. Theory*, 47:498–519.

Lauritzen, S. L., and Spiegelhalter, D., 1988, Local computations with probabilities on graphical structures and their application to expert systems (with discussion), *J. R. Statist. Soc. B*, 50:157–224.

Pearl, J., 1988, *Probabilistic Reasoning in Intelligent Systems: Networks of Plausible Inference*, San Mateo, CA: Morgan Kaufmann. ◆

Shachter, R., Andersen, S., and Szolovits, P., 1994, Global conditioning for probabilistic inference in belief networks, in *Uncertainty in Artificial Intelligence: Proceedings of the Tenth Conference*, pp. 514–522.

Shafer, G. R., and Shenoy, P. P., 1990, Probability propagation, *Ann. Math. Artif. Intell.*, 2:327–352.

Yedidia, J. S., Freeman, W. T., and Weiss, Y., 2001, *Bethe Free Energies, Kikuchi Approximations, and Belief Propagation Algorithms.*, MERL Technical Report 2001–16.

Graphical Models: Structure Learning

David Heckerman

Introduction

The article GRAPHICAL MODELS: PARAMETER LEARNING (q.v.) discussed the learning of parameters for a fixed graphical model. In this article, we discuss the simultaneous learning of parameters and structure. Real-world applications of such learning abound and can be found in, for example, *Proceedings of the Conference on Uncertainty in Artificial Intelligence* (1991 and after). An index to software for parameter and structure learning can be found at http://www.cs.berkeley.edu/murphyk/Bayes/bnsoft.html.

For simplicity, we concentrate on directed-acyclic graphical models (DAG models), but the basic principles described here can be applied more generally. We describe the Bayesian approach in detail and mention several common non-Bayesian approaches.

We use notation that is slightly different from that used in the article on parameter learning. In particular, we use $\mathbf{X} = (X_1, \ldots, X_n)$ to denote the n variables that we are modeling, $\mathbf{x}$ to denote a configuration or observation of $\mathbf{X}$, and $\mathbf{d} = (\mathbf{x}^1, \ldots, \mathbf{x}^N)$ to denote a random sample of N observations of $\mathbf{X}$. In addition, we use $\mathbf{Pa}_i$ to denote the variables corresponding to the parents of X_i in a DAG model and $\mathbf{pa}_i$ to denote a configuration of those variables. Finally, we shall use the terms *model* and *structure* interchangeably. In particular, a DAG model (and hence its structure) is described by (1) its nodes and arcs, and (2) the distribution class of each of its local distributions $p(x_i|\mathbf{pa}_i)$.

The Bayesian Approach

When we learn a model and its parameters, we presumably are uncertain about their identity. When following the Bayesian approach—in which all uncertainty is encoded as (subjective) probability—we encode this uncertainty as prior distributions over random variables corresponding to structure and parameters. In particular, let $\mathbf{m}$ be a random variable having states $\mathbf{m}^1, \ldots, \mathbf{m}^M$ corresponding to the possible models. (Note that we are assuming the models are mutually exclusive.) In addition, let $\theta^1, \ldots, \theta^M$ be random variables corresponding to the unknown parameters of each of the M possible models. Then we express our uncertainty prior to learning as the prior distributions $p(\mathbf{m})$, and $p(\theta^1), \ldots, p(\theta^M)$.

Given data $\mathbf{d}$, a random sample from the true but unknown joint distribution for $\mathbf{X}$, we compute the posterior distributions for each $\mathbf{m}$ and θ^m using Bayes's rule:

$$p(\mathbf{m}|\mathbf{d}) = \frac{p(\mathbf{m})p(\mathbf{d}|\mathbf{m})}{\sum_{m'} p(\mathbf{m}')p(\mathbf{d}|\mathbf{m}')} \tag{1}$$

$$p(\theta^m|\mathbf{d},\ \mathbf{m}) = \frac{p(\theta^m|\mathbf{m})p(\mathbf{d}|\theta^m,\ \mathbf{m})}{p(\mathbf{d}|\mathbf{m})} \tag{2}$$

where

$$p(\mathbf{d}|\mathbf{m}) = \int p(\mathbf{d}|\theta^m, \mathbf{m})p(\theta^m|\mathbf{m})d\theta^m \qquad (3)$$

is called the *marginal likelihood*. Given some hypothesis of interest, h, we determine the probability that h is true given data $\mathbf{d}$ by averaging over all possible models and their parameters:

$$p(h|\mathbf{d}) = \sum_m p(\mathbf{m}|\mathbf{d})p(h|\mathbf{d}, \mathbf{m}) \qquad (4)$$

$$p(h|\mathbf{d}, \mathbf{m}) = \int p(h|\theta^m, \mathbf{m})p(\theta^m|\mathbf{d}, \mathbf{m})d\theta^m \qquad (5)$$

For example, h may be the event that the next case $\mathbf{X}^{N+1}$ is observed in configuration $\mathbf{x}^{N+1}$. In this situation, we obtain

$$p(\mathbf{x}^{N+1}|\mathbf{d}) = \sum_m p(\mathbf{m}|\mathbf{d}) \int p(\mathbf{x}^{N+1}|\theta^m, \mathbf{m})p(\theta^m|\mathbf{d}, \mathbf{m})d\theta^m \qquad (6)$$

where $p(\mathbf{x}^{N+1}|\theta^m, \mathbf{m})$ is the likelihood for the model. It is important to note that, in the Bayesian approach, no single model is learned. Instead, data is used to update the probability that each possible model is the correct one.

Unfortunately, this approach, sometimes called *Bayesian model averaging* or the *full Bayesian approach,* is often impractical. For example, the number of different DAG models for a domain containing n variables grows superexponentially with n. Thus, the approach can only be applied in those few settings where one has strong prior knowledge that can eliminate almost all possible models.

Statisticians, who have been confronted by this problem for decades in the context of other types of models, use two approximations to address this problem: *Bayesian model selection* and *selective Bayesian model averaging.* The former approach is to select a likely model from among all possible models and use it as if it were the correct model. For example, to predict the next case, we use

$$\begin{aligned} p(\mathbf{x}^{N+1}|\mathbf{d}) &\cong p(\mathbf{x}^{N+1}|\mathbf{m}, \mathbf{d}) \\ &= \int p(\mathbf{x}^{N+1}|\theta^m, \mathbf{m})p(\theta^m|\mathbf{d}, \mathbf{m})d\theta^m \end{aligned} \qquad (7)$$

where $\mathbf{m}$ is the selected model. The latter approach is to select a manageable number of good models from among all possible models and pretend that these models are exhaustive. In either approach, we need only the *relative* model posterior—$p(\mathbf{m})p(\mathbf{d}|\mathbf{m})$—to select likely models.

Both approaches can be characterized as *search-and-score* techniques. That is, in these approaches, we search among a large set of models looking for those with good scores. The use of these approximate methods raise several important questions. Do they yield accurate results when applied to graphical model learning? If so, can we compute the model posteriors and perform a search efficiently?

The question of accuracy is difficult to answer in theory. Nonetheless, several researchers have shown experimentally that the selection of a single good hypothesis often yields accurate predictions (e.g., Cooper and Herskovits, 1992; Heckerman, Geiger, and Chickering, 1995) and that selective model averaging using Monte Carlo methods can sometimes be efficient and yield even better predictions (Madigan et al., 1996). These results, which are somewhat surprising, are largely responsible for the considerable interest in learning graphical models.

In the remainder of this section, we address computational efficiency. In particular, we consider situations in which (relative) model posteriors can be computed efficiently as well as efficient search procedures.

We note that model averaging, model selection, and selective model averaging all help avoid overfitting—situations where models perform well on training data and poorly on new data. In particular, the marginal likelihood balances the fit of the model structure to data with the complexity of the model. One way to understand this fact is to note that, when the number of cases N is large and other conditions hold, the marginal likelihood can be approximated as follows:

$$p(\mathbf{d}|\mathbf{m}) \cong p(\mathbf{d}|\hat{\theta}, \mathbf{m}) - \frac{|\theta|}{2} \log N$$

where $\hat{\theta}$ is the maximum-likelihood estimator of the data (e.g., Kass and Raftery, 1995). The first quantity in this expression represents the degree to which the model fits the data, which increases as the model complexity increases. The second quantity, in contrast, penalizes model complexity.

Computation of the Marginal Likelihood

Under certain conditions, the marginal likelihood of a graphical model—and hence its relative posterior—can be computed efficiently. In this section, we examine a particular set of these conditions for structure learning of DAG models. We note that a similar set of conditions holds for the learning of decomposable UG models. For details, see Lauritzen (1996).

Given any DAG model $\mathbf{m}$, we can factor the likelihood of a single sample as follows:

$$p(\mathbf{x}|\theta_m, \mathbf{m}) = \prod_{i=1}^{n} p(x_i|\mathbf{pa}_i, \theta_i, \mathbf{m}) \qquad (8)$$

We shall refer to each term $p(x_i|\mathbf{pa}_i, \theta_i, \mathbf{m})$ in this equation as the *local likelihood for* X_i. Also, in this equation, θ_i denotes the set of parameters associated with the local likelihood for variable X_i.

The first condition in our set of sufficient conditions yielding efficient computation is that each local likelihood is in the exponential family. One example of such a factorization occurs when each variable $X_i \in \mathbf{X}$ is finite, having r_i possible values $x_i^1, \ldots, x_i^{r_i}$, and each local likelihood is a collection of multinomial distributions, one distribution for each configuration of $\mathbf{Pa}_i$—that is,

$$p(x_i^k|\mathbf{pa}_i^j, \theta_i, \mathbf{m}) = \theta_{ijk} > 0 \qquad (9)$$

where $\mathbf{pa}_i^1, \ldots, \mathbf{pa}_i^{q_i}$ ($q_i = \Pi_{X_i \in \mathbf{Pa}_i} r_i$) denotes the configurations of $\mathbf{Pa}_i$, and $\theta_{ij} = ((\theta_{ijk})_{k=2}^{r_i})_{j=1}^{q_i}$ denotes the parameters. The parameter θ_{ij1} is given by $1 - \Sigma_{k=2}^{r_i}\theta_{ijk}$. We shall use this example to illustrate many of the concepts in this article. For convenience, we define the vector of parameters

$$\theta_{ij} = (\theta_{ij1}, \ldots, \theta_{ijr_i})$$

for all i and j. Examples of other exponential families can be found in Bernardo and Smith (1994).

The second assumption for efficient computation is one of parameter independence. In our multinomial example, we assume that the parameter vectors θ_{ij} are mutually independent. Note that, when this independence holds and we are given a random sample $\mathbf{d}$ that contains no missing observations, the parameters remain independent:

$$p(\theta_m|\mathbf{d}, \mathbf{m}) = \prod_{i=1}^{n} \prod_{j=1}^{q_i} p(\theta_{ij}|\mathbf{d}, \mathbf{m}) \qquad (10)$$

Thus, we can update each vector of parameters θ_{ij} independently.

The third assumption is that each independent parameter set has a conjugate prior (e.g., Bernardo and Smith, 1994). In our multinomial example, we assume that each θ_{ij} has a Dirichlet prior $\text{Dir}(\theta_{ij}|\alpha_{ij1}, \ldots, \alpha_{ijr_i})$. In this case, we obtain

$$p(\theta_{ij}|\mathbf{d}, \mathbf{m}) = \mathrm{Dir}(\theta_{ij}|\alpha_{ij1} + N_{ij1}, \ldots, \alpha_{ijr_i} + N_{ijr_i}) \quad (11)$$

where N_{ijk} is the number of cases in $\mathbf{d}$ in which $X_i = x_i^k$ and $\mathbf{Pa}_i = \mathbf{pa}_i^j$. Note that the collection of counts N_{ijk} are sufficient statistics of the data for the model $\mathbf{m}$.

Under these conditions, we can compute the marginal likelihood efficiently and in closed form. For our multinomial example (as first derived in Cooper and Herskovits, 1992), we obtain

$$p(\mathbf{d}|\mathbf{m}) = \prod_{i=1}^{n} \prod_{j=1}^{q_i} \frac{\Gamma(\alpha_{ij})}{\Gamma(\alpha_{ij} + N_{ij})} \cdot \prod_{k=1}^{r_i} \frac{\Gamma(\alpha_{ijk} + N_{ijk})}{\Gamma(\alpha_{ijk})} \quad (12)$$

where $\alpha_{ij} = \sum_{k=1}^{r_i} \alpha_{ijk}$ and $N_{ij} = \sum_{k=1}^{r_i} N_{ijk}$.

Under these same conditions, the integral in Equation 7 also can be computed efficiently. In our example, suppose that, for a given outcome $\mathbf{x}_{N+1}$ of $\mathbf{X}_{N+1}$, the value of X_i is x_i^k and the configuration of $\mathbf{Pa}_i$ is $\mathbf{pa}_i^j$, where k and j depend on i. Using Equations 4, 8, and 9, we obtain

$$p(\mathbf{x}_{N+1}|\mathbf{d}, \mathbf{m}) = \int \left(\prod_{i=1}^{n} \theta_{ijk} \right) p(\theta_m|\mathbf{d}, \mathbf{m}) d\theta_m$$

Because parameters remain independent given $\mathbf{d}$, we get

$$p(\mathbf{x}_{N+1}|\mathbf{d}, \mathbf{m}) = \prod_{i=1}^{n} \int \theta_{ijk}\, p(\theta_{ij}|\mathbf{d}, \mathbf{m}) d\theta_{ij}$$

Finally, because each integral in this product is the expectation of a Dirichlet distribution, we have

$$p(\mathbf{x}_{N+1}|\mathbf{d}, \mathbf{m}) = \prod_{i=1}^{n} \frac{\alpha_{ijk} + N_{ijk}}{\alpha_{ij} + N_{ij}} \quad (13)$$

To compute the relative posterior probability of a model, we must assess the structure prior $p(\mathbf{m})$ and the parameter priors $p(\theta^m|\mathbf{m})$. Unfortunately, when many models are possible, the assessment process will be intractable. Nonetheless, under certain assumptions, we can derive the structure and parameter priors for many models from a manageable number of direct assessments. Several authors have discussed such assumptions and corresponding methods for deriving priors (e.g., Buntine, 1991; Cooper and Herskovits, 1992; Heckerman et al., 1995; Cowell et al., 1999). In the following two sections, we examine some of these approaches.

Priors for Model Parameters

First, let us consider the assessment of priors for the parameters of DAG models. We consider the approach of Heckerman, Geiger, and Chickering (1995)—herein, HGC—who address the case for $\mathbf{X}$ where the local likelihoods are multinomial distributions. A similar approach exists for situations where the local likelihoods are linear regressions (Heckerman and Geiger, 1995).

Their approach is based on two key concepts: Markov equivalence and distribution equivalence. We say that two models for $\mathbf{X}$ are *Markov equivalent* if they represent the same set of conditional-independence assertions for $\mathbf{X}$. For example, given $\mathbf{X} = \{X, Y, Z\}$, the models $X \rightarrow Y \rightarrow Z$, $X \leftarrow Y \rightarrow Z$, and $X \leftarrow Y \leftarrow Z$ represent only the independence assertion that X and Z are conditionally independent given Y. Consequently, these models are equivalent. Another example of Markov equivalence is the set of *complete models* on $\mathbf{X}$. A complete model is one that has no missing edge and that encodes no assertion of conditional independence. When $\mathbf{d}$ contains n variables, there are $n!$ possible complete models, one model structure for every possible ordering of the variables. All complete models for $\mathbf{X}$ are Markov equivalent. In general, two models are Markov equivalent if and only if they have the same structure, ignoring arc directions, and the same v-structures. A *v-structure* is an ordered tuple (X, Y, Z) such that there is an arc from X to Y and from Z to Y, but no arc between X and Z.

The concept of distribution equivalence is closely related to that of Markov equivalence. Suppose that all models for $\mathbf{X}$ under consideration have local likelihoods in the family $\mathcal{F}$. This is not a restriction per se, because $\mathcal{F}$ can be a large family. We say that two model structures $\mathbf{m}_1$ and $\mathbf{m}_2$ for $\mathbf{X}$ are *distribution equivalent with respect to $\mathcal{F}$* if they can represent the same joint probability distributions for $\mathbf{X}$, that is, if, for every θ_{m1}, there exists a θ_{m2} such that $p(\mathbf{x}|\theta_{m1}, \mathbf{m}_1) = p(\mathbf{x}|\theta_{m2}, \mathbf{m}_2)$, and vice versa.

Distribution equivalence with respect to some $\mathcal{F}$ implies Markov equivalence, but the converse does not hold. For example, when $\mathcal{F}$ is the family of generalized linear regression models, the complete model structures for $n \geq 3$ variables do not represent the same sets of distributions. Nonetheless, there are families $\mathcal{F}$—for example, multinomial distributions and linear regression models with Gaussian noise—where Markov equivalence implies distribution equivalence with respect to $\mathcal{F}$ (see HGC). The notion of distribution equivalence is important, because if two model structures $\mathbf{m}_1$ and $\mathbf{m}_2$ are distribution equivalent with respect to a given $\mathcal{F}$, then it is often reasonable to expect that data cannot help to discriminate them. That is, we expect $p(\mathbf{d}|\mathbf{m}_1) = p(\mathbf{d}|\mathbf{m}_2)$ for any data set $\mathbf{d}$. HGC call this property *likelihood equivalence*.

Now let us return to the main issue of this section: the derivation of parameter priors from a manageable number of assessments. HGC show that the assumption of likelihood equivalence combined with the assumption that the θ_{ij} are mutually independent imply that the parameters for any *complete* model $\mathbf{m}_c$ must have a Dirichlet distribution with constraints on the hyperparameters given by

$$\alpha_{ijk} = \alpha p(x_i^k, \mathbf{pa}_i^j|\mathbf{m}_c) \quad (14)$$

where α is the user's equivalent sample size and $p(x_i^k, \mathbf{pa}_i^j|\mathbf{m}_c)$ is computed from the user's joint probability distribution $p(\mathbf{d}|\mathbf{m}_c)$ (discussions of equivalent sample size can be found in, e.g., Heckerman et al., 1995). Note that this result is rather surprising, as the two assumptions leading to the constrained Dirichlet solution are qualitative.

To determine the priors for parameters of *incomplete* models, HGC use the assumption of *parameter modularity*, which says that if X_i has the same parents in models $\mathbf{m}_1$ and $\mathbf{m}_2$, then

$$p(\theta_{ij}|\mathbf{m}_1) = p(\theta_{ij}|\mathbf{m}_2)$$

for $j = 1, \ldots, q_i$. They call this property parameter modularity, because it says that the distributions for parameters θ_{ij} depend only on a portion of the graph structure, namely, X_i and its parents.

Given the assumptions of parameter modularity and parameter independence, it is a simple matter to construct priors for the parameters of an arbitrary model given the priors on complete models. In particular, given parameter independence, we construct the priors for the parameters of each node separately. Furthermore, if node X_i has parents $\mathbf{Pa}_i$ in the given model, then we identify a complete model structure where X_i has these parents, and use Equation 14 and parameter modularity to determine the priors for this node. The result is that all terms α_{ijk} for all model structures are determined by Equation 14. Thus, from the assessments α and $p(\mathbf{d}|\mathbf{m}_c)$, we can derive the parameter priors for all possible model structures. We can assess $p(\mathbf{d}|\mathbf{m}_c)$ by constructing a parameterized model, called a *prior network*, that encodes this joint distribution.

Priors for Model Structures

Now let us consider the assessment of priors on structure. The simplest approach for assigning priors to models is to assume that every model is equally likely. Of course, this assumption is typically inaccurate and is used only for the sake of convenience. A simple refinement of this approach is to ask the user to exclude various structures (perhaps based on judgments of cause and effect), and then impose a uniform prior on the remaining structures. We use this approach in an example described later.

Buntine (1991) describes a set of assumptions that leads to a richer yet efficient approach for assigning priors. The first assumption is that the variables can be ordered (e.g., through a knowledge of time precedence). The second assumption is that the presence or absence of possible arcs are mutually independent. Given these assumptions, $n(n-1)/2$ probability assessments (one for each possible arc in an ordering) determines the prior probability of every possible model. One extension to this approach is to allow for multiple possible orderings. One simplification is to assume that the probability that an arc is absent or present is independent of the specific arc in question. In this case, only one probability assessment is required.

An alternative approach, described by Heckerman et al. (1995), uses the prior network described in the previous section. The basic idea is to penalize the prior probability of any structure according to some measure of deviation between that structure and the prior network. Heckerman et al. (1995) suggest one reasonable measure of deviation.

Search Methods

In this section, we examine search methods for identifying DAG models with high scores. Consider the problem of finding the best DAG model from the set of all DAG models in which each node has no more than k parents. Unfortunately, the problem for $k > 1$ is NP-hard even when we use the restrictive prior given by Equation 14 (Chickering, 1996). Thus, researchers have used heuristic search algorithms, including greedy search, greedy search with restarts, best-first search, and Monte Carlo methods.

One consolation is that these search methods can be made more computationally efficient when the model score is factorable. Given a DAG model for domain $\mathbf{X}$, we say that a score for that model $S(\mathbf{m}, \mathbf{d})$ is *factorable* if it can be written as a product of variable-specific scores:

$$S(\mathbf{m}, \mathbf{d}) = \prod_{i=1}^{n} s(X_i, \mathbf{Pa}_i, \mathbf{d}_i) \quad (15)$$

where $\mathbf{d}_i$ is the data restricted to the variables X_i and $\mathbf{Pa}_i$. An example of a factorable score is Equation 12 used in conjunction with any of the structure priors described previously.

Most of the commonly used search methods for DAG models also make successive arc changes to the graph structure, and employ the property of factorability to evaluate the merit of each change. One commonly used set of arc changes is as follows. For any pair of variables, if there is an arc connecting them, then this arc can either be reversed or removed. If there is no arc connecting them, then an arc can be added in either direction. All changes are subject to the constraint that the resulting DAG contains no directed cycles. We use E to denote the set of eligible changes to a graph, and $\Delta(e)$ to denote the change in $\log p(\mathbf{d}|\mathbf{m})p(\mathbf{m})$ resulting from the modification $e \in E$. Given a factorable score, if an arc to X_i is added or deleted, only $c(X_i, \mathbf{Pa}_i, \mathbf{d}_i)$ need be evaluated to determine $\Delta(e)$. If an arc between X_i and X_j is reversed, then only $c(X_i, \mathbf{Pa}_i, \mathbf{d}_i)$ and $c(X_j, \Pi_j, \mathbf{d}_j)$ need be evaluated.

One simple heuristic search algorithm is greedy hill climbing. We begin with some DAG model. Then, we evaluate $\Delta(e)$ for all $e \in E$, and make the change e for which $\Delta(e)$ is a maximum, provided it is positive. We terminatae search when there is no e with a positive value for $\Delta(e)$. Candidates for the initial model include the empty graph, a random graph, and the prior network used for the assessment of parameter and structure priors.

A potential problem with any local-search method is getting stuck at a local maximum. One method for escaping local maxima

is greedy search with random restarts. In this approach, we apply greedy search until we hit a local maximum. Then we randomly perturb the structure, and repeat the process for some manageable number of iterations. Another method for escaping local maxima is simulated annealing. In this approach, we initialize the system at some temperature T_0. Then we pick some eligible change e at random, and evaluate the expression $p = \exp(\Delta(e)/T_0)$. If $p > 1$, then we make the change e; otherwise, we make the change with probability p. We repeat this selection and evaluation process α times or until we make β changes. If we make no changes in α repetitions, then we stop searching. Otherwise, we lower the temperature by multiplying the current temperature T_0 by a decay factor $0 < \gamma < 1$, and continue the search process. We stop searching if we have lowered the temperature more than δ times. Thus, this algorithm is controlled by five parameters: T_0, α, β, γ, and δ. To initialize this algorithm, we can start with the empty graph, and make T_0 large enough so that almost every eligible change is made, thus creating a random graph. Alternatively, we may start with a lower temperature, and use one of the initialization methods described for local search.

Another method for escaping local maxima is best-first search. In this approach, the space of all models is searched systematically using a heuristic measure that determines the next best structure to examine. Experiments (e.g., Heckerman et al., 1995) have shown that, for a fixed amount of computation time, greedy search with random restarts produces better models than does best-first search.

One important consideration for any search algorithm is the search space. The methods that we have described search through the space of DAG models. Nonetheless, when likelihood equivalence is assumed, one can search through the space of model equivalence classes. One benefit of the latter approach is that the search space is smaller. One drawback of the latter approach is that it takes longer to move from one element in the search space to another. Experiments have shown that the two effects roughly cancel.

Example: College Plans

In this section, we consider an analysis of data, obtained by Sewell and Shah (1968), regarding factors that influence the intention of high school students to attend college. This analysis was given previously by Heckerman in Jordan (1999).

Sewell and Shah (1968) measured the following variables for 10,318 Wisconsin high school seniors: *sex* (SEX): male, female; *socioeconomic status* (SES): low, lower middle, upper middle, high; *intelligence quotient* (IQ): low, lower middle, upper middle, high; *parental encouragement* (PE): low, high; and *college plans* (CP): yes, no. Our goal in this analysis is to understand the relationships among these variables.

The data are (completely) described by the counts in Table 1. Each entry denotes the number of cases in which the five variables take on some particular configuration. The first entry corresponds to the configuration SEX = male, SES = low, IQ = low, PE =

Table 1. Sufficient Statistics for the Sewall and Shah (1968) Study

4	349	13	64	9	207	33	72	12	126	38	54	10	67	49	43
2	232	27	84	7	201	64	95	12	115	93	92	17	79	119	59
8	166	47	91	6	120	74	110	17	92	148	100	6	42	198	73
4	48	39	57	5	47	123	90	9	41	224	65	8	17	414	54
5	454	9	44	5	312	14	47	8	216	20	35	13	96	28	24
11	285	29	61	19	236	47	88	12	164	62	85	15	113	72	50
7	163	36	72	13	193	75	90	12	174	91	100	20	81	142	77
6	50	36	58	5	70	110	76	12	48	230	81	13	49	360	98

low, and CP = yes. The remaining entries correspond to configurations obtained by cycling through the states of each variable such that the last variable (CP) varies most quickly. Thus, for example, the upper (lower) half of the table corresponds to male (female) students.

To generate priors for model parameters, we used the method described earlier in this section with an equivalent sample size of five and a prior network describing a uniform distribution over **X**. (The results we report remain qualitatively the same for equivalent sample sizes ranging from 3 to 40.) For structure priors, we assumed that all models were equally likely, except that we excluded structures (based on causal considerations) where SEX and/or SES had parents, and/or CP had children. We used Equation 12 to compute the marginal likelihoods of the models. The two most likely models that we found after an exhaustive search over all structures are shown in Figure 1. Note that the most likely model has a posterior probability that is extremely close to 1. Both models show a reasonable result: that CP and SEX are independent, given the remaining variables.

Methods for Incomplete Data

Among the assumptions that yield an efficient method for computing the marginal likelihood, the one that is most often violated is the assumption that all variables are observed in every case. In many situations, some variables will be hidden (i.e., never observed) or will be observed for only a subset of the data samples. There are a variety of methods for handling such situations—at greater computational cost—including Monte Carlo (MC) approaches (e.g., DiCiccio et al., 1995), large-sample approximations (e.g., Kass and Raftery, 1995), and variational approximations (e.g., Jordan et al. in Jordan, 1999).

In this section, we examine a simple MC approach called *Gibbs sampling* (e.g., MacKay in Jordan, 1999). In general, given variables $\mathbf{X} = \{X_1, \ldots, X_n\}$ with some joint distribution $p(x)$, we can use a Gibbs sampler to approximate the expectation of a function $f(x)$ with respect to $p(x)$. This approximation is made as follows. First, we choose an initial state for each of the variables in **X** somehow (e.g., at random). Next, we pick some variable $\mathbf{X}_i$, unassign its current state, and compute its probability distribution given the states of the other $n - 1$ variables. Then, we sample a state for $\mathbf{X}_i$ based on this probability distribution, and compute $f(x)$. Finally, we iterate the previous two steps, keeping track of the average value of $f(x)$. In the limit, as the number of cases approach infinity, this average is equal to $E_{p(x)}(f(x))$ provided two conditions are met. First, the Gibbs sampler must be *irreducible*. That is, the probability distribution $p(x)$ must be such that we can eventually sample any possible configuration of **X** given any possible initial configuration of **X**. For example, if $p(x)$ contains no zero probabilities, then the Gibbs sampler will be irreducible. Second, each X_i must be chosen infinitely often. In practice, an algorithm for deterministically rotating through the variables is typically used. An introduction to Gibbs sampling and other Monte Carlo methods, including methods for initialization and a discussion of convergence, is given by Neal (1993).

To illustrate Gibbs sampling, consider again the case where every variable in **X** is finite, the parameters θ_{ij} for a given DAG model **m** are mutually independent, and each θ_{ij} has a Dirichlet prior. In this situation, let us approximate the probability density $p(\theta_m|\mathbf{d}, \mathbf{m})$ for some particular configuration of θ_m, given an incomplete data set **d**. First, we initialize the states of the unobserved variables in each case somehow. As a result, we have a complete random sample $\mathbf{d}_c$. Second, we choose some variable X_{il} (variable X_i in case l) that is not observed in the original random sample D, and reassign its state according to the probability distribution

$$p(x_{il}'|\mathbf{d}_c\backslash x_{il}, \ \mathbf{m}) \ = \ \frac{p(x_{il}', \ \mathbf{d}_c\backslash x_{il}|\mathbf{m})}{\sum_{x_{il}} p(x_{il}'', \ \mathbf{d}_c\backslash x_{il}|\mathbf{m})}$$

where $\mathbf{d}_c\backslash x_{il}$ denotes the data set $\mathbf{d}_c$ with observation x_{il} removed, and the sum in the denominator runs over all states of variable X_{il}. As we have seen, the terms in the numerator and denominator can be computed efficiently (see Equation 12). Third, we repeat this reassignment for all unobserved variables in **d**, producing a new complete random sample $\mathbf{d}_c'$. Fourth, we compute the posterior density $p(\theta_m|\mathbf{d}_c', \mathbf{m})$ as described in Equations 10 and 11. Finally, we iterate the previous three steps, and use the average of $p(\theta_m|\mathbf{d}_c', \mathbf{m})$ as our approximation.

Monte Carlo approximations are also useful for computing the marginal likelihood given incomplete data. One Monte Carlo approach uses Bayes's theorem:

$$p(\mathbf{d}|\mathbf{m}) \ = \ \frac{p(\theta_m|\mathbf{m})p(\mathbf{d}|\theta_m, \ \mathbf{m})}{p(\theta_m|\mathbf{d}, \ \mathbf{m})} \qquad (16)$$

For any configuration of θ_m, the prior term in the numerator can be evaluated directly. In addition, the likelihood term in the numerator can be computed using DAG-model inference (e.g., Kjaerulff in Jordan, 1999). Finally, the posterior term in the denominator can be computed using Gibbs sampling, as we have just described.

Non-Bayesian Approaches

In this section, we consider several commonly used alternatives to the Bayesian approach for structure learning.

One such class of algorithms mimic the search-and-score approach of Bayesian model selection but incorporate a non-Bayesian score. Alternative scores include (1) prediction accuracy on new data, (2) prediction accuracy over cross-validated data sets, and (3) non-Bayesian information criteria such as AIC.

Another class of algorithms for structure learning is the *constraint-based* approach, described by Pearl (2000) and Spirtes, Glymour, and Scheines (2001). In this set of algorithms, statistical tests are performed on the data to determine independence and dependence relationships among the variables. Then, search methods are used to identify one or more models that are consistent with those relationships.

To illustrate this approach, suppose we seek to learn one or more DAG models given data for three finite variables (X_1, X_2, X_3). Assuming each local likelihood is a collection of multinomial distributions, there are 11 possible DAG models that are distinct: (1) a complete model, (2) $X_1 \rightarrow X_2 \rightarrow X_3$, (3) $X_1 \rightarrow X_3 \rightarrow X_2$, (4) $X_2 \rightarrow X_1 \rightarrow X_3$, (5) $X_1 \rightarrow X_2 \leftarrow X_3$, (6) $X_1 \rightarrow X_3 \leftarrow X_2$, (7) $X_2 \rightarrow X_1 \leftarrow X_3$, (8) $X_1 \rightarrow X_2 X_3$, (9) $X_1 \rightarrow X_3 X_2$, (10) $X_2 \rightarrow X_3 X_1$, and (11) $X_1 X_2 X_3$, where $X_i X_j$ means there is no arc between X_i and X_j. There are other possible models that are not listed, but each such model represents a set of distributions that is equivalent to one of the other models

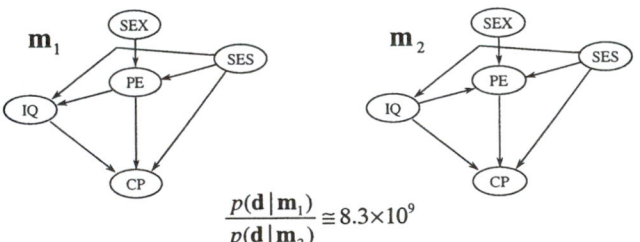

$$\frac{p(\mathbf{d}|\mathbf{m}_1)}{p(\mathbf{d}|\mathbf{m}_2)} \cong 8.3 \times 10^9$$

Figure 1. The a posteriori most likely models.

above. For example, $X_3 \rightarrow X_2 \rightarrow X_1$ and model 2 are distribution equivalent.

Now, suppose that statistical tests applied to the data reveal that the *only* independence relationship is that X_1 and X_3 are independent. Only models 1 and 5 can exhibit only this independence. Furthermore, if we use parameter prior assignments of the form described earlier in this section, then model 1 will exhibit this independence with probability zero. Consequently, we conclude that model 5 is correct (with probability one).

One drawback of the constraint-based approach is that any statistical test will be an approximation for finite data, and errors in the tests may lead the search mechanism to (1) conclude that the found relationships are inconsistent or (2) return erroneous models. One advantage of the approach over most search-and-score methods is that more structures can be considered for a fixed amount of computation, because the results of some statistical tests can greatly constrain model search.

Road Maps: Artificial Intelligence; Learning in Artificial Networks
Background: Graphical Models: Probabilistic Inference
Related Reading: Graphical Models: Parameter Learning

References

Bernardo, J., and Smith, A., 1994, *Bayesian Theory,* New York: Wiley. ◆

Buntine, W., 1991, Theory refinement on Bayesian networks, in *Proceedings of the Seventh Conference on Uncertainty in Artificial Intelligence,* San Mateo, CA: Morgan Kaufmann, pp. 52–60.

Chickering, D., 1996, Learning Bayesian networks is NP-complete, in *Learning from Data* (D. Fisher and H. Lenz, Eds.), New York: Springer-Verlag, pp. 121–130.

Cooper, G., and Herskovits, E., 1992, A Bayesian method for the induction of probabilistic networks from data, *Machine Learn.,* 9:309–347.

Cowell, R., Dawid, A. P., Lauritzen, S., and Spiegelhalter, D., 1999, *Probabilistic Networks and Expert Systems (Statistics for Engineering and Information Science),* New York: Springer-Verlag. ◆

DiCiccio, T., Kass, R., Raftery, A., and Wasserman, L., 1995, *Computing Bayes Factors by Combining Simulation and Asymptotic Approximations,* Technical Report 630, Department of Statistics, Carnegie Mellon University, Pittsburgh, PA.

Heckerman, D., and Geiger, D., 1995, Learning Bayesian networks: A unification for discrete and Gaussian domains, in *Proceedings of the Eleventh Conference on Uncertainty in Artificial Intelligence,* San Mateo, CA: Morgan Kaufmann, pp. 274–284.

Heckerman, D., Geiger, D., and Chickering, D., 1995, Learning Bayesian networks: The combination of knowledge and statistical data, *Machine Learn.,* 20:197–243.

Jordan, M., Ed., 1999, *Learning in Graphical Models,* Cambridge, MA: MIT Press. ◆

Kass, R., and Raftery, A., 1995, Bayes factors, *J. Am. Statist. Assoc.,* 90:773–795. ◆

Lauritzen, S., 1996, *Graphical Models,* Oxford, Engl.: Clarendon Press. ◆

Madigan, D., Raftery, A., Volinsky, C., and Hoeting, J., 1996, Bayesian model averaging, in *Proceedings of the AAAI Workshop on Integrating Multiple Learned Models,* Portland, OR. ◆

Neal, R., 1993, Probabilistic inference using Markov chain Monte Carlo Methods, Technical Report CRG-TR-93-1, Department of Computer Science, University of Toronto.

Pearl, J., Ed., 2000, *Causality: Models, Reasoning, and Inference,* Cambridge, Engl.: Cambridge University Press. ◆

Sewell, W., and Shah, V., 1968, Social class, parental encouragement, and educational aspirations, *Am. J. Sociol.,* 73:559–572.

Spirtes, P., Glymour, C., and Scheines, R., 2001, *Causation, Prediction, and Search,* 2nd ed., Cambridge, MA: MIT Press. ◆

Grasping Movements: Visuomotor Transformations

Giuseppe Rizzolatti and Giacomo Luppino

Introduction

When one attempts to pick up an object, one executes two distinct motor operations. One—reaching—consists of bringing the hand toward an object's location in space, the other—grasping—consists of shaping the hand and fingers in anticipation of the object's size, shape, and orientation (Arbib, 1981; Jeannerod, 1988). This article focuses on grasping. Its aim is to examine where in the cerebral cortex visual information on intrinsic properties of objects is transformed into hand movements and how this transformation occurs.

Motor Areas for Grasping

The agranular frontal cortex of primates consists of several distinct motor areas (Rizzolatti and Luppino, 2001; Picard and Strick, 2001). Their location in the monkey cerebral cortex is shown in Figure 1. Recent data showed that many of them contain distal movement representations (Rizzolatti and Luppino, 2001).

Since the early electrical cortical stimulation experiments, it has been known that the largest and most detailed representation of distal movements is that of the primary motor cortex (F1 or area 4; see Porter and Lemon, 1993). Following lesion of this area, grasping movements, especially those demanding a subtle control of fingers, are lost. The deficit is characterized by a dramatic decrease in force and a loss of the capacity to control individual fingers, but does not affect the mechanisms underlying visuomotor transformation for grasping movements. This view is confirmed by

neurophysiological findings showing that the visual properties (brisk responses to abrupt stimulus presentation) of the few neurons that respond to visual stimuli, do not match those necessary for grip formation.

This last finding raises the problem of which of the areas that have access to the F1 neural machinery also have the visual properties required for organizing grasping movements. Anatomical data and recording studies have shown that this area is F5. This area is richly connected with F1 and many of its neurons respond to the presentation specific visual stimuli (Rizzolatti and Luppino, 2001).

Area F5

Area F5 forms the rostral part of inferior area 6. A fundamental property of F5 is that the discharge of most of its neurons correlates with specific actions (or fragments of a specific action) much better than with elementary movements. A clear instance of this behavior is represented by F5 neurons that discharge when the monkey grasps an object with its right hand, with its left hand, or with its mouth. It is obvious that in this case a description of neuron behavior in terms of elementary movements makes little sense (Rizzolatti et al., 1988).

Using the effective action as classification criterion, F5 neurons were subdivided into various classes. Among them the most represented are "grasping" neurons, "holding" neurons, "tearing" neurons, and "manipulating" neurons. The largest F5 class is related to grasping.

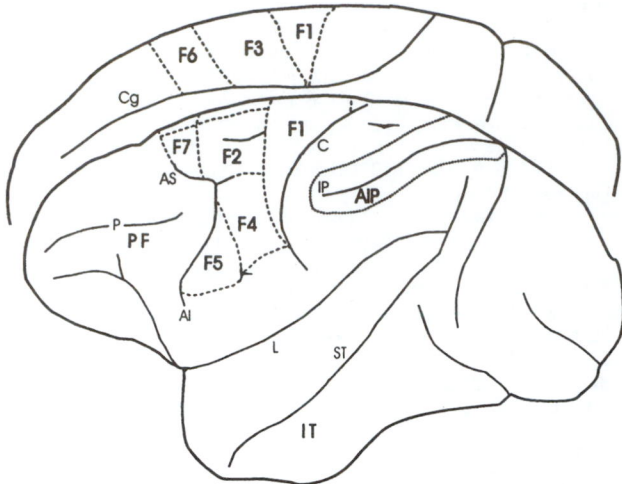

Figure 1. Lateral and mesial views of the monkey cerebral cortex showing the location of the agranular frontal areas and of other cortical areas or sectors referred to in the text. Motor areas in which distal movements are represented are F1, F3, F2, and F5. The intraparietal sulcus (IP) is opened. AI, inferior arcuate sulcus; AS, superior arcuate sulcus; C, central sulcus; Cg, cingulate sulcus; IT, inferotemporal cortex; L, lateral fissure; P, principal sulcus; PF, prefrontal cortex; ST, superior temporal sulcus.

Typically, grasping neurons discharge for actions made with the contralateral as well as the ipsilateral hand. Many of them code specific hand grips. Three basic grip types are extensively represented: precision grip, finger prehension, and whole-hand prehension. Most neurons are selective for one of these types of grasping, the precision grip being the most represented. The temporal relations between neuron discharge and grasping movements vary among neurons. Some of them fire only during the last part of grasping, i.e., during finger flexion. Others start to fire with finger extension and continue to fire during finger flexion. Finally, others are activated in advance of the movement initiation and often cease to discharge only when the object is grasped.

Rizzolatti and co-workers proposed that F5 contains a "vocabulary" of motor acts related to prehension. The "words" of the vocabulary are comprised of populations of neurons related to different motor actions. There are various categories of "words." Some indicate very general commands, e.g., "grasp," "hold," and "tear." Others indicate how the objects have to be grasped, held, or torn (e.g., by precision grip, finger prehension, whole-hand prehension, or their subtypes). Finally, a third group of "words" is concerned with the temporal segments of the actions (e.g., hand aperture, hand closure).

The presence in F5 of a store of "words" or motor schemas (Arbib, 1981) has two important consequences. First, since information is concentrated in relatively few abstract elements, the number of variables to be controlled is much less than it would be if the movements were described in terms of motor neurons or muscles. This solution to the problem of controlling the large number of hand degrees of freedom is remarkably similar to that proposed theoretically (Arbib, Iberall, and Lyons, 1985). Second, the retrieval of the appropriate movement is simplified. Both for internally generated actions and for those emitted in response to an external stimulus, a schema, or a small ensemble of schemas, must be selected. In particular, the retrieval of a movement in response to a visual object is reduced to the task of matching its size and orientation with the appropriate schema.

How can the motor vocabulary of F5 be addressed? The simplest way to examine this issue is to present different types of stimuli—

for example, different objects—and to establish whether the recorded neuron respond to them. Using this approach, "visual" responses are observed in about 20%–30% of F5 neurons. According to the type of stimuli that is effective, two separate classes of neurons have been distinguished. Neurons of the first class (*canonical* neurons) respond to the presentation of graspable objects (Rizzolatti et al., 1988). Neurons of the second class (*mirror* neurons) respond when the monkey sees object-directed actions (Rizzolatti and Luppino, 2001).

The functional properties of canonical neurons and inactivation experiments showed that this class of F5 visuomotor neurons is crucially involved in visuomotor transformations for grasping objects.

The properties of canonical neurons were recently studied in a task in which monkeys were trained to fixate objects of different size and shape and, after a go signal, to grasp them (Murata et al., 1997). The timing of the different phases of the task was such as to allow one to identify the neuron's activity related to object presentation, the preparatory phase preceding the movement, and movement execution. Most neurons were further tested in a task in which monkeys had to fixate an object, but not to grasp it. At the go signal they had only to release a switch. The main result of the experiment was that canonical neurons discharge in response to object presentation even in the absence of any subsequent movement directed toward it. In the majority of neurons the visual discharge was evoked either exclusively by one object or by a small set of objects. Furthermore, the visual responses were evoked only by objects whose size and shape were congruent with the grip coded by the neurons (i.e., neurons visually activated by small objects discharged also selectively during precision grip, while neurons visually activated by large objects, discharged during whole hand prehension).

Recently, a paradigm similar to that described previously was employed to study the effects of inactivation of F5 with muscimol, a GABAergic agonist (Gallese et al., 1997). Small and large inactivations were performed. As a control, in separate sessions, the hand field of F1 was inactivated. The most interesting result was that following F5 inactivations (bank sector of F5) the monkeys were unable to shape the hand according to the intrinsic visual properties of the object. The deficit was particularly evident for small objects, where it was also present following limited inactivations. After large inactivations, however, the prehension of large objects was also affected. An important observation was that the monkeys, in spite of their visuomotor deficit, were still able to grasp and manipulate objects after touching them without any apparent skill impairment. Thus, the execution of individual finger movements was preserved. In contrast, after inactivation of F1 hand field, the monkeys showed a hypotonic paralysis and lack of individual finger movements (Schieber and Poliakov, 1998). Another important difference between F1 and F5 inactivations was that, following F5 inactivation, both hands were affected, not just the hand contralateral to the lesion.

Anterior Intraparietal Area

What is the origin of F5 visual information? Injection of neural tracers in F5 showed that this area receives a strong input from the inferior parietal lobule and, in particular, from an area located in the rostral part of the lateral bank of the intraparietal sulcus—area AIP (Rizzolatti and Luppino, 2001). The functional properties of area AIP have been extensively studied by Sakata and his co-workers (Murata et al., 2000).

The paradigms used by Sakata and colleagues were basically similar to those described for F5. In their initial experiments, monkeys were trained to manipulate four different types of switches, each of which required a peculiar type of grasping. The movements were performed under visual guidance and in the dark. According to each neuron's behavior in the task, neurons were subdivided into three main classes. Neurons of the first class, "motor dominant" neurons, discharged equally well during movements performed in light and in dark. These neurons represented about one-third of the task-related neurons. Neurons of the second class, "visual dominant" neurons, were activated only when the task was performed in the light. They represented about 25% of the studied neurons. Neurons of the third class, "visual and motor" neurons, were less active during movement performed in the dark than in the light. They represented about 40% of the studied neurons.

Neurons belonging to "visual dominant" and "visual and motor" classes typically responded as soon as the object to be grasped was presented. To better study the visual properties of AIP neurons, another series of experiments was carried out by the same authors using a variety of 3D objects. They included spheres, cubes, cones, cylinders, rings, and plates of different sizes and orientations. Furthermore, the neurons were also tested in a condition in which there was no request to act on the presented objects. The results showed that most of the recorded neurons were selective for object shape. Of these, one-third were highly selective, being activated only by one of the six shapes used in the experiment, while half were moderately selective, being activated by two or three different shapes. Many shape-selective neurons were also selective for object size. Finally, in "visual and motor" neurons, a clear congruence was observed between object and motor selectivity.

It is clear from this overview of the functional properties of AIP that the neurons of this area share many common features with F5 neurons. There are also, however, some important differences. First, there are no "visual dominant" neurons in F5. Second, purely motor neurons are much more frequent in F5 than in AIP. Third, most AIP neurons discharge during the whole action leading to the grasping of the objects, often remaining active during the object holding period. In contrast, F5 grasping neurons are typically active only during some of the phases of the grasping/holding action.

Taken together, these data strongly suggest that AIP and F5 form a parieto-frontal circuit devoted to the visuomotor transformation for hand-object interactions (Jeannerod et al., 1995). They predict also that an inactivation of AIP should disrupt the monkey's capacity to preshape the hand and fingers in anticipation of object grasping. This prediction was fully confirmed by experiments in which different sectors of AIP were reversibly inactivated using muscimol microinjections. After inactivation, monkeys showed marked deficits of contralateral hand preshaping without any deficit in arm reaching (Gallese et al., 1997).

Circuit for Grasping in Humans

Earlier brain imaging experiments failed to convincingly demonstrate the existence of a cortical circuit for grasping movements in humans. Recent data by Binkofski et al. (1999) clearly demonstrated that a circuit specifically involved in object manipulation exists also in humans. By using fMRI, they showed that the manipulation of complex objects results in an activation of ventral premotor cortex (BA 44) and of a region in the intraparietal sulcus. If one considers the anatomical location of these areas, and, for area 44, the cytoarchitectonics similarities with F5, it is very likely that this circuit is the human homologue of the monkey circuit formed by F5-AIP.

Discussion

The data described previously indicate that areas AIP and F5 form the key elements in a circuit that transforms visual information on intrinsic properties of objects into grasping movements. Various attempts have been made to explain how AIP and F5 neurons per-

form this transformation (Sakata et al., 1992; Gallese et al., 1997; Fagg and Arbib, 1998).

Common to all these proposals is the idea that "visual dominant" neurons of AIP code the object's intrinsic properties and, then, either directly or via other AIP elements, send this information to specific sets of F5 neurons. F5 neurons transform the received information into patterns of hand movements that are appropriate to the size and shape of the objects to be grasped. Finally, the F5 grasping pattern recruits specific F1 neurons that command grasping execution.

According to Sakata and co-workers, the AIP discharge associated with movements represents a corollary discharge originating in the premotor cortex. Its function is that of creating a reverberatory activity that keeps active AIP neurons. AIP "visual-and-motor" neurons are, therefore, a kind of "memory" that keeps the representation of the object active during the entire movement execution. In this way the representation of the object remains present even when vision of the object is obstructed by the hand movements. Finally, the "motor dominant" neurons would represent an intermediate stage in the transmission of F5 corollary discharge to the AIP "visual-and-motor" neurons.

Sakata's model did not take into consideration the fact that an object may be grasped in several ways and that the chosen grip depends, in addition to the object visual properties, on object semantics and on what the individual who grasps the object wants to do with it. Let us imagine a mug. Once the mug is recognized as a mug, it is grasped by the handle, if one wants to drink from it. However, if one wants to throw the mug at somebody or simply to move it, one will take it by its body or by its upper edge. These possible ways of grasping depend on (1) a preliminary object recognition, and (2) on motor decisions, and obviously not on the visual intrinsic properties of the object. Thus, a more complete model of how F5-AIP circuit works, also requires information (1) from circuits that code object semantics (inferotemporal lobe, IT) and (2) from circuits where decision are taken on what to do. To solve these problems, Fagg and Arbib (1998) proposed that AIP provides F5 not with a single visual description of the object, but with multiple descriptions of the possible way in which a given object may be grasped (affordances). This multitude of possibilities is sent to F5, where the selection of the desired grip is made on the basis of prefrontal inputs that signal the nature of the object as well as the current goals of the organism. Finally, the control exerted by F6 (pre-SMA) on F5 will determine whether the external contingencies allow the action execution.

Fagg and Arbib's model (1998, FARS) is not only physiologically plausible, but has also been computationally implemented. Anatomically, FARS relies heavily on connections between prefrontal cortex and F5. There is evidence, however, that although these connections are very modest, rich connections exist between prefrontal cortex and AIP. Furthermore, AIP, unlike F5, receives a direct input from IT. These findings suggest an alternative possibility, namely that information on object semantics and the goals of the individuals influence AIP rather than F5 neurons. Thus, the fundamental process for selecting an appropriate grip occurs in AIP by biasing those affordances that will lead to the grip appropriate to the individual intention. According to this view, AIP describes several affordances, but information on that bias is able to influence F5. This affordance then activates the F5 neurons for the appropriate grip. The selected action remains a potential action until an appropriate signal comes from F6. A version of the FARS model, modified according to these considerations, is shown in Figure 2.

Road Maps: Mammalian Brain Regions; Mammalian Motor Control
Related Reading: Action Monitoring and Forward Control of Movements; Arm and Hand Movement Control; Eye-Hand Coordination in Reaching Movements; Language Evolution: The Mirror System Hypothesis; Prefrontal Cortex in Temporal Organization of Action

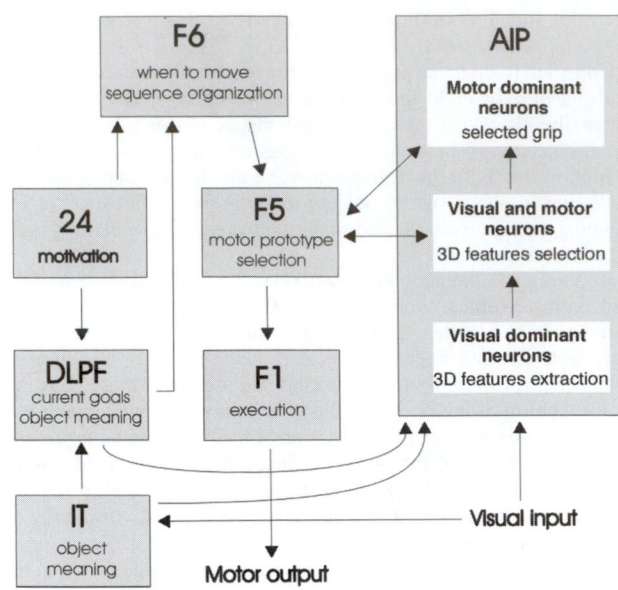

Figure 2. Schematic model of visuomotor transformations for grasping. (From Rizzolatti and Luppino, 2001.)

References

Arbib, M. A., 1981, Perceptual structures and distributed motor control, in *Handbook of Physiology*, sect. 1, vol. 2, part 2 (V. B. Brooks, Ed.), Bethesda. MD: American Physiological Society, pp. 1449–1480.

Arbib, M. A., Iberall, T., and Lyons, D., 1985, Coordinated control programs for movements of the hand, in *Hand Function and the Neocortex* (A. W. Goodman and I. Darian-Smith, Eds.), *Exp. Brain Res.* Suppl 10. Berlin: Springer-Verlag, pp. 111–129.

Binkofski, F., Buccino, G., Posse, S., Seitz, R. J., Rizzolatti, G., and Freund, H.-J., 1999, A fronto-parietal circuit for object manipulation in man: Evidence from an fMRI-study, *Eur. J. Neurosci.*, 11:3276–3286.

Fagg, A. H., and Arbib, M. A., 1998, Modeling parietal-premotor interactions in primate control of grasping, *Neural Networks*, 11:1277–1303.

Gallese, V., Fadiga, L., Fogassi, L., Luppino, G., and Murata, A., 1997, A parietal-frontal circuit for hand grasping movements in the monkey: Evidence from reversible inactivation experiments, in *Parietal lobe contributions to orientation in 3D space* (P. Thier and H.-O. Karnath, Eds.), Heidelberg: Springer, pp. 255–270.

Jeannerod, M., 1988, *The Neural and Behavioral Organization of Goal-Directed Movements*, Oxford: Clarendon.

Jeannerod, M., Arbib, M. A., Rizzolatti, G., and Sakata, H., 1995, Grasping objects: The cortical mechanisms of visuomotor transformation, *Trends Neurosci.*, 18:314–320.

Murata, A., Fadiga, L., Fogassi, L., Gallese, V., Raos, V., and Rizzolatti, G., 1997, Object representation in the ventral premotor cortex (area F5) of the monkey, *J Neurophysiol*, 78:2226–2230.

Murata, A., Gallese, V., Luppino, G., Kaseda, M., and Sakata, H., 2000, Selectivity for the shape, size and orientation of objects in the hand-manipulation-related neurons in the anterior intraparietal (AIP) area of the macaque, *J. Neurophysiol.*, 83:2580–2601.

Picard, N., and Strick, P. L., 2001, Imaging the premotor areas, *Curr. Opin. Neurobiol.*, 11:663–672. ◆

Porter, R., and Lemon, R., 1993, *Corticospinal function and voluntary movement*, Clarendon Press, Oxford, p. 427.

Rizzolatti, G., Camarda, R., Fogassi, L., Gentilucci, M., Luppino, G., and Matelli, M., 1988, Functional organization or inferior area 6 in the macaque monkey, II: Area F5 and the control of distal movements, *Exp. Brain Res.*, 71:491–507.

Rizzolatti, G., and Luppino, G., 2001, The cortical motor system, *Neuron*, 31:889–901. ◆

Sakata, H., Taira, M., Mine, S., and Murata, A., 1992, Hand-movement related neurons or the posterior parietal cortex of the monkey: Their role in visual guidance or hand movements, in *Control of Arm Movement in Space* (R. Caminiti, P. B. Johnson, and Y. Burnod, Eds.), *Exp. Brain Res.* Suppl. 22, Berlin: Springer-Verlag, pp. 185–198.

Schieber, M. H., and Poliakov, A. V., 1998, Partial inactivation of the primary motor cortex hand area: Effects of individuated finger movements, *J. Neurosci.*, 18:9038–9054.

Habituation

Adam S. Bristol, Angela L. Purcell, and Thomas J. Carew

Introduction

Habituation, one of the simplest and most common forms of learning, is typically defined as the progressive decrement in a behavioral response with repeated presentations of the eliciting stimulus. Despite its apparent simplicity, a complete understanding of the underlying neural mechanisms of habituation has not been achieved in any preparation. In this article, we briefly review the fundamental characteristics of habituation and describe several experimental preparations in which the neural basis of habituation has been examined. We conclude by describing attempts to model the habituation process in computational terms, the success and shortcomings of these attempts, and directions for future research.

Characteristics of Habituation

Historically, the unambiguous identification of habituation as a form of learning has been complicated by the necessity of distinguishing it from other causes of response decrement, such as sensory adaptation and motor fatigue. A landmark publication by

Thompson and Spencer (1966) presented nine behavioral criteria for identifying habituation. These criteria have been successfully applied to a wide variety of systems and continue to be used today. They are:

1. Repeated stimuli result in diminishing response (within-session, short-term habituation).
2. After a series of stimuli and a period of rest, the response recovers spontaneously.
3. During repeated series of stimuli separated by spontaneous recovery, habituation occurs more rapidly within each series (savings).
4. The rate and/or magnitude of habituation increases with increases in stimulation frequency.
5. The rate and/or magnitude of habituation decreases with increases in stimulus intensity.
6. When a steady level of habituation has been reached during a series, additional stimuli prolong the time until spontaneous recovery ("subzero" habituation).

7. Habituation to one type of stimulus may result in habituation to other similar stimuli (generalization).
8. The presentation of a strong stimulus different from the habituating stimulus leads to a recovery of the habituated response (dishabituation).
9. Repetition of the dishabituating stimulus leads to successively less dishabituation (habituation of dishabituation).

Two important features of habituation, stimulus generalization and dishabituation (Criteria 7 and 8), are important indicators that the decrease in responding is not due to sensory or effector fatigue. Additionally, the finding that spontaneous recovery occurs more quickly with shorter interstimulus interval (ISI) training (Groves and Thompson, 1970) would not be predicted if sensory adaptation or muscle fatigue were the cause of the response decrement.

Thompson and Spencer's (1966) criteria have been highly influential in the study of habituation, but they have not gone without criticism (for a thorough evaluation, see Hinde, 1970). Moreover, subsequent studies have warranted amendments to these guidelines. First, Davis (1970) questioned the notion that habituation increases with shorter ISIs (Criterion 4) because, within a single training session, training and testing intervals are confounded. That is, when comparing different ISIs (e.g., 2 s and 10 s), both the training and testing intervals for each ISI are different because the response to each stimulus serves as both a training trial and a measure of behavioral habituation. When he controlled for differences in testing conditions, Davis (1970) found that *longer* ISIs resulted in greater and longer-lasting retention, although the rate of habituation was faster with short ISI. This is consistent with the finding that spontaneous recovery occurs more rapidly after short ISIs than long ISIs (Groves and Thompson, 1970) and with the general notion that massed training produces inferior learning relative to spaced training.

Second, the Thompson and Spencer criteria did not distinguish between short-term and long-term forms of habituation. Criterion 3 states that the rate of habituation increases across repeated training sessions, a form of "savings." However, the criteria do not reflect another common feature of multiple habituation trials, namely, that the first response of each repeated session is often progressively diminished, indicating a longer-lasting retention of habituation across sessions. Importantly, short- and long-term forms of habituation have been experimentally dissociated in a number of preparations, including *Aplysia, C. elegans*, crab, and rat.

The third amendment to the Thompson and Spencer criteria comes from work by Christoffersen (1997), who recently conducted a comparative analysis of the kinetics of short-term habituation across a wide variety of species and behaviors. He noted that, despite variability in response types, there is a characteristic learning curve for within-session habituation consisting of a rapid and pronounced early phase of habituation resulting from only a few response activations (from 5 to 15) and a second, slowly declining phase. However, he found that some behaviors do not seem to have a rapid, early phase and that many more stimuli (from 50 to several hundreds) are required to achieve the same absolute level of response decrement. The kinetics of the learning curves could be fitted by the equation:

$$H_{n+1} = H_n(1 + P_n) \qquad (1)$$

in which H_n is the degree of habituation of a normalized reflex before the nth stimulus and P_n is a factor that determines the change in H from stimulus n to $n + 1$. The factor P_n decreases as habituation increases, such that

$$P_n = P_1(H_{max} - H_n) \qquad (2)$$

where H_{max} is the maximum amount of habituation. Interestingly, when Christoffersen (1997) solved for the plasticity parameter, P_1, for numerous cases of habituation, he found that it was many times smaller for slowly habituating reflexes than for rapidly habituating reflexes, suggesting two distinct types of habituation. Thus, this computational approach to examining habituation extends Thompson and Spencer's criteria by indicating that not all reflexes habituate with the same rapidity.

Experimental Preparations and Neural Mechanisms Underlying Habituation

Habituation has been extensively studied in invertebrate preparations, in particular the defensive reflexes of the mollusk *Aplysia* and crayfish, as their relatively simple and accessible nervous systems provide the opportunity to study the neural basis of behavior in considerable detail (see INVERTEBRATE MODELS OF LEARNING: *APLYSIA* AND *HERMISSENDA*). Importantly, these preparations meet many of the criteria put forth by Thompson and Spencer and show short- and long-term forms of habituation. Reflex habituation has also been studied in vertebrate preparations, first in the scratch reflex of the dog and later in the vestibulo-ocular reflex (VOR) in goldfish, and the prey-catching orienting response in frog. (See SCRATCH REFLEX, VESTIBULO-OCULAR REFLEX, and VISUOMOTOR COORDINATION IN FROG AND TOAD for more discussion.)

Neurophysiological studies in invertebrates examining the mechanisms underlying behavioral habituation have led to the widespread notion that habituation results from homosynaptic depression (the activity-dependent decrement in synaptic efficacy) of one or more synapses in a reflex circuit (i.e., an intrinsic mechanism). There are numerous examples showing that synaptic depression occurs during or as a result of a habituation process and that the kinetics of synaptic depression are similar to those of behavioral habituation (for a review, see Christoffersen, 1997). However, even in *Aplysia*, where synaptic depression has been firmly linked to habituation, there is evidence suggesting that other mechanisms may contribute. For example, Stopfer and Carew (1996) found that *facilitation* of the tail sensorimotor synapses accompanied habituation of the tail-elicited siphon withdrawal reflex, suggesting that plasticity at interneuronal sites underlies habituation of this reflex.

Such an "intrinsic" mechanism, where plasticity occurs within the circuit mediating the behavior, is the most popular model, but cases in which habituation also involves modulation from cells extrinsic to the circuit (e.g., heterosynaptic depression) have also been reported. For example, whereas homosynaptic depression of presynaptic sensory cells has been found to contribute to habituation of the crayfish tail-flip reflex, more recent investigations have implicated an increase in tonic descending inhibition as an additional mechanism of habituation in this system (Krasne and Teshiba, 1995). Thus, even within the same animal, homosynaptic and heterosynaptic mechanisms may contribute to habituation in different response systems.

Additional evidence of "top-down" processing in habituation has come from studies of higher vertebrate systems. Frogs with lesions of the medial pallium, a homolog of the mammalian hippocampus, show no habituation of the orienting response to repeated visual stimuli (Finkenstadt, 1989). In a different behavioral paradigm, decerebrate rats failed to show long-term habituation of acoustic startle despite exhibiting short-term habituation (Leaton, Casella, and Borszcz, 1985). These data suggest that short-term and long-term forms of habituation may develop by separate mechanisms, with short-term habituation occurring within the circuit mediating the reflex (perhaps by homosynaptic depression) and long-term habituation occurring via descending modulatory input (perhaps by heterosynaptic depression or tonic synaptic inhibition). Experiments in *Aplysia* have indicated a morphological correlate of long-term habituation: a decreased number of synaptic endings (Bailey and Chen, 1983).

The experiments of Sokolov (1960) on the orienting reflex in humans demonstrate the complex "top-down" control of habituation. For instance, he showed that habituation of the orienting response did not generalize to other stimuli but was stimulus specific, such that any change in the stimulus parameters (e.g., intensity, duration) resulted in a reinstatement of the response (dishabituation). His observation that even *decreases* in stimulus intensities resulted in dishabituation argued against homosynaptic depression of sensory processing. In an incredible demonstration of top-down processing, he showed that habituated responses spontaneously recovered during sleep, became resistant to rehabituation during sleep, and returned to the habituated state when the subject reawakened. These data led him to propose a "comparator theory" of habituation, in which an internal representation, or "template," is created in the brain, to which subsequent external stimuli are compared. Stimuli that "match" the internal representation are habituated, whereas stimuli that are "mismatches" evoke a response (i.e., dishabituation). Sokolov (1960) proposed a neural model of habituation based on his theory in which the cortex, the site of the comparator mechanism, inhibits the reticular formation and, hence, the physiological correlates of the orienting response.

In summary, habituation has been linked to homosynaptic depression within the reflex circuit in a variety of systems. Accordingly, homosynaptic depression continues to be widely regarded as the cellular mechanism underlying habituation, especially short-term forms. However, considerable evidence demonstrating the importance of extrinsic modulatory processes, such as descending cortical input in mammals and tonic inhibition in crayfish, suggests that some forms of habituation may be due to mechanisms both intrinsic and extrinsic to the reflex circuit.

Computational Models of Habituation

Habituation is particularly well-suited for a computational analysis. First, the habituated response is a repeatable behavior, thus allowing for a detailed analysis of the kinetics of learning (i.e., ISI function, trials to criterion, etc.). Second, the habituated behavior is, in many cases, an evoked reflex that relies on a relatively simple neural circuit; for example, in invertebrate preparations such as *Aplysia* and crayfish, many of the individual neural elements in the reflex circuit have been identified. Third, the general underlying assumption guiding computational modeling—namely, that network output is linked to circuit architecture, cellular properties, and synaptic plasticity—also guides physiological studies of behavior, thus allowing the results of computational and biological analyses of habituation to inform each other.

Most attempts at modeling habituation have been top-down and have focused either implicitly or explicitly on short-term, within-session habituation typically involving synaptic plasticity-like learning mechanisms. For example, Horn (1967) put forth a remarkably modern theoretical network model based on synaptic mechanisms very similar to homosynaptic depression and heterosynaptic facilitation. In his model, various features of habituation and dishabituation are accounted for by independent decrementing and facilitating processes, foreshadowing the dual process theory of Groves and Thompson (1970). Stanley (1976) took a similar approach, but added mathematical complexity to his modeling of habituation of the hindlimb flexion reflex in spinal cats. He posited a circuit architecture consisting of two independent pathways, (1) a direct pathway between input and output capable of use-dependent decrement and (2) an indirect pathway with an additional intercalated element between input and output capable of use-dependent enhancement. This simple organization captured the essence of the dual process theory: repetitive low-intensity stimulation of

the direct pathway resulted in synaptic decrement, whereas moderate- and high-intensity stimulation increasingly recruited the indirect, facilitatory pathway, leading to dishabituation (and sensitization). Synaptic change was simulated using a first-order differential equation:

$$\tau \frac{dy(t)}{dt} = \alpha(y0 - y(t)) - S(t) \tag{3}$$

where $y0$ is the initial synaptic strength, $S(t)$ is the effect of external stimulation (which could be habituating or sensitizing), τ is a time constant governing the rate of habituation, and α determines the rate of recovery. This model yielded exponential learning curves typical of the short-term habituation data with varying intensity stimulation but could not account for long-term habituation.

Wang and Arbib (1992) modified the traditional first-order differential equation to include an activity-gated input and included a second equation that, by regulating the rate of recovery, captured the transition from short-term to long-term habituation in their model of habituation of prey-catching behavior in frogs. These two equations took the form:

$$\tau \frac{dy(t)}{dt} = \alpha z(y0 - y(t)) - \beta y(t)S(t) \tag{4}$$

$$\frac{dz(t)}{dt} = \gamma z(t)(z(t) - 1)S(t) \tag{5}$$

where the second term in Equation 4 constitutes activity-gated input with β as a rate parameter. In Equation 5, which regulates recovery, variable $z(t)$ generates an inverse S-shaped curve under constant stimulation $S(t)$. When $z(t)$ is large after few trials, recovery is rapid. In contrast, when $z(t)$ is small, as it is after many trials, recovery is slow. Thus, as habituation progresses, recovery becomes more prolonged, producing longer-lasting habituation. This approach yielded simulated results that resembled experimental data for short recovery times (minutes) but underestimated forgetting for longer recovery times (hours).

Recently, Anastasio (2001) presented a computational model of habituation of the goldfish VOR to sinusoidal stimulation that is conceptually similar to the comparator theory of Sokolov (1960). Structurally, the model is based on a simplified view of vestibular neuroanatomy: a direct excitatory path through the brainstem (BS) to the output of the circuit, the vestibular nucleus (VN), and an inhibitory and plastic indirect path through the vestibulocerebellum (VC) (Figure 1). Behavioral VOR habituation shows frequency-specificity and nonlinearity; the most pronounced habituation occurs at the peak stimulus amplitude and does not occur at the same rate for the two directions of sinusoidal head rotations. These features suggested that the habituation mechanism does not treat the stimulus as a continuous function but as discrete units that habituate independently. Thus, a primary component of the model is that the sinusoidal stimulus is partitioned into segments or patterns. In the model, habituation occurs because of a pattern correlation mechanism in which the VC compares the similarity (the correlation) of the current stimulus (the pattern) with the representation of previous stimuli (a history vector stored in the VC) and weights the inhibition of the VN according to the maximum correlation using the equation:

$$y(t) = x(t) - w_k r_k(t) \tag{6}$$

where $y(t)$ is the output of the VC at time step t, $x(t)$ is the value of the input pattern, and w_k is the weight value corresponding to the pattern having the maximum correlation, r_k, with the history vector. After filtering and dithering the simulation output to mimic neuromuscular dynamics, Anastasio (2001) showed that the model can accurately account for the features of behavioral VOR habituation, thus providing a computational mechanism for producing

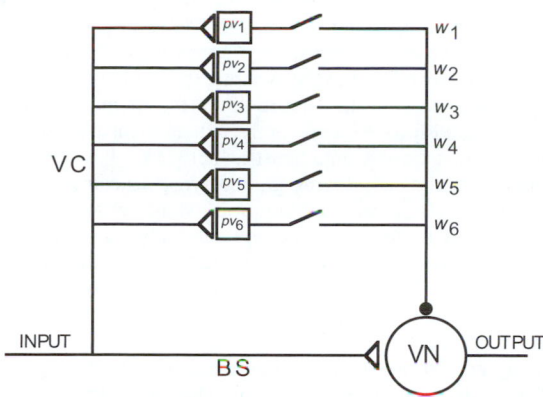

Figure 1. Anastasio's (2001) pattern correlation model of VOR habituation. Open triangles represent excitatory connections. Solid circles represent inhibitory connections. BS, brainstem; VC, vestibulocerebellar nucleus; VN, vestibular nucleus. Pattern vectors and their respective weights are represented by pv_i and w_i ($i = 1, 2, \ldots, 6$). (Adapted from Anastasio, T. J., 2001, A pattern correlation model of vestibulo-ocular reflex habituation, *Neural Netw.*, 14:1–22. Reproduced with permission.)

discontinuous, nonlinear output plasticity from a continuous, elementary function input. Moreover, the pattern correlation model achieves computational instantiations of a Sokolov-like comparator mechanism by storing and matching a history vector to subsequently present stimuli.

Discussion

Habituation continues to be an attractive paradigm in the study of the neural basis of learning and memory. Experimental studies have identified at least two important neural mechanisms of habituation, homosynaptic depression within the reflex circuit and extrinsic descending modulatory input. Although the computational models of habituation described above have achieved success in accounting for important aspects of behavioral habituation in some systems, much work remains to be done in simulating processing in known biological circuitry. There are several well-studied model systems conducive to a biologically realistic computational analysis, such as the tail-flip escape reflex in crayfish and the tap-elicited withdrawal reflex in the nematode. In each of these cases, much of the underlying neural circuitry is known. Habituation in the crayfish tail-flip reflex, due to both afferent depression as well as descending inhibition, is attractive because it offers the opportunity to analyze the interaction and cooperativity of mechanisms intrinsic and extrinsic to the reflex circuit. The nematode *C. elegans* is attractive because of the possibility of a genetic analysis of habituation (see

Rose and Rankin, 2001). Progress in understanding the computational processes of habituation in complex vertebrates and mammals will require greater knowledge of underlying circuitry and neurophysiology. The goal of future work, both experimental and computational, will be to account for the intriguing complexity of this not-so-simple form of learning.

Road Map: Neural Plasticity
Related Reading: Invertebrate Models of Learning: *Aplysia* and *Hermissenda*; Visuomotor Coordination in Frog and Toad

References

Anastasio, T. J., 2001, A pattern correlation model of vestibulo-ocular reflex habituation, *Neural Netw.*, 14:1–22.
Bailey, C. H., and Chen, M., 1983, Morphological basis of long-term habituation and sensitization in *Aplysia, Science*, 220:91–93.
Christoffersen, G. R. J., 1997, Habituation: Events in the history of its characterization and linkage to synaptic depression. A new proposed kinetic criterion for its identification, *Prog. Neurobiol.*, 53:45–66. ◆
Davis, M., 1970, Effects of interstimulus interval length and variability on startle-response habituation in the rat, *J. Comp. Physiol. Psychol.*, 72:177–192.
Finkenstadt, T., 1989, Stimulus-specific habituation in toads: 2DG and lesion studies, in *Visuomotor Coordination: Amphibians, Comparisons, Models, and Robots* (J.-P. Ewert and M. A. Arbib, Eds.), New York: Plenum Press, pp. 767–797.
Groves, P. M., and Thompson, R. F., 1970, Habituation: A dual process theory, *Psychol. Rev.*, 77:419–450.
Hinde, R. A., 1970, Behavioral habituation, in *Short-Term Changes in Neural Activity and Behavior* (G. Horn and R. A. Hinde, Eds.), Cambridge, Engl.: Cambridge University Press, pp. 3–40. ◆
Horn, G., 1967, Neuronal mechanisms of habituation, *Nature*, 215:707–711.
Krasne, F. B., and Teshiba, T. M., 1995, Habituation of an invertebrate escape reflex due to modulation by higher centers rather than local events, *Proc. Natl. Acad. Sci. USA*, 92:3362–3366.
Leaton, R. N., Casella, J. V., and Borszcz, G. S., 1985, Short-term and long-term habituation of the acoustic startle response in chronic decerebrate rats, *Behav. Neurosci.*, 99:901–912.
Rose, J. K., and Rankin, C. H., 2001, Analyses of habituation in *Caenorhabditis elegans, Learn. Mem.*, 8:63–69.
Sokolov, E. N., 1960, Neuronal models and the orienting reflex, in *The Central Nervous System and Behavior* (M. A. B. Brazier, Ed.), Madison, NJ: Madison, pp. 187–276. ◆
Stanley, J. C., 1976, Computer simulation of a model of habituation, *Nature*, 261:146–148.
Stopfer, M., and Carew, T. J., 1996, Heterosynaptic facilitation of tail sensory neuron synaptic transmission during habituation in induced tail and siphon withdrawal reflexes of *Aplysia, J. Neurosci.*, 16:4933–4948.
Thompson, R. F., and Spencer, W. A., 1966, Habituation: A model phenomenon for the study of neuronal substrates of behavior, *Psychol. Rev.*, 73:16–43. ◆
Wang, D., and Arbib, M. A., 1992, Modeling the dishabituation hierarchy: The role of the primordial hippocampus, *Biol. Cybern.*, 67:535–544.

Half-Center Oscillators Underlying Rhythmic Movements

Andrew A. V. Hill, Stephen D. Van Hooser, and Ronald L. Calabrese

Introduction

The half-center oscillator model was first proposed by T. Grahm Brown (1914) to account for the observation that spinal cats could

produce stepping movements even when all dorsal roots were severed, thereby eliminating sensory feedback from the animals' motion. He envisioned pools of interneurons controlling flexor and extensor motor neurons (the half-centers) that had reciprocal inhibitory connections, and that were capable of sustaining alternating oscillatory activity if properly activated. In the model, he assumed that the duration of reciprocal inhibition was limited by some intrinsic factor, e.g., synaptic fatigue, and that the neuron pools (half-centers) showed rebound excitation. In the intervening years we have learned that almost all rhythmic movements of animals are programmed in part by central pattern-generating networks that comprise neural oscillators (MOTOR PATTERN GENERATION; SPINAL CORD OF LAMPREY: GENERATION OF LOCOMOTOR PATTERNS; CRUSTACEAN STOMATOGASTRIC SYSTEM; and LOCOMOTION, VERTEBRATE). In many of these motor pattern-generating networks, in both vertebrates and invertebrates, reciprocal inhibitory synaptic interactions between neurons or groups of neurons are found (Calabrese, 1995). We are beginning to understand how the intrinsic membrane properties of the component neurons interact with reciprocal inhibition to initiate and sustain oscillation in these networks.

Theoretical Framework

A theoretical framework for understanding how reciprocally inhibitory neurons oscillate (i.e. how half-center oscillators work) was developed by Wang and Rinzel (1992) (OSCILLATORY AND BURSTING PROPERTIES OF NEURONS). Their model neurons are minimal. Each contains a synaptic conductance that is a sigmoidal function of presynaptic membrane potential with a set threshold and instantaneous kinetics, a constant leak conductance, and a voltage-gated postinhibitory rebound current, I_{pir}. I_{pir} was originally envisioned to be a T-like Ca^{2+} current (low-threshold, inactivating), but its expression in the model can also accommodate an h current (hyperpolarization activated inward current) (Wang and Rinzel, 1992) or a Ca^{2+} dependent K^+ current (Grillner et al., 2000). Two different modes of oscillation appear in the model, "release" and "escape" (Wang and Rinzel, 1992). For the release mode to occur, the synaptic threshold must be above the steady state membrane potential of the uninhibited neurons. In the release mode, the inactivation of I_{pir} erodes the depolarized or active phase of a neuron so that it falls below threshold for synaptic transmission. Consequently, its partner is released from inhibition and rebounds into the active depolarized state. For the escape mode to occur the synaptic threshold must be below the steady-state voltage of the neurons when uninhibited. This condition can be accomplished simply by increasing g_{pir}. In the escape mode, once inactivation of I_{pir} is removed by the hyperpolarization associated with inhibition, it activates and overcomes the maintained synaptic current so that the neuron escapes into the active phase and thus inhibits its partner.

Skinner, Kopell, and Marder (1994) have extended this analysis using similar model neurons based on the Morris-Lecar equations (low-threshold noninactivating inward current and delayed rectifier current) with a synaptic conductance, which is a steep sigmoidal function of presynaptic membrane potential with a set threshold and instantaneous kinetics. Such model neurons, like the Wang and Rinzel neurons, oscillate between a depolarized plateau and a sustained inhibitory trough. Each of the two modes of oscillation can be further differentiated depending on whether the escape or release is intrinsic or synaptic. If the release is due to a cessation of synaptic transmission (crossing synaptic threshold), it is synaptic release, but if it is due to termination (deactivation of the inward current, activation of the delayed rectifier, or both) of the depolarized plateau, it is intrinsic release. If the escape is due to the commencement of synaptic transmission (crossing synaptic threshold), it is synaptic escape, but if it is due to expression of the depolarized phase (crossing plateau threshold), it is intrinsic escape. Varying the synaptic threshold causes transitions between the modes.

These theoretical studies have been corroborated by hybrid systems studies in which artificial reciprocal inhibitory synapses were introduced between crustacean stomatogastric neurons that are nor-mally unconnected by using dynamic clamp (Sharp, Skinner, and Marder, 1996). To obtain robust oscillations an artificial h current was also added. By adjusting the synaptic threshold of the artificial synapses it was possible to capture all of the richness of the dynamic systems analysis. More recently, a theoretical analysis, based on work in crustacean stomatogastric networks, has shown that even passive neurons employing graded synapses can generate oscillation in the half-center configuration (Manor et al., 1999). Although the models used in the theoretical analyses are simplistic, the major insights that they impart can be transferred to biological neurons, which are connected by simplistic artificial synapses. Real neurons display more complicated intrinsic membrane properties and plastic synaptic interactions that may blur the conclusions of these analyses, but nevertheless they serve as a useful organizing point for the exploration of richer biological systems.

Leech Heartbeat

This review will now focus on the motor pattern generating network that controls heartbeat in the leech. Progress has been made in understanding the role reciprocal inhibitory synaptic interactions and membrane properties play in generating oscillations by combining experimental analyses with realistic modeling.

A network of seven bilateral pairs of segmental heart (HN) interneurons produces rhythmic activity (at about 0.1 Hz) that paces segmental heart motor neurons, which in turn drive the two hearts. The synaptic connections among the interneurons and from the interneurons to the motor neurons are inhibitory. The first four pairs of heart interneurons control the timing of the network. The timing oscillation is dominated by the activity of the third and fourth pairs of heart interneurons. Reciprocally inhibitory synapses between these bilateral pairs of oscillator interneurons, combined with their ability to escape from inhibition and begin firing, pace the oscillation (Figure 1A). Thus, each of these two reciprocally inhibitory heart interneuron pairs can each be considered an elemental half-center oscillator. The first two pairs of heart interneurons act as coordinating fibers, serving to link these two elemental oscillators (Figure 1B).

Several ionic currents have been identified in single electrode voltage-clamp studies that contribute to the activity of oscillator heart interneurons (Calabrese, Nadim, and Olsen, 1995). These include, in addition to the fast Na^+ current that mediates spikes, two low-threshold Ca^{2+} currents [one rapidly inactivating (I_{CaF}) and one slowly inactivating (I_{CaS})], three outward currents [a fast transient K^+ current (I_A) and two delayed rectifier-like K^+ currents, one inactivating (I_{K1}), and one persistent (I_{K2})], a hyperpolarization-activated inward current (I_h) (mixed Na^+/K^+, $E_{rev} = -20$ mV), a low-threshold persistent Na^+ current (I_P) and a leakage current (I_L). The inhibition between oscillator interneurons consists of a graded component that is associated with the low-threshold Ca^{2+} currents and a spike-mediated component that appears to be mediated by a high-threshold Ca^{2+} current. Spike-mediated transmission varies in amplitude throughout a burst according to the baseline level of depolarization (Olsen and Calabrese, 1996). Graded transmission wanes during a burst owing to the inactivation of low-threshold Ca^{2+} currents.

Much of this biophysical data has been incorporated into a detailed conductance-based model of an elemental (two-cell) oscillator (Nadim et al., 1995, Hill et al., 2001). This model uses standard Hodgkin-Huxley representations of each voltage-gated current. Synaptic transmission in the model is complex. A spike-triggered alpha-function is used describe the postsynaptic conductance associated each action potential and the maximal conductance reached is a function of the past membrane potential to reflect the fact that spike-mediated transmission varies in amplitude throughout a burst according to the baseline level of depolarization. Graded

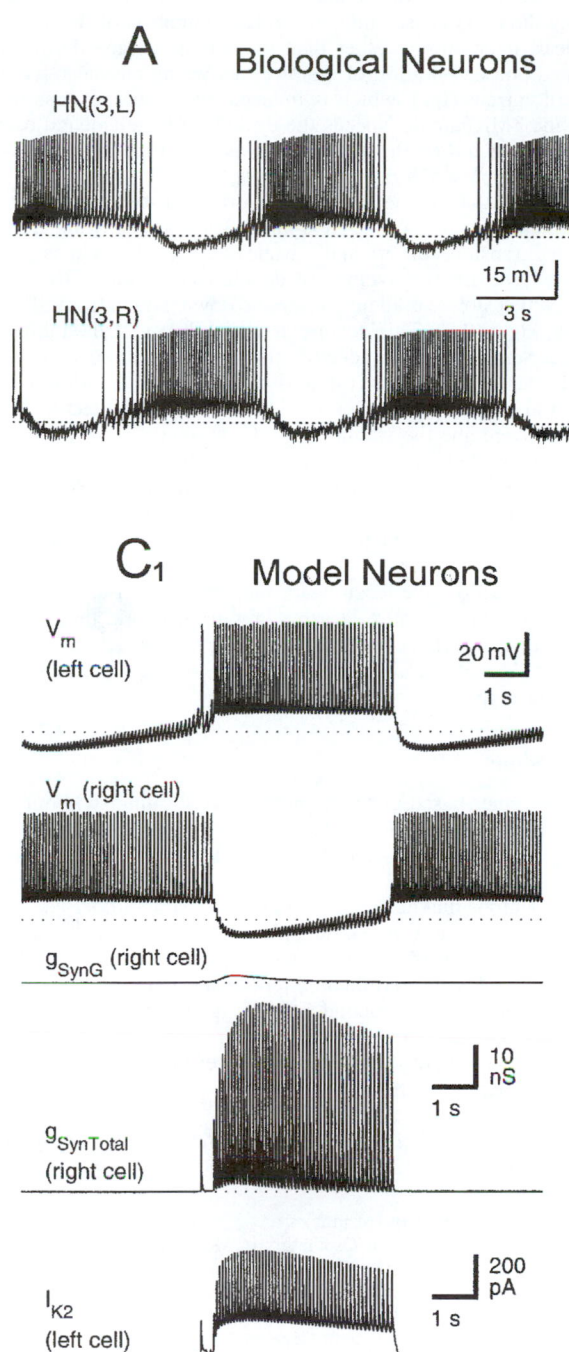

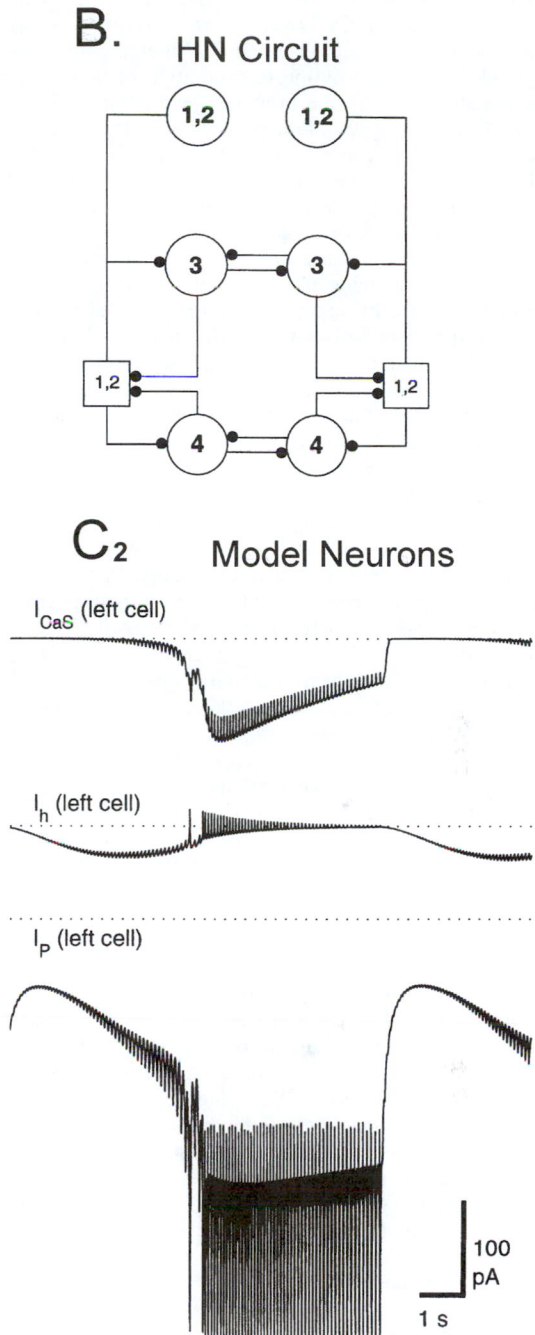

Figure 1. *A*, Simultaneous intracellular recordings showing the normal rhythmic activity of two reciprocally inhibitory heart (HN) interneurons that compose a half-center oscillator in an isolated ganglion preparation. Heart interneurons are indexed by body side (R, L) and ganglion number. *B*, Circuit diagram showing inhibitory synaptic connections among the HN interneurons of the timing network. Coordinating neurons HN(1) and HN(2) are functionally equivalent and are lumped together in the diagram. The HN(1) and HN(2) neurons receive synaptic inputs, initiate action potentials, and make synaptic outputs at sites located in the third and fourth ganglia (open squares). *C1–C2*, Synaptic conductances and some major intrinsic currents that are active during a single cycle of the third-generation model of a two-cell HN interneuron oscillator (half-center). The graded synaptic conductance (g_{SynG}) is shown at the same scale as the total synaptic conductance ($g_{SynTotal}$), which is the sum of the graded and spike-mediated conductances. The slow calcium current (I_{CaS}), the hyperpolarization-activated current (I_h), and the persistent sodium current (I_P) are shown to the same scale. Note that I_P is active throughout the entire cycle period (Hill and Calabrese, unpublished). In *A* and *C* dashed lines indicate −50 mV in voltage traces, 0 nA in current traces, and 0 nS in conductance traces.

synaptic transmission is represented by a synaptic transfer function, which relates postsynaptic conductance (the result of transmitter release) to presynaptic Ca^{2+} build-up and decline, via low-threshold Ca^{2+} currents and a Ca^{2+} removal mechanism, respectively. The model is now in it fouth generation (Hill et al., 2001), having been upgraded each time by the incorporation of new data from experiments suggested by the previous generation of the model (Olsen and Calabrese, 1996). Free parameters in the model are the maximal conductance ($gmax_{ion}$) for each current (voltage-gated or synaptic). The $gmax_{ion}$s were adjusted to be close to the average observed experimentally. The reversal potential, E_{ion}, for each current was determined experimentally and they were considered fixed. Final selection of parameters to form a canonical model was dictated by model behavior under control conditions, passive response of the model to hyperpolarizing current pulses, and reaction of the model to current perturbations. The model cells were tuned by adjusting leak parameters (E_{leak} and $gmax_{leak}$) so that they fire tonically when all inhibition between them was blocked. This tuning was chosen because under conditions of our experiments, which use sharp microelectrodes for recordings, the neurons fire tonically when synaptically isolated with bicuculline (Schmidt and Calabrese, 1992). Recent unpublished work (Gaudry, Cymbalyuk, and Calabrese, Department of Biology, Emory University) suggest that oscillator heart interneurons burst endogenously when isolated with bicuculline. Because the cells must be recorded extracellularly to reveal this bursting, we hypothesize that their bursting behavior is very sensitive to leak parameters that are altered with intracellular recording methods.

The canonical model generates activity, which closely approximates that observed for an elemental half-center oscillator (Figure 1C). Analysis of current flows during this activity (Figure 1C) indicates that graded transmission occurs only at the beginning of the inhibitory period due to inactivation of the low-threshold Ca^{2+} currents that mediate this inhibition. Thus, graded inhibition helps turn off the antagonist neuron, but sustained inhibition of the antagonist neuron is all spike-mediated. The inward currents in the model neurons act to overcome this inhibition and force a transition to burst phase of oscillation. I_P is active throughout the activity cycle, providing a persistent excitatory drive to the system. I_h is slowly activated by the hyperpolarization-associated inhibition, adding a delayed inward current that drives further activation of I_P and eventually the low-threshold Ca^{2+} currents (I_{CaS} and I_{CaF}). These regenerative currents support burst formation. I_P, because it does not inactivate, provides steady depolarization to sustain spiking, while the low-threshold Ca^{2+} currents help force the transition to the burst phase but inactivate as the burst proceeds, thus spike frequency slowly wanes during the burst. Outward currents also play important roles, especially the I_Ks. I_{K2}, which activates and deactivates relatively slowly and does not inactivate, regulates the amplitude of the depolarization that underlies the burst, while I_{K1}, which activates and deactivates relatively quickly and inactivates, controls spike frequency.

Increasing $gmax_{SynS}$ (the maximal spike-mediated synaptic conductance) in the model slows the oscillation while reducing $gmax_{SynS}$ speeds the oscillation. Under canonical conditions graded transmission is suppressed (Nadim et al., 1995). Analysis of state variables (m and h) for low-threshold Ca^{2+} currents indicates that deinactivation of these currents is not effective during the inhibitory period. In the canonical model cells, as in the real cells, the potential for prolonged and intense graded transmission is revealed on rebound from a hyperpolarizing pulse.

The period of the oscillation is sensitive to the level of $gmax_h$, as would be predicted from its key role in forcing the transition from the inhibitory phase to the burst phase. Decreasing $gmax_h$ from canonical levels slows the oscillation proportionately, while increasing it speeds the oscillations. In contrast, increasing $gmax$ of I_P, the other inward current active during the inhibited phase,

slows the oscillation and decreasing $gmax_P$ speeds the oscillation. These observations indicate that the predominate effect of Ip is to prolong the burst phase and concomitant inhibition of the antagonist heart interneuron, rather than to promote escape during the inhibited phase. Addition of a slowly activating and deactivating outward current (I_{KF}), which is induced by the endogenous neuropeptide FMRFamide, speeds the cycling of the elemental oscillator model as it does in the biological oscillator interneurons (Nadim and Calabrese, 1997).

It appears that in the heart interneuron half-center oscillators forces that promote both escape and release are at work. Spike-mediated transmission gradually wanes during a burst because of the slowly declining envelope of depolarization during the burst phase, which slows spike frequency and down modulates IPSP amplitude (Figure 1C). This decline in the inhibition of the inhibited cell represents a release. Indeed, if this decline is eliminated in the model by eliminating inactivation from I_{CaS}, then oscillations cease (Hill et al., 2001). Nevertheless, whenever I_h is sufficiently activated to overcome the waning synaptic current, a transition from the inactive state to the active state occurs, and the "trigger point" for this release is determined by $gmax_h$, which is consistent with an escape mechanism (Hill et al., 2001). Thus this half-center oscillator is not easily categorized, but the theoretical comparisons have been illuminating.

To fully explore the leech heart interneurons half-center model and a model of the entire heartbeat timing network, they can be downloaded from http://calabreselx.biology.emory.edu by anonymous ftp. Various UNIX-based operating systems, including LINUX, are supported.

Conclusions

The half-center-based pattern generators controlling swimming in the pelagic mollusk *Clione* (Arshavsky et al., 1993), in tadpoles (Xenopus) (Roberts et al., 1998), and in lampreys (Grillner et al., 2000), which have also been extensively analyzed and modeled, employ neurons that have pacemaking or bursting properties. Both the *Clione* and the *Xenopus* tadpole swim oscillators appears to operate in the intrinsic release mode (Arshavsky et al., 1993). "Spike" (active state) termination terminates inhibition and allows the antagonist cell to rebound into the active state. Perhaps this mode is more suited to the operational frequency range of these oscillators, which are some ten times faster (about 1 Hz) than the leech heartbeat oscillator.

Acknowledgments. Research in the authors' lab was supported by NIH grant NS24072.

Road Map: Motor Pattern Generators
Related Reading: Chains of Oscillators in Motor and Sensory Systems; Crustacean Stomatogastric System; Locomotion, Invertebrate; Locomotion, Vertebrate; Locust Flight: Components and Mechanisms in the Motor; Oscillatory and Bursting Properties of Neurons; Sensorimotor Interactions and Central Pattern Generators

References

Arshavsky, Y. I., Orlovsky, G. N., Panchin, Y. V., Roberts, A., and Soffe, S. R., 1993, Neuronal control of swimming locomotion: Analysis of the pteropod mollusc Clione and embryos of the amphibian Xenopus, *TINS*, 16:227–233. ◆

Brown, T. G., 1914, On the nature of the fundamental activity of the nervous centres; together with an analysis of the conditioning of rhythmic activity in progression, and a theory of the evolution of function in the nervous system, *J. Physiol.* (Lond.), 48:18–46.

Calabrese, R. L., 1995, Oscillation in motor pattern generating networks, *Curr. Opin. Neurobio.*, 5:816–823.

Calabrese, R. L., Nadim F., and Olsen Ø. H., 1995, Heartbeat control in the medicinal leech: a model system for understanding the origin, coordination, and modulation of rhythmic motor patterns, *J. Neurobiol.*, 27:390–402.

Grillner, S., Cangiano, L., Hu, G-Y., Thompson, R., Hill, R., and Wallen, P., 2000, The intrinsic function of a motor system—from ion channels to networks and behavior, *Brain Res.*, 886:224–236. ◆

Hill, A. A. V., Lu, J., Masino, M. A., Olsen, Ø. H., and Calabrese, R. L., 2001, A model of a segmental oscillator in the leech heartbeat neuronal network, *J. Compu. Neurosci.*, 10:281–302.

Manor, Y., Nadim, F., Epstein, S., Ritt, J., Marder, E., and Kopell, N., 1999, Network oscillations generated by balancing graded asymmetric reciprocal inhibition in passive neurons, *J. Neurosci.*, 19:2765–2779.

Nadim, F., Olsen, Ø. H., De Schutter, E., and Calabrese, R. L., 1995, Modeling the leech heartbeat elemental oscillator: I. Interactions of intrinsic and synaptic currents, *J. Compu. Neurosci.*, 2:215–235. ◆

Nadim, F., and Calabrese, R. L., 1997, A slow outward current activated by FMRFamide in heart interneurons of the medicinal leech, *J. Neurosci.*, 17:4461–4472.

Olsen, Ø. H., and Calabrese, R. L., 1996, Activation of intrinsic and synaptic currents in leech heart interneurons by realistic waveforms, *J. Neurosci.*, 16:4958–4970.

Roberts, A., Soffe, S. R., Wolf, E. S., Yoshida, M. and Zhao, R. L., 1998, Central circuits controlling locomotion in young frog tadpoles, *Ann. NY Acad. Sci.*, 860:19–34. ◆

Schmidt, J., and Calabrese, R. L., 1992, Evidence that acetylcholine is an inhibitory transmitter of heart interneurons in the leech, *J. Exp. Biol.*, 171:339–347.

Sharp, A. A., Skinner, F. K., and Marder, E., 1996, Mechanisms of oscillation in dynamic clamp constructed two-cell half-center circuits, *J. Neurophysiol.*, 76:867–883.

Skinner, F. K., Kopell, N., and Marder, E., 1994, Mechanisms for oscillation and frequency control in reciprocally inhibitory model neural networks, *J. Compu. Neurosci.*, 1:69–87.

Wang, X.-J., and Rinzel, J., 1992, Alternating and synchronous rhythms in reciprocally inhibitory model neurons, *J. Neural Comp.*, 4:84–97. ◆

Hebbian Learning and Neuronal Regulation

Gal Chechik, David Horn, and Eytan Ruppin

Introduction

Since its conception half a century ago, Hebbian learning has become a fundamental paradigm in the neurosciences. The idea that neurons that fire together wire together has become fairly well understood, as in the case of NMDA-dependent long-term potentiation in the hippocampus (Bliss and Collingridge, 1993). However, for both computational and biological reasons, this type of plasticity has to be accompanied by synaptic changes that are not synapse specific but neuron specific; i.e., they involve many synapses of the same neuron. Biologically, such interactions are inevitable as synapses compete for finite resources and are subject to common processes of the same neuron to which they all belong. Computationally, neuron-specific modifications of synaptic efficacies are required in order to obtain efficient learning, or to faithfully model biological systems. Hence, *neuronal regulation,* defined here as a process modulating all synapses of a postsynaptic neuron, is a general phenomenon that complements Hebbian learning.

There exists evidence for cellular mechanisms resulting in normalization of synaptic efficacies, some of which operate to maintain total synaptic strength and others to regulate mean postsynaptic activity (Miller, 1996). Among these mechanisms are cellular regulation of the number of synapses or of trophic factors, competition between synapses for some finite resources, changes in presynaptic and postsynaptic learning thresholds, or activity-dependent regulation of conductances. Normalization of synaptic efficacies is also induced by certain types of plasticity as an emergent phenomenon, for example in the case of spike-time-dependent plasticity (Song, Miller, and Abbott, 2000). Of particular interest are the findings by Turrigiano et al. (1998), who studied cultures of pyramidal neurons of postnatal rats. They observed slow postsynaptic up- or down-regulation of adenosine monophosphate (AMPA)-mediated synaptic currents in a way that maintained the mean firing activity of the neuron. This scaling resulted in overall synaptic normalization through a multiplicative factor that is inversely related to the neuron's activity.

What are the computational consequences of such neuronal-level processes? It turns out that learning through Hebbian learning alone raises many theoretical difficulties and questions, such as: What stops the positive feedback loop of Hebbian learning and guarantees some normalization of the synaptic efficacies of a neuron?

How can a neuron acquire specificity to particular inputs without being prewired? How can memories be maintained throughout life, while synapses suffer degradation due to metabolic turnover? As we will see, neuronal regulation provides a possible answer to all of the above.

We can divide the computational problems to be looked at according to the traditional dichotomy of supervised and unsupervised learning. In unsupervised learning, the important role of neuronal regulation is to allow for *competition* between the various synapses, leading to *normalization* of the synaptic efficacies. This role will be further explained in the next section, where we review some basic learning paradigms, discuss the difference between multiplicative ($\Delta \mathbf{w} \propto \mathbf{w}$) and additive ($\Delta \mathbf{w} = const$) scaling, and identify some applications to biological systems. We will then turn to supervised learning paradigms, and show that neuronal regulation improves the *capacity* of associative memory models and can be used to guarantee the *maintenance* of biological memory systems.

Unsupervised Learning

When Hebbian plasticity operates in a network in an unsupervised manner, a positive feedback loop is created. To illustrate the problem, think of a presynaptic cell A that causes the firing of a postsynaptic cell B. Because of Hebbian plasticity, the efficacy of the synapse w_{BA} from A to B is strengthened. This leads to an increase in the ability of cell A to activate cell B, which in turn leads to strengthening of the same synapse again. When this positive feedback is unconstrained, it leads to synaptic runaway, i.e., the divergence of synaptic efficacies. It seems reasonable to assume that synaptic values are limited by some upper bound that stops this process. Even then a problem emerges: different afferents will activate different synapses of the target neuron B. When all of them get saturated at their upper bounds, the neuron will not have any discrimination ability. This problem may be solved by introducing constraints, such as limiting the total synaptic strength of a neuron, $\Sigma_i w_i^2 = const$. This results in competition between synapses: the increased strength of one synapse causes a decrease in the strength of another, preventing saturation of all synapses.

Multiplicative Versus Additive Constraints

Normalization prevents synaptic divergence; thus, the combined operation of Hebbian learning and normalization induces new dynamics of synaptic efficacies. This combined dynamics was described by Oja (1982), showing that multiplicative weight normalization of a neuron with real-valued stochastic input extracts the first principal component of the input distribution (also known as PRINCIPAL COMPONENT ANALYSIS [q.v.] or Karunen Leove feature extraction).

Whereas PCA extraction follows for multiplicative normalization, the results change if other types of constraints, such as additive normalization, are imposed (Miller and MacKay, 1994). Although multiplicative normalization leads to a graded weight vector that represents even weak correlations in the input (upper plot of Figure 1B), additive normalization yields a sharpened receptive field where weights saturate at their lower and upper bounds in a way that reflects only the maximally correlated inputs (Figure 1B, bottom). Similar results were obtained for competitive learning, where only the weights of the winning unit are changed (Goodhill and Barrow, 1994).

Neuronal Regulation and Synaptic Normalization

What is the relation between synaptic normalization and neuronal regulation? Normalization of synaptic efficacies involves all synapses of a postsynaptic neuron, and thus requires neuronal-level computation. Moreover, in some cases synaptic normalization is an emergent result of synaptic changes that depend on neuronal activity. We approach this idea by discussing two learning models: the Oja learning rule mentioned earlier and the Bienenstock, Cooper, and Munro (BCM) model.

Using the linear perceptron $V = \Sigma_i w_i x_i$, Oja's learning rule can be implemented by $\Delta w_i = \eta V(x_i - V w_i)$. Here, neuronal regulation is explicitly manifested by the second term, which provides a multiplicative correction that is independent of the specific input x_i but is determined by the neuronal output V. Interestingly, this neuronal regulation term guarantees $\Sigma_i w_i^2 = 1$.

The BCM model (Bienenstock, Cooper, and Munro, 1982) is another example of complex interplay of neuronal regulation and synaptic competition. In the BCM approach, both Hebbian potentiation and depression are used in defining the synaptic learning rule: synapses are potentiated when the presynaptic neuron fires frequently, and depressed otherwise. The boundary between potentiation and depression is determined by the activity of the postsynaptic neuron, which is where neuronal regulation comes in. This component of neuronal regulation leads to competition between synapses and introduces statistical correlations (Intrator and Cooper, 1992) that are higher than the second order used in PCA. Thus, the BCM model captures high-order statistical structures in the input and tunes the efficacies of incoming synapses accordingly.

Biological Models

The BCM model was developed to describe the emergence of orientation-selective cells and ocular dominance in the visual cortex and their dependence on the stimuli that the visual system receives during its critical developmental stages. A study that discusses the same issues with particular emphasis on the dynamics of synaptic efficacies under additive and multiplicative normalization schemes is that of Miller and MacKay (1994). They show that when the inputs to a neuron have positive correlations only, additive normalization leads to the convergence of weights to an on-center-off-surround receptive field, or to a bilobed receptive field, depending on the parameter regime. When the cell receives inputs from both eyes, additive normalization leads to ocular dominance through the sharpening of receptive fields. Multiplicative normalization can lead in this case to ocular dominance only if the inputs from both eyes are negatively correlated.

A convenient system for the study of neuronal regulation is the vertebrate neuromuscular junction (NMJ). Its development is characterized by an initial stage of superinnervation (each muscle fiber is innervated by several motor neurons) followed by withdrawal of axon terminals until a state of single innervation is reached. Modeling the NMJ, Willshaw (1993) has shown that competition for postsynaptic resources explains the decrease in innervation, yet fails to account for other experimental findings such as incomplete innervation after artificial partial denervation during development.

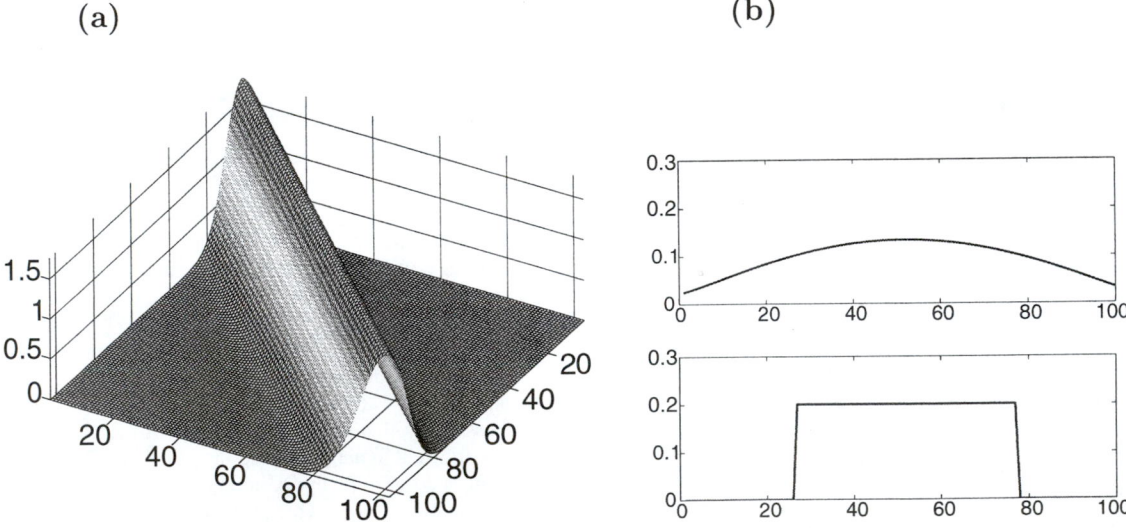

(a)   (b)

Figure 1. Steady states of synaptic weights under multiplicative and additive normalization in a toy example of a neuron with 100 inputs. *A*, The correlation matrix of all inputs. *B*, Under multiplicative constraints, the weights converge onto the first principal component (upper plot), while an additive rule leads to a binary separation of weights that reach their extremal values (bottom plot).

However, a combination of post- and presynaptic competition provides a good account of the data. Indeed, the efficacy of the neuromuscular synapse during the period preceding axonal withdrawal was traced by Colman, Nabekura, and Lichtman (1997), who found changes in quantal content and efficacy. These changes led to continuous strengthening of some synapses with a parallel weakening of the rest, suggesting the operation of a cascade of pre- and postsynaptic processes regulating synaptic efficacies. This is therefore an interesting example in which both pre- and postsynaptic normalization cooperate during early development.

Finally, we wish to point out that competition may arise also through effects other than neuronal regulation. An example is the case of spike-time-dependent synaptic plasticity, in which potentiation of excitatory synapses occurs when the presynaptic spike shortly precedes the postsynaptic spike, and depression occurs when the opposite temporal order holds. Song et al. (2000) assumed that spike-dependent synaptic potentiation is weaker than depression and showed that in a neuron that is driven by net positive input, the excitatory synapses will be weakened. This eventually leads to a balanced input in which the more relevant excitatory synapses are strengthened. Thus, effective competition between synapses may occur even in the absence of an explicit neuronal regulatory term, one that depends on the postsynaptic neuron only.

Supervised Learning

We saw that in unsupervised learning, neuronal regulation solves the problem of synaptic runaway and guarantees specificity of neuronal response through synaptic competition. In supervised learning, normalization constraints introduced by neuronal regulation provide both maintenance of memory systems and high memory capacity.

Memory Maintenance

The concept of neuronal regulation was introduced by Horn, Levy, and Ruppin (1998) in the context of associative memory networks, while these authors were developing a model that could account

for the stability of memory systems in the face of continuous metabolic turnover of synapses. This repetitive process of synaptic degeneration and buildup occurs on a time scale of few days. Under these conditions, one wonders how memories can be stored in synaptic connections for prolonged periods. It turns out that neuronal regulation may play an important role in bringing about the necessary homeostasis of this system, i.e., account for its ability to continue to both learn and retrieve memories (Horn et al., 1998).

To understand this issue, let us consider an associative memory system that is tested through activation by random inputs. Neurons that belong to memories with large basins of attraction will be much more active than those that participate only in memories with small basins of attraction. At this point, we introduce neuronal regulation through multiplicative synaptic corrections that are inversely proportional to the activity of the postsynaptic neuron. This will upregulate weak memories and downregulate strong ones. The multiplicative nature of the correction guarantees that the relative weights of different memories on the same neuron are maintained. The result of this procedure is depicted in Figure 2. As can be seen, repeated synaptic degradation and neuronal regulation leads to normalization of the basins of attraction.

The homeostasis strategy suggested by Horn et al. (1998) involves repeated sessions of random activation, synaptic degradation, and neuronal regulation that provide the required maintenance of the network after it goes through some period of Hebbian learning. It can be shown that the combined effect of synaptic degradation and neuronal regulation also results in the removal of weak synapses, owing to emerging synaptic competition (Chechik, Meilijson, and Ruppin, 1999). This can provide insight into the phenomenon of synaptic pruning that is believed to occur during early development in mammals (see Quartz and Sejnowski, 1997, for a review of the constructive versus selectionist approaches to brain development).

Learning Capacity

Normalization of synaptic efficacies plays a crucial role in producing effective Hebbian learning: Without normalization, Hebbian

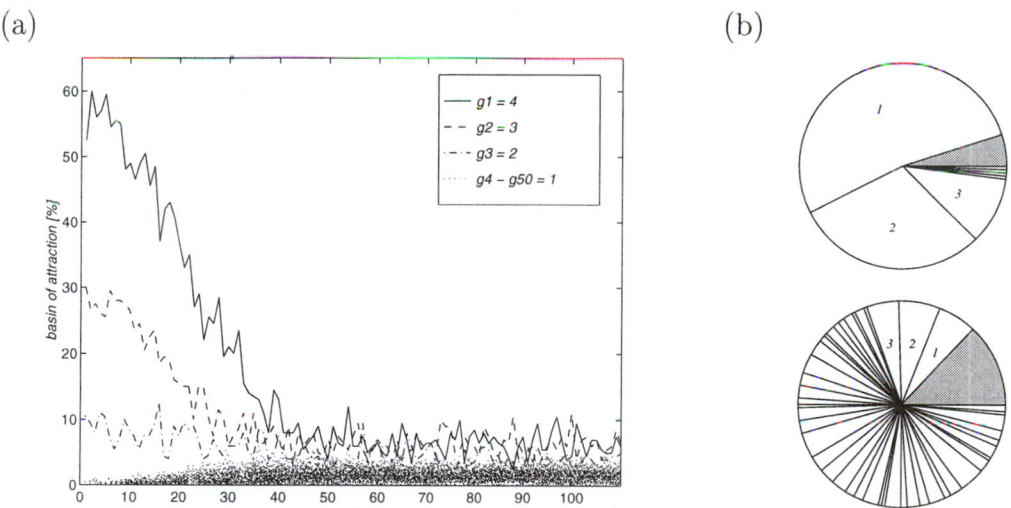

(a)   (b)

Figure 2. *A*, Size of basins of attraction as measured by the percentage of retrievals of specific memories. Fifty memories are stored in a system of a thousand neurons. Three of the memories are stronger (parametrized by *g*) than the rest, overshadowing all others before the corrective dynamic action of NR is introduced. *B*, Shares of memory space (relative sizes of basins of attraction) at the beginning (upper figure) and the end (lower figure) of

the simulation that consists of repeated cycles of synaptic degradation and neuronal regulation. Random inputs lead either to encoded memories or to the null attractor (gray shading) in which all activity stops. (From Horn, D., Levy, N., and Ruppin, E., 1998, Synaptic maintenance via neuronal regulation, *Neural Computat.*, 10:1–18. Reprinted with permission.)

learning leads to poor associative memory capacity that does not grow with the size of the network.

Several authors (e.g., Dayan and Willshaw, 1991; Chechik, Meilijson, and Ruppin, 2001) have studied the space of additive Hebbian learning rules for associative memory networks with low-activity patterns (i.e., patterns where only a low fraction of the neurons fire). Such learning rules determine the changes in synaptic efficacy when a memory pattern is stored, and may be formally written as $\Delta w_{ij} = aS_iS_j + bS_i + cS_j + d$, where $S_i \in \{0, 1\}$ is the activity of the ith neuron of the stored pattern. Analyzing the associative memory capacity of such learning rules shows that only a constrained subspace of learning rules leads to effective memory storage. Figure 3 illustrates this phenomenon, showing the capacity resulting from such rules within a subspace of two parameters. Most learning rules are ineffective and lead to low memory capacity because they create correlations between synaptic weights even when the stored memory patterns are uncorrelated. Moreover, all effective learning rules fulfill a constraint that depends on the fraction of firing neurons within the stored memory patterns (a global network parameter). Unfortunately, small perturbations in the learning rule parameters lead to violation of this constraint, and consequently to memory capacity collapse.

Interestingly, learning with effective learning rules lead to a vanishing sum of synaptic efficacies for each neuron. This is true, for example, for the learning rules on the ridge in Figure 3. More important, the converse also holds: a vanishing synaptic sum guarantees effective learning. Thus, enforcing through neuronal regulation the condition that the sum of synaptic efficacies vanishes yields high memory capacity, irrespective of the generalized Hebbian rule one starts with (Chechik et al., 2001).

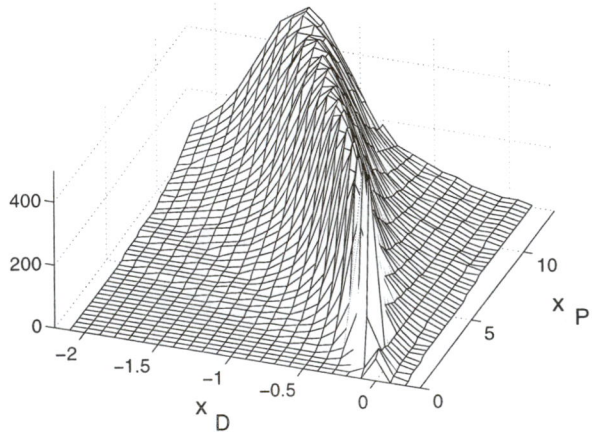

Figure 3. The memory capacity of an associative memory network for various learning rules. The number of memories that can be stored in a 1,000-neurons network and later retrieved from distorted cue is plotted as a function of two parameters: the strength of synaptic potentiation (x_P) and heterosynaptic depression (x_D). These two parameters span the two-dimensional subspace of learning rules $\Delta w_{ij} = x_P S_i S_j + x_D S_i (1 - S_j)$, where $S_i \in \{0, 1\}$ is the activity of the ith neuron. Apparently, only a one-dimensional set of learning rules provides effective learning. (From Chechik, G., Meilijson, I., and Ruppin, E., 2001, Effective learning with ineffective Hebbian learning rules, *Neural Computat.*, 13:817–840. Reprinted with permission.)

Discussion

Hebbian mechanisms per se fail to provide robust and effective learning, both in supervised and in unsupervised scenarios. Although some synapse-specific mechanisms may provide partial remedies for these problems, the current article focused on neuronal regulation of synaptic efficacies and its role in complementing Hebbian learning. Experimental evidence exists for cellular mechanisms that regulate synapses to maintain global constraints on activity or total synaptic strengths (Turrigiano et al., 1998). This evidence suggests that neuronal regulation and Hebbian learning are distinct mechanisms: they are mediated through different receptors (NMDA versus AMPA) and operate on different time scales. From a computational standpoint, the combined operation of Hebbian learning and neuronal regulation provides powerful learning capabilities, ranging from PCA and ICA extraction to robust associative memory learning. We conclude that the functional interplay between synaptic and neuronal mechanisms plays a fundamental role in biological neural networks.

Road Map: Neural Plasticity
Background: Hebbian Synaptic Plasticity
Related Reading: Post-Hebbian Learning Algorithms

References

Bienenstock, E. L., Cooper, L. N., and Munro, P. W., 1982, Theory for the development of neuron selectivity: Orientation specificity and binocular interaction in visual cortex, *J. Neurosci.*, 2:32–48. ■

Bliss, T. V. P., and Collingridge, G. L., 1993, Synaptic model of memory: Long-term potentiation in the hippocampus, *Nature*, 361:31–39.

Chechik, G., Meilijson, I., and Ruppin, E., 1999, Neuronal regulation: A mechanism for synaptic pruning during brain maturation, *Neural Computat.*, 11:2061–2080.

Chechik, G., Meilijson, I., and Ruppin, E., 2001, Effective neuronal learning with ineffective Hebbian learning rules, *Neural Computat.*, 13:817–840.

Colman, H., Nabekura, J., and Lichtman, J. W., 1997, Alterations in synaptic strength preceding axon withdrawal, *Science*, 275:356–361.

Dayan, P., and Willshaw, D. J., 1991, Optimizing synaptic learning rules in linear associative memories, *Biol. Cybern.*, 65:253.

Goodhill, G. J., and Barrow, H. G., 1994, The role of weight normalization in competitive learning, *Neural Computat.*, 6:255–269.

Horn, D., Levy, N., and Ruppin, E., 1998, Synaptic maintenance via neuronal regulation, *Neural Computat.*, 10:1–18.

Intrator, N., and Cooper, L. N., 1992, Objective function formulation theory of visual cortical plasticity: Statistical connections, stability conditions, *Neural Netw.*, 5:3–17.

Miller, K. D., 1996, Synaptic economics: Competition and cooperation in synaptic plasticity, *Neuron*, 17:371–374.

Miller, K. D., and Mackay, D. J. C., 1994, The role of constraints in Hebbian learning, *Neural Computat.*, 6:100–126. ◆

Oja, E., 1982, A simplified neuron model as a principal component analyzer, *J. Math. Biol.*, 15:267–273.

Quartz, S. R., and Sejnowski, T. J., 1997, The neural basis of cognitive development: A constructivist manifesto, *Behav. Brain. Sci.*, 20:537–556.

Song, S., Miller, K. D., and Abbott, L. F., 2000, Competitive Hebbian learning through spike-timing dependent synaptic plasticity, *Nature Neurosci.*, 3:919–926.

Turrigiano, G. G., Leslie, K., Desai, N., and Nelson, S. B., 1998, Activity dependent scaling of quantal amplitude in neocortical pyramidal neurons, *Nature*, 391:892–896.

Willshaw, D. J., 1993, Presynaptic and postsynaptic competition in models for the development of neuromuscular connections, *Biol. Cybern.*, 61:85–93.

Hebbian Synaptic Plasticity

Yves Frégnac

Introduction

Appropriate levels of description must be chosen in order to analyze dynamic changes in brain function during development, learning, and perception. One approach is to go from simple phenomenological rules to complex mechanistic scenarios of synaptic plasticity and to evaluate progressively how each level of complexity affects the processing and adaptive capacities of the overall network. This article briefly summarizes the historical foundations and subsequent elaboration by theoreticians and experimenters of a simple activity-dependent algorithm of synaptic plasticity proposed by Donald Hebb in 1949. The predictions derived from Hebb's postulate can be generalized for different levels of integration (i.e., synaptic efficacy, functional coupling, adaptive change in behavior) simply by adjusting the variables derived from various measures of neural activity and the time scale over which each operates. It is thus interesting to consider to what degree this association law may be independent of the biological substrate that is considered and should be viewed as one of the most general computational principles in brain dynamics.

Five major questions will be addressed:

1. Should the definition of Hebbian plasticity refer to a simple positive correlational rule of learning, or are there biological justifications for including additional pseudo-Hebbian terms (such as synaptic depression due to disuse or competition) in a generalized phenomenological algorithm?
2. What are the spatiotemporal constraints (e.g., input specificity, temporal associativity) that characterize the induction process? In particular, should the Hebbian postulate be interpreted as a co-activity rule, or should it incorporate a causal temporal asymmetry, where presynaptic activity precedes postsynaptic activity by a few milliseconds in order to induce synaptic potentiation?
3. Do the predictions of Hebbian-based algorithms account for most forms of activity-dependent dynamics in synaptic transmission throughout phylogenesis? How do the predictions depend on the complexity of the considered neural network (e.g., direct sensory motor connections in *Aplysia* versus associative networks in neocortex)?
4. On which time scales (perception, learning, epigenesis) and at which stage of development of the organism (embryonic life, critical postnatal developmental periods, adult age) are activity-dependent changes in functional links predicted by Hebb's rule?
5. Are there examples of correlation-based plasticity that contradict the predictions of Hebb's postulate (i.e., those termed anti-Hebbian modifications)?

The Conceptual Framework of Cell Assemblies

Pre-Hebbian Theories

Long before our current knowledge of the synapse-neuron-based structure of the brain, philosophers of antiquity had already theorized how causal relations between external events could be established by the human mind and had pointed out the necessity of repeating sequences of activation in order to link mental representations (Aristotle, ca. 350 B.C.). The application of association theories to the brain can be traced back to as early as 1890: according to William James, the adaptive capacities of our brain depend on mechanistic laws of association that operate under the guidance of central neural structures such as cerebral cortex in higher vertebrates: "When two elementary brain processes have been active together or in immediate succession, one of them, on re-occurring tends to propagate its excitement into the other" (James, 1890). These concepts of association are immediately applicable to the understanding of behavioral learning, and the first extension of classical conditioning in cellular terms was proposed by Jerzy Konorski, a contemporary of Donald Hebb, who assumed that "when the excitation of a given center is synchronous with the rise of excitation in another center, conditioned excitatory connexions are formed from the first of these centers to the latter" (Konorski, 1948).

A second field of application of association theories is the transient formation of mental representations during perception or dreams. In contrast to the previous proposals, the effect produced by repeated associations is no longer restricted to sequences of external events but extends to autonomous activity of the brain. Rather than being transformed under a long-lasting "mnesic" form, the trace of the association is seen here as a reversible facilitation, promoting neural links over the time required for the establishment of the percept (a few hundred milliseconds). In his seminal essay *Le rêve*, Yves Delage hypothesized that each cortical neuron exhibits an intrinsic characteristic periodicity in its activity (Delage, 1919). The relative diversity of the intrinsic frequencies adopted by possible future functional partners (heterochrony) would be dynamically restructured during perception and give place to transient and highly synchronized states (parachrony) among the activated members of the functional assembly.

A Neurophysiological Postulate to Build Assemblies

The physiological association principle proposed by Hebb was in fact just one of several keystones incorporated in a multilevel model of cerebral functioning during perceptual and learning processes. The main concept of a *cellular assembly*, pivotal to his theory, designated an activity process that reverberates in *a set of closed pathways*. The neurophysiological postulate of Hebbian synapses was introduced as one possible way to reinforce functional coupling between co-active cells and thus of growing assemblies. Similar hypotheses were developed at a higher hierarchical level of organization that allowed the linkage between cognitive events and their recall in the form of a temporally organized series of activations of assemblies. Donald Hebb referred to this final binding process as a *phase sequence*. Thus, Hebb's postulate appears simply as a putative low-level biophysical mechanism for establishing the perseverance of activity among assemblies: "When an axon of cell A is near enough to excite cell B, and repeatedly or consistently takes part in firing it, some growth process or metabolic change takes part in one or both cells such that A's efficiency, as one of the cells firing B, is increased" (Hebb, 1949).

The formulation of Hebb's postulate requires not only close temporal coincidence but also the spatial convergence of one neuron onto another, supporting a causal relationship between the afferent activity and the postsynaptic spike. It provides a specific prediction: a period of maintained positive temporal correlation between pre- and postsynaptic activity will lead to an increase in the efficacy of synaptic transmission. Hebb did not elaborate on whether the modifications responsible for this decrease in *synaptic resistance* were presynaptic, postsynaptic, or both. Neither did he describe the biophysical substrate responsible for the modification, leaving the choice open between "metabolic change" and "oriented growth." Both of these options turned out to be true. Historically, Hebb's postulate referred exclusively to excitatory synapses. A symmetric, if not synergetic, version of Hebb's postulate was proposed much later for the case of inhibitory synapses (Stent, 1973), in which functional coupling can be increased by reducing the strength of inhibitory synapses activated at the same time that action potentials are fired in the postsynaptic cell. Some models introduced inhibitory plasticity well before it was proved analytically that the use of negative weights is required for endowing associative memories with an optimal mapping and memory capacity. Thus, the effective gain between input and output, defined at an ideal Hebbian synapse, should be envisioned as a dynamic variable between positive and negative boundaries, depending on whether the net effect induced by the input is excitatory or inhibitory (Figures 1*A* and 1*B*). Some theoretical studies also proposed that synaptic gain could change sign during development (Bienenstock, Cooper, and Munro, 1982), a suggestion later found to apply to inhibitory neocortical or hippocampal circuits.

Post-Hebbian Theories: Dynamic Binding of Assemblies

Peter Milner was probably the first theoretician in the fifties to propose explicit rules for the compositionality of assemblies. The repeated activation of a given cell assembly would reinforce syn-

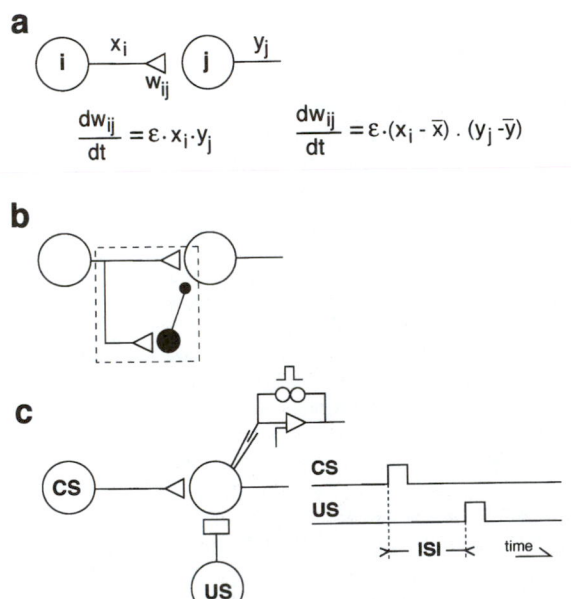

Figure 1. The multiple identities of a Hebbian synapse. *A*, Monosynaptic connection between a presynaptic axon (*i*) and a postsynaptic target cell (*j*). Left, the Hebbian algorithm posits that the change in synaptic efficacy $\Delta\omega_{ij}$ is given by the product (or logical AND) of presynaptic (x_i) and postsynaptic (y_j) activities at any point in time. Right, the "covariance rule" replaces the pre- and postsynaptic terms by the departure of instantaneous pre- and postsynaptic activities from their respective mean values ($\langle\bar{x}\rangle$) and $\langle\bar{y}\rangle$ averaged over a certain time window. *B*, A dual excitatory/inhibitory circuit equivalent to an ideal Hebbian synapse, the gain of which varies between negative and positive boundary values. Open circle indicates an excitatory cell; open triangles indicate synapses. Solid symbols indicate inhibitory cells and synapses. *C*, A cellular analogue of classical conditioning: the Hebbian synapse transmits the neural information fed by the conditioned stimulus (CS). The unconditioned stimulus (US) activates the postsynaptic cell in an all-or-none fashion through a nonmodifiable synapse or through a depolarizing current injection directly applied by the experimenter to the postsynaptic cell. The conditioned response stems from the repeated association of the CS input followed by the US input. The phase of the association (ISI) is defined by the temporal lag between the CS and the US inputs.

aptic links within this assembly, and in addition would "prime" a restricted number of cells, allowing future binding and thus composition with other associative processes. The latent labeled synapses would remain transiently eligible for further potentiation by the contiguous firing of other assemblies, a "tagging" concept that would find its biological counterpart only much later. Repeated sequential activation would reinforce the primed connections so that they became an integral part of the next active assembly, thereby resulting in second-order associations: their firing would thus allow the recall of a complete *phase sequence*. Similar ideas were reworded with the addition of a glue mechanism, namely temporal synchrony, acting on a much faster time scale than that initially proposed by Hebb such as to bind elementary representations into a cognitive whole (Milner, 1974) (see SYNCHRONIZATION, BINDING AND EXPECTANCY). The theoretical work fostered by von der Malsburg and colleagues showed that the combined use of "fast" and reversible Hebbian-like synaptic changes and "slow" Hebbian plasticity provides interesting compositional properties when applied to a specific type of assembly called synfire chains (see SYNFIRE CHAINS). Simultaneous recordings of cortical single-unit activity in behaving monkeys have since shown that a significant fraction of activity correlated with a specific cognitive task can be described as waves of synchrony relayed between sets of co-active neurons, at various delays ranging from a few to several hundred milliseconds. A Lego-like interlacing of dynamic assemblies can be further used to give a neuronal embodiment to abstract compositional models of cognition based on dynamical binding operations between symbols that sit at various levels of a representational hierarchy (reviewed in Frégnac and Bienenstock, 1998; see DYNAMIC LINK ARCHITECTURE).

Theoretical Predictions and Neurobiological Tests of Hebb's Postulate

Ten years after the publication of his *The Organization of Behavior*, Donald Hebb was doubtful whether his theory was definite enough to be testable, not so much because of technical constraints but because of conceptual ones. Most of the premises were based on a number of postulates, each addressing a different level of integration, and failures of tests restricted to the biophysical level of the synapse would not threaten or contradict the theory in itself.

Hebbian Analogs of Cellular Learning

Hebb's postulate was initially applied by cyberneticians and electrophysiologists in the context of supervised learning. In a similar way to the external teacher of the gamma-perceptron, a classifier machine developed by cyberneticians at the end of the sixties that imposes an increase in the gains of active synapses that participate in the "correct" answer (see PERCEPTRONS, ADALINES, AND BACK-PROPAGATION), electrophysiogical tests of Hebbian synapses impose depolarization of the postsynaptic element concomitantly with afferent activity. The exogenous control of postsynaptic activity has been achieved using various technical means (electrical stimulation of an unmodifiable pathway, iontophoresis of excitatory neurotransmitters, intracellular current injection, uncaging of calcium at a dendritic spot) in order to elicit positive reinforcement of the modifiable test response (Figure 1*C*). This strategy has been attempted at a variety of sites in the central nervous system ranging from molluscan neuronal ganglia to the mammalian forebrain (reviewed in Brown et al., 1990; Frégnac and Shulz, 1994; Bi and Poo, 2001). Most success in demonstrating the role of postsynaptic factors has been observed in the vertebrate cortex (hippocampus, neocortex, motor cortex), where synaptic potentiation of various durations can be induced under the cooperative influence of other inputs (as is the case during high-frequency tetanus of afferent pathways) or by forcing the postsynaptic cell to an artificially high level of activity. As we will discuss later, results opposite to the Hebbian prediction have been found in the striatum, in the cerebellum, and in related structures in electric fish (reviewed in Bell, 2001; see CEREBELLUM: NEURAL PLASTICITY).

In spite of some earlier reports that invertebrate synapses possess the capacity for long-term potentiation (LTP), until recently it was assumed that nonassociative and associative forms of behavioral plasticity in *Aplysia* resulted from an activity-dependent presynaptic modulation of the efficacy of sensorimotor synapses (see INVERTEBRATE MODELS OF LEARNING: *APLYSIA* AND *HERMISSENDA*). However, later studies provided strong evidence for a postsynaptic regulation of *Aplysia* sensorimotor synapses in dissociated cell culture. These studies showed a specific influence of the appropriate motor cell in inducing spatial competition and segregation of the locus of termination of the afferent axons corresponding to different presynaptic axons. It also demonstrated that Hebbian pairing protocols induced potentiation of identified sensorimotor synapses.

By which cellular machinery does co-activity exert control over synaptic gain? In vertebrate hippocampus as well as in *Aplysia* sensorimotor co-cultures, evidence implicates the NMDA receptor and its invertebrate homologous form, respectively (see NMDA RECEPTORS: SYNAPTIC, CELLULAR, AND NETWORK MODELS). These receptors are ideally suited to operate conjunctive mechanisms, since they require concomitant presynaptic activation and depolarization of the postsynaptic neuron above a critical level to free their embedded ionophore channel from the magnesium block. However, this mechanism is certainly not unique, since Hebbian forms of plasticity can be observed even during the pharmacological APV blockade of NMDA receptors.

The use of multiple simultaneous whole-cell recordings in vitro has recently improved control of the respective timing of pre- and postsynaptic activity and the ability to patch at different distances from the soma. These experiments suggested that action potentials propagating back into dendrites serve to modify single active synaptic connections (see BACKPROPAGATION: GENERAL PRINCIPLES). Backpropagation can contribute to the induction of synaptic plasticity through three distinct mechanisms. The simplest one relies on the voltage dependency requirements of NMDA receptor activation and remains input specific. The second one, involving voltage-gated calcium channels, will apply to all parts of the dendrite in which the spike is efficiently propagated. A third mechanism involves a chain reaction and depends on the initiation of calcium spikes by otherwise subthreshold distal inputs when the EPSP follows by a 5-ms delay the invasion of the dendrite by a backpropagating action potential (reviewed in Frégnac, 1999). In all cases the backpropagating spike can be seen as the "binding signal" emitted by the soma to differentially modify synapses that are active within a precise temporal window.

A Theoretical Need for Synaptic Depression and Competition: Pseudo-Hebbian Rules

Most algorithms of synaptic plasticity use rules of normalization that require depression of certain synapses in addition to Hebbian reinforcement of active connections (see POST-HEBBIAN LEARNING ALGORITHMS). The "divergence" problem caused by a straightforward application of Hebb's principle was solved by the first modelers using various ad hoc hypotheses: upper bound values (saturation) for individual synaptic weights, forgetting mechanisms slowly activated by disuse, and complementary plasticity rules that operated at the level of synapses fed both by active pathways (associative depression) and by neighboring inactive afferents (heterosynaptic depression). In the latter case, different weight normalization procedures were proposed that gave rise to what is called *competitive learning* in the modeling literature (see COM-

PETITIVE LEARNING). The additional decay terms introduced in the plasticity rule can depend only on local variables, or it can operate as a global constraint that maintains constant the sum (or the sum of the squares) of all the synaptic weights converging onto the same neuron. Gunther Stent proposed a biophysical mechanism inducing a selective decrease in the synaptic efficacy of afferent fibers that were inactive at the time the postsynaptic neuron was discharging under the influence of other inputs (Stent, 1973). He was probably the first theoretician to introduce the concept of a threshold in synaptic plasticity, linked to the local postsynaptic membrane potential, below which synaptic depression occurs. The prediction of this postulate found strong support from later cross-depression studies in visual pathways and from the observation of heterosynaptic depression in the CA1 field and the dentate area of the hippocampus.

The assumption of global constraints in maintaining the total synaptic weight constant onto the recipient neuron has been also made on the basis of more biological grounds, such as the theory of selective stabilization. Correlates to this model were found in simple in vitro systems that allow the culture of specified numbers of pre- and postsynaptic partners, suggesting that the total capacity of the target neuron for synaptic interaction is fixed and divided among the different input lines. Related arguments can also be found during synaptogenesis of neuromuscular junctions and of vertebrate visual pathways.

In spite of their diversity, these different rules have a common implication: they predict spatial and temporal competition between active fibers that impinge on a common target cell; they are referred to as being *pseudo-Hebbian*.

Experimental Support for a Generalized Hebbian Algorithm

Most Hebbian algorithms that were used to model synaptic plasticity in self-organizing networks or behavioral learning, before the concept of spike-timing-dependent plasticity (STDP) arose, are surprisingly uniform and are based on co-activity of pre- and postsynaptic neurons. They may be summarized by the same general equation in which the change of synaptic efficacy with respect to time is equal to the product of a presynaptic term and a postsynaptic term (reviewed in Frégnac and Shulz, 1994). The so-called covariance hypothesis (in visual cortex: Bienenstock et al., 1982) replaces the pre- and postsynaptic terms by the departure of instantaneous pre- and postsynaptic activities from their respective mean values averaged over a certain time window (see Figure 1A). Average values in the covariance product constitute pre- and postsynaptic plasticity thresholds that determine the sign of the modification. They can be replaced by nonlinear functions of past activity (power function with an exponent greater than 1; see Bienenstock et al., 1982). Because of the particular choice of these nonlinearities, synaptic depression will be more readily induced by regimes of high activity during which the plasticity threshold increases faster than the mean postsynaptic activity. Conversely, synaptic potentiation will be promoted following low-activity regimes during which the plasticity threshold decreases slower than mean postsynaptic activity. The "floating threshold" hypothesis predictions agree with the observation of an increased rate of cortical specification in previously deprived animals that are re-exposed to a visually structured environment, when compared with the normal process observed in nondeprived animals. Although most theoretical studies have been concerned with postsynaptic thresholds, experimental evidence (priming protocols, mostly tested in hippocampal slices) suggests as well the existence of a presynaptic averaging mechanism.

The BCM covariance rule in its most general form does account for spatial and temporal competition. In addition to the straightforward Hebbian condition (positive covariance induces an increase in synaptic gain), the covariance hypothesis predicts two forms of depression. The first one is an associative heterosynaptic depression at the level of synapses whose activity was uncorrelated with that of the tetanized pathway (Levy and Steward, 1983). The second form is a homosynaptic depression, when presynaptic activity is associated with repeated failure in synaptic transmission (Frégnac et al., 1988; Frégnac and Shulz, 1999).

Constraints on Spatial and Temporal Specificity

Input Specificity and Cooperativity

A first limitation in the locality of the changes produced by learning depends on the minimal neuroanatomical convergence of input that is necessary to induce a functional change. In the case in which the activity of one afferent alone would be sufficient to induce synaptic change, convergence should be considered to be related to the density and the spatial distribution of boutons made by a single presynaptic axon onto the same target cell. Some studies based on simultaneous dual intracellular recordings failed to observe significant potentiation of individual synaptic connections, whereas their compound activation revealed an increased postsynaptic response. These results suggest the existence of a postsynaptic threshold mechanism controlling the *expression* of LTP: a critical level of depolarization has to be achieved so that the enhancement at the "primed" synapse would be revealed in response to the test input. This nonlinear behavior in the input/output curve of the postsynaptic neuron would have a major consequence: it would greatly increase the spatial input selectivity of LTP by making it conditional on the strength and the convergence of multiple inputs. It could thus prevent temporally unstructured or spatially disperse afferent information from benefiting from the potentiation.

Volume Plasticity

The input specificity of Hebbian schemes of plasticity—i.e., their restriction to active synapses—might suffer strong limitations when the release of retrograde factors and the spatial diffusion of second messengers are considered. Since quantal analysis studies have implicated presynaptic factors in the maintenance of LTP, it is admitted that some feedback signal indicates to the presynaptic terminal that the correlation operation has been accomplished and that potentiation is authorized. Various retrograde messengers have been proposed, including arachidonic acid, nitric oxide, carbon monoxide, and platelet-activating factor. Taking into account the diffusion of messengers in the extracellular medium, the correlation between high levels of the released molecule and active axon terminals could then become the key factor controlling which synapses should be potentiated. This scheme accounts for the observed generalization of potentiation to neighboring synapses belonging to the axon that has initiated the retrograde messenger process, independently of the target neuron. The consequence of this "volume plasticity" is that correlation will be reinforced between elements that are co-active within a given time window and are within some critical volume without being necessarily physically connected. Reasonable estimates of the space constant on which retrograde messenger-induced changes occur are in the order of 50–150 μm, based on dual intracellular recordings of a conditioned cell and a neighbor in vitro, both of which receive parent branches from the same input fiber. More surprisingly, the postsynaptic modification also seems to spread to different presynaptic axons that have or have not been implicated in the induction of the LTP process, regardless of their own history of activation.

More advanced studies have recently been achieved at the level of identified neurons and synapses in low-density hippocampal cultures and have revealed extensive but selective spread of both LTP

and long-term depression (LTD) from the site of induction to other synapses in the network (reviewed in Bi and Poo, 2001). LTD induced at synapses between two glutamatergic neurons can spread to other synapses made by divergent outputs of the same presynaptic neuron (*presynaptic lateral propagation*) or to synapses made by other convergent inputs on the same postsynaptic cell (*postsynaptic lateral propagation*). Furthermore, LTD can spread in a retrograde direction to depress synapses afferent to the presynaptic neuron (*backpropagation*). In contrast, LTP can exhibit only lateral propagation and backpropagation to the synapses associated with the presynaptic neuron. If output synapses of the paired presynaptic neuron undergo LTP/LTD, then the input synapses undergo similar changes. It is interesting to observe that the backpropagation of LTP/LTD observed in cell cultures appears to fit qualitatively the requirement for backpropagation algorithms in multilayer networks. Similar functional effects could operate on a larger scale in vivo if a permanent imbalance in activity is introduced between competing axons, for example altering the spatial grouping of bands of ocular dominance driven by the open eye in monocular deprived visual cortex.

Breaking the Timing Symmetry: Causality Rather than Synchrony

Most applications of Hebbian theories based on pairing protocols indeed stressed the importance of co-activity, ignoring the few-milliseconds step that separates a presynaptic spike from the triggering of postsynaptic activation. The temporal contiguity requirement of Hebbian potentiation in cortex was first estimated in the ± 50 ms range, both in vivo and in vitro, and no temporal ordering was required between pre- and postsynaptic activation. However, the wording of Hebb's principle dictates that presynaptic activity should precede the spike initiation in the postsynaptic element to which it contributes in a causal way ("A's efficiency, as one of the cells firing B"). Temporal asymmetric Hebbian and anti-Hebbian rules (Figure 2B) that have been introduced only in recent years agree in this respect with the original concept.

An overlooked consequence of additional pseudo-Hebbian rules is that their interplay with a purely Hebbian scheme already predicts a loss of symmetry in the temporal domain and a possible narrowing of the critical interval of association. In vitro studies of heterosynaptic plasticity in cocultures of embryonic spinal neurons and myotomal muscles show that synchronous activation of two presynaptic pathways protect them from depression, whereas a delay as short as 100 ms is sufficient to depress one or both pathways. Associative forms of LTD have been observed during contiguous dual-pathway stimulation paradigms or when the test input follows a postsynaptic depolarization induced by a brief current pulse. The exact temporal window during which a recurrent input remains eligible for potentiation depends, however, on the strength of the last unconditioned activation of the cell. These results agree partially with the temporal order requirement in associative heterosynaptic depression reported 20 years ago in the study of the crossed (weak) and uncrossed (strong) entorhinal cortex projection to the dentate gyrus, which still described much more shorter association intervals (20 ms), enabling associative LTP (Levy and Steward, 1983).

Recent work, based in most cases on dual patch recordings in vitro, has been realized in preparations as diverse as cultured hippocampal networks, the developing retinotectal system of the frog, the adult electrosensory lobe of electric fish, and the sensory neocortex of the rat. Results suggest an even tighter temporal contingency rule (10-ms range), where the temporal order of the onset of the postsynaptic subthreshold potential reflecting the arrival of the presynaptic spike and the postsynaptic spike backpropagating in the dendrite decides whether potentiation or depression occurs (re-

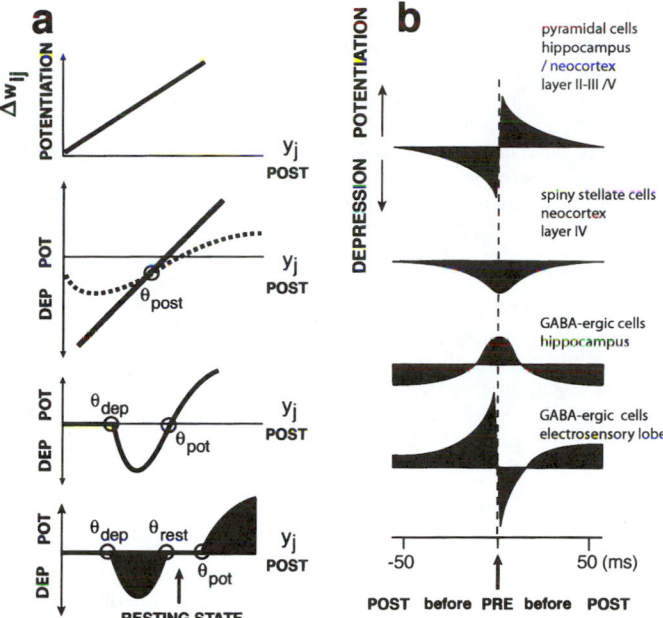

Figure 2. Hebbian synapses and spike-timing-dependent plasticity. *A*, A representation of Hebb's rule (top) and the most commonly observed rules of associative plasticity. Each graph expresses the relationship between the induced synaptic change $\Delta\omega_{ij}$ (positive ordinates for potentiation, negative for depression) and postsynaptic activity (y_j on abscissa) at the time of the association defined by the occurrence of the presynaptic spike. The slope of Hebb's rule is proportional to presynaptic activity. The postsynaptic term (POST) has been equated successively with postsynaptic firing frequency, postsynaptic membrane potential, or calcium influx in the postsynaptic cell. In addition, many authors have confounded, rightly or wrongly, the postsynaptic term with the presynaptic stimulus frequency applied during conditioning, which made these models more manageable in predicting the effects of various input frequencies used more specifically to induce LTD or LTP. From top to bottom: The simple Hebbian rule (top) predicts potentiation only. The covariance rule or BCM rule (second graph from the top) and ABS rule (third graph from the top) predict both depression and potentiation, respectively, with one (ϑ_{post}) or two postsynaptic plasticity thresholds (ϑ_{dep}, ϑ_{pot}). The lower graph is derived from in vivo experiments in which the resting state of the synapse corresponds to a dead zone between depression and potentiation where information is reliably transmitted (Frégnac et al., 1988). *B*, Different forms of spike-timing—dependent plasticity rules established in vitro in cocultures and acute slices. The induced synaptic change is expressed as a function of the temporal delay separating postsynaptic firing from presynaptic firing (taken here as the zero-delay reference), imposed during the pairing protocol. From top to bottom: pyramidal cells in hippocampus or in nongranular layers in neocortex, granular spiny stellate cells in neocortex, GABAergic neurons in hippocampal cultures, GABAergic medium ganglionic layer cells in the electrosensory lobe of the electric fish. Positive ordinates indicate synaptic potentiation and negative ordinates indicate depression.

viewed in Bi and Poo, 2001; Abbott and Nelson, 2000; see Figure 2*B*). An unexpected twist in the story is the claim that the outcome of the rule itself depends on the frequency and the strength of the presynaptic inputs, which could have nontrivial consequences in vivo.

The obvious consequence is that models that incorporate STDP rules account most accurately for the emergence of causal chains within neuronal assemblies and best support phase sequence learning. It is nevertheless possible that both synchrony and causality are required to promote reverberating assemblies rather than the simple build-up of open-ended chains of feedforward activity, as

exemplified by the concept of synfire chains. It is highly plausible that STDP reinforces the progressive establishment of a transmission mode through "pulse packets," since the asymmetric nature of this plasticity rule will indirectly control the jitter that could be observed in the timing spread within each pulse packet.

The most obvious cases of associative learning that depart from Hebbian co-activity or STDP rules are those requiring associations between neural events separated by long delays (see CEREBELLUM AND CONDITIONING), such as the optimal interstimulus intervals (in the range of seconds) of association in classical conditioning (see Figure 1*C*), or between the sample and choice periods in delayed-matching-to-sample comparison tasks (see CORTICAL HEBBIAN MODULES). Predictive rules have been modeled with ad hoc phase-lagged correlation functions (see REINFORCEMENT LEARNING). However, no experimental evidence has yet been obtained to account for the build-up of optimal interstimulus intervals through Hebbian mechanisms. This lack of evidence does not negate the implication of ionic mechanisms responsible for a delayed excitability change, or the slow build-up of a second-messenger-mediated intracellular response.

From Hebbian Synapses to Behavioral Learning

This section addresses the functional and behavioral consequences that Hebbian rules of plasticity induce in biological self-organizing systems.

Unsupervised Learning

Four possible applications of Hebbian processes acting on a long-term scale can be found in the early development or in the forced oriented growth of retinofugal pathways in lower vertebrates, mammals, and primates. These applications exemplify unsupervised learning, or self-organization.

1. The intrinsic synchronous bursting activity ("dark discharge") that arises prenatally from the retina before rods and cones are even formed exerts a structuring influence on the developing retinofugal pathway. The correlated firing among neighboring retinal ganglion cells within one eye and the lack of synchronous firing between ganglion cells of each eye are conditions that allow competition between geniculate afferents according to their ocularity. This correlated input is present in a still stronger way very early in prenatal life, taking the form of spatially organized waves of activity that spread intermittently in random directions across the whole retina. These synchronizing waves could provide the local correlations necessary for the sorting out and topographic refinement of retinal projections onto the lateral geniculate nucleus and, if still present after filtering through the thalamic relay, could be instrumental in the segregation of geniculate afferents in the recipient layer of visual cortex. After the first week of postnatal life in the cat, this intrinsic pattern-generating mechanism will give way to correlated inputs under the guidance of vision (see OCULAR DOMINANCE AND ORIENTATION COLUMNS).

2. Similar activity-dependent rules might apply to the development of intracortical connectivity: the validity of correlational Hebbian rules seems to hold throughout ontogenesis, if one does not restrict the choice of the postsynaptic control variable to spike activity. Indeed, free calcium activity and electrical and glial coupling could act prenatally as a substitute for synaptic transmission to ensure assembly formation in the absence of conventional fast Na^+ action potentials. A more classical form of Hebbian plasticity responsible for the progressive maturation of the horizontal intracortical network occurs during a few weeks following birth in the cat; the process results in a selective activity-dependent pruning and stabilization of horizontal connectivity.

3. Evidence has been obtained for the implication of Hebbian mechanisms during the functional reorganization of cortical processing following anomalous visuomotor behavior. A neuroanatomical and electrophysiological study in divergent strabismic kittens, which compensate misalignment of their eyes by alternate fixation, showed that only territories with the same ocular dominance are linked by tangential intracortical connections, and that synchronized activity is achieved only between cell groups dominated by the same eye. Furthermore, in the case of convergent strabismus, which results behaviorally in a loss of acuity through the eye that is not used for fixation, neurons dominated by the "amblyopic" eye exhibited much weaker synchronized activity than cells driven by the "good" eye. The observed correspondence between alterations in intracortical horizontal connectivity topology, the selective impairment of response synchronization, and the perceptual deficit constitutes probably the best evidence so far for a role of temporal correlation in the functional organization of cortical domains (see SYNCHRONIZATION, BINDING AND EXPECTANCY).

4. A last example illustrates the case of oriented growth of retinal axons that are artificially forced to connect the auditory thalamus after chronic deafferentation from its normal input at an early stage of development (see AUDITORY CORTEX). A combined electrophysiological and optical imaging study in the cortex, which normally should have become a primary auditory area, shows that the thalamic rewiring procedure induces the emergence of an anatomofunctional architecture similar to that observed in normal visual cortex (Sharma, Angelucci, and Sur, 2000): a normal retinotopic projection is formed, an orientation preference map is found with classical pinwheel organization, and, furthermore, the intrinsic intracortical connections show the distinctive patchy pattern along a mediolateral axis that is specific to a V1 area. Sur and colleagues further demonstrated that this rewired cortex can mediate adequate visual behavioral responses in response to visual stimuli. These findings suggest that the specificity found in the columnar organization of a given cortical area and its intrinsic horizontal connectivity are shaped by the particular temporal structure of the sensory input experienced during a critical postnatal period.

In summary, the grouping and sorting out of fibers afferent to cortex, the morphological tuning in the spatial distribution of the terminal boutons of intrinsic and extrinsic axons, the functional expression and possibly silencing of synapses, and the setting of a columnar architecture specific to the sensory modality to be processed could all, at some stage of postnatal development, be under the influence of temporal correlation between presynaptic fibers converging onto the same target, or between pre- and postsynaptic partners. This essential role of co-activity in self-organization was foreseen by theoreticians such as Linsker and Miller, who proposed a unifying role for activity, whether triggered endogenously by the nervous system or evoked by interaction with the environment (see OCULAR DOMINANCE AND ORIENTATION COLUMNS).

Supervised Learning and Cellular Analogues of Visual Cortical Epigenesis

Support for a functional implication of Hebb's postulate has also been found in studies on the neuroanatomical and physiological effects of forced patterns of activity, which simulate the functional effects of anomalous visual experience during critical periods of development (epigenesis, in Frégnac et al., 1988; Frégnac and Shulz, 1999). A differential supervised association protocol was used in vivo to test specific predictions of the covariance rule by imposing opposite changes in the temporal correlation between two test parameters characterizing afferent visual activity and the output signal of the cell. Here, an external supervisor (i.e., the experimenter) helped the cell to respond to one input and blocked the

cell's response to another, different input. The common outcome was that the relative preference between the two test stimulus characteristics was generally displaced toward that which had been paired with imposed increased visual responsiveness.

These pairing-induced modifications of specificity of the visual response have been considered as cellular analogues of epigenesis since they reproduce functional changes occurring during development or following early manipulation of the visual environment (monocular deprivation, rearing in an orientation-biased environment, or optically induced interocular orientation disparity). Surprisingly, the probability of inducing functional changes was found to be comparable in the kitten during the critical period and in older kittens and adults, suggesting that the cellular potential for plasticity might extend well beyond the classical extent of the critical period. Local supervised learning procedures, applied at the cellular level, might bypass the systemic control that normally blocks the expression of plasticity in the mature brain.

Functional Consequences of Spike-Timing-Dependent Plasticity

It has been suggested that, with repeated experience of a sequence of sensory events, spike-timing-dependent plasticity will promote the learning of the sequence and anticipation of future events from past stimuli. Recent tests of this hypothesis have been engineered in vivo in cat primary visual cortex: repetitive sequential presentation of two stimuli, one being the orientation preferred by the recorded cell and the other being either a suboptimal orientation or an electrical stimulation of the cortex, resulted in a compensatory reorganization of orientation tuning, with the direction of the shift in orientation preference depending on the temporal order of the stimulus pair. Furthermore, similar conditioning in human subjects induced a similar shift in perceived orientation, thus mirroring the plasticity described at the single-cell level in cat visual cortex. Thus the relative timing of visual stimulation and cortical activity plays a critical role in dynamic modulations of adult cortical function. In addition, these various adaptive protocols suggest that the susceptibility to adaptive changes is not uniform throughout cortex, and that orientation pinwheel centers may obey plasticity rules differently from their surround.

Gating Signals and Attentional Processes

Both Hebb and Milner were aware of the fact that the expression of synaptic changes could largely depend on the level of preactivation of nonspecific projection systems and arousal. These factors could influence the likelihood of summation at the synapse and thus could affect the amount of correlated input needed to induce synaptic changes. Because of methodological and technical difficulties, the role of the *behavioral context* (i.e., attention, reinforcement) has been often ignored in the study of the synaptic mechanisms underlying learning in mammals. Ahissar and collaborators applied cross-correlation techniques to study the plasticity of "functional connectivity" between simultaneously recorded pairs of neurons in the auditory cortex in awake monkeys performing a sensory discrimination task (reviewed in Ahissar et al., 1998). In order to control the correlation of activity between cells, the auditory stimulus preferred by the presumed postsynaptic cell was applied every time (and immediately after) the presynaptic cell fired spontaneously. The tone used to control the activity of the postsynaptic cell also signaled the reward occurrence. Under these Hebbian conditions, reversible changes in functional coupling could be induced only when the animal was attentive to the tone. These changes lasted for a few minutes and followed the covariance hypothesis predictions. The results indicate that Hebb's requirement is necessary but not sufficient for cortical plasticity in the adult monkey to occur: internal signals indicating the behavioral relevance are also required. More recently, cellular analogues of state-dependent learning have been proposed that show that the recall of a learned association in adult sensory cortex requires the application of the same neuromodulatory signals (Ach) as those present during conditioning in order for the functional changes to be expressed (Shulz et al., 2000).

Anti-Hebbian Forms of Learning

Depending on the neural structure under study (i.e., cerebellum versus cortex) or the time course of the functional effect looked for (i.e., sensory adaptation versus learning), forms of plasticity have been observed that are contrary to the predictions of Hebb's postulate. Such changes are called anti-Hebbian (or reverse Hebbian) and should be unambiguously distinguished from pseudo-Hebbian modifications (see POST-HEBBIAN LEARNING ALGORITHMS). The best-known example of anti-Hebbian plasticity is cerebellar long-term depression (see CEREBELLUM: NEURAL PLASTICITY), which, by its time course and induction requirements, appears similar to Hebbian associative potentiation. The trigger mechanism appears to be the same in both cases: free calcium entry into the postsynaptic cell. In order to explain why in the cerebellar case depression occurs, whereas potentiation is predicted by Hebbian schemes of plasticity, it could be assumed that the sign of the change of the synaptic modification depends on the type of neurotransmission (excitatory/inhibitory) that the postsynaptic neuron will exert on other neuronal targets. Purkinje cells for which Hebbian protocols induce depression are the inhibitory output neurons of the cerebellar cortex. Although no biological basis has been found to support the hypothesis that excitatory and inhibitory cells undergo Hebbian potentiation and depression, respectively, the implications of the hypothesis are very attractive in terms of systems theory: forced co-activity would produce the same type of global positive gain control whatever the neuronal structure under study, either by increasing the transmission of the selected input through a purely excitatory loop or by reducing the excitation fed into the inhibitory efferent pathway.

Other examples of anti-Hebbian plasticity link both cerebellar LTD and fast adaptation processes in perception. In the teleost electric fishes (Mormyridae and Gymnotidae), the cerebellar-like structure that receives primary electrosensory projections is the electrosensory lobe (ELL) (see ELECTROLOCATION). The feedforward sensory input informs the fish of its electrical environment and also provides a reafferent response, owing to the sensory effect of the fish's own electric discharge (EOD). The principal cells of the ELL, like Purkinje cells in cerebellum, receive in addition a diversity of contextual inputs conveyed through parallel fibers. The context can provide a copy of the motor command responsible for the electric discharge ("efferent copy" or "corollary discharge"), proprioceptive cues about movements from the fins or the whole body, or control signals descending from higher integrative areas. The pairing of an electrosensory stimulus at a fixed phase or delay after the EOD motor command, or after the passive bend of the body tail, results, when the contextual signal is reapplied alone, in the recall of a sign-inverted image of the firing pattern evoked by the paired electrosensory stimulus. The plastic changes at the parallel fiber–principal cell synapse can be long-lasting, but the extinction of the effect is an active process depending on the frequency of the recall process. Thus, in the mormyrid ELL, the modifiable corollary discharge elicits the transient storage of a negative image of the temporal and spatial pattern of sensory input that has followed the motor command. Bell and co-workers demonstrated the synaptic nature of the change and its reversibility in GABAergic medium ganglionic cells of the ELL by replacing the sensory input (which affects the whole structure) with an intracellular current pulse affecting only the cell under study (Han, Grant, and Bell, 2000; reviewed in Bell, 2001). Similar findings have been observed with other contextual signals in other cerebellar-like structures, such as the ventilatory motor commands of the fish in the dorsal octaval nucleus of elasmobranchs (sharks and rays).

The application of sign-inverted Hebbian rules to excitatory networks has by itself a straightforward prediction: the output of the association neurons will tend to be reduced in response to input patterns to which the neural system is exposed frequently. Evidence in the visual system has been found for gain control processes acting in the range of hundreds of milliseconds. It is known, for instance, that sensory adaptation in forward masking (the fact that the first presentation of a stimulus can bias the perceived features of a second stimulus or alter its visibility) occurs on a time range too long to be accounted for by direct inhibitory action and too short to be compared with the effects of behavioral learning. Anti-Hebbian plasticity could potentially act in the vertebrate brain to filter out modification of sensory input resulting from motor exploration of the environment, and thus could optimize the detection of new events.

Discussion

The study of memory formation benefits from the use of simple putative elementary principles of plasticity operating at a local level (the synapse) and uniformly across the cell assembly. The large number of experimental attempts to demonstrate the validity of Hebb's postulate prediction during the last 50 years should have inevitably narrowed its fields of application. Surprisingly, Hebbian schemes have survived to become the symbol of an ever-renewed concept of synaptic plasticity, open for more generalization. A variety of experimental networks, ranging from the abdominal ganglion in the invertebrate *Aplysia* to the hippocampus and visual cortex, offer converging validation of the prediction of Hebb's postulate. In these networks, similar algorithms of potentiation can be implemented using different cascades of second messengers triggered by activation of synaptic and/or voltage-dependent conductances. Classes of processes occuring on different time scales—development or epigenesis (days and weeks), learning (minutes or hours), and even perception (milliseconds)—could have similar phenomenological outcomes.

When followed literally, Hebb's postulate refers to the set of direct excitatory synaptic contacts, originating from one presynaptic neuron, onto a postsynaptic neuron that may participate in triggering its activity, and to the correlational rules that predict an increase in efficacy in synaptic transmission. Modelers have often simplified this view to the extreme, using ideal connections between pairs of neurons, and ignoring much of the complexity of different biological implementations of the so-called Hebbian synapse in invertebrates and vertebrates. Most cellular data supporting Hebb's predictions have been derived from electrophysiological measurements of composite postsynaptic potentials or synaptic currents, or from short-latency peaks in cross-correlograms, which cannot always be interpreted simply at the synaptic level. The basic conclusion of these experiments is that covariance between pre- and postsynaptic activity up- and downregulates the "effective" connectivity between pairs of functionnally coupled cells.

It may be concluded that what changes according to a correlational rule is not so much the efficacy of transmission at a given synapse but rather a more general coupling term mixing the influence of polysynaptic excitatory and inhibitory circuits linking the two cells, modulated by the diffuse network background activation. Replacing this composite interaction by a single coupling term defines an ideal Hebbian synapse and has the additional interest for the modeler of providing a weighting function of the input, which can even change sign when inhibition overcomes excitation.

Road Maps: Grounding Models of Neurons; Neural Plasticity
Related Reading: Cerebellum: Neural Plasticity; Dendritic Learning; Hebbian Learning and Neuronal Regulation; NMDA Receptors: Synaptic, Cellular, and Network Models; Post-Hebbian Learning Algorithms

References

Abbott, L. F., and Nelson, S. B., 2000, Synaptic plasticity: Taming the beast, *Nature Neurosci.*, 3(Suppl.):1178–1183. ◆

Ahissar, E., Abeles, M., Ahissar, M., Haidarliu, S., and Vaadia, E., 1998, Hebbian-like functional plasticity in the auditory cortex of the behaving monkey, *Neuropharmacology*, 37:633–655.

Bell, C. C., 2001, Memory-based expectations in electrosensory systems, *Curr. Opin. Neurobiol.*, 11:481–487. ◆

Bi, G., and Poo, M., 2001, Synaptic modification by correlated activity: Hebb's postulate revisited, *Annu. Rev. Neurosci.*, 24:139–166. ◆

Bienenstock, E., Cooper, L. N., and Munro, P., 1982, Theory for the development of neuron selectivity: Orientation specificity and binocular interaction in visual cortex, *J. Neurosci.*, 2:32–48.

Brown, T. H., Ganong, A. H., Kairiss, E. W., and Keenan, C. L., 1990, Hebbian synapses: Biophysical mechanisms and algorithms, *Annu. Rev. Neurosci.*, 13:475–511. ◆

Delage, Y., 1919, *Le Rêve: Etude psychologique, philosophique et litteraire*, Paris: Presses Universitaires de France.

Frégnac, Y., 1999, A tale of two spikes, *Nature Neurosci.*, 2:299–301.

Frégnac, Y., and Bienenstock E., 1998, Correlational models of synaptic plasticity: Develoment, learning and cortical dynamics of mental representation, in *Mechanistic Relationships between Development and*

Learning: Beyond Metaphor (T. Carew, R. Menzel, and C. J. Shatz, Eds.), Chichester: Wiley, pp. 113–148. ◆

Frégnac, Y., and Shulz, D., 1994, Models of synaptic plasticity and cellular analogs of learning in the developing and adult vertebrate visual cortex, in *Advances in Neural and Behavioral Development* (V. Casagrande and P. Shinkman, Eds.), Norwood, NJ: Ablex, pp. 149–235.

Frégnac, Y., and Shulz, D., 1999, Activity-dependent regulation of receptive field properties of cat area 17 by supervised Hebbian learning, *J. Neurobiol.*, 41:69–82. ◆

Frégnac, Y., Shulz, D., Thorpe, S., and Bienenstock, E., 1988, A cellular analogue of visual cortical plasticity, *Nature*, 333:367–370.

Han, V. Z., Grant, K., and Bell, C. C., 2000, Reversible associative depression and non-associative potentiation at a parallel fiber synapse, *Neuron*, 27:611–622.

Hebb, D. O., 1949, *The Organization of Behavior*, New York: Wiley. ◆

James, W., 1890, *Psychology: Briefer Course*, Cambridge, MA: Harvard University Press. ◆

Konorski, J., 1948, *Conditioned Reflexes and Neuron Organization*, London: Cambridge University Press.

Levy, W. B., and Steward, O., 1983, Temporal contiguity requirements for long-term associative potentiation/depression in the hippocampus, *Neuroscience*, 8:791–797.

Milner, P. M., 1974, A model for visual shape recognition. *Psychol. Rev.*, 81:521–535.

Sharma, J., Angelucci, A., and Sur, M., 2000, Induction of visual orientation modules in auditory cortex, *Nature*, 404:841–847. ◆

Shulz, D. E., Sosnik, R., Ego, V., Haidarliu, S., and Ahissar, E., 2000, A neuronal analogue of state-dependent learning, *Nature*, 403:549–553.

Stent, G., 1973, A physiological mechanism for Hebb's postulate of learning, *Proc. Natl. Acad. Sci. USA*, 70:997–1001.

Helmholtz Machines and Sleep-Wake Learning

Peter Dayan

Introduction

Unsupervised learning is largely concerned with finding structure among sets of input patterns such as visual scenes. An important example of structure occurs when the input patterns are generated or caused in a systematic way, for instance when objects with different shapes, surface properties, and positions are illuminated by lights of different characters and viewed by an observer with a digital camera at a particular relative location. Here, the inputs can be seen as living on a manifold that has many fewer dimensions than the space of all possible activation patterns over the pixels of the camera; otherwise, random visual noise in the camera would appear to be a normal visual scene. The manifold should correctly be parameterized by the generators themselves (i.e., the objects, the lights, etc.) (see Hinton and Ghahramani, 1997).

The Helmholtz machine (Dayan et al., 1995; Hinton et al., 1995) is an example of an approach to unsupervised learning called *analysis by synthesis* (see, e.g., Neisser, 1967). Imagine that we have a perfect computer graphics model that indicates how objects appear to observers. We can use this model to synthesize input patterns that look just like the input patterns the observer would normally receive, with the crucial difference that, since we synthesized them, we know in detail how the images were generated. We can then use these pairs of images and generators to train a model that analyzes new images to find out how they too were generated—that is, a model that represents them according to which particular generators underlie them. Conversely, if we have a perfect analysis model that indicates the generators underlying any image, then it is straightforward to use the paired images and generators to train a graphics model. In the Helmholtz machine, we attempt to have an imperfect graphics or generative model train a better analysis or

recognition model, and an imperfect recognition model train a better generative model.

There are three key issues for an analysis by synthesis model. First is the nature of the synthetic or generative model. For the Helmholtz machine, this is a structured belief network (Jordan, 1998; see also BAYESIAN NETWORKS) that is a model for hierarchical top-down connections in the cortex. This model has an overall structure (the hierarchically organized layers, units within a layer, and so on) and a set of generative parameters that determine the probability distribution the model expresses. The units in the lowest layer of the network are observable, in the sense that it is on them that the inputs are presented; units higher up in the network are latent, since they are not directly observable from inputs.

The second issue for an analysis by synthesis model is how new inputs are analyzed or recognized in light of this generative model, i.e., how the states of the latent units are determined so that the input is represented in terms of the way it would be generated by the generative model (see GRAPHICAL MODELS: PROBABILISTIC INFERENCE). For the Helmholtz machine, this is done in an approximate fashion using a second structured belief network (called the recognition model) over the latent units, whose parameters are also learned. The recognition network is a model for the standard, bottom-up connections in cortex.

The third issue is the way that the generative and recognition models are learned from data (see GRAPHICAL MODELS: PARAMETER LEARNING). For the sleep-wake learning algorithm for the stochastic Helmholtz machine, this happens in two phases. In the wake phase, the recognition model is used to estimate the underlying generators (i.e., the states of the latent units) for a particular input pattern, and then the generative model is altered so that those generators are more likely to have produced the input that is actually observed. In the sleep phase, the generative model fantasizes inputs by choosing particular generators stochastically, and then the recognition model is altered so that it is more likely to report those particular generators, if the fantasized input were actually to be observed.

The Generative Model

Figure 1 shows an example Helmholtz machine, involving (for the sake of simplicity) three layers $(\mathbf{x}, \mathbf{y}, \mathbf{d})$ of binary stochastic units. The generative model uses top-down biases and weights $\mathcal{G} = \{g^x, g^y, g^d, \mathbf{G}^{xy}, \mathbf{G}^{yd}\}$ to parameterize a probability distribution over the input units $\mathbf{d} = (d_1, d_2, \dots)$. Consider an example in which the inputs are binary, pixelated, handwritten versions of the digit 9. In this case, we might contrive that x_i represent some relatively abstract features of the handwritten fonts (such as high curvature for circular portions or abnormal lengths for straight portions), and y_j represent some more concrete aspects of a sample character, such as tight corners at the top and bottom of the loops or elongated stems and tails.

In the standard Helmholtz machine model, the units *within* each layer are conditionally independent given the binary states of the layer above (this is called a *factorial* property). In our contrived example, across fonts, the existence of tight curvature is independent of long lengths, i.e.,

$$\mathcal{P}[\mathbf{x}; \mathcal{G}] = \prod_i \mathcal{P}[x_i; \mathcal{G}] \qquad (1)$$

Next, given the particular abstract properties of the font (i.e., given the state of $\mathbf{x}$), the precise concrete realizations (i.e., the y_j) are individually independent:

$$\mathcal{P}[\mathbf{y}|\mathbf{x}; \mathcal{G}] = \prod_j \mathcal{P}[y_j|\mathbf{x}; \mathcal{G}] \qquad (2)$$

Finally, given these concrete properties, pixels are independently inked:

$$\mathcal{P}[\mathbf{d}|\mathbf{y}; \mathcal{G}] = \prod_k \mathcal{P}[d_k|\mathbf{x}; \mathcal{G}] \qquad (3)$$

In sum, by marginalizing, one can write

$$\mathcal{P}[\mathbf{d}; \mathcal{G}] = \sum_{\mathbf{x},\mathbf{y}} \mathcal{P}[\mathbf{x}; \mathcal{G}]\mathcal{P}[\mathbf{y}|\mathbf{x}; \mathcal{G}]\mathcal{P}[\mathbf{d}|\mathbf{y}; \mathcal{G}] \qquad (4)$$

For binary stochastic units,

$$\mathcal{P}[x_i; g_i^x] = \sigma(g_i^x)$$
$$\mathcal{P}[y_j|\mathbf{x}; g_j^y, \mathbf{G}^{xy}] = \sigma\left(g_j^y + \sum_i \mathbf{G}_{ji}^{xy} x_i\right) \equiv \hat{y}_j(\mathbf{x}) \qquad (5)$$

where $\sigma(u) = 1/(1 + \exp(-u))$ is the standard sigmoid function. Although the units $\mathbf{y}$ are conditionally independent given the states of the units $\mathbf{x}$ in the layer above, they are not marginally independent across all the patterns that can be generated. That is, $\mathbf{x}$ can capture statistical structure (i.e., correlations) in the states of $\mathbf{y}$. So, for instance, the abstract curvature property captures the correlation that a tight corner at the bottom of the loop of a 9 is typically associated with a tight corner at the top of the loop. Similarly, $\mathbf{y}$ captures correlations in the states $\mathbf{d}$. The font example is only for illustration. We actually expect the unsupervised learning algorithm itself to find the representations $\mathbf{y}$ and $\mathbf{x}$ that collectively best capture the statistical structure of $\mathbf{d}$.

This top-down generative model is a simple example of a sigmoid belief net (or BAYESIAN NETWORKS). The conditional independence within a layer makes it very straightforward to generate a sample $\mathbf{d}^\bullet$ from $\mathcal{P}[\mathbf{d}|\mathcal{G}]$ by fantasizing a sample $\mathbf{x}^\bullet$, then $\mathbf{y}^\bullet$ given $\mathbf{x}^\bullet$ (both as in Equation 5), and then $\mathbf{d}^\bullet$ given $\mathbf{y}^\bullet$ (using a similar expression).

The Recognition Model

When the generative model is used to create such a complete fantasy, we consider $\mathbf{x}^\bullet$ and $\mathbf{y}^\bullet$ as the *generators* of $\mathbf{d}^\bullet$. The task for the recognition model is to take a new example $\mathbf{d}$ and report the state(s) of $\mathbf{x}$ and $\mathbf{y}$ that might have generated it. In terms of our example, this implies finding a representation for a new image of a handwritten 9 in terms of the settings of the more concrete and more abstract parameters that could have generated it. Using Bayes's theorem, we know that

$$\mathcal{P}[\mathbf{x}, \mathbf{y}|\mathbf{d}; \mathcal{G}] = \mathcal{P}[\mathbf{d}|\mathbf{x}, \mathbf{y}; \mathcal{G}]\frac{\mathcal{P}[\mathbf{x}; \mathcal{G}]\mathcal{P}[\mathbf{y}|\mathbf{x}; \mathcal{G}]}{\mathcal{P}[\mathbf{d}; \mathcal{G}]} \qquad (6)$$

It is straightforward to calculate all the terms on the right-hand side *except* for the denominator $\mathcal{P}[\mathbf{d}; \mathcal{G}]$, which involves a sum over all the possible states of $\mathbf{x}$ and $\mathbf{y}$ (a set that grows exponentially large as the number of elements in $\mathbf{x}$ and $\mathbf{y}$ grows). Thus, an approximation to $\mathcal{P}[\mathbf{x}, \mathbf{y}|\mathbf{d}; \mathcal{G}]$ is usually required. The stochastic version of the Helmholtz machine (the only version we discuss here) uses for approximate recognition a bottom-up belief network (see Figure 1) over exactly the same units. This network instantiates a probability distribution $\mathcal{Q}[\mathbf{x}, \mathbf{y}|\mathbf{d}; \mathcal{R}] = \mathcal{Q}[\mathbf{y}|\mathbf{d}; \mathcal{R}]\mathcal{Q}[\mathbf{x}|\mathbf{y}; \mathcal{R}]$ using a separate set of parameters, the bottom-up biases and weights $\mathcal{R} = \{\mathbf{r}^x, \mathbf{r}^y, R^{dy}, R^{yx}\}$. A critical approximation is that the recognition model is assumed to be factorial in the bottom-up direction, i.e., y_1 is independent of y_2 given $\mathbf{d}$, and so forth. Over the course of learning, it is intended that $\mathcal{Q}[\mathbf{x}, \mathbf{y}|\mathbf{d}; \mathcal{R}]$ should come to be as close to $\mathcal{P}[\mathbf{x}, \mathbf{y}|\mathbf{d}; \mathcal{G}]$ as possible, subject to this approximation. On account of this approximation, it is as easy to generate a sample bottom-up from the recognition model, i.e., to recognize the input in terms of its generators, as it is to generate a sample top-down from the generative model, i.e., to create a fantasy.

Sleep-Wake Learning

As for many unsupervised learning methods (see UNSUPERVISED LEARNING WITH GLOBAL OBJECTIVE FUNCTIONS), the underlying goal of sleep-wake learning is to perform maximum likelihood density estimation by maximizing the log probability of the observed

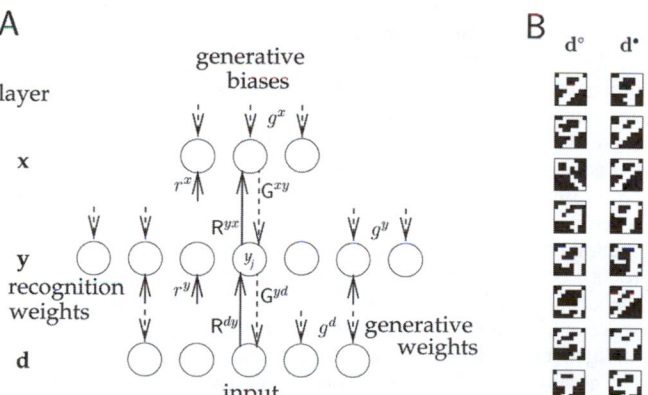

Figure 1. Helmholtz machine. *A*, Structure of a three-layer Helmholtz machine, with generative weights and biases $\mathcal{G}$ (dashed) and recognition weights and biases $\mathcal{R}$ (solid). *B*, Handwritten digit example. The left column shows eight samples from a training set of binarized, 8×8, handwritten 9s; the right column shows eight samples produced by the generative model after training. The training set is as described in Hinton et al. (1995).

data $\mathfrak{D} = \{\mathbf{d}(1), \mathbf{d}(2), \ldots\}$ under the generative model, that is, $E(\mathcal{G}) = \Sigma_t \log P[\mathbf{d}(t)|\mathcal{G}]$. One key idea, due to Neal and Hinton (1998) and Zemel (1994) (see MINIMUM DESCRIPTION LENGTH ANALYSIS), is to take the logarithm of both sides of Equation 4, though using the exact recognition distribution of Equation 6 to swap the order of the log and the sum:

$$\log P[\mathbf{d}; \mathcal{G}] = \sum_{\mathbf{x},\mathbf{y}} P[\mathbf{x}, \mathbf{y}|\mathbf{d}; \mathcal{G}] \log P[\mathbf{x}, \mathbf{y}, \mathbf{d}; \mathcal{G}]$$
$$+ \mathcal{H}[P[\mathbf{x}, \mathbf{y}|\mathbf{d}; \mathcal{G}]] \tag{7}$$

and then to introduce an approximate recognition distribution $\mathcal{Q}[\mathbf{x}, \mathbf{y}; \mathbf{d}, \mathcal{R}]$, with a bounded effect on the expression

$$\log P[\mathbf{d}; \mathcal{G}] \geq \sum_{\mathbf{x},\mathbf{y}} \mathcal{Q}[\mathbf{x}, \mathbf{y}; \mathbf{d}, \mathcal{R}] \log P[\mathbf{x}, \mathbf{y}, \mathbf{d}; \mathcal{G}]$$
$$+ \mathcal{H}[\mathcal{Q}[\mathbf{x}, \mathbf{y}; \mathbf{d}, \mathcal{R}]] \tag{8}$$

that can be quantified using a measure of the discrepancy between approximate and exact recognition distributions:

$$= \log P[\mathbf{d}; \mathcal{G}] - \mathrm{KL}[\mathcal{Q}[\mathbf{x}, \mathbf{y}; \mathbf{d}, \mathcal{R}], P[\mathbf{x}, \mathbf{y}|\mathbf{d}; \mathcal{G}]] \tag{9}$$

$$\equiv -\mathcal{F}[\mathbf{d}; \mathcal{R}, \mathcal{G}] \tag{10}$$

Here, $\mathcal{H}[A] = -\Sigma_{\mathbf{a}} A[\mathbf{a}] \log A[\mathbf{a}]$ is the entropy of probability distribution A, and, in Equation 9, $\mathrm{KL}[A, B] = \Sigma_{\mathbf{a}} A[\mathbf{a}] \log A[\mathbf{a}]/B[\mathbf{a}]$ is the Kullback-Liebler (KL) divergence between two distributions A and B. This KL divergence is greater than or equal to 0, with equality when A and B are essentially equal. Thus, Inequality 8 holds for an arbitrary distribution $\mathcal{Q}[\mathbf{x}, \mathbf{y}; \mathbf{d}, \mathcal{R}]$ over $\mathbf{x}$, $\mathbf{y}$, with equality if $\mathcal{Q}[\mathbf{x}, \mathbf{y}; \mathbf{d}, \mathcal{R}]$ is the true analytical distribution $P[\mathbf{x}, \mathbf{y}|\mathbf{d}; \mathcal{G}]$. Expression $\mathcal{F}[\mathbf{d}; \mathcal{R}, \mathcal{G}]$ can be seen as a Helmholtz free energy; hence the name of the machine.

During the *wake* phase, a single pattern $\mathbf{d}^{\circ}$ is sampled from $\mathfrak{D}$ and presented to the recognition model. This is executed bottom-up to produce a single sample $\mathbf{y}^{\circ}$ given $\mathbf{d}$ and $\mathbf{x}^{\circ}$ given $\mathbf{y}^{\circ}$. Then, the parameters $\mathcal{G}$ of the generative model are changed using stochastic gradient ascent of the lower bound to the log probability, i.e., proportionally to

$$\nabla_{\mathcal{G}} \log P[\mathbf{x}^{\circ}, \mathbf{y}^{\circ}, \mathbf{d}; \mathcal{G}] = \nabla_{\mathcal{G}}\{\log P[\mathbf{x}^{\circ}; \mathcal{G}] + \log P[\mathbf{y}^{\circ}|\mathbf{x}^{\circ}; \mathcal{G}]$$
$$+ \log P[\mathbf{d}^{\circ}|\mathbf{y}^{\circ}; \mathcal{G}]\}$$

For activation functions such as those in Equation 5, this leads to particularly simple "delta" learning rules such as

$$\Delta g_j^y \propto (y_j^{\circ} - \hat{y}_j(\mathbf{x}^{\circ})) \quad \Delta G_{ij}^{xy} \propto (y_j^{\circ} - \hat{y}_j(\mathbf{x}^{\circ}))x_i^{\circ}$$

in which the output of the recognition model is used as the *target* for the generative model instead of vice versa.

The ideal for the *sleep* phase would be to change the recognition weights $\mathcal{R}$ using stochastic gradient descent also of the lower bound in Equation 9. Unfortunately, this procedure is not generally computationally tractable. The second key idea in sleep-wake learning is to attempt during sleep to minimize $\mathrm{KL}[P[\mathbf{x}, \mathbf{y}|\mathbf{d}; \mathcal{G}], \mathcal{Q}[\mathbf{x}, \mathbf{y}; \mathbf{d}, \mathcal{R}]]$ instead. This is not the same, since the KL divergence is not symmetric, although they are equal at their joint minimum where $P[\mathbf{x}, \mathbf{y}|\mathbf{d}; \mathcal{G}] = \mathcal{Q}[\mathbf{x}, \mathbf{y}; \mathbf{d}, \mathcal{R}]$. The KL divergence the wrong way around can be minimized by fantasizing sample $\mathbf{x}^{\bullet}$, $\mathbf{y}^{\bullet}$, and $\mathbf{d}^{\bullet}$ from the generative model (in the way described at the end of the section on that model), and then changing the recognition weights according to

$$\nabla_{\mathcal{R}} \log \mathcal{Q}[\mathbf{x}^{\bullet}, \mathbf{y}^{\bullet}; \mathbf{d}^{\bullet}, \mathcal{R}] = \nabla_{\mathcal{R}}\{\log \mathcal{Q}[\mathbf{y}^{\bullet}|\mathbf{d}^{\bullet}; \mathcal{R}] + \log \mathcal{Q}[\mathbf{x}^{\bullet}|\mathbf{y}^{\bullet}; \mathcal{R}]\}$$

For activation functions such as those in Equation 5, this leads to the same simple delta learning rules as for the generative model, except that the output of the generative model is used as the target for the recognition model.

Since sleep learning involves an approximation, it is only in very special cases (see Neal and Dayan, 1997) that it is possible to prove even that it is appropriately stable. Nevertheless, the model has been shown to work quite well in practice. Figure 1B shows the result of applying sleep-wake learning to a set of input patterns (left column) that are binary images of the handwritten digit 9. The right column shows fantasized samples following learning, and these can be seen to be generated by a distribution close to that in the training distribution.

Discussion

As a directed belief network for analysis by synthesis that is trained according to maximum likelihood density estimation, the Helmholtz machine lives in what has become a rather crowded space (see UNSUPERVISED LEARNING WITH GLOBAL OBJECTIVE FUNCTIONS). In this context, the key property of the Helmholtz machine is that it uses an explicit recognition model that has its own parameters rather than performing recognition by an iterative process involving only the parameters of the generative model. In some ways this is an advantage; in particular, recognition can occur swiftly in a single pass. Learning during the sleep phase can be considered as a way of caching knowledge about how to do recognition effectively. In other ways it is a disadvantage, since the recognition model introduces an extra set of parameters that need to be learned and since, unlike the iterative mean field recognition methods that underlie most of the architectures mentioned earlier, the approximation involved in the recognition model in the Helmholtz machine cannot be tailored on-line to the particular input pattern that is presented. Another key feature is that, unlike many of these methods, the Helmholtz machine is explicitly designed to be hierarchical: units in one layer capture (i.e, both represent and generate) correlations in the layer below. Unlike INDEPENDENT COMPONENT ANALYSIS (q.v.), for instance, units within a layer are not forced to be marginally independent in the generative model, only conditionally independent *given* the activities in the layer above. This potentially allows it a much richer representation of the inputs. Also, the recognition model in the Helmholtz machine allows at least some correlations among the states of the hierarchical generators, a feature denied to mean field methods.

The Helmholtz machine also bears an interesting relationship to the Boltzmann machine (Hinton and Sejnowski, 1986; see also SIMULATED ANNEALING AND BOLTZMANN MACHINES), which can be seen as an undirected belief net. In the Boltzmann machine, which also lacks an explicit recognition model, a potentially drawn-out process of Gibbs sampling is used to recognize and generate inputs, since there is nothing like the simple, one-pass, directed recognition and generative belief networks of the Helmholtz machine. Also, the Boltzmann machine learning rule performs true stochastic gradient ascent of the log likelihood using a contrastive procedure, which, confusingly, involves wake and sleep phases that are quite different from the wake and the sleep phases of the sleep-wake algorithm. The two phases of the Boltzmann machine contrast the statistics of the activations of the network when input patterns are presented with the statistics of the activations of the network when it is running "free." This contrastive procedure involves substantial noise and is therefore slow (a problem rectified in Hinton's (2000) new approximate contrastive divergence learning rule). In the sleep-wake learning procedure for the Helmholtz machine, the wake and sleep phases are not contrastive. Rather, the recognition and generative models are forced to chase each other.

The most important open issue for the Helmholtz machine as a model of top-down and bottom-up connections in the cortex is how to weaken the approximation that the recognition and generative models are factorial within layers, without destroying the simplicity of sampling from and learning the models.

Road Map: Learning in Artificial Networks
Related Reading: Ying-Yang Learning

References

Dayan, P., Hinton, G. E., Neal, R. M., and Zemel, R. S., 1995, The Helmholtz machine, *Neural Computat.*, 7:889–904.

Hinton, G. E., 2000, *Training Products of Experts by Minimizing Contrastive Divergence*, Gatsby Computational Neuroscience Unit Technical Report TR 2000–004, London: Alexandra House.

Hinton, G. E., Dayan, P., Frey, B. J., and Neal, R. M., 1995, The wake-sleep algorithm for unsupervised neural networks, *Science*, 268:1158–1160. ◆

Hinton, G. E., and Ghahramani, Z., 1997, Generative models for discovering sparse distributed representations, *Philos. Trans. R. Soc. B*, 352:1177–1190. ◆

Hinton, G. E., and Sejnowski, T. J., 1986, Learning and relearning in Boltzmann machines, in *Parallel Distributed Processing: Explorations in the Microstructure of Cognition, vol. 1, Foundations* (D. E. Rumelhart, J. L. McClelland, and the PDP Research Group, Eds.), Cambridge, MA: MIT Press, pp. 282–317.

Jordan, M. I., Ed., 1998, *Learning in Graphical Models*, Dordrecht: Kluwer. ◆

Neal, R. M., and Dayan, P., 1997, Factor analysis using delta-rule wake-sleep learning, *Neural Computat.*, 9:1781–1803.

Neal, R. M., and Hinton, G. E., 1998, A view of the EM algorithm that justifies incremental, sparse, and other variants, in *Learning in Graphical Models* (M. I. Jordan, Ed.), Dordrecht: Kluwer, pp. 355–368.

Neisser, U., 1967, *Cognitive Psychology*, New York: Appleton-Century-Crofts.

Zemel, R. S., 1994, A minimum description length framework for unsupervised learning, Ph.D. diss., Toronto: University of Toronto, Computer Science Department.

Hemispheric Interactions and Specialization

James A. Reggia and Svetlana Levitan

Introduction

Currently recognized *hemispheric specializations*, where one cerebral hemisphere performs a task better than the other, include language, handedness, visuospatial processing, emotion and its facial expression, olfaction, and attention (Hellige, 1993). For example, in roughly 95% of people the left cerebral hemisphere is dominant for language, so language is said to be *lateralized* to the left hemisphere in such individuals. Behavioral lateralization in areas such as vocalization and motor preferences has been demonstrated not only in people but also in rodents, birds, primates, and other animals.

The underlying causes of hemispheric specialization/lateralization are not well understood at present. The many anatomical, biochemical, and physiological asymmetries that exist in the brain include a larger left temporal plane in the majority of subjects, greater dendritic branching in speech areas of the left hemisphere, different distributions of important neurotransmitters such as dopamine and norepinephrine between the hemispheres, and a lower left hemisphere threshold for motor-evoked potentials. Understanding which, if any, of these asymmetries actually contribute to hemispheric specialization remains an important problem in neuropsychology and is an instance of the more general issue of how functional modularity arises in the brain (Jacobs, 1997).

Besides the underlying hemispheric asymmetries listed above, another potential factor in function lateralization is hemispheric interactions via pathways connecting the hemispheres, such as the corpus callosum. Callosal fibers are largely but not exclusively homotopic: roughly mirror-symmetric points in each hemisphere are connected to each other. Callosal connections between the hemispheres are excitatory. This, as well as clinical data and split-brain experiments, suggests that transcallosal hemispheric interactions are mainly excitatory in nature, but this hypothesis has long been quite controversial. Transcallosal monosynaptic excitatory effects are subthreshold and followed by stronger, more prolonged inhibition, suggesting to some that transcallosal inhibitory interactions are much more important (Cook, 1986). The case for interhemispheric inhibition/competition has been strengthened recently by transcranial magnetic stimulation studies indicating that activation of one primary motor cortex inhibits the opposite one.

Neural modeling provides a useful way to investigate the implications of hypotheses that complement more traditional methods. In this article, we first consider models of hemispheric interactions that do not incorporate hemispheric differences and, conversely, models examining the effects of hemispheric differences that do not incorporate hemispheric interactions. We then look in more detail at some examples of recent work that studies both hemispheric interactions and differences in the same model, demonstrating how these factors influence the emergence of lateralization in models in which lateralization is not initially present. Finally, we briefly summarize insights gained from simulated damage in these models.

Modeling Hemispheric Interactions/Differences

A number of neural models have examined issues involving hemispheric interactions. In one group of studies, several models were developed representing homotopic left and right hemispheric regions connected via a simulated corpus callosum. For example, one early study demonstrated that oscillatory activity in a simulated hemisphere could be transferred to the other hemisphere via interhemispheric connections (Anninos and Cook, 1988). This was true regardless of assumptions about the excitatory/inhibitory nature of callosal connections, although learning was more rapid when callosal connections were excitatory. Another model, using paired neural networks representing left and right cortical regions, showed that homotopic inhibitory callosal connections produce complementary activity patterns but not lateralization in the two simulated hemispheric regions (Cook, 1986). This was done without postulating intrinsic differences between the cerebral hemispheres. These and other earlier neural models involved simulating hemispheric interactions, but none of them considered underlying asymmetric hemispheric regions or emergent lateralization.

In contrast, other models have simulated single hemispheric regions under differing conditions that are motivated by known asymmetries in the left and right cerebral hemispheres. Although these models have neither paired left and right cortical regions nor callosal connections like those above, they do examine issues related to lateralization.

One study focused on modeling hemispheric differences observed during semantic priming experiments (Burgess and Lund, 1998). Such experiments examine how the occurrence of one word facilitates the subsequent recall from memory of words with similar meanings. This model assumed that each hemisphere has the same representation of semantic information about words, but that the right hemisphere processes this information more slowly. The speed of activation of a target word for a hemisphere was also assumed to be based on a function of the semantic distance between that word and a priming word, and on the word's rate of activation decay. These word-specific quantities were derived from a large corpus of written text. Separate parameterized functions for the rate of activation of a word were determined for left and right hemispheres by evolving the parameters in these functions using a genetic algorithm. The resultant activation functions for each hemisphere, each function having different parameters, were then used successfully to predict the time course of activating word meaning in a number of priming experiments in which stimuli were presented separately to each hemisphere. These results implicitly provide a theory about the underlying differences in left and right hemisphere processing of semantic information.

Another study examining issues related to cerebral specialization without actually simulating paired hemispheric regions, corpus callosum, or the emergence of lateralization focused on the processing of spatial relations (Kosslyn et al., 1992). This investigation hypothesized that receptive field size asymmetries involving low-level visual neurons were responsible for experimental observations that the right cerebral hemisphere is faster at computing coordinate spatial relations involving precise metric information, such as judging distances, while the left hemisphere is faster in evaluating some categorical relations, such as above versus below. The coarse coding provided by error backpropagation neural networks with larger, overlapping receptive fields assumed for the right hemisphere was found to be superior for distance judgments, whereas networks with smaller, nonoverlapping receptive fields assumed for the left hemisphere were found to be superior in judging categorical relations. Conversely, training a network with adaptable receptive fields to do distance judgments led to larger receptive fields than training a network to judge categorical relations (Jacobs and Kosslyn, 1994). A separate model focusing on receptive field asymmetries from a different perspective has also been used to explain several experimentally observed visual processing asymmetries (Ivry and Robertson, 1998).

Simulating the Emergence of Lateralization

A number of neural models of paired left and right cortical regions have been used to examine conditions under which lateralization that was not present initially might emerge during learning. These models incorporate both hemispheric interactions and hemispheric differences. Three examples are given here. The first two incorporate a simulated corpus callosum, and represent end points on a spectrum from supervised to unsupervised learning within which other models fall (Cook, 1999; Shevtsova and Reggia, 1999). The third example illustrates how noncallosal hemispheric interactions can influence lateralization.

Phoneme Sequence Generation

A phoneme sequence generation model, trained using recurrent error backpropagation, was created that takes three-letter words as input and produces the correct temporal sequence of phonemes for the pronunciation of each word as output (Reggia, Goodall, and Shkuro, 1998). Figure 1a schematically summarizes the network architecture, where input elements are fully connected to two sets of neural elements representing corresponding regions of the left and right hemisphere cortex. These regions are connected to each other via a simulated corpus callosum and to output elements representing individual phonemes.

The effects of different hemispheric asymmetries (relative size, excitability, learning rate parameter, etc.) on the emergence of lateralization were examined one at a time. For each hemispheric asymmetry, and for a symmetric control version of the model, the uniform value of callosal connection influences was varied over

a.

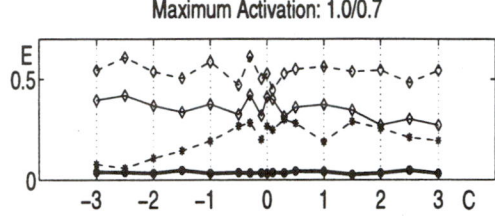

b.

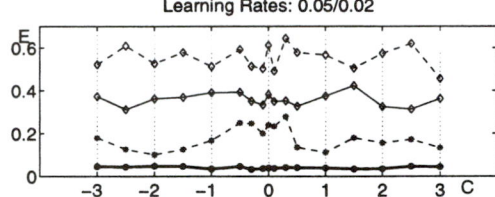

c.

Figure 1. *a*, Network architecture for phoneme sequence generation. I, input elements; LH (RH), left (right) hemisphere cortex region; CC, corpus callosum; O, output elements; S, state elements. In the graphs, error (E) is plotted versus callosal strength (C) for model versions where the left hemisphere (*b*) is more excitable or (*c'*) has more potent synaptic plasticity. In each case the upper dashed curve shows pretraining error and the lowest (thick solid) curve shows post-training error for the full model's output. The two middle curves show post-training output error when the left hemisphere alone (dashed line) or the right hemisphere alone (solid line) controls output.

several excitatory and inhibitory values. Lateralization was measured based on the difference between the output error when the left hemispheric region alone controlled the output versus when the right hemispheric region alone did so. These simulations showed that, within the limitations of the model, it is easy to produce lateralization. For example, lateralization occurred toward the side with higher excitability (Figure 1b) or a higher learning rate parameter (Figure 1c), depending on callosal strength. Lateralization tended to occur most readily and intensely when callosal connections exerted predominantly an inhibitory influence (Figure 1b), but with some asymmetries significant lateralization occurred for all callosal strengths (Figure 1c). In this specific model, the results could be interpreted as a competitive "race-to-learn" involving the two hemispheric regions, with the "winner" (dominant side) determined when the model as a whole acquired the input-output mapping and learning largely ceased. These results suggest that lateralization to a cerebral region can, in some cases, be associated with increased synaptic plasticity in that region relative to its mirror-image region in the opposite hemisphere, a testable prediction.

Self-Organizing Topographic Maps

Topographic maps representing various aspects of the environment are found in primary sensory regions of cortex. Maps in mirror-image regions of sensory cortex exhibit a rich range of patterns of asymmetries and lateralization (Bianki, 1993). A model of corresponding left and right hemispheric regions receiving sensory input has been used to study emergent map asymmetries and lateralization (Levitan and Reggia, 1999). Unlike the phoneme sequence generation model, purely unsupervised competitive learning was used. Map formation was examined while varying the underlying cortical region asymmetries and the assumed excitatory/inhibitory nature of callosal connections.

Figure 2 illustrates pairs of cortical maps appearing in this model where the centers of receptive fields of the cortical elements are plotted in the space of the sensory surface (i.e., these are *not* pictures of the cortical regions involved). Lines between plotted points indicate adjacent cortical elements. In all simulations, cortical maps were initially highly disorganized before learning, owing to randomly assigned initial synaptic strengths (Figure 2a). For excitatory, absent, or weakly inhibitory callosal interactions, complete

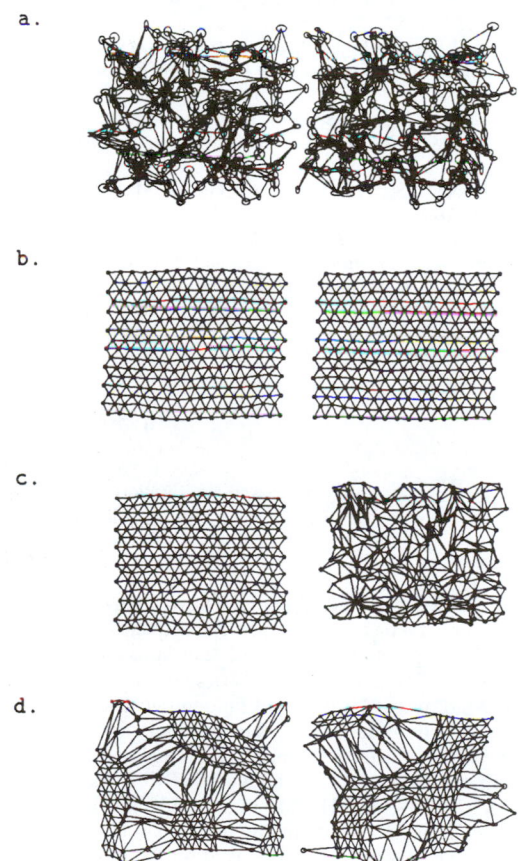

a.

b.

c.

d.

Figure 2. *a,* Unorganized maps bilaterally (e.g., prelearning). *b,* Bilaterally organized maps (e.g., post-training with weak excitatory callosal connections). *c',* Left map more organized than right. *d,* Complementary mosaic maps.

and symmetric mirror-image maps appeared after learning in both hemispheric regions (Figure 2b). In contrast, with stronger inhibitory callosal interactions, after learning, map lateralization tended to occur (Figure 2c; left more organized than right), or the maps became complementary (Figure 2d), reminiscent of "mosaic patterns" described experimentally (Bianki, 1993). Lateralization occurred readily toward the side having higher excitability or a larger cortical region. Unlike with the phoneme sequence generation model, asymmetric plasticity had only a transitory effect on lateralization, indicating that the effects of this factor may differ substantially depending on whether supervised or unsupervised learning is used. In this model, a "phase transition" in behavior occurs at a specific inhibitory callosal strength: above this value, bilateral symmetric maps occur; below it, lateralization and complementary maps occur.

Spatial Relations

Asymmetries in perceptual abilities are sometimes hypothesized to be due to an underlying asymmetry in receptive field sizes in the early visual system: smaller visual receptive fields on the left than on the right. A neural model of two hemispheric regions, represented as multilayer feedforward networks having different afferent pathway receptive field sizes, was implemented to examine the plausibility of this hypothesis (Jacobs and Kosslyn, 1994). This model did not include a simulated corpus callosum but instead had an extra module called a "gating network" that determined the extent to which each hemispheric region controlled the model's output. Each hemispheric region competed to learn each output pattern, and the region whose output most closely matched the correct output pattern "won" and learned more.

In simulations performed with this model, the network was trained to perform both categorical and coordinate tasks, while the left input layer was forced to have smaller receptive field sizes. When the difference in left and right receptive field sizes was sufficiently large, the left hemispheric region became superior at the categorical task, while the right hemispheric region became superior with the coordinate task. These results are consistent with the hypothesis that asymmetric receptive field sizes contribute to hemispheric specialization in processing spatial relations.

Effects of Simulated Damage

Several versions of the above models of interacting left and right hemispheric regions have been subjected to simulated focal damage (Levitan and Reggia, 1999; Shkuro, Glezer, and Reggia, 2000). For example, with the phoneme sequence generation model, an area of focal damage was introduced into an intact model by making part of one simulated hemispheric region nonfunctional. Performance errors of the full model and each hemisphere alone were measured immediately after the damage and then after further training restored the model's performance to normal. During the recovery period, in which performance eventually returned to predamage levels, the undamaged hemispheric region very often participated in and contributed to recovery, more so as the amount of damage increased. These results support the controversial hypothesis that the intact cerebral hemisphere plays a role in adult recovery from damage in the opposite hemisphere. Further, in these simulations of focal damage, when callosal influences were excitatory, the undamaged hemispheric region often had a drop in mean activation and exhibited impaired performance, representing the analog of transcallosal diaschisis (a fall in regional cerebral blood flow and glucose metabolism in the intact cerebral hemisphere following unilateral brain damage). These and other observations following model damage support the view that hemispheric interactions via callosal connections are excitatory.

Discussion

Neural models have recently been used to investigate a variety of issues concerning whether underlying asymmetries can lead to or can explain lateralization and how assumptions about callosal influences affect lateralization. Although these models have been limited in size and scope, and although they are greatly simplified from neurobiological and behavioral reality, they have demonstrated a number of results that are relevant to current issues in brain theory.

First, any one of a variety of underlying hemispheric asymmetries can lead to hemispheric specialization in these models, including asymmetric size, excitability, receptive field sizes, and synaptic plasticity. Such a finding supports past arguments that a single underlying hemispheric asymmetry is unlikely to account for language and other behavioral lateralizations (Hellige, 1993).

Second, resolving the issue of the inhibitory versus excitatory nature of callosal influences remains elusive. Lateralization generally appeared most intensely in models with inhibitory interhemispheric interactions, lending support to past arguments that whatever the actual neurophysiological nature of callosal synaptic *connections*, callosal *influences* are apparently inhibitory in nature, producing competition between the two hemispheres. However, lateralization also occurred in some models with excitatory callosal influences and asymmetric hemispheric regions, and focal damage in these models caused a decrease in activation and sometimes performance in the opposite intact hemispheric region. These latter changes resemble those seen experimentally in stroke patients, supporting past arguments that callosal influences are predominantly excitatory. This conflicting evidence concerning the excitatory versus inhibitory nature of callosal influences may be referred to as the *callosal dilemma*. A possible resolution of this dilemma, excitatory transcallosal influences in the context of subcortical cross-midline inhibitory connections, was recently studied computationally (Reggia et al., 2001). Further examination of this issue would be a fertile topic for future research.

Finally, during the recovery period following focal damage to models, the opposite intact hemispheric region generally contributed to recovery, supporting the controversial hypothesis that the undamaged cerebral hemisphere often contributes to language recovery following unilateral brain damage in adults. This effect increased with increasing damage, suggesting that relevant future experimental studies of recovery from stroke should carefully control for this factor in interpreting data.

Road Map: Cognitive Neuroscience
Related Reading: Lesioned Networks as Models of Neuropsychological Deficits; Neuropsychological Impairments

References

Anninos, P., and Cook, N., 1988, Neural net simulation of the corpus callosum, *Int. J. Neurosci.*, 38:381–391.

Bianki, V., 1993, *The Mechanism of Brain Lateralization*, Newark, NJ: Gordon & Breach.

Burgess, C., and Lund, K., 1998, Modeling cerebral asymmetries in high-dimensional semantic space, in *Right Hemisphere Language Comprehension* (M. Beeman and C. Chiarello, Eds.), Mahwah, NJ: Erlbaum, pp. 215–244.

Cook, N., 1986, *The Brain Code*, New York: Methuen. ◆

Cook, N., 1999, Simulating consciousness in a bilateral neural network, *Consciousness Cognit.*, 8:62–93.

Hellige, J., 1993, *Hemispheric Asymmetry*, Cambridge, MA: Harvard University Press. ◆

Ivry, R., and Robertson, L., 1998, *The Two Sides of Perception*, Cambridge, MA: MIT Press, pp. 225–255.

Jacobs, R., 1997, Nature, nurture and the development of functional specialization, *Psychonom. Bull. Rev.*, 4:299–309.

Jacobs, R., and Kosslyn, S., 1994, Encoding shape and spatial relations, *Cognit. Sci.*, 18:361–386.

Kosslyn, S., Chabris, C., Marsolek, C., and Koenig, O., 1992, Categorical vs. coordinate spatial relations, *J. Exper. Psychol. Hum. Percept. Performance*, 18:562–577.

Levitan, S., and Reggia, J., 1999, Interhemispheric effects on map organization following simulated cortical lesions, *Artific. Intell. Med.*, 17:59–85.

Reggia, J., Goodall, S., and Shkuro, Y., 1998, Computational studies of lateralization of phoneme sequence generation, *Neural Computat.*, 10:1277–1297.

Reggia, J., Goodall, S., Shkuro, Y., and Glezer, M., 2001, The callosal dilemma, *Neurol. Res.*, 23:465–471.

Shevtsova, N., and Reggia, J., 1999, A neural network model of lateralization during letter identification, *J. Cognit. Neurosci.*, 11:167–181.

Shkuro, Y., Glezer, M., and Reggia, J., 2000, Interhemispheric effects of simulated lesions in a neural model of single-word reading, *Brain Lang.*, 72:343–374.

Hidden Markov Models

Hervé Bourlard and Samy Bengio

Introduction

Over the past 20 years, finite-state automata (FSA), and more particularly stochastic finite-state automata (SFSA) and different variants of hidden Markov models (HMMs), have been used successfully to address several complex sequential pattern recognition problems, among them continuous speech recognition, cursive (handwritten) text recognition, time series prediction, and biological sequence analysis.

FSAs allow complex learning problems to be solved by assuming that the sequential pattern can be decomposed into piecewise stationary segments, encoded through the topology of the FSA. Each stationary segment can be parameterized in terms of a deterministic or a stochastic function. In the latter case, it may also be possible that the SFSA state sequence is not observed directly but is a probabilistic function of the underlying finite-state Markov chain. This leads to the definition of the powerful HMMs, involving two concurrent stochastic processes: the sequence of HMM states modeling the sequential structure of the data, and a set of state output processes modeling the (local) stationary character of the data. The Markov model is called hidden because there is an underlying stochastic process (i.e., the sequence of states) that is not observable but that affects the observed sequence of events.

Furthermore, depending on the way the SFSA is parameterized and trained, SFSAs (and HMMs in particular) can be used either as a *production model*, in which the observation sequence is considered to be an output signal produced by the model, or as a *recognition model* (acceptor), in which the observation sequence is considered as being accepted by the model. Finally, it may also be the case that the HMM is used to explicitly model the stochastic relationship between two (input and output) event sequences, resulting in a model usually referred to as an input-output HMM.

The parameters of these models can be trained by different variants of the powerful Expectation-Maximization (EM) algorithm (Baum and Petrie, 1966; Liporace, 1982), which, depending on the criterion being used, is referred to as maximum likelihood (ML) or maximum a posteriori (MAP) training. However, even though they belong to the same family, all of these models exhibit different properties. This article compares some of the variants of these powerful SFSA and HMM models currently used for sequence processing.

Finite-State Automata

In its more general form (Hopcroft, Motwani, and Ullman, 2000) and as summarized in Table 1, an FSA, which will be denoted M in this paper, is defined as an abstract machine consisting of the following:

- A set of states $\mathcal{Q} = \{I, 1, \ldots, k, \ldots, K, F\}$, including the initial state I and final state F, also referred to as accepting state (in the case of recognizers). Variants of this machine include machines having multiple initial states and multiple accepting states. In this article, a specific state visited at time t will be denoted q_t.
- A set $\mathcal{Y}$ of (discrete or continuous) input symbols or vectors. A particular sequence of size T of input symbols/vectors will be denoted $Y = \{y_1, y_2, \ldots, y_t, \ldots, y_T\} = y_1^T$, where y_t represents the input symbol/vector at time t.
- A set $\mathcal{Z}$ of (continuous or discrete) output symbols or vectors. A particular sequence of size T of output symbols/vectors will be denoted $Z = z_1^T$, where z_t represents the output symbol/vector at time t.
- A *state transition function* $q_t = f(y_t, q_{t-1})$, which takes the current input event and the previous state q_{t-1} and returns the next state q_t.
- An *emission function* $z_t = g(q_t, q_{t-1})$, which takes the current state q_t and the previous state q_{t-1} and returns an output event z_t. This automaton is usually know as a *Mealy FSA*, i.e., one producing an output for each input-dependent *transition*. As a variant of this, the emission function of a *Moore FSA* depends only on the current state, i.e., $z_t = g(q_t)$, thus producing an output for each visited state. There is, however, a homomorphic equiv-

alence between Mealy and Moore automata, given an increase and renaming of the states.

Finally, in the case of sequential pattern processing, the processed sequence is often represented as an *observed sequence* of symbols or vectors which, depending on the type of automata and optimization criterion, will sometimes be considered input events and at other times output events. To accommodate this flexibility, we also define the *observed sequence* of size T as $X = x_1^T$, where x_t is the observed event/vector at time t. For example, in the case of speech recognition, x_t would be the acoustic vector resulting from the spectral analysis of the signal at time t, and is equivalent to z_t (since in that case the observations are the outputs of the FSA).

A *deterministic FSA* is one in which the transition and emission functions $f(.)$ and $g(.)$ are deterministic, implying that the output event and next state are uniquely determined by a single input event (i.e., there is exactly one transition for each given input event and state). In comparison, a nondeterministic FSA is one in which the next state is not uniquely determined by the current previous state and input event. However, it is often possible to transform a nondeterministic FSA into a deterministic FSA, at the cost of a significant increase in the possible number of input symbols.

We will not further discuss deterministic FSAs, which have been largely used in language theory (Hopcroft et al., 2000), where FSAs are often used to accept or reject a language (i.e., certain sequences of input events).

Stochastic Finite-State Automata

A *stochastic FSA* (SFSA) is an FSA in which the transition and/or emission functions are probabilistic functions. In the case of Markov models, there is a one-to-one relationship between the observation and the state, and the transition function is probabilistic. In the case of HMMs, the emission function is also probabilistic, and the states are no longer directly observable through the input events. Instead, each state produces one of the possible output events with a certain probability.

Depending on their structure (discussed below), transition and emission (probability density) functions are represented in terms of a set of parameters Θ, which will have to be estimated on repre-

Table 1. Deterministic and Stochastic Finite-State Automata

	Deterministic Finite-State Automata	Stochastic Finite-State Automata			
		Markov Model	HMM	HMM/ANN	IOHMM
States	$k \in \mathcal{Q}$	$x_t = k \in \mathcal{Q}$	$k \in \mathcal{Q}$	$k \in \mathcal{Q}$	$k \in \mathcal{Q}$
Input symbols	$y_t \in \mathcal{Y}$	—	—	$x_t = y_t \in \mathcal{Y}$	$x_t = y_t \in \mathcal{Y}$
Output symbols	$z_t \in \mathcal{Z}$	—	$x_t = z_t \in \mathcal{Z}$	—	$z_t \in \mathcal{Z}$
Transition law	$q_t = f(y_t, q_{t-1})$	Transition probabilities $p(x_t\|x_{t-1})$	Transition probabilities $p(q_t\|q_{t-1})$	Conditional transition probabilities $p(q_t\|x_t, q_{t-1})$	Conditional transition probabilities $p(q_t\|x_t, q_{t-1})$
Emission law					
Mealy	$z_t = g(q_t, q_{t-1})$	—	Emission on transition $x_t = g(q_t, q_{t-1})$ $p(x_t\|q_{t-1}, q_t)$	—	$p(z_t\|q_t, q_{t-1}, x_t, x_{t-1})$
Moore	$z_t = g(q_t)$	—	Emission on state $x_t = g(q_t)$ $p(x_t\|q_t)$	—	$p(z_t\|q_t, x_t)$
Training methodology	Many, often based on heuristics	Relative counts (including smoothing)	EM, Viterbi recurrence	REMAP (GEM)	GEM, EM, GD, Viterbi recurrence
Training criterion	Deterministic	Maximum likelihood	Maximum likelihood	Maximum a posteriori	Maximum a posteriori

Abbreviations: HMM, hidden Markov model; ANN, artificial neural network; IOHMM, input-output HMM; EM, Expectation-Maximization algorithm; GEM, Generalized Expectation-Maximization algorithm; REMAP, recurrent estimation and maximization of a posteriori probabilities

sentative training data. If X represents the whole sequence of training data and M its associated SFSA, the estimation of optimal parameter set Θ^* is usually achieved by optimizing a *maximum likelihood criterion*:

$$\Theta^* = \underset{\Theta}{\operatorname{argmax}}\, p(X \mid M, \Theta) \qquad (1)$$

or a *maximum a posteriori* criterion, which could be either

$$\Theta^* = \underset{\Theta}{\operatorname{argmax}}\, p(M \mid X, \Theta) = \underset{\Theta}{\operatorname{argmax}}\, p(X \mid M, \Theta) p(M \mid \Theta) \qquad (2)$$

or

$$\Theta^* = \underset{\Theta}{\operatorname{argmax}}\, p(M, \Theta \mid X) = \underset{\Theta}{\operatorname{argmax}}\, p(X \mid M, \Theta) p(M, \Theta) \qquad (3)$$

In the first case, we take into account the prior distribution of the model M; in the second case, we take into account the prior distribution of the model M as well as the parameters Θ.

Markov Models

The simplest form of SFSA is a Markov model in which states are directly associated with observations (see the second column in Table 1). We are interested in modeling

$$p(X) = p(F \mid x_1^T) p(x_1 \mid I) \prod_{t=2}^{T} p(x_t \mid x_1^{t-1}, I)$$

which can be simplified, using the kth-order Markov assumption, by

$$p(X) = p(F \mid x_{T-k+1}^T) p(x_1 \mid I) \prod_{t=2}^{T} p(x_t \mid x_{t-k}^{t-1})$$

which leads in the simplest case to the first-order Markov model,

$$p(X) = p(F \mid x_T) p(x_1 \mid I) \prod_{t=2}^{T} p(x_t \mid x_{t-1})$$

where $p(x_1 \mid I)$ is the initial state probability and the other terms can be seen as transition probabilities. Note that any kth-order Markov model can be expressed as a first-order Markov model, at the cost of possibly exponentially more states. Note also that the transition probabilities are time invariant, i.e., $p(x_t = \ell \mid x_{t-1} = k)$ is fixed for all t.

The set of parameters, represented by the $(K \times K)$-transition probability matrix, i.e.,

$$\Theta = p(x_t = \ell \mid x_{t-1} = k), \text{ for all } \ell, k \in \mathcal{Q}$$

is then directly estimated on a large number of possible observation (and, thus, state) sequences such that

$$\Theta^* = \underset{\Theta}{\operatorname{argmax}}\, p(X \mid M, \Theta)$$

and simply amounts to estimating the relative counts of observed transitions, possibly smoothed in the case of undersampled training data, i.e.,

$$p(x_t = \ell \mid x_{t-1} = k) = \frac{n_{k\ell}}{n_k}$$

where $n_{k\ell}$ stands for the number of times a transition from state k to state ℓ was observed, while n_k represents the number of times state k was visited.

It is sometimes desirable to compute the probability of going from the initial state I to the final state F in exactly T steps, which could naively be estimated by summing path likelihoods over all possible paths of length T in model M, i.e.,

$$p(F \mid I) = p(x_1 \mid I) \sum_{\text{paths}} p(F \mid x_T) \prod_{t=2}^{T} p(x_t \mid x_{t-1})$$

although there is a possibly exponential number of paths to explore. Fortunately, a more tractable solution exists, using the intermediate variable

$$\alpha_t(\ell) = p(x_t = \ell, x_1^{t-1}, I)$$

which can be computed using the *forward recurrence*:

$$\alpha_t(\ell) = \sum_k \alpha_{t-1}(k) p(x_t = \ell \mid x_{t-1} = k) \qquad (4)$$

and can be used as follows:

$$p(F \mid I) = \alpha_{T+1}(F)$$

Replacing the sum operator in Equation 4 by the max operator is equivalent to finding the most probable path of length T between I and F.

Although quite simple, Markov models have many uses. For example, they are used in all state-of-the-art continuous speech recognition systems to represent statistical grammars (Jelinek, 1998), usually referred to as N-grams, and for estimating the probability of a sequence of K words

$$p(w_1^K) \approx \prod_{k=N+1}^{K} p(w_k \mid w_{k-N}^{k-1})$$

which is equivalent to assuming that possible word sequences can be modeled by a Markov model of order N.

Hidden Markov Models

In many sequential pattern processing or classification problems (such as speech recognition and cursive handwriting recognition), one of the greatest difficulties is to simultaneously model the inherent statistical variations in sequential rates and feature characteristics. In this respect, HMMs have been one of the most successful approaches used so far. As shown in Table 1, an HMM is a particular form of SFSA in which Markov models (modeling the sequential properties of the data) are complemented by a second stochastic process modeling the local properties of the data. The Markov model is called hidden because there is an underlying stochastic process (i.e., the sequence of states) that is not observable but that affects the observed sequence of events.

Although sequential signals, such as speech and handwriting, are nonstationary processes, HMMs assume that the sequence of observation vectors is a *piecewise stationary* process. That is, a sequence $X = x_1^T$ is modeled as a succession of discrete stationary states $Q = \{1, \ldots, k, \ldots, K\}$, with instantaneous transitions between these states. In this case, an HMM is defined as a stochastic FSA with a particular (generally strictly left-to-right for speech data) topology. An example of a simple HMM is given in Figure 1. In speech recognition, this could be the model of a word or phoneme that is assumed to be composed of three stationary parts. In cursive handwriting recognition, this could be the model of a letter.

Once the topology of the HMM has been defined (usually arbitrarily), the main criterion used for training and decoding is based on the likelihood $p(X \mid M, \Theta)$, i.e., the probability that the observed vector sequence X was produced by Markov model M. In this case, the HMM is thus considered a *production model*, and the observation vectors x_t are considered to be output variables z_t of the HMM. It can be shown that, provided several assumptions are met (Bourlard and Morgan, 1993), the likelihood $p(X \mid M, \Theta)$ can be expressed and computed in terms of *transition probabilities* $p(q_t = \ell \mid q_{t-1} = k, \Theta)$ and *emission probabilities*, which can be of the Mealy type (emission on transitions), $p(x_t \mid q_t, q_{t-1}, \Theta)$, or

Figure 1. A three-state, left-to-right hidden Markov model.

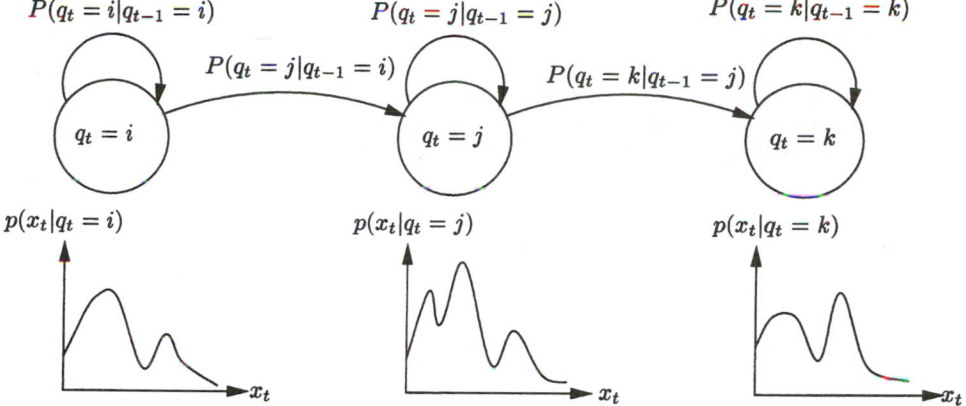

of the Moore type (emission on states), $p(x_t \mid q_t, \Theta)$. In the case of multivariate continuous observations, these emission probabilities are estimated by assuming that they follow a particular functional distribution, usually (mixtures of) multivariate Gaussian densities. In this case, the set of parameters Θ comprises all the Gaussian means and variances, mixing coefficients, and transition probabilities. These parameters are then usually trained according to the maximum likelihood criterion (Equation 1), resulting in the efficient EM algorithm (Liporace, 1982; Gold and Morgan, 2000).

Given this formalism, the likelihood of an observation sequence X given the model M can be calculated by extending the forward recurrence (Equation 4) defined for Markov models to also include the emission probabilities. Assuming a Moore automaton (emission on states), we thus have the *forward recurrence*

$$\alpha_t(\ell) = p(x_1^t, q_t = \ell)$$
$$= p(x_t \mid q_t = \ell) \sum_k \alpha_{t-1}(k) p(q_t = \ell \mid q_{t-1} = k) \quad (5)$$

which will be applied over all possible t, and where Σ_k is applied over all possible predecessor states of ℓ, thus resulting in

$$p(X \mid M, \Theta) = \alpha_{T+1}(F)$$

Replacing the sum operator in Equation 5 by the max operator is equivalent to finding the most probable path of length T generating the sequence X, and then yields the well-known dynamic programming recurrence, also referred to as the *Viterbi recurrence* in the case of HMMs:

$$\bar{p}(x_1^t, q_t = \ell) = p(x_t \mid q_t = \ell)$$
$$\times \max_{\{k\}} \{\bar{p}(x_1^{t-1}, q_{t-1} = k) p(q_t = \ell \mid q_{t-1} = k)]\} \quad (6)$$

where $\bar{p}(x_1^t, q_t = \ell)$ represents the probability of having produced the partial observation sequence x_1^t while being in state ℓ at time t and having followed the most probable path, $\{k\}$ represents the set of possible predecessor states of ℓ (given by the topology of the HMM), and $\bar{p}(X \mid M, \Theta)$ represents the likelihood that the most probable path is obtained at the end of the sequence and is equal to $\bar{p}(x_1^T, F)$.

During training, the HMM parameters Θ are optimized to maximize the likelihood of a set of training utterances given their associated (and known during training) HMM model, according to Equation 1, where $p(X \mid M, \Theta)$ is computed by taking all possible paths into account (forward recurrence) or only the most probable path (Viterbi recurrence). Powerful iterative training procedures based on the EM algorithm exist for both criteria and have been proved to converge to a local optimum. At each iteration of the EM algorithm, the E step estimates the most probable segmentation or

the best state posterior distribution (referred to as hidden variables) based on the current values of the parameters, while the M step reestimates the optimal value of these parameters assuming that the current estimate of the hidden variables is correct.

For further reading about HMM training and decoding algorithms, see Bourlard and Morgan (1993), Deller, Proakis, and Hansen (1993), Gold and Morgan (2000), and Jelinek (1998).

HMM Advantages and Drawbacks

The most successful application of HMMs is in speech recognition. Given a sequence of acoustic signals, the goal is to produce a sequence of associated phoneme or word transcriptions. To solve such a problem, one usually associates one HMM per different phoneme (or word). During training, a new HMM is created for each training sentence as the concatenation of the corresponding target phoneme models, and its parameters are maximized. Over the last few years, a number of laboratories have demonstrated large-vocabulary (at least 1,000 words), speaker-independent, continuous speech recognition systems based on HMMs.

HMMs can deal efficiently with the temporal aspect of speech (time warping) as well as with frequency distortion. They also benefit from powerful and efficient training and decoding algorithms. For training, only the transcription in terms of the speech units that are trained is necessary, and no explicit segmentation of the training material is required. Also, HMMs can easily be extended to include phonological and syntactical rules (at least when these rules use the same statistical formalism).

However, the assumptions that make the efficiency of these models and their optimization possible limit their generality. As a consequence, they also suffer from several drawbacks, including the following:

- Poor discrimination as a result of the training algorithm, which maximizes likelihoods instead of a posteriori probabilities $p(M|X)$ (i.e., the HMM associated with each speech unit is trained independently of the other models).
- A priori choice of model topology and statistical distributions, e.g., assuming that the probability density functions associated with the HMM state can be described as (mixtures of) multivariate Gaussian densities, each with a diagonal-only covariance matrix (i.e., the possible correlation between the components of the acoustic vectors is disregarded).
- Assumption that the state sequences are first-order Markov chains.
- Assumption that the input observations are not correlated over time. Thus, apart from the HMM topology, the possible temporal

correlation across features associated with the same HMM state is simply disregarded.

In order to overcome some of these problems, many researchers have concentrated on integrating artificial neural networks (ANNs) into the formalism of HMMs. In the next section we discuss some of the most promising approaches.

ANN-Based Stochastic Finite-State Automata

The idea of combining HMMs and ANNs was motivated by the observation that HMMs and ANNs have complementary properties. HMMs are clearly dynamic and very well suited to sequential data, but several assumptions limit their generality, whereas ANNs can approximate any kind of nonlinear discriminant functions, are very flexible, and do not need strong assumptions about the distribution of the input data, but they cannot properly handle time sequences (although recurrent neural networks can indeed handle time, they are known to be difficult to train long-term dependencies, and cannot easily incorporate knowledge in their structure, as is the case for HMMs). Therefore, a number of hybrid models have been proposed in the literature.

Hybrid HMM/ANN Systems

HMMs are based on a strict probabilistic formalism, making them difficult to interface with other modules in a heterogeneous system. However, it has indeed been shown (Richard and Lippmann, 1991; Bourlard and Morgan, 1993) that if each output unit of an ANN (typically a multilayer perceptron) is associated with a state k of the set of states $\mathcal{Q} = \{1, 2, \ldots, K\}$ on which the SFSAs are defined, it is possible to train the ANN (e.g., according to the usual least-mean-square or relative entropy criteria) to generate good estimates of a posteriori probabilities of the output classes conditioned on the input. In other words, if $g_k(x_t|\Theta)$ represents the output function observed on the kth ANN output unit when the ANN is presented with the input observation vector x_t, we will have

$$g_k(x_t \mid \Theta^*) \approx p(q_t = k|x_t) \qquad (7)$$

where Θ^* represents the optimal set of ANN parameters.

When using these posterior probabilities (instead of local likelihoods) in SFSAs, the model becomes a recognition model (sometimes referred to as a stochastic finite-state acceptor) where the observation sequence is an *input* to the system and where all local and global measures are based on a posteriori probabilities. It became necessary to revisit the SFSA basis to accommodate this formalism. In Bourlard and Morgan (1993) and Bourlard, Konig, and Morgan (1996), it is shown that $p(M|X, \Theta)$ can be expressed in terms of *conditional transition probabilities* $p(q_t|x_t, q_{t-1})$ and that it is possible to train the optimum ANN parameter set Θ according to the MAP criterion (Equation 2). The resulting training algorithm (Bourlard, Konig, and Morgan, 1994), referred to as REMAP (recursive estimation and maximization of a posteriori probabilities) is a particular form of EM training, directly involving posteriors, in which the M step involves the (gradient-based) training of the ANN and the desired target distribution (required to train the ANN) has been estimated in the previous E step. Since this EM version includes an iterative M step, it is also sometimes referred to as Generalized EM (GEM). As for standard HMMs, there is a full likelihood version (taking all possible paths into account) as well as a Viterbi version of the training procedure.

Another popular solution in using hybrid HMM/ANN as a sequence recognizer is to turn the local posterior probabilities $p(q_t = k|x_t)$ into *scaled likelihoods* by dividing these by the estimated value of the class priors as observed on the training data, i.e.,

$$\frac{p(q_t = k|x_t)}{p(q_t = k)} = \frac{p(x_t \mid q_t = k)}{p(x_t)} \qquad (8)$$

These scaled likelihoods are trained discriminatively (using the discriminant properties of ANN). During decoding, though, the denominator of the resulting scaled likelihoods $p(x_t|q_t = k)/p(x_t)$ is independent of the class and simply appears as a normalization constant. The scale likelihoods can thus be simply used in a regular Viterbi or forward recurrence to yield an estimator of the global scaled likelihood (Hennebert et al., 1997):

$$\frac{p(X \mid M,\Theta)}{p(X)} = \sum_{\text{paths}} \prod_{t=1}^{T} \frac{p(x_t \mid q_t)}{p(x_t)} \, p(q_t \mid q_{t-1}) \qquad (9)$$

where the sum extends over all possible paths of length T in model M.

These hybrid HMM/ANN approaches provide more discriminant estimates of the emission probabilities needed for HMMs without requiring strong hypotheses about the statistical distribution of the data. Since this result still holds with modified ANN architectures, the approach has been extended in a number of ways, including the following:

- Extending the input field to accommodate not only the current input vector but also its right and left contexts, leading to HMM systems that take into account the correlation between acoustic vectors (Bourlard and Morgan, 1993).
- Partially recurrent ANNs (Robinson, Hochberg, and Renals, 1996) feeding back previous activation vectors on the hidden or output units, leading to some kind of higher-order HMM.

Input-Output HMMs

Input-output HMMs (IOHMMs) (Bengio and Frasconi, 1995) are an extension of classical HMMs in which the emission and transition probability distributions are conditioned on another sequence, called the *input sequence*, and notated as $Y = y_1^T$. The emitted sequence is now called the *output sequence*, notated $Z = z_1^T$. Hence, in the simplest case of the Moore model (see Table 1), the emission distribution now models $p(z_t|q_t, y_t)$ while the transition distribution models $p(q_t|q_{t-1}, y_t)$.

Although this looks like an apparently simple modification, it has a structural impact on the resulting model and hence on the hypotheses of the problems to solve. For instance, whereas in classical HMMs the emission and transition distributions do not depend on t (we say that HMMs are homogeneous), this is not the case for IOHMMs, which therefore are called inhomogeneous, as the distributions are now conditioned on y_t, which changes with time t.

Applications of IOHMMs range from speech processing to sequence classification tasks and include time-series prediction and robot navigation. For example, for economic time series, the input sequence could represent different economic indicators while the output sequence could be, for example, the future values of some target assets or the evolution of a given portfolio.

In order to train IOHMMs, an EM algorithm has been developed (Bengio and Frasconi, 1995) that looks very much like the classical EM algorithm used for HMMs, except that all distributions and posterior estimates are now conditioned on the input sequence. Hence we need to implement conditional distributions, either for transitions or emissions, which can be represented, for instance, by ANNs. The resulting training algorithm is thus a generalized EM, which is also guaranteed to converge. For transition probabilities, the output of the ANN would represent the posterior probability of each transition $p(q_t|q_{t-1}, y_t)$, with the constraint that all such probabilities from a given state sum to 1. For emission probabilities, the output of the ANN would represent the parameters of a unconditional probability distribution, such as a classical mixture of

Gaussians. Another implementation option would be to use an ANN to represent only the expectation $E[z_t|q_t, y_t]$ instead of the probability itself. For some applications such as prediction, this is often sufficient and more efficient.

An interesting extension of IOHMMs has been proposed in Bengio and Bengio (1996) in order to handle asynchronous input-output sequences, and thus to match input sequences that might be shorter or longer than output sequences. An obvious application of asynchronous IOHMMs is in speech recognition (or handwritten cursive recognition) where the input sequence represents the acoustic signal and the output sequence represents the corresponding phoneme transcription.

Discussion

We have discussed the use of deterministic and stochastic finite-state automata for sequence processing and have sought to present this information in a unified framework. As a particularly powerful instantiation of SFSAs and one of the most popular tools for the processing of complex piecewise stationary sequences, we also discussed HMMs in more detail. Finally, we described a few contributions of the ANN community to improving those SFSAs, mainly the hybrid HMM/ANN systems and IOHMMs. A more extensive discussion would have taken up related areas, such as transducers, linear dynamical systems, Kalman filters, and so on—all outside the scope of this brief introduction.

Road Maps: Learning in Artificial Networks; Linguistics and Speech Processing
Related Reading: Speech Recognition Technology; Temporal Pattern Processing

References

Baum, L., and Petrie, T., 1966, Statistical inference for probabilistic functions of finite state Markov chains, *Ann. Math. Statist.*, 37:1554–1563.

Bengio, S., and Bengio, Y., 1996, An EM algorithm for asynchronous input/output hidden Markov models, in *Proceedings of the International Conference on Neural Information Processing (ICONIP)*, Hong Kong, pp. 328–334.

Bengio, Y., and Frasconi, P., 1995, An input/output HMM architecture, in *Advances in Neural Information Processing Systems 7*, Cambridge, MA: MIT Press, pp. 427–434.

Bourlard, H., Konig, Y., and Morgan, N., 1994, *REMAP: Recursive Estimation and Maximization of a Posteriori Probabilities*, Technical Report TR-94-064, Berkeley, CA: International Computer Science Institute.

Bourlard, H., Konig, Y., and Morgan, N., 1996, A training algorithm for statistical sequence recognition with applications to transition-based speech recognition, *IEEE Signal Process. Lett.*, 3:203–205.

Bourlard, H., and Morgan, N., 1993, *Connectionist Speech Recognition: A Hybrid Approach*, Boston: Kluwer Academic. ◆

Deller, J., Proakis, J., and Hansen, J., 1993, *Discrete-Time Processing of Speech Signals*, New York: Macmillan. ◆

Gold, B., and Morgan, N., 2000, *Speech and Audio Signal Processing*, New York: Wiley. ◆

Hennebert, J., Ris, C., Bourlard, H., Renals, S., and Morgan, N., 1997, Estimation of global posteriors and forward-backward training of hybrid HMM/ANN systems, in *Proceedings of Eurospeech'97*, pp. 1951–1954.

Hopcroft, J., Motwani, R., and Ullman, J., 2000, *Introduction to Automata Theory, Language and Computations*, 2nd ed., Reading, MA: Addison-Wesley. ◆

Jelinek, F., 1998, *Statistical Methods for Speech Recognition*, Cambridge, MA: MIT Press. ◆

Liporace, L., 1982, Maximum likelihood estimation for multivariate observations of markov sources, *IEEE Trans. Inf. Theory*, IT-28:729–734.

Richard, M., and Lippmann, R., 1991, Neural network classifiers estimate bayesian a posteriori probabilities, *Neural Computat.*, 3:461–483.

Robinson, T., Hochberg, M., and Renals, S., 1996, The use of recurrent neural networks in continuous speech recognition, in *Automatic Speech and Speaker Recognition*, Boston: Kluwer Academic, pp. 233–258.

Hippocampal Rhythm Generation

Péter Érdi and Krisztina Szalisznyó

Introduction

Global brain states in both normal and pathological conditions may be associated with spontaneous rhythmic activities of large populations of neurons. Experimentally, these activities can be detected by recording both from large neural assemblies (as in the EEG) or from a single neuron of the cell population. Two main global hippocampal states that occur normally are known: rhythmic slow activity, called *theta rhythm*, with the associated *gamma oscillation*, and *irregular sharp waves*, with the associated *high-frequency (ripple) oscillation*. A pathological brain state associated with *epileptic seizures* and producing epileptiform patterns also frequently occurs in the hippocampus. This article reviews the basic phenomena and their models. The main hippocampal rhythms are shown in Figure 1.

The general belief is that the different hippocampal rhythms are strongly involved in cognitive functioning. However, the functional significance of these rhythms is mentioned here only briefly (for a fuller discussion, see, e.g., Buzsáki, 1996). The first part of this article describes the most important normal and pathological hippocampal rhythms and the possible underlying mechanisms. In the second part, several different modeling strategies for studying rhythmicity in the hippocampal CA3 region are compared.

Normal Electrical Activity Patterns

Theta Rhythms

The phenomenon. The theta rhythm is a population oscillation with large (1 mV) amplitude and 4–12 Hz frequency. Theta rhythm occurs whenever an animal engages in behaviors such as walking, exploration, or sensory scanning, as well as during REM sleep (Buzsáki, 1996). Single-cell physiological studies showed different relations between the behavior of individual cells and the theta rhythm. Pyramidal cells in the hippocampus proper generally discharge with a very low frequency (0.01–0.5 Hz), although spatially sensitive "place cells" fire at 4–8 Hz when the rat is in its place field, and the position of the animal within a cell's place field may be correlated with the phase of its firing relative to the theta rhythm.

Origin. Discharging neurons phase locked to hippocampal theta waves have been observed in the dorsal raphe nucleus, the nucleus reticularis pontis oralis and caudalis, the supramammillary region, the septum, and the entorhinal cortex. Some of these areas are reciprocally interconnected with the hippocampal formation.

In vitro experiments. Population oscillation at the theta frequency can be induced pharmacologically by instillation of carbachol into

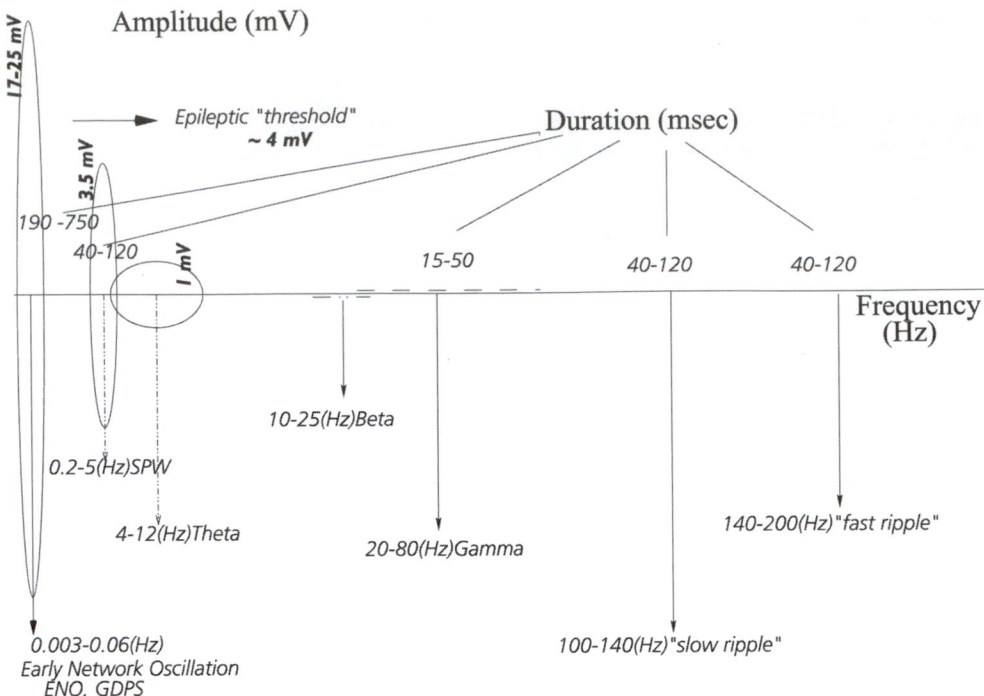

Figure 1. The main hippocampal rhythms occurring during physiological and pathological conditions: their frequency, duration, and amplitude.

hippocampal slices. Based on these and similar findings, it was suggested that theta rhythms may be generated not only extrahippocampally but also by the intrinsic membrane properties of the neurons of the CA3 region. The underlying single-cell firing patterns, however, may be different for in vivo and in vitro carbachol-induced oscillation: the pyramidal cells fire at a much higher frequency than in vivo. Some observations suggest a presence of two, relatively independent theta generators in the hippocampus that are mediated by the entorhinal cortex and the CA3-mossy cell recurrent circuitry, respectively. The CA3-mossy cell theta generator is partially suppressed by the dentate gyrus interneuronal output in the intact brain. Resonant properties of the CA1 neurons were found in the theta frequency range in vitro.

Septohippocampal pathway. The septohippocampal pathway has a cholinergic component, but it is not the only one to contribute to the generation of theta rhythm: atropin, a muscarinic antagonist of acetylcholine, does not entirely abolish the rhythmic slow activity. The GABAergic component of the septal afferents modifies the activity of the principal cells by disinhibition and is also involved in the generation of theta rhythm. These GABAergic cells are located mostly at the border of the medial and lateral septum, and terminate on the GABAergic interneurons of the hippocampus and on the non-GABAergic supramammillary cells, which are known to project to the septal complex and the hippocampus (Figure 2). The cholinergic input into the septum does not show target-selective innervation. There are some backpropagations from the hippocampus to the septum, some of them topographic.

Entorhinal cortex. The timing of the action potentials of pyramidal cells during the theta cycle might be determined by cooperation between the active CA3 neurons and the entorhinal input. Entorhinal excitatory transmitter-containing neurons can also depress the activity of supramammillary theta-generating/regulating cells via septal inhibitory neurons (Figure 2).

Dorsal and medial raphe nuclei. The main neurotransmitter of the raphe projections selectively innervates a subclass of the interneurons in the CA regions. A spatially segregated population of *serotonergic* neurons located caudally in the dorsal raphe nucleus was found to project only to the medial septum, and not to the hippocampus. In addition to the well-known serotonergic effect of the median raphe on hippocampal electrical activity, theta rhythm in the hippocampus may also be modulated by the dorsal raphe nucleus via the medial septum (Figure 2).

Nucleus reticularis pontis oralis, caudalis. A high degree of correlation was observed between theta waves in the nucleus reticularis pontis oralis, hippocampal fields, and nucleus reticularis pontis caudalis. The peak frequency of the theta rhythm, induced by stimulation of the reticularis pontis oralis nucleus in urethane-anesthetized rats, was decreased in aged rats compared with young and mature animals. The cholinergic system showed age-related deterioration in rats, including in the hippocampus (Figure 2).

Supramammillary nucleus. Neurons of the supramammillary nucleus fire phase locked to hippocampal theta rhythm. Stimulation of this area induces theta activity in the hippocampus via the medial septum and facilitates perforant pathway stimulation-evoked population spikes in the dentate gyrus even if the medial septum is inactivated. Most if not all postsynaptic targets of the supramammillary projection are principal cells in both the dentate gyrus and the CA2-CA3a subfields Figure 2).

The functional significance of the theta rhythm, including its possible role in evolution, was recently reviewed by Kahana, Seelig, and Madsen (2001). Studies in rodents have clarified the involvement of theta rhythm in synaptic plasticity and neural coding. Specifically, the phase relationship between theta field activity and single-cell patterns codes the location of the exploring animal. Recently, enhanced theta activity was demonstrated during both verbal and spatial memory tasks.

Figure 2. The interaction of the hippocampus with cortical and subcortical structures. The neurochemical character of the afferent and efferent fibers are visualized.

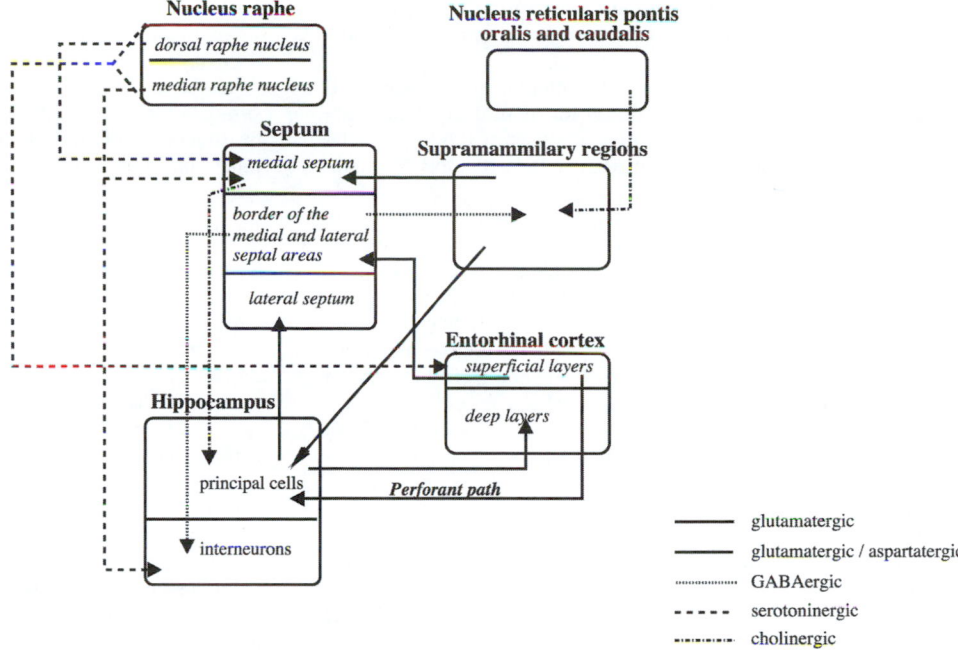

Gamma Oscillations

The phenomenon.   Gamma frequency field oscillations reflect synchronized synaptic potentials in neuronal populations within a range of approximately 10–40 ms. The frequency of this oscillation is in the 20–80 Hz range.

Intrahippocampal origin.   The power of gamma oscillation in the hilus decreased significantly after bilateral removal of the entorhinal cortex but survived after surgical removal of the subcortical inputs of the hippocampus. The GABAergic perforant path input terminates exclusively on the interneurons. This pathway provides a rhythmic hyperpolarization of the interneurons, at theta frequency range, so the hypothesized voltage-dependent gamma oscillation of hippocampal interneurons will be periodically interrupted. Gamma oscillation can emerge independently in each subregion of the hippocampus, including the dentate gyrus, CA3, and CA1 regions, but it occurs with greatest power in the dentate gyrus.

Extrahippocampal origin.   GABAergic neurons in the basal forebrain display a gamma oscillation. These GABAergic cells also project to the GABAergic reticular nucleus of the thalamus and the neocortex, where they preferentially terminate on the GABAergic interneurons. The gamma patterns are modulated by theta activity, and the dominant source of gamma activity after removal of the entorhinal input is the CA3 region.

Underlying mechanisms.   The mechanisms underlying gamma oscillations are not fully understood. Studies of hippocampal formation have suggested that field oscillations in the gamma frequency band reflect synchronous IPSPs on the somata of principal cells. Population oscillation may emerge in interneuronal networks even when individual cells fire at remarkably higher frequencies. At least part of the gamma rhythm recorded in the extracellular space reflects synchronous membrane oscillation in the pyramidal cells brought about by the rhythmic IPSPs. Basket cells innervating the perisomatic region of pyramidal cells discharge at gamma frequency and are phase locked to the field oscillation. These findings indicate that the charges responsible for the rhythmic gamma waves

are mostly carried by chloride ions that enter through GABA$_A$ receptors. Extracellularly observed gamma waves reflect summation of rhythmic EPSPs by the perforant path input at the dendrites (active inward currents) and IPSPs by the oscillating interneurons at the somata (active outward currents) of the granule cell population. Given the spatial segregation of the inward and outward currents (dendrites versus somata), these active currents would summate in the extracellular space. Previous hypotheses suggested that the origin of the synchronized gamma activity may be the mutual excitation among principal cells, or at the single-cell level ("chattering cells"; Traub, Jeffreys, and Whittington, 1999). Simulation studies later showed that interneuronal networks can be synchronized by GABA$_A$ synapses preferentially within gamma frequency range. Resonant properties of pyramidal cells might facilitate network synchrony in the gamma frequency range (Orbán et al., 2001).

The finding that gamma oscillation occurred in different brain regions generated considerable excitement, since gamma oscillation is supposed to be responsible for the binding of perceived and recalled attributes of aspects and events, and for forming memory traces.

Irregular Sharp Waves

The phenomenon.   Sharp waves (SPWs) have a very large amplitude (up to 3 mV), their duration is 40–120 ms, and their frequency can be between 0.2 and 5 Hz. Although maximal SPW frequencies do overlap theta frequencies, theta waves are much more regular than SPWs. SPWs also have behavioral correlates: they occur during awake immobility, drinking, eating, face washing, grooming, and slow wave sleep (Buzsáki, 1996).

Origin.   During SPWs, pyramidal and inhibitory cells fire with increased frequency. Furthermore, there is a partial synchronous cellular activity of both pyramidal and inhibitory neurons. However, the degree of synchrony is below the threshold for induction of epileptic seizures. The amplitude and frequency of SPWs can be increased by high-frequency stimulation of the commissural system and the Schaffer collaterals, suggesting that such stimulation enhances the efficacy of the excitatory synapses. The activity of neurons in the deep layers of entorhinal cortex is also correlated with SPWs.

SPWs are thought to be formed by internal intrahippocampal processes. One important precondition for SPW generation is the occurrence of a population burst in a small set of CA3 pyramidal cells. Their synchronization is mediated by excitatory synaptic connections.

The physiological mechanism of synchronization.   The largest degree of synchronization occurs in the adult hippocampus during an irregular sharp wave under physiological conditions. CA3 pyramidal cells have recurrent excitatory connections that terminate within the CA3 region. The autoexcitation due to these connections produces large excitatory postsynaptic potentials (EPSP), which propagate to the CA1 region through the Schaffer collaterals. Inhibitory connections control the population activity in both regions. Although sharp waves were found in rat hippocampus during consummatory behaviors and slow wave sleep, there is a normal human EEG phenomenon, called small sharp spikes (SSS), that is thought to be analogous to SPW, since it also results from partial synchronous cell firing. Not only "normal" but also epileptiform SPWs can occur. The latter are characterized an amplitude greater than 4 mV or by a less irregular pattern. Their duration is shorter than that of normal SPWs.

During irregular sharp waves, memory traces are supposed to be consolidated and transferred to neocortex.

High-Frequency ("Ripple") Oscillations

The phenomenon.   In conjunction with sharp wave bursts, CA1 pyramidal cells display a high-frequency (200 Hz) network oscillation (ripple) (Ylinen et al., 1995). Similar types of high-frequency oscillation were recorded from the entorhinal cortex and hippocampus of patients with medial temporal lobe epilepsy. The lower-frequency oscillation (80–160 Hz) was regarded as the human equivalent of normal ripples in the rat. The higher-frequency oscillation (250–500 Hz) was found in the epileptogenic regions and may reflect pathological hypersynchronous population spikes of bursting pyramidal neurons. Sleep is characterized by a structured combination of neuronal oscillations. In the hippocampus, slow-wave sleep (SWS) is marked by high-frequency network oscillations, and neocortical SWS activity is organized into low-frequency delta (1–4 Hz) and spindle (7–14 Hz) oscillations. The existence of temporal correlations between hippocampal ripples and cortical spindles is also reflected in the correlated activity of single neurons within these brain structures. This co-activation of hippocampal and thalamocortical pathways may be important for the process of memory consolidation, during which memories are gradually translated from short-term hippocampal to longer-term neocortical stores (Bragin et al., 1999).

Origin and underlying mechanisms.   Single pyramidal cells discharge at a low frequency and are phase locked to the negative peak of the locally derived field oscillation. CA1 basket cells increase their firing rate during the network oscillation and discharged at the frequency of the extracellular ripple. These findings indicate that the intracellularly recorded fast oscillatory rhythm is not solely dependent on membrane currents intrinsic to the CA1 pyramidal cells but is a network-driven phenomenon dependent on the participation of inhibitory interneurons. One of the hypotheses was that fast field oscillation (200 Hz) in the CA1 region reflects summed IPSPs in pyramidal cells as a result of a high-frequency barrage of interneurons (Ylinen et al., 1995). The specific currents responsible for the ripple are believed to be synchronized somatic IPSPs interrupted by synchronous discharges of CA1 pyramidal

neurons every 5–6 ms. Concurrent with the hippocampal sharp wave, ripples are present also in the subiculum, parasubiculum, and deep layers of the entorhinal cortex, but the ripple frequency is fastest in the CA1 region. Recent experimental and computational simulation results suggest that ripple oscillation may be mediated by direct electrotonic coupling of neurons, most likely through gap-junctional connections (Traub et al., 1999).

Oscillation in Developing Hippocampus

Synchronous population activity is present both normally and in pathological conditions such as epilepsy. Low-frequency early network population oscillation (0.006–0.03 Hz), or ENO, was found in the hippocampus proper and in the gyrus dentatus region during the first few weeks of postnatal life. The underlying single-cell activity is the synchronous bursting activity, generated by pyramidal cells and interneurons, via $GABA_A$, NMDA, and AMPA receptors. The oscillation is phase locked to the intracellular Ca^{2+} increase, and the interneuronal network exhibits a Ca^{2+} burst in synchrony with the ENO-associated early pyramidal Ca^{2+} bursts. The ENO is totally blocked by the $GABA_A$ receptor antagonist bicucullin and is reduced by the glutamatergic antagonist. The developmental change of the Cl^- equilibrium potential is responsible for the change of the $GABA_A$ Cl^- ion current direction. The ENO-associated $GABA_A$ LTP and LTD are supposed to be partly responsible for the formation of the interneuronal network, and it is consistent with the theory that the excitatory effect–related synaptic plasticity might play a role even in inhibitory synaptic formation.

Epileptic Seizures

The phenomenon.   Epileptic activity occurs in a population of neurons when the membrane potentials of the neurons are "abnormally" synchronized. A certain degree of synchrony is necessary for normal theta and SPW behavior. However, there are some fundamental questions to be answered. Under what conditions does population firing become synchronized? What factors regulate the extent of synchronization? What are the critical factors that can influence the change from the physiological to the pathological level of the synchronization? Answers obtained in model studies are briefly summarized in the following sections.

In vitro models.   Several in vitro models of seizures have been developed, including models invoking electrical stimulation or low calcium, low magnesium, or elevated potassium levels. (Of course, in vitro models have nothing to do with mathematical models.) The functional removal of some inhibitory interneurons from network activity might be another factor contributing to epileptic phenomena, either because of their inadequate excitatory drive or because of their depolarization blockade. Experiments with ion-selective microelectrodes revealed that a considerable activity of K^+ ions appears temporarily in the extracellular space during enhanced neuronal activity and is removed from the extracellular space by diffusion. The elevated-potassium model of epilepsy suggests that a modest elavation in extracellular potassium ion concentration produces hypersynchronous epileptiform activity. One important element in epileptogenesis may be attenuation of the inhibitory synaptic inputs to pyramidal cells during high-K^+ seizures. A few different epileptic phenomena are found in vitro, such as synchronized bursts, synchronized multiple bursts, and seizure-like events. Synchronized bursts last 50–100 ms, and interburst intervals are generally longer than 1 s. They are analogous to the so-called interictal events found in vivo, and can be elicited by applying a localized $GABA_A$-blocking agent (e.g., picrotoxin, bicucullin, penicillin). Synchronized multiple bursts are characterized by a series of up to about ten synchronized bursts occurring at 65–75 ms intervals. The intervals between the complex events are longer than 10 s. This phenomenon can also be generated by applying GABA$_A$ blocker. Seizure-like events can be generated both with and without the aid of chemical synapses. The latter was demonstrated in slices with low Ca^{2+} solutions. Low Ca^{2+} blocks spike-dependent synaptic transmission, yet spontaneous bursts of population spikes—"field bursts"—with underlying high-frequency firing of pyramidal cells are still evoked.

Computational Models of the CA3 Region: Comparative Studies

1. Compartmental Models

Some detailed single-cell multicompartmental hippocampal pyramidal cell models have been established (Traub et al., 1999, p. 17). Specifically, a 19-compartment pyramidal cable model of a guinea pig CA3 pyramidal neuron was developed and incorporated in several network models. Each compartment contains six active ionic conductances: gNa, gCa, gK(DR) (where DR stands for delayed rectifier), gK(A), gK(AHP), and gK(C). The conductance gCa is of the high-voltage activated type. The model kinetics incorporate voltage-clamp data obtained from isolated hippocampal pyramidal neurons. The model predicts that CA3 pyramidal neurons in media blocking synaptic transmission should fire a burst of action potentials following antidromic stimulation. This was confirmed experimentally in hippocampal slices.

Model reduction.   Multicompartment models could be reduced to allow questions about larger-scale brain regions to be answered while still revealing something about activity at the single-cell level. The 19-compartment Traub model has been reduced to a two-compartment model (Pinsky and Rinzel, 1994). This two-compartment model (soma, dendrite) is able to qualitatively reproduce the salient stimulus-response characteristics of the Traub-Miles (1991) single-cell model, was useful for studying the effect of intercompartmental coupling on the responses generated, and proved to be a computationally effective unit for network simulations. The "slow" and "fast" currents are segregated in the dendrite-like and the soma-like compartments, respectively.

2. Network Studies: Model of an in Vitro CA3 Slice

Physiological synchronized population activities.   Traub and Miles simulated hippocampal (mostly CA3) population activity by building "bottom-up" models from data on anatomic connectivities, ionic conductances, and synaptic properties (Traub and Miles, 1991).

Three basic cell types, pyramidal cells and two types of inhibitory cells, inh(1) and inh(2) cells, were assumed. The postsynaptic effect of the inh(1) cells is mediated by perisomatic GABA$_A$ receptors, while the inhibition of the inh(2) cells is mediated by dendritic GABA$_B$ receptors.

Instead of giving detailed wiring, the strategy for specifying synapses was to define the statistical properties of the topology of the neural structures. Traub and Miles defined both globally and locally random networks. The probabilities of synaptic connections for a given type of cell pair are constant in the former case and decrease with distance in the latter case.

Fully and partially synchronized bursts, multiple bursts, synchronized population oscillations, and interictal epileptic seizures were physiologically measured and reproduced by this model (Traub and Miles, 1991; Whittington, Traub, and Jeffreys, 1995).

Epileptic interictal spikes.   A computer model was constructed of the guinea pig hippocampal region in vitro that contained 100 pyramidal neurons modeled by the 19-compartment model detailed above. This approach has contributed to the understanding of brief (usually less than 100 ms) epileptic events known as interictal spikes. The neurons were randomly interconnected with excitatory synapses, each synapse exerting a fast voltage-independent (AMPA) component and a slower voltage- and ligand-dependent (NMDA) component.

Synchronized gamma oscillations in a hippocampus.   1. *Gamma frequency in the interneuronal network.* Using computer simulations the hypothesis that gamma rhythm can emerge in a random network of interconnected GABAergic fast-spiking interneurons was investigated. The amplitude of spike afterhyperpolarization was above the GABA$_A$ synaptic reversal potential. The ratio between the synaptic decay time constant and the oscillation period was sufficiently large; the effects of heterogeneities were modest because of a steep frequency-current relationship of fast-spiking neurons. It has been demonstrated that large-scale network synchronization requires a critical (minimal) average number of synaptic contacts per cell, and this number is not sensitive to network size. The neuronal firing frequencies could be gradually and monotonically varied by changing the GABA$_A$ synaptic maximal conductance, the synaptic decay time constant, and the mean external excitatory drive to the network, but the network synchronization was found to be high only within a frequency band coinciding with the gamma (20–80 Hz) range. The model predicts that the GABA$_A$ synaptic transmission provides a suitable mechanism for synchronized gamma oscillations in a sparsely connected network of fast-spiking interneurons (Wang and Buzsáki, 1996).

2. *Gamma frequency in the network of interneurons and pyramidal cells.* A network simulation was used to investigate how pyramidal cells, connected to the interneurons and to each other through AMPA-type and/or NMDA-type glutamate receptors, might modify the interneuron network oscillation. With or without AMPA receptor-mediated excitation of the interneurons, the pyramidal cells and interneurons fired in phase during the gamma oscillation. Pyramidal cells caused the interneurons to fire spike doublets or short bursts at gamma frequencies, thereby slowing the population rhythm. Rhythmic synchronized IPSPs allowed the pyramidal cells to encode their mean excitation by their phase of firing relative to the population waves. Recurrent excitation between the pyramidal cells could modify the phase of firing relative to the population waves. This model suggested that pools of synaptically interconnected inhibitory cells are sufficient to produce gamma-frequency rhythms, but the network behavior can be modified by participation of pyramidal cells (Traub, Jeffreys, and Whittington, 1997).

High-frequency oscillation in the hippocampus.   To explore the hypothesis that gap junctions occurring between axons could explain high-frequency oscillations, a network was constructed. It has been shown that in randomly connected networks with an average of two gap junctions per cell or less, synchronized network bursts can arise without chemical synapses, with frequencies in the experimentally observed range (spectral peaks 125–182 Hz). The critical assumptions were that (1) there is a background of ectopic axonal spikes that can occur at low frequency (one event per 25 s per axon), and (2) the gap junction resistance is small enough that a spike in one axon can induce a spike in the coupled axon at short latency. The result of the simulation was that axo-axonal gap junctions, in combination with recurrent excitatory synapses, induced the occurrence of high-frequency population spikes superimposed on epileptiform field potentials.

3. Population Models

There is a long tradition of trying to connect the "microscopic" single-cell behavior to the global "macrostate" of the nervous system, analogously to the procedures applied in statistical physics. Global brain dynamics is handled by using continuous (neural field) description instead of the networks of discrete nerve cells. Both deterministic and statistical approaches have been developed.

Model framework.   In a long series of papers, Ventriglia constructed a neural kinetic theory, i.e., a statistical field theory of large-scale brain activities. He assumed two types of entities, spatially fixed neurons and spatially propagating spikes ("impulses") (Ventriglia, 1994). In the deterministic field-theoretical description, each neuron is represented as a point in the neural layer or field and a neuronal density is defined, while the statistical model describes neural population activity in terms of the probability density functions (p.d.f.'s) of (1) neurons and (2) spikes traveling between the neurons.

Synchronized population oscillation.   A different version of neural kinetic theory has been invoked to simulate a range of epileptiform and nonepileptic rhythms (Barna, Grölber, and Érdi, 1998; Gröbler, Barna, and Érdi, 1998). The synaptic strengths of excitatory and inhibitory synapses have been varied. The degree of pyramidal cell synchronization has been studied, even as single-cell activity (underlying population behavior) was monitored. Phenomena that were reproduced included fully synchronized population bursts, synchronized synaptic potentials, and low-amplitude population oscillation.

Wave propagation.   The spatial pattern of propagation is shown in Figure 3. The model slice is shown with increasing time from top to bottom. High activity appears first in the stimulated subregion, then builds up in the neighboring regions, then propagates through the full length of the slice. The velocity of the simulated wave propagation exhibits a linear increase on the maximal synaptic conductance and is in the interval of 5–10 cm/s.

Discussion

This article reviewed the basic physiological mechanisms and models of normal and pathological hippocampal rhythm generation. The interplay of intrinsic cell properties and synaptic interactions contributes to the generation of rhythms at both single-cell and population levels. Hippocampal rhythms are strongly involved in many areas of cognitive functioning, including navigation (see HIPPOCAMPUS: SPATIAL MODELS), various memory phenomena, such as memory formation, consolidation, and amnesic syndromes.

The hippocampus has an important role in neurological diseases. Alzheimer's disease, epilepsy, and ischemia are characterized by learning and memory impairment and accompanied by selective neuronal death or characteristic changes in the hippocampal circuitry. How the various hippocampal rhythms are involved in these disorders is an open question. Understanding the electrophysiology of the hippocampal area should contribute greatly to the development of pharmacological strategies to overcome the hippocampus-dependent disorders (see NEUROLOGICAL AND PSYCHIATRIC DISORDERS).

Complementary neural models are used to study the generation and control of hippocampal and other cortical rhythms. Multicompartment modeling techniques proved to be an efficient way to simulate the dynamics of even relatively large networks. Statistical population models are proper tools for describing large-scale population phenomena and wave propagation.

Road Maps: Biological Networks; Mammalian Brain Regions
Related Reading: EEG and MEG Analysis; Event-Related Potentials; Hippocampus: Spatial Models; Oscillatory and Bursting Properties of Neurons; Sleep Oscillations

References

Barna, G., Gröbler, T., and Érdi, P, 1998, Statistical model of the hippocampal CA3 region: II. The population framework: Model of rhythmic activity in the CA3 slice, *Biol. Cybern.*, 79:309–321. ◆

Bragin, A., Engel, J., Jr., Wilson, C. L., Fried, I., and Buzsáki, G., 1999, High-frequency oscillations in human brain, *Hippocampus*, 9:137–142.

Buzsáki, G., 1996, The hippocampo-neocortical dialogue, *Cereb Cortex*, 6:81–92.

Buzsáki, G., and Chrobak, J., 1995, Temporal structure in spatially organized neuronal ensembles: A role for interneuronal networks, *Curr. Biol.*, 5:504–510. ◆

Gröbler, T., Barna, G., and Érdi, P., 1998, Statistical model of the hippocampal CA3 region: I. The single-cell module. Bursting model of the pyramidal cell, *Biol. Cybern.*, 79:301–308.

Kahana, M. J., Seelig, D., and Madsen, R., 2001, Theta returns, *Curr. Opin. Neurobiol.*, 11:739–744. ◆

Orbán, G., Kiss, T., Lengyel, M., and Érdi, P., 2001, Hippocampal rhythm generation: Gamma-related theta-frequency resonance in CA3 interneurons, *Biol. Cybern.*, 84:123–132.

Pinsky, P. F., and Rinzel, J., 1994, Intrinsic and network rhythmogenesis in a reduced Traub model for CA3 neurons, *J. Computat. Neurosci.*, 1:39–60.

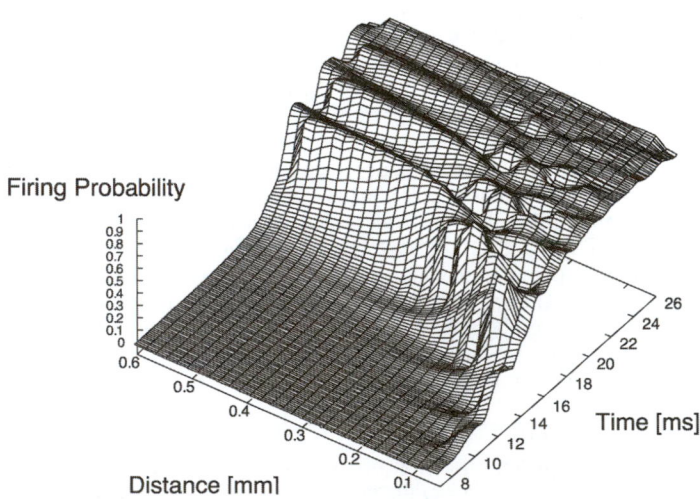

Figure 3. Propagation of activity wave in hippocampal slices. Activity is identified with firing probability.

Traub, R. D., and Miles, R., 1991, *Neuronal Networks of the Hippocampus*, New York: Cambridge University Press. ◆

Traub, R. D., Jeffreys, G. R., and Whittington, M. A., 1997, Simulation of gamma rhythms in networks of interneurons and pyramidal cells, *J. Comput. Neurosci.*, 4:141–150

Traub, R. D., Jeffreys, G. R., and Whittington, M. A., 1999, *Fast Oscillations in Cortical Circuits*, Cambridge, MA: MIT Press. ◆

Ventriglia, F., 1994, Towards a kinetic theory of cortical-like neural fields, in *Neural Modeling and Neural Networks*, New York: Pergamon Press, pp. 217–249.

Wang, X. J., and Buzsáki, G., 1996, Gamma oscillation by synaptic inhibition in a hippocampal interneuronal network model, *J Neurosci.*, 16:6402–6413.

Whittington, M. A., Traub, R. B., and Jeffreys, J. J., 1995, Synchronized oscillations in interneuron networks driven by metabotropic glutamate receptor activation, *Nature*, 370:612–615.

Ylinen, A., Soltesz, I., Bragin, A., Penttonen, M., Sik, A., and Buzsáki, G., 1995, Sharp wave–associated high-frequency oscillation (200Hz) in the intact hippocampus: Network and intracellular mechanisms, *J. Neurosci.*, 15:30–46.

Hippocampus: Spatial Models

Neil Burgess and John O'Keefe

Introduction

The hippocampus is the most-studied part of the brain, attracting interest because of its position (many synapses removed from sensory transducers or motor effectors), its role in human amnesia and Alzheimer's disease, and the discovery of long-term potentiation (LTP, see HEBBIAN SYNAPTIC PLASTICITY) and of spatially coded cell firing. Bilateral damage to the hippocampus and nearby structures in patient H.M., as treatment for epilepsy, produced a profound retrograde and anterograde amnesia, prompting extensive cross-species research to uncover the specific memory deficits that result from hippocampal damage (the most prominent of which, in the rat, appears to be a deficit in spatial navigation). In short, the hippocampus has become the primary region in the mammalian brain for the study of the synaptic basis of memory and learning. Structurally, it is the simplest form of cortex. It contains one projection cell type whose cell bodies are confined to a single layer and which receives inputs from all sensory systems and association areas (Figure 1).

Attempts to model the hippocampus differ both in the level of anatomical detail and in the functionality that they seek to reproduce. Marr (1971) proposed a theory for how the hippocampus could function as an associative memory, from which have grown many extensions, usually focusing on the role of the CA3 recurrent collaterals (see, e.g., McNaughton & Nadel, 1990; for collected works, see Gluck, 1996, and Burgess, Jeffery, and O'Keefe, 1999; for a review, see Burgess et al., 2001; see also ASSOCIATIVE NETWORKS). However, the precise contribution of the hippocampus to memory, as opposed to the contribution of nearby structures, remains controversial. In this article we specifically consider neuronal models of spatial processing in the rat hippocampus, the domain in which the least controversial experimental data are available. We introduce data on the spatial correlates of hippocampal cell firing and the idea of the hippocampus as a spatial map, and describe some models of the firing of hippocampal place cells and their role in navigation.

Basic Data and Issues

Electrophysiology

Single-unit recordings in freely moving rats have revealed "place cells" (PCs) in fields CA3 and CA1 of the hippocampus, so called because their firing is restricted to small portions of the rat's environment (the corresponding "place fields"). There is little topographic organization of PCs relating their positions in CA3 or CA1 to the positions of their firing fields. The firing properties of PCs

A)

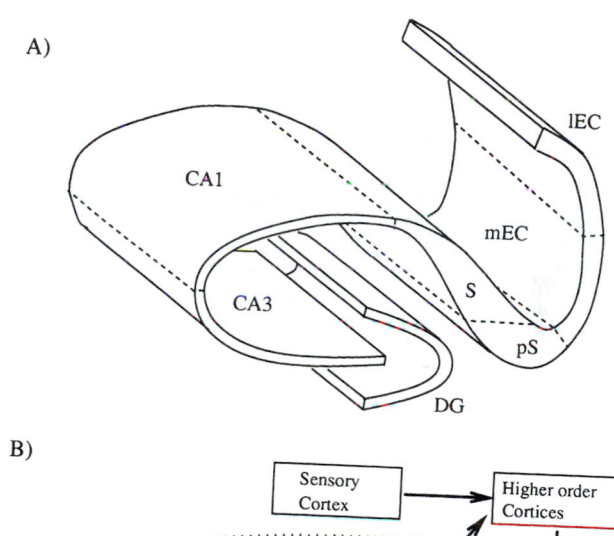

B)

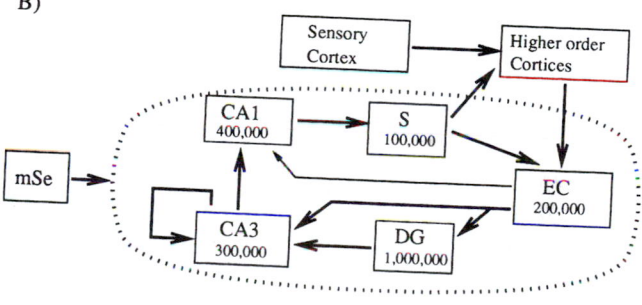

Figure 1. The hippocampus is formed from sheets of cells. *A*, A schematic section cut perpendicular to the longitudinal axis of the hippocampus. EC, entorhinal cortex (mEC, medial EC; lEC, lateral EC); S, subiculum; pS, pre- and parasubiculum; DG, dentate gyrus. *B*, The major projections between subfields (mSe, medial septum), and approximate numbers for the major cell type in each subfield (i.e., pyramidal cells, except for the DG, in which it is granule cells) in the rat. The human hippocampus contains one order of magnitude more cells. In the DG-CA3 projection a single mossy fiber cell projects from each granule cell, making very large synapses onto only 14 or so pyramidal cells. All the other projections have large divergence and convergence (many thousands to 1) and involve the type of synapse in which "Hebbian" LTP has been observed. A variety of interneurons provide feedforward and feedback inhibition. Cells in the mSe project into DG, CA3, and (less strongly) CA1, playing a role in producing the θ rhythm of the hippocampal EEG. Cells in CA3 and CA1 also project out to the lateral septum via the fornix. (Adapted with permission from B. L. McNaughton, 1989, Neuronal mechanisms for spatial computation and information storage, in *Neural Connections, Mental Computation* [L. Nadel, L. A. Cooper, P. Culicover, and R. M. Harnish, Eds.], Cambridge, MA: MIT Press.)

can be manipulated by changing the rat's environment: for example, rotating the major cues in an environment can cause the place fields to rotate. In environments in which direction of movement is restricted (e.g., mazes with narrow arms), PC firing rates appear to depend on the rat's direction of travel as well as its location.

Cells in the entorhinal cortex (the main cortical input to the hippocampus; see Figure 1) also have spatially correlated firing but tend to have larger, less well-defined place fields than those in CA3 or CA1. Cells whose primary behavioral correlate is "head direction" have also been found, in the (dorsal) presubiculum (see Figure 1), anterior thalamus, and mammillary bodies. They fire when the rat points its head in a specific direction relative to the cues in the environment, and independently of its location (see RODENT HEAD DIRECTION SYSTEM and Zhang, 1996, and Sharp, Blair, and Brown, in Gluck, 1996, for models).

The electroencephalogram (EEG) recorded in the hippocampus is the largest electrical signal in the rat brain. One form of the EEG, called the theta (θ) rhythm, is an oscillation of 7–12 Hz. O'Keefe and Nadel (1978) have suggested that in the rat, the θ rhythm coincides with displacement movements. PC firing has been found to have a systematic phase relationship to θ, discovered by O'Keefe and Recce in 1993 (see Burgess and O'Keefe in Gluck, 1996): when a rat on a linear track runs through a place field, the PC tends to fire groups of spikes, with each successive group occurring at an earlier phase of the θ cycle. Consistent with these data, PCs firing at a late phase tend to have place fields centered ahead of the rat, whereas those firing at an early phase tend to have place fields centered behind the rat in open field environments (see Burgess and O'Keefe in Gluck, 1996).

There are two features of PC firing that raise immediate problems for their use in navigation: (1) information about a place in an environment (i.e., the firing of the corresponding PCs) can only be accessed locally (by actually visiting that place), and (2) place fields appear to be no more affected by the location of the goal (which is obviously essential for navigation) than by the location of any other cue. Unfortunately, there are no reports to date of cells that code for the destination of a rat's current trajectory.

Path Integration

An animal may estimate its current position relative to some starting position purely on the basis of internal signals (e.g., vestibular or proprioceptive) relating to its movements in the intervening period. Such a process is often referred to as "path integration" (PI). Many animals appear to be able to use PI to return to a home location in the absence of external stimuli. Interestingly, once a rat has got its orientation from the array of cues, PCs can continue to fire in the correct places after all of the salient cues in an environment have been removed, or after the lights have been switched off (see also the role of PI in the RODENT HEAD DIRECTION SYSTEM). Experiments indicate that PC firing can be supported by visual, auditory, olfactory, tactile, or internal information, as available.

Cognitive Maps

Cognitive maps, or mental representations of the spatial layout of an environment, were first introduced by Tolman to explain place learning in rats, including, for example, their ability to take shortcuts (see COGNITIVE MAPS). An alternative view, suggested by Hull, is that navigation is achieved by following a list of stimulus-response-stimulus steps. O'Keefe and Nadel (1978) proposed that independent neural systems exist in the brain to support a "taxon" system for route navigation and a "locale" system for map-based navigation (for a synopsis, see O'Keefe, 1991). The "map" was taken to be a Euclidean description of the environment in an "allocentric" coordinate system (based on the world and not on some

part of the animal's body). They proposed that the locale navigation system resides in the hippocampus, based on (1) the firing properties of hippocampal PCs, (2) the presence of θ rhythm during displacement movement, (3) deficits in performance of spatial tasks, including the Morris water maze and the Olton eight-arm maze, following hippocampal lesions, and (4) the interpretation of the amnesic syndrome as the loss of episodic memory (memory for specific events set in a spatiotemporal context). Note, however, that the goal independence of PC firing indicates that such cells form only part of a cognitive map, some read-out mechanism being required to guide behavior.

O'Keefe and Nadel (1978) proposed that, while the hippocampal cognitive map was clearly tied to external cues, some form of PI might support its intrinsic distance and direction metric. In their original formulation, a PC could be activated by two independent means. First, PCs could be directly activated by the sensory inputs available to an animal in a particular location. Second, activation of the set of PCs corresponding to one location, coupled with inputs indicating the rat's performance of a movement translating and rotating it by a certain amount, would lead to the activation of the set of PCs corresponding to the new location. Mismatches between the two would provide the signal for exploration, which would bring the two sets of information into correspondence by strengthening some sensory inputs and weakening others (O'Keefe and Nadel, 1978, pp. 220–230).

Models of Place Cell Firing

Sensory Inputs

In this section we describe models of how the spatial firing of PCs develops and is maintained as the rat moves around an environment. Following an earlier mathematical model of PC firing (by Zipser in 1985), Sharp used a simple network with an input layer and two layers of cells governed by "competitive learning" dynamics (see COMPETITIVE LEARNING and Sharp, Blair, and Brown in Gluck, 1996). In this model two types of input (or "neocortical") cells respond to cues placed around the environment: a type 1 cell that "fires" whenever a particular cue is at a given distance from the rat, and a type 2 cell that likewise responds to a particular cue at a given distance, but only if the cue is within a certain range of angles relative to the rat's head. During exploration, competitive learning leads to unsupervised clustering of the input vectors: a PC learns to fire in a portion of the environment in which the inputs (i.e., the distances and angles of cues) are similar. Interestingly, if the simulated rat's exploration is restricted to movements consistent with being in an eight-arm maze, then PC firing tends to be much more strongly correlated with the orientation of the rat (as well as its location) than in the case of unrestricted exploration, which fits well with the experimental data. The place fields in this model are robust to the removal of a subset of the environmental cues. However, the model takes some time to develop realistic place fields, whereas experiments indicate that they are present, and orientation independent, as soon as they can be measured.

Attractors and Path Integration

Touretzky and Redish (in Burgess et al., 1999) proposed a model in which PCs form a coherent representation of location on the basis of estimates of the rat's location from PI and local-view information. The model investigates the interaction of frames of reference supported by different mechanisms and in different brain regions, assuming that resetting the PI system depends on the hippocampus. In a similar approach, Guazzelli, Bota, and Arbib (2001) proposed a feedforward competitive learning model that develops a PC representation by combining PI and sensory inputs, simulating in some detail the effects of darkness, and the deletion or movement of extramaze cues (see also Arbib in Burgess et al., 1999).

Samsonovich and McNaughton (1997) went much farther in placing the hippocampus at the heart of a PI system. They proposed that region CA3 of the hippocampus forms "continuous attractors" (Zhang, 1996) such that sets of place fields form preconfigured "charts," as follows. The recurrent connections between PCs fix the relative locations of place fields within a chart, and also ensure stable and coherent patterns of PC activity (i.e., activity consistent with the rat being in a single location). This system serves as the neural basis of a PI system driven by hardwired motion-related signals that shift PC activity so as to reflect the change in location of the rat corresponding to its movements. A particular chart becomes associated to the sensory stimuli in a particular environment so as to make a correspondence between locations on the chart and locations in reality. This model predicts that hippocampal lesions will impair PI, although the experimental evidence for this is controversial.

Kali and Dayan (2000) showed that continuous attractors could be formed by Hebbian learning in the recurrent connections during exploration. However, to create an attractor of equal depth across an unevenly sampled environment required that learning be mediated by novelty. Hasselmo, Wyble, and Wallenstein (in Gluck, 1996) suggest a mechanism for this. The CA3 representation reflects the expected state of the world, being influenced by the associations learned by the recurrent collaterals, while the CA1 representation reflects direct cortical input. Novelty is detected as a mismatch between the two representations, and mediates learning in CA3 by triggering the release of acetylcholine from the medial septum.

What Inputs Support a Place Cell's Spatially Tuned Firing?

Recording the same PCs in boxes of varying shape and size provides insight into the environment determinants of place fields. In these experiments the location of peak firing tends to maintain a fixed distance from the nearest walls, and a symmetrical, unimodal, place field in a small box may be elongated or multimodal in a larger box. These results are qualitatively fitted by a simple model in which PC firing is a thresholded sum of up to four "boundary vector cell" (BVC) inputs, each tuned to respond maximally whenever there is a wall a given distance away along a given allocentric direction. The tuning to distance is Gaussian, with a width that increases with the distance of the peak response from the wall. (We note that the attractor models discussed earlier can show this behavior only to the extent that the behavior is determined by feedforward BVC inputs.) A random selection of hardwired BVC inputs is sufficient to model the characteristics of populations of place fields, and choosing BVCs to fit a given cell's firing in one set of environments enables prediction of its firing in a novel environment (Hartley et al., 2000).

While the model works well for the initial firing of PCs in an environment, a slow experience-dependent divergence (or "remapping") of the representations of environments of different shape (Lever et al., 2002) indicates an additional role for synaptic plasticity. Because the PC representations in the models of Kali and Dayan (2000) and Gauzzelli et al. (2001) can be incrementally modulated by learning, these models can begin to be used to address the data showing varying degrees of remapping in different experiments, although it is not yet clear what changes will be necessary to provide an accurate model of the dynamics of these data.

Navigation

How could the hippocampus be used to enable navigation? The simplest map-based strategies are based on defining a surface, over the whole environment, on which gradient ascent leads to the goal (see REINFORCEMENT LEARNING). These strategies tend to have a problem, namely, that to build up the surface, the goal must be reached many times, from different points in the environment. A new surface must be computed if the goal is moved, and multiple goals, as in the eight-arm maze, cannot be handled. Learning in these models seems slower and more goal dependent than in rats, and they are unable to perform "latent learning" (e.g., in rats, exploration in the absence of goals improves subsequent navigation). Interestingly, the performance of these models improves somewhat when a spatially diffuse representation (like place fields) rather than a punctate representation is built up during exploration (see Foster, Morris, and Dayan, 2000). Some recent models that have related navigation to the action of individual cells in the hippocampus are described in the following section.

Using the CA3 Recurrent Collaterals

A role in navigation was proposed for the CA3 recurrent collaterals (the axonal projections by which each CA3 PC contacts approximately 5% of the other CA3 PCs) by Muller and Stead (in Gluck, 1996). Given a model of LTP in which pre- and postsynaptic firing within a short time interval leads to a small increase in synaptic "strength," the synaptic strength of a connection between two CA3 PCs can come to depend on the proximity of their place fields. This is also the condition for the formation of a continuous attractor representation, discussed earlier. After brief exploration, the synaptic strengths represent distances along the paths taken by the rat. The model proposes that the rat navigates by moving through the place fields of the cells most strongly connected to the cells with fields at the current and destination positions.

Blum and Abbott (1996) propose a related model in which the temporal asymmetry of LTP (synaptic strengthening can occur when presynaptic activity precedes postsynaptic activity; see TEMPORAL DYNAMICS OF BIOLOGICAL SYNAPSES) is invoked to strengthen recurrent connections from one PC to another if they fire in sequence along the rat's trajectory during exploration. If synaptic modification is also weighted by how soon after the pre- and postsynaptic activity the goal was reached, then the effect of the current collaterals is to shift the location represented by PC firing from the rat's current location toward the goal. This model proposes that the rat navigates by moving from the current location (e.g., read from CA1) to the shifted location in CA3.

Neither of these models makes clear how a direction of motion is actually generated, or if it would be able to generate a shortcut or detour. To build up a true distance metric in complex environments would take a long time and might best be achieved by reinforcement learning (see Foster et al., 2000). Clear experimental support for learned asymmetric connections between PCs comes from the observation that place fields tend to become elongated backward along a path during the first few times that a rat runs along it. Asymmetric recurrent connections have also been invoked to explain the phase precession effect. In these models the spread of activation from cells with fields early in a learned trajectory to cells with fields farther along the trajectory will, later in the θ cycle, cause a PC to fire before reaching the location on the path where its original (externally driven) place field was located. However, recent evidence indicates that blocking LTP blocks the development of asymmetric place fields but does not prevent the phase precession effect.

Local View Model

In 1989, McNaughton proposed that the hippocampus functions as an associative memory, as follows. As the rat explores, it learns to associate each local view and movement made with the local view from the place visited as a result of the movement. Thus, routes through an environment are stored as a chain of local view/ movement associations (see McNaughton and Nadel, 1990). The model is supported by the fact that, in some situations, PC firing depends on the rat's direction (and therefore its "local view"). Some major problems with this theory are the following: (1) simple route-following strategies appear to be the kind of navigation of which hippocampectomized rats are capable (see O'Keefe and Nadel, 1978); (2) it is difficult to know which particular route will lead to the desired goal: solving this problem leads one back to the reinforcement learning approach; (3) the model is not capable of more sophisticated navigation, such as taking shortcuts; and (4) in open fields, PC firing does not seem to depend on direction. It is also not clear whether this scheme is computationally feasible; see Sharp et al. (in Gluck, 1996) for a discussion of the limitations of simple associative nets in a related situation.

Centroid Model

O'Keefe (1991) proposed a navigational mechanism in which environments are characterized by two parameters: the centroid and the slope of the positions of environmental cues, which can be used as the origin and 0° direction of a polar coordinate framework. The firing of a PC could represent the average position of a small number of cues (their minicentroid), while head direction cells could represent the translation vector between pairs of cues. The environmental centroid and slope are then found by averaging the minicentroids and slopes. It was proposed that single cells could represent two-dimensional vectors as phasors: taking the θ rhythm of the EEG as a clock cycle, the amplitude of firing would code for proximity, and the phase of firing within a clock cycle would code for angle. Thus, summing the output of several neurons results in vector addition, and subtraction is equivalent to a phase inversion followed by addition. Thus, the summed PC activity could provide a vector $\vec{v}(t)$ continually pointing to the centroid of the environment, so that, if the "goal" was encountered at time t_g, storing $\vec{v}(t_g)$ (outside the hippocampus) would enable the translation vector $\vec{v}(t) - \vec{v}(t_g)$ from the rat to the goal to be calculated whenever the rat wanted to go to the goal. The advantages of this system include the ability to perform shortcuts, while the disadvantages include the sensitivity of the slope (i.e., small movements of cues could lead to reversal of the coordinate system).

Place Cell Firing and Navigation

The population vector model (see Burgess and O'Keefe in Gluck, 1996) is implemented at the neuronal level but also generates actual movement trajectories for the simulated rat, and aims to surmount some of the difficulties discussed in the previous section. It assumes that the output stage of the hippocampal system is groups of cells that represent the distance and direction from the rat of previously encountered goal locations as it moves around the environment, and that the input to the hippocampus is a set of "sensory cells" with tuning curve responses to the distance of cues from the rat. Each goal location is represented by the firing rates of a group of "goal cells" as a population vector (i.e., the vector sum of cells' preferred directions weighted by their firing rates; see MOTOR CORTEX: CODING AND DECODING OF DIRECTIONAL OPERATIONS), and is used to guide the rat back to a goal location (Figure 2).

The network operates in a feedforward manner. During exploration, a representation of current location is learned in the intermediate layers, entorhinal cells (ECs), PCs, and subicular cells (SCs), which map the sensory input to the population vector output. A type of competitive learning governs the dynamics of the PCs and SCs, similar to that used by Sharp (see Sharp et al. in Gluck, 1996). Latent learning during exploration is expressed as the de-

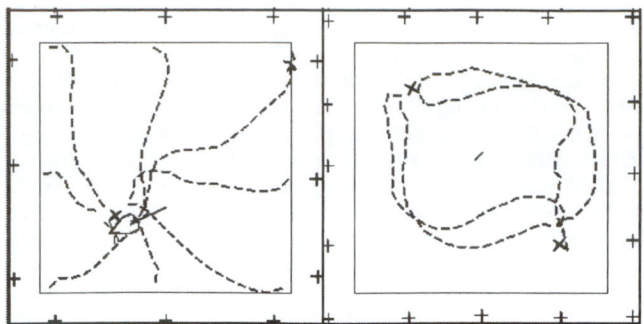

Figure 2. *Left,* Simulated trajectories from eight novel starting positions to a goal encountered after 30 seconds of exploration (at 60 cm/s) in a 135 × 135 cm² environment; the rat is shown to scale. *Right,* Simulated navigation between two goals with an "obstacle" in between. Cues are marked by +, goals by ×, and obstacles by /. (Adapted with permission from Burgess, N., Recce, M., and O'Keefe, J., 1994, *Neural Netw.,* 7:1065–1081.)

velopment of large firing fields in SCs that avoids the locality of information access problem (so that goal cell firing fields cover the whole environment; see later discussion). Upon encountering a goal location, learning by modification of connections to goal cells results in each goal cell having a conical firing rate map whose peak is displaced from the goal position in a particular absolute direction (the "preferred direction" for that cell), creating the appropriate population vector.

The model relies on the phase of firing of SCs (relative to θ) being such that those firing late in a cycle have place fields centered ahead of the rat. This is achieved by making the phase of firing of ECs depend on the angle between the rat's heading direction and the direction of the centroid of the corresponding pair of cues (if the centroid is ahead, the cell fires at a late phase; if behind, it fires early). This property propagates throughout the PC and SC layers. When the rat is at the goal, the goal cell with preferred direction closest to the rat's heading direction receives a strong input, allowing connections to it to be switched on. This signal arrives at a late phase of the θ rhythm, and connections are switched on from those SCs active at that time (which tend to have firing rate maps that peak ahead of the rat). When a goal is encountered, the rat looks around in all directions, so that connections are switched on to goal cells representing each direction.

The direction and proximity (represented by the net firing of the group of goal cells) of interesting objects is the output of the hippocampal "map" and allows the simulated rat to navigate. A small number of obstacles can be avoided during navigation by subtracting the population vector of obstacle cells from the population vector of goal cells. The advantages of this model are that reasonable trajectories, including shortcuts, are performed after one visit to the goal following brief exploration, and its latent learning. The representation of directions is allocentric (e.g., north, south, etc.), and the necessary translation into left-right body turns is assumed to occur in parietal cortex (taking into account the current heading direction and the locations of obstacles) (see also Recce and Harris in Gluck, 1996; Arbib in Burgess et al., 1999; and Burgess et al., 2001).

Brown and Sharp (see Sharp et al. in Gluck, 1996) proposed a similar feedforward model of PC firing and navigation. In their model the output representation (in the nucleus accumbens) is of the egocentric directions (body turns) that lead to the goal. The association from PCs to turn cells is built up over many runs to a goal. As with Blum and Abbott's model, synaptic modification must be weighted by how soon the goal was reached after pre- and postsynaptic activity. This model would not show latent learning, and navigation would be strongly affected if stereotyped routes were used during learning. Foster et al. (2000) suggest that, in addition to a fast learning mechanism related to that used by Burgess and O'Keefe (in Gluck, 1996), a slower process of reinforcement learning might build up an explicit metric representation of the environment over the course of several trials.

Discussion

We have reviewed several simple neuronal models of how the hippocampus takes in sensory information from environmental cues, turns it into a place cell representation of space, and uses this representation to support a spatial memory for where interesting things are located. Several of these models also consider the role of internal signals and recurrent connections in these processes. Together, these models represent some of the clearest examples of neuronal-level explanations of cognitive behavior. As noted earlier, how different environments are distinguished so that where things are in each environment can be remembered separately remains to be well understood, with data on remapping and the roles of the DG and the CA3 recurrent collaterals in providing an associative memory likely to play a part (see Marr, 1971; McNaughton and Nadel, 1990; Gluck, 1996; Burgess et al., 2001; Lever et al., 2002; and ASSOCIATIVE NETWORKS). A related issue is the problem of navigation in complex environments: how can local maps be patched together to guide behavior over long distances (see the "world graph" model of Arbib in Burgess et al., 1999).

With some progress made in understanding the role of the hippocampus in rat navigation, extending these models to include the role of the hippocampus in monkey and human behavior poses an exciting challenge. Recordings in monkey hippocampus that show neurons responding to the performance of actions in places (T. Ono and colleagues) or to the monkey looking in a particular place (see Rolls in Burgess et al., 1999) give an indication of how hippocampal function might generalize from rats to monkeys. In humans, there is evidence that the right hippocampus plays a role in navigation similar to the role it plays in the rat (see, e.g., Burgess et al., 1999, 2001). However, bilateral hippocampal damage in humans causes a general impairment in episodic memory. One idea relating the spatial and mnemonic roles is that a (nonverbal) episodic memory system could be formed in the right hippocampus by the addition of the human sense of linear time to the rat's spatial system; in the left hippocampus, the inputs have been supplemented by verbal information, producing memory for narratives (O'Keefe and Nadel, 1978). These issues, and the relationship between the hippocampus and the parietal cortex (generally considered the primary locus of spatial processing in primates) are explored further in Burgess et al. (1999). Finally, the need to impose

an egocentric point of view on the allocentric representations in long-term memory provides a starting point for modeling the role of the hippocampus and the head-direction system in episodic retrieval (Burgess et al., 2001; see also Recce and Harris in Gluck, 1996).

Road Maps: Mammalian Brain Regions; Mammalian Motor Control
Related Reading: Cognitive Maps; Hippocampal Rhythm Generation; Rodent Head Direction System; Short-Term Memory

References

Blum, K. I., and Abbott, L. F., 1996, A model of spatial map formation in the hippocampus of the rat, *Neural Computat.*, 8:85–93.

Burgess, N., Becker, S., King, J. A., and O'Keefe, J., 2001, Memory for events and their spatial context: Models and experiments, *Philos. Trans. R. Soc. Lond. B*, 356:1493–1503. ◆

Burgess, N., Jeffery, K. J., and O'Keefe, J., Eds., 1999, *The Hippocampal and Parietal Foundations of Spatial Cognition*, Oxford, Engl.: Oxford University Press. ◆

Foster, D. J., Morris, R. G., and Dayan, P., 2000, A model of hippocampally dependent navigation, using the temporal difference learning rule, *Hippocampus*, 10:1–16.

Gluck, M. A., Ed., 1996, *Hippocampus* (Special issue on computational models of the hippocampus), 6:565–762. ◆

Guazzelli, A., Bota, M., and Arbib, M. A., 2001, Competitive Hebbian learning and the hippocampal place cell system: Modeling the interaction of visual and path integration cues, *Hippocampus*, 11:216–239.

Hartley, T., Burgess, N., Lever, C., Cacucci, F., and O'Keefe, J., 2000, Modeling place fields in terms of the cortical inputs to the hippocampus, *Hippocampus*, 10:369–379.

Kali, S., and Dayan, P., 2000, The involvement of recurrent connections in area CA3 in establishing the properties of place fields: A model, *J. Neurosci.*, 20:7463–7477.

Lever, C., Wills, T., Cacucci F., Burgess, N., and O'Keefe, V., 2002, Long-term plasticity in the hippocampal place cell representation of environmental geometry, *Nature*, 416:90–94

Marr, D., 1971, Simple memory: A theory for archicortex, *Philos. Trans. R. Soc. Lond. B*, 262:23–81.

McNaughton, B. L., and Nadel, L., 1990, Hebb-Marr networks and the neurobiological representation of action in space, in *Neuroscience and Connectionist Theory* (M. A. Gluck and D. E. Rumelhart, Eds.), Hillsdale, NJ: Erlbaum, pp. 1–63. ◆

O'Keefe, J., 1991, The hippocampal cognitive map and navigational strategies, in *Brain and Space* (J. Paillard, Ed.), Oxford, Engl.: Oxford University Press, pp. 273–295.

O'Keefe, J., and Nadel, L., 1978, *The Hippocampus as a Cognitive Map*, Oxford, Engl.: Clarendon Press. ◆

Samsonovich, A., and McNaughton, B. L., 1997, Path integration and cognitive mapping in a continuous attractor neural network model, *J. Neurosci.*, 17:5900–5920.

Zhang, K., 1996, Representation of spatial orientation by the intrinsic dynamics of the head-direction cell ensemble: A theory, *J. Neurosci.*, 16:2112–2126.

Hybrid Connectionist/Symbolic Systems

Ron Sun

Introduction

There has been a great deal of research in integrating neural and symbolic processes from either cognitive or engineering standpoints. This research has led to the so-called hybrid systems. Hybrid connectionist-symbolic systems constitute a promising approach for developing more robust, more versatile, and more

powerful systems for modeling cognitive processes as well as for engineering practical intelligent systems. The need for such models has been growing steadily. Events such as the 1992 AAAI Workshop on Integrating Neural and Symbolic Processes, the 1995 IJCAI Workshop on Connectionist-Symbolic Integration, and the 1998 NIPS Workshop on Hybrid Neural Symbolic Integration have brought to light many ideas, issues, controversies, and syntheses in this area. This article provides an overview and a categorization of hybrid systems.

The basic motivation for research on hybrid connectionist-symbolic systems can be summarized as follows:

- Cognitive processes are not homogeneous. A wide variety of representations and processes are likely employed. Some cognitive processes are best captured by symbolic models and others by connectionist models, just as both quantum mechanics and fluid dynamics are needed in order to model physical processes (Dreyfus and Dreyfus, 1987; Smolensky, 1988; Sun, 1994). The need for "pluralism" in cognitive modeling has led to the development of hybrid systems.
- The development of intelligent systems for practical applications would benefit greatly from a proper combination of different techniques, since currently no single technique can do everything successfully. Application domains range from loan approval to process control (Medsker, 1994).

The relative advantages of connectionist and symbolic models have been amply argued for (see, e.g., Feldman and Ballard in Waltz and Feldman, 1986; Smolensky, 1988; Sun, 1994; see also ARTIFICIAL INTELLIGENCE AND NEURAL NETWORKS). Once the relative advantages of each model are understood, the computational benefit of the combination of models is relatively easy to justify. Naturally, one would want to take advantage of both types of models, and especially their synergy. Dreyfus and Dreyfus (1987), Sun and Bookman (1994), and Sun and Alexandre (1997) include detailed justifications for using hybrid systems.

For example, Sun and Peterson (1998) presented a model, CLARION, for capturing human skill learning that went from implicit knowledge to explicit knowledge. By integrating symbolic models (for capturing explicit knowledge) and subsymbolic models (for capturing implicit knowledge), CLARION more accurately captured human data and provided a new perspective on human skill learning.

Issues

In developing hybrid connectionist-symbolic systems, we need to ask the following questions:

1. What types of problems are hybrid systems suitable for?
2. What are the relative advantages and disadvantages of each approach to hybridization?
3. How cognitively plausible is each approach?

Other important issues concern the architecture of hybrid systems and learning in these systems. Hybrid models likely involve a variety of different types of processes and representations, in both learning and performance. Therefore, multiple heterogeneous mechanisms interact in complex ways. Architectures, or ways of structuring these different components, thus occupy a prominent place in this area of research. Some architecture-related issues include the following:

- What type of architecture facilitates what type of process?
- Should hybrid architectures be modular or monolithic?
- For modular architectures, should different representations be used in different modules or should the same representation be used throughout?
- How does an investigator decide whether the representation of a particular part of an architecture should be symbolic, localist, or distributed?
- What are the appropriate representational techniques that bridge the heterogeneity of hybrid systems?

- How do representation and learning interact in hybrid systems? (In such systems, both aspects are likely to be more complex.)
- How should the different parts of a hybrid system be structured to achieve optimal results?

A second matter of concern is the increased difficulty of learning. Although purely connectionist models, which are part of any hybrid system, excel in their learning abilities, hybridization makes it more difficult for a system to perform learning. Very generally, the difficulty hybrid systems have with learning comes from the symbolic side, and that difficulty dilutes the advantage that the connectionist parent brings to learning. Some of the learning-related issues include the following:

- What kind of learning can be carried out in each type of architecture?
- How can complex symbolic structures, such as rules, frames, and semantic networks, be learned in hybrid models?
- How can learning algorithms be developed for (usually knowledge-based) structured connectionist networks?
- What is the relationship among symbolic learning methods, knowledge acquisition methods, and connectionist (neural network) learning algorithms in hybrid systems?
- Can each type of architecture itself be developed with various combinations of the methods listed above?

Although many interesting hybrid models have been developed, a broader understanding of these hybrids awaits future work. Any model proposed should be examined for its cognitive plausibility, application potentials, and its strengths and weaknesses. Such an examination can lead to a synthesis of existing divergent approaches and can provide useful insight for further advances in this area. In the following sections we provide a brief categorization of different existing systems.

Architectures and Representations

Various classification schemes of hybrid systems have been proposed (see, e.g., Sun and Alexandre, 1997). For now, we can divide hybrid systems into two broad categories: *single-module* architectures and *multimodule* architectures (Figure 1).

In single-module systems, the *representation* dimension can be of the following forms (Sun and Bookman, 1994): symbolic (as in conventional symbolic models), localist (with one distinct node for representing each concept; see, e.g., Lange and Dyer, 1989; Shastri and Ajjanagadde, 1993; Barnden in Sun and Bookman, 1994), or distributed (with a set of nonexclusive, overlapping nodes for representing each concept; see, e.g., Pollack, 1990; Miikkulainen in Sun and Bookman, 1994; Plate in Sun and Alexandre, 1997; Sperduti et al. in Sun and Alexandre, 1997; see also CONNECTIONIST AND SYMBOLIC REPRESENTATIONS). Usually it is easier to incorporate prior knowledge into localist models, since their structures can be made to directly correspond to the structure of symbolic

1. **Single-module**
   - Representation: Symbolic, localist, distributed
   - Mapping: Direct translational, transformational
2. **Heterogeneous multimodule**
   - Components: Localist + distributed, symbolic + connectionist
   - Coupling: Loosely coupled, tightly coupled
   - Granularity: Coarse-grained, fine-grained
3. **Homogeneous multimodule**
   - Granularity: Coarse-grained, fine-grained

Figure 1. Classification of hybrid systems.

knowledge. (For more details on localist models, see STRUCTURED CONNECTIONIST MODELS). On the other hand, connectionist learning usually leads to distributed representation, as in the case of backpropagation. Distributed representation has some unique and useful properties. (For more details on distributed models, see PERCEPTRONS, ADALINES, AND BACKPROPAGATION and COMPOSITIONALITY IN NEURAL SYSTEMS.)

A question that may naturally arise is: Why should we use connectionist models (especially localist ones) for symbol processing, instead of symbolic models? Possible reasons for using connectionist models may include the following. (1) Connectionist models are believed to be a more apt framework for capturing a wide variety of cognitive processes (Waltz and Feldman, 1986; Sun, 1994). (2) Some inherent processing characteristics of connectionist models (such as similarity-based processing) make them more suitable for certain tasks (especially in cognitive modeling of human reasoning and learning). (3) Learning processes may be more easily developed in connectionist models, using, e.g., gradient descent and its various approximations, the Expectation-Maximization algorithm, the Baum-Welch algorithm and so on.

For multimodule systems, we can distinguish between *homogeneous* and *heterogeneous* systems. *Homogeneous* systems are similar to single-module systems except that they contain several replicated copies of the same structure, each of which can be used for processing the same set of inputs, to provide redundancy for various reasons. For example, there may be a set of competing experts for the same domain, each of which may vote for a particular solution. Or, each module can be specialized (with regard to content) for processing a particular type of input. For example, there may be different experts with the same structure but with different content knowledge for dealing with different situations.

Heterogeneous multimodule systems are more interesting. This category is the most hybrid of hybrid systems; CONSYDERR (Sun, 1994), SOAR/ECHO (Johnson et al. in Sun and Alexandre, 1997), and SCREEN (Weber and Wermter in Wermter, Riloff, and Scheler, 1996) belong to this category. A variety of distinctions can be made here. The first distinction has to do with *representations* of constituent modules. In heterogeneous multimodule systems, there can be different combinations of different types of constituent modules. For example, a system can be a combination of localist modules and distributed modules (e.g., CONSYDERR: Sun, 1994), or it can be a combination of symbolic modules and connectionist modules (either localist or distributed; e.g., SCRUFFY: Hendler in Barnden and Pollack, 1991). Some of these combinations can be traced to the ideas of Smolensky (1988), who argued for the dichotomy of conceptual and subconceptual processing, and Dreyfus and Dreyfus (1987), who put forward the distinction between analytical thinking and intuitive thinking.

A second distinction that can be made among heterogeneous multimodule systems has to do with the *coupling* of modules. A set of modules can be either loosely coupled or tightly coupled (Medsker, 1994). In loosely coupled situations, modules communicate with each other, primarily through message passing, shared memory locations, or shared files; an example is SCRUFFY (see Hendler in Barnden and Pollack, 1991). Loose coupling enables some loose forms of cooperation among modules. An example of cooperation is pre- and postprocessing versus main processing: while one or more modules take care of pre- and postprocessing, such as transforming input data or rectifying output data, a main module focuses on the main part of the task. Commonly, pre- and postprocessing are done using a neural network, while the main task is accomplished through the use of symbolic methods. Another form of cooperation is a master-slave relationship: while one module maintains control of the task at hand, it can signal other modules to handle some specific aspects of the task. For example, a symbolic expert system, as part of a rule, may invoke a neural network to

perform a specific classification or decision making. Yet another form of cooperation is the equal partnership of multiple modules. In this form, the modules—the equal partners—may consist of (1) complementary processes, such as in SOAR/ECHO (Johnson et al. in Sun and Alexandre, 1997) or (2) multiple functionally equivalent but structurally and representationally different processes, such as in CLARION (Sun and Peterson, 1998); or (3) they may consist of multiple differentially specialized and heterogeneously represented experts, each of which constitutes an equal partner in accomplishing a task.

In tightly coupled systems, on the other hand, the constituent modules interact through multiple channels or may even have node-to-node connections across two modules, as in CONSYDERR (Sun, 1994), in which each node in one module is connected to a corresponding node in the other module. Various forms of cooperation among modules exist, in ways similar to loosely coupled systems.

Yet another distinction that can be made in multimodule systems has to do with the *granularity* of modules in such systems: they can be either coarse-grained or fine-grained. At one end of the spectrum, a multimodule system can be very coarse-grained, so that it contains only two or three modules (such as the examples cited above). At the other end, a system can be so fine-grained that it can contain numerous modules. In an extremely fine-grained system, each tiny module may contain both a (simple and tiny) symbolic component and a (simple and tiny) connectionist component, as exemplified by Kokinov's model or Stevenson's model (see their chapters in Sun and Alexandre, 1997). The computational advantage of such a microlevel integration is that a vast number of simple "processors" can exist that make up an efficient, massively parallel system.

Learning

Learning, which can include learning content (i.e., knowledge) in a certain architecture or learning and developing an architecture itself, is a fundamental issue, and one that is clearly difficult. Learning is necessary not just because it is a fundamental aspect of cognition, but also because it is indispensable if hybrid systems are ever to be scaled up. Earlier work on hybrid models focused mostly on representational issues (see, e.g., Sun and Bookman, 1994). Such a focus might be justified at an early stage of research, since before we learn complex symbolic representations in hybrid models, we need to understand ways of representing complex symbolic structures in the first place. Over the years, some progress on learning has been made. While some have tried to extend neural learning algorithms (such as backpropagation) to learning complex symbolic representations (see PERCEPTRONS, ADALINES, AND BACKPROPAGATION), others have instead incorporated symbolic learning methods into hybrid models.

Let us look at a few models that incorporated symbolic learning methods. Sun and Peterson (1998) presented the two-module model CLARION for sequential decision tasks. In this model, symbolic knowledge is extracted on-line from a reinforcement learning neural network and in turn is used to speed up neural learning and to facilitate transfer of learned knowledge. The work showed not only the synergy between neural and symbolic learning, but also that symbolic knowledge can be learned autonomously on-line, from subsymbolic knowledge, which is essential for developing autonomous agents.

In a similar vein, Johnson et al. (in Sun and Alexandre, 1997) developed a two-module model SOAR/ECHO for abductive reasoning through a combination of symbolic and connectionist learning (symbolic explanation-based learning in SOAR and neural learning in ECHO).

Furthermore, Thrun (1996) developed a method that integrates explanation-based learning and neural learning in a connectionist framework. In his model there is no separate symbolic and connectionist module (thus the model is a single-module one). The model uses initial domain knowledge (in the form of a trained neural network) and an explanation-based learning process to learn a complete domain theory from the initial knowledge (utilizing "explanations" based on the slopes of activation functions of the initial neural network).

There are a variety of other proposals as well (including rule extraction or insertion algorithms). Future advances in hybrid systems are likely to depend heavily on the development of new learning methods for hybrid systems and on the integration of learning and complex symbolic representations. As mentioned earlier, symbolic representation and reasoning may well emerge from subsymbolic processes through learning, and thus an intimate, synergistic combination of symbolic and subsymbolic learning is desirable and should be further pursued.

Application Domains

To see the breadth of the hybrid systems research, let us look at a brief summary of applications.

Cognitive Science

The development of hybrid systems covers most of the traditional topics in cognitive science, among them the following:

- *Reasoning*, which includes work on hybrid models for logical reasoning, case-based reasoning, and schema-based reasoning. Among existing work, Shastri and Ajjanagadde (1993) took a logic-based approach, while Barnden (in Sun and Bookman, 1994) took a case-based approach. Lange and Dyer (1989) performed reasoning based on schemas (frames). Sun (1994) combined logic-based, case-based, and schema-based approaches. These models went beyond existing nonhybrid models in capturing complex cognitive processes involved.
- *Memory*, which is an area where many models, including hybrid models, are being developed by the psychology community.
- *Classification and categorization*, which involve a variety of hybrid models, conceptual or computational (see CONCEPT LEARNING). These hybrid models often more accurately capture human data than their nonhybrid counterparts.
- *Skill learning*, including, e.g., Sun and Peterson (1998) and Johnson et al. (in Sun and Alexandre, 1997). These models have some important advantages. For example, Sun and Peterson (1998) better explained a type of skill learning than any existing nonhybrid models.
- *Word sense disambiguation*, including work by Lange and Dyer (1989), Bookman (in Sun and Bookman, 1994), and Wermter et al. (1996).
- *Natural language processing* in general, including both syntactic and semantic processing. There are many existing models. (See, e.g., Miikkulainen's and Dyer's chapters in Sun and Bookman, 1994, and all relevant chapters in Wermter et al., 1996.)

These hybrid systems use the synergy between connectionist and symbolic processes to more accurately capture human cognitive processes, either quantitatively or qualitatively.

Industrial Applications

Hybrid systems of various sorts have a large variety of practical applications. Because they combine characteristics of connectionist and symbolic models, hybrid systems are often able to perform better at various tasks. For a summary of early work in this area, see Medsker (1994). See also the application-oriented chapters in Sun and Alexandre (1997), and recent issues of various *IEEE Transactions*.

Discussion

Progress in hybrid systems is occurring steadily, if slowly. Because of the many advantages of hybrid systems, there is reason to expect further significant progress in this area. A number of possibilities exist for architectures, representations, and learning. This abundance suggests exciting possibilities in theoretical advances and in applications.

A distillation of the various extant proposals suggests two different approaches, which can be characterized as (1) incorporating symbolic mechanisms and connectionist models, and (2) stretching connectionist models all the way. In the first approach (see, e.g., Hendler in Barnden and Pollack, 1991; Sun, 1994; Wermter et al., 1996), the representation and learning techniques from both symbolic processing models and neural network models are used to tackle problems that neither type of model handles very well alone. Such problems include modeling cognition, which requires dealing with a variety of cognitive capacities. Several researchers (e.g., Smolensky, 1988; Dreyfus and Dreyfus, 1987) have argued that cognition is better captured with a combination of symbolic and neural components. The second approach, stretching connectionist models to their limit (e.g., Pollack, 1990; Giles and Gori, 1998), is predicated on the assumption that one can perform complex symbolic processing using neural networks alone, with, for example, tensor products, RAAM, or holographic models (see relevant chapters in Sun and Alexandre, 1997). Thus far, both approaches have flourished.

Despite the diversity of approaches, there is clearly an underlying theme, namely, the bringing together of symbolic and connectionist models to achieve the synthesis and synergy of two seemingly different paradigms. The various proposed methods, models, and architectures reflect the common belief that connectionist and symbolic methods can be usefully combined and integrated, and that such integration may lead to significant advances in our understanding of cognition.

Road Map: Artificial Intelligence
Related Reading: Artificial Intelligence and Neural Networks; Compositionality in Neural Systems; Connectionist and Symbolic Representations; Decision Support Systems and Expert Systems; Modular and Hierarchical Learning Systems; Schema Theory; Structured Connectionist Models

References

Barnden, J. A., and Pollack, J. B., Eds., 1991, *Advances in Connectionist and Neural Computation Theory*, Hillsdale, NJ: Erlbaum.

Dreyfus, H., and Dreyfus, S., 1987, *Mind Over Machine*, New York: Free Press.

Giles, L., and Gori, M., 1998, *Adaptive Processing of Sequences and Data Structures*, New York: Springer-Verlag. ◆

Lange, T., and Dyer, M., 1989, High-level inferencing in a connectionist network, *Connect. Sci.*, 1:181–217.

Medsker, L., 1994, *Hybrid Neural Networks and Expert Systems*, Boston: Kluwer.

Pollack, J., 1990, Recursive distributed representation, *Artif. Intell.*, 46:77–106.

Shastri, L., and Ajjanagadde, V., 1993, From simple associations to systematic reasoning: A connectionist representation of rules, variables and dynamic bindings, *Behav. Brain Sci.*, 16:417–494.

Smolensky, P., 1988, On the proper treatment of connectionism, *Behav. Brain Sci.*, 11:1–74.

Sun, R., 1994, *Integrating Rules and Connectionism for Robust Commonsense Reasoning*, New York: Wiley. ◆

Sun, R., and Alexandre, F., Eds., 1997, *Connectionist Symbolic Integration*, Hillsdale, NJ: Erlbaum.

Sun, R., and Bookman, L., Eds., 1994, *Architectures Incorporating Neural and Symbolic Processes*, Boston: Kluwer. ◆

Sun, R., and Peterson, T., 1998, Autonomous learning of sequential tasks: Experiments and analyses, *IEEE Trans. Neural Netw.*, 9:1217–1234.

Thrun, S., 1996, *Explanation-Based Neural Network Learning*, Boston: Kluwer.

Waltz, D., and Feldman, J., Eds., 1986, *Connectionist Models and Their Implications*, Norwood, NJ: Ablex.

Wermter, S., Riloff, E., and Scheler, E., Eds., 1996, *Connectionist, Statistical, and Symbolic Approaches to Learning for Natural Language Processing*, Berlin: Springer-Verlag.

Identification and Control

Kumpati S. Narendra

Introduction

System characterization and system identification are fundamental problems in systems theory. The problem of *characterization* is concerned with the mathematical representation of a system as an operator S which maps input signals into output signals. The problem of *identification* is to approximate S using an identification model, along with the measured inputs and outputs to the system. In the past five decades, systems theory has made major advances through a combination of mathematics, modeling, computation, and experimentation. At the same time, there has also been an explosive growth in pure and applied research related to neural networks. This article briefly explores how the concepts and methods developed in the two areas are being combined to generate general principles for the identification and control of complex nonlinear dynamical systems.

Systems can be classified as either continuous time (in which all variables of the systems are defined for all values of time $t \in R$) or discrete time (in which they are defined at integer values, i.e., $t = 0, 1, 2, \ldots$). A very general method of representing multi-input, multi-output continuous-time and discrete-time dynamical systems is by using vector differential and difference equations, as follows:

$$
\begin{array}{ll}
\textit{Continuous-Time Systems} & \textit{Discrete-Time Systems} \\
\dot{x}(t) = f[x(t), u(t)] & x(k + 1) = f[x(k), u(k)] \\
y(t) = h[x(t)] & y(k) = h[x(k)] \qquad (1)
\end{array}
$$

where $u(t)(u(k)) \in R^r$ is an input vector, $x(t)(x(k)) \in R^n$ is the state vector, and $y(t)(y(k)) \in R^m$ is an output vector. From Equation 1 it follows that given the state at time $t_0(k_0)$ and the input (input sequence) for $t(k) \geq t_0(k_0)$, the corresponding state and output can be determined. Equation 1 emphasizes the central role played by the state of the system, since, if the state at time t_0 is known, the past history of the system is not relevant, and the output is determined uniquely by the input from time t_0.

From the very beginning it has been realized by systems theorists that most real dynamical systems are nonlinear. However, linearizations of such systems around equilibrium states yield linear models that are mathematically tractable. For example, the linearization of Equation 1 around an equilibrium state can be described by the equations:

$$
\begin{array}{ll}
\dot{x}(t) = Ax(t) + Bu(t) & x(k + 1) = Ax(k) + Bu(k) \\
y(t) = Cx(t) & y(k) = Cx(k) \qquad (2)
\end{array}
$$

where A, B, and C are constant $n \times n$, $n \times r$, and $m \times n$ matrices, respectively. (In this article, we confine our attention to nonlinear discrete-time dynamical systems of the form given in Equation 1, and to their linearization, given in Equation 2.) The systems given by Equation 2 are said to be time invariant and are completely parameterized by the triple A, B, C. The analytical tractability of the above linear models can be attributed to the fact that the superposition principle applies to them. If any two input sequences $\{u_1(k)\}$ and $\{u_2(k)\}$, when applied to the system at rest, result in output sequences $\{y_1(k)\}$ and $\{y_2(k)\}$, respectively, an input sequence $\{\alpha u_1(k) + \beta u_2(k)\}$ for $\alpha, \beta \in R$ will result in an output sequence $\{\alpha y_1(k) + \beta y_2(k)\}$. Further, in many engineering problems it has been found that most nonlinear systems can be approximated satisfactorily by such linear models in their normal ranges of operation, and this has made the latter attractive in practical contexts as well. It is this combined effect of ease of analysis and practical applicability that accounts for the great success of linear models and has made them the subject of intense study for more than four decades.

The objective of control is to influence the behavior of dynamical system in some desired fashion. The latter includes maintaining the outputs of systems at constant values (regulation) or forcing them to follow prescribed time functions (tracking). Maintaining the altitude of an aircraft or the glucose level in the blood at a constant value are simple examples of regulation; controlling a rocket to follow a given trajectory is a simple example of tracking. For the same reasons given earlier in the context of system representation, the best-developed part of control theory deals with linear time-invariant systems, for which design methods are currently well established.

The demands of a rapidly advancing technology for faster and more accurate controllers have always had a strong influence on the progress of control theory. Applications in new technologies such as robotics, manufacturing, space technology, and medical automation, as well as those in older technologies such as process control and aircraft control, are providing a wealth of new problems in which nonlinearities and uncertainties play a major role and linear approximations are no longer satisfactory. To cope with such problems, research on both identification and control using neural networks has been under way. This article describes why neural networks are attractive in this context, as well as the theoretical assumptions that have to be made when such networks are used as identifiers and controllers.

Artificial Neural Networks

The term artificial neural network (ANN) has come to mean any computing architecture that consists of massively parallel interconnections of simple computing elements. From a systems-theoretic point of view, it can be considered as a conveniently parameterized and easily implementable class of nonlinear maps. In the early 1980s, elaborate ANNs were constructed and empirically demonstrated (using simulation studies) to approximate quite well nearly all functions encountered in practical applications. However, only after numerous authors had demonstrated that such networks are capable of universal approximation in a very precise and satisfactory sense did their study leave its empirical origins to become a mathematical discipline.

Even as these theoretical developments were in progress, empirical investigations continued, and neural networks were used not only for function approximation but also in pattern recognition and optimization problems. In 1990, Narendra and Parthasarathy suggested that feedforward neural networks could also be used as components in feedback systems. The approximation capabilities of such networks could be used in the design of both identifiers and controllers, and their analysis and synthesis could be carried out within a systems-theoretic framework. Following the publication of Narendra and Parthasarathy's paper, there was a frenzy of activity in the area of neural network–based identification and control, and a profusion of methods was suggested for controlling nonlinear systems. Although much of the research was heuristic, it provided empirical evidence that neural networks could outperform traditional methods. However, it soon became evident that more formal methods would be needed to quantitatively assess the scope and limitations of neural network–based control.

MLP and RBFN Networks

The most commonly used network structures for approximating nonlinear maps are the multilayer feedforward networks, also known as the multilayer perceptron (MLP) and the radial basis function network (RBFN). These two classes of neural networks (which are described in greater detail in other articles in this *Handbook*) form the principal building blocks of the dynamical systems considered in the following sections. The n-layer MLP with input u and output y is described by the equation

$$\Gamma[w_n \Gamma[w_{n-1} \cdots \cdot \Gamma[w_1 u + b_1] + \cdots + b_{n-1}] + b_n] = y \tag{3}$$

where w_i is a weight matrix in the ith layer and the vectors b_i represent the threshold value for each node in the ith layer. $\Gamma[\cdot]$ is a nonlinear operator with $\Gamma(x) = [\gamma_1(x), \gamma_2(x), \ldots, \gamma_n(x)]$, where $\gamma_i(\cdot)$ is a smooth activation function (generally a sigmoid). An alternative to the MLP is the RBFN, which can be considered a two-layer network in which the hidden layer performs a nonlinear transformation on the inputs (see RADIAL BASIS FUNCTION NETWORKS). The output layer then combines the outputs of the first layer linearly, so that the output is described by the equation

$$y = f(u) = \sum_{i=1}^{N} w_i R_i(u) + w_0 \tag{4}$$

The functions R_i are termed radial basis functions, and typically these are Gaussian functions.

In both networks, the parameters (weights) are adjusted to decrease the error between the output of the function to be approximated and that of the network, along the negative gradient. Numerous algorithms have been proposed to improve the convergence properties of MLP networks, but invariably all of them are modifications of the gradient approach. When RBFNs are used to approximate an unknown function based only on inputs and outputs, the convergence is substantially faster, since the output error is linear in the parameters.

A question that naturally arises is why neural networks should be preferred to other methods for approximating nonlinear functions in identifiers and controllers. The principal reason, already referred to, is the universal approximating capability of such networks. Empirical evidence is also available that they are fault tolerant and robust in the presence of noise. The fact that they are implementable in hardware makes them attractive in practical applications. However, a convincing theoretical argument was provided by Barron (1993), who showed that the effectiveness of MLPs (in which the output depends nonlinearly on the weights) for approximating a general class of nonlinear functions increases with the dimension of the input space, as compared to networks in which the output depends linearly on the weights. Since the dimension of the input vector used for identification and control in complex dynamical systems is generally quite high, the advantages assured by Barron are very attractive. It must be added here that other authors have taken issue with Barron on this matter by suggesting that RBFNs can enjoy the same advantages if the characteristics of the nonlinear activation functions used in them are also varied.

Identification

If an ANN is to be used for identifying a nonlinear dynamical system, the existence of a dynamic nonlinear map relating the input and output spaces must first be established. In many practical applications, identification has to be carried out using only observed input-output data. In such cases, it is tacitly assumed that there is an underlying nonlinear dynamic map relating the two. An example of such a map is given by the state equation given in Equation 1. The objective would then be to identify the maps f and h. If measurements on the state vector $x(k)$ of the unknown system (generally referred to as the *plant*) are available, a model of the nonlinear system can be set up as

$$\hat{x}(k + 1) = N_f[x(k), u(k)]$$
$$\hat{y}(k) = N_h[x(k)] \tag{5}$$

where N_f and N_h are neural networks approximating f and h, respectively. Since $x(k)$ and $u(k)$ are accessible, standard approximation methods may be used to adjust the parameters of N_f and N_h based on the errors $\tilde{x}(k) = \hat{x}(k) - x(k)$ and $\tilde{y}(k) = \hat{y}(k) - y(k)$, respectively. It must be noted that the state/output of the system $x(k)/y(k)$, rather than $\hat{x}(k)/\hat{y}(k)$ of the network, is used in the right-hand side of the models given in Equation 5. This is generally referred to as a series-parallel model. This makes the identification procedure substantially simpler and hence practically attractive. However, a more realistic model would have the form:

$$\hat{x}(k + 1) = N_f[\hat{x}(k), u(k)]$$
$$\hat{y}(k) = N_h[\hat{x}(k)] \tag{6}$$

Since the estimated state of the system is used to determine $\hat{y}(k)$, we have a feedback system in this case. This implies that the model can be unstable. This model is also referred to as a recurrent network. Determining the gradient of the performance index with respect to the adjustable parameters of the network is no longer simple. Static backpropagation, used in Equation 5, has to be replaced by dynamic backpropagation, which is computationally intensive. A network described by Equation 6 is referred to as a recurrent network, and the stability properties of such networks are not well understood. Hence, the series-parallel networks described by Equation 5 are preferred in practice.

The Nonlinear Autoregressive Moving Average (NARMA) Model

The identification problem using a state representation becomes substantially more complex when the state variables of the plant are unknown, and identification has to be carried out using only input-output data. It is well known that even in the linear case, a unique parameterization of the plant no longer exists. The success of nonlinear identification techniques therefore strongly depends on the specific parameterizations used.

For a single-input single-output (SISO) linear time-invariant system described by the state Equations 2, it can be shown that, if the system is observable, the input and output are related by the equation

$$y(k + 1) = \sum_{i=0}^{n-1} \alpha_i\, y(k - i) + \sum_{j=0}^{n-1} \beta_j u(k - j) \quad (7)$$

where α_i and $\beta_j (i, j = 0, 1, \ldots, n - 1)$ are the parameters of the system. Equation 7 is known as the autoregressive moving average (ARMA) representation of the given plant and expresses the output at any instant as a linear combination of the past n values of the input and the n values of the output. The ARMA representation has found extensive application in linear systems theory.

Motivated by the ARMA model in the linear case, efforts were made in the early 1990s to suggest models for nonlinear system identification. If the linearized system around the equilibrium state of the system in Equation 1 is observable, it was shown (Levin and Narendra, 1993), using the implicit function theorem, that the state $x(k)$ and hence the output $y(k)$ can be determined using n past values of the input and output, as follows:

$$x(k) = G[y(k), y(k - 1), \ldots, y(k - n + 1),$$
$$u(k), \ldots, u(k - n + 1)] \quad (8)$$

and

$$y(k) = F[y(k), y(k - 1), \ldots, y(k - n + 1),$$
$$u(k), \ldots, u(k - n + 1)] \quad (9)$$

where G and F are functions mapping $R^m \times R^{2n}$ into R^n and R, respectively. Equation 9 is an exact mathematical representation of the given system (from Equation 1) in a neighborhood of the equilibrium state. It is referred to as the NARMA model and provides a rigorous mathematical basis for the synthesis of identification models using input-output data.

As mentioned in the Introduction to this article, once the existence of a nonlinear dynamic map from the input space to the output space is established, a neural network can be used to approximate the map using available data. In the present case, identification reduces to the approximation of the function F in Equation 9. A neural network model of the system is then given by

$$\hat{y}(k + 1) = N_F[y(k), y(k - 1), \ldots, y(k - n + 1),$$
$$u(k), \ldots, u(k - n + 1)] \quad (10)$$

where N_F is a neural network whose $2n$ inputs are the past n values of the input and output, respectively. The parameters of the network are adjusted to minimize the error $e_i(k) = \hat{y}(k) - y(k)$, between the output of the network and the output of the given plant. Equation 10, approximating the NARMA model, has been used extensively for the practical identification of nonlinear systems using neural networks.

Comments

The NARMA representation given in Equation 9 and the neural network approximation given in Equation 10 raise numerous theoretical and practical questions.

From a theoretical point of view, one is interested in relating the number of past values of the output and the input needed with the dimension of the state space n of the system (in Equation 9 this is chosen to be n). Also, Equations 9 and 10 describe the evolution of two dynamical systems, and one must establish in what sense the proximity of F and N implies the proximity of the trajectories of the two systems.

From a practical point of view, the choice of the number of nodes and the number of layers in the network to approximate F is important. However, at the present time, this is very much of an art, and the values are chosen by trial and error. There are also numerous gradient-based methods for the adjustment of parameters, but

the performance criterion varies from design to design. A criterion function that has proved effective in applications is one in which the output errors as well as the incremental inputs are weighted over a finite interval of time (i.e., $\sum_k [e_i^2(k) + (u(k) - u(k - 1))^2]$).

Recently, efforts have been made to approximate models of Equation 10 in such a manner that the input $u(k)$ appears linearly. They have the following form:

$$\hat{y}(k + 1) = F_0[y(k), y(k - 1), \ldots, y(k - n + 1)]$$
$$+ \sum_{j=0}^{n-1} F_j[y(k), \ldots, y(k - n + 1)]u(k - j)$$
$$(11)$$

The need for such models is discussed in the following sections in the context of control.

Control

Two distinct classes of problems that are encountered with increasing frequency in industry deserve special attention from the point of view of both the control theorist and the practicing engineer. The first is encountered in the context of systems that are already in existence and that were designed satisfactorily in a small neighborhood of the equilibrium in the state space. In this domain, linear models are used to describe the systems, and linear controllers based on them are found to perform satisfactorily. However, because of the demands of technology, the systems are required to operate in larger regions in the state space, where their characteristics are distinctly nonlinear. Both the identification model and the linear controller are then found to be inadequate to achieve the desired level of performance.

In the second class of problems, mathematical models of the plant (or process) to be controlled cannot be developed from first principles, but the process is known to be distinctly nonlinear. A finite amount of stored input-output data of the plant is available from which an adequate model of the process and a suitable controller are to be determined to satisfy stringent performance criteria.

For both classes of problems stated above, numerous decisions have to be made concerning the representation to be used, the prior information to be obtained to ensure the existence of a controller, the architecture of the identifier and controller, and the algorithms to be used in training their parameters. In the next sections we address some of the theoretical and practical questions that arise in neurocontrol.

Regulation and Tracking

In the Introduction we noted that regulation and tracking are two control problems of general interest. Regulation involves the generalizations of a control input that stabilize the system around an equilibrium state. In the tracking problem, a reference output $y^*(k)$ is specified and the output $y(k)$ of the plant is to approximate it in some sense, e.g., $\lim \sup_{k \to \infty} \|y(k) - y^*(k)\| \leq \varepsilon$. For theoretical analysis, ε is assumed to be zero, so that asymptotic tracking is achieved.

In the following, we assume that linearization of the system around the equilibrium state is both controllable and observable. Controllability implies that the state of the system can be transferred to any other state by the application of a suitable control input. Observability implies that the state of the system can be determined by observing the output over a finite interval of time. If the linearized system is controllable and observable, it follows that the nonlinear system is also locally controllable and observable. Almost all control systems in operation that were designed using linear control principles satisfy the above conditions. This conclusion, in turn, implies that such systems can be controlled as described in the next section, even in regions where their dynamics are nonlinear.

The Identification and Control Procedure

The process of identifying and controlling a plant using neural networks can be summarized as a three-step procedure. In the first step, a neural network is used to approximate the behavior of the given system. In the second step, after a sufficiently accurate model has been obtained, a neural network is designed to control the model (rather than the plant) to achieve the desired performance. In the third step, the same controller is used to control the system. If the performance does not meet specifications, the common procedure is to increase the size(s) of the neural networks used for identification and control, and repeat the entire procedure. If both identification and control are carried out concurrently, we have an adaptive system.

We first consider the dynamical system described by the state Equation 1, in which the entire state vector $x(k)$ is accessible, and attempt to regulate it around the origin. If the linearized system around the origin is controllable, it has been shown (Levin and Narendra, 1993) that $u = g(x)$ (i.e., nonlinear state feedback exists) such that the equilibrium state is stable. Hence, in principle, a neural network can be used to approximate $g(x)$. If $u(k) = N_c[x(k)]$, the overall feedback system is described by the equation

$$x(k + 1) = f[x(k), N_c[x(k)]] \quad (12)$$

The parameters of the neural network are then adjusted using dynamic back propagation. In Levin and Narendra (1993), different methods are described for accomplishing this, based on the measured state $x(k)$. Simulation results indicate that this method is far superior to that obtained using linear theory.

Tracking

The problem of tracking a reference signal when the dynamics of the plant are unknown poses a real challenge to the control engineer. In this case, the principal question that arises is whether an input $u(\cdot)$ exists so that the output of the plant can asymptotically follow the reference input. Assuming that such an input exists, the next problem is to determine a controller structure as well as the inputs to the controller so that the output of the controller is the desired input to the plant.

Various authors have investigated the application of neural networks for tracking. In the pioneering work of Widrow (e.g., Widrow and Wallach, 1996), the nonlinear plant itself is used in place of the identification model while training the controller. In the work of Jordan (1990) and Kawato (1990), inverse modeling using neural networks is used for solving inverse kinematics and inverse dynamics problems. Qin, Su, and McAvoy (1992) have used a similar methodology for process control. More recently, Cabrera and Narendra (1999) studied in detail the conditions that a plant must satisfy for a bounded control to exist in order to achieve asymptotic tracking of any specified bounded signal in the region of interest. In the following paragraphs, we summarize the results contained in the latter that are relevant to the present discussion.

The relative degree and zero dynamics of a nonlinear discrete-time system are important concepts in attempting to determine the control input to a dynamical system to track a desired output. The definitions of relative degree and zero dynamics have been discussed by numerous authors, but the analytical issues involved are for the expert. In qualitative terms, a relative degree d implies that for any arbitrary initial condition in a neighborhood of the origin, the effect of a control input $u(k)$ is felt only at time $k + d$. Hence, for the purposes of our discussion here, the *relative degree* of the

system can be defined as the delay of the system. The *zero dynamics* of the system describe the behavior of the system when the input and the initial conditions are jointly chosen in such a way that the output is identically zero. One of the principal results given by Cabrera and Narendra (1999) is that if the relative degree of a dynamic system is well defined and its zero dynamics are asymptotically stable, the asymptotic tracking problem can be solved using an analytic controller of the form

$$u(k) = \gamma[y(k), y(k - 1), \ldots, y(k - n + 1), u(k - 1), \ldots,$$
$$u(k - n + 1), y^*(k), y^*(k + 1) \ldots y^*(k + d)] \quad (13)$$

where $y^*(k)$ is the desired output at time k, and d is the relative degree of the system. In some cases only the reference input $y^*(k + d)$ may be needed at time k.

The above results have great practical significance, since the existence of a map γ implies that a neural network N_γ can be used to approximate it.

Practical Considerations

Numerous difficulties are encountered when a neural network is used to control a dynamical system. These can be briefly listed as follows:

1. Since the neural network is in a feedback loop with the controlled plant, dynamic rather than static backpropagation is needed to adjust the parameters along the negative gradient. However, in practice, only static backpropagation is used.
2. From both theoretical and practical viewpoints, the best approach in the author's experience is to use the approximate model of Equation 11, in which the control input $u(k)$ can be computed algebraically. To improve the performance further, the parameters of an additional neural network may be adjusted, as in point 1.
3. Because of the complexity of the structure of an MLP neural network and the nonlinear dependence of its map on its parameter values, stability analysis of the resulting system is always very difficult and quite often intractable. However, many interesting results have been obtained by Sanner and Slotine (1992), Jagannathan and Lewis (1996), Polycarpou (1996), and Chen and Khalil (1995), most of which are applicable in specific contexts.
4. In practice, the three-step procedure described earlier is used in industrial problems, to avoid adaptation on-line and the ensuing stability problems. However, if the feedback system is stable, on-line adaptive adjustments can improve performance significantly, provided such adjustments are small.

Conclusions

Numerous control methods have been suggested by different authors over the past decade for the practical control of dynamical systems using neural networks. These methods include supervised control, inverse control, internal model control, and model reference control. In many cases, the authors have attempted to realize identifiers and controllers as static maps using neural networks both to improve convergence and to simplify analysis. In many practical applications, such methods have performed satisfactorily. However, to our knowledge, the identification and control models described in this article are the only ones that have been rigorously derived using theoretical results from nonlinear and adaptive control.

Most of the current interest in the application of neural networks is in static systems, particularly in pattern recognition, where they have been very successful. The need for the control of nonlinear dynamical systems is, however, increasing in new technologies in which nonlinearities, uncertainties, and complexity play a major role. Neural networks are particularly attractive in such situations. However, the results obtained in nonlinear control theory, the concepts and structures provided by linear adaptive control, and the approximating capabilities of neural networks have to be judiciously combined to deal with the control problems that arise in complex dynamical systems (Chen and Narendra, 2001; Jagannathan, 2001).

The presence of a feedback loop in a system implies that stability issues have to be addressed in their design. At present, the neurocontrol problems being attempted in industry are those in which improving performance rather than ensuring stability is the main consideration. However, as faster response is required in industrial applications, stability questions are bound to become more important.

Practical systems design is driven by both cost and operational requirements. Anyone familiar with industrial problems is only too aware that bridging the gap between theoretical principles, on the one hand, and development, testing, and implementation on the other is a slow process. On the basis of theoretical advances made thus far, and the great successes that have already been reported in some cases, there is every reason to believe that neural network–based control systems will be developed in many industries in the next decade.

Road Map: Robotics and Control Theory
Background: Perceptrons, Adalines, and Backpropagation
Related Reading: Motor Control, Biological and Theoretical; Sensorimotor Learning

References

Barron, A. R., 1993, Universal approximation bounds for superpositions of a sigmoidal function, *IEEE Trans. Inform. Theory*, 39:930–945.
Cabrera, J. B. D., and Narendra, K. S., 1999, Issues in the application of neural networks for tracking based on inverse control, *IEEE Trans. Autom. Control*, 44:2007–2027. ◆
Chen, F.-C., and Khalil, H. K., 1995, Adaptive control of a class of nonlinear discrete-time systems using neural networks, *IEEE Trans. Autom. Control*, 40:791–801.
Chen, L. J., and Narendra, K. S., 2001, Nonlinear adaptive control using neural networks and multiple models, *Automatica*, 37:1245–1255.
Jagannathan, S., 2001, Control of a class of nonlinear discrete-time systems using multilayer neural networks, *IEEE Trans. Neural Netw.*, 12:1113–1120.
Jagannathan, S., and Lewis, F. L., 1996, Multilayer discrete-time neural-net controller with guaranteed performance, *IEEE Trans. Neural Netw.*, 7:107–130.
Jordan, M. I., 1990, Learning inverse mappings using forward models, in *Proceedings of the 6th Yale Workshop on Adaptive Learning Systems*, pp. 146–151.
Kawato, M., 1990, Computational schemes and neural networks models for formation and control of multijoint arm trajectory, in *Neural Networks for Control* (W. T. Miller III, R. S. Sutton, and P. J. Werbos, Eds.), Cambridge, MA: MIT Press, pp. 197–228.
Levin, A. U., and Narendra, K. S., 1993, Control of nonlinear dynamical systems using neural networks: Controllability and stabilization, *IEEE Trans. Neural Netw.*, 4:192–206. ◆
Levin, A. U., and Narendra, K. S., 1996, Control of nonlinear dynamical systems using neural networks: Part II. Observability, identification and control, *IEEE Trans. Neural Netw.*, 7:30–42.
Narendra, K. S., and Parthasarathy, K., 1990, Identification and control of dynamical systems using neural networks, *IEEE Trans. Neural Netw.*, 1:4–27.
Polycarpou, M. M., 1996, Stable adaptive neural control scheme for nonlinear systems, *IEEE Trans. Autom. Control*, 41:447–451.
Qin, S., Su, H., and McAvoy, T. J., 1992, Comparison of four neural net learning methods for dynamic system identification, *IEEE Trans. Neural Netw.*, 3:122–130.
Sanner, R. M., and Slotine, J.-J. E., 1992, Gaussian networks for direct adaptive control, *IEEE Trans. Neural Netw.*, 3:837–863.
Widrow, B., and Walach, E., 1996, *Adaptive Inverse Control*, Englewood Cliffs, NJ: Prentice-Hall. ◆

Imaging the Grammatical Brain

Yosef Grodzinsky

Introduction

What do students of language do? Linguists characterize linguistic knowledge; psycholinguists model the algorithms that implement this knowledge in speaking and understanding; and neurolinguists are interested in the neural mechanisms that realize these algorithms. One can imagine a research program in which these perspectives cohere, attempting to understand knowledge of language, its acquisition, processing mechanisms, and neural computation. This is the neurobiological project that attempts to characterize human language. This chapter describes attempts to reconstruct an image of language mechanisms through the analysis of lesion data and functional neuroimaging. I argue that a correct choice of the unit for functional analysis of behavior leads to a clearer image of the linguistic brain.

Innovative technologies have recently made the goal of a coherent, focused picture of the neural basis of language closer than ever before. Linguistic theory provides a sophisticated technology for the analysis of the linguistic signal; instruments that measure neural activity have become less invasive, with high resolution in both time and space; experimental ingenuity may lead to new solutions to old (and new) problems. This research enterprise must thus define brain/language relations in the form of an equation, both sides of which contain complex terms: On the one side there is linguistic behavior, described in the best theoretical vocabulary one can find,

and on the other side there are brain mechanisms, interpreted by whatever techniques neuroscience can offer. The relation between the two sides is also extremely complex, and it is here that disagreements arise. Some neurolinguists study words, some study sentences, and others investigate not linguistic units, but activities, such as speaking, listening, reading, and writing. It is quite difficult to find a unit of analysis on which a consensus (one that would hopefully reflect understanding) exists. In this respect, the study of language is unique. Compare it to the study of the visual system— an uncontroversial success story. Debates in vision exist, yet none regarding the basic unit of analysis. In low-level vision, lines are lines, angles are angles, and edges are edges—elemental parts that quite clearly play a constitutive role in forming our visual experience. Likewise, in visual object recognition, some basic units of analysis—objects organized in hierarchically structured categories—also seem consensual. In the study of language, by contrast, little is agreed upon. This weakness threatens to hinder the effort to image the neural basis of language (Neurolinguistics).

The present perspective sees linguistic capacity as critically involving the pairing of sound sequences and meanings, aided by inventories of combinatorial rules, and stores of complex objects of several types, over which these rules operate as language is practiced through its various modalities. The language faculty, in this view, inheres in a cerebrally represented knowledge base (rule system), and in algorithms that instantiate it in use. It is divided into levels of representation, reflected in language processing: a level for the identification and segmentation of speech sounds (universal phonetics), and a system that enables the concatenation of phonetic units into sequences (phonology), then into words (morphology, where word structure is computed), sentences (syntax), and meaning (lexical and compositional semantics). This rich system of knowledge is cerebrally represented, and has several important properties: At every level beyond phonetics, linguistic units are taken to be discrete; the algorithms that concatenate them do so in keeping with formal rules, some of which are recursive, hence capable of handling strings of arbitrary length; these systems are universal—shared by speakers of all the world's languages. Language-particular rules are encoded in parameters that are embedded within the universal rule system (SPEECH PROCESSING: PSYCHOLINGUISTICS).

Although not all students of language share this view, as should be evident from this handbook (see LANGUAGE PROCESSING; PAST TENSE LEARNING), there is considerable empirical evidence that supports it. This chapter thus briefly reviews some central results emanating from investigations into the brain/language juncture, which support the neural reality of linguistic rules as a constitutive element of the human language faculty. The focus here is on linguistic combinations at the sentence level; but first, some key results in two other successful areas of research are reviewed: the cerebral representation of phonological units, and of word meaning in its isolated and compositional aspects.

Combinatorial Linguistic Systems: The Neural Representation of Sound and Meaning

A central concern of linguists who investigate the phonetic/phonology interface is the nature of the basic building blocks of speech. Rules of concatenation in language typically operate on discrete units, hence the issue of discreteness is critical. Indeed, some recent results suggest that abstracts representations of discrete linguistic objects have neural reality. Experiments in magnetoencephalography (MEG) show that auditory cortex can very rapidly construct abstract representations of discrete linguistic objects that go beyond phonetics. Specifically, representations of discrete phonological categories are available already at the earliest stages of processing. Phillips et al. (2000), for example, have shown this through an "oddball paradigm." They recorded brain activity by MEG, while subjects listened passively to synthetic speech sounds, presented in a phonological and an acoustic condition. The former contrasted stimuli from an acoustic /dæ/-/tæ/ continuum, and elicited a magnetic mismatch field in a sequence of stimuli in which phonological categories occurred in a many-to-one ratio, but no acoustic many-to-one ratio was present. Phillips et al. compared these results to the acoustic condition, where the many-to-one distribution of phonological categories was removed. No such response was elicited, although the stimuli came from an acoustic continuum identical to the phonological condition. Thus, the all-or-nothing property of phonological category membership, as opposed to phonetic stimuli, was demonstrated through MEG, supporting the existence of a neural code for a phonology with discrete categories (see also NEUROLINGUISTICS).

Another issue that neurolinguists are interested in concerns the combination of meaning-bearing units. Some hints regarding this problem may come from a comparison of neural processes involved in the recognition of words in isolation versus sentential context. Posner and Pavese (1998) tried to investigate this question through a paradigm that utilized Evoked Response Potentials (ERPs). They presented sentences like "he ate his food with a____," in which the final word was either an appropriate artifact (fork), or an appropriate natural object (fingers), or an inappropriate artifact/natural object (tub/bush). In one condition, subjects were asked to decide whether the last word referred to an artifact or a natural object (word in isolation); another condition asked whether or not the last word fit the sentential context (sentence task).

Importantly, both conditions focused more on meaning than form. When ERPs obtained in the two tasks were compared, it turned out that left frontal regions were more activated in the lexical task around 120–500 msec into the task, whereas left posterior regions were more activated in the sentence task around half a second into the task. This result suggests that lexical elements are interpreted at different times and locations than sentences, and adds to the growing literature that points to the left frontal and temporal cortices as loci of lexical semantics. It refines the picture in making an initial step toward an identification of regions in which compositional semantic processes take place.

Having discussed sound and meaning in brief, we can now move on to our main topic: how and where in the brain sentences are processed.

Reconstructing the Image of Sentence Grammar: Lesion Data

The nineteenth-century "Connectionist" school, founded by Broca, Wernicke, and Lichtheim, and revived in our time by Geschwind (1979), began modern neuropsychology. This approach emphasized connections between brain regions (rather than the synaptic connections of present-day connectionism), and fortified belief in the existence of cerebral language centers. A clinically oriented approach, it emphasized patients' communicative skills, viewing language as a collection of *activities*, practiced in the service of communication: speaking, listening, reading, writing, naming, repetition, etc. The characterization of the language centers derived from this intuitive theory—each activity was associated with a cerebral locus. Activities are building blocks of the resulting theory of localization, and they are taken to be the essence of human linguistic capacity (NEUROLINGUISTICS).

Since the 1960s, psycholinguists have challenged this view, using theoretical and experimental tools borrowed from linguistics and psycholinguistics (e.g., Goodglass and Berko, 1960; Zurif and Caramazza, 1976). Not denying the relevance of activities, they focused on linguistic distinctions. Language became a structure-dependent piece of knowledge, divided into *levels of representation*. A variety of experiments in the 1970s proved this approach worthwhile, in that results indicated that the brain makes distinctions between types of linguistic information. Such results could not be couched in the standard view, and thus the centers were "redefined" (Zurif, 1980): each anatomical center was now said to contain devices used for the analysis and synthesis of linguistic objects. Roughly, Broca's region (Brodmann's Area BA 44, 45, 47, see Figure 1) was said to house syntax (for both receptive and productive language), while semantics was to reside in Wernicke's area (BA 22, 42, 39). Neuroanatomy also witnessed parallel advances. As large samples of patients became available, it became increasingly clear that language occupies larger areas than previously supposed. As analytic and experimental tools improved, the involvement of both hemispheres in aspects of linguistic activity was documented (cf. Ojemann, 1991).

Yet as findings accumulated—from different tasks, languages, stimulus types, and laboratories—contradictions within the behavioral data began to surface: In some cases, Wernicke's aphasics showed syntactic disturbances; Broca's patients, on the other hand, while failing certain tasks that probe syntactic abilities, succeeded in others. Serious doubts were cast on the new model, in which Broca's (but not Wernicke's) area supports receptive syntactic mechanisms. Attempts to reconcile the findings with the prevailing view argued that regions are organized not just by activities and

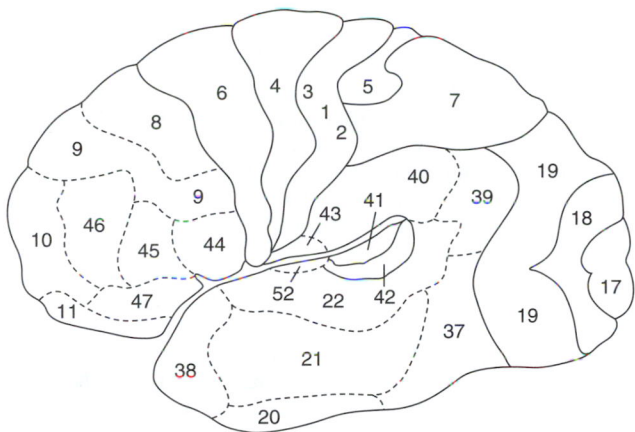

Figure 1. Brodmann's division of the left cortical surface into the areas referred to in the text as BA 22, BA 44, etc.

linguistic levels, but also by *tasks*, saying that "syntactic comprehension is compromised," and "grammaticality judgment is intact."

Upon examination, these analyses share a common thread: Although they were detailed in the description of tasks and activities, they were all rather holistic in their approach to the linguistic signal. Gross distinctions between form and meaning seem sufficient, and hence, less attention is paid to detailed structural properties of linguistic stimuli. Still, the amended neurological model of language could continue and prevail.

An exception to this description is the study of phonology and phonetics (cf. Blumstein (1994), NEUROLINGUISTICS). In these areas fine, theoretically motivated distinctions have long been used, and landmark discoveries of subtle distinctions that the brain makes among informational types have been made. Students working in other domains of language, however, were slower in making connections between matters neuropsychological and linguistic. Yet, when it turned out that the task-oriented approach was incorrect, the next move was to try and argue that the inconsistencies in results discussed previously were just apparent, due to our failure to make distinctions among linguistic types. It was argued that systems of grammatical knowledge are complex, and as such, can experience partial breakdown subsequent to focal brain damage. The next step, then, was to seek linguistic frameworks within which patterns of impairment and sparing in aphasia could be couched, and which in turn would give rise to a more finely grained theory of brain/language relations. This resulted in an investigation into the cerebral localization of *grammatical rule systems*. It was shown that despite the importance of channels through which language is practiced, the correct (in fact most telling) unit of analysis for the interpretation of lesion data is the particular rule type.

It is here that considerations pertaining to the structure of language began to matter heavily. As the most important aspect of our "mental organ for language" is its combinatorial nature, that is, the knowledge base and algorithms for the concatenation of linguistic sequences at all levels. Activities and tasks no doubt play a mediating role in linguistic communication, yet the defining characteristic of the language faculty is its being composed to rule systems. How these rule systems are instantiated in neural tissue thus seems the central question in neurolinguistics.

Thus it was shown that in the domain of language production, the brain makes fine distinctions among rule types: Broca's (but not Wernicke's) aphasics are deficient in producing Tense inflection, but intact in Agreement inflection (as shown in a wide variety of languages). Cross-linguistic studies further indicated that not

only inflection type, but also, the position of the verb in the sentence determines its appearance subsequent to a lesion in Broca's region (Friedmann, 1998). In receptive language, the distinction between transformational and nontransformational sentences, yields a big performance contrast: aphasics with lesions in Broca's region understand active sentences, subject relatives, subject questions and the like normally, yet fail on their transformational counterparts: passives, object relatives and questions, etc. This led to the claim that in receptive language, Broca's aphasics are unable to compute transformational relations. This generalization helps localize this grammatical operation in the brain (Trace-Deletion Hypothesis, TDH, cf. Grodzinsky, 2000). Furthermore, the highly selective character of this deficit has major theoretical ramifications to linguistic theory and the theory of sentence processing. A particularly compelling argument that supports the localization of transformations in Broca's region comes from cross-linguistic comparisons: Chinese, Japanese, German, Dutch, Spanish, and Hebrew have different properties, and the performance of Broca's aphasics is determined by the TDH as it interacts with the particular grammar of each language. In English, aphasics comprehend active sentences properly. Yet the results for Japanese, which has two types of actives, are different. *Taro-ga Hanako-o nagutta* (Taro hit Hanako)—Subject Object Verb], and **Hanako-o** *Taro-ga nagutta*—**Object** Subject Verb. These constructions are simple, they mean the same, and they are identical on every dimension, except in that the latter is derived transformationally, with the bolded element fronted to the left edge of the sentence. Remarkably, Broca's aphasics' comprehension splits: they handle the SOV type properly, and are at chance level on the OSV.

In Chinese, an otherwise SVO language like English, (bolded) heads of relative clauses (1a, 2a) follow the (parenthesized) relative, unlike English (1b, 2b) in which they precede it. Remarkably, this reversed order correlates perfectly with the cross-linguistic results in aphasia: subject relatives (1) are comprehended at chance in Chinese and above chance in English, whereas object relatives (2) yield the opposite pattern:

(1) a. [_ zhuei gou] de **mau** hen da   *chance*
       chase dog that cat very big
   b. **The cat** that [_ chased the dog] was very big   *above chance*
(2) a. [mau zhuei _] de **gou** hen xiao   *above chance*
       cat chased that dog very small
   b. **The dog** that [the cat chased _] was very   *chance*
       small

English and Chinese thus yield mirror-image results, which correlate with a relevant syntactic contrast between the two languages. Other intriguing cross-linguistic contrasts also exist, providing further evidence that Broca's region is critically involved in transformational analysis. Moreover, reflections of the same disruption are also found in the domain of real-time processing (Zurif, 1995). This rich database is further augmented by results regarding grammatical aspects of the mental lexicon. These are also localizable, as they appear retained in Broca's aphasia, but severely disrupted after a lesion in Wernicke's area.

In sum, over the past decade or so, a new, intriguingly complex model of grammar/brain relations has emerged: Aspects of receptive syntax—those dedicated to the computation of transformational relations—are represented in Broca's region, and to some extent in Wernicke's region; the linguistic lexicon is in the latter region, whereas other parts of receptive syntax, while clearly residing in the left hemisphere, are not localizable as of yet; in productive language, Broca's region is dedicated to extremely limited aspects of structure that pertain to the upper, leftmost end of the syntactic tree (Friedmann and Grodzinsky, 2000). Most importantly, linguistic tools appear critical for the analysis of brain/

language relations (for alternative views, see NEUROLINGUISTICS; LESIONED NETWORKS AS MODELS OF NEUROPSYCHOLOGICAL DEFICITS).

Reconstructing the Grammatical Brain: Neuroimaging

The lesion studies story may have an important lesson regarding functional neuroimaging. Early studies that used this experimental methodology grappled with many hard questions, one of which had to do with the choice of experimental materials, determined, to a large extent, by the experimenter's theoretical tastes. One would have expected neuropsychological data to play a central role in this new effort; in practice, functional imaging of language witnessed an attempt to start almost from scratch. Caught by the excitement that swept the field when neuroimaging techniques were introduced, many investigators have largely tended to dismiss aphasia data, rather than seek cross-methodological convergence. Some important mistakes were repeated as a result. Preliminary studies conducted contrastive investigations of *activities and modalities*. The first ones (Petersen et al., 1990) investigated the production versus comprehension of various linguistic stimuli in PET and then fMRI; and although they made a distinction between overt and covert sentence production, the nature of stimuli—their structure—remained unanalyzed and unspecified. No wonder, then, that anatomical overlap among studies was very limited: verb production versus comprehension, for instance, activated the cerebellum and culliculi for Petersen et al., whereas in more recent studies it was localized in the left posterior temporal lobe and the anterior insula bilaterally.

Early studies were also concerned with *cross-language comparisons*, with language once again taken as one unanalyzed whole, leading to great variation in stimuli (and subsequent anatomical variation). Thus, Mazoyer et al. (1993) conducted a PET investigation of the functional anatomy of sentence comprehension in a known (in fact, native) versus unknown language (French vs. Tamil); other authors looked at PET activations during the comprehension of active declarative sentence in spoken language, as compared to similar stimuli in sign language, finding multiple activations in the left frontal lobe, as well as in the temporal lobe bilaterally. Still others compared the fMRI activation during the comprehension of native (Japanese) versus second (English) and an unknown (Hungarian) language in the same speakers. Here, some aspects of the frontal cortex was activated bilaterally, whereas Broca's and Wernicke's regions, as well as some neighboring ones, were activated only on the left side. Similarly, the BOLD response in a comparative fMRI study of English sentences versus sentences in Mandarin Chinese resulted in bilateral activations in the inferior prefrontal cortex (BA 44, 45, 47, Figure 1), bilateral middle prefrontal cortex (BA 6, 8, 9) and secondarily in the left temporal region (BA 22, 21, 38), the left angular gyrus (BA 39), and bilateral activations in the anterior supplementary motor area (BA 8), the superior parietal region (BA 7), and in some occipital regions. So, while most of these studies demonstrated activation in the left Broca's area and around left Wernicke's area, scattered activations in many more regions—in both the left and the right hemispheres—were also recorded, thus blurring the picture, and making it much less stable than we would like it to be.

Yet, when previous neuropsychological data and linguistic considerations are taken into account, it is quite possible that activities or languages may not be the correct units of analysis for a precise characterization of brain/language relations. One possible reason for the lack of anatomical congruence among past studies, then, is that they made incorrect choices of analytic units, and as a consequence, they simply did not use appropriately minimal contrasts in their comparisons. From this perspective, a sentence in sign language is an incorrect control for a condition that contains English

sentences—it may be as inappropriate a control as a Mozart symphony would be for a test for visual object recognition. Psychologists have realized this, and as a next step, set themselves to study more finely grained distinctions. Again, following the neuropsychological tradition, some have attempted to test distinctions among *levels of linguistic description*. Yet here, too, localization has been somewhat disappointing.

Friederici and her colleagues conducted a series of studies that also contrasted syntactic with semantic variables, and sought neural correlates for it, as monitored through MEG. In one study they tried to localize syntactic processes through the measurement of magnetic response during auditory exposure to "syntactically correct" and "syntactically incorrect" sentences. They found that "early syntactic parsing processes" activated temporal regions, possibly the planum polare, as well as fronto-lateral regions. They further comment that "the contribution of the left temporal regions to the early syntactic processes seems to be larger than that of the left fronto-lateral regions." Friederici (2000) summarizes the results from PET and fMRI studies: "The posterior region of the left superior temporal gyrus and the adjacent planum temporale is specifically involved in auditory language comprehension." There is also "an involvement of left inferior frontal regions in phonetic processing," and for syntax there is "maximal activation in the left third frontal convolution . . . but additional activation in the left Wernicke's area as well as some activation in the homotopic areas in the right hemisphere." Another experiment this group conducted sought to dissociate the phonological, semantic, and syntactic subsystems. They presented active declarative sentences along with sentences with the same syntactic "frame" but with nonsense words, and with unstructured word lists and non-word lists. When sentences with real and pseudo words were compared to word and non-word lists (as a reflection of syntax), certain bilateral temporal, parietal, frontal, and subcortical areas were activated.

In a similar vein, Dapretto and Bookheimer (1999) tried to dissociate syntax from semantics through fMRI. They asked subjects to make same/different judgments on sentence pairs of two types: one involving the same sentence structure but with one different word; another involving same meaning but different sentence structure (active versus passive). For both the semantic and syntactic comparisons, they report Broca's region and its vicinity (BA 44, 45, 47) and the superior and middle temporal gyri (BA 42, 22, 21) bilaterally as the main activated area in the comparison, with some more activation on the left for the syntactic comparison (BA 44).

The reader may have noticed that here, too, the anatomical overlap between studies is not very promising. Again, Broca's and Wernicke's regions are activated, providing support to the view—originating in Broca's and Wernicke's writings—that these regions are crucial parts of the language faculty. Yet this is not enough: other regions are activated in a nonoverlapping manner, and we must try and understand what this may mean. Three interpretations are imaginable: either language is widely distributed in the brain, and moreover, linguistic representations are unstable, varying from one individual to the next in a manner that affects findings; or the available imaging technology is unreliable; or experiments do not test what they purport to test.

My own tendency is optimistic, leaning toward the third possibility: while there is clearly individual variation in the precise size, location, and structure of the language areas (cf. Amunts et al., 1999, for compelling cytoarchitectonic evidence), brains appear to be relatively stable in what they represent. A large amount of functional variation and spreading, I would argue, is a consequence of the great variation among experiments at this point, caused mainly by an insufficiently refined view of linguistic structure. The fact that "syntax," "phonology," and the like are undifferentiated is likely an important reason for the wide range of anatomical loci imputed to sentence processing. A linguistic perspective—especially one that seeks to account not just for the functional imaging data, but also the rich body of knowledge that comes from lesion studies—might make matters more uniform.

An attempt to be more detailed psycholinguistically has been made by Caplan and by Just and Carpenter. These groups have attempted to view language processing in the brain from the point of view of the putative processing difficulty of different sentence types. Just et al. (1996) looked at the comprehension of three sentence types in fMRI, and found that they all activated left and right Broca's and Wernicke's regions, yet the magnitude of the effect grew with processing difficulty. Using PET, Stromswold et al. (1996) showed differential activation in left Broca's region for differentially difficult relative clauses; and study by the same group conducted a PET study with similar materials, yet with a slightly different task, and found activations in the centromedian nucleus of the left thalamus, the medial frontal gyrus, Broca's area, and the posterior cingulate gyrus. Differential processing difficulty, used as a marker that delineates the language faculty, again results in poor anatomical overlap. The similarity in the questions posed by most of these studies suggests that discrepancies in anatomical findings may either be due to different imaging devices, or choice of tasks and materials. Still, experience with the linguistic interpretation of lesion data leaves one with a gnawing sense that systematic linguistic description of functional imaging results—and subsequent planning of linguistically motivated experiments—is somewhat lacking. In the case of complexity, the blurred picture may well be due to the fact that the linguistic complexity is not a well-defined notion, and its varying construal affects the nature of experimental materials and the analysis and interpretation of results. It is perhaps advisable to go back to studying aphasia, to try and find some hints there. The strong link between grammatical transformations and the language areas may be a good place to start, if we seek to tease particular components *within* the grammar apart from others.

When transformations are separated from complexity, and tested in fMRI, a fairly clear picture emerges: left Broca's region (BA 44, 45) and to a lesser extent, both Heschl's gyri, are most strongly involved in transformational analysis. Ben-Shachar et al. (2001) have conducted this experiment in Hebrew, searching for a T(ransformational)-effect. They used minimal pairs of equally complex sentences, except that one set contained a transformation (3a) and another did not (3b):

(3) a. I helped the nurse [that John saw __ in the living room]
     b. I told John   [that the nurse slept in the living room]

A T-effect was found in left Broca's area (BA 44, 45): A higher BOLD signal was detected for +Transformation sentences relative to −Transformation sentences (Figure 2). These results suggest a critical role for Broca's region in the analysis of transformations in the healthy brain, and converge on the available lesion data. An ROI approach detected activations in the posterior inferior frontal gyrus and the anterior insula, the posterior superior temporal sulcus and Heschl's complex. Thus, the core computational resource for Movement structures is in areas 44, 45. Auxiliary computations occur at temporal areas bilaterally.

Discussion

We have reviewed results that point to the neurological distinctness and locus of the transformational component of syntax. They also suggest that at least some of the results obtained in the fMRI and PET syntactic complexity experiments could be recast in transformational terms, which may lead to a radical reduction in the amount of variation, and to convergence of cross-linguistic and cross-

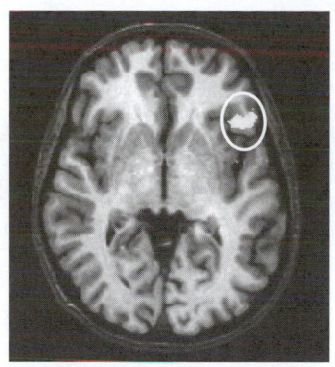

Figure 2. A statistical map associated with +T sentences. Left IFG is the most activated region (Ben-Shachar et al., 2001)

methodological data from lesions studies, as well as from PET and fMRI.

So what is the image of the linguistic brain? We are just beginning to reconstruct it. Whether the somewhat variable anatomy will ever permit precise localization is still an open question; and gross localization, after all, is just a small step toward understanding. Yet our best bet, it seems, is to take linguistic rules as the basic unit of functional analysis of the intricate relationship between language and the brain.

Road Maps: Cognitive Neuroscience; Linguistics and Speech Processing
Related Reading: Imaging the Motor Brain; Imaging the Visual Brain; Lesioned Networks as Models of Neuropsychological Deficits; Neurolinguistics

References

Amunts, K., Schleicher, A., Bürgel, U., Mohlberg, H., Uylings, H. B. M., and Zilles, K., 1999, Broca's region revisited: Cytoarchitecture and intersubject variability, *J. Comp. Neurol.*, 412:319–341. ◆

Ben-Shachar, M., Hendler, T., Kahn, I., Ben-Bashat, D., and Grodzinsky Y., 2001, Grammatical transformations activate Broca's region—An fMRI study. Presented at the Cognitive Neuroscience Society, New York.

Blumstein, S. E., 1994, The neurobiology of the sound structure of language, in *Handbook of Cognitive Neuroscience* (M. Gazzaniga, Ed.), Cambridge, MA: MIT Press.

Dapretto, M., and Bookheimer, S. Y., 1999, Form and content: dissociating syntax and semantics in sentence comprehension, *Neuron*, 24(2):427–432.

Friederici, A., 2000, The neural dynamics of language comprehension, in *Image, Language, Brain* (A. Marantz, Y. Miyashita, and W. O'Neil, Eds.), Cambridge, MA: MIT Press.

Friedmann, N., 1998, *Functional Categories in Agrammatism*, Doctoral dissertation, Tel Aviv University.

Friedmann, N., and Grodzinsky, Y., 2000, Neurolinguistic evidence for split inflection, in *The Acquisition of Syntax* (M. A. Friedemann and L. Rizzi, Eds.), London: Blackwell.

Geschwind, N., 1979, Specializations of the human brain, *Scientific American*, September, 241(3):180–199. ◆

Goodglass, H., and Berko, J., 1960, Agrammatism and inflectional morphology in English, *J. Speech Hear. Res.*, 7:257–267.

Grodzinsky, Y., 2000, The neurology of syntax: language use without Broca's area, *Behav. Brain Sci.*, 23:1–71. ◆

Just, M. A., Carpenter, P. A., Keller, T. A, Eddy, W. F., and Thulborn, K. R., 1996, Brain activation modulated by sentence comprehension, *Science*, 274:114–116.

Mazoyer, B. M., Dehaene, S., Tzourio, N., Frak, V., Murayama, N., Cohen, L., Levrier, O., Salamon, G., Syrota, A., and Mehler, J., 1993, The cortical representation of speech, *J. Cognit. Neurosci.*, 5:467–497.

Ojemann, G. A., 1991, Cortical organization of language, *J. Neurosci.*, 11:2281–2287. ◆

Petersen, S. E., Fox, P. T., Snyder, A. Z., and Raichle, M. E., 1990, Activation of extrastriate and frontal cortical areas by visual words and word-like stimuli, *Science*, 249:1041–1044.

Phillips, C., Pellathy, T., Marantz, A., Yellin, E., Wexler, K. McGinnis, M., Poeppel, D., Roberts, T., 2000, Auditory cortex accesses phonological categories: An MEG mismatch study, *J. Cognit. Neurosci.*, 12:1038–1055.

Posner, M. I., and Pavese, A., 1998, Anatomy of word and sentence meaning, *Proc. Natl. Acad. Sci. USA*, 95:899–905.

Stromswold, K., Caplan, D., Alpert, N. and Rauch, S., 1996, Localization of syntactic comprehension by positron emission tomography, *Brain Lang.*, 52:452–473.

Zurif, E. B., 1980, Language mechanisms: A neuropsychological perspective, *Am. Sci.*, 68:305–311. ◆

Zurif, E. B., 1995, Brain regions of relevance to syntactic processing, in *An Invitation to Cognitive Science*, Vol. I (L. Gleitman and M. Liberman, Eds.), 2nd ed., Cambridge, MA: MIT Press. ◆

Zurif, E. B., and Caramazza, A., 1976, Linguistic structures in aphasia: Studies in syntax and semantics, in *Studies in Neurolinguistics*, Vol. 2 (H. Whitaker and H. H. Whitaker, Eds.), New York: Academic Press.

Imaging the Motor Brain

John Darrell Van Horn

Introduction

Functional imaging of the human brain during the performance of motor tasks examines one of the most basic, as well as one of the most complex, facets of brain function. Early studies assessing regional cerebral blood flow (rCBF), using positron emission tomography (PET), and investigations of blood oxygenation effects, with functional magnetic resonance imaging (fMRI), relied on simple finger opposition tasks to produce large and robust activation patterns in the motor cortex (e.g., Figure 1). However, the results of recent motor neuroimaging studies suggest that the behavioral form and context of a movement are important determinants of functional activity within cortical motor areas and the cerebellum. Unlike the consideration of higher cognitive processes (e.g., memory, learning, vision, etc.), functional imaging of the human motor system is based on the need to understand the interaction of neurological and cognitive processes with the biomechanical characteristics of the limb (e.g., reaching, grasp, rotation, flexion, etc.). This implies a dependency on other neural systems, such as vision (see EYE-HAND COORDINATION IN REACHING MOVEMENTS), to help supply information for the purposes of learning the parameters of motor tasks. Neuroimaging evidence from such studies has accumulated, indicating that multiple neural systems and their functional interactions are needed to successfully perform motor tasks, encode relevant information for motor learning, and update behavioral performance in real time. Thus, more than in any other domain, motor neuroimaging is moving beyond the concept of localization-based modularity and into that of the functional interaction of brain systems for the construction of theories of motor function.

Accompanying the rise in functional neuroimaging as a research tool has been the increase in sophistication of task paradigms employed for probing the motor system. Investigations utilizing both PET and fMRI are now examining complex sequences of finger movements and continuously generated motor behaviors to investigate in finer detail the formation of motor programs, the role of proprioceptive mechanisms, anticipation of movement, and the generation of internal models. For fMRI, in particular, this has necessitated novel approaches to how the behavioral and functional data are collected simultaneously. Also, the mathematical and statistical modeling of these data has required the careful consideration of the temporal characteristics of both the measured blood oxygenation level dependent (BOLD) signal as well as the associated motor behavioral output. These emerging experimental frameworks represent a considerable departure from the traditional "task minus control"-style experimental designs traditionally employed for fMRI. Using such methods, researchers are rapidly gaining insight into motor processes that are hugely dynamic, shaped not only by the demands of the task paradigm itself, but also on the basis of error feedback, behavioral skill acquisition, and automaticity.

In this chapter, the following aspects of the examination of the human motor system with neuroimaging will be discussed: (1) how evidence from functional imaging studies is lending support to current constructs of motor theory concerning the development of internal models of movement, (2) how this information is being functionally integrated by the brain, (3) motor automaticity, and (4) experimental design and data modeling considerations for func-

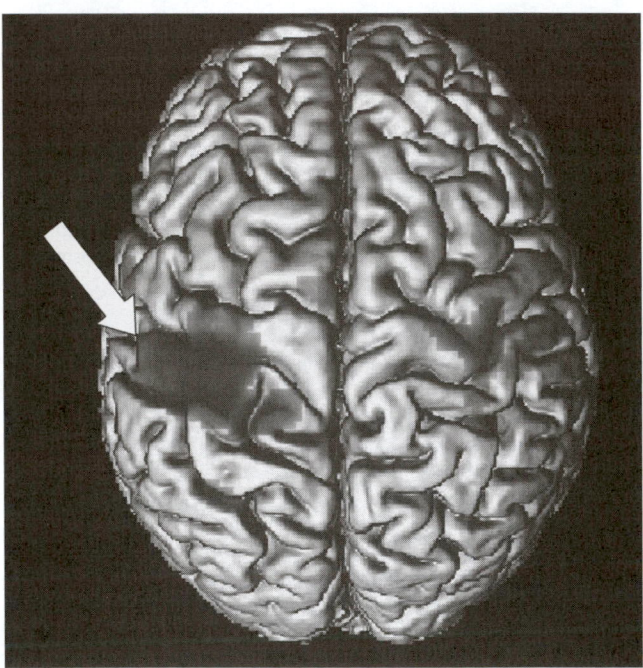

Figure 1. Block-design motor activation. A single male subject alternately rotates a small object in his dominant (right) hand or is at rest in 15-s intervals, over a 4.5-min functional (EPI) scanning session (General Electric Horizon 1.5 Tesla, TR =, 2000 ms, TE = 500 ms, FOV = 24 cm, 27 slices). Significant Student's *t*-test ($p < 0.001$) activation, overlaid on a rendering of the subject's cortex as measured via a high resolution spoiled gradient echo (SPGR) structural scan, is evident in motor and premotor regions, being most extensive contralateral (left; arrow) to the side of movement.

tional imaging of the motor system that bring to bear novel mathematical techniques and extends the scope of functional imaging experimentation.

Mapping the Formation of Internal Models

The notion of internal model formation predicting future motor requirements has emerged as a dominant concept from in vivo studies of the human brain with functional neuroimaging. Reaching, grasping, and tracking objects requires the construction and execution of an internal model of the movements needed for performing the action (Desmurget and Grafton, 2000; Imamizu et al., 2000). Neuroimaging studies of visuomotor tracking, for instance, have been particularly useful for elucidating the development of internal model formation. Several such studies have identified significant changes in regional activity in a network of regions including primary and supplementary motor cortices, basal ganglia, and cerebellum during motor tasks (Grafton, Fagg, and Arbib, 1998; Grafton, Hazeltine, and Ivry, 1998; Turner et al., 1998). Each of these brain areas is directly involved in carrying out motor movements. Turner and colleagues (1998), however, examined rCBF PET images obtained while subjects moved a handheld joystick to track the movement of a target at three different rates of sinusoidal movement. Increases in rCBF during arm movement (relative to an eye tracking only baseline condition) were seen in a distributed pattern of regions, including primary sensorimotor, dorsal and mesial premotor, and dorsal parietal cortices in the left hemisphere and, though not as prominently, the sensorimotor and superior parietal cortices in the right hemisphere. Subcortical activations were observed in left putamen, globus pallidus, and thalamus, in the right basal ganglia, and in the right anterior cerebellum. Left primary motor, left globus pallidus, and right anterior cerebellum had changes in rCBF that correlated positively with the rate of movement. A particularly unique finding was the activation of the globus pallidus with increasing movement velocity. On the other hand, studies of Parkinsonian patients (Nakamura et al., 2001) have revealed increased patterns of rCBF activity in these regions, suggesting a compensation for defective basal ganglia functioning and a failure to correct errors online. This supports the notion that the basal ganglia motor circuit may be involved preferentially in controlling or monitoring the scale and/or dynamics of limb movements needed to minimize movement error. These findings hint at interdependency between distributed brains areas needed for online correction of motor errors leading to internal movement representation.

The Emergence of Motor Automaticity

As subjects gain increased experience with motor tasks they typically display continued improvement in motor execution until those movements have become automatic. In general, motor automaticity is most likely to occur in tasks where performance errors may be readily anticipated and corrected online. Brain imaging studies have demonstrated differential changes in activity in limb motor areas during early motor skill learning, consistent with functional reorganization occurring at the level of motor output. Extensive practice and the emergence of skill automaticity resulted in decreases in the amount of activity in motor and SMA, accompanied by increases in activity in inferior parietal cortex as well as in basal ganglia. These alterations may be further modified over time presumably due to neuronal efficiency and optimization. Therefore, internal models of movements and movement automaticity are tightly linked.

On a simple level, automaticity in the motor system may be indirectly measured when contrasting performance of a motor task using the dominant and nondominant hands. Nondominant hand movements, perhaps being less automatic, appear to require greater cortical BOLD signal activity similar to complex tasks with the dominant hand, and result in greater activation of ipsilateral cortical motor areas and striatum. However, automaticity may be more rigorously examined and manipulated through the use of sensorimotor compatibility task paradigms. Experiments by Grafton, Salidis, and Willingham (2001), for example, assessed motor learning under compatible and incompatible perceptual-motor conditions to identify brain areas involved in different perceptual-motor transformations. Subjects tracked a continuously moving target that moved in a repeating sequence embedded within random movements to block sequence awareness. Psychophysical studies of behavioral transfer from incompatible (joystick and cursor moving in opposite directions) to compatible tracking established that incompatible learning was occurring with respect to target location. rCBF imaging during compatible learning identified increasing activity throughout the precentral gyrus, maximal in the arm area. Incompatible learning also led to increasing rCBF activity in the precentral gyrus, maximal in the putative frontal eye fields. When the incompatible task was switched to a compatible response and the previously learned sequence was reintroduced, there was an increase in activation of the arm region of the motor cortex. These findings indicate that learning-related increases of brain activity leading to motor automaticity are dynamic, with recruitment of multiple motor output areas, contingent on task demands.

Feedback Monitoring

The cerebellum appears to play a critical role in the coordination of movement, being essential in the processing of motor feedback (see CEREBELLUM AND MOTOR CONTROL). Miall, Reckess, and Imamizu (2001) assessed cerebellar involvement using fMRI during visually guided tracking tasks requiring varying degrees of eye-hand coordination. BOLD signal in the cerebellum indicated greater activity during independent rather than coordinated eye and hand tracking. In subsequent tasks, they observed parametric increases in cerebellar activity as eye-hand coordination increased. This demonstrates a nonmonotonic relationship of the cerebellar BOLD signal with tracking performance, showing high activity during both coordinated and independent conditions. In another example, using $H_2^{15}O$ PET, Blakemore, Frith, and Wolpert (2001) examined neural responses to parametrically varied degrees of discrepancy between the predicted and actual sensory consequences of movement. Subjects used their right hand to move a robotic arm. The motion of this robotic arm determined the position of another robotic arm, which made contact with the palm of the subject's left hand. Using this interface, computer-controlled delays were introduced between the movement of the right hand and the tactile stimulation on the left. Activity in the right lateral cerebellar cortex was positively correlated with stimulation delay. These data provide provocative evidence that the cerebellum plays a key role in signaling the sensory discrepancy between the predicted and actual sensory consequences of movements, supporting motor coordination.

Sensorimotor Integration

Sensorimotor integration is the process by which sensory input and motor output signals are combined to provide an internal estimate of the state of both the world and one's own body. Although a single perceptual and motor snapshot can provide information about the current state, computational models show that the state can be optimally estimated by an iterative process in which an internal estimate is maintained and revised by the current sensory and motor signals (see SENSORIMOTOR LEARNING). These theoretical models predict that an internal state system is, indeed, stored in the brain. Reports on patients with lesions of the superior parietal lobe have shown both sensory and motor deficits consistent with an inability to maintain such an internal representation between updates (Wolpert, Goodbody, and Husain, 1998). Such behavioral findings predict that the superior parietal lobe is critical for sensorimotor integration, by maintaining an internal representation of the body's state.

Neuroimaging studies, too, have lent support to this notion. Grafton and co-workers (1992) studied visually guided movements subjects performing visuomotor tracking tasks during PET. Tracking a moving target with the index finger showed a network of focal responses of rCBF observed in the primary motor cortex, dorsal parietal cortex, precuneate cortex, SMA, and ipsilateral anterior cerebellum relative to visual tracking alone. When the temporal complexity of the tracking task was altered by introducing a "no-go" contingency that allowed for greater time for movement preparation, there was a significant increase of rCBF in the SMA. When the spatial complexity was altered by adding a secondary target that provided directional cues for the primary target, there were additional significant increases of rCBF in bilateral dorsal parietal cortex and precuneus. Performing the tracking task with different body parts produced somatotopically distributed responses in only the motor cortex. The results of this study suggest that the SMA plays a role in the sequencing of movements and that medial and dorsal parietal cortices participate in the integration of spatial attributes during movement selection.

Measuring and Modeling the Motor System

PET and fMRI studies have provided ample evidence that activation of motor cortices and online movement error correction repeated over time result in action automaticity and sensorimotor integration. Initial attempts at movements result in widespread activation when the brain is drawing upon numerous systems to approximate the required movement, force, velocity, etc. Successive presentations of the same movements offer the motor system opportunity to tune internal model parameters on the basis of behavioral error and subsequent model updates. A process of reinforcement learning and iterative motor control optimization in this vein has been discussed extensively (see REINFORCEMENT LEARNING IN MOTOR CONTROL). During this process, as the roles of supporting brain systems appear to be no longer required, the pattern of observed activation may be altered, diminishing in extent as the model becomes more accurate, integrated, and automatic. Ultimately, only a minimal set of brain regions necessary for carrying out the needed movement indicate BOLD response activation. Therefore, areas previously involved in the tuning of internal model parameters are now free to devote their neural resources to other cognitive problems.

From a computational point of view, this process resembles that of a control optimization problem (see IDENTIFICATION AND CONTROL). Initially, the parameters governing the system are ill-defined. But through an iterative process of taking errors into account, future errors are minimized as the contribution to performance accuracy from some parameters are minimized and those of others accentuated. At which time, the minimal number of parameters have been identified that minimize overall system error in the presence of system noise (i.e., model equilibrium), thereby indicating that the model has been augmented from that of a purely causal model to that of one also having the ability to forecast the next model state and required motor output (see OPTIMIZATION PRINCIPLES IN MOTOR CONTROL). This, then, forms what is often more broadly referred to in the motor control literature as a "forward model" (Desmurget and Grafton, 2000). From signal processing, such systems may be used to predict system behavior in which the parameter estimation problem involves the identification of complex poles and zeros, along with system gain terms (see also FORECASTING). For example, a simplistic, finite impulse response (FIR) model is presented in Figure 2. This could be used to simulate the forward modeling of visuomotor task performance of the limb, in the presence of system noise, through the use of a switched connectivity between ocular and motor mechanisms.

To achieve the richness of functional imaging data necessary for such modeling purposes, greater sophistication in behavioral paradigms used in the scanning environment is needed. Such paradigms will involve an increased utilization of finely sampled behavioral measurements of motor speed, acceleration and higher derivatives. For example, behavioral paradigms such as that employed by Novak, Miller, and Houk (2000) might be studied with fMRI to measure the neural concomitants of rapid hand and joint movements. These authors attempted to identify overlapping submovements during a rotational target capture task by examining the zero crossings of subject acceleration traces and its derivatives, jerk and snap (the third and fourth derivatives, respectively). Movements without overlapping submovements had, on average, near symmetric, bell-shaped velocity profiles that were independent of speed and consistent with a theoretical minimum jerk velocity

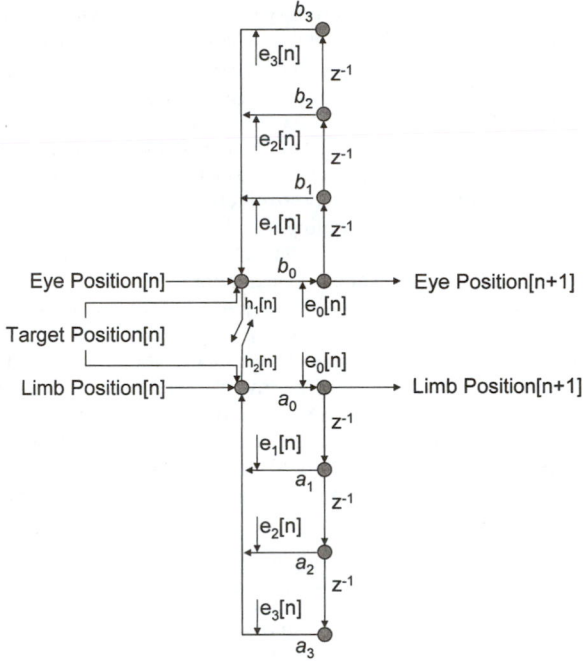

Figure 2. Visuomotor tracking may be modeled computationally using predictive FIR models. This figure shows a FIR model that incorporates separate, butterflied components for visual—and for motor—tracking, connected via a switched line tap. This permits both halves of the model to work independently, when the switch is open, or together using an appropriate cross-system transfer function (h), when the switch is closed. The current state of the limb position enters into the system, is scaled, delayed accordingly using discrete complex exponential delay terms (e.g., $\exp(-i2\pi/N) = z^{-1}$, where $i = \text{sqrt}(-1)$) and aggregated to form the output for the next time step. System error is present at each delay term, which when the parameter estimates have not reached equilibrium may dominate system output. Linear systems theory combined with methods for the analysis of functional and effective connectivity from neuroimaging data permit the construction of dynamic models of brain function in visuomotor control as well as other neural systems. Additionally, these models may be useful in the synthetic simulation of fMRI data as has been previously with PET (see SYNTHETIC FUNCTIONAL BRAIN MAPPING).

model. The authors propose a nonlinearly dampened mass-spring (second-order derivative) model of the wrist as a suitable model governing knob turning. Motor tasks paradigms like this, or ones that utilize a joystick, trackball, or other continuous input device permitting estimation of higher order derivatives, when conducted using whole brain fMRI would help in understanding what brain regions are dynamically involved in the construction of internal models and how they may relate to limb kinematics.

In pursuing this line of investigation, however, new thinking in fMRI experimental methods is needed. Unlike epoch- or event-related paradigms, the use of continuous performance fMRI holds considerable promise for investigation of the dynamic process of motor functioning (Figure 3). Most important in this neuroimaging framework is the performance of the subject in relation to maintaining positional, velocity, and acceleration accuracy rather than the presence or absence of perceptual stimuli. For example, Figure 4 shows the results of a reduced GLM model analysis containing only subject-generated tracking variables indicating significant effect involving visual areas (V1 and V2), cerebellum, primary and supplementary motor cortex with absolute target position; visual areas (V1 and V2), cuneus, and superior frontal gyrus with target velocity; and superior frontal and cingulated gyri with target ac-

celeration. Activation of these visual areas has been previously implicated in attentional networks (Friston and Buchel, 2000; see also VISUAL ATTENTION), underscoring the possible role for these components in visuomotor tracking performance. Subject positional error was significantly correlated with visual areas as well as activation in DLPFC, suggesting a role for the frontal cortex in the organization of action (see PREFRONTAL CORTEX IN TEMPORAL ORGANIZATION OF ACTION). The velocity of subject positional error was significantly correlated with activity in primary motor region, consistent with the aforementioned results of Turner and coworkers (1998). These findings clearly indicate a specific collection of dynamically involved brain regions correlating with target position, velocity, acceleration, and subject-generated variables. Continued investigations of this type can examine more closely how the variables pertaining to visuomanual tracking performance are optimized by the formation of internal models of continuous movement, for instance, over a period of several weeks.

Many cognitive and behavioral models born out of human brain imaging data are often focused on the isolated brain areas associated with statistically high blood flow or BOLD signal response, rather than analyzing the cooperative computation between multiple brain regions. By contrast, the analysis of functional connec-

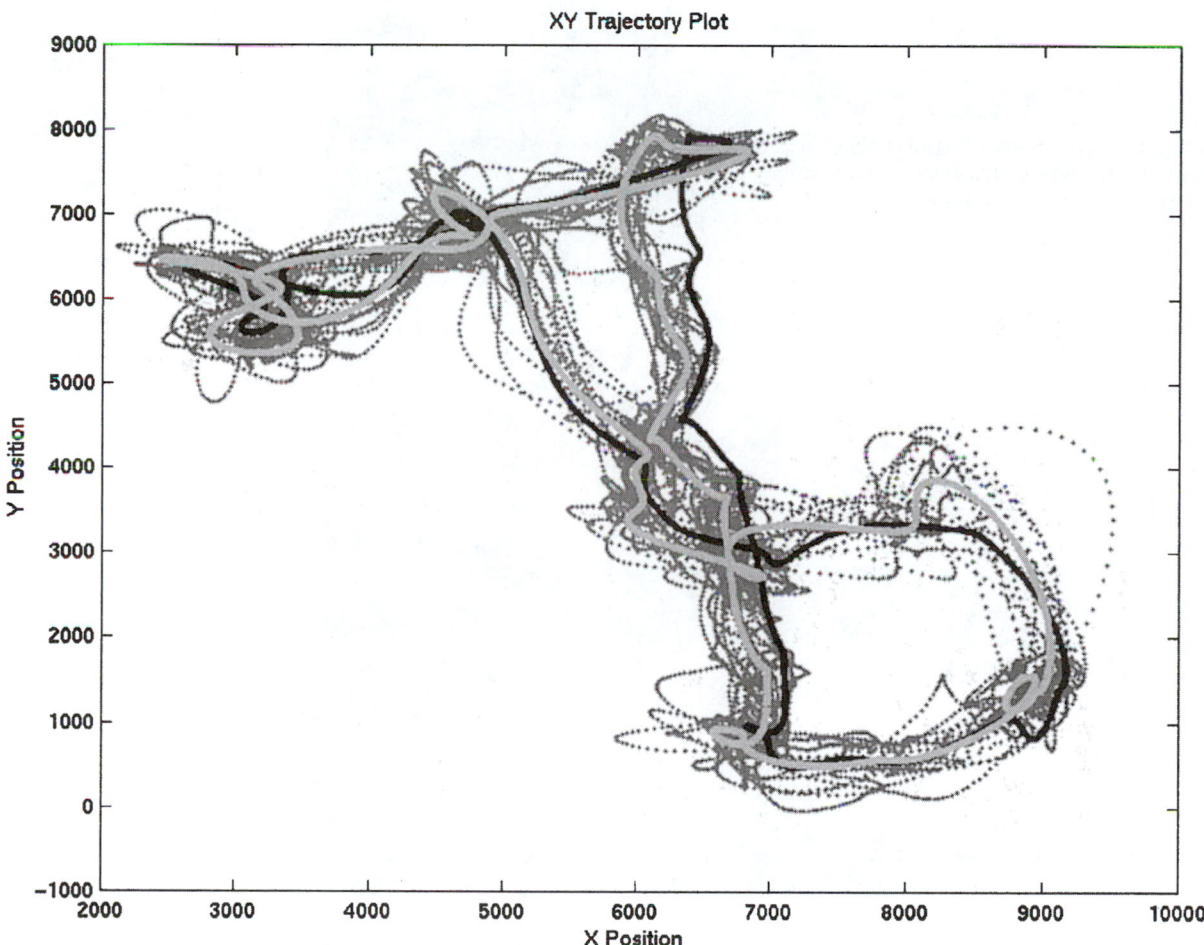

Figure 3. Visuomotor pursuit tracking performance obtained during fMRI in an example subject. The target trajectory presented here was constructed using a 32-point-based complex Fourier spectra having randomized phase-components. Subjects performed six versions of this trajectory, in which four were rotated versions of the same trajectory (0°, +90°, 180°, and −90°); one run was a repeat of the 0° rotated trajectory but in which a 10-time-point temporal lag was imposed on the joystick cursor; and, finally, a different trajectory, comprised of the same frequency magnitudes but having randomized phase relative to the other trajectories. The light gray dotted line represents 16 cycles of an example subject's performance, the black line represents the trajectory followed by the target, and the medium gray line the subject's mean pursuit trajectory taken over the 16 cycles.

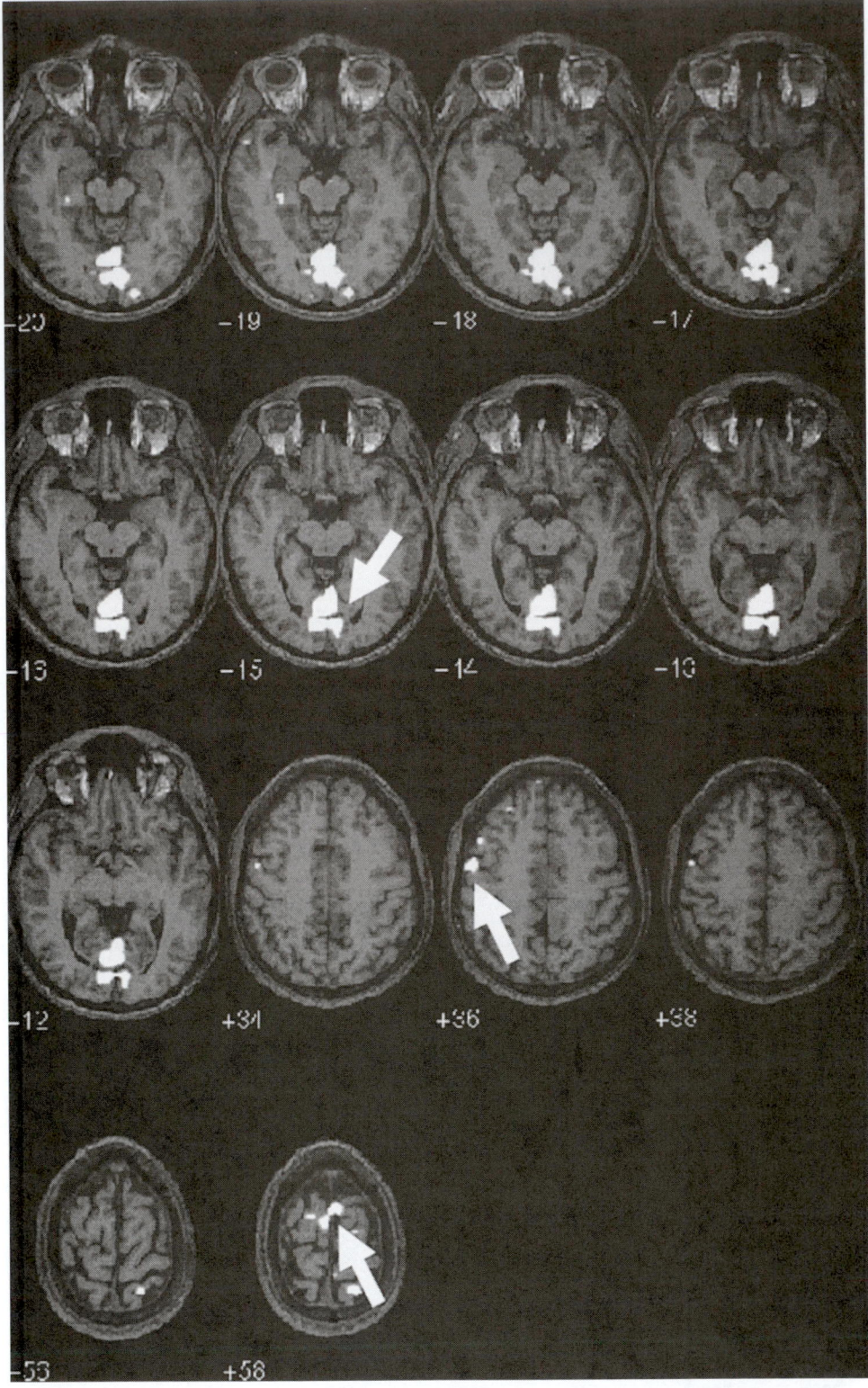

Figure 4. Talairach-space overlay plot of the regression of all continuous visuomotor tracking variables (Reduced Model F(12, 823), $p \leq 0.005$, uncorrected) for an example subject after the removal of run-to-run, linear trend, eye movement, and physiological effects. An all-plastic fiberoptic joystick was specially fabricated for use in the MRI scanner. Subject visuomotor tracking performance, eye position, heart rate, and respiration was continuously measured during collection of BOLD EPI time series (General Electric Horizon 1.5T scanner, TR = 2000 ms, TE = 500 ms, FOV = 24 cm). Scanner and task timing were synchronized using the acquisition of the MR scanner unblank TTL signal from which slice acquisition information was obtained. This information was used to sort both the subject's tracking performance data, as well as physiological monitoring and eye tracking data, into a slice-based experimental design matrix. Additional variates were included in the design matrix to account for run-to-run shifts in baseline as well as within-run linear trends. Voxels from each slice were then subjected to linear regression via the GLM and effects were tested against the Wilk's Lambda criterion and converted to F-statistics. A reduced regression model of only those variables related to subject task performance was obtained after regressing out the effects of physiological, eye tracking, and run-to-run effects. Principle effects of the performance-related variables alone are noted in visual and motor cortices (arrows) as well as in middle frontal gyrus. These results demonstrate the successful activation of principle neural systems during continuous visuomotor tracking in fMRI. Further detail on the relative roles of each of the individual performance variables is the subject of a manuscript in preparation.

tivity provides insight into the functional relationships between distributed brain areas (see COVARIANCE STRUCTURAL EQUATION MODELING). Figure 5 shows a three-dimensional representation of the pattern of inter-regional correlations between BOLD time course activity during visuomotor tracking, indicative of strong

connectivity between visual, motor, and subcortical regions. Such strong interaction between these areas would be expected from current models of internal model formation. The combination of functional connectivity modeling methods for neuroimaging may be combined with techniques for forecasting system behavior thereby

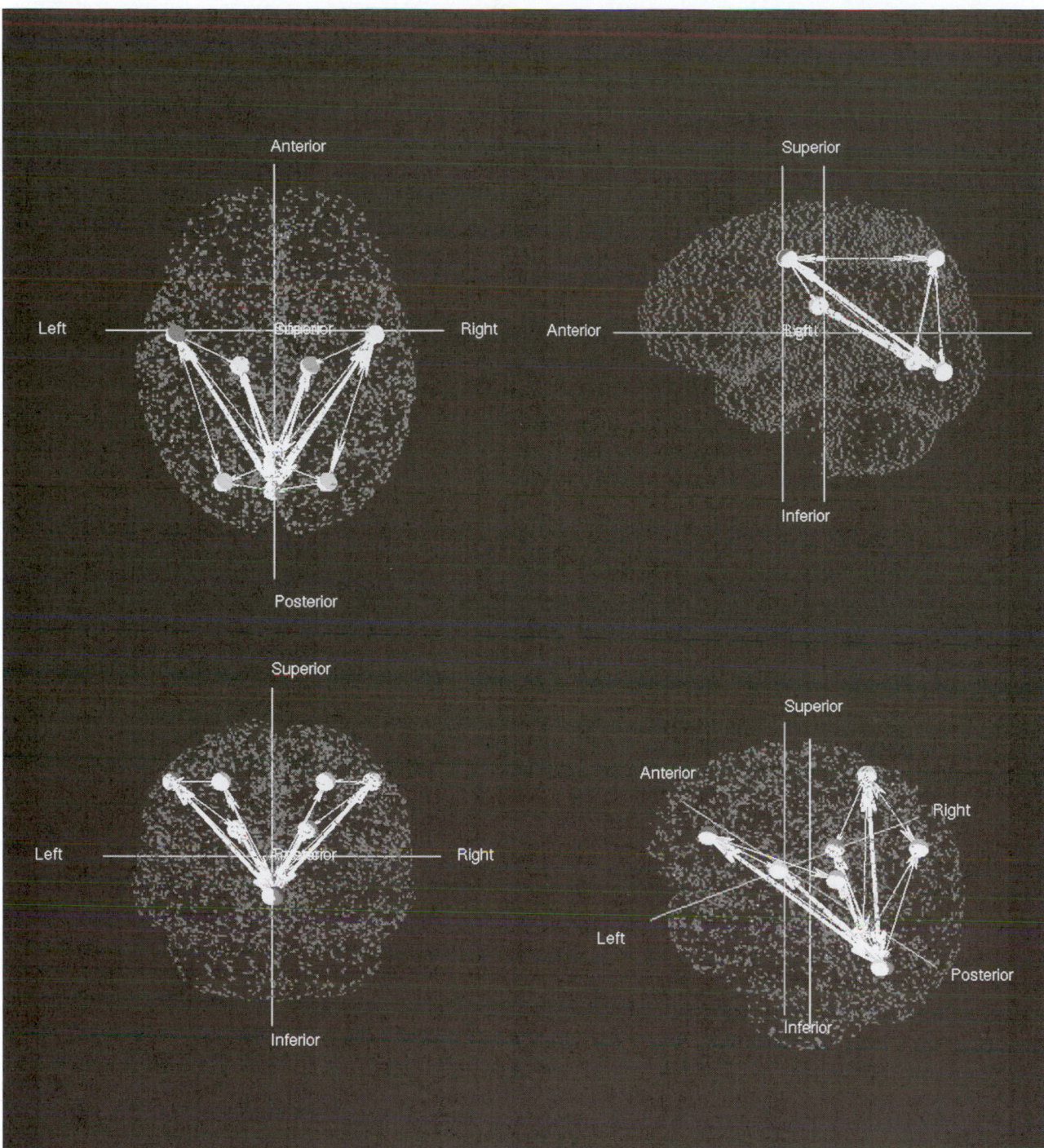

Figure 5. In this figure, multiple views (axial, sagital, coronal, and perspective) of brain regions identified during continuous visuomotor tracking are shown as spheroids in 3D standardized Talairach space. The strength of the correlation is indicated by line thickness and no connectivity is evident where a path connecting two brain regions is not present. The resulting paths indicate bidirectional paths connecting the visual regions, subcortical, parietal, and primary motor regions, with stronger correlations existing between primary visual and motor regions as well as from visual to subcortical regions. Further decomposition of the correlational structure between regions (PCA, structural equation modeling, etc.) can be used to identify the independent contributions that each connection contributes to the region-wise covariance matrix. Inclusion of causal and anticausal lag terms (e.g., as in Figure 2) increases the generality of the model giving it a temporal component similar to that of the hemodynamic lag between stimulus presentation and the BOLD response in fMRI. Moreover, in a connected network it is often useful to identify optimal routes between nodes by which to propagate information through the system. Analytical techniques are available for the assessment of the minimum-cost path (the path in which information loss is minimal or that propagation delay is smallest) between a node in a connected network to other surrounding nodes. For example, Djikstra's minimum-cost path algorithm can be employed to examine the minimum-cost path from V1 to, for instance, the primary motor cortex. The minimum cost path may be further constrained by restricting the number of other regions (nodes) through which it must pass (e.g., the number of hops).

providing an empirically based model for the temporal characteristics of inter-regional connectivity involved during tracking and online error correction. Since the resulting FIR-connectivity model includes temporal delay terms, both causal and anticausal, then feedback and feedforward connections may be estimated. The examination of how the strength of connectivity is altered between regions over time as internal models of motor behavior are formed would also be possible. The analysis of how signals are propagated through the network would identify optimum paths of information flow (see figure caption for discussion). In this manner, the responsibilities of the parietal lobe and cerebellum (Desmurget et al., 2001), as well as the role the basal ganglia (see BASAL GANGLIA), in the formation of internal models and automaticity could be assessed via this modeling process.

Conclusions

The framework of online error correction, automaticity, and integration, gaining support from in vivo functional brain imaging, is helping to explain changes in motor system activation magnitude and spatial extent often accompanying practice and increased skill. In visuomotor tracking, in particular, it is difficult to envision how such behavioral alterations can result in the absence of a predictive internal model. Empirical results from brain imaging have given credence to previously postulated theoretical models of visuomotor coordination (Gauthier et al., 1988) that anticipated such dynamic interaction between motor and visual systems. One can readily expect that the levels of sophistication for examining the domain of the motor system using neuroimaging will continue to improve. In presenting these key examples from the field of neuroimaging, it is clear that there has been and will continue to be much gained from studies imaging the motor brain.

Acknowledgments.   The author is grateful to Dr. Scott T. Grafton for his comments on earlier versions of this chapter. This work was funded by a grant from the National Science Foundation (NSF 01-41, 0121905).

Road Maps: Cognitive Neuroscience; Mammalian Motor Control
Related Reading: Hemispheric Interactions and Specialization; Imaging the Grammatical Brain; Imaging the Visual Brain; Statistical Parametric Mapping of Cortical Activity Patterns; Synthetic Functional Brain Mapping

References

Blakemore, S. J., Frith, C. D., and Wolpert, D. M., 2001, The cerebellum is involved in predicting the sensory consequences of action, *Neuroreport*, 12(9):1879–1884.

Desmurget, M., and Grafton, S., 2000, Forward modeling allows feedback control for fast reaching movements, *Trends Cogn. Sci.*, 4(11):423–431. ◆

Desmurget, M., Grea, H., Grethe, J. S., Prablanc, C., Alexander, G. E., and Grafton, S. T., 2001, Functional anatomy of nonvisual feedback loops during reaching: A positron emission tomography study, *J. Neurosci.*, 21(8):2919–2928.

Friston, K. J., and Buchel, C., 2000, Attentional modulation of effective connectivity from V2 to V5/MT in humans, *Proc. Natl. Acad. Sci. USA*, 97(13):7591–7596.

Gauthier, G. M., Vercher, J. L., Mussa-Ivaldi, F. A., and Marchetti, E., 1988, Oculo-manual tracking of visual targets: Control learning, coordination control and coordination model, *Exp. Brain Res.*, 73:127–137. ◆

Grafton, S. T., Fagg, A. H., and Arbib, M. A., 1998, Dorsal premotor cortex and conditional movement selection: A PET functional mapping study, *J. Neurophysiol.*, 79(2):1092–1097.

Grafton, S. T., Hazeltine, E., and Ivry, R. B., 1998, Abstract and effector-specific representations of motor sequences identified with PET, *J. Neurosci.*, 18(22):9420–9428. ◆

Grafton, S. T., Mazziotta, J. C., Woods, R. P., and Phelps, M. E., 1992, Human functional anatomy of visually guided finger movements, *Brain*, 115(Pt 2):565–587.

Grafton, S. T., Salidis, J., and Willingham, D. B., 2001, Motor learning of compatible and incompatible visuomotor maps, *J. Cogn. Neurosci.*, 13(2):217–231.

Imamizu, H., Miyauchi, S., Tamada, T., Sasaki, Y., Takino, R., Putz, B., Yoshioka, T., and Kawato, M., 2000, Human cerebellar activity reflecting an acquired internal model of a new tool, *Nature*, 403(6766):192–195.

Miall, R. C., Reckess, G. Z., and Imamizu, H., 2001, The cerebellum coordinates eye and hand tracking movements, *Nat. Neurosci.*, 4(6):638–644. ◆

Nakamura, T., Ghilardi, M. F., Mentis, M., Dhawan, V., Fukuda, M., Hacking, A., Moeller, J. R., Ghez, C., and Eidelberg, D., 2001, Functional networks in motor sequence learning: abnormal topographies in Parkinson's disease, *Hum. Brain. Mapp.*, 12(1):42–60.

Novak, K. E., Miller, L. E., and Houk, J. C., 2000, Kinematic properties of rapid hand movements in a knob turning task, *Exp. Brain Res.*, 132(4):419–433. ◆

Turner, R. S., Grafton, S. T., Votaw, J. R., Delong, M. R., and Hoffman, J. M., 1998, Motor subcircuits mediating the control of movement velocity: A PET study, *J. Neurophysiol.* 80(4):2162–2176. ◆

Wolpert, D. M., Goodbody, S. J., and Husain, M., 1998, Maintaining internal representations: the role of the human superior parietal lobe, *Nat. Neurosci.*, 1(6):529–533. ◆

Imaging the Visual Brain

Robert L. Savoy

Introduction

This article describes some of the progress made in functional brain imaging of visual processes and highlights the challenges and opportunities for future progress, especially in the context of testing models and theories. A few key attributes of modern brain-imaging tools are compared. A subset of the many applications to visual processing is described. The primary technology used in the selected studies is functional magnetic resonance imaging (fMRI), which is currently the dominant volumetric imaging technology for studying human brain function. But the emphasis is to describe, independent of the imaging technology, the relevance of particular experimental designs to problems in visual perception and associated issues in higher-level (i.e., necessarily top-down) processing of visual information.

The key features of modern brain-imaging tools as presented here are those features that determine the potential strengths and weaknesses of each tool when the tool is applied to problems in human brain theory. These features include current and likely future limits in spatial and temporal resolution, constraints on subject participation, and trade-offs in experimental design. Within a given imaging modality, such attributes of the various imaging tools are not independent of each other. Lesion data will be mentioned briefly, but as it is not a usable experimental tool with humans, it will not be emphasized, despite its great theoretical and historical importance.

Functional imaging tools have been applied to a wide range of problems associated with low-level and higher-level visual processing. This article will focus on retinotopy (a low-level aspect of the brain's visual architecture), visual motion perception and visual object representation (intermediate-level aspects of vision), and voluntary modulation of attention and visual imagery (higher-level processes that necessarily have top-down components). This list does not come close to covering the full range of applications to the visual system, but it emphasizes some of the areas where modeling and brain theory might be testable using current imaging tools.

Imaging Technologies

Functional imaging technologies can be divided into three categories based on the kind of physical phenomena they can measure. In one group are technologies (EEG, MEG, TMS/rTMS, intracranial electrode recordings) that measure, disrupt, or stimulate the human nervous system by interacting with the electrical properties of active neurons. In a second group are technologies (SPECT, PET, fMRI, NIRS) that measure aspects of blood flow and blood chemistry that change in response to local neural activity. The third category (DOT) may ultimately be able to respond to both aspects of human brain function. For a general overview, see Savoy (2001).

Spatial and Temporal Resolution Limits

Table 1 summarizes the approximate spatial and temporal resolutions for various brain imaging modalities. However, it should be understood that one-number summaries are highly misleading, for at least three reasons. First, the physical resolution limits of the *tool* may be different from the resolution limits implied by the biophysical phenomenon being measured. For example, MRI can collect images in a few milliseconds, and optical techniques like NIRS can collect information in microseconds, but both of these technologies, when applied to functional brain mapping, are constrained by the slower temporal resolution of the neuronally triggered hemodynamic changes. Similar statements can be made about spatial resolution. The second way in which one-number summaries can be misleading is that, for several modalities (notably fMRI), the numbers are moving targets that are changing quickly as improvements are made to the hardware and associated analysis software. Finally, there are often explicit trade-offs available when using these technologies. For example, if one is willing to spend an entire MRI session collecting one brain volume, it is possible to improve the spatial resolution. More generally, there are trade-offs between imaging time, spatial resolution, and signal-to-noise ratio in all modalities, but most dramatically in MRI.

Table 1 lists the current resolutions for typical uses of the modalities in functional brain imaging. At least one specific application is mentioned in the section on retinotopy within which substantially greater spatial resolution is achieved.

Experimental Design and Data Analysis

In addition to the trade-offs with respect to imaging hardware, there are related constraints on available experimental designs. Table 1 includes several columns related to these issues. Most important is the column associated with multiple testing of a single subject. The ability to return, again and again, to the same brain with additional tests is one of the great practical strengths of the minimally invasive technologies that do not use ionizing radiation. This attribute is likely to be of particular importance in testing theories and models in the future.

The information on temporal design types is included in the table to indicate some constraints imposed on experimental design by the various modalities. In block design tests ("BLK"), the subject performs a given task for an extended period of time (say, 1 minute) to get the brain and its associated blood flow in a given state before an image is collected. Other design types refer to the use of single trials. In spaced single trials ("SST"), the responses to individual stimulus presentations are collected and averaged together. SST designs in the domain of blood-based imaging have intertrial intervals on the order of 10–20 s; SST designs in the domain of electrical modalities have intertrial intervals that are much shorter (between 250 and 2,000 ms). Rapid single trial ("RST") designs refer to the use of stimuli that elicit overlapping hemodynamic changes, which are separated via deconvolution during data analysis. This technique is specific to fMRI. Its advantages are the more efficient use of imaging time and the more rapid presentation of stimuli to keep subjects awake and engaged in the tasks; its disadvantages are greater complexity in specifying the design and analyzing the data, as well as less sensitivity. Note that the electrical modalities actually use stimuli that are more "rapid" in the sense that they can be presented at shorter intertrial intervals, but the electrical signals thus stimulated are over much faster than the hemodynamic changes, so they are not generally overlapping, and therefore the term SST is perhaps more appropriate. Both SST and RST, collectively called *event-related designs*, involve the combining of data from different trials within a given trial type. The ultimate, in terms of experimental resolution, is the individual single trial ("IST"), in which data from each individual stimulus presentation are analyzed independently from the rest. In theory, any modality could accomplish this; in practice, only those with sufficient signal-to-noise ratio can be used this way.

Applications in Vision

Retinotopy

The first application of fMRI-based research was in the domain of the early stages of visual processing. Indeed, the very first human fMRI study involved the demonstration that a region of the brain associated with early visual processing, occipital cortex in the calcarine fissure, yielded an NMR signal that varied as flashing lights were presented (or not) to a subject.

This demonstration was exciting, but the excitement was limited, for several reasons. First, nothing new had been demonstrated about human visual cortex. Second, there were a host of technical concerns which, had they been correct, would have meant that the spatial resolution obtainable with fMRI would be seriously compromised. And finally, most of the next simple advances would not

Table 1. Critical Attributes of Current Imaging Modalities

Modality	Spatial Resolution	Temporal Resolution	Temporal Design Types				Many Sessions with Single Subject
			BLK	SST	RST	IST	
O^{15}-PET	8–12 mm	~30–60 s	√	—	—	—	No
SPECT	3–8 mm	~20 s	√	—	—	—	No
TMS, rTMS	~cm	10 s	√	√	—	—	Yes
MEG/EEG	~cm	1 ms	√	√	NA	—	Yes
NIRS	~cm	1 ms	√	√	√	√	Yes
iEEG	μm	1 ms	√	√	NA	√	No
fMRI	1–8 mm	1,000 ms	√	√	√	√	Yes

Abbreviations: BLK: block design; SST: spaced single trials; RST: rapid single trials; IST: individual single trials; PET: positron emission tomography; SPECT: single-photon emission computed tomography; TMS, rTMS: (rapid) transcranial magnetic stimulation; NIRS: near infrared spectroscopy; MEG/EEG: magneto- and electroencephalography; iEEG: intracranial EEG; fMRI: functional magnetic resonance imaging; NA: not applicable.

go beyond what we already know from (invasive) single-cell recordings in nonhuman primates.

However, the development of fMRI in the ensuing years for the study of early visual processing addressed all these concerns, and went far beyond them. First, retinopy was demonstrated for area V1 at a level of spatial resolution that exceeded any previously demonstrated with a noninvasive technique. Second, retinotopy was used to delineate multiple visual areas. Differences between the layout of human visual areas as compared with other primate species were demonstrated, and new visual areas apparently unique to humans were described.

The ability to routinely map retinotopically defined regions of the human brain has enabled progress in number of areas. In one clinically relevant application (Hadjikhani et al., 2001) the visual auras of a migraine headache were mapped for an individual subject as the headache progressed and the auras moved through different portions of the visual field. The ability to objectively observe the physiology underlying what had previously been considered to be purely subjective effects is of obvious practical consequence, especially in the context of evaluating drug treatments and other therapies. In a context perhaps more directly relevant to testing theories and models, several groups have claimed to detect ocular dominance columns in human visual cortex (Cheng, Waggoner, and Tanaka, 2001; Menon et al., 1997). This achievement uses MRI techniques that push the spatial resolution (with associated trade-offs in temporal resolution). If functional imaging of cortical columns in other brain areas is achieved (which is not a trivial extension, as the ocular dominance columns are some of the largest in cerebral cortex), the ability to test increasingly rich and detailed models will be likely.

Motion Processing and the Motion Aftereffect

One of the most robust findings in functional brain imaging is the activation of the cortical area known as V5 or MT by the visual presentation of moving stimuli. This area has been important in at least two types of studies: the popular visual illusion known as the motion aftereffect (MAE), and the documentation of changes in cortical activity in response to voluntary changes of attention.

Virtually concurrent with the earliest studies of retinotopy using fMRI, a classic psychological effect, the MAE, was seen to be associated with detectable brain activity localized to specific parts of the cortex associated with visual motion processing. When subjects looking at moving patterns reported a subjective MAE, specific brain areas—notably area MT/V5—showed increased activity. This initial finding has been extended using behavioral variants of the basic effect to demonstrate particularly tight correlation of MT activity and the subjective perception of the effect. Two studies made use of the fact that the MAE lasts longer (after adaptation) if it is not elicited by the presentation of a stationary test pattern. In one study, subjects were kept in the dark after adaptation. Activity in MT decreased when the subject was in the dark, and returned during subsequent viewing of a stationary target that elicited the subjective impression of motion. In another study, the MAE was generated in only part of the visual field, and MT activity was elicited only when the stationary target was presented to the adapted portion of the field (see Moore and Engel, 1999, for a summary). This collection of work gives some idea of the potential for hypothesis testing associated with functional brain imaging in vision.

Visual Object Representation: General Issues, and Are Faces a Special Case?

One of the most active areas of experimental research and theoretical analysis in the context of functional brain imaging of vision has to do with visual object representation. Numerous imaging and clinical reports have documented localization of cortical function associated with particular classes of visual objects. The category of human faces has received by far the most attention in this regard, but many other categories (from general classes such as living versus inanimate or tools versus animals to highly specific classes such as cows versus horses) have been studied.

One focus of the debate is the meaning of these localized activations per se. Specifically, it has been documented that, for example, the "fusiform face area" responds best to faces in a number of contexts, but the area responds (statistically significantly) to numerous other categories of objects (e.g., Ishai et al., 1999). The question of whether it is best to think of this area as somehow face specific or, alternatively, as specific to any overpracticed category is one of the heated debates in the field. Lesion data are particularly relevant here. There is the relatively rare but well-documented phenomenon of prosopagnosia (a specific impairment of the visual perception of faces), and there is the even rarer case study of an otherwise healthy subject who lost the visual face-processing area of cortex in infancy and continued to show face-specific deficits as an adult. But disentangling the specificity for faces from the possible specificity for a more general overpracticed category has not yet been achieved.

A growing number of quantitative studies are attempting to understand and utilize this cortical specificity to study visual object representation. Discriminating the brain activation responses to different categories has been refined to demonstrating varying degrees of specificity even in areas that are not the best ones for the individual categories. So, for example, it is possible to discriminate houses from scissors even when the imaging data are restricted to areas that are maximally responsive to faces (Haxby et al., 2001).

Independent of the ultimate resolution of these concerns, these cortical areas of reasonable specificity can be exploited to test longstanding questions of theoretical interest in cognitive neuroscience and brain modeling. The following two sections discuss two aspects of visual processing that are necessarily top-down phenomena: voluntary modulation of attention, and imagery. In both cases, the ability to functionally specify an a priori region of interest for analysis (based on the object- or motion-selective specificity outlined above) is crucial for tight experimental and statistical tests.

Visual Attention

Attention is an intensively studied area of cognitive psychology and has been very popular for imaging studies. There are many reviews of visual attention in the context of imaging (e.g., Kanwisher and Wojciulik, 2000). The following discussion focuses on one aspect of this area.

A classic PET study (Corbetta et al., 1990) contrasted the activation of different cortical areas depending on whether the subject needed to attend to a single attribute of the stimuli (size/shape, color, or speed of motion) or to *any* of those three attributes when performing a discrimination task. A more recent study of visual attention took advantage of the known localization of function associated with three categories (motion processing, face processing, and place/building processing) to test an explicit theoretical question of long standing in cognitive psychology and neuroscience. Both of these studies required changes in voluntary attention, with (in some cases) associated changes in behavioral performance measures. But, independent of whether there were detectable changes in behavioral performance on the associated tasks, there were detectable and statistically significant changes in the activity of specific cortical areas. By dint of clever experimental design, these changes were relevant to specific theoretical questions, as elaborated below.

One early fMRI-based study demonstrated that the use of voluntary attention (deciding whether to attend to a subset of moving dots or to a subset of stationary dots in a field of moving and stationary dots) caused detectable changes in MR signals associated with a visual motion-processing area in cortex (O'Craven et al., 1997). This study did not have an overt behavioral measure to provide external evidence that subjects were actually performing their assigned tasks. But the data were sufficiently clean and unambiguous that this study was published and gained considerable attention.

Over the ensuing years the study was replicated and extended in a number of ways by different laboratories around the world. The initial basic demonstration of attentional modulation became the starting point for more subtle experiments, experiments that were more tightly tied to behavioral measures. Importantly, both the qualitative and the quantitative measures of attentional modulation were replicated. For instance, the motion-processing area was active whenever visual movement was present, but that activity increased by about 50% when the subject was attending to the movement, in contrast to when the subject was not attending to the movement. The studies that used analogous tasks as part of their design found quantitatively similar changes.

Taking advantage of the findings that other parts of the brain showed localized activity in response to certain classes of objects (e.g., the so-called fusiform face area [FFA] and parahippocampal place area [PPA]) one study (O'Craven, Downing, and Kanwisher, 1999) addressed the question of whether there was increased processing of the irrelevant attributes of attended objects relative to unattended objects. Stimuli were designed that mixed the attributes of faces, places, and motion on each trial. The discrimination task on a given trial depended on only one of these attributes. Not surprisingly, the three relevant cortical areas (MT/V5, FFA, and PPA) each showed increased activation when the discriminating attribute (motion, faces, or places) was the relevant one for that cortical area. More interestingly, contrasting the imaging data from those trials distinguished by an irrelevant attribute of the stimulus (e.g., whether or not an image was moving in a face discrimination task) led to the demonstration of increased activity in the area responsible for that attribute (e.g., the motion-processing area in the example above), even though the presence or absence of that attribute (motion, in this example) was irrelevant to the discrimination task. This finding was interpreted as supporting models of attentional processing that had an "object-based" component: once the subject is attending to an object for whatever reasons, all attributes of the attended object are enhanced in processing, including those that are not functionally relevant at the time. Thus, brain imaging experiments are being applied to theoretical questions of longstanding interest in cognitive psychology.

Visual Imagery

There have been numerous studies of visual imagery attempting to document changes in brain activity while subjects "imagine," i.e., recreate in their minds, some approximation to the brain state elicited by the physical presentation of various visual stimuli, in the absence of those stimuli. Continuing the thread started with the studies of voluntary visual attention in the previous section, *imagery* shares the property of being necessarily a top-down phenomenon. In at least one study involving the visual imagery of familiar faces or familiar locations, the strength and functional localization of the imagined visual images were sufficient to permit a data analyst looking only at two regions of the cortex (previously localized as being particularly responsive to faces or places, respectively) to estimate, with far greater than chance accuracy, whether the subject was imagining one or the other of the two classes of stimuli *on individual stimulus presentation trials*. That is, it was not necessary

to average across a collection of trials of a given type (e.g., imagining a face) in order to be able to do the discrimination (O'Craven and Kanwisher, 2000). Studies such as this one have obvious potential for both practical applications and the testing of theoretical models of brain function.

Discussion

The present article described some of the lowest-level applications (using the regular retinotopic mapping of multiple visual areas to distinguish those areas), some of the middle-level applications (connected to functional localization associated with object and motion processing), and some of the highest, necessarily top-down applications associated with voluntary attention and imagery. Visual stimulus processing has probably been the most intensively pursued application of functional brain imaging. One reason for this popularity is the wealth of data on the primate visual system, obtained largely through invasive, single-cell recordings and lesion studies. The early dependence on connection to known primate neurophysiology is, in recent times, being turned around. Several laboratories are now developing functional MRI suites designed specifically to study nonhuman primates. The idea is to use the invasive technologies like single-cell recording, adapted for the MR environment, and get a deeper understanding of both the functional brain structures and the relationship between neural activity and hemodynamics, using methods that would be unethical in human subjects.

This article has reviewed some applications in functional brain imaging of the visual modality in which *quantitative* measures of activity were obtained. In analogy with a classic observation in experimental psychology by Paul Meehl (1967), it should be understood that increasing the statistical power of the experimental tool (whether by increasing the number of subjects or by increasing the strength and sensitivity of the imaging hardware) is generally not sufficient to distinguish interesting models of brain function and organization. The fact that brain area X shows a different level of activity in response to task 1 than in response to task 2 has been amply demonstrated for many Xs and pairs of tasks. Increasing the power of the tools will only increase the set of Xs and task pairs for which those differences become statistically significant (Savoy, 2001). Quantitative and parametric observations must be obtained to help functional brain imaging live up to its potential, specifically, the potential to create tight, quantitative tests of theory and causal models. Many experimentalists understand this challenge and the associated dilemmas, and an increasing number of studies go beyond the "boxology" sometimes disparagingly applied to functional imaging studies. Increased communication between brain theorists and functional neuroimagers can only improve the situation.

Road Map: Cognitive Neuroscience; Vision
Related Reading: Covariance Structural Equation Modeling; Statistical Parametric Mapping of Cortical Activity Patterns; Synthetic Functional Brain Mapping

References

Corbetta, M., Miezin, F. M., Dobmeyer, S., Shulman, G. L., and Petersen, S. E., 1990, Attentional modulation of neural processing of shape, color, and velocity in humans, *Science*, 248:1556–1559.

Cheng, K., Waggoner, R. A., and Tanaka, K., 2001, Human ocular dominance columns as revealed by high-field functional magnetic resonance imaging, *Neuron*, 32:359–374.

Hadjikhani, N., Sanches del Rio, M., Wu, O., Schwartz, D., Bakker, D.,

Fischl, B., Kwong, K. K., Cutrer, M. F., Rosen, B. R., Tootell, R. B. H., Sorensen, A. G., and Moskowitz, M. A., 2001, Mechanisms of migraine aura revealed by functional MRI in human visual cortex, *Proc. Natl. Acad. Sci. USA*, 98:4687–4692.

Haxby, J. V., Gobbini, M. I., Furey, M. L., Ishai, A., Schouten, J. L., and Pietrini, P., 2001, Distributed and overlapping representations of faces and objects in ventral temporal cortex, *Science*, 293:2425–2430.

Ishai, A., Ungerleider, L. G., Martin, A., Shouten, J. L., and Haxby, J. V., 1999, Distributed representation of objects in the human ventral visual pathway, *Proc. Natl. Acad. Sci. USA*, 96:9379–9384.

Kanwisher, N., and Wojciulik, E., 2000, Visual attention: Insights from brain imaging, *Nature Rev. Neurosci.*, 1:91–100. ◆

Meehl, P. E., 1967, Theory-testing in psychology and physics: A methodological paradox, *Philos. Sci.*, 34:103–115.

Menon, R. S., Ogawa, S., Strupp, J. P., and Ugurbil, K., 1997, Mapping ocular dominance columns in V1 using fMRI, *J. Neurophysiol.*, 77:2780–2797.

Moore, C., and Engel, S. A., 1999, Visual perception: Mind and brain see eye to eye, *Curr. Biol.*, 9:R74–R76.

O'Craven, K. M., Downing, P. E., and Kanwisher, N., 1999, fMRI evidence for objects as the units of attentional selection, *Nature*, 401:584–587.

O'Craven, K. M., and Kanwisher, N., 2000, Mental imagery of faces and places activates corresponding stimulus-specific brain regions, *J. Cognit. Neurosci.*, 12:1013–1023.

O'Craven, K. M., Rosen, B. R., Kwong, K. K., Treisman, A., and Savoy, R. L., 1997, Voluntary attention modulates fMRI activity in human MT/MST, *Neuron*, 18:591–598.

Savoy, R. L., 2001, History and future directions of human brain mapping and functional neuroimaging, *Acta Psychol.*, 107:9–42. ◆

Imitation

Aude G. Billard

Introduction

Imitation—the ability to recognize and reproduce others' actions—is a powerful means of learning and developing new skills. Species endowed with this capability are provided with fundamental abilities for social learning. In its most complex form, imitation provides fundamental capabilities for social cognition, such as the recognition of conspecifics, the attribution of others' intentions, and the ability to deceive and to manipulate others' states of mind.

Research on imitation builds a bridge between biology and engineering, and between the study and use of imitation. Biology seeks to better understand the cognitive and neural processes behind the different forms of animal imitation, and how these relate to the evolution of social cognition. Engineering uses studies of the biological processes of human imitation to design robot controllers and computational algorithms enabling learning and imitative skills similar in robustness and flexibility to human skills.

There are three major levels of modeling of imitation. *Theoretical modeling* derives models of the cognitive mechanisms behind imitation based on behavioral studies of humans' and other animals' imitation. *Computational modeling* builds models of the neural mechanisms, and their brain correlates, behind imitation learning in human and other animals. *Robotics modeling* designs algorithms for imitation learning, implementable in hardware systems, that allow a robot to be taught by demonstration. Next we briefly describe key findings and issues faced by each of the three levels of imitation modeling.

Theoretical Modeling

The study of animal imitation encompasses a large range of disciplines, including ethology, neuroscience, psychology, and linguistics.

For ethologists, the major issue is to define what behaviors the term *imitation* refers to and in which species these behaviors are exhibited (for reviews, see Whiten, 2000; Heyes, 2001). Animal imitation seems best described in terms of levels of complexity. Imitation (or "true" imitation) is contrasted to mimicry or copying. True imitation is the ability to replicate and, by so doing, learn skills that are not part of the animal's prior repertoire, by observation of those performed by others. Mimicry, in contrast, is the ability to replicate a behavior that is usually part of the usual animal repertoire.

Simple forms of imitation that probably require no understanding of intention or theory of mind are found in, e.g., rats and monkeys. These species' copying ability is considered to be an instance of *social facilitation*, in which the correct behavior is prompted by the social context. This simple imitative behavior relies on a form of associative learning that accepts temporal delays, imprecise timing, and incomplete cues (Heyes, 2001). In this form of imitation, the act of observing enhances learning of a skill by reducing the number of incorrect associations.

More complex forms of imitation are demonstrated by apes and dolphins. Chimpanzees and orangutans can master simple sequential, manipulatory tasks. They are capable of replicating part of the observed behavior in a different context than that in which it was observed. Dolphins can be trained to copy long sequences of body movements following human demonstration, showing an ability to map different body structures to their own (they respond to the demonstrator's movements of the legs and arms with similar movements of their tail and fins, respectively).

These more complex forms of imitation are set apart from simpler ones because they encompass the ability to reproduce *sequences* of actions and the ability to *transform* the actions so as to produce variations (subparts) of the observed behavior in the same or a different context (see, e.g., Byrne and Russon, 1998).

The ability to imitate reaches its fullest complexity in humans. Humans can imitate any actions of the body based on a variety of purposes or goals, such as the goal of reproducing the aesthetic (e.g., dance), efficiency (e.g., sport), or precision (e.g., surgery) aspect of the movement. Imitation can be *immediate* or *deferred*, depending on whether the replication occurs within a short (few minutes) or long (hours, days) time after the demonstration. It may be partial or selective (when only part of the imitative behavior is replicated), goal-directed (when only the means-end of the demonstration is perfectly reproduced), or exact (Bekkering and Prinz in Dautenhahn and Nehaniv, 2002). Imitation in humans extends to verbal and facial expression, and from there to high-level cognitive and behavioral skills. It is a fundamental means to relate socially to others, and people who are impaired in their imitative skills, such as people with autism, also show general impairment in other social skills.

For psychologists, imitation is crucial to the child's growing capacity for representation and symbolization. Meltzoff and colleagues' work contributed to redefining the developmental stages of children's imitation proposed by Piaget in *Play, Dreams and*

Imitation (see Meltzoff and Moore, 1999). In infants, immediate imitation of facial expression appears soon after birth, suggesting an "innate" kinesthetic-visual mapping.* Deferred imitation appears as early as 9 months, implying a growing capacity for internal representation of others' movements. Generalized imitation involving numerous modalities, such as vocal and verbal imitation and the ability to imitate a great variety of actions, begins around 15 to 18 months.

An important body of research in linguistics studies vocal and verbal imitation in birds, with the goal of understanding the role that hearing plays in tuning speech production and how this can relate to similar developmental processes in human infants (see Doupe and Kuhl, 1999). Young birds' songs mature in the presence of a tutor (usually the parent bird) and are species and region specific. Parrots and mynah birds are particularly intriguing because of their ability to reproduce segments of human speech.

Studies of animal imitation show that imitation results not from a single mechanism but from several cognitive mechanisms that are multimodal (audiomotor, visuokinesthetic-motor) in essence and are used for other (nonimitative) behaviors. Visuomotor imitation is better understood at this stage than is vocal imitation, as it can profit from the large body of literature on perception and production of motion. Findings from these studies directly relevant to the study of imitation are briefly summarized next.

Motion Perception

Since Johansson's landmark study in 1973, an abundance of literature has demonstrated the capacity of humans to recognize biological (especially human) motions from a limited number of cues (these studies use point-light display techniques that allow the viewer to see only one point for each moving limb) (for a review, see Dittrich, 1999). Humans can easily make out the general features of the motion, distinguishing the type of gait or the type of action, as well as specific features, such as the weight of an object being lifted or the age and sex of the walker. More important, humans are quite capable of distinguishing between biological and nonbiological motions. This ability relies on powerful visual mechanisms for quickly extracting relevant features from the kinematics of multiple-joint motion. Some of these features are the phase or relationship across limb motion, the orientation, and the speed of limb movement.

Motor Control

Although there is evidence that the brain can recognize motion from a limited number of clues, it is not yet understood which information is used to recognize and to reproduce the motion. Because of the redundancy of multiple-joint motion, the information offered in point-light display experiments is usually not sufficient to lead to a single plausible solution. It seems, therefore, that the mechanisms humans use to assist in visual reconstruction of motion rely on models of the structure of the human body and the dynamics of its possible motion.

Evidence that the central nervous system (CNS) uses models of body dynamics to direct motion also comes from purely motor control studies (see MOTOR CONTROL, BIOLOGICAL AND THEORETICAL). The idea is that, rather than relying on sensory feedback (which is too slow to reach the CNS in time for the next motor command), the CNS uses *feedforward control* to control movements; that is, it uses *inverse forward* models to predict the ex-

pected outcome of a command as well as to estimate the current position and velocity of the moving limbs.

In summary, evidence from psychophysical studies of motion perception and from motion studies suggest that, to achieve a good replication of movements from a paucity of visual cues, the brain uses models of human kinematics and dynamics of motion. Moreover, it is likely that visual and motor representation of movements bear a close relationship for the mapping to be immediate and precise. It is not yet understood how the CNS builds these representations.

Computational Modeling

The challenge faced by computational modeling is to construct a model that can account for all the instances of imitation reported in the literature. The model should provide a means of naming and distinguishing animal imitative abilities, following a list of fundamental cognitive components. Ideally, this hierarchical representation of animal imitation should follow the evolutionary tree, such that the different cognitive processes can be linked to the evolution of specific neural structures. We review next the evidence for neural structures specific to imitation.

Neural Structures Behind Visuomotor Imitation

For a long time imitation has been a topic of research primarily in the cognitive and psychological sciences; only recently has imitation become the explicit topic of a number of neuroscience studies. This new trend started with the discovery of the *mirror neuron* system (Rizzolatti et al., 1996), a neural circuit in F5 area of monkey premotor cortex that is active both when the monkey observes another monkey or a human grasping or manipulating objects and when the monkey performs the same manipulation. The mirror neuron system has been proposed as the link between visual and motor representation that is necessary to learn from the observation and imitation of others' actions. Evidence from brain imaging studies (e.g., Decety et al., 2002) suggests the existence of a similar system in humans involving predominantly Brodmann's areas 44 and 45 (Broca's areas), 40 (parietal lobe), and 21 (superior temporal sulcus).

Evidence that specific areas of the human brain contribute to imitation also comes indirectly from lesion studies. Studies of abnormal imitative behavior can be separated in two groups:

1. Patients suffering from a lack of or strong deficiency in the ability to imitate. Patients with ideomotor apraxia after parietal lesion are unable to make symbolic gestures or to act out the use of an object in response to an oral request (DeRenzi, Motti, and Nichelli, 1980). It is unclear whether ideomotor apraxia results from a deficit in motor imagery mechanisms or in motor execution. Apraxic patients are sometimes also incapable of recognizing a correctly produced gesture when given a stationary (photograph) or moving visual presentation. This suggests that the parietal lobe provides the locus of a neural network responsible for the translation of mental representation into movement production. However, the absence of systematic co-occurrence of ideomotor apraxia and impairment in gesture recognition indicates that motor imagery and motor execution remain two separate processes, even if closely interconnected.

2. Patients displaying obstinate imitation behavior, that is, a compulsive imitation behavior that cannot be stopped easily by command. Patients with frontal lobe damage sometimes display imitation behavior in which they imitate the examiner's gestures without being so instructed (Lhermite, Pillon, and Serdaru, 1986). This type of disorder supports the view that the frontal lobe modulates (mainly inhibits) a subcircuit that continually interprets vi-

---

*Unsuccessful replications of the work led to a large debate that seems now quasi-resolved, thanks to several consecutive successful replications.

sual observation of movements through the activation of motor patterns that would produce the same movements (a typical mirror neuron circuit).

Taken together, evidence from lesion studies and brain imaging suggests a major role for parietomotor connectivity as a basic circuit (possibly the mirror neuron system) behind movement imitation, and it also highlights the importance of frontoparietal connectivity in regulating this circuit.

Since its discovery, the mirror neuron system has led to a number of speculations about its role in imitation. However, evidence to support these hypotheses is still lacking. Research on the human mirror system is still in its early stage and has addressed only simple actions of the arms and hands (fingers). It remains to be shown that mirror neurons exist for driving motion of other limbs, and to understand their role in driving imitation and imitation learning of complex actions (so as to qualify as "true imitation").

Computational modeling investigates some of the possible implications of a high-level representation of movements common to both visual and motor systems (a mirror neuron system) for imitation learning. In this quest, Oztop and Arbib developed a computational model of monkey mirror neuron system (see Arbib et al., 2002, and LANGUAGE EVOLUTION: THE MIRROR SYSTEM HYPOTHESIS). The model accounts for the role of the parietal lobe and F5 area in recognition and control of grasping. In particular, it gives a description of how, through learning of performing grasps, visuomotor (from parietal lobe to F5) connectivity can be built.

At a higher level of abstraction, computational models of the neural and cognitive correlates to human imitation are developed. Demiris and Hayes's model (in Dautenhahn and Nehaniv, 2002) gives an account of the cognitive processes behind imitation, in which the motor system is either active (active imitation) or passive (passive imitation) during perception. The active imitation mode encompasses a motor imagery mechanism (a type of mirror system) in which the same motor structures used in producing motion are used during visual perception for classification and recognition of motion.

Billard's (1999) model gives a high-level, comprehensive, but simplified representation of the visuomotor pathway behind learning by imitation, from processing real video data to directing a dynamic simulation of a humanoid or an actual robot (Figure 1). The model has composite modules whose functionalities were inspired by those of specific brain regions, incorporating abstract models of the superior temporal sulcus (STS), the spinal cord, the primary motor cortex (M1), the dorsal premotor area (PMd), and the cerebellum. Each part is implemented at a connectionist level,

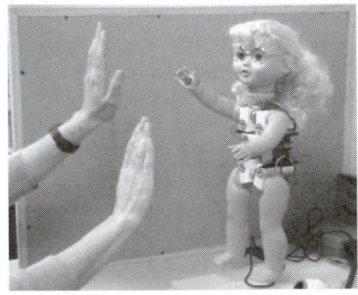

Figure 1. Robota, a minihumanoid, doll-like robot, can mirror the arm and head motion of a human demonstrator by visual tracking of the optical flow. Researchers are investigating its use as an educational toy for normal and handicapped children. (From Billard in Dautenhahn, K., and Nehaniv, C., Eds., 2002, *Imitation in Animals and Artifacts*, Cambridge, MA: MIT Press, Reproduced with permission.)

where the neuron unit is modeled as a *leaky integrator*. Neurons in the PMd module respond both to visual information (from STS) and to corresponding motor commands produced by the cerebellum. The STS-PMd-M1 interconnection is a simplified model of a mirror neuron system. The biological plausibility of the model was validated against kinematic recording of human motion (Billard, 1999) and functional magnetic resonance imaging (fMRI) data of human imitation of finger motion (Arbib et al., 2000).

Robotics Modeling

Robotics investigates the potential of imitation learning as a user-friendly means of human-robot interaction. The goal is to provide robots with the capacity for being reprogrammed in a nonexplicit fashion, that is, through demonstration. The challenge is to determine learning algorithms that are flexible across tasks and across platforms (robots).

An important issue dealt with by computational and robotic modeling is that of determining a measure of the similarity across demonstrator and imitator motions (Schaal, 1999; Dautenhahn and Nehaniv, 2002). For instance, when imitating grasping an object, one can reproduce one, a few, or all characteristics of the movements, and one can in principle reproduce (1) the goal of the movement (grasping the object with any effector following any path), (2) the goal of the movement and the correct effector (grasping the object with the correct hand), and (3) the detail of each joint movement, the motion of subsegments, and even the overall speed of movement. In each case, a different measure of the similarity between demonstrator and imitator movements must be used to account for the correctness of the reproduction. The measure should, in some cases, be qualitative, comparing the relationships across objects (which hand, which object), whereas in other cases it is quantitative, comparing the paths followed by each hand or comparing the angular trajectories of each joint.

In construction imitations of joint motion, the problem is how to transfer human motions into robot motions, insofar as humans and robots have very different dynamics. In other words, the problem is how to compute the inverse kinematics (if working in eccentric coordinates, such as when using visual tracking) or the inverse dynamics (when working in intrinsic coordinates such as when using manipulandum; see ROBOT LEARNING and ROBOT ARM CONTROL).

A large part of robotics research follows a purely engineering perspective, solving assembly task learning from observation (e.g., Friedrich et al., 1996). Typically, the demonstrator's movements are measured either as torques and joint angle displacements through the use of a manipulandum or from visual tracking. The robot is then controlled using classical planning techniques.

More recent efforts, inspired by computational modeling of human imitation, are oriented toward analyzing the underlying mechanisms of imitation in natural systems and modeling those mechanisms in artificial ones. The goal here is to design robot controllers showing similar robustness and adaptability as natural systems. Biologically inspired models of the ability to imitate have been tested in experiments in which the robot could replicate movements of the head and arms of a human (see Schaal, 1999, for a review).

Discussion

Imitation is a concept heavily debated in the biological literature. Modeling can eliminate some of the debate by defining what minimal computation is necessary for each type of imitation. Several theoretical models have been proposed to distinguish between each level of computation, e.g., by differentiating between purely associative imitation (low-level imitation) and sequential imitation (high-level imitation). Although conceptual distinctions are important, they are hard to validate through behavioral studies only. Computational models play a key role in validing these theories by offering an explicit functional description of the computation required for each level of imitation. Realistic modeling that uses real data as input (e.g., video recording of human or animal motion) and physical devices (e.g., robots) or realistic simulation as output is essential to gain a fuller understanding of the mechanisms underlying sensorimotor coordination in imitation.

At this point, there are very few computational or robotic models of imitation. However, the field is currently popular and is bound to grow rapidly within the next years. Its popularity is in part due to recent technological development in robotics that have allowed the design of humanoid robots whose joint complexity approaches that of humans. Modeling of imitation has also benefited from a recent spate of neurological data on human and monkey imitation. Computational and robotic modeling are expected to fill in the gaps between modeling of low-level information (from neurological studies) and modeling of high-level information (from behavioral studies). Modeling of imitation should lead to a better understanding of the neural mechanisms at the basis of social cognition and offer new perspectives on the evolution of animals' ability for social representation.

Road Map: Cognitive Neuroscience
Related Reading: Action Monitoring and Forward Control of Movements; Grasping Movements: Visuomotor Transformations; Language Evolution: The Mirror System Hypothesis; Motor Primitives; Reaching Movements: Implications for Computational Models; Sequence Learning

References

Arbib, M., Billard, A., Iacobonni, M., and Oztop, E., 2000, Mirror neurons, imitation and (synthetic) brain imaging, *Neural Netw.*, 13:953–973.

Billard, A., 1999, Learning motor skills by imitation: A biologically inspired robotic model, *Cybern. Syst.*, 32:155–193.
Byrne, R. W., and Russon, A. E., 1998, Learning by imitation: A hierarchical approach, *Behav. Brain Sci.*, 21:667–721.
Dautenhahn, K., and Nehaniv, C., Eds., 2002, *Imitation in Animals and Artifacts*, Cambridge, MA: MIT Press.
Doupe, A. J., and Kuhl, P. K., 1999, Birdsongs and human speech: Common themes and mechanisms, *Annu. Rev. Neurosci.*, 22:567–631. ◆
Decety, J., Chaminade, T., Grezes, J., and Meltzoff, A. N., 2002, A PET exploration of the neural mechanisms involved in reciprocal imitation, *Neuroimage*, 15:265–272.
DeRenzi, E., Motti, F., and Nichelli, P., 1980, Imitating gestures: A quantitative approach to ideomotor apraxia, *Arch. Neurol.*, 36:6–10.
Dittrich, W. H., 1999, Seeing biological motion: Is there a role for cognitive strategies? in *Lecture Notes in Artificial Intelligence* (A. Braffort et al., Eds.), Berlin: Springer-Verlag, 1739, pp. 3–22.
Friedrich, H., Munch, S., Dillmann, R., Bocionek, S., and Sassin, M., 1996, Robot Programming by demonstration (RPD): Supporting the induction by human interaction, *Machine Learn.*, 23:163–189.
Heyes, C. M., 2001, Causes and consequences of imitation, *Trends Cogn. Sci.*, 5:253–261. ◆
Lhermite, F., Pillon, B., and Serdaru, M., 1986, Human autonomy and the frontal lobes: Part I. Imitation and utilization behavior: A neuropsychological study of 75 patients, *Annu. Neurol.*, 19:326–334.
Meltzoff, A. N., and Moore, M. K., 1999, Resolving the debate about early imitation, in *Reader in Developmental Psychology* (A. Slater and D. Muir, Eds.), Oxford: Blackwell, pp. 151–155. ◆
Rizzolatti, G., Fadiga, L., Gallese, V., and Fogassi, L., 1996, Premotor cortex and the recognition of motor actions, *Cogn. Brain Res.*, 3:131–141.
Whiten, A., 2000, Primate culture and social learning, *Cogn. Sci.*, 24, 2000. ◆
Schaal, S., 1999, Is imitation learning the route to humanoid robots?, *Trends Cogn. Sci.*, 3:233–242. ◆

Independent Component Analysis

Anthony J. Bell

Introduction

Independent component analysis (ICA) is a linear transform of multivariate data designed to make the resulting random vector as statistically independent (factorial) as possible. Despite its relatively short history, it is rapidly becoming a standard technique in multivariate analysis. In signal processing it is used to attack the problem of the blind separation of sources (Haykin, 2000), for example of audio signals that have been mixed together by an unknown process. In the area of neural networks and brain theory, it is an example of an information-theoretic unsupervised learning algorithm, and one that provides one of the most compelling accounts of how early sensory processing may self-organize. That is, when an ICA network is trained on an ensemble of natural images, it learns localized oriented receptive fields (see FEATURE ANALYSIS) qualitatively similar to those found in area V1 of mammalian visual cortex (Bell and Sejnowski, 1997). Finally, in the increasingly important area of analyzing multivariate brain data (multielectrode recordings, electroencephalography, functional magnetic resonance imaging), ICA has been used to pull recordings apart into components of interest to researchers attempting to understand task-related spatial and temporal brain dynamics (Jung et al., 2000; BRAIN SIGNAL ANALYSIS).

Thus we have the pleasingly ironic situation in which the same neural network algorithm is being used both as an explanation of brain properties and as a method of probing the brain.

The idea is as follows. We are given an N-dimensional random vector, $\mathbf{x}$, which could be the instantaneous output of N microphones, N time points of an audio signal, N pixels of an image, the output of N electrodes that record brain potentials, or any other multidimensional signal. Typically there will be many correlations between the elements of the vector $\mathbf{x}$. ICA, like PRINCIPAL COMPONENT ANALYSIS (PCA) (q.v.), is a method of removing those correlations by multiplying the data by a matrix, as follows:

$$\mathbf{u} = \mathbf{Wx} \qquad (1)$$

(Here, we imagine the data are zero-mean; see the next section for details on preprocessing.) But whereas PCA merely uses second-order statistics (the covariance matrix), ICA uses statistics of all orders. PCA attempts to decorrelate the outputs (using an orthogonal matrix $\mathbf{W}$), while ICA attempts to make the outputs statistically independent, and places no constraints on the matrix $\mathbf{W}$. Statistical independence means the joint probability density function (p.d.f.) of the output *factorizes*:

$$p(\mathbf{u}) = \prod_{i=1}^{N} p_i(u_i) \qquad (2)$$

while decorrelation means only that $\langle \mathbf{u}\mathbf{u}^T \rangle$, the covariance matrix of $\mathbf{u}$, is diagonal ($\langle \cdot \rangle$ means average).

Another way to think of the transform in Equation 1 is as follows:

$$\mathbf{x} = \mathbf{W}^{-1}\mathbf{u} \qquad (3)$$

In this, the data are formed by linear superposition of *basis functions* (columns of $\mathbf{W}^{-1}$), each of which is activated by an independent component, u_i. We call the rows of $\mathbf{W}$ *filters* because they extract the independent components. In orthogonal transforms such as PCA, the Fourier transform, and many wavelet transforms, the basis functions and filters are the same (because $\mathbf{W}^T = \mathbf{W}^{-1}$), but in ICA they are different.

The usefulness of a nonorthogonal transform sensitive to higher-order statistics can be seen in Figure 1. Here we plot PCA and ICA basis functions (axes) for a two-dimensional data distribution. Clearly, the ICA axes capture the structure of the data much better. Although this data distribution may look strange, it is actually very common in natural data, much more common than those who like to model data with Gaussians, or mixtures of Gaussians, might suppose. It comes from the nonorthogonal "mixing together" of

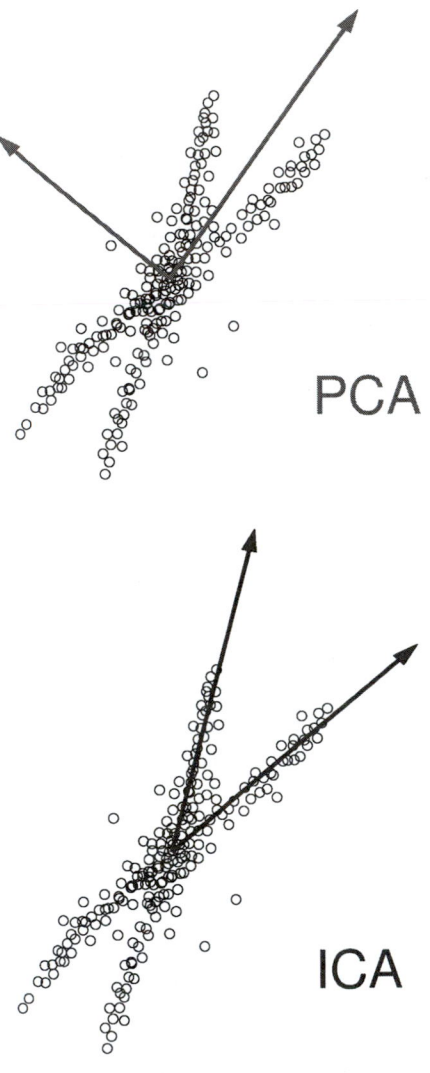

PCA

ICA

Figure 1. The difference between PCA and ICA on a nonorthogonal mixture of two distributions that are independent and highly sparse (peaky with long tails). An example of a sparse distribution is the Laplacian $p(x) \propto e^{1-|x|}$. PCA, looking for orthogonal axes that are ranked in terms of maximum variance, completely misses the structure of the data. Although these distributions look strange, they are very common in natural data. (Courtesy of T.-P. Jung.)

highly sparse independent components, where by *sparse* we typically mean much peakier than a Gaussian, with longer tails. A more technical term for sparse is super-Gaussian. The ICA algorithm we will describe is ideally suited for extracting these sparse independent components.

Before describing the algorithm, we make some remarks regarding the origin of the various algorithms and the relations between them, with pointers to tutorial literature. This is necessary for a balanced treatment, as there is no one ICA algorithm.

The ICA problem was introduced by Herault and Jutten (1986). The results of their algorithm were poorly understood and led to Comon's 1994 paper defining the problem, and to his solution using fourth-order statistics. Much work took place in this period in the French signal processing community, including the maximum likelihood approach (Pham, Garrat, and Jutten, 1992), which subsequently formed the basis of Cardoso and Laheld's (1996) EASI method. These methods are very close to the Infomax approach (Bell and Sejnowski, 1995) so we will refer to this algorithm as Infomax/ML-ICA. Cichocki, Unbehauen, and Rummert (1994) had proposed an algorithm that motivated Amari (1997) and colleagues to show that its success was due to its relation to a "natural gradient" modification of the Infomax/ML-ICA gradient. This modification greatly simplified the algorithm, and made convergence faster and more stable.

This algorithm, which we might, rather clumsily, call NatGrad-Infomax/ML-ICA, is thus derived from multiple authors and is the most widely used adaptive, or on-line (i.e., stochastic gradient), method for ICA. It is also the most neural-network-like. It is the one we will describe in the body of this article, at the risk of underrepresenting other approaches. Useful batch algorithms also exist, such as Hyvärinen's FastICA and many cumulant-based techniques.

Helpful review papers comparing the different algorithms are Lee et al. (1998) and Hyvärinen (1999). The edited collection of Haykin (2000) contains excellent survey papers from many of the authors mentioned above, and the edited collection of Girolami (2000) contains more recent theoretical work and examples of many applications. There have been two international workshops on the topic (ICA 1999 and 2000), the proceedings of which contain much additional material.

An Algorithm for ICA

This section provides enough information for the reader to implement ICA. To follow the full derivations, readers will have to consult the original sources. There is only space here to highlight the mathematics.

Preprocessing

To start with, the linear transform of Equation 1 should actually be an *affine* transform: $\mathbf{u} = \mathbf{W}\mathbf{x} + \mathbf{w}$, where $\mathbf{w}$ is an $N \times 1$ "bias" vector that centers the data on the origin. But if we assume the independent component p.d.f.s, $p_i(u_i)$, are roughly symmetric, then it is simpler to make the data zero-mean beforehand. An additional preprocessing step, one that speeds convergence, is to "sphere" the data beforehand, that is, to diagonalize its covariance matrix. These preprocessing steps are achieved as follows:

$$\mathbf{x} \leftarrow 2\langle \mathbf{x}\mathbf{x}^T \rangle^{-1/2}(\mathbf{x} - \langle \mathbf{x} \rangle) \qquad (4)$$

by which we mean that we subtract the mean of the data, then multiply by twice the inverse square root of its covariance matrix. This yields a decorrelated data ensemble whose covariance matrix satisfies $\langle \mathbf{x}\mathbf{x}^T \rangle = 4\mathbf{I}$, where $\mathbf{I}$ is the identity matrix. This is a useful starting point for further training with the *logistic*-ICA algorithm, which we will describe below. Note that this sphering method is not PCA. It is another decorrelation method called zero-phase whitening, which we have empirically found to be a better starting point for training than PCA-style decorrelation. In fact, there are many decorrelating, or second-order independent transforms, and extra constraints are needed to choose one of them. Zero-phase whitening constrains the matrix **W** to be symmetric, while PCA constrains it to be orthogonal. ICA, also a decorrelation technique, but without any constraints on **W**, finds its constraints in the higher-order statistics of the data.

Natural-Gradient Infomax/ML ICA

Most neural network algorithms have an objective function. ICA is no different. Its objective is to minimize the *redundancy* between the outputs. This is a generalization of the mutual information and is written as follows:

$$I(\mathbf{u}) = \int p(\mathbf{u}) \log \frac{p(\mathbf{u})}{\prod\limits_{i=1}^{N} p_i(u_i)} \, d\mathbf{u} \tag{5}$$

It is easily verified that this redundancy measure has the value of 0 when the p.d.f. $p(\mathbf{u})$ factorizes as in Equation 2.

This is actually a difficult function to minimize directly. The insight that led to the Infomax-ICA algorithm was that $I(\mathbf{u})$ is related to the joint entropy, $H(\mathbf{g}(\mathbf{u}))$, of the outputs passed through a set of sigmoidal nonlinear functions, **g**. The relation is as follows:

$$I(\mathbf{u}) = -H(\mathbf{g}(\mathbf{u})) + E\left[\sum_i \log \frac{|g_i'(u_i)|}{p_i(u_i)} \right] \tag{6}$$

Thus, if the absolute values of the slopes of the sigmoid functions, $|g_i'(u_i)|$, are the same as the independent component p.d.f.s, $p_i(u_i)$, then Infomax (maximizing the joint entropy of the $\mathbf{g}(\mathbf{u})$ vector) will be the same as ICA (minimizing the redundancy in the **u**-vector). The principle of matching the g_i's to the p_is is illustrated in Figure 2, where a single Infomax unit attempts to match an input Gaussian

distribution to a logistic sigmoid unit, for which

$$g(u) = \frac{1}{1 + e^{-u}} \tag{7}$$

The match cannot be perfect, but it does approach the maximum entropy p.d.f. for a distribution bounded between 0 and 1—in other words, the unit distribution—and this is done by maximizing the expected log slope, $E[\log|g'(wx)|]$. The generalization of this idea to N dimensions leads to maximizing the expected log determinant of the Jacobian matrix $[\partial g_i(u_i)/\partial x_j]_{ij}$. This optimization attempts to map the input vectors uniformly into the unit N-cube (assuming that the g-functions are still 0–1 bounded). Intuitively, we can see the following: If our outputs are spread evenly in a cube, then telling you the value along one axis does not tell you anything about the values along the other axes. This is the intuition behind statistical independence.

To cut a long story short, the exact stochastic gradient descent algorithm that maximizes $H(\mathbf{g}(\mathbf{u}))$ is:

$$\Delta\mathbf{W} \propto \mathbf{W}^{-T} + \mathbf{f}(\mathbf{u})\mathbf{x}^T \tag{8}$$

where $-T$ denotes inverse transpose, and the vector function, **f**, has elements

$$f_i(u_i) = \frac{\partial}{\partial u_i} \ln g_i'(u_i) \tag{9}$$

When $g_i'(u_i) = p_i(u_i)$ for all i, then, according to Equation 6, we have an exact ICA algorithm.

This leaves us with the tricky problem. Either we have to estimate the functions **g** on-line during training or we have to hope that the final term in Equation 6 does not interfere with Infomax performing ICA. This is one occasion where hoping actually works, because of the following *robustness conjecture: Any super-Gaussian prior,* $p_i(u_i)$, *will suffice to extract super-Gaussian in-*

(a)

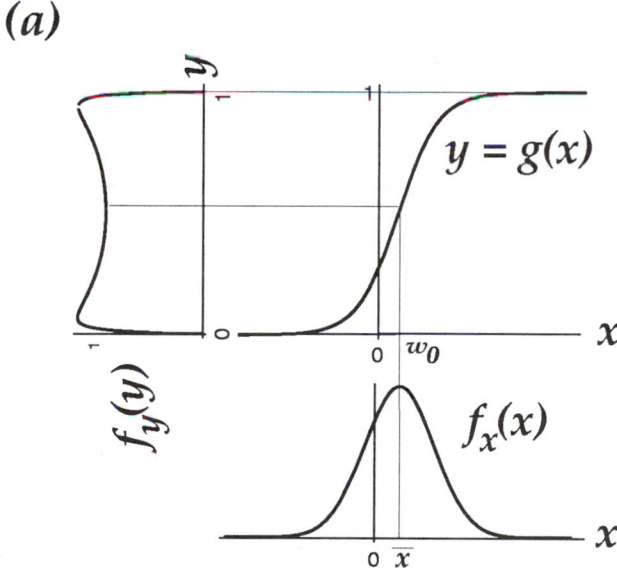

(b)

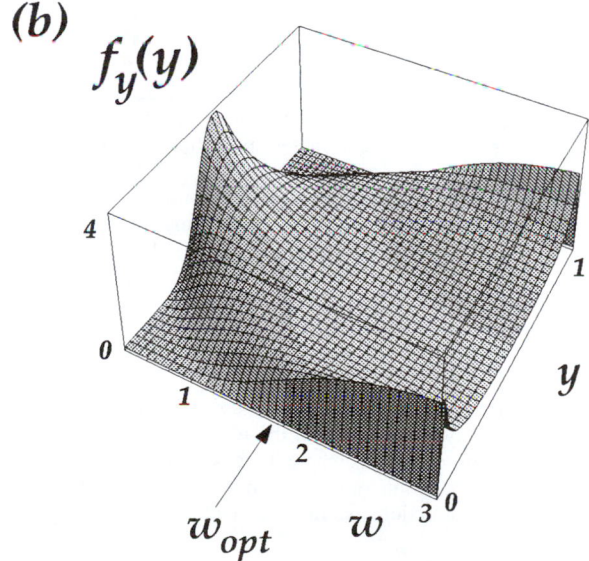

Figure 2. Optimal information flow in sigmoidal neurons. *A*, Input *x*, having probability density function $f_x(x)$ (note: this is $p(x)$ in the text), in this case a Gaussian, is passed through a nonlinear function $g(x)$. The information in the resulting density, $f_y(y)$, depends on matching the mean and variance of *x* to the threshold, w_0, and slope, *w*, of $g(x)$ (Nicol Schraudolph, personal communication). *B*, $f_y(y)$ is plotted for different values of the weight *w*. The optimal weight, w_{opt}, transmits most information. (From Bell, A. J., and Sejnowski, T. J., 1995, An information maximization approach to blind separation and blind deconvolution, *Neural Computat.*, 7:1129–1159. Reproduced with permission.)

dependent components. Any sub-Gaussian prior will suffice to extract sub-Gaussian independent components. Super-Gaussian means peakier than Gaussian, sometimes called *sparse*, and usually signifying positive kurtosis. There are no solid proofs yet of this conjecture; it is more something that has been empirically observed, but it leads to generally successful "extended ICA" algorithms (see Lee et al., 1998) that do on-line switching of the priors, $\hat{p}_i(u_i)$, between super- and sub-Gaussian functions. In practice, because of this robustness, this switching may be all the estimation we need to do. This is also the insight behind "negentropy" approaches to ICA, which maximize the distance of the $p_i(u_i)$ from Gaussian, as described in Hyvärinen (1999) and Lee et al. (1998).

For most natural data (images, sounds, etc.), the independent component p.d.f.s are all super-Gaussian, and many good results can be achieved with what is called logistic ICA, in which our super-Gaussian prior is the slope, $g'(u_i)$, of the common logistic sigmoid function (Equation 7) so often used in neural networks. For this choice of g, the function f in Equation 8 evaluates as $f(u) = 1 - 2g(u)$.

The Infomax-ICA algorithm is almost identical to the maximum likelihood approach (Pham et al., 1992). In maximum likelihood density estimation, we maximize a parameterized estimate of the log of the p.d.f. of the input, $\log\hat{p}(\mathbf{x}|\mathbf{W}, \mathbf{g})$. A simple argument shows that the determinant of the Jacobian matrix, $\det [\partial g_i(u_i)/\partial x_j]_{ij}$, is exactly such a density estimate (for much the same reason that $|g'_i(u_i)|$ is a density estimate for $p_i(u_i)$ in Equation 6). Infomax maximizes this log likelihood, and therefore inherits the useful properties of maximum likelihood methods, while preserving an information-theoretic perspective on the problem.

The final twist in the Infomax/maximum likelihood ICA algorithm comes from Amari and colleagues (Amari, 1997). They observed that a simpler learning rule with much faster and more stable convergence was obtained by multiplying the Infomax gradient of Equation 8 by $\mathbf{W}^T\mathbf{W}$ to obtain the following much simpler rule:

$$\Delta\mathbf{W}_{\text{NatGrad}} = (\Delta\mathbf{W})\mathbf{W}^T\mathbf{W} \propto (\mathbf{I} + \mathbf{f}(\mathbf{u})\mathbf{u}^T)\mathbf{W} \qquad (10)$$

Since $\mathbf{W}^T\mathbf{W}$ is positive definite, it does not change the minima and maxima of the optimization, it just scales the gradient. As luck would have it, it scales the gradient in an optimal fashion, which may be explained by an appeal to information geometry (Amari, 1997) or to equivariance: the gradient vector local to $\mathbf{W}$ is normalized so that it always behaves as it does when $\mathbf{W}$ is close to $\mathbf{I}$. For explanations, see the relevant chapters in Haykin (2000).

Both interpretations reflect the fact that the parameter space of $\mathbf{W}$ is not truly Euclidean, since its axes are entries of a matrix. Technically speaking, the parameter space has the structure of a Lie group.

Equation 10 can be clearly seen to be a nonlinear decorrelation rule, stabilizing when $\langle -\mathbf{f}(\mathbf{u})\mathbf{u}^T \rangle = \mathbf{I}$ (the minus sign is there because the $\mathbf{f}$ functions are typically decreasing). The Taylor series expansion of the $\mathbf{f}$ functions provide information about higher-order correlations necessary to perform the ICA task.

Applications

The blind source separation problem in signal processing has often been considered synonymous with the ICA problem, but ICA can be applied in many situations where there is no clear notion of what constitutes a source. Some of the most interesting results have been achieved in such situations. Here we consider a few.

ICA on Natural Images

From the point of view of computer vision and computational neuroscience, perhaps the most interesting result was the ICA basis vectors obtained for a data set of small image patches drawn from natural images (Bell and Sejnowski, 1997). These basis vectors

consisted of oriented, localized, contrast-sensitive functions, sometimes refered to as edges (though an edge is really something to do with object boundaries).

Figure 3 shows a selection of basis functions (columns of $\mathbf{W}$) and filters (rows of $\mathbf{W}$) obtained from training on 18×18 patches.

The reason why this is interesting is that both the classic experiments of Hubel and Wiesel on orientation-selective neurons in visual cortex and several decades of theorizing about feature detection in vision have left open a question most succinctly phrased by Horace Barlow: "Why do we have edge detectors?" In other words, were there any coding principles that could have predicted the formation of localized, oriented receptive fields?

Barlow was the first to propose that our visual cortical feature detectors might be the end result of a *redundancy reduction* process, in which the activation of each feature detector is supposed to be as statistically independent from the others as possible. Algorithms based on second-order statistics had failed to give clear, robust local filters. In particular, the principal components of natural images are Fourier filters ranked in frequency, quite unlike oriented localized filters.

Several authors proposed projection pursuit-style approaches, culminating in Olshausen and Field's (1997) demonstration of the self-organization of local, oriented receptive fields using a sparseness criterion.

By identifying sparseness with super-Gaussianity (which Olshausen and Field implicitly did), we can readily see why an Infomax/ICA net with the logistic nonlinearity for its $g_i(u_i)$s would produce the filters that produced the sparsest activation distributions when passed over the images. These distributions, furthest from Gaussian on the super-Gaussian side, were the most likely to be as statistically independent as possible, through the central limit theorem argument that any mixture of two independent distributions produces a distribution that is closer to Gaussian. As stated before, it is remarkable that none of the independent components of natural images are sub-Gaussian. This has been verified by using the extended ICA algorithm.

The assumption implicit in both approaches has been that the first layer of visual processing should attempt to invert the simplest possible image formation process, in which the image is formed, just as in Equation 3, by linear superposition of basis vectors (columns of $\mathbf{W}^{-1}$), each activated by independent (or sparse) causes, u_i.

Impressive results have been obtained by van Hateren and Ruderman (1998) on the *basis movies* of moving images. This 1,728-dimensional transform (viewable at http://hlab.phys.rug.nl/demos/ica) is one of the largest ICA applications to date. The resulting spatiotemporal bases are localized, oriented, and moving perpendicular to their orientation direction, just as in monkey visual cortex. And significantly, there are many more with the much lower spatial frequency required to match the profile of monkey visual receptive fields. This helps to answer the complaint that the ICA bases of natural images were clustered around high-frequency (sharp) contrast filters.

Biomedical Applications

This section reports briefly on the work of S. Makeig, T.-P. Jung, M. McKeown, and their colleagues (see Jung et al., 2000, and BRAIN SIGNAL ANALYSIS).

Electroencephalographic (EEG) data are a measure of the brain's electric fields, which are linearly mixed by volume conduction at scalp electrodes with negligible time delays and thus are perfect for ICA analysis. If there were 14 electrical dipoles in the brain, each with independently fluctuating charges, and 14 noiseless electrodes on the scalp, then the dipole signals could be perfectly recovered by ICA. This is, of course, not the case. But the results are interesting nonetheless.

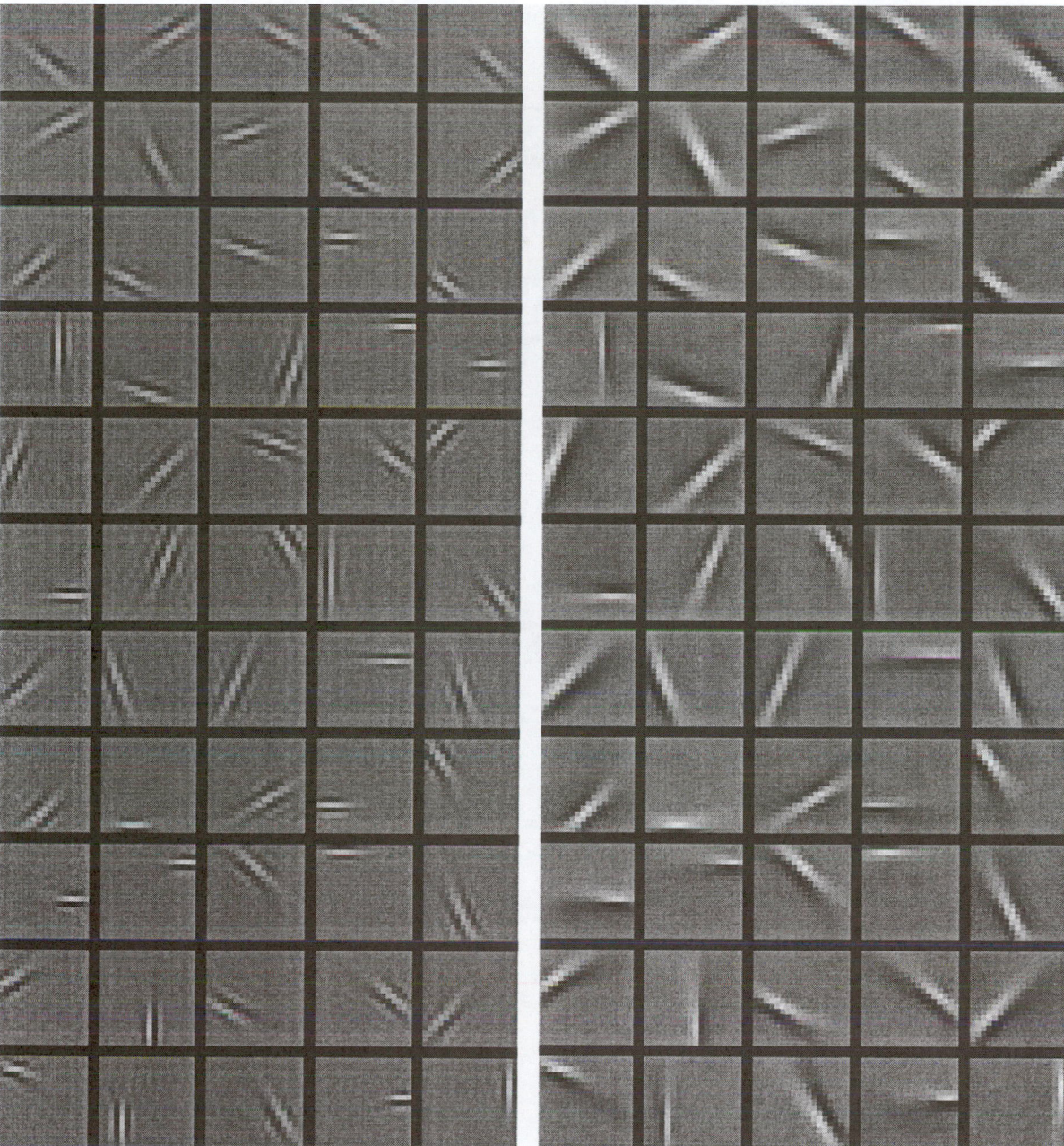

Figure 3. A selection of the 324 independent basis functions (left) and filters (right) obtained by training on 18 × 18 patches drawn from natural images. The results were obtained by van Hateren and van der Schaaf using Hyvärinen's (1999) FastICA method and are similar to those found using Bell and Sejnowski's (1997) Infomax/ML-ICA. (From van Hateren, J. H., and vander Schaaf, *Proc. R. Soc. Lond. B*, 265:359–366. Reprinted with permission.)

As well as decomposing correlated alpha wave activity across electrodes into prominent rhythms in different components with different time courses, many ICA outputs are easy to identify with artifacts known to contaminate brainwave data. In Figure 4, five of these are displayed, corresponding to eye blinks, localized scalp muscle movements, 60-Hz electrical line noise, heartbeat, and a horizontal eye movement. Both their time courses and their scalp maps help support these interpretations. The EEG data can then be cleansed of these artifacts, by zeroing the columns in $\mathbf{W}^{-1}$ corresponding to the artifacts and reconstructing the data using Equation 3.

Another kind of brain recording, functional magnetic resonance imaging (fMRI), monitors humans during the performance of psychomotor tasks and produces a three-dimensional picture of their brain activity with a spatial resolution of about 5 mm^2 and a temporal resolution of about 2 s. The subject is typically asked to alternate between performing a given task and a control task, so that researchers can identify which regions of the brain are differently activated. One of the independent components of the fMRI data studied by McKeown and colleagues was a pattern of spatial brain activation that was activated with a square-wave time course exactly corresponding to the execution of the task. This was true

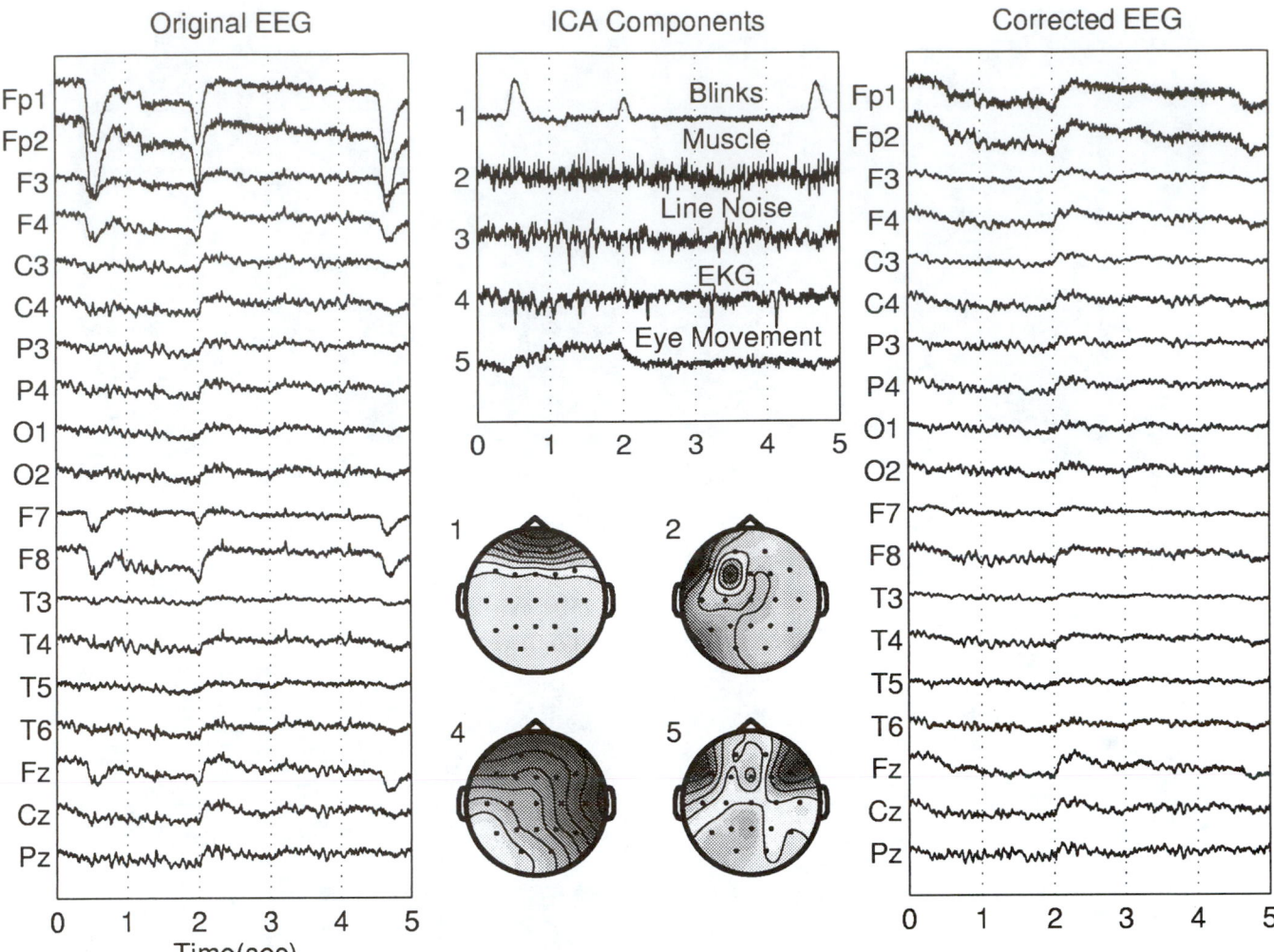

Figure 4. A 5-s portion of the EEG time series (left), ICA components accounting for eye movements, cardiac signals, and line noise sources (center), and the EEG signals corrected for artifacts by removing the five com- ponents (right). (From Jung, T.-P., et al., 1998, *Adv. Neural Inf. Process. Syst.*, 10:894–900. Reprinted with permission.)

over six trials with two subjects. When the independent components were ranked in terms of their strength in the original signal, this time course was ranked between 14th and 41st out of 146, so it was by no means a strong signal in the original data. The brain map associated with it contained activations in relevant areas of the brain corresponding mainly to vision and visual association, but also some in a motor area, and some in prefrontal cortex.

In each case, in focusing on individual time courses, we are looking at on the order of 1/146th of the brain activation data. Thus, the vast majority of the possibly confusing and irrelevant brain activation is stripped away for us, because its brain maps are statistically independent from the ones that concern us.

Discussion

With these descriptions of the application of ICA to image processing and brain recordings, we hope to move the reader away from toy problems to a realization that algorithms of this kind have many applications. In almost every case, the algorithm has yielded surprises. Applications at the ICA 2000 workshop ranged from clustering World Wide Web documents to extracting the earthquake signal on the volcanic island of Stromboli.

On the theoretical side, ICA is in many ways much more interesting than its cousin, PCA, and this success comes from the simultaneous relaxation of two assumptions. The first is geometrical: that coordinate systems in signal transforms should be orthogonal. The second is statistical: that anything interesting in the probability distribution can be captured by the covariance matrix. Progress in this field will be made by further combined statisticogeometrical innovations, such as the identification of group-theoretic symmetries in probability distributions with the subspaces that they are embedded in, but that's another story.

Road Map: Learning in Artificial Networks
Related Reading: Brain Signal Analysis; Feature Analysis; Principal Component Analysis; Unsupervised Learning with Global Objective Functions

References

Amari, S.-I., 1997, Natural gradient works efficiently in learning, *Neural Computat.*, 10:251–276.
Bell, A. J., and Sejnowski, T. J., 1995, An information maximization approach to blind separation and blind deconvolution, *Neural Computat.*, 7:1129–1159.

Bell, A. J., and Sejnowski, T. J., 1997, The "independent components" of natural scenes are edge filters, *Vision Res.*, 37:3327–3338.

Cardoso, J.-F., and Laheld, B. H., 1996, Equivariant adaptive source separation, *IEEE Trans. Signal Process.*, 44:3017–3030.

Cichocki, A., Unbehauen, R., and Rummert, E., 1994, Robust learning algorithm for blind separation of signals, *Electron. Lett.*, 30:1386–1387.

Comon, P., 1994, Independent component analysis: A new concept? *Signal Process.*, 36:287–314.

Girolami, M., Ed., 2000, *Advances in Independent Component Analysis*, New York: Springer-Verlag.

Herault, J., and Jutten, C., 1986, Space or time adaptive signal processing by neural network models, in *Neural Networks for Computing: AIP Conference Proceedings 151* (J. S. Denker, Ed.), New York: American Institute for Physics.

Haykin, S., Ed., 2000, *Unsupervised Adaptive Filtering*, vol. 1: *Blind Separation*, New York: Wiley.

Hyvärinen, A., 1999, Survey on independent component analysis, *Neural Comput. Surv.*, 2:94–128.

Jung, T.-P., Makeig, S., Lee, T.-W., McKeown, M. J., Brown, G., Bell, A. J., and Sejnowski, T. J., 2000, Independent component analysis of biomedical signals, in *Proceedings of ICA 2000*.

Lee, T.-W., Girolami, M., Bell, A. J., and Sejnowski, T. J., 1998, A unifying information-theoretic framework for independent component analysis, *Int. J. Math. Comput. Model.*, 31(11):1–21.

Olshausen, B. A., and Field, D. J., 1997, Sparse coding with an overcomplete basis set: A strategy employed by V1? *Vision Res.*, 37:3311–3325.

Pham, D. T., Garrat, P., and Jutten, C., 1992, Separation of a mixture of independent sources through a maximum likelihood approach, in *Proceedings of the EUSIPCO*, pp. 771–774.

van Hateren, J. H., and Ruderman, D. L., 1998, Independent component analysis of natural image sequences yields spatiotemporal filters similar to simple cells in primary visual cortex, *Proc. R. Soc. Lond. B*, 265:2315–2320.

Information Theory and Visual Plasticity

Nathan Intrator

Introduction

The relevance of information theory to neural networks has become more apparent in recent years. This theory has become important in analyzing and understanding the nature of the neuronal code that is relayed between cortical layers and the nature of the learning goals that guide neuronal learning and synaptic modification. Rapid advances in single- and multiple-electrode recording and other noninvasive techniques have provided a clearer view on neuronal activity and synaptic modification. However, the puzzle is still unsolved. We do not know what neuronal learning goals are, how they are being incorporated, and, most importantly, the nature of the neuronal code and how it is formed and interpreted by successive layers.

Information theory is an excellent tool that tells us how to code the information we want to relay. When studying the brain, we do not exactly know what the brain is coding at a local neuronal neighborhood and, thus, we cannot rely entirely on information theory to understand what neurons do. However, under various assumptions regarding the role of neuronal activity, one can test whether a certain code is optimal. When we try to understand the nature of synaptic learning rules, we should be concerned with possible goals that may underlie synaptic changes. It is conceivable that knowing what could be a useful goal under different input environments could serve for distinguishing between synaptic plasticity theories. Only after this distinction between goals has been achieved can one continue on and distinguish between learning rules aimed at achieving the same objective, on the basis of their detailed mathematical or computational properties. In this article, we briefly indicate possible neuronal goals resulting from various information-theoretic considerations. We are not making a statement about the nature of information relay in the brain or about the nature of information representation, where possible candidates may be action potentials, single spikes, spikes averaged along a time window of few milliseconds, or spike activity averaged over few cells.

For a book on information theory, see *Elements of Information Theory* (Cover and Thomas, 1991). Useful relevances to neuronal activity can be found in Rieke et al. (1996).

Brief Review of Information Theory

Information theory was developed about 50 years ago for the study of communication channels (Shannon, 1948). Shannon considered information as a loss of *uncertainty* and defined it as a function of the probability distribution of the code words. If, for example, the probability distribution $P(X)$ is concentrated on a single value, then the information we can transmit, when choosing values from such distribution, is zero, since there is only one value to transmit. Thus, the amount of information is a function of the variability of the distribution and actually the exact shape of the distribution. This information quantity, which we denote by $H(X)$, should satisfy an additivity constraint, which states that when two random variables are independent, the information contained in both of them should be the sum of the information contained in each of them, namely

$$P(X_1, X_2) = P_1(X_1)P_2(X_2) \Rightarrow H(X_1, X_2) = H(X_1) + H(X_2) \quad (1)$$

Shannon has shown that the only function that is consistent with this condition (and with a few other simple constraints) is the Boltzmann entropy of statistical mechanics. The connection between information theory, statistics, and statistical mechanics is demonstrated in Jaynes (1957). The entropy in continuous and in discrete cases respectively is given by

$$H(X) = -\int_K P(x) \log P(x)dx$$
$$H(X) = -\sum_{i=1}^{K} p(x_i) \log p(x_i) \quad (2)$$

where $p(x_i)$ is the probability of observing the value x_i out of possible K discrete values of the random variable X. (In information theory, it is customary to neglect the Boltzmann constant, which sets up the units correctly, and to use the logarithm of base 2, so that the information is measured in bits.) An intuitive way to look at this function is by considering the average number of bits that is needed to produce an efficient code. It is desirable to use a small number of bits for sending those words that appear with high probability and to use a larger number of bits for sending words that appear with lower probability. In the special case of n words arriving with the same probability, the number of bits that are required for each word is $\log_2 n$.

Shannon formulated this idea for the problem of information flow through a bottleneck, having to optimize the code so as to send the smallest number of bits on average. This led to questions such as how the receiver, given only the transmitted information, maximizes his knowledge about the data available at the sender's end. For our purpose, we formulate the mutual information idea in terms of a neural network of a single layer. Let $\mathbf{d}^i \in R^n$ be an input vector to the network occurring with a probability distribution $P_\mathbf{d}$, and let $\mathbf{c}^i \in R^k$ be the corresponding k-dimensional network activity with its probability distribution P_c. The *relative entropy* or the *Kullback-Leibler distance* between the two probability distributions is defined as

$$D(P_\mathbf{d}\|P_\mathbf{c}) = \sum_{\mathbf{d}_i} P_d(\mathbf{d}_i) \log \frac{P_d(\mathbf{d}_i)}{P_c(\mathbf{c}_i)}$$
$$= E_{P_d}[\log(P_d) - \log(P_c)] \qquad (3)$$

Note that this is not symmetric and does not satisfy the triangle inequality.

Consider now the joint probability distribution of the input and output random variables $P(\mathbf{d}, \mathbf{c})$ such that $P_\mathbf{d}$ and $P_\mathbf{c}$ are the corresponding marginal distributions. The *mutual information* $I(\mathbf{d}, \mathbf{c})$ is the relative entropy between the joint distribution and the product distribution, namely,

$$I(\mathbf{d}, \mathbf{c}) = D(P(\mathbf{d}, \mathbf{c})\|P(\mathbf{d})P(\mathbf{c}))$$
$$= \sum_{\mathbf{d}^i} \sum_{\mathbf{c}^j} P(\mathbf{d}^i, \mathbf{c}^j) \log \frac{P(\mathbf{d}^i, \mathbf{c}^j)}{P(\mathbf{d}^i)P(\mathbf{c}^j)}$$
$$= \sum_{\mathbf{d}^i} \sum_{\mathbf{c}^j} P(\mathbf{d}^i, \mathbf{c}^j) \log \frac{P(\mathbf{d}^i|\mathbf{c}^j)}{P(\mathbf{d}^i)}$$
$$= H(\mathbf{d}) - H(\mathbf{d}|\mathbf{c}) \qquad (4)$$

Additional properties of mutual information can be found in Cover and Thomas (1991). For example, $I(\mathbf{d}, \mathbf{c}) = H(\mathbf{c}) - H(\mathbf{c}|\mathbf{d})$, and $I(\mathbf{d}, \mathbf{c}) = H(\mathbf{c}) + H(\mathbf{d}) - H(\mathbf{d}, \mathbf{c})$.

By maximizing the mutual information, we effectively minimize $H(\mathbf{d}|\mathbf{c})$. Namely, we reduce the uncertainty about the input $\mathbf{d}$ by knowing the output $\mathbf{c}$. Thus, given a constrained situation in which the output $\mathbf{c}$ carries less data than the input $\mathbf{d}$, information theory tells us what the optimal output should be for a given input so as to have, on average, maximal knowledge about the input. Synaptic modification rules can be derived from solving the mutual information maximization problem under various assumptions about the probability distribution of the inputs. The solution to such a learning rule is based on gradient ascent, or other more sophisticated optimization algorithms.

Distributions That Maximize Entropy under Various Constraints

When we observe a certain distribution, it is natural to ask if this distribution represents a redundant coding or if it maximizes entropy under certain constraints. In some cases, we may be interested to recover the constraints under which the distribution maximizes the entropy. This section mentions some of the most common constraints and the distributions that are naturally connected with these constraints. Entropy maximization (or, as it is sometimes called, the MAX-ENT principle) is a powerful statistical inference tool. Given a certain set of constraints on a random variable, it suggests the *only possible* unbiased underlying distribution for the process. If the observed distribution is different, this implies that there are additional or different constraints governing the process. An excellent review with connection to statistical mechanics can be found in Jaynes (1957). Applications of this inference tool are many (see, e.g., Skilling, 1989).

Bounded distributions. The uniform distribution maximizes the entropy of a random variable with bounded values. Note that when discretizing a random variable, its distribution becomes automatically bounded, but it is the nondiscretized distribution that governs

the process. Thus, we would expect a maximal entropy distribution of 8-bit gray-level pictures to have a Gaussian and not a uniform distribution.

Positive valued random variables. Distributions that take only positive values or, more generally, that are bounded from below are a special and important case. They include, for example, distributions of spike counts over a certain measurement window. It turns out that under mean value constraint, the Poisson distribution maximizes the entropy. Under a variance constraint (of positive-valued distribution), the Gibbs distribution maximizes the entropy. This distribution occurs often when a quadratic functional (also called an energy or a Hamiltonian) can be associated with a configuration state of a physical system. A famous example is the annealing process (Brillouin, 1956) and a numerical algorithm called simulated annealing (Kirkpatrick and Gelatt, 1983).

Fixed variance constraint. Under a fixed mean and variance, an unbounded random variable has a normal distribution for entropy maximization. This makes a strong connection between minimizing entropy and searching for distributions that are far from Gaussian. It also shows that a linear layered network receiving Gaussian distributed inputs should extract the projections that maximize the variance, namely, find the principal components of the data in order to maximize the entropy of the projections.

Minimal Description Length

We have seen how information theory can suggest an optimal coding $\mathbf{c}$ for a given input $\mathbf{d}$ based on the probability distribution of the inputs. In this case, the code is transmitted through the bottleneck transmission line to the receiver, which then tries to reconstruct the original inputs. This formulation does not take into account the complexity of the code that is being sent and the complexity of constructing or decoding this code. A different information-theoretic formulation, one that is more appropriate for supervised learning, does take the above considerations into account. This formulation is based on the *minimal description length* (MDL) principle (Rissanen, 1984), which states that the way to choose a better model for data is by minimizing concurrently the cost of describing the model and the cost of describing the misfit between the model and the data. In terms of the information bottleneck (described earlier), we can view the current situation as a teacher-student network in which the teacher is trying to send the student the network to solve a certain problem. Under a supervised setup, the assumption is that both the student and the teacher can see the input data (zero cost), but only the teacher knows what the output should be. For the student to reconstruct the output, he would need to have a good model (network), namely, a small misfit between network output and desired output, and for quick learning, the model should be simple. Both of these properties can be measured by the entropy of sending the information about data misfit and about the model. In classical information theory, it is often assumed that the cost of learning a model can be neglected, as learning takes place only once, whereas data are sent continuously. However, when modeling learning, it is clear that the cost of learning plays an important role and should not be neglected. Hinton and colleagues have presented a formulation based on MDL principles for learning in neural networks (see Zemel and Hinton, 1995). It remains to be seen whether measuring the model (or learning) cost using the cost of sending the model parameters (entropy of the weight distribution) will turn out to be a useful constraint and a useful neuronal learning goal.

Note that measuring model cost by the entropy of its parameters may be radically different from measuring model cost by the actual or effective number of parameters, as has been proposed before (Akaike, 1974).

Projection Pursuit and Cortical Plasticity

Thus far we have discussed maximization of entropy under various conditions. At times, however, minimization of entropy is more relevant. This occurs, for example, when classification is sought and small ambiguity of the outputs is desired. It also occurs when one is searching for independent components (Comon, 1994) and, especially, when one is looking for structure in the data by searching for interesting projections. To see the connection between independent components and the search for structure in the projections, we note that when two (or more) independent components are added together, their combined distribution is more Gaussian than is each of the component's distributions. Thus, seeking projections that are far from Gaussian can find the original distributions, assuming they were non-Gaussian to start with. More generally, the central limit theorem implies that given a list of independent random variables, their mean is normally distributed. Thus, a random projection of high-dimensional data would yield a single-dimensional Gaussian distribution unless there was a strong dependency between the projection vector and the data. A theoretical analysis of properties of projections was done by Diaconis and Freedman (1984). They have shown that for most high-dimensional clouds (of points), most low-dimensional projections are approximately Gaussian. Since entropy is maximized for a Gaussian distribution, searching for minimal entropy amounts to searching for maximal deviation from a Gaussian distribution. In practice, calculating the entropy is computationally expensive and requires knowledge (or robust estimation) of the projected distribution. Therefore, approximations to the entropy are used that rely on polynomial moments. The general framework of exploratory projection pursuit (Friedman, 1987) suggests various ways to seek such non-Gaussian projections. Its supervised version is called *projection pursuit regression* (Friedman and Stuetzle, 1981). It turns out that polynomial moments that are not approximating the entropy are also good candidates for measuring deviation from Gaussian distribution. For example, skewness and kurtosis, which are functions of the first four moments of the distribution, are frequently used in the search for independent components or non-Gaussian projections.

Intrator and Cooper (1992) have shown that a BCM neuron can find structure in the input distribution that exhibits deviation from Gaussian distribution in the form of multimodality in the projected distributions. Since clusters cannot be found directly in the data, owing to its sparsity, this type of deviation, which is measured by the first three moments of the distribution, is particularly useful for finding clusters in high-dimensional data, and thus is useful for classification or recognition tasks. This learning rule has been compared with skewness and kurtosis measures for the purpose of extracting simple-cell receptive fields from natural images (Blais et al., 1998).

Summary

We have demonstrated some features of information theory that are relevant to information relay in cortex. We have presented cases in which information theory considerations led people to seek methods for Gaussianizing the input distribution and, in other cases, led people to seek learning goals for non-Gaussian distributions. The MDL principle was presented as a learning goal that takes into account the complexity of the decoding network. In particular, we have made the connection of entropy-based methods, projection pursuit, and cortical plasticity. Further details on the extraction of information in visual cortex can be found in FEATURE ANALYSIS.

Road Maps: Learning in Artifical Networks; Neural Plasticity
Related Reading: Feature Analysis; Learning and Statistical Inference; Minimum Description Length Analysis; Unsupervised Learning with Global Objective Functions

References

Akaike, H., 1974, A new look at the statistical model identification, *IEEE Trans. Autom. Control*, 19:716–723.
Blais, B. S., Intrator, N., Shouval, H., and Cooper, L. N., 1998, Receptive field formation in natural scene environments: Comparison of single cell learning rules, *Neural Computat.*, 10:1797–1813.
Brillouin, L., 1956, *Science and Information Theory*, New York: Academic Press.
Comon, P., 1994, Independent component analysis: A new concept? *Signal Process.*, 36:287–314.
Cover, T., and Thomas, J., 1991, *Elements of Information Theory*, New York: Wiley. (See especially Chapters 1 and 13.) ◆
Diaconis, P., and Freedman, D., 1984, Asymptotics of graphical projection pursuit, *Ann. Statist.*, 12:793–815.
Friedman, J. H., 1987, Exploratory projection pursuit, *J. Am. Statist. Assoc.*, 82:249–266. ◆
Friedman, J. H., and Stuetzle, W., 1981, Projection pursuit regression, *J. Am. Statist. Assoc.*, 76:817–823.
Intrator, N., and Cooper, L. N., 1992, Objective function formulation of the BCM theory of visual cortical plasticity: Statistical connections, stability conditions, *Neural Netw.*, 5:3–17. ◆
Jaynes, E. T., 1957, Information theory and statistical mechanics: 1, *Phys. Rev.*, 106:620–530, 108:171–190. ◆
Kirkpatrick, S., and Gelatt, C. D., 1983, Optimization by simulated annealing, *Science*, 220:671–680.
Rieke, F., Warland, D., de Ruyter van Steveninck, R., and Bialek, W., 1996, *Spikes: Exploring the Neural Code*. Cambridge, MA: MIT Press.
Rissanen, J., 1984, Universal coding, information, prediction, and estimation, *IEEE Trans. Inf. Theory*, 30:629–636.
Shannon, C. E., 1948, A mathematical theory of communication, *Bell. Syst. Tech. J.*, 27:379–423, 623–656.
Skilling, J., 1989, *Maximum Entropy and Bayesian Methods*, Dordrecht: Kluwer Academic. (See especially Chapters 1 and 13.) ◆
Zemel, R. S., and Hinton, G. E., 1995, Developing population codes by minimizing description length, *Neural Computat.*, 7:549–564.

Integrate-and-Fire Neurons and Networks

Wulfram Gerstner

Introduction

Most biological neurons communicate by short electrical pulses called *action potentials* or *spikes*. In contrast to the standard neuron model used in artificial neural networks, integrate-and-fire neurons do not rely on a temporal average over the pulses. In integrate-and-fire and similar spiking neuron models, the pulsed nature of the neuronal signal is taken into account and considered as potentially relevant for coding and information processing. In contrast to more detailed neuron models, integrate-and-fire models do not explicitly describe the form of an action potential. Pulses are treated as formal events. This is no real drawback, since, in a biological spike train, all action potentials of a neuron have roughly the same form. The time course of an action potential, therefore, does not carry any information.

Integrate-and-fire and similar spiking neuron models are phenomenological descriptions on an intermediate level of detail. Compared to other SINGLE-CELL MODELS (q.v.), they offer several advantages. In particular, coding principles can be discussed in a transparent manner. Moreover, dynamics in networks of integrate-and-fire neurons can be analyzed mathematically. Finally, large systems with thousands of neurons can be simulated rather efficiently. Reviews of integrate-and-fire networks can be found in Maass and Bishop (1998) and in Gerstner and Kistler (2002).

Spiking Neuron Models

Integrate-and-Fire Model

In its simplest form, an integrate-and-fire neuron i consists of a resistor R in parallel to a capacitor C driven by an external current I_i. The voltage u_i across the capacitor is interpreted as the membrane potential. The voltage scale is chosen so that $u_i = 0$ is the resting potential. The temporal evolution of u_i is

$$\tau_m \frac{du_i}{dt} = -u_i + RI_i(t) \tag{1}$$

where $\tau_m = RC$ is the membrane time constant of the neuron.

Spikes are formal events. We say that neuron i has fired a spike if u_i reaches at a time $t = t_i^f$ a threshold ϑ. The form of the action potential is not described explicitly. Immediately after spike firing, the potential u_i is simply reset to a value $u_{\text{reset}} < \vartheta$. Integration of Equation 1 is then resumed with u_{reset} as the initial condition (Stein, 1967). Because the spatial structure of the neuron is neglected, such a model is also called a point model (see SINGLE-CELL MODELS).

In a network of neurons, the input I_i to neuron i is due to the spikes of presynaptic neurons j. Detailed models of synaptic input can be found in SYNAPTIC INTERACTIONS. In the simplest model of a synapse, each presynaptic spike arrival evokes a postsynaptic current with a standard time course α. The total input to neuron i is then

$$I_i = \sum_{j,f} w_{ij} \alpha(t - t_j^f) \tag{2}$$

where the sum runs over all firing times t_i^f of all presynaptic neurons. The factor w_{ij} is the synaptic efficacy of a connection from a presynaptic neuron j to a postsynaptic neuron i. Choices for the postsynaptic current include a delayed δ-pulse, $\alpha(s) = \delta(s - \Delta^{\text{ax}})$, or a double exponential, $\alpha(s) = [e^{-(s-\Delta^{\text{ax}})/\tau_1} - e^{-(s-\Delta^{\text{ax}})/\tau_2}]/(\tau_1 - \tau_2)$, where Δ^{ax} is the axonal transmission delay and τ_1, τ_2 are synaptic time constants.

Spike Response Model

The integrate-and-fire equation (Equation 1) with the synaptic current (Equation 2) can be integrated, either numerically or analytically. Since it is a linear equation, the analytical integration can be done for each term in the sum of Equation 2 separately. The total membrane potential is then the sum of all the postsynaptic potentials (PSPs) caused by presynaptic firing, plus the refractory effect of a negative reset potential. Given the last firing time $\hat{t}_i$ of neuron i, the result of the integration is therefore of the form ($t > \hat{t}_i$)

$$u_i(t) = \eta(t - \hat{t}_i) + \sum_{j,f} w_{ij} \varepsilon(t - \hat{t}_i, t - t_j^f) \tag{3}$$

The next firing of i occurs if the membrane potential u_i approaches the threshold ϑ from below. Equation 3 defines the dynamics of the spike response model (SRM). It was introduced above as an integrated version of the integrate-and-fire model, but the SRM is in fact more general (Figure 1). The function η describes the action potential at $\hat{t}_i$ and the spike afterpotential that follows. The function ε describes the voltage response of neuron i to a presynaptic spike at t_j^f. Let us suppose that the last spike of the postsynaptic neuron i was far back in the past ($t - \hat{t}_i \rightarrow \infty$). Then $\varepsilon(\infty, s)$ as a function of s describes the time course of the PSP caused by a presynaptic spike. If the postsynaptic neuron i has been active in the recent past, then a presynaptic spike is less effective in exciting a postsynaptic response. The first argument of $\varepsilon(t - \hat{t}_i, t - t_j^f)$ describes the dependence on the recent firing history of the postsynaptic neuron. With an appropriate choice of the functions ε and η, about 90% of the firing times of the Hodgkin-Huxley model with time-dependent input can be correctly predicted by the SRM, with a precision of ± 2 ms (Kistler, Gerstner, and van Hemmen, 1997). Moreover, the spatial structure of neurons with a linear dendritic tree can be incorporated by an appropriate choice of ε. For synapses that are farther out on the dendritic tree, the PSP, and hence the function ε, rise more slowly.

Noise

Biological neurons that are driven by a time-dependent intracellular current exhibit a reliable, (nearly) deterministic behavior, just as the models in Equations 1 or 3. On the other hand, neurons that are part of a cortical network emit spikes at irregular intervals. Since the exact spike times cannot be controlled by the experiment, the irregularity is interpreted as noise.

Formally, noise can be introduced into the integrate-and-fire model by adding a fluctuating input $\sigma\xi_i(t)$ on the right-hand side of Equation 1, where σ is a parameter controlling the amplitude of the noise and ξ is a normally distributed random variable with zero mean (see DIFFUSION MODELS OF NEURON ACTIVITY). In the presence of noise, we may ask the following question: Given the last firing time $\hat{t}_i$ of neuron i and the input current $I_i(t')$ for $t' > \hat{t}_i$, what is the probability that the next spike occurs around time t? The answer is given by the conditional interval distribution $P(t|\hat{t}_i, I(\cdot))$. The calculation of $P(t|\hat{t}_i, I(\cdot))$ for the diffusion model is equivalent to the solution of a first-passage-time problem. The general solution to this problem is not known.

Noise can also be introduced into spiking neuron models in a different manner. The voltage $u_i(t)$ is calculated according to Equation 1 or 3. Even before u_i reaches the threshold ϑ, neuron i may fire with an "escape rate," $\rho(t)$, that depends on the momentary distance from threshold and possibly also on the current input I,

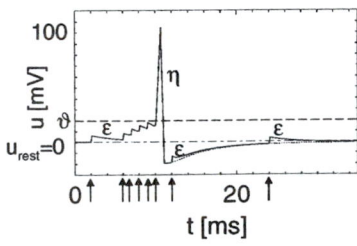

Figure 1. Each input current pulse (arrows) evokes a postsynaptic potential with time course ε. If the sum of the postsynaptic potentials reaches the threshold ϑ, an action potential with time course η is triggered. An input current pulse immediately after the action potential evokes a reduced response because of refractoriness.

viz., $\rho(t) = h(u(t) - \vartheta; I(t))$. In this case, an explicit expression for the conditional interval distribution is known, viz.,

$$P(t|\hat{t}_i, I(\cdot)) = \rho(t) \exp\left[-\int_{\hat{t}_i}^{t} \rho(t')dt'\right] \quad (4)$$

With an appropriate choice of the escape function h, the diffusion model can be approximated by the escape model to a high degree of accuracy For a review of noise models, see Gerstner and Kistler (2002, chap. 5).

Network Dynamics and Population Equations

In many areas of the brain, neurons are organized into groups of cells with similar properties, e.g., pools of motor neurons or columns in the visual cortex. Instead of looking at the firings of individual neurons, we may simply be interested in the fraction of neurons that are active in the population. In each small time window Δt, let us count the number of spikes $n_{sp}(t; t + \Delta t)$ that are emitted across the population, and divide by the number N of neurons and Δt. This procedure defines the population activity or population rate

$$A(t) = \lim_{\Delta t \to 0} \frac{n_{sp}(t; t = \Delta t)}{N\Delta t} = \frac{1}{N}\sum_{j,f}\delta(t - t_j^f) \quad (5)$$

where δ is the Dirac δ function and the sum runs over all spikes of all neurons in the population. The population activity has units of 1 over time and can be seen as the rate at which the total spike count increases. Note that the definition of the population rate (Equation 5) does not involve a temporal average, only a spatial average. What is the temporal evolution of $A(t)$ in a (homogeneous) network of spiking neurons?

The state of each neuron depends on its input *and* on the time $\hat{t}$ of its last spike (see Equation 3). We define a *homogeneous* population by the conditions that (1) lateral coupling has a fixed value $w_{ij} = w_0/N$, and (2) external inputs $I^{stim}(t)$ are the same for all neurons. The total input to any neuron in the network is therefore

$$I(t) = w_0 \int_0^{\infty} \alpha(s)A(t - s)ds + I^{stim}(t) \quad (6)$$

Even though they all receive the same input, different neurons will, in general, have different firing times $\hat{t}$. A neuron that has fired its last spike at $\hat{t}$ and has received an input $I(t')$ for $t' > \hat{t}$ will contribute with weight $P(t|\hat{t}, I(\cdot))$ to the population activity at time t. Hence the expected value of the population activity at time t is

$$A(t) = \int_{-\infty}^{t} P(t|\hat{t}, I(\cdot))A(\hat{t})d\hat{t} \quad (7)$$

For spiking neurons with escape noise $\rho(t)$, $P(t|\hat{t}, I(\cdot))$ is given by Equation 4 and therefore is highly nonlinear. Equation 7 is implicitly contained in Wilson and Cowan (1972) and Knight (1972), and is formally derived in Gerstner (2000) for a homogeneous, fully connected network of spiking neurons in the limit of $N \to \infty$.

In their 1972 paper, Wilson and Cowan proposed transforming the integral Equation 7 into a differential equation of the form

$$\tau \frac{d}{dt}A(t) = -A(t) + g\left[w_0 \int_0^{\infty} \alpha(s)A(t - s)ds + I^{stim}(t)\right] \quad (8)$$

where τ is a time constant, w_0 is the neuronal coupling strength, $I^{ext}(t)$ is a stimulus, and g is a nonlinear transfer function. One of the problems of Equation 8 is that the time constant τ is the result of a process of "time coarse graining," which is necessary for the transition from Equation 7 to Equation 8. Since the time window of coarse graining has to be defined somewhat arbitrarily, the time constant τ is basically ad hoc. Because of the problems inherent in Equation 8, it is preferable to work directly with Equation 7.

For the diffusion noise model, Equation 7 is valid but not very useful, because the conditional interval distribution $P(t|\hat{t}, I(\cdot))$ is not known. As an alternative to Equation 7, the state of the population can be described by the distribution of membrane potentials $P(u, t)$ (Abbott and van Vreeswijk, 1993; Brunel, 2000; Nykamp and Tranchina, 2000). At each moment of time $P(u, t)\Delta u N$ gives the number of neurons in the population with a membrane potential between u and $u + \Delta u$. The equation of the integrate-and-fire model (Equation 1) with additive diffusion noise $\sigma\xi(t)$ can be transformed into a Fokker-Planck equation for the distribution of membrane potentials:

$$\tau \frac{\partial P(u, t)}{\partial t} = \frac{\sigma^2}{2\tau}\frac{\partial^2 P(u, t)}{\partial u^2} + \frac{\partial}{\partial u}\{[u - RI(t)]P(u, t)\} \quad (9)$$

The threshold is treated as an absorbing boundary, so that the probability density vanishes for $u \geq \vartheta$. The probability current across threshold equals the population activity

$$A(t) = \frac{\sigma^2}{2\tau^2}\frac{\partial P(u, t)}{\partial u}\Big|_{u = \vartheta} \quad (10)$$

Since the membrane potential of active neurons is immediately reset to u_{reset}, the population activity $A(t)$ acts a source of probability current at $u = u_{reset}$. For a review, see Gerstner and Kistler (2002, chap. 6).

Application to Coding

Integrate-and-fire models can be used to discuss potential principles of coding and dynamics in a transparent manner (Maass and Bishop, 1998, chaps. 1, 2, 10–14). Before we turn to networks, let us start with two examples of coding on the single-neuron level.

Signal Encoding by Single Neurons

Coherent input is more efficient than incoherent spikes in driving a postsynaptic neuron. To see why, let us consider the SRM (Equation 3). For the sake of simplicity, we assume that the postsynaptic neuron i was inactive in the recent past ($t < 0$) and receives, for $t > 0$, input from two presynaptic neurons $j = 1, 2$, both firing at 100 Hz. We set $w_{i1} = w_{i2} = w_0$. According to Equation 3, each input spike evokes a postsynaptic potential $\varepsilon(-\infty, t - t_j^f)$, where t_j^f is one of the firing times of neuron j. If the two spike trains are out of phase, the summed postsynaptic potential is lower than in the synchronous case (Figure 2). By an appropriate choice of the threshold ϑ, an output spike of the postsynaptic neuron i occurs therefore only in the coherent (or "coincident") case. Quite generally, coincidence detection is possible if the threshold of the postsynaptic neuron is slightly above the mean value, the membrane potential would take for asynchronous input (König, Engel, and Singer, 1996; Kempter et al., 1998). In the auditory system, it is

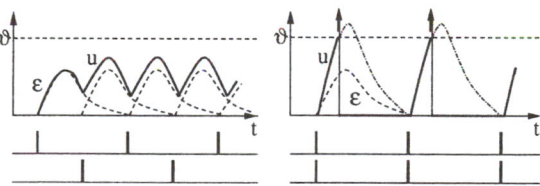

Figure 2. *Left*, Spike trains from two different presynaptic neurons are phase shifted with respect to each other. The summed potential u does not reach the threshold. *Right*, Spikes from the same presynaptic neurons arrive synchronously, so that u reaches the threshold ϑ and evokes the generation of output spikes (arrows). Afterwards, u is reset (schematic figure).

commonly accepted that coincidence detection is used for the localization of sound sources. On the other hand, it is an open question whether *cortical* neurons operate in the regime of coincidence detection (König et al., 1996; see also SINGLE-CELL MODELS).

Coding by Homogeneous Populations

Spiking neurons connected to each other by excitatory or inhibitory synapses exhibit nontrivial dynamical properties. The population may respond rapidly to external signals. The network activity may explode or die away. Neurons may spontaneously develop a tendency to fire synchronously or in groups. All of these phenomena, which can potentially be the basis of various coding schemes, can be understood from an analysis of Equations 6 through 10. Some of the fundamental questions are highlighted in the following.

First, is it possible, in the absence of an external stimulus, to stabilize a population of spiking neurons at a reasonable level of spontaneous activity? For $N \to \infty$, spontaneous activity corresponds to a stationary solution $A(t) \equiv A_0$ of the population dynamics described by Equation 7 or 10. Spontaneous asynchronous firing seems to be a generic feature of cortical tissue, but its role is still unclear. A stability analysis shows that without noise, asynchronous firing is never stable. Thus, the apparent noisiness of cortical neurons is a necessary feature of the system.

Even in the presence of noise, neurons often tend to synchronize their firings and develop collective oscillations. This observation leads to the second question: How is the frequency of collective oscillations related to neuronal parameters? It turns out that there are different oscillatory regimes, depending on the form of the postsynaptic potential, the axonal delay, and the value of the threshold (Abbott and van Vreeswijk, 1993; Brunel, 2000; Gerstner, 2000). The frequency of the collective oscillation may be low (about that of individual neurons) or several times faster. Collective oscillations and synchronization (Maas and Bishop, 1998, chaps. 10 and 11; Gerstner and Kistler, 2002, chap. 12) have been suggested as potential coding schemes in cortex and hippocampus (see SYNCHRONIZATION, BINDING AND EXPECTANCY).

Third, how rapidly does the population activity $A(t)$ respond to changes in the input? An analysis of Equation 7 shows that the response time is not limited by the membrane time constant of the neurons, but can be much faster (Gerstner, 2000). The fast response is due to the fact that, during spontaneous activity, there are always some neurons with a membrane potential just below threshold. A slight increase in the input will make those neurons fire immediately. The fast response of populations of spiking neurons to a new input could be important for an explanation of reaction time experiments (Thorpe, Fize, and Marlot, 1996; cf. FAST VISUAL PROCESSING). The same type of argument also shows that populations of spiking neurons can reliably transmit signals that vary on a time scale that is short compared to the interspike intervals of a neuronal spike train, as is the case in the auditory pathway, for example.

All of the above results hold true for homogeneous networks with either excitatory or inhibitory coupling. Formally, the theory is valid for full connectivity in the limit of $N \to \infty$. It also yields an excellent approximation for networks with random connectivity if the density of connections is either very high or very low. An extension to mixed excitatory/inhibitory populations as found in the cortex is possible (Brunel, 2000).

Coding in Structured Networks

Structure in neuronal networks may arise from a spatial arrangement of neurons or from specific patterns stored in a distributed manner in the network.

In networks with local (or distance-dependent) excitatory connections, traveling waves may occur. In two-dimensional sheets of neurons, wave fronts may have planar or spiral shapes, similar to the ones found in reaction-diffusion systems. Collective oscillations and asynchronous firing are other possible network states. These effects can be described by a direct generalization of the theory of homogeneous systems to a spatially continuous population. Replace $A(t)$ in Equation 7 by $A(x, t)$ where x is the spatial location. Instead of Equation 6, we use $I(x, t) = \int dx' w(|x - x'|) \int ds \, \alpha(s) A(x', t - s)$, where $w(\cdot)$ is the distance-dependent coupling strength. Activity waves have been reported in slice cultures. It has also been suggested that similar activity waves could account for some of the trial-to-trial variability in cortical spike train recordings.

In the previous example, neurons that are strongly connected are located next to each other. Activity spreads from one group of neurons to its neighbors, which is easily recognizable by an external observer as a traveling wave of activity. Let us now keep the connections between the same neurons as before, but move all neurons to a new random location on the two-dimensional sheet. Apart from the fact that connection lines are longer, nothing has changed. What used to be a propagating wave in the original spatial arrangement now looks like asynchronous firing of neurons all over the sheet. Nevertheless, it is a specific, nearly deterministic spatiotemporal spike pattern. These "hidden" waves of activity have been termed SYNFIRE CHAINS (q.v.) (Abeles, 1991). Although the existence and stability of synfire chains can be shown by simulation or analysis of model networks, this does not necessarily imply that real brains make use of synfire chains for coding.

Discussion

What is the code used by cortical neurons? What is signal, what is noise in neuronal spike trains? Although the final answers to these questions have to come from additional experiments, modeling on the level of integrate-and-fire networks can contribute to answering, because models allow researchers to explore potential coding schemes and to identify relevant operating regimes.

In populations of integrate-and-fire neurons, a rate code can be a very fast code, if rate is defined by a population average ("population activity") rather than by a temporal average (Knight, 1972; Gerstner, 2000). In contrast to widespread belief, the speed of signal transmission is not limited by the membrane time constant of the neuron. Moreover, with appropriate spike-based learning rules (Maass and Bishop, 1998, chap. 14), spiking neurons can work, in principle, at a very high temporal precision (Abeles, 1991). Large-scale simulations of integrate-and-fire networks provide a link between theory and experiments.

One of the points that has been stressed in recent models of integrate-and-fire neurons in the relevance of the subthreshold regime. If neuronal and network parameters are chosen so that the mean membrane potential stays just below threshold, then several interesting properties emerge. First, neurons act as coincidence detectors. They are sensitive to fluctuations in the input and can therefore "read out" the coherent aspects of the input signal (König et al., 1996; Kempter et al., 1998). Second, neurons in this regime respond rapidly to changes in the input (Gerstner, 2000). This might be relevant for explaining fast reaction times (Thorpe et al., 1996). Third, to stabilize a highly recurrent network of spiking neurons in the subthreshold regime, a certain amount of noise is necessary (Abbott and van Vreeswijk, 1993; Gerstner, 2000). From that point of view, it comes as no surprise that cortical neurons appear to be noisy. Whether this apparent noisiness is due to intrinsic noise sources in the neuronal dynamics, to noise in the synaptic transmission, or to deterministic chaos in a network is not clear. Model studies have shown that noise itself can arise as a network effect if neurons are in the subthreshold regime. Although individual neurons behave more or less deterministically, the same neurons show large firing variability when part of a random network of excitatory and inhibitory neurons with sparse connectivity (Brunel, 2000). Such networks can represent past input in their spatiotemporal firing pattern (see TEMPORAL INTEGRATION IN RECURRENT MICROCIRCUITS). Thus, the study of integrate-and-fire networks may shed new light on the burning questions of brain theory.

Road Maps: Biological Networks; Neural Coding
Background: Single-Cell Models
Related Reading: Pattern Formation, NeuralRate Coding and Signal ProcessingSpiking Neurons, Computation with

References

Abbott, L. F., and van Vreeswijk, C., 1993, Asynchronous states in a network of pulse-coupled oscillators, *Phys. Rev. E*, 48:1483–1490.
Abeles, M., 1991, *Corticonics*, Cambridge, Engl.: Cambridge University Press.
Brunel, N., 2000, Dynamics of sparsely connected networks of excitatory and inhibitory neurons, *Computat. Neurosci.*, 8:183–208. ◆
Gerstner, W., 2000, Population dynamics of spiking neurons: Fast transients, asynchronous states and locking, *Neural Computat.*, 12:43–89.

Gerstner, W., and Kistler, W. M., 2002, *Spiking Neuron Models: Single Neurons, Populations, Plasticity*, Cambridge, Engl.: Cambridge University Press. ◆
Kempter, R., Gerstner, W., van Hemmen, J. L., and Wagner, H., 1998, Extracting oscillations: Neuronal coincidence detection with noisy periodic spike input, *Neural Computat.*, 10:1987–2017.
Kistler, W. M., Gerstner, W., and van Hemmen, J. L., 1997, Reduction of Hodgkin-Huxley equations to a single-variable threshold model, *Neural Computat.*, 9:1015–1045.
Knight, B. W., 1972, Dynamics of encoding in a population of neurons, *J. Gen. Physiol.*, 59:734–766.
König, P., Engel, A. K., and Singer, W., 1996, Integrator or coincidence detector? the role of the cortical neuron revisited, *TINS*, 19:130–137. ◆
Maass, W., and Bishop, C., Eds., 1998, *Pulsed Neural Networks*, Cambridge, MA: MIT Press. ◆
Nykamp, D., and Tranchina, D., 2000, A population density approach that facilitates large-scale modeling of neural networks: Analysis and application to orientation tuning, *J. Computat. Neurosci.*, 8:19–50.
Stein, R. B., 1967, Some models of neuronal variability, *Biophys. J.*, 7:37–68.
Thorpe, S., Fize, D., and Marlot, C., 1996, Speed of processing in the human visual system, *Nature*, 381:520–522.
Wilson, H. R., and Cowan, J. D., 1972, Excitatory and inhibitory interactions in localized populations of model neurons, *Biophys. J.*, 12:1–24.

Invertebrate Models of Learning: *Aplysia* and *Hermissenda*

John H. Byrne and Terry Crow

Introduction

Certain invertebrates lend themselves to the study of learning and memory because of their relatively simple central nervous systems. In many cases, a fairly complete "wiring diagram" can be specified and modeled. Many neurons are relatively large and can be uniquely identified, which permits the examination of the functional properties of an individual cell and the ability to correlate those properties with a specific behavior mediated by the cell. Biophysical and molecular events underlying the changes in cellular properties can then be elucidated and mathematically modeled. This chapter summarizes the progress that has been made toward a mechanistic analysis of learning in the gastropod mollusks *Aplysia* and *Hermissenda*.

Nonassociative Modifications of Defensive Siphon and Tail Withdrawal Reflexes in *Aplysia*

Behaviors and Neural Circuits

The siphon-gill and tail-siphon withdrawal reflexes of *Aplysia* have been used to analyze the neuronal mechanisms contributing to nonassociative and associative learning (see Carew, 2000; Kandel, 2001; Byrne, 2002). The siphon-gill withdrawal reflex is elicited when a stimulus is delivered to the siphon and results in withdrawal of the siphon and gill (Figure 1*A*). The tail-siphon withdrawal reflex is elicited by stimulation of the tail, which results in a coordinated set of defensive responses composed of a reflex withdrawal of the tail and the siphon (Figure 1*B*).

Defensive reflexes in *Aplysia* exhibit three forms of nonassociative learning: habituation, dishabituation, and sensitization. Habituation is defined as a decrement in response caused by repeated delivery of a stimulus (see HABITUATION). Dishabituation is defined as a restoration of a habituated (decremented) response by

delivery of another stimulus. Finally, sensitization is defined as an enhancement of a nondecremented response by delivery of another stimulus to the animal. With repeated stimulation, the reflexes undergo both short-term (minutes) and long-term (days) habituation. Applying a noxious stimulus to the head or tail can produce restoration of a habituated response (dishabituation) or sensitization of a nonhabituated response. Short-term sensitization lasts minutes, whereas long-term sensitization lasts days to weeks depending on the type of sensitization training. Although not described here, *Aplysia* also exhibits forms of associative learning such as classical conditioning and operant conditioning, which have been analyzed at the mechanistic level. Some of these mechanisms have been mathematically modeled and simulated by using a series of coupled ordinary differential equations (Byrne et al., 1990).

The afferent limb of the siphon-gill withdrawal reflex consists of sensory neurons with somata in the abdominal ganglion. The sensory neurons monosynaptically excite gill and siphon motor neurons, which are also located in the abdominal ganglion. Excitatory, inhibitory, and modulatory interneurons in the withdrawal circuit have also been identified.

The afferent limb of the tail-siphon withdrawal reflex consists of a cluster of 200 sensory neurons located in the pleural ganglion. These sensory neurons make monosynaptic excitatory connections with motor neurons in the adjacent pedal ganglion (Figure 2). The motor neurons produce withdrawal of the tail. In addition to their connections with tail motor neurons, sensory neurons form synapses with various identified interneurons. Some of these interneurons provide a parallel pathway to activate the tail motor neurons. These same interneurons activate motor neurons in the abdominal ganglion that control reflex withdrawal of the siphon (Figure 2). Several additional neurons modulate the reflex (not shown in Figure 2). Aspects of the neural circuit controlling tail withdrawal and its plasticity have been mathematically modeled and simulated us-

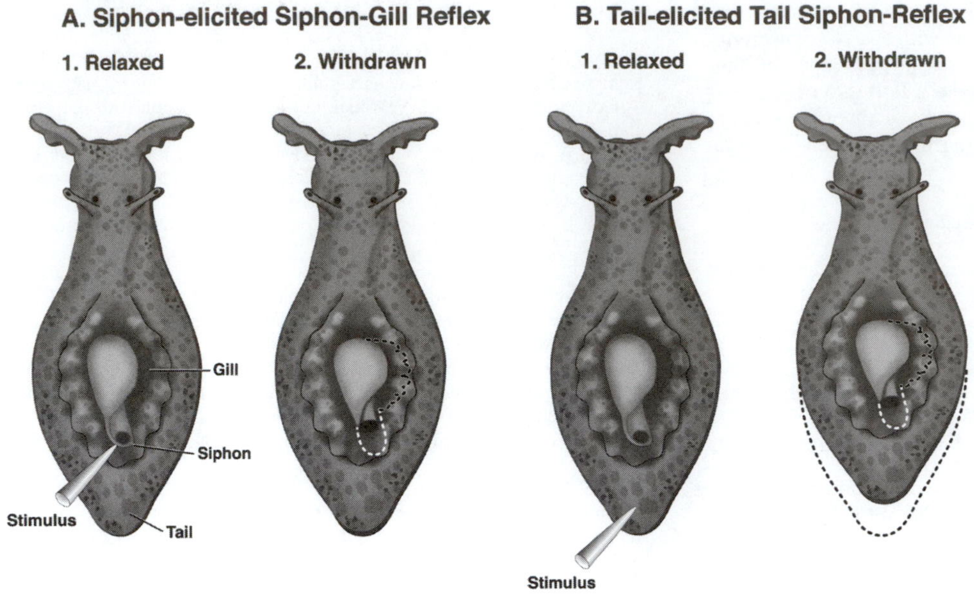

A. Siphon-elicited Siphon-Gill Reflex

1. Relaxed   **2. Withdrawn**

Gill

Siphon

Stimulus   Tail

B. Tail-elicited Tail Siphon-Reflex

1. Relaxed   **2. Withdrawn**

Stimulus

Figure 1. Siphon-gill and tail-siphon withdrawal reflexes of *Aplysia*. *A*, Siphon-gill withdrawal. Dorsal view of *Aplysia*. (1) Relaxed position. (2) A stimulus (e.g., a water jet, brief touch, or weak electric shock) applied to the siphon causes the siphon and the gill to withdraw into the mantle cavity. *B*, Tail-siphon withdrawal reflex. (1) Relaxed position. (2) A stimulus (e.g., touch or weak electric shock) applied to the tail elicits a reflex withdrawal of the tail and siphon.

ing the conductance-based simulator package SNNAP (White et al., 1993; see also NEUROSIMULATION: TOOLS AND RESOURCES).

The sensory neurons for both the siphon-gill and tail-siphon withdrawal reflexes are similar and appear to be key plastic elements in the neural circuits. Changes in their membrane properties and synaptic efficacy are associated with sensitization and the procedures that mimic short- and long-term sensitization training (see below).

Cellular Mechanisms in Sensory Neurons Associated with Short- and Long-Term Sensitization in Aplysia

Short-term sensitization.   Short-term sensitization is induced when a single brief train of shocks to the body wall results in the release

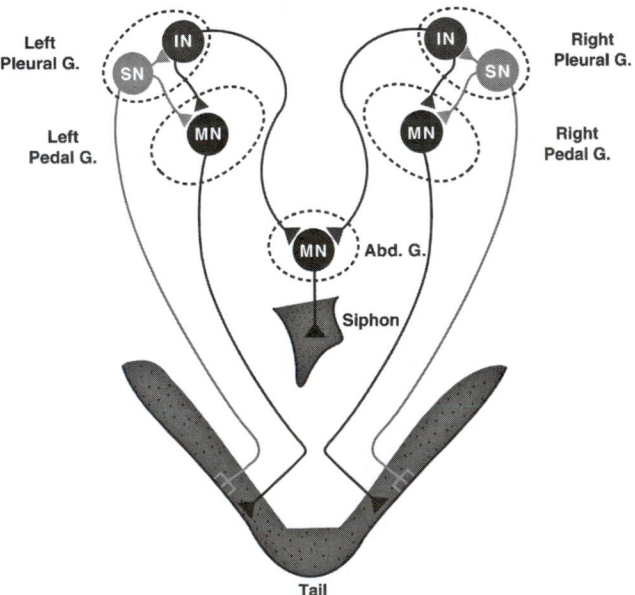

Figure 2. Simplified circuit diagram of the tail-siphon withdrawal reflex (see text for details).

of modulatory transmitters such as serotonin (5-HT) from facilitatory neurons that innervate the sensory neurons. The binding of 5-HT to receptors activates adenylyl cyclase, raising the level of the second messenger cAMP in sensory neurons. The increase in cAMP activates cAMP-dependent protein kinase (protein kinase A, PKA), which adds phosphate groups to specific substrate proteins and consequently alters their functional properties. One result of this protein phosphorylation is an alteration of the properties of membrane channels. Specifically, the increased levels of cAMP lead to a modulation of the S-K$^+$ current ($I_{K,S}$), the delayed K$^+$ channel ($I_{K,V}$), and the calcium-activated K$^+$ current ($I_{K,Ca}$). These changes in membrane currents lead to depolarization of the membrane potential, enhanced excitability, and an increase in the duration of the action potential. Cyclic AMP also appears to activate a membrane-potential- and spike-duration-independent process of facilitation, which may be due to the translocation of transmitter vesicles from a storage pool to a releasable pool. This process would result in more vesicles available for release with subsequent action potentials in the sensory neuron. These combined effects contribute to the short-term cAMP-dependent enhancement of transmitter release. Serotonin also appears to act through another receptor to increase the level of second messenger diacylglycerol (DAG), which in turn activates protein kinase C (PKC). Like PKA, PKC modulates the delayed K$^+$ channel ($I_{K,V}$) and activates the spike-duration-independent process of facilitation. This modulation of $I_{K,V}$ also contributes to the increase in duration of the action potential. Serotonin can also activate mitogen-activated protein kinase (MAPK). One substrate for MAPK is the synaptic-vesicle-associated protein synapsin, which tethers synaptic vesicles to cytoskeletal elements and thus helps to control the reserve pool of vesicles in synaptic terminals. Of general significance is the observation that a single modulatory transmitter (i.e., 5-HT) activates at least three kinase systems. The consequences of the activation of these multiple messenger systems and multiple modulations of cellular processes occur when test stimuli elicit action potentials in the sensory neuron at various times after the presentation of the sensitizing stimuli. The enhanced release of transmitter from the sensory neuron leads to an enhanced activation of follower interneurons and motor neurons and an enhanced behavioral response (i.e., sensitization).

Aspects of the modulation of membrane channels and the dynamics of second messenger systems, calcium regulation, and transmitter storage and release have been mathematically modeled and simulated (Gingrich and Byrne, 1987; Baxter et al., 1999). The details of these biophysical and biochemical processes were necessary to simulate the features of the empirical data, which could not be captured by less detailed models (see Baxter and Byrne, 1993).

Long-term sensitization. Repetition of the sensitizing stimuli leads to the induction of long-term facilitation. Repeated training leads to a translocation of PKA to the nucleus, where it phosphorylates the transcriptional activator CREB1 (cAMP-responsive element-binding protein). CREB1 binds to a regulatory region of genes known as the cAMP-responsive element (CRE). Next, this bound and phosphorylated form of CREB1 leads to increased transcription. cAMP also leads to the activation of MAPK, which phosphorylates the transcriptional repressor CREB2. Phosphorylation of CREB2 by MAPK leads to a derepression of CREB2 and therefore promotes CREB1-mediated transcriptional activation. The combined effects of activation of CREB1 and derepression of CREB2 lead to changes in the synthesis of specific proteins.

One protein whose synthesis is regulated in this manner is *Aplysia* tolloid/BMP-like protein (ApTBL-1). Tolloid and the related molecule BMP-1 appear to function as secreted Zn^{2+} proteases. In some preparations, they activate members of the transforming growth factor β (TGF-β) family. Indeed, in sensory neurons, TGF-β mimics the effects of 5-HT in that it produces long-term increases in synaptic strength of the sensory neurons. Interestingly, TGF-β activates MAPK in the sensory neurons and induces its translocation to the nucleus. Thus, ApTBL-1 and TGF-β could be part of an *extracellular* positive feedback loop possibly leading to another round of protein synthesis to further consolidate the memory.

Prolonged stimulation and increased cAMP also activate a process that decreases the level of PKA regulatory subunits, further prolonging PKA activation (Greenberg et al., 1987). With fewer regulatory subunits to bind to catalytic subunits, the catalytic units would be persistently active and could contribute to long-term facilitation of transmitter release through the same cAMP-dependent processes that are seen in the short term. Some of these cAMP-PKA-induced changes include a decrease in $I_{K,S}$ and enhanced excitability, perhaps as well as a change in the synthesis of an $I_{K,S}$ channel protein or protein associated with the channel.

The downregulation of a homolog of a neuronal cell adhesion molecule (NCAM) ApCAM also plays a key role in long-term facilitation. This downregulation has two components. First, the synthesis of ApCAM is reduced. Second, preexisting ApCAM is internalized via increased endocytosis. The internalization and degradation of ApCAM allow for the restructuring of the axon arbor. The sensory neuron can now form additional connections with the same postsynaptic target or make new connections with other cells. As with short-term sensitization, the enhanced release of transmitter from existing contacts of sensory neurons onto motor neurons and interneurons contributes to the enhanced long-term responses of the animal to test stimuli (i.e., sensitization). However, unique to long-term sensitization, increases in axonal arborization and synaptic contacts may contribute to the enhanced activation of follower interneurons and motor neurons (e.g., Figure 2).

In addition to the cellwide changes in protein synthesis described above, recent work by Martin, Kandel, and their colleagues indicates that protein synthesis also occurs at the sites of synaptic contacts between sensory neurons and motor neurons. This local protein synthesis appears to be important in synapse-specific changes in synaptic efficacy.

Other temporal domains for the memory of sensitization. Historically, memory has been divided into two temporal domains: short term and long term. It has become increasing clear from stud-

ies of a number of memory systems that this distinction is overly simplistic. For example, in *Aplysia*, Carew and his colleagues and Kandel and his colleagues have recently discovered an intermediate phase of memory that has distinctive temporal characteristics and a unique molecular signature. The intermediate-phase memory for sensitization is expressed at times approximately 30 minutes to three hours after the beginning of training. It declines completely prior to the onset of long-term memory. Like long-term sensitization, its induction requires protein synthesis, but unlike long-term memory, it does not require mRNA synthesis. The expression of the intermediate-phase memory requires the persistent activation of PKA.

Associative Learning in *Hermissenda*

Pavlovian Conditioning

Pavlovian (or classical) conditioning of *Hermissenda* involves changes in light-elicited locomotion and foot length (conditioned responses, CRs) produced by stimulation of the visual and vestibular systems with their adequate stimuli (see Sahley and Crow, 1998). The Pavlovian conditioning procedure consists of pairing light, the conditioned stimulus (CS), with high-speed rotation, the unconditioned stimulus (US). After conditioning, the CS suppresses normal light-elicited locomotion and elicits foot shortening (see Figure 3). Retention of conditioned behavior persists for several days to weeks depending on the number of conditioning trials used in initial acquisition (Alkon, 1989; Sahley and Crow, 1998). Pavlovian conditioning in *Hermissenda* exhibits CS specificity and is dependent on the association of the two sensory stimuli involving both contiguity and contingency. Nonassociative contributions to behavior are expressed in the initial trials of the conditioning session and decrement rapidly following the termination of multiple-trial conditioning. In addition to multiple-trial conditioning of suppression of light-elicited locomotion and foot contraction, one-trial conditioning also modifies light-elicited locomotion (Crow and Forrester, 1986). Pairing the CS with direct application of 5-HT (nominal US) to the exposed nervous system of otherwise intact *Hermissenda* produces suppression of light-elicited locomotion when the animals are tested 24 hours after the one conditioning trial. One-trial conditioning also produces enhanced excitability of type B photoreceptors (see Figure 4), a component of the CS pathway that expresses cellular plasticity produced by multiple-trial Pavlovian conditioning (see below).

Cellular and Synaptic Plasticity Associated with Pavlovian Conditioning

Certain sites of intrinsic modifications of cellular and synaptic plasticity in classically conditioned animals are associated with both enhanced excitability and synaptic facilitation, which have been localized to the primary sensory neurons (photoreceptors) of the pathway mediating the CS (Alkon, 1989; Frysztak and Crow, 1994). Enhanced excitability in identified photoreceptors of conditioned *Hermissenda* is expressed by a significant increase in spike activity elicited by the CS or extrinsic current, an increase in the input resistance, an alteration in the amplitude of light-elicited generator potentials, decreased spike frequency accommodation, and a reduction in the peak amplitude of voltage-dependent (I_A, I_{Ca}) and Ca^{2+}-dependent ($I_{K,Ca}$) currents (for reviews, see Alkon, 1989; Sahley and Crow, 1998). The enhanced excitability, expressed by an increase in both the amplitude of CS-elicited generator potentials and the number of action potentials elicited by the CS, may be a major contributor to changes in the duration and amplitude of CS-elicited complex postsynaptic potentials (PSPs) and enhanced CS-elicited spike activity observed in postsynaptic targets. How-

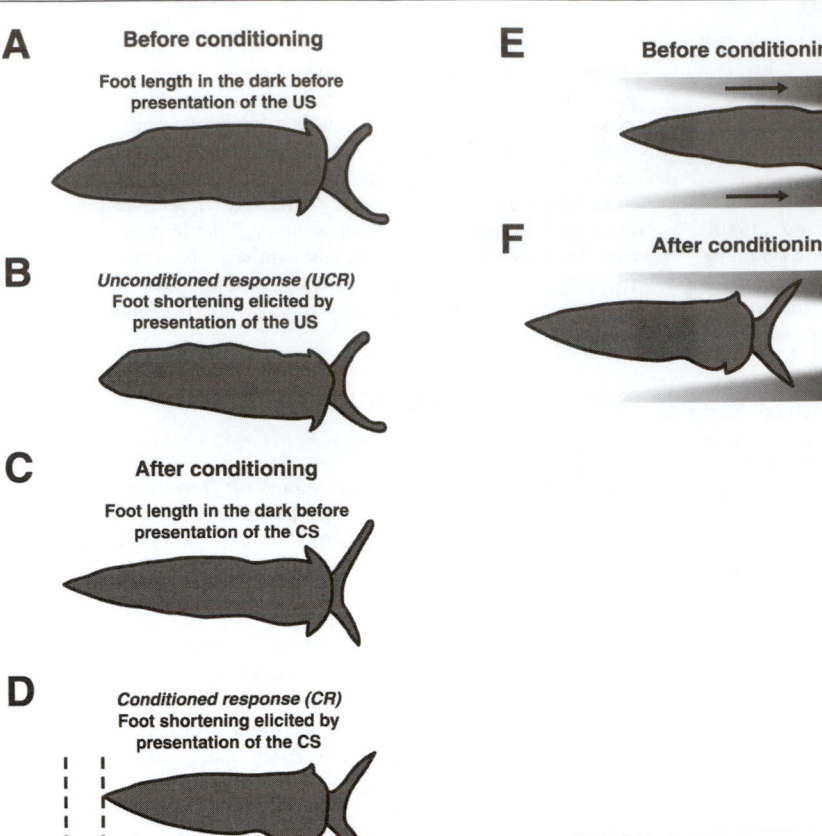

A **Before conditioning**
Foot length in the dark before
presentation of the US

B *Unconditioned response (UCR)*
Foot shortening elicited by
presentation of the US

C **After conditioning**
Foot length in the dark before
presentation of the CS

D *Conditioned response (CR)*
Foot shortening elicited by
presentation of the CS

E **Before conditioning**

F **After conditioning**

Figure 3. Pavlovian conditioned foot shortening and conditioned suppression of light-elicited locomotion of *Hermissenda. A,* Foot length in the dark before presentation of the unconditioned stimulus (US). *B,* The unconditioned response (UCR) elicited by rotation (US) of the animal in the dark. *C,* Foot length in the dark after Pavlovian conditioning and before presentation of the light (CS). *D,* Conditioned response (CR), foot shortening elicited by presentation of the CS. The area indicated between the dashed lines represents the magnitude of foot shortening elicited by the CS after conditioning. *E,* Light-elicited locomotion toward a light source assessed before conditioning. *F,* Suppression of light-elicited locomotion detected after Pavlovian conditioning. Pseudorandom or random presentations of the CS and US do not result in the development of suppression of either light-elicited locomotion or CS-elicited foot shortening.

ever, changes in the strength of synaptic connections between type B photoreceptors and other components of the CS pathway have also been detected following conditioning. Facilitation of the amplitude of monosynaptic inhibitory postsynaptic potentials (IPSPs)

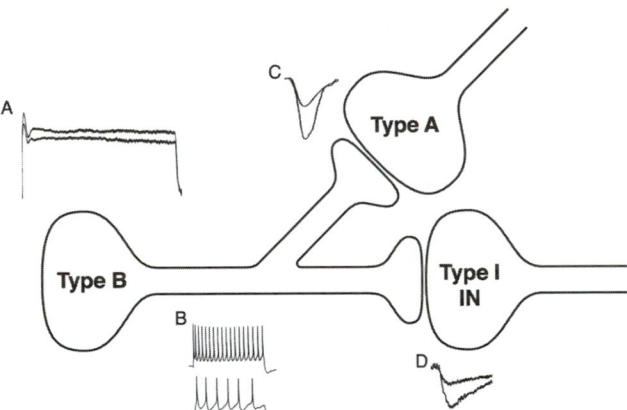

Figure 4. Components of the CS pathway that express plasticity in conditioned *Hermissenda. A,* The CS elicits a larger amplitude generator potential (upper trace) recorded from type B photoreceptors of conditioned animals as compared to pseudorandom controls (lower trace). *B,* An extrinsic current pulse elicits more action potentials in type B photoreceptors from conditioned preparations as compared to pseudorandom controls. *C,* Conditioning results in facilitation of the synaptic connections between type B photoreceptors and type A photoreceptors and type B photoreceptors and type I interneurons (*D*) as compared to control animals that received pseudorandom presentations of the CS and US.

elicited by single spikes in type B photoreceptors is detected in type A photoreceptors and type I interneurons of conditioned animals (Figures 4*C* and 4*D*). A second site of cellular plasticity in conditioned animals is the type A photoreceptor. Lateral type A photoreceptors of conditioned animals exhibit an increase in CS-elicited spike frequency, a decrease in generator potential amplitude, and enhanced excitability and decreased spike frequency accommodation to extrinsic current (for a review, see Sahley and Crow, 1998). The evidence for localization of cellular changes in the CS pathway indicates that multiple sites of plasticity involving changes in excitability and synaptic strength exist in the type B photoreceptors of conditioned animals (see Figure 4). Anatomical studies of type B photoreceptors indicate the existence of spatially segregated compartments (Alkon, 1989). Phototransduction occurs in the soma-rhabdomeric compartment, spike generation in the distal axon, and synaptic interactions in the axon terminal regions within the cerebropleural neuropil. Therefore, a decrease in K^+ conductances of type B photoreceptors could contribute both directly and indirectly to enhanced excitability by increasing the amplitude of CS-elicited generator potentials and increasing CS-elicited spike activity in the spike-generating zone by modification of conductances that influence the interspike interval.

Mechanisms of Pavlovian Conditioning

Recent modeling studies utilizing a Hodgkin-Huxley type analysis of membrane conductances and the SNNAP simulator (see NEUROSIMULATION: TOOLS AND RESOURCES) have shown that modulation of several K^+ currents (I_A, I_h, $I_{K,Ca}$) can account for both the enhanced excitability of type B photoreceptors and enhancement of monosynaptic IPSPs detected in conditioned animals (Cai, Baxter, and Crow, 2001; see also Fost and Clark, 1996). In addition, modeling studies incorporating an analysis of membrane conductances in the phototransduction compartment, spike-generating zone, and synaptic terminals are providing insights into determining the relative contribution of changes in excitability and synaptic strength to modifications of complex PSP amplitude in postsynaptic neurons of the CS pathway.

Studies of the signal transduction pathways responsible for the modification of diverse K^+ currents of type B photoreceptors of conditioned animals have identified several second messenger systems. Both protein kinase C (PKC) and extracellular signal-regulated protein kinase (ERK) contribute to the conditioned modification of excitability and synaptic efficacy of *Hermissenda* (Alkon, 1989; Sahley and Crow, 1998; Muzzio et al., 2001).

Studies of one-trial conditioning have provided insights into the mechanisms of memory consolidation. One-trial conditioning (see above) produces short-, intermediate-, and long-term memory for enhanced excitability in identified type B photoreceptors. Associated with intermediate memory is the phosphorylation of a 24-kDa protein (CSP24) that exhibits a sequence identity to the β-thymosin family of actin-binding proteins (Crow and Xue-Bian, 2000). The regulation of CSP24 by one-trial conditioning occurs in neurons of the CS pathway and not in either the pedal or cerebropleural ganglia. Cytoskeletal-related proteins such as CSP24 may contribute to long-term structural remodeling in the CS pathway by regulating the turnover of actin filaments during the intermediate-term transition period between short- and long-term memory.

Discussion

The possibility of relating cellular changes to complex behavior in invertebrates is encouraged by the progress that has already been made in examining the neural mechanisms of simple forms of non-associative and associative learning. The results of these analyses have shown that (1) learning involves changes in existing neural circuitry (at least for the short-term, the growth of new synapses and the formation of new circuits for learning and memory are not necessary); (2) learning involves the activation of second messenger systems; (3) the second messenger affects multiple subcellular processes to alter the responsiveness of the neuron (at least one locus for the storage of memory is the alteration of specific membrane currents); (4) long-term memory requires new protein synthesis, whereas short-term memory does not; and (5) long-term memory may be associated with structural changes in the nervous system.

Road Map: Neural Plasticity
Related Reading: Conditioning; Habituation; Neuromodulation in Invertebrate Nervous Systems

References

Alkon, D. L., 1989, Memory storage and neural systems, *Sci. American*, 261(1):42–50. ◆

Baxter, D. A., and Byrne, J. H., 1993, Learning rules for neurobiology, in *The Neurobiology of Neural Networks* (D. Gardner, Ed.), Cambridge, MA: MIT Press, pp. 71–105.

Baxter, D. A., Canavier, C. C., Clark, J. W., and Byrne, J. H., 1999, Computational model of the serotonergic modulation of sensory neurons in *Aplysia*, *J. Neurophysiol.*, 82:2914–2935.

Byrne, J. H., 2002, Learning and memory: Basic mechanisms, in *Fundamental Neuroscience*, 2nd ed. (L. R. Squire, F. E. Bloom, J. L., Roberts, M. J. Zigmond, S. K. McConnell, and N. C. Spitzer, Eds.), San Diego: Academic Press. ◆

Byrne, J. H., Baxter, D. A., Buonomano, D. V., and Raymond, J. L., 1990, Neuronal and network determinants of simple and higher-order features of associative learning: Experimental and modeling approaches, *Cold Spring Harbor Symposium on Quantitative Biol.*, 40:175–186.

Cai, Y., Baxter, D. A., and Crow, T., 2001, A computational study of enhanced excitability in *Hermissenda* type B photoreceptor underlying one-trial conditioning: Role of conductances modulated by serotonin, *Soc. Neurosci. Abstr.*, 27:2532.

Carew, T. J., 2000, *Behavioral Neurobiology*, Sunderland, MA: Sinauer Associates, chap. 10. ◆

Crow, T., and Forrester, J., 1986, Light paired with serotonin mimics the effects of conditioning on phototactic behavior in *Hermissenda*, *Proc. Natl. Acad. Sci. USA*, 83:7975–7978.

Crow, T., and Xue-Bian, J. J., 2000, Identification of a 24 kDa phosphoprotein associated with an intermediate stage of memory in *Hermissenda*, *J. Neurosci.*, 20:1–5.

Fost, J. W., and Clark, G. A., 1996, Modeling *Hermissenda*: I. Differential contributions of I_A and I_C to type B cell plasticity, *J. Computat. Neurosci.*, 3:137–153.

Frysztak, R. J., and Crow, T., 1994, Enhancement of type B- and type A-photoreceptor inhibitory connections in conditioned *Hermissenda*, *J. Neurosci.*, 14:1245–1250.

Gingrich, K. J., and Byrne, J. H., 1987, Single-cell neuronal model for associative learning, *J. Neurophysiol.*, 57:1705–1715.

Greenberg, S. M., Castellucci, V. F., Bayley, H., and Schwartz, J. H., 1987, A molecular mechanism for long-term sensitization in *Aplysia*, *Nature*, 329(6134):62–65.

Kandel, E. R., 2001, Cellular mechanisms of learning and the biological basis of individuality, in *Principles of Neuroscience*, 4th ed. (E. R. Kandel, J. H. Schwartz, and T. M. Jessell, Eds.), New York: McGraw-Hill, pp. 1247–1279.

Muzzio, I. A., Gandhi, C. C., Manyam, U., Pesnell, A., and Matzel, L. D., 2001, Receptor-stimulated phospholipase A(2) liberates arachiodonic acid and regulates neuronal excitability through protein kinase C, *J. Neurophysiol.*, 85:1639–1647.

Sahley, C., and Crow, T., 1998, Invertebrate learning: Current perspectives, in *Neurobiology of Learning and Memory* (J. Martinez and R. Kesner, Eds.), New York: Academic Press, pp. 171–209. ◆

White, J. A., Ziv, I., Cleary, L. J., Baxter, D. A., and Byrne, J. H., 1993, The role of interneurons in controlling the tail-withdrawal reflex in *Aplysia*: A network model, *J. Neurophysiol.*, 70:1777–1786.

Ion Channels: Keys to Neuronal Specialization

José Bargas, Lucía Cervantes, Elvira Galarraga, and Andrés Fraguela

Introduction

Neurons code information and communicate by firing voltage spikes called action potentials (APs). Firing of APs is due to the presence of voltage-gated ion channels. Charge movement through them produces transient electrical currents that generate spikes. Ligand-gated ion channels activated during synaptic functioning produce patterns of voltage changes (see TEMPORAL DYNAMICS OF BIOLOGICAL SYNAPSES) that bring membrane voltage to the activation range of different sets of voltage-gated ion channels. The latter promote or restrain the firing of APs following certain patterns (coding). Patterning is nonlinear and is not the simple summation of excitatory and inhibitory influences. This article summarizes why: the operation of voltage-gated channels.

Hodgkin and Huxley (1952) established a model to explain how ion channels generate APs (see AXONAL MODELING). APs link cellular and systems neurophysiology: they are the feature extracted to design formal neurons (Arbib, 1964) (see CANONICAL NEURAL MODELS); they encode the physical properties of stimuli, motor commands, and working memory, and they correlate with behavior and perception (see section on MAMMALIAN BRAIN REGIONS and COGNITIVE DEVELOPMENT). However, diverse combinations of different voltage-gated ion channels are possible. Each neuron is endowed with a different combination (Llinás, 1988; Huguenard and McCormick, 1994). Therefore, each cell responds with a distinct set of firing patterns on synaptic activation: plateaus with repetitive firing, bistability, frequency adaptation, tonic firing, bursting, spontaneous pacemaking, etc. There is a "neuronal specialization" that reflects different functions of neural nets (locationism) supported by variations in firing (Llinás, 1988), morphology (Cajal, 1899), and the distribution of afferents with transmitters and modulators (Nicoll, 1988) (see BIOPHYSICAL MOSAIC OF THE NEURON) (Fig. 1).

More than 50 genes encode the pore-forming domains (α-subunits) of K^+ channels (KCN). More than 10 genes encode Na^+ channels (SCN), and at least 10 genes encode pores for Ca^{2+} channels (CACN). Five genes encode cation or pacemaking channels (HCN). And α-subunits are not alone. Auxiliary subunits, β, γ, $\alpha_2\delta$, and δ, encoded by other genes, change the kinetics and voltage dependence of channels. Thousands of channel types can theoretically arise from subunit combination and alternative splicing (proteomics from genomics). How can we make functional sense of this complexity? One way is to take *firing* as the crucial property. Since neurons are specialized, we should extract, as simply as possible, their different firing properties (e.g., Suri, Bargas, and Arbib, 2001). We need to know which are the main ion channels that contribute to different firing patterns.

The roles for ion channels are (1) to generate APs and (2) to set a particular pattern, rhythm, oscillation, threshold, adaptation, pa-

cemaking, bursting, etc. for the firing of APs. This is the coding process that produces a distinct input-output function (I/O function) for a neuron in a certain condition (see SINGLE-CELL MODELS).

Operation of Ion Channels

Figure 2 simplifies the operations of an ion channel, and Figure 3 illustrates basic firing patterns. Ion currents through channels follow Ohm's law,

$$I_i = (G_{MAX} \cdot m^n h) \cdot (V - E_i) \tag{1}$$

where I_i = current, $G_{MAX} m^n h$ = conductance ($g(V)$), and $V - E_i$ = voltage (ΔV). Channels can be closed (C), open (O), or inactive (I) (Figure 2). Only the O-state produces an I_i. To be in any state, C, O, or I, depends on voltage and time: $I(V, t)$. A voltage change (ΔV) modifies the probability of being in any state. But velocity of change, or *time dependence*, is a main difference between ion channels, which is assessed by extracting time constants (τ_s) from current (I_i) records represented by (for example):

$$I_i(t) = r_1(1 - \exp(-t/\tau_m))^n \exp(-t/\tau_h) + r_2 \tag{2}$$

where τ_m is an activation time constant, τ_h is an inactivation time constant, r_1 and r_2 are constants, and n is the exponent that fits nonlinear kinetics (Figure 2). τ_s (h or m above) depend on voltage. Fitting I_i records for different voltages (I-V plots) with Equation 2 produces a family of τ_s (Figure 2) where $\tau \approx 1/(\alpha + \beta)$ and α is the forward rate constant, whereas β is the backward rate constant for changing state (Figure 2). Differences in *time dependence* dictated by τ_s make currents *transient, fast, slow, persistent*, or *slowly inactivating*.

Conductance, $g(V)$, measurements are also obtained from I-V plots, where Equation 1 is applied to each record to obtain $g(V)$,

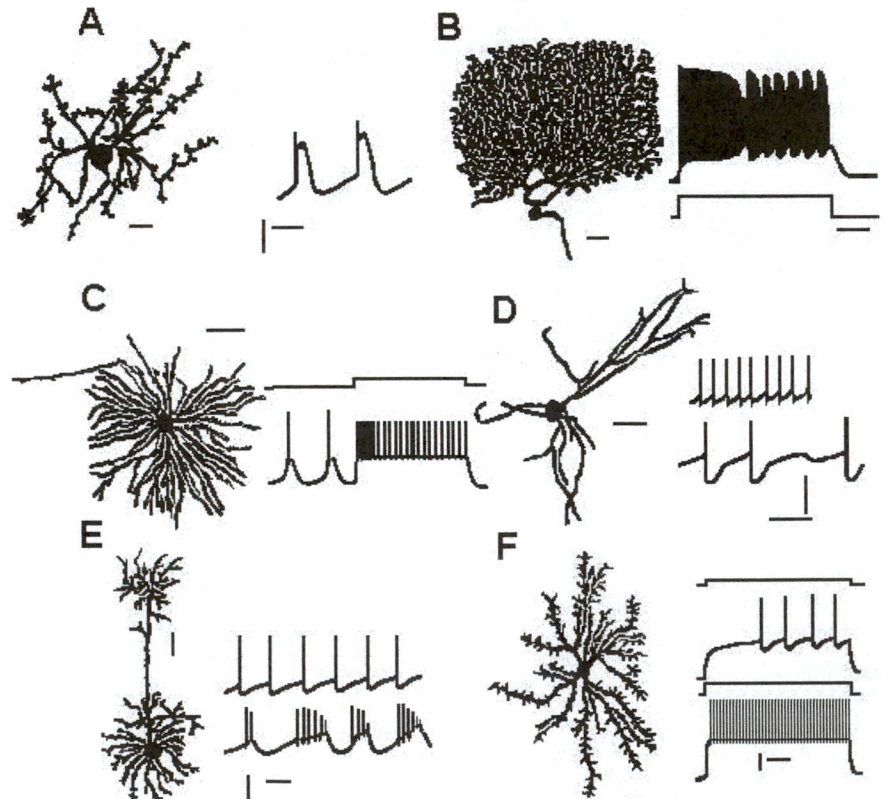

Figure 1. Neurons differ in morphology and firing pattern (see NEOCORTEX-BASIC NEURON TYPES). *A*, Inferior olive neuron. *B*, Cerebellar Purkinje cell. *C*, Thalamic relay neuron. *D*, Subtantia nigra compacta neuron. *E*, Cortical pyramidal neuron. *F*, Spiny neuron of the neostriatum.

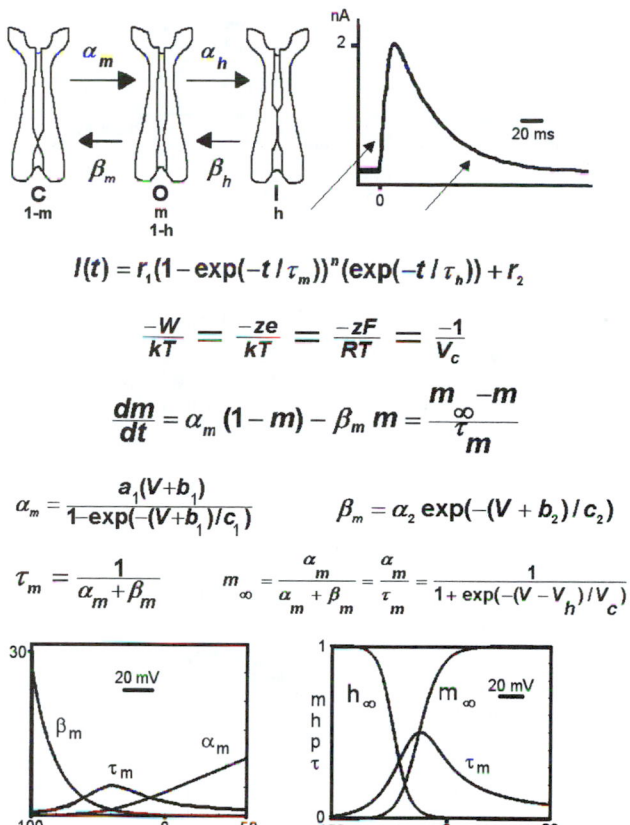

$$I(t) = r_1(1 - \exp(-t/\tau_m))^n(\exp(-t/\tau_h)) + r_2$$

$$\frac{-W}{kT} = \frac{-ze}{kT} = \frac{-zF}{RT} = \frac{-1}{V_c}$$

$$\frac{dm}{dt} = \alpha_m(1-m) - \beta_m m = \frac{m_\infty - m}{\tau_m}$$

$$\alpha_m = \frac{a_1(V+b_1)}{1-\exp(-(V+b_1)/c_1)} \qquad \beta_m = \alpha_2 \exp(-(V+b_2)/c_2)$$

$$\tau_m = \frac{1}{\alpha_m + \beta_m} \qquad m_\infty = \frac{\alpha_m}{\alpha_m + \beta_m} = \frac{\alpha_m}{\tau_m} = \frac{1}{1+\exp(-(V-V_h)/V_c)}$$

Figure 2. Channel function. At the top, a closed channel (C) may open (O) following rate constant α_m (below). The channel may close again following rate constant β_m or may inactivate (I) following rate constant α_h. Deinactivation follows rate constant β_h. $\tau_{m,h} \approx 1/\alpha + \beta$. Activation ($m_\infty$) and inactivation ($h_\infty$) functions can be obtained by plotting the conductance obtained from I-V plots. The bottom graph depicts relations between m_∞, τ, α, and β. Once α and β are obtained, a differential equation (dm/dt) describes the kinetics of a channel. Channels differ in voltage and time dependence.

which, plotted against V, forms a sigmoid function (Figure 2) called the *activation* (or *inactivation*) function (m_∞ and h_∞). $g(V)$ dictates the *voltage dependence* of the current and is the other main difference between ion channels, which are then *threshold, subthreshold,* or *suprathreshold* in respect to firing. $g(V)$ can be fitted to:

$$g(V) = G_{MAX}/(1 + \exp(\pm(V - V_h)/V_c)) \qquad (3)$$

(activation: $-$; inactivation $+$ sign). Where $G_{MAX} = g$ when all channels are open, V denotes voltage, V_h is the voltage at which half the channels are open, and V_c is the slope factor of the sigmoid equivalent to a Boltzmann exponent (RT/F or kT/e -in mV; ≈ 26 mV at 25°C), z denotes valence, $V - V_h$ is ΔV, and F, R, T, k, T, and e have their usual meaning (Figure 2). $g(V)$ is a cumulative Boltzmann distribution (Figure 2) but, normalizing $G_{MAX} = 1.0$, becomes a probability (P) function where m is the P to open and $1 - m$ is the P to close (Figure 2). *Inactivation* is denoted by h (Figure 2 uses p for both).

α and β define first-order kinetics: simple exponential solutions multiplied by constants (Figure 2) (Jack, Noble, and Tsien, 1975) or Boltzmann distributions. $g(V)$ is proportional to permeability

$(P(I, V))$, which can be obtained transforming I-V plots with the Goldman-Hodgkin-Katz equation for current,

$$P(I, V) = \frac{I}{V} \cdot \frac{RT}{(zF)^2} \cdot \left(\frac{\exp(-zFV/RT) - 1}{[C]_o \cdot \exp(-zFV/RT) - [C]_i} \right) \quad (4)$$

where $[C]_i$ denotes internal ion concentrations, $[C]_o$ denotes external ion concentrations, I is current, and V is voltage. $g(V)$ can also be obtained by differentiating the I-V plot or by using instantaneous I-V plots (tail currents).

In summary, V_h, V_c, and τ_s *characterize* ion conductances, i.e., $g(V)/\tau_m = \alpha_m$, etc., giving their time and voltage dependence. Neurons use an array of ion conductances differing in time, voltage dependence, and the ion carried. The concerted work of them makes up the firing properties or coding.

The activation function m (Equations 1 and 3) is raised to an n power, where n is the order of the kinetic reaction. Thus, nonlinearity arises by the parallel action of n first-order processes. Each represents the movement of a protein (channel) subunit or domain. All of them move for the whole channel molecule to change state. The sigmoidal delay to change may be viewed as the many "closed states" ($C_1, C_2, \ldots, C_n$) that have to be crossed before entering the "open state." Note that, since each channel is composed of several domains, nonlinearity arises at the molecular level. Imagine then what happens when many of such molecules combine to produce a firing pattern, when neurons possessing different arrays of these channels combine to form a neural net, and when nuclei possessing different nets arrange to produce a nervous system.

Inward or outward ion currents depend on the value of E_i or equilibrium potential of the ion (Equation 1). If E_i is less than firing threshold, I is a hyperpolarizing outward current that will tend to arrest firing (Figure 3). If E_i is greater than firing threshold, I is a depolarizing inward current that will promote firing. When a neuron increases firing, there is no a priori way to know whether an inward current was facilitated or an outward current was restrained.

Neuronal Specialization

Each neuronal class has a different set of ion conductances. The original HH model (see AXONAL MODELING), consisting of a transient inward current (Figures 3*B*1, 3*C*1), a persistent outward current (Figures 3*B*3, 3*C*2), and a leak current (Figure 3*A*2) (I_{Na}, I_K, and I_{leak}), gives a *basic firing mechanism* (BFM). Leak currents are made up of a family of K$^+$ channels with a double pore-forming domain in tandem (KCNK1-7, 9, 10, 12, 13, 16, 17) with 13 members. These channels make up the electrotonic structure or cable properties.

A good exercise using a simulator (e.g., Huguenard and Mc-Cormick, 1994) is to begin with the BFM (Figure 3*A*3) and then add one class of conductance at a time to see how the BFM is modified (column *A* in Figure 3). From top to bottom, the records in column *A* of Figure 3 show the BFM (Figure 3*A*3) with one auxiliary current at a time (Figures 3*A*4–9). Any firing pattern is due to a sum of conductances,

$$C\frac{Vd}{dt} = -\sum_i^n (I_i) = -(I_{Na} + I_k + I_{leak} + I_{to} + I_{so} + I_{ti} + I_{si} + \cdots + I_n) \quad (5)$$

where *to* denotes transient outward, *so* denotes slowly inactivating outward, *ti* denotes transient inward, *si* denotes slowly inactivating inward, and so on; C denotes capacitance. Column *D* shows a modeling experiment adding several auxiliary conductances in sequence.

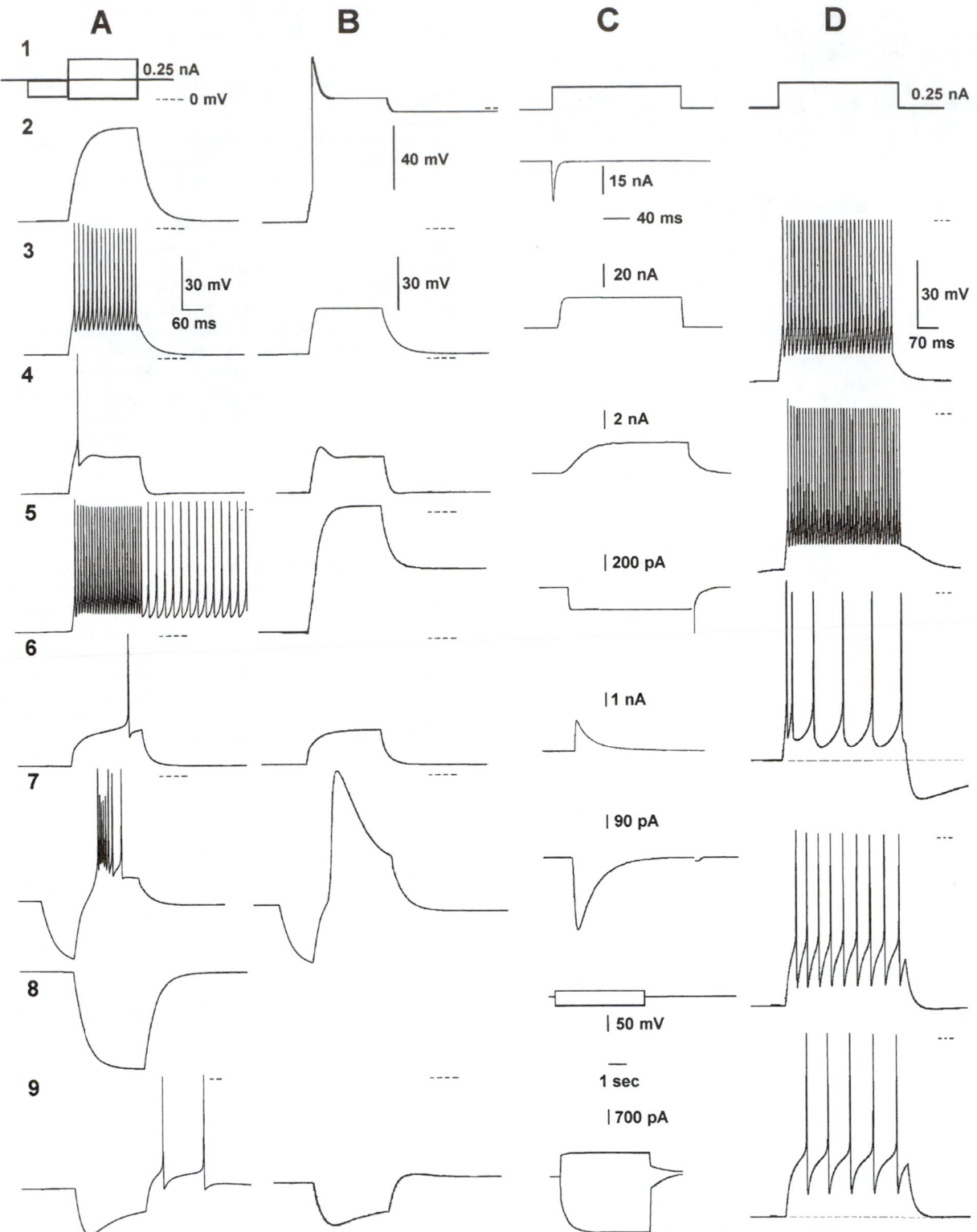

Figure 3. Firing patterns. Columns *A*, *B*, and *D* are voltage recordings; column *C* shows current recordings. *A1*, Stimuli. The main stimulus is a depolarizing current step. *A2*, I_{leak} produces RC responses. *A3*, I_{Na} and I_K are added to produce a basic firing mechanism (BFM). *A4*, BFM plus I_{SO} produces adaption. *A5*, BFM plus I_{SI} produces a plateau potential and increases firing. *A6*, BFM plus I_{TO} delays firing. *A7*, BFM plus I_{TI} produces bursting after a hyperpolarization. *A8*, Hyperpolarizing RC response (cf. *A2*). *A9*, BFM plus I_h produces rebound excitation. *B*, RC response plus-

$I_{Na}(B2)$, $I_K(B3)$, $I_{SO}(B4)$, $I_{SI}(B5)$, $I_{TO}(B6)$, $I_{TI}(B7)$, and $I_h(B9)$. *C*, A depolarizing command (*C1*) evokes $I_{Na}(C2)$, $I_K(C3)$, $I_{SO}(C4)$, $I_{SI}(C5)$, $I_{TO}(C6)$, $I_{TI}(C7)$, and hyperpolarizing and depolarizing commands (*C8*) elicit $I_h(C9)$. *D*, BFM after a depolarizing step (*D3*), plus subthreshold I_{Ca} (firing increases: *D4–5*), I_{SK} (AHP and adaptation increase while frequency decreases: *D6*), I_{BK} (frequency increases and there is less adaptation: *D7–8*), and I_D (frequency decreases and becomes regular; AHPs look smaller than *D9*) added in sequence.

Functional Classification

- Activated by depolarization
  Inward
    Transient (I_{ti})
    Slowly or incompletely inactivating (I_{si})
  Outward
    Transient (I_{to})
    Slowly or incompletely inactivating (I_{so})
- Activated by hyperpolarization
  Inward
    Cationic currents (pacemaking) (I_h)
  Outward
    Inward rectifiers (K_{ir})

Transient inward (l_{it}) currents are sodium currents (I_{Na} in Figure 3*C*2; Goldin, 2001) that inactivate quickly and produce the depolarizing phase of the spike (Figures 3*A*3, 3*B*2). One class, Nav1.1 to 1.9 or SCN1–11, is blocked by tetrodotoxin and saxitoxin, although some of them need high concentrations (SCN10, 11). A second class, Nav2.1 (SCN6, 7: SNS and NaN), is tetrodotoxin resistant. Certain types allow a small percentage of the current (<10%) without inactivation, generating a persistent current (e.g., Nav 1.6).

Another I_{ti} are calcium "T-currents" ($\alpha_{1G,H,I}$, I_T, or CACNA, blocked by kurtoxin) (Randal and Benham, 1999), which produce "low-threshold spikes" (sinoatrial node) (Figure 3*B*7) that trigger sodium spikes (in neurons), producing bursts (Figure 3*A*7). A previous hyperpolarization—an afterhyperpolarization (AHP) or an inhibitory synaptic potential (IPSP)—de-inactivates T-channels (Figure 3*A*7). Thalamic, nigral, pallidal, pontine, cortical, and many other neurons use I_T to fire in bursts after an IPSP, producing rebound excitation, postinhibitory afterdischarges, augmentation responses, and slow rhythmic bursting, like that seen in spindle waves (see Oscillatory and Bursting Properties of Neurons). At depolarized potentials, T-channels are inactive.

Thus, neurons are able to respond differently depending on previous membrane potential. This allows a net to behave differently at different moments, while using the same neuronal elements (multitask networks). Since APs can be evoked from two different membrane potentials, the neuron has two functionally different firing thresholds. A neuron may have more than one threshold, and different firing patterns may be evoked from each threshold.

Transient outward (I_{to}) currents are potassium currents or I_A (e.g., Kv1 and Kv4 families, or KCN1,4, blocked by dendrotoxin and aminopyridines) (Figure 3*C*6). They oppose I_T. Inactivating between spikes, they set a stereotyped behavior between APs pacing tonic firing (Figure 3*D*9) at low frequencies. When subthreshold, they oppose any depolarization (Figure 3*B*6), so that membrane potential reaches threshold with a delay: I_A "retards" membrane trajectory toward threshold (Figure 3*A*6). A "conditioning" stimulus inactivates I_A, increasing responses with time, so that a previous subthreshold stimulus may reach threshold after a delay (*facilitation*).

A number of genes, differing in τ_h, code for I_A (Shieh et al., 2000). Hence, firing latency and rhythmic firing depend on voltage and time, expanding the I/O function (see column *D* of Figure 3).

Slowly inactivating inward (I_{si}) currents inactivate after several hundreds of milliseconds or seconds. On a short time scale they may be viewed as persistent. They are calcium currents, or persistent components of some sodium currents, or cationic currents. Their activation produces a depolarization that adds to the stimulus, enhancing it (Figure 3*B*5; cf. Figure 3*A*2) and increasing firing (Figure 3*A*5). Calcium channels come in two families, L ($\alpha_{1S,C,D,F}$ or CACNA-S,C,D,F) and non-L ($\alpha_{1A,B,E}$ or CACNA-A,B,E). L channels are blocked by calciseptine and dihydropyridines. Their inactivation depends on intracellular Ca^{2+} and voltage: Ca^{2+} en-

ters and shuts down the channel (feedback). Inactivation of the non-L family depends mainly on voltage (except for P).

I_{si} produce "plateau potentials" that sustain repetitive firing (Figure 3*D*5; cf. Figure 3*D*3) and bistable properties, i.e., two stable membrane potentials that alternate. There is a gain in the I/O function during plateaus. In the dendrites, slow synaptic depolarizations (NMDA) boost plateaus produced by I_{si}.

Activated during the spike, I_{si} contribute to it and to activating the potassium conductances that generate the AHP (Figure 3*D*6). Plateau potentials, bistability, dendritic spikes, and activation of outward currents are only some roles of I_{si}. Calcium entry has many other roles: in transmitter release, muscle contraction, cytoskeleton function, enzyme and gene activation, and so on.

Slowly inactivating outward (I_{so}) potassium currents (Figure 3*C*4) consist of (1) Kv channels as Kv2,3 or KCNA–D, 1–4; (2) KvLQT or KCNQ1–5, HERG or KCNH1–4, which are blocked by TEA, noxiustoxin, etc. (Shieh et al., 2000); (3) SK and IK channels or KCNN1–3 and KCNN4, respectively, which are blocked by apamin and charybdotoxin and activated by intracellular calcium; and (4) slow channels, BK or KCNMA1, which are blocked by TEA, iberiotoxin, and charybdotoxin (Shieh et al., 2000) and activated by voltage and intracellular calcium. All tend to maintain a quiet membrane-opposing depolarizing stimulus (Figure 3*B*4), spikes, inward currents, and plateau potentials. They decrease excitability, decrease or arrest firing frequency, and augment firing threshold. Depolarization activates I_{so}, it hyperpolarizes the membrane and then shuts down again (feedback). The BFM (Figure 3*A*3) becomes adapting firing (Figure 3*A*4) if a slow outward current (Figure 3*C*4) is superimposed. Conversely, when I_{so} is blocked, a frequency gain occurs. Note that several I_{so} depend on calcium accumulation. Ca^{2+} enters with each spike, allowing a short-time memory. Calcium-dependent gating of AHP opens a fraction of channels, depending on the number of spikes fired (digital to analog conversion) (Figure 3*D*6). The AHP fixes the time interval between spikes or trains of spikes and ends episodes of increased excitability, sets the pace for rhythmic firing and bursting, and allows frequency control and adaptation (see Thalamus). Firing depends on calcium dynamics (see column *D* in Figure 3) because all neurons posses some variety of a calcium-dependent I_{so}. Thus, firing mechanisms have to simulate calcium dynamics to be realistic.

Inward currents activated by hyperpolarization (I_h) or HCN1–4 blocked by cesium (Kaupp and Seifert, 2001) activate when the membrane potential hyperpolarizes below firing threshold, producing voltage "sags" ($E_i \approx -35$ mV) that oppose the same hyperpolarization (Figure 3*B*9). They contribute to rebound "humps" that may attain firing (Figure 3*A*9) when the hyperpolarization is over. I_h, I_T, and I_A, acting in concert, produce rhythmic bursting (see Sleep Oscillations). I_h are "pacemaking currents" that allow spontaneous firing: an AP produces an AHP; the AHP activates I_h, which then depolarizes the membrane back to fire another AP, which is followed by another AHP that repeats the cycle, keeping the cell firing. When I_h reaches the threshold for T-channels during rebound, a low-threshold Ca spike and bursting may ensue. Since the cycle (e.g., the orbit in the phase plane) is initiated by a hyperpolarization, the cell has a "threshold" going in the hyperpolarizing direction (an unstable singular point that initiates the entire orbit).

Outward currents activated by hyperpolarization ($K_{ir}s$) are inward rectifier potassium channels composed of four domains, each with only two transmembrane segments. Strong activation by a hyperpolarization produces inward potassium currents (K_{ir} or KCNJ1–15, blocked by cesium and barium) (Shieh et al., 2000), but no physiological stimulus hyperpolarizes the cell beyond E_K. Thus, the role of these channels is to *close* when the cell is depolarized. At rest, some channels are open and participate in the resting membrane potential and cable properties. When synaptic entries depolarize the cell, K_{ir} current shuts down and all inputs increase their value abruptly, since electrotonic length has shrink.

The threshold is dynamic. It depends on $K_{ir}s$, which act as a gate, requiring a convergence of inputs to pass the signal. A sum of synaptic inputs is not responsible for firing, but a complex interaction of intrinsic and synaptic conductances change the I/O function. Activation of $K_{ir}s$ depends on the potential and on extracellular potassium, which depend on the excitability level (synchronicity).

Discussion

Brain neuronal circuits are complex and dynamic. Ion channels endow neurons with properties such as multiple thresholds, different firing patterns associated with each threshold, the possibility of switching between different firing patterns, timing, multiple time constants for spike frequency adaptation, a changing electrotonic length, pacemaking, intrinsic facilitation, gating, bistable properties, short memory traces, etc. Each ion current contributes to a set of properties. Many ion conductances modify the BFM. Different firing patterns are shaped by previous activity and modulation. Accordingly, neuronal nets dynamically switch between different firing states and different configurations of synaptic weights: n thresholds and n firing levels due to n ion conductances activated at each level. A different pattern at each level will reach synaptic terminals differently. Each pattern encompasses a different I/O function. An I/O function may favor learning, while others may favor consolidation. Some would be preferred by sensory neurons, others by intermediate or motor neurons. Some net-states induce resonance between a set of nuclei. Other net-states decouple these nuclei but may couple other nuclei.

The simple picture used here to hint into this complexity is an abstraction. Nonlinearities produce many counterintuitive outcomes. One example is shown in column D of Figure 3, in which several conductances were added in sequence (from top to bottom) to the BFM (in Figures 3D3–4): a subthreshold Ca current (Figures D4–5)-enhanced evoked discharge, a Ca-activated SK-type current (Figure 3D6) decreased firing frequency and increased AHPs and adaptation, but addition of a BK type of current did not decrease firing (Figure 3D8) but, surprisingly, increased firing and produced less adaptation. The addition of I_A (with a rather slow τ_h) produced

tonic firing with very low firing frequencies never reached by BFM alone (e.g., as in a neostriatal spiny neuron). Comparing the AHPs of records in Figure 3D6 and Figure 3D9, one would not imagine that the firing in Figure 3D9 involved more outward current.

Road Map: Biological Neurons and Synapses
Related Reading: Activity-Dependent Regulation of Neuronal Conductances; Biophysical Mechanisms in Neuronal Modeling; Biophysical Mosaic of the Neuron; Neocortex: Chemical and Electrical Synapses

References

Arbib, M. A., 1964, *Brains, Machines, and Mathematics*, New York: McGraw-Hill.
Cajal, S. R., 1899, *Textura del Sistema Nervioso del Hombre y de Los Vertebrados*, Madrid: Universidad de Alicante.
Goldin, A. L., 2001, Resurgence of sodium channel research, *Annu. Rev. Physiol.*, 63:871–894.
Hodgkin, A. L., and Huxley, A. F., 1952, A quantitative description of membrane current and its application to conduction and excitation in nerve, *J. Physiol. (Lond.)*, 117:500–544.
Huguenard, J., and McCormick, D. A., 1994, *Electrophysiology of the Neuron*, New York: Oxford University Press. ◆
Isomoto, S., Kondo, C., and Kurachi, Y., 1997, Inwardly rectifying potassium channels: The molecular heterogeneity and function, *Jpn. J. Physiol.*, 47:11–39.
Jack, J. J. B., Noble, D., and Tsien, R. W., 1975, *Electric Current flow in Excitable Cells*, Oxford: Clarendon Press. ◆
Kaupp, U. B., and Seifert, R., 2001, Molecular diversity of pacemaker ion channels, *Annu. Rev. Physiol.*, 63:235–257.
Llinás, R., 1988, The intrinsic electrophysiological properties of mammalian neurons: Insights into central nervous system function, *Science*, 242:1654–1664.
Nicoll, R. A., 1988, The coupling of neurotransmitter receptors to ion channels in the brain, *Science*, 241:545–451.
Randall, A., and Benham, C. D., 1999, Recent advances in the molecular understanding of voltage-gated Ca^{2+} channels, *Mol. Cell. Neurosci.*, 14:255–272.
Shieh, C.-C., Coghlan, M., Sullivan, J. P., and Gopalakrishnan, M., 2000, Potassium channels: Molecular defects, diseases, and therapeutic opportunities, *Pharmacol. Rev.*, 52:557–593
Suri, R. E., Bargas, J., and Arbib, M. A., 2001, Modeling functions of striatal dopamine modulation in learning and planning, *Neuroscience*, 103:65–85.

Kalman Filtering: Neural Implications

Simon Haykin

Introduction

The time-domain description of a system by a *state-space model*, depicted in Figure 1, is of profound importance. The notion of state plays a key role in the formulation of this model. The *state*, denoted by the vector $\mathbf{x}(n)$, is defined as any set of quantities that would be sufficient to uniquely describe the unforced dynamic behavior of the system at discrete time n. The model of Figure 1 is not only mathematically convenient, it also offers a close relationship to physical/neurobiological reality and a basis for accounting for the statistical behavior of the system.

The state-space model of Figure 1 embodies two basic equations:

1. *Process equation*

$$\mathbf{x}(n+1) = \mathbf{F}(n+1, n)\mathbf{x}(n) + v_1(n) \qquad (1)$$

where $\mathbf{F}(n+1, n)$ is a transition matrix and the vector $v_1(n)$ is an additive dynamic noise.

2. *Measurement equation*

$$\mathbf{y}(n) = \mathbf{C}(\mathbf{n})\mathbf{x}(n) + v_2(n) \qquad (2)$$

where the vector $\mathbf{y}(n)$ is the *observation*, $\mathbf{C}(n)$ is a *measurement matrix*, and the vector $v_2(n)$ is an additive *measurement noise*.

Typically, the state $\mathbf{x}(i)$ is hidden and therefore unknown, and the requirement is to estimate it using a sequence of observations $\mathbf{y}(1), \mathbf{y}(2), \ldots, \mathbf{y}(n)$. The sequential estimation problem is called *filtering* if $i = n$, *prediction* if $i > n$, and *smoothing* if $1 \le i < n$. Unlike smoothing, both filtering and prediction are real-time operations. In this article, we only consider prediction and filtering, which are closely related.

Kalman Filters

In a classic paper, Kalman (1960) derived a general solution for the *linear* filtering problem, and with it the celebrated *Kalman filter*

Figure 1. Signal-flow graph representation of a linear, discrete-time dynamical system.

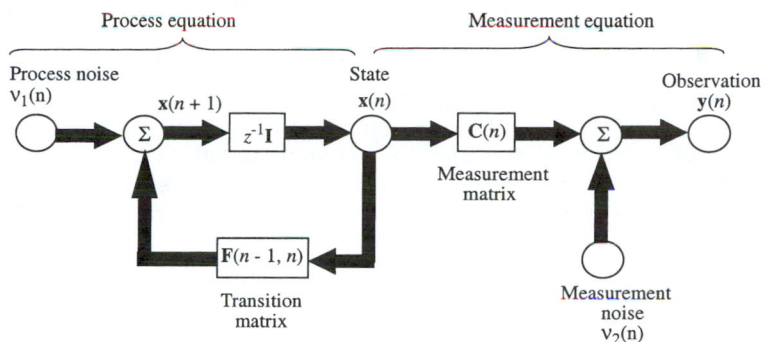

was born. Assuming that the dynamic noise $v_1(n)$ and measurement noise $v_2(n)$ are independent, white, and Gaussian processes, the Kalman filter is a recursive estimator that is optimum in the minimum mean-square error or, equivalently, maximum likelihood sense (Jazwinski, 1970).

Let $\mathbf{Y}_{n-1}$ denote the subspace spanned by the observations $\mathbf{y}(1)$, $\mathbf{y}(2), \ldots, \mathbf{y}(n-1)$. Given the new observation $\mathbf{y}(n)$, the current estimate of the state denoted by $\hat{\mathbf{x}}(n|\mathbf{Y}_{n-1})$ is recursively updated as follows:

$$\hat{\mathbf{x}}(n+1|\mathbf{Y}_n) = \mathbf{F}(n+1, n)\hat{\mathbf{x}}(n|\mathbf{Y}_{n-1}) + \mathbf{G}(n)\alpha(n) \quad (3)$$

where $\mathbf{G}(n)$ is the *gain matrix*, and the vector

$$\alpha(n) = \mathbf{y}(n) - \mathbf{C}(n)\hat{\mathbf{x}}(n|\mathbf{Y}_{n-1}) \quad (4)$$

is the *innovation*, representing the part of $\mathbf{y}(n)$ that is new. Equations 3 and 4 show that the underlying structure of the Kalman filter is in the closed-loop form of a *predictor-corrector*, consisting of two steps:

1. *Measurement update*, which uses the current observation $\mathbf{y}(n)$ to compute the innovation $\alpha(n)$.
2. *Time update*, which uses $\alpha(n)$ to update the past estimate $\hat{\mathbf{x}}(n|\mathbf{Y}_{n-1})$.

In addition to Equations 3 and 4, the Kalman filter involves three other basic steps (Haykin, 2002):

1. *Computation* of the gain matrix $\mathbf{G}(n)$ in terms of an error covariance matrix $\mathbf{K}(n, n-1)$, where the error refers to the difference between the true state $\mathbf{x}(n)$ and the current estimate $\hat{\mathbf{x}}(n|\mathbf{Y}_{n-1})$.
2. *Time updating* of the error covariance matrix $\mathbf{K}(n, n-1)$ via the so-called *Riccati equation*.
3. *Initialization* of the filter by setting $\hat{\mathbf{x}}(1|\mathbf{Y}_0) = \mathbf{0}$ and $\mathbf{K}(1, 0) = \Pi_0$, where $\mathbf{0}$ is the null vector and Π_0 is a prescribed diagonal matrix.

The computational complexity of the Kalman filter is of order M^2, where M is the dimensionality of the state space.

A serious limitation of the standard Kalman filter is that it is prone to unstable behavior that may arise due to model mismatch and use of finite-precision arithmetic. The origin of the problem is traced to the fact that in situations of this kind, the Riccati equation may *not* result in a non-negative definite solution for the error covariance matrix $\mathbf{K}(n, n-1)$, which is unacceptable. (An important property of a covariance matrix is that it must be non-negative definite.) The unstable behavior of the Kalman filter is referred to as the *divergence phenomenon*.

To overcome this phenomenon, we may use *square-root filtering*, whereby the square root of the error covariance matrix rather than the error covariance matrix itself is propagated through the filter. According to the *Cholesky factorization*, we may write

$$\mathbf{K}(n, n-1) = \mathbf{K}^{1/2}(n, n-1)\mathbf{K}^{T/2}(n, n-1) \quad (5)$$

where $\mathbf{K}^{1/2}(n, n-1)$ is a lower triangular matrix (i.e., all the elements above the main diagonal are zero), and $\mathbf{K}^{T/2}(n, n-1)$ is its transpose. The important thing to note here is that the product of a lower triangular matrix and its transpose is unlikely to become indefinite.

The discussion up to this point rests on the premise that the state-space model of Equations 1 and 2 is linear. What if the model is nonlinear, as shown by the equations

$$\mathbf{x}(n+1) = \mathbf{f}(n, \mathbf{x}(n)) + v_1(n) \quad (6)$$

$$\mathbf{y}(n) = \mathbf{c}(n, \mathbf{x}(n)) + v_2(n) \quad (7)$$

where $\mathbf{f}$ and $\mathbf{c}$ are time-varying, vector-valued functions? The explicit dependence on time n accounts for a possibility that the equations are time varying. To deal with this new situation, we may extend the use of the standard Kalman filter. Specifically, the nonlinear process equation (Equation 6) and the nonlinear measurement equation (Equation 7) are linearized at each iteration of the filter around most recent estimates of the state, which is achieved by retaining the first-order terms in the Taylor series expansions of the nonlinear functions $\mathbf{f}$ and $\mathbf{c}$. For obvious reasons, the resulting filter is referred to as the *extended Kalman filter*, or EKF (Jazwinski, 1970; Haykin, 2002).

Supervised Training of Neural Networks

The Kalman filter offers two important properties: (1) estimation of the state using the entire past sequence of observations, and (2) use of second-order information in the form of an error covariance matrix. These two properties make the Kalman filter into a powerful tool for the supervised training of neural networks. The issue of concern here is how to proceed with this approach in a computationally feasible manner without compromising the application of Kalman filter theory. The answer lies in using a *decoupled* form of the extended Kalman filter, in which the computational complexity is made to suit the requirements of a particular application and available computational resources (Puskorius and Feldkamp, 2001).

In this article, we consider the supervised training of a recurrent multilayer perceptron (RMLP), for which the decoupled extended Kalman filter (DEKF) has established itself as an enabling technology by solving some difficult signal processing and control problems.

Let the vector $\mathbf{w}(n)$ denote the synaptic weights of the entire RMLP at iteration n. With adaptive filtering in mind and $\mathbf{w}(n)$ viewed as a state of the RMLP, we may formulate the state-space model of the network as (Haykin, 1999)

$$\mathbf{w}(n + 1) = \mathbf{w}(n) + v_1(n) \qquad (8)$$

$$\mathbf{d}_0(n) = \mathbf{c}(\mathbf{w}(n), \mathbf{u}(n), \mathbf{v}(n)) + v_2(n) \qquad (9)$$

Equation 8 describes a diffusion process. The vector-valued function $\mathbf{c}$ accounts for the overall nonlinearity from the input layer to the output layer of the RMLP. The arguments $\mathbf{u}(n)$ and $\mathbf{v}(n)$ of the function $\mathbf{c}$ denote the signal vector applied to the input layer and the vector of recurrent activation potentials at internal nodes of the RMLP, respectively. The vector $v_1(n)$ denotes noise *artificially* introduced into the process equation, and the vector $v_2(n)$ denotes additive noise in the measured data. The vector $\mathbf{d}_0(n)$ is the desired response of the RMLP.

There are two contexts in which the term "state" is used here:

- The network's weights, $\mathbf{w}(n)$, which are adjusted during training.
- The recurrent activation functions, $\mathbf{v}(n)$, which continue to evolve nonlinearly with time once the training ends.

By comparing the model of Equations 8 and 9 for the RMLP with the linear dynamical model of Equations 1 and 2, we see that the difference between these two models is in the nonlinear form of the measurement equation (Equation 9). This matter is taken care of through linearization, thereby facilitating application of the EKF. This linearization requires the partial derivatives of the output(s) of the RMLP with respect to its weights. (Backpropagation through time provides an efficient algorithm for computing these partial derivatives.) Decoupling is introduced into the extended Kalman filtering algorithm by assuming that the interactions between the estimates of certain weights in the RMLP can be ignored, the effect of which is to introduce zeros into the error covariance matrix. If the weights are decoupled so that certain subgroups of weights are mutually exclusive of one another, then the error covariance matrix can be arranged into a block-diagonal form, thereby reducing the computational burden of the algorithm (Puskorius and Feldkamp, 2001).

Two noteworthy points on the use of Kalman filtering for the supervised training of recurrent networks are:

1. Introduction of the artificial noise $v_1(n)$ in the process equation (Equation 8) has the desirable effects of accelerating the convergence process and enhancing the likelihood of reaching a global minimum of the error performance surface. Through the use of an annealing procedure, the effect of $v_1(n)$ can be gradually reduced as the network approaches an equilibrium condition.
2. The presence of second-order information in the form of error covariance matrix has the desirable effect of overcoming the vanishing gradients problem that arises when a recurrent network is trained with a gradient-based algorithm such as the real-time recurrent learning algorithm (Haykin, 1999).

Dynamic Model of Visual Recognition

The visual cortex is endowed with two key anatomical properties:

- *Abundant use of feedback.* The connections between any two connected areas of the visual cortex are bilateral, thereby accommodating the transmission of forward as well as feedback signals between the interconnected cortical areas.
- *Hierarchical multiscale structure.* The receptive fields of lower-area cells in the visual cortex span only a small fraction of the visual field, whereas the receptive fields of higher-area cells increase in size until they span almost the entire visual field. It is this constrained network structure that makes it possible for the fully connected visual cortex to perform prediction in a high-

dimensional data space with a reduced number of free parameters and therefore in a computationally efficient manner.

Rao and Ballard (1997) exploit these two properties of the visual cortex to build a dynamic model of visual recognition, recognizing that vision is fundamentally a nonlinear dynamic process. The motivation for building the model was to explain the way in which the responses of cells in the visual cortex are significantly modulated by stimuli from beyond the classical receptive field. This modulation can be exerted from multiple sources, including the higher-level systems that are activated when an animal views a natural scene.

The Rao-Ballard model of visual recognition is a hierarchically organized neural network, with each intermediate level of the hierarchy receiving two kinds of information: bottom-up information from the preceding level, and top-down information from the higher level. For its implementation, the model uses a multiscale estimation algorithm that may be viewed as a hierarchical form of the extended Kalman filter. In particular, the EKF is used to simultaneously learn the feedforward, feedback, and prediction parameters of the model using visual experiences in a dynamic environment. The resulting adaptive processes operate on two different time scales:

- A *fast* dynamic state-estimation process, which allows the dynamic model to anticipate incoming stimuli.
- A *slow* Hebbian learning process, which provides for synaptic weight adjustments in the model.

In a subsequent study, Patel, Becker, and Racine (2001) studied the use of an RMLP trained with the DEKF algorithm to deal with high-dimensional signals, namely, moving visual images. The particular problem dealt with is the tracking of objects that vary in both shape and location, which is a challenging problem. By making use of short-term continuity, Patel et al. show that their model is capable of tracking a mixture of different geometric shapes (circles, squares, and triangles). As with the Rao-Ballard dynamic model of visual recognition, the Patel-Becker-Racine model is designed with a hierarchical structure; specifically, the first hidden layer of neurons in the RMLP was connected to relatively small, local regions of the visual field applied to the input layer, and a subsequent hidden layer spanned the entire visual field. The Patel-Becker-Racine model may be viewed as a first step toward modeling the dynamic mechanism by which the human brain might be simultaneously recognizing and tracking moving stimuli.

Hypothesis That the Cerebellum Is a Neural Analog of a Dynamic State Estimator

The cerebellum has an important role to play in the control and coordination of movements, which are ordinarily carried out in a very smooth and almost effortless manner. The fundamental issue to be resolved here is whether the cerebellum plays the role of a controller or a dynamic state estimator, in light of what we know about modern control theory. Unfortunately, this issue cannot be resolved solely on the basis of the evidence that cerebellar damage or disease causes inaccuracy or instability of movements.

The key point in support of the dynamic state-estimation hypothesis is embodied in the following statement, the validity of which has been confirmed by decades of work on the design of automatic tracking and guidance systems: *Any system, be it a biological or artificial system, required to predict and/or control the trajectory of a stochastic multivariate dynamic system, can only do so by using or invoking the essence of Kalman filtering in one way or another.*

Building on this key point, Paulin (1997) presented several lines of evidence that favor the hypothesis that the cerebellum is a neural analog of a dynamic state estimator. A particular line of evidence presented therein relates to the vestibulo-ocular reflex (VOR), which is part of the oculomotor system. The function of the VOR is to maintain visual (i.e., retinal) image stability by making eye rotations that are opposite to head rotations. This function is mediated by a neural network that includes the cerebellar cortex and vestibular nuclei. Now, from modern control theory we know that a Kalman filter is an optimum linear system with minimum mean-square error for predicting the state trajectory of a dynamic system using noisy measurements; it does so by estimating the particular state trajectory that is most likely, given an assumed model for the underlying dynamics of the system. A consequence of this strategy is that when the dynamic system deviates from the assumed model, the Kalman filter makes estimation errors of a predictable kind, which may be attributed to the filter believing in the assumed model rather than the actual sense data. According to Paulin (1997), estimation errors of this kind are observed in the behavior of the VOR.

The important point to note, in this brief discussion of the hypothesis that the cerebellum is a neural analog of a Kalman filter, is that the hypothesis is *not* to be taken to imply that the cerebellum physically resembles a Kalman filter. Rather, the cerebellum may provide information in the nervous system, which is analogous to state estimation in a Kalman filter.

From Kalman Filters to Particle Filters

Many dynamical phenomena, whether biological or physical, that are encountered in practice are inherently very complex, involving one or more of the following elements: nonlinearity, non-Gaussianity, and high dimensionality. The EKF deals with the first two elements by doing two things:

- Localized linearization of the nonlinear functions in the process and measurement equations by retaining first-order terms in their Taylor series expansions.
- Approximations of the process and measurement processes by Gaussian processes that are propagated analytically through the first-order approximations of the nonlinear functions.

The practical limitation of this approach is that it may produce large errors in the state estimates.

An analytic approach to circumvent this problem is to use the unscented Kalman filter, which builds on the *unscented transformation* due to Julier, Uhlmann, and Durrant-Whyte (1995). In this new transformation, the input stochastic process is again approximated by a Gaussian process, but the nonlinear transformation is treated in a special way involving a carefully chosen set of sample points. To be specific, let the vector $\bar{\mathbf{x}}$ and the matrix $\mathbf{K_x}$ respectively denote the mean and covariance of a stochastic process $\mathbf{x}(n)$ whose dimensionality is M. Let $\mathbf{x}(n)$ be propagated through a nonlinear function: $\mathbf{y} = \mathbf{f}(x)$. To calculate the mean and covariance of the output vector $\mathbf{y}(n)$, we first form a set of $2M + 1$ *sigma vectors*, defined by

$$
\left.
\begin{aligned}
\chi_0 &= \bar{\mathbf{x}} \\
\chi_i &= \bar{\mathbf{x}} + \sqrt{M + \lambda}(\mathbf{K_x}^{1/2})_i \quad i = 1, 2, \ldots, M \\
\chi_i &= \bar{\mathbf{x}} - \sqrt{M + \lambda}(\mathbf{K_x}^{1/2})_i \quad i = M + 1, M + 2, \ldots, 2M
\end{aligned}
\right\}
$$

$$(10)$$

where λ is a scaling factor under the designer's control, and $(K_x^{1/2})_i$ is the ith column of the square root of matrix $\mathbf{K_x}$ (i.e., lower triangular matrix in the Cholesky factorization of $\mathbf{K_x}$). The mean and covariance of the nonlinearly transformed vector $\mathbf{y}(n)$ are ob-

tained by using weighted sums of a new vector $\mathbf{y}_i$ related to the sigma vectors as

$$\mathbf{Y}_i = \mathbf{f}(\chi_i), \quad i = 1, 2, \ldots, M$$

For an arbitrary nonlinearity, the deceptively simple unscented transformation produces approximations that are accurate to third order for Gaussian inputs, and at least second order for non-Gaussian inputs. The *unscented Kalman filter* (UKF) is a straightforward extension of the unscented transformation (Wan and van der Merwe, 2001). It is a derivative-free state estimator in that, by using multiple forward propagations, the need for explicit computation of Jacobians is avoided; hence, differentiable nonlinear functions are no longer a necessary requirement. The computational complexity of the UKF is, in general, $O(M^3)$; but under special conditions the computation can be restructured to be $O(M^2)$, which is essentially the same as that for the EKF.

The EKF and UKF rely on the use of approximations to ensure mathematical tractability. To avoid approximations, we have to sacrifice mathematical tractability. This is precisely what is done in particle filters, which are rooted in Bayesian theory (Bernardo and Smith, 1998) and Monte Carlo simulation (Robert and Casella, 1999).

Particle filters provide a tool for recursive computation of a stochastic point-mass approximation to the posterior distribution of the hidden states of a nonlinear dynamic system, given a set of observations related to the states. These filters are based on the following stochastic model (Andrieu, Doucet, and Punskaya, 2001):

1. The hidden states are described by the initial distribution $p(\mathbf{x}(0))$ and transition distribution $p(\mathbf{x}(n)|\mathbf{X}_{n-1})$.
2. The observations $\mathbf{y}(1), \mathbf{y}(2), \ldots, \mathbf{y}(n)$ are conditionally independent, given the likelihood $p(\mathbf{y}(n)|\mathbf{Y}_{n-1}, \mathbf{x}(n))$.

The goal of particle filtering is to recursively estimate the *posterior distribution* $p(\mathbf{X}_n|\mathbf{Y}_n)$, the *filtering distribution* $p(\mathbf{x}(n)|\mathbf{Y}_n)$, and certain expectations such as the conditional mean and conditional covariance of $\mathbf{x}(n)$, where $\mathbf{X}_n$ denotes the sequence $\mathbf{x}(0), \mathbf{x}(1), \ldots, \mathbf{x}(n)$, and $\mathbf{Y}_n$ denotes the sequence $\mathbf{y}(1), \mathbf{y}(2), \ldots, \mathbf{y}(n)$. Note that the model described under points 1 and 2 defines a generic dynamic model, embodying hidden Markov models as a special case.

In Monte Carlo simulation, a set of weighted, independent, and identically distributed particles (i.e., samples) is drawn from the posterior distribution, thereby mapping integrals to discrete sums. Typically, it is not possible to sample directly from the posterior distribution; hence the recourse to *importance sampling* from an arbitrary *proposal distribution*. The choice of the proposal is a major design issue. In this context, we may use approximations based on the EKF or UKF to generate Gaussian proposal distributions. Basically, the use of UKF here leads to the formulation of the unscented particle filter (Wan and van der Merwe, 2001). Some nice results on image tracking using the unscented particle filter are reported in Rui and Chen (2001).

A limitation of importance sampling is that it does not lend itself to recursive estimation. To get around this problem, we may use a constrained version of importance sampling known as *sequential importance sampling*. The use of this approach yields a set of parameters known as *normalized importance weights*; they are involved in recursively computing the conditional expectations of interest.

Unfortunately, sequential importance sampling has a serious limitation of its own: The variance of the normalized importance weights increases stochastically over time. Typically, after a few iterations the normalized weights of a large number of particles (samples) become practically insignificant, with the result that they are removed from the sample set, in which case the algorithm no longer adequately represents the posterior distribution of interest. This degeneracy problem is avoided by using a *bootstrap filter*, which involves the elimination of samples with small weights and the multiplication of samples with large weights. The bootstrap filter is essentially modular in extent and therefore simple to implement.

A particle filter may be made highly efficient (i.e., the variance of the estimation error is reduced) by using the so-called Rao-Blackwellization procedure (Robert and Casella, 1999). In so doing, each particle is replaced by a Gaussian distribution propagated through a Kalman filter. The Rao-Blackwellized particle filter represents a stochastic bank (i.e., mixture) of standard Kalman filters (de Freitas, 2002).

To sum up, particle filters offer a powerful tool for sequential state estimation under full nonlinear and non-Gaussian conditions. Although it is computationally intensive, it lends itself to straightforward implementation on a parallel computer.

Discussion

Kalman filtering is a powerful idea rooted in modern control theory and adaptive signal processing; it has withstood the test of time since 1960. Under the ideal conditions of linearity and Gaussianity, the Kalman filter produces an estimate of the hidden state of a dynamic system, with the estimate being optimum in the mean-square-error sense or, equivalently, the maximum likelihood sense. The state-estimation procedure is recursive, which makes it well suited for implementation on a digital computer.

In practical terms, the Kalman filter provides an indispensable tool for the design of automatic tracking and guidance systems, and an enabling technology for the design of recurrent multilayer perceptrons that can simulate any finite-state machine. In the context of neurobiology, Kalman filtering provides invaluable insight into visual recognition and motor control.

The classic Kalman filter and its extensions, namely, the extended Kalman filter and the unscented Kalman filter, offer mathematical tractability by invoking certain approximations and Gaussian assumptions. When the issue of approximations and Gaussian assumptions is of serious concern, we may resort to another powerful tool, particle filters, which are rooted in Bayesian theory and Monte Carlo simulation. Again, particle filters are computationally intensive, but with a parallel computer, they can be implemented in a straightforward modular fashion.

Acknowledgments. Input from Michael Arbib, Sue Becker, Nando de Freitas, and Ron Racine is much appreciated.

Road Maps: Applications; Vision
Related Reading: Filtering, Adaptive; Sensorimotor Learning

References

Andrieu, C., Doucet, A., and Punskaya, E., 2001, Sequential Monte Carlo methods for optimal filtering, in *Sequential Monte Carlo Methods in Practice* (A. Doucet, N. de Freitas, and N. Gordon, Eds.), New York: Springer-Verlag. ◆

Bernardo, J. M., and Smith, A. F. M., 1998, *Bayesian Theory*, New York: Wiley.

de Freitas, N., 2002, Rao-Blackwellised particle filtering for fault diagnosis, presented at a meeting of the IEEE AC, paper no. 493.

Haykin, S., 2002, *Adaptive Filter Theory*, 4th ed., Englewood Cliffs, NJ: Prentice-Hall. ◆

Haykin, S., 1999, *Neural Networks: A Comprehensive Foundation*, 2nd ed., Englewood Cliffs, NJ: Prentice-Hall.

Jazwinski, A. H., 1970, *Stochastic Processes and Filtering Theory*, New York: Academic Press.

Julier, S. J., Uhlmann, J. K., and Durrant-Whyte, H., 1995, A new approach for filtering nonlinear systems, in *Proceedings of the American Control Conference*, pp. 1628–1632.

Kalman, R. E., 1960, A new approach to linear filtering and prediction problems, *Trans. ASME J. Basic Engn.*, 82:35–45.

Patel, G. S., Becker, S., and Racine, R., 2001, Learning shape and motion from image sequences, in *Kalman Filtering and Neural Networks* (S. Haykin, Ed.), New York: Wiley, pp. 69–81.

Paulin, M. G., 1997, Neural representations of moving systems, *Int. Rev. Neurobiol.*, 41:515–533. ◆

Puskorius, G. V., and Feldkamp, L. A., 2001, Parameter-based Kalman filter training: Theory and implementation, in *Kalman Filtering and Neural Networks* (S. Haykin, Ed.), New York: Wiley, pp. 23–67.

Rao, R. P. N., and Ballard, D. H., 1997, "Dynamical model of visual recognition predicts response properties in the visual cortex," *Neural Computation*, vol. 9, pp. 721–763. ◆

Robert, C. P., and Casella, G., 1999, *Monte Carlo Statistical Methods*, New York: Springer-Verlag.

Rui, Y., and Chen, Y., 2001, Better proposed distributions: Object tracking using unscented particle Filter, *IEEE CPVR*, vol. II, pp. 786–793.

Wan, E. A., and van der Merwe, R., 2001, The unscented Kalman filter, in *Kalman Filtering and Neural Networks* (S. Haykin, Ed.), New York: Wiley, pp. 221–280.

Laminar Cortical Architecture in Visual Perception

Stephen Grossberg

Introduction

The cerebral cortex is the seat of the highest forms of biological intelligence in all sensory and cognitive modalities. Neocortex has an intricate design that exhibits a characteristic organization into six distinct cortical layers. Differences in the thickness of these layers and in the sizes and shapes of neurons led the German anatomist Korbinian Brodmann to identify more than 50 divisions, or areas, of neocortex. This classification has been invaluable as a basis for classifying distinct functions of different parts of neocortex. The functional utility of the laminar organization itself in the control of behavior has, however, remained a mystery until recently. Several models of visual cortex (e.g., Li, 1998; Stemmler, Usher, and Niebur, 1995; Somers et al., 1998; Yen and Finkel, 1998) have clarified aspects of cortical dynamics, but have not articulated how the laminar architecture of cortex contributes to visual perception. A LAMINART model has recently proposed clear functional roles for these layers for the purposes of visual perception (Grossberg, 1999a; Grossberg and Raizada, 2000). The present article uses this model as an organizing theme with which to integrate the analysis and explanation of a variety of data about visual perception and neuroscience. Additional recent research suggests that the functional roles for cortical layers that are proposed by the model may also generalize, with appropriate specializations, to other forms of sensory and cognitive processing.

Bottom-up, top-down, and horizontal interactions are well known to occur within and between the cortical layers. The model proposes how these interactions help the visual cortex to realize (1) the binding process whereby cortical groups distributed data into coherent object representations, (2) the attentional process whereby cortex selectively processes important events, and (3) the developmental and learning processes whereby cortex shapes its circuits to match environmental constraints. It is suggested that the mechanisms that achieve the third property imply the first and second properties. That is, constraints that control stable cortical self-organization in the infant seem to strongly constrain properties of learning, perception, and attention in the adult.

Perceptual Grouping and Attention

During visual perception, the visual cortex can generate perceptual groupings and can focus attention on objects of interest. *Perceptual grouping* is the process whereby the brain organizes image contrasts into emergent boundary structures that segregate objects and their backgrounds in response to texture, shading, and depth cues in scenes and images. Perceptual grouping is a basic step in solving the "binding problem," whereby spatially distributed features are bound into representations of objects and events in the world. Vivid perceptual groupings, such as illusory contours, can form over image positions that do not receive contrastive bottom-up inputs from an image or scene. Perceptual groupings can form *preattentively* and automatically, without requiring the conscious attention of a viewing subject.

Attention enables humans and other animals to selectively process information that is of interest to them. In contrast to perceptual grouping, top-down attention typically does not form visible percepts over positions that receive no bottom-up inputs. Attention can modulate, sensitize, or prime an observer to expect an object to occur at a given location or with particular stimulus properties. But were attention by itself able to routinely generate fully formed perceptual representations at positions that did not receive bottom-up inputs, then we could not easily tell the difference between external reality and internal fantasy, and we would experience hallucinations all the time. In fact, it has been proposed that a breakdown in this modulatory property of attention can give rise to hallucinations in patients with mental disorders like schizophrenia.

Despite the fact that perceptual grouping and attention make opposite requirements on bottom-up inputs, many recent experiments have shown that perceptual grouping and attention can occur simultaneously within the same circuits of the visual cortex, notably cortical areas V1 and V2 (see Grossberg, 1999a, and Grossberg and Raizada, 2000, for reviews). How is this possible? How does cortical circuitry form perceptual groupings that can complete a boundary grouping over locations that receive no bottom-up visual inputs, whereas top-down attention cannot do so? Why should attention be deployed throughout the visual cortex, including cortical areas that previously were thought to accomplish purely preattentive processing? An answer can be found by exploring the link between attention and learning.

Attention and Learning

Top-down attention has been proposed to be a key mechanism whereby the brain solves the *stability-plasticity* dilemma (Grossberg, 1999b). The stability-plasticity dilemma concerns that fact that our brains can rapidly learn enormous amounts of information throughout life, without just as rapidly forgetting what they already know. Brains are *plastic* and can rapidly learn new experiences, without losing the *stability* that prevents catastrophic forgetting. How are attentive processes realized within neocortex in order to stabilize the learning process?

An improper solution to this problem could easily lead to an infinite regress. This is true because perceptual groupings can form preattentively and provide the substrate on which higher-level attentional processes can act. How can the preattentive grouping mechanisms develop in a stable way, before higher-order attentional processes can develop with which to stabilize them? How can you use attentional mechanisms to stabilize the formation of preattentive grouping circuits, if these attentional mechanisms cannot develop until the preattentive grouping mechanisms do? This is called the *attention-preattention interface problem*. Below we discuss the possibility that the laminar circuits of visual cortex enable preattentive grouping processes to use some of the same circuitry that attentive mechanisms use, even before attentive mechanisms come into play, in order to stabilize their own cortical development and learning. Preattentive grouping uses top-down *intra*cortical feedback between the layers, whereas attention uses top-down *inter*cortical feedback between them. Both feedback processes converge on a shared decision circuit that helps to determine which perceptual groupings will be perceived.

A solution to the attention-preattention interface problem can be derived from earlier efforts to understand how attention helps to solve the stability-plasticity dilemma: bottom-up signals activate top-down expectations, whose signals are matched against bottom-up data. Both the bottom-up and the top-down pathways contain adaptive weights, or long-term memory traces, that can be modified by experience. The learned top-down expectations "focus attention" on information that matches them. They select, synchronize, and amplify the activities of cells within the attentional focus while suppressing the activities of irrelevant cells, which could otherwise be incorporated into previously learned memories and thereby destabilize them. The cell activities that survive such top-down attentional focusing rapidly reactivate bottom-up pathways. The amplified, synchronized, and prolonged activation of cells within the bottom-up and top-down signal exchanges form a *resonant* state. Such resonances rapidly bind distributed information at multiple levels of brain processing into context-sensitive representations of objects and events. The greater activity, duration, and synchrony of these resonances can support slower processes of learning; hence the term *adaptive* resonance. ADAPTIVE RESONANCE THEORY (q.v.), or ART, has been developed to quantitatively explain how processes of learning, expectation, attention, synchronization, memory search, and consciousness are linked in both healthy subjects and clinical patients. A rapidly growing body of neurobiological data has begun to confirm the predicted links between learning, top-down matching, attention, synchronization, and consciousness.

Learning can easily lead to catastrophic forgetting in response to a changing world. Many popular neural models experience such catastrophic forgetting, notably feedforward models such as backpropagation. ART shows how top-down attention can stabilize learning if it satisfies four properties that together are called the ART matching rule:

1. *Bottom-up automatic activation:* A cell, or cell population, can become active enough to generate output signals if it receives a large enough bottom-up input, other things being equal. Such an input can drive the cell to supraliminal levels of activation.
2. *Top-down priming:* A cell becomes subliminally active if it receives only a large top-down expectation input. Such a top-down priming signal can sensitize, or modulate, the cell and thereby prepare it to react more quickly and vigorously to subsequent bottom-up inputs that match the top-down prime. The top-down prime by itself, however, cannot generate supraliminal output signals from the cell.
3. *Match:* A cell is activated if it receives large convergent bottom-up and top-down inputs. Such a matching process can generate enhanced activation as resonance takes hold.

4. *Mismatch:* A cell's activity is suppressed, even if it receives a large bottom-up input, if it also receives only a small, or zero, top-down expectation input.

Recent data analyses have suggested that variants of the simplest circuit (Figure 1), a top-down on-center off-surround network, is used by the brain (Grossberg, 1999b). In such a circuit, when only bottom-up signals are active, all cells can fire that receive large enough inputs. When only top-down attention is active, cells in the off-surround that receive inhibition but no excitation can be strongly inhibited, while cells in the on-center that receive a combination of excitation and inhibition can become at most subliminally activated, owing to the balance between excitation and inhibition. When bottom-up and top-down inputs match (pathway 2 in Figure 1*C*), the two excitatory sources of excitation (bottom-up and top-down) that converge at the cell can overwhelm the one inhibitory source; it is a case of two against one. When bottom-up and top-down inputs mismatch (pathway 1 in Figure 1*C*), the top-down inhibition can neutralize the bottom-up excitation; it is a case of one against one.

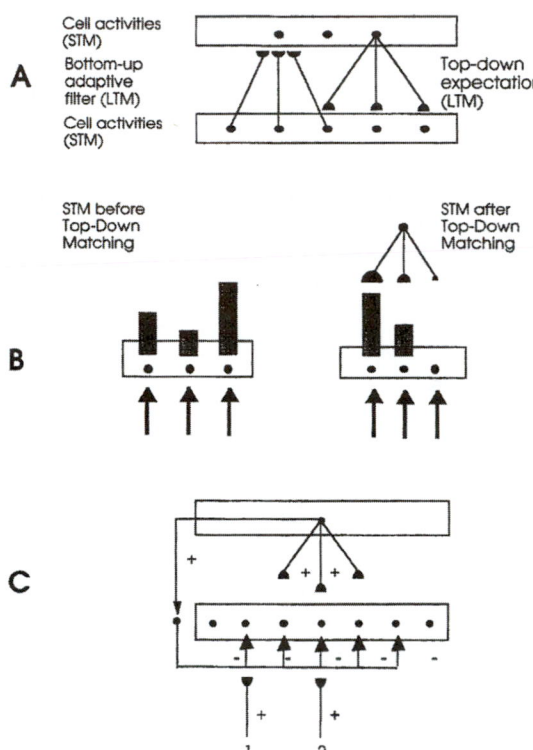

Figure 1. *A,* Patterns of activation, or short-term memory (STM), on a lower processing level send bottom-up signals to a higher processing level. These signals are multiplied by adaptive weights, or learned long-term memory (LTM) traces, which influence which cells are activated at the higher processing level. These latter cells, in turn, activate top-town expectation signals that are also multiplied by learned LTM traces. These top-down expectations are matched against the STM pattern that is active at the lower level. *B,* This matching process selects, amplifies, and synchronizes STM activations that are supported by large LTM traces in an active top-down expectation, and suppresses STM activations that do not get top-down support. The size of the hemidisks at the end of the top-down pathways represents the strength of the learned LTM trace that is stored in that pathway. *C,* The ART matching rule can be realized by a modulatory top-down on-center off-surround network, as discussed in the text. (From Grossberg, S., 1999a, How does the cerebral cortex work? Learning, attention, and grouping by the laminar circuits of visual cortex, *Spatial Vision,* 12:163–185. Reprinted with permission.)

Attention Is Modulatory

The ART matching rule predicted that top-down attention is part of a modulatory *priming* and *matching* process. By itself, attention cannot supraliminally activate cells, so they cannot generate output signals. Data compatible with this prediction have gradually been reported over the years. For example, Zeki and Shipp (1988, p. 316) wrote that "backward connections seem not to excite cells in lower areas, but instead influence the way they respond to stimuli." Likewise, the data of Sillito et al. (1994) on attentional feedback from V1 to the lateral geniculate nucleus (LGN) led them to conclude that "the cortico-thalamic input is only strong enough to exert an effect on those dLGN cells that are additionally polarized by their retinal input . . . the feedback circuit searches for correlations that support the 'hypothesis' represented by a particular pattern of cortical activity." Their experiments demonstrated all of the properties of the ART matching rule, since they found in addition that "cortically induced correlation of relay cell activity produces coherent firing in those groups of relay cells with receptive-field alignments appropriate to signal the particular orientation of the moving contour to the cortex . . . this increases the gain of the input for feature-linked events detected by the cortex." In other words, top-down priming by itself cannot fully activate LGN cells; it needs matched bottom-up retinal inputs to do so, and those LGN cells whose bottom-up signals support cortical activity get synchronized and amplified by this feedback. In addition, anatomical studies have shown that the top-down V1 to LGN pathway realizes a top-down on-center off-surround network.

How to Stabilize Cortical Development and Learning

The preceding discussion suggests that top-down attentional mechanisms should be present in *every* cortical area in which self-stabilizing learning can occur, since without top-down learned expectations that focus attention, any such learned memories could easily be degraded due to catastrophic forgetting.

These analyses should, in particular, apply to the perceptual grouping process, because the cortical horizontal connections that support perceptual grouping in cortical areas like V1 develop through a learning process that is influenced by visual experience (e.g., Calloway and Katz, 1990; Antonini and Stryker, 1993). It is also known that many developmental and learning processes, including those that control horizontal cortical connections, are stabilized dynamically and can be reactivated by lesions and other sources of cortical imbalance (Das and Gilbert, 1995); and that adult learning uses the same types of mechanisms as the infant developmental processes on which it builds (Kandel and O'Dell, 1992). What cortical mechanisms ensure this type of dynamical stability?

This is a particularly challenging problem for perceptual groupings because they can generate suprathreshold responses over positions that do not receive bottom-up inputs. They therefore seem to violate the ART matching rule. How, then, can the horizontal connections that generate perceptual groupings maintain themselves in a stable way? Why are they not washed away whenever an illusory contour grouping forms over positions that do not receive a bottom-up input? The LAMINART model proposes an answer to this question that clarifies how attention, perceptual grouping, development, and perceptual learning work and interact within the laminar circuits of visual cortex.

Preattentive Mechanisms of Perceptual Grouping

Four circuit properties summarize this proposal of how the visual cortex, notably areas V1 and V2, uses its laminar design to generate coherent perceptual groupings that maintain their analog sensitivity to environmental inputs, the so-called property of *analog coherence*. Four additional circuit properties will then be summarized whereby attention, development, and learning may be integrated into this laminar design. Each of these design constraints is supported by neurophysiological, anatomical, and psychophysical data.

Analog Sensitivity to Bottom-Up Sensory Inputs

Bottom-up inputs from the retina go through the LGN on their way to cortex. LGN outputs directly excite layer 4. LGN inputs also excite layer 6, which then indirectly influences layer 4 via an on-center off-surround network of cells, as in Figure 2A. The net effect of LGN inputs on layer 4 cells is thus via an on-center off-surround network. Such a feedforward on-center off-surround network of cells can preserve the analog sensitivity of, and normalize, the activities of target cells if these cells obey the membrane equations of neurophysiology. Such a network can preserve the analog sensitivity of layer 4 cells in response to LGN inputs that may vary greatly in intensity.

Bipole Boundary Grouping

The active layer 4 cells input to pyramidal cells in layer 2/3. These cells initiate the formation of perceptual groupings. They generate excitatory signals among themselves using monsynaptic long-range horizontal connections, and inhibition using short-range disynaptic inhibitory connections, as in Figure 2B. These interactions support inward perceptual groupings between two or more boundary inducers, as in the case of illusory contours, but not outward groupings from a single inducer, which would fill the visual field with spurious groupings.

These grouping properties may be ensured as follows. When a single active pyramidal cell sends horizontal monosynaptic excitation to other pyramidal cells, this excitation is inhibited by the disynaptic inhibition that it also generates; this balance between excitation and inhibition is a case of one against one. Model simulations have shown that such an approximate balance between excitation and inhibition is needed to stabilize the development of horizontal connections. A different result obtains when two or more pyramidal cells are activated at positions that are located at opposite sides of a target pyramidal cell, and all the cells share approximately the same orientation preference and are approximately collinear across space. Then the excitation from the active pyramidal cells summates at the target cell, thereby generating a larger total excitatory input than a single pyramidal cell could. In addition, the active cells excite a single population of disynaptic inhibitory interneurons, which generates a saturating, or normalized, inhibitory output to the target cell. Thus, excitation is bigger than inhibition in this case, so that grouping can occur; it is a case of two against one. This combination of constraints is called the *bipole* property. Layer 2/3 pyramidal cells may thereby become active either because of direct inputs from layer 4, or because of bipole boundary groupings that form in response to other active layer 2/3 cells.

Folded Feedback and Analog Coherence

The active cells in layer 2/3 can form groupings on their own in response to unambiguous visual inputs. In response to scenes wherein multiple groupings are possible but only a few of them are correct, intracortical feedback helps to select the correct cells, and also binds them together in a coherent way. This selection happens when active cells in layer 2/3 send excitatory feedback signals to layer 6 via layer 5, as in Figure 2C. Layer 6 then activates the on-center off-surround network from layer 6 to 4. This feedback process is called *folded feedback*, because feedback signals from layer

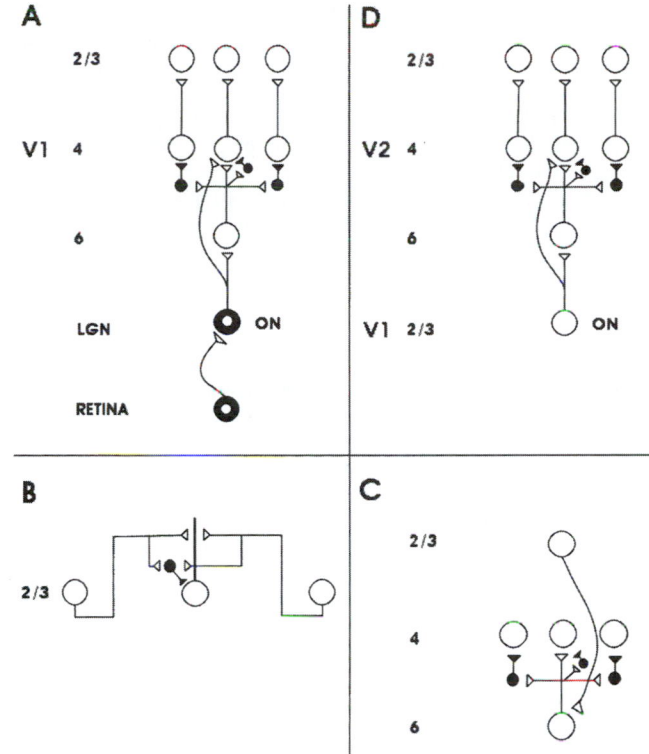

Figure 2. *A* model circuit of retinal, lateral geniculate nucleus (LGN), and cortical V1 interactions. Open symbols indicate excitatory interactions and closed symbols indicate inhibitory interactions. *A*, Feedforward circuit from retina to LGN to cortical layers 4 and 6. Retina: Retinal ON cells have an on-center off-surround organization. Retinal OFF cells have an off-center on-surround organization. LGN: The LGN ON and OFF cells receive feedforward ON and OFF cell inputs from the retina. Layer 4: Layer 4 cells receive feedforward inputs from LGN and layer 6. LGN ON and OFF cell excitatory inputs to layer 4 directly establish oriented simple-cell receptive fields. Layer 6 cells excite layer 4 cells with a narrow on-center and inhibit them using inhibitory interneurons that span a broader off-surround, which includes cells in the on-center (not shown). Like-oriented layer 4 simple cells with opposite-contrast polarities compete (not shown) before generating half-wave rectified outputs that converge on layer 2/3 pyramidal (complex) cells. Layer 2/3: The converging simple cell outputs enable complex cells to respond to both polarities. They thereby full-wave rectify the image. *B*, Horizontal grouping interactions in layer 2/3: After being activated by inputs from layer 4, layer 2/3 pyramidal (complex) cells excite each other monosynaptically via horizontal connections, primarily on their apical dendrites. They also inhibit one another via disynaptic inhibition that is mediated by model smooth stellate cells. Multiple horizontal connections share a common pool of stellate cells near each target pyramidal cell. This ensures that boundaries form inwardly between pairs or greater numbers of boundary inducers, but not outwardly from a single inducer. *C*, Cortical feedback loop from layer 2/3 to layer 6: Layer 6 cells receive excitatory inputs from layer 2/3. The long-range cooperation thereby engages the feedforward layer 6-to-4 on-center off-surround network, which then reactivates layer 2/3 cells. This "folded feedback" loop can select winning groupings without a loss of analog coherence. *D*, Outputs from layer 2/3 to area V2 directly excite layer 4 cells and layer 6 cells, which indirectly influence layer 4 cells via an on-center off-surround network, as in area V1. (From Grossberg, 1999a).

2/3 to layer 6 get transmitted in a feedforward fashion back to layer 4; that is, feedback is "folded" back into the feedforward flow of bottom-up information within the laminar cortical circuits.

Folded feedback turns the cortex into a feedback network that binds the cells throughout layers 2/3, 4, and 6 into functional columns. The on-center off-surround network also helps to select the strongest groupings that are formed in layer 2/3 and to inhibit weaker groupings, while preserving the analog values of the selected groupings. In particular, the on-center signals from layer 6-to-4 support the activities of those pyramidal cells in layer 2/3 that are part of the strongest horizontal groupings. The off-surround signals can inhibit inputs to layer 4 that were supporting less active groupings in layer 2/3. In this way, signals from layer 4 to the less active groupings in layer 2/3 are removed, and thus these groupings collapse.

Self-Similar Hierarchical Boundary Processing

Converging evidence suggests that area V2 replicates aspects of the structure of area V1, but at a larger spatial scale. Thus, layer 2/3 in area V1 sends bottom-up inputs to layers 4 and 6 of area V2, much as LGN sends bottom-up inputs to layers 4 and 6 of area V1, as in Figure 2D. This input pattern from V1 to V2 can preserve the analog sensitivity of layer 4 cells in V2 for the same reason that the LGN inputs to V1 can preserve the analog sensitivity of layer 4 cells in V1. The shorter perceptual groupings in layer 2/3 of area V1 are proposed to group together, and enhance the signal-to-noise ratio of, nearby V1 cells with similar orientation and disparity selectivity. The longer perceptual groupings in area V2 are proposed to build long-range boundary segmentations that separate figure from background; generate 3D groupings of the edges, textures, shading, and stereo information that go into object representations; and complete boundaries across gaps in bottom-up signals due to the retinal blind spot and veins (Grossberg, 1994).

Attention, Development, and Learning

The following four circuit properties are proposed to integrate top-down attention into the preattentive grouping process in a way that solves the attention-preattention interface problem and enables grouping circuits to develop and learn in a stable way.

Top-Down Feedback from V1 to LGN

As noted above, layer 6 of area V1 sends a top-down on-center off-surround network to the LGN, as in Figure 3A. This top-down pathway automatically gain-controls and focuses attention on those LGN cells whose activities succeed in activating V1 cells. Data of Sillito et al. (1994) are compatible with the hypothesis that this feedback obeys the ART matching rule, and thus can only subliminally activate, or modulate, LGN cells. Matched bottom-up inputs are needed to supraliminally activate LGN cells while top-down signals are active. This process is predicted to help stabilize the development of receptive fields in V1, including disparity-tuned complex cells, during the visual critical period.

Folded Feedback from Layer 6 of V2 to Layer 4 of V1

A similar top-down process seems to occur at all stages of visual cortex, and probably beyond. Layer 6 in a given cortical area, such as V2, generates top-down cortical signals to layer 6 of lower cortical areas, such as V1, where they activate the layer 6-to-4 folded feedback network in the lower area (Figure 3B). One such known top-down pathway exits layer 6 in V2 and activates V1 via layer 1, then layer 5, then layer 6, as in Figure 3C. Top-down feedback can thereby activate a top-down on-center off-surround circuit, as required by the ART matching rule. Intercortical attention is herewith suggested to use outputs from layer 6 of a given cortical area to activate layer 4 of a lower cortical area via layer 6-to-4 folded feedback.

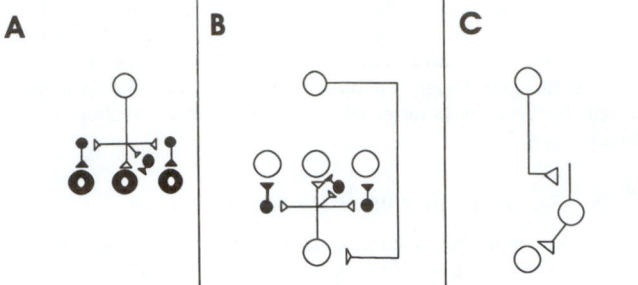

Figure 3. *A*, Top-down corticogeniculate feedback from layer 6: LGN ON and OFF cells receive topographic excitatory feedback from layer 6 in V1, and more broadly distributed inhibitory feedback via LGN inhibitory interneurons that are excited by layer 6 signals. The feedback signals pool outputs over all cortical orientations and are delivered equally to ON and OFF cells. Cortiogeniculate feedback selects, gain-controls, and synchronizes LGN cells that are consistent with the cortical activation that they cause, thereby acting like a type of automatic attentional focus. *B*, Attentional feedback from V2 to V1: Layer 6 in V2 activates layer 6 in V1, which then activates the layer 6-to-4 on-center off-surround network that attentionally primes layer 4 cells. *C*, One feedback pathway arises from layer 6 cells in V2 and activates apical dendrites in layer 1 of V1. Cells in layer 5 are activated through these apical dendrites and thereupon activate layer 6 cells. Layer 6 in V2 can also modulate layer 2/3 of V1 by activating layer 1 dendrites of both excitatory and inhibitory cells in layer 2/3. (From Grossberg, 1999a).

Layer 6-to-4 Signals Are Subliminal

The ART matching rule predicts that this top-down pathway subliminally activates, or modulates, cells in layer 4. This modulatory property is predicted to be due to the fact that the excitatory and inhibitory signals within the on-center from layer 6-to-4 are approximately balanced, so that at most, a weak excitatory effect occurs after activating the circuit via top-down feedback. Consistent data show that "feedback connections from area V2 modulate but do not create center-surround interactions in V1 neurons" (Hupé et al., 1997, p. 1031) and that top-down connections have an on-center off-surround organization (Bullier et al., 1996). Model simulations have shown that that this approximate balance is needed to achieve stable development of interlaminar 6-to-4 connections.

Although it is modulatory, this top-down circuit can have a major effect on cortical cell activations when the cortex is activated bottom-up by visual inputs: it can strongly inhibit activities of layer 4 cells whose layer 2/3 cell projections are not bound into strong groupings, and amplify the strongest groupings until they can resonate. A competitive effect of top-down attention has been reported in the neurophysiological experiments of Reynolds, Chelazzi, and Desimone (1999). Its laminar substrates have not yet been tested, however. By using such an attentional mechanism, higher-level influences such as figure-ground separation or even learned object prototypes can bias the cortex to select consistent groupings at lower cortical levels. In this way, automatic early vision filtering, 3D boundary and surface processing, and higher-order knowledge constraints can mutually influence one another.

Two Bottom-Up Input Sources to Layer 4

A simple functional explanation can now be given of a ubiquitous cortical design; namely, why there are direct bottom-up inputs to layer 4, as well as indirect bottom-up inputs to layer 4 via layer 6 (e.g., Figures 2A and 2D). Why are these two separate input pathways not just a gigantic waste of wire? In particular, why is the indirect layer 6-to-4 pathway not sufficient to fully activate layer 4 cells *and* to maintain their analog sensitivity using its on-center off-surround network? The proposed explanation is that the indirect layer 6-to-4 inputs need to be modulatory to preserve the stability of cortical development and learning. Direct inputs to layer 4 are therefore also needed to fully activate layer 4 cells.

Taken together, these eight cortical design principles lead to the circuit diagram in Figure 4 for perceptual grouping, attention, development, and learning within and between areas LGN, V1, and V2. The generality of the constraints that lead to this design poses the intriguing possibility that the same cortical circuits may explain data at multiple levels and modalities of neocortical sensory and cognitive processing.

The Preattentive Perceptual Grouping Is Its Own Attentional Prime

These circuit constraints suggest how the horizontal connections within cortical area V1 and V2 can develop and learn stably in response to visual inputs, and thereby solve the preattention-attention interface problem: both preattentive perceptual groupings within V1 and attentive feedback from V2 to V1 generate feedback signals to layer 6 of V1, one via intracortical pathways from layer 2/3 of the same cortical area, and the other via intercortical pathways from layer 6 of a higher cortical area. Both types of feedback activate the folded feedback circuit from layer 6-to-4. Top-down attention uses this circuit to focus attention within V1 by inhibiting layer 4 cells that are not supported by excitatory 6-to-4 feedback. Perceptual grouping uses it to select the correct grouping by inhib-

iting layer 4 cells that would otherwise form incorrect groupings. In both cases, folded feedback prevents the wrong combinations of cells in layers 4 and 2/3 from being active simultaneously. In the adult, this selection process defines perceptual grouping properties. In the infant, and also during adult perceptual learning, it prevents incorrect horizontal connections from being learned, since "cells that fire together wire together." This sharing of the layer 6-to-4 selection circuit by both grouping and attention clarifies how attention can propagate along a boundary grouping and can thereby selectively prime an object representation (Grossberg and Raizada, 2000; Roelfsema, Lamme, and Spekreijse, 1998).

The folded feedback circuit from layer 6-to-4 gets activated by perceptual grouping signals from layer 2/3 at *all* positions of the grouping, even positions that do not receive bottom-up inputs. The ART matching rule is thus satisfied at all positions, and the source of the "top-down expectation" is intracortical top-down signals from the perceptual grouping itself. In summary, the *preattentive perceptual grouping is its own attentional prime* because it can use the modulatory 6-to-4 circuit to stabilize its own development using *intra*cortical feedback, even before attentional *inter*cortical feedback can develop.

Discussion

All sensory and cognitive neocortical areas share key laminar properties. For example, long-range horizontal connections are known to occur in many areas of neocortex, such as the auditory and language areas of the human temporal cortex. Ongoing research suggests that the above principles of how to achieve stable cortical development and learning, to bind together distributed cortical data through a combination of bottom-up adaptive filtering and horizontal associations, and to modulate it with top-down attention generalize to other neocortical areas.

Acknowledgments.   Work was supported in part by grants from the Defense Advanced Research Projects Agency and the Office of Naval Research (ONR N00014-95-1-0409), the National Science Foundation (NSF IRI-97-20333), and the Office of Naval Research (ONR N00014-95-1-0657 and ONR N00014-01-1-0624).

Road Maps: Mammalian Brain Regions; Vision
Background: Adaptive Resonance Theory
Related Reading: Contour and Surface Perception; Visual Attention; Visual Cortex: Anatomical Structure and Models of Function

References

Antonini, A., and Stryker, M. P., 1993, Functional mapping of horizontal connections in developing ferret visual cortex: Experiments and modeling, *J. Neurosci.*, 14:7291–7305.

Bullier, J., Hupé, J. M., James, A., and Girard, P., 1996, Functional interactions between areas V1 and V2 in the monkey, *J. Physiol. (Paris)*, 90:217–220.

Calloway, E. M., and Katz, L. C., 1990, Emergence and refinement of clustered horizontal connections in cat striate cortex, *J. Neurosci.*, 10:1134–1153.

Das, A., and Gilbert, C. D., 1995, Long-range horizontal connections and their role in cortical reorganization revealed by optical recording of cat primary visual cortex, *Nature*, 375:780–784.

Grossberg, S., 1994, 3-D vision and figure-ground separation by visual cortex, *Percept. Psychophys.*, 55:48–120.

Grossberg, S., 1999a, How does the cerebral cortex work? Learning, attention, and grouping by the laminar circuits of visual cortex, *Spatial Vision*, 12:163–185. ◆

Grossberg, S., 1999b, The link between brain learning, attention, and consciousness, *Consciousness Cognit.*, 8:1–44. ◆

Grossberg, S., and Raizada, R. D. S., 2000, Contrast-sensitive perceptual grouping and object-based attention in the laminar circuits of primary visual cortex, *Vision Res.*, 40:1413–1432.

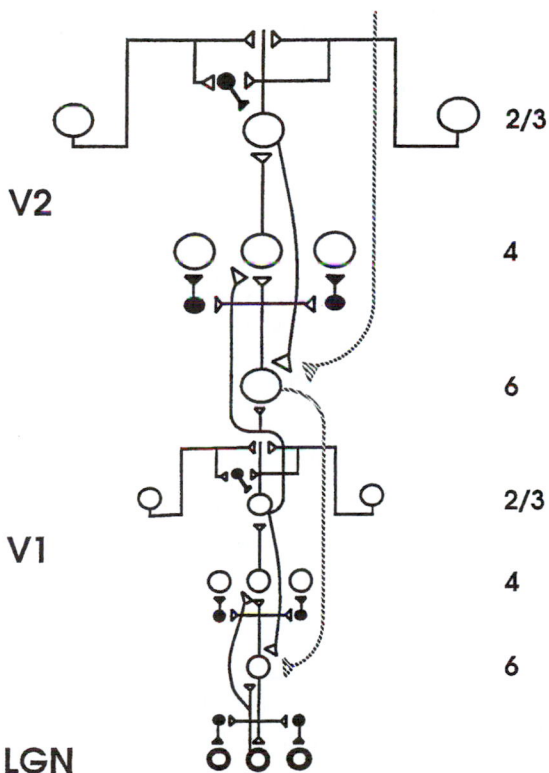

Figure 4. A model synthesis of bottom-up, top-down, and horizontal interactions in LGN, V1, and V2. Cells and connections with open symbols denote preattentive excitatory mechanisms that are involved in perceptual grouping. Closed symbols denote inhibitory mechanisms. Gray denotes top-down attentional mechanisms. (From Grossberg, 1999a).

Hupé, J. M., James, A. C., Girard, P., and Bullier, J., 1997, Feedback connections from V2 modulate intrinsic connectivity within, *Soc. Neurosci. Abstr.*, 23:1031, abstr. 406.15

Kandel, E. R., and O'Dell, T. J., 1992, Are adult learning mechanisms also used for development? *Science*, 258:243–245.

Li, Z., 1998, A neural model of contour integration in the primary visual cortex, *Neural Computat.*, 10:903–940.

Reynolds, J., Chelazzi, L., and Desimone, R., 1999, Competitive mechanisms subserve attention in macaque areas V2 and V4, *J. Neurosci.*, 19:1736–1753.

Roelfsema, P. R., Lamme, V. A. F., and Spekreijse, H., 1998, Object-based attention in the primary visual cortex of the macaque monkey, *Nature*, 395:376–381. ◆

Sillito, A. M., Jones, H. E., Gerstein, G. L., and West, D. C., 1994, Feature-linked synchronization of thalamic relay cell firing induced by feedback from the visual cortex, *Nature*, 369:479–482. ◆

Somers, D. C., Todorov, E. V., Siapas, A. G., Toth, L. J., Kim, D., and Sur, M., 1998, A local circuit approach to understanding integration of long-range inputs in primary visual cortex, *Cereb. Cortex*, 8:204–217.

Stemmler, M., Usher, M., and Niebur, E., 1995, Lateral interactions in primary visual cortex: A model bridging physiology and psychophysics, *Science*, 269:1877–1880.

Yen, S. C., and Finkel, L. H., 1998, Extraction of perceptually salient contours by striate cortical networks, *Vision Res.*, 38:719–741.

Zeki, S., and Shipp, S., 1988, The functional logic of cortical connections, *Nature*, 335:311–317. ◆

Language Acquisition

Brian MacWhinney

Introduction

Language is a uniquely human achievement. All of the major social achievements of human culture—architecture, literature, law, science, art, and even warfare—rely on the use of language. Although there have been attempts to teach language to primates, the ability to learn language is a distinctive mark of the human species. This view of language led Chomsky (1965) to voice this assessment:

> It is, for the present, impossible to formulate an assumption about initial, innate structure rich enough to account for the fact that grammatical knowledge is attained on the basis of the evidence available to the learner. Consequently, the empiricist effort to show how the assumptions about a language acquisition device can be reduced to a conceptual minimum is quite misplaced. The real problem is that of developing a hypothesis about initial structure that is sufficiently rich to account for acquisition of language, yet not so rich as to be inconsistent with the known diversity of language.

To address this challenge, neural network researchers have explored a wide variety of network architectures and linguistic problems. This work has shown how children can learn language without relying on specifically linguistic, innate initial structure. However, several problems must be addressed before we can say that neural networks have answered Chomsky's challenge.

An Example

Let us consider, as an example of this type of research, the neural network developed by MacWhinney et al. (1989). This model was designed to explain how German children learn to select one of the six different forms of the German definite article. In English, we have a single word "the" that serves as the definite article. In German, the article can take the form *der*, *die*, *das*, *des*, *dem*, and *den*, as indicated in Table 1. The choice of a particular form of the article depends on three additional features of the noun: its gender (masculine, feminine, or neuter), its number (singular or plural), and its role within the sentence (subject, possessor, direct object, prepositional object, or indirect object). There are 16 cells in the paradigm for the four cases and four genders (masculine, feminine, neuter, plural), but there are only six forms of the article. This means that a given form of the article, such as *der* can be used for either masculine-nominative-singular or feminine-genitive-singular, and so on.

To make matters worse, assignment of nouns to gender categories in German is quite nonintuitive. For example, the word for

"fork" is feminine, the word for "spoon" is masculine, and the word for "knife" is neuter. Acquiring this system of arbitrary gender assignments is particularly difficult for adult second language learners. Mark Twain expressed his consternation at this aspect of German in a treatise entitled "The aweful German language" in which he accuses the language of unfairness and capriciousness in its treatment of young girls as neuter, the sun as feminine, and the moon as masculine. Along a similar vein, Maratsos and Chalkley (1980) argued that, because neither semantic nor phonological cues can predict which article accompanies a given noun in German, children could not learn the language by relying on simple surface cues.

These relations are so complex that a careful linguistic description of the system occupies well over 200 pages. However, MacWhinney et al. (1989) show that it is possible to construct a connectionist network that learns this system from the available cues (see Figure 1). The model uses a simple feedforward architecture. The input is structured into two pools of units. The first pool has 143 phonological units and 5 token meaning units. The second pool has 17 case cues from syntactic structure and 11 phonological cues from endings on the noun. These two input pools feed into two separate pools of collector units that then feed together into a second level of hidden units. The output is a set of six nodes for the six possible forms of the German article. It is important to remember that each of these six articles must serve several functions to fill up the 16 cells of the declensional paradigm.

The network was trained using the backpropagation algorithm. After 40 epochs of training on a set of 102 real German nouns, the network was able to choose the correct article 98% of the time. This meant that it not only succeeded in getting the gender of the noun right, but also figured out how to use the case cues to correctly select one of the 16 cells of the paradigm. To test the network's generalization abilities, we presented it with old nouns in new case roles. In these tests, the network chose the correct article in 92% of trials. This type of cross-paradigm generalization provides clear evidence that the network went far beyond rote memorization during the training phase. In fact, the network quickly succeeded in learning the whole of the basic formal paradigm for the marking of German case, number, and gender on the noun.

In addition, the simulation was able to generalize its internalized knowledge to solve the problem that had so perplexed Mark Twain—guessing at the gender of entirely novel nouns. We presented the network with 48 new high-frequency German nouns in a variety of sentence contexts. On this completely novel set, the simulation chose the correct article from the six possibilities in 61%

Figure 1. A network model of the acquisition of German declensional marking

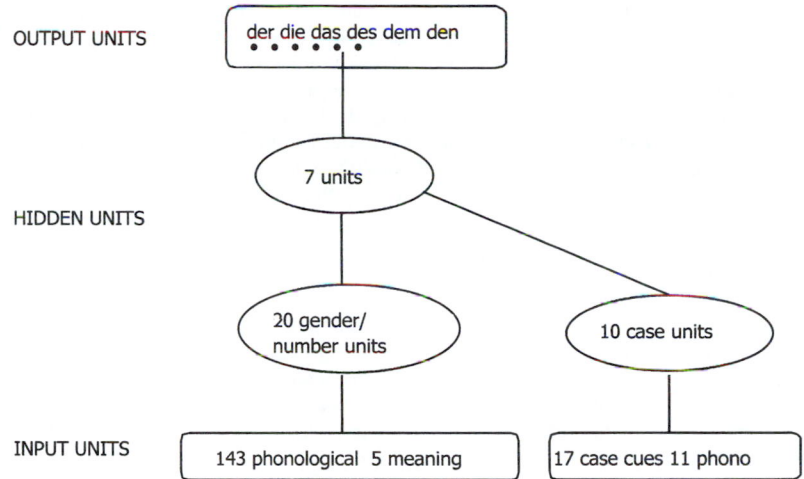

of trials, versus 17% expected by chance. Thus, the system's learning mechanism, together with its representation of the noun's phonological and semantic properties and the context, produced a good guess about what article would accompany a given noun, even when the noun was entirely unfamiliar. In a subsidiary simulation, we showed that, when the model only has to guess the gender of the noun, and not its position in the paradigm, it achieves over 70% accuracy on new nouns. This is a level that comes close to that achieved by native speakers.

The network's learning paralleled children's learning in a number of ways. Like real German-speaking children, the network tended to overuse the articles that accompany feminine nouns. The reason for this is that the feminine forms of the article have a high frequency, because they are used both for feminines and for plurals of all genders. The simulation also showed the same type of overgeneralization patterns that are often interpreted as reflecting rule use when they occur in children's language. For example, although the noun "Kleid" (clothing) is neuter, the simulation used the initial "kl" sound of the noun to conclude that it was masculine. Because of this, it invariably chose the article that would accompany the noun if it were masculine. Interestingly, the same article-noun combinations that are the most difficult for children were also the most difficult for the network.

Demonstrations of this type illustrate how children can acquire linguistic knowledge without relying on stipulated, hard-wired constraints of the type envisioned by Chomsky. Similar demonstrations have been produced in a wide variety of areas including: the English past tense, Dutch word stress, universal metrical features, German participle acquisition, German plurals, Italian articles, Spanish articles, English derivation for reversives, lexical learning from perceptual input, deictic reference, personal pronouns, polysemic patterns in word meaning, vowel harmony, historical change, early auditory processing, the phonological loop, early phonological output processes, ambiguity resolution, relative clause processing, word class learning, speech errors, bilingualism, and the vocabulary spurt.

Challenges

Researchers have contested the logic underlying these demonstrations. Some of the problems that have been raised relate only to minor implementational features of the earliest models (MacWhinney and Leinbach, 1991), but others are more fundamental. The five most fundamental challenges are:

Dual route. Neural networks provide a good account of associative processes, but fail to account for the learning of regular rules.

Lexical learning. Neural networks have problems learning large numbers of words.

Syntax. Neural networks have problems dealing with the compositional aspects of complex syntax.

Neuronal realism. Some neural network architectures make inappropriate assumptions regarding neural processing.

Embodiment. Neural networks have not been able to model the ways in which the mind is linked to the body.

Let us look at responses to each of these five challenges in greater detail.

Dual Route

Pinker (1999) has been a key proponent of the application of a dual-route model to language acquisition. He contends that irregular forms, such as *fell*, *went*, *feet*, or *broken*, are processed through an associative memory grounded on neural networks, but that regular forms, such as *jumped*, *wanted*, *cats*, and *dropped*, are produced by rule. Pinker views his defense of the psychological reality of linguistic rules as a part of a general defense of the linguistic theory of generative grammar.

The fact that irregulars are processed differently from regulars does not prove the existence of symbolic rules. Neural networks have no problem representing both regular and irregular patterns in a single network. For example, the network developed by Kawamoto (1994) encodes regular forms as nodes in competition with less regular nodes. In that homogeneous recurrent network architecture, regular and irregular forms display quite different temporal activation patterns, in accord with empirical observations. Kawamoto's model also accords with the fact that even the most regular patterns display phonological conditioning and patterns of gradience (Bybee, 1995) of the type modeled by neural networks.

Lexical Learning

Neural networks have problems learning large numbers of words. Typically, neural network architectures have been used primarily as methods for extracting and classifying patterns. Word learning differs from classification in two ways. First, the association between a word's meaning and its sound is almost entirely arbitrary. There is nothing in the specific sounds of *table* that depicts the shape or purpose of a table. This means that the learning of words cannot rely on the methods for pattern detection that are so important in neural network research. Second, the number of words that a speaker must learn is extremely large. If we look just at word stems, adult English speakers control between 10,000 and 50,000 words. Many of these words have multiple meanings and many can be further combined into compounds and rote phrases. Thus, the effective lexicon of an adult English speaker is from 20,000 to 80,000 words.

Self-organizing maps (SOMs) (Farkas and Li, 2001) offer a promising framework for dealing with the encoding of lexical items. Precision of encoding can be obtained by increasing the dimensionality of the coding space and then recompressing the additional dimensions. Conflicts between related words that are close on the lexical map can trigger a process of focused learning that concentrates specifically on words that are being confused. Catastrophic interference can be avoided by adding new nodes without forgetting older patterns (Hamker, 2001).

Because SOMs provide a relatively local encoding of words, they then allow us to address four additional problems that stem from problems of representing words in neural networks.

U-shaped learning.   Children often produce a form like *went* correctly for several weeks or months and then shift to occasionally saying *go-ed*. Later, they move back to saying *went* consistently. This pattern, known as *U-shaped learning*, requires an ability to learn some forms first by rote. Backpropagation networks are good at producing overgeneralizations like *go-ed* but weak at producing and holding on to a rote form like *went* (Plunkett and Marchman, 1993). By default, SOMs place an emphasis on early rote learning and are slower to generalize out the regular patterns.

Homophony.   Because most neural network models do not have discrete representations for lexical items, they have problems distinguishing homophonous forms. Consider what happens to the three homophones of the word *ring* in English. We can say *the maid wrung out the clothes*, *the soldiers ringed the city*, or *the choirboy rang the bell*. These three different words all have the same sound /rIN/ in the present, but each takes a different form in the past. In SOMs, these three words have clearly different representations in semantic space.

Compounds.   Without discrete representations for lexical items, neural networks have problems with compound words. The fact that the past tense of *undergo* is *underwent* depends on the fact that *undergo* is a variant of the stem *go*. When the compound itself is high enough in frequency, the network can learn to treat it as an irregular. Networks have problems learning the past tense of low-frequency irregular compounds. However, if the network can detect the present of "go" inside "undergo," it can solve this problem.

Derivational status.   Neural networks have problems utilizing information regarding the derivational status of lexical items. In English, the past tense forms of denominal verbs always receive the regular past tense suffix. For example, the word *ring* can be used as a verb in *the groom ringed her finger*, but we would never say *the groom rung her finger*. Without an ability to know that a word derives from a noun, neural networks cannot encode this pattern. German provides even clearer examples of the importance of derivational status. All German nouns that derive from verbs are masculine. For example, the noun *der Schlag* ("blow"; "cream") derives from the verb *schlagen* ("to hit"). However, there is no motivated way of indicating this in the model. In general, the model includes no independent way of representing morphological relationships between words. Thus, no distinction is made between true

phonological cues such as final /e/ or initial /kn/ and derivational markers for the diminutive, such as *-chen* or *-ett*. This leads to some very obvious confusions. For example, masculines such as *der Nacken* ("neck") and *der Hafen* ("harbor") end in phonological /en/, whereas neuters such as *das Wissen* ("knowledge") and *das Lernen* ("learning") end in the derivational suffix *-en*. Confusion of these two suffixes leads to inability to correctly predict gender for new nouns ending in /en/. Without having a way of representing the fact that derivational morphemes have an independent lexical status, neural networks cannot process these patterns.

These four difficulties reflect a single core problem. By working with neural networks that flexibly encode lexical items, we can begin to address these additional features of word structure.

Syntax

Elman (1990) has provided demonstrations of the ability of neural networks to process complex syntactic structures. His model uses recurrent connections to update the network's memory after it listens to each word. The network's task is to predict the next word. This framework views language comprehension as a highly constructive process in which the major goal is trying to predict what will come next. Psycholinguists recognize the importance of prediction, but they view the major task of language processing as the construction of mental models. It is not clear how understanding prediction will help us understand the construction of mental models, although the two processes are certainly related.

An alternative to the predictive framework relies on the older neural network mechanisms of spreading activation and competition. For example MacDonald, Perlmutter, and Seidenberg (1994) have presented a model of ambiguity resolution in sentence processing that is grounded on competition between lexical items. Models of this type do an excellent job of modeling the temporal properties of sentence processing. Such models assume that the problem of lexical learning in neural networks has been solved. They then proceed to use localist representations to control interactive activation during sentence processing. Until we have indeed solved the problem of lexical learning, this is a very effective way of advancing the research agenda.

Another approach that makes similar assumptions uses a linguistic framework known as Construction Grammar. This framework emphasizes the role of individual lexical items in early grammatical learning (Tomasello, 2000). Early on, children learn to use simple frames such as *my* + *X* or *his* + *X* to indicate possession. As development progresses, these frames are merged into general constructions, such as the possessive construction. In effect, each construction emerges from a lexical gang. Sentence processing then relies on the child's ability to combine constructions online. When two alternative constructions compete, errors appear. An example would be **say me that story*, instead of *tell me that story*. In this error, the child has treated *say* as a member of the group of verbs that forms the dative construction. In the classic theory of generative grammar, recovery from this error is supposed to trigger a learnability problem, since such errors are seldom overtly corrected and, when they are, children tend to ignore the feedback. Neural network implementations of Construction Grammar address this problem by emphasizing the direct competition between *say* and *tell* during production. The child can rely on positive data to strengthen the verb *tell* and its link to the dative construction, thereby eliminating this error without corrective feedback. In this way, models that implement competition provide solutions to the logical problem of language acquisition.

These various approaches to syntactic learning must eventually find a way of dealing with the compositional nature of syntax (Valiant, 1994). A noun phrase such as "my big dog and his ball" can be further decomposed into two segments conjoined by the "and."

Each of the segments is further composed of a head noun and its modifiers. Our ability to recursively combine words into larger phrases stands as a major challenge to connectionist modeling. One likely solution would use predicate constructions to activate arguments that are then combined in a short-term memory buffer during sentence planning and interpretation. To build a model of this type, we need to develop a clearer mechanistic link between constructions as lexical items and constructions as controllers of the on-the-fly process of syntactic combination.

Neuronal Realism

Some researchers have criticized neural network models in the area of language acquisition for a failure to properly represent basic facts about the brain. To the degree that the backpropagation algorithm relies on reciprocal connections between units, this criticism is well founded. However, work in this area has begun to rely on models such as self-organizing feature maps, adaptive resonance, and Hebbian learning that have closer mappings to the features of neural organization. In fact, Elman (1999) has shown how the imposition of biologically realistic assumptions, such as the brain's preference for short connections, can lead to more effective language learning. Thus, this particular challenge to neural network theory may end up being more of a searchlight than a barrier.

Neural networks must also achieve a closer match to what we are now learning about functional neural circuitry. We know that auditory cortex, Broca's area, temporal word storage, and frontal attentional areas are all involved in various ways in language processing. However, we have not yet figured out exactly how these separate brain structures map onto separate aspects of lexical and syntactic processing.

Embodiment

The final challenge to neural network modeling comes from researchers who have begun to explore the ways in which the mind is grounded on the body. This relatively new line of research emphasizes the importance of findings that mental imagery makes use of the reactivation of perceptual systems to recreate physically grounded images. A convergence of work in neuroscience, psychology, and cognitive linguistics points to the view of language use not as disembodied symbol processing, but as indirectly grounded on basic mechanisms for perception and action, which themselves operate on the human body. Neural network models have just begun to deal with this new challenge. One approach emphasizes the ways in which distal learning processes can train action patterns such as speech production on the basis of their perceptual products (Plaut and Kello, 1999). Another approach, adopted by the NTL (Neural Theory of Language) group (Bailey et al., 1997) relies on the higher-order formalism of Petri nets to represent the control structure of body motions such as *pull* or *stumble*. The architecture then includes transparent methods of linking the higher-level representation to a neural network implementation.

One trend that will facilitate this work, as well as all modeling of language acquisition is the increasing availability of transcript and multimedia data from children interacting with their caretakers. The Child Language Data Exchange System (CHILDES) at http://childes.psy.cmu.edu now provides thousands of hours of transcripts of child language data, much of it linked to audio and some to video. In the context of the broader TalkBank Project at http://talkbank.org, this data is being recoded in XML format and linked to a variety of computational tools for analyzing gestural, phonological, morphological, and syntactic structure. This growing database provides increasingly rich targets for neural network modeling.

Conclusions

Neural networks have addressed many aspects of Chomsky's challenge. They have been used to develop useful models of virtually all aspects of language learning and processing. However, further challenges lie ahead. Of these, the most pressing is the need to develop methods for simulating the learning of a realistically sized lexicon of several thousand words. If this problem can be solved, it will have further positive consequences for models of syntactic development that emphasize the importance of item-based learning. It is likely that a good solution to this problem will need to rely on an improved understanding of the ways in which the brain stores and processes lexical items. An even greater challenge will be developing models that express the ways in which language processing is grounded on embodied cognition. Together, these challenges guarantee vitality in this area for years to come.

Road Map: Linguistics and Speech Processing
Related Reading: Cognitive Development; Constituency and Recursion in Language; Developmental Disorders; Language Evolution and Change; Language Evolution: The Mirror System Hypothesis

References

Bailey, D., Feldman, J., Narayanan, S., and Lakoff, G., 1997, Modeling embodied lexical development, *Proceedings of the 19th Meeting of the Cognitive Science Society*, pp. 18–22. ◆

Bybee, J., 1995, Regular morphology and the lexicon, *Lang. Cognit. Proc.*, 10:425–455.

Chomsky, N., 1965, *Aspects of the Theory of Syntax*, Cambridge, MA: MIT Press.

Elman, J., 1990, Finding structure in time, *Cogni. Sci.*, 14:179–212. ◆

Elman, J. L., 1999, The emergence of language: A conspiracy theory, in *The Emergence of Language* (B. MacWhinney, Ed.), Mahwah, NJ: Lawrence Erlbaum Associates, pp. 1–28.

Farkas, I., and Li, P., 2001, Modeling the development of lexicon with a growing self-organizing map, in *Processing of the Sixth Joint Conference on Information Science* (H. J. Caulfield, Ed.), New York: Association for Intelligent Machines, pp. 553–556.

Hamker, F. H., 2001, Life-long learning cell structures—continuously learning without catastrophic interference, *Neural Networks*, 14:551–573.

Kawamoto, A., 1994, One system or two to handle regulars and exceptions: How time-course of processing can inform this debate, in *The Reality of Linguistic Rules* (S. D. Lima, R. L. Corrigan, and G. K. Iverson, Eds.), Amsterdam: John Benjamins, pp. 389–416.

MacDonald, M. C., Perlmutter, N. J., and Seidenberg, M. S., 1994, Lexical nature of syntactic ambiguity resolution, *Psychol. Rev.*, 101(4):676–703. ◆

MacWhinney, B., and Leinbach, J., 1991, Implementations are not conceptualizations: Revising the verb learning model, *Cognition*, 29:121–157. ◆

MacWhinney, B. J., Leinbach, J., Taraban, R., and McDonald, J. L., 1989, Language learning: Cues or rules? *J. Mem. Lang.*, 28:255–277. ◆

Maratsos, M., and Chalkley, M., 1980, The internal language of children's syntax: The ontogenesis and representation of syntactic categories, in *Children's Language: Volume 2* (K. Nelson, Ed.), New York: Gardner, pp. 127–214.

Pinker, S., 1999, *Words and Rules: The Ingredients of Language*, New York: Basic Books.

Plaut, D. C., and Kello, C. T., 1999, The emergence of phonology from the interplay of speech conrephension and production: A distributed connectionist approach, in B. MacWhinney (Ed.), *The Emergence of Language* (B. MacWhinney, Ed.), Mahwah, NJ: Lawrence Erlbaum Associates, pp. 381–416.

Plunkett, K., and Marchman, V., 1993, From rote learning to system building, *Cognition*, 49:21–69.

Tomasello, M., 2000, The item-based nature of children's early syntactic development, *Trends Cognit. Sci.*, 4:156–163. ◆

Valiant, L., 1994, *Circuits of the Mind*, Oxford, UK: Oxford University Press.

Language Evolution and Change

Morten H. Christiansen and Rick Dale

Introduction

No direct evidence remains from before the emergence of writing systems to inform theories about the evolution of language. Only as evidence is amassed from many different disciplines can theorizing about the evolution of language be sufficiently constrained to remove it from the realm of pure speculation and allow it to become an area of legitimate scientific inquiry. To go beyond existing data, rigorously controlled thought experiments can be used as crucial tests of competing theories. Computational modeling has become a valuable resource for such tests because it enables researchers to test hypotheses about specific aspects of language evolution under controlled circumstances (Cangelosi and Parisi, 2002; Turner, 2002). With the help of computational simulations, it is possible to study various processes that may have been involved in the evolution of language, as well as the biological and cultural constraints that may have shaped language into its current form (see EVOLUTION AND LEARNING IN NEURAL NETWORKS).

Connectionist models have played an important role in the computational modeling of language evolution. In some cases, the networks are used as simulated agents to study how social transmission via learning might give rise to the evolution of structured communication systems. In other cases, the specific properties of neural network learning are enlisted to help illuminate the constraints and processes that may have been involved in the evolution of language. This article surveys this connectionist research, starting from the emergence of early syntax and continuing to the role of social interaction and constraints on network learning in subsequent evolution of language and to linguistic change within existing languages.

Emergence of Simple Syntax

Models of language evolution focus on two primary questions: how language emerged, and how languages continue to change over time. An important feature of the first question is the emergence of syntactic communication. Cangelosi (1999) studied the evolution of simple communication systems, but with an emphasis on the emergence of associations not only between objects (meaning) and symbols (signal), but also between the symbols themselves (syntax). In particular, the aim was to demonstrate that simple syntactic relations (a verb-object rule) could evolve through a combination of communicative interactions and cross-generational learning in populations of neural networks.

In Cangelosi's simulations, populations of networks evolved based on their ability to forage in an environment consisting of a two-dimensional 100×100 array of cells. About 12% of the cells contained randomly placed mushrooms that served as food. Three types of mushrooms were edible, increasing a network's fitness if collected, whereas another three types were poisonous, decreasing the network's fitness if collected. The networks had a standard feedforward architecture with a single hidden unit layer and were trained using backpropagation (see BACKPROPAGATION: GENERAL PRINCIPLES). Input was represented in terms of three sets of input units encoding the location of a mushroom, the visual features of the mushroom, and words naming objects or actions. The output contained sets of units representing actions (*approach, avoid, discriminate*) and words with the latter units organized into two winner-take-all clusters (object and verb). Populations consisted of 80 networks, each with a life span of 1,000 actions. The 20 networks with the highest fitness level were selected for asexual reproduc-

tion, each producing four offspring through random mutation of 10% of its starting weights. During the first 300 generations, the populations evolved an ability to discriminate between edible and poisonous mushrooms without the use of words. In subsequent populations, parents provided teaching input for the learning of words denoting the different mushrooms (objects) and the proper action to take (verbs). The simulations were repeated with different random starting populations. Sixty-one percent of the simulations resulted in optimal vocabulary acquisition, with different "verb" symbols used with edible (*approach*) and poisonous (*avoid*) mushrooms, and different "noun" symbols used for the different types of mushrooms.

The simulations indicate how a simple noun-verb communication system can evolve in a population of networks. Because the features of a mushroom were perceived only 10% of the time, paying attention to the parental language input provided a selective advantage with respect to foraging, thus reinforcing successful linguistic performance.

Another approach to the emergence of elementary syntax has been offered by Batali (1998). He suggested that a process of negotiation between agents in a social group may have given rise to coordinated communication. Whereas Cangelosi's model involved the emergence of rudimentary verb-object syntax in a foraging environment, Batali's networks were assigned the task of mapping meaning onto a sequence of characters for the purpose of communication in a social environment. The networks in this simulation did not start out with a predetermined syntactic system. Instead, a process of negotiation across generations engendered the evolution of a syntactic system to convey common meanings.

Each agent in the simulation was a simple recurrent network (SRN; Elman, 1990), capable of processing input sequences consisting of four characters and producing an output vector representing a meaning involving a subject and a predicate. In a negotiation round, one network was chosen as a learner, and ten randomly selected teachers conveyed a meaning converted into a string of characters. The learner then processed the string produced by the teacher, and was trained using the difference between the teacher's and the learner's meaning vectors. Batali described this interaction between learners and teachers as a kind of negotiation, since each must adjust weights in accordance with its own cognitive state and that of others. At the start of the simulations the networks generated only very long strings that were unique to each meaning. After several thousand rounds of negotiation, the agents developed a more efficient and partially compositional communication system, with short sequences of letters used for particular predicates and referents. To test whether novel meanings could be encoded by the communication system, Batali omitted ten meanings, and reran the simulations. After training, networks performed well at sending and processing the omitted meaning vectors, demonstrating that the rudimentary grammar exhibited systematicity capable of accommodating a structured semantics.

Batali's model offers illuminating observations for the evolution of language. An assumption of this model was that social animals can use their own cognitive responses (in this case, translating meaning vectors into communicable signals) to predict the cognitive state of other members of their community. Batali compared this ability to one that may have arisen early in hominids and contributed to the emergence of systematic communication. Once such an elementary communication system is in place, migration patterns may have promoted dialectical variations. The next section explores how linguistic diversity might arise as a result of geographical separation between groups of communicating agents.

Linguistic Diversity

The diversity of the world's many languages has offered puzzling questions for centuries. Computational simulations allow for the investigation of factors influencing the distribution and diversity of language types. An intuitive approach, considered in the next section, is that languages assume an adaptive shape governed by various constraints in the organism and environment. Livingstone and Fyfe (1999) have proposed an alternative perspective based on simulations in which linguistic diversity arises simply as a consequence of spatial organization and imperfect language transmission in a social group.

The social group in the simulation consisted of networks with two layers of three input and output units, bidirectionally connected and randomly initialized. As in Batali's simulations, agents were given the task of mapping a meaning vector onto an external "linguistic" signal. For each generation, a learner and a teacher were randomly selected. The output of the teacher was presented to the learner, and the error between meaning vectors was used to change the learner's weights. Each successive generation had agents from the previous generation acting as teachers. The agents were spatially organized along a single dimension and communicated only with other agents within a fixed distance. By comparing agents across this spatial organization, performance akin to a dialect continuum was observed: small clusters of agents communicated readily, but as the distance among them increased, error in communication increased. When the simulation was implemented without spatial organization (i.e., each agent was equally likely to communicate with all others), the entire population quickly negotiated a global language, and diversity was lost. This model supports the position that diversity is a consequence of spatial organization and imperfect cultural transmission.

The results of Livingstone and Fyfe's as well as Batali's simulations may not rely directly on the properties of neural network learning, but rather on the processes of learning-based social transmission. However, when it comes to explaining why certain linguistic forms have become more frequent than others, the specific constraints on learning in such networks come to the fore. The next section discusses how limitations on network learning can help explain the existence of certain so-called linguistic universals.

Learning-Based Linguistic Universals

Despite the considerable diversity that can be observed across the languages of the world, it is also clear that languages share a number of relatively invariant features in the way words are put together to form sentences. Spatial organization and error in transmission cannot account for these widespread commonalities. Instead, the specific constraints on neural network learning may offer explanations for these consistent patterns in language types. As an example, we can consider heads of phrases, that is, the particular word in a phrase that determines the properties and meaning of the phrase as a whole (such as the noun *boy* in the noun-phrase *the boy with the bicycle*). Across the world's languages, there is a statistical tendency toward a basic format in which the head of a phrase consistently is placed in the same position—either first or last—with respect to the remaining clause material. English is considered to be a head-first language, meaning that the head is most frequently placed first in a phrase, as when the verb is placed before the object noun-phrase in a transitive verb phrase such as *eat curry*. In contrast, speakers of Hindi would say the equivalent of *curry eat*, because Hindi is a head-last language.

Christiansen and Devlin (1997) trained SRNs with eight input and eight output units encoding basic lexical categories (i.e., nouns, verbs, prepositions, and a possessive genitive marker) on corpora generated by 32 different grammars with differing amount of head-

order consistency. The networks were trained to predict the next lexical category in a sentence. Importantly, these networks did not have built-in linguistic biases; rather, they were biased toward the learning of complex sequential structure. Nevertheless, the SRNs were sensitive to the amount of head-order inconsistency found in the grammars, such that there was a strong correlation between the degree of head-order consistency in a given grammar and the degree to which the network had learned to master the grammatical regularities underlying that grammar. The higher the inconsistency, the more erroneous the final network performance was. The sequential biases of the networks made the corpora generated by consistent grammars considerably easier to acquire than the corpora generated by inconsistent grammars. Christiansen and Devlin further collected frequency data concerning the specific syntactic constructions used in the simulations. They found that languages incorporating fragments that the networks found hard to learn tended to be less frequent than languages the network learned more easily. This suggests that constraints on basic word order may derive from nonlinguistic constraints on the learning and processing of complex sequential structure. Grammatical constructions incorporating a high degree of head-order inconsistency may simply be too hard to learn, and would therefore tend to disappear.

More recently, Van Everbroeck (1999) presented network simulations in a similar vein in support of an explanation for language-type frequencies based on processing constraints. He trained recurrent networks (a variation on the SRN) to produce the correct grammatical role assignments for noun-verb-noun sentences that were presented one word at a time. The networks had 26 input units, providing distributed representations of nouns and verbs as well as encodings of case markers, and 48 output units, encoding the distributed noun-verb representation according to grammatical role. Forty-two different language types were used to represent cross-linguistic variation in three dimensions: word order (e.g., subject-verb-object), and noun and verb inflection. The results of the simulations coincided with many observed trends in the distribution of the world's languages. Subject-first languages, both of which make up the majority of language types (51% and 23%, respectively), were easily processed by the networks. Object-first languages, on the other hand, were not well processed and have very low frequency among the world's languages (object-verb-subject: 0.75%; object-subject-verb: 0.25%). Van Everbroeck argued that these results were a predictable product of network processing constraints. Not all results, however, were directly proportional to actual language-type frequencies. For example, verb-subject-object languages account for only 10% of the world's language types, but the model's performance on these exceeded performance on the more frequent subject-first languages. Van Everbroeck suggested that making the simulations more sophisticated (incorporating semantics or other aspects of language) might allow network performance to better approach observed frequencies. Together, the simulations by Van Everbroeck and by Christiansen and Devlin provide preliminary support for a connection between learnability and frequency in the world's languages based on the learning and processing properties of connectionist networks. The next section discusses additional simulations that show how similar network properties may also help explain linguistic change within a particular language.

Linguistic Change

The English system of verb inflection has changed considerably over the past 1,100 years. Simulations by Hare and Elman (1995) demonstrate how neural network learning and processing constraints may help explain the observed pattern of change. The morphological system of Old English (ca. 870) was quite complex, involving at least ten different classes of verb inflection (with a minimum of six of these being "strong"). The simulations involved several "generations" of neural networks, each of which received as input the output generated by a trained net from the previous generation. The first net was trained on data representative of the verb classes from Old English. However, training was stopped before learning could reach optimal performance. This reflected the causal role of imperfect transmission in language change. The imperfect output of the first net was used as input for a second generation net, for which training was also halted before learning reached asymptote. Output from the second net was then given as input to a third net, and so on, until seven generations were trained. This training regime led to a gradual change in the morphological system. These changes can be explained by verb frequency in the training corpus, and internal phonological consistency (i.e., distance in phonological space between prototypes). The results revealed that membership in small classes, inconsistent phonological characteristics, and low frequency all contributed to rapid morphological change. As the morphological system changed through generations in these simulations, the pattern of results closely resembled the historical change in English verb inflection from a complex past tense system to a dominant "regular" class and small classes of "irregular" verbs.

Discussion

This article has surveyed the use of neural networks for the modeling of language evolution and change. The results discussed here are encouraging, even though neural network modeling of language evolution is very much in its infancy. However, it is also clear that the current models suffer from obvious shortcomings. Most of them are highly simple and do not fully capture the vast complexity of the issues at hand. For example, the models of the emergence of verb-object syntax and linguistic diversity incorporated very simple relationships between meaning and form. Moreover, although the simulations of the influence of processing constraints on the shape of language involved relatively complex grammars, they did not include any relationship between the language system and the world. Nevertheless, these models demonstrate the potential for exploring the evolution of language from a computational perspective.

Both connectionist and nonconnectionist models (e.g., Nowak and Komarova, 2001) have been used to provide important thought experiments in support of theories of language evolution. Connectionist models have become prominent in such modeling, both for their ability to simulate social interaction in populations and for their demonstrations of how learning constraints imposed on communication systems can engender many of the linguistic properties we observe today. Together, the models point to an important role

for cultural transmission in the origin and evolution of language. This perspective receives further support from neuroscientific considerations, suggesting a picture of language and brain that argues for their co-evolution (e.g., Deacon, 1997). The studies discussed here highlight the promise of neural network approaches to these issues. Future studies will likely seek to overcome current shortcomings and move toward more sophisticated simulations of the origin and evolution of language.

Road Maps: Linguistics and Speech Processing; Neuroethology and Evolution
Background: Language Processing
Related Reading: Constituency and Recursion in Language; Evolution and Learning in Neural Networks; Language Evolution, The Mirror System Hypothesis

References

Batali, J., 1998, Computational simulations of the emergence of grammar, in *Approaches to the Evolution of Language: Social and Cognitive Bases* (J. R. Hurford, M. Studdert-Kennedy, and C. Knight, Eds.), Cambridge, Engl.: Cambridge University Press, pp. 405–426.
Cangelosi, A., 1999, Modeling the evolution of communication: From stimulus associations to grounded symbolic associations, in *Advances in Artificial Life: Proceedings of the ECAL99 European Conference on Artificial Life* (D. Floreano, J. Nicoud, and F. Mondada, Eds.), Berlin: Springer-Verlag, pp. 654–663.
Cangelosi, A., and Parisi, D., 2002, Computer simulation: A new scientific approach to the study of language evolution, in *Simulating Language Evolution* (A. Cangelosi and D. Parisi, Eds.), London: Springer-Verlag, pp. 3–28. ◆
Christiansen, M. H., and Devlin, J. T., 1997, Recursive inconsistencies are hard to learn: A connectionist perspective on universal word order correlations, in *Proceedings of the 19th Annual Cognitive Science Society Conference*, Mahwah, NJ: Erlbaum, pp. 113–118.
Deacon, T., 1997, *The Symbolic Species: The Co-evolution of Language and the Brain*, New York: Norton. ◆
Elman, J. L., 1990, Finding structure in time, *Cogn. Sci.*, 14:179–211.
Hare, M., and Elman, J. L., 1995, Learning and morphological change, *Cognition*, 56:61–98.
Nowak, M. A., and Komarova, N. L., 2001, Towards an evolutionary theory of language, *Trends Cognitive Sci.*, 5:288–295.
Livingstone, D., and Fyfe, C., 1999, Modelling the evolution of linguistic diversity, in *Advances in Artificial Life: Proceedings of the ECAL99 European Conference on Artificial Life* (D. Floreano, J. Nicoud, and F. Mondada, Eds.), Berlin: Springer-Verlag, pp. 704–708.
Turner, H., 2002, An introduction to methods for simulating the evolution of language, in *Simulating Language Evolution* (A. Cangelosi and D. Parisi, Eds.), London: Springer-Verlag, pp. 29–50. ◆
Van Everbroeck, E., 1999, Language type frequency and learnability: A connectionist appraisal, in *Proceedings of the 21st Annual Cognitive Science Society Conference*, Mahwah, NJ: Erlbaum, pp. 755–760.

Language Evolution: The Mirror System Hypothesis

Michael A. Arbib

Introduction

What is the evolutionary path leading to language in humans, and what are the relevant data on brain mechanisms? Since the fossil record offers no trace of brain structure beyond clues from ancient skulls on brain size and perhaps some fissures of the brain, the answers to these questions are varied and controversial (Wilkins and Wakefield, 1995). The present article emphasizes the *mirror system hypothesis* (MSH). The "mirror system" for grasping in

monkey, which contains *mirror neurons* that are active both when the monkey executes a specific hand action and when it observes a human or other monkey carrying out a similar action, is the homologue of Broca's area, a crucial speech area in humans. MSH asserts that the matching of neural code for execution and observation of hand movements is present in the common ancestor of monkey and human and is the precursor of the crucial language property of *parity*, namely, that an utterance usually carries similar meaning for speaker and hearer (using these terms neutrally for spoken and signed languages). This provides a neurobiological "missing link" for the hypothesis that communication based on manual gesture preceded speech in language evolution (e.g., Stokoe, 2001).

Where the present article focuses on brain mechanisms for vision, action, and language, the article LANGUAGE EVOLUTION AND CHANGE, focuses on the use of connectionist modeling to test hypotheses (usually more psychological than neurological in nature) about specific aspects of language evolution.

What Does the Biology of the Brain Provide?

Chomsky (e.g., 1975) has argued that since children acquire language rapidly despite the "poverty of the stimulus," the basic structures of language must be innate, forming a universal grammar encoded in the human genome. For example, universal grammar would encode the knowledge that sentences in a human language could be ordered as subject-verb-object, subject-object-verb, or one of a few other options, so that the child simply needs to hear a few sentences of his first language to "set the parameter" for the preferred order of that language. Against this, others have argued that the child has both a rich set of language stimuli linked to action and perception and powerful learning mechanisms, so that a child can indeed learn from its social interactions aspects of syntax which Chomsky would see as genetically prespecified (see LANGUAGE ACQUISITION). There is no argument against the view that human evolution yielded genetic specification of some of the structures which *support* language. Humans have hands, a larynx, and facial mobility suited for generating gestures that can be used in language, and the brain mechanisms needed to produce and perceive rapidly generated sequences of such gestures (Lieberman, 1991). In this sense, the human brain and body is *language ready*. The term *language readiness* was, I believe, my coinage (Arbib, 2002), but of course I was not the first to assert that the biological evolution that took us to ancestors with a language-ready brain (by some other name) had to be followed by a cultural evolution that took us from rudimentary manual-vocal communication to full language capability.

Although it is a matter of ongoing debate to delimit what constitutes language readiness and how it differs from language, we offer here a tentative list of criteria as a basis for future research.

Language Readiness

The first three properties support communication system without necessarily yielding language, while the last four properties are more general:

Symbolization: The ability to associate an arbitrary symbol with a class of events, objects, or actions, etc. At first, these symbols may not have been words in the modern sense, nor need they have been vocalized.
Intentionality: Communication is *intended* by the utterer to have a particular effect on the recipient.
Parity (mirror property): What counts for the speaker (or producer) must count for the listener (or receiver).
Hierarchical structuring: Production and recognition of components with subparts. This relates to basic mechanisms of action-oriented perception with no necessary link to the ability to communicate about these components and their relationships.
Temporal ordering: Temporal activity coding these hierarchical structures.
Beyond the here-and-now: The ability to recall past events or imagine future ones.

Paedomorphy and sociality: The prolonged immaturity of the infant and the prolonged caregiving of adults combine to create conditions for complex social learning.

Deacon (1997) makes symbolization central to his account of the co-evolution of language and the human brain. He stresses the componential homology that allows us to learn from relations between the brains of monkeys and humans. His more recent writings stress the role of self-organization as the child's brain adapts to the cultural environment in which the child develops. Where Deacon places most emphasis on the enlargement of frontal cortex, we place more emphasis on the differential development of specific subsystems that support language readiness. Interestingly, Semendeferi et al. (2002) argue that magnetic resonance imaging shows that human frontal cortices are not disproportionately large in comparison to those of the great apes. They thus suggest that the special cognitive abilities of humans may be due to differences in individual cortical areas and to a richer interconnectivity, rather than to an increase in the overall relative size of the frontal lobe during human evolution.

Language

We now turn to criteria for language, which we here hypothesize as what cultural evolution and learning add to the brain's capabilities for language readiness. Note that nothing in this list rests on the medium of exchange of the language, and that the list applies both to spoken language and to sign language.

Symbolization: The symbols become words in the modern sense, interchangeable and composable in the expression of meaning.
Syntax and semantics: The matching of syntactic to semantic structures co-evolves with the fractionation of utterances. This includes the ability to build utterances recursively (see CONSTITUENCY AND RECURSION IN LANGUAGE).
Beyond the here-and-now: Verb tenses (or alternative syntactic constructs) arise to express recall of past events and imagination of future ones.
Learnability: To qualify as a human language, it must contain a *significant subset* of symbolic structures learnable by most human children (but children do not master a language completely by 5 or 7 years of age).

Bickerton (1995) characterizes *protolanguage* as a form of communication whose users can only string together a small handful of words at a time, may leave out words arbitrarily, may often depart from customary word order, cannot form any complex structures, and use only a tiny fraction of the inflections and "grammatical words" that make up 50% of true language utterances. Bickerton then makes two distinct claims: (1) that the productions of apes who have been taught to use signs, early-stage pidgin languages, and the speech of children under 2 share enough properties in common that they can all be characterized as examples of a common entity, "protolanguage"; and (2) that this same entity, protolanguage, characterizes the "prelanguage" of early hominids. The counterhypothesis advanced here is that the prelanguage of early hominids was not a protolanguage in Bickerton's sense, but rather was made up of "one-word utterances" in which the "words" were *holophrastic*, i.e., more like today's complete phrases or sentences, with modern-sense words and syntax later co-evolving culturally.

Neurobiological Foundations

With this, we turn to the neurobiology of the monkey to ground claims as to the brain of the common ancestor of monkeys and humans of perhaps 20 million years ago, and hypotheses on how such brains changed to become language ready.

Brain Mechanisms for Grasping

Parietal area AIP and ventral premotor area F5 anchor the cortical circuit in monkey that transforms visual information on intrinsic properties of an object into hand movements for grasping it (see GRASPING MOVEMENTS: VISUOMOTOR TRANSFORMATIONS). Discharge in most F5 neurons correlates with an action rather than with the individual movements that form it, so that one may relate F5 neurons to various motor schemas (see SCHEMA THEORY) corresponding to the action associated with their discharge.

The FARS model (Fagg and Arbib, 1998) provides a computational account of the system centered on the AIP → F5 pathway (Figure 1): AIP cells encode "affordances"—visual features of the object relevant to action—for grasping and send (neural codes for) these on to area F5, which selects one of these for action. Inferotemporal cortex (IT) and prefrontal cortex (PFC) modulate F5's selection of an affordance. However, the dorsal stream via AIP does not know "what" the object is, it can only see the object as a set of possible affordances. The ventral stream (from primary visual cortex to IT), by contrast, is able to recognize what the object is (see DISSOCIATIONS BETWEEN VISUAL PROCESSING MODES). This information is passed to PFC, which can then, on the basis of the current goals of the organism and the recognition of the nature of the object, bias F5 to choose the affordance appropriate to the task at hand. (See GRASPING MOVEMENTS: VISUOMOTOR TRANSFORMATIONS for recent neuroanatomical data suggesting that PFC may act on action selection at the level of parietal cortex rather than premotor cortex.)

Figure 1 gives only a partial view of the FARS model, which also provides mechanisms for sequencing actions. It segregates the F5 circuitry that encodes unit actions from the circuitry encoding a sequence, possibly the part of the supplementary motor area called pre-SMA (Rizzolatti, Luppino, and Matelli, 1998). The administration of the sequence (inhibiting extraneous actions, while priming imminent actions) is then carried out by the basal ganglia (see BASAL GANGLIA and SEQUENCE LEARNING).

The Mirror System for Grasping

Further study revealed a class of F5 neurons that discharged not only when the monkey grasped or manipulated objects, but also when the monkey observed the experimenter make a gesture similar to the one that, when actively performed by the monkey, involved activity of the neuron. Neurons with this property are called *mirror neurons* (Gallese et al., 1996). Mirror neurons respond only to an interaction between the agent and the object of an action. The simple presentation of objects, even when held by hand, does not evoke the neuron discharge.

Not all F5 neurons respond to action observation. We thus distinguish mirror neurons from *canonical neurons* in F5, which are active only when the monkey itself performs the relevant actions. Mirror neurons receive input from the PF region of parietal cortex encoding observations of arm and hand movements. This is in contrast to the canonical F5 neurons, which receive object-related input from AIP. It is the canonical neurons, with their input from AIP, that are modeled in the FARS model.

Bridging from Action to Language

A Mirror System for Grasping in Humans

The notion that a mirror system might exist in humans was tested by PET experiments, which showed that grasp observation significantly activated the superior temporal sulcus (STS), the inferior parietal lobule, and the inferior frontal gyrus (area 45). All activations were in the left hemisphere. The last area is of special interest: areas 44 and 45 in the left hemisphere of the human constitute Broca's area. F5 in monkey is generally considered (see analysis by Matelli in Rizzolatti and Arbib, 1998) to be the homologue of Broca's area in humans; i.e., it can be argued that these areas of monkey and human brain are related to the same region of the common ancestor. Thus, the cortical areas active during action observation in humans and monkeys correspond very well, indicating that there is a fundamental primate mechanism for action recognition: we argue that individuals recognize actions made by others because the neural pattern elicited in their premotor areas during action observation is similar to a part of that internally generated to produce a similar action. Note, however, that "understand-

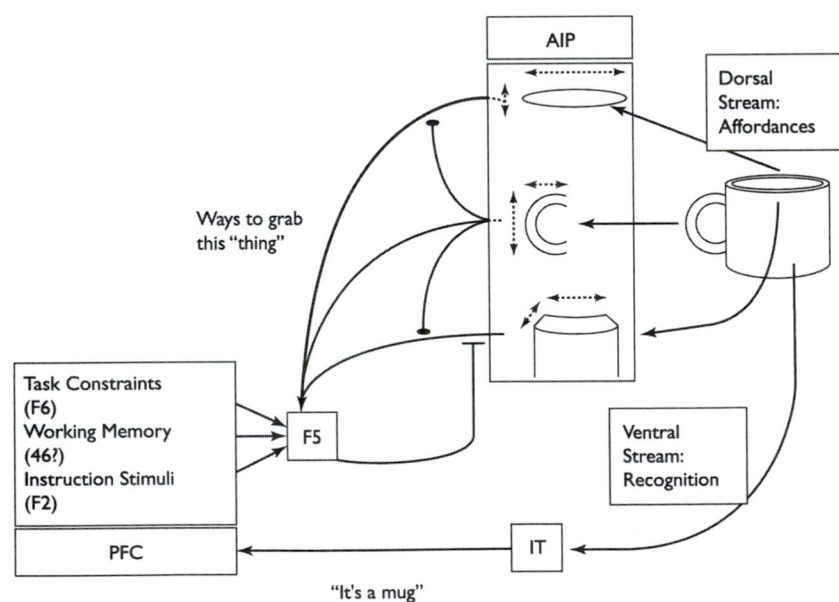

Figure 1. The role of IT (inferotemporal cortex) and PFC (prefrontal cortex) in modulating F5's selection of an affordance from the repertoire forwarded by AIP.

ing" involves the cooperation of many brain systems and cannot be reduced to just the activity in a subset of F5 neurons.

Primate Vocalization

Monkeys exhibit a primate call system (a limited set of species-specific calls) and an orofacial (mouth and hand) gesture system (a limited set of gestures expressive of emotion and related social indicators). This communication system is *closed* in the sense that it is restricted to a specific repertoire. This is to be contrasted with the open nature of human languages. (Although each human language is open as to, e.g., nouns and verbs, it is [almost] closed with respect to prepositions and grammatical markers.) Strikingly, the neural substrate for primate calls is in a region of cingulate cortex distinct from F5, which we have seen to be the monkey homologue of Broca's area in the human. One challenge, then, is to understand why it is F5, rather than the cingulate area already involved in monkey vocalization, that is homologous to the human's frontal substrate for language. Note that the claim is not that Broca's area is genetically preprogrammed for language, but rather that the development of a human child in a language community normally adapts this brain region to play a crucial role in language performance.

The Mirror System Hypothesis

What turns a movement into an action is that it is associated with a goal, so that initiation of the movement is accompanied by the creation of an expectation that the goal will be met. We distinguish "pragmatic action," in which the hands are used to interact physically with objects or the bodies of other creatures, and "gestures" (both manual and vocal), whose purpose is communication. Our assumption is that monkeys use hand movements only for pragmatic actions. The mirror system allows other monkeys to understand these actions and act on the basis of this understanding. Similarly, the monkey's orofacial gestures register emotional state, and primate vocalizations can also communicate something of the current situation of the monkey.

Stokoe (2001) provides a recent summary of the argument, rooted in the analysis of sign language, that communication based on manual gesture played a crucial role in human language evolution, preceding communication by speech. In this regard, we stress that the "openness" or "generativity" that some see as the hallmark of language is present in manual behavior, which can thus supply the evolutionary substrate for its appearance in language. With our understanding that the mirror system in monkeys is the homologue of Broca's area in humans, we can now appreciate the mirror system hypothesis.

The mirror system hypothesis: Language evolved from a basic mechanism *not* originally related to communication: the *mirror system for grasping*, with its capacity to generate *and* recognize a set of actions. More specifically, Broca's area in the human contains a mirror system for grasping that is homologous to the F5 mirror system of monkey, and this provides the evolutionary basis for *language parity*; i.e., an utterance means roughly the same for both speaker and hearer.

However, having a mirror system is not equivalent to having language. Monkeys have mirror systems but do not have language, and we expect that many species have mirror systems for varied socially relevant behaviors.

Simple and Complex Imitation Systems for Grasping

It is unclear whether the mirror system for grasping is sufficient for the copying of actions. It is one thing to recognize an action

using the mirror system and another thing to use that representation as a basis for repeating the action. In any case, the ability to copy *single* actions is just the first step toward imitation, since imitation involves "parsing" a complex movement into more or less familiar pieces and then performing the corresponding composite of (variations on) familiar actions. Myowa-Yamakoshi and Matsuzawa (1999) observed that chimpanzees typically took 12 trials to learn to "imitate" a behavior, and in doing so paid more attention to where the manipulated object was being directed rather than to the actual movements of the demonstrator. This may involve using one or both hands to bring two objects into relationship or to bring an object into relationship with the body. Thus the form of imitation reported for chimpanzees is a long and laborious process compared to the rapidity with which humans can acquire novel sequences. I have called this the contrast between "simple" imitation and "complex" imitation (Arbib, 2002) and assert that monkeys have neither, chimpanzees have simple imitation, and humans have complex imitation (not all primatologists accept this distinction; see IMITATION for further discussion).

If we assume (1) that the common ancestor of monkeys and apes had no greater imitative ability than present-day monkeys and (2) that the ability for simple imitation shared by chimps and humans was also possessed by their common ancestor, but that (3) only humans possess a talent for "complex" imitation, then we have established a case for the claim that brain mechanisms for simple imitation developed in the 15 million-year evolution from the common ancestor of monkeys and apes to the common ancestor of apes and humans, and that a complex imitation system—acquiring (longer) novel sequences of more abstract actions in a single trial—developed in the 5 million-year evolution from the common ancestor of apes and humans along the hominid line that led, in particular, to *Homo sapiens*. The argument, then, is that extension of the mirror system from recognition of single actions to imitation of compound actions was one of the key innovations in the brains of hominids relevant to language readiness.

A Manual-Based Communication System

Given a creature with the ability for complex imitation, how might further hominid evolution have yielded a manual-based communication system that could lead to the further evolution of brain and body mechanisms supporting language readiness? Our hypothetical sequence leading to manual gesture and beyond is the following:

1. Pragmatic action directed toward a goal object
2. Imitation of such actions
3. Pantomime in which similar actions are produced in the absence of any goal object

In terms of observable movements, imitation of an action and pantomime of an action may appear the same. However, imitation is the generic attempt to reproduce movements performed by another, whether to master a skill or simply as part of a social interaction. By contrast, pantomime is essentially communicative, performed with the intention of getting the observer to think of a specific action or event. Thus, even though the movements may be similar, the actions (movement + goal) are very different.

4. Abstract gestures divorced from their pragmatic origins (if such existed). In pantomime it might be hard to distinguish a grasping movement signifying "grasping" from one meaning "a [graspable] raisin," thus providing an "incentive" for coming up with an arbitrary gesture to distinguish the two meanings.

This suggests that *arbitrary* symbols emerged when the communicative capacities of pantomiming were exhausted. This can be illustrated with modern American Sign Language, in which, for example, noun/verb pairs may be differentiated by movement. For example (Stokoe, 2001), the AIRPLANE/FLY pair of signs uses the same handshape, but the noun has short, repeated movements, whereas the verb has a single prolonged movement.

We thus distinguish *complementary roles for imitation* in the posited evolution of manual-based communication: extending imitation to pantomime to provide "natural" gestures that may convey a situation to the observer; and extending the mirror system from the grasping repertoire to mediate imitation of gestures that provide "conventionalized" symbols that can reduce ambiguity and extend the semantic range.

My current hypothesis is that stages (2) and (3) and a rudimentary (presyntactic) form of (stage 4) were present in prehuman hominids, but that the explosive development of linked symbols that we know as language depended on cultural evolution, well after biological evolution had formed modern *Homo sapiens*.

The Path to Protospeech Is Indirect

Earlier we noted that the neural substrate for primate calls is in a region of cingulate cortex distinct from F5, which latter is the monkey homologue of Broca's area in the human. Rizzolatti and Arbib (1998) suggest two evolutionary stages:

1. A *distinct* manuobrachial (hand-arm) communication system evolved (as just described) to complement the primate calls/ orofacial communication system. At this stage, the "speech" area (i.e., the area of the hominid brain presumably homologous to monkey F5) mediated only orofacial and manuobrachial communication.
2. The manual-orofacial symbolic system then "recruited" vocalization. The association of vocalization with manual gestures allowed it to assume a more open referential character, yielding "protospeech" (but not full-blown spoken language). This yields the MSH explanation of why F5, rather than the primate call area, provides the evolutionary substrate for language readiness.

However, language and vocalization systems are nonetheless linked. Lesions centered in the anterior cingulate cortex and supplementary motor areas of the brain can also cause mutism in humans, similar to the effects produced in muting monkey vocalizations. Conversely, a patient with a Broca's area lesion may nonetheless swear when provoked. But note that "emitting an imprecation" is more like a monkey vocalization than like the syntactically structured use of language. Lieberman (1991) suggests that the primate call made by an infant separated from its mother not only survives in the human infant, but in humans develops into the breath group, i.e., the pattern of breathing in and breathing out that is shaped to provide the contour for each continuous sequence of a spoken utterance. This suggests that the evolution of speech yielded the pathways for cooperative computation between cingulate cortex and Broca's area, with cingulate cortex involved in breath groups and emotional shading and Broca's area involved in providing (in concert with, e.g., the basal ganglia) motor control for rapid production and interweaving of elements of an utterance.

From Protospeech to Language

The cultural evolution of *Homo sapiens* may have involved an increased ability to name actions and objects to create a rapidly growing set of verb-argument structures, and the ability to compound those structures in diverse ways. Earlier I suggested that many grammatical structures would have been "postbiological" in their origin (Arbib, 2002). We might then see as ingenious human

discoveries that the one word *ripe* halves the number of fruit names to be learned, or that separating action names from object names requires one to learn only $m + n$ words (m nouns and n verbs) to be able to form $m*n*m$ of the most basic utterances.

The spread of these innovations resided in the ability of other humans not only to imitate the new actions and compounds of actions demonstrated by the innovators, but also to do so in a way that related increasingly general classes of symbolic behavior to the classes, events, behaviors, and relationships they were to represent. Indeed, consideration of the spatial basis for "prepositions" may help show how visuomotor coordination underlies some aspects of language, while variations in the use of corresponding prepositions, even in English and Spanish, show how the basic, functionally grounded semantic-syntactic correspondences have been overlaid by a multitude of later innovations and borrowings.

Toward a Mirror System–Based Neurolinguistics

The monkey needs many brain regions for the mirror system for grasping. We will need many more brain regions for a full neurolinguistic model that extends the linkages far beyond the F5 ≈ Broca's area homology. To set the stage for the future development of such a model, we briefly link our view of AIP and F5 in monkey to data on human abilities. Studies of the visual system of monkey led to the distinction between IT mechanisms for object recognition ("what") and posterior parietal (PP) mechanisms for localizing objects ("where"). Others extended this to a dichotomy between human "what" (IT) and "how" (PP): a patient with damage to the IT pathway could grasp and orient objects appropriately for manipulating them but could not report, either verbally or by pantomime, how big an object was or what the orientation of a slot was; another patient with damage to the PP pathway could communicate the size of a cylinder but not preshape appropriately (see DISSOCIATIONS BETWEEN VISUAL PROCESSING MODES).

Let us now try to reconcile these observations with our mirror system–based approach to language. Our evolutionary theory suggests a progression from action to action recognition to language, as follows:

1. Object → AIP → F5$_{canonical}$ pragmatics
2. Action → PF → F5$_{mirror}$ action recognition
3. Scene → Wernicke's → Broca's   utterance

The "zero-order" model of the above PP/IT data is:

4. Parietal "affordances" → preshape
5. IT "perception of object" → pantomime or verbally describe size

However, step 5 implies that one cannot directly pantomime or verbalize a parietal affordance; one needs the "unified view of the object" (IT) before one can communicate attributes. The problem with this is that the "language" path as shown in step 3 is independent of the IT system. To resolve this paradox, we note the experiments of Bridgeman and his colleagues (DISSOCIATIONS BETWEEN VISUAL PROCESSING MODES). When an observer sees a target in one of several possible positions and a frame either centered before the observer or deviated left or right, verbal judgments of the target position are altered by the background frame's position, but "jabbing" at the target never misses. The point is that communication must be based on the size estimate generated by IT, presumably for overall planning of movement, and not on that generated by PP, which provides precise parameters for motor control.

Given these data, we may now recall (Figure 1) that although AIP extracts a set of affordances, it is IT and PFC that are crucial to F5's selection of the affordance to execute, and then offer the scheme shown in Figure 2 (from Arbib in Cangelosi and Parisi,

Figure 2. An early pass on a mirror system–based neurolinguistics. (From Arbib, 2002.)

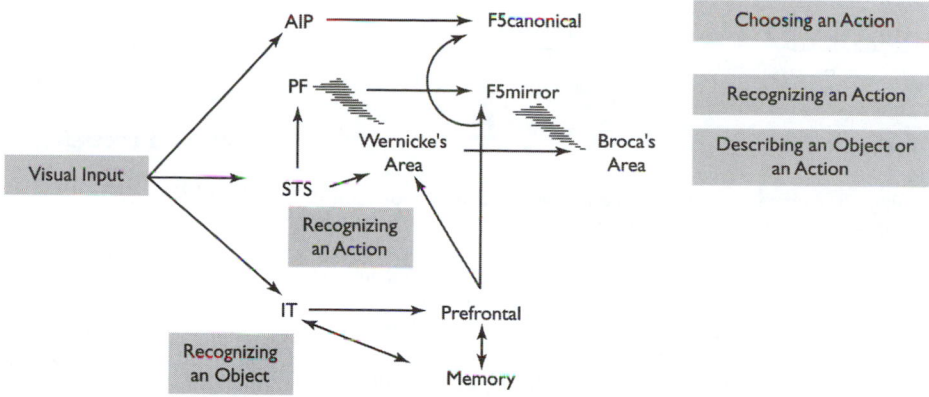

2001). Here we emphasize the crucial role of IT-mediated functioning of PFC in the activity of Broca's area. This is the merest of sketches. For example, we do not tease apart the roles of different subdivisions of PFC in modulating $F5_{canonical}$, $F5_{mirror}$, and Broca's area. However, the crucial suggestion is that, just as $F5_{mirror}$ receives its parietal input from PF rather than AIP, so Broca's area receives its size data as well as object identity data from IT via PFC, rather than via a side path from AIP. This is just the beginning.

Discussion

The approach taken here has rich implications for the study of human evolution and NEUROLINGUISTICS (q.v.).

1. It is a mistake to assume that features common to modern-day languages must be biological in nature. Work on brain mechanisms of language must seek to distinguish the biological givens of language readiness from the cultural extensions that define the world's languages today.
2. We must be open to multiple hypotheses about the nature of hominid "prelanguage," seeking to evaluate the claims of Bickerton's protolanguage hypothesis against the claims for fractionation and imitation-based symbolization advanced here.
3. MSH offers a clear explanation for why Broca's area is homologous to an area for grasping in the human brain rather than to the cingulate area involved in primate vocalizations.
4. MSH also explains why language is multimodal, so that a deaf child can acquire sign language as readily as a hearing child acquires speech.

Even the canonical system (the FARS model) involves multiple regions in the monkey's brain (including AIP, F5, IT, pre-SMA, and basal ganglia), and the mirror system involves many more (including STS and PF). As we seek to understand the extensions of these that mediate complex imitation and undergird language readiness, we see that there is far more to the human brain's unique capability to master language than "F5 becomes Broca's area to provide parity." Building on Figure 2, or on other hypotheses grounded in the comparative study of primate brains, to develop a rich model of language readiness—and developing an integrated view of syntax and semantics to build upon it—will require both analysis of neurological data and subtle modeling that links neurolinguistics to the basic neural mechanisms for the recognition of the interactions of actors and objects, and for the elaboration of suitable motor plans for interacting with the environment so perceived. A further challenge is to explore the extent to which MSH

constrains the structure of modern languages, despite the great variations wrought by cultural evolution. One such example (Arbib and Jean-Roger Vergnaud, in prep.) is the assertion that sentences are canonically structured as

$$[_S NP_s [_{vP} v [_{VP} \times NP_O]]]$$

v-V being the analysis of the verb in the sentence, because the canonical system of F5 binding action to object underlies the merging of the V-component with the object NP_O, while the mirror system of F5 binding agent to action underlies the merging of the subject NP_s with the complex v-VP.

Road Maps: Linguistics and Speech Processing; Neuroethology and Evolution
Related Reading: Evolution of Artificial Neural Networks; Evolution of the Ancestral Vertebrate Brain; Grasping Movements: Visuomotor Transformations; Imitation; Language Evolution and Change; Neuroethology, Computational

References

Arbib, M. A., 2002, The mirror system, imitation, and the evolution of language, in *Imitation in Animals and Artifacts* (C. Nehaniv and K. Dautenhahn, Ed.), Cambride, MA: MIT Press, pp. 229–280. ◆
Bickerton, D., 1995, *Language and Human Behavior*, Seattle: University of Washington Press.
Cangelosi, A., and Parisi, D., Eds., 2001, *Simulating the Evolution of Language*, London: Springer-Verlag.
Chomsky, N., 1975, *Reflections on Language*, New York: Pantheon.
Deacon, T. W., 1997, *The Symbolic Species: The Co-evolution of Language and the Brain*, New York: Norton.
Fagg, A. H., and Arbib, M. A., 1998, Modeling parietal-premotor interactions in primate control of grasping, *Neural Netw.*, 11:1277–1303.
Gallese, V., Fadiga, L., Fogassi, L., and Rizzolatti, G., 1996, Action recognition in the premotor cortex, *Brain*, 119:593–609.
Lieberman, P., 1991, *Uniquely Human: The Evolution of Speech, Thought, and Selfless Behavior*, Cambridge, MA: Harvard University Press.
Myowa-Yamakoshi, M., and Matsuzawa, T., 1999, Factors influencing imitation of manipulatory actions in chimpanzees (Pan troglodytes), *J. Comp. Psychol.*, 113:128–136.
Rizzolatti, G., and Arbib, M. A., 1998, Language within our grasp, *Trends Neurosci.*, 21:188–194. ◆
Rizzolatti, G., Luppino, G., and Matelli, M., 1998, The organization of the cortical motor system: New concepts, *Electroencephalogr. Clin. Neurophysio.*, 106:283–296.
Semendeferi, K., Lu, A., Schenker, N., and Damasio, H., 2002, Humans and great apes share a large frontal cortex, *Nature Neurosci.*, 5:272–276.
Stokoe, W. C., 2001, *Language in Hand: Why Sign Came Before Speech*, Washington, DC: Gallaudet University Press. ◆
Wilkins, W. K., and Wakefield, J., 1995, Brain evolution and neurolinguistic preconditions, *Behav. Brain Sci.*, 18:161–226.

Language Processing

Richard Shillcock

Introduction

Language has provided some of the most important opportunities and challenges for connectionist cognitive modeling. There is a wealth of human behavioral data, from cognitive psychology experiments, from observations of children acquiring language, and from studies of developmental or acquired language disorders. There are also comprehensive insights from formal domains, such as phonology and syntax. Since McClelland and Rumelhart's (1981) Interactive Activation Model of visual word recognition, connectionist modeling has been applied to most areas of language processing. For instance, neural network architectures have been employed to discover syllable structure from waveforms, to manage constraint satisfaction with different categories of linguistic information in parsing, and to simulate data from historical linguistics and language typology. Even in formal syntax, the connectionist paradigm shift has provoked notions such as the graded application of rules (see OPTIMALITY THEORY IN LINGUISTICS). In the following paragraphs we review a number of models that capture detailed behavioral data and simulate the brain's discovery and manipulation of structure in spoken and written language.

This modeling was conducted against the backdrop, within psychology and cognitive science, of two related concerns: modularity and top-down feedback. Researchers have asked whether the functional architecture of cognition is modular: Are certain kinds of processing autonomous and encapsulated from other kinds of information, or do different types of information freely interact? The paradigm example has been the claimed autonomy of syntactic processing. Researchers have also asked whether genuine top-down feedback occurs: Is more sophisticated, higher-order, contextual information ever used to enhance the processing of lower-order, more peripheral representations, or is cognition fundamentally "bottom-up"? The paradigm example here has been the relationship between a word and its constituent letters or speech segments (see SPEECH PROCESSING: PSYCHOLINGUISTICS).

Many classical box-and-arrow cognitive models have become very elaborate in an attempt to accommodate additional human data, and have often been limited in their ability to generate interesting emergent behavior that might be tested against human subjects. Finally, there has been a fierce debate over the nature of representation in the brain, the status of rules, and the extent of any specific genetic endowment underlying human language learning. Despite the insights gained from the formal study of language, the formal approach has allowed researchers to say relatively little about learning and development. Thus, the "connectionist program" for understanding language has concentrated on the process of *change*, exploring topics such as language development (see LANGUAGE ACQUISITION; PAST TENSE LEARNING); language breakdown (see LESIONED NETWORKS AS MODELS OF NEUROPSYCHOLOGICAL DEFICITS; NEUROLINGUISTICS); the dynamics of representation in complex systems, which themselves may be receiving changing input (see SPEECH PROCESSING: PSYCHOLINGUISTICS); and, more recently, the evolution of language (see LANGUAGE EVOLUTION AND CHANGE). Despite the fact that connectionist models of language have often been built to cover restricted domains, such as learning the past tense, a common goal has been to show the *emergence* of complex linguistic behavior from more basic foundations, which may not themselves be specifically linguistic in nature.

Lexical Processing

Reading Single Words

Models of single-word reading and pronunciation have perhaps been the most compelling of any connectionist models of cognition. McClelland and Rumelhart's Interactive Activation Model (IAM) is an enduring example of a large-scale model producing illuminating and testable emergent behaviors through the management of very large numbers of interactions. It identifies four-letter words from an input of visual features in the four-letter positions. This input level is connected to a level containing a representation of each letter in each position, which is connected to a level containing a representation of each word. The model was handwired so that excitatory connections between levels cause features to activate the relevant letter representations, which then activate all of the words in which they occur. Each activated word node sends supportive activation to its constituent letters. Inhibitory connections between and within levels suppress inconsistent representations. This localist model accurately simulated human data concerning the perception of letters in briefly presented words, such as the apparent top-down support of "gangs" of similar words for shared letters in particular positions. The model has been incorporated as a proper part of Coltheart and colleagues' (1993) symbolic/connectionist hybrid model of pronunciation.

Recognizing Spoken Words

Top-down feedback similar to the IAM's appeared in McClelland and Elman's TRACE model of spoken word recognition, in which an interactive activation network was replicated across subsequent time slices to capture the flow of activation from phonetic features to segments to words. Interesting behaviors were observed, such as the trading of different cues to segment identity and an emergent segmentation of the continuous speech stream into a single string of words simply by the activation of all possibly implicated words, combined with winner-take-all competitions. Top-down feedback in TRACE is computationally effective, but in the long-running controversy over the existence of such feedback, Norris, McQueen, and Cutler (2000) have argued that it is unwarranted and unnecessary in a model of spoken word recognition. In related models of spoken word recognition and of phoneme recognition in speech (Norris et al., 2000), interactive activation principles have been employed in purely bottom-up architectures.

Distributed Lexical Representations

The modeling of normal and impaired single-word reading is the flagship of the connectionist cognitive modeling enterprise (Seidenberg and McClelland, 1989; Plaut et al., 1996). Seidenberg and McClelland (1989) characterized lexical processing in terms of a triangle of mappings between orthographic, phonological, and semantic representations, using three-layer networks trained by the backpropagation of error. (Only in later developments of this model has semantic processing been implemented.) An identity mapping from orthographic representations to orthographic representations was used to model the capturing of a secure visual representation of the word. The model did not possess a discretely structured lexicon; instead, information about a particular word was distributed across the many weighted connections between the three sets of representational units as the model learned the words in its training set. The goal has been to simulate the reading of regular words, irregular words (e.g., *pint*), and nonwords (e.g., *tenk*) within the same homogeneous architecture, and to explore an emergent division of labor between orthographic and semantic contributions to the pronunciation of different word types (see READING). An important improvement in later versions of this model involved employing local orthographic and phonological representations that respected the formal distinctions of the onset, nucleus, and coda of monosyllabic words (e.g., the *d*, *e*, and *sk* of *desk*). This innovation illustrates a criticism heard on both sides of the debate over connectionist cognitive modeling. Critics have stated that specifying the input and output representations relies on the formal insights of the classical, symbol-processing tradition and takes the crucially hard work out of solving the problem. Quartz and Sejnowski (1997), arguing a "constructivist" case for concentrating on the role of activity and growth in development, make the related point that it is the identification of the problem in the first place that is critical in learning and development. We might add that employing representations developed by formal linguists, such as phonemes, distinctive features, or syntactic categories, brings both advantages and disadvantages; all such categories involve ambiguity at their boundaries, even in the formal domains for which they were developed. All symbolic distinctions made about natural language are graded, in the limit.

Further improvements in the modeling of lexical processing have come from using recurrent architectures trained to settle into steady states, each corresponding to a desired output. Such attractor networks allow a feedforward model to map initially to an approximate output, which is then "cleaned up" appropriately if the initial approximation falls within the "basin of attraction" of the desired output. This innovation has been crucial in mapping between orthographic and semantic representations (Hinton and Shallice, 1991), where the relationship is essentially arbitrary. It has also allowed better generalization in the quasi-regular mapping between orthographic and phonological form, as such attractors have been shown to behave componentially in generating pronunciations.

The modeling of lexical processing has been important because of its psychologically realistic scale. The benchmark has been the pronunciation of a more or less complete slice of the lexicon, such as all the four-letter words or all the monosyllabic words of English. (Modeling with polysyllabic words has been limited.) A further aspect of the models' scale is that they involve the full repertoire of letters and speech segments. In these respects, such modeling is psychologically grounded in a way that cannot be claimed for small models with unrepresentative training sets. The modeling of other language domains, such as morphology, syntax, or semantics, has typically not achieved this rich, realistic scale and coverage.

The folk interpretation of the mental lexicon as a dictionary suggests a discrete lexical entry for each word, and it is surprising that models based on superpositional storage can achieve so much. Models of visual and spoken word recognition employing distributed representations of words have largely superseded the localist, handwired models such as the IAM and TRACE, which cannot capture the phenomena of learning and development and that are also relatively large architectures to build if they are to achieve wide coverage. Nevertheless, both types of connectionist model continue to generate important, experimentally testable predictions, and there has been eloquent advocacy of the merits of localist representation.

Less attention has been given to semantic processing in lexical models, partly because the central ability of connectionist models to generalize is maladaptive, given the arbitrary relationship between form and meaning, and partly because of the inherent difficulties of representing the meanings of words. However, when semantic representations have been studied, they have been based either on hand-crafted (sometimes dictionary-derived) semantic features (e.g., "+edible" or "+living"), or on corpus-derived context vectors, which specify the lexical contexts in which words are found. It is easier to see the latter type of semantic representation as being psychologically grounded: the context vectors are derived from very large corpora of real language, and wide coverage of the lexicon is more feasible than with an approach that uses semantic features.

Word Production

Research on word production has been overwhelmingly concerned with slips of the tongue and with dysphasia resulting from strokes, but there has been a growing interest in the priming of syntactic structure. Connectionist modeling of word production has not been extensive and has centered on Dell's interactive activation model (Dell, 1986). In this model, activation initially flows downward from a lexical node to levels representing linguistic units—syllables, onsets and rimes, phonemes, and phonological features. Activation also feeds back upward, and after a set time the most activated nodes are selected for the onset, vowel, and coda slots. In a later version, semantic units activate word units and, in a second phase, word units activate phoneme units. Dell and colleagues have simulated both slips of the tongue and dysphasic errors within this framework, and have also developed learning models based on recurrent networks to avoid the limitations of hand-coded interactive activation models.

Learning Rules

Researchers have explored the analogy between a connectionist model learning the structure of a linguistic domain and an infant acquiring language. Formal theories of language acquisition had led to the conclusion that a universal grammar had to be genetically specified in some detail. Within this approach, symbol-based rules are explicitly implemented. Connectionist modeling has held out the prospect that language learning could arise from more general-purpose cognitive processing, with rule-like behavior emerging from distributed representations. The learning of morphology has attracted the most research, but attention has recently centered on the abilities of very young infants to learn the regularities present in very simple "artificial grammars" and on the capabilities of connectionist models to simulate these data.

Rumelhart and McClelland began this debate about development with their model of past tense acquisition (see PAST TENSE LEARNING). Their model attracted robust criticism, but later modeling of morphological processing, even involving the apparently problematic case of minority default forms in German, has revealed a more detailed developmental picture that has supported Rumelhart and McClelland's original insight that a quasi-regular mapping can be captured by a model with a single mechanism operating with distributed representations of words. However, the broader debate continues, with one side exploring the capacity of models with a homogeneous architecture to account for the data while the other side argues for "dual-route" models containing explicit rules and stored exceptions to those rules.

Higher-Level Processing

Higher-level, sentential processing involves syntax and semantics and immediately differs from lexical processing in terms of productivity: a speaker can produce an infinite number of different sentences. Syntactic processing is the paradigm example of symbolic behavior: the usage of the word *John* is determined by the category to which it belongs, proper nouns, rather than by features intrinsic to that particular word, so that being able to process *John sees Kim* necessarily implies being able to process *Kim sees John*. It has been claimed that connectionist models cannot transcend their inherent capacities to associate and to generalize between similar items so as to be able to capture the productivity and systematicity of natural language. Nevertheless, a variety of models have been developed to show that the principles of the connectionist modeling of cognition can be applied to sentence processing.

There is a long history of using the constraint satisfaction abilities of localist connectionist models to parse strings of words when syntactic and semantic categories are given. Such approaches implement insights such as the role of the frequency of particular transitions or the competition between possible parses. However, they take for granted the discreteness of the given formal categories, they can say little about development, and they cannot arbitrate the psychological issue of whether any particular category or type of information (typically syntax) has priority in processing.

An important departure came with Elman's simple recurrent network (SRN) and the demonstration that such models could discover and use syntactically relevant information in sentences (Elman, 1990). The SRN was developed to take account of temporal context in a sequence of inputs with no length restriction. In a three-layer network, the state of the hidden units at a particular point in time is recycled back to the hidden units simultaneously with the new input at the next point in time. Thus, the hidden units are affected by the previous inputs and states of the network. Elman required SRN models to predict the identity of the next word in a novel sentence as a means of testing whether the models had learned syntactic and semantic generalizations from the training corpus. Elman and others have shown, using this approach, that SRNs can capture some of the processing behavior observed in human readers, involving difficulties with particular construction types. Christiansen and Chater have shown that such models are capable of behavior that resembles the human ability to use words in accordance with their constituent nature, such as using *boy* in a novel syntactic position appropriate for a noun.

These approaches to higher-level structure in language have been shown to be capable of at least beginning the process of language learning (see CONSTITUENCY AND RECURSION IN LANGUAGE). Further work has been directed to extending the complexity of the input; more construction types have been covered, and the effects of memory constraints on syntactic processing have been revealed, with implications for the observed distribution of different language types.

An influential approach to modeling adult parsing competence has been based on Pollack's Recursive Auto-Associative Memory (RAAM), in which the hidden units of the model are made to develop distributed representations of successive layers of a parse tree. The model is required to autoassociate these patterns, which are provided by the modeler. The hidden unit activations may be stored and read back off a stack, when they may be used to recreate the parse across the output units. In addition, the trained model may generalize its parsing behavior to novel inputs. A recurrent version of this model has been developed that, like the SRN, discovers sequential dependencies in its inputs that correlate with syntactic roles.

In general, parsing models that have been claimed to learn structured syntactic relationships between words also discover a variety of other types of information relevant to parsing. In the real world, potential clues to syntactic structure may include prosody, phonosyntactic regularities, punctuation, semantic attributes of words, argument structure, discourse context, and real-world knowledge; it is a strong claim to say that any potentially useful information is ignored by the brain in assigning a parse. Some brain imaging studies suggest autonomous syntactic processing of unproblematic input and fast interaction with other types of information when ambiguity is encountered. The debate about the autonomy of syntax continues even with the advent of sophisticated imaging techniques (see IMAGING THE GRAMMATICAL BRAIN).

Overall, the period from the mid-1980s has seen an explosion in the increasingly sophisticated application of connectionist methods to the discovery and/or management of higher-level structure in language, from syntax and morphosyntax through to semantics and discourse structure. Researchers have simulated processing in such subdomains as parsing, variable binding, question answering, sentence generation, topic identification, anaphora resolution, application of world knowledge to language understanding, translation, grammaticality judgment, text compression, information retrieval, and discourse understanding. Some researchers have dealt with the more ambitious combinations of tasks using completely connectionist modular architectures, and others have augmented connectionist architectures with more traditional computational approaches, creating hybrid models. (For coverage of some of this growing field, see Reilly and Sharkey, 1992; Wermter, Riloff, and Scheler, 1996; Dale, Moisl, and Somers, 2000; and Christiansen and Chater, 2001.)

Finally, the last decade has seen growing interest in modeling the evolution of language. Connectionist architectures have been used, along with other statistical models, to simulate the evolution, by iterative learning, of simple "languages" by successive generations of individuals. The goal has been to elicit the emergence of compositional structure and other attributes of natural language.

Starting Small

One set of studies addressing development has attracted wide attention across a range of disciplines. Elman captured in network terms the intuition from language learning research that the cognitive constraints found in the developing infant may actually be advantageous to learning. Elman trained an SRN to learn syntactic dependencies separated by different numbers of intervening words in a sequential input and found that constraints that were intended to mimic the memory and attention limitations of infants acted to structure the training regimen by focusing learning on the shorter dependencies before the longer ones. The model that began with constraints that were subsequently relaxed outperformed the model that began with "adult" abilities. However, even though the notion of "starting small" still has deep implications for understanding development, Rohde and Plaut have shown that this principle may not be so unambiguously demonstrated using SRNs.

Anatomical Reality

Models have not typically incorporated observable anatomical detail beyond the general claims regarding interactivity, distributed representations, and superpositional storage (although some researchers have explored giving priority to short connections in cortical processing). Arguably there is little, if any, discrete brain anatomy exclusively dedicated to language processing, unlike the areas and pathways responsible for vision, for instance. Some neuroimaging research suggests that although some language activities may be closely associated with certain brain areas, it may be truer to say that those areas specialize in particular subtasks (e.g., Broca's area and sequence storage) that are not exclusively linguistic. Furthermore, task difficulty seems to affect the configurations of activation seen (e.g., Broca's area may be only minimally activated by syntactically undemanding language), perhaps reflecting the redundancy present in language. These observations may mean that for a very long time, our best understanding of language processing may still come from relatively high-level connectionist modeling.

However, the largest anatomical distinction, the hemispheric division of the brain, indisputably has an impact on language processing. Reggia, Goodall, and Shkuro have modeled hemispheric lateralization of phonological processing during development, and Shillcock and Monaghan (2001) have modeled single-word reading based on the observation that the fovea in the human retina is vertically split and projects contralaterally to the two hemispheres.

The issue of anatomical reality is closely connected to attempts to model cognitive impairment by lesioning trained connectionist models. Indeed, a critical part of the validation of models of normal processing has been to study their ability to capture impaired processing. The modeling of dyslexia is the most developed part of this field. Some of the lesions applied to the relevant models may be interpreted anatomically, but the range of possible instantiations of such damage is large. Thus, "impairment to the orthographic representations" could refer to anything from ocular problems to hemispheric desynchronization. Finally, a different approach to anatomical specificity comes from Miikkulainen (1997), who shows how the development and subsequent lesioning of a self-organizing feature map of word meanings can result in the category-specific impairment observed in deep dyslexia, in which particular semantic categories (e.g., furniture, tools, fruit) are disproportionately affected.

Discussion

Perhaps the most important outcome of this expanding field of research is that testable predictions have been made about normal and impaired language processing in human subjects. The resulting experiments tell us more about the phenomena concerned. Some of the models represent the state-of-the-art theory about their domain, vying with nonconnectionist models for best coverage of the data; other models remain principled existence proofs of the application of soft constraint satisfaction or distributed representations, for instance, to language processing problems. However, the major debates—over top-down feedback, over the capacity of connectionist models to capture the productivity and systematicity of human language, and over the degree of modularity in language processing—have not been settled by this combination of modeling and human experimentation. The terms of the debates may well change before any such resolution is manifest. For instance, much still remains to be understood about the nature of the brain's pervasive recurrent connectivity. In addition, we are becoming aware of the speed with which visual input makes contact with sophisticated stored cortical representations.

The most secure results have arguably come from modeling that possesses psychologically realistic dimensions. Some aspect of the model might be full-scale; for instance, the number of words in a lexical model might be large enough to approach the real ambiguities of word recognition. Or the model might contain the full repertoire of representations found in a particular domain, such as the full range of phonemes. Alternatively, the model might contain a comprehensive range of *types* of representation. For instance, lexical models containing implemented semantic representations are more convincing than those that do not. Plaut and Shallice's (1993) model of deep dyslexia captures seemingly disparate data by virtue of the range of representations it contains: it simulates visual, semantic, and mixed visual/semantic errors, together with category-specific errors and a concreteness effect (see LESIONED NETWORKS AS MODELS OF NEUROPSYCHOLOGICAL DEFICITS). A

further dimension of psychological reality involves how the model is tested. For example, in modeling the pronunciation of a written word, the error over the representation of the whole word at the output of the model may be an inappropriate measure of the difficulty of naming that word if pronunciation can commence on the strength of the processing of the first part of the word alone. Finally, models of language processing can be psychologically grounded by extending them to other languages. Individual human languages differ substantially as to where their complexity resides, and lexical, morphological, and syntactic categories may not be closely comparable across languages. Thus, it is possible to apply some of the insights present in connectionist models of the pronunciation of English words to the pronunciation of Chinese characters and words (indeed, Perfetti and Tan discuss a nonimplemented interaction activation model), but the orthographies are so different that only the major themes of the modeling of English pronunciation survive. Nonetheless, such a cross-linguistic perspective can provide valuable insights into the nature of language impairments and into the parameter space within which models of normal processing may exist.

When a model comprehensively covers a domain, the connectionist approach may have more in common with the conventional statistical analysis of that domain. Connectionist modeling may allow the researcher to avoid making certain representational decisions, and lesioning the trained model can be a convenient means of producing a picture of impairment. Nonetheless, the behaviors of such models will typically be relatively opaque, and they are usually most convincingly explained in terms of the statistics of the training regimen, once the researcher knows the relevant statistic to look for. Accordingly, connectionist modeling and the conventional statistical exploration of language corpora may often be complementary: the former demonstrates mechanisms but often cannot be full-scale, and the latter confirms that the training regimen was representative of the language in its fullest extent.

Finally, the relationships between production and perception, and between spoken and written language, are critical areas for further research. The continuing uncertainty about just what representations and processes are shared across these major divides speaks to the difficulties of these issues. It is also testament to the flexibility of the brain in incorporating the daunting cognitive task of reading, a recent cultural innovation, into the brain's older mastery of spoken communication.

In summary, there has been important progress in many areas of connectionist-based research into language processing, and this modeling continues to influence psychological and neuropsychological experimentation and observation.

Road Map: Linguistics and Speech Processing
Related Reading: Constituency and Recursion in Language; Language Acquisition; Neurolinguistics; Optimality Theory in Linguistics; Past Tense Learning

References

Christiansen, M. H., and Chater, N., 2001, *Connectionist Psycholinguistics*, Westport, CT: Ablex. ◆

Coltheart, M., Curtis, B., Atkins, P., and Haller, M., 1993, Models of reading aloud: Dual-route and parallel-distributed-processing approaches, *Psychol. Rev.*, 100:589–608.

Dale, R., Moisl, H., and Somers, H., 2000, *Handbook of Natural Language Processing*, New York: Marcel Dekker. ◆

Dell, G. S., 1986, A spreading activation theory of retrieval in language production, *Psychol. Rev.*, 93:283–321.

Elman, J. L., 1990, Finding structure in time, *Cognit. Sci.*, 14:179–211.

Hinton, G. E., and Shallice, T., 1991, Lesioning an attractor network: Investigations of acquired dyslexia. *Psychol. Rev.*, 98:74–95.

McClelland, J. L., and Rumelhart, D. E., 1981, An interactive activation model of context effects in letter perception: Part 1. An account of basic findings, *Psychol. Rev.*, 88:375–407.

Miikkulainen, R., 1997, Dyslexic and category-specific aphasic impairments in a self-organizing feature map model of the lexicon, *Brain Lang.*, 59:334–366.

Norris, D., McQueen, J. M., and Cutler, A., 2000, Merging information in speech recognition: Feedback is never necessary, *Behav. Brain Sci.*, 23:352–363.

Plaut, D. C., McClelland, J. L., Seidenberg, M. S., and Patterson, K., 1996, Understanding normal and impaired word reading: Computational principles in quasi-regular domains, *Psychol. Rev.*, 103:56–115.

Plaut, D. C., and Shallice, T., 1993, Deep dyslexia: A case study of connectionist neuropsychology, *Cognit. Neuropsychol.*, 10:377–500.

Quartz, S. R., and Sejnowski, T. J., 1997, The neural basis of cognitive development: A constructivist manifesto, *Behav. Brain Sci.*, 20:537–596.

Reilly, R. G., and Sharkey, N. E., 1992, *Connectionist Approaches to Natural Language Processing*, Hove, Engl.: Erlbaum. ◆

Seidenberg, M. S., and McClelland, J. L., 1989, A distributed, developmental model of word recognition and naming, *Psychol. Rev.*, 96:523–568.

Shillcock, R. C., and Monaghan, P., 2001, The computational exploration of visual word recognition in a split model, *Neural Computat.*, 13:1171–1198.

Wermter, S., Riloff, E., and Scheler, G., 1996, *Connectionist, Statistical and Symbolic Approaches to Learning for Natural Language Processing*, New York: Springer-Verlag. ◆

Layered Computation in Neural Networks

Hanspeter A. Mallot

Introduction

Layering is a common architectural feature of many neural subsystems, both in vertebrate and in invertebrate brains. It is best studied in the mammalian neocortex but can be found in regions as diverse as the optic tectum, the avian visual wulst, or the cephalopod optic lobe. In a broader sense, layered neural areas with strong vertical connectivity and topographic organization of input and output may be called *cortical* in all these different structures.

Neural layers are characterized by various anatomical and physiological parameters, such as relative abundance of cell classes, soma size, pharmacology, and both intrinsic and interarea connectivity (Braitenberg and Schüz, 1991; see also NEUROANATOMY IN A COMPUTATIONAL PERSPECTIVE). These parameters remain constant within a two-dimensional sheet but vary between sheets. In contrast, the "layers" of artificial neural networks are defined by topology only (block structure of the connectivity matrix), leaving no room for geometrical concepts such as two-dimensional extent. Some important properties of cortical layering are as follows:

1. Both intralayer and interlayer connectivity are largely determined by spatial constraints, such as nearness. In particular, the two-dimensional topology of layers is important.
2. Connections between two neurons can be mediated by multiple synapses located in different layers. If detailed timing is considered, this multiplicity of connections can be functionally significant, owing to differences in propagation time.
3. Layers can be void of nerve cell somata, mediating fiber contacts of neurons whose somata are located elsewhere (e.g., the molecular layer of the neocortex).
4. Feedback connections can occur even within each layer.

This article deals with three aspects of layering: quantitative descriptions of layered or cortical organization, the activation dynamics of network models incorporating this organization, and applications to problems of information processing and computation. Although the concepts are general, examples will repeatedly be drawn from (primate) visual cortex.

Quantitative Anatomy

Uniformity and Continuous Models

Given the vast numbers of cells found in layered cortical areas, it seems appropriate to build spatially continuous models (neural "fields") where each point in space corresponds to a neuron (Korn and von Seelen, 1972; Amari, 1977; see also the references in Mallot and Giannakopoulos, 1992). Besides being a good approximation of large neuron numbers, the continuous description allows for a natural modeling of position and distance of neurons. In a continuous model, a "neuron" consists of (1) a point on the sheet at the position of its soma, (2) a cloud or density function of postsynaptic (dendritic) sites specifying the input sensitivity for each point on the sheet, (3) a density function of postsynaptic (axonal) sites, and (4) an appropriate activation function (see the discussion that follows). The usefulness of these model features rests on two assumptions:

- The strength (or likelihood) of a connection between two neurons is proportional to the overlap of their dendritic and axonal clouds and the efficiencies of the presynaptic and postsynaptic sites involved. This assumption is discussed at length by Braitenberg and Schüz (1991), who have termed it "Peters's rule" (see also Peters, 1985:64*ff*).
- Intrinsic connectivity is largely uniform; i.e., the fiber clouds of the neurons are shifted versions of each other.

While space variance (nonuniformity) presents a problem to the sketched continuous approach, some common cases can be dealt with rather easily: e.g., by topographic maps between brain areas and modulations of neuron density within single layers. Topographic mapping can be modeled in terms of piecewise, continuous, point-to-point coordinate transforms. Explicit mathematical functions have been derived from known or assumed distributions of areal magnification by integrating the "mapping-magnification equation" in one or two dimensions (Schwartz, 1980, log *z*; Mallot and Giannakopoulos, 1992). Point-to-point models have also been proposed for columnar input patterns, such as ocular dominance stripes (Mallot, von Seelen, and Giannakopoulos, 1990). An important case of intrinsic space variance is the columnar pattern of cell densities such as the one revealed by the cytochrome oxidase stain. In the continuous model, this can be accounted for by a space-variant density factor.

Populations, Layers, and Areas

In the continuous approach, the unit of modeling is the neural population, i.e., a set of neurons from the same anatomical class with a space-invariant connectivity pattern. Examples of such populations in the visual system (see VISUAL CORTEX: ANATOMICAL STRUCTURE AND MODELS OF FUNCTION) are the spiny stellate cells in layer 4a, the GABAergic cells in layer 3, the pyramidal cells of layer 6 connecting to the lateral geniculate nucleus, and so on. The neural population is characterized by a number of variables that fall into three groups. *Anatomical variables* include the dendritic and axonal fiber clouds, $\delta(\mathbf{x})$, $\alpha(\mathbf{x})$; cell density, $\rho(\mathbf{x})$; and topographic output maps, $\mathscr{R}(\mathbf{x})$. Physiological variables include a nonlinear compression function, $f(u)$; time delays for the propagation of activity, T; synaptic integration time, τ; and gain factors. Activity is described by three *state variables*: input, $s(\mathbf{x}, t)$; potential, $u(\mathbf{x}, t)$; and output, $e(\mathbf{x}, t)$, where $\mathbf{x} \in \mathbb{R}^2$.

When connecting neural populations into networks, it is convenient (although slightly redundant) to keep the two separate state variables for input and output, the somatic activity $e(\mathbf{x}, t)$, and the "synaptic" activities $s(\mathbf{x}, t)$. The idea is that the output of one population is not the immediate input to some other population. Rather, several outputs from different populations are accumulated into one distribution of presynaptic activity, which then feeds into all neural populations with an appropriate dendritic port. We call the support of the presynaptic activity *connection planes*; they are indexed by $l \in \{1, \ldots, L\}$ in Equations 1 and 3 in the next section. Connection planes are reminiscent of the *blackboard* structure in multi-agent computer systems (see MULTIAGENT SYSTEMS) in that they collect activity from several populations without keeping track of the original source of the activity. When in turn a neural population "reads" from the connection plane, it cannot know whose activity it is reacting to; this lack of labeling of the activities is a direct consequence of Peters's rule.

Using the idea of connection planes, we can now give a definition of the terms layer and area. A *layer* is a connection plane together with all neuron populations whose somata are located in that plane. (The number of populations in a layer may be zero, as is the case in the molecular layer of the cortex. There may also be just one population allowing for specific circuitry; in this case, the pooling effect of the connection planes is bypassed and the distinction between layers and populations becomes obsolete.) An *area* is a set of layers connected without topographic maps (other than the identity). That is to say, in the case of modeling a visual system, just one retinotopic map, $\mathscr{R}_i$, is assigned to each visual area A_i, which is valid for all its layers. For projections between different areas—e.g., from A_i to A_j—a mapping of the form $\mathscr{R}_j \circ \mathscr{R}_i^{-1}$ is required to connect points representing the same retinal location.

Activation Dynamics

Network Equations

Consider a network of P neural populations (index p, state variables $e_p(\mathbf{x}, t)$ and $u_p(\mathbf{x}, t)$) connected via L connection planes (index l, state variable $s_l(\mathbf{x}, t)$). The activation dynamics of the resulting network can be formulated in three steps (cf. Figure 1 and Mallot and Giannakopoulos, 1992):

1. Dendritic summation ($s_l \rightarrow u_p$): For each population p, inputs from different connection planes $s_l, \ldots, s_L$ are accumulated according to dendritic arborizations, δ_{pl}; delays, T_l^δ; and synaptic integration time, τ:

$$\frac{\partial}{\partial t} u_p(\mathbf{x}, t) = \frac{u_p(\mathbf{x}, t)}{\tau}$$
$$+ \sum_{l=1}^{L} \int s_l(\mathbf{x}', t - T_l^\delta) \delta_{pl}(\mathbf{x} - \mathbf{x}') d\mathbf{x}' \quad (1)$$

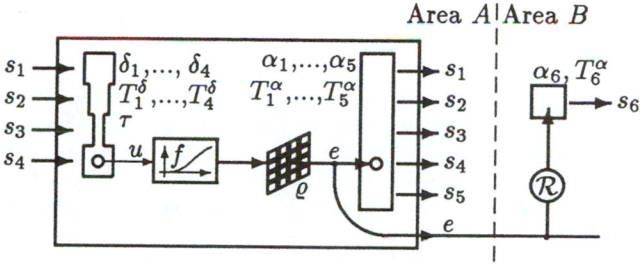

Figure 1. Activation transfer function of a neural population modeling dendritic summation, somatic point operations, and axonal spreading of activity. In Equations 1–3 (explained in the text), an additional index p is used to distinguish between different populations.

2. Somatic point operations ($u_p \rightarrow e_p$): The resulting intracellular potential is passed through a nonlinearity f_p and locally weighted with the density of the cell population $\rho_p(\mathbf{x})$. For example, if we consider a cell population in the magnocellular stream, $\rho_p(\mathbf{x})$ reflects the pattern of cytochrome oxidase blobs (see VISUAL CORTEX, ANATOMICAL STRUCTURE AND MODELS OF FUNCTION)

$$e_p(\mathbf{x}, t) = \rho_p(\mathbf{x}) f_p(u_p(\mathbf{x}, t)) \quad (2)$$

3. Axonal spread ($e_p \rightarrow s_l$): The resulting excitation is spread over the axonal densities α_{lp} and added to the activity of the connection layer to which the axon projects, again with appropriate delays (propagation times) T_l^α. For axons from population p projecting to a connection layer l in another cortical area, a point-to-point mapping $\mathscr{R}_{lp}$ has to be considered.

$$s_l(\mathbf{x}, t) = \sum_{p=1}^{P} \int e_p(\mathbf{x}', t - T_l^\alpha) \alpha_{lp}(\mathbf{x} - \mathscr{R}_{lp}(\mathbf{x}')) d\mathbf{x}' \quad (3)$$

Integro-differential equations of the leaky integrator type, such as the equations just given, have been studied extensively. One important special case is the interaction of two populations—one excitatory and one inhibitory—with all of the space-variant terms in Equations 1–3 omitted (e.g., Amari, 1977; Ermentrout and Cowan, 1979; Chipalkatti and Arbib, 1988; Murray, 1989). The formulation given here allows for space variances, both in the inter-area connections (topographic mapping functions $\mathscr{R}_{lp}$ in Equation 3) and in the cell densities (ρ_p in Equation 2). In addition, cell populations can be multiply connected via different cortical layers so that each path has its own spatiotemporal characteristic (Krone et al., 1986; Mallot et al., 1990; Mallot and Giannakopoulos, 1992).

Receptive Fields and Point Images

When stimulated with an external signal, $s_{\text{ext}}(\mathbf{x}, t)$, the network reacts with a distribution of activity $e(\mathbf{y}, t)$ that corresponds to the neural representation of the stimulus. As an example, let $\mathbf{x}$ denote retinal and $\mathbf{y}$ cortical coordinates. In neurophysiological experiments, the relation between stimulus and excitation is often described by two so-called characteristic functions that can easily be modeled in continuous neural networks:

- The point image, point spread function, or impulse response, $p_{ps}(\mathbf{y}, t)$, is the distribution of activity resulting from stimulation with a spatiotemporal Dirac function, $\delta(\mathbf{x}, t)$, e.g., a briefly flashed spot of light in the visual system. If the system were linear, space invariant, and stationary, responses to arbitrary stimuli could be predicted by superposition of appropriately shifted, delayed, and weighted impulse responses (convolution).

- The receptive field profile $p_{rf}(\mathbf{x}, t)$ of a cortical unit at position $\mathbf{y}$ describes the influence that each input site $\mathbf{x}$ at each instant in time has on the unit in question. In linear, space-invariant, and stationary systems, point spread function and receptive field are identical up to a mirroring in spatial and temporal coordinates (e.g., while p_{rf} "looks backward in time," p_{ps} "looks forward"). In general linear systems, they are the kernels of adjoint operators (Mallot et al., 1990).

Point images and receptive fields are most useful in linear systems, where they completely describe the stimulus-response behavior by way of superposition. In order to interpret neurophysiological measurements of these functions, nonlinear approaches are required. Possible choices are (1) cascades of linear systems with stationary nonlinearities, (2) Wiener-Volterra expansions (usually terminated after order 2), and (3) nonlinear network equations, such as presented earlier in Equations 1–3.

Receptive Field Properties

Figure 2 shows four steps for increasing realism in the modeling of receptive fields. Figure 2A illustrates the space- and time-

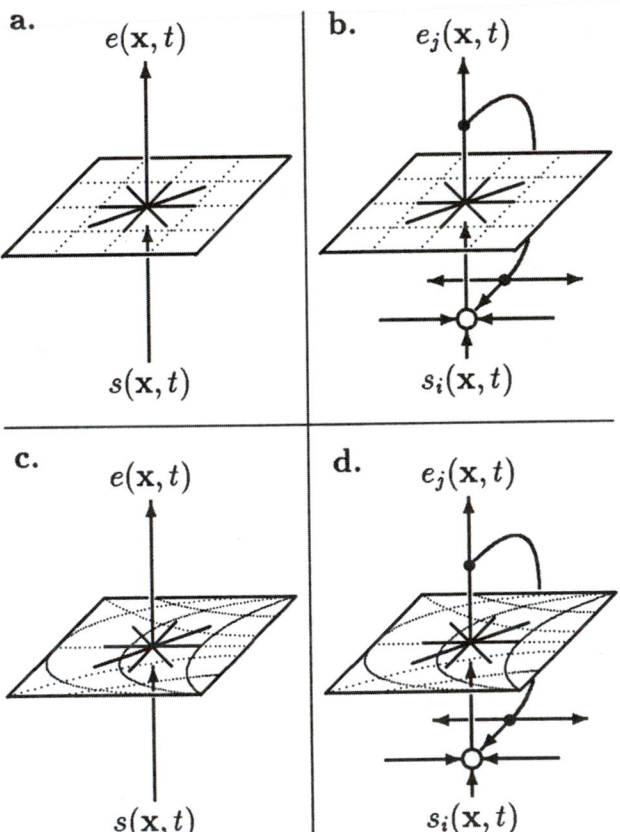

Figure 2. Continuous layers as models of receptive fields. *A*, Space-invariant, feedforward (spatiotemporal convolution). *B*, Space-invariant network of continuous layers. *C*, Space-variant, feedforward. *D*, Space-variant network of continuous layers.

invariant feedforward system, where the spatiotemporal version of linear systems theory can be applied (Korn and von Seelen, 1972). Since the early work on lateral inhibition in the compound eye of the chelicerate *Limulus*, a number of filter functions have been discussed as models of both receptive fields and spatial vision (difference of Gaussians, various derivatives of Gaussians, Gabor functions). Many of these are now used as filters in image processing. In the feedforward case, the spatial and temporal parts of the neural "filter function" are usually considered separable, equivalent to a cascade of two steps, one of which is temporal only and the other of which is spatial only. Simple nonseparability can be introduced by adding several of these cascades (e.g., one for the on-center and another for the off-surround of a retinal ganglion cell; see Dinse, Krüger, and Best, 1990). One important computational application of the resulting spatiotemporal filters is the processing of visual motion (Korn and von Seelen, 1972). Interestingly, many more can be found, if receptive fields specifically responding to other stimulus parameters (orientation, velocity, spectra, etc.) are considered (Adelson and Bergen, 1991; Mallot et al., 1990).

Parts *B* and *C* of Figure 2 show simple extensions of the space-invariant feedforward situation. In Figure 2*B*, many layers with feedback connections are considered (Krone et al., 1986). The main effects of this architecture include (1) increased width of receptive fields, since point stimuli can be signaled through the entire network by feedback connections, and (2) full nonseparability of spatial and temporal aspects of the receptive field. The first of these effects has been used by Horn (1974) in the deconvolution step of the "retinex" scheme for recovering lightness from image intensities. This article also introduces the idea of resistive networks for image processing which links the continuous Equations 1–3 to discrete implementations, as well as to diffusion-type equations in which spatial interaction is modeled by partial derivatives rather than by integral kernels.

In Figure 2*C*, the feedforward situation is extended by allowing for space variance by retinotopic mapping (Mallot et al., 1990). The combination of mapping and feedback illustrated in Figure 2*D* has not yet been studied in detail. Its activation dynamics is described by Equations 1–3 cited earlier.

Information Processing Capabilities of Neural Layers

The filter operations discussed earlier exploit the neighborhood relations in a neural layer. Other features that can be used for computational purposes are nonlinear activation dynamics and neural maps. Some examples include the following:

1. *Lateral cooperativity.* Lateral interactions between neural activities in a layer can have cooperative and/or inhibitory effects, leading to filling-in or related kinds of shaping of the activity pattern (Murray, 1989). One important application of this principle is the solution of the correspondence problem in stereovision by means of cooperative dynamics in a disparity map (for a review, see Blake and Wilson, 1991; see also Chipalkatti and Arbib, 1988, and STEREO CORRESPONDENCE). Other examples of nonlinear lateral interactions include various winner-take-all or nonmaximum-suppression schemes that are widely used in artificial neural networks.

2. *Topographic mapping.* While the continuity of neural representations is a prerequisite for neighborhood operations, such as filtering, the smooth distortions introduced by topographic mapping can simplify subsequent information processing tasks. Examples include the allocation of cortical neurons to different parts of the visual field (fovea/periphery), and the simplified processing of images with systematic space variances, such as optic flow patterns. The optic flow resulting from translation in a plane can be compensated for by so-called inverse perspective

mapping of the input images. Obstacles in the way of the observer lead to uncompensated changes in the flow field that are easily detected. A review of applications of topographic mapping to image processing problems is given elsewhere (Mallot et al., 1990).

3. *Feature maps and population coding.* While the examples presented so far apply to sensory input, analogous results have been obtained for motor pathways. Here, the distribution of activity on a neural layer has to be interpreted in terms of the "motor fields" of its active neurons. If this is done, the flow of activity in the appropriate motor areas predicts the initiated movements.

Discussion

The type of cortex model sketched in this article has the advantage of modeling a prominent structural unit of the vertebrate nervous system, the neural layer, on a rather high level. It can easily deal with geometrical features, such as maps, columns, dendritic and axonal arborization patterns, varying cell densities, and the like. This level of modeling is required to understand large-scale activation dynamics of cortical networks as have been made accessible by recently developed imaging techniques. The continuity limit seems appropriate when entire cortical areas are to be represented in a neural network model. On the other hand, it is not very well suited to model properties that differ from one cell to the next. For example, synaptic plasticity is not easily included. It is, therefore, most useful for the modeling of rather short time scales, where plasticity may be excluded, and for systems in steady states.

[Reprinted from the First Edition]

Road Map: Biological Networks
Background: I.3. Introducing the Neuron
Related Reading: Directional Selectivity; Gabor Wavelets and Statistical Pattern Recognition; Pattern Formation, Neural; Thalamus

References

Adelson, E. H., and Bergen, J. R., 1991, The plenoptic function and the elements of early vision, in *Computational Models of Visual Processing* (M. S. Landy and J. A. Movshon, Eds.), Cambridge, MA: MIT Press, pp. 3–20. ◆

Amari, S.-I., 1977, Dynamics of pattern formation in lateral-inhibition type neural fields, *Biol. Cybern.*, 27:77–87.

Blake, R., and Wilson, H. R., 1991, Neural models of stereoscopic vision, *Trends Neurosci.*, 14:445–452. ◆

Braitenberg, V., and Schüz, A., 1991, *Anatomy of the Cortex: Statistics and Geometry*, Berlin: Springer-Verlag. ◆

Chipalkatti, R., and Arbib, M. A., 1988, The cue integration model of depth perception: A stability analysis, *J. Math. Biol.*, 26:235–262.

Dinse, H. R., Krüger, K., and Best, J., 1990, A temporal structure of cortical information processing, *Concepts Neurosci.*, 1:199–238.

Ermentrout, G. B., and Cowan, J. D., 1979, A mathematical theory of visual hallucination patterns, *Biol. Cybern.*, 34:137–150.

Horn, B. K. P., 1974, Determining lightness from an image, *Comput. Vis. Graph. Image Proc.*, 3:277–299.

Korn, A., and von Seelen, W., 1972, Dynamische Eigenschaften von Nervennetzen im visuellen System, *Kybernetik*, 10:64–77.

Krone, G., Mallot, H. A., Palm, G., and Schüz, A., 1986, The spatio-temporal receptive field: A dynamical model derived from cortical architectonics, *Proc. R. Soc. Lond. B Biol. Sci.*, 226:421–444.

Mallot, H. A., and Giannakopoulos, F., 1992, Activation dynamics of space-variant continuous networks, in *Neural Network Dynamics* (J. G. Taylor, E. R. Caianiello, R. M. J. Cotterill, and J. W. Clark, Eds.), Berlin: Springer-Verlag, pp. 341–355.

Mallot, H. A., von Seelen, W., and Giannakopoulos, F., 1990, Neural mapping and space-variant image processing, *Neural Netw.*, 3:245–263.

Murray, J. D., 1989, *Mathematical Biology*, Berlin: Springer-Verlag, chap. 16. ◆

Peters, A., 1985, Visual cortex of the rat, in *Cerebral Cortex*, vol. 3, *Visual Cortex* (A. Peters and E. G. Jones, Eds.), New York: Plenum Press, pp. 19–80. ◆

Schwartz, E. L., 1980, Computational anatomy and functional architecture of striate cortex: A spatial mapping approach to perceptual coding, *Vis. Res.*, 20:645–669.

Learning and Generalization: Theoretical Bounds

Ralf Herbrich and Robert C. Williamson

Introduction

The fundamental difference between a system that learns and one that merely memorizes is that the learning system *generalizes* to unseen examples. In order to understand the performance of learning machines and to gain insight helpful for designing better ones, it is useful to have theoretical bounds on the generalization ability of the machines. The determination of such bounds is the subject of this article. In order to formulate the bounds it is first necessary to formalize the learning problem and turn the question of how well a machine generalizes into a mathematical question. In the next section we introduce one possible formalization, the one adopted in the field of statistical learning theory.

Formalization of the Learning Problem

To study the learning problem in a mathematical framework, we assume the existence of an *unknown* distribution $\mathbf{P}_{XY}$ over an *input space* $\mathcal{X}$ (e.g., $\mathbb{R}^n$) and an *output space* $\mathcal{Y}$ (e.g., $\{0, 1\}$). We are given only a *sample* $z = ((x_1, y_1), \ldots, (x_m, y_m)) \in (\mathcal{X} \times \mathcal{Y})^m = \mathcal{Z}^m$, which is assumed to be drawn *iid* (independent identically

distributed) from $\mathbf{P}_{XY}$; we define $\mathbf{P}_Z := \mathbf{P}_{XY}$. (In this article, random variables are always written sans-serif, e.g., X.)

In an attempt to discover the unknown relation $\mathbf{P}_{Y|X=x}$ between inputs and outputs, a *learning algorithm* $\mathcal{A}$ chooses a deterministic *hypothesis* $h: \mathcal{X} \to \mathcal{Y}$ solely on the basis of a given training sample $z \in \mathcal{Z}^m$. Formally,

$$\mathcal{A} : \bigcup_{i=1}^{\infty} \mathcal{Z}^i \to \mathcal{H},$$

where $\mathcal{H} \subseteq \mathcal{Y}^{\mathcal{X}}$ is the *hypothesis space* used by the algorithm. (Recall that $\mathcal{Y}^{\mathcal{X}}$ denotes the set of maps from $\mathcal{X}$ to $\mathcal{Y}$.) Some of the bounds take account of more information regarding $\mathcal{A}$ than just $\mathcal{H}$.

The performance of the learning algorithm is judged according to a *loss function* $l: \mathcal{Y} \times \mathcal{Y} \to \mathbb{R}^+$, which measures the cost of the prediction $\hat{y}$ if y is the correct output. The choice of the loss function is a key part of the formal specification of the learning problem. The *learning problem* is to find an hypothesis, $h : \mathcal{X} \to \mathcal{Y}$, such that the *expected risk*, $R[h] := \mathbf{E}_{XY}[l(h(X), Y)]$, is minimized.

Pattern recognition. In this case, $|\mathcal{Y}| < \infty$. Typically one is interested in the misclassification error $\mathbf{P}_{XY}(h(X) \neq Y)$. This can be modeled by the *zero-one loss*, $l_{0-1}(\hat{y}, y) := \mathbb{1}_{\hat{y} \neq y}$. (Here $\mathbb{1}$ denotes the indicator function.) More complex loss functions are obtained by using a cost matrix $\mathbf{C} \in \mathbb{R}^{|\mathcal{Y}| \times |\mathcal{Y}|}$.

Function learning. Here, $\mathcal{Y} = \mathbb{R}$. The classical regression scenario utilizes squared loss, $l_2(\hat{y}, y) := (\hat{y} - y)^2$. Other loss functions are the ℓ_1 loss function, $l_1(\hat{y}, y) := |\hat{y} - y|$, and the ε-insensitive loss, $l_\varepsilon(\hat{y}, y) := \max\{|\hat{y} - y|, \varepsilon\} - \varepsilon$.

If we knew $\mathbf{P}_Z$, the solution of the learning problem would be straightforward:

$$h_{\text{opt}}(x) := \underset{y \in \mathcal{Y}}{\operatorname{argmin}} \ \mathbf{E}_{Y|X=x}[l(y, Y)]. \tag{1}$$

The fact that h_{opt} cannot be identified only on the basis of the training sample z is the motivation for studying *theoretical bounds* on the generalization error of learning algorithms. These bounds are only valid for most random draws of the training sample. Formally, they read as follows:

$$\mathbf{P}_{Z^m}(R[\mathcal{A}(\mathbf{Z})] \leq \varepsilon_{\mathcal{A}}(\mathbf{Z}, \ldots, \delta)) \geq 1 - \delta. \tag{2}$$

In the analysis of such bounds, it is convenient to think of the loss function induced function class

$$\mathcal{L}_{\mathcal{H}} := \{(x, y) \mapsto l(h(x), y) \mid h \in \mathcal{H}\}.$$

For simplicity, we will mostly consider the pattern recognition case and the zero-one loss; the reasoning in the function learning case is conceptually similar.

Consistency of Learning Algorithms

Consistency is a property of a learning algorithm that guarantees that in the limit of an infinite amount of data, the learning algorithm will achieve the minimum possible expected risk. The definition is relative to a fixed hypothesis space $\mathcal{H} \subseteq \mathcal{Y}^{\mathcal{X}}$ and requires

$$\forall \varepsilon > 0: \ \lim_{m \to \infty} \mathbf{P}_{Z^m}(R[\mathcal{A}(\mathbf{Z})] - \inf_{h \in \mathcal{H}} R[h] > \varepsilon) = 0. \tag{3}$$

For the results stated below (Vapnik, 1998), a more complex notion of *nontrivial consistency* is needed. In particular, this notion requires that Equation 3 holds even if $\mathcal{H}$ is replaced by $\mathcal{H}_c := \{h \in \mathcal{H} \mid R[h] \geq c\}$ for all $c \in \mathbb{R}$. Note that in this case, $\inf_{h \in \mathcal{H}_c} R[h] = c$. It is known that for the class of *empirical risk minimization* (ERM) algorithms

$$\mathcal{A}_{\text{ERM}}^{\mathcal{H}}(z) := \underset{h \in \mathcal{H}}{\operatorname{argmin}} \ \underbrace{\frac{1}{m} \sum_{i=1}^{m} l(h(x_i), y_i)}_{\hat{R}[h, z] \quad \text{(the empirical risk)}}$$

consistency is equivalent to uniform one-sided convergence of empirical risks to expected risk; that is,

$$\forall \varepsilon > 0: \ \lim_{m \to \infty} \mathbf{P}_{Z^m}(\sup_{h \in \mathcal{H}} (R[h] - \hat{R}[h, \mathbf{Z}]) > \varepsilon) = 0 \tag{4}$$

A slightly stronger condition than that in Equation 4, namely uniform two-sided convergence, is equivalent to

$$\forall \varepsilon > 0: \ \lim_{m \to \infty} \frac{\ln(\mathbf{E}_{Z^m}[\mathcal{N}(\varepsilon, \mathcal{L}_{\mathcal{H}}, \mathbf{Z})])}{m} = 0 \tag{5}$$

where $\mathcal{N}(\varepsilon, \mathcal{L}_{\mathcal{H}}, z)$ is the *covering number* of $\mathcal{L}_{\mathcal{H}}$ on the sample z at scale ε. This is the smallest number of functions $\hat{g}: \mathcal{X} \to \mathbb{R}$ such that for every induced loss function $g \in \mathcal{L}_{\mathcal{H}}$ there exists a function $\hat{g}$ with

$$\frac{1}{m} \sum_{i=1}^{m} |g(z_i) - \hat{g}(z_i)| \leq \varepsilon.$$

In the case of the zero-one loss, l_{0-1}, the covering number $\mathcal{N}(1/m, \mathcal{L}_{\mathcal{H}}, z)$ equals the number of different error patterns $(g(z_1), \ldots, g(z_m)) \in \{0, 1\}^m$ incurred by induced loss functions $g \in \mathcal{L}_{\mathcal{H}}$.

This *characterization* result (that consistency of $\mathcal{A}_{\text{ERM}}^{\mathcal{H}}$ is "almost" equivalent to Equation 5) is the justification for the central place that covering numbers play in statistical learning theory. It is important to note that the results are only for $\mathcal{A}_{\text{ERM}}^{\mathcal{H}}$. It is still an open problem to characterize consistency for algorithms other than $\mathcal{A}_{\text{ERM}}^{\mathcal{H}}$, and thus it is not known what their "right" technical parameters are.

Theoretical Bounds for Learning Algorithms

The starting point of all the analysis presented here is the observation that for a *fixed* hypothesis $h: \mathcal{X} \to \mathcal{Y}$ (and induced loss function g, $g((x, y)) := l(h(x), y)$), we know that

$$\mathbf{P}_{Z^m}(R[h] - \hat{R}[h, \mathbf{Z}] > \varepsilon) = \mathbf{P}_{Z^m}\left(\mathbf{E}_Z[g(Z)] - \frac{1}{m} \sum_{i=1}^{m} g(Z_i) > \varepsilon\right)$$
$$< \exp(-c \cdot m\varepsilon^\beta) \tag{6}$$

where c is some constant and $\beta \in [1, 2]$, if the loss is bounded or has bounded moments. This is due to well-known results in large deviation theory (see Devroye and Lugosi, 2001, chap. 1).

The second tool is the *union bound*, which states that for events A and B,

$$\mathbf{P}(A \cup B) = \mathbf{P}(A) + \mathbf{P}(B) - \mathbf{P}(A \cap B) \leq \mathbf{P}(A) + \mathbf{P}(B)$$

As a consequence, if we consider a hypothesis space of finite size, say n, then the chance that for at least one of the hypotheses the expected risk is larger than the empirical risk by more than ε is of order $n \cdot \exp(-m\varepsilon^\beta)$. The general application of this simple inequality for learning theory is that given n *high-probability bounds* $\Upsilon_i: \mathcal{Z}^m \times \ldots \times [0, 1] \to \{\text{false, true}\}$ such that

$$\forall i \in \{1, \ldots, n\}: \forall \delta \in [0, 1]:$$
$$\mathbf{P}_{Z^m}(\Upsilon_i(\mathbf{Z}, \ldots, \delta)) \geq 1 - \delta, \tag{7}$$

then

$$\forall \delta \in [0, 1]:$$
$$\mathbf{P}_{Z^m}\left(\Upsilon_1\left(\mathbf{Z}, \ldots, \frac{\delta}{n}\right) \wedge \ldots \wedge \Upsilon_n\left(\mathbf{Z}, \ldots, \frac{\delta}{n}\right)\right) \geq 1 - \delta.$$

There are two conceptual simplifications that aid the study of the generalization performance of learning algorithms:

1. *Algorithm independence*: Motivated by Equation 4, consider the uniform convergence and bound this probability. This automatically gives a bound which holds for all hypotheses, including the one learned with a given learning algorithm. Although this is a very crude step, it has largely dominated statistical learning theory for the past 30 years; the whole analysis is independent of the learning algorithm used except via $\mathcal{H}$.
2. *Data independence*: If the training sample is entering the bound only via the empirical risk, we call the analysis *sample independent*, as we are unable to exploit the serendipity of the training sample to obtain a better bound.

Algorithm-Independent Bounds

Algorithm-independent analysis has historically been the most common. Below we examine the Vapnik-Chervonenkis framework, data-dependent structural risk minimization, and the PAC-Bayesian framework.

The Vapnik-Chervonenkis framework. The Vapnik-Chervonenkis (VP) framework, established in 1971, studies $\mathcal{A}_{\text{ERM}}^{\mathcal{H}}$ via uniform convergence (see Vapnik, 1998, and Anthony and Bartlett, 1999, for more details). The bounds are sample independent in the sense defined above. The only extra tool required is the *basic lemma*. This result makes precise the idea that whenever it is likely that two empirical risks measured on a training sample and a *ghost sample* (another sample of the same size drawn independently) are close to each other, then it must also be likely that the empirical risk on a training sample is close to the expected risk. A result of this is a generalization bound in terms of $\mathbf{E}_{Z^{2m}}[\mathcal{N}(1/2m, \mathcal{L}_{\mathcal{H}}, \mathbf{Z})]$, where the $2m$ is a consequence of the basic lemma. However, this is still not really useful, since computing $\mathbf{E}_{Z^{2m}}[\mathcal{N}(1/2m, \mathcal{L}_{\mathcal{H}}, \mathbf{Z})]$ requires knowledge of the distribution $\mathbf{P}_Z$. For l_{0-1} loss, use is made of the inequalities

$$\mathbf{E}_{Z^{2m}}\left[\mathcal{N}\left(\frac{1}{2m}, \mathcal{L}_{\mathcal{H}}, \mathbf{Z}\right)\right] \leq \sup_{z \in \mathfrak{L}^{2m}} \mathcal{N}\left(\frac{1}{2m}, \mathcal{L}_{\mathcal{H}}, z\right) \leq \left(\frac{2em}{d_{\mathcal{H}}}\right)^{d_{\mathcal{H}}},$$

where $d_{\mathcal{H}}$ is known as the *VC-dimension* of $\mathcal{H}$:

$$d_{\mathcal{H}} := \max\left\{m \in \mathbb{N} \,\middle|\, \sup_{z \in \mathfrak{L}^{2m}} \mathcal{N}\left(\frac{1}{2m}, \mathcal{L}_{\mathcal{H}}, z\right) = 2^m\right\}.$$

The generalization bound for the zero-one loss l_{0-1} then reads as follows: *With probability at least $1 - \delta$ over the random draw of the training sample $z \in \mathfrak{L}^m$, for all hypotheses $h \in \mathcal{H}$, $R[h] \leq \varepsilon_{\mathrm{VC}}(z, d_{\mathcal{H}}, \delta)$, where*

$$\varepsilon_{\mathrm{VC}}(z, d_{\mathcal{H}}, \delta) := \hat{R}[h, z] + \sqrt{\frac{8}{m}\left(\underbrace{d_{\mathcal{H}} \ln\left(\frac{2em}{d_{\mathcal{H}}}\right)}_{\text{effective complexity}} + \ln\left(\frac{4}{\delta}\right)\right)}. \quad (8)$$

The key term in this bound is labeled the *effective complexity* and in this case is essentially determined by the VC-dimension $d_{\mathcal{H}}$. Note that for general loss functions $l: \mathcal{Y} \times \mathcal{Y} \to \mathbb{R}^+$, similar results are obtained by studying the family $\{(\hat{y}, y) \mapsto \mathbb{I}_{l(\hat{y}, y) > \theta} \mid \theta \in \mathbb{R}\}$ of zero-one loss functions.

There are many results bounding the VC-dimension for specific hypothesis spaces (see VAPNIK-CHERVONENKIS DIMENSION OF NEURAL NETWORKS and PAC LEARNING AND NEURAL NETWORKS). Since the result in Equation 8 is uniform, it automatically provides a bound on the generalization error of any algorithm that chooses its hypotheses from some fixed hypothesis space $\mathcal{H}$.

Data-dependent structural risk minimization. An application of the union bound allows the combination of several VC bounds for different hypothesis spaces $\mathcal{H}_1 \subseteq \mathcal{H}_2 \subseteq \ldots \subseteq \mathcal{H}_k \subseteq \mathcal{Y}^{\mathcal{X}}$. This is the idea underlying *structural risk minimization* (SRM): using the combination of VC bounds, an SRM algorithm aims to minimize the bound directly. It is thus applicable to regularized risk-minimization learning algorithms. The bound, however, requires that the series of hypothesis spaces be defined *independently* of the training sample. Hence, we cannot directly use the training sample to control the effective complexity (only implicitly via the resulting training error).

We can relax this assumption by introducing an ordering among the hypotheses to be covered for a given sample $z \in \mathfrak{L}^m$. Such a function, $L: \cup_{i=1}^{\infty} \mathfrak{L}^i \times \mathcal{H} \to \mathbb{R}$, is called a *luckiness* (see Shawe-Taylor et al., 1998). For each luckiness function it is required that a value measured on the training sample allows one to bound the covering number on the training sample *and* ghost sample of hypotheses that increase the luckiness. This property is called *probable smoothness* with respect to a function $\omega: \mathbb{R} \times \mathbb{N} \times [0, 1] \to \mathbb{N}$.

The main result (which is data dependent in the sense used above) for the zero-one loss l_{0-1} reads as follows: *For all luckiness functions L that are probably smooth with respect to ω, with probability at least $1 - \delta$ over the random draw of the training sample*

$z \in \mathfrak{L}^m$, *for all hypotheses $h \in \mathcal{H}$ such that $\hat{R}[h, z] = 0$, $R[h] \leq \varepsilon_{\mathrm{DSRM}}(z, h, \omega, L, \delta)$ where*

$$\varepsilon_{\mathrm{DSRM}}(z, h, \omega, L, \delta) := \frac{2}{m}$$
$$\times \left(\underbrace{\log_2\left(\omega\left(L(h, z), m, \frac{\delta}{2m}\right)\right)}_{\text{effective complexity}} + \log_2\left(\frac{2m}{\delta}\right)\right). \quad (9)$$

The result can also be stated for non-zero training error and general loss functions shown by Equation 8. Each probably smooth luckiness function defines a data-dependent structuring $\mathcal{H}_1(z) \subseteq \mathcal{H}_2(z) \subseteq \ldots \subseteq \mathcal{H}_m(z) \subseteq \mathcal{H}$ of the hypothesis space $\mathcal{H}$ by

$$\mathcal{H}_i(z) := \left\{h \in \mathcal{H} \mid \omega\left(L(h, z), m, \frac{\delta}{2m}\right) \leq 2^i\right\}.$$

The choice of the luckiness function is not unique; it is best compared to the choice of a prior in a Bayesian analysis (see BAYESIAN METHODS AND NEURAL NETWORKS).

PAC-Bayesian framework. The PAC-Bayesian framework (McAllester, 1998) studies only Bayesian learning algorithms. The main ideas are very similar to the luckiness framework. One of the motivations is to capture an important feature of Bayesian confidence intervals—their width depends on the sample itself and not just its size.

A direct application of the union bound with factors different from $1/n$ leads to the following result: *For all measures $\mathbf{P}_H$ and $\mathbf{P}_Z$, with probability at least $1 - \delta$ over the random draw of the training sample $z \in \mathfrak{L}^m$, for all hypotheses $h \in \mathcal{H}$ such that $\mathbf{P}_H(h) > 0$, $R[h] \leq \varepsilon_{\mathrm{PB}}(z, h, \mathbf{P}_H, \delta)$, where*

$$\varepsilon_{\mathrm{PB}}(z, h, \mathbf{P}_H, \delta) := \hat{R}[h, z] + \sqrt{\frac{1}{2m}\left(\underbrace{\ln\left(\frac{1}{\mathbf{P}_H(h)}\right)}_{\text{effective complexity}} + \ln\left(\frac{1}{\delta}\right)\right)}.$$

If the likelihood function $\mathbf{P}_{Z|H=h}((x, y))$ equals $\mathbb{I}_{h(x)=y}$, then the bound maximizer is given by the *maximum a posteriori* estimator $h_{\mathrm{MAP}} := \mathrm{argmax}_{h \in \mathcal{H}} \mathbf{P}_{H|Z^m=z}(h)$.

Using a tool known as the *quantifier reversal lemma*, it is possible to study the *Gibbs classification strategy*, which uses a randomly drawn hypothesis for each new data point to be classified:

$$\mathcal{A}_{\mathrm{Gibbs}}^H(x) := h(x), \quad h \sim \mathbf{P}_{H|H \in H}$$

The quantifier reversal lemma is a high-probability equivalent of the union bound: *Given n high-probability bounds Υ_i (see Equation 7) and any distribution $\mathbf{P}_l$ over the numbers $\{1, \ldots, n\}$,*

$$\forall \alpha \in [0, 1]: \forall \delta \in [0, 1]:$$
$$\mathbf{P}_{Z^m}(\mathbf{P}_l(\Upsilon_l(\mathbf{Z}, \ldots, \alpha\delta) \geq 1 - \alpha) \geq 1 - \delta.$$

The proof is very simple and makes use of Markov's inequality. Noticing that for all loss functions $l: \mathcal{Y} \times \mathcal{Y} \to [0, 1]$,

$$R[\mathcal{A}_{\mathrm{Gibbs}}^H] = \mathbf{E}_{H|H \in H}[R[H]] \leq c \cdot \mathbf{P}_{H|H \in H}(R[H] \leq c)$$
$$+ 1 \cdot \mathbf{P}_{H|H \in H}(R[H] > c)$$

it is possible to prove the following result: *Given a prior measure $\mathbf{P}_H$, with probability at least $1 - \delta$ over the random draw of the training sample $z \in \mathfrak{L}^m$, for all subsets $H \subseteq \mathcal{H}$, the generalization error of the Gibbs classification strategy $\mathcal{A}_{\mathrm{Gibbs}}^H$ satisfies*

$$R[\mathcal{A}_{\mathrm{Gibbs}}^H(z)] \leq \mathbf{E}_{H|H \in H}[\hat{R}[H, z]]$$
$$+ \sqrt{\frac{1}{2m}\left(\underbrace{\ln\left(\frac{1}{\mathbf{P}_H(H)}\right)}_{\text{effective complexity}} + \ln\left(\frac{m^2}{\delta}\right)\right)} + \frac{1}{m}.$$

The effective complexity scales inversely with $\mathbf{P}_H(H)$, which in the case of the likelihood function $\mathbf{P}_{Z|H=h}((x, y)) = \mathbb{I}_{h(x)=y}$ and the Bayesian posterior $\mathbf{P}_{H|Z^m=z}$ equals the *evidence* $\mathbf{E}_H[\mathbf{P}_{Z^m|H=h}(z)]$ (see BAYESIAN METHODS AND NEURAL NETWORKS). The complexity term is minimized if we choose H such that $\mathbf{P}_H(H) = 1$. However, for a small overall bound value, it is also required that the expected empirical risk $\mathbf{E}_{H|H\in H}[\hat{R}[H, z]]$ be small. It is worth mentioning that the results are still algorithm independent, since they hold not only for the Bayesian posterior but for all hypotheses $h \in \mathcal{H}$ and all subsets $H \subseteq \mathcal{H}$.

Algorithm-Dependent Bounds

We now summarize three distinct but related approaches to the analysis of learning algorithms that utilize particular properties of the algorithm apart from the space $\mathcal{H}$ it draws its hypotheses from.

The compression framework. The compression framework (Floyd and Warmuth, 1995) is based on the idea that a good learning algorithm is able to reconstruct its hypothesis using only a small fraction of the training sample z. It is assumed that the learning algorithm can be written as

$$\mathcal{A}(z) := \mathcal{R}(z_{\mathcal{C}(z)}) \tag{10}$$

where $\mathcal{C}: \cup_{m=1}^{\infty} \mathcal{Z}^m \to \mathcal{I}$ maps the training sample to indices $\mathbf{i} \in \mathcal{I}$, $\mathcal{I} = \{(i_1, \ldots, i_n) \mid n \in \mathbb{N}, i_1 \neq \ldots \neq i_n\}$, $z_{\mathbf{i}} := (z_{i_1}, \ldots, z_{i_n})$, and $\mathcal{R}: \cup_{m=1}^{\infty} \mathcal{Z}^m \to \mathcal{Y}^{\mathcal{X}}$ computes the final hypothesis using only the subsample indexed by $\mathcal{C}(z)$. A typical example of such an algorithm is the perceptron learning algorithm (see PERCEPTRONS, ADALINES, AND BACKPROPAGATION), which can reconstruct its hypothesis using only the training patterns on which it needed to update the weight vector.

The mathematical tool needed to study this class of learning algorithms is again the union bound:

$$\mathbf{P}_{Z^m}(R[\mathcal{A}(\mathbf{Z})] - \hat{R}[\mathcal{A}(\mathbf{Z}), \mathbf{Z}] > \varepsilon)$$
$$\leq \mathbf{P}_{Z^m}(\exists \mathbf{i} \in \mathcal{I}: R[\mathcal{R}(\mathbf{Z}_{\mathbf{i}})] - \hat{R}[\mathcal{R}(\mathbf{Z}_{\mathbf{i}}), \mathbf{Z}] > \varepsilon)$$
$$\leq \sum_{\mathbf{i}\in\mathcal{I}} \mathbf{P}_{Z^m}(R[\mathcal{R}(\mathbf{Z}_{\mathbf{i}})] - \hat{R}[\mathcal{R}](\mathbf{Z}_{\mathbf{i}}), \mathbf{Z}] > \varepsilon)$$

Interestingly, for any index vector $\mathbf{i}$ the sample $z\backslash z_{\mathbf{i}}$ is an iid test sample on which the fixed hypothesis $\mathcal{R}(z_{\mathbf{i}})$ is assumed to have a difference in empirical and expected risk of more than ε. Using Equation 6—which holds independent of $\mathbf{i}$—and the fact that there are no more than $\binom{m}{d} \leq (em/d)^d$, $d = |\mathbf{i}|$, many different index sets for a training sample z of size m, leads to the main result of the compression framework: *For the zero-one loss l_{0-1} and any learning algorithm that can be written in the form of Equation 10, with probability at least $1 - \delta$ over the random draw of the training sample $z \in \mathcal{Z}^m$, $R[\mathcal{A}(z)] \leq \varepsilon_{cr}(z, |\mathcal{C}(z)|, \delta)$, where for $d = |\mathcal{C}(z)|$*

$$\varepsilon_{cr}(z, d, \delta) := \frac{m}{m-d} \cdot \hat{R}[\mathcal{A}(z), z]$$
$$+ \sqrt{\frac{1}{2m-d}\left(\underbrace{d \ln\left(\frac{em}{d}\right) + \ln\left(\frac{m^2}{\delta}\right)}_{\text{effective complexity}}\right)}. \tag{11}$$

A similar result can be stated for general loss functions. Note that this bound is data dependent, since $|\mathcal{C}(z)|$ depends both on the learning algorithm $\mathcal{A}$ and on the training sample z.

The compression framework has its roots in the theory of on-line learning (Littlestone, 1988). An *on-line learning algorithm* proceeds in trials. In each trial, the algorithm is presented with a training sample $x_i \in \mathbf{x}$ and makes a prediction $\hat{y} \in \mathcal{Y}$. It then receives the desired output $y_i \in \mathbf{y}$ and incurs a mistake whenever $\hat{y} \neq y_i$. The performance measure of an on-line learning algorithm

is the number of mistakes it incurs on a training sample z. If the on-line algorithm is *mistake driven*, that is, if it only updates the hypothesis whenever a mistake is incurred, then any mistake bound is also an upper bound on $|\mathcal{C}(z)|$. This scheme allows the determination of generalization error bounds for on-line learning algorithms applied in batch mode (see, e.g., Cesa-Bianchi et al., 1997).

The Algorithmic Stability Framework. In the algorithmic stability framework (Bousquet and Elisseeff, 2001), it is assumed that any additional training example has a limited influence on the function learned insofar as the prediction on any possible test point is concerned. Such algorithms are called *uniformly stable* and have the property that for all $i \in \{1, \ldots, m\}$:

$$\forall z \in \mathcal{Z}^m : \forall (x, y) \in \mathcal{Z}: |l(\mathcal{A}(z)(x), y) - l(\mathcal{A}(z_{\backslash i})(x), y)| \leq \beta(m),$$

where $z_{\backslash i} := (z_1, \ldots, z_{i-1}, z_{i+1}, \ldots, z_m)$. The $\beta(\cdot)$-stability of learning algorithms can be determined if the loss function is *Lipschitz continuous* with (Lipschitz) constant C_l: the difference $|l(\hat{y}, \cdot) - l(\hat{y}, \cdot)|$ is bounded from above by $C_l \cdot |\hat{y} - \tilde{y}|$. The ℓ_1 loss l_1 and the ε-insensitive loss l_ε are both Lipschitz continuous with constant $C_l = 1$.

Given a Lipschitz continuous loss function l and a reproducing kernel Hilbert space $\mathcal{H}$ with kernel $k: \mathcal{X} \times \mathcal{X} \to \mathbb{R}$, the class of regularized risk minimization learning algorithms

$$\mathcal{A}_{RRM}^{\mathcal{H}, \lambda} := \underset{h\in\mathcal{H}}{\text{argmin}} \left(\hat{R}[h, z] + \lambda\|h\|^2\right)$$

is $\beta(\cdot)$-stable with $\beta(m) \leq C_l \sup_{x\in\mathcal{X}} k(x, x)/2\lambda m$. Intuitively, the larger $\lambda > 0$, the smaller the influence of the empirical term $\hat{R}[h, z]$, and hence the more stable the learning algorithm (see also GENERALIZATION AND REGULARIZATION IN NONLINEAR LEARNING SYSTEMS).

In order to exploit the $\beta(\cdot)$-stability of a learning algorithm, a result from the theory of large deviations of functions of random variables known as *McDiarmid's inequality* is used (Devroye and Lugosi, 2001). This inequality asserts that the probability of a deviation of ε between the value of a function f of m iid variables and the expected value of that function decays as $\exp(-\varepsilon^2/mc^2)$, where c is the maximal deviation of the function's value when exchanging one variable. In this sense, McDiarmid's inequality is a generalization of Equation 6 for nonpointwise loss functions. Considering the deviation between the expected risk and the empirical risk of the function learned by $\mathcal{A}$ as a function of m iid random variables leads to the following result: *For any $\beta(\cdot)$-stable learning algorithm $\mathcal{A}$ and a bounded loss function $l: \mathcal{Y} \times \mathcal{Y} \to [0, 1]$, with probability at least $1 - \delta$ over the random draw of the training sample $z \in \mathcal{Z}^m$, $R[\mathcal{A}(z)] \leq \varepsilon_{AS}(z, \beta, \delta)$, where*

$$\varepsilon_{AS}(z, \beta, \delta) := \hat{R}[\mathcal{A}(z), z] + 2\beta(m)$$
$$+ \sqrt{\frac{2(4\beta(m) \cdot m + 1)^2 \ln\left(\frac{1}{\delta}\right)}{m}}. \tag{12}$$

There are three interesting observations to make:

1. In order for the result to be nontrivial, it is required that $\beta(m)$ decay faster than $1/m$. This readily tells us the range of λ values to consider for $\mathcal{A}_{RRM}^{\mathcal{H},\lambda}$.
2. The result as stated in Equation 12 is not directly applicable to the zero-one loss l_{0-1}, as the difference in the latter cannot decay at a rate of $1/m$ but is fixed to the values $\{0, 1\}$. Noticing that in practice we often use thresholded real-valued functions $h(\cdot) = \text{sign}(f(\cdot))$ for classification, it is possible to overcome this limitation by bounding the zero-one loss function from above. In particular, if $\mathcal{Y} = \{-1, +1\}$ then

$$l_{\text{margin}}(f(x), y) := \min(\max(0, 1 - yf(x)), 1) \geq l_{0-1}(f(x), y)$$
$$:= \mathbb{1}_{yf(x) \leq 0},$$

that is, any upper bound on the expected risk $\mathbf{E}_{XY}[l_{\text{margin}}(f(X), Y)]$ is by definition an upper bound on $R[h]$ for the zero-one loss l_{0-1} and the associated binary classification function h.

3. The result is data independent, as the stability $\beta(m)$ needs to be known before the training sample arrives. Recent developments in this area aim to overcome this problem by the notion of a stability measured on the given training sample.

The algorithmic luckiness framework. Finally, we present a recently developed algorithm-dependent framework (Herbrich and Williamson, 2002) that builds on ideas of the data-dependent structural risk-minimization framework. The key observation is that the basic lemma is true not only when one considers the maximum deviation between the expected and empirical risk, it is also true for the deviation between the expected and empirical risk of the *one* function learned using a fixed learning algorithm $\mathcal{A}$. As a consequence, for any double sample $zz' \in \mathcal{Z}^{2m}$ (training sample z and ghost sample z'), one need only consider the set $\mathcal{H} \subseteq \mathcal{Y}^{\mathcal{X}}$ of functions that can be learned by a fixed learning algorithm $\mathcal{A}$ from any subsample of size m. If the learning algorithm under consideration is permutation-invariant, then this set cannot be larger than $|H| \leq 2^{2m}$, regardless of the loss function considered.

The notion of *luckiness* changes in that it now maps a given learning algorithm $\mathcal{A}$ and a given training sample z to a real value, which effectively measures the extent to which the given data align with an encoded prior belief. In accordance with the data-dependent structural risk-minimization framework, it is required that the measured value of the luckiness on a random training sample z can be used to upper bound the number of subsets of a double sample that will lead to an increase in the luckiness value. This rather technical condition is known as ω-smallness and is best compared to the probable smoothness of luckiness functions earlier. Using the union bound together with the refined basic lemma leads to the following generalization error bound for all loss function $l: \mathcal{Y} \times \mathcal{Y} \to [0, 1]$: *For all algorithmic luckiness functions L which are ω-small, with probability at least $1 - \delta$ over the random draw of the training sample $z \in \mathcal{Z}^m$, $R[\mathcal{A}(z)] \leq \varepsilon_{\text{AL}}(z, \mathcal{A}, \omega, L, \delta)$*

$$\varepsilon_{\text{AL}}(z, \mathcal{A}, \omega, L, \delta) := \hat{R}[\mathcal{A}(z), z]$$
$$+ \sqrt{\frac{8}{m}\left(\underbrace{\log_2\left(\omega\left(L(\mathcal{A}, z), \frac{\delta}{2m}\right)\right)}_{\text{effective complexity}} + \log_2\left(\frac{2m}{\delta}\right)\right)}.$$

The main difference from Equation 9 is in the definition of the luckiness function. In contrast to Equation 9, we can now exploit properties of the learning algorithm in the definition of the ω-smallness. As an easy example, consider the luckiness function $L_0(\mathcal{A}, z) := -|\mathcal{C}(z)|$ for algorithms of the form given by Equation 10. Then, given a value $d = -L_0(\mathcal{A}, z)$ of the luckiness function on any training sample, there cannot be more than $\binom{2m}{d}$ distinct subsets of the training sample and ghost sample, which shows that $\omega(L_0, m, \delta) = \binom{2m}{-L_0}$ is a valid ω function. Note that this example removes the factor $m/(m - d)$ in front of the empirical term in Equation 11 at the cost $2m$ rather than m in the complexity term d $\ln(2em/d)$.

Discussion

Our presentation of the theory of learning and generalization is nonstandard, since we sought to present many, seemingly different approaches. For standard presentations with more details, see Devroye, Györfi, and Lugosi (1996), Vapnik (1998), Anthony and Bartlett (1999), Herbrich (2002), and Schölkopf and Smola (2002). A fairly comprehensive overview is given in Kulkarni, Lugosi, and Venkatesh (1998). In this article, we have assumed that the genuine interest is in bounds on the generalization error (see Equation 2). It is worth mentioning that another way to quantify generalization behavior of learning algorithms is in terms of bounds on the leave-one-out error (for further details, see Devroye et al., 1996).

Although we would like to use theoretical bounds directly for model selection and model validation, it currently seems that the potential value of these results is to provide insight into the design of learning algorithms. For example, the question of consistency says that covering numbers are the "right" quantities to look at for ERM algorithms.

For other algorithms the situation is less clear, although there are now several variants on classical VC analysis methods that use the same formal learning problem setup. The various bounds we presented ($\varepsilon_{\text{VC}}(z, d_{\mathcal{H}}, \delta)$, $\varepsilon_{\text{DSRM}}(z, h, \omega L, \delta)$, $\varepsilon_{\text{PB}}(z, h, \mathbf{P}_{\text{H}}, \delta)$, $\varepsilon_{\text{cr}}(z, |\mathcal{C}(z)|, \delta)$, $\varepsilon_{\text{AS}}(z, \beta, \delta)$, $\varepsilon_{\text{AL}}(z, \mathcal{A}, \omega, L, \delta)$) were in terms of a range of parameters; we still do not really know what the "right" ones are. Recent work (Mendelson, 2001) has shown the power of alternative geometric approaches to develop certain classes of generalization bounds. We expect that these and other approaches will lead to deeper understanding of the generalization ability of learning machines.

Road Maps: Computability and Complexity; Learning in Artificial Networks
Related Reading: PAC Learning and Neural Networks; Vapnik-Chervonenkis Dimension of Neural Networks

References

Anthony, M., and Bartlett, P., 1999, *Neural Network Learning: Theoretical Foundations,* Cambridge, Engl.: Cambridge University Press. ◆

Bousquet, O., and Elisseeff, A., 2001, Algorithmic stability and generalization performance, in *Advances in Neural Information Processing Systems* (T. K. Leen, T. G. Dietterich, and V. Tresp, Eds.), Cambridge, MA: MIT Press, vol. 13, pp. 196–202.

Cesa-Bianchi, N., Freund, Y., Haussler, D., Helmbold, D. P., Schapire, R. E., and Warmuth, M. K., 1997, How to use expert advice, *J. ACM,* 44:427–485.

Devroye, L., Györfi, L., and Lugosi, G., 1996, *A Probabilistic Theory of Pattern Recognition,* No. 31 in *Applications of Mathematics,* New York: Springer-Verlag, 1996. ◆

Devroye, L., and Lugosi, G., 2001, *Combinatorial Methods in Density Estimation,* New York: Springer-Verlag.

Floyd, S., and Warmuth, M., 1995, Sample compression, learnability, and the Vapnik Chervonenkis dimension, *Machine Learn.,* 27:1–36.

Herbrich, R., 2002, *Learning Kernel Classifiers: Theory and Algorithms,* Cambridge, MA: MIT Press. ◆

Herbrich, R., and Williamson, R. C., 2002, Algorithmic luckiness, *Machine Learn.,* 3:175–212.

Kulkarni, S., Lugosi, G., and Venkatesh, S., 1998, Learning pattern classification: A survey, *IEEE Trans. Inform. Theory,* 44:2178–2206. ◆

Littlestone, N., 1988, Learning quickly when irrelevant attributes abound: A new linear-threshold algorithm, *Machine Learn.,* 2:285–318.

McAllester, D. A., 1998, Some PAC Bayesian theorems, in *Proceedings of the Annual Conference on Computational Learning Theory,* Madison, WI: ACM Press, pp. 230–234.

Mendelson, S., 2001, Geometric methods in the analysis of Glivenko-Cantelli classes, in *Proceedings of the 14th Annual Conference on Computational Learning Theory COLT* (D. Helmbold and B. Williamson, Eds.), pp. 256–272.

Schölkopf, B., and Smola, A. J., 2002, *Learning with Kernels,* Cambridge, MA: MIT Press. ◆

Shawe Taylor, J., Bartlett, P. L., Williamson, R. C., and Anthony, M., 1998, Structural risk minimization over data-dependent hierarchies, *IEEE Trans. Inform. Theory,* 44:1926–1940.

Vapnik, V., 1998, *Statistical Learning Theory,* New York: Wiley. ◆

Learning and Statistical Inference

Shun-ichi Amari

Introduction

Neural networks, real or artificial, have an ability to learn from examples. Learning takes place under stochastic fluctuations, because learning from examples in neural networks is of a stochastic nature in the sense that examples are randomly generated and a network's behavior is intrinsically fluctuating owing to noise. Statistical estimation identifies the mechanism underlying stochastic phenomena and has a long tradition and history of research. Promising approaches to the study of learning problems from the statistical point of view include such concepts as the Fisher information measure, Bayesian loss, and sequential estimation. Information geometry (Amari and Nagaoka, 2000) affords a more advanced approach connecting statistics and neural networks (see NEUROMANIFOLDS AND INFORMATION GEOMETRY).

Nonlinear neurodynamics, learning, and self-organization, among others, are key concepts leading to new developments in statistical science. Consequently, many statisticians have recently become interested in neural network technology (see, e.g., Bishop, 1995; Ripley, 1996). The present article reviews various aspects of neural learning from the statistical point of view.

Neural Networks and Statistical Models

We first describe stochastic behaviors of single neurons, and then those of networks. A mathematical neuron receives a number of input signals $\{x_1, \ldots, x_n\}$, summarized in an input vector $\mathbf{x} = (x_0, x_1, \ldots, x_n)$, and emits an output z. Here, $x_0 = 1$ is added to set the bias or the threshold term. The neuron calculates the weighted sum of inputs

$$u = \mathbf{w} \cdot \mathbf{x} = \sum w_i x_i \tag{1}$$

where w_i are the synaptic efficacies or connection weights. The output z is determined stochastically, depending on u. When z takes analogue values, representing the firing rate of a neuron, it is given by a sigmoidal nonlinear function $f(u)$ of u, disturbed by additive noise,

$$z = f(u) + n \tag{2}$$

Since the noise n is random, let $r(n)$ be its probability density function. The expectation of n is assumed to be zero. When input $\mathbf{x}$ is applied, z is determined stochastically, and its conditional probability density is given by

$$p(z|\mathbf{x}) = r\{z - f(\mathbf{w} \cdot \mathbf{x})\}$$

The expectation of z is

$$E[z|\mathbf{x}] = \int z p(z|\mathbf{x}) dz = f(\mathbf{w} \cdot \mathbf{x}) \tag{3}$$

where $E[z|\mathbf{x}]$ denotes the coditional expectation of z under the condition that the input is $\mathbf{x}$ (White, 1989). That is, the output z is fluctuating around $f(\mathbf{w} \cdot \mathbf{x})$.

In the binary neuron model, z takes on the binary values 0 and 1, representing nonfiring and firing of a neuron, respectively. A widely used stochastic neuron model is specified by the following probability:

$$p(z|\mathbf{x}) = \frac{\exp\{\beta z \mathbf{w} \cdot \mathbf{x}\}}{1 + \exp\{\beta \mathbf{w} \cdot \mathbf{x}\}}, \quad z = 0, 1 \tag{4}$$

Here, $\beta > 0$ is a constant, and, when β is large, the probability of firing ($z = 1$) is very large for $\mathbf{w} \cdot \mathbf{x} > 0$. When β is small, the probability of firing is almost fifty-fifty, that is, randomness dominates. For this reason, β is called the "inverse temperature," in analogy with statistical physics. In this case,

$$E[z|\mathbf{x}] = f(\mathbf{w} \cdot \mathbf{x})$$

with the sigmoidal function

$$f(u) = \frac{\exp\{\beta u\}}{1 + \exp\{\beta u\}}$$

A multilayer perceptron is a neural network with feedforward connections (see PERCEPTRONS, ADALINES, AND BACKPROPAGATION). It consists of input neurons, hidden neurons, and output neurons. It receives an input $\mathbf{x}$ from the input neurons and emits an output vector signal $\mathbf{z} = (z_1, \ldots, z_m)$ from the m output neurons. Even when the hidden neurons behave deterministically, noise is added to the output neurons. Hence, the behavior of a network is stochastic and represented by the conditional probability distribution $p(\mathbf{z}|\mathbf{x})$. Since the network includes a large number of modifiable parameters (synaptic efficacies and thresholds of component neurons), we summarize all of them in a vector $\mathbf{w} = (w_1, \ldots, w_k)$. The conditional probability is expressed in the form $p(\mathbf{z}|\mathbf{x}; \mathbf{w})$, showing that it depends on the parameters $\mathbf{w}$. The conditional expectation of $\mathbf{z}$ is represented by $\mathbf{f}(\mathbf{x}, \mathbf{w}) = E[\mathbf{z}|\mathbf{x}; \mathbf{w}]$.

Let $(\mathbf{x}_t, \mathbf{z}_t)$, $t = 1, \ldots, T$, be observed examples of input-output pairs. Learning as well as statistical estimation is carried out based on the training set

$$D_T = \{(\mathbf{x}_1, \mathbf{z}_1), \ldots, (x_T, \mathbf{z}_T)\} \tag{5}$$

to identify the true $\mathbf{w}$ from which the data are generated. In many cases, $\mathbf{x}_t$ are generated independently, subject to an unknown probability distribution $q(\mathbf{x})$, and $\mathbf{z}_t$ is the desired output provided from the "teacher," which has the true parameter $\mathbf{w}$. In the case of self-organization or unsupervised learning, the desired outputs $\mathbf{z}_t$ are missing, so that D_T consists of only $\mathbf{x}_t$s. Statistical estimation uses all the data D_T to estimate the true parameter, whereas on-line learning assumes that data come in one by one. The current candidate for $\hat{\mathbf{w}}$ is modified by a new input-output pair when it arrives. The old data are discarded and are not used again. Hence, on-line learning is a procedure to modify the network parameters $\mathbf{w}$ sequentially, based on the series of training data D_T, such that the trained network performs sufficiently well to simulate the true network from which the training data are obtained.

Different from on-line learning, batch learning uses all the data D_T, modifies the current estimate $\hat{\mathbf{w}}$, and repeats the procedure until it converges. Hence, batch learning is an interactive estimation procedure.

Information Measures

Data $(\mathbf{x}_t, z_t)$ include information to identify the probability distribution $p(z|\mathbf{x}; \mathbf{w})$ or its parameters $\mathbf{w}$. How can one measure it? R. A. Fisher argued this problem, and proposed the Fisher information measure, which is defined soon. This is different from the Shannon information measure, which measures uncertainty by using the entropy of random variables. However, there are certain connections between them. We briefly summarize these information measures and their relations.

Let $p(x, \mathbf{w})$ be the probability density function of a random variable x parameterized by $\mathbf{w}$. In the case of neural networks, x represents a pair $(x, \mathbf{z})$. The family $M = \{p(x, \mathbf{w})\}$ is called a statistical model. Let $x_1, \ldots, x_T$ be T independent observations, and let $\hat{\mathbf{w}}$ be an estimator of the true $\mathbf{w}$. How much information is included in the training data concerning $\mathbf{w}$? The Fisher information matrix $G = (g_{ij})$ represents such information. It is defined in component form by

$$g_{ij}(\mathbf{w}) = E\left[\frac{\partial}{\partial w_i} \log p(x, \mathbf{w}) \frac{\partial}{\partial w_j} \log p(x, \mathbf{w})\right] \quad (6)$$

where E denotes the expectation with respect to $p(x, \mathbf{w})$. In vector matrix notation, this can be rewritten as

$$G(\mathbf{w}) = E[\nabla \log p(x, \mathbf{w}) \nabla \log p(x, \mathbf{w})^T] \quad (7)$$

where $\nabla f(\mathbf{w})$ is the gradient (column) vector of f

$$\nabla f = \left[\frac{\partial f}{\partial w_1}, \ldots, \frac{\partial f}{\partial w_n}\right]^T \quad (8)$$

T denoting transposition.

When we measure the accuracy of an estimator $\hat{\mathbf{w}}$ by its error covariance matrix $V = (v_{ij})$,

$$v_{ij} = E[(\hat{w}_i - w_i)(\hat{w}_j - w_j)] \quad (9)$$

the Cramér-Rao theorem shows that

$$V \geq \frac{1}{T} G^{-1} \quad (10)$$

implying that the error covariance matrix is at best as small as the inverse of the Fisher information measure divided by the number T of observations. One of the most popular estimates is the maximum likelihood estimator $\hat{\mathbf{w}}_{mle}$, which maximizes the likelihood $p(x_1, \mathbf{w}) \ldots p(x_T, \mathbf{w})$, that is, the probability of obtaining the observed data $x_1, \ldots, x_T$ when the underlying distribution is $p(x, \mathbf{w})$. This estimate attains the bound asymptotically, that is, $V \approx G^{-1}/T$ for large T. When G is large, the error $V = G^{-1}/T$ is small, so it is natural to regard G as the measure of information. This topic is covered in standard textbooks (e.g., Cox and Hinkley, 1974).

Another important quantity is the divergence measure between two probability distributions $p(x)$ and $q(x)$. How different are they? The Kullback-Leibler divergence, or the relative entropy, defined by

$$KL(p\|q) = \int p(x) \log \frac{p(x)}{q(x)} dx \quad (11)$$

is a frequently used measure in statistics and information theory (Cover and Thomas, 1991). It is related to both Shannon and Fisher information measures, as follows. Let $p_{XY}(x, y)$ be the joint probability of X and Y, and let $p_X(x)$ and $p_Y(y)$ be their marginal distributions. Then the mutual information between X and Y, defined by Shannon, is

$$I(X : Y) = KL\{p_{XY}(x, y)\|p_X(x)p_Y(y)\} \quad (12)$$

When $\mathbf{w}$ and $\mathbf{w} + d\mathbf{w}$ are infinitesimally close, the divergence between $p(x, \mathbf{w})$ and $p(x, \mathbf{w} + d\mathbf{w})$ is given by

$$KL(p(x, \mathbf{w})\|p(x, \mathbf{w} + d\mathbf{w})) = \frac{1}{2} \sum g_{ij}(\mathbf{w})dw_i dw_j \quad (13)$$

so that the KL divergence is measured locally by the quadratic form of the Fisher information measure.

The behavior of a parameterized network is given by the conditional probability $p(\mathbf{z}|\mathbf{x}; \mathbf{w})$. When $\mathbf{x}$ is generated subject to $q(\mathbf{x})$, the input-output joint distribution is $p(\mathbf{x}, \mathbf{z}; \mathbf{w}) = q(\mathbf{x})p(\mathbf{z}|\mathbf{x}; \mathbf{w})$. Consider the set $M = \{p(\mathbf{x}, \mathbf{z}; \mathbf{w})\}$ of all such probability distributions related to neural networks specified by parameter $\mathbf{w}$. This is identified with the space of parameters $\mathbf{w}$.

Given data D_T, the maximum likelihood estimator $\hat{\mathbf{w}}_{mle}$ is the one that maximizes the likelihood of the data, $P(D_T; \mathbf{w}) = \Pi p(\mathbf{x}_t, \mathbf{z}_t; \mathbf{w})$ or its logarithm

$$\log P(D_T; \mathbf{w}) = \sum \log q(\mathbf{x}_t) + \sum \log p(\mathbf{z}_t|\mathbf{x}_t; \mathbf{w})$$

The $\hat{\mathbf{w}}_{mle}$ is a consistent estimator in the sense that $\hat{\mathbf{w}}_{mle}$ converges to the true parameter $\mathbf{w}_0$ from which the training data are derived, or its optimal approximation in M. More precisely, $\hat{\mathbf{w}}_{mle}$ is asymptotically normally distributed with mean $\mathbf{w}_0$ and covariance matrix G^{-1}/T (Cox and Hinkley, 1974), where G is the Fisher information matrix, defined in this case by

$$G = E[\nabla \log p(\mathbf{z}|\mathbf{x}, \mathbf{w})\{\nabla \log p(\mathbf{z}|\mathbf{x}, \mathbf{w})\}^T] \quad (14)$$

As T becomes large, the error term G^{-1}/T converges to 0.

Since the Fisher information matrix plays a fundamental role in the accuracy of estimation and learning, some examples are shown here. In the first case, the output $\mathbf{z}$ is a noise-contaminated version of $\mathbf{f}(\mathbf{x}; \mathbf{w})$, which is the output of a multilayer perceptron with analogue activation function:

$$\mathbf{z} = \mathbf{f}(\mathbf{x}; \mathbf{w}) + \mathbf{n}$$

where $\mathbf{n}$ is Gaussian noise with mean 0 and covariance matrix $\sigma^2 I$, I being the identity matrix. From the statistical viewpoint, this is the nonlinear regression problem of observed data D_T to the nonlinear model $f(\mathbf{x}, \mathbf{w})$. By simple calculations, the Fisher information matrix is given by

$$G = \frac{1}{\sigma^2} E[\nabla \mathbf{f}(\mathbf{x}; \mathbf{w})\{\nabla \mathbf{f}(\mathbf{x}; \mathbf{w})\}^T] \quad (15)$$

where the expectation is taken over the distribution $q(\mathbf{x})$. This shows that the Fisher information tends to infinity, and the estimation error tends to 0, as the noise term σ^2 becomes 0.

In the case of binary neurons given by Equation 4, the Fisher information is calculated as

$$G = \frac{2\beta e^{\beta f}}{1 + e^{\beta f}} \nabla\nabla f + \frac{\beta^2 e^{\beta f}}{(1 + e^{\beta f})^2} \nabla f(\nabla f)^T \quad (16)$$

It should also be noted that G tends to ∞ as the temperature term β^{-1} tends to 0.

Stochastic Descent On-Line Learning and the Bayesian Standpoint

The aim of learning is not to estimate $\mathbf{w}$ but to obtain a network with good information-processing performance. The Bayesian standpoint (Berger, 1985) assumes that we have prior knowledge concerning the probability of $\mathbf{w}$ to be estimated. After observing data, it is modified to the posterior distribution of $\mathbf{w}$. It also suggests using the notion of a risk or loss function that is to be minimized through learning.

Let $l(\mathbf{x}, \mathbf{z}, \mathbf{w})$ be a loss when an input signal $\mathbf{x}$ is processed by a network of parameter $\mathbf{w}$, where $\mathbf{z}$ is the desired output given by the teacher. A simplest example is the squared error,

$$l(\mathbf{x}, \mathbf{z}; \mathbf{w}) = \frac{1}{2} |\mathbf{z} - \mathbf{z}(\mathbf{x}, \mathbf{w})|^2 \quad (17)$$

where $\mathbf{z}(\mathbf{x}, \mathbf{w})$ is the output from the network specified by $\mathbf{w}$. In the case when $\mathbf{z}(\mathbf{x}, \mathbf{w})$ is given by

$$\mathbf{z}(\mathbf{x}, \mathbf{w}) = \mathbf{f}(\mathbf{x}, \mathbf{w}) + \mathbf{n} \tag{18}$$

where $\mathbf{n}$ is a Gaussian noise subject to $N(0, I)$, this $l(\mathbf{x}, \mathbf{z}; \mathbf{w})$ coincides with the negative of the log likelihood $l(\mathbf{x}, \mathbf{z}, \mathbf{w}) = -\log p(\mathbf{x}, \mathbf{z}; \mathbf{w})$ except for a constant term $-\log q(\mathbf{x})$ not depending on $\mathbf{w}$. Hence, minimizing the loss is equivalent to maximizing the likelihood in this case.

Sometimes, a function $F(\mathbf{w})$ of $\mathbf{w}$ is added to the loss in order to penalize a complex network. The function $F(\mathbf{w})$, called the regularization term, takes a large value when the network with parameter $\mathbf{w}$ is complex (Poggio, Torre, and Koch, 1985). One typical example is

$$F(\mathbf{w}) = \sum w_i^2$$

which penalizes large w_i. Another one is

$$F(\mathbf{w}) = \sum \frac{w_i^2}{1 + w_i^2} \tag{19}$$

which penalizes the number of nonzero w_is when w_i are large.

The risk function $R(\mathbf{w})$ is the expected loss

$$R(\mathbf{w}) = E[l(\mathbf{x}, \mathbf{z}; \mathbf{w})] \tag{20}$$

where expectation is taken with respect to the distribution given by the teacher. When the teacher generates $\mathbf{z}$ by using the network with parameter $\mathbf{w}_0$, the distribution of $(\mathbf{x}, \mathbf{z})$ is $q(\mathbf{x})p(\mathbf{z}|\mathbf{x}; \mathbf{w}_0)$. The function $R(\mathbf{w})$ is called the generalization error, since the behavior of the network specified by $\mathbf{w}$ is evaluated by the expectation with respect to a new example $(\mathbf{x}, \mathbf{z})$ subject to the same distribution. The best network is supposed to be the one that minimizes $R(\mathbf{w})$.

However, we do not know the risk function $R(\mathbf{w})$, since the true $\mathbf{w}_0$ which is used in Equation 20 for taking expectation is unknown. Instead, we have a training set D_T generated from the true distribution. This gives us the empirical risk function

$$R_{\text{train}}(\mathbf{w}) = \frac{1}{T} \sum_{t=1}^{T} l(\mathbf{x}_t, \mathbf{y}_t; \mathbf{w}) \tag{21}$$

which is an estimate of $R(\mathbf{w})$ by using the training data themselves. It is called the training error, and it converges to $R(\mathbf{w})$ as T tends to infinity.

The penalty term may be derived from the Bayesian standpoint. Assume that we have prior knowledge of $\mathbf{w}$ such that $\mathbf{w}$ is subject to a prior distribution $p_{pr}(\mathbf{w})$. Then, the joint probability of $(\mathbf{x}, \mathbf{z}, \mathbf{w})$ is given by

$$p_{pr}(\mathbf{w})q(\mathbf{x})p(\mathbf{z}|\mathbf{x}, \mathbf{w}) \tag{22}$$

Therefore, the joint probability of data D_T and the parameter $\mathbf{w}$ is

$$p_{pr}(\mathbf{w}) \prod p(\mathbf{x}_t, \mathbf{z}_t; \mathbf{w}) \tag{23}$$

When data D_T are obtained, the posterior probability of $\mathbf{w}$ is

$$p_{\text{post}}(\mathbf{w}|D_T) = \frac{p_{pr}(\mathbf{w})P(D_T|\mathbf{w})}{P(D_T)} \tag{24}$$

A good candidate for $\mathbf{w}$ suggested by data D_T is the maximum posterior estimate that maximizes $p_{\text{post}}(\mathbf{w}|D_T)$. This reduces to the maximum likelihood estimator when $p_{pr}(\mathbf{w})$ is uniform. Minimizing $-\log p_{\text{post}}(\mathbf{w}|D_T)$ is equivalent to minimizing

$$R_{\text{train}} = \frac{1}{T} \sum r(\mathbf{x}_t, \mathbf{z}_t; \mathbf{w}) \tag{25}$$

where

$$l(\mathbf{x}, \mathbf{z}; \mathbf{w}) = -\log p(\mathbf{x}, \mathbf{z}, \mathbf{w}) - \frac{1}{T} \log p_{pr}(\mathbf{w}_t) \tag{26}$$

In this case, the penalty term is given by $-(1/T) \log p_{pr}(\mathbf{w})$.

Learning is a procedure to estimate the optimal $\mathbf{w}$ based on a given data set D_t. Batch learning uses all the stored data D_T repeatedly. The batch gradient learning method modifies the current estimate $\mathbf{w}_t$ at time t into $\mathbf{w}_{t+1} = \mathbf{w}_t + \Delta\mathbf{w}_t$ by

$$\Delta\mathbf{w}_t = -\eta_t \nabla R_{\text{train}}(\mathbf{w}_t) \tag{27}$$

Here, ∇R_{train} is the gradient vector of R_{train} whose components are $(\partial/\partial w_i)R_{\text{train}}(\mathbf{w})$, and η_t is a learning rate. This is called the *gradient descent method*, because $\mathbf{w}_t$ is modified in the direction of the gradient of R_{train}. For an adequate sequence η_t, $\mathbf{w}_t$ converges to the minimizer of $R_{\text{train}}(\mathbf{w})$. Hence, when l is the negative log likelihood, $\mathbf{w}_t$ converges to the maximum likelihood estimator.

On-line learning, on the other hand, cannot use all the data D_T at once. Instead, one input-output training pair $(\mathbf{x}_t, \mathbf{z}_t)$ becomes available at time t. The current estimator $\mathbf{w}_t$ is updated to $\mathbf{w}_{t+1}$ by using this. The data $(\mathbf{x}_t, \mathbf{z}_t)$ are then discarded so that they cannot be used again. On-line learning provides a simple learning rule, and its behavior is flexible even when the behavior of the teacher is changing.

The stochastic descent on-line learning procedure updates $\mathbf{w}_t$ by

$$\Delta\mathbf{w}_t = -\eta_t \nabla l(\mathbf{x}_t, \mathbf{z}_t; \mathbf{w}_t) \tag{28}$$

This simple stochastic descent learning was proposed by Amari (1967) and was later called the *generalized delta rule* (Rumelhart, Hinton, and Williams, 1986). When it is applied to the multilayer perceptron, the calculation of ∇l is performed through error propagation in the backward direction. This is a nice interpretation (Rumelhart et al., 1986), and the algorithm is called the *error backpropagation method* (see BACKPROPAGATION: GENERAL PRINCIPLES).

For a deterministic neural network without stochastic fluctuations, the squared error (Equation 17) is not related to the negative log probability. This corresponds to the case with $\sigma^2 \to 0$. However, the gradient descent learning algorithm does not directly include σ^2. This method was proposed in the deterministic case, and its relation to statistics became clear only later (White, 1989).

The backpropagation learning method has been widely used and is one of the standard engineering tools. However, it is not free from a number of flaws. It is not Fisher efficient; that is, the estimation error of $\mathbf{w}_t$ does not satisfy the Cramér-Rao bound, which the maximum likelihood estimator does. There exist a large number of local minima in R_{train} so that $\mathbf{w}_t$ converges to one of the local minima, which might be different from the global minima. Further, its convergence has been found very slow because of "plateaus."

It is known that the error decreases quickly in the beginning of learning, but its rate of decrease becomes extremely slow. After surprisingly many steps, the error again decreases rapidly. This is understood as showing that $\mathbf{w}_t$ is trapped in a plateau. A *plateau* is a critical point of $R_{\text{train}}(\mathbf{w})$, but it is not a local minimum. However, it takes a long time for learning to escape from it. The statistical physical method makes clear that plateaus exist because of the "symmetry" existing in the hidden units in the multilayer perceptron (Saad and Solla, 1995).

Various acceleration methods for the backpropagation learning rule have been proposed, but they cannot eliminate plateaus. The natural gradient method (Amari, 1998), based on the Riemannian structure of a neuromanifold, not only eliminates plateaus but is Fisher efficient, as will be shown in the next section.

We should mention that this type of learning is applicable to any parameterized family $p(\mathbf{z}|\mathbf{x}, \mathbf{w})$ of stochastic behaviors as well as to deterministic behaviors. The idea is also used in the self-organization scheme, where there are no desired outputs $\mathbf{z}_{\text{true}}$ but the network modifies its structure depending only on the input data $D_T = \{\mathbf{x}_1, \ldots, \mathbf{x}_T\}$. For example, if the loss function is put equal to

$$l(\mathbf{x}, \mathbf{w}) = a|\mathbf{w}|^2 - \frac{1}{2}|\mathbf{w} \cdot \mathbf{x}|^2 \qquad (29)$$

for a single neuron, the connection weight vector $\mathbf{w}$ of the neuron converges to the principal eigenvector of the correlation matrix

$$V = \int q(\mathbf{x})\mathbf{x}\mathbf{x}^T d\mathbf{x} \qquad (30)$$

of the input signals, if $|\mathbf{w}|$ is normalized. This fact was pointed out in more general perspectives on neural learning by Amari (1977) and studied in detail by Oja (1982) (see PRINCIPAL COMPONENT ANALYSIS).

Another example of self-organization is Kohonen's learning vector quantizer (see LEARNING VECTOR QUANTIZATION). Let us consider a set of k neurons whose connection weights are $\mathbf{w}_1, \ldots, \mathbf{w}_k$. The neurons receive a common input $\mathbf{x}$ and calculate the distance $|\mathbf{w}_i - \mathbf{x}|$. The neuron whose weight $\mathbf{w}_i$ is closest to $\mathbf{x}$ is called the winner, and its output is assigned $z_k = 1$, while all the other $z_j = 0$. This is called the *winner-take-all rule*. Let us put

$$l(\mathbf{x}, \mathbf{w}) = \frac{1}{2} \min_i |\mathbf{w}_i - \mathbf{x}|^2$$

where $\mathbf{w} = (\mathbf{w}_1, \ldots, \mathbf{w}_k)$. Then the risk is given by

$$R(\mathbf{w}) = \frac{1}{2} \int \min_i |\mathbf{w}_i - \mathbf{x}|^2 q(\mathbf{x}) d\mathbf{x} \qquad (31)$$

The learning rule (Equation 28) in this cases leads to the Kohonen learning vector quantizer.

Natural Gradient Learning

The natural (Riemannian) gradient learning method based on the Fisher information matrix was proposed by Amari (1998) to eliminate plateau phenomena and to accelerate convergence. The gradient $-\nabla l(\mathbf{w})$ is usually believed to be the steepest descent direction of a scalar function $l(\mathbf{w})$. However, in a parameter space M of multilayer perceptrons, it is natural to define

$$\tilde{\nabla} r(\mathbf{w}) = G^{-1}(\mathbf{w})\nabla r(\mathbf{w}) \qquad (32)$$

Here, G^{-1} is the inverse of the Fisher information matrix $G = (g_{ij})$. This is called the natural gradient.

The natural gradient learning algorithm was proposed as the steepest descent method in a Riemannian space where G is the metric,

$$\Delta \mathbf{w}_t = -\eta_t G^{-1}(\mathbf{w}_t)\nabla l(\mathbf{x}_t, \mathbf{z}_t; \mathbf{w}_t) \qquad (33)$$

It has two remarkable properties. First, it avoids plateaus, so that it has an optimal dynamic rate of convergence. Second, the accuracy of estimator $\mathbf{w}_t$ by the natural gradient is Fisher efficient when $\eta_t = 1/t$, that is, it has the same asymptotic property as the best batch estimator. The natural gradient method is also successfully applied to INDEPENDENT COMPONENT ANALYSIS (q.v.). The natural gradient method does not eliminate local minima. There are a number of techniques to overcome this problem (see NEUROMANIFOLDS AND INFORMATION GEOMETRY).

Learning Curves and Generalization Errors

A learning curve shows how quickly a learning network improves its behavior evaluated by the generalization error. This is related to the dynamical behavior of neural learning and the complexity of neural networks. We analyze this important problem in this section.

The stochastic approximation guarantees that $\hat{\mathbf{w}}_t$ converges to the optimal parameter $\mathbf{w}_0$ with probability 1, when the learning

constant η_t tends to 0 in an adequate speed. However, when η_t is too small, learning becomes ineffective. What learning is for, in many cases, is to adjust the network parameters in a changing environment. In this case, η_t should be kept at least to a small constant ε. When η_t is put equal to a small constant ε, the dynamical behavior of $\hat{\mathbf{w}}_t$ is studied in an old paper (Amari, 1967), where the stochastic descent learning rule was proposed for the multilayer perceptron from the Bayesian standpoint.

Let us analyze the accuracy of estimator $\mathbf{w}_t$ obtained by Equation 28. We assume the case that the initial value $\mathbf{w}_1$ is in a neighborhood of the (local) optimal value $\mathbf{w}_0$ such that it converges to $\mathbf{w}_0$. Let us define two matrices, the Hessian and the covariance of the gradient of l,

$$A = E[\nabla\nabla l(\mathbf{w}_0)] \qquad (34)$$

$$B = E[\nabla l(\nabla l)^T] \qquad (35)$$

The expected value of $\hat{\mathbf{w}}_t$ converges to $\mathbf{w}_0$ exponentially, and the covariance of the error $\hat{\mathbf{w}}_t - \mathbf{w}_0$ also converges exponentially to εV, where V is a matrix obtained from A and B (Amari, 1967). The dynamical behavior of $\mathbf{w}_t$ was also studied when the environment, that is, the optimal $\mathbf{w}_0$, is periodically changing over time slowly.

Since the behavior of the net is evaluated by $R(\hat{\mathbf{w}}_t)$, but not directly by $\hat{\mathbf{w}}_t$, it is important to know how fast $R(\hat{\mathbf{w}}_t)$ approaches its optimum value. Here, $R(\hat{\mathbf{w}}_t)$ is the expectation of the loss $l(\mathbf{x}, \mathbf{z}; \hat{\mathbf{w}}_t)$ with respect to a new example pair $(\mathbf{x}, \mathbf{z})$. This is the generalization error, which evaluates the behavior of the net by a new example $(\mathbf{x}, \mathbf{z})$ that is not included in the training set D_T. This is different from the training error in Equation 25, which is an evaluation of $\hat{\mathbf{w}}_t$ based on the training data D_T. We can calculate the latter, but it is difficult to know the generalization error $R(\hat{\mathbf{w}}_T)$ because we do not know the function $R(\mathbf{w})$ itself. If we know the relation between R_{train} and R, we can then evaluate R through R_{train}.

A standard technique of asymptotic statistical inference (Cox and Hinkley, 1974) can be applied to this problem. Let us fix the training data D_t, and let $\hat{\mathbf{w}}_t$ now be the best estimator obtained therefrom, where t is assumed to be a large number. It maximizes R_{train}, so that it satisfies

$$0 = \nabla R_{\text{train}}(\hat{\mathbf{w}}_t)$$

On the other hand, the optimal $\mathbf{w}_0$ satisfies $\nabla R(\mathbf{w}_0) = 0$. From this we have, by mathematical analysis,

$$E[R(\hat{\mathbf{w}}_t)] = R(\mathbf{w}_0) + \frac{1}{2t}\,\text{tr}(B^{-1}A) \qquad (36)$$

Mathematical analysis also gives

$$E[R_{\text{train}}(\hat{\mathbf{w}}_t)] = R(\mathbf{w}_0) - \frac{1}{2t}\,\text{tr}(B^{-1}A) \qquad (37)$$

The relation between the training error and generalization error $E[R(\hat{\mathbf{w}}_t)]$ is given from Equations 36 and 37 by

$$E[R(\hat{\mathbf{w}}_t)] = E[R_{\text{train}}(\hat{\mathbf{w}}_t)] + \frac{1}{t}\,\text{tr}(B^{-1}A)$$

The term $\text{tr}(B^{-1}A)$ shows the difference between the training error and the generalization error. When this term is large, R_{train} is much smaller than R because of overfitting. That is, the estimated network fits too much to the observed examples, but it fails to capture the mechanism generating the examples. If a complex network is used, the observed data D_t are easily overfitted. Therefore, this term represents the penalty due to the use of a complex network. This is a generalization of the Akaike information criterion, which is widely used in statistical inference. When the loss is the negative log likelihood and the model includes the true one, both A and B are equal to the Fisher information matrix, so that we have an evaluation of complexity by the number of modifiable parameters, $\text{tr}(B^{-1}A) = \text{tr}(I) =$ the number of modifiable parameters. This is the result first obtained by Akaike for selecting a reasonable model. This is universal in the sense that the complexity (overfitting factor) depends only on the number of parameters, independently of the architecture of the network. Universal properties of this type are more or less known in various situations concerning learning machines (Amari and Murata, 1993). One more remarkable fact is the t^{-1} convergence of the learning error in learning curves. As the number t of training examples increases, the generalization decreases in proportion to $1/t$. This was first remarked on by T. Cover in his doctoral thesis in 1964. This result is proved in Amari and Murata in a general situation. Learning attracts researchers from algorithmic, information-theoretic, and physics points of view because of its general and flexible ability for information processing related to the human ability.

Discussion

We have focused on neural network learning from the viewpoint of statistical inference. Learning is a sequential estimation from the statistical point of view. The accuracy of learning was shown in terms of the Fisher information measure. We are interested in the dynamical behaviors of a learning network under a general loss criterion. The natural gradient learning algorithm was introduced in this respect. The behavior of learning curves was shown, and the complexity of a neural network was introduced to elucidate the discrepancy between the training and generalization errors.

Road Map: Learning in Artificial Networks
Related Reading: Bayesian Methods and Neural Networks; Data Clustering and Learning; Generalization and Regularization in Nonlinear Learning Systems; Graphical Models: Probabilistic Inference; Independent Component Analysis; Perceptrons, Adalines, and Backpropagation; Stochastic Approximation and Efficient Learning

References

Amari, S., 1967, Theory of adaptive pattern classifiers, *IEEE Trans. Electron. Comput.*, 16:299–307.
Amari, S., 1977, Neural theory of association and concept-formation, *Biol. Cybern.*, 26:175–185.
Amari, S., 1998, Natural gradient works efficiently in learning, *Neural Group*, 10:251–276.
Amari, S., and Murata, N., 1993, Statistical theory of learning curves under entropic loss, *Neural Comp.*, 5:140–153.
Amari, S., and Nagaoka, H., 2000, *Introduction to Information Geometry*, London: AMS and Oxford University Press. ◆
Berger, J. O., 1985, *Statistical Decision Theory and Bayesian Analysis*, 2nd ed., New York: Springer-Verlag. ◆
Bishop, C. M., 1995, *Neural Networks for Pattern Recognition*, Oxford: Clarendon Press.
Cover, T. M., and Thomas, J. A., 1991, *Elements of Information Theory*, New York: Wiley.
Cox, D. R., and Hinkley, D. V., 1974, *Theoretical Statistics*, London: Chapman and Hall. ◆
Oja, E., 1982, A simplified neuron model as a principal component analyzer, *J. Math. Biol.*, 15:267–273.
Poggio, T., Torre, V., and Koch, C., 1985, Computational vision and regularization theory, *Nature*, 317:314–319.
Ripley, B. D., 1996, *Pattern Recognition and Neural Networks*, Cambridge, Engl.: Cambridge University Press. ◆
Rumelhart, D. E., Hinton, G. E., and Williams, R. J., 1986, Learning internal representation by error backpropagation, in *Parallel Distributed Processing* (D. E. Rumelhart, J. L. McClelland, and PDP Group, Eds.), Cambridge, MA: MIT Press.
Saad, D., and Solla, S. A., 1995, On-line learning in soft committee machines, *Phys. Rev. E*, 52:4225–4243.
White, H., 1989, Learning in artificial neural networks: A statistical perspective, *Neural Comp.*, 1:425–464. ◆

Learning Network Topology

Chuck P. Lam and David G. Stork

Introduction

To create a neural network, a designer typically fixes a network topology and uses training data to tune its parameters such as connection weights. The designer, however, often does not have enough knowledge to specify the ideal topology. It is thus desirable to learn the topology from training data as well.

Traditional learning can be viewed as a search in the space of parameters. This article looks at topology learning as a search in the space of topologies. In particular, we define in general terms a measure that quantifies the "goodness" of a topology and some search strategies over the space of topologies to find the best one. This framework is applied to learning the topologies of the two forms of networks that have found use in pattern recognition, feedforward neural networks, and BAYESIAN NETWORKS (q.v.).

Objectives of Learning

Learning is the automated process of modifying a system to improve its performance on its given task. When learning is restricted to modifying a network's weights, performance is generally measured as just the network's ability to model a set of input samples. However, this performance measure alone is problematic when one can choose arbitrary topologies, since a large enough network can model a given data set arbitratily well, leading to overfitting. Therefore, for topology learning, a bias is added to prefer smaller models. It is often found that this bias produces a network that has better generalization and is more interpretable.

A principled approach to topology selection is to find the most probable topology T given training data D (Cheeseman, 1990). Applying Bayes's rule, one is thus searching for the topology that maximizes $p(T|D) \propto p(T)p(D|T)$. Here $p(T)$ is a *prior* probability that expresses one's belief about the probabilities of various topologies to be a "good" topology. One can express one's *bias* for smaller topologies through $p(T)$. Viewed another way, $p(T)$ allows one to impose a *penalty* on larger topologies. Next, $p(D|T)$ is interpreted as how well a topology models the data, and this measure generally has a higher maximum as T gets bigger and more complex. Most topology learning algorithms follow this framework at least in spirit, somehow incorporating the trade-off between a topology's fit to data, measured as the output error, and the desirability of that topology, measured as some penalty term. This framework expresses a simple, explicit trade-off between how well a model predicts the data and our belief in the goodness of that model. As we shall see subsequently, learning the topology of Bayes nets often follow this framework explicitly (Buntine, 1996).

Using a measure that takes into account a topology's fit to data and one's preference for smaller networks, one can search for the topology with the highest value. Except for certain unique cases, a greedy search is used over this topology space. For feedforward neural networks there are two dominant approaches to this searching, growing, and pruning (Figure 1). In *growing*, a small network is created initially, and nodes are added through learning. The search space is constrained by the particular method and its way of adding nodes. In some cases the search space is limited to the set of neural networks with a single hidden layer. Conversely, *pruning* starts with a sufficiently large network specified by the designer and proceeds to eliminate "unimportant" weights or nodes. The search space is thus limited to pruned versions of the initial network. In Bayesian networks, all the nodes of the network are given and set, and one searches for a topology by adding or deleting links.

Growing

In network growing, nodes are added and the network is retrained iteratively until it reaches satisfactory performance. Adding nodes to a network can always improve the network's fit to the training data. The penalty/bias to prevent overly large networks can be expressed as a stopping criterion. One stops adding nodes once the network has satisfactory performance or when adding more nodes does not improve performance further.

Cascade-Correlation Learning Architecture

Fahlman and Lebiere (1990) developed a growing algorithm that searches in the topology space of *cascade architectures*. A cascade architecture is a special type of feedforward neural network in which each hidden layer has only one unit and each layer gets input from all the nodes in all the input and hidden layers before it. Thus each output node is connected to all the input nodes and all the hidden nodes of the network (see the top left of Figure 1).

In this algorithm, the network is frozen before the addition of each node. A pool of candidate nodes is trained to predict the current residual error. The best of the candidates is then connected to the network's output nodes, thereby reducing the residual error. The rest of the candidates are discarded. This is repeated until the network's error rate is satisfactory. Conceptually, this is like a Tay-

lor approximation, in which early nodes express lower-order terms while later nodes are like higher-order terms that add to making a finer approximation.

Dynamic Node Creation

Ash (1989) introduced the dynamic node creation (DNC) method for adding hidden nodes to a three-layer feedforward neural network. The algorithm starts with a network with only one hidden node. The given network is then trained normally to reduce its average squared error E. A new hidden node is added whenever learning has slowed down. Specifically, the algorithm adds a node when the reduction in error in the previous T epochs is less than some threshold Δ set by the designer, given that no nodes were added during those T epochs. The algorithm stops when another user-defined criterion (e.g., average or maximum output error) is met.

A major difference between cascade-correlation learning and DNC is that cascade-correlation learning freezes the network before the addition of each node. Ash (1989) argued in favor of DNC, claiming that since all weights are continuously adjusted as each node is added, a more complete search is done in the lower-dimensional weight space. For this reason, DNC can often find smaller acceptable networks than can cascade correlation. On the other hand, Fahlman and Lebiere (1990) believe that a significant amount of time in weight learning is due to the weights trying to adjust to each other. Freezing the network before each node addition enables the weights to learn in a stable context and focuses the learning effort on reducing the output error. Therefore, overall training should be faster.

Pruning

Pruning entails removing weights or nodes from a trained network. When growing a network, one knows that adding nodes will always decrease a network's training error. Conversely, pruning nearly always increases a network's training error. A good pruning algorithm should thus start with a fairly large network with low training error, and should prune the weights or nodes whose removal will

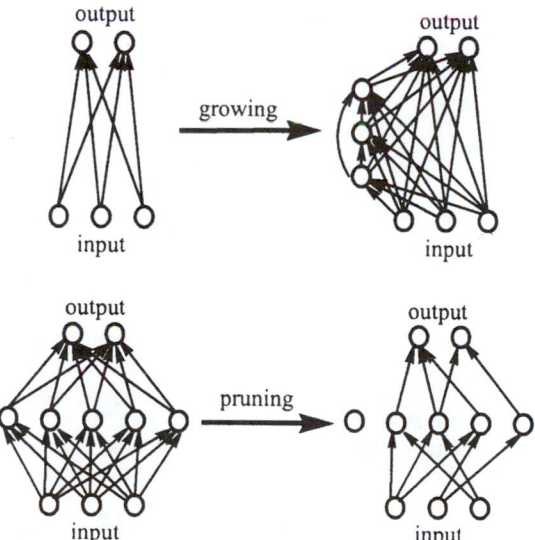

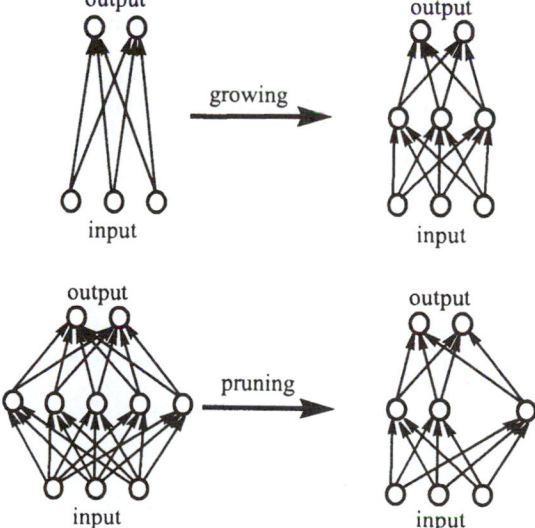

Figure 1. The figure shows network growing and pruning. At the top left, hidden nodes are added in a cascade topology. At the top right, hidden nodes are added in a three-layer topology. At the bottom right, nodes are pruned from a network. At the bottom left, individual weights are pruned. Note that if all weights are eliminated from a node, then that node has been effectively pruned from the network.

increase a network's training error the least (Reed, 1993). After such removal one may elect to retrain the network for better performance. Some pruning methods were designed to remove individual weights, while others remove entire nodes. Pruning all of a node's input weights or all of its output weights is equivalent to pruning the node itself.

Various researchers have developed approximations to a weight or a node's *saliency*, which is defined as the increase in training error from that weight/node's removal. Those algorithms then proceed to prune weights/nodes with low saliency. Other researchers have worked under the magnitude-based pruning paradigm. In this approach, weight-learning algorithms (generally backpropagation) are modified such that the magnitude of weights (or some other parameters) are trained to become good indicators of saliency. After such training, low-magnitude weights are then pruned.

Magnitude-based Pruning

A weight with zero magnitude can be pruned without any effect on the network. This leads to the intuitive notion that weights with small magnitude can be pruned away without affecting training error too much. This simple version of *magnitude-based pruning* often does not work, however. Consider a neuron working in the linear region of its input-output function. The same function can be expressed either as a neuron with small input weights and large output weights, or as a neuron with medium input weights and medium output weights. The magnitude of each individual weight alone does not necessarily tell one about its saliency.

However, many researchers have added bias terms to the network error in weight-learning algorithms to penalize "complex" networks (Chauvin, 1989; Hanson and Pratt, 1989; Ji, Snapp, and Saltis, 1990). These biases are designed to favor networks in which magnitude-based pruning makes sense. The topological bias is thus embedded in the weight-learning algorithm.

Ji et al. (1990) proposed a penalty term to reduce the number of hidden units and the magnitude of weights. Their effect was to impose a smoothness constraint on the network's input-output function. Chauvin (1989) proposed a penalty term to reduce the sum of "energy" from all the hidden nodes, in which "energy" is some positive monotonic function of the square of a node's output. Examples of energy function include o^2, $\log(1 + o^2)$, and $o^2/(1 + o^2)$, where o is the output of a node. Hanson and Pratt (1989) proposed a penalty term that is the sum of biases from all units. They specifically examined the hyperbolic bias, $w_i/(1 + \lambda w_i)$, and the exponential bias, $1 - e^{-\lambda w_i}$ (where λ is an adjustable parameter and $w_i = \Sigma_j \|w_{ij}\|$). Kruschke and Movellan (1991) proposed a penalty term that eliminates hidden nodes that are functionally redundant, as when the correlation between their input weights is high. Some authors (Hanson and Pratt, 1989; Ji et al., 1990) have noted that the addition of a penalty term significantly slows learning.

Skeletonization

Mozer and Smolensky (1989) developed skeletonization, a technique that prunes one node at a time. They introduce an *attentional strength* α_j for each node j. The output of node i is then

$$o_i = f\left(\sum_j \alpha_j w_{ij} o_j \right)$$

If $\alpha_j = 1$, then node j is just a conventional node. If $\alpha_j = 0$, then node j is considered pruned. The saliency of a node is then just the difference between the network's output error when α_j is 1 and when α_j is 0. They note that this saliency is an approximation to the derivative of the output error function with respect to α_j,

$$E_{\alpha_j=0} - E_{\alpha_j=1} \approx -\left.\frac{\partial E}{\partial \alpha_j}\right|_{\alpha_j=1}$$

Conversely, they use the derivative to approximate saliency for pruning. The approximation can be computed with a backpropagation-like algorithm. In practice, $\partial E/\partial \alpha$ fluctuates strongly in time, and the saliency estimate is smoothed by exponentially decay time averaging. Mozer and Smolensky also use a linear error function in assessing saliency while using the traditional squared error for training.

When tested over a set of logic problems, skeletonization showed that it could correctly identify the salient input and hidden nodes. The skeleton network can also learn with comparable or fewer number of training epochs than a standard network (Mozer and Smolensky, 1989).

Optimal Brain Damage and Optimal Brain Surgeon

The effect of a weight change on output error, which we have defined before as saliency, can be approximated by a Taylor-series expansion,

$$\delta E = \left(\frac{\partial E}{\partial \mathbf{w}}\right)^T \cdot \delta \mathbf{w} + \frac{1}{2} \delta \mathbf{w}^T \cdot \mathbf{H} \cdot \delta \mathbf{w} + O(\|\delta \mathbf{w}\|^3)$$

where $\mathbf{H} \equiv \partial^2 E/\partial \mathbf{w}^2$ is the Hessian matrix, $\delta \mathbf{w}$ is a small candidate weight change, and the superscript T denotes vector transpose. When the network is trained to a local optimum on the error surface, the first term on the right-hand side becomes zero. In the quadratic approximation, cubic and higher-order terms are ignored. One is left with just the second term and can then solve for $\delta \mathbf{w}$ such that (at least) one of the weights become zero in $\mathbf{w} + \delta \mathbf{w}$ yet the predicted increase in error, $\frac{1}{2}\delta \mathbf{w}^T \cdot \mathbf{H} \cdot \delta \mathbf{w}$, is minimum. In addition to finding the weight whose removal increases error the least, this approach also finds an adjustment for the remaining weights to compensate for the weight removal.

The full algorithm follows:

1. Train a "reasonably large" network to minimum error.
2. Compute $\mathbf{H}^{-1}$. Optimal Brain Damage (OBD) (Le Cun, Denker, and Solla, 1990) assumes $\mathbf{H}$ to be diagonal, which has a simple inverse. Optimal Brain Surgeon (OBS) (Hassibi and Stork, 1993) gives an efficient recursive algorithm to calculate the inverse of the full Hessian.
3. Find the candidate weight (indexed by j) that gives the smallest saliency

$$L_j = \frac{w_j^2}{2[\mathbf{H}^{-1}]_{jj}}$$

If this candidate error increase is greater than a user-specified threshold, go to step 5.
4. Delete the candidate weight. Update the remaining weights by

$$\delta \mathbf{w} = -\frac{w_j}{[\mathbf{H}^{-1}]_{jj}} \mathbf{H}^{-1} \cdot \mathbf{u}_j$$

where $\mathbf{u}_j$ is the unit vector corresponding to j, the index of the weight that was deleted. Go back to step 2.
5. No more weights can be deleted without a large increase in network error. At this point one may want to retrain the network.

OBS is more effective than OBD at finding the correct weights to prune and is suitable for small and medium-size networks. For large networks, however, the computational and storage requirement for deriving the full $\mathbf{H}^{-1}$ may be infeasible, and OBD should be used instead.

Topology Learning in Bayes Nets

Topology learning in Bayes nets has become a significant research area (Buntine, 1996). Since the usage of Bayes nets can be quite different from that of feedforward neural networks, topology learning for Bayes nets operates under a different set of assumptions.

Typically, each node in a Bayes net stands for a random variable that has some specific meaning in the real world. Adding or deleting a node in a Bayes net changes the semantics of the underlying domain, and neither growing nor pruning nodes is therefore done in Bayes nets. Furthermore, the direction of the links in a feedforward neural network denotes information flow and is predetermined (i.e., going from input layer to the hidden layers to the output layer), whereas the direction of links in a Bayes net establishes parent-child relationships to imply certain conditional independencies.

As with neural nets, topology learning in Bayes nets relies on a trade-off between network complexity and accuracy in modeling training data. In Bayes net topology learning, this trade-off is often expressed explicitly in a single metric. One of the more popular metrics is minimum description length (MDL) (Lam and Bacchus, 1994). Heckerman, Geiger, and Chickering (1995) derived another metric, BDe, from methods of Bayesian statistics. The MDL metric is simply the sum of a network's complexity and its accuracy in modeling data, while the BDe is a measure of prior belief plus data. These two metrics converge asymptotically as more data are given (under certain technical assumptions).

As expected, searching over the topology space to optimize a metric is computationally expensive. One usually has to resort to greedy searches. Fortunately, both metrics mentioned above are decomposable into a sum of scores for each node. That is, for nodes labeled $X_1, \ldots, X_n$, the metric for the network can be written as $\Sigma_i \, Score(X_i, Parents(X_i))$. When an arc is added or deleted, i.e., when a parent is added or deleted, the action affects only one term in the summation. The overall metric can thus be quickly recalculated for each step of the search.

Discussion

This article has highlighted two main issues in topology learning. One is the trade-off between network complexity and fit to data, the other is the selection of a search strategy over the topology space. Growing is a search strategy that adds nodes, while pruning deletes parameters or nodes. In learning Bayesian networks, any efficient greedy search strategy can be used. In practice, when a "good" topology is highly problem dependent and the practitioner has little guideline on how to select a "good" topology, it makes sense to learn it from available data.

Road Map: Learning in Artificial Networks
Related Reading: Bayesian Networks; Graphical Models: Structure Learning

References

Ash, T., 1989, Dynamic node creation in backpropagation networks, *Connect. Sci.*, 1:365–375.

Buntine, W., 1996, A guide to the literature on learning probabilistic networks from data, *IEEE Trans. Knowledge Data Eng.*, 8:195–210. ◆

Chauvin, Y., 1989, A back-propagation algorithm with optimal use of hidden units, in *Advances in Neural Information Processing Systems*, vol. 1 (D. S. Touretzky, Ed.), San Mateo, CA: Morgan Kaufmann, pp. 519–526.

Cheeseman, P., 1990, On finding the most probable model, in *Computational Models of Scientific Discovery and Theory Formation* (J. Shrager and P. Langley, Eds.), San Mateo, CA: Morgan Kaufmann, pp. 73–95. ◆

Fahlman, S. E., and Lebiere, C., 1990, The Cascade-Correlation learning architecture, in *Advances in Neural Information Processing Systems*, vol. 2 (D. S. Touretzky, Ed.), San Mateo, CA: Morgan Kaufmann, pp. 524–532.

Hanson, S. J., and Pratt, L. Y., 1989, Comparing biases for minimal network construction with backpropagation, in *Advances in Neural Information Processing Systems*, vol. 1 (D. S. Touretzky, Ed.), San Mateo, CA: Morgan Kaufmann, pp. 177–185.

Hassibi, B., and Stork, D. G., 1993, Second order derivatives for network pruning: Optimal Brain Surgeon, in *Advances in Neural Information Processing Systems*, vol. 5 (S. J. Hanson, J. D. Cowan, and C. L. Giles, Eds.), San Mateo, CA: Morgan Kaufmann, pp. 164–171.

Heckerman, D., Geiger, D., and Chickering, D., 1995, Learning Bayesian networks: The combination of knowledge and statistical data, *Machine Learn.*, 20:197–243. ◆

Ji, C., Snapp, R. R., and Psaltis, D., 1990, Generalizing smoothness constraints from discrete samples, *Neural Computat.*, 2:188–197.

Karnin, E. D., 1990, A simple procedure for pruning back-propagation trained neural networks, *IEEE Trans. Neural Netw.*, 1:239–242.

Kruschke, J. K., and Movellan, J. R., 1991, Benefits of gain: Speeded learning and minimal hidden layers in back-propagation networks, *IEEE Trans. Syst. Man Cybern.*, 21:273–280.

Lam, W., and Bacchus, F., 1994, Learning Bayesian belief networks: An approach based on the MDL principle, *Computat. Intell.*, 10:269–293.

Le Cun, Y., Denker, J. S., and Solla, S. A., 1990, Optimal brain damage, in *Advances in Neural Information Processing Systems*, vol. 2 (D. S. Touretzky, Ed.), San Mateo, CA: Morgan Kaufmann, pp. 598–605.

Mozer, M. C., and Smolensky, P., 1989, Skeletonization: A technique for trimming the fat from a network via relevance assesssment, in *Advances in Neural Information Processing Systems*, vol. 1 (D. S. Touretzky, Ed.), San Mateo, CA: Morgan Kaufmann, pp. 107–115.

Reed, R., 1993, Pruning algorithms—a survey, *IEEE Trans. Neural Netw.*, 4:740–747. ◆

Learning Vector Quantization

Teuvo K. Kohonen

Introduction

Neural network models are often applied to statistical pattern recognition problems, in which the class distributions of pattern vectors usually overlap and one must pay attention to the optimal location of the decision borders. The *learning vector quantization* (*LVQ*) algorithms discussed in this article define very good approximations for the optimal decision borders. These algorithms are computationally very light.

In the basic competitive learning neural networks to which the LVQ belongs, all cells may be thought to form an input layer, while there also exist mutual feedbacks or other types of lateral interaction between the cells. All cells receive the same external input, and by means of comparisons made in the lateral direction of the layer, an active response is switched on at the cell with the highest activation (the "winner"), while the responses of all the other cells are suppressed; this is called the *winner-take-all* (*WTA*) *function* (cf. Didday, 1970, 1976; Grossberg, 1976; Amari and Arbib, 1977).

Although many competitive learning neural networks have been based on nonlinear dynamic neural models, the decision or classification functions that ensue from their collective behavior are simply described by a formalism that was originally developed for signal analysis, namely, *vector quantization* (*VQ*). (For a general review of VQ, see Makhoul, Roucos, and Gish, 1985.) Thus, VQ and the neural network models of competitive learning are not alternative methods: the former is an idealized description of the latter on the signal-space level.

Vector Quantization

As in simple neural network models, we assume a signal vector $x = (\xi_1, \xi_2, \ldots, \xi_n) \in \mathbb{R}^n$ and a set of units or cells, each provided with a parametric vector (called *codebook vector*) $m_i = (\mu_{i1}, \mu_{i2}, \ldots, \mu_{in})^T \in \mathbb{R}^n$. The winner in the category of VQ problems is usually defined as the unit c whose codebook vector has the smallest Euclidean distance from x:

$$\|x - m_c\| = \min_i \{\|x - m_i\|\} \tag{1}$$

If x is a natural, stochastic, continuous-valued vectorial variable, we need not consider multiple minima: the probability for $\|x - m_i\| = \|x - m_j\|$ for $i \neq j$ is then zero.

The VQ methods were originally developed to compress information. The m_i had to be placed into the input signal space such that the average expected quantization error E was minimized:

$$E = \int \|x - m_{c(x,m_i,\ldots,m_k)}\|^2 p(x)dx = \min! \tag{2}$$

where $p(x)$ is the probability density function of x, and dx is a hypervolume differential in the signal space. Notice that c, the index of the winner, depends on x and all the m_i. It has been shown by Zador (1982), for example, that the point density of the m_i values that minimize E is proportional to $[p(x)]^{n/(n+2)}$. Since in practical problems usually $n \gg 2$, it can then be said that the distribution of the m_i approximates $p(x)$.

Optimal Decision

Assume that all samples of x are derived from a finite set of classes $\{S_k\}$, the distributions of which are allowed to overlap. The problem of optimal decision or statistical pattern recognition is usually discussed within the framework of the Bayes theory of probability (for a textbook account, see, e.g., Kohonen, 1989, chap. 7.2). Let

$P(S_k)$ be the a priori probability of class S_k, and $p(x|x \in S_k)$ be the conditional probability density function of x on S_k, respectively. In this method the so-called *discriminant functions* are defined as

$$\delta_k(x) = p(x|x \in S_k)P(S_k) \tag{3}$$

It can be shown that the average rate of misclassifications is minimized if the sample x is determined to belong to class S_c according to

$$\delta_c(x) = \max_k \{\delta_k(x)\} \tag{4}$$

Learning Vector Quantization Algorithms

The LVQ1

Consider now Figure 1. In the LVQ approaches we assign *a subset of codebook vectors to each class* S_k and then search for the codebook vector m_i that has the smallest Euclidean distance from x. This assignment can be made in such a way that codebook vectors belonging to different classes are not intermingled, although the class distributions overlap. The sample x is then thought to belong to the same class as the closest m_i. As only codebook vectors closest to the class borders define the decision borders, a good approximation of $p(x|x \in S_k)$ is not necessary everywhere. We must place the m_i into the signal space in such a way that the nearest-neighbor rule (Equation 1) minimizes the average expected misclassification probability. Notice that in considering the average expected classification accuracy, the quantization errors can be large in regions where $p(x)$ has small values.

Let

$$c = \arg \min_i \{\|x - m_i\|\} \tag{5}$$

define the index of the nearest m_i to x, denoted by m_c; x is then determined to belong to the same class to which the nearest m_i belongs.

Let $x = x(t)$ now be a time-series sample of input, and let the $m_i(t)$ represent sequential values of the m_i in the discrete-time domain, $t = 0, 1, 2, \ldots$, obtained in the following process. Starting with properly defined initial values $m_i(0)$, Equation 6 shall define the basic learning vector quantization process (Kohonen, 1988; Kohonen, Barna, and Chrisley, 1988); this particular algorithm is called LVQ1.

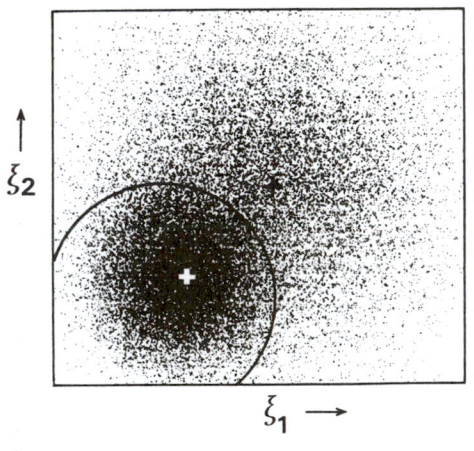

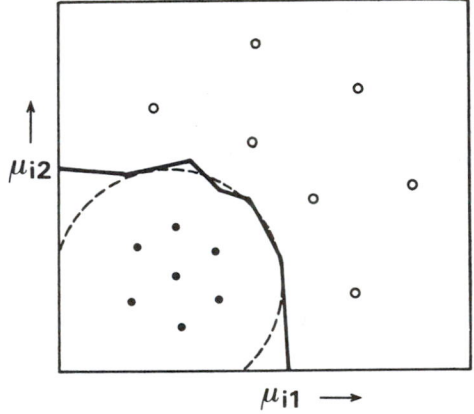

Figure 1. *A*, The probability density function of $x = [\xi_1, \xi_2]^T$ is represented here by its samples, the small dots. The superposition of two symmetric Gaussian density functions corresponding to two different classes S_1 and S_2, with their centroids shown by the white and dark cross, respectively, is shown. Solid curve denotes the theoretical optimal Bayes decision surface. *B*, Large black dots denote codebook vectors of class S_1; open circles denote codebook vectors of class S_2; the solid curve indicates a decision surface obtained by LVQ1; the broken curve indicates a Bayes decision surface.

A

B

$$m_c(t + 1) = m_c(t) + \alpha(t)[x(t) - m_c(t)]$$
$$\text{if } x \text{ and } m_c \text{ belong to the same class}$$
$$m_c(t + 1) = m_c(t) - \alpha(t)[x(t) - m_c(t)] \quad (6)$$
$$\text{if } x \text{ and } m_c \text{ belong to different classes}$$
$$m_i(t + 1) = m_i(t) \text{ for } i \neq c$$

It will be shown that the asymptotic values of m_i obtained in this process define a vector quantization for which the rate of misclassifications is approximately minimized. Here $0 < \alpha(t) < 1$, and $\alpha(t)$ (learning-rate factor) is usually made to decrease monotonically with time. It is recommended that α should initially be rather small, say, smaller than 0.1. If only a restricted time is available for learning, the exact law $\alpha = \alpha(t)$ is not crucial, especially also if only a restricted set of training samples is available; they may be applied cyclically, and $\alpha(t)$ may even be made to decrease linearly to zero.

It is in general difficult to show what the exact convergence limits of Equation 6 are. The following discussion is based on the idea that VQ tends to approximate density functions such as $p(x)$. Instead of $p(x)$, we may also consider any non-negative function $f(x)$ in Equation 2.

The Bayes decision borders defined by Equations 3 and 4 divide the signal space into class regions B_k such that the rate of misclassifications is minimized. All such borders together are defined by the condition $f(x) = 0$, where, for $x \in B_k$ and $h \neq k$,

$$f(x) = p(x|x \in S_k)P(S_k) - \max_k \{p(x|x \in S_h)P(S_h)\} \quad (7)$$

Notice that $f(x)$ is piecewise continuous and non-negative. For each $x \in B_k$, $f(x)$ has a positive hump, and these humps are separated by the Bayes borders at which $f(x) = 0$.

If we approximate $f(x)$ by the point density of codebook vectors defined by classical VQ, this point density must then also tend to zero at all borders.

In order to find the minimum of E in Equation 2 and the optimal values for the m_i in VQ by gradient descent, we need an expression for the gradient of E. From Kohonen (1991, Equations A1 through A14) we obtain the result

$$\nabla_{m_i} E = -2 \int \delta_{ci} \cdot (x - m_i)p(x)dx \quad (8)$$

where δ_{ic} is the Kronecker delta, and c is the index of the m_i that is closest to x (i.e., the winner). The gradient step of vector m_i is

$$m_i(t + 1) = m_i(t) - \lambda \cdot \nabla_{m_i(t)} E \quad (9)$$

where λ defines the step size, and

$$\nabla_{m_i(t)} E = -2\delta_{ci}[x(t) - m_i(t)] \quad (10)$$

If $p(x)$ in E is now replaced by $f(x)$, we get by substitution:

$$\nabla_{m_i} E = -2 \int \delta_{ci}(x - m_i)f(x)dx$$
$$= -2 \int \delta_{ci}(x - m_i)[p(x|x \in S_k)P(S_k)$$
$$- \max_k \{p(x|x \in S_h)P(S_h)\}]dx \quad (11)$$

The gradient steps must be computed separately in the event that the sample $x(t)$ belongs to S_k, and in the event that $x(t) \in S_h$. In the event that $x(t) \in S_k$, we obtain

$$\nabla_{m_i(t)} E = -2\delta_{ci}[x(t) - m_i(t)] \quad (12)$$

with the a priori probability $P(S_k)$.

The class with $\max_h\{p(x|x \in S_h)P(S_h)\}$ is the runner-up class signified by index r. In the event that $x(t) \in S_r$, the following expression for $\nabla_{m_i} E$ is obtained with the a priori probability $P(S_r)$:

$$\nabla_{m_i(t)} E = +2\delta_{ci}[x(t) - m_i(t)] \quad (13)$$

The different cases are collected into the following set of equations, rewritten with $\alpha(t) = 2\lambda$:

$$m_c(t + 1) = m_c(t) + \alpha(t)[x(t) - m_c(t)]$$
$$\text{for } x(t) \in B_k \text{ and } x(t) \in S_k$$
$$m_c(t + 1) = m_c(t) - \alpha(t)[x(t) - m_c(t)] \quad (14)$$
$$\text{for } x(t) \in B_k \text{ and } x(t) \in S_r$$
$$m_c(t + 1) = m_c(t) \text{ for } x(t) \in B_k \text{ and } x(t) \in S_h, h \neq r$$
$$m_i(t + 1) = m_i(t) \text{ for } i \neq c$$

If the m_i of class S_k are already within B_k, the VQ will further attract them to the hump corresponding to B_k, at least if the learning steps are small. With a sufficiently large number of codebook vectors in each class region B_k, the closest codebook vectors in adjacent regions B_k will be arbitrarily close to the Bayes border. Thus, VQ and Equation 7 have been shown to define the Bayes borders with arbitrarily good accuracy.

Near equilibrium, close to the borders at least, Equations 6 and 14 can be seen to define almost similar corrections; notice that in Equation 6, *the classification of x was approximated by the nearest-neighbor rule*, and this approximation will be improved during learning. However, notice too that in Equation 6 the minus sign corrections were made every time when x was classified incorrectly, whereas Equation 14 only makes the corresponding correction if x is exactly in the runner-up class. The error thereby made is often insignificant. As a matter of fact, the algorithms called LVQ2 and LVQ3 (Kohonen, 1990) are even closer to Equation 14 in this respect.

The Optimized-Learning-Rate LVQ1 (OLVQ1)

If an individual learning rate $\alpha_i(t)$ is assigned to each m_i, we obtain the following modified learning process (Kohonen, 1992). Let c be defined by Equation 5. Then

$$m_c(t + 1) = m_c(t) + \alpha_c(t)[x(t) - m_c(t)]$$
$$\text{if } x \text{ is classified correctly}$$
$$m_c(t + 1) = m_c(t) - \alpha_c(t)[x(t) - m_c(t)] \quad (15)$$
$$\text{if } x \text{ is classified incorrectly}$$
$$m_i(t + 1) = m_i(t) \text{ for } i \neq c$$

We may try to determine the $\alpha_i(t)$ for fastest convergence of Equations 15. Let us express Equations 15 in the shorter form

$$m_c(t + 1) = [1 - s(t)\alpha_c(t)]m_c(t) + s(t)\alpha_c(t)x(t) \quad (16)$$

where $s(t) = +1$ if the classification is correct, and $s(t) = -1$ if the classification is wrong. It may be obvious that the *statistical accuracy* of the learned codebook vector values is approximately optimal if all samples have been used with equal weight, i.e., if the effects of the corrections made at different times, when referring to the end of the learning period, are of approximately equal magnitude. Notice that $m_c(t + 1)$ contains a trace of $x(t)$ through the last term in Equation 16, and traces of the earlier $x(t')$, $t' = 1, 2, \ldots, t - 1$, through $m_c(t)$. In a learning step, the magnitude of the last trace of $x(t)$ is scaled down by the factor $\alpha_c(t)$, and, for instance, during the same step the trace of $x(t - 1)$ becomes scaled down by $[1 - s(t)\alpha_c(t)] \cdot \alpha_c(t - 1)$. Now we first stipulate that these two scalings must be identical:

$$\alpha_c(t) = [1 - s(t)\alpha_c(t)]\alpha_c(t - 1) \quad (17)$$

If this condition is made to hold for all t, by induction it can be shown that the traces collected up to time t of all the earlier $x(t')$ will be scaled down by an equal amount at the end, and thus the "optimal" values of $\alpha_i(t)$ are determined by the recursion

$$\alpha_c(t) = \frac{\alpha_c(t - 1)}{1 + s(t)\alpha_c(t - 1)} \quad (18)$$

For fast learning, the OLVQ1 algorithm can be started with the $\alpha_i(0)$ in the range of 0.3 to 0.5.

General Considerations

Initialization of the Codebook Vectors

A rather good strategy is to start with the same number of codebook vectors in each class. An upper limit to the total number of codebook vectors is set by the restricted recognition time and computing power. An identical number of codebook vectors per class is justifiable, since for optimal approximation of the borders the average distances between the adjacent codebook vectors (which depend on their numbers per class) ought to be the same in each class. Because the final placement of the codebook vectors and thus their distances are not known until the end of the learning process, equalization of the distances in the various classes ought to be made iteratively.

Once the numbers of codebook vectors have been fixed, one may use first samples of the real training data for their initial values. Referring to the derivation of Equation 9, however, the codebook vectors should always remain inside the respective class regions. For the initial values one can then accept only samples that are not misclassified. In other words, a sample is first tentatively classified against all the other samples in the training set, for instance by the traditional k-nearest-neighbor (kNN) method, and accepted for a possible initial value only if this tentative classification is the same as the class identifier of the sample. (In the learning algorithm itself, however, no samples must be excluded; they are applied independently of whether they fall on the correct side of the class border or not.)

Overall Learning Strategy

One may start the learning with the OLVQ1 algorithm, which has fast convergence; its final recognition accuracy will approximately be achieved after a number of learning steps that is about 30 to 50 times the total number of codebook vectors. In an attempt to ultimately improve recognition accuracy, one may try to continue with the basic LVQ1, or with the other LVQ versions, using a low initial value of learning rate, which is then the same for all classes.

The neural network algorithms often "overlearn"; i.e., when the learning and test phases are alternated, the recognition accuracy is first improved until an optimum is reached. After that point, the accuracy often starts to decrease slowly. A possible explanation in the present case is that when the codebook vectors become very specifically tuned to the training data, the ability of the algorithm to generalize with respect to new data suffers. It is therefore necessary to stop the additional learning process after some optimal number of steps, say, 50 to 200 times the total number of the codebook vectors. Such a stopping rule can only be found by experience.

Comparison with Other Methods

LVQ and SOM

Another related algorithm, the *self-organizing map* (*SOM*) (Kohonen, 1989, 1990, 1993; see also SELF-ORGANIZING FEATURE MAPS) should be mentioned in this context. It is an unsupervised learning method, whereas supervised training is used in the LVQ. In LVQ, only one or two winner cells are updated during each adaptation step, whereas in the SOM, a block of neighboring cells around the winner *relating to the physical network* is updated simultaneously. The main application areas of these algorithms are also different: LVQ is used for the classification of stochastic data, whereas the SOM is more useful for the visualization of high-dimensional data on a two-dimensional display.

Table 1. Error Percentages in Phonemic Classification

Parametric Bayes	kNN	LVQ1
12.1	12.0	10.2

Relative Performance of LVQ as a Classifier

The number of different applications of LVQ (and SOM) is for the present at least on the order of many hundreds, and it is very difficult to make any comparative survey. Just to give a feeling of the relative performance, Table 1 (Kohonen, 1990) compares the classification accuracies achievable by a couple of classical methods as well as by LVQ1. The data, 15-channel acoustic spectra representing 19 different phonemic classes, were collected from Finnish speech. A total of 1,550 samples were used for training, and another set of 1,550 independent samples for testing, respectively. There were in total 117 codebook vectors.

The term *parametric Bayes* in Table 1 means a Bayesian classification method in which the discriminant functions are approximated by multivariate normal distributions, and kNN is the classical k-nearest-neighbor method, i.e., comparison of each test sample against all the training samples and voting over k closest ones (here $k = 5$). It is generally known that the kNN algorithm gives a very good approximation of the theoretical Bayes limit; but LVQ1 is still better, and here more than ten times faster computationally.

[Reprinted from the First Edition]

Road Map: Learning in Artificial Networks
Related Reading: Competitive Learning; Coulomb Potential Learning; Data Clustering and Learning; Self-Organizing Feature Maps

References

A list of over 5,000 literature references to analyses and applications of LVQ and SOM algorithms is available on the Internet, at the address http://www.icsi.berkeley.edu/~jagota/NCS. Extensive software packages of LVQ and SOM algorithms, diagnostic programs, and exemplary data can be found at http://www.cis.hut.fi/research.

The following works have been referred to in this article:

Amari, S., and Arbib, M. A., 1977, Competition and cooperation in neural nets, in *Systems in Neuroscience* (J. Metzler, Ed.), New York: Academic Press, pp. 119–165. ◆

Didday, R. L., 1970, The simulation and modelling of distributed information processing in the frog visual system, PhD diss., Stanford University.

Didday, R. L., 1976, A model of visuomotor mechanisms in the frog optic tectum, *Math. Biosci.*, 30:169–180.

Grossberg, S., 1976, Adaptive pattern classification and universal recoding: I. Parallel development and coding of neural feature detectors, *Biol. Cybern.*, 23:121–134; II. Feedback, expectation, olfaction, illusions, *Biol. Cybern.*, 23:187–202.

Kohonen, T., 1988, An introduction to neural networks, *Neural Netw.*, 1:3–16. ◆

Kohonen, T., 1989, *Self-Organization and Associative Memory*, 3rd ed., Berlin: Springer-Verlag.

Kohonen, T., 1990, The self-organizing map, *Proc. IEEE*, 78:1464–1480. ◆

Kohonen, T., 1991, Self-organizing maps: Optimization approaches, in *Artificial Neural Networks* (T. Kohonen, K. Makisara, O. Simula, and J. Kangas, Eds.), Amsterdam: Elsevier, vol. 2, pp. 1677–1680.

Kohonen, T., 1992, New developments of learning vector quantization and the self-organizing map, in *Symposium on Neural Networks: Alliances and Perspectives in Senri 1992 (SYNAPSE'92)*, Osaka, Japan.

Kohonen, T., 1993, Physiological interpretation of the self-organizing map algorithm, *Neural Netw.*, 6:895–905.

Kohonen, T., Barna, G., and Chrisley, R., 1988, Statistical pattern recognition with neural networks: Benchmarking studies, in *Proceedings of the IEEE International Conference on Neural Networks*, vol. 1, New York: IEEE, pp. 61–68.

Makhoul, J., Roucos, S., and Gish, H., 1985, Vector quantization in speech coding, *Proc. IEEE*, 73:1551–1588. ◆

Zador, P. L., 1982, Asymptotic quantization error of continuous signals and the quantization dimensions, *IEEE Trans. Inform. Theory*, IT-28:139–149.

Lesioned Networks as Models of Neuropsychological Deficits

John A. Bullinaria

Introduction

Cognitive neuropsychology uses the patterns of performance observed in brain-damaged patients to constrain our models of normal cognitive function. Historically, this methodology was rooted in simple "box-and-arrow" models, with particular cognitive deficits being taken to indicate selective breakdown of corresponding "boxes" or "arrows." Studying patients with complementary patterns of deficit allows us, in principle, to piece together a complete model of mental structure (Shallice, 1988). Of particular importance in this process has been the concept of *double dissociation*, which has been taken to imply modularity within many systems. If one patient can perform task 1 better than task 2 and another can perform task 2 better than task 1, then a natural explanation is in terms of separate modules for the two tasks.

In recent years, connectionist techniques have been employed to model the operation and interaction of these "modules" in increasing detail (Farah, 1994). Networks of simplified processing units loosely based on real neurons are set up with general architectures based on known physiology, trained to perform appropriately simplified versions of the human tasks, and iteratively refined by checking their performance against humans'. Such network models can clearly be wired together in the manner of the old box-and-arrow models, with all the old explanations of patient data carrying through. The obvious advantage now is that we can look at the details of the degradation of the various components and, by removing neurons or connections in our models, construct natural analogues of real brain damage. Moreover, in addition to elaborating previous models, we can also question the validity of the old assumptions of neuropsychological inference and explore the possibility that processing is actually more distributed and interactive than the older models implied.

This article reviews the general issues involved in lesioning neural network models to simulate neuropsychological deficits. I shall point out potential sources of misleading results, clarify apparent contradictions in the literature, and discuss some representative models.

Lesioning Simple Feedforward Networks

Many neural network models of human performance are based on simple feedforward networks that map between conveniently simplified input and output representations via a single hidden layer, or that have such systems as identifiable subcomponents. An important feature of these models is that they *learn* to perform the relevant tasks by iteratively adjusting their connection weights (e.g., by some form of gradient descent algorithm) to minimize the output errors for an appropriate training set of input-output pairs. Generally, we simply assume that the quick and convenient learning algorithms we choose will generate results similar to those produced by more biologically plausible procedures. Comparisons between backpropagation and contrastive Hebbian learning by Plaut and Shallice (1993) provide some justification for this assumption. We can then compare the development of the networks' performance during training and their final performance (e.g., their output errors, generalization ability, reaction times, priming effects, speed-accuracy trade-offs, robustness to damage, etc.) with the performance of human subjects to narrow down the correct architecture, representations, and so on, to generate increasingly accurate models.

An obvious feature of network learning is that performance on one pattern will be affected by training on other patterns. It follows straightforwardly from adding up the network weight change contributions resulting from individual training patterns that:

1. Regular items will be learned more quickly than irregular items, because consistent weight changes combine and inconsistent weight changes cancel.
2. High-frequency items will be learned more quickly than low-frequency items, because the appropriate weight changes get applied more often.
3. Ceiling effects will arise as sigmoids saturate and weight changes tend to zero.

These fundamental properties of neural network learning not only result in human-like *age of acquisition* effects but indirectly account for realistic patterns of reaction times, speed-accuracy trade-off effects, and so on (Bullinaria, 1997). After training our networks and confirming that they are performing in a sufficiently human-like manner, we can then set about inflicting simulated brain damage on them. Small (1991) considered the various ways in which connectionist networks might be lesioned, and discussed their neurobiological and clinical neurological relevance. He identified two broad classes of lesion: *diffuse*, such as those created by globally scaling or adding noise to all the weights, and *focal*, such as those created by removing adjacent subsets of connections and/or hidden units. Which class we choose will depend on the type of patient we are modeling. Focal lesions would be appropriate for stroke patients, whereas diffuse lesions would be required for diseases such as Alzheimer's. Generally, for our simplified models, it is appropriate to examine all these possibilities. Finally, we should be aware that relearning after damage may affect the observed pattern of deficits, and so we must check this also (Plaut, 1996).

The relevant issues have been explored in an abstract setting by Bullinaria (1999), who trained a simple feedforward network (with 10 inputs, 100 hidden units, and 10 outputs, with binary inputs and output targets) on two sets of 100 regular items (different permuted identity mappings) and two sets of 10 irregular items (random mappings). One regular set and one irregular set appeared during training 20 times more frequently than the others. Figure 1 shows that both regularity and frequency do indeed affect the speed of learning in the expected manner.

Bullinaria and Chater (1995) explored the effects of damage on fully distributed, homogeneous connectionist systems and investigated the possibility that double dissociation between regular and irregular items could arise without modularity. They found that lesioning trained networks by removing random hidden units, removing random connections, globally scaling the weights, or adding random noise to the weights all led to very similar patterns of deficits. They concluded that, assuming one successfully avoids small-scale artifacts and controls for all other factors, only single dissociations were possible. Moreover, these single dissociations were seen to be a natural consequence of the ease with which the mappings were originally learned. Plotting the patterns of activation feeding into the output units revealed why this should be the case. Each form of damage results in these activations either drifting in a random direction or falling to zero. For every output unit there will be some correct response threshold, and the items that are learned first during training will end up furthest past the thresholds when the training is stopped. They will consequently tend to be the last to cross over again and hence be the last to result in output errors as more damage is incurred. Thus we get clear dissociations, with the regulars more robust than frequency-matched irregulars and high-frequency items more robust than regularity matched low-frequency items. Figure 2 shows this pattern explicitly for the network of Figure 1.

These basic effects extend easily to more realistic models, for example, surface dyslexia in the reading model of Bullinaria (1997). Here we successfully simulate not only the relative error proportions for the various word categories (i.e., regular/irregular, high/low frequency) but also the types of errors that are produced. The closest threshold to an irregularly pronounced letter will be that of regular pronunciation, and hence the errors will be predominantly regularizations of the lowest-frequency irregular items, exactly as is observed in acquired human surface dyslexia.

Figures 1 and 2 also reveal what is behind a potential source of confusion. Bullinaria and Chater (1995) argued that network lesions would always result in single dissociations with the regular items more robust. Marchman (1993), however, studied models of past tense production and seemingly found dissociations, with the irregular items more robust than the regulars. It is easy to see from the figures that sufficiently high-frequency irregulars can be more robust than regulars. The English language has evolved to leave the irregulars with much higher frequencies than the regulars; otherwise, they would have been lost from the language. Marchman built this into her models, with the expected consequences. This illustrates how important it is to control for all confounding factors when describing dissociations and drawing conclusions from them. Lavric et al. (2001) provide a review of the issues involved in understanding the dissociations of verb morphology.

It is also evident from Figure 2 that, if the frequencies and regularities are carefully matched, performance on the high-frequency irregulars can cross performance on the lower-frequency regulars. Initially there is a dissociation with better performance on the irregulars, and later the opposite dissociation. Such a "double dissociation" is a form of *resource artifact* that is well known not to imply underlying modularity (Shallice, 1988, p. 234). Patterns of deficits of this type are actually rather easily obtainable in neural network models. Devlin et al. (1998) present an interesting example involving a connectionist account of category-specific semantic deficits. The finer grain of detail that connectionist modeling affords here allows explicit accounts of human deficits that older box-and-arrow models could accommodate only with difficulty.

The general point one can make about single, fully distributed subsystems is that some items are naturally learned more quickly and more accurately than others, and the effects of subsequent network damage follow automatically from these patterns of learning. There are actually many factors, in addition to regularity and frequency, that can cause differing learning and damage rates. We can explore them all in a similar manner and use them in models of neuropsychological data in the same way. Consistency and neighborhood density are the factors most closely related to regularity and are commonly found in models of language tasks such as reading and spelling (e.g., Plaut et al., 1996; Bullinaria, 1997). Representation sparseness or pattern strength are often used to distinguish between concrete and abstract semantics, as in models of deep dyslexia (e.g., Plaut and Shallice, 1993). Correlation, redundancy, and dimensionality are commonly used in models to distinguish the semantics of natural things versus artifacts, as in models of category-specific semantic deficits (e.g., Devlin et al., 1998). At some level of description, all of these factors act in a similar manner as frequency and regularity, and their effects can easily be confounded. Which we use will depend on exactly what we are attempting to model. If we want to make claims about neuropsychological deficits involving one of them, however, we need to be careful to control for all the others.

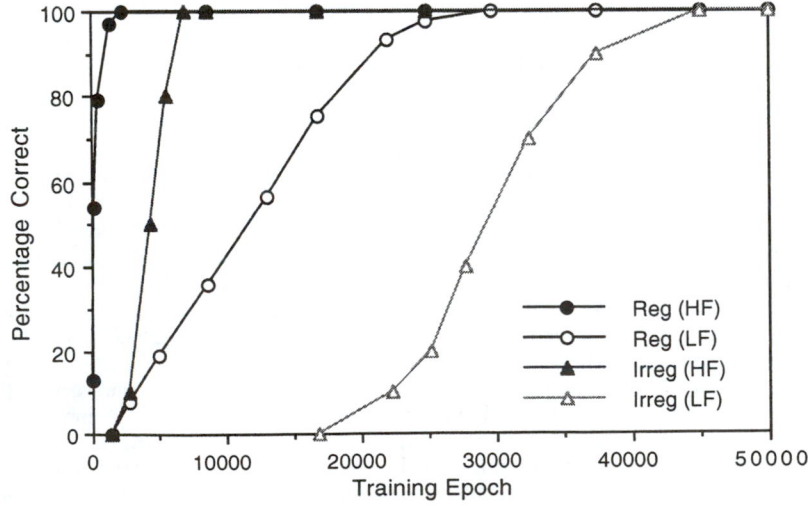

Figure 1. Regularity and frequency effects during the course of learning. HF, high frequency; LF, low frequency.

Figure 2. Regularity and frequency effects with increasing degrees of network damage. HF, high frequency, LF low frequency.

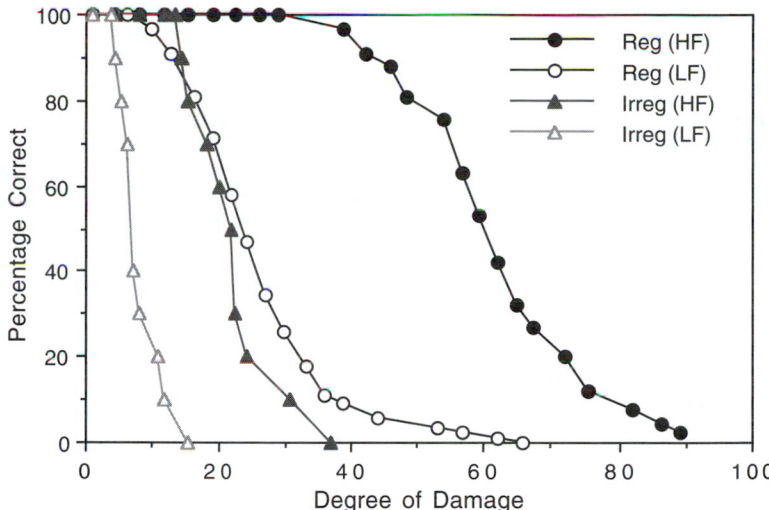

Following brain damage, patients often show a rapid improvement in performance. This is important to connectionist modelers for two reasons. First, if relearning occurs automatically and quickly in patients, then we need to be sure that the same effects are observed in our models, and that we are comparing patient and model data at equivalent stages of the relearning process. Second, our models may be of assistance in formulating appropriate remedial strategies for brain-damaged patients (Plaut, 1996). Since learning and damage have the same underlying regularity and frequency effects, relearning from the original training data is unlikely to reverse this pattern; indeed, it is likely to enhance it (Bullinaria and Chater, 1995). However, if some rehabilitation regime is employed that involves a very different set of training examples from that of the original learning process, it is possible for different results to arise (Plaut, 1996). Here the models can be used to predict or refine appropriate relearning strategies, and the patients' responses can be used to validate our models.

Small-Scale Artifacts

One should never forget that modeling massively parallel brain processes by simulating neural networks on serial computers is rendered feasible only by abstracting the essential details and scaling down the size of the networks. It is clearly important not to take the abstraction and scaling process so far that we miss important fundamental properties of the systems we are modeling, or introduce features that are nothing but small-scale artifacts. The damage curves of Figure 2 are relatively smooth because our network has many more hidden units and connections than are actually required to perform the given mappings, and individual connections or hidden units make only small contributions to the network's outputs. For smaller networks, however, the effect of individual damage contributions can be large enough to produce wildly fluctuating performance on individual items, and this can result in dissociations in arbitrary directions. Often these small-scale artifacts are sufficient to produce convincing-looking double dissociations (Shallice, 1988, p. 254). Bullinaria and Chater (1995) showed that as we scale up to larger networks, the processing becomes more distributed, and apparent double dissociations dissolve into single dissociations.

Our modeling endeavors would be much easier if some independent procedure could determine when networks were sufficiently distributed to obtain reliable results. In effect, we need to make sure that individual processing units are not acting as "mod-

ules" in their own right, and the obvious way to do this is by checking that all the individual contributions feeding into each output unit are small compared to the total. In this case, many such lost contributions must conspire to result in an output change large enough to be deemed an error. This is the brain-like resilience to damage often known as *graceful degradation*. Fortunately, this distribution of information processing tends to occur automatically if the network is supplied with a sufficiently large number of hidden units. However, in general, it seems that we do need many hidden units to avoid small-scale artifacts—many times the minimal number required to learn the given task (Bullinaria, 1999). So, what can be done if limited computational resources make this impossible? Obviously, after removing a random subset of the hidden units or connections, the number of contributions will be reduced by some factor, but in large, fully distributed networks, the mean contribution will not change much, and so the total contribution after damage is simply reduced by the same factor. We can achieve the same result simply by globally scaling all the weights by the same factor. In smaller networks, this equivalence breaks down because the means tend to suffer relatively large random fluctuations during damage. However, since global weight scaling does not suffer from such random fluctuations, it can be used to simulate a smoothed form of lesioning and give a reasonable approximation in small networks to what will happen in more realistic networks. Alternatively, if one wants to claim that each hidden unit corresponds to a number of real neurons, then the weight scaling can be regarded as removing a fraction of those neurons.

Lesioning Attractor Networks

Many successful models of human performance and their associated neuropsychological deficits have been based on attractor networks (see COMPUTING WITH ATTRACTORS) rather than simple feedforward networks. These are recurrent networks that develop *attractors* to appropriate patterns of activity; i.e., they have points in the *state space* of output activations to which the network settles. Lesions of this type of network can alter the settling behavior by distorting or shifting the *basins of attraction*. Here the errors correspond to the network settling into the wrong attractor, rather than an output unit activation failing to reach a particular threshold. Nevertheless, the resilience to damage still follows directly from how the particular items were originally learned.

One of the earliest applications of attractor networks to neuropsychology was the Mozer and Behrmann (1990) model of *neglect dyslexia*. But perhaps the most successful models of this type are the Plaut and Shallice (1993) models of *deep dyslexia*, which were extensions of earlier work by Hinton and Shallice (1991) showing how both visual and semantic errors could arise from a single lesion. These attractor networks mapped from orthography to semantics via a layer of hidden units, and then from semantics to phonology via another set of hidden units, with layers of *clean-up units* at the semantics and phonology levels. One particular model was trained on 40 words, using backpropagation through time, until it settled into the correct semantics and phonology when presented with each orthography. Lesions at two different locations in the trained network were then found to produce a double dissociation between concrete and abstract word reading, where concreteness was coded as the proportion of activated semantic microfeatures. Specifically, removal of orthographic to hidden layer connections resulted in preferential loss of abstract word reading, whereas removal of connections to the semantic clean-up units primarily impaired performance on the concrete words. Although the two damage locations do not constitute modules in the conventional sense, it is not difficult to understand how they contribute to the processing of the two word types to different degrees, and give opposite dissociations when damaged. It is simply a consequence of the sparser representations of the abstract words making less use of the semantic clean-up mechanism, and depending more on the direct connections, than the richer representations of the concrete words (Plaut and Shallice, 1993). This does not conflict with the claim of Bullinaria and Chater (1995) that only single dissociations are possible. The robustness of each location in the attractor network is fully consistent with the general discussion above, and the only disagreement concerns the appropriateness of using the word "module" to describe the two damage locations. As Plaut himself points out (Plaut, 1995), one of the problems when discussing modularity is that different authors define the term differently. This is fine, but to avoid confusion one should be careful to quote the definitions along with the conclusions.

Discussion

This article has covered the basic issues and complications involved in lesioning neural network models to provide accounts of neuropsychological deficits, and has provided pointers to a range of representative case studies. It seems clear that, despite all the abstractions and simplifications involved, connectionist modeling has a lot to offer in fleshing out the details of, or even replacing, earlier box-and-arrow models to provide a more complete picture of cognitive processing. The resulting enhanced models and the

new field of connectionist neuropsychology not only are producing good accounts of existing empirical data, but are also beginning to suggest more appropriate experimental investigations for further fine-tuning of these models, and an ethical approach for exploring potential remedial actions for neuropsychological patients.

Road Map: Cognitive Neuroscience
Related Reading: Neurological and Psychiatric Disorders; Neuropsychological Impairments

References

Bullinaria, J. A., 1997, Modelling reading, spelling and past tense learning with artificial neural networks, *Brain Lang.*, 59:236–266.
Bullinaria, J. A., 1999, Connectionist dissociations, confounding factors and modularity, in *Connectionist Models in Cognitive Neuroscience* (D. Heinke, G. W. Humphreys, and A. Olsen, Eds.), London: Springer-Verlag, pp. 52–63.
Bullinaria, J. A., and Chater, N., 1995, Connectionist modelling: Implications for cognitive neuropsychology, *Lang. Cognit. Proc.*, 10:227–264. ◆
Devlin, J. T., Gonnerman, L. M., Andersen, E. S., and Seidenberg, M. S., 1998, Category-specific semantic deficits in focal and widespread brain damage: A computational account, *J. Cognit. Neurosci.*, 10:77–94.
Farah, M. J., 1994, Neuropsychological inference with an interactive brain: A critique of the locality assumption, *Behav. Brain Sci.*, 17:43–104.
Hinton, G. E., and Shallice, T., 1991, Lesioning an attractor network: Investigations of acquired dyslexia, *Psychol. Rev.*, 98:74–95.
Lavric, A., Pizzagalli, D., Forstmeir, S., and Rippon, G., 2001, Mapping dissociations in verb morphology, *Trends Cognit. Sci.*, 5:301–308.
Marchman, V. A., 1993, Constraints on plasticity in a connectionist model of the English past tense, *J. Cognit. Neurosci.*, 5:215–234.
Mozer, M. C., and Behrmann, M., 1990, On the interaction of selective attention and lexical knowledge: A connectionist account of neglect dyslexia, *J. Cognit. Neurosci.*, 2:96–123.
Plaut, D. C., 1995, Double dissociation without modularity: Evidence from connectionist neuropsychology, *J. Clin. Exp. Neuropsychol.*, 17:291–321. ◆
Plaut, D. C., 1996, Relearning after damage in connectionist networks: Towards a theory of rehabilitation, *Brain Lang.*, 52:25–82.
Plaut, D. C., McClelland, J. L., Seidenberg, M. S., and Patterson, K. E., 1996, Understanding normal and impaired word reading: Computational principles in quasi-regular domains, *Psychol. Rev.*, 103:56–115.
Plaut, D. C., and Shallice, T., 1993, Deep dyslexia: A case study of connectionist neuropsychology, *Cognit. Neuropsychol.*, 10:377–500. ◆
Shallice, T., 1988, *From Neuropsychology to Mental Structure*, Cambridge, Engl.: Cambridge University Press. ◆
Small, S. L., 1991, Focal and diffuse lesions in cognitive models, in *Proceedings of the Thirteenth Annual Conference of the Cognitive Science Society*, Hillsdale, NJ: Erlbaum, pp. 85–90.

Limb Geometry, Neural Control

Francesco Lacquaniti, Mauro Carrozzo, Yuri P. Ivanenko, and Myrka Zago

Introduction

Sensorimotor transformations.   Motor control involves the problem of transforming sensory inputs into motor outputs. The outputs are the motor commands that act on muscles and the inputs are derived from sensory feedback and efference copy of the motor commands. The simplest solution would be to encode similar parameters at both input and output levels, such as the kinetic parameters of muscle forces and joint torques. The problem of motor

control would then simplify to one of specifying patterns of time-varying muscle activity, and causality would dictate the ensuing limb motion. Some sensory inputs reflect kinetics (e.g., Golgi tendon organs), but many others reflect kinematics. For instance, muscle spindles encode changes in muscle length, and retinal or auditory signals encode target motion. Moreover, motor planning requires the ability to predict the limb motion resulting from the application of a given torque. Prediction is straightforward only for a limited class of movements, those restricted to a single joint; in such cases, angular acceleration is simply proportional to joint torque. However, this simple relation does not hold for movements involving multijointed coordination.

Multijointed control. Consider the case of arm movements involving shoulder and elbow rotations. The activation of an elbow flexor will always contribute a flexor torque at the elbow, but the resulting elbow movement can be flexion, extension, or no motion at all, depending on the actively produced torque at the shoulder. In general, the relation between joint torque and angular acceleration of each limb segment depends in a complex manner on limb inertia, angular velocity, and limb geometrical configuration (Soechting and Flanders, 2002; see GEOMETRICAL PRINCIPLES IN MOTOR CONTROL). Limb geometry, in turn, affects limb inertia and determines the gravitational loads that need to be opposed. Because limb inertia, geometry, and velocity may all vary during a movement, the central nervous system (CNS) should be able to estimate each of these parameters by means of feedback or feedforward, to predict the motion resulting from the application of a given torque. However, the time delays in position and velocity feedback and the uncertainties in the estimate of the starting position of the limb may prevent accurate estimates.

Kinematic and kinetic variables. Although in principle, a coordinated motor action could be planned muscle by muscle, a more parsimonious solution is to plan more global goals at higher levels of organization and let the lower-level controllers specify the implementation details. Global goals often encompass both kinematics and kinetics. Thus, reaching or walking require the specification of the spatial location and contact force of the respective end point (hand or foot). According to hierarchical control, kinematic and kinetic plans could be fed as inputs to limb controllers; the latter would transform these plans into the appropriate motor commands. A kinematic plan could involve the mere specification of target position, and therefore of the limb end point that matches the target. In addition, however, the plan could include a specification of the path and law of motion of the end point from start to target. Kinematic transformations (inverse kinematics) convert the desired end-point trajectory into the angular motion of each limb segment. Dynamic transformations (inverse dynamics) convert limb motion into the appropriate commands to generate muscle forces and torques. A kinetic plan could involve the specification of the force field at the end point (see MOTOR PRIMITIVES), or it could specify directly the arm and muscle dynamics (Nakano et al., 1999).

Implementation problems. Despite the apparent simplicity of this cascade of events, their actual implementation can be very demanding from a computational standpoint and can result in substantial errors. In a redundant limb, such as the arm or leg, that involves many more degrees of freedom at the level of muscles and joints than at the end point, inverse transformations generally are ill defined. Unique solutions can be imposed by introducing kinematic and/or kinetic constraints, or by using optimization principles. In the following sections we briefly review some issues related to the kinematic aspects of limb geometry control for arm movements and for posture and gait.

Arm Movements

Sensorimotor Transformations for Reaching to a Target

End-point specification. To reach a visual target requires transforming information about target location into commands that specify the patterns of muscle activity that bring the hand to the target. Psychophysical evidence suggests that the specification of the final position of the hand depends on a cascade of sensorimotor transformations that remaps target location from the initial two-dimensional (2D) retinal frame of reference to a three-dimensional (3D) binocular viewer-centered frame to arm- and hand-centered frames (Flanders, Helms Tillery, and Soechting, 1992; Gordon, Ghilardi, and Ghez, 1994; McIntyre et al., 2000; see also EYE-HAND COORDINATION IN REACHING MOVEMENTS). Remapping depends on the combination of retinal and extraretinal signals with somatic signals to update target and end-point spatial representations as the eyes, head, trunk, or limb move. Exactly how this remapping occurs is a matter of controversy, but an emerging view is that the frame of reference used to specify the end point may be task and context dependent. Moreover, different spatial dimensions of the end point (e.g., direction and distance) are not treated in a unitary manner but are processed in parallel and largely independently of each other, according to principles of modular organization (see Georgopoulos, 1991; Gordon et al., 1994).

Egocentric frames. The spatial patterns of hand errors have been studied extensively in pointing to actual or remembered targets that are presented visually or proprioceptively, the movements being performed with or without visual guidance (Baud-Bovy and Viviani, 1997; Flanders et al., 1992; Gordon et al., 1994; McIntyre et al., 2000). Constant and variable errors may reveal the presence of bias and random noise, respectively, in internal representations of the end point, whereas local distortions may reveal transformations between different frames of reference (McIntyre et al., 2000). Thus, in pointing to a continuously visible virtual target, the presence of radial noise and contraction of distance along the sightline indicates the representation of the target and limb end point in a 3D binocular viewer-centered frame, the anisotropy resulting from fusion of eye position signals with retinal disparity signals and from a coupling of uncompensated eye movements. When vision of the hand is prevented, head- and shoulder-centered distortions characterize end-point distribution and denote the transformation of information into the corresponding frames. The increase in head/shoulder-centered local contraction for increasing delays (up to 8 s) for movements performed toward previously visible then memorized targets indicates that memory storage of the intended end point is held within these frames, with separate storage of distance and direction, the distance information decaying faster than the directional information. Additional variability along the movement direction suggests that target information is combined with hand information to form a hand-centered vectorial plan of the intended movement trajectory as an extent and direction relative to the starting hand position (Gordon et al., 1994). Extent and direction also adapt differentially during motor learning (Krakauer et al., 2000). By contrast, when targets are presented kinesthetically instead of visually, subjects underestimate the perceived target distance relative to the shoulder (Baud-Bovy and Viviani, 1997).

Allocentric frames. The evidence reviewed so far indicates that, when targets are immersed in an otherwise neutral space, end-point position is specified in egocentric frames of reference, that is, relative to some body parts (eyes, head, or arm). However, when targets are embedded in a geometrically structured space, the visual or cognitive context can shape pointing errors and reveal the use of allocentric reference frames to represent end-point position. Thus, the final position of a pointing movement toward a remembered target is biased by the position of a surrounding frame (Bridgeman, Peery, and Anand, 1997; see DISSOCIATIONS BETWEEN DIFFERENT VISUAL PROCESSING MODES).

Limb Kinematics

Kinematic regularities. A different issue is whether kinematic plans also include a specification of the path and law of motion of the limb. Moreover, is limb kinematics planned at the level of the end point or at the level of joint and limb segments? There is no consensus on these issues. A number of lawful relationships have been described for the kinematic trajectories of the hand in external space and of individual limb segments in the angular coordinates of the joints. Thus, the spatial trajectories of both the hand and the joints are essentially unaffected by wide changes in speed and load. In point-to-point movements the velocity profile of the hand tends to be bell-shaped, while the velocity profiles of shoulder and elbow angular motions tend to be temporally correlated. In curved movements (such as those of drawing and handwriting), the instantaneous tangential velocity of the hand is inversely related (by a power law) to the local curvature of the path (Lacquaniti, 1997).

Optimum principles.   Although these kinematic regularities are compatible with the existence of a kinematic plan, they do not prove it. Nevertheless, kinematic optimization principles are able to predict the time course of reaching and drawing (see OPTIMIZATION PRINCIPLES IN MOTOR CONTROL). Optimization may involve end-point trajectory or joint angular trajectories. The minimum jerk principle, for instance, constrains hand reaching to follow a maximally smooth time course. Superposition of smooth harmonic oscillations of joint angular motion predicts the power law for drawing.

Kinematic regularities could also result from optimizing kinetic criteria instead of kinematic ones. Nakano et al. (1999) have been able to account for a variety of reaching trajectories by assuming that the commanded change in torque is minimized. In a similar vein, Soechting and Flanders (2002) showed that for reaching to a given target starting from different locations, the final posture of the arm minimizes the amount of work that must be done to transport the arm from start to end.

Planning Dynamic Interactions

In interceptive tasks, such as catching, information about the relative motion between limbs and objects must be preprocessed in order to plan the dynamic interaction in advance of its occurrence. Time, location, and momentum of the impact need be accurately estimated, and limb kinematics and kinetics controlled accordingly. A priori knowledge of the most likely path and law of motion of the object is used in conjunction with visual on-line information. Thus, catching movements are time-locked to time-to-contact computed by combining optic flow information with an internal estimate of the acceleration of gravity (Lacquaniti, 1997). Also, the compliant relation between hand and object appears to be internally modeled by the CNS, resulting in prospective tuning of limb geometry and compliance. This control scheme is adaptive: the response to the dynamic interaction predicted by the internal model is compared with the actual response of the limb (as monitored by kinesthetic and cutaneous signals), and the resulting error is used to calibrate the parameters of the neural controller and to update the internal model.

Processes of trajectory formation have also been shown to undergo adaptive changes in response to novel force fields experienced at the hand; adaptation is based on the progressive changes of the internal models of limb dynamics, initially defined in the intrinsic coordinates of the joints and muscles. Proprioceptive information is essential to maintain internal models (Ghez, Gardon, and Ghilardi, 1995). Indeed, deafferented (as a result of large-fiber neuropathies) subjects are unable to compensate for workspace anisotropies in limb inertia and produce pointing errors that are direction dependent.

Neural correlates

Positional and directional codes.   Electrophysiological recordings from single neurons in frontal and parietal cortical areas have been related to kinematic parameters of reaching in different frames of reference (see MOTOR CORTEX: CODING AND DECODING OF DIRECTIONAL OPERATIONS; REACHING MOVEMENTS: IMPLICATIONS FOR COMPUTATIONAL MODELS). In general, many neurons are broadly tuned to both the target location and the direction of the hand movement (Georgopoulos, 1991). Target location and movement direction can be defined in eye-centered or arm-centered coordinates, depending on the cerebral area and the task (Batista et al., 1999). The combination of retinal, eye-, and hand-related signals occurs at early stages of cortical processing, as revealed by the activity pattern of parieto-occipital neurons (Battaglia-Mayer et al., 2001). Directional signals of many such neurons for hand reaching are spatially congruent with those for eye saccades. These activity patterns are modulated by context (presence or absence of visual feedback of hand movement, memory delay), in agreement with the psychophysical data reported above.

Velocity codes.   The time-varying changes in length and direction of the population vectors in M1 parallel the corresponding changes in the vector of tangential velocity in reaching and drawing. In drawing, the virtual changes in movement velocity predicted by the population vectors are related to path curvature by the same power law that applies to actual movement velocity.

Kinematics or kinetics?   Neural codes of limb kinematics can occur independently of limb kinetics, or there may be an interaction. Thus, when the same movement is performed in the presence of different loads pulling the arm in different directions, some neurons are very sensitive to the applied load and appear to encode parameters related to movement kinetics, whereas other neurons are relatively insensitive to loads and appear to encode movement kinematics, and still other neurons fall in between, exhibiting both kinematic and kinetic tuning.

Limb geometry configuration.   Another possible interaction is between the movement direction and the geometrical configuration of the limb and the participating muscles. Thus, the directional tuning of wrist muscles for flexion/extension and abduction/adduction depends on forearm pronation/supination. Directional tuning of some motor cortical neurons changes in parallel with the changes in directional tuning of the muscles (compatible with a kinetic code), whereas the tuning of other neurons changes in parallel with changes in posture (compatible with a kinematic code of limb geometrical configuration), and the tuning of still other neurons is not affected (compatible with a kinematic code of abstract movement direction independent of limb configuration and muscle activity; Kakei, Hoffman, and Strick, 1999).

Posture

Control of Limb Geometry in Posture

Postural control is often equated with stabilization of the body against gravity, i.e., a kinetic control problem. In fact there is now ample evidence that limb geometry can be controlled largely independent of the ground contact forces. Thus, when cats standing on a platform are pitched by variable angles, the resulting distribution of ground contact forces and joint torques is idiosyncratic to each animal and condition, whereas the geometry of both forelimbs and hindlimbs is much more stereotyped (Lacquaniti, 1997). The length and the angle of orientation of the limb axis relative to the vertical change little despite wide changes in platform tilt. Limb geometry is also preserved unmodified after the application of external loads, at the expense of marked changes in the distribution of weight and effort between forelimbs and hindlimbs. The CNS controls postural geometry directly rather than balance (distribution of contact forces), presumably because it has learned that the preferred posture is stable under normal operating conditions. On the other hand, not only has posture largely evolved to oppose gravity for the maintenance of balance, it is also organized in a reference frame that is anchored to the direction of gravity. As was noted earlier, limb orientation is controlled relative to the vertical.

Modular Organization.

In contrast to limb orientation, limb length is not significantly affected by tilt of the visual surround or by application of abnormal somesthetic stimuli. This and the differential dynamic behavior of the changes in limb length and orientation in response to dynamic pitch suggest that these two geometrical variables might be controlled independently of each other. This modular organization is reminiscent of that reported above for the control of direction and distance in arm reaching. Note further that limb length and orientation are encoded independently in the responses of dorsal spinocerebellar neurons to applied changes in lower-limb posture in the anesthetized cat spinal cord (Poppele, Bosco, and Rankin, 2002).

Coordinate Transformations for the Control of Posture

Length and orientation specify the position of the foot relative to the hip in a global manner, leaving the detailed geometrical configuration undetermined. There is an additional processing stage that transforms limb length and orientation into the angular coordinates of the joints (Lacquaniti, 1997). The changes of these angles under both static and dynamic conditions are not independent, but covary close to one plane. The orientation of this plane is essentially the same in all animals (despite wide differences in their biomechanical parameters), and is also the same at the forelimbs and at the hindlimbs. The latter invariance is especially remarkable, considering that the forelimbs differ considerably from the hindlimbs in terms of the length and orientation of the individual corresponding segments. A related planar covariation has also been found in the case of whole-body motion in man (postural responses to external perturbations and anticipatory responses prior to voluntary trunk axial bending). Moreover, these kinematic strategies remain unchanged under microgravity, that is, in the absence of equilibrium constraints.

Neural Network Implementation of Coordinate Transformation

How might a nervous system learn to map limb length and orientation into joint angles? A forward model of the controlled system could be learned by monitoring both the input and the output of the system. The forward model would map the expected relationship between the set of joint angles and the resulting end-point position. This forward model would not need to be learned in its most general and exact manner by the postural system. In fact, although the forward mapping from joint angles to limb length and orientation is generally nonlinear, we find that the latter two parameters can be estimated simply and accurately using linear compounds of the joint angles, at least within the range of postures normally adopted. After the forward model has been learned, the desired movement trajectory (sequence of end-point positions) could be fed to the inverse model to derive the feedforward motor command (sequence of joint angles). The resulting error in end-point position is propagated through the forward model to derive the corresponding error in the motor command space (joint angle space). The latter error represents the signal to train the inverse model. Parameterized constraints, such as the planar constraint on the joint angles for the postural control, could be incorporated into

the learning procedure, and could thereby bias the choice of a particular inverse function.

Locomotion

Kinematic Coordination

A law of planar covariation also applies to the changes of elevation angles of lower limb segments during locomotion (Lacquaniti, Grasso, and Zago, 1999). The fact that similar laws of intersegmental coordination apply to the control of posture and locomotion is functionally significant, inasmuch as locomotion must ensure a forward progression compatible with dynamic equilibrium, adapting to potentially destabilizing factors (e.g., changes in body posture or load, uneven terrain, obstacles) in an anticipatory fashion by means of coordinated synergies of the whole body (see LOCOMOTION, VERTEBRATE).

In walking, the patterns of limb segment angular motion are remarkably simple and consistent. Each segment of the lower limbs oscillates forward and backward, with a waveform that mainly differs in timing and amplitude among different segments. The temporal changes of the elevation angles of lower limb segments do not evolve independently of each other, but they are tightly coupled. When the elevation angles are plotted one versus the others, they describe regular loops constrained close to a plane, common to both stance and swing phases. The specific orientation of the plane of angular covariation reflects the phase relationships between the elevation angles of the lower limb segments, and therefore the timing of the intersegmental coordination. Because the degrees of freedom of limb angular motion in the sagittal plane are reduced to two by the planar constraint, they match the corresponding degrees of freedom of linear motion of the center of body mass (CM).

Relation to Energy Expenditure

Saving the mechanical energy of the body during walking depends to a large extent on the exchange between the forward kinetic energy and the gravitational potential energy of CM. The selection of the elevation angles of each limb segment with respect to the direction of gravity and that of forward progression as the controlled variables may help predict the energetic consequences of the desired kinematics. Moreover, the planar covariation of the elevation angles is instrumental in reducing the degrees of freedom of limb motion to those of CM, where most mechanical energy is expended in walking. There is an additional, important mechanism embedded in the law of kinematic coordination that contributes to the control of mechanical energy expenditure. The net mechanical power tends to increase rapidly with speed, because the changes in potential energy are roughly independent of speed, whereas the changes in kinetic energy increase with speed, and therefore less and less energy is conserved by means of the energy exchange. However, there is a compensatory mechanism that reduces the oscillations of CM. The phase coupling between the instantaneous changes of the elevation angles of the limb segments shifts systematically with increasing speed both in humans and in cats. In humans, it has been shown that the phase shift translates into a reduction in the increment of the net mechanical power with increasing speed. This mechanism is not equally developed in all human subjects, however. Trained subjects generally exhibit a more pronounced phase shift with increasing speed than untrained subjects. Accordingly, the mechanical power output at intermediate and high speeds is significantly lower in the former than in the latter subjects.

Interaction Between Posture and Locomotion

Human erect locomotion is unique among living primates. Evolution selected specific biomechanical features that make human locomotion mechanically efficient. These features are matched by the motor patterns generated in the CNS. But what happens when humans walk stooped (as it happens in a low tunnel)? Are normal motor patterns of erect locomotion maintained, or are locomotor patterns completely reorganized? Walking has been compared in bent postures, either knee-flexed or knee- and trunk-flexed. These postures imply large differences in the position of the CM compared with its position in the standard erect posture: the CM is displaced downward and forward (outside the body), and its oscillations are reduced because the legs cannot fully extend. Thus, the exchange of kinetic and potential energy is much more limited than usual.

In bent posture, ground reaction forces differ prominently from those of erect posture, displaying characteristics intermediate between those typical of walking and those of running. Amplitudes and waveforms of the muscle activities also are deeply affected by the adopted posture. By contrast, the waveforms of the elevation angles along the gait cycle remain essentially unchanged, irrespective of the adopted postures. Thigh, shank, and foot angles covary close to a plane in all conditions, but the plane orientation is systematically different in bent versus erect locomotion. This is explained by the changes in the temporal coupling (phase shift) among the three segments.

An integrated control of gait and posture is made possible because these two motor functions share some common principles of spatial organization. Thus, the kinematic reference frame seems to be anchored to the vertical for both postural responses and locomotion. Also, the planar law of intersegmental kinematic coordination applies to both tasks.

Adaptation to Changes in Body Load

Body weight unloading is compatible with accurate control of limb kinematics in human locomotion. Changing the amount of body weight support (BWS) between 0% and 95% while subjects walk results in drastic changes in kinetic parameters but in limited changes in kinematic coordination. In particular, the peak vertical contact forces decrease proportionally to BWS; at 95% BWS they are 20-fold smaller than at 0% and are applied at the forefoot only. Also, there are considerable changes in the amplitude of EMG activity of most lower limb muscles and a complex reorganization of the pattern of activity of limb muscles. By contrast, the corresponding variation in the parameters that describe shape and variability of the foot path is very limited, always less than 30% of the corresponding values at 0% BWS. Moreover, the planar covariation of the elevation angles is obeyed at all speed and BWS values. At 100% BWS, subjects step in the air, their feet oscillating back and forth just above the treadmill but never contacting it. In this case, step-to-step variability of foot path is much greater than at all other BWS levels, but it is restored to lower values when minimal surrogate contact forces are provided during the "stance" phase. Thus, the detection of minimal contact forces is sufficient for accurate limb trajectory control.

Reversal of Walking Direction

Reversal of walking direction from forward to backward is a key test for studying locomotor patterns. According to the influential scheme put forth by Grillner, backward walking could be produced by switching the sign of the phase coupling among unit oscillators (see MOTOR PATTERN GENERATION). As a result, the controlled output patterns would simply be the time-reversed copy of those of forward gait. If we consider the patterns of muscle activities, there is no way we can superimpose those of backward gait onto those of forward gait, irrespective of whether the waveforms are plotted in normal forward time or reversed in time (Lacquaniti et al., 1999). This is perhaps not so surprising given that the mechanical requirements of backward walking are very different from those of forward walking. Stance is characterized by an inverted plantigrade-digitigrade sequence in the two movement directions. Forward stance begins with heel contact and ends with toe-off. Backward stance begins with toe contact and ends with heel-off. The anatomical and functional asymmetry of foot and leg muscles along the anteroposterior axis also imposes different biomechanical constraints on forward and backward gait. Forward thrust is mainly provided by ankle plantar flexors, whereas the backward thrust is provided by hip and knee extensors.

However, the time-reversed waveforms of backward gait are almost perfectly superimposable onto those of forward gait (Lacquaniti et al., 1999). Accordingly, the planar covariation is the same; the loop is simply traversed in the opposite direction, owing to a switching of the thigh-shank phase. Thus, kinematic patterns follow Grillner's predictions of a phase switch among unit oscillators. It appears as though the same kinematic templates can be output by CPGs in either direct or time-reversed form (like a motor tape), depending on the direction (forward or backward) of gait.

Mechanisms for Kinematic Coordination in Locomotion

The planar law of intersegmental coordination may emerge from the coupling of neural oscillators between each other and with limb mechanical oscillators. Muscle contraction intervenes at variable times to reexcite the intrinsic oscillations of the system when energy is lost. The hypothesis that a law of coordinative control results from a minimal active tuning of the passive inertial and viscoelastic coupling among limb segments is congruent with the idea that movement has evolved according to minimum energy criteria.

It is known that multisegment motion of mammals locomotion is controlled by a network of coupled oscillators (CPGs; see HALF-CENTER OSCILLATORS UNDERLYING RHYTHMIC MOVEMENTS). Flexible combinations of unit oscillators give rise to different forms of locomotion. Interoscillator coupling can be modified by changing the synaptic strength (or polarity) of the relative spinal connections. As a result, unit oscillators can be coupled in phase, out of phase, or with a variable phase, giving rise to different behaviors, such as speed increments or reversal of gait direction (from forward to backward). Supraspinal centers may drive or modulate functional sets of coordinating interneurons to generate different walking modes (or gaits).

Although it is often assumed that CPGs control patterns of muscle activity, an equally plausible hypothesis is that they control patterns of limb segment motion instead. According to this kinematic view, each unit oscillator would directly control a limb segment, alternately generating forward and backward oscillations of the segment. Intersegmental coordination would be achieved by coupling unit oscillators with a variable phase. Intersegmental kinematic phase plays the role of global control variable previously postulated for the network of central oscillators. In fact, intersegmental phase shifts systematically with increasing speed both in humans and in cats. Because this phase shift is correlated with the net mechanical power output over a gait cycle, phase control could be used for limiting the overall energy expenditure with increasing speed. Adaptation to different walking conditions, such as changes in body posture, body weight unloading, and backward walking, also involves intersegmental phase tuning, as does the maturation of limb kinematics in toddlers.

Conclusion

There is ample evidence that movement trajectories are controlled for tasks as diverse as arm reaching, drawing, catching, and walking. Also, limb kinematics can be controlled independently of kinetics. Ill-defined inverse transformations from end point to joint coordinates can be solved by introducing kinematic constraints, such as the law of planar intersegmental coordination, or by means of optimization principles (see OPTIMIZATION PRINCIPLES IN MOTOR CONTROL). To simplify, control, and reduce errors, hybrid feedback/feedforward control schemes are presumably used whenever possible (see MOTOR CONTROL, BIOLOGICAL AND THEORETICAL). In addition internal models that map motor commands onto their sensory consequences and vice versa are used to improve estimates and to learn new tasks (see SENSORIMOTOR LEARNING). However, we still do not know how the kinematic control is obtained, and in particular, we ignore whether it arises from explicit trajectory planning or is derived implicitly from implementation of intrinsic neural dynamics.

Road Map: Mammalian Motor Control
Related Reading: Arm and Hand Movement Control; Geometrical Principles in Motor Control; Optimization Principles in Motor Control

References

Batista, A. P., Buneo, C. A., Snyder, L. H., and Andersen, R. A., 1999, Reach plans in eye-centered coordinates, *Science*, 285:257–260.
Battaglia-Mayer, A., Ferraina, S., Genovesio, A., Marconi, B, Squatrito, S., et al., 2001, Eye-hand coordination during reaching: II. An analysis of visuomanual signals in parietal cortex and of their relationship with parieto-frontal association projections, *Cereb. Cortex*, 11:528–544.
Baud-Bovy, G., and Viviani, P., 1997, Pointing to kinesthetic targets in space, *J. Neurosci.*, 18:1528–1545.
Bridgeman, B., Peery, S., and Anand, S., 1997, Interaction of cognitive and sensorimotor maps of visual space, *Percept. Psychophysics*, 59:456–469.
Flanders, M., Helms Tillery, S. I., and Soechting, J. F., 1992, Early stages in a sensorimotor transformation, *Behav. Brain Sci.*, 15:309–362.
Georgopoulos, A. P., 1991, Higher order motor control, *Ann. Rev. Neurosci.*, 14:361–377. ◆
Ghez, C., Gordon, J., and Ghilardi, M. F., 1995, Impairments of reaching movements in patients without proprioception: II. Effects of visual information on accuracy, *J. Neurophysiol.*, 73:361–372.
Gordon, J., Ghilardi, M. F., and Ghez, C., 1994, Accuracy of planar reaching movements: I. Independence of direction and extent variability, *Exp. Brain Res.*, 99:97–111.
Kakei, S., Hoffman, D. S., and Strick, P., 1999, Muscle and movement representations in the primary motor cortex, *Science*, 285:2136–2139.
Krakauer, J. W., Pine, Z. M., Ghilardi, M. F., and Ghez, C., 2000, Learning of visuomotor transformations for vectorial planning or reaching trajectories, *J. Neurosci.*, 20:8916–8924.
Lacquaniti, F., 1997, Frames of reference in sensorimotor coordination, in *Handbook of Neuropsychology* (F. Boller and J. Grafman, Eds.), vol. 11, Amsterdam: Elsevier, pp. 27–64. ◆
Lacquaniti, F., Grasso, R., and Zago, M., 1999, Motor patterns for walking, *News Physiol. Sci.*, 14:168–174.
McIntyre, J., Stratta, F., Droulez, J., and Lacquaniti, F., 2000, Analysis of pointing errors reveals properties of data representations and coordinate transformations within the central nervous system, *Neural Computat.*, 12:2823–2855.
Nakano, E., Imamizu, H., Osu, R., Uno, Y., Gomi, H., Yoshioka, T., and Kawato, M., 1999, Quantitative examinations of internal representations for arm trajectory planning: Minimum commanded torque change model, *J. Neurophysiol.*, 81:2140–2155.
Poppele, R. E., Bosco, G., and Rankin, A. M., 2002, Independent representations of limb axis length and orientation in spinocerebellar response components, *J. Neurophysiol.*, 87:409–422.
Soechting, J. F., and Flanders, M., 2002, Movement regulation, in *Encyclopedia of the Human Brain* (V. S. Ramachandran, Ed.), San Diego: Academic Press. ◆

Localized Versus Distributed Representations

Simon J. Thorpe

Introduction

What happens in the brain when you recognize a familiar stimulus such as your grandmother's face? Most researchers accept that recognition involves activating some sort of internal representation, but there is little agreement about how such representations are physically implemented in neuronal hardware. According to the localist coding view, recognizing an object involves activating neurons tuned to that particular object—an idea often described as "grandmother cell" coding. Alternatively, the presence of a particular object might never be made explicit at the single-cell level. Instead, the final representation of one's grandmother might be distributed across large populations of cells, none responding selectively to grandmothers alone.

Suppose we need to represent four different stimuli—green and red bars that can be either horizontal or vertical. Figure 1 illustrates three options: a local coding scheme using separate units to code each stimulus (Figure 1A), a semilocal scheme with color and orientation encoded separately (two active units are needed to represent each stimulus; Figure 1B), and a distributed coding scheme representing all four stimuli with just three units (Figure 1C). In the last case, someone listening to the response of any individual unit would have difficulty making sense of the activity. Such situations arise both in so-called Hopfield networks (see COMPUTING WITH ATTRACTORS) and in the hidden layer of backpropagation-trained networks that have fewer units than the number of stimuli that need to be represented.

So, what does the brain do? It is likely that the brain uses a range of coding strategies; there are several possibilities. Few neuroscientists have gone so far as to suggest that individual neurons might explicitly represent particular objects, Jerzy Konorski and Horace Barlow being two notable exceptions (Konorski, 1967; Barlow, 1985). Most prefer some form of sparse representation in which a relatively low percentage of active cells represents each object but none is tuned to that particular object (see SPARSE CODING IN THE PRIMATE CORTEX), as in the semilocal scheme illustrated earlier. However, many connectionists have used localist representations to model phenomena that include word and letter perception (see CONNECTIONIST AND SYMBOLIC REPRESENTATIONS) (Grainger and Jacobs, 1998; Page, 2000), and although they generally insist that the units in their models are not real neurons, there is no obvious reason why such models might not map directly to the neural level.

How might we determine the nature of the strategy used by the brain to represent objects? In the first section of this article we examine neurophysiological evidence that both distributed coding and local coding are used in high-order visual areas. In the second section we examine some computational reasons for preferring representations that are more distributed or localist. Finally, we ex-

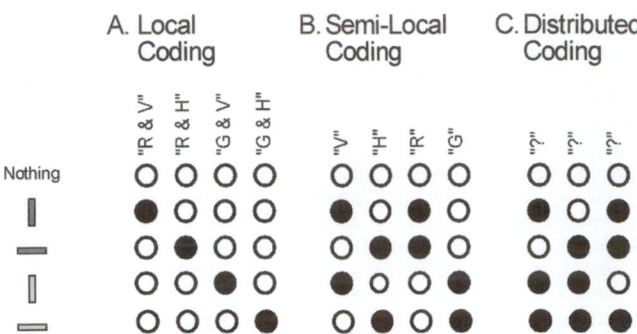

Figure 1. Three ways of representing four stimuli. Filled circles correspond to active units. *A*, Local coding. Each stimulus is explicitly coded by dedicated units. *B*, Semilocal coding. The different features—red (R), green (G), vertical (V), and horizontal (H)—are represented by separate units. *C*, Distributed coding.

amine how work on temporal coding schemes has changed the nature of the local versus distributed debate.

Neurophysiological Evidence

The best way to analyze how neurons represent objects is to record responses to a wide range of stimuli and determine their selectivity. This should be done at the highest levels of the sensory pathways, in areas such as inferotemporal (IT) cortex (see OBJECT RECOGNITION, NEUROPHYSIOLOGY). In the early 1970s, Charles Gross and his colleagues at Princeton described cells in IT with selectivity for complex shapes such as monkey paws. At the time, many scientists read such reports with incredulity, but by the early 1980s, researchers such as Bob Desimone, David Perrett, and Edmund Rolls had started to provide incontrovertible evidence for neurons responding selectively to faces (Perrett, Mistlin, and Chitty, 1987) (see FACE RECOGNITION: NEUROPHYSIOLOGY AND NEURAL TECHNOLOGY). Although most such cells respond to a range of faces, there have been reports of much higher degrees of selectivity. For example, one study described a cell that responded to only one of a set of 27 photographs of Japanese male faces (Young and Yamane, 1992).

Some researchers feel that the high selectivity for faces constitutes a special case, but highly selective responses to a range of visual stimuli have now been found. Nikos Logothetis and coworkers trained monkeys to respond to arbitrary "paper clip" forms from a range of views. Following training, some cells responded only to particular shapes seen from a limited range of viewing angles (Logothetis, Pauls, and Poggio, 1995). Rufin Vogels (1999) studied neuronal responses to photographs of natural objects in monkeys performing a categorization task and found that 17% responded to less than four out of a set of 60 images. And in a study in which 100 different photographs were presented repeatedly to a large number of IT cells, half of the cells responded to seven or less of the stimulus set (Tamura and Tanaka, 2001). Indeed, the most selective cell responded over five times more to the best stimulus (a photograph of a chair) than to the next best one, and showed significant responses to only three of the 100 photographs.

Some of the most intriguing data have come from single-cell recordings in humans undergoing investigation for intractable epilepsy. Such studies have provided tantalizing hints that in humans, too, neurons are remarkably selective to categories of visual stimuli that include faces, natural scenes and houses, famous people, and animals (Kreiman, Koch, and Fried., 2000).

Clearly, at least some IT neurons show strong selectivity. But there is also plenty of evidence for more broadly tuned cells re-

sponding to many different objects, and some authors have argued strongly for distributed coding (Rolls and Deco, 2002). However, the data are also perfectly consistent with a hybrid model using both distributed and local coding. It is important to realize that neuronal selectivity in IT appears strongly experience dependent, the most selective responses being found in monkeys trained with particular sets of stimuli many hours a day for weeks or even months. Furthermore, the response properties of IT cells are plastic: even a few seconds of visual exposure can change selectivity (Tovee, Rolls, and Ramachandran, 1996). It could be that while most cells are relatively broadly tuned, experience might produce small numbers of increasingly specialized cells. Although allowing specialized cells for all possible objects would be impossible, it might not be so unreasonable to devote neural hardware to the relatively small number of objects that are particularly critical. In the next section, we will look at some of the computational reasons why the brain might prefer to opt for more explicit local coding in certain cases.

Computational Pros and Cons

If it is possible to represent objects with a pattern of activity across a large population of cells, why would the brain ever move to more localist representations? After all, distributed codes have certain clear advantages. They allow large numbers of different stimuli to be represented with a relatively small number of units, as in the case of the ASCII code, where seven binary nodes can encode 128 (or 2^7) different characters (a localist version would need 128 nodes). By using relatively broad tuning, distributed coding guarantees some sort of activity pattern even for stimuli never experienced before, and it has been claimed that distributed codes have a greater capacity for generalization and graceful degradation in the event of damage to the system (see Rolls and Deco, 2002).

On the other hand, localist representations also have some computational advantages. For example, efficient learning requires organisms to estimate the relative frequencies of events in the outside world, which in turn requires some sort of counting mechanism. It could be considerably easier to estimate the frequency of events represented with a local code than when the representation is distributed across a large number of neurons (Gardner-Medwin and Barlow, 2001). Imagine trying to estimate the frequency of the character E by examining the frequency of activation of the individual bits of the ASCII code. The problem would be trivial with a neuron that responded every time the letter E was presented.

Localist representations are also largely immune to the classic "binding problem" that results when two or more different objects or events need to be represented simultaneously. All three coding schemes in Figure 1 are fine for representing the four different objects as long as only one object is present at a time, but when both a red vertical bar and a green horizontal bar are present, only the local representation can provide reliable information. For the semilocal code, there is no way to decide which color goes with which orientation, and the fully distributed code would be completely unable to generate a meaningful response.

Interestingly, detecting the presence of red vertical bars in a field composed of green vertical and red horizontal distractors is a difficult and time-consuming task. In contrast, even relatively complex visual forms such as animals can be easy to detect in complex natural scenes (see FAST VISUAL PROCESSING). Why would such high-level objects "pop out" when other, apparently simpler combinations of features pose such problems? One possibility is that only stimuli that are explicitly coded at the single-unit level can be processed in parallel. Our difficulty with certain stimulus conjunctions might stem from the fact that we rarely, if ever, need to use a simple combination of vertical and red to define an object. Perhaps units at the earlier levels of the visual system that would be useful for explicitly coding such combinations are no longer sufficiently plastic in adults to allow such low-level features to be used. In contrast, richer combinations of features of the type that could be encoded in IT cortex might be easier to group together as a result of experience in adults.

The Impact of Temporal Coding

In this final section, we will examine how the debate over local versus distributed representations has been influenced by the development of ideas concerning temporal coding in neural processing. Many earlier discussions of coding schemes were based on the premise that neurons effectively use a firing rate code. For instance, in Barlow's 1972 formulation, firing rate represents the probability that a particular stimulus configuration is present. But the situation changes radically if we introduce the idea that information can also be contained in the temporal pattern of spikes. There is now considerable evidence that synchronization across populations of cells can help bind features together (see SYNCHRONIZATION, BINDING AND EXPECTANCY and DYNAMIC LINK ARCHITECTURE), and this could provide an alternative solution to the binding problem mentioned earlier. With the semilocal coding scheme in Figure 1B, the simultaneous presence of a red vertical bar and a green horizontal bar would cause problems. But synchronization could be used to link the different features together by making the "red" neuron fire synchronously with the "vertical" neuron, and the "green" neuron fire with the "horizontal" neuron. This is a clear case of a distributed representation, because analyzing the firing of the four single cells in isolation would fail to disambiguate the stimuli.

Another particularly clear example of a distributed code is rank-order coding that uses the order in which a population of neurons fire to encode information (Thorpe, Delorme, and Van Rullen, 2001). It uses the fact that the time taken for a neuron to reach threshold and fire a spike depends on the strength of the input: the stronger the input, the shorter the latency (Figure 2A). Under such conditions, the order of activation across a population of neurons can encode the stimulus (Figure 2B). In a sense, this is the ultimate illustration of a distributed code, because listening to each neuron on its own provides no information whatsoever about the stimulus. It is only when the relative ordering across neurons is taken into account that an observer can derive information about the stimulus.

Interestingly, decoding order-related information can be done quite simply using a biologically plausible circuit involving feedforward excitatory synapses coupled with shunting inhibition. In one step, it is possible to go from a representation of the input pattern that is fully distributed to one in which the information is made explicit in the firing of a single cell. The power of the coding scheme is illustrated by recent results showing that simple feedforward architectures based on these principles can produce outputs that are effectively grandmother cells, responding to different views of only one particular face (Delorme and Thorpe, 2001). This demonstrates that switching from a fully distributed to a local representation can be done efficiently and with limited hardware.

Discussion

The suggestion that our brains might contain "grandmother cells" is a very controversial one, but it is a suggestion that should not be rejected without good reason. In recent years, neurophysiological evidence for highly selective neurons has become increasingly difficult to ignore. Furthermore, several computational arguments make local coding attractive in certain situations. But it is also clear that it would be impracticable to use local coding to represent all objects. Common sense would seem to favor hybrid systems with both distributed and local representations, thus allowing the best

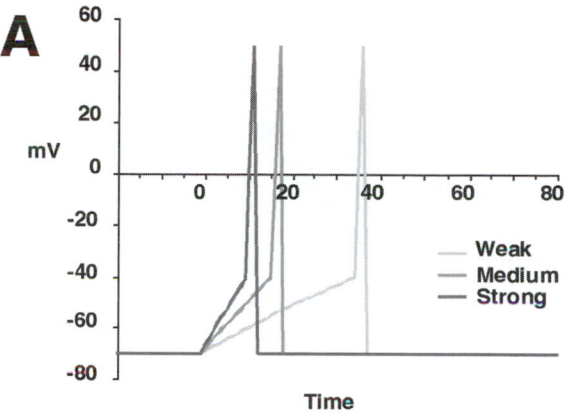

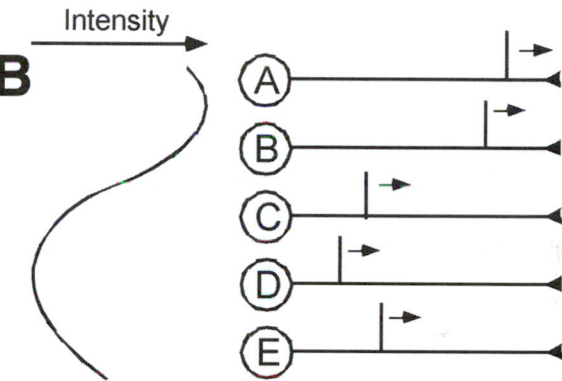

Figure 2. *A* distributed representation based on rank-order coding. *A,* Spike latency varies with the intensity of the input. *B,* With several units, the order of firing (in this case A > B > E > C > D) provides information about the input pattern.

of both worlds. Indeed, even if neurons at the top end of the visual system do explicitly code the presence of particular objects and stimuli, representations of these objects earlier in the system have to be distributed.

The fact that selective neurons are typically found in animals following extensive training suggests that the move toward more explicit, local representations is experience dependent. It might be that high-capacity sparse distributed representations are often sufficient; it may be worth dedicating neurons to the representation of stimuli that are particularly significant. Such local coding could increase reliability and allow such stimuli to be detected in parallel without the need for time-consuming attention-based search.

Road Map: Neural Coding
Related Reading: Connectionist and Symbolic Representations; Feature Analysis; Object Recognition, Neurophysiology; Sparse Coding in the Primate Cortex

References

Barlow, H. B., 1985, The Twelfth Bartlett Memorial Lecture: The role of single neurons in the psychology of perception, *Q. J. Exp. Psychol. A,* 37:121–145
Delorme, A., and Thorpe, S. J., 2001, Face identification using one spike

per neuron: Resistance to image degradations, *Neural Netw.*, 14:795–803.

Gardner-Medwin, A. R., and Barlow, H. B., 2001, The limits of counting accuracy in distributed neural representations, *Neural Computat.*, 13:477–504.

Grainger, J., and Jacobs, A. M., 1998, *Localist Connectionist Approaches to Human Cognition*, Mahwah, NJ: Erlbaum.

Konorski, J., 1967, *Integrative Activity of the Brain: An Interdisciplinary Approach*, Chicago: University of Chicago Press.

Kreiman, G., Koch, C., and Fried, I., 2000, Category-specific visual responses of single neurons in the human medial temporal lobe, *Nature Neurosci.*, 3:946–953.

Logothetis, N. K., Pauls, J., and Poggio, T., 1995, Shape representation in the inferior temporal cortex of monkeys, *Curr. Biol.*, 5:552–563.

Page, M., 2000, Connectionist modelling in psychology: A localist manifesto, *Behav. Brain Sci.*, 23:443.

Perrett, D. I., Mistlin, A. J., and Chitty, A. J., 1987, Visual neurons responsive to faces, *Trends Neurosci.*, 10:358–364.

Rolls, E. T., and Deco, G., 2002, *Computational Neuroscience of Vision*, Oxford: Oxford University Press.

Tamura, H., and Tanaka, K., 2001, Visual response properties of cells in the ventral and dorsal parts of the macaque inferotemporal cortex, *Cereb. Cortex*, 11:384–399.

Thorpe, S., Delorme, A., and Van Rullen, R., 2001, Spike-based strategies for rapid processing, *Neural Netw.*, 14:715–725.

Tovee, M. J., Rolls, E. T., and Ramachandran, V. S., 1996, Rapid visual learning in neurones of the primate temporal visual cortex, *Neuroreport*, 7:2757–2760.

Vogels, R., 1999, Categorization of complex visual images by rhesus monkeys: Part 2. Single-cell study, *Eur. J. Neurosci.*, 11:1239–1255.

Young, M. P., and Yamane, S., 1992, Sparse population coding of faces in the inferotemporal cortex, *Science*, 256:1327–1331.

Locomotion, Invertebrate

Randall D. Beer and Hillel J. Chiel

Introduction

Locomotion can be defined as an animal's ability to move its body along a desired path, making it fundamental to many other animal behaviors (Dickinson et al., 2000). Given the diversity of ecological niches that animals inhabit, and the variety of body plans that they possess, it is not surprising that their modes of locomotion are equally diverse. Types of locomotion include walking, swimming, flying, crawling, and burrowing.

Despite this diversity, certain common principles can be discerned. All locomotion systems must solve the twin problems of *support* and *progression*. The problem of support arises because in many modes of locomotion (e.g., flight), the gravitational attraction of the earth must be overcome. The problem of progression arises because an animal must generate propulsive forces that overcome not only its body's inertia, but also any drag from the density and viscosity of the medium or the friction of the substrate.

Both support and progression involve the generation of forces. This is accomplished by the contraction of muscles attached to either flexible hydrostatic skeletons or rigid skeletons. In addition, many animals have specialized body structures and appendages that facilitate locomotion, such as fins, wings, and legs. Thus, the detailed design of an animal's body is a crucial component of its locomotion system. As a result of the nature of these specializations, the problems of support and progression are rarely independent. Wings, for example, are used to generate both lift and propulsion in flying animals.

In order to provide support and progression, the movements of these specialized body structures must be coordinated by an animal's nervous system. The diverse modes of locomotion and the variety of body plans lead to equally diverse neural circuitry mediating locomotion. However, once again, certain basic principles can be discerned. Underlying many forms of locomotion are basic oscillatory patterns of movement generated by neural circuits that are referred to as *motor pattern generators* (MOTOR PATTERN GENERATION). Even when these circuits contain dedicated neurons that autonomously produce rhythmic outputs (so-called *central pattern generators*), this central pattern is often strongly shaped by sensory feedback, fundamentally involving the body and environment in the generation of a locomotor pattern. In fact, sensory feedback can play such a fundamental role that it sometimes makes no sense to speak of a distinct central pattern generator.

Researchers have begun to use computer modeling to understand the neural basis of locomotion. In contrast to most work in computational neuroscience, models of animal bodies are playing an important role in understanding locomotion systems. Increasingly, experimental evidence suggests that motor systems cannot be fully understood without considering the biomechanical properties of the bodies in which they are embedded (Chiel and Beer, 1997). Modeling of both an animal's body and the neural circuitry underlying its behavior has been termed *computational neuroethology* (NEUROETHOLOGY, COMPUTATIONAL). This chapter will focus on invertebrate locomotion systems for which quantitative modeling has been done, reviewing computer models of swimming, flying, crawling, and walking.

Swimming

In swimming, support is less of a problem than it is in other modes of locomotion. However, unless an animal is neutrally buoyant, it must still make efforts to keep from either sinking or rising. Progression requires much more effort as a result of the drag from water's density and viscosity. Thus, the bodies of swimming animals are streamlined. Swimming invertebrates utilize one of two mechanisms, either hydraulic propulsion or rhythmic undulations of the body.

Although models of swimming in leeches, mollusks, and nematodes have been constructed (Pearce and Friesen, 1988; Niebur and Erdös, 1991), perhaps the most modeled swimming system is not that of an invertebrate but that of a primitive vertebrate known as the lamprey. Lampreys swim using coordinated contractions of muscles on each side of the body. These contractions produce a traveling wave along the body, with a wavelength of approximately one body length across a wide range of swimming speeds. Although the lamprey possesses much of the basic vertebrate neural architecture, the experimental accessibility of its nervous system has allowed a level of neurophysiological analysis that is more typically applied to invertebrate systems. Earlier work used mathematical analysis and simulation of chains of model oscillators to study intersegmental coordination in the lamprey spinal cord (SPINAL CORD OF LAMPREY: GENERATION OF LOCOMOTOR PATTERNS; CHAINS OF OSCILLATORS IN MOTOR AND SENSORY SYSTEMS). Recent work has focused on more realistic models of the underlying neuronal circuit and models of the relevant mechanics of the lamprey body and the water through which it swims.

Ekeberg and Grillner (1999) have reviewed much of the recent work in this area. The rhythm-generation circuit consists of populations of motor neurons, excitatory interneurons, and two distinct types of inhibitory interneurons repeated in each segment. Models of this circuitry have demonstrated that oscillations are relatively easy to generate, but details of the pattern (e.g., burst termination) depend on biophysical details of the nerve cells. The generation and propagation of the traveling wave along the segments has been studied by coupling chains of model segmental oscillators. This work revealed that if the rostral segments receive stronger excitation, they become the source of the traveling wave, and variation of this extra excitation allows the spatial wavelength of the swimming pattern to be controlled separately from its temporal frequency.

Mechanical aspects of swimming have been investigated by coupling pattern-generation circuitry to a segmented body model actuated by linear viscoelastic model muscles and embedded in a model of the static drag force produced by the surrounding water. By varying the level and asymmetry of tonic input, this neuromechanical model could produce swims at a range of speeds, turns, and rolls. In addition, two kinds of sensory feedback have been modeled. Incorporating feedback from intraspinal stretch receptors led to improved robustness of the swim pattern against unpredictable changes in water flow. Feedback from vestibular receptors was incorporated in order to model roll and pitch stabilization.

Flying

In many ways, flying is similar to swimming. However, because of the much lower density of air, considerably faster motions are required for powered flight than for swimming. While quasi-steady-state aerodynamic analyses of the sort used to understand aircraft have been successfully applied to larger animals, they have not been very successful for small flying insects. According to steady-state theory, many insects should be unable to generate sufficient lift to hold themselves aloft!

A recent model by Dickinson and colleagues has begun to shed considerable light on insect flight (Dickinson, Lehmann, and Sane, 1999). Because of the delicate size and high speed of insect wings, direct measurement of the forces involved is extremely difficult. For this reason, a robotic model was used to explore unsteady flows during hovering by the fruit fly *Drosophila melanogaster*. The model was submerged in mineral oil and scaled both in space and time so as to reproduce the Reynolds number (ratio of inertial to viscous forces) relevant to small insects flying in air. Dickinson and colleagues found that three major mechanisms contributed to lift generation in the model. First, vortices formed at the leading edge of the wing produce lift during much of the power stroke. Second, additional lift is produced by circulation of air around the wings resulting from rapid rotation at the beginning and end of each stroke. Third, further forces are produced at the start of each upstroke and downstroke as a result of collisions of the wings with the swirling wake produced by the previous stroke, a mechanism termed *wake capture*. Because of the sensitivity of the latter two mechanisms to the timing of wing rotation, the model suggests that the control of small details of wing motion can used in steering flight.

Crawling

In crawling, locomotion occurs along the bottom surface of an aquatic environment or the surface of the earth via rhythmic contact between the body and the substrate. Invertebrates generate propulsive forces for crawling by changing body shape in one of three

ways: contract-anchor-extend (as in the leech), pedal locomotion (as in molluscs), or peristaltic locomotion (as in earthworms). Crawling invertebrates typically utilize either hydrostatic skeletons or muscular hydrostatic structures to accomplish these movements.

A detailed neuromechanical model of crawling in the leech has been constructed by Kristan et al. (2000). This model assumes that the cross-sectional geometry of each body segment is elliptical, that the volume of body segments remains constant during movement, and that the animal's shape minimizes total potential energy. Kristan et al.'s simulations incorporate relatively realistic models of the circular and longitudinal muscles found in the leech body wall. Driving the model body with activation patterns deduced from the kinematics of intact animals produces crawling movements that are considerably more realistic than those produced by activation patterns derived from reduced preparations. These results suggest that sensory feedback plays a critical role in providing appropriate timing of activation of longitudinal and circular muscles.

Walking

In legged animals, the body is raised above the ground and propelled by a sequence of leg movements. During walking, each leg cycles between a *stance phase*, in which the leg is providing support and propulsion, and a *swing phase*, in which the leg is off the ground and swinging forward. Swing phase duration is often nearly constant, while stance phase duration varies considerably with the speed of progression. Because the legs provide both support and propulsion and must be lifted after each stance, their movements must be coordinated so that the center of mass of the body remains within a polygon of support formed by the stancing legs (static stability). Otherwise, the animal must dynamically stabilize its body. Another coordination problem arises because adjacent legs must not interfere with one another. In many-legged animals, avoiding interference between adjacent legs is the crucial coordination problem, whereas the maintenance of stability is more important for animals with fewer legs.

Insect locomotion is remarkably flexible and robust. Insects can walk over a variety of terrains, as well as vertically and upside-down. In addition, they can also adapt their gait to the loss of up to two legs without severe degradation of performance (Delcomyn, Chapter 2 in Beer, Ritzmann, and McKenna, 1993) and sometimes even utilize dynamically stable gaits (Full, Chapter 1 in Beer et al., 1993). Most modeling has focused on statically stable walking across flat, horizontal surfaces. Even under these conditions, insects exhibit different gaits depending on their speed of locomotion.

Slowly walking insects show distinct *metachronal waves* on each side of the body: each leg begins its swing immediately following the termination of the swing of the leg behind it, with a 180° phase relationship between the pair of legs in each segment. Fast-walking insects utilize a *tripod gait*, in which the front and back legs on each side of the body step in unison with the middle leg on the opposite side. In one of the earliest theoretical models of insect walking, Wilson (1966) suggested that the entire range of observed insect gaits could be explained by assuming that fixed, antiphasic metachronal waves on each side of the body increasingly overlap as walking speed increases.

We developed a neural network model based on work by Pearson and colleagues on the neural organization of the American cockroach's walking system (Beer and Chiel, Chapter 12 in Beer et al., 1993). In this model, each leg controller has a pacemaker neuron whose output rhythmically oscillates due to a voltage-dependent intrinsic current. These pacemakers implement the swing burst-generators that Pearson hypothesized. A pacemaker burst initiates a swing by inhibiting the foot and backward swing motor neurons and exciting the forward swing motor neurons, causing the foot to lift and the leg to swing forward. Between bursts, the foot is down and tonic excitation from a command neuron moves the leg backward. Feedback from two sensors that signal when a leg is nearing its extreme forward or backward position fine-tunes pacemaker output. Forward angle sensor inhibition encourages burst termination, whereas backward angle sensor excitation encourages burst initiation. The forward angle sensor also makes direct connections to the motor neurons, modeling leg reflex pathways described by Pearson.

In order to generate statically stable gaits, the swings of the individual legs must be coordinated in some way. Following Pearson, we inserted mutually inhibitory connections between the pacemaker neurons of adjacent legs. We also added an entrainment mechanism for generating metachronal waves: slightly increasing the angle ranges of the rear legs lowers the burst frequency of the rear pacemakers, causing the pattern generators on each side of the body to phase-lock into a stable metachronal relationship.

In simulations of this circuit in a kinematic hexapod body model, a continuous range of statically stable gaits similar to those described by Wilson (1966) were observed. This range of gaits was produced simply by varying the tonic level of excitation of the command neuron. Smooth transitions between gaits could be generated by continuously varying this excitation. We found that the ability of this circuit to generate statically stable gaits was quite robust to lesions. For example, removing any single sensor or interpacemaker connection did not generally disrupt locomotion. These studies also demonstrated that sensory feedback was crucial for the maintenance of the slower metachronal gaits, but was relatively unimportant in the tripod gait.

The stick insect *Carausius morosus* has also been a major focus of legged locomotion research. Cruse (1990) reviewed leg coordination influences in both the stick insect and the crayfish *Astacus leptodactylus*. In the stick insect, there are three major influences: (1) a swinging leg inhibits the swing of a more anterior leg; (2) when a leg begins its stance phase, it excites the swing of a more anterior leg; and (3) as a stancing leg nears the end of its stance, it increasingly excites the swing of a more posterior leg. Some of these influences also operate between pairs of legs in the same segment.

Dean (1991) simulated these and other coordination mechanisms. The pattern generator for each leg was modeled as a relaxation oscillator with two states corresponding to stance and swing. The positions of each of the six legs were the state variables for a kinematic model of walking. The coordination mechanisms modified the position at which an affected leg began its swing, with inhibitory influences producing a posterior shift and excitatory influences producing an anterior shift. Dean's simulations demonstrated that these coordination mechanisms were sufficient to generate a continuous range of gaits, including the wave gait at low stepping frequencies and the tripod gait at high stepping frequencies. The model also exhibited distinct asymmetries in stepping pattern observed in the stick insect, in which the phase relationship between legs in the same segment is consistently lower or higher than 180°. A good review of earlier models of stick insect walking can also be found in Dean (1991).

Dean also explored the robustness of these coordinating mechanisms to various perturbations, including variations in starting configurations, perturbations of individual leg velocities, and obstructions to the swing of individual legs. He found that the gaits generated by these mechanisms were quite robust to such perturbations and that, in most cases, the model's responses were similar to those of the insect. Discrepancies between the model and the insect could be traced to the need for dynamic variables in addition to kinematic ones. Dean varied the strength and form of the coordination mechanisms. He found that influence (3) was the most important to maintaining proper coordination due to its graded nature, though the model was quite robust to substantial variations in the strengths of individual mechanisms.

Biorobotics

The remarkable flexibility and robustness of animal locomotion has intrigued roboticists. Biologically inspired locomotion controllers offer a number of advantages over more classical approaches, including their distributed nature, their robustness, and their computational efficiency. Likewise, robots can serve as an important new modeling methodology for testing biological hypotheses. Thus, a number of researchers have begun to explore the interface between biology and robotics (Beer et al., 1998; Webb, 2000). Raibert and Hodgins (Chapter 14, in Beer et al., 1993) have argued for the importance of leg and actuator design in locomotion, designing a series of dynamically stable hopping and running robots based on the biomechanical design of animal limbs. For example, we implemented both the locomotion circuit and the stick insect coordination mechanisms described previously in hexapod robots and found that they could generate a range of gaits similar to those observed in simulations and were equally robust to perturbations (Beer et al., 1997), and more recent work has successfully incorporated significantly more biological realism into the latest robot (Quinn and Ritzmann, 1998). Thus, models of animal locomotion may not only yield insights into the neural control of motor behavior, but may also have significant technological applications.

Discussion

We have touched on several successful examples of quantitative modeling of locomotion. It is notable that the different simulations utilize very different neural models. More fundamentally, it is striking that very different neural architecture can be utilized to generate locomotion. Undoubtedly, this variety is a result of the diverse body plans of animals and the many different ecological niches that they occupy. One consistent theme that does emerge, however, is the complex interplay of sensory input and central circuitry in the generation of locomotion. This complex interplay is responsible for the adaptive flexibility of animal locomotion.

Road Map: Motor Pattern Generators
Related Reading: Biologically Inspired Robotics; Chains of Oscillation in Motor and Sensory Systems; Half-Center Oscillators Underlying Rhythmic Movements; Locomotion, Vertebrate; Locust Flight: Components and Mechanisms in the Motor; Spinal Cord of Lamprey: Generation of Locomotor Patterns

References

Beer, R. D., Quinn, R. D., Chiel, H. J., and Ritzmann, R. E., 1997, Biologically-inspired approaches to robotics, *Comm. ACM*, 40:31–38.

Beer, R. D., Chiel, H. J., Quinn, R. D., and Ritzmann, R. E., 1998, Biorobotic approaches to the study of motor systems, *Curr. Op. Neuro.*, 8:777–782. ◆

Beer, R. D., Ritzmann, R. E., and McKenna, T., Eds., 1993, Biological neural networks in invertebrate neuroethology and robotics, Academic Press.

Chiel, H. J., and Beer, R. D., 1997, The brain has a body: Adaptive behavior emerges from interactions of nervous system, body and environment, *Trends Neurosci.*, 20:553–557.

Cruse, H., 1990, What mechanisms coordinate leg movement in walking arthropods? *Trends Neurosci.*, 13:15–21.

Dean, J., 1991, A model of leg coordination in the stick insect, *Carausius morosus*. II. Description of the kinematic model and simulation of normal step patterns, *Biol. Cybern.*, 64:393–402.

Dickinson, M. H., Farley, C. T., Full, R. J., Koehl, M. A. R., Kram, R., and Lehman, S., 2000, How animals move: An integrative view, *Science*, 288:100–106. ◆

Dickinson, M. H., Lehmann, F.-O., and Sane, S. P., 1999, Wing rotation and the aerodynamic basis of insect flight, *Science*, 284:1954–1960.

Ekeberg, O., and Grillner, S. 1999, Simulations of neuromuscular control in lamprey swimming, *Phil. Trans. R. Soc. Lond. B*, 354:895–902.

Kristan, W. B., Jr., Skalak, R., Wilson, R. J. A., Skierczynski, B. A., Murray, J. A., Eisenhart, F. J., and Cacciatore, T. W., 2000, Biomechanics of hydroskeletons: Studies of crawling in the medicinal leech, in *Biomechanics and Neural Control of Posture and Movement* (J. M. Winters and P. E. Crago, Eds.), New York: Springer-Verlag, pp. 206–218.

Niebur, E., and Erdös, P., 1991, Theory of the locomotion of nematodes:

Dynamics of undulatory progression on a surface, *Biophys. J.*, 60:1132–1146.

Pearce, R. A., and Friesen, W. O., 1988, A model for intersegmental coordination in the leech nerve cord, *Biol. Cybern.*, 58:301–311.

Quinn, R. D., and Ritzmann, R. E., 1998, Construction of a hexapod robot with cockroach kinematics benefits both robotics and biology, *Conn. Sci.*, 10:239–254.

Webb, B., 2000, What does robotics offer animal behaviour? *Anim. Behav.*, 60:545–558. ◆

Wilson, D. M., 1966, Insect walking, *Annu. Rev. Entomol.*, 11:103–122.

Locomotion, Vertebrate

Auke Jan Ijspeert

Introduction

Locomotion is a fundamental skill for animals. It is required for a large variety of actions, such as finding food, encountering a mate, and escaping predators. Among the various forms of vertebrate locomotion are swimming, crawling, walking, flying, and the more idiosyncratic movements such as hopping, brachiation, and burrowing.

Animal locomotion is characterized by rhythmic activity and the use of multiple degrees of freedom (i.e., multiple joints and muscles). In vertebrates, motion is generated by the musculoskeletal system, in which torques are created by antagonistic muscles at the joints of articulated systems composed of rigid bones. All types of vertebrate locomotion rely on some kind of rhythmic activity to move forward: undulations or peristaltic contractions of the body, oscillations of fins, legs, or wings. As the animal rhythmically applies forces to the environment (ground, water, or air), reaction forces are generated that move the body forward.

This type of locomotion is in contrast to the motion of most man-made machines, which usually relies on few degrees of freedom (e.g., a limited number of powered wheels, propellers, or jet engines) and continuous rather than rhythmic actuation. From a technological point of view, animal locomotion is significantly more difficult to control than most wheeled or propelled machines. The oscillations of the multiple degrees of freedom need to be well coordinated to generate efficient locomotion. However, as can be observed from the swimming of a dolphin or the running of a goat over irregular terrain, animal locomotion presents many interesting features, such as energy efficiency (for swimming) and agility. The next sections review the neural and mechanical mechanisms underlying vertebrates' fascinating locomotor abilities.

Neural Control of Locomotion

Despite diversity in types of locomotion, the general organization of the vertebrate locomotor circuit appears to be highly conserved. Locomotion is controlled by the interaction of three components: (1) spinal central pattern generators (CPGs), (2) sensory feedback, and (3) descending supraspinal control. The combination of these three components is sometimes called the motor pattern generator (MPG).

Central Pattern Generators

Central pattern generators are circuits that can generate rhythmic activity without rhythmic input (see HALF-CENTER OSCILLATORS UNDERLYING RHYTHMIC MOVEMENTS and MOTOR PATTERN GEN-

ERATION). The rhythms can often be initiated by simple tonic (i.e., nonoscillating) electrical or pharmacological stimulation. In vertebrates, the CPGs are located in the spinal cord and distributed in different oscillatory centers. In the lamprey, for instance, the swimming CPG is a chain of approximately 100 segmental oscillators distributed from head to tail (see CHAINS OF OSCILLATORS IN MOTOR AND SENSORY SYSTEMS and SPINAL CORD OF LAMPREY: GENERATION OF LOCOMOTOR PATTERNS). In tetrapods, the locomotor CPG appears to be composed of different centers, one for each limb, that are themselves decomposed into different oscillatory subcenters for each joint (Grillner, 1981). Recent evidence from intracellular recordings in the mudpuppy suggests that joint subcenters can be decomposed even further into distinct oscillatory centers for flexor and extensor muscles (Cheng et al., 1998).

Experiments in completely isolated spinal cords and in deafferented animals (i.e., animals without sensory feedback) have shown that the patterns generated by the CPG are very similar to those recorded during intact locomotion. This demonstrates that sensory feedback is not necessary for generating and coordinating the oscillations underlying locomotion during stationary conditions.

Sensory Feedback

Although sensory feedback is not necessary for rhythm generation, it is essential for shaping and coordinating neural activity with actual mechanical movements. The main sensory feedback to the CPGs is provided by sensory receptors in joints and muscles (see MOTOR CONTROL, BIOLOGICAL AND THEORETICAL). Rhythmically moving the tail or a limb of a decerebrate vertebrate is often sufficient to initiate the rhythmic patterns of locomotion. The frequency of oscillations then matches that of the forced movement, illustrating the strong influence of peripheral feedback on pattern generation.

Sensory feedback is especially important in higher vertebrates with upright posture such as mammals (as opposed to vertebrates with sprawling postures, like certain amphibians and reptiles), because the limbs of those vertebrates play an important role in posture control—supporting the body—in addition to locomotion.

A whole set of reflexes exists to coordinate neural activity with mechanical activity. One example is the stretch reflex, which generates the contraction of a muscle when the muscle is lengthened and which therefore helps maintain posture. The reflex pathways often share many of the interneurons that participate in locomotion control, and the action of reflexes is therefore not fixed. During locomotion, the action of reflexes can be modulated by central commands and in some cases even reversed, depending on the timing within the locomotor cycle (see Pearson and Gordon, 2000, and

Descending Supraspinal Control

Locomotion is initiated and modulated by descending pathways
from diencephalic and mesencephalic locomotor centers. (For reviews, see Donkelaar, 2001, and Rossignol in Rowell and Shepherd, 1996, chap. 5). Some of these pathways are direct; an example
is the pathway from the vestibular nuclei and the cerebellum to the
spinal neurons. Other pathways are relayed by centers in the brainstem, in particular the red nucleus and the reticular nuclei. In all
vertebrates, the reticulospinal tract plays a crucial role in generating
the drive for the basic propulsive body and limb movements. In
the lamprey, for instance, reticulospinal neurons control both the
speed and direction of locomotion (Grillner et al., 1995). In mammals, additional direct pathways exist between the motor cortex
and the spinal cord—the corticospinal tracts. These tracts are
unique to mammals and play an important role in visuomotor coordination, such as accurate foot placement in uneven terrain.

Interestingly, the input signals to the brainstem do not need to
be complex to generate locomotion. It has been known since the
1960s that simple electrical stimulation of the brainstem initiates
the walking gait in a decerebrate cat, and progressively increasing
the amplitude of the stimulation leads to an increase in the oscillation frequency, accompanied by a switch from walking to trotting
and eventually to galloping (Shik, Severin, and Orlovsky, 1966).
This demonstrates that the brainstem and the spinal cord contain
most of the circuitry necessary for locomotion, including complex
phenomena such as gait transitions (see GAIT TRANSITIONS).

The Biomechanics of Locomotion

Locomotion is the result of an intricate coupling between neural
dynamics and body dynamics, and many fundamental aspects of
locomotion control, including gait transition, control of speed, and
control of direction, cannot be fully understood by investigating
the locomotor circuit in isolation from the body it controls. A body
has its own dynamics and intrinsic frequencies with complex nonlinear properties, to which the neural signals must be adapted for
efficient locomotion control. As observed by roboticist Marc Raibert, the central nervous system (CNS) does not control the body,
it can only make suggestions.

The body is a redundant system, with many muscles per joint
and several muscles acting on more than one joint. Muscles serve
as actuators, brakes, stiffness regulators, and stores of elastic energy. During locomotion, the frequencies, amplitudes, and phases
of the signals sent to the multiple muscles must be well orchestrated. In most vertebrates, complex coordination is required not
only between different joints and limbs but also between antagonist
muscles, which combine periods of co-activation for modulating
the stiffness of the joint and periods of alternation for actuating the
joint.

In legged locomotion, the dynamics of a leg can be approximated
by a pendulum model during walking and by a spring-mass model
during running. These models allow one to relate several features,
such as resonance frequencies, to the length and stiffness of the
legs, and are able to describe the mechanics of legged locomotion
surprisingly well in many animals.

The importance of the mechanical properties of the body is illustrated by research on passive walkers. Passive walkers are legged machines (some with knees and arms) that transform potential
energy from gravity into kinetic energy when walking down a gentle slope. When correctly designed, these machines do not require
any actuation or control for generating a walking gait, which in
some cases can be strikingly human-like.

Numerical Simulations of Locomotor Circuits

Although the general organization of the vertebrate locomotor circuit is known, much work remains to be done to elucidate how its
different components are implemented and how they interplay to
generate the complex patterns underlying locomotion. This is a
complex task because (1) these patterns are due to the interaction
of the CNS and the body in movement, (2) numerous neurons in
the brainstem and the spinal cord are involved, and (3) in most
vertebrates, the same circuits appear to be involved in generating
very different patterns of activity (e.g., different gaits in tetrapods).
For the moment, the best decoded locomotor circuits are probably
the swimming circuits in the lamprey and the frog embryo. For
other vertebrates, in particular tetrapods, significant parts of the
structure and functioning of the locomotion circuitry remain
unknown.

Numerical simulations have an important role to play in evaluating whether a potential model of a neural circuit is adequate and
sufficient to reproduce the rhythmic patterns observed through intracellular and/or EMG measurements. Several important issues
can be investigated in simulation, such as the general stability of
the patterns and the effect of modulating the tonic drive on the
frequencies and phases of the oscillations. Simulations do not need
to be restricted to the CNS. An interesting approach to understanding locomotion control is to couple the simulations of the locomotor circuits to physics-based simulations of the body (or to a
robot). Such *neuromechanical* simulations are particularly useful
because they embed the neural circuits in a body in interaction with
the environment, therefore allowing one to close the sensing-acting
loop and to investigate the complete resulting motor patterns (as
opposed to only the patterns produced by the isolated CPGs).

Some Models of Vertebrate Locomotor Systems

This section presents some results of modeling of vertebrate locomotion, with a special focus on neuromechanical simulations.

Swimming

Vertebrate swimming has been most studied in the lamprey (see
SPINAL CORD OF LAMPREY: GENERATION OF LOCOMOTOR PAT-
TERNS), an eel-like fish using *anguilliform* swimming, in which a
traveling wave is propagated along the whole elongated body.
Ekeberg developed a neuromechanical simulation composed of a
connectionist neural network representing the lamprey's 100-
segment spinal locomotor circuit and a simplified model of the
body in interaction with water (Ekeberg, 1993). The neural network
produces oscillating activity when tonic input is provided to the
neurons, with the frequency of oscillation being proportional to the
level of excitation. When extra excitation is provided to the most
rostral (i.e., closest to the head) segments, a traveling wave is propagated from head to tail. The extra excitation determines the wavelength, independent of the frequency. With these settings, the
model therefore replicates the fact that a swimming lamprey can
cover a large range of frequencies while maintaining the wavelength constant at approximately one body length.

The mechanical simulation is a two-dimensional articulated rigid
body actuated by muscles simulated as spring and dampers. Although the hydrodynamics of the model is simplified, it produces
swimming gaits very similar to those of lamprey swimming (Figure
1). The mechanical simulation allowed Ekeberg to investigate the
effect of modulating the locomotor pattern on the speed and direction of locomotion, as well as the effect of sensory feedback from
spinal stretch–sensitive cells. The model demonstrated that the
speed of swimming can be varied by changing the frequency of
oscillation through the level of tonic input, whereas the direction

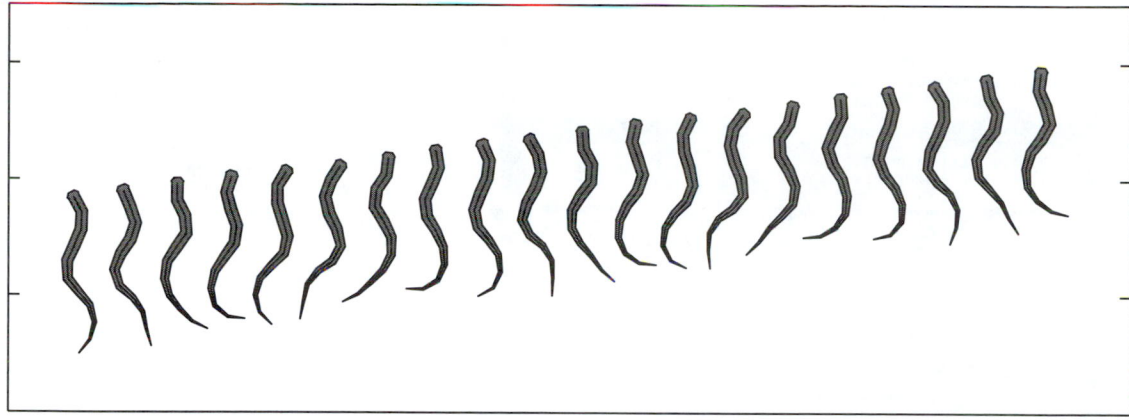

Figure 1. Neuromechanical simulation of lamprey swimming. (Reimplementation by the author of the model presented in Ekeberg, Ö, 1993, A combined neuronal and mechanical model of fish swimming, *Biol. Cybern.*, 69:363–374.)

of swimming can be varied by applying asymmetric tonic drive between left and right sides of the locomotor circuit.

Vertebrate swimming has inspired several underwater vehicles, such as eel-like robots that use anguilliform swimming (REEL, at the University of Pennsylvania) and a lamprey-based undulatory robot (at the Marine Science Center of Northeastern University), and caranguiform swimming in the RoboTuna (at the Massachusetts Institute of Technology).

From Swimming to Walking

One of the most important changes during vertebrate evolution has been the transition from aquatic to terrestrial habitats. Our own work investigated the transition from swimming to walking in the salamander, an animal that is believed to be one of the modern animals closest to the first vertebrates that made this transition during evolution.

The salamander swims like a lamprey by propagating an undulation from head to tail. On ground, it switches to a stepping gait, usually with the phase relation of a trot. Although the locomotor circuit of the salamander has not yet been decoded, it has been found to share many similarities with the swimming circuit of the lamprey (Cohen, 1988; Delvolvé, Bem, and Cabelguen, 1997).

Our work sought to demonstrate that a lamprey-like swimming circuit could be extended to produce the swimming and stepping gaits of the salamander, with, in particular, a traveling wave along the body during swimming and a standing wave during stepping. The neural configuration of the model is illustrated in Figure 2. It is composed of a lamprey-like body CPG, extended by forelimb and hindlimb CPGs (Ijspeert, 2001). These limb centers have been identified just rostral to the anterior and posterior girdles, respectively. The mechanical simulation was an extension of Ekeberg's model of the lamprey (see Ijspeert, 2001, for a detailed description).

The model is able to (1) generate stable traveling waves and standing waves, depending on simple tonic input, (2) quickly switch between them, and (3) coordinate body and limb movements so as to produce swimming and walking gaits very similar to those recorded in salamanders. Gait transition is obtained as follows: when only the body CPG receives tonic input, the limb CPGs remain silent (limbs are maintained tonically against the body) and the body CPG produces a traveling wave that propels the salamander forward in water, whereas when tonic input is applied to both the body CPG and the limb CPGs, the body CPG is forced by the limb CPGs to produce a standing wave for stepping. The body then makes a standing S-shaped wave with the nodes at the girdles that

is coordinated with the movements of the limbs so as to increase the reach of the limbs during the swing phase (Figure 3, bottom).

Much as in Ekeberg's model of the lamprey, the speed and direction of locomotion can be modulated by respectively varying the level and the asymmetry (between left and right) of tonic input applied to the CPGs. Experiments involving the tracking of a randomly moving target show that locomotion is stable even when the input signals change rapidly and continuously (Ijspeert and Arbib, 2000). In collaboration with Richard Woesler and Gerhard Roth, we are currently extending this work to investigate visuomotor coordination (see VISUOMOTOR COORDINATION IN SALAMANDER).

Quadruped Locomotion

Quadruped locomotion in vertebrates has evolved from the sprawling posture found in salamanders and lizards to the upright posture found in mammals. During that evolution, the limbs gradually moved under the body, and movements in the body evolved from lateral to mainly sagittal (i.e., ventrodorsal) undulations.

The upright posture means that limbs serve both for locomotion and for maintaining balance. Gaits can either be *statically stable*, in which the center of mass is maintained at all times above the polygon formed by the contact points of the limbs with the ground, or *dynamically stable*, when this rule is not maintained at all times and stability is achieved as a limit cycle that balances moments, gravitational forces, and inertial forces over time. Depending on the phase relation between limbs, a large variety of gaits can be distinguished, such as the walk, the trot, the pace, and the gallop. Mammals can usually switch between these gaits very quickly (see GAIT TRANSITIONS).

The neural mechanisms underlying quadruped locomotion have not yet been decoded, but investigations in the cat have shown that the rhythmic patterns for locomotion are generated by spinal CPGs, while control of posture and accurate placement of feet are under control of the cerebellum and motor cortex. Decerebrate cats, for instance, can produce normal-looking gaits on a treadmill, but need to be supported to do so. The mechanisms underlying intra- and interlimb coordination, however, are still far from understood, especially in relation to gait transition.

Kimura, Akiyama, and Sakurama (1999) present a model of quadruped locomotion that emerges from the coupling of a neural controller with a quadruped robot with 12° of freedom. The neural controller is composed of four coupled oscillators, one for each limb, and several types of reflexes. Kimura and colleagues investigated several schemes of how feedback from load sensors, touch

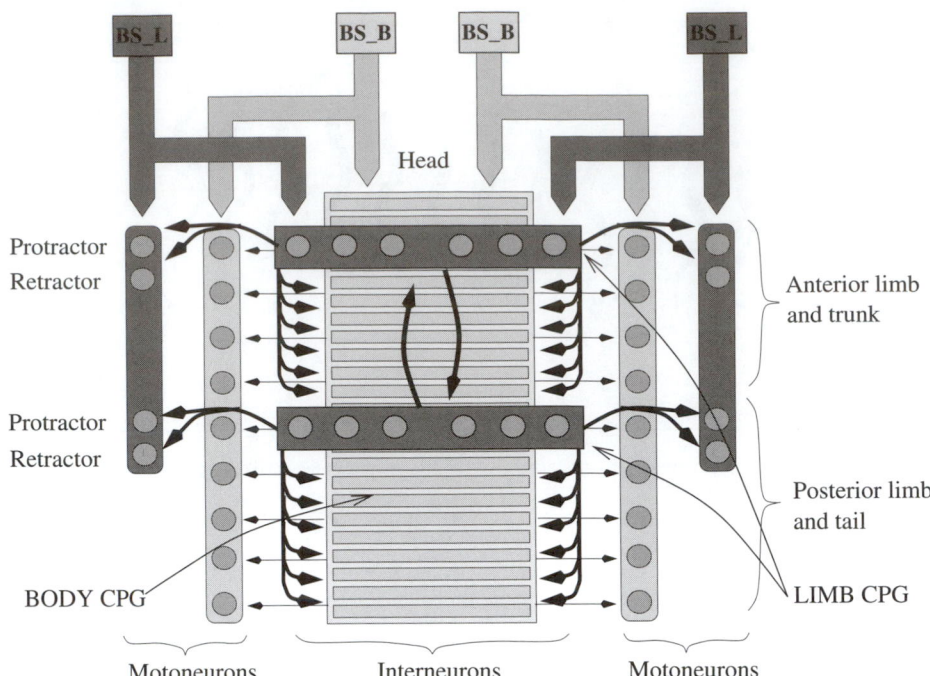

Figure 2. Potential model for the central pattern generator responsible for locomotion in the salamander. (From Ijspeert, A., 2001, A connectionist central pattern generator for the aquatic and terrestrial gaits of a simulated salamander, *Biol. Cybern.*, 85:331–348. Reprinted with permission.)

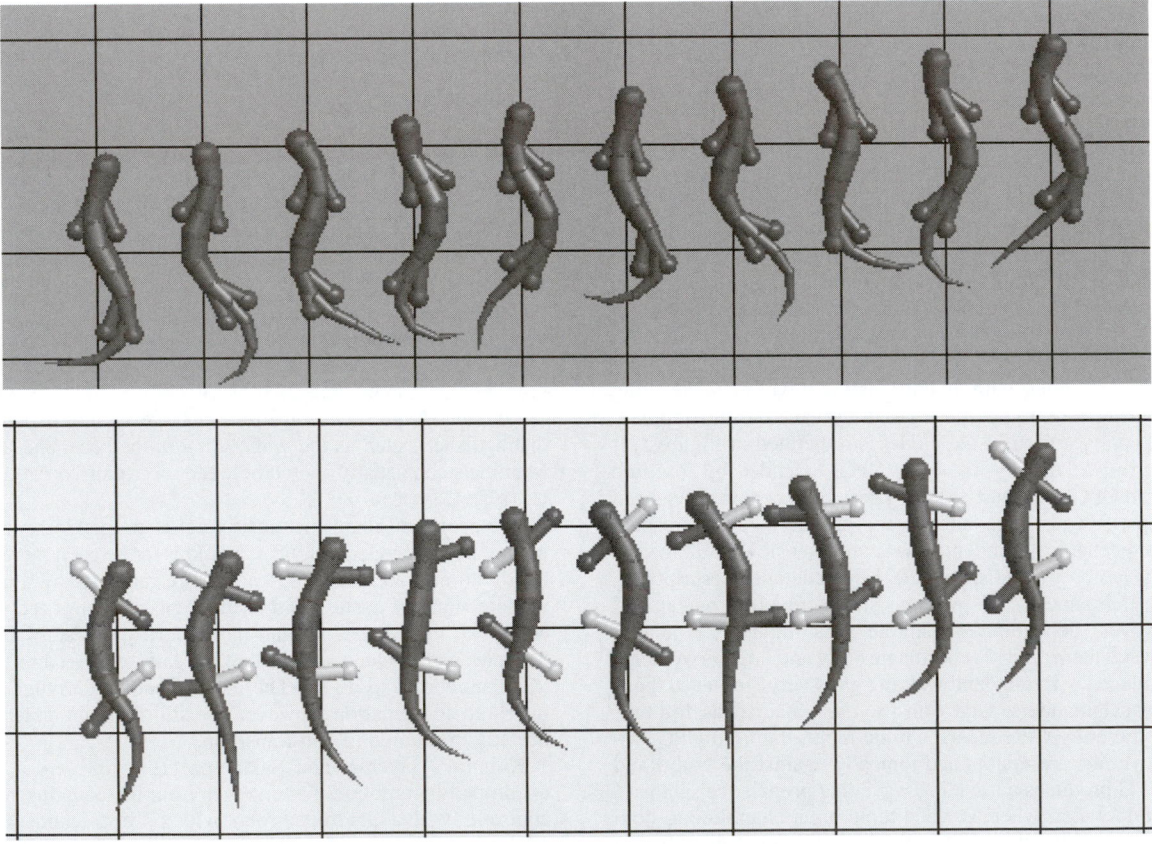

Figure 3. Neuromechanical simulation of salamander locomotion. *Top*, swimming; *bottom*, stepping. (From Ijspeert, A., 2001, A connectionist central pattern generator for the aquatic and terrestrial gaits of a simulated salamander, *Biol. Cybern.*, 85:331–348. Reprinted with permission.)

sensors, and a vestibular system (a rate gyro) could be coupled to the CPG. The schemes in which the feedback was fed into and gated by the CPGs (as opposed to being independent of the CPGs) were found to generate significantly more stable gaits on irregular terrain. This strongly resembles the modulation of reflex signals by CPGs found in vertebrates and described earlier under Sensory Feedback. Other examples of impressive running and hopping robots can be found in Raibert and Hodgins (1993), for instance.

Biped Locomotion

Biped locomotion, such as human locomotion, is usually a dynamically stable gait. Humans use mainly two gaits: walking, in which at least one foot is in contact with the ground during the whole locomotor cycle, and running, which has a flight phase without foot contact.

The control of posture is essential in biped locomotion because of the erect posture. In humans, the motor cortex and the cerebellum play a crucial role in locomotion, much more so than in lower vertebrates. As in other vertebrates, there seems to be good evidence that the locomotor pattern can be generated at the spinal level, most likely driven from reticulospinal pathways. Clearly, the postural problem involves an important role of the cerebellum for behaviorally successful locomotion, with the corticospinal pathway playing, in addition, a role in the step-to-step modification (e.g., visually guided) of the locomotor cycle. See Horak and Mac-Pherson in Rowell and Shepherd (1996, chap. 7) for a review.

In a series of papers, Gentaro Taga developed an interesting two-dimensional model of human locomotion (motion in the sagittal plane) in which stable locomotor patterns emerged from the interaction of a set of neural oscillators coupled to a musculoskeletal system composed of eight rigid segments (e.g., Taga, 1998). Taga's work was seminal in showing potential mechanisms of global entrainment between two highly nonlinear systems, the neural oscillators and the body. Balance in the model is maintained by a posture controller that regulates the impedance of the joints in parallel to the oscillators. The patterns are sufficiently stable to generate gaits even in unpredictable environments. In the latest version of the model, the locomotion controller is extended with a discrete movement generator for anticipatory adaptation for stepping over obstacles. The discrete movement generator modifies the stepping by generating a sequence of discrete motor signals, changing the gains of specific muscles. The functional role of the discrete movement generator is therefore comparable to the modulatory effect of the motor cortex observed during obstacle avoidance tasks in cats and humans.

Discussion

Vertebrate locomotion control is organized such that neural networks in the spinal cord generate the basic rhythmic patterns necessary for locomotion, and higher control centers interact with the spinal circuits for posture control and accurate limb movements. This means that, in general, the control signals sent to the spinal cord do not need to specify all the details of when and how much the muscles must contract, but rather specify higher-level commands such as stop and go signals, speed, and heading of motion. This type of distributed control has provided an interesting inspiration for robotics, as it implies (1) a reduction in the amount of information that has to be communicated back and forth, and (2) a reduction in the time delays between sensing, command generation, and acting.

Locomotor circuits are the result of evolution, which means that there exists a chain of changes from the ancestral vertebrate to all vertebrates. An important question that remains open is to determine which modifications have occurred in the locomotor circuits

from the generation of traveling waves for swimming (the most ancestral vertebrates were close to the lamprey) to the generation of standing waves for walking, to the generation of multiple gaits for quadruped locomotion, and finally to the generation of biped locomotion (not to forget all the other forms of vertebrate locomotion mentioned in the Introduction). This is an important issue, since the mechanisms of locomotion in modern vertebrates are strongly shaped by this evolutionary heritage and might not be fully understood without taking evolution into account. In particular, we will need to determine to what extent the three components of locomotion control—CPGs, sensory feedback, and supraspinal descending commands—have changed. It is clear that important morphological changes have significantly modified the patterns of sensory feedback. However, for lower vertebrates, it is likely that most of the changes are due to modifications of the CPGs, since CPGs are able to generate relatively normal gaits without sensory feedback, and comparative studies show that descending pathways are in general strikingly conserved (Donkelaar, 2001). In higher vertebrates such as mammals, changes of the CPGs have been accompanied by important modifications of the descending pathways under the requirements of complex posture control and accurate limb movements, although the extent of the respective changes remains unknown. In addition to neurophysiological experiments and comparative studies, computer models, in particular models that combine neural models with biomechanical models, have an important role to play in answering these fascinating questions.

Road Maps: Motor Pattern Generators; Neuroethology and Evolution
Related Reading: Evolution of Artificial Neural Networks; Spinal Cord of Lamprey: Generation of Locomotor Patterns; Visuomotor Coordination in Salamander

References

Cheng, J., Stein, R., Jovanovic, K., Yoshida, K., Bennett, D., and Han, Y., 1998, Identification, localization, and modulation of neural networks for walking in the mudpuppy (*Necturus maculatus*) spinal cord, *J. Neurosci.*, 18:4295–4304.

Cohen, A., 1988, Evolution of the vertebrate central pattern generator for locomotion, in *Neural Control of Rhythmic Movements in Vertebrates* (A. H. Cohen, S. Rossignol, and S. Grillner, Eds.), New York: Wiley.

Delvolvé, I., Bem, T., and Cabelguen, J.-M., 1997, Epaxial and limb muscle activity during swimming and terrestrial stepping in the adult newt, *Pleurodeles waltl, J. Neurophysiol.*, 78:638–650.

Donkelaar, H. ten, 2001, Evolution of vertebrate motor systems, in *Brain Evolution and Cognition* (G. Roth and M. Wullimann, Eds.), New York: Wiley Spectrum, pp. 77–112.

Ekeberg, Ö., 1993, A combined neuronal and mechanical model of fish swimming, *Biol. Cybern.*, 69:363–374.

Grillner, S., 1981, Control of locomotion in bipeds, tetrapods and fish, in *Handbook of Physiology: The Nervous System, 2, Motor Control* (V. Brooks, Ed.), Bethesda, MD: American Physiology Society, pp. 1179–1236. ◆

Grillner, S., Degliana, T., Ekeberg, Ö., El Marina, A., Lansner, A., Orlovsky, G., and Wallén, P., 1995, Neural networks that co-ordinate locomotion and body orientation in lamprey, *Trends Neurosci.*, 18:270–279.

Ijspeert, A., 2001, A connectionist central pattern generator for the aquatic and terrestrial gaits of a simulated salamander, *Biol. Cybern.*, 85:331–348.

Ijspeert, A., and Arbib, M., 2000, Visual tracking in simulated salamander locomotion, in *Proceedings of the Sixth International Conference of the Society for Adaptive Behavior (SAB2000)* (J. Meyer, A. Berthoz, D. Floreano, H. Roitblat, and S. Wilson, Eds.), Cambridge, MA: MIT Press, pp. 88–97.

Kimura, H., Akiyama, S., and Sakurama, K., 1999, Realization of dynamic walking and running of the quadruped using neural oscillators, *Auton. Robots*, 7:247–258.

Pearson, K., and Gordon, J., 2000, Spinal reflexes, in *Principles of Neural*

Science, 4th ed. (E. Kandel, J. Schwartz, and T. Jessel, Eds.), New York: McGraw-Hill. ◆

Raibert, M., and Hodgins, J., 1993, Legged robots, in *Biological Neural Networks in Invertebrate Neuroethology and Robotics* (R. Beer, R. Ritzmann, and T. McKenna, Eds.), San Diego, CA: Academic Press, pp. 319–354.

Rowell, L., and Shepherd, J., Eds., 1996, *Handbook of Physiology*, sect.

12: *Exercise: Regulation and Integration of Multiple Systems, Neural Control of Movement*. New York: Oxford University Press. ◆

Shik, M., Severin, F., and Orlovsky, G., 1966, Control of walking by means of electrical stimulation of the mid-brain, *Biophysics*, 11:756–765.

Taga, G., 1998, A model of the neuro-musculo-skeletal system for anticipatory adjustment of human locomotion during obstacle avoidance, *Biol. Cybern.*, 78:9–17.

Locust Flight: Components and Mechanisms in the Motor

R. Meldrum Robertson

Introduction

The locust flight motor provides an excellent model system for investigations of constraints and mechanisms of MOTOR PATTERN GENERATION at the neuronal level. In locusts the neural elements involved in generating the patterns of flight motor activity are individually identifiable (see Comer and Robertson, 2001, for a review of identified neurons controlling insect behaviors). It is thus possible to describe the operation of networks of identified neurons, connected by identified synapses, and to determine how these networks contribute to the computational task of producing rhythmical motor patterns capable of keeping the locust aloft in an unpredictable environment.

The flight systems of other insects have attracted research interest in their neural control mechanisms. Indeed, the visuomotor control of dipteran flight has received notable attention (VISUAL COURSE CONTROL IN FLIES). Nevertheless, it is only for the locust that enough is known of the circuitry underlying the form and timing of the wingbeat that it can be useful as a model of central nervous system function.

The Motor Output

The locust flight system (Figure 1) creates a spatiotemporal pattern of electrical activity in about 80 flight motoneurons that activate muscles controlling the four wings (a pair of forewings and a pair of hindwings) and cause beating of the wings at around 22 cycles/s. Telemetric techniques now exist to monitor the activity of identified flight muscles during free flight under conditions that require the generation of different combinations of rotational and translational flight forces (Kutsch, 1999). Particular features of the motor pattern can be correlated with specific flight parameters that are modified to effect adaptive flight maneuvers (i.e., natural behaviors). It was originally demonstrated that a version of the motor pattern, albeit slower (around 12 cycles/s), could be generated by a central nervous system deafferented from phasic timing information emanating from wing proprioceptors and other sense organs. This discovery was influential in establishing the central pattern generator concept (MOTOR PATTERN GENERATION). An important question is to what extent the central pattern generator is responsible for controlling the *behavior*, particularly given that afferent input can change the set of active flight interneurons in the locust. There is no doubt that a rhythmic central pattern can be generated, but it is conceivable that this pattern is the output of a network artificially created by the act of deafferentation, i.e., a malformed, degenerate pattern that has no real bearing on the generation of the functional flight motor pattern. There is little evidence for this extreme position, and the extent to which sensory feedback supersedes the role of the central pattern generator in normal intact

flight remains unclear. Nevertheless, it is quite clear that proprioceptive feedback is necessary for appropriate timing of the wingbeat phase transitions. The tegulae are external sense organs stimulated by depression of each wing and they can initiate the subsequent elevator phase by excitation of elevator motoneurons and interneurons. The stretch receptors are internal, at the wing base, and activated by wing elevation. They promote the occurrence of the subsequent depression by opposing the hyperpolarization between the bursts of action potentials in depressor moto-

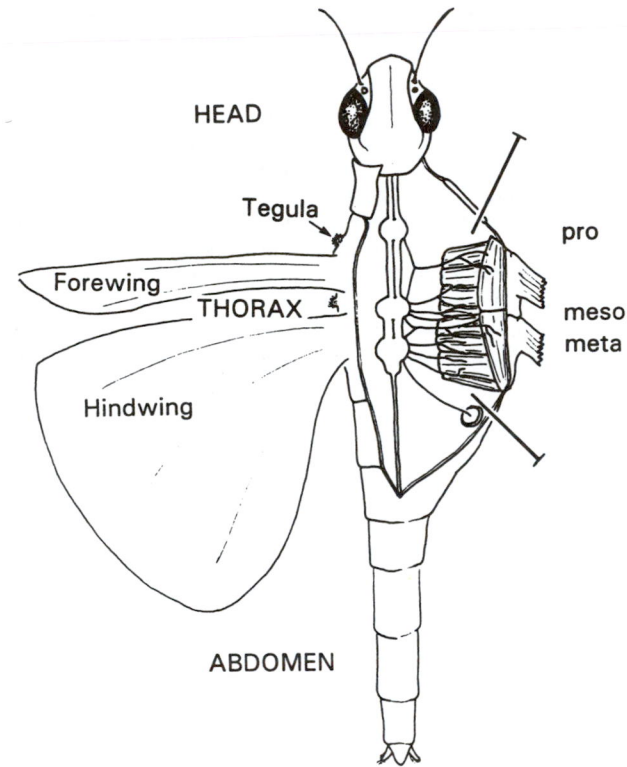

Figure 1. The locust flight system. Diagrammatic representation of a locust showing on the left side the form of the forewing and hindwing and the position of the fore and hind tegulae (only the forewing tegula is labeled). On the right side the thorax has been pinned open to reveal the bank of flight muscles that power the wings and the three thoracic ganglia (pro-, meso-, and metathoracic) that contain the motoneurons and interneurons involved in generating flight motor patterns.

neurons. A simple model describing how the stretch receptors regulate wing beat frequency has been described but would benefit from a quantitative implementation (Figure 2) (Pearson and Ramirez, 1990).

The Neuronal Components and Their Organization

The centrally generated rhythm arises as a result of the cellular properties of interneurons in the three thoracic ganglia (pro-, meso-, and metathoracic) and the interactions between these neurons. Numerous interneurons have been described. They are connected into circuits via standard, short latency, synaptic interactions probably mediated by gamma-aminobutyric acid (inhibitory) and glutamate (excitatory) (Robertson, 1989). This central circuit operates essentially as a unit distributed throughout six serially homologous, segmental neuromeres (Robertson, Pearson, and Reichert, 1982). A

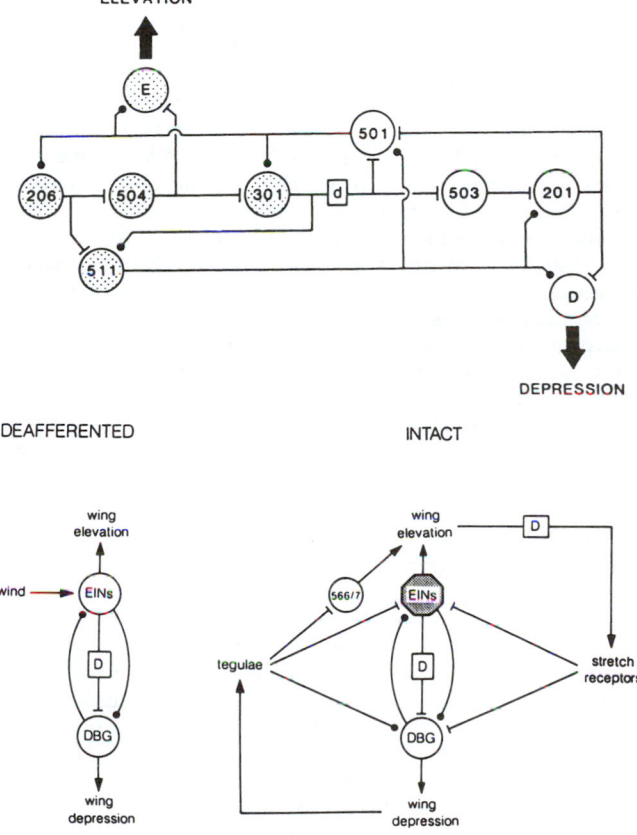

Figure 2. Circuit models of the locust flight system. *A,* Model illustrating the role of proprioceptive feedback in generating the flight motor pattern. The deafferented system (left) consists of a depressor burst generator (DBG) with reciprocal inhibitory interactions with elevator interneurons (EINs). These interneurons also pass excitation from wind input to the DBG through a delay (D) pathway. In intact animals (right), feedback from proprioceptors can recruit interneurons (e.g., 566/7) as well as interacting with the elements of the central rhythm generator. Stippling indicates that the activity pattern of the EINs is altered by the feedback. Filled circles, inhibitory connections; 'T'-bars, excitatory connections. Taken from Pearson and Ramirez, 1992. *B,* Model illustrating some of the connections between flight interneurons that may contribute to generating the central flight rhythm. Elevator interneurons are stippled. Interneuron 206 receives excitation from wind input. Note the similarity with the deafferented model in A. The heart of the circuit is delayed excitation (301 to 501) and feedback inhibition (501 to 301). Taken from Robertson, 1986.

simple conceptual model of the circuitry described to date has at its heart a circuit of delayed excitation and feedback inhibition that would result in an elevator-depressor burst sequence (Figure 2*B*) (Robertson and Pearson, 1985).

Transection and hemisection experiments have demonstrated a multiplicity of patterning elements that may aid in stabilizing the output pattern, an extremely important role for sensory elements in timing and coordination of the four wings during intact flight, and a preeminent role for the metathoracic ganglion, compared with the role of the mesothoracic ganglion, in central pattern generation. There are many oscillator mechanisms contributing to the generation of the rhythm, such that rhythm generation survives much experimental manipulation (see the section, "Modeling in the Locust Flight System," later in this article). However, there is not yet any strong evidence to support the notion that the central rhythm generator is organized as a coupled oscillator system in the sense that each wing, or pair of wings, is controlled by a separate central oscillator with the relative phasing determined by the nature of the coupling between them. This makes the locust flight system apparently unique among locomotor pattern generators, most of which do seem to be organized as coupled central oscillators.

Circuitry Underlying Steering

An important feature of any motor pattern generator for locomotion is that it must control the direction of movement through space, as well as simple translation (VISUAL COURSE CONTROL IN FLIES and SENSORIMOTOR INTERACTIONS AND CENTRAL PATTERN GENERATORS). This entails both maintaining a course in the face of environmental factors tending to displace the animal, and changing the course to enable movement toward or away from biologically relevant stimuli. Most information has accumulated for course correction behaviors—mechanisms of the "autopilot." It is only for the course correction circuitry that there is a model, at the cellular level, explaining how multimodal sensory input signaling deviation from course can be integrated into the operation of the central circuitry to cause the asymmetries in the motor output that would be necessary to compensate for an unintended change in the direction of flight (e.g., Reichert, Rowell, and Griss, 1985). The basis of the model is that continuous signals from exteroceptors, such as the ocelli (simple light detectors) or wind-sensitive head hairs, excite premotor interneurons that are rhythmically activated by the central circuits at the same time. Thus, the course deviation signal is gated through these premotor interneurons and transmitted to the motor neurons at the appropriate phase for an effective change in the motor pattern. Much of the asymmetry in the form of the wingbeat that generates steering torques occurs during the downstroke (the power stroke) of the wings, while the upstroke remains relatively symmetrical. The deviation signal can be gated so that it affects only those motoneurons involved in controlling the form of the downstroke, and it need not interact directly with the central rhythm generator.

Neuromodulation and Plasticity

The neural networks that control motor patterns are not static entities (Pearson, 2000; also see NEUROMODULATION IN INVERTEBRATE NERVOUS SYSTEMS). The mix of circulating transmitters and neuromodulators controls the particular set of circuit components and characteristics at any one time. Octopamine has a multifaceted role in the control and coordination of locust flight (Orchard, Ramirez, and Lange, 1993). From mobilization of energy resources to the modification of flight muscle properties, octopamine has influences throughout the locust enabling it to fly efficiently and, equally, to respond to the metabolic demands of flight. Indeed octopamine released from specific subgroups of DUM (*dor-*

sal *un*paired *me*dian) neurons may orchestrate the peripheral reconfigurations required by different motor programs such as walking or flight (Duch and Pflüger, 1999). Local injection of octopamine at specific sites in the thoracic ganglia is sufficient to release flight-like activity from the nervous system. Similarly, topical application of octopamine to exposed nervous systems can generate flight-like motor patterns, even in immature stages of the locust that normally do not generate such patterns. The basis for these observations is likely the fact that octopamine can induce intrinsic bursting properties (plateau potentials; OSCILLATORY AND BURSTING PROPERTIES OF NEURONS) in identified flight interneurons, and there are good reasons for supposing that this experimental manipulation reflects a physiological role for octopamine in the generation of normal flight motor patterns. It also seems likely that, in addition to the described interneuronal circuits, cellular properties and the generation of bistable plateau potentials contribute to the generation of the motor pattern in the absence of octopamine.

A short-term plasticity in the output of the flight system has been described and is ascribed to associations between muscle-specific proprioceptive input and exteroceptive input signaling deviation from course (Möhl, 1993). The interesting concept proposed by this work is that the central circuits provide a motor framework that is subsequently sculpted by the immediately preceding flight experience to provide the output that is most effective in controlling flight (e.g., maintaining a straight and level orientation). Thus, the operating circuit can be tailored to the current condition of the animal and its flight system. The specific synaptic mechanisms underlying this short-term plasticity remain to be determined. In contrast, there is some information on the synaptic mechanisms involved in a longer-term plasticity underlying functional recovery after a specific deafferentation (Wolf and Büschges, 1997). Ablation of the hindwing tegulae impairs the operation of the flight system, and this is reflected in a reduced wingbeat frequency. However, the system recovers during the subsequent two weeks due to the forewing tegulae taking over the function of the ablated hindwing tegulae. The basis for the recovery is the formation of new connections between the afferents and specific flight interneurons, accompanied by sprouting and growth of both the axonal branches of afferent fibers and the dendritic arbors of the interneurons. The synaptic connections are in a dynamic equilibrium that is disrupted by the lesion, and it is particularly interesting that different, though serially homologous, sense organs can replace those ablated.

Finally, locusts do not physiologically regulate body temperature but exist in a harsh ecological niche where ambient temperatures often exceed 45°C. Adaptive mechanisms exist to condition the circuitry by prior exposure to high temperatures and thus to extend the operating range by 5°–7°C. The current model proposes that heat stress-mediated long-term reduction of potassium conductance delays the failure of action potentials as temperature is increased by preventing potassium currents from overwhelming sodium currents at high temperatures (Wu and Robertson, 2001). Given the evolutionary conservation of cellular protective responses (e.g., the heat shock response), the mechanisms underlying thermoprotection of circuit function in this system could have implications for the development of therapeutic strategies to combat thermal failure of mammalian circuits (e.g., the hyperthermic failure of respiratory rhythm generation that has been proposed as an explanation for some cases of SIDS).

Modeling in the Locust Flight System

Insect flight lends itself to modeling at several different levels. The construction of flapping machines and flying robots is well advanced and our understanding of the aerodynamics of flapping insect flight has been greatly improved by biomechanically modeling the wing kinematics of functionally two-winged fliers (dipteran flies and moths). Extending this approach to functionally four-winged locusts remains a challenge. Robotic and virtual models of the processing and integration of sensory information to control a search strategy (e.g., olfactory stimuli) or avoid collisions (e.g., looming visual stimuli) are well established. However, the modeling of circuit and cellular mechanisms generating flight motor rhythms is unsophisticated compared with that of many other rhythm generating systems.

Initial attempts to model the locust flight circuits used electronic Lewis "neuromimes," which simulate the behavior of neural membranes and can be connected into networks (Wilson and Waldron, 1968). An arrangement of neuromimes into positively coupled subsets interconnected with reciprocal inhibition successfully mimicked several features of the flight motor pattern. Unfortunately, successive families of detailed models have not followed this early success. What mostly exist in the literature are conceptual circuit models of the common "ball and stick" type (e.g., Figure 2). One notable exception is the computer simulation of the central flight circuit performed with BioSim 3.0 (Grimm and Sauer, 1995). This simulation was rudimentary by current standards and introduced numerous simplifications; nevertheless, it clearly demonstrated the following: that the known circuit could produce acceptable flight-like rhythms; that subloops of the complete circuit could generate comparable rhythms; that circuit operation was relatively resistant to "synaptic strength"; and that the addition of plateau potential generating properties did not greatly affect the output of the circuit or the robustness of the rhythm generating mechanism.

Knowledge of the flight system is currently at a stage at which more detailed models would be beneficial. Could changing the parameters of a model central circuit, according to the known effects of temperature on conduction velocities and synaptic interactions, replicate the known effects of temperature on the motor patterns? Is it possible to generate a model that mimics the coordination of the four wings using a single depressor burst generator located primarily in the metathoracic ganglion? Can the effect of specific ablations and recoveries be accurately modeled? The list here, as for any other nontrivial system, is endless.

Discussion

Locust flight motor patterns are generated by an interactive mixture of the intrinsic properties of flight neurons, the operation of complex circuits, and phase-specific proprioceptive input. These mechanisms are subject to the concentrations of circulating neuromodulators and are also modulated according to the demands of a constantly changing sensory environment to produce adaptive behaviors. The system is flexible and plastic in the short term and in the long term, able to operate in spite of severe ablations and subsequently to recover from these lesions, and able to cope with extreme environmental conditions.

Without a doubt, the neural processes involved in higher brain functions will not be first described in the locust. However, the basis for these higher functions is likely due both to the generation of patterns of electrical activity in time and space and to the modulation of these patterns by the extracellular environment, by the periphery, and by experience—the control of such spatiotemporal patterning can profitably be investigated in the locust flight system.

Road Maps: Motor Pattern Generators; Neuroethology and Evolution
Related Reading: Half-Center Oscillators Underlying Rhythmic Movements; Locomotion, Invertebrate; Motor Pattern Generation; Respiratory Rhythm Generation

References

Comer, C. M., and Robertson, R. M., 2001, Identified nerve cells and insect behavior, *Prog. Neurobiol.*, 63:409–439. ◆

Duch, C., and Pflüger, H.-J., 1999, DUM neurons in locust flight: A model system for amine-mediated peripheral adjustments to the requirements of a central motor program, *J. Comp. Physiol.*, 184:489–499.

Grimm, K., and Sauer, A. E., 1995, The high number of neurons contributes to the robustness of the locust flight-CPG against parameter variation, *Biol. Cybern.*, 72:329–335.

Kutsch, W., 1999, Telemetry in insects: The "intact animal approach," *Theory Biosci.*, 118:29–53. ◆

Möhl, B., 1993, The role of proprioception for motor learning in locust flight, *J. Comp. Physiol.*, 172:325–332.

Orchard, I., Ramirez, J.-M., and Lange, A. B., 1993, A multifunctional role for octopamine in locust flight, *Annu. Rev. Entomol.*, 38:227–249.

Pearson, K. G., 2000, Neural adaptation in the generation of rhythmic behavior. *Annu. Rev. Neurosci.*, 62:723–753. ◆

Pearson, K. G., and Ramirez, J.-M., 1990, Influence of input from the forewing stretch receptors on motoneurones in flying locusts, *J. Exp. Biol.*, 151:317–340.

Pearson, K. G. and Ramirez, J.-M., 1992, Parallels with other invertebrate and vertebrate motor systems, in *Dynamic Biological Networks* (R. M. Harris-Warrick, E. Marder, A. I. Selverston, and M. Moulins, Eds.), Cambridge, MA: MIT Press, pp. 263–281

Reichert, H., Rowell, C. H. F., and Griss, C., 1985. Course correction circuitry translates feature detection into behavioural action in locusts, *Nature (Lond.)*, 315:142–144.

Robertson, R. M., 1986, Neuronal circuits controlling flight in the locust: Central generation of the rhythm. *Trends Neurosci.*, 9:278–280

Robertson, R. M., 1989, Idiosyncratic computational units generating innate motor patterns: Neurones and circuits in the locust flight system, in *The Computing Neurone* (R. Durbin, R. C. Miall, and G. Mitchison, Eds.), London: Addison-Wesley, pp. 262–277. ◆

Robertson, R. M., and Pearson, K. G., 1985, Neural circuits in the flight system of the locust, *J. Neurophysiol.*, 53:110–128.

Robertson, R. M., Pearson, K. G., and Reichert, H., 1982, Flight interneurons in the locust and the origin of insect wings, *Science*, 217:177–179.

Wilson, D. M., and Waldron, I., 1968, Models for the generation of the motor output pattern in flying locusts, *Proc. IEEE*, 56:1058–1064

Wolf, H., and Büschges, A., 1997, Plasticity of synaptic connections in sensory-motor pathways of the adult locust flight system, *J. Neurophysiol.*, 78:1276–1284.

Wu, B. S., and Robertson, R. M., 2001, Heat shock-induced thermoprotection of action potentials in the locust flight system, *J. Neurobiol.*, 49:188–199.

Markov Random Field Models in Image Processing

Anand Rangarajan and Rama Chellappa

Introduction

Markov random field (MRF) models have become useful in several areas of image processing. The success of MRFs can be attributed to the fact that they give rise to good, flexible, stochastic image models. The goal of image modeling is to find an adequate representation of the intensity distribution of a given image. What is adequate often depends on the task at hand, and MRF image models have been versatile enough to be applied in the areas of image and texture synthesis (Zhu, Wu, and Mumford, 1997), image restoration (Geman and Geman, 1984), tomographic reconstruction (Lee, Rangarajan, and Gindi, 1995), image and texture segmentation (Krishnamachari and Chellappa, 1997), flow field segmentation (Konrad and Dubois, 1992), surface reconstruction (Geiger and Girosi, 1991), and object recognition (Gold and Rangarajan, 1996). Our aim in this article is to highlight the central ideas of this field using illustrative examples and to provide pointers to the many applications.

A guiding insight underlying most of the work on MRFs in image processing is that the information contained in the local spatiotemporal structure of images or image sequences is sufficient to obtain a good, global representation. This notion is captured by means of a local, *conditional* probability distribution. Here, the image intensity at a particular location depends only on a *neighborhood* of pixels. The conditional distribution is called an MRF. For example, a typical MRF model assumes that the image is locally smooth except for relatively few intensity gradient discontinuities corresponding to region boundaries or edges. The MRF image models are defined on the image intensities and on a further set of *hidden* attributes (edges, texture, and region labels). The observed quantities are usually noisy, blurred images, feature vectors, or projection data (in the case of emission tomography). The intensity image underlying the observations is needed in applications such as restoration and tomographic reconstruction, whereas region, boundary, and texture labels are sought in applications such as texture segmentation.

Once the local, conditional probability distribution of the MRF is specified, there are five remaining steps involved. First, the joint

distribution of the MRF is obtained. In this way, the image is represented in one global, joint probability distribution. Next, the process by which the observations are generated from the image is captured in a *degradation* probability distribution. In image restoration, for example, the degradation corresponds to a (typically uniform) blur. Then, Bayes's theorem is invoked to obtain the posterior probability distribution of the image given the observations. The posterior distribution gives us the probability that an image (with smooth regions and sharp region boundaries, for example) could have been degraded to obtain the particular observed noisy, blurred image. Once the posterior probability distribution is obtained, we can associate a cost with each configuration in the posterior. For example, if only the true underlying image will do, the cost penalizes all other images equally. The cost is formulated, keeping in mind the task at hand. A measure of the cost is minimized with respect to the image intensities (in image recovery tasks) or image attributes (in labeling tasks). Finally, since MRFs are specified with model parameters, these are estimated from a training set (if one exists) or adaptively, along with the cost minimization phase alluded to earlier. The overall MRF framework fits well within a Bayesian estimation/inference paradigm. In the next section, we step through all five phases of MRF modeling.

A Framework for Estimation and Inference

MRF image models represent knowledge in terms of local probability distributions. Specifically, the kinds of probability distributions generated by MRFs have a local neighborhood structure. Neighborhood systems commonly used by MRFs are depicted in Figure 1A.

Let us associate an image with a random process X whose element is X_s, where $s \in S$ refers to a site in the image. The local conditional distribution can be written as follows:

$$\Pr(X_s = x_s | X_t = x_t, t \neq s, t \in S) = \Pr(X_s = x_s | X_t = x_t, t \in G_s) \quad (1)$$

where X and x denote the random field and a particular realization, respectively, and G_s is the local neighborhood at site s. Note that

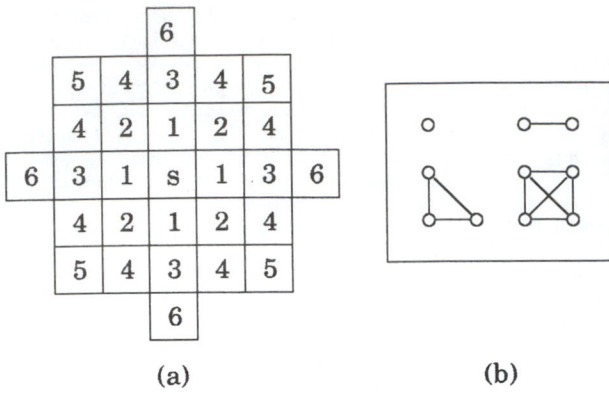

(a)   **(b)**

Figure 1. A, Neighborhood systems for MRFs. B, Cliques in MRFs.

in general, G_s can be large or small, but it is usually a local neighborhood, in keeping with the spirit of MRF modeling.

Let s be the site (i, j) and let the local neighborhood be a first-order neighborhood ($G(s)$ is the collection $(i, j + 1)$, $(i, j - 1)$, $(i + 1, j)$, $(i - 1, j)$). Then, let the conditional density take the form

$$p(X_s = x_s | X_t, t \in G_s) = \frac{1}{\sqrt{2\pi}}$$
$$\times \exp\left[-\frac{1}{2}\left(x_{ij} - \frac{1}{4}[x_{i,j+1} + x_{i,j-1} + x_{i+1,j} + x_{i-1,j}]\right)^2\right] \quad (2)$$

This is a very simple special case of the first-order Gauss-Markov model (Besag, 1974). The Gauss-Markov model has been widely used in image processing tasks (Dubes and Jain, 1989).

The MRF model consists of a set of *cliques*. A clique is a collection of sites such that any two sites are neighbors. Different orders of cliques are shown in Figure 1B. The order of a clique refers to the number of distinct sites that appear multiplicatively. We now calculate the clique energies involving the site x_{ij} by expanding the conditional probability density and collecting the terms. There are cliques of order one and two. They are

$$\frac{x_{ij}^2}{2}, \quad -\frac{x_{ij}x_{i,j+1}}{4}, \quad \text{and} \quad -\frac{x_{ij}x_{i+1,j}}{4} \quad (3)$$

The first term in Equation 3 is of order one and the latter two terms are of order two.

MRF-Gibbs equivalence

We now ask the following question: Given the conditional probability structure $\Pr(X_s = x_s | X_t = x_t, t \in G_s)$, what is the joint probability distribution $\Pr(X = x)$? This is of utmost importance, since it is the joint probability distribution and not the conditional distribution that contains the complete image representation.

Before relating the conditional and joint distributions, we introduce the concept of a Gibbs distribution, which will turn out to be crucial in specifying the relationship. A Gibbs distribution is specified by an *energy function* $E(x)$ and can be written as

$$\Pr(X = x) = \frac{1}{Z} \exp(-E(x)) \quad (4)$$

where the *partition function*

$$Z = \sum_x \exp(-E(x)) \quad (5)$$

is a normalizing constant and involves a summation over all possible configurations of X. Energy functions have been widely used

in spin-glass models of statistical physics. The minimum energy configuration corresponds to an ordered system of spins. $E(x)$ cannot take infinite values.

Our detour into Gibbs distributions is justified for the following reason. The Hammersley-Clifford theorem (Besag, 1974; Geman and Geman, 1984) states that any conditional distribution has a joint distribution, which is Gibbs (Dubes and Jain, 1989) if the following conditions hold.

Positivity: $\Pr(X = x) > 0$.
Locality: $\Pr(X_s = x_s | X_t = x_t, t \neq s, t \in S) = \Pr(X_s = x_s | X_t = x_t, t \in G_s)$.
Homogeneity: $\Pr(X_s = x_s | X_t = x_t, t \in G_s)$ is the same for all sites s.

The locality condition is the same as the Markov property described by Equation 1. The Hammersley-Clifford theorem allows us to shuttle between the conditional probability structure in Equation 1 and the joint probability in Equation 4.

The recipe for obtaining the joint density function is as follows: (1) assemble the different clique energies from the conditional probability, and (2) compute the energy function by adding up the clique energies.

We calculate the energy function for the simple first-order Gauss-Markov model:

$$E(x) = \frac{1}{2}\left(\sum_{ij}\left[x_{ij}^2 - \frac{x_{ij}x_{i,j+1}}{2} - \frac{x_{ij}x_{i+1,j}}{2}\right]\right)$$
$$= \frac{1}{8}\sum_{ij}[(x_{ij} - x_{i,j+1})^2 + (x_{ij} - x_{i+1,j})^2] \quad (6)$$

It can be seen from the energy function $E(x)$ and the conditional density that the essence of the Hammersley-Clifford theorem lies in the clique energies. We examined the conditional density and teased apart the different orders of cliques (first and second order) and the associated clique energies. Then, all clique energies were summed (taking care to count each clique only once), yielding the energy function $E(x)$. Our presentation has been quite terse, and further details on cliques and the transition from the conditional to the joint probability distribution can be found in Besag (1974), Geman and Geman (1984), and Dubes and Jain (1989).

The Prior and Degradation Models

Naturally, we are not content with merely obtaining MRF-Gibbs image models. These models can be used in a variety of image processing and analysis tasks. As mentioned previously, MRF modeling fits perfectly into a Bayesian estimation/inference paradigm. A Bayesian setup consists of two ingredients—the prior and the degradation model. The prior model is defined on the set of image attributes X that are of interest. In edge-preserving image restoration (Geman and Geman, 1984), for example, X includes the set of image intensities and a further set of binary-valued edge labels. In texture segmentation (Lakshmanan and Derin, 1989), X includes the image intensities and a set of texture labels at each location. The degradation model is a model of the physical process by which the observations are generated. Usually, we are faced with noisy and incomplete observations. Denote the set of observations by Y, and let the degradation model also be a Gibbs-Markov distribution:

$$\Pr(Y = y | X = x) = \frac{1}{Z_D(x)} \exp(-E_D(x, y)) \quad (7)$$

where

$$Z_D(x) = \sum_y \exp(-E_D(x, y)) \quad (8)$$

In general, the partition function $Z_D(x)$ is a function of the image attributes x. $E_D(x, y)$ is the energy function corresponding to the degradation model. For example,

$$E_D(x, y) = \frac{1}{2} \sum_s \left(y_s - \sum_t \mathcal{H}_{st} x_t \right)^2$$

yields a Gaussian degradation model wherein Y is obtained by blurring X with a *blur function* $\mathcal{H}$ and adding additive Gaussian noise at each site s. This type of degradation model routinely occurs in image restoration (Geman and Geman, 1984) and (with some modifications) in tomographic reconstruction (Lee et al., 1995).

A Bayesian Posterior Energy Function

Given the degradation and prior models, Bayesian estimation/inference proceeds as follows. The posterior distribution $\Pr(X = x|Y = y)$ is obtained by using Bayes's theorem:

$$\Pr(X = x|Y = y) = \frac{\Pr(Y = y|X = x)\Pr(X = x)}{\Pr(Y = y)} \quad (9)$$

Once the posterior distribution is obtained, an estimate $(\hat{X})$ of X is found by minimizing the expected cost, which is a measure of the distance between the true and estimated values:

$$C = \sum_x C(x, x^*)\Pr(X = x|Y = y) \quad (10)$$

where x^* is the true value. When the familiar squared-error cost is used, the estimator (MMSE) turns out to be the conditional mean $\mathcal{E}(X|Y = y)$ ($\mathcal{E}$ denotes the expectation operator). If the cost *equally* penalizes all x different from $x^*(C(x, x^*) = \delta_{x,x^*})$, the maximum a posteriori (MAP) estimator results.

When the degradation and prior models are Gibbs, the posterior is Gibbs as well. To see this, assume a prior energy function $E_P(x)$ giving $\Pr(X = x) = (1/Z_p) \exp(-E_P(x))$. The posterior distribution (using Equation 9) is

$$\Pr(X = x|Y = y)$$
$$= \frac{\exp(-E_D(x, y) - \log(Z_D(x)) - E_P(x))}{\sum_x \exp(-E_D(x, y) - \log(Z_D(x)) - E_P(x))} \quad (11)$$

The posterior energy function $E(x) = E_D(x, y) + \log(Z_D(x)) + E_P(x)$. In the case of the MAP estimate, the entire Bayesian estimation engine reduces to minimizing just this posterior energy function $E(x)$, since the partition function of the posterior is independent of x. However, when the MMSE estimate is desired, the expected value of X in the posterior distribution needs to be computed. This computation is usually intractable, since it involves computing the partition function of the posterior distribution.

MAP Estimation

Restricting our focus to MAP estimation, we observe that MAP estimation reduces to minimizing the posterior energy function $E(x)$. This minimization involves the different kinds of processes that make up X. For example, in edge-preserving image restoration (Geman and Geman, 1984), the process X includes both continuous-valued image intensities and binary-valued edge variables. Consequently, the minimization of the posterior objective function is a difficult problem, owing to the presence of nontrivial local minima. A general technique for finding global minima is simulated annealing (Geman and Geman, 1984; Lakshmanan and Derin, 1989) or, more recently, Markov chain Monte Carlo (MCMC) (Zhu et al., 1997), but these methods are usually computationally very intensive. A lot of effort has been expended in obtaining good suboptimal solutions to the MAP estimation problem (Yuille and

Kosowsky, 1994; Lee et al., 1995; Gold and Rangarajan 1996). Deterministic annealing (DA) is a general method that has emerged. Deterministic annealing methods begin with a modified posterior:

$$\Pr(X = x|Y = y) = \frac{1}{Z(\beta)} \exp(-\beta E(x)) \quad (12)$$

where $\beta > 0$ is the inverse temperature. Note that the partition function is now a function of the inverse temperature. The terminology is inherited from statistical physics. The idea of cooling a system slowly to reach a minimum energy configuration has a computational parallel in MRFs. The basic idea is to embed the posterior in a β exponentiated manner and to track the maximum of this posterior through a gradual increase in β. In this manner, the posterior energy function is increasingly closely approximated by a sequence of smooth, continuous energy functions.

The main reason for doing this is based on the following statistical mechanics identity:

$$F(\beta) \stackrel{def}{=} -\frac{1}{\beta} \log Z(\beta) = \mathcal{E}(E(x)) - \frac{1}{\beta} S(\beta) \quad (13)$$

where S is the entropy (defined as $-\sum_x \Pr(X = x|Y = y) \log(\Pr(X = x|Y = y))$). The entropy is proportional to the logarithm of the total number of configurations, and as the temperature is reduced (and fewer configurations become likely), it gradually goes to zero. Also, the expected value of the posterior energy goes to the minimum value of the energy. The key idea in deterministic annealing is to minimize the *free energy* F instead of $E(x)$ while reducing the temperature to zero. The free energy (at low β) is a smooth approximation to the original, nonconvex energy function and approaches $E(x)$ as β tends to infinity. However, the free energy involves the logarithm of the partition function, which is intractable! An approximation to the free energy (usually called the naive mean field approximation) is minimized instead. Although the details are beyond the scope of this article (see Geiger and Girosi, 1991; Yuille and Kosowsky, 1994; Lee et al., 1995; and Gold and Rangarajan, 1996), we present an example illustrating the method. Let the energy function contain only binary-valued variables and take the following form:

$$E(x) = \sum_{ij} T_{ij} x_i x_j + \sum_i h_i x_i, \; x_i \in \{0, 1\} \quad (14)$$

The free energy F is given by

$$F(v) = \sum_{ij} T_{ij} v_i v_j + \sum_i h_i v_i + \frac{1}{\beta} \sum_i [v_i \log(v_i)$$
$$+ (1 - v_i) \log(1 - v_i)] \quad (15)$$

where $v_i \in [0, 1]$. The free energy consists of two terms. The first term can be seen as an approximation to the expected value of the energy once the identification $v_i \approx \mathcal{E}(x_i)$ is made. Now,

$$\mathcal{E}(E(x)) = \sum_{ij} T_{ij} \mathcal{E}(x_i x_j) + \sum_i h_i \mathcal{E}(x_i) \quad (16)$$

When the expected value of the product $x_i x_j$ is replaced by the product of the expected values ($v_i v_j$), the naive mean field approximation results. The third term in Equation 15 is an approximation to the entropy. At each setting of β, Equation 15 is minimized with respect to v, after which β is increased. In this manner, a deterministic network is obtained. There are questions regarding the choice of annealing schedules and the quality of the minima obtained, and for the most part, except for very specific posterior energy functions, there is a dearth of analytical results in this area. However, the method is quite general and has been applied with varying degrees of success to a variety of image processing and analysis tasks, such as tomographic reconstruction (Lee et al., 1995), flow field segmentation (Konrad and Dubois, 1992), surface reconstruction (Geiger and Girosi, 1991), and object recognition (Gold and Rangarajan, 1996).

Parameter Estimation

So far we have concentrated on estimating X given the noisy observations Y. We have emphasized that Gibbs-Markov models are specified by local clique energies (from which the global distribution can be obtained). Consider a prior distribution

$$\Pr(X = x|\theta) = \frac{1}{Z(\theta)} \exp \left(-\frac{1}{2} \sum_k \sum_{\langle s,t \rangle_k} \theta_k (x_s - x_t)^2 \right) \quad (17)$$

where θ_k is a parameter associated with clique $\langle s, t \rangle$. Since pairwise interactions are used, a clique between pixels s and t is denoted by $\langle s, t \rangle$. This is the general form of the Gauss-Markov model. The model is a generalization of our earlier model (Equation 6) since it has the same clique form, although with a more general neighborhood structure. The partition function involves a sum over the configurations of X and is a function of θ. Other than the estimation/inference problem, we are also saddled with the problem of parameter estimation.

The parameters can be estimated by maximizing the joint probability of X with respect to the unknown parameters (Lakshmanan and Derin, 1989). In most cases, this computation is intractable in its pure form, and approximations have to be devised. The typically available approximations are pseudo-likelihood, mean-field, and MCMC. The computational requirements of the different methods range from low for pseudo-likelihood to moderate for mean-field to high for MCMC. The availability of a suitable training set is critical to both likelihood and pseudo-likelihood parameter estimation. When a training set is not available, parameter estimation and cost minimization proceed in lockstep, resulting in the so-called joint MAP procedure wherein the parameters θ and the states X are bootstrapped (Lakshmanan and Derin, 1989). From a theoretical standpoint, there are important issues of consistency and efficiency of the parameter estimates; for details, see Kashyap and Chellappa (1983).

Discussion

The MRF framework is well suited to a wide variety of image processing and analysis tasks. Our exposition has been brief, and we have ignored important issues such as validation, choice of the order of MRF models, and sizes of training sets. Validation, for example, takes us into the bias/variance dilemma (Geman, Bienenstock, and Doursat, 1992). MRF models, being parametric, introduce a certain kind of bias into the image representation. This seems to be the right kind of bias (in terms of reducing variance) for tasks like image restoration, tomographic reconstruction, and texture segmentation. However, if the order of the chosen model is incorrect, high bias could result. It is in bias/variance terms that MRF image models should be compared alongside "mechanical" (as opposed to probabilistic) models such as splines, generic representations like radial basis functions (RBFs), and tabula rasa, feedforward neural networks. Also, there are interesting similarities between Gauss-Markov models and thin-plate splines (Lee et al.,

1995; Wahba, 1990); see GENERALIZATION AND REGULARIZATION IN NONLINEAR LEARNING SYSTEMS). For example, the simple case of the first-order Gauss-Markov model with the parameters $\theta_1 = \theta_2 = (1/4)$ is identical to the discrete membrane (first-order thin-plate spline in two dimensions). Correspondences of this sort should be expected, since MRF models, splines, and RBFs impose local smoothness constraints, although in different ways. In recent years there has been increased interest in scale-space and multiresolution image processing and analysis methods. Although there are deep unresolved issues in integrating scale into Markov models, this situation has not deterred researchers from using multiresolution MRFs in specific applications (Lakshmanan and Derin, 1989; Krishnamachari and Chellappa, 1997). Finally, and very recently, interesting interrelationships have been discovered between Bayesian MAP estimation on Gibbs posterior energy functions and Bayesian belief propagation algorithms (Weiss, 2000; see GRAPHICAL MODELS: PROBABILISTIC INFERENCE).

Road Map: Vision
Related Reading: Hidden Markov Models; Probabilistic Regularization Methods for Low-Level Vision

References

Besag, J., 1974, Spatial interaction and the statistical analysis of lattice systems, *J. R. Statist. Soc. B*, 36:192–236. ◆
Dubes, R. C., and Jain, A. K., 1989, Random field models in image analysis, *J. Appl. Statist.*, 16:131–164. ◆
Geiger, D., and Girosi, F., 1991, Parallel and deterministic algorithms from MRFs: Surface reconstruction, *IEEE Trans. Pattern Anal. Machine Intell.*, 13:401–412.
Geman, S., Bienenstock, E., and Doursat, R., 1992, Neural networks and the bias/variance dilemma, *Neural Computat.*, 4:1–58.
Geman, S., and Geman, D., 1984, Stochastic relaxation, Gibbs distributions and the Bayesian restoration of images, *IEEE Trans. Pattern Anal. Machine Intell.*, 6:721–741.
Gold., S., and Rangarajan, A., 1996, A graduated assignment algorithm for graph matching, *IEEE Trans. Pattern Anal. Machine Intell.*, 18:377–388.
Kashyap, R. L., and Chellappa, R., 1983, Estimation and choice of neighbors in spatial interaction models of images, *IEEE Trans. Inform. Theory*, 29:60–72.
Konrad, J., and Dubois, E., 1992, Bayesian estimation of motion vector fields, *IEEE Trans. Pattern Anal. Machine Intell.*, 9:910–926.
Krishnamachari, S., and Chellappa, R., 1997, Multiresolution Gauss-Markov random field models for texture segmentation, *IEEE Trans. Image Proc.*, 6:251–267. ◆
Lakshmanan, S., and Derin, H., 1989, Simultaneous parameter estimation and segmentation of Gibbs random fields using simulated annealing, *IEEE Trans. Pattern Anal. Machine Intell.*, 8:786–799.
Lee, S. J., Rangarajan, A., and Gindi, G., 1995, Bayesian image reconstruction in SPECT using higher order mechanical models as priors, *IEEE Trans. Med. Imaging*, 14:669–680.
Wahba, G., 1990, *Spline Models for Observational Data*, Series in Applied Mathematics, vol. 59, Philadelphia, PA: SIAM.
Weiss, Y., 2000, Correctness of local probability propagation in graphical models with loops, *Neural Computat.*, 12:1–41.
Yuille, A. L., and Kosowsky, J., 1994, Statistical physics algorithms that converge, *Neural Computat.*, 6:341–356. ◆
Zhu, S. C., Wu, Y. N., and Mumford, D., 1997, Minimax entropy principle and its application to texture modeling, *Neural Computat.*, 9:1627–1660.

Memory-Based Reasoning

David L. Waltz

Introduction

Memory-based reasoning (MBR) refers to a family of nearest-neighbor-like methods (Dasarthy, 1991) for making decisions or classifications. MBR differs from other nearest-neighbor methods primarily in its metrics for computing the distance between examples, and in MBR's suitability for use with symbolic-valued features. Nearest-neighbor methods generally use a simple overlap distance metric, which defines distance as the number of mismatched features between two instances. MBR uses metrics related to the value distance metric (VDM), introduced in Stanfill and Waltz (1986). Considerable effort on recoding training cases is generally required in order to use neural nets on symbolic problems. In general, symbolic items need to be mapped to numerical values, feature vectors, or some related form. MBR is specifically designed to handle such cases directly; MBR uses the statistical similarity of outcomes to automatically generate similarity metrics for symbolic inputs, without the need for recoding. MBR has been used for software recommendation agents such as the Firefly (Maes and Kozierok, 1993), classification of news articles (Linoff, Masand, and Waltz, 1992) and U.S. Census Bureau long forms (Creecy et al., 1992), computational biology (Zhang, Mesirov, and Waltz, 1992; Yi and Lander, 1993; Cost and Salzberg, 1993), and a variety of other tasks. See Aha (1997) for a survey of MBR and related systems and applications, and discussions of trade-offs in case-based system design.

Comparisons of MBR and Neural Nets

Several projects have compared MBR with backpropagation neural nets. In terms of decision accuracy, MBR has often outperformed neural nets, and in some cases all the other learning methods with which it has been compared (Zhang et al., 1992; Cost and Salzberg, 1993; Rachlin et al., 1994); results for MBR are generally comparable with the best other learning methods. MBR has also been applied to cases that are beyond the representational reach of current neural net methods, such as the classification of free-text examples of arbitrary lengths (Creecy et al., 1992). Like neural nets, MBR systems can be built easily and quickly, with very little programming required. Unlike neural nets, no learning phase is necessary. Updating is therefore simple, requiring only additions, deletions, and modifications to MBR's database of examples, and decisions are always based on all known data, even the most recent. Also, unlike neural nets, MBR does not generally require elaborate re-representation schemes. MBR provides "justifications" for decisions, namely the nearest example(s) from the database, whereas considerable analysis effort is generally required to understand why a neural net system behaves as it does. Thus, debugging and tuning tend to be easier with MBR. And finally, MBR methods can provide confidence levels.

MBR does have a major disadvantage: although it does not require a training phase, MBR's decision phase is computationally expensive, and MBR systems have high memory requirements. In general, the entire database of examples is kept, whereas with neural nets, the total storage requirements for a trained net are generally much smaller than the training set used to create it. Because of this, early MBR systems were implemented on massively parallel computers or special-purpose hardware.

"Eager" Versus "Lazy" Systems

Lazy systems (such as MBR) defer classification decisions until a case is presented, while eager systems (like backpropagation and other learning systems) do most of their classification work ahead of time in a training phase (Aha, 1997). Systems intermediate between eager and lazy often have attractive properties (Kasif et al., 1998).

How Does MBR Work?

Every MBR system requires a similarity metric for judging the distance between an item to be classified and all items in the example database. If the MBR system uses k-nearest neighbors, then a scheme for combining the information from k examples is also needed. We can illustrate the idea with a simple metric, the modified value difference metric (MVDM) (Cost and Salzberg, 1993), which is similar to the ones that have been most commonly used in MBR applications. Assume the database is relational, with n-tuples consisting of $n - 1$ predictor fields ($p_1, p_2, \ldots, p_{n-1}$) plus a goal field G. (This is not the fully general case, but it is the simplest and most common one, and serves well for purposes of illustration.) Each case in the database is a vector of predictor values ($a_1, a_2, \ldots, a_{n-1}$), plus a goal G that can take on any of a finite set of values: G is an element of ($g_1, g_2, \ldots, g_m$). Then the distance between a novel situation $B = (b_1, b_2, \ldots, b_{n-1})$ and a case A from the database $A = (a_1, a_2, \ldots, a_{n-1})$, is:

$$\sum_j \left[\sum_i |\text{Prob}(g_j|b_i) - \text{Prob}(g_j|a_i)| \right]$$

where j ranges over all possible values for the goal field and i ranges over all predictor fields. To keep computation tractable, the set of goal fields may be limited, for example by only indexing over goals that correspond to database instances with non-zero overlap metrics (which are much cheaper to compute).

The MVDM metric basically compares the distribution of cases for each pair of predictor field values of A and B. The distance between A and B is small if these two-predictor field values are associated with similar distributions of goal field values.

The result of applying this metric is a rank-ordered list of cases from the database, with distance values for each. The classification proposed for the novel situation is then the goal field value of the case with the minimum distance (single neighbor case), or the goal field value whose weighted sum of distances over the k closest cases is the smallest (k-nearest-neighbor case).

NETtalk Task

MBRtalk, the first MBR system (Stanfill and Waltz, 1986), used as its main example the NETtalk database, and compared its performance with NETtalk (Sejnowski and Rosenberg, 1987). The NETtalk task is to produce pronunciations for all English words, based on a small (700-word) training set. Sejnowski and Rosenberg's NETtalk, a backpropagation system (with some special output processing), achieved a 78% letter-by-letter generalization performance. MBRtalk produced a 78% letter-by-letter generalization performance on the original NETtalk database, the same as that reported by Sejnowski and Rosenberg. MBRtalk demonstrated a 93% correct generalization using a 16,000-word corpus, a task that has not been attempted with a neural net system and one that would probably require very long training times. MBR does not require training, although it is possible to do some precalculation in order make the MBR decision phase run faster.

Protein Structure Prediction

For several years, the best protein secondary structure prediction systems were based on neural nets (Qian and Sejnowski, 1988). After considerable experimentation and tuning, Zhang et al. (1992) showed that MBR outperforms backpropagation on this task, albeit by a small margin—64.5% correct for MBR, versus 63.5% for a three-layer backpropagation system and 64.0% for a cascaded backpropagation system (Qian and Sejnowski, 1988), all using eight-way cross-validation on the same 19,861-residue database. Interestingly, MBR and neural nets agreed with each other only about 80% of the time, and both methods agreed with a statistical system with 63.5% performance about as often. A hybrid system was constructed that used a backpropagation net to combine the outputs of the three methods, yielding a performance of 66.4%, an improvement that is better than any of the others alone, with high statistical significance (Zhang et al., 1992). Current methods, often combining recurrent neural nets with MBR-like methods, perform significantly better, in the range of 76% (Baldi et al., 1999), although a considerable portion of this improvement may be the result of more complete and accurate protein databases.

Tests on UCI Repository of Machine Learning Databases

Several papers have reported results on data sets from the University of California–Irvine (UCI) repository that allow us to compare MBR, specifically the widely used PEBLS system (Cost and Salzberg, 1993), with backpropagation neural nets.

As reported in Kasif et al. (1998), PEBLS outperformed or equaled both a Bayes classifier and a Hamming distance nearest-neighbor system on six of eight tasks, and was within 1.1% on the other two tasks. This paper also showed that MBR always outperforms a Bayes classifier in domains with nonplanar decision boundaries. Neural nets outperformed MBR on small databases (soybean disease with 289 examples, iris database with 150 examples).

Discussion

MBR as a Neural Model?

It has been suggested that the cerebellum stores many examples of motor movements that can then be interpolated to provide smooth motor movements (Atkeson, Moore, and Schaal, 1997). MBR, as a variant of case-based reasoning (CBR), has been proposed as an associative memory implementation.

Why Do These Methods Perform Differently?

Generally stated, MBR and neural nets form decision surfaces differently, and so will perform differently. MBR can become arbitrarily accurate if large numbers of cases are available, and if these cases are well-behaved and properly categorized. Neural nets cannot respond well to isolated cases but tend to be good at smooth extrapolation. To give an example, consider training a NETtalk

system to pronounce the letter *p*, and assume that all *p*s are either pronounced *P* (as in *pig*) or *F* (as in *photo*) except for one example, where *p* is silent (*psychology*). Given that there are many *P* and *F* examples, these will statistically dominate the hidden units for a backpropagation net, and it is very unlikely that words beginning with *p*s will be correctly pronounced. But MBR is able to pronounce a *ps* word correctly, even with only a single near example.

For other examples, different MBR metrics can be used for systems for tasks that cannot be currently handled by neural nets. In Creecy et al. (1992), for example, a text similarity metric ("vector similarity"—basically normalized weighted word overlap) allowed an MBR system to assign keywords to Census Bureau data with free-text fields. Such a task is beyond current neural net training methods.

Road Map: Artificial Intelligence
Related Reading: Data Clustering and Learning; Pattern Recognition

References

Aha, D., Ed., 1997, *Lazy Learning* (special issue), *Artif. Intell. Rev.*, 11:7–423.

Atkeson, C., Moore, A., and Schaal, S., 1997, Locally weighted learning for control, *Artif. Intell. Rev.*, 11:75–113.

Baldi, P., Brunak, S., Frasconi, P., Pollastri, G., and Soda, G., 1999, Exploiting the past and the future in protein secondary structure prediction, *Bioinformatics*, 15:937–946.

Cost, S., and Salzberg, S., 1993, A weighted nearest neighbor algorithm for learning with symbolic features, *Machine Learn.*, 10(1):57–78. ◆

Creecy, R., Masand, B., Smith, S., and Waltz, D., 1992, Trading MIPS and memory for knowledge engineering, *Commun. ACM*, 35(8):48–64.

Dasarthy, B., 1991, *Nearest Neighbor (NN) Norms*, Washington, DC: IEEE Computer Society Press.

Kasif, S., Salzberg, S., Waltz, D., Rachlin, J., and Aha, D., 1998, A probabilistic framework for memory-based reasoning, *Artif. Intell.*, 104:287–311.

Linoff, G., Masand, B., and Waltz, D., 1992, Classifying news stories using memory based reasoning, in *Proceedings of the SIGIR Conference*, Copenhagen, pp. 59–65.

Maes, P., and Kozierok, R., 1993, Learning interface agents, in *Proceedings of the Eleventh National Conference on Artificial Intelligence*, Cambridge, MA: MIT Press, pp. 459–465.

Qian, N., and Sejnowski, T., 1988, Predicting the secondary structure of globular proteins using neural network models, *J. Mol. Biol.*, 202:865–884.

Rachlin, J., Kasif, S., Salzberg, S., and Aha, D., 1994, Towards a better understanding of memory-based and Bayesian classifiers, in *Proceedings of the Eleventh International Conference on Machine Learning*, New Brunswick, NJ, pp. 242–250.

Sejnowski, T., and Rosenberg, C., 1987, Parallel networks that learn to pronounce English text, *Complex Systems*, 1:145–168.

Stanfill, C., and Waltz, D., 1986, Toward memory-based reasoning, *Commun. ACM*, 29(12):1213–1228. ◆

Yi, T.-M., and Lander, E., 1993, Protein secondary structure prediction using nearest neighbor methods, *J. Mol. Biol.*, 232:1117–1129.

Zhang, X., Mesirov, J., and Waltz, D., 1992, A hybrid method for protein secondary structure prediction, *J. Mol. Biol.*, 225:1049–1063.

Minimum Description Length Analysis

Richard S. Zemel

Introduction

In this article, we review a variety of ways in which ideas relating to minimum description length (MDL) have been applied to neural networks. We begin with a brief introduction to the historical roots of MDL, and then describe the direct relationship between MDL and Bayesian model selection methods. We divide the applications of MDL to neural networks into two categories corresponding to the two main classes of learning in networks: supervised and unsupervised.

Historical Background

The underlying approach in MDL—applying coding theory to determine simplicity—grew out of work from the mid-1960s, when Kolmogorov, Solomonoff, and Chaitin introduced theories concerning the information content of an object. Instead of relating information to probabilities, as Shannon had (e.g., Shannon, 1948), they adopted a computational approach. They defined the information in a binary string to be the length of the shortest program with which a general-purpose computer can generate the string. The resulting algorithmic theory of information has significant implications in many areas, but it has not had much impact on the practical construction of programs, because the proposed form of information is not computable in its pure form. However, a number of learning techniques (including MDL) have been derived by making approximations to this information measure. The interested reader should consult Li and Vitanyi (1993) for a detailed mathematical review of the history of MDL and its relationship to many other current inductive inferencing techniques.

Defining the Minimum Description Length Principle

MDL can be seen as a principled version of Occam's razor, where the goal is to find the simplest accurate description of a set of data. An informal definition of the MDL principle (Rissanen, 1989) is that the best model to explain a set of data is the one that minimizes the summed length, in bits, of (1) the description of the model and (2) the description of the data, when encoded with respect to the model.

In algorithmic information theory, the model is a general computational model, i.e., a Turing machine. The MDL approach makes the problem tractable by considering particular classes of models. For example, if the goal is to infer decision trees, then the model is a decision tree, while if the goal is to learn the weights of a neural network, the model may be a network with a particular architecture. In this article, a model refers to various aspects of a network, such as its weights and activities.

It is useful to formulate MDL based on a communication protocol in which these terms are unified into a single encoded message that must be decoded in order to reproduce the data. The sender transmits a message, encoded in the description language $\mathcal{L}$, that conveys both the model M and the data D with respect to the model; this second term can be seen as the residuals, i.e., aspects of the data not predicted by the model. The standard goal of inferring an optimal M from the data is then equivalent to minimizing the length of this encoded message:

$$|\mathcal{L}(M, D)| = |\mathcal{L}(M)| + |\mathcal{L}(D \text{ using } M)| \qquad (1)$$

The notion of comparing models based on simplicity can equivalently be expressed from a Bayesian perspective. The goal is to infer a model M from a set of observations D. Bayes's theorem states that the posterior probability of a model is:

$$p(M|D) = \frac{p(M)p(D|M)}{p(D)} \qquad (2)$$

The most plausible model is then inferred by comparing these posterior probabilities:

$$\arg\max_{M} [p(M)p(D|M)] = \arg\max_{M} [\log p(M) + \log p(D|M)] \qquad (3)$$

The trade-off inherent in both these approaches between simpler, more constrained networks and more complex, general networks echoes the *bias-variance dilemma* in statistics: introducing many parameters incurs high variance, while restricting the number of parameters incurs high bias in the set of possible solutions (Geman,

Bienenstock, and Doursat, 1992). MDL and Bayesian analysis (see BAYESIAN METHODS AND NEURAL NETWORKS) offer an approach to this dilemma by formalizing the Occam's razor idea—a complex network is preferred only when its predictions are sufficiently more accurate—as an inference rule.

The link between the two objectives (Equations 1 and 3) is provided by the *optimal coding theorem* (Shannon, 1948), which states that x can be communicated at a cost that is bounded below by $-\log_2 p(x)$ bits.

Applying this theorem produces the general MDL equation:

$$-\log p(M, D) = -\log p(M) - \log p(D|M) \qquad (4)$$

Shannon's theorem describes the optimal code if the true probability distribution for a set of discrete alternatives is known. In general, however, one does not know the true distribution; so, because coding from a description language based on the wrong probability distribution will always take more bits on average, selecting an appropriate probability distribution for the codes is a key aspect of MDL applications. MDL provides a method of comparing these choices based on the resulting code lengths.

The distribution must be chosen to suit the nature of the task. For example, in a classification task, the data (given the model) consist of a number of discrete alternatives, each with some probability of occurrence. Here we can save bits by simply communicating the fact that the model output is correct on the correctly classified examples. When the information to be encoded takes on real values, a continuous distribution is required. A coding distribution that is often (implicitly) selected is a Gaussian. In this case, if we assume that the residuals (the second term in Equation 1) are independent and have a zero-mean, fixed-variance Gaussian distribution, then, if the values are encoded to some fixed accuracy, the code length is the familiar summed-squared-error cost function.

An Example of Applying MDL to Neural Networks

One of the standard approaches to improving generalization in neural networks can be formulated as an MDL technique. This approach adds an extra term to the error function that penalizes the complexity of the network, so that the objective function used to train the network involves a trade-off between the data misfit and the network complexity:

$$\text{Cost} = \alpha \text{ Complexity} + \text{Error} \qquad (5)$$

If we regard each possible weight vector of the network as a potential model, then this complexity term is simply the cost of specifying the model in the definition of MDL above.

Applying Shannon's theorem then equates the complexity of a network to the negative log probability of its weights. Thus the critical question becomes the choice of encoding scheme, or prior distribution on the weights. A simple prior is a radially symmetric, mean-zero Gaussian. Setting the variance of this Gaussian to $1/\alpha$ yields an often used complexity term—the sum of the squares of the weights, $\Sigma_j w_j^2$. Differentiating this measure produces simple weight decay in the learning rule, which forces weights with small gradients from the error term to decay away, leaving only the required weights for the task. This example points out the key role of probability distributions in MDL; now we consider other encoding distributions and see how this choice affects the models that MDL favors.

Applications of MDL to Neural Networks

The MDL principle has been applied in a wide variety of areas over the past couple of decades. With respect to neural networks, the duality between Bayesian analysis and MDL means that a range of applications of Bayesian techniques to neural networks may also be expressed in MDL terms. Few neural network methods have referred directly to minimal length encoding, but this relationship to Bayesian techniques makes many network methods relevant to this article.

We separate MDL applications into two classes involving fundamentally different formulations in terms of the communication protocol. In supervised learning, each data item consists of an input-output pair. The sender and receiver both have access to the inputs. The task of the sender is to succinctly communicate the desired outputs for each input. The network is a generative model of the output given the input; this model includes the network architecture and weights, while the data are the residuals.

In unsupervised learning, the receiver does not have access to the input, and the sender must provide enough information to allow an accurate input reconstruction. For example, in a clustering task, the sender first communicates the cluster centers (i.e., the weights of a competitive learning network). Then she only needs to say which cluster each input belongs to, and the residual error, or the distance to the cluster center. Given this information, the receiver can recover the actual input. Thus, here the network is a generative model of the input itself.

Note that this communication protocol formulation is only a device to derive an MDL objective function that can be used to train a neural network. The algorithms described below are not actually interested in sending the message, but rather in developing good models of a data set.

Supervised Learning

In supervised learning, the primary application of MDL techniques has been to improve the generalization performance of networks. Good generalization requires that the amount of information required to specify the output vectors of the training cases must be considerably larger than the number of independent parameters of the network. When only a small amount of labeled training data is available, a large network will not readily produce a good solution.

A range of techniques have been proposed to address this problem. These include weight sharing, weight/unit pruning (see LEARNING NETWORK TOPOLOGY), and cross-validation training. MDL techniques offer an alternative approach to this problem. In this section, we highlight two types of techniques. The first class assumes that the network architecture is given, and uses MDL to limit the complexity of the network weights. The second class uses MDL to select between potential network architectures.

Using MDL to determine network weights. The standard neural network training problem of finding the appropriate set of weights can usefully be formulated in MDL terms. We showed above that a radially symmetric Gaussian prior on the weights produces a weight decay term in the learning rule. Many different types of priors have been discussed in the literature. MacKay (1992) compared several priors for a single learning problem. He showed that for this problem, using the simple weight-decay prior with a different α for separate weight classes—weights into hidden units, hidden unit biases, and weights into output units—achieves better generalization than using a single α for all the weights.

More complicated priors on the weights can produce better generalization. For example, the prior could be a mixture of two zero-mean Gaussian distributions, a very wide one and a narrow one. The narrow Gaussian encourages small weight values to approach zero; the broader distribution takes responsibility for larger weights, and provides little pressure to change these values. The combined effect is to simplify the network by eliminating small weights.

The prior may also be adapted to the data. For many problems, such as translation-invariant recognition, improved network performance can be achieved by constraining particular subsets of the weights to share the same value. Nowlan and Hinton (1992) accomplished this by fitting a mixture of Gaussians to the weights, allowing the network to decide which weights should be tied together.

Finally, Hinton and van Camp (1993) extended this work to consider the general MDL objective where the cost function is the sum of two encoding costs: the weights of the network and the output error residuals. On a sample problem, coding the weights using an adaptive mixture-of-Gaussians prior allowed the network to find three sharp clusters for the weights. Discovering this structure avoided overfitting the data, as the network was able to generalize even though the number of training cases was less than the dimensionality of the input vector.

Note that the MDL objectives described above involve several hyperparameters, such as the regularization constant α controlling the trade-off between the error and the complexity terms. Several methods have been proposed for determining hyperparameters (MacKay, 1992; Neal, 1996).

Recent work has extended MDL to include hyperparameters, which allows the application of MDL principles to a different class of learning methods. MDL formalizes the Occam's razor idea of finding the simplest model for a given data set. Yet the simplest model is not always one with few parameters. Neal (1996) showed that a particular neural network in the limit of an infinite number of parameters is a Gaussian process, which is actually a simple model that can be handled tractably. Other function approximation methods use a very large set of basis functions to model the data. Rasmussen and Ghahramani (2001) show that learning using these large models can also be expressed in MDL terms, where the model description applies not to parameters but instead to the functions included in the model.

Using MDL methods to determine a network architecture. MDL methods have also been applied to evaluate network architectures (see BAYESIAN METHODS AND NEURAL NETWORKS). The weights for various network architectures are learned using an MDL objective, and then these networks are compared based on the same data fit/complexity trade-off. MacKay (1992) demonstrated how this MDL/Bayesian procedure accurately predicts the appropriate number of hidden units on a small interpolation problem, where the target is determined by examining how well the various architectures generalize to an unseen test set.

Kendall and Hall (1993) proposed an MDL approach to network construction in which the model and data misfit are encoded over a discrete space. They computed the code length of the network parameters from a histogram of the weight values; since the task is assumed to be classification, the data code length is simply the cost of specifying which training cases are incorrectly predicted by the model. The authors found that using a genetic optimization algorithm to minimize the total description length succeeded in finding optimal network architectures on some simple problems.

MDL methods have been applied to architecture selection in other areas relevant to neural networks. Stolcke and Omohundro (1993) described an algorithm for inferring the structure of a hidden Markov model that involves a Bayesian/MDL approach. The algorithm begins with a model that directly encodes the training data, and then successively merges states based on a description length criterion that penalizes models according to the number of transitions and output values at each state. In addition, the MDL principle has been applied to learn the structure and parameters of BAYESIAN NETWORKS (q.v.), (e.g., Suzuki, 1999). Roughly speaking, a Bayesian network can be viewed as a form of neural network in which the nodes correspond to random variables and the weights encode conditional distributions. Encoding a Bayesian network with n nodes entails encoding the parents of each node and its set of conditional probabilities. The MDL approach formalizes the trade-off between the simplicity of the Bayesian network structure and its ability to model the data.

Unsupervised Learning

For unsupervised learning networks, in which the goal of learning can be viewed as a form of probability density estimation, MDL techniques have been applied in several ways. The most popular approach is to use MDL to learn the number of distributions in the estimate, as well as the parameters of those distributions. A second approach involves applying MDL methods not only to the weights of the network, but also to the activities of the hidden units.

MDL and finite mixture models. A standard statistical technique for unsupervised classification can be formulated in an MDL framework. In finite mixture models, each datum in a training set is assumed to be drawn from one of J different classes. While learning the class parameters, we can also determine the optimal J by maximizing the posterior distribution of this number given the data set. This search for J resembles the architecture selection approach described above.

AutoClass (Cheeseman et al., 1988) is an unsupervised classification system based on this approach. It determines J by starting with more classes than are believed to be present and iteratively eliminating them. A prior that makes classes accounting for little data improbable can be seen as a description length prior on the model complexity. Similar approaches have been used in clustering algorithms, where a complexity term penalizing complex clusterings (based on measures such as their summed entropy) is added to create an MDL-style objective trading of data fit for model simplicity (see DATA CLUSTERING AND LEARNING).

MDL and autoencoders. In the unsupervised schemes described above, the model cost was some function of the number of underlying components in the clustering or mixture model algorithm, while the data cost was simply the summed-squared error. This represents one type of MDL objective function. If we adopt a more general viewpoint, we see that a wide range of other objective functions is possible.

In particular, we can view unsupervised learning in terms of an autoencoder (i.e., a network that attempts to reproduce its inputs on its outputs) where the MDL objective is to minimize the total cost of communicating the input vectors to a receiver. There are three terms in the description length:

- The *representation cost* is the number of bits required to communicate the representation (the hidden unit activities) that the algorithm assigns to each input vector.
- The *model cost* is the number of bits required to specify the hidden-to-output weights of the network, which provide an estimate of the input from its representation.
- The *reconstruction cost* is the number of bits required to fix up errors in the estimate of the input.

The sum of these three terms provides an objective function for training the autoencoder.

We can view many unsupervised algorithms in terms of this framework by understanding how they encode each of these three terms. For example, in competitive learning, the representation is the identity of the winning hidden unit, so the average representation cost is at most the logarithm of the number of units, while the reconstruction cost is proportional to the squared difference of the winner's weight vector and the input. Standard competitive learning algorithms minimize this latter cost, while algorithms that attempt to limit the number of clusters can be seen as trading off

representation cost for reconstruction cost. Principal Component Analysis (PCA) can be viewed as a version of MDL in which we ignore the model cost and the representation cost and minimize the reconstruction cost. Factor analysis can be viewed as a version of MDL in which we ignore the model cost but minimize the representation cost and reconstruction cost.

Many new algorithms can be derived by adopting new assumptions about the structure of the data and using them to formulate different methods of encoding the three terms in this MDL cost function. Any method that communicates each hidden activity independently will tend to lead to factorial representations, because any mutual information between hidden units will cause redundancy in the communicated message, so the pressure to keep the message short will squeeze out the redundancy. Zemel (1994) and Hinton and Zemel (1994) describe algorithms derived from this MDL approach for learning factorial representations; Zemel and Hinton (1995) describe how this MDL approach can also be used to develop population codes in which the activities of hidden units are locally correlated so as to form a topographical map. See UNSUPERVISED LEARNING WITH GLOBAL OBJECTIVE FUNCTIONS for a discussion of other algorithms that can be expressed within the MDL framework.

Discussion

MDL methods have been applied in a variety of neural network training paradigms, both for learning the weights and for assembling the architecture. These methods involve selecting a class of models and an encoding scheme for the two terms in the description: the model and the data. Given these elements, an appropriate objective function can be constructed for either an unsupervised or a supervised learning problem. Because of a common underlying framework, many Bayesian inferencing methods can also be viewed in MDL terms.

Many important issues remain to be explored in this area. One key issue concerns when it is better to use other methods of improving generalization, such as stopping training based on performance on a validation set, versus using an MDL-based regularization. In the unsupervised learning area, an open problem concerns formulating appropriate priors for learning hierarchical representations. Finally, an area that is ripe for MDL applications is temporal learning, in which MDL can be used to develop concise models that can accurately predict sequential events.

Road Map: Learning in Artificial Networks
Related Reading: Bayesian Methods and Neural Networks; Helmholtz Machines and Sleep-Wake Learning; Learning Network Topology; Unsupervised Learning with Global Objective Functions

References

Cheeseman, P., Kelly, J., Self, M., Stutz, J., Taylor, W., and Freeman, D., 1988, AutoClass: A Bayesian classification system, in *Proceedings of the Fifth International Conference on Machine Learning*, pp. 54–62.

Geman, S., Bienenstock, E., and Doursat, R., 1992, Neural networks and the bias/variance dilemma, *Neural Computat.*, 4:1–58.

Hinton, G. E., and van Camp, D., 1993, Keeping neural networks simple by minimizing the description length of the weights, in *Sixth ACM Conference on Computational Learning Theory*, Santa Cruz, CA.

Hinton, G. E., and Zemel, R. S., 1994, Autoencoders, minimum description length, and Helmholtz free energy, in *Advances in Neural Information Processing Systems 6* (J. D. Cowan, G. Tesauro, and J. Alspector, Eds.), San Mateo, CA: Morgan Kaufmann, pp. 3–10.

Kendall, G., and Hall, T., 1993, Optimal network construction by minimum description length, *Neural Computat.*, 5:210–212.

Li, M., and Vitanyi, P. M. B., 1993, *An Introduction to Kolmogorov Complexity and Its Applications*, Reading, MA: Addison-Wesley.

MacKay, D., 1992, A practical Bayesian framework for backpropagation networks, *Neural Computat.*, 4:448–472.

Neal, R., 1996, *Bayesian Learning for Neural Networks*, New York: Springer-Verlag. ◆

Nowlan, S. J., and Hinton, G. E., 1992, Simplifying neural networks by soft weight sharing, *Neural Computat.*, 4:173–193.

Rasmussen, C. E., and Ghahramani, Z., 2001, Occam's razor, in *Advances in Neural Information Processing Systems 13* (T. Leen, T. Dietterich, and V. Tresp, Eds.), Cambridge, MA: MIT Press, pp. 294–300.

Rissanen, J., 1989, *Stochastic Complexity in Statistical Inquiry*, Singapore: World Scientific Publishing.

Shannon, C. E., 1948, A mathematical theory of communication, *Bell System Tech. J*, 27:379–423, 623–656.

Stolcke, A., and Omohundro, S., 1993, Hidden Markov model induction by Bayesian model merging, in *Advances in Neural Information Processing Systems 5* (S. J. Hanson, J. D. Cowan, and C. L. Giles, Eds.), San Francisco: Morgan Kaufmann, pp. 11–18.

Suzuki, J., 1999, Learning Bayesian belief networks based on the minimum description length principle: Basic properties, *IEICE Transactions, Fundamentals*, E82-A, 9.

Zemel, R. S., 1994, A minimum description length framework for unsupervised learning, Ph.D. diss., University of Toronto.

Zemel, R. S., and Hinton, G. E., 1995, Developing population codes by minimizing description length, *Neural Computat.*, 7:549–564.

Model Validation

Joachim M. Buhmann

Introduction

Mathematical models of interacting neuronal assemblies occur in brain theory and neural networks research in various ways. In *computational neuroscience*, highly sophisticated and detailed computer models of neurobiological phenomena are developed to gain insight into the complex nonlinear behavior of interacting neuronal populations and synaptic circuitry. The key question—how well does a selected neural network model describe the neurobiology of a neuronal population studied in vivo, i.e., the interactions and the dynamics of living neurons?—should be answered in the tradition of the biological sciences and of scientific investigations into neurobiological phenomena (see PERSPECTIVE ON NEURON MODEL COMPLEXITY). In artificial neural networks, assemblies of neuronal units are combined to represent statistical estimators for supervised learning tasks, i.e., classification and regression, or they model the data source under investigation in an unsupervised fashion by self-organizing maps (see SELF-ORGANIZING FEATURE MAPS), recurrent networks (see RECURRENT NETWORKS), or even more complicated structures.

In both situations the data analyst tries to infer functional dependencies from empirical data (Vapnik, 1982). The usefulness of a model is determined by its ability to capture those properties of the real world that are of interest to the data analyst. Mathematically, we have to measure or estimate the difference between the neurobiological system under investigation and our model simulation. A good model fit should reproduce the behavior of the studied system in the relevant parameter range that is supposed to be explained by the model study. Outside of this parameter range we tolerate large deviations between the model system and the real system. In computational neuroscience as well as in artificial neural networks (ANNs), the model complexity has to be controlled to avoid the following two modeling errors: too simplistic models usually miss essential features of the considered process or system (underfitting), whereas too complicated models adapt to stochastic fluctuations in the data without revealing reliable and useful knowledge (overfitting).

The trade-off between too simple and too complex models is systematically studied in statistics. The statistical literature on simulation (see Deaton, 1988) distinguishes the following five steps in the design of a well-planned simulation study: (1) system identification, (2) model development, (3) model verification, (4) model validation, and (5) model analysis. The first three items in the list summarize the necessary design steps to build a qualitatively correct model. After identifying the essential functional dependencies of a system and their parametric description, the modeler is in a position to develop a conceptual abstraction of these relations. It is important for the success of a simulation study, in particular for model development, to explicitly state the scientific questions that should be answered by the conceptual model. The complexity of reality is never fully captured by the model world, and the modeler should ensure that the conceptual abstraction is appropriate to understand the relevant scientific issues under discussion. In step 3, an implementation of this abstraction has to be verified to guarantee that the computer simulation reflects the behavior and properties of the model. After ensuring the correctness of the implementation, we validate the model in the fourth step by comparing the simulated behavior with observations of the real system. The last step describes the indirect study of real-world phenomena by studying the behavior of the simulation model. The crucial step (step 4) between the model synthesis part (steps 1–3) and the analysis part (step 5) assesses how appropriate the model is to gain insight in the real-world system. In the most likely case of an imperfect model with deviations between model and reality, the *model quality* must be measured by an appropriate weighting according to the relevance of these deviations for answering the scientific questions under investigation. Models might even be developed for one scientific question but be found, on validation, to be more appropriate for another phenomenon than originally intended. For example, the Ising model was supposed to capture the essential collective features of magnetism, but it seems to work even better in studies of surface adhesion, while the wide use of Ising models in neural network theory was never anticipated by his designer.

Model Quality

How should we compare the model's behavior with the real-world system? We will look into this question first for simulation models in general and then for the more restricted class of probabilistic models for classification and regression.

The deviation of a simulation model from its counterpart in the real world is difficult to quantify, since it strongly depends on the purpose of the model. For the sake of concreteness, let us assume that we have implemented a network of locally coupled neurons of the FitzHugh-Nagumo type (Koch, 1999), a simplified version of the Hodgkin-Huxley equations for neuronal dynamics. This level of detail—two coupled nonlinear ordinary differential equations per neuron—is likely too crude for an experimental physiologist who studies depolarization effects in the cell membrane of neurons at the level of ion channel dynamics, but the same model might be more than adequate to analyze collective synchronization phenomena, even at a quantitative level. It is important to emphasize that the fine details of neural dynamics should be taken into consideration in the case of a physiological study, and therefore deviations between simulations and experiments should be weighted more strongly than in a simulation study of the collective behavior of many coupled BvP oscillators.

The underlying scientific issue of the sufficient explanatory power of a model and its necessary simplicity is traditionally studied in the philosophy of science. The limits—how scientific theories should be designed and compared with reality—are investigated in the *theory of knowledge*, also known as epistemology. Different concepts and ideas have been proposed to explain how general laws can be inducted from a finite number of empirical observations. Since a logically conclusive inductive principle is considered to be impossible, philosophers of empiricism, in particular Karl Popper (1968), have focused on the concept of falsifiability of theories. Models and theories should be designed in such a way that they can be tested, and the degree of empirical testability should allow us to measure how well a theory has been confirmed by experimental observations. In the case of very complex models, the *Turing test* provides a crude experimental procedure to quantify the appropriateness of a model. A panel of experts is asked to distinguish between the real system and its model on the basis of the respective outputs or measurements of system parameters. Statistical tests can then be used to quantify the significance of the experts' answers and their deviations from chance events. A perfect simulation is reached if the experts are unable to distinguish between the real system and its simulation model in a statistically significant way.

A much simpler situation exists in *supervised learning* of classifiers and regression functions. The model quality of regression is defined by the expected deviation between the regression function $f(x; \theta)$ and the random variable y, which characterizes the noise-perturbed functional dependency under consideration. The regression function $f(x; \theta) \in \mathcal{H}$ is an element of an application-dependent hypothesis (function) class $\mathcal{H}$, which is indexed by θ. The true model θ_0 is often assumed to be perturbed by additive noise $y(x) = f(x; \theta_0) + \eta(x)$ with $\mathbf{E}[\eta(x)] = 0$, $\mathbf{E}[\eta(x)^2] = \sigma^2$ in regression, or by classification noise $y(x) = f(x; \theta_0)$ with probability $1 - p$ and $y(x) = 1 - f(x; \theta_0)$ with probability p. The joint probability $\Pr(x, y)$ of the data point x and the random variable y weights the influence of data on the model quality and determines the expected risk:

$$R(\theta) = \int \ell(y, f(x; \theta)) \Pr(x, y) dx dy \qquad (1)$$

The most popular choices of loss functions for regression and classification are the quadratic loss $\ell(x, f) = (y - f(x; \theta))^2$ and the classification error $\ell(x, f) = \mathbf{1}(y \neq f(x; \theta))$ (0–1 loss), respectively. The goal of regression validation is to estimate the minimum $\theta^* = \arg \min_\theta \mathbf{E}[R(\theta)]$ on the basis of a training sample set $\mathscr{X} := \{(x_1, y_1), \ldots, (x_n, y_n)\}$ without explicit knowledge of the joint distribution $\Pr(x, y)$. The true model $f(x; \theta_0)$ does not necessarily have to be an element of $\mathcal{H}$. The induction principle *empirical risk minimization* (ERM) advocates calculating the minimum of the empirical risk:

$$\hat{R}(\theta; \mathscr{X}) = \frac{1}{n} \sum_{i=1}^{n} \ell(y_i, f(x_i; \theta)) \qquad (2)$$

i.e., the empirical risk minimizer $\hat{\theta} := \arg \min_\theta \hat{R}(\theta; \mathscr{X})$ is used as an estimate of the expected risk minimizer θ^*.

Model Complexity and Model Selection

The validation of models in statistical learning of classifiers and regression curves is inspired by Popper's philosophy of science and the requirement that scientific theories be falsifiable. Vapnik and Chervonenkis (see Vapnik, 2000) have analyzed the nature of statistical learning and have identified necessary and sufficient conditions for learning classifiers by empirical risk minimization. They analyzed the probability $\Pr(R(\hat{\theta}) - R(\theta^*) > \varepsilon)$ that the expected risk of the classifier with minimal empirical risk $\hat{\theta}$ exceeds the best classifier in the hypothesis class θ^* by more than a constant ε in costs or risk. In the case of a finite hypothesis class, the probability of this large deviation is bounded by the cardinality of $\mathcal{H}$ times a fit factor that decays exponentially fast with the size n of the sample set (see Devroye, Györfi, and Lugosi, 1996), i.e.,

$$\Pr(R(\hat{\theta}) - R(\theta^*) > \varepsilon) \leq$$
$$|\mathcal{H}| \sup_{f(.;\theta) \in \mathcal{H}} \Pr(|\hat{R}(\theta) - R(\theta)| > \varepsilon/2) \equiv \delta \qquad (3)$$

where the probability on the right-hand side scales as $\mathbb{O}(\exp(-\lambda n))$. The trade-off between the complexity term $|\mathcal{H}|$ and the model-fitting factor $\sup_{f(.;\theta) \in \mathcal{H}} \Pr(|\hat{R}(\theta) - R(\theta)| > \varepsilon/2)$ allows us to determine a necessary sample size $n_0(\varepsilon, \delta)$ of the training set given the hypothesis class $\mathcal{H}$. Too complex hypothesis classes yield very loose bounds on the large deviations, despite the fact that we have used the best-performing classifier on the training data. Too simple hypothesis classes, on the other hand, introduce a significant model mismatch or bias, and they constrain the parameter space so severely that the signal in the data might not be captured by the learning algorithm.

How can we measure the complexity of a model when the cardinality is infinite, e.g., the space of polynomial discriminant functions of degree p or smaller? Obviously, the complexity depends on the degrees of freedom that are available to adapt to signal properties of the data set. To measure the complexity of a model, statisticians have developed sophisticated mathematical techniques from combinatorics and functional analysis. A very crude but for many practical applications sufficient rule of thumb counts the number of parameters in the model and requires that we provide at least ten data points per parameter to estimate the model. This rule implicitly assumes that all parameters increase the complexity of the model by an approximately constant amount. Consequently, applied statisticians have advocated adding a complexity penalty to the quality measure, which is linear in the number of parameters, like the AIC or the BIC criterion (see Hastie, Tibshirani, and Friedman, 2001). From estimating regression curves, however, we know that the slope of a linear regression function and the frequency of a trigonometric function add a vastly different amount of complexity to the model class. That is, oscillatory functions with a sufficiently high frequency allow us to approximate all data points in a bounded range with arbitrarily high precision, whereas linear functions cannot in general interpolate more than two points. The concept of covering numbers of function spaces measures this effect and relates the fitting power of functions to general properties of the underlying hypothesis (function) class. The *Vapnik-Chervonenkis dimension* and the *fat-shattering dimension* (Anthony and Bartlett, 1999) (see VAPNIK-CHERVONENKIS DIMENSION OF NEURAL NETWORKS) are derived parameters that measure the complexity of a hypothesis class for classification and regression independent of the probability distribution of the data.

Cross-Validation and Bootstrap

Cross-Validation

Apart from analytical techniques to derive bounds on the validity of models, a large number of numerical techniques have been developed to validate statistical models. Numerical methods for model validation split the data into three different subsets, the training set for parameter estimation, the validation set for selection of the model class, and the test set for estimation of the prediction error. The validation set is used for training if the model class has been selected a priori. One of the most widely used techniques in classification and regression is the *k-fold cross-validation* method, which gains statistical precision at the expense of computation. The data set is split into k subsets of approximately equal size. The learning algorithm uses $k - 1$ of these subsets to estimate the model parameters, e.g., to find the empirical risk minimizer based on the data of these $k - 1$ subsets. The data of the kth subset, which have been set aside for model testing, are then used to estimate the model quality on future data. This procedure can be repeated k times, resulting in k different estimators. There exists a rich literature on how these different estimators can be combined, ranging from averages with different weighting schemes in regression (model averaging) to majority votes in classification. Popular versions of cross-validation are fivefold or tenfold cross-validation.

The validation set is required in cases where we not only have to estimate model parameters but also have to select an appropriate model order, e.g., to decide whether we should use a model with four parameters or one with five or more parameters. In such a data analysis scenario, we first train the model on the basis of the training data, then we validate our choice of the model order based on the estimated prediction error for the validation data. The model order with the best performance on the validation data is then selected. At the end of the data analysis process, the test data set is used to estimate the prediction error of the selected model, e.g., how well the selected model performs on future data. Using the test data rather than the validation data for model order selection—an unfortunately common practice among applied data analysts—usually leads to an overly optimistic estimate of the model error, since a selection bias in favor of low errors obscures the true error of the model.

Bootstrap

One of the drawbacks of cross-validation is the loss of training data for validation and testing. In the small-sample-size scenario, which occurs quite often in practical data analysis problems, we have too few data compared to the desired model complexity, and therefore we cannot afford to set aside some data exclusively for testing. Efron (see Efron and Tibshirani, 1993; Davison and Hinkley, 1997) has proposed a *resampling scheme with replacements*, called *bootstrap*, which is schematically summarized in Figure 1. Conceptually, we replace the unknown true probability distribution of the

data with the available empirical distribution. Sampling from this empirical distribution generates B bootstrap sample sets $Z^{*b} = \{(x_1^{*b}, y_1^{*b}), \ldots, (x_n^{*b}, y_n^{*b})\}$, $1 \le b \le B$. A reasonable number B of bootstrap samples is between 25 and 200. Note that the bootstrap samples are not just permutations of each other, since we sample with replacements. Each of these bootstrap sample sets allows us to fit a model by estimating the model parameters with statistics S, e.g., the sample means, variances, or medians for mixture models. Finally, we combine these B bootstrap models by an appropriate averaging or merging procedure to derive an averaged model with supposedly more robust behavior than any single model.

To estimate the quality of the models fitted by bootstrapping, we choose those data in the training samples for testing that have not been selected for the bootstrap sample. Using the complete training sample set Z for testing would result in an overly optimistic model quality, since a fraction of approximately $(1 - 1/e)n \approx 0.632n$ of the data have been used in the bootstrap sample for model fitting. Improved and more robust estimators of model quality have been suggested by Efron and others, which are known as the $S^{(.632)}$ estimator and variants of it (Hastie et al., 2001).

Discussion

Model validation in inference defines the core problem in learning and statistical estimation. When we induce a general model from a finite number of samples, we have to consider the complexity of the model in relation to the amount of data available for inference. Too complex models feign a high quality on small sample sets that is not confirmed on (future) test data. Analytical and numerical methods have been proposed over the last 40 years of neural network research to bound the deviations between empirical and expected risk of a statistical model. Bounds of the VC type usually contain a complexity term that accounts for the richness and flexibility of the hypothesis class, and a fitting term that measures the contraction of measure due to the large number of samples. Both influences have to be controlled, either by numerical methods like cross-validation and bootstrap or by analytical techniques from computational learning theory. The trade-off between model complexity and goodness of fit and its relation to the computational complexity of learning remains one of the deep challenges for future research on learning.

Road Map: Learning in Artificial Networks
Related Reading: Data Clustering and Learning; Vapnik-Chervonenkis Dimension of Neural Networks

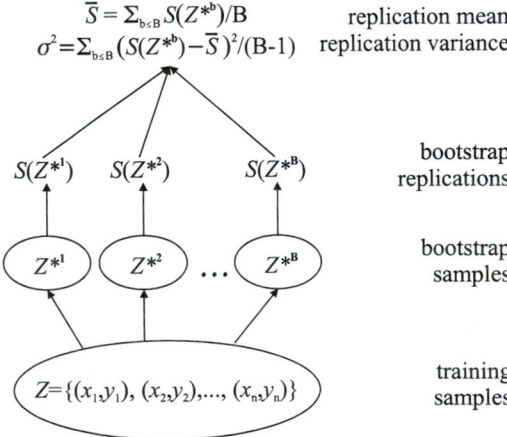

$$\overline{S} = \Sigma_{b \le B} S(Z^{*b})/B \qquad \text{replication mean}$$
$$\sigma^2 = \Sigma_{b \le B}(S(Z^{*b}) - \overline{S})^2/(B-1) \qquad \text{replication variance}$$

$S(Z^{*1}) \quad S(Z^{*2}) \quad S(Z^{*B})$ — bootstrap replications

$Z^{*1} \quad Z^{*2} \ldots Z^{*B}$ — bootstrap samples

$Z = \{(x_1, y_1), (x_2, y_2), \ldots, (x_n, y_n)\}$ — training samples

Figure 1. Processing pipeline of bootstrap estimation via bootstrap samples Z^{*b} and their associated statistics $S(Z^{*b})$.

References

Anthony, M., and Bartlett, P. L., 1999, *Neural Network Learning: Theoretical Foundations*, Cambridge, Engl.: Cambridge University Press.
Davison, A. C., and Hinkley, D. V., 1997, *Bootstrap Methods and Their Application*, Cambridge, Engl.: Cambridge University Press.
Deaton, M. L., 1988, Validation of simulation models, in *Encyclopedia of Statistical Sciences*, (S. Kotz and N. L. Johnson, Eds.), New York: Wiley, vol. 8, pp. 481–484.
Devroye, L., Györfi, L., and Lugosi, G., 1996, *A Probabilistic Theory of Pattern Recognition*, New York: Springer-Verlag. ◆
Efron, B., and Tibshirani, R., 1993, *An Introduction to the Bootstrap*, London: Chapman and Hall. ◆
Hastie, T., Tibshirani, R., and Friedman, J., 2001, *The Elements of Statistical Learning*, New York: Springer-Verlag. ◆
Koch, C., 1999, *Biophysics of Computation*, Oxford, Engl.: Oxford University Press.
Popper, K., 1968, *The Logic of Scientific Discovery*, New York: Harper.
Vapnik, V. N., 1982, *Estimation of Dependences Based on Empirical Data*, New York: Springer-Verlag.
Vapnik, V. N., 2000, *The Nature of Statistical Learning Theory*, 2nd ed., New York: Springer-Verlag.

Modular and Hierarchical Learning Systems

Michael I. Jordan and Robert A. Jacobs

Introduction

In this article we discuss the problem of learning in modular and hierarchical systems. Modular and hierarchical systems allow complex learning problems to be solved by dividing the problem into a set of subproblems, each of which may be simpler to solve than the original problem. Within the context of supervised learning—our focus in this article—modular architectures arise when we assume that the data can be well described by a collection of functions, each of which is defined over a relatively local region of the input space. A modular architecture can model such data by allocating different modules to different regions of the space. Hierarchical architectures arise when we assume that the data are well described by a multiresolution model—a model in which regions are divided recursively into subregions.

Modular and hierarchical systems present an interesting credit assignment problem—it is generally the case that the learner is not provided with prior knowledge of the partitioning of the input space. Knowledge of the partition would correspond to being given "labels" specifying how to allocate modules to data points. The assumption we make is that such labels are absent. The situation is reminiscent of the unsupervised clustering problem in which a classification rule must be inferred from a data set in which the class labels are absent, and indeed, the connection to clustering has played an important role in the development of the supervised learning algorithms that we present here.

The learning algorithms that we describe solve the credit assignment problem by computing a set of values—posterior probabilities—that can be thought of as estimates of the missing "labels." These posterior probabilities are based on a probabilistic model associated with each of the network modules. This approach to learning in modular systems was developed by Jacobs et al. (1991). Jordan and Jacobs (1994) extended the modular system to a hierarchical system, made links to the statistical literature on classification and regression trees (Breiman et al., 1984), and developed an Expectation-Maximization (EM) algorithm for the architecture. We describe these developments in the remainder of the article, emphasizing the probabilistic framework.

The Mixture-of-Experts (ME) Architecture

The modular architecture that we consider is shown in Figure 1. The architecture is composed of N modules referred to as *expert networks*, each of which implements a parameterized function $\mu_i = f(\mathbf{x}, \theta_i)$ from inputs $\mathbf{x}$ to outputs μ_i, where θ_i is a parameter vector. We attach a probabilistic interpretation to each of the expert networks by assuming that the experts generate outputs $\mathbf{y}$ with probability $P(\mathbf{y}|\mathbf{x}, \theta_i)$, where μ_i is the mean of the conditional density P.

Because we assume that different expert networks are appropriate in different regions of the input space, the architecture requires a mechanism that identifies, for any given input $\mathbf{x}$, that expert or blend of experts that is most likely to produce the correct output. This is accomplished via an auxiliary network, known as a *gating network*, that produces as output a set of scalar coefficients g_i that serve to weight the contributions of the various experts. These coefficients are not fixed constants but vary as a function of the input $\mathbf{x}$.

The probabilistic interpretation of the gating network is as a *classifier*, a system that maps an input $\mathbf{x}$ into the probabilities that

the various experts will be able to generate the desired output (based on knowledge of $\mathbf{x}$ alone). These probabilities (the g_i) are constrained to be nonnegative and sum to one (for each $\mathbf{x}$).

There are many ways to enforce the probabilistic constraints on g_i. One approach is to utilize the *softmax* function, defined as follows. Let ξ_i denote an intermediate set of variables that are parameterized functions of the input $\mathbf{x}$:

$$\xi_i = \xi_i(\mathbf{x}, \eta) \tag{1}$$

where η is a parameter vector, and define the outputs g_i in terms of ξ_i as follows:

$$g_i = \frac{e^{\xi_i}}{\sum_j e^{\xi_j}} \tag{2}$$

It is readily verified that the g_i are nonnegative and sum to one for each $\mathbf{x}$. This approach has the virtue of having a simple probabilistic interpretation: the ξ_i can be viewed as discriminant surfaces for a classification problem in which the class-conditional densities are members of the exponential family of probability distributions (Jordan and Jacobs, 1994).

The Mixture Model

Let us now specify the probabilistic model underlying the mixture-of-experts architecture more precisely. We assume that the training set $\mathcal{X} = \{(\mathbf{x}^{(l)}, \mathbf{y}^{(l)})\}_{l=1}^L$ is generated in the following way. Given the choice of an input $\mathbf{x}$, a label i is chosen with probability $P(i|\mathbf{x}, \eta^0)$ (where the superscript 0 denotes the putative true values of the parameters). Given the choice of the label and given the input, the target output $\mathbf{y}$ is assumed to be generated with probability $P(\mathbf{y}|\mathbf{x}, \theta_i^0)$. Each such data point is assumed to be generated independently in this manner.

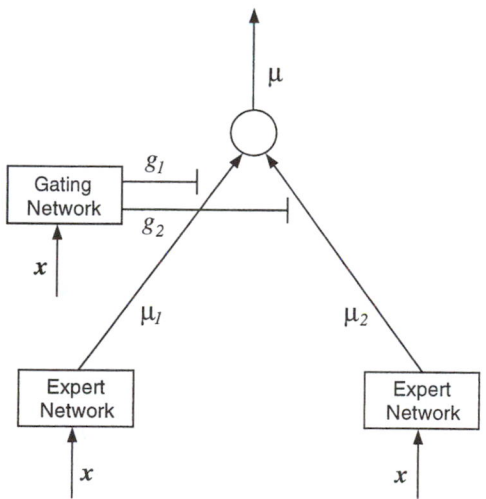

Figure 1. A mixture-of-experts architecture. The output μ is the conditional mean of $\mathbf{y}$ given $\mathbf{x}$ (see text).

Note that a given output **y** can be generated in N different ways, corresponding to the N different choices of the label i. Thus, the total probability of generating **y** from **x** is given by the sum over i:

$$P(\mathbf{y}|\mathbf{x}, \Theta^0) = \sum_i P(i|\mathbf{x}, \eta^0)P(\mathbf{y}|\mathbf{x}, \theta_i^0) \qquad (3)$$

where Θ^0 denotes the vector of all of the parameters ($\Theta^0 = [\theta_1^0, \theta_2^0, \dots, \theta_N^0, \eta^0]^T$). The density in Equation 3 is known as a *mixture density*. It is a mixture density in which the mixing proportions, $P(i|\mathbf{x}, \eta^0)$, are conditional on the input **x**.

It is the task of the gating network to model the probabilities $P(i|\mathbf{x}, \eta^0)$, which can be construed as class probabilities in a multiway classification problem of the input **x**. We parameterize these probabilities via Equations 1 and 2, identifying the gating network outputs g_i with $P(i|\mathbf{x}, \eta)$.

It is straightforward to compute moments of the mixture density. For example, the conditional mean $\mu = E(\mathbf{y}|\mathbf{x}, \Theta)$ is readily obtained by taking the expected value of Equation 3:

$$\mu = \sum_i g_i \mu_i$$

where μ_i is the conditional mean associated with the probability distribution $P(\mathbf{y}|\mathbf{x}, \theta_i^0)$. The conditional mean is quite commonly used as the output of supervised learning systems, and this is reasonable in the mixture-of-experts setting as well, but only when no more than one value g_i is significantly different from zero for a given input **x**. When more than one expert has a large value of $\mathbf{g}_i$, however, the conditional distribution of **y** given **x** is multimodal, and it is important to make fuller use of the entire mixture density in such cases.

A Gradient-Based Learning Algorithm

To develop an algorithm for estimating the parameters of a mixture-of-experts architecture, we make use of the maximum likelihood (ML) principle. That is, we choose parameters for which the probability of the training set given the parameters (a function known as the *likelihood*) is largest. Taking the logarithm of the product of N densities of the form of Equation 3 yields the following log likelihood:

$$l(\mathcal{X}, \Theta) = \sum_l \log \sum_i P(i|\mathbf{x}^{(l)}, \eta)P(\mathbf{y}^{(l)}|\mathbf{x}^{(l)}, \theta_i) \qquad (4)$$

a function that we wish to maximize with respect to Θ. One approach to maximizing the log likelihood is to use gradient ascent (a better approach is to use the EM algorithm, as discussed in a later section). Computing the gradient of l with respect to μ_i and ξ_i yields:

$$\frac{\partial l}{\partial \mu_i} = \sum_l h_i^{(l)} \frac{\partial}{\partial \mu_i} \log P(\mathbf{y}^{(l)}|\mathbf{x}^{(l)}, \theta_i) \qquad (5)$$

and

$$\frac{\partial l}{\partial \xi_i} = \sum_l (h_i^{(l)} - g_i^{(l)}) \qquad (6)$$

where $h_i^{(l)}$ is defined as $P(i|\mathbf{x}^{(l)}, \mathbf{y}^{(l)})$. In deriving this result, we have used Bayes' rule:

$$P(i|\mathbf{x}^{(l)}, \mathbf{y}^{(l)}) = \frac{P(i|\mathbf{x}^{(l)})P(\mathbf{y}^{(l)}|\mathbf{x}^{(l)}, i)}{\sum_j P(j|\mathbf{x}^{(l)})P(\mathbf{y}^{(l)}|\mathbf{x}^{(l)}, j)}$$

where we have omitted the parameters to simplify the notation. This suggests that we define $h_i^{(l)}$ as the *posterior probability* of the

ith label, conditional on the input $\mathbf{x}^{(l)}$ and the output $\mathbf{y}^{(l)}$. Similarly, the probability $g_i^{(l)}$ can be interpreted as the *prior probability* $P(i|\mathbf{x}^{(l)})$, the probability of the ith label, given only the input $\mathbf{x}^{(l)}$. Given these definitions, Equation 6 has the natural interpretation of moving the prior probabilities toward the posterior probabilities.

An interesting special case is an architecture in which the expert networks and the gating network are linear and the probability density associated with the experts is a Gaussian with identity covariance matrix. In this case, Equations 5 and 6 yield the following on-line learning algorithm (on-line meaning that we have dropped the summation across l):

$$\Delta\theta_i = \rho h_i^{(l)}(\mathbf{y}^{(l)} - \mu_i^{(l)})\mathbf{x}^{(l)^T} \qquad (7)$$

and

$$\Delta\eta_i = \rho(h_i^{(l)} - g_i^{(l)})\mathbf{x}^{(l)^T} \qquad (8)$$

where ρ is a learning rate. Note that both of these equations have the form of the classical LMS rule, with the updates for the experts in Equation 7 being modulated by their posterior probabilities.

It is also of interest to examine the expression for the posterior probability in the Gaussian case:

$$h_i^{(l)} = \frac{g_i^{(l)}e^{-1/2(\mathbf{y}^{(l)} - \mu_i^{(l)})^T(\mathbf{y}^{(l)} - \mu_i^{(l)})}}{\sum_j g_j^{(l)}e^{-1/2(\mathbf{y}^{(l)} - \mu_j^{(l)})^T(\mathbf{y}^{(l)} - \mu_j^{(l)})}} \qquad (9)$$

This is a normalized distance measure that reflects the relative magnitudes of the residuals $\mathbf{y}^{(l)} - \mu_i^{(l)}$. If the residuals for expert i are small relative to those of the other experts, then $h_i^{(l)}$ is large, otherwise, $h_i^{(l)}$ is small. Note, moreover, that the $h_i^{(l)}$ are positive and sum to one for each $\mathbf{x}^{(l)}$; this implies that credit is distributed to the experts in a competitive manner.

It is straightforward to utilize other members of the exponential family of densities as component densities for the experts, to allow dispersion (e.g., covariance) parameters to be incorporated in the model and to estimate the dispersion parameters via the learning algorithm (Jordan and Jacobs, 1994; Jordan and Xu, 1995).

The Hierarchical Mixture-of-Experts (HME) Architecture

The ME architecture solves complex function approximation problems by allocating different modules to different regions of the input space. This approach can have advantages for problems in which the modules are simpler than the large network that would be required to solve the problem as a whole. If we now inquire about the internal structure of a module, however, we see that the same argument can be repeated. Perhaps it is better to split a module into simpler submodules rather than to use a single module to fit the data in a region. This suggests a thoroughgoing divide-and-conquer approach to supervised learning in which a tree-structured architecture is used to perform multiple nested splits of the input space (Figure 2). The splitting process terminates in a set of expert networks at the leaves of the tree, which, because they are defined over relatively small regions of the input space, can fit simple (e.g., linear) functions to the data. This hierarchical architecture, suggested by Jordan and Jacobs (1994), has close ties to the classification and regression tree models in statistics and machine learning (e.g., Breiman et al., 1984). Indeed, the architecture can be viewed as a probabilistic variant of such models.

The mathematical framework underlying the HME architecture is essentially the same as that underlying the ME architecture. We simply extend the probability model to allow nested sequences of labels to be chosen, corresponding to the nested sequence of re-

Figure 2. A two-level binary hierarchical architecture. The top-level gating network produces coefficients g_i that effectively split the input space into regions, and the lower-level gating networks produce coefficients $g_{j|i}$ that effectively split these regions into subregions. The expert networks fit surfaces within these nested regions. Deeper trees are formed by expanding the expert networks recursively into additional gating networks and subexperts.

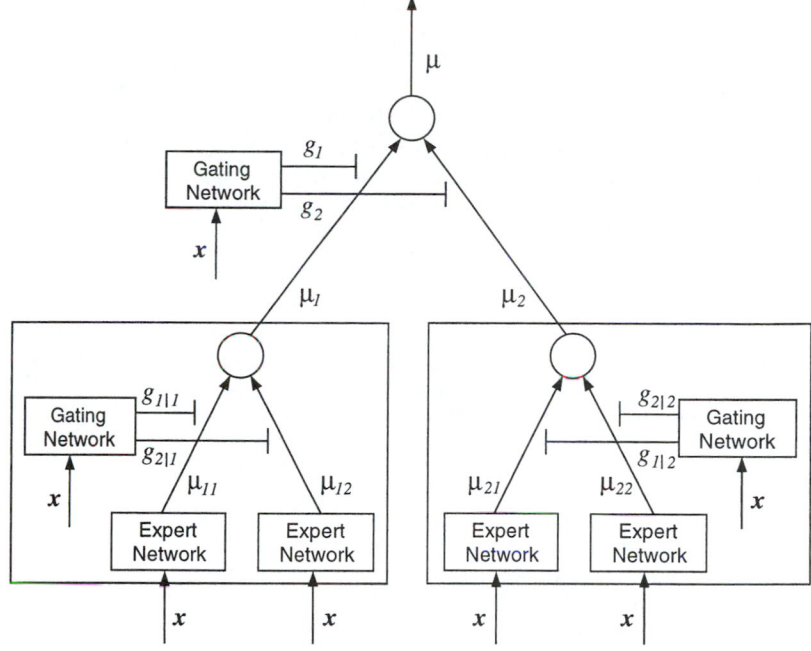

gions needed to specify a leaf of the tree. The probability model for a two-level tree is as follows:

$$P(\mathbf{y}|\mathbf{x}, \Theta) = \sum_i P(i|\mathbf{x}, \eta) \sum_j P(j|i, \mathbf{x}, \mathbf{v}_i) P(\mathbf{y}|\mathbf{x}, \theta_{ji}) \quad (10)$$

which corresponds to a choice of label i with probability $P(i|\mathbf{x}, \eta)$, followed by a conditional choice of label j with probability $P(j|i, \mathbf{x}, \mathbf{v}_i)$. This probability model yields the following log likelihood function:

$$l(\mathcal{X}, \Theta) = \sum_l \log \sum_i P(i|\mathbf{x}^{(l)}, \eta) \sum_j P(j|i, \mathbf{x}^{(l)}, \mathbf{v}_i) P(\mathbf{y}^{(l)}|\mathbf{x}^{(l)}, \theta_{ji}) \quad (11)$$

where, as in the one-level case, the prior probabilities $g_i^{(l)} = P(i|\mathbf{x}^{(l)}, \eta)$ and $g_{j|i}^{(l)} = P(j|i, \mathbf{x}^{(l)}, \mathbf{v}_i)$ are defined in terms of underlying variables ξ_i and ξ_{ij} using the softmax function (cf. Equation 2). We also use Bayes' rule to define posterior probabilities in the obvious way:

$$h_i^{(l)} = \frac{g_i^{(l)} \sum_j g_{j|i}^{(l)} P(\mathbf{y}^{(l)}|\mathbf{x}^{(l)}, \theta_{ij})}{\sum_j g_j^{(l)} \sum_k g_{k|j}^{(l)} P(\mathbf{y}^{(l)}|\mathbf{x}^{(l)}, \theta_{jk})} \quad (12)$$

and

$$h_{j|i}^{(l)} = \frac{g_{j|i}^{(l)} P(\mathbf{y}^{(l)}|\mathbf{x}^{(l)}, \theta_{ij})}{\sum_j g_{j|i}^{(l)} P(\mathbf{y}^{(l)}|\mathbf{x}^{(l)}, \theta_{ij})} \quad (13)$$

The posterior probability $h_i^{(l)}$ can be viewed as the credit assigned to the ith nonterminal in the tree, and the posterior probability $h_{j|i}^{(l)}$ is the credit assigned to the branches below the nonterminals. The product $h_i^{(l)} h_{j|i}^{(l)}$ is therefore the credit assigned to expert (i, j).

A recursive relationship is available to compute the posterior probabilities efficiently in deep trees. The recursion proceeds upward in the tree, passing the denominator of the conditional posterior upward, multiplying by the priors, and normalizing (cf. the computation of h_i from $h_{j|i}$ in Equations 12 and 13).

We obtain a gradient ascent learning algorithm by computing the partial derivatives of l. If, as in the previous section, we assume linear experts and a linear gating network, as well as Gaussian probabilities for the experts, we obtain the following LMS-like learning algorithm:

$$\Delta\theta_{ji} = \rho h_i^{(l)} h_{j|i}^{(l)} (\mathbf{y}^{(l)} - \mu_{ij}^{(l)}) \mathbf{x}^{(l)T} \quad (14)$$

$$\Delta\eta_i = \rho(h_i^{(l)} - g_i^{(l)}) \mathbf{x}^{(l)T} \quad (15)$$

and

$$\Delta\mathbf{v}_{ji} = \rho h_i^{(l)} (h_{j|i}^{(l)} - g_{j|i}^{(l)}) \mathbf{x}^{(l)T} \quad (16)$$

Each of these partial derivatives have a natural interpretation in terms of credit assignment. Credit is assigned to an expert by taking the product of the posterior probabilities along the path from the root of the tree to the expert (cf. Equation 14). The updates for the gating networks move the prior probabilities at a nonterminal toward the corresponding posterior probabilities, weighting these updates by the product of the posterior probabilities along the path from the root of the tree to the nonterminal in question (cf. Equation 16).

An EM Algorithm

Jordan and Jacobs (1994) have derived an Expectation-Maximization (EM) algorithm for estimating the parameters of the ME and HME architectures. (See McLachlan and Krishnan, 1997, for a general treatment of the EM algorithm.) This algorithm, an alternative to gradient methods, is particularly useful for models in which the expert networks and gating networks have simple parametric forms. Each iteration of the algorithm consists of two phases: (1) a recursive propagation upward and downward in the tree to compute posterior probabilities (the *E-step*), and (2) solution of a set of local weighted maximum likelihood problems at the nonterminals and terminals of the tree (the *M-step*). Jordan and Jacobs (1994) tested this algorithm on a nonlinear system identification problem (the forward dynamics of a four-degrees-of-freedom robot arm) and reported that it converges rapidly, converging nearly two orders of magnitude faster than backpropagation in a comparable multilayer perceptron network.

Discussion

Mixtures of experts should be compared to ensemble methods such as bagging and boosting (see ENSEMBLE LEARNING), which provide another general approach to building a supervised learning architecture out of collections of simple learners. In bagging and boosting, the overall input-output mapping is a convex combination of the members of the ensemble, much as in the case of mixtures of experts (in which the conditional mean is a convex combination of the outputs of the experts). However, the weights in this convex combination are constants in the case of bagging and boosting, whereas they are functions of the input for mixtures of experts. Moreover, in the mixture of experts, the weights have an interpretation as prior probabilities under a probabilistic mixture model and are explicitly parameterized as such. In particular, under this model, a single expert is assumed to be associated with each data point, an assumption that is not made for the ensemble methods. In essence, the mixture of experts approaches the supervised learning problem via a divide-and-conquer methodology reminiscent of unsupervised clustering, whereas ensemble methods approach the problem via superposition and averaging.

We conclude with a brief list of pointers to additional papers. The problem of model selection for HME architectures has been addressed by a number of authors. Several papers propose the use of greedy search procedures combined with some form of penalization for model complexity (Ramamurti and Ghosh, 1996; Saito and Nakano, 1996; Fritsch, Finke, and Waibel, 1997). Bayesian approaches for model selection or model averaging have also been presented, including methods based on Gibbs sampling (Jacobs, Peng, and Tanner, 1997) and variational approximation (Waterhouse, MacKay, and Robinson, 1994).

Theoretical analyses of the approximation and estimation rates for the ME (Zeevi, Meir, and Maiorov, 1998) and the HME (Jiang and Tanner, 1998) are available. A basic result is that the HME achieves an approximation rate of $O(m^{-2/s})$, where m is the number of experts and s is the dimensionality of the input vector. Jordan and Xu (1995) present an analysis of the convergence rate for the EM algorithm for the HME. Kang and Oh (1997) provide an analysis of the HME using tools from statistical physics; in particular, they show that successive partitions in the HME can be analyzed as phase transitions.

There is a broad literature on engineering applications of the HME architecture, including applications to state-space filtering, optimization, control, vision, speech recognition, speaker identification, and time series analysis. Recent biological applications of the ME architecture have been presented by Haruno, Wolpert, and Kawato (2001), who describe an architecture for human motor control based on a mixture of experts in which each expert is a paired forward-inverse model, and by Erickson and Kruschke (1998), who used the mixture of experts to build a model of human category learning that combines rule-based and exemplar-based representations.

Road Map: Learning in Artificial Networks
Related Reading: Competitive Learning; Sensorimotor Learning

References

Breiman, L., Friedman, J. H., Olshen, R. A., and Stone, C. J., 1984, *Classification and Regression Trees*, Belmont, CA: Wadsworth International.
Erickson, M. A., and Kruschke, J. K., 1998, Rules and exemplars in category learning, *J. Exp. Psychol. Gen.*, 127:107–140.
Fritsch, J., Finke, M., and Waibel, A., 1997, Adaptively growing hierarchical mixtures of experts, in *Advances in Neural Information Processing Systems*, vol. 9 (M. Mozer, M. Jordan, and T. Petsche, Eds.), Cambridge, MA: MIT Press.
Haruno, M., Wolpert, D. M., and Kawato, M., 2001, MOSAIC model for sensorimotor learning and control, *Neural Computat.*, 13:2201–2220.
Jacobs, R. A, Jordan, M. I., Nowlan, S. J., and Hinton, G. E., 1991, Adaptive mixtures of local experts, *Neural Computat.*, 3:79–87. ◆
Jacobs, R. A., Peng, F., and Tanner, M. A., 1997, A Bayesian approach to model selection in hierarchical mixtures-of-experts architectures, *Neural Netw.*, 10:231–241.
Jiang, W., and Tanner, M. T., 1998, Hierarchical mixtures-of-experts for exponential family regression models: Approximation and maximum likelihood estimation, *Ann. Statist.*, 27:987–1011.
Jordan, M. I., and Jacobs, R. A., 1994, Hierarchical mixtures of experts and the EM algorithm, *Neural Computat.*, 6:181–214. ◆
Jordan, M. I., and Xu, L., 1995, Convergence properties of the EM approach to learning in mixture-of-experts architectures, *Neural Netw.*, 8:1409–1431.
Kang, K., and Oh, J.-H., 1997, Statistical mechanics of the mixture of experts, in *Advances in Neural Information Processing Systems*, vol. 9 (M. Mozer, M. Jordan, and T. Petsche, Eds.), Cambridge, MA: MIT Press.
McLachlan, G. J., and Krishnan, T., 1997, *The EM Algorithm and Extensions*, New York: Wiley.
Ramamurti, V., and Ghosh, J., 1996, Structural adaptation in mixture of experts, in *Proceedings of the 13th International Conference on Pattern Recognition*, Los Alamitos, CA: IEEE Computer Society Press.
Saito, K., and Nakano, R., 1996, A constructive learning algorithm for an HME, in *Proceedings of the IEEE International Conference on Neural Networks*, pp. 1268–1273.
Waterhouse, S., MacKay, D., and Robinson, T., 1994, Bayesian methods for mixtures of experts, in *Advances in Neural Information Processing Systems*, vol. 8 (D. S. Touretzky, M. C. Mozer, and M. E. Hasselmo, Eds.), Cambridge, MA: MIT Press.
Zeevi, A., Meir, R., and Maiorov, V., 1998, Error bounds for functional approximation and estimation using mixtures of experts, *IEEE Trans. Inform. Theory*, 44:1010–1025.

Motion Perception, Elementary Mechanisms

David C. Burr

Introduction

Visual motion is essential for many aspects of biological function, including rapidly detecting predators and prey, navigating through the visual environment, and constructing a three-dimensional visual representation from two-dimensional retinal input. However, motion information is not provided by the instantaneous retinal signal, but has to be computed from temporal variations in luminance over the image. Although the neural mechanisms that achieve this vary considerably throughout the animal kingdom, the underlying principles of the algorithms seem to be very similar.

Models of Motion Perception

In biological visual systems, motion is initially analyzed in parallel by arrays of local motion detectors that exhibit certain basic properties: they require at least two spatially separate sampling units, one delayed with respect to the other, that are combined (usually nonlinearly) to create directional selectivity. Werner Reichardt (1961) was the first to provide a formal model of a motion detector based on these principles, in what has become know as a "correlator-type" model, or more simply, the *Reichardt detector*. The detector, at its simplest, is illustrated in Figure 1. The response of two spatially separated units ($\Delta\varphi$ apart) are multiplied together (at M), after one has been delayed by ϵ. The figure illustrates two such units arranged as mirror images, symmetrically, using the same input. The unit on the left will respond best to rightward motion, maximally for speeds of $\Delta\varphi/\epsilon$; that on the right will respond best to leftward velocities of $\Delta\varphi/\epsilon$. Each unit M can be considered to be an elementary motion detector, in that it shows a direction preference. However, by combining the output of two such mirror-symmetrical units (subtractively in this case), the direction selectivity is further enhanced, to produce what is referred to as the *full Reichardt detector*.

The essential components of the Reichardt detector—spatial and temporal asymmetries and cross-correlation—can be implemented in many different ways. The initial model was inspired by the fly visual system, in which the two sampling points are adjacent ommatidia, and the temporal delay ϵ is introduced by some form of delay line, typically a low-pass filter. Models of human motion have been heavily influenced by the application of Fourier analysis to vision research, showing spatial and temporal filtering of the visual input at early stages. For moving stimuli, detectors are tuned in both space and time, leading to spatiotemporally oriented filters, or receptive fields. This concept has proven invaluable, not only in constructing physiologically plausible models of motion perception, but also in explaining how the form of moving objects is encoded (Burr and Ross, 1986).

One specific example of a model based on this concept is shown in Figure 2. The model starts with spatiotemporally oriented receptive fields tuned to a finite band of spatial and temporal frequencies, and hence to motion in a given direction (corresponding to a preferred orientation in the spatiotemporal plane). The orientation in space-time is readily achieved by linear combination of filters with appropriate spatial and temporal phase-shifts. In the particular model shown in Figure 2, the output of two such filters in quasi-quadrature phase in space and time, is squared then summed, to produce what has been termed "unidirectional motion energy." This model responds to a drifting sinusoidal grating with a constant response, strongest when the velocity of the sinusoid corresponds to the orientation of the spatiotemporal receptive field,

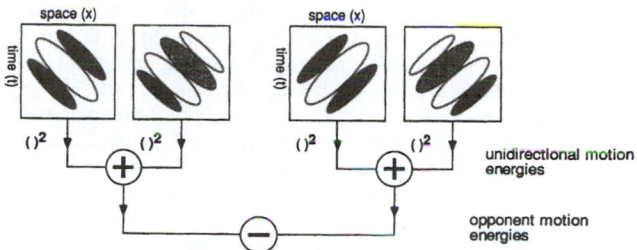

Motion Energy Model

space (x)   time (t)   unidirectional motion energies   opponent motion energies

Figure 2. An example of a motion detector based on filters oriented in space-time. (Reproduced with permission from Adelson and Bergen, 1985.)

and weakest when in the orthogonal orientation (opposite direction). However, like the simple Reichardt detector, such a motion unit is not in itself a true motion detector, in that it will respond to many stationary transient stimuli, such as to a briefly flashed pattern of appropriate spatial frequency. Further specificity is achieved by inhibition between opponent motion energies, either by subtraction, as shown here, or by division. Interestingly, the full version of the motion energy model is formally equivalent to the full Reichardt motion detector, elaborated to include a spatial and temporal filtering stage, even though no part of the Reichardt detector corresponds to the unidirectional motion energy extractors (Adelson and Bergen, 1985).

Physiological measurements of neurons in macaque monkey visual cortex have identified plausible neural substrates for the two stages of the motion energy model (Qian and Andersen, 1994). Cells in the primary visual cortex V1 show directional selectivity, but also respond well to bidirectional motion; this is consistent with the expected performance of the first stage. However, cells in the middle temporal area (MT) show a strong inhibition by motion in the nonpreferred direction, consistent with opponent motion stage of the model. FMRI studies in humans provide support for this suggestion: V1 responds more strongly to counterphased sinusoidal gratings (that can be considered as the sum of two opposing drifting gratings) than to a single component drifting grating; whereas in MT complex, the result is reversed, with a much stronger response to the single component (Heeger et al., 1999).

Velocity Tuning

The selectivity to speed of the two motion detectors of Figures 1 and 2 can be varied by changing either the temporal or the spatial characteristics. For the Reichardt detector, the preferred speed can be increased either by increasing the spacing $\Delta\varphi$ between the two sampling points, or by decreasing the delay ϵ. Similarly, for the energy model, where the spatial and temporal offsets are given by phase shifts, preferred speed will depend on both spatial and temporal frequency preference. In humans, it is possible to measure spatial and temporal selectivity, using a variety of techniques, including "masking," in which one measures contrast sensitivity to a "test" stimulus in the presence of a high-contrast "mask." The assumption is that the mask will cause maximum desensitization when its spatiotemporal characteristics match that of the detector responding to the test. To study motion perception, the test stimuli were drifting sinusoidal gratings of variable spatial and temporal frequency, displayed together with mask gratings, also varying in spatial and temporal frequency (Anderson and Burr, 1985). Over a wide range of spatial frequencies (0.025 c/deg to 15 c/deg), maximal masking occurs when the frequency of the mask matches that of the test. This suggests that there exist a battery of detectors with

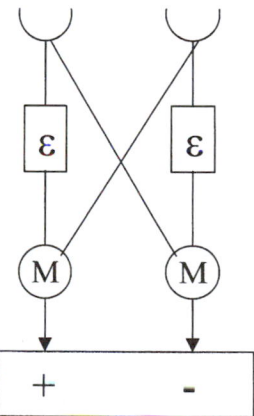

Figure 1. Simplified "full Reichardt detector." (Adapted from Reichardt, 1961.)

preferred spatial frequency varying over this entire range, so that for any given test frequency the most sensitive detector will be tuned to that frequency; the most effective mask will therefore also be of that spatial frequency. For test frequencies lower than 0.025 c/deg or higher than 15 c/deg, maximum masking occurs not at the frequency of the test, but at 0.025 and 15 c/deg, respectively, suggesting that there do not exist motion detectors tuned to frequencies outside these bounds; a test of 0.01 c/deg will be detected by a mechanism tuned to 0.025 c/deg, so the most effective mask will be tuned to 0.025 c/deg, not 0.1 c/deg. In the temporal domain, the results are quite different. Maximal masking always occurs for masks near 10 Hz, irrespective of the temporal frequency of the test, implying that there is not a range of temporal tuning, but all detectors have similar temporal properties. Taken together, the results imply that in human vision, the variation in speed tuning is achieved not by varying temporal characteristics of the motion detector, but by varying spatial frequency preference, over a 600-fold range.

What is the range of speeds to which humans are sensitive? The lowest speed at which direction can accurately be discriminated is about 1 min/s for small stimuli moving over the fovea. This threshold increases steadily with eccentricity, reaching 8–10 min/s at 90° eccentricity (largely explained by the optical degradation in the periphery). However, the upper limit of motion detection is not a fixed speed but, as may be expected from the previous paragraph, varies considerably with the spatial frequency content of the stimuli (Burr and Ross, 1982). This is brought out clearly in Figure 3, showing contrast sensitivity (inverse of contrast thresholds) for biphasic bars (signal cycles of sinusoid) of various sizes, as a function of drift speed (abscissa). The small bars were seen best (required least contrast to discriminate their direction) when moving slowly, and could not be resolved at all at speeds above 100 deg/s. The largest bars, however, were best seen when moving at 500 deg/s, and could still be reliably resolved at 10,000 deg/s. Thus, the upper limit of motion perception is not so much a speed limit as a temporal frequency limit. The large variation in receptive field size ensures that human motion perception can operate over an extremely wide range of speeds, spanning nearly six orders of magnitude (0.015 to 10,000 deg/s).

Apparent Motion

Much of the motion we view daily at the cinema and on television is not real motion but an illusion created by displaying a series of still pictures in rapid succession (24 Hz for cinema, 60 Hz for NSTC television). This type of motion is referred to as "apparent motion," "stroboscopic motion," or, most accurately, "sampled motion." For some time it was thought that apparent motion may be detected by different processes from those detecting real motion, but recent studies find little justification for this view. Most motion detectors that incorporate spatiotemporal filtering will respond well to sampled motion, provided the sampling rate is sufficiently high. The spatiotemporal trajectory for apparent motion is a row of dots in space-time. If the spatiotemporal receptive fields (Figure 2) are oriented parallel to this trajectory, they will integrate the discrete samples, effectively causing the motion to become continuous (Burr and Ross, 1986).

The minimum theoretical sampling rate is given by the Nyquist limit, which requires that the image be sampled at at least twice the temporal frequency of image motion. Sampling below this frequency will cause *aliasing*, well-illustrated by the so-called "wagon-wheel" effect: periodic moving stimuli, such as wagon wheels in Westerns, are seen to stop and reverse direction as the wagon accelerates. When the repetition frequency of spokes exceeds half the sampling frequency (12 Hz for cinema), it will be undersampled, creating strong aliasing in the form of erroneous motion. The conditions under which sampled motion is indistinguishable from smooth motion can be predicted quantitatively from measurements of contrast sensitivity and linear systems analysis (Burr, Ross, and Morrone, 1986). Sampling a motion signal introduces spurious artifacts, whose frequency and amplitude depend on the sampling rate. Psychophysical measurements show that subjects are able to distinguish sampled from smooth motion if and only if the spurious frequencies produced by the sampling regime are not resolvable, as determined by measuring their thresholds for isolated sinusoids.

The spatiotemporally oriented receptive fields not only allow for the perception of discontinuous motion, but can also cause the image to be interpolated between the positions where it is displayed on each sample. The extrapolation is extremely accurate, and works over long ranges. Indeed, this property can be used to generate complex spatial forms from temporal information alone (Burr and Ross, 1986). When moving forms pass behind a "virtual slatted fence" (allowing information to be displayed only at discrete points), the visual system interpolates between the display points to give the impression of complete spatial forms. Thus, motion detectors not only encode velocity information about moving objects, but also participate in their spatial analysis.

Chromatic and Second-Order Motion

The examples discussed so far refer to motion of objects or images defined by luminance, typically bright or dark lines, sinusoidal grat-

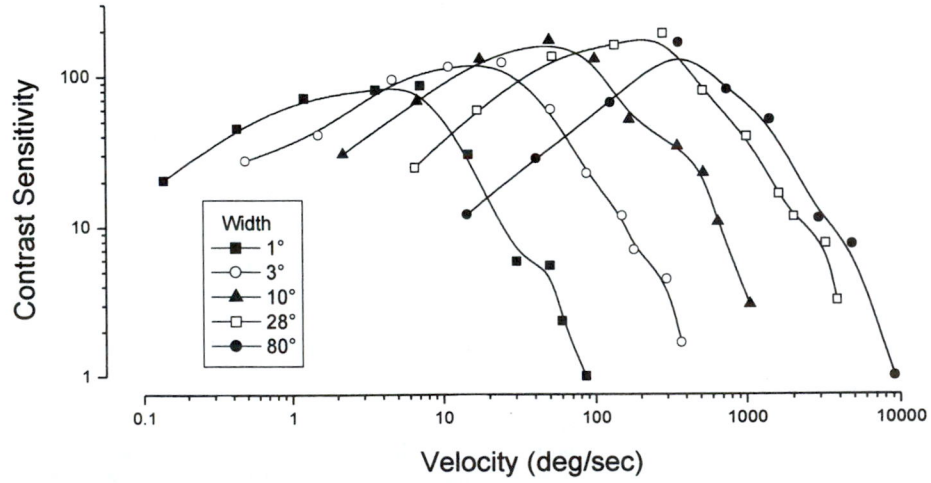

Figure 3. Contrast sensitivity for detecting the direction of motion biphasic bars of various sizes, as a function of speed. (Reproduced from Burr and Ross, 1982).

ings, or random dot patterns. However, luminance is not the only way to delineate objects: others include color, texture, and depth, and all these attributes can support motion. A well-studied example is the equiluminant class of stimuli, defined only by chromatic contrast. Movement of these stimuli yields a sensation of motion, albeit slower and jerkier than that for luminance patterns (Cavanagh, 1991).

Another very common stimulus in recent years is the class defined by variations in contrast, rather than luminance, giving rise to what is now called "second-order" motion (Chubb and Sperling, 1988). A typical example of second-order motion is a field of random dots multiplied (or amplitude-modulated) by a broad moving stimulus, typically a sinusoid. The interesting aspect of this stimulus is that although it gives rise to a strong and compelling sense of motion, neither the Reichardt detector of Figure 1 nor the motion-energy detector of Figure 2 would respond to it. However, a fairly simple extension can render both models sensitive to second-order motion: all that is needed is a "texture detector," a filter responding to contrast instead of luminance, at the front stage, and the model will respond to amplitude-modulated motion. The "texture detector" need not be complicated: a simple half- or full-wave rectifier would suffice. It is still a debated point whether first- and second-order motions are detected by different neural structures, or by essentially the same mechanism with an add-on front-end texture detector. Evidence exists for both possibilities, such as mutual induction of aftereffects between the different types of motion, and differential selective activation during fMRI.

Two-Dimensional Motion

The models shown previously are essentially one-dimensional, discriminating leftward from rightward motion. There are various ways of extending these models to cover the two spatial dimensions, such as constructing many such units with spatial subfields oriented in various directions. Further spatial selectivity can be achieved by extending the spatial filters, or receptive fields, orthogonally to their direction of motion selectivity, emulating the physiological characteristics of receptive fields of mammalian vision. However, these two-dimensional motion units will demonstrate an inherent ambiguity about stimulus direction, usually referred to as the "aperture problem." This stems from the fact that motion along a given trajectory can be decomposed into vectors spanning a range of 180°, so a vast range of detectors will be stimulated by any given trajectory (Figure 4). Various schemes have

been proposed for disambiguating the problem, usually involving the combination of signals from more than one detector, either in the form of a "vector sum" of motion units, or "intersection of constraints." There is physiological evidence that the primate visual system adopts one of these schemes (Movshon et al., 1985). When stimulated with "plaids" (two orthogonal sinusoidal gratings) drifting in various directions, neurons in primary visual cortex V1 respond best when the direction of drift is such as to orient one or other of the components appropriately for that neuron, irrespective of the pattern drift. However, in the motion-specialized area MT, neurons respond best when the global motion of the plaid is in the appropriate direction, even though each component is then 45° off-axis. This suggests that as well as being responsible for the opponent stage of the motion detector, MT may help to disambiguate the two-dimensional direction of motion signals.

Other solutions have been proposed for the aperture problem, including the novel suggestion of Bill Geisler (1999; see also Burr, 2000). Geisler points out that given the temporal integration of the visual system, a small, localized target will leave a motion streak, much like the "speed lines" used by cartoonist to caricaturize motion. These static streaks provide potential information to disambiguate direction. A series of masking and motion aftereffect studies suggests that this spatial information is in fact integrated with motion information, and may help disambiguation. Another quite different class of experiment has shown that spatial structure of a certain type of moiré pattern can bias otherwise truly apparent motion, showing the influence of static structure on motion direction. Interestingly, however, although the moving streaks may be used to help sense motion, they are not perceived as streaks by the visual system. Although we integrate over time for 120 ms or so, the smear left by moving objects is far less, quite unlike what a camera with that shutter speed would record (Burr and Ross, 1986). Our motion detectors are based on receptive fields that are oriented in space-time, aligning themselves with the motion trajectory, and this should reduce the perceived blur.

This article has concentrated on basic motion mechanisms, the early mechanisms that analyze motion locally. Local-motion signals are combined in various ways, depending on the task. Analysis of optic flow requires integration of local-motion signals over large areas and complex trajectories. On the other hand, the ability to see transparent motion, and to localize accurately the position of small moving objects, requires that the local signals are kept distinct. How these conflicting goals are achieved is the subject of much modern research into motion perception.

Road Map: Vision
Related Reading: Directional Selectivity; Global Visual Pattern Extraction; Motion Perception: Navigation; Visual Cortex: Anatomical Structure and Models of Function

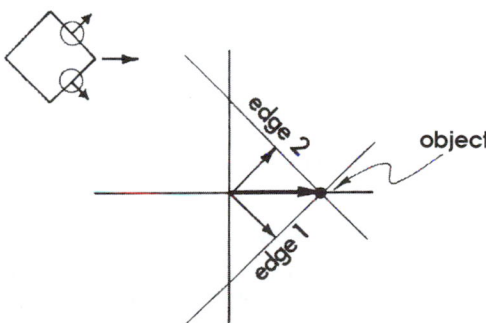

Figure 4. Illustration of the inherent ambiguity of two-dimensional motion. As the diamond moves rightward, the motion of the edges, within the receptive fields indicated by the circles, is diagonally upward or downward. In primate cortex, cells in V1 respond to the "component motion" of the edges, while some (but not all) cells in motion area MT respond to the direction of global motion (rightward).

References

Adelson, E. H., and Bergen, J. R., 1985, Spatiotemporal energy models for the perception of motion, *J. Opt. Soc. Am.*, A2:284–299.

Anderson, S. J., and Burr, D. C., 1985, Spatial and temporal selectivity of the human motion detection system, *Vision Res.*, 25:1147–1154.

Burr, D. C., 2000, Motion vision: Are "speed lines" used in human visual motion? *Curr. Biol.*, 10(12):R440–R443. ◆

Burr, D. C., and Ross, J., 1982, Contrast sensitivity at high velocities, *Vision Res.*, 23:3567–3569.

Burr, D. C., and Ross, J., 1986, Visual processing of motion, *Trends in Neuroscience*, 9:304–306. ◆

Burr, D. C., Ross, J., and Morrone, M. C., 1986, Smooth and sampled motion, *Vision Res.*, 26:643–652.

Cavanagh, P., 1991, Vision at equiluminance, in *Visual Function and Dys-*

function: Volume 5 (J. Cronly-Dillon, Ed.), London: Macmillan, pp. 234–250. ◆

Chubb, C., and Sperling, G., 1988, Drift-balanced random stimuli: A general basis for studying non-Fourier motion perception, *J. Opt. Soc. Am.*, A5:1986–2007.

Geisler, W. S., 1999, Motion streaks provide a spatial code for motion direction, *Nature*, 400:65–69.

Heeger, D. J., Boynton, G. M., Demb, J. B., Seidemann, E., and Newsome, W. T., 1999, Motion opponency in visual cortex, *J. Neurosci.*, 19:7162–7174.

Movshon, J. A., Adelson, E. H., Gizzi, M. S., and Newsome, W. T., 1985, The analysis of moving visual patterns, in *Pattern Recognition Mechanisms* (R. G. C. Chagas and C. Gross, Eds.), The Vatican, Pontificiae Academiae Scientiarum Scripta Varia, pp. 117–151.

Qian, N., and Andersen, R., 1994, Transparent motion perception as detection of unbalanced motion signals. II. Physiology, *J. Neurosci.*, 14:7367–7380.

Reichardt, W., 1961, Autocorrelation, a principle for evaluation of sensory information by the central nervous system, in *Sensory Communications* (W. Rosenblith, Ed.), New York: John Wiley, pp. 303–317.

Motion Perception: Navigation

Constance S. Royden and Ellen C. Hildreth

Introduction

When an observer moves through the world, the resulting image motion on the retina, known as *optical flow*, can inform the observer about his own motion through space and about the three-dimensional (3D) structure and motion of objects in the scene. This information is essential for tasks such as the visual guidance of locomotion through the environment and the manipulation and recognition of objects.

This article focuses on the recovery of observer motion from optical flow. We include strategies for detecting moving objects and avoiding collisions, discuss how this information may be used to control actions, and describe the neural mechanisms underlying heading perception.

The Image Flow Field

This section describes the relationship between two-dimensional (2D) image motion and the 3D translation and rotation of the observer relative to the scene. The mechanisms for deriving the 2D image velocities that result when the observer or objects move are described elsewhere (Hildreth and Koch, 1987; Mitiche and Bouthemy, 1996; see also MOTION PERCEPTION: ELEMENTARY MECHANISMS).

Consider an observer moving relative to a stationary scene, with a coordinate system fixed to the observer and the *z*-axis directed along the optical axis. The instantaneous translation of the observer can be expressed in terms of translation along three orthogonal directions, given by the vector $\mathbf{T} = (T_x, T_y, T_z)^T$. Observer rotation can be expressed in terms of rotation around each of these axes, given by $\mathbf{R} = (R_x, R_y, R_z)^T$. Let $\mathbf{P} = (X, Y, Z)^T$ be the position of a point in space, as shown in Figure 1. The 3D velocity of $\mathbf{P}$ in the observer's coordinate frame is given by

$$\mathbf{V} = (\dot{X}, \dot{Y}, \dot{Z})^T = -\mathbf{T} - \mathbf{R} \times \mathbf{P}$$

where

$$\dot{X} = -T_x - R_y Z + R_z Y$$
$$\dot{Y} = -T_y - R_z X + R_x Z$$
$$\dot{Z} = -T_z - R_x Y + R_y X$$

If we assume perspective projection onto the image plane, using a focal length of 1, the projection of $\mathbf{P}$ onto the image (x, y) is given by

$$x = X/Z, \quad y = Y/Z$$

The projected velocities in the image plane (v_x, v_y) are therefore

$$v_x = (-T_x + xT_z)/Z + R_x xy - R_y(x^2 + 1) + R_z y$$
$$v_y = (-T_y + yT_z)/Z + R_x(y^2 + 1) - R_y xy - R_z x$$

The first term represents the component of image velocity due to observer translation and depends on the depth Z of each point in the scene. The remaining terms represent the component of image velocity due to the observer's rotation and do not depend on depth. The translational component yields a radial pattern of velocity (Figure 2*A*) that emanates from a single location in the image, called the *focus of expansion* (FOE). The FOE corresponds to the observer's heading and occurs at the location $(T_x/T_z, T_y/T_z)$ in the image. In contrast, the image flow field that results from a pure rotation of the observer is nearly constant over this region of the image. The image flow field for combined translation and rotation of the observer (Figure 2*B*) is the vector sum of the two flow fields from translation and rotation.

For observer translation, one can locate the FOE by finding the point of intersection of lines through the velocity vectors in the image. This simple strategy fails for combined translation and rotation, which occurs when the observer moves along a curved path or rotates his eyes or head, because the additional rotation components of velocity eliminate the FOE. This strategy also fails for nonrigid scenes that contain moving objects whose paths of motion deviate from the radial translational flow lines.

The Perception of Heading

Perceptual studies show that people judge 3D motion accurately under many conditions (Hildreth and Royden, 1998; Warren, 1998a; van den Berg, in Lappe, 2000). When translating toward a stationary scene, people exhibit discrimination thresholds as low as 0.2° when the heading is near the line of sight. Thresholds rise with more peripheral headings. Heading judgments are performed successfully with sparse, discontinuous flow fields, and require a relatively small field of view if the rotational flow is small. For pure translation, people recover heading with moderate accuracy

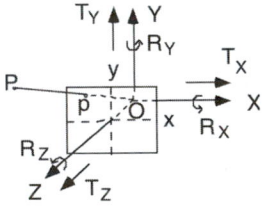

Figure 1. Coordinate system for a moving observer who is located at the origin.

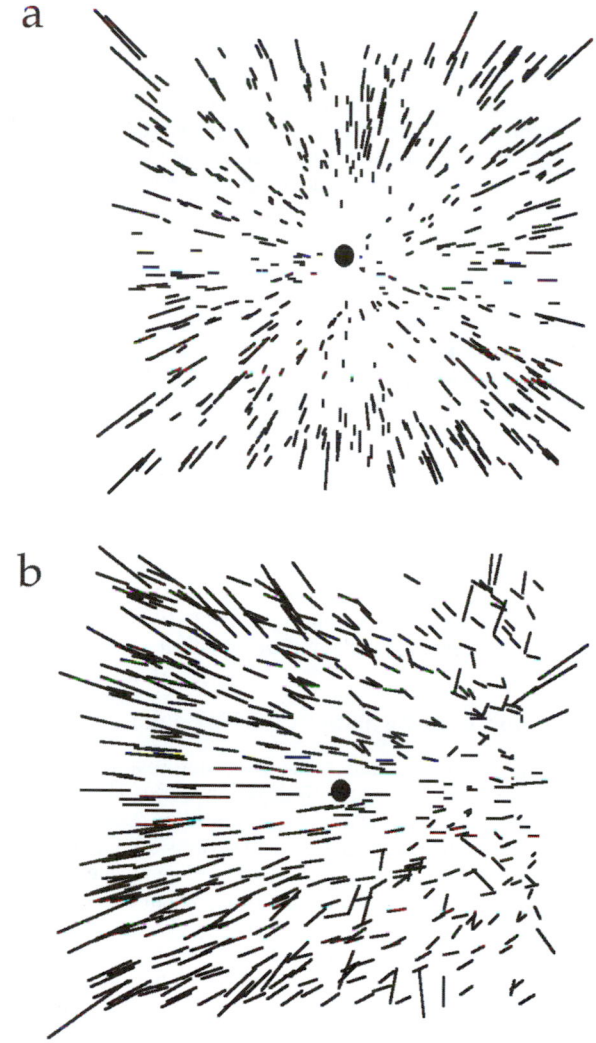

a

b

Figure 2. *A*, Radial flow field resulting from an observer moving in a straight line through a 3D cloud of dots. *B*, Flow field resulting from an observer translating and rotating (about a vertical axis) through a 3D cloud of dots. The solid circles indicate the direction of observer translation.

from only a 90 ms presentation, but improve up to about 300 ms of viewing time. Heading judgments remain accurate in the presence of moderate amounts of noise in the image flow field. The addition of other static and stereoscopic depth cues can enhance the accuracy of heading judgments in the presence of added noise or observer rotations.

People judge their translational heading accurately in the presence of small rotational rates generated by slow eye movements. Faster eye movements require extraretinal information about the speed of eye movement for accurate heading recovery (Hildreth and Royden, 1998; Warren, 1998a). In contrast, people accurately judge their motion along curved paths at low and high rotation rates (Warren, 1998a; van den Berg, in Lappe, 2000).

Under many conditions, a moving object has no effect on heading judgments. However, when the object crosses the observer's path, small biases in observer heading judgments result (Royden and Hildreth, 1996; Warren, 1998a). The ability to judge heading does not deteriorate when observers attend a second, object-related task (Hildreth and Royden, 1998).

These observations suggest that the human mechanism for judging heading from visual stimuli is remarkably robust and performs well under a variety of nonoptimal conditions.

Models of Observer Motion Recovery

Computational approaches for recovering heading can be divided into several categories, as described in this section. Many models fit more than one category; we present individual models within a category that best represents the particular approach.

Discrete Models

In discrete models, image features are tracked over time. Their sequence of positions forms the input to a system of equations whose solution yields the parameters of 3D structure and motion, assuming that the features move in a rigid configuration relative to the observer. Computer experiments indicate that such algorithms are vulnerable to error in the image motion measurements, although the use of motion measurements over an extended time can yield better performance (Martin and Aggarwal, 1988).

Differential Models

These models recover 3D motion and structure parameters from first and second spatial derivatives of the image flow field. One approach uses the *differential invariants* of the flow field, divergence (expansion/contraction), curl (rotation), and two components of deformation, dilation and shear (for references see Hildreth and Royden, 1998). Divergence and deformation depend only on the observer's translation and surface slant, and are invariant under observer rotations. In principle, these measures can be used to recover the observer's translation and the 3D shape of object surfaces. Most models that use differential invariants require a continuous, smooth optical flow field. In contrast, the human system can recover heading reliably from a few, sparse features that are sampled from a discontinuous flow field.

Motion Parallax Models

Motion parallax models use the fact that the translational components of the image velocities depend on the depth of the points in the scene, while the rotational components are independent of depth (Longuet-Higgins and Prazdny, 1980). Consequently, subtracting the image velocities from two points located at a depth discontinuity eliminates the rotational components. One can locate the translational heading using the resulting "difference vectors" by calculating the best point of intersection of lines through these vectors.

These models provide a method for quickly assessing heading, independent of the recovery of observer rotation and 3D scene structure. Because they combine information from multiple velocity vectors, they work fairly well in the presence of noisy velocity inputs. Simulations with a motion parallax model developed by Hildreth (1992) show behavior consistent with that observed in earlier perceptual studies. Motion differences computed by neurons in the middle temporal (MT) area of the primate visual system may be used to compute observer translation in the presence of rotations (Royden, 1997).

Error Minimization Models

Error minimization models compute observer motion and 3D structure parameters that yield a flow field that best fits the measured optical flow. For example, Bruss and Horn use this approach to derive observer motion parameters and surface structure that best account for the measured flow field in a least-squares sense (see Hildreth and Royden, 1998). The error minimization strategy, together with spatial pooling of motion measurements over an extended image region, allows the algorithm to tolerate substantial error in the individual image motion measurements. Many models proposed for recovery of observer motion incorporate some form of error minimization. Notably, Heeger and Jepson (1992) presented an error minimization model that has been implemented in a neural network form by Lappe and Rauschecker (in Lappe, 2000).

Template Models

Template models use special-purpose computational mechanisms, such as a family of templates, tailored to detect patterns of optical flow corresponding to specific observer motion parameters. For example, a template for detecting forward motion along the line of sight would respond optimally to a radially expanding pattern of image velocities whose FOE is located at the center of the visual field. Template models deal effectively with noise in the input velocity measurements by integrating over a large area. Perrone and Stone (1994) proposed a template model that computes heading using components that respond to motion similarly to neurons in the primate visual area MT.

Eye Movement Models

In addition to retinal information, the human visual system can use the oculomotor signal to obtain information about eye rotation, either from an efference copy of the signal or from proprioceptive feedback from the extraocular muscles. Royden, Crowell, and Banks suggest that this information is essential for recovering heading accurately in the presence of fast eye rotations. The flow field corresponding to a known eye rotation could be subtracted from the overall flow field before the observer's heading is calculated (Hildreth and Royden, 1998). Lappe (in Lappe, 2000) and van den Berg and Beintema (see Lappe, in Lappe, 2000) have developed neural models that explicitly incorporate eye movement signals.

Cutting (1986) noted that when an observer fixates a point in space, the most rapidly moving objects in the vicinity of the fixation point can be used to judge heading relative to the fixation direction. One can locate the heading with successive fixations on objects in the scene. This model requires little computation from the flow field itself; however, it fails for certain configurations of scenes and eye fixations. It also requires multiple saccades to locate heading, something that is not essential for human heading judgments.

Neural Network Models

Several neural network models use training algorithms to learn to compute heading from optic flow input (Lappe, in Lappe, 2000). Hatsopoulos and Warren created a two-layer neural network that is trained using the Widrow-Hoff learning rule to recognize the correct translational heading for an observer moving along a straight line. The input layer consists of units tuned to direction and speed of motion. After training, the weights connecting the input and output layers adapt so that the output neurons detect radial patterns of motion corresponding to particular headings. The network only interprets flows derived from pure observer translation. Zemel and Sejnowski developed a learning network that segments the scene according to the motion of objects relative to the observer. Heading can be estimated from the resulting encoding.

Motion on a Curvilinear Path

When an observer moves along a curvilinear path, his instantaneous translation and rotation are the same as those for an observer pursuing straight-line motion with eye movement, resulting in an ambiguity. Distinguishing these situations requires an analysis of the flow field over an extended time. Alternatively, eye movement information may be used to disambiguate these conditions. Human observers distinguish curved from straight paths with high accuracy and judge the path curvature well. This finding suggests that the visual system computes both translation and rotation components of observer motion (Warren, 1998a; van den Berg, in Lappe, 2000).

Coping with Moving Objects

For most models, the presence of moving objects in the scene can adversely affect the derivation of observer motion. Image points associated with moving objects may move in a direction inconsistent with the observer's motion, causing errors in the heading estimate. Some models first detect moving objects and then compute heading from the remaining stationary components of the scene. Another approach computes an initial estimate of observer motion by combining all available data or by performing separate computations within limited image regions. One can then identify moving objects by finding areas of the scene for which the image motion differs significantly from that expected from these initial motion parameters (e.g., Hildreth, 1992). See Hildreth and Royden (1998) for a review of models of moving object detection.

Visuomotor Transformations for Navigation

Successful navigation requires that visual information be used to control motor actions to move through the world. This requires a transformation between the retinocentric heading coordinates computed by the models described in the previous section to a body-centered coordinate system, taking into account eye and head movements. It seems likely that the visual system uses extraretinal information, such as eye movement and vestibular signals, to account for rotations of the head and eyes. Neurons in the medial superior temporal (MST) area of visual cortex may combine these extraretinal signals with visual information to compute the body-centric heading (see Andersen et al., in Lappe, 2000).

The mechanisms for transformation of the visual information into motor control commands are not yet understood, but several approaches have been described. In one approach, motor planning takes place based on the computed heading of the observer. For example, to reach a desired goal, the motor system could initiate turning commands that minimize the error between the computed heading and the direction to the goal. Visual feedback allows constant refinement of the motor strategy to keep errors in heading from accumulating (Warren, 1998b).

Another approach is based on specific tasks the observer must perform to navigate through the environment. Such tasks include steering toward a goal, pursuing prey, braking, avoiding obstacles, or computing time to contact with an approaching surface. It has been suggested that each of these tasks may be accomplished through a task-specific subsystem that uses only the information in the flow field necessary to complete the task (Aloimonos, 1997; Warren, 1998b). For example, time to contact can be computed from the ratio, τ, given as the ratio of size/(rate of size change). The coupling between the task-specific information and the resulting action can be modeled as a nonlinear dynamical system. For example, when steering toward a goal, visual information provides the angle, β, between the FOE and the direction of the goal. This angle can be used to control the observer's rate of turning. The result is a system with a stable fixed point at $\beta = 0$, corresponding to the observer heading toward the goal. Complex motor behavior may emerge through interactions between loosely coupled subsystems underlying different tasks (Warren, 1998b).

Neural Mechanisms of Heading Computation

In primates, visual area MST is probably involved in computing heading (Duffy, in Lappe, 2000). Neurons in MST respond well to large motion patterns and receive direct input from cells in area MT, which is known to process motion (see also MOTION PERCEPTION: ELEMENTARY MECHANISMS). Some MST neurons prefer expanding or contracting radial patterns of motion, as would be generated by an observer moving in a straight line forward or backward. These cells have different preferred centers of expansion, so they could be involved in finding the FOE in an optical flow field. Other cells respond well to uniform motion in a single direction, and yet others respond to rotating patterns of motion. Many cells respond to some combination of these.

It is unclear how these cell responses contribute to the computation of heading in the presence of rotations; however, several models have been developed that could explain this. Hatsopoulos and Warren (Warren, 1998a) and Perrone and Stone (1994) proposed template models that use components that behave similarly to neurons in area MT in their response to motion. In both models, these components connect to another layer of cells with properties similar to the cells in MST. The connection patterns are such that the cells in the second layer respond to spatial patterns that mimic the flow fields that result from particular observer motion parameters. The Hatsopoulos and Warren model deals only with pure observer translation. Perrone and Stone used templates that deal with combinations of translations and the rotations that result when the observer makes eye movements to track an object in the scene. This model also recovers the relative depths of surfaces in the scene.

Royden (1997) developed a model that makes use of the motion-opponent properties of MT neurons to deal with observer rotations. Many neurons in MT have both excitatory and inhibitory regions within their receptive fields. The Royden model uses operators with this receptive-field layout to eliminate the observer rotation at the initial processing stage. These cells project to a second layer of cells, similar to those in MST, that are tuned to radial patterns of input. As with the motion parallax models described earlier, the centers of these radial patterns correspond to observer headings.

Finally, Lappe (in Lappe, 2000) and van den Berg and Beintema (cited by Lappe, in Lappe, 2000) developed neural models that explicitly incorporate eye movement signals to deal with rotations generated by eye movements. In Lappe's model, extraretinal input compensates for the image motion induced by eye movements. In van den Berg and Beintema's model, the responses of template cells tuned to retinal flow are multiplied by a "rate-coded" measure of eye velocity, producing a layer of cells that have a preferred flow field that changes dynamically to compensate for eye movements.

Currently, there is insufficient physiological or psychophysical data to distinguish among these models of neural computation of heading. It seems likely that some compensation for eye movements occurs in area MST (see Andersen et al., in Lappe, 2000); however, this compensation could be incorporated into the models that do not currently use it. The models are all reasonably consistent with the known behavior of MT and MST cells. Determination of which, if any, most accurately describes the neural computation awaits further experimentation.

Discussion

People judge heading well under many conditions; however, it is still uncertain how the visual system accomplishes this task. Superficially, most of the models cited here exhibit general biological plausibility, in that they can be implemented by a network of simple, local processing mechanisms operating in parallel. Physiological observations reveal the general properties of the representation of optic flow information and provide some indication that heading computations take place in areas MT and MST of the primate visual system. It remains a challenge to incorporate all of the important aspects of recovery of 3D observer motion into a neuronal model that exhibits a broad range of human behavior and incorporates the details of physiological observations.

Road Map: Vision
Related Reading: Motion Perception: Elementary Mechanisms; Robot Navigation

References

Aloimonos, Y., Ed., 1997, *Visual Navigation: From Biological Systems to Unmanned Ground Vehicles*, Mahwah, NJ: Erlbaum.

Cutting, J. E., 1986, *Perception with an Eye for Motion*, Cambridge, MA: Bradford/MIT Press.

Heeger, D. J., and Jepson, A. D., 1992, Subspace methods for recovering rigid motion: I. Algorithm and implementation, *Int. J. Comput. Vision*, 7:95–117.

Hildreth, E. C., 1992, Recovering heading for visually-guided navigation, *Vision Res.*, 32:1177–1192.

Hildreth, E. C., and Koch, C., 1987, The analysis of visual motion: From computational theory to neuronal mechanisms, *Annu. Rev. Neurosci.*, 10:477–533.

Hildreth, E. C., and Royden, C. S., 1998, Computing observer motion from optic flow, in *High-Level Motion Processing: Computational, Neurobiological and Psychophysical Perspectives* (T. Watanabe, Ed.), Cambridge, MA: MIT Press, pp. 269–293. ◆

Lappe, M., Ed. 2000, *Neuronal Processing of Optic Flow, Int. Rev. Neurobiol.* vol. 44. (special issue),

Longuet-Higgins, H. C., and Prazdny, K., 1980, The interpretation of a moving retinal image, *Proc. R. Soc. Lond. B*, 208:385–397.

Martin, W. N., and Aggarwal, J. K., Eds., 1988, *Motion Understanding: Robot and Human Vision*, Boston: Kluwer.

Mitiche, A., and Bouthemy, P., 1996, Computation and analysis of image motion: A synopsis of current problems and methods, *Int. J. Comput. Vision*, 19:29–55. ◆

Perrone, J. A., and Stone, L. S., 1994, A model of self-motion estimation within primate extrastriate visual cortex, *Vision Res.*, 34:2917–2938.

Royden, C. S., 1997, Mathematical analysis of motion-opponent mechanisms used in the determination of heading and depth, *J. Opt. Soc. Am. A*, 14:2128–2143.

Royden, C. S., and Hildreth, E. C., 1996, Human heading judgments in the presence of moving objects, *Percept. Psychophy.*, 58:836–856.

Warren, W. H., 1998a, The state of flow, in *High-Level Motion Processing: Computational, Neurobiological and Psychophysical Perspectives* (T. Watanabe, Ed.), Cambridge, MA: MIT Press, pp. 315–358. ◆

Warren, W. H., 1998b, Visually controlled locomotion: 40 years later, *Ecol. Psychol.*, 10:177–219.

Motivation

Alan G. Watts

Introduction

Motivated or goal-directed behaviors are sets of motor actions that direct an animal toward a particular goal object, an interaction that promotes the survival of an individual or maintains the species. Goal-directed behaviors consist of sleep/wake, ingestive, reproductive, thermoregulatory, and aggressive/defensive behaviors. At the simplest level, motivated behaviors can be considered the behavioral adjuncts of those physiological (i.e., homeostatic) processes concerned with maintaining the composition of the internal environment. They are often accompanied by emotion or affect.

Despite their apparent utility, defining the terms *drive, instinct,* and *motivation* with respect to the neural substrates of behavior has always been controversial (Grossman, 1979; Pfaff, 1982). Although the most rigorous use of the terms drive and motivation has been as intervening variables between stimulus and behavioral response, there is an attraction to trying to assign particular brain regions responsibility for putting the motivation into behavior. However, "neuralizing" drive, and particularly motivation, has often been criticized because it has been thought impossible to identify and measure their specific neural properties (e.g., Hinde, 1970).

With this in mind, a neural systems approach will be adopted here that downplays the notion of associating motivation with specific neural mechanisms. To this end, this article will concentrate more on discussing what and how particular parts of the brain contribute to the expression of behaviors that have a motivated character. The framework adopted here is based to a large extent on Hullerian incentive models of motivation (see Bindra, 1978, and Toates, 1986, for further discussion), where the probability of a particular behavior being expressed at any one time is dependent on the integration of sets of afferent information: information from systems that control circadian timing and regulate arousal state, inputs derived from interosensory information that encode internal state (e.g., hydration state, plasma glucose, leptin), modulatory hormonal inputs such as gonadal steroids that mediate sexual behavior, and inputs derived from classic sensory modalities (i.e., exterosensory information). The advantage of this approach for identifying neural substrates is that it allows us to utilize the common experimental paradigm of tracing how information derived from sensory inputs known to generate specific behaviors is distributed within the brain (e.g., Swanson and Mogenson, 1981). With the advent of sophisticated functional neuroanatomical methods, this approach is proving quite useful (Watts, 2001; Watts and Swanson, 2002).

Temporal Organization of Motivated Behavior

A scheme describing the temporal organization of motivated behavior was first outlined by Wallace Craig in 1918, and later elaborated by Mogenson and colleagues (Swanson and Mogenson, 1981). Here, behavior is initiated following interactions among sensory information, the neural systems that control arousal state, and those systems that control sensory object representation. These interactions determine the value of the "drive" associated with a particular behavior. In turn, the integral of competing drives then determines which series of actions will generate the most appropriate procurement (or appetitive) phase, where the goal object is actively sought. The motor events expressed during the procurement phase involve foraging behavior, are individualized for the particular situation, and can be quite complex.

When the goal object has been located, the subsequent consummatory phase involves more stereotypic rhythmic movements—licking, chewing, copulating, etc.—that allow the animal to interact directly with the goal object. During the consummatory phase, how the animal structures the interaction (e.g., determines the duration and the amount consumed during a feeding episode, or the duration of the intermeal interval) is an important function that arises from the dynamic interaction of sensory inputs and the central neural networks that control motor function. Furthermore, reward/aversion functions, together with learning and memory, are also critical processes, particularly during the procurement phase; a previously rewarded or an aversive experience of a particular goal object, remembering where it is located, and remembering how to get there are important considerations that contribute to the integrative process. Finally, as the consummatory phase continues, interosensory feedback signals are generated that increase the probability of its termination, most likely using inhibitory networks. Termination may also occur at any time following new exterosensory signals (e.g., the presence of a predator) that override an ongoing behavior and allow the animal to switch immediately to another, more appropriate behavior (McFarland and Sibly, 1975).

Neural Substrates

At the simplest level, four broad-ranging neural systems are concerned with generating motivated behaviors: those involved with the transduction and processing of sensory signals, those that control arousal state and circadian timing, those involved with motor control, and those that process the types of information concerned with sensory object representation. These systems are represented at the simplest level in Figure 1 without reference to anatomical locus.

The notion of drive and the idea that particular behaviors are selected to reduce the level of specific drive states have together been very influential if somewhat controversial concepts in neuroscience. From the perspective of delineating neural systems, it is useful to think of drives as being dynamic properties within different sets of neural networks, each of which is concerned with regulating a specific motivated behavior. In this way, drives are properties of behaviorally specific networks within the motor control module of Figure 1. Drive states are determined by the inputs from sensory processing, arousal state control, and object representation systems. The values of drive states within these networks are altered by these inputs in a way that increases or decreases the probability of a particular behavior being expressed at any one time.

Figure 2 expands the scheme shown in Figure 1 to illustrate specific components within the object representational and motor control networks. It shows that there are four principal inputs that can activate motor systems. The most complex motor control processes are those that generate anticipatory behaviors. In some instances, information from systems controlling arousal state—for example, circadian timing—provide the predominant signals (input 1, Figure 2). But this type of anticipatory control often derives from interactions between processed sensory information and those forebrain systems concerned with encoding object representation, particularly learning and memory, reward, and spatial orientation and navigation. The integrated output of these regions then regulates motor control systems (input 2, Figure 2). However, increased drives for motivated behaviors can also be produced by hormones or internally generated deficit signals (e.g., the thirst arising from dehydration, or the hunger from starvation) that access motor control networks more directly (input 3, Figure 2).

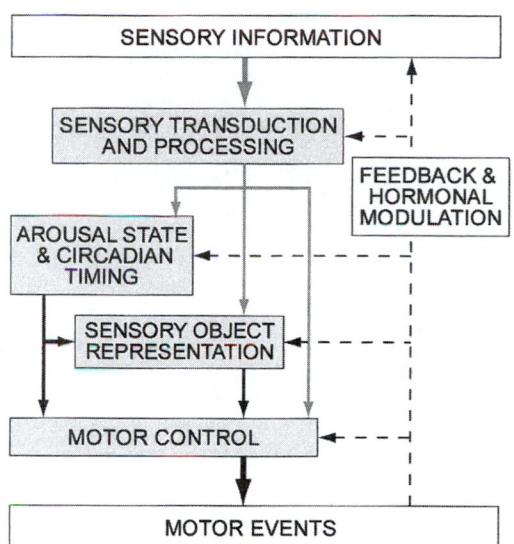

Figure 1. A schematic representation of the neural systems and their interactions involved with controlling motivated behaviors. Sensory inputs are shown in gray, central neural connections in black, and hormonal and feedback signals as dashed lines.

Collectively, inputs 1, 2, and 3 to the motor control networks can be thought of as "drive-determining" interactions. Mechanisms then integrate outputs from different drive networks to select the behavioral action most appropriate for reducing the drive state with the highest value, so initiating the appropriate procurement phase.

Finally, simple reflex actions are generated by direct sensory inputs to the premotor and motor networks with little higher-order processing (input 4, Figure 2). However, although these reflex actions lack any motivated character, they make important contributions to the consummatory phase of motivated behaviors.

Sensory Information

Neural systems that control motivated behaviors are regulated by a host of sensory inputs, which are defined either as interosensory signals encoding internal state or as exterosensory inputs that encode features of the goal object such as smell, taste, temperature, tactile properties, and appearance. Each of these sensory modalities has specific receptors, transduction mechanisms, and "labeled line" access to central processing networks located throughout the brain. Although important sensory processing occurs within the telencephalon, particularly sensory cortex, the initial sensory processing that occurs subcortically has important implications for controlling motivated behaviors; for example, altered sensitivity to the taste of sodium occurs in the hindbrain of hyponatremic animals and is an important adjunct to increased sodium appetite.

Some sensory signals directly access drive networks, as typified by the drinking initiated by increasing plasma osmolality or angiotensin II (A-II), or the deficit-induced feeding activated by adiposity signals (primarily leptin and insulin), which have direct hypothalamic actions (Elmquist, Elias, and Saper, 1999). In both of these cases, however, it is not clear whether the outcome of processing the deficit signal in the hypothalamus requires close interaction with the object representation networks. The fact that hypothalamic regions involved with this type of sensory transduction project directly to regions concerned with ingestive motor control (Elmquist et al., 1999) suggests that they may not.

Circadian Timing and Arousal State Control

Parts of the brain provide critical circadian timing information and control arousal state that enable motor command networks to generate anticipatory behaviors. The circadian timing system originates in the hypothalamic suprachiasmatic nucleus, which generates the signal that entrains virtually all neural activity within limits determined by the prevailing photoperiod. Catecholamine cell groups in the hindbrain (e.g., the locus coeruleus), histaminergic neurons in the tuberomammillary nucleus, the ventrolateral preoptic nucleus, and the recently identified hypocretin/orexin neurons in the lateral hypothalamic area (LHA) supply information that is of critical importance for controlling arousal state.

Object Representation

Those systems that generate neural representations of sensory objects are important for controlling motivational behaviors. These include learning and memory mechanisms in the telencephalon and cerebellum; reward/aversion systems in the midbrain ventral tegmentum, parts of the basal forebrain (particularly the nucleus accumbens), amygdala, and parts of the cortex, particularly prefrontal regions; and systems in the hippocampus and parts of the parietal cortex responsible for allocentric and egocentric spatial representation. A great deal of exterosensory information is processed

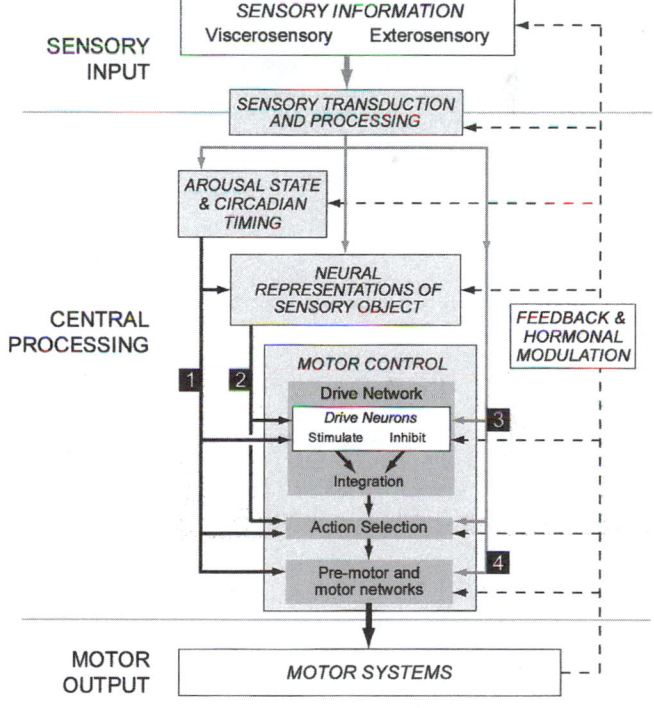

Figure 2. Motor control networks are organized at three levels: drive networks, which can either stimulate or inhibit behaviors; action selection networks, which integrate the outputs of drive networks with those of other systems; and executive premotor and motor neuron networks. The generation of motivated behavioral actions by motor control networks can be initiated by four different sets of inputs: (1) from systems controlling arousal state and circadian timing; (2) from systems that generate representations of sensory objects; (3) directly from modulatory hormone and the sensory signals that encode physiological deficits; and (4) from sensory signals that generate reflex actions by interacting directly with premotor and motor neuron networks. Sensory inputs are shown in gray, central neural connections in black, and hormonal and feedback signals as dashed lines.

through these networks, parts of which collectively assign what has been called "incentive value" to a particular goal object. Neural pathways mediating the interactions between the object representation and motor networks are not fully understood, but sets of bidirectional connections between the hypothalamus and cortical structures such as the prefrontal cortex and hippocampus, together with subcortical regions such as the amygdala, septal nuclei, bed nuclei of the stria terminalis, and basal ganglia, are all likely to be critical for the integrative operations that designate and coordinate these aspects of motivated behaviors (Saper, 1985; Risold, Thompson, and Swanson, 1997; Swanson and Petrovich, 1998).

Motor Control

Figure 2 shows that motor control systems operate at three levels: a series of drive networks that set up and coordinate the motor events associated with specific behaviors; regions that are concerned with action selection; and the premotor/motor neuron networks that execute the actions. Figure 2 also shows a clear distinction between drive networks and object representation systems. This derives from the fact that object representation systems appear, at least at the systems level, to be behaviorally nonspecific, whereas drive networks are explicitly concerned with specific behaviors. For example, an animal uses the same parts of the telencephalon for spatial navigation whether it is looking for food, a mate, or shelter, whereas parts of the hypothalamus are concerned specifically with feeding or sexual behavior. However, with regard to other neural structures (for example, cell groups in the basal ganglia), this distinction may not be so clear-cut, and here it may prove difficult to determine to which system particular sets of neurons belong.

The concept of drive networks as defined here evolved from the idea of discretely localized hypothalamic satiety and hunger centers that was popular during the 1950s and 1960s. With elaboration of these pioneering studies over the ensuing 30 years, the idea of isolated centers has been replaced with a scheme whereby sets of more widely distributed but highly interconnected motor control networks direct the motor responses for particular behaviors. Each drive network contain sets of command circuits that stimulate, inhibit, or disinhibit a particular motor event (Figure 2). The exact nature of the expressed behavior, or whether it is expressed at all, is determined by the integrated output of these circuits.

Determining how the neural substrates of specific drive networks are distributed throughout the brain has proved quite difficult. Lesion and electrical stimulation experiments identified some time ago that the hypothalamus was a key structure for the expression of motivated behaviors. More recently, a wealth of neurochemical data has revealed that many neuropeptides have either stimulatory or inhibitory effects on particular motor functions. In turn, the fact that many of these neuropeptides are synthesized in hypothalamic neurons, which in some cases project quite widely throughout the brain, has focused attention on this forebrain region as a key locus of specific drive network components. Furthermore, a synthesis of results from lesion, microinjection, and neuroanatomical tracing studies has identified specific regions of the hypothalamus—particularly cell groups in the medial zone of the hypothalamus (Risold et al., 1997; Watts and Swanson, 2002)—as being principal components of individual drive networks.

One critical point that has emerged from these studies is that it is often difficult to place individual hypothalamic cell groups within specific command circuits (Figure 2). This is because traditionally defined cell groups such as the LHA, arcuate (ARH), or paraventricular (PVH) nuclei appear to contain elements that, in terms of function, belong to more than one type of command circuit; it seems unlikely that there is a tight "one cell group–one command circuit" relationship in the hypothalamus.

A well-documented example of a stimulatory circuit is the one activated by circulating A-II to stimulate drinking. A-II is detected by a central sensory transducer, the subfornical organ (SFO), which then directly and specifically stimulates water intake. The SFO provides efferents, most of which also contain A-II (Swanson, 1987), to a relatively limited set of structures, including parts of the prefrontal cortex, substantia innominata, medial preoptic area, bed nuclei of the stria terminalis, zona incerta, PVH, supraoptic nucleus, and LHA (Swanson, 1987), and presumably it is these regions that constitute part of the stimulatory circuit that initiates the motor aspects of drinking. Neuropeptide Y (NPY) neurons in the ARH contribute to a well-known example of a stimulatory eating mechanism; results from many studies show that NPY contributes to a circuit that directly stimulates food intake. In terms of inhibitory circuits, feeding again provides good examples of hypothalamic components. For example, α-MSH, a peptide synthesized in ARH neurons, provides an inhibitory signal to feeding by way of melanocortin 4 receptors expressed by LHA and PVH neurons (Elmquist et al., 1999).

Finally, interactions between different drive networks, particularly in the hypothalamus, are of paramount importance. For example, the effects of starvation are not limited just to increasing the drive to eat, they also reduce reproductive capacity. Similarly, dehydration leads to severe anorexia, as well as increasing the drive to drink (Watts, 2001). This cross-behavioral coordination is part of the mechanism that selects the drive with the highest priority, and most likely involves hormonal modulation acting together with the divergent neuroanatomic outputs from individual drive networks.

Those parts of the brain concerned with the planning, selection, and the moment-to-moment execution of particular motor actions include parts of the motor cortex, basal ganglia, midbrain, and hindbrain. Like the object representational systems, these regions at a systems level are generally behaviorally nonspecific. Although they express topography with regard to the mapping of particular motor actions, they do not seem to be organized in the behaviorally specific manner of the drive networks. To organize the appropriate behavior, regions controlling action selection must receive the integrated outputs of the drive networks. Although not well understood, complex sets of projections from the hypothalamus are most likely involved with this function.

Alpha-motor neurons in the ventral horn of the spinal cord control the striate musculature and hence the expression of all behavior. In turn, sets of premotor networks directly control oscillatory and the more complex patterns of motor neuron firing. Simple rhythmic movement patterns develop from an interaction between oscillatory rhythm generators, which directly involve the motor neurons, and networks of premotor CPGs located somewhat more distally in the spinal cord and hindbrain. A critical feature of these pattern generators is that they are capable of producing rhythmic output without sensory input. In turn, pattern generator output is modulated further by afferents from those parts of the appropriate command networks in the diencephalon and telencephalon. These often highly varied inputs provide the critical drive and contextual information that select the most appropriate motor program at any particular time.

Hormonal Modulation

Hormones have been known for many years to be critical modulators of motivated behaviors that influence a variety of neural structures at all brain levels (Figure 2). In this manner, because they are not encoding aspects of internal state, they are not feedback signals, but act more as permissive factors. Steroid hormones, particularly gonadal steroids, are important signals of this type.

Feedback

Finally, feedback is a critical feature of behavioral motor control, and sensory signals encoding the magnitude and consequences of generated motor actions can control the length of a motivated behavioral episode. For example, postabsorptive humoral feedback (e.g., increasing CCK or decreasing plasma osmolality) and interosensory signals (e.g., gastric distension, oropharyngeal metering) lead to the termination of ingestive behaviors and subsequent behavioral refractoriness.

Discussion

Sophisticated neuroanatomical and molecular techniques are beginning to clarify the organization of those neural circuits that are responsible for controlling motivated behaviors. They emphasize that understanding how motivated behaviors are controlled requires the interaction of neural systems distributed throughout the brain that are both behaviorally specific and nonspecific. Although the structure of the different hypothalamic drive networks is reasonably well established, future work will need to clarify how each drive network interacts with others, with other forebrain systems concerned with complex sensory object representation, and with those hindbrain circuits concerned more directly with reflex actions and motor execution.

Road Map: Psychology
Related Reading: Conditioning; Emotional Circuits; Reinforcement Learning

References

Bindra, D., 1978, How adaptive behaviour is produced: A perceptual-motivational alternative to response reinforcement, *Behav. Brain Sci.*, 1:41–91.

Elmquist, J. K., Elias, C. F., and Saper, C. B., 1999, From lesions to leptin: Hypothalamic control of food intake and body weight, *Neuron*, 22:221–232.

Grossman, S. P., 1979, The biology of motivation, *Annu. Rev. Psychol.*, 30:209–242. ◆

Hinde, R. A., 1970, *Animal Behaviour: A Synthesis of Ethology and Comparative Psychology*, 2nd ed., New York: McGraw-Hill. ◆

McFarland, D. J., and Sibly, R. M., 1975, The behavioural final common path, *Philos. Trans. R. Soc. Lond. B*, 270:265–293.

Pfaff, D. W., 1982, Motivational concepts: Definitions and distinctions, in *The Physiological Mechanisms of Motivation* (D. W. Pfaff, Ed.), New York: Springer-Verlag, pp. 3–24. ◆

Risold, P. Y., Thompson, R. H., and Swanson, L. W., 1997, The structural organization of connections between hypothalamus and cerebral cortex, *Brain Res. Rev.*, 24:197–254.

Saper, C. B., 1985, Organization of cerebral cortical afferent systems in the rat: II. Hypothalamocortical projections, *J. Comp. Neurol.*, 237:21–46.

Swanson, L. W., 1987, The hypothalamus, in *Handbook of Chemical Neuroanatomy*, vol 5. (A. Bjorklund, T. Hökfelt, and L. W. Swanson, Eds.), Amsterdam: Elsevier, pp. 1–124.

Swanson, L. W., and Mogenson, G. J., 1981, Neural mechanisms for the functional coupling of autonomic, endocrine and somatomotor responses in adaptive behavior, *Brain Res.*, 228:1–34.

Swanson, L. W., and Petrovich, G. D., 1998, What is the amygdala? *Trends Neurosci.*, 21:323–331.

Toates, F., 1986, *Motivational Systems*, Cambridge, Engl.: Cambridge University Press. ◆

Watts, A. G., 2001, Neuropeptides and the integration of motor responses to dehydration, *Annu. Rev. Neurosci.*, 24:357–384.

Watts, A. G., and Swanson, L. W., 2002, Anatomy of motivational systems, in *Stevens' Handbook of Experimental Psychology*, 3rd ed. (C. R. Gallistell, Ed.), New York: Wiley, vol. 3, pp. 563–632. ◆

Motoneuron Recruitment

Daniel Bullock

Introduction

Motoneurons are neurons that directly innervate muscle fibers. When motoneuron discharges cause muscle fibers to contract, the resultant forces oppose static loads, and produce active accelerations and decelerations of limb segments. Moreover, co-contractions of opposing muscles allow us to stiffen joints and thereby maintain desired postures despite perturbations of unexpected magnitude and direction. Because of the direct anatomical link between motoneurons and contractile fibers, there is a close relationship between motoneuron activity and force production.

A motoneuron together with the contractile fibers that it innervates constitutes a *motor unit*. The range of forces producible by one motor unit is small. To make it possible to generate large forces, motor units must be combined into larger aggregates, and the results of such aggregation are the muscles. Immediately associated with each muscle is a population or pool of motoneurons. Muscles are therefore composite structures, and their force-generating components, the motor units, are typically heterogeneous. For example, muscle fibers differ systematically in fatiguability and the associated motoneurons differ systematically in their size. How are these heterogeneous aggregates of force-generating elements recruited in the service of reflexes, voluntary movement,

and posture? Such task-dependent recruitment is achieved by a combination of motor unit and neural network specializations.

Consider the simple question of control of force magnitude. If any excitatory input were sufficient to cause simultaneous excitation of all motor units, then the minimum force produced by the aggregate would be much too large for most purposes. To produce accurate movements, forces must be finely graded in response to the input to the motoneuron pool. The fine grading of forces required for accuracy favors a design that allows both partial activation of the motoneuron/fiber pool and finely graded changes, up or down, from preexisting states of activation.

Such force grading by a cells/fibers aggregate provides a functional context for understanding the *size principle* of motoneuron recruitment proposed in 1965 by Henneman, Somjen, and Carpenter (see Burke, 1998, for a review). The size principle encompasses many aspects of the design of motoneuron pools and their embedding within the sensorimotor system. In this design, an excitatory input often reaches all elements of the motoneuron pool at the same time. However, elements of the motoneuron pool differ in their activation thresholds. Because there is a distribution of threshold values from small to large, the larger the excitatory input to the pool, the more elements become active. This enables a continuously varying input signal to produce a graded force response from the muscle. As the excitatory input to the pool grows, motoneurons are recruited in order by size from smallest to largest, because motoneurons with larger somatic volumes also have higher thresholds. As excitatory input declines, or inhibitory input increases, motoneurons are derecruited in order by size, from largest to smallest.

The grading of force by recruitment, which is necessarily quantal, is supplemented by finer grading through firing rate modulation of individual cells, because each cell's firing rate is sensitive to input fluctuations in its suprathreshold range. This design affords finely graded increments and decrements in force over the entire range of muscle force capability.

It might appear that the size principle serves to make each spinomuscular force generator a fixed-gain, near-linear, amplifier of excitatory inputs. However, many factors complicate the situation. First, the gain is not fixed because muscle force can become decoupled from motoneuron pool activation if a contraction-opposing load causes muscle yielding, or if the muscle fatigues. Second, the amplification function is often faster-than-linear because motoneurons with larger cell bodies, and thus higher recruitment thresholds, typically project by larger, faster-conducting axons to more muscle fibers, each of which exhibits shorter twitch contraction times. Third, twitch contractions of muscle fibers are slow relative to rapid fluctuations of excitatory inputs to motoneurons. Fourth, muscle obeys a *force-velocity law*: force output from a muscle decreases as its shortening velocity increases. Fifth, the conventional delimitation of a motor unit, although minimal, is somewhat arbitrary. Several other closely linked neural and sensory constituents appear in most mammalian muscle control systems as part of the apparatus for force generation (cf. Burke, 1998). For example, before exiting the spinal cord, the axons of most alpha-motoneurons give off collaterals that excite Renshaw cells (RCs), which inhibit those same alpha-motoneurons. Sixth, the net torque developed at a joint depends on both mechanical advantage and the balance of forces created by groups of muscles arranged into synergistically antagonistic sets. Each of these considerations reveals a need for network control of recruitment, to ensure that opponent muscle sets generate the right force balances through time.

Compensations for Fatigue and Yielding

Muscle fatigue and yielding make the functional relation between pool activation and force inherently variable, and network interactions provide compensations that reduce the variability in this linkage. Nichols and Houk (1973) argued that two feedbacks from muscle receptors to spinal motoneuron pools cooperate to reduce variability in *muscle stiffness*, the ratio of muscle force changes to muscle length changes. Muscle yielding events reduce stiffness while also increasing the activity of stretch-sensitive receptors, the spindles, and decreasing the activity of tension-sensitive receptors, the Golgi tendon organs (GTOs). Because spindle feedback directly excites alpha-motoneurons via type Ia sensory fibers, whereas GTOs can inhibit motoneurons via Ib interneurons, both feedbacks are compensatory. It is often noted that GTO feedback also has appropriate characteristics to compensate for muscle fatigue. Bullock and Grossberg (1989) argued that the covariation of motor unit sizes and contraction rates is also compensatory for yielding.

Linearization or Equalization of Pool Responses

By itself, the covariation of recruitment threshold, number of fibers contacted, and fiber contraction rates with motoneuron size can produce a faster-than-linear relationship between excitatory input to the motoneuron pool and the force output of the muscle, at least under isometric conditions when the system is not approaching saturation. Akazawa and Kato (1990) and Bullock and Grossberg

(1989) independently proposed that Renshaw feedback improves this transduction. The Akazawa and Kato analysis (1990) treated a single motor unit pool, and showed that inhibitory Renshaw feedback may be able to linearize the relationship between excitatory inputs and force outputs. Bullock and Grossberg (1989) sought to explain how spinal circuitry enabled the higher brain to achieve independent control of joint angle and joint stiffness. Accordingly, these authors analyzed the "FLETE" circuit (Figure 1), which encompassed a lumped pair of motor unit pools associated with biomechanically opposed muscles. By Factoring the LEngth and TEnsion properties of muscle, the FLETE network allows a descending co-contraction signal to stiffen and thereby stabilize the joint at any desired angle. Available data (Humphrey and Reed, 1983) indicate that voluntary stiffness adjustments are achieved by varying an excitatory signal relayed to both opponent motoneuron pools. Bullock and Grossberg (1989) showed that in the absence of Renshaw feedback, a descending co-contractive signal would generally be unequally amplified by recruitment events within opposing motoneuron pools. Such unequal amplification would lead to an undesired joint rotation as well as to a change in joint stiffness. They then showed that Renshaw-mediated feedback could help guarantee independent control of joint stiffness and joint angle by equalizing the two pools' amplifications of the co-contractive signal. This equalization, which need not involve global linearization of recruitment, is achieved by a local circuit that incorporates mutual inhibition between opponent Renshaw pools and between Ia reciprocal inhibitory interneurons, which, like alpha-motoneurons, are inhibited by Renshaw cells (RCs).

This view of the role of RCs is consistent with data that contradict alternative views. Pratt and Jordan (1987) showed that RCs fired in phase with alpha-motoneurons during fictive locomotion, but that they were not needed for generation of the locomotor cycle. This disconfirmed the hypothesis that they were an integral part of the spinal locomotor generator. Lindsay and Binder (1991) observed that although steady-state Renshaw inhibition caused similar synaptic currents in alpha-motoneurons of different sizes, IPSP amplitudes did correlate with cell size. They concluded that "the

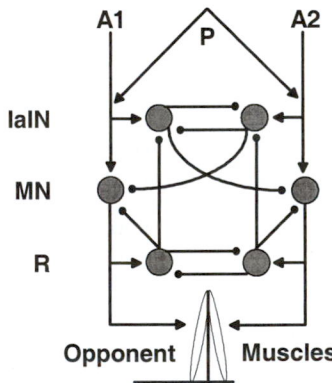

Figure 1. Partial connectivity of the FLETE model for independent control of joint angle and joint stiffness. To set desired joint angle, the higher brain reciprocally adjusts descending signals A1 and A2 directed to two opposing alpha motoneuron (MN) pools that project to opposing muscles. Descending signal P to both motoneuron pools adjusts joint stiffness without modifying joint angle if increments in P lead to equal increments in the force outputs of the two opposing muscles. Renshaw (R) cell feedbacks, among others, compensate for nonlinearities in the motoneuron response function and thereby help assure equal force increments in the two muscles affected by P. Renshaw feedback disinhibits opponent MNs via the Ia interneurons (IaIN). Arrow and dot line-endings, respectively, indicate excitatory and inhibitory synapses.

biggest impact of [RC] inhibition will be on the force output of motoneurons firing on the steep part of their force-frequency curve" (p. 176).

A subsequent extension of the FLETE model showed that the *triphasic* EMG bursts characteristic of rapid self-terminated joint rotations *emerge* within an arm-controlling network activated by *monophasic* descending control signals, if the network incorporates velocity-sensitive muscle spindles. Contreras-Vidal, Grossberg, and Bullock (1997) showed that the FLETE model is applicable to multi-joint arm movement control using both mono- and bi-articular muscles, and that the independent control property is enhanced by the incorporation of sensory feedbacks from spindle (Ia), GTO, and joint receptors. Moreover, van Heijst, Vos, and Bullock (1998) showed that connection weights consistent with the independent-control property will self-organize in the circuit of Figure 1 if local synapses are adjusted by a Hebbian learning process while the circuit is stimulated by a rhythmic input. Their developmental simulation modeled how such spinal circuits self-tune during prenatal episodes of rhythmic activity in avian and mammalian embryos.

Adaptive Central Control of Motoneuron Gain

Renshaw cells also mediate descending modulation of the motoneuron recruitment process. Stimulation in nucleus interpositus (NIP) of the cerebellum, or in its target, the Red Nucleus (RN), which projects to spinal pools via the rubrospinal pathway, enhances the gain of the monosynaptic stretch reflex by inhibiting RCs, thereby releasing alpha-motoneurons from recurrent inhibition. The NIP or RN stimulation also excites motoneurons. Bullock and Grossberg (1989) proposed that the implied bivalent rubral projection to RCs and alpha-motoneurons afforded adaptive, i.e., learning-based, control of the "gain" of movement commands directed to motoneuron pools. Contreras-Vidal et al. (1997) introduced a neural network comprising a central trajectory generator, an extended FLETE model, and a model cerebellar network capable of learning to modulate motoneuron recruitment via a bivalent output to RCs and alpha-motoneurons. Simulations of the circuit (Figure 2) showed that if the cerebellum received both a desired velocity signal and an error feedback routed from spindles to cerebellum via the inferior olive, then a learning-adjusted cerebellar output substantially enhanced the dynamic tracking characteristics of the limb by transiently exciting, and removing inhibition from, the agonist motoneuron pool (Figure 1). This model is consistent with recent biophysics-based models of cerebellar adaptive timing (e.g., Fiala, Grossberg, and Bullock, 1996), and with common observations of phasic RN and interpositus activity during learned movements. A closely related modeling treatment, encompassing cerebellar modulation of the Figure X circuit in the context of realistic sensory lags, has recently appeared (Spoelstra, Schweighofer, and Arbib, 2000).

Roles of Motor Cortex in Motoneuron Recruitment

Many cells in the primary motor cortex (M1) of primates excite motoneurons via mono- or short polysynaptic pathways, and the pathway for the long-loop stretch reflex traverses M1. Moreover, cooling of the dentate nucleus of the cerebellum, which affects M1 via the thalamus, eliminates anticipatory, force-related, components of normal M1 activity. Many studies have strongly implicated M1 in load compensation achieved by direct recruitment of motoneurons, although a subset of M1 cells are relatively load insensitive (Kalaska et al., 1989). Yet other studies have appeared to implicate M1 in a high-level representation of the direction of movement in Cartesian space. Recently, two models have begun

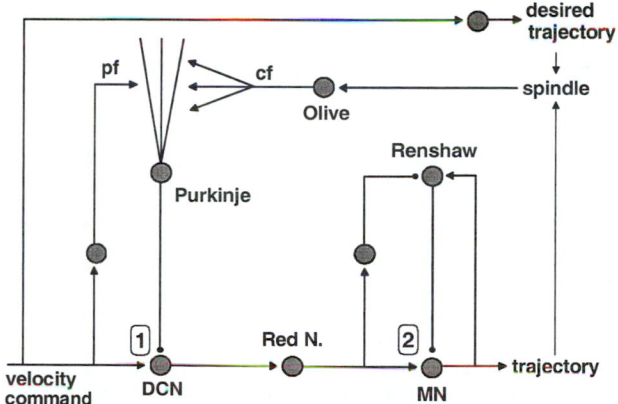

Figure 2. Network model incorporating two sites for controlling motorneuron excitation by release from inhibition. Prior to learning, a velocity control signal directed toward a muscle via the deep cerebellar nuclear (DCN) pathway will have a negligible effect due to Purkinje (P) cell inhibition of DCN sites and Renshaw cell inhibition of alpha-motoneurons (MN). However, trajectory errors detected by muscle spindles activate the inferior olive, whose climbing fibers (cf) reach the dendrites of Purkinje cells. Climbing fiber activity causes long term depression of coactive parallel fiber (pf) synapses that excite Purkinje cells. Depression of Purkinje excitation causes disinhibition of DCN sites. This "opens the gate" for the velocity control signal to activate the Red Nucleus. The Red Nucleus both excites alpha-motoneurons and inhibits Renshaw cells.

to address the dilemma posed by these observations. The extended Vector Integration To Endpoint (VITE) model of Bullock, Cisek, and Grossberg (1998) proposed a circuit involving 6 electrophysiologically identified cell types in M1 and parietal area 5 to explain the distinct computational roles of load-sensitive and load-insensitive cells in both arm trajectory generation *and* load compensation. This model's relatively load-insensitive cells have polysynaptic links to alpha-motoneurons, whereas the most load-sensitive cells have monosynaptic links. Todorov (2000) proposed a model (pertinent primarily to load-sensitive cells) based on the assumption that M1 recruitment compensates for the negative effects of the force-velocity law on the ability of muscle to sustain force when shortening at a significant velocity.

If some M1 cells directly control motoneuron recruitment, and thus force generation, then theories of sensorimotor transformations (e.g., Barreca and Guenther, 2001) predict that the preferred spatial directions of such M1 cells must be strongly posture dependent—and they are. Several recent simulations based on this premise have succeeded in predicting posture- and trajectory-dependent tuning properties of M1 cells and the muscles to which they project (Ajemian, Bullock, and Grossberg, 2001; Scott and Kalaska, 1997).

Discussion

Neural network analyses have begun to clarify how local spinal circuits cooperate with central adaptive circuits for task-dependent control of motoneuron recruitment, but many basic questions remain to be addressed. Too little is known about the pathways for descending control of gamma- versus alpha-motoneurons. Also, the behavioral functions of many known aspects of the recruitment system, such as motoneuronal plateau potentials, remain to be elucidated by computational analyses. Models must also be elaborated to accommodate the unique connectivities that govern recruitment in different species, which differ dramatically in biomechanical, behavioral, and neuronal specializations.

Road Map: Mammalian Motor Control
Related Reading: Cerebellum and Motor Control; Equilibrium Point Hypothesis; Limb Geometry, Neural Control; Muscle Models; Vestibulo-Ocular Reflex

References

Ajemian, R., Bullock, D., and Grossberg, S., 2001, A model of movement coordinates in motor cortex: Posture-dependent changes in the gain and direction of single cell tuning curves, *Cerebral Cortex*, 11:1124–1135.

Akazawa, K., and Kato, K., 1990, Neural network for control of muscle force based on the size principle of motor unit, *Proc. IEEE*, 78:1531–1535.

Barreca, D. M., and Guenther, F. H., 2001, A modeling study of potential sources of curvature in human reaching movements, *J. Motor Behav.*, 33:387–400.

Bullock, D., Cisek, P. E., and Grossberg, S., 1998, Cortical networks for control of voluntary arm movements under variable force conditions, *Cerebral Cortex*, 8:48–62.

Bullock, D., and Grossberg, S., 1989, VITE and FLETE: Neural modules for trajectory formation and postural control, in *Volitional Action* (W.A. Hershberger, Ed.), Amsterdam: North-Holland/Elsevier, pp. 253–298. ◆

Burke, R. E., 1998, Spinal cord: Ventral horn, in *The Synaptic Organization of the Brain* (G.M. Shepherd, Ed.), New York: Oxford, pp. 77–120. ◆

Contreras-Vidal, J. L., Grossberg, S., and Bullock, D., 1997, A neural model of cerebellar learning for arm movement control: Cortico-spino-cerebellar dynamics, *Learning and Memory*, 3:475–502.

Fiala, J. C., Grossberg, S., and Bullock, D., 1996, Metabotropic glutamate receptor activation in cerebellar Purkinje cells as substrate for adaptive timing of the classically conditioned eye blink response, *J. Neurosci.*, 16:3760–3774.

Humphrey, D. R., and Reed, D. J., 1983, Separate cortical systems for control of joint movement and joint stiffness: Reciprocal activation and coactivation of antagonist muscles, *Adv. Neurol.*, 39:347–372. ◆

Kalaska, J. F., Cohen, D. A. D., Hyde, M. L., and Prud'homme, M. J., 1989, A comparison of movement direction-related versus load direction-related activity in primate motor cortex, using a two dimensional reaching task, *J. Neurosci.*, 9:2080–2102.

Lindsay, A. D., and Binder, M. D., 1991, Distribution of effective synaptic currents underlying recurrent inhibition in cat triceps surae motoneurons, *J. Neurophysiol.*, 65:168–177.

Nichols, T. R., and Houk, J. C., 1973, Reflex compensation for variations in the mechanical properties of a muscle, *Science*, 181:182–184.

Pratt, C. A., and Jordan, L. M., 1987, Ia inhibitory interneurons and Renshaw cells as contributors to the spinal mechanisms of fictive locomotion, *J. Neurophysiol.*, 57:56–71.

Scott, S. H., and Kalaska, J. F., 1997, Reaching movements with similar hand paths but different arm orientations. I. Activity of individual cells in motor cortex, *J. Neurophysiol.*, 77:826–852.

Spoelstra, J., Schweighofer, N., and Arbib, M. A., 2000, Cerebellar learning of accurate predictive control for fast reaching movements, *Biol. Cybernetics*, 82:321–333.

Todorov, E., 2000, Direct cortical control of muscle activation in voluntary arm movements: A model, *Nature Neurosci.*, 3:391–398.

van Heijst, J. J., Vos, J. E., and Bullock, D., 1998, Development in a biologically inspired spinal neural network for movement control, *Neural Networks*, 11:1305–1316.

Motor Control, Biological and Theoretical

R. Christopher Miall

Introduction

Biological motor control can be characterized as a problem of controlling nonlinear, unreliable systems whose states are monitored with slow and sometimes low-quality sensors. In response to changing sensory inputs, internal goals, or motor errors, the motor system must solve several basic problems: selection of an appropriate action and transformation of control signals from sensory to motor coordinate frameworks; coordination of the selected movement with other ongoing behaviors and with postural reflexes; and monitoring the movement to ensure its accuracy. These stages may be interlinked, so that separation of any one particular problem into these individual stages may not be possible. This article describes some of the ways we think that biological motor systems solve these tasks, based on principles (and terminology) whose origins are in engineering and cybernetics. The field of cybernetics has developed from Norbert Wiener's initial ideas on communication and control theory in complex mechanical and biological systems, which focused on feedback mechanisms.

A motor control system acts by sending motor commands to a controlled object, often called the "plant," which in turn acts on its local environment (Figure 1). The plant or the environment has one or more variables that the motor system attempts to regulate, either to maintain them at a steady reference level in the face of disturbances (a "regulator") or to follow some changing reference value (a "controller"). The motor control system may make use of sensory signals from the environment, from its reference inputs, and from the plant to determine what actions are required. Sensory inputs from the plant can provide information about the *state* of

the controlled object. Here, the state can be considered as all relevant variables that adequately describe the controlled object. But note that the sensory inputs to the controller do not necessarily provide direct measures of the true state of the system: they may be inaccurate or delayed, as discussed later. If controller output is based on signals that are unaffected by the plant output, it is said to be a *feedforward controller*: the feedforward control path is the thick line from left to right in Figure $1A_1$, which requires no return signals. If the controller output is instead based on a comparison between the reference and the controlled variables, it is a *feedback controller* (Figure $1B_1$): the control pathway is a closed loop. One can add more complex control strategies to these simple systems (Figure $1A_2$, $1B_2$), as described in more detail below.

The advantage of feedforward control is that it can, in the ideal case, give perfect performance with no error between the reference and the controlled variable. The main disadvantages for biological systems include the potential difficulty in generating an accurate controller for a complex system and the lack of error corrections. If the controller is not accurate, if the plant is unreliable, or if unexpected external disturbances occur, output errors go unchecked. Since no biological system can be both perfectly accurate and perfectly free of external disturbances, error correction is usually necessary. In contrast, the major advantage of negative feedback control lies in its very simple, robust strategy. The controller drives the plant so as to cancel the feedback error signaled by the comparator. Because it constantly seeks to cancel the error, it operates well, even without exact knowledge of the controlled object and despite internal or external disturbances. But feedback control strategies also have disadvantages: errors cannot be avoided but

Figure 1. *Feedforward control*: A_1, The black arrows represent the on-line control signals; the dotted lines are off-line signals used to update controller. A_2, Adaptive controllers using off-line information can adjust parameters of the feedforward controller to reflect changes in the plant properties. *Negative feedback control*: B_1, The black circle represents a comparison between the reference and feedback signals. The black arrows now form a closed control loop; the crossed circle is a comparator. B_2, An internal model of the controlled object can replace the external feedback loop with a rapid feedback estimate.

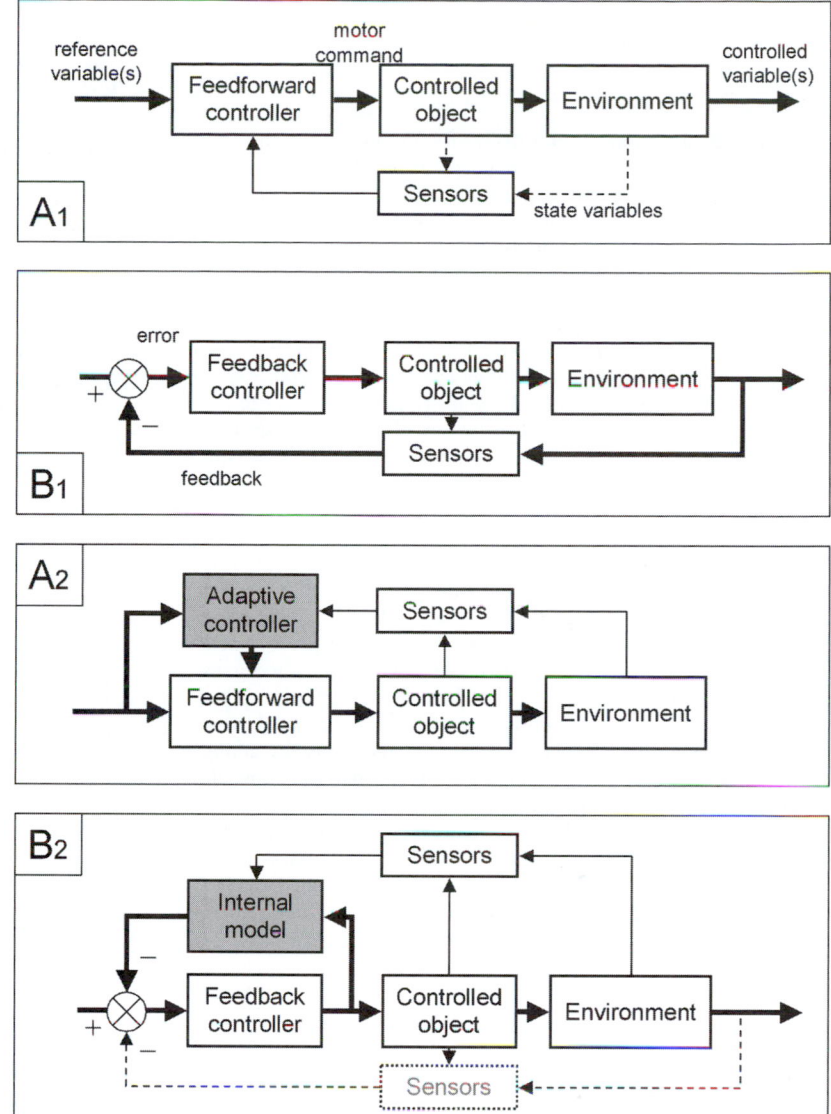

Feedback Control

The design criteria for negative feedback control are dominated by the closed-loop gain. Gain is defined as the ratio of a system's output to its input. For a linear servo controller, the gain should be close to unity, so that a given input (the reference value) evokes an output of almost equal magnitude. In a feedback circuit (Figure $1B_1$), one can define both open-loop and closed-loop gains. The open-loop gain K_o is given by the ratio of the response to the error; it gives the response expected if the feedback path shown in Figure $1B_1$ is cut, thus opening the loop. The closed-loop gain K_c is given by the ratio of response to reference amplitudes. The closed-loop gain K_c is determined by the open-loop gain where $K_c = K_o/(1 + K_o)$. For ideal control, K_c should be unity under all conditions; thus the open-loop gain K_o should be as high as possible, ensuring that K_c approaches unity. In practice, K_o is usually frequency dependent and can never reach infinity; hence K_c is also frequency dependent and less than unity.

must occur and be corrected, and feedback control—especially in biological systems—tends to be slow.

The design of nonlinear and multidimensional feedback systems is beyond the scope of this article, except to note that, in many instances, complex control problems can be simplified and linearized around the current state of the system. This may be particularly true of biological systems, in which control is often only approximate.

Notice that the comparison of the reference value with the controlled variable to give an error signal (Figure $1B_1$) is affected by the dynamics of the motor control and sensory systems. When a command is issued by the controller, its effects are not immediately apparent to the comparator, but are delayed by the plant and sensor dynamics and by transport delays on both the forward and feedback paths. In biological systems, where sensor delays are inevitable, the comparison is always out of date. Hence in any feedback system there will be a frequency at which these delays combine to impart a 180° phase lag. The open-loop gain K_o at that frequency now only needs to be unity (instead of very large) to make $K_c > 1.0$, forcing the system into instability. Any small error or disturbance will be overcorrected and result in even bigger errors, leading to yet bigger corrections. Human examples of instability are indeed seen when control delays are artificially increased in man-machine interfaces

(Miall and Wolpert, 1996) or as a result of increased neural transport delays in neuropathies such as multiple sclerosis.

Physiological Feedback Circuits

Although feedback control circuits are found throughout physiology, let us consider just two examples from vertebrate motor systems. The major tension-producing fibers of the vertebrate muscle, known as extrafusal fibers, contract following excitation by alpha motor neurons. However, the amount of tension produced by the muscle in response to a motor command varies with the length of the muscle, its speed of contraction, level of fatigue, and so on. The muscles are therefore provided with numerous sensory structures, muscle spindles, that signal back to the CNS the length and rate of stretch of the muscle. Spindles are complex sensorimotor structures combining contractile elements (intrafusal fibers, excited by specialized gamma motor neurons) with a central stretch-sensitive region. Their axons project onto alpha motor neurons in the spinal cord that serve the same muscle and synergistic muscles. This circuit (the stretch reflex) is a feedback controller for muscle length. If the muscle is stretched, the spindles respond, exciting the alpha motor neurons, and the resulting reflex contraction of the extrafusal fibers restores the muscle to its original length, silencing the spindles again. Thus the spindles signal a deviation from their regulated length, and the controller (the alpha motor neuron) acts to cancel the error. The muscles also contain Golgi tendon organs (GTOs), which are attached to the tendons of muscle and respond to increased tension in the tendon. They excite interneurons that inhibit motor neurons of that muscle and other muscles acting around the same joint, and also act in a feedback manner. If muscle tension increases due to an external load, for example, the GTOs are activated and, via the inhibitory interneuron, inhibit the motor neurons, causing the muscle to relax. This reduces tension, and thus the negative feedback loop serves to maintain a controlled level of tension. This description of the spindle and GTO is oversimplified, ignoring aspects such as control of muscle stretch velocity, but emphasizes their basic control properties. Together, they act to maintain a muscle in its current state: changes in length or in tension will be automatically opposed.

Feedforward Control

Feedforward control schemes may be grouped as those based on direct control and those based on indirect control using internal models. Here, direct control means control without *explicit* knowledge of the behavior of the plant (see REINFORCEMENT LEARNING IN MOTOR CONTROL). In practice, a controller that can store and issue appropriate motor programs must have implicitly, if not explicitly, captured knowledge of the plant. Hence feedforward controllers must be matched to the properties of the plant they control. As a physiological example, the equilibrium point hypothesis (see EQUILIBRIUM POINT HYPOTHESIS) makes use of the spring-like properties of muscles. For any set of springs pulling across the multiple joints of a limb, there will be a stable position into which the limb passively settle. Thus, the CNS could define the "end-point" muscle tensions and the limb would move to the desired position without the controller's knowing either its starting position or its behavior during the movement. An alternative direct scheme is to generate the appropriate commands—a temporal sequence of required changes in muscle force, acquired and stored as a motor program—but again without any explicit knowledge of the plant. In the limit one could use a memorized lookup table to store appropriate motor commands for each input-output pair. However, the memory demands grow explosively if a motor command is stored for every possible pairing. Some form of generalization is assumed to avoid this problem (see SENSORIMOTOR LEARNING)

such that a coarse-grained representation is achieved, with interpolation.

Physiological Feedforward Control

Muscle spindles and GTOs are used to ensure that actions occur as planned. By sending motor commands both to the alpha and to the gamma motor neurons, both the force-producing extrafusal fibers of the muscle and the much weaker intrafusal fibers of the spindle co-contract. If the joint fails to move fast enough owing to an unexpected load, the spindle contractile elements shorten within the main muscle, the stretch-sensitive sensory region is stimulated, and additional excitatory drive is reflexively added to the spinal alpha motor neurons to overcome the load. The original position control theory proposed by Merton has had to be supplemented by tension and velocity control; but this simple description, while incomplete, highlights the main principles. Note that by co-activating alpha and gamma motor neurons, the reference values of the feedback circuit described earlier are predictively modified. Thus for the supraspinal centers driving the movement, the spinal circuits can be treated as a feedforward controller, autonomously regulating the muscles without the need for feedback to these higher centers. Of course, if errors become large, cortical control can be invoked. This demonstrates an important principle: biological motor circuits are often hierarchical, with lower levels regularizing the behavior of the controlled object and higher systems providing increasingly indirect control (Loeb, Brown, and Cheng, 1999).

Another example of feedforward control is found in the oculomotor system (see COLLICULAR VISUOMOTOR TRANSFORMATIONS FOR GAZE CONTROL). Human eye muscles have muscle spindles, but they do not seem to have a functional stretch reflex: passive movements of the eyes are not reflexively adjusted, and even seem to be ignored. As Helmholtz noted, if one pushes on the side of one's own eye, the resulting retinal movement is reported by the visual system as movement of the external world. The reason the oculomotor system may be able to operate in feedforward mode is that the mechanical load (the spherical eyeball) is relatively constant, unaffected by external weights or gravity, and is therefore more easily controlled than a multi-jointed limb. Functionally, of course, there is powerful *visual* feedback: if the eyes drift from the target of gaze, the error is reported as slip of the visual image over the retina. Retinal slip drives "on-line" corrective velocity adjustment during smooth eye movement. Because saccades are of short duration, errors are corrected "off-line" with a secondary saccade. Consistent saccadic under- or overshooting errors lead to long-term changes in the feedforward controller, an example of adaptive control.

Adaptive Control and Internal Models

Adaptive Control

Adaptive control relies on monitoring performance over a longer time scale than that used by negative feedback control to generate a measure of average performance rather than of moment-to-moment error. The adaptive controller is then used to adjust the motor responses, for example, by modulating the feedforward controller as indicated in Figure $1A_2$ or by modulating the open-loop gain of a feedback controller. The advantage of adaptive control is that it can compensate for gradual changes in the motor performance of the controlled object. Controllers can also be designed to track predictable changes in the reference value. Because the performance of physiological systems (as well as the goals of behavior) changes over time, all biological control systems are to some extent adaptive through mechanisms as diverse as evolutionary change, growth, or learning and memory. In control of eye movements, there is good evidence that the cerebellum is involved in adaptation (Robinson and Fuchs, 2001).

Internal Models

Two forms of internal model can be distinguished. An ideal feedforward controller will ensure that the plant output (the controlled variable) is always identical to the reference value. Thus it inputs the reference value (and often also the state signals, Figure $1A_1$) and outputs a motor command; the motor command shifts the plant into a new state, which should equal the reference value. Thus one can describe the ideal feedforward controller as an *inverse* of the plant: the plant translates commands into states whereas the inverse controller translates desired states into commands. If the transfer function of the plant is represented as P, its inverse is P^{-1}, and the transfer function of the complete system (from reference value to controlled variable) is $P \cdot P^{-1} = 1$. Again, this implies that the perfect system has a gain of unity. Inverse modeling is covered in more detail in Jordan (1994).

The alternative type of internal model is known as a forward model of the plant (Figure $1B_2$). Its inputs are a copy of the motor command being sent to the plant and also the current feedback of the plant state, and its output is an estimate of the next state of the plant or of the controlled variables. This estimate is available to the feedback controller more rapidly than actual feedback. Thus, the external feedback loop can be replaced by an internal loop, which avoids the feedback delays mentioned above. A negative feedback loop with negligible delay and a high open-loop gain will rapidly and accurately drive its plant in a direction to minimize the comparator error. Thus, a fast internal loop including a forward model is functionally equivalent to an inverse dynamic model. Of course, viewed from outside the loop, it functions as a feedforward controller: it disregards the actual feedback and hence is no longer error correcting. The oculomotor feedforward controller may be an inverse model like that shown in Figure $1A_2$ (Krauzlis and Lisberger, 1989); an alternative proposal suggests an internal forward model as in Figure $1B_2$ (Robinson, 1975).

Schemes that combine feedback with feedforward control (Hoff and Arbib, 1992; Miall et al., 1993) depend on estimation of the expected feedback signal, including its delay. Recent theories have proposed combined forward and inverse models, working in pairs for system identification, control, and adaptation (Wolpert, Miall, and Kawato, 1998).

Physiological Internal Models

Visual guidance of the human arm is based on sensory information from the visual system with processing delays of up to 100 ms. Motor commands issued by the CNS may take 50 ms to initiate muscle contraction, and these changes are signaled by vision and by proprioceptors with delays of perhaps 50 to 100 ms. So feedback signals from the environment will lag significantly behind the issue of each motor command. Despite this, we control our limbs skillfully and accurately with movement durations of well under half a second. Thus, our motor control cannot be based entirely on feedback signals; we also employ feedforward control. It is likely (although not yet certain) that control is based on internal representations of the motor system—internal models (Miall and Wolpert, 1996).

Can we identify these internal models in the brain? The cerebellum is a strong contender for internal model representations (Ito, 1984; Wolpert et al., 1998). The model should receive as inputs either the motor goal or an efferent copy of the motor command, and also receive proprioceptive information about the current state of the body. There must be a mechanism to allow the model to adapt to predict accurately the behavior of the limb, i.e., a neural learning mechanism. And the output of the model must form either the motor command or a sensory prediction of the action outcome. The cerebellum can satisfy all these constraints, but this alone is not proof. Other possible sites are the motor cortex, parietal cortex,

and the spinal cord, although a spinal representation would probably be more closely related to individual muscles than a model of the whole arm.

There are strong connections from the motor cortical areas and posterior parietal cortex to the lateral hemispheres of the cerebellum, and from there, ascending paths back to premotor and motor cortices or descending to brainstem nuclei. Spinocerebellar tracts provide a large array of proprioceptive signals, updating the cerebellum on the current state of the limb. For adaptation, we know that coincident activity in climbing fiber and parallel fiber inputs to Purkinje cells results in a sustained change in the strength of the parallel fiber:Purkinje cell synapse (see CEREBELLUM: NEURAL PLASTICITY). Some researchers therefore suspect that the cerebellum acts as an adaptive inverse model on the feedforward control pathway (Figure $1A_2$; Ito, 1984; Kawato and Gomi, 1992). Ito viewed the cerebellum as an adaptive side path to the descending systems, modulating the feedforward commands issued by cerebral control centers. Kawato views it as an alternative to these cerebral systems, replacing their control function. The alternative forward model-based scheme (Figure $1B_2$) is also valid; hence the cerebellum may represent an adaptive forward model on a feedback pathway (Miall et al., 1993). This Smith predictor theory places the forward model within the closed cerebrocerebellar loop as the controller and incorporates feedback via an adaptive delay module. Each module is learned independently, with different time courses. It is difficult to distinguish between inverse dynamics models (Figure $1A_2$) and internal feedback loops containing forward models (Figure $1B_2$) unless one can get access to their internal structure. One might block the internal feedback loop needed for a forward model or decoding the input and output signals. However, many recent psychophysical, electrophysiological, and functional imaging experiments have generated strong evidence of the use of internal models for motor control, for state estimation, and for planning and interpretation of actions.

Road Maps: Mammalian Motor Control; Robotics and Control Theory
Related Reading: Action Monitoring and Forward Control of Movements; Cerebellum and Motor Control; Optimization Principles in Motor Control; Sensorimotor Learning

References

Hoff, B., and Arbib, M. A., 1992, A model of the effects of speed, accuracy and perturbation on visually guided reaching, in *Control of Arm Movement in Space: Neurophysiological and Computational Approaches*, vol. 22, *Experimental Brain Research Series* (R. Caminiti, Ed.), Berlin: Springer-Verlag, pp. 285–306.
Ito, M., 1984, *The Cerebellum and Neural Control*, New York: Raven Press.
Jordan, M., 1994, Computational aspects of motor control and motor learning, in *Handbook of Motor Control* (H. Heuer and S. Keele, Eds.), Berlin: Springer-Verlag, pp. 1–65.
Kawato, M., and Gomi, H., 1992, The cerebellum and VOR/OKR learning models, *Trends Neurosci.*, 15:445–453.
Krauzlis, R. J., and Lisberger, S. G., 1989, A control systems model of smooth pursuit eye movements with realistic emergent properties, *Neural Computation*, 1:116–122.
Loeb, G. E., Brown, I. E., and Cheng, E. J., 1999, A hierarchical foundation for models of sensorimotor control, *Exp. Brain Res.*, 126:1–18.
Miall, R. C., and Wolpert, D. M., 1996, Forward models for physiological motor control, *Neural Networks*, 9:1265–1279. ◆
Miall, R. C., Weir, D. J., Wolpert, D. M., and Stein, J. F., 1993, Is the cerebellum a Smith predictor? *J. Motor Behav.*, 25:203–216.
Robinson, D. A., 1975, Oculomotor control signals, in *Basic Mechanisms of Ocular Motility and Their Clinical Implications* (G. Lennerstrand and P. Bach-y-Rita, Eds.), Oxford: Pergamon Press, pp. 337–374.
Robinson, F. R., and Fuchs, A. F., 2001, The role of the cerebellum in voluntary eye movements, *Annu. Rev. Neurosci.*, 24:981–1004.
Wolpert, D. M., Miall, R. C., and Kawato, M., 1998, Internal models in the cerebellum, *Trends Cogn. Sci.*, 2:338–347.

Motor Cortex: Coding and Decoding of Directional Operations

Bagrat Amirikian and Apostolos P. Georgopoulos

Introduction

Two fundamental issues—how does the brain work, and how can we build intelligent machines?—are the leitmotifs of this *Handbook*. There are many strategies for attacking these questions, depending on what particular aspects of these broad issues we are interested in. One approach lies in the behavioral-neurophysiological domain. The recording of the activity of single cells in the brain of behaving animals provides a tool for directly studying how a particular behavioral pattern is represented and generated. Studies along this line intend to answer the first question: How does the brain work?

In the framework of this approach, the firing of a single neuron or a population of neurons can be correlated with one or several behavioral variables changing in time. The main challenge is to solve a pair of complementary problems: the coding/specification problem and the decoding/implementation problem. The former addresses the question of how the information about a particular behavioral variable is encoded in the neuronal activity being produced (see POPULATION CODES). The latter concerns the neural mechanisms by which encoded variables generate a behavioral pattern unfolding in time.

In the behavioral-neurophysiological domain, the constructive framework for attacking the issue of building "intelligent" machines could be formulated in the context of the decoding problem, namely: How can we design adaptive systems that would transform neuronal signals recorded in the brain of behaving animals into the physiologically appropriate behavioral pattern generated by an artificial machine? (see BRAIN-COMPUTER INTERFACES).

The work reported here summarizes a series of studies based on experimental work and abstract modeling. It exemplifies the successful application of the above-mentioned paradigms to the study of the arm motor system of the monkey and to the design of adaptive systems that transform chronically recorded brain signals into the motor output of artificial actuators. For that purpose, relatively simple but behaviorally meaningful motor actions such as a reaching movement and an exertion of force were chosen. We address the question of how movement variables are encoded in the motor cortex and how this information could be used to drive a simulated actuator that mimics the primate arm.

Cortical Representation of Movement

Coding by Single Cells

A common and behaviorally meaningful movement is reaching to targets in space. Reaching involves well-coordinated motion about the shoulder and elbow joints for transporting the hand in space and bringing it to a desired location. A reaching movement can be regarded as a vector, pointing from its origin to its target, with direction and amplitude.

A relation between the direction of reaching, **M**, and the cell discharge rate, *d*, has been established for several brain areas, including the motor cortex, the premotor cortex, area 5, the cerebellar cortex, and the deep cerebellar nuclei (Georgopoulos, 1996). This relation is characterized by a broad tuning function, *d*(**M**), the peak of which denotes the "preferred" direction of the cell, **C**, that is, the direction of movement for which the cell's activity would be highest (Figure 1). Typically, cell activity (discharge rate) varies

as a linear function of the cosine of the angle, θ_{MC}, between the preferred direction of the cell **C** and the direction of reaching **M**:

$$d(\mathbf{M}) = b + k \cos\theta_{MC} \qquad (1)$$

where *b* and *k* are cell-specific regression coefficients. (Although other functions could fit the data [Amirikian and Georgopoulos, 2000], the cosine function is a simple one that explains a good percentage of variation in cell activity.) Equation 1 holds both for reaching movements in a two-dimensional (2D) plane and for free reaching movements performed in three-dimensional (3D) space (Georgopoulos, 1996). Preferred directions of single cells range over the directional continuum and are multiply represented in the motor cortex.

Broad directional tuning of motor cortical cells was also observed with respect to the force pulses exerted by the monkey arm against an immovable object (Georgopoulos et al., 1992). A monkey was trained to exert forces in a 2D plane on an isometric handle in the presence of a constant force bias. First, the monkey was required to exert a postural (static) force **P**, which compensated a given bias force **B** (**P** + **B** = 0). After a holding period, a cue instructed the monkey to exert a force **S** such that the net force **N** acting on the handle (i.e., the force exerted by the monkey **S** *plus* the bias force applied to the handle **B**) would be in a visually specified (instructed) direction. Note that the net force **N** is congruent to the incremental (dynamic) component **I** of the force **S** exerted by the animal: **I** = **S** − **P** = **S** + **B** = **N**. Eight instructed directions and eight bias force directions evenly distributed in the 2D plane were employed. Recordings of neuronal activity in the motor cortex revealed that when the arm exerted a force without moving, the activity of single cells showed approximately the same broad directional tuning properties as when the arm moved through space. Cells were tuned not to the direction of force **S** exerted by the animal but to the direction of the dynamic component **I** of the force **S**.

Fu, Suarez, and Ebner (1993) investigated the relations between neuronal activity at the single-cell level and the amplitude of motor action. In these studies monkeys moved a handle over a planar working surface in eight directions (0–360°, in 45° intervals) and six amplitudes (1.4–5.4 cm, in 0.8-cm increments) in a pseudo-random order. The activity of cells in the motor and premotor cortex was directionally tuned in a cosine fashion, as described previously; the preferred direction was very similar for movements of different amplitudes. Cell activity generally increased with movement amplitude. Two aspects of this latter finding are noteworthy: first, the highest increase in neuronal activity with movement amplitude was not always along the cell's preferred direction; and second, the strongest relations with movement amplitude were observed for cell activity during but not before the movement (in the latter case, the direction of movement is the most important factor). These findings indicate that the motor cortex is involved primarily in the *specification* of movement direction, as the movement is planned during the reaction time, and in *monitoring* movement amplitude, as the movement evolves during the movement time.

The relationship of ongoing cell activity to evolving movement variables such as position, speed, and acceleration was also studied (Ashe and Georgopoulos, 1994; Schwartz and Moran, 2000). It was found that cell activity was related to all these parameters, although movement velocity and target direction provided the main contribution. Therefore, the activity of motor cortical cells can be tuned to several movement parameters.

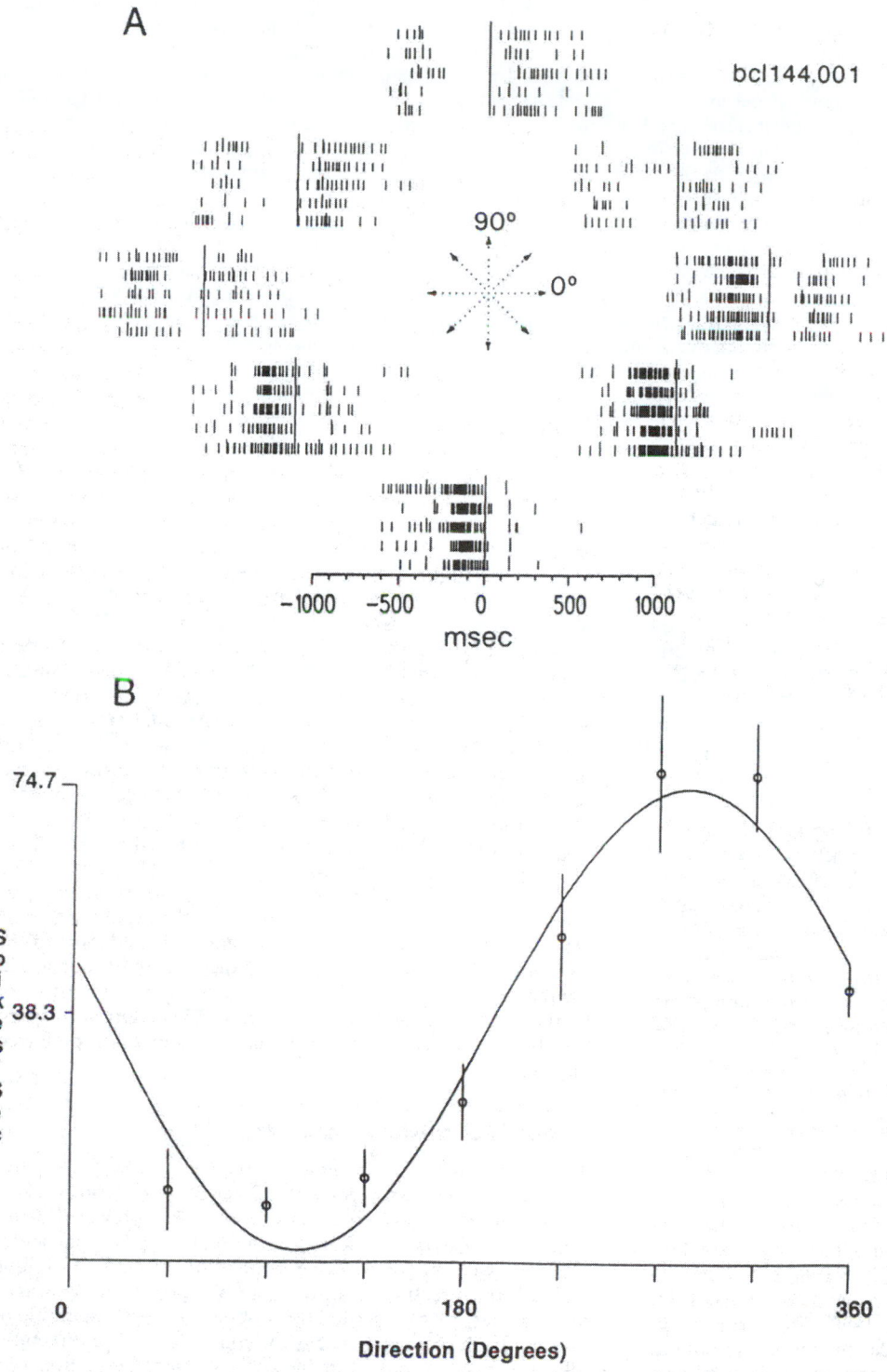

Figure 1. Discharge patterns during the center-out task. *A*, Rasters are arranged schematically at each target location around the center start position. Each raster is aligned to the time of exit from the center start position (zero time). The first long tickmark of each trial is the target onset time, the second is the time of movement onset, and the third is the time of target acquisition. *B*, The cosine tuning function was derived from the average rate of discharge (circles) between target onset and target acquisition for each movement. The error bars show the standard deviation of the discharge rate. The regression coefficients (see Equation 1 in the text) were as follows: $b = 37.9$ spikes/s, $k = 36.1$ spikes/s. The proportion of variance in discharge rate explained by the regression was $R^2 = 0.95$. (From Schwartz, A. B., 1992, Motor cortical activity during drawing movements: Single-unit activity during sinusoid tracing, *J. Neurophysiol.,* 68:528–541. Reprinted with permission.)

The findings of the studies reviewed above regard discrete reaching movements. Schwartz (1992) studied the neural mechanisms of continuous, drawing movements by recording the activity of single cells in the motor cortex while the monkey traced on a touch screen sinusoids of various amplitudes and spatial frequencies. Under these conditions, the direction and speed of movement changed continuously in time. In another task, monkeys made equal-amplitude movements from a central point to peripheral targets (center-out task). The following were found: (1) in the center-out task, cell activity varied in a cosine fashion with the direction of the movement, as found previously; (2) in the tracing task, the ongoing direction of movement explained most of the variance in ongoing cell activity; and (3) a good proportion of the remaining, nondirectional variance could be accounted for by the ongoing speed of the movement. This relation to speed was best observed for movements near the cell's preferred direction.

Recently, a thorough assessment of single-cell recording studies in primates (Johnson, Mason, and Ebner, 2001) emphasized the idea of a multiparametric control of movement. Particularly, it was pointed out that the activity of single cells in central motor structures relates to several motor parameters (e.g., end-point force, acceleration, velocity, position), the relative contribution of which may vary in time and is influenced by the motor behavioral context.

Coding by Neuronal Populations

The broad directional tuning of single-cell activity indicates that a given cell participates in movements of various directions; from this result, and from the fact that preferred directions range widely, it follows that a movement in a particular direction will engage a whole population of cells. A unique code for the direction of movement (Georgopoulos, 1996) regards this population of directionally tuned cells as an ensemble of vectors in which each vector stands for the contribution of an individual cell. Specifically, the ith cell is represented by a vector that points in the cell's preferred direction $\mathbf{C}_i$ and has a length $w_i(\mathbf{M})$ proportional to the change in cell activity associated with a particular movement direction $\mathbf{M}$. The vector sum of these neuronal contributions is the "population vector":

$$\mathbf{P}(\mathbf{M}) = \sum_{i=1}^{N} w_i(\mathbf{M})\mathbf{C}_i \qquad (2)$$

where N is the number of cells in the population. The population vector points in the direction of the movement for discrete movements in 2D and 3D space.

The length of the population vector is proportional to the instantaneous speed of the movement (Schwartz and Moran, 2000). The time series of population vectors calculated during the movement were added successively tip-to-tail, resulting in a "neural" trajectory that predicted well the ensuing trajectory of the actual movement by an average time lead of approximately 120 ms. Therefore, the population vector carries information concerning the unfolding movement trajectory.

The population vector algorithm was also used to retrieve information encoded in the ensemble of directionally tuned cells recorded while the monkey executed the isometric force task (Georgopoulos et al., 1992) described above. It turned out that the time-varying population vector reflected neither the force $\mathbf{S}$ exerted by the animal, which changed appreciably in direction and magnitude during individual trials, nor the static component $\mathbf{P}$ of the force $\mathbf{S}$, which compensated for the constant force bias $\mathbf{B}$. Instead, the direction of the population vector remained invariant during the trial and pointed in the direction of the dynamic component $\mathbf{I}$ of the force $\mathbf{S}$ exerted by the monkey. Based on this analysis, it was hypothesized (Georgopoulos et al., 1992) that the motor cortex provides the dynamic component of the force signal during force

development, while other, possibly subcortical structures provide the static compensatory signal. These signals could converge in the spinal cord and provide an ongoing integrated signal to the motor neuronal pools.

It is important to realize that the population vector is a simple algorithm that retrieves an encoded variable from the activity of cells tuned to that variable, without making any assumptions about how the tuning itself emerges. There is controversy, however, as to what kind of variables these cells are coding: low-level variables such as muscle forces, or high-level variables such as end-point velocity (Flash and Sejnowski, 2001; Johnson et al., 2001). The matter has been recently sharpened by Todorov (2000), who proposed a simple model that (under certain assumptions) explicitly related cell activity to end-point force, acceleration, velocity, and position during small-amplitude movements. Interestingly, the model is consistent with experimental observations of multiparametric tuning of motor cortical cells (Johnson et al., 2001), and directly states that a *required* directional cell tuning is defined by a linear combination of end-point force, acceleration, velocity, and position terms. The relative contribution of each of these terms to the tuning depends on model parameters as well as experimental conditions (e.g., external loads). The main emphasis of Todorov's paper, however, is the "reinterpretation of the population vector." Since model cells were not explicitly related to high-level parameters but directly controlled low-level parameters (muscle forces), it was claimed that the view that motor cortex codes low-level variables "is in principle correct." Conversely, experimentally observed correlations with high-level motor variables (Johnson et al., 2001) is an epiphenomenon rather than a true neural code (Scott, 2000).

Todorov's model, however, does not allow one to make such far-reaching claims. The point is that the model is not "closed": the directional tuning is not an emergent property of the model but rather is built into it. Therefore, the derived expression for cell activity (Equation 2, Todorov, 2000), which is a starting point for all of Todorov's results, specifies a *required* activity of directionally tuned cells in order to generate a particular movement. The model, however, does not concern itself with *how* this required time-varying activity is produced in the course of movement. Note that cortical cell activity is a response to dynamic inputs received from cells in a local environment as well as inputs received from remote cortical areas. None of these factors is present in the model. Therefore, whether the information conveyed to individual cells via these inputs is related to low- or high-level motor variables cannot be answered in the framework of the model. The question of a *true* code is simply beyond the scope of this model. In a sense, the situation is similar to experimental studies in which cell activity, but not the cause of this activity, is recorded.

Decoding Motor Cortical Signals

The population vector code, by combining activities of broadly tuned cells, provides an unambiguous and reliable estimation (see POPULATION CODES) of the upcoming motor output (movement or force). However, the population vector allows only reading out as a single vector the cortical representation of distributed motor commands. It does not answer the question of how the motor commands, encoded in the cell activities, are translated into coordinated contraction of limb muscles to generate a desired motor action. This problem is closely related to the design of adaptive systems that transform neuronal signals chronically recorded from the motor cortex into physiologically appropriate motor output of artificial actuators such as multijoint prosthetic limbs (Schwartz, Taylor, and Helms Tillery, 2001; see BRAIN-COMPUTER INTERFACES).

Despite apparent similarities between these two problems, the approaches suitable for attacking each one pursue different goals.

The methods used to solve the first problem are heavily based on anatomical, neurophysiological, and biomechanical properties of the actual biological structures involved. The ultimate goal of this data-driven approach is to understand how real biological systems implement motor control. In contrast, the methods used to solve the second problem are usually based on theoretical analysis, the ultimate goal of which is to develop a computational algorithm that utilizes the raw biological signals to drive an artificial actuator. Here, the computational scheme does not try to be biologically realistic. Any control algorithm that successfully solves the problem is acceptable. Despite the difference in goals, the importance of interplay between the data- and theory-driven approaches should not be underestimated. The ideas and concepts developed in one field drive the other, and vice versa.

This was illustrated by Lukashin, Amirikian, and Georgopoulos (1996a, 1996b), who addressed the question of how neuronal signals might be used to drive an artificial actuator so that its motor output would correspond to the performance of a real limb. They suggested a computational scheme that transformed impulse activity recorded from the monkey motor cortex during performance of the isometric force task to the force produced by a simulated actuator. Although this computational model is not an accurate realization of biological motor control, it is biologically plausible. The model was inspired by, and based on, experimental findings obtained in anatomical, neurophysiological, and psychophysical studies conducted on three different organisms: (1) experiments on microstimulation of the frog's spinal cord (see MOTOR PRIMITIVES); (2) studies of human arm stiffness characteristics (Mussa-Ivaldi, Hogan, and Bizzi, 1985; see also references in EQUILIBRIUM POINT HYPOTHESIS); and (3) single-cell recordings in the motor cortex of monkey (Georgopoulos, 1996).

Transformation of Spiking Activity into Isometric Force Exerted by an Actuator

The motor cortical activity used in Lukashin et al., (1996b) as command signals came from single-cell recording experiments (Georgopoulos et al., 1992), discussed above, when there was no force bias applied ($\mathbf{B} = 0$). In this case, the force $\mathbf{S}$ exerted by the monkey had only the dynamic component $\mathbf{I}$ and was the only force acting on the isometric handle. Therefore, the force $\mathbf{S}$ developed over time had to be in the instructed direction and had to increase in magnitude in order to exceed a required threshold. The bottom left part of Figure 2 shows an example of impulse activity of $N = 15$ different cells. These spike trains were recorded in different trials but for the same instructed direction of force (180° in the 2D workspace, Figure 2, top left). The key idea is that these cortical signals must now drive a simulated actuator (Figure 2, top right) in such a way that it would exert an isometric force in the same direction as the monkey did.

The actuator is a planar two-joint, six-muscle model of the arm. The transformation of cortical signals into motor output of the actuator is performed by an artificial neural network (Figure 2, bottom right) connected to the actuator. The network receives experimentally measured impulse activity as a time-varying input to the input layer and transforms it into a time-varying pattern of activity at the output layer. This results in contraction of actuator "muscles" by means of changing the muscle rest lengths. Finally, a set of the muscle rest lengths unambiguously defines the direction and magnitude of the end-point force exerted by the actuator against an immovable object. Thus the motor control algorithm realized in this model transformed a neural field, i.e., cortical activity, to a force field, i.e., end-point force (see GEOMETRICAL PRINCIPLES IN MOTOR CONTROL).

In the framework of this computational scheme, the performance of the model (i.e., the relation between the input cortical signals

and the force exerted) depends mainly on the network connectivity, which must provide a synergistic activation of all muscles to generate a required motor action. To ensure physiologically normal motor output of the actuator, the network was trained (Lukashin et al., 1996a) on experimental data obtained from studies of human arm stiffness (Mussa-Ivaldi et al., 1985). As a result, the stiffness properties of the model arm were similar to those measured for the human arm. Moreover, the biological relevance of this model was further independently tested (Lukashin et al., 1996a) by simulating experiments on microstimulation of frog spinal cord (see MOTOR PRIMITIVES). The model was fully consistent with experimentally observed vector summation of active force fields, realizing the idea of a linear combination of a small number of force field primitives to produce a large repertoire of motor behaviors (see MOTOR PRIMITIVES).

After training, the underlying set of synaptic weights was fixed and the performance of the model was tested against the whole neurophysiological data set (Georgopoulos et al., 1992), which included both experimentally measured motor cortical commands and resulting motor actions. An important issue of the performance is the robustness of the decoding scheme with respect to (1) the size of the population of cells generating neuronal signals, (2) variations in the composition of cells included in the population of a given size, and, finally, (3) changes in the cell activity from trial to trial.

The uniformity of the distribution of the cells' preferred directions throughout space is of particular importance in reconstructing the directional signal encoded in the population activity (see POPULATION CODES). Therefore, all other factors being equal, the best performance for a fixed-size population is expected for such a composition of cells whose preferred directions form a nearly uniform distribution. Lukashin et al., (1996b) found that when the uniformity requirement is fulfilled, the performance and robustness of the model improve gradually as the size of the population (N) increases, revealing a tendency for saturation as N approaches 15–20 cells.

Typical results for $N = 15$ demonstrating the time-evolving performance of the model are displayed in Figure 3. The forces exerted by the monkey and by the actuator are shown for four instructed directions, together with the corresponding motor cortical activity. It can be seen (Figure 3, templates $A1$, $B1$, $C1$, $D1$) that directional tuning of cortical impulse activity is barely perceptible, owing to the large variability in cell discharge. However, the computation scheme successfully decodes these signals, and the time-varying forces developed by the actuator (Figure 3, templates $A3$, $B3$, $C3$, $D3$) are very similar to those developed by the monkey arm (Figure 3, templates $A2$, $B2$, $C2$, $D2$). Following an initial period of time, which lasts 100–200 ms, the direction of force exerted by the actuator stabilizes and the magnitude of force increases. The stabilized direction of force is close to the instructed direction for which the cortical activity was recorded. This was also observed for the remaining four instructed directions for this particular ensemble of cells and for other ensembles of cells ($N \geq 15$) and trials, thus suggesting a high degree of robustness of the decoding algorithm.

Discussion

One of the major challenges of brain theory is to elucidate the neural basis of behavior. Significant progress has been made over the past decade in determining functional properties of single motor cortical cells with respect to relatively simple yet behaviorally meaningful motor actions. The finding that neurons are broadly tuned to behavioral variables led to the key idea of distributive coding. The population vector algorithm allows a read-out of this code by transforming aggregates of purely temporal spike trains into a spatiotemporal vector. The neuronal population vector has

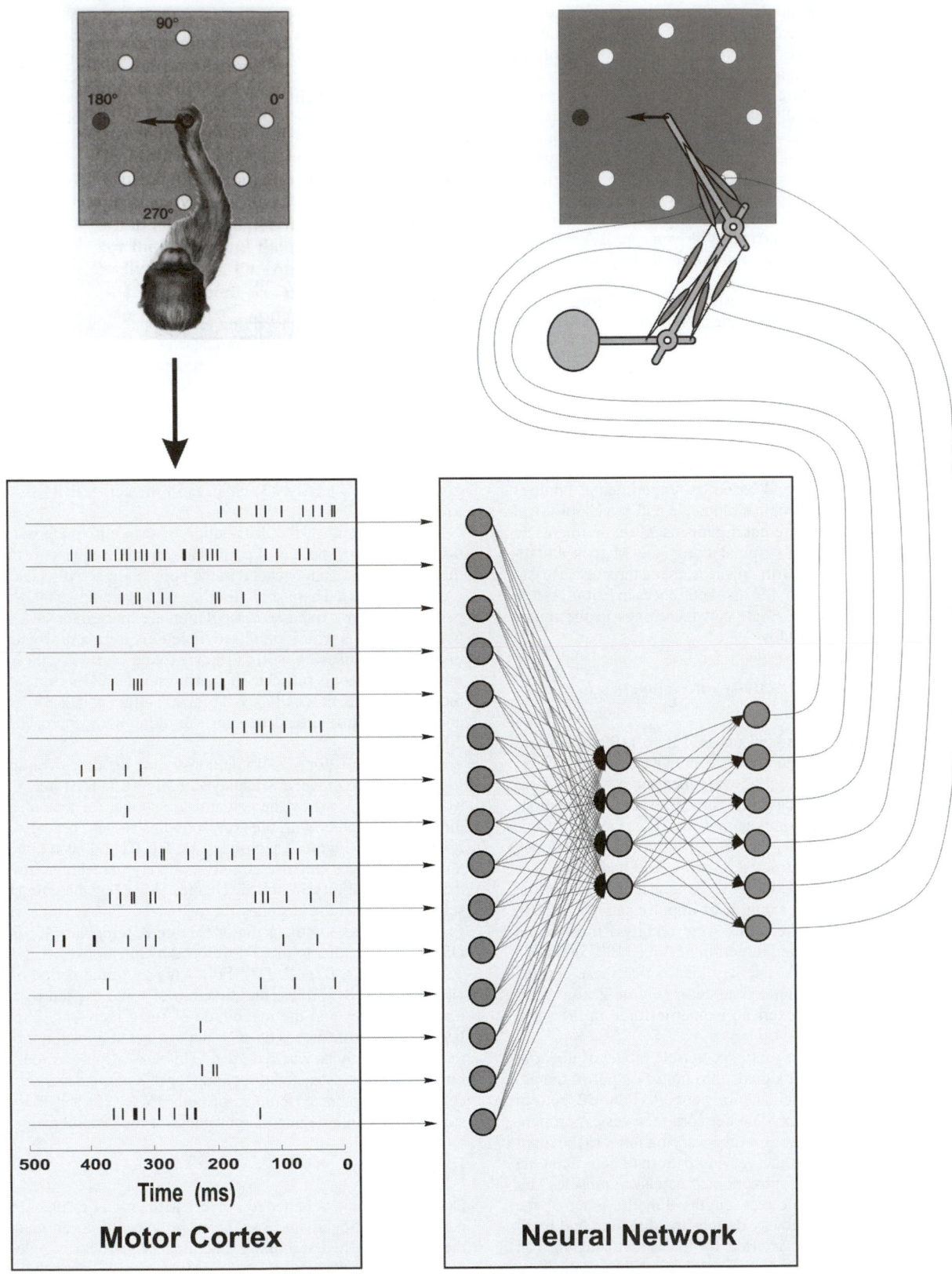

Figure 2. The decoding computation scheme used to transform neuronal commands encoded in a series of action potentials into a force exerted by the simulated actuator. The top left part of the figure illustrates a monkey exerting a force against the immovable handle in one (180°) of eight instructed directions. An example of the motor cortical activity recorded while the animal performed this task is represented in the bottom left panel. These neuronal signals drive the simulated actuator sketched in the top right part of the figure. A three-layered feedforward neural network (the directed connections are shown by thin arrows) transforms cortical signals into coordinated activation of actuator muscles.

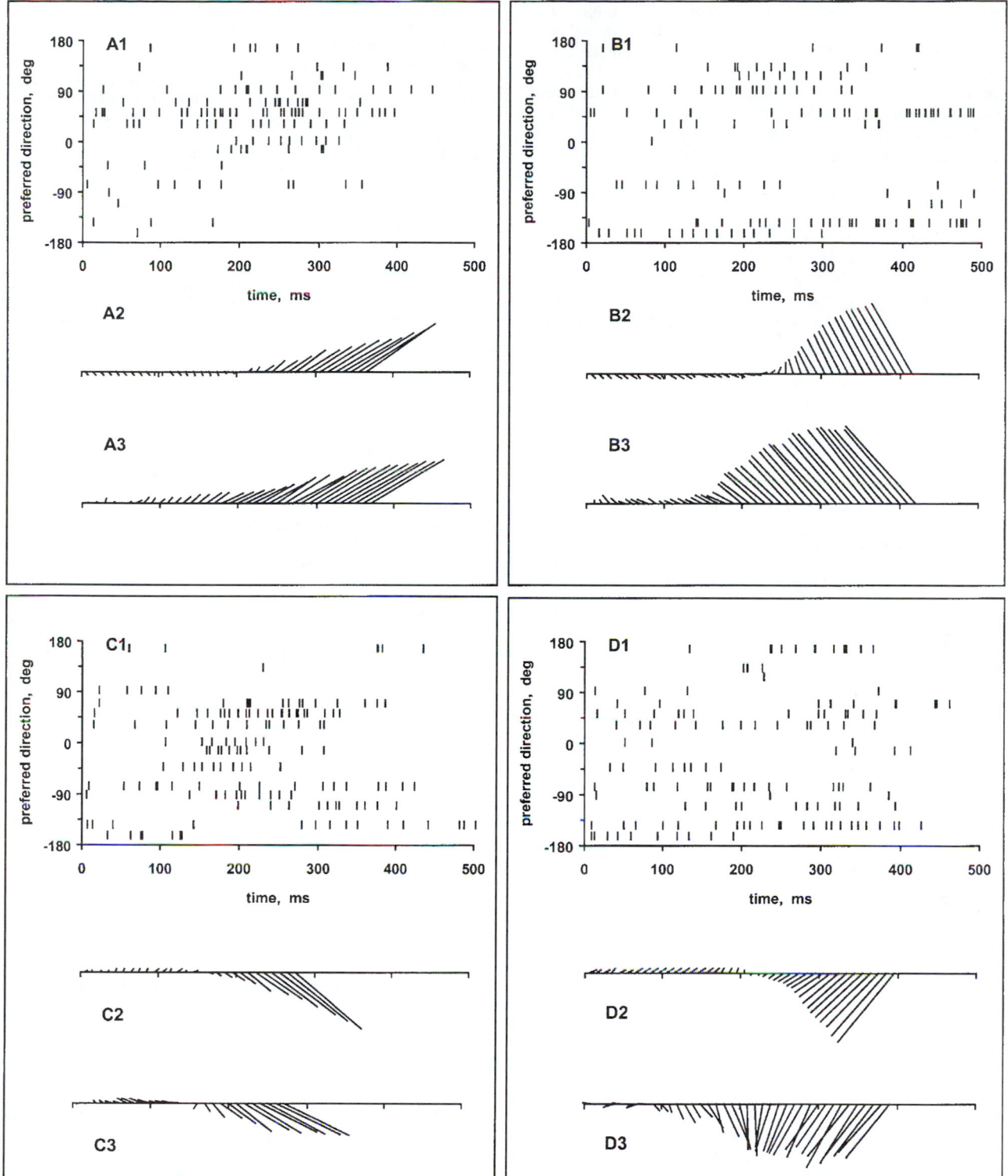

Figure 3. The motor cortical activity and the forces exerted by a monkey and by a simulated actuator. Four rasters, *A*1, *B*1, *C*1, and *D*1, show spiking activity recorded while the monkey developed isometric forces in four different instructed directions (45°, 135°, −45°, and −135°, respectively). The spike trains are aligned to the time of visual stimulus (zero time) instructing the monkey to begin the motor action. Each raster includes spike trains for the same 15 cells ordered along the vertical axis in accordance with their preferred directions. The time-varying forces developed by the monkey are depicted in *A*2, *B*2, *C*2, and *D*2. The force vectors measured every 10 ms are displayed as line segments; the tails of force vectors are aligned along the time axis (the horizontal line). The time scale is the same as shown in the rasters above. Finally, *A*3, *B*3, *C*3, and *D*3 show forces exerted by the actuator in response to the neuronal activity presented in the rasters. The forces were calculated using the decoding algorithm described (see text and Figure 2) with a 10-ms time step and were arranged along the time axis in the same way as experimentally measured forces. The measured and calculated forces are normalized to the same magnitude, assigned arbitrarily.

proved to be a robust and accurate measure of the directional tendency of a neuronal ensemble in different brain structures and under a variety of conditions. The discovery of cortical representation of motor commands, combined with the elucidation of neural mechanisms by which these commands generate a particular behavioral pattern unfolding in time, should further advance our understanding of neural basis of motor behavior.

The research in this direction also provides an impetus to the field of neuroprosthetics (see PROSTHETICS, NEURAL) and the design of adaptive systems that transform neuronal signals recorded from the brain into physiologically accurate motor output of multi-joint prosthetic limbs (see BRAIN-COMPUTER INTERFACES). The feasibility of this idea was demonstrated by Lukashin et al. (1996b) in a particular case when the required motor output was an exertion of isometric force. The simulated actuator, which mimicked the primate arm, responded to the experimentally recorded motor cortical commands with surprising fidelity, generating forces in quantitative agreement with those exerted by a trained monkey in both the temporal and spatial domains. An important finding was that even a small ensemble of cortical cells can reliably control relatively complex motor output. Recent studies (Schwartz et al., 2001, and references therein) have made further progress toward the cortical control of arm prosthetics.

Road Maps: Mammalian Brain Regions; Mammalian Motor Control; Neural Coding
Related Reading: Arm and Hand Movement Control; Brain-Computer Interfaces; Motor Primitives; Population Codes; Reaching Movements: Implications for Computational Model

References

Amirikian, B., and Georgopoulos, A. P., 2000, Directional tuning profiles of motor cortical cells, *Neurosci. Res.*, 36:73–79.

Ashe, J., and Georgopoulos, A. P., 1994, Movement parameters and neuronal activity in motor cortex and area 5, *Cereb. Cortex*, 6:590–600.
Flash T., and Sejnowski T. J., 2001, Computational approaches to motor control, *Curr. Opin. Neurobiol.*, 11:655–662.
Fu, Q. G., Suarez, J. I., and Ebner, T. J., 1993, Neuronal specification of direction and distance during reaching movements in the superior precentral premotor area and primary motor cortex of monkeys, *J. Neurophysiol.*, 70:2097–2116.
Georgopoulos, A. P., 1996, Arm movements in monkeys: Behavior and neurophysiology, *J. Comp. Physiol. A*, 179:603–612. ◆
Georgopoulos, A. P., Ashe, J., Smyrnis, N., and Taira, M., 1992, The motor cortex and the coding of force, *Science*, 256:1692–1695.
Johnson, M. T. V., Mason, C. R., and Ebner, T. J., 2001, Central processes for multiparametric control of arm movements in primates, *Curr. Opin. Neurobiol.*, 11:684–688. ◆
Lukashin, A. V., Amirikian, B. R., and Georgopoulos, A. P., 1996a, Neural computations underlying the exertion of force: A model, *Biol. Cybern.*, 74:469–478.
Lukashin, A. V., Amirikian, B. R., and Georgopoulos, A. P., 1996b, A simulated actuator driven by motor cortical signals, *NeuroReport*, 7:2597–2601. ◆
Mussa-Ivaldi, F. A., Hogan, N., and Bizzi, E., 1985, Neural, mechanical, and geometric factors subserving arm posture in humans, *J. Neurosci.*, 5:2732–2743.
Schwartz, A. B., 1992, Motor cortical activity during drawing movements: Single-unit activity during sinusoid tracing, *J. Neurophysiol.*, 68:528–541.
Schwartz, A. B., and Moran, D. W., 2000, Arm trajectory and representation of movement processing in motor cortical activity, *Eur. J. Neurosci.*, 12:1851–1856. ◆
Schwartz, A. B., Taylor, D. M., and Helms Tillery, S., 2001, Extraction algorithms for cortical control of arm prosthetics, *Curr. Opin. Neurobiol.*, 11:701–707.
Scott, S. H., 2000, Population vectors and motor cortex: neural coding or epiphenomenon? *Nature Neurosci.*, 3:307–308.
Todorov, E., 2000, Direct cortical control of muscle activation in voluntary arm movements: A model, *Nature Neurosci.*, 3:391–398.

Motor Pattern Generation

Jeffrey Dean and Holk Cruse

Introduction

Movement is central to the survival of animals and the performance of machines. The elegance of animals moving in complex environments has long aroused curiosity and the desire to emulate this ability. Animals move using muscles that produce force, sensory systems that signal the state of the organism and its surroundings, and a nervous system that links the two and contributes its own intrinsic activity. All possess some characteristics unattractive to engineers. Muscles are relatively slow and their force varies with muscle length, its rate of change, and the pattern of activation (see MUSCLE MODELS). Most sense organs conflate information about a parameter's value and its rate of change (see ADAPTIVE SPIKE CODING). Most neurons transmit information slowly using a pulse code of limited bandwidth. Response variability necessitates feedback supervision (see MOTOR CONTROL, BIOLOGICAL AND THEORETICAL), but inherent transmission delays, component variability, and limited coding precision force feedback gains to be low to avoid instability and unwanted oscillations.

The contrast between component quality and exquisite motor performance raises major unsolved puzzles. One is whether component characteristics actually simplify control. For example, the spring-like properties of muscles might reduce movement planning to end-point specification (see EQUILIBRIUM POINT HYPOTHESIS).

Others lie in the distributed, highly parallel organization of biological control systems.

Metaphors and Tools

Since Descartes reduced animals to machines, biologists have applied metaphors from contemporary technology to the brain and motor control. As technology advanced, metaphors progressed from clock mechanisms and pneumatic actuators through card readers and magnetic tape to current computer-based concepts. For example, the orchestration of complex muscle activity was attributed to a central motor score that could be stored and replayed like magnetic tape: Graham Hoyle envisioned both a motor tape for motor neuron activation (*motor output* in Figure 1) and a sensory tape for the sensory signals expected during unperturbed execution (*efference copy* in Figure 1).

Currently dominant is *motor program*, analogous to the instructions for a computer (Keele, Cohen, and Ivry, 1990). Varying usage led to alternative suggestions (e.g., *coordinated control program*: see SCHEMA THEORY; *motor control structure*: Cruse et al., 1990). *Motor program* is still apt if program is understood very generally as code that can generate complex output in the absence of input, vary its output depending on inputs, and modify itself. The important caveat is that the term not imply classical von Neumann ar-

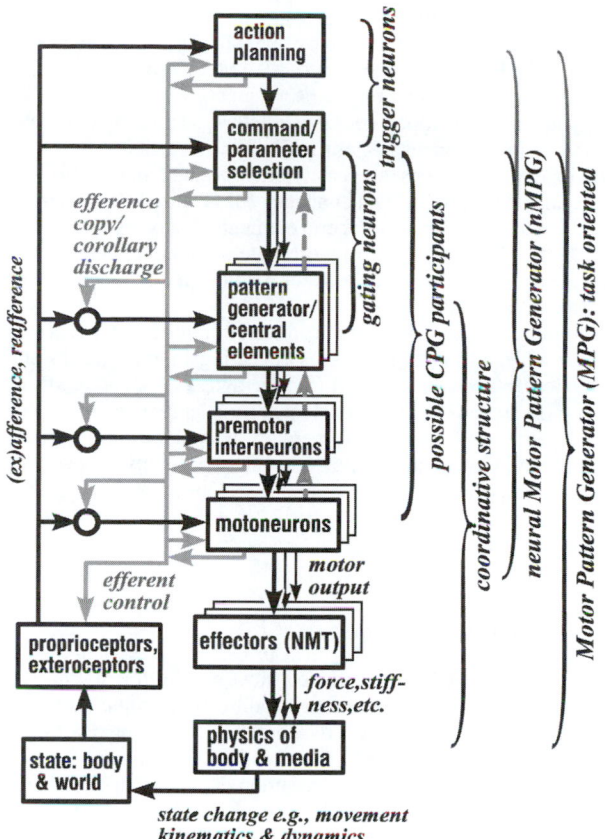

Figure 1. A hierarchical description of motor pattern generation showing potential interactions between efferent (motor), afferent (sensory), and central elements. nMPG is the set of neural elements, together with their states and interactions, that produces patterned motor output for a particular behavior; MPG includes the properties of effectors, body, and substrate. Sensory information can modify activity at all levels, but may itself be modified by central activity (efference copy, corollary discharge). Particularly in vertebrates, recurrent connections or corollary pathways may equal or exceed forward connections. For simplicity, the gray pathway (left) combines ascending (recurrent, internal loop) and descending interactions. Not shown are multi-element recurrent loops that implicitly or explicitly implement internal representations, models, and model-reference control. In complex behavioral sequences, planning instances participate in nMPGs. Even in simple nervous systems, functional hierarchies need not correspond to separate anatomical levels: individual neurons may participate in several functions (three leftmost brackets) and transmit signals forward and backward across several levels. NMT, neuromuscular transform.

chitectures with one processor working through sequences of instructions stored in separate memory. Instead, motor programs represent states established in the nervous system that produce coherent, task-related patterns of intrinsic activity and responses to stimuli. Like schemas, they are high-level shorthand for the function of parallel, distributed physiological systems (e.g., Figure 1).

This article focuses on the biological implementation of motor programs. Biomechanics and neurophysiology, supported by neuroanatomy, modeling, and molecular techniques, provide data. Cybernetics, the formal analysis of a system's input-output characteristics whereby systems can range from single neurons to whole animals (see MOTOR CONTROL, BIOLOGICAL AND THEORETICAL), provides systems-level analytical tools. So does the theory of dynamic systems (see COOPERATIVE PHENOMENA), which seeks collective variables summarizing emergent properties of complex systems and control parameters influencing their behavior.

Motor Pattern Generation

Like any physical system, animals move subject to the forces acting within and upon them. Animals actively control muscle forces, so generating movement is equivalent to generating appropriate patterns of muscle activity. As Sherrington noted, regardless of the complexity of the central nervous system (CNS), all motor influences must converge on or before the motor neurons, the final common path. *Motor output*—activity in this final common path recorded as muscle electrical activity (EMG), efferent activity in peripheral nerves, or activity in identified motor neurons—is often a convenient measure when experimental conditions preclude movement.

Although typical hierarchical descriptions of motor control (Figure 1) depict effectors, usually muscles, transforming into action a plan represented in motor output, the relationship between motor output and muscle force or movement is not simple (Hooper and Weaver, 2000; see MUSCLE MODELS). Nonmuscular forces like gravity or tendon and substrate elasticity strongly influence many movements. The characteristics of the body as a physical plant and the body–environment interaction may already be incorporated into motor output (Chiel and Beer, 1997), further obscuring the relationship between movement and neural activity.

Movement itself and motor output are called motor patterns, but we will focus on active control and use *neural motor pattern generator* (*nMPG*) for the system producing (neural) motor output that in appropriate contexts causes natural behavior. nMPGs can include simple and complex reflexes as well as intrinsic CNS activity. Many scientists would combine the nMPG, the body realizing its output, and the environment into a single dynamical system, arguing that each can contribute equally to molding the movement (Chiel and Beer, 1997); we will use *motor pattern generator* (*MPG*) for this dynamical system.

MPGs are conventionally linked to particular behaviors or actions, but defining units of behavior and thus MPGs is a matter of taste and inherently recursive (see SCHEMA THEORY). Investigators adopting whole-animal, functional perspectives might choose walking and a walking MPG as convenient initial units, so that refining the analysis to consider single legs or joints leads to models with many subunits in a walking MPG (e.g., Figure 1). Other investigators might begin with joint flexion and a flexion MPG, so that expanding the scope leads to models with many MPGs interacting to produce walking.

Regardless of the choice, similar questions arise. First, how is a particular motor pattern generated? Which system properties are necessary? Which are sufficient? Is the output stable with respect to external disturbances? Next, how is the pattern switched on and off? How are movement speed, form, and amplitude specified and adapted to task demands? How are external and internal state variables reflected within the nMPG? Finally, in ontogeny and evolution, do genes encode precise circuits—specifying each element and its connections—or crude circuits plus general measures of activity that engage plasticity mechanisms to achieve appropriate behavior (see ACTIVITY-DEPENDENT REGULATION OF NEURONAL CONDUCTANCES), and how do MPGs for similar behaviors compare in different species?

A Brief History of Theories of Motor Pattern Generation

When physiological study of the nervous system began in earnest, the easily accessible parts—peripheral sensory and motor elements and their combination in elementary reflexes—were investigated first. Because theories are built on what is known, reflexes assumed central roles, making animals into reactive, reflex driven machines. In biology, motor patterns were explained as chains of reflexes in which each movement creates appropriate sensory stimuli to elicit the next movement, leading to complex behavioral sequences or, if the chain is closed, rhythmic behaviors. Timing and continuation of leg movements in walking were attributed to reflexes based on changes in leg position, loading, and equilibrium signals during the step, but such conceptual models were never simulated quantitatively. In psychology, the analogous theory was *response chaining*. Such reaction-based formulations were extended in ethology to interactions between individuals and in psychology to behaviorism.

The rigidity of reflex or response chain theories caused their downfall (e.g., Lashley, 1951; Keele et al., 1990). Both had to postulate subtle stimulus differences to account for different behaviors under seemingly identical conditions and were unable to explain rule-based behavior in novel situations. Response chains based on reflex loops cannot explain rapid sequences when event intervals are shorter than minimum response latencies. Chains based on internal loops have difficulty explaining concurrency of preparatory movements and their dependence on preceding *and* succeeding actions.

A new theory was needed, one incorporating generalized representations of behaviors—plans or schemas (Lashley, 1951; see SCHEMA THEORY) or motor programs—which are modifiable by external and internal influences. In psychology, neurological findings implicate specific brain structures in planning (see BASAL GANGLIA; CEREBELLUM AND MOTOR CONTROL), but the details are unclear. In biology, motor programs acquired physiological foundations, beginning with the realization that the CNS alone can produce patterned motor output. T. Graham Brown showed that cats deprived of sensory inputs could still produce coordinated stepping; he envisioned a neural oscillator producing alternating activity in flexor and extensor muscles. His experimental approach—deafferentation—and his conceptual model both remain current (see HALF-CENTER OSCILLATORS UNDERLYING RHYTHMIC MOVEMENTS). Later, von Holst's (see Delcomyn, 1980) quantitative analyses of rhythmic behaviors were best explained by interactions among multiple intrinsic rhythm generators.

As physiological techniques improved, intrinsic motor patterns were traced within the CNS. Individual neurons or networks able, in the absence of patterned sensory inputs, to produce patterned motor output related to natural behaviors are generally called *central pattern generators* (*CPGs*). *Neural oscillator* or *central oscillator* are terms also used, particularly for rhythmic patterns, but CPG includes discrete movements. (Naming CPGs again raises questions of system boundaries. CPGs in the lobster stomatogastric system originally distinguished according to anatomical segment and function were later found to interact in complex ways within what in a broader view is an ingestion CPG; see CRUSTACEAN STOMATOGASTRIC SYSTEM.)

For a time, the importance of CPGs was overemphasized at the expense of peripheral elements. Wilson's demonstration of basic flight rhythms in the efferent motor fibers of deafferented locusts was particularly influential (see LOCUST FLIGHT: COMPONENTS AND MECHANISMS IN THE MOTOR). Sensory influences were relegated to providing tonic excitation rather than cycle-by-cycle patterning. Initial physiological descriptions of neural oscillators reinforced this emphasis, especially when evidence for CPGs was found in virtually all rhythmic behaviors (Delcomyn, 1980). Besides the physiological data, however, a willingness to overlook differences between natural motor patterns and those in deafferented preparations contributed to the emphasis on CPGs (Pearson, 1993).

The necessary correction occurred when it was shown that sensory inputs, besides influencing frequency, timing, and form of rhythmic activity, often fulfill both criteria for CPG inclusion (Pearson, 1993): (1) rhythmic activity correlated with the behavior and (2) the ability to shift or "reset" the phase of ongoing rhythms when appropriately stimulated. For example, actual wing movement and loading, visual stimuli, and changes in air flow past the head modulate and stabilize locust wing movement on a cycle-by-cycle basis (see LOCUST FLIGHT: COMPONENTS AND MECHANISMS IN THE MOTOR). Similar entrainment by sensory inputs occurs in many systems with well-developed neural oscillators, as does modulation of transitions in sequences of nonrhythmic movements.

Peripheral influences are easily incorporated into motor programs and similar high-level concepts; MPG and nMPG inherently include both central and peripheral elements. Many researchers also expand the CPG concept to incorporate sensory influences when available, but this disrupts the natural congruity of functional and anatomical boundaries.

In summary, most MPGs incorporate both intrinsic CNS activity (CPGs) and peripheral influences reflecting biomechanical characteristics, reflexes, and proprioceptive and exteroceptive afferent activity (Pearson, 1993). As strategies for adaptive behavior, these two elements are analogous to network adaptation via genetic algorithms and via learning or developmental plasticity, respectively. The balance is subject to evolutionary selection, depending on the cost of errors and the predictability of motor command outcomes; it remains a subject of debate and research.

Central Pattern Generators

Understanding of CPGs progressed most rapidly for rhythmic behaviors. Initial conceptual models addressed simple two-phase rhythms, such as alternation between stance and swing. Half-center oscillator models contain two functional units connected by reciprocal inhibition and subject to a common excitatory drive, whereby functional units can be either single neurons or groups of neurons synchronized by reciprocal excitatory synapses. This bistable circuit oscillates if the inhibition decays or if other functionally equivalent changes occur (see Camhi, 1984). George Szekely demonstrated that multiphase rhythms can be generated by neurons or functional groups in a ring with recurrent inhibition (e.g., Camhi, 1984).

Early physiological findings distinguished two kinds of neural oscillators. In *cellular oscillators* (*pacemakers*; see OSCILLATORY AND BURSTING PROPERTIES OF NEURONS), rhythms depend on complex, nonlinear membrane properties and continue when the cell is isolated from the nervous system, whereas in *network oscillators* they depend on the connectivity of cells incapable of rhythmic activity on their own. Connectivity was emphasized initially because it was easier to characterize and because several vertebrate and invertebrate networks contained reciprocal or recurrent inhibition, providing a satisfying agreement with theoretical simulations using simple model neurons.

Subsequent results blurred the distinction and emphasized the contribution of cellular properties (Selverston et al., 1997). First, time delays necessary for half-center models require nonlinear properties. Second, some neurons within putative network oscillators, and even some motor neurons, possess nonlinear membrane properties, allowing them to oscillate or exhibit *plateau potentials*, switching between inactivity and prolonged high activity (see OSCILLATORY AND BURSTING PROPERTIES OF NEURONS; NEUROMODULATION IN INVERTEBRATE NERVOUS SYSTEMS). Unexpected pacemakers turned up within putative network oscillators. Third, synaptic interactions show similar complexity, changing in strength or even sign, depending on time or on the relative potentials of sender and recipient (see TEMPORAL DYNAMICS OF BIOLOGICAL SYNAPSES). Fourth, besides simple recurrent inhibition, real networks include positive feedback or mixtures of circuits. Even the five-neuron recurrent ring initially identified as the swim CPG of the leech contains reciprocal inhibitory connections within and diagonally across the ring (see Camhi, 1984). Finally, real CPGs incorporate both cellular and network properties, with redundancy contributing to robust rhythmicity.

Complexity and redundancy impede attribution of function to particular elements even in simple invertebrate networks with few neurons. CPG simulations using realistic synaptic interactions and membrane characteristics are absolutely necessary. The practical difficulty is the ever-increasing list of properties of possible significance. Consideration of neuronal morphology adds further complexity (see DENDRITIC PROCESSING). Morphology influences responses according to both the timing and the location of inputs. Thus, simulation of even a single real neuron, let alone a network, is a formidable problem (see SINGLE-CELL MODELS). Even some well-studied CPGs lack definitive models. Although the optimism following early successful simulations using simplistic neurons dissipated, newer, more realistic models provide grounds for renewed optimism (e.g., Selverston et al., 2000).

Network simulations and physiological data do show that systems can perform appropriately even when some connections appear nonfunctional or even dysfunctional (e.g., excitatory connections to neurons normally silent when the sender is active). Such "rogue" elements (Robinson, 1992) occur even in simple resistance and withdrawal reflexes. Because natural selection works most directly on behavior, eliminating all rogue elements may not be possible or necessary: motor output is an emergent property of the whole CPG.

CPGs may drive normal movements or merely facilitate particular modes of motor output. They avoid peripheral delays at the expense of adaptability to bodily and environmental changes. They represent predictions for suitable motor output, or a kind of *internal model* for adaptive behavior in a given context. Given the incomplete understanding of simple CPGs and their somewhat stereotyped outputs, moving beyond these to understand flexible motor control presents major challenges. Recurrent connections prominent in higher vertebrates presumably contribute to more elaborate internal models supporting flexible nMPGs (see ACTION MONITORING AND FORWARD CONTROL OF MOVEMENTS; REACHING MOVEMENTS: IMPLICATIONS FOR COMPUTATIONAL MODELS).

Switching Patterns On and Off

Functionally, pattern generators are controlled by a switch. Neural elements implementing the switch were labeled *command neurons* (see Figure 1) (Kupfermann and Weiss, 2001). Activity in command neurons should be both necessary and sufficient for producing behavior. If action potentials are required, the neuron's threshold determines the behavioral threshold. In practice, few neurons fulfill both criteria (Camhi, 1984). More often, control is distributed among many neurons, reflecting the redundancy common in biological systems. As a result, the concept has been extended to "command systems" containing multiple "command elements" (see COMMAND NEURONS AND COMMAND SYSTEMS).

Two kinds of switches have been identified. Some behaviors continue only as long as an appropriate stimulus is present; others continue after it ends. A similar distinction applies to command neurons: activity in *trigger neurons* initiates a longer-lasting behavior, while activity in *gating neurons* determines the duration of the behavior. Command neurons turning on one behavior may also turn off or inhibit command neurons for interfering behaviors and excite those for functionally linked behaviors—an architecture replicated in P. Maes's ANN. If not actively turned off, gating neuron activity may simply decay below threshold, terminating the behavior.

Real nervous systems often mix command, coordination, and pattern generation, and behavioral choice involves multiple functional levels. Activity in some gating neurons oscillates with the output rhythm. Some can reset the rhythm and fulfill criteria for CPG inclusion. Some leech gating neurons are functionally outside the CPG, but the recurrent, excitatory pathways modulating their activity help prolong this activity. In *Tritonia*'s escape system, the command signal reflects membrane properties of CPG neurons: depending on stimulus strength the network produces either a single longitudinal contraction or multicycle dorsoventral flexions. Thus, one anatomical network may be a *polymorphic network* producing qualitatively different motor patterns; in other words, individual neurons participate in multiple behaviors, and command is a population code (Kristan and Shaw, 1997).

Command signals often work via nonlinear effects of neural activity (see ACTIVITY-DEPENDENT REGULATION OF NEURONAL CONDUCTANCES) or modulatory transmitters and hormones (see NEUROMODULATION IN INVERTEBRATE NERVOUS SYSTEMS) that modify membrane properties, producing qualitative changes in outputs or even functional reconfigurations of nMPGs. Thus, biological nMPGs show a protean variability compared to artificial neural networks, where unit properties are usually static and output changes reflect input changes or connectivity changes through learning.

Sensory Influences

nMPGs usually incorporate feedforward and feedback using sensory information about the surroundings and motor performance. Formally, feedback depends on the consequences of motor activity. Negative feedback acts to reduce deviations ("errors") from a reference value, as in resistance reflexes, whereas positive feedback (with suitable limiting nonlinearities) maintains or accentuates ongoing movements. Feedforward pathways help select actions or set parameters in advance, such as specifying the size of a saccade or an escape turn. However, in natural, continuous streams of behavior, distinguishing error-correcting feedback from parameter-setting feedforward mechanisms is not always clear (Cruse et al., 1990). For example, learning can be described as delayed negative feedback that adjusts future parameter setting.

Sensory signals can be modified at various levels (see Figure 1). Sensory activity can be modulated peripherally through efferent control or centrally at the output synapses of the primary afferent fibers. Reflexes occurring in one situation can be reversed or replaced by wholly new responses (Pearson, 1993). In invertebrates, resistance reflexes—negative feedback opposing leg displacement during posture—are replaced as stance begins by assistance reflexes to boost propulsion. At other times they remain active, opposing deviations from normal trajectories. Phase-dependent reflex modulation may be a natural consequence of spike thresholds in neurons (see LOCUST FLIGHT: COMPONENTS AND MECHANISMS IN THE MOTOR).

The relative importance of central and peripheral components varies considerably. For example, central elements appear weaker in walking than in flying and swimming, where the substrate is more forgiving. In flying, variability in wing movements affecting lift and steering can be corrected over several subsequent cycles, whereas in walking, not finding a foothold or tripping over an obstruction must be corrected immediately. When stick insects walk, movement of the leg itself, as signaled by sensory inputs, determines the state of the step CPG (Bässler, 1986; Dean et al., 1999); isolated CPGs produce slow, fragmentary, irregular motor output. Our work shows that a simple step rhythm can arise from a four-unit, recurrent nMPG in which two units represent the state and two units represent position criteria for changing state. Recurrent connections provide positive feedback to reinforce the current state, causing each movement to continue to its endpoint.

Other Peripheral Influences on Motor Patterns

Physical characteristics of muscles, tendons, skeletal elements, and the environment modify or even create movement. Motor behaviors are often studied using motor output, but the transformation between this activity and movement is not trivial. Different neural rhythms in the lobster CPG controlling chewing were characterized long before their functional significance was determined (see CRUSTACEAN STOMATOGASTRIC SYSTEM). Modeling the transformation from neural activity to muscle force is difficult but improving (Hooper and Weaver, 2000). Motor neuron activity is difficult to relate to movement, partly owing to the sophistication with which animals use passive and elastic properties of their muscles and skeletons. According to one hypothesis for limb movements to a target (see EQUILIBRIUM POINT HYPOTHESIS, but also ARM AND HAND MOVEMENT CONTROL), muscle activity is not related to movement as such but to the target, the allowable deviation, and an estimate of possible and allowable errors.

Including the periphery in MPG models is particularly important when it strongly affects movement. Algorithms for step coordination simulated using a simplified representation of leg position will be unable to control a machine with real legs if they try to place legs in unreachable positions. Behavioral data on limb interactions, the basis of many coordination models, actually represent the total effect of internal activity, reflexes, and the physics of animal and environment. Dynamical systems theory, using collective variables like phase, can sometimes provide a succinct encapsulation of this system behavior.

In extreme cases, significant aspects of movements are determined by the physical system. Treating bipedal walkers simply as a system of passive, damped pendulums explains many characteristics, suggesting that muscle activity is only occasionally necessary to maintain the pendular motion or correct disturbances (McGeer, 1990). In some insects, flight muscles require general activation, but individual wing beats result from mechanical oscillations involving the muscles' intrinsic response to stretch.

In summary, biological movement is not always driven rigidly by nMPG output (see CEREBELLUM AND MOTOR CONTROL). Taking advantage of physical properties may enable adequate control using neural approximations of exact algorithms and internal models (e.g., Dean et al., 1999), especially when animals are small or compliances are high, so that impacts or stresses arising from inaccuracies can be absorbed without injury. This may not be true of large, powerful robots in an environment where safety is an essential concern.

Coordinating Multiple Motor Patterns

Many behaviors contain distinct elements that occur concurrently or sequentially, requiring spatial and temporal coordination of body parts (e.g., EYE-HAND COORDINATION IN REACHING MOVEMENTS; LOCOMOTION, INVERTEBRATE) or the completion of one action before another begins. For this purpose, several MPGs or subunits within one MPG can be structured hierarchically or in parallel, depending on task requirements (see Figure 1). For speaking and typing, the kinds of errors and time delays, the concurrence of preparatory and execution phases, and the modulation of elements depending on earlier and later elements indicate a hierarchical arrangement, whereas relative coordination of concurrent rhythms indicates a parallel arrangement.

In these cases, interactions among and within MPGs can occur at many levels, ranging from overall planning through parameter setting and CPG activity to peripheral loops involving mechanical coupling and reafference. Network models offer natural simulations of these interactions. Rhythm coordination has been studied extensively (see CRUSTACEAN STOMATOGASTRIC SYSTEM; CHAINS OF OSCILLATORS IN MOTOR AND SENSORY SYSTEMS). Coordination mechanisms within MPGs are often highly redundant and thus robust. In insect walking, multiple centrally mediated mechanisms

are augmented by multiple locally mediated (intraleg) mechanisms sensitive to leg position, state, and load (Dean et al., 1999).

Discussion

In the near future, interactions between theoreticians and experimentalists should be fruitful in many but not all respects. Neuroscience clearly needs computational neuroscientists using simulations of biological nMPGs to represent acquired knowledge and test its completeness. Artificial neural networks provide new tools and, more important, reemphasize several concepts that have important implications for interpreting physiological experiments (e.g., Robinson, 1992): (1) the common currency in neural networks is neuronal activity; (2) this activity need not be simply related to physical parameters; (3) processing is distributed and parallel; (4) redundancy contributes robustness; and (5) approximations may suffice.

Neural engineers naturally look to animals for inspiration in improving technical systems, expecting concise lists of biological solutions for different computational problems. Because animals are so diverse, neuroscience provides only rudimentary guidelines. Each species has its own answer to a very complex and specialized problem, an important part of which is reproduction. Genes and development constrain animals to evolve in small steps that are themselves adaptive, or at least not seriously detrimental. In contrast, technological innovation can create radically new machines; prototypes hopelessly outperformed by existing technologies are not doomed to extinction.

Nevertheless, the very diversity of biological solutions enhances what biology has to offer. Better understanding of biological MPGs should help algorithm selection for technical applications, especially as artificial networks approach the complexity of biological networks in size, connectivity, unit properties, and plasticity. Optimization techniques based on biological learning or evolution already help adapt control systems (see LOCOMOTION, INVERTEBRATE). *Animat research*, by studying real robots, shows that implementing MPGs in real robots sometimes simplifies control and representation issues. Purely reactive robots, with integration at the effectors and no explicit world models, can generate astonishingly complex behavior. Optimally balancing reactive control with implicit and explicit representations is a current challenge for animat research; understanding biological implementations is a challenge for neuroscience.

Road Map: Motor Pattern Generators
Related Reading: Command Neurons and Command Systems; Motor Control, Biological and Theoretical; Sensorimotor Learning

References

Bässler, U., 1986, On the definition of central pattern generator and its sensory control, *Biol. Cybern.*, 54:65–69. ◆
Camhi, J. M., 1984, *Neuroethology: Nerve Cells and the Natural Behavior of Animals*, Sunderland, MA: Sinauer. ◆
Chiel, H. J., and Beer, R. D., 1997, The brain has a body: Adaptive behavior emerges from interactions of nervous system, body and environment, *Trends Neurosci.*, 20:553–557.
Cruse, H., Dean, J., Heuer, H., and Schmidt, R. A., 1990, Utilization of sensory information for motor control, in *Relationships Between Perception and Action: Current Approaches* (O. Neumann and W. Prinz, Eds.), Berlin: Springer-Verlag, pp. 43–79. ◆
Dean, J., Kindermann, T., Schmitz, J., Schumm, M., and Cruse, H., 1999, Control of walking in the stick insect: From behavior and physiology to modeling, *Auton. Robots*, 7:271–288.
Delcomyn, F., 1980, Neural basis of rhythmic behavior in animals, *Science*, 210:492–498.

Hooper, S. L., and Weaver, A. L., 2000, Motor neuron activity is often insufficient to predict motor response, *Curr. Opin. Neurobiol.*, 10:876–682.

Keele, S. W., Cohen, A., and Ivry, R., 1990, Motor programs: Concepts and issues, in *Attention and Performance: XIII. Motor Representation and Control* (M. Jeannerod, Ed.), Hillsdale, NJ: Erlbaum, pp. 77–110. ◆

Kristan, W. B., Jr., and Shaw, B. K., 1997, Population coding and behavioral choice, *Curr. Opin. Neurobiol.*, 7:826–831.

Kupfermann, I., and Weiss, K. R., 2001, Motor program selection in simple model systems, *Curr. Opin. Neurobiol.*, 11:673–677.

Lashley, K. S., 1951, The problem of serial order in behavior, in *Cerebral Mechanisms in Behavior: The Hixon Symposium* (L. A. Jeffress, Ed.), New York: Hafner, pp. 112–136.

McGeer, T., 1990, Passive dynamic walking, *Int. J. Robot. Res.*, 9:62–82.

Pearson, K. G., 1993, Common principles of motor control in vertebrates and invertebrates, *Annu. Rev. Neurosci.*, 16:265–297.

Robinson, D. A., 1992, Implications of neural networks for how we think about brain function, *Behav. Brain Sci.*, 15:644–655. ◆

Selverston, A. I., Panchin, Y. V., Arshavsky, Y. I., and Orlovsky, G. N., 1997, Shared features of invertebrate central pattern generators, in *Neurons, Networks, and Motor Behavior* (P. S. G. Stein, S. Grillner, A. I. Selverston, and D. F. Stuart, Eds.), Cambridge, MA: MIT Press, pp. 105–117. ◆

Selverston, A. I., Rabinovich, M. I., Abarbanel, H. D. E., Elson, R., Szücs, A., Pinto, R. D., Huerta, R., and Varona, P., 2000, Reliable circuits from irregular neurons: A dynamical approach to understanding central pattern generators, *J. Physiol. (Paris)*, 94:357–374.

Motor Primitives

Simon F. Giszter

Introduction

The concept of a modular organization of spinal motor systems dates back to Sherrington (1910) or earlier (see citation in Giszter et al., 2001a). Recently, a new perspective on motor system modularity (and especially spinal cord) has developed as a result of a series of experiments on the spinal cords of frog, rat, and cat. It has been proposed that a set of motor elements termed "motor primitives" are implemented in the spinal cord. These are recruited by central pattern generators to construct spinal motor acts. Data from the frog have been especially significant in this framework (see SCRATCH REFLEX). The frog wiping behaviors have been utilized in the study of motor control since the nineteenth century. The advantages of these behaviors are the clear adjustments documented, the simplicity of aspects of frog motor organization, and the robustness of the behaviors. The frog's wiping responses are largely organized in the spinal cord: they persist unaltered following spinal transection (i.e., in the isolated spinal cord). Examination of wiping movements and microstimulation of frog spinal cord (and more recently an examination of descending controls) has generated a framework for describing the basis of spinal construction of motor behavior. Movements are constructed as a sequencing and combination of a collection of force-field motor primitives or fundamental elements. Although controversial, because the biological circuit underpinnings are not yet well established, this framework is proving promising, and to date, it is holding up under careful experimental scrutiny and implementation in robots (see Schaal, 1999).

Properties of Force-Field Motor Primitives

Microstimulation of frog spinal cord in intermediate gray regions using low currents (1–10 μA, 0.5-ms pulses at 40 Hz for 300 ms) activates a few hundred or thousand cells and elicits specific groups of muscle responses. With the spinal frog held immobile in an isometric apparatus, these muscle responses could be characterized as an endpoint (ankle) force vector and a vector of associated joint torques (see Giszter, Mussa-Ivaldi, and Bizzi, 1993). This measurement was repeated at multiple limb configurations and stimulus strengths. At a single configuration, over time, and at increasing stimulation strength up to 15 μA, the orientation of force elicited from a single site remained fixed, while the amplitude was modulated. By moving the limb to new positions, the effects of muscle-length-dependent viscoelastic properties, moment arms, and the ef-

fects of linkage kinematics on endpoint force and joint torques could be assessed. These effects were summarized by expressing the endpoint force as a function of endpoint position, or the joint torque vectors as a function of limb configuration (see, e.g., force fields measured in this way for a behavioral response in Figures 1F through 1H). When data were expressed in this way, it was discovered that the magnitude ratios and relative orientations of vectors across the range of positions remained fixed for a single site (Figure 1H). Force measured in isometric conditions could be expressed as a function of stimulus amplitude (s), configuration (r), and time (t) as

$$F(r,\ s,\ t)\ =\ A(s)\cdot a(t)\cdot \phi(r) \tag{1}$$

where $A(s)$ was a scalar function of stimulus strength and $a(t)$ was a scalar function of time; $\phi(r)$ was a fixed field structure that was simply scaled, was conservative, and was often convergent in both limb joint and limb endpoint coordinates. The function $a(t)$ varied with site of stimulation. There were phasic, tonic, and phasic/tonic sites (Giszter et al., 1993).

When the electrode was moved a small distance in spinal cord a similar field $\phi(r)$ was obtained. However, for larger changes in position of the electrode in spinal cord, the force pattern could alter significantly. Over a sampling of the lumbar spinal cord intermediate gray using microstimulation (see Bizzi et al., 2000; Giszter et al., 2001b), chemical stimulation (Saltiel, cited in Bizzi et al., 2000), or combined skin and microstimulation, a small set of force-field types was found. About six force-field patterns were found in all, separated in middle and deep intermediate zones by relatively silent areas (Giszter et al., 2001b).

Combination of stimuli applied to ipsilateral areas producing different force-field types resulted in one of two effects for costimulation: (1) In 85% of combinations, linear superposition or vector summation occurred (see Equation 2); (2) in 15% of combinations, winner-take-all occurred with one site dominating response (see Equation 3). Graded motion of a limb could be obtained by controlled costimulation. The combinations observed are consistent with modular construction of reflex responses; and see Mussa-Ivaldi (cited in Bizzi et al., 2000) and the section below entitled "Wiping Motor Pattern Construction and Control Using Force-Field Primitives." In summary, for ipsilateral costimulation, either linear or winner-take-all combinations occur:

$$
\begin{aligned}
F(r,\ S_1,\ S_2)\ &=\ B\cdot [\Phi_1(r,\ S_1)\ +\ \Phi_2(r,\ S_2)] \\
&=\ B\cdot [A(S_1)\phi_1(r)\ +\ a(S_2)\phi_2(r)]
\end{aligned} \tag{2}
$$

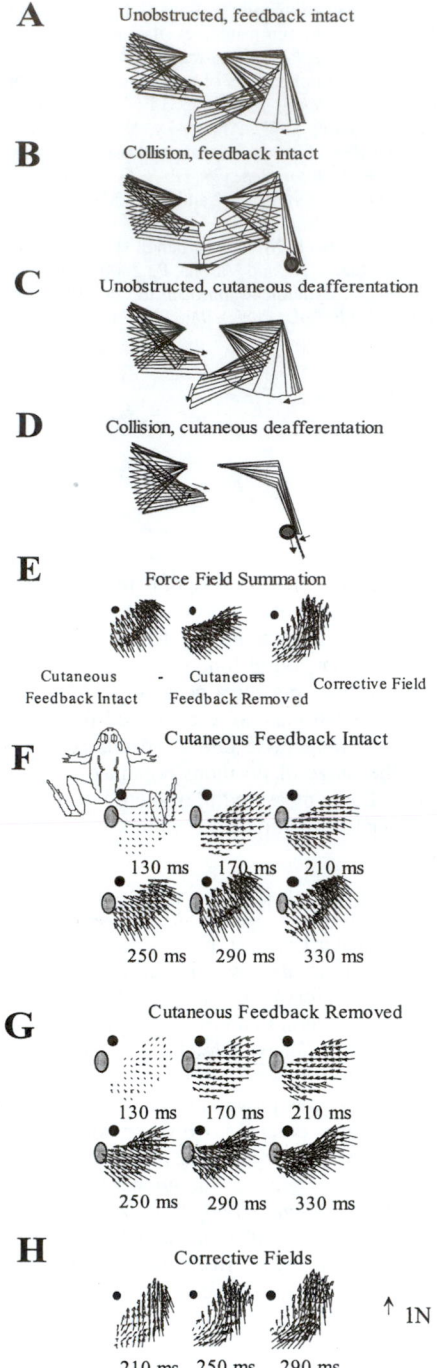

A Unobstructed, feedback intact

B Collision, feedback intact

C Unobstructed, cutaneous deafferentation

D Collision, cutaneous deafferentation

E Force Field Summation

Cutaneous   -   Cutaneous   Corrective Field
Feedback Intact   Feedback Removed

F Cutaneous Feedback Intact

130 ms   170 ms   210 ms

250 ms   290 ms   330 ms

G Cutaneous Feedback Removed

130 ms   170 ms   210 ms

250 ms   290 ms   330 ms

H Corrective Fields

↑ 1N

210 ms   250 ms   290 ms

Figure 1. Examples of spinally organized responses and their force-field bases (redrawn from Giszter et al., 2000a; Kargo and Giszter, 2000). Upper panels: free-limb kinematics; lower panels: isometric force-field measurements. *A*, normal wipe trajectory. *B*, corrections to obstacles. *C*, loss of skin feedback from the effector limb (right limb) does not alter free trajectory. *D*, Corrections for collisions are abolished by loss of skin feedback. *E*, At each of a grid of ankle locations, the isometric force production is measured at the ankle. The correction response pattern is hypothesized to be due to vector summation of a corrective force-field primitive with the unperturbed pattern. *F*, field pattern with collision detection. *G*, field pattern without correction. *H*, Corrective primitive obtained by subtraction (i.e., *G* from *F* as described in panel *E*). The force pattern is a scaled version of a single pattern at each time point shown, consistent with definitions used for a force-field primitive (see text). Data collected and published in Kargo and Giszter (2000), with support of NIH NS34640 and NS40412.

or

$$F(r, S_1, S_2) = B \cdot [\Phi_1(r, S_1)] \quad (3)$$

where B is a scalar scaling parameter and A and a are scalar functions of stimulus strength.

More recently, costimulation between contralateral sites has also been tested (Giszter et al., 2000a). For bilateral costimulation, some spinal cord regions do show nonlinear responses to costimulation while the remainder obey the combination rules above (Giszter et al., 2000a). Taken in total, these effects are consistent with microstimulation providing access to primitives and parts of the CPGs that can be combined in various ways.

Localization and Circuit Underpinnings of Motor Primitives

It is worth considering how microstimulation recruits cells and what the underpinnings of the functional relations observed above might be. The next sections demonstrate the functional uses of primitives in theory and real behavior, but the circuit underpinnings of these primitives are poorly understood, and the initial microstimulation that was used remains extremely controversial. Microstimulation as a technique of mapping has often been used. However, the laminar, nucleated, and segmentally organized spinal cord, such maps are harder to interpret and understand than, for example, in cortical columns. Spinal cord's recursive or looped projections, as opposed to simple output cascades, are confounding factors. Thus, although mappings with microstimulation or chemical stimuli reveal topographies, they may not reveal the localization (if any) that can be ascribed to primitives (Bizzi et al., 2000, and Giszter et al., 2001b). Rather, they are hot spots for more or less pure access to (and control of) primitives, which is entirely different. The circuit underpinning of the primitive may be discretely localized, broadly distributed, or an emergent pattern or mode of the spinal circuitry. Nonetheless, the fact that the circuitry supports these computational and functional primitives and that they may be accessed and combined in different ways through different localized sites is an important contribution. It may affect understanding of both motor control and neuroprostheses. Important future tasks are discovering how the circuitry supports primitives and how to link this meta-organization of primitives to the enormous body of exquisite physiology and anatomy of the spinal cord elaborated in the last 50 years by groups in Sweden, Denmark, Russia, Britain, Canada, and the United States. Some of the recent findings provide a series of strong hypotheses for this future work.

Capabilities of a System of Primitives: Theory

Important theoretical issues for motor primitives are (1) how to build time-varying field structures from motor primitives to support movement, (2) discovering the motor primitive basis sets that best provide general approximations and stability guarantees, and (3) discovering how appropriate basis sets might be constructed and modified by developmental or learning mechanisms.

Initially, Mussa-Ivaldi (1992, cited in Giszter et al., 2000b) showed that arbitrary fields were readily approximated by using a linear combination of conservative and circulating (or rotational) radial vector field primitives. In biological testing, circulating fields accounted for less than 5% of the variance of field structures observed. This concept has now been applied in the frog and in human biomechanics (see EQUILIBRIUM POINT HYPOTHESIS). The coefficients of these basis-field elements could be found by standard methods.

Mathematically, the force field $F(x)$ relating force to position x can be approximated by using k basis fields $q_i(x)$ and control parameters c_i:

$$F(x) = \sum_{i=1}^{k} c_i q_i(x) \qquad (4)$$

The k basis fields $q_i(x)$ are subdivided into two groupings. These two groupings consist of **k/2** conservative or irrotational fields and $k/2$ solenoidal or circulating fields. Thus,

$$F(x) = C(x) + R(x) = \sum_{i=1}^{k/2} q_i(x) + \sum_{i=k/2+1}^{k} q_i(x) \qquad (5)$$

where $C(x)$ is a pure conservative field and $R(x)$ a pure solenoidal field. Circulating fields have curl and can be used to generate energy in closed cycles. In biological measures to date, $R(x)$ is generally found to be sufficiently small that it can be neglected.

Given a set of j sampled (or planned/desired) force vectors $\mathbf{P}_i$ at locations x_i the task of a planner is to find the control vector $\mathbf{c}$, which minimizes the error e given by

$$e = \sum_{i=1}^{j} [F(x_i) - P_i]^2 \qquad (6)$$

Depending on the number of samples (j), a minimum norm, an exact, or a least squares approximate solution can be found.

Applying the Mussa-Ivaldi vector field work to the motor system in the nonredundant limb allows approximation of arbitrary smooth vector fields. However, it follows that the planning and choice of the control fields to be approximated must be obtained in some other manner.

Serially redundant manipulators might pose difficulty for the use of this class of models in many biological systems. A study of how far the mechanism of basis field summation might apply to serially redundant planar linkages Mussa-Ivaldi and Gandolfo suggested that in serially redundant linkages a close approximation to vector summation may occur among a large fraction of randomly chosen control primitives. Mussa-Ivaldi (1997) extended these analyses to human-like movement trajectory construction. Use of force-field construction for motion generation in a nonconvex work space can be used for obstacle avoidance and navigation (see Khatib et al., 1999, and POTENTIAL FIELDS AND NEURAL NETWORKS).

More recently, Kargo and Giszter (2000) have proposed on experimental grounds that the primitives should ideally be considered as viscoelastic fields of specific durations (therefore wavelet-like in behavior) and that the approximation problem for biological motor control can be formulated as

$$F(r, \dot{r}, t) = \sum_i A_i \cdot a(b_i t + \tau_i) \cdot \Phi_i(r, \dot{r}) \qquad (7)$$

where A_i are scalar amplitude parameters, parameters b_i control frequency of a fixed waveform given by function a, τ_i is a phase parameter, and $\phi_i(r, r')$ are the viscoelastic force-field primitives.

Collections of primitives might be used in several ways. Planning and calculating how to combine primitives to approximate a desired field structure is one task that the CNS could perform for each behavior and perhaps each individual instance. In principle, arbitrary field structures and field time courses can be generated by the techniques of basis field approximation. However, as discussed, this flexibility implies that planning the details of these processes must be deferred to other mechanisms. In biological terms, collections of primitives could also be used in low-level motor behaviors driven by CPG oscillators, reflex stimuli, and simpler reinforcement and decision systems to elaborate simple protective actions and perhaps to bootstrap higher motor organization in mammals. Alternative models can be developed in this framework (Giszter et al., 2000b; see also Eliasmith and Anderson, 2000). Clearly, motor primitives could be used in each of these ways in biological systems.

Ideal primitives should provide specific stability guarantees in movement construction and execution. The biologically identified motor primitives simulate passive systems. When they are examined in viscoelastic terms, it is speculated that they may also represent contracting systems, which provide specific stability guarantees when combined in different arrangements (see Slotine and Lohmiller, 2001). The relationship of primitives to contracting systems awaits experimental testing.

It is also important to relate the motor primitives and elements discussed above to rhythmicity and CPGs (see Kiehn, Hounsgaard, and Sillar, 1997). Recently, Sternad et al. (2001) have strongly argued the need for use of limit cycle oscillating "primitives" in human and robot movement construction to synthesize timing. CPGs and limit cycle systems (see MOTOR PATTERN GENERATION) are a huge area that can be mentioned only briefly in this context. The relationship of timing or phasing systems to the force-field primitives discussed above is unclear in the biological data. The role of oscillation and timing in motor learning is clearly significant (Sternad et al., 2001). Kargo and Giszter (2000) have argued for a separation of rhythm and sequence generation from the force-field motor primitives used in execution. Several investigators are actively examining oscillating or "limit cycle primitives" and stability guarantees for these (e.g., Slotine and Lohmiller, 2001; Eliasmith and Anderson, 2000). It is possible that a hierarchy of different types of modules may form the basis of rapid motor development, flexible movement construction, and motor learning.

How force-field primitives are initially constructed and established in a motor system is an important issue that has also recently been considered. Todorov and Ghahramani have advanced the notion that the biological primitives that have been observed can be predicted as the result of a developmental process of system identification of a compact basis. The basis set that is obtained is able to jointly represent the limb dynamics and sensorimotor relationships in the neural control (unpublished work in progress; see also Mataric, Zordan, and Williamson, 1999, and Fod, Mataric, and Chadwicke Jenkins, 2002).

Motor Primitives in Real Behaviors: Biological Motor Control

Wiping Motor Pattern Construction and Control Using Force-Field Primitives

The task of wiping movements consists of locating a stimulus on the body surface and executing an action that removes it. The task involves many elements of sensorimotor behavior seen in more complex and voluntary acts. The animal subdivides the task as follows: (1) It moves together the body segment on which the target stimulus is located and the effector limb, closing the kinematic chain, and (2) it executes a movement that removes the irritant. These subtasks require the frog to transform skin location, limb configuration, and body scheme to (a) select an appropriate effector, (b) select a set of postures and limb trajectories for the effector, and (c) generate a set of appropriate muscle activations to control and move the effector through these postures and trajectories. Each stage involves ill-posed problems; that is, there is a set of many possible solutions to the problem, from which one must be selected.

A wiping strategy normally consists of a sequence of trajectories and postures. As an example, the kinematic postures and transitions (note, for example, placing and aiming) that are observed in wipes to the opposite hindlimb are summarized in Figure 1A. For some types of wipes, particular phases are optional and need not be executed during each cycle. Thus, in wiping to the back, extension may be omitted, flexion may be omitted, and whisk and flexion may be blended in both intact and spinal frogs (see Berkinblit, Feldman, and Fookson, 1986). It is clear that body scheme information is used to control wiping. This frequently involves active posturing of target limbs. Initial experiments on force-field primitives suggested a linkage of force-field primitives and elements of reflex behaviors such as wiping (Giszter et al., 1993). This linkage is now much more firmly established. Both flexion withdrawal and wiping (Giszter et al., 2000b) have been shown to be composed of sequences and combinations of force-field primitives. In wiping, hip and knee extensor deletions in the motor pattern (which were first observed by Stein's group in turtle scratch; see SCRATCH REFLEX) represent deletions of specific force-field primitives (Kargo and Giszter, 2000). An example of kinematic corrections and the isometrically measured correction force-fields taking this form are redrawn from Giszter et al. (2000b) (based on original work in Kargo and Giszter, 2000) and shown in Figure 1.

Rapid online corrections of wiping trajectories (Figure 1*B*) can be shown to occur by inserting specific force-field primitives into the ongoing behavior as a result of obstacle collisions (Figure 1*F*; Kargo and Giszter, 2000). The fields without correction (Figure 1*G*) can be subtracted from those in Figure 1*F* (e.g., as in Figure 1*E*) and lead to a fixed structure field (Figure 1*H*). Setup and adjustment of the motor pattern and trajectory and response to muscle vibration can all be described as amplitude or phase modulation of force-field primitives that are combined by the spinal cord of spinalized frogs according to the rule in Equation 7 above with parameter *b* fixed for all primitives, that is,

$$F(r, \dot{r}, t) = \sum_i A_i \cdot a(t + \tau_i) \cdot \Phi_i(r, \dot{r}) \qquad (8)$$

Descending Control and Force-Field Primitives

d'Avella and Bizzi have extended the spinal results to less reduced or intact preparations and have shown that a small basis set of muscle patterns and force patterns observed in the spinal frog represent a major fraction of the basis for vestibular correction (Bizzi et al., 2000) and intact behaviors.

Force-Field Primitives in Mammals

Force-field primitives of properties closely resembling the frog data are found in rat (Tresch and Bizzi, 1999) and cat, respectively. This framework in mammals suggests a new generation of functional electrical stimulation neuroprostheses stimulating either motor pools or interneuron pools to recruit single muscles or ensemble primitives (see Giszter et al., 2000b, for review). The relationship identified interneuron systems such as the C3–C4 and L3–L4 interneurons (found in the cervical [C3–C4] and lumbar [L3–L4] segments of mammalian spinal cord) remains to be explored.

Primitives in Voluntary Movement and in Motor Adaptation

Decomposition of human motor acts into a few summed elements has now been achieved by various laboratories (see publications of Sanger et al., cited in Kargo and Giszter, 2000). The use of the idea of motor primitives in describing effects in motor learning has gained support from the work of Thoroughman and Shadmehr and of Matsuoka and Bizzi (see Giszter et al., 2001a). How these elements used in learning and adaptation relate to spinal structures remains to be seen. The relationship of the primitives used to approximate and generalize the control of a trajectory in a novel environment and the primitives that are established as a basis set in reflexes in spinal cord of "lower" animals is clearly an important area. The higher-level elements of motor learning may represent more spatially localized patterns of recruitment, activation, and combination of the whole limb spinal primitives. However, it is also likely that completely novel primitives are elaborated in development and learning, for example, in motor cortex and cerebellum, to augment the spinal "bootstrap" or reflex behaviors and ex-

pand the domain of movement possibilities through life in a variety of ways (see Giszter et al., 2001a). How the construction and plasticity of primitives are organized in mental development and then later during the learning of novel motor acts or after trauma in adults is a fascinating and important area of investigation.

Road Maps: Motor Pattern Generators; Neuroethology and Evolution
Related Reading: Command Neurons and Command Systems; Equilibrium Point Hypothesis; Geometrical Principles in Motor Control; Locomotion, Vertebrate; Motor Pattern Generation; Potential Fields and Neural Networks; Radial Basis Function Networks; Scratch Reflex; Visuomotor Coordination in Frog and Toad; Visuomotor Coordination in Salamander

References

Berkinblit, M. B., Feldman, A. G., and Fookson, O. I., 1986, Adaptability of innate motor patterns and motor control mechanisms, *Behav. Brain Sci.*, 9:585–638. ◆

Bizzi, E., Tresch, M., Saltiel, P., and d'Avella, A., 2000, New perspectives on spinal motor systems, *Nature Rev. Neurosci.*, 1:101–108. ◆

Eliasmith, C., and Anderson, C. H., 2000, Rethinking central pattern generators: A general approach, *Neurocomputing*, 32–33:735–740.

Fod, A., Mataric, M. J., and Chadwicke Jenkins, O., 2002, Automated derivation of primitives for movement classification, *Autonomous Robots*, 12(1):39–54.

Giszter, S. F., Grill, W., Lemay, M., Mushahwar. V., and Prochazka, A., 2000a, Intraspinal microstimulation: Techniques, perspectives and prospects for FES, in *Neural Prostheses for Restoration of Sensory and Motor Function* (K. A. Moxon and J. K. Chapin, Eds.), Boca Raton, FL: CRC Press, pp. 101–138. ◆

Giszter, S. F., Moxon, K. A., Rybak, I., and Chapin, J. K., 2000b, A neurobiological perspective on design of humanoid robots and their components, *IEEE Intelligent Systems*, 15(4):64–69. ◆

Giszter, S. F., Moxon, K. A., Rybak, I., and Chapin, J. K., 2001a, Neurobiological and neurorobotic approaches to design of a controller for a humanoid motor system, *Robotics and Autonomous Systems*, 37:219–235. ◆

Giszter, S. F., Mussa-Ivaldi, F. A., and Bizzi, E., 1993, Convergent force field organized in the frog's spinal cord, *J. Neurosci.*, 13:467–491.

Giszter, S. F., Loeb, E., Mussa-Ivaldi, F. A., and Bizzi, E., 2001b, Repeatable spatial maps of a few force and joint torque patterns elicited by microstimulation applied throughout the lumbar spinal cord of the spinal frog, *Human Movement Sci.*, 19:597–626.

Kargo, W. J., and Giszter, S. F., 2000, Rapid corrections of aimed movements by combination of force-field primitives, *J. Neurosci.*, 20:409–426.

Khatib, O., Yokoi, K., Brock, O., Chang, K., Casal, A., 1999, Robots in human environments: Basic autonomous capabilities, *Int. J. Robotics Res.*, 18(7):684–696.

Kiehn, O., Hounsgaard, J., and Sillar, K., 1997, Basic building blocks of vertebrate spinal central pattern generators, in *Neurons, Networks, and Motor Behavior* (P. Stein, S. Grillner, A. Selverston, and D. Stuart, Eds.), Cambridge, MA: MIT Press, pp. 47–60. ◆

Mataric, M. J., Zordan, V. B., and Williamson, M. M., 1999, Making complex articulated agents dance: An analysis of control methods drawn from robotics, animation, and biology, *Autonomous Agents and Multi-Agent Systems*, 2(1):23–44.

Mussa-Ivaldi, F. A., 1997, Nonlinear force fields: A distributed system of control primitives for representing and learning movements, *Proceedings of the IEEE International Symposium on Computational Intelligence in Robotics and Automation*, pp. 84–90.

Schaal, S., 1999, Is imitation learning the route to humanoid robots?, *Trends Cogn. Sci.*, 3(6):233–242. ◆

Slotine, J. J., and Lohmiller, W., 2001, Modularity, evolution, and the binding problem: A view from stability theory, *Neural Networks*, 14(2):137–145.

Sternad, D., Duarte, M., Katsumata, H., and Schaal, S., 2001, Dynamics of a bouncing ball in human performance, *Phys. Rev. E Stat. Nonlin. Soft Matter Phys.*, 63(1, Pt 1):011902.

Tresch, M. C., and Bizzi, E., 1999, Responses to spinal microstimulation in the chronically spinalized rat and their relationship to spinal systems activated by low threshold cutaneous stimulation, *Exp. Brain Res.*, 129:401–416.

Motor Theories of Perception

Carol A. Fowler, Bruno Galantucci, and Elliot Saltzman

Introduction

Motor theories of perception propose that there is recruitment of the motor system or of motor competence (i.e., knowledge) in perception. Perhaps the best known motor theory of perception is Liberman's motor theory of speech perception (see Liberman, 1996, for a history and overview of the motor theory). Within speech science, despite its prominence, the theory has been judged implausible on several grounds. However, in the larger field encompassing studies of perception, action, and their coupling, it is given more credence. It is instructive to consider why the judgments differ between speech experts and experts in the broader domain.

In the following, we outline the motor theory of speech perception and describe some of the findings underlying its development. Next we offer reasons why speech scientists have doubted especially one of its two central claims, namely, that the speech motor system participates in speech perception. Then we suggest why the reasons are not sufficient to refute the claim, and we show that it acquires credibility when it is set in the larger context of investigations of perception, action, and their coupling. In addition, we summarize research that suggests a neural system consistent with Liberman's largely undeveloped ideas about neural support for speech perception. The discovery of mirror neurons in primates (Rizzolatti and Arbib, 1998) provides an existence proof of neuronal perceptuomotor couplings.

The Motor Theory of Speech Perception

Although in alphabetic script, consonants and vowels are discrete, their expression in acoustic speech signals is not. This is because speakers coarticulate speech gestures; that is, they produce the articulatory gestures of successive consonants and vowels in a temporally and spatially overlapping manner. Gestures are linguistically significant actions of the vocal tract. More specifically, they are equivalence classes of articulatory patterns controlled with respect to linguistically significant goals defined in an abstract task space. Consequences of coarticulation are evident, for example, during production of the word *to* when activation of the vowel /u/'s lip protrusion gesture overlaps the activation of the consonant /t/'s lingual gesture (compare *tea*). Due to coarticulation, acoustic speech signals are highly context sensitive, and they lack a discrete segmental structure.

Liberman developed a motor theory of speech perception when he and his colleagues found that speech percepts track articulation more closely than the acoustic signals to which articulation gives rise. Two experimental findings were especially telling. One was that, in the synthesized syllables /di/ and /du/, the critical acoustic cues for /d/ were quite different, owing to the effects of coarticulation by the different vowels. Indeed, the cues were audibly distinct when presented in isolation to listeners. However, the gestures for /d/ are the same in natural productions of the two syllables, and the consonants sound alike. A complementary finding was that the same acoustic cue was identified as /p/ before /i/ and /u/, but as /k/ before /a/. Because of coarticulation, to generate the cue before /i/ or /u/ requires production of /p/, whereas to generate it before /a/ requires production of /k/.

Both findings suggested to Liberman that when articulation and acoustic patterns diverge due to coarticulation, perception tracks articulation, a central claim of the motor theory. Subsequently, many other findings (see Liberman, 1996, for a review) converged

on the same conclusion. A notable one is the McGurk effect (McGurk and MacDonald, 1976), in which a video of a speaker mouthing one syllable, say, /da/, is dubbed with a different acoustic syllable, say, /ma/. Listeners hear a syllable (/na/ in the example) that reflects integration of gestural information from both modalities.

In Liberman's view, recovery of articulation in speech perception implies recruitment of the motor system. Such motor recruitment is required because of coarticulation in speech production. Speech information must be transmitted rapidly, and the gestural overlap provided by coarticulation permits efficient packaging of consonants and vowels. However, coarticulation has other consequences, including context sensitivity in acoustic information for phonetic segments. Therefore, two specializations, one for coarticulating and one for perceiving coarticulated speech, are needed, and, because neither specialization is useful without the other, they had to coevolve. Moreover, given the motor character of the percept, and Liberman's view that this reflects recruitment of the motor system in perception, the inference was plausible that the specializations were one and the same: a phonetic module. By using gestures as a common currency for talkers and listeners, the module helps guarantee achievement of parity between them—that is, sufficient equivalence between phonological messages sent and received, a necessity for successful communication.

Speech Science: The Implausiblity of the Motor Theory

Following are grounds on which the motor theory of speech perception has been judged implausible, and then some reasons why we reject each argument.

1. Many speech scientists (e.g., Ohala, 1996) deny that speech percepts have a motor character, and they have no other reasons to suppose that the speech motor system is involved in perceiving speech.
2. Liberman and colleagues wrote very little about how the speech motor system might participate in speech perception, and the mechanism that they typically alluded to (analysis by synthesis) is not obviously workable at the rates at which consonants and vowels are perceived.
3. Listeners' perception of speech gestures need not imply that the speech motor system is recruited in speech perception. This is because the acoustic signal, having been caused by the gestures, and taking distinctive forms for distinct gestures, provides information about them. Listeners perceive gestures because that is what the information in acoustic speech signals is about.

We will address the first objection here only by remarking that, in our opinion as in Liberman's, evidence in favor of perceiving motor gestures is substantial and unrefuted. For example, we know of no studies that refute the evidence we cited in the previous section in favor of the claim that, when articulation and acoustic patterns diverge, perception tracks articulation. As for the other two objections, however accurate they may be, neither refutes the motor theory's claim of motor system recruitment in speech perception. As for the second objection, even if the particular mechanisms proposed by Liberman and colleagues are not the ones that support speech perception, it does not follow that no mechanism involving a production-perception link does the job. As for the last objection, even though acoustic speech signals provide information about speech gestures, that does not preclude a perceptual mechanism in which the speech motor system or motor competence participates in decoding the acoustic signal.

The Broader Scientific Field: The Necessity for Motor Theories?

In the broader scientific field, central theoretical ideas of Liberman's motor theory recur (e.g., Viviani and Stucchi, 1992), and there are research findings suggesting motor involvement in perception. We review one example of a theoretical view that shares critical ideas with those of Liberman and then summarize a few of the research findings.

A Related Idea

Prinz (e.g., 1997) addresses an issue that arises in the study of perceptually guided action and that is very much like the one we have labeled parity. In speech, *parity* refers to the relation between messages sent and perceived. The messages must characteristically be the same; otherwise communication fails. Prinz has raised the same issue in asking how perception can guide action under the common assumption that percepts are representations of sensory information, and planned actions are coded in purely motor terms; that is, they lack a common currency. He proposes instead that percepts and actions share a common code. Further, consistent with the motor theory's identification of gestures as the common currency of talkers and listeners, and with the hypothesis that gestures are represented in the task spaces of talkers and listeners (SPEECH PRODUCTION), Prinz's *action effect principle* invokes a common code that represents not the proximal stimulus, but the relevant distal event properties. (*Proximal* refers to the signals that stimulate the sense organs, whereas *distal* refers to the environmental events that causally structure the proximal stimuli). Prinz's research shows, for example, that when stimuli that guide responses in some tasks share distal features with responses, response times are affected.

Research Findings

The larger context of evidence, to which we alluded earlier, in which the motor theory gains plausibility includes evidence from communication systems of other animals, evidence of motor recruitment in perception of motion, and findings of mirror neurons. In each domain, we provide illustrative examples.

Communication systems of other animals.   Male crickets produce mating calls to attract females. Females respond to the calls by moving toward the male, but they do not produce calls themselves. However, males and females show a remarkable symmetry. Different varieties of crickets produce different calls, and females prefer the calls of their own type. When crickets are hybridized by mating the male of one type to the female of another, the male's call exhibits components from the calls of both parental types. Remarkably, female hybrids prefer the hybrid call to the call of either parental type (Hoy, Hahn, and Paul, 1977). This suggests a genetic correspondence between neural systems supporting call production in males and call perception in females.

Evidence of perception-action coupling can be found within individuals as well as between them. In zebra finches, the neural system supporting call production also responds to components of auditorily presented songs (Williams and Nottebohm, 1985). A major path for song production in the zebra finch brain begins at a "higher vocal center" (HVc), which projects to the robustus archistriatum (RA) and from there to the tracheosyringeal portion of the hypoglossal nerve (nXIIts). nXIIts innervates the muscles of the syrinx. The HVc and nXIIts both respond to tone bursts, and motor neurons in nXIIts are differentially responsive to different components of perceived songs. Hauser (1996) concludes that "in order for birds to perceive the proper acoustic features of a song syllable, the percept must be converted into a series of motor actions required to produce the sound" (pp. 148–149).

Evidence in humans for motor recruitment in perception outside the speech domain.   The tangential velocity of curved movements made by humans is proportional to curvature according to a two-thirds power law, decreasing with increases in curvature (e.g., Viviani and Stucchi, 1989). Viviani and Stucchi have shown that observers' judgments of the shapes of ellipses being drawn on a computer screen (judgments as to whether the major axis is oriented vertically or horizontally) are affected not only by the form's shape, but also by its velocity profile. When ellipses were drawn with constant velocity—a profile characteristic, in natural drawing, of a circular form—perceivers' judgments were poor. Tracings of ellipses that adhered to the two-thirds power law were judged accurately. An implicit proprioceptive-motor, rather than visual, task (Viviani, Baud-Bovy, and Redolfi, 1997) provided similar results. Blindfolded participants' right arms were moved in elliptical trajectories that did or did not preserve the two-thirds power law. With the left arm, participants tried to reproduce the movement of the right arm. Shapes of reproduced trajectories were more accurate when ellipses traced by the right arm conformed to the two-thirds power law than when they did not. Together, these data show that motor competence, here knowledge about velocity constraints on biological movements, is brought to bear on perception of motion.

Other evidence for linkages between the motor and perceptual systems comes from experiments that manipulate the similarity between a stimulus-response pair and measure its facilitatory or inhibitory influence on motor performance (see Prinz, 1997, for a review). For example, Stürmer, Aschersleben, and Prinz (2000) had participants produce a grasping gesture (first close the hand, then open it) or a spreading gesture (first open then close). The task-relevant stimuli for the movements were color changes on a hand that was displayed on a computer monitor, with different colors signaling each task. The visible hand also produced a task-irrelevant gesture on each trial, starting and ending from a neutral half-open position. In one case, it closed and then opened; in the other, it opened and then closed. Although participants were told to ignore the irrelevant information, selecting their responses only on the basis of the color change, their response latencies were faster when their movements matched the irrelevant ones. That perception of a hand gesture interacts with the execution of a similar or dissimilar hand gesture provides strong evidence that the perceptual and the motor systems share a common currency.

Mirror neurons.   The foregoing evidence, like the evidence underlying the motor theory of speech perception, suggests access to the motor system or to motor knowledge in perception. Recent findings of mirror neurons may reveal part of a neural mechanism that permits and promotes such access.

Rizzolatti and colleagues (see Rizzolatti and Arbib's, 1998 review) have found neurons in the premotor cortex of the monkey (area F5) that respond both when the monkey performs a given action and when it perceives a similar action performed by another monkey or by a human. Many mirror neurons are quite specific in firing during the performance of, say, one manual grasping movement but not another. Many of them exhibit the same specificity in the observed actions that stimulate them to fire.

There is evidence for mirror neurons in humans. Fadiga et al. (1995) used transcranial magnetic stimulation (TMS) of the motor area, in which stimulation provoked muscle activity in the fingers. During TMS, participants observed several events or situations: someone grasping an object, the stationary object itself, someone tracing shapes in the air with the arm, or the dimming of a light. The investigators found more TMS-induced muscle activity in the fingers when participants were observing grasping than when they were observing any other of the events. The modulation of muscle activity was specific to the actions observed. Fadiga et al. concluded that "in humans there is a neural system matching action observation and action execution" (p. 2609).

The finding of mirror neurons reveals neural systems that underlie perception-action coupling in monkeys and perhaps in humans as well. From the perspective of the motor theory of speech perception, it is intriguing that the neurons were found in an area of the monkey brain that includes the homologue of Broca's area in humans, which is involved in language use. The findings, therefore, lend credence to the motor theory's claim of a production-perception coupling in speech.

Discussion

The motor theory of speech perception has inspired analogous theories in other domains. Yet the theory was motivated by requirements of speaking and listening that Liberman considered special to speech. Is speech special in respects that should discourage efforts to generalize some of its proposals to other domains? We suspect not.

As we have noted, talkers and listeners must characteristically achieve parity to communicate successfully (Liberman, 1996), and parity achievement requires use of a common currency by talkers and listeners. That the speech percept has a motor character suggests that this common currency is defined in gestural task space: listeners *detect* the proximal acoustic signal, but they *perceive* the distal gestural activities of talkers. According to the motor theory, gesture perception is fostered by motor recruitment in perception.

This is not very different from what is required for successful nonlinguistic transactions with the environment, including those with other actors. Although proximal energy patterns stimulate the sense organs, animals must perceive the distal possibilities afforded for action (e.g., Gibson, 1979; see also GRASPING MOVEMENTS: VISUOMOTOR TRANSFORMATIONS). For actions to be felicitous, parity is required among perceived possibilities for action, real possibilities for action, and action itself. This is real-world, functional perception-action coupling. Plausibly, neural-motor recruitment in

perception fosters achievement of these parities as well as those of linguistic communication.

In much cognitive science research, perception and action are assumed to be sufficiently distinct and autonomous that they can be studied independently. However, consideration of the relations between animals and their environments uncovers no principled way to draw such a sharp distinction. Perception-action couplings are central to the design of animals. Understanding the real-world settings in which cognitive activity occurs reveals that it could not be otherwise.

Road Map: Linguistics and Speech Processing
Related Reading: Language Evolution: The Mirror System Hypothesis; Language Processing; Optimality Theory in Linguistics; Speech Production

References

Fadiga, L, Fogassi, L., Pavesi, G., and Rizzolatti, G., 1995, Motor facilitation during action observation: A magnetic stimulation study, *J. Neurophysiol.*, 7:2608–2611.

Gibson, J. J., 1979, *The Ecological Approach to Visual Perception*, Boston: Houghton Mifflin. ◆

Hauser, M., 1996, *The Evolution of Communication*, Cambridge, MA: MIT Press. ◆

Hoy, R., Hahn, J., and Paul, R., 1977, Hybrid cricket auditory behavior: Evidence for genetic coupling in animal communication, *Science*, 195:82–84.

Liberman, A. M., 1996, *Speech: A Special Code*, Cambridge, MA: MIT Press. ◆

McGurk, H., and MacDonald, J., 1976, Hearing lips and seeing voices, *Nature*, 264:746–748.

Ohala, J., 1996, Listeners hear sounds not tongues, *J. Acoust. Soc. Am.*, 99:1718–1728.

Prinz, W., 1997, Perception and action planning, *Eur. J. Cogn. Psychol.*, 9:129–154. ◆

Rizzolatti, G., and Arbib, M., 1998, Language in our grasp, *Trends Neurosci.*, 21:188–194. ◆

Stürmer, B., Aschersleben, G., and Prinz, W., 2000, Correspondence effect with manual gestures and postures: A study of imitation, *J. Exp. Psychol. Hum. Percept. Perform.*, 26:1746–1759.

Viviani, P., Baud-Bovy, G., and Redolfi, M., 1997, Perceiving and tracking kinesthetic stimuli: Further evidence of motor-perceptual interactions, *J. Exp. Psychol. Hum. Percept. Perform.*, 23:1232–1252.

Viviani, P., and Stucchi, N., 1989, The effect of movement velocity on form perception: Geometrical illusions in dynamic display, *Percept. Psychophys.*, 46:266–274.

Viviani, P. and Stucchi, N., 1992, Motor-perceptual interactions, in *Tutorials in Motor Behavior II* (G. Stelmach and J. Requin, Eds.), Amsterdam: North Holland.

Williams, H., and Nottebohm, F., 1985, Auditory responses in avian vocal motor neurons: A motor theory for song perception in birds, *Science*, 229:279–282.

Multiagent Systems

José M. Vidal and Edmund H. Durfee

Introduction

Natural systems are based on parallel, distributed processing at many different levels. At the neural level, interconnected and concurrently acting neurons propagate signals among themselves such that coherent behavior emerges from their joint activity. Within the

brain, different neural subsystems combine and exchange signals to work together to yield an overall intelligent nervous system. Beyond the boundaries of a single intelligent entity are other such entities, which together make up societies that achieve more than the individual entities can. Thus, what constitutes an "individual" can be highly subjective: what is an individual to one researcher may, to another, be a complex distributed system comprised of finer-grained agents. In this context, an agent's "granularity" corresponds to the amount of processing it does between interactions with others.

Research in artificial neural networks (ANNs) has concentrated on the finer-grained levels of intelligence evidenced in the brain, drawing on neurophysiology and psychology as sources of inspiration when trying to build computational models of such natural systems. Research in brain theory has dealt with different levels, from neurons to brain regions to humans. Finally, research in multiagent systems has focused on coarse-grained levels of individuality and interaction, where the goal is to draw on sociological, political, and economic insights to develop multiagent systems composed of autonomous interacting agents (Weiss, 1999). As such, there is ample room for comparison between the ANN, brain theoretic, and multiagent systems approaches. Much can be gained by comparing the different techniques used in these fields of study. Specifically, agents in multiagent systems must interact with each other. This interaction is often facilitated by the use of agent models. That is, agents either have or learn models of the agents with which they interact. Agents that learn models of other agents can do so by observing their past behavior. These models allow agents to avoid dealing with malicious or broken agents. In a system with many learning agents, we can expect agents to build nested models of the other agents—that is, models that include an agent's models of other agents, and so on. We might expect agents to build deeper and deeper nested models of each other in an effort to outguess each other. However, while there is some amount of deep-model escalation—agents building nested models of each other to greater and greater depths—some research (Vidal and Durfee, 1998) shows that these deeper models exhibit decreasing returns. By using their models of each other, the agents loosely organize themselves into self-reinforcing communities of trust.

Learning agents can use any type of learning, including ANNs. Although there has been very little research into this topic, ANNs seem like a promising learning technique because of their flexibility and ability to generalize. An agent that uses ANNs could learn about the "tags" that identify a cheating agent by extrapolating from a few examples. This would allow the agent to avoid unproductive future interactions with other agents that it has never met. Such behavior, when enacted by all the agents in the system, would speed up system convergence and discourage cheating agents more rapidly. Furthermore, the dynamics generated by a system composed of many learning agents are not unlike the dynamics of an ANN. Some of the same problems of credit assignment and propagation of rewards arise in both of these systems, even if the protocol details are different.

Brain theory can be related to multiagent systems at many levels. At one level brain theory considers neurons as agents. That is, it considers them as a basic behavior unit. Unlike agents in a system, neurons do not engage in complex interactions with other neurons. However, neurons have predefined rules of encounter. For example, a neuron can "count on" the signals of a particular input line carrying specific information. These simple rules enable coordination of the system of neurons. Similar rules are often used by multiagent systems to achieve coordination. At a higher level, brain theory considers brain regions as agents. These agents are more complex and might start to derive a benefit by considering other brain regions as agents and trying to build models of them or trying to interact with them using multiagent techniques. At an even higher level, brain theory considers people as agents. At this level we might wonder if the theories developed for the construction and control of artificial multiagent systems might be useful in either explaining or guiding collective human behaviors.

We can also contrast the various abstraction levels in brain theory to the two organizational varieties in multiagent systems: top-down and bottom-up. In a top-down approach, one or a few agents monitor the global performance of the organization and detect when a particular organizational structure is needed. Most typically, roles in the new organization are assigned (often through a contracting style of protocol) and the new organization is adopted (Corkill and Lesser, 1983). Alternatively, in a bottom-up approach, an agent monitors its own performance, decides when a change (such as to the tasks it itself performs) is in order, and unilaterally makes that change. This in turn could cause other agents to change what they are doing, and reorganization propagates throughout the network (Ishida, Gasser, and Yokoo, 1992). These techniques are similar to the brain theory studies of bottom-up organizational emergence as seen in neurons and the top-down organizational rules as developed and imposed by humans in their organizations.

In this article we will begin by categorizing the different types of agent interaction protocols that are being studied in multiagent systems, from cooperative problem solving among cooperative agents to coordination protocols for autonomous selfish agents. These will be explained in detail in later sections of this article, including brief overviews of the latest research in these areas. We conclude this article by summarizing some of the similarities and differences between multiagent systems and the fields of brain theory and neural networks, highlighting some potentially important areas for cross-fertilization between them.

Agent Coordination

A central concern in distributed artificial intelligence (DAI) is the development of interaction protocols for the coordination of agents. System designers build protocols that determine how, when, and what the agents will communicate to each other. A good protocol should achieve the expected global goals while maintaining some independence between agents. The degree of independence depends on the particular application. For example, if the agents are robots in a large field, then we can expect them not to interfere with each other as long as they keep their distance. However, if these same robots are charged with the task of lifting a large object, then much tighter coordination will be needed. The amount of independence depends on the type of tasks the agents must achieve and on their interaction opportunities within the environment.

Agents often use commitments and conventions in order to coordinate (Jennings, 1994). *Commitments* are pledges from an agent that it will try to achieve a specified task. Commitments help other agents plan their actions without interfering with each other. *Conventions* specify when commitments can be broken and what the agents should do when this happens. In a typical system we can expect that unforeseen circumstances might force an agent to drop certain commitments, especially if the world the agent inhabits is changing. Conventions tell the agent how it can renege on its commitments without causing undue distress to the system.

DAI systems can be roughly separated into two categories: systems in which all agents share a common goal, and systems in which each agent has its own goals. When all agents have the same goal, the interaction protocol enables balanced task decomposition and allocation. That is, the interaction protocol divides and distributes the tasks among the agents so as to avoid overloading any resource or agent, handing agents overlapping or conflicting tasks, and leaving tasks unhandled. When all the agents have different goals, then a coordination protocol must be designed to align their interests with the designer's global system goal. We discuss these types of systems, and their protocols, in the next sections.

Cooperative Problem-Solving Systems

In a cooperative distributed problem-solving system (Bond and Gasser, 1988), agents work together to solve problems that require them to cooperate. Research in this area takes two major forms.

One of these forms is represented by the functionally accurate/ cooperative (FAC) paradigm (Corkill and Lesser, 1983), where problem solvers individually solve their local subproblems and share their partial results so that, over time, increasingly complete results get formed and the system solves the entire problem. Success is achieved when one or more agents construct and share a hypothesis that satisfies the solution criteria. Of course, the wholesale exchange of all partial results can bog down a system quickly, and so substantial effort has gone into the development of techniques by which cooperating agents could model each other to be smart about which results to share. These models have included organizational structures (Corkill and Lesser, 1983), partial global plans (Durfee and Lesser, 1991), and the TAEMS framework (Decker and Lesser, 1995). Another approach is to include team considerations from the beginning, which has led to research into team-oriented programming (Tambe and Zhang, 1998).

A complementary perspective on cooperative problem solving has viewed the process as sharing tasks rather than results. As embodied in the Contract-Net protocol (Smith, 1980), the task-sharing perspective sees the coordination problem as associating tasks to be done with the right agents to do them. In Contract-Net, for example, an agent with a large task to do would decompose it into smaller tasks, and then attempt to contract these out to the most suitable agents by announcing each subtask, collecting bids, and awarding the subtask. Because agents choose to bid on the tasks they receive, the assignment of tasks to agents involves mutual selection. A similar specialization occurs in the evolutionary structuring of the brain into specialized regions. Task sharing can also be coupled with result sharing, such that organizational roles could be contracted out, FAC would follow, and then tasks to implement the solution could be contracted out.

Continuing research in cooperative distributed problem solving has served to extend and refine the basic paradigms of task and result sharing, involving, among other things, the introduction of planning to the process, and the formulation of negotiation strategies for reaching a compromise between what different agents want that maximizes the overall system performance. Note, however, that in this discussion the emphasis has been on the overall system rather than an individual. The assumption is that agents in these systems are built with an implicit goal of doing whatever they need in order to improve the performance of the entire system. Although this assumption is often reasonable when building real systems, since we can design such agents, it does neglect the issue of how to get individual agents, each with its own selfish goals, to solve problems cooperatively. This issue has been the focus of a variety of research activities more recently, as the next section explains.

Selfish Agents

Cooperative problem solving has been shown to be generally beneficial from a systemwide perspective, but many DAI researchers are concerned with how such cooperation might emerge when an agent can only see benefits to itself. In other words, what is the knowledge and reasoning that agents employ in making smart decisions about when to work together? Once they have adopted the goal of working together, then they can employ cooperative problem solving techniques to actually accomplish their joint activities.

One of the most fruitful fields for insights when investigating how selfish agents can still work together for their mutual benefit is economics. In fact, the use of economic techniques for coordinating multiagent systems is a very active area of research. The techniques used include voting, bargaining, and auctions (Weiss, 1999, chap. 9). Each technique has different strengths and weaknesses. They are all concerned with the making of rational decisions by a group of distributed agents, each with its own goals. These techniques usually involve several communication steps as

well as rational decision making by the agents. They are very useful techniques for structuring the interactions between agents because they aggregate the individual agents' desires to form a global decision or allocation.

Auctions, for example, are very efficient methods for matching buyer and seller agents that are interested in the same good or service. The use of a single exchange currency allows an agent to externalize its utility with a single number that is understood by all other agents. If there are enough agents participating in the auction, then both buyers and sellers are generally guaranteed a fair price. Finally, the auction acts as a location service where all agents that are interested in the item can find each other and interact using the auction's bidding protocol, thereby eliminating the need for agents to find and try to talk directly to each other.

There are, however, some problems with auctions that echo the problems studied by economists. For example, just like their human counterparts, intelligent agents might be able to collude with each other and manipulate the auction's price to their benefit. This problem can be circumvented by changing the type of auction or by increasing the number of participants. A lying auctioneer who does not assign the winnings to the correct agent might also break an auction. Finally, auctions assume that all agents are trading exact instances of the same item. That is, they do not consider the possibility that one agent's products are of a higher quality than another agent's products. Economists often ignore minor differences in the quality of a good or, if the difference is great enough, they state that the different quality goods should simply be considered different goods altogether.

Even in the presence of agents that cheat or offer different quality goods, a stable system can often be achieved by allowing agents to use models of other agents. For example, if the agents see each other as rational, then they can make a deal allowing them to cooperate (Rosenschein and Genesereth, 1985). Alternatively, they can evaluate the performance of alternative strategies to select the cooperative strategy from a purely selfish view (Gmytrasiewicz, Durfee, and Wehe, 1991), leading to self-organization for their mutual benefit. Finally, they can use learning techniques to build models of other agents (Vidal and Durfee, 1998) and use these models to guide interactions.

Organization theory (Malone, 1987) has also looked at the problem of how organizations form and why individuals are willing to become parts of an organization. In joining an organization, an individual forgoes some of his freedom because he has now committed to performing some set of actions for others in the organization. He has also accepted dependencies on others. The positive side of the resulting web of commitments (Gasser, 1991) is that, when the agents abide by their responsibilities and while the circumstances under which the organization was formed hold, the payoff to members of the successful organization is higher than those members could have gained individually. So organization, under the right circumstances, is the rational thing to do. The remaining challenge, then, is in developing computational mechanisms by which individuals can detect that the circumstances are right for organizing and for performing the organizational self-design.

Discussion

Given the information above, and the larger context in which this article is written, we now wish to delve deeper into the relation between multiagent systems, brain theory, and ANNs. They differ in many respects. One respect is clearly the granularity of computation relative to communication. Multiagent systems generally assume that communication is time consuming, error prone, and costly. Thus, communication decisions are made judiciously, and messages among entities in multiagent systems are at the symbol rather than signal level, encoding much richer semantic content.

Because communication is at such a premium, and because envisioning the impact of a message requires a model of the hearer of that message, agents in multiagent systems usually have explicit models of other agents, including their interests, abilities, and expectations. Decision making in agents is thus a complex process of mapping potential actions (including communication acts) into explicit models of the anticipated activities of others, leading to a wide range of behaviors. Often, to anticipate the actions of another, an agent will execute its inferencing processes on its model of that other agent, drawing conclusions about what the other agent could be thinking or doing by "putting itself in the other's shoes."

In brain theory, this implies that an agent should be able to ignore its current state and instead to "think" as if it were another agent. Because such projection requires an agent to be able to disconnect from its own reality and superimpose that assumed of another, this implies that models of the mind must provide a higher-level override capability to control the processing of the parallel brain regions and schemas. In this way, the same machinery that an agent uses to control its own actions can be used to predict those of others.

In ANNs the individual units are generally simpler, signal-processing elements, and the complexities arise from the sheer number of interconnections and the ways that those interconnections evolve over time. In multiagent systems, the primary concern has been to endow agents with knowledge about protocols, conventions, common goals, and so on right from the start, so that they can immediately interact efficiently; interaction is usually too expensive and slow to depend on "learning" how to interact. In many approaches to ANNs, the focus is precisely on learning, because interaction is cheap and fast in the tightly coupled, signal-propagating architecture assumed. Thus, in ANNs, important performance criteria include trainability, convergence, and robustness. Multiagent systems share the robustness criterion, but rather than the capability to learn, they focus on performance in terms of correctly and quickly coordinating activity to work as an effective team from the outset, making maximum use of resources at all times.

For example, having mobile robots learn to coordinate their movements by allowing them to learn from colliding is generally infeasible, since collisions can lead to disablement of the robots. In a multiagent approach (Montgomery and Durfee, 1993), the robots each plan their behaviors and then engage in a dialogue to efficiently isolate and resolve conflicting actions. Following a predominant paradigm in AI, the robots essentially engage in a distributed search through the space of joint behaviors, using a hierarchical representation to focus their search. Through the distributed hierarchical search, the agents can balance the costs of coordination with its benefits, to attain an appropriate level of coordination. As problems scale up, moreover, the agents can employ abstractions to represent teams of agents as single entities. Mobile robots performing deliveries, for example, are clustered into geographic teams such that a robot models only the other members of its team, and coordinates with other teams through the decisions of team leaders. Properties of the task and of the agents, known ahead of time by the agents, dictate appropriate decomposition and task-abstraction strategies that, in the best case, can reduce the time to solution from exponential in the single-agent case to logarithmic in the multiagent case.

However, even thought agents are usually endowed with the needed interaction protocols, it is often the case that these protocols leave the agent with many possible choices. For example, the fact that agents must interact using a Contract-Net protocol says nothing about which tasks the agents should bid on, or how much they should bid. In fact, the correct choice might depend on the current state of the system and of the other agents. These problems have

led to the study of learning agents within multiagent systems. As mentioned earlier, this is an area where multiagent systems and ANNs share some similarities. Both of them try to understand the behavior of systems composed of adaptive agents. In the multiagent case the agents are more complex and loosely connected, whereas in ANNs the units are simpler and have fixed connections but can interact much more often. Still, many of the same mathematical tools used to understand the emergent behaviors in ANNs could be used to understand and engineer multiagent systems.

Another critical similarity between multiagent systems and ANNs is an emphasis on emerging intelligence—on the whole being more than the sum of its parts. From relatively simple neural units, complex patterns of activity can arise in neural networks; from cooperation and competition among schemas, intelligent behavior results; from rational choices among individuals, societies and civilizations (to anthropomorphize) emerge. As was alluded to at the outset of this article, all systems are distributed if you look closely enough, and it is the fact that the collection is more than the sum of its parts that allows us to call it a system rather than a collection of component parts. Whether simple or complex, communicating signals or symbols, distributed systems are a ubiquitous framework encompassing all of these studies. As such, these studies have common ground for sharing ideas and insights.

As a specific example of the opportunities in a cross-disciplinary study, a key concern in multiagent systems, as in ANNs, is in how to propagate global feedback such that individual entities can modify their behavior correctly. Multiagent systems suffer from the same credit/blame assignment problems as neural networks and schema systems. If the system as a whole performs well or poorly, which entities, and which interactions among entities, were responsible?

Propagation algorithms that have been developed for neural networks, multiagent systems composed of learning agents, and feedback loops that support reorganization in multiagent systems raise many common concerns. So far, the similarities and potential overlaps between the multiagent systems and ANN algorithms have not been widely studied.

Similarly, multiagent systems, brain theory, and ANNs are all concerned with timely and appropriate communication among computational units. The thresholding computations used in neural networks and the cooperative/competitive links among brain regions have analogues in multiagent systems that decide when a result is good enough to share, and how much to believe results received from others. Such analogies are, to date, not firmly understood, and represent opportunities for cross-fertilization.

Road Map: Artificial Intelligence
Related Reading: Artificial Intelligence and Neural Networks; Competitive Queuing for Planning and Serial Performance; Decision Support Systems and Expert Systems; Hybrid Connectionist/Symbolic Systems; Schema Theory; Speech Recognition Technology

References

Bond, A. H., and Gasser, L., Eds., 1988, *Readings in Distributed Artificial Intelligence*, San Mateo, CA: Morgan Kaufmann. ◆

Corkill, D. D., and Lesser, V. R., 1983, The use of meta-level control for coordination in a distributed problem solving network, in *Proceedings of the Eighth International Joint Conference on Artificial Intelligence*, San Francisco: Morgan Kauffman, pp. 748–756.

Decker, K., and Lesser, V. R., 1995, Designing a family of coordination mechanism, in *Proceedings of the First International Conference on Multi-Agent Systems*, Cambridge, MA: AAAI Press, pp. 73–80.

Durfee, E. H., and Lesser, V. R., 1991, Partial global planning: A coordination framework for distributed hypothesis formation, *IEEE Trans. Syst. Man. Cybern.*, 21:1167–1183.

Gasser, L., 1991, Social conceptions of knowledge and action: DAI foundations and open systems semantics, *Artif. Intell.*, 47:107–138.

Gmytrasiewicz, P. J., Durfee, E. H., and Wehe, D. K., 1991, A decision-theoretic approach to coordinating multiagent interactions, in *Proceedings of the Twelfth International Joint Conference on Artificial Intelligence*, San Francisco: Morgan Kauffman, pp. 62–68.

Ishida, T., Gasser, L., and Yokoo, M., 1992, Organization self-design of distributed production systems, *IEEE Trans. Knowledge Data Eng.*, 4:123–134.

Jennings, N. U., 1994, Commitments and conventions: The foundation of coordination in multi-agent systems, *Knowledge Eng. Rev.*, 8:223–250.

Malone, T. W., 1987, Modeling coordination in organizations and markets, *Manage. Sci.*, 33:1317–1332.

Montgomery, T. A., and Durfee, E. H., 1993, Search reduction in hierarchical distributed problem solving, *Group Decis. Negotiat.*, 2:301–317.

Rosenschein, J. S., and Genesereth, M. R., 1985, Deals among rational agents, in *Readings in Distributed Artificial Intelligence* (A. H. Bond and L. Gasser, Eds.), San Mateo, CA: Morgan Kaufmann, pp. 227–234.

Smith, R. G., 1980, The contract net protocol: High-level communication and control in a distributed problem solver, *IEEE Trans. Comput.*, C-29:1104–1113.

Tambe M., and Zhang W., 1998, Towards flexible teamwork in persistent teams, in *Proceedings of the Third International Conference on Multi-Agent Systems*, Cambridge, MA: AAAI Press.

Vidal, J. M., and Durfee, E. H., 1998, Learning nested models in an information economy, *J. Exp. Theoret. Artif. Intell.*, 10:291–308.

Weiss, G., Ed., 1999, *Multiagent Systems*, Cambridge, MA: MIT Press. ◆

Muscle Models

Thomas G. Sandercock, David C. Lin, and W. Zev Rymer

Introduction

Muscle is a remarkable mechanical actuator that transduces chemical energy into force and motion, thereby providing power to move the skeleton. Because of the complexity of this transduction and the intricacies of muscle microstructure and architecture, no comprehensive models have yet been able to predict muscle performance completely. For this reason, muscle models are widely used to fulfill a variety of more narrowly defined objectives, ranging from attempts to promote understanding at the molecular level to more practical simulations of whole-muscle behavior. These practical simulations are typically used as part of a broader study of basic musculoskeletal biomechanics or for issues of understanding neural control mechanisms.

Muscle models can be usefully classified in order of increasing complexity. The more elaborate models generally have a wider range of application and can give more accurate results. However, this increase in fidelity is achieved at the cost of an increase in the mathematical complexity, involving parameters that are often not known initially and are not readily measured. Aside from the mechanisms of force generation, many other processes, such as activation, potentiation, and fatigue, also play an important role. In the absence of a single model that captures all these features, models are usually simplified to include only those behaviors that are deemed of interest in a particular application. This article outlines three major model classes and provides guidelines for their application:

1. *Input-output models*. The simplest of models are "black box" input-output models that attempt to capture very specific behavior over a restricted range of operation. Such models commonly use linear transfer function descriptors to transform neural excitation into force.

2. *Lumped parameter mechanical models*. The next level in complexity is typified by lumped parameter mechanical models. These are often composed of combinations of linear mechanical elements such as springs and dashpots to create fairly simple viscoelastic analogs of muscle. Nonlinear relations representing hyperbolic force-velocity behavior and tendon properties can also be incorporated. Such models are usually termed "Hill models." The parameters characterizing the elements of these models are usually directly measurable by experiments. Model inputs may be neural excitation or length and force perturbations, while outputs may include muscle force, stiffness, and the time course of muscle length changes.

3. *Cross-bridge models*. More sophisticated "cross-bridge" models attempt to reproduce the dynamics of molecular processes that are responsible for force generation in muscle. These models incorporate mathematical descriptions of the dynamics of cross-bridge populations, their driving chemical reactions, and the resulting mechanical consequences. Such models usually require knowledge of numerous parameters and rate functions for the underlying reactions. Most of these parameters are not directly measurable, making the fitting of the model to a specific muscle or experimental situation difficult. Again, inputs can consist of neural excitation pulses or mechanical perturbations, while various outputs can be obtained from such a model, ranging from mechanical variables to thermodynamic information.

We next summarize briefly the relevant basic physiology of muscle. See McMahon (1984) for more details.

Muscle Architecture

A muscle is composed of many long, thin cells, or fibers, arranged parallel to each other. Most fibers terminate in microtendons, which merge to form a common tendon that connects to the skeleton. Because of this parallel organization, the total force a muscle can produce is proportional to the summed cross-sectional area of all the fibers. The fibers are, in turn, composed of several thousand parallel myofibrils. Each myofibril is composed of repeating microscopic units (2–3 μm in length) called sarcomeres, which are the basic contractile units of muscle. Since sarcomeres within a fiber are linked in series and contract together, many key muscle properties, such as the maximum speed at which a muscle can shorten, are proportional to the length of the fiber. For this reason, muscle contractile properties are often normalized by both the muscle cross-sectional area and the fiber length (Zajac, 1989).

Muscles come in an array of sizes and shapes, reflecting differences in fiber length, fiber number, and fiber orientation. There are also systematic differences in biochemistry and metabolic properties. See Alexander (1981) for a discussion of muscle and tendon architecture and Burke (1981) for a discussion of muscle fiber and motor unit specialization.

Input-Output (System) Models

At the simplest level, muscle may be treated as a linear system, usually of second order, with a single input and single output (SISO). In fact, since muscle has many simultaneous inputs—primarily neural activation, but also length, force, temperature, and so on—additional constraints on the system are required to apply linear systems approaches.

For example, Mannard and Stein (1973) modeled isometric cat soleus muscle as a linear system, with a neural pulse train input and a force output. Here, motor axons were excited by a random electrical pulse train, and the resulting force data were well fitted by a critically damped, linear, second-order system. Essentially, this muscle acted as a low pass filter, with a cutoff of 5 Hz. Difficulties with the linear systems approach became apparent when slight changes were made in the experiment. By changing the amplitude of the input (mean stimulus rate to the ventral roots), system gain changed by more than a factor of 4, and the cutoff frequency ranged from 8 to 2 Hz. Changing muscle length also changed the system parameters. Thus, the linear approximation assumed by this model holds true only for closely specified conditions.

There are several other nonlinearities in muscle that limit the usefulness of the linear systems approach. First, active muscle behaves quite differently when it is shortening than when it is lengthening—behavior that is inconsistent with linear system properties. For example, if active muscle is stretched rapidly, force may drop precipitously after an initial region of high stiffness, giving rise to muscle "yield." Second, muscle force shows marked hysteresis when measured during increasing neural activation compared with decreasing activation.

Because a SISO linear system model is at best an approximation, the model must be identified for the specific application for which it is used. Attempts to identify a more broadly applicable model by using nonlinear system techniques generally fail because muscle is quite nonstationary and the system changes before it can be fully characterized. Advances in nonlinear techniques may make this a viable approach. For now, the linear systems approach has the advantage of its well-developed theoretical background, which allows relatively simple system identification techniques to be implemented.

Lumped Parameter Models

The earliest experimentally based descriptions of muscle resulted in muscle models that were composed of viscoelastic elements. The most widely applicable of these models is that of A.V. Hill and can be described as follows: Muscle is composed operationally of three elements: (1) a contractile element (CE) that acts as an active force generator, (2) an elastic element (SE) that represents the combined stiffness of tendon and cross-bridges in series with the force generator, and (3) a second elasticity in parallel with the previous two elements (PE) that represents the passive tissue contributions to muscle force (Figure 1A).

Hill (1938) characterized the CE by applying a series of constant force inputs (i.e., an "isotonic load") to active muscle. Muscle responds to such an input by shortening with an initially constant velocity. Smaller loads result in larger velocities. Plotting a number of such force-velocity pairs demonstrates this trade-off (Figure 1B), which can be fitted well with a hyperbola of the form

$$V_{CE} = \frac{b(P_o - F)}{F + a}, \qquad F \le P_o \qquad (1)$$

where F is the applied isotonic force, V_{CE} is the resulting initial velocity of shortening, P_o is the maximum isometric (velocity equal to zero) force, and a and b are empirical constants. Equation 1 has been found to describe the steady-state force-velocity behavior of a wide variety of skeletal muscles during shortening. The constitutive relation for the CE embodies this hyperbolic force-velocity trade-off.

The series elasticity is usually modeled as a purely linear spring of stiffness k, and the passive elasticity often takes the form of an exponential function that increases with extension. The total muscle length is the sum of the lengths of the CE and SE. The contribution of the PE depends on the precise muscle geometry but is often important only at long muscle lengths and is thus frequently neglected in practice. When passive tension is neglected, a single, first-order, ordinary differential equation expresses the dynamics of this model with force, F, as an output:

$$\frac{dF}{dt} = k_{SE}(V_M - V_{CE}) \qquad (2)$$

where V_M is the velocity of the end of the whole muscle, V_{CE} is the contractile element velocity from Equation 1, and k_{SE} is the series elastic stiffness. The V_{CE} property described by Equation 1 applies only to shortening muscle and only when the muscle is operating in a length range at which isometric force does not vary. Modifications to this standard model extend its applicability to situations in which large length excursions occur. For example, length dependence (Figure 1C) can be incorporated into the force-velocity relation (Equation 1) by changing P_o to reflect the isometric force available at the current muscle length and scaling the parameters a and b by this factor as well. A length-dependent nonlinear SE stiffness can also be included.

In contrast, it is necessary to define an entirely new force-velocity relation to describe behavior during lengthening contraction, that is, when the muscle is forced to lengthen by an external load that exceeds its active force-generating capacity. One such relation (Mashima et al., 1972) is given by

$$V_{EC} = \frac{b'(P_o - F)}{2P_o - F + a'}, \qquad F > P_o \qquad (3)$$

where a' and b' are empirical constants. Such an extended model has been shown to perform well for complex motions involving both eccentric and concentric contractions at full activation (Krylow and Sandercock, 1997).

Cross-Bridge Models

The main components of the sarcomere are two sets of interdigitating protein filaments called thin filaments (made up partly of actin) and thick filaments (made up largely of myosin) (Squire, 1981). When suitably activated by calcium ions and in the presence of adenosine triphosphate (ATP), large populations of molecular projections (cross-bridges) on the thick filaments interact with receptor sites on the actin to produce force and relative motion between the two sets of filaments. Each cross-bridge is believed to act independently, interacting cyclically with successive actin sites to produce a ratchet-like action. The forces thus produced between the two filaments are in a direction to cause each sarcomere to shorten. The actin and myosin filaments are approximately inextensible, and sarcomere shortening occurs because of the relative sliding of the filaments past each other (sliding filament theory).

Muscle force exhibits a pronounced length dependence that can be explained by the sliding filament theory. As muscle length changes, the relative overlap of the actin and myosin filaments in each sarcomere changes because of telescoping of the sarcomere structure, and this overlap determines the maximum number of available cross-bridges at any given muscle length. Figure 1C shows the idealized length-tension curve measured during steady-state isometric contraction when the muscle is fully active.

In contrast to lumped parameter models, which try to reproduce macroscopic behavior with discrete mechanical elements, cross-bridge models strive to incorporate the known microstructure of the sarcomere together with biochemical kinetics of muscle protein to predict macroscopic variables such as whole muscle force, stiffness, shortening velocity, energy consumption, heat liberation, and

Figure 1. Schematic representations of (*A*) Hill model structure, (*B*) the force-velocity relation for both concentric and eccentric regions, and (*C*) isometric force-length relation and the corresponding sarcomere geometry responsible for this effect.

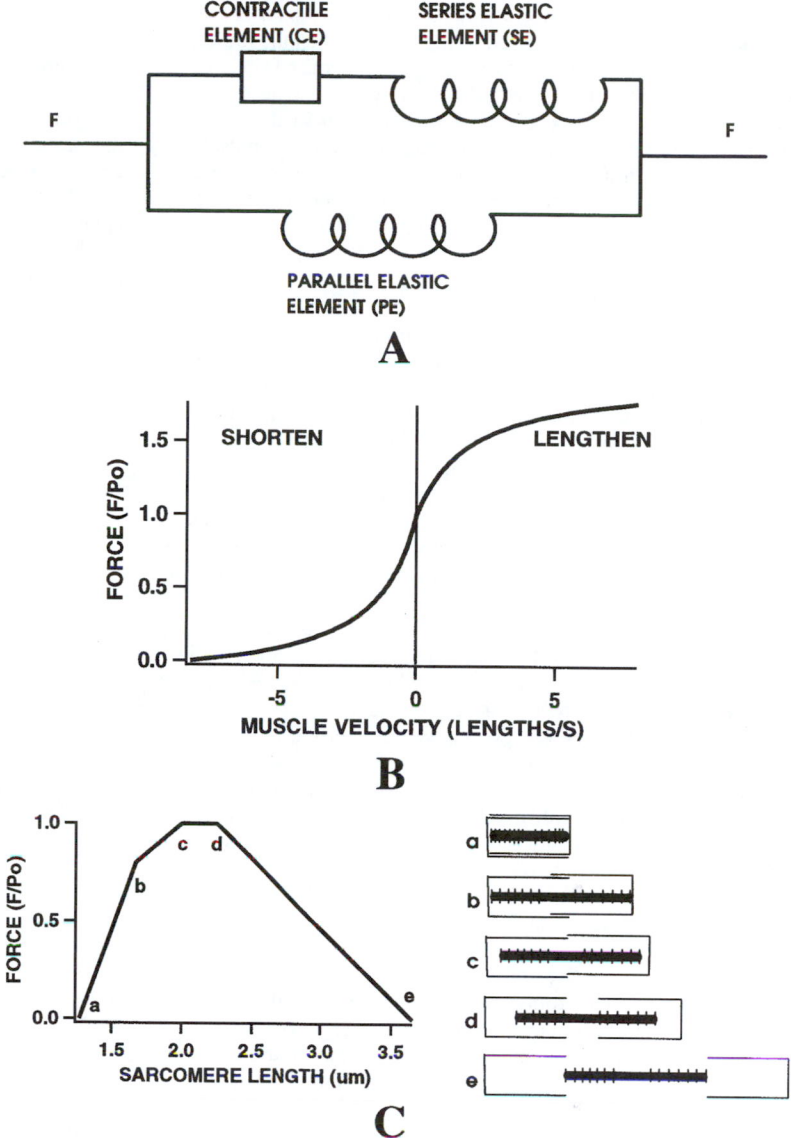

so on. The prototypical scheme for this type of model (Huxley, 1957) idealizes the interaction of actin and myosin as consisting of two possible cross-bridge states—either bound or unbound—and derives equations that describe the evolution of the distribution of bond lengths for the population of bound cross-bridges. The cross-bridges are assumed to act independently as linear springs, producing force in proportion to their extension, when bound to actin. It is necessary to define simplified chemical reactions that describe the transitions between the states and the form of the rate functions that determine the extent and directions of these reactions. Since the chosen rate functions depend explicitly on the cross-bridge length, the reactions are coupled directly to mechanical events of the cross-bridge cycle as well as to external perturbations imposed on the muscle by loading conditions. See McMahon (1984) and Zahalak (1981, 1992) for more details.

Tendon Properties

An idealized structure is often assumed for the tendon, in which muscle is connected to a linear series elastic element with high stiffness. In fact, the tendon is far from being simply an inextensible link, and its mechanics modify muscle output significantly. For example, under some conditions, the muscle fibers can shorten while the complete muscle-tendon structure lengthens. The tendon can be used to store energy, as was demonstrated in the Achilles tendon of the wallaby (Alexander, 1981), where its energy storage plays an integral role in efficient jumping locomotion. Although tendon is often simply modeled as an ideal spring, the mechanical properties of tendon are more complex. Its force-length curve depicts an initial compliant region, followed by a reduced compliance, and is often described as exponential, exponential-linear, or a quadratic function of length. When a tendon is stretched and released, the measured force shows a pronounced hysteresis that is a complex function of its history. Nonlinear tendons have been incorporated as the series elastic elements in Hill-type models, providing some improvement in model accuracy.

The cross-bridges that generate force in a muscle are themselves often modeled as ideal springs. They can be lumped together and modeled as an elasticity in series with the tendon to define a global muscle stiffness. For example, in cat soleus muscle, which is considered to have a short, stiff tendon, half of its compliance (the reciprocal of stiffness) is attributed to the tendon when the muscle is fully activated. In muscles with longer tendons, the compliance of the tendon even predominates at high activation. At lesser activation levels, fewer attached cross-bridges result in the sarcomeres becoming the primary source of compliance in the muscle. Experiments show muscle stiffness increases approximately linearly with activation. This important mechanical property of muscle is often incorrectly represented in lumped parameter models.

Models of Activation

Muscle receives neural input in the form of discrete action potentials. Through a complex sequence of events, each action potential results in a release of calcium from stores in the sarcoplasmic reticulum. This calcium binds to regulatory proteins and allows cross-bridge cycling to proceed. The calcium is quickly sequestered, deactivating the actin-binding sites and allowing the muscle to relax. The frequency of action potential arrival at the muscle determines the degree of muscle activation. At low frequencies, muscle responds with discrete force transients (twitches). At high frequencies, isometric force fuses into a smooth contraction (tetanus) that rises to maximal levels (Figure 2).

The muscle models presented earlier need to be coupled with a model of activation to be fully comprehensive. These models fall into two basic categories: (1) models based on an estimated mean level of neural excitation to the muscle and (2) models that translate a sequence of discrete action potentials into muscle activation. When simulating voluntary movement, models based on estimated mean excitation are preferable because the true excitation is never known, and little is accomplished by trying to estimate the action potential sequence to all motor units in the muscle. However, when muscle is stimulated by a known action potential train, modeling of the discrete action potentials is necessary to reproduce the ripple occurring in an unfused tetanus.

The most widely used activation model uses the rectified and filtered electromyogram (REMG) to estimate the input to a muscle (Deluca, 1979). The electromyogram signal is recorded by using either surface or intramuscular electrodes and results from the complex summation of electric fields produced by each muscle fiber action potential. The REMG provides a measure of the total number

of action potentials to the muscle. It often has a linear or exponential relationship to isometric force, and the output of this relationship can serve as the input to a Hill-type or cross-bridge model. Unfortunately, the relationship between the REMG and force varies in different muscles, for different recording electrodes, or even with the placement of the electrodes. Furthermore, because of its stochastic properties, an ensemble average of the REMG is needed for rapidly changing levels of excitation. At best, REMG is a crude approximation of neural drive.

The second approach to modeling activation is to approximate the physiological events after the arrival of an action potential at the muscle. Unfortunately, the complexity of the events precludes an accurate and simple model. In addition, activation is strongly influenced by muscle length. Well-documented activation-related phenomena can more than double or halve the force measured from a muscle stimulated by identical pulse trains. See Burke (1981) for discussions of potentiation, doublets, sag, and fatigue.

A simple model to transform a time sequence of action potentials into activation for a Hill-type model is described by

$$x(t) = \sum_n \delta(t - t_n)$$
$$\dot{r}(t) = -C_1 r(t) + C_2 x(t)$$
$$\dot{y}(t) = \begin{cases} -C_3 y(t) + r(t), & y(t) \le 1 \\ -C_3(t), & y(t) > 1 \end{cases} \qquad (4)$$

where $x(t)$ is the input, $\delta(t)$ are unit impulses representing action potentials at times t_n, and C_1, C_2, and C_3 are constants. Activation, $y(t)$, is used to scale the force-velocity relationship: P_o, a, b, a', and b' in Equations 1 and 3 are multiplied by $y(t)$. The results of the model applied to cat soleus (Figure 2) show good agreement with the experimental data measured during isometric conditions. However, the model shows substantial errors (up to 50% of maximal muscle force) with low firing rates and high velocity length changes. The largest errors can be attributed to the separation of activation and contractile properties inherent in a Hill-type model (Sandercock and Heckman, 1997). More sophisticated activation models coupled with a cross-bridge model (Zahalak, 1992) address this problem but have not yet been shown to reduce the overall error for widely varying muscle conditions.

Furthermore, during natural contraction of a muscle, slow-fatigue-resistant motor units are active at low forces, and fast-fatigable motor units are recruited only for stronger contractions (Burke, 1981). Because the mechanical properties of these motor units are strikingly different, the overall mechanical properties of a muscle probably change substantially with activation. A muscle model might address this by changing the muscle parameters with increasing activation or by treating the fast and slow motor unit populations separately and combining the results. This problem has received little attention, yet is likely to be a significant source of error in existing models.

Discussion

As we outlined in the Introduction, the choice of a particular type of model is determined by the intended use of the resulting information. Linear system-type muscle models can provide intuitive insights in the frequency domain that are not easily obtained from the other methods, but muscle's inherent nonlinearities make such models locally applicable at best. Cross-bridge-type models are essentially the only choice to study molecular mechanisms. To study whole muscle or multiple muscle systems, both cross-bridge and Hill-type models offer possibilities, although Hill-type models are much more accessible. Cross-bridge models are capable of a wider range of behaviors, but they pay the price by needing more parameters. Because of the difficulty in estimating these parameters, cross-bridge models are rarely used to study control of mul-

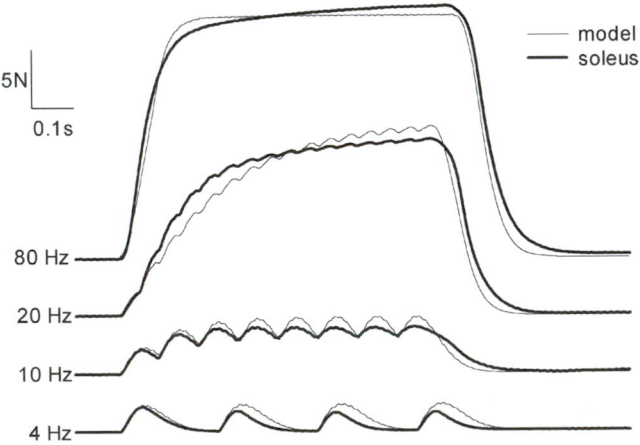

Figure 2. Cat soleus force responses for increasing rates of synchronous stimulation. At low stimulus rates, force pulses are responses to individual stimulus pulses. Force pulses fuse to produce smooth traces as the rate approaches 40 Hz. Simple Hill model predictions using the activation scheme given by Equation 4 show similar behavior.

timuscle movement. Hill-type models are by far the most widely used for this application.

A Hill model that is extended to include eccentric contraction and large muscle length changes does a fair job predicting muscle behavior and is the most practical solution for many requirements but has at least two major weaknesses. First, the extensions to Hill-type models for lengthening contractions fit well only under limited conditions and cannot predict muscle "yield." Second, when activation is coupled with the Hill model, the model has no mechanism to handle varying cross-bridge persistence observed with different movement histories. Systematic methods to identify the parameters in a simplified cross-bridge-type model could make it the method of choice.

It is not known how accurate a muscle model must be to effectively study control of movement. Since muscle is a nonstationary system, with crucial time- and history-dependent properties, it is difficult, even under carefully controlled laboratory conditions, to get the identical response to the same input. Perhaps neural control systems make such differences unimportant. Conversely, Lehman (1990) has shown that predicted neural control signals are very sensitive to the muscle model structure. Here, activations necessary to reproduce experimental wrist motions were calculated by using three different muscle models: a linear viscoelastic model, a Hill model with constant SE stiffness, and a Hill model with activation-dependent stiffness. The most complex muscle model predicted control signals that most closely resembled the actual EMG signals. Other nonlinear properties of muscle, the very ones that make modeling difficult, may be advantageous for function and thus may be required to help us understand the control of movement.

In Memoriam: The authors gratefully acknowledge the major contributions of Andrew Krylow and wish to dedicate this chapter in his memory.

Road Map: Mammalian Motor Control
Related Reading: Motoneuron Recruitment; Prosthetics, Motor Control

References

Alexander, R. M., 1981, Mechanics of skeleton and tendons, in *Handbook of Physiology, Section L: The Nervous System*, vol. 2, *Motor Control, Part I* (V. B. Brooks, Ed.), Bethesda, MD: American Physiological Society, pp. 17–42.

Burke, R. E., 1981, Motor units: Anatomy, physiology, and functional organization, in *Handbook of Physiology, Section 1: The Nervous System*, vol. 2, *Motor Control, Part I* (V. B. Brooks, Ed.), Bethesda, MD: American Physiological Society, pp. 345–422. ◆

Deluca, C. J., 1979, Physiology and mathematics of myoelectric signals, *IEEE Trans. Biorned. Eng.*, BME-26:313–326.

Hill, A. V., 1938, The heat of shortening and the dynamic constants of muscle, *Philos. Trans. R. Soc. Lond. B Biol. Sci.*, 126:136–195.

Huxley, A. F., 1957, Muscle structure and theories of contraction, *Prog. Biophys.*, 7:255–318.

Krylow, A. M., and Sandercock, T. G., 1997, Test of a modified Hill model in reproducing force responses involving eccentric contraction, *J. Biomech.*, 30, 27–33.

Lehman, S. L., 1990, Input identification depends on model complexity, in *Multiple Muscle Systems: Biomechanics and Movement Organization* (J. M. Winters and S. L.-Y. Woo, Eds.), New York: Springer-Verlag, pp. 94–100.

Mannard, A., and Stein, R. B., 1973, Determination of the frequency response of isometric soleus muscle in the cat using random nerve stimulation, *J. Physiol.*, 229:275–296.

Mashima, H., Akazawa, K., Kushima, H., and Fujii, K., 1972, The force-load-velocity relation and the viscous-like force in the frog skeletal muscle, *Jpn. J. Physiol.*, 22:103–120.

McMahon, T. A., 1984, *Muscles, Reflexes, and Locomotion*, Princeton, NJ: Princeton University Press.

Sandercock, T. G., and Heckman, C. J., 1997, Force from cat soleus muscle during locomotor-like movements: Experimental data versus Hill-type model predictions, *J. Neurophysiol.*, 77, 1538–1552. ◆

Squire, J., 1981, *The Structural Basis of Muscular Contraction*, New York: Plenum.

Zahalak, G. I., 1981, A distribution-moment approximation for kinetic theories of muscular contraction, *Math. Biosci.*, 55:89–114.

Zahalak, G. I., 1992, An overview of muscle modeling, in *Neural Prostheses: Replacing Motor Function After Disease or Disability* (R. B. Stein, P. Hunter Peckham, and D. B. Popovic, Eds.), New York: Oxford University Press, pp. 17–57. ◆

Zajac, F. E., 1989, Muscle and tendon: Properties: Models, scaling, and application to bio-mechanics and motor control, *CRC Crit. Rev. Biomed. Eng.*, 112:52–62.

Neocognitron: A Model for Visual Pattern Recognition

Kunihiko Fukushima

Introduction

The *neocognitron* (Fukushima, 1980, 1988b, 1991) is a neural network model for deformation-resistant visual pattern recognition.

In primary visual cortex, neurons respond selectively to local features of a visual pattern, such as lines or edges in particular orientations. In the inferotemporal cortex, cells exist that respond selectively to certain figures such as circles, triangles, or squares, or even human faces. Thus, the visual system seems to have a hierarchical architecture in which simple features are first extracted from a stimulus pattern, then integrated into more complicated ones. In this hierarchy, a cell in a higher stage generally has a larger receptive field and is more insensitive to the position of the stimulus. This kind of physiological evidence suggested the network architecture for the neocognitron.

The neocognitron is a hierarchical network consisting of many layers of neuron-like cells. There are forward connections between cells in adjoining layers. Some of these connections are variable and can be modified by learning. The neocognitron can acquire the ability to recognize patterns by learning. Since it has a large power of generalization, presentation of only a few typical examples of deformed patterns (or features) is enough for the learning process to be successful. It is not necessary to present all of the deformed versions of the patterns that might appear in the future. After learning, the neocognitron can recognize input patterns robustly, with little effect from deformation, changes in size, or shifts in position. It is even able to correctly recognize a pattern that has not been presented before, provided the pattern resembles one of the training patterns.

The principle of the neocognitron can be used in various kinds of pattern recognition systems, such as systems recognizing handwritten characters (Fukushima, 1988b, 2002; Fukushima and Wake, 1991).

The Network Architecture

The neocognitron has a multilayered architecture, as shown in Figure 1, in which each rectangle represents a two-dimensional array of cells. Each cell receives its input connections from only a limited number of cells situated in a small area on the preceding layer. The density of cells in each layer is designed to decrease with the order of the stage.

The lowest stage of the hierarchical network is an input layer U_0, consisting of a two-dimensional array of receptor cells. Each succeeding stage has a layer U_S consisting of "S-cells," followed by another layer U_C consisting of "C-cells." Thus, in the whole network, layers of S-cells and C-cells are arranged alternately.

Each layer of S-cells or C-cells is divided into subgroups, called "cell-planes," according to the features to which they respond. The cells in each cell-plane are arranged in a two-dimensional array. Each rectangle drawn with heavy lines in Figure 1 represents a cell-plane. The connections converging to the cells in a cell-plane are homogeneous and topographically ordered. In other words, the connections have a translational symmetry such that each of the cells of a cell-plane shares the same set of input connections. This condition of translational symmetry holds for both fixed and variable connections. The modification of variable connections is always done under this condition.

S-cells are feature-extracting cells. They resemble simple cells in the visual cortex in their response. Connections converging to these cells may be modified by learning. After learning, S-cells are able to extract features from input patterns. In other words, an S-cell is activated only when a particular feature is presented in its receptive field. The features extracted by the S-cells are determined during the learning process. Generally speaking, local features, such as lines in particular orientations, are extracted in the lower stages. More "global" features, such as parts of a training pattern, are extracted in higher stages.

C-cells, which resemble complex cells in the visual cortex, are inserted in the network to allow for positional errors in the features of the stimulus. The connections from S-cells to C-cells are fixed and invariable. Each C-cell receives signals from a group of S-cells that extract the same feature, but from slightly different positions (Figure 2). The C-cell is activated if at least one of these S-cells is active. Even if the stimulus feature is shifted in position and another S-cell is activated instead of the first one, the same C-cell keeps responding. Hence, the C-cell's response is less sensitive to shifts in the position of the input pattern.

The layer of C-cells at the highest stage is the recognition layer: the response of the cells in this layer is the final result of pattern recognition by the neocognitron.

Principles of Deformation-Resistant Recognition

In the whole network, with its alternate layers of S-cells and C-cells, the process of feature extraction by the S-cells and toleration of positional shift by the C-cells is repeated. During this process, local features extracted in lower stages are gradually integrated into more global features. Finally, each C-cell of the recognition layer at the highest stage integrates all the information of the input pattern and responds only to one specific pattern. Figure 2 illustrates this situation schematically.

Tolerating positional error a little at a time at each stage, rather than all in one step, plays an important role in endowing the network with the ability to recognize even distorted patterns. Figure 3 illustrates this situation. Let an S-cell in an intermediate stage of the network have already been trained to extract a global feature consisting of three local features of a training pattern "A," as shown in Figure 3A. The cell tolerates a positional error of each local feature if the deviation falls within the dotted circle. Hence, the S-cell responds to any of the deformed patterns shown in Figure 3B. The toleration of positional errors should not be too large at this stage. If large errors are tolerated at any one step, the network may come to respond erroneously, such as by recognizing a stimulus like Figure 3C as an "A" pattern.

Since errors in the relative position of local features are thus tolerated in the process of extracting and integrating features, the same C-cell responds in the recognition layer at the highest stage, even if the input pattern is deformed, changed in size, or shifted in position.

Self-Organization of the Neocognitron

The neocognitron can be trained to recognize patterns through either unsupervised or supervised learning. Various training methods have been proposed, and this section introduces two of them.

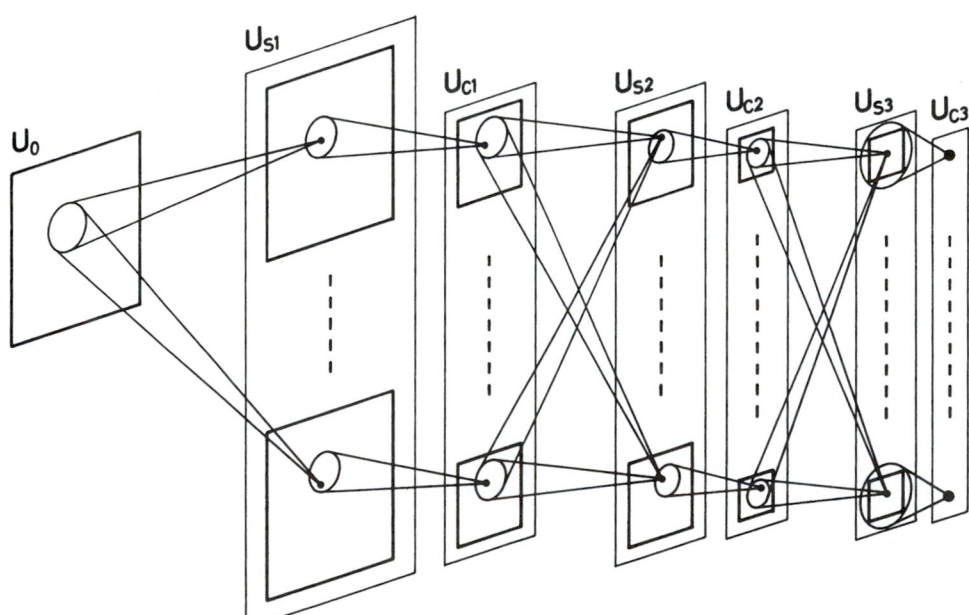

Figure 1. The network architecture of the neocognitron. Each rectangle drawn with heavy lines represents a "cell-plane." The cells in each cell-plane are arranged in a two-dimensional array.

Figure 2. Illustration of the process of pattern recognition in the neocognitron (Fukushima, 1980). As shown in the upper half of the figure, local features extracted in lower stages are gradually integrated into more "global" features. The lower half of the figure is an enlarged illustration of a part of the network. The cell-plane with $k = 1$ in layer U_{S1} consists of S-cells that extract ∧-shaped features. Since the stimulus pattern "A" contains the ∧-shaped feature at the top, an S-cell near the top of this cell-plane is active. A C-cell in the succeeding cell-plane ($k = 1$) in U_{C1} has excitatory input connections from S-cells situated in the circle and is activated if one of these S-cells is active. Only one cell-plane is shown in U_{S2} in this enlarged illustration. Each S-cell in this cell-plane detects the existence of features $k = 1, 2, 3$ in U_{C1}, and at the same time the absence of features $k = 4, 5$.

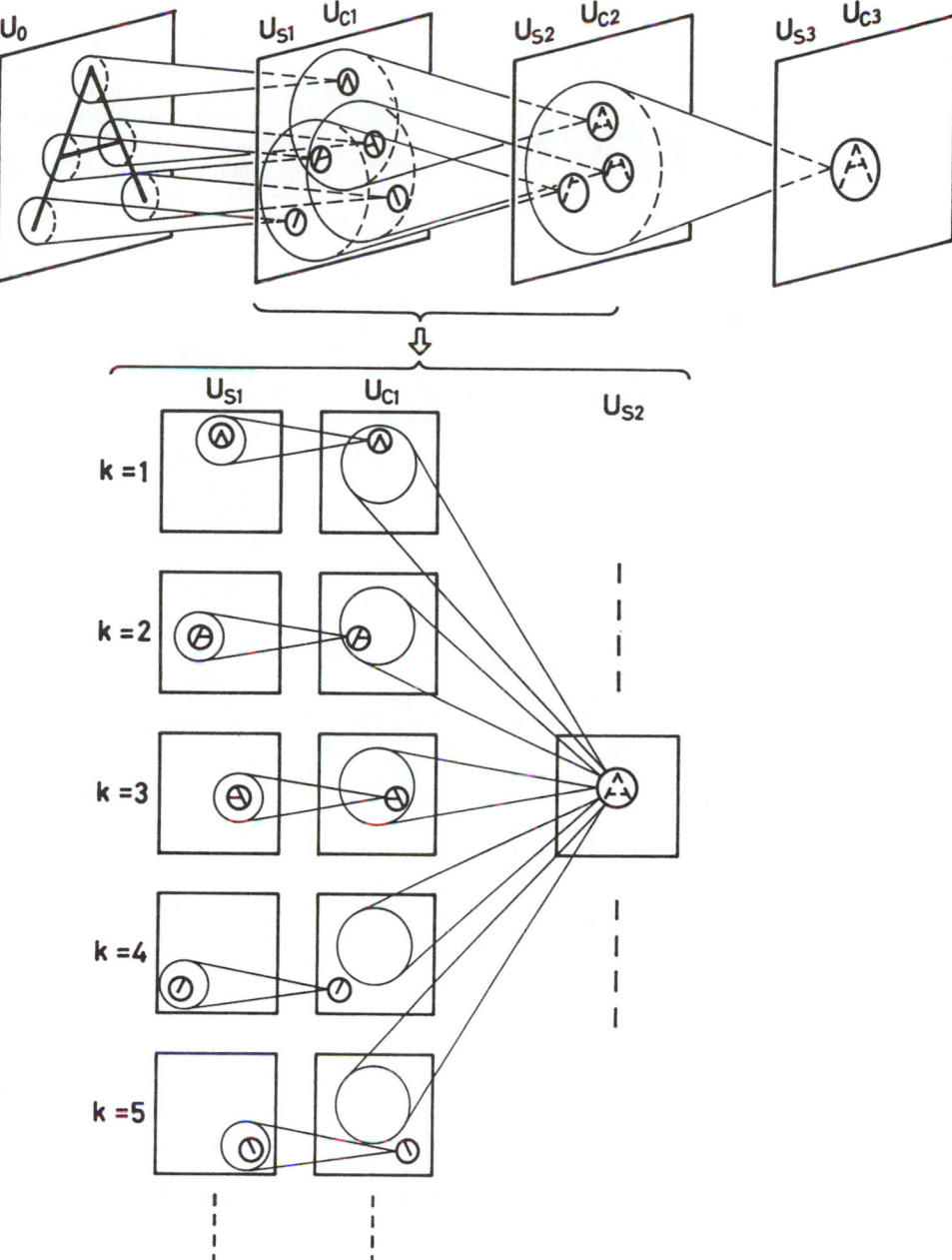

In the case of unsupervised learning, the self-organization of the network is performed using two principles. The first principle is a kind of "winner-take-all" rule (see WINNER-TAKE-ALL NET-WORKS): among the cells situated in a certain small area, only the one responding most strongly has its input connections reinforced. The change of each input connection to this maximum-output cell is proportional to the intensity of the response of the cell from which the relevant connection leads.

Figure 4 illustrates this process, showing only the connections converging to an S-cell. The S-cell receives variable excitatory connections from a group of C-cells of the preceding stage. The cell also receives a variable inhibitory connection from an inhibitory cell, called a V-cell. The V-cell receives fixed excitatory connections from the same group of C-cells as does the S-cell, and always responds with the average intensity of the output of the C-cells.

The initial strength of the variable connections is very weak and nearly zero (Figure 4A). Suppose the S-cell responds most strongly of the S-cells in its vicinity when a training stimulus is presented (Figure 4B). According to the winner-take-all rule just described, variable connections leading from activated C- and V-cells are reinforced, as shown in Figure 4C. The variable excitatory connections to the S-cell grow into a "template" that exactly matches the spatial distribution of the response of the cells in the preceding layer. The inhibitory variable connection from the V-cell is also increased at the same time, but not strongly, because the output of the V-cell is not as large.

After the learning, the S-cell acquires the ability to extract a feature of the stimulus presented during the learning period. Through the excitatory connections, the S-cell receives signals indicating the existence of the relevant feature to be extracted. If an

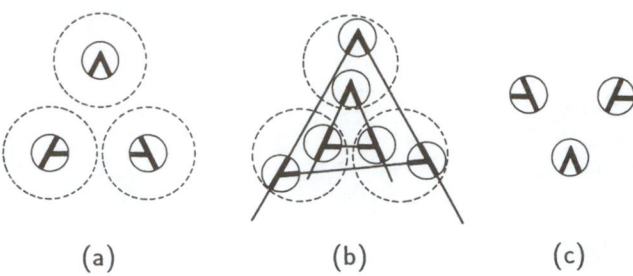

Figure 3. Illustration of the principle for recognizing deformed patterns (Fukushima, 1988a). An S-cell, which has already been trained to extract a global feature consisting of three local features as shown in part *a*, tolerates a positional error of each local feature if the deviation falls within the dotted circle. Hence, the S-cell responds to any of the deformed patterns shown in part *b*. The toleration of positional errors should not be too large at this stage. If large errors are tolerated at any one step, the network may come to respond erroneously, such as by recognizing a stimulus like the one in part *c* as an "A" pattern.

irrelevant feature is presented, the inhibitory signal from the V-cell becomes stronger than the direct excitatory signals from the C-cells, and the response of the S-cell is suppressed (Fukushima, 1989).

Once an S-cell is thus selected and reinforced to respond to a feature, the cell usually loses its responsiveness to other features. When a different feature is presented, a different cell usually yields the maximum output and has its input connections reinforced. Thus, a "division of labor" among the cells occurs automatically.

The second principle for learning is introduced in order that the connections being modified always preserve translational symmetry. The maximum-output cell not only grows by itself, it also controls the growth of neighboring cells, working, so to speak, like a seed in crystal growth. To be more specific, all of the other S-cells in the cell-plane, from which the "seed cell" is selected, follow the seed cell, and have their input connections reinforced by having the same spatial distribution as that of the seed cell.

Although the neocognitron can thus be trained by unsupervised learning, supervised learning is still useful when we want to train a system to recognize, for instance, handwritten characters, which should be classified not only on the basis of similarity in shape but also on the basis of certain conventions. In the case of supervised learning, the "teacher" presents training patterns to the network and points out the positions of the features that should be extracted.

The cells whose receptive field centers coincide with the positions of the features take the place of the "maximum-output cells" and become seed cells. The other process of reinforcement is identical to that of the unsupervised learning and occurs automatically.

It is another advantage of the neocognitron that these learning methods, both supervised and unsupervised, require extremely short training times compared with other learning algorithms such as backpropagation. In an extreme case of unsupervised learning, for example, three presentations of a training set consisting of one training pattern from each category was sufficient to train the network to recognize 10 numeric characters robustly (Fukushima and Wake, 1992).

The optimal scale of the neocognitron changes depending on the set of patterns to be recognized. If the complexity of the patterns is high, the total number of stages in the hierarchical network needs to be large. Conversely, the necessary number of cell-planes in each stage of the network increases with the number of categories of patterns to be recognized. However, the increase in scale is not proportional. For example, if we compare a system recognizing 35 alphanumeric characters with a system recognizing 10 numerals, the number of characters to be recognized increases 3.5 times, but the number of cells increases only 1.9 times (Fukushima and Wake, 1991). This results from the fact that the local features extracted in the lower stages are common, and they usually are contained in many patterns of different categories. Although the number of cells is large in these systems, the number of parameters required to describe the network is quite small, because all of the cells in each cell-plane share the same set of input connections.

Selective Attention Model (SAM)

Although the neocognitron has considerable ability to recognize deformed patterns, it does not always recognize patterns correctly when two or more patterns are presented simultaneously. The *selective attention model* (SAM) has been proposed to eliminate these defects (Fukushima, 1986, 1987, 1988a). In the SAM, backward (i.e., top-down) connections were added to the conventional neocognitron-type network, which had only forward (i.e., bottom-up) connections.

When a composite stimulus consisting of two patterns or more is presented, the SAM focuses its attention selectively on one of the patterns, segments it from the rest, and recognizes it. After the identification of the first segment, the SAM switches its attention to recognize another pattern. The SAM also has the function of associative recall. Even if noise or defects affect the stimulus pattern, the SAM can recognize it and recall the complete pattern from

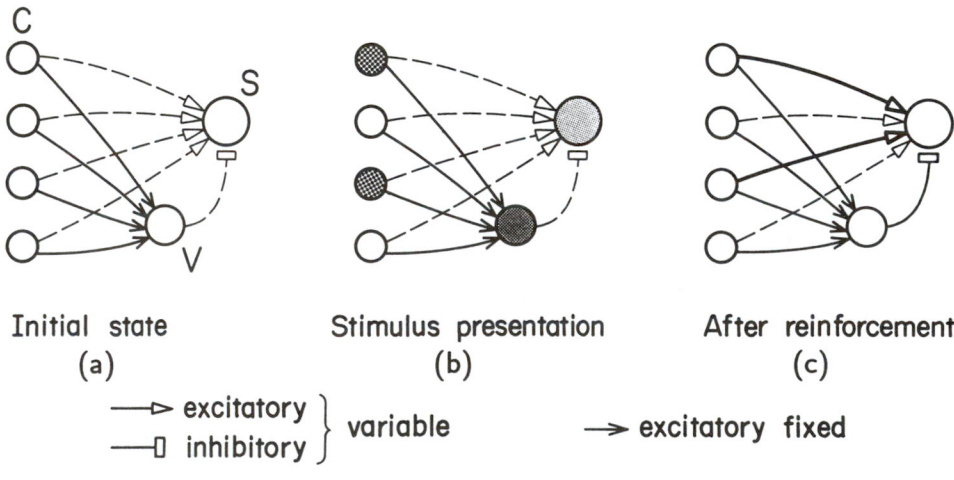

Initial state
(a)

Stimulus presentation
(b)

After reinforcement
(c)

⟶▷ excitatory ⎫
⟶▢ inhibitory ⎬ variable
⟶ excitatory fixed

Figure 4. The process of reinforcement of the forward connections converging to a feature-extracting S-cell (Fukushima, 1988a). The density of the shadow in the circle represents the intensity of the response of the cell. *a*, The initial state before training. *b*, Stimulus presentation during the training. *c*, The connections after reinforcement.

which the noise has been eliminated and defects corrected. These functions can be successfully performed even for deformed versions of training patterns that have not been presented during learning.

The SAM has some similarity to the ADAPTIVE RESONANCE THEORY model (q.v.; see also Carpenter and Grossberg, 1987), but the most important difference between the two is the fact that the SAM has the ability to accept patterns deformed in shape and shifted in position, while the adaptive resonance theory does not, in principle, have such functions. With the SAM, not only the recognition of the patterns but also the filling-in process for defective parts of imperfect input patterns work on the deformed and shifted patterns themselves. The SAM can repair the deformed pattern without changing the basic shape and location of the deformed input pattern. The deformed patterns themselves can be repaired at their original locations, thus preserving their deformation.

The principles of the SAM can be extended to be used for several applications: for example, the recognition and segmentation of connected characters in cursive handwriting of English words (Fukushima and Imagawa, 1993), and the recognition of Chinese characters (Fukushima, Imagawa, and Ashida, 1991).

[Reprinted from the First Edition]

Road Maps: Learning in Artificial Networks; Vision
Background: Dynamics and Bifurcation in Neural Nets
Related Reading: Convolutional Networks for Images, Speech, and Time Series; Object Recognition; Visual Scene Perception

References

Carpenter, G. A., and Grossberg, S., 1987, ART 2: Self-organization of stable category recognition codes for analog input patterns, *Appl. Opt.*, 26:4919–4930.

Fukushima, K., 1980, Neocognitron: A self-organizing neural network model for a mechanism of pattern recognition unaffected by shift in position, *Biol. Cybern.*, 36:193–202.

Fukushima, K., 1986, A neural network model for selective attention in visual pattern recognition, *Biol. Cybern.*, 55:5–15.

Fukushima, K., 1987, A neural network model for selective attention in visual pattern recognition and associative recall, *Appl. Opt.*, 26:4985–4992.

Fukushima, K., 1988a, A neural network for visual pattern recognition, *IEEE Computer*, 21(3):65–75. ◆

Fukushima, K., 1988b, Neocognitron: A hierarchical neural network capable of visual pattern recognition, *Neural Netw.*, 1:119–130.

Fukushima, K., 1989, Analysis of the process of visual pattern recognition by the neocognitron, *Neural Netw.*, 2:413–420.

Fukushima, K., 1991, Neural networks for visual pattern recognition, *IEICE Trans.*, E74:179–190. ◆

Fukushima, K., 2002, Neocognitron for handwritten digit recognition, *Neurocomputing*, in press.

Fukushima, K., and Imagawa, T., 1993, Recognition and segmentation of connected characters with selective attention, *Neural Netw.*, 6:33–41.

Fukushima, K., Imagawa, T., and Ashida, E., 1991, Character recognition with selective attention, in *Proceedings of the International Joint Conference on Neural Networks, 1991*, vol. 1, New York: IEEE, pp. 593–598.

Fukushima, K., and Wake, N., 1991, Handwritten alphanumeric character recognition by the neocognitron, *IEEE Trans. Neural Netw.*, 2:355–365.

Fukushima, K., and Wake, N., 1992, Improved neocognitron with bend-detecting cells, in *Proceedings of the International Joint Conference on Neural Networks, 1992*, vol. 4, New York: IEEE, pp. 190–195.

Neocortex: Basic Neuron Types

Maria Toledo-Rodriguez, Anirudh Gupta, Yun Wang, Cai Zhi Wu, and Henry Markram

Introduction

The neocortex is functionally parcellated into vertical columns (~0.5 mm in diameter) traversing all layers (layers I–VI). These columns have no obvious anatomical boundaries, and the topographic mapping of afferent and efferent pathways probably determines their locations and dimensions as well as their functions (Peters and Jones, 1984; White, 1989). Multiple columns overlap, suggesting that the underlying neural microcircuits are designed to enable universal computation. These apparently omnipotent and stereotypical microcircuits are composed of a daunting variety of precisely and intricately interconnected neurons (Douglas and Martin, 1998; Somogyi, 1998; White, 1989), that differ in terms of their anatomical, electrophysiological, and molecular properties (Cauli et al., 1997; DeFelipe, 1993; Gupta, Wang, and Markram, 2000; Kawaguchi and Kubota, 1997; Peters and Jones, 1984; Thomson and Deuchars, 1997). This neuronal diversification may provide a foundation for maximizing the computational abilities of the neocortex.

Basic Neuron Types—Anatomy

Excitatory Neurons

Excitatory neurons constitute by far the majority of neocortical cells (70–80%) and consist mainly of two types of neurons (Peters and Jones, 1984; Somogyi, 1989; White, 1989):

- *Pyramidal cells* (PC; Figure 1A1), the most commonly occurring neocortical neuron (located in layers II–VI), are characterized by a single, prominent, vertically oriented dendrite emerging from the apex of their mainly pyramidal-shaped somata (apical dendrite), several (~4–6) more or less horizontally radiating basal dendrites, and long descending axons that project to other cortical and subcortical areas. The apical dendrite traverses through several layers, allowing PCs to sample multiple layer-specific inputs, before fanning out into a terminal tuft (often reaching layer I). The basal dendrites mainly remain within the layer of the cell body (sometimes entering adjacent layers), spanning the full diameter of the cortical column. PC axons give rise to a local columnar cluster that may spill over into neighboring columns before continuing to the white matter. Additionally, long vertical and horizontal collaterals project across layers and columns, sometimes forming secondary axonal clusters. PCs are therefore "local circuit neurons" as well as "projection neurons."

- *Spiny stellate cells* (SSC; Figure 1A1), found almost exclusively in layer IV of the primary sensory areas, are characterized by multiple short dendrites (contained within a layer and column) radiating from spherical somata (stellate appearance). Their axons produce a local axonal cluster of columnar extent within layer IV, before projecting either loosely or in tight bundles to arborize extensively in layers II/III. Some collaterals descend toward layers V/VI. SSCs are mainly "local circuit neurons," al-

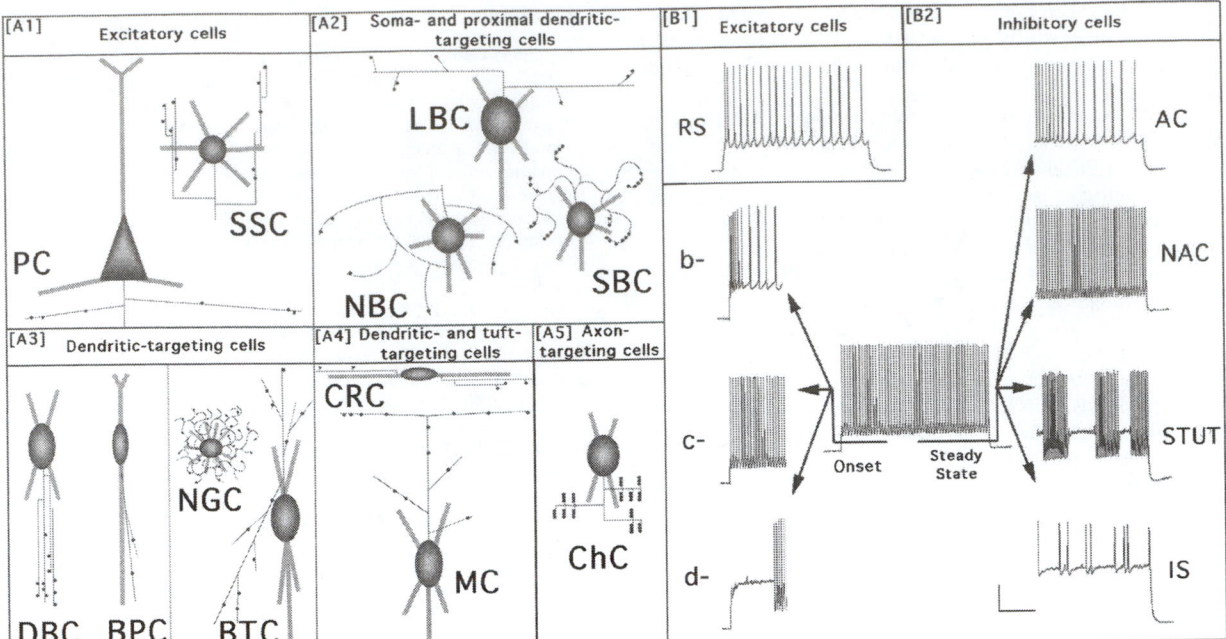

Figure 1. Anatomical and Electrophysiological Diversity of Neocortical Neurons. *A*, Schema, summarizing the main anatomical properties of neocortical excitatory (A1) and inhibitory (A2–5) neurons. Each neuron type is labeled by three-letter abbreviation (for explanation, see text). Dendrites: thick, light gray; axon: thin, black lines; black dots: axonal boutons. Spines omitted for clarity. Neurons oriented with pia facing upward and white matter (WM) downward. Note the presence of a prominent, vertical dendrite directed toward WM on some interneurons (A2–4). Inhibitory interneurons (A2–5) are mainly distinguished by the structure of their axonal arbor (see text) and typically innervate selective domains [A2: (peri-) so-matic; A3,4 dendritic; A5: axonal] of their target cells. *B*, Representative samples of the most common discharge responses of neocortical excitatory (B1) and inhibitory (B2) neurons to standardized intrasomatic step-current injections. B1: Excitatory cells typically display regular-spiking (RS) discharge behavior. B2: Inhibitory interneurons display a vast repertoire of discharge responses, displaying either bursts (b-), delays (d-), or neither burst/delay (classical, c-) at step-onset, and accommodation (AC), non-accommodation (NAC), stuttering (STUT), or irregular spiking (IS) at steady-state. Scale bar (20 mV; 500 ms) applies to all traces.

though in few cases they have been shown to project to other cortical areas (Douglas and Martin, 1998).

Whereas PCs and SSCs are easily distinguished by multiple morphological features, both types of excitatory neurons share several *functional* properties, that have been amply used to distinguish them from inhibitory neurons (White, 1989): (1) their dendrites are typically densely studded with small membranous protuberances known as spines (hence they are also known as spiny neurons; see DENDRITIC SPINES); (2) they release glutamate from their presynaptic terminals (boutons), which form asymmetric (excitatory) synapses mainly onto the spines of other excitatory neurons (see NEO-CORTEX: CHEMICAL AND ELECTRICAL SYNAPSES); (3) their somata invariably receive *only* symmetrical (inhibitory) synapses.

Inhibitory Neurons

Inhibitory neurons constitute 20–30% of the neocortical cells and are highly heterogeneous (Peters and Jones, 1984; Somogyi, 1989; White, 1989; Figure 1A2–5). They are easily distinguished from excitatory neurons by their lack of an apical dendrite, low spine densities (hence they are also known as smooth and/or sparsely spiny neurons), beaded dendrites, and axonal arbors that remain almost exclusively within a column (hence they are also known as local circuit neurons or interneurons; but see exceptions discussed later in this article). Instead of an apical dendrite projecting toward the pia, many interneurons have a prominent dendrite (with more branches) extending toward the white matter (WM). Moreover, the initial course of their axons, which either originate from the soma

or a primary dendrite, is often toward the pia (instead of toward the WM, which characterizes the axon trajectory of excitatory neurons). Inhibitory neurons release GABA at their symmetric synapses, and their cell bodies invariably receive *both* excitatory and inhibitory synapses. Most types of interneurons may display various soma shapes (ovoid, spindle-shaped, triangular, inverted pyramidal) and dendritic morphologies (bipolar, bitufted, and multipolar), but each type characteristically displays unique features in its axonal structure. Details of the axonal arborization (White, 1989), as well as the preferential placement of synapses onto different target-cell domains (Somogyi, 1989; Somogyi et al., 1998), have therefore provided the foundation for classifying interneurons. This selective innervation allows each type of interneuron to effect its target cells in a compartment-specific and potentially independent manner (see PERSPECTIVE ON NEURON MODEL COMPLEXITY).

Inhibitory neurons that selectively innervate:

- the (peri-) somatic region of their target cells, may affect the strength and gain of summated synaptic potentials (see SINGLE-CELL MODELS), the timing of action potential (AP)-generation and hence the concerted action of populations of target cells (see SYNCHRONIZATION, BINDING AND EXPECTANCY)
- the dendrites of their target cells, may influence dendritic processing and integration of synaptic inputs (see DENDRITIC PRO-CESSING), generation and propagation of dendritic APs, and synaptic plasticity (see HEBBIAN SYNAPTIC PLASTICITY)
- the axon initial segment of their target cells, may affect both the generation and the "gating" of APs (see AXONAL MODELING)

Most interneuron types, although mainly studied in layers II–V, are also found in layer VI, whereas layer I is characterized by its own distinct set of interneurons (see discussion later in this article). Moreover, it is currently not known whether additional subtypes, specific to layer VI, exist, although this lamina is characterized by a multitude of ill-defined local circuit neurons (~8–12 types) that still await precise description (Peters and Jones, 1984). The following describes the most common types of interneurons located in rat somatosensory cortex (layers II–V), based on a very large data set with considerable emphasis on quantitative morphometric analysis (see, for example, Wang et al., 2002). These basic interneuron types are found across different neocortical areas and species. Minor structural variations of these interneuron types (depending on neocortical layers, regions, age, and species) will not be considered here.

Interneurons that preferentially target somata and proximal dendrites. Basket cells (BCs), probably the most frequently encountered neocortical interneurons, are distinguished by their preferential innervation of somata (20–40%) and proximal dendrites (onto shafts and spines) (Kisvarday, 1992). BCs in general give rise to several beaded, mainly aspiny, dendrites. They are composed of three main subclasses, that differ in the structure of their axonal arborizations (Wang et al., 2002), each of which appears to be differentially distributed throughout layers II–VI.

- *Large basket cells* (LBC, Figure 1A2) produce a *sparse* local, mainly intralaminar and intracolumnar, axonal cluster composed of few, long and straight branches of low bouton density (BD) before generating their characteristic conspicuous long-range horizontal collaterals, that traverse multiple columns and some vertically projecting collaterals that may cross all layers (Somogyi, 1989). LBCs are therefore "local circuit" as well as inhibitory "projection" neurons.
- *Small basket cell* (SBC, Figure 1A2) give rise to a characteristic *dense* local, intralaminar and intracolumnar, axonal cluster composed of frequent, short, and curvy axonal branches with high BD. Occasionally SBCs may generate a few far-reaching collaterals projecting across layers and columns. A special subtype of SBC, termed *Clutch Cell*, has been observed in layer IV of the visual cortices of cat/monkey (Kisvarday, 1992). These cells are medium-sized, multipolar cells that typically produce large bulbous terminals, which often "clutch" somata of their target cells.
- *Nest basket cell* (NBC, Figure 1A2) give rise to a *sparse to dense* local, mainly intralaminar and intracolumnar, axonal cluster composed of infrequent, long, and smoothly bending axonal branches of low BD. They may occasionally produce a few far-reaching collaterals projecting across layers and columns. In addition, NBCs exhibit a characteristically simple dendritic arbor with few short and infrequently branching dendrites (Gupta et al., 2000; Wang et al., 2002).

Interneurons that preferentially target dendrites. Interneurons that preferentially target dendrites, usually give rise to beaded, aspiny, or sparsely spiny dendrites. Importantly, their overall "axonal fields" are preferentially vertically oriented (except NGCs, see the following discussion).

- *Bitufted cells* (BTC, Figure 1A3) display ovoid somata that emit two dendritic tufts from opposite poles that are preferentially vertically oriented and may emit an additional oblique dendrite (Somogyi, 1989). Their axonal arborizations are characterized by long, vertically oriented collaterals of low BD that may extend through all layers and mainly branch in a bifurcating manner. Their axonal ramification is mostly intracolumnar, although in some cases they may extend into neighboring columns.

- *Bipolar cells* (BPC, Figure 1A3) typically produce the simplest dendritic and axonal arborization of all interneurons, as both dendrites and axons branch very infrequently at shallow angles. The two long, vertically oriented, primary dendrites of BPCs are emitted from the opposite poles of their small spindle-shaped somata, and may span all cortical layers occasionally forming a dendritic tuft in layer I (Peters and Jones, 1984). The axon of BPCs typically emerges from a primary dendrite (usually the lower dendrite) before ramifying vertically across multiple or all layers. It is characterized by a very low number of boutons that are typically placed onto the dendritic shafts of rather restricted population of target neurons. Some BPCs in layers II–V have been shown to form asymmetrical synapses, preferentially onto spines, suggesting that they are excitatory (eBPCs, not shown; White, 1989).
- *Double bouquet cells* (DBC, Figure 1A3) are interneurons that like BPCs appear to consist of two classes. Inhibitory DBCs, that appear to be preferentially located in layers II/III, display bitufted or multipolar dendritic morphologies and typically produce a thin axon that bifurcates to give rise to a characteristic, mainly descending, "horsetail-like," tight fascicular axonal bundle. The collaterals forming these narrow columnar bundles of high BD are typically much thicker than the main stem, and may extend across all layers. A local axonal ramification of different densities may occasionally be formed. Some double bouquet cells in layers II–V that generate *both* ascending and descending axonal collateral bundles have been shown to form asymmetrical synapses onto target cells, suggesting that they are excitatory (eDBCs, not shown; White, 1989).
- *Neurogliaform cells* (NGC, Figure 1A3) are very small cells that produce dense, spherical dendritic, and axonal fields confined within a single layer and column (densest fields of all interneuron types). They typically produce a large number of thin, radiating dendrites that are short, aspiny, finely beaded, and rarely branched. Their very thin axons, branches intricately to produce a very dense and highly intertwined arborization (spiderweb-like appearance) that is studded with tiny boutons. NGCs target mainly dendritic shafts (Somogyi, 1989) and are also found in layer I.

Interneurons that preferentially target dendrites and dendritic tufts

- *Martinotti cells* (MC, Figure 1A4) display a more elaborate dendritic arbor than most interneurons, which is formed by beaded and sparsely- to medium-spiny dendrites. Their local and quite dense axonal cluster (mainly intralaminar and intracolumnar) is formed by collaterals that branch at wide angles before projecting up to layer I, where they spread across many columns, forming *spiny boutons*. MCs are "similar" to LBCs in that they are "local circuit" as well as inhibitory "projection" neurons. However, due to their innervation of distal dendrites and tufts, the form of their inhibitory impact is expected to differ substantially from that of LBCs.
- *Neurons exclusive to layer I* are believed to mainly innervate the dendritic tufts of target neurons and encompass several interneuron types. *Cajal-Retzius cells* (CRC, Figure 1A4) display large somata, long horizontal dendrites, and horizontally projecting axons, which characteristically give rise to numerous short ascending and some descending terminal fibrils. *Small layer I cells* (not shown) are neurons with short processes that constitute a heterogeneous group of multipolar interneurons with varying axonal arborizations. These have been subdivided into small neurons with poor or rich axonal plexus, respectively (Peters and Jones, 1984).

Interneurons that preferentially target axons

- *Chandelier cells* (ChC, Figure 1A5) are characterized by a local axonal cluster with a "chandelier-like" appearance resulting from the terminal axonal portions forming short vertical bouton arrays ("candlesticks") onto the axon initial segments of target neurons (mainly PCs; Somogyi et al., 1998). Their local axonal clusters—mainly confined within a single layer and column—are formed by collaterals of high BD that frequently branch at shallow angles. ChCs give rise to mostly aspiny, beaded, infrequently branching dendrites that may span one or several layers.

Basic Neuron Types—Electrophysiology

Neocortical neurons display diverse intrinsic electrophysiological properties that result mainly from differences in their ion channel composition and constellation. Ion channels are state dependent and therefore a neuron's passine and active properties may change according to different conditions (see ION CHANNELS: KEYS TO NEURONAL SPECIALIZATION). However, for standardized stimulation and recording conditions, neuronal discharge responses are stable and can serve as a reliable "marker" of their biophysical identity. Electrophysiological diversity indicates that identical spatiotemporal patterns of synaptic inputs will be differentially integrated and transformed into fundamentally different AP-patterns (and hence different synaptic outputs) and may therefore profoundly increase the computational repertoire of neural circuits (see SPIKING NEURONS: COMPUTATION WITH).

Excitatory Neurons

Excitatory neurons have been shown to display limited diversity in their discharge responses. Differences in their discharge properties have been described by three distinct features: (1) kinetic properties of single APs, (2) discharge response to intrasomatic threshold, and (3) supra-threshold current injections (Amitai and Connors, 1995; Connors and Gutnick, 1990; see Table 1). Discharge responses to supra-threshold current injections have proven to be the most useful parameter in distinguishing subclasses of both excitatory as well as inhibitory neurons (see the following discussion).

By far the most common discharge response observed for both PCs and SSCs has been described as *regular-spiking* (RS, see Figure 1B1). Sustained supra-threshold currents cause these cells to fire repetitively with a progressive decrease in firing frequency [progressive increase in inter-spike intervals (ISIs)], generally referred to as *spike train adaptation* or *accommodation*. Differences in the degree of accommodation have led to subclassification into RS1 (weak accommodation; *most common behavior*; see Figure 1B1) and RS2 cells (strong accommodation; behavior of PC- and SSC-subpopulations; see Table 1) (Connors and Gutnick, 1990). Some PCs and SSCs have been shown to display *intrinsic bursting* behavior (IB; not shown; see Connors and Gutnick, 1990). These neurons discharge with a cluster of three to five APs riding on a slow depolarizing wave (referred to as a burst), followed by an after-hyperpolarization, and then by either single spikes or bursts at more or less regular intervals (referred to as regular spiking and repetitive bursting, respectively). Other much less common discharge behaviors have been observed for subpopulations of PCs (see Table 1), including *chattering* (CHTs; not shown; Gray and McCormick, 1996) and *rhythmic firing* (RF; not shown; Amitai and Connors, 1995). CHT-cells usually display repetitive long clusters of APs to sustained supra-threshold current injections that, when made audible, sound like chattering. RF-cells discharge continually without accommodation.

Inhibitory Neurons

Inhibitory neurons display a much larger repertoire of discharge behaviors compared to excitatory neurons (see Figure 1B2; see Table 1), and their electrophysiological (sub-) classification has been gradually refined over the last decade. Initially only a single discharge behavior, known as *fast-spiking* (FS), was described for *smooth or sparsely spiny neurons* throughout layers II-VI. FS-cells generate *single* APs with characteristics distinct from that of spiny (excitatory) neurons (faster rise rates (RR) and fall rates (FR), distinct fast afterhyperpolarizing potentials (fAHP); Connors and Gutnick, 1990) and discharge *repetitively* at high frequencies with little or negligible accommodation to sustained supra-threshold currents. Since other discharge behaviors were not observed initially for smooth cells, it was believed that interneurons represent a homogenous population of characteristically fast-spiking (referring to both the brevity of single APs and the resulting high discharge rate) neurons. Subsequent studies, mainly carried out in layers II/III and V, however, gradually demonstrated, that interneurons could display several other discharge patterns: (1) *burst spiking nonpyramidal* cells (BSNP) originally described as *low-threshold spiking* cells (LTS), typically display burst-like discharges after a hyperpolarizing pre-pulse (see Kawaguchi and Kubota, 1997); (2) *late-spiking* cells (LS) respond with a slow ramp depolarization and a late onset of discharge after a step current pulse (Kawaguchi and Kubota, 1997); (3) *regular spiking nonpyramidal* cells (RSNP) displaying discharge patterns similar to the RS response of PCs (Kawaguchi and Kubota, 1997); and (4) *irregular spiking* cells (IS) typically discharge with an initial burst of APs followed by an irregular spiking response (Cauli et al., 1997). IS cells have been further divided into two subclasses (IS1 and IS2) according to the duration of the initial burst.

Attempts to assign distinct electrophysiological discharge patterns to specific anatomical interneuron types have been made (Kawaguchi and Kubota, 1997; Thomson and Deuchars, 1997). Unfortunately, in many cases, the precise morphological identites of the electrophysiologically classified neurons could only be determined in *fractions* of the recorded cells: some MCs and DBCs were shown to display BSNP behavior, whereas LS behavior was observed for some NGCs and IS behavior for some interneurons with bipolar morphology (Cauli et al., 1997). Finally, DBCs, MCs, and BPCs may also display RSNP behavior, indicating that the same anatomical type may display more than one discharge pattern (see Table 1).

Interneuron discharge patterns, however, display an even richer diversity of behaviors. Recent studies—aimed at understanding the *functional* position of a large number of morphologically identified interneurons within the neocortical microcrocuitry—adopted a simple classification scheme that encompasses previous schemes (Gupta et al., 2000; see Table 1) and considers both the *steady-state* and the *onset* response to sustained somatic current injections (Figure 1B2). According to this scheme, neocortical interneurons are categorized into five main classes with three subclasses each, according to the discharge response at steady-state and onset phase, respectively. These interneuronal discharge patterns are stable for (1) different baseline membrane potentials and (2) durations and amplitudes (several times threshold) of step current injections (Gupta et al., 2000; Wang et al., 2002):

- *Nonaccommodating* cells (NAC, Figure 1B2) fire repetitively without frequency accommodation (no or minimial change in ISIs). The steady-state discharge frequency increases steeply as a function of the injected current amplitude, allowing NACs to reach very high firing frequencies. Their APs are very brief and characteristically display a deep fAHP. NACs are the most frequently encountered cells in all layers

Table 1. Electrophysiological Classes of Neocortical Excitatory and Inhibitory Neurons

Electrophysiological Classes of Excitatory Neurons			
Supra-Threshold Responses	AP Characteristics	Threshold Responses	Morphological Type of Excitatory Neuron (*)
RS1	fast RR and fast FR	single AP	PC (layer II–VI); SSC
RS2	fast RR and fast FR	single AP	subpopulations of PC (layer IV–VI) and SSC
IB	fast RR and fast FR	burst	subpopulations of PC (layer V)
CHAT	nd	nd	subpopulations of PC (layer II/III)
RF	nd	bistable: no or nonaccommodating response	subpopulations of PC (layer V)

Electrophysiological Classes of Inhibitory Neurons			
Main Classes	Subclasses	Other Classification Schemes	Morphological Type of Interneuron (*)
NAC (layers I–VI)	b-NAC	FS	LBC, NBC
	d-NAC	FS; LS	LBC, NBC, SBC, BTC, NGC, ChC
	c-NAC	FS	LBC, NBC, SBC, BTC, MC
AC (layer II–VI)	b-AC	BSNP	NBC, BTC, MC, ChC,
	d-AC	FS(**); LS	LBC, NBC, ChC,
	c-AC	RSNP	LBC, NBC, SBC, BTC, BPC, DBC, MC, ChC
STUT (layers II–VI)	b-STUT	BSNP	NBC, BTC, MC
	d-STUT	FS; LS	LBC, NBC
	c-STUT	FS	LBC, NBC, BPC
IS (layers II–V)	b-IS	IS-1, IS-2	BPC
	c-IS	—	BPC, MC
	d-IS (nd)	—	—
BST (layers II–V)	r-BST	—	ChC
	s-BST	BSNP	BPC, DBC
	I-BST	BSNP	BPC, DBC

Interneuron classification: main classes and subclasses defined according to discharge responses at steady-state and onset-phase to intrasomatic current injections, respectively (see text; see Figure 1B2). Abbreviations explained in text; nd: not determined/detected so far; (*) morphological types listed according to sequence of description in text and not according to frequency of occurrence; (**) some authors have suggested to distinguish between accommodating FS-cells (FS-cells) and non-accommodating FS-cells (classical FS-cells or CFS; see Thomson and Deuchars, 1997).

- *Accommodating* cells (AC, see Figure 1B2) fire repetitively with a decrease in discharge frequency (the gradual increase in ISIs preventing high firing rates) and are the second most frequently observed electrophysiological class.
- *Stuttering* cells (STUT, see Figure 1B2) fire high frequency AP-clusters (with no or minimal accommodation) intermingled with unpredictable periods of silence ("morse-code"-like discharges). Cells displaying stuttering near threshold and fast spiking at slightly higher depolarizations are not considered STUTs.
- *Irregular spiking* cells (IS, see Figure 1B2) discharge single APs in a random manner throughout a depolarizing pulse, but do not form distinct clusters of APs.

Each of these main classes displays an array of stereotypical onset responses, which have been used for subclassification. They either discharge with:

- a *burst* (a high-frequency cluster of three or more APs), that *seamlessly* merges into the steady-state response (b-subclass, see Figure 1B2),
- a distinct *delay* before discharging to a current pulse (d-subclass, see Figure 1B2). The duration of the delay decreases progressively as the amplitude of current injection increases. Delayed discharging cells characteristically show significantly higher action potential thresholds than the b- and c-subclasses, or
- neither a burst nor a delay (referred to a *classical* response). The "onset" phase of these cells (c-subclass, see Figure 1B2) is therefore indistinguishable from the steady-state phase.

A fifth main class of *bursting* cells (BST; less frequent than the above main classes), with three subclasses, was recently observed (not shown). The onset response of BST cells is characterized by a high-frequency cluster of three to five APs riding on a slow *de-*

polarizing wave followed by a strong *slow* AHP, that causes a *clear separation* of the onset burst response from the consecutive steady-state responses, even at high current injections. The peak amplitudes of these APs decrease during the bursts in most cells. These burst properties differ fundamentally from those that define the b-subclasses of NAC-, AC-, STUT-, and IS-cells. BST-cells may be subclassified according to their steady-state discharge response into

- *r-BST* cells, which characteristically discharge *repetitive* burst (r = repetitive),
- *s-BST* cells, which characteristically fail to discharge after their initial burst due to a more pronounced, complex of powerful AHP (s = single), or
- *i-BST* cells, which characteristically discharge an accommodating train of APs (i = initial).

Recent computational studies have addressed the mechanisms of bursting behavior in neocortical PCs (see OSCILLATORY AND BURSTING PROPERTIES OF NEURONS). Similar studies for the other types of discharge behaviors in both excitatory and inhibitory neurons are eagerly awaited, especially in light of the profound effects, that different discharge properties may have on the behavior of neural circuits (i.e., van Vreeswijk and Hansel, 2001).

Basic Neuron Types—Molecular

Neocortical neurons express a variety of intracellular molecules including classical neurotransmitters (glutamate, GABA, acetylcholine, and catecholamines), neuropeptides, and calcium-binding proteins (CaBPs), as well as a multitude of different cell-surface molecules (neurotransmitter receptors, etc.). While these molecular species are found throughout the neocortex, each neuron only expresses some of these molecules and in specific combinations

Table 2. Molecular Classes of Excitatory and Inhibitory Neocortical Neurons

Molecular Classes of Excitatory Neurons (Glutamate +)			
Calcium Binding Proteins	Neuropeptides	Anatomical Identity	Electrophysiological Identity
CB	—	PC	RS
—	SOM	PC	RS
—	CCK	PC	RS
CB	CCK	PC	RS

Molecular Classes of Inhibitory Neurons (GABA +)			
Calcium Binding Proteins	Neuropeptides	Anatomical Identity	Electrophysiological Identity
CB	—	LBC, NBC, BTC, MC, DBC	c-AC, c-NAC, d-NAC
PV	—	ChC, LBC, NBC	c-NAC, d-NAC, c-STUT, d-STUT
CR	—	BPC, DBC, CRC	c-AC
CB + PV	—	LBC, NBC	d-NAC
—	NPY	LBC, MC, NBC	c-AC, c-NAC, d-NAC, c-STUT
—	VIP	DBC, BPC, SBC	c-AC, b-NAC, c-IS, b-IS
—	SOM	MC, BTC, NBC	c-AC, c-NAC, b-AC
—	CCK	LBC, BTC, MC, NBC, SBC	b-NAC, c-AC, c-NAC, c-STUT
CB	SOM	MC	c-AC
PV	SOM (*)	NBC	c-AC
CR	VIP	BPC, BTC	b-IS
CB	NPY + SOM	MC	c-AC

Excitatory neurons (shown to express glutamate) and inhibitory neurons (shown to express GABA or GABA producing enzymes GAD 65 and/or GAD 67), located throughout layers II–VI, have been sorted according to the detection of CaBPs, neuropeptides, and their co-expression. Abbreviations explained in text. In all cases listed, consistent expression profiles have been determined at both the protein and mRNA level, except (*), in which co-expression of SOM and PV was only detected at the mRNA level (compare Cauli et al., 1997, Wang et al., 2002, with Kawaguchi and Kubota, 1997). Note that the expression profiles are listed separately for *either* the anatomical *or* electrophysiological identities of the inhibitory neurons. Detailed information regarding expression profiles of SSCs not available to date.

(DeFelipe, 1993), allowing the use of expression and co-expression patterns for neuronal classification. Of these "molecular markers," the (co-) expression of the most common CaBPs (calbindin, CB, parvalbumin, PV and calretinin, CR) and neuropeptides (neuropeptide Y, NPY, vasoactive intestinal peptide, VIP, somatostatin, SOM, cholecystokinine, CCK) has been most extensively studied (Cauli et al., 1997; DeFelipe, 1997; Kawaguchi and Kubota, 1997; Wang et al., 2002). The functional significance of this molecular diversity is currently not fully understood, although some of the above-mentioned "markers" (i.e., synaptically released neuropeptides) have been implicated in modulating synaptic transmission and/or neuronal excitability.

Table 2 summarizes molecular expression profiles of neocortical neurons (mainly layers II–VI; except CRC, see previous discussion) for the most commonly investigated CaBPs and neuropeptides, based on studies of protein- or mRNA-expression (mainly rodent neocortex). Whereas, *every* molecular expression profile detected at the protein level has been confirmed at the mRNA level, some mRNA-expression profiles have not been detected at the protein level (compare Cauli et al., 1997 and Wang et al., 2002, with Kawaguchi and Kubota, 1997). In general, neocortical excitatory neurons (mainly PCs) have been shown to differ from inhibitory neurons, (1) in that the percentage of PCs expressing CaBPs and/or neuropeptides is considerably lower and (2) in that they typically display a much more restricted set of expression profiles.

Discussion

This article outlines the main properties defining the basic cell types in the neocortex. The most striking feature of neocortical neurons is their immense anatomical, electrophysiological, and molecular diversity. All anatomical cell types can display multiple discharge patterns and molecular expression profiles. Different cell types are synaptically interconnected according to complex organizational principles to form intricate stereotypical microcircuits.

It is still unknown how afferent and efferent pathways determine the locations, dimensions, and functions of these seemingly omnipotent microcircuits that underlie the formation of functional columns. The major challenge for neural network models is to incorporate and account for the cellular diversity, which may explain the universal computational capability of these stereotypical microcircuits.

Road Map: Biological Neurons and Synapses
Related Reading: Biophysical Mosaic of the Neuron; Dendritic Processing; Ion Channels: Keys to Neuronal Specialization; Neocortex: Chemical and Electrical Synapses; Single-Cell Models; Temporal Integration in Recurrent Microcircuits; Visual Cortex: Anatomical Structure and Models of Function

References

Amitai, Y., and Connors, B. W., 1995, Intrinsic physiology and morphology of single neurons in neocortex, in *Cerebral Cortex, Vol 11: The Barrel Cortex of Rodents* (E. G. Jones and I. T. Diamond, Eds.), New York: Plenum Press, pp. 299–331.

Cauli, B., Audinat, E., Lambolez, B., Angulo, M. C., Ropert, N., Tsuzuki, K., Hestrin, S., and Rossier, J., 1997, Molecular and physiological diversity of cortical nonpyramidal cells, *J. Neurosci.*, 17:3894–3906.

Connors, B. W., and Gutnick, M. J., 1990, Intrinsic firing patterns of diverse neocortical neurons, *Trends Neurosci.*, 13:99–104. ◆

DeFelipe, J., 1993, Neocortical neuronal diversity: Chemical heterogeneity revealed by colocalization studies of classic neurotransmitters, neuropeptides, calcium binding proteins, and cell surface molecules, *Cereb. Cortex*, 3:273–289.

DeFelipe, J., 1997, Types of neurons, synaptic connections and chemical characteristics of cells immunoreactive for calbindin-D28K, parvalbumin and calretinin in the neocortex, *J. Chem. Neuroanat.*, 14:1–19.

Douglas, R., and Martin, K. A. C., 1998, Neocortex, in *The Synaptic Organization of the Brain* (G. M. Shepherd, Ed.), New York: Oxford University Press, pp. 459–509.

Gray, C. M., and McCormick, D. A., 1996, Chattering cells: Superficial pyramidal neurons contributing to the generation of synchronous oscillations in the visual cortex, *Science*, 274:109–113.

Gupta, A., Wang, Y., and Markram, H., 2000, Organizing principles for a diversity of GABAergic interneurons and synapses in the neocortex, *Science*, 287:273–278. ◆

Kawaguchi, Y., and Kubota, Y., 1997, GABAergic cell subtypes and their synaptic connections in rat frontal cortex, *Cereb. Cortex*, 7:476–486. ◆

Kisvarday, Z. F., 1992, GABAergic networks of basket cells in the visual cortex, *Prog. Brain. Res.*, 90:385–405.

Peters, A., and Jones, E. G., 1984, *Cerebral Cortex, Vol. 1: Cellular Components of the Cerebral Cortex*, New York: Plenum Press.

Somogyi, P., 1989, Synaptic organization of GABAergic neurons and GABA-A receptors in the lateral geniculate nucleus and visual cortex, in *Neural Mechanisms of Visual Perception. Proceedings of the Retina*

Research Foundation Symposia (D. K.-T. Lam and C. D. Gilbert, Eds.), The Woodlands: Portfolio Publications, pp. 35–63.

Somogyi, P., Tamas, G., Lujan, R., and Buhl, E. H., 1998, Salient features of synaptic organisation in the cerebral cortex, *Brain Res.Rev.*, 26:113–135. ◆

Thomson, A. M., and Deuchars, J., 1997, Synaptic interactions in neocortical local circuits: Dual intracellular recordings in vitro, *Cereb. Cortex*, 7:510–522. ◆

van Vreeswijk, C., and Hansel, D., 2001, Patterns of synchrony in neural networks with spike adaptation, *Neural Comput.*, 13:959–992.

Wang, Y., Gupta, A., Toledo-Rodriguez, M., Wu, C. Z., and Markram, H., 2002, Anatomical, physiological, molecular and circuit properties of nest basket cells in the developing somatosensory cortex, *Cereb. Cortex*, 12:395–410.

White, E., 1989, *Cortical Circuits: Synaptic Organization of the Cerebral Cortex; Structure, Function, and Theory*, Berlin: Birkhauser Verlag. ◆

Neocortex: Chemical and Electrical Synapses

Jay R. Gibson and Barry W. Connors

Introduction

Synapses are specialized sites of communication between neurons. Our goal here is to summarize the diverse functional properties of synapses in neocortex. Synapses in the neocortex tend to be small, but their structure and biochemistry are complex. This intricacy befits their rich and highly dynamic functions. Short-term dynamics allow synapses to serve as temporal filters of neural activity; long-term synaptic plasticity provides specific, localized substrates for various forms of memory; modulation of synaptic function by neurotransmitters provides a mechanism for globally altering the properties of a neural circuit during changes of behavioral state. An important point is that each of these functions—short- and long-term plasticity and modulation—has diverse forms that vary between synapses, depending on their site within the cortical circuit.

Synapses come in two distinctly different types, chemical and electrical, both of which exist in neocortex. Chemical synapses are by far the most abundant. They use a chemical neurotransmitter that is packaged presynaptically into vesicles, released in quantized (vesicle-multiple) amounts, and binds to postsynaptic receptors that either open an ion channel directly or activate a G protein–coupled receptor. Electrical synapses are simpler in both structure and function. Their essential element is a protein called a *connexin;* 12 connexins form a single intercytoplasmic ion channel, and a cluster of such channels constitutes a *gap junction*. Electrical synapses provide a direct pathway that allows ionic current or small organic molecules to flow from the cytoplasm of one cell to that of another.

Our description of the neurons and synapses in the neocortex will follow the very simplified diagram shown in Figure 1. This represents only the input stage of the circuit, but it serves to outline the range of synapse functions seen throughout neocortex; we neglect synaptic connections between cortical layers and areas, as well as the output pathways. Most of the data discussed here originated in studies of sensory and motor neocortices of adolescent and adult rats, mice, guinea pigs, and cats.

Excitatory and Inhibitory Cells

To make sense of the diversity of neocortical synapses, it is essential to understand the nature of the neurons that they interconnect. Neocortical neurons are either excitatory or inhibitory; i.e., their axons form presynaptic terminals that release the excitatory transmitter glutamate or the inhibitory transmitter γ-aminobutyric acid

(GABA). Excitatory neurons include virtually all pyramidal cells and the spiny stellate cells of layer 4 (Figure 1, center). The somata of pyramidal cells exist in all layers below layer 1, and they extend an apical dendrite toward, and often into, layer 1. Pyramidal cells are the output neurons of the neocortex, and their axons often project to other brain areas. Spiny stellate cells are small, locally interacting cells confined to layer 4. Excitatory cells usually produce action potentials that have "regular spiking" characteristics, although subsets may have intrinsic bursting properties (Connors and Gutnick, 1990; see also OSCILLATORY AND BURSTING PROPERTIES OF NEURONS).

The inhibitory neurons tend to have relatively few spines on their dendrites (Thomson and Deuchars, 1997). Many classification schemes have been proposed for inhibitory interneurons based on

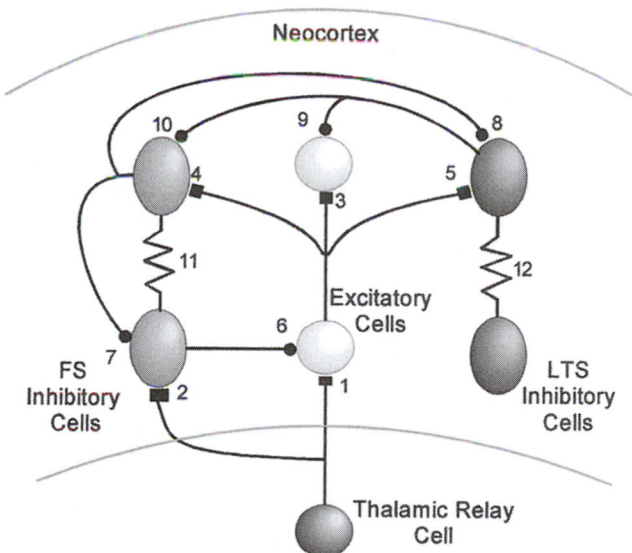

Figure 1. A simplified diagram of the neuronal circuitry in the primary input layer of sensory neocortex. Chemical synapses are represented by rectangles (for excitatory synapses) or dots (for inhibitory synapses), and electrical synapses are represented by zig-zags. The numbers refer to specific synaptic connections that are described in the text.

their dendritic and axonal morphology, the genes they express, their electrophysiological properties, and their synaptic physiology (e.g., Kawaguchi and Kubota, 1997; Gupta, Wang, and Markram, 2000; see also NEOCORTEX: BASIC NEURON TYPES). The number of inhibitory cell types and the criteria for distinguishing them are not universally agreed upon.

The majority of inhibitory neurons can be divided into three basic classes. The first expresses the Ca^{2+}-binding protein parvalbumin, and constitutes about 50% of all GABAergic neurons. Physiologically these cells are often called "fast spiking" (FS) because of their exceptionally short-duration action potentials, which can fire at high rates with little or no adaptation (Figure 1, left). Morphologically, many FS cells are either classical basket cells, with axons that make synaptic contacts onto somata or proximal dendrites, or chandelier (axo-axonic) cells, which synapse exclusively onto the initial axon segments of pyramidal cells. The second largest class of inhibitory neurons expresses the Ca^{2+}-binding protein calbindin, as well as the neuroactive peptide somatostatin; these neurons constitute about 17% of GABAergic neurons. Physiologically, at least some are "low-threshold spiking" (LTS) cells; their tonic firing shows adaptation, and they can fire rebound spikes in response to hyperpolarization (Figure 1, right). LTS cells often have vertically oriented dendritic patterns, and probably include many of the sparsely spiny, bitufted cells and Martinotti cells. A third class of cells stains for the Ca^{2+}-binding protein calretinin and for vasoactive intestinal polypeptide (VIP), and they also constitute about 17% of GABAergic neurons. Their physiological properties include irregular or intermittent firing patterns in response to steady current stimuli, and morphologically they are usually vertically oriented bipolar cells.

Neurotransmitters and Their Receptors

The excitatory neurotransmitter glutamate binds to two types of iontropic receptors: non-NMDA and NMDA (Ozawa, Kamiya, and Tsuzuki, 1998). The binding of glutamate induces a conformational change in the receptor, which biases an ion channel toward an open state, allowing the passage of ions. Currents passing through these channels usually have a reversal potential around 0 mV. Because the transmembrane potential of a cell is usually much more negative than this, channel opening results in net inward current flow and transient membrane depolarization: the excitatory postsynaptic potential (EPSP). Usually, both types of glutamate receptors exist at the same excitatory synapse. Non-NMDA receptors can be further subdivided into AMPA receptors and kainate receptors. AMPA receptors mediate the vast majority of fast glutamatergic EPSPs, while the functions of kainate receptors are poorly understood. Most AMPA receptor channels are permeable to Na^+ and K^+ and have linear current-voltage relationships, but many excitatory synapses on inhibitory cells also include AMPA receptor subtypes that are permeable to Ca^{2+} and have a more nonlinear current-voltage relationship. In response to synaptically released glutamate, AMPA receptor-mediated currents have an extremely fast onset, and a decay time constant of roughly 3 ms.

NMDA receptor-mediated responses, in contrast, are slow; their decay time constants are about 40 ms. They are also highly permeable to Ca^{2+}, in addition to K^+ and Na^+. NMDA receptors have a nonlinear voltage dependence, with highest conductance at potentials positive to about -30 mV. The voltage dependence of the NMDA channel is caused by extracellular Mg^{2+} ions, which block the channel due to electrostatic attraction; membrane depolarization releases this attraction. As a consequence, at standard excitatory synapses containing both NMDA and AMPA receptors, synaptic release of glutamate always opens AMPA receptors, whereas NMDA receptors are open only during the conjunction of glutamate release and relative depolarization of the postsynaptic

membrane. This property allows NMDA receptors to act as coincidence detectors, sensing the simultaneous activation of presynaptic glutamate release and postsynaptic activation of the cell through other synaptic inputs. The opening of NMDA receptors, and the subsequent influx of postsynaptic Ca^{2+} they provide, is thought to mediate many forms of long-term synaptic change.

Fast inhibitory synaptic transmission in neocortex seems to be exclusively mediated by the neurotransmitter GABA (Connors, 1992). GABA binds to ionotropic $GABA_A$ receptors, inducing the opening of channels permeable to Cl^-. Cl^- reversal potentials tend to be about -70 mV in mature neocortical neurons. If the postsynaptic membrane is positive to this potential, inhibitory activation evokes a transient hyperpolarization—an inhibitory postsynaptic potential (IPSP)—owing to the influx of Cl^-. An inhibitory effect may result either from this shift in membrane potential, or from a current "shunt" caused by the increase in membrane conductance to Cl^-. Synaptically triggered $GABA_A$ currents have a decay time constant of about 10 ms in cerebral cortex.

So far, we have only discussed synaptic transmission mediated by ionotropic receptors, i.e., receptors that are also ion channels. There are also many examples of synaptic transmission mediated by metabotropic receptors, i.e., receptors that activate G proteins, which in turn interact with downstream effector proteins. All neurotransmitters known to exist in neocortex activate specific metabotropic receptors. These include the two most important neurotransmitters that activate ionotropic receptors, glutamate and GABA, as well as other neuromodulators. Metabotropic responses tend to start more slowly than ionotropic responses (tens to hundreds of milliseconds versus fractions of a millisecond), last much longer (hundreds of milliseconds to seconds versus a few milliseconds), and can occur in both postsynaptic cells and presynaptic terminals. Postsynaptically, responses can be inhibitory, excitatory, or both. Most notable is the slow IPSP mediated by the $GABA_B$ receptor, which is generated by an increase in K^+ conductance (Connors, 1992). Presynaptic metabotropic effects modify, and usually depress, the subsequent release of neurotransmitter.

Functional Properties of Chemical Synapses

The effectiveness of a chemical synapse is determined by several factors, including the probability of transmitter release (which can range widely, from near zero to almost one), the mean number of transmitter quanta released (which for many neocortical synapses is a maximum of one quantum per presynaptic terminal), the dynamics of the release process, and the history of prior activity. These factors often interact. We will describe how the functional properties of synapses vary between different pathways in neocortex; numbers in boldface refer to specific synapses in Figure 1. When we speak of a "unitary" synaptic response we mean the postsynaptic response to the firing of a single presynaptic cell or axon. One axon may make multiple synaptic contacts onto a single postsynaptic cell, so the strength of a unitary response is strongly determined by the number of synaptic contacts per axon, in addition to the physiological factors listed above. The "short-term dynamics" of a synapse refers to its time-varying changes in strength during repetitive activation over relatively brief intervals (milliseconds to seconds). Synapses may show short-term depression or facilitation, or a combination of the two.

Thalamic Input

Thalamic inputs are the conduit by which all specific information enters the neocortex. Thalamocortical axons form relatively strong excitatory synapses onto excitatory cells (**1**) and FS inhibitory cells (**2**), but not LTS cells (Figure 1; Gibson, Beierlein, and Connors, 1999). The strongest responses are generated in cortical layers 4 and 6, where most thalamic axons terminate. Unitary thalamocortical connections generate relatively large-amplitude EPSPs, with high reliability and practically no failures, and the responses show pronounced short-term depression (Figure 2A; Gil, Connors, and Amitai, 1999). Unitary thalamocortical EPSPs onto excitatory cells activate an average of roughly seven synaptic release sites, but unitary inputs to FS cells are twice as strong, with occasional single-axon responses surpassing 12 mV (FS mean = 4 mV, excitatory cell mean = 2 mV). Electron microscopic observations show that thalamocortical synapses terminate primarily on the soma and proximal dendrites of FS cells, and on the proximal dendritic spines of excitatory spiny stellate cells in layer 4 (Somogyi et al., 1998).

Intracortical Excitatory Synapses

The probability and strength of excitatory synaptic contacts vary widely and depend on the nature of the targets. Estimates suggest that the typical unitary connection between two excitatory cells (**3**) comprises about two to eight synaptic contacts, on average about half that of the average thalamocortical connection (Gil et al., 1999). These synapses target mostly dendritic spines (85%). There are exceptions. For example, a specific population of layer 6 spiny cells projects only 30% of its synapses onto spines (Somogyi et al., 1998). The amplitude of unitary intracortical EPSPs range from less than 0.5 mV up to 9 mV. The larger the response, the more reliable it tends to be. Failure rates are higher in connections with relatively small unitary responses (Thomson and Deuchars, 1997).

The dynamics of synapses between excitatory cells range from moderately depressing to weakly facilitating. The short-term dynamics of these intracortical connections depend on the maturity

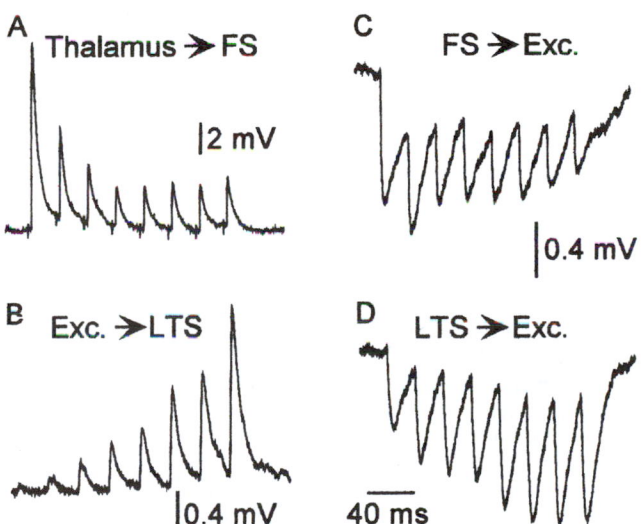

Figure 2. Variability in the strength and short-term dynamics of specific synaptic connections. In each case the presynaptic cell was activated at 40 Hz to test the dynamics of the postsynaptic response. *A,* The excitatory synapses from thalamocortical axons onto FS inhibitory cells (connection **2** in Figure 1) tend to be relatively strong and reliable, but depress during activation at high frequencies. *B,* The intracortical synapses from excitatory cells onto LTS inhibitory cells (**5**) tend to be quite unreliable when first activated, but strongly facilitate at frequencies above about 20 Hz. *C,* Inhibitory synapses from FS cells onto excitatory neurons (**8**) tend to be strong and reliable, and show moderate depression. *D,* Inhibitory synapses from LTS cells onto excitatory neurons (**9**) are moderately strong, and often facilitate during high-frequency activation. (Data from M. Beierlein, J. R. Gibson, and B. W. Connors.)

of the cortex. For instance, in the adolescent rat (14–17 days postnatal), excitatory synapses between layer 5 pyramidal cells show clear depression, but by postnatal day 28 the same synapses are either weakly depressing or slightly facilitating.

Excitatory cells also synapse onto inhibitory cells, but the properties of the synapses vary with the postsynaptic inhibitory cell type. When excitatory axons fire at a rate above 5 Hz, EPSPs onto FS inhibitory cells (**4**) generally depress (Thomson and Deuchars, 1997). At low frequencies of stimulation (<0.2 Hz), unitary EPSPs onto FS cells are relatively reliable, with low failure rates. Unitary EPSP sizes can range from a few μV to 12 mV, and they have a distinctly shorter duration than EPSPs in excitatory cells (Thomson and Deuchars, 1997). Axons from excitatory cells make about one to four synapses onto a single FS cell, and yield a response about 1 mV in amplitude. Most of these synapses terminate on dendrites, with fewer onto the soma.

The intracortical excitatory synapses that terminate on LTS inhibitory cells (**5**) have unusual dynamics, showing very strong short-term facilitation when activated at frequencies above 20 Hz (Figure 2B). At low-frequency stimulation (<1 Hz), EPSPs onto LTS cells have high failure rates, despite the likelihood that unitary connections are mediated by as many as three to 12 synapses. At higher frequencies, after facilitation develops, unitary EPSPs can be as large as 3 mV. Thus, inhibitory LTS cells may be activated only when local excitatory cells fire at high and sustained rates, suggesting that they serve as a "governor" on the cortical circuit, helping to prevent runaway excitation.

Metabotropic glutamate receptors (mGluRs) are expressed by various types of neurons in neocortex, both pre- and postsynaptically. Postsynaptic effects mediated by these receptors presumably require relatively large rates of glutamate release. Electron microscopy has localized mGluRs to the marginal regions of the subsynaptic membrane (Somogyi et al., 1998). Responses mediated by mGluRs are relatively slow, lasting hundreds of milliseconds. Some types of excitatory cells apparently depolarize when mGluRs are activated, while others hyperpolarize; it may be that responses vary with the neurons' laminar location. Activating mGluRs depolarizes FS and LTS cells, but LTS cells are more strongly excited. Glutamate can also act on mGluRs expressed on presynaptic terminals. Activation of presynaptic mGluRs usually inhibits further transmitter release, reducing the amplitude of the postsynaptic response.

Fast, ionotropic excitatory synaptic transmission in neocortex is subject to long-term synaptic plasticity. Long-term potentiation (LTP) and long-term depression (LTD) occur primarily at excitatory synapses onto excitatory cells, but generally not at synapses onto inhibitory cells. Some forms of LTP and LTD depend on the opening of NMDA channels, while other forms of LTD depend on activation of the metabotropic glutamate channel.

Inhibitory Synapses

Inhibitory cells may inhibit excitatory neurons or other inhibitory neurons. The connection specificity depends on the cell types involved (Thomson and Deuchars, 1997; Kawaguchi and Kubota, 1997; Somogyi et al., 1998). Calretinin-expressing interneurons preferentially inhibit other interneurons in visual cortex, but the functional properties of their synapses are unknown. FS (parvalbumin-expressing) cells frequently synapse onto excitatory cells (**6**), other FS cells (**7**), and onto LTS cells (**8**), where they tend to form synapses on the soma or dendritic shafts. Unitary axonal connections of up to 20 synapses have been described, from a single basket (FS) cell onto the soma and proximal dendrites of spiny cells and other inhibitory interneurons. Responses mediated by FS-derived synapses are very reliable, but tend to depress during repetitive activation (Figure 2C). The unitary IPSPs of these synapses have peak amplitudes of about 2 mV when the postsynaptic cell's membrane potential is just below firing threshold. Some neocortical areas have an FS-like interneuron, called the axo-axonic cell, whose synapses exclusively and precisely target the axonal initial segments of pyramidal cells. The IPSPs of the axo-axonic connection have not been characterized in neocortex, but a similar connection in hippocampus displays short-term depression (Thomson and Deuchars, 1997).

Anatomical studies show that LTS-like (somatostatin-expressing) cells tend to synapse on the more distal dendritic shafts and spines of excitatory cells (**9**) and on distal dendritic shafts of FS cells (**10**). In one example, an LTS cell made ten synapses onto a single pyramidal cell—six onto spines and four onto dendritic shafts. Interestingly, recordings from neurons in layer 4 imply that LTS cells rarely make chemical synapses upon one another. The short-term dynamics of inhibitory synapses from LTS cells differ from those of FS cells. LTS-to-spiny cell IPSPs are fairly stable at 10 Hz and slower, while at 40 Hz and above they often show moderate facilitation (Figure 2D).

The computational consequences of inhibitory synapses can be complex, and synaptic location can play a role (Vu and Krasne, 1992). For example, activation of distal inhibition may shift the preferred input of the postsynaptic cell to a more proximal position. Proximally placed inhibition may be most effective for controlling the precise timing of action potentials and subthreshold activity. Postsynaptic inhibition can be divisive or subtractive in overall quality, depending on whether the inhibitory synapse is near the soma or farther out on the dendrites, respectively.

Activation of single inhibitory neurons tends to induce pure $GABA_A$ receptor-mediated IPSPs in both excitatory and inhibitory cells. However, strong stimulation, which activates multiple inhibitory cells and yields large quantities of GABA release, can evoke an additional, and much longer-lasting, IPSP that is mediated by $GABA_B$ receptors (Connors, 1992). Most $GABA_B$-mediated inhibition has been studied in excitatory cells, and its possible role in regulating inhibitory neurons is unknown. $GABA_B$ receptors are also located presynaptically on both GABA- and glutamate-releasing terminals. When these receptors are activated, they inhibit evoked transmitter release.

Electrical Synapses

Electrical synapses have been directly demonstrated only between inhibitory neurons in the neocortex (Gibson et al., 1999; Galarreta and Hestrin, 2001), although there is indirect evidence that they may be more widespread early in development. Electrical synapses allow ionic current to pass directly between cells, equally well in both directions, with little or no voltage or time dependence. Recordings from two electrically coupled LTS cells are shown in Figure 3. Current steps of opposite polarity applied to LTS_1 induced either depolarization plus a train of action potentials, or a hyperpolarization (V_1); the voltage of LTS_2 responded in parallel with either strongly attenuated action potentials riding on a slower depolarization, or a slow hyperpolarization, respectively (V_2). The electrical synapses of inhibitory cells have an average "coupling coefficient," or attenuation factor, of about 0.1 for low-frequency signals; this decreases to about 0.01 for faster signals such as action potentials. Thus, a single presynaptic spike of 90 mV induces an electrical PSP that is typically less than 1 mV at its peak.

The functional significance of electrical synapses in neocortex is currently being studied. In general, electrical synapses promote synchronous electrical activity among the interneurons they connect. The electrical synapses between interneurons are located at dendrodendritic or dendrosomatic sites of contact (Tamas et al., 2000). This constrains them to closely neighboring cells, and indeed the most strongly connected inhibitory cells have somata

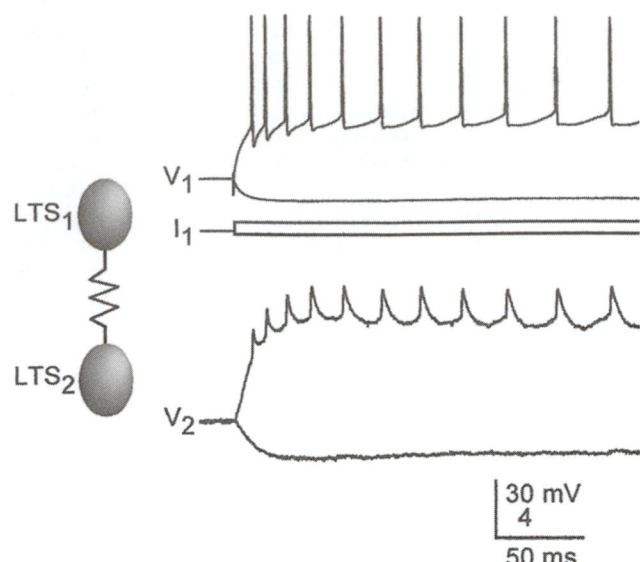

Figure 3. An electrical synapse between two LTS inhibitory neurons. Recordings on the top right show the superimposed responses of the first cell (LTS_1) as it was directly stimulated by two steps of injected current, depolarizing and hyperpolarizing. Responses from the second cell (LTS_2), on the lower right, were generated by current flowing through the electrical synapse from LTS_1. Notice that action potentials were more strongly attenuated than low-frequency voltage components. Voltage calibration is 30 mV for top traces, 4 mV for lower traces. (Data from J. R. Gibson, M. Beierlein, and B. W. Connors.)

within 100 μm of each other. Extensive sampling of neuron pairs in layer 4 (Gibson et al., 1999) showed that, with rare exceptions, FS cells formed electrical synapses only with other FS cells (**11**), and LTS cells only with LTS cells (**12**). Thus, electrical synapses are a molecular and functional marker that serves to define and distinguish the boundaries between the FS and LTS inhibitory networks. It is also possible that the connexin-based channels of electrical synapses mediate the passage of small organic signaling molecules between interneurons.

Neuromodulation

Modulators such as acetylcholine, norepinephrine, serotonin, dopamine, and histamine can modulate presynaptic and postsynaptic neocortical function via G protein–coupled receptors. In general, these modulators are released throughout most or all of the neocortex from synaptic terminals whose axons originate extracortically, and the rates of modulator release depend strongly on behavioral state (Steriade, McCormick, and Sejnowski, 1993).

The two best-studied neuromodulators are acetylcholine and norepinephrine, and many of their effects are similar. Via postsynaptic actions, they can both depolarize and hyperpolarize excitatory cells, depending on the receptor subtypes that they activate, and they can also modulate spiking patterns via more subtle actions. Acetylcholine and norepinephrine depolarize both FS and LTS interneurons, but they are more effective at inducing LTS cells to surpass action potential threshold. Presynaptic effects of these modulators usually suppress transmitter release, resulting in smaller PSPs together with a reduction in short-term depression.

Discussion

There seem to be distinct rules governing the synaptic connections among neurons in the neocortex. First, connections are specific; for example, thalamocortical synapses are strong and common onto FS interneurons but quite weak and rare onto LTS interneurons, and electrical synapses only interconnect interneurons of similar type. Second, the functional characteristics of synapses, such as efficacy, short-term dynamics, and location, vary with the identity of the pre- and postsynaptic neurons that participate in making the synapse. Third, synaptic function can be modulated by the common transmitters intrinsic to neocortex, glutamate and GABA, and by transmitters such as acetylcholine and norepinephrine that are mainly released by extrinsic neurons whose activity depends on behavioral state. The computational consequences of these complex synaptic properties are rich (e.g., Markram et al., 1998; see also TEMPORAL INTEGRATION IN RECURRENT MICROCIRCUITS and TEMPORAL DYNAMICS OF BIOLOGICAL SYNAPSES), although far from fully understood.

Road Map: Biological Neurons and Synapses
Related Reading: Neocortex: Basic Neuron Types; Neuromodulation in Mammalian Nervous Systems; Synaptic Interactions

References

Connors, B. W., 1992, GABA$_A$- and GABA$_B$-mediated processes in visual cortex, *Prog. Brain Res.*, 90:335–348. ◆
Connors, B. W., and Gutnick, M. J., 1990, Intrinsic firing patterns of diverse neocortical neurons, *Trends Neurosci.*, 13:99–104. ◆
Galarreta, M., and Hestrin, S., 2001, Electrical synapses between GABA-releasing interneurons, *Nature Rev. Neurosci.*, 2:425–433. ◆
Gibson, J. R., Beierlein, M., and Connors, B. W., 1999, Two networks of electrically coupled inhibitory neurons in neocortex, *Nature*, 402:75–79.
Gil, Z., Connors, B. W., and Amitai, Y., 1999, Efficacy of thalamocortical and intracortical synaptic connections: Quanta, innervation, and reliability, *Neuron*, 23:385–397.
Gupta, A., Wang, Y., and Markram, H., 2000, Organizing principles for a diversity of GABAergic interneurons and synapses in the neocortex, *Science*, 287:273–278.
Kawaguchi, Y., and Kubota, Y., 1997, GABAergic cell subtypes and their synaptic connections in rat frontal cortex, *Cereb. Cortex*, 7:476–486.
Markram, H., Gupta, A., Uziel, A., Wang, Y., and Tsodyks, M., 1998, Information processing with frequency-dependent synaptic connections, *Neurobiol. Learn. Mem.*, 70:101–112.
Ozawa, S., Kamiya, H., and Tsuzuki, K., 1998, Glutamate receptors in the mammalian central nervous system, *Prog. Neurobiol.*, 54:581–618. ◆
Somogyi, P., Tamas, G., Lujan, R., and Buhl, E. H., 1998, Salient features of synaptic organisation in the cerebral cortex, *Brain Res. Rev.*, 26:113–135. ◆
Steriade, M., McCormick, D. A., and Sejnowski, T. J., 1993, Thalamocortical oscillations in the sleeping and aroused brain, *Science*, 262:679–685. ◆
Tamas, G., Buhl, E. H., Lorincz, A., and Somogyi, P., 2000, Proximally targeted GABAergic synapses and gap junctions synchronize cortical interneurons, *Nature Neurosci.*, 3:366–371.
Thomson, A. M., and Deuchars, J., 1997, Synaptic interactions in neocortical local circuits: Dual intracellular recordings in vitro, *Cereb. Cortex*, 7:510–22.
Vu, E. T., and Krasne, F. B., 1992, Evidence for a computational distinction between proximal and distal neuronal inhibition, *Science*, 255:1710–1712.

Neural Automata and Analog Computational Complexity

Hava T. Siegelmann

Introduction

Computational theory has developed hand in hand with the field of neural computation. The Turing machine was suggested in 1935 as a model of a mathematician who solves problems by using a specifiable algorithm. McCulloch and Pitts demonstrated the first computational model of a neuron, where they explicitly sought to provide a "brain" for the Turing machine. They proposed to model the nervous system as a finite interconnection of logical devices. Following the development of von Neumann's universal model of computation based on the principle of the McCulloch-Pitts neuron, the digital approach prevailed in the field of cybernetic research.

In the last few decades, continuous, rather than digital, neural network models have been emphasized. Unlike the output values 0, 1 of the McCulloch-Pitts neuron, these models calculate continuous values. This was key to the development of the backpropagation algorithm that learns neural parameters; it enabled the foundation of machine learning, engineering tools such as optimal controllers, and adaptive technologies.

The connection between neural networks and computation, or more generally between physical systems and computation, is formalized by computational theories that describe features and capabilities of computational process. Automata are the basic mathematical abstractions used in such formalization.

A digital automaton has a set of internal states Ω, it receives a string of input symbols belonging to an alphabet Σ, and it moves from state to state according to the transition rules until the computation ends. Current neural automata are quite different from classical automata. Whereas classical automata describe digital machines, neural models frequently require a framework of analog

computation. In these terms, a physical system, beginning from an initial state (input), evolves in its state space according to an update equation (the computation process) until it reaches some designated state (the output).

Properties that distinguish analog from digital computation include the following:

1. Analog models are defined on a continuous phase space, while the phase space of a digital model is inherently discrete.
2. Physical dynamics is characterized by the existence of real constants that influence the macroscopic behavior of the system. In contrast, in digital computation all constants are in principle accessible to the programmer.
3. The motion of a physical system has local continuity. Unlike the flow in digital computation, analog models do not include locally discontinuous statements such as if $x > 0$ then compute one thing and if $x > 0$ continue in another computation path.
4. Continuous time dynamics is part of some analog systems.
5. A system composed of analog components may be sensitive to external noise.

In this article, we first review some work on analog and neural computation, and then focus on analog computation under noise. The fundamental question is, how should computational models described by networks of continuous neurons be characterized? The need for theories describing the operations and capabilities of machines that are analog or adaptive arises when one wants to describe and analyze nature's computation, as well as the already developing analog chips and adaptive technologies.

Analog Computation

Blum, Shub, and Smale (1989) introduced a discrete-time computational model that operates in each time step on real-valued registers. The BSS model is considered a model of computation over the real numbers, rather than a model of analog computation, because it lacks the property of local continuity (item 3 above). Hybrid models of computation behave similarly. These models combine discrete- and continuous-time dynamics, usually by means of ODEs that are governed by finite automata. Because of their finite automaton component, hybrid systems also do not adhere to local continuity. A coupled map lattice is the analog version of a cellular automaton. This model is composed of an infinite lattice of variables with a local homogeneous transition rule, and can be defined generally enough to include practically any discrete-time model. The general-purpose analog computers, by Shannon (1941) and by Pour-el (1974), are based on continuous-time operators and include integrators. Unlike their name, these models are not universal and not very general.

Of special interest in physical computation are analog systems based on dissipative dynamics. Dynamical systems are called dissipative if their dynamics converge to attractors. When a dissipative system has energy (Lyapunov) functional, the attractors are fixed points; otherwise, more complex attractors may appear. Dissipative systems are mainly popular in neural modeling of memory, such as in the Hopfield and other related models. The meaningful attractors of these networks, where information is stored, are all simple: either stable fixed points or limit cycles. There are various models of neural activity that report chaos, such as in the olfactory, though they are typically not being considered in computational terms.

The dynamics of dissipative systems can be thought of as computation: either the initial state or parameter values can be considered the input to a computational problem, the evolution along the trajectory is the computation process, and the attractor describes the solution. We realized (Siegelmann and Fishman, 1998) that while fixed points can be computed efficiently, chaotic attractors could only be computed efficiently by means of nondeterminism. The inherent difference between fixed points and chaotic attractors led us to propose that, in the realm of dynamical systems, efficient deterministic computation differs from efficient nondeterministic computation: Pd <> NPd.

A general theory of computation for dissipative dynamical systems was developed in Siegelmann, Ben-Hur, and Fishman (1999). This theory interprets the evolution of dissipative dynamical systems, both discrete and continuous in state space and in time, as a process of computation, and it relates the computational complexity to the true relaxation time. Prior to this work, no tool existed with which to analyze continuous-time algorithms and analog VLSI systems; ODE-based algorithms could only be analyzed by means of time discretization, which could result in loss of the main characteristics of these systems. We exemplified our theory with popular computer science problems, showing, e.g., a continuous algorithm for the maximum network flow problem that has linear time complexity, an algorithm for MAX that converges in logarithmic time, and a probabilistic continuous algorithm for the linear programming problem, which for a Gaussian distribution over instances of LP converges in linear time.

The analog recurrent neural network consists of a finite assembly of simple processors (or neurons), each of which computes a scalar—real-valued, continuous function, or activation, of an integrated input (Siegelmann and Sontag, 1994). This activation function is nonlinear and monotonic with bounded range, reminiscent of neural responses to input stimuli. The scalar value produced by a neuron is, in turn, broadcast to the successive neurons involved in a given computation. The existence of feedback loops in the interconnection graph allows the processing of arbitrarily long data with a fixed size network. A related model is the network of spiking neurons (see SPIKING NEURONS, COMPUTATION WITH, and INTEGRATE-AND-FIRE NEURONS AND NETWORKS). There, the neurons output binary values only, but the time intervals between consecutive spikes are considered exact analog value. The computational analysis of the two models is similar under the transformation of neural value and time interval.

Neural Automata

Unlike the von Neumann computer model, the structure of neural networks is not separated into a memory region and a processing unit; memory and processing are strongly coupled. Each neuron is part of the processing unit, and the memory is implicitly encoded in the mutual influence between any pair of neurons. The influence can be represented by a real number weight. The status of the weights prompts two different views of the neural mode according to whether the weights are perceived as unknown parameters or as fixed constants. When the weights are considered unknown parameters, the network is a semiparametric adaptive technology, able to approximate input-output mappings by means of parameter estimation/learning. When the weights are considered constant (after or without a process of adaptation), the networks can perform exact computations rather than mere approximations. We next consider the latter case.

In the McCulloch-Pitts neuron, the potential is updated by

$$u_i(t) = \sum_{j \in \text{in}(i)} w_{ij} x_j(t - 1) \tag{1}$$

where $\text{in}(i)$ is the set of presynaptic neurons of i and $w_{ij} \in \mathbb{R}$ is the weight on the edge directed from neuron j to neuron i. The activation value is updated by

$$x_i(t) = \mathcal{H}(u_i(t) - c_i) \tag{2}$$

where c_i is the firing threshold of neuron i and $\mathcal{H}$ is the binary response function

$$\mathcal{H}(x) = \begin{cases} 0, & x < 0 \\ 1, & x \geq 0 \end{cases}$$

In the analog recurrent network, the activation function is continuous, e.g., the sigmoid $\sigma(x) = 1/(1 + e^{-x})$, or the *saturated-linear function*:

$$\sigma(x) = \begin{cases} 0, & x \leq 0 \\ x, & 0 < x < 1 \\ 1, & x \geq 1 \end{cases} \tag{3}$$

The update equation of the basic analog neuron is

$$x_i(t) = \sigma(u_i(t) - c_i) \tag{4}$$

where u_i is defined as in Equation 1. Despite the similarity to the McCulloch-Pitts neurons, these two models are very different in their dynamical behavior and their computational power.

An asynchronous version of the analog neuron uses a potential, as in spiking neurons or integrate and fire neurons. Let $\mathcal{F}_j(t)$ be the set of firing times of neuron j until time t, and let ε_{ij} be a kernel function. The update equation of the neuronal potential is

$$u_i(t) = \sum_{j \in \text{in}(i)} \sum_{\tau \in \mathcal{F}_j(t)} w_{ij} \varepsilon_{ij}(t - \tau) \tag{5}$$

Some variants of this model take into account the refractory period as well.

Preliminaries: Language Recognition

The computer science approach of characterizing the discernibility between different inputs employs the concept of formal languages.

Let Σ be a set of symbols, e.g., $\{0, 1\}$, called an *alphabet*. Finite sequences of symbols in Σ are called *strings*. The set of all strings over Σ is denoted by Σ^*. A subset of Σ^* is called a *formal language*.

There are various ways to associate languages with automata, which are mostly equivalent. In this chapter we focus on language recognition. A *recognizer* reads an input string and decides whether the string is a correctly formed string of its language. Such a device has two types of halting states: accepting states and rejecting states. The language recognized or accepted by the automaton is the set of all input strings for which a computation ends in an accepting state. Thus, each automaton defines a language. Languages are divided into classes according to the type of automata that are needed to recognize them or the "difficulty" of recognizing them. Two types of automata are said to be equivalent if they accept the same class of languages.

A finite network of McCulloch-Pitts neurons has a finite memory only. This is far less than what one expects from a general digital computer. Even tasks like "decide whether there are more 0's or more 1's in a given binary input string" is not possible in a predefined size of memory. The formal description of a digital computer is in terms of the Turing machine. This consists of a control box with a finite memory coupled to a tape that is indefinitely expandable. The input is given by the initial state of the tape; the output is read off the tape if and when the Turing machine halts. Only with this extra tape are the languages recognized by digital machines captured mathematically.

To perceive neural automata as language recognition machines one needs to define an input-output convention. Two possibilities are outlined here. In the first the input is static, appearing in a designated set of neurons at the beginning of the computation. In the case of Boolean neurons, a finite network cannot encode an arbitrary number of symbols. (In this input convention one needs to consider a series of networks with an increasing number of input neurons.) In this article we consider mainly another input convention, where input arrives as a stream of symbols appearing consecutively on the input channels. This allows us to use a single network to recognize a language with strings of arbitrary length. In this convention, Equation 1 for the potential becomes

$$u_i(t) = \sum_{j \in in(i)} w_{ij} x_j(t - 1) + \sum_{j \in I} b_{ij} I_j(t - 1) \qquad (6)$$

where I is the set of input channels, $I_j(t)$ is the value of input channel j at time t, and b_{ij} are the weights that connect the input channels to the rest of the network. There are various possible conventions for halting a computation of an analog machine, such as convergence to a fixed point, or, as we will consider here, a designated neuron reaching some value. Acceptance is then decided from the value of another neuron. In asynchronous models, the input stream arrives in a predetermined sequence of times t_{in}^1, t_{in}^2, . . . at the input neurons.

Computational Power

Deterministic networks of Boolean McCulloch-Pitts neurons were studied first. Minsky (1967) showed that Boolean networks can simulate any combination of Boolean gates, and thus in particular, finite automata. Sima and Wiedermann (1998) have quantified the size of a network required to recognize a particular regular language. They also characterized the Hopfield languages—the languages recognized by Boolean automata with symmetric interconnections—as a strict subset of regular languages. If a series of Hopfield networks is considered in the static input convention, the computational power is much higher.

Analog recurrent neural networks have been analyzed in a series of papers and in Siegelmann (1999). Although the structure and dynamics of analog recurrent neural automata are very different from those of the von Neumann machine, the automata were found to compute exactly like the digital computer when their parameters took rational values. Moreover, in the absence of noise, and if the networks took real-valued weights, they became more powerful than digital computers and recognized nonrecursive (super-Turing) languages. In particular, the efficient computation class is "P/poly."

To explain the extra power stemming from the real weights, two more results were obtained (Siegelmann, 1999). In one, the complexity, or information content, of the weights was measured by a variant of resource-bounded Kolmogorov complexity, taking into account the time required for constructing the numbers. With Balczar and Gavald, we showed a full and proper hierarchy of nonuniform complexity classes associated with networks having weights of increasing Kolmogorov complexity, of which the classes "P" and "P/poly" are the two extreme cases.

Second, we proposed a new model that, although it seems digital, is still hypercomputational. This model is a network with rational weights only. In addition to the neurons, it includes a binary coin that outputs 0/1 with a probability p that is a real number. Although p is a real number, it is never accessed by any neuron (the coin is binary, so the other neurons receive from it digital values only). The computational power of this type of network is still hypercomputational (though less than "P/poly"). That is, the real value does not have to be explicit, but any process that is affected by a real number brings on nonrecursive computation.

All of the results mentioned in this section assume a noise-free environment.

Noisy/Probabilistic Analog Automata

The two classes of language that have arisen in noisy analog models are known as *regular* and *definite*. *Regular* languages are those accepted by finite automata. A language is called *definite* if for some integer r, any two strings coinciding on the last r symbols are either both or neither in the language. Definite languages are reminiscent of short-term memory. If the alphabet is finite, then definite languages are also regular; otherwise, they are not comparable with them.

Models of noisy analog neural networks were recently examined (e.g., Casey, 1996; Maass and Orponen, 1998; Maass and Sontag, 1999). The networks appeared to compute either regular or definite languages. Similarly, earlier models of probabilistic automata and circuits (e.g., Rabin, 1970; Paz, 1971; Pippenger, 1990) were found to compute sometimes regular and sometimes definite languages, depending on the properties of the probabilistic transition rules. These results make one wonder which details of the stochastic systems are essential for the computational power and which details are "accidental" aspects of the specific models. In particular, can one describe a general mechanism leading to the generation of these two classes of languages?

This challenge was partially met by Roitershtein and Siegelmann (1999), who proposed a general framework of stochastic computation. This framework, called *Markov computational systems* (MCS), includes all of the models just mentioned. Furthermore, it provides a natural way to introduce probabilistic counterparts of many diverse computational systems, such as topological automata, networks with nonfixed (e.g., growing) dimensions, hybrid systems that combine discrete and continuous variables, cellular automata, coupled map lattices, and the Blum, Shub, and Smale (1989) model.

In our generalization, the internal states of an automaton are substituted by distributions of states, and the transition function that guides the movement is substituted by operators, using an "operator theoretic" framework. The alphabet can be any set (e.g., real numbers) and so is the state space (e.g., not necessarily Euclidean or even metric).

Definition 1. An operator P acting in the space of finite measures defined on a measurable space $(\Omega, \mathcal{B})$ is said to be a *Markov operator* if for any probability measure μ, the image $P\mu$ is again a probability measure. A *Markov system* is a set of Markov operators defined on an alphabet Σ : $T = \{P_u : u \in \Sigma\}$.

A Markov system $T = \{P_u : u \in \Sigma\}$ is associated with a computational system, as follows. At each computational step $t = 0, 1, \ldots$, the system receives an input symbol, $u_t \in \Sigma$, and updates its state, $x_t \in \Omega$. Let $\mu_t(A)$ be the probability of finding x_t in the set A. The evolution of the system is governed by the update equation, $\mu_{t+1} = P_{u_t}\mu_t$.

For an input sequence $w = w_0 w_1 \cdots w_n \in \Sigma^{n+1}$, define a Markov operator $P_w = P_{w_n} \ldots P_{w_1} P_{w_0}$. If the probability distribution on the initial states is given by the probability measure μ_0, then the distribution of states after $n + 1$ computational steps on the input $w = w_0, w_1, \ldots, w_n$ is defined by

$$P_w \mu_0(A) = P_{w_n} \cdots P_{w_1} P_{w_0} \mu_0 \qquad (7)$$

Let $\mathcal{A}$ be the set of "accepting" probability distributions, and let $\mathcal{R}$ be the set of "rejecting" probability distributions. We need the condition

$$\mathrm{dist}(\mathcal{A}, \mathcal{R}) = \inf_{\mu \in \mathcal{A}, v \in \mathcal{R}} \|\mu - v\|_1 = \rho > 0 \qquad (8)$$

where $\|\cdot\|_1$ is the total variation norm $\|\mu\|_1 = \sup_A \mu(A) - \inf_A \mu(A)$. Then, a Markov computational system is defined to accept or reject the input according to the distribution it has after reading the input string.

Quasi-compactness and Regular Languages

$T = \{P_w : w \in \Sigma^*\}$ is considered quasi-compact when:

1. The alphabet Σ is finite.
2. The operators P_w are "close to being compact" in the sense that there exist $r > 0$ and $\delta < 1$ such that for every input string w of length r, there exists a compact operator Q_w, which satisfies $\|P_w - Q_w\|_1 \le \delta$.

We proved the correlation between quasi-compact operators and the recognition of regular languages. Special cases of automata that satisfy the above condition are the probabilistic automata of Rabin (1970) and the noisy model of Maass and Orponen (1998). Various conditions leading to quasi-compactness were shown.

Weak Ergodicity and Definite Languages

Probabilistic computational models with the power to recognize definite languages have their roots in Rabin's (1970) pioneering work on probabilistic automata. Paz (1971) generalized the method and introduced the notion of weak ergodicity for automata having a denumerable state space. Maass and Sontag (1999) focused on analog recurrent neural nets perturbed with additive Gaussian-like noise of a certain type. We pinpointed the underlying connection

of this chain and formalized its ultimate generalization. For this, we redefined weak ergodicity to describe all probabilistic systems that mix their probability distributions to the extent that they approach the uniform distribution. More formally,

Definition 2. A Markov system $\{P_u, u \in \Sigma\}$ is called *weakly ergodic* if for every $\alpha > 0$, there is an integer $r = r(\alpha)$ such that for any string w with length larger than r and any two probability distributions μ, v,

$$\|P_w \mu - P_w v\|_1 \le \alpha \qquad (9)$$

Let $\mathcal{M}$ be defined with a weakly ergodic operator set. Then it recognizes only definite languages.

Remark 1. Weakly ergodic systems are robust with respect to perturbations of the system parameters and under some types of external noise.

Road Map: Computability and Complexity
Background: I.1. Introducing the Neuron
Related Reading: Analog Neural Nets: Computational Power

References

Blum, L., Shub, M., and Smale, S., 1989, On a theory of computation and complexity over the real numbers: NP completeness, recursive functions, and universal machines, *Bull. AMS*, 21:1–46.

Casey, M., 1996, The dynamics of discrete-time computation, with application to recurrent neural networks and finite state machine extraction, *Neural Computat.*, 8:1135–1178.

Maass, W., and Orponen, P., 1998, On the effect of analog noise in discrete time computation, *Neural Computat.*, 10:1071–1095.

Maass, W., and Sontag, E., 1999, Analog neural nets with Gaussian or other common noise distribution cannot recognize arbitrary regular languages, *Neural Computat.*, 11:771–782.

Minsky, M., 1967, *Computation: Finite and Infinite Machines*, Englewood Cliffs, NJ: Prentice Hall.

Paz, A., 1971, *Introduction to Probabilistic Automata*, London: Academic Press.

Pippenger, N., 1990, Developments in: The synthesis of reliable organisms from unreliable components, *Proc. Symp. Pure Math.*, 5:311–324.

Pour-El, M. B., 1974, Abstract computability and its relation to the general purpose analog-computer (some connections between logic, differential equations and analog computers), *Trans. AMS*, 199:1–29.

Rabin, M., 1970, Probabilistic automata, *Inform. Control*, 41:539–550.

Roitershtein, A., and Siegelmann, H. T., 1999, On Markov computational systems, Information Systems Engineering, Haifa, Israel, typescript.

Shannon, C. E., 1941, Mathematical theory of the differential analyzer, *J. Math. Phys. MIT*, 20:337–354.

Siegelmann, H. T., 1999, *Neural Networks and Analog Computation: Beyond the Turing Limit*, Boston: Birkhauser.

Siegelmann, H. T., Ben-Hur, A., and Fishman, S., 1999, Computational complexity for continuous time dynamics, *Phys. Rev. Lett.*, 83:1463–1466.

Siegelmann, H. T., and Fishman, S., 1998, Computation by dynamical systems, *Physica D*, 120:214–235.

Siegelmann, H. T., and Sontag, E. D., 1994, Analog computation via neural networks, *Theoret. Comput. Sci.*, 131:331–360.

Sima, J., and Wiedermann, J., 1998, Theory of neuromata, *J. ACM*, 45:155–178.

Neuroanatomy in a Computational Perspective

Almut Schüz

Introduction

This article is intended to help the modeler get a feel for real brains. It provides an introduction to basic principles of brain organization and to network structures within the brain. By focusing especially on the cerebral cortex, the article shows how quantitative neuroanatomy can contribute to brain theory.

The Role of Neuroanatomy in Brain Theory

In simple organisms in which the sensory organs are connected by direct pathways and effectors (muscles, glands), tracing such pathways may provide a sufficient explanation of behavior. However, in the course of evolution, the number of neurons has increased considerably and the pathways between input and output have become less and less direct.

The human brain contains between 7×10^{10} and 8×10^{10} neurons (Haug, 1986). Most of them belong to the cerebellar cortex (approximately 5×10^{10}) and the cerebral cortex (approximately 1.5×10^{10}). Many other parts of the human brain, such as the first relay station of the optic nerve in the thalamus, contain about 10^6 neurons. The corpus callosum, the main fiber bundle that connects the two hemispheres, consists of about 10^8 fibers. For a comprehensive collection of neuroanatomical measures, see Blinkov and Glezer (1968).

In small mammals, the numbers of neurons are reduced by a factor of about 1000 compared to the human brain. The cerebral cortex of the mouse, for example, contains about 10^7 neurons, and the corpus callosum of the mouse contains about 10^5 fibers. But even with these reduced numbers, a complete assessment of the neuronal network would be a hopeless undertaking.

However, the high number of neurons is not the main obstacle to understanding the neural mechanisms underlying higher brain functions. The situation is complicated by the fact that most connections in the brain are not one to one. In most nerve networks, it is beyond practical means to trace the anatomical pathways in detail. Many neurons receive input from thousands of other neurons and distribute their output to just as many. Physiologically, even if a direct anatomical connection between two neurons were demonstrated, whether the activity of neuron A leads to the activation of neuron B largely depends on what else is going on in the network.

Thus, in complex nerve networks, the task of neuroanatomy is not so much to study all of the connections in detail, but rather to show the typical structural properties that characterize a specific part of the brain. These properties provide clues to the understanding of its specific function, as will be shown later for the cerebral cortex.

White and Gray Matter: Projection Versus Computation

One general principle of construction in the brain is the spatial separation of long axons (composing the "white" matter) from the synaptic tissue in which the signal exchange between neurons occurs—the "gray" matter. Over short axons running within the gray matter, a neuron can reach other neurons within a radius of a few hundred microns, up to a few millimeters at most; but through the white matter, neurons can reach cells located in the centimeter range and in distant regions of the brain and spinal cord.

The largest mass of white matter in the human brain is that of the cerebral cortex. The white matter of the hemispheres consists largely of fibers that connect different parts of the cortex to each other. Apparently, one of the principles of cortical connectivity is the rich projection of the cortex onto itself. In contrast, the thin sheet of white matter accompanying the cerebellar cortex indicates that local computation plays a major role in this part of the brain (Braitenberg, Heck, and Sultan, 1997).

White Matter, Brain Size, and Connectedness

Large brains have comparatively more cortical white matter than do small brains. For example, 42% of the human neocortex (white and gray matter taken together) is white matter, while in the hedgehog the white matter content is only 13% (Frahm, Stephan, and Stephan, 1982). Clearly, if one wants to connect a large cortex in a style similar to one with fewer neurons, the fiber mass has to increase more than proportionately to the number of neurons. The question is whether the increase in white matter with brain size indicates an increasing, decreasing, or constant degree of interconnectedness. The answer is either decreasing or constant, depending on whether one is focusing on individual neurons or on groups of neurons. The percentage of neurons of the cortex reached by an individual neuron is definitely lower in larger cortices than in smaller ones. However, if one defines compartments the size of the largest dendritic trees in each species, and if one postulates a complete set of connections between all the compartments, the relative increase in white matter corresponds to a roughly constant interconnectedness (Braitenberg, 2001).

In a similar way, Mitchison (1992) showed that if the neurons in the cortex were not organized into spatially distinct areas connected through the white matter, but were merged into one huge piece of gray matter, the volume of the human cortex would have to increase by a factor of 10 to maintain the same degree of connectedness.

Not only the number of connections but also time delays play a role in the interconnectedness of various parts of a network. In a large brain, distant elements may not be able to collaborate efficiently owing to delays in the transmission from one point to the other. Since conduction velocity depends on the thickness of an axon, this problem could theoretically be solved by an appropriate increase in the diameter of the longer axons in larger brains. However, this remedy is self-defeating; thicker fibers would further increase brain size and therefore increase time delays, which would in turn require thicker fibers, and so on. Starting with a brain as large as the human one, such a series would converge at a volume approximately 50% larger if one wanted interhemispheric signals to travel twice as fast as they do (Ringo et al., 1994). As a way out of this dilemma, Ringo et al. (1994) have proposed a higher degree of functional specialization of cortical regions in larger brains.

Overall Connectivity of the Brain

There are no isolated parts of the brain; there are fiber connections, direct or indirect, from any part of the brain to every other. Nevertheless, the brain is highly structured. Some parts (e.g., the cerebral cortex and the thalamus) interact directly with each other by way of reciprocal connections. Other parts may be arranged in loops, such as (1) the cerebral cortex–basal ganglia–thalamus (ventral anterior nucleus)–cerebral cortex loop and (2) the cerebral cortex–pontine nuclei–cerebellum (ventral lateral nucleus)–thalamus–cerebral cortex loop.

Such loops may traverse the same part of the brain and remain separate, as is the case for the two loops just mentioned when they pass through the thalamus. At other places, cross-talk may occur.

As a matter of fact, the cortical regions involved in these two loops overlap (Rouiller et al., 1994). In addition, shortcuts to the main stream may exist, parallel routes through further relay stations may accompany part of a loop, or subloops may be added to the main loop (see BASAL GANGLIA). Depending on the neurons involved, a signal can be fed back either negatively or positively onto the place of its origin. Positive feedback can also be transmitted by way of disinhibition when two inhibitory stations are connected in series. This type of positive feedback characterizes the cortico-cortical loop through the basal ganglia.

The projections between the various parts of the brain mostly suggest parallel processing in the sense that large regions of one part are connected to large regions of another by thousands or millions of fibers.

Sometimes, the projections from one part of the brain to another form patterns that suggest special kinds of computation. For example, the projections may be organized such that neighborhood relationships are maintained (e.g., the retinotopic projections in the visual system). In other cases, complex, patchy divergent, or convergent patterns may occur, suggesting a combination of inputs from different sources and/or distribution of inputs to disparate loci (e.g., projections from the various regions of the cerebral cortex to the basal ganglia).

The projections can also differ in that they may be point to point in some cases (sometimes one point to several points), while in others the terminal arbors of the axons may be smeared over large regions of the target structure. In a sense, this anatomical distinction corresponds to an important functional difference. Relatively restricted terminal arbors are typical for pathways that are involved in computation, such as those between the specific thalamic nuclei and the cerebral cortex or between cortical neurons. In contrast, huge terminal arbors extending over large portions of the brain and coming from small nuclei in the brainstem (e.g., the locus coeruleus) are involved in the global regulation of the level of activity, providing the background on which the information processing takes place (see EMOTIONAL CIRCUITS).

Geometry of the Gray Matter

Some of the structural features of the various parts of the brain are easily recognized at both the macroscopic and the microscopic level. The gray matter can either form lumps (often called nuclei) or show a two-dimensional, layered arrangement as in the so-called cortices. With respect to function, the latter type suggests that the same kind of operation is performed over the whole surface. One would expect such an arrangement, for example, in the processing of two-dimensional pictures. Indeed, this type of arrangement is found in centers for visual processing in all vertebrates, as well as in many invertebrates. Among the cortices, further distinctions can be made (Figure 1). In the cerebral cortex, the plane is isotropic in the sense that different directions cannot be distinguished in the histological picture. In contrast, in the cerebellar cortex, two perpendicular dimensions of the cortical plane are organized in completely different ways. Most of the axons run in a laterolateral direction, while the dendritic trees of the same layer extend in planes perpendicular to this.

A mixture of these two types also exists. In the hippocampus, the dendrites and some axonal systems are spread in all directions of the plane, while other axonal systems (mossy fibers, Schaffer collaterals) superimposed onto these run in one direction only. Furthermore, the serial reentrant arrangement of the latter is suggestive of cyclic operation (Figure 1C).

In contrast to cortices, geometry does not seem to play an important role in many nuclei. Their fine structure appears to be isotropic in all directions (Figure 1D).

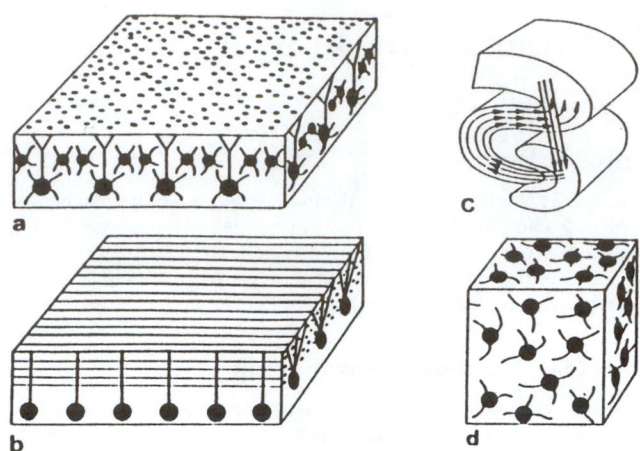

Figure 1. Different types of geometry in the gray matter. *A*, The structure in the horizontal plane is isotropic and different from that in the vertical plane (as in the cerebral cortex). *B*, All three planes of sectioning are different from each other (as in the cerebellar cortex). *C*, In the hippocampus, the horizontal (folded) plane is isotropic, but overlaid by a subpopulation of fibers that run in one direction only. These are, furthermore, arranged such that a cyclic operation is suggested. *D*, All three dimensions are equal. [Modified from Braitenberg, V., and Schüz, A., 1993, Allgemeine Neuroanatomie, in *Neuro- und Sinnesphysiologie* (R. F. Schmidt, Ed.), Berlin: Springer.]

Histology and Connectivity

Different parts of the brain differ with respect to density and size of neurons, shape of axonal and dendritic trees, or arrangement in layers. But in spite of our detailed knowledge of such structural features, it is difficult to grasp the underlying principles of connectivity. What are the rules, for example, behind the felt of axons stained in Figure 2? To how many neurons do they belong and where do they come from? Is what we see in Figure 2 an intermingling of separate circuits, or are these fibers part of the same network?

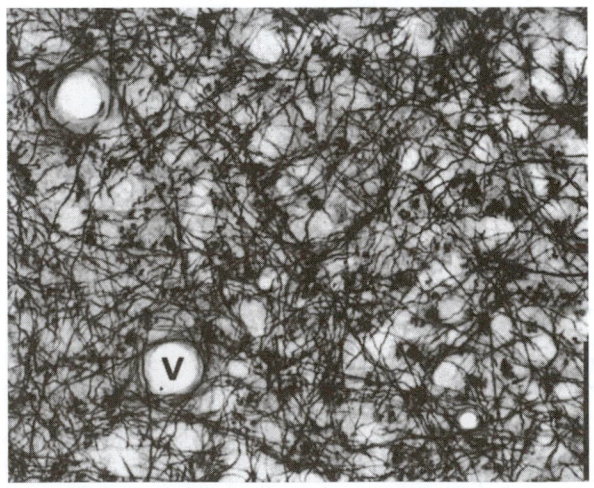

Figure 2. Axonal net. Light micrograph of the visual cortex of a monkey (area 17). A horizontal section is shown through layer IV. Only axons are stained. V indicates a blood vessel. The bar equals 50 μm.

Specific Versus Statistical Connectivity

One crucial problem springs to mind in view of a fiber felt as shown in Figure 2: the degree to which the target of an individual fiber is defined. This question is relevant to the anatomist in determining at what level of detail to analyze the structure. The theoretician, too, must decide whether to base a model on a certain well-defined connectivity or on a random network. (For a more comprehensive treatment of this topic, see Arbib, Érdi, and Szentágothai, 1998).

In Figure 3, three possibilities are depicted. In Figure 3A, neurons of type A connect to neurons of type B in a strictly defined manner. There is specificity between types (A, B) and between individual neurons ($A_{1/1}$ and $A_{2/1}$ to B_1; $A_{1/2}$ and $A_{2/2}$ to B_2; etc.). A prerequisite for this kind of connectivity is that the neurons can be labeled individually, either by their geometric arrangement or by some other means, such as a chemical marker. On the other hand, the specificity could be restricted to types of neurons (e.g., A connects to B only) without further specification, as shown in Figure 3B. In this case, it is no longer crucial whether a certain neuron A connects to a particular neuron B rather than to its neighbor.

In the third case (Figure 3C), there is no specificity whatsoever. The neurons of both types are intermingled and connect to the cells they happen to meet.

All three types of connectivity are realized in nature. An example of the first kind is the visual system of the fly. There, the photoreceptors are arranged in strict geometric order and connect to the first optic ganglion in a completely determined manner.

The second kind of network describes the situation in the cerebellar cortex. There, it is determined how the various types of neurons are connected. The granule cells, for example, connect to the other four cell types of the cerebellar cortex, but not to other granule cells; basket cells contact only Purkinje cells; and so on.

The network in Figure 3C comes close to the situation in the cerebral cortex. With the exception of the chandelier cells, which have been found to connect to pyramidal cells only, pyramidal and nonpyramidal cells connect to each other and often in the expected proportion, although interesting biases also occur (see White, 1989). The overall connectivity depends, then, on the density of neurons, on their ramification patterns, on the location of their terminal arbors, and on the relative numbers of the various cell types. These constraints, which are of a probabilistic nature, are in part genetically determined and in part refined by activity-dependent self-organization (see SELF-ORGANIZATION AND THE BRAIN).

Statistical Neuroanatomy

One approach to the question of connectivity in complex nerve networks is a quantitative assessment of the various components shown by the different histological methods (cell bodies, synapses, axons, etc.). How such data can be used to determine the structural properties of a network and to constrain neural models accordingly was shown in detail for the cerebral cortex (see Braitenberg and Schüz, 1998, and references therein). The main points are briefly summarized here.

Basic Structure of the Cerebral Cortex

Some of the quantities that have been measured are shown in Table 1 (*a–m*). They refer to the mouse cortex and are corrected for tissue shrinkage. The letters *n–s* show further quantities that can be derived from those. A number of these quantities require some explanation.

The *relative density of axons* (Table 1, *q*) is defined as follows. Imagine a piece of cortex punched out perpendicularly to the cortical surface and just large enough to contain the local axonal tree of an individual neuron within the gray matter. If the total length of this individual axon is divided by the sum of the lengths of all axons within this volume, the relative axonal density is obtained. It quantifies the axonal contribution of an individual neuron to the

Table 1. Quantitative Anatomy of the Mouse Cerebral Cortex

Measured quantities

a: Volume (iso- and allocortex)	2×87 mm^3
b: No. of sensory input fibers	$<10^6$
c: Density of neurons	9.2×10^4/mm^3
d: Percent pyramidal cells	85%
e: Density of synapses	7.2×10^8/mm^3
f: Percent type I synapses	89%
g: Percent synapses on spines	75%
h: Density of axons	4 km/mm^3
i: Density of dendrites	0.4 km/mm^3
j: Length of axonal tree	10–40 mm
k: Length of dendritic tree	4 mm
l: Range of axonal tree (pyramidal cell)	1 mm
m: Range of dendritic tree	0.2 mm

Deduced quantities

n: (a, c) Total no. of neurons	1.6×10^7
o: (c, e) Synapses/neuron	8000
p: (e, h) Synapses/length of axon	200/mm
q: (h, j, l) Relative density of axons (pyramidal cells)	10^{-5}
r: (i, k, m) Relative density of dendrites (pyramidal cells)	10^{-3}
s: (p, q, r) Probability of synapses between two pyramidal cells 0.2–0.3 mm apart	0 synapses, $p = 0.9$
	1 synapse, $p = 0.09$
	2 synapses, $p = 0.004$

Conclusions

t: (b, n) No. of neurons $\gg$ no. of input fibers
u: (d, f, g) Most connections between neurons of one kind
v: (f) Most connections excitatory
w: (o, s) Great divergence and convergence
x: (s) Connections very weak
y: (u–x) Mixing machine
z: (t, u, g) Memory rather than computation
z': (y, z) Associative memory with formation of cell assemblies

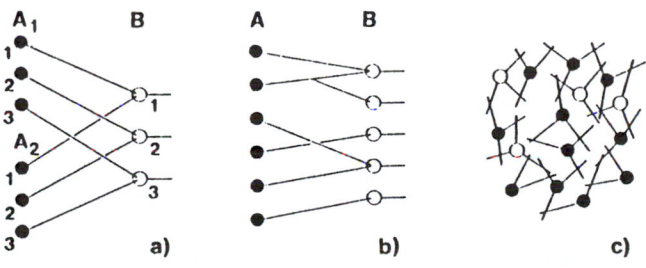

a)   b)   c)

Figure 3. Three networks illustrating various degrees of specificity. *A*, All connections are determined. *B*, The connections are specified only with respect to type, not with respect to individual neurons. *C*, There is no specificity. [From Schüz, A., 1992, Randomness and constraints in the cortical neuropil, in *Information Processing in the Cortex* (A. Aertsen, and V. Braitenberg, Eds.), Berlin: Springer, fig. 1, p. 4. Reprinted with permission.]

Modified from Braitenberg and Schüz (1998). The numbers represent measurements on light and electron micrographs from the cortex of the mouse (*a–m*), quantities that can be deduced from those measurements (*n–s*), and conclusions that can be drawn for the connectivity (*t–x*), as well as the functional interpretation (*y–z'*). The letters in parentheses indicate from which other quantities the corresponding quantity or conclusion can be derived.

neuropil within which it ramifies and is a measure for the intermingling of axons belonging to different neurons. The *relative density of dendrites* (r) is derived similarly by dividing the dendritic length of an individual neuron by the sum of the lengths of all dendrites present in the volume within which the dendritic arbor ramifies.

The *probability of synapses between two pyramidal cells* (s) is determined on the basis of $p–r$ and the assumption that a synapse between two neurons is made wherever the axon of one touches a dendrite of the other. The probability of this occurrence decreases with distance, i.e., with decreasing overlap between the two neurons.

From these data, some properties of cortical connectivity can be inferred (Table 1, $t–x$). A functional interpretation is also given in Table 1 ($y–z'$).

In short, the network of the cortex consists mainly of one type of neuron, the pyramidal cells (including the spiny stellate cells), which are connected by excitatory synapses. Most of these synapses are located on dendritic spines. Since synapses on spines are assumed to be modifiable in strength, one may conclude that one of the main tasks of the cortex is storage of information.

Nonpyramidal cells (about 15%) are interspersed among the pyramidal cells. They are inhibitory. Pyramidal and most kinds of nonpyramidal cells connect onto each other. The inhibitory neurons, however, contribute only about 11% of the synapses in the cortex. The number of synapses contributed by input fibers is small compared with the number of synapses that connect cortical neurons to each other. Most pyramidal cells have a local axonal tree, which connects them to other neurons in their neighborhood, as well as a far-reaching axonal tree, which, in most cases, connects them to another region of the cortex through the white matter.

The low relative axonal and dendritic densities have interesting implications. In the mouse, the local axonal tree of an individual pyramidal cell is interwoven with the dendrites of 10^5 other neurons and competes with axons from approximately 5×10^5 other neurons ramifying in the same territory. Geometric considerations suggest that multiple synapses (more than 2 or 3 between any pair of neurons) account for only a small percentage of the whole synaptic population of a neuron. This makes it probable that the 8000 synapses of a pyramidal cell connect to thousands of different neighbors. Thus, theories based on a probabilistic connectivity, as sketched in Figure 3*C*, seem to be appropriate.

For the most part, the knowledge gained from the mouse cortex applies to mammals in general. Some of the numbers in Table 1 differ with brain size according to known rules *(a–c, j–m)*; others seem to be constant *(d–i)*. For some, the dependence on brain size is not yet clear *(q–s)*, but the differences and uncertainties are not strong enough to affect the conclusions about the basic connectivity and function of the cortex.

Basic Function of the Cortex

This description of cortical structure fits Hebb's theory of cell assemblies remarkably well. This theory postulates that meaningful events are represented by groups of neurons that are connected more strongly to each other than to other neurons. These groups are formed through a learning process (see HEBBIAN SYNAPTIC PLASTICITY). The learning is assumed to strengthen the connections between neurons that are often activated together, a process known as *associative storage* (see ASSOCIATIVE NETWORKS).

For such cell assemblies to form, a large number of neurons of the same type must be connected into a network. What is crucial is an initial connectivity that is sufficiently rich to allow as many constellations of neuronal activity as possible to be detected and learned in the connections. The fact that the individual pyramidal cell seems to strive toward a large number of different synaptic neighbors, together with the large mass of corticocortical fibers,

indicates that the cortex is well suited for this task. The excitatory and modifiable synapses that are implicit in Hebb's theory are also present in the cortex. The fact that individual neurons are weakly connected through one or only a few synapses implies that only correlated activity of many neurons can activate another neuron. This implication is also in agreement with the theory of cell assemblies.

The linkage of the structure of the cortex with the theory of cell assemblies has led to more precise formulations of this concept. It permits estimates of the storage capacity of the cortex and the size and internal structure of cell assemblies (Palm, 1993) and allows concrete ideas to develop about the regulation of their dynamics through the hippocampus (Miller, 1991) or the striatum (Miller and Wickens, 1991).

Other Basic Principles of Connectivity

The connectivity of the cortex contrasts with that of other parts of the brain. The *cerebellar cortex* differs from the cerebral cortex primarily in its complete lack of positive feedback connections within the cortex and in its strict geometric order, which indicates computation along quasi-one-dimensional lines (Figure 1). These and other structural features suggest that the cerebellar cortex plays a role in the detection of sequences, a view supported by recent experimental evidence (Braitenberg et al., 1997). In addition, the cerebellar cortex stands out by virtue of its very large number of granule cells, which exceeds the number of neurons in the rest of the brain. Their small size and large numbers suggest a combinatorial richness of mossy fiber inputs that may be essential for the subtleties of motor coordination (Arbib et al., 1998).

Another contrasting network is the *striatum*. Although the cerebral cortex and the striatum have a number of features in common, a fundamental difference is that the cortex operates primarily on the basis of mutual excitation of neurons, while mutual inhibition seems to play an essential role in the striatum. There, more than 90% of the neurons (the medium spiny neurons) are GABAergic and, in addition to providing the output, make axon collaterals within the striatum. Thus, while the dominating principle in the cortex seems to be cooperation, the internal connectivity of the striatum suggests competition between neurons (Miller and Wickens, 1991; Wickens and Oorschot, 2000).

A basic difference also exists between cortex and *thalamus*. As in the cortex, most of the neurons in the thalamic relay nuclei are excitatory. However, in contrast to the neurons in the cortex, the lack of axon collaterals within the relay nuclei indicates that the excitatory neurons in the thalamus do not make synapses with each other (Steriade, Jones, and Llinás, 1990).

Homogeneity Versus Heterogeneity of Brain Structures

Some parts of the brain show local anatomical variations; others do not. For example, the cerebellar cortex exhibits no obvious differences over its whole extent.

In the striatum, compartments known as striosomes can be detected with histochemical methods. They differ from the surrounding matrix not only in their histochemistry but also in their input-output organization. The medium spiny neurons, the main cell type, are located in both regions but tend to avoid crossing the boundaries between striosomes and matrix (Penny, Wilson, and Kitai, 1988).

In the cerebral cortex, local differences on a large scale are the basis of its division into areas. These differences are of a kind that influences the statistics of the connectivity between neurons (density of neurons in the various layers; size, shape, and density of dendritic and axonal fields). Cortical areas can differ along two coordinates: the coordinate of hierarchy and the coordinate of modality. Hierarchy is reflected, for example, in the degree of myelination. Overall myelination diminishes with increasing distance from the primary sensory and motor areas. The existence of a well-developed layer IV in primary sensory fields is another example. In addition, the size of the local axonal fields of pyramidal cells, as well as the size of basal dendritic trees, increases with distance from the periphery, at least in the visual system (for details, see Schüz and Miller, 2002). The coordinate of modality is reflected in the fact that primary areas not only share commonalities that set them apart from higher cortical areas, but also differ one from the other. Such differences characterize the most conspicuous neocortical areas: the primary visual cortex in primates, with its particularly prominent layering; the somatosensory cortex in some rodents, with the barrel field (see SOMATOSENSORY SYSTEM); and the primary motor cortex, with its huge corticospinal neurons.

Some histological methods, particularly the cytochromoxidase method and tracer methods, also reveal substructure *within* cortical areas—usually, bands or patches a few hundred microns in diameter, which are best known in the visual system (Arbib et al., 1998; see also OCULAR DOMINANCE AND ORIENTATION COLUMNS; VISUAL CORTEX: ANATOMICAL STRUCTURE AND MODELS OF FUNCTION). To a large extent, this phenomenon is the result of the alternating insertion of input bundles from different sources (via the white matter) into a relatively homogeneous internal network. Intracortical axonal ramifications of pyramidal cells, however, may also exhibit a patchy distribution, particularly in large brains. These patches connect columns with similar functional properties. In contrast to the situation in the striatum, the dendritic trees seem to freely cross borders between columns, an arrangement that suggests a maximization of diversity in neuronal connections (Malach, 1994; see also Dinse and Schreiner in Schüz and Miller, 2002).

Road Map: Mammalian Brain Regions
Related Reading: Basal Ganglia; Cerebellum and Motor Control; Cortical Hebbian Modules; Neocortex: Basic Neuron Types; Visual Cortex: Anatomical Structure and Models of Function

References

Arbib, A. M., Érdi, P., and Szentágothai, J., 1998, *Neural Organization: Structure, Function, and Dynamics*, Cambridge, MA: MIT Press. ◆
Blinkov, S. M., and Glezer, I. I., 1968, *The Human Brain in Figures and Tables: A Quantitative Handbook*, New York: Plenum.
Braitenberg, V., 2001, Brain size and number of neurons: An exercise in synthetic neuroanatomy, *J. Computational Neurosci.*, 10:71–77.
Braitenberg, V., and Schüz, A., 1998, *Cortex: Statistics and Geometry of Neuronal Connectivity* (2nd edition of *Anatomy of the Cortex: Statistics and Geometry*), Berlin: Springer-Verlag. ◆
Braitenberg, V., Heck, D., and Sultan, F., 1997, The detection and generation of sequences as a key to cerebellar function: Experiments and theory, *Behav. Brain Sci.*, 20(2):229–277.
Frahm, H. D., Stephan, H., and Stephan, M., 1982, Comparison of brain structure volumes in insectivora and primates, I: Neocortex, *J. Hirnforsch.*, 23:375–389.
Haug, H., 1986, History of neuromorphometry, *J. Neurosci. Methods*, 18:1–17.
Malach, R., 1994, Cortical columns as devices for maximizing neuronal diversity, *Trends Neurosci.*, 17(3):101–104.
Miller, R., 1991, *Cortico-hippocampal Interplay and the Representation of Contexts in the Brain*, Berlin: Springer. ◆
Miller, R., and Wickens, J. R., 1991, Corticostriatal cell assemblies in selective attention and in representation of predictable and controllable events: A general statement of corticostriatal interplay and the role of striatal dopamine, *CINS (Concepts Neurosci.)*, 2:65–95.
Mitchison, G., 1992, Axonal trees and cortical architecture, *Trends Neurosci.*, 15:122–126.
Palm, G., 1993, On the internal structure of cell assemblies, in *Brain Theory: Spatio-temporal Aspects of Brain Function* (A. Aertsen, Ed.), Amsterdam: Elsevier, pp. 261–270.
Penny, G. R., Wilson, C. J., and Kitai, S. T., 1988, Relationship of the axonal and dendritic geometry of spiny projection neurons to the compartmental organization of the neostriatum, *J. Comp. Neurol.*, 269:275–289.
Ringo, J. L., Doty, R. W., Demeter, S., and Simard, P. Y., 1994, Time is of the essence: A conjecture that hemispheric specialization arises from interhemispheric conduction delay, *Cereb. Cortex*, 4:331–343.
Rouiller, E. M., Liang, F., Babalian, A., Moret, V., and Wiesendanger, M., 1994, Cerebellothalamocortical and pallidothalamicocortical projections to the primary and supplementary motor cortical areas: A multiple tracing study in macaque monkeys, *J. Comp. Neurol.*, 345:185–213.
Schüz, A., and Miller, R. (Eds.), 2002, *Cortical Areas: Unity and Diversity*, London: Taylor & Francis.
Steriade, M., Jones, E. G., and Llinás, R. R., 1990, *Thalamic Oscillations and Signaling*, New York, Chichester: John Wiley & Sons.
White, E. L., 1989, *Cortical Circuits: Synaptic Organization of the Cerebral Cortex—Structure, Function and Theory*, Boston: Birkhäuser. ◆
Wickens, J., and Oorschot, D. E., 2000, Neural dynamics and surround inhibition in the neostriatum, in *Brain Dynamics and the Striatal Complex* (R. Miller and J. Wickens, Eds.), Australia, Canada: Harwood Academic Publishers.

Neuroethology, Computational

Dave Cliff

Introduction

Over the past decade, a number of neural network researchers have used the term *computational neuroethology* to describe a specific approach to neuroethology. *Neuroethology* is the study of the neural mechanisms underlying the generation of behavior in animals, and hence it lies at the intersection of neuroscience (the study of the nervous systems) and ethology (the study of animal behavior); for an introduction to neuroethology, see Simmons and Young (1999). The definition of computational neuroethology is very similar, but is not quite so dependent on studying animals: animals just happen to be biological *autonomous agents*. But there are also non-biological autonomous agents, such as some types of robots and some types of simulated embodied agents operating in virtual worlds. In this context, autonomous agents are self-governing entities capable of operating (i.e., coordinating perception and action) for extended periods of time in environments that are complex, uncertain, and dynamic. Thus, computational neuroethology can be characterized as the attempt to analyze the computational principles underlying the generation of behavior in animals and in artificial autonomous agents. For the sake of brevity, in the rest of this article autonomous agents will be referred to simply as agents, and computational neuroethology will be abbreviated to CNE.

CNE can be distinguished from classical computational neuroscience by its increased emphasis on studying the neural control of behavior within the context of neural systems that are both embodied and situated within an environment. The "computational" nature of CNE comes not so much from treating neural systems as inherently computational devices, but rather in the use of sophisticated computer-based simulation and visualization tools for exploring issues in neuroethology.

Put most simply, CNE involves the use of computational modeling in trying to understand the neural mechanisms responsible for generating "useful" behaviors in an agent. The word useful is rather imprecise; it is more common to talk of *adaptive* behaviors. In the ethology literature, an adaptive behavior is usually defined as a behavior that increases the likelihood that an animal will survive long enough to produce viable offspring. Often implicit in this definition is the assumption that the animal's environment is sufficiently unforgiving (or hostile) that if the animal does nothing, it will die before it can reproduce. In studying artificial agents, the utility of behavior is frequently evaluated by less harsh criteria, such as observed behaviors scored according to some metric that indicates how close they come to satisfying some set of performance objectives or criteria.

Neural networks that generate adaptive behavior should not be confused with adaptive neural networks, where connection strengths may alter as a result of experience. Adaptation or plasticity may itself give rise to new or improved adaptive behaviors, but there are many cases of adaptive behaviors that are genetically determined (e.g., "hardwired" behaviors such as reflexes and instincts).

When CNE is approached in the context of adaptive behavior research, it becomes clear that the neural system is just one component in the *action-perception cycle*, where an agent's actions may alter what information it perceives concerning its environment, and where those alterations in perceived information may lead to changes in the agent's internal state, and where those changes in state may in turn affect further actions, thereby affecting what information is subsequently perceived, and so on. Thus, crucially, the agent's nervous system, body, and environment all combine to form a tightly coupled dynamical system. This is a notion long stressed by Arbib:

> In speaking of human perception, we often talk as if a purely passive process of classification were involved—of being able, when shown an object, to respond by naming it correctly. However, for most of the perception of most animals and much of human behavior, it is more appropriate to say that the animal perceives its environment to the extent that it is *prepared* to *interact* with that environment in some reasonably structured fashion (1972, p. 16).

As defined thus far, CNE may not seem to be particularly distinguishable from most work in neural network research. After all, many people in computational neural network research might argue that their work will, ultimately, lead to understanding of the neural mechanisms underlying the generation of (some) adaptive behaviors. For example, face recognition is an adaptive behavior in humans and could probably be classed as an adaptive behavior in, say, a security robot. So why can't a backpropagation network that learns to distinguish between photographs of human faces (for example) be classed as work in CNE?

Motivations

Typically, artificial neural network models employ homogeneous groups of highly idealized and simplified neuron models (called *units*), connected in a regular fashion, that exhibit some form of "learning" or adaptation. The large majority of such models can be described in essence as mapping or transforming between representations: input data are presented to the network in a particular format, and the network is judged successful when its outputs can be interpreted as a correct representation of the results of performing the desired transformation. In almost all cases, the input and output representation formats are prespecified by the experimenter

(although this is not entirely true of unsupervised learning networks, and there are a number of artificial neural network models that draw inspiration from biological data in their choice of input and output representations). If such networks are to be employed in artificial agents, or are to be of use in understanding biological agents, then this can only be so under the (often unspoken) assumption that, eventually, it will be possible to assemble a "pipeline" of such input-output transducer networks that links sensory inputs to motor outputs, and produce adaptive behavior. The most significant issue here is the heavy dependence on a priori intermediate representations, which may not be justifiable: neural sensorimotor pathways generating adaptive behaviors might not be neatly partitioned into representation-transforming modules; such pathways may not exhibit any patterns of activity identifiable as a representation in the conventional sense, and even if they do, there is no guarantee that they will be in strong accordance with representations chosen a priori by modelers.

This should not be mistaken for an argument against representation or for a denial of the vital role played by internal states in the generation of adaptive behaviors; it is simply an awareness of the dangers of being misled by a priori notions of representation. One of the safest ways of avoiding these dangers is to model, as far as is possible, *entire* sensorimotor pathways (i.e., the complete sequence of neural processing, from sensory input to motor output) involved in the generation of adaptive behavior. This requires that the agent be studied *while situated in an environment*: most sensorimotor processing for adaptive behavior involves dynamic interaction with the environment, and a situated agent is part of a closed-loop system, because certain actions can affect subsequent sensory inputs. Thus, the sensorimotor pathway should not be viewed as a "pipeline" transforming from a given input representation to a desired output representation, but rather as one link in the action-perception cycle.

When such an approach is adopted, the true nature of the representations and processing necessary for the generation of relatively complex adaptive behaviors is more likely to be revealed, and the validity of any a priori assumptions is clarified.

Naturally, it is beyond the state of the art to attempt to model complete sensorimotor pathways in humans or other large mammals, but experimental work in the neuroethology literature provides a wealth of data from less intellectually able animals, such as arthropods (the animal class that includes insects, spiders, and crustacea), amphibia, and other "simple" vertebrates such as eels or salamanders. Such animals are used as the domains of study in some CNE research, but in other work, simple idealized models are rigorously studied, in a manner akin to Galileo's models of perfect spheres rolling down inclined frictionless planes.

The argument that a priori commitment to certain representations or architectures for sensorimotor processing can lead to surprisingly wrong conclusions can be illustrated by reference to a classic series of thought experiments devised by Braitenberg (1984). Braitenberg described specifications for a series of simple mobile vehicles operating in a world with simplified kinematics. The series of vehicles starts with an elementary device that performs primitive heat-seeking behavior and progresses through vehicles that exhibit positive or negative taxes (i.e., orientation toward or away from a directional stimulus) and primitive forms of learning, pattern detection, and movement detection, culminating in vehicles that exhibit chaotic dynamics and predictive behavior. The internal control mechanisms of all the vehicles are rigorously minimal. The simpler vehicles contain nothing more than wires connecting sensors to actuators, while the more advanced ones employ nonlinear threshold devices with delays and pseudo-Hebbian adaptation.

Braitenberg notes that the psychological language indicative of intentional mental states has compelling intuitive appeal in describing the observed behavior of the vehicles. He ascribes *fear, aggression, love, values and taste, rules, trains of thought, free will, foresight, egotism,* and *optimism* to his vehicles. But he also demonstrates that whereas such terms may be very useful at the level of description of an external observer, the internal causal mechanisms could be surprisingly simple and, crucially, could contain nothing that can meaningfully be said to either "represent" or "implement" these intentional mental states. That is to say, the intentionality is in the eye of the beholder, not in the workings of the agent. For further discussion of these issues, see Cliff and Noble (1997).

While Braitenberg's vehicles are nothing more than thought experiments, they provide insight into possible organizational principles in natural and artificial creatures, and demonstrate the limits of applicability of intentional terminology. Further discussion of the utility of agent models in biology can be found in Dean (1998).

To summarize, research in CNE can be characterized as placing increased emphasis on modeling entire adaptive behavior–generating sensorimotor pathways in embodied agents, where those agents are situated in environments that supply sensorimotor feedback. Such an approach lessens the chances of making untenable assumptions concerning issues of representation and processing. Moreover, in order to study such pathways where there is reliable biological data, it may often be necessary to focus attention on relatively simple animals, such as arthropods or amphibia. For further discussion of the rationale for CNE, see Beer (1990) and Cliff (1990).

It is important to note that there is a tradition of related work in the artificial neural network literature. Research on reinforcement learning for control tasks is most close; see REINFORCEMENT LEARNING IN MOTOR CONTROL.

Selected Current Research Projects

Two specific longstanding CNE research programs are discussed in this section: the work of Arbib's research group on visuomotor behavior in simple vertebrates, and Beer's work on the neural foundations of adaptive behavior in even simpler agents (i.e., cockroaches) and in abstract idealized agents. Before delving into these bodies of work, it is useful to consider where they sit in the CNE canon, and to point to CNE research that resides at other points in that space.

For the purposes of framing, there are three major axes along which work in CNE can be categorized. In no particular order, they are the degree of reliance on computer software simulation, the degree of concentration on a specific animal species or class, and the extent to which semiautomated design techniques are employed.

The degree of reliance on computer simulation in CNE research projects varies from the complete, where all work is carried out using software simulations, to the minimal, where the CNE model takes the form of an operational physical robot, with the model neurons (individually or at the network level) being constructed from electronic circuits. Examples of the former include work by Arbib (1987) and Beer (1990), while many examples of the latter are discussed by Webb (2001). Note also that Beer went on to use robot platforms in continuations of his work that was initially software-only (Beer et al., 1992) while Arkin (see REACTIVE ROBOTIC SYSTEMS) made similar use of Arbib's works. A comprehensive review of the merits of using physical robots (rather than computer software) as simulations of animals has recently been published by Webb (2001), with copious references to work in this field; see also BIOLOGICALLY INSPIRED ROBOTICS.

The extent to which CNE research projects concentrate on a specific animal species or class varies from, at one extreme, CNE studies of one specific species (e.g., Beer, 1990) through generic CNE studies of several species of animals within the same order (e.g., Arbib's 1987 work on anuran visual control of action), to the other extreme, where neural mechanisms underlying the generation

of adaptive behavior in wholly abstract and idealized agents is explored within the CNE methodology (e.g., Beer, 2002).

Finally, with the continuing falls in the real cost of processor power and memory and disk storage, there has been an increased tendency over the past decade to move away from hand-designed computational/robot models and toward models that are the product of automated or semiautomated design processes. The use of evolutionary computation techniques such as genetic algorithms in particular (see EVOLUTION OF ARTIFICIAL NEURAL NETWORKS) has proved fruitful. At the hands-on extreme, there are CNE models where each artificial neuron's parameters (e.g., its time constants, thresholds, and connectivity to other components) are specified by the designer of the model (see, e.g., Arbib, 1987; Beer, 1990), whereas at the hands-off extreme the modeler sets up a (usually truly vast) space of possible network designs and then uses an evolutionary search process to identify points in that design space that best satisfy some performance metric (i.e., the fitness evaluation function). Examples of this latter approach include Isjpeert (2001) and Beer (2002).

Computational Frogs, Toads, and Salamanders

Probably the most mature body of work in CNE is the research program led by Arbib for two decades on a family of models of visually mediated behavior in simple vertebrates. In the initial years of this project the focus was on visuomotor activity in frogs and toads; see Arbib's 1987 paper for a review of the project with peer commentary and his 1997 publication for a discussion of how this work integrates with studies of monkeys and of rats. Arbib named his simulation model *Rana computatrix*, the computational frog, in homage to W. Grey Walter's seminal *Machina Speculatrix* robots from the 1950s.

The *R. computatrix* models are faithful to the known biology, and there is an interplay between the experimental and theoretical work: an initial first approximation model was extended and refined in a number of stages, leading to a family of models.

Arbib's approach involves defining a number of functional *schemas*. Schemas can be modeled by interacting layers of neuron-like elements or by nets of intermediate-level units; the network models can be related to experimental data concerning neural circuitry, and the development process iterates (Arbib, 1987, p. 411 *ff.*). Further details can be found in SCHEMA THEORY.

The primary focus in the *R. computatrix* models has been on how frogs and toads use vision to detect and catch prey, in environments that include obstacles and barriers. Arbib has developed a series of schema-based models that account for depth perception as interaction between accommodation and binocular clues, and at the lowest level the schemas are plausibly based on known details of the relevant neurological data.

One of the more striking results from this work, with reference to Marr's well-known theory of vision, is the indication that, at least in frogs and toads, there are different perceptual mechanisms for different visual stimuli. That is, the depths to prey and to barriers are extracted from the optic array by different processing channels and are integrated in the sensorimotor pathways much later than Marr's theory might suggest. Arbib and Liaw (1995) went on to demonstrate how lessons learned from the *R. computatrix* project could inform the design of visually guided robot systems.

In more recent work, Ijspeert and Arbib (2000) have reported on experiments in which a sophisticated simulation of a 3D multi-segmented biomechanical model of a salamander's body is controlled by a complex neural network model. The network is composed of separate central pattern generators (CPGs; see LOCOMOTION, VERTEBRATE) for the body and the limbs, each of which may be activated and modulated by descending tonic inputs. Ijspeert and Arbib use this simulation system to explore the neural circuitry underlying the generation of visually steerable salamander locomotion behaviors in water and on land. One notable aspect of this work in relation to the earlier studies of anuran circuitry is that, while the gross morphology of the CPG circuits is decided by the experimenters, a genetic algorithm is used to determine the fine details of the CPG circuits' internal connectivity and parameter values, the intersegmental coupling, and the coupling between the limb CPG and the body CPG. Thus, unlike the hands-on incremental modeling employed in the *R. computatrix* models, the salamander model is the product of a semiautomatic evolutionary design process.

Computational Cockroaches and Vehicles *Redux*

Beer's 1990 book, *Intelligence as Adaptive Behavior*, contains both methodological arguments for CNE and details of experimental work on his model of a computational cockroach, *Periplaneta computatrix*, which is a simulated hexapod agent embedded in an environment, inspired by neuroethological studies of the cockroach *Periplaneta americana*. The real cockroach uses chemotaxis as one of several strategies to locate food sources. If its path along an odor gradient is blocked by an obstacle, it performs stereotyped "edge-following" behavior. The artificial cockroach is controlled by a heterogeneous neural network that was inspired by biological data and has been used to study issues in locomotion, guidance, and behavioral choice.

The primary external sensory input was simulated chemosensory information: patches of food in the environment gave off odor gradients detectable under an inverse square law relating distance to odor intensity. The neural nets also received mechanosensory input from proprioceptors in the limbs and tactile sensors that signaled the presence of food under the mouth. The simulation model included elementary kinematics: if the artificial cockroach failed to adopt a stable position for a sufficient length of time, it fell down.

Results from the simulation sessions demonstrated behavior in the model that was highly similar to behavior in the real animal, and Beer subsequently performed "lesion" experiments by selectively deleting connections or units from the *P. computatrix* control network. Again, the results obtained with the artificial system were in agreement with the biological data.

P. computatrix was inspired by biological data, but it was not intended as a biological model. The various behaviors were generated by heterogeneous neural networks. The neuron model employed by Beer was more faithful to biology than many of the "formal neurons" used in conventional artificial neural network research: the units involved differential equations modeling membrane potentials, which gave his model neural assemblies a rich intrinsic dynamics. For further details, see LOCOMOTION, INVERTEBRATE.

The central focus in Beer's (1990) work was on designing architectures composed from such neural units that could act as controllers for the various behaviors that *P. computatrix* should exhibit. Thus, there was no treatment of learning in the initial body of work on the cockroach. Subsequently, Beer reported on work that extended the original *P. computatrix* simulation model, testing it by allowing it to control walking in a real hexapod robot (Beer et al., 1992).

In the robot implementation, the control network was still simulated (i.e., the units in the neural network were not realized physically), but the sensorimotor connections to the artificial neural network were interfaced to physical sensors and actuators by means of analog-digital and digital-analog converters. Beer et al. reported that in all cases, the response of the physical robot was highly similar to that previously observed in simulation. The implementation did, however, reveal one problem in the controller that had not been examined in the simulation. This problem, involving disturbances in the crossbody phasing of the legs, was easily rectified,

but nevertheless this demonstrates that simulation models cannot be trusted to perfectly replicate any physical implementation they may ultimately be intended for.

For a wider unified perspective on this work, see LOCOMOTION, INVERTEBRATE; VISUOMOTOR COORDINATION IN FROG AND TOAD; and LOCOMOTION, VERTEBRATE.

Subsequent to his work on *P. computatrix*, one line of research that Beer has pursued is, in comparison, radically simplified, divorced from any specific animal, and yet in its simplicity it reaches to the core of fundamental issues in cognitive science and adaptive behavior research. Rather than be constrained (and potentially confused) by biology, Beer (2002) developed a series of simple idealized embodied and embedded model agents, each of which is capable of "minimally cognitive" behaviors. Beer defines a minimally cognitive behavior as one that is just above the threshold for raising issues of genuine interest to cognitive science (see also COGNITIVE MODELING: PSYCHOLOGY AND CONNECTIONISM).

Beer's minimal agents exist in a two-dimensional world, but can only move along a bounded horizontal baseline. Various geometric shapes such as circles or diamonds drop from above, toward the agent's baseline. In each experiment, the intention is that the minimal agents use their sensors to detect the nature of whatever geometric shape or shapes is or are currently falling toward it, and thereby generate behavior "appropriate" to the current situation. The definition of appropriate behavior depends on the experiment but may, for example, be as apparently trivial as "intercept circular objects and avoid diamond-shaped ones." To achieve this sensorimotor coordination, each minimal agent is equipped with a small continuous-time recurrent neural network (CTRNN) (see RECURRENT NETWORKS: LEARNING ALGORITHMS).

The CTRNN for each minimal agent has a small number (e.g., seven) of fixed-orientation ray-casting "visual" proximity sensors (each of which sends a straight limited-length ray out at a particular angle to the agent's body and reports on how far the ray traveled before it intercepted an object, if at all). Each sensor feeds onto a small number (e.g., five) of fully interconnected "interneurons," and all of these in turn feed onto a small number (e.g., two) of "output" neurons—one for moving to the left and one for moving to the right. Thus, a typical minimal agent may have 14 units and perhaps 70 connection weights in its CTRNN.

Any particular design for a CTRNN sensorimotor controller for one of Beer's minimal agents specifies the time-constant, bias, gain, and input weights for each neuron. Rather than design appropriate networks by hand, Beer employs a "hands-off" genetic algorithm to explore a very large space of possible network designs, evaluating each design on a measure of its observed behavior. To halve the size of the search space, Beer imposed a bilateral symmetry requirement. Other than this enforcement of symmetry, there is very little a priori commitment to any particular CTRNN solution. Over a reasonably small evolutionary experiment (e.g., 2,000 generations with a population size of 100), minimal agents evolve that reliably score well on the experiment's evaluation function, and that also generalize well to situations not encountered in the evolutionary adaptation period.

So far, so simple. Yet, in a series of papers published since 1996, Beer and his colleagues have reported on the evolution of CTRNNs for sensorimotor control in minimally cognitive agents that have been evaluated on the basis of their ability to perform a variety of increasingly sophisticated behaviors. These behaviors include orientating toward and reaching for objects, discriminating between objects, judging the passability of openings relative to the agent's own body size, discriminating between visible parts of the agent's body and other objects in the agent's environment, predicting and remembering the future location of falling objects so that they can later be intercepted "blind," and switching attention between multiple objects as they fall. All of these behaviors are achieved with the same simple agent CTRNN architecture outlined above.

This array of cognitively interesting behaviors achieved by Beer's minimally cognitive agents prompts the question of what, precisely, is happening at the mechanistic level within the evolved CTRNNs to generate these behaviors. And at this point we return to the arguments and issues explored in the opening sections of this article. Beer presents concrete analyses of the CTRNNs of these agents, demonstrating a full understanding of their mechanistic activity from a *dynamical systems* perspective; and yet, as he points out, this analysis is of little or no use in attempts at elucidating an understanding from a *computational* (and hence *representational*) perspective: there is nothing readily identifiable in the CTRNNs that represents a circle or a diamond, or the action of intercepting or of avoiding. Rather, a full explanation of the behavior exhibited by one of Beer's minimally cognitive agent's CTRNNs can only be given in the context of the dynamics of that agent's embodiment and of the environment in which it is situated. See Beer (2002) and Cliff and Noble (1997) for further details.

Discussion

Computational neuroethology studies neural mechanisms that generate adaptive behaviors, and hence requires that embodied agents be studied within the situated context of their environmental and behavioral niches.

From the descriptions given in this article, some patterns emerge: the animal-specific CNE projects mentioned are dependent on the availability of fairly detailed neuroethological data. Such data invariably come from invasive in vivo experimentation, and the neuroanatomy of "simpler" animals such as arthropods or simpler vertebrates is particularly amenable to such techniques. For arthropods in particular, certain neurons performing particular functions are readily locatable in different individual animals of the same species. Although there are manifest obstacles preventing the collection of such data from more complex vertebrate subjects, research in these areas is making significant progress. Furthermore, by definition, any truly *general* principles underlying the neural generation of adaptive behaviors are those that are common to a number of species, so only cross-species studies will help identify general principles (Cliff, 1990, p. 37).

Yet surely the most general principles of all are those that apply to all agents within a certain class of cognitive or behavioral niches, regardless of the hardware (or software) that those agents are implemented in. In this respect, Beer's minimally cognitive agents are highly cogent. Until the representation-manipulating explanatory language that has traditionally been brought to bear on the supposed neural behavior-generating mechanisms of "complex" animals (including humans) can be demonstrated to be routinely applicable to "simpler" agents (including Beer's *vehicle*-like minimal

agents), the rigor and limits of that explanatory language will remain in doubt.

Road Map: Neuroethology and Evolution
Related Reading: Action Monitoring and Forward Control of Movements; Arm and Hand Movement Control; Eye-Hand Coordination in Reaching Movements; Motor Cortex: Coding and Decoding of Directional Operations; Pursuit Eye Movements; Reaching Movements: Implications for Computational Models; Sensorimotor Learning; Vestibulo-Ocular Reflex

References

Arbib, M. A., 1972, *The Metaphorical Brain: An Introduction to Cybernetics as Artificial Intelligence and Brain Theory*, New York: Wiley-Interscience. ◆

Arbib, M. A., 1987, Levels of modelling of mechanisms of visually guided behavior, *Behav. Brain Sci.*, 10:407–465.

Arbib, M. A., 1997, From visual affordances in monkey parietal cortex to hippocampal-parietal interactions underlying rat navigation, *Philos. Trans. R. Soc. Lond. B*, 352:1429–1476.

Arbib, M. A., and Liaw, J., 1995, Sensorimotor transformations in the worlds of frogs and robots, *Artif. Intell.*, 72:53–79.

Beer, R. D., 1990, *Intelligence as Adaptive Behavior: An Experiment in Computational Neuroethology*, New York: Academic Press. ◆

Beer, R. D., 2002, The dynamics of active categorical perception in an evolved model agent, *Behav. Brain Sci.*, in press; available: http://vorlon.cwru.edu/~beer/Papers/BBSpaper.pdf.

Beer, R. D., Chiel, H. J., Quinn, R. D., Espenschied, K., and Larsson, P., 1992, A distributed neural network architecture for hexapod robot locomotion, *Neural Comput.*, 4:356–365.

Braitenberg, V., 1984, *Vehicles: Experiments in Synthetic Psychology*, Cambridge, MA: MIT Press/Bradford Books. ◆

Cliff, D., 1990, Computational neuroethology: A provisional manifesto, in *From Animals to Animats: Proceedings of the First International Conference on Simulation of Adaptive Behavior (SAB90)* (J.-A. Meyer and S.W. Wilson, Eds.), Cambridge, MA: MIT Press/Bradford Books, pp. 29–39.

Cliff, D., and Noble, J., 1997, Knowledge-based vision and simple visual machines, *Philos. Trans. R. Soc. Lond. B*, 352:1165–1175. ◆

Dean, J., 1998, Animats and what they can tell us, *Trends Cognit. Sci.*, 2:60–67.

Ijspeert, A. J., 2001, A connectionist central pattern generator for the aquatic and terrestrial gaits of a simulated salamander, *Biol. Cybern.*, 84:331–348.

Ijspeert, A. J., and Arbib, M. A., 2000, Visual tracking in simulated salamander locomotion, in *From Animals to Animats 6: Proceedings of the Sixth International Conference of the Society for Adaptive Behavior (SAB2000)* (J.-A. Meyer, A. Berthoz, D. Floreano, H. Roitblat, and S. W. Wilson, Eds.), Cambridge, MA: MIT Press, pp. 88–97.

Simmons, P., and Young, D., 1999, *Nerve Cells and Animal Behaviour*, Cambridge, Engl.: Cambridge University Press. ◆

Webb, B., 2001, Can robots make good models of biological behavior? *Behav. Brain Sci.*, 24(6).

Neuroinformatics

Michael A. Arbib

Introduction

Some define the term "neuroinformatics" as the use of databases, the World Wide Web, and visualization for the storage and analysis of neuroscience data, but we here broaden the definition to include the role of computational models in structuring masses of data. From the perspective of this *Handbook*, the key challenge for neuroinformatics is to integrate insights from synthetic data obtained

from running a model with data obtained empirically from studying the animal or human brain. Moreover, we must integrate all levels from molecules to compartments and neurons up to biological neural networks and on to the behavior of organisms. One must thus maintain an architecture for a federation of empirical databases in which the results from diverse laboratories can be integrated, providing an environment in which we can make quantitative verifiable or disprovable predictions from the model to the database.

Neuroscience integrates anatomy, behavior, physiology, and chemistry. Each vertebrate has hundreds of brain regions, discriminated from other regions by gross anatomy, cytoarchitectonics, input and output connections of the region, and detailed neurophysiology. Then, for a variety of behaviors—whether they be eye movements, aspects of motor control, performance on memory tasks, and so on—we may seek to characterize the regions of the brain that are most involved in such behaviors and then characterize the firing of particular populations of neurons in temporal correlation with different aspects of the task. In such modeling studies, we seek to understand what must be added to the available database on neural responsiveness and connectivity to explain the time course of cellular activity, and the way in which they mediate between sensory data, the animal's intention, and behavior. But we also seek to use insights from these studies to better understand the human brain.

Shepherd et al. (1998) review the contribution to neuroinformatics tools for integrating, searching, and modeling multidisciplinary neuroscience data made by researchers supported by the Human Brain Project, a consortium of U.S. federal research agencies led by the National Institute of Mental Health. Kötter (2001) reviews current issues in the representation, integration, and analysis of neuroscience data from molecular to brain systems levels, including issues of implementation, standardization, management, quality control, copyright, confidentiality, and acceptance, with particular emphasis on integrative neuroinformatics approaches for exploring structure-function relationships in the brain. Arbib and Grethe (2001; hereafter *CtB*) present an integrated approach to neuroinformatics whose delineation will structure much of this article.

Federating a Variety of Databases

A database on the neurochemistry of synaptic plasticity might be constructed as a view of plasticity data within various databases for different brain regions. An atlas of brain regions can be used to structure data both on the location of single cells (a link to a neurophysiology database) and for standardizing slice-based data (such as stains of receptor activity in a neurochemistry database). In short, neuroinformatics requires a *federation* of databases with tools for linking data from diverse databases to answer complex questions (Heimbigner and McLeod, 1985; Liao and McLeod, Chapter 5.1 of *CtB*). Databases in such a federation may be of one or more of the following types.

Article Repositories

Many publishers now offer their journals on-line. Even if articles migrate from linear text to hypertext, such narratives about the data—"This is the recent experiment that I did," "Here is my review," and so on—will often provide the way for humans to get started in understanding what is going on in some domain, even if they will eventually search specific data sets of the kind described below.

Repositories of Empirical Data

This is where we get data from different laboratories and make them generally available by linking each data set to the *protocol* that produced it: information (like that in the Methods section of an article but in a more algorithmic form) on the hypotheses being tested, the experimental methods used, and so on.

Summary Databases

In these databases are assembled the assertions, summaries, hypotheses, tables, and figures that encapsulate the state of knowledge in a particular domain. Assertions in summary databases can be linked through the database federation not only to primary literature, but also to models or empirical data. However, in many fields, there is no consensus as to just which hypotheses have been firmly established. Different reviewers may therefore assign different confidence levels to different primary data, and these will affect the confidence level of assertions in the summary database.

Model Repositories

These repositories will not only provide access to computational models, but also link each model to empirical and summary databases to provide evidence for hypotheses in the model or data to test predictions from simulation runs made with the model. We have viewed the protocol as a way to delineate the structure of an experiment. When we design a model, we often give an interface that mimics the protocol so that operations on the model capture the manipulations the experimenter might have made on the nervous system. This makes it easy for somebody who is not expert in modeling to nonetheless evaluate a model by seeing how it runs in a variety of situations.

NeuroCore and Time Series Databases

Neuroscience provides many examples of time series data. For example, the time series data for a single experiment for a study of classical conditioning of a rabbit's eyeblink (see CEREBELLUM AND CONDITIONING) might include for each trial traces showing the movement of the eyelid and a display of firing of a single neuron. The firing data might then be aggregated across trials in a histogram. This example motivates the database issues: How do we store time series? How do we register data with time stamps to facilitate interesting processing of sets of data? How do we link each firing pattern to the position in the brain of the neuron it is taken from? We again see the need to store the protocol as well as, making explicit what hypotheses were being tested, what experimental methods were used, and what conditions were required to elicit each data set.

NeuroCore (Grethe, Mureika, and Merchant, Chapter 3.2, in *CtB*) provides a core schema, an extendible object-relational database schema implemented in Informix. The schema (structure of data tables, etc.) for each NeuroCore database is an extension of the core database schema that has links to repositories of neuroanatomical and neurochemical concepts and provides an extendible specification of items needed in most experimental records, such as research subject, experimental manipulation, structure of the research data, and the statistics performed on the data. There is a slot for research data and a standard extension for handling time series data. NeuroCore comes with a Java applet called the Schema Browser, which allows one to learn the structure of a particular laboratory's database by showing, for each familiar core table, the extensions particular to that laboratory.

Mediator Systems and Common Ontologies

In a cooperative federated database system, the challenge is to provide conceptual links between data sources to begin to address the problem of data integration: assisting users by selecting, restructuring, and merging information from different databases and providing an integrated view of the information. Each database in the federation has its own *ontology* (the collection of concepts and their relationships used to describe information units in the database). But these ontologies may use terms differently (a "cell" in one may be a "neuron" in another and a "neuron" or a "glia cell" in yet another). If we seek a direct translation between each pair of ontologies, then n ontologies require $n(n - 1)$ translators. However, if we can define a common ontology and translate back and forth between it and the other ontologies, then only $2n$ translators are required. With a common ontology that serves the basis of mutual understanding among participants in the federation, information is shared via what are called *mediators*. These support import (folding remote information into local environments), export (registering information to share), discovery (searching for relevant information), and browsing (navigating through information sources).

Kahng and McLeod (Chapter 5.1 of *CtB*) show one way to dynamically build a common ontology. Their motivation is that it is extremely difficult to reach total agreement on an ontology if there are many participants and that the ontology should be allowed to change dynamically as the federation evolves.

The model-based mediation architecture offered by Ludaescher, Gupta, and Martone (2001) employs F-logic as a data and knowledge representation and reasoning formalism. Integrated database views are defined and executed at the level of conceptual models rather than at the usual level of database schemas or XML. To semantically correlate across databases with little or no overlap in their schemas, they introduce domain maps, which are semantic nets of terms and relationships used to mediate across sources; for example, Purkinje cell "is a" neuron; cerebellum "has a" cerebellar cortex. The mediator then uses these rules to navigate through the various levels of brain analysis to allow for complex queries that span multiple levels of resolution and multiple data sources. Sources of domain knowledge include existing ontologies such as those provided by brain atlases and the Unified Medical Language System (UMLS) project of the National Library of Medicine (http://www.nlm.nih.gov/research/umls/), but the aim is to provide tools to allow different groups of users to tailor their own extensions to the ontology.

Modeling and Simulation

Consider modeling the role of neural circuitry of certain brain regions in a given set of tasks. For each brain region, a survey of the neurophysiological data calls attention to a few basic cell types with firing characteristics that are strongly correlated with some aspect of that task. For example, in eye movement tasks, some cells fire most strongly near the onset of the target stimulus, others seem to be active during a delay period, and others are more active near movement initiation. The data tell the modeler what the activity of the cells should be in a variety of situations, but in many cases, experimenters do not know in any quantitative detail the way in which the cell responds to its synaptic inputs, nor do they know the action of the synapses in great detail. In short, the available empirical data might not be rich enough to define a *causally complete* model. Therefore, to get the model to run, the modeler has to make a number of hypotheses about some of the unknown connections, weights, time constants, and so on. The modeler may even have to postulate cell types that experimenters have not yet looked for and show by computer simulation that the resulting network will indeed perform in the observed way when known experiments are simulated, in which case it must match both external behavior and the key data on model populations that were based on cell populations with measured physiological responses. What raises the ante is that (1) the modeler's hypotheses suggest new experiments on neural dynamics and connectivity and (2) the model can be used to simulate experiments that have never been conducted with real nervous systems.

A few years from now, new models will both examine the interactions of a larger number of brain regions and analyze cells within each region in increasing detail. There is no way we would be able to keep cognitive track of these models if we had to look at everything at once. One approach (e.g., Arbib, Chapter 2.1, in *CtB*) is to represent complex models in an object-oriented way, using a hierarchy of interconnected modules. A module might be an interconnected set of brain regions; each region in turn might itself be a module composed of yet smaller modules that represent

arrays of neurons sharing some common anatomical or physiological property. In any case, a module is either decomposable, in which case this "parent module" is decomposed into submodules known as its child modules, or the module is a "leaf module" that is not decomposed further but is directly implemented in the chosen programming language. There are basically two ways to proceed for a complex model. We can get a hierarchical view of the overall model, or we can zoom in on subsystems and study them in detail.

Multilevel Simulation

As recently as 2000, a detailed model of chemicals reacting and diffusing around a single synapse could require a full day of workstation processing to simulate just a few seconds of synaptic activity. There may be of the order of 10,000 synapses on a "typical" neuron, millions of neurons in a single region, and hundreds of regions in a brain. Clearly, any simulation methodology that required one to simulate every synapse in such detail would be doomed to failure. No short-term increase in computer power will allow us to reduce the simulation of a second's activity in a system with 10^{15} synapses from 10^{15} hours or minutes down to a single second. A major challenge for work in multilevel simulation is thus to undertake detailed simulation at one level to validate a (possibly context-dependent) approximation that can be used in far more efficient large-scale simulations at the next level.

Neurosimulation: Tools and Resources, NSL Neural Simulation Language, GENESIS Simulation System, and NEURON Simulation Environment present tools bridging from circuits in interacting brain regions down to compartmental models of individual neurons. For example, a NSL model might employ a neuron module that is far simpler than a corresponding compartmental model developed in NEURON but that has been validated by careful studies to yield an economical but effective approximation to it. Or a GENESIS modeler might want to check that a model of a compartment provides a satisfactory approximation to a far more detailed model of neurochemical details for the neuron. All this raises two important challenges for the neural simulation community. One is to increase the range of tools currently available for comparing model to model as well as model to data (with the parameter search methods that this implies). The other is to develop "wrapping" technology so that modules developed by using one simulator can indeed be used to replace objects (whether to simplify them or attend to crucial new details) in an existing model developed by using another simulator.

Young, Hilgetag, and Scannell (2000) offer one example of modeling at the highest level, far removed from the details of neural circuits (see also Covariance Structural Equation Modeling). They developed a formal framework for inferring function from structure in which knowledge of connectivity is necessary but not sufficient. They applied this framework to inferences about a simple network that reproduces intact, lesioned, and paradoxically restored orienting behavior. Lesion effects could be used to infer which structures contributed to particular functions in this simple network. Clearly, such an approach can complement, but not replace, attempts to link high-level data from lesion effects or brain imaging to the analysis of detailed neural circuitry. Synthetic Functional Brain Mapping reviews methods for calibrating human brain imaging against simulations of monkey neurophysiology; while Kötter et al. (2002) simulate activity propagation in the primate visual cortex with the aim of relating neuronal activity to cortical activation patterns and relating onset response latencies to the structure of the underlying anatomical network.

Usui (2002) describes the NRV (Neuroinformatics Research in Vision) project, which aims to construct mathematical models for each level of the visual system (single neuron, retinal neural circuit, visual function), build resources for neuroinformatics, and develop a new vision device based on brain-type information-processing principles. A mathematical model of a retinal neural circuit will be constructed from neurophysiological experimental data and from the characteristics of single neurons. This circuit will form the basis for a "virtual retina" that encompasses everything from the light energy conversion mechanism in a photoreceptor to the encoding mechanism of impulse sequence in a ganglion cell, which is the retinal output. The results of this project will be made available in a database, the VISIOME Platform, that integrates morphological and physiological knowledge and mathematical models with related studies and references.

Arbib (1995) formulated the challenge of building databases that link models developed with different simulators to each other and to empirical databases, and Bischoff-Grethe, Spoelstra, and Arbib (Chapter 6.2 in *CtB*) explore the integration of one such model repository, Brain Models on the Web, with a summary database. Goddard et al. (2001) further develop the theme that software tools are needed that support discussion, development, and exchange of computational models. They describe methodologies that focus on these tasks and discuss the use of templates, declarative forms of model description equivalent to object-oriented classes and database schemas, to describe models ranging from neuron cell membranes to neural networks. The paper introduces NeuroML, a markup language for neuroscience that is defined syntactically using templates, with a component designed to support communication between modeling-related tools.

Neuroanatomy

One way to integrate data from diverse experiments on the brains of a given species is to register the data—whether the locations of cells recorded neurophysiologically, the tract tracings of an anatomical experiment, or the receptor densities revealed on a slice of brain in a neurochemical study—against a standard brain atlas. Just as people have different faces, so do rats and other animals have different brains, and therefore there is a registration problem: Given a location in an individual brain, what is the best bet as to the corresponding location in the "standard" brain?

Part 4 of Arbib and Grethe (2001) offers a number of approaches to atlas-based databases. The core of the work is NeuARt, a neuroanatomical viewer for the rat brain based on the Swanson atlas (Swanson, 1998). It also present NeuroSlicer, a tool for registering 2D slice data against a 3D model of the rat brain reconstructed from the Swanson atlas, as well as the design of an atlas-based database of neurochemical data. The Swanson atlas contains 73 plates representing cross sections of one-half of the rat brain. These are not uniformly spaced but rather were chosen to exhibit many crucial features of the rat's neuroanatomy. Each plate contains a photomicrograph of a stained brain section on the left and Swanson's representation of that section on the right, in which he draws boundaries separating different brain regions and labels the regions. Many of the curves dividing one nucleus from another correspond obviously to boundaries in the cell densities visible on the micrograph. Others cannot be seen from that particular micrograph and can be revealed only by a variety of staining techniques or by the incorporation of physiological and other data. It therefore requires great skill on the part of the anatomist to draw those nonobvious divisions, and in fact even expert neuroanatomists may disagree. Therefore, although there is much agreement between the Swanson atlas and the other leading atlas of the rat brain, the Paxinos-Watson atlas (Paxinos and Watson, 1998), there are also disagreements. Thus we have the future challenge not only of registering data against a particular choice of atlas, but also of facing the issue of how to update such data sets as future anatomical research resolves certain disagreements and leads to more reliable demarcation of boundaries.

NeuARt allows one to view any template of the Swanson atlas through a Web browser, together with any data overlays retrieved from the database. A Display Manager allows one to see these different results, and a Viewer Manager allows one to customize the Display Manager to one's needs. The Query Manager provides forms that make it easy to request anatomical information from the Informix database; the results of these queries are described textually by a Results Manager, and the user can maintain a set of results of interest. The Level Manager allows one to choose which level (template) of the brain to examine, and the Active Set Manager then shows which results of the query have data that are relevant for that set. These can then be displayed by clicking on the appropriate elements.

Another approach to preparing neuroanatomical data is to flatten computer images of monkey or human cerebral cortex. As we know from atlases of the world, such flattening requires cuts if it is to preserve areas of the surface and then can preserve only local, but not global, spatial relationships. Nonetheless, when data about cortex rather than deep brain structures is paramount, display of data on such a flattened map of cortex allows one to take in patterns at a glance in a way that is impossible if one must scroll slice by slice through the pages of a conventional brain atlas. Van Essen et al. (2001) describe three software programs for carrying out surface-based analyses of cerebral cortex: SureFit (Surface Reconstruction by Filtering and Intensity Transformations) is used primarily for cortical segmentation, volume visualization, and initial surface generation; Caret (Computerized Anatomical Reconstruction and Editing Toolkit) provides a range of surface visualization and analysis options plus capabilities for surface flattening, surface-based deformation, and other surface manipulations; and SuMS (Surface Management System) provides a version control system that is capable of handling large numbers of surface and volume data sets. With built-in database management system support, SuMS provides rapid search and retrieval capabilities across all the data sets while also incorporating multiple security levels to regulate access.

Of course, the problem of linking data to neuroanatomy is not limited to vertebrates, let alone mammals. Jacobs and Theunissen (2000) examine the anatomical basis for the representation of stimulus parameters within a neural map and examine the extraction of these parameters by sensory interneurons in the cricket cercal sensory system. Their modeling of the cricket cercal system makes crucial use of their identified neuron database (http://cns.montana.edu/research/neurosys/).

We close this section with the work of Toga and Thompson (2002) on the collection of images of normal and diseased human brains brain in vivo and post vivo. They stress that the design of appropriate reference systems for human brain data presents considerable challenges, since these systems must capture how brain structure and function vary in large populations, across age and gender, in different disease states, and across imaging modalities, not to mention comparison across species. This work requires new approaches in computer vision, partial differential equations, and statistical field theory to detect and visualize disease-specific patterns. They survey the types of maps relevant to mental disorders, including maps that capture dynamic patterns of brain change in dementia.

The NeuroHomology Database

The term "homology" is a central one in comparative biology, referring to characteristics of different species that are inherited from a common ancestor. Defining homologies between brain structures requires a process of inference from distinct clusters of attributes. Bota and Arbib (Chapter 6.4 of *CtB*) introduce the concept of *degree of homology*. To define a neural structure, neuroscientists use numerous attributes, including gross morphology, relative location, cytoarchitecture, types of cell responses to different ways of stimulation, and function. In similar fashion, Bota and Arbib employ eight criteria for determining the degree of homology of two brain structures: the morphology of cells within each brain structure and the relative position, cytoarchitecture, chemoarchitecture (neurotransmitters that are found within a brain structure), myeloarchitecture, afferent and efferent connections, and function of each of a pair of brain structures from two species. If two brain structures have common cell types, chemoarchitectonics, and cytoarchitectonics and common connectivity patterns, then one should expect that those two brain structures have the same function or related functions. This is the case for the primary visual area (area 17). In each major mammalian species, area 17 can be delimited on the basis of myeloarchitecture (heavy myelination) and cytoarchitecture (the presence of a granular layer IV), the presence of a single and systematic visuotopic map, a well-defined pattern of subcortical afferents, small receptive fields, and the presence of many orientation-selective neurons with simple receptive fields. Bota and Arbib not only discuss the homology criteria that can be established between pairs of brain structures across species, but also introduce the NeuroHomology (NHDB) summary database. This database contains three interconnected entities: Brain Structures, Connections, and Homologies. A user who wants to find whether there is any homology between structures X and Y from two different species can also find the definitions of structures X and Y according to different sources, as well as the afferents and efferents of these two structures. More important, the latest version of NHDB has three inference engines: one for combining data of differing reliability on the connections between two brain regions, one for comparing neuroanatomical data for a given species when the data come from the different parcellations provided by different brain atlases, and one for estimating the degree of homology according to multiple criteria.

Discussion

The full development of neuroinformatics will provide an environment that helps the user pass back and forth between empirical data and related models, even though these are distributed across a federation of databases. Mediation technology will help to integrate these databases despite their diversity of ontologies and database schemas. In particular, a variety of brain atlases will provide reference platforms for a host of data within a species, with the analysis of homologies supporting the linkage of data across species. Future standards activity will provide modelers using a variety of simulation environments with tools to develop interfaces that make it easy for nonprogrammers to run basic "experiments" with the models and add to the database comments on the comparison of simulation results with available empirical data, to install models, to create versions of both models and parameter sets, and to freeze models in various interesting states for later analysis under varying conditions. A crucial aspect in all this is to catalyze a truly cumulative style of modeling in neuroscience by facilitating the *reus-*

ability of modules within current neural models, with the pattern of reuse fully documented and tightly constrained by the linkage with a federation of databases of empirical neuroscientific data.

Road Map: Implementation and Analysis
Related Reading: Databases for Neuroscience; Neurosimulation: Tools and Resources

References

Arbib, M. A., 1995, Brain models on the Web, in *Computational Intelligence, A Dynamic Systems Perspective* (M. Palaniswami, Y. Attikouzel, R. J. Marks II, D. Fogel, and T. Fukuda, Eds.), New York: IEEE Press, pp. 219–231.

Arbib, M. A., and Grethe, J. S. (Eds.), 2001, *Computing the Brain: A Guide to Neuroinformatics*, San Diego: Academic Press. ◆

Goddard, N. H., Hucka, M., Howell, F., Cornelis, H., Shankar, K., and Beeman, D., 2001, Towards NeuroML: Model description methods for collaborative modeling in neuroscience, *Philos. Trans. R. Soc. Lond. B Biol. Sci.*, 356(1412):1209–1228.

Heimbigner, D., and McLeod, D., 1985, A federated architecture for information management, *ACM Transactions on Office Information Systems*, 3(3):253–278.

Jacobs, G. A., and Theunissen, F. E., 2000, Extraction of sensory parameters from a neural map by primary sensory interneurons, *J. Neurosci.*, 20(8):2934–2943.

Kötter, R., 2001, Neuroscience databases: Tools for exploring brain structure-function relationships, *Philos. Trans. R. Soc. Lond. B.*, 356:1111–1120. ◆

Kötter, R., Nielsen, P. D., Johnsen, J., Sommer, F. T., and Northoff, G., 2002, Multi-level neuron and network modeling in computational neuroanatomy, in *Computational Neuroanatomy: Principles and Methods* (Ascoli, G., Ed.), Totowa, NJ: Humana, pp. 359–382.

Ludaescher, B., Gupta, A., and Martone, M. A., 2001, Model-based mediation with domain maps, *17th International Conference on Data Engineering (ICDE)*, IEEE Computer Society, Heidelberg, Germany, pp. 81–90.

Paxinos, G., and Watson, C., 1998, *The Rat Brain in Stereotaxic Coordinates*, 2nd ed., San Diego, CA: Academic Press.

Shepherd, G. M., Mirsky, J. S., Healy, M. D., Singer, M. S., Skoufos, E., Hines, M. S., Nadkarni, P. M., and Miller, P. L., 1998, The Human Brain Project: Neuroinformatics tools for integrating, searching, and modeling multidisciplinary neuroscience data, *Trends Neurosci.*, 21:460–468.

Swanson, L. W., 1998, *Brain Maps: Structure of the Rat Brain*, Amsterdam: Elsevier Science Publishers.

Toga, A. W., and Thompson, P. M., 2002, New approaches in brain morphometry, *Am. J. Geriatr. Psychiatry*, 10(1):13–23. ◆

Usui, S., 2002, The NRV project (Neuroinformatics Research in Vision), http://www.neuroinformatics.gr.jp/.

Van Essen, D. C., Dickson, J., Harwell, J., Hanlon, D., Anderson, C. H., and Drury, H. A., 2001, An integrated software system for surface-based analyses of cerebral cortex, *JAMA (Special issue on the Human Brain Project)*, 41:1359–1378.

Young, M. P., Hilgetag, C. C., and Scannell, J. W., 2000, On imputing function to structure from the behavioural effects of brain lesions, *Philos. Trans. R. Soc. Lond. B Biol. Sci.*, 355(1393):147–161.

Neurolinguistics

Barry Gordon

Introduction

Neurolinguistics began as the study of the language deficits occurring after brain injuries but now encompasses all aspects of language and the brain, normal as well as disturbed. To help place neural modeling efforts in perspective, this chapter is intended as an overview of current understanding of language and its putative neural bases.

Recent reviews of neurolinguistics and its methods can be found in Berndt (2001) and Brown and Hagoort (1999). Speech perception is reviewed in SPEECH PROCESSING: PSYCHOLINGUISTICS; speech production in LANGUAGE PROCESSING, SPEECH PRODUC-

TION and Levelt (2001). Gordon (1997) provides an example of a detailed, multilevel analysis of one language function, the visual naming task.

First-Order Model of Speech/Language and Neuroanatomy

There is now general agreement concerning what constitutes actual language and what does not, what major functional abilities underlie speech and language, how these are interconnected, and their approximate neuroanatomic dependencies. Collectively, this first-order model can summarize many features of normal ability as well as developmental and acquired disorders. A century and a half of intensive study has also identified many errors that might occur in the experimental and theoretical analysis of behavior-brain relationships. Understanding these pitfalls is useful for interpreting current evidence and for modeling attempts in the future.

Language and Language Development

Babbling, grunts, shouts, and other emotional expressions are not language; they occur in non-human primates and are not affected by the same brain lesions that may abolish almost all language abilities. Even curses, idiomatic expressions, and singing may also be spared by such lesions. The language and related speech capabilities that are the focus of this chapter are propositional (i.e., both symbolic or referential, and created from combinations of elements). Although language can express concepts and reasoning, concept formation and reasoning do not necessarily depend on language.

All normal individuals have the capability to rapidly acquire language (LANGUAGE ACQUISITION). Some of this capability is expressed neonatally and even in utero. An extensive search for genes that might be responsible for language capabilities has produced several candidates and much controversy.

Until recently, it was thought that this facile ability to acquire language might atrophy in most people after approximately five years of age. New evidence, both empirical and theoretical, suggests that at least some of the apparent loss of plasticity could be the result of entrapment by the first-learned language. With special training or stimuli, some phonological limitations may be overcome.

Functional Architecture

It is generally agreed that the complex overt functions of language and speech are the byproduct of various combinations of internal subprocesses (stages). Different overt functions may use these stages in different arrangements, and with different demands. Figure 1 is a schematic of these stages and their inputs, outputs, and interconnections. Every normal auditory/oral language user has functional modules for auditory phonemic perception, auditory word recognition (phonologic word-form recognition), lexical-semantics, abstract word form retrieval (which may or may not involve syntactic information, depending on the account), phonological word-form retrieval, and production of articulatory patterns. The process of learning to read and to write also establishes language-specific capabilities within the visual and motor systems. In the case of an alphabetic language such as English, this includes stages that perform abstract visual letter- and word-form recognition. These stages are connected to phonemic, phonologic word-form, and lexical-semantic processes. Output (in English) maps from phonologic and subphonologic word-forms to the written forms. Language communicated by gesture (such as American Sign Language) requires its own specialized visual recognition and manual production mechanisms, which also communicate with core language faculties (Crone et al., 2001). Figure 2 shows the approximate neuroanatomic associations of some of these stages in normal right-handed individuals.

In normal right-handed individuals, core functions required for speech and language are almost always (>99%) the responsibility of the left (dominant) hemisphere. In left-handed individuals (who make up ~13% of the population), or even those who are right-handed but with a family history of left-handedness, the core functions can be in the right hemisphere, or more bilaterally distributed. The lateralization of speech and language is under genetic control.

Lesion Effects and Classic Syndromes

A large part of the evidence for this lateralization, parcellation, and mapping of language functions has come from individuals with

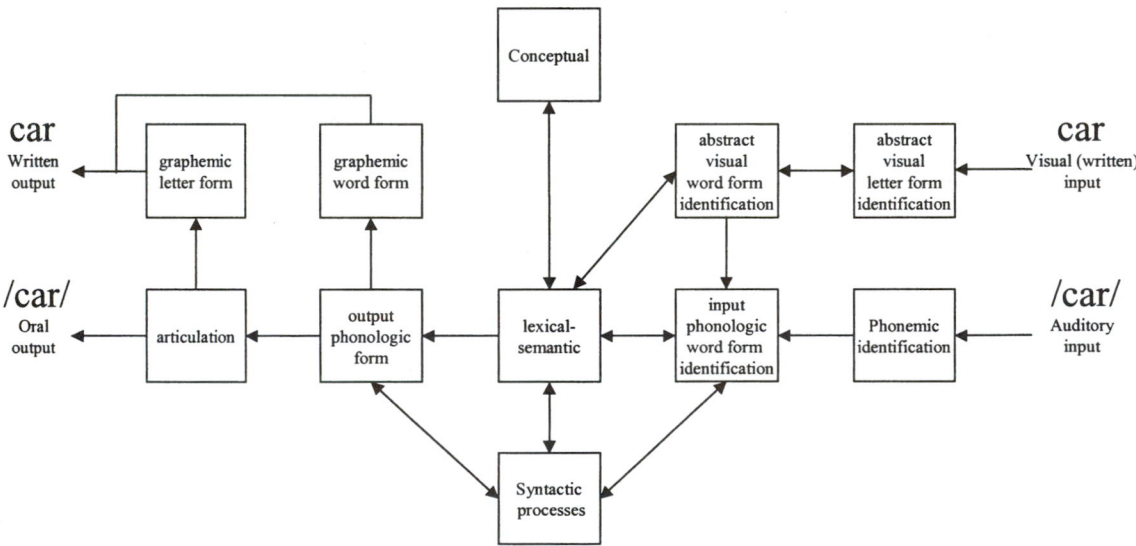

Figure 1. Schematic of larger-scale functional modules and interconnections involved in speech/language and related functions. Visual confrontation naming uses visual inputs analogous to those used for reading; see Figure 4. (Copyright IA, Inc. Used with permission.)

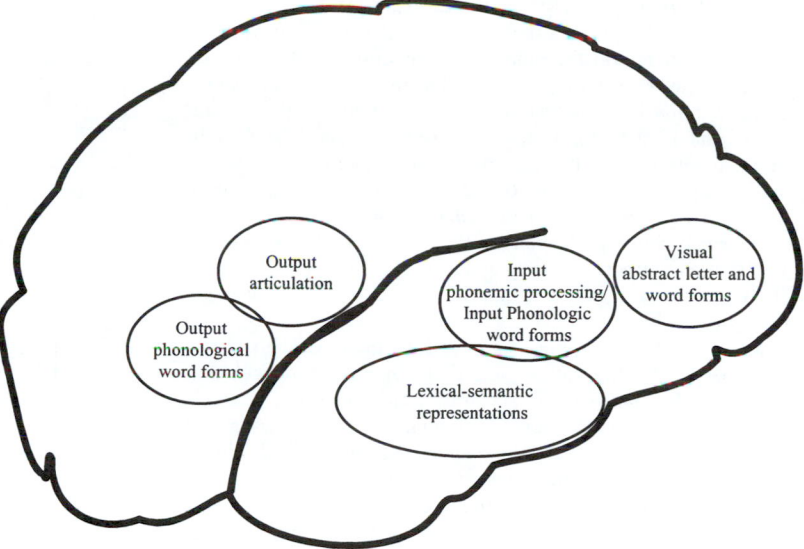

Figure 2. Neuroanatomic associations in the left (dominant) hemisphere of some of the functional modules shown in Figure 1. Note that these are approximate, and that there is also considerable individual variation; see text. (Copyright IA, Inc. Used with permission.)

acquired brain injuries. The common forms of brain injury that occur in adults tend to produce somewhat distinctive patterns of impairment in language and speech (collectively termed "aphasia"), particularly in the late (>6 month) period after the injury. *Broca's aphasia* is typified by slow, effortful, halting speech, frequently described as telegraphic and agrammatic because function words and grammatical endings are often omitted. These individuals may appear to have good comprehension of speech, but it is now appreciated that their comprehension of syntax is also impaired. Lesions associated with Broca's aphasia are typically in the anterior regions of the left hemisphere, including the posterior inferior frontal lobe (Broca's area), but are more extensive than this area. The pattern of deficits in Broca's aphasia contrasts with that of *Wernicke's aphasia*, in which speech is fluent and well articulated but often empty of specific meaning (as in "Jabberwocky"). Content words (nouns and verbs) are often misused or not recognizable (neologisms). Grammatical function words and endings are present but used incorrectly (with errors in inflections, and with nongrammatical (paragrammatic) constructions). These deficits are found in both production and comprehension as well as in reading. Individuals with Wernicke's aphasia are usually found to have lesions that include the posterior superior temporal lobe and adjacent parietal lobe (Wernicke's area) of the dominant hemisphere. In addition to these syndromes, a number of other relatively distinctive ones have been described, with varying degrees of anatomic lesion specificity.

Aphasic deficits reveal themselves as either complete failures to perform a function or as delays and/or errors in performance. Among the errors commonly observed are those that sound like the intended target (such as "bot" for "dot") (*phonemic paraphasias*) and those with a meaning similar to the intended target (as in "door" for "exit") (*lexical* or *semantic paraphasias*). Normal individuals also make most, if not all, of the errors made by aphasic individuals, as Freud and others pointed out, but aphasic individuals make them with a much higher frequency.

The Expanded First-Order Model

Aphasic syndromes and the errors that normal and aphasic individuals may make have not changed in the past hundred years. As a

result, the basic block diagrams of the models explaining them have not changed much (compare Figure 3), but critical details are now different. Methodological errors have been identified, and additional methods and subject groups have been used. As a result, finer details have been added. In addition, speech and language are now recognized as the products of interactive dynamic systems, with major implications for modeling normal and abnormal performance and for understanding their neural substrates.

Methodological Refinements

Broca's aphasia, Wernicke's aphasia, and the other aphasic syndromes are now understood to be collections of more than one fundamental deficit. For example, Broca's aphasia is a variable mix of difficulties in comprehension of syntax (IMAGING THE GRAMMATICAL BRAIN) and deficits in word retrieval, production of syntax, and articulation. These independent functions happen to co-occur in Broca's aphasia because the typical brain injury that causes the syndrome, vascular infarction, affects all the different regions responsible at once. Similarly, Wernicke's aphasia has now been reinterpreted as a variable mixture of deficits in phonemic speech

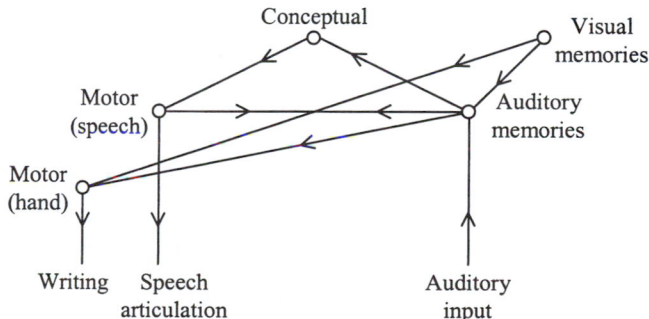

Figure 3. An example of a classical model of speech/language functions: Lichtheim's 1885 model, redrawn and labeled for brevity. Note that the modern meanings of the labels may not correspond exactly to the meanings Lichtheim originally intended. (Copyright IA, Inc. Used with permission.)

perception, the input phonological word system, lexical semantics, and word retrieval processes, perhaps also with syntactic deficits.

It is now understood that analysis of functions and functional architecture must to be strictly separated from analysis of the neural structures and mechanisms that may be responsible for those functions, at least in the initial stages of investigation. The flaw in assuming otherwise can be seen even with machines that are designed to perform basic functions. It is likely to be even more necessary to keep functions and structures separate for systems such as speech/language, which evolved from simpler beginnings by mutation and opportunistic adaptation. The correspondence between functional and neural levels in such cases is likely to be extremely convoluted.

Lesions remain a valuable source of information. Their utility has increased with the investigation of hyperacute strokes and follow-up studies (Hillis et al., 2002) and with the use of methods for inducing temporary "lesions" in humans, such as intracarotid amobarbital injection, transcranial magnetic stimulation, and direct cortical electrical stimulation (Berndt, 2001). However, it is now clear that lesions do not produce simple effects on neural tissue or on function. For example, functional and neuroanatomic reorganization often occurs in the minutes to months after a lesion, blurring lesion effects and neuroanatomic associations.

Besides lesion methods, there are now observational (correlational) methods for identification of the neural activity associated with language performance. These include regional cerebral metabolic studies (PET), regional cerebral blood flow (PET and functional MRI), and electrophysiological methods, such as evoked potentials, magnetoencephalographic recording, and direct cortical electrical recording (Berndt, 2001). To use these methods effectively, it is necessary to determine how the quantities measured correspond to brain activities, and in turn how brain activities are related to task performance. These methods allow examination of the whole brain (or large portions) at once and most involve little or no risk, so they can be performed in normal subjects as well as those with cerebral injuries.

Neurolinguistics now draws on a wide range of subject groups. Normal subjects have been studied more intensively, because it is now better understood that there are wide variations in normal abilities, that different languages may make different demands on mental functions, and that special training (such as literacy) can affect language and related functions. Individuals with developmental disorders that cause language functions to be affected disproportionately (e.g., autism) or relatively spared (e.g., William's syndrome) have provided valuable data concerning what components comprise language abilities and what sequence of steps is required to learn language (DEVELOPMENTAL DISORDERS).

Tasks used to probe language functions have been refined in light of the theoretical understanding of what it takes to accomplish a particular task and what components are of interest in any particular experiment. Traditional subtractive logic and additive factors logic have been found to have limitations. More subtle manipulations, such as word frequency, may be needed to affect a single stage of interest (Levelt, 2001). Techniques such as speeded reaction can induce informative errors and response patterns.

Amplifications and Controversies

The schematics presented in Figures 1 and 2 need to be expanded in several ways to be brought into conformity with current understanding. The parcellation of functions at large scale remains correct, and so do their approximate neuroanatomic associations. However, it is clear that even the classical processing chains have many more subfunctions than once thought. Furthermore, in many normal individuals, the nondominant hemisphere can perform many language-related functions. Figure 4 gives an outline of the

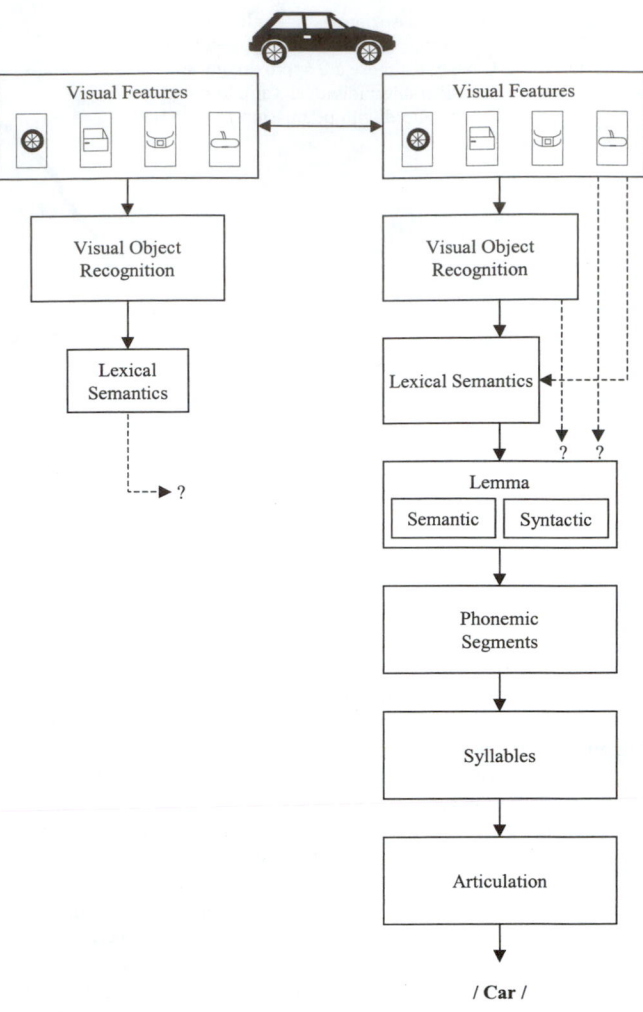

Figure 4. Supplemental detail for Figure 1, for the visual confrontation naming task. The processes identified here are used by other tasks as well; see Gordon, 1997. The bihemispheric distribution of these processes is illustrated. (Copyright IA, Inc. Used with permission.)

subprocesses involved in the relatively straightforward task of naming visual objects and of their hemispheric associations. Moreover, processes and regions apart from those traditionally thought to be involved in language are now known to contribute to language abilities. For instance, metaphor and emotion are important for language but are not affected by lesions in left hemisphere language areas; instead, they seem to depend on the non-dominant hemisphere.

What functions are subdivided, the nature of the processing performed in these subfunctions, and the neuroanatomic associations of any particular subfunction, are all active areas of inquiry. Some important current debates include the following:

Speech perception and its functional anatomy alone are far more complex than presented here; additional information can be found in Hickok and Poeppel (2000) and in SPEECH PROCESSING: PSYCHOLINGUISTICS. Figure 1 separates input phonology from output phonology, although some have argued these are identical (Martin, Lesch, and Bartha, 1999). Working memory and sensory-specific memory stores (such as auditory-verbal memory) are also important for speech and language processing (but see Martin et al., 1999).

Syntactic functions are clearly important for both comprehension and production. Some consider syntactic abilities to be the product of a relatively small set of functions (IMAGING THE GRAMMATICAL BRAIN), whereas others have suggested that syntactic abilities are the product of a much larger and more variegated collection of processes (Dick et al., 2001).

There is no consensus on the nature of conceptual and semantic abilities. Much evidence favors the existence of modality-specific semantic capabilities, connecting to an amodal repository of additional semantic knowledge. However, both extremes (only modality-specific semantic processes, or only an amodal semantic system) have also been argued.

It is also now understood that, in any one individual, the areas devoted to specific language functions are likely to be smaller in extent, and more variable in location, than the maps derived from chronic studies of large numbers of individuals (Gordon et al., 2001). As a result, when it is necessary to have precise localization in any one individual (as in patients requiring focal cerebral excisions for treatment of seizures or tumors), detailed, individualized mapping is necessary (Gordon et al., 2001).

Dynamic Processing Considerations

Perhaps the most important addition to the modern understanding of how language is represented and processed in the brain is an understanding of its dynamic properties. That language is the product of complex, interacting, dynamic systems may explain the richness of language abilities and hitherto intractable problems such as how word and sentence information might be integrated online. Furthermore, what is known or should be known about these dynamics will need to be explained by any theory of the neural processes responsible for them. What follows is a synthesis of the inferences and assumptions that have been made concerning the dynamics of processing of the cognitive information relevant to speech/language and related functions.

Between-Stage Information Flow

The approximate sequence of the flow of information between stages is shown in Figure 1. Auditory speech perception somewhat precedes lexical semantic comprehension; visual perception of a picture somewhat precedes its comprehension and the generation of its name. However, the times involved in each stage are relatively long compared to the time required for the overall process, so there is considerable overlap in processing between stages (cascaded processing).

In addition, there is almost certain to be extensive feedback between stages (only shown for the most likely ones in Figure 1), both at adjacent levels and at greater psychological (and neural) distances. Many potential neuroanatomic mechanisms for such feedback are known to exist, and some have been shown to be operational (with the most compelling examples coming from the visual domain).

Dynamics of Within-Stage Processing

There is fair agreement that processing within a stage is not a step function; it has a rise and fall that can be measured by behavioral as well as by more interventional techniques (Hart et al., 1998). Although the data on durations of processing are difficult to interpret, it certainly appears that speech perceptual processes can be accomplished in as little as 20–50 ms (or less), whereas lexical-semantic selection involved in a function such as naming may take 200–400 ms.

Unitary Representations and Activation

It has been widely assumed that the contents of any particular stage are some form of unitized, independent representations. The terminology of these unitized representations is confusing (Gordon, 1997). In cognitive science, they are often termed "nodes." However, these are not the nodes of connectionist networks. Nor do these unitized representations almost ever correspond to the activity of single neurons, either in actuality or in theory (although they could, if there really were "grandmother cells"). Here, we will use the standard cognitive science terminology of "nodes."

What information these unitized representations convey has not been settled. They may correspond to features that have already been psychologically identified (e.g., the /ba/ part of the phonological representation of /bat/, or the {round} semantic feature of a lexical-semantic representation of {ball}). Others have assumed that what they represent is much less transparent.

Nodes are generally assumed to have a number of characteristics and properties (although not every theorist who uses nodes necessarily endorses or uses all of the ones listed here; see Gordon, 1997):

Except for perhaps very basic perceptual and motor features, nodes are not preexisting; they must be created by experience.

Once created, nodes persist in latent form, available for activation.

The latent strength of a node is greater, depending on its experiential frequency. Experiential frequency is probably a surrogate for memory; the strength of a node is a form of memory, increased by frequency of exposure and by all the other mechanisms that consolidate learning (such as salience).

Nodes can be converted from a latent to an active (activated) state.

Nodes are activated by virtue of their connections to other nodes ("spreading activation").

The degree to which a node is activated is determined by several factors:

By how well the input(s) match the node's receptive pattern. Inputs can be inhibitory as well as facilitatory.

By the node's latent strength

By a random component (noise). Noise may be absolute, or it may be correlated with the degree of activation, or both.

Activation of a node grows over time to the maximum determined by the factors listed previously.

After a node has reached maximal activation, its activation may persist for a time or may decay.

It is likely that there is some degree of control over nodal properties, both internal and external to each stage: how easily they are formed, how they activate and decay, and how they can be altered by experience.

There is little direct evidence for nodes, but there are several lines of indirect support. Postulating nodes with properties such as those listed previously has proven to be very useful for understanding many otherwise puzzling phenomena of normal and brain-injured performance (Gordon, 1997). Some brain injuries can be interpreted as though they selectively destroy some nodal representations within a stage (see Gordon, 1997). In other cases, focal brain injuries have been successfully modeled in terms of changes in nodal properties or connection strengths, as in the Dell et al. (1997) and Foygel and Dell (2000) simulations discussed later in this article.

Processing by Constraint Satisfaction

The input information available to a stage is very likely to underspecify the correct output, particularly at the beginning of processing. Evidence exists from several different levels of language processing (speech perception, reading, and sentence-level comprehension, among others) that all possible candidate representations are activated initially. With continued input, and with input from other stages, the candidate set is winnowed down to the correct one. The specifics of this process are debated, but it is likely that such dynamic, interactive computation plays a critical role in many known examples of language processing. Dynamic processing by interactive constraint satisfaction may also explain how multiple sources of information can interact in the course of comprehension and production. See, for example, Arbib and Caplan (1979), LESIONED NETWORKS AS MODELS OF NEUROPSYCHOLOGICAL DEFICITS, and OPTIMALITY THEORY IN LINGUISTICS.

Possible Neural Bases

As depicted in the schematic of Figure 2, some stages or collections of stages seem to be the product of relatively discrete areas of the cerebral cortex. Connections between stages seem to correspond to short- and long-range subcortical white matter pathways.

How the cognitive elements (nodes) of psychological theorizing correspond to actual neuronal activity is not known for certain. However, the attractor states that can occur in neuronal networks with feedback are viable candidates for behaving as nodes are posited to behave (LESIONED NETWORKS AS MODELS OF NEUROPSYCHOLOGICAL DEFICITS). A single neural network can have multiple attractor states. The sculpting of connections to create an attractor can be equated with the learning of a node. The width of a basin of attraction of a neural activity state may be the neural counterpoint of a node's similarity relations (its receptive field). The depth of a basin of attraction, as well as its width, may correspond to frequency ("strength"). The process of "activation" of a cognitive node may correspond to the evolution of neural activity toward the attractor. Attractor dynamics have proven to be very useful in modeling a number of language and related functions (see, for example, McLeod, Shallice, and Plaut, 2000; also COMPUTING WITH ATTRACTORS; NEUROLOGICAL AND PSYCHIATRIC DISORDERS). However, attractors are not the only emergent features of neural network activity that might be candidates for nodes (see, for example, STRUCTURED CONNECTIONIST MODELS).

Models of Speech/Language Functions

Many modeling efforts in neurolinguistics have been concerned with the consequences of relatively large-scale assumptions about stages and connections. Examples of models that have incorporated both stage- and substage-level assumptions are those used by Dell et al. (1997) and by Foygel and Dell (2000). Dell et al. (1997) simulated picture naming using semantic, lexical, and phonologic stages. Each level represented its information as nodes, with properties similar to those discussed earlier. Spreading activation drove production. Parameters that replicated normal performance were derived from control data. Then, to model the picture naming performance of aphasic subjects, two parameters were altered for each aphasic subject: one governed how much activation spread, and one determined how rapidly activation declined. There was a "fairly good" fit between simulated and actual performance with just these assumptions (as characterized by Foygel and Dell, 2000). In addition, Dell et al. (1997) were able to capture much of the pattern of recovery of patients in terms of changes in these same parameters back to their normal values. Even so, Foygel and Dell (2000) have suggested that the data used by Dell et al. (1997), and other cases in the literature, might be better explained by alterations in two other parameters: the connection strengths (weights) be-

tween semantic and lexical units, and those between lexical and phonological units.

Modeling efforts by Dell and his colleagues represent one motivation for this chapter's method of review. Modeling efforts are likely to be most productive when they are informed by a good knowledge of existing data and theoretical explanations and also by a realistic understanding of when those data and explanations may be incomplete or arguable. LESIONED NETWORKS AS MODELS OF NEUROPSYCHOLOGICAL DEFICITS provides additional perspectives on modeling attempts.

Discussion

The emergent complexity of language functions is a daunting challenge for both its experimental investigation and for modeling attempts. However, it is also encouraging, because it makes it more likely that the same fundamental building blocks and processes that are identified in other domains of brain function will be applicable to understanding language, and vice versa.

Road Maps: Cognitive Neuroscience; Linguistics and Speech Processing
Related Reading: Imaging the Grammatical Brain; Language Evolution: The Mirror System Hypothesis; Language Processing; Lesioned Networks as Models of Neuropsychological Deficits

References

Arbib, M. A., and Caplan, D., 1979, Neurolinguistics must be computational, *Behav. Brain Sci.*, 2:449–483.

Berndt, R. S., 2001, *Language and Aphasia* (2nd ed.), Amsterdam, Netherlands: Elsevier. ◆

Brown, C. M., and Hagoort, P., 1999, *The Neurocognition of Language*, Oxford, UK: Oxford University Press. ◆

Crone, N. E., Hao, L., Hart, J., Jr., Boatman, D., Lesser, R. P., Irizarry, R., and Gordon, B., 2001, Electrocorticographic gamma activity during word production in spoken and sign language, *Neurology*, 57(11):2045–2053.

Dell, G. S., Schwartz, M. F., Martin, N., Saffran, E. M., and Gagnon, D. A., 1997, Lexical access in aphasic and nonaphasic speakers, *Psychol. Rev.*, 104(4):801–838.

Dick, F., Bates, E., Wulfeck, B., Utman, J. A., Dronkers, N., and Gernsbacher, M. A., 2001, Language deficits, localization, and grammar: Evidence for a distributive model of language breakdown in aphasic patients and neurologically intact individuals, *Psychol. Rev.*, 108(4):759–788.

Foygel, D., and Dell, G. S., 2000, Models of impaired lexical access in speech production, *J. Mem. Lang.*, 43:182–216. ◆

Gordon, B., 1997, Models of naming, in *Anomia: Neoroanatomical and Cognitive Correlates* (H. Goodglass and A. Wingfield, Eds.), San Diego, CA: Academic Press, pp. 31–64. ◆

Gordon, B., Boatman, D., Hart, J., Jr., Miglioretti, D., and Lesser, R. P., 2001, Direct cortical electrical interference (stimulation), in *Language and Aphasia*, 2nd ed., Vol. 3 (R. S. Berndt, Ed.), Amsterdam: Elsevier Science B.V., pp. 375–391.

Hart, J., Jr., Crone, N. E., Lesser, R. P., Sieracki, J., Miglioretti, D. L., Hall, C., Sherman, D., and Gordon, B., 1998, Temporal dynamics of verbal object comprehension, *Proc. Natl. Acad. Sci. USA*, 95(11):6498–6503.

Hickok, G., and Poeppel, D., 2000, Towards a functional neuroanatomy of speech perception, *Trends Cogn. Sci.*, 4(4):131–138.

Hillis, A. E., Kane, A., Tuffiash, E., Ulatowski, J. A., Barker, P., Beauchamp, N. J., and Wityk, R. J., 2001, Reperfusion of specific brain regions by raising blood pressure restores selective language functions in subacute stroke, *Brain Lang.*, 79(3):495–510

Levelt, W. J., 2001, Inaugural Article: Spoken word production: A theory of lexical access, *Proc. Natl. Acad. Sci. USA*, 98(23):13464–13471. ◆

Martin, R. C., Lesch, M. F., and Bartha, M. C., 1999, Independence of input and output phonology in word processing and short-term memory, *J. Mem. Lang.*, 41(1):3–29.

McLeod, P., Shallice, T., and Plaut, D. C., 2000, Attractor dynamics in word recognition: Converging evidence from errors by normal subjects, dyslexic patients and a connectionist model, *Cognition*, 74(1):91–114.

Neurological and Psychiatric Disorders

Eytan Ruppin and James A. Reggia

Introduction

In the last decade it has become natural to ask how neural modeling may be harnessed to investigate the pathogenesis and potential treatment of brain disorders, and in what ways it may complement more traditional research methodologies. Indeed, early attempts in this direction have been extensively developed in recent years.

The interest of the psychiatric and neurological communities in neural network modeling probably reflects the belief that, although the gathering of neurobiological data has led to much progress in our understanding of basic brain mechanisms, we do not appear to have come much closer to understanding how these mechanisms result in behavior. Neural modeling is a methodology that is precisely aimed at bridging this gap, by studying the relation between the "microscopic" pathological alterations of the underlying neural networks and the "macroscopic" functional and behavioral disease manifestations that characterize the network's function.

To study brain or cognitive disorders computationally, one first has to construct a model network that is capable of performing some basic functions, such as controlling movements or storing and retrieving information. Thereafter, by lesioning the intact network's structural components or disrupting its dynamic mechanisms, the specific neuroanatomical and neurophysiological findings assumed to characterize the pathogenesis of the disease can be modeled, and the resulting changes in the behavior of the network can be examined. It is then also possible to search for mechanisms that may counteract the damaging effects of the simulated pathological alterations.

Neural models are limited in that they necessarily simplify the biological phenomena occurring in the nervous system and are generally constrained in size. The simulated lesions in such models are substantial simplifications of abnormal events occurring within the brain and/or in cognitive processes. Nevertheless, such computer-based models complement traditional methods of studying brain disorders in substantial and important ways. The size and location of simulated brain damage can be controlled precisely and can be systematically varied over arbitrarily large numbers of experimental "subjects" and information processing tasks. Further, the computational experiments are open to detailed inspection in ways that biological systems are not.

Neural models of brain and cognitive disorders, like neural network models in general, vary widely in the level of realism with which they aim to model the underlying phenomena. This is true both with regard to the level of biological detail employed in describing the individual building blocks themselves (the neurons and their interactions), and also with regard to the description level of the network's architecture, i.e., to the extent the latter aims to reconstruct a specific brain region. In general, computational studies addressing neuropsychological or cognitive disorders tend to describe more abstract models, fairly removed from specific brain architectures, compared with the models addressing neurological and psychiatric disorders. Models of neuropsychological disorders are reviewed in LESIONED NETWORKS AS MODELS OF NEUROPSYCHOLOGICAL DEFICTS. Here we review some computational studies of a few major neurological and psychiatric disorders. In addition to studies of Alzheimer's disease, Parkinson's disease, and stroke reviewed in this chapter, neurological modeling studies have addressed a wide variety of other disorders, including multi-infarct dementia, migraine, and delirium. Our review of psychiatric disorders focuses on schizophrenia and affective disorders, but preliminary computational modeling studies have also addressed paranoid disorders, dissociative disorders, and others. For recent papers describing these studies the interested reader is referred to Reggia, Ruppin, and Berndt (1996); Reggia, Ruppin, and Glanzman (1999); and Parks, Levine, and Long (1998).

Neurological Disorders

Many models of memory impairment have addressed various aspects of Alzheimer's disease (Horn et al., 1993, Hasselmo, 1994), the most common dementing illness. The essential clinical feature of Alzheimer's disease is a broad-based intellectual decline from previous levels of functioning, but memory impairment is a major clinical hallmark of the disease. These models have examined two main hypotheses concerning the pathogenesis of the disease. One hypothesis has been that *failure of neuronal synaptic compensatory mechanisms* (which in normal subjects successfully counteracts synaptic degenerative changes) plays a primary role in Alzheimer's pathogenesis (Horn et al., 1993). Variations on the rate and exact functional form of synaptic compensation were used to define various compensation strategies, and these could account for the observed variation in the severity and progression rate of Alzheimer's disease. The second hypothesis has focused on *synaptic runaway*, a pathological exponential growth of synaptic connections that may occur due to interference by previously stored memory patterns during the storage of new patterns (Hasselmo, 1994). Several factors can lead to the initiation of synaptic runaway, but once it occurs, its increased metabolic demands or excitotoxic effects could presumably be sufficiently severe to cause neuronal degeneration, parallel to that found in Alzheimer's disease. Interestingly, the pattern of spread of pathological damage in Alzheimer's disease fits well the hypothesis of synaptic runaway.

Recent work on modeling Alzheimer's disease has focused on more realistic models incorporating spiking neurons. These models share the view that the hippocampus (and more generally, medial temporal lobe structures) plays a primary role in consolidation of memories in the cortex. Extending their previous work, Hasselmo and his co-workers have studied a fairly realistic model of the hippocampus, both in terms of its subdivision into various substructures and in terms of accounting for several known neuromodulatory effects on hippocampal memory processing. The latter enables one to address the cholinergic disturbances that are assumed to play an important role in memory and learning dysfunction in Alzheimer's disease. The possible role of cholinergic neuromodulation of the hippocampus in Alzheimer's disease has also been recently addressed by Menschick and Finkel (1998). Their work is performed in a realistic compartmental model of associative memory, and discusses the pathogenesis of memory decline in Alzheimer's disease in dynamic terms that emerge from such spiking models, identifying a cascade of malfunctions occurring at multiple levels.

Models of stroke (sudden focal brain damage due to impaired regional blood flow) have been developed to address the events occurring immediately following the acute stroke event, and also later on during the chronic, reorganization phase. Naturally, these models differ in the kind of computational framework involved. Models of acute focal stroke encompass a combined neural/metabolic description that traces the temporal evolution of several variables that play a critical role in ischemic stroke (Revett et al., 1998). This work has examined the hypothesis that *cortical spreading depression* waves play a primary role in the spread of damage into the penumbral perinfarct region from the infarct core. It successfully reproduced several experimental dependencies and has made testable predictions about the number, velocity, and duration of spreading depression waves. In contrast, studying chronic reorganization after focal stroke has been based on models simulating map formation in the cortex (Goodall et al., 1997). These models involve the projection of high-dimensional data on a two-dimensional cortical surface, and generate computational maps that mimic cortical "maps" representing relevant aspects of the external world (e.g., the homunculus in primary somatosensory or motor cortex). When a lesion is introduced into the simulated map, the model reorganizes such that the sensory surface originally represented by the lesioned area spontaneously reappears in adjacent cortical areas, as has been seen experimentally in animal studies. Two key hypotheses emerged from this modeling work. First, that postlesion map reorganization is a two-phase process, consisting of a rapid phase due to the dynamics of neural activity and a longer-term phase due to synaptic plasticity. Second, that increased perilesion excitability is necessary for useful map reorganization to occur. Similar self-organizing models, but based on cortical deafferentation, have been used recently to support a theory of *phantom limb* experiences (Spitzer et al., 1994). This latter work presented an interesting solution, in neural network terms, to the ongoing controversy about the relative weight of central versus peripheral nervous system alterations in the pathogenesis of these disturbing symptoms.

Parkinson's disease is an important motor and cognitive degenerative disorder. Its primary pathology has been traced to the degeneration of nigral dopaminergic neurons projecting on the striatum, and it has been a subject of quite a few modeling studies in recent years (see BASAL GANGLIA and DOPAMINE, ROLES OF). Again, the pathogenesis of the disease can be studied at different levels. In a more high-level model, Contreras-Vidal, Teulings, and Stelmach (1998) describe the activation of many of the pathways known to exist in basal ganglia in terms of a system of coupled differential equations, composing a gross-scale representation of basal ganglia structures as single dynamical variables. This model was able to produce handwriting patterns that were comparable to handwriting changes observed in Parkinson's patients before and after L-DOPA treatment. On a lower-level of description, Kotter and Wickens (1998) have presented a more detailed, realistic model of the striatum, including effects of dopamine on the various receptor subtypes. This work suggests that dopamine therapy would tend to reverse only a subset of the changes produced by dopamine depletion, resulting in striatal dynamics that are significantly different from those encountered in the normal, premorbid state.

Psychiatric Disorders

Neural models have been created for a wide range of psychiatric disorders, but most of the work has focused on schizophrenia and affective disorders.

Schizophrenia is a clinically heterogeneous disorder with a broad spectrum of manifestations. Its symptoms include both "positive symptoms," such as hallucinations, delusions, disorganized speech and behavior, and "negative symptoms," such as loss of fluency of thought and speech, impaired attention, abnormalities in the expression and observation of emotion, and loss of volition and drive. The course of the illness tends to be marked by exacerbations and remissions, but the persistence of the impairment may give the disease a "dementia-like" quality in more advanced stages. The pathogenesis of schizophrenia is unknown. Perhaps the most enduring biochemical explanation of the pathophysiology of schizophrenia is the dopamine hypothesis, which postulates the coexistence of hypodopaminergic activity in the mesocortical system, resulting in negative symptoms, and hyperdopaminergic activity in the mesolimbic system, resulting in positive symptoms. Structural and functional imaging and neuroanatomical postmortem studies are providing converging evidence of the involvement of specific brain regions in schizophrenia, such as the prefrontal areas, temporal lobes and the temporo-limbic circuitry, and subcortical circuitry. Integrative pathophysiological hypotheses have been proposed, but so far no single explanatory mechanism has prevailed.

Neural modeling of schizophrenia has taken two main paths, reflecting the view of schizophrenia as composed of positive symptoms that arise due to temporo-frontal pathology, and negative symptoms that are a result of prefrontal abnormalities. The first avenue has concentrated on modeling schizophrenic positive symptoms in the framework of an associative memory attractor network (Hoffman, 1987). In this framework, pathological alterations in an attractor neural network modeling excessive synaptic pruning can lead to the formation of *parasitic attractors*, whose cognitive and perceptual manifestations may play an important role in the emergence of schizophrenic delusions and hallucinations, by altering speech perception and production processes. In this line of research, Ruppin, Reggia, and Horn (1996) have modeled a frontal module as an associative memory neural network receiving its inputs from degenerating temporal projections and undergoing reactive synaptic regeneration. They have shown that while preserving memory performance, compensatory synaptic regenerative changes coupled with Hebbian activity-dependent synaptic changes may eventually lead to a *biased* retrieval distribution that is strongly dominated by few memory patterns, resembling the concentration of psychotic delusions and hallucinations on very few cognitive and perceptual themes.

Building upon their work on modeling the neuromodulatory effects of catecholamines on information processing, Cohen and Servan-Schreiber (1992) have presented a modeling study of the performance of normal subjects and schizophrenics in three attentional and language processing tasks. These tasks are important indices of cognitive dysfunction in schizophrenia, and are related to schizophrenic negative symptoms. In all of the tasks modeled, a backpropagation algorithm was used to train the networks to simulate normal performance. Although each task was modeled by a network designed specifically for that task, the networks used rely on similar information processing principles and share a common module for representing context, which is identified with the prefrontal cortex. The hypothesized neuromodulatory effects of dopamine on information processing were modeled as a global change of the input gain. Simulations demonstrated that a change in the gain of neurons in the context module can quantitatively account for the differences between normal and schizophrenic performance in the tasks examined. Postulating that the prefrontal cortex plays a central role in establishing context (see Braver and Cohen in Reggia et al., 1999), it has been proposed that dopamine might regulate context information in prefrontal cortex by providing an appropriate gating signal. Their model provides a mechanism for flexible updating of stored information, and is able to accurately simulate the performance breakdown of schizophrenics in the Continuous Performance Test.

More recently, Hoffman et al. have addressed the pathogenesis of schizophrenic positive symptoms from a neurodevelopmental perspective. They show that although the process of synaptic pruning can improve generalization of previously learned information, when taken to excess it would result in spontaneous percepts (hallucinations) and in "hyperpriming," both seen in schizophrenia (Hoffman and McGlashan, 1997). This provides an interesting view of the pathogenesis of a disease by a normal developmental process that is taken "much too far." Recent work has investigated the role of the prefrontal cortex in the pathogenesis of schizophrenia using more biologically realistic spike response neurons (see Reid and Willshaw in Reggia et al., 1999). They show that the ability of the prefrontal cortex to hold working memory information may be disrupted by changes in dopaminergic activity, reduced GABAergic activity, and reduced prefrontal connectivity, which have all been implicated in schizophrenia. As in the case of neural models of dementia and Alzheimer's disease, the general trend is to move from simplistic models employing McCulloch-Pitts binary neurons to networks using compartmental models of neurons and more realistic descriptions of synaptic transmission.

Attractor neural networks have also been considered as a framework for modeling cognitive manifestations of manic-depressive disorder. Manic bouts are characterized by a distinctly elevated, expansive or irritable mood, accompanied by "hyperactivity" symptoms. In contradistinction to schizophrenic positive symptoms, Hoffman (1987) has suggested that manic "hyperactivity" arises not as a result of structural damage leading to the formation of pathological attractors, but due to an increase in the noise levels resulting in enhanced rate of transition between attractors.

Past work related to major depression has concentrated on modeling learned helplessness, an experimental psychological model of depression, in an adaptive resonance network. More recently, a general model aimed at explaining how cognitive, emotional, and motor processes might influence one another has been presented (see Grossberg, in Reggia et al., 1999). Grossberg postulated opponent processing modules to control reinforcement learning in response to positive and negative reenforcers. Taking yet another approach to modeling major depression, it has recently been shown that the affective interference of depression might produce network overtraining and result in a network that responds excessively to negative stimuli and reinforces the dark obsessions characteristic of rumination.

Discussion

The conceptual and methodological challenges tackled by the studies surveyed here serve to illustrate the early stages of coalescence of a field that ambitiously endeavors to study the pathogenesis of brain disorders computationally. There is a large gap between the conceptual and modeling levels utilized in "realistic" computational studies of brain disorders versus more abstract ones. This gap arises in part because of the different disorders and phenomena addressed. It also reflects the long-standing controversy in the literature between more realistic "bottom-up" models and simpler, conceptual "top-down" models. In our current state of knowledge of the workings of the brain there is certainly room for both kinds of models.

The work reviewed in this paper demonstrates that neural models are a potentially useful methodological tool for examining the feasibility of theoretical hypotheses within a computational context. They can offer new insights into the experimental data, and may unify previously unrelated observations. Even the much simplified models reviewed here are sufficiently complicated to generate interesting and nontrivial predictions, as the feedback structure of the systems and processes involved makes the study of lesioned models a difficult and considerable challenge.

Future challenges and prospects of modeling brain disorders include:

1. *Modeling new experimental data*: Recent advances in several experimental techniques have yielded a number of promising developments. Of special interest to neural modelers are the developments in techniques that provide information on neural and synaptic degenerative processes. Those include neuroanatomical morphometric and immunochemical methods and magnetic resonance spectroscopy. Much hope for further advancement relies on the rapid development of functional imaging techniques, but a significant discrepancy remains between the scale of the distributed networks of brain activation revealed by current functional imaging studies and the scale of current neural models.

2. *Developing neural models of more complex cognitive functions*: current work has concentrated on making use of available neural modeling tools. This has restricted the cognitive phenomena studied to memory-related processes, and to learning relatively simple tasks in a supervised manner. The development and incorporation of more sophisticated neural models is probably an essential step towards capturing more complex phenomena. Promising venues include models of reinforcement learning, multimodular associative memories, and multilayered recurrent networks.

The studies reviewed here are just the "end of the beginning." As more becomes known about the normal functioning of brain and cognitive systems, we shall be in a much better position to model their abnormalities. Some of the research projects in this field demonstrate another, perhaps not less promising, potential value of computational studies of brain disorders: to use the constraints imposed by such studies to learn more about the normal functioning of the brain by way of "reverse engineering." Computational modeling helps us to formulate our ideas precisely and study their consequences by making them explicit within simulation and analytical models. As such, we believe it will continue to develop as a fundamental research approach, working in a complementary manner with other research methodologies.

Road Map: Cognitive Neuroscience
Related Reading: Developmental Disorders; Dopamine, Roles of; EEG and MEG Analysis; Neuromodulation in Mammalian Nervous Systems

References

Cohen, J. D., and Servan-Schreiber, D., 1992, Context, cortex, and dopamine: A connectionist approach to behavior and biology in schizophrenia, *Psychol. Rev.*, 99(1):45–77.

Contreras-Vidal, J. L., Teulings H. L., and Stelmach G. E., 1998, Neural dynamics of short and medium-term motor control effects of levodopa therapy in parkinson's disease, *Artif. Intell. Med.*, 13(1–2):57–80.

Goodall, S., Reggia, J., Chen, Y., Ruppin, E., and Whitney, C., 1997, A computational model of acute focal cortical lesions, *Stroke*, 28:101–109.

Hasselmo, M. E., 1994, Runaway synaptic modification in models of the cortex: Implications for Alzheimer's disease, *Neural Networks*, 7(1):13–40.

Hoffman, R. E., 1987, Computer simulations of neural information processing and the schizophrenia-mania dichotomy, *Arch. Gen. Psychiatry*, 44:178.

Hoffman, R. E., and McGlashan, T. H., 1997, Synaptic elimination, neurodevelopment and the mechanism of hallucinated voices in schizophrenia, *Am. J. Psychiatry*, 154:1683–1689.

Horn, D., Ruppin, E., Usher, M., and Herrmann, M., 1993, Neural network modeling of memory deterioration in alzheimer's disease, *Neural Computation*, 5:736–749.

Kotter, R., and Wickens, J., 1998, Striatal mechanisms in parkinson's disease: New insights from computer modeling, *Arti. Intell. Med.*, 13(1–2):37–56.

Menschick, E. D., and Finkel, L. H., 1998, Neuromodulatory control of hippocampal function: towards a model of Alzheimer's disease, *Artif. Intell. Med.*, 13:99–121.

Parks, R. W., Levine, D. S., and Long, D. L., 1998, *Fundamentals of Neural Network Modeling: Neuropsychology and Cognitive Neuroscience*, Cambridge, MA: MIT Press. ◆

Reggia, J., Ruppin, E., and Berndt, R., 1996, *Neural Modeling of Brain and Cognitive Disorders*, Singapore: World Scientific. ◆

Reggia, J., Ruppin, E., and Glanzman, D., 1999, *Brain, Behavioral and Cognitive Disorders: The Neurocomputational Perspective*. Progress in Brain Research Series, Amsterdam: Elsevier Science Publishers. ◆

Revett, K., Ruppin, E., Goodall, S., and Reggia, J., 1998, Spreading depression in focal ischemia: A computational study, *J. Cerebral Blood Flow Metab.*, 18(9):998–1007.

Ruppin, E., Reggia, J., and Horn, D., 1996, A neural model of positive schizophrenic symptoms, *Schizophrenia Bull.*, 22(1):105–123.

Spitzer, M., Bohler, P., Weisbrod M., and Kischka, U., 1994, A neural network model of phantom limbs, *Biol. Cybernet.*, 72:197–206.

Neuromanifolds and Information Geometry

Shun-ichi Amari

Introduction

A neural network is specified by its architecture and by a number of parameters consisting of connections or synaptic weights, together with bias terms or thresholds. These parameters are modifiable, and learning or self-organization is carried out by changing them. Let us denote all of these parameters by a vector $\boldsymbol{\theta} = (\theta_1, \ldots, \theta_n)$, where n is the number of the parameters, and consider the parameter space where $\boldsymbol{\theta}$ is its coordinate system. Any neural network of this architecture is specified by a point $\boldsymbol{\theta}$ in the parameter space, so that we identify the parameter space with the set of all the neural networks.

Neural networks are regarded as stochastic nonlinear systems. Some models are intrinsically stochastic, because of the stochastic nature of neural firing. These models include Boltzmann machines (see SIMULATED ANNEALING AND BOLTZMANN MACHINES) and Bayesian or belief-propagation networks (see BAYESIAN NETWORKS). Some are deterministic but work in the noisy environment, so that its behaviors are not free from stochastic fluctuations. A typical example is a multilayer perceptron.

Learning takes place in the parameter space, and a learning process is represented by a trajectory. Here an important problem arises: What is the geometrical structure of the parameter space, and how do learning behaviors depend on its structure? Information geometry, which originated in studies of the manifolds of probability distributions, can be used to answer these questions (Amari and Nagaoka, 2000). It defines a Riemannian metric and a pair of dual affine connections. It gives a geometrical framework to elucidate problems related to stochastic phenomena, so that it is useful not only for statistical inference and information theory but also for neural networks.

This article introduces geometrical structures in the parameter space of neural networks known as neuromanifolds and elucidates how the dynamical behaviors of neural learning are related to the underlying geometrical structures. We use multilayer perceptrons and Boltzmann machines as examples. Geometrical ideas are also applied to support vector machines (Burges, 1999; Amari and Wu, 1999), boosting methods (Lebanon and Lafferty, 2001), and many others. The principles and practical implementations of natural gradient learning (Amari, 1998) are described first.

Neuromanifold of Multilayer Perceptrons

Let us consider a multilayer perceptron consisting of one hidden layer with h hidden neurons and one output neuron. Let its inputs, $x_1, \ldots, x_k$, be denoted by an input vector $\mathbf{x} = (x_1, \ldots, x_k)$. The ith hidden neuron receives $\mathbf{x}$ and calculates its weighted sum, $u_i = \mathbf{w}_i \cdot \mathbf{x} = \Sigma w_{ij} x_j$, where $\mathbf{w}_i = (w_{i1}, \ldots, w_{ik})$ is the synaptic weight vector. It then emits a nonlinear sigmoidal function $\varphi(u_i)$ as its output, where $\varphi(u) = \tanh(u)$ is the hyperbolic tangent.

The output neuron summarizes all the outputs of the hidden neurons with weights $\mathbf{v} = (v_1, \ldots, v_h)$, and emits its output. The sum is disturbed by Gaussian noise n, so that the overall input-output relation is written as

$$y = \sum_{i=1}^{h} v_i \varphi(\mathbf{w}_i \cdot \mathbf{x}) + n \qquad (1)$$

The parameter space of the multilayer perceptron is specified by the set of all the parameters $\boldsymbol{\theta} = (w_{11}, \ldots, w_{1k}, w_{21}, \ldots, \ldots, w_{hk}; v_1, \ldots, v_h)$. It can be seen that each point $\boldsymbol{\theta}$ corresponds to the nonlinear function $f(\mathbf{x}, \boldsymbol{\theta}) = \Sigma v_i \varphi(\mathbf{w}_i \cdot \mathbf{x})$ of the perceptron. However, since the behavior of each perceptron is represented by the probability distribution of the output y given $\mathbf{x}$,

$$p(y|\mathbf{x}, \boldsymbol{\theta}) = \frac{1}{\sqrt{2\pi}} \exp \left\{ -\frac{1}{2} (y - f(\mathbf{x}, \boldsymbol{\theta}))^2 \right\} \qquad (2)$$

we may identify each point $\boldsymbol{\theta}$ with the above probability distribution.

We first address the problem of the identifiability of the parameters of neural networks. When two networks with different parameters $\boldsymbol{\theta}$ and $\boldsymbol{\theta}'$ have the same input-output behavior, it is not possible to identify the parameters from the behaviors. Such networks are said to be equivalent. Two types of unidentifiability are known (Chen, Lu, and Hecht-Nielsen, 1993):

1. *Permutation*: Permutation of the number of hidden units does not change a network's behavior.
2. *Sign change*: Sign change of both $\mathbf{w}_i$ and v_i at the same time does not change its behavior, because $v_i \varphi(\mathbf{w}_i \cdot \mathbf{x}) = -v_i \varphi(-\mathbf{w}_i \cdot \mathbf{x})$.

The above transformation induces the following equivalent networks (Rüger and Ossen, 1997): When the synaptic weight vectors $\mathbf{w}_i$ and $\mathbf{w}_j$ are equal, the two hidden neurons can be merged into one neuron, where $v' = v_i + v_j$ gives a new connection weight to the output neuron without changing its behavior. Hence, on the submanifold defined by $\mathbf{w}_i = \mathbf{w}_j$, two networks are equivalent when $v_i + v_j$ are equal. It also happens that, in the submanifold defined by $v_i = 0$, whatever value $\mathbf{w}_i$ takes, $v_i \varphi(\mathbf{w}_i \cdot \mathbf{x}) = 0$. Hence, whatever $\mathbf{w}_i$ is, the behaviors are the same, and this neuron can be removed. The same holds when $\mathbf{w}_i = 0$. We call these submanifolds defined by $\mathbf{w}_i = \mathbf{w}_j$ or $v_i |\mathbf{w}_i| = 0$ the critical submanifolds. Parameters are not identifiable on critical submanifolds.

When we consider equivalent networks as one object, the equivalent points in the neuromanifold will be merged into one point. For example, the submanifold defined by $v_i = 0$ reduces to one point. The reduced manifold has singularities on which dimensions are reduced. This causes a singular topological structure in the reduced neuromanifold.

It is usual to use the Kullback-Leibler divergence (Cover and Thomas, 1991) as a measure of divergence defined by two probability distributions $p(\mathbf{x})$ and $q(\mathbf{x})$:

$$KL[p(\mathbf{x}) : q(\mathbf{x})] = E_p \left[\log \frac{p(\mathbf{x})}{q(\mathbf{x})} \right] = \int p(\mathbf{x}) \log \frac{p(\mathbf{x})}{q(\mathbf{x})} \, d\mathbf{x} \qquad (3)$$

where E_p is expectation with respect to $p(\mathbf{x})$. This quantity is nonnegative and is equal to 0 when and only when $p(\mathbf{x}) = q(\mathbf{x})$, but it is not symmetric; that is, $KL[p : q] \neq KL[q : p]$ in general. The KL divergence is related to information theory. Let X, Y be two random variables whose joint probability is $p(x, y)$ and whose marginal distributions are $p_X(x)$ and $p_Y(y)$, respectively. The probability distribution $p_X(x)p_Y(y)$ is different from $p(x, y)$ except for the case in which X and Y are independent. How much are the random variables X and Y related? This is measured by the Shannon mutual information $I[X : Y]$, which is equal to the KL divergence, in this way:

$$I[X : Y] = KL[p(x, y) : p_X(x)p_Y(y)] \quad (4)$$

When the probability distribution is given by a parametric form $p(\mathbf{x}, \boldsymbol{\theta})$ (or conditional distribution $p(y|\mathbf{x}, \boldsymbol{\theta})$, in the present case), the KL divergence $D(\boldsymbol{\theta} : \boldsymbol{\theta}')$ is given in the parameter space by

$$D[\boldsymbol{\theta} : \boldsymbol{\theta}'] = KL[p(y|\mathbf{x}, \boldsymbol{\theta}) : p(y|\mathbf{x}, \boldsymbol{\theta}')] \quad (5)$$

When the two points are close, we put $\boldsymbol{\theta}' = \boldsymbol{\theta} + d\boldsymbol{\theta}$. Then, by Taylor expansion, we have the quadratic form

$$KL[p(y|\mathbf{x}, \boldsymbol{\theta}) : p(y|\mathbf{x}, \boldsymbol{\theta} + d\boldsymbol{\theta})] = \tfrac{1}{2}\, d\boldsymbol{\theta}^T G d\boldsymbol{\theta} \quad (6)$$

where

$$G(\boldsymbol{\theta}) = E\left[\frac{\partial}{\partial\boldsymbol{\theta}} \log p(y|\mathbf{x}, \boldsymbol{\theta}) \frac{\partial}{\partial\boldsymbol{\theta}} \log p(y|\mathbf{x}, \boldsymbol{\theta})^T\right] \quad (7)$$

is a matrix called the Fisher information matrix, and the quadratic form is regarded as the square of the distances between two nearby points $\boldsymbol{\theta}$ and $\boldsymbol{\theta} + d\boldsymbol{\theta}$. Here, $\partial/\partial\boldsymbol{\theta}$ is the gradient and T denotes transposition of a column vector.

The Fisher information matrix is a measure concerning how much information is obtained by observing a random variable, in order to estimate the underlying distribution. On the other hand, the Shannon information matrix is a measure concerning how much information is obtained concerning random variable X when another random variable Y is observed. Hence, they are used for different purposes, although they are derived from the same KL divergence.

A manifold is said to be Riemannian when the square of the distance between two nearby points is given by a quadratic form like that in Equation 6, based on a symmetric positive matrix G. The matrix is called the Riemannian metric.

The neuromanifold is a Riemannian space, having the Fisher information matrix G as its Riemannian metric. It is positive-definite in general, but it degenerates on the critical submanifolds of the neuromanifold of multilayer perceptrons, that is,

$$d\boldsymbol{\theta}^T G d\boldsymbol{\theta} = 0 \quad (8)$$

on a critical submanifold, when $d\boldsymbol{\theta}$ is the direction of unidentifiability. This reflects the fact that the distance between two equivalent points is 0. Such a manifold may be said to be pseudo-Riemannian. Hence, the Riemannian structure accounts for the topological singularity in the reduced manifold.

The gradient of a function $f(\boldsymbol{\theta})$ represents the direction of the steepest change of the function f in a Euclidean space. "The steepest" implies that, when $\boldsymbol{\theta}$ changes by $d\boldsymbol{\theta}$ with a small fixed length, say $|d\boldsymbol{\theta}|^2 = \varepsilon^2$, the change of f, $\Delta f = f(\boldsymbol{\theta} + d\boldsymbol{\theta}) - f(\boldsymbol{\theta})$, is largest in the direction of the gradient $d\boldsymbol{\theta} \propto \nabla f(\boldsymbol{\theta})$. In the case of a Riemannian space, the distance is defined by the quadratic form given in Equation 6. The steepest direction is then given by the natural or Riemannian gradient (Amari, 1998).

$$\tilde{\nabla} f = G^{-1}\nabla f \quad (9)$$

Natural Gradient Learning in a Neuromanifold

Learning takes place in a neuromanifold by modifying the current parameters $\boldsymbol{\theta}$, depending on the current input and output pair $(\mathbf{x}_t, y_t)$ at time $t = 1, 2, \ldots$, in a training set of examples. Let $l(\mathbf{x}, y; \boldsymbol{\theta})$ be a loss function that is to be minimized through learning. A popular loss is the square of errors of the outputs. The backpropagation learning rule is given by the gradient method

$$\Delta\boldsymbol{\theta} = -\eta\nabla l(\mathbf{x}, y; \boldsymbol{\theta}) \quad (10)$$

However, backpropagation learning is very slow. The error rate decreases quickly in the early stages of learning, but soon the decrement becomes very small. Such a position is called a plateau, and it takes a long time to get rid of it. Plateaus are not local minima but saddle points.

It is known from the statistical-physical method that plateaus result from the permutation symmetry of the hidden neurons and thus are ubiquitous (Rattray and Saad, 1999). Moreover, a learning trajectory is usually attracted to such a saddle point, and convergence slows greatly. Such a phenomenon is caused by the geometrical structure of the neuromanifold, corresponding to its topological and metrical properties.

Plateaus mostly occur on critical submanifolds where the parameters are not identifiable. A change in the parameters around a critical submanifold causes only a negligibly small improvement in its behaviors. However, if we take the metrical structure into account, the gradient should be replaced by the Riemannian one, the natural gradient. Then, the plateau phenomenon given rise to by unidentifiability disappears. The natural gradient learning rule is given by

$$\Delta\boldsymbol{\theta} = -\eta G^{-1}\nabla l(\mathbf{x}, y; \boldsymbol{\theta}) \quad (11)$$

where η is a learning rate (Amari, 1998). It should be noted that G is singular on a critical submanifold, so that G^{-1} diverges there. This has an effect of preventing the parameters $\boldsymbol{\theta}$ from approaching critical submanifolds, thus avoiding plateaus.

This method is equivalent locally to the Newton method, implying superlinear convergence. However, the merit of natural gradient learning lies not only in the speed with which local convergence can be achieved but also in the avoidance of plateaus in the learning process, which is the main obstacle slowing convergence. In general, natural gradient learning differs from a second-order method such as Newton's in that natural gradient learning depends on both the Riemannian structure and the cost function, while the second-order method takes only the second derivatives of the cost function.

In general, it is difficult to calculate and invert the Fisher information matrix G. In order to overcome this difficulty, the *adaptive natural gradient method* has been proposed (Amari, Park and Fukumizu, 2000) in which the inverse G^{-1} is estimated by an adaptive method, by changing the current G^{-1} into $G^{-1} + \Delta G^{-1}$,

$$\Delta G^{-1} = \eta' G^{-1}\nabla l (G^{-1}\nabla l)^T \quad (12)$$

where η' is another learning rate.

In the special case of the squared loss, the adaptive natural gradient method is equivalent to the adaptive version of the Gauss-Newton method, although the motivation is quite different. However, the adaptive natural gradient method is used for many other types of learning problems, including the Kullback-Leibler loss (Park, Amari, and Fukumizu, 2000), INDEPENDENT COMPONENT ANALYSIS (q.v.) (Hyvarinen et al., 2001), and others.

Information Geometry of Boltzmann Machines and EM Algorithm

We now introduce a more advanced theory of information geometry, in which a manifold has a pair of dual affine connections in addition to the Riemannian metric (Amari and Nagaoka, 2000). We will defer the mathematical details in favor of an intuitive explanation. For the manifold consisting of probability distributions, a Riemannian metric is given by the Fisher information matrix. How is a geodesic defined in such a manifold? The Riemannian geodesic is given by the shortest path connecting two points. Two other types of geodesics, called the e-geodesic and m-geodesic, are introduced as follows:

Given two probability distributions $p(x)$ and $q(x)$, the e-geodesic connecting them is a curve $r_e(x, t)$ given by

$$\log r_e(x, t) = (1 - t) \log p(x) + t \log q(x) + c(t) \quad (13)$$

where t is the parameter of the curve and c is a normalization constant. In other words, an e-geodesic connects two distributions linearly in the logarithmic scale. Such a curve is an exponential family. The m-geodesic connecting them is given by

$$r_m(x, t) = (1 - t)p(x) + tq(x) \quad (14)$$

In other words, it connects two distributions linearly, giving a mixture family.

We next define the orthogonality. In a Riemannian manifold, two curves $\theta_1(t)$ and $\theta_2(t)$ that intersect at $t = 0$, $\theta_1(0) = \theta_2(0)$ are orthogonal at the intersection when the inner product of their tangents $\dot{\theta}_1(0)$ and $\dot{\theta}_2(0)$ is 0:

$$\langle \dot{\theta}_1, \dot{\theta}_2 \rangle = \dot{\theta}_1^T G \dot{\theta}_2 = 0 \quad (15)$$

Here $\dot{\theta}_i = (d/dt)\theta_i(t)$ represents the tangent of curve $\theta_i(t)$. In the present case, the two curves $r(x, t)$ and $q(x, t)$, $r(x, 0) = q(x, 0)$ are orthogonal when

$$\langle \dot{r}(x, 0), \dot{q}(x, 0) \rangle = \int \frac{\dot{r}(x, 0)\dot{q}(x, 0)}{r(x, 0)} \, dx = 0 \quad (16)$$

The following is a fundamental theorem of a dually flat manifold (Figure 1).

Generalized Pythagoras Theorem. For three distributions $p(x)$, $q(x)$, and $r(x)$, when the m-geodesic connecting p and q intersects the e-geodesic connecting q and r orthogonally at q,

$$KL[p : q] + KL[q : r] = KL[p : r] \quad (17)$$

The Boltzmann machine (see SIMULATED ANNEALING AND BOLTZMANN MACHINES) is a recurrently connected stochastic neural network whose behavior is directly connected with a probability distribution. Hence, its performance is elucidated by information geometry. The state of a Boltzmann machine is specified by vector $\mathbf{x} = (x_i)$, where x_i is 1 when the ith neuron is excited and is 0 otherwise. The state changes stochastically at discrete times. The next state $\mathbf{x}'$ is determined as follows. Choose one neuron, say j, randomly. Then, x'_j (the jth component of $\mathbf{x}'$) is determined to be equal to 1 with probability related to $u_j = \Sigma w_{ji}x_i$, where $\mathbf{w} = (w_{ji})$ are the connection weights between neurons i and j. Here, $w_{ji} = w_{ij}$ and $w_{ii} = 0$ are assumed. The state transition of a Boltzmann machine is described by a symmetric Markov chain. Its stable distribution is explicitly given by

$$p(\mathbf{x}; \mathbf{w}) = c \exp \{-E(\mathbf{x})\} \quad (18)$$

$$E(\mathbf{x}) = -\frac{1}{2} \sum w_{ij}x_i x_j \quad (19)$$

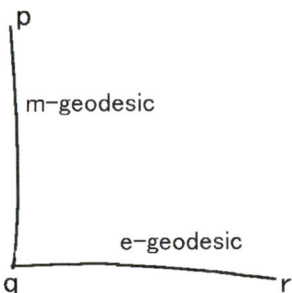

Figure 1. Pythagorean relation in information geometry.

When the Boltzmann machine is working for a long period, state $\mathbf{x}$ appears with relative frequency $p(\mathbf{x}; \mathbf{w})$. A Boltzmann machine is used to simulate an environmental information source that generates signal $\mathbf{x}$ with relative frequency $q(\mathbf{x})$. To this end, we need to train a Boltzmann machine by modifying the synaptic connections $\mathbf{w} = (w_{ij})$ such that $p(\mathbf{x}; \mathbf{w})$ approximates $q(\mathbf{x})$, by using the training data $D_T = \{\mathbf{x}_1, \ldots, \mathbf{x}_T\}$.

A Boltzmann machine has visible neurons and hidden neurons, where the hidden neurons control the behaviors of the visible neurons. We first explain the simplest case without hidden neurons. Let S be the set of all the probability distributions over the state set $X = \{\mathbf{x}\}$. Since there are 2^n states over n neurons, a probability distribution $q = \{q(\mathbf{x})\}$ over these states specifies 2^n probabilities $q(\mathbf{x})$ for all $\mathbf{x} \in X$. Since

$$\sum_{\mathbf{x} \in X} q(\mathbf{x}) = 1 \quad (20)$$

holds, q has $2^n - 1$ degrees of freedom. Geometrically, this implies that S is a $(2^n - 1)$-dimensional manifold. The probability distributions $p(\mathbf{x}; \mathbf{w})$ realized by Boltzmann machines are of the form given by Equation 18, having only $0.5n(n + 1)$ degrees of freedom $\mathbf{w} = (w_{ij})$. Therefore, the set B of the probability distributions realized by Boltzmann machines is a $0.5n(n + 1)$-dimensional submanifold included in the larger manifold S.

Given a training set D_T from the environment distribution q, we need to obtain $p \in B$, which approximates q best. The criterion of approximation is to minimize the Kullback divergence or relative entropy of q and p:

$$D(q\|p) = \sum_{\mathbf{x}} q(\mathbf{x}) \log \frac{q(\mathbf{x})}{p(\mathbf{x})} \quad (21)$$

Information geometry elucidates the geometrical structure of S and B, and the optimal approximator is easily obtained (Amari, Kurata, and Nagaoka, 1992). Let $\hat{p} \in B$ be the minimizer of $D(q\|p)$. Then, from the Pythagoras theorem, the m-geodesic connecting q and $\hat{p}$ is orthogonal to B, that is, orthogonal to any curves in B. Such a point is called the m-projection or q to B. Hence the optimal approximator of q is given by its m-projection.

In the general case, neurons are divided into two parts, hidden neurons and visible neurons. The state $\mathbf{x}$ is also divided into two parts, $\mathbf{x}_V$ and $\mathbf{x}_H$, $\mathbf{x} = (\mathbf{x}_V, \mathbf{x}_H)$. The stable distribution of $\mathbf{x}_V$ is

$$p(\mathbf{x}_V; \mathbf{w}) = \sum_{\mathbf{x}_H} p(\mathbf{x}_V, \mathbf{x}_H; \mathbf{w}) \quad (22)$$

which is more general than those specified by Boltzmann machines (cf. Equation 18) without hidden units.

The training data D_T are given only to the visible neurons, and no information is available for the states of the hidden neurons. However, it is more flexible to adjust $p(\mathbf{x}_V)$ to fit $q(\mathbf{x}_V)$ of the environment, by modifying the connection weights, including the hidden neurons. Let S be the set of all the joint probability distributions $q(\mathbf{x}_V, \mathbf{x}_H)$. Let B be the joint distributions $p(\mathbf{x}_V, \mathbf{x}_H; \mathbf{w})$ realized by the Boltzmann machines. Since the training data D_T specify relative frequencies $q(\mathbf{x}_V)$ of the visible part only, the marginal distribution $q(\mathbf{x}_V)$ is available from D_T. Let $\tilde{D}$ be the set of all the probability distributions $q(\mathbf{x}_V, \mathbf{x}_H)$ whose marginal distribution is specified by the training data D_T. We can prove that $\tilde{D}$ is an m-flat submanifold in S.

The best approximation is to minimize $D\{q(\mathbf{x}_V)\|p(\mathbf{x}_V; \mathbf{w})\}$. A recursive procedure to obtain the best approximation is shown (Amari, 1995). Starting from any initial guess $p_1 \in B$, project it by the e-geodesic to $\tilde{D}$, obtaining $q_1 \in B$. Then, project q_1 to B by the m-geodesic, obtaining a new candidate $p_2 \in B$. Here, two dualistic notions of the e-geodesic and m-geodesic play a fundamental role. It is interesting that this coincides with the Expectation-Maximization (EM) algorithm known in statistics. Here, the e-

projection part corresponds to taking the expected value of the unknown (hidden) frequencies of $q(\mathbf{x}_V, \mathbf{x}_H)$ when the candidate is p, as is given by the E procedure in the EM algorithm. The m-projection part is maximization of the likelihood, deriving the maximum likelihood estimator p from q.

Conclusion

Information geometry provides a mathematical structure that originated in the study of the intrinsic geometry of manifolds of probability distributions. It gives a Riemannian metric together with a dual pair of affine connections, where generalizations of the Pythagoras theorem and projection theorem hold. It is applied to various stochastic models in many fields of research, including neural networks. Further developments can be found in Watanabe (2001).

Road Map: Learning in Artificial Networks
Related Reading: Data Clustering and Learning; Learning and Statistical Inference; Model Validation; Simulated Annealing and Boltzmann Machines; Support Vector Machines

References

Amari, S., 1995, Information geometry of the EM and em algorithms for neural networks, *Neural Netw.*, 8:1379–1408.

Amari, S., 1998, Natural gradient works efficiently in learning, *Neural Computat.*, 10:251–276.

Amari, S., Kurata, K., and Nagaoka, H., 1992, Information geometry of Boltzmann machines, *IEEE Trans. Neural Netw.*, 3:260–271.

Amari, S., and Nagaoka, H., 2000, *Methods of Information Geometry*, New York: AMS and Oxford University Press. ◆

Amari, S., Park, H., and Fukumizu, K., 2000, Adaptive method of realizing natural gradient learning for multilayer perceptions, *Neural Computat.*, 12:1399–1409.

Amari, S., and Wu, S., 1999, Improving support vector machine classifiers by modifying kernel functions, *Neural Netw.*, 12:783–789.

Burges, C. J. C., 1999, Geometry and invariance in kernel based methods, in *Advances in Kernel Methods* (B. Schölkopf, et al., Eds.), Cambridge, MA: MIT Press, pp. 89–116.

Cover, T. M., and Thomas, J. A., 1991, *Elements of Information Theory*, New York: Wiley. ◆

Chen, A. M., Lu, H., and Hecht-Nielsen, R., 1993, On the geometry of feedforward neural network error surfaces, *Neural Computat.*, 5:910–927.

Hyvärinen, A., Karhunen, J., and Oja, E., 2001, *International Component Analysis*, New York: Wiley.

Lebanon, G., and Lafferty, J., 2001, *Boosting and Maximum Likelihood for Exponential Models*, Technical Report CMU-CS-01-144, Pittsburgh, PA: Carnegie Mellon University, School of Computer Science.

Park, H., Amari, S., and Fukumizu, K., 2000, Adaptive natural gradient learning algorithms for various stochastic models, *Neural Netw.*, 13:755–764.

Rattray, M., and Saad, D., 1999, Analysis of natural gradient descent for multilayer neural networks, *Phys. Rev. E*, 59:4523–4532.

Rüger, S. M., and Ossen, A., 1997, The metric of weight space, *Neural Process. Lett.* 5:63–72.

Watanabe, S., 2001, Algebraic analysis for non-identifiable learning machines, *Neural Computat.*, 13:899–933.

Neuromodulation in Invertebrate Nervous Systems

Patsy S. Dickinson

Introduction

Because animals live in changing environments, behavior and hence nervous system output must be flexible. This flexibility manifests itself in several ways that are important when using either experimental studies or modeling to understand neural network function. First, neurons are not all alike; they show a rich variety of conductances that endow them with different functional properties. Second, these properties and hence the collective activity of the networks to which the neurons belong are not fixed, but are subject to modulation that can change their characteristics and output. Modulation as a result of both locally released neuromodulators and more widely acting hormones differs qualitatively from the moment-to-moment integration of synaptic excitation and inhibition that a neuron receives. Neuromodulators can provoke dynamic changes in neurons or circuits on time scales ranging from seconds to days.

Neuronal membrane properties and synapses, neuromuscular junctions, and muscle properties are all subject to modulation. Together, these modulations allow the same groups of neurons to generate diverse arrays of behaviors and to respond appropriately to a wide variety of sensory stimuli. Frequently, the same modulators act at multiple levels to influence or bias motor output. Because of their relative simplicity and accessibility, invertebrate nervous systems have provided the clearest examples of modulation and its importance to neuronal output.

Temporal and Spatial Dynamics of Neuromodulation

Neuromodulators act on a variety of both temporal and spatial scales owing to the nature of release and breakdown as well as the mechanisms through which they exert their effects (Figure 1). Some modulators are hormones; thus, they are spatially widespread and show relatively slow temporal changes. In *Aplysia*, for example, the bag cells release several peptides that change the activity of numerous other neurons, and of themselves via autoreceptors, for up to 18 hours (Levitan and Kaczmarek, 2002). Alternatively, other modulators are released at defined neuropilar locations and may be rapidly broken down. In addition to the amines, which often function as modulators, some peptides, such as proctolin in the crustacean stomatogastric nervous systems, are rapidly broken down by peptidases (Nusbaum et al., 2001). Moreover, the same transmitter substance may be released both hormonally and neuronally. At the same time, the cellular mechanisms by which modulators act may selectively potentiate the effects of some modulators. For example, some modulators activate second messengers, which may outlast the presence of the modulator itself. Others may act on relatively short time scales, so cellular properties in a rhythmic network, for example, may vary over the course of each cycle. Because of these dynamics, networks are continuously refined and reconfigured during behavior (Marder, 1997), and such dynamics must be incorporated into models if they are to explain the flexibility observed in behaving animals.

Factors Determining Variability in Neuromodulator Effects

The effects of a given neuromodulator on its target neuron(s) or network(s) depend on a number of other factors. First, many neuromodulator influences may be dependent on the concentration of

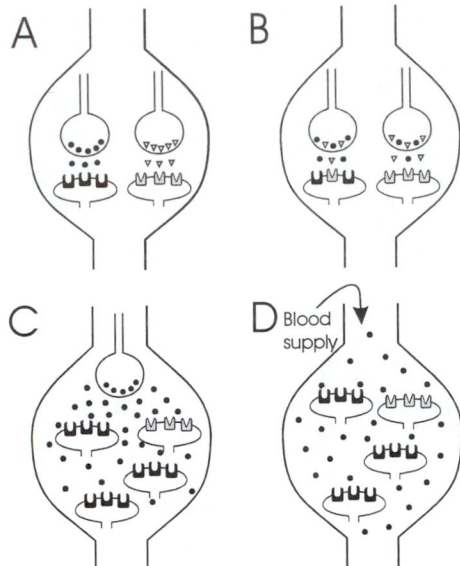

Figure 1. Modulatory transmitters can affect other neurons on a number of spatial scales and in a variety of combinations. For example, each of two different modulatory neurons could release a modulator into specific neuropilar regions, resulting in "pointwise" modulation that is limited in both time and space (*A*). Alternatively, two or more co-transmitters (one or both of which are modulatory) could be released from the same synaptic terminals (*B*). The two substances need not act simultaneously on the same postsynaptic terminals. Instead, they could be released by differential spiking frequencies or patterns; moreover, not all postsynaptic neurons necessarily have receptors for both modulatory compounds. A third alternative (*C*) is more widespread release from nonsynaptic sites, such that the transmitter diffuses to influence a larger group of neurons, with a gradient as a function of distance from the presynaptic release site. Finally, modulators can be released into the bloodstream and thus delivered to all neurons (*D*), although they affect only those with appropriate receptors.

transmitter present. In most experiments using bath application, there is a dose-dependent effect. When modulators are released from neurons, the amount of transmitter released can be a function not only of spike frequency in the modulatory neuron, but also of the pattern with which the neuron fires. For example, small molecule transmitters may be released with each spike, but peptides and amines, which are frequently modulatory, may be released only when the neuron fires in high-frequency bursts. Thus, the effect of a modulatory neuron firing tonically at 10 Hz may differ both qualitatively and quantitatively from the effects of the same neuron firing 0.5-s, 40-Hz bursts every 2 s, even though the average spike frequency is unchanged. In the *Aplysia* motor neuron B15, for example, acetylcholine is released with each action potential, but the modulatory peptides (small cardioactive peptides, SCPs) that it contains are released only with elevated (e.g., 25–50 Hz) spike frequencies (Whim, Church, and Lloyd, 1994). Peptide release from this neuron does not depend on spike frequency alone, but rather on complex interactions between spike frequency, burst duration, and interburst interval. Additionally, it should be noted that while peptide release is often pattern sensitive, this is not always the case, as illustrated by another motor neuron in *Aplysia*, which likewise releases the SCPs, but does so even at very low firing frequencies (<1 Hz; Whim et al., 1994).

Second, many modulatory neurons contain more than one transmitter. These co-transmitters may be released differentially as a function of neuronal firing pattern, as described above. Likewise, they may be released differentially at different neuronal terminals

(Nusbaum et al., 2001). Additionally, they may act differentially on different postsynaptic neurons as a function of the availability of different postsynaptic receptors. The situation becomes even more complex when we realize that the same neuron can contain co-transmitters that exert opposing effects on the same postsynaptic targets, so they may be excitatory under certain conditions yet be inhibitory under other firing regimes. Finally, the release of modulatory peptides may itself be modulated by other neurotransmitters. In *Aplysia* motor neuron B1, for example, serotonin increases excitability but simultaneously decreases the amount of the SCPs it releases (Whim et al., 1994).

Third, the effect of a given modulator frequently depends on the state of the system when the modulator is applied. Modulators themselves may affect this state, thereby altering the responses of the network to other inputs. In the lobster stomatogastric system, for example, the peptide proctolin by itself has no effect on the cardiac sac pattern. However, if proctolin is applied shortly after red pigment-concentrating hormone (RPCH) is applied, it elicits strong cardiac sac bursting (Dickinson et al., 1997). In formulating models of such systems, it should be remembered that the response of a system to one modulator may not always be identical, but instead may be a longer-term function of the modulatory history of the animal.

Modulation of Sensory Systems

The sensory information that an animal needs depends on a number of factors, including its activity patterns and motivational state. Thus, the sensitivities of many sensory receptors can be modulated, as is seen for a stretch receptor, the oval organ, in crustaceans. This organ contains three sensory afferents and provides proprioceptive feedback to the gill ventilatory system. Proctolin increases the amplitude of the receptor potential and hence the number of action potentials produced in two of these afferents, whereas octopamine and serotonin decrease these responses. Interestingly, the dendrites within the oval organ itself contain proctolin, suggesting that receptor activity might automodulate receptor sensitivity in that increased activity would induce greater proctolin release, thereby increasing receptor gain (Pasztor, 1989).

In addition to receptor sensitivity itself, the extent to which sensory information is conveyed to central and motor systems is subject to modulatory control. This has been extensively examined in the sensorimotor synapses of *Aplysia* in the context of learning, but is also prevalent on shorter time scales associated with ongoing activity of many motor systems. In a number of locomotive systems in arthropods, for example, it has been shown that reflexes that stabilize posture in a quiet animal can change not only in magnitude, but also in direction when the animal begins to move. Such reflex reversal involves a number of mechanisms at both the presynaptic and postsynaptic levels (Clarac, Cattaert, and LeRay, 2000). Moreover, the strength of the reflex can vary cyclically as a function of the ongoing movement, again underscoring the importance of temporal dynamics in neuromodulation.

Modulation at Central Levels

Modulators can activate, terminate, or modify rhythmic pattern-generating networks. The detailed outputs of many rhythmic patterns are highly variable; frequency, phase relationships within the pattern, and number of participating neurons are subject to change. Additionally, many neurons and/or muscles participate in more than one behavior. Thus, in modeling networks, the mechanisms by which modulators sculpt specific patterns of activity from more generalized pattern generators must be considered. Getting and Dekin (reviewed in Harris-Warrick and Marder, 1991), who first described such networks as "polymorphic," showed that the same network could be reconfigured by modulatory inputs to produce either escape swimming or reflexive withdrawal in the mollusk *Tritonia*.

Intrinsic Versus Extrinsic Neuromodulation

Until recently, most modulators studied were located in control centers removed from the target network, and hence the release of transmitter was independent of the network and neurons being modulated. It is now clear, however, that neurons within a network may release modulators that act on the same network (Katz, 1998). With such "intrinsic neuromodulation," the pattern of modulator release thus depends on the activity of the network of neurons being modulated. In the CPG network controlling swimming in *Tritonia*, for example, one neuronal type, the dorsal swim interneurons, releases the transmitter serotonin. Serotonin not only reciprocally inhibits the ventral swim interneurons within the pattern generator, but also modulates the strength of other synapses within the network (Katz, 1998). Serotonin levels thus fluctuate dynamically during the course of a swim, and recent models have shown that this intrinsic modulation is a critical component in the production of the swim motor pattern (Frost et al., 1997).

Alteration of Intrinsic Properties of Neurons

Many neurons have voltage-dependent conductances that allow them to generate rhythmic bursts of action potentials in the absence of synaptic input (see OSCILLATORY AND BURSTING PROPERTIES OF NEURONS for further details). However, many of these conductances are activated only in the presence of an appropriate neuromodulator. For example, the Anterior Burster neuron in the lobster pyloric network does not oscillate when completely isolated from its network partners and modulatory inputs. However, the isolated neuron oscillates strongly when superfused with any of several neuromodulators (Harris-Warrick and Marder, 1991). The characteristics of these oscillations (burst period, duration, amplitude) are different for each modulator. This diversity results at least partly from the fact that bursting in this neuron can be driven by a number of different voltage-dependent currents, a finding that has subsequently been confirmed by modeling studies (Marder, 1997). Each amine activates a different subset of conductances, resulting in different bursting patterns (Harris-Warrick and Marder, 1991).

Similarly, dopamine and serotonin modulate different currents in *Aplysia* neuron R15 to produce superficially similar changes in bursting, in this case the cessation of spontaneous bursting. However, when silenced by serotonin but not by dopamine, a brief depolarizing input provokes sustained bursting. A modeling study of this system showed that by modulating different currents, both amines silence R15, but dopamine prevents other input signals from activating the neuron, whereas serotonin amplifies synaptic inputs (reviewed in Fellous and Linster, 1998).

Modulators also alter the ability of neurons to generate plateau potentials, the regenerative switch between two stable membrane potentials. At one, the cell is hyperpolarized and silent; at the other, it is depolarized and fires action potentials. Shifts between the two levels occur abruptly when the neuron's membrane potential crosses a threshold value in response to current injection or postsynaptic potentials. The abilities of neurons to generate plateau potentials can be enhanced or suppressed by modulatory inputs. In the stomatogastric system, for example, activity in the Anterior Pyloric Modulator neuron enhances or suppresses the abilities of different neurons to generate plateau potentials. One effect of the changes in plateau capability is an altered sensitivity to synaptic inputs. When plateaus are generated, inputs strong enough to trigger the regenerative shift from one level to the other have greater effects than they would otherwise have, whereas those that are too

weak to trigger the shift have little effect (Dickinson and Nagy, 1983). Once the threshold is reached, further increases in synaptic strength have little effect. In network computations, this characteristic effectively decreases the importance of synaptic strength (Marder, 1993). Consequently, the postsynaptic response becomes nonlinear. In addition, the effective duration of synaptic inputs is changed, since, once shifted, the postsynaptic neuron remains at its new level; hence, the effect of inputs sufficient to induce a switch from one plateau level to another long outlasts the stimulus duration (Figure 2).

Changes in the abilities of neurons to generate plateau potentials can have far-reaching effects on network activity. For example, when the plateau properties of the ventricular dilator (VD, a pyloric neuron), are suppressed, the VD no longer fires with the pyloric pattern. Instead, if the much slower cardiac sac pattern is active, the VD fires with this network (reviewed in Harris-Warrick and Marder, 1991).

The roles of different conductances in determining the firing patterns of nonoscillatory neurons have now been examined in the stomatogastric nervous system both in models and in experiments using the dynamic clamp technique. The LP neuron, for example, is modulated by proctolin, and adding the proctolin conductance to the model alters both its activity and other membrane currents in ways that reflect the peptide's biological effects. Modeling has confirmed that even small currents that produce minor changes in membrane potential may have profound effects (Marder, 1993).

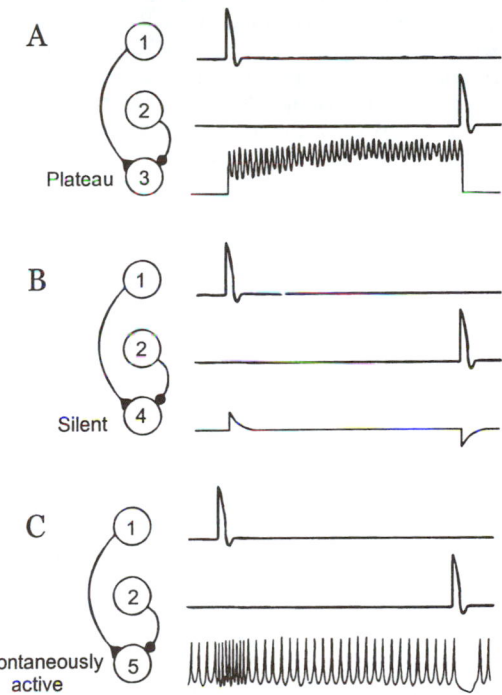

Figure 2. Plateau properties in a postsynaptic neuron increase the duration of its response to synaptic input. *A,* When the follower cell, 3, has plateau properties, an excitatory postsynaptic potential (from 1, triangle) triggers a shift to a depolarized plateau, whereas an inhibitory postsynaptic potential (from 2, circle) terminates the plateau. When the follower cell (4, 5) is silent but does not have plateau properties (*B*) or is spontaneously active (*C*), the effect of the same excitatory or inhibitory postsynaptic potential lasts for only a short time after the input. (Source: Marder, E., 1993, Modulating membrane properties of neurons: Role in information processing, in *Exploring Brain Functions: Models in Neuroscience* (T.A. Poggio and D.A. Glasser, Eds.), Chichester, Engl.: Wiley, p. 30. Copyright 1993. Reprinted by permission of John Wiley & Sons, Ltd.)

Similarly, it has been possible to determine which K currents are most important for provoking the changes in postinhibitory rebound, and hence phasing of the pyloric pattern, when dopamine is applied to the stomatogastric system (Harris-Warrick et al., 1998).

An intriguing recent finding is the observation that many different modulators, including the peptides proctolin, RPCH, CabTRP, and TNRNFLRFamide and the muscarinic agonist pilocarpine, activate the same membrane current in neurons of the lobster STG. However, while all these modulators activate the pyloric pattern, each produces a different variant of the pattern, owing to the fact that a different subset of pyloric neurons contains receptors for each modulator (Nusbaum et al., 2001).

When modeling networks subject to neuromodulation, one must consider that although a modulator may act on only a subset of neurons in the network, neurons that are not direct targets of the modulator can likewise be affected and can influence the output of the system through their synapses within the network (for further discussion, see CRUSTACEAN STOMATOGASTRIC SYSTEM).

Alteration of Synaptic Efficacy by Neuromodulators

The efficacy of both chemical and electrical synapses can be changed by neuromodulator actions. For chemical synapses, changes in the amount of transmitter released or in the responsiveness of postsynaptic neurons can contribute to modulation. In *Aplysia*, for example, changes in synaptic efficacy are largely responsible for the long-term changes that underlie learning (see INVERTEBRATE MODELS OF LEARNING: *APLYSIA* AND *HERMISSENDA*). In the stomatogastric system, RPCH increases the efficacy of the synapses from a single presynaptic neuron onto its follower cells; this increase in synaptic efficacy is sufficient to cause a functional rewiring of two pattern generators and to provoke the generation of a novel rhythm (reviewed in Harris-Warrick and Marder, 1991).

Many synapses in invertebrates release transmitter not only in response to action potentials, but also as a graded function of membrane potential. It has recently been found that graded and spike-mediated transmitter release can be differentially modulated. Thus, for example, dopamine enhances graded synaptic transmission but decreases spike-evoked transmission at the LP-PD neuron synapse of the pyloric network (Harris-Warrick et al., 1998).

Electrical synapses are likewise subject to modulation. Serotonin, octopamine, and dopamine alter electrical coupling in the lobster pyloric system, with coupling at some synapses increased while at other synapses it is decreased. Because the same modulators can change the efficacies of both chemical and electrical synapses between the same neurons, the effective sign of a synapse can be changed. Dopamine, for example, alters synaptic efficacy between several pairs of pyloric neurons that are connected by dual synapses. Under control conditions, the electrical component dominates, and the synapses are largely excitatory. Under dopamine, however, the chemical component dominates, and the synapses are largely inhibitory (Harris-Warrick et al., 1998).

Modulation of Neuromuscular Junctions and Muscles

Neuromodulators in many systems exert effects on neuromuscular junctions or on muscles themselves. These effects are often consistent with central or sensory effects of the same modulators. Modulators, which are released both from motor neurons and from exogenous sources, can change the amplitude, duration, or speed of muscle contraction or relaxation. These effects result from changes at one or more of three levels: presynaptic effects resulting in altered transmitter release from motor terminals, electrical properties and excitability of the muscle fibers themselves, and excitation-contraction coupling (Harris-Warrick and Marder, 1991).

These multiple steps have recently been incorporated into a model of the "neuromuscular transform" (NMT) by Brezina et al. (Brezina, Orekhova, and Weiss, 2000), who used a dynamical systems approach to examine modulation of feeding muscles in *Aplysia*, both theoretically and in this model neuromuscular system. These authors show that the NMT, which acts as a dynamic, nonlinear filter, limits the range of behaviors that can be produced. In particular, they find that many rhythmic behaviors break down at the level of the NMT when the neuronal cycle frequency driving the muscles increases beyond certain limits. However, neuromodulators in *Aplysia* modify a number of characteristics of the neuromuscular system, including the amplitude of contraction and rate of relaxation in response to neuronal stimulation, thereby altering the constraints on the system. Both intrinsic and extrinsic peripheral neuromodulation occur in this system, and the theoretical framework developed by these authors has shown that intrinsic modulation, which varies with the motor pattern itself, optimizes the performance of a single behavior. In contrast, extrinsic modulation, which is independent of the motor pattern, allows multiple contraction shapes to be generated and hence allows multiple behaviors to be produced using the same neuromuscular system.

Discussion

Modulation is prevalent in both invertebrate and vertebrate nervous systems, and it occurs at all levels: sensory, central, and motor. Neuromodulators alter the output of a system by changing membrane properties of neurons, synaptic interactions, and intracellular properties such as excitation-contraction coupling in muscles. Moreover, modulatory inputs can act on time scales ranging from seconds to days. Consequently, the properties of individual neurons, as well as the nature and extent of their interactions within networks, are dynamic rather than static, and so the temporal dynamics of such changing properties must be considered if we are to fully understand and appreciate the flexibility of the nervous system. Moreover, these dynamics must be incorporated into models if they are to fulfill their promise in illuminating principles of neuronal functioning. Additionally, the responses of a given system to a specific neuromodulator are not always the same and may depend on the state of the preparation when the modulator is applied or activated. Because a range of substances modulates invertebrate systems, this variability can have important consequences.

Moreover, because the neural circuits that are subject to modulation differ substantially, the same modulator can cause different effects on different systems. Serotonin, for example, enhances swimming behavior in leeches, *Tritonia*, and the pteropod *Clione*. In both leeches and *Tritonia*, one component of this increase is enhanced presynaptic transmitter release. In *Tritonia* and *Clione*, the excitability of pattern-generating neurons is enhanced. In the lobster STG, serotonin causes an overall activation of the pyloric pattern but an inhibition of a number of neurons within the network, so the circuit is effectively limited to three of the eight neuronal types (Levitan and Kaczmarek, 2002).

The specific effects of a given neuromodulator are determined by numerous factors, including (1) the array of neurons expressing receptors for that modulator, (2) the membrane channels (often voltage-dependent) that are altered by the modulator, (3) the membrane potentials of neurons in the circuit, and (4) the interactions of those neurons within the network.

At least partly because of the dynamic nature and complexity brought to nervous systems by modulation, models are being successfully used to test fundamental assumptions underlying mechanisms of neuronal and network function and modulation. Modeling studies have, for example, confirmed that neuromodulators are able to increase and control the computational complexity of networks without increasing their structural complexity. However, it is important to consider neuromodulation as an integral part of models rather than simply as an "add-on" (Fellous and Linster, 1998). Moreover, models will ultimately need to incorporate the more complex aspects of neuromodulation that are now being found experimentally, including, for example, interactions amongst modulators, and the actions of modulators at multiple levels.

Road Map: Biological Networks
Related Reading: Crustacean Stomatogastric System; Neuromodulation in Mammalian Nervous System

References

Brezina, V., Orekhova, I., and Weiss, K., 2000, Optimization of rhythmic behaviors by modulation of the neuromuscular transform, *J. Neurophysiol.*, 83:260–279.

Clarac, C., Cattaert, D., and LeRay, D., 2000, Central control components of a "simple" stretch reflex, *Trends Neurosci.*, 23:199–208. ◆

Dickinson, P. S., Fairfield, W. P., Hetling, J. R., and Hauptman, J., 1997, Neurotransmitter interactions in the stomatogastric system of the spiny lobster: One peptide alters the response of a central pattern generator to a second peptide, *J. Neurophysiol.*, 77:599–610.

Dickinson, P. S., and Nagy, F., 1983, Control of a central pattern generator by an identified modulatory interneurone in Crustacea: II. Induction and modification of plateau properties in pyloric neurones, *J. Exp. Biol.*, 105:59–82.

Fellous, J.-M., and Linster, C., 1998, Computational models of neuromodulation, *Neural Comput.*, 10:771–805. ◆

Frost, W. N., Lieb, J., Jr., Tunstall, M. J., Mensh, B. D., and Katz, P. S. 1997, Integrate-and-fire simulations of two molluscan neural circuits, in *Neurons, Networks, and Motor Behavior* (P. G. Stein, S. Grillner, A. I. Selverston, and D. Stuart, Eds.), Cambridge, MA: MIT Press, pp. 173–179.

Harris-Warrick, R. M., Johnson, B. R., Peck, J. H., Kloppenburg, P., Ayali, A., and Skarbinski, J., 1998, Distributed effects of dopamine modulation in the crustacean pyloric network, *Ann. N.Y. Acad. Sci.*, 860:155–167. ◆

Harris-Warrick, R. M., and Marder, E., 1991, Modulation of neural networks for behavior, *Annu. Rev. Neurosci.*, 14:39–57. ◆

Katz, P. S., 1998, Comparison of extrinsic and intrinsic neuromodulation in two central pattern generator circuits in invertebrates, *Exp. Physiol.*, 83:281–292. ◆

Levitan, I., and Kaczmarek, L., 2002, *The Neuron: Cell and Molecular Biology*, Oxford, Engl.: Oxford University Press. ◆

Marder, E., 1993, Modulating membrane properties of neurons: Role in information processing, in *Exploring Brain Functions: Models in Neuroscience* (T. A. Poggio and D. A Glaser., Eds.), New York: John Wiley, pp. 27–42. ◆

Marder, E., 1997, Computational dynamics in rhythmic neural circuits, *The Neuroscientist*, 3:295–302. ◆

Nusbaum, M. P., Blitz, D. M., Swensen, A. M., Wood, D., and Marder, E., 2001, The roles of co-transmission in neural network modulation, *Trends Neurosci.*, 24:146–154. ◆

Pasztor, V. M., 1989, Modulation of sensitivity in invertebrate sensory receptors, *Semin. Neurosci.*, 1:5–14. ◆

Whim, M. D., Church, P. J., and Lloyd, P. E., 1994, Functional roles of peptide cotransmitters at neuromuscular synapses in *Aplysia, Molec. Neurobiol.*, 7:335–347. ◆

Neuromodulation in Mammalian Nervous Systems

Michael E. Hasselmo, Bradley P. Wyble, and Erik Fransen

Introduction

Neuromodulators change the way in which neural circuits process information. The term *neuromodulation* usually refers to the effect of neurochemicals such as acetylcholine (ACh), dopamine, norepinephrine, and serotonin, and other substances, including neuropeptides (see Hasselmo, 1995; Fellous and Linster, 1998; Katz, 1999; Doya, Dayan, and Hasselmo, 2002). The term neuromodulation does not refer to the rapid transmission of information through the nervous system by excitatory and inhibitory synaptic potentials. Rapid synaptic potentials are caused by neurotransmitters such as glutamate or γ-aminobutyric acid (GABA) acting on receptor proteins containing ion channels (ionotropic receptors), which cause fast changes in the conductance of the cell membrane to specific ions. In contrast, the neuromodulators primarily activate receptor proteins that do not contain an ion channel (metabotropic receptors). These receptors activate enzymes that change the internal concentration of substances called second messengers. Second messengers cause slower and longer-lasting changes in the physiological properties of neurons, resulting in changes in the processing characteristics of the neural circuit.

The effect of a neurochemical is receptor dependent (Table 1). Thus, a single neuromodulator such as serotonin can have dramatically different effects on different neurons, depending on the type of receptor it activates. Even the distinction between neurotransmitters and neuromodulators has exceptions based on receptor effects: glutamate and GABA can activate slower metabotropic receptor subtypes (mGluR and $GABA_B$), whereas some receptors for ACh and serotonin are ionotropic (nicotinic ACh and 5-HT_3).

Neural network models are important for understanding the function of neuromodulatory influences, because neuromodulation causes effects that may appear subtle and contradictory in recordings from single neurons but have a significant effect on dynamical properties when distributed throughout a network (Hasselmo, 1995; Fellous and Linster, 1998; Katz, 1999; Doya et al., 2002). The anatomical distribution of fibers releasing neuromodulatory substances in the brain is usually very diffuse, as shown in Figure 1. This allows the activity of a small number of neuromodulatory neurons to influence the functional properties of broad regions of the brain. Neuromodulatory effects are usually slower than effects at ionotropic receptors, causing longer-term changes in functional state.

This review falls into two main sections, the cellular effects of neuromodulators and the functional modeling of neuromodulation. The first section summarizes some of the physiological effects of neuromodulation, including effects on (1) the resting membrane potential of pyramidal cells and interneurons, (2) spike frequency adaptation, (3) synaptic transmission, and (4) long-term potentiation. The second section reviews several different theories of the function of modulatory influences in neural circuits, including (1) noradrenergic modulation of attentional processes, (2) dopaminergic modulation of working memory, (3) cholinergic modulation of input versus internal processing, and (4) modulation of oscillatory dynamics in cortex and thalamus.

Modeling Cellular Effects of Neuromodulation

A range of different neuromodulatory effects have been modeled in compartmental simulations of cortical pyramidal cells, including

Table 1. Some Receptor-Dependent Effects of a Subset of Neuromodulatory Substances

| Neuromodulator | Receptor Subtype | Resting Potential | | Spike Adaptation | Synaptic Transmission | | | Long-Term Potentiation |
		Pyramidal Cell	Interneuronal		Inhibition	Afferent Input	Feedback	
Acetylcholine	Muscarinic	↑	↑	↓	↓		↓	↑
	Nicotinic	↑	↑			↑		
Dopamine	D_1		↑		↑		↑	
	D_2				↓			
Norepinephrine	α				↓		↓	
	β		↑	↓			↑	↑
Serotonin	$5\text{-}HT_1$	↓	↓					
	$5\text{-}HT_2$			↓				
	$5\text{-}HT_3$	↑	↑					
Opioids	μ		↓					

changes in resting membrane potential, spike frequency adaptation, synaptic transmission, and long-term potentiation. Many of these effects are described in more detail in reviews of neuromodulation (McCormick, Wang, and Huguenard, 1993; Hasselmo, 1995; Fellous and Linster, 1998; Katz, 1999).

Pyramidal Cell Membrane Potential

Some neuromodulatory agents cause slow changes in resting membrane potential owing to changes in the resting membrane conductance to individual ions. For example, activation of muscarinic ACh receptors causes a slow depolarization of pyramidal cells by decreasing the leak potassium conductance. In contrast, GABA activation of $GABA_B$ receptors and serotonin activation of $5\text{-}HT_{1A}$ receptors causes a slow hyperpolarization by increasing potassium conductance. The time course of this $GABA_B$ effect is modeled in SYNAPTIC INTERACTIONS (q.v.).

Inhibitory Interneuron Membrane Potential

Many neuromodulators have a strong effect on the membrane potential of inhibitory interneurons. Depolarization of interneurons as a result of activation of dopaminergic, noradrenergic, cholinergic, and serotonergic receptors has been detected, whereas opioid receptors have a strong hyperpolarizing effect on interneurons.

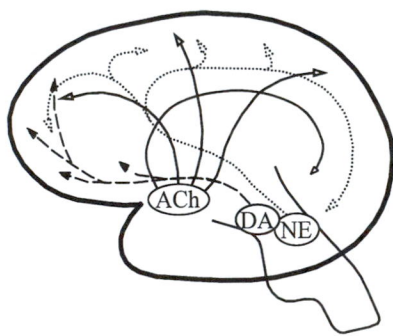

Figure 1. Example of the anatomy of neuromodulatory systems. Neurons producing acetylcholine (ACh) are clustered in nuclei of the basal forebrain. This relatively small population of neurons sends diffuse projections to a broad range of brain regions. Similarly, noradrenergic neurons (NE) are clustered in the locus coeruleus, and send diffuse connections throughout the brain. Dopaminergic neurons (DA) are in the ventral tegmental area and substantia nigra and project to nucleus accumbens, striatum, and frontal cortex.

Spike Frequency Adaptation

When injected with current, cortical pyramidal cells fire action potentials initially at high frequencies, but neurons show a rapid decrease in firing frequency, referred to as *accommodation* or *adaptation*. ACh, norepinephrine, and serotonin reduce spike frequency adaptation, allowing higher frequency firing. In models, spike frequency adaptation can be modeled with an increase in intracellular calcium, because of the voltage-dependent calcium influx caused by each action potential. The increasing intracellular calcium concentration activates calcium-dependent potassium currents (also known as $I_{K(AHP)}$), which are reduced by the above neuromodulators.

Synaptic Transmission

Many neuromodulatory substances activate presynaptic receptors, which alter the release of neurochemicals, including glutamate and GABA. Receptors that cause presynaptic inhibition at glutamatergic synapses include the α-adrenergic receptors (which are a subtype of norepinephrine receptors), muscarinic ACh receptors, $GABA_B$ receptors, neuropeptide Y receptors, and adenosine receptors. As shown in Table 1, these effects can be selective for specific synapse types.

Long-Term Potentiation

Neuromodulators have been shown to induce long-term potentiation and to enhance long-term potentiation induced by synaptic stimulation. β-adrenergic receptors and muscarinic receptors appear to actively induce long-term potentiation at specific synaptic connections. Activation of dopamine receptors, muscarinic ACh receptors, metabotropic glutamate receptors, opioid receptors, and $GABA_B$ receptors appears to influence the magnitude of long-term potentiation caused by synaptic stimulation.

Functional Modeling of Neuromodulation

The cellular effects of neuromodulators can dramatically alter the functional dynamics of neural circuits, in contradiction to the common notion that neuromodulation only slightly increases or decreases the normal function of the network (Hasselmo, 1995; Fellous and Linster, 1998; Katz, 1999). The essential functional role of neuromodulation is illustrated by the breakdown of normal cognitive function by high doses of drugs such as scopolamine (which blocks ACh receptors) and by the important clinical effects of selective serotonin reuptake inhibitors (SSRIs).

Modulator effects are often described in simple colloquial terms such as "memory," "attention," or "reward," but the techniques of computational neuroscience allow a more sophisticated assessment of the specific functional influence of modulators on neural circuits (Hasselmo, 1995; Fellous and Linster, 1998; Doya et al., 2002). This will allow data from specific behavioral tasks to be addressed directly in terms of the dynamics of neural circuits rather than as simple verbal hypotheses.

Norepinephrine

Drugs that enhance the release of norepinephrine and other monoamines have been shown to enhance performance on tests of sustained attention, such as the continuous performance task, in which subjects must detect an infrequent target stimulus in a long series of distractor stimuli. In recordings from monkeys, the enhancement of performance on these tasks has been linked to activity of noradrenergic neurons. The role of norepinephrine in this regard has been modeled using a hybrid model with detailed representation of the spiking activity of noradrenergic neurons in the locus coeruleus, coupled with a more abstract representation of cortical circuits performing the visual detection task (Usher et al., 1999). The cortical model regulates the behavioral response to individual stimuli using competing processing units with sigmoid input-output functions. The gain (slope) of these sigmoid units is increased by noradrenergic modulation. In this model, noradrenergic neurons have a low baseline firing rate, ensuring low gain in the cortical network, and a low false alarm rate. However, these neurons show a brief response to the target stimulus, which transiently increases the gain of the cortical units, increasing the likelihood of generating a response. The phasic level of noradrenergic neuron activity correlates with greater performance accuracy in the model and in experiments (Usher et al., 1999). A tonic increase in noradrenergic activity enhances the response to all stimuli, consistent with general arousal, which allows orienting to all stimuli but decreases visual detection performance.

The change in input-output functions described above could be a reasonable representation of the changes in circuit dynamics caused by norepinephrine. On a cellular level, norepinephrine activates β-adrenergic receptors, which decrease spike frequency adaptation and enhance postsynaptic responses (see Table 1). At the same time, norepinephrine activates presynaptic α-adrenergic receptors, which suppress excitatory transmission. In network simulations of piriform cortex, these effects enhance the response of pyramidal cells to afferent input while decreasing the background activity caused by excitatory transmission between pyramidal cells in the cortex (Hasselmo et al., 1997). Norepinephrine has the apparently contradictory effects of decreasing excitatory synaptic input to interneurons while directly depolarizing these same interneurons. These effects decrease the activity of local circuits in response to weak input but increase their activity in response to strong input, an effect that resembles the change in gain of sigmoid input-output functions utilized in the model described above.

Dopamine

Models of dopamine function include research on reinforcement learning as well as working memory. Dopamine has traditionally been viewed as a neuromodulator signaling reinforcement, but electrophysiological recording of the activity of dopaminergic neurons in the ventral tegmental area demonstrates activity dependent on the expectation of reward rather than on the reward itself. This pattern of activity appears similar to the error signal used in temporal difference learning. Models of the role of dopamine in reinforcement learning are described in more detail in REINFORCEMENT LEARNING and DOPAMINE, ROLES OF.

Experimental data also indicate a role for dopamine in working memory (the capacity to hold information in short-term memory

for performance of tasks). Working memory may involve sustained spiking activity in populations of neurons within the prefrontal cortex. This sustained spiking activity can be maintained by excitatory recurrent connectivity or by the intrinsic properties of individual neurons. Detailed biophysical modeling demonstrates how dopaminergic modulation could contribute to both the transition between different activity states, as well as the maintenance of stable spiking activity (Durstewitz, Seamans, and Sejnowski, 2000). In this model, dopamine enhances the maintenance of individual stored items through enhancement of persistent voltage-sensitive sodium currents and the NMDA current. At the same time, dopamine reduces AMPA currents and depolarizes inhibitory interneurons through activation of the D_1 subtype of receptor. In the model, this serves to prevent activation of other task-irrelevant memories. Other work from that group showed that the initial response to dopaminergic modulation involved a D_2 receptor-mediated suppression of inhibitory synaptic transmission, which could serve to allow activation of prefrontal cortex by multiple inputs, and exploration of the input space. This effect is transient, while the more persistent effects at D_1 receptors could allow selection and maintenance of a single memory for a more extended period.

Acetylcholine

The cellular effects of ACh play an important role in the function of cortical networks (Hasselmo, 1995). For example, muscarinic cholinergic antagonists such as scopolamine impair the encoding of new words but not the retrieval of previously encoded words. Models demonstrate how ACh could be important for enhancing encoding of new information in the cortex. As shown in Figure 2, computational modeling demonstrates how cholinergic activation of a calcium-sensitive cation current in layer II pyramidal cells in entorhinal cortex could cause sustained spiking activity such as that observed during the delay period of a delayed non-match-to-sample task (Fransen, Alonso, and Hasselmo, 2002). These mechanisms could allow maintenance of novel information for encoding and working memory.

Computational modeling also demonstrates how the cellular effects of ACh can enhance the encoding of new information patterns by selectively enhancing the response to external sensory stimuli

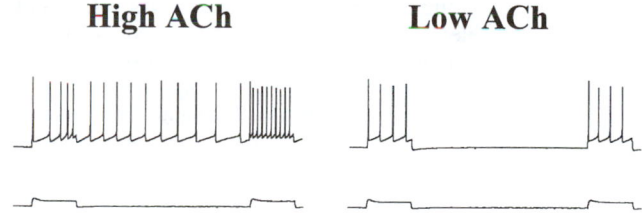

High ACh   **Low ACh**

500 msec

Figure 2. A biophysical simulation of an entorhinal cortex layer II pyramidal cell demonstrates that cholinergic enhancement of a calcium-sensitive cation current could allow maintenance of sustained spiking without afferent input. Bottom traces show the timing of depolarizing input, which causes spiking for 500-ms periods separated by a 2,500-ms delay. When cholinergic modulation is present (in a condition of high ACh, left side), the calcium influx during initial spiking causes activation of the cation current. This causes further depolarization, which causes additional spiking and calcium influx. This causes regenerative spiking activity even in the absence of external input. With lower ACh levels (right side), the current is not sufficiently activated and the neuron does not fire during the delay period.

versus internal retrieval (Hasselmo, 1995). This results from cholinergic suppression of glutamatergic transmission at feedback synapses but not at feedforward synapses, coupled with cellular depolarization, which makes neurons more likely to spike in response to afferent input. This causes activity to be clamped to the pattern of afferent input, allowing accurate storage of input patterns without interference from retrieval of previously stored patterns. Cholinergic enhancement of long-term potentiation offsets the reduction of synaptic input at excitatory intrinsic connections, allowing Hebbian synaptic modification of these connections for autoassociative storage of input patterns. On a faster time scale, similar transitions could occur in different phases of each cycle of hippocampal theta rhythm oscillations (Hasselmo, Bodelon, and Wyble, 2002). Theta rhythm appears when an animal is actively exploring the environment or attending to relevant stimuli. The phase with strong afferent input could allow encoding of new sequences without interference from retrieval, while a separate phase of dominant feedback connections could allow retrieval. Loss of this oscillatory modulation could underlie the learning impairments caused by fornix lesions, which damage the modulatory influences pacing theta rhythm.

Low ACh levels allow strong feedback transmission for consolidation. During quiet waking and slow-wave sleep, there is a dramatic decrease in ACh level, which is accompanied by the appearance of sharp wave events in the EEG (Buzsaki, 1989). During sharp waves, associations encoded in hippocampus are theorized to be reactivated, causing activity in hippocampus and neocortex that could mediate the formation of additional traces of the same memory (Buzsaki, 1989; Shen and McNaughton, 1996). The generation of sharp waves becomes more robust and drives neocortical activity more strongly when low levels of ACh release the suppression of excitatory feedback connections, allowing a shift from tonic theta rhythm oscillations to bursts of activity due to excitatory positive feedback.

Modulation and Network Oscillations

Changes in modulatory levels play an important role in setting the oscillatory properties of the EEG and functional properties important for behavior. Microdialysis of neuromodulators during different stages of waking and sleep show dramatic changes in their levels associated with changes in the cortical EEG. High levels of ACh, NE, and 5-HT are present during waking, very low levels of ACh are present during slow-wave sleep, and very low levels of NE and 5-HT coupled with high levels of ACh are present during REM sleep. Computational models have illustrated potential mechanisms for these modulatory influences on cortical dynamics.

Neuromodulation alters the way in which thalamic circuitry regulates low-frequency synchronous oscillations that appear in the neocortex during sleep, including spindle activity and delta waves. Modeling demonstrates that the fundamental frequency of spindle activity could result from the interaction of intrinsic currents in thalamic reticular neurons, which fire bursts due to a low-threshold calcium current and hyperpolarize due to a calcium-activated potassium current. These cells provide rhythmic inhibitory input to thalamocortical relay cells, which then repolarize because of the hyperpolarization-activated nonspecific cation current and fire bursts because of the activation of the low-threshold calcium current (Terman, Bose, and Kopell, 1996; also see SYNAPTIC INTERACTIONS). Cholinergic innervation of thalamic circuits could prevent the generation of spindle and delta wave oscillations by depolarizing neurons through blockade of potassium currents, thereby inactivating the low-threshold calcium current underlying bursting (McCormick et al., 1993). Decreases in cholinergic depolarization would initially cause spindles when both thalamocortical neurons and thalamic reticular neurons are active, but as reticular neurons become less depolarized, their activity decreases, and thalamocortical neurons can oscillate synchronously at delta wave frequencies (Terman et al., 1996).

Neuromodulation plays an essential role in generating the hippocampal theta rhythm (see HIPPOCAMPAL RHYTHM GENERATION). Theta rhythm is primarily paced by rhythmic input from the medial septum, but it can also arise from intrinsic mechanisms in local circuits. In slice preparations of the hippocampus, cholinergic modulation has been demonstrated to induce theta rhythm oscillations (Tiesinga et al., 2001). Simulations demonstrate that the appearance of oscillations in the slice could result from slow depolarization of pyramidal cells, causing spiking activity, which is then synchronized by excitatory synaptic connections, with a time course dependent on the calcium-activated potassium current (Traub, Miles, and Buzsaki, 1992; Tiesinga et al., 2001). Computational modeling provides a means for understanding the role of neuromodulation in regulating a wide range of oscillatory dynamics.

Discussion

Neuromodulation plays an important role in brain function, as demonstrated by the dramatic behavioral effects of drugs that influence the release of neuromodulators or activate receptors for neuromodulators. Neuromodulators do not just cause slight quantitative changes in network function but can qualitatively alter neural circuits to a completely different functional state. Computational modeling helps us understand the functional role of modulatory effects that may appear contradictory at a cellular level (for example, many modulators simultaneously depolarize neurons while suppressing synaptic transmission). Computational modeling will prove essential to understanding the functional role of diffuse modulatory effects with complex effects on multiple components of neural circuits.

Road Map: Biological Networks
Related Reading: Dopamine, Roles of; Neuromodulation in Invertebrate Nervous Systems

References

Buzsaki, G., 1989, Two-stage model of memory trace formation: A role for "noisy" brain states, *Neuroscience*, 31:551–570.

Doya, K., Dayan, P., and Hasselmo, M. E., Eds., 2002, Special issue on neuromodulation, *Neural Netw.*, 15.

Durstewitz, D., Seamans, J. K., and Sejnowski, T. J., 2000, Dopamine-mediated stabilization of delay-period activity in a network model of prefrontal cortex, *J. Neurophysiol.*, 83:1733–175.

Fellous, J. M., and Linster, C., 1998, Computational models of neuromodulation, *Neural Computat.*, 10:771–805. ◆

Fransen, E., Alonso, A. A., and Hasselmo, M. E., 2002, Simulations of the role of the muscarinic-activated calcium-sensitive non-specific cation current I(NCM) in entorhinal neuronal activity during delayed matching tasks, *J. Neurosci.*, 22:1081–1097.

Hasselmo, M. E., 1995, Neuromodulation and cortical function: Modeling the physiological basis of behavior, *Behav. Brain Res.*, 67:1–27.

Hasselmo, M. E., Bodelon, C., and Wyble, B. P., 2002, A proposed function for hippocampal theta rhythm: Separation of encoding and retrieval enhances reversal of prior learning, *Neural Computat.*, 14:793–817.

Hasselmo, M. E., Linster, C., Ma, D., and Cekic, M., 1997, Noradrenergic suppression of synaptic transmission may influence cortical "signal-to-noise" ratio, *J. Neurophysiol.*, 77:3326–3339.

Katz, P. S., 1999, *Beyond Neurotransmission: Neuromodulation and Its Importance for Information Processing*, New York: Oxford University Press. ◆

McCormick, D. A., Wang, Z., and Huguenard, J., 1993, Neurotransmitter control of neocortical neuronal activity and excitability, *Cerebr. Cortex*, 3:387–398.

Shen, B., and McNaughton, B. L., 1996, Modeling the spontaneous reactivation of experience-specific hippocampal cell assembles during sleep, *Hippocampus*, 6:685–692.

Terman, D., Bose, A., and Kopell, N., 1996, Functional reorganization in thalamocortical networks: Transition between spindling and delta sleep rhythms, *Proc. Natl. Acad. Sci. USA*, 93:15417–15422.

Tiesinga, P. H., Fellous, J. M., Jose, J. V., and Sejnowski, T. J., 2001, Computational model of carbachol-induced delta, theta, and gamma oscillations in the hippocampus, *Hippocampus*, 11:251–274.

Traub, R. D., Miles, R., and Buzsaki, G., 1992, Computer simulation of carbachol-driven rhythmic population oscillations in the CA3 region of the in vitro rat hippocampus, *J. Physiol. (Lond.)*, 451:653–672.

Usher, M., Cohen, J. D., Servan-Schreiber, D., Rajkowski, J., and Aston-Jones, G., 1999, The role of locus coeruleus in the regulation of cognitive performance, *Science*, 283:549–554.

Neuromorphic VLSI Circuits and Systems

Stephen P. DeWeerth and Andreas G. Andreou

Introduction

Biological systems excel at sensory perception, motor control, and sensorimotor coordination by sustaining high computational throughput with minimal energy consumption. Research in electronic neuromorphic engineering (Mead, 1989) has had two intertwined objectives. The first objective is the use of very large-scale integrated (VLSI) technology as a modeling tool aimed at capturing the behavior of living neurons, networks of neurons, and the complex mechanical-electrical-chemical information processing present in biological systems. The second objective—the subject of this article—is the development of engineered systems based on abstractions of sensory, motor, and brain function.

Neuromorphic VLSI systems employ distributed and parallel representations and computation akin to those found in their biological counterparts. The hardware implementations combine analog and digital circuits to realize a variety of computational primitives and architectures. Unlike traditional analog computing, neuromorphic representations are not linearized a priori, but rather exploit the inherent nonlinearities and dynamics that arise from the physics of the devices and circuits. The bio-inspired approach to the engineering of VLSI microsystems results in the embodiment of computation in complex, *physical* systems that exploit biological inspiration and lie beyond digital computing and that have a wide range of industrial applications (Vittoz, 2002).

The high levels of system integration offered in VLSI technology make it attractive for the implementation of highly complex artificial neuronal systems, even though the physics of the liquid-crystalline state of biological structures is different from the physics of the solid-state silicon technologies. Silicon complementary metal oxide semiconductor (CMOS) transistors are used in their subthreshold region of operation (Vittoz, 1985; Mead, 1989) because in this regime the primary constraint of highly integrated microsystems, power consumption, is all but eliminated. Circuits operating in their subthreshold region also exhibit a diverse set of computational primitives that are continuous, analog functions of time, space, voltage, current, and charge.

In this article, we discuss neuromorphic VLSI viewed at three hierarchical levels: the *device* level, the *circuit/network* level, and the *systems* level. Given the space limitations, we focus primarily on the circuit/network level. We describe a design style that employs mixed-signal (analog/digital), current-mode CMOS circuits that have minimal complexity (Andreou et al., 1991). Our presentation is not a comprehensive overview of the field, even within the bounds of circuits and networks. Rather, it provides a basic foundation in device physics and presents a set of specific circuits that implement certain essential functions that exemplify the breadth possible within this design paradigm.

Devices

Neuromorphic VLSI circuits and systems are designed with two basic device building blocks available in CMOS technology—transistors and capacitors.

The transistors used in most neuromorphic implementations are devices operating in their *subthreshold* regime. In this regime, the current through the device is an *exact difference* of exponential functions of the drain and source voltages (Vittoz, 1985; Mead, 1989; Andreou et al., 1991). For an *n*MOS transistor, the current is given by

$$I_{DS} = I_{n0} \cdot S \cdot e^{\kappa_n V_{GB}}(e^{-V_{SB}} - e^{-V_{DB}}) \tag{1}$$

and for a *p*MOS transistor by

$$I_{SD} = I_{p0} \cdot S \cdot e^{-\kappa_p V_{GB}}(e^{V_{SB}} - e^{V_{DB}}) \tag{2}$$

The terminal voltages V_{GB}, V_{SB}, and V_{DB}, in these equations are normalized to the thermal voltage $U_t = kT/q$, which is approximately equal to 25 mV at room temperature. The constants I_{n0} and I_{p0} depend on the mobility of the carriers (electrons and holes) and other physical properties of the silicon, and are typically in the range of 10^{-15} A. The geometry factor, $S = W/L$, where W and L are the width and length of the device, respectively. The constants κ_n and κ_p take values between 0.6 and 0.9. All of these parameters are fixed by the fabrication process, and thus cannot be modified by the designer or user with the exception of the variable S, which can be modified by designing the geometry of the device, and U_1, which is a function of operational temperature.

The MOS transistor has excellent circuit properties as a voltage-input, current-output device (a *transconductance amplifier*) with good fan-out capabilities (high transconductance, $g_m = \partial I_{DS}/\partial V_{GS}$) and good fan-in capability (extremely high input impedance). Additionally, the exponential voltage-current relationships depicted in Equations 1 and 2 facilitate a powerful synthesis (and analysis) procedure, the *translinear principle* that has also been generalized for MOS circuits (Andreou and Boahen, 1996; Gilbert, 1996).

In addition to CMOS transistors, neuromorphic VLSI systems also utilize capacitors extensively. These capacitors, which are implemented as parallel-plate devices between fabrication layers (e.g., vertically adjacent layers of polysilicon), endow the systems with temporal properties based on the capacitor's ability to store charge (energy). The capacitor equation

$$I = C\frac{dV}{dt} \quad V = \frac{1}{C}\int I dt \tag{3}$$

demonstrates that the capacitor integrates input current and represents this integrated value as a voltage.

Circuits and Networks

The synthesis of computational structures begins at the circuit level and manifests itself as the emergence of *networks*. At the circuit level, conservation laws—the conservation of charge (Kirchoff's current law), $\Sigma_n I_n = 0$, and the conservation of energy (Kirchoff's voltage law), $\Sigma_n V_n = 0$—are used to realize simple constraint equations. These laws, combined with the integration of charge on capacitors, provide a means of implementing functions of both space and time.

The important concept of *negative feedback* is also exploited to implement the inverse of natural functions in the technology and to trade off the gain in the active elements for precision and speed in the circuits. The simplest circuit that exploits the high-gain transconductance of the MOS transistor, its exponential characteristics, and negative feedback is the *diode-connected* transistor. This circuit uses negative feedback to invert the exponential characteristic of the transistor to create a logarithmic current-in, voltage-out configuration.

Current replication and scaling are two additional operations that are used in the implementation of many systems. Current replication is implemented using the *current mirror,* which uses an input transistor to convert an input current logarithmically to a voltage. This voltage is distributed to one or more output transistors, each of which converts this voltage exponentially back into a current that is equal (modulo fabrication offsets and second-order effects) to the input current. Scaling can be accomplished in multiple ways, including transistor sizing and using an additional parameter to control the source of a transistor.

In the remainder of this circuits section, we focus on three computational functions in space and time that are essential to and exemplify the breadth of neuromorphic microsystems: (1) signal aggregation, (2) normalization, and (3) signal quantization. These particular choices certainly do not represent a complete itemization of all of the important neuromorphic circuits/networks, but rather are a representative list. For each of these functions, we discuss both spatial and temporal implementations, and in some cases show circuit schematics and describe the corresponding operation. Finally, we present the issue of the representation and communication of signals among subsystems, which is essential in the implementation of large-scale systems. Throughout this section, we discuss systems that utilize these circuits, networks, and representations as fundamental elements in their implementation.

Signal Aggregation

Signal aggregation is the collection and processing of signals over space and/or time. Spatial aggregation can take many forms, including simple summation, computation of global attributes, and localized aggregation. Temporal aggregation is typically formulated as the integration of charge over time on a capacitor, and includes many temporal filtering functions. The representation of analog signals as currents facilitates the elegant implementation of both spatial and temporal aggregation as a direct result of Kirchoff's current law; thus, aggregation is implemented primarily using currents.

Spatial aggregation.   One particularly useful circuit for local spatial aggregation is the resistive network (Mead, 1989, chap. 6). It performs linear addition of signals over a confined region of space, such as that observed throughout the nervous system. The basic resistive network depicted in Figure 1A employs voltages and currents. Its node equation is

$$I_j = G \cdot (V_i + V_k - 2V_j) \cong G\nabla^2 V \qquad (4)$$

Note that the term $V_i + V_k - 2V_j$ is a first-order approximation to the Laplacian operator $\nabla^2 = \partial^2/\partial x^2 + \partial^2/\partial y^2$, with the internode distance normalized to unity.

The resistive network in Figure 1A, although simple, is not amenable to compact VLSI integration because conductances G with a large linear range typically consume large amounts of both area and power. However, MOS transistors provide a natural way to exploit the underlying device physics to implement analog VLSI aggregation networks that can be applied to systems, including silicon retinas (Andreou et al., 1995; Vittoz, 2002).

The exponential functions of V_{SB} and V_{DB} in Equations 1 and 2 correspond to Boltzmann-distributed charges at the source and drain diffusing through the channel. For the *n*MOS transistor, the exponentials can be conveniently represented as dimensionless quantities of charge

$$Q_S \equiv e^{-V_{\text{SB}}} \quad Q_D \equiv e^{-V_{\text{DB}}} \qquad (5)$$

and diffusivity

$$D \equiv S \cdot e^{V_{\text{GB}}} \qquad (6)$$

so that the Equation 1 becomes

$$I_{DS} = I_{n0} \cdot D^\kappa \cdot (Q_S - Q_D) \qquad (7)$$

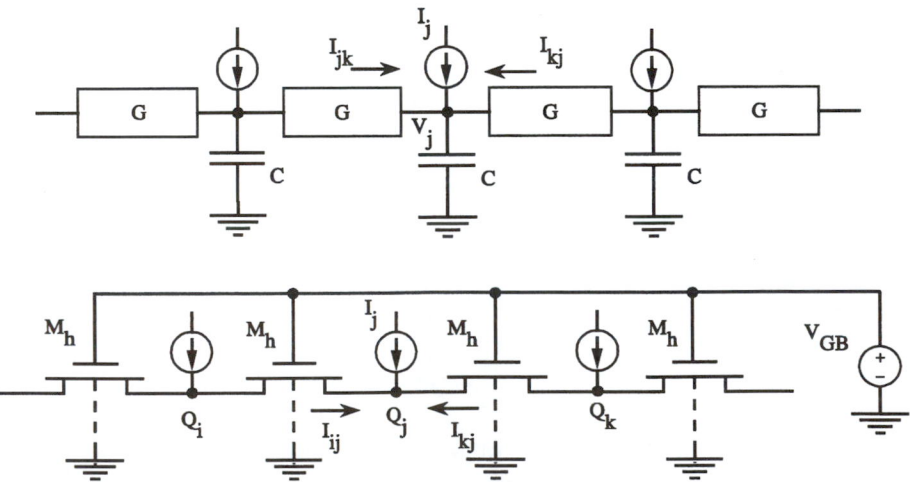

Figure 1. *A*, Signal aggregation in space using a linear resistive network. *B*, A network of nonlinear conductances implemented using MOS transistors.

The charge-based representation depicted in Equation 10 suggests that the MOS transistor in subthreshold is a highly linear device in the charge domain. This property can be used to implement the resistive network using MOS transistors, as shown in Figure 1B. This network employs charges (positive) and currents through *n*MOS transistors operating in their subthreshold regime. The node equation is

$$I_j = I_{n0} \cdot D \cdot (Q_i + Q_k - 2Q_j) \cong I_{n0}D\nabla^2Q \qquad (8)$$

assuming that S and V_{GB} are identical for all transistors in the network. The diffusivity D can be controlled by setting the voltage at the gate of transistor M_h at the desired value.

Temporal integration. The aggregation of signals in time is performed using temporal integration circuits that combine a device or circuit that generates a current with a capacitor that integrates that current. The diode capacitor integrator shown in Figure 2 is one of the simplest and most useful of these circuits. The input to this circuit can take the form of a continuously varying current or of a pulse stream generated by quantization circuits such as those described in a subsequent section.

Given subthreshold bias voltages, the input current, I_1, and output current, I_2, are related as follows:

$$Q\frac{dI_2}{dt} = I_2 \cdot \left(I_1 - \frac{I_2}{A}\right) \qquad (9)$$

where $Q = CU_t/\kappa$ and $A = e^{V_E/U_t}$. This equation demonstrates that the time constant of the circuit can be modified separately from the input current by changing V_E.

When a steady-state train of pulses of width w and frequency $f = 1/T$ is applied to this integrator, the nonlinear behavior of the diode capacitor integrator has the following interesting properties: (1) the steady-state current is proportional to pulse-stream frequency f, (2) the steady-state current is proportional to pulse width w, (3) the steady-state current ripple (error) is independent of current level, and (4) the steady state is reached, for a given precision, after a constant number of pulses.

The diode capacitor integrator has been used in many systems, including silicon retinas that compute motion (Sarpeshkar et al., 1996) and the receiver sections for multichip neuromorphic systems (Boahen, 2000).

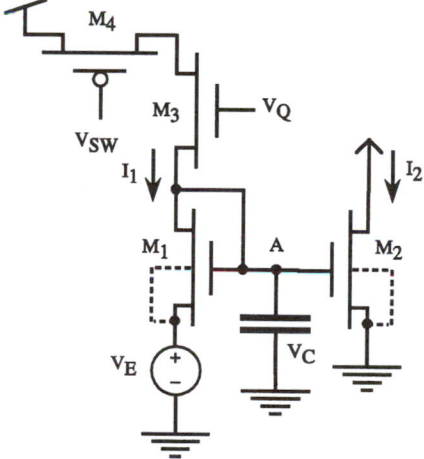

Figure 2. Diode capacitor integrator. The input and output signals are currents. The circuit is basically a current mirror with scaling, with the integrating capacitor at node A providing a time history of the input signals.

Gain Control

Gain control is an important function in biological systems. Many biological signals, especially those in the sensory periphery (e.g., visual and auditory signals), exhibit orders of magnitude of dynamic range. In order to process these signals, it is necessary to modify the dynamic range while not diminishing the information embedded in the signal. This type of normalization occurs in both space and time. Spatial normalization is used to bring a spatially distributed set of signals into a common or prescribed range that is matched to further processing. Temporal normalization typically takes the form of adaptation in which a slow variable that sets the gain of a circuit or network is modified over time to adapt to changes in signal magnitude.

Spatial normalization. Spatial normalization can be divided into *global* and *local* operations. Global normalization modifies the gain of all of the signals in a network, serving to shift the global level of these signals. Local normalization serves to perform similar processing but controls gain based on the activity in a local region.

One example of global normalization is the linear, current-mode normalizing circuit (Gilbert, 1996). Using the translinear principle, it can be shown that the output currents of this circuit are related to its input currents through the following expression:

$$I_{On} = \frac{I_T}{\sum I_{In}} \cdot I_{In} \qquad (10)$$

Thus an output current I_{On} in the array is proportional to the corresponding input current I_{In} normalized to the sum of all input currents. The current I_T is a scaling parameter that can be controlled externally. This circuit demonstrates the basic formulation of global normalization: the gain of individual elements is modified based on a global aggregate, in this case the sum (or average) of the input currents. Similar circuits have been created to compute a wide variety of nonlinear normalization functions using the same principle. Local normalization can also be implemented via the addition of resistive elements between the individual nodes, resulting in localized sums of input currents against which the input signals are compared.

Temporal adaptation. Normalization in time is accomplished through the combination of "fast" input variables normalized by "slow" adaptation variables. As in the case of spatial normalization, the basic premise of temporal adaptation is the averaging of the input signal—in this case, averaged over time using the slow variable—and the scaling of the input based on this average.

One of the simplest and most widely used adaptive circuits that implements temporal gain control is the adaptive photoreceptor (Delbruck and Mead, 1996). This circuit provides an analog output that has low gain for static signals and high gain for transient signals that vary about an operating point. The circuit's adaptive function allows the output to represent a large dynamic range of absolute intensities while retaining sensitivity to small inputs. The adaptive photoreceptor has been used extensively in vision chips, including those that compute motion (Sarpeskar et al., 1996) and visual attention (Morris and DeWeerth, 1999).

Signal Quantization

Signal quantization is seen throughout the nervous systems of animals. Information is transmitted using action potentials, which are temporally quantized forms of the analog membrane potentials from which they are derived. Spatial quantization is also widespread, taking forms such as the *place codings* found in motor maps in areas including colliculus and primary motor cortex. Such quantization is essential to system operation because multidimensional signals must be represented by sets of individual neurons, each of which encodes one piece of a quantized signal.

Spatial quantization. One example of spatial quantization is the current-mode winner-take-all circuit (Lazzaro et al., 1989; Andreou et al., 1991), a variation of which is shown in Figure 3. In this circuit, pairs of MOS transistors (M_{1n} and M_{2n}) configured as *current conveyors* compete for current supplied to a common line. Each current conveyor sees a voltage V_T at its common node. Consequently, for conveyor n, if $I_n < I_0 Se^{\kappa V_T}$, M_{1n} enters its linear region ($V_{DS} < 4$), turning M_{2n} off at that element. This condition occurs in all but one of the conveyors. At the element with the largest input, negative feedback in transistor M_{2n} adjusts V_T so that $I_n = I_0 Se^{\kappa V_T}$. Thus, the conveyor with the largest input sets the voltage on the common node and conveys the common current I_T to its output. The result is a network that, for normal operation, selects the largest input by generating a non-zero output at only that element. Variants of the basic winner-take-all circuit have been used extensively in systems such as attention-based imagers (Morris and DeWeerth, 1999) and large classifier arrays (Pouliquen et al., 1997).

Temporal quantization. Temporal quantization is exemplified by the creation of neural "spikes" (action potentials) as a function of a continuous input current (Mead, 1989, chap. 12). For example, integrate-and-fire neurons convert continuous-value representations of signals into a discrete-value representation. Spiking neuron circuits are used widely in interface circuits to communicate information among different subsystems and is an essential component of the address event representation discussed in the next section. They have also been used extensively as the primary output devices in the pulse-modulated control of motor systems.

Representation and Communication

To construct systems from the circuits and networks described previously, we must have a paradigm for representing and communicating signals over long distances (including between VLSI chips) with potentially significant fan-in and fan-out. The massive connectivity of the brain is impossible to implement directly using VLSI because of wiring limitations within and between microchips. We can, however, exploit the temporally sparse nature of spike codes and the high bandwidth of VLSI systems in order to overcome this connectivity problem by time-multiplexing signals from many connections onto a single high-speed data bus. The resulting

address-event representation (AER) (Lazzaro et al., 1993) has emerged as a general paradigm for communicating large amounts of data in distributed spatiotemporal architectures. The core paradigm represents individual local activity that is encoded by neural spikes as *events*. Each of these events represents the origin/destination and timing information of a single spike, and is communicated on high-speed data buses throughout the network.

Because AER was originally formulated to emulate the optic nerve and the auditory nerve (Lazzaro et al., 1993), it implements a one-to-one connection topology. To implement more complex neural circuits, convergent and divergent connections are required. For example, architectures have been developed for emulating short and long connections along the spinal cord (DeWeerth et al., 1997), and for memory-based projective field mappings that enable the projection of an address event to multiple receiver locations (Boahen, 2000).

Discussion

Neuromorphic engineering represents a design paradigm that combines biological inspiration with microsystems technology to facilitate the design and implementation of systems that address a wide variety of tasks that are presently beyond the abilities of today's computer systems but appear accessible and even trivial to the nervous systems of the simplest animals. The field is based on the premise that it is the nonlinearities and dynamics, the circuit architectures, and the basic computational paradigms present in these biological systems—most of which are foreign to traditional engineered systems—that make them successful. The ultimate goal of this field is to abstract these organizational principles by implementing them in real, physical systems in order to create artificial systems that exploit the power of biological computation.

In this article we have discussed neuromorphic electronic systems at three levels of organization: devices, circuits/networks, and systems, with an emphasis on the intermediate level. At the device level, we presented the basic devices—transistors and capacitors—that form the foundation for the other levels. At the circuit/network level, we described a set of essential circuits and networks that are employed as building blocks for a wide variety of systems. A full appreciation of the value of these circuits can be attained only by studying their use in larger systems. For more detailed coverage of this rapidly developing field, readers are referred for such excellent journals as *IEEE Transactions on Circuits and Systems, IEEE Transactions on Neural Networks, IEEE Journal of Solid-State Circuits, Analog Integrated Circuits and Signal Processing, Neural*

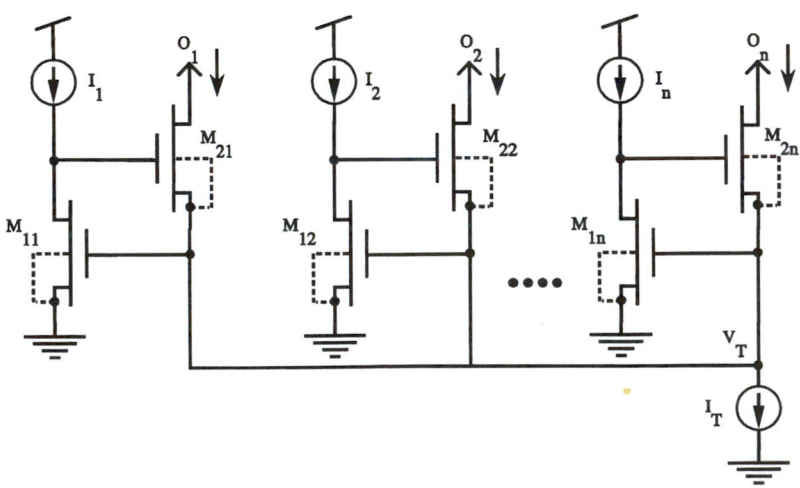

Figure 3. Winner-take-all circuit with current input and current output signals.

Computation, and *Neural Networks,* which carry regular articles and have special issues on hardware implementations of neuromorphic microsystems.

Road Map: Implementation and Analysis
Related Reading: Analog VLSI Implementation of Neural Networks; Digital VLSI for Neural Networks; Photonic Implementations of Neurobiologically Inspired Networks

References

Andreou, A., and Boahen, K., 1996, Translinear circuits in subthreshold CMOS, *Analog Integr. Circuits Sign. Process.,* 9:141–166.

Andreou, A. G., and Boahen, K. A., 1991, Current-mode subthreshold MOS circuits for analog VLSI neural systems, *IEEE Trans. Neural Netw.,* 2:205–213.

Andreou, A. G., and Meitzler, R. C., 1995, Analog VLSI neuromorphic image acquisition and pre-processing systems, *Neural Netw.,* 8:1323–1347.

Boahen, K. A., 2000, Point-to-point connectivity between neuromorphic chips using address events, *IEEE Trans. Circuits Syst. II Analog Digital Sign. Process.,* 47:416–434.

Delbruck, T., and Mead, C. A., 1996, *Analog VLSI Phototransduction by Continuous-Time, Adaptive, Logarithmic Photoreceptor Circuits,* technical report, Caltech CNS Memo No. 30.

DeWeerth, S. P., Patel, G. N., Simoni, M., Schimmel, D., and Calabrese, R., 1997, A VLSI architecture for modeling intersegmental coordination,

in *Proceedings of the 17th Conference on Advanced Research in VLSI,* pp. 182–200, Los Alamitos, CA.

Gilbert, B., 1996, Translinear circuits: An historical overview, *Analog Integr. Circuits Sign. Process.,* 9:95–118.

Lazzaro, J., Ryskebusch, S., Mahowald, M. A., and Mead, C. A., 1989, Winner-take-all circuits, in *Advances in Neural Information Processing Systems,* vol. 1 (D. S. Touretzky, Ed.), San Mateo, CA: Morgan Kaufmann, pp. 703–711.

Lazzaro, J., Wawrzynek, J., Mahowald, M., Sivilotti, M., and Gillespie, D., 1993, Silicon auditory processors as computer peripherals, *IEEE Trans. Neural Netw.,* 4:523–528. ◆

Mead, C. A., 1989, *Analog VLSI and Neural Systems,* Reading, MA: Addison-Wesley. ◆

Morris, T. G., and DeWeerth, S. P., 1999, A smart-scanning analog VLSI visual-attention system, *Int. J. Analog Integr. Circuits Sign. Process.,* 21:67–78.

Pouliquen, P. O., Andreou, A., and Strohbehn, K., 1997, Winner-takes-all associative memory: A hamming distance vector quantizer, *Analog Integr. Circuits Sign. Process.,* 13:211–222.

Sarpeshkar, R., Kramer, J., Indiveri, G., and Koch, C., 1996, Analog VLSI architectures for motion processing: From fundamental limits to system applications, *Proc. IEEE,* 84:969–987. ◆

Vittoz, E. A., 1985, The design of high-performance analog circuits on digital CMOS chips, *IEEE J. Solid State Circuits,* 20:657–665.

Vittoz, E. A., 2002, Present and future industrial applications of bio-inspired VLSI systems, *Analog Integr. Circuits Sign. Process.,* 30:173–184.

NEURON Simulation Environment

Michael L. Hines and N. Ted Carnevale

Introduction

NEURON is designed to be a convenient and efficient environment for simulating models of biological and artificial neurons, individually and in networks. Great care has been exercised at every point in its development to achieve computational efficiency and robustness while helping users maintain conceptual clarity, i.e., the knowledge that what has been instantiated in the computer is an accurate implementation of one's conceptual model. NEURON's application domain extends beyond continuous system simulations of models of individual neurons with complex anatomical and biophysical properties, and includes discrete-event and hybrid simulations that combine biological and artificial neuronal models. Here we review features of NEURON that are of special interest to prospective users.

Who Uses NEURON, and Why?

Presently, more than 300 papers have reported research performed with NEURON (see http://www.neuron.yale.edu/neuron/bib/usednrn.html). Among the research topics are descriptions of models of individual neurons and networks of neurons with properties such as complex branching morphology, multiple channel types, inhomogeneous channel distribution, ionic diffusion and buffering, active transport, second messengers, and use-dependent synaptic plasticity. At the cellular level, NEURON has been used to investigate pre- and postsynaptic mechanisms involved in synaptic transmission, the roles of dendritic architecture and active membrane properties in synaptic integration, spike initiation and propagation in dendrites and axons, the effects of developmental changes of anatomy and biophysics, the functional genomics of ion channels, and extracellular stimulation and recording, among other topics.

Network models implemented with NEURON have been used to address issues such as the origin of cortical and thalamic oscillations, the role of gap junctions in neuronal synchrony, information encoding in biological networks, visual orientation selectivity, mechanisms of epilepsy, and the actions of anticonvulsant drugs.

NEURON is also being used in neuroscience education at the undergraduate and graduate level at numerous universities across the United States and around the world. Many of these courses are completely homegrown, but one lab manual with exercises has already appeared in print (Moore and Stuart, 2000), and we are involved in a collaboration to develop another set of laboratory exercises for publication. NEURON is particularly well suited to educational applications, since special expertise in numerical methods or programming is not required for its productive use. Furthermore, NEURON runs under MacOS, MSWindows, and UNIX/Linux, and can execute research-quality simulations with reasonable run times on entry-level hardware.

How Does NEURON Work?

Historically, NEURON's primary domain of application was in simulating empirically based models of biological neurons with extended geometry and biophysical mechanisms that are spatially nonuniform and kinetically complex. In the past decade its functionality was enhanced to include extracellular fields, linear circuits to emulate the effects of nonideal instrumentation, models of artificial (integrate-and-fire) neurons, and networks that can involve any combination of artificial and biological neuron models. The following sections outline how these capabilities have been implemented so as to achieve computational efficiency while maintaining conceptual clarity, i.e., the knowledge that what has been instantiated in the computer model is an accurate representation of the user's conceptual model.

Representing Biological Neurons

Information processing in the nervous system involves the spread and interaction of electrical and chemical signals within and between neurons and glia. These signals are continuous functions of time and space and are described by the diffusion equation and the closely related cable equation (Rall, 1977; Crank, 1979). To simulate the operation of biological neurons, NEURON uses the tactic of discretizing time and space, approximating these partial differential equations by a set of algebraic difference equations that can be solved numerically (numerical integration) (Hines and Carnevale, 1997).

Discretization is often couched in terms of compartmentalization, but it is perhaps better to regard it as an approximation of the original continuous system by another system that is discontinuous in time and space. Simulating a discretized model results in computation of the values of spatiotemporally continuous variables over a set of discrete points in space ("nodes") for a finite number of instants in time. If NEURON's second-order-correct integration method is used, these values are a piecewise linear approximation to the continuous system, so that second-order-accurate estimates of continuous variables at intermediate locations can be found by linear interpolation (Hines and Carnevale, 2001).

In one form or another, spatial discretization lies at the core of all simulators used to model biological neurons, e.g., GENESIS SIMULATION SYSTEM (q.v.). Unlike other simulators, however, NEURON does not force users to deal with compartments. Instead, NEURON's basic building block is the section, an unbranched, continuous cable whose anatomical and biophysical properties can vary continuously along its length. The branched architecture of a cell is reconstructed by connecting sections together, each section having its own anatomical dimensions, biophysical properties, and discretization parameter nseg, which specifies the number of nodes at which solutions are computed. This strategy makes it easier to manage anatomically detailed models, since each section in the model is a direct counterpart to a branch of the original cell (Figure 1). Furthermore, neuroscientists naturally tend to think in terms of axonal or dendritic branches rather than compartments.

But even in topologically simple cases, there is still the problem of how to treat variables that are continuous functions of space. Thinking in terms of compartments leads to representations that require users to keep track of which compartments correspond to which anatomical locations. If we change the size or number of compartments, e.g., in order to see whether spatial discretization is adequate for numerical accuracy, we must also abandon the old mapping between compartments and locations in favor of a completely new one.

This is the motivation for another strategy that helps NEURON users maintain conceptual clarity: *range* and *range variables*. Range variables are continuous functions of position along a branch of a cell, e.g., diameter, membrane potential, or ion channel density. NEURON deals with range variables in terms of arc length (normalized distance) along the centroid of each section. This normalized distance, which is called range, is a continuous parameter that varies from 0 at one end to 1 at the other. In NEURON's programming language hoc, the membrane potential at a point 700 μm down the length of a 1,000-μm-long axon would be called axon.v(0.7), regardless of the value of the axon's discretization parameter nseg. Range and range variables allow NEURON itself to take care of the correspondence between nodes and anatomical location. This avoids the tendency of compartmental approaches to confound representation of the physical properties of neurons, which are biologically relevant, with implementational

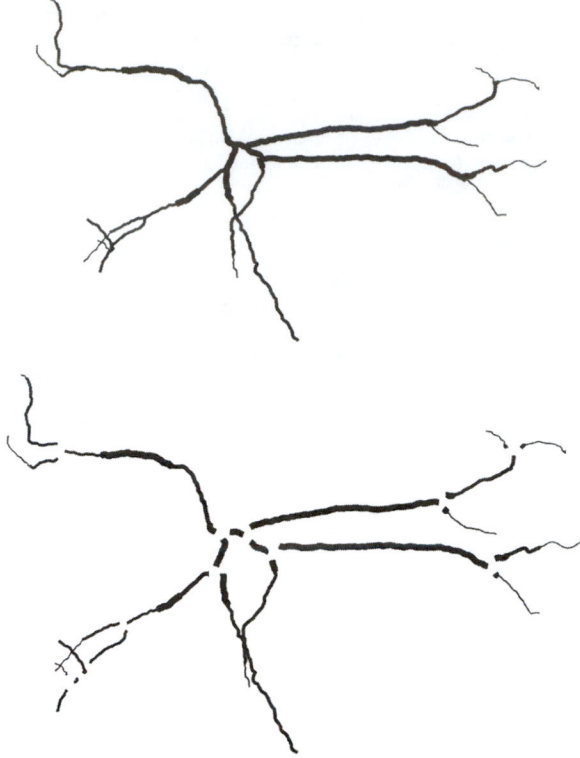

Figure 1. *Top*, Morphometric reconstruction of a hippocampal interneuron (data from A. I. Gulyás). *Bottom*, An "exploded" view, in which individual, unbranched neurites have been separated from each other at branch points.

details such as compartment size, which are mere artifacts of having to use a digital computer to emulate the behavior of a distributed physical system that is continuous in time and space.

Representing Artificial Neurons

In NEURON, the basic difference between biological and artificial neuron models is that the former may have arbitrarily complex anatomical and biophysical complexity, while the latter have no spatial extent and employ highly simplified kinetics. Indeed, the three built-in classes of artificial spiking neurons are so simple that they are simulated using a discrete-event method, which executes hundreds of times faster than numerical integration methods. If an event occurs at time t_1, all state variables are computed from the state values and time t_0 of the previous event. Since computations are performed only when an event occurs, total computation time is proportional to the number of events delivered and independent of the number of cells, number of connections, or problem time. Thus, handling 100,000 spikes in 1 hour for 100 cells requires the same time as handling 100,000 spikes in 1 s for one cell. This takes advantage of NEURON's event delivery system, which was originally implemented to facilitate efficient network simulations of biological neurons (see following section).

Three different classes of integrate-and-fire models are built into NEURON. The simplest is IntFire1, a leaky integrator that treats input events as weighted delta functions. When an IntFire1 cell receives an input event of weight w, its "membrane potential" state m jumps instantaneously by an amount equal to w and thereafter resumes its decay toward 0 with time constant τ_m.

A step closer to the behavior of a biological neuron is the IntFire2 mechanism, which differs in that m integrates a net synaptic current i. An input to an IntFire2 cell makes the synaptic current jump by an amount equal to the synaptic weight, after which i continues to decay toward a steady level i_b with its own time constant τ_s, where $\tau_s > \tau_m$. Thus a single input event produces a gradual change in m with a delayed peak, and cell firing does not obliterate all traces of prior synaptic activation. The firing rate is $\sim i/\tau_m$ if $i \gg 1$ and $\tau_s \gg \tau_m$.

Although IntFire2 can emulate a wide range of relationships between input pattern and firing rate, all inputs produce responses with the same kinetics, regardless of whether they are excitatory or inhibitory. The fact that synaptic excitation in biological neurons is generally faster than inhibition inspired the design of IntFire4. IntFire4 integrates two synaptic current components that have different dynamics, depending on whether the input event is excitatory or inhibitory (Figure 2). Excitatory inputs add instantaneously to an excitatory synaptic current e, which otherwise decays toward 0 with a single time constant τ_e; this is analogous to IntFire2 with $i_b = 0$. However, the inhibitory synaptic current i_2 is described by the reaction scheme

$$i_1 \xrightarrow{1/\tau_{i1}} i_2 \xrightarrow{1/\tau_{i2}} \text{bath} \qquad (1)$$

where an inhibitory input (weight $w < 0$) adds instantaneously to i_1, so that i_2 follows a biexponential course (a slow rise followed by an even slower decay).

These are not the only kinds of artificial neurons that can be simulated using discrete events. The only prerequisite for discrete event simulations is that all state variables of a model cell can be

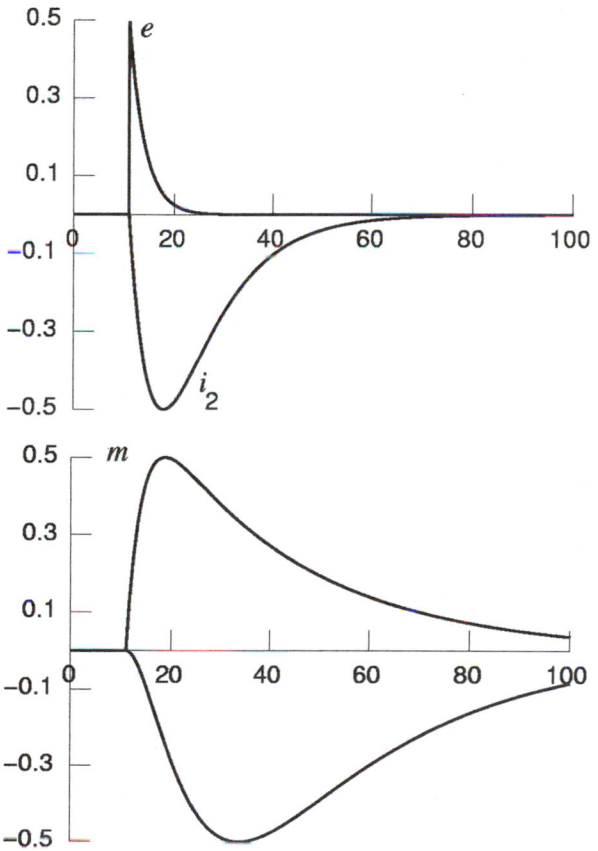

Figure 2. *Top,* Current generated by a single input event to an IntFire4 cell with weight 0.5 (e) or -0.5 (i_2). *Bottom,* The corresponding response of m. Parameters are $\tau_e = 3$, $\tau_{i1} = 5$, $\tau_{i2} = 10$, and $\tau_m = 30$ ms.

computed analytically from a new set of initial conditions. Users who have special needs can add other kinds of artificial neuron classes to NEURON with the NMODL language (discussed later).

Representing Networks

NEURON can handle networks that involve gap junctions or graded transmitter release, but this discussion is restricted to spiking networks. NEURON's NetCon class and event delivery system are used to manage synaptic communication between any combination of artificial and biological model neurons in a network. The event delivery system can also serve other purposes, such parameter changes on the fly, and it is a key part of the implementation of the built-in integrate-and-fire models, but these topics are beyond the scope of this article.

NEURON's strategy for dealing with synaptic connections emerged from techniques initially developed by Destexhe, Mainen, and Sejnowski (1994) and Lytton (1996). This strategy is based on a very simple conceptual model of synaptic transmission: arrival of a spike at the presynaptic terminal causes transmitter release, which in turn perturbs some mechanism in the postsynaptic cell (e.g., a membrane conductance or second messenger) that is described by a differential equation or kinetic scheme. All that matters is whether or not a spike has occurred in the presynaptic cell; mechanistic details in the presynaptic and postsynaptic cells do not affect transmitter release. This conceptual model separates the specification of the connections between cells from the specification of the postsynaptic mechanisms that the connections activate.

A presynaptic spike triggers an event that, after a delay to account for conduction along the axon, transmitter release, and diffusion time, is delivered to the postsynaptic mechanism, where it causes a change in some variable (e.g., a conductance). Event delivery is computationally efficient because of how synaptic divergence ("fan out") and convergence ("fan in") are handled. Synaptic divergence from model biological neurons is efficient because threshold detection is performed on a per source basis rather than a per connection basis. That is, if a neuron projects to multiple targets, the presynaptic variable is checked only once per time step, and when it crosses threshold an event is generated for each of the targets. Fan-out from artificial neurons is also very efficient, since their discrete event mechanisms do not have to be checked at each time step. However, the greatest computational savings are offered by synaptic convergence onto model biological neurons. Suppose a neuron receives multiple synaptic inputs that are close to each other and of the same type, i.e., each synapse has the same kind of postsynaptic mechanism. Then the total effect of all these synapses can be represented by a single kinetic scheme or set of equations driven by multiple input streams, each of which has its own weight.

The implementation of the event delivery service in NEURON takes into account the fact that the delay between initiation and delivery of events is different for different streams. Consequently, the order in which events are generated by a set of sources is rarely the order in which they are received by a set of targets. Furthermore, the delay may be 0 or 10^9 or anything in between.

As noted earlier, NEURON separates specification of the connections between cells from specification of the postsynaptic mechanisms that the connections activate. This separation means that NEURON models are compatible with other event delivery systems, such as the parallel discrete event delivery system used by NeoSim (Goddard et al., 2001).

Integration Methods

Users can choose among several different integration methods, but the "best" method for any given problem depends on many factors and may require empirical testing. Every choice involves trade-offs between accuracy, on the one hand, and stability and/or run time, on the other. For more extensive treatments of this topic, see Hines and Carnevale (1995, 1997, 2001).

Two methods use fixed time steps: backward Euler, and a Crank-Nicholson variant. NEURON's default integrator is backward Euler, which is first-order accurate in time, inherently stable, and generally produces good qualitative results even with large time steps. Used with extremely large Δt, it will find the steady-state solution of a linear ("passive") model in one step, and quickly converge to a steady state for nonlinear models. The Crank-Nicholson (CN) variant employs a staggered time step in order to provide second-order accuracy without having to iterate nonlinear equations. The computational cost of a single time step is practically the same as for backward Euler, but much shorter run times are possible with CN because it can use a larger Δt for a given degree of accuracy. However, CN cannot be used with models that involve purely algebraic relations between states, and it can produce spurious oscillations if Δt is too large or if the model includes a fast voltage clamp.

Models that work with CN are generally also amenable to CVODE (Cohen and Hindmarsh, 1984), the variable order, variable time step method offered by NEURON. For a given run time, CVODE often yields greater accuracy than CN. CVODE is usually the best choice for network models that involve artificial neurons. NEURON also offers a local variable order, variable time step method in which each cell has its own time step. This can be advantageous for network models in which most cells are silent most of the time.

Development Environment

Constructing and managing models and controlling simulations can be accomplished with an object-oriented interpreter, a set of GUI tools, or a combination of both. Most common tasks can be performed with the GUI tools, which are especially convenient for exploratory simulations during model development. Where the GUI is inadequate, users can resort to the interpreter, which is based on hoc (Kernighan and Pike, 1984). The interpreter is also appropriate for noninteractive simulations, such as production runs that generate large amounts of data for later analysis. Even so, several of the GUI tools are quite powerful in their own right, offering functionality that would require significant effort for users to recreate in hoc. This is particularly true of the optimization and electrotonic analysis tools. Thus, the most flexible and productive use of NEURON is to combine the GUI and hoc programming, taking advantage of the strengths of both.

Because of the ever-growing number and diversity of ligand- and voltage-gated ionic currents, pumps, buffers, etc., NEURON has a special facility for expanding its library of biophysical mechanisms (Hines and Carnevale, 2000). A user can write a text file that contains a description of the mechanism in NMODL, a programming language whose syntax for expressing nonlinear algebraic equations, differential equations, and kinetic reaction schemes closely resembles familiar notation. This file is then converted into C by a translator that automatically generates code for handling details such as mass balance for each ionic species. The translator output, which includes code that is suitable for each of NEURON's integration methods, is then compiled for computational efficiency. This achieves tremendous conceptual leverage and savings of effort because the high-level mechanism specification in NMODL is much easier to understand and far more compact than the equivalent C code, and the user is not bothered with low-level programming issues like how to interface the code with other mechanisms and with NEURON itself.

NEURON runs under MacOS, MSWindows, and UNIX/Linux, with a similar X11-based look and feel on all platforms. Further-more, the same hoc and NMODL code works under all these operating systems without modification. This facilitates collaborations in a heterogeneous computing environment.

Distribution, Documentation, and Support

NEURON is available free of charge from http://www.neuron .yale.edu/, along with extensive documentation and tutorials. The UNIX/Linux distribution includes full source code; the MSWin and MacOS distributions employ an identical computational engine and come with the hoc code that implements the GUI and the NMODL definitions of the built-in biophysical mechanisms and artificial neuron classes.

The web site also has a sign-up page for joining the NEURON Users' Group, a moderated mailing list for questions and answers, and pertinent announcements such as program updates and courses on NEURON. For the past several years we have presented "executive summary" and intensive hands-on courses at sites in the United States and Europe, and we plan to continue this in the future. NEURON is actively supported by a development team that responds to bug reports and questions about program usage. Indeed, much of the program's current functionality has been stimulated by requests and suggestions from users, and we are grateful to them for their continued interest and encouragement.

Discussion

The level of detail included in NEURON models can extend from a single compartment with linear membrane, to intricate extended architectures with membrane and cytoplasm that have complex biophysical properties. There are also several classes of artificial spiking neurons. Networks can involve biological neurons, artificial neurons, or both. Models can be simulated with fixed time step or with variable order, variable time step methods. With the variable time step integrator, the built-in artificial neurons are simulated as discrete event models, executing orders of magnitude faster than models of biological neurons do. Users can add new kinds of biophysical mechanisms and artificial neuron classes to NEURON's built-in library. NEURON runs on a wide variety of platforms, is actively supported, and is under continuous development, with revisions and updates that address the evolving needs of users. Because of these features, NEURON is employed in research on topics that range from the biophysical basis of neuronal function at the subcellular level to the operation of large-scale networks involved in consciousness, perception, learning, and memory. It is also increasingly being adopted for neuroscience education.

Road Map: Implementation and Analysis
Related Reading: Neurosimulation: Tools and Resources; Perspective on Neuron Model Complexity

References

Cohen, S. D., and Hindmarsh, A. C., 1984, *CVODE User Guide*, Livermore, CA: Lawrence Livermore National Laboratory.

Crank, J., 1979, *The Mathematics of Diffusion*, 2nd ed., London: Oxford University Press. ◆

Destexhe, A., Mainen, Z. F., and Sejnowski, T. J., 1994, An efficient method for computing synaptic conductances based on a kinetic model of receptor binding, *Neural Computat.*, 6:14–18.

Goddard, N., Hood, G., Howell, F., Hines, M., and De Schutter, E., 2001, NEOSIM: Portable large-scale plug and play modelling, *Neurocomputing*, 38:1657–1661. ◆

Hines, M., and Carnevale, N. T., 1995, Computer modeling methods for neurons, in *Handbook of Brain Theory and Neural Networks* (M. A. Arbib, Ed.), Cambridge, MA: MIT Press, pp. 226–230. ◆

Hines, M. L., and Carnevale, N. T., 1997, The NEURON simulation environment, *Neural Computat.*, 9:1179–1209. ◆

Hines, M. L., and Carnevale, N. T., 2000, Expanding NEURON's repertoire of mechanisms with NMODL, *Neural Computat.*, 12:839–
851. ◆

Hines, M. L., and Carnevale, N. T., 2001, NEURON: A tool for neuroscientists, *Neuroscientist*, 7:123–135. ◆

Kernighan, B. W., and Pike, R., 1984, Appendix 2: Hoc manual, in *The
UNIX Programming Environment*, Englewood Cliffs, NJ: Prentice-Hall,
pp. 329–333. ◆

Lytton, W. W., 1996, Optimizing synaptic conductance calculation for network simulations, *Neural Computat.*, 8:501–509.

Moore, J. W., and Stuart, A. E., 2000, *Neurons in Action: Computer Simulations with NeuroLab*, Sunderland, MA: Sinauer.

Rall, W., 1977, Core conductor theory and cable properties of neurons, in
Handbook of Physiology, vol. 1, part 1, *The Nervous System* (E. R. Kandel, Ed.), Bethesda, MD: American Physiological Society, pp. 39–
98. ◆

Neuropsychological Impairments

Martha J. Farah

Why Model Neuropsychological Impairments?

Neuropsychological impairments are an important source of evidence about the organization of cognition in the normal brain. For
example, the finding that amnesic patients retain the ability to learn
certain kinds of implicit information led to the idea of multiple
memory systems and the distinction between explicit and implicit
learning, both key insights in modern memory research (Squire,
1987). However, the inferences that link a neuropsychological impairment to a particular theory in cognitive neuroscience are not as
direct as one might first assume. A patient's behavior following
brain damage is not necessarily determined by a simple subtraction
of one or more components of the mind or brain, with those that
remain functioning normally. The brain is a distributed and highly
interactive system, such that local damage to one part can unleash
new modes of functioning in the remaining parts of the system.
Thus, the link between neuropsychological impairments and models of the normal system must take into account not only the subtraction of one of more components of that system, but also changes
in the functioning of other components that had previously been
influenced by the missing components.

Neural network models of cognition and the brain provide a
framework for reasoning about the effects of local lesions in distributed, interactive systems (Farah, 1994). Computer simulations
of such models allow us to test hypotheses concerning the normal
cognitive system using data from neurological patients, by simulating the candidate systems. The simulations of normal systems
can be "lesioned," for example by removing their neuron-like units,
or connections between units, and the behavior of the lesioned system can be compared with the behavior of patients.

In many cases a model's behavior after lesioning is somewhat
counterintuitive. Indeed, it is often very different from what one
would expect by reasoning in terms of simple deletion of parts from
a normal system, with minimal interactions among the parts. For
this reason, the use of neural networks when interpreting neuropsychological impairments can lead to very different interpretations
regarding the nature of the normal system.

Examples of Neural Network Models in Neuropsychology

The remainder of this article will back up these statements with
some specific examples of well-known neuropsychological impairments whose interpretations vis-à-vis the normal brain have
been changed dramatically by neural network modeling. In each
example the neural networks are highly simplified models of real
brain tissue, in the tradition of parallel distributed processing (PDP;
Rumelhart and McClelland, 1986).

PDP systems consist of a large number of highly interconnected
neuron-like units. These units are connected to one another by
weighted connections that determine how much activation from
one unit flows to another. Each part of the network functions locally
and in parallel with the other parts; hence the first P in PDP. Representations consist of the pattern of activation distributed over a
population of units, and long-term memory knowledge is encoded
in the pattern of connection strengths distributed among a population of units; hence the D. There are many types of PDP networks
with different computational properties. Among the features that
determine network type are the activation rule, connectivity, and
the learning rule.

PDP models differ from real neural networks, including the human brain, in numerous ways. Even the biggest PDP networks are
tiny compared with the brain. PDP models have just one kind of
unit, compared with a variety of types of neurons, and just one kind
of activation (which can act excitatorily or inhibitorily) rather than
a multitude of different neurotransmitters, and so on. Of course, all
models are simplifications of reality and possess both theory-
relevant and theory-irrelevant features. Among the theory-relevant
features of PDP models are the use of distributed representations,
the large number of inputs to and outputs from each unit, the modifiable connections between units, the existence of both inhibitory
and excitatory connections, summation rules, bounded activations,
and thresholds. PDP models allow us to find out what aspects of
behavior, normal and pathological, can be explained by this set of
theory-relevant attributes. The three examples that follow demonstrate the explanatory work that can be done in neuropsychology
with such models.

Interpreting Error Types: The Case of Deep Dyslexia

Neuropsychologists have long assumed that the nature of the damaged component could be inferred from the kind of errors made.
In a syndrome known as deep dyslexia, patients make two kinds
of errors. They make semantic errors, that is, errors that bear a
semantic similarity to the correct word, such as reading *cat* as *dog*.
They also make visual errors, that is, errors that bear a visual similarity to the correct word, such as reading *cat* as *cot*. The most
straightforward interpretation would seem to be that deep dyslexics
have at least two lesions, with one affecting the visual system and
another affecting semantic knowledge. However, a consideration
of the effects of single lesions in a neural network with attractor
states suggests that a single lesion is sufficient to account for these
patients' errors. Furthermore, it suggests that mixtures of error
types will be the rule rather than the exception when the system
that has been damaged normally functions to tranform the stimulus
representation from one form that has one set of similarity relations
(e.g., visual, in which *cot* and *cat* are similar) to another form with
different similarity relations (e.g., semantic, in which *cot* and *bed*
are similar).

Hinton and Shallice (1991) trained the recurrent network shown in Figure 1 to produce semantic representations of a set of words, given their printed orthography as input. The grapheme-to-"sememe" (their term for elements of semantic representation) mapping is carried out with the aid of hidden units, and the sememes are interconnected among themselves and connected to a final layer of semantic representation that connects, recurrently, back to the sememes. This pattern of connectivity in the semantic layers creates attractor states for the network. The input to the semantic layers need not be perfectly on target for the semantics of a particular word; as long as it is sufficiently similar to the correct semantics, which is an attractor state, it will be pulled in (i.e., as long as it falls in a region of activation space that slopes downward to the correct activation pattern, it will be transformed into that pattern). Damage to the network, from the removal of units or connections, distorts the shape of the activation space. Figure 2 illustrates the normal attractor structure of a region of activation space containing *cot*, *cat*, and *bed*, and the altered structure following damage to semantics. Whereas before damage, "cat" fell into the *cat* basin of attraction, after damage the edges of the basins have shifted and "cat" falls into the *cot* basin of attraction. Thus, one need not hypothesize damage to visual representations to account for the visual errors in deep dyslexia.

Plaut and Shallice (1993) have demonstrated the generality of Hinton and Shallice's account by replicating their simulation results with a variety of different networks, with different patterns of connectivity and different training procedures. As long as there are attractors that serve to transform input patterns whose similarity relations are based on visual appearance into semantic representations whose similarity relations are based on meaning, the landscape of the activation space will be organized by both visual and semantic similarity, and distortions of that landscape due to network damage will result in both visual and semantic errors.

Determining a Processing Sequence: The Example of Neglect Dyslexia

Patients with left visual neglect omit or misidentify letters on the left side of letter strings. When the letter string is a word, this pattern of performance is termed neglect dyslexia. Surprisingly, neglect dyslexics are more likely to report the initial letters of a word than of a nonword letter string, even when the initial letters of the word cannot simply be guessed on the basis of the end of the word. This seems to have a fairly specific, though surprising, implication for the order in which word recognition and spatial attention occur in the brain. If lexical status (word versus nonword) affects the allocation of attention, then it would seem that word recognition occurs before attention is allocated.

The concept of attractors is helpful here too, in understanding how an impairment in a prelexical attentional process could nevertheless show a lexicality effect. Mozer and Behrmann (1990) simulated neglect dyslexia by damaging the attentional mechanism in a computational model of printed word recognition so that attention was distributed asymmetrically over letter strings. In their model, attention *preceded* word recognition. In fact, it gated the flow of information out of early visual feature maps. Neglect therefore resulted in full information from the right side of a letter string, but only partial information from the left, being transmitted to word representations.

According to this model, the errors that occur with nonword letter strings result from partial visual information about the letter features on the left side of the string, which is not sufficient to identify precisely which letters are present. In contrast, the same partial information about the initial letters of a word, with good-quality information about the remaining letters of a word, will result in an activation pattern that is similar to the activation pattern for that word. Because known words are attractors, the network will settle into the pattern of the word, complete with initial letters. In this way, it is possible to explain why neglect dyslexics read words better than nonwords, without giving up the hypothesis that neglect is a disorder of visual perception that affects stimulus processing prior to the recognition stage.

It is worth noting that computational models make predictions that can be tested empirically. According to this model of neglect dyslexia, if the asymmetry of attention is too extreme, no information about the initial letters will get through to word representations, and the resulting activation state will not fall within the basin of attraction for the word. Behrmann et al. (1990) tested this prediction with a patient who had severe neglect. As predicted, he did not show better perception of the initial letters of words than nonwords. Furthermore, when his attention was drawn to the left, and the attentional asymmetry thereby made less extreme, he

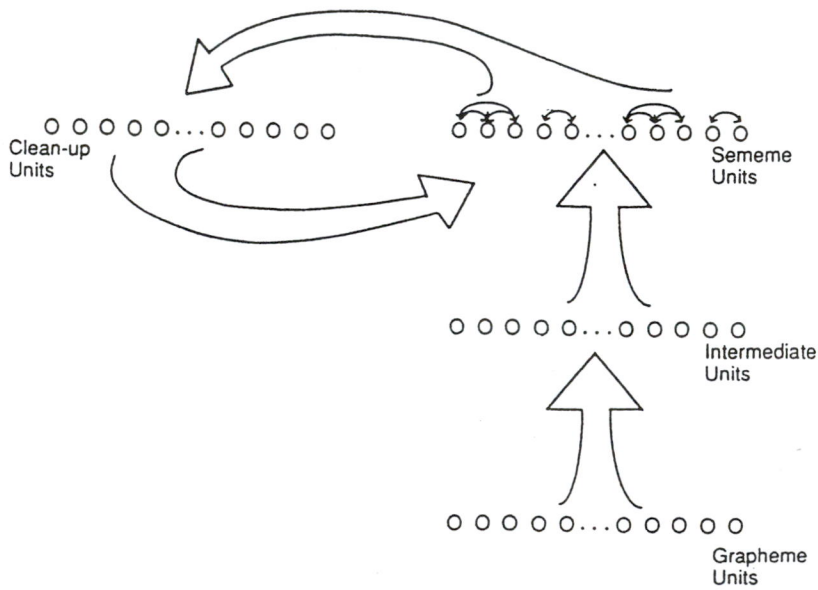

Figure 1. Hinton and Shallice's (1991) PDP model of reading, in which visual graphemic representations are associated with semantic representations. Single lesions in this model produce a mixture of visual and semantic errors.

Figure 2. Part of the activation space of the Hinton and Shallice model as represented by Plaut and Shallice (1993), showing attractors for three words. After damage to semantic units, the basins of attraction shift from those shown in solid lines to those shown in dotted lines, resulting in visual errors.

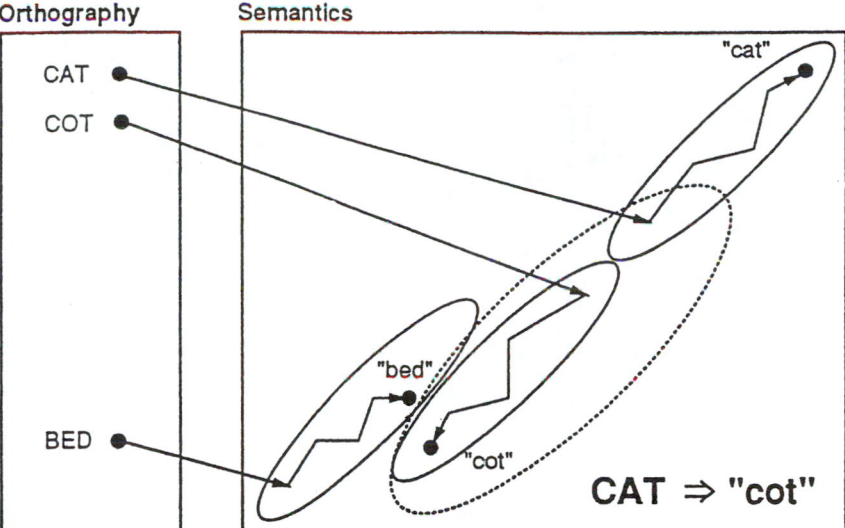

showed the usual difference between word and nonword letter strings. Conversely, a patient who normally showed this difference between words and nonwords was stopped from doing so by attentional manipulations that increased his attentional asymmetry.

Dissociation Without Separate Systems: The Example of Covert Face Recognition

Prosopagnosia is an impairment of face recognition that can occur relatively independently of impairments in object recognition. The behavior of some prosopagnosic patients (described below) seems to suggest that recognition and awareness depend on dissociable and distinct brain systems (Figure 3). My colleagues and I built a computer simulation that is able to account for covert recognition in a number of different tasks (Farah, O'Reilly, and Vecera, 1993; O'Reilly and Farah, 1999). The network is shown in Figure 4 and consists of face recognition units, semantic knowledge units, and name units (embodying knowledge of people's facial appearance, general information about them, and their names, respectively). Hidden units were interposed between these layers to assist the network in learning to associate faces and names by way of semantic information. No part of the network is dedicated to awareness.

The first finding to be simulated was that some prosopagnosics can learn to associate facial photographs with names faster when the pairings are true (e.g., Harrison Ford's face with Harrison Ford's name) than when they are false (e.g., Harrison Ford's face with Michael Douglas's name; De Haan, Young, and Newcombe, 1987). This result was initially taken to imply that these patients were recognizing the faces normally, and that the breakdown in processing lay downstream from vision, as shown in Figure 3. However, when some of the face units were eliminated from our model, thus simulating a lesion in the visual system, the network also relearned old face-name pairings faster than new ones. Why should this be? We can think of learning as a process of moving through weight space. After damage, the network is in a high-error region of weight space for both old face-name pairings and new ones, and therefore the network cannot overtly associate any faces with any names. However, that region of weight space is closer to a low-error region for the old pairings than for the new ones, because the residual weights (connecting intact units) have the correct values for the old pairings, and the learning process is therefore shorter.

A second finding, that previously familiar faces are perceived more quickly in the context of a same/different matching task, has also been interpreted as evidence for intact visual face processing (De Haan et al., 1987). However, after lesions to the face units in our model, the remaining face units settled into a stable state faster for previously familiar face patterns. This can be understood in terms of the distortion of the network's attractor structure after damage. The original structure was designed to take familiar face patterns as input and settle quickly to a stable state. After damage,

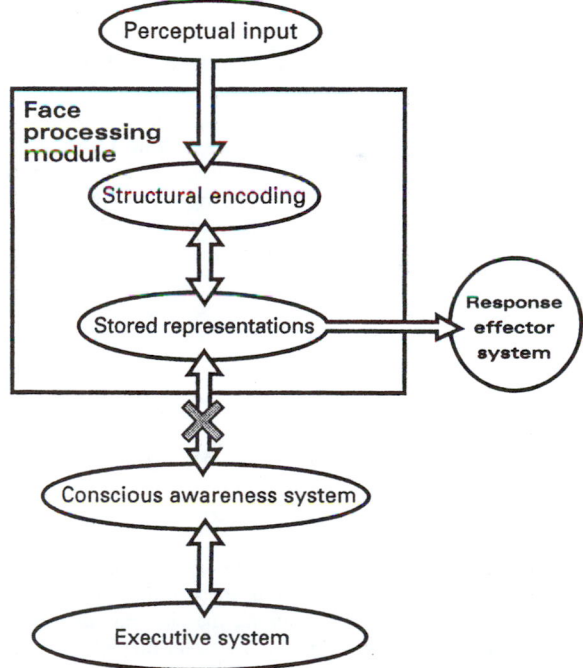

Figure 3. A model proposed by De Haan, Bauer, and Greve (1992) to account for covert face recognition in prosopagnosia. A separate mechanism for conscious awareness is hypothesized, distinct from the mechanisms of face recognition, and covert recognition is explained by a lesion at location ×, disconnecting the two parts of the model.

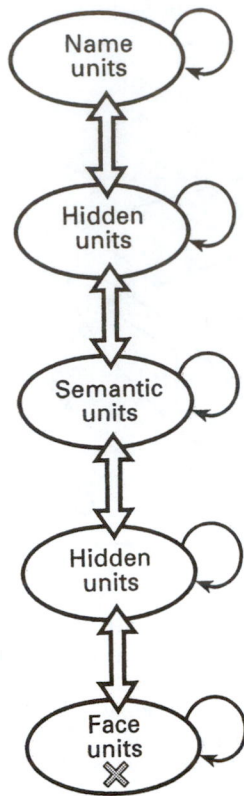

Figure 4. A model proposed by Farah, O'Reilly, and Vecera (1993) to account for covert face recognition in prosopagnosia. The dissociation between overt and covert face recognition emerges when the face recognition system is damaged.

these patterns will still find themselves on downward-sloping parts of the energy landscape more often than novel patterns, even if the energy minima into which they roll have changed.

In yet another task, one that requires classifying a printed name as belonging to an actor or a politician, both normal subjects and prosopagnosics are influenced by a face from the opposite occupation category shown in the background, again implying that the face is recognized despite prosopagnosia (De Haan et al., 1987).

To simulate this finding, we removed face units until the network's overt performance at classifying faces according to occupation was as poor as the patient's. At this level of damage, wrong-category faces slowed performance in the name classification task. This can be understood in terms of the distributed nature of representation in neural networks, which allows for partial representation of information when some but not all units representing a face have been eliminated. The partial information generally raises the activation of the appropriate downstream occupation units, thus biasing their responses to the printed names, but is not generally able to raise their activations above threshold to allow an explicit response to faces.

Road Map: Cognitive Neuroscience
Related Reading: Cognitive Development; Developmental Disorders; Face Recognition: Psychology and Connectionism; Reading

References

Behrmann, M., Moscovitch, M., Black, S., and Mozer, M., 1990, Perceptual and conceptual mechanisms in neglect dyslexia: Two contrasting case studies, *Brain*, 113:1163–1183.

De Haan, E. H. F., Bauer, R. M., and Greve, K. W., 1992, Behavioral and physiological evidence for covert recognition in a prosopagnosic patient, *Cortex*, 28:77–95. ◆

De Haan, E. H. F., Young, A. W., and Newcombe, F., 1987, Face recognition without awareness, *Cogn. Neuropsychol.*, 4:385–415.

Farah, M. J., 1994, Neuropsychological inference with an interactive brain: A critique of the locality assumption, *Behav. Brain Sci.*, 17:43–61.

Farah, M. J., O'Reilly, R. C., and Vecera, S. P., 1993, Dissociated overt and covert recognition as on emergent property of lesioned attractor networks, *Pychol. Rev.*, 100:571–588. ◆

Hinton, G. E., and Shallice, T., 1991, Lesioning an attractor network: Investigations of acquired dyslexia, *Psychol. Rev.*, 98:96–121.

Mozer, M. C., and Behrmann, M., 1990, On the interaction of selective attention and lexical knowledge: A connectionist account of neglect dyslexia, *J. Cogn. Neurosci.*, 2:96–123.

O'Reilly, R. C., and Farah, M. J., 1999, Simulation and explanation in neuropsychology and beyond, *Cogn. Neuropsychol.*, 16:49–72.

Plaut, D. C., and Shallice, T., 1993, Deep dyslexia: A case study of connectionist neuropsychology, *Cogn. Neuropsychol.*, 10:377–500.

Rumelhart, D. E., and McClelland, J. L., 1986, *Parallel Distributed Processing: Explorations in the Microstructure of Cognition*, Cambridge, MA: MIT Press.

Sieroff, E., Pollatsek, A., and Posner, M. I., 1988, Recognition of visual letter strings following injury to the posterior visual spatial attention system, *Cogn. Neuropsychol.*, 5:427–449. ◆

Squire, L. R., 1987, *Memory and Brain*, New York: Oxford University Press.

Neurosimulation: Tools and Resources

Randall D. Hayes, John H. Byrne, and Douglas A. Baxter

Introduction

In all scientific fields, including neuroscience, experimental hypotheses are based on models. Often, these models only qualitatively describe the relationships among the elements of a system, such as the molecules that make up a second-messenger cascade or the neurons that make up a network. Mathematical models provide a more rigorous framework within which investigators can organize large amounts of empirical data, test whether current data can account for the behavior of the system, identify critical features that warrant additional experimental investigation, and discover dynamic properties that are not intuitively obvious.

This article reviews neurosimulators, that is, programs designed to reduce the time and effort required to build models of neurons and neural networks. We include programs for modeling networks of spiking neurons as well as programs for kinetic modeling of intracellular signaling cascades and regulatory genetic networks. A comprehensive description of all neurosimulators is beyond the scope of this chapter (see also GENESIS SIMULATION SYSTEM, NEURON SIMULATION ENVIRONMENT, and NSL NEURAL SIMULATION LANGUAGE). Instead, we provide a general picture of the capabilities of several neurosimulators, highlighting some of the best features of the various programs, and refer the reader to more specific information (Bower and Bolouri, 2002; Skrzypek, 1994; Koch and Segev, 1998; De Schutter, 2001). We do not list connectionist simulators in this chapter (see Murre, 1995).

This article also describes ongoing efforts to increase compatibility among the various programs, which serve two purposes. First, compatibility allows models built with one neurosimulator to be independently evaluated and extended by investigators using different programs, thereby reducing duplication of effort. Second, compatibility allows for models describing different levels of complexity (i.e., molecular, cellular, network) to be related to one another.

General Considerations

General considerations in selecting a simulator program include the hardware capabilities and programming expertise of the lab. Complicated models require fast workstations or networks of desktop computers running portions of the model in parallel (Hammarlund and Ekeberg, 1998). For investigators with limited resources, it may be necessary to simplify a model so that a less powerful computer can run a simulation in a reasonable amount of time. Building a model takes more time than simulating one, so using a simple program to build a simple model can speed up the process even further.

Hardware Issues

Platform requirements for various neurosimulators are listed in Tables 1 to 3. We include a few programs that can run on older, less expensive computers (e.g., *Nodus, MetaModel*). Programs written in Java or Perl (e.g., *CATACOMB, NSL, SNNAP, StochSim*) can run on multiple platforms without modification. Another solution to the problem of computer compatibility is to separate the simulator code, which is less platform sensitive, from the user interface code (e.g., *NEST/SYNOD, CONICAL*). For some simulators, the user can log onto a centralized network server through a web browser (e.g., *iCell, CMISS, Vcell*).

Level of Tech Support

An important issue is how much support the developers provide to the first-time user (see Tables 1 to 3). Most programs distribute manuals, which vary greatly in how complete and up-to-date they are. Buyers of commercial packages may receive personal instruction (e.g., *In Silico Cell, ModelMaker, SABER*). Another option is to attend short courses at workshops or national meetings (e.g., *GENESIS, Mcell, NEURON, SNNAP*). Many developers maintain e-mail lists or bulletin boards, where users can ask questions. Es-

pecially useful to the beginner are templates of possible conductances, cells, or circuits. These allow the user to start modeling immediately by modifying an existing file rather than beginning from scratch.

Numerical Methods

Discrete events.   Connectionist simulators generally use continuous scalar variables to represent firing rate and synaptic weight (see SINGLE-CELL MODELS). The integrate-and-fire units used by discrete event neurosimulators (e.g., *NeuroImitator, SpikeNET*) are more realistic. They have a membrane potential that sums the cell's inputs over time; a spiking threshold, which determines when the cell will fire; and often a refractory hyperpolarization after the spike. When threshold potential is exceeded, a time-stamped spike event (not an action potential waveform) is generated, and the membrane potential is reset. After some fixed delay representing axonal conduction, the spike event triggers synaptic conductances in postsynaptic target cells. Note that most of the programs that calculate a waveform for each action potential by one of the methods described below also default to fixed axonal delays, rather than propagating the action potential (see AXONAL MODELING), to save computing time.

By adjusting the free parameters that control threshold and refractory period, the user can reproduce the firing rates and spike frequency adaptation of a wide range of biological neurons. Because individual conductances contributing to the membrane potential are ignored, discrete event simulators are suitable for studying network behaviors but not the intracellular mechanisms that produce them (see INTEGRATE-AND-FIRE NEURONS AND NETWORKS).

Ordinary differential equations (ODE).   Most simulators represent individual neurons as systems of ODEs, which represent the average change in a dependent variable (usually membrane voltage or concentration) in a well-mixed spatial compartment over one time step of the simulation (Cobelli and Foster, 1998). The dependent variable is recalculated at regular intervals, with the intervals chosen to capture the fastest dynamics of the model (often tens of microseconds). In addition, some simulators (e.g., *BIOQ, NEURON, Surf-Hippo, XNBC*) provide variable time-step algorithms, which recalculate the dependent variable more often when it is changing rapidly and less often when it is changing slowly. These algorithms can shorten the computer time required to simulate large networks.

Monte Carlo methods.   Other simulators explicitly follow each molecule in the simulation over time (e.g., *BIOQ, CKS, MCELL, StochSim*). At each time step, random numbers are chosen for the

Table 1. Programs Suitable for Demonstration and Teaching

Name	Topics	Control	Platform	Support	Web Site
ArtMem/MemPot/MemCable $	P I A C	G	W, DOS	M	http://www.med.unsw.edu.au/PHBSoft/
cLabs $	P I A C	G W	W		http://www.clabs.de/clabs.htm
Computational Neuroscience $	P I A C N	G	M, W	T M	http://www.compneuro.org/
iCell	A C	W	M, W		http://ssd1.bme.memphis.edu/icell/
NerveWorks	P I A C N	S G	M, U, W	T M	http://nerve-works.com/
NeuroDynamix $	P I A C N	G		T M	http://www.people.virginia.edu/~wof/pub
NeuroSim $	P I A C N	G	W	T M	http://biology.st-and.ac.uk/sites/neurosim/
Vclamp/Cclamp	A C	C	W, DOS	T M	http://tonto.stanford.edu/~john/
Electrophysiology o/t Neuron $	P I A C N	G	M, W	T M	http://tonto.stanford.edu/eotn/

$ indicates that software must be purchased. Abbreviations under Topics: P = Passive membrane, I = Ion channel, A = Action potential, C = Cell, N = Network of multiple neurons. Abbreviations under Control: C = Command line, S = Scripts, G = Graphical user interface, W = Web browser. Abbreviations under Platform: M = MacOS, U = Unix, W = Windows. Abbreviations under Support: T = Templates, C = Courses, M = Manual, L = List.

Table 2. Packages Specialized for Neurobiological Modeling

Name	Spiking Neurons	Chemical Kinetics	Control	Platform	Support	Web Site
BioPSE	ODE		G W	U	T M L	http://www.sci.utah.edu/ncrr/software/biopse.html
BIOSIM	ODE		G	U, W	T M	ftp://ftp.uni-kl.de/pub/bio/neurobio/
CATACOMB	ODE	ODE	G	M, U, W	T	http://www.compneuro.org/catacomb/index.shtml
CONICAL	ODE		C S	M, U, DOS		http://www.strout.net/conical/
GENESIS	ODE	ODE	C S G	U	T C M L	http://www.genesis-sim.org/GENESIS/
Maxsim	ODE		C S G	U	M	http://ibcmsg6.unil.ch/staff/tettoni/maxsim/
Mcell	MC	MC	C S	U	T C M L	http://www.mcell.cnl.salk.edu/
NeMoSys	ODE	ODE	S G	U	T M	http://cns.montana.edu/research/nemosys
NEST/SYNOD	ODE InF		C S	U	T M	http://www.synod.uni-freiburg.de/
Neurolmitator $	InF		G	W	T M	http://www.cellmc.com/ni/ni.html
NEURON	ODE InF	ODE	C S G	M, U, W	T C M L	http://www.neuron.yale.edu/
NeuronC	ODE InF	ODE	G	U, DOS		http://retina.anatomy.upenn.edu/~rob/neuronc.html
Nodus	ODE		G	M	M	http://bbf-www.uia.ac.be/SOFT/downloads.shtml
NSL	ODE InF		S G	U, W	T M	http://www-hbp.usc.edu/Projects/nsl.htm
Neurosys	ODE		C S G	M, U, W	T	http://nexus.cs.usfca.edu/neurosys/
SEE	ODE	ODE	S G	U, Cray		http://debian.nada.kth.se/sans.php?cont=tools
SNNAP	ODE InF	ODE	S G	M, U, W	T C M	http://snnap.uth.tmc.edu/
SONN	ODE InF	ODE	G	U, W	M	http://www.ls.huji.ac.il/~litvak/Sonn/sonn.html
SpikeNET	InF		S	U	M	http://www.cnl.salk.edu/~arno/SpikeNET
Surf-Hippo	ODE InF	ODE	C S G	U	T M L	http://www.cnrs-gif.fr/iaf/iaf9/surf-hippo.html
XNBC	ODE InF	ODE	G	U, W	M	http://www.u444.jussieu.fr/xnbc/
BIOQ		ODE MC	G	U, W	M	http://www.ls.huji.ac.il/~litvak/Bioq/bioq.html
CKS		MC	G	M, W, OS/2	T M	http://www.almaden.ibm.com/st/msim/index.html
DBSolve		ODE	C G W	U, W	T	http://websites.ntl.com/~igor.goryanin/
Gepasi		ODE	G	W	T C M	http://www.gepasi.org/
In Silico Cell $		ODE	G	W	M	http://www.physiome.com/
Jarnac/Indigo		ODE	C S G	W	T M L	http://www.sys-bio.org
KinSim/FitSim		ODE	S G	M, U, W	M	http://www.biochem.wustl.edu/cflab/message.html
MacKinetics		ODE	S	M, W	M	http://members.dca.net/leipold/mk/advert.html
MetaModel		ODE	C	DOS		http://bip.cnrs-mrs.fr/bip 10/modeling.htm
StochSim		MC	G	U, W	M	http://www.zoo.cam.ac.uk/comp-cell/StochSim.html
Vcell	ODE	ODE	G W	M, U, W	M L	http://www.nrcam.uchc.edu/index.html

Packages that simulate the electrical activity of cells are in the top half of the table. Packages that simulate chemical reactions are in the bottom half of the table. Methods abbreviated under Spiking Neurons and Chemical Kinetics: ODE = Ordinary differential equations, MC = Monte Carlo, InF = Integrate-and-fire. Abbreviations under Control, Platform, and Support are identical to those in Table 1.

direction and distance each individual molecule diffuses (Stiles and Bartol, 2001). If two or more molecules happen to collide, another random number is compared to a rate constant to determine whether a chemical reaction occurs. These methods are more accurate than ODEs when well-mixed assumptions are violated, such as when a simulation involves small numbers of molecules per spatial compartment. Monte Carlo methods can also be faster than ODEs when complicated three-dimensional structure requires a large number of compartments to meet the well-mixed assumptions of ODEs. The major disadvantage of Monte Carlo methods is the amount of memory required to track every element of a simulation.

Progression of Complexity

In our experience, users generally prefer to start out using a program through a graphical user interface (GUI), in which the number of choices is restricted and approachable. As they become more proficient, users often dispense with the GUI and begin to interact with the program at the more flexible command-line level or through scripts (lists of commands saved in text files). This allows them to automate common tasks that would otherwise have to be performed step by step. In keeping with this progression, we divide the simulators into three levels of complexity: demonstration pro-

Table 3. General Modeling Tools for Detailed Analysis

Name	Control	Platform	Support	Web Site
CMISS	C S G W	U	T M	http://www.cmiss.org
CONTENT $	G	U, W	M	http://www.cwi.nl/ftp/CONTENT/
JSIM/XSIM	G	U, W	T C M	http://nsr.bioeng.washington.edu/index.html
Madonna $	S G	M, W	M	http://www.berkeleymadonna.com/
MatLab $	C S	M, U, W	C M	http://www.mathworks.com/products/
ModelMaker $	G	W	T C M	http://www.modelkinetix.com/
SAAM $	G	W	T M	http://www.saam.com/software/saam2
SABER $	G	U, W	C M	http://www.analogy.com/products/simulation/
ScoP $	C S G	U, W, DOS	T C M	http://www.simresinc.com/
SPICE	C S G	U	M	http://bwrc.eecs.berkeley.edu/Classes/IcBook/SPICE/
XPP-AUT	C S G	U, W	M L	http://www.math.pitt.edu/~bard/xpp/xpp.html

Abbreviations under Control, Platform, and Support are identical to those in Table 1.

grams, modeling packages specialized for neurobiology, and generalized modeling tools. Each level has its advantages, as described in more detail below.

Demonstration Programs

Demonstration programs are particularly appropriate for students, for researchers who are approaching modeling for the first time, and for quick explorations of experimental hypotheses. They are limited to a few general examples (see Table 1), although those examples can be rich, with parameters for temperature and other common experimental variables (Friesen and Friesen, 1994; Huguenard and McCormick, 1994). Several demonstration programs use virtual experimental rigs, including electronic components such as amplifiers and analog-to-digital converters, perfusion pumps for drugs, and oscilloscopes; this allows users to become comfortable with using the equipment before proceeding to simulated or real experiments (e.g., *cLabs, NerveWorks*). Some programs allow the preset simulations to be modified (e.g., *NeuroSim, VClamp/CClamp*). For example, *NeuroSim* allows the teacher to simplify simulations by hiding irrelevant parameters; this feature can also hide the values of parameters so that students have to deduce them experimentally. A drawback for experimenters is that these demonstration programs generally do not include automated tools to analyze their output or to save their output so that third-party software could analyze it (but see GENESIS SIMULATION SYSTEM and NEURON SIMULATION ENVIRONMENT).

Packages Specialized for Simulating Spiking Neurons

A number of specialized packages are available to simulate the electrical activity of neurons and neural circuits. These packages are more flexible than the demonstration programs discussed above. The trade-off for this richness is an increase in complexity of the software used to build models. For example, *SNNAP* uses a hierarchical parameter tree composed of 26 parameter file types, including conductances (voltage-gated or ligand-gated), modulators, and intracellular pools of ions (Ziv, Baxter, and Byrne, 1994). Each parameter file consists of a single equation, chosen from a list of possibilities. Simulations are controlled through the GUI, although the text of the parameter files can be accessed through an ASCII text editor, a faster and more flexible option for experienced users.

Individual cells.   Packages vary in the detail with which individual neurons are modeled. The simplest ODE package (*SONN*) models each cell as a single-compartment isopotential sphere, using a fixed set of four differential equations, sufficient to describe the minimal soma capable of bursting behavior. Most other neurosimulators divide a cell into many compartments, each with its own parameters. For example, a dendritic compartment might be electrically passive, whereas an axonal compartment would contain the Na^+ and K^+ conductances necessary to support spiking. Certain packages can automate creation of multicompartmental three-dimensional structures to some extent by importing anatomical files, either with built-in tools (e.g., *Maxsim, NeMoSys, Surf-Hippo*) or through the use of third-party applications (e.g., *GENESIS, NEURON*).

Packages vary in their analytical capabilities, as well. Most packages can run batches of simulations to systematically vary parameters, saving the results in files to be examined by other tools. Some can also optimize model parameters to fit experimental data (e.g., *GENESIS, NEURON, NeuronC, Surf-Hippo*). *Surf-Hippo* runs scripts that detect spikes or other events in the output of a cell. *XNBC* has menu-based tools for time series analysis.

Small circuits.   Most packages, whether based on discrete events, ODEs, or Monte Carlo, come with built-in synaptic conductances

that can be used to connect neurons into a circuit. The most common "alpha function" synapse has a maximal conductance, a reversal potential, and an exponential time course (see SYNAPTIC INTERACTIONS). In many packages, synaptic conductances can be modulated by intracellular second messengers to produce various profiles of synaptic plasticity (see the "Chemical Kinetics" column in Table 2). Built-in electrical synapses that simulate gap junctions are relatively uncommon (however, see *NeuronC, SNNAP*). *NeuronC* is unusual in that it models the synapse as a series of filters that determine how presynaptic voltage affects postsynaptic voltage to study information transfer across the synapse. In addition to graphs of membrane voltage over time in individual neurons, several packages allow the user to visualize the entire network as a grid of icons in order to examine spatial patterns of activity, such as waves that sweep through the network (e.g., *BioSim, NeuroImitator, XNBC*).

Large networks.   Some packages allow for abstraction beyond integrate-and-fire neurons to reduce the number of network elements. For example, a group of neurons whose interactions form an oscillator or a filter function can be represented as a single unit (e.g., *NSL, SpikeNET*). In some packages (e.g., *SEE, SpikeNET, XNBC*), the user can define populations of identical neurons that project topographically to other populations, which reduces effort in wiring up large networks.

Detailed compartmental modeling of many thousands of neurons requires a package optimized for that purpose, usually running on parallel processors, because of the large number of calculations involved (e.g., *GENESIS, NEST/SYNOD, NEURON, Parallel Neurosys, SEE*). A program for simulation at even larger scales is *BioPSE*, which models electrical field potentials in biological tissue.

Specialized Biochemical Packages

Many of the packages described above can simulate intracellular processes such as diffusion of ions and second-messenger cascades (see the top half of Table 2). Other packages, designed to study metabolic or genetic networks (see the bottom half of Table 2), have additional analytical capabilities that may benefit neural researchers. For example, some (e.g., *Gepasi, Jarnac/Indigo*) are capable of metabolic control analysis. This sensitivity analysis measures the relative control exerted by each enzyme on the system's fluxes and metabolite concentrations (Wildermuth, 2000). A convenient feature of *BIOQ* allows the user to check closed-form reactions, such as the opening and closing of an ion channel, for violations of the law of conservation of energy.

Most of these biochemical modeling packages can compile a kinetic description of a reaction into differential equations. Some packages incorporate a GUI that allows the user to build a "biochemical network" using icons of molecules and reaction schemes. The equations are then generated by the program and presented for the user's inspection.

General Modeling Tools

The powerful programs described in this section can potentially be used to simulate any dynamical system (Table 3). However, they are less likely to have built-in model templates relevant to a particular neurobiological system. For example, *SABER* and *SPICE* are electrical circuit simulators that have been used to simulate biological neurons (Bove et al., 1994). *MatLab* is commonly used by connectionist modelers but has no official support for compartmental neuron simulations. With the advent of model databases, this may be less of a restriction on the usefulness of general modeling tools, because individual users of a particular package may have models to share (see DATABASES FOR NEUROSCIENCE).

One advantage of these general tools is their analytical power. For instance, *MatLab* has many functions for analyzing time series data such as spike trains. *XXP-AUT* and *CONTENT* are specialized for analyzing dynamical phenomena, such as nullclines, singularity points, bifurcations, and steady states (Ermentrout, 2002; see PHASE-PLANE ANALYSIS OF NEURAL NETS). Currently, perhaps the best compromise is to analyze models built in more specialized packages with these general tools. Ready examples of this type of synergy between programs are *GENESIS* and the biochemical simulator *Jarnac/Indigo*, which can export their output in *MatLab* format.

Increasing Cooperation among Modelers

Some of the most exciting developments in neurosimulation technology will allow modelers to compare and modify models, verify one another's simulations, and extend models with their own tools. We examine two of these enabling technologies below (see also DATABASES FOR NEUROSCIENCE).

Brokering Agents

One way to coordinate the actions of multiple simulation packages is through software called a brokering agent. For example, a model can be built by using a biophysically detailed neuron model from one simulator, an integrate-and-fire network from a different simulator, and a number of individualized Java or C++ components for visualization or analysis. Each component runs independently, receiving input from the broker and sending back its output.

A brokering agent can also support the distribution of a single model onto multiple processors without the need to modify the model description. This last point is crucial, as some parallel simulation tools (such as *GENESIS*) require the model itself to be a parallel program, which is not a trivial modification. This "transparent parallelism" is possible if the model is specified as a number of entities that communicate using discrete events, a strategy that is employed to some extent by many neurosimulators.

Three brokering agents are currently under development for use in neural simulation. *Bio/Spice* (http://www.darpa.mil/ipto/research/biocomp/index.html) and the *Systems Biology Workbench* (http://www.cds.caltech.edu/erato/the_project.html) interface between biochemical simulators. *NEOSIM* (http://www.neosim.org/) is designed to work at the level of neuronal networks. An existing example of the possibilities for a brokering agent, *ISYS*, provides interfaces between genomic databases (Siepel et al., 2001).

Open-Source Development

Another approach to collaborative modeling is taken by five cooperating laboratories in producing *NEST/SYNOD* (Diesmann and Gewaltig, in press). In an open-source project, registered users can modify the software. A centralized server automatically updates the software and distributes the latest version to users. The large number of reviewers ensures that bugs will be found and repaired quickly. This is unlike most neurosimulators, for which a single laboratory controls the development of the software, albeit with suggestions from users, and individual users are responsible for their own updates. It remains to be seen whether the open-source approach will spread to other neurosimulator packages.

Discussion

Understanding the brain requires an enormous amount of data about its individual components and their interactions. Because of the sheer volume of data and the nonlinear nature of the interactions, it becomes impossible to understand the system without computational modeling.

No single monolithic simulation package can fulfill all of the diverse requirements of individual neuroscientists doing quantitative simulations. At the same time, developers are challenged to encourage collaboration by increasing interoperability among the many neurosimulators and by building tools to manage the ever-increasing number of models and simulations. As these challenges are met, models that span levels of neural organization, ranging from genetic regulatory networks to large-scale brain structures, will become possible.

Road Map: Implementation and Analysis
Related Reading: Databases for Neuroscience; Neuroinformatics; Perspective on Neuron Model Complexity

References

Bove, M., Massobrio, G., Martinoia, S., and Grattarola, M., 1994, Realistic simulations of neurons by means of an ad hoc modified version of SPICE, *Biol. Cybern.*, 71(2):137–145. ◆

Bower, J. M., and Bolouri, H., 2002, *Computational Modeling of Genetic and Biochemical Networks*, Cambridge, MA: MIT Press.

Cobelli, C., and Foster, D. M., 1998, Compartmental models: Theory and practice using the SAAM II software system, *Adv. Exp. Med. Biol.*, 445:79–101.

De Schutter, E. (Ed.), 2001, *Computational Neuroscience: Realistic Modeling for Experimentalists*, Boca Raton, FL: CRC Press. ◆

Diesmann, M., and Gewaltig, M.-O., in press, NEST: An environment for neural systems simulations, in *Forschung und wissenschaftliches Rechnen* (V. Macho, Ed.), Gottingen, Germany: Gesselschaft für Wissenschaftliche, Datenverarbeitung.

Ermentrout, B., 2002, *Simulating, Analyzing and Animating Dynamical Systems: a Guide to XPPAUT for Researchers and Students*, Philadelphia, PA: Society for Industrial and Applied Mathematics.

Friesen, W. O., and Friesen, J. A., 1994, *NeuroDynamix: Computer Models for Neurophysiology*, New York: Oxford University Press.

Hammarlund, P., and Ekeberg, O., 1998, Large neural network simulations on multiple hardware platforms, *J. Comput. Neurosci.*, 5(4):443–459. ◆

Huguenard, J., and McCormick, D., 1994, *Electrophysiology of the Neuron: An Interactive Tutorial*, Oxford, Engl: Oxford University Press.

Koch, C., and Segev, I. (Eds.), 1998, *Methods in Neuronal Modeling: From Ions to Networks*, Cambridge, MA: MIT Press.

Murre, J. M. J., 1995, Neurosimulators, in *Handbook of Brain Theory and Neural Networks* (M. A. Arbib, Ed.), Cambridge, MA: MIT Press, pp. 634–639.

Siepel, A., Farmer, A., Tolopko, A., Zhuang, M., Mendes, P., Beavis, W., and Sobral, B., 2001, ISYS: A decentralized, component-based approach to the integration of heterogeneous bioinformatics resources, *Bioinformatics*, 17(1):83–94.

Skrzypek, J. (Ed.), 1994, *Neural Network Simulation Environments*, Dordrecht, The Netherlands: Kluwer Academic Publishers.

Stiles, J. R., and Bartol, T. M., 2001, Monte Carlo methods for simulating realistic synaptic microphysiology using Mcell, in *Computational Neuroscience: Realistic Modeling for Experimentalists* (E. De Schutter, Ed.), Boca Raton, FL: CRC Press, pp. 87–127.

Wildermuth, M. C., 2000, Metabolic control analysis: Biological applications and insights, *Genome Biol.*, 1(6):REVIEWS1031. ◆

Ziv, I., Baxter, D. A., and Byrne, J. H., 1994, Simulator for neural networks and action potentials: Description and application, *J. Neurophysiol.*, 71(1):294–308.

NMDA Receptors: Synaptic, Cellular, and Network Models

Michel Baudry, Jean-Marie Bouteiller, Jim-Shih Liaw, and Theodore W. Berger

Introduction

NMDA receptors are subtypes of receptors for the excitatory neurotransmitter, glutamate, that are selectively activated by the agonist *N*-methyl-D-aspartate (NMDA), a glutamate analog. They are involved in diverse physiological as well as pathological processes such as visual perception, motor pattern generation, learning and memory, and epilepsy- or stroke-induced neuronal damage (Dingledine et al., 1999).

NMDA receptors have three unique properties that distinguish them from other ligand-gated channels (channels activated by molecules that bind to them). First, they mediate a relatively "slow" excitatory postsynaptic potential (EPSP). Second, their activation requires not only the binding of an agonist (a molecule that mimics the effect of the endogenous neurotransmitter), but also the depolarization of the postsynaptic membrane to remove the voltage-dependent blockade of the channel by Mg^{2+} ions. Thus, NMDA receptors act as coincidence-detectors of presynaptic and postsynaptic activity. Third, NMDA receptors are 10 times more permeable to Ca^{2+} ions than to Na^+ or K^+. They often are colocalized with other receptor channels that conduct "fast" EPSPs (e.g., the α-amino-3-hydroxy-5-methyl-4-isoxazole proprionic acid, or AMPA, receptor). The interactions between the slow NMDA-mediated and fast AMPA-mediated currents provide the basis for a range of interesting dynamic properties, which contribute to a diversity of neuronal processes.

NMDA receptors have attracted a lot of interest in neuroscience because of their role in learning and memory. Their properties of coincidence detectors make them an ideal molecular device for producing Hebbian synapses, that is, synapses whose strength is modified depending on the correlation of presynaptic and postsynaptic activity. Furthermore, the influx of Ca^{2+} ions through the NMDA receptor channel triggers cascades of molecular processes that lead to various forms of synaptic plasticity, including short-term potentiation, long-term potentiation, and long-term depression (Malenka and Nicoll, 1999), as well as to pathological processes, including neuronal death. As a result, they have been a subject of intense investigation by both experimentalists interested in understanding the features of the protein that result in its functional properties and theorists/modelers attempting to incorporate NMDA receptors into models of synapses, neurons, or circuitries. We will briefly review here data related to the biological characteristics of NMDA receptors and to models that have been used to describe their function in isolated membrane patches, in neurons, and in complex circuits.

Biological Characteristics of NMDA Receptors

Cloning techniques have provided evidence for the existence of a multiplicity of NMDA receptor subunits conferring distinct properties for the NMDA receptors (see Cull-Candy, Brickley, and Farrant, 2001, for a review). The NR1 subunits is required in combination with at least one member of the NR2 family (four distinct genes), and NR1/NR2 complexes may also co-assemble with a member of the NR3 family (two genes). NMDA receptor activation requires not only the presence of glutamate, but also the presence of another amino acid, glycine, which therefore has been called a co-agonist and binds to NR1 subunits, while glutamate binds to NR2 subunits. A number of other binding sites for Mg^{++}, Zn^{++},

and polyamines are also present on the subunits, and their occupation modifies receptor properties. It is generally assumed that the NMDA receptors are multimeric entities (i.e., composed of several subunits), possibly pentameric proteins by analogy with the acetylcholine nicotinic receptor. Moreover, as different combinations of receptor subunits produce receptors with different physiological and pharmacological properties, it is likely that several functional classes of NMDA receptors exist in adult neurons, and a major challenge remains to determine their cellular distributions and the mechanisms regulating subunit expression and receptor assembly and turnover.

A major avenue of research over the last five years has focused on the mechanisms underlying NMDA receptor targeting and anchoring in postsynaptic sites. Thus a very large complex of proteins, including receptor molecules, PSD-95, cytoskeletal proteins, and associated protein kinases has been shown to be localized in postsynaptic densities and to play critical roles in mediating multiple effects of NMDA receptor activation (Kennedy, 1998).

Kinetic Models of NMDA Receptors

The behavior of a receptor can be described by the kinetic scheme of its transition between various discrete states representing the occupancy of the different binding sites and the functional states of the channel (a simple example is $A + R \leftrightarrow AR \leftrightarrow AR^*$, where A, R, AR, and AR^* represent agonist, receptor, and receptor-agonist complex in closed state and open state, respectively; additional desensitized states of the receptors correspond to receptor occupied by agonists but with closed channels). Several kinetic models of the NMDA receptors have been developed to study various aspects of the nature of the receptor and the dynamics of its behavior.

Glycine Binding

Glycine is a necessary co-agonist of the receptor, and various models of NMDA receptors have been developed to study the number of glycine binding sites and the interaction between glutamate and glycine on the receptors. Recordings in outside-out patches from cultured hippocampal neurons were used to measure the rate constants for agonist binding, open/close transitions, and desensitization of the NMDA receptor. The measured rate constants were used in models assuming one, two, or three agonist binding sites. For both glutamate and glycine binding, a two-site model provided a superior fit for the time course of NMDA channel activation. Desensitization was also studied in excised outside-out patches and was interpreted as an interaction between the glutamate and the glycine site such that glycine binding produced a decreased affinity of glutamate for its binding site (Lester, Tong, and Jahr, 1993). Note that binding experiments also suggest a strong positive allosteric effect between glutamate and glycine binding (Marvizon and Baudry, 1993).

Number of States of the NMDA Receptor

Jahr and Stevens (1990) developed a model of NMDA receptor-channel kinetics to address the issue of the number of states of the receptor. They assumed that the NMDA receptor exists in three states: closed (C), open (O), and blocked (B). The kinetic behavior of the NMDA receptor-channel was characterized by four experimentally measured quantities: open time (T_o), interruption time (T_i), number of interruptions (N), and burst length (T_b). The predictions made by the model failed to match several key experimental data, and these shortcomings suggested an extension to include a second blocked state in addition to the Mg^{2+} block. The four-state model could describe NMDA receptor behavior in all conditions except the low-amplitude, second-exponential component in T_o, which occurred in low Mg^{2+} concentrations and positive voltage. A theory based on the four-state model postulates that the interruptions could be the result of a voltage-dependent conformational change, which could be facilitated by the binding of Mg ions to some sites on the NMDA receptor.

NMDA Receptors in Models of Neurons

NMDA receptor models have been incorporated in several models of synapses/neurons developed to answer questions related to short-term as well as long-term synaptic plasticity and to mechanisms of synaptic integration. As was mentioned in the introduction, a major focus is on the role of the voltage-dependent Mg^{2+} blockade, which gives rise to the property of coincidence detection and Ca^{2+} influx through the NMDA receptor, in initiating the molecular events leading to changes in synaptic strength. Furthermore, the interplay between the slow NMDA-mediated and fast AMPA-mediated currents leads to important features in the timing of synaptic inputs required to induce long-term potentiation (LTP)

Short-Term Synaptic Plasticity

Pongrácz et al. (1992) used a compartmental model to study short-term changes in excitability of a hippocampal pyramidal neuron. The pyramidal neuron was represented by five compartments for the apical and basal dendrites, one compartment for the soma, and a layer representing extracellular K^+ concentration. The model included intrinsic membrane conductances and excitatory (NMDA and AMPA) and inhibitory ($GABA_A$ and $GABA_B$) synaptic conductances distributed in the apical dendrite compartment. The voltage dependency of NMDA receptors (due to the Mg^{2+} blockade of the channel) resulted in a weak conductance by single stimulation, but the conductance increased with increasing number and intensity of repeated stimulation. The model suggested that such cumulative activation of NMDA-mediated synaptic conductances contributed to the frequency-dependent EPSP potentiation, a form of short-term plasticity, of hippocampal neurons.

Long-Term Synaptic Plasticity

Holmes and Levy (1990) developed a compartmental model of a granule cell from the dentate gyrus to study the role of Ca^{2+} and the subsequent biochemical events involved in triggering LTP. In particular, they were interested in understanding the mechanisms amplifying the calcium signal and the relative timing of presynaptic and postsynaptic activation. An 11-compartment model was constructed to represent a spine and a small patch of the neighboring dendrite. Calcium dynamics, including Ca^{2+} influx, buffering, pumping, and diffusion were computed over this domain. One glutamate binding site and the voltage-dependent Mg^{2+} block were included in the NMDA receptor kinetics. The amplitude of the peak intracellular-free Ca^{2+} concentration was regarded as the critical parameter for the induction of LTP at a particular synapse. When few synapses were activated, Ca^{2+} influx was small, even with high input frequency. When a large number of synapses were activated simultaneously, a steep rise in Ca^{2+} influx was seen with increasing frequency due to the voltage dependency of the NMDA-mediated conductance. However, total Ca^{2+} influx never increased by more

than fourfold, which is too small an amount to account for the selective induction of LTP. The threefold to fourfold increase could be amplified 20- to 30-fold by transient saturation of the fast Ca^{2+} buffering system. When a weak input was paired with a strong one, the largest increase in peak $[Ca^{2+}]_i$ was seen in cases in which the weak stimulation preceded the strong input by 1–8 ms, because of the slow rate constant of NMDA receptor kinetics. De Schutter and Bower (1993) extended this model to evaluate the effect of Ca^{2+} permeability of the NMDA receptor channel. Maximum amplification of $[Ca^{2+}]_i$ was obtained at permeability close to values reported in the literature and decreased significantly when permeability was reduced by more than 50%. Furthermore, simulations showed that $[Ca^{2+}]_i$ was up to 80% higher at distal spines than at proximal ones.

Synaptic Integration

In addition to synaptic plasticity, NMDA receptors are also involved in the integration of spatiotemporal patterns of inputs by a neuron. Fox and Daw (1992) developed an electrical model of a neuron in area 17 of the visual cortex to study neuronal responses to visual stimuli. The model was composed of two compartments: a somatic component and a dendritic compartment with NMDA and AMPA receptors. The model showed that instead of switching on only at a higher level of contrast, the NMDA receptor-mediated conductance contributed to the response to visual stimuli in a graded fashion, all the way from near threshold to saturation. This property of the NMDA receptor could not be accounted for solely by its voltage dependency. In addition, the higher affinity (binding rate) of NMDA receptors for glutamate, in comparison to the non-NMDA receptor, was involved.

A compartmental model was developed to study the integrative behavior of a complex dendritic tree with particular focus on the role of NMDA receptors in the generation of neuronal responses (Mel, 1993). An anatomically characterized cortical pyramidal cell was represented by a model consisting of 903 electrically coupled compartments. A glutamatergic synapse was placed on the distal end of a spine containing both AMPA and NMDA receptors. The major finding from the simulation of the model was that when the NMDA receptors constituted a large portion of the synapse, the neuron responded preferentially to spatially clustered, rather than randomly distributed activated synapses. This was due to the voltage dependency of the NMDA receptors that were more effective when activated in group than individually. As a result of activity-dependent synaptic modifications, synapses on a dendritic tree were organized in such a way that stimuli that activated a similar set of synapses as those activated by patterns presented during the learning period had a higher probability of eliciting a neuronal response. Therefore, manipulating the spatial ordering of afferent activation of a dendritic tree provides a biological strategy for storing and classifying patterned information.

Metaplasticity

Considerable attention has been devoted to understanding mechanisms that could account for changes in rate of learning, a phenomenon referred to as metaplasticity. Several models of neurons or of networks of neurons have introduced various parameters to incorporate metaplasticity. The most popular model is the so-called modification threshold or sliding rule introduced by Bienenstock, Cooper, and Munro (1982). In their model of synaptic plasticity, activity-dependent changes in NMDA receptors could account for such a rule.

NMDA Receptors in Models of Neuronal Circuits

The role of NMDA receptors in neuronal networks has been studied in various systems. In this section, we briefly review their roles in generating evoked field potentials, oscillatory or epileptiform activity in neuronal networks, in working memory and learning of temporal sequences. In all these cases, the interactions between excitatory and inhibitory synapses shape the dynamics of the neural network.

NMDA Receptors and Evoked Field Potentials

A recent compartment model of a hippocampal network comprising pyramidal neurons, inhibitory interneurons, and feedback and feed-forward inhibition explored the contribution of NMDA receptor-mediated synaptic currents to evoked field potentials (Wang et al., in press). As predicted from the kinetics of the receptors, the NMDA receptors contribute significantly to the late phase of the evoked potentials, and their influence becomes more important with repeated stimulation as in paired-pulse or burst of stimulation. This effect is illustrated in Figure 1, which clearly indicates that NMDA receptors contribute significantly to burst-evoked synaptic depolarization. Likewise, compartment model simulation indicated that the amplitude of NMDA receptor-mediated calcium signals is greatly increased with increased frequency of stimulation. Furthermore, several experimental and model studies have now shown that the presence of NMDA receptors at synapses could account for low-pass temporal frequency tuning in several sensory pathways (Krukowski and Miller, 2001).

Role of NMDA Receptors in Oscillators

A network of interneurons conformed to experimentally identified cell types was constructed to simulate the spinal locomotor pattern generation in lamprey (Trävén et al., 1993). Excitatory synapses displayed both NMDA and AMPA receptors, while the inhibitory

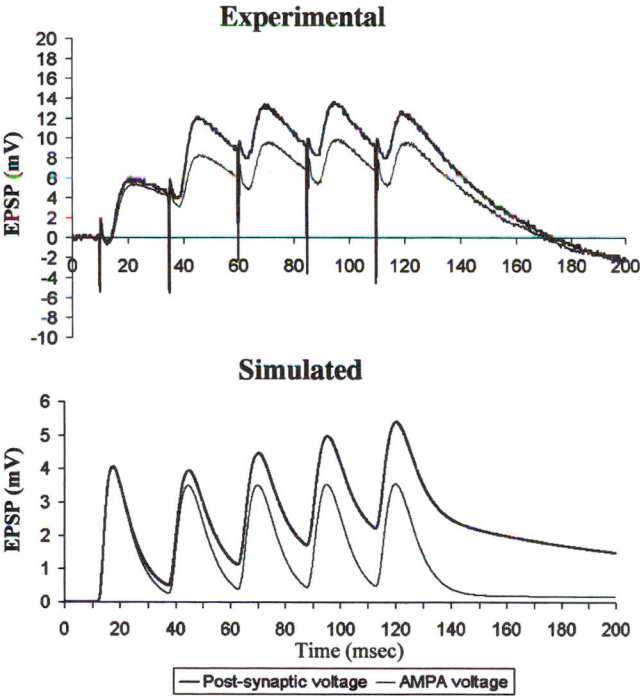

Figure 1. Contribution of NMDA receptors to postsynaptic depolarization elicited by a train of five pulses (40 Hz) in field CA1 (*Top*) and in a simulated computational model (*Bottom*). In both cases, the top trace represents total depolarization, and the bottom trace represents depolarization in the presence of the NMDA receptor blocker, APV.

synaptic transmission was glycinergic and mediated by chloride ions. The NMDA receptor current was modeled as a product of channel conductance, the difference of the membrane potential and the equilibrium potential and a state variable, which accounted for the voltage-dependent Mg^{2+} block of the channel. Oscillatory bursts could be evoked in a postsynaptic cell driven by NMDA receptor-mediated synaptic currents, but the presynaptic neuron had little effect on oscillation frequency. The presynaptic control of oscillation frequency increased when AMPA receptors were added. A continuous range of network burst rate could be produced by the NMDA and AMPA receptor-mediated conductances. The simulations suggested that spinal locomotor network could be modulated by controlling the balance between NMDA and AMPA receptor-mediated synaptic input. The NMDA receptor-containing synapses mainly served to stabilize the rhythmic motor output, whereas the AMPA receptor-containing synapses provided direct phasic control of the burst pattern.

NMDA Receptors and Epileptiform Activity

Traub, Miles, and Jefferys (1993) developed a computer model of hippocampal CA3 region consisting of pyramidal neurons and inhibitory interneurons. Each pyramidal neuron was composed of 19 compartments with six voltage-dependent ionic conductances. Each pyramidal neuron was randomly connected to 20 other pyramidal neurons via excitatory (NMDA and AMPA) receptors and to 20 interneurons via inhibitory ($GABA_A$ and $GABA_B$) receptors. The computation of NMDA receptor-mediated current involved a scaling factor, a synaptic conductance term with a slow decay time constant, and a term representing the voltage-dependent Mg^{2+} blockade. The simulation suggested the following conditions for the occurrence of population oscillations: (1) The strength of excitatory synapses falls within a limited range, (2) the after-hyperpolarization conductance is significantly reduced, (3) the inhibitory postsynaptic potentials are blocked, and (4) the apical dendrites of the pyramidal neurons are depolarized. The NMDA receptor conductance was not necessary for the population oscillation. The model generated synchronized population bursts that resemble experimental data obtained from hippocampal slices perfused with a $GABA_A$ receptor blocker and predicted that dendritic calcium spikes occurred during each secondary burst generated by the AMPA receptor current. However, with sufficiently high NMDA receptor conductance, synchronized bursts could occur in the absence of AMPA receptor current.

NMDA Receptors and Memory

Experimental evidence has strongly implicated NMDA receptors in various forms of learning and memory. Although it is generally assumed that this is a consequence of the role of NMDA receptors in activity-dependent changes in synaptic transmission in various networks, the specific roles of NMDA receptors in memory has also been more formally evaluated in various simulations of network activity and dynamics. In particular, several groups have shown that the properties of NMDA receptors are well suited for learning of sequences of information. This is particular true for networks exhibiting both theta and gamma activities, allowing recall of stored sequence by presentation of the initial element of the sequence (Jensen and Lisman, 1996).

Another interesting role of NMDA receptors has been recently proposed to account for the persistent activity in prefrontal cortex, which is assumed to be the basis for working memory (Compte et al., 2000). In this case, stable and persistent activity could be observed when recurrent synaptic excitation was mediated principally by NMDA receptor-mediated currents.

Discussion

This review of the various models of NMDA receptors at the synaptic, cellular, and network levels illustrates that the three unique properties of these receptors (i.e., slow conductance, voltage and transmitter dependency, and calcium permeability) provide the basis for their involvement in a large variety of fundamental dynamic properties of synaptic transmission, including not only short-term and long-term plasticity at individual synapses, but also complex network properties such as synaptic integration, motor pattern generation, and epileptiform activity.

The review also indicates the usefulness of this approach to investigate the contribution of different characteristics of the receptors at the functional level. In particular, the recent suggestion that metaplasticity could be accounted for by changes in NMDA receptor subunit composition and function needs to be emphasized. A number of issues still remain unresolved, in part because of the limited knowledge concerning the exact number of binding sites for the various effectors of the receptors, the mechanisms underlying desensitization, and the anatomical distribution of the different types of receptors. Interestingly, developmental switches in the subunit composition of NMDA receptors have been shown to dramatically alter network properties and information processing in these networks. Therefore, as the understanding of the characteristics and properties of NMDA receptors continue to be resolved in greater details, new models will need to be generated to capture these properties and to evaluate their contributions to the computational properties of individual neurons as well as to complex circuitries.

Road Map: Neural Plasticity
Related Reading: Biophysical Mosaic of the Neuron; Hebbian Synaptic Plasticity; Temporal Dynamics of Biological Synapses; Ion Channels: Keys to Neuronal Specialization

References

Bienenstock, E. L., Cooper, L. N., and Munro, P. W., 1982, Theory for the development of neuron selectivity: Orientation, specificity, and binocular interaction in visual cortex, *J. Neurosci.*, 2:32–48.

Compte, A., Brunel, N., Goldman-Rakic, P. S., and Wang, X. J., 2000, Synaptic mechanisms and network dynamics underlying spatial working memory in a cortical network model, *Cereb. Cortex*, 10:910–923.

Cull-Candy, S., Brickley, S., and Farrant, M., 2001, NMDA receptor subunits: Diversity, development and disease, *Curr. Opin. Neurobiol.*, 11:327–335.

De Schutter, E., and Bower, J. M., 1993, Sensitivity of synaptic plasticity to the Ca^{2+} permeability of NMDA channels: A model of long-term potentiation in hippocampal neurons, *Neural Computation*, 5:681–694.

Dingledine, R., Borges, K., Bowie, D., and Traynelis, S. F., 1999, The glutamate receptor ion channels, *Pharmacol. Rev.*, 51:7–61.

Fox, K., and Daw, N., 1992, A model for the action of NMDA conductances in the visual cortex, *Neural Comput.*, 4:59–83.

Holmes, W. R., and Levy, W., 1990, Insights into associative long-term potentiation from computational models of NMDA receptor-mediated calcium influx and intracellular calcium concentration changes, *J. Neurophysiol.*, 63:1148–1168.

Jahr, C. E., and Stevens, C. F., 1990, A quantitative description of NMDA receptor-channel kinetic behavior, *J. Neurosci.*, 10:1830–1837.

Jensen, O., and Lisman, J. E., 1996, Theta/gamma networks with slow NMDA channels learn sequences and encode episodic memory: Role of NMDA channels in recall, *Learn. Mem.*, 3:264–278.

Kennedy, M. B., 1998, Signal transduction molecules at the glutamatergic postsynaptic membrane, *Brain Res. Rev.*, 26:243–257.

Krukowski, A. E., and Miller U. D., 2002, Thalamo-cortical NMDA conductances and intracortical inhibition can explain cortical temporal tuning, *Nature Neurosci.*, 4:429–430.

Lester, R. J. A., Tong, G., and Jahr, C. E., 1993, Interaction between the glycine and glutamate binding sites of the NMDA receptor, *J. Neurosci.*, 17:1088–1098.

Malenka, R. C., and Nicoll, R. A., 1999, Long-term potentiation: A decade of progress?, *Science*, 285:1870–1874.

Marvizon, J. C., and Baudry, M., 1993, Receptor activation by two agonists: Analysis by nonlinear regression and application to *N*-Methyl-D-Aspartate receptors, *Anal. Biochem.*, 213:3–11.

Mel, B. W., 1993, NMDA-based pattern discrimination in a modeled cortical neuron, *Neural Comput.*, 4:502–516.

Pongrácz, F., Poolos, N. P., Kocsis, J. D., and Shepherd, G. M., 1992, A model of NMDA receptor-mediated activity in dendrites of hippocampal CA1 pyramidal neurons, *J. Neurophysiol.*, 68:2248–2259.

Traub, R. D., Miles, R., and Jefferys, J. G. R, 1993, Synaptic and intrinsic conductances shape picrotoxin-induced synchronized after-discharges in the guinea-pig hippocampal slice, *J. Physiol.*, 461:525–547.

Träven, H., Brodin, L., Lansner, A., Ekeberg, Ö., Wallén, P., and Grillner, S., 1993, Computer simulations of NMDA and non-NMDA receptor-mediated synaptic drive: Sensory and supraspinal modulation of neurons and small network, *J. Neurophysiol.*, 70:695–709.

Wang, Z., Song, D., and Berger, T. W., 2002, Contribution of NMDA receptor channels to the expresion of LTP in hippocampal dentate gynus, *Hippocampus* (in press).

NSL Neural Simulation Language

Alfredo Weitzenfeld

Introduction

Neural simulation plays an essential role in understanding the brain. While many neural simulators exist today (see NEUROSIMULATION: TOOLS AND RESOURCES for a listing of the most important ones), design considerations can be quite different. For example, systems supporting very detailed neural elements can simulate only a few neurons at a time (see NEURON SIMULATION ENVIRONMENT and GENESIS SIMULATION SYSTEM), while systems supporting coarser elements can usually simulate larger neural populations. In this article, we describe the Neural Simulation Language (NSL) (Weitzenfeld, Arbib, and Alexander, 2002), an *object-oriented* system (Wegner, 1990) primarily designed to support simulation of large neural networks. The system addresses the needs of a wide range of users, from novice users requiring friendly user interfaces to advanced users requiring advanced programming and integration to other systems. Two versions of the system exist today, one in Java (Gosling et al., 2000) and the other in C++ (Stroustrup, 2000). Both of these can run on a wide range of computer platforms, making the system quite independent from the actual computing environment.

Modularity in Neural Systems

A particular aspect that distinguishes NSL from comparable simulators is its special focus on *modularity*, a well-known software development strategy in dealing with large and complex systems. As neural models become large and complex, they become hard to manage. Moreover, modularization of biological neural networks is further motivated by taking into consideration the way we analyze the brain as a set of different brain regions, as seen by the example shown in Figure 1.

The general methodology for understanding a complex neural system involves two basic approaches. One is to focus on some particular brain region or module and carry out studies of that region in detail. The other is to step back and look at higher levels of organization in which the details of particular modules are hidden. Full understanding comes as we cycle back and forth between different levels of detail in analyzing different subsystems, sometimes simulating modules in isolation, at other times designing computer experiments that help us follow the dynamics of the interactions between the various modules.

Modeling in NSL

There are two ways to describe a model in NSL: (1) by direct programming in NSLM, the NSL (compiled) modeling language, and (2) by using the Schematic Capture System (SCS), a visual programming interface to NSLM supporting the description of module assemblages. In general, NSL supports the two levels of modeling, *modules* and *neural networks*, as described next.

Modules

Modules in NSL are hierarchical structures organized in a tree fashion having a root module, the *model*, and multiple levels of *module assemblages*. Modules may be implemented in different ways and independently from each other in a top-down and a bottom-up fashion, an important benefit from modular design. In particular, *neural modules* are implemented with neural networks, corresponding to leaves on a tree. In general, the external interface to a module is described by a set of unidirectional input and output *data ports*, representing module entry or exit points, where data are sent or received, usually in the form of numerical values with varying dimension, that is, a single scalar, a one-dimensional array of values (*vector*), a two-dimensional array (*matrix*), or higher ones. To communicate, modules require interconnections among ports belonging to different modules. The following is sample NSLM code describing module assemblages:

```
nslModel Model ()
{
    private StimulusModule stimulus ();
    private MainModule main ();
    private OutputModule output ();
    public void makeConn () {
        nslConnect (stimulus.sout, main.in);
        nslConnect (stimulus.sout, output.sin);
        nslConnect (main.out, output.oin);
    }
}
```

The description is analogous to a class specification in object-oriented programming. The attribute section describes a three-module assemblage consisting of a "stimulus," "main," and "output" modules, while the *makeConn* method specifies module interconnections using the *nslConnect* statement (see Weitzenfeld et al., 2002, for a more extensive description of all NSLM commands.) This sample NSLM code could be automatically generated from SCS as well. Figure 2 shows sample schematics for a module assemblage within a higher-level module.

Neural Networks

Modules representing brain regions can be anatomically or physiologically divided to obtain *neural modules*, modules described by

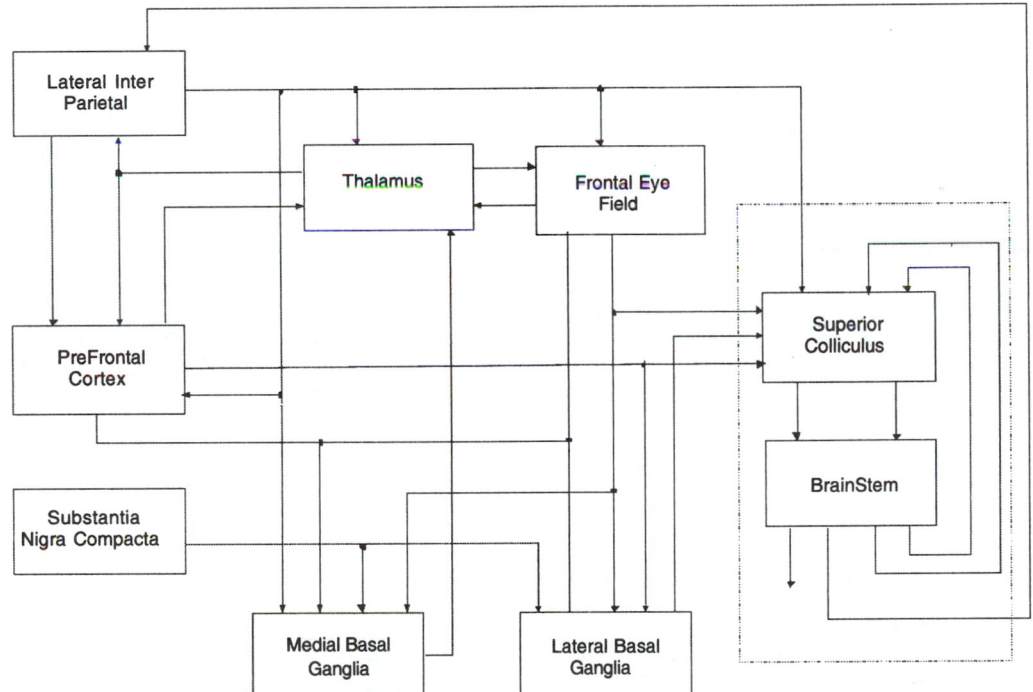

Figure 1. The smaller outlined diagram shows a basic model for control of eye movements consisting of a superior colliculus {XE "Superior Colliculus"} (sc) and brainstem {XE "Brainstem"} modules, each representing a single brain region, responsible for generation of saccades (see COLLICULAR VISUOMOTOR TRANSFORMATIONS FOR GAZE CONTROL). As an example of the benefits of modularization, the SC and Brainstem modules can be embedded into the much larger and far more complex model of interacting brain regions, such as the Crowley-Arbib model of BASAL GANGLIA (Crowley, Oztop, and Mármol, 2002).

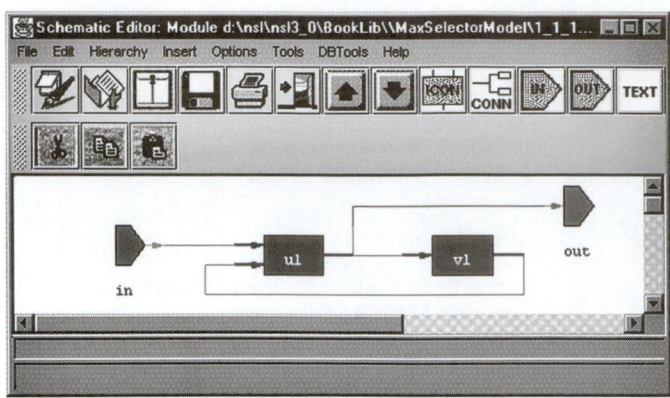

Figure 2. The window shows the Schematic Capture System (SCS) view of the schematics of a sample module consisting of a two-module assemblage and two data ports. Modules are represented by rectangles, while entry (left) and exit (right) ports are represented by pentagon-shaped icons.

neural arrays. To model a complete neural network, it is necessary to describe (1) the particular neuron model, that is, the desired neural level of detail, (2) the neurons making up the network, (3) the set of interconnections among neurons, and (4) network parameters, such as inputs and connection weights. Without disregarding the importance of other neural models, we focus here on the *leaky integrator* (Arbib, 1989) neuron model, a single-compartment neuron having one output and many inputs. The internal state of the neuron is described by a single scalar quantity, its membrane potential *mp*, which depends on the neuron's inputs and past history. The output is described by another single scalar quantity, its firing rate *mf*, and may serve as input to multiple neurons, including itself. As the input to a neuron varies, the membrane potential and firing rate vary as well.

In NSL, two numerical structures (**NslDouble0** data type) are required to represent such a neuron, one corresponding to the membrane potential and the other one to its firing rate:

private NslDouble0 mf ();
private NslDouble0 mp ();

In many cases, we may want the value of *mf* to be communicated to other modules. If such is the case, the declaration for *mf* should be modified from a private variable to a public output port (note the *Dout* keyword):

public NslDoutDouble0 mf();

The *membrane potential* for *mp* is described by a first-order differential equation with dependence on its previous history and input S_m:

$$\tau_m \frac{dmp(t)}{dt} = f(s_m, mp, t)$$

Variable τ_m represents the time constant, while the choice of f defines the particular neural model utilized. The *leaky integrator* model is described by $f(s_m, mp, t) = -mp(t) + s_m(t)$, or

$$\tau_m \frac{dmp(t)}{dt} = -mp(t) + s_m(t)$$

In addition to the membrane potential and firing rate descriptions, we also need to specify the input to the neuron, s_m, internal to the module or obtained from another module. In the latter case, input s_m would be specified as an input port (note the "Din" keyword):

public NslDinDouble0 sm();

where *sm* holds a weighted spatial summation of all input to the corresponding neuron.

While neural networks are continuous in their nature, their simulated state is approximated by discrete-time computations. For this reason, we must specify an integration or approximation method to generate as faithfully as possible the corresponding neural state. The dynamics for *mp* are described by the following statement:

mp = **nslDiff** (mp, tau, −mp + sm);

Function *nslDiff* defines a first-degree differential equation equal to "$-mp + sm$" as described by the leaky integrator model. Different methods can be used to approximate the differential equation, such as Euler and Runge-Kutta. The choice of method may affect both the computation time and its precision. The specific method to use is chosen during simulation and not as part of the model architecture.

The firing rate *mf*, the output of the neuron, is obtained by applying a *threshold*, typically a *ramp, step, saturation,* or *sigmoidal* function, to the neuron's membrane potential:

$$mf(t) = \sigma(mp(t))$$

where σ is usually a nonlinear function.

For example, if σ is set to a *step* threshold function, the equation for the firing rate *mf* would be described by

mf = **nslStep** (mp);

where *nslStep* is the corresponding NSL *step* threshold function.

The previous definition specifies a single neuron without any interconnections. An actual neural network is made of a number of interconnected neurons in which the output of one neuron serves as input to the others. In the leaky integrator neural model, interconnections are very simple structures. On the other hand, *synapses*, the links among neurons, are—in biological systems—complex electrochemical systems and may be modeled in exquisite detail. However, many models have succeeded with a very simple synaptic model in which each synapse carries a connection weight that describes how neurons affect each other. The most common formula for the input *sv* to a neuron *v* is given by

$$sv_j = \sum_{i=0}^{n-1} w_{ji}uf_i$$

where uf_i is the firing of neuron u_i whose output is connected to the *j*th input line of neuron v_j and w_{ji} is the weight for that link, as shown in Figure 3 (*up* and *vp* are analogous to *mp*, while *uf* and *vf* are analogous to *mf*).

Expanding the summation, input to neuron v_j (identified by its corresponding membrane potential vp_j) is given by sv_j, which is defined as

$$sv_j = w_{j0}uf_0 + w_{j1}uf_1 + w_{j2}uf_2 + \cdots + w_{jn-1}uf_{n-1}$$

Figure 3. The diagram shows a sample two-layer fully connected neural organization (see BACK-PROPAGATION: GENERAL PRINCIPLES for an example of networks using such architectures). Each neuron is described by a single compartment represented by a value *up* or *vp*, its membrane potential, and a value *uf* or *vf*, to its firing, the output from the neuron. Input to the first neural layer is represented by *s*. Additionally, weights *w* have been added to the different connections.

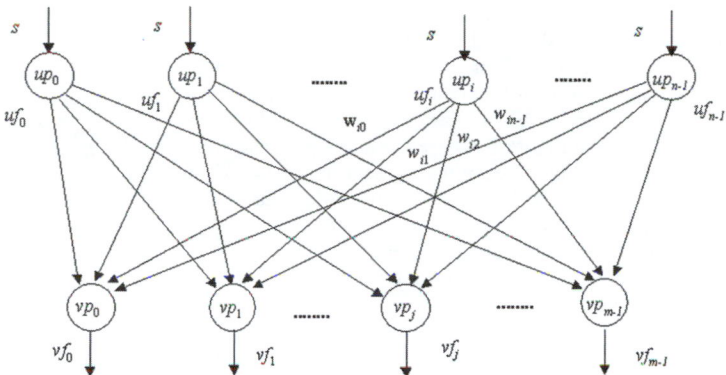

While module interconnections are specified in NSL via a *nslConnect* method call, doing this with neurons would in general be prohibitively expensive, considering that there may be thousands or millions of neurons and even more connections in a single neural network. Instead, we use mathematical expressions similar to those used for their representation. For example, the input to neuron v_j, represented by sv_j, would be the sum for all outputs of neuron uf_i multiplied (using the * operator) by connection weight wji, correspondingly, as shown next:

$$sv_j = wj0*ufo + wj1*uf1 + wj2*uf2 + \cdots;$$

Note that there exist *m* such equations in the network. We could describe each membrane potential and firing rate individually, or else we could make all u_i and v_j neuron vector structures. The first approach would be very long, inefficient, and prone to typing errors; therefore, we present the second approach, using *neuron arrays* and *connection masks* representing spatial arrangements among homogeneous neurons and their connections, respectively. We consider uf_i the output from a single neuron in an array of neurons and sv_j the input to a single neuron in another array of neurons.

If mask w_{jk} (for $-d \leq k \leq d$) represents the synaptic weights from the uf_{j+k} (for $-d \leq k \leq d$) elements to v_j, for every j, we then have

$$sv_j = \sum_{k=-d}^{d} w_{jk} uf_{j+k}$$

where the same mask *w* is applied to the output of each neuron uf_{i+k} to obtain input sv_j. In NSL, the *convolution* operation is described by a single symbol '@':

$$sv = w@uf;$$

This kind of representation results in great conciseness, an important concern in working with large numbers of interconnected neurons. Note that this is possible as long as connections are regular. Otherwise, single neurons would still need to be connected separately, one by one. This also suggests that the operation is best defined when the number of *v* and *u* neurons matches, although a nonmatching number of units can be processed by using a more complex notation.

Simulation in NSL

Simulation involves interactively specifying aspects of the model that tend to change, in particular parameter values, input patterns, simulation control, and visualization. It is important not only to design a good model, but also to design good graphical interfaces, both input and output. In terms of input, NSL offers a number of approaches: (1) by interactively writing code in NSLS, the NSL (interpreted) scripting language, (2) by loading NSLS scripts stored in files, and (3) by designing custom input interfaces. In terms of output, NSL enables the user to specify various forms of graphical and textual output, including temporal and spatial 2D and 3D graphics (see Weitzenfeld et al., 2002, for input and output visualization examples as well as more extensive description of NSLS commands).

Discussion

In this article we have overviewed modeling and simulation using NSL, a system primarily designed to simulate modular neural systems, both biological and artificial (see BACKPROPAGATION: GENERAL PRINCIPLES for an example of artificial neural networks). The underlying NSL computational model is based on the Abstract Schema Language (ASL) (Weitzenfeld, 1993) inspired by the work on SCHEMA THEORY (q.v.), on actors (Agha, 1986), and more generally on object-based concurrent programming (Yonezawa and Tokoro, 1987).

There are a number of issues worth discussing from our experience with NSL. While user interactivity plays an essential role while creating and testing new neural models, as model becomes more stable, simulation efficiency becomes a primary concern. This is a very important issue if we consider that neural network execution can consume extensive amounts of processing time, possibly hours or even days depending on the size and architecture of the network. For example, we have processed in NSL "simple" biological network, such as the retina model (see RETINA) involving 10,000 neurons, consuming just a few seconds. On the other hand, a more complex network such as the one described in Figure 1 could take several minutes if implemented by "faithful" neural components. The general solution to this problem is to use parallelism and distributed computing facilities in speeding up computation. While a number of neural systems have been ported to supercomputers, we are currently developing a distributed simulation environment to run on networks of low-cost computers (Weitzenfeld, Peguero, and Gutiérrez, 2000). In general, the client-server distributed architecture has become quite pervasive, thanks to the Internet.

A web-based simulation interface (Alexander, Arbib, and Weitzenfeld, 1999) brings additional possibilities to the process of neural modeling. For example, users could be offered shared model repositories in creating new models or in addressing experimental data linked to it. These two thrusts are part of a project known as Brain Models on the Web (BMW), a model repository in which model assumptions, empirical data, and simulation results are stored (see DATABASES FOR NEUROSCIENCE).

An important issue arising from the sharing of module libraries is how to reuse portions of different models in creating new ones. An important consideration is to provide a general module interconnection specification to be followed by all modelers. This specification should deal with issues such as "edges" in the block diagrams as the one shown in Figure 1, where module interconnections and the corresponding ports are designed to deal only with primitive data without any temporal considerations. Additionally, the specification could address the relationship to the particular experimental protocol on which the model is based. These aspects need to be defined and then specified as a "meta-level" that will separate the internal module characteristics from the external ones.

Another consideration is the extensibility the system. Since not all users use similar simulation systems, it is important to offer interoperability of data and model descriptions to be shared by multiple simulation systems and applications in general. Additionally, integration with simulated or real-time REACTIVE ROBOTIC SYSTEMS (q.v.) is of particular interest, in particular BIOLOGICALLY INSPIRED ROBOTICS (q.v.), as exemplified by a number of NSL-based neural architectures developed to control mobile robots (Fagg et al., 1992; Weitzenfeld, 2000). Since many approaches exist today to mobile robotics, it is an interesting challenge to design new architectures integrating nonneural and neural-based approaches (Arkin et al., 2000).

Road Map: Implementation and Analysis
Related Reading: Neurosimulation: Tools and Resources; Schema Theory; Single-Cell Models

References

Agha, G., 1986, *Actors: A Model of Concurrent Computation in Distributed Systems*, Cambridge, MA: MIT Press.

Alexander, A., Arbib, M. A., and Weitzenfeld, A., 1999, Web simulation of brain models, in *Proceedings of SCS 1999 International Conference on Web-Based Modelling and Simulation*, January 17–20, San Francisco, CA.

Arbib, M. A., 1989, *The Metaphorical Brain 2: Neural Networks and Beyond*, New York: Wiley. ◆

Arkin, R. C., Ali, K., Weitzenfeld, A., and Cervates-Perez, F., 2000, Behavioral models of the praying mantis as a basis for robotic behavior, *J. Robotics and Autonomous Systems*, 32(1):39–60.

Crowley, M., Oztop, E., and Mármol, S., 2002, Crowley-Arbib saccade model, in *The Neural Simulation Language: A System for Brain Modeling* (A. Weitzenfeld, M. Arbib, and A. Alexander, Eds.), Cambridge, MA: MIT Press.

Fagg, A. H., King, I. K., Lewis, M. A., Liaw, J. S., and Weitzenfeld, A., 1992, A neural network based testbed for modeling sensorimotor integration in robotics applications, in *Proceedings of IJCNN '92*, Baltimore, MD.

Gosling, J., Joy, B., Steele, G., and Bracha., G., 2000, *The Java Language Specification*, 2nd ed., Reading, MA: Addison-Wesley.

Stroustrup, B., 2000, *The C++ Programming Language*, Special Edition, Reading, MA: Addison-Wesley.

Wegner, P., 1990, Concepts and paradigms of object-oriented programming, *SIGPLAN OOPS Messenger*, 1(1):7–87. ◆

Weitzenfeld, A., 1993, ASL: Hierarchy, composition, heterogeneity, and multi-granularity in concurrent object-oriented programming, in *Proceedings on Neural Architectures and Distributed AI: From Schema Assemblages to Neural Networks Workshop*, Oct. 19–20, Center for Neural Engineering, USC, Los Angeles, CA.

Weitzenfeld, A., 2000, A multi-level approach to biologically inspired robotic systems, in *Proceedings of NNW 2000 10th International Conference on Artificial Neural Networks and Intelligent Systems*, Prague, Czech Republic, July 9–12.

Weitzenfeld, A., Arbib, M. A., and Alexander, A., 2002, *The Neural Simulation Language, A System for Brain Modeling*, Cambridge, MA: MIT Press. ◆

Weitzenfeld, A., Peguero, O., and Gutiérrez, S., 2000, NSL/ASL: Distributed simulation of modular neural networks, in *Proceedings of MICAI 2000: Advances on Artificial Intelligence*, Acapulco, Mexico, April 10–14, LNCS 1796.

Yonezawa, A., and Tokoro, M. (Eds.), 1987, *Object-Oriented Concurrent Programming*, Cambridge, MA: MIT Press.

Object Recognition

Bosco S. Tjan

Introduction

Visual object recognition is a classification task that assigns a behaviorally relevant label to a region of an image. It is one of the most important functions carried out by the human visual system. Understanding how it is achieved is almost as great a task as understanding visual processing in its entirety (Marr, 1982; Ullman, 1997; Rolls and Deco, 2002). Object recognition is a special case of PATTERN RECOGNITION (q.v.) in which the pattern to be classified is a two-dimensional (2D) projection of a three-dimensional (3D) structure. The 3D structure in question can be a single object (e.g., a car), an arrangement of objects (a convoy of cars), or even a space surrounding the observer (the interior of a car). For the same object, the assigned label depends on the task. A car may be recognized as "an obstacle" (along with garbage cans, lampposts) when one tries to maneuver through parked cars or "an approaching hazard" when one tries to cross the street. The level of classification also varies. An object can be recognized at what cognitive psychologists call the *basic* level (e.g., "a car"), a coarser *superordinate* level ("a vehicle"), or a finer *subordinate* level ("VW Beetle"). In general, object recognition is a mapping, $\mathbf{G}:\{x\} \rightarrow \{c\}$, from a set of input images $\{x\}$ to a set of task-dependent class labels $\{c\}$.

Ideally, the mapping should be achieved by selecting the class label $c \in \{c\}$ that *best* explains the image in a probabilistic sense (i.e., by maximizing the posterior probability $\Pr(c|x)$; see BAYESIAN NETWORKS). The challenge lies in the fact that the 2D image of a 3D structure changes dramatically under different *imaging conditions*: variations in lighting, position of the observer, presence or absence of other objects in the foreground and background, etc. A theory of object recognition must therefore explain (1) how a system may retain constancy in object classification in spite of large image variability, and (2) how such a system may learn and generalize. Among all the varying imaging parameters, the one that has received most attention is *viewpoint*, i.e., viewing position and direction of the observer relative to an object.

In this article, we review a number of computational theories of object recognition. The review, which is neither exhaustive nor comprehensive, is meant to show a broad range of the approaches. Space limitations prevent us from discussing the psychological validity of each approach—a difficult issue that is hotly debated. We emphasize computational theories over their neurological implementations, relying on other articles in this *Handbook* to bridge the two (see OBJECT RECOGNITION, NEUROPHYSIOLOGY; OBJECT STRUCTURE, VISUAL PROCESSING). Our discussion of the computational theories of object recognition leads to a language of decision complexity, which we will use to characterize the trade-offs chosen by each theory. We will argue that a general-purpose object recognition system, such as the human brain, must be able to represent an object in multiple ways, and we outline a computational framework for such a system.

Matching: A Core Operation

Object recognition is about matching an input *image* (2D array of luminance and chromaticity values) to a stored *representation* of an object. A very rudimentary form of object recognition is *template matching* performed at (or near) the image level, in which an input image is matched pixel to pixel to a set of stored images. The input image may be preprocessed to reduce the variability in luminance, size, 2D position, and/or image-plate rotation. A degree of mismatch is computed with some knowledge about the noise processes in image acquisition and preprocessing. For example, the commonly used mean-square error, or L2-norm, between an image and a stored template is appropriate if the imaging noise is an identically and independently distributed Gaussian in pixel value. A match is found when the degree of mismatch is less than some threshold.

The obvious advantage of image-level template matching is that little preprocessing is required, and few assumptions about the utility and detectability of certain image features are needed to transform the input image into a template. On the other hand, small variations in imaging conditions, such as changes in viewpoint or illumination direction, can produce a large mismatch between an input image and a restored template. As a result, image-level template matching methods are of little use for general-purpose object recognition.

On the other hand, it is not difficult to see that template matching is at the core of every object recognition theory. Superficially, the final decision stage that matches a processed input to a stored representation of an object is a template matcher operating at the level of the representation. A more fundamental role of template matching can be seen as follows. Let $v_c(\mathbf{g})$ be a view of object c in some representation, where $\mathbf{g}$ is a vector of imaging parameters (i.e., viewpoint, illumination, occlusion, etc.). The posterior probability, $\Pr(c|x)$, of object c being present in the image x can be expressed in terms of all the possible views of c by integrating over the generic variable $\mathbf{g}$. With Bayes's rule, we have:

$$\Pr(c|x) = \int_{\mathbf{g}} p(v_c(\mathbf{g})|x)d\mathbf{g} = \int_{\mathbf{g}} \frac{p(x|v_c(\mathbf{g}))p(v_c(\mathbf{g}))}{p(x)}\,d\mathbf{g} \quad (1)$$

where $p(v_c(\mathbf{g}))$ is prior probability density of a view, $p(x|v_c(\mathbf{g}))$ is the likelihood of $v_c(\mathbf{g})$ being the cause of the input image x, and $p(x)$ is the probability density of seeing the input image x, which, for our purposes, is simply a normalization constant independent of c and $\mathbf{g}$. The decision rule that is most accurate on average is to select c that maximizes $\Pr(c|x)$. That is,

$$\arg \max_{c} \Pr(c|x) = \arg \max_{c} \int_{\mathbf{g}} p(x|v_c(\mathbf{g}))p(v_c(\mathbf{g}))d\mathbf{g} \quad (2)$$

If the view $v_c(\mathbf{g})$ is represented as an N-pixel image, the likelihood function $p(x|v_c(\mathbf{g}))$ is simply the probability density function describing the imaging noise. For example, if the imaging noise is an identically and independently distributed Gaussian pixel noise, then $p(x|v_c(\mathbf{g})) = 1/(\sigma\sqrt{2\pi})^N \exp(-\|x - v_c(\mathbf{g})\|^2/2\sigma^2)$. The L2-norm term $\|x - v_c(\mathbf{g})\|^2$ in the exponent represents image-level template matching. In other words, object constancy could in theory be achieved with image-level template matching, provided one has the space and time to store and compare the input image against all views of all objects of interest (or according to Tjan and Legge

[1998], a large but finite set of random views would suffice). Moreover, the decision rule of Equation 2 evaluated at the image level, with unlimited memory for object views, achieves the theoretical maximum in average accuracy.

Theories of Object Recognition

Theoretical ideals notwithstanding, if object constancy is to be achieved practically, a visual system must explore regularities in the mapping between an input image and the intended output label. This is often done in two steps. First, photometric and geometric regularities inherent in the image-formation process are explored by extracting image features that remain constant (or nearly so) with respect to changes in imaging conditions. The extracted features then form a *representation* of the input. Second, this representation of the input is compared to the stored representations of different objects to identify a match. This decision process explores the statistical regularities inherent in the mapping between the representation (as opposed to the input image) and the output label. Theories of object recognition differ in their respective emphases on the representation or decision step. In their succinct discussion of the computational theories of object recognition, Trucco and Verri (1998) mentioned two general approaches to object recognition. If a system constructs a representation that does not vary (i.e., is *invariant*) with respect to imaging parameters but is sufficiently *discriminating* to tell one object from another, then the decision step will be relatively trivial. This type of approach is referred to as being *invariant based*. However, finding features that are both invariant and discriminatory is often difficult. The alternative is to rely less on an invariant representation and more on statistical inference to implicitly capture the regularities between the stimuli and the output labels. Because such an approach often makes object decisions using a representation closely resembling the input image, it is termed *appearance based*. A third type of approach, which does not fit neatly into either category described by Trucco and Verri, is to store a 3D model for each object. Recognition proceeds by trying to align a 3D model to match the input image. We will refer to this type of approach as *model based*.

Invariant-Based Object Recognition

For an invariant-based object recognition system, the primary objective of visual processing is to extract and construct features that are constant relative to imaging conditions. For example, the presence of an *edge* often signals a discontinuity in surface orientation, mostly independent of lighting conditions. Hence, edge detection and contour formation are often proposed as the first steps of visual processing. The position, orientation, length, and curvature of a contour, however, vary with respect to an observer's viewpoint. Quantization is sometimes used to gain an additional degree of invariance. Within sensory acuity, many edges appear straight. Classifying the curvature of an edge as "straight" or "curved" makes the (qualitative) curvature of an edge invariant to viewpoint. Quantization represents a trade-off between discriminability and invariance. For example, a circle could not be discriminated from an ellipse if edges were classified solely as either straight or curved.

Another important means to attain invariance is to form compound features from elementary ones. For example, if there exist four identifiable points, $P_1, \ldots, P_4$, on a straight edge (perhaps due to surface markings), then the *cross ratio*, defined as $(|P_1 - P_2| \cdot |P_3 - P_4|)/(|P_1 - P_3| \cdot |P_2 - P_4|)$, is a quantity invariant to viewpoint under perspective projection (Duda and Hart, 1973). The cross-ratio of four collinear points can therefore be treated as a discriminating "feature" invariant to viewpoint. Other invariants based on configurations of points, lines, and conics have been proposed for the purpose of object recognition (Mundy and Zisserman,

1992). Like feature quantization, discriminability in object shape is often reduced when object identification relies on invariant features. For example, if shapes are represented by cross-ratios alone or any invariant derived from them, objects that are an affine (linear) transformation away from one another will be indistinguishable. In particular, a cube would be indistinguishable from a rectangular box or a parallelepiped.

Human observers are unaware of most of the geometric invariants, such as cross-ratios. However, a few spatial arrangements of features, such as collinearity of edges, parallelism, closure, or symmetry, are perceptually conspicuous. It has been proposed that such feature arrangements are ecologically significant, useful for segmenting an object from a cluttered environment. Lowe (1987) demonstrated an object recognition system that relies on perceptual organization of features to achieve invariant object recognition in a cluttered scene. Specifically, line segments were hypothesized to belong to the same object if they could be grouped based on proximity, parallelism, or collinearity.

Another well-known example of achieving invariance by feature grouping is the recognition by components theory (RBC; Beiderman, 1987). Beiderman argued that some 50 elementary 3D volumes (called *geons*) could be uniquely identified from their 2D images over a range of viewpoints by expressing edge configurations in terms of their qualitative (quantized) properties: straight versus curve, parallel versus converging, and type of intersection ("fork," "arrow," "L," or "T"). General-purpose object recognition proceeded by first identifying the geons then the spatial relationships between the geons. Spatial relationships were also identified in quantized terms, such as "on," "next-to," "left-of," etc. In short, RBC proposes that an object is represented by the qualitative spatial relationship between its parts, and the parts are represented as geons.

In general, an invariant-based object recognition theory proposes to construct, through stages of feature extraction, combination, and quantization, a set of higher-order features that are largely unaffected by imaging conditions. The final set of invariant features is then compared to those stored in memory as object models. Recognition results when a reasonably good match is found between the invariant representation of the input and that of a known object.

Model-Based Object Recognition

Instead of combining features or quantizing feature attributes to achieve invariance, a visual system can factor out image variability by making explicit use of the 3D structure of an object. Lowe (1987) and later Huttenlocher and Ullman (1990) proposed the alignment method for object recognition, in which a small number (three or more) of identifiable features (parallel line segments, corners, junction types) were first hypothesized to be in correspondence with the compatible features of a stored 3D object model. The hypothesized correspondence was used to compute an orientation of the object (called a *pose*) that could bring the 3D model features into alignment with the corresponding 2D image features. The validity of the proposed object model was determined by the degree of match between the rest of the image and the projection of the model onto the image using the computed pose.

Common to most model-based approaches is an explicitly 3D representation of the objects, which allows the appearance of an object to be determined from any viewpoint, thus achieving invariance. Acquiring such a representation, however, can be challenging, especially if the 3D representation is to be derived from 2D inputs. Fortunately, an object's 3D structure is implicitly captured in its 2D images. Techniques have since been developed to exploit the three-dimensionality using image-to-image operations, bypassing the need to explicitly construct or store any 3D object model. Such techniques are often referred to as being appearance based.

Appearance-Based Object Recognition

The most basic (and least plausible) form of appearance-based object recognition is the image-level template matching described earlier. It typifies one prominent feature of the appearance-based object recognition theories, namely, that decisions are made based on representations that closely resemble the raw input image. This is in sharp contrast to the invariant-based approach, which relies on higher-order features designed to be invariant to imaging conditions. Making object decisions near the image level relieves the system from depending on the complicated and often noisy feature extraction and construction processes, which results in higher tolerance to input noise and better discrimination. In addition, operations needed for learning new objects (model acquisition) are usually more robust and straightforward. The obvious challenge, however, is to achieve a reasonable level of viewpoint invariance for the technique to be useful.

An N-pixel image view $\mathbf{v}_c(\mathbf{g})$ can be expressed as a vector of N pixel values. This vector denotes a point in the *image space*. Over all the continuously varying imaging parameters (e.g., viewpoint, illumination), the set of points $\mathbf{v}_c(\cdot)$ form an *object manifold* embedded in the image space, which implicitly captures the 3D structure of the object. The process of object recognition in the image space can be thought of as determining which object manifold $\mathbf{v}_c(\cdot)$ is the "closest to" the input image. Because the input is a single point in the image space, but a manifold is a set of points, the distance between the two can take many forms. Equation 2 expresses one such form, which maximizes the average recognition accuracy. A brute-force implementation of Equation 2, however, would require storing too many images and would take too long to compute to be practical. Most of the appearance-based theories try to approximate Equation 2 by exploiting various regularities of the object manifolds, in order to significantly reduce storage and computation requirements.

An object manifold $\mathbf{v}_c(\cdot)$ can be arbitrarily complex and not necessarily smooth, even if the imaging parameters vary smoothly. There exist conditions, however, where the object manifold has a simple analytic form with parameters that can be determined from a sparse set of images. For example, if the only allowable variations in imaging conditions are the direction and intensity of illumination, then the object manifold will be piecewise linear (ignoring cast shadow). This means that images of the same object over a range of illumination changes can be synthesized by linearly combining three known images. Moreover, recent analysis has shown that the entire object manifold under illumination changes is "flat," residing close to a nine-dimensional subspace embedded in the image space of a few million dimensions. A practical appearance-based recognition system needs to store only nine images per object to achieve invariance over lighting variations (Basri and Jacobs, 2001; Lee, Ho, and Kriegman, 2001).

Another important case is when the image $\mathbf{v}_c(\mathbf{g})$ is not a vector of luminance values but a list of 2D coordinates of feature points. Furthermore, it is assumed that the correspondence between feature points across different views has been established. Object manifolds in this *correspondence space* (as opposed to the image space) are piecewise linear, if the viewing distance is large compared to object size. Ullman and Basri (1991) explored this property and pointed out that the views of an object over a range of viewpoints could be synthesized by linearly combining the coordinates of corresponding features between two views, thus avoiding the need for storing a large number of views. Other means of correspondence-space view interpolation, such as one using RADIAL BASIS FUNCTION NETWORKS (q.v.) (Poggio and Edelman, 1990), have also shown promise.

If the analytical form of an object manifold is not known, as is often the case, a visual system can still exploit the regularity of the manifold implicitly. For example, it could (1) use an inexact matching operation, (2) reduce the dimensionality of the manifolds, or (3) increase the distance between manifolds by mapping them to an even higher-dimensional space.

Von der Malsburg and colleagues (Lades et al., 1993) adapted DYNAMIC LINK ARCHITECTURE (q.v.) to perform elastic graph matching for object recognition. An object from a given viewpoint was represented by a grid of sparsely sampled image features, each being a vector (called a "jet") representing the local spatial frequency spectrum. To match an input image, the grid was allowed to deform mildly in search of the best-matched feature points. Recognition can be invariant over a modest range of viewpoints because a small change in viewpoint tends to displace feature points without significantly altering their local spatial frequency spectrum.

The set of images an appearance-based system can possibly store for a given object is usually a very sparse sample of the object manifold. Therefore, it is often advantageous to reduce the dimensionality of the object manifold to make the stored images more representative. The eigenspace method (Murase and Nayar, 1995; see PRINCIPAL COMPONENT ANALYSIS and INDEPENDENT COMPONENT ANALYSIS) is a principled way of achieving this. The idea is to express a set of n known images of an object in terms of a weighted sum of their principal components $\mathbf{e}_1 \ldots \mathbf{e}_n$. This mounts to a coordinate transformation from the image space (of pixel values) to an eigenspace via rigid rotation. If the principal components are arranged in descending order of their associated eigenvalues, then the weighted sum of the first k principal components ($k < n$) is the "best" k-dimensional approximation of the image set, in the sense of having the minimum mean-square error. That is, if $\mathbf{v}_c(\mathbf{g})$ is an image of the object c in some imaging condition $\mathbf{g}$, then

$$\mathbf{v}_c(\mathbf{g}) = w_1\mathbf{e}_1 + w_2\mathbf{e}_2 + \cdots + w_k\mathbf{e}_k + \cdots + w_n\mathbf{e}_n$$
$$\approx w_1\mathbf{e}_1 + w_2\mathbf{e}_2 + \cdots + w_k\mathbf{e}_k = [\mathbf{e}_1, \ldots, \mathbf{e}_k]*\mathbf{w}_c(\mathbf{g}) \quad (3)$$

where $\mathbf{w}_c(\mathbf{g}) = [w_1, w_2, \ldots, w_k]^T$. In practice, k can often be much smaller than n. This means that an image $\mathbf{v}_c(\mathbf{g})$ in a high-dimensional image space can be approximated with a k-dimensional weight vector $\mathbf{w}_c(\mathbf{g})$ in an eigenspace. Furthermore, the only images that need to be stored are the first k eigenvectors $\mathbf{e}_1, \ldots, \mathbf{e}_n$, which jointly define the eigenspace.

The eigenspace method seeks to reduce the dimensionality of an object manifold. Some recent appearance-based theories, however, take exactly the opposite approach, realizing that if the manifolds of different objects can be made far apart from each other, there will be no need to represent the manifolds in any detail. A simple hyperplane (a plane in a high-dimensional space) will be sufficient to partition the decision space into regions, with each containing at most one object manifold. SUPPORT VECTOR MACHINES (q.v.), for example, first map a set of known images to a high-dimensional *feature* space by passing them through a nonlinear transformation ψ. The dimensionality of this feature space can be arbitrarily high, making it possible for a hyperplane to separate one object's manifold from another. For each object, a support vector machine finds the *optimal* hyperplane in the feature space by maximizing the distance between the hyperplane and the object manifolds it tries to separate. Because such a hyperplane is fully determined by the points on the object manifolds that are closest to it, only those points, which are simply images, need to be stored. These images that determined the optimal hyperplanes are called *support vectors*. Conceptually, object recognition proceeds by first mapping an input image to a point in the feature space via ψ, and then deciding on which sides of the hyperplanes the input resides. Mathematically, this two-step process is equivalent to comparing the input image with the set of stored images (support vectors) using an *inner product kernel* function K, which relates to the nonlinear feature map ψ as $K(\mathbf{v}, \mathbf{v}_s) = \psi(\mathbf{v})^T\psi(\mathbf{v}_s)$. The inner product kernel $K(\mathbf{v}, \mathbf{v}_s)$ returns a scalar and can be thought of as a generalized similarity measure in the feature space between the unknown input image $\mathbf{v}$ and a set of stored image $\mathbf{v}_s$.

Two key features of an appearance-based theory distinguish it from the invariant-based approach. First, the stored representation of an object is often very close to the images of the object and does not possess a high degree of invariance. Second, invariant object decisions are achieved with some distance measure between the unknown input image and a sizable set of image-like representations that jointly define an object.

Decision Complexity and Representations

Each theory reviewed in the preceding section proposes one "final" representation used for object recognition. The theories differ in the amount of details the final representation retains. There is generally a trade-off between invariance (with an abstract representation) and discriminability (with an image-specific representation).

Regardless of the approach, an object recognition system has to decide which object manifold an input image belongs to. The decision task is easy if the object manifolds are (1) simple *and* (2) far apart. Historically, most object recognition theories, especially the invariant-based ones, have pursued the first factor. If successful, such an approach would have produced a general-purpose object representation that is appropriate regardless of the task or objects involved. However, if the manifolds for different objects intertwine, an attempt to reduce the manifolds' dimensionality can also make them indistinguishable from one another. Furthermore, the ever-present noise in the input can perturb the transformation processes required to map the input image to its final representation, leading to misidentification.

We refer to the extent to which object manifolds intertwine in the decision space as the *decision complexity*. Decision complexity is a function of the recognition task and the *set* of objects to be recognized. The decision complexity of telling two chickens apart is clearly different from that of recognizing a chicken from a fish. Tjan and Legge (1998) used a random sampling method to estimate the decision complexity in the image space for different sets of objects. Specifically, they measured the number of unprocessed raw images that an *ideal observer* operating according to Equation 2 would need to store in order to fully represent a set of objects. They found that decision complexity in the image space varied over two orders of magnitude across different types of objects and was highly dependent on what other objects were involved in the task. This result matches qualitatively to humans' varying difficulty in achieving viewpoint-invariant recognition across object sets.

In a practical object recognition system, the mapping between the image space and the decision space is highly nonlinear. Hence, decision complexity in the image space does not necessarily dictate decision complexity in the decision space. Intuition and practical experiences, however, suggest that the two are coupled. How intertwined the object manifolds are in the image space limits the minimum decision complexity one can practically attain in a decision space, after the noise in the input and visual processing has been accounted for. The wide range of image-space decision complexities observed by Tjan and Legge therefore implies that a general-purpose object recognition system cannot rely on a single form of representation for a wide range of tasks and objects.

Adaptive Selection of Representations

The idea that the human visual system may use multiple forms of representations is uncontroversial, but details are lacking. Specifically, what are the representations used by the human visual system, and how does the system decide which representation to use for a particular task? We make two observations (Tjan, 2001). First, to obtain a representation with a high degree of invariance, a series of processing stages are needed for feature extraction and the construction of higher-order features. This hierarchical processing architecture is common to most invariant- or model-based theories and is consistent with neurological findings about the visual system (Rolls and Deco, 2002). The intermediate output of each processing stage is in fact a representation at a particular level of abstraction. Thus, in the process of forming a representation with high degree of invariance, we obtain as "byproducts" a series of intermediate representations, each making a different trade-off between discriminability and invariance, each suitable for a recognition task of a different decision complexity. Second, if object decisions are made by the optimal strategy of maximizing posterior probabilities (i.e., Equation 2), or are approximately so, the magnitude of posterior probability $Pr(c|x)$ of the best choice can serve as a confidence measure regarding the decision (because posterior probabilities sum to one). The confidence of a decision can be low if (1) the representation is not detailed enough to make the discrimination, or (2) the representation is too detailed to attain a sufficient level of invariance for recognizing a novel input. Such a confidence measure can therefore be used to determine on-the-fly which level of representation is most appropriate for a given task.

Tjan (2001) proposed a simple architecture for object recognition that adaptively selects the most appropriate level of representation for a given task and objects. The architecture consists of a single visual processing pathway, loosely modular. Decision sites with local memory are attached to the processing modules along this pathway. Object-identity decision is made independently and in parallel at every decision site. The response latency of a site decreases with the maximum posterior probability evaluated at the site, but increases with the site's effective memory size. The first-arriving response from any site is taken to be the system's response. Simulation results showed that, although the intermediate representations were generic, the effective representation revealed behaviorally by the system appeared to be specific to the object category and task. The system showed an efficient trade-off between speed and accuracy, indicating that the object decisions were made at the appropriate level of abstraction.

Discussion

A great number of object recognition theories have been proposed in the past 30 years. While not all of them are biologically feasible, each provides important insight into the range of possible computations and representations for recognizing objects. Each theory makes a particular trade-off between discriminability and invariance. A system designed to discriminate similar objects is generally more sensitive to imaging conditions and requires a larger memory footprint to represent the objects than a system designed to discriminate highly dissimilar objects. Our analysis of decision complexity shows that it is unlikely for a single form of representation to be suitable for all kinds of object recognition tasks a human or other visual animals encounter each day. A key ingredient in a comprehensive brain theory for object recognition is therefore a computational framework that allows on-demand selection or adaptation of representations based on the task. To this end, we proposed a simple confidence-driven horse-racing scheme (a sort of first past the post, temporal winner-take-all scheme) for self-selecting the most appropriate level of abstraction, given a finite set of available representations along a visual processing pathway. Simulation results suggested that the framework is consistent with known behavioral and neurological data. We believe this framework is sufficiently simple and concrete for it to be biologically viable.

Road Map: Vision
Related Reading: Feature Analysis; Object Recognition, Neurophysiology; Object Structure, Visual Processing; Pattern Recognition; Visual Scene Perception

References

Basri, R., and Jacobs, D., 2001, Lambertian reflectance and linear subspaces, in *Proceedings of the IEEE 8th International Conference on Computer Vision*, Los Alamitos, CA: IEEE Computer Society Press, pp. 383–390.
Biederman, I., 1987, Recognition-by-components: A theory of human image understanding, *Psychol. Rev.*, 94:115–147.
Duda, R. O., and Hart, P. E., 1973, *Pattern Classification and Scene Analysis*, New York: Wiley.
Huttenlocher, D. P., and Ullman, S., 1990, Recognizing solid objects by alignment with an image, *Int. J. Comput. Vision*, 5:195–212.
Lades, M., Vorbrüggen, J. C., Buhmann, J., Lange, J., Von der Malsburg, C., Würtz, R. P., Konen, W., 1993, Distortion invariant object recognition in the dynamic link architecture, *IEEE Trans. Comput.*, 42:300–311.
Lee, K. C., Ho, J., and Kriegman, D., 2001, Nine points of light: Acquiring subspaces for face recognition under variable lighting, in *Proceedings of the IEEE Conference on Computer Vision and Pattern Recognition*, Los Alamitos, CA: IEEE Computer Society Press, pp. 519–526.
Lowe, D. G., 1987, Three-dimensional object recognition from single two-dimensional images, *Artif. Intell.*, 31:355–395.
Marr, D., 1982, *Vision*, New York: Freeman.
Mundy, J. L., and Zisserman, A., 1992, *Geometric Invariance in Computer Vision*, Cambridge, MA: MIT Press.
Murase, H., and Nayar, S. K., 1995, Visual learning and recognition of 3-D objects from appearance, *Int. J. Comput. Vision*, 14:5–24.
Poggio, T., and Edelman, S., 1990, A network that learns to recognize three-dimensional objects, *Nature*, 343:263–266.
Rolls, E. T., and Deco, G., 2002, *Computational Neuroscience of Vision*, New York: Oxford University Press.
Tjan, B. S., 2001, Adaptive object representation with hierarchically-distributed memory sites, in *Advances in Neural Information Processing Systems 13*, San Mateo, CA: Morgan Kaufmann, pp. 66–72.
Tjan, B. S., and Legge, G. E., 1998, The viewpoint complexity of an object recognition task, *Vision Res.*, 38:2335–2350.
Trucco, E., and Verri, A., 1998, *Introductory Techniques for 3-D Computer Vision*, Upper Saddle River, NJ: Prentice Hall.
Ullman, S., 1997, *High-level Vision*, Cambridge, MA: MIT Press.
Ullman, S., and Basri, R., 1991, Recognition by linear combinations of models, *IEEE Trans. Pattern Anal. Machine Intell.*, 13:992–1005.

Object Recognition, Neurophysiology

Guy Wallis and Heinrich H. Bülthoff

Introduction

As viewing distance, viewing angle, or lighting conditions change, so too does the image of an object that we see. Despite the seemingly endless variety of images that objects can project, the human visual system is able to rapidly and reliably identify those objects. How humans achieve this feat of recognition has long been a source of debate. Researchers have still not agreed on even the most fundamental questions of how objects are represented in cortex. This article provides a brief overview of some theoretical approaches in the context of mainly neurophysiological evidence. It also considers the related question of objects within a physical context, that is, the analysis of visual scenes. Scene analysis is relevant to the question of object recognition because scenes are initially recognized at a holistic, object-like level, providing a context or "gist" that itself influences the speed and accuracy of recognition of the constituent objects (Rensink, 2000). A precise characterization of gist remains elusive, but it may well include information such as global color patterns, spatial frequency content, correlational structure, or anything that is useful for categorizing or recognizing the scene.

To provide an anatomical framework for this chapter it is instructive to review the major functional divisions of visual cortex. Visual processing begins at the back of neocortex, in the occipital lobe. From there, information flows down into the temporal lobe, forming the ventral stream, and up into the parietal lobe, forming the dorsal stream (Figure 1). On the basis of neuropsychological and single-cell recording data, theorists have proposed a functional division between these streams. The dorsal stream is considered to process deciding "where" an object is and the ventral stream "what" an object is (Ungerleider and Haxby, 1994). In this article we mainly focus on the "what" stream, since it is seen as the center of object recognition, but an integrated model of scene perception will almost certainly require a broader approach encompassing all four lobes.

The Ventral Stream

The path from primary visual cortex to the inferior temporal lobe (IT) passes through as many as ten neural areas before reaching the last wholly visual areas (Figure 1). Early recordings of the temporal lobe indicated neurons selective for faces, and from later recordings workers were able to verify that these cells could not be excited by simple visual stimuli or as part of an emotional response to seeing a particular face (Rolls, 1992; Logothetis and Sheinberg, 1996).

One striking feature of the response properties of neurons in the IT is that the farther down the ventral stream one looks, the more specialized and selective the neurons become. Of special interest

to the field of object recognition was the discovery that along with increasing selectivity, many neurons become tolerant to shifts in stimulus position; changes in viewing angle, size/depth, or illumination; or the spatial frequencies present in the image (Rolls, 1992).

A great deal of this work originally had to do with neurons selective for faces, but although face cells account for as much as 20% of neurons in some regions of the IT and STS, they account for only about 5% of all cells present in IT cortex. In the early 1990s, Tanaka and his colleagues (Tanaka et al., 1991) showed that many of the remaining neurons are selective for complex combinations of features, including a basic shape with bounded light and shaded or colored bounded regions, and that these neurons also demonstrate useful invariance properties. This work has dispelled the idea of a special stream designed specifically for face recognition.

Recent work has focused on the issue of how the cellular response properties of temporal lobe neurons change over time. Several studies have shown that repeated exposure to a particular object class results in changes in the number of neurons selective for that stimulus (e.g., Rolls, 1992; Miyashita, 1993; Logothetis and Sheinberg, 1996). In humans, we should not be surprised to learn that a car enthusiast has neurons tuned to the appearance of a yellow VW Beetle, or that a lepidopterist has neurons tuned to an Orange Tip butterfly.

The Dorsal Stream

Abstracting an object's form from its precise location, size, or orientation is clearly important for tasks such as recognition and categorization. However, there are plenty of situations in which an object's location and orientation are important, not least when we want to interact with that object by picking it up or manipulating it. The processing of location and orientation appears to be the major concern of neurons in the parietal lobe. These neurons form part of the dorsal stream. In humans, damage to the parietal lobe severely affects the localization of objects within a scene, leading to disorders such as visual neglect, and it appears that the dorsal stream is intrinsically linked to the control of visual attention and eye movements (Ungerleider and Haxby, 1994).

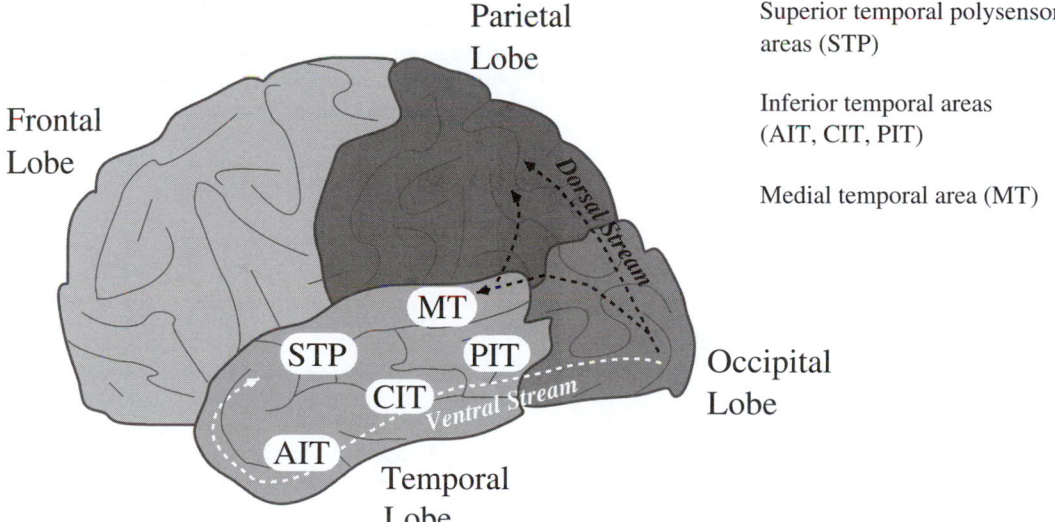

Superior temporal polysensor areas (STP)

Inferior temporal areas (AIT, CIT, PIT)

Medial temporal area (MT)

Figure 1. Principle divisions of neocortex, including the main areas of the temporal lobe. Dark arrows indicate information flow along the dorsal stream. Light arrow indicates flow along the ventral stream.

Of course, many tasks require the interaction of the two types of information, both where and what an object is. Our lepidopterist would like to be able to net a Tortoiseshell fluttering among Red Admirals. This raises an as yet unanswered question, namely, how these types of information interact and where various representations are held. It turns out that there are plenty of routes that information could take between the temporal and parietal lobes, including a direct route, via the occipital lobe or the frontal lobe. It has been shown, for example, that regions AIT and CIT of IT (see Figure 1) connect to the frontal lobe, and CIT and PIT connect to the parietal lobe (Webster, Bachevalier, and Ungerleider, 1994). One aim of any modeling work must be to investigate the possible siginificance of these connections.

A Processing Hierarchy

One of the striking features of the ventral stream is its hierarchical structure. Neurons in the regions of the temporal lobe furthest from the retina can be thought of as sitting on top of a processing pyramid (Figure 2). Receptive field size grows steadily larger the farther up this pyramid one looks, and the response times of neurons also rise systematically (Rolls, 1992).

One possible explanation for the presence of such a hierarchy is that the visual system is gradually building representations of ever-increasing complexity to produce neurons that respond to combinations of inputs, themselves forming the effective stimuli for later neurons. By responding to local combinations of neurons co-active in the previous layer, arbitrary spatial arrangements of the same features should fail to activate the same neuron. This should then reduce the chance of finding the trigger features supporting recognition in random arrangements of the features, an issue often referred to as the "feature-binding problem." Some of the most selective and view-invariant responses belong to cells in the superior temporal areas. These neurons appear to pool the outputs of view-selective AIT cells. One explanation of how the STPa neurons know which AIT neurons to group together is discussed in the next section.

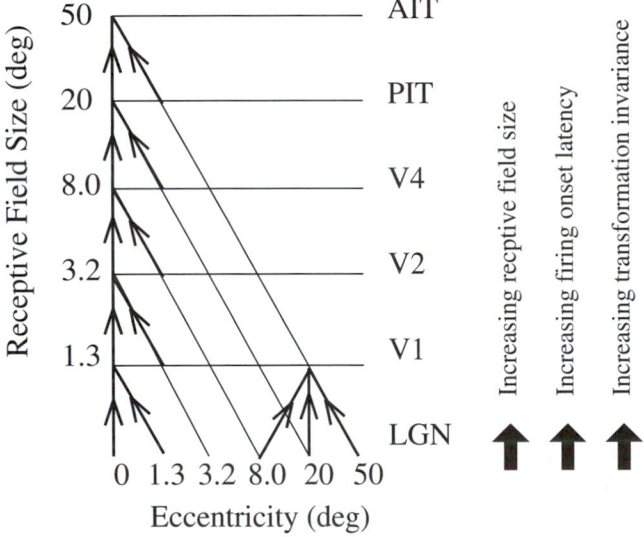

Figure 2. Schematic of convergence in the ventral processing stream. The steady growth in receptive field size suggests that neurons in one layer of the hierarchy receive input from a select group of neurons in the preceding layer. The time taken for the effects of seeing a new visual stimulus increases systematically through the hierarchy, supporting the notion of a strictly layered structure.

Neuroanatomists tell us that there are at least as many connections running back as there are running forward in the ventral stream, and this is important when one comes to devise models. The precise use of these connections remains unclear. Some theorists have argued that they are used in recall, and it is true that the act of remembering visual events causes activity to spread into primary visual areas. They may also control visual attention. Certainly attending to specific regions of the visual environment has been shown to facilitate the processing of signals in topographically matched regions of visual cortex, which may well be due to selectively raising the activity (or lowering the activation thresholds) of neurons along the processing hierarchy. One important role that the connections almost certainly do play is in relaying "top-down" influences on recognition, due to expectations or selective attention, perhaps prompted by the gist of a scene. Such influences include contextual priors, which in this case are functions that govern the likelihood of seeing a particular object in a particular context. Our lepidopterist will implicitly change these priors with habitat, improving the chances of correctly distinguishing a Caper White in the rocky bush of South Australia from a Cabbage White on the meadows of southern England.

Some have argued that the backward-projecting connections, apart from their role in relaying attentional mechanisms, play an integral role in normal visual processing. Some have gone so far as to suggest that each neural region forms a recurrent attractor network, each connected through the cortex, up to and including the temporal lobe. Although such models may be needed to deal with confusing or low-quality images, there is good evidence that timing constraints prohibit such a model from acting during the rapid recognition of everyday, familiar objects (Thorpe, Fize, and Marlot, 1996).

Encoding Objects in the Temporal Lobe

Despite the apparent selectivity of temporal lobe neurons, it is important to realize that they are not "grandmother cells" selective for a single entity (such as your grandmother) in the manner proposed in early theories of object representation. On the contrary, many of the cells reported in the literature responded to several examples of objects within their particular object category. Evidence is emerging that object encoding is achieved via small ensembles of firing cells that efficiently and robustly code for individual objects.

Under a distributed scheme, many hundreds or thousands of neurons, each selective for its specific feature, would act together to represent an object. Although many of these features represent only small regions of an object, others appear to represent an object's outline, or some other global but general property. In addition, the neural representation of these features is more sophisticated than a simple template, since they may exhibit invariance to scale and size, something typical of temporal lobe neurons.

Implementing representation in a distributed code brings with it several advantages. First, the representations are robust to cell damage: since hundreds or thousands of neurons react to the presence of a single object, the death of one neuron within the ensemble will not adversely affect recognition accuracy or speed. Second, a distributed representation provides immediate recognition generalization to novel stimuli: a new object can be represented distinctly from all other stimuli by using a unique combination of the many well-established feature-selective neurons already present. In so doing, each neuron brings knowledge of how its feature changes in appearance with changes in viewpoint. The numerous beneficial, emergent properties of a distributed representation have long been realized by neural network theorists (see POPULATION CODES).

In addition to the general encoding and topological organization of IT cortex, work has also been carried out to establish what functional organization might be present. Some researchers have made moves to describe the functional organization of IT. Cells were tested and their key stimulating features characterized, revealing a columnar structure in which groups of neurons appear to respond to similar though subtly different collections of features. Neighboring columns seem to have less in common. This work in part replicates the findings of other researchers who have described localized "clusters" or "patches" of face cells (see Rolls, 1992), and the findings have been taken by some as evidence for local excitatory and more diverse inhibitory connections within the processing layers, akin to those used in competitive networks (see Wallis and Bülthoff, 1999; Riesenhuber and Poggio, 2000).

Models of Object Representation and Recognition

A huge number of systems for object recognition have been proposed over the years. Some were inspired by the desire to build intelligent machines, others by the desire to describe human recognition processes. This section summarizes some of the popular models and their relevance, or otherwise, to human object recognition. Extensive reference lists can be found in review articles on the topic by Wallis and Bülthoff (1999) and Riesenhuber and Poggio (2000).

One family of models, which owes its heritage to artificial intelligence research in the 1970s, sees the need to extract cues to three-dimensional (3D) structure. Using texture gradients, linear perspective, structure from motion, and so on, models in this family seek to transform the retinal image into a full-fledged internal 3D model capable of rotation, scaling, and translation and therefore matching to a store of known objects. Various means for achieving this reconstruction have been proposed, although perhaps the most preeminent is the geon theory of Biedermann and its associated network model, called JIM (see OBJECT STRUCTURE, VISUAL PROCESSING). Unfortunately, although there are plenty of neurons sensitive to cues such as terminated edges or complex forms of motion, neurophysiologists have yet to find evidence for large quantities of the types of neural analyzers that this type of models would predict, and even less evidence for the set of 36 3D volumetric building blocks that Biederman's theory claims are combined to represent all objects. What is more, there is only limited evidence for the neural synchronization mechanism that it uses to bind elements of activated geons, and there is no evidence of neurons purely selective for the spatial relationships of parts, such as "left of," "above," and so on. Nonetheless, some form of structural representation must surely exist, particularly in defining object categories for distinguishing a quadruped from a biped, or a telephone from an elephant. The JIM model is one of the very few models focused on human object recognition that provides a principled means of extracting and representing structure.

As an alternative to this type of bottom-up object reconstruction, a number of approaches to object recognition have considered the possibility of matching the incoming image to a large collection of 2D images or whole 3D objects. This process takes a number of different forms. In some models the image of the object is normalized for size and location and then simply matched pixel by pixel to a stored set of images. Of course, simple 3D transformations such as depth rotation lead to nontrivial changes in the 2D projected image. To compensate for this, some models have employed local distortions of the incoming image in the matching process. Others have presupposed an ability to extract 3D anchor points in the image that allow stored 3D representations to be rotated and scaled in 3D before the matching process begins. In practice, most of these models work well on predefined sets of objects and small changes in appearance, but they are prone to errors if the incoming image changes considerably. Models that employ local distortion or rotation algorithms are more robust, but this robust-

ness comes at a cost. The models are slow and become slower the more objects are stored in the internal library. The simplest form of 2D template matching is at least fast, and if the process proceeds in parallel, it can scale extremely well as the number of objects increases. However, where all of these models fall down is in explaining our ability to categorize and generalize recognition of new objects to changes in viewing direction.

A possible solution to this final problem is based on a further alternative model for how objects are represented and recognized. This approach once again suggests that objects are stored as images or multiple views (Bülthoff and Edelman, 1992). However, rather than being stored as a single template, each view is represented as a collection of small picture elements, each tolerant to small view changes (Wallis and Bülthoff, 1999; Riesenhuber and Poggio, 2000). Such a system immediately reaps the benefits of a distributed encoding system in terms of robustness and transformation generalization for novel objects; it also accords with the types of neural response properties known to exist in the ventral stream.

In practice, many systems base recognition on a combination of pictorial features. Some have simply attempted to look across the entire image for telltale features, irrespective of relative position, as evidence for the presence of one object rather than another. Of course, models that throw away spatial information in this way run into the problem of "recognizing" random rearrangements of the features triggering recognition. This is not the case for real neurons responsive to faces, which often reduce their response to faces in which the features appear jumbled up (Rolls, 1992; Logothetis and Sheinberg, 1996). Nor is it true for cells responsive to more abstract features (Tanaka et al., 1991); indeed, this is an example of the feature-binding problem. As described earlier in this article, one solution to this problem is to combine features gradually over a series of stages, achieving translation invariance step by step. This has inspired many theorists to take this approach in object recognition. One of the first to construct a truly hierarchical model was Fukushima (1980). His neocognitron is an elegant example of how piecewise combinations of features can lead to comprehensive translation and scale invariance while at the same time retaining object specificity, thereby avoiding one form of the feature-binding problem. Fukushima's ideas accord well both with elements of the known neurophysiology of the ventral stream and a view-based scheme of object representation, and has inspired a whole series of models (see Wallis and Rolls, 1997; Riesenhuber and Poggio, 2000). The Riesenhuber and Poggio paper also describes their development of Fukushima's model and how it predicts the use of a nonlinear weighting mechanism on the inputs to neurons of each layer. Wallis and Rolls describe their own model, which is once again hierarchical and convergent but simpler in structure. Despite its simplicity, it has been shown to be able to learn invariant representations of objects without recourse to nonlocal learning mechanisms, supervised learning, specialist neural populations, or specific, prescribed connectivity. An important omission from such models is any explicit representation of object structure. As mentioned earlier, structure may well be important for higher levels of categorization, for distinguishing broad categories such as insects from mammals. Image-based approaches, on the other hand, are probably of more importance for within-category discrimination, such as discriminating a Peacock butterfly from a Meadow Brown. For more on this and related issues, see OBJECT RECOGNITION.

Another aspect that the hierarchical feedforward models lack is an account of the effects of top-down information due to expectation or selective attention. As such they really only deal with recognition within the high-acuity center of the visual field and would require some other mechanism for locating and fixating objects. One hierarchical model that does consider this has been described by Olhausen, Anderson, and van Essen (1993). It selects targets by controlling the breadth and number of pathways present in the model's hierarchy. Recognition is achieved using a classical object-matching algorithm, which suffers from the disadvantages noted earlier, but the model does provide insight into a possible mechanism for object selection, and with it an additional solution to the problem of translation and scale invariance.

Temporal Order

Although it is possible to conceive of the ventral stream building features to represent individual views of objects, the question still remains as to how neurons learn to treat their preferred feature as the same, irrespective of size or location. Indeed, ultimately, one would like to understand how neurons learn to recognize objects as they undergo nontrivial transformations, perhaps due to changes in viewing direction or lighting.

One solution to this problem is to assume that each neuron receives some external information as to the identity of a particular stimulus. Of course, this simply begs the question of where this information originates in the first place. To describe a potential solution, it is worth reflecting on what clues our environment gives us about how to associate the stream of images that we see in everyday life. Recently, several theorists have argued that our natural environment provides a temporal cue to object identity. This cue emerges from the simple fact that we often study objects for extended periods. This then provides us with a simple heuristic for deciding how to associate novel images of objects with stored object representations. Since objects are often seen over extended periods, any unrecognized view coming straight after a recognized one is most probably of the same object. This heuristic will work as long as accidental associations from one object to another are random and associations from one view of an object to another are experienced regularly. There is every reason to suppose that this is actually what will happen under normal viewing conditions, and that by approaching an object, watching it move, or rotating it in our hand we will receive a consistent associative signal capable of bringing all of the views of the object together.

It was Miyashita (1993) who discovered that many neurons within IT cortex had developed selectivity for small sets of fractal images that he had been using in a short-term memory task. Although this task did not explicitly require the overall test sequence to be remembered, Miyashita noted that these neurons consistently responded well to single images that neighbored one another in the test sequence. For example, one neuron might respond preferentially to images 5, 6, and 7, whereas another neuron responded to images 37, 38, and 39. The fact that the images were generated randomly meant that there was no particular reason—on the grounds of spatial similarity—why these images should have become associated together by a single neuron. Instead, the results indicate the importance of temporal order in controlling the learning of neural selectivity. Recent studies of human recognition learning have found evidence for such a mechanism as well (Wallis and Bülthoff, 2001). Taken together, the two sources of evidence provide important preliminary support for the temporal association hypothesis (Wallis and Bülthoff, 1999). Several network models have made successful use of the temporal cue to view association, and it forms the core of learning in the model described by Wallis and Rolls (1997).

Discussion

This article has reviewed much of the current thinking on object recognition. In particular, it has proposed the presence of a distributed, view-based representation in which objects are recognized on the basis of multiple, 2D feature-selective neurons. Specialist cells appear to play a role in associating such feature combinations into

certain nontrivial image transformations, coding for a certain percentage of all stimuli in a largely view-invariant manner. The article has also pointed to evidence that a convergent hierarchy is used to build invariant representations over several stages, and that at each stage lateral competitive processes are at work between the neurons.

We have argued that temporal association could act as a cue for associating views of objects. If such a mechanism exists, it could only work in the ventral stream, since it would *not* be appropriate in the dorsal visual system, where motion and location are processed (Ungerleider and Haxby, 1994). Indeed, the importance of using temporal association in invariant object recognition, and the importance of not making such associations in the part of the visual system involved in processing motion and location, might be a fundamental reason for keeping these two processing streams apart.

We have touched on the analysis of visual scenes both within and beyond the ventral stream. Although much has been said about the roles of the parietal and temporal lobes, relatively little has been said about the frontal lobe. We do know that it acts as a temporary or working memory store, and that neurons within the frontal lobe are responsive to combinations of both where and what an object is. It may well turn out that the frontal lobe acts as a running store of objects currently being represented within a scene (Rensink, 2000). A challenge for models in the future will be to integrate the frontal lobe into the overall picture of scene analysis.

Road Map: Vision
Related Reading: Cortical Hebbian Modules; Fast Visual Processing; Object Recognition; Object Structure, Visual Processing; Visual Scene Perception, Neurophysiology

References

Bülthoff, H., and Edelman, S., 1992, Psychophysical support for a two-dimensional view interpolation theory of object recognition, *Proc. Natl. Acad. Sci. USA*, 92:60–64. ◆

Fukushima, K., 1980, Neocognitron: A self-organizing neural network model for a mechanism of pattern recognition unaffected by shift in position, *Biol. Cybern.*, 36:193–202.

Logothetis, N. K., and Sheinberg, D. L., 1996, Visual object recognition, *Annu. Rev. Neurosci.*, 19:577–621. ◆

Miyashita, Y., 1993, Inferior temporal cortex: Where visual perception meets memory, *Annu. Rev. Neurosci.*, 16:245–263. ◆

Olhausen, B. A., Anderson, C. H., and van Essen, D. C., 1993, A neurobiological model of visual attention and invariant pattern recognition based on dynamic routing of information, *J. Neurosci.*, 13:4700–4719.

Rensink, R. A., 2000, The dynamic representation of scenes, *Vis. Cognit.*, 7:17–42. ◆

Riesenhuber, M., and Poggio, T., 2000, Models of object recognition, *Nature Neurosci.*, 3:1199–1204.

Rolls, E. T., 1992, Neurophysiological mechanisms underlying face processing within and beyond the temporal cortical areas, *Philos. Trans. R. Soc. Lond. B*, 335:11–21.

Tanaka, K., Saito, H., Fukada, Y., and Moriya, M., 1991, Coding visual images of objects in the inferotemporal cortex of the macaque monkey, *J. Neurophysiol.*, 66:170–189.

Thorpe, S., Fize, D., and Marlot, C., 1996, Speed of processing in the human visual system, *Nature*, 381:520–522.

Ungerleider, L. G., and Haxby, J. V., 1994, "What" and "where" in the human brain, *Curr. Opin. Neurobiol.*, 4:157–165. ◆

Wallis, G., and Bülthoff, H. H., 1999, Learning to recognize objects, *Trends Cognit. Sci.*, 3:22–31. ◆

Wallis, G., and Bülthoff, H. H., 2001, Effects of temporal association on recognition memory, *Proc. Natl. Acad. Sci.*, 98:4800–4804.

Wallis, G., and Rolls, E. T., 1997, A model of invariant object recognition in the visual system, *Progr. Neurobiol.*, 51:167–194.

Webster, M. J., Bachevalier, J., and Ungerleider, L. G., 1994, Connections of inferior temporal areas TEO and TE with parietal and frontal-cortex in macaque monkeys, *Cerebr. Cortex*, 4:470–483.

Object Structure, Visual Processing

Shimon Edelman and Nathan Intrator

A Functional Characterization of Structure Processing

A computational-level analysis of the processes dealing with object and scene structure requires that we first identify the common functional characteristics of structure-related behavioral tasks. In other problems in high-level vision, effective functional characterization typically led to advances in the computational understanding, and to better modeling, of the relevant aspects of the human visual system. In the study of visual motion, for example, realization of the central role of the correspondence problem constituted just such an advance. Likewise, object recognition tasks, such as identification or categorization, have at their core a common operation, namely, the matching of the stimulus against a stored memory trace.

For the structure-processing tasks, a good candidate for the signature common characteristic is the *restriction of the spatial scope* of at least some of the operations involved to some fraction of the visual extent of the object or scene under consideration. In other words, a task should qualify for the label "structural" only if it calls for a separate treatment of some *fragment(s)* of the stimulus (and not merely of the whole). Here are a few examples of behavioral tasks that qualify as structural according to this criterion:

- *Given two objects, or an object and a class prototype, identify their corresponding regions*. The correspondence here may be based on local shape similarity (find the eyes of a face in a Cubist painting), or on similar role played by the regions in the global structure (find the eyes in a smiley icon).
- *Given an object and an action, identify a region in the object toward which the action can be directed*. Similarities between objects vis à vis this task are defined functionally (as in the parallel that can be drawn between the handle of a pan and a door handle: both afford grasping).
- *Given an object, describe its structure*. This explicitly structural task arises in the context of trying to make sense of an unfamiliar object (as in perceiving a hot-air balloon, upon seeing it for the first time, as a pear-like shape over a box-like one).

The characterization of structure processing in terms of scope-restricted spatial analysis mechanisms has two immediate implications. Consider, on the one hand, the *appearance-based* computational approaches to recognition and categorization, according to which objects are represented by collections of entire, spatially unanalyzed views. Because of the holistic nature of the representations they rely on, these approaches are seen to be incapable, in principle, of supporting structure processing (Hummel, 2000). On the other hand, the "classical" *structural decomposition* approaches (Biederman, 1987) have the opposite tendency: the recursive symbolic structure they impose on objects seems too rigid and too elaborate, compared to the basic principle of spatial analysis proposed above, which requires merely that the spatial scope of each of its operators be limited to a fragment of the visual scene.

Object Form Processing in Computer Vision

Until recently, the attainment of classical structural descriptions has been widely considered to be the ultimate goal of object form processing in computer vision. The specific notion that the structural descriptions are to be expressed in terms of volumetric parts, popularized by Marr (1982), was subsequently adopted by Biederman (1987), who developed it into a (psychological) theory of recog-

nition by components (RBC). In Biederman's formulation, the representation is explicitly *compositional*: it consists of symbols that stand for generic parts (called "geons"); the symbols are drawn from a small repertoire and are bound together by categorical symbolically coded relations (such as "above" or "to the left of"). RBC's compositional nature is explicit in a sense stressed by Fodor and McLaughlin (1990): a classical structural description of an entire object necessarily contains *tokenings* of its (stipulated) constituent parts, in the same sense that a sentence considered as a concatenation of some words necessarily contains each and every of its words in their original, unchanged format (see COMPOSITIONALITY IN NEURAL SYSTEMS).

By virtue of their compositionality, the classical structural descriptions meet the two main challenges in the processing of structure: productivity and systematicity. A visual system is productive if it is open-ended, that is, if it can deal effectively with a potentially infinite set of objects. A visual representation is systematic if a well-defined change in the spatial configuration of the object, such as swapping top and bottom parts, causes a principled change in the representation, such as the interchange of the representations of top and bottom parts. Compositionality, however, has its cost. The requirement that object parts be "crisp" and relations syntactically compositional is a principle that may be appealing (by analogy with an intuitive view of the language faculty that it embodies), but is difficult to adhere to in practice. Indeed, in computer vision, a panel of experts deemed the structural analysis of raw images (as opposed to the analysis of symbolically specified line drawings of Biederman's examples) to be unpromising: "the principal problems with this approach seem to be the difficulty in extracting sufficiently good line drawings, and the idealized nature of the geon representation" (Dickinson et al., 1997, p. 284).

Both of these problems can be effectively neutralized by giving up the classical compositional representation of shape by a fixed alphabet of crisp "all-or-none" explicitly tokened primitives (such as geons) in favor of a fuzzy, superpositional coarse-coding by an open-ended set of image fragments. This alternative approach has met with considerable success in computer vision. For example, the system described by Nelson and Selinger (1998) starts by detecting contour segments, then determines whether their relative arrangement approximates that of a model object. Because none of the individual segment shapes or locations is critical to the successful description of the entire shape, this method does not suffer from the brittleness associated with the classical structural description models of recognition. Moreover, the tolerance for moderate variation in the segment shape and location data allows it to categorize novel members of familiar object classes (Nelson and Selinger, 1998).

In a similar fashion, the method of Burl, Weber, and Perona (1998) combines "local photometry" (shape primitives that are approximate templates for small snippets of images) with "global geometry" (the probabilistic quantification of spatial relations between pairs or triplets of primitives). In general, such methods use snippets of images taken from objects to be recognized to represent these objects; recognition is declared if at least some of the fragments are reliably detected, and if the spatial relations among these fragments conform to the stored description of the target. In all of these methods, the interplay of loosely defined local shape ("what") and approximate location ("where") information leads to robust algorithms supporting both recognition and categorization. These same methods may also lead to the development of an effective alternative to the classical structural description approach to object form, provided that they can be extended to support hierarchical treatment of shape details across spatial scales.

Mechanisms Implicated in Structure Processing in Primate Vision

In theoretical neuroscience, ideas advanced to explain structure processing by the primate visual system can be roughly divided into two groups, following the distinction made in the preceding discussion between the classical crisp part-based compositional methods and the fuzzy fragment-based *what + where* approach. The two kinds of theories invoke distinct neural mechanisms to explain the manner in which object constituents (whether explicitly tokened crisp parts or fuzzy superimposed fragments) are (1) represented individually and (2) bound together to form the whole.

Consider the classical theories built around the syntactic compositionality idea (Biederman, 1987). First, these theories require that "crisply" defined geon-like parts and categorical relations be explicitly represented on the neural level. Although no evidence seems to exist for the neural embodiment of geons as such, there are reports that cells in the inferotemporal (IT) cortex exhibit a higher sensitivity to "nonaccidental" visual features than to "metric" properties of the stimuli; nonaccidental features such as curvature sign or parallelism of contours are used to define geons, because of their diagnosticity and invariance to viewpoint changes. Second, the classical theories hold that symbols representing the parts are bound into the proper structure dynamically, by the synchronous firing of the neurons that code each symbol. Thus, a mechanism capable of supporting dynamic binding must be available; it is possible that this function is fulfilled by the synchronous or phase-locked firing of cortical neurons (see SYNCHRONIZATION, BINDING, AND EXPECTANCY), although the status of this phenomenon in primates has been disputed.

The alternative theory, proposed by Edelman and Intrator (2000), calls for an open-ended set of fuzzy fragments instead of geons. The role of fragment detectors may be fulfilled by those neurons in the IT cortex that respond selectively to some particular views of an object or to a specific shape irrespective of view (Logothetis and Sheinberg, 1996). This very kind of shape-selective response may also constitute the neural basis of *binding by retinotopy*, an idea based on the observation (Edelman, 1994) that the visual field itself can serve as the frame encoding the relative positions of object fragments, simply because each such fragment is already localized within that frame when it is detected. The binding by retinotopy is possible if the receptive field of each cell is confined to some relatively limited portion of the entire visual field (as per the definition of the signature characteristic of structural processing proposed in the Introduction). Neurons with such response properties have been found in the IT cortex (Op de Beeck and Vogels, 2000) and in the prefrontal cortex, where they were called *what + where* cells (Rao, Rainer, and Miller, 1997).

Neuromorphic Models of Visual Structure Processing

We now proceed to outline two implemented models of structure representation in primate vision. The first of these, JIM.3 (Hummel, 2001), exemplifies the classical compositional approach, and the second, Chorus of Fragments, or CoF (Edelman and Intrator, 2000), the alternative one just discussed.

The JIM.3 model is structured as an eight-layer network (Figure 1). The first three layers extract local features: contours, vertices and axes of symmetry, and surface properties. Surfaces are represented in terms of five categorical properties: (1) elliptical or not; (2) possessing parallel, expanding, convex, or concave axes of symmetry; (3) possessing a curved or a straight major axis; (4) truncated or pointed; and (5) planar or curved in 3D. Units coding these

local features group themselves into representations of geons by synchrony of firing. These representations are then routed by the units of layer 4 to two distinct destinations in layer 5. The first of these is a population of units coding for geons and spatial relations that are independent or "disembodied" in the sense that each of them may have originated from any location within the image. Within this population, the emergence of a representation of the object's structure requires dynamic binding, which the model stipulates to be carried out under attentional guidance and to take a relatively long time (a few hundred milliseconds).

The second destination of the outgoing connections of layer 4 is a population of geon units arranged in the form of a retinotopic map. Here, the relations between the geons are coded implicitly, by virtue of each representation unit residing in the proper location within the map, which reflects the location of the corresponding geon in the image. In contrast to the attention-controlled stream, this one can operate much faster, and is postulated to be able to form a structural representation in a few tens of milliseconds. This speed and automaticity have a price: because of the fixed spatial structure imposed by the retinotopic map, the representation this stream supports is more sensitive to object transformations such as rotation in depth and reflection (Hummel, 2001).

The other implemented model we outline here, the Chorus of Fragments (CoF) model, exemplifies the coarse-coded fragment-based approach to the representation of structure (Edelman and Intrator, 2000, 2001). It simulates cells with *what + where* receptive fields to represent object fragments and uses attentional *gain fields*, such as those found in area V4 (Connor et al., 1997), to decouple the representation of object structure from its location in the visual field (the gain field of a neuron refers to those locations where the presence of a secondary stimulus modulates the cell's response to the primary stimulus shown within the classical receptive field; in this case, the modulation is exerted by shifting the focus of attention).

Unlike JIM.3, the CoF system operates directly on gray-level images, preprocessed by a front end that is a rough simulation of the primary visual cortex. The system illustrated in Figure 2 contains two *what + where* units, one (labeled "above center") responsible for the top fragment of the object (as extracted by an appropriately configured Gaussian gain field), and the other (labeled "below center") responsible for the bottom fragment. The units are trained jointly for three-way discrimination, for translation tolerance, and for autoassociation. Figure 3 shows the performance of a CoF system charged with learning to reuse fragments of the members of the training set (three bipartite objects composed of numeral shapes) in interpreting novel composite objects. The gain field mechanism allowed it to respond largely systematically to the learned fragments shown in novel locations, both absolute and relative.

The CoF model offers a unified framework for understanding the functional significance of *what + where* receptive fields and of attentional gain modulation. It extends the previous use of gain fields in the modeling of translation invariance, and highlights a parallel between *what + where* cells and probabilistic fragment-based approaches to structure representation in computer vision, such as that of Burl et al. (1998). The representational framework it embodies is both productive and effectively systematic. It is capable, as a matter of principle, of recognizing such objects that are related through a rearrangement of "middle-scale" fragments, without the need for dynamic binding, and without being taught those fragments individually. When coupled with statistical inference methods such as the Minimum Description Length principle, this model may be capable of unsupervised learning of useful fragments, an issue that is currently under investigation (Edelman and Intrator, 2001). Further testing is also needed to determine whether or not the CoF model can be scaled up to learn larger collections

Figure 1. The architecture of the JIM.3 model (Hummel, 2001). The model had been trained on a single view (actually, a line drawing) of each of 20 objects—hammer, scissors, and so on—as well as on some "nonsense" objects. It was then tested on translated, scaled, reflected, and rotated (in the image plane) versions of the same images. The model exhibited a pattern of results consistent with a range of psychophysical data obtained from human subjects (Hummel, 2001). Specifically, the categorization performance was invariant with respect to translation and scaling, and was reduced by rotation. Moreover, because of the dual nature of the binding process in JIM.3—dynamic and static/retinotopic—the model behaved differently when given attended and unattended objects: reflected images primed each other in the former case, but not in the latter case. (Figure courtesy of J. E. Hummel.)

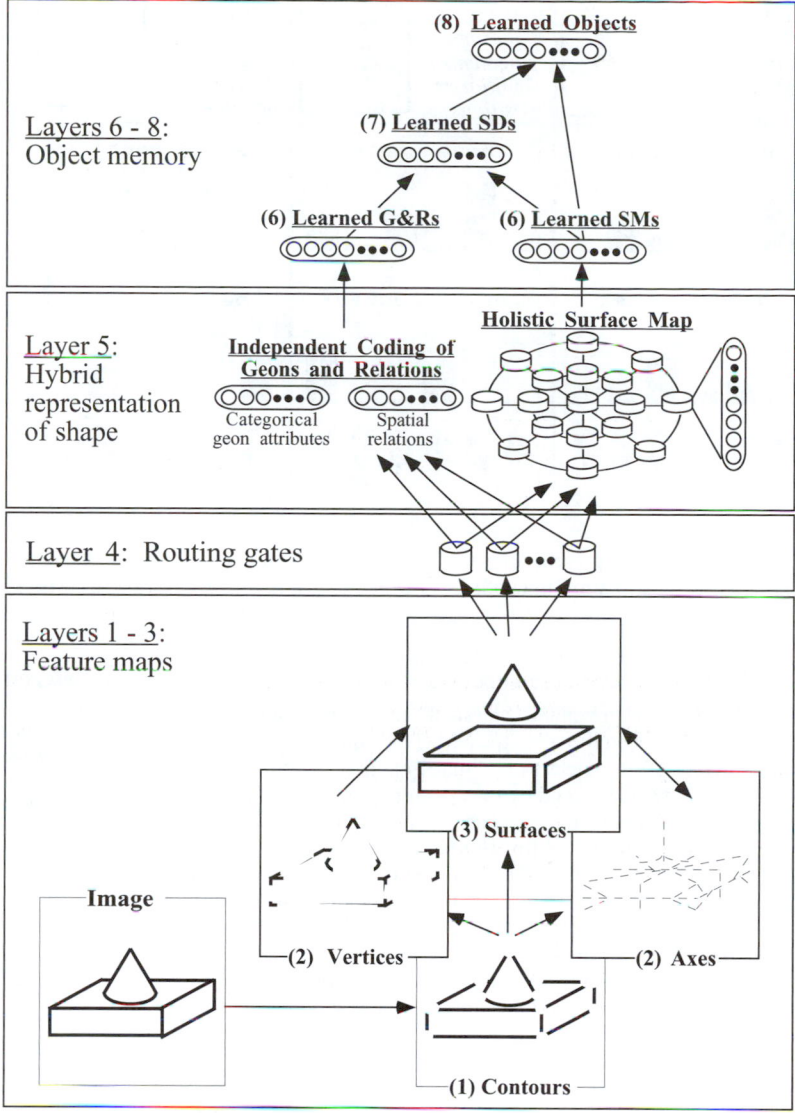

Figure 2. The CoF model, trained on three composite objects (numerals 4 over 5, 3 over 6, and 2 over 7). The model consists of two *what* + *where* units, responsible for the top and the bottom fragments of the stimulus, respectively. Gain fields (boxes labeled "below center" and "above center") steer each input fragment to the appropriate unit. The learning mechanism (R/C, for Reconstruction and Classification) can be implemented either as a multilayer perceptron or as a radial basis function network. The reconstruction error (Δ) modulates the classification outputs and helps the system learn binding (a co-activation pattern over units of the preceding stage will have a small reconstruction error only if both its *what* and *where* aspects are correct).

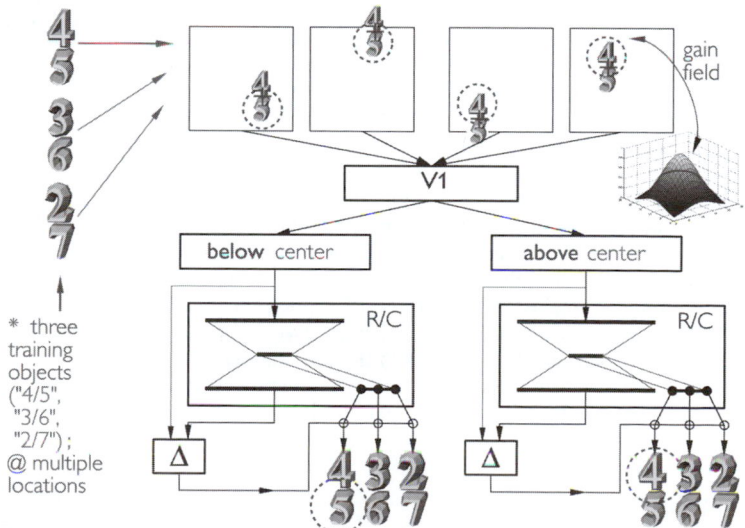

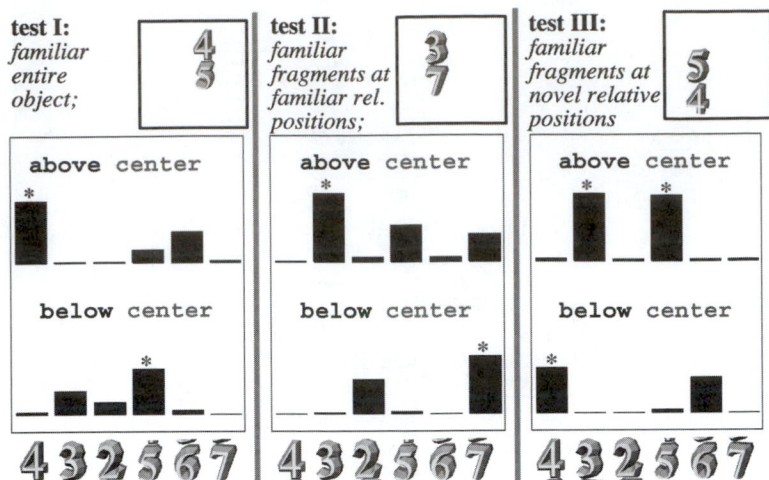

Figure 3. The response of the CoF model to a familiar composite object at a novel location (test I) and to novel compositions of fragments of familiar objects (tests II and III). In the test scenario, each unit ("above" and "below") must be fed each of the two input fragments ("above" and "below"); hence the 12 bars in the plots of the model's output.

of objects, and to represent finer structure, under realistic transformations such as rotation in depth.

Conclusions

For decades, the prevalent "classical" theory of visual structure processing has been rooted in the perceived computational need for the structure of an object to be "made explicit" to enable its recognition (Marr, 1982), and by the apparent uniqueness of the compositional solution to the problems of productivity and systematicity (Fodor and McLaughlin, 1990).

The first of these two issues is made moot by recent advances in computer vision, which indicate that neither recognition nor categorization requires a prior derivation of a classical structural description. Moreover, making structure explicit may not be a good idea, either from a philosophical viewpoint or from a practical one. On the philosophical level, it embodies a gratuitous ontological commitment to the existence of object parts, which are presumed to be waiting for detection by the visual system; on the practical level, reliable detection of such parts has proved to be an elusive goal. The second issue, focusing on productivity and systematicity of structure processing, is also being transformed at present by claims that a system can be productive and systematic without relying on representations that are compositional in the classical sense (Edelman and Intrator, 2000).

The alternative stance on these issues, discussed in the preceding sections, holds that structure can be represented by a coarse code based on image fragments that are bound together by retinotopy. This notion is supported by the success of computer vision methods (such as "local photometry, global geometry"), by data from neurophysiological studies in primates (such as the discovery of *what + where* cells), and by psychological findings and metatheoretical considerations not mentioned in this article (Edelman and Intrator, 2000). In the field of neuromorphic modeling, these developments have brought about a curious convergence between an approach initially grounded in classical structural description theory (Hummel, 2001) and that derived from a holistic view of object representation (Edelman and Intrator, 2001). In this rapidly changing field, the theoretical and factual aspects of structure processing (but, we believe, not the metatheoretical ones) are likely to require reconsideration on a regular basis.

Road Map: Vision
Background: Feature Analysis

Related Reading: Object Recognition; Object Recognition, Neurophysiology; Synchronization, Binding and Expectancy

References

Biederman, I., 1987, Recognition by components: A theory of human image understanding, *Psychol. Rev.*, 94:115–147.

Burl, M. C., Weber, M., and Perona, P., 1998, A probabilistic approach to object recognition using local photometry and global geometry, in *Proceedings of the 4th European Conference on Computing and Vision* (H. Burkhardt and B. Neumann, Eds.), LNCS series, vol. 1406–1407, Berlin: Springer-Verlag, pp. 628–641.

Connor, C. E., Preddie, D. C., Gallant, J. L., and Van Essen, D. C., 1997, Spatial attention effects in macaque area V4, *J. Neurosci.*, 17:3201–3214.

Dickinson, S., Bergevin, R., Biederman, I., Eklundh, J., Munck-Fairwood, R., Jain, A., and Pentland, A., 1997. Panel report: The potential of geons for generic 3-d object recognition, *Image Vision Comput.*, 15:277–292.

Edelman, S., 1994, Biological constraints and the representation of structure in vision and language, *Psycoloquy*, 5(57). FTP host: ftp.princeton.edu; FTP directory: /pub/harnad/Psycoloquy/1994.volume.5/; file name: psyc.94.5.57.language-network.3.edelman.

Edelman, S., and Intrator, N., 2000, (Coarse coding of shape fragments) + (retinotopy) ~ representation of structure, *Spat. Vision*, 13:255–264.

Edelman, S., and Intrator, N., 2001, A productive, systematic framework for the representation of visual structure, in *Advances in Neural Information Processing Systems 13* (T. K. Leen, T. G. Dietterich, and V. Tresp, Eds.), Cambridge, MA: MIT Press, pp. 10–16.

Fodor, J., and McLaughlin, B., 1990, Connectionism and the problem of systematicity: Why Smolensky's solution doesn't work, *Cognition*, 35:183–204.

Hummel, J. E., 2000, Where view-based theories of human object recognition break down: The role of structure in human shape perception, in *Cognitive Dynamics: Conceptual Change in Humans and Machines* (E. Dietrich and A. Markman, Eds.), Hillsdale, NJ: Erlbaum, chap. 7.

Hummel, J. E., 2001, Complementary solutions to the binding problem in vision: Implications for shape perception and object recognition, *Vis. Cognit.*, 8:489–517.

Logothetis, N. K., and Sheinberg, D. L., 1996, Visual object recognition, *Annu. Rev. Neurosci.*, 19:577–621. ◆

Marr, D., 1982, *Vision*, San Francisco, CA: Freeman. ◆

Nelson, R. C., and Selinger, A., 1998, Large-scale tests of a keyed, appearance-based 3-D object recognition system, *Vision Res.*, 38:2469–2488.

Op de Beeck, H., and Vogels, R., 2000, Spatial sensitivity of macaque inferior temporal neurons, *J. Comp. Neurol.*, 426:505–518.

Rao, S. C., Rainer, G., and Miller, E. K., 1997, Integration of what and where in the primate prefrontal cortex, *Science*, 276:821–824.

Ocular Dominance and Orientation Columns

Kenneth D. Miller

Introduction

The classic example of activity-dependent neural development is the formation of ocular dominance columns in the cat or monkey primary visual cortex (reviewed in Miller and Stryker, 1990; Crair et al., 2001; Katz and Crowley, 2002). The primary visual cortex (V1) receives signals from the lateral geniculate nucleus of the thalamus (LGN), which in turn receives input from the retinas of the two eyes (Figure 1).

To describe ocular dominance columns, several terms must be defined. First, the *receptive field* of a cortical cell refers to the area on the retina in which appropriate light stimulation evokes a response in the cell, and also to the pattern of light stimulation that evokes such a response. Second, a *column* is defined as follows. V1 extends many millimeters in each of two "horizontal" dimensions. Receptive field positions vary continuously along these dimensions, forming a *retinotopic* map, a continuous map of the visual world. In the third, "vertical" dimension, the cortex is about 2 mm in depth, and consists of six layers. Receptive field positions do not significantly vary through this depth. Such organization, in which cortical properties are invariant through the vertical depth of cortex but vary horizontally, is called *columnar* organization and is a basic feature of cerebral cortex. Finally, *ocular dominance*, or eye preference, describes the degree to which a cortical cell's responses are better driven by stimulation of one eye or the other. Like retinotopy, ocular dominance has a columnar organization: alternating stripes or patches of cortex are dominated throughout the cortical depth by a single eye, and are known as *ocular dominance columns*.

The anatomical basis for ODCs is the segregated pattern of termination of the LGN inputs to V1 (Figures 1 and 2A). Inputs serving a single eye terminate in alternating stripes or patches of cortex. This segregation arises early in development. Although the exact time at which ocular dominance columns emerge is currently controversial (compare Crair et al., 2001, with Katz and Crowley, 2002, noting that 2 weeks of age in cat corresponds developmentally to about 5 weeks of age in ferret), it is clear that they begin

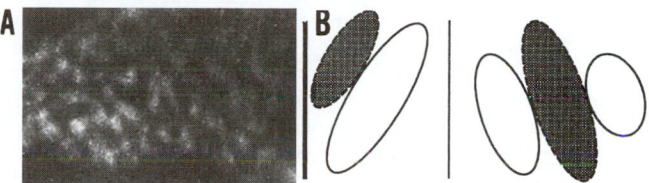

Figure 2. *A*, Ocular dominance columns from cat V1. A horizontal cut through the LGN-recipient layer of V1 is shown. Terminals serving a single eye are labeled white. Dark regions at edges are out of plane containing LGN terminals. Region shown is 5.3 × 7.9 mm. (Photograph courtesy of Dr. Y. Hata.) *B*, Two examples of simple cell-receptive fields (RFs). Regions of the visual field from which a simple cell receives ON-center (white) or OFF-center (dark) input are shown. Note: Ocular dominance columns (*A*) represent an alternation, across cortex, in the type of input (left or right eye) received by different cortical cells, while a simple cell RF (*B*) represents an alternation across visual space in the type of input (ON- or OFF-center) received by a *single* cortical cell.

to form at least a week before the beginning of the critical period. The *critical period* is the time during which the structure of the ocular dominance columns is susceptible to alteration by altered patterns of visual experience. For example, closure of one eye during the critical period will cause that eye's patches to shrink and the open eye's patches to expand.

A longstanding hypothesis is that the formation of ocular dominance columns results from an activity-instructed competition between the geniculate terminals serving the two eyes. Under this hypothesis, the signal indicating that different terminals represent the same eye is the correlation in their neural activities (reviewed in Weliky, 2000). These correlations exist because of both spontaneous activity, which is locally correlated within each retina, and visually induced activity, which correlates the activities of retinotopically nearby neurons within each eye and, to a lesser extent, between the eyes. An attractive feature of this hypothesis is that it suggests that the same mechanisms underlie both the formation of ocular dominance columns and their subsequent susceptibility to alteration by visual experience. However, one must then explain why ocular dominance columns begin forming *before* the beginning of the critical period, that is, at a time when alterations in visual experience do not influence ocular dominance column development. A possible explanation (Crair et al., 2001) is that before the critical period, the loop between cortex and LGN may dominate over the retinal input in determining LGN activities (see Weliky, 2000), so that alterations in retinal activity would have minimal effect on activity-instructed development of connections from LGN to cortex. Alternatively, it has been proposed that the initial formation of ocular dominance columns may be guided by molecular cues in cortex that label the regions appropriate for each eye's innervation (no such molecules have yet been found), and that activity only comes to play an instructive role in ocular dominance column development at the onset of the critical period (Katz and Crowley, 2002). In this article, we shall consider models of ocular dominance column formation under the first scenario, in which the initial formation of ocular dominance columns is instructed by activity.

At least during the critical period, the process guiding the segregation of ocular dominance columns is *competitive*—the two eyes compete for cortical territory based on their patterns of activity

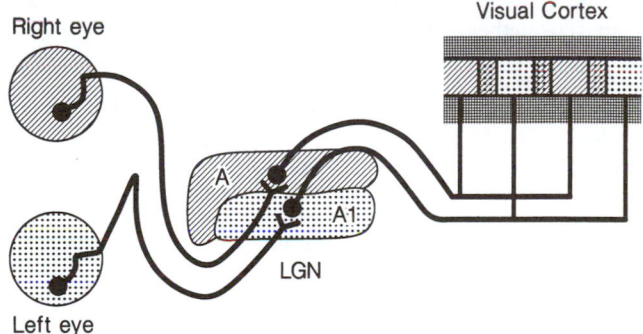

Figure 1. Schematic of the mature visual system. Retinal ganglion cells from the two eyes project to separate layers of the lateral geniculate nucleus (LGN). Neurons from these two layers project to separate patches or stripes within visual cortex (V1). Binocular regions (receiving input from both eyes) are depicted at the borders between the eye-specific patches. (From Miller, K. D., Keller, J. B., and Stryker, M. P., Ocular column dominance development: Analysis and simulation, *Science*, 245:605–615. © 1989 by the AAAS. Reprinted with permission.)

(reviewed in Miller and Stryker, 1990). If one eye is caused to have less activity than the other during the critical period, the more active eye takes over most of the cortical territory; but the eye with reduced activity suffers no loss of projection strength in retinotopic regions in which it lacks competition from the other eye. Thus, the fate of one eye's projection is not determined solely by its own activity, but rather by its activity *relative* to that of the opposite eye.

Orientation columns are another striking feature of visual cortical organization. Most V1 cells are orientation selective, responding selectively to light/dark edges over a narrow range of orientations. The preferred orientation of cortical cells varies regularly and periodically across the horizontal dimension of cortex, and is invariant in the vertical dimension. The initial development of orientation selectivity often begins before eye opening and is unaffected by whether the eyes are open or closed, but depends on normal spontaneous patterns of neural activity, while the later maturation of orientation selectivity depends on vision (reviewed in Miller, Erwin, and Kayser, 1999). The dependence of orientation selectivity on vision begins at about the same time that the critical period for ocular dominance plasticity begins, suggesting that a single set of changes renders both systems vulnerable to visual experience.

The inputs from LGN to V1 serving each eye are of two types: ON-center and OFF-center. Both kinds of cells have circularly symmetric receptive fields that are relatively insensitive to stimulus orientation, and respond to contrast rather than uniform luminance. ON-center cells respond to light against a dark background, or to light onset; OFF-center cells respond to dark against a light background, or to light offset. In the cat, the orientation-selective V1 cells that receive the bulk of LGN input are *simple cells*: cells with receptive fields consisting of alternating oriented subregions that receive exclusively ON-center or exclusively OFF-center input (Figure 2*B*). One theory for the development of orientation selectivity is that, like ocular dominance, it develops through a competition between two input populations: in this case, a competition between the ON-center and the OFF-center inputs (Miller, 1994).

Correlation-Based Models

To understand ocular dominance and orientation column formation, two processes must be understood:

1. The development of *receptive field structure*: Under what conditions do receptive fields become monocular (drivable only by a single eye) or orientation selective?
2. The development of *periodic cortical maps* of receptive field properties: What leads ocular dominance or preferred orientation to vary periodically across the horizontal dimensions of cortex, and what determines the periodic length scales of these maps?

Typically, the problem is simplified by consideration of a two-dimensional model cortex, ignoring the third dimension, in which properties such as ocular dominance and orientation are invariant.

One approach to addressing these problems is to begin with a hypothesized mechanism of synaptic plasticity and to study the outcome of cortical development under such a mechanism. Most commonly, theorists have considered a Hebbian synapse (see HEBBIAN SYNAPTIC PLASTICITY): a synapse whose strength is increased when pre- and postsynaptic firing are correlated, and possibly decreased when they are anticorrelated. Other mechanisms can lead to similar dynamics, in which synaptic plasticity depends on the correlations among the activities of competing inputs. We refer to models based on such mechanisms as correlation-based models.

Von der Malsburg's Model of V1 Development

Von der Malsburg (1973; von der Malsburg and Willshaw, 1976) first formulated a correlation-based model for the development of visual cortical receptive fields and maps. His model had two basic elements. First, synapses of LGN inputs onto cortical neurons were modified by a Hebbian rule that is *competitive*, so that some synapses were strengthened only at the expense of others. He enforced the competition by holding constant the total strength of synapses converging on each cortical cell (conservation rule). Second, cortical cells tended to be activated in *clusters*, due to intrinsic cortical connectivity, e.g., short-range horizontal excitatory connections and longer-range horizontal inhibitory connections.

The conservation rule leads to competition among the inputs to a single target cell. Inputs that tend to be coactivated—that is, that have correlated activities—are mutually reinforcing, working together to activate the postsynaptic cells and thus to strengthen their own synapses. Different patterns that are mutually un- or anticorrelated compete, since strengthening of some synapses means weakening of others. Cortical cells eventually develop receptive fields responsive to a correlated pattern of inputs.

The clustered cortical activity patterns lead to competition between different groups of cortical cells. Each input pattern comes to be associated with a cortical cluster of activity. Overlapping cortical clusters contain many coactivated cortical cells, and thus become responsive to overlapping, correlated input patterns. Adjacent, nonoverlapping clusters contain many anticorrelated cortical cells, and thus become responsive to un- or anticorrelated input patterns. Thus, over distances on the scale of an activity cluster, cortical cells will have similar response properties, while on the scale of the distance between nonoverlapping clusters, cortical cells will prefer un- or anticorrelated input patterns. This combination of local continuity and larger-scale heterogeneity leads to continuous, periodic cortical maps of receptive field properties.

In computer simulations, this model was applied to the development of orientation columns (von der Malsburg, 1973) and ocular dominance columns (von der Malsburg and Willshaw, 1976). For orientation columns, inputs were activated in oriented patterns, each pattern consisting of a stripe of inputs through a common center position. Individual cortical cells then developed selective responses corresponding to one such oriented pattern, with nearby cortical cells preferring nearby orientations. For ocular dominance columns, inputs were activated in monocular patterns consisting of a localized set of inputs from a single eye. Individual cortical cells came to be driven exclusively by a single eye, and clusters of cortical cells came to be driven by the same eye. The final cortical pattern consisted of alternating stripes of cortical cells preferring a single eye, with the width of a stripe approximately set by the diameter of an intrinsic cluster of cortical activity.

In summary, a competitive Hebbian rule leads individual receptive fields to become selective for a correlated pattern of inputs. Combined with the idea that the cortex is activated in intrinsic clusters, this suggests an origin for cortical maps: coactivated cells in a cortical cluster tend to become selective for similar, coactivated patterns of inputs. These basic ideas are used in most subsequent models.

Mathematical Formulation

A typical correlation-based model is mathematically formulated as follows (von der Malsburg, 1973; Linsker, 1986; Miller and Stryker, 1990). Let $x, y, \ldots$ represent retinotopic positions in V1, and let $\alpha, \beta, \ldots$ represent retinotopic positions in the LGN. Let $S^\mu(x, \alpha)$ be the synaptic strength of the connection from α to x of the LGN projection of type μ, where μ may signify left eye, right eye, ON-center, OFF-center, etc. Let $B(x, y)$ represent the synaptic strength and sign of connection from the cortical cell at y to that at x. For simplicity, $B(x, y)$ is assumed to take different signs for a fixed y as x varies, but alternatively, separate excitatory-projecting and inhibitory-projecting cortical neurons may be used. Let $a(x)$ and $a^\mu(\alpha)$ represent the activity of a cortical or LGN cell, respectively.

The activity $a(x)$ of a cortical neuron is assumed to depend on a linear combination of its inputs:

$$a(x) = f_1\left(\sum_{\mu,\alpha} S^\mu(x, \alpha)a^\mu(\alpha) + \sum_y B(x, y)a(y)\right) \quad (1)$$

Here, f_1 is some monotonic function such as a sigmoid or linear threshold.

A Hebbian rule for the change in feedforward synapses can be expressed

$$\Delta S^\mu(x, \alpha) = A^\mu(x, \alpha)f_2[a(x)]f_3[a^\mu(\alpha)] \quad (2)$$

Here, $A(x, \alpha)$ is an "arbor function," expressing the number of synapses of each type from α to x; a minimal form is $A(x, \alpha) = 1$ if there is a connection from α to x, $A(x, \alpha) = 0$ otherwise. A typical form for the functions f_2 and f_3 is $f(a) = (a - \langle a \rangle)$, where $\langle a \rangle$ indicates an average of a over input patterns. This yields a *covariance rule*: synaptic change depends on the covariance of postsynaptic and presynaptic activity.

Next, the Hebbian rule must be made *competitive*. This can be accomplished by conserving total synaptic strength over the postsynaptic cell (von der Malsburg, 1973), which in turn may be done either subtractively or multiplicatively (Miller and MacKay, 1994). The corresponding equations are

$$\frac{d}{dt}S^\mu(x, \alpha) = \Delta S^\mu(x, \alpha) - \varepsilon(x)A(x, \alpha) \quad \text{(Subtractive)} \quad (3)$$

$$\frac{d}{dt}S^\mu(x, \alpha) = \Delta S^\mu(x, \alpha) - \gamma(x)S^\mu(x, \alpha) \quad \text{(Multiplicative)} \quad (4)$$

where $\varepsilon(x) = [\sum_{\kappa,\alpha}\Delta S^\kappa(x, \alpha)]/[\sum_{\kappa,\alpha}A(x, \alpha)]$, and $\gamma(x) = [\sum_{\kappa,\alpha}\Delta S^\kappa(x, \alpha)]/[\sum_{\kappa,\alpha}S^\kappa(x, \alpha)]$. Either form of constraint ensures that $\sum_{\mu,\alpha}(d/dt)S^\mu(x, \alpha) = 0$. Alternative approaches have been developed that lead Hebbian rules to be competitive (Miller and MacKay, 1994; Song, Miller, and Abbott, 2000).

Finally, synaptic weights may be limited to a finite range, $s_{min}A(x, \alpha) \le S^\mu(x, \alpha) \le s_{max}A(x, \alpha)$. Typically, $s_{min} = 0$ and s_{max} is some positive constant.

Semilinear Models

In semilinear models, the fs in Equations 1 and 2 are chosen to be linear. Then, after substituting for $a(x)$ from Equation 1 and averaging over input patterns (assuming that all inputs have identical mean activity and that changes in synaptic weights are negligibly small over the averaging time), Equation 2 becomes

$$\Delta S^\mu(x, \alpha) = \lambda A(x, \alpha) \sum_{y,\beta,\kappa} I(x - y)[C^{\mu\kappa}(\alpha - \beta) - k_2]$$
$$\times S^\kappa(y, \beta) + k_1 A(x, \alpha) \quad (5)$$

Here, $I(x - y)$ is an element of the intracortical interaction matrix $\mathbf{I} \equiv (\mathbf{1} - \mathbf{B})^{-1} = \mathbf{1} + \mathbf{B} + \mathbf{B}^2 + \cdots$, where the matrix $\mathbf{B}$ is defined in Equation 1. This summarizes intracortical synaptic influences, including contributions via 0, 1, 2, . . . synapses. The sum over κ is a sum over input types. The covariance matrix $C^{\mu\kappa}(\alpha - \beta) = \langle(a^\mu(\alpha) - \bar{a})(a^\kappa(\beta) - \bar{a})\rangle$ expresses the covariation of input activities. The factors λ, k_1, and k_2 are constants. Translation invariance has been assumed in both cortex and LGN.

When there are two competing input populations, Equation 5 can be further simplified by transforming to sum and difference variables: $S^S \equiv S^1 + S^2$, $S^D \equiv S_1 - S_2$. Assuming equivalence of the two populations (so that $C^{11} = C^{22}$, $C^{12} = C^{21}$), Equation 5 becomes

$$\Delta S^S(x, \alpha) = \lambda A(x, \alpha) \sum_{y,\beta} I(x - y)[C^S(\alpha - \beta) - 2k_2]$$
$$\times S^S(y, \beta) + 2k_1 A(x, \alpha) \quad (6)$$

$$\Delta S^D(x, \alpha) = \lambda A(x, \alpha) \sum_{y,\beta} I(x - y)C^D(\alpha - \beta)S^D(y, \beta) \quad (7)$$

Here, $C^S \equiv C^{11} + C^{12}$, $C^D \equiv C^{11} - C^{12}$. A similar transformation to one sum and three difference coordinates can be made in the case of four competing input populations, such as ON and OFF inputs from left and right eyes (Erwin and Miller, 1998).

How Semilinear Models Behave

Linear equations like Equations 6 and 7 can be understood by finding the eigenvectors or "modes" of the operators on the right side of the equation. The eigenvectors are the synaptic weight patterns that grow independently and exponentially, each at its own rate. The fastest-growing eigenvectors typically dominate development and determine basic features of the final pattern, although the final pattern ultimately is stabilized by nonlinearities such as the limits on the range of synaptic weights or the nonlinearity involved in multiplicative renormalization (Equation 4).

I will focus on the behavior of Equation 7 for S^D. S^D describes the difference in the strength of two competing input populations. Thus, it is the key variable describing the development of ocular dominance segregation, or development under an ON-center/OFF-center competition. It also is sensible to imagine that S^D is initially small, and that the dynamics do not intrinsically favor either of the competing input types; under these assumptions, the initial development of S^D will be described by linear equations, giving some justification for studying linear equations for the development of S^D.

Equation 7 can be simply solved in the case of full connectivity from the LGN to the cortex, when $A(x, \alpha) \equiv 1$ for all x and α. Then modes of $S^D(x, \alpha)$ of the form $e^{ikx}e^{il\alpha}$ grow exponentially and independently, with rate proportional to $\tilde{I}(k)\tilde{C}^D(l)$, where $\tilde{I}$ and $\tilde{C}^D$ denote the Fourier transforms of I and C^D, respectively. The wave number k determines the wavelength $2\pi/|k|$ of an oscillation of S^D across cortical cells, while the wave number l determines the wavelength $2\pi/|l|$ of an oscillation of S^D across geniculate cells. The fastest-growing modes, which will dominate early development, are determined by the k and l that maximize $\tilde{I}(k)$ and $\tilde{C}^D(l)$, respectively. The peak of a function's Fourier transform corresponds to the cosine wave that best matches the function, and thus represents the "principal oscillation" in the function.

To understand these modes (Figure 3), consider first the set of inputs received by a single cortical cell, that is, the shape of the mode for a fixed cortical position x. This can be regarded as the "receptive field" of the cortical cell. Each receptive field oscillates with wave number l. This oscillation, of $S^D \equiv S^1 - S^2$, is an oscillation between receptive field subregions dominated by S^1 inputs and subregions dominated by S^2 inputs. Thus, in ocular dominance competition, monocular cells (cells whose entire receptive fields are dominated by a single eye) are formed only by modes with $l = 0$ (no oscillation). Monocular cells thus dominate development if the peak of the Fourier transform of the C^D governing left/right competition is at $l = 0$, which occurs if this $\tilde{C}^D(\alpha)$ is a nonnegative, monotonically decreasing function of $|\alpha|$ such as a Gaussian. Now instead consider an ON/OFF competition: S^1 and

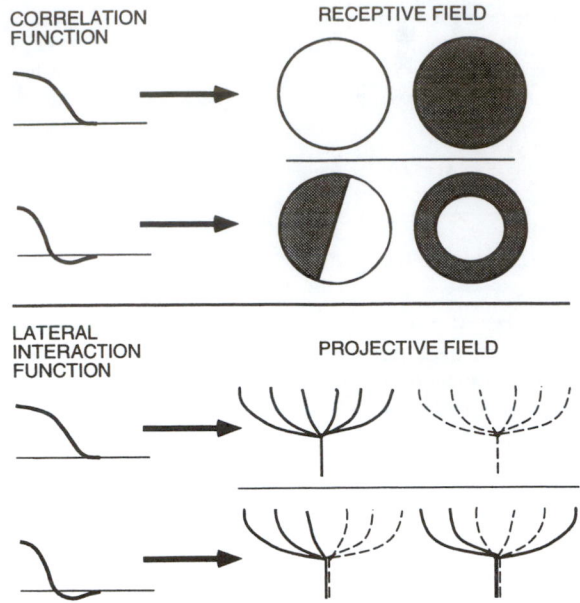

CORRELATION FUNCTION   RECEPTIVE FIELD

LATERAL INTERACTION FUNCTION   PROJECTIVE FIELD

Figure 3. Schematic of the outcome of semilinear correlation-based development. *Top*, The correlation function (C^D) determines the structure of receptive fields (RFs). White RF subregions indicate positive values of S^D; dark subregions indicate negative values. If C^D oscillates, there is a corresponding oscillation in the type of input received by individual cortical cells, as in simple cell RFs. Alternative RF structures could form, as shown, but oriented simple-cell-like outcomes predominate for reasonable parameters (Miller, 1994). When C^D does not oscillate, individual cortical cells receive only a single type of input, as in ocular dominance segregation. *Bottom*, The intracortical interactions (I) similarly determine the structure of projective fields. Here, solid lines indicate positive values of S^D, dotted lines indicate negative values.

S^2 represent ON- and OFF-center inputs from a single eye. Then the receptive fields of modes with non-zero l resemble simple cells: they receive predominantly ON-center and predominantly OFF-center inputs from successive, alternating subregions of the visual world. Thus, simple cells can form if the C^D governing ON/OFF competition has its peak at a non-zero l, which occurs if this $C^D(\alpha)$ oscillates from positive to negative with increasing $|\alpha|$.

Now consider the arborizations or "projective fields" projecting from a single geniculate point, that is, the shape of the mode for a fixed geniculate position α. These oscillate with wave number k. In ocular dominance competition, this means that left- and right-eye cells from α project to alternating patches of cortex. When monocular cells form ($l = 0$), these alternating patches of cortex are the ocular dominance columns: alternating patches of cortex receiving exclusively left-eye or exclusively right-eye input, respectively. Thus, the width of ocular dominance columns—the wavelength of alternation between right-eye-dominated and left-eye-dominated cortical cells—is determined by the peak of the Fourier transform of the intracortical interaction function I. In ON/OFF competition, with $l \neq 0$, the identity of the cortical cells receiving the ON-center or OFF-center part of the projection varies as α varies, so individual cortical cells receive both ON- and OFF-center input, but from distinct subregions of the receptive field.

In summary, there is an oscillation across receptive fields, with wave number l determined by the peak of $\tilde{C}^D$, and an oscillation across arbors, with wave number k determined by the peak of $\tilde{I}$ (Figure 3). These two oscillations are "knit together" to determine the overall pattern of synaptic connectivity. The receptive field oscillation, which matches the receptive field to the correlations, is

the quantitative generalization of von der Malsburg's finding that individual receptive fields become selective for a correlated pattern of inputs. Similarly, the arbor oscillation matches projective fields to the intracortical interactions, and thus to the patterns of cortical activity clusters. This quantitatively generalizes the relationship between activity clusters and maps. Note that the factor e^{ikx} can be regarded as inducing a phase shift, for varying x, in the structure of receptive fields. Thus, cortical cells that are nearby on the scale of the arbor oscillation have similar receptive fields, while cells ½ wavelength apart have opposite receptive fields.

The competitive, renormalizing terms (Equations 3 and 4) do not substantially alter this picture, except that multiplicative renormalization can suppress ocular dominance development in some circumstances (Miller and MacKay, 1994). These results hold also for localized connectivity (finite arbors), and thus generally characterize the behavior of semilinear models (Miller and Stryker, 1990). The major difference in the case of localized connectivity is that, if k or l corresponds to a wavelength larger than the diameter of connectivity from or to a single cell, then it is equivalent to $k = 0$ or $l = 0$, respectively.

Understanding Ocular Dominance and Orientation Columns with Semilinear Models

This understanding of semilinear models leads to simple models for the development of ocular dominance columns (Miller and Stryker, 1990), orientation columns (Miller, 1994), and their codevelopment (Erwin and Miller, 1998), as follows.

Monocular cells develop through a competition of left- and right-eye inputs in a regime in which $\tilde{C}^D(l)$ is peaked at $l = 0$. The wavelength of ocular dominance column alternation is then determined by the peak of $\tilde{I}(k)$.

Orientation-selective simple cells develop through a competition of ON-center and OFF-center inputs in a regime in which $\tilde{C}^D(l)$ is peaked at $l \neq 0$. The mean wavelength of alternation of ON-center and OFF-center subregions in the simple cells' receptive fields is determined by the peak of $\tilde{C}^D(l)$. This wavelength corresponds to a cell's preferred spatial frequency under stimulation by sinusoidal luminance gratings. In individual modes, all cortical cells have the same preferred orientation, but their spatial phase varies periodically with cortical position. The mixing of such modes of all orientations, along with the saturating nonlinearities limiting the sizes of individual synaptic weights, leads to a periodic variation of preferred orientation across cortex.

For ocular dominance and orientation selectivity to codevelop, the two eyes must be sufficiently uncorrelated to allow ocular dominance segregation, but sufficiently correlated that preferred orientations match in the two eyes on binocular cells and that the map of preferred orientations is continuous across ocular dominance boundaries. The requirements for this to occur turn out to be simple generalizations of the above two requirements, plus an additional requirement that between-eye correlations be specific for center type (e.g., between-eye ON-ON and ON-OFF correlations should be distinct, in a manner that varies over a receptive field diameter).

This model of ocular dominance column formation is similar to that of von der Malsburg (von der Malsburg and Willshaw, 1976). The latter model assumed anticorrelation between the two eyes; this assumption was required because of the use of multiplicative renormalization (Equation 4). With subtractive renormalization (Equation 3), ocular dominance column formation can occur even with partial correlation of the two eyes (Miller and MacKay, 1994).

The model of orientation-selective cell development is quite different from that of von der Malsburg (1973). Von der Malsburg postulated that oriented input patterns lead to the development of orientation-selective cells. The ON/OFF model instead postulates that ON/OFF competition results in oriented receptive fields in the absence of oriented input patterns; the circular symmetry of the input patterns is spontaneously broken. This symmetry-breaking potential of Hebbian development was first discovered by Linsker (1986). In all of these models, the continuity and periodic alternation of preferred orientation is due to the intracortical connectivity.

The models can be compared to experiment most simply by measuring activity correlations in the LGN, such as to determine whether the ON/OFF C^D has the predicted oscillation or whether the between-eye correlations have the predicted structure. Progress toward such tests is reviewed in Weliky (2000).

Related Semilinear Models

Linsker (1986) proposed a model that was highly influential in two respects. First, he pointed out the potential of Hebbian rules to spontaneously break symmetry, yielding orientation-selective cells given approximately circularly symmetric input patterns. Second, he demonstrated that Hebbian rules could lead to segregation *within* receptive fields, so that a cell would come receive purely excitatory or purely inhibitory input in alternating subregions of the receptive field. Two factors underlay the results. One factor was that oscillations in a correlation function can induce oscillations in a receptive field, as described earlier. The other factor was a constraint in the model fixing the percentage of positive or negative synapses received by a cell; this constraint forced an alternation of positive and negative subregions even when the correlation function did not oscillate.

Tanaka has independently formulated models of ocular dominance (Tanaka, 1991) and orientation columns (Miyashita and Tanaka, 1992) that are similar to those described above. The major difference is that in his regime, each cortical cell comes to receive only a single LGN input. (The reason is that he works in a regime in which, on each postsynaptic cell, (1) total synaptic weight is conserved, (2) the only stable outcome is if all or all-but-one synapses are saturated at either the lower or upper bounds on synaptic weights [this is also true for linear rules with subtractive weight normalization—see Miller and MacKay, 1994—although Tanaka's rule is slightly different], and (3) there is a lower bound on synaptic weights at zero, but no upper bound. The result is that the only stable configuration is one in which one synapse acquires all of the conserved weight, and all of the other synapses are forced to the lower bound at zero.) Tanaka defines cortical receptive fields as the convolution of the input arrangement with the intracortical interaction function. This definition means that a cortical cell's receptive field is due to its single input from the LGN, plus its input from all other cortical cells within reach of the intracortical interaction function. Thus, orientation selectivity in this model arises from the breaking of circular symmetry in the pattern of inputs to different cortical cells rather than to individual cortical cells.

The Problem of Map Structure

The models described to this point account well for basic features of primary visual cortex, including the structure of individual receptive fields and local continuity across cortex of receptive field properties. However, certain details of real orientation maps are not replicated by these models (reviewed in Erwin, Obermayer, and Schulten, 1995; Swindale, 1996). One reason may be the simplicity of the model of cortex: the real cortex has three dimensions rather than two, has cell-specific connectivity rather than connectivity that depends only on distance, and has plastic rather than fixed intracortical connections. Another reason is that the details of map structure inherently involve nonlinearities, by which the fastest-growing modes interact and compete, whereas the semilinear framework primarily focuses on early pattern formation, in which the fastest-growing modes emerge and mix randomly without interacting.

Some simple models that focus on map development rather than on receptive field development and that use reduced, feature-based representations of the input yield maps that strikingly match the structures observed in monkey visual cortex (Erwin et al., 1995; Swindale, 1996). One such model uses the self-organizing feature map (SOFM) of Kohonen (see SELF-ORGANIZING FEATURE MAPS). In the SOFM, only a single cluster of cortical cells is activated in response to a given input pattern. This is an abstraction of the idea that the cortex responds in localized activity clusters. In addition, an abstract representation of the input is used. Correlation-based models are "high-dimensional" models: the vector of input weights received by a cell has hundreds or thousands of dimensions, one for each input cell. The SOFM model of visual cortex is instead a "low-dimensional" or "feature-based" model: the vector of input weights received by a cell has only five dimensions, representing features of the visual input (two dimensions represent retinotopic position and one each represent ocular dominance, orientation selectivity, and preferred orientation). Assumptions are made as to the relative "size" of, or variance of the input ensemble along, each dimension. There is no obvious biological interpretation for this comparison between dimensions. Under certain such assumptions, Hebbian learning in the feature space leads to maps of orientation and ocular dominance that are, in detail, remarkably like those seen in macaque monkeys (Erwin et al., 1995; Swindale, 1996). (SOFMs with high-dimensional input representations have also been studied, but it is not clear whether they are any better at capturing map structure than other high-dimensional models.)

The SOFM and other feature-based models, such as those based on the "elastic net" algorithm (Erwin et al., 1995; Swindale, 1996), lead to locally continuous mappings in which a constant distance across the cortex corresponds to a roughly constant distance in the reduced "input space." This means that, when one input feature is changing rapidly across cortex, the others are changing slowly. Thus, the models predict that orientation changes rapidly where ocular dominance changes slowly, and vice versa. This feature may be key to replicating the details of macaque maps. However, recent results suggest that this relationship may not hold between retinotopy and orientation in cat visual cortex (Das and Gilbert, 1997).

A possibly related approach to map organization supposes that the structure of maps is determined by evolutionary pressure to minimize the wire length of neuronal connections (Chklovskii and Koulakov, 2000; Koulakov and Chklovskii, 2001). Assuming a certain "connectivity function," specifying probabilistically which cells should connect to which, a feature map that allows such connectivity to be achieved with minimal wire length is computed. For certain forms of the connectivity function, orientation maps are obtained with pinwheels—point singularities around which preferred orientation rotates by 180 degrees—much as in real maps (Koulakov and Chklovskii, 2001). The model predicts that the ocular dominance map should go from a stripe-like structure to a patch-like structure when one eye contributes less than 40% of the total innervation, and just such a transition at about the appropriate point is seen in monkey visual cortex (Chklovskii and Koulakov, 2000).

Another approach to studying map development is based on very general assumptions as to symmetries of the map-formation process. It was shown that any of a large class of developmental models of orientation selectivity that obey a few basic symmetries and that produce a periodic map of preferred orientation with period λ should produce an initial density of pinwheels of at least π per λ^2 (Wolf and Geisel, 1998). Comparison with actual maps showed a range of densities from 2 to 4, suggesting that if real maps develop by a self-organizing process, those with densities less than π must undergo reorganization involving pinwheel annihilation during early development. It will be exciting if such pinwheel annihilation should be observed, although it is possible that such annihilation might occur only before maps become visible with current methods.

Open Questions

Among the many open questions in the field are these: How can biologically interpretable developmental models replicate the details of cortical maps? How might more realistic models of Hebbian learning and of competition (e.g., Song et al., 2000) modify the basic insights into development obtained by studying simple semi-linear models? How will these insights, which apply to development of feedforward connections, be modified by considering codevelopment of feedforward and intracortical synaptic innervations? (See Song and Abbott, 2001, and Kayser and Miller, 2002.) How will they be modified by developing models that learn on temporal as well as spatial correlations? The simple models have yielded real insights, but the field now seems prepared to enter more complex terrain.

Road Maps: Neural Plasticity; Vision
Related Reading: Development of Retinotectal Maps; Hebbian Synaptic Plasticity; Pattern Formation, Biological; Visual Cortex: Anatomical Structure and Models of Function

References

Chklovskii, D. B., and Koulakov, A. A., 2000, A wire length minimization approach to ocular dominance patterns in mammalian visual cortex, *Physica A*, 284:318–334.

Crair, M., Horton, J., Antonini, A., and Stryker, M., 2001, Emergence of ocular dominance columns in cat visual cortex by 2 weeks of age, *J. Comp. Neurol.*, 430:235–249.

Das, A., and Gilbert, C. D., 1997, Distortions of visuotopic map match orientation singularities in primary visual cortex, *Nature*, 387:594–598.

Erwin, E., and Miller, K. D., 1998, Correlation-based development of ocularly-matched orientation maps and ocular dominance maps: Determination of required input activity structures, *J. Neurosci.*, 18:9870–9895.

Erwin, E., Obermayer, K., and Schulten, K., 1995, Models of orientation and ocular dominance columns in the visual cortex: A critical comparison, *Neural Computat.*, 7:425–468.

Katz, L. C., and Crowley, J. C., 2002, Development of cortical circuits: Lessons from ocular dominance columns, *Nature Rev. Neurosci.*, 3:34–42. ◆

Kayser, A. S., and Miller, K. D., 2002, Opponent inhibition: A developmental model of layer 4 of the neocortical circuit, *Neuron*, 33:131–142.

Koulakov, A., and Chklovskii, D., 2001, Orientation preference patterns in mammalian visual cortex: A wire length minimization approach, *Neuron*, 29:519–527.

Linsker, R., 1986, From basic network principles to neural architecture (series), *Proc. Natl. Acad. Sci. USA*, 83:7508–7512, 8390–8394, 8779–8783.

Miller, K. D., 1994, A model for the development of simple cell receptive fields and the ordered arrangement of orientation columns through activity-dependent competition between ON- and OFF-center inputs, *J. Neurosci.*, 14:409–441.

Miller, K. D., Erwin, E., and Kayser, A., 1999, Is the development of orientation selectivity instructed by activity? *J. Neurobiol.*, 41:44–57. ◆

Miller, K. D., and MacKay, D. J. C., 1994, The role of constraints in Hebbian learning, *Neural Comput.*, 6:100–126.

Miller, K. D., and Stryker, M. P., 1990, The development of ocular dominance columns: Mechanisms and models, in *Connectionist Modeling and Brain Function: The Developing Interface* (S. J. Hanson and C. R. Olson, Eds.), Cambridge, MA: MIT Press/Bradford, pp. 255–350.

Miyashita, M., and Tanaka, S., 1992, A mathematical model for the self-organization of orientation columns in visual cortex, *NeuroReport*, 3:69–72.

Song, S., and Abbott, L., 2001, Cortical development and remapping through spike timing–dependent plasticity, *Neuron*, 32:339–350. ◆

Song, S., Miller, K. D., and Abbott, L. F., 2000, Competitive Hebbian learning through spike-timing-dependent synaptic plasticity, *Nature Neurosci.*, 3:919–926.

Swindale, N. V., 1996, The development of topography in the visual cortex: A review of models, *Network*, 7:161–247. ◆

Tanaka, S., 1991, Theory of ocular dominance column formation: Mathematical basis and computer simulation, *Biol. Cybern.*, 64:263–272.

von der Malsburg, C., 1973, Self-organization of orientation selective cells in the striate cortex, *Kybernetik*, 14:85–100.

von der Malsburg, C., and Willshaw, D. J., 1976, A mechanism for producing continuous neural mappings: Ocularity dominance stripes and ordered retino-tectal projections, *Exp. Brain Res.*, Suppl. 1:463–469.

Weliky, M., 2000, Correlated neuronal activity and visual cortical development, *Neuron*, 27:427–430.

Wolf, F., and Geisel, T., 1998, Spontaneous pinwheel annihilation during visual development, *Nature*, 395:73–78.

Olfactory Bulb

Andrew P. Davison and Gordon M. Shepherd

Introduction

The olfactory bulb is the second stage in the olfactory pathway. It receives input from the sensory neurons in the olfactory epithelium and sends its outputs to the olfactory cortex, among other brain regions. The bulb is of special interest to neural modelers. It was one the first regions of the brain for which compartmental models of neurons were constructed, which led to some of the first computational models of functional microcircuits. The aim of this article is to give an overview of (1) olfactory bulb cells and circuits, (2) current ideas about the computational functions of the bulb, and (3) modeling studies to investigate these functions. Together with the article on the OLFACTORY CORTEX (q.v.), this material provides an introduction to the nature of information processing in the olfactory system.

Cells and Circuits

Olfactory Sensory Input

The first stage in the vertebrate olfactory pathway is the detection of odor molecules by olfactory sensory neurons (OSNs). Odor molecules bind to olfactory receptor proteins (ORs), leading to the generation of receptor potentials, which are converted into action potentials. There are genes for several hundred to more than a thousand ORs in mammalian genomes. Each OSN expresses only one of these proteins. The axons of OSNs project to the olfactory bulb, where they form synapses with the dendrites of olfactory bulb neurons in spherical regions of neuropil called glomeruli. There are 1,000–2,000 glomeruli in a rodent olfactory bulb. The subset of OSNs expressing the same OR type all project their axons to the same glomeruli, generally one on the medial side and one on the lateral side of the bulb. Furthermore, since it appears that each glomerulus receives axons from only a single type of receptor neuron, there is a one-to-one mapping between a glomerulus and an OR type.

An odor molecule typically binds to many ORs, with varying affinities, and therefore activates many glomeruli to different degrees. Since the olfactory bulb is a laminar structure, there is a mapping from 1,000-dimensional odor space (one dimension per OR) to two-dimensional neural space.

The Basic Circuit of the Olfactory Bulb

There are two distinct levels of synaptic interactions in the olfactory bulb, the glomerular layer and the external plexiform layer (EPL) (Figure 1). These layers can be regarded as levels of input processing and output control, respectively.

Within the glomeruli, OSN axons make excitatory synapses onto the distal dendritic tuft of mitral, tufted, and periglomerular (PG) cells. Mitral and tufted (M/T) cells make excitatory dendrodendritic synapses onto PG cells. PG cells make inhibitory dendrodendritic synapses onto M/T cells and probably onto other PG cells. PG cells also send axons to neighboring glomeruli, where they form inhibitory synapses onto M/T cell dendrites.

The secondary dendrites of M/T cells extend long distances laterally in the EPL, up to half of the circumference of the bulb for mitral cells. There is evidence that action potentials can propagate from the soma to the very tips of these dendrites. M/T secondary dendrites make reciprocal, dendrodendritic synapses with granule cells, which are axonless interneurons. These reciprocal synapses consist of an excitatory synapse from M/T cells onto granule cell spines paired with an inhibitory synapse from the spine onto the M/T cell dendrite.

The effects of the dendrodendritic synapses are strongly affected by the intrinsic properties of the cells, particularly the granule cells.

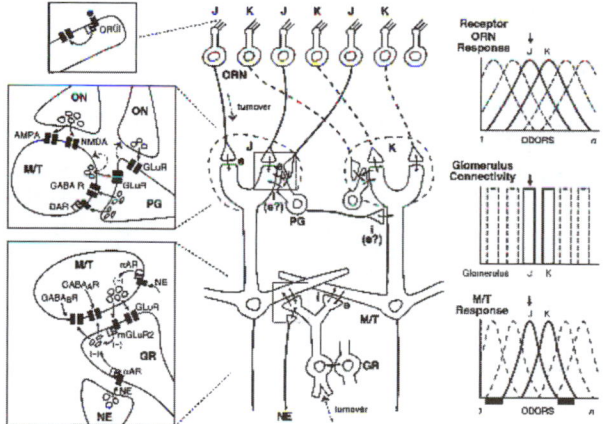

Figure 1. Basic circuit for the olfactory bulb. Abbreviations (left, molecular components): OR, olfactory receptor; ON, olfactory nerve; AMPA, 2-amino-5-phosphonovaleric acid; NMDA, *N*-methyl-D-aspartate; M/T, mitral/tufted cell; PG, periglomerular cell; GluR, ionotropic glutamate receptor; GABA R, γ-aminobutyric acid receptor; DAR, dopamine receptor; NE, norepinephrine; αAR, α-adrenoreceptor; mGluR2, metobotropic glutamate receptor; GR, granule cell. Middle (synaptic circuit): ORN, olfactory receptor neuron; J, K, ORN subsets; e, excitatory; i, inhibitory. Right (structure-function relations) top: overlapping response spectra of ORNs to a range of odors (1 − *n*); middle: connectivity of subsets to individual glomeruli; bottom: response spectra of M/T cells show less overlap because of lateral inhibition (black bars below abscissa).

First, the synapses are onto spines, so a small current can produce a large local membrane depolarization. Second, the granule cell dendrites contain an A-type potassium current, which prevents short-duration synaptic inputs from producing an action potential. Granule cell action potentials may not be required for recurrent inhibition of the M/T cells; glutamate released by the M/T cell depolarizes the granule cell spine sufficiently to produce GABA release, which then inhibits the M/T cell. In mitral cells, subthreshold membrane potential oscillations may interact with postsynaptic potentials to gate the times at which action potentials occur.

M/T cells exhibit autoexcitation due to diffusion of synaptically released glutamate to extrasynaptic ionotropic and metabotropic receptors on both primary and secondary dendrites. This can lead to very prolonged responses to excitatory input. M/T cells do not make chemical synapses with other M/T cells. However, several studies have recently demonstrated functional excitatory connections between mitral cells, probably due again to glutamate spillover to extrasynaptic receptors. M/T cells give off collaterals in the granule cell layer.

Mitral cells send axons to several basolateral brain regions, including the piriform cortex (primary OLFACTORY CORTEX) and the amygdala. The projections of tufted cells are more limited. Centrifugal inputs from several brain areas include cholinergic, serotonergic, and noradrenergic pathways. These inputs mostly terminate on granule and PG cells to influence neuronal excitability and neurotransmitter release. They are critical in setting the behavioral state of the whole system.

Compartmental Models of Olfactory Bulb Neurons

Wilfrid Rall introduced the compartmental method for computational modeling of neurons in 1964 (see PERSPECTIVE ON NEURON MODEL COMPLEXITY). Motoneurons in the spinal cord and mitral and granule cells in the olfactory bulb (Rall and Shepherd, 1968) were the first neurons to be modeled using this approach. Both active and passive dendritic properties were explored in these models. These studies have been extended by compartmental models in which the distribution of active properties in the dendritic trees has been assessed by systematic parameter searches (Bhalla and Bower, 1993). A limitation of earlier studies is that the physiological data were obtained from single-point recordings in the soma, so distal parts of the neurons (e.g., the mitral cell primary dendrite tuft) are much less well constrained than the soma and proximal parts.

Recently, more tightly constrained models have been made possible by experimental data obtained from single- and dual-patch recordings from the soma and from distal sites on the primary dendrite. These studies have shown that full action potentials are generated throughout the primary dendrite, supported by an even distribution of fast Na and K conductances. The M/T cell primary dendrite supports the backpropagation of action potentials from the soma to the tuft. Under conditions of moderate to strong ON input and/or somatic inhibition, action potentials can be initiated in the tuft and propagate in the forward direction to the soma.

These properties have been closely simulated by a tightly constrained compartmental model of the mitral cell (Shen et al., 1999). The results provide one of the best models, in a vertebrate central neuron, of the shifting sites of action potential initiation dependent on the integration of excitatory and inhibitory synaptic inputs with active membrane properties. They support a wide range of studies giving evidence of the importance of active properties of distal dendrites in neuronal function. This gives added emphasis to the importance of the contributions of distal dendrites to the basic circuits for different brain regions, which need to be incorporated into neural networks in order to fully capture the mechanisms used by the real nervous system.

Compartmental models of granule cells have shown that high-input-resistance spines and low levels of activity favor reciprocal over lateral inhibition; conversely, lower-input-resistance spines and high levels of activity favor lateral inhibition (Antón, Granger, and Lynch, 1993), and that with entirely passive membrane in a morphologically detailed model, "the degree of spread of synaptic potentials can define functionally related subsets of spines within the dendritic tree . . . that can mediate discrete localized inhibition onto subsets of mitral or tufted cell secondary dendrites" (Woolf, Shepherd, and Greer, 1991).

The Computational Functions of the Olfactory Bulb

As the first stage of synaptic processing in the olfactory pathway, the olfactory bulb carries out several key functions.

Glomeruli Contribute to Odor Detection

A mechanism that has long been recognized for supporting odor detection is the tremendous convergence of OSNs onto glomeruli. In mammals, the convergence ratio is of the order 10,000:1. As noted earlier, it is believed from axon-labeling studies that all of the OSNs expressing a given OR converge onto one or two common target glomeruli. Thus, at the lowest concentrations, when only the highest-affinity receptor type is activated, all odor responses are concentrated on a single pair of glomeruli.

Spatial Maps Mediate Odor Recognition

A given odor activates a particular set of OR types. The set of activated ORs is mapped onto a two-dimensional pattern of activated glomeruli. These patterns have been visualized by a large number of imaging techniques (see Xu, Greer, and Shepherd, 2000, for a review). The responses to different odor stimuli have also been characterized. These studies have shown that odor molecules that are structurally similar activate glomeruli that are near one another, and the patterns of activation for different odorants generally overlap considerably. There is thus increasing support for the hypothesis that odor recognition is based on patterns characteristic for given odors.

Odor Maps Encode Odor Concentration

Odor mapping methods show that increasing odor concentration recruits increasing numbers of activated glomeruli, as the higher concentrations cause binding of additional ORs with lower affinities in OSNs projecting to other glomeruli (see Xu et al., 2000). Thus, odor concentration appears to be encoded at least in part by the number of activated glomeruli, and probably also by the intensity of their activation. Modeling studies have suggested that odor intensity could additionally be encoded by the number of M/T cells within a glomerulus that are firing (Antón, Lynch, and Granger, 1991). Experimentally, there is a gradient of decreasing excitability from tufted to mitral cells, so that increasing odor intensity will recruit additional neurons to fire. An argument against this hypothesis is the observation that M/T cells have different projection patterns and so are not a single population for the purpose of transmitting information to cortex.

Temporal Structure Encodes Odor Concentration

Time may also be used as a dimension for encoding stimulus intensity. First, the temporal firing pattern of M/T cells changes as odor concentration is increased. Second, time delays may be used to encode odor intensity. White et al. (1998) developed a network model of the olfactory bulb that receives input from an array of fiber-optic chemodetectors constituting an artificial nose. The network functions as a delay line neural network in which odor identity is encoded by spatial pattern and odor intensity by response delay. This network outperforms standard feedforward neural networks in discriminating odors when limited training sets are used. This work represents an important practical application of neural networks in the olfactory system for artificial chemosensing systems, with applications in industry and for detecting narcotics and hidden explosives.

Lateral Inhibition Mediates Odor Discrimination

A critical function of olfactory bulb circuits is to contribute to the neural basis for discrimination between different odors. As we have seen, the responses to different odors are carried in some 2,000 parallel glomerular pathways. Discrimination between odors requires circuits that can compare the patterns of responses across the pathways and extract the differences.

A key operation for mediating odor discrimination is reducing the overlap between the representations of different odors. Strongly activated mitral cells suppress the activity of more weakly activated mitral cells by lateral inhibition, mediated through the dendrodendritic synapses with granule and periglomerular cells. This sharpens the tuning curves of mitral cells connected to a given glomerulus. This is equivalent to reducing the overlap between the affinity spectra (the molecular receptive ranges) of the individual glomeruli. This was demonstrated experimentally by Yokoi, Mori, and Nakanishi (1995), who found that affinity spectra for a series of aldehydes were broadened by blocking lateral inhibition, presumably mediated through granule cells.

The distinction between the roles of granule and PG cells in mediating lateral inhibition has been investigated in an olfactory bulb model developed by Linster and Hasselmo (1997): PG cell activity affects the number of active mitral cells, while granule cell activity determines the response intensity of active mitral cells. Both granule and PG cell activities may be controlled by centrifugal inputs. The result of the two levels of lateral inhibition is to make the odor representation more sparse.

A complementary mechanism for reducing overlap is to add temporal structure to the responses (i.e., two odors may activate the same ensembles of cells, but at different times) by way of the lateral interactions. Adding time as an extra dimension gives more space in which to separate out odors. Experimentally, the response patterns of mitral cells have complex temporal structures. Laurent et al. (2001) have introduced a dynamical systems model of the olfactory bulb/antennal lobe in which the state of the system, represented by the instantaneous firing rates of the projection neurons, follows a heteroclinic orbit in phase space. Orbits starting from nearby starting points (representing similar odorants) diverge rapidly, thus allowing easier discrimination between them. Experimentally, they provide evidence in zebrafish that an initially "clustered" representation becomes declustered with time.

Temporal Correlations May Contribute to Odor Discrimination

It has been suggested that one function of the bulb is to introduce temporal correlations, such as spike synchronization, between the signals from different receptors responding to the same odor (Laurent et al., 2001). If the olfactory cortex has cells that are tuned as "coincidence detectors," this could increase the salience of mitral cells that are synchronized relative to unsynchronized cells. Gamma-frequency, odor-induced oscillations in local field potential (LFP) recordings have been reported in the olfactory bulbs of vertebrates and in the antennal lobes of insects. These oscillations are thought to reflect the rhythmical, synchronous firing of populations of neurons. In insects and rabbits, the spiking of individual neurons is phase-locked to the LFP, and spiking in simultaneously recorded pairs of neurons is often closely synchronized. Oscillations with different (sometimes harmonically related) frequencies may be elicited in different regions of the olfactory bulb. In insects, different subpopulations of neurons may be synchronized with the global oscillation at different periods during the response (see Laurent et al., 2001). In honeybees, oscillatory synchronization has been shown to have functional relevance: pharmacologically induced desynchronization impairs the ability to discriminate between similar odorants but has no effect on discrimination of dissimilar odorants (see Laurent et al., 2001).

Synaptic Modification Produces a Transformation of Odor Space

Not all synapses are equal in strength. Therefore, the firing of some cells will have a larger influence on bulb output than others. The strength of synapses may be changed by mechanisms of synaptic plasticity during learning experiences. For example, recordings of mitral cell activity in the olfactory bulb of sheep before and after giving birth showed that before parturition, the majority of cells responded preferentially to food odors, and after parturition, the majority responded preferentially to lamb odors (Kendrick, Lévy, and Keverne, 1992). Accompanying this change in preference were increases in neurotransmitter release in the bulb. It appears, therefore, that a function of the bulb is to produce a mapping between the input, physical/chemical odor space and the output, neural odor space, such that behaviorally important odors cover a larger region of output space, enhancing the ability of the system to discriminate between similar odors. Odors with less behavioral significance would be mapped to a reduced region of output space. Changes in synaptic strengths can alter this mapping. In the case of the sheep, synaptic changes in the bulb increased the representation of lamb odors in output space at the expense of the extent of output space representing food odors.

Realistic Network Models

Several models have been developed that attempt to reproduce the anatomy and physiology of real cells and synapses and the connectivity of the real olfactory bulb network without any a priori idea of how the network should behave.

White et al. (1992) have investigated how responses of olfactory bulb neurons to electrical or odor stimulation may be shaped by microcircuit interactions in the salamander olfactory bulb. The total number of cells in the model is 1,000-fold fewer than found in the real system, but the ratios between the populations are maintained. Mitral cells are modeled with three compartments (soma and two dendritic tufts) using standard cable equations. Granule and PG cells are represented by single compartments. Presynaptic spikes and/or subthreshold increases in membrane potential trigger postsynaptic conductance changes. In simulations, each of the major types of response seen in electrophysiological recordings of salamander cells is reproduced by varying the spatial pattern of activity applied to the receptor cells (Figure 2).

Davison, Feng, and Brown (2003) simulated a network of 100 mitral cells and 15,000 granule cells using simplified versions of the models of Bhalla and Bower (1993) and realistic synaptic conductances. This model network displayed properties of center-surround inhibition that are consistent with the experimental findings of Yokoi et al. (1995) (Figures 3A–D). The model also displayed synchronization between mitral cells in response to odor inputs, as seen in the rabbit olfactory bulb and similar to the synchronization seen in the insect antennal lobe (Figure 3E). Weakly activated mitral cells fire less frequently than, but always synchronously with, strongly activated cells. Nearby cells synchronize more readily than widely separated ones. These findings also dem-

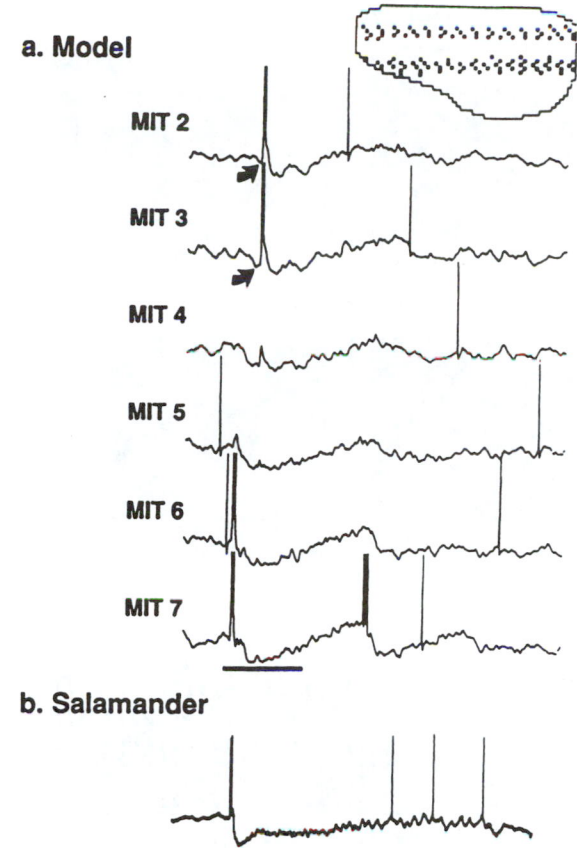

a. Model

MIT 2

MIT 3

MIT 4

MIT 5

MIT 6

MIT 7

b. Salamander

Figure 2. Odor stimulation of modeled mitral (MIT) cell responses (MIT 2–7) (*A*) compared with experimental recordings (*B*). Note the pattern of excited receptor cells in the receptor sheet in the inset at top. Arrows in *A* indicate a brief hyperpolarization that is also seen in experimental recordings. (From White, J., Hamilton, K. A., Neff, S. R., and Kauer, J. S., 1990, Emergent properties of odor information coding in a representational model of the salamander olfactory bulb, *J. Neurosci.*, 12:1772–1780. Reprinted with permission.)

onstrate the central role of the dendrodendritic synapses in generating both the spatial and the temporal properties of the network behavior.

Bazhenov et al. (2001) have developed a realistic model of the locust antennal lobe based on single-compartment cell models with ionic currents chosen to generate realistic firing profiles. The model reproduces the phenomena of transient oscillatory synchronization and slow temporal patterning seen in experimental recordings. The fast excitatory/inhibitory connections between local neurons (LNs) and projection neurons (PNs) were found to be necessary for network oscillations, while inhibitory connections between LNs were needed to make the synchronization transient. Adding slow inhibitory synapses from LNs to PNs was sufficient to produce the slow temporal patterns.

Discussion

The olfactory bulb has a simple structure that has made it attractive for analysis of microcircuit organization and models of neural circuits. For brain theorists, its organization offers examples of information processing without impulses and of output functions of dendrites, which has forced new concepts of the neuron as a complex computational unit. It provides unique opportunities for correlating

Before stimulus

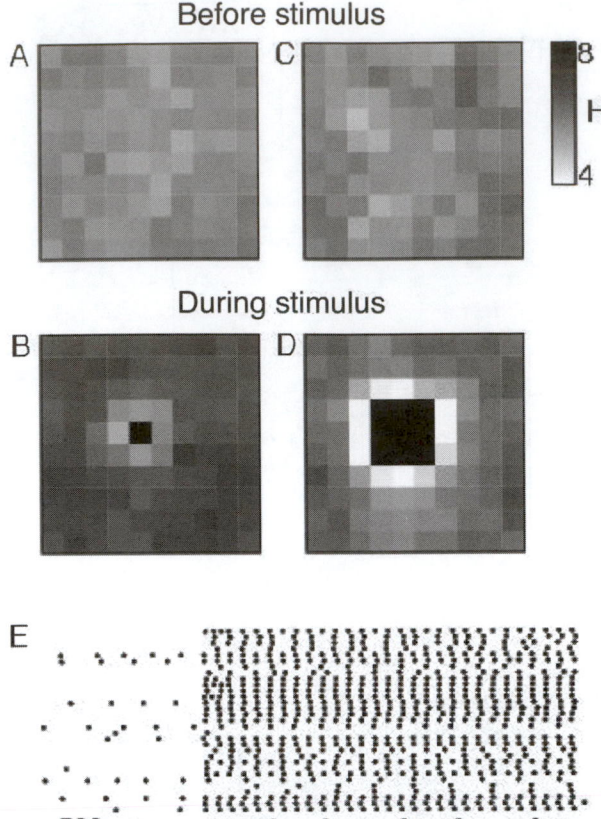

During stimulus

Figure 3. Lateral inhition and stimulus-induced synchronization in an olfactory bulb model. (*A–D*), 10 × 10 array of mitral cells with uniform background activity. The gray-scale value of each square represents the mean firing rate, averaged over 2 s of simulation. Firing rates above 8 Hz are represented by black. Firing rates below 4 Hz are represented by white. *A* and *C*, The background firing rate, before stimulus onset. *B*, Stimulation of a single mitral cell. The firing rates of neighboring cells are depressed by about 1.5 Hz relative to the bulk of the mitral cell population. *D*, Stimulation of a 3 × 3 block of mitral cells. The firing rates of cells neighboring this block are depressed by about 3 Hz relative to the bulk of the population. *E*, Raster plot for a 6 × 6 array of mitral cells. Each dot represents an action potential. Each line is a different mitral cell. The cells are unsynchronized prior to stimulus onset. The stimulus increases the degree of synchronization in the network. (From Davison, A. P., Feng, J., and Brown, D., 2003, Dendrodendritic inhibition and simulated odor responses in a detailed olfactory bulb network model, *J. Neurophysiol.* (submitted).

derstand how the spatial and temporal aspects of the olfactory responses interact in olfactory information processing.

Road Maps: Mammalian Brain Regions; Other Sensory Systems
Related Reading: Dendritic Processing; Olfactory Cortex

References

Antón, P. S., Granger, R., and Lynch, G., 1993, Simulated dendritic spines influence reciprocal synaptic strengths and lateral inhibition in the olfactory bulb, *Brain Res.*, 628:157–165.

Antón, P. S., Lynch, G., and Granger, R., 1991, Computation of frequency-to-spatial transform by olfactory bulb glomeruli, *Biol. Cybern.*, 65:407–414.

Bazhenov, M., Stopfer, M., Rabinovich, M., Abarbanel, H., Sejnowski, T., and Laurent, G., 2001, Model of cellular and network mechanisms for odor-evoked temporal patterning in the locust antennal lobe, *Neuron*, 30:569–581.

Bhalla, U. S., and Bower, J. M., 1993, Exploring parameter space in detailed single cell models: Simulations of the mitral and granule cells of the olfactory bulb, *J. Neurophysiol.*, 69:1948–1965.

Davison, A. P., Feng, J., and Brown, D., 2001, Spike synchronization in a biophysically-detailed model of the olfactory bulb, *Neurocomputing*, 38–40:515–521.

Davison, A. P., Feng, J., and Brown, D., 2003, Dendrodendritic inhibition and simulated odor responses in a detailed olfactory bulb network model, *J. Neurophysiol.* (submitted).

Kendrick, K. M., Lévy, F., and Keverne, E. B., 1992, Changes in the sensory processing of olfactory signals induced by birth in sheep, *Science*, 256:833–836.

Laurent, G., Stopfer, M., Friedrich, R. W., Rabinovich, M. I., Volkovskii, A., and Abarbanel, H. D. I., 2001, Odor encoding as an active, dynamical process: Experiments, computation, and theory, *Annu. Rev. Neurosci.*, 24:263–297. ◆

Linster, C., and Hasselmo, M., 1997, Modulation of inhibition in a model of olfactory bulb reduces overlap in the neural representation of olfactory stimuli, *Behav. Brain Res.*, 84:117–127.

Rall, W., and Shepherd, G. M., 1968, Theoretical reconstruction of field potentials and dendrodendritic synaptic interactions in olfactory bulb, *J. Neurophysiol.*, 31:884–915.

Shen, G. Y., Chen, W. R., Midtgaard, J., Shepherd, G. M., and Hines, M. L., 1999, Computational analysis of action potential initiation in mitral cell soma and dendrites based on dual patch recordings, *J. Neurophysiol.*, 82:3006–3020.

White, J., Dickinson, T. A., Walt, D. R., and Kauer, J. S., 1998, An olfactory neuronal network for vapor recognition in an artificial nose., *Biol. Cybern.*, 78:245–251.

White, J., Hamilton, K. A., Neff, S. R., and Kauer, J. S., 1992, Emergent properties of odor information coding in a representational model of the salamander olfactory bulb, *J. Neurosci.*, 12:1772–1780.

Woolf, T. B., Shepherd, G. M., and Greer, C. A., 1991, Local information processing in dendritic trees: Subsets of spines in granule cells of the mammalian olfactory bulb, *J. Neurosci.*, 11:1837–1854.

Xu, F., Greer, C. A., and Shepherd, G. M., 2000, Odor maps in the olfactory bulb, *J. Comp. Neurol.*, 422:489–495. ◆

Yokoi, M., Mori, K., and Nakanishi, S., 1995, Refinement of odor molecule tuning by dendrodendritic synaptic inhibition in the olfactory bulb, *Proc. Natl. Acad. Sci. USA*, 92:3371–3375.

membrane and cellular properties with network functions, thus pointing the way toward a deeper understanding of the neural basis of network functions. The main challenge for the future is to un-

Olfactory Cortex

Christiane Linster, Michael E. Hasselmo, Matthew A. Wilson, and Gordon M. Shepherd

Introduction

The olfactory cortex has traditionally played an important role in theoretical studies of cortical function. It is the earliest cortical region to differentiate in the evolution of the vertebrate forebrain. It is the only region within the forebrain to receive direct sensory input. The olfactory input processed by the cortex dominates the behavior of most vertebrate species. Thus, the role of the olfactory cortex is critical for the evolution of much of vertebrate behavior. Finally, the olfactory cortex has the simplest organization among the main types of cerebral cortex. These features have suggested that the olfactory cortex may serve as a model for understanding basic principles underlying cortical organization.

The olfactory pathway begins with the olfactory receptor neurons in the nose, which project their axons to the olfactory bulb. The function of the OLFACTORY BULB (q.v.) is to perform the initial stages of sensory processing of the olfactory signals before sending this information to the olfactory cortex. The olfactory cortex is defined as the region of the cerebral cortex that receives direct connectons from the olfactory bulb (Figure 1). It is subdivided into several areas that share a basic organization but are distinct in terms of details of cell types, lamination, and sites of output to the rest of the brain. The main area involved in olfactory perception is the piriform (also called prepiriform) cortex (Figure 1), which projects to the mediodorsal thalamus, which in turn projects to the frontal neocortex. This is often regarded as the main olfactory cortex, and is the subject of this article.

Evolutionary Significance of the Olfactory Cortex

For brain theorists interested in principles of cortical organization, the early appearance of the olfactory cortex in phylogeny deserves attention. The cerebral cortex first appears in vertebrate evolution in fishes as a simple structure composed of three layers: a superficial layer containing incoming nerve fibers, dendrites of intrinsic and output neurons, and scattered cell bodies of interneurons; a layer of the large cell bodies of output neurons; and a deep layer of interspersed input and output fibers, and scattered cell bodies of interneurons. This is the classical three-layered cortex. The cortex on the ventrolateral surface that receives direct olfactory input from the olfactory bulb is termed *paleocortex*, which is the olfactory cortex as described above. On the medial surface is another part related to the septum, termed *archicortex*; this is the anlage of the hippocampus in higher vertebrates. On the dorsal surface is the so-called dorsal cortex, generally believed to be the anlage of neocortex.

During phylogeny, the paleocortex and archicortex develop in extent and complexity but retain their three-layered character. Neocortex, however, emerges in mammals as a five- to six-layered structure. It is controversial among evolutionary neurobiologists whether the dorsal cortex can in fact be considered an early representation of neocortex or whether it is more properly considered an anlage, i.e., a predecessor of true neocortex. In reptiles, such as turtles, this dorsal cortex has become sufficiently differentiated to serve as the visual cortex for visual input relayed from the thala-

mus. Whether this can be regarded as a true "primary" visual cortex, homologous to primary visual cortex in the mammal, or whether it is only a primitive anlage of primary visual cortex is a matter for debate.

With the rise of modern studies of synaptic organization, it was hypothesized that comparisons between brain cortical regions in phylogeny should focus less on the numbers of layers and more on the particular types of circuits that are present and the functions that they mediate (Shepherd, 1998). We will therefore identify the main types of circuits that are present in the olfactory cortex. We will then describe compartmental and network models, and discuss the insights gained from these models into olfactory processing and their relevance for understanding general properties of cortical networks.

Basic Circuit for Olfactory Cortex

The concept of a basic or "canonical" circuit is of critical importance for computational neuroscience and brain theory. The basic circuit combines the results of anatomical, physiological, neurochemical, and computational studies into a consensus representation of the main circuits in a particular region (Shepherd, 1998). This objective is facilitated by the extent to which the region in question has distinct layers, clearly differentiated cell types, and readily characterizable inputs. Of all cortical regions, the olfactory cortex best satisfies these criteria.

Our current understanding of the olfactory cortex basic circuit has arisen from a series of anatomical, physiological, and pharmacological studies. The current consensus model is summarized in Figure 2. The main features of the basic circuit include the following.

The primary sensory input (through the lateral olfactory tract from the olfactory bulb) makes its synapses on the most distal parts of the apical dendrites of the pyramidal neurons. This continues the pattern present in the earlier stages of the olfactory pathway, in which primary sensory input is delivered to the most distal parts of the dendrites of the sensory neurons, and their axons in turn make synapses on the most distal dendrites of their targets, the mitral/tufted cells of the olfactory bulb. Thus, distal dendrites, rather than being sites for weak background modulation of neuronal activity, are the preferred sites for rapid transmission of specific sensory transmission from neuron to neuron in this pathway. This fact is critically important for brain theorists and neural modelers, because it means that the specific properties of distal dendrites must be included in network models in order to represent the mechanisms of processing. The properties of dendrites are discussed in PERSPECTIVE ON NEURON MODEL COMPLEXITY.

The distal inputs in olfactory cortex are made exclusively onto dendritic spines of the apical dendrites. These are very small branches, only a micron or so in length and 0.1–0.2 μm in diameter, terminating in a head (1–2 μm across) that receives an excitatory synapse. Spines are of considerable current interest as sites for activity-dependent mechanisms, such as long-term potentiation (LTP), that may underlie learning (reviewed in Shepherd, 1998). Both the afferent excitatory inputs and the recurrent excitatory inputs are made to spines, and both show properties of LTP.

The intrinsic cortical circuits for processing information consist of inhibitory and excitatory local circuits. The inhibitory circuits are of two types: those for feedforward inhibition and those for feedback (lateral) inhibition, as indicated in Figure 2. A given interneuron may be involved exclusively in one of these types, or it may be a node for convergence and integration of both types. The excitatory circuits provide not only for the excitation of the inhibitory interneurons in the feedback (lateral) pathway, but also for direct recurrent excitation of other pyramidal neurons. These intrinsic excitatory and inhibitory inputs are made to different regions

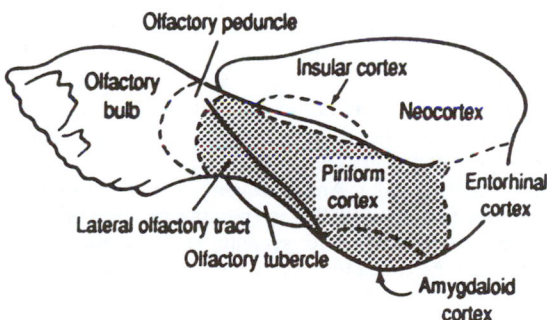

Figure 1. The relation of the olfactory cortex to the main components of the olfactory pathway. (From Haberly, L. B., 1990, Olfactory cortex, in *The Synaptic Organization of the Brain* (G. M. Shepherd, Ed.), New York: Oxford University Press. Reprinted with permission.)

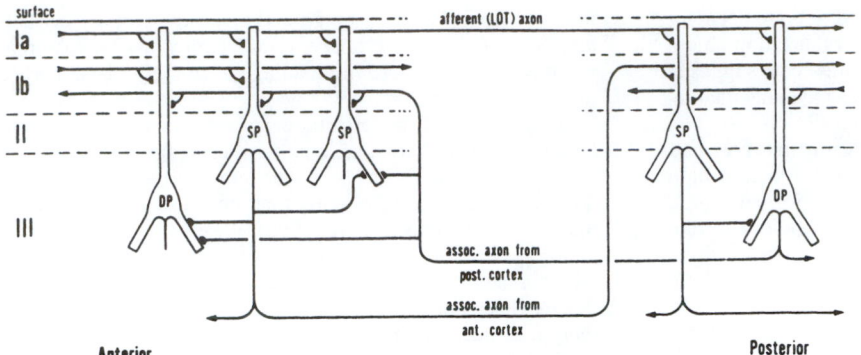

Figure 2. The basic circuit of the olfactory cortex. FF, feedforward; FB, feedback; P, pyramidal neurons, superficial (S) and deep (D). (From Haberly, L. B., 1990, Olfactory cortex, in *The Synaptic Organization of the Brain* (G. M. Shepherd, Ed.), New York: Oxford University Press. Reprinted with permission.)

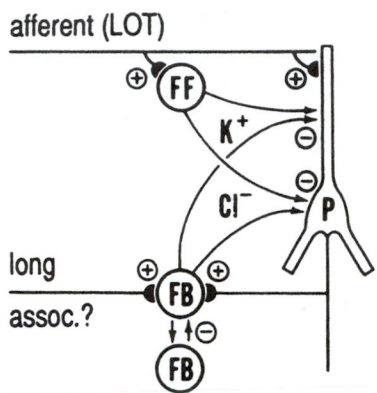

and levels of the apical and basal dendritic trees of the pyramidal neurons. Thus, in the case of apical dendrites, these inputs can gate the transfer of the specific sensory responses in the distal dendrites to the soma.

The essential elements of the olfactory cortex basic circuit can thus be summarized as follows: (1) pyramidal output neurons, with apical and basal dendritic fields; (2) differentiation of pyramidal neurons into subtypes in sublayers; (3) reception of excitatory inputs by dendritic spines; (4) different modes of input driving: direct excitation, feedforward inhibition; (5) intrinsic recurrent axon collaterals for feedback and lateral inhibition; (6) intrinsic recurrent axon collaterals for feedback and lateral excitation; and (7) lamination of inputs to the dendritic trees of pyramidal neurons. Taken together, these constitute a unique set of circuit elements that not only is characteristic of olfactory cortex but also is shared with the other type of three-layered cortex, the dentate-hippocampal complex. Furthermore, these elements are also embedded in most regions of neocortex, where they are further elaborated into additional layers, additional subtypes of neurons and internal circuits, and additional types of inputs and outputs (see Shepherd, 1998).

Network Models of Olfactory Cortex

The first suggestion that olfactory cortex could serve as a simple model for learning and memory in cortical networks was made by Lewis Haberly. In a landmark paper (Haberly, 1985), he described the features of the olfactory cortex outlined above, and pointed out that this organization, distributed in a broad sheet, would subserve the functions of a cortex with content-addressable memory. The critical features were the widespread distribution of inputs by the input fibers and the presence of recurrent excitation, providing for a wealth of combinatorial possibilities for activation and reactivation of the cortical circuits. He further pointed out the possible

similarities between processing of the olfactory input by olfactory cortex and processing of complex visual stimuli in the face area of the neocortex.

These suggestions stimulated studies by several laboratories that have established the olfactory cortex as an attractive subject for network models of cortical functions. We will summarize briefly some of the main studies to date.

Ambros-Ingerson, Granger, and Lynch (1990) drew on the basic olfactory circuit to discuss the principles of a model of piriform (olfactory) cortex that would function as an associative memory network having the ability to identify conjunctions of odor components that constitute complex odors. The role of piriform cortex in olfactory memory was contrasted with the role of the hippocampus in maintaining or enabling the establishment of long-term olfactory associations. A reduced model of the basic olfactory circuit was described that incorporated properties of LTP and that implements a "combinatorial memory system." In this model, during learning, novel combinations of stimulus features result in unique representations. Complex stimuli composed of previously experienced odor components produce a response that is biased toward the existing representations within the cortex. It was proposed that piriform cortex could be regarded as a model for a general cortical memory representational system of this type.

In pursuing this model, Ambros-Ingerson et al. (1990) obtained results that led to a proposal that interactions between the olfactory bulb and olfactory cortex, with synaptic modification in the input pathway, could result in a form of hierarchical clustering that could serve to construct perceptual hierarchies used for storage and recognition of complex olfactory stimuli. This was a departure from earlier models, which had explored the role of intrinsic excitatory connections in associative memory functions. In this model, the olfactory cortex selectively inhibits previously active olfactory bulbar neurons. The response to subsequent odor presentations leads to responses that reflect the differences between stimuli. While experimental work reported a tendency for cortical response generalization following the presentation of a number of similar stimuli, supporting the type of clustering predicted by this model, this intriguing hypothesis awaits further experimental testing.

Building on the work of Haberly and his collaborators, Wilson and Bower (1992) used the piriform cortex to approach the investigation of cortical function on two fronts. First, compartmental models of pyramidal neurons based on anatomical and physiological data, as reviewed above, were used to simulate intracellular potentials, extracellular field potentials, and ensemble impulse activity as recorded experimentally in response to orthodromic volleys in the lateral olfactory tract. Second, this network model, constrained by physiological response properties, was used for simulations that attempted to demonstrate computational properties that would underlie its functions as an associative memory. The results of this study showed the ability to store and retrieve patterned impulse information in a network that displayed the physiological responses and temporal dynamics of the real cortex, using only a local Hebbian-type rule for modification of intrinsic excitatory synaptic interactions (Figure 3).

An interesting aspect of these simulations was the suggestion of a role for oscillatory phenomena, such as the prominent gamma range (30–100 Hz) extracellular oscillations. It was proposed that these oscillations coordinate computational processes that directly underlie the associative memory function of piriform cortex (Wilson and Bower, 1992). Oscillatory phenomena have become one of the chief subjects of interest among workers pursuing models of piriform cortex.

Based on this model, Liljenstrom (1991) drew on the work of Hopfield to develop further a model that used simplified sigmoidal output units. The local circuits for feedforward and feedback inhibition, together with the excitatory interactions between pyramidal neurons, were critically important for the input-output dynamics. The model demonstrated simultaneous slow theta and rapid gamma oscillations characteristic of olfactory cortex. It reproduced the experimental effects of acetycholine, both on the modulation of these oscillations by selectively increasing excitability and suppressing intrinsic synaptic transmission and on associative memory functions (reviewed in Hasselmo and Linster, 1999).

Hasselmo developed both simplified network models and compartmental network simulations to investigate learning mechanisms (see Hasselmo and Linster, 1999). These models explored the effects of selective modification of both input and intrinsic excitatory connections. Associative memory performance was enhanced by the combination of suppression of intrinsic fiber transmission and increased excitability during learning, as seen with cholinergic modulation. The model could also exhibit effective associative memory properties under these conditions. This work represents a synthesis of abstraction and physiological detail in modeling of cortical function. It was proposed that this model could represent a basic unit for learning and memory in cortical circuits. This model has helped to guide subsequent experimental studies on the suppressive modulatory actions of cholinergic inputs and intepret their implications for the associative memory functions of the network (see Linster and Hasselmo, 2001, for review). Based on this modeling, several behavioral experiments on cholinergic modulation from Hasselmo's group have shown that cholinergic modulation is indeed involved in the processing and learning of overlapping olfactory stimuli (Linster and Hasselmo, 2001). This group has also proposed a possible role for the neuromodulator noradrenaline (NA) in signal-to-noise enhancement in piriform cortex; in that study, data on noradrenergic suppression of synaptic transmission in piriform cortex slices were combined with a model of odor processing in piriform cortex.

This illustrates a noteworthy aspect of olfactory cortical models: their close application to guiding and interpreting experimental

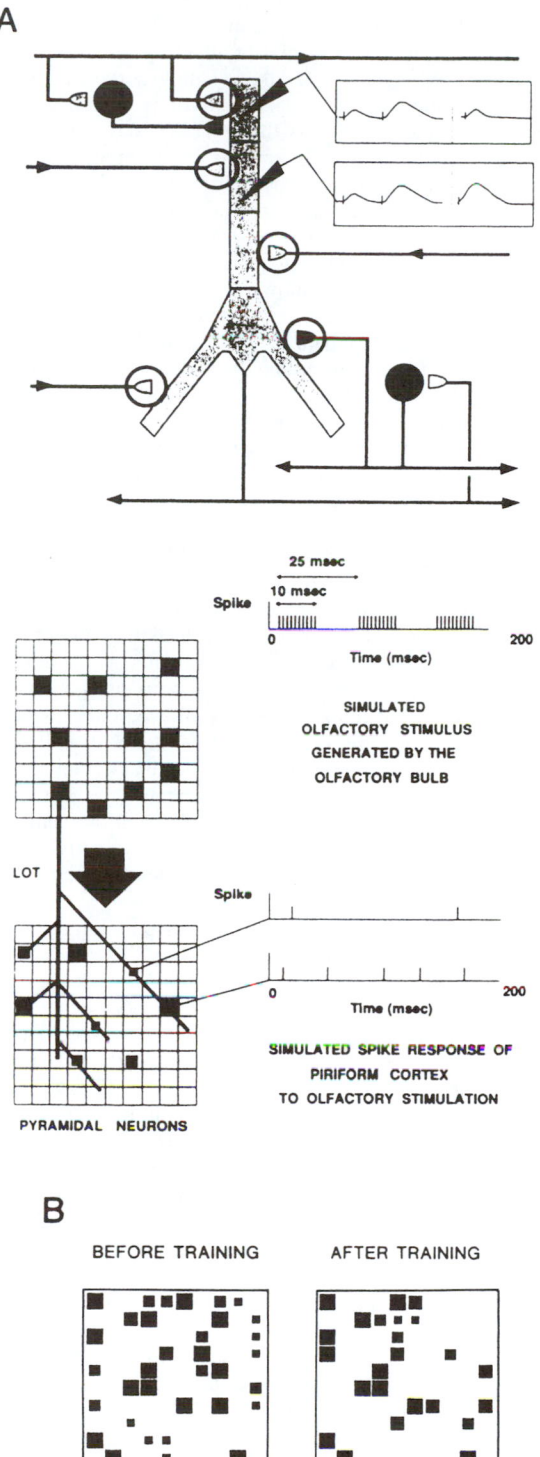

Figure 3. Autoassociation memory functions of a network model based on the basic circuit of Figure 2. *A*, Top, pyramidal neuron model with excitatory (open) and inhibitory (filled) synaptic inputs. Circles indicate synapses where Hebbian modification rules applied during learning. Middle, bulbar input patterns to the cortex (spike activity indicated by size of square). *B*, Responses of pyramidal neurons before and after learning produced a stable activity pattern. (Modified from Hasselmo et al., 1990.)

studies of olfactory cortex. Cattarelli and her colleagues (Litaudon, Datiche, and Cattarelli, 1997) have also used this approach to identify different functional regions within the olfactory cortex.

Nonlinear and chaotic properties of olfactory cortex were studied by Freeman (1987), who showed that a simple cortical model could display the chaotic properties of EEG rhythms; he proposed that a feedback gain parameter Q sets the level of arousal of the cortex. It is this factor that appears to be sensitive to the modulatory actions of acetycholine, as described above. Simulated actions of acetycholine on this parameter in the simplified olfactory cortical model produce point attractor, limit cycle attractor, and strange chaotic or nonchaotic attractor behavior (Liljenstrom, 1991). Recently, several theoretical papers have shown that the neural dynamics observed in olfactory cortex can be modeled to encode odor stimuli in spatiotemporal activity patterns (corresponding to limit cycles) (Li and Hertz, 2000) that resemble those described experimentally (Freeman, 1987) in the olfactory bulb.

An important development in studies of olfactory cortical networks is the realization that their operations are closely interrelated with those of the olfactory bulb, so that they function as an integrated system. An analogy with thalamocortical systems may be made in this regard. This has been recognized in both experimental and computational approaches. Fukai (1996) analyzed the importance of mutual feedback interactions between the olfactory bulb and cortex in a model that represented both structures as chained oscillators. The models incorporated the backprojection from cortical units to the bulbar oscillators in particular ways. Both structures exhibited rapid and robust synchronous oscillations in the presence of odorant stimuli, while they showed either nonoscillatory states or propagating waves in the absence of stimuli, depending on the values of model parameters. Feedback interactions between the two structures were shown to enhance the establishment of large-scale synchrony. The results suggest, in agreement with experimental data, that the modulation of neural activity through centrifugal inputs may play an important role at the early stage of cortical information processing.

A second example of combined olfactory bulb–olfactory cortex networks is the model of Li and Hertz (2000). They postulated that olfactory bulb to olfactory cortex transmission encodes recognition of an odor, while feedback from cortex to bulb generates odor segmentation by producing adaptation that is odor specific. As discussed in OLFACTORY BULB (q.v.), this allows the system to recognize a subsequent novel odor. Independently, Wilson (2000) has provided experimental evidence in single-unit recordings from olfactory cortex that cell responses do habituate to a given odor, that this habituation is associated with a decrease in amplitude of excitatory postsynaptic potentials (EPSPs) from the olfactory bulb, and that this habituation is odor specific. Other examples of analysis of the distributed system that includes olfactory bulb and olfactory cortex include Chabaud et al. (1999).

Running through much of current studies, both experimental and theoretical, of odor processing is the question of the relative importance of spatial and temporal patterns in encoding the information contained in different odorous compounds. The presence of spatial patterns, forming virtual internal "odor images" within the olfactory bulb, has been demonstrated by many methods. However, these patterns are not seen in the olfactory cortex. Temporal patterns are seen in both the responses of single cells and summed EEG potentials, and a strong case has been made on both experimental and computational grounds for their role in encoding odors (see Freeman, 1987). It is important to recognize that both space and time are involved in encoding odors, at all stages of odor processing, as in the processing of other senses; construction of networks is not complete without incorporation of both aspects.

In view of the similarities in organization of the olfactory bulb of vertebrates and the antennal lobe of insects (Hildebrand and Shepherd, 1997), it is of interest to inquire into possible similarities between olfactory cortex and the next stage in the insect olfactory pathway, the mushroom bodies. Several properties that may be involved have been identified experimentally; these properties include long-lasting inhibitory potentials, synaptic plasticity, and wide interconnectivity. It has been proposed that these properties, incorporated into a network model, are well suited for decoding temporal patterns specific for given odors in the dendrites of Kenyon cells in the mushroom bodies.

The models of olfactory cortical function discussed here have been at the neuronal or circuit/network level. The behaviors at these levels depend in turn on properties at the membrane and synaptic level, and on the differential properties of cell bodies and dendrites. An initial step toward assessing these has been made by constructing compartmental models of apical dendrites and their spines and analyzing their responses to excitatory and inhibitory inputs. Basic logic operations of AND, OR, and NOT-AND were found to arise from spine interactions when active membrane properties were placed in the spines or the dendritic branch (Shepherd, Woolf, and Carnevale, 1989). These studies support the idea, discussed earlier, that distal dendrites of pyramidal neurons receive and process rapid, precise input information, rather than mediating only slow and weak background modulation. They emphasize the importance of including apical and dendritic properties in network models to represent the full complexity of cortical circuits and cortical functions.

Summary

The organization of the olfactory cortex can be summarized by a basic circuit composed of a unique set of elements, which may be embedded and elaborated in more complicated cortical regions. Models of olfactory cortex emphasize the importance of cortical dynamics, including the interactions of intrinsic excitatory and inhibitory circuits and the role of oscillatory potentials, in generating the computations performed by the cortex. This replaces earlier interpretations of simple modulation or synchronization of activity within the cortex. In this way, the olfactory cortex, and neural networks based on it, may serve as a useful approach to the study of computations defined by cortical dynamics. It is also recognized that the olfactory cortex functions in close interaction with the olfactory bulb, forming a bulbar-cortical system, in processing odor inputs.

Acknowledgments.   C. L. is supported by a fellowship from the Alfred P. Sloan foundation and M. H. by grants NIH60013, NIH61492, and NIH60450. M. W. has been supported by grants from the NSF and ONR. G. M. S. is supported by RP1 DC 00086-34; PO1 DC 04732-02 under the Human Brain Project; and the Department of Defense under a Multiple University Research Initiative.

Road Maps: Mammalian Brain Regions; Other Sensory Systems
Related Reading: Evolution of the Ancestral Vertebrate Brain; Hippocampal Rhythm Generation; Olfactory Bulb; Perspective on Neuron Model Complexity

References

Ambros-Ingerson, J., Granger, R., and Lynch, G., 1990, Simulation of paleocortex performs hierarchical clustering, *Science*, 247:1344–1348.

Chabaud, P., Ravel, N., Wilson, D. A., and Gervais, R., 1999, Functional coupling in rat central olfactory pathways: A coherence analysis, *Neurosci. Lett.*, 276:17–20.

Freeman, W. J., 1987, Simulation of chaotic EEG patterns with a dynamic model of the olfactory system, *Biol. Cybern.*, 56:139–150.

Fukai, T., 1996, Bulbocortical interplay in olfactory information processing via synchronous oscillations, *Biol. Cybern.*, 74:309–317.

Haberly, L. B., 1985, Neuronal circuitry in olfactory cortex: Anatomy and functional implications, *Chem. Senses*, 10:219–238. ◆

Hasselmo, M. E., and Linster, C., 1999, Modeling the piriform cortex, *Cereb. Cortex*, 13:525–560. ◆

Hildebrand, J. G., and Shepherd, G. M., 1997, Mechanisms of olfactory discrimination: Converging evidence for common principles across phyla, *Annu. Rev. Neurosci.*, 20:595–631.

Li, Z., and Hertz, J., 2000, Odour recognition and segmentation by a model of olfactory bulb and cortex, *Netw. Comput. Neural Syst.*, 11:83–102.

Liljenstrom, H., 1991, Modeling the dynamics of olfactory cortex using simplified network units and realistic architecture, *Int. J. Neural Syst.*, 2:1–15.

Linster, C., and Hasselmo, M. E., 2001, Neuromodulation and the functional dynamics of piriform cortex, *Chem. Senses*, 26:585–594, Review. ◆

Litaudon, P., Datiche, F., and Cattarelli, M., 1997, Optical recording of the rat piriform cortex activity, *Prog. Neurobiol.*, 52:485–510.

Shepherd, G. M., Ed., 1998, *The Synaptic Organization of the Brain*, 4th ed., New York: Oxford University Press. ◆

Shepherd, G. M., Woolf, T. B., and Carnevale, N. T., 1989, Comparisons between active properties of distal dendritic branches and spines: Implications for neuronal computations, *J. Cogn. Neurosci.*, 1:273–286.

Wilson, D. A., 2000, Odor specificity of habituation in the rat anterior piriform cortex, *J. Neurophysiol.*, 83:139–145.

Wilson, M., and Bower, J. M., 1992, Cortical oscillations and temporal interactions in a computer simulation of piriform cortex, *J. Neurophysiol.*, 67:981–995.

Optimal Sensory Encoding

Li Zhaoping

Introduction

What is optimal depends on computational tasks. Many recent works define optimality in information-theoretic terms, such as information transmission rates. This can be particularly revelant in the early stages of vision, which are mainly concerned with transmitting information indiscriminately. In this article we focus on the better-known visual system to discuss optimal sensory encoding, although encoding in other sensory systems can be addressed by similar avenues.

Consider a simplified visual input model with, say, 1,000 × 1,000 pixels arranged in a regular grid at one byte per pixel and 20 images per second. This model provides many megabytes per second of raw data. Given the information bottleneck in the long optic nerve from retina to thalamus and the limited firing rates (thus limited data capacity) of cortical neurons (see SENSORY CODING AND INFORMATION TRANSMISSION), early vision can greatly benefit from a data encoding that reduces the rate of data transmission without significant information loss. Since nearby image pixels tend to convey similar signals (e.g., luminance values) and thus carry redundant information, significant savings can be achieved by avoiding transmitting the information redundantly. If, within a particular time window, each original pixel codes one byte of information, 80% of which is redundant information shared with neighboring pixels, then one million pixels code only 200 kilobytes of nonredundant information. One way to avoid redundancy is to transform the original signal $\mathbf{S} = \{S_1, S_2, \ldots, S_N\}$ in the N neurons (e.g., photoreceptors) to signals $\mathbf{O} = \{O_1, O_2, \ldots, O_M\}$ in another M (more/fewer) neurons (e.g., the retinal ganglion cells or cortical neurons), such that signals in O_i and O_j for all i, j are not significantly redundant. Consequently, 200 kilobytes of information in $\mathbf{S}$ could be coded by only 0.2 bytes in each neuron O_i if $M = N$, which needs a much reduced firing rate. Lossless encoding means that, if needed, $\mathbf{S}$ can be reconstructed from $\mathbf{O}$. Such observations have led to the *Infomax* proposal, namely, that early vision constructs an optimal coding of input to allow maximum information transmission from retina to cortex under limited channel capacity of the optic nerve or neural activities (Attneave, 1954; Barlow, 1961; Linsker, 1990; Atick, 1992). This principle has provided many insights into the properties of the receptive fields in early vision.

Optimal Encoding Illustrated by Stereo Vision

Consider the redundancy and encoding of stereo signals (Li and Atick, 1994a). Let S_L and S_R be the signals to the left and right eyes

(Figure 1). They may be the average luminance in the images or the Fourier components (of a particular frequency) of the images. Assume that they have zero mean (for simplicity) and equal variance (or signal power) $\langle S_L^2 \rangle = \langle S_R^2 \rangle$ ($\langle .. \rangle$ denotes average over the input ensemble). The redundancy is seen in the correlation matrix:

$$R^S \equiv \begin{pmatrix} \langle S_L^2 \rangle & \langle S_L S_R \rangle \\ \langle S_R S_L \rangle & \langle S_R^2 \rangle \end{pmatrix} = \langle S_L^2 \rangle \begin{pmatrix} 1 & r \\ r & 1 \end{pmatrix}$$

where $0 \leq r \leq 1$ is the correlation coefficient between S_L and S_R. The value of r is high, $r \to 1$, for mean luminance signals $S_{L,R}$, but low, $r \to 0$, if $S_{L,R}$ are a high spatial frequency Fourier component of the respective images. A simplifying assumption is that $\mathbf{S}$ are Gaussian signals, which are defined to have a probability distribution $P(\mathbf{S}) \propto exp(-\Sigma_{ij}S_iS_j(R^S)_{ij}^{-1}/2)$. An encoding

$$O_+ = S_+ \equiv (S_L + S_R)/\sqrt{2}, \quad O_- = S_- \equiv (S_L - S_R)/\sqrt{2}$$

gives zero correlation $\langle O_+ O_- \rangle$ in $\mathbf{O}$, leaving output probability $P(\mathbf{O}) = \Pi_i P(O_i)$ factorized, as is easily verified. The transform $\mathbf{S} \to \mathbf{O}$ is linear, which approximates the cell response properties in the retina and, to a less degree, in primary visual cortex. The cell coding O_+ is a binocular cell, owing to the binocular summation of inputs, while the cell coding O_- is monocular or ocularly opponent. Note that $S_\pm$ are the eigenvectors of the correlation matrix R^S, or the principal components of the signals, and their signal power $\langle S_\pm^2 \rangle = (1 \pm r)\langle S_L^2 \rangle$ is the corresponding

S^L $\qquad\qquad$ S^R

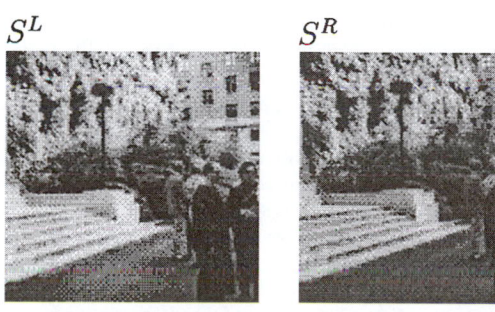

Figure 1. A stereo pair input to the two eyes.

eigenvalues. In reality, input noise $\mathbf{N}$ is added on $\mathbf{S}$, and the coding transform introduces additional noise $\mathbf{N}_o$; hence, $O_\pm = [(S_L + N_L) \pm (S_R + N_R)]/\sqrt{2} + N_{o,\pm}$, giving effective output noise $N_\pm = (N_L \pm N_R)/\sqrt{2} + N_{o,\pm}$. For simplicity, the noise terms are assumed to be independent of each other and of the signals. Let $\langle N^2 \rangle \equiv \langle N_L^2 \rangle = \langle N_R^2 \rangle$, and $\langle N_o^2 \rangle \equiv \langle N_{o,+}^2 \rangle = \langle N_{o,-}^2 \rangle$. Input $S_{L,R} + N_{L,R}$ has

$$I_{L,R} = \frac{1}{2} \log_2 \frac{\langle S_{L,R}^2 \rangle + \langle N^2 \rangle}{\langle N^2 \rangle}$$

bits of (mutual) information about $S_{L,R}$, since, for Gaussian signals and noise, the information amount is $(\frac{1}{2})\log_2$ (signal-to-noise), whereas $O_\pm$ has

$$I_\pm = \frac{1}{2} \log_2 \frac{\langle O_\pm^2 \rangle}{\langle N_\pm^2 \rangle} = \frac{1}{2} \log_2 \frac{\langle S_\pm^2 \rangle + \langle N^2 \rangle + \langle N_o^2 \rangle}{\langle N^2 \rangle + \langle N_o^2 \rangle}$$

bits of information about $S_{L,R}$ or $S_\pm$. Note that the redundancy between S_L and S_R causes higher or lower signal powers $\langle O_+^2 \rangle$ or $\langle O_-^2 \rangle$ in O_+ or O_-, respectively, leading to a higher or lower information rate I_+ or I_-. As an initial choice, define cost as the total signal power, although there can be many other cost considerations (discussed later). Since $I_\pm = (\frac{1}{2})\log_2(\langle O_\pm^2 \rangle) + \text{constant} = (\frac{1}{2})\log_2 (\text{cost}) + \text{constant}$, we note that the gain in information per unit cost ($\Delta I/\Delta$ cost) is smaller in the O_+ than in the O_- channel. This motivates a reduction (increment) of costs in the $O_+(O_-)$ channels by introducing the gains $V_\pm$, such that $O_\pm = V_\pm[(S_L + N_L) \pm (S_R + N_R)]/\sqrt{2} + N_{o,\pm}$, at the expense (benefit) of the information transmitted:

$$I_\pm = \frac{1}{2} \log_2 \frac{V_\pm^2(\langle S_\pm^2 \rangle + \langle N^2 \rangle) + \langle N_o^2 \rangle}{V_\pm^2 \langle N^2 \rangle + \langle N_o^2 \rangle} \quad (1)$$

Hence, the optimal encoding, balancing the cost and information extraction, is to find the gains $V_\pm$ to minimize

$$E(V_\pm) \equiv \sum_a (\langle O_a^2 \rangle) - \lambda \sum_a (I_a)$$
$$= \text{cost} - \lambda \cdot \text{Information} \quad (2)$$

where λ is the Lagrange multiplier whose value determines the balance. The optimal gains can be obtained by $\partial E/\partial V_\pm = 0$ to give

$$V_\pm^2 \propto \text{Max}\left\{ \left[\frac{1}{2} \frac{\langle S_\pm^2 \rangle}{\langle S_\pm^2 \rangle + \langle N^2 \rangle} \right. \right.$$
$$\left. \left. \times \left(1 + \sqrt{1 + \frac{4\lambda}{\log 2 \langle N_o^2 \rangle} \frac{\langle N^2 \rangle}{\langle S_\pm^2 \rangle}} \right) - 1 \right], 0 \right\} \quad (3)$$

In the zero noise limit, when $(\langle S_\pm^2 \rangle/\langle N^2 \rangle) \gg 1$, $V_\pm^2 \propto \langle S_\pm^2 \rangle^{-1}$. As expected, this suppresses the stronger ocular summation signal S_+ and amplifies the weaker ocular contrast signal S_-, in order to save the cost, since the cost increases linearly with $V_\pm^2$, but the extracted information increases only logarithmically with $V_\pm^2$. Hence, for instance, when the coding noise $\mathbf{N}_o$ is negligible (i.e., $(\langle N_o^2 \rangle/V_\pm^2 \langle N^2 \rangle) \ll 1$), output $\mathbf{O}$ and the original input $\mathbf{S} + \mathbf{N}$ contain the same amount of information about the true signal $\mathbf{S}$, but $\mathbf{O}$ consumes much less power with $V_+ \ll V_- < 1$, when $r \sim 1$. This gain $V_\pm \propto \langle S_\pm^2 \rangle^{-1/2}$ also equalizes output power $\langle O_+^2 \rangle \approx \langle O_-^2 \rangle$, since $\langle O_\pm^2 \rangle = V_\pm^2 \langle S_\pm^2 \rangle + \text{noise power}$, making the output correlation matrix R^o (with elements $R_{ab}^o = \langle O_a O_b \rangle$) proportional to an identity matrix (since $\langle O_+ O_- \rangle = 0$). Such a transform $\mathbf{S} \rightarrow \mathbf{O}$, which leaves output channels decorrelated and equally powered, is called *whitening*. Any rotation $\mathbf{O} \rightarrow \mathbf{UO}$ via a rotation or unitary transform $\mathbf{U}(\mathbf{UU}^T = 1)$, by angle θ in the two-dimensional space

$\mathbf{O}$, multiplexes the channels O_+ and O_- to give two alternative channels

$$\begin{pmatrix} O_1 \\ O_2 \end{pmatrix} = \begin{pmatrix} \cos(\theta) & \sin(\theta) \\ -\sin(\theta) & \cos(\theta) \end{pmatrix} \begin{pmatrix} O_+ \\ O_- \end{pmatrix} = \begin{pmatrix} \cos(\theta)O_+ + \sin(\theta)O_- \\ -\sin(\theta)O_+ + \cos(\theta)O_- \end{pmatrix}$$

which are also decorrelated ($\langle O_1 O_2 \rangle = 0$). Furthermore, note from Equations 2 and 1 that cost $= \text{Tr}(R^o)$ and Information $= (\frac{1}{2}) \log (\det R^o)/(\det R^N)$, where R^N is the correlation matrix of the noises in the output channel and Tr(.) and det(.) denote the trace and determinant of a matrix. Since both the trace and the determinant are invariant to unitary transforms (rotations), the optimized objective function $E = (\text{cost} - \lambda \text{ Information})$ is invariant to this rotation $O_\pm \rightarrow O_{1,2}$. Hence, both encoding schemes $S_{L,R} \rightarrow O_\pm$ and $S_{L,R} \rightarrow O_{1,2}$, with the former a special case of the latter, are equally optimal in making the output decorrelated (nonredundant), in extracting information about $S_{L,R}$, and in saving the coding cost $\Sigma_a \langle (O_a)^2 \rangle$. Since

$$\begin{pmatrix} O_1 \\ O_2 \end{pmatrix} = \begin{pmatrix} S_L(\cos(\theta)V_+ + \sin(\theta)V_-) + S_R(\cos(\theta)V_+ - \sin(\theta)V_-) \\ S_L(-\sin(\theta)V_+ + \cos(\theta)V_-) + S_R(-\sin(\theta)V_+ - \cos(\theta)V_-) \end{pmatrix}$$

in general O_1 and O_2 prefer different eyes. In particular, $\theta = -45°$ gives $O_{1,2} \propto S_L(V_+ \mp V_-) + S_R(V_+ \pm V_-)$. The visual cortex indeed has neurons of a whole spectrum of ocularities.

Variations of Optimal Encodings

It is now apparent that infomax coding as defined in Equation 2 is related to whitening, decorrelation, principal component analysis, and *factorial codes*, defined as when probabilities of signals factorize $P(\mathbf{O}) = \Pi_a P(O_a)$. Among the many other relatives of optimal codings are *minimum entropy* or *minimum description length*, since minimizing $\langle O_1^2 \rangle + \langle O_2^2 \rangle$ reduces the total output entropy $H(O_1) + H(O_2)$ (H(.) stands for entropy) for Gaussian signals O_a; *independent component analysis*, since principal components are independent components for Gaussian signals; *redundancy reduction*, since the well-known inequality $\Sigma_a H(O_a) > H(\mathbf{O})$ means that minimizing $\Sigma_a H(O_a)$ reduces the redundancy, intuitively defined as $\Sigma_a H(O_a)/H(\mathbf{O}) - 1 \geq 0$ (equal to zero when there is no redundancy), between output channels; *sparse coding*, since it is defined as lowering the coding bits $H(O_a)$ for all channels a; *maximum entropy code*, since $H(\mathbf{O})$ is maximized given $\Sigma_a H(O_a)$ when redundancy is removed; *predictive codes*, since the code effectively predicts or explains away S_R from S_L to achieve minimum $\Sigma_a \langle O_a^2 \rangle$ for given $I(\mathbf{O}; \mathbf{S})$ (information in $\mathbf{O}$ about $\mathbf{S}$); and *minimum predictability codes* or *least mutual information* between output channels, since $\Sigma_a H(O_a) = H(\mathbf{O})$ means zero mutual information between output channels O_a and O_b. All of these variations of "optimal encoding" often mean approximately or exactly the same (Nadal and Parga, 1997), depending on their precise definitions and the statistics of the signals concerned, and should not be thought of as independent coding principles.

Optimal Visual Encoding in Space, Time, Color, and Scale

In general, for simple linear encoding of approximately Gaussian signals $\mathbf{S}$, a recipe for optimal coding is visualized in Figure 2. Given input signal $\mathbf{S}$ with noise $\mathbf{N}$, the encoding transform $\mathbf{K}$ and additional coding noise $\mathbf{N}_o$ gives output signal $\mathbf{O} = \mathbf{K}(\mathbf{S} + \mathbf{N}) + \mathbf{N}_o$. The optimal transform $\mathbf{K}$ is dictated by the input statistics characterized by the correlation matrix R^S. The first step is principal component analysis, transforming $\{S_a\}$ via a matrix $\mathbf{K}_o$ to the principal components $\{S_k\}$, i.e., $S = K_o S$. The powers of the components S are the eigenvalues of R^S. Next, the optimal gain V_k to S_k is determined by S_k's signal-to-noise ratio via Equation 3. A particular optimal coding transform is $\mathbf{K} = \mathbf{VK}_o$, where $\mathbf{V}$ is a diag-

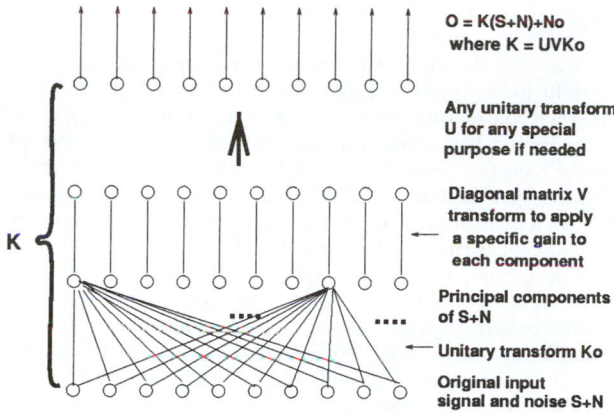

$$O = K(S+N) + No$$
where $K = UVK_o$

Any unitary transform U for any special purpose if needed

Diagonal matrix V transform to apply a specific gain to each component

Principal components of S+N

Unitary transform Ko

Original input signal and noise S+N

Figure 2. A schematic of the steps to obtain infomax (linear) code for Gaussian signals.

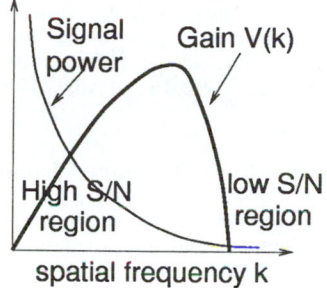

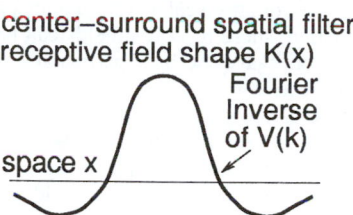

Figure 3. The contrast gain $V(k)$ as a function of spatial frequency k, determined from the signal-to-noise ratio (S/N) of the inputs (S + N) at that frequency. The corresponding spatial filter $K(x)$ is the Fourier inverse of $V(k)$, adopted by the retinal ganglion cells on the photoreceptor inputs.

onal matrix with diagonal elements equal to the optimal gains V_k or $V(k)$. The resulting $\mathbf{O}$ have decorrelated components and retain the maximum information about $\mathbf{S}$ given output cost $\Sigma_a \langle O_a^2 \rangle$. Furthermore, any transform in the class $\mathbf{K} = \mathbf{UVK_o}$, where $\mathbf{U}$ is any unitary transformation (rotation, $\mathbf{UU}^T = 1$), is equally optimal, since it leaves the outputs $\mathbf{O}$ with the same information extraction and cost, and, in the zero noise limit, the same decorrelation. The conceptual steps above correspond mathematically to finding the (degenerate) solution $\mathbf{K}$ of $\partial E / \partial \mathbf{K} = 0$, where $E(\mathbf{K}) = \text{cost} - \lambda$ Information.

In spatial coding (Atick, 1992), the signal at visual location x is S_x. Since the signal correlation is translation invariant, i.e., $\langle S_x S_{x'} \rangle$ is a function of only $x - x'$, the principal components are Fourier modes, and K_o is the Fourier transform $K_o^{kx} \sim e^{-ikx}$ such that $S_x \to S_k \sim \Sigma_x K_o^{kx} S_x \sim \Sigma_x e^{-ikx} S_x$. Field (1987) measured the power spectrum as $\langle S_k^2 \rangle \sim 1/k^2$ with Fourier frequency k. Assuming white noise power $\langle N^2 \rangle$, the high signal-to-noise ratio S^2/N^2 in the low-k region leads to the gain V_k or $V(k) \propto k$ that increases with k. However, for high k, where S^2/N^2 is low, $V(k)$ quickly decays with increasing k to zero, according to Equation 3, in order not to amplify noise. This gives a bandpass $V(k)$ as a function of k (Figure 3). If $\mathbf{U}$ is the inverse Fourier transform $U^{x'k} \sim e^{ikx'}$, then the whole transform $\mathbf{K} = \mathbf{UVK_o}$ transforms signal S_x to activities $O_{x'}$ of a neuron with a receptive field at location x' as a bandpass filter, i.e., $O_{x'} \sim \Sigma_k V(k) \Sigma_x e^{ik(x'-x)} S_x + \text{noise}$. This is roughly what retinal output (ganglion) cells do, achieving a center-surround transform on the input image and emphasizing the intermediate-frequency band where the signal-to-noise ratio is of order 1. Function $V(k)$ is the well-known contrast sensitivity function. When the visual environment dims down, reducing the overall signal-to-noise ratio $\langle S_k^2 \rangle / \langle N^2 \rangle$ in all frequencies, say from $(\langle S_k^2 \rangle / \langle N^2 \rangle) \sim 100/k^2$ to $(\langle S_k^2 \rangle / \langle N^2 \rangle) \sim 1/k^2$, the bandpass region should shift toward lower frequencies, effectively making $V(k)$ a low pass. This explains the dark adaptation of the retinal ganglion cells' receptive fields, from a center-surround contrast-enhancing (bandpass) filter to a Gaussian-like smoothing (low-pass) filter, to integrate signals and smooth out noise.

Encoding in time is analogous to encoding in space. Image statistics in time (Dong and Atick, 1995) determine the temporal frequency sensitivities $V(\omega)$ (of frequency ω) of the optimal temporal filter. Given a sustained input $S(t)$ over time t, the output $O(t)$ may be more sustained or transient depending on whether the filter is more low pass or band pass. By an appropriate choice of the rotation transform $\mathbf{U}$ (Dong and Atick, 1995; Li, 1996), the temporal filter can be made causal, i.e., the output $\mathbf{O}$ depends only on input $\mathbf{S}$ of the past but not the future.

Visual color encoding (Atick, 1992) is analogous to stereo encoding. The inputs are three-dimensional (3D), S_r, S_g, and S_b, for red, green, and blue signals. The principal components include a strong luminance channel, a weighted summation of the cone inputs, and two weaker chrominance channels, one roughly red-green opponency and another yellow-blue opponency. Optimal encoding then involves appropriate gains to these channels and additional multiplexing of them as needed. Physiologically, color and space codings are coupled, resulting, for instance, in the red-center, green-surround receptive fields (Figure 4) of the retinal ganglion cells. This can be understood in a simplified two-cone system, red and green. The high signal-to-noise luminance channel ($S_r + S_g$) needs a center-surround or bandpass spatial filter, while the low signal-to-noise chromatic channel ($S_r - S_g$) needs a smoothing or low-pass filter. The multiplexing of these two channels, a rotational operation $\mathbf{U}$ in the 2D color space, leads to addition or subtraction

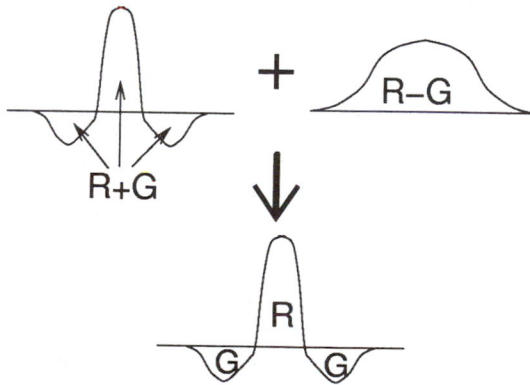

Figure 4. Multiplexing the center-surround achromatic (R + G) filter with the chromatic (R − G) Gaussian-like filter gives a red-center, green-surround double (in space and in color) opponency receptive field observed in retina.

of these two filters. The results are the red-center, green-surround or green-center, red-surround receptive fields. In the retina and/or primary visual cortex, codings in space, time, color, and stereo are all coupled together (Atick, 1992; Li and Atick, 1994a,b; Li, 1996).

Multiscale Encoding in the Primary Visual Cortex

Primary visual cortex receives retinal outputs via the lateral geniculate nucleus. Its receptive fields are orientation selective in the shape of small bars or edges. Different receptive fields have different orientations and different sizes (or tuned to different spatial frequency bands), in a multiscale fashion such that receptive fields of different sizes are roughly scaled versions of each other, also called wavelet coding. These receptive fields can be seen as components of another optimal code by a particular choice of the rotation (unitary) matrix U in the coding transform $K = UVK_o$. Retinal receptive fields are given when $U = K_o^{-1}$, and are theoretically the same for all retinal ganglion cells except for a spatial translation. Another optimal code, apparently not adopted anywhere in our visual system, is when $U = \mathbb{I}$, an identity matrix. The receptive fields would be infinitely large, and each would be unique and a particular principal component (Fourier component) with a particular gain. The U transform for the multiscale coding is when U is somewhere in between the two extremes $U = K_o^{-1}$ and $U = \mathbb{I}$. To construct a cortical receptive field, U multiplexes the principal components (Fourier waves) within a finite frequency range $k \in (k_1, k_2)$ such that the resulting receptive field is responsive only to a restricted range of orientations and spatial frequencies k. The code can be viewed as an intermediate between the Fourier wave code, where each receptive field is infinitely large and responds to only one frequency and orientation, and the retinal code, where each receptive field is small and responsive to all frequencies k and all orientations. Different cortical units cover different ranges of frequencies to give a complete sampling (Li and Atick, 1994b).

It has been argued (reviewed by Simoncelli and Olshausen, 2001) that the multiscale code, which should be as good as the retinal code if the visual inputs assume Gaussian statistics, is actually better in light of the actual non-Gaussian nature of the signals. Oriented receptive fields have been argued to capture the nontrivial third-order statistics, in particular the third-order correlation $\langle S_a S_b S_c \rangle$ between signals from three image pixels a, b, and c, that are not accounted for by Gaussian statistics. Previous works (Simoncelli and Olshausen, 2001) argued that the cortical orientation-selective reflective fields match the orientation features in inputs, and that the neurons are inactive unless those matches happen. The code is thus argued to be a sparser code, since the activities of different cells are supposedly less correlated (see SPARSE CODING IN THE PPRIMATE CORTEX). Why doesn't retina adopt this code? One reason could be that the cortical representation is in addition overcomplete, i.e., the number M of cortical units (output units O_a) is orders of magnitude larger than the number N of the retinal units (input units S_a). The overcompleteness has been argued to improve sparseness, though at the expense of the neural proliferation, because cells tuned to different image features cannot be active together. However, it should be noted that if cortical activities O depend linearly on visual input S, the O units are necessarily (mathematically) dependent on, or correlated with, each other in an overcomplete representation where $M > N$ (Li, 1996). Cortical response O depends on visual input S nonlinearly, by rectification, thresholding, saturation, and normalization, etc. (Simoncelli and Olshausen, 2001). The observed nonlinearity is unlikely to be sufficient to achieve decorrelation. However, the nonlinearity and the overcomplete representation are more likely to serve nontrivial cognitive computations (Li, 2002) beyond the traditional coding considerations.

Discussion

It is clear that maximizing information transmission alone is not enough to specify optimal codes. One may prefer one code or another when considering other costs and benefits (see, e.g., Levy and Baxter, 1996). The retinal code has the advantage of small and identical receptive field shapes that involve shorter neural wiring and easier specifications. It also has stronger correlation between output signals than the Fourier wave codes outside the zero noise limit (both codes should have zero second-order correlation in zero noise limit), making it easier for error correction purposes. Its translation invariance also allows an object translated laterally to induce the same pattern of neural activities except for a change in the responding neurons. When this invariance is extended to objects moving in depth (when images of objects change sizes), the cortical multiscale code is preferred. In this case many different receptive fields are scaled and/or translated versions of each other, leading to translation invariance within a scale and scale invariance between scales (Simoncelli et al., 1992).

More significant are optimality measures not based on information measures. For example, to give a best estimation $\hat{S}$ of input S from $O = K(S + N) + N_o$, the optimal coding transform K to minimize the estimation error $\langle (S - \hat{S})^2 \rangle$ given output power $\langle O^2 \rangle$ certainly does not satisfy infomax. Another example is afforded by the two classes of the retina ganglion cells. Whereas the infomax principle explains well the receptive fields of the more numerous class of retinal ganglion cells, the P cells in monkeys or X cells in cats, another class of ganglion cells, M cells in monkeys or Y cells in cats, have receptive fields that are relatively larger, color unselective, and tuned to higher temporal frequencies. These M cells do not extract the maximum information possible (infomax) about input S, but can serve to extract the information as fast as possible (Li, 1992), i.e., the temporal outputs $(O(t = -\infty), \ldots O(t - 1), O(t))$ should contain some information about $S(t' \le t)$ with a shortest possible delay $t - t'$. This observation should have significant implications for how P and M pathways should interact at later stages of processing.

Information theory provides excellent means to *quantify the amount* of information to design optimal coding for *information transmission*. Cognitive functions often require a selection of the *quality or modality* of information, which is beyond information theory. Information theory is more likely to find application in the early stages of sensory processing, before information is selected or discriminated for any specific cognitive task, when general purpose information transmission is the main concern. This explains the success of information theory in the retina and partly in the primary visual cortex, to the extent that there is quantitative agreement with experimental results and to the extent that information theory has predictive power for new data (Dong and Atick, 1995; Chen and Li, 1998). Optimal sensory coding in later stages of sensory pathways is expected to depend on cognitive tasks beyond simple information transmission, and should require applications of alternative theories in future research.

Road Map: Neural Coding
Related Reading: Feature Analysis; Information Theory and Visual Plasticity; Sensory Coding and Information Transmission; Unsupervised Learning with Global Objective Functions

References

Atick, J. J., 1992, Could information theory provide an ecological theory of sensory processing? *Network: Computat. Neural Syst.*, 3:213–251. ◆

Attneave, F., 1954, Informational aspects of visual perception, *Psychal. Rev.*, 61:183–193.

Barlow, H. B., 1961, Possible principles underlying the transformations of sensory messages, in *Sensory Communication* (W. A. Rosenblith, Ed.), Cambridge, MA: MIT Press, pp. 217–234. ◆

Chen, D., and Li, Z., 1998, A psychophysical experiment to test the efficient stereo coding theory, in *Theoretical Aspects of Neural Computation* (K. M. Wong, I. King, and D. Y. Yeung, Eds.), New York: Springer-Verlag.

Dong, D. W., and Atick, J. J., 1995a, Temporal decorrelation: A theory of lagged and non-lagged responses in the lateral geniculate nucleus, *Network: Computat. Neural Syst.*, 6:159–178.

Dong, D. W., and Atick, J. J. 1995b, Statistics of natural time-varying images, *Network: Computat. Neural Syst.*, 6:345–358.

Field, D. J., 1987, Relations between the statistics of natural images and the response properties of cortical cells, *J. Opt. Soc. Am.* A, 4:2379–2394.

Levy, W. B., and Baxter, R. A., 1996, Energy efficient neural codes, *Neural Computat.*, 8:531–543.

Li, Z., 1992, Different retinal ganglion cells have different functional goals, *Int. J. Neural Syst.*, 3:237–248.

Li, Z., 1996, A theory of the visual motion coding in the primary visual cortex, *Neural Computat.*, 8:705–730.

Li, Z., and Atick, J. J., 1994a, Efficient stereo coding in the multiscale representation version *Network: Computat. Neural Syst.*, 5:157–174. ◆

Li, Z., and Atick, J. J., 1994b, Towards a theory of striate cortex, *Neural Computat.*, 6:127–146. ◆

Li, Z., 2002, A saliency map in primary visual cortex, *Trends Cog. Sci.*, 6:9–16. ◆

Linsker, R., 1990, Perceptual neural organization: Some approaches based on network models and information theory, *Annu. Rev. Neurosci.*, 13:257–281.

Nadal, J.-P., and Parga, N., 1997, Redundancy reduction and independent component analysis: Conditions on cumulants and adaptive approaches, *Neural Comput.*, 9:1421–1456.

Simoncelli, E. P., Freeman, W. T., Adelson, E. H., and Heeger, D. J., 1992, Shiftable multiscale transforms, *IEEE Trans. Inf. Theory*, 38:587–607.

Simoncelli, E., and Olshausen, B., 2001, Natural image statistics and neural representation, *Annu. Rev. Neurosci.*, 24:1193–1216. ◆

Optimality Theory in Linguistics

Kie Zuraw

Introduction

Prince and Smolensky (1993) introduced Optimality Theory (OT) as a framework for linguistic analysis. Kager (1999) gives an entry-level introduction to OT, McCarthy (2001) surveys advanced topics, and the Rutgers Optimality Archive (http://ruccs.rutgers.edu/roa.html) contains hundreds of OT papers. Within phonology, OT has largely supplanted rule-based frameworks. OT has also been applied to syntax and semantics, although not as widely; Legendre, Grimshaw, and Vikner (2001) provide an overview of current work in OT syntax.

Rule-based frameworks account for linguistic patterns through the sequential application of transformations to lexical entries. Variation between two pronunciations of the English plural suffix—[s] in *cats* but [z] in *dogs*—is explained by a rule that devoices the suffix after voiceless consonants (like [t]). The input *cat* + /z/, assembled from entries in the speaker's mental dictionary, is transformed by rule into the output *cat[s]*. In OT, the output is instead chosen through competition with other candidates: a constraint requiring adjacent consonants to match in voicing favors *cat[s]* over *cat[z]*.

Generation of utterances in OT involves two functions, *Gen* and *Eval*. *Gen* takes an input and returns a (possibly infinite) set of output candidates. Some candidates might be identical to the input, others modified somewhat, others unrecognizable. *Eval* chooses the candidate that best satisfies a set of ranked constraints; this optimal candidate becomes the output.

The constraints of *Eval* are of two types. *Markedness* constraints enforce well-formedness of the output itself, prohibiting structures that are difficult to produce or comprehend, such as consonant clusters or phrases without overt heads. *Faithfulness* constraints enforce similarity between input and output, for example, requiring all input consonants to appear in the output, or all morphosyntactic features in the input to be overtly realized in the output. Markedness and faithfulness constraints can conflict, so the constraints' ranking, which differs from language to language, determines the outcome. One language might eliminate consonant clusters by deleting consonants, despite the resulting faithfulness violations; another might retain all input consonants, violating the markedness constraint.

In standard OT, constraints are strictly ranked and violable. *Strict ranking* means that a candidate violating a high-ranked constraint cannot redeem itself by satisfying lower-ranked constraints (constraints are not numerically weighted, and lower-ranked constraints cannot gang up on a higher-ranked constraint). *Violability* means that the optimal candidate need not satisfy all constraints. *Eval* can be viewed as choosing the subset of candidates that best satisfy the top-ranked constraint, then, of this subset, selecting the sub-subset that best satisfies the second-ranked constraint, and so on. Another way of describing *Eval* is that a candidate *i* is optimal if and only if, for any constraint that prefers another candidate *j* to *i*, there is a higher-ranked constraint that prefers *i* to *j*.

The *tableau* (a standard expositional device in OT) in Figure 1 illustrates output selection for the input /ilp/ in a hypothetical mini-language. Each of the four output candidates is flawed: *c*, the most faithful, has a consonant cluster, violating the markedness constraint *CC, as indicated by the asterisk at the intersection of *CC's column and *c*'s row. Candidate *b* has deleted a segment, and *a* has inserted a segment; these candidates violate the faithfulness constraints DON'TDELETE and DON'TINSERT, respectively (phonologists' MAX and DEP). Candidate *d* has inserted a segment without breaking up the consonant cluster, violating both DON'TINSERT and *CC.

*CC is the highest-ranked constraint (ranking is indicated by left-to-right ordering of the constraints' columns; we can also write

/ilp/		*CC	DON'T DELETE	DON'T INSERT
a	☞ [ilip]			*
b	[il]		*!	
c	[ilp]	*!		
d	[ilpi]	*!		*

Figure 1. Optimality Theory tableau.

*CC ≫ DON'TDELETE ≫ DON'TINSERT). *Eval* first eliminates *c* and *d* from the competition (an exclamation point represents elimination) because they alone violate *CC. The shading in the cells to the right represents the irrelevance of *c*'s and *d*'s performance on any lower-ranked constraints. *Eval* next eliminates *b*, because it violates DON'TDELETE. The remaining candidate, *a*, is optimal, as indicated by the pointing finger. In this language, an input string /ilp/ is pronounced [ilip]; in another language the constraint ranking, and thus the output, might be different. There are rankings that would choose *a* or *b* as the optimal candidate. Candidate *d*, however, is *harmonically bounded* by *a*, and by *c*: its violations are a proper superset of both *a*'s and *c*'s. Therefore, *d* cannot be the optimal candidate under any ranking of just these three constraints, although it could be optimal with a larger constraint set.

Wilson (2001) proposes an alternative formulation of *Eval* in which markedness constraints are "targeted": they compare only candidates that are maximally perceptually similar and impose only pairwise preferences on candidates. For each constraint, starting with the highest ranked, *Eval* adds any new pairwise preferences that do not contradict those imposed by higher-ranked constraints, and constructs the transitive closure.

OT in Linguistic Theory

This section reviews why OT has been so widely adopted, and its advantages and disadvantages (see McCarthy, 2001).

OT was developed as a response to a "conceptual crisis at the center of phonological thought" (Prince and Smolensky, 1993, p. 1) concerning the role of output constraints. In a 1970 *Linguistic Inquiry* article, Charles Kisseberth identified a "conspiracy" in Yawelmani: rules of vowel insertion and deletion conspire to place every consonant adjacent to a vowel. Kisseberth proposed introducing constraints (such as *CCC, forbidding three-consonant clusters) to block or trigger rules, which could then be simplified and made more similar across languages. Output constraints were increasingly exploited in the literature, but many aspects of their use were unclear. How should a constraint be designated to block or trigger a rule? What if output constraints conflicted? How could nonabsolute preferences be expressed? For example, Yawelmani allows the sequences C*i*CC and CC*i*C, but underlying CCC is repaired to C*i*CC. Therefore, in addition to the constraint *CCC and the rule of *i*-insertion, there must be a constraint preferring C*i*CC over CC*i*C. But this second constraint is violable, because CC*i*C sequences do occur. OT addressed these problems by eliminating rules entirely in favor of constraints, and specifying how constraints interact.

One advantage of OT over rule-based theories is that it predicts the emergence of the unmarked (TETU): a markedness constraint that is frequently violated in a language may still affect outputs. The constraint favoring C*i*CC over CC*i*C in Yawelmani, for example, is not surface-true (CC*i*C sequences do occur, because high-ranking faithfulness constraints preserve them), but when *CCC forces a vowel to be inserted, C*i*CC is preferred over CC*i*C. A major contribution of OT has been to focus attention on TETU, of which many new cases have been found.

Another advantage of OT is its straightforward account of what McCarthy calls "homogeneity of target/heterogeneity of process." A rule specifies the structure to which it applies (the target) and the operation to be performed on that structure (process). It has long been observed, however, that rules applying different processes to the same target tend to occur, both across languages and within the same language. A rule-based theory has no explanation for why a structure should be a recurring target. In OT, however, the explanation is straightforward: there is a markedness constraint against the target, but whether and how the target is repaired depends on interaction with other constraints. In Figure 1, for example, permuting the constraint ranking yields three minilanguages: one that allows CC clusters, one that eliminates them by vowel insertion, and one that eliminates them by consonant deletion. The set of predicted languages that results from permuting the ranking of a group of constraints is its *factorial typology*. A proposed set of interacting constraints is considered viable only if its factorial typology matches the typology of observed languages—that is, it predicts all existent and no nonexistent patterns.

In some cases, OT's prediction of heterogeneity of process may be overly exuberant. For example, all else being equal, languages that resolve intervocalic CC clusters by deletion delete the first consonant, not the second. Wilson's targeted constraints close this gap and others in the factorial typology: with targeted constraints, deleting the second consonant cannot be optimal under any constraint ranking.

OT is at a disadvantage in dealing with opacity. In a rule-based framework, opacity occurs when a later rule either eliminates the structure that caused an earlier rule to apply (obscuring why the earlier rule applied) or creates a structure that would have caused an earlier rule to apply (obscuring why the earlier rule failed to apply). Standard OT, however, is unable to capture most opacity. Several additional proposals have therefore been made, including harmonic serialism, turbid output representations, output-output faithfulness, sympathy, targeted constraints, and constraint conjunction (see McCarthy, 2001, chap. 3, for a survey). The computability consequences of these proposals, in learning and/or generation, remain to be established.

Computability of OT

Generation

In rule-based frameworks, generation—mapping input to output, the speaker's task—is straightforward. Each rule identifies target structures in a representation, makes the required change, and passes the result to the next rule. In OT, generation presents a computational challenge, because the candidate set may be infinite (in phonology, it is always infinite, because insertions are unlimited). In that case, *Eval* cannot proceed in the obvious way, by first going through all candidates and totaling violations of the highest-ranked constraint, because that first step would never end.

Eisner (1997), building on earlier work by Mark Ellison, proposes a simple way of dealing with the infinite candidate set. At every point in his generation algorithm, the candidate set is represented as a finite-state automaton (FSA), rather than as a list. This is possible if the candidates and constraints are expressed in Eisner's Primitive Optimality Theory (OTP) formalism.

The winning candidate in OTP can be defined recursively. *Repns* is an FSA that accepts all syntactically well-formed OTP representations of input-output mappings. *Input* is an FSA that accepts mappings from the given input to any output. Intersecting *Repns* and *Input* produces an FSA, S_0, that accepts well-formed mappings from the given input. S_0 is the initial candidate set.

Further, define an FSA C_i for each of the *n* constraints in the hierarchy, where C_1 corresponds to the highest-ranked constraint. Each C_i accepts any mapping, but the arcs that a mapping traverses when it violates CONSTRAINT*i* are weighted. C_1 is intersected with S_0 to produce an FSA that accepts S_0, but with the arcs corresponding to violations of CONSTRAINT1 weighted. Dijkstra's Best Paths algorithm, which finds the least-weighted path(s) through an FSA, is then applied to $C_1 \cap S_0$ to yield an FSA (S_1) that accepts the representations in S_0 that minimally violate CONSTRAINT1—i.e., the set of candidates left after CONSTRAINT1 has applied. Repeating this procedure for all *n* constraints, the winning candidate (or set of candidates, if there are not enough constraints to select a unique winner) is S_n.

Comprehension

Comprehension—the listener's task—has been little addressed for standard OT, although Eisner (2000) proposes an algorithm for comprehension under "directional constraint evaluation." A comprehension algorithm would yield, for a given output form, the (possibly infinite) set of inputs that would map to that output under the given grammar. The problem is not trivial: the input may contain a markedness violation not found in the output just in case the constraint ranking is such that the violation would have been repaired by a higher-ranking faithfulness constraint, and the result of the repair would be the observed output.

Learning

Learning—the child's task—includes (at least) two subtasks: building a lexicon and determining the constraint ranking of the target language. If the constraint set is not universal, the learner must also determine what the constraints of her language are; see Boersma (1998) for a model of learning articulatory and acoustic constraints, and Albright and Hayes (1999) for an algorithm that learns morphophonological constraints.

Little work exists on the learnability of the lexicon. Prince and Smolensky (1993) propose "lexicon optimization": where possible, learners construct lexical representations that are identical to the surface representations they hear. When the learner encounters alternations, such as the different pronunciations of the English plural suffix, she must construct a single lexical representation. Curtin (2001) presents evidence that children's early lexical representations are phonetically detailed and do not strip out redundancies; this suggests that lexical consolidation of different pronunciations of the same morpheme occurs relatively late in learning, perhaps after most of the constraint ranking is established.

The problem of establishing a constraint ranking has been addressed more thoroughly. Tesar and Smolensky's (2000) Constraint Demotion Algorithm and its variants rank a set of constraints given a set of outputs. The algorithm compares an observed output (presumed to come from a mature speaker) to any candidate erroneously rated as optimal under the learner's current constraint ranking. In order to make the observed output optimal, for every constraint B that prefers the spurious output, some higher-ranked constraint A must prefer the observed output. If this is not already the case, the learner demotes B below A. The learner must know the input form in order to evaluate faithfulness constraints; in a more realistic model, some interleaving of input-learning and ranking-learning would be necessary. Variants of the algorithm accommodate the common proposal that the learner ranks markedness above faithfulness unless she encounters evidence to the contrary.

The Constraint Demotion Algorithm finds a ranking consistent with the learning data, if one exists. The algorithm has not been successfully generalized to learn variable grammars (discussed below), however, and is not robust to occasional errors in the learning data.

Probabilistic and Variable OT

Intraspeaker variation is common in language: a speaker may produce an utterance differently on different occasions. For example, American English speakers optionally produce [nt] as a nasalized flap (so that "winter" sounds similar to "winner"). The desire to capture variability in OT has led to proposals of variable constraint ranking.

Anttila (1997) proposes that a "stratified" constraint ranking is equivalent to all the linear rankings that are consistent with it, and the predicted frequency of a variant is the proportion of linear rankings that generate it. Suppose a language has the stratified ranking $A \gg \{B, C, D\}$ (i.e., B, C, and D are freely ranked, but below A), and a candidate a is optimal only under $A \gg B \gg C \gg D$ and $A \gg B \gg D \gg C$. The stratified ranking collapses six linear rankings, two of which produce a, so a should be observed 33% of the time. In a corpus study of Finnish genitive plurals, Anttila found a good match between predicted and observed frequencies of variants. No learning algorithm has been proposed, however, for grammars with free rankings.

Boersma (1998) proposes stochastic constraint ranking—ranking that is neither absolutely fixed nor absolutely free, but probabilistic. Each constraint in an individual's grammar has a ranking value in arbitrary units. For every utterance, the speaker generates effective values for each constraint by randomly perturbing each ranking value slightly. Each constraint is thus associated with a probability density function centered on its ranking value. Figure 2 illustrates a minigrammar in which constraint C_1 is nearly always top ranked, and C_4 is nearly always bottom ranked, but C_2 and C_3 are variably ranked, with a preference for the ranking $C_2 \gg C_3$.

Stochastic constraint ranking captures fine-grained frequencies. In an Anttilian grammar with three variably ranked constraints, a variant can occur only 0%, 33%, 67%, or 100% of the time, depending on which rankings produce that variant. In a Boersmian grammar with the same three constraints, the variant can occur at any frequency, depending on the ranking values of the constraints. Boersma and Hayes (2001) suggest some cases of very infrequent variants that would be difficult to capture in an Anttilian model, although firm data remain to be gathered.

An advantage of Boersma's model is its learnability. Boersma's Gradual Learning Algorithm can learn stochastic grammars from variable learning data (if the learning data are not variable, the ranking values learned are so far apart that the ranking is effectively fixed). In each learning trial of the algorithm, the learner compares its production to an adult target form. If there is a mismatch, the learner increments the ranking values of all constraints that prefer the learner's incorrect form, and decrements the ranking values of all constraints that prefer the adult form. The algorithm is robust to errors in the learning data; if an erroneous learning datum nudges a constraint in the wrong direction, subsequent data push it back. The Gradual Learning Algorithm can also model the course of acquisition. Curtin (2001) shows how, for the acquisition of prosody, the Gradual Learning Algorithm successfully models variability in children's productions, stage-like progression, and the order in which markedness constraints are demoted.

The Gradual Learning Algorithm can learn rates of variation because conflicting variants exert opposite influences on ranking values. The more frequent variant occurs in more learning trials, so the relevant constraints' ranking values are separated to the degree that the variants differ in frequency. The algorithm is also able to learn rates of lexical variation (situations in which each word's pronunciation is stable, but certain words display a phonological phenomenon and others do not), as shown in Zuraw (2000). In Zuraw's model, the resulting grammar has high-ranking faithfulness constraints that ensure the correct pronunciation of existing words, with lexical variation encoded in low-ranked constraints that come into play in the production and comprehension of new words.

Discussion

OT was partly inspired by neural networks. The ideas of optimization, parallel evaluation, competition, and soft, conflicting constraints are familiar. Prince and Smolensky (1997) discuss the implementation of OT in a neural network. Constraints are implemented as connection weights, and the network implements a Lya-

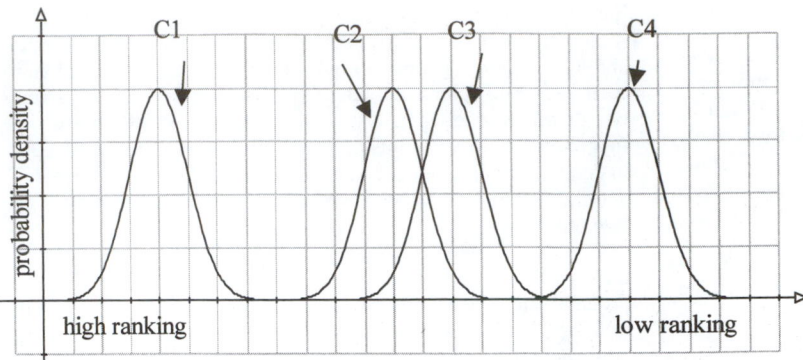

Figure 2. Stochastic constraint ranking.

punov function that maximizes "harmony" ($\Sigma_{ij}\, a_i w_{ij} a_j$: the sum, for all pairs i, j of neurons, of the product of the neurons' activations and their connection weight). Hierarchically structured representations (e.g., consonants and vowels grouped into syllables) can be represented as matrices of neurons, where each matrix is the tensor product of a vector for a linguistic unit and a vector for its position in the hierarchy. Implementing strict domination (rather than the usual numerical weighting) of constraints remains unsolved, however, so translation between OT grammars and neural networks is not in general possible.

Road Map: Linguistics and Speech Processing
Related Reading: Speech Production

References

Albright, A., and Hayes, B., 1999, An automated learner for phonology and morphology, UCLA Working Paper in Linguistics, University of California, Los Angeles.

Anttila, A., 1997, Deriving variation from grammar: A study of Finnish genitives, in *Variation, Change, and Phonological Theory* (F. Hinskens, R. van Hout, and L. Wetzels, Eds.), Amsterdam: John Benjamins, pp. 35–68.

Boersma, P., 1998, *Functional Phonology*, The Hague: Holland Academic Graphics.

Boersma, P., and Hayes, B., 2001, Empirical tests of the Gradual Learning Algorithm, *Ling. Inquiry*, 32:45–86. ◆

Curtin, S., 2001, Enriched lexical representations and constraint organization in a developing system, Ph.D. diss., University of Southern California.

Eisner, J., 1997, Efficient generation in primitive Optimality Theory, in *Proceedings of the 35th Annual Meeting of the Association for Computational Linguistics and the 8th Conference of the European Association for Computational Linguistics*, San Francisco: Morgan Kaufmann, pp. 313–320.

Eisner, J., 2000, Directional constraint evaluation in Optimality Theory, in *Proceedings of the 18th International Conference on Computational Linguistics (COLING 2000)*, San Francisco: Morgan Kaufmann, pp. 257–263.

Kager, R., 1999, *Optimality Theory*, Cambridge, Engl.: Cambridge University Press. ◆

Legendre, G., Grimshaw, J., and Vikner, S., Eds., 2001, *Optimality-Theoretic Syntax*, Cambridge, MA: MIT Press. ◆

McCarthy, J., 2001, *A Thematic Guide to Optimality Theory*, Cambridge, Engl.: Cambridge University Press.

Prince, A., and Smolensky, P., 1993, *Optimality Theory: Constraint Interaction in Generative Grammar*, New Brunswick, NJ: Rutgers Center for Cognitive Science Technical Report TR-2. (See Kager, 1999, for textbook treatment.)

Prince, A., and Smolensky, P., 1997, Optimality: From neural networks to universal grammar, *Science*, 275:1604–1610. ◆

Tesar, B., and Smolenksy, P., 2000, *Learnability in Optimality Theory*, Cambridge, MA: MIT Press.

Wilson, C., 2001, Consonant cluster neutralisation and targeted constraints, *Phonology*, 18:147–197.

Zuraw, K., 2000. Patterned exceptions in phonology, Ph.D. diss., University of California, Los Angeles.

Optimization, Neural

Carsten Peterson and Bo Söderberg

Introduction

Many combinatorial optimization problems require a more or less exhaustive search to achieve exact solutions, with the computational effort growing exponentially or worse with system size. Hence, for large problems, the quest for an exact solution has to be abandoned. Instead, various kinds of heuristic methods have been developed that yield reasonably good approximate solutions.

Artificial neural network (ANN) methods in general fall within this category. Particularly interesting in the context of optimization are *recurrent network* methods based on *deterministic annealing*. In contrast to most other methods, these are not based on a direct exploration of the given discrete state space; instead, they utilize an interpolating continuous (analogue) space, allowing for shortcuts to good solutions. Key concepts here are the *mean-field* (MF) approximation (Hopfield and Tank, 1985; Peterson and Söderberg, 1989) and *annealing*.

Although early versions were confined to problems encodable with a quadratic energy in terms of a set of binary variables, in the past decade the method has been extended to deal with more general problem types in terms of both variable types and energy functions, and has evolved to a general-purpose heuristic for combinatorial optimization. An appealing feature is that the basic MF dynamics is directly implementable in VLSI (see ANALOG VLSI IMPLEMENTATIONS OF NEURAL NETWORKS), facilitating hardware implementations.

Recurrent Networks

Recurrent networks appear in the context of associative memories (Hopfield, 1982) and difficult optimization problems (Hopfield and Tank, 1985; Peterson and Söderberg, 1989). Such networks resemble statistical models of magnetic systems ("spin glasses"), with an atomic spin state (up or down) seen as analogous to the "firing" state of a neuron (on or off). This similarity has been the source of much inspiration for neural network studies.

The archetype of a recurrent network is the Hopfield model (Hopfield, 1982), which is based on an energy function of the form

$$E(s) = -\frac{1}{2} \sum_{ij} w_{ij} s_i s_j \tag{1}$$

in terms of binary variables (or Ising spins, as used in magnetic models), $s_i = \pm 1$ (in some contexts, equivalent 0,1 spins are preferred), with symmetric weights w_{ij}. Owing to the identity $s_i^2 = 1$, diagonal components w_{ii} are redundant and can be assumed to vanish.

With an appropriate choice of weights determined by a set of stored patterns, the latter appear as local minima, satisfying

$$s_i = \text{sgn} \left(\sum_j w_{ij} s_j \right) \tag{2}$$

With a simple asynchronous dynamics based on iterating Equation 2, this system turns into a recurrent ANN, having the local minima as stationary points. In effect, this model serves as an associative memory (see COMPUTING WITH ATTRACTORS).

Update Modes

Note the importance of *asynchronous* update (in random order or sequentially), in which case $E(s)$ is a Lyapunov function and cannot increase. This guarantees the convergence toward a fixed point defining a local energy minimum.

Attempting to iterate Equation 2 in *synchrony* would not necessarily yield convergence to a local minimum. The system could wind up in a two-cycle instead, with a subset of the spins flipping signs on every update.

This behavior can be understood by viewing two consecutive synchronous updates of the N spins as a single sequential update of a system of $2N$ spins, $\{x_i, y_i\}$, where first the x are updated based on y (as $x_i = \text{sgn} \sum_j w_{ij} y_j$), and then the y are updated based on the new x. The corresponding energy $\hat{E}(x, y) = -\sum_{ij} x_i w_{ij} y_j$ is a Lyapunov function, and the extended system must converge to a fixed point (x^*, y^*). If x^* and y^* are equal, they define a fixed point s^* (a local energy minimum) of the original system; otherwise a two-cycle results with s alternating between x^* and y^*. If x^* and y^* are maximally different ($x^* = -y^*$), they define two equivalent local *maxima* of E. Other, mixed cases can be seen as saddle points.

Consider also the related problem of minimizing $-E$ (i.e., maximizing E), obtained by flipping all signs in w. In terms of x, y, the corresponding update equations differ from the original only by replacing, say, y by $-y$. Thus, there is a one-to-one correspondence between sequences of states for s obtained for $-E$ and for E: one is obtained from the other by flipping the signs of every second state. This shows that with synchronous update, the system cannot really tell the difference between minimizing and maximizing E.

The undesirable behavior of synchronous update can be avoided by introducing stabilizing *self-couplings* in the form of positive diagonal elements large enough to make w a positive-definite matrix (and $E(s)$ a concave function); this, however, has the negative side effect of adding a multitude of stationary states that are not local minima.

Below the sequential update mode without self-couplings will be assumed where not otherwise stated.

Optimization with Recurrent Networks

Many types of optimization problems can be encoded in terms of a Hopfield model, with the energy function adapted to a specific problem by a dedicated choice of weights, such that global minima of $E(s)$ correspond to solutions. For simple problems, the recurrent network dynamics of iterating Equation 2 can be used to find a solution. For more difficult problems, however, the system will most likely get trapped in a nonoptimal local minimum close to the starting point, which is not desired. A more refined approach is needed to reach the global minimum, or at least a low-lying local minimum.

Stochastic Methods

A possible strategy is to employ a stochastic algorithm that allows for uphill moves, such as simulated annealing (SA) (see SIMULATED ANNEALING AND BOLTZMANN MACHINES). In this approach, a stochastic neighborhood search method is used in an attempt to generate a sequence of configurations distributed according to a Boltzmann distribution, $P(s) \propto e^{-E(s)/T}$, where T is an artificial temperature representing the noise level of the system, which is slowly decreased (annealing). With a very slow annealing rate, the system can avoid getting stuck in a local minimum, and produce a global minimum as $T \rightarrow 0$. Such a procedure can be very CPU-consuming, however.

The Mean-Field Equations

An alternative is given by MF annealing, where the stochastic SA method is approximated by a deterministic dynamics based on the MF approximation, defined as follows for a system of Ising spins.

The true Boltzmann distribution $P(s)$ is approximated by the direct product of single-spin distributions, $\Pi_i p_i(s_i)$. Such a factorized distribution is characterized by the absence of correlations between the spins and is completely determined by the single-spin averages $v_i \equiv \langle s_i \rangle = p_i(1) - p_i(-1) \in [-1, 1]$. The parameters v_i are variationally determined so as to minimize the *free energy*,

$$F(v) = E(v) - TS(v) \tag{3}$$

where $E(v) \equiv \langle E(s) \rangle = -(\frac{1}{2}) \sum_{i \neq j} w_{ij} v_i v_j$ is the average energy, while $S(v) \equiv -(\frac{1}{2}) \sum_i [(1 + v_i) \log(1 + v_i) + (1 - v_i) \log(1 - v_i)]$ is the entropy associated with the approximating distribution. Minimization of F with respect to v_i directly yields the *MF equations*,

$$v_i = \tanh(u_i/T), \text{ with} \tag{4}$$

$$u_i \equiv -\frac{\partial E(v)}{\partial v_i} \equiv \sum_j w_{ij} v_j \tag{5}$$

The analog *MF variables* v_i take values in the interval $[-1, 1]$, interpolating between the discrete spin states ± 1, which is natural since they approximate the thermal spin averages $\langle s_i \rangle_T$.

Analog Network

The MF equations (Equation 4) can be solved by asynchronous iteration, analogously to the discrete Equation 2. The only difference is the replacement of the sharp step function $\text{sgn}(u_i)$ by a smooth sigmoid $\tanh(u_i/T)$, with an adjustable parameter $1/T$ controlling the gain: high T corresponds to very smooth sigmoids, while in the low-T limit the stepfunction of Equation 2 is recovered.

Most of the discussion on update modes in the context of Equation 2 also applies to the MF dynamics; thus, with asynchronous updating, the free energy $F(v)$ of Equation 3 defines a Lyapunov function guaranteeing the convergence to a fixed point defined by a local minimum of F.

Mean-Field Annealing

In MF (or deterministic) annealing, the fixed-T MF dynamics is slowly modified by lowering an initially high T, using, for example, a geometric annealing schedule.

For the quadratic Hopfield energy, the dynamics then will exhibit a behavior with two phases. At large temperatures, the system relaxes to a trivial fixed point v^o, with $v_i^o = 0$. As the temperature sinks below a critical value T_c, v^o becomes unstable and nontrivial fixed points emerge; as $T \to 0$ these are pushed toward discrete (± 1) values, representing a specific decision made as to the solution of the problem in question.

The position of the bifurcation point T_c can be determined by linearizing Equation 4 around v^o, that is, replacing the sigmoid function (tanh) by its argument. With sequential updating without self-couplings, this yields a smooth tangent bifurcation at a temperature given by the largest positive eigenvalue of w (Peterson and Söderberg, 1989) (see also DYNAMICS AND BIFURCATION IN NEURAL NETS).

For an energy without the exact symmetry under $v \to -v$, as results, for example, from adding a linear energy term, a distinct bifurcation might be absent; then the high-T fixed point is only approximately zero, with the MF variables evolving continuously from smaller to larger values over a finite T interval. This is not a problem: a suitable initial T can still be estimated. Alternatively, an auxiliary spin variable can be introduced and multiplied by the linear term to restore symmetry.

Deterministic annealing yields a more efficient method for finding low-lying energy minima than setting $T = 0$ from the start (i.e., iterating Equation 2). Tracking a local minimum as T is lowered can guide the system to better low-T minima (see STATISTICAL MECHANICS OF NEURAL NETWORKS).

The Graph Bisection Problem

As an example application illustrating the abstract discussions heretofore presented, we will use graph bisection (GB). A graph with an even number N of nodes is to be divided into two halves of $N/2$ nodes each, such that the cut-size (the number of connections between the halves) is minimal (Figure 1A). The encoding is particularly transparent here because of the binary nature of the problem: with each node i a binary spin s_i is associated, to be assigned a value ± 1 representing whether the node will wind up in the left or right partition of Figure 1A. The graph is given in terms of a symmetric connection matrix J, such that an element J_{ij} equals 1 if vertices i, j are connected, and 0 if not (or if $i = j$). With this notation, the product $J_{ij}s_is_j$ is non-zero only for a connected pair of nodes i, j, yielding 1 if they are put in the same partition and -1 if not. Thus, the cut-size is proportional to $-(1/2)\Sigma_{ij}J_{ij}s_is_j$ plus an unimportant constant.

In addition, one needs to take into account the global constraint of equal partition of the nodes, requiring $\Sigma_i s_i = 0$. This can be done by adding to the energy function a term that penalizes an illegitimate partition. A term proportional to $(\Sigma s_i)^2$ will do the trick. Discarding the constant diagonal part $\Sigma_i s_i^2 = N$, we obtain a Hopfield energy function, Equation 1, with $w_{ij} = J_{ij} - \alpha(1 - \delta_{ij})$:

$$E = -\frac{1}{2}\sum_{ij} J_{ij}s_is_j + \frac{\alpha}{2}\left(\left(\sum_i s_i\right)^2 - \sum_i s_i^2\right) \quad (6)$$

where the constraint coefficient α sets the relative strength of the penalty term.

Equation 6 has a structure common in combinatorial optimization problems: $E = \text{Cost} + \text{Global constraint}$. The origin of the difficulty inherent in this kind of problem is very transparent here: the conflict associated with minimizing the two competing terms makes the system frustrated, which often leads to the appearance of many local minima.

For large random GB problems, MF annealing yields a distinctively better performance than simple iteration of Equation 2.

Recurrent Potts Networks

For GB and many other optimization problems, an encoding in terms of binary elementary variables is natural. However, there are many problems where the natural elementary decisions are of the type one-of-K with $K > 2$.

Early attempts to approach such problems with recurrent network methods were based on *neuron multiplexing* (Hopfield and Tank, 1985), where for each elementary K-fold decision, a set of K binary 0/1 neurons was used, with a *syntax* constraint requiring that precisely one of them be on (i.e., equal to 1) implemented in a soft way with a penalty term. In the original work on the traveling salesman problem, as well as in subsequent investigations on the graph partition problem (Peterson and Söderberg, 1989), this approach did not yield high-quality solutions in a parameter-robust way.

A more efficient encoding is based on K-state *Potts spins* with the syntax constraint built in. This confines the dynamics to the relevant parts of solution space and leads to a drastically improved performance.

MF Annealing with Potts Spins

A K-state Potts spin is a variable that has K possible values (states). For our purposes, the best representation is in terms of a K-dimensional vector $\mathbf{s} = (s_1, s_2, \ldots, s_K)$, with the ath state given by the ath principal unit vector, defined by $s_a = 1$, $s_b = 0$ for $b \neq a$. These vectors point to the corners of a regular K-simplex (see Figure 2 for the case of $K = 3$). They are all normalized and mutually orthogonal, and fulfill in addition the syntax constraint $\Sigma_a s_a = 1$.

The MF equations for a system of Potts spins $\mathbf{s}_i$ with a given energy function $E(\mathbf{s})$ in multilinear form ($\partial^2 E/\partial s_{ia}\partial s_{ib} = 0$) are derived in analogy to the Ising case: Approximate the Boltzmann distribution with a factorized Ansatz, $P(\mathbf{s}) = \Pi_i p_i(\mathbf{s}_i)$, parameterized by the single-spin averages $\mathbf{v}_i \equiv \langle \mathbf{s}_i \rangle$. These are determined so as to minimize an associated free energy,

$$F(\mathbf{v}) = \langle E(\mathbf{s}) \rangle - TS(\mathbf{v}) = E(\mathbf{v}) - TS(\mathbf{v}) \quad (7)$$

where the last equality follows from multilinearity; the entropy S is given by $-\Sigma_{ia}v_{ia}\log(v_{ia})$. A local minimum of F satisfies the MF equations

$$v_{ia} = \frac{e^{u_{ia}/T}}{\sum_b e^{u_{ib}/T}} \quad (8)$$

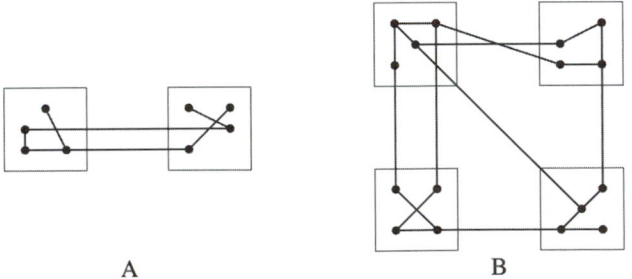

Figure 1. *A*, A graph bisection problem. *B*, A $K = 4$ graph partition problem.

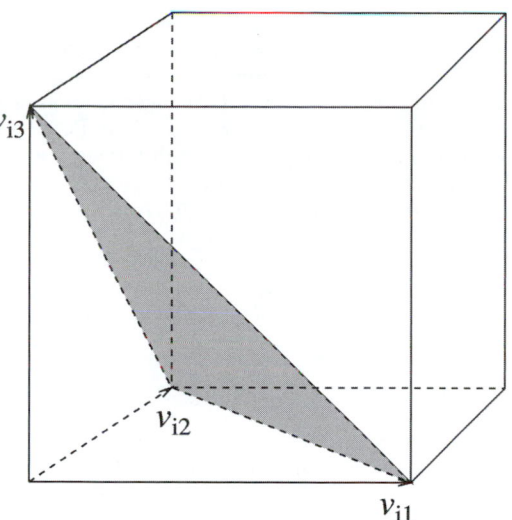

Figure 2. The cubic solution space corresponding to the neuron multiplexing encoding for $K = 3$, interpolating between the eight allowed spin states at the corners of the cube. With a Potts encoding, the solution space is restricted to the shaded triangle, interpolating between the three allowed Potts spin states at its corners.

with

$$v_{ia} \equiv -\frac{\partial E(\mathbf{v})}{\partial v_{ia}} \quad (9)$$

These result in *Potts MF neurons* $\mathbf{v}_i$, approximating the thermal average of $\mathbf{s}_i$, and satisfying $v_{ia} \geq 0$, $\Sigma_a v_{ia} = 1$ (for $K = 3$ the shaded region in Figure 2). A component v_{ia} represents a probability for the ith spin to be in state a. For $K = 2$ one recovers the formalism of the Ising case (with $v_i = v_{i1} - v_{i2} \in [-1, 1]$). As $T \to 0$, each MF neuron $\mathbf{v}_i$ is forced to approach a sharp spin state, defined by the index of the largest component of $\mathbf{u}_i$ in Equation 8 (see also WINNER-TAKE-ALL NETWORKS).

Asynchronous iteration of the Potts MF equations in combination with annealing yields a deterministic annealing approach for Potts systems. As for an Ising system, a suitable initial temperature can be obtained, for example by means of a linear stability analysis.

The Graph Partition Problem

An illustration is given by K-fold *graph partition* (GP): The N nodes of a graph, defined by a symmetric connection matrix $J_{ij} = 0, 1, i \neq j = 1, \ldots, N$, are to be grouped in K subsets of N/K nodes each, with a minimal cut-size (i.e., the number of connections between distinct subsets; see Figure 1B).

GP is naturally encoded with Potts spins, as follows. With each node $i = 1, \ldots, N$, a K-state Potts spin, $\mathbf{s}_i = (s_{i1}, \ldots, s_{iK})$, is associated, where a single nonvanishing component $s_{ia} = 1$ is to be chosen to represent the choice of subset a for node i. A suitable quadratic energy function (cf. Equation 6) is

$$E(\mathbf{s}) = -\frac{1}{2} \sum_{i,j=1}^{N} J_{ij} \mathbf{s}_i \cdot \mathbf{s}_j + \frac{\alpha}{2} \left(\left(\sum_{i=1}^{N} \mathbf{s}_i \right)^2 - \sum_{i=1}^{N} \mathbf{s}_i^2 \right) \quad (10)$$

where the first term is a cost term (cut-size), while the second is a penalty term with a minimum when the nodes are equally partitioned into the K subsets. Note that the diagonal contributions are subtracted in the second term to secure multilinearity.

Writing E as $-(1/2)\Sigma_{ij} w_{ij} \mathbf{s}_i \cdot \mathbf{s}_j$, we have for the input $\mathbf{u}_i = \Sigma_j w_{ij} \mathbf{v}_i$, in analogy to Equation 5.

Refinements and Generalizations

In this section, we discuss modifications and extensions of MF annealing, as well as complications that may arise in optimization applications and that require special care in one way or another.

Continuous-Time Methods

An alternative method for solving, say, the Ising MF equations (Equations 4 and 5) is to use a continuous-time formalism, based on $\dot{u}_i = -u_i + \Sigma_j w_{ij} v_j$, with $v_j \equiv \tanh(u_j/T)$. Indeed, such a formulation was used in the original work of Hopfield and Tank (1985). It is easily generalized to the Potts case. In both cases such a dynamics can also be directly implemented in VLSI.

A continuous-time formalism facilitates an alternative method for implementing a global constraint, such as $\Sigma_i s_i = 0$ in GB, with a linear term $\lambda \Sigma_i s_i$, where λ is a *Lagrange multiplier* to be dynamically adjusted such that a balanced stationary state results. Such methods are discussed in Platt and Barr (1988).

A naive discretization of the continuous-time system with a unit time step results in synchronous updating of Equation 4, with problems like an absent Lyapunov function and two-cycle behavior. However, with a small enough time step $\varepsilon \ll 1$, a stabilized discrete-time approach results, corresponding to synchronous updating of the inputs u according to $u_i = (1 - \varepsilon)u_i + \varepsilon \Sigma_j w_{ij} v_j$, defining a parallelizable alternative to the standard asynchronous discrete-time dynamics. For a sequential software implementation, however, the latter is far more efficient.

Nonquadratic Energy Functions

With a quadratic Potts energy $E(\mathbf{s})$, self-couplings can be avoided and multilinearity secured by removing all diagonal terms, $s_{ia}s_{ib} \to \delta_{ab}s_{ia}$; such a procedure can be generalized to any polynomial E. Although in principle any energy function of a finite number N of spins can be rewritten as a polynomial of at most degree N, this may be difficult in practice for large N with an energy in nonquadratic form.

An efficient and general alternative method for disarming self-couplings in a Potts system with a given generic energy function E is to simply replace the derivative in Equation 9 for the input by a difference:

$$u_{ia} = -\frac{1}{T} \left(E(\mathbf{v})|_{\mathbf{v}_i = \mathbf{e}_a} - E(\mathbf{v})|_{\mathbf{v}_i = 0} \right) \quad (11)$$

where $\mathbf{e}_a$ is a unit vector in the a-direction. Whenever E is multilinear, Equations 9 and 11 are equivalent.

Inequality Constraints

In the optimization problems mentioned above, the constraints considered were all of the *equality* type, $g(s) = 0$, that could be implemented with quadratic penalty terms $\propto g(s)^2$. However, in many optimization problems, especially those of the resource allocation type, one has to deal with *inequalities*. An inequality constraint, $g(s) \leq 0$, can be implemented with a penalty term proportional to, e.g.,

$$\Phi(g) = g\Theta(g) \quad (12)$$

with Θ the Heaviside step function: $\Theta(x) = 1$ if $x > 0$ and 0 otherwise. Of course, such a nonpolynomial term in the energy requires the use of Equation 11.

Inequality constraints appear, for example, in the *knapsack problem*, where one has a set of N items i, with associated utilities c_i and loads a_{ki}. The goal is to fill a "knapsack" with a subset of the items such that their total utility is maximized, subject to a set of

M load constraints. In terms of binary spins $s_i \in \{1, 0\}$, representing whether or not item i goes into the knapsack, the total utility can be expressed as

$$U = \sum_{i=1}^{N} c_i s_i \qquad (13)$$

and the load constraints as

$$\sum_{i=1}^{N} a_{ki} s_i \leq b_k, \quad k = 1, \ldots, M \qquad (14)$$

where $b_k > 0$ define load capacities, which can be seen as representing distinct limiting aspects of the knapsack (its height, width, etc.).

In Ohlsson, Peterson, and Söderberg (1993), a set of difficult random knapsack problems were successfully approached with an MF annealing method based on the energy function

$$E = -\sum_{i=1}^{N} c_i s_i + \alpha \sum_{k=1}^{M} \Phi\left(\sum_{i=1}^{N} a_{ki} s_i - b_k\right) \qquad (15)$$

Scheduling and Constraint Satisfaction

Scheduling problems have a natural formulation in terms of Potts spins and can be approached with Potts MF annealing. A pure scheduling problem can have the following simple structure: For a given set of events, a time slot and a location are to be chosen, each from a set of allowed possibilities, such that no clashes occur. Such a problem consists entirely in fulfilling a set of basic no-clash constraints, $g = 0$, each of which can be handled with a non-negative penalty term, e.g., $\propto g^2$, that will vanish for a legal schedule.

In realistic scheduling applications, there often exist additional preferences within the set of legal schedules that lead to the appearance also of *cost terms*. A set of real-world scheduling problems was successfully dealt with in Gislén, Peterson, and Söderberg (1992), using a straightforward MF Potts formalism.

Pure scheduling is a special type of *constraint satisfaction* problem (CSP) where the entire object is to satisfy a set of constraints. Such problems have been much studied in computer science. *INN* is a modified MF annealing approach dedicated to CSP, where a particular kind of nonpolynomial penalty term is used, based on an information-theoretic analysis. In Jönsson and Söderberg (2001), INN was applied to a set of difficult K-SAT problems and shown to outperform a conventional MF annealing approach based on polynomial penalty terms.

For constrained optimization, a *hybrid approach* might be advantageous, using a conventional polynomial energy term for the cost part and nonpolynomial INN-type penalty terms for the constraints.

Routing Problems

Many network routing problems can be conveniently handled using a Potts MF approach. The basic idea can be illustrated with a simple shortest-path problem: Given a network of N nodes connected by arcs of given lengths, find the shortest path between nodes a and b, i.e., the shortest sequence of arcs leading from a to b.

This problem can be solved in polynomial time using, e.g., the Bellman-Ford (BF) algorithm (Bellman, 1958), where every node i estimates its distance D_{ib} to b, minimized with respect to the choice of a continuation node j among its neighbors (nodes directly connected to i via an arc of length d_{ij}):

$$D_{ib} = \min_j (d_{ij} + D_{jb}), \quad i \neq b \qquad (16)$$

while $D_{bb} = 0$. Iteration of Equation 16 gives convergence in less than N steps, and D_{ab} can be read off.

Also, more complex routing problems, such as ones with several competing routing requests, can be formulated in terms of optimal neighbor choices that can be encoded by a set of Potts spins. The resulting system can then be handled with a Potts MF annealing algorithm. An appealing feature of such an approach is the *locality* inherited from BF: all information required for the neighbor choice is local to the node and its neighbors.

In Häkkinen et al. (1998) a set of complex routing problems in finite-capacity networks was approached in this manner, aided by a *propagator* formalism for monitoring global topological aspects of the fuzzy MF routes.

Mutual Assignment Problems

In certain classes of problems, one seeks an optimal one-to-one assignment between the elements in two sets of equal size N. Such an assignment can be encoded with a doubly stochastic 0/1-matrix s,

$$s_{ij} \in \{0, 1\}, \quad i, j = 1, \ldots, N \qquad (17)$$

$$\sum_j s_{ij} = 1 \qquad (18)$$

$$\sum_i s_{ij} = 1 \qquad (19)$$

such that $s_{ij} = 1$ represents the mutual assignment of element i in the first set with element j in the other.

An example is the traveling salesman problem, where the goal is to minimize the total length of a closed tour connecting a set of N cities with given pairwise distances. This can be seen as finding an optimal mutual assignment between cities and positions in the tour.

In an early approach Hopfield and Tank (1985) to the traveling salesman problem, each component of s was considered an independent binary 0/1 spin, and the row and column sum constraints on s were softly implemented by means of penalty terms. In a refined MF annealing approach (Peterson and Söderberg, 1989), each row of s was taken as a separate Potts spin, while penalty terms were used for the column sum constraints (*row-Potts*; the opposite, *column-Potts*, is of course also possible), yielding a noticeable increase in performance.

Ideally, however, one would prefer a dedicated MF method for mutual assignments. Such an approach can indeed be devised, by using a single Potts spin with $N!$ components, one for each possible assignment. A problem with this approach is the inevitably non-polynomial time consumption for large N, which makes it infeasible for large problems.

For large mutual assignment problems, the best recurrent network method around appears to be *Softassign* (Yuille and Kosowski, 1994; Rangarajan, Gold, and Mjolsness, 1996), where both row and column sum constraints are formally implemented in an exact manner by means of Lagrange multipliers, yielding a formalism that can be seen as a synthesis between the row- and column-Potts MF approaches, although not strictly derived from a proper MF formalism. Softassign requires synchronous updating, in contrast to the row-Potts approach, where one row at a time can be updated; this yields instability problems that have to be remedied, such as with positive self-couplings. At low temperatures, it also suffers an inevitable slowing down of the row and column normalization procedure.

Hybrid Approaches

A large class of optimization problems can be viewed as *parametric assignment* problems, containing elements of both discrete assignment and parametric fitting to given data, e.g., by using templates with a known structure. Then the assignment part can be encoded in terms of Potts neurons while the template part can be formulated in terms of a set of continuous adjustable parameters.

Also, certain pure assignment problems with a well-defined geometric structure can be cast in this form; a nice example is the *elastic net* algorithm (Durbin and Willshaw, 1987; Simic, 1990; Yuille, 1990) for planar traveling salesman problem, where a closed curve is allowed to move and deform elastically in the plane, with each city choosing a nearby point on the curve by means of an analog Potts MF neuron. As $T \to 0$, each chosen point is attracted to the respective city, while the remaining points on the curve are adjusting to form straight segments in between.

Discussion

For a large class of combinatorial optimization problems, a straightforward MF annealing approach can be used, based on an encoding in terms of Ising or Potts spins, with the following basic steps:

- Map the problem onto a recurrent network by a suitable encoding of solution space (in terms of a set of binary or Potts spins) and an appropriate choice of energy function, and derive the associated MF equations.
- Compute a suitable starting temperature (e.g., by means of a linear stability analysis of the asynchronous MF dynamics).
- Solve the MF equations iteratively while slowly lowering T.
- When the system has settled, the solutions are checked with respect to constraint satisfaction, if applicable. If needed, one may perform a simple corrective postprocessing or rerun the system (possibly with modified constraint coefficients).

This very general approach has been numerically explored for many different problem types, resulting in the following general picture. The MF annealing method, without excessive fine-tuning, consistently performs roughly in parity with dedicated problem-specific heuristics, designed to perform well for a particular problem class. Convergence is consistently achieved after a modest number (typically 50–100) of iterations, independently of problem size.

Modified variants of this method have been defined for specific problem types, such as INN for pure constraint satisfaction problems and Softassign for mutual assignment problems. For parametric assignment problems and for certain low-dimensional geometrical assignment problems such as the planar traveling salesman problem, hybrid methods can be used in which Potts MF neurons are combined with conventional analog parameters.

Road Map: Dynamic Systems
Background: Computing with Attractors
Related Reading: Cortical Hebbian Modules; Energy Functionals for Neural Networks; Phase-Plane Analysis of Neural Nets; Statistical Mechanics of Neural Networks

References

Bellman, R., 1958, On a routing problem, *Q. Appl. Math.*, 16:87–90.
Durbin, R., and Willshaw, D., 1987, An analog approach to the traveling salesman problem using an elastic net method, *Nature*, 326:689–691. ◆
Gislén, L., Peterson, C., and Söderberg, B., 1992, Complex scheduling with Potts neural networks, *Neural Computat.*, 4:805–831.
Häkkinen, J., Lagerholm, M., Peterson, C., and Söderberg, B., 1998, A Potts neuron approach to communication routing, *Neural Computat.*, 10:1587–1599.
Hopfield, J. J., 1982, Neural networks and physical systems with emergent collective computational abilities, *Proc. Natl. Acad. Sci. USA*, 79:2554–2558.
Hopfield, J. J., and Tank, D. W., 1985, Neural computation of decisions in optimization problems, *Biol. Cybern.*, 52:141–152.
Jönsson, H., and Söderberg, B., 2001, An information-based neural approach to constraint satisfaction, *Neural Computat.*, 13:1827–1838. ◆
Ohlsson, M., Peterson, C., and Söderberg, B., 1993, Neural networks for optimization problems with inequality constraints: The knapsack problem, *Neural Computat.*, 5:331–339.
Platt, J. C., and Barr, A. H., 1988, Constrained differential optimization, in *Neural Information Processing Systems* (Anderson, D. Z., ed.), New York: AIP, p. 55.
Peterson, C., and Söderberg, B., 1989, A new method for mapping optimization problems onto neural networks, *Int. J. Neural Syst.*, 1:3–22.
Rangarajan, A., Gold, S., and Mjolsness, E., 1996, A novel optimizing network architecture with applications, *Neural Computat.*, 8:1041–1060.
Simic, P., 1990, Statistical mechanics as the underlying theory of "elastic" and "neural" optimizations, *Network*, 1:89–103. ◆
Yuille, A. L., 1990, Generalized deformable models, statistical physics, and matching problems, *Neural Computat.*, 2:1–24.
Yuille, A. L., and Kosowski, J. J., 1994, Statistical physics algorithms that converge, *Neural Computat.*, 6:341–356.

Optimization Principles in Motor Control

Tamar Flash, Neville Hogan, and Magnus J. E. Richardson

Introduction

Optimization theory has become an important research tool in our attempts to discover organizing principles that guide the generation of goal-directed motor behavior. It provides a convenient way to formulate a coarse-grained model of the underlying neural computation, without requiring specific details of the way those computations are carried out. Generally speaking, this application of optimization theory consists of defining an objective function that quantifies what is to be regarded as optimum (i.e., best) performance and then applying the tools of variational calculus to identify the specific behavior that achieves that optimum. This forces us to make explicit, quantitative hypotheses about the goals of motor actions and allows us to articulate how those goals relate to observable behavior. Not all motor behaviors are necessarily optimal, but attempts to identify optimization principles can be useful for developing a taxonomy of motor behavior and gaining insight into the neural processes that produce motor behavior.

Ill-Posed Problems in Motor Behavior

Many optimization-based models in the literature have been developed to address the "excess degrees-of-freedom" problem. How does the motor system select the behavior it uses from the infinite number of possibilities open to it? In mathematical parlance, this is an "ill-posed" problem in the sense that many solutions are possible. For example, most limb segments are moved by a larger number of muscles than appear to be necessary. To reach for a cup of coffee, the hand may move along many different paths. The same figural form (e.g., the letter Z or an ellipse) may be drawn using a wide variety of time profiles for the pen's position. The central question is how the nervous system chooses values for the large number of parameters that can be controlled. One appealing possibility is that the nervous system has evolved to select solutions that maximize the organism's fitness, i.e., that are optimal in some sense. More specifically, the hypothesis is that in performing a motor task, the brain produces coordinated actions that minimize some measure of performance (such as effort, smoothness, etc.). In this article we review several studies in which the validity of such ideas was examined in the context of planar upper limb movements. Similar ideas have been explored in the context of other effector systems and motor actions, such as whole body posture, gait, and various sporting activities, but they will not be considered here. The interested reader is referred to Winters and Crago (2000) for further information.

Arm Trajectory Formation

Our first topic is the kinematic aspects of movement. *Kinematics* refers to the time course of limb position, velocity, etc., while *dynamics* refers to variables such as forces and torques. In principle, even a single-degree-of-freedom movement (e.g., elbow rotation) can be performed in many different ways. Thus, while the hand path is constrained to follow a circular arc, its speed along the path may follow many different time profiles. One way to gain insight into the processes responsible for the selection of specific limb trajectories is to experimentally observe human movements. Patterns or invariances in the observed behavior suggest hypotheses about the way these movements are organized. Optimization theory provides a mathematical tool for concisely formulating and testing these hypotheses. The key step is the identification of an *objective function* that defines a measure of performance by assigning a cost to each member of the class of possible behaviors under study (e.g., arm trajectories). One member of this class (e.g., one trajectory) will then be selected to maximize or minimize that function. How the objective function is defined determines what aspects of the motor behavior are considered important.

Kinematic Versus Dynamic Objective Functions

In this article we will consider two different types of objective functions that have been proposed (out of the multitude of possibilities) as they reflect two major competing theories of how motor computations are organized. The first type of objective function is based solely on kinematic variables (e.g., limb position and its time derivatives). If a kinematic objective function can be found that leads to optimal trajectories that accurately reproduce the patterns of observed behavior, it implies that the brain ignores nonkinematic factors in selecting and producing that behavior. This would be consistent with a theory that, to produce movement, neural computations are organized hierarchically and executed by proceeding from the abstract (i.e., move to that light over there) to the particular (i.e., activate that set of motor neurons in this manner). The most compelling evidence supporting this idea is the observation that similar kinematic patterns are observed even when widely different musculoskeletal systems are involved in producing motor behavior. One's signature on paper is equally as recognizable and distinctive as one's signature on a blackboard, despite the enormous differences in the mechanics and physiology of the body parts used to produce it. Nevertheless, a troubling aspect of this theory is that it seems to imply that, at least at the higher levels of the postulated hierarchy, the brain does not take into account *any* dynamic considerations, such as the energy required, the loads on the limb segments, or the force and fatigue limitations of its peripheral neuromuscular system.

To circumvent this problem within the framework of optimization theory, a second type of objective function may be formulated based on dynamic variables (e.g., joint torques, muscle forces, etc., and their time derivatives). If a dynamic objective function can be found that leads to optimal trajectories that accurately reproduce the patterns of observed behavior, it implies that the brain considers dynamic factors in selecting and producing that behavior. It is also consistent with a theory that neural computations to produce movement are executed in parallel, taking all relevant factors (e.g., dynamics as well as kinematics) into account simultaneously.

Single-Joint Movements

As has been frequently observed, single-joint movements are characterized by single-peaked, bell-shaped speed profiles. This finding and the tendency of natural movements to be characteristically smooth and graceful led Hogan (1984) to suggest that motor coordination can be mathematically modeled by postulating that voluntary movements are made, at least in the absence of any other overriding concerns, to be as smooth as possible. For mathematical convenience (there are many other plausible measures of smoothness), maximizing smoothness was expressed as minimizing mean-squared average jerk, the third time derivative of position. In the single-joint case,

$$C = \int_{t_0}^{t_f} \left(\frac{d^3\theta}{dt^3}\right)^2 dt \qquad (1)$$

where $\theta(t)$ is the joint angle, and t_0 and t_f are the initial and final movement times, respectively. Using variational calculus, the unique time history of joint positions that minimizes this performance measure may be derived analytically. It is described by the following quintic polynomial in time:

$$\theta(t) = c_0 + c_1 t + c_2 t^2 + c_3 t^3 + c_4 t^4 + c_5 t^5 \qquad (2)$$

where c_i, $i = 0, \ldots, 5$ are unspecified coefficients whose values are determined by the conditions at the beginning and end of the movement (boundary conditions). Originally, Hogan (1984) analyzed movements that start and end at rest and therefore assumed zero initial and final velocities and accelerations. Consequently, the predicted trajectories were characterized by symmetric bell-shaped speed profiles. For movements of different amplitudes and durations, the ratio of peak speed to average speed was invariant at 1.88. For a repetitive sequence of movements, speed profiles were again symmetric and this ratio was again invariant, but with a value of 1.57. These predictions appear to be in good agreement with observation. A constant ratio of peak speed to average speed has been reported by several researchers, with values between 1.60 and 1.90, depending on the conditions of measurement. However, a distinctive feature of these minimum-jerk movements is their symmetric speed profile, and that is not always observed experimentally. For example, when enhanced accuracy of target acquisition is demanded, an asymmetric speed profile is typically observed, with the peak speed occurring earlier in the movement. This indicates that the simple minimum-jerk theory may need to be modified. One possible way to account for this asymmetry is by adding (to the objective function) a term to minimize hand-to-target error integrated across the movement. An alternative is to modify the boundary conditions.

Another alternative is to use a dynamic objective function. This requires formulation of a model of neuromuscular and skeletal mechanics to relate dynamic variables (e.g., forces) to kinematics. Hasan (1986) proposed a minimum-effort theory of single-joint movement generation based on a model that described neuromuscular behavior as equivalent to a "spring-like" element driving the limb toward a neurally defined "equilibrium position," determined by simultaneous activation of agonist and antagonist muscle groups. Minimization of effort was expressed as follows:

$$C = \int_{t_0}^{t_f} \left(\sigma(t) \left(\frac{d\beta}{dt}\right)^2 \right) dt \qquad (3)$$

where σ is the joint stiffness (describing the rate of change of the restoring force generated by the "spring-like" element with its displacement from equilibrium) and $d\beta/dt$ is the time derivative of the equilibrium position. Thus, for single-joint movements, optimization theories using both kinematic and dynamic objective functions have been applied with success. A more telling test of these theories is found in multijoint movements.

Multijoint Movements and the Question of Coordinates

The kinematics of multijoint arm movements may be represented in a number of different ways, e.g., as a series of hand positions, joint angles, or muscle lengths. Each of these may be considered as alternative "coordinate frames" for describing the movement. The neural computations underlying multijoint arm movements may make use of any one (or even several) of these representations. Experimental observations of unconstrained human reaching movements are characterized by approximately straight hand paths and symmetric bell-shaped speed profiles that remain nearly invariant despite changes in movement direction, speed, and starting position. Because these features are evident only in the motions of the hand, and not in the movements of individual limb segments, it was proposed that the neural computations underlying movement production take place in terms of hand motion through extracorporeal space and not in terms of joint rotations.

Flash and Hogan (1985) showed that the maximum-smoothness theory reproduced all of these features, provided the objective function was expressed in terms of the Cartesian coordinates of the hand as follows:

$$C = \int_{t_0}^{t_f} \left(\left(\frac{d^3x}{dt^3}\right)^2 + \left(\frac{d^3y}{dt^3}\right)^2 \right) dt \qquad (4)$$

where $x(t)$, $y(t)$ describe the hand position coordinates and t_f is the movement duration.

Minimizing this objective function yielded analytic expressions for the hand trajectories. For unrestrained point-to-point movements starting and ending at rest, the model predictions agreed closely with experimental data and successfully accounted for the invariance of hand trajectories under translation, rotation, amplitude and speed scaling.

In more complex curved movements, patterns were again evident in hand kinematics, but not in joint kinematics. When subjects were instructed to generate curved or obstacle-avoidance movements, although the hand paths appeared smooth, movement curvature was not uniform; the trajectories displayed two or more curvature maxima. The hand speed profiles also had two or more maxima, and the minima between adjacent peaks temporally corresponded to the peaks in curvature.

To describe curved and obstacle-avoidance movements, the maximum-smoothness model was extended by assuming that a small number of points along the path through which the hand should pass are specified (Flash and Hogan, 1985). The time of passage through those "via" points and the hand velocity at that time were not specified a priori but were predicted by the model. For the simplest case of one via point between the initial and final positions, the theory yielded explicit mathematical expressions for the hand motion (Flash and Hogan, 1985) that reproduced all the features of the experimental observations: distinct maxima in the speed profile with a minimum between them which coincided temporally with a curvature maximum; trajectory shape invariant under

translation, rotation, amplitude, and time scaling; and nearly equal durations of movement from the initial position to the via point, and from the via point to the final position. The latter observation was referred to as the *isochrony principle* (Viviani and Terzuolo, 1982), or the phenomenon that movement durations of large and small segments of a trajectory are roughly equal.

Minimum Torque Change Models

In contrast to the maximum-smoothness model, Uno, Kawato, and Suzuki (1989) postulated that movement selection optimizes the rate of change of actuator efforts, e.g., joint torques. Although minimizing jerk and minimizing the rate of change of joint torques appear conceptually similar (in a single-joint system with predominantly inertial dynamics they are proportional to one another), there are important differences. First, the objective function is based on dynamic variables: the rate of change of torque. Therefore, the predicted motion depends sensitively on the modeled dynamic behavior of the musculoskeletal system. Second, the objective function was formulated in terms of joint torques rather than functions of the hand's coordinates, as is the case for minimum jerk. This implies that motor computations are based on a joint-space representation of behavior. Although (as outlined above) kinematic patterns are most evident in hand motions in extracorporeal space, approaches based on either joint or muscle spaces have the advantage that they can generate solutions to important aspects of the ill-posed motor control problems, such as kinematic redundancy (the apparent excess degrees of freedom) or actuator redundancy (the apparent excess of muscles). The maximum-smoothness model expressed in hand coordinates does not address these issues.

Initially, Uno et al. (1989) reported that the performance of the minimum torque change model surpassed that of the maximum-smoothness model. It appeared to account for the small but systematic curvature seen in point-to-point movements, and also for the larger curvature seen in movements that pass from the side to the front of the body. However, an independent study (Flash, 1990) and a later reappraisal co-authored by some of the original proponents of the minimum torque change model (Nakano et al., 1999) invalidated these conclusions: it was shown that a combination of too large an inertia and too small a viscosity contingently led to predictions compatible with experimental results.

However, in Nakano et al. (1999), a variant of the minimum torque change model, the minimum *commanded* torque change model, was introduced. In this model the commanded torque includes non-zero viscous terms that arise from biochemical and mechanical reaction processes within the muscles, and in this way both the muscles and the link dynamics are considered as controlled objects. Using more realistic, measured physical parameters, this second model was again able to reproduce the experimentally verified effects of curvature.

Motor Adaptation Studies

The most critical comparison of these two models arises from their fundamental differences. According to kinematically based optimization models, neural computations specify intended motions independently of movement dynamics or external load conditions. In contrast, dynamically based optimization models imply that external loads profoundly influence intended motions. For example, according to the minimum torque change models, movements in the presence of elastic loads should be more curved than unloaded movements, whereas the maximum-smoothness model predicts no effect.

Investigating motor adaptation to elastic loads, Uno et al. (1989) concluded that the behavior in the presence of the load was different from the unloaded case. Completely different results, however, were obtained in another study in which static elastic loads were unexpectedly introduced during human reaching toward visual targets (Flash and Gurevich, 1997). In the first few trials following load application, movements were found to be misdirected and to miss the target, but after a small number of practice trials (five to seven), the loaded movements tended to follow straight hand paths with symmetric velocity profiles. In another study (Shadmehr and Mussa-Ivaldi, 1994), velocity-dependent force fields were used to perturb the motion, and the perturbed trajectories performed in the presence of the new force fields were again found to converge toward the ones seen in the unloaded case. In a third related study, Wolpert, Ghahramani, and Jordan (1995) used altered visual feedback conditions that caused an increase in the perceived curvature of aiming movements. This led to significant corrective adaptation of the movements actually produced: the hand movements became curved, thereby reducing the visually perceived curvature. These results support the notion that arm trajectories follow a kinematic plan formulated in extrinsic visual space, independent of movement dynamics or external force conditions. They are incompatible with the assumptions of dynamically based optimization models formulated in terms of intrinsic coordinates.

Furthermore, it should be noted that small deviations from straight-line movements do not necessarily imply planning in joint coordinates. Such phenomena are compatible with planning in kinematic space, but with perturbations due to the dynamics of the arm and neuronally controlled muscles at the implementation stage (Flash, 1990). Conclusions with respect to the sensorimotor mapping that associate desired trajectories to motor commands were drawn based on motor adaptation studies. Shadmehr and Mussa-Ivaldi (1994) have analyzed the aftereffects observed when, after training in one region of the work space, subjects were asked to perform reaching movements at a nearby space. The patterns of aftereffects suggested that generalization from learning was in terms of intrinsic joint-based coordinates.

Relation to Physiology

The kinematic and dynamic objective functions discussed above are based on measures of smoothness in different coordinate frames. Both of these models have in common that they are *phenomenological* approaches. The controller (nervous system) and plant (arm) are treated as a *black box*, with the input the experimental task and the output the goal-fulfilling movement. The success (or otherwise) of phenomenological theories in fitting experiment affords insight into which variables the central nervous system (CNS) might consider important in the movement planning process. Results have been presented above that support the idea that the high-level planning processes in the CNS might be in the coordinates of the hand's position.

The fact that movements are smooth, whether in hand or joint coordinates, has been interpreted as compatible with increasing the predictability of the trajectory or reducing the amount of information needed to internally represent motor plans (Hogan, 1984; Flash and Hogan, 1985). Smoothness maximization and the superposition of elemental movements to generate more complicated arm trajectories are also closely related to regularization-based approaches to learning from examples. Those approaches view learning as equivalent to identifying a function from sparse and noisy data. The trade-off between accurate data reproduction and "well-behavedness" of the mapping is achieved by maximizing the smoothness of the function.

Work has also been done on how the CNS might implement an optimization procedure such as minimum jerk. For example, it has been shown that a minimum-jerk movement planner can be directly implemented by a radial basis function (RBF) network. Another implementation scheme was described by Hoff and Arbib (1992), who showed how the minimum-jerk principle could be converted into a real-time controller in which delays and noise effects could explain a number of experimental observations beyond the fitting of simple point-to-point trajectories. However, looking for neural circuits that can reproduce explicitly the calculations inherent in the phenomenological theories of minimum jerk and minimum torque might be a too literal interpretation of the success of such theories in reproducing experiment. The kinematic and psychophysical observations reported to date do not sufficiently constrain the possible movement-generating algorithms to distinguish the finer details of neural implementation. Nevertheless, these phenomenological theories serve as background, coarse-grained descriptors to which deeper, more biologically detailed theories must conform.

Recently, some effort has been made in grounding the optimization approach to motor control in a neurobiological context. It was noted that biological systems are corrupted by noise, the variance of which increases with the size of the signal (Harris and Wolpert, 1998). Hence, any preplanned movement is likely to be off-target when the motor program is run through the noisy neuromuscular system. As each goal-directed movement has some characteristic level of error, this suggests a natural optimization criterion: the CNS chooses movements that minimize the final error in the achievement of the motor task.

Harris and Wolpert (1998) analyzed the predictions of this hypothesis in the context of saccadic eye movements. The error in the final eye position was functionally minimized with respect to the control signal (using a linear model of the plant). It was found that small final error was achieved by low-bandwidth neuronal signals, corresponding to the smooth velocity profiles seen experimentally. This approach was also extended to arm movements in the particular case of two-joint motions in the plane (Harris and Wolpert, 1998). A large range of experimental results were successfully reproduced, including the small curvature seen in point-to-point movements. Furthermore, it was claimed that the predicted trajectory of the hand was, to a large degree, independent of the specifics of the model of the plant: the controlling neuronal signal adapts to produce similar output.

The role of noise in the coordination of movement has been further examined in the context of *optimal feedback control* (Todorov and Jordan, 2001). It was noted that the variability and redundancy inherent in, for example, the control of the human arm are often treated as problems to be overcome in the planning process. In their work on optimal feedback control, Todorov and Jordan showed that increased accuracy in the goal-specific parameters of movement can be obtained by allowing the variance to increase in the redundant variables. In fact, their model does not enforce a desired trajectory but corrects only those deviations that interfere with the task, a principle of *minimum intervention*. Despite this minimal formulation, experimentally observed features such as simplifying rules, control parameters, and synergies emerge as epiphenomena of the control process. The theory is supported by a number of exemplary experimental results and provides a satisfying interpretation of the role of variability and the so-called degrees-of-freedom problem.

Motion Planning for Three-Dimensional Movements

For completeness, we briefly mention recent work on motion in three dimensions (i.e., not confined to a plane). Compared with the success of optimization techniques in two dimensions, the use of cost function analysis is still in the investigative phase for this more general class of motion. It is known that point-to-point motions in three dimensions are considerably more curved than in the plane. Nevertheless, there has been some success in predicting this more complex behavior using the techniques of the optimization approach. Hypothesized cost functions have included minimum kinetic energy (Soechting et al., 1995), in which it was also shown that a simple Donder's law rule that expresses a kinematic constraint on eye orientation does not apply to arm motions. Other models that incorporate a description of muscle dynamics and hypothesize the minimization of a metabolic energy cost or consider the effect of final posture of the arm have also been developed, representing attempts to deal with the acute degrees-of-freedom problem found in three-dimensional movements.

Discussion

One of the exciting challenges of brain theory is the need to deal with reality at the level of whole, functioning systems. Traditionally, scientific endeavor has advanced our state of knowledge by delving into finer and finer details of isolated pieces of reality—the essence of the reductionist approach. However, because of the limited amount known of these fine details and the difficulties involved in studying complex systems of many neurons, this bottom-up approach is severely limited in its ability to describe systemwide behavior: large-scale, strongly interacting systems exhibit characteristics that emerge primarily from interactions among their parts. To understand them, a top-down approach is far more effective, beginning at a coarse-grained macroscopic level and proceeding to finer levels of detail as their structure is discerned. Optimization theory provides a powerful set of mathematical tools that lend themselves well to a top-down approach to studying the brain. As we have reviewed in this article, optimization theory facilitates a rigorous approach, based on macroscopic observations of psychophysical behavior, to some fundamental and far-reaching questions about the structure of neural computations.

Road Map: Mammalian Motor Control
Background: Motor Control, Biological and Theoretical
Related Reading: Equilibrium Point Hypothesis; Limb Geometry, Neural Control; Sensorimotor Learning

References

Flash, T., 1990, The organization of human arm trajectory control, in *Multiple Muscle Systems: Biomechanics and Movement Organization* (J. Winters and S. Woo, Eds.), New York: Springer-Verlag, pp. 282–301.

Flash, T., and Gurevich, I., 1997, Arm trajectory generation and stiffness control during motor adaptation to external loads, in *Self-Organization, Computational Maps and Motor Control* (P. G. Morasso and V. Sanguinetti, Eds.), Amsterdam: Elsevier, pp. 423–482.

Flash, T., and Hogan, N., 1985, The coordination of arm movements: An experimentally confirmed mathematical model, *J. Neurosci.*, 5:1688–1703. ◆

Harris, C. M., and Wolpert, D. M., 1998, Signal-dependent noise determines motor planning, *Nature*, 394:780–784. ◆

Hasan, Z., 1986, Optimized movement trajectories and joint stiffness in unperturbed inertially loaded movements, *Biol. Cybern.*, 53:373–382.

Hoff, B., and Arbib, M. A., 1992, A model of the effects of speed, accuracy, and perturbation on visually guided reaching, in *Control of Arm Movement in Space: Neurophysiological and Computational Approaches* (R. Caminiti, P. B. Johnson, and Y. Burnod, Eds.), *Experimental Brain Research* Series 22:285–306.

Hogan, N., 1984, An organizing principle for a class of voluntary movements, *J. Neurosci.*, 4:2745–2754. ◆

Nakano, E., Imamizu, H., Osu, R., Uno, Y., Gomi, H., Yoshioka, T., and Kawato, M., 1999, Quantitative examinations of internal representations for arm trajectory planning: Minimum commanded torque change model, *J. Neurophysiol.*, 81:2140–2155.

Shadmehr, R., and Mussa-Ivaldi, F. A., 1994, Adaptive representation of dynamics during learning of a motor task, *J. Neurosci.*, 14:3208–3224. ◆

Soechting, J. F., Buneo, C. A., Hermann, U., and Flanders, M., 1995, Moving effortlessly in three dimensions: Does Donder's law apply to arm movements? *J. Neurosci.*, 15:6271–6280. ◆

Todorov, E., and Jordan, M. I., 2001, Optimal feedback control as a theory of motor coordination, available: http://www-rcf.usc.edu/etodorov/. ◆

Uno, Y., Kawato, M., and Suzuki, R., 1989, Formation and control of optimal trajectory in human multijoint arm movement: Minimum torque-change model, *Biol. Cybern.*, 61:89–101. ◆

Viviani, P., and Terzuolo, C., 1982, Trajectory determines movement dynamics, *Neuroscience*, 7:431–437.

Winters, J. M., and Crago, P., 2000, *Biomechanics and Neural Control of Posture and Movement*, New York: Springer-Verlag. ◆

Wolpert, D. M., Ghahramani, Z., and Jordan, M. I., 1995, Are arm trajectories planned in kinematic or dynamic coordinates? An adaptation study, *Exp. Brain Res.*, 103:460–470. ◆

Orientation Selectivity

Robert Shapley, David McLaughlin, and Michael Shelley

Introduction

The detection of edge information from within a visual scene is an essential component of visual processing. This processing is believed to be initiated in the primary visual cortex, where individual neurons are known to act as feature detectors of the orientation of edges within the visual scene. Individual neurons can have an *orientation preference* (which states that neuron's preferred orientation of the angle of edges) and an *orientation selectivity* (which measures the neuron's sensitivity as a detector of orientation).

This article considers mechanisms of orientation selectivity in the visual cortex. In V1 there is a transformation to orientation-tuned elements (Hubel and Wiesel, 1962). Along the visual pathway prior to V1, in the retina and lateral geniculate nucleus (LGN) of the thalamus, there is weak or no orientation selectivity in single cells. It has been thought from the time of its discovery that orientation selectivity, as an emergent property in visual cortex, must be an important clue to how the cortex works and why it is built

the way it is. Much has been learned about the basic principles of cortical neurophysiology through intense investigations of orientation selectivity.

Models of Orientation Selectivity

Feedforward Models

There are two schools of thought about the explanation for cortical orientation selectivity: feedforward filtering, on the one hand, and strong excitatory corticocortical feedback on the other. The models of the latter, with sufficiently strong excitatory feedback, possess "attractor states" that are intrinsic to the nonlinear cortical dynamics.

Our view, based on experimental results and also on our own modeling, is somewhere in the middle; perhaps a good label for our view of the cause of orientation selectivity in V1 would be *recurrent network filtering*. However, the first view proposed his-

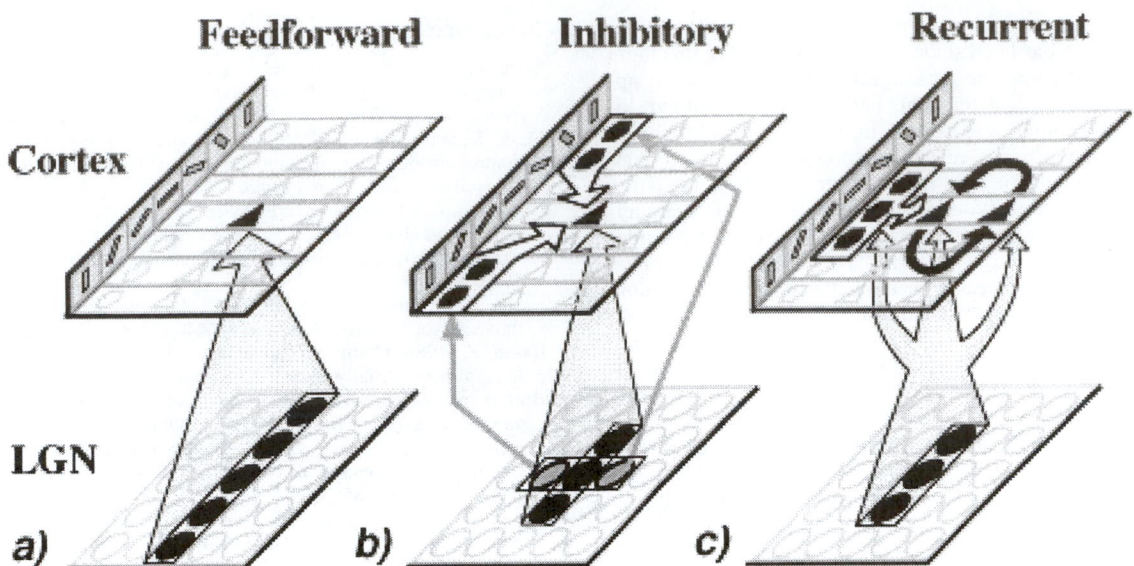

Figure 1. Sketch of different models for cortical orientation selectivity. At the cortical level, hexagonal shapes stand for inhibitory neurons and triangular shapes stand for excitatory neurons. The LGN cells are depicted as the circular shapes at the LGN level in the models. *A*, Feedforward. All cortical cells receive input from a row of LGN cells aligned in space. *B*, In inhibitory models, there is inhibitory input from orientation-tuned cortical neurons, indicated by the outlined white arrows. *C*, Recurrent excitatory and inhibitory feedback models have both corticocortical inhibition (white arrows) and corticocortical excitation (black arrows) impinging on all cortical cells. These corticocortical interactions are supposed to greatly sharpen a broadly tuned input from LGN (indicated by the shorter row of aligned LGN cells). (From Somers, D. C., Nelson, S. B., and Sur, M., 1995, An emergent model of orientation selectivity in cat visual cortical simple cells, *J. Neurosci.*, 15:5448–5465. Reprinted with permission.)

torically and the first one discussed here is the feedforward view, which descended from the pioneering work of Hubel and Wiesel (1962). From the time of its publication, Hubel and Wiesel's feedforward model has been a dominant idea in this field. Figure 1, from Somers, Nelson, and Sur (1995), compares and contrasts the feedforward model in panel *A* with cortical interaction models in panels *B* and *C*. As shown in the figure, the HW model involves the addition of signals from LGN cells that are aligned in a row along the long axis of the receptive field of the orientation-selective neuron. In the HW model, this collection of LGN cells, taken together, sets the orientation preference and selectivity of that cortical cell onto which the LGN cells converge. The experiment on the cooling of cat V1 by Ferster, Chung, and Wheat (1996) is an important result that was interpreted to mean that there is substantial orientation tuning of the collective thalamic input to a cortical neuron, consistent with the HW model. In spite of this evidence, several authors agree that the HW model predicts rather little orientation selectivity, and therefore does not account for the visual properties of V1 cells (Sompolinsky and Shapley, 1997; Troyer et al., 1998; McLaughlin et al., 2000).

The reason for the shortfall of orientation selectivity in the HW model can be stated as follows. LGN cells have a low spontaneous rate but are quite responsive to visual stimuli, so their firing rate during visual stimulation clips at zero spikes per second. Because of this rectification, LGN cells act like nonlinear excitatory subunits as inputs to their cortical targets. Since the HW model simply adds up the LGN sources, and each of these responds to every orientation, the model's summation of the clipped LGN inputs would cause it to have a non-zero response at 90° from the optimal orientation. In fact, the HW model predicts that the total number of spikes elicited by a stimulus could be the same at 90° as at 0°, although the spikes would be more spread out in time at 90° (Sompolinsky and Shapley, 1997; Troyer et al., 1998). Computational simulations of the HW model have demonstrated that this analysis is correct (Sompolinsky and Shapley, 1997; McLaughlin et al.,

2000), as illustrated in Figure 2, where the orientation selectivity of an HW model is shown. But experimental observations establish that many cortical cells respond little or not at all at 90° from peak orientation, so we must conclude that the HW convergence mechanism is only part of the story of cortical orientation selectivity. In the literature on orientation selectivity, it is often stated that the nonlinearity of the neuronal spike threshold could cause major sharpening of the orientation tuning curve in the cortical cell response even if the convergent LGN input is as broad as in Figure

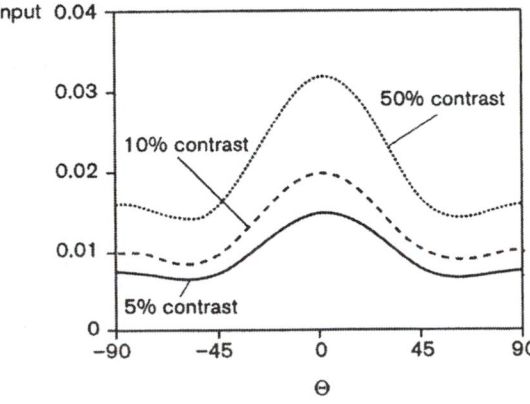

Figure 2. Orientation tuning of a feedforward model. Many LGN elements are assumed to converge via excitatory synapses onto single cortical cells in this model. No corticocortical excitation or inhibition modifies the feedforward excitation. Responses at three contrast levels are shown: 5% 10%, and 50% contrast. At all levels of contrast, there is a non-zero voltage generated 90° away from the preferred orientation. (After Sompolinsky and Shapley, 1997.)

2. This sharpening based on nonlinear thresholding is sometimes termed the iceberg effect. The iceberg effect is not a practical way to obtain sharpening, however. If the threshold is set so high that it causes the requisite significant sharpening, it will also diminish response magnitude a great deal, causing a loss of sensitivity. Also, thresholding works only at one stimulus contrast level. To obtain orientation tuning that does not broaden a great deal at high contrast, one needs another kind of mechanism.

One may wonder why the experiments of Ferster et al. (1996) are not decisive pieces of evidence for the hypothesis that LGN convergence causes a large amount of orientation selectivity. Here is our analysis of these experiments. The cooling experiments of Ferster et al. measured the first-order temporal Fourier component (F1) in the intracellular voltage response to a drifting grating from a neuron in a cooled cortex, and found it to be as tuned for orientation as in the warm cortex. But this does not account for the tuning of the mean spike rate, which is tuned as much as the F1 component of the spike rate. Also, the mean spike rate during a stimulus is the most often measured component of the neuron's response, and thus it is important to explain the tuning of this component. It is known from the work of Ferster et al. and others that the mean spike rate is an approximately linear function of mean membrane voltage (above a threshold value). So, to attempt to account for the orientation selectivity that is observed in the mean spike rate, it would have been necessary for Ferster et al. to measure also the orientation selectivity of the mean intracellular voltage response in the cooled cortex. They did not do this in the cooling experiments reported in 1996, probably for technical reasons. But suppose they had measured the DC response in the cooled cortex, and suppose the HW model does describe the LGN input to V1 neurons. Then we can predict that Ferster et al. would have found the mean (or DC) intracellular voltage response to be only weakly selective for orientation (based on the analysis of the HW model in the previous paragraph and Figure 2). Because the HW model predicts substantial membrane voltage response at 90° from peak, it cannot account for the sharp tuning of mean spike rate that is observed in experiments.

One can go further and analyze why Ferster et al. found so much orientation tuning for the F1 component. The only mechanism for orientation-selective response for an F1 response in the HW model is different spatial frequency resolution along the two axes of the elliptical receptive field. The reason is, the HW model has no inhibition; it is a purely excitatory model. Thus (if indeed the HW model applied), Ferster et al. probably observed orientation selectivity in the cooled cortex only because the spatial frequency of the grating they used was too high for the elliptical LGN array to resolve it along the long axis. However, the spatial frequency was not too high for the summed LGN input to resolve it along the minor axis. To put it another way, if orientation selectivity for the F1 Fourier component depended on feedforward LGN convergence as in the HW model, it would be very strongly dependent on spatial frequency, but in the normally functioning cortex, it is not, as reported 20 years ago by Jones and Palmer and then a few years after that by Webster and DeValois. The conclusion of all these considerations of the cooling experiment is that it is not decisive evidence for a feedforward explanation of orientation selectivity.

Cortical Inhibition

One possible addendum to the HW model that increases the orientation selectivity greatly is to add inhibition, either push-pull inhibition (Troyer et al., 1998) or some other kind of inhibition that is broadly distributed in orientation (Somers et al., 1995; Ben-Yishai, Bar-Or, and Sompolinsky, 1995; McLaughlin et al., 2000). But given what is known about V1, this inhibition must come through cortical interneurons rather than directly from the thalamic afferents. Such a model is diagrammed in Figure 1, panel *B*. Ex-

periments on intracortical inhibition in V1 have given mixed results. Initially, Adam Sillito's experiments with bicuculline suggested that intracortical inhibition might be necessary for orientation tuning. However, subsequent experiments by Sacha Nelson and colleagues at MIT, involving blocking inhibition intracellularly, have been interpreted to mean that inhibition of a single neuron is not necessary for that neuron to be orientation tuned. However, the role of intracortical inhibition has been supported by the work of A. B. Bonds and his collaborators. They have studied interactions between stimuli at different orientations, the effects of blocking activity in infragranular layers, and the effects of GABA on orientation selectivity. More recently, Ulf Eysel and his collaborators in Germany have accumulated a body of evidence in cat cortex for the important role of inhibition in causing a sharpening of orientation selectivity. Eysel and co-workers have blocked the lateral spread of cortical inhibition with local injection of inhibitory agonists that block local activity. When they do this, they often observe broadening of orientation tuning curves.

A theory of orientation tuning in cat cortex offered by Troyer et al. (1998) attempts to explain orientation tuning in terms of specific "push-pull" inhibition in which there is phase-specific inhibition superimposed on phase-specific excitation of the opposite sign. However, the main mechanism for sharpening of orientation tuning in the Troyer model is corticocortical inhibition that is broadly tuned for orientation. In the Troyer model there is moderately tuned LGN-convergent excitation from an HW mechanism, and then more broadly tuned inhibition that cancels out the wide-angle responses but leaves the tuning curve around the peak orientation relatively unchanged. Therefore, this model is one of a class of corticocortical interaction models for orientation selectivity.

More recently, we have developed a large-scale model of four hypercolumns in layer 4cα of macaque V1. The hypercolumn, a compact cortical region approximately 0.5 mm × 0.5 mm in area, is the unit of cortical processing. All orientations are represented in a hypercolumn, by arrays of neurons of similar orientation preference arranged as if they were spokes of a pinwheel around a central singularity, the pinwheel center. This architecture has been deduced from the results of experiments with intrinsic optical imaging by Bonhoeffer and Grinvald (1993). Our model incorporates known facts about the physiology and anatomy of V1. This model accounts for many visual properties of V1 neurons, especially orientation selectivity. Inspired by the Somers et al. (1995) and Ben-Yishai et al. (1995) models, it seeks to account for the same set of phenomena as these models but with more biological realism. One novelty in our model is that the spatial strength of connections between neurons is taken to be the spatial density of synaptic connections revealed by anatomical investigations of cortex. The model places the "footprints" of synaptic excitation and inhibition on the pinwheel latticework that is revealed by optical imaging (Bonhoeffer and Grinvald, 1993). In our model the spatial scale of corticocortical excitation exceeds that of inhibition, as indicated by cortical neuroanatomy. In its focus on the visual-functional consequences of the pinwheel organization, our model is novel and original. Our model causes significant sharpening and also diversity of orientation selectivity, and produces simple cells. The most significant difference between this model and that of Troyer et al. (1998) is that in our model (the McLaughlin model), the inhibitory conductance input to a cell is phase-insensitive (the opposite of push-pull). This happens because inhibition of a model cell is a sum from many neural sources, and it is likely that each of these sources is a cortical inhibitory cell with a fixed phase preference different from those of neighboring neurons. It is also consistent with the measured phase insensitivity of measured inhibition (Borg-Graham, Monier, and Fregnac, 1998; Anderson, Carandini, and Ferster, 2000). Anderson et al. (2000) state that their data support a push-pull, that is, phase-sensitive inhibition model. However, a close scrutiny of their data reveals that much of the measured inhibitory conductance (in response to drifting gratings) is a phase-insensitive elevation of inhibition, as predicted by the McLaughlin model (a point discussed in Wielaard et al., 2001).

Cortical Excitation and Attractor Models

The idea that corticocortical excitatory feedback plays a crucial role in orientation tuning has been put forward most forcefully by theorists of brain function. Several well-known papers make the case for this corticocortical feedback. One, by Somers et al. (1995), presents an elaborate computational model for orientation tuning. Another paper in this genre is by Ben-Yishai et al. (1995), who offer an analytical model from which they make several qualitative and quantitative predictions. One of their important theoretical results is that one cannot predict contrast invariance of orientation tuning with feedforward models, but the feedback model of Ben-Yishai et al., with recurrent excitation and inhibition, does exhibit contrast invariance. Another of their results is that if recurrent feedback is strong enough, one will observe the "marginal phase" state in which V1 behaves like a set of attractors for orientation. Using a ring model that resembles the architecture of the Ben-Yishai model, Pugh et al. (2000) demonstrated that they could account for some of the important features of orientation dynamics that could not be explained by feedforward models, features such as the Mexican-hat tuning in orientation.

The attractor states of recurrent excitatory models are discussed not only by Ben-Yishai et al. (1995) but also by Tsodyks et al. (1999). Using intrinsic optical imaging of visual cortex, Tsodyks et al. found that there were patterns of spontaneous activity that resembled the patterns evoked during stimulation with oriented gratings. This provided some evidence for the idea that there were active states of cortical activity associated with orientation selectivity. The concept is that very weakly orientation-selective feedforward signals can be massively sharpened by strong recurrent excitatory feedback, causing the cortex to respond to any visual signal by relaxing into a state of activity governed by the pattern of corticocortical feedback. We believe that this theory, like the pure feedforward theory, has trouble explaining some important data, for instance, the existence of simple cells in which response waveforms follow the time course of the stimulus faithfully.

Bandwidth and Circular Variance

There are different ways to measure orientation selectivity, and they can tell us about different aspects of orientation selectivity. A traditional method is to determine the half-bandwidth of the tuning curve around the peak of the tuning. This indicates the shape of the tuning curve near the peak. However, there are important ques-

tions about mechanisms that depend on the global shape of the tuning curve at all orientations. Various vector-averaging measures have been devised by different investigators. We favor the use of circular variance, a measure that is used in circular statistics. If we write the spike rate as a function of angle as $m(\theta)$, the circular variance of $m(\theta)$ is:

$$CV[m] = 1 - \left| \frac{\int m(\theta) \exp(2i\theta)d\theta}{\int m(\theta)d\theta} \right|$$

Circular variance is $1 - \{$relative modulation of $m(\theta)$ as a function of $\theta\}$. The relative modulation is the ratio of the best-fitting Fourier component of the orientation tuning curve (with period equal to 180°), divided by the average response. For a flat tuning curve, CV $= 1$. For a very highly tuned tuning curve, CV approaches 0. CV reflects wide-angle responses that the bandwidth does not. Other investigators have also used global measures for selectivity that are related to circular variance.

Response Dynamics

In an attempt to provide a database to test models of orientation selectivity, Ringach, Hawken, and Shapley (1997) applied the subspace reverse correlation method. The idea was to measure the time evolution of orientation selectivity extracellularly in single V1 neurons. One main result from the use of this technique is that there is evidence for a slightly delayed inhibition or suppression in orientation selectivity's time evolution. Also, in a few neurons one observes a progressive shift of the peak orientation with time. The presence of shifter cells provides a realization of the "marginal mode" (a name for one of the attractor states referred to above) predicted by Ben-Yishai et al. (1995), and thus provides some confirmation of the attractor states of the recurrent models with strong corticocortical excitation. However, such neurons are found to be the exception, not the rule, in the reverse correlation observations. What one does observe often are highly selective cells in the output layers of the cortex in whose activity there is the following pattern: a delayed suppression at the orientation that is the peak orientation early in the response. The suppression causes it to become the least preferred orientation late in the response. Thus, in neurons with such delayed suppression, one observes a change in the preferred orientation later in the response, also. But unlike the shifter neurons, the suppressed neurons have a rather sudden flip in preferred orientation, usually by as much as 90°.

The time dependence of orientation tuning is illustrated for one macaque 4cα neuron in Figure 3, row *a*. This neuron, like many

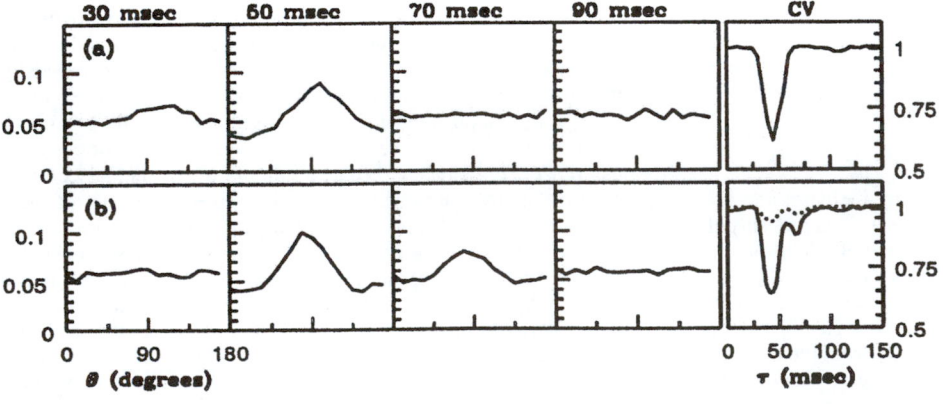

Figure 3. Time dependence of orientation tuning in a macaque 4cα neuron and in the large-scale model of McLaughlin et al. (2000). In the first four panels, $p(\theta, \tau)$ is graphed. In the fifth panel the circular variance (CV) is shown. Row *a* is for a typical 4cα neuron; row *b* is from the model. The dotted line in the rightmost panel of row *b* is the CV versus time for a pure feedforward model.

cells in the input layer $4c\alpha$, does not exhibit much late suppression. Figure 3 also illustrates that a feedforward model would produce little orientation selectivity in the reverse correlation experiment. This is illustrated in the rightmost panel of row *b*, in which circular variance (CV) is drawn for the full model (solid line) and for a pure feedforward model (dotted line).

Discussion

In our view, corticocortical inhibition is a crucial ingredient in the emergence of orientation selectivity in the visual cortex. The orientation preference of each neuron, and the orderly orientation preference map, are likely to be consequences of the pattern of feedforward convergence. However, the selectivity observed in steady-state experiments, and even more so in orientation dynamics experiments, cannot be achieved by a purely feedforward model. At present, we cannot yet evaluate the relative importance of corticocortical excitation in enhancing orientation selectivity. It may play a role for some neurons. For cortical simple cells, the results of our modeling indicate that corticocortical inhibition dominates, and that in simple cells, cortical excitation has to be relatively weak compared to the LGN excitation (see Wielaard et al., 2001). However, it is highly likely that corticocortical excitation is much more significant for the function of complex cells in V1.

Road Map: Vision
Related Reading: Ocular Dominance and Orientation Columns; Visual Cortex: Anatomical Structure and Models of Function

References

Anderson, J. S., Carandini, M., and Ferster, D., 2000, Orientation tuning of input conductance, excitation, and inhibition in cat primary visual cortex, *J. Neurophysiol.*, 84:909–926.
Ben-Yishai, R., Bar-Or, R. L., and Sompolinsky, H., 1995, Theory of orientation tuning in visual cortex, *Proc. Natl. Acad. Sci. USA*, 92:3844–3848.
Bonhoeffer, T., and Grinvald, A., 1993, The layout of iso-orientation domains in area 18 of cat visual cortex: Optical imaging reveals a pinwheel-like organization, *J Neurosci*, 13:4157–4180.
Borg-Graham, L. J., Monier, C., and Fregnac, Y., 1998, Visual input evokes transient and strong shunting inhibition in visual cortical neurons, *Nature*, 393:369–373.
Ferster, D., Chung, S., and Wheat, H., 1996, Orientation selectivity of thalamic input to simple cells of cat visual cortex, *Nature*, 380:249–252.
Hubel, D. H., and Wiesel, T. N., 1962, Receptive fields, binocular interaction and functional architecture in the cat's visual cortex, *J. Physiol.*, 160:106–154.
Mclaughlin, D., Shapley, R., Shelley, M., and Wielaard, J., 2000, A neuronal network model of sharpening and dynamics of orientation tuning in an input layer of macaque primary visual cortex, *Proc. Natl. Acad. Sci. USA*, 97:8087–8092.
Pugh, M. C., Ringach, D. L., Shapley, R., and Shelley, M. J., 2000, Computational modeling of orientation tuning dynamics in monkey primary visual cortex, *J. Comput. Neurosci.*, 8:143–159.
Ringach, D., Hawken, M., and Shapley, R., 1997, The dynamics of orientation tuning in the macaque monkey striate cortex, *Nature*, 387:281–284.
Somers, D. C., Nelson, S. B., and Sur, M., 1995, An emergent model of orientation selectivity in cat visual cortical simple cells, *J. Neurosci.*, 15:5448–5465.
Sompolinsky, H., and Shapley, R., 1997, New perspectives on the mechanisms for orientation selectivity, *Curr. Opin. Neurobiol.*, 7:514–522. ◆
Troyer, T. W., Krukowski, A. E., Priebe, N. J., and Miller, K. D., 1998, Contrast-invariant orientation tuning in cat visual cortex: Thalamocortical input tuning and correlation-based intracortical connectivity, *J. Neurosci.*, 18:5908–5927.
Tsodyks, M., Kenet, T., Grinvald, A., and Arieli, A., 1999, Linking spontaneous activity of single cortical neurons and the underlying functional architecture, *Science*, 286:1943–1946.
Wielaard, J., Shelley, M., Mclaughlin, D. M., and Shapley, R. M., 2001, How simple cells are made in a nonlinear network model of the visual cortex, *J. Neurosci.*, 21:5203–5211.

Oscillatory and Bursting Properties of Neurons

Xiao-Jing Wang and John Rinzel

Introduction

Rhythmicity is a common feature of temporal organization in neuronal firing patterns. Historically, when recordings from *isolated* nerves became possible in the 1930s, systematic study of repetitive firing behaviors ensued. Arvanitaki (1939) and Hodgkin (1948, see citation in Rinzel and Ermentrout, 1998) identified three categories of crustacean axons by their rhythmic discharge patterns: those that fire repetitively over a wide (I) or narrow (II) range of frequencies and those whose firing hardly repeats (III). Later, Arvanitaki also pioneered the *Aplysia* preparation and discovered *bursting* oscillations, in which impulse clusters occur periodically, separated by phases of quiescence.

Since then, many other stereotypical single-neuron firing patterns, including a fascinating variety of endogenous oscillations, have been identified (Llinás, 1988; Connors and Gutnick, 1990). One wonders anew about categorizing neuronal firing modes and the criteria on which to base such a classification. In 1952, Hodgkin and Huxley showed that many spiking properties could be explained in terms of various active ionic currents across the cell membrane. Today, many types of ion channels are known, and some particular neuronal rhythms have been linked to selected subsets of channels. However, membrane potential oscillations with apparently similar characteristics can be generated by different ionic mechanisms and by other biophysical factors, such as cable properties. In addition, a given cell type may display several different firing patterns under different neuromodulatory conditions. For these reasons, the visual appearance of particular voltage time courses and the presence of certain ionic mechanisms are insufficient bases for classification. A rational scheme should consider a cell's complete *repertoire* of dynamical modes and the nature of the transitions between modes.

Here we apply the mathematics of dynamical systems to describe precisely the dynamical modes of neuronal firing and the transformations between them. The approach was pioneered by FitzHugh (1961) with his phase space analysis of nerve membrane excitability. In this theoretical framework, membrane dynamics is described by coupled *differential equations*, e.g., à la Hodgkin and Huxley (cf. Rinzel and Ermentrout, 1998), the behavior modes by *attractors*, and the transitions between modes by *bifurcations*. The rest state is represented by a time-independent *steady state* and repetitive firing by a *limit cycle*. The transition from resting to oscillating typically occurs via either a *Hopf bifurcation* or a *homoclinic bifurcation* (Figure 1) (see, e.g., Rinzel and Ermentrout, 1998). The firing frequency versus applied current curves are qualitatively different in the two cases (minimum frequency being non-

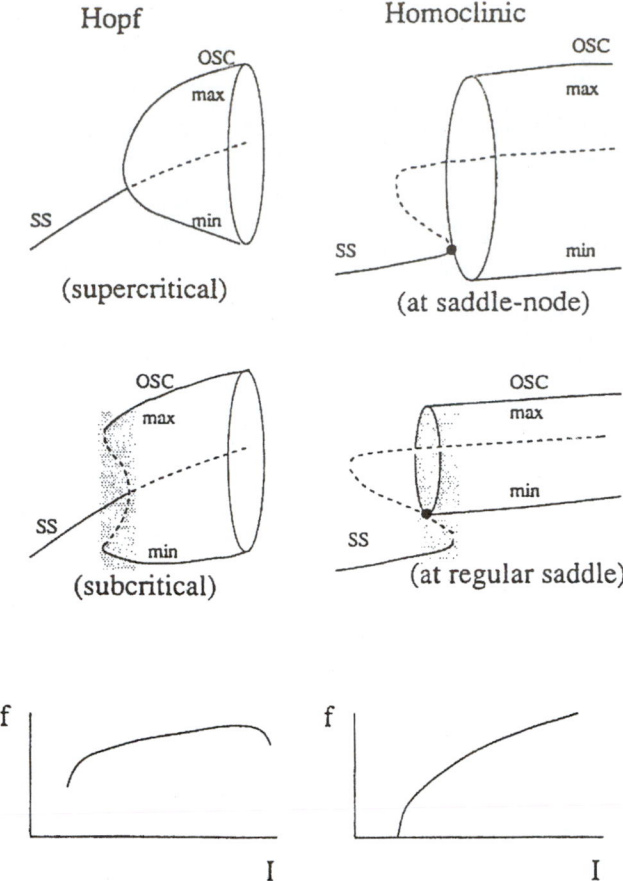

Figure 1. Schematic bifurcation diagrams from a steady state (SS) to an oscillatory firing state (OSC). The abscissa is a control parameter, such as the applied current intensity. The ordinate corresponds to the membrane potential, the repetitive firing state being indicated by the maximal and minimal amplitudes of the oscillatory membrane potential. The solid curve indicates stable and the dashed curve unstable. In the lowermost panels, the ordinate (f) is the frequency of repetitive firing. The left panels show *Hopf bifurcation.* At the onset of oscillation, the rhythmic amplitude is small and the frequency is finite. The bifurcation may be *supercritical,* where the new oscillatory branch is stable, or *subcritical,* where the new oscillatory branch is unstable and becomes stable at a turning point. The right panels show *homoclinic bifurcation.* It corresponds to the coalescence of an oscillatory state with an unstable steady state. This steady state can be either of saddle-node or saddle type. As this bifurcation point is approached, the amplitude of oscillation remains finite, while the rhythmic frequency tends to zero (the period diverging to infinity). In the case of a subcritical Hopf bifurcation or a normal homoclinic bifurcation, there is a range of parameter values where a steady-state attractor and an oscillatory attractor coexist (bistability, shaded region).

zero or zero, respectively) and might subserve an abstract basis for the distinction between the Arvanitaki-Hodgkin type II and type I axons. Our review generalizes this theoretical methodology to characterize various *bursting* oscillations in single neurons, elaborating on a qualitative classification scheme for bursting mechanisms proposed by Rinzel (1987).

Neuronal Bursting: Examples

We summarize some qualitative features of observed bursting patterns and then relate these to our classification scheme. We briefly mention conductance mechanisms that are *sufficient* to produce

some of these bursting oscillations. Although network synaptic interactions and dendritic cable properties influence bursting behavior, for the most part our discussion concerns an isolated, isopotential neuron. The main biophysical idea is that rhythmicity is generated by a depolarization process that is autocatalytic (positive feedback), followed by a *slower* repolarization process (negative feedback). These opposing processes may involve activation and slow inactivation of an inward ionic current, or a fast inward current and a slower outward current. Such features underlie action potential generation, and for bursting, there is at least another, *slower* negative feedback process.

The burst pattern of Figure 2A has a *square-wave* form, with abrupt periodic switching between rest (silent phase) and depolarized repetitive firing (active phase). Spiking here is due primarily to a *high-threshold* fast calcium current and a Hodgkin-Huxley-like potassium current. A minimal biophysical mechanism for square-wave bursting involves a calcium-activated potassium current, as originally proposed by Chay and Keizer in 1983. During the active phase, each calcium spike slightly increases $[Ca^{2+}]_i$, slowly turning on this current and eventually repolarizing the membrane to terminate the active phase. During the silent phase, the Ca^{2+} channels are closed, $[Ca^{2+}]_i$ decreases, and, as the potassium conductance deactivates, the cell slowly depolarizes until threshold for the next active phase is reached. Suggested alternative mechanisms for this type of bursting include slow inactivation by Ca^{2+} or by voltage of the Ca^{2+} current. Here, if spikes are abolished by pharmacologically blocking the calcium current, bursting is lost.

Although the dopamine-secreting neuron (Figure 2B) superficially appears to be a square-wave burster, we would not classify it as such. Its underlying slow wave persists even when action potentials are blocked. It appears to be of dendritic origin, and it drives somatic spiking via electrotonic interaction.

The bursting patterns of Figure 2C and 2D exhibit brief spike bursts riding on a slow *triangular wave*. Thalamocortical relay cells (Figure 2C) burst at the delta wave frequency (3 Hz) of quiet sleep (Steriade, McCormick, and Sejnowski, 1993), while the 5-Hz oscillation in inferior olivary cells (Figure 2D) is probably involved with movement tremor (see Llinás, 1988). Remarkably, in both cases, rhythmic bursting occurs for maintained hyperpolarizing rather than depolarizing stimuli. The underlying slow wave (due to a low-threshold calcium current) is unmasked when the fast action potentials are blocked, and is sometimes seen for modest hyperpolarizing inputs, even without blocking spikes. The Ca^{2+} current activates rapidly, below the voltage threshold for action potentials. Its inactivation by voltage, with a time scale like that of the triangular wave's depolarization, provides the slow negative feedback.

The *Aplysia* R15 neuron (Figure 2E) is the quintessential experimental model of an endogenous burster. The sodium spike rate during a burst first increases and then decreases; hence there is *parabolic* bursting. Blocking these spikes reveals an underlying quasi-sinusoidal slow wave that is generated primarily by a Ca^{2+} current. This current activates more slowly and at lower depolarizations than that associated with the square-wave bursting of Figure 2A. Its slow activation and the slower $[Ca^{2+}]_i$ that inactivates it provide the two variables for a minimal model of a parabolic burster's underlying slow oscillator (see the next section).

Parabolic burst-like features are seen in the 10-Hz oscillations of mammalian thalamic reticular neurons (Figure 2F) during the spindle waves of quiet sleep (Steriade et al., 1993). The oscillation depends on a low-threshold calcium current, like that of triangular bursting. In addition to this current's slow inactivation, there is likely a second slow variable to support the parabolic pattern, e.g., $[Ca^{2+}]_i$ for activating a calcium-dependent potassium current in these cells.

A quite different kind of burst pattern consists of spike clusters interspersed with epochs of small-amplitude subthreshold oscilla-

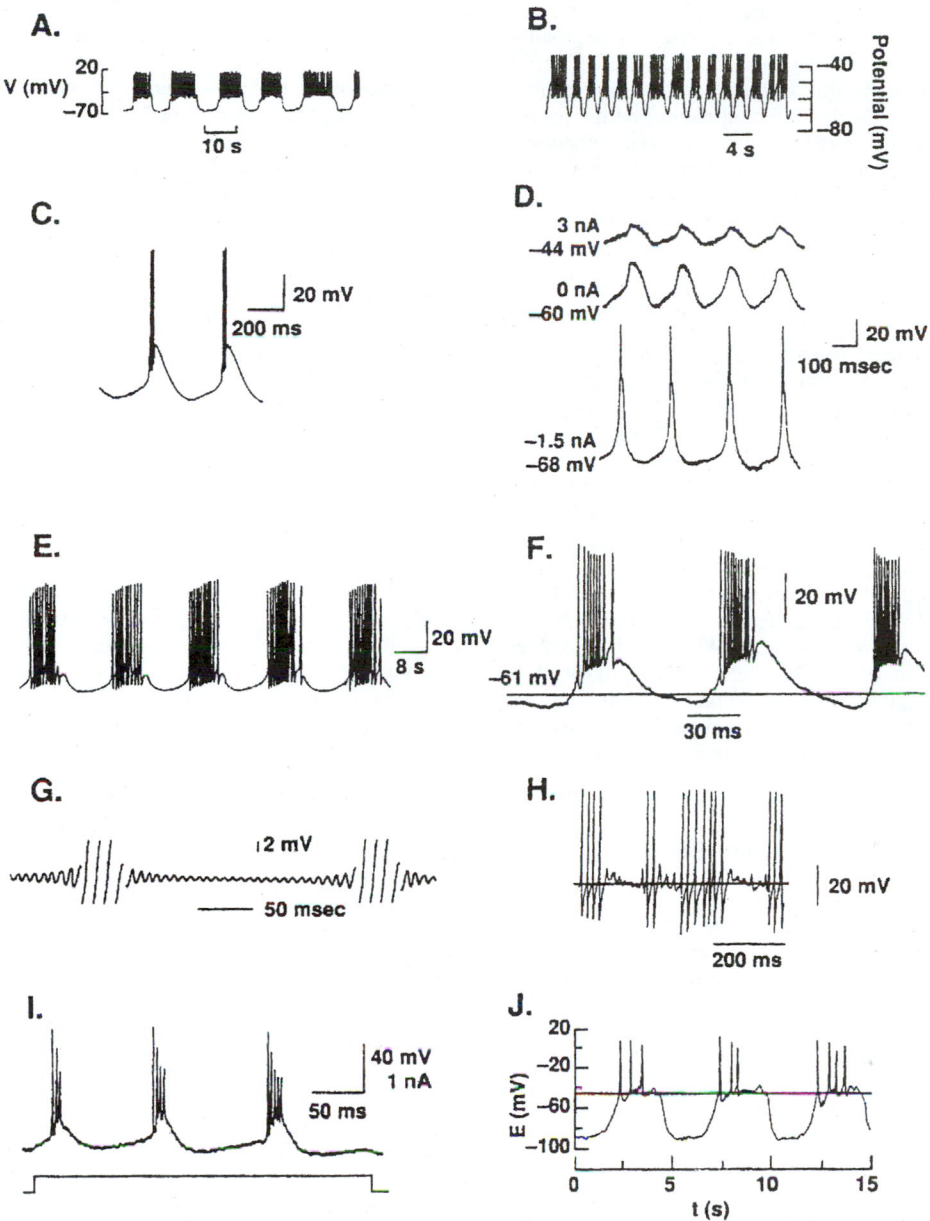

Figure 2. Examples of rhythmic bursting, showing the time courses of membrane potential, with the exception of *G*, which is extracellular voltage. See text for explanations. *A*, Pancreatic *β*-cell (From Sherman, A., Carroll, P., Santos, R. M., and Atwater, I., 1990, Glucose dose response of pancreatic beta-cells: Experimental and theoretical results, in *Transduction in Biological Systems* (C. Hidalgo et al. Eds.), New York: Plenum, p. 123; reprinted with permission.) *B*, Dopamine-containing neurons in the rat midbrain. (From Johnson, S. W., Seutin, V., and North, R. A., 1992, Burst firing in dopamine neurons induced by *N*-methyl-D-aspartate: Role of electrogenic sodium pump, *Science*, 258:665–667; reprinted with permission. Copyright 1992 by the AAAS.) *C*, Cat thalamocortical relay neuron. (From McCormick, D. A., and Pape, C.-H., 1991, Properties of a hyperpolarization-activated cation current and its role in rhythmic oscillation in thalamic relay neurons, *J. Physiol. Camb.*, 431:291–318; reprinted with permission.) *D*, Guinea pig inferior olivary neuron. (From Benardo, L., and Foster, R. E., 1986, Oscillatory behaviors in inferior olive neurons: Mechanism, modulation, cell aggregates, *Brain Res. Bull.*, 17:773–784; copyright 1986; reprinted with permission from Elsevier Science Ltd.) *E, Aplysia* R15 neuron. (From Lotshaw, D. P., Levitan, E. S., and Levitan, I. B., 1986, Fine tuning of neuronal electrical activity: Modulation of several ion channels by in-

tracellular messengers in a single identified nerve cell, *J. Exp. Biol.*, 124:302–322; reprinted with permission of Company of Biologists Ltd.) *F*, Cat thalamic reticular neuron. (From Mulle, C., Madariaga, A., and Deschênes, M., 1986, Morphology and electrophysiological properties of reticularis thalami neurons in cat: In vivo study of a thalamic pacemaker, *J. Neurosci.*, 6:2134–2145; reprinted with permission of the Society for Neuroscience.) *G, Sepia* giant axon. (From Arvanitaki, A., 1939, Recherche sur la réponse oscillatoire locale de l'axone géant isolé de *Sepia*, *Arch. Int. Physiol.*, 49:209–256; reprinted with permission.) *H*, Rat thalamic reticular neuron. (From Pinault, D., and Deschênes, M., 1992, Voltage-dependent 40 Hz oscillations in rat reticular thalamic neurons in vivo, *Neuroscience*, 51:245–258; copyright 1992; reprinted with permission from Elsevier Science Ltd.) *I*, Mouse neocortical pyramidal neuron. (From Agmon, A., and Connors, B. W., 1989, Repetitive burst-firing neurons in the deep layers of mouse somatosensory cortex, *Neurosci. Lett.*, 99:137–141; reprinted with permission.) *J*, Rat pituitary gonadotropin-releasing cell. (From Tse, A., and Hille, B., 1993, Role of voltage-gated Na$^+$ and Ca^{2+} channels in gonadotropin-releasing hormone-induced membrane potential changes in identified rat gonadotropes, *Endocrinology*, 132(4):1475–1481; reprinted with permission. © The Endocrine Society.)

tions (Figures 2*G* and 2*H*). The envelope of fast events slowly waxes and wanes, forming an approximate spindle or ellipse; hence the term, *elliptic bursting*. Here, the inactive phase is not totally silent but often shows small oscillations. The frequency of intra-burst spiking is comparable to that of the interburst subthreshold oscillations. Only recently has this bursting pattern been reported for mammalian neurons and associated with important functional roles, such as the limbic system's theta rhythm (not shown), and the gamma fast oscillations (about 40 Hz) that occur intermittently with increased alertness and focused attention (Figure 2*H*). Experimental (Llinás, Grace, and Yarom, 1991) and computational (Wang, 1993) studies indicate that the 40-Hz elliptic bursts involve a persistent Na^+ conductance and a specific voltage-dependent transient K^+ conductance.

Some oscillations (Figures 2*I* and 2*J*) depend on the electrical cable properties of neuronal dendrites and intracellular sources of regenerative ion fluxes. The bursting behavior of some pyramidal neurons (Figure 2*I*) in neocortex (Connors and Gutnick, 1990) and in the hippocampus depends on high-threshold calcium channels located on the distal dendrites, while the faster sodium spikes are generated primarily in the perisomatic region (Williams and Stuart, 1999). Computer simulations suggest that a one-compartment description is inadequate, and that electrotonically distinct compartments must be explicitly modeled and analyzed (Traub et al., 1991; Pinsky and Rinzel, 1994). Figure 2*J* displays the bursting pattern of a pituitary gonadotropin-releasing cell. Although it resembles the square-wave form of Figure 2*A*, here the underlying slow rhythm is generated by a cytoplasmatic second messenger system that leads to nonlinear, time-dependent calcium fluxes across the endoplasmic reticulum (ER) membrane and to oscillations in $[Ca^{2+}]_i$.

Bursting Systems Analysis: Fast/Slow Phase Space Dynamics

Since different bursters may have qualitatively similar patterns, a qualitative classification should not depend on quantitative properties such as the rhythm's period or its precise biophysical bases. Our general framework involves a *geometrical* analysis of the bursting dynamics for a model's differential equations (Rinzel, 1987; Rinzel and Ermentrout, 1998; Izhikevich, 2000). The model for an isopotential neuron may be written as:

$$\frac{dX}{dt} = F(X, Y) \qquad (1)$$

$$\frac{dY}{dt} = G(X, Y) \qquad (2)$$

where the vectors X and Y represent the variables with fast and slow time scales, respectively. Typically, the membrane potential is a fast variable, so Equation 1 might be the membrane's current balance equation:

$$C_m \frac{dV}{dt} = -\sum_i I_i + I_{app}$$

The other dynamic variables include the gating variables for specific ionic channels plus relevant second-messenger variables and ionic concentrations. Here we consider only one or two slow variables Y_k, which might be a slow voltage-dependent gating variable or $[Ca^{2+}]_i$, or both.

The fast/slow phase space dissection method (Rinzel, 1987; Rinzel and Ermentrout, 1998; Izhikevich, 2000) exploits the presence of two disparate time scales. For simplicity, suppose there is only one slow variable, Y. One first treats Y as a *control parameter* and considers the dynamics of Equation 1 as a function of Y. The fast

subsystem's various behavioral states are then summarized in a bifurcation diagram, plotting response amplitude, say V, versus Y, as in Figure 1, but where Y (instead of I) is the parameter. When the full system is considered, Y evolves slowly in time according to Equation 2, slowly sweeping through a range of values, while the fast subsystem slowly tracks its stable states (*attractors*). For example, an oscillatory state of the fast subsystem corresponds to the repetitive firing of a burst's active phase. During a silent phase, the fast subsystem would be following a pseudo-steady state of hyperpolarized V. To complete the description, one must understand the slow dynamics from Equation 2 in order to know where on the fast subsystem's bifurcation diagram Y will be increasing or decreasing. When the full system, Equations 1 and 2, is integrated and the resulting burst trajectory is projected onto the (V, Y) plane, it coincides with portions of the bifurcation diagram. Through visualization of this geometrical representation, one can make predictions about the qualitative behavior of bursting and the effects of various parameter changes.

1. *Square-wave bursting.* The prototypical fast/slow phase plane (Figure 3*A*) was originally developed for the Chay-Keizer model of β-cell bursting, where $[Ca^{2+}]_i$ was the slow, negative-feedback variable. For the fast/slow dissection, one first constructs the fast subsystem's bifurcation diagram by treating Y as a parameter. This yields the Z-shaped curve of steady states. The oscillatory state "surrounding" the upper branch corresponds to repetitive spiking of an active phase. It terminates by contacting the unstable middle steady-state branch, at a homoclinic bifurcation. The Z-curve's lower branch represents a stable steady state of hyperpolarization, as tracked during a burst's silent phase. In an intermediate range of Y values, there is bistability of the depolarized oscillation and the hyperpolarized steady state.

Next, Y is allowed to vary according to its kinetics. Bursting occurs if the slow kinetics dictate that Y increases (decreases) when the fast spike-generating subsystem is in its upper (lower) state, where the voltage-dependent channels are (are not) activated. The slow Y modulation induces abrupt switching between the two co-existing states and thus temporal alternation between a train of spikes and a resting phase, as seen in Figure 2*A*.

2. *Triangular bursting.* Figure 3*B* shows fast/slow phase planes associated with triangular bursting. A minimal model has one slow variable, and its fast subsystem has regimes of bistability, as in the square-wave case. Here, however, the steady-state curve has five branches, composed of *two* S-shaped portions in different V ranges. These S-curves correspond to the two sets of regenerative currents active in the subthreshold voltage ranges, such as in thalamic relay or inferior olivary cells. The depolarized oscillatory state (repetitive spiking) joins the middle steady-state branch at its right knee (a saddle-node homoclinic bifurcation). Different oscillation patterns occur, depending on whether the lower S's right knee extends rightward beyond that of the upper S's right knee. If this is not the case (Figure 3*B*, left), a slow subthreshold oscillation without fast spikes may occur. The alternative case (Figure 3*B*, right) corresponds to more intense hyperpolarizing input, when triangular bursting arises (Figure 2*D*). "Triangular" refers to the gradually falling V time course of the active phase, related to the middle branch's steep slope (Figure 3*B*).

3. *Parabolic bursting.* This bursting type has a smooth underlying slow subthreshold wave. Its generation requires at least two slow variables, one for positive feedback and the other for negative feedback. The minimal fast/slow phase plot has three dimensions: V and the two slow variables (Figure 3*C*, originally constructed for a model of the *Aplysia* R15 neuron; see Rinzel, 1987). Steady states of the fast subsystem are now represented by a *Z-surface*. Similarly, a surface describes the fast oscillatory (repetitive spiking) attractors. These periodic solutions disappear via homoclinic bifurcation as they contact the Z-surface, precisely at its lower knee, a saddle-

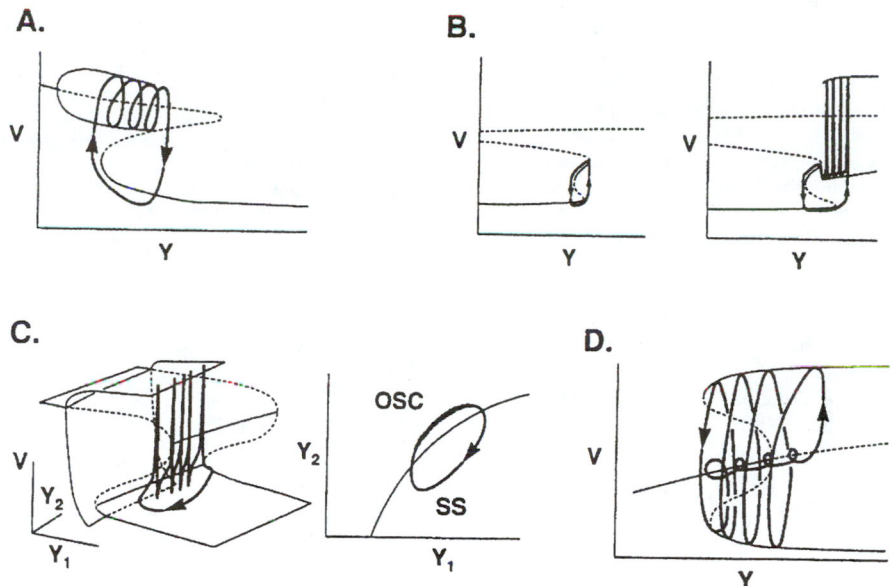

Figure 3. Fast- and slow-phase plot of bursting dynamics. The variable *Y* is a slow variable (there are two slow variables, Y_1 and Y_2, in part *C*). In each case the bifurcation diagram is computed for the fast subsystem, with *Y* treated as a parameter and plotted in terms of the membrane potential (*V*) behavior as a function of *Y*. The solid curve shows stable and the dashed curve unstable branches. The oscillatory state of repetitive firing is represented by its maximum and minimum of *V* (cf. Figure 1). The heavy curves with arrows are bursting trajectories of the full system plotted on the (*V*, *Y*) plane or the (*V*, Y_1, Y_2) space. *A*, Square-wave bursting is based on a bistability of a steady state and a repetitive firing state in the fast subsystem and periodic switching between the two, induced by the slow-variable dynamics. *B*, Triangular bursting has a similar phase plot as in part *A*, but the fast subsystem's steady-state curve is quintic rather than cubic, with two branches of stable steady states. Depending on whether the stable repetitive firing state overlaps with the lowermost steady-state branch, oscillations of the full system may be either purely subthreshold (left panel) or bursting (right panel). For simplicity, the repetitive firing state is shown only on the right panel, not on the left panel. *C*, Parabolic bursting is generated by an oscillation in a two-variable (Y_1 and Y_2) slow subsystem (right panel) that induces smooth periodic switching between a steady state (SS) and a repetitive spiking state (OSC) (which do not overlap) of the fast subsystem. *D*, Elliptic bursting involves a subcritical Hopf bifurcation in the fast subsystem. Bursting involves slow switching between a steady state and a repetitive firing state that are bistable in the fast subsystem. The silent phase exhibits damped or growing small oscillations as its trajectory passes through the Hopf bifurcation point. (Parts *A* and *C–D* are adapted from Rinzel, 1987; Part *B* from Rush, M., and Rinzel J., 1994, *Biol. Cybern.*, 71:281–291.)

node coalescence (cf. Figure 1). Here, the fast subsystem is monostable. The slow-variable phase plane is divided into two non-overlapping regions: one for the resting steady state and the other for the repetitive spiking regime of the fast subsystem.

Now, when the slow variables are allowed to vary, an oscillation may occur in this two-variable slow system (Figure 3C, right). If the slow oscillatory trajectory visits both of the fast subsystem's regimes, bursting occurs, with repetitive smooth switching between the resting and spiking states. As a burst begins and ends, its trajectory crosses a homoclinic bifurcation of the fast subsystem and spike frequency drops dramatically; hence the parabolic nature.

4. *Elliptic bursting.* A minimal model has only one slow variable (Figure 3D, originally constructed for a modified FitzHugh-type model; see Rinzel, 1987). The fast subsystem has bistability because of a *subcritical* Hopf bifurcation (cf. Figure 1) of periodic solutions from a monotonic steady-state curve. As in the square-wave case, during bursting the full system operates in the (*V*, *Y*) regime of bistability, repetitively switching between the steady state and the spiking state. A distinguishing feature, however, is that the "silent phase," when the fast subsystem operates near its steady state, is no longer truly silent: it can display small oscillations that damp and then grow as the trajectory slowly passes through the Hopf bifurcation point, where the steady state is a spiral-type fixed point.

5. *Complex bursting.* The theoretical study of certain bursting types (Figures 2I and 2J) is relatively recent, and mathematical understanding of their mechanisms is just emerging. For analyzing the case of Figure 2I, one requires a minimal model of at least two

electrotonically separated compartments (Pinsky and Rinzel, 1994). Such a model can still be analyzed by the fast/slow dissection method, which shows that complex bursting of neocortical pyramidal cells can be described as the square-wave type (Kepecs and Wang, 2000). As for Figure 2J, one must take into account the interaction between second-messenger-mediated calcium fluxes from intracellular pools and voltage-dependent plasma membrane calcium currents.

The classification discussed here is based on various fast/slow phase plots. Although consistent with some of the wave-form phenomenology, the two may sometimes disagree. For instance, a system with the fast/slow phase plot of Figure 3C may burst with a slow wave that is less sinusoidal and more rectangular if one slow variable is much slower than the other. However, in contrast to a square-wave burster (Figures 2A and 3A), its slow wave may persist, even with the fast action potentials blocked.

Discussion

We have reviewed various neuronal bursting oscillations and, by using notions and analytic tools from the mathematics of dynamical systems, we discussed how these bursting patterns might be theoretically described and classified. Our examples are minimal for these categories. Indeed, one can imagine subcategories based on differences in the fast subsystem's bifurcation diagram. In summary, bursting in a single-compartment model typically involves some slow processes that induce repetitive switching between a relatively quiescent state and an active state of repetitive spiking of a faster system. In the cases of square-wave, triangular, and elliptic bursting, one slow variable is sufficient, and the fast subsystem must be bistable. In the parabolic bursting case, the fast subsystem need not display bistability, and two slow variables are required.

The geometrical analysis by fast/slow dissection illustrates how novel and powerful theoretical approaches can emerge from fruitful interactions between neurobiology and the science of dynamical systems. Possible extensions might consider cable-like distributed systems with local burst-generating dynamics, or systems with many slow variables, or systems with complicated bifurcation diagrams, perhaps involving chaotic attractors. One can expect that dynamical systems methods, including fast/slow dissection, may also play a role in our understanding of neural networks with many synaptically coupled neurons, as long as there are disparate time scales in the system (Tabak et al., 2000).

Road Map: Biological Neurons and Synapses
Background: Dynamics and Bifurcation in Neural Nets
Related Reading: Hippocampal Rhythm Generation; Neuromodulation in Mammalian Nervous Systems; Sleep Oscillations

References

Arvanitaki, A., 1939, *Les Variations graduées de la polarization des systèmes excitables,* Paris: Hermann.

Chay, T. R., and Keizer, J., 1983, Minimal model for membrane oscillations in the pancreatic beta-cell, *Biophys. J.,* 42:181–190.

Connors, B. W., and Gutnick, M. J., 1990, Intrinsic firing patterns of diverse neocortical neurons, *Trends Neurosci.,* 13:99–104. ◆

FitzHugh, R., 1961, Impulses and physiological states in models of nerve membrane, *Biophys. J.,* 1:445–466.

Izhikevich, E. M., 2000, Neural excitability, spiking, and bursting, *Int. J. Bifurcat. Chaos,* 10:1171–1266. ◆

Kepecs, A., and Wang, X.-J., 2000, Analysis of complex bursting in cortical pyramidal neuron models, *Neurocomputing,* 32:181–187.

Llinás, R., 1988, The intrinsic electrophysiological properties of mammalian neurons: Insights into central nervous system function, *Science,* 242:1654–1664. ◆

Llinás, R. R., Grace T., and Yarom, Y., 1991, *In vitro* neurons in mammalian cortical layer 4 exhibit intrinsic oscillatory activity in the 10- to 50-Hz frequency range, *Proc. Natl. Acad. Sci. USA,* 88:897–901.

Pinsky, P., and Rinzel, J., 1994, Intrinsic and network rhythmogenesis in a reduced Traub model for CA3 neurons, *J. Computat. Neurosci.,* 1:39–60.

Rinzel, J., 1987, A formal classification of bursting mechanisms in excitable systems, in *Proceedings of an International Congress of Mathematicians* (A. M. Gleason, Ed.), Providence, RI: American Mathematical Society, pp. 1578–1594.

Rinzel, J., and Ermentrout, G. B., 1998, Analysis of neural excitability and oscillations, in *Methods in Neuronal Modeling: From Ions to Networks,* 2nd ed. (C. Koch and I. Segev, Eds.), Cambridge, MA: MIT Press, pp. 251–291. ◆

Steriade, M., McCormick, D. A., and Sejnowski, T. J., 1993, Thalamocortical oscillations in the sleep and aroused brain, *Science,* 262:679–685. ◆

Tabak J., Senn W., O'Donovan, M. J., and Rinzel, J., 2000, Modeling of spontaneous activity in developing spinal cord using activity-dependent depression in an excitatory network, *J. Neurosci.,* 20:3041–3056.

Traub, R., Wong, R., Miles, R., and Michelson, H., 1991, A model of a CA3 hippocampal pyramidal neuron incorporating voltage-clamp data on intrinsic conductances, *J. Neurophysiol.,* 66:635–649.

Wang, X.-J., 1993, Ionic basis for intrinsic 40 Hz neuronal oscillations, *NeuroReport,* 5:221–224.

Williams, S. R., and Stuart, G. J., 1999, Mechanisms and consequences of action potential burst firing in rat neocortical pyramidal neurons, *J. Physiol.,* 521:467–482.

PAC Learning and Neural Networks

Martin Anthony and Norman Biggs

Introduction

In this article, we discuss the "probably approximately correct" (PAC) learning paradigm as it applies to artificial neural networks. The PAC learning model is a probabilistic framework for the study of learning and generalization. It is useful not only for neural classification problems but also for learning problems more often associated with mainstream artificial intelligence, such as the inference of Boolean functions. In PAC theory, the notion of successful learning is formally defined using probability theory. Very roughly speaking, if a large enough sample of randomly drawn training examples is presented, then it should be likely that, after learning, the neural network will classify most other randomly drawn examples correctly. The PAC model formalizes the terms "likely" and "most." Furthermore, the learning algorithm must be expected to act quickly, since otherwise it may be of little use in practice.

There are thus two main emphases in PAC learning theory. First, there is the issue of how many training examples should be presented. Second, there is the question of whether learning can be achieved using a fast algorithm. These are known, respectively, as the *sample complexity* and *computational complexity* problems. This article provides a brief introduction to these problems. We highlight the importance of the Vapnik-Chervonenkis dimension, a combinatorial parameter that measures the expressive power of a neural network, and describe how this parameter quantifies fairly precisely the sample complexity of PAC learning. In discussing the computational complexity of PAC learning, we shall present a re-

sult that illustrates that in some cases, the problem of PAC learning is inherently intractable.

There are many variations on the basic PAC model that is the topic of this article, but there is insufficient space to explore these variations here. However, our discussion of the basic model serves as an introduction to the considerations that form the basis of recent extensions.

PAC Learning

Basic Definitions

In this section, we describe the basic PAC model of learning introduced by Valiant (1984). This model is applicable to neural networks with one output unit that outputs either the value 0 or 1; thus, it applies to *classification* problems. In the PAC model, it is assumed that the neural network receives a sequence of *examples* x, each labeled with the value $t(x)$ of the particular *target function* that is being "learned." A fundamental assumption of this model is that these examples are presented independently and at random according to some fixed (but unknown) probability distribution on the set of all examples.

We first explain how to formalize the notion of generalization. Suppose that the set of all possible examples is $X = \mathbb{R}^n$ or $X = \{0, 1\}^n$, where n is the number of inputs to the network, and that the target function t can be computed by the neural network in some state. A *training sample* for t of length m is an element $\mathbf{s}$ of $(X \times \{0, 1\})^m$, of the form

$$\mathbf{s} = ((x_1, t(x_1)), (x_2, t(x_2)), \ldots, (x_m, t(x_m)))$$

We shall denote by $S(m, t)$ the set of all training samples of length m for t. The learning algorithm accepts the training sample $\mathbf{s}$ and alters the state of the network in some way in response to the information provided by the sample. It is desired that the function computed by the network when in the resulting state be an approximation to the target function.

Probability and Approximation

If $L(\mathbf{s})$ is the function computed by the network after training sample $\mathbf{s} \in S(m, t)$ has been presented and learning algorithm L has been applied, one way in which to assess the success of the learning process is to measure how close $L(\mathbf{s})$ is to t. Since there is assumed to be some probability distribution P on the set of all examples, and since t takes only the values 0 or 1, we may define the *error*, $\mathrm{er}_P(h, t)$, of a function h (with respect to t) to be the P probability that a randomly chosen example is classified incorrectly by h. In other words,

$$\mathrm{er}_P(h, t) = P(\{x \in X : h(x) \neq t(x)\})$$

The aim is to ensure that the error of $L(\mathbf{s})$ is "usually small." Since each of the m examples in the training sample is drawn randomly and independently according to P, the sample vector $\mathbf{x}$ is drawn randomly from X^m according to the product probability distribution P^m. Thus, more formally, we want it to be true that with high P^m probability, the sample $\mathbf{s}$ arising from $\mathbf{x}$ is such that the function $L(\mathbf{s})$ computed after training has small error with respect to t. This leads us to the following formal definition of PAC learning.

The learning algorithm L is a *PAC learning algorithm* for the network if *for any* given $\delta, \varepsilon > 0$ there is a sample length $m_0(\delta, \varepsilon)$ such that *for all* target functions t computable by the network and *for all* probability distributions P on the set of examples, we have

$$m \geq m_0(\delta, \varepsilon) \Rightarrow P^m(\{\mathbf{s} \in S(m, t) : \mathrm{er}_P(L(\mathbf{s}), t) > \varepsilon\}) < \delta$$

In other words, provided the sample has length at least $m_0(\delta, \varepsilon)$, then it is "probably" the case that after training on that sample, the function computed by the network is "approximately" correct. (We should note that the product probability distribution P^m is really defined not on subsets of $S(m, t)$ but on sets of vectors $\mathbf{x} \in X^m$. However, this abuse of notation is convenient and is unambiguous: for a fixed t, there is a clear one-to-one correspondence between vectors $\mathbf{x} \in X^m$ and training samples $\mathbf{s} \in S(m, t)$.) Note that the probability distribution P occurs twice in the definition: first in the requirement that the P^m probability of a sample be small, and again in the fact that the error of $L(\mathbf{s})$ is measured with reference to P. The crucial feature of the definition is that we require that the sample length $m_0(\delta, \varepsilon)$ be independent of P and of t. It is not immediately clear that this is possible, but the following informal arguments explain why it can be done. If a particular example has not been seen in a large sample $\mathbf{s}$, the chances are that this example has low probability (with respect to P), and therefore misclassification of that example contributes little to the error of the function $L(\mathbf{s})$. In other words, the penalty paid for misclassification of a particular example is its probability, and, very loosely speaking, the two occurrences of the probability distribution in the definition can therefore "balance" or "cancel" each other.

The Finite Case

We shall show that if the network computes only a finite number of functions (for example, when the weights of a neural network

are restricted to a finite set of allowed values), then there is a PAC learning algorithm for the network.

We say that the learning algorithm L is *consistent* if, given any training sample $\mathbf{s} = ((x_1, t(x_1)), (x_2, t(x_2)), \ldots, (x_m, t(x_m)))$, the functions $L(\mathbf{s})$ and t agree on x_i, for each i between 1 and m. Such a condition seems quite natural. We should note, however, that neither the standard on-line perceptron learning algorithm nor the on-line backpropagation algorithm is, in general, consistent. But the batch versions of these algorithms, in which one repeatedly cycles through the training sample until no further changes are required, *are* consistent algorithms.

Suppose that the network is capable of computing a total of M different functions, and let t be any one of these. If h is computable by the network and has error $\varepsilon_h \geq \varepsilon$ with respect to t and P, then the probability (with respect to the product distribution P^m) that h agrees with t on a random sample is clearly at most $(1 - \varepsilon_h)^m$. This is at most $\exp(-\varepsilon_h m)$, using a standard approximation. Thus, since there are certainly at most M such functions h, the probability that *some* function computable by the network has error at least ε *and* is consistent with a randomly chosen sample $\mathbf{s}$ is at most $M \exp(-\varepsilon m)$. Here we have used the "union bound" (see LEARNING AND GENERALIZATION: THEORETICAL BOUNDS). For any fixed positive δ, this probability is less than δ, provided that

$$m \geq m_0(\delta, \varepsilon) = \frac{1}{\varepsilon} \log\left(\frac{M}{\delta}\right)$$

This bound is independent of both the distribution and the target function.

This analysis shows that if a network computes only a finite number of functions, then there is a PAC learning algorithm for the network; moreover, *any* consistent learning algorithm for the network is a PAC learning algorithm. The argument fails if the network in question computes infinitely many functions, and it is not immediately clear that PAC learning is possible in such circumstances. In the next section, we present a theory that shows that, in many such cases, it is possible.

PAC Learning and the Vapnik-Chervonenkis Dimension

The Vapnik-Chervonenkis Dimension

In this section, we show how the problem of PAC learning can be addressed by means of a combinatorial parameter known as the Vapnik-Chervonenkis dimension (henceforth called the VC-dimension) (see also VAPNIK-CHERVONENKIS DIMENSION OF NEURAL NETWORKS). Suppose $\mathcal{N}$ is a neural network that outputs 0 or 1, and suppose that $\mathcal{N}$ accepts examples from a set X (for example, $X = \mathbb{R}^n$, where n is the number of inputs). We say that a set T of examples is *shattered* by $\mathcal{N}$ if for each of the $2^{|T|}$ possible ways of dividing T into two disjoint sets T_1 and T_0, there is *some* function f computable by $\mathcal{N}$ such that $f(x) = 1$ if $x \in T_1$ and $f(x) = 0$ if $x \in T_0$. In what follows, it is sometimes convenient to say that x is a positive (respectively, negative) example of f if $f(x) = 1$ (respectively $f(x) = 0$). The *VC-dimension* of $\mathcal{N}$, denoted $\mathrm{VCdim}(\mathcal{N})$, is defined to be the largest size of a set of examples shattered by $\mathcal{N}$. The VC-dimension may be thought of as a measure of the "expressive power" of the network, although Vapnik and Chervonenkis (1971) defined this parameter in a more general context and not specifically in the context of neural networks. It should be noted that the notion of Vapnik-Chervonenkis dimension is, in a sense, an extension to that of linear (or vector-space) dimension. Dudley (1978) proved that if $\mathcal{F}$ is a vector space of real functions defined on a set X and if, for $f \in \mathcal{F}$, we define $f_+ : X \to \{0, 1\}$ by $f_+(x) = 1 \Leftrightarrow f(x) > 0$, then the VC-dimension of $\{f_+ : f \in \mathcal{F}\}$ is the linear dimension of $\mathcal{F}$.

It is instructive at this stage to determine the VC-dimension of the simplest neural network, the *simple real perceptron* $\mathcal{P}_n$ on n inputs. This network consists of n real-valued inputs, each of which is connected by a weighted connection to the single, linear threshold, output unit. (The weights can be any real numbers.) It is clear that, for functions computable by $\mathcal{P}_n$, the sets of positive examples and negative examples are separated by a hyperplane.

Theorem 1. For any positive integer n, let $\mathcal{P}_n$ be the simple real perceptron with n inputs. Then

$$\text{VCdim}(\mathcal{P}_n) = n + 1$$

Proof. Let T be *any* set of $n + 2$ examples. It can be shown that there is a nonempty subset T_1 of T such that, if $T_0 = T \backslash T_1$, then $\text{conv}(T_1) \cap \text{conv}(T_0) \neq 0$, where $\text{conv}(A)$ denotes the convex hull of A. (This follows from Radon's theorem, which may be found in Grunbaum [1967], for instance.) It follows immediately that the sets T_1 and T_0 cannot be separated by a hyperplane; in other words, there can be no function f computable by $\mathcal{P}_n$ such that $f(x) = 1$ if $x \in T_1$ and $f(x) = 0$ if $x \in T_0$. Therefore T is not shattered and the VC-dimension of $\mathcal{P}_n$ must be at most $n + 1$. It remains to prove the reverse inequality. Let o denote the origin of $\mathbb{R}^n$ and, for $1 \leq i \leq n$, let e_i be the point with a 1 in the ith coordinate and all other coordinates 0. Then $\mathcal{P}_n$ shatters the set $T = \{o, e_1, e_2, \dots, e_n\}$ of $n + 1$ examples. To see this, suppose that $T_1 \subseteq T$. For $i = 1, 2, \dots, n$, let α_i be 1 if $e_i \in T_1$ and -1 otherwise, and let θ be $-1/2$ if $o \in T_1$, $1/2$ otherwise. Then it is straightforward to verify that if h is the function computed by the perceptron when the threshold is θ and the weights are $\alpha_1, \alpha_2, \dots, \alpha_n$, then $h(x) = 1$ if $x \in T_1$ and $h(x) = 0$ if $x \in T_0$. Therefore, T is shattered and, consequently, $\text{VCdim}(\mathcal{P}_n) \geq n + 1$. $\square$

Finite VC-Dimension Characterizes PAC Learning

We have observed that if $\mathcal{N}$ computes only a finite number of functions, then any consistent learning algorithm is a PAC algorithm, and a value of $m_0(\delta, \varepsilon)$ involving the number of computable functions can be determined. It turns out that, as far as PAC learning is concerned, it is not the size of the set of computable functions that is crucial but the *VC-dimension* of the network. More precisely, we have the following key result, due to Blumer et al. (1989) and Ehrenfeucht et al. (1989).

Theorem 2. If a neural network $\mathcal{N}$ has finite VC-dimension $d \geq 1$, then any consistent learning algorithm L for $\mathcal{N}$ is a PAC learning algorithm. Moreover, there is a constant K such that a sufficient sample length $m_0(\delta, \varepsilon)$ for any such algorithm is

$$K\varepsilon^{-1}(d \ln(\varepsilon^{-1}) + \ln(\delta^{-1}))$$

On the other hand, there is a constant c such that for any PAC learning algorithm for $\mathcal{N}$, the sufficient sample length $m_0(\delta, \varepsilon)$ must be at least $c\varepsilon^{-1}(d + \ln(\delta^{-1}))$, for all $\varepsilon \leq 1/8$ and $\delta \leq 1/100$.

In fact, an analogue of Theorem 2 holds for general classes of $\{0, 1\}$-valued functions, and not simply those computable by neural networks.

VC-Dimension of Neural Networks

We now discuss some results on the VC-dimensions of certain types of network. A more detailed treatment of this topic may be found in VAPNIK-CHERVONENKIS DIMENSION OF NEURAL NETWORKS. First, we start with the feedforward linear threshold net-

work. The first part of the following result is due to Baum and Haussler (1989) and the second part is due to Maass (1993).

Theorem 3. There is $K > 0$ such that, if $\mathcal{N}$ is any feedforward linear threshold network having W variable weights and thresholds and N threshold units, then $\text{VCdim}(\mathcal{N}) \leq KW \log N$. Furthermore, there is $c > 0$ such that some feedforward linear threshold networks having W weights and N threshold units have VC-dimension at least $cW \log N$; in other words, the upper bound is tight to within a constant.

Recent important work on the VC-dimension of neural networks includes that of Goldberg and Jerrum (1993) and Karpinski and MacIntyre (1995). In these papers, techniques from geometry and logic are used to study the VC-dimension of neural networks of certain types. In particular, the paper of Karpinski and MacIntyre, among other things, provides bounds on the VC-dimension of feedforward networks in which the output unit is a linear threshold and all other computational units have the standard sigmoid activation function given by $f(x) = 1/(1 + e^{-x})$. They obtain the following result.

Theorem 4. Suppose $\mathcal{N}$ is a feedforward network with a linear threshold unit as output unit, and with the remaining N computational units having the standard sigmoid activation. If $\mathcal{N}$ has W variable weights and thresholds, then

$$\text{VCdim}(\mathcal{N}) \leq (WN)^2 + 11WN \log_2(18WN^2)$$

The Computational Complexity of PAC Learning

Efficiency with Respect to Accuracy, Example Size, and Sample Length

Thus far, a learning algorithm has been defined as a function that maps training samples into hypotheses. We shall now be more specific about the computational effectiveness of this function. If the process of PAC learning by an algorithm L is to be of practical value, it should be possible to implement the algorithm quickly. We wish to quantify the behavior of a learning algorithm for a particular neural network architecture with respect to the size of the network. In particular, we wish to consider how the running time of the algorithm varies with the number n of inputs to the network: for a learning algorithm to be efficient, this running time should increase polynomially with n. However, there is another important consideration in any discussion of efficiency. Until now, we have regarded the accuracy parameter ε as fixed but arbitrary. It is clear that decreasing this parameter makes the learning task more difficult, and therefore the time taken to produce a probably approximately correct output should be constrained in some appropriate way as ε decreases; the appropriate condition is that the running time must be polynomial in $1/\varepsilon$. Formally, we say that a learning algorithm L is *efficient with respect to accuracy ε, example size n and sample length m* if its running time is polynomial in the length m of the training sample and if there is a value of $m_0(\delta, \varepsilon)$ sufficient for PAC learning that is polynomial in n and ε^{-1}.

Hardness Results

In complexity theory, two important classes of problems, RP and NP, are defined. The class RP is the class of all problems that can be solved by "randomized" algorithms in polynomial time, while NP is the class of problems that can be solved by nondeterministic Turing machines in polynomial time. (We refer the reader to the book by Cormen, Leiserson, and Rivest, 1990.) It is conjectured, and widely believed, that these classes are not the same; more precisely, it is believed that RP is a strict subset of NP. This is known as the "RP ≠ NP" conjecture. For fixed k, for each n, let $\mathcal{P}_n^k$ be the neural network that consists of k linear threshold units, each connected to all of n inputs, the outputs of these threshold networks then being combined together by a hardwired AND gate. Thus, the network outputs 1 if and only if all k threshold units output 1. Blum and Rivest (1988) proved (essentially) the following result. (See also Anthony and Biggs, 1992.)

Theorem 5. Let $\mathcal{P}_n^k$ be as described, where $k \geq 2$. If there is a PAC learning algorithm for $\mathcal{P}_n^k$ that is efficient with respect to accuracy, example size, and number of inputs, then the "RP ≠ NP" conjecture is false.

Thus, it is extremely unlikely that there is an efficient PAC learning algorithm for this surprisingly simple class of neural networks.

The point of this section has been to define what we might mean by an efficient algorithm, and to illustrate an approach (via computational complexity) to showing that certain learning problems are difficult. Therefore, we have presented a "negative" result. However, it should not be supposed that there are no positive results on efficient neural network learning. For example, there are efficient algorithms for perceptron learning, and also for more complex networks, including those in which the output of the network is a real number (and where we have to modify the definition of efficient learning from that given above, but in a fairly straightforward way). For instance, see Chapter 26 of Anthony and Bartlett (1999) for an efficient algorithm (due to Lee, Bartlett, and Williamson) for certain types of two-layer neural networks with linear threshold hidden units and a linear output unit.

Discussion

We have considered basic PAC learning as it applies to learning in artificial neural networks. There are two distinct aspects: the length of training sample to be used and the efficiency of learning. In other words, we have the *sample complexity* problem and the *computational complexity* problem. The Vapnik-Chervonenkis dimension of a neural network determines in a fairly precise way the length of sample sufficient for PAC learning. This dimension can, in many cases, be related to the structure of the network, as in the examples presented here. Techniques from computational complexity theory can be applied to show that in a number of cases, *efficient* algorithmic PAC learning is impossible unless the NP ≠ RP conjecture is false.

There are a number of recent important extensions and generalizations of the PAC model that can be applied to artificial neural networks. For example, much attention has focused on PAC-type models of learning for networks in which the output is a real number rather than simply 0 or 1. The paper by Haussler (1992) was an important part of this development, and much work has subsequently been carried out on extending the PAC model to regression

and to classification by real-output neural networks. This involves generalized notions of VC-dimension. There is insufficient space here to do these recent developments justice, but the reader can consult the book by Anthony and Bartlett (1999) for details.

Road Map: Computability and Complexity
Related Reading: Learning and Generalization: Theoretical Bounds; Vapnik-Chervonenkis Dimension of Neural Networks

References

Anthony, M., and Bartlett, P. L., 1999, *Neural Network Learning: Theoretical Foundations,* Cambridge, Engl.: Cambridge University Press. ◆
Anthony, M., and Biggs, N., 1992, *Computational Learning Theory: An Introduction,* Cambridge, Engl.: Cambridge University Press. ◆
Baum, E. B., and Haussler, D., 1989, What size net gives valid generalization? *Neural Computat.,* 1:151–160.
Blum, A., and Rivest, R. L., 1988, Training a 3-node neural network is NP-complete, in *Proceedings of the 1988 Workshop on Computational Learning Theory,* San Mateo, CA: Morgan Kaufmann, pp. 9–18. (See also *Neural Netw.,* 1992, 5:117–127.)
Blumer, A., Ehrenfeucht, A., Haussler, D., and Warmuth, M. K., 1989, Learnability and the Vapnik-Chervonenkis dimension, *J. ACM,* 36:929–965.
Cormen, T. H., Leiserson, C. E., and Rivest, R. L., 1990, *Introduction to Algorithms,* Cambridge, MA: MIT Press. ◆
Dudley, R., 1978, Central limit theorems for empirical measures, *Ann. Probab.,* 6:899–929.
Ehrenfeucht, A., Haussler, D., Kearns, M., and Valiant, L., 1989, A general lower bound on the number of examples needed for learning, *Inform. Computat.,* 82:247–261.
Goldberg, P., and Jerrum, M., 1993, Bounding the Vapnik-Chervonenkis dimension of concept classes parameterized by real numbers, in *Proceedings of the Sixth Annual ACM Conference on Computational Learning Theory,* New York: ACM Press, pp. 361–369. (See also Goldberg, P., and Jerrum, M., 1995, Bounding the Vapnik-Chervonenkis dimension of concept classes parameterized by real numbers, *Machine Learn.,* 18(2/3):131–148.)
Grunbaum, B., 1967, *Convex Polytopes,* London: Wiley.
Haussler, D., 1992, Decision theoretic generalizations of the PAC model for neural net and other learning applications, *Inform. Computat.,* 100:78–150.
Karpinski, M., and MacIntyre, A. J., 1995, Polynomial bounds for VC dimension of sigmoidal neural networks, in *Proceedings of the 27th Annual ACM Symposium on Theory of Computing,* New York: ACM Press, pp. 200–208. (See also Karpinski, M., and Macintyre, A. J., 1997, Polynomial bounds for VC dimension of sigmoidal and general Pfaffian neural networks, *J. Comput. Syst. Sci.,* 54:169–176.)
Maass, W., 1993, Bounds on the computational power and learning complexity of analog neural nets, in *Proceedings of the Twenty-Fifth Annual ACM. Symposium on the Theory of Computing,* New York: ACM Press, pp. 335–344. (See also Maass, W., 1994, Neural nets with superlinear VC-dimension, *Neural Computat.,* 6:877–884.)
Valiant, L. G., 1984, A theory of the learnable, *Commun. ACM,* 27:1134–1142.
Vapnik, V. N., and Chervonenkis, A. Ya., 1971, On the uniform convergence of relative frequencies of events to their probabilities, *Theory Probab. Appl.,* 16:264–280.

Pain Networks

Marshall Devor

Introduction

Pain is an unpleasant sensory and emotional experience that arises in a conscious brain, typically in response to noxious stimuli. There is a growing consensus that the classical conception of how the

pain system works is incomplete, notably for its failure to adequately account for sensory abnormalities seen in patients with chronic pain. For example, people with nerve injury often report bizarre symptoms such as electric shock-like paroxysms, or severe burning pain in skin that is numb to the touch. In this article, I outline a new synthesis, now emerging, that builds on the old scheme by addressing both normal and pathophysiological pain processes. There are many unsolved problems that could benefit from computational analysis but very little computational work has been done on pain to date.

The Pain System: Normal Functioning

Stimulus-Response Variability

The pain system encodes information on the intensity, location, and dynamics of strong, tissue-threatening stimuli. This sensory-discriminative function is shared with all sensory systems. Where pain differs is in the degree to which emotional-motivational and cognitive-evaluative variables can modulate the basic sensory message. The sight of blood may frighten you, but fright doesn't make red look like blue. In contrast, emotional and cognitive factors can render strong noxious stimuli painless. Consider, for example, the wounded soldier pulling his unconscious buddy out of the line of fire, or the placebo effect, in which belief that an inert pill contains analgesic ingredients is often enough to relieve pain. Even under everyday conditions, shifts of attention and expectation cause normal, rational people to display wide variability in pain sensation. For this reason, pain professionals usually avoid speaking of pain stimuli (or pain receptors), preferring instead *noxious stimuli* (or *nociceptors*). A noxious stimulus may evoke more or less pain, depending on context; the degree of pain felt depends as much on system variables as it does on the stimulus itself (Wall, 1999).

Stimulus Encoding by Sensory Receptor Endings

The first step in sensory signaling is to encode the quality and location of the stimulus. This is done with spatial arrays of sensory receptor endings, each responsive to a specific type of stimulus at a specific location. Sensory receptors are the ends of axons of primary somatosensory neurons (primary afferents), the cell bodies of which are located near the spine (but not in the spinal cord), in the dorsal root ganglia (DRGs, Figure 1*B*). Each DRG neuron has a peripheral axon that travels in a nerve and terminates in a sensory transducer ending in skin, muscle, viscera, etc., and a central axon that travels in a dorsal root and ends synaptically in the spinal cord and/or the brainstem. The cell body itself is offset from the main

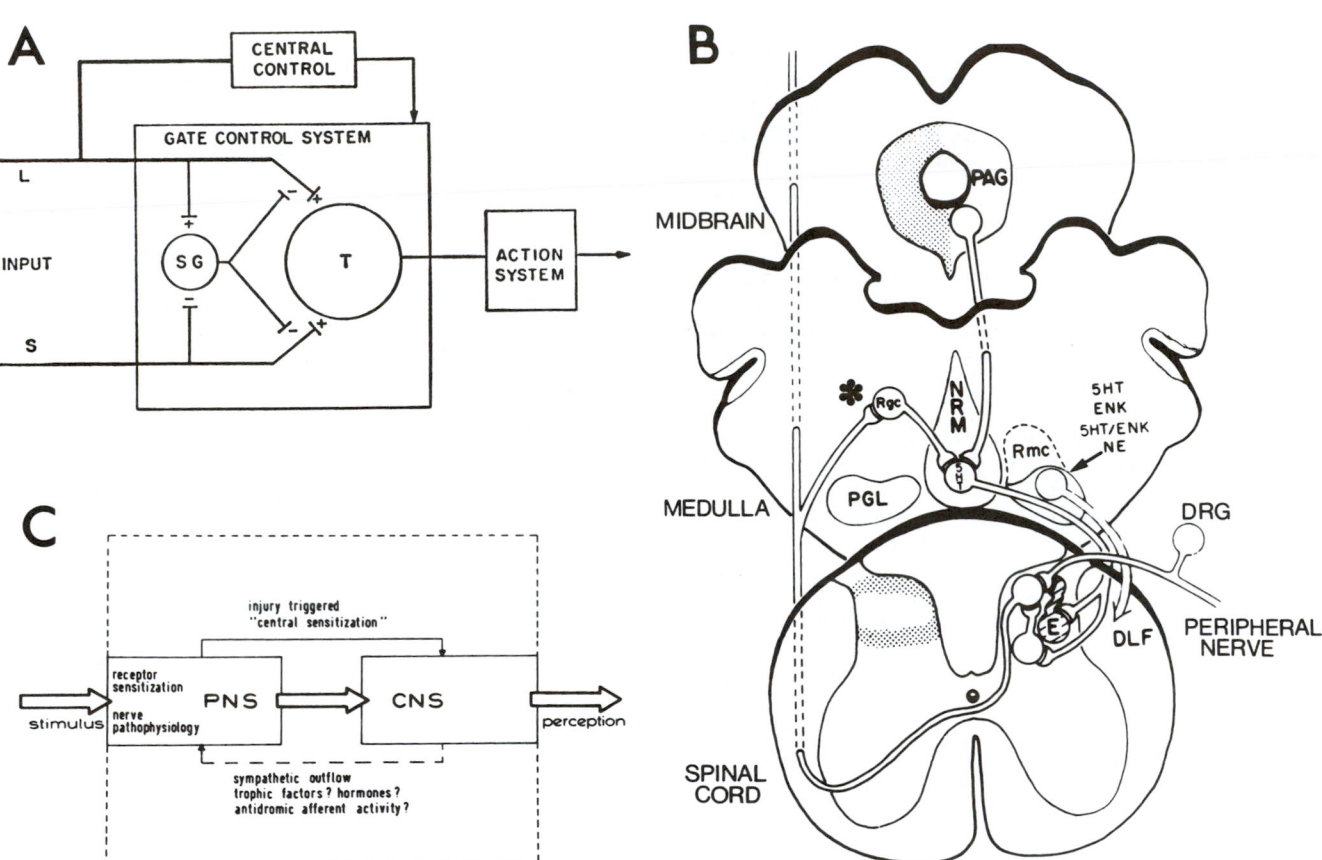

Figure 1. Three circuits for the modulation of pain signals. *A*, The original gate control system of Melzack and Wall (1965). Input from low-threshold (L) afferents and nociceptors (S) activates WDR transmission neurons (T) in the dorsal horn of the spinal cord. The former, but not the latter, activate substantia gelatinosa (SG) interneurons, which presynaptically inhibit the nociceptive input. Central control is also noted. *B*, Subsequently discovered details of the central control system (Fields and Basbaum, 1999). Activity in the midbrain PAG, relayed through specific medullary nuclei, including the nucleus raphe magnus (NRM) and the reticular magnocellular nucleus (Rmc), evokes synaptic inhibition on ascending pain-signaling neurons in the spinal cord partly via enkephalinergic (E) spinal interneurons. The descending axons of the NRM and Rmc, which use as neurotransmitters 5-hydroxytryptamine (5-HT), enkephalin (ENK), and/or norepinephrine (NE), travel in the dorsolateral funiculus (DLF). A collateral branch of the ascending WDR pain-signaling neurons (T) contributes to descending inhibition via nucleus reticularis gigantocellularis (Rgc, asterisk) in a negative feedback loop. *C*, Pain amplification mechanisms associated with tissue and nerve damage. The pain signal is modulated in the PNS and CNS by the local processes noted, and by a combination of feedback and feedforward. (From Devor, M., and Seltzer, Z., 1999, Pathophysiology of damaged nerves in relation to chronic pain, in *Textbook of Pain*, 4th ed. [P. D. Wall and R. Melzack, Eds.], London: Churchill Livingstone, pp. 129–164.)

axon by a small stem. Nerve impulses run from the receptor ending, past the DRG, and on into the CNS without pause. Curiously, the cell is specially designed so that spikes will invade it. Given that there are no synapses in the DRG, why has nature gone to the trouble of arranging for this spike invasion?

Somatosensory afferents are modality specific. Some, *low-threshold mechanoreceptors* (LTMs), respond to gentle touch and vibration. Others, *nociceptors*, respond only to strong stimuli. Some nociceptors respond to a particular submodality, e.g., mechanical (pinch) or thermal (hot, cold), but most encode the combined intensity of strong mechanical, thermal, and irritant chemical stimuli. These *polymodal nociceptors* pose the dilemma of how we distinguish a pinprick from a bee sting. Some nociceptors do not respond to any stimuli at all unless they have been sensitized by tissue inflammation (*silent nociceptors*). LTMs mostly have heavily myelinated, fast-conducting $A\beta$ axons. Nociceptors have slow-conducting axons either with thin myelin ($A\delta$ fibers) or with no myelin (C-fibers).

Within each modality, firing frequency encodes stimulus strength. LTMs, for example, respond to increasing pressure by accelerating their firing rate. LTMs also respond to noxious pinch. But since their firing rate saturates below the noxious range, they do not encode the intensity of noxious stimuli. Direct electrical microstimulation of LTM axons evokes a sensation of touch or pressure, but it does not (normally) evoke pain even at very high frequency (Vallbo et al., 1979). *Normally*, pain is felt only when activity is recruited in nociceptors; when stimulus strength approaches the noxious range, encoding is handed off from LTMs to nociceptors. I stress "normally" because there are system states where activity in LTMs does evoke pain (discussed in the next section).

Central Convergence

The spatial information inherent in the arrays of sensory receptor endings—in the skin, for example—is preserved by topographic (*somatotopic*) mapping of primary afferent axons onto the spinal cord, and thence onto all subsequent waystations up to the cortex. The coding of sensory quality is more complicated.

Extrapolating from the specificity of primary afferents, many investigators concluded in the past (and some still believe) that each somatosensory modality, including pain, remains separate and pathway-specific all the way to consciousness. This idea, the classical specificity theory of pain, should have been shaken by the discovery that most neurons in the spinal cord that receive synaptic input from nociceptors also receive low-threshold input; they are modality-convergent *wide dynamic range* (WDR) neurons. Indeed, some combine low-threshold and nociceptive skin input with proprioceptive and/or visceral input and hence are *multireceptive* neurons. Specificity theory was saved by the discovery of a small population of neurons in the most superficial part of the spinal dorsal horn that are (normally) nociceptive selective. But if these alone signal pain, what of the large majority of spinal WDR neurons that have convergent nociceptor input?

In fact, there is now abundant evidence that activity in WDR neurons can evoke pain sensation. But with the modality multiplexing of WDR neurons, how are the specific touch and pain sensations that we feel decoded? A number of schemes have been advanced. For example, the comparator model holds that activity in WDR neurons is interpreted as pain only if nociceptive-selective neurons are also active. Another proposal posits that stimulus quality is coded in discharge patterning. The most likely scheme, however, is that spike frequency is the key parameter. Touch is felt when WDR neurons fire slowly; pain is felt when they fire rapidly. Since each WDR neuron has its own encoding function (firing rate as a function of stimulus strength), increasingly strong stimuli pro-

gressively recruit WDR neurons with sequentially overlapping encoding functions. In this model, any given stimulus would produce a unique aggregate of neuronal activity when viewed across the entire population of neurons that map a particular patch of skin. Somatosensation is a symphony.

Ascending Pathways and Cephalic Representation

Textbook representations of ascending somatosensory pathways typically show two compact routes, the spinothalamic (anterolateral column) system for pain and temperature, and the dorsal column-medial lemniscus system for touch and vibration, each relaying through nuclei of the ventrobasal thalamus and ending mapwise in the somatosensory cortex. This vision, virtuous for being easy to teach and learn, corresponds to the ideology of specificity theory. It is also fundamentally misleading. Although some axons of the anterolateral column system reach the thalamus directly, most branch extensively, dropping terminals en route in numerous spinal, medullary, pontine, and mesencephalic structures. There are also massive projections to the cerebellum, and directly or indirectly to widespread areas of the limbic forebrain. In other words, much of the brain receives direct or nearly direct synaptic input from spinal cord WDR neurons. Ascending pain pathways are also dynamic. For example, cutting the anterolateral column usually relieves pain felt below the cut, but the pain usually returns within a few months. Any successful pain theory must take these facts into account.

Modulation and Gate Control

Peripheral Nervous System Sensitization

Sensory modulation is obvious from everyday experience. In sunburned skin, for example, gentle warming is painful. This primary hyperalgesia apparently results from peripheral sensitization, the fact that tissue inflammation can increase the gain (sensitivity) of the transduction process in nociceptive endings in skin, muscle, joints, and so forth, rendering them responsive to previously innocuous stimuli. Much of modern pain research is devoted to working out the molecular details of peripheral sensitization (Levine and Reichling, 1999; Woolf and Salter, 2000). Tissue inflammation is usually self-limiting, and hence the resulting pain is acute or subacute. Sustained inflammation, such as in rheumatoid arthritis, causes chronic pain. Most simple over-the-counter analgesics work by reducing peripheral sensitization. However, recent evidence suggests that these drugs may also have a significant CNS action.

Modulation in the CNS

Although peripheral sensitization yields pain in response to normally nonpainful stimuli (*allodynia*), it does not violate the spirit of the specificity theory in the sense that the signaling lines for the various modalities remain specific and independent. In 1965 Melzack and Wall presented the first real challenge to the specificity theory with their famous gate control theory of pain (Figure 1A). This theory began with the radical idea that pain is signaled primarily by populations of convergent WDR neurons, and added that the convergence itself is dynamic and modulated in an ongoing fashion by afferent input from the periphery, and by descending control from the brain. For example, input along low-threshold $A\beta$ afferents inhibits the response of WDR neurons to simultaneously arriving nociceptive input, "closing a gate on pain." This explains the relief obtained from gently rubbing tender skin. Central control was also a key feature of the original gate control model (Figure 1A), but the details emerged only later (Fields and Basbaum, 1999). Although ideas about the circuitry of spinal gating/modulation have changed over the years, the fundamental concept has been vindicated by a great richness of CNS modulatory processes that form the basis of the new synthesis.

Descending Inhibition

The midbrain periaqueductal gray matter (PAG in Figure 1*B*) is a nodal point for a descending inhibitory control circuit through which the brain gates ascending nociceptive information. Electrical stimulation of the PAG, or microinjection of opiates (e.g., morphine), activates nuclei in the medulla that contain cells rich in the neurotransmitters serotonin (5-HT; e.g., NRM in Figure 1*B*) and norepinephrine (NE). These cell groups in turn give rise to a compact bundle of axons that descend in the dorsolateral part of the spinal cord (DLF in Figure 1*B*). Activity in these descending axons inhibits the response of dorsal horn WDR neurons to noxious input, while responses to innocuous input are largely unaffected. Activation of this midbrain-medullospinal inhibitory circuit by morphine or by endogenous morphine-like neurotransmitters (enkephalin, endorphin) appears to be largely responsible for the antinociception obtained from opiates. Moreover, there is accumulating evidence that this system is also responsible for the stress-induced analgesia shown by the heroic soldier noted earlier, and for the placebo effect (Benedetti, Arduino, and Amanzio, 1999). We are talking about the neurology of belief and anticipation.

Central Sensitization

Spinal gating involves excitation and not just inhibition. For example, I noted the fact that inflammation may sensitize nociceptor endings, yielding primary hyperalgesia. However, tenderness around such injuries often spreads to a much larger area of surrounding skin where there is no inflammation and no nociceptor sensitization. There has long been evidence that such "secondary hyperalgesia" is due to impulses entering the CNS along LTM Aβ touch afferents. This idea of Aβ pain was strongly resisted, as it violates the most fundamental dogma of specificity theory, namely, that pain can only be evoked by Aβ and C nociceptors. However, in recent years the evidence has become increasingly compelling.

It turns out that a momentary noxious input is enough to trigger a system state, called *central sensitization*, in which Aδ touch input transiently elicits pain (Raja et al., 1999; Woolf and Salter, 2000). Moreover, this state can be maintained indefinitely so long as a persistent source of nociceptive input is present (Gracely, Lynch, and Bennett, 1992). Central sensitization is particularly important as an amplifier in touch/brush-evoked pain (in contrast to thermal-evoked pain). It now appears that most of the tenderness we feel after everyday bumps and scrapes is due to Aβ touch afferents. A working model of central sensitization is given in Figure 2 (see legend).

Neuropathic Pain

The strongest impetus for revising classical ideas about pain came from observations of chronic pain in patients, particularly the bizarre and intractable pain associated with damage to peripheral nerves, dorsal roots, and the CNS. Such *neuropathic pain* is paradoxical in the sense that when a sensory conduction channel is compromised, sensation is expected to be reduced, not augmented. Perhaps the most striking example is phantom limb pain in amputees, but neuropathic pain also includes such common conditions as limb pain in diabetics (diabetic neuropathy), postherpetic neuralgia (shingles), sciatica, and many instances of cancer pain.

Nerve Pathophysiology/Ectopia

The key to understanding neuropathic pain is the realization that nerves do not behave like copper telephone cables. When an axon is cut across, or stripped of its myelin, the neuron reacts with path-

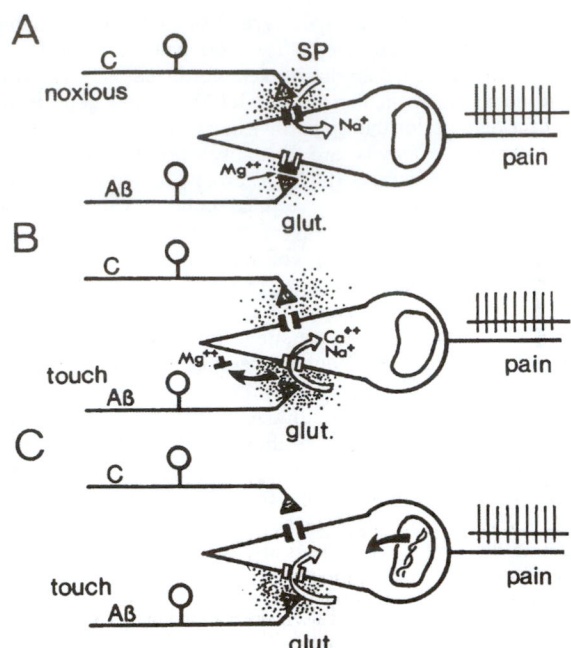

Figure 2. A proposed central sensitization mechanism for triggering touch-evoked pain (Woolf and Salter, 2000). *A*, Normally, activity in peripheral C-nociceptors activates spinal WDR neurons by means of excitatory amino acid and peptide neurotransmitters, probably including substance P (SP). This triggers an ascending pain signal. Touch input, carried along low-threshold Aβ afferents, evokes release of the neurotransmitter glutamate (glut). However, this drives the WDR neurons minimally because the NMDA-type (*N*-methyl *d*-aspartate) glutamate receptors on the postsynaptic dendrites are blocked at normal membrane potentials by Mg^{2+} ions. *B*, Intense noxious C-input produces prolonged (tens of seconds) SP-evoked depolarization. This displaces the Mg^{2+} block, enabling the NMDA receptors. Now, glutamate released from Aβ touch afferents can strongly activate the WDR neurons and hence evoke pain and tenderness. Ca^{2+} entering the WDR neurons through the enabled NMDA receptor channels may trigger phosphorylation of the channels, due to activation of a Ca^{2+}-dependent protein kinase (PKA), sustaining the touch-evoked pain state for hours. *C*, More speculatively, a change in gene expression triggered by tissue or nerve injury could prolong the central sensitization state indefinitely.

ophysiological changes that may render it intrinsically resonant (Amir et al., 2002) and electrically hyperexcitable (Figure 3). The result is ongoing and stimulus-evoked firing that originates at abnormal (ectopic) sites, notably in the region of injury and/or the sensory cell body in the DRG. Other pathophysiological processes, such as nonsynaptic neuron-to-neuron coupling, may augment the ectopia (Devor and Seltzer, 1999)

Ectopic hyperexcitability appears to result primarily from injury-provoked remodeling of membrane electrical properties in the axon and/or sensory cell body, due to changes in gene expression and vectorial trafficking of expressed proteins (Devor and Seltzer, 1999; Waxman et al., 1999). Early simulations of the process indicated the potential importance of Na$^+$ channel accumulation (Figure 3*C*), but ultimately, excitability is due to the complex integrated action on numerous channel types and subtypes (Amir et al. 2002). Ectopic firing in injured afferents contributes to pain in two ways. First, it injects an abnormal afferent impulse barrage into the CNS. Second, it may trigger and maintain central sensitization. In the sensitized state, Aβ touch input from the skin, and also Aβ activity from ectopic sources, is felt as pain (tenderness to touch and spontaneous pain).

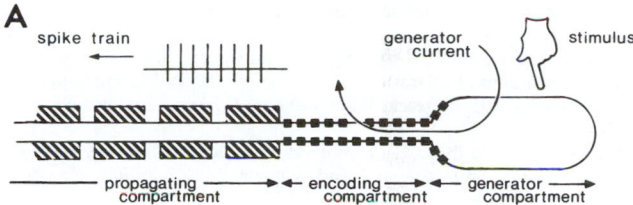

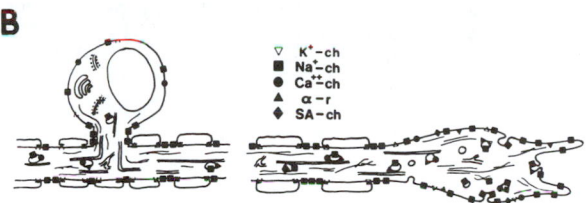

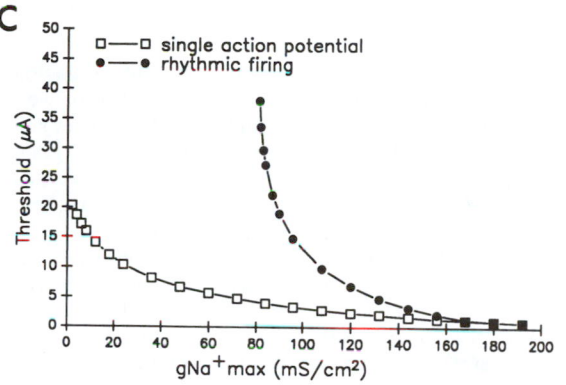

Figure 3. Stimulus transduction and encoding at normal sensory endings, and ectopic electrogenesis at sites of nerve injury, depends on the precise regulation of membrane electrical properties in the cell body and at the axon end. *A*, Applied stimuli create a generator current that is encoded into a spike train in a patch of membrane rich in Na^+ channels (black squares in encoding compartment). *B*, The membrane channels (-ch), receptors (-r), and other proteins responsible for electrogenesis are synthesized in the cell body and transported down the axon. These include K^+, Na^+, and Ca^{2+} ion channels, α-adrenoreceptors (α-r), and mechanosensitive stretch-activated (SA) channels, among others. In the presence of nerve injury, channels and receptors accumulate in the membrane of the cut axon end and sprouts (right), rendering them hyperexcitable and a source of ectopia and neuropathic pain. *C*, Numerical simulation demonstrating that the accumulation of voltage-sensitive Na^+ channels (gNa^+ max) sharply reduces the threshold for rhythmic firing, but has less of an effect on the threshold for evoking individual nerve impulses. (From Devor, M., and Seltzer, Z., 1999, Pathophysiology of damaged nerves in relation to chronic pain, in *Textbook of Pain*, 4th ed. [P. D. Wall and R. Melzack, Eds.], London: Churchill Livingstone, pp. 129–164.)

Where Is Pain?

I opened this article by characterizing pain as an unpleasant percept aroused in a conscious brain by noxious stimuli. So far I have referred to the signal acquisition apparatus of the pain system, and to neural pathways that transmit and modulate nociceptive signals. But where does the experience of pain actually occur?

First, it is safe to exclude the PNS and spinal cord, on the grounds that quadriplegics experience pain, including pain referred to anesthetic parts of the body (phantom body pain). Surprisingly, the somatosensory cortex also appears nonessential, despite the fact that cortical neurons in a number of different regions respond to noxious stimuli (Peyron, Laurent, and Garcia-Larrea, 2000). For example, while lesions in the occipital cortex produce blindness, even extensive damage to the postcentral gyrus and other cortical projections does not preclude pain sensation, even in parts of the body whose cortical representation has been destroyed. More important, cortical seizure activity, and direct electrical stimulation of the somatosensory cortex, rarely evoke pain.

A part of the anterior cingulate gyrus has been implicated recently in pain perception on the grounds that the magnitude of activations there correlates with felt pain rather than with stimulus intensity when the pain percept is manipulated by hypnosis and distraction (Rainville et al., 1997). However, this correlation may simply reflect the operation of descending spinal modulatory pathways (Figure 1*B*) and hence attentional modulation of the ascending nociceptive signal. A final candidate is the collection of brain-stem and subcortical forebrain regions that receive and modulate nociceptive signals (Devor and Zalkind, 2001). Few would argue that pain behavior, both withdrawal reflexes and more complex escape responses, may be organized subcortically. But can perception occur outside of the cortex? Might pain experience have arisen early in vertebrate evolution, in parallel with pain behavior and before cortical domination of the brain?

Perspective

Pain, particularly persistent pain, remains a medical health problem of the first order: witness the prominence of alternative approaches to treating pain, built largely on the therapeutic failures of conventional medicine. It is also a remarkable basic science challenge. Situated at the interface of body and mind, only a few synapses intervene between the biophysics of stimulus transduction and the magic of conscious perception (Devor and Zalkind, 2001).

At each level of analysis there are problems that could be fruitfully approached using computational methods. For example, in the periphery, the fine diameter of C-fiber endings precludes direct electrophysiological measurement. Testable hypotheses concerning the ionic mechanisms of transduction, encoding, sensitization (e.g., during inflammation), and ectopia could be provided by theoretical analysis. At the level of spinal processing are issues such as the modes of convergence that go into synthesizing natural receptive fields, the problem of how WDR neurons encode specific sensations, and mechanisms of functional plasticity (e.g., gate control and central sensitization). Finally, theoretical analysis might provide insights into the higher-level functions that control descending pain inhibition and ultimately pain experience. In the visual pathway, the extraction of meaning (Is it a passing cloud or a rhinoceros charging?) requires a massive analytical apparatus. In the pain system, meaning is much closer at hand.

Road Map: Other Sensory Systems
Related Reading: Emotional Circuits; Motivation; Somatosensory System; Somatotopy: Plasticity of Sensory Maps

References

Amir, R., Liu, C.-N., Kocsis, J. D., and Devor, M., 2002, Oscillatory mechanism in primary sensory neurons, *Brain*, 125:421–435.

Benedetti, F., Arduino, C., and Amanzio, M., 1999, Somatotopic activation of opioid systems by target-directed expectations of analgesia, *J. Neurosci.*, 19:3639–3648.

Devor, M., and Seltzer, Z., 1999, Pathophysiology of damaged nerves in relation to chronic pain, in *Textbook of Pain*, 4th ed. (P. D. Wall and R. Melzack, Eds.), London: Churchill Livingstone, pp. 129–164. ◆

Devor, M., and Zalkind, V., 2001, Reversible analgesia, atonia, and loss of consciousness on bilateral intracerebral microinjection of pentobarbital, *Pain*, 94:101–112.

Fields, H. L., and Basbaum, A. I., 1999, Central nervous system mechanisms of pain modulation, in *Textbook of Pain*, 4th ed. (P. D. Wall and R. Melzack, Eds.), London: Churchill Livingstone, pp. 309–329. ◆

Gracely, R., Lynch, S., and Bennett, G., 1992, Painful neuropathy: Altered central processing, maintained dynamically by peripheral input, *Pain*, 51:175–194.

Levine, J., and Reichling, D., 1999, Peripheral mechanisms of inflammatory pain, in *Textbook of Pain*, 4th ed. (P. Wall and R. Melzack, Eds.), London: Churchill Livingstone, pp. 59–84.

Melzack, R., and Wall, P., 1965, Pain mechanisms: A new theory, *Science*, 150:971–979.

Peyron, R., Laurent, B., and Garcia-Larrea, L., 2000, Functional imaging of brain responses to pain: A review and meta-analysis, *Neurophysiol. Clin.*, 30:263–288.

Rainville, P., Duncan, G. H., Price, D. D., Carrier, B., and Bushnell, M. C.,

1997, Pain affect encoded in human anterior cingulate but not somatosensory cortex, *Science*, 277:968–971.

Raja, S. N., Meyer, R. A., Ringkamp, M., and Campbell, J. N., 1999, Peripheral neural mechanisms of nociception, in *Textbook of Pain*, 4th ed. (P. D. Wall and R. Melzack, Eds.), London: Churchill Livingstone, pp. 13–44.

Vallbo, A. B., Hagbarth, K. E., Torebjork, H. E., and Wallin, B. G., 1979, Somatosensory, proprioceptive, and sympathetic activity in human peripheral nerves, *Physiol. Rev.*, 59:919–957.

Wall, P. D., 1999, *Pain: The Science of Suffering*, London: Weidenfeld and Nicholson. ◆

Waxman, S. G., Dib-Hajj, S., Cummins, T. R., and Black, J. A., 1999, Sodium channels and pain, *Proc. Natl. Acad. Sci. USA*, 96:7635–7639.

Woolf, C. J., and Salter, M. W., 2000, Neuronal plasticity: Increasing the gain in pain, *Science*, 288:1765–1769.

Past Tense Learning

Amit Almor

Introduction

The English past tense, a seemingly simple linguistic phenomenon that has come to epitomize the latest round in the centuries-old debate between rationalists and empiricists, exemplifies the processes that more generally handle the formation of words and their structure. These processes have been traditionally studied by the linguistics field of "morphology," which has assumed a level of representation that is based on the smallest meaning-bearing linguistic units, called *morphemes*. The main goal of linguistic morphology has been to systematically identify morphemes and describe the principles that govern the way they are used to form words (see Spencer and Zwicky, 1998, for current issues in linguistic morphology). Morphemic representation lies in between the phonological level, where the basic representations consist of individual sounds (phonemes), and whole words. Some morphemes are identical to whole words. For example, each of the words *base* and *ball* consists of one morpheme (/base/ and /ball/, respectively), and the word *baseball* consists of these two morphemes combined. Not all morphemes are words, however; the word *dislike* consists of the non-word morpheme /dis/ and the word morpheme /like/, and the word *liked* consists of the stem morpheme /like/ and the non-word past tense morpheme /ed/. The relation between meaning and word form is not always transparent. One reason is that the meaning of some morphemes can only be traced etymologically. For example, the meaning of *-mit* in *permit, submit,* and *remit* is not transparent to modern day English speakers but can be traced back to the Latin suffix *mittêre* (roughly meaning, "to let go"). Moreover, even when the meanings of the component morphemes are known and can be ascertained (as in /break//fast/, i.e., the meal that breaks the fast) it is not clear that these meanings are transparent and accessible enough to affect actual word use. Finally, even when the meanings of the component morphemes are transparent and readily accessible, the meaning of the resulting compound is not consistently entailed. Although there is much regularity in how the meanings of morphemes are related to word meanings (e.g., *housedog* is a kind of dog and a *doghouse* is a kind of house) there are many exceptions. *Hotdog* is not a kind of dog, *sweetbread* is not a kind of bread, and *hammerhead* is not a kind of head. Thus, although the relation between word form, word meaning, and morphemes seems to encompass much regularity, it is not trivial and cannot be easily captured by simple combinatorial rules.

This may be differentially true for different kinds of morphological processes. Most morphological theories distinguish between inflectional and derivational processes. Inflectional processes generally involve elements of word structure that are related to grammar, such as markings for tense, number, gender, and case. Languages vary in the extent to which this grammatical information is morphologically encoded. In Hebrew, verbs are marked for tense, number, gender, and argument structure, resulting in a complex and highly regular verbal inflectional system. In English, verbs are only marked for tense and number, and in Mandarin Chinese, verbs are marked for neither tense nor number. Inflectional processes apply in accordance with sentence structure (in English, the subject noun of a sentence has to agree in number with the verb; a failure to do so results in ungrammaticality) and do not alter the core meaning or grammatical class of the inflected stem. Inflectional processes can be viewed as generating classes of systematically related word forms from a basic stem/root form via a small set of morphological operations. Inflectional processes are also highly productive in the sense that they apply to all the words in the language with new words "automatically" receiving a so-called regular "default" treatment. For example, all verbs in English are marked for tense and new verbs generally receive the regular *-ed* past tense suffix (e.g., *faxed, emailed*).

In contrast, derivational processes are more open ended and involve the creation of new words from other words and morphemes, often resulting in changes in grammatical category. For example, in English, the suffix *-ly* can be used to form adverbs from adjectives: *glad-gladly, poor-poorly*, etc. Derivational processes do not apply across the board (e.g., the suffix *-ly* cannot be added to adjectives such as *tall, old, young*).

Historically, the more regular nature of inflectional processes suggested that the relation between morphemes, meanings, and word forms could be more easily explained in the area of inflectional morphology than in the area of derivational morphology. It also suggested that the underlying computational machinery might involve rules. Although in recent years derivational processes have begun to attract as much attention as inflectional processes, it has been in the area of inflectional morphology that most current ideas and theories were formed.

Regulars and Rules

Indeed, for many years, regular inflection such as the *-ed* English past tense suffix was used as the showcase example for symbolic rules in mental computation. Two main observations were most often cited. The first is that speakers readily apply the regular rule to new words they haven't heard before, regardless of the new words' similarity to other words that conform to the regular pattern. This observation has received much empirical support from numerous studies using variants of Berko's (1958) well-known "Wug test" in which a subject is asked to complete a fragment like: "Here is one *wug*. These are two___." Adults and children from about age three usually apply the regular English plural suffix and respond "wugs" despite never having heard the word *wug* before. Similar results have been obtained with the English past tense in that subjects aged three and older readily inflect a novel verb with the regular -*ed* suffix. The second observation thought to support symbolic rules was children's over-regularization errors. It has long been observed that children exhibit what may seem like a paradoxical decline in language performance starting at around three years of age. At this age, children who may have previously used irregular forms correctly suddenly start inappropriately regularizing many irregular forms. A child who may have already used the past tense form *went* in her speech might suddenly start using *goed* or *wented*. This over-regularization lasts well into the elementary school years. This learning pattern is usually referred to as a "U-shaped learning curve" because when plotted against age, children's performance worsens and then improves, thus resembling the shape of the letter U. U-shaped learning was believed to reflect children's switch from rote memorization of both regular and irregular past tense forms to the use of symbolic rules. By this account, at around age three, children's ability to use rules matures and they start applying rules across the board, occasionally producing over-regularization errors.

The Past Tense Debate

The view that regular inflection shows the working of an underlying rule was challenged by Rumelhart and McClelland's (1986) landmark connectionist model. This model was trained to map phonological representations of stem forms into output phonological representations of past tense forms. By using a general error-correcting learning algorithm, the statistical relations between the input stem phonemes and the output past form phonemes were encoded in the weights of the links. These learned associations enabled the model to generalize and produce the regular past tense form for novel verbs it was not trained on, thus exhibiting behavior that could be described as rule-governed even though no rules were involved in producing this behavior. Remarkably, without implementing any underlying rules, the model's course of learning mimicked the U-shaped curve characteristic of children. The model thus illustrated how the generalization ability previously thought to be the signature of an underlying rule mechanism can arise in a connectionist network without explicit rules. This model had a substantial effect on the fields of psycholinguistics and cognitive science. After two decades in which statistical learning was considered inadequate as an explanation of language (mainly due to an influential critique of statistical learning by Chomsky, 1959), Rumelhart and McClelland's work showed that statistical learning can provide a viable alternative to symbolic rules.

Rumelhart and McClelland's challenge to symbolic rules met with considerable criticism, starting with Pinker and Prince (1988). Critics argued that the behavior of the model diverges in important ways from human behavior. For example, unlike humans, the model did not generalize well to novel forms that have an unusual sound (e.g., the model mapped the stem *tour*, which was not in the training set, to the past tense *toureder*.) Critics also argued that the most impressive feat of the model, its U-shaped learning curve, is the result of an implausible and carefully engineered training regime that does not parallel the input to the child or the child's own

output. Indeed, many critics argued that in order for a connectionist model to properly handle regular inflections, it must implement rules albeit using connectionist machinery. While this view concedes that such "implementation models" can help explain how rules are represented and executed by the brain, it nevertheless maintains that such models do not provide a theoretical alternative to rule based theories (for a summary of the criticism of Rumelhart and McClelland's model, see Pinker, 1999).

The combination of successes and problems of the Rumelhart and McClelland model led many researchers to propose that while connectionist models may provide an adequate account for how irregularly inflected forms are processed, the processing of regular inflections must be driven by a rule-based mechanism. This "dual mechanism" approach maintains both a rule-based mechanism and a connectionist memory system living side by side. The latter contains memorized mappings from stem to inflected forms for all the irregular mappings but, being nonselective, may also include frequently encountered (and possibly irregular sounding) regular mappings. To explain how processing in the two components is coordinated, this view also stipulates a "blocking mechanism" that allows an activated memorized inflected form to block the usage of the default rule (for a detailed presentation of the dual route model, see Pinker, 1999.)

The critique of Rumelhart and McClelland's model and the subsequent development of the dual mechanism approach provided the road map for much of the research that has followed since. A new generation of connectionist models attempted to address the design flaws and empirical shortcomings of the original Rumelhart and McClelland model as well as to broaden the scope of the empirical data covered. Many models added hidden layers and clean-up units to allow for a wider range of learnable mappings. Other models included semantic representations, which enabled them to address more than one type of inflection and to assign different inflections to homophonic stems. For example, MacWhinney and Leinbach (1991) developed a model that handled both noun plurals and verb past tenses and that could further distinguish past tense forms of homophones (*break-broke* vs. *brake-braked*). Plunkett and Marchman's (1993) model addressed many of the developmental issues related to the U-shaped learning curve.

Although these and many other models have successfully addressed many of the problems in the original Rumelhart and McClelland model, they nevertheless met with new criticism from dual mechanism theorists. One line of criticism continued to be directed at specific design aspects of various models, with some models accused of stealthily implementing the past tense rule. For example, the MacWhinney and Leinbach's (1991) model was accused of implementing a rule because, in addition to the regular input to output connections, it had special connections between the corresponding phonological units in the input and output (Pinker, 1999). The value of this line of criticism is questionable because, as connectionist theorists are quick to admit (e.g., Seidenberg, 1997), implemented models require many simplifying assumptions. Broadly criticizing models for making these assumptions without considering their specific implications risks missing important insights about the connection between behavior and underlying computation.

Moreover, this kind of criticism can be equally directed at the dual mechanism account, which makes its own set of problematic assumptions. In particular, it does not make clear how the blocking mechanism works, how and why it develops, and why is it not triggered by the many regulars that were already learned before the rule mechanism matured. As is often the case with theoretical constructs that are hard to explain or motivate, blocking is assigned the status of an innate mechanism. This not only relieves the theory from having to explain how this mechanism works and develops, but also adds one more marvel to the bag of wonders that cannot be explained without an arsenal of highly specialized language-specific mental machinery.

Besides debating details of implementation, much research has focused on behavioral and neuropsychological differences between the processing of regulars and irregulars and on the implications of such differences for the single and dual mechanism theories.

Frequency of Inflected Forms

One way in which regulars and irregulars differ has to do with how the frequency of inflected forms affects their processing. The use of irregularly inflected forms is strongly affected by their frequency, and to the extent that regularly inflected forms show frequency effects, these effects are quite small (see Pinker, 1999, for details). According to the dual mechanism view, these differences indicate that regulars and irregulars are processed by two separate mechanisms. This is because the memorized irregular mappings are strengthened each time an irregularly inflected form is encountered, but the application of the regular symbolic rule is not sensitive to the properties of the individual stems or inflected forms. The small frequency effects with regularly inflected forms found in some experiments is explained as a result of special circumstances that encourage the use of the memory system, for example when subjects are presented with a list containing an unnaturally high number of irregular forms.

Single mechanism accounts can also explain differences in the frequency dependence of regulars and irregulars. In these systems, frequency by regularity interactions can arise because "regular" input to output mappings, which are shared by a large number of different inputs, are less dependent on the frequency of individual input-output mappings, whereas "irregular" mappings that are shared by only a small number of inputs are more sensitive to the frequency of individual mappings (Seidenberg and McClelland, 1989). By this account, regularity itself, and by extension frequency effects, fall along a continuum defined by the number and similarity of input-output mappings.

A frequency effect that can better distinguish between the two theories is related to whether the frequency of regular forms makes their production less or more prone to interference by similarly sounding irregulars. Empirical evidence shows that such irregularization errors are more likely for low frequency regular verbs than for high frequency regular verbs and that the latency of correct regular production for high frequency regulars is less affected by interference from phonologically similar irregulars than the latency of correct responses for low frequency regulars (Long and Almor, 2000). These findings are compatible with a single mechanism view in which regulars and irregulars are processed similarly such that more frequent items are processed more quickly and with fewer errors than less frequent items. These results are not compatible with the dual mechanism view. Because, by this account, the only kind of *regularly* inflected forms that are stored in the memory system and are therefore prone to interference are high frequency regulars, this account falsely predicts that competition between similarly sounding irregular and regular stems would only occur for high frequency regulars but not for low frequency regulars (Pinker, 1999, page 303, fn 22). Obviously, the dual mechanism account can be easily modified to say that regular past tense production can benefit from (rather than be hindered by) the existence of a stored mapping in the associative network. Alternatively, the dual mechanism account could be modified to say that regular mappings of stems that rhyme with irregularly inflected stems are stored in the associative network regardless of frequency. The apparent ease with which such post hoc modifications can be applied to the theory highlights its underspecification and in particular the vagueness of the blocking mechanism.

Further frequency-related arguments have been made on the basis of inflectional systems in other languages such as German and Hebrew in which, unlike English, the default inflection was argued not to apply to the majority of stems (see Pinker, 1999, chapter 8, for details). According to dual mechanism theorists, an inflection that applies to a minority of the stems in the language but that is productively applied to new forms is not compatible with the statistical learning of connectionist models. Some of the relevant data, however, has been called into question (Bybee, 1995). In particular, even if the stems that undergo the so-called regular inflection are not the majority of stems, the combined instances of these stems can still be more frequent than the instances of other inflections. Although to date the implications of inflections in other languages have not been fully explored, they may eventually help resolve some of these issues in ways that are not possible using the morphologically impoverished English.

Neurological Impairments and Imaging

Findings from different neurological impairments that selectively affect the processing of either regulars or irregulars, as well as imaging findings of different brain activation patterns associated with processing regulars vs. irregulars, have also been cited as evidence for separate mechanisms. Marslen-Wilson and Tyler (1997) found that although some aphasic patients seem to lose the knowledge that regular stems and inflected forms are related (exposure to *walked* did not speed their subsequent response to *walk*) but not the knowledge that uninflected regular forms are related to their stems (exposure to *found* speeded their subsequent response to *find*), other aphasic patients show exactly the opposite loss pattern. Other researchers found similar double dissociations in other neurological disorders. Aphasic patients with agrammatism, patients with Parkinson's disease, and children with Williams syndrome have been reported to have more trouble with regulars than irregulars, while anomic aphasics, patients with Alzheimer's disease, and some children with SLI have been reported to have more trouble with irregulars than regulars (see Pinker, 1999, chapter 9; and Ullman, 2001, for details). Functional imaging studies have also revealed temporal as well as location differences in the brain activation accompanying the processing of regulars vs. irregulars. Although the exact temporal patterns and brain areas vary from study to study (and sometimes from one experiment to the next within the same study), it seems that the processing of regulars more strongly involves left frontoparietal cortex, whereas the processing of irregulars involves temporoparietal areas in both hemispheres. Dual mechanism supporters have interpreted these dissociations as indicating that the grammar areas in the brain handle regular processing, and lexical semantics areas handle irregular processing. An interesting variation of this account has been proposed by Ullman (2001), who views regular processing as relying on procedural memory, the mental storage for skills and other routine mental operations, and irregular processing as relying on declarative memory, the storage for events and idiosyncratic facts. Ullman's view differs from that of many other dual mechanism theorists because inflectional rules are not considered a specialized language mechanism any more than bicycle riding skills are considered a specialized bicycling mechanism. Arguably, the only language-specific machinery in Ullman's account is the blocking mechanism.

Although these neurological dissociations seem to favor the dual mechanism view, connectionist models that include both semantic and phonological representations can also show selective impairments to regulars or irregulars as a result of certain artificial lesions. These dissociations occur because irregulars depend more on semantics than on phonology, whereas regulars depend more on phonology than on semantics. By this argument, brain impairments that affect regulars more than irregulars simply involve more damage to phonological than to semantic representations while brain impairments that affect regulars more than irregulars involve more damage to semantic than to phonological representations (Joanisse and Seidenberg, 1999).

Discussion

Despite the active controversy surrounding the mental processing of regular inflections, most researchers agree that the mental processing of irregular inflections is not rule governed but rather works much like a connectionist network. It is therefore important to remember that Rumelhart and McClelland's model and its successors are important even if dual mechanism theories are correct and regular inflection is rule based.

Despite failing to flesh out important parts of their models, dual mechanism proponents enjoy the advantage that rules provide an intuitively appealing explanation to regular behavior. Rules, however, need not be part of the language processing mechanism, as is assumed by the dual mechanism account. Instead, rules could be meta-linguistic. People are clearly able to consciously identify regularities and describe them with explicit rules that can then be deliberately followed. This is often used in second-language learning when students are explicitly instructed about certain "rules." Meta-linguistic rules may also be used in tasks that require overt responses such as the "Wug" test, which requires people to inflect a novel form. The underlying language processing system may be only involved insofar as it supplies probabilistic input to the meta-linguistic rule (as in the "Wug" test), or as it is modified as a result of being exposed to the output of the explicit rule (as in second-language learning). This means that the linguistic processes underlying inflection should be studied by tasks that do not require making a choice of inflection but that instead rely on activation-based measures such as priming between inflected and stem forms. Comparing the results of such studies to the results of explicit response tasks would provide a better assessment of whether rules are meta-linguistic.

Road Map: Linguistics and Speech Processing
Related Reading: Connectionist and Symbolic Representations; Imaging the Grammatical Brain; Language Processing; Speech Processing: Psycholinguistics

References

Berko, J., 1958, The child's learning of English morphology, *Word*, 14:150–177.
Bybee, J., 1995, Regular morphology and the lexicon, *Lang. Cognit. Proc.*, 10(5):425–455.
Chomsky, N., 1959, Review of B. F. Skinner's *Verbal Behavior*, *Language*, 35:26–58.
Joanisse, M. F., and Seidenberg, M. S., 1999, Impairments in verb morphology after brain injury: a connectionist model, *Proc. Natl. Acad. Sci. USA*, 96(13):7592–7597.
Long, C., and Almor, A., 2000, Irregularization: The interaction of item frequency and phonological interference in regular past tense production, in *Proceedings of the Twenty-Second Annual Conference of the Cognitive Science Society*, Hillsdale, NJ: Lawrence Erlbaum Associates, pp. 310–315.
MacWhinney, B., and Leinbach, J., 1991, Implementations are not conceptualizations: Revising the verb learning model, *Cognition*, 40(1–2):121–157.
Marslen-Wilson, W. D., and Tyler, L. K., 1997, Dissociating types of mental computation, *Nature*, 387(6633):592–594.
Pinker, S., 1999, *Words and Rules: The Ingredients of Language* (1st Ed.), New York: Basic Books. ◆
Pinker, S., and Prince, A., 1988, On language and connectionism: Analysis of a parallel distributed processing model of language acquisition, *Cognition*, 28(1–2):73–193.
Plunkett, K., and Marchman, V., 1993, From rote learning to system building: Acquiring verb morphology in children and connectionist nets, *Cognition*, 48(1):21–69.
Rumelhart, D. E., and McClelland, J. L., 1986, On learning the past tenses of English verbs, in *Parallel Distributed Processing: Explorations in the Microstructure of Cognition*, vol. 2, *Psychological and Biological Models*, (J. L. McClelland, D. E. Rumelhart, and P. R. Group, Eds.), Cambridge, MA: MIT Press. ◆
Seidenberg, M. S., 1997, Language acquisition and use: Learning and applying probabilistic constraints, *Science*, 275(5306):1599–1603. ◆
Seidenberg, M. S., and McClelland, J. L., 1989, A distributed, developmental model of word recognition and naming, *Psychol Rev*, 96(4):523–568.
Spencer, A., and Zwicky, A. M., 1998, *The Handbook of Morphology*, Malden, MA: Blackwell. ◆
Ullman, M. T., 2001, A neurocognitive perspective on language: The declarative/procedural model, *Nature Rev. Neurosci.*, 2(10):717–726.

Pattern Formation, Biological

James D. Murray

Introduction

The generation of biological spatial patterns is fundamental to many disciplines, among them bacteriology, developmental biology, physiology, neurobiology, epidemiology, ecology, and tumor growth. In population biology, patchiness in population densities is the norm rather than the exception. In developmental biology, groups of previously identical cells follow different developmental pathways, depending on their position. The rich spectrum of mammalian coat patterns and the patterns found on fishes, reptiles, molluscs, and butterflies reflect developmental processes that are still not fully understood; Figure 1 shows some examples. Stationary patterns as well as a wide variety of waves have been observed in chemical reactions. Ocular dominance stripes reflect patterns in the connectivity of the visual cortex, while hallucination patterns can be partially explained as activity patterns in the visual cortex. These patterns have been used by shamans for millennia.

The discovery in 1998 of anti-angiogenic drugs, such as Angiostaten and Endostatin, opened up exciting new possibilities for anticancer therapy. The new therapy is based on a revolutionary idea put forward by Dr. Judah Folkman in the 1970s, namely, that if tumors are starved of nutrients, they will die, and that starvation could be achieved if angiogenesis (genesis of blood vessels) in the tumor could be prevented. Only recently (1998) has the success of this concept been reported: anti-angiogenic drugs stopped tumor growth in mice. This result refocused attention on the patterning process of angiogenesis and network formation of endothelial cells in extracellular matrix; it is one of the exciting research areas in pattern formation. In this article we briefly discuss a mechanical model for generating such networks. The model's mechanism is firmly based on known biology. A comparison of the model's predictions with experimental results shows remarkable correlations. The book on vascular morphogenesis edited by Little, Mironov,

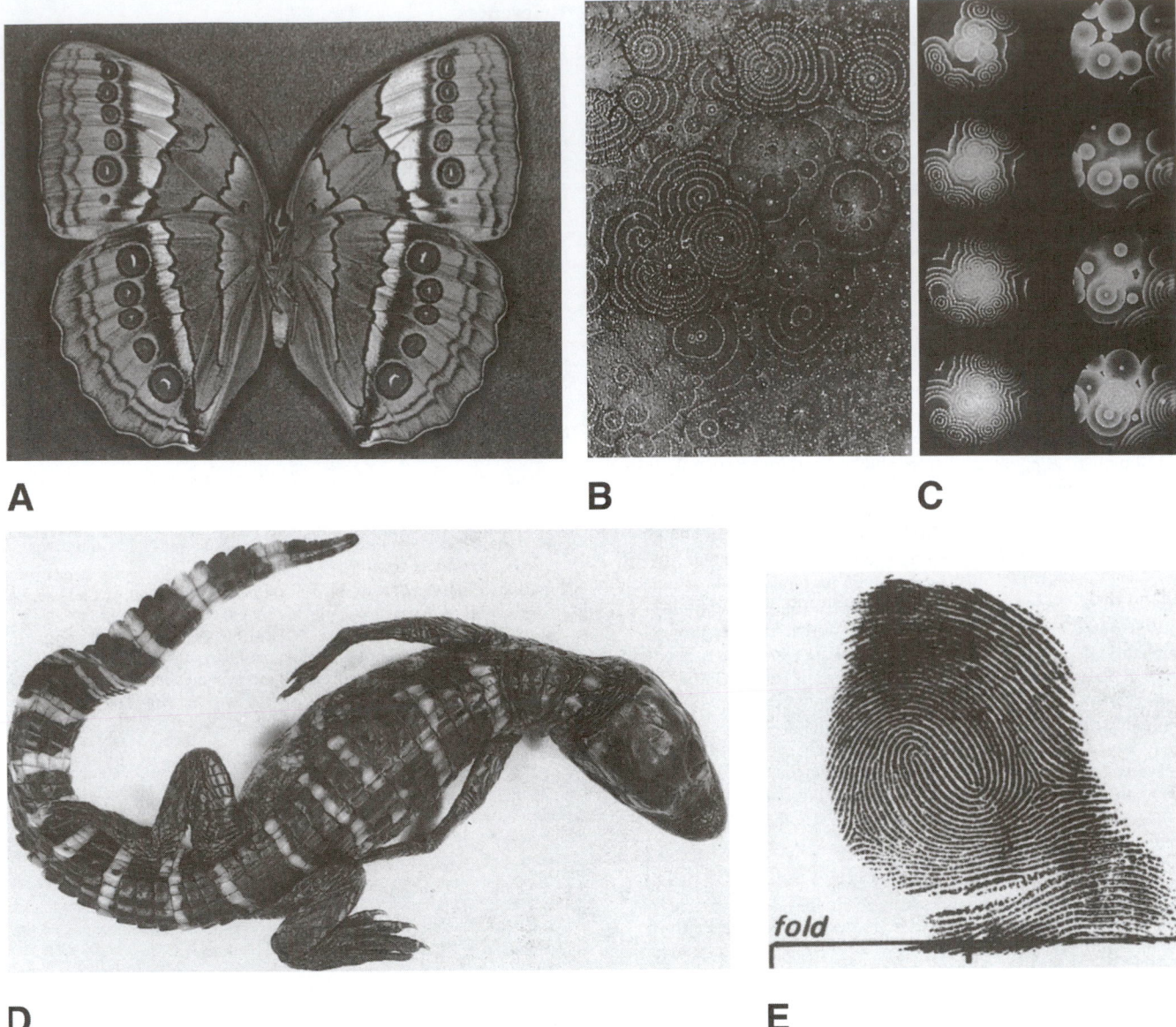

Figure 1. A small sampling of the diverse spatial patterns for which model mechanisms have been proposed. *A*, The butterfly *(Stichophthalama camadeva)* shown exhibits most of the basic pattern elements observed in butterfly wings. (Photograph courtesy of H. F. Nijhout.) *B*, Example of moving and stationary bands of amoebae of the slime mold *Dictyostelium* *discoideum*. (Photograph courtesy of P. C. Newell.) *C*, Circular and spiral waves in the Belousov-Zhabotinskii reaction (Photograph courtesy of A. T. Winfree.) *D*, Stripes on an alligator *(Alligator mississipiensis)*. (Photograph courtesy of M. W. J. Ferguson.) *E*, Typical human fingerprint.

and Sage (1998), with a foreword and brief description by Folkman (1998) of anti-angiogenic therapy as opposed to conventional therapy, provides an extensive review of current knowledge in the field. In this article we also touch on a new approach for predicting brain tumor growth in which angiogenesis does not play a role.

Although biological patterns occur on a wide range of spatial scales, spanning the molecular, cellular, individual, and population levels, a common feature is that macroscopic patterns result from microscopic interactions. Although genes play a crucial role in developmental outcomes, they do not actually produce the pattern. Mathematical models have been proposed for the mechanisms that generate these biological patterns, based on the principle of interactions between the relevant components. We describe two of the main classes, reaction-diffusion models and mechanical models,

and briefly mention some others. Each model can exhibit spontaneous pattern formation; that is, patterns develop in homogeneous environments without particular initial conditions, boundary conditions, or other external forces to drive them. The patterns are therefore self-organizing and symmetry breaking. The cancer cell patterns discussed in the brain tumor diffusion model are closely related, but there the patterns are not self-organizing.

Our goal is to develop a mechanism from knowledge of biology and to determine (1) the range of parameters attending this mechanism in which pattern formation is expected, (2) the nature of the pattern (steady, oscillating, or moving through space), (3) the scale of the pattern, and (4) perhaps the most important, the relation of the theoretical results, conclusions, and predictions to the actual biomedical problem. Relating model predictions to actual problems frequently suggests new experimental avenues and new biological insights. One of the major strategies to investigate such a relationship is as follows. First, a suggested biological mechanism is translated into a set of mathematical equations (the model). An appreciation of the pattern formation potential of existing models is invaluable here, and we hope that this brief survey will be useful in that regard. Once the model has been specified, we determine a homogeneous steady state and use linear stability analysis to determine whether perturbations of such an unpatterned state will grow or decay. For parameters supporting pattern formation, we isolate unstable modes and use the dominant modes to predict the scale and shape of the pattern. Although we generally cannot estimate all the parameters from the experiment, nevertheless we can use our knowledge of the biology to suggest broad ranges for some of the key parameters. The development of sophisticated mathematical models bearing little or no relation to the underlying biology, even if they are interesting mathematically, is of scant interdisciplinary value.

Reaction-Diffusion Models

To date, reaction-diffusion models have been the most widely studied of the models we discuss. They have been applied with effect, for example, in developmental biology, tumor growth, wound healing, population biology, epidemiology, neurophysiology, chemistry, and physics (see Murray, 2002). The variables, which depend on time and space, may be a type of molecule or cell; we refer to them generally as species. Species disperse and react, and these two processes are independent. Developing expressions for local interactions between species and their flux, and invoking conservation laws, we obtain the general form

$$\frac{\partial n}{\partial t} = f(n) + D\nabla^2 n \qquad (1)$$

where $n(x, t)$ is the vector of species densities, f is the vector of reaction terms, D is the diffusion coefficient matrix, and ∇^2 is the diffusion operator in one, two, or three space dimensions; t denotes time. Initial conditions and boundary conditions must also be specified.

The patterns we are most interested in are stable, stationary ($\partial n/\partial t = 0$), inhomogeneous solutions to Equation 1. For a single species in a single spatial dimension, it can be shown that a homogeneous steady state cannot be destabilized by diffusion: in two dimensions this is not always the case. Two-species models are very much more interesting, while three-species (and higher) models have not been studied in any depth, even though in most pattern formation situations several species are involved. The aim in practical modeling is to isolate the key dependent variables.

Two-Species Models

In 1952, Alan Turing (of Turing machine fame) suggested that the differential diffusion of two interacting species could act to destabilize a homogeneous steady state. Since diffusion is usually thought of as a stabilizing (or smoothing) force, this was a startlingly original idea. It has since been supported both mathematically and experimentally (see Murray, 2002, who describes many applications and gives numerous references).

Consider the two-species system in one dimension, x, given by

$$\frac{\partial A}{\partial t} = f(A, B) + d_A\left(\frac{\partial^2 A}{\partial x^2}\right), \quad \frac{\partial B}{\partial t} = g(A, B) + d_B\left(\frac{\partial^2 B}{\partial x^2}\right) \qquad (2)$$

in which a steady state exists at (A_0, B_0), where $f(A_0, B_0) = g(A_0, B_0) = 0$. Linearizing around (A_0, B_0), we get

$$\frac{\partial A}{\partial t} = f_A A + f_B B + d_A\left(\frac{\partial^2 A}{\partial x^2}\right),$$
$$\frac{\partial B}{\partial t} = g_A A + g_B B + d_B\left(\frac{\partial^2 B}{\partial x^2}\right) \qquad (3)$$

where $f_A = \partial f/\partial A$ is evaluated at (A_0, B_0), and so on. We assume that the steady state is stable in the absence of spatial interaction (diffusion) and therefore that $g_B < 0$ without loss of generality.

We look for solutions of the form $e^{\lambda t + ikx}$ and generate a *dispersion relation* relating eigenvalues, λ, to modes, k (the growth rate of mode k is $Re(\lambda(k))$. The dispersion relation provides conditions for unstable modes to exist (see Murray, 2002, vol. II, for a full exposition and many other practical uses of dispersion relations):

$$f_A + g_B < 0 \quad \Delta = f_A g_B - f_B g_A > 0$$

($g_B < 0$ without loss of generality)

$$d_A > 0, \quad \delta f_A + g_B > 0, \quad (\delta f_A + g_B)^2 > 4\delta\Delta \qquad (4)$$

where $\delta = d_B/d_A$

Some necessary conditions for Turing instability are (1) the self-inhibiting species, $B(g_B < 0)$, must diffuse at the higher rate, and (2) A must be self-activating ($f_A > 0$). Also, f_B and g_A must have opposite signs. The species that promotes growth of the other is the *activator*, and the other species is the *inhibitor*. The two possible cases are illustrated schematically in Figure 2. In case 1, A is the activator (which is also self-activating), while the inhibitor, B, diffuses at a higher rate and inhibits not only A but also itself. In case 2, B is the activator, again self-inhibiting, and again diffuses at a higher rate. It can be shown that in case 1 the two species occur at high or low density together (Figure 2C), whereas in case 2, A is at high density where B is low, and vice versa (Figure 2D).

We now give two analogies, one ecological for conceptual simplicity, for the mechanisms underlying Turing instabilities and the evolution of spatial patterns. Consider case 1, and refer to Figure 3A, which are sketches of the local phase plane. Let A be prey to a predator, B. How can patterns arise as in Figure 2C when predators disperse more rapidly than their prey? Suppose there were an area of increased prey density. In the absence of diffusion, this would be damped out after a temporary increase in both populations. However, with high predator dispersal, it is possible that the local increase in predators partially disperses and hence is not strong enough to push the prey population back toward equilibrium. Furthermore, when predators disperse, they lower the prey density in neighboring regions and cause the opposite effect. It is thus possible to have alternating clumps of high and low population density of both species.

Consider the second type of dynamics (Figures 2B, D, and 3B). Suppose now that A is a slowly dispersing, autocatalytic ($f_A > 0$) predator and B is its prey. In an area of high prey density, without diffusion, predator numbers would increase at the expense of prey, and eventually both populations would return to the steady state. However, there is a transient increase in the predator population and a reduction in the prey population to below its steady-state value. The resulting net influx of rapidly dispersing prey from neighboring regions would cause the predator population to drop in those regions while prey flourished. A pattern can become established in which areas of few predators and many prey supply prey to areas that contain few prey and large numbers of predators.

The dispersion relation also indicates the scale on which a pattern occurs, through the wavelength, l_c, of the fastest growing mode:

$$l_c = \frac{2\pi(d_B - d_A)^{1/2}}{[(\delta + 1)((-f_B g_A)/\delta)^{1/2} - f_A + g_B]^{1/2}}, \quad \text{where } \delta = \frac{d_B}{d_A} \qquad (5)$$

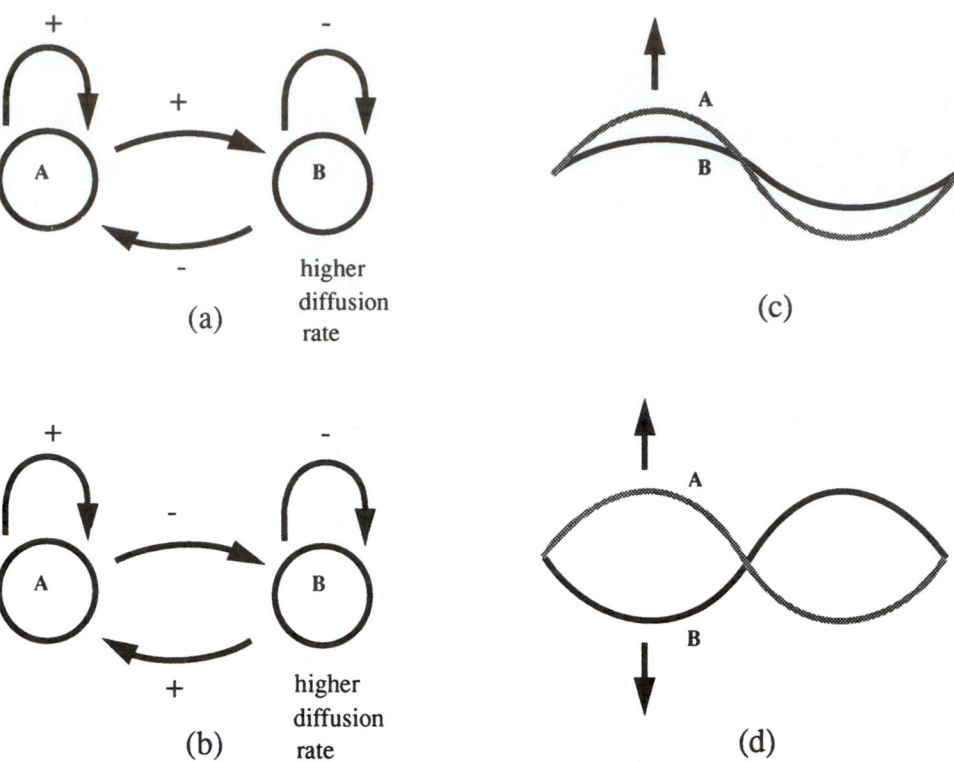

Figure 2. Some interactions support diffusion-driven instabilities. In part *A*, self-activing *A* also activates *B*, which inhibits both species. The resulting spatial pattern is shown schematically in part *C*. In part *B*, self-activitating *A* now inhibits *B* but is itself activated by *B*. The resulting pattern is shown in part *D*. Corresponding reaction phase planes are shown in Figure 3.

(see Murray, 2002, vol. II). Equation 5 indicates that Turing instabilities can occur on a broad range of spatial scales. For large δ, $l_e \approx 2\pi[(d_A d_B)/(-f_B g_A)]^{1/4}$.

Mathematical analysis can also provide insight into the effect of boundary size and shape on pattern formation. In models for animal coat patterns (Murray, 2002, vol. II, and references there), one finds that only crosswise stripes can occur in long narrow domains, whereas spots can occur on wider domains. This is a possible explanation for why animals that have spots over most of their bodies (e.g., leopards) tend to have hooped patterns, or no pattern at all, on their tails; it also explains why a striped animal cannot have a spotted tail. The qualitative form of the pattern is governed by the size and shape of the animal at the time the pattern is determined.

In Turing's theory of morphogenesis, the developmental concept is that a chemical two-species system generates a landscape of chemical concentration to which cells react differentially and hence form spatial patterns. These chemicals are referred to as morphogens. Although these types of models have prompted enlightening experiments, their use has been limited because of the illusive nature of the morphogens in real biological situations. This view is changing; see the important paper by Lander, Nie, and Wan (2002).

Virtual Brain Tumors: Predicting Growth and Enhancing Medical Imaging

A medical use of classical diffusion models is that of predicting the growth (and control) of brain tumors (gliomas). This involves the spatial spread from an initial source of cancerous cells. Gliomas differ from most other cancers by their diffuse invasion of the surrounding normal tissue. Although medical imaging has increased the detection of gliomas, it has still a long way from defining accurately enough the degree of tumor cell invasion peripheral to the bulk of the tumor mass. This inadequacy of current medical imaging is substantiated by the fact that even extensive surgical re-

moval (resection) or local irradiation of gliomas is followed by tumor recurrence at or near the edge of the resection bed.

Since the mid-1990s, E. C. Alvord, M.D. (neuropathology), J. D. Murray (applied mathematics), and their research group at the University of Washington have developed mathematical models to quantify the spatiotemporal growth and invasion of gliomas in three dimensions throughout a virtual human brain with a resolution of 1 mm^3 in which, latterly, the anatomically correct distributions of gray and white matter have been defined (Swanson, Alvord, and Murray, 2000, 2002; see also Murray, 2002, vol. II, for a full review). These mathematical models quantify the extent of tumorous invasion of individual gliomas to a degree beyond the capability of present medical imaging, including even microscopy. They also quantify the consequences of certain control therapies such as chemotherapy and resection.

We briefly describe their approach here. Our basic model can vary the two key characteristics, proliferation and cell motility (diffusion), in heterogeneous, anatomically accurate brain tissue. We allow the motility coefficient to differ depending on the local tissue composition.

Our basic mathematical model quantifying the differential motility of gliomas in gray and white matter is quantified mathematically by

$$\frac{\partial c}{\partial t} = \nabla \cdot (D(\mathbf{x})\nabla c) + \rho c, \tag{6}$$

where $c(\mathbf{x}, t)$ is the concentration of tumor cells at location $\mathbf{x}$ and time t. $D(\mathbf{x})$, a function of position $\mathbf{x}$ in the brain, is the diffusion coefficient defining the random motility of the glioma cells with $D(\mathbf{x}) = D_g, D_w$, constants for $\mathbf{x}$ in gray and white matter, respectively. ρ represents the net proliferation rate of the glioma cells. This term predicts exponential growth of the cancer cells, but within the survival period of the patient it has been shown to be a very good approximation. The diffusion coefficient in white matter

Figure 3. Reaction phase planes for diffusion-driven instabilities. Part *A* shows the phase plane corresponding to parts *A* and *C* of Figure 2. Part *B* shows the phase plane corresponding to parts *B* and *D* of Figure 2. The steady state is at the intersection of the two null clines. Arrows represent the direction of change due to local species interaction.

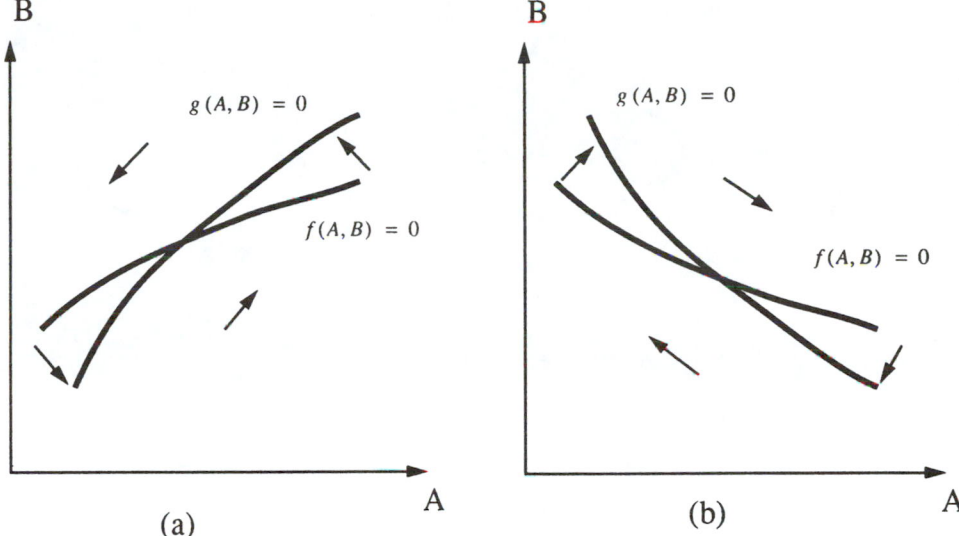

(a)

(b)

is larger than that in gray matter; that is, $D_w > D_g$. The model assumes that the tumor has grown to about 4,000 cells as a local mass before it begins to diffuse and the model Equation 6 applies.

For every medical imaging technique there is a threshold of detection below which glioma cells are not detectable. A tumor boundary detected by enhanced computed tomography (CT) corresponds to a tumor cell concentration of only about 8,000 cells/mm³. Mathematically, of course, in our virtual tumor, we can set the detection at any level we choose.

Based on the medical literature, the models assumed that a medical diagnosis is made when the volume of an enhanced CT–detectable tumor has reached a size equivalent to an average 3 cm in diameter and that death occurs when the volume reaches an average 6 cm in diameter. The difference between these two times can be defined as the survival time of the hypothetical or virtual patient. We can estimate these times from the model results, and they agree well with the average survival times for each grade of gliomas we have studied.

Crucial to the models' use is the ability to determine reasonable estimates of the critical parameters, the growth rate ρ and the diffusion coefficient D. We have estimates, but they vary quite widely. Some of the current research is focused on determining the values for individual patients, and these values can be then used in prognosis and treatment protocols.

Figure 4 shows three perpendicular cross-sections (coronal, sagittal, and horizontal or axial) of the virtual human brain, intersecting in a point marked by an asterisk in the superior frontal region where the virtual tumor originates. The gray and white matters of the brain domain appear gray and white, respectively. In each image, a single thick black curve defines the edge of the tumor that the model suggests would be detectable on enhanced CT, associated with a threshold of detection of 8,000 cells/mm³. The outermost profile corresponds to an arbitrary threshold of detection 80 times more sensitive than enhanced CT (i.e., 100 cells/mm³). The left column of images in Figure 4 represents the tumor at the time of detection, defined as an enhanced CT–detectable tumor with average diameter of 3 cm, while the right column represents the tumor at the time of death, defined by an enhanced CT–detectable tumor with average diameter of 6 cm. The simulations clearly reveal the subthreshold invasion of the tumor well beyond the detectable portion of the tumor. No matter the extent of resection, the mathematical model indicates that the gross tumor will ultimately recur and kill.

Unlike real patients with real gliomas, virtual patients with virtual gliomas can be analyzed by letting any particular factor vary while keeping all the other determining factors constant. Such isolation techniques, of course, require a mathematical model that has sufficient complexity to contain a realistic number of variables. The recent availability of simulated MRI, with proportions of gray and white matter accurately indicated, permitted the development of this model, which is sufficiently complex to allow different diffusion rates in gray and white matter (e.g., a 5-fold increase in diffusion or migration in white matter).

Murray-Oster Mechanical Models

The Murray-Oster mechanical theory is based on the fact that mesenchymal cells exert significant traction forces on the surrounding extracellular matrix, thereby influencing their movement and the density of the surrounding matrix. The model simply consists of conservation equations for the cells and matrix and a force balance equation for the interaction between the cell-generated forces and the viscoelastic resistive properties of the matrix. An extensive pedagogical review is given in Murray (2002, vol. II). Harris, Stopak, and Warner (1984) first presented graphic experimental confirmation of some of the predictions made with the original model system.

The overriding feature of the Murray-Oster mechanical theory of pattern formation is its simplicity (in spite of its relative mathematical complexity): complicated patterns arise solely as a consequence of the interaction of the cell traction forces and the viscoelastic properties of a deformable matrix in which they are embedded. We give an intuitive description of the process below. The theory has been widely used in a variety of problems, especially in wound healing studies (for example, Tranquillo and Murray, 1993; Olsen, Maini, and Sherratt, 1998; and the review by Sherratt and Dallon, 2002).

The cell-matrix network patterns found experimentally (Vernon et al., 1995) when vascular endothelial cells are placed on a basement extracellular membrane provide a unique theoretical and experimental opportunity to determine the important components in the morphogenetic process of the complex network formation. Figure 5 shows an example of typical patterns obtained from the model mechanism and experiment. In these experiments, endothelial cells were placed on a gelled basement membrane matrix (BMM, Ma-

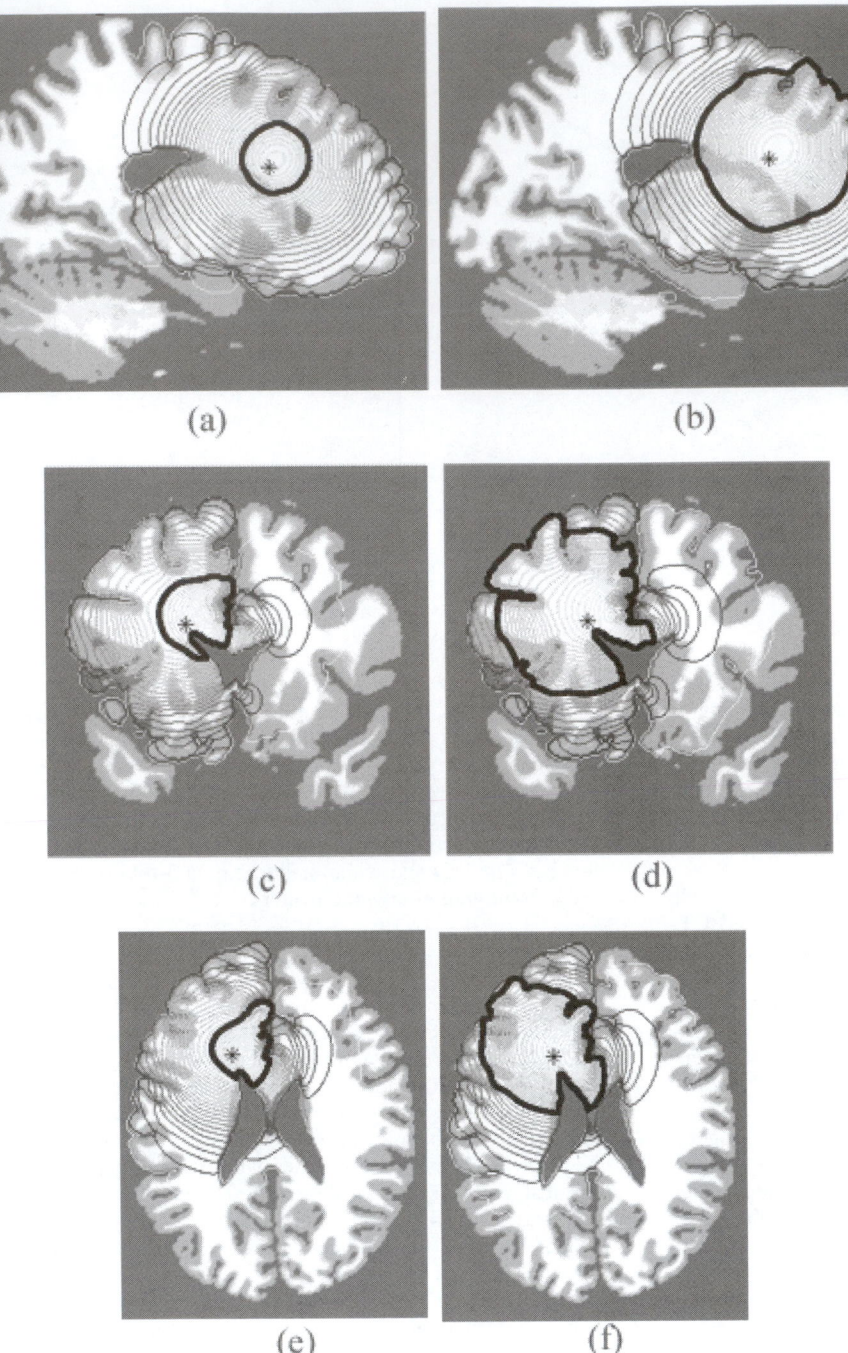

(a)

(b)

(c)

(d)

(e)

(f)

Figure 4. Sections of the virtual brain in sagittal, coronal, and horizontal planes that intersect at the site of the brain tumor (glioma) originating in the thalamus denoted by an asterisk. A thick black contour defines the edge of the tumor detectable by enhanced computed tomography. Cell migration was allowed to occur in an anatomically accurate three-dimensional representation of the human brain.

trigel). In the course of a few hours, aggregates started to form, and after 24 hours all of the BMM had been pulled into an aggregate network.

In view of the importance of angiogenesis in cancer therapy, we describe a version of the theory that generates networks of cells and matrix and that has been suggested (Manoussaki et al., 1996; Murray et al., 1998) as the possible mechanism of network formation (Vernon et al., 1995). The model shows unequivocably that cell-matrix contact guidance plays a crucial role. There is no cell proliferation in the case of the cell-Matrigel patterns mimicking early network patterns of angiogenesis, in which the complex strand-like structures of matrix are formed. The pattern forms purely from cellular traction forces and their interaction with the fibrous matrix: there are no external forces, cell proliferation, or other complicating factors. We can thus isolate, in our models, the central mechanical interaction underlying a range of biological phenomena in development and other contexts. There are a number of well-determined parameters, such as cell density, matrix density, matrix thickness, pattern wave number, time scale, and some parameters that we can confine to a range of possible values, as well as the Young modulus and the magnitude of cellular traction forces.

The conservation equations in this (experimental) situation are

$$\frac{\partial n}{\partial t} + \nabla \cdot [nv - D(\varepsilon)\nabla n] = 0, \quad \frac{\partial \rho}{\partial t} + \nabla \cdot (\rho v) = 0 \quad (7)$$

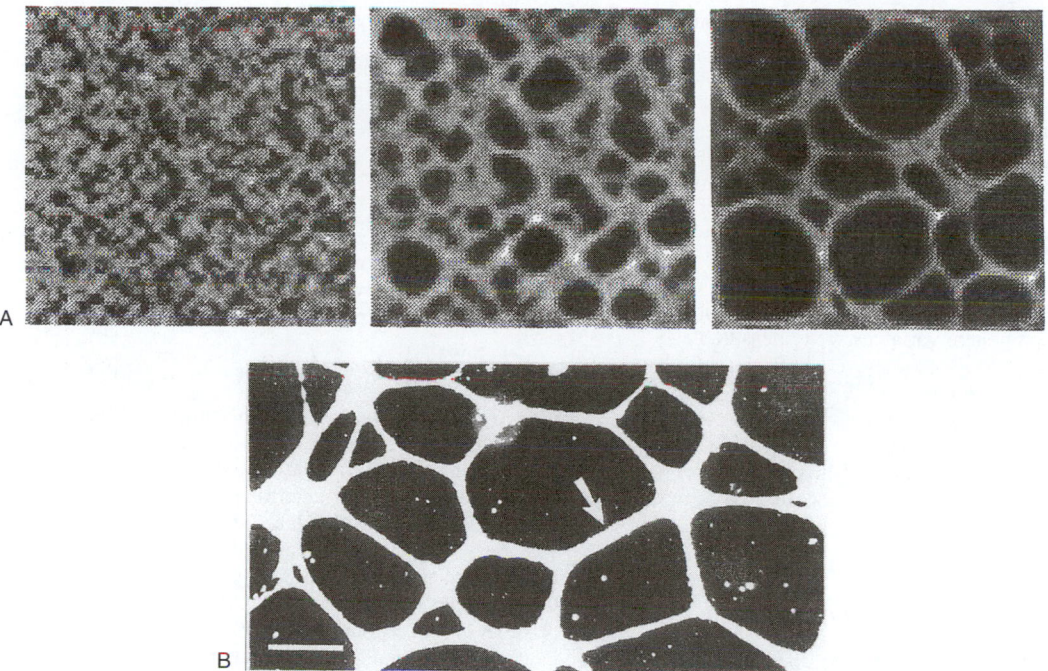

Figure 5. Cell density network formation when cells are embedded in a matrix gell: white areas denote high cell densities. *A*, Initially the cells were uniformly distributed and the model equations simulated numerically with the parameters obtained from the literaure and related experiments: the time scale for the pattern formation is 24 hours: the complete square is 800 μm.

B, Experimental patterns obtained with bovine aortic endothelial cells cultured on Matrigel. Each cord (example arrow) consists of many cells; the image is viewed by darkfield illumination (bar = 200 μm). (Photograph courtesy of R. B. Vernon.)

where cells (n) and matrix (ρ) convect as a single phase with material velocity $v = Du/Dt$. $D(\varepsilon)$ is the cell motility tensor, dependent on the matrix strain, ε, defined by

$$\varepsilon = \tfrac{1}{2} (\nabla \cdot u + \nabla \cdot u^T)$$

where u is the vector of matrix displacement and u^T its transpose.

The force balance equation simply says that the traction forces generated by the cells, $T(n, \rho)$; the induced response stress of the matrix, σ; and the substrate anchoring, $(s/\rho)(\partial u/\partial t)$, where s is the strength of the fluid-like drag force of the matrix attachment, are in equilibrium, namely

$$\nabla \cdot [\sigma + T(n, \rho)] = \frac{s}{\rho} \frac{\partial u}{\partial t} \qquad (8)$$

The detailed form of $D(\varepsilon)$ and each term in the force equation have to be specified; they are crucial elements in the modeling.

This particular model is analyzed in detail by Manoussaki et al. (1996) and by Murray et al. (1998). They took

$$\sigma = \tau \frac{n}{1 + \alpha n^2}$$

where α is a positive parameter: this form reflects the reduction in traction as the cell density becomes large. Tranqui and Tracqui (2000; see earlier references there) have developed experimental techniques to determine the detailed form and estimate the parameters.

The derived biased diffusion $D(\varepsilon)$ is

$$D(\varepsilon) = D_0 \begin{pmatrix} 1 + \dfrac{\varepsilon_{xx} - \varepsilon_{yy}}{2} & \dfrac{\varepsilon_{xy} + \varepsilon_{yx}}{2} \\ \dfrac{\varepsilon_{xy} + \varepsilon_{yx}}{2} & 1 - \dfrac{\varepsilon_{xx} - \varepsilon_{yy}}{2} \end{pmatrix}$$

where D_0 is the motility coefficient when there is no strain present.

The viscoelastic matrix stress must account for the density and reorientation of the matrix fibers as well as their strength. This was taken to be made up of a viscous and an elastic part given by a Voigt form, namely

$$\sigma = \frac{E(\varepsilon)}{1 + v} \left(\varepsilon + \frac{v}{1 - 2v} \theta I \right) + \left(\mu_1 \frac{\partial \varepsilon}{\partial t} + \mu_2 \frac{\partial \theta}{\partial t} I \right)$$

where E is the strain-dependent elastic modulus and v is the Poisson ratio, which measures how a strip of gel will contract in one direction when stretched in the transverse direction. μ_1, μ_2 are the shear and bulk visosities, $\theta(= \nabla \cdot u)$ is the dilation tensor, and I is the unit tensor.

Intuitively we can see how the mechanism generates the observed complex cellular and matrix patterns. Cells initially uniformly distributed on the matrix (essentially a two-dimensional geometry in the experiments) pull the matrix and hence cause stress lines to appear, resulting in realignment of the matrix fibers. The cells can move more easily along the directions of stress and form regions of higher cell density. These clusters of cells in turn generate higher traction forces because of their higher cell density, which in turn increases the deformation of the matrix and enhances "highways" of matrix along which the cells move more freely. In this way a network of fiber bundles is formed, giving rise to the quasi-hexagonal network observed in experiments (see Figure 5). The formation of these fiber bundles/highways we associate with the process of angiogenesis, or, in the context here, vasculogenesis.

Murray et al. (1998) analyzed the model using parameters estimated from the literature. Figure 5 illustrates some time-evolving network patterns together with one of the typical networks found experimentally by Vernon et al. (1995). Various other hypothetical scenarios were studied that also compared well with subsequent experiments. Clearly, no patterns form if there is no cell traction, as found experimentally. The case for such a mechanical model of cell-matrix network patterns is further strengthened by the way the patterns are formed in vitro and mathematically. The evolution is from irregular polygons that increase in size and decrease in number, with the smallest polygons pinching off and disappearing. Also, on thicker gels, larger polygons form. They also found, surprisingly, that if the cell traction is sufficiently high, networks formed even in the *absence* of biased diffusion. The effect of matrix thickness on the patterns also reflected what was observed experimentally.

This mechanical model was the first mathematical description of cell-matrix interactions for the formation of network patterns in which all of the component variables were measurable.

Discussion

We have seen how two fundamentally different types of model can give rise to patterns. Here we briefly mention other mechanisms that have been studied.

Negative and Long-Range Diffusion

If, in a reaction-diffusion equation, the diffusion coefficient was negative, this would intuitively cause clumping (imagine viewing a movie of diffusion in reverse). Although such a problem is ill-posed mathematically, this can be rescued by adding a biharmonic term, as in the Cahn-Hilliard equation (Cahn, 1968). Murray (2002, vol. I) shows that a biharmonic term is a natural practical modification when fluxes have a long-range component (they depend on densities in a neighborhood of the reference point). Such long-range effects are present in the Murray-Oster mechanical model via the extracellular matrix and the finger-like filapodia of the cells.

Chemotaxis

Chemotaxis is the name given to the process whereby cells move up or down a chemical (chemoattractant or chemorepellent) gradient. Typically, chemoattractant (c) is secreted and degraded by cells (n), and the cells respond to gradients in c with a convection speed of $\chi(\partial c/\partial x)$, with typical equations, in one dimension, given by

$$\frac{\partial n}{\partial t} = D_n \frac{\partial^2 n}{\partial x^2} - \frac{\partial}{\partial x}\left(n\chi\frac{\partial c}{\partial x}\right), \quad \frac{\partial c}{\partial t} = f(n,\,c) + D_c\frac{\partial^2 c}{\partial x^2} \quad (9)$$

where χ is the chemotactic parameter (in fact usually a function of c), the Ds are diffusion coefficients, and $f(n,\,c)$ is the source function of c. For spatial patterns to form, cells must diffuse at a lower rate than the chemoattractant, and the chemoattractive (destabilizing) force need only be slightly stronger than the diffusive (stabilizing) force. There is a single dimensionless parameter that determines whether or not a pattern will form.

Bacteria such as *E. coli* and *Salmonella* exhibit strong chemotactic respones and have been the subject of intense study since the early 1990s. The experimental work of Budrene and Berg (1995; see earlier references therein) graphically illustrates the complex regular patterns that can be formed. This work was the basis for the mathematical models that reflect the detailed biology by Tyson and her colleagues, including the experimentalists (Tyson, Lubkin, and Murray 1998; see other references there and Murray, 2002, vol. II, for a full survey). This specific paper shows the minimum requirements a model and the biology must have to produce the observed patterns.

Cross-Taxis

Two species can exhibit taxis with respect to one other:

$$\begin{aligned}\frac{\partial A}{\partial t} &= D_1\frac{\partial^2 A}{\partial x^2} - \chi_1\frac{\partial}{\partial x}\left(A\frac{\partial B}{\partial x}\right),\\[4pt]\frac{\partial B}{\partial t} &= D_2\frac{\partial^2 B}{\partial x^2} - \chi_2\frac{\partial}{\partial x}\left(B\frac{\partial A}{\partial x}\right)\end{aligned} \quad (10)$$

(if $\chi_1 > 0$ and $\chi_2 > 0$, for example, constant here, the two species move up each other's gradient). Although not greatly studied, such models are known to be susceptible to blow-up (see Murray, 2002, vol. II, for references and a brief analysis).

Mathematical Techniques

We have barely scratched the surface of the mathematical analysis of pattern formation. Close to bifurcation (loss of stability), it is possible to analyze the behavior of small-amplitude patterns. For example, one can determine whether two basic spatial patterns, hexagonal and striped, are stable with respect to each other (Murray, 2002, vol. II). We have only briefly confronted the fact that pattern formation generally takes place on a finite domain, perhaps with a particular geometry. At the very least, this reduces the number of modes that can occur: we refer the reader to Murray's (2002, vol. II) modeling of mammalian coat pattern formation as a graphic example. The most important aspect of mathematical models for biological pattern formation must remain, however, their close relation to the real world of biology.

Road Map: Dynamic Systems
Related Reading: Cooperative Phenomena

References

Budrene, E. O., and Berg, H. C., 1995, Dynamics of formation of symmetrical patterns by chemotactic bacteria, *Nature*, 376:49–53.

Cahn, J. W., 1968, Spinodal decomposition: The 1967 Institute of Metals Lecture, *Trans. Metall. Soc. AIME*, 242:167–180.

Folkman, J., 1998, Foreword, in *Vascular Morphogenesis: In Vivo, In Vitro, In Mente* (C. D. Little, V. Mironov, and E. H. Sage, Eds.), Boston: Birkhäuser, pp. vi–ix.

Harris, A. K., Stopak, D., and Warner, P., 1984, Generation of spatially periodic patterns by a mechanical instability: A mechanical alternative to the Turing model, *J. Embryol. Exp. Morphol.*, 80:1–20.

Lander, A. D., Nie, Q., and Wan, F. Y. M., 2002, Do morphogen gradients arise by diffusion? *Devel. Cell*, 2:786–796.

Little, C. D., Mironov, V., and Sage, E. H., Eds., 1998, *Vascular Morphogenesis: In Vivo, In Vitro, In Mente*, Boston: Birkhäuser.

Manoussaki, D., Lubkin, S. R., Vernon, R. B., and Murray, J. D., 1996, A mechanical model for the formation of vascular networks in vitro, *Acta Biotheoret.*, 44:271–282.

Murray, J. D., 2002, *Mathematical Biology*, 3rd ed., vol. I: *An Introduction*; vol. II: *Spatial Models and Biomedical Applications*, New York: Springer-Verlag. ◆

Murray, J. D., Manoussaki, D., Lubkin, S. R., and Vernon, R. B., 1998, A mechanical theory of *in vitro* vascular network formation, in *Vascular Morphogenesis: In Vivo, In Vitro, In Mente* (C. D. Little, V. Mironov, and E. H. Sage, Eds.), Boston: Birkhäuser, pp. 178–188.

Olsen, L., Maini, P. K., and Sherratt, J. A., 1998, Simple modelling of extracellular alignment in dermal wound healing, *J. Theor. Med.*, 1:175–192.

Sherratt, J. A., and Dallon, J. C., 2002, Theoretical models of wound healing: Past successes and future challenges, *Compt. Rend. Acad. Sci. (Paris) (Life Sciences)* (in press).

Swanson, K. R., Alvord, E. C., and Murray, J. D., 2000, A quantitative model for differential motility of gliomas in grey and white matter, *Cell Prolif.*, 33:317–329.

Swanson, K. R., Alvord, E. C., and Murray, J. D., 2002, Virtual brain tumors (gliomas) enhance the reality of medical imaging and highlight inadequacies of current therapy, *Br. J. Cancer*, 86:14–18. ◆

Tranqui, L., and Tracqui, P., 2000, Mechanical signalling and angiogenesis: The integration of cell–extracellular matrix couplings, *Compt. Rend. Acad. Sci. (Paris) (Life Sciences)*, 323:31–47.

Tranquillo, R. T., and Murray, J. D., 1993, Mechanistic model of wound contraction, *J. Surg. Res.*, 55:233–247.

Turing, A. M., 1952, The chemical basis of morphogenesis, *Philos. Trans. R. Soc. Lond. B Biol. Sci.*, 237:37–72.

Tyson, R., Lubkin, S. R., and Murray, J. D., 1998, A minimal mechanism for bacterial patterns, *Proc. R. Soc. Lond. B*, 266:299–304. ◆

Vernon, R. B., Lara, S. L., Drake, C. J., Iruela-Arispe, M. L., Angello, J. C., Little, C. D., Wight, T. N., and Sage, E. H., 1995, Organized type I collagen influences endothelial patterns during "spontaneous angiogenesis in vitro": Planar cultures as models of vascular development, *In Vitro Vasc. Dev. Biol.*, 31:120–131.

Pattern Formation, Neural

Paul C. Bressloff and Jack D. Cowan

Introduction

In studying the large-scale functional and anatomical structure of cortex, two distinct questions naturally arise: How did the structure develop and what forms of spontaneous and stimulus-driven neural dynamics are generated by such a cortical structure? It turns out that in both cases, the Turing mechanism for spontaneous pattern formation plays an important role. Turing originally considered the problem of how animal coat patterns develop. He suggested that chemical markers in the skin make up a system of diffusion-coupled chemical reactions among substances called morphogens. Turing showed that in a two-component reaction-diffusion system, a state of uniform chemical concentration can undergo a diffusion-driven instability, leading to the formation of a spatially inhomogeneous state (see PATTERN FORMATION, BIOLOGICAL). Wilson and Cowan (1973) proposed a nonlocal version of this mechanism based on competition between short-range excitation and longer-range inhibition. In the neural context, interactions are mediated not by molecular diffusion, but by long-range axonal connections; hence the term *nonlocal*. Since then, this neural version of the Turing instability has been applied to many problems concerning the dynamics (Bressloff and Cowan, 2002; see also DYNAMICS AND BIFURCATION IN NEURAL NETS) and development (Swindale, 1980) of cortex. In the former case, pattern formation occurs in neural activity; in the latter, it occurs in synaptic weights. In most cases, there exists some underlying symmetry in the model that plays a crucial role in the selection and stability of the resulting patterns.

Feature Selectivity and Tuning

Probably the simplest example of neural pattern formation is that of orientation tuning in the ring model of a cortical hypercolumn (Somers, Nelson, and Sur, 1995). The one-population version of this model consists of a continuous distribution of neural populations labeled by their orientation preference $\phi \in [0, \pi)$. The state of the network is expressed in terms of an activity variable $a(\phi, t)$ evolving according to the equation

$$\tau \frac{\partial a}{\partial t} = -a + w \circ \sigma[a] + h \tag{1}$$

where τ is a time constant, $w \circ \sigma$ signifies the convolution

$$(w \circ \sigma[a])(\phi) = \int_0^\pi w(\phi - \phi')\sigma[a(\phi')] \frac{d\phi'}{\pi} \tag{2}$$

and σ denotes a firing rate function (typically taken to be a smooth sigmoid function of activity). The weight distribution w represents nonlocal neural interactions within the hypercolumn, whereas h denotes an external drive generated by some oriented visual stimulus.

First, consider the case of constant external drive, $h(\phi) = h_0$, and suppose that $\bar{a}$ is a homogeneous fixed-point solution of Equation 1, that is, $\bar{a} = w \circ \sigma[\bar{a}] + h_0$. Linearizing about this fixed point by setting $a(\phi, t) = \bar{a} + u(\phi)e^{\lambda t/\tau}$ leads to the eigenvalue equation

$$(\lambda + 1)u(\phi) = \mu \, w \circ u(\phi) \tag{3}$$

where $\mu = \sigma'[\bar{a}]$. Expanding the π-periodic functions $u(\phi)$ and $w(\phi)$ as Fourier series

$$w(\phi) = \sum_{n=-\infty}^{\infty} W_n e^{2in\phi}, \quad u(\phi) = \sum_{n=-\infty}^{\infty} U_n e^{2in\phi} \tag{4}$$

we can diagonalize the eigenvalue equation to find the discrete set of eigenvalues

$$\lambda_n = -1 + \mu W_n \tag{5}$$

for integer n, with corresponding eigenfunctions $U_n e^{2in\phi}$. We assume that $w(\phi)$ is a real, symmetric function of ϕ so that $W_{-n} = W_n$ with W_n real. It follows that for sufficiently small μ (corresponding to a low activity state $\bar{a}$), $\lambda_n < 0$ for all n, and the fixed point $\bar{a}$ is stable. However as μ increases beyond a critical value μ_c, the fixed point becomes unstable, owing to excitation of the eigenfunctions associated with the largest Fourier component of w. We refer to such eigenfunctions as *excited modes*.

Two examples of Fourier spectra are shown in Figure 1. In the first case, W_1 is maximal, so $\mu_c = W_1^{-1}$, and the excited modes are of the form

$$u(\phi) = ze^{2i\phi} + z^*e^{-2i\phi} = |z| \cos(2[\phi - \phi_0]) \tag{6}$$

with complex amplitude $z = |z| e^{-2i\phi_0}$. Since these modes have a single maximum around the ring, the network supports an activity profile consisting of a tuning curve centered about the point ϕ_0 (see Figure 1C). The location of this peak is arbitrary and depends only on random initial conditions, reflecting the rotation invariance or *symmetry* of the weight distribution w. This follows from the assumption that w depends only on the difference between the orientation preferences ϕ and ϕ' as in Equation 2. Such a symmetry is said to be spontaneously broken by the action of the pattern-forming instability. Also note that since the dominant component is W_1, the distribution w is excitatory (inhibitory) for neurons with sufficiently similar (dissimilar) orientation preferences. (This is analogous to the Wilson-Cowan "Mexican hat" function; see below.) On the other hand, when the inhibitory component is weakened such that W_0 is maximal, the network undergoes a bulk instability at the critical point $\phi_c = W_0^{-1}$ in which no particular orientation ϕ_0 is favored, since the excited eigenmode reduces to U_0.

So far, we have shown how linear stability analysis can be used to establish the growth of an inhomogeneous state from a homogeneous state through a pattern-forming instability. However, as

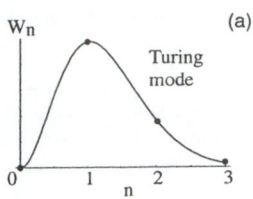
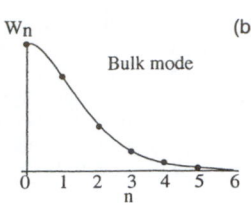
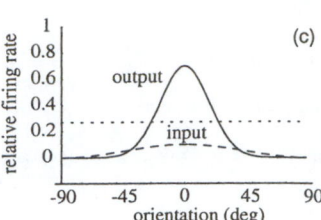

Figure 1. Orientation tuning in the ring model. Fourier spectrum W_n of local weight distribution $w(\phi)$ with (A) a maximum at $n = 1$ (Turing mode) and (B) a maximum at $n = 0$ (bulk mode). C, Tuning curve generated by a pattern-forming instability. Recurrent excitation and inhibition amplifies a weakly biased external input. The dotted line is baseline output without orientation tuning.

the new state increases in amplitude, the linear approximation breaks down, so one has to use nonlinear theory to investigate whether or not a stable pattern ultimately forms. Sufficiently close to the bifurcation point at $\mu = \mu_c$, where the homogeneous state becomes unstable, we can treat $\varepsilon = \mu - \mu_c$ as a small parameter and carry out a perturbation expansion of Equation 1 in powers of $\varepsilon^{1/2}$ (see DYNAMICS AND BIFURCATION IN NEURAL NETS). First, Taylor expand the nonlinear term $\sigma[a]$ about the fixed point $\bar{a}$:

$$\sigma[a] = \sigma[a_0] + \gamma_1(a - a_0) + \gamma_2(a - a_0)^2 + \gamma_3(a - a_0)^3 + \cdots$$

where $\gamma_n = n!^{-1} d^n \sigma[a_0]/da^n$. Second, substitute the series expansion

$$a(\phi, t) = a_0 + \varepsilon^{1/2}[z(t)e^{2im\phi} + z^*(t)e^{-2im\phi}] + O(\varepsilon)$$

into Equation 1 and equate equal powers of $\varepsilon^{1/2}$. A standard perturbation calculation then yields a nonlinear ordinary differential equation at order $\varepsilon^{3/2}$ for the amplitude $z(t)$ of the excited modes (Bressloff and Cowan, 2002):

$$\frac{dz}{dt} = z(\mu - \mu_c - \Lambda|z|^2) \tag{7}$$

where

$$\Lambda = -\frac{3\gamma_3}{\gamma_1^2} - \frac{2\gamma_2^2}{\gamma_1^2}\left[\frac{W_2}{1 - \gamma_1 W_2} + \frac{2W_0}{1 - \gamma_1 W_0}\right] > 0 \tag{8}$$

It follows that if $\mu > \mu_c$, then the fixed point $z = 0$ is unstable, and there is a new branch of stable tuning curves with arbitrary phase and steady-state amplitude $|z| = (\mu - \mu_c)/\Lambda$.

Now suppose that there is a weakly biased external drive of the form

$$h(\phi) = h_0[(1 - \kappa) + \kappa \cos(2[\phi - \Phi])] \tag{9}$$

representing a visual stimulus with orientation Φ. Assuming that $\kappa = O(\varepsilon^{3/2})$, one finds that there is an additional term $h_0\kappa e^{-2i\Phi}$ on the right-hand side of the $O(\varepsilon^{3/2})$ amplitude equation (Equation 7). The phase of the stable inhomogeneous state is now equal to Φ. Hence, when the network is operating in the tuned or *Turing mode*, recurrent interactions amplify a weakly biased input, leading to an orientation tuning curve whose peak coincides with the stimulus orientation; the circular symmetry of the network is now explicitly broken by the presence of a biased input. This amplification mechanism has received recent experimental support in that optical imaging of visual cortical responses in the presence of voltage-sensitive dyes reveals responses sharply tuned for orientation whose amplitude then grows in a manner consistent with the onset of the Turing mode (Sharon and Grinvald, 2002).

It is also possible to extend the above ideas to incorporate other stimulus features for which cortical neurons exhibit tuned responses, including spatial frequency, color, and motion. An interesting question then arises, namely, "What is the appropriate symmetry of the associated pattern forming instability?" For example, it has recently been suggested that orientation and spatial frequency preferences can be combined by replacing the ring network, which

has circular symmetry, by a network with the topology of the surface of a sphere (Bressloff and Cowan, 2002). Motivated by recent optical imaging data on orientation and spatial frequency preference maps (Issa, Trepel, and Stryker, 2000), such feature preferences are represented by angular coordinates on the sphere. (Note that such a coordinate system refers to the feature preferences; it does not imply that the actual distribution and connections of visual cortex neurons fit on a sphere—in fact, they fit on a plane.) High and low spatial frequency preferences are located at the poles of the sphere, which are identified with the singularities of the orientation preference map, commonly referred to as *orientation pinwheels*. Cortical amplification through spontaneous breaking of spherical (rather than circular) symmetry leads to a sharply tuned, contrast-invariant response to both stimulus features.

Geometric Visual Hallucinations

Geometric visual hallucinations are seen by many observers after taking hallucinogens such as LSD, cannabis, or mescaline; on viewing bright flickering lights; on waking up or falling asleep; in "near death" experiences; and in many other syndromes. The Chicago neurologist Klüver organized such images into four groups called *form constants*: (I) tunnels and funnels, (II) spirals, (III) lattices, including honeycombs and triangles, and (IV) cobwebs, all of which contain repeated geometric structures. Figure 2A shows their appearance in the visual field. Note in particular the difference between the first two *noncontoured* images, which consist of alternating regions of light and dark, and the *contoured* nature of the last two images.

Ermentrout and Cowan (1979) provided a first account of the generation of visual hallucinations, based on the idea that some disturbance such as a drug or flickering light can destabilize the primary visual cortex (V1), inducing spontaneous pattern of cortical activity that reflects the underlying architecture of V1. They studied interacting populations of excitatory and inhibitory neurons distributed within a two-dimensional cortical sheet. Modeling the evolution of the network in terms of a set of Wilson-Cowan equations, they showed how spatially periodic patterns such as stripes, squares, and hexagons bifurcate from a low-activity homogeneous state via a Turing instability. They then noted that there is an orderly retinotopic mapping of the visual field onto the surface of cortex, with the left and right halves of visual field mapped onto the right and left cortices, respectively. Except close to the fovea (the center of the visual field), this map can be approximated by a complex logarithm (Schwartz, 1977) as illustrated in Figure 2B. Applying the inverse of this retinocortical map, they showed that when the periodic cortical patterns are mapped back into visual field coordinates, noncontoured hallucinatory images such as the form constants (I) and (II) of Figure 2A are reproduced.

Interestingly, the model cannot reproduce the contoured images (III) and (IV), since there is no information in it regarding the orientation selectivity of neurons in V1. Recently, a much more detailed model of the functional and anatomical structure of V1 has been developed that treats the cortex as a continuum of interacting hypercolumns, each of which has the internal structure of the ring

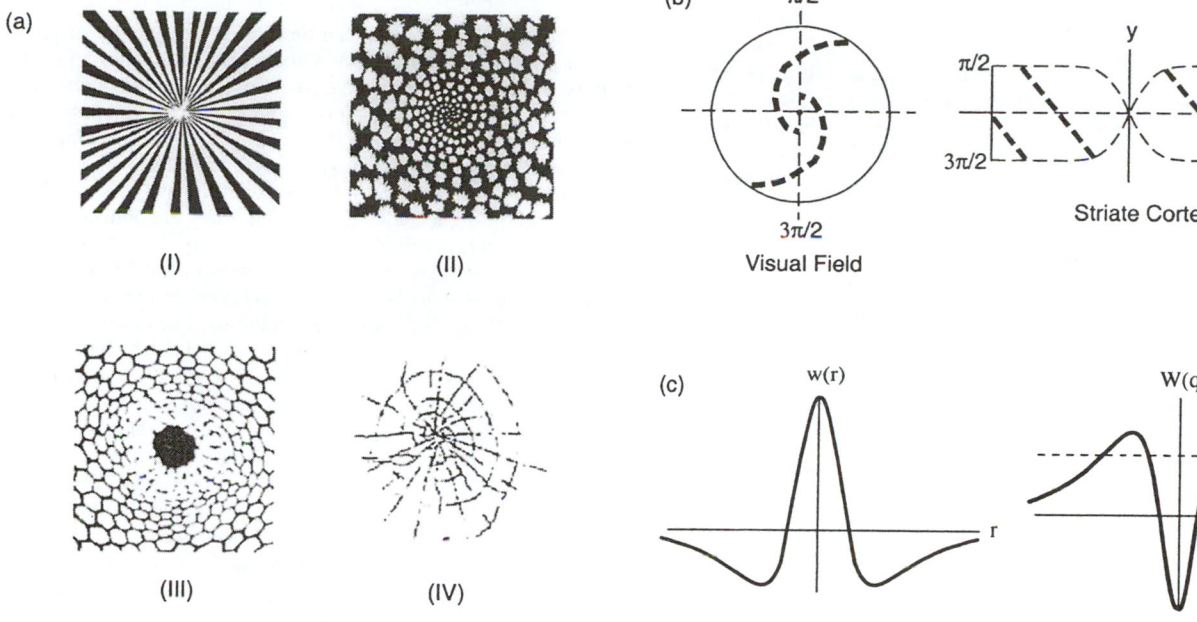

Figure 2. *A*, Hallucination form constants: (I) funnel and (II) spiral images seen following ingestion of LSD, (III) Honeycomb generated by marijuana, (IV) cobweb petroglyph. *B*, Retinocortical map showing how a spiral image in visual field is mapped to a stripe of activity in cortex. *C*, Mexican hat interaction function $w(r)$ showing short-range excitation and long-range inhibition together with its Fourier transform $W(q)$.

model for orientation tuning (Bressloff et al., 2001). In this new model, both contoured and noncontoured hallucinatory images can be generated depending on whether each isolated hypercolumn undergoes a local Turing or bulk instability with respect to orientation (see Figure 1*A*).

We now consider the theory of cortical pattern formation in more detail. For simplicity, we describe the earlier version due to Ermentrout and Cowan. Let $a_E(\mathbf{r}, t)$ be the activity of excitatory neurons in a given volume element of a slab of neural tissue located at $\mathbf{r} \in R^2$, and let $a_I(\mathbf{r}, t)$ be the corresponding activity of inhibitory neurons; a_E and a_I can be interpreted as local spatiotemporal averages of the membrane potentials or voltages of the relevant neural populations. When neuron activation rates are low, they can be shown to satisfy nonlinear evolution equations of a similar form to Equation 1:

$$\tau \frac{\partial a_l}{\partial t} = -a_l + \sum_{m=E,I} w_{lm} \cdot \sigma[a_m] + h_l \qquad (10)$$

where $w \cdot \sigma$ now signifies the convolution

$$(w \cdot \sigma[a])(\mathbf{r}) = \int_{R^2} w(|\mathbf{r} - \mathbf{r}'|)\sigma[a(\mathbf{r}', t)]d\mathbf{r}' \qquad (11)$$

with $w_{lm}(|\mathbf{r} - \mathbf{r}'|)$ giving the weight per unit volume of all synapses to the lth population from neurons of the mth population a distance $|\mathbf{r} - \mathbf{r}'|$ away. Note that $w_{IE} > 0$ and $w_{II} < 0$ and the external input h_l is assumed to be constant. An important property of the weight distributions w_{lm} is that they are invariant under the action of the planar Euclidean group—the group of rigid motions in the plane consisting of translations, rotations, and reflections. This symmetry plays a crucial role in determining the types of pattern that emerge through a Turing instability.

For a sigmoid firing rate function σ, it can be shown that there exists at least one fixed-point solution $\bar{a}_l$ of Equation 10:

$$\bar{a}_l = \sum_{m=E,I} W_{lm} \cdot \sigma[\bar{a}_m], \quad W_{lm} = \int_{R^2} w_{lm}(\mathbf{r})d\mathbf{r} \qquad (12)$$

If the external input h_l is sufficiently small relative to the threshold for firing, then this fixed point is unique and stable. There are thus two ways to increase the excitability of the network and thus destabilize the fixed point: either by increasing the external input or reducing the threshold. The latter can occur through the action of drugs on certain brainstem nuclei, which therefore provides a mechanism for generating geometric visual hallucinations. The local stability of the fixed point is found by linearization. Setting $a_l(\mathbf{r}, t) = \bar{a}_l + u_l(\mathbf{r})e^{\lambda t/\tau}$ leads to the eigenvalue equation

$$(\lambda + 1)u_l(\mathbf{r}) = \sum_{m=E,I} \mu_m(w_{lm} \cdot u_m)(\mathbf{r}) \qquad (13)$$

where $\mu_l = \sigma'(\bar{a}_l)$. This can be diagonalized by introducing Fourier transforms $W_{lm}(\mathbf{k})$ and $U_m(\mathbf{k})$ and using the convolution theorem. The result is a matrix dispersion relation for λ as a function of $q = |\mathbf{k}|$ given by solutions of the characteristic equation det $([\lambda + 1]\mathbf{I} - \Lambda(q)) = 0$, where $\Lambda_{lm}(q) = \mu_m W_{lm}(|\mathbf{k}|)$ and $\mathbf{I}$ is the unit matrix. One can simplify the formulation by assuming that $w_{EE} = w_{IE}$ and $w_{II} = w_{EI}$ so that the dispersion relation reduces to $\lambda(q) = -1 + \mu W(q)$, where $W(q)$ is the Fourier transform of $w(\mathbf{r}) = [\mu_E w_{EE}(\mathbf{r}) + \mu_I w_{II}(\mathbf{r})]/\mu$.

It is then relatively straightforward to set up the conditions under which the homogeneous state undergoes a Turing instability, namely, that $W(q)$ be *bandpass*. This can be achieved with the "Mexican hat" function shown in Figure 2*C*, representing short-range excitation and long-range inhibition. It is simple to establish that λ then passes through zero at the critical value $\mu_c = 1/W(q_c)$, signaling the growth of spatially periodic patterns with wave number q_c, where $W(q_c) = \max_q\{W(q)\}$. Close to the bifurcation point, these patterns can be represented as linear combinations of plane waves:

$$u(r) - \sum_{n=1}^{N} [z_n e^{i\mathbf{k}_n \cdot \mathbf{r}} + z_n^* e^{-i\mathbf{k}_n \cdot \mathbf{r}}] \qquad (14)$$

where the sum is over all wave vectors with $|\mathbf{k}_n| = q_c$. Rotation symmetry implies that the space of such modes is infinite dimensional. That is, all plane waves with wave vectors on the critical circle $|\mathbf{k}_n| = q_c$ are allowed (see Figure 3A). However, translation symmetry means that we can restrict the space of solutions to that of doubly periodic functions corresponding to regular tilings of the plane. The symmetry group is then reduced to that of certain crystal lattices: square, rhomboid, and hexagonal lattices (see Figure 3B). The sum over n in Equation 14 is now finite with $N = 2$ (square, rhomboid) or $N = 3$ (hexagonal), and depending on the boundary conditions, various patterns of stripes or spots can be obtained as solutions. Amplitude equations for the coefficients z_n can then be obtained by using the perturbation approach described in the discussion of orientation tuning. Here the rotation and translation symmetries introduced above restrict the structure of the amplitude equations. In the case of a square or rhombic lattice, we can take $\mathbf{k}_1 = q_c(1, 0)$ and $\mathbf{k}_2 = q_c(\cos \varphi, \sin \varphi)$ such that

$$\frac{dz_n}{dt} = z_n\left[\mu - \mu_c - \gamma_0|z_n|^2 - 2\gamma_\varphi \sum_{m \neq n} |z_m|^2\right] \quad (15)$$

for $n = 1, 2$, where γ_φ depends on the angle φ. In the case of a hexagonal lattice, we can take $\mathbf{k}_n = q_c(\cos \varphi_n, \sin \varphi_n)$ with $\varphi_1 = 0$, $\varphi_2 = 2\pi/3$, and $\varphi_3 = 4\pi/3$ such that

$$\frac{dz_n}{dt} = z_n[\mu - \mu_c - \gamma_0|z_n|^2 - \eta z_{n-1}^* z_{n+1}^*]$$
$$- 2\gamma_{\varphi_2} z_n(|z_{n-1}|^2 + |z_{n+1}|^2) \quad (16)$$

where $n = 1, 2, 3 \pmod 3$.

These ordinary differential equations can then be analyzed to determine which particular types of pattern are selected and to calculate their stability. The results can be summarized in a bifurcation diagram as illustrated in Figure 3C for the hexagonal lattice with $\eta > 0$ and $2\gamma_{\varphi_2} > \gamma_0$. (Note that such patterns have also been observed in fluids in the form of convection rolls and honeycombs as well as in animal coat markings in the form of stripes and spots. This indicates that although the physics may be very different, the interactions in all these phenomena are such that they can all be represented within the framework of the Turing mechanism.)

Cortical Development

Essentially the same analysis can be applied to a variety of problems concerning the neural development of feature maps and connectivity patterns (see also OCULAR DOMINANCE AND ORIENTATION COLUMNS). Consider, for example, the development of topographic maps from eye to brain (von der Malsburg and Willshaw, 1977; DEVELOPMENT OF RETINOTECTAL MAPS). Such maps develop by a process that involves both innate and activity-dependent factors. The actual growth and decay of connections are activity dependent, involving synaptic plasticity. However, the final solution is constrained by innate factors in the form of gene products acting as *morphogens* (see PATTERN FORMATION, BIOLOGICAL), which act like boundary conditions. The key insight was provided by von der Malsburg (1973), who showed that pattern formation can occur in a developing neural network whose synaptic connectivity or weight matrix is activity dependent and modifiable, provided that some form of *competition* is present. Thus, Haüssler and von der Malsburg (1983) formulated the topographic mapping problem (in the case of a one-dimensional cortex) as follows: let w_{rs} be the weight of connections from the retinal point r to the cortical point s, and let $\mathbf{w}$ be the associated weight matrix. An evolution equation for $\mathbf{w}$ embodying synaptic plasticity and competition can then be written as

$$\frac{d\mathbf{w}}{dt} = \alpha\mathbf{J} + \beta\mathbf{w} \cdot C(\mathbf{w}) - \mathbf{w} \cdot B[\alpha\mathbf{J} + \beta\mathbf{w} \cdot C(\mathbf{w})] \quad (17)$$

where $\mathbf{J}$ is a matrix with all elements equal to unity, $C_{rs}(\mathbf{x}) = \Sigma_{rs}c(r - r', s - s')x_{r's'}$, and

$$B(\mathbf{x}) = \frac{1}{2}\left[\frac{1}{N}\sum_{r'} x_{r's} + \frac{1}{N}\sum_{s'} x_{rs'}\right] \quad (18)$$

One can easily show that $\mathbf{w} = \mathbf{J}$ is an unstable fixed point of Equation 17. Linearizing about this fixed point leads to an equation that can be written as

$$\tau\frac{d\mathbf{v}}{dt} = -\mathbf{v}(\mathbf{r}, t) + \tau(I - B)[(I + C)(\mathbf{v})] \quad (19)$$

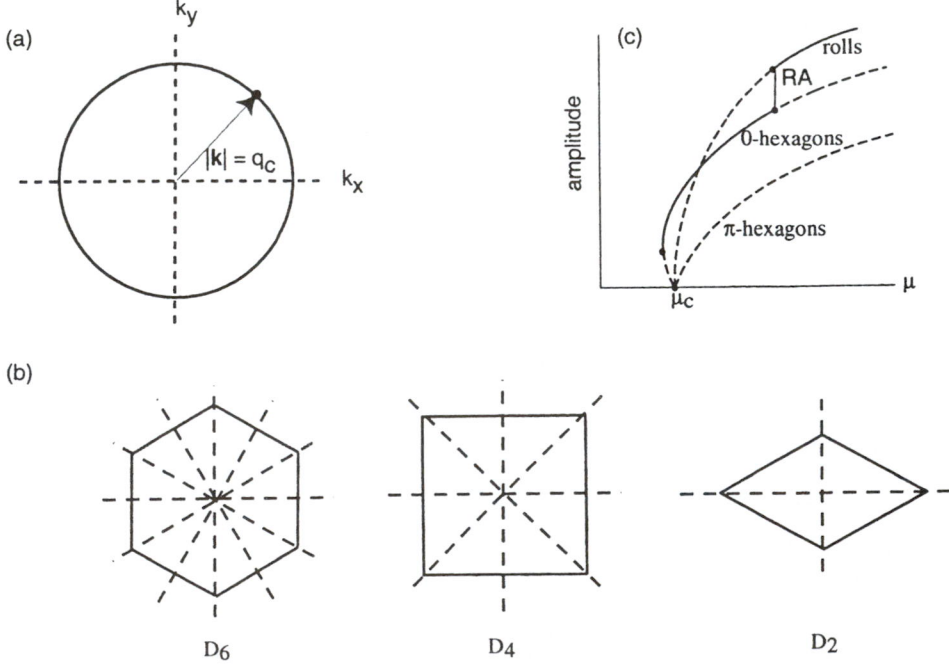

Figure 3. *A*, Critical circle for Turing instability. *B*, Crystal lattice groups: hexagonal (D_6), square (D_4), and rhomboid (D_2). *C*, Bifurcation diagram showing the variation in amplitude C with parameter μ for patterns on a hexagonal lattice. Solid and dashed curves indicate stable and unstable solutions, respectively. The different patterns are distinguished by the coefficients $\mathbf{z} = (z_1, z_2, z_3)$ with $\mathbf{z} = (1, 0, 0)$ for roll or stripe patterns, $\mathbf{z} = (1, 1, 1)$ for 0-hexagons, and $\mathbf{z} = (1, 1, -1)$ for π-hexagons. It is also possible for additional patterns to form through secondary bifurcations (such as rectangular (RA) patterns). However, higher-order contributions to the amplitude equation (Equation 16) are needed to determine such bifurcations.

where $\tau = (1 - \alpha)^{-1}$. It is not too difficult to see that the term $(I - B)[(I + C)(\mathbf{v})]$ is equivalent to the action of an effective convolution kernel of the form $w(\mathbf{r}) = w_+(\mathbf{r}) - w_-(\mathbf{r})$, so Equation 19 can be rewritten in the familiar form:

$$\tau \frac{d\mathbf{v}}{dt} = -\mathbf{v}(\mathbf{r}, t) + \tau \int_{\mathbf{R}^2} w(\mathbf{r} - \mathbf{r}')v(\mathbf{r}', t)d\mathbf{r}' \quad (20)$$

where in this case $\mathbf{r} = \{r, s\}$ and $\mathbf{v}$ is a matrix. Once again there is a dispersion relation of the form $\lambda = -1 + \mu W(\mathbf{k}) \equiv \lambda(\mathbf{k})$, where $k = \{k, l\}$, and given appropriate boundary conditions, it is the Fourier transform $W(\mathbf{k})$ of $w(\mathbf{r})$ that determines which of the eigenmodes

$$\sum_{kl} c_{kl} \exp\left[i \frac{2\pi}{N}(kr + ls)\right]$$

emerges at the critical wave number $\mathbf{k}_C = \{k_C, l_C\}$. It can be shown that in the rs plane, $w(\mathbf{r})$ looks like a circular Mexican hat except that the inhibitory surround is in the form of a cross. This forces the eigenmodes emerging from the Turing instability to be diagonal in the rs plane. If $\mathbf{k}_C$ is selected so that only one wave is present, and if the initial conditions or some morphogen favor the NW → SE diagonal rather than the NE → SW one, then this corresponds to an ordered and correctly oriented retinocortical map. Figure 4 shows details of the emergence of such an eigenmode.

A second example involves the development of ocular dominance maps (Swindale, 1980). Let $n_R(\mathbf{r}, t)$ and $n_L(\mathbf{r}, t)$ be the normalized right and left eye densities of synaptic connections to the visual cortex modeled as a two-dimensional sheet of neurons. Such densities are assumed to evolve according to the equation

$$\frac{\partial u_l(\mathbf{r}, t)}{\partial t} = \sum_{m=R,L} \int_{\mathbf{R}^2} w_{lm}(|\mathbf{r} - \mathbf{r}'|)\sigma[u_m(\mathbf{r}', t)]d\mathbf{r}' \quad (21)$$

where $u_m = \log n_m - \log(1 - n_m)$ so that $\sigma[u_m] = n_m$, and the coupling matrix $\mathbf{w}$ is given by

$$\mathbf{w}(|\mathbf{r}|) = w(r)\begin{pmatrix} +1 & -1 \\ -1 & +1 \end{pmatrix}.$$

With the additional constraint $n_R + n_L = 1$, Equation 21 reduces to a one-variable form in n_R:

$$\frac{\partial n_R(\mathbf{r}, t)}{\partial t} = \left[2 \int_{\mathbf{R}^2} w(|\mathbf{r} - \mathbf{r}'|)n_R(\mathbf{r}', t)d\mathbf{r}' - \int_{\mathbf{R}^2} w(|\mathbf{r}'|)d\mathbf{r}'\right]$$
$$\times \ n_R(\mathbf{r}, t)(1 - n_R(\mathbf{r}, t)) \quad (22)$$

The fixed points of this equation are easily seen to be 0, 1, and 0.5. The first two are stable; however, the third is unstable to small perturbations. Linearizing about this fixed point generates the dispersion relation $\lambda = 0.5W(|\mathbf{k}|)$. Once again, the Fourier transform of the interaction kernel $w(|\mathbf{r}|)$ controls the emergence of the usual eigenmodes, in this case plane waves of the form $\exp(i\mathbf{k} \cdot \mathbf{r})$ in the

cortical plane. Note that the fixed point $n_R = n_L = 0.5$ corresponds to $u_R = u_L = 0$ and is a point of reflection symmetry of the function $\sigma[u]$. It is this additional symmetry that generates stripes rather than spots or blobs when the fixed point destabilizes.

Discussion

It will be seen that many examples of both spontaneous and stimulus-driven neural pattern formation can be formulated and analyzed within the framework of the Turing instability. Many other examples exist of the role of this instability in visual neuroscience, such as stereopsis (Dev, 1975; Marr and Poggio, 1976; see STEREO CORRESPONDENCE) and the development of iso-orientation patches (Swindale, 1982; see OCULAR DOMINANCE AND ORIENTATION COLUMNS). All such models contain the same basic mechanism of competition between excitation and inhibition, and most have some underlying symmetry that plays a crucial role in the selection and stability of the ensuing patterns. It is an interesting question as to how universal this mechanism is for neural pattern formation.

Road Map: Dynamic Systems
Related Reading: Amplification, Attenuation, and Integration; Cooperative Phenomena; Dynamics and Bifurcation in Neural Nets; Pattern Formation, Biological

References

Bressloff, P. C., and Cowan, J. D., 2002, Spontaneous pattern formation in primary visual cortex, in *Nonlinear Dynamics: Where Do We Go from Here?* (A. Champneys and S. J. Hogan, Eds.), Bristol, Engl.: IOP. ◆

Bressloff, P. C., Cowan, J. D., Golubitsky, M., Thomas, P. J., and Wiener, M. C., 2001, Geometric visual hallucinations, Euclidean symmetry, and the functional architecture of striate cortex, *Philos. Trans. R. Soc. Lond. B Biol. Sci.*, 356:299–330. ◆

Dev, P., 1975, Perception of depth surfaces in random-dot stereograms: A neural model, *Int. J. Man-Machine Studies*, 7:511–528.

Ermentrout, G. B., and Cowan, J. D., 1979, A mathematical theory of visual hallucination patterns, *Biol. Cybernetics*, 34:137–150.

Häussler, A., and von der Malsburg, C., 1983, Development of retinotopic projections: An analytical treatment, *J. Theoret. Neurobiol.*, 2:47–73.

Issa, N. P., Trepel, C., and Stryker, M. P., 2000, Spatial frequency maps in cat visual cortex, *J. Neurosci.*, 20:8504–8514.

Marr, D., and Poggio, T., 1976, Cooperative computation of stereo disparity, *Science*, 194:283–287.

Schwartz, E., 1977, Spatial mapping in the primate sensory projection: Analytic structure and relevance to projection, *Biol. Cybernetics*, 25:181–194.

Sharon, D., and Grinvald, A., 2002, Dynamics and constancy in cortical spatiotemporal patterns of orientation processing, *Science*, 295:512–515.

Somers, D. C., Nelson, S., and Sur, M., 1995, An emergent model of orientation selectivity in cat visual cortex simple cells, *J. Neurosci.*, 15:5448–5465.

Swindale, N. V., 1980, A model for the formation of ocular dominance stripes, *Proc. R. Soc. Lond. B Biol. Sci.*, 208:243–264.

Swindale, N. V., 1982, A model for the formation of orientation columns, *Proc. R. Soc. Lond. B Biol. Sci.*, 215:211–230.

von der Malburg, C., 1973, Self-organization of orientation-selective cells in striate cortex, *Kybernetik*, 14:85–100.

von der Malsburg, C., and Willshaw, D., 1977, How to label nerve cells so that they can interconnect in an ordered fashion, *Proc. Natl. Acad. Sci. USA*, 74:5176–5178.

Wilson, H. R., and Cowan, J. D., 1973, A mathematical theory of the functional dynamics of cortical and thalamic nervous tissue, *Kybernetik*, 13:55–80. ◆

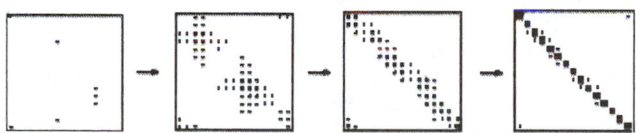

Figure 4. Stages in the development of an ordered and correctly oriented retinotopic map. A single stripe develops in the rs-plane. (Redrawn from Häussler and von der Malsburg, 1983.)

Pattern Recognition

Yann LeCun and Yoshua Bengio

Introduction

Pattern recognition (PR) addresses the problem of classifying objects, often represented as vectors or as strings of symbols, into categories. The difficulty is to synthesize, and then to efficiently compute, the *classification function* that maps objects to categories, given that objects in a category can have widely varying input representations. In most instances, the task is known to the designer through a set of example patterns whose categories are known, and through general, a priori knowledge about the task, such as "the category of an object is not changed when the object is slightly translated or rotated in space."

Historically, the field of PR started with the early efforts in neural networks (perceptrons, adalines, etc.; see PERCEPTRONS, ADALINES, AND BACKPROPAGATION). Whereas in the past, neural networks (NNs) sometimes played the role of an outsider in PR, recent progress in learning algorithms and the availability of powerful hardware have made them the method of choice for many PR applications.

Because most PR problems are too complex to be solved entirely by handcrafted algorithms, machine learning has always played a central role in PR. Learning automatically synthesizes a classification function from a set of labeled examples. Unfortunately, no learning algorithm can be expected to succeed unless it is guided by prior knowledge. The traditional way of incorporating knowledge about the task is to divide the recognizer into a feature extractor and a classifier. Since most learning algorithms work better in low-dimensional spaces with easily separable patterns, the role of the feature extractor is to transform the input patterns so that they can be represented by low-dimensional vectors, or short strings of symbols, that (1) can be easily compared or matched, and (2) are relatively invariant to transformations that do not change the nature of the input objects. The feature extractor contains most of the prior knowledge and is rather specific to the task. It also requires most of the design effort because it is often handcrafted, although unsupervised learning methods, such as PRINCIPAL COMPONENT ANALYSIS (q.v.), can sometimes be used. The classifier, on the other hand, is often general purpose and trainable. One of the main problems with this approach is that the recognition accuracy is largely determined by the ability of the designer to come up with an appropriate set of features. This turns out to be a daunting task which, unfortunately, must be redone for each new problem.

One of the main contributions of NNs to PR has been to provide an alternative to this design: properly designed multilayer networks can learn complex mappings in high-dimensional spaces without requiring complicated handcrafted feature extractors. Networks containing hundreds of inputs and tens of thousands of parameters can be trained on databases containing several hundreds of thousands examples. This allows designers to rely more on learning and less on detailed engineering of feature extractors. Crucial to success is the ability to tailor the network architecture to the task, which allows incorporating prior knowledge and therefore learning complex tasks without requiring excessively large networks and training sets.

The success of multilayer networks relies on one surprising fact: gradient-based minimization techniques can be used to learn very complex nonlinear mappings. Generalizations of the concept of gradient-based learning have allowed one to view many PR techniques, neural and nonneural, in a unified way, including not only traditional multilayer feedforward nets with sigmoid units and dot products but also many other structures such as radial basis functions, hidden Markov models (HMMs), vector quantizers, etc. Many recent efforts have been directed toward combining adaptive modules of different types into a single system and training them cooperatively by propagating gradients through them, particularly for recognizing composite objects such as handwritten or spoken words (see LeCun et al., 1998, for a review and applications).

Learning and Generalization

Owing to the presence of noise, the high dimension of the input, and the complexity of the mapping to be learned, PR applications create some of the most challenging problems in machine learning. Most learning methods are trained by minimizing a *cost function* computed over a set of training examples. The cost function is generally of the form

$$C(W) = \sum_X Q(X, F(X, W)) + H(W) \qquad (1)$$

where X is a training example, $F(X, W)$ is the recognizer output for pattern X and "parameters" W, $Q(X, F(X, W))$ is a cost function (the training error), and $H(W)$ is a measure of "capacity" of the recognizer (the *regularizer*). Such cost functions attempt to model the real measure of performance, i.e., the *testing error* (error rate on a test set disjoint from the training set) (see LEARNING AND GENERALIZATION: THEORETICAL BOUNDS).

System designers have to strike the right balance between learning the training set (by using powerful learning architectures) and minimizing the difference between the training error and the test error (by limiting the capacity of the machine). Large machines can learn the training set but may perform poorly if the training set is not large enough, a problem known as overparameterization, or overfitting. On the other hand, too little capacity yields underfitting—i.e., large error on both training and test sets.

Most adaptive recognizers stand between two extremes of a continuous spectrum. At one end, parameter-based methods, in which a set of learned parameters determines the input-output relation, put the emphasis on minimizing the first term in Equation 1 with a fixed H (e.g., multilayer neural networks). At the other end, memory-based methods, which rely on matching or comparing the incoming pattern with a set of learned or stored prototypes, keep the first term close to zero, and attempt to minimize the regularizer (e.g., nearest-neighbor algorithms).

Although in principle, any appropriate functional form for F, Q, and H can be used, the choice is largely determined by (1) the belief that it is well suited to the task and (2) the efficiency of the available minimization algorithms. There is a strong incentive to choose smooth and well-behaved functions whose gradient can be computed easily, so that gradient-based minimization algorithms can be used, as opposed to inefficient combinatorial search methods. Preferably, F will be a smooth real-valued function (e.g., layers of sigmoid units) rather than a discrete function (e.g., layers of threshold units); Q is often chosen to be the mean square error between the actual output and a target, rather than the number of misclassified patterns, which would be more relevant but is practically impossible to minimize.

A Few Basic Classification Methods

Linear and Polynomial Classifiers

A linear classifier is essentially a single neuron. An elementary two-class discrimination is performed by comparing the output to a threshold (multiple classes use multiple neurons). Training algorithms for linear classifiers are well studied (see PERCEPTRONS, ADALINES, AND BACKPROPAGATION). Their limitations are well known: the likelihood that a partition of P vectors of dimension N is computable by a linear classifier decreases very quickly as P increases beyond N (Duda and Hart, 1973). One method to ensure separability is to represent the patterns by high-dimensional vectors (large N). If necessary, the dimension of original input vectors can be enlarged using a set of basis functions ϕ_i:

$$F(X, W) = \sum_i w_i \phi_i(X) \qquad (2)$$

A simple example is when the basis functions are cross-products of K or fewer coordinates of the input vector X (F is a polynomial of degree K). Such polynomial classifiers have been studied since the early 1960s and have been "renamed" in the context of NNs as sigma-pi units or high-order nets. Unfortunately, polynomial classifiers are often impractical because the number of features scales like N^K. Nevertheless, *feature selection* methods can be used to reduce the number of product terms, or to reduce the number of original input variables.

Local Basis Functions

Another popular kind of space expansion (Equation 2) uses *local* basis functions, which are activated within a small area of the input space. A popular family consists of the radial basis functions (RBFs; see RADIAL BASIS FUNCTION NETWORKS): $\phi_i(X) = e^{-(X - P_i)^2}$, where the P_i are a set of appropriately chosen "prototypes." Methods based on such expansions can cover the full spectrum between parameter-based and purely memory-based methods by varying the number of prototypes, the way they are computed, and the classifier that follows the expansion (which can be more complex than a simple weighted sum). At one extreme, each training sample is used as a prototype, to which the sample's label is attached. In the K-nearest neighbors algorithms, the K nearest prototypes to an unknown pattern vote for its label. In the Parzen windows method, the normalized sum of all the $\phi_i(X)$ associated with a particular class is interpreted as the conditional probability that X belongs to that class (Duda and Hart, 1973). In the RBF method the output is a (learned) linear combination of the outputs of the basis functions. Associating a prototype with each training sample can be very inefficient and increases the complexity term. Therefore, several methods have been proposed for *learning* the prototypes. One way is to use unsupervised clustering techniques such as K-means to put prototypes in regions of high sample density, but supervised methods can also be used (see RADIAL BASIS FUNCTION NETWORKS). An important one is LVQ2, in which prototypes that are near a training sample are moved away from it if its assigned class differs from the sample's, and moved toward it if its class is equal to the sample's (see LEARNING VECTOR QUANTIZATION). Another important supervised method for RBF networks is simply gradient descent. The partial derivatives of the cost function with respect to the parameters of the basis functions (the prototype vectors) can be computed using a form of backpropagation: in the same way that gradients can be backpropagated through sigmoids and dot products, they can be backpropagated through exponentials and Euclidean distances. The parameters can then be adjusted using the gradient. It has been argued that the local property leads to faster learning than standard multilayer nets, and to good rejection properties (Lee, 1991). Several authors enhance the power of prototype-based systems by using distance measures that are more complex than just Euclidean distance between the prototypes and the input patterns (such as general bilinear forms with learned coefficients). Methods that add prototypes as needed have also been proposed, notably the RCE algorithm.

Support Vector Machines

A recently proposed and elegant way of avoiding the curse of dimensionality in polynomial and local classifiers rests on the fact that, if the w_i in Equation 2 are computed to maximize the *margin* (the minimum distance between training points and the classification surface), the W obtained after training can be written as a linear combination of a small subset of the expanded training examples (Boser, Guyon, and Vapnik, 1992). Points in this subset are called *support vectors*, hence the name support vector machines (SVMs). This leads to a surprisingly simple way of evaluating high-degree polynomials in high-dimensional spaces without having to explicitly compute all the terms of the polynomial. For example, maximum-margin polynomials of degree K can be computed using

$$F(X) = \sum_{j \in S} \alpha_j (X \cdot P_j + 1)^K \qquad (3)$$

where the P_j are the support points (subset of the training set) and the α_j are coefficients that uniquely determine the weights W. Learning the α_j amounts to solving a quadratic programming problem with linear inequality constraints. Besides polynomial kernels, SUPPORT VECTOR MACHINES (q.v.) can be built for a variety of kernels, such as RBFs and neuron-like kernels. SVMs have also been extended beyond classification problems to regression and density estimation. Excellent results for the classification of handwritten digit images have been obtained with a fourth-degree polynomial computed using this method (Bottou et al., 1994). The number of multiply-adds per recognition was a few hundred thousands, much less than the $O(400^4)$ multiply-adds required to directly evaluate the polynomial.

Complex Distance Measures

Although many memory-based methods use simple distance measures (Euclidean distance) and large collections of prototypes, some applications can take advantage of more complex, problem-dependent, distance measures and use fewer prototypes. Ideal distance measures should be invariant with respect to transformations of the patterns that do not change their nature (e.g., translations and distortions for characters, time or pitch distortion for speech). With invariant distances, a single prototype can potentially represent many possible instances of a category, reducing the number of necessary prototypes. An important family of invariant distance measures entails *elastic matching*. Elastic matching comes down to finding the point closest to the input pattern on the surface of all possible deformations of the prototype. Naturally, the exhaustive search approach is prohibitively expensive in general. However, if the surface is smooth, better search techniques can be used, such as gradient descent or conjugate gradient. If the deformations are along one dimension (as in speech), dynamic programming can find the best solution efficiently. Simard, LeCun, and Denker (1993) approximated the surface of a deformed prototype by its tangent plane at the prototype. The matching problem reduces to finding the minimum distance between a point and a plane, which can be done efficiently. This has been applied to handwritten character recognition with great success.

Multilayer Networks and Gradient-Based Learning

The vast majority of applications of NNs to PR are based on multilayer feedforward networks trained with backpropagation. At first it seems almost magical that an algorithm as simple as gradient descent works at all to learn complex nonlinear mappings (nonconvex, ill-conditioned error surfaces). Minsky and Selfridge's warning about the limitations of "hill-climbing" methods for machine learning in the late 1950s is an indication of the general belief that it could not work. Surprisingly, experiments show that local minima are rarely a problem with large networks. As evidence of the success of backpropagation, all but two of the entries in the last NIST character recognition competition used some form of backpropagation network.

PR problems are often characterized by large and redundant training sets with high-dimensional inputs, which translates into large networks and long learning times. Much effort has been devoted to speeding up training using refined nonlinear optimization methods (conjugate gradient, quasi-Newton methods, and so on). These are essentially batch methods (the weights are updated after a complete pass through the training set) and can rarely compete with "carefully tuned" stochastic (on-line) gradient descent (where the weights are updated after each pattern presentation). This is due to the presence of redundancy in large natural training sets. On typical large-scale image or speech recognition tasks, stochastic gradient descent converges in one to a few dozen epochs. To avoid overlearning, a validation set should be set aside, and training should be stopped when the error rate on the validation set stops decreasing. An important limitation to the popularity of NN techniques for PR is that certain simple tricks must be used and many common pitfalls must be avoided that are part of the "oral culture" rather than scientific facts.

Once backpropagation with feedforward networks of sigmoid units and dot products established the value of gradient-based learning, it seemed natural to extend the idea to other structures. Minimizing a cost function through gradient-based learning can be seen as the unifying principle behind many methods: RBFs or mixtures of Gaussians, learning vector quantization, HMMs, and many prototype-based methods that use various distance measures. Experiments have shown the advantage of using different types of modules in different parts of a learning system. In particular, sigmoids and dot products seem better for processing large amounts of high-dimensional and low-level information (early feature extraction), while RBFs or other more local modules seem better suited for final classification, a more memory-intensive task. With the gradient-based learning framework, modules of different types can be connected in any configuration and trained cooperatively by backpropagating gradients through them. To achieve this, one needs only to be able to compute the partial derivatives of each output of a module with respect to each input and each parameter of the module (see MODULAR AND HIERARCHICAL LEARNING SYSTEMS). In addition, many cost functions can be considered as just another module (with a scalar output) through which gradients can be backpropagated. Examples include the mean squared error, modified LVQ cost functions, maximum likelihood, maximum mutual information, cross-entropy, classification figure of merit, and several types of statistical or graphical postprocessors (LeCun et al., 1998).

Local/Global and Modular Methods

It has recently been suggested that good PR systems should behave differently in different parts of the input space. For example, parts of the input space may be very sparsely populated, requiring a low-capacity learner, while denser areas may require a more complex one. A simple idea is to use a collection of modules, each of which is activated when the input lies in a particular region. A separate module called a *gater* decides which module should be activated. When the gater is differentiable, the whole system (modules plus gater) can be trained cooperatively (see MODULAR AND HIERARCHICAL LEARNING SYSTEMS). In such multimodular systems, parameters are relatively decoupled across modules, which is believed to allow faster training (or better scaling of training time). In another interesting "semilocal" method, a simple network (e.g., single layer) is trained each time a new test pattern is presented, using training patterns in the neighborhood of this test pattern; training is done "on demand" during recognition (Bottou and Vapnik, 1992).

In general, local methods learn fast, but they are expensive at runtime in terms of memory and, often, of computation. In addition, they may not be appropriate for problems with high-dimensional inputs. Global methods, such as multilayer networks, take longer to train, but they are quite compact, and they execute quickly. They can handle high-dimensional inputs, particularly when specialized architectures are used.

Specialized Architectures, Convolutional Networks

The great hope that multilayer networks brought with them was the possibility of eliminating the need for a separate handcrafted feature extractor, relying on the first layers to automatically learn the right set of features. Although fully connected networks fed with "raw" character images (or speech spectra) have very large numbers of free parameters, they have been applied with some success (Martin and Pittman, 1991). This can be explained as follows. With small initial weights, a multilayer network is almost equivalent to a single-layer network (each layer is quasilinear). As incremental learning proceeds, the weights gradually increase, thereby progressively increasing the effective capacity of the system (to the authors' knowledge, this explanation was first suggested by Léon Bottou in 1988).

On the other hand, using a specialized network architecture instead of a fully connected net can reduce the number of free parameters and facilitate the learning of invariances. In certain applications, the need for a separate handcrafted feature extractor can be eliminated by wiring the first few layers of the network in a way that forces it to learn relevant features and eliminate irrelevant variability. Convolutional networks, including time-delay neural networks (TDNNs), are an important class of specialized architectures well suited for dealing with one- or two-dimensional signals such as time series, images, or speech (see CONVOLUTIONAL NETWORKS FOR IMAGES, SPEECH, AND TIME SERIES). Convolutional networks use the techniques of local receptive fields, shared weights, and subsampling (loosely based on the architecture of the visual cortex) to ensure that the first few layers extract and combine local features in a distortion-invariant way. Although the wiring of the convolutional layers is designed by hand, the values of all the coefficients are learned with a variant of the backpropagation algorithm. The main advantage of this approach is that the feature extractor is totally integrated into the classifier and is produced by the learning process rather than by the hand of the designer (LeCun et al., 1990). Because of the weight-sharing technique, the number of free parameters in a convolutional network is much less than in a fully connected network of comparable power, which has the effect of reducing the complexity term in Equation 1 and improving the generalization. The success of convolutional nets of various types has had a major impact on several application domains, among them speech recognition, character recognition, and object spotting. On handwriting recognition tasks they compare favorably with other techniques (Bottou et al., 1994) in terms of accuracy, speed, and memory requirements. Character recognizers using convolutional nets have been deployed in commercial applications. A very promising feature of convolutional nets is that they can be efficiently replicated, or scanned, over large input fields, resulting in the so-called *space displacement neural net* (SDNN) architecture (see below, and CONVOLUTIONAL NETWORKS FOR IMAGES, SPEECH, AND TIME SERIES).

Networks with recurrent connections can be used to map input sequences to output sequences, while taking long-term context into account. The main advantage of recurrent networks over TDNNs for analyzing sequences is that the span of the temporal context

Figure 1. A multimodule architecture combining a convolutional NN with a postprocessor such as an HMM.

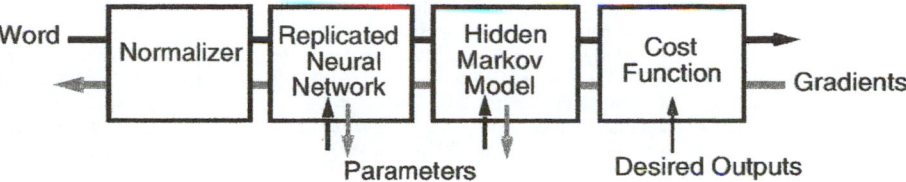

that the network can take into account is not hard-wired within a fixed temporal window by the architectural choices but can be learned by the network. However, theoretical and practical hurdles (Bengio, Simard, and Frasconi, 1994) limit the span of long-term dependencies that can be learned efficiently.

Recognition of Composite Objects

In many real applications, the difficulty is not only to recognize individual objects but also to separate them from context or background. For example, one approach to handwritten word recognition is to *segment* the characters out of their surrounding and *recognize* them in isolation. A typical handwritten word recognizer uses heuristics to form multiple, possibly overlapping character candidates by cutting the word or by joining nearby strokes. Then the recognizer must either classify each candidate as a character or reject it as a noncharacter. In many applications, such as cursive handwriting or continuous speech, it is difficult or even impossible to devise robust segmentation heuristics. One approach to avoid explicit segmentation is simply to scan the recognizer over all possible locations on the input (character string or spoken sentence) and collect the sequence of corresponding recognizer outputs. Although this is very computationally expensive in general, replicated convolutional networks (SDNNs or TDNNs) can be used to do that very efficiently. In the case of handwriting recognition, an SDNN output will contain a well-identified label when centered on a character. Between characters, the output should indicate a reject. However, combinations of off-center characters may cause ambiguous outputs (e.g., *cl* labeled as *d*). Since both methods, explicit segmentation and scanning, generate many extraneous candidates, a postprocessor is required to resolve ambiguities and pull out the most consistent interpretation, retaining genuine characters and rejecting erroneous stroke combinations, possibly taking linguistic constraints into account (a lexicon or grammar) Figure 1. For this to succeed, the recognizer must be trained not only to classify characters but also to reject noncharacters. The search for the best interpretation is easily done within the framework of graph transducers (LeCun et al., 1998), which generalize HMMs. A graph is built in which each path corresponds to a possible interpretation of the input and in which each node is given probabilities of matching recognizer outputs. Dynamic programming can be used to find the path of highest probability, which yields the most likely interpretation. Furthermore, it is possible to backpropagate errors through this graph in order to train the system to maximize the a posteriori probability of the correct sequence of labels.

Multimodule Architectures and Cooperative Training

Such combinations of neural networks and HMMs (or other graph-based postprocessors) have been proposed by several authors, mostly for speech recognition (see SPEECH RECOGNITION TECHNOLOGY), but also for handwriting recognition (see LeCun et al., 1998, and CONVOLUTIONAL NETWORKS FOR IMAGES, SPEECH, AND TIME SERIES).

The main technical difficulty is in training such hybrid systems. Training the recognizer exclusively on presegmented characters is

neither sufficient nor always possible, since (1) the recognizer must be trained to reject noncharacters and (2) in many cases, such as cursive handwriting, segmented characters are not available, only whole words are. The solution is to simultaneously train the recognizer and the postprocessor to minimize an error measure at the *word level*. This means being able to backpropagate gradients through the postprocessor, down to the recognizer, or to generate desired outputs for the recognizer using the best path in the graph (see Franzini, Lee, and Waibel, 1990, and SPEECH RECOGNITION TECHNOLOGY). Simultaneous training of such hybrids has been reported to yield large reductions in error rates over independent training of the modules in speech recognition (for TDNN/dynamic time warping, see Driancourt, Bottou, and Gallinari, 1991, and Haffner, Franzini, and Waibel, 1991; for TDNN/HMM, see Bengio et al., 1992), and on-line handwriting recognition (for SDNN/HMM, see Bengio, LeCun, and Henderson, 1994). See LeCun et al. (1998) for a review and applications to document analysis.

Discussion

Neural networks, particularly multilayer backpropagation NNs, provide simple yet powerful and general methods for synthesizing classifiers with minimal effort. However, most practical systems combine NNs with other techniques for pre- and postprocessing. On isolated character recognition tasks, multilayer nets trained with variants of backpropagation have approached human accuracy, at speeds of about 1,000 characters per second using NN hardware. NNs have allowed workers to minimize the role of detailed engineering and maximize the role of learning. Despite the recent advances in multimodule architectures and gradient-based learning, several key questions are still unanswered, and many problems are still out of reach. How much has to be built into the system, and how much can be learned? How can one achieve true transformation-invariant perception with NNs? Convolutional nets are a step in the right direction, but new concepts will be required for a complete solution (see DYNAMIC LINK ARCHITECTURE). How to recognize compound objects in their context? The accuracy of the best NN/HMM hybrids for written or spoken sentences cannot even be compared with human performance. Topics such as the recognition of three-dimensional objects in complex scenes are totally out of reach. Human-like accuracy on complex PR tasks such as handwriting and speech recognition may not be achieved without a drastic increase in the available computing power. Several important questions may simply resolve themselves with the availability of more powerful hardware, allowing the use of brute-force methods and very large networks.

Road Map: Learning in Artificial Networks
Related Reading: Concept Learning; Feature Analysis; Perceptrons, Adalines, and Backpropagation; Statistical Mechanics of On-line Learning and Generalization

References

Bengio, Y., Simard, P., and Frasconi, P., 1994, Learning long-term dependencies with gradient descent is difficult, in *Recurrent Neural Networks* (special issue), *IEEE Trans. Neural Netw.*, 5:157–166.

Bengio, Y., LeCun, Y., and Henderson, D., 1994, Globally trained hand-written word recognizer using spatial representation, space displacement neural networks and hidden Markov models, in *Advances in Neural Information Processing Systems 6* (J. Cowan, G. Tesauro, and J. Alspector, Eds.), San Mateo, CA: Morgan Kaufmann, pp. 937–944.

Bengio, Y., Mori, R. D., Flammia, G., and Kompe, R., 1992, Global optimization of a neural network-hidden Markov model hybrid, *IEEE Trans. Neural Netw.*, 3:252–259.

Boser, B., Guyon, I., and Vapnik, V., 1992, An algorithm for optimal margin classifiers, in *Fifth Annual Workshop on Computational Learning Theory*, Pittsburgh, pp. 144–152.

Bottou, L., 1998, Online algorithms and stochastic approximations, in *Online Learning in Neural Networks* (D. Saad, Ed.), Cambridge, U.K.: Cambridge University Press. ◆

Bottou, L., Cortes, C., Denker, J., Drucker, H., Guyon, I., Jackel, L., LeCun, Y., Muller, U., Sackinger, E., Simard, P., and Vapnik, V., 1994, Comparison of classifier methods: A case study in handwritten digit recognition, in *Proceedings of an International Conference on Pattern Recognition*, Los Alamitos, CA: IEEE Computer Society Press.

Bottou, L., and Vapnik, V., 1992, Local learning algorithms, *Neural Computat.*, 4:888–900. ◆

Driancourt, X., Bottou, L., and Gallinari, P., 1991, Learning vector quantization, multi-layer perceptron and dynamic programming: Comparison and cooperation, in *Proceedings of an International Joint Conference on Neural Networks*, vol. 2, Piscataway, NJ: IEEE Press, pp. 815–819.

Duda, R., and Hart, P., 1973, *Pattern Classification and Scene Analysis*, New York: Wiley. ◆

Franzini, M., Lee, K., and Waibel, A., 1990, Connectionist Viterbi training: A new hybrid method for continuous speech recognition, in *Proceedings of an International Conference on Acoustics, Speech and Signal Processing*, Piscataway, NJ: IEEE Press, pp. 425–428.

Haffner, P., Franzini, M., and Waibel, A., 1991, Integrating time alignment and neural networks for high performance continuous speech recognition, in *Proceedings of an International Conference on Acoustics, Speech and Signal Processing*, Piscataway, NJ: IEEE Press, pp. 105–108.

LeCun, Y., Boser, B., Denker, J., Henderson, D., Howard, R., Hubbard, W., and Jackel, L., 1990, Handwritten digit recognition with a back-propagation network, in *Advances in Neural Information Processing Systems 2* (D. Touretzky, Ed.), San Mateo, CA: Morgan Kaufmann, pp. 396–404.

LeCun, Y., Bottou, L., Bengio, Y., and Haffner, P., 1998, Gradient-based learning applied to document recognition, *Proc. IEEE*, 86(11):2278–2324.

Lee, Y., 1991, Handwritten digit recognition using K nearest neighbor, radial-basis function, and backpropagation neural network, *Neural Computat.*, 3:441–449.

Martin, G., and Pittman, J., 1991, Recognizing hand-printed letters and digits using back-propagation learning, *Neural Computat.*, 3:258–267.

Minsky, M., and Selfridge, O. G., Learning in random nets, in *Information Theory* (C. Cherry, Ed.), London: Butterworths, pp. 335–347.

Simard, P., LeCun, Y., and Denker, J., 1993, Efficient pattern recognition using a new transformation distance, in *Advances in Neural Information Processing Systems 5* (S. J. Hanson, J. D. Cowan, and C. L. Giles, Eds.), San Mateo, CA: Morgan Kaufmann, pp. 50–58.

Perception of Three-Dimensional Structure

James T. Todd

Introduction

Human observers have a remarkable ability to perceive the three-dimensional (3D) layout of the environment from patterns of light that project onto the retina. Were it not for the facts of our day-to-day experiences, it would be tempting to conclude that the perception of 3D form is a mathematical impossibility, because the properties of optical stimulation appear to have so little in common with the properties of real objects encountered in nature. Whereas real objects exist in 3D space and are composed of tangible materials, an optical image of an object is confined to a two-dimensional (2D) projection surface and consists of nothing more than flickering patterns of light. Nevertheless, for many animals, including humans, these seemingly uninterpretable patterns of light are the primary source of sensory information about the layout of surfaces in the surrounding environment.

There are many different aspects of optical stimulation that are known to provide perceptually salient information about 3D form. Some of these properties—the so-called pictorial depth cues—are available within individual static images. These include texture gradients, contour configurations, and patterns of shading. Others are defined by systematic transformations among multiple images, including the disparity between each eye's view in binocular vision and the optical deformations that occur when objects are observed in motion.

There are two important issues that need to be considered in evaluating any computational model of 3D form perception. The first of these issues involves how 3D structure is perceptually represented. After all, in order to compute an object's shape from visual information, one must first define precisely what shape is. There are numerous attributes of 3D structure that could potentially be represented by the visual system (e.g., curvature, relative depth, local orientation), and the relative computational complexity of an-

alyzing these different attributes can vary dramatically. It is much more difficult, for example, to determine the precise euclidean distance between a pair of visible points than to merely assess which point is closer in depth.

A second related issue concerns ambiguities that are inherent in the nature of visual information. The primary goal of all 3D vision problems is to invert (or partially invert) a function of the following form: $\Lambda = f(\phi)$, where ϕ is the space of environmental properties that can influence patterns of ambient light and Λ is the space of measurable image properties at a point of observation. What can make these problems so difficult is that this is a many-to-one mapping: for any give pattern of optical structure, there is often an infinity of possible 3D structures that could potentially have produced it.

For many problems in 3D vision, it can be useful to separate the properties of environmental structure into two distinct categories. There are some aspects of environmental structure that are invariant over the transformation $\Lambda = f(\phi)$. These properties can be determined with relative ease by measuring the appropriate relationships within available image data. Other properties that are not invariant over this transformation are much more difficult to estimate. Because these properties are inherently ambiguous, a computational analysis must restrict the set of possible interpretations by assuming the existence of environmental constraints. Unfortunately, many of the constraints that have been employed for this purpose seem to have been adopted more for their mathematical convenience than for their ecological validity. The problem with this approach is that the resulting analyses of 3D form may only function effectively within narrowly defined contexts, which have a small probability of occurrence in the natural environments of real biological organisms.

This article reviews various computational models that have been proposed in the literature for analyzing an object's 3D structure from different types of optical information, both individually and in combination. It also examines how the performance of these models compares with the capabilities and limitations of actual human observers in judging different aspects of 3D structure under varying viewing conditions. The goal is to identify the specific representations and computational mechanisms by which 3D form is perceptually analyzed within the human visual system.

Shape from Shading

The most basic type of information available to any visual system is the light that stimulates different regions of the retina from illuminated surfaces in the environment. Smooth gradations in surface luminance are often referred to as shading, and they are one of the primary cues used by artists for the pictorial representation 3D form. The analysis of image shading is made especially difficult because the luminance of any visible surface region can depend on several factors, including the positions and spectral composition of its sources of illumination, the local reflectance and orientation of the surface, and the position of the observer. In order to compute shape from shading it is necessary to somehow decompose these different factors. Most existing algorithms for analyzing 3D shape from shading achieve this decomposition by making several strong assumptions to constrain the structure of an observed scene (Horn and Brooks, 1989). It is typically assumed, for example, that a scene is composed of smoothly curved surfaces that have a known uniform reflectance function, with no specular components, and that there is a uniform pattern of illumination with a known direction and spectral composition.

An important limitation on theoretical analyses of 3D shape from shading is that an image of a surface with homogeneous lambertian reflectance has an infinity of possible 3D interpretations that are all related by an affine transformation (Belhumeur, Kriegman, and Yuille, 1999). Thus, a pattern of image shading provides sufficient information to specify the affine properties of an object, such as the parallelism of local surface patches or relative distance intervals in parallel directions, but it does not allow a unique determination of metric properties involving relative distance intervals in different directions. A similar ambiguity is also evident in judgments of 3D shape from shading by human observers. Recent psychophysical experiments have shown that these judgments are often idiosyncratic and task dependent (Koenderink et al., 2001), such that the correlations between observers or response tasks can in some cases be close to zero. Despite these variations in judged metric structure, however, the affine properties of perceived shape from shading have a high degree of reliability.

A fundamental assumption of almost all existing models of the perception of 3D shape from shading is that illumination and reflectance remain constant throughout a scene, such that all variations in shading can be attributed to the geometry of an observed surface. The problem with this approach, however, is that these assumptions are seldom satisfied in an unconstrained natural environment. Other common factors that can produce variations of image shading include the attenuation of light with distance, interreflections among different surfaces, variations in surface reflectance, cast shadows, specular highlights, and transparency. Existing computational models of 3D shape from shading cannot cope with any of these phenomena, yet human observers seem to have little difficulty in correctly identifying them.

Shape from Surface Contours and Texture

It has long been recognized that a convincing pictorial representation of an object can sometimes be achieved by drawing just a few critical lines, and there have been numerous attempts in both human and machine vision to analyze how line drawings of 3D scenes might be perceptually interpreted. The earliest models to address this issue were developed for interpreting line drawings of simple plane-faced polyhedra whose vertices are all formed by the junction of three faces. The different types of vertices that can arise in line drawings of these objects were exhaustively catalogued, and then used to label which lines in a drawing correspond to convex, concave, or occluding edges. Similar procedures were later developed to label line drawings of arbitrary polyhedral scenes (Malik, 1987), and to deal with other types of lines corresponding to shadows or cracks.

Another type of image feature that provides useful information for the perception of 3D shape is the contour that separates the visible and occluded parts of a smoothly curved surface. Indeed, an occlusion contour presented in isolation can often provide sufficient information to recognize an object, and to reliably segment it into distinct parts. Koenderink (1984) has shown that the relative sign of curvature at each point on a smooth occlusion contour uniquely specifies the sign of Gaussian curvature of visible surface regions in its immediate local neighborhood. More recent research has combined this analysis with earlier work on polyhedral objects to perform edge labeling on complex surfaces with both smoothly curved and faceted regions (Malik, 1987).

Still another important source of information for the perception of 3D shape comes from patterns of reflectance on smoothly curved surfaces, which are often referred to as texture. Some popular textures that are used in optical art for creating an appearance of 3D shape include random patterns of polka dots or networks of roughly parallel contours (see Todd and Oomes, 2002). Several potential models have been proposed for the computational analysis of these patterns. Some of these models are based on the assumption that all texture elements are approximately circular. Others assume that the depicted surface is singly curved, and that the contours lie along lines of curvature or surface geodesics (e.g., Knill, 2001). The empirical evidence suggests, however, that these assumptions are too restrictive to account for the perceptions of human observers (Todd and Oomes, 2002). A more general approach to this problem has recently been developed by Malik and Rosenholtz (1997). This approach computes local surface structure by measuring the affine distortions between texture patches in neighboring image regions, based on a more ecologically reliable assumption about texture homogeneity.

Shape from Binocular Disparity

Some of the most powerful analyses for estimating 3D shape from visual information are designed to exploit the systematic transformations of optical structure that occur when an object is viewed over multiple vantage points. For example, human observers have two eyes with overlapping visual fields, such that each eye receives a slightly different view of the same scene. It is especially interesting to note that binocular overlap reduces the size of the combined visual field relative to what would otherwise be possible if the two eyes faced in opposite directions, as is the case with many other animals. For the ecology of human observers, however, this cost is apparently outweighed by the useful information that is provided by the disparities between each eye's view in the region of overlap.

In order to compute 3D shape from binocular disparity, it is first necessary to determine the correspondence relations between the patterns of stimulation in each eye. The difficulty of this problem is demonstrated most clearly by the ability of observers to perceive 3D structure from random dot stereograms, in which each stereoscopic half-image contains a dense configuration of small dots. For any given dot presented to one eye, the visual system must somehow determine a single corresponding dot with which it should be matched among the many possible targets presented to the other.

Numerous computational models have been developed for solving this stereo correspondence problem, many of which are designed to simulate the physiological properties of the primate visual system (see Anderson and Julesz, 1995, for a recent review).

Like other sources of visual information, the horizontal disparity between each eye's view is inherently ambiguous with respect to the metric structure of an observed scene. The ambiguity in this case arises from the fact that the disparity produced by a given depth interval varies with viewing distance. In principle, there are a variety of ways that disparity could be scaled based on other sources of information, such as knowledge of the convergence angle or an analysis of vertical disparities, but there is considerable evidence to indicate that human observers are incapable of doing so with any reasonable degree of accuracy. Although observers can make accurate judgments about some aspects of 3D shape from stereoscopic vision, their judgments of metric structure typically exhibit large systematic distortions, even when viewing real 3D scenes in a fully illuminated natural environment (see Hecht, van Doorn, and Koenderink, 1999).

A fundamental assumption for most existing models of binocular stereopsis is that the corresponding features in each eye's view are projectively related to the same physical points in 3D space. This assumption is generally valid for certain types of image structures, such as those that arise from discontinuities of surface orientation or surface reflectance, but there other types of optical phenomena for which this assumption can be violated. There are two important cases that need to be considered in this regard. One is the occurrence of features that are occluded in one eye but not the other, which are sometimes referred to as half-occlusions. These would be treated as noise by most existing models of binocular stereopsis, but there is a growing body of evidence to indicate that they provide an important source of information for human perception (Anderson and Julesz, 1995). A second important case to consider is the occurrence of optical structures such as smooth occlusion contours or specular highlights, whose location on a surface varies with viewing direction. Because each eye sees these structures at a different surface location, their binocular disparities should therefore provide misleading information about 3D shape. Recent evidence suggests, however, that highlights and smooth occlusions provide perceptually useful information that enhances the appearance of stereoscopic depth (Todd et al., 1997).

Shape from Motion

Another relevant source of information for the perceptual analysis of 3D shape includes the systematic transformations of optical structure that occur when an object is observed in motion. The analysis of structure from motion is similar in some respects to the analysis of shape from binocular disparity in that it generally requires two distinct stages of processing. The first of these stages is to compute an optical flow field from changing patterns of light on the retina, and numerous models have been proposed to describe how this process is accomplished within the primate visual system (see Watanabe, 1998, chaps. 4–6).

The next stage of the problem is to incorporate these motion measures to estimate the 3D structure of an observed scene. When an object rotates in depth under appropriate conditions, its pattern of projected motion over three or more views provides sufficient information to determine its complete metric structure. However, there is a growing body of evidence that human observers have low sensitivity to this information and that the perception of 3D structure from motion is primarily determined by first-order relations between pairs of views (Watanabe, 1998, chap. 12). First-order motion measures under weak perspective are similar to shading in that they allow an infinity of possible 3D interpretations that are all related by an affine transformation (Koenderink and van

Doorn, 1991). Thus, they can uniquely specify the affine structure of an object, while being inherently ambiguous with respect to metric structure. A similar distinction between these structural attributes is also characteristic of human perception. Observers are often quite accurate at judging structural properties that are uniquely specified by first-order motion measures, whereas judgments of metric structure are inaccurate and unreliable.

Another similarity between models for computing 3D shape from motion or binocular disparity is their dependence on a limited subset of the possible optical structures that can occur under natural conditions. Most shape-from-motion algorithms are based on a strong assumption that moving features within a visual image remain projectively attached to fixed locations on an object's surface, but a wide variety of common optical phenomena violate this assumption. These phenomena include the deformations of smooth occlusion contours and specular highlights, which do not remain fixed on an object's surface when it is observed in motion. Similarly, when an object moves relative to its sources of illumination, then the optical deformations of shadows and lambertian shading will violate this assumption as well. Although these aspects of optical motion are degenerate for most current models, they are easily interpretable for human observers (Norman and Todd, 1994).

Shape from Multiple Sources

All of the models considered thus far are designed to be used with a particular source of information presented in isolation. Under natural viewing conditions, of course, it is likely that these different sources of information would occur in combination with one another, thus providing a certain degree of redundancy for the perceptual specification of 3D shape. The presence of these redundancies could be potentially quite useful for resolving ambiguities that are often inherent in visual information. If two sources of information allow different families of possible interpretations, then their simultaneous occurrence could be used to mutually constrain those interpretations in order to obtain a more accurate estimate of 3D metric structure. There is some disagreement in the literature about the extent to which this strategy can be exploited in human perception. A majority of investigators have found, however, that observers' judgments of 3D metric structure are inaccurate and unreliable even when multiple sources of information are available simultaneously (e.g., Tittle et al., 1995).

Discussion

A fundamental problem for the computational analysis of 3D shape from various aspects of optical stimulation is that most known sources of visual information are inherently ambiguous with respect to the precise metric structure of an observed scene. There are two general strategies for dealing with problems. One is to incorporate prior assumptions about environmental constraints to limit the set of possible interpretations. The primary weakness of this approach is that it will produce large systematic errors when objects are observed in an unconstrained natural environment, in which these assumptions may frequently be violated. An alternative strategy that seems to be more characteristic of human perception is to limit the analysis of shape to those structural properties that can be estimated with a higher degree of confidence. Depending on the particular source of information being analyzed, this could involve a perceptual representation of affine, ordinal, or topological relations. The evidence suggests that biological visual systems prefer robustness over precision.

Another important problem for the computational analysis of 3D shape from visual information is that changes in image intensity can be caused by a wide variety of environmental phenomena, including surface occlusions, specular highlights, transparency, variations in surface reflectance, variations in the pattern of illumination, and smooth or abrupt changes in surface orientation. Because all current models of 3D shape perception are appropriate for just a limited subset of these phenomena, their successful application in an unconstrained environment would seem to require an early-level process for labeling image intensity changes. It is interesting to note that contour labeling is one of the oldest problems in computational vision, but the successes in this area have been largely limited to line drawings (see Malik, 1987). In order to develop more robust models of 3D shape estimation, it is important that this work be extended to include natural scenes with shading and texture.

Road Map: Vision
Related Reading: Object Structure, Visual Processing; Stereo Correspondence; Tensor Voting and Visual Segmentation

References

Anderson, B. L., and Julesz, B., 1995, A theoretical analysis of illusory contour formation in stereopsis, *Psychol. Rev.*, 102:705–743.

Belhumeur, P. N., Kriegman, D. J., and Yuille, A. L., 1999, The bas-relief ambiguity, *Int. J. Comput. Vision*, 35:33–44.

Hecht, H., van Doorn, A., and Koenderink, J. J., 1999, Compression of visual space in natural scenes and in their photographic counterparts, *Percept. Psychophys.*, 61:1269–1286.

Horn, B. K. P., and Brooks, M. J., 1989, *Shape from Shading*, Cambridge, MA: MIT Press.

Knill, D. C., 2001, Contour into texture: Information content of surface contours and texture flow, *J. Opt. Soc. Am. A*, 18:12–35.

Koenderink, J. J., 1984, What does the occluding contour tell us about solid shape? *Perception*, 13:321–330.

Koenderink, J. J., and van Doorn, A. J., 1991, Affine structure from motion, *J. Opt. Soc. Am. A*, 8:377–385.

Koenderink, J. J., van Doorn, A. J., Kappers, A. M. L., and Todd, J. T., 2001, Ambiguity and the "mental eye" in pictorial relief, *Perception*, 30:431–448.

Malik, J., 1987, Interpreting line drawings of curved objects, *Int. J. Comput. Vision*, 1:73–103.

Malik, J., and Rosenholtz, R., 1997, Computing local surface orientation and shape from texture for curved surfaces, *Int. J. Comput. Vision*, 23:149–168.

Norman, J. F., and Todd, J. T., 1994, The perception of rigid motion in depth from the optical deformations of shadows and occlusion boundaries, *J. Exp. Psychol. Hum. Percept. Perform.*, 20:343–356.

Tittle, J. S., Todd, J. T., Perotti, V. J., and Norman, J. F., 1995, The systematic distortion of perceived 3D structure from motion and binocular stereopsis, *J. Exp. Psychol. Hum. Percept. Perform.*, 21:663–678.

Todd, J. T., Norman, J. F., Koenderink, J. J., and Kappers, A. M. L., 1997, Effects of texture, illumination and surface reflectance on stereoscopic shape perception, *Perception*, 26:806–822.

Todd, J. T., and Oomes, A. H. J., 2002, Generic and nongeneric conditions for the perception of surface shape from texture, *Vision Res.*, 42:837–850.

Watanabe, T., 1998, *High-Level Motion Processing: Computational, Neurobiological, and Psychophysical Perspectives*, Cambridge, MA: MIT Press.

Perceptrons, Adalines, and Backpropagation

Bernard Widrow and Michael A. Lehr

Introduction

The field of neural networks has enjoyed major advances since 1960, a year which saw the introduction of two of the earliest feedforward neural network algorithms: the perceptron rule (Rosenblatt, 1962) and the LMS algorithm (Widrow and Hoff, 1960). Around 1961, Widrow and his students devised Madaline Rule I (MRI), the earliest learning rule for feedforward networks with multiple adaptive elements. The major extension of the feedforward neural network beyond Madaline I took place in 1971, when Paul Werbos developed a backpropagation algorithm for training multilayer neural networks. He first published his findings in 1974 in his doctoral dissertation (see BACKPROPAGATION: GENERAL PRINCIPLES). Werbos's work remained almost unknown in the scientific community until 1986, when Rumelhart, Hinton, and Williams (1986) rediscovered the technique and, within a clear framework, succeeded in making the method widely known.

The development of backpropagation has made it possible to attack problems requiring neural networks with high degrees of nonlinearity and precision (Widrow and Lehr, 1990; Widrow, Rumelhart, and Lehr, 1994). Backpropagation networks with fewer than 150 neural elements have been successfully applied to vehicular control simulations, speech generation, and undersea mine detection. Small networks have also been used successfully in airport explosive detection, expert systems, and scores of other applications. Furthermore, efforts to develop parallel neural network hardware are advancing rapidly, and these systems are now becoming available for attacking more difficult problems such as continuous speech recognition.

The networks used to solve the above applications varied widely in size and topology. A basic component of nearly all neural networks, however, is the adaptive linear combiner.

The Adaptive Linear Combiner

The adaptive linear combiner has as output a linear combination of its inputs. In a digital implementation, this element receives at time k an input signal vector or input pattern vector $\mathbf{X}_k = [x_0, x_{1_k}, x_{2_k}, \ldots, x_{n_k}]^T$ and a desired response d_k, a special input used to effect learning. The components of the input vector are weighted by a set of coefficients, the weight vector $\mathbf{W}_k = [w_{0_k}, w_{1_k}, w_{2_k}, \ldots, w_{n_k}]^T$. The sum of the weighted inputs is then computed, producing a linear output, the inner product $s_k = \mathbf{X}_k^T \mathbf{W}_k$. The components of $\mathbf{X}_k$ may be either continuous analog values or binary values. The weights are essentially continuously variable and can take on negative as well as positive values.

During the training process, input patterns and corresponding desired responses are presented to the linear combiner. An adaptation algorithm automatically adjusts the weights so the output responses to the input patterns will be as close as possible to their respective desired responses. In signal processing applications, the most popular method for adapting the weights is the simple LMS (least mean square) algorithm (Widrow and Hoff, 1960), often called the Widrow-Hoff Delta Rule (Rumelhart et al., 1986). This algorithm minimizes the sum of squares of the linear errors over the training set. The linear error ε_k is defined to be the difference between the desired response d_k and the linear output s_k during presentation k. Having this error signal is necessary for adapting the weights. Both the LMS rule and Rosenblatt's perceptron rule will be detailed in later sections.

An important element used in many neural networks is the ADaptive LInear NEuron, or *adaline* (Widrow and Hoff, 1960). In the neural network literature, such elements are often referred to as *adaptive neurons*. The adaline is an adaptive threshold logic element. It consists of an adaptive linear combiner cascaded with a hard-limiting quantizer that is used to produce a binary ± 1 output, $y_k = \text{sgn}(s_k)$. A bias weight, *threshold*, w_{0_k}, which is connected to a constant input, $x_0 + 1$, effectively controls the threshold level of the quantizer. Such an element may be seen as a McCulloch-Pitts neuron augmented with a learning rule for adjusting its weights.

In single-element neural networks, the weights are often trained to classify binary patterns using binary desired responses. Once training is complete, the responses of the trained element can be tested by applying various input patterns. If the adaline responds correctly with high probability to input patterns that were not included in the training set, it is said that generalization has taken place. Learning and generalization are among the most useful attributes of adalines and neural networks.

With n binary inputs and one binary output, a single adaline is capable of implementing certain logic functions. There are 2^n possible input patterns. A general logic implementation would be capable of classifying each pattern as either $+1$ or -1, in accordance with the desired response. Thus, there are 2^{2^n} possible logic functions connecting n inputs to a single binary output. A single adaline is capable of realizing only a small subset of these functions, known as the linearly separable logic functions or threshold logic functions. These are the set of logic functions that can be obtained with all possible weight variations. With two inputs, a single adaline can realize 14 of the 16 possible binary logic functions. The two it cannot learn are exclusive OR and exclusive NOR functions. With many inputs, however, only a small fraction of all possible logic functions are realizable, i.e., linearly separable. Combinations of elements or networks of elements can be used to realize functions that are not linearly separable.

Nonlinear Neural Networks

One of the earliest trainable layered neural networks with multiple adaptive elements was the *Madaline I* structure of Widrow and Hoff. In the early 1960s, a 1,000-weight Madaline I was built out of hardware and used in pattern recognition research (Widrow and Lehr, 1990). The weights in this machine were memistors—

electrically variable resistors, developed by Widrow and Hoff, that are adjusted by electroplating a resistive link in a sealed cell containing copper sulfate and sulfuric acid.

Madaline I was configured in the following way. Retinal inputs were connected to a layer of adaptive adaline elements, the outputs of which were connected to a fixed logic device that generated the system output. Methods for adapting such systems were developed at that time. An example of this kind of network is shown in Figure 1. Two adalines are connected to an AND logic device to provide an output. With weights suitably chosen, the separating boundary in pattern space for the system can implement any of the 16 two-input binary logic functions, including the exclusive OR and exclusive NOR functions.

Madalines were constructed with many more inputs, with many more adaline elements in the first layer, and with various fixed logic devices such as AND, OR, and majority vote-taker elements in the second layer. Those three functions are all threshold logic functions.

Multilayer Networks

The madaline networks of the 1960s had an adaptive first layer and a fixed threshold function in the second (output) layer (Widrow and Lehr, 1990). The feedforward neural networks of today often have many layers, all of which are usually adaptive. The backpropagation networks of Rumelhart et al. (1986) are perhaps the best-known examples of multilayer networks. A three-layer feedforward adaptive network is illustrated in Figure 2. It is "fully connected" in the sense that each adaline receives inputs from every output in the preceding layer.

During training, the responses of the output elements in the network are compared with a corresponding set of desired responses. Error signals associated with the elements of the output layer are thus readily computed, so adaptation of the output layer is straightforward. The fundamental difficulty associated with adapting a layered network lies in obtaining *error signals* for hidden-layer adalines, that is, for adalines in layers other than the output layer. The backpropagation algorithm provides a method for establishing these error signals.

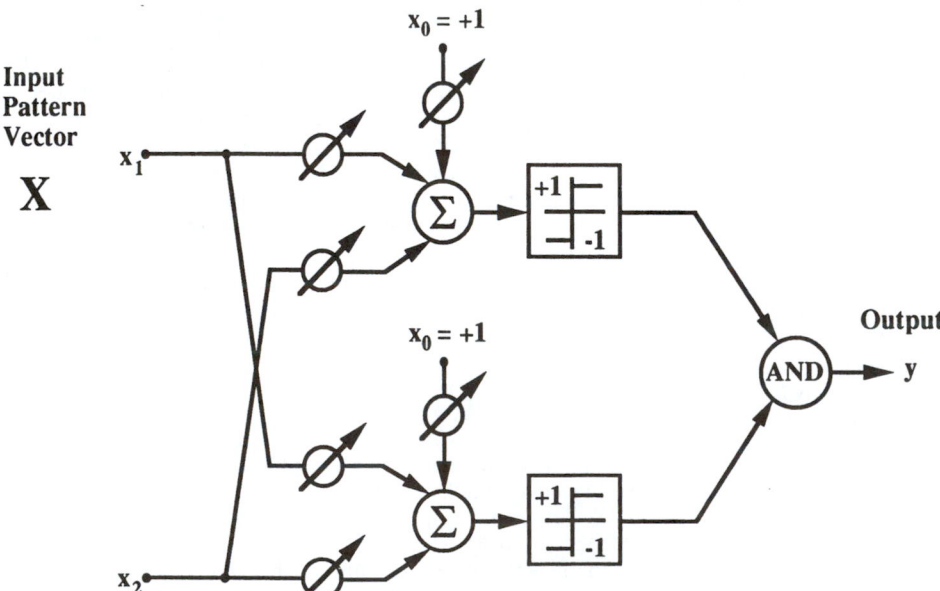

Figure 1. A two-adaline form of madaline.

Figure 2. A three-layer adaptive neural network.

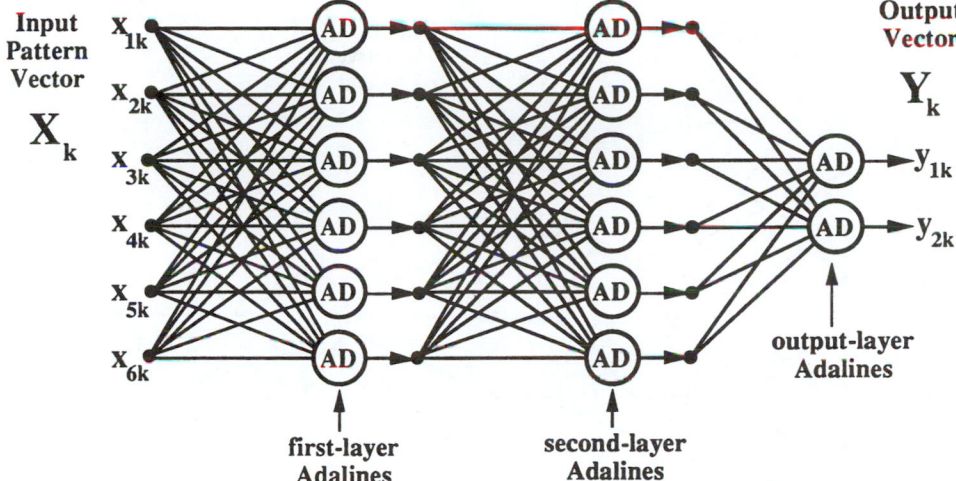

Learning Algorithms

The iterative algorithms described here are all designed in accord with the *Principle of Minimal Disturbance: Adapt to reduce the output error for the current training pattern, with minimal disturbance to responses already learned.* Unless this principle is practiced, it is difficult to simultaneously store the required pattern responses. The minimal disturbance principle is intuitive. It was the motivating idea that led to the discovery of the LMS algorithm and the madaline rules. In fact, the LMS algorithm had existed for several months as an error reduction rule before it was discovered that the algorithm uses an instantaneous gradient to follow the path of steepest descent and minimizes the mean square error of the training set. It was then given the name LMS (least mean square) algorithm.

The LMS Algorithm

The objective of adaptation for a feedforward neural network is usually to reduce the error between the desired response and the network's actual response. The most common error function is the mean square error (MSE), averaged over the training set. The most popular approaches to mean-square-error reduction in both single-element and multielement networks are based on the method of gradient descent.

Adaptation of a network by gradient descent starts with an arbitrary initial value $\mathbf{W}_0$ for the system's weight vector. The gradient of the mean-square-error function is measured and the weight vector is altered in the direction opposite to the measured gradient. This procedure is repeated, causing the MSE to be successively reduced on average and causing the weight vector to approach a locally optimal value.

The method of gradient descent can be described by the relation

$$\mathbf{W}_{k+1} = \mathbf{W}_k + \mu(-\nabla_k) \qquad (1)$$

where μ is a parameter that controls stability and rate of convergence and ∇_k is the value of the gradient at a point on the MSE surface corresponding to $\mathbf{W} = \mathbf{W}_k$.

The LMS algorithm works by performing approximate steepest descent on the mean-square-error surface in weight space. This surface is a quadratic function of the weights and is therefore convex and has a unique (global) minimum. An instantaneous gradient based on the square of the instantaneous error is

$$\hat{\nabla}_k = \frac{\partial \varepsilon_k^2}{\partial \mathbf{W}_k} = \begin{Bmatrix} \dfrac{\partial \varepsilon_k^2}{\partial w_{0k}} \\ \vdots \\ \dfrac{\partial \varepsilon_k^2}{\partial w_{nk}} \end{Bmatrix} \qquad (2)$$

LMS works by using this crude gradient estimate in place of the true gradient ∇_k. Making this replacement into Equation 1 yields

$$\mathbf{W}_{k+1} = \mathbf{W}_k = \mu(-\hat{\nabla}_k) = \mathbf{W}_k - \mu \frac{\partial \varepsilon_k^2}{\partial \mathbf{W}_k} \qquad (3)$$

The instantaneous gradient is used because (1) it is an unbiased estimate of the true gradient (Widrow and Stearns, 1985) and (2) it is easily computed from single data samples. The true gradient is generally difficult to obtain. Computing it would involve averaging the instantaneous gradients associated with all patterns in the training set. This is usually impractical and almost always inefficient.

The present error or *linear* error ε_k is defined to be the difference between the desired response d_k and the linear output $s_k = \mathbf{W}_k^{\mathrm{T}} \mathbf{X}_k$ before adaptation:

$$\varepsilon_k \overset{\Delta}{=} d_k - \mathbf{W}_k^{\mathrm{T}} \mathbf{X}_k \qquad (4)$$

Performing the differentiation in Equation 3 and replacing the linear error by the definition in Equation 4 gives

$$\mathbf{W}_{k+1} = \mathbf{W}_k - 2\mu\varepsilon_k \frac{\partial(d_k - \mathbf{W}_k^{\mathrm{T}} \mathbf{X}_k)}{\partial \mathbf{W}_k} \qquad (5)$$

Noting that d_k and $\mathbf{X}_k$ are independent of $\mathbf{W}_k$ yields

$$\mathbf{W}_{k+1} = \mathbf{W}_k + 2\mu\varepsilon_k \mathbf{X}_k \qquad (6)$$

This is the LMS algorithm. The learning constant μ determines stability and convergence rate (Widrow and Stearns, 1985).

The Perceptron Learning Rule

The Rosenblatt α-perceptron (Rosenblatt, 1962), diagrammed in Figure 3, processed input patterns with a first layer of sparse, randomly connected, fixed-logic devices. The outputs of the fixed first layer fed a second layer, which consisted of a single adaptive linear threshold element. Other than the convention that its input signals and its output signal were {1,0} binary and that no bias weight was included, this element was equivalent to the adaline element. The learning rule for the α-perceptron was very similar to LMS, but its behavior was in fact quite different.

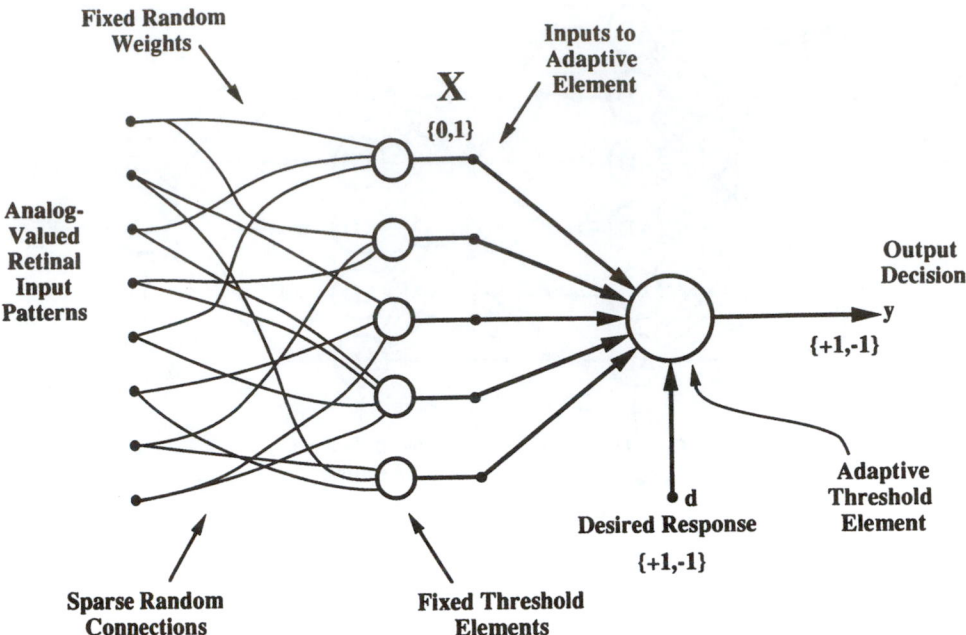

Fixed Random Weights

Inputs to Adaptive Element

Figure 3. Rosenblatt's α-perceptron.

X

{0,1}

Analog-Valued Retinal Input Patterns

Output Decision

y

{+1,-1}

Adaptive Threshold Element

Desired Response

{+1,-1}

d

Sparse Random Connections

Fixed Threshold Elements

Adapting with the perceptron rule makes use of the *quantizer* error $\tilde{\tilde{\varepsilon}}_k$, defined to be the difference between the desired response and the output of the quantizer

$$\tilde{\tilde{\varepsilon}}_k \overset{\Delta}{=} d_k - y_k \qquad (7)$$

The perceptron rule, sometimes called the *perceptron convergence procedure*, does not adapt the weights if the output decision y_k is correct, i.e., if $\tilde{\tilde{\varepsilon}}_k = 0$. If the output decision disagrees with the binary desired response d_k, however, adaptation is effected by adding the input vector to the weight vector when the error $\tilde{\tilde{\varepsilon}}_k$ is positive, or subtracting the input vector from the weight vector when the error $\tilde{\tilde{\varepsilon}}_k$ is negative. Note that the quantizer error $\tilde{\tilde{\varepsilon}}_k$ is always equal to either 1, 1, or 0. Thus, the product of the input vector and the quantizer error $\tilde{\tilde{\varepsilon}}_k$ is added to the weight vector. The perceptron rule is identical to the LMS algorithm, except that with the perceptron rule, one-half of the quantizer error, $\tilde{\tilde{\varepsilon}}_k/4$, is used in place of the linear error ε_k of the LMS rule. The perceptron rule is nonlinear, in contrast to the LMS rule, which is linear. Nonetheless, it can be written in a form which is very similar to the LMS rule of Equation 6:

$$\mathbf{W}_{k+1} = \mathbf{W}_k + 2\mu \frac{\tilde{\tilde{\varepsilon}}_k}{2} \mathbf{X}_k \qquad (8)$$

Rosenblatt normally set μ to 1. In contrast to LMS, the choice of k does not affect the stability of the perceptron algorithm, and it affects convergence time only if the initial weight vector is nonzero. Also, while LMS can be used with either analog or binary desired responses, Rosenblatt's rule can be used only with binary desired responses.

The perceptron rule stops adapting when the training patterns are correctly separated. There is no restraining force controlling the magnitude of the weights, however. The direction of the weight vector, not its magnitude, determines the decision function. The perceptron rule has been proved capable of separating any linearly separable set of training patterns (Rosenblatt, 1962; Nilsson, 1965). If the training patterns are not linearly separable, the perceptron algorithm goes on forever, and in most cases the weight vector gravitates toward zero. As a result, on problems that are not linearly separable, the perceptron often does not yield a low-error solution, even if one exists.

This behavior is very different from that of the LMS algorithm. Continued use of LMS does not lead to an unreasonable weight solution if the pattern set is not linearly separable. Nor, however, is this algorithm guaranteed to separate any linearly separable pattern set. LMS typically comes close to achieving such separation, but its objective is different, i.e., error reduction at the linear output of the adaptive element.

"Backpropagation" for the Sigmoid Adaline

A *sigmoid adaline* element incorporates a sigmoidal nonlinearity. The input-output relation of the sigmoid can be denoted by $y_k = \text{sgm}(s_k)$. A typical sigmoid function is the hyperbolic tangent

$$y_k = \tanh(s_k) = \left(\frac{1 - e^{-2s_k}}{1 + e^{-2s_k}} \right) \qquad (9)$$

We shall adapt this adaline with the objective of minimizing the mean square of the *sigmoid error* $\tilde{\varepsilon}_k$, defined as

$$\hat{\varepsilon}_k \overset{\Delta}{=} d_k - y_k = d_k - \text{sgm}(s_k) \qquad (10)$$

The method of gradient descent is used to adapt the weight vector. By following the same line of reasoning used to develop LMS, the instantaneous gradient estimate obtained during presentation of the kth input vector $\mathbf{X}_k$ can be found to be

$$\hat{\nabla}_k = \frac{\partial(\tilde{\varepsilon}_k)^2}{\partial \mathbf{W}_k} = 2\tilde{\varepsilon}_k \frac{\partial \tilde{\varepsilon}_k}{\partial \mathbf{W}_k} = -2\tilde{\varepsilon}_k \, \text{sgm}'(s_k)\mathbf{X}_k \qquad (11)$$

Using this gradient estimate with the method of gradient descent provides a means for minimizing the mean square error even after the summed signal s_k goes through the nonlinear sigmoid. The algorithm is

$$\mathbf{W}_{k+1} = \mathbf{W}_k + \mu(-\hat{\nabla}_k) = \mathbf{W}_k + 2\mu\delta_k\mathbf{X}_k \qquad (12)$$

where δ_k denotes $\tilde{\varepsilon}_k \, \text{sgm}'(s_k)$. The algorithm of Equation 12 is the *backpropagation* algorithm for the single adaline element, although the backpropagation name makes sense only when the algorithm is utilized in a layered network, which will be studied later.

If the sigmoid is chosen to be the hyperbolic tangent function (Equation 9), then the derivative $sgm'(s_k)$ is given by

$$sgm'(s_k) = \frac{\partial(\tanh(s_k))}{\partial s_k}$$
$$= 1 - (\tanh(s_k))^2 = 1 - y_k^2 \qquad (13)$$

Accordingly, Equation 12 becomes

$$\mathbf{W}_{k+1} = \mathbf{W}_k + 2\mu\tilde{\varepsilon}_k(1 - y_k^2)\mathbf{X}_k \qquad (14)$$

The single sigmoid adaline trained by backpropagation shares some advantages with both the adaline trained by LMS and the perceptron trained by Rosenblatt's perceptron rule. If a pattern set is linearly separable, the objective function of the sigmoid adaline, the mean square error, is minimized only when the pattern set is separated. This is because, as the weights of the sigmoid adaline grow large, its response approximates that of a perceptron with weights in the same direction. The sigmoid adaline trained by backpropagation, however, also shares the advantage of the adaline trained by LMS: it tends to give reasonable results even if the training set is not separable.

Backpropagation training of the sigmoid adaline does have one drawback, however. Unlike the linear error of the adaline, the output error of the sigmoid adaline is a nonlinear function of the weights. As a result, its mean square error surface is not quadratic, and may have local minima in addition to the optimal solution. Thus, unlike the perceptron rule, it cannot be guaranteed that backpropagation training of the sigmoid adaline will successfully separate a linearly separable training set. Nonetheless, the single sigmoid adaline performs admirably in many filtering and pattern classification applications. Its most important role, however, occurs in multilayer networks, to which we now turn.

Backpropagation for Networks

The backpropagation technique is a substantial generalization of the single sigmoid adaline case discussed in the previous section. When applied to multilayer feedforward networks, the backpropagation technique adjusts the weights in the direction opposite to the instantaneous gradient of the sum square error in weight space. Derivations of the algorithm are widely available in the literature (Rumelhart et al., 1986; Widrow and Lehr, 1990). Here we provide only a brief summary of the result.

The instantaneous sum square error ε_k^2 is the sum of the squares of the errors at each of the N_y outputs of the network. Thus

$$\varepsilon_k^2 = \sum_{i=1}^{N_y} \varepsilon_{ik}^2 \qquad (15)$$

In its simplest form, backpropagation training begins by presenting an input pattern vector $\mathbf{X}$ to the network, sweeping forward through the system to generate an output response vector $\mathbf{Y}$, and computing the errors at each output. We continue by sweeping the effects of the errors backward through the network to associate a *square error derivative* δ with each adaline, computing a gradient from each δ, and finally updating the weights of each adaline based on the corresponding gradient. A new pattern is then presented and the process is repeated. The initial weight values are normally set to small random values. The algorithm will not work properly with multilayer networks if the initial weights are either zero or poorly chosen non-zero values.

The δs in the output layer are computed just as they are for the sigmoid adaline element. For a given output adaline,

$$\delta = \tilde{\varepsilon}\, sgm'(s) \qquad (16)$$

where $\tilde{\varepsilon}$ is the error at the output of the adaline and s is the summing junction output of the same unit.

Hidden-layer calculations, however, are more complicated. The procedure for finding the value of $\delta^{(l)}$ the value of δ associated with a given adaline in hidden layer l, involves respectively multiplying each derivative $\delta^{(l+1)}$ associated with each element in the layer immediately downstream from the given adaline by the weight connecting it to the given adaline. These weighted square error derivatives are then added together, producing an error term $\varepsilon^{(l)}$, which in turn is multiplied by $sgm'(s^{(l)})$, the derivative of the given adaline's sigmoid function at its current operating point. Thus, the δ corresponding to adaline j in hidden layer l is given by

$$\delta_j^{(l)} = sgm'(s_j^{(l)}) \sum_{i \in N^{(l+1)}} \delta_i^{(l+1)} w_{ij}^{(l+1)} \qquad (17)$$

where $N^{(l+1)}$ is a set containing the indices of all adalines in layer $l+1$ and $w_{ij}^{(l+1)}$ is the weight connecting adaline i in layer $l+1$ to the output of adaline j in layer l.

Updating the weights of the adaline element using the method of gradient descent with the instantaneous gradient is a process represented by

$$\mathbf{W}_{k+1} = \mathbf{W}_k + \mu(-\hat{\mathbf{V}}_k) = \mathbf{W}_k + 2\mu\delta_k\mathbf{X}_k \qquad (18)$$

where $\mathbf{W}$ is the adaline's weight vector and $\mathbf{X}$ is the vector of inputs to the adaline. Thus, after backpropagating all square error derivatives, we complete a backpropagation iteration by adding to each weight vector the corresponding input vector scaled by the associated square error derivative. Equations 16, 17, and 18 comprise the general weight update rule of the back propagation algorithm for layered neural networks.

Many useful techniques based on the backpropagation algorithm have been developed. One popular method, called *backpropagation through time*, allows dynamical recurrent networks to be trained. Essentially, this is accomplished by running the recurrent neural network for several time steps and then "unrolling" the network in time. This results in a virtual network with a number of layers equal to the product of the original number of layers and the number of time steps. The ordinary backpropagation algorithm is then applied to this virtual network and the result is used to update the weights of the original network. This approach was used by Nguyen and Widrow (1989) to enable a neural network to learn without a teacher how to back up a computer-simulated trailer truck to a loading dock (Figure 4). This is a complicated and highly nonlinear steering task. Nevertheless, with just six inputs providing information about the current position of the truck, a two-layer neural network with only 26 sigmoid adalines was able to learn of its own accord to solve this problem. Once trained, the network could successfully back up the truck from any initial position and orientation in front of the loading dock.

Discussion

Although this article has focused on pattern classification issues, nonlinear neural networks are equally useful for such tasks as interpolation, system modeling, state estimation, adaptive filtering, and nonlinear control. Unlike their linear counterparts, which have a long track record of success, nonlinear neural networks have only recently begun proving themselves in commercial applications. The capabilities of multielement neural networks have improved markedly since the introduction of Madaline Rule I. This has resulted largely from development of the backpropagation algorithm, easily the most useful and popular neural network training algorithm currently available. As we have seen, backpropagation is a generalization of LMS that allows complex networks of sigmoid adalines to be efficiently adapted. Backpropagation and related algorithms

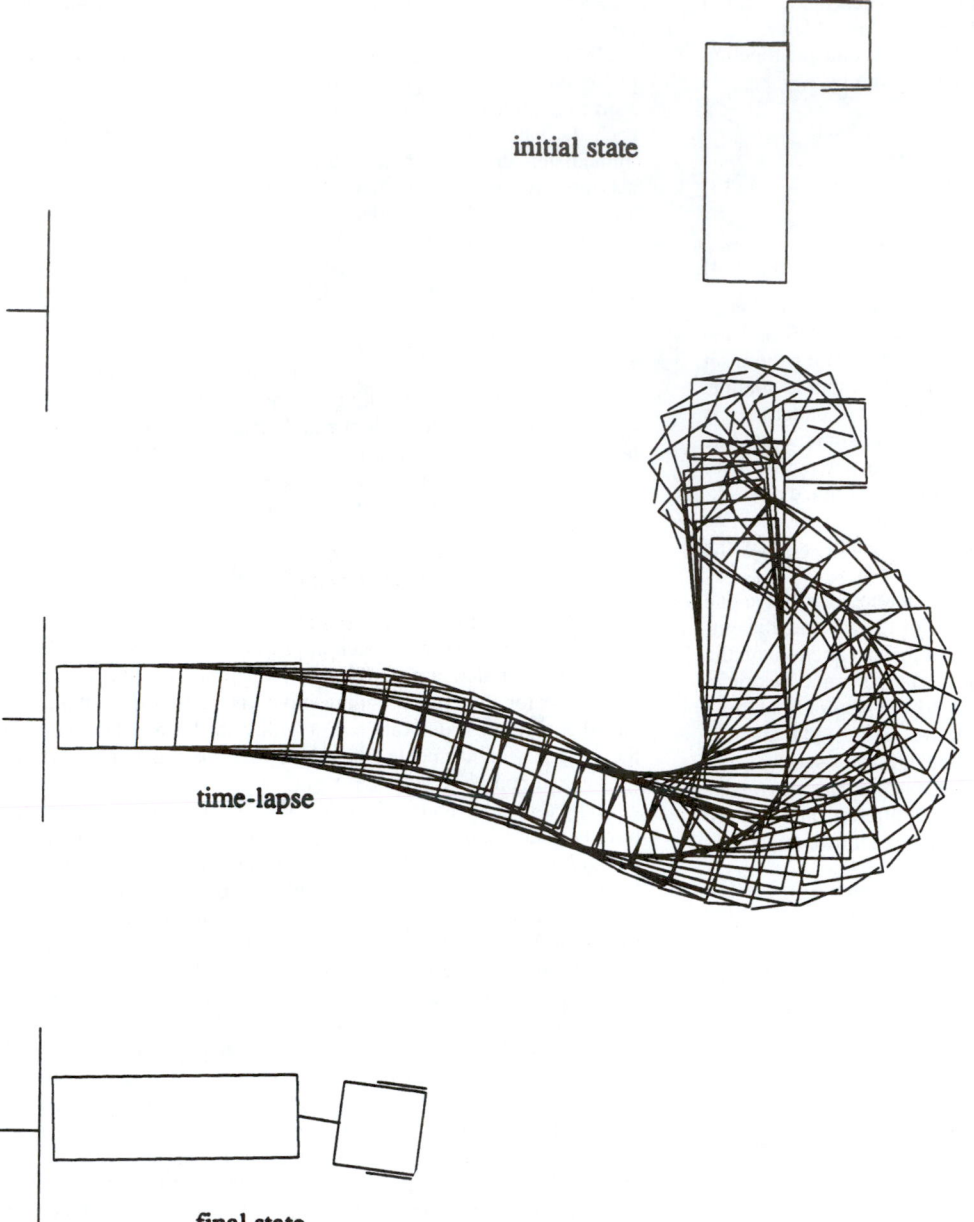

initial state

time-lapse

final state

Figure 4. Example of a truck backup sequence.

are in large part responsible for the dramatic growth the field of neural networks is currently experiencing.

The timing of the current boom in the field of neural networks is also due to the rapid advance in computer and microprocessor performance, which continues to improve the feasibility and cost-effectiveness of computationally expensive techniques in relation to classical approaches of engineering and statistics. Although single-element linear adaptive filters are still used more extensively than nonlinear multielement neural networks, the latter are potentially applicable to a much wider range of problems. Furthermore, the applications for which multielement neural networks are best suited often involve complicated nonlinear relationships for which classical solutions are either ineffective or unavailable. The continued advancement of neural network algorithms and techniques, in conjunction with improvements in the special and general purpose computer hardware used to implement them, sets the stage for a future in which neural networks will play an increasing role in commercial and industrial applications.

[Reprinted from the First Edition]

Road Maps: Grounding Models of Networks; Learning in Artificial Networks
Background: Dynamics and Bifurcation in Neural Nets
Related Reading: Identification and Control; Filtering, Adaptive

References

Nilsson, N., 1965, *Learning Machines*, New York: McGraw-Hill. ◆
Nguyen, D., and Widrow, B., 1989, The truck backer-upper: An example of self-learning in neural networks, in *Proceedings of the International*

Joint Conference on Neural Networks, vol. 2, New York: IEEE, pp. 357–363.

Rumelhart, D. E., Hinton, G. E., and Williams, R. J., 1986, Learning internal representations by error propagation, in *Parallel Distributed Processing: Explorations in the Microstructure of Cognition*, vol. 1, *Foundations*, (D. E. Rumelhart, J. L. McClelland, and PDP Research Group, Eds.), Cambridge, MA: MIT Press, chap. 8. ◆

Rosenblatt, F., 1962, *Principles of Neurodynamics: Perceptrons and the Theory of Brain Mechanisms*, Washington, DC: Spartan.

Widrow, B., and Hoff, M. E., Jr., 1960, Adaptive switching circuits, in *1960 IRE WESCON Convention Record*, Part 4, New York: IRE, pp. 96–104.

Widrow, B., and Lehr, M. A., 1990, 30 years of adaptive neural networks: Perceptron, madaline, and backpropagation, *Proc. IEEE*, 78:1415–1442. ◆

Widrow, B., Rumelhart, D., and Lehr, M. A., 1994, Neural networks: Applications in industry, business, and science, *Commun. ACM*, 37(3):93–105.

Widrow, B., and Stearns, S. D., 1985, *Adaptive Signal Processing*, Englewood Cliffs, NJ: Prentice-Hall. ◆

Perspective on Neuron Model Complexity

Wilfrid Rall

Introduction

There is a wide range of choice in model complexity, from very simple to rather complex neuron models. Which model to choose depends, in each case, on the context. How much information do we already have about the neurons under consideration? What questions do we wish to explore?

Sometimes we wish to model a particular biological neuron whose anatomy and physiology are known in considerable experimental detail. In such cases, we may choose to specify a model that includes at least some of the dendritic branching of the neuron, because synapses from one source may be distributed preferentially to either a distal or a proximal dendritic location, while synapses from another source may end mainly at the soma, or on a different dendritic tree of the same neuron. Also, there may be a functionally significant nonuniformity in the distribution of channel densities of several ion channel types over the surface of the soma and dendrites. How much detail is needed depends on the biological experiments to be simulated and the questions asked.

Conversely, many network modelers are not constrained by anatomical or physiological data. For some network modeling, this is partly justified by a paucity of available data. However, more often, network modelers are constrained by their mathematical methods, which lead them to focus on abstract networks composed of extremely simple units. The simplest units are two-state, binary units, analogous to atomic spin, previously studied for condensed matter physics (see, e.g., OPTIMIZATION, NEURAL). Such binary units do not resemble neurons, but they do have a strong appeal for nerve-net modelers, who have generated an extensive literature. That literature lies outside the scope of the current article.

When simple binary units are compared with a dendritic neuron model (especially with nonuniform distributions of synapses and ion channels), it becomes apparent that one dendritic model neuron can perform tasks that would require a network of many simple units to duplicate. For the purpose of machine design, it may seem quite appropriate to consider the trade-offs in cost and flexibility (between the one realistic model and the many binary units), but for functional insights and understanding of biological nervous systems, I freely state my bias for the more realistic neuron models. I do not choose the most complex, in the sense of including all known anatomical and physiological details; I favor an intermediate level of complexity that preserves the most significant distinctions between regions (soma, proximal dendritic, distal dendritic, different trees), especially when further justified by nonuniform distributions of synapses and ion channels (see also Segev, 1992).

The claim is sometimes made that network properties depend primarily on the connectivity between the units, and not on the properties of the units. Although this may be true for some gross network properties, I do not believe it to be true for many of the actual biological networks that perform important, complicated tasks. I regard it as a worthwhile challenge for like-minded neural modelers to provide interesting demonstrations in support of this belief. The challenge is to demonstrate a useful computation or discrimination that can be accomplished with a dendritic neuron model, or a network composed of such models, and then show that this useful capacity is lost when all of the dendritic membrane is lumped with the soma, and all of the inputs to each neuron are now delivered to that lumped membrane. There are valuable examples that already meet this challenge, several of which are presented in three later sections of this article. Other examples can be found in a review by Borst and Egelhaaf (1994; see also VISUAL COURSE CONTROL IN FLIES).

Brief Historical Notes

Neurons are biological cells, and their electrical properties depend on ions and the cell membrane, in a manner brilliantly elucidated by Hodgkin, Huxley, and Katz during the period 1948–1952. It is a fascinating historical coincidence that two seeds of their important insights can be found in a single 1902 volume of *Pfluegers Archiv*, in pioneering articles by Bernstein and by Overton. Following the earlier theoretical insights of Nernst and Planck, Bernstein recognized the importance of the potassium ion concentration difference across the membrane in determining a non-zero resting potential; he regarded excitation as a brief breakdown of the membrane, a concept that prevailed until 1948, when Hodgkin and Katz showed that the key is a sudden overwhelming increase in membrane permeability to sodium ions. Overton's 1902 paper had correctly emphasized the importance of the external sodium ion concentration to the excitability properties of nerve, but no one put these ideas together in 1902. Between 1900 and 1914, several investigators, including Hermann, Lucas, and Lapique, recognized the importance of membrane capacitance; the concept of nerve membrane as a leaky integrator, with a threshold for an action potential, was used to understand the strength-duration curve for a threshold stimulus. During the 1930s, several investigators, including Rashevsky, Hill, and Monnier, developed mathematical models of excitation and inhibition; Rashevsky's textbook *Mathematical Biophysics* (1948) includes many examples of network modeling by himself; by Householder, Landahl, and others; and by McCulloch and Pitts, whose famous 1943 paper arose in the context of Rashevsky's research seminars at the University of Chicago (see also the historical notes in Schwartz, 1990). Ever since that time, many neuron modelers have been content with the leaky integrator neuron model, which reduces a neuron to a single node that integrates synaptic excitation (+) and synaptic inhibition (−) delivered to it by other neurons. Several errors caused by these oversimple assumptions were demonstrated by compartmental computations in 1962; see Rall's chapter in Reiss (1964) or in Segev, Rinzel, and Shepherd (1995). Other chapters in Reiss (1964) also provide several interesting early perspectives on neural modeling. The mathematical modeling of nonlinear membrane properties has been presented and discussed in an outstanding early review by FitzHugh (1969), and in a chapter by Rinzel and Ermentrout that appears in Koch and Segev (1989).

The concept of a nerve axon as an extended core conductor (i.e., membrane cylinder with ionic conducting media inside and outside) goes back to the 1870s, when it was treated mathematically by Hermann and Weber; both the concept of passive electrotonus in membrane cylinders and the mathematics (of passive cable theory) were explored over the years, culminating in classic papers by Hodgkin and Rushton and by Davis and Lorente de Nó, both around 1946–1947; see references in Rall (1977). Before 1900, neuroanatomical studies by Ramón y Cajal demonstrated the extensiveness of dendritic branching for most neuron types; this was confirmed by many anatomists, and later (in the 1950s), use of the electron microscope made it possible to verify the existence of very many synapses on the dendritic branches and on the dendritic spines of neurons. These anatomical facts, together with the introduction of intracellular microelectrode recording from single dendritic neurons (in the 1950s), made it urgent to extend cable theory to the dendrites of individual neurons. This was begun in the late 1950s and carried forward into the 1960s and 1970s; for a review, see Jack, Noble, and Tsien (1975) or Rall (1977); see also Koch and Segev (1989), McKenna, Davis, and Zornetzer (1992), Rall et al. (1992), Segev et al. (1995), and DENDRITIC PROCESSING.

Dendritic Neuron Model Complexity: Geometric Versus Membrane Complexity

The concept of complexity in dendritic neuron models can be explored quite efficiently by making a two-dimensional chart. One dimension would be membrane complexity, ranging from the simple case of a passive linear membrane to that of postsynaptic membrane models with time-varying ion permeability (or conductance), and then to excitable membrane models with voltage-dependent ion conductances as described by Hodgkin and Huxley (see AXONAL MODELING), or as now described with increasing detail in terms of many different species of ion channels whose voltage and time dependence are currently being characterized (see ION CHANNELS: KEYS TO NEURONAL SPECIALIZATION). The other dimension would be geometric complexity, ranging from the simple case of an isopotential region of membrane (a soma, or a space-clamped section of a cylinder) to that of a uniform membrane cylinder with two sealed ends (or with one end voltage clamped, or current clamped), and then to several dendritic trees attached to a soma (with or without an axon), where the soma may be shunted and the branching of the trees may be specified to varying degrees of arbitrariness. The most complicated geometric case, with arbitrary branching and shunted soma, has recently been solved analytically (for transients, assuming passive membrane) in a mathematical tour de force by Major, Evans, and Jack (1993); see also Holmes, Segev, and Rall (1992). The less complicated, but illuminating, case of idealized branching with a point soma was solved earlier by Rall and Rinzel; see the 1973 and 1974 papers reprinted in Segev et al. (1995). However, these analytical methods do depend on the assumption of linear membrane properties. When nonlinear membrane complexity is combined with geometric complexity, the transient solutions can be obtained computationally by using compartmental models; see 1964 and 1968 papers reprinted in Se-

gev et al. (1995); see also DENDRITIC PROCESSING and several chapters in Koch and Segev (1989) and in McKenna et al. (1992).

Dendritic Model Can Provide Spatiotemporal Discrimination

Figure 1 summarizes a demonstration of how a dendritic neuron model could perform a discrimination between two contrasting spatiotemporal patterns of synaptic input (i.e., possible movement detection); this discrimination is lost if the compartments and inputs are lumped together. A neuron is represented by a chain of ten compartments; compartment 1 represents the soma, while compartments 2 to 10 represent dendritic membrane of the same neuron, with increasing cable distance from the soma. One spatiotemporal input sequence, A-B-C-D, has the proximal dendritic input first, followed in time by progressively more distal dendritic input locations. The other input pattern, D-C-B-A, is opposite in having the most distal input first, followed in time by progressively more proximal input locations. Comparison of the resulting computed voltage transients (EPSP at the soma), shown in Figure 1, reveals that input sequence D-C-B-A yields a significantly larger voltage amplitude than does input sequence A-B-C-D. Intuitive understanding of this computed result is obtained by noting that the delayed proximal input builds on membrane depolarization that has spread to the soma (with delay) from the distal dendrites (which were activated earlier). If the voltage threshold for spiking at the soma were tuned between these two peak amplitudes, a spike would be produced by sequence D-C-B-A, but a spike would not be produced by sequence A-B-C-D; this would constitute a discrimination between these two sequences. The dashed curve in the figure shows the computed result when the compartments are lumped together; either sequence of input synapse activation then produces the same intermediate result, and no discrimination would be possible.

Models for Mitral and Granule Cell Populations in Olfactory Bulb

A rather different example is provided by the neuron models used for the mitral cell and granule cell populations in simulating experiments on the OLFACTORY BULB (q.v.) of rabbit; see the 1968 paper of Rall and Shepherd in Segev et al. (1995); or see figures 2.11 and 2.12 in Koch and Segev (1989). Here, the task was to model and compute extracellular field potentials that matched those observed experimentally in olfactory bulb when the mitral cell population was activated in near synchrony by means of an antidromic volley. Compartmental models were used; a nine-compartment model (three axonal, one somatic, and five dendritic) was used to simulate antidromic activation of a mitral cell, while a ten-compartment model was used to simulate nonspiking activity in the dendrites of an axonless granule cell. The dendritic compartments were absolutely essential for the computation of electric current flow between different dendritic regions of each granule cell and between the dendrites and soma of each mitral cell; without these currents, it would have been impossible to compute the field potentials generated by the synchronously activated neuron populations. Also, this modeling led to a critically important distinction in the depth distribution of the two fields: the larger, longer-lasting field potentials generated by the very large population of granule cells extended to significantly greater depth in the olfactory bulb than did the earlier, smaller, briefer field potentials generated by the mitral cell population. The difference between these two fields was such that neither population could have generated the other field. This provided the key to our prediction of (and the functional interpretation of subsequent electron microscopic evidence for) dendrodendritic synaptic interactions between the mitral secondary dendrites and the distal dendrites of the granule cells, which are

Figure 1. Effect of spatiotemporal dendritic pattern of synaptic input on the computed EPSP at the soma, for a ten-compartment model. Upper diagram indicates the mapping of a soma and dendritic tree into a chain of ten equal compartments. Compartment 1 represents the soma membrane, while compartments 2 to 10 represent dendritic membrane, from proximal to distal locations. The middle diagram (at left) shows the synaptic input sequence A-B-C-D, meaning proximal dendritic input location active first, followed by successive activation at increasingly more distal input locations; this input pattern produced the soma voltage transient (computed composite EPSP) labeled A-B-C-D at lower left. The middle diagram (at right) shows the opposite synaptic input sequence D-C-B-A, meaning distal dendritic input location first, followed by successively more proximal input locations; this input pattern produced a significantly different soma voltage transient (computed composite EPSP), having a delayed rise to a larger peak amplitude, labeled D-C-B-A. In both cases, each input compartment (shown in black) received a synaptic excitatory conductance pulse ($G_e = G_r$, for a duration 0.25τ) during one of the four labeled periods. The same total amount of synaptic input produced the dashed curve when the spatiotemporal pattern was eliminated by smearing the synaptic conductance in space and time ($G_e = 0.25\ G_r$, in eight compartments (compartments 2 to 9) for the full time duration from $t = 0$ to $t = \tau$). The membrane equivalent circuit (upper right) holds for each compartment. Further details can be found in the 1964 chapter by Rall in Reiss (1964), reprinted in Segev et al. (1995).

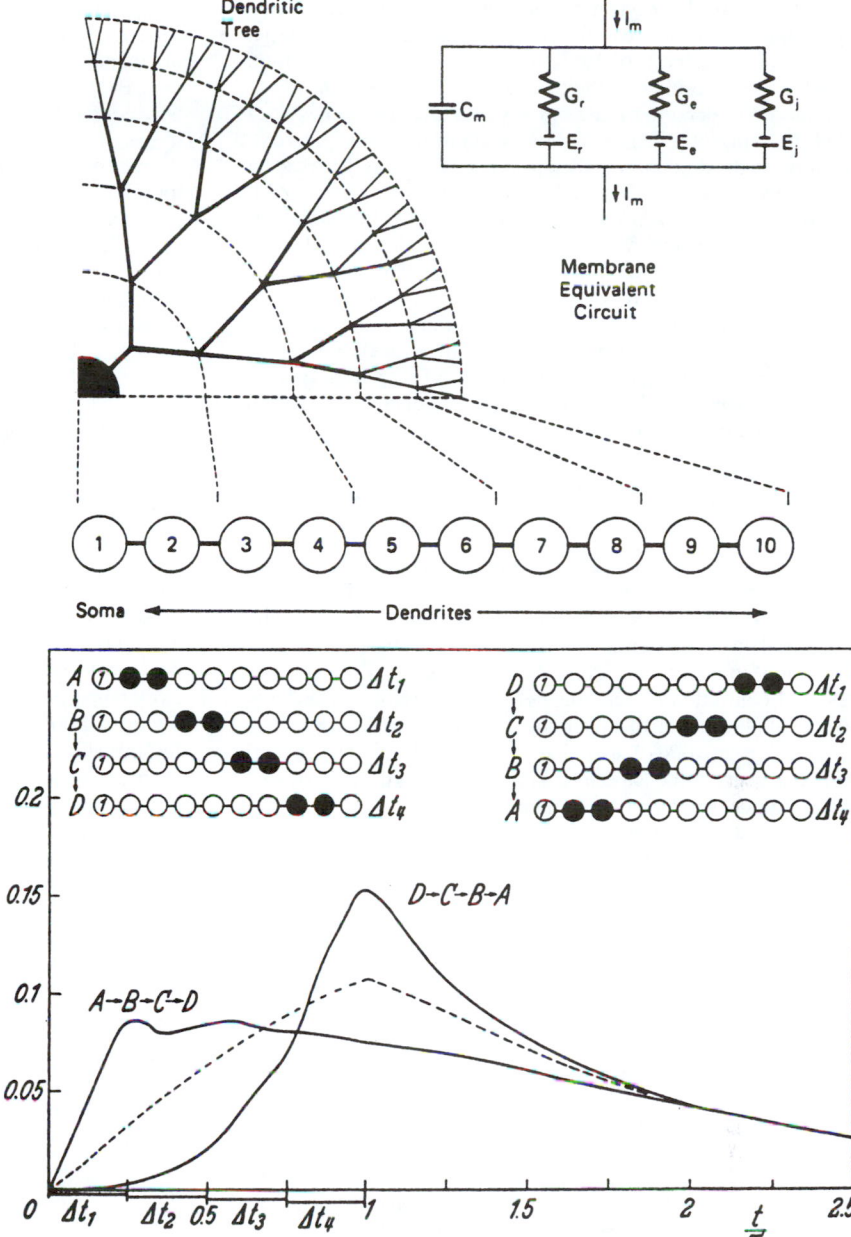

intermingled in the external plexiform layer of the bulb. If these cells had been modeled as lumped somas, without dendrites, neither the successful simulation of the experimental field potentials nor the exciting new insights about a dendrodendritic pathway for recurrent inhibition would have been possible.

Similarly, for the earlier simulations and insights obtained for motor neurons of cat spinal cord, we found that observations made at the soma seemed paradoxical until they were understood in terms of synaptic events that occur in distal dendrites (see the 1967 paper in Segev et al., 1995); these results and insights would not have been possible without dendritic compartments in the neuron field.

Comment on Functional Aspect of Dendrodendritic Interactions

To highlight an important functional difference, note first that motor neurons do exhibit the classical functional polarity envisaged by Ramón y Cajal and Sherrington (as well as most modelers). The dendrites receive inputs from many sources (their effects converge on the soma); the output (when spike threshold is exceeded) is an all-or-nothing action potential propagated by the axon to muscle units that may be quite distant; i.e., classically, input is received by the dendrites and output is delivered by the axon. In contrast, the dendrites of both the mitral cells and the granule cells are functionally different, because they both send as well as receive synaptic information, locally. The mitral secondary dendrites, which are smooth and spineless, send nonspiking synaptic excitatory output, which is received as input by the spines (see DENDRITIC SPINES) of the adjacent granule cells. The granule cells have no axons and perhaps no action potentials; their spines receive graded synaptic excitatory input and then send graded synaptic output that is inhibitory to the adjacent mitral cell dendrites. It is important to emphasize that this is not a rare anomaly found only in the olfactory bulb; evidence for dendrodendritic synapses and for graded local synaptic interactions is now found in many parts of the brain (e.g., retina and inferior olive). In 1965, when we (Rall et al.; see 1966 and 1968 papers reprinted in Segev et al., 1995) first presented our interpretations of dendrites that send as well as receive, some critics resisted this concept as heretical; however, our functional interpretation of these dendrodendritic synapses is now widely accepted by physiologists and anatomists. This kind of graded two-way synaptic interaction is very different from the classical functional polarity just described for motor neurons; it provides graded functional coupling between neurons (without axonal impulses). The implications have so far hardly been explored in theoretical networks. Such exploration will require explicit modeling of dendritic compartments; a point neuron model would be useless for this. Note also that computational exploration of localized plastic changes at synapses and at dendritic spines depends on neuron models that include dendritic compartments.

Network Rhythmogenesis Using the Traub Model and a Reduced Model

A 19-compartment cable model for the pyramidal cells of the CA3 region of guinea pig hippocampus was developed by Traub et al. (1991; see also the chapter by Traub and Miles in McKenna et al., 1992). Based on experimental measurements, parameters were chosen for each compartment, using up to six active ionic conductances, and controlled by ten-channel gating variables. They succeeded in finding a set of physiologically reasonable parameters for which the network of model neurons could simulate several important aspects of the experimental repertoire of the slightly disinhibited hippocampal slice preparation. Although Traub et al. recognized that their successful simulations of network behavior depended on specifying significantly different ion channel densities for the soma and for the dendrites, the critical importance of this difference was made starkly clear by the modeling of Pinsky and Rinzel (1994); they obtained essentially the same behavioral repertoire by using a network composed of a severely reduced neuron model consisting of only two compartments per pyramidal cell. One compartment represented the soma and proximal dendrites, while the other compartment represented the distal dendrites. To be more specific, the ion channels for fast-spiking currents (inward sodium, and delayed rectifier) were restricted to the soma-like compartment, and the ionic channels for the slower calcium currents (calcium-inward and calcium-modulated currents) were restricted to the dendrite-like compartment. I hasten to add that these results also show that at least two compartments are needed for simulations of this behavior; a single lumped compartment, with all of the ion channels in parallel, could not produce the same behavior, especially the rhythm, which basically involves an alternating flow of current between the two coupled compartments. A special advantage of the reduced neuron model is that much simpler computations can explore how much the interesting behavior depends on the values of key parameters, especially the parameter that defines the tightness of coupling between the two compartments. Also, the behavior of very large networks can be explored more efficiently using such a reduced neuron model. Further study may show that the two-compartment model cannot match the fuller model in certain important tests, but, in any case, these findings so far represent a very satisfying example that illustrates the thesis of this article.

Discussion

In an earlier essay offering perspective on neural modeling (a chapter in Binder and Mendell, 1990), I provided a completely different set of examples. One of these provided a detailed consideration of the number of degrees of freedom to be found in a neuron model composed of a thousand compartments. Such models exist today because of tremendous improvements in anatomical methods and in computation facilities now available to experimental investigators. Because they have the morphological data and a computer, why not put everything into the model? The answer is that you can if you wish to, but you should be aware of the huge number of degrees of freedom implied by the large number of parameters that must be specified; as someone once pointed out, given enough free parameters, he could fit an elephant. Is the membrane uniform, or do we know the density of every channel species in every membrane compartment? How are the inputs distributed to the many compartments? Today, the data needed for such detailed specifications are largely missing; however, such data are beginning to become at least partly available for some neurons. Where the data are not available, the modeler must make reasonable guesses. If it seems reasonable to assign the same parameter values to many neighboring compartments, one should consider lumping those compartments together to produce a simpler model with fewer compartments. Nevertheless, one important merit of the larger model is that it can be used to test whether it can perform some interesting task that cannot be performed by the reduced model.

As stated earlier, my preference is for intermediate levels of complexity; I vote for the smallest number of compartments that can preserve what one judges to be the functionally important differences between dendritic regions with regard to ion channel densities and to distributions of synapses from different sources. If a five-compartment model can provide a good approximation of the interesting properties of a 1,000-compartment model, I would prefer the smaller model, for two important reasons: (1) it helps sharpen our intuitive understanding about what is essential to obtaining the behavior of interest, and (2) it can greatly facilitate computations with networks composed of such neuron models. I expect modeling of this kind will continue to be particularly fruitful in the near future (see also the discussion by Segev, 1992).

Concluding Comment

As when drawing, painting, sculpting, or composing music, so too, when deeply engaged in neural modeling, I believe that much of the fun and satisfaction comes from interactions between my conscious mind and my subconscious sources of creativity. It seems that preliminary sketching serves to plant seeds in the subconscious, where they can grow, if nurtured. Conscious pursuit of the problem can then stimulate differentiation and development in the subconscious and may produce fruits that can reach conscious awareness (popping up like mushrooms produced by an underground mycelium). Such fruits may provide exciting new insights for the conscious mind. Indeed, the pleasure of such creative discovery can become almost addictive for those fortunate enough to have both the interest and the opportunity for creative activity. I hasten to add that a lot of hard work is usually required to test and polish before one can produce a finished product. Pioneering in dendritic neuron modeling provided me with such an opportunity; now [at the time of the First Edition], with retirement upon me, I hope to persist by sculpting, painting, and by designing a house for a natural mountain setting.

[Reprinted from the First Edition]

Road Maps: Biological Neurons and Synapses; Grounding Models of Neurons
Background: I.1. Introducing the Neuron
Related Reading: Dendritic Processing

References

Binder, M. D., and Mendell, L. M., Eds., 1990, *The Segmental Motor System*, Oxford: Oxford University Press.

Borst, A., and Egelhaaf, M., 1994, Dendritic processing of synaptic information by sensory interneurons, *Trends Neurosci.*, 17:257–263.

FitzHugh, R., 1969, Mathematical models of excitation and propagation in nerve, in *Biological Engineering* (H. P. Schwann, Ed.), New York: McGraw-Hill. ◆

Holmes, W. R., Segev, I., and Rall, W., 1992, Interpretation of time constant and electrotonic length estimates in multi-cylinder or branched neuronal structures, *J. Neurophysiol.*, 68:1401–1420.

Jack, J. J. B., Noble, D., and Tsien, R. W., 1975, *Electric Current Flow in Excitable Cells*, Oxford: Oxford University Press. ◆

Koch, C., and Segev, I., 1989, *Methods in Neuronal Modeling: From Synapses to Networks*, Cambridge, MA: MIT Press. ◆

Major, G., Evans, J. D., and Jack, J. J. B., 1993, Solutions for transients in arbitrarily branching cables: I. Voltage recording with a somatic shunt, *Biophys. J.*, 65:423–449.

McKenna, T., Davis, J., and Zornetzer, S. F., 1992, *Single Neuron Computation*, San Diego, CA: Academic Press. ◆

Pinsky, P. F., and Rinzel, J., 1994, Intrinsic and network rhythmogenesis in a reduced Traub model for CA3 neurons, *J. Computat. Neurosci.*, 1:39–60.

Rall, W., 1977, Core conductor theory and cable properties of neurons, in *Handbook of Physiology: The Nervous System: Cellular Biology of Neurons*, sect. 1, vol. I, part 1, chap. 3, Bethesda, MD: American Physiological Society, pp. 39–97. ◆

Rall, W., Burke, R. E., Holmes, W. R., Jack, J. J. B., Redman, S. J., and Segev, I., 1992, Matching dendritic neuron models to experimental data, *Physiol. Rev.*, 72:S159–S186. ◆

Rashevsky, N., 1948, *Mathematical Biophysics*, Chicago: University of Chicago Press; reissued 1960, New York: Dover.

Reiss, R., Ed., 1964, *Neural Theory and Modeling*, Stanford, CA: Stanford University Press.

Schwartz, E. L., 1990, *Computational Neuroscience*, Cambridge, MA: MIT Press. ◆

Segev, I., 1992, Single neurone models: Oversimple, complex and reduced, *Trends Neurosci.*, 15:414–421. ◆

Segev, I., Rinzel, J., and Shepherd, G. M., Eds., 1995, *The Theoretical Foundation of Dendritic Function: Selected Papers of Wilfrid Rall with Commentaries*, Cambridge, MA: MIT Press. ◆

Traub, R., Wong, R., Miles, R., and Michelson, H., 1991, A model of a CA3 hippocampal pyramidal neuron incorporating voltage-clamp data on intrinsic conductances, *J. Neurophysiol.*, 66:635–649.

Phase-Plane Analysis of Neural Nets

Bard Ermentrout

Introduction

Models of neural networks often involve the solutions to differential equations that describe the time evolution of these complex systems. The dynamical behavior of these networks ranges from the convergence to an equilibrium (generally desired in connectionist applications) to oscillatory behavior (in models of central pattern generators and bursting) through possibly chaotic behavior. There are many ways to analyze these models; the most commonly used techniques entail simulation. In this article I will give an overview of an alternative technique for studying the *qualitative* behavior of small systems of interacting neural networks. One form that the models take is (Ellias and Grossberg, 1975; Hopfield, 1984; Wilson and Cowan, 1972):

$$\tau_i \frac{dx_i}{dt} = -x_i + f_i\left(\sum_{j=1}^{n} w_{ij}x_j + s_i\right) \quad i = 1, \ldots, n \quad (1)$$

where x_i represents the activity or firing rate of the ith neuron, τ_i is the time constant, w_{ij} are the connection weights, s_i are inputs, and f_i are typically saturating nonlinear functions that have the form shown in Figure 1. That is, the nonlinear functions are increasing and bounded. Some typical examples are:

$$f(x) = \tanh(x) \quad (2)$$

$$f(x) = \tan^{-1}(x) \quad (3)$$

$$f(x) = \frac{1}{1 + \exp(-x)} \quad (4)$$

Often, a slightly different form of (1) is chosen where the nonlinearities are inside the sums. The transformation from one to the other is elementary and all of the following holds for either type of model.

A complete analysis of networks of the form in Equation 1 is obviously impossible. However, if $n \leq 2$, then a fairly complete description of Equation 1 can be given. Thus, the goal of this article is to introduce the reader to the qualitative theory of differential equations in the plane. In particular, I will analyze two neuron networks that consist of (1) two excitatory cells, (2) two inhibitory cells, and (3) an excitatory and an inhibitory cell. The advantages of restricting the analysis to these small networks are the special topology of the plane, the completeness of the analysis possible, and finally the case of exposition. Indeed, an overview of nonlinear dynamics can be obtained through these simple examples. Beer (1995) has attempted to exhaustively study the dynamics in the case $n = 2$ and gives a nearly complete overview of the possible types of behavior that can be expected. However, he does miss several interesting examples (Ermentrout, 1998, pp. 371–373). Another more general approach for the analysis of large numbers of coupled systems is to use bifurcation methods that enable one to *reduce* the dimensionality of the resulting equations and then apply techniques such as those used here. While planar systems may seem to be a rather extreme simplification, there is some justification for it. For example, in some local cortical circuits, there is no structure in the connectivity and there are essentially two types of neurons, excitatory and inhibitory. Thus, we can view the simple planar system as representing a population of coupled excitatory and inhibitory neurons. This approach was used successfully to study cortical processing in the rodent somatosensory system (Pinto et al., 1996) and to explain the effects of altering inhibitory interneurons in the hippocampus (Tsodyks et al., 1997).

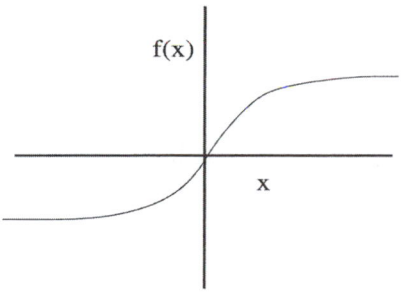

Figure 1. Typical nonlinear input-output function of a single model neuron.

The approach of this article is not restricted to neural networks and can be applied to a variety of other systems such as positive-feedback biochemical models (Segel, 1984), activator-inhibitor systems (Edelstein-Keshet, 1988), population and disease models (Murray, 1989), and membrane models of the action potential (Rinzel and Ermentrout, 1998). The techniques are powerful and provide insights into the behavior of these systems that would otherwise only be accessible through simulation. Computational methods are a very powerful adjunct to this type of analysis and, together with the qualitative analysis of this article, enable the researcher to understand his or her system.

In the next section, I will describe a pair of neurons coupled with mutual inhibition and mutual excitation. The penultimate section is devoted to a summary of the rich behavior of an excitatory-inhibitory pair. Finally, some comments on numerical methods and software close the review. In DYNAMICS AND BIFURCATION IN NEURAL NETS (q.v.), a systematic analysis of a particular case is given in order to illustrate alternative techniques.

Two Coupled Cells of the Same Type

In this section, we analyze the behavior of two cells that act via mutual inhibition or mutual excitation. I will use phase-plane analysis to draw a complete picture of the phase space.

General Considerations

Before analyzing the two-component neural network, I will first give a brief description of phase-plane techniques in general. Consider a planar differential equation:

$$x' = f(x, y) \qquad (5)$$

$$y' = g(x, y) \qquad (6)$$

At each point (x_0, y_0) there is a solution $(x(t), y(t))$ such that $(x(0), y(0)) = (x_0, y_0)$ and such that the tangent to the trajectory is $(f(x(t), y(t)), g(x(t), y(t)))$. Thus, at any point in the plane, one can easily determine the direction of the trajectory by simply evaluating f and g at that point. These directions enable one to paint a qualitative picture of the dynamics of Equations 5 and 6; i.e., I can determine where x and y are increasing and decreasing with time. The most crucial points are those values of x and y at which the direction of the trajectory changes. Thus, setting $f(x, y) = 0$ defines a curve in the plane where x does not change and breaks the plane into regions where x is either increasing or decreasing. This curve is called the x-nullcline. The curve $g(x, y) = 0$ defines the y-nullcline. The two curves together usually break the plane into regions of four distinct types: (1) x and y are increasing, (2) x and y are decreasing, (3) x increases and y decreases, and (4) x decreases and y increases. The intersection of the two nullclines occurs at points where both x and y are not changing, that is, at equilibria or rest states of Equations 5 and 6.

The behavior of trajectories away from equilibria is straightforward and is found by simply looking at the signs of f and g. Near the equilibria, one can look at the linearization of (f, g) about the equilibrium. This results in a two-by-two matrix called the Jacobian:

$$A = \begin{pmatrix} \dfrac{\partial f}{\partial x} & \dfrac{\partial f}{\partial y} \\ \dfrac{\partial g}{\partial x} & \dfrac{\partial g}{\partial y} \end{pmatrix} \equiv \begin{pmatrix} a & b \\ c & d \end{pmatrix} \qquad (7)$$

where the partial derivatives are evaluated at the equilibrium. The eigenvalues of A determine the behavior of the equilibria. If they both have negative real parts, the equilibrium is stable, and if any have positive real parts, the equilibrium is unstable. If both are real

and of the same sign, the point is called a *node*. Nodes consist of infinitely many trajectories emanating from (unstable) or entering (stable) the equilibrium. If both eigenvalues are complex, the rest state is a *vortex*, and trajectories spiral into (stable) or out of (unstable) the rest point. If the eigenvalues have opposite signs, the rest state is a *saddle point*. Then a single pair of trajectories that define the *stable manifold* or *set* enter the rest point, and a single pair of trajectories, defining the *unstable manifold*, leave the equilibrium. When the determinant of A (i.e., $ad - bc$) is negative, the rest point is a saddle; if it is positive and the trace of $A(a + d)$ is non-zero, the equilibrium is a node or vortex. Cases for which the real part is zero do not persist for small changes in the parameters and often indicate the appearance of new equilibria or periodic solutions. A simple necessary and sufficient criterion for linear stability is that the trace $a + d$ be negative and the determinant of A, $ad - bc$, be positive. A complete description of phase-plane methods can be found in Edelstein-Keshet (1988) and in most texts on ordinary differential equations.

Crossed Excitatory and Inhibitory Networks

The first result I want to establish in systems that have mutual coupling of the same sign is that periodic solutions are impossible. Once this is established, then a complete characterization can be made simply by studying the intersections of the nullclines.

Theorem 1. Suppose that $w_{21}w_{12} \geq 0$. Then there are no periodic solutions to

$$\tau_1 x_1' = -x_1 + f(w_{11}x_1 + w_{12}x_2 + s_1) \qquad (8)$$

$$\tau_2 x'_2 = -x_2 + f(w_{21}x_1 + w_{22}x_2 + s_2) \qquad (9)$$

As the proof of this theorem was given in the previous edition of the *Handbook* (p. 733, Theorem 1), I will not prove it again here.

All solutions to Equations 8 and 9 are bounded, and Theorem 1 implies that trajectories are monotone, so this means that all solutions tend to equilibria. This in turn means that the time constants can be set to 1 without loss of generality, as the dynamics is completely trivial. The intersections of the nullclines and some observations on the signs of the coefficients in the linearized matrix based on the nullclines allow one to completely determine the number and stability type of the equilibria.

Recall that f is increasing and bounded. Without loss of generality, one can assume that the minimum of f is 0 and the maximum is 1. f is invertible, and the inverse is also monotone, with asymptotes at 0 and 1. The formula for the x_1-nullcline is

$$x_2 = (-w_{11}x_1 - s_1 + f^{-1}(x_1))/w_{12} \qquad (10)$$

The x_2-nullcline satisfies:

$$x_1 = (-w_{22}x_2 - s_2 + f^{-1}(x_2))/w_{21} \qquad (11)$$

If $h(x) = (-w_s x - s + f^{-1}(x))/w_c$, then h is monotone if w_s is either positive or small and negative. However, if w_s is large enough, h develops a kink and is "cubic"-shaped (Figure 2A). If w_c is positive (mutual excitation) then $h \to -\infty$ as $x \to 0$ and $h \to \infty$ as $x \to 1$ (Figure 2A). When w_c is negative (mutual inhibition), the asymptotes are switched (Figure 2B). Finally, the stimulus parameter s merely translates the nullclines up and down in the case of the x_1-nullcline and left-right for the x_2-nullcline. The phase plane is easy to construct with these observations.

In both cases, there can be up to nine different equilibria, and there is always at least one. Figure 3 shows some typical configurations for mutually inhibitory interactions. To assess the stability of the equilibria, one need only look at the positions of the nullclines at the equilibria. Referring to Equation 7, I will use the nullclines to determine the signs and relative magnitudes of the entries

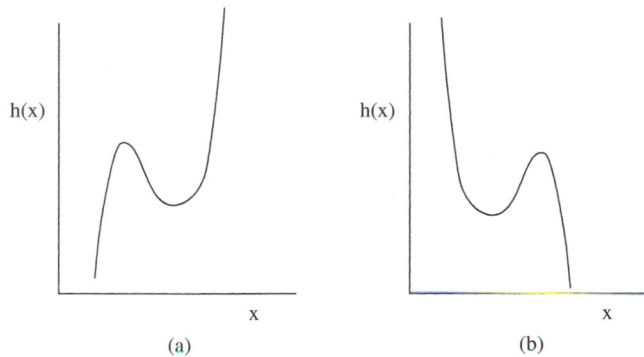

Figure 2. Nullcline shape for (A) mutual excitation and (B) mutual inhibition.

in this matrix. For mutually inhibiting cells, the following are necessary and sufficient for stability:

1. The slope of both nullclines is negative through an equilibrium.
2. The slope of the x_1 nullcline is steeper than the x_2 nullcline through the equilibrium.

If either of these is violated, the equilibrium is unstable.

For mutually excitatory cells, the conditions for stability are:

1. The slope of both nullclines is positive through an equilibrium.
2. The slope of the x_1 nullcline is steeper than the x_2 nullcline through the equilibrium.

Tangential intersections are saddle nodes and, as some parameter varies, will lead either to two new equilibria or to the disappearance of the pair. The matrix A has a zero eigenvalue when there are tangential crossings, for then the slopes of the nullclines are the same. That is, $-a/b = -c/d$, so $ad - bc = 0$. A bit of counting shows that when there are nine equilibria, four are stable nodes,

four are saddle points, and one is an unstable node. As the parameters vary, a pair of equilibria is lost, a saddle point and either a stable node or the unstable node, leaving seven equilibria. Further losses of equilibria (or gains, up to a maximum of nine) are obtained as the parameters vary, ending in the minimum of a single globally stable equilibrium.

When there are several stable equilibria, it is important to determine what initial conditions lead to which of the equilibria. The set of all initial data that tend to a particular equilibrium point is called the *domain of attraction* of the equilibrium point. For the present networks, this is very easy to determine geometrically. Figure 3 depicts a network of mutually inhibitory cells that has five equilibria (labeled *a–e*). The above discussion allows one to conclude that *a*, *c*, and *e* are stable nodes and *b* and *d* are saddle points. Each saddle point has associated with it one positive eigenvalue and one negative eigenvalue. Corresponding to this negative eigenvalue is the stable manifold for the saddle point. It consists of the set of all initial conditions that tend to the equilibrium point as $t \to \infty$. For two-dimensional neural nets, this is a one-dimensional set and is then often called a *separatrix*. I have drawn it for each of the two saddle points in Figure 3 as the dashed lines pointing into *b* and *d*. These curves divide the two-dimensional plane into three regions, which I have labeled *A*, *C*, and *E*. All initial data in *A* tend to equilibrium point *a*, and so on. Thus, although the saddle points are unstable, their stable manifolds provide the boundaries that determine the final states of the network given the initial state. From this description the reader should be able to construct complete qualitative pictures for other configurations of the nullclines for mutually excitatory or inhibitory nets.

Summarizing, I have used phase-plane analysis to show that for a pair of coupled neurons with mutual excitation or inhibition, the only stable solutions are equilibria. The stable manifolds of the saddle points divide the plane into domains of attraction for each of the stable equilibria. All equilibria are approached monotonically, and there can be up to four stable steady states.

A Pair of Excitatory and Inhibitory Cells

In many regions of cortex, and in fact throughout the central nervous system, many of the coupled excitatory and inhibitory cells

Figure 3. Phase plane for two mutually inhibitory neurons. Nullclines are solid lines and the stable manifolds of the saddle points *b* and *d* are shown dashed. *a*, *c*, and *e*, are stable nodes with domains of attraction *A*, *C*, and *E*, respectively. Insets show other some other possible nullcline configurations.

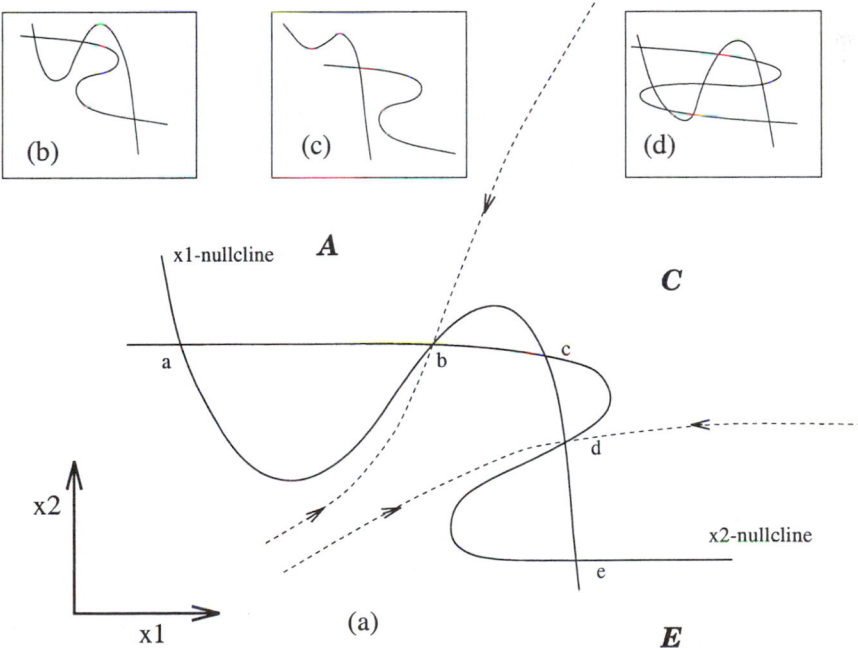

constitute a local neural network. These networks have been the subject of numerous mathematical and computational investigations (Wilson and Cowan, 1972; Ellias and Grossberg, 1975; Ermentrout and Cowan, 1979; Beer, 1995; Pinto et al., 1996). One can view such systems either as two neurons acting in isolation (a difficult experiment to imagine) or, more reasonably, as a two-layer network with spatially homogeneous activity. Then each component is the activity of a *pool* of cells rather than the activity of a single cell.

I will consider a network of the form:

$$x'_1 = -x_1 + f(w_{11}x_1 - w_{12}x_2 + s_1) \tag{12}$$

$$x'_2 = (-x_2 + f(w_{21}x_1 - w_{22}x_2 + s_2))/\tau \tag{13}$$

where all of the weights are non-negative. I have introduced a time constant for the inhibitory neurons because one cannot expect them to have the same temporal behavior as the excitatory cells. The Jacobian matrix $A = [\partial x'_i / \partial x_j]$ at an equilibrium point $(\bar{x}_1, \bar{x}_2)$ has coefficients:

$$a = -1 + w_{11}f'(w_{11}\bar{x}_1 - w_{12}\bar{x}_2 + s_1) \tag{14}$$

$$b = -w_{12}f'(w_{11}\bar{x}_1 - w_{12}\bar{x}_2 + s_1) < 0 \tag{15}$$

$$c = (w_{21}f'(w_{21}\bar{x}_1 - w_{22}\bar{x}_2 + s_2))/\tau > 0 \tag{16}$$

$$d = (-1 - w_{22}f'(w_{21}\bar{x}_1 - w_{22}\bar{x}_2 + s_2))/\tau < 0 \tag{17}$$

It is clear that all of the coefficients except for a have a fixed sign independent of the parameters. If $w_{11}f' > 1$, then $a > 0$, and the system is called an *activator-inhibitor* system, since x_1 activates both itself and x_2, while x_2 inhibits everything to which it connects. Activator-inhibitor models occur ubiquitously in biology, and their dynamics is rich and varied (see, e.g., PATTERN FORMATION, BIOLOGICAL). Oscillations, excitability, and multiple steady states are among the possible behaviors of these networks. Since a very complete analysis of these systems as applied to neural excitation is given in Rinzel and Ermentrout (1998), I only sketch some of the dynamic behavior possible for this network.

The qualitative behavior of any planar model can be understood by combining nullcline analysis with local stability analysis of the equilibria, which depends on the coefficients of the Jacobian A. The neural model studied in Rinzel and Ermentrout (1998) has exactly the same nullcline structure and has a Jacobian matrix with the same structure as the neural net model. Hence, I will only outline the dynamics of this system; details can be extracted from the aforementioned article.

It is instructive to first consider the effects of parameters on the shapes of the nullclines. A typical nullcline configuration is shown in Figure 4 for Equations 12 and 13. The x_2-nullcline is always monotonically increasing; w_{21} sharpens it, while w_{22} makes it shallower and s_2 shifts it left and right. As described earlier, the effect of w_{11} is to kink the x_1-nullcline, while w_{12} makes it less kinked; s_1 shifts it up and down. Finally, the parameter τ has no effect on the nullclines but dramatically alters the dynamics and stability of the equilibria. Changing τ has no effect on the determinant of A (so a saddle point cannot become a node), but it can switch the sign of the trace of A and so change a point from a stable node to an unstable node.

The positions of the nullclines make it clear that there can be up to five equilibria and at least one equilibrium point. Furthermore, all equilibria that occur on the "unkinked" part of the x_1-nullcline are necessarily asymptotically stable, since then $a < 0$ in Equation 14. Thus, the trace, $a + d < 0$, and the determinant, $ad - bc > 0$. If w_{11} is sufficiently small so that the x_1-nullcline is monotone, then there is only one equilibrium point, and it is globally stable. This statement follows from the facts that all solutions are bounded and from application of Bendixson's negative criterion (Edelstein-Keshet, 1988), which eliminates periodic orbits when $a + d < 0$. Any time the inhibitory nullcline has a lesser slope than the excit-

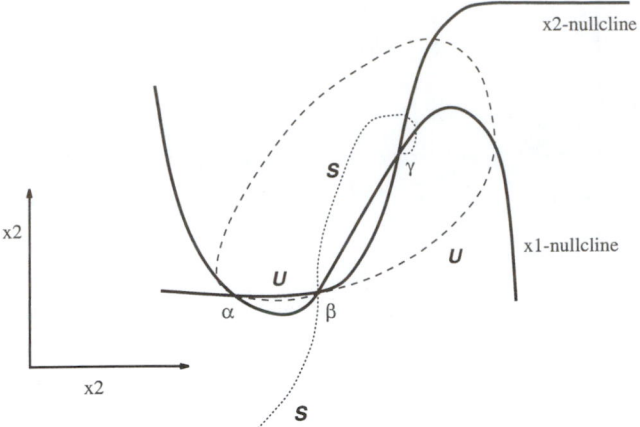

Figure 4. Typical phase plane for an excitatory-inhibitory pair. Nullclines and a typical trajectory are shown. There is a unique globally attracting equilibrium point.

atory nullcline, the equilibrium is a saddle point. These considerations, along with the preceding discussion, show how the parameters affect the local existence and stability of various rest states. The global dynamics is much more complicated since one cannot eliminate the possibility of limit cycle solutions.

Excitability

One important difference between networks consisting of one excitatory and one inhibitory layer and the networks described earlier in this article is the possibility of excitable dynamics. As was shown earlier, trajectories of the activity of cells are necessarily monotone. Thus, if, say, x_1 is increasing, then it can never decrease again. However, in mixed networks, no such restriction occurs, and it is possible for x_1 to initially increase before decreasing again. In particular, a network is said to be *excitable* if there is a *unique globally stable* rest state with the following property: Small perturbations from rest decay monotonically back to rest, but perturbations larger than some *threshold* continue to grow before decaying back to the stable rest state (Figure 5). There are at least two qualitatively different types of excitability for networks with the present structure. In type I excitability there are three equilibria, while in type II there is one. These two cases are described in Rinzel and Ermentrout (1998). In the context of neural networks, this type of behavior has been called an *active transient*. It can be viewed

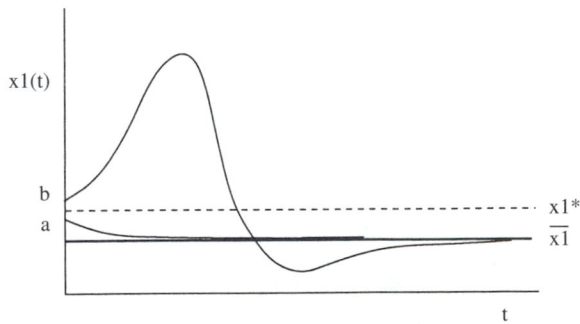

Figure 5. Excitable dynamics. $\bar{x}_1$ is the globally stable rest state and x_1^* is the threshold. Trajectory a is subthreshold and b is superthreshold.

as a transient excitatory activity due to a stimulus that is eventually quelled by the inhibitory interneuronal feedback.

Periodic Solutions

Periodic solutions occur generally (although not strictly) when there is a single rest state on the middle branch and it is unstable. This point must necessarily be a node, and the boundedness of solutions thus implies that a limit cycle exists. If some parameter (say τ) is varied in such a way as to make the unique equilibrium go from a stable point to an unstable point (without introducing any new rest states), then a *Andronov-Hopf bifurcation* generically occurs, and this implies that a periodic solution exists near the rest state. For planar systems, easily checked necessary conditions for an Andronov-Hopf bifurcation are that the determinant of A remain positive and the trace change from negative to positive as the parameter is varied. If this new limit cycle is unstable, then there can be regimens in parameter space where there are two stable behaviors: (1) a stable rest state and (2) a stable *large-amplitude* periodic solution (Figure 6). This is known as *bistability*.

Other Behavior

In addition to excitability, multiple equilibria, oscillations, and bistability, other types of dynamic behavior can be found in these simple models. Infinite period oscillations and homoclinic trajectories can be obtained in some parameter regimens. (A *homoclinic* trajectory is one that leaves a saddle point from one side and enters it from another, and can occur as the period of a limit cycle tends to infinity.) Homoclinics are important because they separate qualitatively different types of behavior. Furthermore, when one periodically stimulates a system with homoclinics, it is possible to obtain a complex irregular behavior called *chaos* that cannot occur in planar systems without forcing (see Guckenheimer and Holmes, 1983.)

There are many other pictures possible with this simple model and I urge the reader to explore the phase-plane dynamics of this excitatory inhibitory net. Phase-plane methods provide a powerful analytic and qualitative tool for studying small neural networks. When combined with sophisticated numerical tools, a complete understanding of the global dynamics is possible.

In systems with more than two components, it is difficult to make any general comments on behavior. For symmetrically coupled networks with no self-connections, a complete analysis can be given (Hopfield, 1982). Weakly coupled systems of intrinsically oscillatory networks can be analyzed with the techniques described in CHAINS OF OSCILLATORS IN MOTOR AND SENSORY SYSTEMS. Bifurcation methods and averaging techniques can often be used to reduce higher-dimensional systems to a simpler set of equations that is in a much lower dimension (see Hoppensteadt and Izhikevich, 1997; see also CANONICAL NEURAL MODELS).

Numerical Methods

The computer is a valuable adjunct in the exploration of systems of differential equations. For this article, I have used a program called XPPAUT that is available for both Windows 95/NT/98 computers (Winpp) and Unix workstations. Both are available through http://www.pitt.edu/~phase. To get *global* pictures of the dynamics as one or two parameters are varied, a powerful numerical package written by Doedel et al. (1997) called AUTO can be used. A version is available at http://indy.cs.concordia.ca/auto/.

Road Map: Dynamic Systems
Related Reading: Canonical Neural Models; Cortical Population Dynamics and Psychophysics; Dynamics and Bifurcation in Neural Nets; Pattern Formation, Neural

References

Beer, R. D., 1995, On the dynamics of small continuous time recurrent neural networks, *Adapt. Behav.*, 3:469–509. ◆

Doedel, E., Champneys, A., Fairgrieve, T., Kuznetsov, Y., Sandstede, B., and Wang, X. J., 1997, AUTO97: Continuation and bifurcation software for ordinary differential equations (with HomCont), Montreal: Computer Science Department, Concordia University.

Edelstein-Keshet, L., 1988, *Mathematical Models in Biology*, New York: Random House. ◆

Ellias, S. A., and Grossberg, S., 1975, Pattern formation, contrast control, and oscillations in the short-term memory of shunting on-center off-surround networks, *Biol. Cybern.*, 20:69–98.

Ermentrout, G. B., 1998, Neural networks as spatio-temporal pattern-forming systems, *Rep. Prog. Phys.*, 61:353–430. ◆

Ermentrout, G. B., and Cowan, J. D., 1979, Temporal oscillations in neuronal nets, *J. Math. Biol.*, 7:265–280.

Guckenheimer, J., and Holmes, P. J., 1983, *Nonlinear Oscillations, Dynamical Systems, and Bifurcations of Vector Fields*, Heidelberg: Springer-Verlag.

Hopfield, J. J., 1982, Neural networks and physical systems with emergent collective computational abilities, *Proc. Natl. Acad. Sci. USA*, 79:2554–2558.

Hopfield, J. J., 1984, Neurons with graded responses have collective computational properties like those of two-state neurons, *Proc. Natl. Acad. Sci. USA*, 81:3088–3092.

Hoppensteadt, F., and Izhikevich, E., 1997, *Weakly Connected Neural Networks*, New York: Springer-Verlag. ◆

Murray, J. D., 1989, *Mathematical Biology*, Heidelberg: Springer-Verlag.

Pinto, D., Brumberg, J., Simons, D., and Ermentrout, B., 1996, A quantitative population model of whisker barrels: Re-examining the Wilson-Cowan equations, *J. Comput. Neurol.* 3:247–264.

Rinzel, J., and Ermentrout, G. B., 1998, Analysis of neural excitability and oscillations, in *Methods of Neuronal Modelling: From Synapses to Networks*, 2nd ed. (C. Koch and I. Segev, Eds.), Cambridge, MA: MIT Press.

Segel, L. A., 1984, *Modelling Dynamic Phenomena in Molecular and Cellular Biology*, New York: Cambridge University Press.

Shepherd, G. M., 1990, *The Synaptic Organization of the Brain*, Oxford, Engl.: Oxford University Press.

Tsodyks, M. V., Skaggs, W. E., Sejnowski, T. J., and McNaughton, B. L., 1997, Paradoxical effects of external modulation of inhibitory interneurons, *J. Neurosci.*, 17:4382–4388.

Wilson, H. R., and Cowan, J. D., 1972, Excitatory and inhibitory interactions in localized populations of model neurons, *Biophys. J.*, 12:1–24.

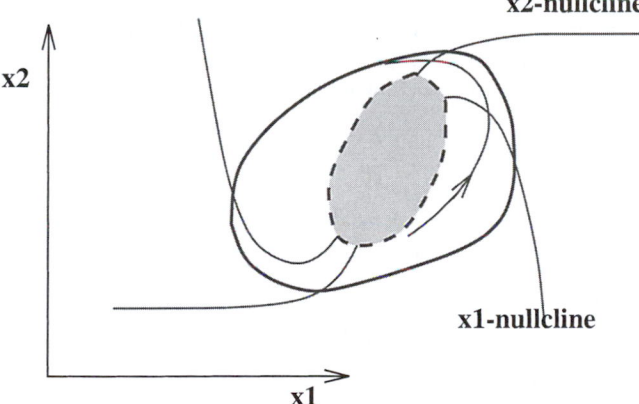

Figure 6. Phase plane for bistable regimen of parameters. Nullclines are shown, as is the stable periodic orbit (dark line), the unstable periodic orbit (dashed line), and representative trajectories (thin lines). The gray area denotes the domain of attraction for the fixed point. The rest of the plane is attracted to the stable periodic orbit.

Philosophical Issues in Brain Theory and Connectionism

Andy Clark and Chris Eliasmith

Introduction

In this article, we highlight three questions: (1) Does human cognition rely on structured internal representations? (2) How should theories, models, and data relate? (3) In what ways might embodiment, action, and dynamics matter for understanding the mind and the brain?

The first question concerns a fundamental assumption of most researchers who theorize about the brain. Do neural systems exploit classical compositional and systematic representations, distributed representations, or no representations at all? The question is not easily answered. Connectionism, for example, has been criticized for both holding and challenging representational views. The second question concerns the crucial methodological issue of how results emerging from the various brain sciences can help to constrain cognitive scientific models. Finally, the third question focuses attention on a major challenge to contemporary cognitive science: the challenge of understanding the mind as a controller of embodied and environmentally embedded action.

Does Cognition Need Representations?

This question is the most difficult and least well defined of our three questions. But it addresses one of the most philosophically interesting features of many connectionist models, especially those most closely related to brain theory. The intuition is that connectionism poses a challenge to the classical view of the brain as a syntax-sensitive engine. This idea involves depicting all or most of human cognition as involving something akin to logical operations applied to something akin to linguistic (sentential) structures. The prime philosophical exponent of the identification of genuine cognitive processes with such operations on quasi-sentential entities is Fodor (see Fodor, 1987; Fodor and Pylyshyn, 1988). Fodor argues in favor of an innate symbolic code (the *language of thought*) and mental processes involving operations defined over the syntactically structured strings of that code. The underlying image is of an inner economy in which symbol strings are operated on by procedures sensitive to the structure of the string.

In contrast, a typical trained-up network does not employ grammatical strings or, a fortiori, processing operations sensitive to the structure of such strings. Instead, we find prototypical complexes of properties represented in a high-dimensional space (see Churchland, 1995). The space is highly organized in the sense that data items that need to be treated in closely related ways become encoded in neighboring regions of the space. It is this *semantic metric* that allows the network to generalize and to respond well under conditions of noise, for example. But this organization of the encoded knowledge does not amount to the provision of a genuine syntax. One way to see this difference is to ask what rules of combination of represented elements apply, and in what systematic ways we can operate on complexes of represented items. As Fodor and Pylyshyn (1988) point out, there is no analog in distributed representations for the logical operations of detaching an element from one string (complex representation) and adding it to another.

Nevertheless, a variety of connectionist techniques have been developed to allow for structure-sensitive processing, but such techniques have been described (van Gelder, 1990) as providing *functional*, as opposed to *concatenative*, compositional structure. A complex representation has concatenative structure if it embeds the individual constitutive elements unaltered within it. It has functional compositional structure if such components are usable or

retrievable, but the complex expression does not itself embed unaltered tokens of these parts. Most connectionist schemes for dealing with compositional structure are functionally compositional (e.g., RAAM architectures, tensor product encodings, holographic reduced representations [HRRs]), although synchrony binding is concatenative. (For a review, see CONNECTIONIST AND SYMBOLIC REPRESENTATIONS.) Of these, HRRs are perhaps best suited to bridging the traditional gap between connectionist and symbolicist approaches to understanding language-like processing. HRRs are supremely structure sensitive, do not suffer from the dimensional increases of tensor products, and can be implemented in standard connectionist networks, yet they are not concatenative (Eliasmith and Thagard, 2001).

In our opinion, a major benefit of exploring the space of connectionist cognitive models is that it may help us expand our sense of the possible nature of internal representation and hence better understand what is truly essential to notions such as *structure, syntax*, and *complex representation*. Doing so, we may discover which aspects of our models are simply artifacts of our (over)familiarity with one representational format, viz., the format of atomic elements and grammar common to language and logic.

How Do Theories, Models, and Data Relate?

As a computational formalism, connectionism is quite powerful, allowing us to approximate nearly any function or performance profile that we desire. However, the mere fact that some input-output pattern P is found in human cognition and can be mimicked using some connectionist model is, in itself, of only marginal psychological interest. The demands of cognitive science, unlike those of artificial intelligence, require more. Ideally, we must provide models that are both consistent with neurological data and comprehensible. However, the relation between data and models is not unidirectional. Models are constrained by data, but they also help us determine what sorts of experiments to use in looking for more relevant details. The role of theory in unifying the brain sciences and connectionism is an important but (for the time being) mysterious one (but see Eliasmith and Anderson, 2002, chap. 1, for one possibility).

The data that constrain models come largely from two sources: higher levels (i.e., from the mind "down") from work in disciplines such as psychology and psycholinguistics, and lower levels (i.e., from the neuron "up"), from work in neuroscience and brain theory with behavior as the meeting ground for these diverse approaches. From psychology and psycholinguistics we can extract vast bodies of constraining data that go far beyond the mere specification of a task-specific input-output mapping. Such data can concern, for example, the relative difficulty of parsing certain sentences or solving certain problems, the time course of problem solving, the developmental profile of skill acquisition, and the way in which new and old knowledge interact in the context of new learning (for detailed examples, see Karmiloff-Smith, 1992; see also DEVELOPMENTAL DISORDERS).

For current purposes, however, it is the lower-level constraints that we seek to highlight. The question here concerns the proper relation between connectionist-computational modeling and the detailed constraints emerging from the various brain sciences. Such sciences include neuroanatomy, neurochemistry, lesion studies, and research at the single-cell, circuit, and systems level. It seems clear that any acceptable model of human information processing must respect the results of such studies. To do so, some intelligible relation must exist between the theories put forward by, for example, connectionist-computational modeling and the entities and lawful interactions studied by the brain sciences. It is a duty sadly neglected by both classical artificial intelligence and a great deal of connectionist work to make some effort to display the precise nature of such relations.

Such a task is complicated by the variety of levels of interest that may characterize the brain sciences. These include the levels of biochemical specification: single cells, circuits, subsystems, and networks of subsystems. Marr's suggestion that studies at each level can be independently pursued is highly dubious. Our top-level decomposition of a task into subtasks appropriate for computational modeling may be challenged once we become familiar with the distribution of information-processing resources in the brain. What we originally thought of as two distinct functions may actually share circuitry in the brain (see Arbib, 1989). Such a result will not be devoid of psychological significance, since it will figure in an explanation of the breakdown profile as revealed by, for example, lesion studies of the system.

How, then, should we conceive the bridge between idealized artificial intelligence models and brain theory? It is precisely the complex relations between implementation and function that have spawned a recent surge of interest in computational neuroscience. With the explicit goal of taking biological constraints as seriously as computational ones, computational neuroscience has begun to explore a vast range of realistic neural models. For example, Reike et al. (1997) provide an information-theoretic analysis of spike trains, allowing accurate stimulus signal reconstruction. The combination of such spike train analyses and, for example, Abbott's higher-level discussions of basis function representations can provide valuable insights into the functioning of populations of neurons (see Eliasmith and Anderson, 2002). Though preliminary, the tools developed by such research are promising candidates for generating biologically realistic connectionist models.

Such models should prove useful in providing constraints of their own. Insights from basis function analyses suggest new experiments for neurophysiologists. In particular, it seems that neurons may have higher-dimensional tuning profiles than previously imagined. Although neurological techniques for determining complex profiles have yet to be perfected, connectionist modeling suggests that such tuning properties are important to the everyday functioning of neurons. So, not only does biology inform the construction of computational models, but, ideally, those same models can help suggest important experiments for neuroscientists to perform. In this sense, models and data can be mutually beneficial. Of course, the benefits are highly constrained by assumptions of both the model and the experimental design.

Although no model can be expected to do justice to all aspects of its target, what justice it can do depends on the biological realism of the assumptions behind the model. Biological realism, of course, can be incorporated into a model in many ways, such as by including neurochemical diffusion, single neuron morphology, spike train statistics, neuroanatomical constraints, population dynamics, or system-level organization (see Eliasmith and Anderson, 2002, for examples). In any case, what we can and should expect from a modeler is a clear statement of what aspects of the target phenomenon are supposed to be explained, and (if it is a computational model) at what level the computational story is intended to capture real neurophysiological facts. Successful attempts to exploit the close relation between experiment and model are still something of a rarity. This is largely because theoreticians (typically mathematicians, physicists, and engineers) and experimentalists (typically neuroscientists and biologists) do not yet have many conceptual tools in common. In order to reap the benefits of mutual, interlevel constraint, this will likely have to be rectified.

In What Ways Might Embodiment Matter for Understanding the Mind and the Brain?

In recent years, an important challenge has been issued to cognitive science. It stems from the work of researchers espousing the *dynamicist hypothesis* (van Gelder, 1995). The dynamicist commitment to making time central to cognitive modeling is inspired by the broader realization that cognitive systems are real physical systems acting in the real world in real time. Given the finite, though vast, computational resources of the brain, it also seems that evolution has often off-loaded complex computational tasks to the body and to the environment. This double "situatedness" of cognitive systems needs to be reckoned with if we are to develop an accurate picture of precisely the kinds of computation neural systems perform. Connectionism and brain theory must conspire to explain this kind of representational and computational economy. Thus, while looking *inside* to the brain and the results of neuroscience, we can not afford to turn a blind eye to constraints and resources that come from the *outside*, from the gross body and environment of a cognitive system (Clark, 1997).

Consider vision. There is now a growing body of work devoted to so-called animate vision (Ballard, 1991). The key insight here is that the task of vision is not to build rich inner models of a surrounding three-dimensional reality, but rather to use visual information efficiently and cheaply in the service of real-world, real-time action. Animate vision thus rejects Marr's analysis, what Churchland et al. nicely dub the paradigm of "pure vision"—the idea (associated with work in classical AI and in the use of vision for planning) that vision is largely a means of creating a world model rich enough to let us "throw the world away," targeting reason and thought to the inner model instead. Real-world action, in these "pure vision" paradigms, functions merely as a means of implementing solutions arrived at by pure cognition.

The animate vision paradigm, by contrast, gives action a starring role. Computational economy and temporal efficiency are purchased by a variety of bodily actions and local environment–exploiting tricks and ploys, including

- the use of cheap, easy-to-detect (possibly idiosyncratic) environmental cues (e.g., searching for Kodak film in a drug store: Seek "Kodak yellow");
- the use of active sensing (e.g., use motor action, guided by rough perceptual analysis, to seek further inputs yielding *better* perceptual data—move head and eyes for better depth perception, etc.); and
- the use of repeated consultations of the world in place of rich, detailed inner models.

Ballard et al. (1997) have recently demonstrated that subjects do not bind color and location information in a block-copying task until it is absolutely required by current problem solving. As a result, changes made to the display (such as switching the color of blocks during a saccade) are very often undetected.

Vision, this body of work suggests, is a highly active and intelligent process. It is not the passive creation of a rich inner model so much as the active retrieval (typically by moving the high-resolution fovea in a saccade) of useful information *as it is needed* from the constantly present real-world scene. Ballard et al. speak of "just-in-time representation," while the roboticist Rodney Brooks coined the phrase, "The world is its own best model" (Brooks, 1991). The combined moral is clear: Vision makes the most of the persisting external scene, and gears its computational activity closely and sparingly to the task at hand.

The general thrust of the animate vision research program, however, is not to reject the ideas of internal models and representations so much as to reconfigure them in a sparser and more interactive image. We thus read of inner databases that associate objects (such as car keys) and locations (on the kitchen table) of internal feature representations, of indexical representations, and so on. What is being rejected is not the notion of inner content-bearing states per se, but only the much stronger notion of rich, memory-intensive, all-purpose forms of internal representation.

The crucial distinction, it seems to us, is thus not between representational and nonrepresentational solutions so much as between rich and action-neutral forms of internal representation (which may increase flexibility but require additional computational work to specify a behavioral response) and sparse and action-oriented forms (which exploit the body and world and which begin to build the response into the representation itself).

Discussion

Our vision of basic biological reason is changing rapidly. There is a growing emphasis on the computational economies afforded by real-world action, and an increasing appreciation of the way larger structures (of agent and artifacts) both scaffold and transform the shape of individual reason. These twin forces converge on a rather more minimalist account of individual cognitive processing, an account that tends to eschew rich, all-purpose internal models and sentential forms of internal representations. Such minimalism, however, has its limits. Despite some ambitious arguments, there is currently no reason to doubt the guiding vision of individual agents as loci of internal representations and the individual agents as users of a variety of inner models. Rather than opposing representationalism against interactive dynamics, we should be embracing a broader vision of the inner representational resources themselves.

The sciences of the mind are thus in a state of productive flux, the product of multiple converging influences coming from real-world robotics, systems-level neuroscience, cognitive psychology, evolutionary theory, AI, and philosophical analysis. This flux has forced us to reconsider earlier accounts of the relation between theory, models, and data relevant to cognitive systems. More important, we can see a new vision of mind emerging. The point at which many of these influences currently converge is captured by seeing mind as in essence a controller of embodied and environmentally embedded action. Mind is an organ for orchestrating real-time responses to a real world.

One major player in these recent events has been the explosion of work on artificial neural networks (ANNs). Such networks amounted to an existence proof of the possibility of adaptive intelligent behavior without reliance on explicitly formulated rules or language-like data structures. Moreover, the networks integrated representation and action in a very direct manner: knowledge became encoded in a form dictated by its use in a particular type of problem solving. But the neural networks revolution was incomplete. It was incomplete because it was still burdened with much of the unnecessary baggage of the previous, disembodied, symbol-crunching approach to understanding cognition. Mind was still treated as an essentially timeless locus of abstract problem-solving capacities.

All this changed with the surge of interest, in the late 1980s and early 1990s, in what became known as autonomous agent research (see, e.g., essays in Beer, Ritzmann, and McKenna, 1993). This research aimed to model and understand the adaptive success of single, complete, embodied systems: insects that walk and seek food, the cockroach's amazingly sophisticated mechanisms for detecting and evading attackers, robots that learn to swing from branch to branch using real mechanical arms, and many other kinds

of systems. Many of these models exploit ANNs as control systems. But the constraints on success became very different.

Finally, the constraints on computation using ANNs are very different from the constraints on real biological computation. It is here that the relation among theory, model, and data again becomes pivotal. Interestingly, reconceptualizing mind in each of these previous cases has depended on rethinking the relevant constraints (i.e., linguistic versus nonlinguistic symbols, partial versus full-bodied systems). Introducing the complexities of natural neural computation is bound to have a similar impact on our concept of mind.

Many important questions remain open. Can work in ANNs come to grips with the real complexity of biological computation? What kinds of systems-level models can help make sense of the complex balance between specialization and cooperation that we find in real brains? Can a representation-sparse approach make headway with all aspects of human cognition, or is it limited to cases of perceptuomotor control and on-line reasoning? How does the command of public language impact and transform human thought and reason?

The cognitive science of the biological, embodied mind is still in its infancy, and the full power and scope of the new vision remain to be determined. But the issues raised will, we believe, shape the agenda of the next decade of research into mind and its place in nature.

Road Map: Psychology
Related Reading: Artificial Intelligence and Neural Networks; Consciousness, Neural Models of; Perspective on Neuron Model Complexity; Structured Connectionist Models

References

Arbib, M. A., 1989, *The Metaphorical Brain 2: Neural Networks and Beyond*, New York: Wiley-Interscience.
Ballard, D., 1991, Animate vision, *Artif. Intell.*, 48:57–86.
Ballard, D., Hayhoe, M., Pook, P., and Rao, R., 1997, Deictic codes for the embodiment of cognition, *Behav. Brain Sci.*, 20:723–767.
Beer, R., Ritzmann, R., and McKenna, T., Eds., 1993, *Biological Neural Networks in Invertebrate Neuroethology and Robotics*, London: Academic Press. ◆
Brooks, R., 1991, Intelligence without representation, *Artif. Intell.*, 47:139–159.
Churchland, P. M., 1995, *The Engine of Reason, The Seat of the Soul*, Cambridge, MA: MIT Press. ◆
Clark, A., 1997, *Being There: Putting Brain, Body, and World Together Again*, Cambridge, MA: MIT Press. ◆
Eliasmith, C., and Anderson, C. H., 2002, *Neural Engineering: Computation, Representation, and Dynamics in Neurobiological Systems*, Cambridge, MA: MIT Press. ◆
Eliasmith, C., and Thagard, P., 2001, Integrating structure and meaning: A distributed model of analogical mapping, *Cognit. Sci.*, 25:245–286.
Fodor, J., 1987, *Psychosemantics: The Problem of Meaning in the Philosophy of Mind*, Cambridge, MA: MIT Press. ◆
Fodor, J., and Pylyshyn, Z., 1988, Connectionism and cognitive architecture: A critical analysis, *Cognition*, 28:3–71.
Karmiloff-Smith, A., 1992, *Beyond Modularity: A Developmental Perspective on Cognitive Science*, Cambridge, MA: MIT Press.
Reike, F., Warland, D., de Ruyter van Steveninck, R., and Bialek, W., 1997, *Spikes: Exploring the Neural Code*, Cambridge, MA: MIT Press.
van Gelder, T., 1990, Compositionality: A connectionist variation on a classical theme, *Cognit. Sci.*, 14:355–384.
van Gelder, T., 1995, What might cognition be, if not computation? *J. Philos.*, 91:345–381.

Photonic Implementations of Neurobiologically Inspired Networks

B. Keith Jenkins and Armand R. Tanguay, Jr.

Introduction

Technological implementations of neural networks in both software and hardware forms have been largely motivated by biological neural networks, but also include network topologies, synaptic interconnection rules, and neuron unit functionalities that combine to yield novel system-level properties. Software implementations of such networks are highly flexible in design and reconfiguration but are time-, power-, and computational-resource-consumptive for even modest numbers of neuron units and interconnections. Neural network implementations in both electronic and photonic hardware are designed to circumvent these limitations in applications that require compact systems, low latencies, and high computational throughputs.

In VLSI-based neural networks (Mead, 1989), the neuron units and weighted (synaptic) interconnections are incorporated on one or more planar microelectronic chips (see NEUROMORPHIC VLSI CIRCUITS AND SYSTEMS; ANALOG VLSI IMPLEMENTATIONS OF NEURAL NETWORKS; DIGITAL VLSI FOR NEURAL NETWORKS; SILICON NEURONS). An important advantage of this approach is the capability for near-term technology insertion, with leverage provided by a well-established technology base. An equally important limitation, however, is the difficulty of scaling up or interconnecting multiple neural chips to incorporate large numbers of neuron units in highly interconnected architectures without significantly increasing the computational time. This inherent trade-off derives from the limited pin counts, off-chip communication bandwidths, and on-chip interconnection densities available in both current generation and projected chip designs.

In this article we consider the photonic implementation of neurobiologically inspired networks, in which optical (free-space or through-substrate) techniques are utilized to enable an increase in the number of neuron units and the interconnection complexity by using the off-chip (third) dimension (Jenkins and Tanguay, 1992; Wagner and Psaltis, 1993; Jutamulia, 1994). This merging of optical and photonic devices with electronic circuitry provides additional features such as parallel weight implementation, adaptation, and modular scalability.

General Principles Extracted from Biological Systems

In this section, we discuss the key general principles that can be extracted from neurobiological systems and then crafted in hybrid electronic/photonic form, a base technology substrate that exhibits wide-ranging differences with respect to human wetware (Hubel, 1988). Although the discussion below is framed within the human visual system (retina through early visual cortex), these architectural principles apply throughout the mammalian brain to a large extent, and can potentially be used to advantage in biologically inspired neural systems.

Biological vision systems exhibit a number of common themes that have pertinence to hardware implementations, including (1) a propensity for layering of the processing architecture (Wandell, 1995), (2) the employment of massive parallelism with simple local processing units and minimal local storage within each processing unit, (3) the use of a multiplicity of neuron unit types and associated fan-out and fan-in patterns, (4) the incorporation of dense synaptic/dendritic interconnections at all scales (from local to global, among multiple brain regions) with a high degree of fan-out and fan-in at each processing node, (5) adaptivity on multiple time scales as exhibited by both short- and long-term plasticity, (6) distributed storage of information, and (7) an associative memory organizational construct.

Although many of these themes can be individually incorporated into hardware implementations using existing technology, to our knowledge no implementation has included all of these themes together using a single technology base. Primate visual systems, for example, use several types of photoreceptors and neurons at the lowest levels of vision processing, with primarily local, fixed, and weighted interconnections among multiple layers within the retina (Dowling, 1992). The photoreceptors are densely packed, ranging from about $1–3 \times 10^7$ cm^{-2} in the fovea (1-μm-diameter cones) to 4×10^6 cm^{-2} in the periphery, with a mixture of 4- to 10-μm-diameter cones separated by a much higher density of 1-μm-diameter rods (Wandell, 1995). This density can be instructively compared with the current pixel densities of solid-state imaging sensor arrays (including focal plane arrays in the visible, infrared, and ultraviolet frequencies; CCD arrays; and active pixel sensor (APS) arrays), which range from about 1×10^6 cm^{-2} to 4×10^6 cm^{-2}. Current smart pixel arrays have not yet achieved even these densities because of the incorporation of local processing circuitry within each pixel.

The biological propensity for incorporation of dense interconnections is evident within the retina and the lateral geniculate nucleus, and extends into the lowest levels of the visual cortex. Throughout, the interconnection mappings tend to be local, highly regular (retinotopic), and only partially adaptive. Higher up the processing stream (within the primate visual cortex), interconnections tend to become gradually less local, less regular, and more adaptive, with a degree of interconnectivity (fan-out from and fan-in to a given neuron) that is typically 10^3 to 10^4 (Hubel, 1988; Dowling, 1992; Wandell, 1995).

The biological imperative for layering is also of considerable interest to examine further. In primate visual systems, layering accomplishes a number of computationally important functions. (1) Layering provides a convenient mechanism for the implementation of multiple concatenated operations comprising nonlinearities and weighted fan-out/fan-in functions. The latter operation can be viewed as the convolution of a 2D input function with a set of 2D kernels (weighting functions), and provides the basis for implementing both space-invariant and space-variant operations across multiple spatial scales. The separation of a given complex operation into several sequential steps of nonlinearity/convolution also allows access to intermediate scale results for both feedforward and feedback connections that project beyond intervening layers, as observed throughout biological vision systems. (2) Layering also provides for the implementation of higher-order complexity (hierarchical) operations that can be derived from simple primitives implemented over multiple spatial scales. (3) Layering naturally provides for the hierarchical buildup of the size of the receptive field, so that nonlocal operations such as contrast enhancement and color constancy can be implemented with invariance to object size. (4) Finally, layering carries with it the potential for increased algorithmic efficiency, in that certain operations (e.g., even certain linearly decomposable convolutions at a given kernel size) can be performed in multiple layers with less cost in computational resources (e.g., fan-out from neurons via axons, synapses, and dendrites; total number of equivalent primitive operations; computational energy).

The Holographic Paradigm

With these general principles in mind, in this section we consider the potential implementation of neurobiologically inspired networks based on the holographic recording and readout of weighted interconnection patterns. In volume holography, the storage of a set of recorded holographic images in a volume holographic optical element by means of the coherent interference between a set of image-bearing signal beams and a corresponding set of reference beams (multiplexed in angle, wavelength, or position) can also be thought of as the storage of a set of weighted interconnection patterns; each input pixel (picture element) in a given reference beam is connected to a given output pixel in the reconstructed image with a weight (diffraction efficiency) that governs the brightness or intensity of the reconstructed pixel. Sets of weighted interconnection patterns can be read out in parallel to form multiple inputs to each output pixel, providing a dense interconnection network with a high degree of fan-out from each reference beam pixel and fan-in to each output image pixel.

The storage of such weighted interconnection patterns in volume holographic optical elements exhibits a number of characteristics that are similar to characteristics observed in the neurobiological processes of memory and learning as well as in many neural networks (Pribram, 1991). For example, the information (memory) associated with the set of holographically stored weighted interconnection patterns is distributed over a significant portion of the volume hologram; such distributed memory storage is also characteristic of neural networks. Holographically stored weighted interconnection patterns can implement dense interconnections at all scales from local to global, and can exhibit degrees of fan-out and fan-in from unity (a point-to-point connection) to upward of 10^3 or 10^4. Recall of such stored patterns can be configured in many ways, including both retinotopic-like (highly structured) and associative-memory-like mappings, and can provide for both feedforward and feedback connections, depending on the specific network architecture.

If appropriate real-time recording and readout materials are employed, such as photorefractive crystals or polymers, the interconnection weights can be updated by means of holographic recording principles, so that weight updates analogous to those characteristic of adaptivity and learning in certain neural network models can be performed. These weights will typically decay with time (and also with multiple exposures), suggestive of short-term memory. In many such real-time materials, the capability exists to "fix" all or part of the recorded interconnection patterns, thereby greatly extending the storage time, suggestive in turn of long (or at least longer) term memory. In addition, the properties of real-time holographic recording lead naturally to the incorporation of a dependence for weight updates on temporal correlations between the signal and reference beams (as derived, for example, from two temporally correlated neuron units).

In the following sections, we describe several approaches for implementing photonic neurobiologically inspired networks. All such architectures incorporate dense fan-out/fan-in interconnections but range in the type and degree of connectivity from compact photonic multichip modules with local interconnections between layers to photonic neural networks that incorporate global holographic interconnections. Descriptions of the various photonic components that comprise such architectures can be found in the previous edition of the *Handbook* (Jenkins and Tanguay, 1995).

Compact Photonic Multichip Modules for Layered Networks

A conceptual diagram of one possible three-dimensional (3D) integrated electronic/photonic multichip module (PMCM) structure is shown in Figure 1 (Veldkamp, 1993; Tanguay et al., 2000; Tanguay and Jenkins, 2002). Multiple layers of pixellated silicon VLSI chips (chips that are divided into arrays of nearly identical functional regions) are densely interconnected by a combination of electronic, optical, and photonic devices to produce either a space-invariant or space-variant degree of fan-out and fan-in to each individual pixel (neuron unit, or processing node). These weighted fan-out/fan-in interconnections are suggestive of the axonal projections, synapses, and dendritic tree structures that characterize biological organisms. The use of optical and photonic devices in particular allows for the implementation of these interconnections *between* adjacent physical layers within the stack of chips. In addition, the use of silicon VLSI for neuron units or processing elements allows considerable flexibility in the neuron model or neuron-unit function implemented.

In one such implementation (Tanguay et al., 2000; Tanguay and Jenkins, 2002), shown schematically in Figure 2, two-dimensional (2D) arrays of bottom-emitting vertical-cavity surface-emitting lasers (VCSELs) fabricated on a gallium arsenide (GaAs) substrate provide optical outputs from a given integrated layer of the structure. These VCSEL arrays are flip-chip bonded on a pixel-by-pixel basis to the silicon VLSI chips, which typically incorporate local optical detectors (for optical inputs from the previous layer) and electronics comprising processing elements (either acting alone or in concert with electrical inputs from nearest and next-nearest neighbors within the plane), memory elements (in the analog or digital domain), and VCSEL drivers. Proximity-coupled diffractive optical element (DOE) arrays, designed to incorporate both focal power (lens) and weighted fan-out functions, are used to establish interconnections that are modulated (temporally varied) in intensity by each individual VCSEL element and its associated silicon driver circuit. Alternatively, separate concatenated DOE and microlens arrays can be used.

Other implementations of compact photonic multichip modules include a similar 3D stacked structure using a different materials system and an array of one-to-one (digital) photonic interconnections between adjacent chips (Bond et al., 1999); and a set of

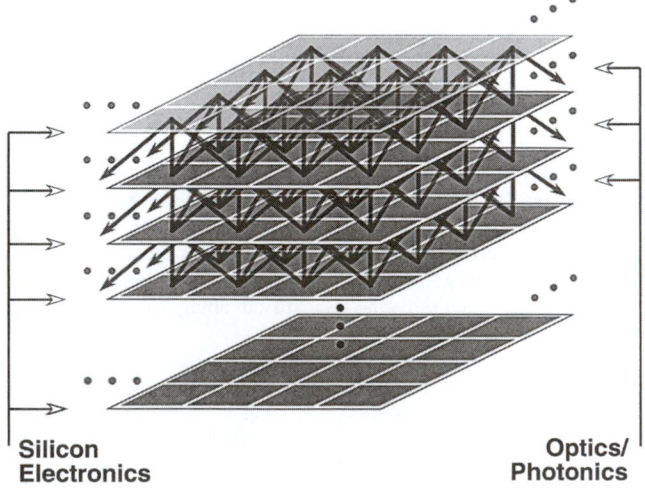

Figure 1. Three-dimensional photonic multichip module concept.

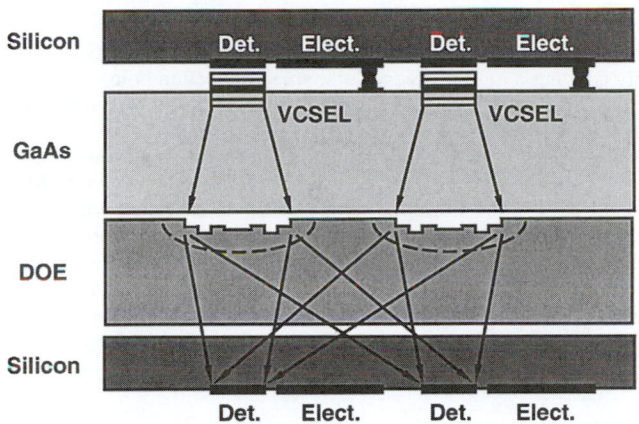

Figure 2. Multilayer compact photonic multichip module. Only two cells within an $N \times N$ array are shown, as well as only two (of M) silicon chip layers.

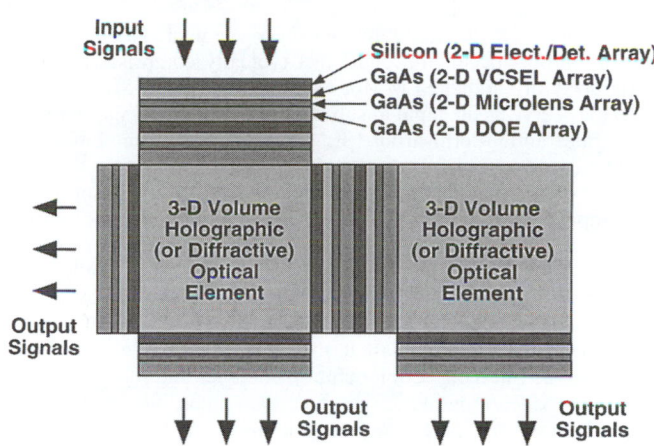

Figure 3. Densely interconnected extended photonic multichip module.

chips laid out on a planar substrate, with neural network interconnections implemented in the third dimension using photonics (Fey et al., 2000).

For the specific case of adaptive vision sensors, the design of the individual silicon VLSI chips, and in particular the use of spatiotemporal multiplexing techniques for network implementation and signal processing functions, is motivated by the recent development of several promising neurobiologically inspired vision algorithms that can potentially be mapped onto the emerging 3D PMCM platform (Tanguay et al., 2000, and references therein).

Extended Photonic Multichip Modules for Layered Networks

As the level of representation extends from low-level vision through mid-level vision to high-level vision operations, interconnections tend to become both more sparse and more global; in some cases, particularly between functionally partitioned vision processing modules, dense global interconnections may be required. Both local and global interconnection cases can potentially be accommodated within the PMCM architecture by incorporating novel stratified volume diffractive optical elements (SVDOEs; Tanguay et al., 2000, and references therein) as shown schematically in Figure 3. These SVDOEs consist of multiple layers of proximity-coupled and aligned DOEs that implement either space-variant or space-invariant interconnection patterns with properties characteristic of volume holograms. They also offer the advantages of planar fabrication methods compatible with VLSI design rules.

In Figure 3, several sets of compact PMCMs that implement primarily local interconnections, and perhaps also implement hierarchical functions, are interconnected across the faces of a cubic submodule by each SVDOE, offering the potential for more global interconnectivity. The mappings might be retinotopic in some cases, and columnar or fully space-variant in others.

Volume Holographic Systems for Large-Scale Adaptive Networks

Volume holographic optical elements are capable of global, dense interconnections that are adaptive at the hardware level. The potential exists for the implementation of large numbers of weighted

interconnections (e.g., 10^{10} in one module) that adapt by means of outer-product learning algorithms (e.g., Hebbian learning, or single- or multiple-layer least-mean squares [backpropagation], including weight decay). These learning algorithms exploit the physics of holographic (typically photorefractive) materials, the properties of which currently limit both adaptation and retention times. Such holographic interconnection systems for adaptive neural network implementations are not yet practical, but have been extensively researched (e.g., Jenkins and Tanguay, 1992; Wagner and Psaltis, 1993; Li et al., 1996; and references therein).

A conceptual diagram of one particular optical implementation of a large-scale artificial neural network with both local and global fan-out/fan-in adaptive interconnections is given in Figure 4. Many related implementations are possible, with similar overall characteristics. Two smart pixel spatial light modulators (SLMs, such as pixellated silicon VLSI chips mated to GaAs chips that comprise arrays of optical modulators rather than arrays of lasers; see also Jenkins and Tanguay, 1995, p. 679; Worchesky et al., 1996) are used to implement a 2D array of training term generators (SLM$_1$) and a 2D array of neuron units (SLM$_2$). A volume holographic

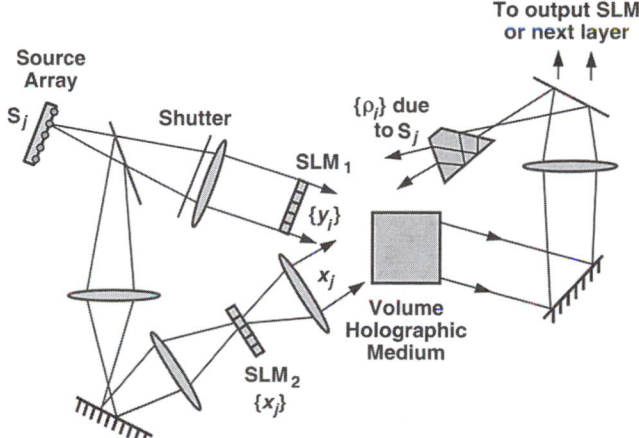

Figure 4. Photonic volume holographic system for large-scale adaptive networks; the Hebbian case is depicted. Beams from the source array on the left serve to read out the signals generated by both SLMs; the neuron-unit inputs to SLM$_2$ are not shown.

medium serves as the key interconnection element. The interconnection outputs occur in a plane that typically comprises the detector array of another SLM (for example, the output SLM). This SLM may serve as the input to subsequent signal processing stages, or as the training-term array (SLM_1) or input neuron-unit-array (SLM_2) in the case of a system with feedback.

In the computing phase (i.e., hologram readout), the beam from each input-neuron-unit pixel of SLM_2 (x_j) illuminates the holographic medium at a unique position, angle, and/or wavelength. The selective nature of volume holograms then allows only the appropriate interconnection weights w_{ij} to be multiplied by each input beam, yielding the set of products $w_{ij}x_j$. The output beam optics then sums over j of these terms at the location of each output term ρ_i in the interconnection output plane, yielding $\rho_i = \Sigma_j w_{ij} x_j$.

During the learning phase (i.e., hologram recording), each pixel of SLM_1 generates the appropriate training term, δ_i. An exposure is made of the interference pattern between beams emanating from the two SLMs in Figure 4. With appropriate choices of parameters, this exposure can increment the value of each interconnection weight w_{ij} by an amount that is approximately proportional to $\delta_i x_j$. In the Hebbian case, for example, $\delta_i = y_i$, in which y_i is the output-neuron-unit signal. It should be noted that when designing an architecture that will generate and record these weight increments, care must be taken to ensure that the appropriate interference terms are recorded with minimal crosstalk. One of the key differences among full-scale optical neural network architectures is the technique used to avoid such crosstalk (Wagner and Psaltis, 1993). In addition, the actual weight increment that physically occurs in holographic systems depends on the particular architecture employed (Wagner and Psaltis, 1993; Petrisor et al., 1996).

The interconnections within the particular implementation depicted in Figure 4 are based on a technique for multiplexed volume holography that uses double angular multiplexing and incoherent/coherent recording and readout (Jenkins and Tanguay, 1992). This interconnection technique exhibits an advantageous combination of total number of channels and interchannel crosstalk, in the case of high total optical throughput efficiency. One of its key features is the use of a source array that consists of an array of lasers, each of which generates light independently of the others. Because of this independence, a pair of beams from *different* lasers is not capable of interfering and recording a hologram, whereas a pair of beams generated from the *same* laser can interfere and thereby record a hologram in a holographic medium. From this source array, a set of coherent beam pairs is formed, one pair from each laser, that can record holograms pairwise.

In the computing phase of most volume hologram–based implementations of neural networks, the overall computing time is determined by the SLM response time. During learning, the holographic material sensitivity or response time typically limits the weight increment rate, which in turn puts an upper bound on the achievable learning gain constant; such holographic material response times depend on the material and vary over many orders of magnitude from one material to another. Similarly, the minimum decay rate (or maximum retention time) of holograms in read/write holographic materials puts a lower bound on the weight decay constant, and is similarly material dependent.

Large-scale optical *nonadaptive* networks are important as well. In this case the interconnection hologram need not be recorded in accordance with a specific learning algorithm. If the weights are known a priori, then any standard technique can be used to pre-record the hologram. In many cases, however, the weights may not be known. A common scenario may involve the training of a "master" network; once it has been trained, multiple copies of the network would be produced. If the network is large, and particularly if it utilizes volume holographic interconnections, then making direct copies of the volume hologram may be more practical than

probing the values of all of the weights and then loading those weight values into a recording system. Thus, the capability of rapidly copying a multiplexed volume interconnection hologram may be important (Jenkins and Tanguay, 1995, and references therein, especially to Piazzolla et al.).

Most optical and photonic neural network architectures (or "modules") of this class can be generalized in the following additional ways. First, multiple modules can be cascaded with fully parallel communication. Second, multiple neural network layers can be implemented either by adding feedback capability to the single module described or by cascading multiple modules. And finally, smart pixel SLMs can be employed to implement various neuron-unit models.

Discussion

Research to date on optical and photonic neural network implementations has included the development and analysis of new architectures, analysis of scalability issues, development of the technology base for near-optimal individual components, and experimental proof-of-concept demonstrations. Additional research and development directions that are key for the eventual realization of physically small, high-performance, reasonable-cost photonic neural networks include increased focus on the manufacturability of the photonic and optical components, development of packaging and miniaturization techniques for hybrid electronic/photonic systems, and increased design automation and flexibility. Substantial progress has already been made along these lines. Significant leverage is also provided by rapid advances in the related areas of photonic digital interconnection systems, digital volume holographic memory systems, and components for early vision.

As the technology base evolves, photonic neural network implementations inspired by more sophisticated neuron, synapse, dendrite, axon, and network models should become feasible (e.g., models that include temporal correlations or dynamic synapses; see DYNAMIC LINK ARCHITECTURE; SELF-ORGANIZATION AND THE BRAIN; and SYNCHRONIZATION, BINDING AND EXPECTANCY). Furthermore, the eventual implementation of photonic neural networks will likely engender a concomitant development of application areas for large-scale networks, and a deeper understanding of their properties.

Road Map: Implementation and Analysis
Related Reading: Analog VLSI Implementations of Neural Networks; Digital VLSI for Neural Networks

References

Bond, S.W., Vendier, O., Myunghee, L., Jung, S., Vrazel, M., Lopez-Lagunas, A., Chai, S., Dagnall, G., Brooke, M., Jokerst, N. M., Wills, D. S., and Brown, A., 1999, A three-layer 3-D silicon system using through-SI vertical optical interconnections and SI CMOS hybrid building blocks, *IEEE J. Selected Topics in Quantum Electronics*, 5:276–286.

Dowling, J. E., 1992, *Neurons and Networks: An Introduction to Neuroscience*, Cambridge, MA: Belknap Press/Harvard University Press. ◆

Fey, D., Erhard, W., Gruber, M., Jahns, J., Bartelt, H., Grimm, G., Hoppe, L., and Sinzinger, S., 2000, Optical interconnects for neural and reconfigurable VLSI architectures, *Proc. IEEE*, 88:838–848.

Hubel, D. H., 1988, *Eye, Brain, and Vision*, New York: Freeman. ◆

Jenkins, B. K., and Tanguay, A. R., Jr., 1992, Photonic implementations of neural networks, in *Neural Networks for Signal Processing* (B. Kosko, Ed.), Englewood Cliffs, NJ: Prentice Hall, pp. 287–382. ◆

Jenkins, B. K., and Tanguay, A. R., Jr., 1995, Optical architectures for neural network implementations, and optical components for neural network implementations, in *Handbook of Brain Theory and Neural Net-*

works, 1st ed. (M. Arbib, Ed.), Cambridge, MA: MIT Press, pp. 673–682. ◆

Jutamulia, S., Ed., 1994, *Selected Papers on Optical Neural Networks*, Bellingham, WA: SPIE Press. ◆

Li, Y., Tanida, J., Tooley, F., and Wagner, K., Eds., 1996, *Optical Computing* (special issue), *Appl. Opt.*, 35:1177–1380. ◆

Mead, C., 1989, *Analog VLSI and Neural Systems*, Reading, MA: Addison-Wesley. ◆

Petrisor, G. C., Goldstein, A. A., Jenkins, B. K., Herbulock, E. J., and Tanguay, A. R., Jr., 1996, Convergence of backward-error-propagation learning in photorefractive crystals, *Appl. Opt.*, 35:1328–1343.

Pribram, K. H., 1991, *Brain and Perception: Holonomy and Structure in Figural Processing*, Hillsdale, NJ: Erlbaum.

Tanguay, A. R., Jr., and Jenkins, B. K., 2002, Hybrid electronic/photonic multichip modules for vision and neural prosthetic applications, in *Toward Replacement Parts for the Brain: Implantable Biomimetic Elec-*

tronics as the Next Era in Neural Prosthetics (T. W. Berger and D. L. Glanzman, Eds.), Cambridge, MA: MIT Press (in press). ◆

Tanguay, A. R., Jr., Jenkins, B. K., von der Malsburg, C., Mel, B., Holt, G., O'Brien, J., Biederman, I., Madhukar, A., Nasiatka, P., and Huang, Y., 2000, Vertically integrated photonic multichip module architecture for vision applications, in *Optics in Computing 2000* (R.A. Lessard and T. Galstian, Eds.), *Proc. SPIE*, 4089:584–600. ◆

Veldkamp, W. B., 1993, Wireless focal planes "on the road to amacronic sensors," *IEEE J. Quant. Electron.*, 29:801–813. ◆

Wagner, K., and Psaltis, D., 1993, Eds., *Optical Implementations of Neural Networks* (special issue), *Appl. Opt.*, 32:1249–1476. ◆

Wandell, B. A., 1995, *Foundations of Vision*, Sunderland, MA: Sinauer. ◆

Worchesky, T. L., Ritter, K. J., Martin, R., and Lane, B., 1996, Large arrays of spatial light modulators hybridized to silicon integrated circuits, *Appl. Opt.*, 35:1180–1186.

Population Codes

Alexandre Pouget and Peter E. Latham

Introduction

Many sensory and motor variables in the brain are encoded by coarse codes, i.e., by the activity of large populations of neurons with broad tuning curves. For example, the direction of visual motion is believed to be encoded in the medial temporal (MT) visual area by a population of cells with bell-shaped tuning to direction, as illustrated in Figure 1*A*. Other examples of variables encoded by populations include the orientation of a line, the contrast in a visual scene, the frequency of a tone, and the direction of intended movement in motor cortex. These encodings extend to two dimensions—a single set of neurons might contain information about both orientation and contrast—or more.

Population codes are computationally appealing for at least two reasons. First, the overlap among the tuning curves allows precise encoding of values that fall between the peaks of two adjacent tuning curves (Figure 1*A*). Second, bell-shaped tuning curves provide basis functions that can be combined to approximate a wide variety of nonlinear mappings. This means that many cortical functions, such as sensorimotor transformations, can be easily modeled with population codes (see Pouget, Zemel, and Dayan, 2000, for a review).

In this article we focus on decoding, or reading out, population codes. Decoding is the simplest form of computation that one can perform over a population code, and as such, it is an essential step

toward understanding more sophisticated computations. It is also important for accurately identifying which variables are encoded in a particular brain area and how they are encoded.

A key element of population codes—and the main reason why decoding them is difficult—is that neuronal responses are noisy, meaning that the same stimulus can produce different responses. Consider, for instance, a population of neurons coding for a one-dimensional parameter: the direction, θ, of a moving object. An object moving in a particular direction produces a *noisy* hill of activity across this neuronal population (Figure 1*C*). On the basis of this noisy activity, one can try to come up with a good guess, or estimate, $\hat{\theta}$, of the direction of motion, θ. In the second and third sections of this article we review the various estimators that have been proposed, and in the fourth section we consider their neuronal implementations.

Additional sources of uncertainty, beside neuronal noise, can come from the variable itself. For example, there is intrinsically more variability in one's estimate of, say, motion on a dark night than motion in broad daylight. In cases such as this, it is not unreasonable to assume that population activity codes for more than just a single value, and in the extreme case the population activity could code for a whole *probability distribution*. The goal of decoding is then to recover an estimate of this probability distribution. We consider an example of this later in the article.

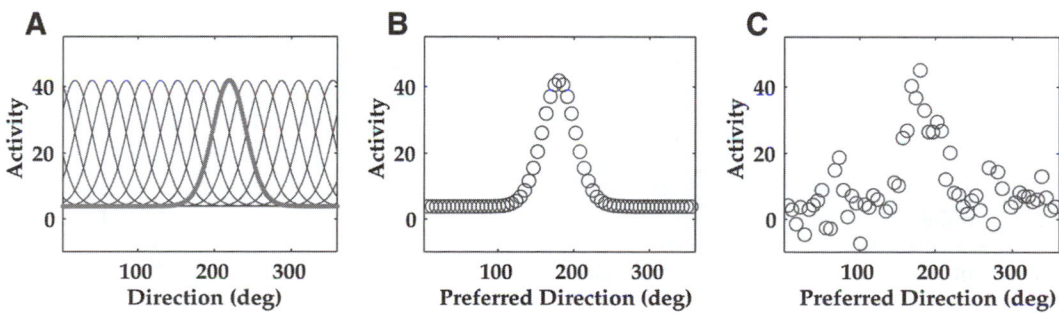

Figure 1. *A*, Idealized tuning curves for 16 direction-tuned neurons. *B*, Noiseless pattern of activity (○) from 64 simulated neurons with tuning curves like the ones shown in *A*, when presented with a direction of 180°.

The activity of each neuron is plotted at the location of its preferred direction. *C*, Same as *B*, but in the presence of Gaussian noise.

Models of Neuronal Noise and Tuning Curves

To read a population code, it is essential to have a good understanding of the relation between the patterns of activity and the encoded variables. One common assumption, particularly in sensory and motor cortex, is that patterns of activity encode a single value per variable at any given time. This is a reasonable assumption in many situations (although there are exceptions, as discussed later). For example, an object can move in only one direction at a time, so the neurons encoding its direction of motion have only one value to encode.

Under the assumption of a single value, neuronal responses are generally characterized by tuning curves, noted $f_i(\theta)$, which specify the mean activity of cell i as a function of the encoded variable. These tuning curves are typically bell shaped, and are often taken to be Gaussian for nonperiodic variables and circular normal for periodic ones.

Simply measuring the mean activity, however, is not sufficient for performing estimation. A neuron may fire at a rate of 20 spikes/s on one trial but only 15 spikes/s on the next, even though the same stimulus was presented both times. This trial-to-trial variability is captured by the noise distribution, $P(a_i = a|\theta)$, where a_i is the activity of cell i. The noise distribution is often assumed to be Gaussian, either with fixed variance or with a variance proportional to the mean (the latter being more consistent with experimental data), and independent. Such a distribution has the form

$$P(a_i = a|\theta) = \frac{1}{\sqrt{2\pi\sigma_i^2}} \exp\left(-\frac{(a - f_i(\theta))^2}{2\sigma_i^2}\right) \quad (1)$$

where σ_i^2 is either fixed or equal to the mean, $f_i(\theta)$. Another popular choice, especially useful if one is counting spikes, is the Poisson distribution:

$$P(a_i = k|\theta) = \frac{f_i(\theta)^k e^{-f_i(\theta)}}{k!} \quad (2)$$

Figure 1C shows a typical pattern of activity with Gaussian noise and σ_i^2 fixed.

Estimating a Single Value

We now consider various approaches to reading out a population code under the assumptions that (1) a single value is encoded at any given time, and (2) the only source of uncertainty is the neuronal noise. Most of these methods, known as estimators, seek to recover an estimate, $\hat{\theta}$, of the encoded variable. We first discuss how one assesses the quality of an estimator in general; we then provide descriptions of common estimators used for decoding population activity.

Fisher Information

An estimate, $\hat{\theta}$, is obtained by computing a function of the observed activity $\mathbf{A}$, where $\mathbf{A} \equiv (a_1, a_2, \ldots)$. Because of neuronal noise, $\mathbf{A}$ is a random variable and thus so is $\hat{\theta}$. This means that $\hat{\theta}$ will vary from trial to trial even for identical presentation angles. The best estimators are ones that are unbiased and efficient. An unbiased estimator is right on average: the conditional mean, $E[\hat{\theta}|\theta]$, is equal to the encoded direction, θ, where E denotes an average over trials. An efficient estimator, on the other hand, is consistent from trial to trial: the conditional variance, $E[(\hat{\theta} - \theta)^2|\theta]$, is minimal.

In general, the quality of an estimator depends on a compromise between the bias and the conditional variance. In this chapter, however, we consider unbiased estimators only, for which the conditional variance is the important measure because it fully determines how well one can discriminate small changes in the encoded variable based on observation of the neuronal activity. There exists a theoretical lower bound on the conditional variance, which is known as the Cramér-Rao bound. For an unbiased estimator, this bound is equal to the inverse of the Fisher information (Paradiso, 1988; Seung and Sompolinsky, 1993), which leads to the inequality

$$E[(\hat{\theta} - \theta)^2|\theta] \geq \frac{1}{I_{\text{Fisher}}}$$

where

$$I_{\text{Fisher}} \equiv E\left[-\frac{\partial^2}{\partial\theta^2} \log P(\mathbf{A}|\theta)\right]$$

An efficient estimator is one whose conditional variance is equal to the Cramér-Rao bound, $1/I_{\text{Fisher}}$. When $P(\mathbf{A}|\theta)$ is known, it is often straightforward to compute I_{Fisher}. For example, for the Gaussian distribution given in Equation 1,

$$I_{\text{Fisher}} = \sum_{i=1}^{N} \frac{f_i'(\theta)^2}{\sigma_i^2}$$

and for the Poisson distribution given in Equation 2,

$$I_{\text{Fisher}} = \sum_{i=1}^{N} \frac{f_i'(\theta)^2}{f_i(\theta)}$$

(Seung and Sompolinsky, 1993).

In both of these expressions, the neurons that contribute most strongly to the Fisher information are those with a large slope (large $f_i'(\theta)$). Therefore, the most active neurons are not the most informative ones. In fact, they are the *least* informative: the most active neurons correspond to the top of the tuning curve, where the slope is zero, so these neurons make no contribution to Fisher information.

Voting Methods

Several estimators rely on the idea of interpreting the activity of a cell, normalized or not, as a vote for the preferred direction of the cell. For instance, the optimal linear estimator is given by

$$\hat{\theta}_{\text{OLE}} = \sum_{i=1}^{N} \theta_i a_i$$

where θ_i is the preferred direction of cell i, that is, the peak of the function $f_i(\theta)$. A variation on this theme is the center of mass estimator, defined as

$$\hat{\theta}_{\text{COM}} = \frac{\sum_{i=1}^{N} \theta_i(a_i - \gamma)}{\sum_{i=1}^{N} (a_i - \gamma)}$$

where γ is the spontaneous activity of the cells.

A third variation is known as a population vector estimator (Figure 2A). This has been extensively used for estimating periodic variables, such as direction, from real data (Georgopoulos et al., 1982). It is equivalent to fitting a cosine function through the pattern of activity and using the phase of the cosine as the estimate of direction:

$$\hat{\theta}_{\text{COMP}} = \text{phase}(z)$$

where

$$z = \sum_{j=1}^{N} a_j e^{i\theta_j}$$

The first two methods work best for nonperiodic variables; the third one can only be used when the variables are periodic. All

Figure 2. *A*, The population vector estimator uses the phase of the first Fourier component of the input pattern (solid line) as an estimate of direction. It is equivalent to fitting a cosine function to the input. *B*, The maximum likelihood estimate is found by moving an "expected" hill of activity (dashed line) until the squared distance with the data is minimized (solid line).

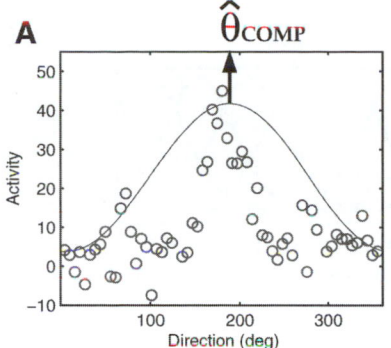

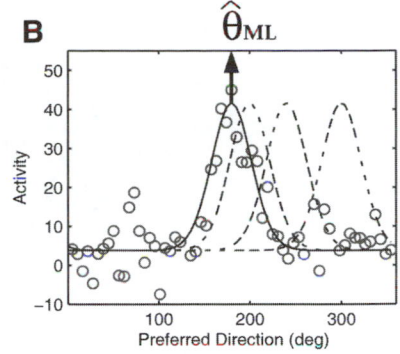

three estimators are subject to biases, although careful tuning of the parameters can often correct for them. More important, all three methods are almost always suboptimal (the variance of the estimator exceeds the Cramér-Rao bound). The exceptions occur for a very specific set of tuning curves and noise distributions (Salinas and Abbott, 1994): the center of mass is optimal only with Gaussian tuning curves and Poisson noise, and the population vector is optimal only for cosine tuning curves and Gaussian noise of fixed variance.

Maximum Likelihood

A better choice than the voting methods, at least from the point of view of statistical efficiency, is the maximum likelihood (ML) estimator

$$\hat{\theta}_{ML} = \arg \max_{\theta} P(\mathbf{A}|\theta)$$

When there are a large number of neurons, this estimator is unbiased and its variance is equal to the Cramér-Rao bound for a wide variety of tuning curve profiles and noise distribution (Paradiso, 1988; Seung and Sompolinsky, 1993). The term maximum likelihood comes from the fact that $\hat{\theta}_{ML}$ is obtained by choosing the value of θ that maximizes the conditional probability of the activity, $P(\mathbf{A}|\theta)$, also known as the likelihood of θ.

Finding the ML estimate reduces to template matching (Paradiso, 1988), i.e., finding the noise-free hill that is closest to the activity, as illustrated in Figure 2*B*. If the noise is independent and Gaussian, then "closest" is with respect to the Euclidean norm, $\Sigma_i(a_i - f_i(\theta))^2$. For other distributions the norm is more complicated. Template matching involves a nonlinear regression, which is typically performed by moving the position of the hill until the distance from the data is minimized, as shown in Figure 2*B*. The position of the peak of the final hill corresponds to the ML estimate.

The main difference between the population vector and the ML estimator is the shape of the template being matched to the data. Whereas the population vector matches a cosine, the ML estimator uses a template that is directly derived from the tuning curves of the neurons that generated the activity (Figures 2*A* and 2*B*). (When all neurons have identical tuning curves, as for our examples, the template has the same profile as the tuning curves.) It is because the ML estimator uses the correct template that its variance reaches the Cramér-Rao bound. There is, however, a cost: one needs to know the profile of all tuning curves to use ML estimation, whereas only the preferred directions, θ_i, are needed for the population vector estimator.

Bayesian Approach

An alternative to ML estimation is to use the full posterior distribution of the encoded variable, $P(\theta|\mathbf{A})$. This is related to the distribution of the noise, $P(\mathbf{A}|\theta)$, through Bayes's theorem:

$$P(\theta|\mathbf{A}) = \frac{P(\mathbf{A}|\theta)P(\theta)}{P(\mathbf{A})}$$

where $P(\mathbf{A})$ and $P(\theta)$ are the prior distributions over $\mathbf{A}$ and θ. The value that maximizes $P(\theta|\mathbf{A})$ can then be used as an estimate of θ. This is known as a maximum a posteriori estimate, or MAP estimate. The main advantage of the MAP estimate over the ML estimate is that prior knowledge about the encoded variable can be taken into account. This is particularly important when the conditional distribution, $P(\mathbf{A}|\theta)$, is not sharply peaked compared to the prior, $P(\theta)$. This happens, for example, when only a small number of neurons are available, or when one observes only a few spikes per neuron. The MAP estimate is close to the ML estimate if the prior distribution varies slowly compared to the conditional, and the two are exactly equal when the prior is flat. Several authors have explored and/or applied applied this approach to real data (Foldiak, 1993; Sanger, 1996; Zhang et al., 1998).

Neuronal Implementations

Methods such as the voting schemes or ML estimator are biologically implausible, for one simple reason: they extract a single value, the estimate of the encoded variable. Such explicit decoding is very rare in the brain. Instead, most cortical areas and subcortical structures use population codes to encode variables. This means that, throughout the brain, population codes are mapped into population codes. Hence, V1 neurons, which are broadly tuned to the direction of motion, project to MT neurons, which are also broadly tuned, but in neither area is the direction of motion read out as a single number. The neurons in MT are nevertheless confronted with an estimation problem: they must choose their activity levels on the basis of the noisy activity of V1 neurons.

What is the optimal strategy for mapping one population code into another? We cannot answer this question in general, but we can address it for the broad class of networks depicted in Figure 3. In these networks, the input layer is a set of neurons with wide tuning curves, generating noisy patterns of activity like the one shown in Figure 1*C*. This activity, which acts transiently, is relayed to an output layer through feedforward connections. In the output layer the neurons are connected through lateral connections.

An update rule (discussed later) causes the activity in the output layer to evolve in time. In the next section we consider networks in which the update rule leads to a smooth hill. The peak of that hill can be interpreted as an estimate of the variable being encoded. As previously, we can assess how well the network did by looking at the mean and variance of this estimate.

We will consider two kinds of networks: those with a linear activation function and those with a nonlinear one.

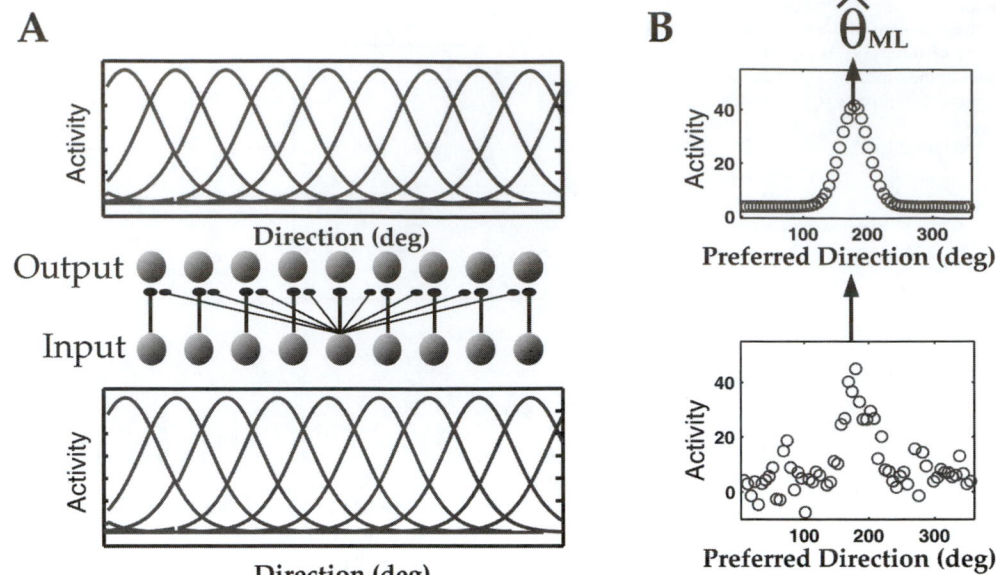

Figure 3. *A*, A set of units with broad tuning to a sensory variable (in this case direction) projects to another set of units also broadly tuned to the same variable. This type of mapping between population codes is very common throughout the brain. In this particular network, the output layer is fully interconnected with lateral connections, and receives feedforward connections from the input layer. *B*, Temporal evolution of the activity in the output layer for a nonlinear network. The activity in the output layer is initiated with a noisy hill generated by the input units (bottom). For an appropriate choice of weights and activation function, these activities converge eventually to a smooth hill (top), which peaks close to the location of the maximum likelihood estimate of direction, $\hat{\theta}_{ML}$. This network is performing the template-matching procedure used in maximum likelihood and illustrated in Figure 2*B*.

Linear Networks

We first consider a network with linear activation functions in the output layer, so that the dynamics is governed by the difference equation

$$\mathbf{O}_t = ((1 - \lambda)I + \lambda W)\mathbf{O}_{t-1} \tag{3}$$

where λ is a number between 0 and 1, I is the identity matrix, and W is the matrix for the lateral connections. The activity at time 0, $\mathbf{O}_0$, is initialized to $W\mathbf{A}$, where $\mathbf{A}$ is an input pattern (like the one shown in Figure 1*C*) and W is the feedforward weight matrix (for simplicity, the feedforward and lateral weights are the same, although this is not necessary).

The dynamics of such a network is well understood: each eigenvector of the matrix $(1 - \lambda)I + \lambda W$ evolves independently, with exponential amplification for eigenvalues greater than 1 and exponential suppression for eigenvalues less than 1. When the weights are translation invariant ($W_{ij} = W_{i-j}$), the eigenvectors are sines and cosine. In this case the network amplifies or suppresses independently each Fourier component of the initial input pattern, **A**, by a factor equal to the corresponding eigenvalue of $(1 - \lambda)I + \lambda W$. For example, if the first eigenvalue of $(1 - \lambda)I + \lambda W$ is more than 1 (respectively less than 1), the first Fourier component of the initial pattern of activity will be amplified (respectively suppressed). Thus, W can be chosen such that the network amplifies selectively the first Fourier component of the data while suppressing the others.

As formulated, the activity in such a network would grow forever. However, if we stop after a large yet fixed number of iterations, the activity pattern will look like a cosine function of direction with a phase corresponding to the phase of the first Fourier component of the data. The peak of the cosine provides the estimate of direction. That estimate turns out to be the same as the one provided by the population vector discussed above.

The unchecked exponential growth of a purely linear network can be alleviated by adding a nonlinear term to act as gain control. This type of network was proposed by Ben-Yishai, Bar-Or, and Sompolinsky (1995) as a model of orientation selectivity. Although such networks keep the estimate in a coarse code format, they suffer from two problems: it is not immediately clear how to extend them to periodic variables, such as disparity, and they are suboptimal, since they are equivalent to the population estimator.

Nonlinear Networks

To obtain optimal performance, one needs a network that can implement template matching with the correct template—the one used by the ML estimator (see Figure 2*B*). This requires templates that go beyond cosines to include curves that are consistent with the tuning curves of the input units (see Figure 2*B*).

Nonlinear networks that admit line attractors have this property (Deneve, Latham, and Pouget, 1999). In such networks, the line attractors correspond to smooth hills of activity, with profiles determined by the patterns of weights *and* the activation functions. For a given activation function, it is therefore possible to select the weights to optimize the profile of the stable state. Pouget et al. (1998) demonstrated that this extra flexibility allows these networks to act as ML estimators (see Figure 3*B*).

More recent work by Deneve et al. (1999) has shown that the ML property is preserved for a wide range of nonlinear activation functions. In particular, this is true for networks using divisive normalization, a nonlinearity believed to exist in cortical microcircuitry. It is therefore possible that all cortical layers are close approximations to ML estimators.

Estimating a Probability Distribution

So far we have reviewed decoding methods in which only one value is encoded at any given time and the only source of uncertainty comes from the neuronal activity. Situations exist, however, in which either (or both) of these assumptions are violated. For instance, imagine that you are lost in Manhattan on a foggy day, but you can see, faintly, the Empire State building and the Chrysler building in the distance. Because of the poor visibility, the views of these landmarks are not sufficient to specify your exact position, but they are enough to provide a rough idea of where you are (Harlem versus Little Italy). In this situation, it would be desirable to compute the probability distribution of your location given that you are seeing the landmarks; i.e., compute $P(\theta|w)$ where θ is the position (now a two-dimensional vector) in Manhattan and w represents the views of the buildings. Here, the uncertainty about θ comes from the fact that you do not have enough information to tell precisely where you are. In such a situation, the neurons could encode the *probability distribution, $P(\theta|w)$*.

Because the encoded entity is a probability distribution rather than a single value, we can no longer use either Equation 1 or Equation 2 as a model for the responses of the neurons; these equations provide only the likelihood of θ, $P(\mathbf{A}|\theta)$. What we need instead is a model that specifies the likelihood of the whole encoded probability distribution, $P[\mathbf{A}|P(\theta|w)]$. Note that $P(\theta|w)$ plays the same role as θ previously, which is to be expected, now that $P(\theta|w)$ is the encoded entity. It is beyond the scope of this discussion to provide equations for such models, but examples can be found in Zemel, Dayan, and Pouget (1998).

Since $\mathbf{A}$ is now a code for the probability distribution, the relevant quantity to estimate is $P(\theta|w)$, which we denote $\hat{P}(\theta|w)$. This is still within the realm of estimation theory, so we can use the same tools that we used for the simpler case, such as ML decoding (see Zemel et al., 1998).

To see the difference between encoding a single value and encoding a probability distribution, it is helpful to consider what happens when the neurons are deterministic—that is, when the neuronal noise goes to zero. In this case, the encoded variable can be recovered with infinite precision, since the only source of uncertainty, the neuronal noise, is gone. Thus the ML estimate would be exactly equal to the encoded value, and the posterior distribution, $P(\theta|\mathbf{A})$, would be a Dirac function centered at θ. If the activity encodes a probability distribution, on the other hand, one would recover the *distribution* with infinite precision. However, the uncertainty about θ may still be quite large (as was the case in our Manhattan example), potentially far from a Dirac function.

It is too early to tell whether neurons encode probability distributions; more empirical as well as theoretical work is needed. But if the cortex has the ability to represent probability distributions, it might be possible to determine how, and whether, the brain performs Bayesian inferences. Bayesian inference is a powerful method for performing computation in the presence of uncertainty. Many engineering applications rely on this framework to perform data analysis or to control robots, and several studies are now suggesting that the brain might be using such inferences for perception and motor control (see, e.g., Knill and Richards, 1996).

Conclusions

Understanding how to decode patterns of neuronal activity is a critical step toward developing theories of representation and computation in the brain. This article concentrated on the simplest case, a single variable encoded in the firing rates of a population of neurons. There are two main approaches to this problem. In the first, the population encodes a single value, and decoding can be done with Bayesian or maximum likelihood estimators. The underlying assumption in this case is that neuronal noise is the only source of uncertainty. We also saw that within this framework, one can design neural networks that perform decoding optimally. In the second approach, the population encodes a full probability distribution over the variable of interest. Here both the variable and its uncertainty can be extracted from the population activity. This scheme could be used to perform statistical inferences—a powerful way to perform computations over variables whose value is not known with certainty. The challenge for future work will be to determine whether the brain uses this type of code, and, if so, to understand how realistic neural circuits can perform statistical inferences over probability distributions.

Road Map: Neural Coding
Related Reading: Cortical Population Dynamics and Psychophysics; Motor Cortex: Coding and Decoding of Directional Operations

References

Ben-Yishai, R., Bar-Or, R. L., and Sompolinsky, H., 1995, Theory of orientation tuning in visual cortex, *Proc. Natl. Acad. Sci. USA*, 92:3844–3848.

Deneve, S., Latham, P. E., and Pouget, A., 1999, Reading population codes: A neural implementation of ideal observers, *Nature Neurosci.*, 2:740–745. ◆

Foldiak, P., 1993, The "ideal homunculus": Statistical inference from neural population responses, in *Computation and Neural Systems* (F. H. Eeckman and J. M. Bower, Eds.), Norwell, MA: Kluwer Academic, pp. 55–60. ◆

Georgopoulos, A. P., Kalaska, J. F., Caminiti, R., and Massey, J. T., 1982, On the relations between the direction of two-dimensional arm movements and cell discharge in primate motor cortex, *J. Neurosci.*, 2:1527–1537.

Knill, D. C., and Richards, W., 1996, *Perception as Bayesian Inference*, New York: Cambridge University Press.

Paradiso, M. A., 1988, A theory of the use of visual orientation information which exploits the columnar structure of striate cortex, *Biol. Cybern.* 58:35–49. ◆

Pouget, A., Zhang, K., Deneve, S., and Lathan, P., 1998, Statistically efficient estimation using population codes, *Neural computation*, 10:373–401.

Pouget, A., Zemel, R. S., and Dayan, P., 2000, Information processing with population codes, *Nature Rev. Neurosci.*, 1:125–132.

Salinas, E., and Abbott, L. F., 1994, Vector reconstruction from firing rate, *J. Computat. Neurosc.*, 1:89–107. ◆

Sanger, T. D., 1996, Probability density estimation for the interpretation of neural population codes, *J. Neurophysiol.*, 76:2790–2793.

Seung, H. S., and Sompolinsky, H., 1993, Simple model for reading neuronal population codes, *Proc. Natl. Acad. Sci. USA*, 90:10749–10753.

Zemel, R. S., Dayan, P., and Pouget, A., 1998, Probabilistic interpretation of population code, *Neural Computat.*, 10:403–430. ◆

Zhang, K., Ginzburg, I., McNaughton, B. L., and Sejnowski, T. J., 1998, Interpreting neuronal population activity by reconstruction: Unified framework with application to hippocampal place cells, *J. Neurophysiol.*, 79:1017–1044.

Post-Hebbian Learning Algorithms

Péter Érdi and Zoltán Somogyvári

Post-Hebbian Learning Rules: A Retrospective

Hebb's introduction of his learning rule inaugurated a new era and resulted in the appearance of many new branches of theory and new models of learning. Two characteristics of the original postulate (Hebb, 1949) played key roles in the subsequent development of post-Hebbian learning rules. First, despite being biologically motivated, Hebb's learning rule was a verbally described, *phenomenological* rule, unlinked to detailed physiological mechanisms. Second, because the learning rule was extremely convincing, it was widely adopted both as a theoretical framework and as a formal tool in the field of neural networks.

As a result, the etiolation of Hebb's idea occurred in two principal directions. First, the postulate inspired an intense and long-lasting search for the molecular and cellular basis of learning phenomena, which were assumed to be Hebbian; thus, this particular development has been absorbed by neurobiology. Second, because of its computational usefulness, many variations of the *biologically inspired* learning rules appeared and were applied to a huge number of very different problems in artificial neural networks, without any relation to a biological foundation being claimed. Several families of rules sprouted from the original idea. Before discussing them, we should note that what we consider a Hebbian, post-Hebbian, or non-Hebbian learning rule to be is subjective and time varying.

This *Handbook* includes a broad overview of the subject in the article Hebbian Synaptic Plasticity (q.v.). Here we focus predominantly on computational implementations of Hebbian rules. First, however, we discuss the different roots and new developments related to Hebb's hypothesis, such as psychologically motivated conditioning, neural development, and physiologically realistic cellular level learning phenomena. Thereafter families of formal Hebbian learning, or *algorithms*, are considered.

Variations on the Hebbian Theme: Motivations

Conditioning

Since the end of the nineteenth century, physiologists have known that mature nerve cells cannot divide (though in the late 20th century they changed their minds!). Thus, because learning could not result from the proliferation of new neurons, the locus of learning had to be *the connections between cells*. Such phenomena are related to the neural basis of classical conditioning. The first attempt to model conditioning in terms of synaptic change was by Hebb.

Hebb's original intent was to connect the behavior of whole organisms to neural mechanisms by using concepts represented by cell assemblies. Specifically, classical conditioning involves the development of an association between two otherwise unrelated events over a number of trials in which the events are temporally paired. Typically, a neutral stimulus, one that does not naturally provoke behavior, is presented, immediately followed by an unconditioned stimulus, or an event that does not require training to produce a response, resulting in the eliciting of an unconditioned response.

Classical conditioning (see Conditioning) has been described by Rescorla and Wagner's (1972) model. They proposed a formal model of conditioning that expresses the capacity of a conditioned stimulus (CS) to become associated with an unconditioned stimulus (US) at any given time. The fulcrum of the Wagner-Rescorla model is that learning occurs if and when events violate expectations. More specifically, learning occurs whenever the actual level of US received during a trial differs from the level expected. The Rescorla-Wagner rule can be interpreted as saying that the discrepancy between expected and actual values determines the measure of reinforcement. So, the rule and its many later modifications act over the unsupervised learning paradigm. One drawback of the Rescorla-Wagner model, however, is that it completely ignores the temporal sequence in which information is presented.

Development

The formation and refinement of neural circuits involves both the establishment of new connections and the elimination of already existing connections. The leading mechanism in synaptic elimination is considered to be *axonal* or *synaptic competition*. Neuromuscular junctions and the visual system are the two best investigated examples in which synaptic competition plays an important role.

A large variety of generalized Hebbian learning rules have been applied to neural development (see review by van Ooyen, 2001). An example is the different mechanisms of competition elaborated in the context of population biology that have been adopted in the neural context. In *consumptive competition* in systems of consumers and resources (e.g., predators and prey), each individual consumer tries to avoid other consumers and hinders other consumers solely by consuming resources that they might have consumed. In other words, consumers hinder each other because they draw on the same resources. In neurobiology, competition is commonly associated with this dependence on shared resources. In *interference competition*, instead of hindrance through dependence on shared resources, there is direct interference between individuals. Such interference occurs, for example, if there are direct negative interactions (e.g., aggressive or toxic interactions) between individuals. In axonal competition, nerve terminals could seek to destroy each other by releasing proteases.

Long-Term Potentiation—Long-Term Depression

Long-term potentiation (LTP) was first discovered in the hippocampus and is very prominent there. LTP is an increase in synaptic strength that can be rapidly induced by brief periods of synaptic stimulation. It has been reported to last for hours in vitro, and for days to weeks in vivo.

LTP (and later long-term depression, or LTD) became regarded as the physiological basis of Hebbian learning. Subsequently, the properties of LTP and LTD became clearer, and the question then arose as to whether LTP and LTD could really be considered the microscopic basis of the phenomenological Hebbian type of learning. Formally, the question is how to specify the general function F to serve as a learning rule with the known properties of LTP and LTD. Recognizing the existence of this gap between biological mechanisms and the long-used Hebbian learning rule, many workers have attempted to derive the corresponding phenomenological rule based on more or less detailed neurochemical mechanisms.

The time course of LTP may be insufficient to sustain long-term memory, but there appear to be multiple LTP mechanisms, and one dependent on protein synthesis might serve long-term memory: inhibition of protein synthesis disrupts the maintenance of LTP but leaves the induction of LTP relatively or totally intact. It is possible to relate the properties and mechanisms of long-term synaptic plasticity in the mammalian brain to learning and memory.

An example of the new synaptic bidirectional Hebbian rules was introduced by Grzywacz and Burgi in 1998. When this rule was compared with physiological homosynaptic conditions in the hippocampus, the results indicated that this rule was consistent with LTP and LTD phenomenologies. The phenomenologies considered included the reversible dynamics of LTP and LTD and the effects of N-methyl-D-aspartate (NMDA) blockers and phosphatase inhibitors.

Timing

Studies in cortical and hippocampal slices have shown that back-propagating action potentials may contribute to the induction of persistent synaptic potentiation or depression. The timing of presynaptic and postsynaptic action potentials plays a decisive role in determining the sign of synaptic modification (Markram et al., 1997). The temporal order of the synaptic input and the postsynaptic spike within a narrow window of time determines whether LTP or LTD is elicited, according to a temporally asymmetric Hebbian learning rule.

Bi and Poo (1998) showed that postsynaptic spiking that peaked within 20 ms *after* synaptic activation resulted in LTP, whereas spiking within 20 ms *before* synaptic activation led to LTD. They suggested that a narrow and asymmetric window for the induction of synaptic modification should be taken into account.

Most generalized Hebbian rules are based on the statistical properties of presynaptic and postsynaptic activity (e.g., activity product, activity covariance) and do not consider the detailed temporal structure of the spike patterns. Relative spike timing, however, had been taken into account as early as 1981 by Sutton and Barto.

Since changes in synaptic efficacy can depend on the precise temporal relations of pre- and postsynaptic spikes, phenomenological "temporal learning rules" generate opposite changes in synaptic efficiency, depending on whether the postsynaptic spike occurs before or after the presynaptic spike. Roberts (1999) attempted to show that differential Hebbian learning could take into account the timing effects.

Generalized Hebbian Rules and Their Phenomenological Derivations

Hebb's idea has been formalized in many variations. The first and simplest versions of the Hebbian learning rule have the important properties of being *local* and *interactive* (specifically, *conjunctional* and *time dependent*), as we will now explain. We will consider what happens when we attempt to preserve these properties in the course of generalizing the Hebbian learning rule.

The most general form of Hebb's rule is that the synaptic weight from neuron i to neuron j changes according to

$$\frac{d}{dt} w_{ij}(t) = F(a_i, a_j) \qquad (1)$$

where F is a functional, and a_j and a_i are presynaptic and postsynaptic activity functions (i.e., they may include activity levels over some period of time and not just the current activity values). To define specific learning rules (i.e., the form of F), a few points should be clarified.

1. What are the assumptions about the *locality* of the modifying signal? In many cases the modification of a synapse between neurons i and j depends on the state of these two cells alone; i.e., the mechanism is local. In this case, teacher or external reinforcement signals are not explicitly involved: local synapses are the bases of the unsupervised learning.
2. How, if at all, do the presynaptic and postsynaptic cells *interact?* Consider first the potential answers for the "if at all" part of the question. The modification can be interactive if both the pre-

and postsynaptic cells are involved, and noninteractive if either the pre- or postsynaptic cell alone influences the modification. The mechanism of the interaction may be conjunctional or correlational. In the first case, co-occurrence of pre- and postsynaptic activity is sufficient to cause synaptic change, while in the second case, covariance of the two activities must be taken into account. (From a formal point of view, additive interactions, such as those given by the function $F(a_i \pm a_j)$, could have been defined, but they are considered as noninteractive rules. In other words, not only an entire rule but each term of it can be evaluated as interactive or noninteractive.)

3. What are the assumptions about the form of the *time-dependent* activity functions? In the simplest case, only the actual activity values are involved. In somewhat more complex situations, short-term averaged activity values determine the synaptic change. More generally, the history of the activity values plays a role in the modification process.

The simplest Hebbian learning rule can be formalized as

$$\frac{d}{dt} w_{ij}(t) = ka_i(t)a_j(t), \qquad k > 0 \qquad (2)$$

This rule expresses the conjunction among pre- and postsynaptic elements (using neurobiological terminology) or associative conditioning (in psychological terms), by a simple product of the actual states of pre- and postsynaptic elements, $a_j(t)$ and $a_i(t)$.

A characteristic and unfortunate property of the simplest Hebbian rule in Equation 1 is that the synaptic strengths are ever increasing (see HEBBIAN LEARNING AND NEURONAL REGULATION for solutions to the problems this property raises).

$$\frac{d}{dt} w_{ij}(t) = kg(a_i(t))h(a_j(t)) \qquad (3)$$

where g and h, functions of the actual activity, serve as some measure of the post- and presynaptic activity (i.e., $g, h > 0$), and

$$\frac{d}{dt} w_{ij}(t) = kg(a_i(\cdot))h(a_j(\cdot)) \qquad (4)$$

where g and h are now functionals of the activity function. A special case is

$$\frac{d}{dt} w_{ij}(t) = k \int_0^t a_i(t)dt \int_0^t a_j(t)dt \qquad (5)$$

which takes into account the total activity history.

There is a particular time-dependent, local, and conjunctional rule that does not increase the synaptic weight. This is the case in which the pre- and postsynaptic activities are negatively correlated:

$$\frac{d}{dt} w_{ij}(t) = ka_i(t)a_j(t), \qquad k < 0 \qquad (6)$$

This "anti-Hebbian" rule (there is some confusion in the literature concerning this terminology; here it is used in the sense that $k < 0$) or "decorrelation" rule was suggested to describe features of dissociations of patterns (Barlow and Földiak, 1989).

There are both brutal and sophisticated methods to eliminate the unpleasant property of ever-increasing weights, which, unless compensated for, yield a network with saturated synaptic weights, and thus no effective pattern discrimination. The adjective "brutal" was adopted for the situation in which some external constraint (somehow taking into account the finiteness of resources) is applied to the internal mechanism. First, a predetermined upper bound can be given, such as the maximal value of the synaptic strength. Second, the so-called normalization procedure (described in Rochester et al., 1956) gives a finite-sum constraint on all synaptic strengths, and can be interpreted as a competition of the presynaptic elements for postsynaptic resources (therefore, it violates locality). Such rules may explain some aspects of neural development

More sophisticated methods decrease the synaptic strengths selectively. Brown, Kairiss, and Keenan (1990) use the expression *generalized Hebbian synaptic mechanism* for cases in which interactive synaptic increase is combined with activity-dependent synaptic depression. The underlying mechanism behind synaptic depression may be of interactive or noninteractive type.

Instead of giving a formal derivation of the rules that are able to describe selective decrease, we will mention two important special cases. First, the rule

$$\frac{d}{dt} w_{ij}(t) = kg(a_i(t))(h(a_j(t)) - \theta(t)) \quad (7)$$

implements synaptic increase only if the $h(a_j(t))$ presynaptic activity is larger than the $\theta(t)$ modification threshold. If the presynaptic activity is smaller than the threshold, the synaptic weight decreases. Second,

$$\frac{d}{dt} w_{ij}(t) = k(g(a_i(t)) - \theta(t))h(a_j(t)) \quad (8)$$

implements a postsynaptic control mechanism on the modification process.

The learning rules in Equations 8 and 9 can be written in the form $kgh - k\theta g$ and $kgh - k\theta h$, respectively. Each of these expressions may be interpreted as the sum of a Hebbian interactive term and a noninteractive term. In the first case, the decrease is due to postsynaptic activity g and is called *heterosynaptic depression*, while in the second case it depends on the presynaptic activity h and is called *homosynaptic depression*. Learning rules of the form of Equation 9 were suggested by Bienenstock, Cooper, and Munro (1982) and so are sometimes referred as the BCM theory; they are used to model the plasticity of visual cortex. $\theta(t)$ was identified with a nonlinear function of the averaged postsynaptic activity:

$$\theta(t) = [g(t)]^2 \quad (9)$$

where $[\cdot]$ is the average taken for a period of time. The suggestion that the occurrence of either homosynaptic LTP or LTD depends on the strength of the depolarizing current induced by an NMDA blocker (which increases the modification threshold) in the visual cortex seemed to be justified experimentally.

The learning expression has also been described in the form $\phi(g, [g])h$, where the two-variable function ϕ depends on an actual value and an averaged quantity, so an underlying microscopic stochastic mechanism should exist behind the phenomenological and deterministic formalism.

The weaker form of the interactive rule (namely, when correlational and nonconjunctional interactions were assumed), or

$$\frac{d}{dt} w_{ij}(t) = k(a_i(t) - [a_i(t)])(a_j(t) - [a_j(t)]) \quad (10)$$

was offered by Rochester et al. (1956). Depending on the sign of the correlation, the rule is capable of describing either synaptic enhancement or decrease. Covariance was suggested to induce associative LTD in the hippocampus.

Another way to describe the decrease of synaptic weights is the introduction of a spontaneous decay (or "forgetting") term. The original Hebbian rule (Equation 2) supplemented with a decay term reads as

$$\frac{d}{dt} w_{ij}(t) = -k_1 w_{ij}(t) + k_2 a_i(t)a_j(t) \quad (11)$$

(Instead of first-order decay, a quadratic forgetting term was also introduced and studied to improve the stability properties of the

learning rule.) If the decay is not spontaneous but modulated with the postsynaptic activity, the rule has the form

$$\frac{d}{dt} w_{ij}(t) = -k_1 w_{ij}(t)a_i(t) + k_2 a_i(t)a_j(t)$$
$$\equiv a_i(t)(k_2 a_j(t) - k_1 w_{ij}(t)) \quad (12)$$

and describes the phenomenon called competitive learning. Postsynaptic neurons compete for incoming resources: the larger the postsynaptic activity, the larger the measure of learning:

$$\frac{d}{dt} w_{ij}(t) = k \frac{d}{dt} a_i(t) \frac{d}{dt} a_j(t) \quad (13)$$

This rule is an example of a differential learning mechanism (Klopf, 1986). Obviously, the rate of change of activities may be positive or negative; that is, both synaptic increase and decrease may occur. The differential competitive rule,

$$\frac{d}{dt} w_{ij}(t) = \frac{d}{dt} a_i(t)(k_2 a_j(t) - k_1 w_{ij}(t)) \quad (14)$$

implements the "learn only if change" principle.

In some cases, the time delay due to signal transmission is explicitly taken into account; consequently, earlier presynaptic activities, rather than current activities, are in conjunction:

$$\frac{d}{dt} w_{ij}(t) = ka_i(t)a_j(t - \tau) \quad (15)$$

This spirit of "timing sensitivity" is materialized in the rule

$$\frac{d}{dt} w_{ij}(t) = k_1 \frac{d}{dt} a_i(t)[a_j(t)] \quad (16)$$

used to describe conditioning (see, e.g., Sejnowski and Tesauro, 1990).

Hebbian Mechanisms and Hebbian Algorithms

Hebb proposed that the connection between two neurons will increase if activity in the neurons is temporally paired. More specifically, the Hebbian model proposes that the strength of a particular connection will increase if use of the synapse contributes to the occurrence of an action potential in the postsynaptic neuron. This account critically depends on coincidence detectors in the postsynaptic neuron.

The underlying biophysical mechanisms and algorithms of even generalized Hebbian synaptic modification were reviewed by Brown et al. (1990). Over the next several years, system-level computational models of the neural bases of learning and memory began to proliferate.

The general question has been, and still is, how to connect the formal algorithms of the neural basis of learning phenomena. Although many commonly used learning rules lead to successful models of plasticity and learning, they are inconsistent with what is known about neurophysiology. Other, more physiologically plausible rules fail to specify relevant properties, such as bidirectionality and the biological mechanism that prevents synapses from changing from excitatory to inhibitory, and vice versa. More recent attempts have tried to overcome these difficulties.

Discussion: Over the Hebbian Paradigm

It is certainly not true that all learning rules could be interpreted in even a generalized Hebbian sense. It is difficult, however, to discriminate precisely between Hebbian and non-Hebbian frameworks. One way to do so might be to consider a learning rule Hebbian if only two elements, one presynaptic, one postsynaptic, are involved. If we accept this limitation, we know by exclusion what a non-Hebbian learning rule is. Many types of supervised learning rules used in artificial neural networks, such as delta rules, and their variations certainly belong to this category. Heterosynaptic plasticity and the modifiability of synaptic triads and glomeruli, in which more than two cells are explicitly involved in the modification process, could also be understood as non-Hebbian. Such a choice, however, would also exclude rules with the normalization procedure.

What is the relationship between homosynaptic (or Hebbian activity–dependent) and heterosynaptic (or modulatory input–dependent) plasticity? It has often been suggested (see, e.g., Bailey et al., 2000) that Hebbian mechanisms are used primarily for learning and for forming short-term memory traces, but they are not sufficient to recruit the events required to maintain a long-term memory. In contrast, heterosynaptic plasticity commonly recruits long-term memory mechanisms that lead to transcription and to synaptic growth. When jointly recruited, homosynaptic mechanisms ensure that learning is effectively established and heterosynaptic mechanisms ensure that memory is maintained.

The spirit of the Hebbian idea survived more than half a century. It will be interesting to see what kinds of phenomenological learning rules will be derived in the next several years, starting from cellular level experimental and modeling studies of synaptic modifiability.

Road Map: Neural Plasticity
Background: Hebbian Synaptic Plasticity
Related Reading: Hebbian Learning and Neuronal Regulation

References

Bailey, C., Giustetto, M., Huang, Y., Hawkins, R., and Kandel, E., 2000, Is heterosynaptic modulation essential for stabilizing Hebbian plasticity and memory? *Nature Rev. Neurosci.*, 1:11–20.

Barlow, H., and Földiak, P., 1989, Adaptation and decorrelation in the cortex, in *The Computing Neuron* (R. Durbin, C. Miall, and G. Mitchison, Eds.), Wokingham, Engl.: Addison-Wesley, pp. 54–72.

Bi, G., and Poo, M., 1998, Synaptic modifications in cultured hippocampal neurons: Dependence on spike timing, synaptic strength, and postsynaptic cell type, *J. Neurosci*, 18:10464–10472.

Bienenstock, E., Cooper, L., and Munro, P., 1982, Theory for the development of neuron selectivity: Orientation specificity and binocular interaction in visual cortex, *J. Neurosci.*, 2:32–48.

Brown, T., Kairiss, E., and Keenan, C., 1990, Hebbian synapses: Biophysical mechanisms and algorithms, *Annu. Rev. Neurosci.*, 13:475–511. ◆

Grzywacz, N., and Burgi, P., 1998, Toward a biophysically plausible bidirectional Hebbian rule, *Neural Computat.*, 10:499–520.

Hebb, D., 1949, *The Organization of the Behavior*, New York: Wiley.

Klopf, A., 1986, A drive-reinforcement model of single neuron function: An alternative to the Hebbian neuronal mode, in *Proceedings of the American Institute of Physics: Neural Networks for Computing*, New York: American Institute of Physics pp. 265–270.

Markram, H., Lubke, J., Frotscher, M., Roth, A., and Sakmann, B., 1997, Physiology and anatomy of synaptic connections between thick tufted pyramidal neurones in the developing rat neocortex, *J. Physiol.*, 500(Pt. 2):409–440.

Rescorla, R., and Wagner, A., 1972, A theory of Pavlovian conditioning: Variations in the effectiveness of reinforcement and nonreinforcement, in *Classical Conditioning II* (A. Black and W. Prokasy, Eds.), New York: Appleton-Century-Crofts.

Roberts, P., 1999, Computational consequences of temporally asymmetric learning rules: I. Differential Hebbian learning, *J. Comput. Neurosci.*, 7:235–246.

Rochester, N., Holland, J., Haibt, L., and Duda, W., 1956, Tests on a cell assembly theory of the action of the brain, using a large scale digital computer, *IRE Trans. Inform. Theory*, IT-2:80–93.

Sejnowski, T., and Tesauro, G., 1990, Building network learning algorithms for Hebbian synapses, in *Brain Organization and Memory Cells, Systems, and Circuit* (N. McGaugh, N. Weinberger, and G. Lynch, Eds.), New York: Oxford University Press. ◆

Sutton, R., and Barto, A., 1981, Toward a modern theory of adaptive networks: Expectation and prediction, *Psychol. Rev.*, 88:135–170. ◆

van Ooyen, A., 2001, Competition in the development of nerve connections: A review of models, *Network*, 12:R1–R47.

Potential Fields and Neural Networks

Jiming Liu and Oussama Khatib

Introduction

In this article, we review the ideas and observations involved in the concept of potential fields. *Potential fields* are often defined to characterize the vector-field output of a behavior module, the impedance of a structure, or the external constraints of an environment. Such a characterization is useful for modeling motor behavior control in humans and robots. Here we also examine how neural networks are related to potential fields, as underlying architectures for enabling sensorimotor control and behavior learning.

Biological Relevance of Potential Fields in Behavior Modeling

In biological studies, potential fields offer a way to represent and measure the motor output behavior of a physiological mechanism. Many of the reported biological studies that have taken into account potential fields have sought to understand how the neural circuits in the frog's spinal cord are organized and how the motor behaviors of the frog, such as postures, are governed by the neural control modules.

Complex Motor Behaviors and Vector Fields

The theoretical work of Mussa-Ivaldi and Giszter (e.g., 1992), known as vector-field approximation, characterizes the elicited outputs of distinct postural control modules as basis fields. Simple motor tasks can therefore be described by the specific features of vector fields, such as stable equilibrium, impedance, unstable equilibrium, saddle point, uniform field, and circulation. In their simulations, they show that a repertoire of convergent force patterns can readily be approximated based on the superposition of basis fields (as training examples). Furthermore, by combining the field features, it is possible to produce a variety of more complex control patterns.

Linear Combination of Force Fields

In relation to vector-field approximation and complex pattern generation, Mussa-Ivaldi, Giszter, and Bizzi (1994) have tested the hypothesis that vectorial superposition—that is, linear combination—of the motor primitives in the neural circuits of the frog's spinal cord can lead to a variety of motor behaviors. They conducted experiments to measure the force fields in the workspace of the frog's leg while stimulating the premotor sites in the frog's spinal cord. Their experimental results have shown that simultaneously stimulating two regions in the spinal cord generates the vector summation of the end-point forces generated by the separate stimulation of each spinal region (see MOTOR PRIMITIVES).

Adaptive Combination of Motor Primitives

Based on results achieved in the linear combination of force fields, we might ask whether motor behavior learning can also be modeled in terms of changes in the primitive combination. Thoroughman and Shadmehr (2000) believe that a flexible combination of human motor primitives provides a model for experience-based complex movement learning. They suggest that the human brain builds a state-dependent internal model of muscle forces for generating the dynamic trajectories of movements. This internal model is essentially a sensorimotor map that is constructed by combining a set of motor primitives. The primitives have Gaussian-like turning functions for encoding arm velocities. The experience-based learning of a movement is therefore reflected in the adaptive adjustment of the weight matrix that defines the primitive combination.

Designing Force-Field Motor Primitives

Insights into the organization of motor primitives and their role in the generation of force fields not only enhance our understanding of how biological neural circuits produce motor patterns, they also provide guidance in designing behavior-based robotic systems.

One of the earliest studies demonstrating the use of motor primitives in robot motion control was reported by Arkin in 1989. The object was to develop an experimental mobile robot system that would perform path planning and execution in a way resembling the Arbib and House (1987) model of detour behavior in the frog. The Arbib and House model is an abstraction that characterizes prey acquisition behavior in an obstacle-strewn environment, with primitive vector fields resulting from the frog's perception of its environment. The primitive vector fields are the prey-attractant field, barrier repellent field, and frog representation field. The path-determining vectors can therefore be calculated based on the summation of the primitive vector fields. In autonomous robot architecture (ARA), the path execution mechanism employs a set of concurrently activated motor behaviors called motor schemas. These schemas include *move-to-goal* (similar to the Arbib and House prey-attractant field), *avoid-static-obstacles* (similar to the Arbib and House repellant field), *stay-on-path*, *avoid-moving-obstacles*, *find-intersection*, and *find-landmark* behaviors (see REACTIVE ROBOTIC SYSTEMS).

Force-Field Motor Primitives in a Humanoid

Mataric et al. (1998), drawing on biological findings concerning the organization of force-field motor primitives, have investigated the idea of generating complex motion based on a collection of basic motion primitives, and have demonstrated such a behavior-based motion control approach to a 20-degrees-of-freedom simulated humanoid torso. In their simulation, three behavior primitives are defined as a basic behavior set: *move-to-point, get-posture*, and *avoid*. *Move-to-point* is implemented using impedance control such that the arm of the humanoid, as if connected to virtual springs and dampers, can interact with complex environments with stability. *Get-posture* resembles the spinal field of the frog, which is generated by the spring-like muscles in the leg. Running concurrently with other two behavior primitives, *avoid* follows the virtual repulsive forces generated from the obstacles in the torso's environment. Based on the basic behavior primitives, more complex motor behaviors can be produced, such as *touch right hand to top of left shoulder*.

Behavior Templates and Anchors

With the demonstration that complex motor behaviors can be induced in both animals and animats by incorporating various motor primitives, a new question concerning generalizing the concept of motor primitives arises: Can the dynamically coupled interactions between an organism and its environment, such as locomotion on land, be decoded as the neural control of motor primitives?

Full and Koditschek (1999) have suggested a neuromechanical approach to characterizing legged locomotion on land. Their approach involves the notions of template and anchor. The former provides a minimal behavioral model for guiding the control of locomotion; the latter offers elaborated morphological and physiological mechanisms for a template. Full and Koditschek hypothesize that the control of locomotion incorporates both neural and mechanical systems. During slow, variable-frequency locomotion, the neural system dominates. In the case of rapid, rhythmic locomotion, the mechanical system plays a key role.

Artificial Potential Fields in Modeling External Task Constraints

The problem of robot motion planning has traditionally been treated as an optimization problem in which the configuration of a robot is represented in a parameter space and a solution to this problem is computed by searching the parameter space in an attempt to satisfy a predefined cost function, such as the distance between the robot and a goal point. The limitation of this approach is that it is computationally too costly to generate new plans when dealing with dynamic environments that involve unexpected obstacles. As a more practical approach to the real-time planning of collision-free motions for manipulators and mobile robots, the concept of an artificial potential field (APF) was proposed by Khatib (1986). The APF approach incorporates dynamic sensing feedback into robot control, and hence overcomes the aforementioned limitation by extending the reactiveness of the low-level motion control.

APF theory states that for any goal-directed robot in an environment that contains stationary or moving obstacles, an APF can be formulated and computed, taking into account an attractive pole at the goal position of the robot and repulsive surfaces of the obstacles in the environment. This potential field can be expressed as follows:

$$U_{\text{art}}(x) = U_{\text{goal}}(x) + U_{\text{obs}}(x) \tag{1}$$

where $U_{\text{art}}(x)$, $U_{\text{goal}}(x)$, and $U_{\text{obs}}(x)$ denote the APF, the attractive potential from the goal, and the repulsive potential from the obstacles, respectively, and x denotes a set of independent parameters, called operational coordinates, that describe the position and orientation of the robot end-effector.

Generally speaking, U_{obs} is chosen such that U_{art} is a non-negative continuous and differentiable function that tends to infinity when x approaches the surface of an obstacle and tends to zero when x approaches the goal position, x_{goal}.

Given Equation 1, the force resulting from the APF at x can therefore be derived as follows:

$$F_{\text{art}} = -\nabla[U_{\text{art}}(x)] \tag{2}$$

where ∇ denotes a gradient.

Potential Fields for Guiding Motion

Equation 2 tells us that applying APF $U_{\text{art}}(x)$ to a robot end-effector can here be realized by using F_{art} as a command vector to control the end-effector in operational space (because the motion of the end-effector can be decoupled in operational space; Khatib, 1986). In so doing, the joint forces corresponding to F_{art} must be obtained using the Jacobian matrix. Under such a control, the robot will be able to avoid obstacles (as the repulsive force in the potential field "pushes" it away into the valleys of the field) and at the same time move toward a goal position (as the attractive force in the potential field "pulls" it in the direction of a global zero-potential pole).

By following the potential field that models the spatial constraints in an environment, a robot will be able to avoid obstacles and at the same time achieve stable configurations in its operational space. However, the stable configurations may not be guaranteed to include the goal configuration. In this case, a global motion plan may be used to guide the robot out of a local stable configuration and set it moving toward a goal position. Another alternative is to define an APF function that does not contain a local minimum. An example is a harmonic function defined in the configuration space of a robot where the boundaries of all obstacles and goals are treated as the boundary for the domain of the function.

Other Forms of Potential Fields for Modeling External Task Constraints

Artificial potential fields for modeling external task constraints can take various forms. In the following discussion we consider two generalized APF formulations, *elastic bands* and *elastic strips*, that draw on and generalize the previous work on APF-oriented robot planning and control. These two approaches effectively allow real-time planning and control of robot motion that is both locally *reactive* to any dynamically changing obstacles and globally *optimal* with respect to any motion criteria for attaining a predefined goal.

Elastic Bands

As implemented by Quinlan and Khatib (1993) in a mobile manipulation system, an elastic band has its own internal contraction force when it is in a stretched configuration; at the same time, it receives an external repulsive force if it is close to an obstacle. A *global* collision-free path corresponds to an elastic band at equilibrium that connects initial and goal locations. Whenever a new obstacle approaches, the elastic band will *react* to the situation by deforming itself until a new equilibrium is reached. To compute its artificial forces, an elastic band is represented as a series of consecutive *bubbles*. A bubble at a certain configuration is a spherical free subspace whose radius corresponds to the minimum distance between the configuration and the environment. The total force on the bubble is calculated as follows: The internal contraction force is created by a series of springs connecting the bubbles, whereas the repulsive force is exerted by an obstacle that pushes away the bubble and increases its size. Based on the calculated artificial forces, the position of the bubble will be locally updated, and hence the elastic band deforms.

Elastic Strips

That elastic strips approach real-time motion planning and control was demonstrated by Brock and Khatib (1998). Their work generalizes the notion of bubbles centered at via points into protective hulls that consist of bubbles centered on the spines covering the individual rigid bodies of the manipulator and its mobile platform. Next, an elastic strip is formed by connecting consecutive configurations of the robot on its trajectory, and a tunnel of local free subspace is formed by connecting a series of consecutive protective hulls. With such a representation, it is possible to find the internal contraction force on the elastic strip by calculating the tension between two consecutive configurations for each respective joint of

the robot. It is also possible to find the external repulsive force on the elastic strip by calculating the force acting on the bubbles of a protective hull. Hence, we can determine the deformation of the strip by taking into account the total force acting on the strip, and joint displacements by computing the respective joint torques. The equilibrium elastic strip provides a global collision-free trajectory for the robot that connects the initial and the goal configurations.

Potential Fields in Interaction Controllers

So far we have discussed how potential fields are useful for representing the spatial constraints of a robot task environment in such a way as to effectively guide real-time motion planning and control. Another effective use of potential fields is in the design of robot dynamics that exhibit certain behaviors as if governed by a potential field.

This idea has been part of control systems theory for some time. For instance, Colgate and Hogan (1988) proposed designing a controller for a manipulator that would be capable of dynamically interacting with a diverse set of environments of unknown dynamics and parametric uncertainty. Their specifications for an *interaction controller* emphasize both coupled stability (in addition to nominal stability) and desirable interactive behavior (in addition to command following). The interactive behavior can be established by controlling the impedance of the manipulator as if it were connected with virtual springs and dampers. The stability of a linear system coupled to a passive environment can be guaranteed by making sure the driving point impedance of the system is real and positive.

Artificial Neural Networks

Artificial neural networks (ANNs) are biologically inspired computational models. Each network is composed of a set of neurons connected by fixed synapses. A neuron receives stimuli from external input sources and exchanges messages with other neurons through the connecting synapses. As the strengths of connections between neurons are varied, the neural network builds an associative map between input data patterns and output values. With this computational capability, neural networks have been widely used to solve recognition and classification problems in control, pattern analysis, function learning, feature pattern extraction, and signal processing.

Depending on the homogeneity of neurons, the layered structure of networks, the algorithms for learning input-output associations, and the error propagation mechanisms, different ANNs can be developed, such as the multilayer perceptron, Hopfield networks, backpropagation networks, and Kohonen networks.

APF versus ANN Approaches

Both APF and ANN approaches have been applied to solving practical problems ranging from robot motion planning and control to conceptual mapping and learning.

Given a certain geometric model of a physical environment, it is possible to derive an analytical form of APF for the environment as a function of operational coordinates. An advantage to having an analytical form of APF is that the analytical expression is easier to update if changes occur in the environment. An ANN, on the other hand, builds a numerical input-output map for a set of empirical observations based on a weight-updating and error-correction algorithm. When new empirical data arrive, it is necessary to update the existing ANN by iterating the learning algorithm with each sample of the new data set. As a result of such step-by-step relearning, the weights of an ANN will be modified to some extent, reflecting the discovery and acquisition of new patterns from the data.

With an APF, a robot can reach a stable configuration in its environment by following the negative gradient of its potential field. In this case, locally stable configurations are inevitable. Nevertheless, they can be readily overcome by either incorporating a global motion planner, or utilizing a harmonic function that does not contain any local minima, or applying generalized APF formulations such as elastic bands and elastic strips. The APF approach is particularly advantageous when dealing with robots with many degrees of freedom in dynamically changing environments.

Similarly, an ANN offers another practical way to solve optimization problems, especially when the search space is of high dimension. With an ANN, the goal is to build an optimal association from given input data patterns to desirable output values. Thereafter the optimal association can be incrementally obtained as the network evolves toward a stable equilibrium state. Unlike the case of an APF, where a stable configuration is approached through updating the configurations following a potential field, the evolution of the neural network relies on updating connection weights and error corrections for the network in accordance with a learning algorithm.

Artificial Neural Network–Based Potential Field Motor Control

An important challenge in the practical applications of APF methodology is to formulate a potential field. For a given robot environment, this task can be decomposed into the subtasks of identifying geometrical primitives in the environment, calculating individual repulsive potential functions for the primitives, and composing a global potential field function based on the individual potential functions. The question that remains is how the APF methodology can be used if the robot environment concerned is not given as a priori knowledge. In such a situation, it would be essential to dynamically derive a numerical potential field representation based on the sensory data obtained during the interaction between the robot and its environment. As mentioned earlier, the ANN methodology is well suited to derive associative maps from certain available input data. In this respect, the ANN approach enables the application of APF in unknown environments.

Operational Space Motor Control

In the past, several researchers have focused on the research question of how to build an operational space potential field map based on real-time sensory measurements. For instance, Prassler (1995) has proposed the use of a massively parallel network of simple processing elements, arranged in a rectangular grid structure, for computing and manipulating a two-dimensional (2D) potential field. The structure is of three layers: a long-term map (LTM) that describes the stationary parts in the environment, a short-term map (STM) that describes a more recent state of the environment, and an occupancy grid representation of the current sensory readings.

Collective Self-Organization

One of the practical concerns in merging APF with an ANN approach is input data requirement. Generally speaking, evolving a stable APF is a time-consuming learning process that requires a large amount of input data coming from the robot-environment interaction. In order to overcome this shortcoming, Liu and Wu (2001) have proposed an evolutionary self-organization learning approach that can efficiently build a potential field map by determining and collecting locally most informative sensory measurements from an unknown environment. This approach can readily

be used by a group of cooperative robots for collective exploration and world modeling.

Joint-Space Motor Control

Besides developing an APF that explicitly models the geometrical characteristics (e.g., clearance) of a robot environment, some studies have focused on how to acquire an APF map directly encoded in the joint space of a robot. Falling into this category are efforts to enable the robot to learn reactive joint activation strategies in response to different external sensory conditions.

An example of such studies is the work on the operant conditioning–based learning of approach and avoidance behaviors in a mobile robot by Chang and Gaudiano (1998). In their study, a wheeled mobile robot is developed that uses a form of self-supervised learning based on an operant conditioning neural network. The output of this neural network is a one-dimensional (1D) population of neurons that encodes the robot's angular velocities, called an angular velocity map, for its left and right wheels. The robot learns its avoidance behavior through "punishment" signals produced by the collision of the robot during random exploratory motion. As a result, a given pattern of sensory inputs will tend to suppress movements that would yield punishment. On the other hand, an excitatory association may be acquired by the robot as it receives a reward such as higher light intensity, with the result that the robot reinforces its movements toward light sources. Unlike the aforementioned 2D operational space APF, the acquired angular velocity map is a 1D representation that directly encodes the potential fields in the joint space of the robot's two wheels.

Artificial Neural Network–Based Perception and Inverse Kinematics for Navigation

Neural networks have been applied not only to build a robot's internal representation of its task environment but also to acquire the control strategies for its collision-free motion. In a vision-based manipulator navigation system, Blase, Pauli, and Bruske (1998) have shown the use of two layers of radial basis function (RBF) networks in the three-dimensional (3D) reconstruction of obstacles from their optical flow vectors. The RBF networks in the first layer are trained for respective image areas to give the depth coordinate z. The depth coordinate z is in turn used by the second layer to generate the corresponding x and y coordinates of the obstacle. In addition, their system also uses one layer of RBF networks to construct the inverse kinematics of a manipulator. Based on the 3D models of obstacles and the inverse kinematics built, the manipulator knows where the obstacles are and how to reach a goal position. While navigating toward the goal position, it also avoids the detected obstacles. In so doing, it dynamically constructs and follows a vector field of simulated forces generated by repulsive forces encoding the obstacle constraints and attractor forces encoding the desired goal.

Summary

In this article, we have examined some of the important biological findings in the use of potential fields to characterize the control and learning of motor primitives. Such biological insights can lead to the development of primitive motor behavior–based robots capable of interacting with dynamic environments. Similarly, the concept of potential fields can be incorporated to model the externally induced constraints as well as the internally constructed sensorimotor maps for robot motion control. Apart from its biological relevance, potential field–based motion control can benefit from the use of ANN-based learning.

Road Map: Robotics and Control Theory
Related Reading: Cognitive Maps; Hippocampus: Spatial Models; Motor Primitives; Reactive Robotic Systems

References

Arbib, M., and House, D., 1987, Depth and detours: An essay on visually guided behavior, in *Vision, Brain and Cooperative Computation* (M. A. Arbib and A. R. Hanson, Eds.), Cambridge, MA: A Bradford Book/MIT Press, pp. 129–163. ◆

Arkin, R., 1989, Neuroscience in motion: The application of schema theory to mobile robotics, in *Visuomotor Coordination: Amphibians, Comparisons, Models, and Robots* (J.-P. Ewert and M. Arbib, Eds.), New York: Plenum Press, pp. 649–672.

Blase, W., Pauli, J., and Bruske, J., 1998, Vision-based manipulator navigation using mixtures of RBF neural networks, in *Proceedings of the International Conference on Neural Networks and Brain*, Peking, China, pp. 531–534.

Brock, O., and Khatib, O., 1998, Executing motion plans for robots with many degrees of freedom in dynamic environment, in *Proceedings of the IEEE International Conference on Robotics and Automation*, pp. 1–6. ◆

Chang, C., and Gaudiano, P., 1998, Application of biological learning theories to mobile robot avoidance and approach behaviors, *J. Complex Syst.*, 1:79–114.

Colgate, J. E., and Hogan, N., 1988, Robust control of dynamically interacting systems, *Int. J. Control*, 48:65–88.

Full, R. J., and Koditschek, D. E., 1999, Templates and anchors: Neuromechanical hypotheses of legged locomotion on land, *J. Exp. Biol.*, 202:3325–3332.

Khatib, O., Spring 1986, Real-time obstacle avoidance for manipulators and mobile robots, *Int. J. Robot. Res.*, 5:90–98.

Liu, J., and Wu, J., 2001, *Multi-Agent Robotic Systems*, Boca Raton, FL: CRC Press.

Mataric, M. J., Williamson, M., Demiris, J., and Mohan, A., 1998, Behavior-based primitives for articulated control, in *From Animals to Animats 5: Proceedings of the Fifth International Conference on Simulation of Adaptive Behavior (SAB-98)* (R. Pfeifer, B. Blumberg, J.-A. Meyer, and S. W. Wilson, Eds.), Cambridge, MA: MIT Press.

Mussa-Ivaldi, F. A., and Giszter, S. F., 1992, Vector field approximation: A computational paradigm for motor control and learning, *Biol. Cybern.*, 67:491–500.

Mussa-Ivaldi, F. A., Giszter, S. F., and Bizzi, E., 1994, Linear combination of primitives in vertebrate motor control, *Proc. Natl. Acad. Sci. USA*, 91:7534–7538.

Prassler, E., 1995, Robot navigation: A simple guidance system for a complex changing world, in *Modeling and Planning for Sensor Based Intelligent Robot Systems* (H. Bunke, T. Kanade, and H. Noltemeier, Eds.), Singapore: World Scientific, pp. 86–103.

Quinlan, S., and Khatib, O., 1993, Elastic bands: Connecting path planning and control, in *Proceedings of the IEEE International Conference on Robotics and Automation*, pp. 802–807. ◆

Thoroughman, K. A., and Shadmehr, R., 2000, Learning of action through adaptive combination of motor primitives, *Nature*, 407:742–747. ◆

Prefrontal Cortex in Temporal Organization of Action

Joaquín M. Fuster

Introduction

The prefrontal cortex is the association cortex of the frontal lobes. It is one of the cortical regions to develop last and most in the course of evolution (Figure 1). In the human brain it constitutes nearly one-third of the totality of the neocortex. Also in the course of individual ontogeny, the prefrontal cortex is one of the cortices to develop last and most. The cellular and connective architecture of the human prefrontal cortex does not reach full maturity until young adulthood. Presumably, the reason for the late morphological development of this cortex, in both phylogeny and ontogeny, is its support of higher cognitive functions related to the capacity to execute novel and complex actions, which reaches its maximum in the adult human brain. The prefrontal cortex of primates can be anatomically subdivided into three major regions: inferior or orbital, medial-cingulate, and lateral. Of the three, the lateral prefrontal cortex, that is, the association cortex of the convexity of the frontal lobe, is the one that undergoes the most development phylogenetically and ontogenetically and is the most implicated in cognitive functions. In the human it is appropriate to label it "the organ of creativity."

In primates, the cortex of the frontal lobe in its entirety can be considered *motor cortex* in the broadest sense of the term, for it is cortex dedicated to the representation and execution of all manner of actions of the organism: actions in the skeletal domain, in the oculomotor domain, in the visceral domain, in the language domain, and in the domain of complex cognitive operations, such as reasoning and problem solving. The inferior (orbital) and medial regions of the prefrontal cortex are involved in the representation and enactment of emotional behavior and related visceral and autonomic manifestations. The lateral region, on the other hand, is involved in the representation and temporal organization of sequential behavior and, in the human, of speech and reasoning. In this article I consider, in particular, the physiological functions of the lateral prefrontal cortex in the temporal organization of behavior.

Anatomy and Connections

By anatomical definition, the prefrontal cortex of the primate is comprised of three major regions (Figure 2), each with a somewhat different cytoarchitecture (Petrides and Pandya, 1994): the *lateral* prefrontal cortex (LPC), or association cortex of the frontal convexity (Brodmann's area 46, and lateral parts of areas 8, 9, 10, and 11); the *medial* and *cingulate* prefrontal cortex, which is nearly flat and faces the medial surface of the contralateral frontal pole (areas 12, 24, and 32, and medial parts of areas 8, 9, 10, and 11); and the *inferior* or *orbital* prefrontal cortex, directly above the orbit of the eye (areas 13, 47, and inferior parts of 10, 11, and 13). The lateral region is bordered in the back by the premotor cortex (area 6); the medial and orbital prefrontal cortices lie anterior to the corpus callosum and limbic structures (piriform cortex and amygdala, cingulate cortex, septum, and hypothalamus).

The prefrontal cortex is one of the best connected of all cortices (Fuster, 1997). It maintains reciprocal fiber connections with a wide range of subcortical and cortical structures. Especially prominent are its connections with the anterior, medial, and dorsal nuclei of the thalamus. In addition, all three prefrontal regions are connected with several limbic structures, especially the hippocampus, the amygdala, and the hypothalamus. Further, the lateral region sends important efferents to the basal ganglia, notably the caudate nucleus, the globus pallidus, and the substantia nigra. Finally, the prefrontal cortex—especially its lateral component—is topologically and reciprocally connected with other frontal areas (premotor,

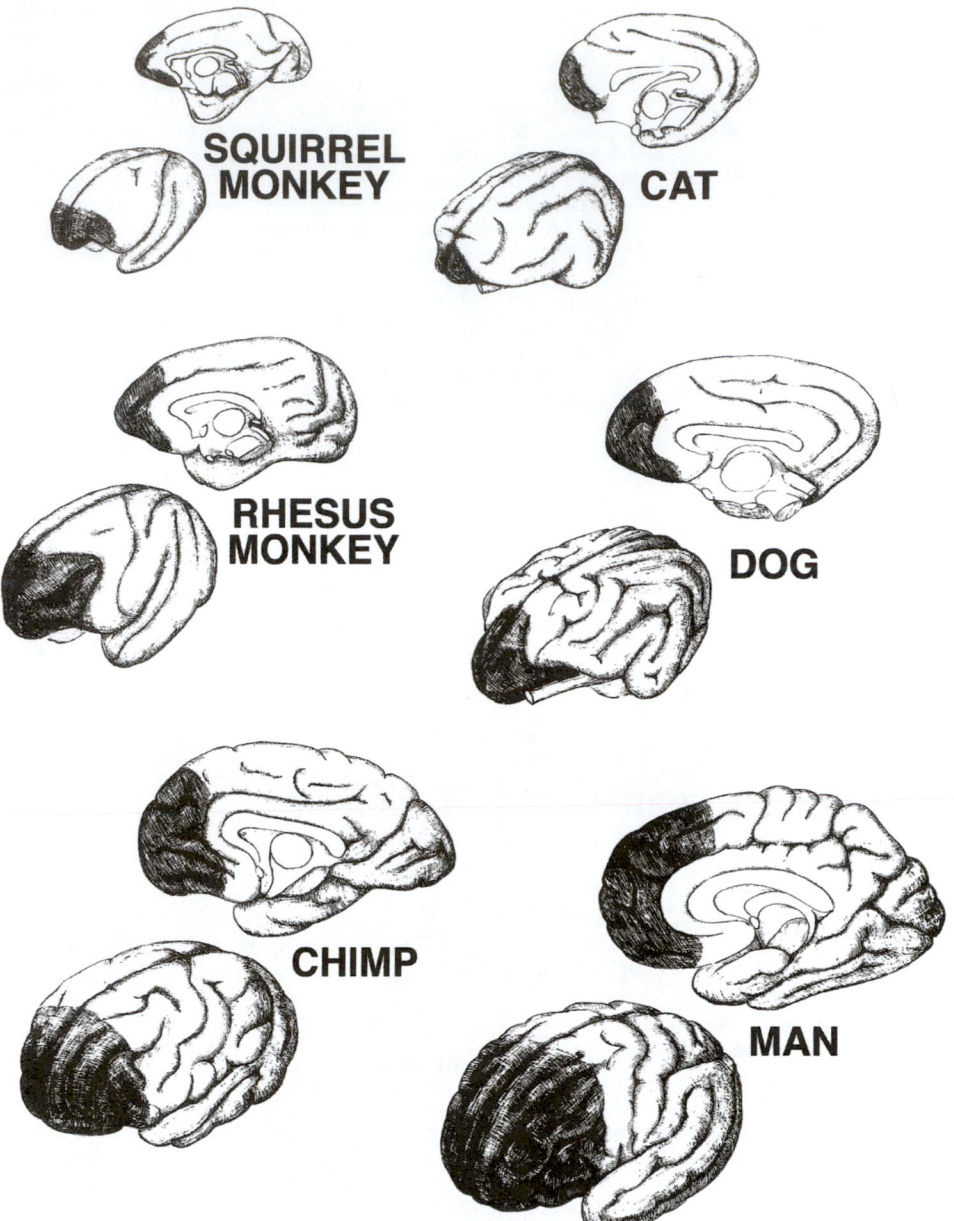

Figure 1. The prefrontal cortex (dark shading) in six mammalian species.

SQUIRREL MONKEY

CAT

RHESUS MONKEY

DOG

CHIMP

MAN

motor cortices) and with areas of posterior cortex, that is, with posterior cortical areas of association in the parietal and temporal lobes (Pandya and Yeterian, 1985).

The connections of the prefrontal cortex with the thalamus mediate inputs from the brainstem and limbic structures to that cortex, as well as inputs from itself (reentrant) and from other cortical regions. However, the functional role of the thalamic connectivity of the prefrontal cortex is still largely unknown. The direct limbic connections of the prefrontal cortex, especially with the amygdala and the hippocampus, are most likely essential for the formation of executive (motor) memory in that cortex, as well as for its retrieval. Connections of ventral and medial prefrontal cortex with limbic and brainstem structures probably serve the functions of the prefrontal cortex in drive, motivation, and the control of emotional behavior. Its outputs to basal ganglia are part of reentry loops that, beyond these nuclei, course through the thalamus and return to frontal cortex; those connective loops play a major, though still

poorly understood, role in motor control. All the corticocortical connections of the prefrontal cortex, especially the lateral region, are important for the cognitive functions of that cortex in the temporal organization of behavior and, presumably, also speech and reasoning.

Physiology

The medial and orbital prefrontal areas are involved in motivation, emotional behavior, and visceral functions. The precise nature of those involvements and their mechanisms is unknown, especially because the relevant evidence derives almost exclusively from the study of the effects of lesions. Large lesions of the medial prefrontal cortex in the human cause apathy and lack of spontaneity in speech, behavior, and reasoning. The orbital prefrontal cortex is essential for the inhibitory control of internal drives and instinctual behavior. Animals or humans with orbitofrontal lesions commonly manifest

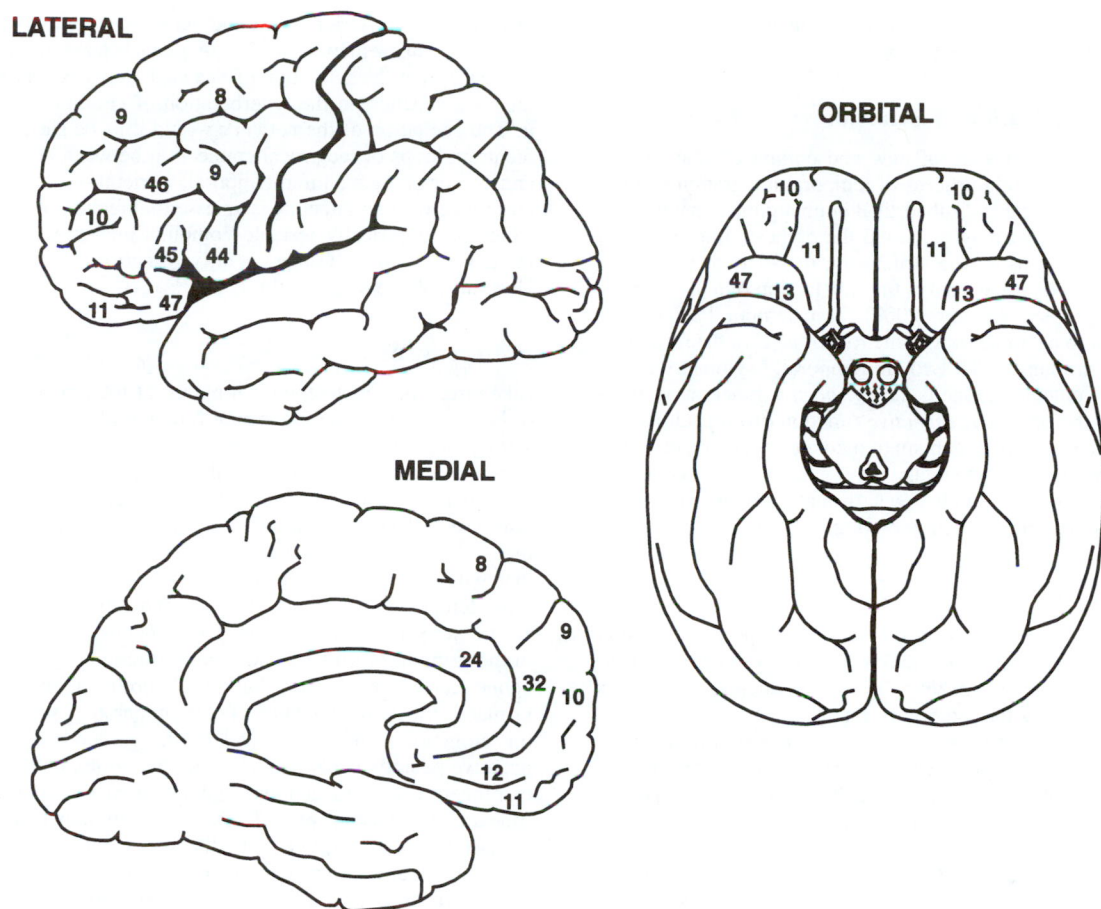

Figure 2. Three views of the frontal lobe. Prefrontal areas designated by numbers in accord with Brodmann's cytoarchitectonic map.

disinhibition of eating, sex, and aggression, as well as abnormal social behavior related to those disinhibitions. The human subject with lesions of that cortex is prone to impulsivity, risk taking, gross humor, and lack of moral judgment. Insofar as appropriate drive and impulse control are essential to sustain attention, the orbitomedial prefrontal cortex is important for the general role of the prefrontal cortex in rational decision making and the organization of cognition and behavior.

The prefrontal cortex of the lateral convexity plays a role in the representation as well as the execution of temporally organized sequences of behavior and cognition (Fuster, 1997); that role extends to language and reasoning. Those representations can be generally categorized as motor or executive memory. This form of memory includes, in particular, the representations of new and complex schemes of sequential action. After they have been learned and automatized, sequential behaviors become part of procedural executive memory and are no longer represented or enacted by the prefrontal cortex (Grafton et al., 1992) but by other structures at lower stages of the neural hierarchy for the organization of movement (e.g., premotor cortices, basal ganglia).

Anatomical, physiological, and neuropsychological studies have led some investigators to infer areas within LPC that specialize in various aspects of cognitive information. In the human as in the monkey, the so-called frontal eye field of area 8 is implicated in visual attention. Further, single-cell studies in the monkey support the commitment of that and other lateral areas to the representation of separate categories of visual information, such as spatial location

or shape (Goldman-Rakic, 1995). Other studies, however, point to the supramodal associative characteristics of cells in all prefrontal areas. Lateral prefrontal cells have been found to associate information across sensory modalities and across time (Fuster, Bodner, and Kroger, 2000). Some of those cells associate sensory stimuli with subsequent motor actions (Rainer, Assad, and Miller, 1998) or rewards (Hikosaka and Watanabe, 2000). These associative properties of lateral prefrontal cells emphasize their integrative functions. Their apparent sensory or motor specificity may be determined by the specificity of their inputs from sensory structures or outputs to motor structures. That specificity seems subservient and secondary to their functions of cognitive integration, which are essential for the temporal organization of behavior.

The connections of the prefrontal cortex with the hippocampus may be critical for the formation of the procedural memory of behavioral sequences in that cortex, in a similar manner as connections between hippocampus and posterior cortex play an important role in the formation of so-called declarative memory (episodic and semantic). The procedural or executive memory networks of the cortex of the frontal lobe seem hierarchically organized (see Cortical Memory). The primary motor cortex, which is the lowest stage of that organization, represents the elementary motor "memories" of somatic movements executed by synergistic muscle groups. Above the motor cortex, the premotor cortex represents movements by goal and trajectory. At the summit of the cortical motor hierarchy, the LPC represents schemes and sequences of goal-directed action. In addition to representing those schemes and sequences, the LPC plays a critical role in their execution, especially if they are novel and complex.

Temporal Organization of Behavior

The execution of a sequence of new and complex behavior is a highly elaborate, dynamic process of temporal integration that engages numerous cortical and subcortical brain regions. That process takes place under what may be called the orchestrating functions of the LPC, which ensure the structuring of behavior toward its ultimate goal, whether that goal is the satisfaction of a drive or the solution of a problem (Fuster, 2001). Two temporal integrative functions seem to be at the root of the role of LPC in the formation of behavioral structures. The two are temporally symmetrical and mutually complementary. One is a *retrospective* function of short-term memory, the other a *prospective* function of preparatory set. The two together help the organism to mediate cross-temporal contingencies of behavior. Both engage the executive networks of LPC in functional interactions with lower frontal cortices, subcortical structures, and posterior association cortex.

Short-Term Memory

The LPC function of short-term memory in support of temporal integration approximately coincides with what in cognitive psychology has been named *working memory* (Baddeley, 1992). This function is essentially the temporary retention—"on-line"—of information, old or new, for the execution of an action in the short term, as required for complex behavior or the solution of problems. There is a wealth of evidence that the LPC is critically involved in this process of active short-term memory toward a goal (Fuster, 1997). Selective cortical lesion (or inactivation) of LPC induces deficits in the performance of "delay" tasks (e.g., delayed response, delayed matching). In these tasks, the animal is presented on successive trials with an item of sensory information (which varies from trial to trial) and is required to retain it in memory for executing a given motor response seconds or minutes later. Monkeys with lesions of LPC seem unable to keep the working memory of the stimulus for each trial, as they make many errors, even with short delays. Further evidence for prefrontal short-term memory derives from single-cell recording in animals performing delay tasks. Neurons of LPC fire persistently, and often at stimulus-specific frequency, during the delay (memory period) of every trial (Fuster and Alexander, 1971; Niki, 1974; Funahashi, Bruce, and Goldman-Rakic, 1989). These observations indicate the importance of the neuronal dynamics of LPC for working memory and for the performance of delay tasks that depend on this form of memory.

The function of the prefrontal cortex in active short-term memory is essentially defined by its teleological quality, that is, by the presence of an objective in the near future, which is the construction of prospective action toward a goal. As noted above, some prefrontal areas seem to specialize in the sensory and motor aspects of the information retained in working memory. That apparent specialization may derive from different concentrations of specific inputs and outputs in those areas. In general terms, however, each area is probably engaged in the temporary activation of specific sensory-sensory or sensory-motor associations leading to organized sequential action. In those terms, the cell groupings and areas of LPC are components of teleological associations, the mnemonic paths to prospective action.

The precise neural mechanism of working memory is still unknown. Based on physiological evidence from the monkey (summary review in Fuster, 1997), it appears that working memory is maintained by the persistent activation of the widely distributed cortical network that represents its content (see CORTICAL MEMORY). The network contains neuronal assemblies of sensory representation in posterior cortex and neuronal assemblies of motor or executive representation in LPC. A plausible assumption, still unproved, is that the activation of one such network serving working memory depends on the reverberation of neural excitation within it. The excitation of the network would thus be sustained through reentrant loops of reciprocal connection between lateral prefrontal and posterior—e.g., inferotemporal, parietal—cortex. Hence, recurrent cortical architecture is an essential feature of the most plausible and empirically testable computational models of working memory, as well as of other cognitive functions (Zipser et al., 1993; Duncan, 2001; Wang, 2001).

Prospective Set

Likewise, from the teleological nature of the temporal structuring of behavior derives the prefrontal function of readiness to act. The setting of sensory receptors and motor effectors for prospective actions is, in the time domain, the mirror image of active short-term memory. This complementary integrative function of preparatory set is the counterpart of working memory. It serves to prepare the subject for anticipated actions; it is the "memory of the future" that will complement retrospective memory in the bridging of a cross-temporal contingency. The neural mechanisms of prospective set are not yet well understood. These mechanisms probably result in the priming of sensory and motor structures by way of efferent connections of the prefrontal cortex. In both human and nonhuman primates, the involvement of LPC in preparatory set is reflected by the progressive increase in cell discharge and the slow surface-negative potentials that take place in that cortex before a stimulus-contingent act. Both memory and set seem to occur at the same time and in the same areas of LPC, both simultaneously during the interval that separates two mutually contingent events. While some prefrontal neurons engage in the memory of the cue, others engage in the preparation of the consequent and subsequent behavioral response. Neuronal recording from the LPC shows that, while the memory of the sensory information wanes, the representation of the response in preparation increases (Quintana and Fuster, 1999).

The selection of an action among many is the motor equivalent of focusing sensory attention. Consequently, the prefrontal function of prospective set may be appropriately considered *motor attention*, that is, the selective focusing of attention on a motor act to ensure the prompt and efficient execution of that act in the near future. In conclusion, the symmetry of the two temporal integrative functions of the LPC, active memory and set, parallels the symmetry of attentive processes, one sensory and the other motor. Active short-term memory is attention focused on the representation of a recent sensory stimulus, while prospective set is attention focused on a subsequent and consequent act. Whereas attention, in particular sensory attention, is commonly associated with conscious awareness, neither of the two temporal integrative functions of the LPC, active memory or set, need be conscious to accomplish their objective.

Perception-Action Cycle

The temporal organization of complex behavior requires a continuous succession of sensorimotor integrations, that is, a succession of temporal mediations of contingencies between sensory events and consequent motor acts. To some degree, each integration depends on previous ones. Each sensorimotor integration induces certain changes in the environment that will determine and modify subsequent sensory inputs, and these will determine and modify subsequent acts, and so on. This cybernetic cycle of interactions of the organism with its environment, through a series of sensorimotor integrations, is a fundamental principle in biology: the perception-action cycle.

The neural operations of the perception-action cycle ensure that mutually contingent percepts and acts are properly integrated in the progression of behavior toward its goal. The attainment of that goal requires the attainment of lesser or subordinate goals, each dependent on a particular translation of perception to action and its consequent change in the environment. Innumerable neural structures participate in the mediation of perception-action contingencies that one such sequence requires. These structures, both on the sensory side and on the motor side, are hierarchically organized throughout the nerve axis, from the spinal cord to the cerebral cortex, and also within the latter. Figure 3 shows highly schematically the cortical layers of the perception-action cycle. If the behavior is new, all layers of that cycle are involved in its temporal organization, up to and including the cortex. Routine and automatic sequences, such as walking, are relegated to and organized at lower levels. The cortex remains involved even if the behavioral sequence is old and well rehearsed but contains uncertainties or ambiguities.

Goal-directed behavioral sequences may contain delays or temporary interruptions imposed by the subject or by the environment. Such is the case with the so-called delay tasks, where time intervenes between a percept and an action that are contingent from each other. Because that contingency must be mediated cross-temporally, the correct performance of those tasks depends on the LPC. The LPC, through the two temporally integrative functions of short-term memory and prospective set, integrates perception with action across time at the highest level of the hierarchy of neural structures serving the perception-action cycle. There is considerable empirical evidence that the LPC performs those temporal integrative functions in dynamic cooperation with posterior cortical areas of association, which constitute the highest substrate for the perceptual side of the cycle. The highest and most characteristically human operations of the perception-action cycle take place in the

construction of the spoken language. Given what we know about the role of posterior cortex (Wernicke's area) and LPC in the perceptual and motor aspects of language, respectively, it is reasonable to view those cortices as the highest levels of the perception-action cycle for speech. At the neural root of a dialogue between two persons, it is appropriate to hypothesize a dynamic interaction of the cycles of the two interlocutors. The action of one is the perception of the other, and vice versa. The frontal and postcentral cortices of the two subjects would thus interact reciprocally in the coordination of two perception-action cycles organizing the dialogue in the temporal domain.

Discussion

The association cortex of the frontal lobe, or prefrontal cortex, is highly heterogeneous, anatomically as well physiologically. Further, this cortex is widely connected with many other brain structures, cortical and subcortical. The heterogeneity and diverse connectivity of the prefrontal cortex serve a variety of functions related to the organization of actions in the temporal domain. This article has focused on the temporal organizing functions of the LPC, the prefrontal region that undergoes the greatest phylogenetic and ontogenetic development in primates. Two of those functions have been highlighted that are especially evident in the primate: active short-term memory (working memory) and prospective set. The two cooperate toward temporally integrating sensory and motor information by mediating cross-temporal contingencies of behavior. This integrative role of the prefrontal cortex covers a wide range of sensory inputs and motor outputs; hence the apparent sensory or motor specificity of certain prefrontal areas. Temporal integration seems to be the overarching function that, despite their heterogeneity, unifies the many activities and functions of the LPC.

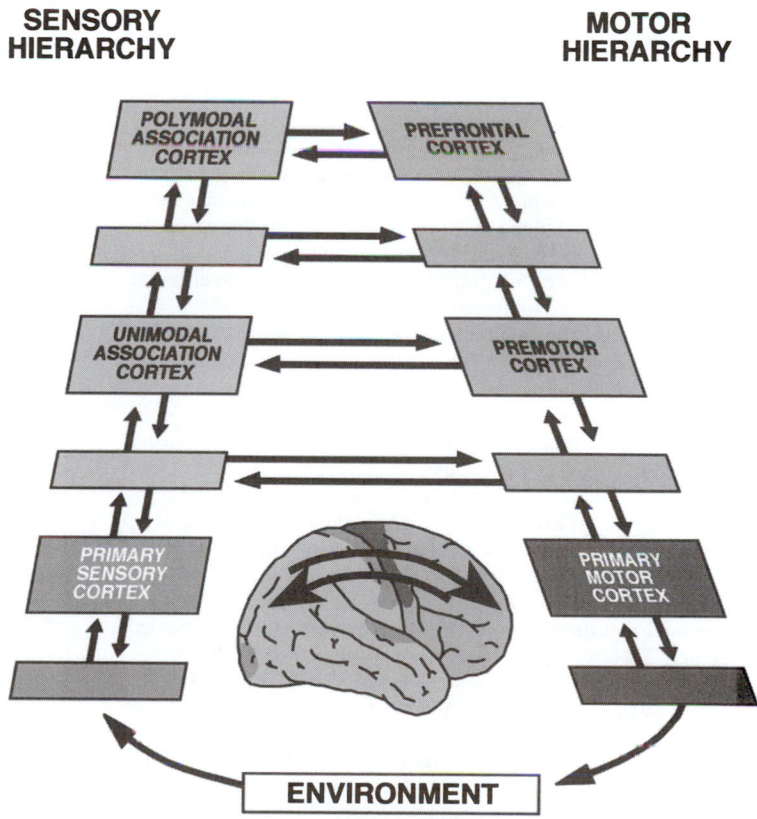

Figure 3. The cortical hierarchies of the perception-action cycle depicted around a lateral view of the human brain. Unlabeled cortical entities represent subareas of labeled regions or areas interposed between them. The arrows represent connections that have been demonstrated in the monkey.

Temporal integration, through memory and set, supports the goal-directed performance of the perception-action cycle. It is a role that extends to the temporal organization of higher cognitive operations, including spoken language.

Road Map: Mammalian Brain Regions
Related Reading: Basal Ganglia; Competitive Queuing for Planning and Serial Performance; Grasping Movements: Visuomotor Transformations; Sequence Learning; Thalamus; Visual Scene Perception

References

Baddeley, A., 1992, Working memory, *Science*, 255:556–559.

Duncan, J., 2001, An adaptive coding model of neural function in prefrontal cortex, *Nature Neurosci.*, 2:820–829. ◆

Funahashi, S., Bruce, C. J., and Goldman-Rakic, P. S., 1989, Mnemonic coding of visual space in the monkey's dorsolateral prefrontal cortex, *J. Neurophysiol.*, 61:331–349.

Fuster, J. M., 1997, *The Prefrontal Cortex*, 3rd ed., Philadelphia: Lippincott-Raven. ◆

Fuster, J. M., 2001, The prefrontal cortex—an update: Time is of the essence, *Neuron* ◆

Fuster, J. M., and Alexander, G. E., 1971, Neuron activity related to short-term memory, *Science*, 173:652–654.

Fuster, J. M., Bodner, M., and Kroger, J., 2000, Cross-modal and cross-temporal association in neurons of frontal cortex, *Nature*, 405:347–351.

Goldman-Rakic, P. S., 1995, Architecture of the prefrontal cortex and the central executive, *Proc. Natl. Acad. Sci. USA*, 769:71–83. ◆

Grafton, S. T., Mazziotta, J. C., Woods, R. P., and Phelps, M. E., 1992, Human functional anatomy of visually guided finger movements, *Brain*, 115:565–587.

Hikosaka, K., and Watanabe, M., 2000, Delay activity of orbital and lateral prefrontal neurons of the monkey varying with different rewards, *Cereb. Cortex*, 10:263–271.

Niki, H., 1974, Prefrontal unit activity during delayed alternation in the monkey: I. Relation to direction of response, *Brain Res.*, 68:185–196.

Pandya, D. N., and Yeterian, E. H., 1985, Architecture and connections of cortical association areas, *Cereb. Cortex*, 4:3–61. ◆

Petrides, M., and Pandya, D. N., 1994, Comparative architectonic analysis of the human and the macaque frontal cortex, in *Handbook of Neuropsychology* (F. Boller and J. Gafman, Eds.), Amsterdam: Elsevier, pp. 17–58.

Quintana, J., and Fuster, J. M., 1999, From perception to action: Temporal integrative functions of prefrontal and parietal neurons, *Cereb. Cortex*, 9:213–221. ◆

Rainer, G., Assad, W. F., and Miller, E. K., 1998, Selective representation of relevant information by neurons in the primate prefrontal cortex, *Nature*, 393:577–579.

Wang, X., 2001, Synaptic reverberation underlying mnemonic persistent activity, *Trends Neurosci.*, 24:455–463.

Zipser, D., Kehoe, B., Littlewort, G., and Fuster, J., 1993, A spiking network model of short term active memory, *J. Neurosci.*, 13:3406–3420. ◆

Principal Component Analysis

Erkki Oja

Introduction

Principal Component Analysis (PCA) and the closely related Karhunen-Loève transform, or the Hotelling transform, are standard techniques in feature extraction and data compression (see, e.g., Devijver and Kittler, 1982; Oja, 1983). In general terms, the input vectors in PCA are random vectors x with K elements. In PCA, no assumptions on the probability density of the vectors are needed, as long as their means and covariances are known or can be estimated from a sample. This is in contrast to another well-known statistical technique, factor analysis, that is based on an explicit Gaussian model. Typically the elements of x are measurements such as pixel gray levels or the values of a signal at different time instants. They are mutually correlated.

In the PCA transform, vector x is linearly transformed to another vector y with N elements, $N < K$, so that the redundancy induced by the correlations is removed. This is done by finding a rotated coordinate system such that the elements of x in the new coordinates become uncorrelated. For instance, if x has a Gaussian density that is constant over ellipsoidal surfaces in the K-dimensional space, then the rotated coordinate system coincides with the principal axes of the ellipsoid. Even if the density is not Gaussian, similar principal axes can be computed. For most practical data, the density is not spherical but strongly elongated, and thus the axes have very different lengths. A considerable number of the axes are so small that the components they represent can be discarded altogether. Those components that are left constitute vector y.

As an example, take a sequence of small 32 × 32 digital images of hand-written characters. In real-time digital video transmission, it would be essential to reduce such images as much as possible without losing too much of the visual quality, because the total amount of data is very large: 1024 pixels for each image. Using PCA, a compressed representation vector is obtained for each image, which can be stored or transmitted. Figure 1 shows two examples of such characters from a large database and the reconstruction from the compressed PCA representation. This is the fundamental idea behind practical image and signal compression methods like the discrete cosine transform.

In mathematical terms, consider a linear combination

$$y_1 = \sum_{k=1}^{K} w_{k1}x_k = w_1^T x$$

of the elements $x_1, \ldots, x_K$ of vector x, where $w_{11}, \ldots, w_{K1}$ are scalar coefficients or weights, elements of a K-dimensional vector w_1, and w_1^T denotes the transpose of w_1. Usually it is assumed that x has zero mean; if not, then the mean vector is estimated separately and subtracted from x to obtain a zero mean vector.

The factor y_1 is the first principal component of x if the variance of y_1 is maximally large under the constraint that the norm of w_1 is constant (see, e.g., Devijver and Kittler, 1982). Then the weight vector w_1 maximizes the PCA criterion

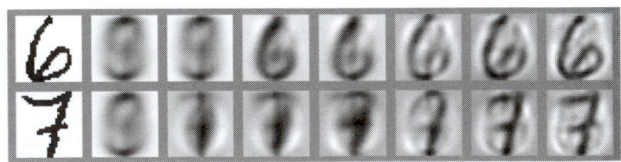

Figure 1. Results of using PCA to compress images. In the leftmost column are two digital images in a 32 × 32 grid. The next column shows the mean of all the samples. The remaining columns show the images as reconstructed by PCA when 1, 2, 5, 16, 32, or 64 principal components (out of the total of 1024) were used in the expansion.

$$J_1^{PCA}(w_1) = E\{y_1^2\} = E\{(w_1^T x)^2\} = E\{(w_1^T x)(x^T w_1)\}$$
$$= w_1^T E\{xx^T\} w_1 = w_1^T C w_1, \quad \|w_1\| = 1 \qquad (1)$$

where $E\{\cdot\}$ is the expectation over the density of input vector x, and the norm of w_1 is defined as

$$\|w_1\| = (w_1^T w_1)^{1/2} = \left[\sum_{k=1}^{K} w_{k1}^2 \right]^{1/2}$$

The matrix C in Equation 1 is the $K \times K$ covariance matrix defined by

$$C = E\{xx^T\} \qquad (2)$$

The solution is given in terms of the unit-length eigenvectors c_1, . . . , c_K of the matrix C. With $\lambda_1, \ldots, \lambda_K$ the corresponding eigenvalues in decreasing order (or nonincreasing, in case of multiple eigenvalues), the solution is given by

$$w_1 = c_1$$

Thus the first principal component of x is given by $y_1 = c_1^T x$.

The criterion J_1^{PCA} in Equation 1 can be generalized to N principal components, with N any number between 1 and K. Denoting the nth ($1 \le n \le N$) principal component by $y_n = w_n^T x$ with w_n the corresponding weight vector, the variance of y_n is maximized under the constraints

$$\|w_n\| = 1, \quad w_n^T w_m = 0, \quad m < n \qquad (3)$$

Note that compared to the first principal component, there is now the extra constraint that the weight vector w_n must be orthonormal with all the previous weight vectors. The solution is

$$w_n = c_n$$

thus the nth principal component is $y_n = c_n^T x$. It follows that

$$E\{y_n^2\} = E\{c_n^T xx^T c_n\} = c_n^T C c_n = \lambda_n$$

This can often be used in advance to determine N, if the eigenvalues are known. The eigenvalue sequence $\lambda_1, \lambda_2, \ldots$ is usually sharply decreasing, and it is possible to set a limit below which the eigenvalues, hence principal components, are insignificantly small. This limit determines how many principal components are used.

Another possible extension of Equation 1 is:

$$J_N^{PCA}(w_1, \ldots, w_N) = E\left\{ \sum_{n=1}^{N} y_n^2 \right\} = E\left\{ \sum_{n=1}^{N} (w_n^T x)^2 \right\}$$
$$= \sum_{n=1}^{N} w_n^T C w_n = max \qquad (4)$$
$$w_m^T w_n = \delta_{mn} \qquad (5)$$

This criterion determines the subspace spanned by vectors w_1, . . . , w_N in a unique way as the subspace spanned by the N first eigenvectors $c_1, \ldots, c_N$, but does not specify the basis of this subspace at all.

To use the closed-form solutions given above, the eigenvectors of the covariance matrix C must be known. This is rarely true in practice. In an on-line data compression application like image or speech coding, it is usually not possible to solve the eigenvector-eigenvalue problem for computational reasons. The PCA solution is then replaced by suboptimal standard transformations. Another alternative is to derive gradient ascent algorithms for the maximization problems above. The algorithms will then converge to the solutions of the problems, i.e., to the eigenvectors. This approach is the basis of the neural network learning rules.

PCA Learning Algorithms and Neural Networks

Neural networks provide a novel way for parallel on-line computation of the PCA expansion. The PCA network (Oja, 1992) is a layer of parallel linear artificial neurons (Figure 2). The output of the nth unit ($n = 1, \ldots, N$) is $y_n = w_n^T x$, with x denoting the K-dimensional input vector of the network and w_n denoting the weight vector of the nth unit. The number of units, N, will determine how many principal components the network will compute. Sometimes this can be determined in advance for typical inputs, or N can be equal to K if all principal components are required.

The PCA network learns the principal components by unsupervised learning rules, by which the weight vectors are gradually updated until they become orthonormal and tend to the theoretically correct eigenvectors. The network also has the ability to track slowly varying statistics in the input data, maintaining its optimality when the statistical properties of the inputs do not stay constant. Because of their parallelism and adaptivity to input data, such learning algorithms and their implementations in neural networks are potentially useful in feature detection and data compression tasks.

Some basic learning algorithms are listed here. In the following, k denotes discrete time; thus $x(k)$ is a stream of input data vectors (e.g., image windows or segments of a time-varying signal) entering the learning neural network. The learning weight vectors are $w_j(k), j = 1, \ldots, N$.

The Stochastic Gradient Ascent (SGA) Algorithm

This algorithm (Oja, 1983) is obtained from the maximum variance criterion by taking the gradients with respect to weight vector w_j and using the normalization constraints. Denoting

$$\Delta w_j(k - 1) = w_j(k) - w_j(k - 1) \qquad (6)$$

the learning rule is

$$\Delta w_j(k - 1) = \gamma(k) y_j(k)[x(k) - y_j(k) w_j(k - 1) - 2 \sum_{i<j} y_i(k) w_i(k - 1)] \qquad (7)$$

There, $\gamma(k)$ are the step sizes in the gradient ascent, typically a sequence of small numbers tending slowly to zero.

The first term on the right contains the product $y_j(k)x(k)$, which is a Hebbian term—note that $y_j(k) = w_j(k - 1)^T x(k)$ is the output of the jth neuron at time k, and $x(k)$ is the input—and the other terms are implicit orthonormality constraints. The case $j = 1$ gives

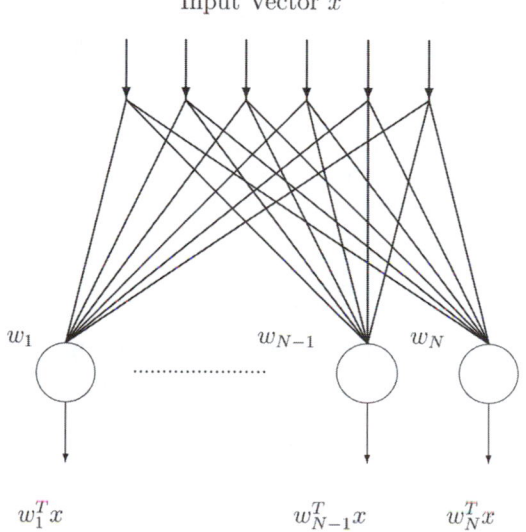

Figure 2. The basic linear PCA layer.

the constrained Hebbian learning rule of the basic PCA neuron introduced by Oja (1982). The convergence of the vectors $w_1(k)$, ..., $w_N(k)$ to the eigenvectors $c_1, ..., c_N$ was established by Oja (1983). A modification called the generalized Hebbian algorithm (GHA) was presented by Sanger (1989), who also applied it to image coding, texture segmentation, and the development of receptive fields.

The algorithm may have significance in hierarchical clustering of learned cues in the cerebral cortex. Ambros-Ingerson, Granger, and Lynch (1990) performed simulations on the olfactory paleocortex receiving inputs from the olfactory bulb. They used a network model resembling the SGA algorithm in which the first neuron (in their case, a competitive subnet) learned the input as such, and consequent neurons (subnets) learned progressively masked versions of the input. Masking corresponds to subtracting from the input the previous weight vectors, as in Equation 7. The simulation revealed how perceptual hierarchies may arise for recognizing environmental cues.

The Subspace Network Learning Algorithm

The subspace network learning algorithm (Oja, 1983; Williams, 1985) is formulated as follows:

$$\Delta w_j(k - 1) = \gamma(k)y_j(k)[x(k) - \sum_{i=1}^{N} y_i(k)w_i(k - 1)] \quad (8)$$

It is obtained as a gradient ascent maximization of criterion 4. The network implementation is analogous to the SGA algorithm but still simpler, because the feedback term, depending on the other weight vectors, is the same for all neuron units. Thus, learning at an individual connection weight w_{ji} is local, as it depends only on y_i, x_j, and the feedback term, all of which are easily accessible at that position in a hardware network. The convergence was studied by Williams (1985), who showed that the weight vectors $w_1(k)$, ..., $w_N(k)$ will not tend to the eigenvectors $c_1, ..., c_N$ but only to a rotated basis in the subspace spanned by them, in analogy with the subspace criterion discussed earlier. A global convergence analysis was given by Yan, Helmke, and Moore (1994).

The Recursive Least Squares Algorithm and Extensions

On-line algorithms typically suffer from slow convergence. The learning rate would have to be tuned optimally. One way of doing this is to use recursive least squares methods. It is well known that they converge much faster at the expense of a somewhat larger computational cost. An efficient algorithm called the Projection Approximation Subspace Tracking (PAST) was introduced by Yang (1996).

Also, minor components defined by the eigenvectors corresponding to the smallest eigenvalues can be computed by similar algorithms (see Oja, 1992). A recent overview of these and related neural network realizations of signal processing algorithms is given by Cichocki and Unbehauen (1993) and Diamantaras and Kung (1996). Extensions to nonlinear PCA learning rules are given in Hyvärinen, Karhunen, and Oja (2001).

Learning PCA by Backpropagation Learning

Another possibility for PCA computation in neural networks is the multilayer perceptron network, which learns by the backpropagation algorithm in unsupervised autoassociative mode. This network was suggested for data compression by Cottrell, Munro, and Zipser (1987).

In the three-layer autoassociative perceptron net, the input and output layers have K units and the one hidden layer has $N < K$ units. The outputs of the hidden layer are given by

$$h = \sigma(W_1 x + w_1) \quad (9)$$

where W_1 is the input-to-hidden layer weight matrix, w_1 is the corresponding bias vector, and σ is the usually nonlinear activation function, to be applied elementwise. The output y is an affine linear function of hidden layer outputs:

$$y = W_2 h + w_2 \quad (10)$$

with obvious notation. In autoassociative mode, the same vectors x are used both as inputs and as desired outputs in backpropagation learning. If σ is linear, then the hidden layer outputs will become the principal components of x.

For the linear net, backpropagation learning is especially feasible because it was shown by Baldi and Hornik (1989) that the "energy" function has no local minima. The nonlinear case was analyzed by Japkowitz, Hanson, and Gluck (2000). The three-layer net has been used for image compression by Cottrell et al. (1987).

Discussion

The algorithms reviewed in this article are typical learning rules for adaptive PCA extraction, and they are especially suitable for neural network implementations. In numerical analysis and signal processing, many other algorithms have been reported for different computing hardware (for a review, see Comon and Golub, 1990). PCA is a useful technique for, e.g., spatial decorrelation and denoising. Experimental results on the PCA algorithms both for finding the eigenvectors of stationary training sets and for tracking the slowly changing eigenvectors of nonstationary input data streams have been reported by Oja (1983) and Sanger (1989). An obvious extension of PCA neural networks would be to use nonlinear units, such as perceptrons, instead of the linear units, as suggested by Xu (1991). Such nonlinear PCA networks will in some cases give the independent components of the input x, instead of just uncorrelated components. This is due to the higher-order statistics that are induced by the nonlinearities. The technique of INDEPENDENT COMPONENT ANALYSIS (q.v.) is very useful in blind source separation (Hyvärinen et al., 2001). In fact, a useful preprocessing step in ICA is whitening, which means performing PCA followed by variance normalization.

Road Map: Learning in Artificial Networks
Related Reading: Data Clustering and Learning; Independent Component Analysis; Learning Vector Quantization; Perceptrons, Adalines, and Backpropagation

References

Ambros-Ingerson, J., Granger, R., and Lynch, G., 1990, Simulation of paleocortex performs hierarchical clustering, *Science*, 247:1344–1348.

Baldi, P., and Hornik, K., 1989, Neural networks and principal components analysis: Learning from examples without local minima, *Neural Netw.*, 2:52–58.

Cichocki, A., and Unbehauen, R., 1993, *Neural Networks for Optimization and Signal Processing*, New York: Wiley. ◆

Comon, P., and Golub, G., 1990, Tracking a few extreme singular values and vectors in signal processing, *Proc. IEEE*, 78:1327–1343. ◆

Cottrell, G. W., Munro, P. W., and Zipser, D., 1987, *Image Compression by Back-propagation: A Demonstration of Extensional Programming*, Technical Report 8702, University of California, San Diego, Institute of Cognitive Science.

Devijver, P. A., and Kittler, J., 1982, *Pattern Recognition: A Statistical Approach*, London: Prentice-Hall. ◆

Diamantaras, K., and Kung, S., 1996, *Principal Component Neural Networks: Theory and Applications*, New York: Wiley. ◆

Hyvärinen, A., Karhunen, J., and Oja, E., 2001, *Independent Component Analysis*, New York: Wiley. ◆

Japkowitz, N., Hanson, S. J., and Gluck, M. A., 2000, Nonlinear autoassociation is not equivalent to PCA, *Neural Computat.*, 12:531–545.

Oja, E., 1982, A simplified neuron model as a principal components analyzer, *J. Math. Biol.*, 15:267–273.

Oja, E., 1983, *Subspace Methods of Pattern Recognition*, Letchworth, Engl.: Research Studies Press and Wiley. ◆

Oja, E., 1992, Principal components, minor components, and linear neural networks, *Neural Netw.*, 5:927–935. ◆

Sanger, T. D., 1989, Optimal unsupervised learning in a single-layer linear feedforward network, *Neural Netw.*, 2:459–473.

Williams, R., 1985, *Feature Discovery Through Error-Correcting Learn-*

ing, Technical Report 8501, University of California, San Diego, Institute of Cognitive Science.

Xu, L., 1991, Least mean square error reconstruction principle for self-organizing neural nets, *Neural Netw.*, 6:627–648.

Yan, W., Helmke, U., and Moore, J., 1994, Global analysis of Oja's flow for neural networks, *IEEE Trans. Neural Netw.*, 5:674–683.

Yang, B., 1996, Asymptotic convergence analysis of the Projection Approximation Subspace Tracking algorithm, *Signal Process.*, 50:123–126.

Probabilistic Regularization Methods for Low-Level Vision

Jose L. Marroquin and Mariano Rivera

Introduction

Current research in computational vision follows two main paradigms. In the first paradigm, the primary task that a visual system must solve is considered to be reconstructing, from the set of images that constitute the sensory input, a set of fields that represent, on the one hand, the physical properties of the three-dimensional surfaces around the viewer, and on the other, the boundaries between patches that "belong together" in some sense and thus may correspond to the outlines of plausible physical objects in the scene. This process, which is usually called early or low-level vision, is supposed to be performed in natural systems by a set of loosely coupled neural networks (computational modules), each specializing in the reconstruction of a particular field. Thus, specific modules have been proposed for the computation of brightness edges; depth (from stereo, shading, and motion); color, lightness and albedo; velocity and optical flow; spatial and spatiotemporal interpolation and approximation, and so on.

In the second paradigm, many of the problems to be solved using vision are thought not to need a complete reconstruction of the three-dimensional world; for a given task, it may be possible to feed the raw sensory data to a network (such as a multilayer perceptron) that directly generates the desired control commands. The plausibility of this approach is illustrated, for example, in Pomerlau (1991), where such a network is used for an autonomous navigation task. In this case, however, it is also necessary to determine a set of fields defined on the same lattice as the observations: these fields represent the weights that indicate the relative importance of each pixel value for the subnetwork of the corresponding hidden unit.

In both cases, the determination of the corresponding fields exhibits an important common characteristic due to the loss of information inherent to imaging and sensory transduction processes and, in the second case, to the fact that one usually has a limited number of available examples to train the network: the values of the fields are constrained by the data but are not determined in a unique and stable way (i.e., the reconstruction problems are mathematically ill-posed). This means that the networks that implement the solutions must incorporate in their structure prior knowledge about the reconstructed fields.

For the sake of clarity, this article is focuses on the reconstruction (multimodule) paradigm, although most of the results may be extended to the action-oriented case as well. The general problem that we consider is the following.

Suppose that we are given sensory measurements in the form of a set of observed fields g at the nodes of a regular lattice L (usually a square lattice is assumed, although other arrangements are possible). From these measurements, we wish to reconstruct a field f

$= \{ f_i, i \in L \}$, given the "direct" equations that model g in terms of f and some noise process n:

$$\phi(g, f, n) = 0 \qquad (1)$$

The simplest instance of this problem is image filtering, in which g consists of a single field (the noisy observed image), f is the desired reconstructed image, and the observation model is

$$g - f - n = 0 \qquad (2)$$

Another example is the recovery of depth from stereoscopic pairs of images. Here, the observations $g = (g_L, g_R)$ are the gray levels measured in the left and right retinas, respectively, and f is the associated disparity between pairs of corresponding points (if this "correspondence problem" is solved, and if the geometry of the sensors is known, the actual recovery of depth is a matter of simple geometric computations). If the sites of the lattice are identified by a two-dimensional (2D) index $i = (i_x, i_y)$, and assuming horizontal epipolar lines, a simplified direct equation is

$$g_L(i_x, i_y) - g_R(i_x + f_i, i_y) - n_i = 0$$

for each $i \in L$.

Another example is image segmentation. Here, the input lattice is partitioned into a set of nonoverlapping regions $\{R_1, \ldots R_M\}$ so that the spatial variation of the observed images is represented by a parametric model $\Psi(i, \theta_k)$ inside region R_k:

$$g_i = \sum_{k=1}^{M} \Psi(i, \theta_k) f_{ik} + n_i \qquad (3)$$

where f_{ik} is the indicator variable of region R_k: $f_{ik} = 1$ iff $i \in R_k$ and $\{\theta_1, \ldots, \theta_M\}$ are the parameter vectors.

In the first example, the field f is underconstrained, because the noise field is not known. In the second example, even in the absence of noise, the field f is not uniquely determined, because there may be many points in the right image with the same gray level of a given point in the left one. Finally, in the third example, nonuniqueness arises because of measurement noise and because neither the parameter vectors nor the indicator variables are known. Similar ambiguous situations arise in other early vision problems for different reasons, and in all these cases it is necessary to introduce additional prior constraints.

In this article we present systematic ways for adding prior constraints, and for embedding the solution algorithms in suitable networks.

Probabilistic Regularization

The classical way of finding solutions to ill-posed problems is based on regularization methods, where stability and uniqueness of the solution are enforced by the introduction of prior smoothness constraints in the solution. A more general approach, and one that includes the classical solution as a particular case, is probabilistic, and considers f and g as realizations of random fields, so that the reconstruction of f is understood as an estimation problem. The prior knowledge about the solution is expressed in the form of a joint probability distribution for f that specifies the desired dependencies between values at neighboring sites. In this way, one may specify not only global smoothness constraints (as in standard regularization) but also piecewise smoothness, as well as constraints on the shape of the discontinuities.

The basic tool in this approach is Bayes's rule, which specifies the way in which prior information (i.e., the prior distribution P_f) is to be combined with the constraints generated by the observations (i.e., the conditional distribution $P_{g|f}$) to generate the posterior distribution $P_{f|g}$:

$$P_{f|g}(f;\ g) = \frac{P_f(f)P_{g|f}(f;\ g)}{P_g(g)} \qquad (4)$$

Note that since the observations g are given, $P_g(g)$ is a constant. The optimal estimator $\hat{f}*$ is then obtained as the minimizer of the expected value (taken with respect to the posterior distribution) of an appropriate cost function $C(f, \hat{f})$.

This approach, then, requires the specification of three basic components (besides the cost function): the observation model $P_{g|f}$, the prior distribution P_f, and the network that will effect the reconstruction. We will now analyze them in detail.

The Observation Model

The form of the constraints that sensor measurements impose on the reconstructed field depends on the particular assumptions that are made about the image formation process. If the random variables n_i, $i \in L$, are assumed to be independent, identically distributed with distribution P_n, then the conditional distribution is found by solving for n in Equation 1: $n_i = \phi^{-1}(f, g)$ and setting

$$P_{g|f}(f;\ g) = \prod_{i \in L} P_n(\phi^{-1}(g, f))$$

which can be written in the general form:

$$P_{g|f}(f;\ g) = \exp\left[\sum_{i \in L} -\Phi_i(f, g)\right] \qquad (5)$$

In most cases, the functions Φ_i are quadratic—i.e., the noise is assumed to be Gaussian—although other forms that reduce the influence of gross measurement errors have also been used (see Black and Rangarajan, 1996).

Prior Distributions

The success of the Bayesian approach depends on the specification of a probability distribution $P_f(f)$ that models the desired behavior of the solution. In particular, one would like to be able to specify a distribution in which fields where neighboring sites exhibit the appropriate dependencies are more probable than those in which these local constraints are violated. A general way of constructing such distributions is by defining an "energy" function $U(f)$, which is formed by a sum of terms that measure the violation of the local constraints. The probability distribution of the field is then given by the Gibbs measure:

$$P_f(f) = \frac{1}{Z} \exp[-U(f)] \qquad (6)$$

where Z is a normalizing constant.

More precisely, if we define a neighborhood system $\{N_i, i \in L\}$, that is, a collection of subsets of sites indexed by the sites of L: $\{N_i \subset L, i \in L\}$ with the properties:

$$i \notin N_i$$

$$i \in N_j \Leftrightarrow j \in N_i$$

its *cliques* consist of either single sites or subsets of sites such that any two belonging to the same clique are neighbors of each other. With this definition, the energy may be written as:

$$U(f) = \sum_C V_C(f) \qquad (7)$$

where C ranges over all the cliques of the neighborhood system, and each "potential function" V_C depends only on $\{f_i, i \in C\}$.

A random field F whose probability distribution is given by Equations 5 and 6 is called a *Markov random field* on L (Geman and Geman, 1984; Chellapa and Jain, 1993; Li, 2001). From (4), (5) and (7), one can see that the posterior distribution is also of the form (6), but now the energy includes the data term:

$$U(f) = \sum_{i \in L} -\Phi_i(f, g) + \sum_C V_C(f)$$

so that the Maximum a Posteriori (MAP) optimal estimator for f is obtained by minimizing this function.

The potential functions represent the "user interface" of the model, since through them one may specify the desired characteristics of the sample fields. Although they may be arbitrarily specified, there are four basic types that are generally used, depending on the characteristics of the desired reconstruction:

1. *Piecewise constant fields*: Here, each f_i may take only a finite (usually small) number of values. These fields are mostly used in segmentation problems, in which case it is often convenient that each f_i takes the form of a binary unit vector whose elements correspond to the indicator variables in Equation 3. The most widely used potential is the generalized Ising potential for cliques of size 2:

$$V_C(f_i, f_j) = -\beta, \quad \text{if } f_i = f_j$$
$$= \beta, \quad \text{otherwise}$$

2. *Globally smooth fields*: This case corresponds to standard regularization; the potentials are obtained as the squares of finite difference approximations of differential operators. For first-order differences, one obtains the "membrane" model:

$$V_C(f_i, f_j) = (f_i - f_j)^2 \qquad (8)$$

where i and j denote a pair of nearest neighbor sites in the lattice.

If one adopts the observation model (Equation 2) and assumes that P_n is a zero-mean Gaussian distribution, the posterior energy becomes equivalent to the discretized functional of standard regularization, and its (unique) maximizer corresponds to the MAP estimator (see below).

3. *Piecewise smooth fields*: This is a very important and general case. There are two basic approaches for the construction of the potentials. In the first case, the discontinuities of the field are explicitly modeled by means of an auxiliary "line field" s (originally introduced by Geman and Geman, 1984), which is defined on a "dual" lattice whose sites are between each pair of (horizontal or vertical) neighboring sites of L; s is thus indexed by a pair of indices corresponding to sites of L. Each line element s_{ij} may take values on the set $\{0, 1\}$, indicating, respectively, the absence or presence of a line (discontinuity) (in some models, s is allowed to take noninteger values in the interval $[0, 1]$ as well; see Geman and Reynolds, 1992; Black and Rangarajan, 1996).

The prior energy takes the form:

$$U(f, s) = \sum_{\langle i,j \rangle} [(f_i - f_j)^2 s_{ij} + \Psi(s_{ij})] + \sum_D W_D(s) \qquad (9)$$

where $\Psi(s_{ij})$ is a function that assigns a penalty for the introduction of a discontinuity between pixels i and j.

The line potentials $W_D(s)$ assign penalties to different local line configurations. They are summed over the cliques D of a neighborhood system defined on the dual lattice, and they are used to favor, for example, piecewise smooth lines, and to prevent the formation of smooth patches that are too thin or too small.

In the second case, the discontinuities are implicitly modeled by nonquadratic potentials $\rho(f_i - f_j)$, where ρ behaves like a quadratic function for small values of its argument but grows at a smaller rate as its argument becomes large. The derivatives of these potentials are related to influence functions of robust statistical estimators, and are therefore called *robust potentials*.

If the term $\Sigma_D W_D(s)$ is omitted, it is always possible to express Equation 9 in the form of a sum of robust potentials, simply by putting

$$\rho(f_i - f_j) = \inf_{s_{ij}} [(f_i - f_j)^2 s_{ij} + \Psi(s_{ij})]$$

where the right-hand side may be explicitly evaluated in many cases. If certain technical conditions on the ρ function are fulfilled, it is also possible to write a robust potential in the line field form (Charbonnier et al., 1997). Being able to go from one representation to the other, one may add spatial interaction terms to robust potentials, or use continuation methods that have been developed for robust potentials in the line field case (see Blake and Zisserman, 1987; Black and Rangarajan, 1996).

4. *Piecewise parametric models*: In this case the smooth patches are assumed to follow a parametric model with a relatively small number of parameters; for example, in the case of the reconstruction of the velocity field (optical flow) from a sequence of images, an affine model for the velocity of the form $f_i = A_i + b$ is often used, e.g., Black, Fleet, and Yakoob, 2000. In other cases, spline models with controlled stiffness are more appropriate (Marroquin et al., 2000). The problem here is that not only the parameters for each model have to be determined, but also the domain of validity of each model, i.e., a field of indicator variables, as in Equation 3. The prior constraints refer in this case to the spatial coherence of these domains, and may be enforced by Ising potentials.

Other examples of the application of these approaches to a variety of problems, as well as extensions and theoretical results, may be found in Chellapa and Jain (1993), Li (2001), and Marroquin et al. (2000, 2001).

Networks

Since the reconstruction is needed at the sites of the pixel lattice L, it is very natural to model the reconstructing network as a cellular automaton that consists of an array of processors or cells also located at the sites of L. The state of these processors at a given time t is denoted by $\xi^{(t)} = \{\xi_i^{(t)}, i \in L\}$. The interconnection pattern between processors is specified by the defined neighborhood system. The state of each processor changes from time to time with a rule that depends on its own state and that of its neighbors:

$$\xi_i^{(t+1)} = R(\xi_j^{(t)}, j \in N_i \cup \{i\})$$

Cellular automata (CA) may be deterministic (DCA) or stochastic (SCA), depending on the nature of the rule R.

Given this model for the architecture of a computational module, the important question is how to specify R, so that, in the deterministic case, the DCA has a fixed point and the reconstructed field f is obtained from it, and in the stochastic case, the automaton is regular and f is obtained from time averages of functions of its state.

In the case of globally smooth reconstructions, the energy function is usually convex, and the best estimator is obtained by min-

imizing this energy. The reconstructing networks are in this case equivalent to distributed iterative methods for matrix inversion (Bertsekas and Tsitsiklis, 1989). They may also be implemented analogically with pure resistor networks (see Marroquin, Mitter, and Poggio, 1987).

In the case of piecewise smooth potentials, when these are represented in the line field form and the term $\Sigma_D W_D(s)$ is not included, the energy function becomes quadratic in f for a given value of s, and therefore it may be minimized by the methods described in Bertsekas and Tsitsiklis (1989). On the other hand, if f is kept fixed, one may find the value of the s variables that minimizes U in closed form. By alternating these two steps, one gets an effective algorithm for the computation of the optimal estimator (Geman and Reynolds, 1992; Charbonnier et. al., 1997). If the energy is represented in terms of robust potentials, often local descent schemes combined with continuation methods are most effective (Blake and Zisserman, 1987).

An important issue in all these cases is the determination of the parameters included in the energy function. In many cases these are hand-adjusted for a given class of images; it is better, however, to determine them automatically, as in Zhang (1993) or Chen, Chen, and Zhou, (2000).

Discussion

The key idea of this article is that Bayesian Estimation Theory, using prior MRF models, constitutes a general method that permits the formulation of many reconstruction problems in computational vision, so that they become equivalent to the minimization of an energy function that includes two terms: one that requires the solution to be consistent with the data (the likelihood term), and another that embodies prior constraints about its behavior. For the case of piecewise constant fields, however, the best estimator is not necessarily obtained by minimizing the posterior energy (i.e., the maximum a posteriori or MAP estimator). It has been shown that the estimator that maximizes the posterior marginal probabilities (the MPM estimator) has better behavior, particularly for low signal-to-noise ratios (Marroquin et al., 1987). In both cases, the cost for the exact computation of the optimal estimators is too high, so that approximations must be made. The most precise approximations are obtained with stochastic cellular automata, which mathematically correspond to regular Markov chains whose invariant measures correspond to the posterior distribution $P_{f|g}$. In this case, one can estimate the posterior marginals, by counting the number of times a given cell is in each state, from which the MPM estimator may be obtained. It is also possible to approximate the MAP estimator by introducing a "temperature" parameter that goes slowly to zero (a procedure known as simulated annealing; see SIMULATED ANNEALING AND BOLTZMANN MACHINES and Geman and Geman, 1984).

The main drawback of these stochastic methods is their computational complexity, since many iterations are needed to obtain accurate results. This is especially important in the case of the estimation of piecewise parametric models, since here the most effective procedures consist of two steps that are performed alternately in an iterative manner until convergence is achieved. These steps are:

1. Estimate the best segmentation (i.e., the f indicator variables in Equation 3), given the model parameters.
2. Estimate the model parameters given the segmentation.

An appropriate initialization step is also required. Instances of these procedures are found in Marroquin et al. (2000) and Black et al. (2000).

To perform step 1, it is necessary to have efficient estimators for piecewise constant fields. One way to obtain them is derived from mean-field (MF) theory of statistical physics. The MF-based estimation algorithm may be implemented by a deterministic cellular automaton with M layers, where each unit corresponds to a specific marginal probability. The update rule for each node involves the computation of the exponential of the sum of the local contributions of neighboring sites plus a normalization step (see Zhang, 1993).

A different approach is based on the idea of constructing a random field of discrete probability distributions using a Gauss-Markov model, so that the mean value of this field corresponds to the posterior marginal probabilities. Since this field is Gaussian, its mean value is found by the minimization of a quadratic form, which, because of the Markovian property, has a particularly simple structure. The network that computes the optimal estimator is shown in Figure 1. Note that, unlike the MF network, in this case there is no need either of exponentiation or of normalization; as a result, one can get better results at a fraction of the computational cost (see Marroquin et al., 2000, 2001).

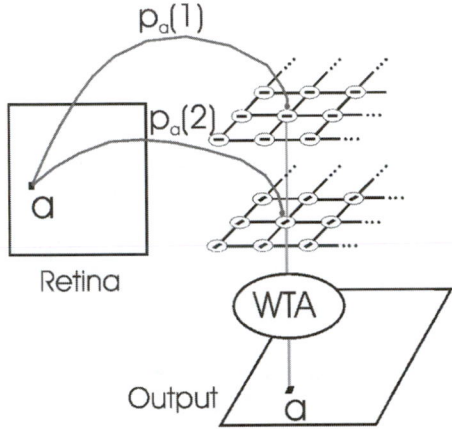

Figure 1. Network that computes the optimal estimator for a discrete-valued field. Each layer corresponds to a valid value for the field (in this example, orientation). Each cell computes the average of the state of its neighbors and the corresponding likelihood p_a obtained from the retina. A Winner Takes All mechanism outputs the most probably state at each time. Note that the layers are decoupled; they must, however, be synchronized for the system to work properly.

Road Map: Vision
Related Reading: Generalization and Regularization in Nonlinear Learning Systems; Hidden Markov Models; Statistical Mechanics of Neural Networks

References

Bertsekas, D. P., and Tsitsiklis, J. N., 1989, *Parallel and Distributed Computation: Numerical Methods*, Englewood Cliffs, NJ: Prentice Hall. ◆

Black, M. J., Fleet, D. J., and Yakoob, Y., 2000, Robustly estimating changes in image appearance, *Comput. Vision Image Understand.*, 78:8–31.

Black, M. J., and Rangarajan, A., 1996, On the unification of line processes, outlier rejection, and robust statistics with applications in early vision, *Int. J. Comput. Vision*, 19:57–91. ◆

Blake, A., and Zisserman, A., 1987, *Visual Reconstruction*, Cambridge, MA: MIT Press. ◆

Charbonnier, P., Blanc-Feraud, L., Aubert, G., and Barlaud, M., 1997, Deterministic edge-preserving regularization in computer imaging, *IEEE Trans. Image Proc.*, 6:298–311. ◆

Chellapa, R., and Jain, A., Eds., 1993, *Markov Random Fields: Theory and Practice*, Boston: Academic Press.

Chen, W., Chen, M., and Zhou, J., 2000, Adaptively regularized constrained total least-squares image restoration, *IEEE Trans. Image Proc.*, 9:588–596.

Geman, D., and Reynolds, G., 1992, Constrained restoration and the recovery of discontinuities, *IEEE Trans. Image Proc.*, 14:367–383.

Geman, S., and Geman, D., 1984, Stochastic relaxation, Gibbs distributions and the Bayesian restoration of images, *IEEE Trans. Pattern Anal. Machine Intell.*, 6:721–741.

Li, S. Z., 2001, *Markov Random Field Modeling in Image Analysis*, New York: Springer-Verlag. ◆

Marroquin, J. L., Botello, S., Calderon, F., and Vemuri, B. C., 2000, The MPM-MAP algorithm for image segmentation, *Proceedings of the 15th International Conference in Pattern Recognition (ICPR-2000)*, IEEE Computer Society, Barcelona, Spain, pp. 303–308.

Marroquin, J. L., Mitter, S., and Poggio, T., 1987, Probabilistic solution of ill-posed problems in computational vision, *J. Am. Statist. Assoc.*, 82:76–89. ◆

Marroquin, J. L., Velasco, F., Rivera, M., and Nakamura, M., 2001, Gauss-Markov measure field models for low-level vision, *IEEE Trans. Pattern Anal. Machine Intell.*, 23:337–348.

Pomerlau, D. A., 1991, Efficient training of artificial neural networks for autonomous navigation, *Neural Computat.*, 3:88–97.

Zhang, J., 1993, The mean field theory in EM procedures for blind Markov random field image restoration, *IEEE Trans. Image Proc.*, 2:27–40.

Programmable Neurocomputing Systems

Krste Asanović

Introduction

General-purpose personal computers and workstations are the most popular computing platforms used by researchers to simulate artificial neural network (ANN) algorithms. They provide a convenient and flexible programming environment, and advances in technology have been rapidly increasing their performance and reducing their cost. But large ANN simulations can still overwhelm the capabilities of even the most powerful workstations. For example, computations may require more than 10^{15} arithmetic operations and may operate on data sets containing several gigabytes of data (Ellis and Morgan, 1999).

Many neural net algorithms are highly parallelizable, allowing simulation speed to be improved by employing a network of workstations (NOW) (Anderson et al., 1995). Compared with more specialized hardware, a NOW can be an expensive solution. Fast network hardware increases the cost per node, and parallelization overheads reduce the performance per node.

For constrained application domains, fixed-function neural computing circuits can provide extremely high compute speeds at low cost, but they do not have the flexibility required to support experimentation with ANN algorithms.

To meet the need for high performance on large ANN simulations with flexible software control and reasonable cost/performance ratio, several groups have proposed and built *programmable neurocomputers*. Programmable neurocomputers (hereafter abbreviated to "neurocomputers") attempt to maintain most of the flexibility of a general-purpose computer system while improving the cost/performance ratio by specializing processors for neural computation.

This article reviews the most significant neurocomputer architectures, discusses their design and use, and concludes with predictions of future trends.

Survey of Neurocomputer Architectures

Programmable neurocomputers can be classified into four major categories. The first category uses commercial digital signal processors (DSP); the last three categories are based on custom-designed silicon.

Commercial DSP Arrays

Several neurocomputers have been built using arrays of commercial DSPs. Two notable examples are the RAP (Ring Array Processor), developed at the International Computer Science Institute (Morgan et al., 1992), and the MUSIC system, developed at the Swiss Federal Institute of Technology. (Muller et al., 1992). Both of these systems connect the DSPs in a unidirectional ring topology with communication circuitry built from field-programmable gate arrays (FPGAs). The RAP supports up to 40 Texas Instruments TMS320C30 floating-point DSPs, with a peak performance of 32 MFLOPS per node. The MUSIC system connects up to 45 Motorola DSP96002 floating-point DSPs, with a peak performance of 60 MFLOPS per node.

Both of these systems have distributed memories and are programmed using a Single Program Multiple Data (SPMD) model, in which all nodes run identical programs but operate on different portions of the data. A separate host computer manages the overall program flow and handles data input and output.

SIMD Processor Arrays

Another popular approach in neurocomputer design is a Single Instruction Multiple Data (SIMD) array of processors with some limited form of interprocessor interconnect. In these SIMD designs, a central sequencer broadcasts instructions that are executed simultaneously by all processors. The processors in a SIMD system can be much simpler than those in a SPMD system because they do not have to fetch and decode instructions. Also, SIMD processing elements do not require separate synchronizing operations because all processors work in lockstep.

Example SIMD neurocomputers include the CNAPS systems, from Adaptive Solutions (Hammerstrom, 1990), and the SNAP system, from HNC (Means and Lisenbee, 1991). The CNAPS system is built around large custom chips containing an array of 64 SIMD processing elements. Each processing element contains a fixed-point 16-bit $\times$ 8-bit multiplier, a 24-bit accumulator, a set of 32 16-bit registers, and 4 Kbytes of local on-chip memory. The processing elements are connected by two 8-bit broadcast busses and a 2-bit interprocessor ring connect. The HNC system is built from SNAP chips, each of which contains four 32-bit floating-point multiply-add datapaths with access to local off-chip memory. Both of these systems allow multiple chips to be interconnected and controlled by the same central sequencer.

Systolic Processor Arrays

Several neurocomputers have been built around systolic processor arrays that perform the matrix operations at the heart of most neural algorithms. A systolic processor contains an array of interconnected pipelines through which operands flow in a regular rhythmic fashion.

The most advanced of these systems is the Synapse-1, constructed and sold by Siemens (Ramacher et al., 1991). This system is based on a custom systolic multiply-accumulate chip, the MA-16, which integrates 16 16-bit fixed-point multipliers. The Synapse-1 system employs multiple-chained MA-16 chips to give higher throughput. Large quantities of off-chip memory are provided, split into several disjoint memory areas. Operands must be located in the correct memory region before performing a given systolic matrix operation. Additional special-purpose fixed-point datapath hardware is provided to support ANN node activation functions not provided by the MA-16 chips, and Motorola 68040 CISC processors are used to perform all other operations. The entire system is controlled by a host workstation.

Another example of a systolic neural net engine is the Mantra machine, built at EPFL, Switzerland (Ienne and Viradez, 1994). Mantra can have up to 1600-bit serial processing elements arranged in a 40 $\times$ 40 systolic mesh. A commercial DSP acts as system controller.

Vector or SIMD Coprocessor

The machines discussed to this point all rely on some form of off-chip control sequencer or host computer to manage the matrix computations occurring on the parallel processor arrays. An alternative approach is to tightly integrate the control processor with the parallel execution units on the same die. Two examples of this type of design are the T0 vector microprocessor (Wawrzynek et al., 1996) and the L-Neuro 2.3 multi-DSP (Duranton, 1996).

The T0 vector microprocessor integrates an industry-standard MIPS-II 32-bit integer scalar RISC processor with a tightly coupled fixed-point vector coprocessor. The vector coprocessor contains a central vector register file with 16 vector registers each holding 32 elements of 32 bits, two vector arithmetic units, and a vector memory unit. The two vector arithmetic units each contain eight parallel pipelines and can produce up to eight 32-bit results per clock cycle. One of the arithmetic units contains 16-bit fixed-point multipliers, but otherwise the two pipelines are identical. The memory unit connects to off-chip memory over a 128-bit data bus. T0 has a single flat memory space equally accessible by the scalar unit and any element in the vector unit. T0 is similar in design to vector supercomputers (Russel, 1978), and scalar and vector instructions can be freely intermixed in the single instruction stream. The instruction set was designed to enable object-code compatibility with future higher-performance implementations.

The L-Neuro 2.3 design contains a 16-bit RISC controller plus an array of 12 DSP datapaths. The DSP datapaths are controlled via a writable microinstruction store indexed by the RISC controller macroinstructions. The wide microinstruction words allow pairs of DSP datapaths to perform different functions, and a flexible inter-DSP communication network is provided. The L-Neuro 2.3 supports an off-chip memory connection for each DSP datapath.

Neurocomputers Versus General-Purpose Processors

Neurocomputers are distinguished from general-purpose processors by their specialization for neural computations. If we examine the range of neurocomputers above, we find that three features specific to neural computation have been exploited to improve cost/performance:

- *Limited numeric precision*. Many neural algorithms can be coded to require only 8–16 bits of fixed-point arithmetic precision (Asanović and Morgan, 1991). The reduced precision allows reductions in the area required for arithmetic circuits, particularly multipliers, and also reduces the bandwidth required to transfer operands.

- *Data parallelism.* Most neural algorithms are inherently highly data parallel, where the same operation is performed across large arrays of data. Data parallelism is the simplest form of parallelism to exploit because a single block of control hardware can be shared over many datapaths.
- *Restricted communication patterns.* Broadcast buses or unidirectional rings are sufficient to support parallel execution of many common neural network algorithms. These simplified communication networks reduce the cost of interconnecting large numbers of parallel processing elements.

All neurocomputers aim to achieve high performance on the matrix computations at the heart of many neural algorithms by exploiting these features. But real-world neural net programs require operations other than these basic matrix operations. For example, an ANN training run may require significant disk I/O to retrieve training patterns and to checkpoint trained weights. Also, the training patterns may need preprocessing before being presented to the network, and the network outputs may require postprocessing to obtain results. If the neurocomputer is too slow at performing these other nonmatrix tasks, then the overall system performance will be dominated by these nonneural components. This result is well known in general-purpose computing as Amdahl's law (Amdahl, 1967):

$$S = \frac{1}{(1 - f) + f/E}$$

where E is the factor by which performance is improved by some new technique, f is the fraction of the program execution time for which the new technique is applicable, and S is the resulting overall speedup. For example, if 90% of the execution time of a computation is taken by matrix arithmetic, then even an infinitely fast matrix computation engine will never achieve an overall speedup greater than 10. Some neural computer designs have exacerbated this problem by imposing a *slowdown* for nonneural computations by requiring slow communication to a remote host processor to implement the required functionality. Ideally, fast general-purpose computing should be tightly integrated with the special-purpose processing units.

Another related issue is that the existing neurocomputers have been primarily designed to accelerate neural algorithms with dense connectivity (e.g., backpropagation), which can be expressed using dense matrix-vector operations. However, researchers are also interested in algorithms that explore sparse connectivity and sparser activation. These require fast scatter/gather memory operations and support for rapid irregular communications.

Flexible software support is perhaps the most important aspect of a successful neurocomputer design. Most neurocomputers are intended to be programmed using libraries of optimized matrix-vector functions. This approach is adequate for the computation portion of the code provided the libraries are extensive and are easy to compose in arbitrary ways. In particular, difficulties can arise if the libraries place constraints on the location of operands when the machine has multiple distributed memories.

To support experimentation with new ANN models, it is important to provide tools to allow users to extend the libraries to provide missing functionality. Ideally, this would consist of an optimizing high-level language compiler, but in practice, assembler or microcode programming is usually required. Some of the neurocomputers have extremely complicated microarchitectures that are difficult to program efficiently at this low level. The features that complicate the task of the low-level programmer include:

- *Multiple distributed memories.* These require the programmer to carefully position data and to manage movement of data between memories.

- *Deep exposed execution pipelines.* These require the programmer to explicitly schedule operations occurring over many clock cycles.
- *Multiple levels of control flow.* Some systems have several levels of control flow (e.g., controller macroinstructions, microcontroller microinstructions, nanocontroller nanoinstructions) that must be jointly scheduled for peak performance.

Architectures that expose many details of an implementation to a programmer incur a significant programming overhead. If the same programmer-visible architecture is not preserved in subsequent machines, the software investment in low-level library code cannot be carried forward to new technology.

It is also important to provide libraries for I/O functions as well as computation, as often the amount of code required to manage data input and output dwarfs that required for matrix computation.

Discussion

The development of programmable neurocomputers was based on the premise that neurocomputing was significantly different from general-purpose computing and thus that a new type of computer architecture was warranted. But the preceding sections outlined many concerns shared with conventional computer architectures, namely, the need for flexible software development, high-performance library code, reasonable performance on arbitrary code, and fast I/O.

The primary distinguishing characteristics, namely, limited numeric precision and large-scale data parallelism, are features not only of ANN algorithms but also of many other algorithms in the areas of digital signal processing and multimedia. In recent years, many general-purpose microprocessors have added multimedia processing extensions (Lee and Smith, 1996) that provide support for data-parallel fixed-point processing. Typically, these multimedia extensions partition an existing 64-bit-wide datapath into a short vector of lower-precision subword components, e.g., 4 × 16-bit values, with new instructions that operate on all subword components simultaneously, e.g., adding two vectors of 4 × 16-bit operands to produce a vector of 4 × 16-bit results. Microprocessors with multimedia extensions are very similar to the vector or SIMD coprocessor-based neurocomputer architectures, and share the same advantage of a tightly coupled general-purpose scalar unit.

Although the multimedia extensions implemented to date provide only a limited boost to the performance of general-purpose processors on fixed-point matrix code, they signal an intent by commercial microprocessor manufacturers to perform well on these types of code. As commercial design teams incorporate multimedia-style kernels into the workloads they consider during the design of new microprocessors, we can expect performance to increase rapidly also for ANN algorithms. The continuing tremendous investment placed in high-volume microprocessors ensures that these devices will use the most advanced fabrication technologies and the most aggressive circuit design styles yielding the highest clock rates. Given these trends, there will be greatly reduced interest in future special-purpose neurocomputers.

In attempting to optimize microprocessors for these multimedia codes, microprocessor architects will face many of the same challenges that confronted neurocomputer architects. Perhaps the greatest limitation on performance of highly data-parallel codes is sustainable memory bandwidth. Sustaining high bandwidth to off-chip memory requires both high raw memory bandwidth and the ability to tolerate long memory latencies by overlapping many concurrent memory requests. New off-chip memory architectures and packaging techniques will help improve raw memory bandwidths, but significant improvements in on-chip processor architecture will be required to provide sufficient parallelism to tolerate large off-chip memory latencies. The current multimedia extensions provide only very limited data parallelism of four or eight elements at a time. It is likely that future designs will exploit much longer vectors to increase the level of parallelism supported without incurring additional instruction bandwidth costs. In addition, although current microprocessor multimedia extensions have no support for scatter/gather operations, it is likely that these will eventually be added to accelerate the large set of applications that rely on sparse matrix calculations.

A promising future direction is to integrate processor and main memory together on the same die, as in the Berkeley IRAM project (Kozyrakis et al., 1997). The IRAM project is placing a vector processor similar to T0 on the same die as a large DRAM-based main memory. The vector processor is a simple hardware scheme for controlling a large degree of parallelism, while the on-chip memory both reduces latencies and dramatically increases available memory bandwidths. The vector unit provides fast scatter/gather operations from multiple on-chip memory banks. The combination should provide high sustained performance at low cost for data-parallel codes, including both dense and sparse ANN algorithms.

Road Map: Implementation and Analysis
Background: Digital VLSI for Neural Networks
Related Reading: Neuromorphic VLSI Circuits and Systems; Neurosimulation: Tools and Resources

References

Amdahl, G. M., 1967, Validity of the single processor approach to achieving large scale computing capabilities, in *AFIPS Conference Proceedings*, Reston, VA: AFIPS Press, pp. 483–485. ◆
Anderson, T. E., Culler, D. E., Patterson, D. A., and the NOW Team, 1995, A case for NOW (networks of workstations), *IEEE Micro.*, 15(1):54–64.
Asanović, K., and Morgan, N., 1991, Experimental determination of precision requirements for back-propagation training of artificial neural networks, in *Proceedings of the 2nd International Conference on Microelectronics for Neural Networks*, Munich: Kyrill & Method Verlag.
Duranton, M., 1996, Image processing by neural networks, *IEEE Micro.*, 16(5):12–19.
Ellis, D., and Morgan, N., 1999, Size matters: An empirical study of neural network training for large vocabulary continuous speech recognition, in *Proceedings of an International Conference on Acoustics, Speech, and Signal Processing*, Piscataway, NJ: IEEE Press.
Hammerstrom, D., 1990, A VLSI architecture for high-performance, low-cost, on-chip learning, in *Proceedings of an International Joint Conference on Neural Networks*, Piscataway, NJ: IEEE Press, pp. II-537–II-543.
Ienne, P., and Viredaz, M. A., 1994, Implementation of Kohonen's self-organizing maps on MANTRA-I, in *Proceedings of the Fourth International Conference on Microelectronics for Neural Networks and Fuzzy Systems*, IEEE Computer Society Press, pp. 273–279.
Kozyrakis, C., Perissakis, S., Patterson, D., Anderson, T., Asanović, K., Cardwell, N., Fromm, R., Golbus, J., Gribstad, B., Keeton, K., Thomas, R., Treuhaft, N., and Yelick, K., 1997, Scalable processors in the billion-transistor era: IRAM, *IEEE Comput.*, 30(9):75–78.
Lee, R. B., and Smith, M. D., 1996, Special issue on media processing, *IEEE Micro.*, 16(4):6–9.
Means, R., and Lisenbee, L., 1991, Extensible linear floating-point SIMD neurocomputer array processor, in *Proceedings of the International Joint Conference on Neural Networks*, Piscataway, NJ: IEEE Press, pp. 587–592.
Morgan, N., Beck, J., Kohn, P., Bilmes, J., Allman, E., and Beer, J., 1992, The Ring Array Processor (RAP): A multiprocessing peripheral for connectionist applications, *J. Parallel Distrib. Comput.*, 14:248–259. ◆
Muller, U. A., Baumie, B., Kohler, P., Gunzinger, A., and Guggenbuhl, W., 1992, Achieving supercomputer performance for neural net simulation with an array of digital signal processors, *IEEE Micro.*, 12(5):55–64. ◆
Ramacher, U., Beichter, J., Raab, W., Anlauf, J., Bruls, N., Hachmann, M., and Wesseling, M., 1991, Design of a 1st generation neurocomputer, in *VLSI Design of Neural Networks*, Boston: Kluwer.
Russel, R. M., 1978, The CRAY-1 computer system, *Commun. ACM*, 21:63–72.
Wawrzynek, J., Asanović, K., Kingsbury, B., Beck, J., Johnson, D., and Morgan, N., 1996, Spert-II: A vector microprocessor system, *IEEE Comput.*, 29(3):79–86. ◆

Prosthetics, Motor Control
Gerald E. Loeb and Ning Lan

Introduction

This article deals with the subset of neural prosthetic interfaces that employ electrical stimulation to alter the function of motor systems, either directly or indirectly. The general biophysical considerations and technology are described in PROSTHETICS, NEURAL (q.v.).

Clinical Applications

Therapeutic Electrical Stimulation

Therapeutic electrical stimulation (TES) is an electrically produced exercise in which the beneficial effect occurs primarily off-line as a result of trophic effects on muscles and perhaps the central nervous system (CNS). One simple example is periodic exercise of the shoulder muscles to prevent disuse atrophy after a stroke (Faghri et al., 1994), which otherwise often results in chronically painful subluxation of the joint. TES effects have also been used to reduce spasticity following spinal cord injury (Stefanovska et al., 1989), presumably by downregulating the gain of hyperactive spinal reflex circuits. TES systems are relatively simple to implement because the patient chooses when and where to administer the treatment and does not require any immediate effects from the stimulation. Stimulation programs are usually devised by the caregiver, but some parameters may be adjusted manually by the patient during self-treatment sessions.

Neuromodulatory Stimulation

Neuromodulatory stimulation (NMS) involves preprogrammed stimulation that directly triggers or modulates a function without ongoing control or feedback from the patient. Perhaps the oldest clinically successful neural prosthesis is phrenic nerve pacing to provide respiration in patients with central hypoventilation (Glenn and Phelps, 1985). More recently, sacral nerve stimulation has been used successfully to empty the bladder (Brindley and Rushton, 1990) and to reduce detrusor spasticity in patients with urge incontinence (Dijkema et al., 1993). NMS systems must be portable and reliable, but they function mostly autonomously.

Functional Electrical Stimulation

Functional electrical stimulation (FES) involves precisely controlled muscle contractions that produce specific movements required by the patient to perform a task. Much motor prosthetic research has been aimed toward permitting paraplegic patients to walk, a high-risk, high-energy activity that requires sophisticated interactions among the patient's immediate intentions, the pattern of stimulation applied to multiple muscles, and the ongoing movement elicited in the limbs. There have been some laboratory demonstrations of relatively complex but still crude systems that permit slow locomotor progress, but none is yet available clinically. The WalkAide is an FDA-approved (but not widely available) prosthesis that uses transcutaneous stimulation of the peroneal nerve to correct foot drop (Wieler et al., 1999). Research emphasis has shifted to FES-assisted grasp in quadriplegic patients, using residual motor function in the proximal and contralateral limb to control stimulation of finger muscles (Prochazka et al., 1997; Smith et al., 1998; Figure 1). Most of the subsystems described in the next section are in development to improve on-line control of FES.

Subsystems

Muscle Stimulation

Most research has been performed with skin surface electrodes, percutaneous wire electrodes, and implanted multichannel stimulators (Figure 1). The development of advanced stimulation techniques that require less extensive surgery (e.g., intramuscular

BIONs, Figure 2; Loeb et al., 2001) promises to improve the practicality of FES systems that require specific and reliable control of large numbers of individual muscles. Electrical activation of muscles by any route does not replicate the natural orderly recruitment of different types of muscle fibers, which gives rise to the high efficiency and fatigue resistance of normal force production. However, artificially stimulated muscles gradually undergo fiber-type conversions as a result of trophic effects that improve their aerobic capacity (Peckham, Mortimer, and Van der Meulen, 1973).

Active muscle has complex intrinsic mechanical properties that complicate attempts to develop feedforward control strategies based on predicting joint torques and movements. Muscle force depends nonlinearly on the number and frequency of firing of recruited muscle units and on the length and velocity of the muscle fibers. Many muscles have substantial amounts of series-elastic connective tissue (tendon and aponeurosis), which means that the length and velocity of the muscle fibers depend, in turn, on the amount of stretch that they produce in that connective tissue, as well as on the trajectory of the limb. While difficult to model mathematically, these complexities appear to play an important role in stabilizing the limb during rapid perturbations (Brown and Loeb, 2000) and in storing and releasing energy to improve the efficiency of cyclical movements such as walking. Many muscles cross more than one joint, further complicating their effects on the overall trajectory of movements.

The NeuroControl Freehand System

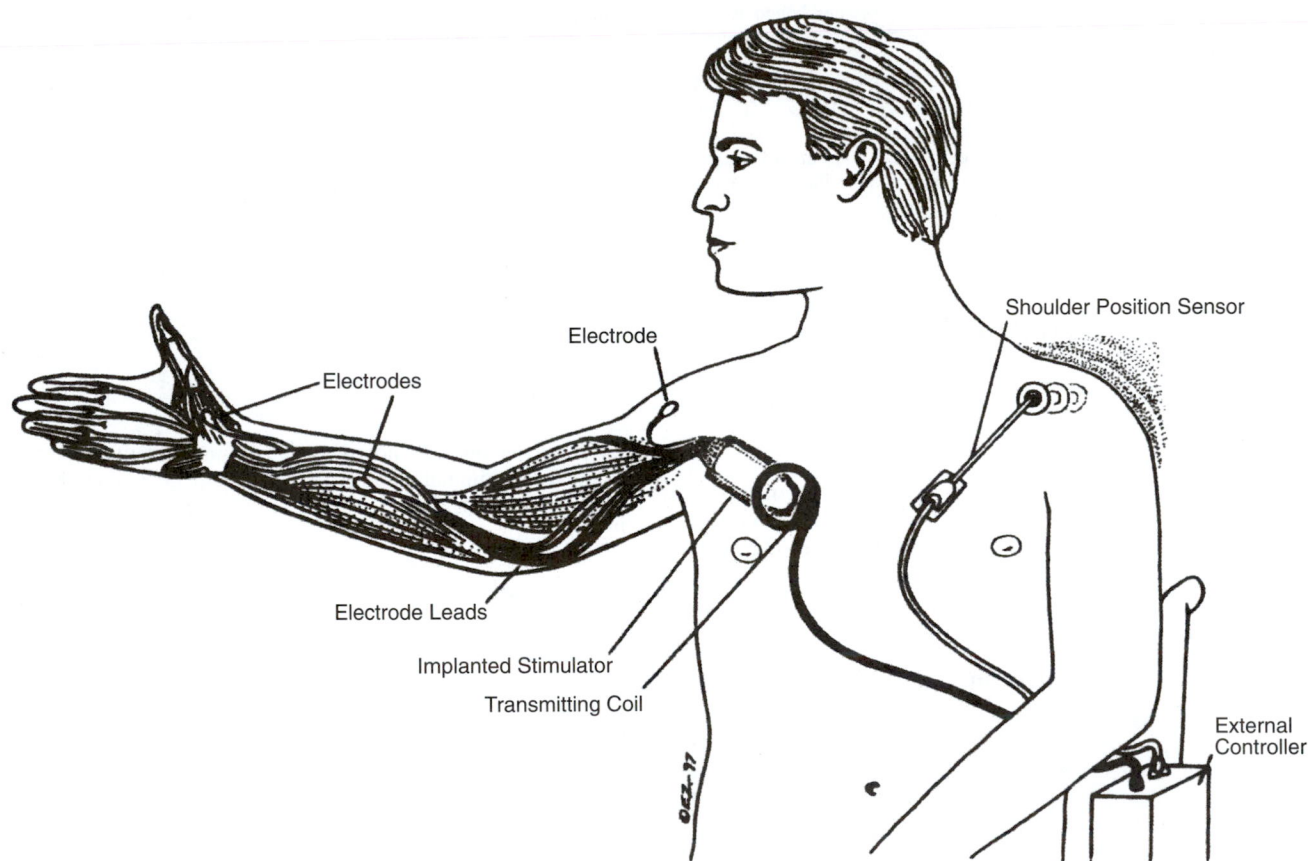

Figure 1. Freehand multichannel implanted stimulation system, approved by the U.S. Food and Drug Administration for control of grasp in spinal cord–injured patients. Voluntary shoulder motion detected by the external sensor triggers a stimulation control program that is transmitted to the implanted stimulator and routed to epimysial electrodes implanted near the nerve entry zones of various muscles operating the wrist and digits. (From Smith et al., 1998; photograph courtesy of the manufacturer, NeuroControl Corp., Cleveland, Ohio.)

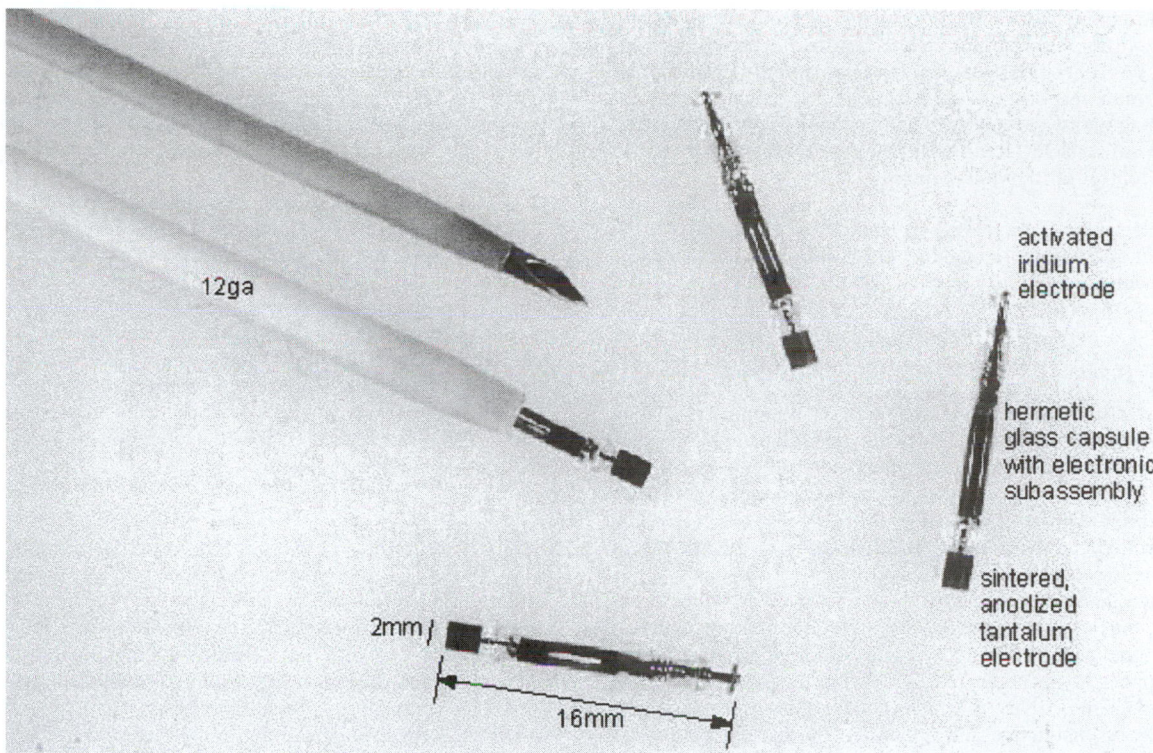

activated
iridium
electrode

hermetic
glass capsule
with electronic
subassembly

sintered,
anodized
tantalum
electrode

12ga

2mm

16mm

Figure 2. BION injectable microstimulators, now in clinical trials of TES to prevent shoulder subluxation due to muscle atrophy following stroke. Each implant (2 mm diameter × 16 mm long) receives power and digital command signals from an amplitude-modulated 2 MHz magnetic field cre-ated by an externally worn controller and transmitter coil. Each command specifies the address of one BION, the stimulus current (0.2–30 mA, in 30 steps), and the pulse width (4–514 μs, in 512 steps).

Sensory Feedback

In biological sensorimotor control, an order of magnitude more neural information comes from intramuscular proprioceptors (muscle spindle and tendon organ afferents) than goes out to control motor units. When this information is absent, both animals and humans have a great deal of difficulty making stable and accurate movements. For tasks requiring manipulation of objects, information from cutaneous mechanoreceptors is even more important. Most rehabilitation therapists believe that an insensate hand is actually less useful than a paralyzed hand.

There are three general approaches to providing sensory feedback signals to implement biological-like control systems:

- Recording the proprioceptive and cutaneous signals that are still largely present in the peripheral nerves and dorsal root ganglia of patients with upper motor lesions. Microelectrode arrays have been implanted long term into these structures in animals (Loeb, Bak, and Duysens, 1977), but the technology is not yet robust enough for clinical use. Nerve cuff electrodes can record the aggregate activity of the large-diameter fibers in peripheral nerves, which can be useful in nerves with fairly homogeneous populations of afferents such as those innervating the digits (Haugland et al., 1999).
- Affixing various electromechanical sensors to the surface of the skin or to worn components of the prosthetic system, such as braces and gloves. While useful as research tools, such external appliances generally result in unacceptable problems related to mechanical maintenance, donning time, and physical appearance.
- Implanting artificial sensors into the sites where they are needed. In addition to the design problems inherent in protecting electro-mechanical sensors from body fluids, such systems also require electrical leads or wireless communication to handle data and power requirements from large numbers of distributed transducers.

Sensorimotor Regulation

It has long been known that biological systems use a form of servocontrol. Mechanical perturbations sensed by mechanoreceptors give rise to specific reflex responses that tend to stabilize posture and force in the limb (e.g., the stretch reflex). More recently, spinal neurophysiologists have made substantial progress in unraveling the complexities of the spinal interneuronal circuitry and its role in coordinating descending commands with continuous sensory feedback.

The peripheral motor control system is substantially different in its organization from the servocontrollers used in robots. Spinal interneurons receive convergent input from many different modalities and origins of proprioceptive and cutaneous afferents, and they tend to project directly and indirectly to motor neurons controlling many different muscles and joints. Furthermore, most of the descending command signals from the brain that control limb movements terminate on these interneurons rather than directly on motor neurons. This has three important implications for the design of biological control systems (the ramifications for FES control remain unclear):

- The effects of command signals are essentially continuously modulated by the background activity from somatosensory afferents converging on the spinal interneurons.

- The brain can achieve a particular pattern of muscle activation via many different programs of interneuronal activation and inhibition, with each program resulting in potentially different patterns of reflex responses to perturbations.
- Descending pathways appear to be organized to produce various synergies of muscle recruitment and derecruitment rather than specific control of individual muscles.

FES control systems are starting to employ state-dependent logic to switch among different regulatory algorithms as different phases of the movement are detected from patterns in the signals from sensors (Kostov et al., 1995).

Control Systems

Controllers convert a given volitional command signal into a set of time-varying outputs from which the instantaneous intensities of muscle stimulation can be computed. Robotic engineering approaches that are based on complete knowledge of the sensorimotor plant have proved difficult to apply to the many degrees of freedom to be controlled and the number and complexity of the muscles to be stimulated for an FES task. An alternative approach may be to duplicate the adaptive control strategies of the CNS, which tends to perform much better in the low-precision but unpredictable demands of most activities of daily living. Biological sensorimotor systems appear to be organized in a hierarchical manner (Loeb, Brown, and Cheng, 1999), in which each layer of information processing plays a distinctive and important role in achieving goals with reasonable accuracy, stability, and energy efficiency. It remains to be elucidated how a motor goal is translated into a pattern of muscle activation through this hierarchical process, and what the organizing principles behind the formation of motor programs are. Given a sufficiently rich set of sensory feedback and informative commands, it may be possible to create interneuron-like networks for sensorimotor regulation and to use neural networks to learn how to control them to achieve similar goals for FES. For this strategy to be acceptable clinically, however, it will have to minimize the sort of trial-and-error sensorimotor learning that occupies so much of an infant's first few years of life.

Command Signals

Command signals convey the intent of the user to the control system of the prosthetic device. The control system senses and interprets the user's intent and computes an appropriate pattern of muscle stimulation. The controllers of all current FES systems and motorized artificial limbs obtain command signals from the myoelectrical activity or mechanical motion produced by those muscles that the subject can still control voluntarily. There is a general paradox in prosthetic motor control, however: the higher the level of the injury, the more degrees of freedom the prosthetic system must control, but the fewer the sources of voluntary command signals. For FES control of grasp, contralateral shoulder motion and residual wrist movement have been used to provide relatively simple commands (Smith et al., 1998). Subjects are able to produce reasonably high information rates on one channel by modulating rapidly among several distinguishable positions, probably because these muscles are still equipped with proprioceptive feedback. Other command sources, such as EMG and voice, tend to be slower and/or less precise. It remains to be seen whether systems can be designed to command the multiple simultaneous degrees of freedom involved in tasks such as coordinated reach and grasp.

An alternative approach to sensing residual voluntary muscle activity is to record command signals directly from the CNS above the level of the lesion. Attempts to record "brainwaves" via EEG and gross electrocortical electrodes have produced only very low data rates (McFarland, McCane, and Wolpaw, 1998), probably because they reflect the aggregate activity of millions of neurons carrying very different signals simultaneously. Chronic unit recording techniques have been used for many years as a research tool to understand the role of the sensorimotor cortex in controlling natural motor behaviors; technologies feasible for clinical use are starting to emerge (Rousche and Normann, 1998). Limited functional use of such signals has been demonstrated in animals (Chapin et al., 1999) but the ultimate potential is likely to depend on the representation of complex movement in the brain, a subject that is still hotly debated by neurophysiologists. For example, it has been variously proposed that the primary motor cortex (Brodman's area 4) contains a representation of the desired position in space of the hand, the angles of the joints required to achieve a desired posture, the amount of force required from the individual muscles, and the states of the spinal interneurons. These have very different implications for the design of a controller required to respond to and interpret such command signals.

Conclusions

At one extreme, motor prostheses require only very simple exercise of one or a few muscles. At the other extreme, they require sophisticated bidirectional interfaces with the patient and on-line solution of problems in motor coordination that are normally solved by complex and poorly understood circuitry in the brain and spinal cord. FES applications provide particularly interesting challenges to our theoretical understanding of the normal roles of muscles, proprioceptors, spinal reflex pathways, and trajectory planning by the brain. They have also sparked attempts to reconcile traditional engineering approaches for the control of robotic manipulators with the very different but still obscure strategies for adaptive sensorimotor control in living organisms.

Road Maps: Applications; Mammalian Motor Control
Related Reading: Motor Control, Biological and Theoretical; Motoneuron Recruitment; Muscle Models; Prosthetics, Neural; Prosthetics, Sensory Systems

References

Brindley, G. S., and Rushton, D. N., 1990, Long-term follow-up of patients with sacral anterior root stimulator implants, *Paraplegia*, 28:469–475.

Brown, I. E., and Loeb, G. E., 2000, A reductionist approach to creating and using neuromusculoskeletal models, in *Neuro-Control of Posture and Movement* (J. Winters and P. Crago, Eds.), New York: Springer. Verlag, pp. 148–163.

Chapin, J. K., Moxon, K. A., Markowitz, R. S., and Nicolelis, M. A. L., 1999, Real-time control of a robot arm using simultaneously recorded neurons in the motor cortex, *Nature Neurosci.*, 2:664–670.

Dijkema, H. E., Weil, E. H. J., Mijs, P. T., and Janknegt, R. A., 1993, Neuromodulation of sacral nerves for incontinence and voiding dysfunctions: Clinical results and complications, *Eur. Urol.*, 24:72–76.

Faghri, P. D., Rodger, M. M., Glaser, R. M., Bors, J. G., Ho, C., and Akuthota, P., 1994, The effects of functional electrical stimulation on shoulder subluxation, arm function recovery, and shoulder pain in hemiplegic stroke patients, *Arch. Phys. Med. Rehabil.*, 75:73–79.

Glenn, W. W. L., and Phelps, M. L., 1985, Diaphragm pacing by electrical stimulation of the phrenic nerve, *Neurosurgery*, 17:974–984.

Haugland, M., Lickel, A., Haase, J., and Sinkjaer, T., 1999, Control of FES thumb force using slip information obtained from the cutaneous electroneurogram in quadriplegic man, *IEEE Trans. Rehabil. Eng.*, 7(2):215–227.

Kostov, A., Andrews, B. J., Popovic, D., Stein, R. B., and Armstrong, W. W., 1995, Machine learning in control of functional electrical stimulation systems for locomotion, *IEEE Trans. Biomed. Eng.*, 42:541–551.

Loeb, G. E., Bak, M. J., and Duysens, J., 1977, Long-term unit recording from somatosensory neurons in the spinal ganglia of the freely walking cat, *Science*, 197:1192–1194.

Loeb, G. E., Brown, I. E., and Cheng, E., 1999, A hierarchical foundation for models of sensorimotor control, *Exp. Brain Res.*, 126:1–18.

Loeb, G. E., Peck, R. A., Moore, W. H., and Hood, K., 2001, BION system for distributed neural prosthetic interfaces, *Med. Eng. Phys.*, 23:9–18. ◆

McFarland, D. J., McCane, L. M., and Wolpaw, J. R., 1998, EEG-based communication and control: Short-term role of feedback, *IEEE Trans. Rehabil. Eng.*, 6:7–11.

Peckham, P. H., Mortimer, J. T., and Van der Meulen, J. P., 1973, Physiologic and metabolic changes in white muscle of cat following induced exercise, *Brain Res.*, 50:424–429.

Prochazka, A., Gauthier, M., Wieler, M., and Kenwell, Z., 1997, The bionic glove: An electrical stimulator garment that provides controlled grasp and hand opening in quadriplegia, *Arch. Phys. Med. Rehabil.*, 78:608–614.

Rousche, P. J., and Normann, R. A., 1998, Chronic recording capability of the Utah Intracortical Electrode Array in cat sensory cortex, *J. Neurosci. Methods*, 82:1–15.

Smith, B., Tang, Z., Johnson, M. W., Pourmehdi, S., Gazdik, M. M., Buckett, J. R., and Peckham, P. H., 1998, Externally powered, multichannel, implantable stimulator-telemeter for control of paralyzed muscle, *IEEE Trans. Biomed. Eng.*, 45:463–475. ◆

Stefanovska, A., Vodovnik, L., Gros, N., Rebersek, S., and Acimovic-Janezic, R., 1989, FES and spasticity, *IEEE Trans. Biomed. Eng.*, 36:738–745.

Wieler, M., Stein, R. B., Ladouceur, M. Whittaker, M., Smith, A. W., Naaman, S., Barbeau, H., Bugaresti, J., and Aimone, E. 1999, Multicenter evaluation of electrical stimulation systems for walking, *Arch. Phys. Med. Rehabil.*, 80:495–500.

Prosthetics, Neural

Gerald E. Loeb

Introduction

This article provides an overview of the physical components that tend to be common to all neural prosthetic systems. It emphasizes the biophysical factors that constrain the sophistication of those interfaces. Specific applications to neural prosthetic systems for sensory replacement and motor control are covered in PROSTHETICS, SENSORY SYSTEMS (q.v.) and PROSTHETICS, MOTOR CONTROL (q.v.), respectively. Electrical stimulation of the nervous system is also being used to treat other disorders; examples include spinal cord stimulation to control pain and basal ganglia stimulation to control parkinsonian dyskinesias.

Electroneural Interfaces

Two types of physical system are known to be capable of real-time information processing: electronic circuits, in which information is carried by the flow of electrons in metal conductors, and neural circuits, in which information is carried by ions in water. Much contemporary research in computational neurobiology is concerned with discovering or exploiting common principles of information processing in these two systems. Thus, it is natural that real-time interfaces between these systems have been developed so that electronic instrumentation can be used to study neural systems. Neural prosthetics are clinical applications of neural control interfaces whereby information may be exchanged between neural and electronic circuits. Their technology to date has been derived largely from cardiac pacemakers, which themselves have evolved from the fixed-rate, single-channel stimulators of the 1950s to become programmable and adaptive systems equipped with sensors and sophisticated data processing.

In principle, information could be transferred into and out of the nervous system by any of several means, including chemical, magnetic, optical, and ultrasonic. In practice, neural prostheses require temporospatial resolution and physical portability, which have only been achieved with the types of electrical signals that are familiar to most electrophysiologists. Thus, the future of neural prosthetics depends heavily on the well-understood biophysical properties of excitable membranes and on the development of technology that can approach physical limits that are readily predictable from those properties.

In addition to the obvious goal of restoring function to patients with disabilities, the field of neural prosthetics offers important opportunities for pure research:

- The clinical and commercial value of neural prostheses justifies the development of technology that is also useful in basic research.
- The implantation of sophisticated neural control interfaces in sentient observers creates unique opportunities for a new class of psychophysical research into neural computation.
- The development of functional replacement parts for the nervous system forces researchers to examine and test theories of neural computing more rigorously than they might do otherwise.
- The development of neural prosthetic controllers that can deal successfully with the exigencies of daily life will almost certainly require advancement of principles and methods for neural networks and other forms of adaptive control.

Stimulation

Most neural prosthetic devices operate by injecting electrical current into the extracellular fluids surrounding excitable neurons in order to elicit action potentials in those neurons. Action potentials so elicited are indistinguishable from those that arise through the natural mechanisms of sensory transduction or synaptic input. When these action potentials arrive at their destinations, the receiving cells respond to and interpret the signals as if they arose from naturally occurring neural activity. Thus, the goal of the neural prosthetic device is to recreate the temporospatial pattern of activity that would have occurred normally during the particular function that is being replaced or augmented prosthetically (see PROSTHETICS, SENSORY SYSTEMS, for a discussion of these factors in cochlear implants).

Biophysics. Topologically, a neuron in its resting state is essentially a charged spherical capacitor with elongated deformations comprising its axon and dendrites. The cell membrane is the dielectric, the ionic solutions on either side of the membrane constitute the plates, and differences in the concentrations of ions on each side generate the charging potential of about -70 mV (inside versus outside). In order to generate an action potential, the membrane capacitance must be discharged by about 15 mV in a small region. This results in a brief sequence of openings and closings of sodium and potassium channels in the membrane, which results in the flow of the action current. The action current depolarizes and then repolarizes adjacent regions of the cell membrane, giving rise to the propagating wave of activity known as an action potential or spike.

The process of evoking an action potential through extracellular stimulation is somewhat counterintuitive. In order to depolarize a capacitor, it is necessary to pass charge across the dielectric, i.e., into the cell body. However, neither the source nor the sink electrode of the stimulator is actually inside the cell. Instead, the stimulator creates a voltage gradient in the tissues surrounding the target cell. This gradient induces charge to flow across the cell membrane by capacitive conductance in response to the rate of change of the voltage gradient, i.e., *dV/dt*. The amount and extent of the depolarization so produced depend on the intensity and time course of the pulse of stimulation current, its propagation through the various conductances in the tissues through which it diffuses, and the physical dimensions and consequent electrical properties of the excitable target cell (Ranck, 1975).

The most important physical dimension of highly elongated neurons is their diameter, which affects the ratio of membrane surface area (which determines capacitance) to axonal cross-sectional area (which determines resistance to current spread inside the cell). The presence, thickness, and disposition of myelin are also important because myelin greatly reduces the capacitance that must be discharged in order to reach threshold depolarization. It should also be remembered that electrical current must form a complete circuit, so that any capacitive stimulation current that enters a cell at one point, depolarizing its cell membrane locally, must be balanced by equal current leaving the cell and causing some degree of local hyperpolarization in other regions.

In order to predict accurately the effects of stimulating a complex structure such as a part of the cerebral cortex or a muscle with embedded sensory and motor axons, it is necessary to have a great deal of quantitative information about the neural architecture and the disposition of the stimulating electrodes. There are some useful rules of thumb, however, that cover most of the important phenomena:

- The most important consequence of a stimulation pulse is the steepness of the extracellular field gradient that it produces in the vicinity of the target neurons. Small electrodes positioned close to excitable processes are most effective.
- The important stimulus variable is the charge of a pulse, which is current times duration. Voltage is not important, as most of the voltage tends to be dissipated across the metal-electrolyte interface (see below) rather than contributing to the voltage gradient in the tissue surrounding the neurons.
- Stimulation pulses are most efficient when they have a duration that is somewhat shorter than the membrane time constant of the target cells, which is usually on the order of 100–200 μs for myelinated axons and 500–1,000 μs for unmyelinated axons and cell bodies.
- The first recruited elements tend to be the largest, most elongated, and most myelinated elements, namely large-diameter myelinated axons and large cell bodies attached to myelinated axons.
- Most body tissues (including bone and scar tissue) are sufficiently conductive that they tend, in aggregate, to act as volume conductors in which stimulus current density steadily decreases with distance from the electrode.
- Stimulation electrodes must be used in pairs (source and sink), but each contact tends to function as an independent monopolar electrode unless the two contacts are positioned closer together than to the target neurons.

Electrochemistry.   The rise of safe and effective neural prosthetic devices over the past 30 years is a consequence of the gradual elucidation of the electrochemical processes involved in converting electrical current from flow of electrons in a metal conductor to flow of ions in an aqueous one. In order for this to occur without cumulative deterioration of the electrodes or damage to the tissues,

it is necessary that this be accomplished by entirely reversible chemical reactions. The typical reactions of electrolysis result in irreversible breakdown of water molecules into gases and acid or alkali solutions and shifts of the neutral valence of metals into positive-valence oxides with very different electrical, chemical, and biotoxic properties (reviewed by Loeb, McHardy, and Kelliher, 1982).

The most obvious fully reversible reaction is the charging and discharging of the capacitance between the metal electrode and the body fluids. Because the irreversible reactions of electrolysis all have minimal working voltages that must be exceeded before they occur (usually about ± 0.8 VDC), stimulating current can be passed into and out of the electrode safely as long as capacitive charging never reaches these working voltages. Thus, repeated brief pulses of electrical current can be applied safely, as long as an equal and opposite amount of charge flows in the opposite direction between each stimulating pulse.

The amount of charge that can be passed by this double-layer charging depends on the capacitance of this interface, which depends on the surface area of the electrode and the thickness of the effective dielectric boundary of the interface. A metal that forms little or no surface oxide, such as platinum, has a dielectric boundary thickness that depends on the thermodynamics of molecules bouncing off its surface. Metals that form stable nonconductive oxides, such as tantalum, can be anodized to build up their oxide thickness, reducing the capacitance but providing a barrier to inadvertent electrolytic reactions (Guyton and Hambrecht, 1974) and permitting them to sustain much higher voltages during stimulation pulses. Other reversible reactions available on some metal surfaces include absorption and desorption of hydrogen and oxygen. Iridium provides the highest charge density limit (about 3 mC/cm^2) of any biocompatible electrode material because it can be "activated" by growing a multilayer surface oxide that is electrically conductive and porous to ions (Robblee, Lefko, and Brummer, 1983). Iridium exhibits a range of stable positive valences from about $+3$ to $+4.8$, so that each atom in the oxide layer can absorb or release about two electrons, with concomitant release or absorption of two hydroxyl ions.

Electrochemical considerations are particularly important to attempts to extend neural prosthetic technology to provide denser multichannel interfaces with the nervous system. In order to provide more independent channels of stimulation in a given neural pathway, it is necessary to make the electrodes smaller and position them closer to their target neurons (Loeb, Peck, and Martyniuk, 1995). Such a microelectrode produces sufficient current density to activate local neurons selectively, while minimizing the spread of stimulation current to adjacent sites under the control of other microelectrodes. Unfortunately, the surface area of such electrodes tends to decrease faster than the amount of charge required to activate local neurons, pushing electrode materials to their safe charge density limits.

Recording

Electrophysiological recordings of interest to the control of neural prosthetics range from the potentials generated by large populations of cells (such as those measured in EEG and EMG) to the action potentials generated by individual neurons. All of these signals are small-amplitude AC signals (typically less than 1 mV) that must be detected against a background of interfering signals from other bioelectrical sources and various sources of noise. In most parts of the central and peripheral nervous systems, the activity of adjacent neurons is often quite distinctive, making it necessary to record and distinguish the action potentials of single units to use them as command and control signals. This has been accomplished for brief periods of time in many research applications, but techniques remain to be developed for stable, long-term recordings from human patients.

The action potentials generated by individual neurons are produced by action currents of 1–10 nA lasting 0.2–2 ms, depending on the size and myelination of the cell. As in the case of the currents produced by electrical stimulation, the current density and the resulting potential gradient in the surrounding tissues drop rapidly with distance from the current source (Rall, 1962). Microelectrodes usually must be within 100 μm of a neuron to record a usable action potential. In order to be positioned that close to a neuron, such a microelectrode must be physically small, with a small surface area. For a metal microelectrode, double-layer charging of the metal-electrolyte interface provides the mechanism for converting a biopotential from ion fluxes in water to electron motion in a metal conductor. The small surface area of the exposed metal surface provides only a small capacitance, resulting in a relatively high impedance in the frequency band of the action potential (typically 100–1,000 kΩ at 0.5–5 kHz). The resistivity of the saline in the immediate vicinity of the microelectrode also presents a substantial impedance. High impedance is associated with high thermal noise, which adds to and obscures any biopotentials to be recorded.

Usually microelectrodes pick up signals from several adjacent neurons, which may need to be discriminated based on small differences in their waveforms. Even relatively low noise levels may degrade the reliability of such discrimination. Small movements of the microelectrode with respect to the neurons are likely to distort the relative amplitude and shape of the single unit potentials or change the sampled population entirely.

Systems Hardware

Power and Data Management

In order to improve the sophistication and capabilities of neural prosthetic interfaces, larger numbers of stimulating and recording channels must be positioned closer to their neural targets. This raises the problem of how to transmit more data to and from arrays of small electrodes located in delicate neural tissues.

One approach is to combine many electrodes into an array that includes active electronic processing so that a large number of separate signals can be multiplexed onto one data connection (Najafi, Ji, and Wise, 1990). Stimulation pulses are usually relatively brief ($\sim$100 μs) compared to their interpulse intervals ($\sim$10–100 ms), making it possible for a single stimulus channel to be multiplexed among many electrodes. Bioelectrical potentials are more difficult to multiplex because they usually have high concurrent bandwidths (1–10 kHz) on each channel, resulting in very high aggregate sampling rates.

Any active circuitry for multiplexing or demultiplexing requires DC power. Electrical leads and connectors carrying DC voltages are particularly difficult to insulate because even tiny amounts of saline leakage result in electrolytic corrosion (see below). The very low power consumption of some integrated circuit technologies has led to interest in the wireless transmission of power. Radio-frequency (RF) inductive coupling is now used routinely in cochlear implants and has been developed for injectable muscle stimulators (Troyk and Schwan, 1992). Infrared transmission and photoelectric conversion may also be possible over short distances.

Packaging

Active microelectronic circuitry is generally contained within a hermetic enclosure to protect it from moisture. This adds greatly to the physical bulk of the circuitry, particularly if large numbers of input-output channels must be routed through feedthroughs and connectors incorporated into the package. The design of the package and the selection of hermetic materials (metals, ceramics, and glasses) are likely to be further complicated by the need to transmit RF or infrared energy to power and control the electronics. Embedding in epoxy, silicone, and other nonhermetic polymers was commonplace in the early cardiac pacemaker industry, but it is difficult to perform reliably on complex circuits. There is much interest in passivating monolithic integrated circuits so that they can be implanted directly into the nervous system with few or no attached leads.

Nonhermetic encapsulation and passivation depends on adhesion of the coating material to the substrate electronic components rather than impermeability. Water in the vapor phase tends to diffuse through all polymeric materials, but it does not cause electronic problems until it condenses onto the circuitry itself. Once condensation occurs, the water vapor forms an ionic solution by dissolving surface contaminants or the materials themselves. This solution represents an osmotic attractant, pulling additional water vapor out of the surrounding polymer and pressurizing itself so that it dissects along the surface, eventually bridging electrical conductors and resulting in corrosion and circuit failure. Condensation on hydrophilic surfaces can be prevented only if there are no voids and there is sufficient adhesive force between the encapsulant and all substrate materials. Even trace surface contaminants tend to interfere with adhesion, which usually depends on electrostatic bonding (Donaldson, 1987).

An alternative approach to chemical adhesion for certain geometries is to use hydrostatic pressure. This has proved useful in preventing electrical shorting from condensed water within connectors that must be opened and closed in the body. The encapsulant is pressurized mechanically as the connector is closed so that its hydrostatic pressure exceeds the maximal osmotic pressure of salt solutions (typically 200–250 psi) (Loeb et al., 1983).

Conclusions

Serious attempts to build functional neural prostheses have been under way for about 35 years. Progress has been limited because it depended on concurrent developments in microelectronic and biomaterial technologies as well as on advances in understanding the neurophysiology of the functions to be restored. Once these thresholds have been passed for a given application (e.g., cochlear implants for the deaf; see PROSTHETICS, SENSORY SYSTEMS), dramatic functional restoration has been achieved, although the development of these complex and highly regulated medical devices remains much slower than that of comparable consumer electronics. As the armamentarium of applicable technology and basic neurophysiology enlarges, there should be a steady acceleration in the clinical application of neural prostheses.

Road Map: Applications
Related Reading: Brain-Computer Interfaces; Brain Signal Analysis; Prosthetics, Motor Control; Prosthetics, Sensory Systems

References

Donaldson, P. E., 1987, Twenty years of neurological prosthesis-making, *J. Biomed. Eng.*, 9:291–298. ◆
Guyton, D. L., and Hambrecht, F. T., 1974, Theory and design of capacitor electrodes for chronic stimulation, *Med. Biol. Eng.*, 12:613–619.
Loeb, G. E., Byers, C. L., Rebscher, S. J., Casey, D. E., Fong, M. M., Schindler, R. A., Gray, R. F., and Merzenich, M. M., 1983, The design and fabrication of an experimental cochlear prosthesis, *Med. Biol. Eng. Comput.*, 21:241–254.

Loeb, G. E., McHardy, J., and Kelliher, E. M., 1982, Neural prosthesis, in *Biocompatibility in Clinical Practice*, vol. II (D. F. Williams, Ed.), Boca Raton: CRC Press, pp. 123–149. ◆

Loeb, G. E., Peck, R. A., and Martyniuk, J., 1995, Toward the ultimate metal microelectrode, *J. Neurosci. Methods*, 63:175–183.

Najafi, K., Ji, J., and Wise, K. D., 1990, Scaling limitations of silicon multichannel recording probes, *IEEE Trans. Biomed. Eng.*, 37:1–11.

Rall, W., 1962, Electrophysiology of a dendritic neuron model, *Biophys. J.*, 2:145–167.

Ranck, J. B., Jr., 1975, Which elements are excited in electrical stimulation of mammalian central nervous system: A review, *Brain Res.*, 98:417–440. ◆

Robblee, L. S., Lefko, J. L, and Brummer, S. B., 1983, Activated Ir: An electrode suitable for reversible charge injection in saline solution, *J. Electrochem. Soc.*, 130:731–733.

Troyk, P. R., and Schwan, M. A., 1992, Closed-loop class E transcutaneous power and data link for microimplants, *IEEE Trans. Biomed. Eng.*, 39:589–599.

Prosthetics, Sensory Systems

Gerald E. Loeb and Blake Wilson

Introduction

This article concerns sensory prostheses, in which information is collected by electronic sensors and delivered directly to the nervous system by electrical stimulation of pathways in or leading to the parts of the brain that normally process a given sensory modality. In principle, all of the senses could be replaced or even augmented by such technology. In practice, only some sensory modalities seem amenable to currently available approaches; the status for each sense is summarized below:

- Hearing—widespread clinical success with the use of cochlear implants over the past decade.
- Vision—long-standing goal, with a recent resurgence in preclinical research plus some pilot human experiments.
- Touch—some clinical research on peripheral restoration in conjunction with functional electrical stimulation (FES; see PROSTHETICS, MOTOR CONTROL).
- Proprioception—little research under way, despite eventual importance to FES.
- Balance—some theoretical potential and early-stage analysis of feasibility.
- Smell—some theoretical interest because of the clinical significance of anosmia in the elderly, but hampered by the complexity of the natural senses and the unavailability of prosthetic sensors.
- Taste—no research under way; little clinical interest.

The general problem in constructing and implementing sensory prostheses is to understand and emulate the relevant parts of the neural code used by normal sense organs to encode and transmit sensory information to the brain. In practice, this means identifying a surgically accessible site through which to apply a complex temporospatial pattern of electrical stimulation. The general biophysical and electronic considerations can be found in PROSTHETICS, NEURAL. This article describes current research on auditory and visual prostheses.

Cochlear Prostheses

Current Technology

Cochlear prostheses use direct electrical stimulation of auditory nerve cells to bypass absent or defective hair cells that normally transduce acoustic vibrations into neural activity. They are the most sophisticated and the most successful neural prostheses to date, and they are still evolving. The currently available devices generally use multicontact electrodes inserted into the scala tympani of the cochlea so that they can differentially activate auditory neurons that normally encode different pitches of sound (for a historical review,

see Loeb, 1990). A much smaller number of patients with bilateral degeneration of the auditory nerve have been treated with modest success by stimulation of the cochlear nucleus in the brainstem. In all currently available systems, an external, wearable control unit (Figure 1) determines a pattern of electrical stimulation in which the stimulus amplitude in each channel depends on the spectral content in the acoustic input and a previously stored map of auditory sensations that can be elicited by electrical stimulation of each channel in that patient. Many algorithms have been developed over the years, employing both analog and pulsatile electrical waveforms delivered sequentially and/or simultaneously to fixed or dynamically changing channels.

Clinical results with cochlear implants have improved steadily, to the point that they are the treatment of choice for most cases of severe to profound sensorineural hearing loss in both adults and children. Most patients with adult-onset deafness are devastated by the loss of social interactions and find it difficult to develop alternatives such as lip-reading and sign language. Cochlear implants provide essentially immediate restoration of awareness of sound in all patients and functional levels of speech recognition in the majority, suggesting that the goal of replicating the salient natural encoding of sound has been achieved in most but not all patients (see below).

For prelinguistically deafened children, the trend is to implant a cochlear prosthesis at an early age, generally under 6 and increasingly under 2 years old. Young children appear to benefit from the increased plasticity of the young nervous system and the ability to participate in conventional verbal educational programs (Svirsky et al., 2001). In general, they acquire language skills at the same rate as normal children, but they remain delayed by the preimplantation period. Individuals who have received no acoustic stimulation in the first few years of life appear to lose much of their ability to learn to process such information by adolescence (Busby et al., 1991), consistent with the notion of "critical periods" in the training of biological neural networks.

Current Research

Improved temporospatial representations of speech sounds. The replacement of 10,000 independent hair cell transducers with 8 to 20 sources of stimulation current necessarily results in distortions of both the temporal and spatial patterns of neural activity received by the brain. The spatial problem is further aggravated by the tendency of stimulus currents to spread radially from their source in the volume-conductive tissues of the cochlea, resulting in "crosstalk," whereby a stimulus targeted to one spatial subgroup of spiral ganglion cells exerts modulatory effects on distant subgroups that are the target of another stimulation channel. The extent of this problem has been appreciated relatively recently through both clini-

Figure 1. Clarion cochlear prosthesis showing external (left foreground) and implanted (right) components. The implanted components include a 16-contact intracochlear electrode (wedged into the spiral shape of the first one-and-a-half turns of the scala tympani by the dark blue positioner; see insert) and hermetically encased electronics (labeled implant: 25 mm wide by 6 mm thick). The external sound processor contains patient-operated controls, a rechargeable battery, a microprocessor, and a digital signal processor, and connects to a headpiece with a microphone and the antenna that transmits power and data to the implant. Acoustic signals from the microphone are filtered and converted into 8 to 16 channels of stimulus waveforms; these are delivered by the electrode contacts to recruit tonotopically arranged subsets of the spiral ganglion cells that comprise the auditory nerve. (Photograph courtesy of the manufacturer, Advanced Bionics Corp., Valencia, Calif.)

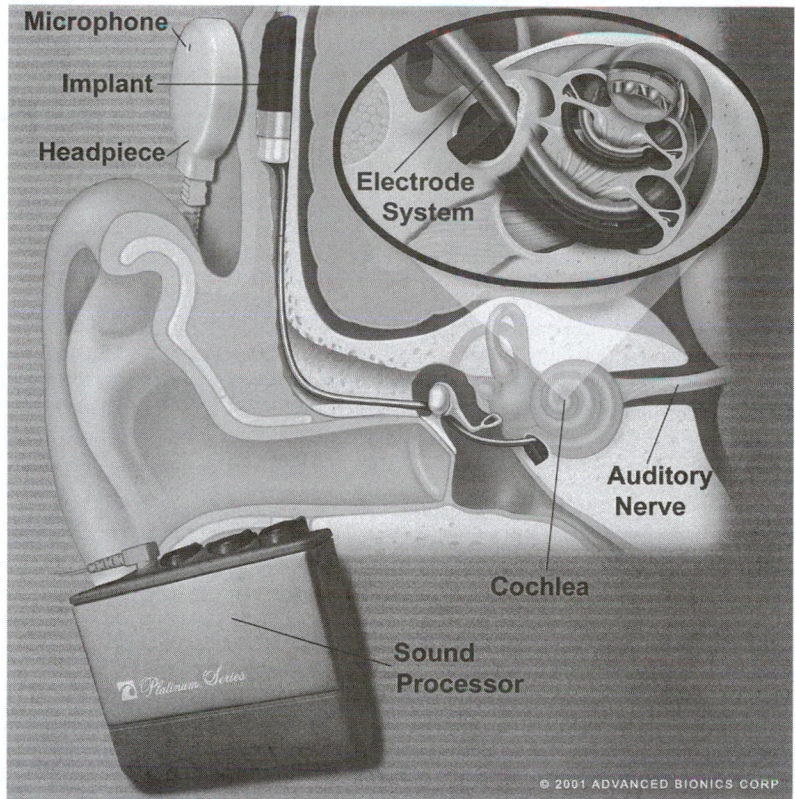

cal studies (Lawson et al., 1996) and computer modeling (Frijns, Briaire, and Grote, 2001). It is particularly severe for apical (low-frequency) sites. This has led to renewed development and testing of novel cochlear electrode arrays intended to position the contacts closer to the target spiral ganglion cells and reduce spread of stimulation currents.

The temporal distortions are more complex and their significance and amelioration less obvious. As the strength of an electrical stimulus is increased to represent increasing loudness, it recruits more and more auditory neurons, as would occur with an acoustic stimulus, but the electrically evoked activity tends to be much more highly synchronized. This results in a form of "beating" or "aliasing" among the repetition rates of the stimulation pulses (typically 400–800 pps), the modulation bandwidths of the acoustic information (typically 100–400 Hz), and the relative refractory periods of auditory neurons (probably 1–3 ms, corresponding to 300–1,000 Hz). The effect is most severe for low-frequency (apical) percepts, which are normally decoded from both temporal and spatial cues in the neural activity. It appears to be possible and useful to break up such beating by employing stimulation pulse rates that are far higher than those that can be followed by individual neurons (e.g., 1,500 up to 5,000 pps). This reduces beating and aliasing and results in a more randomized temporospatial representation, which many patients find to be subjectively less annoying and functionally more useful (Wilson et al., in press).

Combined electrical and acoustic stimulation in patients with residual hearing. There are many more patients with severe than with profound hearing loss, and most of these tend to have preferential preservation of low-frequency (apical) acoustic perception. This is the band in which cochlear implants tend to produce the greatest spatial and temporal distortions (see above). Clinical testing in a limited number of such subjects suggests that it is usually

possible to preserve acoustic hearing apical to an electrode array that has been inserted shallowly into the scala tympani. The simultaneous presentation of amplified low-frequency acoustic information together with a multichannel electrical representation of the higher frequencies produces substantial improvements in performance, particularly for complex tasks such as perception of speech in highly noisy environments (Wilson et al., in press).

Bilateral cochlear implants. Individuals with normal hearing use binaural cues to distinguish desirable signals from noise sources that are located at different positions. Differences in relative loudness and arrival time at the two ears are decoded in the auditory brainstem so that the cognitive centers of the cortex can focus on spectral information from a single source. At least some of the few patients who have received cochlear implants in both ears have experienced substantial improvements in speech perception in noisy environments (Wilson et al., in press). This has motivated additional research on methods to synchronize the stimulation of the corresponding channels in the two ears, which might lead to performance that would warrant the additional expense and invasiveness of two cochlear implants.

Psychophysical correlates of performance variability. The development and testing of cochlear implants has been plagued by large variability of results among patients with no distinguishing characteristics. This complicates the design and interpretation of studies comparing the performance of different devices and speech-processing strategies. It also makes it difficult to justify implantation in the many patients whose residual hearing provides function comparable to that obtained by the poorest implant recipients. Enhanced psychophysical tests enabled by more flexible stimulation systems have started to identify neurophysiological correlates of cochlear implant performance (Wilson et al., in press). This bodes well for the development of speech-processing strategies to overcome these individual limitations and to fit them to the appropriate patients.

Fully implanted systems. Cochlear implants have been following a development track similar to that of hearing aids, their technological predecessors. Both started with relatively large and power-hungry circuitry that had to be worn on the body, including large, heavy, rechargeable batteries. Both used improvements in low-power integrated circuitry and battery technologies to miniaturize the sound-processing systems so they could be worn behind the ear (or even in the ear canal, in the case of hearing aids). Because one component of a cochlear prosthetic system must be surgically implanted, an obvious goal is to eliminate the external components entirely. This poses three major challenges that seem likely to be overcome within the next 2–3 years:

- The power consumed by the stimulation pulses themselves is substantial in a high-speed, multichannel implant, necessitating the development of high-performance batteries that can be recharged rapidly and frequently by inductive coupling of RF energy applied outside the body. More efficient electrodes closer to the spiral ganglion cells should also help.
- The microphone in present cochlear implant systems is usually located with the external headpiece that transmits power and data to the implanted electrodes. Novel technologies are in development for an implanted microphone that will function electrically and acoustically in a surgically suitable site.
- The dynamic range of electrical stimulation (from perceptual threshold to uncomfortably loud) is very narrow compared with that of acoustic hearing (6–20 dB versus 100 dB). Speech processors employ sophisticated digital algorithms for dynamic gain control and stimulus intensity mapping, but many patients find it necessary to make frequent adjustments to the manual loudness control on their externally worn speech processors. An alternative strategy is to have the implant monitor the electromyographic activity associated with the stapedius reflex and use it to make automatic adjustments of stimulation intensity. This is a protective reflex that comes on when the brain perceives the sound to be uncomfortably loud; it is intact in most cochlear implant recipients.

Visual Prostheses

As in the early days of auditory prostheses, there is not yet any general agreement on the most promising site to apply electrical stimulation to the visual pathways. Sites that have been considered include subretinal (microelectronic array of photocells between the retina and the sclera), epiretinal (thin film electrode array on the vitreous surface of the retina), optic nerve (nerve cuff electrode), optic radiations (probes with multiple contacts inserted stereotactically), surface of striate cortex (arrays of contacts on the pial surface), and striate intracortical (see below). The obvious difference between auditory and visual prostheses is that auditory information requires a small number of channels with high data rates while the visual system requires a large number of channels with low data rates. This would seem to favor the two sites described below, which offer large, fairly flat surfaces on which to deploy retinotopically mapped electrode arrays.

Cortical Approach

Attempts to provide useful visual sensations in the blind by direct electrical stimulation of visual cerebral cortex began in 1966 (Brindley and Lewin, 1968). The initial devices used arrays of small electrodes (about 1 mm diameter) on the pial surface. Relatively high stimulus currents (about 1 mA for a 200 μs pulse) were required to produce sensations of light called phosphenes. Because of current spread by volume conduction, such stimulation presented to a single electrode presumably recruits neurons scattered over many adjacent cortical columns, but the surround inhibitory mechanisms actually result in a surprisingly small, well-formed dot of light. This seems to suggest that a complete, if coarse-grained, picture could be built up from a sufficient number of such phosphenes. The problem is that the processes responsible for the focusing operate quite slowly, so that stimulus trains presented concurrently but interleaved between even two such sites produce unpredictable, nonlinear interactions (Girvin, 1988). A useful image will require hundreds, if not thousands, of independently controllable phosphenes.

More recently, intracortical microelectrodes have been employed successfully to create similar phosphenes with stimulus currents (5–20 μA) that would tend to recruit only a few neurons within the immediately vicinity of the electrode tip (Bak et al., 1990). When two sites spaced less than a millimeter apart are stimulated concurrently, their phosphenes seem to combine and fuse in a predictable and desirable manner. Silicon fabrication (Wise and Najafi, 1991; Normann et al., 1996) may make it feasible to build dense arrays of contacts and associated electronic circuitry that are safe to implant and operate continuously for long periods of time.

Retinal Approach

Recent improvements in low-power integrated circuitry and intraocular surgical techniques have sparked interest in the possibility of placing an array of microelectrodes on the inner retinal surface. This approach requires viable retinal ganglion cells, so it is limited to blindness caused by photoreceptor degeneration, such as retinitis pigmentosa and macular degeneration.

Human research to date has employed intraoperative probes and small electrode arrays to determine suitable stimulation parameters and the percepts that they evoke. Data are inconclusive because of the severe limitations on intraoperative experiments and because of uncertainties about the positioning of the electrodes and the condition of the retinal circuitry. The following is a tentative interpretation of the biophysics of retinal stimulation and their implications for the design of a functional visual prosthesis.

In the intact retina, photoreceptors maintain a polarization level that maximizes sensitivity to incident photons, which results in changes in the release of transmitter and in the background spontaneous activity of bipolar and ganglion cells. Even tiny transretinal currents in the μA range can change the bias levels of these photoreceptors, resulting in perceptions of light and dark phosphenes. In the absence of photoreceptors, electrical stimulation pulses must produce sufficiently intense voltage gradients to depolarize neurons from the resting potential to the threshold for the propagation of action potentials. Retinal neurons are relatively small and unmyelinated, so they would be expected to have high thresholds and long membrane time constants. The output axons of retinal ganglion cells are the largest structures and lie on the vitreous surface of the retina, immediately under the stimulating electrodes, so they would be expected to have the lowest thresholds. However, the axons at a given location originate from a wedge-shaped sector of the retina, so their activation would be expected to produce elongated and overlapping phosphenes. Bipolar cells are more localized and tend to be preserved in most retinopathies, but their electrical thresholds are unclear. Because bipolar cells have longer membrane time constants than ganglion cells (1–2 ms versus 0.5 ms), they can be activated selectively by long-duration pulses (Greenberg et al., 1999). However, such stimulation applied to a large array may result in cross-talk between channels and unacceptable levels of power dissipation.

Information Processing

The introduction of information directly into the CNS, bypassing the natural sensory encoding, raises interesting questions about how that information will be interpreted by the CNS.

Temporal Patterning

Classical neurophysiology is grounded in the notion that the output of each individual neuron represents an independent channel in which the mean spike rate encodes unidimensional information. There have been various theories regarding the encoding and decoding of information in the fine temporal details of activity patterns in ensembles of neurons. One theory of pitch perception held that the acoustic frequency information encoded in the phase-locked activity of auditory afferents could be decoded by cross-correlation of delayed and undelayed versions of this signal. However, patients reported pitch sensations that were dominated by place of electrical stimulation rather than frequency for stimulation rates above about 500 Hz (Eddington et al., 1978). Electrical stimulation of the visual cortex would seem to offer a powerful technique to test current theories regarding the significance of widespread synchronization among neurons responding to a single object in a complex scene.

Neuronal Plasticity

There have been dramatic demonstrations of remapping of both sensory maps and motor representations in primary cortex in response to various surgical, electrical, and behavioral modifications of cortical input (Merzenich and Grajski, 1990). Abrupt or gradual loss of signals from failing sense organs is likely to induce various reorganizations of the ascending pathways, as well as the general atrophy that has been noted. The use of electrical stimulation to restore sensory information inevitably results in somewhat unphysiological temporospatial patterns of neural activity that are likely to induce further reorganizations. For example, recent evidence suggests that the tendency of cochlear implants to produce a better representation of high (basal) versus low (apical) acoustic frequencies may result in a remapping of the central representations and consequent improvements in speech perception (Svirsky et al., 2001). Because of the complex precortical processing of auditory information, the locus of such plasticity will be difficult to identify. Similar experiments in the much simpler visual system have the potential to provide important insights into cortical information processing.

Conclusions

The growing clinical application of neural prosthetics should provide a major catalyst for the expansion of basic knowledge about the nervous system. The devices themselves provide unique opportunities for psychophysical testing of current theories of neural computing and immediate incentives for improving those theories when their limitations are revealed. The technology that is being developed to build these prostheses has considerable spin-off potential as neurophysiological research tools. Conversely, the nervous system embodies tried and proven solutions to computational problems that have resisted conventional algorithmic approaches of robotics and artificial intelligence. It is difficult to imagine a more appropriate application of electronic neural networks than in the repair of the biological systems that have inspired them.

Road Maps: Applications; Other Sensory Systems
Related Reading: Prosthetics, Motor Control; Prosthetics, Neural

References

Bak, M., Girvin, J. P., Hambrecht, F. T., Kufta, C. V., Loeb, G. E., and Schmidt, E. M., 1990, Visual sensations produced by intracortical microstimulation of the human occipital cortex, *Med. Biol. Eng. Comput.*, 28:257–259.

Brindley, G. S., and Lewin, W. S., 1968, The sensations produced by electrical stimulation of the visual cortex, *J. Physiol.*, 196:479–493.

Busby, P. A., Roberts, S. A., Tong, Y. C., and Clark, G. M., 1991, Results of speech perception and speech production training for three prelingually deaf patients using a multiple-electrode cochlear implant, *Br. J. Audiol.*, 25:291–302.

Eddington, D. K., Dobelle, W. H., Brackmann, D. E., Mladejovsky, M. G., and Parkin, J., 1978, Place and periodicity pitch by stimulation of multiple scala tympani electrodes in deaf volunteers, *Trans. Am. Soc. Artif. Intern. Organs*, 24:1–5.

Frijns, J. H. M., Briaire, J. J., and Grote, J. J., 2001, The importance of human cochlear anatomy for the results of modiolus-hugging multichannel cochlear implants, *Otol. Neurotol.*, 22:340–349. ◆

Girvin, J. P., 1988, Current status of artificial vision by electrocortical stimulation, *Neuroscience*, 15:58–62.

Greenberg, R. J., Velte, T. J., Humayun, M. S., Scarlatis, G. N., and de Juan, E., Jr., 1999, A computational model of electrical stimulation of the retinal ganglion cell, *IEEE Trans. Biomed. Eng.*, 46:505–514.

Lawson, D. T., Wilson B. S., Zerbi, M., and Finley, C. C., 1996, *Speech Processors for Auditory Prostheses: 22 Electrode Percutaneous Study. Results for the First Five Subjects*, Quarterly Progress Report 3, NIH project N01-DC-5-2103, Neural Prosthesis Program.

Loeb, G. E., 1990, Cochlear prosthetics, *Annu. Rev. Neurosci.*, 13:357–371. ◆

Merzenich, M. M., and Grajski, K., 1990, Cortical network changes underlying representational plasticity, *Cold Spring Harbor Symp. Quant. Biol.*, 55:873–887.

Normann, R. A., Maynard, E. M., Guillory, K. S., and Warren, D. J., 1996, Cortical implants for the blind, *IEEE Spectrum*, 54–59. ◆

Svirsky, M. A., Silveira, A., Suarez, H., Neuburger, H., Lai, T. T., and Simmons, P. M., 2001, Auditory learning and adaptation after cochlear implantation: A preliminary study of discrimination and labeling of vowel sounds by cochlear implant users, *Acta Otolaryngol.*, 121:262–265.

Wilson, B. S., Brill, S. M., Cartee, L. A., Cox, J. H., Lawson, D. T., Schatzer, R., Wolford, R. D., Muller, J. M., Schon, F., Tyler, R. S., Kiefer, J., Pfennigdorff, T., and Gstottner, W. (in press), From the 2001 Conference on Implantable Auditory Prostheses: Some likely next steps in the further development of cochlear implants, *Ear Hearing*. ◆

Wise, K. D., and Najafi, K., 1991, Microfabrication techniques for integrated sensors and microsystems, *Science*, 254:1335–1342.

Pursuit Eye Movements

Richard J. Krauzlis and Leland S. Stone

Introduction

When viewing objects, primates use a combination of saccadic and pursuit eye movements to stabilize the retinal image of the object of regard within the high-acuity region near the fovea. Although these movements involve widespread regions of the nervous system, they mix seamlessly in normal behavior. Saccades are discrete movements that quickly direct the eyes toward a visual target, thereby translating the image of the target from an eccentric retinal location to the fovea. In contrast, pursuit is a continuous movement that slowly rotates the eyes to compensate for the motion of the visual target, minimizing blur that can compromise visual acuity. Whereas other mammalian species can generate smooth optokinetic eye movements—which track the motion of the entire visual surround—only primates can smoothly pursue a single small element within a complex visual scene, regardless of any extraneous motion on the retina. This difference likely reflects the greater ability of primates to segment the visual scene, to identify individual visual objects, and to select targets of interest.

Basic Features of Pursuit Behavior

The basic features of pursuit can be illustrated by considering the *ramp paradigm*, in which a target initially at rest moves at a constant speed (Figures 1A and 1B). Pursuit is often interrupted by initial "catch-up" saccades, because the delay in the eye movement response makes the eye lag behind the target. However, if the onset of target motion is accompanied by a position step in the opposite direction, pursuit can be elicited without any catch-up saccades (Rashbass, 1961). The eye movement records obtained with this paradigm can be divided roughly into four phases (Figure 1B). During the latent phase (1), the target is moving, but the eyes have not yet begun to move. During the initiation of pursuit (2), eye speed increases at a nearly constant rate related to the constant image motion experienced during the latent phase. This is followed by a transition phase (3), as eye speed continues to increase and often overshoots target speed slightly. During sustained pursuit (4), eye speed settles to a steady-state value that often oscillates around a value near target speed.

The ramp paradigm illustrates several features of the pursuit system. The first feature is that, as Rashbass (1961) demonstrated, the pursuit response is dominated by target motion; pursuit rotates the eyes in the direction of target motion, even if this is away from the current position of the target. Although subordinate to motion, position offsets can also contribute to the visual drive for pursuit (Pola and Wyatt, 1979).

A second feature is that, because the retina is part of the eye, there is a reciprocal relationship between the motion of the target's retinal image and the motion of the eyes. During the latent phase, the retinal *image speed* (the difference between target and eye speeds) is equal to target speed. Afterward, image speed decreases and then oscillates near zero during sustained pursuit. Pursuit therefore acts like a negative feedback system; its eye-movement output tends to reduce its visual motion input.

A third feature is the relatively long delay (~100 ms) associated with sensory and motor processing. Combined with negative feedback, this delay tends to make the system unstable; in fact, under certain conditions, pursuit can exhibit large-amplitude oscillations. To compensate for this inherent problem, pursuit uses predictive mechanisms. For example, pursuit can maintain a constant speed in the absence of visual motion, perhaps by retaining an *eye velocity memory*. Visual motion is therefore an indicator of how eye speed should change and is correlated with future *eye acceleration* (compare Figures 1C and 1D; see also Lisberger et al., 1981).

A fourth feature is that pursuit provides a steadily changing *muscle force* to produce a constant-speed eye movement (Figure 1E). The required changes in muscle force are a function of eye position in the orbit and can be approximated by taking the mathematical integral of eye speed. This integration process, believed to be common to all eye movements, is accomplished by an *oculomotor integrator* contained within the brainstem.

A fifth feature is that pursuit largely compensates for the mechanical effects on movement dynamics caused by the eye "plant": the collective term for the inertial mass of the eye and

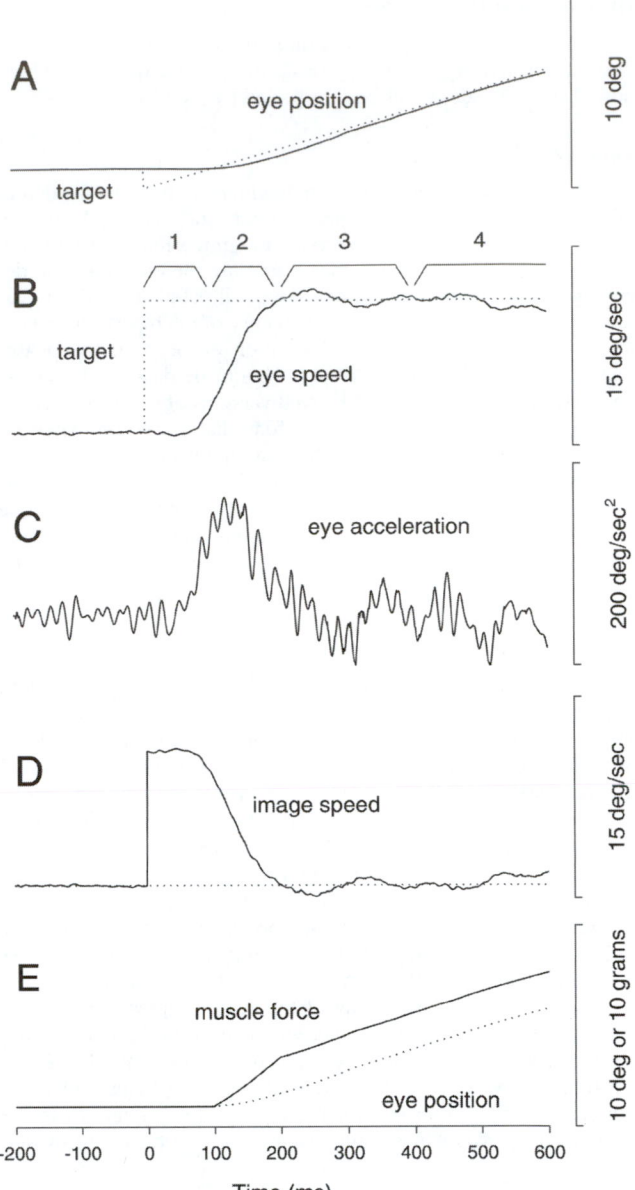

Figure 1. Basic features of pursuit are illustrated with the ramp paradigm. The target jumps to an eccentric position (step) and moves at a constant speed of 10°/s (ramp) that is matched by the human's smooth eye movement after a few hundred milliseconds.

the viscoelastic properties of the eye muscles. As indicated by the initial offset between muscle force and eye position, the applied force begins with an additional boost to overcome the sluggish dynamics of the eye (Robinson, 1965). Without this initial extra force, it would take three to four times longer for pursuit eye speed to match target speed. Pursuit therefore provides an eye movement command that is neurally filtered to compensate for the dynamics of the eye plant.

Pursuit as a Negative Feedback System

Pursuit was originally viewed as a negative feedback velocity-servo system, driven primarily by retinal image motion error signals and sustained by an internal positive feedback loop to enhance performance (Figure 2A). The contribution of several neural sites to pursuit can be understood within this framework. Areas within the extrastriate cortex that are specialized for processing visual motion, such as the middle temporal area (MT) and the medial superior temporal area (MST), are the major source of the visual-motion information used to guide pursuit (Dursteler and Wurtz, 1988). These cortical regions provide outputs to motor regions in the brainstem and cerebellum that form the motor commands for pursuit. In these subcortical pathways for pursuit, there are reciprocal connections between the ventral paraflocculus of the cerebellum and its target nuclei in the brainstem. This anatomical loop has been suggested to form an eye-command feedback circuit that implements the *velocity memory* for pursuit (Stone and Lisberger, 1990). Purkinje cells in the ventral paraflocculus discharge during pursuit even when there is no image motion on the retina. This discharge, if updated by visual error information from extrastriate cortical areas ($\Delta\dot{E}_d$), could continuously provide a command to change the current eye speed ($\dot{E}_c$). Although appealing because of its simplicity, there is now abundant evidence that the simple control strategy outlined in Figure 2A cannot account for some of the known physiological and behavioral features of the pursuit system.

Gain Control in the Pursuit System

Contradicting the essentially linear control strategy outlined previously, there is abundant evidence that the pursuit system displays major nonlinear behaviors. One such nonlinearity is demonstrated by the dramatic changes in efficacy of visual stimuli with behavioral context. For example, it has been shown that rapid displacements of a target can cause a smooth eye acceleration if they are imposed during pursuit of a moving target, but not if they are imposed during fixation of a stationary target. Models of pursuit have simulated these nonlinear effects by including a variable gain element (Krauzlis and Lisberger, 1994). The observation that steady-state eye speed can exceed target speed requires that the proposed variable gain element affect not only the sensitivity to the visual inputs driving the initiation of pursuit, but also the signals maintaining steady-state eye speed.

The behavioral effects of altering activity at different neural sites (Table 1) have helped identify the location of a gain element in the pursuit pathways. Electrical stimulation applied within area MST or the pons can produce changes in smooth eye speed, but only if applied when the monkey is already engaged in pursuit, suggesting that these structures probably lie upstream of a variable gain element. In contrast, stimulation of the ventral paraflocculus elicits smooth eye movements even during fixation, consistent with the proximity of this structure to the final motor pathways for pursuit and its likely placement downstream of the gain element. Finally, microstimulation of the Superior Colliculus (SC) or the pursuit area within the Frontal Eye Fields (FEF) modifies pursuit speed, suggesting that these areas might directly influence a variable gain element (Basso, Krauzlis, and Wurtz, 2000; Tanaka and Lisberger, 2001).

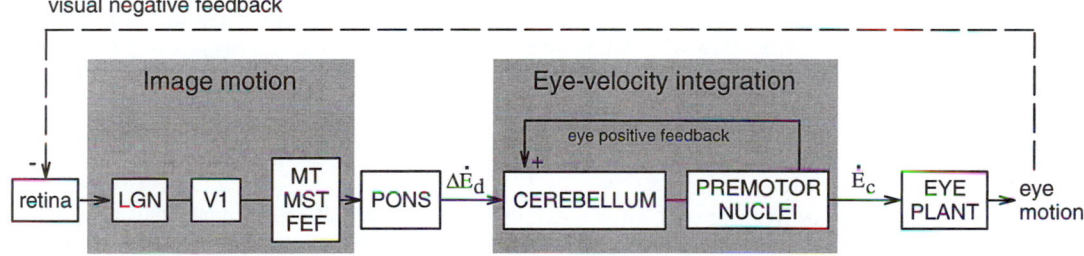

A   Image-motion model

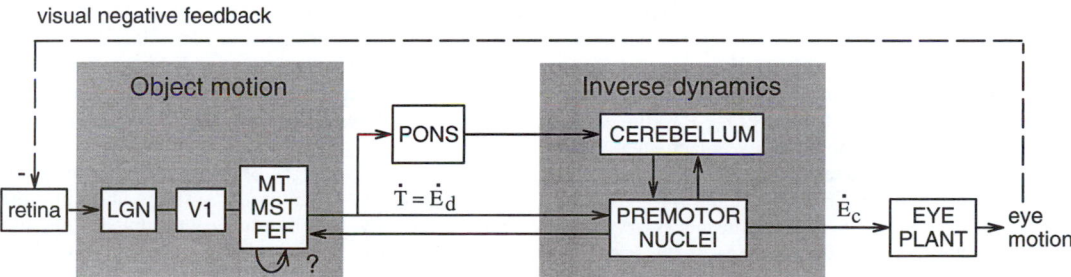

B   Object-motion model

Figure 2. Two models of pursuit that relate system functions to physiology. (A) The "image-motion model" assumes that the cortex provides an image-motion signal encoding pursuit error. The subcortical pathways integrate the descending visual error signals or correction commands ($\Delta\dot{E}_d$) to generate a command for smooth eye movement ($\dot{E}_c$). (B) The "object-motion model" assumes that the cortex provides a combined visual and extra-retinal signal encoding the target object's motion. The cerebellar loop transforms this object-motion signal ($\dot{T}$) or desired eye motion signal ($\dot{E}_d$) into a plant compensated eye-velocity command ($\dot{E}_c$), whereas the brainstem provides the required neural integration to generate the eye-position command.

Table 1. Summary of Physiological Studies

Structure	A. Lesions	B. Microstimulation	C. Neuronal recording
1. V1	Retinotopic deficits in saccades and pursuit		
2. Extrafoveal MT	Retinotopic deficits in the initiation of pursuit		Visual responses tuned for direction/speed of small stimuli
3. Foveal MT	Retinotopic deficits in initiating pursuit; directional deficits for ipsiversive sustained pursuit	Ipsiversive eye acceleration if applied during sustained pursuit	Visual responses tuned for direction/speed of small stimuli
4. MST	Deficits in initiating pursuit; directional deficits for ipsiversive sustained pursuit	Ipsiversive eye acceleration if applied during sustained pursuit	Visual responses to small- and large-field motion; extraretinal responses during sustained pursuit
5. 7a, VIP			Visual responses to stimulus motion; extraretinal responses
6. FEF	Deficits in sustained and predictive or anticipatory pursuit	Eye acceleration, often ipsiversive	Visual responses to stimulus motion; responses during pursuit
7. Rostral SC		Contraversive saccades, contraversive eye acceleration if applied during pursuit	Visual responses to stimulus position; responses during fixation, pursuit and saccades
8. DLPN	Deficits in initiating pursuit; deficits for ipsiversive sustained pursuit	Ipsiversive eye acceleration if applied during sustained pursuit	Visual responses best for moving large stimuli; extraretinal responses
9. DMPN, NRTP	Deficits in pursuit		Visual responses to large-field motion
10. NOT	Deficits in ipsiversive pursuit	Ipsiversive eye acceleration	Visual responses to large-field motion
11. LTN			Visual responses to large-field motion
12. Ventral paraflocculus	Deficits in pursuit	Ipsiversive eye acceleration	Responses to eye and head velocity; transient responses during pursuit initiation and changes in eye speed
13. Oculomotor vermis	Deficits in pursuit	Ipsiversive saccades if applied during fixation, ipsiversive eye acceleration or saccades if applied during pursuit	Responses to eye and head velocity; passive visual responses
14. VN, FN, NPH	Deficits in pursuit and saccades		

Abbreviations: V1, primary visual cortex; MT, middle temporal area; MST, medial superior temporal area; VIP, ventral intraparietal area; FEF, frontal eye fields; DLPN, dorsolateral pontine nucleus; DMPN, dorsomedial pontine nucleus; NRTP, nucleus reticularis tegmenti pontis; NOT, nucleus of the optic tract; LTN, lateral terminal nucleus; VN, vestibular nucleus; FN, fastigial nucleus; NPH, nucleus prepositus hypoglossi; SC, superior colliculus.

The Role of the Cerebellum: Velocity Memory or Plant Compensation?

The command signal provided by the central nervous system compensates for the lagging dynamics of the eye plant (Figure 1); this compensation appears to be included in the output signal of the ventral paraflocculus of the cerebellum. One line of evidence has shown that the time-varying profiles of individual Purkinje cell firing rates can be replicated by a weighted average of eye position, eye velocity, and eye acceleration (Shidara et al., 1993). The fits provided by this model suggest that the output of the ventral paraflocculus could represent an inverse dynamic signal. In a more direct test, it has been shown that when the average Purkinje cell output is provided as the input to a model of eye mechanics, the output matches the observed time course of eye velocity (Krauzlis, 2000). These results demonstrate that neural circuits through the ventral paraflocculus are capable of providing the necessary dynamic compensation for the mechanical properties of the eyeball and surrounding orbital tissues.

The evidence in favor of plant compensation suggests an alternative functional role for the brainstem-cerebellar loop. Rather than forming a velocity memory for pursuit, this circuit may be responsible for ensuring that the movement of the eyes matches that of the target as specified by descending signals (i.e., by converting $\dot{E}_d$

to $\dot{E}_c$ in Figure 2B). This interpretation is consistent with evidence that information about image and eye motion already appears to be combined within cortical areas such as MST, thereby obviating the need to combine them downstream. In fact, the sustained output of MST neurons during perfect steady-state pursuit in the absence of visual motion (Newsome, Wurtz, and Komatsu, 1988) casts doubt on the original interpretation of the similar finding within the ventral paraflocculus (Stone and Lisberger, 1990), which reinforced the view of pursuit shown in Figure 2A. More explicitly, if the cerebellar input from MST is not reduced to zero during perfect steady-state pursuit, then the sustained activity observed at the level of the cerebellum may simply reflect this sustained descending input, rather the presence of eye-velocity feedback from brainstem structures.

Additional advantages of the plant-compensation view are that it generalizes to other motor systems and simplifies the overall control strategy. All motor systems must contend with the mechanical properties of the body part they control. Rather than attempting to tailor individual sensory signals appropriately for each body part or movement type, the strategy of plant compensation makes it possible for the same input signal to control multiple body parts synergistically—the same object-motion signal could be used in several different ways, allowing one's eyes or one's pointed finger to simultaneously track the same object. This generalization

The Role of the Cerebral Cortex: Retinal Motion or Object Motion?

The pursuit behaviors that led to the development of the view in Figure 2A were mostly studied with small spots moving over a featureless background. However, one of the distinguishing features of pursuit, as compared to phylogenetically older smooth eye-movement systems, is that, by performing a global analysis of the visual scene, it can track complex objects over textured backgrounds—even when those objects are only partially visible. Experiments using more complex visual stimuli suggest that the descending cortical signal driving pursuit is not a 2D *image motion* signal that relays ongoing eye-movement errors ($\Delta\dot{E}_d$ in Figure 2A), but rather a 3D *object motion* signal that relays the current estimate of the target's trajectory ($\dot{T}$ in Figure 2B), or in motor terms, the desired eye trajectory ($\dot{E}_d$ in Figure 2B). For example, more than two decades ago, Steinbach (1976) provided qualitative evidence that humans can pursue the horizontal motion of a wagon wheel defined only by the cycloidal motion of a few illuminated points along its circumference. More recently, it has been shown that humans can pursue the motion of partially occluded line-figure objects (Stone, Beutter, and Lorenceau, 2000). These stimuli were designed such that the object's motion could only be recovered by selectively grouping its local component line segments (i.e., deciding which pieces belong together) and performing a global motion-integration (i.e., combining the disparate local motions to compute a single object-motion vector). Furthermore, when the static luminance of such line-figure stimuli is altered to induce a percept of independent line segments, rather than of a single moving object, pursuit can no longer accurately follow the object despite the identical image motion. These parallel effects on both motion perception and pursuit cannot be accounted for by any linear system, so future models of both perception and pursuit must contend with this inherently nonlinear processing. They will also have to incorporate the fact that the visual signals driving pursuit are time-varying, initially reflecting image motion and converging towards object motion only after a few hundred milliseconds (Pack and Born, 2001). Finally, the close relationship between smooth eye movement and 3D perception is further supported by the findings that humans can generate smooth vergence eye movements in response to the kinetic depth effect, i.e., perceived motion in depth from global motion integration in the absence of disparity (Ringach, Hawken, and Shapley, 1996). These results imply that the sustained steady-state pursuit previously attributed to an *eye-velocity memory* within a brainstem-cerebellar loop, might actually result from an *object-motion memory* within the cortex, most probably in area MST, derived either from local cortical circuits or ascending feedback from brainstem oculomotor structures (question mark in Figure 2B). Modulation of this object motion signal by nonvisual factors could account for the frequently observed effects of attention and cognitive expectations on pursuit movements (e.g., Kowler, 1989; Barnes, 1993).

Another component of the analysis required for pursuit in real world conditions is the selection of the visual target from within the visible scene. The presence of a moving distractor stimulus can alter the latency or direction of pursuit made to a target stimulus. Although similar effects have been observed with microstimulation of area MT, single-unit studies of MT neurons in selection tasks have produced variable and often only small effects (Ferrera and Lisberger, 1997), suggesting that the process of target selection occurs elsewhere. The role of target selection in pursuit has a close

affinity to the idea of a variable gain element described previously—both putative mechanisms regulate how sensory information accesses the motor pathways for pursuit. Given that the SC and the FEF are involved in saccade target selection, it is tempting to postulate that these areas play a similar role in pursuit (Krauzlis and Dill, 2002).

Pursuit and Saccades: Separate Motor Systems or Coordinated Motor Outputs?

Pursuit and saccades have been viewed as functionally and anatomically distinct eye movement systems, but recent studies have begun to question this assumption. The pursuit-related areas of the cerebral cortex are not restricted to those processing visual motion, but can also be found adjoining each of the saccade-related eye fields; these pursuit and saccade areas have overlapping connections with several subcortical structures. Accordingly, several regions in the brainstem that have been traditionally considered part of the saccadic system now appear to be involved in pursuit as well (Krauzlis and Stone, 1999). Recent single-unit and microstimulation studies show that the SC is involved in the programming of pursuit, in addition to its well-known role in the control of saccades, perhaps by processing target signals that are common to the two types of movements (Krauzlis and Dill, 2002; Basso, Krauzlis, and Wurtz, 2000). The firing rate of some saccade-related "burst" neurons is related to eye speed during pursuit, as well as during saccades (Missal et al., 2000). These new findings suggest the presence of direct pathways through the brainstem for the control of pursuit, in addition to the established pathways through the cerebellum. As we learn more about these alternate pathways, the organization of the pursuit system may more nearly resemble that of the saccade system, consisting of direct pathways from the cerebral cortex to the brainstem and pre-motor nuclei, with a critical but less direct pathway involving the cerebellum.

Discussion

This brief review has outlined in broad strokes old and new frameworks for understanding the sensorimotor processing and control strategy of the pursuit eye-movement system. Control theory models and experiments using small-spot stimuli have helped frame some of the basic organizational principles of the pursuit system. However, the fundamentally linear models that have resulted from this approach cannot account for more recent behavioral and physiological data obtained under more realistic visual stimulus conditions. The growing evidence that inherently nonlinear processes such as image segmentation, selective motion integration, target identification and selection, prediction, and even cognitive and attentional factors play essential roles in pursuit, highlights the critical need for new pursuit models to transcend traditional linear or quasi-linear system control theory. Moreover, the growing evidence of interactions between the pursuit and saccade systems raise basic questions about the overall control strategy employed during tracking eye movements. The operation of pursuit is clearly not limited to the narrow goal of minimizing retinal image motion, but—together with saccadic eye movements—has the broader goal of acquiring and using visual information about real objects in the 3D world to guide motor behavior.

Road Maps: Mammalian Motor Control; Vision
Related Reading: Collicular Visuomotor Transformations for Gaze Control; Eye-Hand Coordination in Reaching Movements; Vestibulo-Ocular Reflex

References

Barnes, G. R., 1993, Visual-vestibular interaction in the control of head and eye movement: The role of visual feedback and predictive mechanisms, *Prog. Neurobiol.*, 41:435–472.

Basso, M. A., Krauzlis, R. J., and Wurtz, R. H., 2000, Activation and inactivation of rostral superior colliculus neurons during smooth-pursuit eye movements in monkeys, *J. Neurophysiol.*, 84:892–908.

Dursteler, M. R., and Wurtz, R. H., 1988, Pursuit and optokinetic deficits following chemical lesions of cortical areas MT and MST, *J. Neurophysiol.*, 60:940–965.

Ferrera, V. P., and Lisberger, S. G., 1997, Neuronal responses in visual areas MT and MST during smooth pursuit target selection, *J. Neurophysiol,* 78(3):1433–1446.

Kowler, E., 1989, Cognitive expectations, not habits control anticipatory smooth oculomotor pursuit, *Vision Res.*, 29:1057–1094.

Krauzlis, R. J., 2000, Population coding of movement dynamics by cerebellar Purkinje cells, *NeuroReport*, 11:1045–1050.

Krauzlis, R. J., and Dill, N., 2002, Neural correlates of target choice for pursuit and saccades in the primate superior colliculus, *Neuron*, 35:355–363.

Krauzlis, R. J., and Lisberger, S. G., 1994, A model of visually-guided smooth pursuit eye movements based on behavioral observations, *J. Comp. Neurosci.*, 1:265–283.

Krauzlis, R. J., and Stone, L. S., 1999, Tracking with the mind's eye, *Trends Neurosci.*, 22:544–550. ◆

Lisberger, S. G., Evinger, C., Johanson, W., and Fuchs, A. F., 1981, Relationship between eye acceleration and retinal image velocity during foveal smooth pursuit in man and monkey, *J. Neurophysiol.*, 46:229–249.

Missal, M., De Brouwer, S., Lefevre, P., and Olivier, E., 2000, Activity of mesencephalic vertical burst neurons during saccades and smooth pursuit, *J. Neurophysiol.*, 83:2080–2092.

Newsome, W. T., Wurtz, R. H., and Komatsu, H., 1988, Relation of cortical areas MT and MST to pursuit eye movements. II. Differentiation of retinal from extraretinal inputs, *J. Neurophysiol.*, 60:604–620.

Pack, C. C., and Born, R. T., 2001, Temporal dynamics of a neural solution to the aperture problem in visual area MT of macaque brain, *Nature*, 409:1040–1042.

Pola, J., and Wyatt, H. J., 1979, Target position and velocity: The stimuli for smooth for pursuit eye movements, *Vision Res.*, 20:523–534.

Rashbass, C., 1961, The relationship between saccadic and smooth tracking eye movements, *J. Physiol. Lond.*, 159:326–338.

Ringach, D. L., Hawken, M. J., and Shapley, R., 1996, Binocular eye movements caused by the perception of three-dimensional structure from motion, *Vision Res.*, 36:1479–1492.

Robinson, D. A., 1965, The mechanics of human smooth pursuit eye movement, *J. Physiol. Lond.*, 180:569–591.

Shidara, M., Kawano, K., Gomi, H., and Kawato, M., 1993, Inverse-dynamics model eye movement control by Purkinje cells in the cerebellum, *Nature*, 365:50–52.

Steinbach, M., 1976, Pursuing the perceptual rather than the retinal stimulus, *Vision Res.*, 16:1371–1376.

Stone, L. S., Beutter, B. R., and Lorenceau, J., 2000, Visual motion integration for perception and pursuit, *Perception*, 29:771–787.

Stone, L. S., and Lisberger, S. G., 1990, Visual responses of Purkinje cells in the cerebellar flocculus during smooth pursuit eye movements in monkeys. I. Simple spikes, *J. Neurophysiol.*, 63:1241–1261.

Tanaka, M., and Lisberger, S. G., 2001, Regulation of the gain of visually guided smooth-pursuit eye movements by frontal cortex, *Nature*, 409:191–194.

Q-Learning for Robots

Claude F. Touzet

Introduction

Robot learning is a challenging—and somewhat unique—research domain. If a robot behavior is defined as a mapping between situations that occurred in the real world and actions to be accomplished, then the supervised learning of a robot behavior requires a set of *representative* examples (situation, desired action). In order to be able to gather such a learning base, the human operator must have a deep understanding of the robot-world interaction (i.e., a model). However, in many application domains, such models cannot be obtained, either because detailed knowledge of the robot's world is unavailable (e.g., spatial or underwater exploration, nuclear or toxic waste management), or because it would be too costly. In this context, the *automatic* synthesis of a representative learning base is an important issue. It can be sought using reinforcement learning techniques—in particular, Q-learning, which does not require a model of the robot-world interaction. Compared to supervised learning, Q-learning examples are triplets (situation, action, Q value), where the Q value is the *utility* of executing the action in the situation. A supervised learning base is obtained through the selection by the human operator of the triplets with the highest utility. Robot Learning avoids human operator involvement: an important step toward automatic learning.

Because it allows the synthesis of behaviors despite the absence of a robot-world interaction model, Q-learning (Watkins and Dayan, 1992) has become one of the most used learning algorithms for autonomous robotics. Although the convergence theorem does not apply to the robotics domain (due to the limited number of situation-action pairs that can be explored during the lifetime of robot batteries), heuristically adapted Q-learning has proved successful in applications such as obstacle avoidance, wall following, go-to-the-nest, etc. This is mostly due to *neural-based* implementations, such as multilayer perceptrons trained with backpropagation, or self-organizing maps. Such implementations provide an efficient generalization, i.e., fast learning, and designate the critic—the reinforcement function definition—as the real issue. The articles REINFORCEMENT LEARNING and REINFORCEMENT LEARNING IN MOTOR CONTROL provide background information on reinforcement learning. Kaelbling, Littman, and Moore (1996), Sutton and Barto (1998) and Wiering, Salustowicz, and Schmidhuber (1999) are three other sources of information. For more detailed treatments, the reader should consult Touzet (1997).

Q-Learning

Figure 1 shows a functional decomposition of Q-learning. Three different functions are involved: *evaluation, memorization,* and *updating.* Using the information stored in the robot memory, the current situation is evaluated to select the *best* action to accomplish (i.e., the most reward-promising action). This proposition is modified to allow exploration of the situation-action space. The new situation, entered as a consequence of the execution of the action, is qualified by the reinforcement function. Its qualitative criterion (reinforcement) is used by the updating algorithm to adjust the Q values in the following way:

$$Q(s, a)_{\text{new}} = Q(s, a)_{\text{old}} + \beta(r + \gamma \cdot \text{Max}(Q(s', a)) - Q(s, a)_{\text{old}}) \quad (1)$$

where s is the situation, a is the action, r is the reinforcement, and s' represents all situations that can be reached from s. β and γ are positive coefficients less than 1.

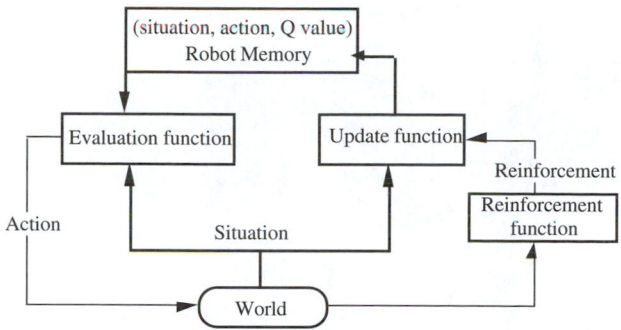

Figure 1. Q-learning method functional decomposition. In response to the present situation, an action is proposed by the robot memory. This action is the one that has the best probability of reward (relatively to the robot memory). However, this proposition may be modified by the evaluation function to allow an extensive exploration of the situation-action space. After the execution of the action by the robot in the real world, a reinforcement function provides a reinforcement value. This value—a simple qualitative criterion (e.g., +1, 1, or 0)—is used by the updating algorithm to adjust the utility value associated with the situation-action pair.

Convergence

Recent developments in the theory of reinforcement learning have allowed proof of asymptotic convergence. These proofs rely on several assumptions that do *not* apply to robots facing real-world tasks. In particular, the asymptotic convergence requires a discrete coding of the situation-action pairs (look-up table storage) and requires attempting every action for every situation an infinite number of times. A robot is a mechanical device that needs at least a few hundred microseconds to execute any action. Therefore, because robot battery life typically lasts less than 10 hours, only a few thousand situation-actions can be visited during a given experiment. This is an extremely small number when compared to the potential number of situation-action pairs (e.g., 10^{26} for the Khepera miniature mobile robot (basic module with eight IR sensors and two wheels), today the most common research robot). Thus, generalization between similar situation-action pairs is *mandatory*.

Generalization

Improvements emphasizing generalization have been proposed by Mahadevan and Connell (1992) who used weighted Hamming distance to generalize between similar situations. This simple method is limited to *syntactic* situation criteria (i.e., it is dependent on the coding of the situations). A second method, proposed by the same authors, adds the action into the syntactic criteria, using clusters to generalize across similar situation-action sets. One of the problems is that the clusters must be handpicked.

Neural Q-Learning

Neural implementations offer a *compact* representation (i.e., limited memory requirement) and good generalization performance (as demonstrated by numerous connectionist applications). The memorization function uses the weight set of the neural network: the memory size required by the system to store the knowledge is defined, a priori, by the number of connections in the network. It is independent of the number of explored situation-action pairs. The proposed action is the processing result of the situation by the network, plus the addition of a random component for the exploration. The update function uses the weight modification algorithm to store the utility values computed by the Q-learning rule (1).

The ideal neural implementation would provide, in a given situation, the best action to undertake and its associated Q value. However, training of such a network requires the definition of an error on the output layer, i.e., knowledge of the best action to undertake in every situation. Such knowledge can be inferred if there are only two different possible actions for the robot, as in the cart pole balancing problem. However, in the general case, the number of actions is larger. Lin (1993)—who proposed the first multilayer perceptron implementation of the Q-learning (Q-Con)—uses as many perceptrons as there are actions, each network output coding for the utility of accomplishing this action in the current situation. Therefore, only one Q-Con network is updated at every time step, and generalization between networks (i.e., actions) is impossible. Other multilayer perceptron implementations have been proposed (Ackley and Littman, 1991; Touzet, 1997), but they do not yet solve the output error definition problem.

Q-Kohon

Unsupervised learning models—such as SELF-ORGANIZING FEATURE MAPS (q.v.), RADIAL BASIS FUNCTION NETWORKS (q.v.), and ADAPTIVE RESONANCE THEORY (ART; q.v.)—do not require an error definition for updating their weight values. Q-Kohon, a Kohonen map implementation of the Q-learning, is a method of state grouping involving syntactic similarity and locality (McCallum, 1995). Each neuron codes a particular triplet (situation, action, Q value); therefore the number of neurons equals the number of stored associations. The neighborhood property of the self-organizing map accounts for the generalization across similar situation-action pairs.

Q-Kohon uses the self-organizing map as an *associative memory*. This associative memory stores triplets. Part of a triplet is used to probe the self-organizing map in search of the corresponding information. Here, situation and Q value are used to find the action: the best action to undertake in a world situation is given by the neuron that has the minimal distance to the input situation and to a Q value of value +1. The selected neuron corresponds to a triplet (situation, action, Q). It is this particular action that should offer the best reward in the world situation. To update the Q value, equation (1) requires the maximum Q value of the new entered situation. This is easily obtained by probing the map with the new situation and a Q value of value +1. The selected neuron Q value will be the maximum possible value.

A nice side effect of using clustering techniques to implement the Q-learning is that the learned behavior can be interpreted by looking (see SELF-ORGANIZING FEATURE MAPS) at the network weights (something extremely difficult with multilayer implementations). Also, because the neurons of the self-organizing map approximate the probability density function of the inputs, one can predict that if a correct behavior is learned, all neurons will code positive Q values. This is most useful to determine when a correct behavior has been learned. This last fact results in the *optimization* of the stored knowledge.

Comparisons

Experiments aimed at comparing various implementations of the Q-learning in a task of synthesizing an *obstacle avoidance behavior* for the miniature robot Khepera (Touzet, 1997) demonstrate that neural Q-learning implementations require a lot less memory and less learning examples, and learn faster (Table 1). The Q-Kohon implementation also exhibits the best behavior after learning, i.e., less negative reinforcements received than all the other implementations.

Table 1. Comparison of Various Implementation.

	Q-learning	+Hamming	+Clustering	Q-Comp	Q-Kohon
Time length	55 mn	25 mn	30 mn	8 mn	2 mn
# iterations	7500	3500	4000	2000	500
Memory size	6400	6400	$1.6 \cdot 10^6$	56	176

The learning time is the time in seconds needed to synthesize an obstacle avoidance behavior. It reflects the number of real world experiments required. The number of learning iterations is the number of updates to the memory (look-up table or neural network). The memory size is the number of floats required to store the information.

Reinforcement Function Design

The reinforcement function quality is intrinsically limited by the expert's abilities. When a reinforcement learning experiment does not converge, it is impossible to know if this is due to the fact that the experiment was too short and more examples are needed, or if the intrinsic nature of the reinforcement function forbids convergence. Today, reinforcement learning researchers use a slow and painful *trial-and-error* approach to define the reinforcement function. In the meantime, efforts have been devoted to find ways to automatically define such functions. Santos and Touzet (1999) have proposed an Update Parameter Algorithm (UPA) to automatically adjust the threshold values: θ_+ and θ_- within a particular definition of the reinforcement function:

$$RF(s_1, \ldots, s_u) = \begin{cases} +1 & \text{if } g_1(s_1, \ldots, s_u) > \theta_+ \\ -1 & \text{if } g_2(s_1, \ldots, s_u) < \theta_- \\ 0 & \text{otherwise} \end{cases} \quad (2)$$

where $(s_1, \ldots, s_u)$ is the output readings of the sensors, $g_1()$ and $g_2()$ are any functions linking the sensor data to the rewards.

The resulting effect is to *optimize* the exploration part of the learning phase by achieving and maintaining predefined ratios of positive and negative rewards. If there is no positive reward, the evaluation function built during the learning phase will have "0" as a maximum value and the policy cannot select effective actions. If there is no negative reward, the robot can remain in a dead-end situation forever. If there is no null reward, the evaluation function will be noncontinuous at the frontier between positive and negative situation-action pairs.

A dynamic version of UPA (Santos and Touzet, 1999) updates the threshold values during the learning phase—exploration and exploitation (to take into account the improvement of the robot policy). It allows behavior performance improvements without the need of some sort of external supervisor, capable of ranking situations by difficulty and of choosing tasks of increasing difficulty. (Dorigo and Colombetti, 1998). Santos et al. have been able to synthesize a wall-following behavior by using reinforcement learning (Figure 2), demonstrating support for reinforcement function design techniques.

Discussion

Q-learning is one of the most used (reinforcement) learning technique for behavior-based robots (see REACTIVE ROBOTIC SYSTEMS). Neural-based Q-learning implementations provide compactness and generalizability. Clustering-based neural methods, such as Q-Kohon, allow drastic reduction of the learning time and number of examples required. Their efficiency puts forward the definition of the reinforcement function as a major issue.

Another major issue involves the ability to overcome the exponentially growing number of required learning examples that comes with target behaviors of greater complexity. Battery lifetime seems

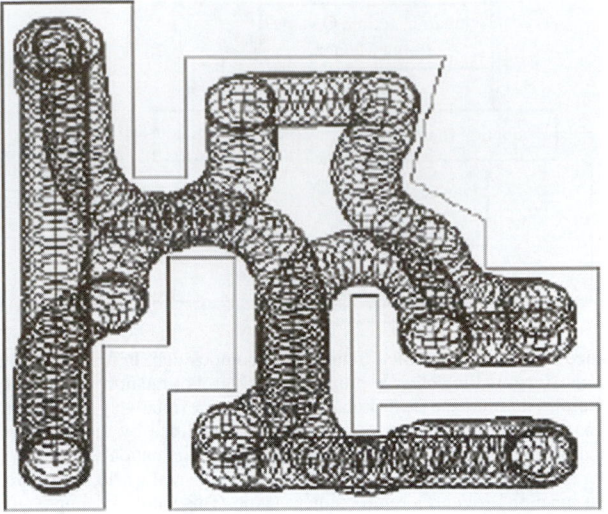

Figure 2. The trace of the miniature Khepera robot after the synthesis of a wall following behavior using a RBF implementation of the Q-learning and Dynamic-UPA in a new environment. Only about 2000 learning iterations are needed.

to impose a definite limit, and researchers tend to promote knowledge incorporation as a speed-up mechanism. The goal is to bias the exploration toward "rewarding" part of the search space—at the expense of *tabula rasa* methods. The drawback is that new—unforeseen—solutions *cannot* be discovered.

Lazy learning (Aha, 1997), also called instance-based learning, provides a way to add samples without implying bias. In a lazy learning approach, computation of the inputs is delayed until the necessity arises. Lazy learning samples the situation-action space, storing the succession of events in memory and, when needed, probes the associative memory for the best move. The sampling process stores the successive situation-action pairs generated by a random action selection policy. The exploration phase is done only once, stored, and used later by all future experiments. The probing of the memory involves complicated computations: clustering, pattern matching, and so forth.

By storing situation-action pairs, a lazy memory builds a nonexplicit model of the situation transition function, that is used as a bias to leverage the model-free following learning phase (i.e., Q-learning). Sheppard and Salzberg (1997) propose to mix lazy learning and reinforcement learning, probing the memory with the reinforcement function. Their objective is to provide a method for predicting the rewards for some state-action pairs without explicitly generating them. They call their algorithm *lazy Q-learning*. For the current real-world situation, a situation matcher locates all the states in the memory that are within a given distance. If the situation matcher has failed to find any nearby situations, the action comparator selects an action at random. Otherwise, the action comparator examines the expected rewards associated with each of these situations and selects the action with the highest expected reward. This action is then executed, resulting in a new situation. There is a fixed probability of generating a random action, regardless of the outcome of the situation matcher. New situation-action pairs are added to the memory, along with their Q values computed in the classical way. Among similar situation-action pairs in the memory, an update of the stored Q values is made. There is a limit to the generalizability of this lazy memory because the Q values associated with the situation-action pairs only apply for a particular application.

Learning is not restricted to single robots. Learning in *cooperative robotics* is intriguing: this would be a way to program a set of robots without having to explicitly model their interactions with the world—including the other team members—to achieve cooperation. To achieve this goal, mechanisms that relay the *unique* information associated with the team behavior (reinforcement value) to the individual robots have to be found (see Parker, Touzet, and Fernandez, 2001). Results from the multi-agent research community cannot be applied since they are usually symbolic methods, where robot Q-learning requires a sub-symbolic approach.

Despite all the efforts and success around Q-learning, several drawbacks are associated with supervised and reinforcement learning when it comes to real applications. First, the time needed to achieve the synthesis of any behavior is *prohibitive,* and determining good initial approximations that reduce wasted exploration is not recommended, since it may forbid the finding of unsuspected solutions. Second, the robot behavior during the learning phase is—by definition—bad, and it may even be *dangerous.* To put constraints that preclude dangerous moves implies that there exists a complete model of the robot-world interactions (which by definition does not exist). Third, except within the lazy learning approach, a new behavior implies a *new* learning phase. What is needed is a learning that instantaneously synthesizes any behavior, and which leads to improvement in performance resulting from the mere repetition of this behavior (for a first step in this direction see Touzet, 1999).

Road Map: Robotics and Control Theory
Related Reading: Reinforcement Learning in Motor Control; Robot Arm Control; Robot Learning

References

Ackley, D., and Littman, M., 1991, Interactions between learning and evolution, in *Artificial Life II,* SFI Studies Sc. Complexity, vol. X (C. G.

Langton, C. Langton, C. Taylor, J. D. Farmer, and S. Rasmussen, Eds.), Reading, MA: Addison-Wesley, pp. 487–509.

Aha, D., Ed., 1997, *Lazy Learning,* Dordrecht, Netherlands: Kluwer Academic Publishers (reprinted from *Artif. Intell. Rev.,* 11:1–5). ◆

Dorigo, M., and Colombetti, M., 1998, *Robot Shaping: An Experiment in Behavior Engineering,* Cambridge, MA: MIT Press. ◆

Kaelbling L., Littman, M., and Moore, A., 1996, Reinforcement learning: A survey, *J. Artif. Intell. Res.,* 4:237–285. ◆

Lin, L-J., 1993, *Reinforcement Learning for Robots Using Neural Networks,* Ph.D. thesis, Carnegie Mellon University, Pittsburgh, CMU-CS-93-103.

Mahadevan, S., and Connell, J., 1992, Automatic programming of behavior-based robots using reinforcement learning, *Artif. Intell.,* 55(2–3):311–365.

McCallum, R. A., 1995, Instance-based state identification for reinforcement learning, in *Advances in Neural Information Processing Systems 7* (G. Tesauro, D. Touretzky, and T. Leen, Eds.), Cambridge, MA: MIT Press.

Parker, L. E., Touzet, C., and Fernandez, F., 2001, Techniques for learning in multi-robot teams, in *Robot Teams: From Diversity to Polymorphism* (T. Balch and L. E. Parker, Eds.), Natick, MA: A. K. Peters. ◆

Santos, J. M., and Touzet, C., 1999, Dynamic update of the reinforcement function during learning, *Connection Science,* special issue on adaptive robots (C. Torras, Ed.), 11(3–4):267–290.

Sheppard, J. W., and Salzberg, S. L., 1997, A teaching strategy for memory-based control, in *Lazy Learning* (D. Aha, Ed.), Dordrecht, Netherlands: Kluwer Academic Publishers, pp. 343–370.

Sutton, R., and Barto, A., 1998, *Reinforcement Learning,* Cambridge, MA: MIT Press. ◆

Touzet, C., 1997, Neural reinforcement learning for behaviour synthesis, *Robotics and Autonomous Systems,* special issue on learning robots: The new wave (N. Sharkey, Ed.), 22(3–4):251–281.

Touzet, C., 1999, Programming robots with associative memories, in *Proceedings of International Joint Conference on Neural Networks,* Washington, DC, July 10–16.

Watkins, C. J. C. H., and Dayan, P., 1992, Technical note: Q-learning, *Machine Learning,* 8(3–4):279–292.

Wiering, M., Salustowicz, R., Schmidhuber, J., 1999, Reinforcement learning soccer teams with incomplete world models, *J. Autonomous Robots,* 7(1):77–88.

Radial Basis Function Networks

David Lowe

Introduction

The radial basis function (RBF) network is conceptually a very simple yet intrinsically powerful network structure. Recent reviews of the RBF approach from a mathematical perspective of function interpolation can be found in Buhmann (2000), from a perspective of regularization and connections to support vectors machines in Evgeniou, Pontil, and Poggio (2000; see also SUPPORT VECTOR MACHINES), and in relation to ideas in statistical analysis in Lowe (1999).

We can motivate the basic idea of the RBF network and reveal its difference from the multilayer perceptron by considering Figure 1. This figure conceptually illustrates a simple classification example in which the distribution of data points exhibits a simple clustering. There are primarily two ways to separate these clusters. One is by segregating the space into polygonal cells. The straight lines in the figure illustrate this decomposition of the pattern space into regions, as would be obtained by a simple multilayer perceptron, where the lines represent the class boundaries. An alternative is to describe the clusters of data themselves as if they were generated according to an underlying probability density function, modeled here in the figure by elliptical distributions. Thus, one

method concentrates on class boundaries and the other focuses on regions where the data density is highest. These are complementary approaches, with respective disadvantages and advantages. The latter alternative is the RBF approach.

The RBF constructs global approximations to functions using combinations of basis functions centered on weight vectors (Figure 2), whereas a multilayer perceptron constructs an architecture out of separating hyperplanes. These weight vectors could be actual data points in the training set, as they are in the basic interpolation model of RBF networks, or they could be chosen according to a utility function, such as a clustering criterion, in density modeling, or a separation criterion, as in support vector machines and regularization. An extra distinction is that the RBF employs a distance function to convert the vector input pattern into a scalar at the hidden layer, as opposed to a vector dot product such as is used in the multilayer perceptron. The network's strength derives from a rich interpretational foundation because it lies at the confluence of a variety of established scientific disciplines. Thus, although the original motivation of this particular network structure was in terms of function approximation techniques (Broomhead and Lowe, 1988; Powell, 1992), the network may be derived on the basis of statistical pattern processing theory (Lowe, 1999), regression and

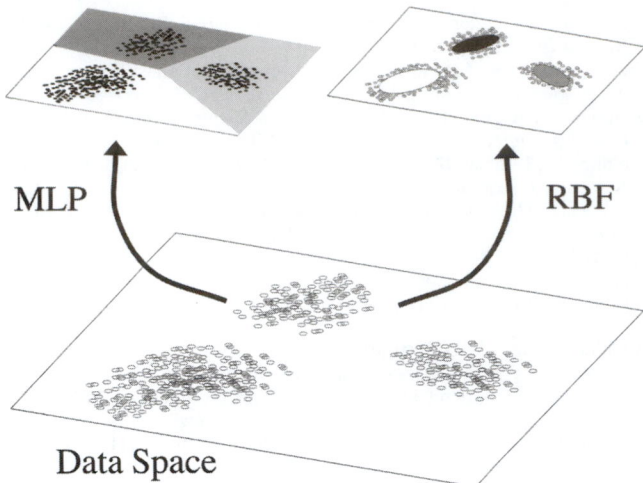

MLP   RBF

Data Space

Figure 1. Dissection of pattern space by clusters and hyperplanes. The multilayer perceptron (MLP) exploits the logistic nonlinearity to create combinations of hyperplanes to dissect pattern space into separable regions. Subsequent layers combine these regions to allow the formation of nonconvex class boundaries. The radial basis function (RBF) dissects pattern space by modeling *clusters* of data directly and so is more concerned with data distributions.

regularization (Evgeniou et al., 2000), biological pattern formation (Logothetis, Pauls, and Poggio, 1995), mapping in the presence of noisy data and, more recently, in terms of kriging approximations (Wan and Bone, 1997) and kernel methods, particularly support vector machines (see SUPPORT VECTOR MACHINES). However, in addition to exhibiting a range of useful theoretical properties, the RBF network structure is above all a practical construct, as it may be applied efficiently to problem domains in discrimination (such as speaker verification), time series prediction (such as economic modeling), and feature extraction or even topographic mapping problem domains (such as encoding the sensory space of an artificial nose in chemical vapor analysis). Some studies have even suggested that RBF topology developed in nature as an evolutionary functional counterpart to object views for vision, where the

basis functions correspond to cell aggregates tuned to particular views of familiar objects (Logothetis et al., 1995). This idea supports Edelman's "chorus of prototypes" and is reflected in the approach adopted in Moody and Darken (1989) using locally tuned processing units, although understanding of the biology in this area is presently insufficient to support generalizations.

The Basic RBF Structure

The RBF is a single-hidden-layer feedforward network with linear output transfer functions and nonlinear transfer functions, $\phi_j(\ldots)$, on the hidden layer nodes. Many types of nonlinearities may be used. There is also typically a bias on each output node. The primary adjustable parameters (see Figure 2) are the final layer weights, $\{\lambda_{jk}\}$, connecting the jth hidden node to the kth output node. There are also weights $\{\mu_{ij}\}$ connecting the ith input node with the jth hidden node, and occasionally a "smoothing" factor matrix, $\{\Sigma_j\}$. It often helps to think of the weights $\{\mu_{ij}\}$ as representing "prototypes" of patterns in the input space, either as cluster centers or as pattern exemplars that are in some sense representative of the distribution of input patterns. Similarly, the weights $\{\Sigma_j\}$ that govern the regularization of the network (after the model order complexity of the number of basis functions) are sometimes considered to represent the range of influence of these prototypes (though this intuition can break down for some of the nonlocal basis functions that can be employed).

The mathematical embodiment of the RBF takes the following form. The kth component of the output vector $\mathbf{y}_p$ corresponding to the pth input pattern $\mathbf{x}_p$ is expressed as

$$[\mathbf{y}(\mathbf{x}_p)]_k = \sum_{j=0}^{h} \lambda_{jk} \phi_j\left(\|\mathbf{x}_p - \boldsymbol{\mu}_j\|; \sum_j\right) \qquad (1)$$

where $\phi_j(\ldots)$ denotes the nonlinear transfer function of hidden node j, $(\phi_0(\ldots) \equiv 1$ is the bias node), and the possible dependence on a smoothing matrix is left explicit. The most common example of the smoothing factor is in the use of a general Gaussian transfer function, i.e., $\phi(z) \approx \exp -[z^T\Sigma^{-1}z]$. Since the general expression is an analytic function of the variables corresponding to the basis function positions and smoothing factors, it is possible to adapt them by a full nonlinear least squares process if required (Moody and Darken, 1989). This is usually not necessary. As can be seen from Equation 1, the main difference from a multilayer perceptron is that the output of the hidden node j, h_j is given as a *radial* function of the distance between each pattern vector and each hidden node weight vector (or prototype), $h_j^{RBF} = \phi_j(\|\mathbf{x} - \boldsymbol{\mu}_j\|)$, rather than as a scalar product, $h_j^{MLP} = \phi_j(\mathbf{x} \cdot \boldsymbol{\mu}_j)$.

One of the advantages of the RBF is that the first-layer weights $\{\boldsymbol{\mu}_j, \Sigma_j; j = 1, \ldots h\}$ may often be determined or specified by a judicious use of prior knowledge, or adapted by simple techniques. Early work (Broomhead and Lowe, 1988) found it sufficient to position the basis functions at data points sampled randomly according to the distribution of the data. This ensured that network resources were concentrated in regions of higher data density. Another early technique (Moody and Darken, 1989) was to position the centers of the basis functions according to a K-means clustering process on the data points, and then set the smoothing parameters of the assumed Gaussian basis functions to be the average distance between cluster centers. Over the past decade, many variations on these themes have been introduced that employ some form of prior knowledge expressed as a utility function, which the choice of prototypes should try to optimize. Therefore, once the weights associated with the first layer have been specified, the major problem in training an RBF network is focused on determining the final layer weights. Since the RBF network is typically employed to perform a *supervised* discrimination or prediction task, such as time

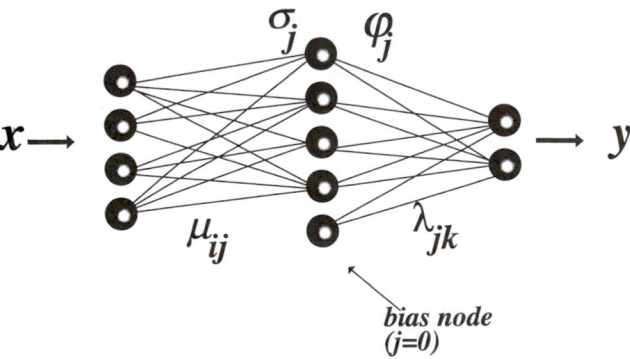

$\sigma_j \quad \varphi_j$

$x \longrightarrow$

y

$\mu_{ij} \qquad \lambda_{jk}$

bias node
(j=0)

Figure 2. The basic radial basis function structure. A nonlinear basis function $\phi_j(\ldots)$ is centered on each hidden node weight vector $\boldsymbol{\mu}$, which also has a (possibly) adaptable "range of influence" σ_j. The output of the hidden node j, h_j is given as a *radial* function of the distance between each pattern vector and each hidden node weight vector, $h_j = \phi_j(\|\mathbf{x} - \boldsymbol{\mu}_j\|/\sigma_j)$. This is the main difference from a multilayer perceptron. The network outputs are evaluated by a traditional scalar product between the vector of hidden node outputs and the weight vector attached to output node k, as $o_k = \mathbf{h}.\lambda_k$.

series forecasting, this training usually takes the form of optimizing a cost function requiring the outputs of the network to somehow closely approximate a set of known target values. It is common to attempt to minimize a standard residual sum-of-squares cost function, although other cost functions may be employed. Because this is a linear optimization process (the parameters $\{\lambda_{jk}\}$ occur linearly when minimizing the residual sum-squared-error measure), the RBF is computationally more attractive in applications than a multilayer perceptron, even though they are both computationally universal architectures (Park and Sandberg, 1991).

RBFs for Classification

One of the more common uses for an RBF network is as a semiparametric classification model capable of modeling nonlinear boundaries between clusters. This problem can be analyzed statistically and may be motivated from the perspective of kernel-based density estimation (Tråvén, 1991). Here we outline how the RBF architecture emerges from this statistical perspective, although historically it first emerged from interpolation theory.

In classification, we are primarily interested in the posterior, $p(c|x)$, the probability that class c is present given the observation x. However, it is easier to model other related aspects of the data, such as the unconditional distribution of the data, $p(x)$, and the likelihood of the data, $p(x|c)$, which is the probability that the data were generated given that the data came from a specific class c. We can then recreate the posterior from these quantities according to Bayes's theorem, $p(c_i|x) = p(c_i)p(x|c_i)/p(x)$. The distribution of the data is modeled as if it were generated by a mixture distribution, i.e., a linear combination of parameterized states or of basis functions such as Gaussians. Since individual data clusters for each class are not likely to be approximated by a single Gaussian distribution, we need several basis functions per cluster. We assume that the likelihood and the unconditional distribution can both be modeled by the same set of distributions, $q(x|s)$, but with different mixing coefficients, i.e., $p(x) = \Sigma_s \hat{p}(s)q(x|s)$ and $p(x|c_i) = \Sigma_s p(s; i)q(x|s)$. Then the quantity we are interested in $p(c_i|x) = p(c_i)p(x|c_i)/p(x)$ is given by

$$p(c_i|x) = \sum_s \frac{p(c_i)p(s; i)}{\hat{p}(s)} \frac{\hat{p}(s)q(x|s)}{\sum_{s'} \hat{p}(s')q(x|s')} \equiv \sum_j \lambda_{ij}\phi(x|j)$$

where $\lambda_{ij} = p(c_i)p(j; i)/\hat{p}(j)$ relates the overall significance of state j to class i, and $\phi(x|j)$ is a normalized basis function, $\hat{p}(j)q(x|j)/\Sigma_j\hat{p}(j)q(x|j)$.

This gives an RBF architecture. For a total of h functions used to approximate the likelihood and the unconditional density, there are h hidden nodes corresponding to the normalized basis functions, and the final layer weights relate the significance of the hidden nodes to the c output class nodes, providing the class-conditional information. Of course, the positions and possibly also the ranges of influence of each of these basis functions need to be specified or adapted to allow an adequate model of each data cluster. This can be achieved by unsupervised clustering techniques.

In this manner, the RBF is an ideal network for use in classification problems. Note that the architecture of RBF networks for density estimation is more general than was indicated in the discussion of motivation. In particular, it is not essential that each basis function itself should be a probability density function.

RBFs for Prediction

In the previous section, the RBF was motivated by a statistical interpretation of data distributions. In that case, the underlying generator of the data (the probability density function) was sampled

stochastically. However, the original formulation of the RBF network was developed in order to produce a deterministic mapping of data by exploiting links with traditional function approximation. This approach attempted to introduce the notion that the training of neural networks could be described as curve fitting. Hence, "generalization" consequently has a natural interpretation as interpolating along this fitting surface.

The basic idea was as follows. Assume that we have a set of input/output pairs of input/target patterns representing data from an unknown but smooth surface in $\mathbb{R}^n \times \mathbb{R}^c$. As a simple example, consider a set of (x, y) pairs generated according to $y = x^2$. In this approach, the problem is to choose a function $y : \mathbb{R}^n \to \mathbb{R}^c$, which satisfies the interpolation conditions $y(x_p) = t_p, p = 1, 2, \ldots, P$. This is *strict* interpolation, in which the function is constrained to pass through all the known data points. The strategy in interpolation theory was to construct a linear function space spanned by a set of nonorthogonal basis functions that depended on the positions of the known data points. The radial basis function expansion mapping to one dimension was originally expressed as $y(x) = \Sigma_{j=1}^P \lambda_j \phi(\|x - x_j\|)$. By using the interpolation conditions, the fitting parameters λ may be determined by matrix inverse methods. The approach was generalized to higher-dimensional mappings, to incorporate bias terms, and to account for the fact that strict interpolation is not a good strategy for real-world noisy data, leading to the feedforward neural network topology already discussed.

In the case of the simple $y = x^2$ example mentioned above, the inputs are x values, the targets are specific y values, and the RBF network is constructed so as to produce a fitting surface to the parabola $y = x^2$, which is a surface in $\mathbb{R}^1 \times \mathbb{R}^1 = \mathbb{R}^2$. Note that this is curve fitting to the *parabola* in the product space, not the data samples themselves. This parabola may be interpreted as the *generator* of the observed data, as locations on the parabola "produce" or "generate" the (x, y) input/output pairs. As long as the generator of the data is smooth and nonlinear, we should be able to arbitrarily closely approximate it with an RBF network. This explains why networks can be successful in predicting deterministically chaotic time series: although the time series themselves may exhibit apparent randomness, the underlying map that produces the samples is itself usually very smooth.

Miscellaneous Topics

Many topics related to RBF networks cannot be addressed in detail here. Among them are the issues of how many centers to use, what types of nonlinearities may be employed, Bayesian approaches to choosing the smoothing parameters, how to optimize the various weights, how to assist generalization through regularization, and how to determine confidence intervals. A few of these topics are briefly discussed below.

Choice of Kernel Function

The theory of statistical density estimation produces many recommended bounded kernels that may or may not be density functions themselves. Examples of $\phi(z)$ are the Epanechnikov ($3/4[1 - z^2/5]/\sqrt{5}$ for $|z| < \sqrt{5}$, and 0 otherwise), the triangular ($1 - |z|$ for $|z| < 1$ and 0 otherwise), and of course the Gaussian. From interpolation theory the following choices are common: cubic (z^3), thin-plate spline ($z^2 \log z$), inverse multiquadric ($[z^2 + c^2]^{-1/2}$), multiquadric ($[z^2 + c^2]^{1/2}$), and again the Gaussian. Note that these functions do not have finite support, and indeed, some of the choices are *unbounded* functions, contrary to intuition and common belief that network basis functions are localized. However, despite this unbounded nature, it is correct that the parameters of the network may be chosen such that $y(x) \to 0$ as $x \to \infty$ so that the network as a whole achieves a localized response, even if the individual basis functions do not.

Regularization

Various schemes have emerged to discourage overfitting of the training data points. Such options include (1) choosing a small set of initial centers and adapting the positions and spreads to best describe the data in some sense; (2) regularization—having a center located at each data point, but adding a smoothing term that is an effective constraint on the possible weight values, the magnitude of this extra term governing the amount of smoothing applied to the fitting surface (see GENERALIZATION AND REGULARIZATION IN NONLINEAR LEARNING SYSTEMS); (3) selecting centers over a subset of the data points in the training set incrementally to maximize the descriptive power of the data variance obtained by adding each new basis function; and (4) Bayesian approaches of using the evidence to estimate the hyperparameters and weights. Because of its importance, we outline the regularization approach. Extensive and useful reviews of this approach, along with further references, can be found in Haykin (1999) and Evgeniou et al. (2000).

In regularization we wish to interpolate a finite data set using an approximation $y(x)$. Of all possible approximators, we wish to choose the one that minimizes the augmented functional

$$H[y] = \sum_{p=1}^{P} (t_p - y(x_p))^2 + \eta \|\hat{O}y\|^2$$

where $\hat{O}$ is an operator such as $\partial/\partial x$, which is a mathematical embodiment of our prior knowledge on desired smoothness constraints. For example, this particular choice of operator gives an extra component to the overall cost function that represents curvature of the resulting map (it is an approximation to the expected Hessian or matrix of second derivatives of the map). So, high curvature solutions will incur a higher penalty than lower curvature solutions. Overall, then, there will be an interplay between the desire to produce a very-low-curvature RBF mapping and the desire to produce a surface that exactly passes through each data point. This latter objective usually requires very high curvature surfaces, since there will be random noise on the data points. η is the regularization parameter that embodies the degree to which the constraint should dominate the data. Interestingly (Lowe, 1999), the functional that formally minimizes $H[y]$ takes the form of an RBF, i.e., $y(x) = \sum_{p=1}^{P} \lambda_p G^{\dagger}(x, x_p)$. Here, $G^{\dagger}(x, x_p)$ denotes a Green function that is a solution of an equation determined by the regularization operator. If the operator $\hat{O}^{\dagger}\hat{O}$ is rotationally and translationally invariant, then the Green function is only a function of the radial differences of its arguments, i.e., $G(\|x - x_p\|)$. Thus, once again the form of the RBF may be derived, but this time from the perspective of preventing overfitting by regularization. In this case the form of the basis function is determined by the type of smoothness constraint we have imposed. As in the previous interpolation case, the weighting coefficients, λ_p, may be determined by the solution of a linear equation. Again, strictly speaking, this approach requires a center or basis function located at each data point, and overfitting is avoided by imposing the smoothing constraint. However, in practice the number of centers may also be chosen to vary, in which case these precise mathematical relationships no longer hold.

Discussion

This article has discussed the motivation and application of the radial basis function network from a variety of perspectives. We have chosen to concentrate on contrasting a statistical pattern processing perspective with a function approximation perspective. However, both perspectives have the common philosophical basis that the aim of the network is to approximate the underlying structure that generated the observed data, rather than the data itself. This is also how a multilayer perceptron operates. However, the RBF was introduced to make this link with curve fitting and interpolation explicit.

The RBF may be employed in classification tasks, time series prediction, and both unordered and topographic feature extraction. Because of its computational tractability, the RBF has been applied to many diverse real-world problems, and there is some evidence that its structure may have similarities to biological aspects of vision processing. But above all, its strength and utility derive from its simplicity and from a close relationship with other areas of signal and pattern processing and other neural network architectures. These connections and interpretations are still being uncovered, as recent work on support vector machines (see SUPPORT VECTOR MACHINES), Gaussian processes, and kriging has demonstrated.

Road Maps: Grounding Models of Networks; Learning in Artificial Networks
Related Reading: Bayesian Methods and Neural Networks; Support Vector Machines

References

Broomhead, D. S., and Lowe, D., 1988, Multivariable functional interpolation and adaptive networks, *Complex Syst.*, 2:321–355.
Buhmann, M. D., 2000, Radial basis functions, *Acta Numerica* (A. Dsertes, Ed.), 9:1–38.
Evgeniou, T., Pontil, M., and Poggio, T., 2000, Regularization networks and support vector machines, *Adv. Computat. Math.*, 13:1–50.
Haykin, S., 1999, *Neural Networks: A Comprehensive Foundation*, 2nd ed., Englewood Cliffs, NJ: Prentice Hall, chap. 5. ◆
Logothetis, N. K., Pauls, J., and Poggio, T., 1995, Shape recognition in the inferior temporal cortex of monkeys, *Curr. Biol.*, 5:552–563.
Lowe, D., 1999, Radial basis function networks and statistics, in *Statistics and Neural Networks: Advances at the Interface* (J. W. Kay and D. M. Titterington, Eds.), New York: Oxford University Press, pp. 65–95.
Moody, J., and Darken, C., 1989, Fast learning in networks of locally tuned processing units, *Neural Computat.*, 1:281–294.
Park, J., and Sandberg, I. W., 1991, Universal approximation using radial basis function networks, *Neural Computat.*, 3:246–257.
Powell, M. J. D., 1992, The theory of radial basis function approximation in 1990, in *Advances in Numerical Analysis*, vol. 2, *Wavelets, Subdivision Algorithms and Radial Basis Functions* (W. A. Light, Ed.), Oxford. Engl.: Oxford University Press, pp. 105–210.
Tråvén, H. G. C., 1991, A neural network approach to statistical pattern classification by "semiparametric" estimation of probability density functions, *IEEE Trans. Neural Netw.*, 2:366–377.
Wan, E., and Bone, D., 1997, Interpolating earth science data using RBF networks and mixtures of experts, *Adv. Neural Inf. Process. Syst.*, 8:988–994.

Rate Coding and Signal Processing

Fabrizio Gabbiani

Introduction

In the peripheral and central nervous system, many neurons encode information and pass it on to other neurons by generating irregular sequences of short voltage pulses, typically less than 1 ms in duration, called action potentials. The shape of these action potentials, or spikes, is usually quite stereotyped over the course of time. The sequence of spike occurrence times generated by the cell, often called the *spike train*, is therefore thought to carry most of the information that a neuron communicates to its targets. When studying how sensory information might be encoded in neuronal spike trains, one is faced with the fact that spike trains are often quite variable under seemingly identical stimulation conditions (Figure 1). Is this variability simply noise, perhaps due to uncontrolled changes in the state of some internal variable, or does it carry information about the stimulus? Answering this question in a particular case would require a thorough knowledge of the biophysical mechanisms of spike generation and of stimulus coding—knowledge that is out of reach at present.

Although no universal definition exists, the term *rate coding* is applied in situations where the precise timing of spikes is not thought to play a significant role in carrying sensory information. Rate codes have been identified in many sensory systems and are probably the best understood means by which neurons encode information. In many cases, rate codes have been shown to play an important role in determining behavioral responses of animals.

Rate coding comes in two flavors: mean firing rate codes and instantaneous firing rate codes. The sensory information conveyed by these two types of codes can be studied rigorously by applying classical methods of statistical signal processing borrowed from the engineering literature. In the next two sections, we will show how these methods can be carried over to the analysis of neuronal spike trains. Before turning to more general examples in the third section, we will illustrate them in the case of electrical field amplitude–sensitive neurons of weakly electric fishes. These animals possess an unusual sense for the electrical properties of their environment that is favorable to computational investigations (see Electrolocation).

Rate coding is not the only mean by which neurons convey information. In weakly electric fishes and in other auditory-like sensory systems, the role played by spike timing information is well documented (see Electrolocation and Echolocation: Cochleotopic and Computational Maps). Two articles address the

issue of spike timing in cortical circuits (Synfire Chains; Synchronization, Binding and Expectancy). Finally, the role of rate coding in the context of neuronal populations is examined in Population Codes (q.v.) and Motor Cortex (q.v.), Coding and Decoding of Directional Operations (q.v.).

Mean Firing Rate Coding

An increase in firing rate is typically the most conspicuous change recorded from sensory neurons in response to external stimuli. It is therefore natural to ask how well the spike count observed in a single trial from such a cell can predict the presence of the stimulus. Let us take the example of a neuron having a mean spontaneous rate $\bar{\lambda}_0 = 30$ spk/s that fires at a rate of $\bar{\lambda}_s = 50$ spk/s under stimulus presentation (Figure 1*B*). We will first assume for simplicity that spikes are generated completely independently of each other (i.e., following a Poisson process) and thus do not carry any additional information beyond their mean rate of occurrence.

Figure 2*A* illustrates the distribution of spike counts observed during a 200 ms window in the baseline and stimulus condition for this model neuron. The overlap between these two distributions indicates that guessing the presence of the stimulus from the spike count observed in a single trial will lead to a significant fraction of errors. A simple method to decide between the two alternatives "stimulus present" or "no stimulus" consists in choosing a threshold number of spikes, k_{thres}, and classifying the observed responses, n, as baseline activity or stimulus-induced activity according to whether the threshold is exceeded or not:

$$n < k_{\text{thres}} \Rightarrow \text{baseline activity}$$
$$n > k_{\text{thres}} \Rightarrow \text{stimulus present} \tag{1}$$

This decision strategy leads to two types of errors. On the one hand, we might call for the stimulus to be present in a trial during which spontaneous activity was unusually high. This type of error is called a false alarm. On the other hand, we might confuse an unusually low stimulus response with spontaneous activity, an error called a false miss. Clearly, the proportion of false alarms to false misses depends on the choice of the threshold k_{thres}: high (low) threshold values correspond to low (high) probabilities of false alarms with higher (lower) fractions of false misses. It is customary to characterize the performance of this detection algorithm by varying the threshold from low to high values and plotting the probability of correct detection, p_D (i.e., 1 minus the probability of false

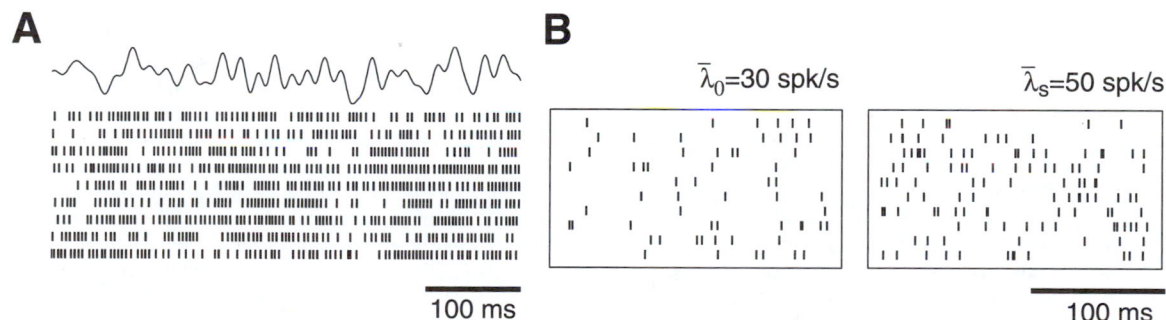

Figure 1. *A*, Nine spike trains recorded from an amplitude-sensitive afferent in the weakly electric fish *Eigenmannia* in response to repeated presentations of the same random electrical field amplitude modulation (shown on top). (Adapted from Kreiman et al., 2000.) *B*, Ten spike trains (200 ms long) obtained from a Poisson process with mean firing rate $\bar{\lambda}_0 = 30$ spk/s (spontaneous rate, left) and $\bar{\lambda}_s = 50$ spk/s (stimulus-induced rate, right).

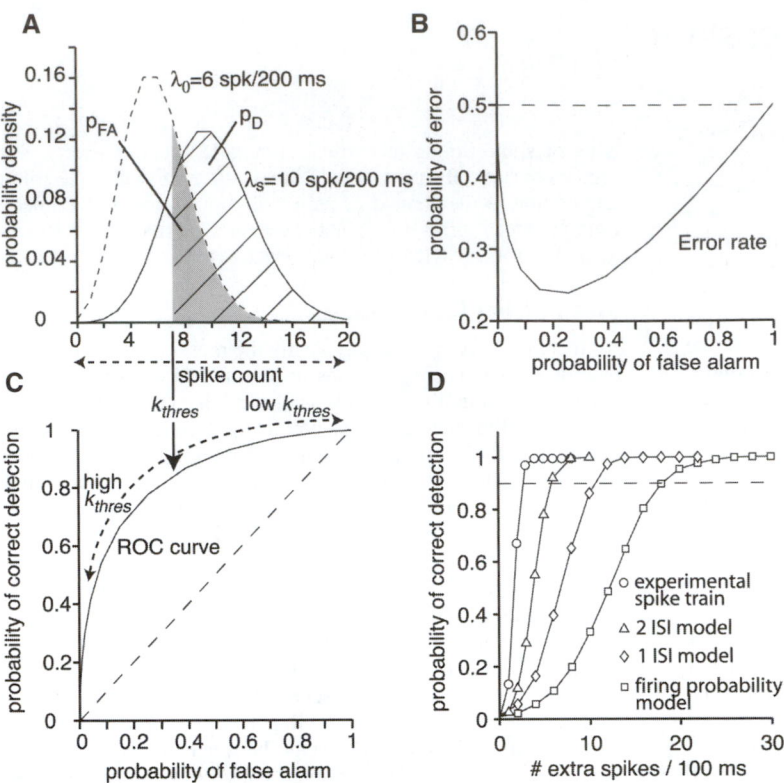

A

B

C

D

Figure 2. *A*, Probability distributions of the spike count observed in a 200 ms window for the two Poisson processes illustrated in Figure 1*B*. Choosing a threshold number of spikes (k_{thres}) to discriminate between the presence or absence of the stimulus leads to errors because of the overlap of the distributions. The probability of false alarm (p_{FA}) and of correct detection (p_D) are illustrated by the gray and hatched areas, respectively. *B*, Plot of p_D versus p_{FA}, called an ROC curve. Different thresholds will correspond to different values of p_D and p_{FA} (dashed double arrows in *A* and *B*). *C*, Overall probability of error (see Equation 2), computed from the ROC curve in *B*. *D*, Probability of correct detection obtained from the spike trains of an amplitude-sensitive afferent neuron as a function of the number of spikes above spontaneous activity generated by the cell (circles). Note that the cell can discriminate with more than 90% accuracy increases of three spikes or more, corresponding to a 1% increase in firing rate. Different models that take into account only the mean firing rate (squares), the mean firing rate and the interspike interval distribution (diamonds), or in addition the joint properties of successive intervals (triangles) are unable to match the experimental performance. (Adapted from Ratnam and Nelson, 2000.)

misses), as a function of the probability of false alarms, p_{FA} (i.e., 1 minus the probability of correct rejections; Figure 2*B*).

This curve is called the receiver operating characteristic (ROC) curve of the detection algorithm (a term originating from early applications to radar observations). The dashed diagonal line $p_D = p_{FA}$ corresponds to chance performance (i.e., independent of the threshold, k_{thres}, the probability, p_D, of correctly detecting the stimulus is as good as the probability, p_{FA}, of incorrectly mistaking spontaneous activity with stimulus-induced activity). Thus, the higher the ROC curve lies above the diagonal, the better the performance of our detection algorithm and, in the limit of perfect performance, $p_D = 1$ over the entire interval $0 \leq p_{FA} \leq 1$.

From the ROC curve, one can obtain the values of p_{FA} and $p_D(p_{FA})$ that minimize the overall probability of stimulus detection error (comprising both false alarms and false misses). If the stimulus is presented on average in one-half of the trials, the error rate is given, for a fixed value of p_{FA}, by

$$\varepsilon(p_{FA}) = \frac{1}{2} p_{FA} + \frac{1}{2} (1 - p_D(p_{FA})) \qquad (2)$$

The minimum of $\varepsilon(p_{FA})$ as a function of p_{FA} can be easily found by numerical methods (see Figure 2*C*). The corresponding threshold k_{thres} may then be obtained from $p_{FA}(k_{thres})$. Thus, in our example the minimal error rate $\varepsilon = 0.24$ is achieved for $p_{FA} = 0.26$, corresponding to a detection threshold k_{thres} of 8.5 spk/s.

One important question remains: Given the simplicity of this algorithm, could it be outperformed by a more sophisticated one? Remarkably, this is not the case: under fairly general assumptions, the threshold condition of Equation 1 is equivalent to a similar condition on the likelihood ratio, $l(n) = p_s(n)/p_0(n)$, where $p_s(\cdot)$ and $p_0(\cdot)$ are the probability distributions of the spike count in the presence and absence of the stimulus, respectively (Figure 2*A*). The likelihood ratio is a quantity central to signal detection theory, and this equivalence shows that, for a fixed value of p_{FA}, no other al-

gorithm taking into account only the probability distributions of Figure 2*A* can outperform the threshold test. Thus, the ROC curve defines the performance of an ideal observer of the mean rate code, having complete access to $p_0(\cdot)$ and $p_s(\cdot)$. Whether neurons or neuronal networks in the brain adopt similar algorithms to read out information about the external world remains an open question.

The performance of the ideal observer algorithm will be affected by at least two additional factors, the first being the length of the time window over which spikes are registered. Longer windows typically lead to better performance by averaging out the noise component of the spike rate that causes deviations from the mean. In the case of the Poisson process discussed above, for a fixed mean firing rate $\bar{\lambda}$, the mean number of spikes observed in a time window T is given by $\bar{n} = \bar{\lambda}T$, whereas the standard deviation is $\sigma = \sqrt{\bar{\lambda}T}$. Thus, $\bar{n}/\sigma \propto \sqrt{T}$, and the signal grows as $\sqrt{T}$ with respect to noise over the course of time. Currently, the time interval that is relevant for behavioral responses often is only weakly constrained by experimental observations.

The second factor is the regularity of the spike train or, in other words, the amount of noise that is present to start with. While many neurons in cortical areas have highly variable responses resembling those obtained from Poisson processes, other neurons can be much more regular. In the weakly electric fish *Apteronotus*, for example, the spike trains of primary sensory afferent neurons sensitive to amplitude modulations of the electrical field have a variability that is almost an order of magnitude smaller than that expected from a Poisson spike train on behaviorally relevant time scales (Ratnam and Nelson, 2000). These neurons are thought to encode information necessary for the detection of small prey, such as the water fleas on which the fish feeds. Computer simulations, behavioral observations, and electrophysiological recordings suggest that the firing rate of these cells will increase by only a few spikes per second during the 200 ms needed to detect the prey. An ROC analysis reveals that increases of 2–3 spk/s above baseline activity can be detected with greater than 90% accuracy even if the probability of a false alarm is very low, 0.1% (Figure 2D). Such low false alarm rates ($p_{FA} \leq 0.001$) are constrained from behavioral observations showing that fishes almost never strike a nonexistent prey. As illustrated in Figure 2D, three spike trains of models designed to reproduce the short-term variability of the experimental spike trains cannot reproduce these results. The first model (squares) reproduces only the mean firing rate of the afferents, while the second and third models also reproduce the interspike interval distribution (diamonds) or the joint statistical distribution of two successive interspike intervals (triangles), respectively. The regularity and statistical structure of the spike trains over at least three firing cycles is therefore responsible for this unusually low detection threshold.

Instantaneous Rate Coding

Stimuli that vary on a fast time scale—comparable to the 200 ms observation window introduced in the last section—cannot be encoded by the mean spike count alone. Such stimuli are ubiquitous in the sensory environment of many animals. Motion of an object or self-motion, for example, result in rapid changes in light intensity across the visual field. Sound stimuli used for communication or localization correspond to rapidly varying changes in air pressure. In the case of weakly electric fishes considered in the last section, time-varying electrical field amplitude modulations occur as the fish moves through an electrically dense environment in water.

Such time-varying stimuli could be encoded by time-varying changes in the instantaneous firing rate of a neuron, even if the precise timing of spikes does not play an essential role in the process (Gabbiani and Koch, 1999). Consider, for example, the Poisson spike train model of the previous section with a spontaneous rate $\bar{\lambda} = 30$ spk/s. We assume that changes in the instantaneous firing rate from its mean value, $\bar{\lambda}$, are caused by changes of the stimulus, $s(t)$, from its mean value, $\bar{s}$,

$$\lambda(t) = \alpha(s(t) - \bar{s}) + \bar{\lambda} \qquad (3)$$

The constant α is a conversion factor between stimulus and firing rate, and $\lambda(t)$ is assumed to be positive. In the following discussion the stimulus will usually be assumed to have zero mean, i.e., $\bar{s} = 0$.

How much information does such a spike train convey about the stimulus? Using an approach analogous to that introduced in the last section, this question can be addressed by presenting a random stimulus $s(t)$ and estimating it from the spike train (Figure 3A). Because $s(t)$ varies randomly in time, the estimate $s_{est}(t)$ will also have to vary in time to track $s(t)$. Thus, this estimation problem is more complex than the detection problem considered in the last section. It is customary to minimize the root mean square error between the stimulus and its estimate,

$$\varepsilon = \langle (s(t) - s_{est}(t))^2 \rangle^{1/2} \qquad (4)$$

where the average is taken over the stimulus presentation interval (Figure 3A). It is much more difficult to find an optimal estimate $s_{est}(t)$ from the spike train than it is to find an optimal classification strategy based on the spike count. A simplification is therefore

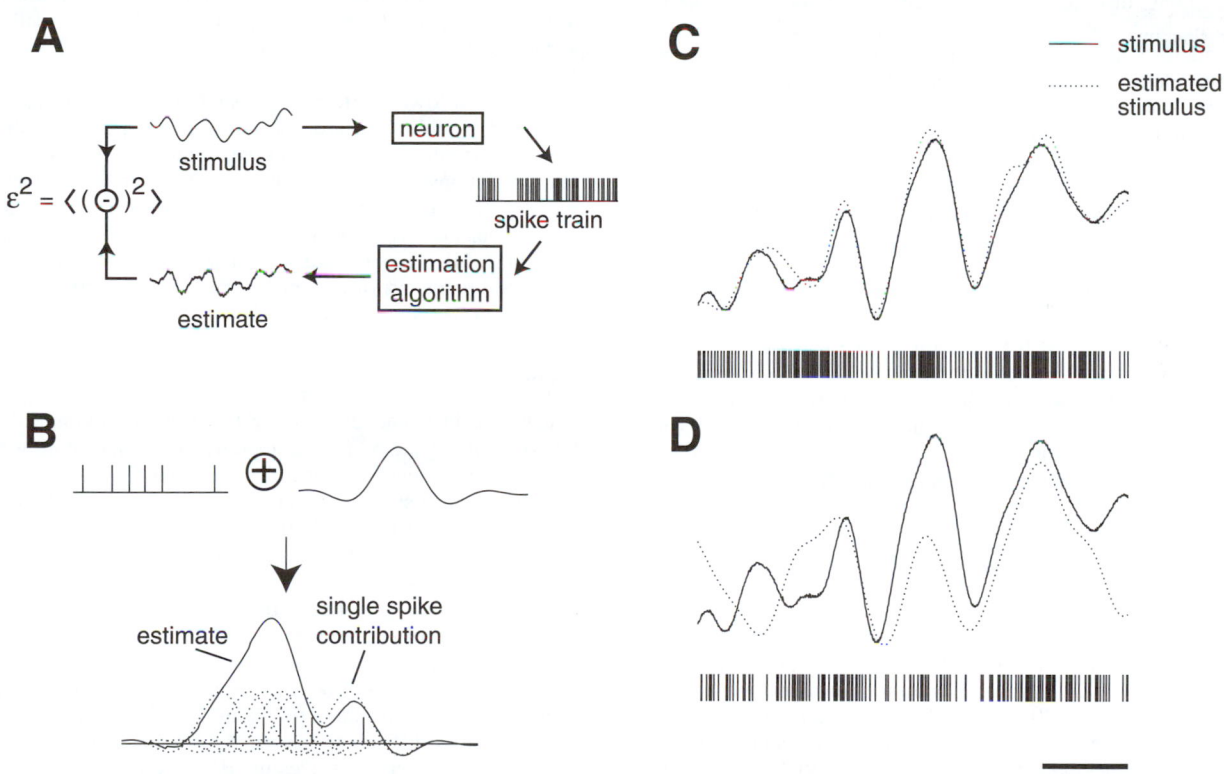

Figure 3. A, Stimulus estimation is performed using a linear algorithm (see B) that is based on a comparison of the stimulus and its estimate aimed at minimizing the mean square error between the two (Equation 4). B, The linear algorithm consists in taking a spike train (left) and placing a waveform (right) around each spike. Linear superposition of these waveforms (bottom) yields the estimate. The waveform is chosen to minimize the mean square error between stimulus and estimate (see A). C, Estimation of a random amplitude modulation from the spike train of an amplitude sensitive afferent neuron in *Eigenmannia* (mean firing rate 314 spk/s). D, Same stimulus estimated from a Poisson spike train encoding the stimulus according to Equation 3 at the same mean firing rate as in C.

made by looking only at estimates obtained from linear superpositions of a waveform, $h(t)$, around each spike. If $r(t) = \sum_i \delta(t - t_i)$ is a sum of delta functions representing the sequence of spikes at times $\{t_i\}$, the estimated stimulus is assumed to be of the form

$$
\begin{aligned}
s_{\text{est}}(h, t) &= \int h(t - t_0)r(t_0)dt_0 - \bar{r} \int h(t_0)dt_0 \\
&= \sum_i h(t - t_i) - \bar{r} \int h(t_0)dt_0 \quad (5)
\end{aligned}
$$

where $\bar{r}$ is the mean firing rate of the cell and the second term ensures that $s_{\text{est}}(t)$ has zero mean value, as was assumed for $s(t)$ (Figure 3B). Under this assumption, the optimal waveform, $h(t)$, minimizing the root mean square error in Equation 4 can be obtained by standard statistical and Fourier transform techniques. The minimum value obtained for the root mean square error, ε, is usually normalized by the stimulus standard deviation, σ, which corresponds to chance guessing (i.e., to the error obtained in Equation 4 when $s_{\text{est}}(t) = \bar{s} = 0$). Figure 3C illustrates the result of this estimation procedure using the spike train of an amplitude-sensitive afferent obtained in response to a random electrical field amplitude modulation in a second species of weakly electric fishes, *Eigenmannia*. From the spike train, the amplitude modulation could be estimated with an error $\varepsilon/\sigma = 0.17$. Equivalently, our ideal linear observer could reproduce 83% of the stimulus standard deviation using a single spike train.

In contrast, estimation of the same stimulus using a spike train generated using a Poisson process and Equation 3 is considerably less accurate (only 25% of the stimulus standard deviation is recovered; Figure 3D), because a Poisson process is more variable than the spiking of *Eigenmannia* afferents (Kreiman et al., 2000). Thus, as in the signal detection case, spike train variability plays an important role in stimulus estimation. Other factors that play a significant role in the encoding capacity of the instantaneous firing rate are the contrast of the stimulus (or its standard deviation σ; typically, higher contrasts result in larger firing rate modulations and thus better encoding), the mean firing rate of the cell (higher mean firing rates lead to a finer temporal sampling of the stimulus), and the cutoff frequency of the stimulus (accurate encoding is possible only when temporal stimulus frequencies are well below the mean firing rate of the cell).

The assumption relating spike train and stimulus estimate by a linear transform embodied in Equation 5 works very well in practice when the encoding of the stimulus by the spike train can be described by equations analogous to Equation 3. This result can be justified theoretically (Gabbiani and Koch, 1999). In contrast, no systematic studies have been carried out on the effect of nonlinear relations between stimulus and firing rate; only a few scattered examples have been examined (Gabbiani and Koch, 1999; Haag and Borst, 1998).

Rate Coding in Neural Systems

Instantaneous and mean firing rate codes have been extensively characterized in a variety of different neuronal systems. In the following discussion, we will highlight a few directions of investigation and some open questions relevant to the subject.

Starting in the late 1940s, signal detection methods have been applied to characterize the information conveyed by neuronal spike trains, along the lines prescribed earlier in this article (see Parker and Newsome, 1998). The investigation of neuronal signals carried by optic nerve fibers of the horseshoe crab *Limulus* was one of the earliest examples of work on this topic (see Parker and Newsome, 1998). Over the next 30 years, signal detection methods were extended to the activity of sensory neurons in the early auditory, somatosensory, and visual pathways of vertebrates. The variability of retinal ganglion cell spike trains, for example, has been exten-

sively investigated in an attempt to explain its impact on the encoding reliability of visual signals (Parker and Newsome, 1998).

More recently, signal detection methods have been applied to neurons in cerebral cortical areas (visual and somatosensory, for instance) of monkeys trained to perform discrimination tasks. In some cases, the reliability of neuronal firing could be compared to the behavioral accuracy of the animal performing the task. These results, together with analyses of variability and correlation across cells, have led to neural models of signal encoding that can account for the animal's behavior (see Parker and Newsome, 1998). The neural mechanisms underlying behavioral selection in those discrimination tasks, however, remain difficult to test experimentally.

In the cockroach, directional escape responses to wind stimuli are thought to rely on the mean firing rate of 14 giant interneurons (GIs). Several models that could in principle explain escape behaviors on the basis of the mean firing rate of GIs have been tested by directly manipulating them through current injections (Levi and Camhi, 2000). The results of these experiments suggest that a directional average of the GIs' mean firing rate is the most accurate description of the behavior. Mean firing rate codes across population of neurons have also been shown to play similar roles in vertebrate neurons, in the generation of visual saccades in the superior colliculus of monkeys, and in the generation of limb movements in motor cortical areas (Sparks, Kristan, and Shaw, 1997).

Given that in the engineering literature signal estimation is usually considered a close relative of signal detection (Poor, 1994), it is perhaps surprising that it has been applied to neural spike trains only within the past 10 years. Estimation of time-varying stimuli along the lines developed earlier in this article has shown that single spike trains of sensory neurons can accurately convey information about time-varying stimuli, although the results are usually less spectacular than those shown in Figure 3B (Borst and Theunissen, 1999). At present, these methods have been applied mainly to invertebrate and lower vertebrate preparations. Mechanisms of encoding across multiple neurons and their relation to behavior have received little attention so far (but see Stanley, Li, and Dan, 1999).

In contrast, instantaneous firing rate codes have been extensively studied by characterizing how stimulus attributes are encoded in the instantaneous firing rate of neurons through generalizations of Equation 3. Such models are particularly well developed for the early visual pathways of mammals, from the retina to early visual cortical areas (Dayan and Abbott, 2001).

Discussion

Mean and instantaneous firing rate codes are undoubtedly the best documented and best understood way by which neurons transmit information. Several other codes have also been studied, among them the mechanisms of coincidence detection in auditory processing (Pena and Konishi, 2001). More elaborate coding schemes are likely to be found, particularly across populations of neurons, although the highly sophisticated codes at the heart of information theory seem unlikely to find a place in describing the signaling repertoire of sensory and motor neurons.

One question that has long intrigued neuroscientists is whether the spike train variability usually observed in neurons using rate coding also carries further sensory information (Bullock, 1970). This question is difficult to answer rigorously. In the case of the cockroach, the pattern of spikes in GIs does not appear to play a role in determining escape behaviors (Liebenthal, Uhlmann, and Camhi, 1994). On the other hand, it has been suggested that in electric fishes, coincidence detection could be used to integrate the information conveyed by the amplitude-sensitive receptors described in this article and in Berman and Maler (1999). Thus, neurons might use a combination of different codes simultaneously at different levels of a neuronal circuit.

Road Map: Neural Coding
Related Reading: Population Codes; Sensory Coding and Information Transmission

References

Borst, A., and Theunissen, F. E., 1999, Information theory and neural coding, *Nature Neurosci.*, 2:947–957. ◆

Berman, N. J., and Maler, L., 1999, Neural architecture of the electrosensory lateral line lobe: Adaptations for coincidence detection, a sensory searchlight and frequency-dependent adaptive filtering, *J. Exp. Biol.*, 202:1243–1253.

Bullock, T. H., 1970, The reliability of neurons, *J. Gen. Physiol.*, 55:565–584. ◆

Dayan, P., and Abbott, L. F., 2001, *Theoretical Neuroscience*, Cambridge, MA: MIT Press. ◆

Gabbiani, F., and Koch, C., 1999, Principles of spike train analysis, in *Methods in Neuronal Modeling: From Synapses to Networks*, 2nd ed. (C. Koch and I. Segev, Eds.), Cambridge, MA: MIT Press, pp. 313–360. ◆

Haag, J., and Borst, A., 1998, Active membrane properties and signal encoding in graded potential neurons, *J. Neurosci.*, 18:7972–7986.

Kreiman, G., Krahe, R., Metzner, W., Koch, C., and Gabbiani, F., 2000, Robustness and variability of neuronal coding by amplitude-sensitive afferents in the weakly electric fish *Eigenmannia*, *J. Neurophysiol.*, 84:189–204.

Levi, R., and Camhi, J. M., 2000, Population vector coding by the giant interneurons of the cockroach, *J. Neurosci.*, 20:3822–3829.

Liebenthal E., Uhlmann, O., and Camhi, J. M., 1994, Critical parameters of the spike trains in a cell assembly: Coding of turn direction by the giant interneurons of the cockroach, *J. Comp. Physiol. A*, 174:281–296.

Parker, A. J., and Newsome, W. T., 1998, Sense and the single neuron: Probing the physiology of perception, *Annu. Rev. Neurosci.*, 21:227–277. ◆

Pena, J. L., and Konishi, M., 2001, Auditory spatial receptive fields created by multiplication, *Science*, 292:249–252.

Poor, H. V., 1994, *An Introduction to Signal Detection and Estimation*, New York: Springer-Verlag. ◆

Ratnam, R., and Nelson, M. E., 2000, Nonrenewal statistics of electrosensory spike trains: Implications for the detection of weak sensory signals, *J. Neurosci.*, 20:6672–6683.

Sparks, D. L., Kristan, W. B., and Shaw, B. K., 1997, The role of population coding in the control of movement, in *Neurons, Networks, and Motor Behavior* (P. S. G. Stein, S. Grillner, A. I. Selverston, and D. G. Stuart, Eds.), Cambridge, MA: MIT Press, pp. 21–32. ◆

Stanley, G. B., Li, F. F., and Dan, Y., 1999, Reconstruction of natural scenes from ensemble responses in the lateral geniculate nucleus, *J. Neurosci.*, 19:8036–8042.

Reaching Movements: Implications for Computational Models

Paul Cisek and John F. Kalaska

Introduction

Computational models are playing an increasingly important role in the study of biological motor control. In the first edition of this *Handbook*, the article on reaching movements (Kalaska, 1995) reviewed a range of computational models of visually guided movements and discussed their implications for cerebral cortical mechanisms of motor control. Here, we take the opposite approach. We discuss a number of issues that are emerging from neurophysiological studies of motor control and their implications for model development. We present these issues and implications as a set of challenges for computational models that hope to meet the demands of both functional competence and biological plausibility.

Planning Movement

Much of the theoretical background for computational models of the motor control system comes from engineering. Engineering practice usually solves a problem by breaking it down into a set of subproblems, each solved by a dedicated and distinct module. For example, a central distinction that motor control models inherit from engineering is that between planning and execution (Figure 1A). However, while this distinction may appear obvious from a robotics perspective because it is implied by the statement of the problem of control, it is not necessarily the most appropriate description for the organization of the biological motor system.

Neurophysiological evidence does not support a rigid separation between planning and execution at either the single-cell level or the population level (Kalaska, Sergio, and Cisek, 1998). Neurons that become active during movement preparation are distributed throughout the premotor and motor regions as well as in parietal regions, and those same cortical areas exhibit movement-related activity during execution. Motor imaging studies show that many of the same cortical areas are activated whether the subject is actually performing a movement or merely imagining it. Furthermore, even during execution of the movement itself, extensive representations of higher-order movement parameters and "early" sensorimotor transformations can be seen, especially in areas outside of primary motor cortex (Shen and Alexander, 1997a, b; Wise et al., 1997). Finally, correlates of both motor planning and execution processes can often be found in the activity of single cells, whose association with motor output changes in time from more abstract aspects of the task to more limb movement–related parameters (Crammond and Kalaska, 2000; Shen & Alexander, 1997a, b), as if single cells tended to shift functionally from the planning to the execution boxes of traditional models.

The functional distinctions most useful in understanding the organization of the biological motor control system may not be those that have proved most useful for traditional engineering methods. The general organization of the motor control system may in fact not resemble the serial input-to-output hierarchy of traditional models (Figure 1A) but instead may consist of parallel systems for *action specification* and *action selection* (Kalaska et al., 1998) (Figure 1B). Action specification includes all mechanisms involved in the computation of the parameters of motor actions. For a reaching movement, this begins with the processing of sensory information defining parameters such as distance to target and required grip size, and continues even during movement execution with on-line modification of the hand trajectory and joint torques. Because it continues even during movement itself, action specification incorporates processes that are often separated into the planning and execution stages of many computational models. Action selection includes all the mechanisms that choose between the various actions that are possible at a given moment. For a reaching movement, it encompasses such processes as attentional mechanisms that orient the eyes toward potential targets and select the ones most relevant at a given moment, cognitive mechanisms which decide the most appropriate response based on prior reinforcement, and

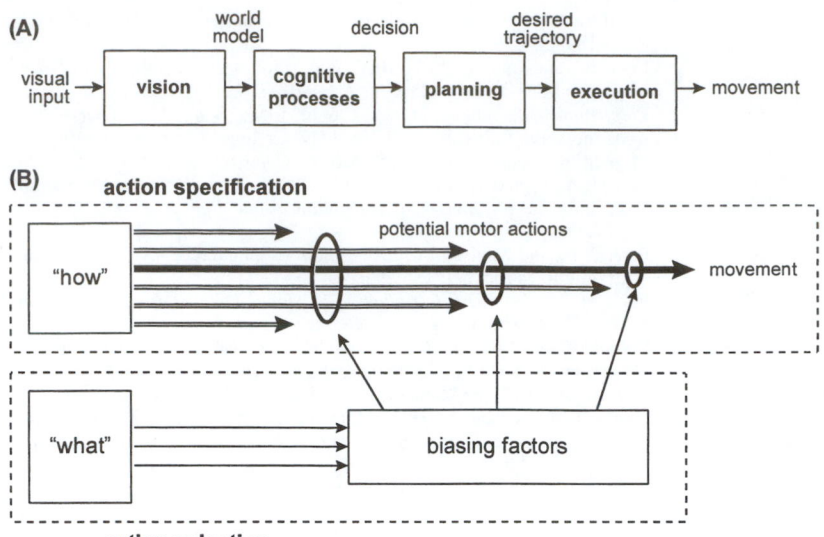

(A)

visual input → **vision** → world model → **cognitive processes** → decision → **planning** → desired trajectory → **execution** → movement

(B)   action specification

"how" → potential motor actions → movement

"what" → biasing factors

action selection

Figure 1. *A,* The traditional "sequential processing" model of visually guided behavior. In this model, visual input is used to construct a model of the world that is used to make decisions. After decisions are made, a desired trajectory is generated and executed. *B,* Schematic representation of the "specification and selection" architecture for visually guided behavior. Under this view, visual information has two different roles: specifying the parameters of potential motor actions, and defining criteria that bias competition among those potential actions until a single action is selected. These biasing factors include attention, behavioral relevance, prior reinforcement, required effort, behavioral context, learned associations, motivations, long-term behavioral objectives, desired outcomes, and any other factor that influences action selection. The processes of specification and selection occur in parallel and continue even during overt movement. A striking feature of this architecture is the absence of a central model of the visual world.

even mechanisms that abort or switch ongoing actions if the need arises.

The processes of selection and specification need not occur in a serial order but can instead both operate in parallel. Several potential motor actions may begin to be specified by the available sensory information through parallel sensorimotor transformations, allowing multiple responses to be "primed" for action (Cisek and Kalaska, 2002). At the same time, selection mechanisms using information on object identity and the organism's objectives influence attentional and decision-making mechanisms, which select out the action most appropriate at the time. While the selected action is performed, other alternatives may not be discarded but instead may be maintained and updated in case the need arises to switch the course of action. Such a parallel architecture allows the flexibility of behavior required by the changing demands of a natural environment. This perspective argues against computational models with a strict sequential hierarchical structure and supports models that emphasize dynamic interactions between different brain regions.

Because the tasks of action specification and action selection impose different demands on the processing of sensory information, they likely involve at least partially independent neuronal systems. Action specification requires information about the spatial relationships between body segments and objects in the environment with which the organism is interacting. In contrast, action selection emphasizes information about the nature and identity of external objects in order to evaluate the possible consequences of acting on these objects. These differing demands correspond well to the differing properties of the dorsal and ventral visual streams (Milner and Goodale, 1995), suggesting that these sensory systems evolved initially to serve the needs of the motor system, not to generate an internal representation of the world.

The general architecture of action specification and selection has much in common with Arbib's SCHEMA THEORY (q.v.). According to schema theory, visual information activates perceptual mechanisms ("perceptual schemas"), such as object localization and size recognition, that provide the information required to prepare specific action-oriented mechanisms ("motor schemas"), such as hand transport and hand preshaping, which are selected and released for execution according to learned contextual clues. Instead of a serial decomposition of action into planning and execution modules, schema theory suggests that behavior consists of the interplay between different parallel perception-action schemas that the organism applies when interacting with its environment.

Trajectory Generation

Another consequence of assuming separate planning and execution systems is the assumption that there must exist a representation of the motor plan that links them together. Different theories subscribe to this assumption to different degrees. For example, some theories propose that the motor plan takes the form of a representation of the complete time sequence of states that the execution system will pass through, a "desired trajectory" that is prespecified before movement begins. This is particularly important for explicit optimization models, which must know about the final states of movement before adjusting parameters of the intermediate states (see OPTIMIZATION PRINCIPLES IN MOTOR CONTROL).

To date, however, there has been no compelling neurophysiological evidence for an explicit representation of desired trajectories prior to the execution phase of motor tasks. One simple way to assess trajectory preplanning is to compare activity between instructed-delay tasks in which complete information about the metrics of an upcoming movement is presented prior to the instruction to initiate movement ("Go signal"), and reaction-time tasks in which the metrics are specified at the same time as the Go signal. One expects that during instructed-delay tasks, preplanning can take place as soon as movement metrics are specified, and need not be recapitulated after the Go signal. Although some of the predicted "neural savings" can be seen, especially in premotor cortex, most of the movement-related activity in premotor and primary motor cortex is relatively unaltered by the prior information, suggesting that most of the spatiotemporal details of the trajectory are generated dynamically as the movement unfolds (Crammond and Kalaska, 2000).

This is supported by another study (Shen and Alexander, 1997a, b), which dissociated the direction of limb movement and the direction of visual feedback guiding action (cursor motion on a screen). It was found that most of the activity in premotor and primary motor cortex during the delay period reflected the direction of cursor motion, and that a representation of the direction of limb motion became prominent only after the Go signal. This implies that only a relatively abstract representation of motor output is preplanned, even during well-practiced behaviors, whereas limb-specific signals are expressed at the time of movement. This implication does not contradict the possibility that certain high-level aspects of complex movements such as via points or sequence elements can be preplanned (see SEQUENCE LEARNING).

One might also question the concept of preplanned trajectories from an evolutionary perspective. It is unlikely that very primitive creatures preplanned and optimized the details of their actions before executing them. Instead, they generated movement on-line, adjusting movement details based on information fed back in real time. This kind of solution can produce acceptable results for many kinds of movements without requiring complex internal models of the dynamics of the controlled object. With a closed-loop system, the dynamics of the controlled object directly participate in the modification of the time course of the control signals. It is likely that such a simple strategy set the ancestral foundation for motor control.

Indeed, recent evidence suggests that movements are fine-tuned and adjusted using on-line sensory information during the movement itself. When a target of a reaching movement unexpectedly jumps during the course of the reach, subjects adjust automatically, even when the jump is not consciously perceived (Desmurget et al., 1999). Such on-line correction processes appear to involve the parietal cortex (Milner and Goodale, 1995; Desmurget et al., 1999) and are presumed to operate at all times during natural movements. In fact, without on-line correction, most normal activity would be very inaccurate because the world around us is always changing. For example, one could never catch a baseball by preplanning one's position and glove placement only when the ball is first hit or thrown. Instead, constant adjustments are necessary as the ball approaches, with the subject using sensory information about the ball's motion as well as feedback about the subject's own movements.

Nevertheless, the ability of the motor system to adjust movements on-line does not imply that it operates purely in the closed-loop manner of a standard feedback controller. That would not be possible with the conduction delays inherent in the system. To compensate for such delays, the motor system is able to learn specific movement contexts and to predict the state of the system when performing in each context (see SENSORIMOTOR LEARNING). For example, the system may learn an internal "forward model" that predicts, for a given movement context, what the outcome of a particular set of motor commands will be. With such a forward model, compensation for an expected perturbation can occur even before the perturbation causes any overt movement errors. As the system becomes more and more familiar with a given movement context, its dynamics will converge on the production of those commands that minimize the errors most relevant for the given task. However, although the resulting trajectory may be described as optimal (with respect to some criterion such as end-point error), this optimization arises slowly over a series of repeated action-perception cycles. It does not occur before movement begins through the explicit optimization of a desired trajectory. Instead, trajectories are produced during movement through the interplay of dynamics involving overt feedback and forward models, and it is the set of parameters implicitly defining these dynamics that is optimized during learning over many repeated movements.

Temporal Features of Cortical Activity

Many motor control models are described in terms of abstract computational elements whose activity over time does not clearly correspond to any of the neural activity profiles observed in the nervous system. However, the temporal features of cell activities in movement-related cortical areas should be very informative about the evaluation and modification of motor control models.

Neural activities in primary motor cortex exhibit a variety of complex shapes that appear to be importantly related to the kinematic and kinetic requirements of the task at hand (Kalaska et al., 1989; Fetz, 1992; Sergio and Kalaska, 1998). Since even the cells that project directly to spinal motor neurons exhibit complex temporal response profiles that do not explicitly code the ensuing EMG, it is clear that the descending command is not simple. These studies demonstrate that many details of the time-varying aspects of movement are already evident at the cortical level and thus are not all computed at the spinal cord, despite the elegance of proposed schemes for doing so (see EQUILIBRIUM POINT HYPOTHESIS).

These various temporal response profiles must certainly be informative for computational models. For example, area 4 cells exhibit several different kinds of response profiles, including phasic, tonic, and phasic-tonic responses (Kalaska et al., 1989; Fetz, 1992). The phasic-tonic cells are the most load sensitive of these and are most often found in the deeper layers from which the pyramidal tract projection originates. They form the largest proportion of corticomotor-neuronal (CM) cells that directly project to spinal motor neurons (Fetz, 1992). Their temporal response pattern is clearly related to the dynamical requirements of different tasks (Sergio and Kalaska, 1998). In contrast, phasic cells tend to show much less load sensitivity, are more often found in superficial layers, and are almost never CM cells. There are also important differences between the activities of cortical neurons in different regions and different layers, as well as during different movement contexts. For example, cells in parietal area 5 exhibit much less sensitivity to loads than do cells in primary motor cortex, especially at the population level (Kalaska et al., 1990).

Such observations led Bullock, Cisek, and Grossberg (1998) to outline a circuit model that incorporates neural elements whose activity resembles these observed temporal patterns. According to this model, the load-sensitive phasic-tonic cells in area 4 assemble a descending command by integrating a directional signal from phasic cells and combining it with launching and braking pulses. Area 5 tonic cells combine a load-sensitive corollary discharge signal from area 4 and a load-sensitive feedback from stretch receptors to yield a load-insensitive position representation. In the model, interactions between area 4 and area 5 cells result in the on-line generation of reaching trajectories. By assigning specific functional roles to observed cell profiles, such models make specific predictions that can be tested in future neurophysiological experiments.

Overlapping Polymodal Gradients

Motor control models usually consist of discrete functional modules, with specific computational roles assigned to specific elements. However, a striking feature of cortical neurophysiology, at least in the motor system, is the absence of well-delineated borders separating populations of cells with different functional properties. Instead, one observes gradual transitions in cell properties as one moves across the cortical surface.

Within a local area, cells do not neatly partition into separate classes or "types," but rather form a complex continuum exhibiting different mixtures of properties (Caminiti, Ferraina, and Battaglia-Mayer, 1998). As we move along the cortical surface, the mixture of cell properties changes gradually. Moving medially or laterally in the motor cortex, we find cells whose activity relates to different body parts. Moving rostrally from the central sulcus over the precentral gyrus, we find progressively more phasic and less load-sensitive cells and more correlation with abstract task information than with the details of movement kinematics or dynamics. In the postcentral gyrus, there is a reciprocal gradient of progressively less movement-related and more preparation-related activity as we move caudally along area 5 and into the deep intraparietal sulcus. These opposing gradients in pre- and postcentral areas are paralleled by a connectivity pattern, with neurophysiologically similar regions across the central sulcus being reciprocally connected. As already mentioned, gradual transitions are also observed in the time domain, with cell properties changing during the course of a movement trial.

In addition to smooth gradients of changing cell properties, some movement-related cortical areas also exhibit a great deal of polymodality. For example, in premotor and posterior parietal areas, cells are found that are sensitive to a variety of sensory and motor information. Cells respond to different degrees to salient retinal inputs, especially to objects and motion in the region of space near the monkey, and are modulated by direction of gaze, direction of attention, direction of intended movement, limb configuration, and cutaneous contact, among other factors (Caminiti et al., 1998). Modeling studies suggest that these combinations of signals converging on single cells are appropriate to effect a sensorimotor coordinate transformation. However, neurophysiological studies routinely fail to find a significant population of cells whose activity explicitly encodes the output of that transformation in a unique coordinate system. Instead, the output may be implicitly embedded in the distributed pattern of activity across the population, and extracted by appropriate decoding mechanisms (Pouget and Sejnowski, 1997). This diversity of polymodal properties indicates that computational models based on strict engineering principles and homogeneous coordinate systems (for instance, inverse differential kinematics from instantaneous hand velocity to instantaneous rates of change of muscle lengths) may have some heuristic value but do not capture the true nature of cerebral cortical motor control processes.

A model being developed by Yves Burnod and colleagues (Burnod et al., 1999) takes on the challenge of addressing the distributed nature of movement-related information in the cerebral cortex. In their framework, learned associations between combinations of sensory information (such as target position, gaze direction, and current limb configuration) and motor commands (such as gaze shifts or arm movements) are retrieved by "match" units, and the combination defining the movement that is most appropriate to the given task is selected by "condition" units on the basis of prior reinforcement. These match and condition units are distributed throughout the cortex in a continuum reflecting the possible combinations of information necessary to guide movement in various contexts. Thus, the model suggests that the overlapping gradients of polymodal activities in frontal and parietal regions are not merely a biological nuisance masking the true functional decomposition of motor control but are instead the basis of the motor system's strategy for flexibly integrating information for the demands of different tasks.

Discussion

Models that attempt both to solve interesting computational problems and to explain biological data face many challenges. These challenges come from diverse directions, including constraints imposed by the laws of physics, neurophysiological data, psychophysics, the evolution and development of the nervous system, and the impressive flexibility and adaptability of movement. The best way for progress to be made in such an endeavor is through a combined modeling and empirical approach. Models should be viewed as stepping stones in such a process, complementary to the experiments that they help to guide and that in turn help to modify and refine the models.

Road Map: Mammalian Motor Control
Related Reading: Arm and Hand Movement Control; Cerebellum and Motor Control; Eye-Hand Coordination in Reaching Movements; Limb Geometry, Neural Control; Robot Arm Control

References

Bullock, D., Cisek, P., and Grossberg, S., 1998, Cortical networks for control of voluntary arm movements under variable force conditions, *Cereb. Cortex*, 8:48–62.

Burnod, Y., Baraduc, P., Battaglia-Mayer, A., Guigon, E., Koechlin, E., Ferraina, S., Lacquaniti, F., and Caminiti, R., 1999, Parieto-frontal coding of reaching: An integrated framework, *Exp. Brain Res.*, 129:325–346.

Caminiti, R., Ferraina, S., and Battaglia-Mayer, A., 1998, Visuomotor transformations: Early cortical mechanisms of reaching, *Curr. Opin. Neurobiol.*, 8:753–761. ◆

Cisek, P., and Kalaska, J. F., 2002, Simultaneous encoding of multiple potential reach directions in dorsal premotor cortex, *J. Neurophysiol.*, 87:1149–1154.

Crammond, D. J., and Kalaska, J. F., 2000, Prior information in motor and premotor cortex: Activity during the delay period and effect on premovement activity, *J. Neurophysiol.*, 84:986–1005.

Desmurget, M., Epstein, C. M., Turner, R. S., Prablanc, C., Alexander, G. E., and Grafton, S. T., 1999, Role of the posterior parietal cortex in updating reaching movements to a visual target, *Nature Neurosci.*, 2:563–567.

Fetz, E. E., 1992, Are movement parameters recognizably coded in the activity of single neurons? *Behav. Brain Sci.*, 15:679–690. ◆

Kalaska, J. F., 1995, Reading movements: Implications of connectionist models, in *The Handbook of Brain Theory and Neural Networks* (M. A. Arbib, Ed.), Cambridge, MA: The MIT Press, pp. 788–793. ◆

Kalaska, J. F., Cohen, D. A. D., Hyde, M. L., and Prud'homme, M. J., 1989, A comparison of movement direction-related versus load direction-related activity in primate motor cortex, using a two-dimensional reaching task, *J. Neurosci.*, 9:2080–2102.

Kalaska, J. F., Cohen, D. A. D., Prud'homme, M. J., and Hyde, M. L., 1990, Parietal area 5 neuronal activity encodes movement kinematics, not movement dynamics, *Exp. Brain Res.*, 80:351–364.

Kalaska, J. F., Sergio, L. E., and Cisek, P., 1998, Cortical control of whole-arm motor tasks, in *Sensory Guidance of Movement: Novartis Foundation Symposium No. 218* (M. Glickstein, Ed.), Chichester, UK: Wiley, pp. 176–201. ◆

Milner, A. D., and Goodale, M. A., 1995, *The Visual Brain in Action*, London: Oxford University Press. ◆

Pouget, A., and Sejnowski, T. J., 1997, Spatial transformations in the parietal cortex using basis functions, *J. Cogn. Neurosci.*, 9:222–237.

Sergio, L. E., and Kalaska, J. F., 1998, Changes in the temporal pattern of primary motor cortex activity in a directional isometric force versus limb movement task, *J. Neurophysiol.*, 80:1577–1583.

Shen, L., and Alexander, G. E., 1997a, Neural correlates of a spatial sensory-to-motor transformation in primary motor cortex, *J. Neurophysiol.*, 77:1171–1194.

Shen, L., and Alexander, G. E., 1997b, Preferential representation of instructed target location versus limb trajectory in dorsal premotor area, *J. Neurophysiol.*, 77:1195–1212.

Wise, S. P., Boussaoud, D., Johnson, P. B., and Caminiti, R., 1997, Premotor and parietal cortex: Corticocortical connectivity and combinatorial computations, *Annu. Rev. Neurosci.*, 20:25–42. ◆

Reactive Robotic Systems

Ronald C. Arkin

Introduction

Reactive systems are a relatively recent development in robotics that has redirected artificial intelligence (AI) research. This new approach grew out of a dissatisfaction with existing methods for producing intelligent robotic response and a growing awareness of the importance of studying biological systems as a basis for constructing intelligent behavior. Reactive robots are often referred to as behavior-based robots: they are instructed to perform through the activation of a collection of low-level primitive behaviors. Complex physical behavior emerges through the interaction of the behavioral set and the complexities of the environment in which the robot finds itself, resulting in more rapid and flexible responses than are attainable through traditional methods of robotic control.

Some of the hallmark characteristics of purely reactive robotic systems include (Arkin, 1998):

1. *Behaviors are the basic building blocks.* A behavior in these systems is often a simple sensorimotor circuit, where sensory activity consists of providing necessary information to support low-level reactive motor response, such as avoiding obstacles, escaping from predators, being attracted to goals, etc.
2. *Abstract representational knowledge is avoided.* Creating and maintaining accurate representations of the world is a time-consuming error-prone process. Purely reactive systems do not maintain world models, instead reacting directly to the stimuli the world presents. This is particularly useful in highly dynamic and hazardous worlds, where the environment is unpredictable and potentially hostile.
3. *Animal models of behavior are often used as a basis for these systems.* Models from neuroscience, cognitive psychology, and ethology are used to capture the nature of the behaviors that are necessary for a robot's safe interaction with a hostile world.
4. *Demonstrable robotic results have been achieved.* These techniques have been applied to a wide range of robots, including six-legged walking robots, pipe-crawling robots, military robots, entertainment robots such as Sony's AIBO, mobile manipulators, dextrous hands, and entire herds of mobile robots. Because these systems are highly modular, they can be constructed incrementally from the bottom up by adding new behaviors to an existing repertoire. From an engineering perspective, this property is quite desirable, as it facilitates the growth and application of existing software and hardware systems to new domains.

Even more recently, hybrid reactive/deliberative robotic architectures have emerged that combine aspects of more traditional AI symbolic methods and their use of abstract representational knowledge with the responsiveness, robustness, and flexibility of purely reactive systems. Both purely reactive and hybrid architectures are discussed in this article.

Biological Basis for Reactive Robotic Systems

Many of the designers of reactive systems look to biology as a source of models for use in robots. Although these efforts are quite diverse, ranging from traditionally engineered systems to those dedicated to faithfully replicating biological behavior, this article reports on a few exemplars that have affected reactive and hybrid system design.

Action-oriented perception. Neuroscientists and psychologists, especially in the cognitive and ecological communities, have provided models for the relationships between perceptual activities and behaviors required for a particular task. One excellent example is presented in Arbib (1972). His model of action-oriented perception shows that what an agent needs to perceive is based on its need to act. This is a primary guiding principle in the design of reactive robots. The traditional computer vision community often views perception as a disembodied perceiver that interprets images without consideration for what the knowing agent needs to do. In contrast, the strong coupling between action and perception is one of the hallmarks of purely reactive robotic systems. Neisser has further developed these ideas in the context of cognitive psychology (see Arkin, 1998, for a review of those aspects relevant to robotic systems).

Ethological studies. A pressing question for reactive robotic system designers is just what behaviors are necessary or sufficient for a particular task and environment. Many of these researchers have turned to ethological studies as a source for behaviors that are relevant in certain circumstances. Specific models used in reactive robotic systems have been quite varied, including bird flocking, ant foraging, fish schooling, and cockroach escape, among others. One example involving toad detour behavior (Arbib and House, 1987) provided motivation and justification for the use of vector fields in reactive schema-based robot navigation (Arkin, 1998).

Coexistence of parallel planning and execution systems (hybrid systems). Norman and Shallice (1986) have modeled the coexistence of two distinct systems concerned with controlling human behavior. One system models "automatic" behavior and is closely aligned with reactive systems. This system handles automatic action execution without awareness, starts without attention, and consists of independent parallel activity threads (schemas). The second system controls "willed" behavior and expresses an interface between deliberate conscious control and the automatic system.

While purely reactive robotic systems are compatible with the modeled automatic system (e.g., Brooks, 1986), most hybrid robotic systems (e.g., Arkin, 1990; Gat, 1992) incorporate both willed (deliberative) and automatic (reactive) components in a manner somewhat consistent with the above model.

One problem confronting the reactive robotic systems designer is that much of the data reported by biological scientists is often presented statistically. Although this approach may be useful within the context of their home disciplines, it is important for process models to be constructed whenever possible to facilitate the adoption of this work into intelligent robotic systems (see NEUROETHOLOGY, COMPUTATIONAL).

Purely Reactive Robotic Systems

Reactive robotic systems originated in the cybernetic movement of the 1940s. Grey Walter (1953) developed an electronic "tortoise" capable of moving about the world, avoiding perceived threats and attracted to certain goals. Of special interest was the inclusion of changing goals regarding the robot's recharging station. When power was low, the tortoise was attracted to and docked with the recharger. When sufficient energy was acquired, it lost its "appetite" (charger attraction) and was repelled by it. There was no use of abstract representational constructs as later found in traditional AI; perception directly controlled motor action. Simple behaviors were created: head toward weak light, back away from strong light, and turn-and-push to avoid obstacles.

Braitenberg (1984) revived interest in this class of creatures. Using simple analog circuitry, he demonstrated that "creatures" could be built that manifested behaviors comparable to those found in animals, such as cowardice, aggression, love, exploration, and logic. These thought experiments in "synthetic psychology" showed that seemingly complex behavior could result from a collection of simple sensorimotor transformations.

Brooks (1986) was an early leader of the purely reactive robotic paradigm. His group pursued this approach with the development of subsumption architecture. He articulated the departure from classical AI and broke away from the sense-plan-act paradigm that dominated AI in the 1970–1980s as typified by robots like Shakey that used resolution theorem proving as its primary reasoning mechanism. This new position brought into question the role of representational knowledge in AI altogether. The subsumption architecture was biologically motivated only in the behaviorist sense, as it produced overt results that resembled the behaviors of certain insect systems but was unconcerned for the underlying biological mechanisms that produced them.

At about the same time that subsumption architecture appeared, other researchers were interested in pursuing parallels in biological and mechanical systems. A sort of cybernetics revival occurred. Studies produced by ethologists, neuroscientists, and others provided models that were used within reactive robotic systems. These researchers' goals varied. For example, Arkin (1990) exploited these models for the purpose of constructing intelligent robotic systems, using interacting schemas as a basis for reactive robotic control systems design (see SCHEMA THEORY). Beer, alternatively, used robotic systems to demonstrate the fidelity of neuroscientific models (see LOCOMOTION, INVERTEBRATE). Significant conferences now exist dedicated to animal and computational systems relationships; an example is the conference whose proceedings are regularly published as *Simulation of Adaptive Behavior: From Animals to Animats*, by MIT press.

Figure 1 presents a simple reactive control system example. A robot controlled by this system wanders around avoiding collisions until it finds a path, which it then follows until it locates its goal. It consists of four behaviors: *avoid-obstacle* prevents the robot from colliding with anything; *wander-about* ensures movement in the absence of goal or path attraction; *stay-on-path* guides the robot down a hall or road to find the goal near the path's end; and *move-to-goal* attracts the robot to the final goal. The perceptual strategies for each behavior are also depicted. The behavior coordination mechanism can be of several forms. Arbitration or action-selection mechanisms are typically found in subsumption-style architectures where only one behavior is active at any given time. This action-selection mechanism can be complex, involving extensive connections between behaviors for inhibition/suppression. The schematic representation of this mechanism is greatly simplified in this figure. Other coordinators may involve blending, as in schema-based reactive control systems, where all active behaviors contribute somewhat to the overall coordinated motion. Even combinations of different coordination mechanisms can be used to compose intelligent robotic behavior.

Hybrid Reactive/Deliberative Robotic Systems

Hybrid architectures permit reconfiguration of reactive control systems based on available world knowledge, adding considerable flexibility over purely reactive systems. Dynamically reconfiguring the control system based on deliberation (reasoning over world models) is an important addition to the overall competence of general-purpose robots.

It should be recognized that purely reactive robotic systems are not appropriate for every robotic application. In situations where the world can be accurately modeled, where there is restricted uncertainty, and where there exists some guarantee of virtually no change in the world during execution (such as an engineered assembly workcell), deliberative methods are often preferred, since a plan can most likely be effectively carried out. In the real world, in which biological agents function, these prerequisites for purely deliberative planners do not exist. If roboticists hope to have their machines functioning in the same environments that we do, methods like reactive control are required. Many feel that hybrid systems capable of incorporating both deliberative reasoning and reactive execution are needed to deliver the full potential of robotic systems.

Arkin was among the first to advocate the use of both deliberative (hierarchical) and reactive (schema-based) control systems within the Autonomous Robot Architecture. Incorporating a traditional planner that could reason over a flexible and modular reactive control system, specific robotic configurations could be constructed that integrated behavioral, perceptual, and a priori environmental knowledge (Arkin, 1990). This system was tested on a wide range of applications, both indoors and outdoors.

Gat (1992) proposed a three-level hybrid system (Atlantis) incorporating a Lisp-based deliberator, a sequencer that handled failures of the reactive system, and a reactive controller. This system was fielded and tested successfully on Mars rover prototypes.

Perception and Reactivity

A fundamental guiding principle for purely reactive systems is that perceptual activities should always be viewed on the basis of motor needs (i.e., a *need-to-know basis*). A large body of mainstream computer vision research is concerned with the abstract task of image understanding, which usually is considered independently of a particular agent's needs. Proponents of purely reactive control advocate that perception serves motor action, and that image interpretation algorithms must take this into account. Sensing strategies should be constructed that take advantage of the knowledge of underlying behavioral requirements. This eliminates the need to construct global representations of the world, an activity avoided in purely reactive robotic systems. By creating perceptual algorithms that extract only relevant information and that exploit expectations of what is necessary and sufficient to be perceived, efficient sensor processing is a natural consequence.

Hybrid approaches, nonetheless, are more consistent with the views of neuroscientists (e.g., Mishkin, Ungerleider, and Macko

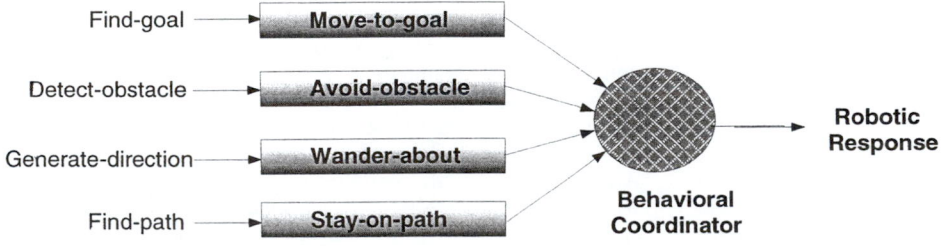

Figure 1. Example of a reactive control system.

1983) on *what* + *where* visual systems that account for the maintenance of spatial relationships in a more than purely reactive manner (see VISUAL SCENE PERCEPTION).

There are three ways in which reactive systems can utilize perceptual information: perceptual channeling (sensor fission), action-oriented sensor fusion, and perceptual sequencing. Perceptual channeling is straightforward: a motor behavior requires a particular stimulus for it to be invoked, so a single sensor system is created. A simple sensorimotor circuit results. There are numerous examples (e.g., Maes, 1990; Brooks, 1991).

Action-oriented sensor fusion (Arkin, 1993) permits the construction of representations (percepts) that are local to individual behaviors. Restricting the representation to the requirements of a particular behavior provides the benefits of reactive control while permitting more than one sensor to provide input, resulting in increased robustness.

Sometimes fixed action patterns require varying stimuli to support them over separations in time and space. As a behavioral response unfolds, it may be modulated by different sensors or different views of the world. Perceptual sequencing supports the coordination of multiple perceptual algorithms over time in support of a single behavioral activity. Perceptual algorithms are phased in and out, based on the needs of the agent and the environmental context in which it is situated.

Discussion

Space prevents an extensive survey of the wide range of reactive robotic systems; the reader is referred to Maes (1990), Brooks (1991), Mataric (1992), Efken and Shaw (1993), and Arkin (1998) for additional information and alternative perspectives. These methods have gained dramatically in popularity and utility since the mid-1980s and are being applied to robotic systems throughout the world.

Hybrid reactive/deliberative architectures have been created to address several of the potential shortcomings of purely reactive systems. They permit the incorporation of world knowledge and the construction of global representations, yet preserve the strength of reactive execution and responsiveness to environmental change.

Road Map: Robotics and Control Theory
Related Reading: Potential Fields and Neural Networks; Visuomotor Coordination in Frog and Toad

References

Arbib, M. A., 1972, *The Metaphorical Brain: An Introduction to Cybernetics as Artificial Intelligence and Brain Theory*, New York: Wiley.
Arbib, M., and House, D., 1987, Depth and detours: An essay on visually guided behavior, in *Vision, Brain, and Cooperative Computation* (M. Arbib and A. Hanson, Eds.), Cambridge, MA: MIT Press, pp. 139–163.
Arkin, R. C., 1990, Integrating behavioral, perceptual, and world knowledge in reactive navigation, *Robotics and Autonomous Systems*, 6:105–122.
Arkin, R. C., 1993, Modeling neural function at the schema level: Implications and results for robotic control, in *Biological Neural Networks in Invertebrate Neuroethology and Robotics* (R. Beer, R. Ritzmann, and T. McKenna, Eds.), San Diego: Academic Press, pp. 383–410.
Arkin, R. C., 1998, *Behavior-Based Robotics*, Cambridge, MA: MIT Press. ◆
Braitenberg, V., 1984, *Vehicles: Experiments in Synthetic Psychology*, Cambridge, MA: MIT Press.
Brooks, R., 1986, A robust layered control system for a mobile robot, *IEEE J. Robot. Automat.*, 2:14–23.
Brooks, R., 1991, New approaches to robotics, *Science*, 13 Sept., pp. 1227–1232. ◆
Efken, J., and Shaw, R., 1993, Ecological perspectives on the new artificial intelligence, *Ecol. Psychol.*, 4:247–270. ◆
Gat, E., 1992, Integrating planning and reacting in a heterogeneous asynchronous architecture for controlling real-world mobile robots, *Proc. AAAI-92*, pp. 809–815.
Maes, P., Ed., 1990, *Designing Autonomous Agents*, Cambridge, MA: MIT Press/Elsevier, 1990. ◆
Mataric, M., 1992, Integration of representation into goal-driven behavior-based robots, *IEEE Trans. Robot. Automat.*, 8:304–312.
Mishkin, M., Ungerleider, L. G., and Macko, K. A., 1983, Object vision and spatial vision: Two cortical pathways, *Trends Neurosci.*, 6:414–417.
Norman, D., and Shallice, T., 1986, Attention to action: Willed and automatic control of behavior, in *Consciousness and Self-Regulation: Advances in Research and Theory*, vol. 4 (R. Davidson, G. Schwartz, and D. Shapiro, Eds.), New York: Plenum Press, pp. 1–17.
Walter, W. G., 1953, *The Living Brain*, New York: Norton.

Reading

John G. Holden and Guy C. Van Orden

Introduction

A skilled reader can recognize many thousands of printed words, each in a fraction of a second, with no noticeable effort. A child who is developmentally dyslexic does not easily acquire this skill. For a dyslexic child, recognizing a printed word as a particular word can be effortful to the point of frustration. Dyslexia may plague an otherwise bright and articulate child, and the fact of dyslexia illustrates how recognition of printed words as words is the crux of reading. Reading is not exclusively the recognition of printed words, but it is word recognition that sets reading apart from natural language. In effect, to become a reader is to master this special skill (Perfetti, 1985). A vast empirical literature concerns word recognition, and most "neural" networks of reading are models of word recognition.

One tool with which to diagnose dyslexia is a naming task that presents individual *pseudoword spellings*, such as "glurp," to be read aloud. A dyslexic child may have great difficulty with this task, and success in this nonword task is generally correlated with word reading skill. Trouble decoding the pronunciations of letter strings is a symptom of the most common form of dyslexia (Pennington, 1991). In this form, dyslexia is a specific problem in translating words' spellings into their phonology (roughly, their sounds or pronunciations). And the key to word recognition would seem to lie in the derivation of phonology from words' printed forms.

All written languages have systematic relationships between words' printed and spoken forms (Mattingly, 1992), so perhaps word recognition includes an analytic letter-by-letter process that translates spelling into phonology. This possibility has preoccupied reading scientists for over 100 years. Nevertheless, word recognition is not simply analytic. Evidence that supports an analytic hypothesis has always existed side by side with evidence that word recognition is synthetic (or holistic). The consequent synthetic/analytic debate defined reading theory throughout the twentieth century, and it provides the organizing theme for this article.

Early Reading Research

Nineteenth century studies introduced almost all topics of current reading research (Rayner and Pollatsek, 1989). A key early finding from eye-movement studies was that readers' eyes make a series of jumps in moving across a line of text, pausing for about a quarter of a second when fixated. Discrete eye movements implied the *fixation* (recognition) of individual printed words in natural reading. Another key development was the invention of the t-scope (or tachistoscope). A t-scope can flash individual words for a few milliseconds at a time, well within the range of fixation times observed in eye movements.

More recent t-scope studies, in the second half of the twentieth century, perpetuated the synthetic/analytic debate. Ulric Neisser's seminal book *Cognitive Psychology* (1967) includes a review of this debate concerning word recognition. For example, pseudoword spellings, such as "glurp," that obey the letter-to-sound pronounceability patterns of English are more easily recognized and recalled than are random strings of letters. The advantage for pronounceable letter strings suggests an analytic process. A more contemporary finding, however, indicates that word recognition could be synthetic. Words that are flashed for a fraction of a second (and then replaced by a "pattern mask" of letter features) are more accurately reported than are their component letters presented individually under the same extreme conditions, a phenomenon known as the *word superiority effect*.

Dual-Route Theories

Dual-route theories emerged in the 1970s with the advent of cognitive psychology. As the name implies, traditional dual-route theories were an ad hoc resolution of the synthetic/analytic debate. Both options were included as separate processing modules (mechanisms). Early dual-route theories were important in this regard because they moved past a contentious theoretical debate that could not be resolved empirically.

The two modules of dual-route theories accomplish word recognition in two different ways. Skilled readers reading frequently encountered words rely on a fast, synthetic, lexical module to translate a visual representation into an entry in the lexicon, the mind's dictionary. The speed of access to dictionary entries in the lexical module is determined by the relative frequency with which a word appears in print. Word frequency is estimated by counting the occurrence of each word (per million words) in large samples of text. Higher-frequency words are more readily available in the lexicon. (Different dual-route theories propose different frequency-sensitive mechanisms.)

By contrast, novice readers and skilled readers who encounter a novel word recognize words via a slow, analytic, sublexical module. At the heart of the sublexical module are rules to translate minimum units of spelling (graphemes) into minimum units of phonology (phonemes). A combination of phonemes may guide assembly of pronunciation for completely novel letter strings, such as "glurp," or may achieve lexical access when the unfamiliar spelling translates into the phonology of a familiar word. Access to a lexical entry allows access, in turn, to lexical representations of words' pronunciations and conventional meanings, as one would find in a dictionary. (Different dual-route theories propose different representations and translation procedures.)

Word Naming

Word naming experiments measure the time required to pronounce individually presented words. At one time, dual-process theories provided a sufficient account of results from naming experiments, with skilled readers as participants. Low-frequency regular words, such as "mint," that obey sublexical grapheme-phoneme corre-

spondence rules are named faster than low-frequency exception words, such as "pint," that entail exceptions to the rules. No regularity effect was found to high-frequency words. Hence, naming of low-frequency words is accomplished by the sublexical module, but naming of all other words is accomplished by the lexical module. Eventually, however, this categorical regular/exception distinction was contradicted. New studies found graded effects of semiregular relationships between spelling and phonology, not simply the regular versus exception distinction predicted by traditional dual-route theories. For instance, although both "wave" and "wade" obey the grapheme-phoneme rules, the existence of "have," an exception "neighbor" to "wave," induces slower naming times to "wave" itself.

Lexical Decision

Word recognition is also studied by using the *lexical decision task*. Lexical decision experiments measure the time required to indicate that an individually presented word is a word (with catch trials that present pseudoword spellings). Previously, lexical decision time did not appear to be affected by regularity, only by relative frequency. High-frequency words are recognized faster than low-frequency words. Regularity effects arise in the sublexical module, and frequency effects arise in the lexical module. Hence, recognition for lexical decisions appeared to rely on the lexical module, exclusively. New studies contradicted this hypothesis, however. Key findings were subcategories of exception words, such as "weird" or "choir," called *strange words*, that produced slow and error-prone performance, reliably worse performance than that to ordinary exception words such as "pint." These findings, like the graded-regularity effects in naming experiments, contradict the categorical regularity distinction of dual-route theories.

Patient Studies

At one time, dual-process theories also provided a reasonable account of neuropsychological findings. Lexical and sublexical modules were corroborated in the patterns of naming errors, described in case studies of brain-damaged individuals. For example, surface dyslexics incorrectly regularize exception words ("pint" is pronounced to rhyme with "mint") but correctly name regular words. Regularized pronunciations of exception words dissociate the sublexical module (the source of regularization errors) from the damaged or absent lexical module (the source of correct pronunciations). Alternatively, deep dyslexics produce visual errors ("bush" is pronounced as "brush") and semantic errors ("bush" is pronounced as "tree"). These errors were attributed to a dissociated but damaged lexical module.

Evidence from patient studies proved to be problematic, however. No general agreement emerged concerning which patients' deficits actually counted as dissociated components of word recognition. All of the patient case studies that concerned reading were challenged by competing theorists, who claimed that they did not actually dissociate synthetic versus analytic components or that they simply did not pertain to reading (Van Orden, Pennington, and Stone, 2001). More recent brain-imaging studies appear to have arrived at a similar impasse. No general agreement has emerged in the brain-imaging literature that uniformly implicates specific brain regions in a large sample of reading tasks. Indeed, small differences in reading tasks and experimental methods appear to implicate different brain regions in what appear, intuitively, to be very similar reading acts.

Additive Factors Method

As we have noted, dual-process theories emerged in the 1970s, when cognitive psychology was predominantly concerned with information processing. Within that framework, the mind was conceived as an information-processing device that could be described in a way much like a flowchart of information processing in a computer program. Simon (1973) described how complex systems, such as cognitive systems, could be partly decomposed if the system's components interact approximately linearly. If interactions (exchanges) between components are linear in their effect, then the components can be identified even if their internal dynamics are nonlinear. Cognitive components thus described work as a chain of single causes—a metaphorical extension of domino causality. Push the first domino in a chain of standing dominoes, and each will fall in its turn.

The previous theoretical rationale coincided with a methodological tool to individuate cognitive components: the *additive factors method*, proposed by Sternberg (1969). Factorial experiments allow simultaneous manipulations of candidate variables that may influence distinct hypothetical components. The main effects of two or more manipulations are additive if they add up to the total behavioral effect. In this idealization, separate experimental manipulations selectively influence (e.g., slow) the falling times of separate "dominoes." Alternatively, when nonadditive interaction effects are observed, manipulations do not satisfy the assumption of selective influence and influence (at least) one component in common. Thus, to Sternberg's lasting credit, his method included an empirical failure point: ubiquitous nonadditive interaction effects.

Additive main effects are rarely observed in reading experiments. It is not possible to manipulate all factors simultaneously in one experiment, but it is possible to trace chains of nonadditive interactions across published experiments that preclude the assignment of any factors to distinct components. For example, factorial manipulations of word frequency and regularity yield nonadditive interaction effects. This raises the question of whether the respective effects actually arise from separate synthetic and analytic processes.

Parallel Distributed Processing Models

Parallel distributed processing (PDP) models allowed a new position in the debate, because they did not require distinct synthetic and analytic processes (Seidenberg, 1995). PDP models are connectionist models in which constraints (connection weights) determine the activation values of nodes. Nodes represent words' spellings, pronunciations, or meanings, and patterns of response times are simulated in a model's *error term* (the difference between a model's pronunciation, for example, and an ideal correct pattern of pronunciation-node activation). A learning algorithm shapes a matrix of connection weights to reflect statistical relationships among node representations. This is referred to as statistical or *covariant learning*. PDP models introduced covariant learning algorithms to a broad audience of cognitive scientists. PDP models were equally important as existence proofs, which advanced the synthetic/analytic question. Covariant learning may reflect, in a single process, both subword (analytic) and whole-word (synthetic) covariation, as we illustrate next.

Distinctions in the relationships among English spellings and pronunciations, at a variety of scales, may all be construed as statistical relationships. Covariant learning tracks all scales of covariation, simultaneously, in the connection weights of a PDP model (Plaut et al., 1996). For example, consonant spellings and pronunciations are more reliably correlated than vowel spellings and pronunciations, and in both cases, there are statistically dominant and subordinate relationships. "Regular" words, comprising dominant relationships, are named more quickly than "exception" words that include subordinate relationships. Likewise, spelling bodies (e.g., the spelling pattern "-uck" in "duck") and pronunciation rimes (e.g., pronunciation /uk/ in /duk/) are invariantly correlated; but some other body-rime relationships are dominant though less

strongly correlated ("-int" pronounced as in "mint"); and still other body-rimes are subordinate and only weakly correlated ("-int" pronounced as in "pint"). This rank order is corroborated in naming times; words like "duck" are named faster than words like "mint," and words like "mint" are named faster than words like "pint" (all other things being equal). Finally, a word's relative frequency estimates the strength of the relationship between the word's (whole-word) spelling and pronunciation; high-frequency words are named faster than low-frequency words.

As the examples illustrate, the outcome of covariant learning will be determined by the pattern of statistical relationships in a *training set*—the sample of words used to train the model. Each training set entails a sample of constraints (relationships between spelling, phonology, and meaning) from the body of constraints in a literate culture, and covariant learning attunes the network to the sampled constraints. Thus, implicit in the training set is a description of the cultural artifact—a particular language's pattern of relationships—that is crucial for cognitive theory. Jared (1997) used this implication of PDP models to derive a nonintuitive empirical test. Careful attention to statistical relationships among the spellings and pronunciations of high-frequency words predicted a statistical advantage for high-frequency words with invariant body-rime relationships. Jared subsequently corroborated this prediction—a previously unobserved "regularity" effect in naming for high-frequency words. However, no such effect was observed in a lexical decision experiment.

Hybrid, partially recurrent, connectionist models moved the PDP approach further in the direction of fully recurrent, iterative, "neural" network models. In a hybrid model, the output of nonrecurrent (strictly feedforward) portions of a PDP network sets the initial conditions in a recurrent subnetwork that includes feedback connections. The recurrent portion behaves as an attractor network, tuned to fixed points that correspond to word pronunciations (for example), and pronunciation times are simulated in the number of iterations before the network reaches a "stable" attractor.

Partly "damaged" hybrid networks simulated the bizarre semantic and visual errors of deep dyslexic patients as well as the regularization errors of surface dyslexics. Simulated lesions have been implemented in several ways, including (a) random cutting of some connections between nodes, (b) random changes in connection weights, and (c) random selection of nodes whose values are fixed at zero. The various patterns of dyslexic patient's naming errors have been mimicked by using one or combinations of these simulated lesions.

Iterative Network Models

Hybrid feedforward PDP models were actually proposed as a first step toward fully recurrent, iterative networks. Iterative networks are attractor networks simulated as nonlinear iterative maps. A nonlinear iterative map may approximate solutions of a system of nonlinear differential equations. Thus, iterative network models, as dynamical systems, invoke the most sophisticated mathematical framework available to scientists (Farmer, 1990). An iterative map takes its output at one time step as input on the next time step until a stable pattern of node activity emerges—an attractor state. A stable attractor state corresponds to an iterative model's naming response.

Iterative network models may include covariant learning algorithms that reflect relationships that map from patterns of spelling to pronunciations and from pronunciations to spelling patterns (and meanings). Invariant, bidirectional relationships correspond to stable attractors in the network, which extends the previous view of statistical relationships among spellings and pronunciations. Some consonants have invariant bidirectional relationships with their pronunciations. For example, the grapheme B at the beginning of a word is always pronounced /b/, and the /b/ pronunciation is always spelled B. Likewise, some spelling-body pronunciation-rime relationships are invariant (e.g., "-uck" and /uk/, as in "duck," always co-occur). And most words have a bidirectional invariant relationship between their particular whole-word spelling and their particular pronunciation. As we noted, invariant bidirectional relationships correspond to stable attractor states in an iterative network. By contrast, ambiguous spelling-pronunciation relationships correspond to multiple, mutually inconsistent *multistable*, or more precisely *metastable*, attractor states in an iterative network.

Empirical studies of nonlinear systems typically focus on their less stable behavioral regimes, because very stable regimes reveal less of system dynamics. Pioneering studies have examined how ambiguous relationships between spelling and pronunciation affect empirical patterns in naming performance. By definition, the relationship between spelling and phonology is ambiguous if more than one reliable pronunciation is elicited by the same spelling. For example, a homograph, such as "wind," has two legitimate pronunciations and is thus an ambiguous spelling. In the case of "wind," its "regular" pronunciation (to rhyme with "pinned") is produced faster than its "exception" pronunciation (to rhyme with "find"). Thus, the dynamics of word naming must unfold in a way that respects this ordering.

Kawamoto and Zemblidge (1992) simulated homograph naming using an iterative network. Relationships (connections) among letter, phoneme, and semantic node families were recurrent (including both feedforward and feedback connections) and excitatory, but within each node family, recurrent connections were (predominantly) inhibitory. The multistable unfolding of homograph pronunciations was simulated as a transcritical bifurcation. In a transcritical bifurcation, for example, the two possible pronunciations of "wind" exchange stability at a bifurcation point. That is, initial dynamics unfold in favor of one potential solution, but over successive iterations, additional constraints (which may unfold on a slower time scale) begin to favor an alternative solution. In the case of "wind," the faster "regular" pronunciation reflected a strong local attractor between letter and phoneme nodes. However, coherent interactive activation among phoneme and semantic nodes slowly emerged to favor the "exception" pronunciation. The bifurcation point occurred when the balance of constraints switched to favor the "exception" pronunciation. At the bifurcation point, the "regular" pronunciation (attractor) exchanged stability with the "exception" pronunciation.

Discussion

The previous simulation of ambiguous homograph pronunciations as bifurcation phenomena illustrates how nonlinear dynamical systems theory has been applied to reading performance. However, empirical methods that are appropriate to nonlinear analysis are not widely applied. In large part, connectionism has inherited the empirical methods of information-processing psychology. However, statistical analyses that assume the general linear model and theories to be implemented as strongly nonlinear dynamical systems may be incompatible because they entail different notions of causality.

Previously, we discussed how the factorial logic of additive factors method assumes a one-way, domino-effect notion of causality. In contrast, bifurcation phenomena entail *circular causality*. Circular causality requires a strategic (not morphological) reduction of system behavior, due to emergent properties. In a strategic reduction, generic emergent properties may be found at multiple levels of systems, but emergent properties at "higher" levels do not reduce to causal properties of "lower" levels.

Plausible nonlinear models allow that it may not be productive, for scientific purposes, to view word recognition (or reading) as a component process, but linear methods are directed at the discovery of component processes. Moreover, the results of a vast linear analysis actually raise the question of whether a distinct process of word recognition may be distinguished. All reading tasks would seem to include word recognition, but they do not yield any converging pattern of word recognition effects.

Consider the word frequency effect in the lexical decision task, for example. The same set of words that produce a large word frequency effect in the lexical decision task may produce a reduced, or statistically unreliable, word frequency effect in naming (or other tasks). Within the lexical decision task itself, it is possible to modulate the word frequency effect by making the non-words more or less word-like (and, in turn, modulate nonadditive interaction effects among word frequency, regularity, and other variables). Across languages, Hebrew produces a larger word frequency (familiarity) effect than English, and English produces a larger effect than Serbo-Croatian (which tracks the analytic transparency of their print-to-sound relationships—less transparent equals larger frequency effect).

All empirical phenomena of word recognition appear to be conditioned by task, task demands, and reference language (Frost and Katz, 1992; Lukatela and Turvey, 1998). These nonadditive interactions allow the question of whether "word recognition effects" may be attributed to a distinct process of word recognition. Consider the previous examples together, within the guidelines of additive factors logic. Word recognition factors cannot be individuated from each other, and they cannot be individuated from the context of their occurrence (task, task demands, and language). Because additivity of task effects or language effects is never observed, we lack evidence that may individuate word recognition.

Despite these problems, most theorists, including connectionist theorists, share the intuition that a distinct separable component of word recognition may yet exist. We speculate, however, that the intuition persists because most cognitive theorists were trained exclusively in linear methods. If we are correct, then rigorous tests of iterative network models await a reliable logic of nonlinear analysis that is consistent with nonlinear dynamical systems theory and appropriate to reading performance. Thus, the historical question of analytic versus synthetic processes with which we began is replaced by the question of linear versus nonlinear dynamics—a question motivated in part by the success of nonlinear iterative network models.

Road Map: Linguistics and Speech Processing
Related Reading: Constituency and Recursion in Language; Developmental Disorders; Motor Theories of Perception

References

Farmer, J. D., 1990, A Rosetta Stone for connectionism, *Phys. D*, 42:153–187.
Frost, R., and Katz, L. (Eds.), 1992, *Orthography, Phonology, Morphology, and Meaning*, Amsterdam: North Holland. ◆
Jared, D., 1997, Spelling-sound consistency affects the naming of high-frequency words, *J. Mem. Lang.*, 36:505–529.
Kawamoto, A. H., and Zemblidge, J. H., 1992, Pronunciation of homographs, *J. Mem. Lang.*, 31:394–374.
Lukatela, G., and Turvey, M. T., 1998, Reading in two alphabets, *Am. Psychol.*, 53:1057–1072. ◆
Mattingly, I. G., 1992, Linguistic awareness and orthographic form, in *Orthography, Phonology, Morphology, and Meaning* (R. Frost and L. Katz, Eds.), Amsterdam: North-Holland, pp. 11–26.
Neisser, U., 1967, *Cognitive Psychology*, Englewood Cliffs, NJ: Prentice Hall. ◆
Perfetti, C. A., 1985, *Reading Ability*, New York: Oxford University Press. ◆
Pennington, B. F., 1991, *Diagnosing Learning Disorders: A Neuropsychological Framework*, New York: Guilford Press. ◆
Plaut, D. C., McClelland, J. L., Seidenberg, M. S., and Patterson, K., 1996, Understanding normal and impaired word reading: Computational principles in quasi-regular domains, *Psychol. Rev.*, 103:56–115.

Rayner, K., and Pollatsek, A., 1989, *The Psychology of Reading*, Englewood Cliffs, NJ: Prentice Hall. ◆

Seidenberg, M. S., 1995, Visual word recognition: An overview, in *Speech, Language, and Communication* (J. L. Miller and P. D. Eimas, Eds.), New York: Academic Press, pp. 137–179.

Simon, H. A., 1973, The organization of complex systems, in *The Chal-lenge of Complex Systems* (H. H. Pattee, Ed.), New York: George Braziller, pp. 1–27.

Sternberg, S., 1969, The discovery of processing stages: Extensions of Donders' method, *Acta Psychol.*, 30:276–315.

Van Orden, G. C., Pennington, B. F., and Stone, G. O., 2001. What do double dissociations prove? *Cogn. Sci.*, 25:111–172.

Recurrent Networks: Learning Algorithms

Kenji Doya

Introduction

The backpropagation algorithm for feedforward networks (Figure 1A) has been successfully applied to a wide range of problems, from neuroscience to consumer electronics (see BACKPROPAGATION: GENERAL PRINCIPLES). However, what can be implemented by a feedforward network is just a static mapping of the input vectors. The human brain, however, is not a stateless input-output system but a high-dimensional nonlinear dynamical system. In order to model dynamical functions of the brain, or to design a machine that performs as well as a brain does, it is essential to utilize a system that is capable of storing internal states and implementing complex dynamics.

This is why learning algorithms for *recurrent neural networks* (Figure 1B), which have feedback connections and time delays, have been studied with enthusiasm. In a recurrent network, the state of the system can be encoded in the activity pattern of the units and a wide variety of dynamical behaviors can be programmed by the connection weights.

A popular subclass of recurrent networks is those with symmetric connection weights. In this case, the network dynamics is guaranteed to converge to a minimum of "energy" function (see ENERGY FUNCTIONALS FOR NEURAL NETWORKS and COMPUTING WITH ATTRACTORS). Typical examples are associative memory networks (see ASSOCIATIVE NETWORKS), optimization networks (see OPTIMIZATION, NEURAL), and WINNER-TAKE-ALL NETWORKS (q.v.).

However, steady-state solutions are only a limited portion of the capabilities of recurrent networks. A recurrent network can serve as a sequence recognition system (see LANGUAGE PROCESSING) or as a sequential pattern generator (see MOTOR PATTERN GENERATION and SEQUENCE LEARNING). More generally, it is capable of transforming an input sequence into some other output sequence (see TEMPORAL PATTERN PROCESSING). It can be used as a nonlinear filter (see KALMAN FILTERING: NEURAL IMPLICATIONS), a nonlinear controller (see IDENTIFICATION AND CONTROL), or a finite-state machine (see LANGUAGE PROCESSING).

This article reviews the learning algorithms for training recurrent networks. There are three major frameworks of learning: *supervised learning*, based on the output error signal, *reinforcement learning*, based on the scalar reward signal, and *unsupervised learning*, based on the statistical feature of the input signal. Our main focus will be on supervised learning algorithms for recurrent networks. We also provide a brief overview of reinforcement and unsupervised learning algorithms.

Supervised Learning Algorithms

The problem setup of supervised learning in recurrent networks is similar to the case of feedforward networks: a network is given a desired output for an input. An error function is defined and its gradient with respect to the weights is derived. However, the major difference is that the input and output are not static vectors but *time sequences*.

For example, in the recurrent network shown in Figure 1B, units 1 and 2 are output units; units 3, 4, and 5 are hidden units; and units 6 and 7 are input units. A small change of a connection weight, say w_{43} (shown as black dot), affects the output units, say unit 1, not only through the direct connection from unit 4 to 1 (thick black line), but also through indirect connections, through units 2, 3, and 5 (thick gray lines), and through infinitely many multistep paths with multiple delays. It makes exact calculation of output error gradient rather complex.

One simple strategy is to neglect all the indirect paths. In this case, although the network state evolves according to the recurrent network, as in Figure 1B, a simple backpropagation algorithm is

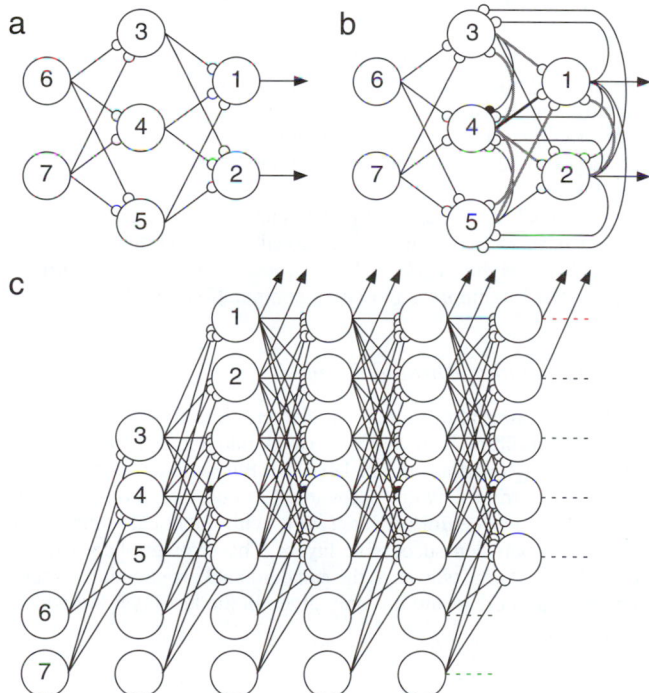

Figure 1. Examples of a feedforward network (*A*) and a recurrent network (*B*), where units 1 and 2 are output units; units 3, 4, and 5 are hidden units; and units 6 and 7 are input units. The multistep operation of a recurrent network (*B*) can be unrolled as a multilayer feedforward network (*C*).

applied by regarding it as a feedforward network, as in Figure 1A. Such coarse approximation methods turned out to be effective in work on language acquisition using *simple recurrent networks* that have recurrent connections between hidden units (see LANGUAGE PROCESSING).

There are two basic ways to calculate the exact gradient of the output with respect to the weights: forward methods and backward methods. Forward methods estimate the effects of a small change in a weight on the network state trajectory in the form of a linear dynamical equation system. This can be calculated concurrently with the network dynamic, and thus is useful for on-line learning. A drawback is the amount of computation needed to update a set of dynamical equations for each weight.

Backward methods estimate the causes of the output error backward in time. In discrete-time case, this method is realized by "unrolling" the multistep evolution of the network state as a multilayer feedforward network, as in Figure 1C, and applying the standard backpropagation algorithm (Rumelhart, Hinton, and Williams, 1986). In continuous-time cases it is done by running a set of "adjoint systems" backward in time. Although the method requires asynchronous operation, with the evolution and storage of the state trajectory done first and the error gradient calculation done afterwards, the amount of computation is much less than in the forward methods (see Pearlmutter, 1995, for a comprehensive review). In the following sections, we formulate these algorithms for both discrete-time and continuous-time models, and then discuss technical problems in using them.

Discrete-Time Model

We will start with a discrete-time recurrent network with n units and m inputs. We denote the state of the ith unit by y_i and the connection weights from the jth to the ith unit by w_{ij}. Both external inputs u_j and recurrent inputs y_j are represented as z_j for convenience:

$$y_i(t + 1) = f\left(\sum_{j=1}^{n+m} w_{ij} z_j(t)\right) \quad (i = 1, \ldots, n)$$

$$z_j(t) = \begin{cases} y_j(t), & j \leq n \\ u_{j-n}, & j > n \end{cases} \quad (1)$$

The output nonlinearity $f(\ )$ is usually a squashing function, such as $f(x) = 1/(1 + e^{-x})$ and $f(x) = \tanh x$, whose derivatives are conveniently given by $f'(x) = f(x)(1 - f(x))$ and $f'(x) = 1 - f(x)^2$, respectively. We can introduce a bias parameter by assuming that one of the inputs u_j is constant.

The goal of learning is to set the parameters w_{ij} so that the output trajectory $(y_1(t), \ldots, y_n(t))$ follows a desired trajectory $(d_1(t), \ldots, d_n(t))(t = 1, \ldots, T)$ with a given initial state $(y_1(0), \ldots, y_n(0))$ and an input sequence $(u_1(t), \ldots, u_m(t))(t = 0, \ldots, T - 1)$. We define the error function

$$E = \sum_{t=1}^{T} \sum_{i=1}^{n} \mu_i(t) \tfrac{1}{2} (y_i(t) - d_i(t))^2 \quad (2)$$

and perform gradient descent on E with respect to the weights w_{ij}. The masking function $\mu_i(t)$ specifies which components of the trajectory are to be supervised at what time. In a typical case, $\mu_i(t) \equiv 1$ for output units and $\mu_i(t) \equiv 0$ for hidden units. When only the end point of the trajectory is specified, $\mu_i(T) = 1$ and $\mu_i(t) = 0$ for $t < T$.

Real-Time Recurrent Learning

The effect of weight change on the network dynamics can be seen by simply differentiating the network dynamics equation (Equation 1) by a weight w_{kl} (Williams and Zipser, 1989).

$$\frac{\partial y_i(t + 1)}{\partial w_{kl}} = f'(x_i(t))\left[\sum_{j=1}^{n} w_{ij} \frac{\partial y_j(t)}{\partial w_{kl}} + \delta_{ik} z_l(t)\right]$$
$$(i = 1, \ldots, n) \quad (3)$$

where $x_i(t) = \sum_{j=1}^{n+m} w_{ij} z_j(t)$ is the net input to the unit and δ_{ik} is Kronecker's delta ($\delta_{ik} = 1$ if $i = k$ and otherwise 0). The term $\delta_{ik} z_l(t)$ represents an *explicit* effect of the weight w_{kl} on the unit k, and the term $\sum_{j=1}^{n} w_{ij}(\partial y_j(t)/\partial w_{kl})$ represents an *implicit* effect on all the units because of network dynamics.

Equation 3 for each unit $i = 1, \ldots, n$ constitutes an n-dimensional linear dynamical system (with time-varying coefficients), where $((\partial y_1/\partial w_{kl}), \ldots, (\partial y_n/\partial w_{kl}))$ is taken as a dynamical variable. Since the initial state $y_i(0)$ of the network is independent of the connection weights, the appropriate initial condition for Equation 3 is

$$\frac{\partial y_i(0)}{\partial w_{kl}} = 0 \quad (i = 1, \ldots, n)$$

Thus, we can compute $\partial y_i(t)/\partial w_{kl}$ *forward in time* by iterating Equation 3 simultaneously with the network dynamics (Equation 1). From this solution, we can calculate the error gradient as follows:

$$\frac{\partial E}{\partial w_{kl}} = \sum_{t=1}^{T} \sum_{i=1}^{n} \mu_i(t)(y_i(t) - d_i(t)) \frac{\partial y_i(t)}{\partial w_{kl}} \quad (4)$$

A standard *batch* gradient descent algorithm is to accumulate the error gradient by Equation 4 and update each weight w_{kl} by

$$w_{kl} := w_{kl} - \varepsilon \frac{\partial E}{\partial w_{kl}} \quad (5)$$

where $\varepsilon > 0$ is a learning rate parameter.

An alternative update scheme is the gradient descent of *current* output error $\sum_{i=1}(\tfrac{1}{2})\mu_i(t)(y_i(t) - d_i(t))^2$ at each time step, namely,

$$w_{kl}(t + 1) = w_{kl}(t) - \varepsilon \sum_{i=1}^{n} \mu_i(t)(y_i(t) - d_i(t)) \frac{\partial y_i(t)}{\partial w_{kl}} \quad (6)$$

Note that we assumed that w_{kl} is a constant, not a dynamical variable, in deriving Equation 3, so we have to keep the learning rate ε small enough. However, this on-line update scheme was shown to be effective on a number of temporal learning tasks (Williams and Zipser, 1989), and it is often called *real-time recurrent learning*.

A drawback to this error gradient calculation forward in time is that we have to solve an n-dimensional system (Equation 3) for each of the weights $w_{kl}(k = 1, \ldots, n; l = 1, \ldots, n + m)$. It requires $O(n^3)$ memories and $O(n^4)$ computations.

Backpropagation Through Time

Another learning algorithm for a discrete-time model can be derived by "unfolding" a recurrent network into a multilayer network (Figure 1C) (Rumelhart et al., 1986). In this scheme, T-step iteration of a recurrent network is regarded as one sweep of operation in a T-layered feedforward network with identical connection weights w_{ij} between successive layers. The error gradient can be derived in the same way as in the standard backpropagation, except that the output errors are not only given in the last layer but added in each layer:

$$\frac{\partial E}{\partial y_i(t)} = \sum_{j=1}^{n} \frac{\partial E}{\partial y_j(t + 1)} f'(x_j(t))w_{ji} + \mu_i(t)(y_i(t) - d_i(t))$$
$$(i = 1, \ldots, n) \quad (7)$$

Since the error E is independent of the state at $t > T$, the boundary condition for Equation 7 is given at the final time step as

$$\frac{\partial E}{\partial y_i(T + 1)} = 0 \quad (i = 1, \ldots, n)$$

Thus, the learning equation (Equation 7) can be iterated *backward in time* from $t = T$ to 1.

From the solution $\partial E/\partial y_i$, the error gradients are given by

$$\frac{\partial E}{\partial w_{ij}} = \sum_{t=1}^{T} \frac{\partial E}{\partial y_i(t)} f'(x_i(t - 1))z_j(t - 1) \quad (8)$$

and the weights are updated in a batch using Equation 5.

The advantage of this algorithm is that we have to solve only one n-dimensional system, Equation 7, for adjusting all the weights. Therefore, only $O(n^2)$ computations are required. However, since the learning equation, Equation 7, has to be solved *backward* in time, we cannot update the weights on-line, and we have to store the history of the network state $y_i(t)$ ($i = 1, \ldots, n; t = 1, \ldots T$), which requires $O(nT)$ memories.

Continuous-Time Model

A continuous-time model is a natural choice for modeling systems that are governed by differential equations. Time constants of continuous-time models are convenient parameters for setting local memory spans for individual units. They can also be adjusted by learning, as discussed later.

Slightly different versions of continuous-time models have been studied. Here, we focus on the following model (Pearlmutter, 1989),

$$\tau_i \dot{y}_i(t) = -y_i(t) + f\left(\sum_{j=1}^{n+m} w_{ij}z_j(t)\right) \quad (i, = 1, \ldots, n)$$

$$z_j(t) = \begin{cases} y_j(t), & j \le n \\ u_{j-n}, & j > n \end{cases} \quad (9)$$

However, similar derivations apply to other models as well (Doya and Yoshizawa, 1989).

We define an error integral

$$E = \int_0^T \sum_{i=1}^n \mu_i(t) \, \tfrac{1}{2} \, (y_i(t) - d_i(t))^2 dt \quad (10)$$

and derive a gradient descent algorithm for minimizing E for a desired trajectory $(d_1(t), \ldots, d_n(t))(0 \le t \le T)$ with a given initial state $(y_1(0), \ldots, y_n(0))$ and an input sequence $(u_1(t), \ldots, u_m(t))$.

Variation Method

The effect of a change in a weight w_{kl} on the state $y_i(t)$ can be estimated by differentiating Equation 9, the network dynamics equation, as follows:

$$\tau_i \frac{d}{dt}\left(\frac{\partial y_i}{\partial w_{kl}}\right) = -\frac{\partial y_i}{\partial w_{kl}} + f'(x_i(t))\left[\sum_{j=1}^n w_{ij}\frac{\partial y_j}{\partial w_{kl}} + \delta_{ik}z_l(t)\right] \quad (i = 1, \ldots, n) \quad (11)$$

This forms an n-dimensional linear differential equation system with the state variable $((\partial y_1/\partial w_{kl}), \ldots, (\partial y_n/\partial w_{kl}))$ and is called a *variation system* of the network dynamics equation, Equation 9. The initial condition for this system is given by

$$\frac{\partial y_i(0)}{\partial w_{kl}} = 0 \quad (i = 1, \ldots, n)$$

because the initial state of the network is independent of the weights. We can numerically integrate Equation 11 forward in time concurrently with the network dynamics in Equation 9.

From the solution $(\partial y_i(t)/\partial w_{kl})(0 \le t \le T)$, the error gradient is given by

$$\frac{\partial E}{\partial w_{ij}} = \int_0^T \sum_{i=1}^n \mu_i(t)(y_i(t) - d_i(t)) \frac{\partial y_i(t)}{\partial w_{kl}} dt \quad (12)$$

We can use either the batch update scheme (Equation 5) at the end of a sequence, or the on-line update scheme

$$\dot{w}_{kl} = -\varepsilon \sum_{i=1}^n \mu_i(t)(y_i(t) - d_i(t)) \frac{\partial y_i(t)}{\partial w_{kl}} \quad (13)$$

with sufficiently small learning rate $\varepsilon > 0$.

The error gradient for a time constant τ_k is given by the following variation equation:

$$\tau_i \frac{d}{dt}\left(\frac{\partial y_i}{\partial \tau_k}\right) = -\frac{\partial y_i}{\partial \tau_k} + f'(x_i(t))\left[\sum_{j=1}^n w_{ij}\frac{\partial y_j}{\partial \tau_k} - \delta_{ik}\dot{y}_k(t)\right] \quad (i = 1, \ldots, n) \quad (14)$$

Adjoint Method

The backward algorithm for a continuous-time model can be derived in several ways, for example, by finite difference approximation (Pearlmutter, 1989). Here we derive the algorithm as an "adjoint" system of the forward learning equation, Equation 11.

A pair of n-dimensional linear systems

$$\dot{p} = A(t)p + b(t) \quad \text{and} \quad \dot{q} = -A^*(t)q - c(t)$$

are called *adjoint* to each other, where A^* denotes the transpose of matrix A. A useful property of adjoint systems is that their solutions satisfy the following *Green's equality*:

$$\int_0^T q(t) \cdot b(t)dt - \int_0^T c(t) \cdot p(t)dt = q(T) \cdot p(T) - q(0) \cdot p(0)$$

We can actually compose an adjoint system of the variation equation, Equation 11,

$$\dot{q}_i = \frac{q_i(t)}{\tau_i} - \sum_{j=1}^n \frac{f'(x_j(t))}{\tau_j} w_{ji}q_j(t) - \mu_i(t)(y_i(t) - d_i(t)) \quad (15)$$

where we put $p_i = (\partial y_i/\partial w_{kl})$, $A_{ij}(t) = (f'(x_i(t))/\tau_i)w_{ij} - (\delta_{ij}/\tau_i)$, $b_i(t) = (f'(x_i(t))/\tau_i)\delta_{ik}y_l(t)$, and $c_i(t) = \mu_i(t)(y_i(t) - d_i(t))$. With the boundary conditions $p_i(0) = (\partial y_i(0)/\partial w_{kl}) = 0$ and $q_i(T) = 0$, Green's equality becomes

$$\int_0^T \sum_{i=1}^n q_i(t) \frac{f'(x_i(t))}{\tau_i} \delta_{ik}y_l(t)dt =$$
$$\int_0^T \sum_{i=1}^n \mu_i(t)(y_i(t) - d_i(t)) \frac{\partial y_i}{\partial w_{kl}} dt \quad (16)$$

Note that the right-hand side is identical to the error gradient (Equation 12). Thus, we have an alternative form of the error gradient

$$\frac{\partial E}{\partial w_{kl}} = \int_0^T q_k(t) \frac{f'(x_k(t))}{\tau_k} z_l(t)dt \quad (17)$$

Similarly, the error gradient for a time constant is given by

$$\frac{\partial E}{\partial \tau_k} = \int_0^T q_k(t) \frac{f'(x_k(t))}{\tau_k} (-\dot{y}_k(t))dt \quad (18)$$

As in the discrete-time case, we first run the network dynamics (Equation 9) forward in time and then run the adjoint system (Equation 15) backward in time with the terminal condition $q_i(T) = 0$. The weights are updated in batch by Equation 5.

Technical Remarks

Forward or Backward?

The forward algorithms require $O(n^4)$ computations. Therefore, it is not suitable for a fully connected network with tens or hundreds of units. However, for a small-sized network or a network with only local connections, on-line weight update can be an advantage.

In order to allow on-line weight update with the efficiency of the backward algorithm, a truncated version of the backpropagation-through-time algorithm has been proposed (Schmidhuber, 1992)

Teacher Forcing

The so-called teacher forcing technique has been shown to be helpful, especially in training a network into an autonomous dynamical system (Doya and Yoshizawa, 1989; Williams and Zipser, 1989). In this scheme, the desired output $d_i(t)$ is used to drive the network dynamics in place of the feedback of its actual output $y_i(t)$.

The reasons for needing teacher forcing are:

- The state of the network is assigned to the desired one of the many attractor domains.
- In learning oscillatory patterns, unless the phase of the network output is synchronized to the teacher signal, there will be an apparently large error (Doya and Yoshizawa, 1989).
- It will avoid a local minimum solution of static output at the mean value of the dynamic teacher signal (Williams and Zipser, 1989).
- The linearized equation for a limit cycle trajectory is not asymptotically stable if the system is running autonomously (Doya, 1992).

One problem with this technique is that the trajectory learned with teacher forcing may not be stable when the network is run autonomously after learning. Several heuristics have been proposed for enhancing the stability of the nonforced trajectory:

Noisy forcing: Add some noise to the forcing input.
Partial forcing: Use a mixed input $z_i(t) = y_i(t) + \alpha(d_i(t) - y_i(t))$ with $0 < \alpha < 1$ and decrease the forcing rate α with the progress of learning.
Part-time forcing: Turn on forcing to synchronize the network to the teacher, and then turn off forcing to train the autonomous trajectory.

Bifurcation Boundaries

In many learning tasks, the goal is not only to replicate particular sample trajectories but to reconstruct some *attractors* in the state space, such as fixed points, limit cycles, and chaotic attractors.

For example, when a network is trained as a finite-state machine, it must have distinct attractors in order to represent discrete states. As another example, when a network is trained as a periodic oscillator, it must have a limit cycle attractor. When we gradually change network parameters, we expect that the shape and location of the attractors will change continuously. However, that is not always true. At some points in the parameter space, attractors can emerge, disappear, or change their stability. Such a phenomenon is known as *bifurcation* in nonlinear systems theory (see DYNAMICS AND BIFURCATION IN NEURAL NETS and CANONICAL NEURAL MODELS).

With some kinds of bifurcation, such as saddle-node bifurcation, the state of the network changes drastically. Even if the equilibrium or the trajectory persists, the linearized equations that are used for gradient computation can lose asymptotic stability. Accordingly, when the network goes through a bifurcation point, the solution of the learning equation can grow rapidly, and the gradient descent algorithm can be unstable (Doya, 1992).

Although this might sound like a rare, pathetic situation, bifurcation is actually an inevitable step in many learning tasks (Doya,

1992). If the connection weights w_{ij} are initialized with small random values, the network dynamics has a single global attractor point. In order to have multiple attractor domains or a limit cycle, the network must go through some bifurcation boundary. Conversely, until the network goes through an appropriate bifurcation, even a simple memory task can be very difficult, owing to exponential decay of the error gradient.

Incremental Training

It has been reported that gradual increase in the complexity of training examples is critical for successfully training a network as a finite-state machine (see LANGUAGE ACQUISITION). A possible reason for this is that a network can acquire memory mechanisms only gradually, by going through bifurcation boundaries. If we impose examples that require many internal states with a long time delay from the beginning, we might simply mess up the network. This problem of the developmental capability of recurrent networks needs further examination.

Discussion

A fully connected recurrent neural network is potentially a very powerful system for temporal information processing. Based on the universal approximation theorem for three-layered networks (see UNIVERSAL APPROXIMATORS), it has been shown that a recurrent network can, with enough units, approximate any dynamical system (Funahashi and Nakamura, 1993). It has also been shown that a recurrent neural network, with its analog-valued computation, can have super-Turing computational power (see NEURAL AUTOMATA AND ANALOG COMPUTATIONAL COMPLEXITY). However, these theories do not guarantee that such a network can be readily realized by error gradient descent learning.

As already mentioned, the error gradient can decay or expand exponentially in time, which makes gradient descent more difficult than in the case of feedforward networks. Convergence of learning depends critically on the choice of network topology, initial weights, and the choice of training samples. These are some of the reasons why networks with specialized architectures have been crafted for specific problems, for example, networks with tapped delay-lines or local recurrent loops.

In a recent study of grammar learning (see LANGUAGE PROCESSING), recurrent neural networks were successfully trained to predict strings from context-free and context-sensitive languages (Rodriguez, 2001). In these examples, fractal structures in the network state space were utilized to approximate multiple "counters," which are necessary for processing complex grammatical structures such as palindromes. Interesting findings in such studies were that recurrent networks can generalize in terms of the depth of embedding.

Bayesian approaches have recently been applied to the learning of dynamics in recurrent networks (see BAYESIAN METHODS AND NEURAL NETWORKS; BAYESIAN NETWORKS; GRAPHICAL MODELS). A recurrent network can be trained by the method of extended Kalman filtering, which has properties similar to the RTRL algorithm with teacher forcing (Williams, 1992). EM methods for estimating the states of the hidden units and the weight parameters have been formulated (Ghahramani and Hinton, 2000). This seems to be a theoretically more sound way of nonlinear dynamical system estimation. However, since EM is essentially a local optimization process, whether this new wave of modeling methods can escape from the issue of bifurcation remains to be seen. Many recent approaches to temporal sequence processing are reviewed in Sun (2001) and other articles in the same book.

Figure 2. Network architectures of the cerebellum (*A*), the basal ganglia (*B*), and the cerebral cortex (*C*).

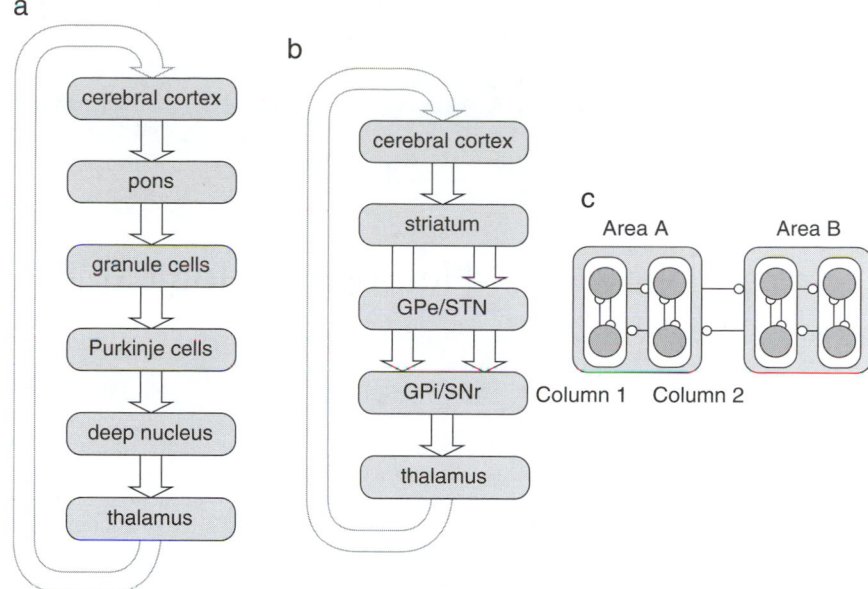

Biologically Inspired Learning Methods

It has been suggested that the network architectures of the cerebellum, the basal ganglia, and the cerebral cortex are specialized for different frameworks of learning, namely, the cerebellum for supervised learning, the basal ganglia for reinforcement learning, and cerebral cortex for unsupervised learning (Doya, 1999). The circuits of the cerebellum (Figure 2*A*) and the basal ganglia (Figure 2*B*) have roughly feedforward structures. While learning in the cerebellum is characterized by specific error signals carried by the climbing fibers to the Purkinje cells, learning in the basal ganglia is characterized by the reward signal broadcasted by the dopaminergic input to the striatum (see CEREBELLUM AND MOTOR CONTROL and BASAL GANGLIA). They both form long recurrent loops starting from and ending in the cerebral cortex. The circuit of the cerebral cortex is characterized by massive recurrent connections, within and between functional columns, and between cortical areas (Figure 2*C*). Learning in the cerebral cortex is characterized by Hebbian learning (see CORTICAL HEBBIAN MODULES). Since the cerebral cortex embodies the most successful application of recurrent networks, both within the cortex and in the corticocerebellar and cortico–basal ganglia recurrent loops, it is natural to try to draw insights from the cortical network architecture.

The combination of recurrent excitation and lateral inhibition can implement a winner-take-all mechanism (see WINNER-TAKE-ALL NETWORKS). In combination with Hebbian plasticity and certain regulatory mechanisms, self-organization of feature detectors can be achieved (see SELF-ORGANIZATION AND THE BRAIN; COMPETITIVE LEARNING; HEBBIAN LEARNING AND NEURONAL REGULATION). This basic framework is shared by recent studies of receptive field formation and INDEPENDENT COMPONENT ANALYSIS (q.v.), which combine bottom-up Hebbian plasticity with lateral or top-down anti-Hebbian plasticity (see PATTERN FORMATION, NEURAL; INDEPENDENT COMPONENT ANALYSIS; UNSUPERVISED LEARNING WITH GLOBAL OBJECTIVE FUNCTIONS).

The Boltzmann Machine (see SIMULATED ANNEALING AND BOLTZMANN MACHINES) with its wake and sleep modes, is another basic model of cortical processing. Its extension to layered recurrent networks, the Helmholtz machine, is capable of extracting the hidden structure of sensory data and reproducing the data by top-down processing (see HELMHOLTZ MACHINES AND SLEEP-WAKE LEARNING).

One of the main open issues in REINFORCEMENT LEARNING (q.v.) is how to learn a good behavior when the environmental states are not perfectly observable (see IDENTIFICATION AND CONTROL). In such a case, the agent should store a certain "belief state" and update it according to the model of the environment. Actions are chosen according to the predicted future reward based on the belief state. Such complex operations could be implemented in the corticocerebellar and corticobasal ganglia loops, with the cerebral cortex representing the belief state, the cerebellum implementing the internal model of the environment, and the basal ganglia predicting the future reward. Better understanding of the corticocerebellar–basal ganglia system may give some clue for designing an adaptive agent under uncertainty.

Road Map: Learning in Artificial Networks
Related Reading: Computing with Attractors; Dynamics and Bifurcation in Neural Nets; Dynamics of Association and Recall; Helmholtz Machines and Sleep-Wake Learning; Recurrent Networks: Neurophysiological Modeling; Simulated Annealing and Boltzmann Machines

References

Doya, K., 1992, Bifurcations in the learning of recurrent neural networks, in *Proceedings of the 1992 IEEE International Symposium on Circuits and Systems*, vol. 6, New York: IEEE, pp. 2777–2780.
Doya, K., 1999, What are the computations in the cerebellum, the basal ganglia, and the cerebral cortex? *Neural Netw.*, 12:961–974.
Doya, K., and Yoshizawa, S., 1989, Adaptive neural oscillator using continuous-time backpropagation learning, *Neural Netw.*, 2:375–386.
Elman, J. L., 1990, Finding structure in time, *Cognit. Sci.*, 14:179–211.
Funahashi, K., and Nakamura, Y., 1993, Approximation of dynamical systems by continuous time recurrent neural networks, *Neural Netw.*, 6:801–806.
Ghahramani, Z., and Hinton, G. E., 2000, Variational learning for switching state-space models, *Neural Comput.*, 12:831–864.
Pearlmutter, B. A., 1989, Learning state space trajectories in recurrent neural networks, *Neural Comput.*, 1:263–269.
Pearlmutter, B. A., 1995, Gradient calculations for dynamic recurrent neural networks: A survey, *IEEE Trans. Neural Netw.*, 6:1212–1228. ◆
Rodriguez, P., 2001, Simple recurrent networks learn context-free and context-sensitive languages by counting, *Neural Comput.*, 13:2093–2118.
Rumelhart, D. E., Hinton, G. E., and Williams, R. J., 1986, Learning representations by back-propagating errors, *Nature*, 323:533–536.

Schmidhuber, J., 1992, A fixed size storage $O(n^3)$ time complexity learning algorithm for fully recurrent continually running networks, *Neural Computat.*, 4:243–248.

Sun, R., 2001, Introduction to sequence learning, in *Sequence Learning: Paradigms, Algorithms, and Applications* (R. Sun and C. L. Giles, Eds.), New York: Springer-Verlag, pp. 1–10. ◆

Williams, R. J., 1992, Training recurrent networks using the extended Kalman filter, in *Proceedings of the International Joint Conference on Neural Networks*, vol. 4, Piscataway, NJ: IEEE, pp. 241–250.

Williams, R. J., and Zipser, D., 1989, A learning algorithm for continually running fully recurrent neural networks, *Neural Computat.*, 1:270–280.

Recurrent Networks: Neurophysiological Modeling

Eberhard E. Fetz and Larry E. Shupe

Introduction

Dynamic recurrent network models can provide invaluable tools to help systems neurophysiologists understand the neural mechanisms mediating behavior. They can help overcome the limitations of biological experiments, which typically provide limited samples of the system, such as anatomical structures and their connections, the effects of lesions on behavior, or the activity of single neurons in behaving animals. The missing element required to synthesize these pieces can be provided by neural network models of the complete system. New algorithms make it possible to derive networks that simulate dynamic sensorimotor behavior and incorporate anatomically appropriate recurrent connectivity. The resulting networks determine the remaining free parameters based on examples of the behavior itself.

Training procedures initially developed for feedforward networks have been extended to dynamic recurrent networks, which differ from other modeling approaches in three key properties. First, the units are *dynamic*, meaning they can exhibit time-varying activity that can represent the mean firing rates of single or multiple neurons, membrane potentials, or some relevant time-varying stimulus or motor parameter. Second, the networks can have *recurrent* connectivity, including feedback and cross-connections. Third, the network connections required to simulate a particular dynamic behavior can be derived from examples of the behavior by *gradient descent* methods, such as backpropagated error correction. The resulting models provide complete neural network solutions of the behavior, insofar as they determine all the connections and activations of the units that simulate the behavior.

Neural networks that emulate particular dynamic behaviors basically transform spatiotemporal inputs into appropriate spatiotemporal outputs. These networks are usually comprised of interconnected "sigmoidal" units (units whose outputs are sigmoidal functions of their inputs); this mimics a biological neuron's property of saturating at maximal rates for large inputs and decreasing to zero for low inputs.

To illustrate the training procedure, Figure 1 shows a representative network of such units, with input and output patterns that simulate a target-tracking task. Four input units carry signals representing the step changes in target locations; eight output patterns represent the firing rates of motor units in monkeys tracking such targets. To train the network, the synaptic weights between units are initially assigned randomly and the output response of the network is determined. The difference between network output patterns N(t) and the desired target output activations T(t) is the error E(t). The backpropagation algorithm calculates the weight changes that would reduce this error, and therefore implements a "gradient descent" of the error as a function of the weights (Figure 1, inset). The process of presenting input patterns and changing the weights to reduce the remaining error is iterated until the network converges on a solution with minimal error. Various training methods for recurrent networks are presented in Williams and Zipser (1989) (see also RECURRENT NETWORKS: LEARNING ALGORITHMS). It should be recognized that backpropagation is not a model for biological learning, simply an effective method of obtaining a solution. Biologically plausible learning algorithms will also find the same solutions, but usually take longer (Mazzoni, Andersen, and Jordan, 1991; see also REINFORCEMENT LEARNING IN MOTOR CONTROL).

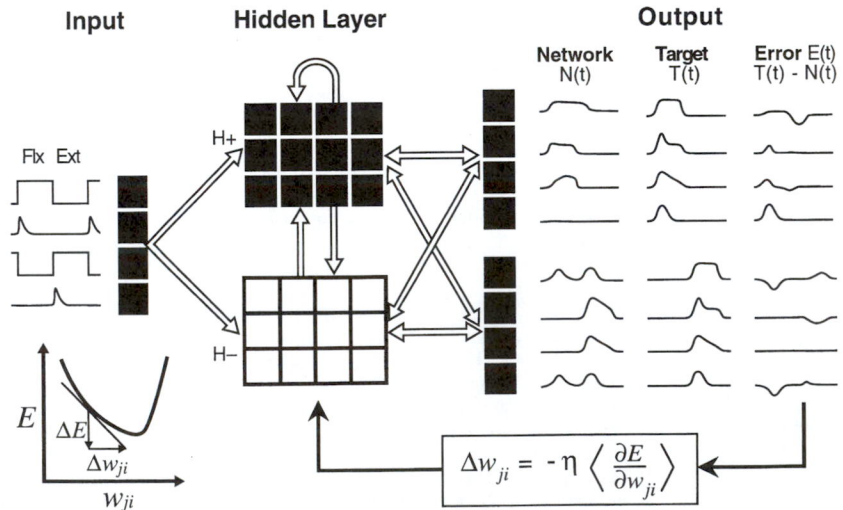

Input **Hidden Layer** **Output**

Network N(t)   Target T(t)   Error E(t) T(t) - N(t)

Flx Ext

H+

H−

E ΔE Δw_{ji} w_{ji}

$$\Delta w_{ji} = -\eta \left\langle \frac{\partial E}{\partial w_{ji}} \right\rangle$$

Figure 1. Typical network architecture and training procedure used with dynamic recurrent networks. This network simulates the step-tracking task. The network input consists of four representations of the step target position and target change; the output represents the firing patterns of eight representative motor units in flexor and extensor muscles. The intervening hidden units consist of excitatory and inhibitory groups, with distributed connections indicated by the open arrows. Network training proceeds by calculating the difference between the network output [N(t)] and the desired target activations [T(t)], and changing the connection weights in such a way as to reduce the error [E(t)]. Inset at lower left illustrates the error as a function of one weight, and how the gradient of this function is used to determine the appropriate weight change.

Other algorithms, such as genetic algorithms (see LOCOMOTION, VERTEBRATE) or random weight perturbations (Arnold and Robinson, 1991), can also be applied when the unit input-output functions are not differentiable.

Applications

The applications of these dynamic recurrent networks fall into three general categories:

1. *Pattern recognition* applications involve sorting of spatiotemporal input patterns into discrete categories. A set of input units receiving time-varying signals can represent a spatiotemporal pattern, and the output codes the appropriate categories.

2. *Pattern generation* networks produce temporal patterns in one or more output units, either autonomously or under the control of a gating input. These include oscillating networks (Williams and Zipser, 1989) and simulations of central pattern generators (Tsung, Cottrell, and Selverston, 1990; Rowat and Selverston, 1993; Lansner, Kotaleski, and Grillner, 1998; see also ACTIVITY-DEPENDENT REGULATION OF NEURONAL CONDUCTANCES).

3. *Pattern transformation* networks convert spatiotemporal input patterns into spatiotemporal outputs. Examples include simulations of the leech withdrawal reflex (Lockery and Sejnowski, 1992), step target tracking in the primate (Fetz, 1993), the vestibulo-ocular reflex (Arnold and Robinson, 1991; Lisberger and Sejnowski, 1992) and short-term memory tasks (Zipser, 1991; Moody et al., 1998). Recurrent networks can also simulate analytical transforms such as integration and differentiation of input signals (Munro, Shupe, and Fetz, 1994).

Oscillating Networks

Among the many examples of autonomously generated periodic motor activity to be found in biological systems are locomotion, mastication, and respiration. The neural circuitry underlying cyclic periodic movements has been called a *central pattern generator* (CPG). Williams and Zipser (1989) first trained dynamic recurrent networks to generate oscillatory activity with various frequencies. The smallest circuit that sustained quasi-sinusoidal oscillations consisted of two interconnected sigmoidal units.

Tsung et al. (1990) trained a network with the connectivity and sign constraints of neurons in the lobster gastric mill circuit to simulate their oscillatory activity. This network replicated the correct phase relations of the biological interneurons. If its activity was perturbed, the network reverted to the original pattern, indicating that the weights found by the learning algorithm represented a strong limit cycle attractor. Dynamic recurrent networks simulating the oscillatory activity of the gastric mill circuit have shown remarkably robust abilities to mimic the observed patterns (Rowat and Selverston, 1993; see also ACTIVITY-DEPENDENT REGULATION OF NEURONAL CONDUCTANCES).

Primate Target Tracking

We used dynamic networks to simulate the neural circuitry controlling forelimb muscles of the primate. In monkeys performing a step-tracking task, physiological experiments documented the discharge patterns and output connections of task-related neurons. Premotoneural (PreM) cells were identified by postspike facilitation of target muscle activity in spike-triggered averages of EMG. During alternating wrist movements, the response patterns of different PreM cells—corticomotorneuronal (CM), rubromotorneuronal (RM), dorsal root afferents, and PreM interneurons—as well as of single motor units (MU) of agonist muscles fall into specific classes (Fetz et al., 1989). All groups include cells that exhibit phasic-tonic, tonic, or phasic discharge, as well as cells with

unique firing properties. Many MUs show decrementing discharge through the static hold period. Some RM cells fire during both flexion and extension, and some are unmodulated with the task.

To investigate the function of these diverse cells and to determine what other types of discharge patterns might be required to transform a step signal to the observed output of motor neurons, we derived dynamic networks that generated as outputs the average firing rates of motor units recorded in monkeys performing a step-tracking task (Figure 1). Changes in target position are represented by step inputs to the network and/or by brief transient bursts at the onset of target changes. The input signals are transformed to eight output patterns by intervening hidden units consisting of interconnected excitatory and inhibitory units.

The activation patterns and connection matrix of units in such networks are illustrated elsewhere (Fetz, 1993). In these simulations the network solutions have features that resemble biological situations but that were not explicitly incorporated: (1) Divergent connections of hidden units to different co-activated motor units are representative of divergent outputs of physiological PreM neurons (Fetz et al., 1989). (2) Some hidden units have counterintuitive discharge patterns also seen in biological neurons, e.g., bidirectional and sustained activity. (3) Different network simulations with the same architecture but initialized with different weights often converged on different solutions, comparable to the diversity of neural relations seen in biological networks

A useful heuristic feature of these networks is the ability to quickly probe their operation with manipulations (Fetz, 1993). The contributions of hidden units can be tested by making selective *lesions* and analyzing the behavior of the remaining network. The output effects of a given unit can also be tested by delivering a simulated *stimulus* and analyzing the propagated network response. Because of changing activation levels, the effect of a stimulus depends on the time it is delivered, as is also observed in physiological experiments. These networks can also be trained to scale their responses, that is, to generate output activation patterns proportional to the size of the input. Their ability to generalize can be quickly tested by presenting different inputs.

To generate more realistic models of the primate motor system, the same approach has been used with networks incorporating additional biological features (Maier, Shupe, and Fetz, 1993): (1) the connectivity of central and segmental neurons was included with appropriate conduction delays; (2) the known activity of some central units was required to be part of the solution; and (3) in addition to the active target-tracking task, the network was required to simulate reflex responses to peripheral perturbations of the limb. The resulting networks can generate both types of behaviors and have more realistic properties. Some complex activity patterns seen in PreM neurons of monkeys, such as bidirectional responses of RM cells, also appear in the networks. Even some apparently paradoxical relations seen in monkeys, such as PreM units that covary with muscles that they inhibit, appear in networks and make contributions that are understandable in terms of other units: their activity subtracts out inappropriate components of bidirectional activity patterns. Thus, network simulations have proved useful in elucidating the function of many puzzling features of biological networks.

In contrast to such simulations of a specific neuronal system, others have modeled the representation of reaching movements, as described in REACHING MOVEMENTS: IMPLICATIONS FOR CONNECTIONIST MODELS.

Short-Term Memory Tasks

Neural mechanisms of short-term memory have been investigated in many experiments by recording cortical cell activity in animals performing instructed delay tasks. A common type of instructed delay task involves the requirement to remember the value of a particular stimulus. Zipser (1991) trained recurrent networks to simulate short-term memory of an analog value during the delay; the resulting network implements a sample-and-hold function. The network has two inputs: an analog signal representing the stimulus value to be remembered and a gate signal specifying the times to take samples. The network output is the value of the analog input at the time of the previous gate. During the delay between gate signals, the activity of many hidden units resembles the response patterns of cortical neurons recorded in monkeys performing comparable instructed delay tasks. The activity patterns of hidden units, like those of cortical neurons, fall into three main classes: sustained activation proportional to the remembered analog value, often with a decay or rise; transient modulation during the gate signal; and combinations of the two. The network simulations allow the function of the patterns observed in the animal to be interpreted in terms of their possible role in the memory task.

We investigated such short-term memory networks to further analyze their operation. To elucidate the underlying computational algorithm, we constrained units to have either excitatory or inhibitory output weights, and reduced the network to the minimal essential network. A larger network was initially trained, then reduced by (1) combining units with similar responses and connections into one equivalent unit and (2) eliminating units with negligible activation or weak connections, then (3) retraining the smaller networks to perform the same operation. A reduced network performing the sample-and-hold function (Figure 2) consists of three excitatory and one inhibitory unit. The two inputs are the sample gate signal (S) and the analog variable (A); the output (O) is the value of A at the last sample gate. This reduced version reveals a computational algorithm that exploits the nonlinear sigmoidal input-output function of the units. The first excitatory unit (SA) carries a transient signal proportional to the value of A at the time of the gate. This signal is derived by clipping the sum of the analog and gating inputs with a negative bias, as shown by the input weights to SA in the first column. This input sample is then fed to two excitatory units (M1 and M2) that maintain their activity by reciprocal connections and also feed their summed activity to the output (M1 and M2 could also be replaced by a single self-connected M unit). The inhibitory unit (SM) carries a transient signal proportional to the previous value of A. Its value is derived from a clipped sum of the gate S and the previous values held in M1 and M2. The function of SM is to subtract the previously held value from the integrating hidden units and from the output. Thus, the network uses nonlinearity and integration to yield the appropriate remembered value.

More sophisticated recurrent networks have been derived that perform delayed matching-to-sample tasks (Moody et al., 1998). These networks identified test stimuli presented at the location of a previous sample and ignored intervening distractor stimuli. In reduced networks, the hidden units performed either storage or comparator functions. Another form of spatial memory is involved in making delayed saccades to remembered targets. This function can be simulated in networks whose inputs represent visual targets in space and eye position, and whose hidden units have recurrent connections. The outputs can represent either motor error (Xing and Andersen, 2000) or stored locations in retinal and head-centered coordinates that remain stable in the face of intervening saccades (Mitchell and Zipser, 2001).

Neural Integration

In biological motor systems, neural integrators have been postulated to transform transient commands into sustained activity and to mediate the vestibulo-ocular reflex (VOR) (see VESTIBULO-OCULAR REFLEX). Arnold and Robinson (1991) modeled the VOR integrator with a recurrent network whose connections resembled those of the vestibulo-ocular system. Two input signals represented the reciprocal responses of opposed vestibular afferents to head movement; these connected to four interneurons that were interconnected to each other and to motor neurons. Since vestibular afferents carry tonic activity in the absence of head movement, the integrator had to be configured so as to integrate only deviations from baseline, but not the baseline activity itself. The authors used units with intrinsically sustained activity with decay and a nondifferentiable rectifying input-output characteristic. To train the networks, they tweaked individual weights, and used the effect on the error to update the weights. Integration was performed through positive recurrent connections between the interneurons. The networks could mimic physiological responses to lesions and postsaccadic drift.

Lisberger and Sejnowski (1992) used dynamic networks to investigate mechanisms of learning in the vestibulo-ocular system. The network was constructed to include many anatomical and physiological constraints, including pathways through the cerebellar flocculus, with appropriate delays. The two inputs to the network, head velocity and target velocity, were converted to a single output: eye velocity. The network was initially trained to simulate three behaviors: smooth pursuit of a moving visual target, the VOR to head movement, and suppression of the VOR (when head and target move together). Then the network was required to change the gain of the VOR (as occurs after wearing magnifying or minifying goggles) and also to maintain accurate smooth pursuit visual

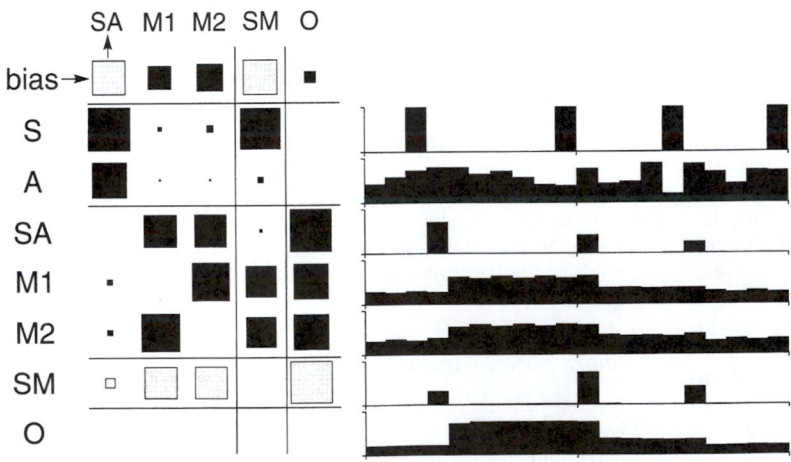

Figure 2. Reduced network performing a sample-and-hold function, simulating short-term memory. The units are indicated by abbreviations and representative activation patterns at right. The weights are indicated by squares (black = excitatory; gray = inhibitory) proportional to the connection from row unit to column unit (e.g., arrows). The two inputs are the sample signal (S) and a random analog value (A); the output (O) is the sustained value of the last sampled analog value.

tracking. Performing these functions required changes in the connection weights at both of two specific sites: the vestibular input to the flocculus and to the brainstem neurons controlling oculomotor neurons. This study exemplifies the insights gained from a biologically constrained dynamic model that can incorporate the time course of neural activity observed under different behavioral conditions, and shows the power of such simulations to reveal novel network mechanisms.

Discussion

The unique insights provided by neural network simulations assures their continued use in elucidating the operations of neural systems. The basic limitation of conventional physiological and antomical data is that they provide a selective sample of a complex system, leaving a gap between particular glimpses of neural activity or anatomical structure and the behavior of the overall system. This gap is usually bridged by intuitive inferences, often based on selective interpretations of the data (Fetz, 1992). A more objective approach would be to derive neural network models that simulate the behavior. These models can incorporate the observed responses of units and can help explain the functional meaning of neural patterns. Thus, integrative neurophysiologists can profitably use a combination of unit recording and neural modeling to elucidate network mechanisms. To the extent that models can incorporate anatomical and physiological constraints, they can provide plausible explanations of the biological neural mechanisms mediating behavior.

Acknowledgments.   Work was supported by ONR (grant No. N18-89-J-1240) and NIH grants NS12542 and RR00166.

Road Map: Biological Networks
Related Reading: Layered Computation in Neural Networks; Recurrent Networks: Learning Algorithms; Short-Term Memory

References

Arnold, D. B., and Robinson, D. A., 1991, A learning network model of the neural integrator of the oculomotor system, *Biol. Cybern.*, 64:447–454.

Fetz, E. E., 1992, Are movement parameters recognizably coded in the activity of single neurons? *Behav. Brain Sci.*, 15:679–690. ◆

Fetz, E. E., 1993, Dynamic neural network models of sensorimotor behavior, in *The Neurobiology of Neural Networks* (D. Gardner, Ed.), Cambridge, MA: MIT Press, pp. 165–190. ◆

Fetz, E. E., Cheney, P. D., Mewes, K., and Palmer, S., 1989, Control of forelimb muscle activity by populations of corticomotoneuronal and rubromotoneuronal cells, *Prog. Brain Res.*, 80:437–449. ◆

Lansner, A., Kotaleski, J. H., and Grillner, S., 1998, Modeling of the spinal neuronal circuitry underlying locomotion in a lower vertebrate, *Ann. N. Y. Acad. Sci.*, 860:239–249.

Lisberger, S. G., and Sejnowski, T. J., 1992, Computational Analysis Suggests a New Hypothesis for Motor Learning in the Vestibulo-ocular Reflex, Technical Report INC-9201, Institute for Neural Computation, University of California at San Diego.

Lockery, S. R., and Sejnowski, T. J., 1992, Distributed processing of sensory information in the leech: A dynamical neural network model of the local bending reflex, *J. Neurosci.*, 12:3877–3895.

Maier, M., Shupe, L. E., and Fetz, E. E., 1993, A spiking neural network model for neurons controlling wrist movement, *Soc. Neurosci. Abstr.*, 19:993.

Mazzoni, P., Andersen, R. A., and Jordan, M. I., 1991, A more biologically plausible learning rule than backpropagation applied to a network model of cortical area 7a, *Cereb. Cortex*, 1:293–307.

Mitchell, J., and Zipser, D., 2001, A model of visual-spatial memory across saccades, *Vision Res.*, 41:1575–1592.

Moody, S. L., Wise, S. P., di Pellegrino, G., and Zipser, D., 1998, A model that accounts for activity in primate frontal cortex during a delayed matching-to-sample task, *J. Neurosci.*, 18:399–410.

Munro, E., Shupe, L., and Fetz, E., 1994, Integration and differentiation in dynamic recurrent neural networks, *Neural Computat.*, 6:405–419.

Rowat, P. F., and Selverston, A. I., 1993, Modeling the gastric mill central pattern generator of the lobster with a relaxation-oscillator network, *J. Neurophysiol.*, 70:1030–1053.

Tsung, F.-S., Cottrell, G. W., and Selverston, A. I., 1990, Experiments on learning stable network oscillations, *Proceedings IJCNN-90*, vol. 1, pp. 169–174.

Williams, R. J., and Zipser, D., 1989, A learning algorithm for continually running fully recurrent neural networks, *Neural Computat.*, 1:270–280.

Xing, J., and Andersen, R. A., 2000, Memory activity of LIP neurons for sequential eye movements simulated with neural networks, *J. Neurophysiol.*, 84:651–665.

Zipser, D., 1991, Recurrent network model of the neural mechanism of short-term active memory, *Neural Computat.*, 3:179-193.

Reinforcement Learning

Andrew G. Barto

Introduction

The term *reinforcement* comes from studies of animal learning in experimental psychology, where it refers to the occurrence of an event, in the proper relation to a response, that tends to increase the probability that the response will occur again in the same situation. Although not used by psychologists, the expression *reinforcement learning* has been widely adopted by theorists in artificial intelligence and engineering to refer to learning tasks and algorithms based on this principle of reinforcement. The simplest reinforcement learning methods use the commonsense idea that if an action is followed by a satisfactory state of affairs, or an improvement in the state of affairs, then the tendency to produce that action is strengthened, i.e., reinforced. The ideas of reinforcement learning have been present in engineering for many decades (e.g., Mendel and McClaren, 1970) and in artificial intelligence since its earliest days (Turing, 1950; Minsky, 1954, 1961; Samuel, 1959). It is only relatively recently, however, that the development and

application of reinforcement learning methods have occupied a significant number of researchers in these fields. Fueling this interest are two basic challenges: (1) designing autonomous robotic agents that can operate under uncertainty in complex dynamic environments, and (2) finding useful approximate solutions to very-large-scale dynamic decision-making problems.

Reinforcement learning is usually formulated as an *optimization problem* with the objective of finding a strategy for producing actions that is optimal, or best, in some well-defined way. In practice, however, it is usually more important for a reinforcement learning system to continue to improve than it is for it to actually achieve optimal behavior. Reinforcement learning differs from the more commonly studied paradigm of supervised learning, or "learning with a teacher," in significant ways that we discuss in the course of this article. It also differs significantly from various forms of unsupervised learning. The article REINFORCEMENT LEARNING IN MOTOR CONTROL (q.v.) contains additional information. For a more detailed introductory treatment, the reader should consult Sutton and Barto (1998); for a more in-depth mathematical treatment, the reader should consult Bertsekas and Tsitsiklis (1996).

The Reinforcement Learning Problem

Think of an agent interacting with its environment over a potentially infinite sequence of discrete-time steps $t = 1, 2, 3, \ldots$. At each time step t, the reinforcement learning agent receives some representation of the environment's current *state*, $s_t \in S$, where S is the set of possible states, and on that basis executes an *action*, $a_t \in A(s_t)$, where $A(s_t)$ is the set of actions that can be executed in state s_t. One time step later, the agent receives a *reward*, r_{t+1}, a real number, and finds itself facing a new state, $s_{t+1} \in S$ (Figure 1). The reward and new state are influenced not only by the agent's action, they are also influenced by the state, s_t, in which the action was taken, and they can depend on random factors as well. Throughout this article we assume that S and $A(s)$, $s \in S$, are finite sets, but extension to infinite sets is possible, as is extension to continuous-time formulations.

The rule the agent uses to select actions is called its *policy*. It is a function, often denoted π, that for each state assigns a probability to each possible action: for all $s \in S$ and all $a \in A(s)$, $\pi(s, a)$ is the probability that the agent executes a when in state s. While interacting with its environment, a reinforcement learning agent adjusts its policy based on its accumulating experience to try to improve the the amount of reward it receives over time. More specifically, it tries to maximize the *return* it receives after each time step. The most commonly studied type of return is the *discounted return*. If $r_{t+1}, r_{t+2}, r_{t+3}, \ldots$, denotes the sequence of rewards received after time step t, then the discounted return for step t is

$$\sum_{k=0}^{\infty} \gamma^k r_{t+k+1} \tag{1}$$

where $\gamma \in [0, 1)$ is the *discount factor*. A reinforcement learning agent adjusts its policy to try to maximize the expected value of this quantity for all $t \geq 0$.

The discount factor determines the present value of future rewards. If $\gamma = 0$, the agent is only concerned with maximizing immediate rewards: its objective would be to learn how to act at each time step t so as maximize only r_{t+1}. But in general, acting to maximize immediate reward can reduce access to future rewards, so that a longer-term return may actually be reduced. As γ approaches one, the objective takes future rewards into account more strongly: the agent becomes more far-sighted. Discounting is used because it is mathematically the simplest way to deal with cases in which the agent and environment can interact for an unbounded

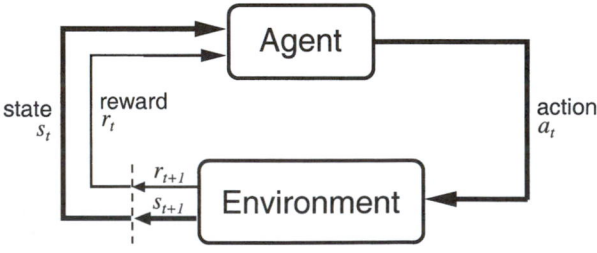

Figure 1. A reinforcement learning model. A reinforcement learning agent and its environment interact over a sequence of discrete-time steps. The *actions* are the choices made by the agent, the *states* provide the agent's basis for making the choices, and the *rewards* are the basis for evaluating these choices. (From Sutton, R. S., and Barto, A. G., 1998, *Reinforcement Learning: An Introduction*, Cambridge, MA: MIT Press.)

number of time steps. In many problems only finite numbers of steps can ever happen in each learning trial, so that γ can be set to one. These are called *episodic* problems. Other definitions of return have been extensively studied as well.

This model of the reinforcement learning problem is based on the theory of *Markov decision processes* (MDPs), which has been extensively developed in decision theory and stochastic control (see, e.g., Bertsekas, 1987). An MDP has the property that the environment satisfies the Markov property, which means that environment state at any time step $t > 0$ provides the same information about what will happen next as would the entire history of the process up to step t. A full specification of an MDP includes the probabilistic details of how state transitions and rewards are influenced by states and actions, i.e., a full probabilistic model of the environment and how it is influenced by the agent's actions. The objective is to compute an *optimal policy*, i.e., a policy that maximizes the expected return from each state. In theory, this can be done using any of several stochastic dynamic programming algorithms, although their computational complexity makes them impractical for large-scale problems.

Reinforcement learning has much in common with this traditional study of MDPs, but it emphasizes approximating optimal behavior during on-line behavior instead of computing optimal policies off-line on the basis of known probabilistic models. In particular, the objective in reinforcement learning is actually not to compute an optimal policy; it is instead to allow the agent to receive as much reward as possible during its behavior. This does not always require a policy that is optimal for all possible states, since the agent may not visit all of these states while it is behaving.

Following are some key observations about the reinforcement learning problem:

1. *Uncertainty* plays a central role in reinforcement learning. The agent's environment and its own behavior can be subject to random fluctuations, so that the outcomes of decisions cannot be known beforehand with complete certainty. An accurate probabilistic model of the these uncertainties may or may not be available to the agent.

2. The reward input to the agent can be any scalar signal evaluating the agent's behavior. It might indicate just success when a goal state is reached or just failure while not reaching a goal state; or it might provide moment-by-moment evaluations of ongoing behavior (as, for example, in giving the amount of energy currently being consumed while a task is being accomplished). Moreover, multiple evaluation criteria can be combined in various ways to form the scalar reward signal (for example, via a weighted sum).

3. An important difficulty faced by a reinforcement learning system is the *credit-assignment problem* (Minsky, 1961): How do you distribute credit for success among the many decisions that may have been involved in producing it? (see also REINFORCEMENT LEARNING IN MOTOR CONTROL).

4. A reinforcement learning system often has to forgo immediate reward in order to obtain more reward later or over the long run. This kind of "sacrificing" behavior arises because the agent's actions influence not only each reward input but also the environment's state transitions. An action may be preferred because it sets the stage for a large reward later rather than for its immediate reward.

5. The reward signal does not directly tell the agent what action is best; it only evaluates the action taken. A reward input also does not directly tell the agent how to change its actions. These are key features distinguishing reinforcement learning from supervised learning, and we discuss them further below.

6. Reinforcement learning algorithms are *selectional* processes. There must be *variety* in the action-generation process so that

the consequences of alternative actions can be compared to select the best. Behavioral variety is called *exploration*; it is often generated through randomness, but it need not be.

7. Reinforcement learning involves a conflict between *exploitation* and *exploration*. In deciding which action to take, the agent has to balance two conflicting objectives: it has to exploit what it has already learned to obtain high rewards, and it has to behave in new ways—explore—to learn more. Because these needs ordinarily conflict, reinforcement learning systems have to somehow balance them. In control engineering, this is known as the conflict between control and identification.

8. Some researchers think of reinforcement learning as a form of supervised learning (because the reward input is a kind of supervision), and others think of it as a form of unsupervised learning (because the reward input is not like the label of an example). There is some truth to each of these views, but reinforcement learning is really different from both. A key distinguishing feature is the presence in reinforcement learning of the conflict between exploitation and exploration. This is absent from supervised and unsupervised learning unless the learning system is also engaged in influencing which training examples it sees.

Value Functions

The most commonly studied reinforcement learning algorithms are based on estimating *value functions*, which are scalar functions of states, or of state-action pairs, that tell how good it is for the agent to be in a state, or to take an action in a state. The notion of "how good" is the return expected to accumulate over the future, which is well-defined if the Markov property holds and the agent's policy is specified.

If the agent uses policy π, then the state value function V^π gives the *value*, $V^\pi(s)$, of each $s \in S$, which is the return expected to accumulate over the time period after visiting s, assuming that actions are chosen according to π. For the discounted return defined by Equation 1, the value of state s is

$$V^\pi(s) = E_\pi \left[\sum_{k=0}^{\infty} \gamma^k r_{t+k+1} \middle| s_t = s \right]$$

where E_π is the expected value given that policy π is followed. A state's *optimal value*, $V^*(s)$, is the return expected after visiting s, assuming that actions are chosen optimally; i.e., it is the largest expected return possible after visiting s.

Similarly, the *action value* of taking action a in state s under a policy π, denoted $Q^\pi(s, a)$, is the expected return starting from s, taking the action a, and thereafter following policy π:

$$Q^\pi(s, a) = E_\pi \left[\sum_{k=0}^{\infty} \gamma^k r_{t+k+1} \middle| s_t = s, a_t = a \right]$$

The *optimal action value* of taking action a in state s, denoted $Q^*(s, a)$, is the expected return starting from s, taking the action a, and thereafter following an optimal policy.

Value functions are useful because of several properties of MDPs. If V^* is known, optimal policies can be found by looking ahead only one time step. That is, if s_t is the state at step t, then an optimal action is any $a \in A(s_t)$ that maximizes the expected value of $r_{t+1} + \gamma V^*(s_{t+1})$. Thus, given V^* and an accurate model of the immediate effects on the environment of all of the actions, acting optimally does not require deep look-ahead because V^* summarizes the effects of future behavior. If Q^* is known, then finding optimal actions is even easier. An optimal action at step t is any action that maximizes $Q^*(s_t, a)$. In this case, it is not necessary to look ahead one step, so that no model is needed of the effect of actions on the environment. This is what makes reinforcement

learning algorithms that use action-value functions a popular choice in many applications. Any such one-step-ahead maximizing action for a state value function, or a maximizing action for an action value function, is called a *greedy* action with respect to that function.

Value functions that depend on a policy, that is, V^π and Q^π, are useful for improving behavior because of the *policy improvement property*. Suppose the agent is deciding which action to execute in a state. It could pick an action using its current policy, π, or it could select some other action. If it picks an action that is greedy with respect to V^π, and otherwise follows π, then its performance is guaranteed to be at least as good as it would have been under π, and possibly better. This fact is the basis of the policy improvement, or policy iteration, dynamic programming algorithm, and it motivates many reinforcement learning algorithms, as we explain below.

A fundamental property of value functions is that they satisfy particular consistency conditions if the Markov property holds. For any policy π and any state s, the following is true (for the discounted return case):

$$V^\pi(s) = E_\pi \left[\sum_{k=0}^{\infty} \gamma^k r_{t+k+1} \middle| s_t = s \right]$$
$$= E_\pi \left[r_{t+1} + \gamma \sum_{k=0}^{\infty} \gamma^k r_{t+k+2} \middle| s_t = s \right]$$
$$= E_\pi \left[r_{t+1} + \gamma V^\pi(s_{t+1}) | s_t = s \right] \qquad (2)$$

An analogous consistency condition holds for values of Q^π. Similarly, V^* satisfies the following equation for all $s \in S$:

$$V^*(s) = \max_a E[r_{t+1} + \gamma V^*(s_{t+1}) | s_t = s, a_t = a]$$

and Q^* satisfies

$$Q^*(s, a) = E[r_{t+1} + \gamma \max_{a'} Q^*(s_{t+1}, a') | s_t = s, a_t = a]$$

for all pairs (s, a), $s \in S$, $a \in A(s)$.

If a model is available giving the probabilistic details of how the environment responds to actions, then these equations (or, more precisely, these *sets* of equations) are completely specified and can in principle be solved using one of a variety of methods for solving systems of linear equations (to obtain V^π or Q^π) or nonlinear equations (to obtain V^* or Q^*). These are often called *Bellman equations*, after Richard Bellman, who introduced the term *dynamic programming* to refer to a collection of solution methods (Bellman, 1957). There are many books that explain dynamic programming (e.g., Bertsekas, 1987).

Solving Bellman equations is therefore one route to finding optimal policies. Unfortunately, in many problems of interest one does not have the complete Markov model of the environment needed to fully define the Bellman equations, or the state set may be so large that it is not computationally feasible to exactly solve the Bellman equations. Unless some special additional structure can be exploited, one has to settle for approximate solutions.

Reinforcement Learning Based on Value Functions

Value functions are used in several different ways in reinforcement learning. One approach uses the *actor-critic architecture*, which maintains a representation of both a value function and a policy (Figure 2). To select actions, an agent using this architecture consults its current policy, represented by the *actor* component. The policy might be represented by a lookup table, by an artificial neural network, with its input coding the current state and its output coding the action to be taken, or by some other means. To evaluate the action just taken, the *critic* component is consulted, which

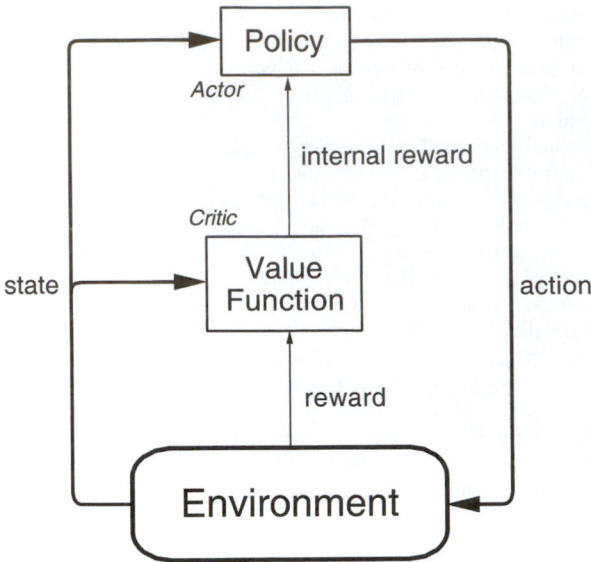

Figure 2. Actor-critic architecture. The *critic* provides an internal reward signal to an *actor*, which learns a policy for interacting with the environment.

maintains an estimate of the value function of the current policy. The action is considered to be "good" ("bad") to the extent that it leads to a next state with a value higher (lower) than that of *s*, both state values being estimated by the critic. Upon receiving this evaluation, the actor updates the policy by making a good action more likely to be selected on revisiting *s*, or a bad action less likely, thus implementing a version of Edward Thorndike's famous Law of Effect (Thorndike, 1911). The critic component then updates its value function estimate using a temporal difference learning algorithm of the kind described below.

Barto, Sutton, and Anderson (1983) used this architecture for learning to balance a simulated pole mounted on a cart. Their perspective was that the critic provides an internal reinforcement signal—changes in estimated values—that provides *immediate* action evaluations, even though the goal is to maximize reward over the long term. To the extent that the critic's value estimates are correct given the actor's current policy, the actor actually learns to increase the total amount of future reinforcement. This method thus relies on the policy improvement property. Although not a fail-safe approach from a theoretical perspective, it is often successful in improving the agent's behavior.

Another type of reinforcement learning algorithm that uses value functions maintains an estimate of the current policy's value function but does not keep an explicit representation of the current policy. Instead, it selects actions solely by consulting its current value function estimate. At each time step, the agent selects an action that is either greedy with respect to its current estimate of the value function or is an exploratory action chosen on some other basis (see below). If state values are being estimated, finding a greedy action requires projecting ahead one step using an environment model; if action values are being estimated, no look-ahead is required, as explained above. Like actor-critic methods, this approach also relies on the policy improvement property, but since there is no separate policy representation and no separate policy update rule, it is more closely related to various dynamic programming algorithms and is therefore somewhat easier to understand.

Estimating Value Functions

The simplest method for estimating the value function of the current policy while the agent is behaving is to average an ensemble of returns actually observed. For example, if an agent follows policy π and maintains, for each state *s* encountered, an average of the actual returns that have followed that state, then the averages will converge to $V^\pi(s)$ as the number of times that state is encountered approaches infinity. If separate averages are kept for each action, *a*, taken in a state, then these averages will similarly converge to the action values, $Q^\pi(s, a)$. This is easiest to do in episodic problems, where return is accumulated over finite numbers of time steps. Methods like this are sometimes called *simple Monte Carlo* value estimation methods.

Another class of value estimation methods are called *temporal difference* (TD) algorithms (Sutton, 1988). The most basic TD algorithm, called *tabular TD(0)*, estimates V^π while the agent is behaving according to π and is applicable when the state set is small enough to store the state values in a lookup table with a separate entry for the value of each state. Suppose the agent is in state *s*, executes action *a*, and then observes the resulting reward *r* and the next state *s'*. TD(0) updates the current estimate of the value of state *s*, $V(s)$, using the following update:

$$V(s) \leftarrow V(s) + \alpha[r + \gamma V(s') - V(s)] \qquad (3)$$

where α is a positive step-size parameter. TD algorithms are based on the consistency condition expressed by the Bellman equations. This TD algorithm is designed to move the term $r + \gamma V(s') - V(s)$, called the *TD error*, toward zero for every state. If the expected TD error could be made to equal zero for every state, then the corresponding Bellman equation (Equation 2) would be satisfied. An update of this general form is often called a *backup* because the value of a state is moved toward the current value of a successor state, plus any reward that is received on the transition.

This algorithm converges to the correct state values under certain conditions (Sutton, 1988). This and other TD algorithms have been extended to include *eligibility traces*, which allow values to be backed up over more than one time step. When so extended, these are called TD(λ) algorithms, where λ is a parameter determining the temporal characteristics of the backups: λ ranges from zero (no eligibility traces as above) to one (resulting in a simple Monte Carlo method). Forms of this TD algorithm are also known as *adaptive critic algorithms*.

Another TD algorithm, known as *Q-learning*, was proposed by Watkins in 1989 (see Sutton and Barto, 1998). This algorithm directly estimates Q^* without relying on the policy improvement property. Its tabular form works as follows. Suppose the agent is in state *s*, executes action *a*, and then observes the resulting reward *r* and the next state *s'*. The Q-learning algorithm updates the action value estimate, $Q(s, a)$, of the pair (s, a) using the following backup:

$$Q(s, a) \leftarrow Q(s, a) + \alpha[r + \gamma \max_{a'} Q(s', a') - Q(s, a)] \qquad (4)$$

where α is a positive step-size parameter. If α decreases appropriately with time and each state-action pair is visited infinitely often in the limit, then this algorithm converges to $Q^*(s, a)$ for all $s \in S$ and $a \in A(s)$ with probability one. Unless it is known that the environment is deterministic, the "infinitely often" requirement is necessary for this kind of strong convergence of any method that is based, as this one is, on sampling environment state transitions and rewards. Letting the agent sometimes select actions randomly from a uniform distribution is one simple way to help the agent maintain enough variety in its behavior to try to satisfy this condition. Otherwise, the agent executes actions that are greedy with respect to its current estimate of Q^*.

Closely related to Q-learning is the *Sarsa* algorithm. Suppose the agent is in state *s*, executes action *a*, observes reward *r* and the next state *s'*, and then executes action *a'*. Then the Sarsa update is

$$Q(s, a) \leftarrow Q(s, a) + \alpha[r + \gamma Q(s', a') - Q(s, a)]$$

which is the same as the Q-learning update (Equation 4) except that instead of taking the maximum over the actions available in s', it uses the action, a', which was actually executed. (This requirement of s, a, r, s', a' is what accounts for the algorithm's name.) Notice that if actions are always greedy with respect to the current estimate of Q^*, then Sarsa is the same as Q-learning. Despite this similarity, Sarsa and Q-learning have somewhat different properties (see Sutton and Barto, 1998). Whereas Q-learning converges to Q^* independently of the agent's behavior (as long as the conditions for convergence are satisfied), Sarsa converges to an action value function that is optimal given the agent's mode of exploration. Like the TD algorithm for state values described above, both Q-learning and Sarsa can be extended to include eligibility traces.

TD algorithms are closely related to dynamic programming algorithms, which also use backup operations derived from Bellman equations. There are two main differences. First, a dynamic programming backup computes the expected value of successor states using the state-transition distribution of the MDP, whereas a TD backup uses a sample from this distribution. (TD backups are sometimes called *sample backups*, in contrast to the *full backups* of dynamic programming.) A second difference is that dynamic programming uses multiple exhaustive "sweeps" of the MDP's state set, whereas TD algorithms operate on states as they occur in actual or simulated experiences. These differences make it possible to use TD algorithms on problems for which it is not feasible to use dynamic programming.

Function Approximation

Instead of storing the estimated values of states or state-action pairs in lookup tables, it is possible to represent them more compactly. This is an important feature of reinforcement learning because it enables its use for problems whose state sets are too large to allow explicit representation of each value estimate, and hence too large for textbook dynamic programming algorithms to be feasible. Very large state sets often arise due to combinatorial explosions in representing states that are configurations of discrete objects. They also arise when multidimensional continuous spaces are discretized (prompting Bellman to coin the familiar phrase, "the curse of dimensionality"). For example, the game of backgammon, to which reinforcement learning has been applied with striking success (Tesauro, 1992), has more than 10^{20} states.

Any of the TD backup rules described above can be used to derive an update rule for a parameterized function approximation method of the type developed for supervised learning. Many reinforcement learning applications have used multilayer artificial neural networks and error backpropagation (see BACKPROPAGATION: GENERAL PRINCIPLES). To do this requires representing states or state-action pairs as feature vectors. Training examples are extracted from the agent's behavioral trajectory. For example, suppose one approximated the value of any state s by a function of a feature vector $\vec{\phi}(s)$ and parameter vector $\vec{\theta}$: $V(s) = f(\vec{\phi}(s), \vec{\theta})$. Then the agent's experience of observing state s, followed by reward r and successor state s', would yield the training example consisting of input vector $\vec{\phi}(s)$ and the target output $r + \gamma f(\vec{\phi}(s'), \vec{\theta}_t)$. A gradient-descent update of $\vec{\theta}$ derived from Equation 7 is

$$\vec{\theta}_{t+1} = \vec{\theta}_t + \alpha[r + \gamma f(\vec{\theta}(s'), \vec{\theta}_t) - f(\vec{\phi}(s), \vec{\theta}_t)]\nabla_{\vec{\theta}_t} f(\vec{\phi}(s), \vec{\theta}_t)$$

Notice that unlike the case in supervised learning, the target output also depends on the parameter vector. This complicates the behavior and analysis of this type of learning rule. Convergence results have been derived for TD(λ) algorithms in the case of function approximators that are linear in $\vec{\theta}$, and counterexamples to convergence have been presented for Q-learning (see Sutton and Barto, 1998, and Bertsekas and Tsitsiklis, 1996, for discussions of these

results). Despite a shortage of theoretical guarantees, many reinforcement learning systems using nonlinear function approximators have demonstrated good performance, and much current research is examining these issues.

Exploration

Reinforcement learning agents have to explore: they have to sometimes select actions that appear to be suboptimal according to their current state of knowledge (e.g., current value and/or policy estimates). Otherwise, behavior can become irretrievably suboptimal as the knowledge base comes to reflect only limited experiences. Balancing exploration with the exploitation of current knowledge is a subtle problem that has been extensively studied. In principle, it is possible to optimally balance exploration and exploitation by solving an MDP whose states are *belief states* that summarize the agent's entire history of observations and actions. But this approach is not feasible for most tasks of interest.

Several simple heuristic exploration methods are usually used in applications of reinforcement learning. In the simplest, the agent selects ε-*greedy* actions. This means that with probability $1 - \varepsilon$, the agent exploits its current knowledge by selecting a greedy action, that is, an action that is optimal given its current value estimates, and with probability ε, it selects an action at random, uniformly, independently of its of its current value estimates. Somewhat more complicated is the *softmax* method, which selects actions according to a Boltzmann distribution based on the current action values. This gives actions with higher estimated values higher probabilities of being selected, with a "temperature" parameter determining how much an action's estimated value influences its selection probability. More sophisticated methods monitor the degree of certainty involved in action choices and direct exploration accordingly. How to design methods for balancing exploration and exploitation that are practical, effective, and amenable to theoretical treatment is an important research area.

Direct Policy Search

Not all reinforcement learning methods use value functions. It is possible to search directly in the space of policies. For example, the amount of reward that a policy yields can be estimated by running the policy for some number of time steps, possibly repeating many times from different initial states. This provides an evaluation of the entire policy that can be used to direct the search in policy space. The success of the approach usually depends on suitably parameterizing policies by vectors of real numbers so that the search can be conducted in parameter space using any of a large number of optimization algorithms. Some of these algorithms require estimates of the gradient of the policy evaluation with respect to the parameters, which can also be extracted from sample policy executions.

If the agent-environment interaction is approximately Markov, TD methods can take advantage of local consistency conditions to obtain state-localized information about how to improve a policy. On the other hand, direct policy search does not depend on the Markov property and so can be used when state information is not close to being available. Direct policy search methods also do not require the use of function approximation methods to represent value functions. Offsetting these advantages of direct policy search methods, however, is the more coarse form of credit assignment that is possible and the difficulty of efficiently evaluating entire policies. Which type of method is to be recommended is highly problem dependent. The actor-critic architecture can be considered to combine aspects of value function and direct policy search algorithms, and there is considerable interest in this hybrid approach.

Using Environment Models

Algorithms like Q-learning and Sarsa do not need a model of the agent's environment. They can learn from the agent's actual experience as the agent behaves in the real world. However, many reinforcement learning systems do take advantage of environment models. For example, algorithms like Q-learning and Sarsa are often applied to experience generated as the agent interacts with a simulation of its environment. This not only allows much faster learning (since simulations can run much faster than real time), it eliminates the potential of catastrophic consequences that can occur in some domains when a learning system is given control over a real system.

Sutton and Barto (1998) called models that can support learning from simulations *sample models*. In contrast, stochastic dynamic programming algorithms need *distribution models*, which explicitly represent the environment's state-transition and reward probabilities. Since sample models can sometimes be much easier to construct than distribution models, their ability to form policies through simulation is an important advantage of reinforcement learning methods for some applications. It is also easy to devise algorithms that learn from both real and simulated experience. Other reinforcement learning algorithms take advantage of distribution models by using full, instead of sample, backups, while still applying backups to states encountered along simulated or actual behavioral trajectories. This approach makes each backup more informative than a sample backup but avoids the exhaustive sweeping of dynamic programming.

Determining a policy from an environment model, either a distribution or a sample model, is a form of *planning*. Reinforcement learning algorithms that use models are not clearly distinct from some types of planning algorithms. Their main distinguishing characteristic is probably that they often do not fully complete a planning process before committing to actions. The planning process is extended over time, with knowledge in the form of a value function and/or a policy accumulating as behavior continues. Model-based reinforcement learning is closely related to *decision-theoretic planning* in artificial intelligence, which also makes use of the MDP formalism.

Elaborations and Extensions

Among the many topics being addressed by current reinforcement learning research are (1) extending theoretical results to include parameterized function approximation methods; (2) understanding how exploratory behavior is best introduced and controlled; (3) learning under conditions in which the environment state cannot be fully observed (related to the theory of partially observable MDPs, or POMDPs); (4) exploiting the structure present when states and/or actions are represented as vectors giving the values

of descriptive variables (formalized in terms of *factored* or *structured* MDPs); and (5) introducing various forms of abstraction such as temporally extended actions and hierarchy (which rely strongly on the theory of semi-Markov decision processes, or SMDPs). Finally, researchers are studying the relationship of computational reinforcement learning theories to brain reward mechanisms. Strong parallels exsit between TD learning and the activity of dopamine neurons (Schultz, 1998; see also DOPAMINE, ROLES OF).

Road Maps: Grounding Models of Neurons; Learning in Artificial Networks
Related Reading: Dopamine, Roles of; Q-Learning for Robots; Reinforcement Learning in Motor Control

References

Barto, A. G., Sutton, R. S., and Anderson, C. W., 1983, Neuronlike elements that can solve difficult learning control problems, *IEEE Trans. Syst. Man Cybern.*, 13:835–846. Reprinted in *Neurocomputing: Foundations of Research* (J. A. Anderson and E. Rosenfeld, Eds.), Cambridge, MA: MIT Press, 1988, pp. 535–549.

Bellman, R. E., 1957, *Dynamic Programming*, Princeton, NJ: Princeton University Press.

Bertsekas, D. P., 1987, *Dynamic Programming: Deterministic and Stochastic Models*, Englewood Cliffs, NJ: Prentice-Hall. ◆

Bertsekas, D. P., and Tsitsiklis, J. N., 1996, *Neuro-Dynamic Programming*, Belmont, MA: Athena Scientific. ◆

Mendel, J. M., and McLaren, R. W., 1970, Reinforcement learning control and pattern recognition systems, in *Adaptive Learning and Pattern Recognition Systems: Theory and Applications* (J. M. Mendel and K. S. Fu, Eds.), New York: Academic Press, pp. 287–318.

Minsky, M. L., 1954, Theory of neural-analog reinforcement systems and its application to the brain-model problem, Ph.D. diss., Princeton University.

Minsky, M. L., 1961, Steps toward artificial intelligence, *Proc. Inst. Radio Eng.*, 49:8–30. Reprinted in *Computers and Thought* (E. A. Feigenbaum and J. Feldman, Eds.), New York: McGraw-Hill, 1963, pp. 406–450.

Samuel, A. L., 1959, Some studies in machine learning using the game of checkers, *IBM J. Res. Dev.*, 3:210–229. Reprinted in *Computers and Thought* (E. A. Feigenbaum and J. Feldman, Eds.), New York: McGraw-Hill, 1963, pp. 71–105.

Schultz, W., 1998, Predictive reward signal of dopamine neurons, *J. Neurophysiol.*, 80:1–27.

Sutton, R. S., 1988, Learning to predict by the method of temporal differences, *Machine Learn.*, 3:9–44.

Sutton, R. S., and Barto, A. G., 1998, *Reinforcement Learning: An Introduction*, Cambridge, MA: MIT Press. ◆

Tesauro, G. J., 1992, Practical issues in temporal difference learning, *Machine Learn.*, 8:257–277.

Thorndike, E. L., 1911, *Animal Intelligence*, Darien, CT: Hafner.

Turing, A. M., 1950, Computing machinery and intelligence, *Mind*, 59:433–460. Reprinted in *Computers and Thought* (E. A. Feigenbaum and J. Feldman, Eds.), New York: McGraw-Hill, 1963, pp. 11–35.

Reinforcement Learning in Motor Control

Andrew G. Barto

Introduction

How do we learn motor skills such as reaching, walking, swimming, or riding a bicycle? There is a large literature on motor skill acquisition that is full of controversies (for an introduction to human motor control, see Schmidt and Lee, 1999), but there is general agreement that motor learning requires the learner, human or not,

to receive response-produced feedback through various senses providing information about performance. Careful consideration of the nature of the feedback used in learning is important for understanding the role of reinforcement learning in motor control (see REINFORCEMENT LEARNING). One function of feedback is to guide the performance of movements. This is the kind of feedback with which we are familiar from control theory, where it is the basis of servocontrol, although its role in guiding animal movement is more complex. Another function of feedback is to provide information useful for improving *subsequent* movement. Feedback having this function has been called *learning feedback*. Note that this functional distinction between feedback for control and feedback for learning does not mean that the signals or channels serving these functions need to be different.

Learning Feedback

When motor skills are acquired without the help of an explicit teacher or trainer, learning feedback must consist of information automatically generated by the movement and its consequences on the environment. This has been called *intrinsic feedback* (Schmidt and Lee, 1999). The "feel" of a successfully completed movement and the sight of a basketball going through the hoop are examples of intrinsic learning feedback. A teacher or trainer can augment intrinsic feedback by providing *extrinsic feedback* (Schmidt and Lee, 1999) consisting of extra information added for training purposes, such as a buzzer indicating that a movement was on target, a word of praise or encouragement, or an indication that a certain kind of error was made.

Most research in the fields of machine learning and artificial neural networks has focused on the learning paradigm called *supervised learning*, which emphasizes the role of training information in the form of desired, or "target," network responses for a set of training inputs (see PERCEPTRONS, ADALINES, AND BACKPROPAGATION). However, motor learning is more complex than supervised learning, even when it involves extrinsic feedback provided by a trainer. For example, a trainer can tell or show us what to do, explicitly guide our movements, give us hints on how to deal with difficult parts of a skill, tell us when we have improved or done badly, etc. The aspect of real training that corresponds most closely to the supervised learning paradigm is the trainer's role in telling or showing the learner what to do, or explicitly guiding his or her movements. These activities provide standards of correctness that the learner can try to match as closely as possible by reducing the error between his or her behavior and the standard. Supervised learning can also be relevant to motor learning when there is no trainer, because intrinsic feedback can be used to learn various kinds of *models* that are useful for motor control. Kawato (1999) and Desmurget and Grafton (2000) discuss some of the uses of models in motor control.

In contrast to supervised learning, *reinforcement learning* emphasizes learning feedback that *evaluates* the learner's performance without providing standards of correctness in the form of behavioral targets (see REINFORCEMENT LEARNING). Although the most obvious evaluative feedback is extrinsic feedback provided by a trainer, most evaluative feedback is probably intrinsic, being derived by the learner from sensations generated by a movement and its consequences on the environment: the kinesthetic and tactile feel of a successful grasp or the swish of a basketball through the hoop. Evaluative feedback is often called *reinforcement* feedback (and it need not involve pleasure or pain). A reinforcement learning system has to actively try alternatives, compare the resulting evaluations, and use some kind of selection mechanism to guide behavior toward the better alternatives. This basic idea follows Thorndike's classical law of effect (Thorndike, 1911) and is commonly called learning by trial and error (not to be confused with error-correction, or supervised, learning).

The great Russian physiologist Nikolai Bernstein discussed the role of trial-and-error learning in motor control in his classic 1967 book (Bernstein, 1967). He distinguished his view from the concept of random undirected search, which he attributed to the behaviorists. According to Bernstein, the process must be an active search involving "gradient extrapolation" by probabilistic sampling so that each attempt is informed by previously acquired information about

"how and where the next step must be taken." This is very much in accord with modern concepts of reinforcement learning, where randomness is often used to generate behavioral variety, but action selections are strongly constrained by evaluations of earlier experience (see REINFORCEMENT LEARNING). To Bernstein, this kind of search was important for motor behavior, especially for movements requiring high levels of coordination. Another motor control theorist, Jack Adams, provided an interesting discussion of the role of the law of effect in motor control in a 1978 article (Adams, 1978). Although he called into question some of the details of Thorndike's theories, he affirmed the importance of reinforcement learning in motor control.

Motor learning involves feedback carrying many different kinds of information. Consequently, it is incorrect to view motor learning strictly in terms of supervised, reinforcement, or any other learning paradigms that have been formulated for theoretical study. Aspects of all of these paradigms play interlocking roles, with their relative importance undoubtedly varying with the type of task as well as the developmental stage. However, reinforcement learning may be an essential component of motor learning simply because evaluative feedback is more easily obtained than many other kinds of learning feedback.

Learning from Consequences

To illustrate how reinforcement learning applies to motor learning, we first discuss it within the general context of control. Then we describe several special cases related to motor control. Figure 1, panel *A*, is a variation of the classical control system diagram. A controller provides control signals to a controlled system. The behavior of the controlled system is influenced by disturbances, and feedback from the controlled system to the controller provides information on which the control signals can depend. Commands to the controller specify aspects of the control task's objective.

In Figure 1, panel *B*, the control loop is augmented with another feedback loop that provides learning feedback to the controller. In accordance with common practice in reinforcement learning, a

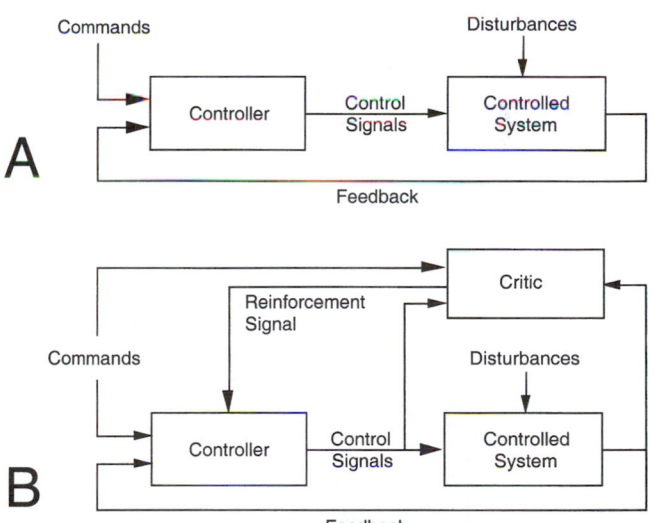

Figure 1. *A*, A basic control loop. A controller provides control signals to a controlled system, whose behavior is influenced by disturbances. Feedback from the controlled system to the controller provides information on which the control signals can depend. Commands to the controller specify aspects of the control task's objective. *B*, A control system with learning feedback. A *critic* provides the controller with a reinforcement signal evaluating its success in achieving the control objectives.

critic is included that generates evaluative learning feedback on the basis of observing the control signals and their consequences on the behavior of the controlled system. The critic also needs to know the command to the controller because its evaluations must be different depending on what the controller should be trying to do. The critic is an abstraction of whatever process supplies evaluative learning feedback, both intrinsic and extrinsic, to the learning system. It is often said that the critic provides a *reinforcement signal* to the learning system. In most artificial reinforcement learning systems, the critic's output at any time is a number that scores the controller's behavior: the higher the number, the better the behavior. Assume for a moment that the behavior being scored is the immediately preceding unit of behavior. (We discuss what a unit of behavior might be, as well as more complex temporal relationships, in later sections.) For this process to work, there must be some *variability* in the controller's behavior so that the critic can evaluate many alternatives. A learning mechanism can then adjust the controller's behavior so that it tends toward behavior that is favored by the critic.

A learning rule particularly suited to reinforcement learning control systems implemented as artificial neural networks was developed by Gullapalli (1990) in the form of what he called a Stochastic Real-Valued (SRV) unit. An SRV unit's output is produced by adding a random number to the weighted sum of the components of its input pattern. The random number is drawn from a zero-mean Gaussian distribution. This random component provides the unit with the variability necessary for it to "explore" its activity space. When the reinforcement signal indicates that something good happened just after the unit emitted a particular output value in the presence of some input pattern, the unit's weights are adjusted to move the activation in the direction in which it was perturbed by the random number. This has the effect of increasing the probability that future outputs generated for that input pattern (and similar input patterns) will be closer to the output value just emitted. If the reinforcement signal indicates that something bad happened, the weights are adjusted to move future output values away from the value just emitted. Another part of the SRV learning rule decreases the variance of the Gaussian distribution as learning proceeds. This decreases the variability of the unit's behavior, with the goal of making it eventually stick (i.e., become deterministic) at the best output value for each input pattern. Using this learning rule, an SRV unit learns to produce the best output in response to each input pattern (given appropriate assumptions). Unlike more familiar supervised learning units, it is never given target outputs; it has to discover what outputs are best through an active exploration process.

Overcoming the Distal Error Problem

As a simple illustration of how reinforcement learning can be useful in motor learning, consider the problem of learning to reach to specific points in space starting from a variety of initial hand positions. Lipitkas et al. (1993) proposed a particularly straightforward method (although not as a model of the human learning process, which is much more complex). Their controller is an artificial neural network receiving inputs coding the initial spatial location and the desired, or target, spatial location of the hand (ignoring hand orientation). The six outputs of the network provide parameters to a torque generator that generates time-varying signals for driving the joint actuators of a dynamic arm model (Figure 2). The time-varying signals are parameterized by six numbers determining characteristics of their wave-like shapes (e.g., giving the magnitudes and relative timing of the half-waves). During each movement, the controller operates in open-loop mode, generating the torque time functions without the aid of sensory feedback. The problem for the network is to learn a function associating each pair of hand starting and target positions with the values of the six torque-generator parameters that will accomplish the movement.

A straightforward application of supervised learning is not possible here because the required training examples are not available: it is not known what parameters will work for any pair of starting and target positions (except possibly the trivial cases in which the starting position is already the target position, but these are not useful as training examples). This is an instance of what has been called the *distal error problem* (Jordan and Rumelhart, 1992) for supervised learning. This problem is present whenever the standard of correctness required for supervised learning is available in a coordinate system that is different from the one in which the learning system's activity must be specified for learning. In the case of learning how to move the hand from a starting position to a target position, the standard of correctness is the target position, but what must be learned is the control signals to the joint actuators, that is, to the muscles. The hand position error is distal to the output of the controller that has to be learned. Although a non-zero distal error vector indicates that the controller made an error, it does not tell the controller how it should change its output in order to reduce the error.

The distal error problem can be solved by using a model of the controller's influence on the arm's movement (possibly learned via supervised learning) to translate distal error vectors into error vectors required for supervised learning (Jordan and Rumelhart, 1992). Another approach is to learn an inverse model of the controller's influence on the arm's movement (Jordan and Rumelhart, 1992; Kawato, 1999). Reinforcement learning offers another way to overcome the distal error problem because it does not need learning feedback in the form of error vectors. Continuing with the reaching example, Lipitkas et al. (1993) defined a reinforcement signal that attains a maximum value of 1 if the hand reaches the desired position and stops there. The signal decreases, depending on the distance between the hand's final position and the target position and on its tangential velocity as it passes the target position. The reinforcement signal could include other criteria of successful move-

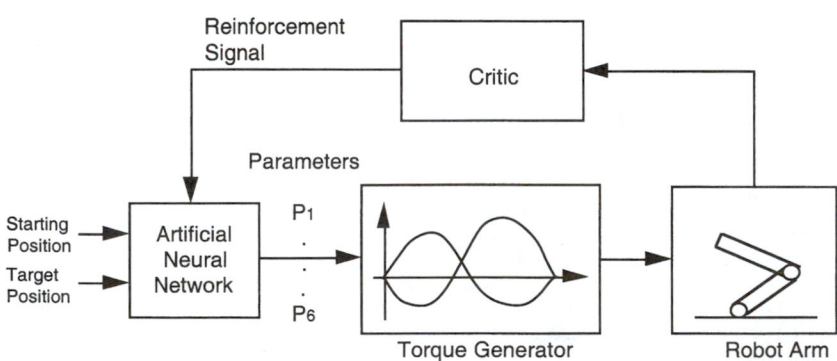

Figure 2. Block diagram of a reinforcement learning controller of an arm. Given inputs coding the starting and target positions of the hand, the network controller learns to provide correct parameters to a torque generator that generates, in open-loop mode, time-varying torque signals to the arm. The reinforcement signal evaluates the success of each movement after its completion. (Modified from Lipitkas et al., 1993, Figure 1.)

ments as well. With inputs coding starting and target hand positions, the network employs SRV units to generate six parameter values using its current weights. The torque generator generates a movement using these parameter values. When the movement is completed, it is scored by the reinforcement signal, and the network's weights are changed according to Gullapalli's SRV learning rule. After a few thousand movements with different starting and target hand positions, the system could move with reasonable accuracy for new pairs of starting and target positions as well as for the pairs on which it was trained. This amount of practice is required because the system effectively has to search the six-dimensional parameter space for each starting and target position. A more complicated example of reinforcement learning using SRV units is the work on biped walking by Benbrahim and Franklin (1997).

The relative advantages and disadvantages of supervised and reinforcement learning approaches to the distal error problem have been discussed by many researchers. It is clear that reinforcement learning approaches are simpler, but reinforcement learning is usually slower in terms of the amount of experience required for learning. This is true because reinforcement learning methods extract less information from each experience than do the model-based supervised approaches. However, in some problems it is easier to learn the right actions than it is to model their effects on a complicated process. Reinforcement learning methods are also more plausible from the perspective of neuroscience (see below), while the backpropagation process often used by supervised approaches is more difficult to reconcile with what we know about neural mechanisms. In practical terms, which approach is more advantageous will depend on aspects of the specific problem being considered.

Collective Behavior

Another property of reinforcement learning that might be relevant to motor control is the ability of a "team" of reinforcement learning systems to learn to cooperate so that the team as a whole improves performance. Here is an example presented in a 1965 lecture by the cybernetician Mikhail Tsetlin (Tsetlin, 1973), a pioneer in the study of simple reinforcement learning systems called learning automata. He presented the basic idea as follows in terms of human players (the so-called Goore game). Suppose there is a referee and some number of players. The referee can see the players, but the players cannot see one another. At the sound of a buzzer, each player is to raise one or two fingers. The referee determines what percentage of players raised one finger, then pays each player a fixed amount with a probability that depends only on this percentage (and is the same for each player). The process repeats each time the buzzer sounds. It turns out that for any number of players each implementing a sufficiently competent reinforcement learning rule, eventually each player will settle on raising either one or two fingers, so that the percentage of those raising one finger is (with probability close to 1) a local maximum of whatever payoff function the referee uses. This occurs with no direct communication among the players and no agreements of any kind among them.

It is possible to extend this result to one in which the referee provides payments based not just on the percentage of players raising one finger, but on *any function whatsoever* of the pattern of players' fingers. One can see how this is an instance of the problem of learning with a distal teacher, with the added complication that the payoff, or reinforcement signal, to each player is extremely noisy due to the noise introduced by the actions of the other players (in addition to the referee's probabilistic payoff method).

Tsetlin speculated that the recruitment of motor units can be reduced to this type of problem. Here, the problem would be to activate the right number of motor units to obtain a pull of a given force. The referee corresponds to a process that evaluates the results of the collective behavior of the entire pool of motor units on the resulting force. The collective behavior of reinforcement learning systems has been studied by many researchers (e.g., Narendra and Thathachar, 1989; Barto, 1985), although no modern work following up Tsetlin's suggestion about motor unit recruitment appears to exist.

Credit Assignment Problems

The challenge of reinforcement learning is often summed up as various kinds of *credit assignment* problems. A scalar evaluation of a complex mechanism's behavior does not indicate which of its many action components, both internal and external, were responsible for the evaluation. This makes it difficult to determine which of these components deserve the credit (or the blame) for the evaluation. This problem is sometimes referred to as the *structural* credit assignment problem: How is credit assigned to the internal workings of a complex structure? One approach is to assign credit equally to *all* the components, so that, through a process of averaging over many variations of the behavior, the components that are key in producing laudable behavior end up gaining the most strength, while inappropriate components are weakened. This is the general approach illustrated above by the Goore game.

The fact that reinforcement learning can work under these circumstances makes neural implementation quite plausible. A single reinforcement signal uniformly *broadcasted* to all the sites of learning, either neurons or individual synapses, is consistent with anatomical and physiological evidence showing the existence of diffusely projecting neural pathways by which neuromodulatory chemicals can be widely and nonspecifically distributed. It has been suggested that some of these pathways may play a rule in reward-mediated learning. A specific hypothesis is that dopamine mediates synaptic enhancement in the corticostriatal pathway in the manner of a broadcasted reinforcement signal (see DOPAMINE, ROLES OF). This may be one of the ways in which reinforcement learning is implemented for motor control.

Another aspect of the credit assignment problem occurs when the temporal relationship between a system's behavior and evaluations of that behavior is not as simple as assumed above. How can reinforcement learning work when the learner's behavior is temporally extended and evaluations occur at varying and unpredictable times? Under these more realistic conditions, it is not always clear what elements of behavior are being evaluated. This has been called the *temporal* credit assignment problem. It is especially relevant in motor control because movements extend over time and evaluative feedback may become available only after the end of a movement. An approach to this problem that is receiving considerable attention is the use of methods by which the critic itself can learn to provide useful evaluative feedback immediately after the evaluated event. According to this approach, reinforcement learning is not only the process of improving behavior according to given evaluative feedback; it also includes learning how to improve the evaluative feedback itself. The strong parallels between algorithms for adapting evaluative feedback (temporal difference methods; see REINFORCEMENT LEARNING) and the properties of dopamine-producing neurons in the brain (see DOPAMINE, ROLES OF) make it plausible that the brain uses similar methods for dealing with the temporal credit assignment problem.

The modern view of reinforcement learning developed by machine learning researchers uses the framework of stochastic optimal control to study the temporal credit assignment problem (see REINFORCEMENT LEARNING). From this perspective, reinforcement learning algorithms are methods for approximating solutions to complex stochastic optimal control problems via relatively simple mechanistic learning rules. Because optimality principles have played significant roles in theories of motor control (Engelbrecht, 2001), and because stochasticity may be an important element of motor control (Harris, 1998), the modern theory of reinforcement may prove to be of great utility in extending our understanding of motor learning.

Discussion

As this article has emphasized, motor learning is too complex to be viewed strictly in terms of either supervised learning or reinforcement learning. Feedback used in motor learning ranges from specific standards of correctness to nonspecific evaluative information, and many learning mechanisms with differing characteristics probably interact to produce the motor learning capabilities of animals. However, reinforcement learning principles may be indispensable for motor learning because they seem necessary for improving motor performance when the standards of correctness required by supervised learning are not available.

Road Maps: Mammalian Motor Control; Robotics and Control Theory
Background: Reinforcement Learning
Related Reading: Basal Ganglia; Dopamine, Roles of; Q-Learning for Robots

References

Adams, J. A., 1978, Theoretical issues for knowledge of results, in *Information Processing in Motor Control and Learning* (G. E. Stelmach, Ed.), New York: Academic Press, pp. 229–240.

Barto, A. G., 1985, Learning by statistical cooperation of self-interested neuron-like adaptive elements, *Hum. Neurobiol.*, 4:229–256.

Benbrahim, H., and Franklin, J. A., 1997, Biped dynamic walking using reinforcement learning, *Robot. Auton. Systems*, 22:283–302.

Bernstein, N., 1967, *The Co-ordination and Regulation of Movements*, Oxford, Engl.: Pergamon Press.

Desmurget, M., and Grafton, S., 2000, Forward modeling allows feedback control for fast reaching movements, *Trends Cognit. Sci.*, 4:423–431. ◆

Engelbrecht, S. E., 2001, Minimum principles in motor control, *J. Math. Psychol.*, 45:497–542. ◆

Gullapalli, V., 1990, A stochastic reinforcement algorithm for learning real-valued functions, *Neural Netw.*, 3:671–692.

Harris, C. M., 1998, On the optimal control of behavior: A stochastic perspective, *J. Neurosci. Methods*, 83:73–88.

Jordan, M. I., and Rumelhart, D. E., 1992, Supervised learning with a distal teacher, *Cognit. Sci.*, 16:307–354.

Kawato, M., 1999, Internal models for motor control and trajectory planning, *Curr. Opin. Neurobiol.*, 9:718–727.

Lipitkas, J., D'Eleuterio, G. M. T., Bock, O., and Grodski, J. J., 1993, Reinforcement learning and the parametric motor control hypothesis applied to robotic arm movements, in *Proceedings of the DND Workshop on Advanced Technologies*, Ottawa, CDN, 1993.

Narendra, K., and Thathachar, M. A. L., 1989, *Learning Automata: An Introduction*, Englewood Cliffs, NJ: Prentice Hall.

Schmidt, R. A., and Lee, T. D., 1999, *Motor Control and Learning: A Behavioral Emphasis*, 3rd ed., Champaign, IL: Human Kinetics Publishers. ◆

Thorndike, E. L., 1911, *Animal Intelligence*, Darien, CT: Hafner.

Tsetlin, M. L., 1973, *Automata Theory and Modeling of Biological Systems*, New York: Academic Press.

Respiratory Rhythm Generation

Richard J. A. Wilson, John E. Lewis, and John E. Remmers

Introduction

After several decades of intense debate, fueled by exciting experimental advance, a number of fundamental issues regarding the neuronal mechanisms that synthesize normal breathing (eupnea) remain unresolved. This article examines recent data and evaluates insights from modeling studies. We begin by discussing potential neuronal components of the respiratory rhythmogenic network and then assess current models of the respiratory oscillator in the context of the mechanisms of rhythmogenesis.

The apparent simplicity and reliability of breathing are enticing to the experimenter and modeler alike. During inspiration, activity in the phrenic nerve contracts the diaphragm, sucking air into the lungs. During expiration, passive recoil of the lungs, diaphragm, and ribs almost suffices for stale air expulsion. However, a closer look reveals a fascinating and complex behavior involving recruitment of many muscles (facial, upper airway, thoracic, abdominal, postural), modulation from many different sources (mechanosensory, chemosensory, descending), and coordination with many other behaviors (e.g., swallowing, locomotion).

In light of this complexity, perhaps one of the most remarkable ideas to arise in the field over the last decade is that only a small kernel of brainstem neurons (perhaps as few as 1,200) are responsible for the rudimentary respiratory rhythm (Gray et al., 2001). This idea originated from studies in vitro. If this idea is correct, then in vivo these neurons should meet *all* the following criteria: (1) have activity correlated with breathing, (2) be necessary for breathing (i.e., breathing is abolished if they are functionally

ablated), and (3) be sufficient for breathing (functionally defined as capable of accelerating breathing when stimulated). Unfortunately, demonstrating all but the last criterion experimentally has proved to be very difficult, as reviewed below.

Possible Components of Rhythm Generator

Correlation

Respiratory neurons are generally defined by and categorized in relation to inspiratory phrenic discharge. At least six categories have been identified (e.g., Richter, Ballanyi, and Schwarzacher, 1992): pre-inspiratory (PreI), early inspiratory (EI), throughout inspiratory (I), late inspiratory (LateI), post-inspiratory (PostI), and expiratory (E2). These categories are found across different species and, some claim, experimental preparations. Note, however, that while the phrenic discharge during eupnea consists of augmenting bursts, phrenic activity changes dramatically during other behaviors such as hiccuping, coughing, and gasping. For unambiguous identification of eupneic respiratory neurons therefore, the *pattern* of the phrenic discharge must be considered.

Correlation is but one of the three criteria that should be applied before a neuron can be given a functional definition. A neuron that fires in relation to the eupneic rhythm could conceivably be more important (i.e., necessary) for some other behavior. Furthermore, despite the presence of several categories of respiratory neurons, the generation of the eupneic rhythm may require but a subset of the types found.

Further details of the data discussed below may be found in the papers by Ballanyi, Onimaru, and Homma (1999); St. Jacques and St. John (1999); and St. John, (1996). Further information on models is given by Smith et al. (2000).

Sufficiency and Necessity

The brainstem alone can produce the respiratory rhythm. Rhythmic augmenting bursts in cranial nerves, a characteristic of eupnea, continues in vagotomized animals after transections at the midcollicular level and at the obex. Several regions in the brainstem cause acceleration of respiratory rhythm when stimulated (i.e., are sufficient). Two of these areas in the medulla, the pre-Bötzinger complex (preBötC) and the pre-inspiratory region have received particularly intense study.

The preBötC is situated rostral to the ventral respiratory group and ventral to the nucleus ambiguous (Rekling and Feldman, 1998). Gray et al. (2001) determined that the preBötC can be defined anatomically according to the distribution of Substance P receptors. The pre-inspiratory region lies just rostral and ventral to the preBötC (see Ballanyi, Onimaru, and Homma, 1999).

The preBötC contains the complete suite of respiratory neurons, and several groups have shown it to be necessary for eupnea. Ramirez et al. showed that in anesthetized, artificially ventilated, vagotomized cats, irreversible inactivation of this region with tetrodotoxin caused the cessation of the eupneic motor pattern but not anoxia-induced gasping. Gray et al. (2001) demonstrated that in awake rats, four to five days after injection of poison-conjugated Substance P into the preBötC, blood gases and breathing were abnormal, with ablated cells concentrated in, though not limited to, the preBötC.

Other in vivo experiments have generated contrasting results. Huang et al. have reported that lesioning both preBötC and pre-inspiratory regions of anesthetized, artificially ventilated, vagotomized neonatal rats with kainic acid had no effect on eupnea but eliminated anoxia-induced gasping. Lucid histological boundaries of the preBötC have been identified only recently. Therefore, discrepant results between lesion studies may reflect ablations in different regions. While this explanation may explain why some studies failed to eliminate eupnea following ablation of sites in the ventral medulla, in other studies, the lesions seem too extensive to have spared the preBötC. St. Jacques and St. John (1999) found that massive kainic acid injections (whether ipsilateral or bilateral) in the vicinity of the preBötC eliminate eupnea but only transiently. Gasping, however, was permanently abolished. While these results support the importance of the preBötC for eupnea, they also suggest that it may not be necessary, at least in the strictest sense, and that sites other than the preBötC can produce the eupneic rhythm. Where might these sites be?

One candidate is the pre-inspiratory area. This area contains large numbers of neurons that begin firing before inspiration (e.g., PreI and PostI) and, when stimulated with single shocks, can reset the respiratory rhythm. In addition, brainstem areas rostral to the medulla (i.e., in the pons) may also be necessary for eupnea. The pons also contains large numbers of respiratory neurons and may have an inherent rhythm-generating capability (St. John, 1996). It is possible that this pontine rhythm generator may interact with that in the medulla to generate breathing. Indeed, transecting the brainstem at the pontine-medulla level causes profound changes in phrenic nerve activity, to a pattern that is no longer eupneic and therefore could be produced by a different brainstem circuit (see St. John, 1996).

In summary, there is mounting evidence that the preBötC plays an important role in respiratory rhythmogenesis (Rekling and Feldman, 1998). However, we are of the opinion that the preBötC might not act alone to produce the respiratory rhythm: other areas, most notably the pons, may also be necessary for eupnea. Slices containing the preBötC complex are capable of producing rhythmic activity. However, elevated extracellular $[K^+]$ is usually required, and some argue that the rhythm produced is more gasp-like than eupneic (St. John, 1996). The ability to generate a rhythm when isolated from other neuronal structures does not dictate that the preBötC is solely responsible for the eupneic rhythm in the intact animal. In our thinking, we allow for the possibility that sites other than the preBötC may be necessary and that rhythmogenesis may be distributed.

Mechanism of Rhythm Generation

Despite the difficulty of localizing categorically the necessary and sufficient components responsible for the eupneic rhythm, models have been proposed for the mechanism by which the rhythm is generated. These models fall into two distinct groups: (a) *hybrid-pacemaker models*, in which the basic rhythm is generated by the endogenous pacemaker-like membrane properties of a small subset of respiratory neurons (Figure 1A), and (b) *network models*, in which the rhythm is generated by synaptic interactions within a large network (Figure 1B). These models are based largely on different data, obtained from in vitro and in vivo experiments, respectively.

Hybrid-Pacemaker Models

These models predict that the basic rhythm stems from a small population of respiratory neurons. These neurons, when synaptically isolated, burst as a result of inherent membrane properties (e.g., Ramirez and Richter, 1996; Reckling and Feldman, 1998; Smith et al., 2000). In these models, synaptic interactions between respiratory neurons are not necessary for rhythmogenesis per se but function primarily to elaborate, shape, and transmit the basic rhythm to generate the eupneic motor pattern.

Evidence that some respiratory neurons have pacemaker-like membrane properties arises mainly from in vitro neonatal preparations. For example, I and PostI neurons in the pre-inspiratory area of the in vitro neonatal rat brainstem-spinal cord preparation retained rhythmic bursts of action potentials after blocking inhibitory synaptic transmission either with GABA and glycine antagonists

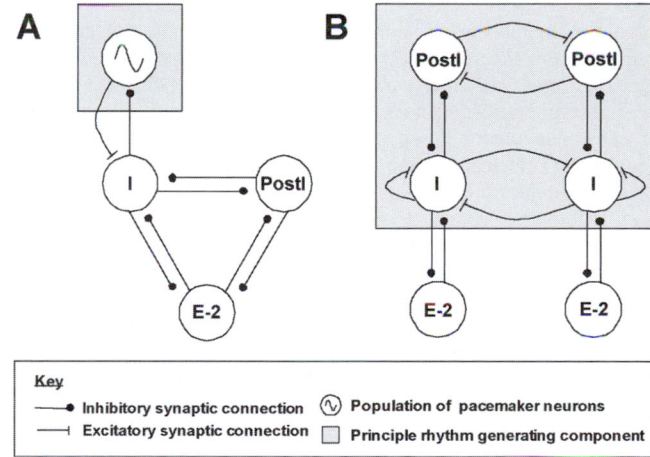

Figure 1. Two different models of the eupneic respiratory rhythm generator. *A*, Hybrid pacemaker model. *B*, Network model. Shaded boxes encapsulate key rhythm-generating components. Each circle represents a population of neurons.

or by bathing the preparation in a low Cl⁻ solution (Ballanyi et al., 1999). Similarly, in the transverse slice preparation from the neonatal rat, rhythmic bursts persisted in I and E2 preBötC neurons despite blocking of chemical synaptic connections with low Ca^{2+} (Johnson et al., 1994).

These important experiments suggest that some respiratory neurons have endogenous bursting properties, at least under certain conditions. However, Johnson et al. (1994) identified a third class of cell whose activity was transformed from tonic to bursts when exposed to low Ca^{2+}. This illustrates the difficulty of ascertaining the normal properties of neurons when they are examined outside their usual ionic and synaptic realms. In this light, one should note that the in vitro neonatal rat brainstem-spinal cord preparation has an anoxic, acidic (pH ~6.5) core that compromises synaptic inhibition and produces a gasp-like motor pattern (see St. John, 1996). One should also note that the preBötC in the in vitro slice preparation has lost many synaptic inputs and usually requires elevated $[K^+]$ for rhythmogenesis. Therefore, bursting cells in vitro may operate at membrane potentials that are not normally encountered. Whether endogenous bursting drives eupnea in vivo will be an important question for future research.

The hybrid-pacemaker model was first implemented by using conductance-based Hodgkin-Huxley-type model neurons, each with up to nine ionic conductances (see Smith et al., 2000). The early simulations consisted of a kernel of endogenous bursting neurons, which fired during the inspiratory phase. Burst initiation was determined largely by a subthreshold activating persistent Na^+ conductance ($I_{Na(p)}$), whereas a persistent K^+ conductance was critical for burst termination. These neurons provided drive to both inhibitory interneurons and premotor neurons. Interactions between interneurons and premotor neurons form the basis of the pattern-forming network, appropriately phasing the motor output. It should be emphasized that feedback from the inhibitory interneurons onto the endogenous bursters, while not necessary for eupneic rhythmogenesis per se, nonetheless makes an important contribution to the eupneic rhythmogenesis by both controlling baseline membrane potential (which influences burst frequency) and facilitating burst termination. Increasingly elaborate hybrid pacemaker-type simulations are now being used. Although the voltage clamp data to support the use and magnitude of specific conductances are extremely sparse, these second-generation simulations benefit from recent work to characterize the voltage-dependent behavior of preBötC neurons. They also involve much larger numbers of neurons to account for heterogeneous cellular properties within given neuronal populations. As such, the output of these simulations is becoming increasingly realistic, but more important, they are now being used to formulate experimentally testable hypotheses about how rhythmicity in vitro is generated (Del Negro et al., 2001). With the third generation of models, we can look forward to simulation of (1) conductances based on voltage clamp data from preBötC neurons, (2) electrical synaptic connections, and (3) effects of neuronal modulation.

A different approach to using conductance-based modeling is to use more abstract components, which make the analysis of dynamic behavior more tractable. For example, Matsugu, Duffin, and Poon (1998) considering a minimal respiratory network consisting of two mutually inhibitory elements (representing I and E neurons) that were driven by different periodic inputs (representing "pacemaker" neurons). By varying the nature of the coupling between elements, the authors found that 1:1 entrainment to the "pacemaker" required a number of specific conditions. The simplified nature of this model, while allowing a rigorous analysis, does not allow an easy transfer of these predictions to practical experimental tests. However, an important aspect of this study is that it aimed specifically at evaluating the class of hybrid-pacemaker model in the context of respiratory rhythmogenesis.

Network Models

By far the most common feature of neuronal networks that generate rhythmic output is the presence of cells with mutually inhibitory synaptic connections. Such networks have an inherent tendency to generate rhythmic outputs without the need for cells with endogenous bursting properties. The network models for respiratory rhythm generation can be thought of as an elaboration on this basic theme (Figure 1B). These models have been constructed by analyzing the activity and phase of synaptic inputs of various types of respiratory neurons (see Richter et al., 1992). The data necessary to construct these models come from cross-correlation and spike-triggered averaging from single-unit recordings largely from in vivo preparations.

Data supporting inhibitory synaptic interactions in rhythmogenesis include the following:

1. Reduced Cl⁻ solutions caused cessation of eupneic bursts in an adult arterially perfused rodent preparation (Hayashi and Lipski, 1992).
2. GABA and glycine antagonists injected bilaterally into the preBötC of the in vivo cat abolished eupnea (Pierrefiche et al., 1998).

These data are consistent with a role for phasic inhibition in rhythmogenesis. However, these manipulations may have had direct effects on membrane potential and/or removed tonic inhibition, either of which could silence pacemaker neurons.

Paton and Richter (1995), using both in vivo and in vitro preparations, showed comparable results blocking inhibitory synaptic transmission in postnatal animals. However, in neonates, they found that blocking inhibitory synaptic transmission did not eliminate rhythmic motor output, in line with previous results from experiments on neonates (e.g., Ballanyi et al., 1999; Johnson et al., 1994). The authors conclude that inhibitory synaptic connections are necessary for respiratory rhythmogenesis, but only in postnatal (>15 days) animals. Others have found no dependence of rhythmicity on postnatal age (Ramirez in Ramirez and Richter, 1996). These dichotomous results might be explained by the fact that the preparations used by Paton and Richter included the pons. Some have argued that a late-developing pontine input negates the bursting properties of pacemaker neurons, making inhibitory connections in the ventral medulla necessary for eupneic rhythmogenesis (Pierrefiche et al., 1998).

These data have motivated a number of modeling efforts. Early network models took the view that each population of respiratory neurons could be considered as a homogenous group, often described with a few simple equations, with connections between populations as the underlying mechanism of rhythmogenesis (Lewis, 1995). More recent simulations have used individual conductance-based model neurons. In one study, by balancing the relative contributions of six different channels, two different types of neurons were modeled. The first type shows an "adapting" response to synaptic excitation (resembling Early I, PostI), while the second type exhibits a "ramping" response to release from inhibition (resembling I, Late I, E2). Modeling demonstrated that the ratio of high- and low-threshold Ca^{2+} channels was the principle factor in determining type. The greater the high-threshold Ca^{2+} conductance, the more likely the neuron would have an adaptive firing pattern. This prediction remains to be tested experimentally. Using these two types of "canonical" neurons, the authors then constructed a network consisting of seven cells representing seven classes of respiratory neurons—those described in the classification of Richter et al. (1992) plus an additional class of expiratory neuron. The model also includes inputs from pulmonary stretch receptors. The authors used various network configurations (based on experimental data) to show how intrinsic membrane properties interact with synaptic (network) properties to control the firing patterns of individual neurons as well as the dynamics involved in changing between inspiratory and expiratory phases.

Discussion: A Hybrid-Pacemaker or a Network-Based Rhythm Generator?

We have outlined experimental data from two types of preparations that lead to very different predictions about the mechanisms of respiratory rhythmogenesis. In vivo data point to the importance of network interactions in generating the basic rhythm, whereas results from in vitro experiments indicate the importance of endogenous bursting neurons. Most recent modeling studies retain this polarity, concentrating on one or the other data set, resulting in models in which rhythmogenesis is either pacemaker driven or network driven. By providing a quantitative framework, these modeling studies have been invaluable in helping to understand the cellular basis of each of these mechanisms. In listing the assumptions they require to make the models, they also illustrate the need for more voltage clamp data from respiratory neurons.

An important use of modeling in the future will likely be to determine how to distinguish experimentally between pacemaker-driven and network-driven rhythmogenesis. Rybak, St. John, and Paton (2001) recently published a study demonstrating the possibility of using models in this way. Using a conductance-based pacemaker model as a starting point, they shifted the voltage dependence of $I_{Na(p)}$ by -9 mV (which they considered more physiological) and added a transient K^+ current (I_{kA}). These modifications did not affect the model neuron's ability to burst under the simulated conditions of elevated extracellular K^+ (9 mM) used in vitro. However, when $[K^+]$ was reduced toward levels closer to those in vivo (6 mM), the model neuron lost its ability to generate spontaneous bursts, owing to suppression of $I_{Na(p)}$ by I_{kA}. Furthermore, simulations suggested that bursting was disrupted by phasic synaptic inhibition. The authors suggest that rhythmogenesis in vitro represents a "switching" from a network-driven mechanism. They speculate that in vivo, the $I_{Na(p)}$ in conditional pacemakers is suppressed, but in vitro, the $I_{Na(p)}$ is released from suppression, owing to higher extracellular $[K^+]$ and the loss of synaptic inhibition. The authors tested this hypothesis in an artificially perfused preparation by blocking I_{kA} (using 4-AP), reducing inhibitory synaptic transmission (with a low dose of strychnine), and elevating extracellular K^+ (10 mM). The eupneic bursts were transformed to gasp-like events similar to those produced by in vitro preparations. While the details of Rybak et al.'s model are likely to be debated and the effects of their experimental manipulations should be scrutinized, the elegance of this study demonstrates the true potential of modeling and its growing importance in the study of respiratory rhythm generation.

Road Map: Motor Pattern Generators
Related Reading: Chains of Oscillators in Motor and Sensory Systems; Half-Center Oscillators Underlying Rhythmic Movements; Spinal Cord of Lamprey: Generation of Locomotor Patterns

References

Ballanyi, K., Onimaru, H., and Homma, I., 1999, Respiratory network function in the isolated brainstem-spinal cord of newborn rats, *Prog. Neurobiol.*, 59:583–634. ◆

Del Negro, C. A., Johnson, S. M., Butera, R. J., and Smith, J. C., 2001, Models of respiratory rhythm generation in the pre-Botzinger complex: III. Experimental tests of model predictions, *J. Neurophysiol.*, 86:59–74.

Gray, P. A., Janczewski, W. A., Mellen, N., McCrimmon, D. R., and Feldman, J. L., 2001, Normal breathing requires preBotzinger complex neurokinin-1 receptor-expressing neurons, *Nat. Neurosci.*, 4:927–930.

Hayashi, F., and Lipski, J., 1992, The role of inhibitory amino acids in control of respiratory motor output in an arterially perfused rat, *Resp. Physiol.*, 89:47–63.

Johnson, S. M., Smith, J. C., Funk, G. D., and Feldman, J. L., 1994, Pacemaker behavior of respiratory neurons in medullary slices from neonatal rat, *J. Neurophysiol.*, 72:2598–2608.

Lewis, J. E., 1995, Respiratory rhythm generation, in *Handbook of Brain Theory and Neural Networks*, 1st ed. (M. A. Arbib, Ed.), Cambridge, MA: MIT Press, pp. 813–816.

Matsugu, M., Duffin, J., and Poon, C.-S., 1998, Entrainment, instability, quasi-periodicity, and chaos in a compound neural oscillator, *J. Comput. Neurosci.*, 5:35–51.

Paton, J. F., and Richter, D. W., 1995, Role of fast inhibitory synaptic mechanisms in respiratory rhythm generation in the maturing mouse, *J. Physiol.*, 484:505–521.

Pierrefiche, O., Schwarzacher, S. W., Bischoff, A. M., and Richter, D. W., 1998, Blockade of synaptic inhibition within the pre-Bötzinger complex in the cat suppresses respiratory rhythm generation *in vivo*, *J. Physiol. (Lond.)*, 509:245–254.

Ramirez, J. M., and Richter, D. W., 1996, The neuronal mechanisms of respiratory rhythm generation, *Curr. Opin. Neurobiol.*, 6:817–825. ◆

Rekling, J. C., and Feldman, J. L., 1998, PreBotzinger complex and pacemaker neurons: Hypothesized site and kernel for respiratory rhythm generation, *Annu. Rev. Physiol.*, 60:385–405. ◆

Richter, D. W., Ballanyi, K., and Schwarzacher, S., 1992, Mechanisms of respiratory rhythm generation, *Curr. Opin. Neurobiol.*, 2:788–793.

Rybak, I. A., St. John, W. M., and Paton, J. F. R., 2001, Models of neuronal bursting behavior: Implications for *in vivo* versus *in vitro* respiratory rhythmogenesis, *Adv. Exp. Med. Biol.*, 499:159–164.

Smith, J. C., Butera, R. J., Koshiya, N., Del Negro, C., Wilson, C. G., and Johnson, S. M., 2000, Respiratory rhythm generation in neonatal and adult mammals: The hybrid pacemaker-network model, *Respir. Physiol.*, 122:131–147. ◆

St. John, W. M., 1996, Medullary regions for neurogenesis of gasping: Noeud vital or noeuds vitals, *J. Appl. Physiol.*, 81:1865–1877. ◆

St. Jacques, R., and St. John, W. M., 1999, Transient, reversible apnoea following ablation of the pre-Botzinger complex in rats, *J. Physiol. (Lond.)*, 520:303–314.

Retina

Robert G. Smith

Introduction

At the most basic level, the retina transduces spatial and temporal variations in light intensity and transmits them to the brain. However, instead of directly coding intensity, the retina transforms visual signals in a multitude of ways to code properties of the visual world such as contrast, color, and motion. This article develops a conceptual theory to explain why the retina codes visual signals and how the structure of the retina is related to its coding function.

The vertebrate retina reliably responds to light contrast as low as 1% (Shapley and Enroth-Cugell, 1984). Yet as the delicate visual signal is amplified in its passage through the retina, the biological limitations of neural processing add distortion and noise. The ease with which we see fine details in the presence of such biological limitations suggests that one function of retinal circuitry is to maintain the signal's quality by removing redundant signals (Laughlin, 1994). This hypothesis predicts that much of the retina's signal coding and structural detail is derived from the need to optimally amplify the signal and eliminate noise.

Structure

Layers and Cell Classes

The retina is a thin (100–200 μm) tissue at the rear surface of the eye consisting of three layers of neurons and glial cells (Figure 1) (see Dowling, 1987; Sterling, 1997; Rodieck, 1998). Neurons in the *outer nuclear layer* (ONL) are exclusively photoreceptors. The *inner nuclear layer* (INL) (i.e., the middle layer) contains the cell bodies of horizontal cells (H), bipolar cells (B), and amacrine cells (A). Between these two layers lies the *outer plexiform layer* (OPL), in which bipolar and horizontal cells extend dendritic processes laterally to receive synaptic contacts from photoreceptors. The innermost cell layer, called the *ganglion cell layer* (GCL), contains cell bodies of ganglion cells and amacrine cells. Between the INL and GCL lies the *inner plexiform layer* (IPL), where bipolar, amacrine, and ganglion cells are synaptically connected. Ganglion cells send their output to the brain through axons that lie on the inner surface of the retina.

Cell Types: Specificity in Form and Function

Each class of neuron described above comprises several cell types, and overall the retina comprises several dozen (Sterling, 1997; Rodieck, 1998). A cell type is defined by a distinctive morphology, distribution, synaptic connection pattern, physiology, and/or immunocytochemical staining pattern (Rodieck, 1998). That distinct cell types exist suggests that each has a specific function. Although

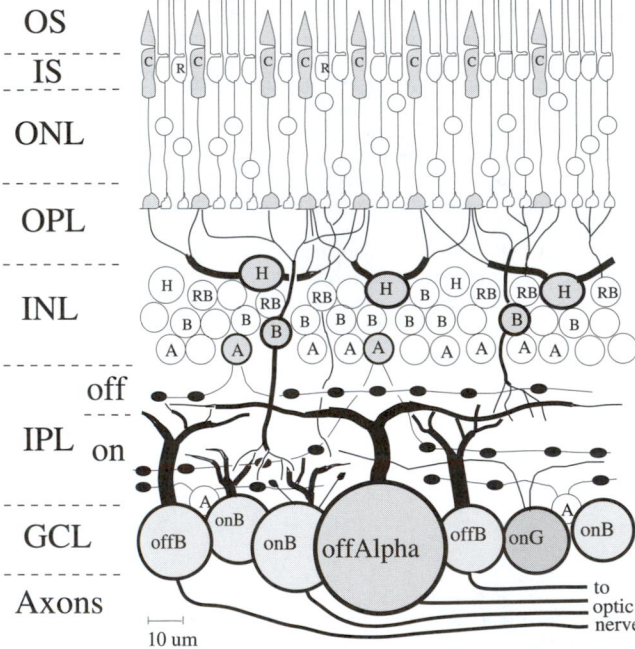

Figure 1. Structure of the retina, showing the outer segments (OS), inner segments (IS), outer nuclear layer (ONL), outer plexiform layer (OPL), inner nuclear layer (INL), inner plexiform layer (IPL), ganglion cell layer (GCL), horizontal cells (H), bipolar cells (B), amacrine (A), and rod bipolar (RB) cells.

the retina of one species may contain cell types not present in another, the same five retinal cell classes exist in all vertebrate species (Dowling, 1987; Masland, 1988; Sterling, 1997; Rodieck, 1998; Kandel, Schwartz, and Jessel, 2000). Therefore all vertebrates likely share similar neural circuit organization.

Receptive Fields and Connectivity

Neurons of each type are spaced in a regular array across the retina (see Figure 1), so the key to understanding retinal function is to identify the processing strategies of repeating functional circuits or modules (Sterling, 1997). To understand a retinal neuron's physiological function, investigators measure its *receptive field*, the region in space and time over which it responds to light. Receptive fields of retinal neurons consist of a sensitive circular region in visual space, called the *center*, and a larger but weaker antagonistic region concentric with the center, called the *surround* (Rodieck, 1998). These receptive fields are determined by intrinsic and presynaptic mechanisms. For example, a ganglion cell's receptive field shape and properties reflect its morphology and biophysical properties (Kandel et al., 2000), and also the receptive field properties of its presynaptic bipolar and amacrine cells, which in turn originate to some extent in the receptive field properties of photoreceptors and horizontal cells (Dowling, 1987; Sterling, 1997; Rodieck, 1998).

Although receptive field analysis is a powerful method for studying the function of a neural circuit (see Rodieck, 1998; Shapley and Enroth-Cugell, 1984), the origin of a receptive field in a circuit that includes several layers of neurons is difficult to grasp. The difficulty is to separate the effects of cell morphology, synaptic connectivity, and membrane channels on the receptive field (see, e.g., DIRECTIONAL SELECTIVITY). However, by computationally simulating these biophysical details based even on partial knowledge, it is possible to test specific hypotheses about neural circuit connectivity (Teeters and Arbib, 1991; Smith, 1995).

Functional Circuits

Photoreceptors and Adaptation

The outer segment (OS) of a vertebrate photoreceptor transduces light via a multistep biochemical cascade (Rodieck, 1998; Kandel et al., 2000) into an electrical signal that is conducted through the photoreceptor's axon to its terminal in the OPL. In response to a flash of light, ion channels close, hyperpolarizing the photoreceptor proportionally over a limited range of stimulus intensity. The advantage of this coding function is that a photoreceptor responds well to low-contrast signals common in the visual world. The disadvantage is that outside this limited range the photoreceptor responds poorly. At lower intensities, the photoreceptor's transduction gain (i.e., proportion of change in its output signal to a change in light) tends to be insufficient, and at higher intensities the photoreceptor's response tends to saturate. To solve such saturation problems, the photoreceptor adjusts its gain in a process called *adaptation*, which in some species can modulate transduction gain by up to 4 log units.

The two classes of photoreceptors, rods and cones (Rodieck, 1998), differ in that rods are sensitive to single photons and are bleached by daylight, but cones are less sensitive and can regenerate their pigment in daylight (photopic intensity range). At twilight (the mesopic intensity range), rods are coupled via gap junctions to neighboring cones, causing the rod signal to pass directly into cones, where it is carried by the lower-gain cone pathway (Rodieck, 1998). At night (scotopic intensity range), a special *rod bipolar* pathway (RB in Figure 1) carries quantal *single-photon* signals, removes dark noise, and adapts over an extra 3 log units of intensity (Sterling, 1997; Rodieck, 1998; Smith and van Rossum, 1998).

Outer Plexiform Layer

The axon terminal of a cone transmits its signal to bipolar cells with a chemical synapse, increasing signal gain at the cost of extra noise and a reduction in the intensity range over which the bipolar cell can respond (Laughlin, 1994). To reduce the tendency of the cone signal to saturate its synapse, the OPL filters the signal (Laughlin, 1994). The filter consists of two components, a spatial low-pass filter constructed from lateral electrical connections (gap junctions) between cones, and a spatiotemporal high-pass filter constructed by horizonal cells. Cone coupling removes uncorrelated noise from the cone's response, and consequently causes cone synaptic release to be more correlated. Although the coupling also causes "neural blur," it is useful to provide an anti-aliasing filter for the next stage of processing in the IPL.

The OPL's high-pass filter is constructed by subtracting a local average from the cone. Horizontal cells, also coupled laterally by gap junctions, sum inputs from many cone terminals and provide negative feedback to each via a feedback synapse. The negative feedback mechanism in some cases is a GABA-ergic synapse (Dowling, 1987; Sterling, 1997), but has also recently been postulated to be a form of electrical feedback. The synaptic structure that performs this function, called a *triad*, has both feedforward and feedback contacts, so it is termed *reciprocal* (Dowling, 1987; Rodieck, 1998). This type of coding has been termed *predictive* (Laughlin, 1994) because the ideal signal to subtract would be a *local average* of signals from neighboring cones (Smith, 1995).

Synaptic Function and Noise: Signal-Processing Mechanisms

The glutamatergic synapse that transmits a cone's signal to bipolar and horizontal cells adds noise originating in the random fluctuation of synaptic vesicle release rate (Sterling, 1997; Kandel et al., 2000). To reduce the amount of noise relative to the signal, vesicles are released at a high rate by a ribbon that functions as a docking site and reservoir for vesicles (Sterling, 1997; Rodieck, 1998; Kandel et al., 2000). The synapse that relays rod signals to rod-bipolar cells in starlight has a special challenge because noise generated by the rod's transduction cascade and synapse would swamp the tiny single-photon signal. A computer simulation suggested the solution (recently verified by in vitro recordings): a nonlinear threshold in the postsynaptic second-messenger system removes the noise (Smith and van Rossum, 1998).

IPL: Bipolar and Amacrine Circuits

The retina contains about 10 types of bipolar cell and more than 20 types of amacrine cell (Kolb, Nelson, and Mariana, 1981; Masland, 1988; Sterling, 1997; Rodieck, 1998). Bipolar cell dendrites arborize in the OPL to receive multiple synaptic contacts from photoreceptors, and their axons terminate in the IPL. Amacrine cells extend their dendrites laterally in the IPL to contact bipolar, amacrine, and ganglion cells.

Bipolar cells respond as photoreceptors do with a voltage proportional to light intensity, but their response range is narrower and they adapt over a wider range of stimuli. Adaptation occurs at the dendritic tip from changes in gain at a second-messenger biochemical cascade, at the membrane by voltage-gated ion channels, or at the axon, where gain of output synapses is regulated in several ways by feedback. Bipolar cells contact ganglion cells with glutamatergic ribbon synapses to allow high release rates and reduce noise. A bipolar cell may contact several ganglion cell types, each

with a different characteristic number of synapses, which implies a specific coding of the bipolar signal (Teeters and Arbib, 1991; Sterling, 1997).

Function of Amacrine Cells

Amacrine cells are a diverse group in both morphology (Kolb et al., 1981; Rodieck, 1998) and neurochemistry (Masland, 1988). Many have a large (0.5–2 mm) but sparse dendritic field with very fine dendritic processes (0.2 μm diameter) that stretch between small swellings, called *varicosities*, where synaptic connections are made (Kolb et al., 1981; Dowling, 1987). Most amacrine cells contain voltage-gated Na^+ channels and fire action potentials, which allows them to transmit signals laterally over the extent of their dendritic field (Masland, 1988). Amacrine cells are generally either GABAergic (Rodieck, 1998; Kandel et al., 2000) or glycinergic, which implies that they perform subtractive or shunting control functions. Some, such as the cholinergic "starburst" amacrine, are involved in temporal processing and respond transiently to light (Masland, 1988). Amacrine circuitry is thought to be responsible for accentuating the surround, directional selectivity in ganglion cells (see DIRECTIONAL SELECTIVITY), excitatory transient and peripheral effects, and several types of gain control (Shapley and Enroth-Cugell, 1984; Dowling, 1987; Rodieck, 1998).

Amacrine cells receive synaptic contacts from bipolar cells at a *dyad*, where a bipolar ribbon synapse contacts two postsynaptic neurons, usually ganglion and amacrine cells (Rodieck, 1998). The similarity between the synaptic dyad in the IPL and the triad in the OPL is striking (Rodieck, 1998). Both contain synaptic ribbons, and both include reciprocal feedback from a lateral neuron. The reason may be the identical problem of noise. The reciprocal feedback from an amacrine varicosity to its presynaptic bipolar cell can process the signal, reducing its dynamic range before transmission to ganglion cells (Masland, 1988; Dowling, 1987; Rodieck, 1998).

Gap Junction Coupling in Amacrine and Bipolar Cells

Amacrine and bipolar cells, like many types of neuron in the brain, are widely coupled by gap junctions to their neighbors. Bipolar cell coupling, like cone coupling, correlates neighboring cells' signals to enhance synchronous vesicle release. Since many amacrines fire action potentials, one possibility is that gap junctions allow them to synchronize their firing. But their diversity emphasizes the complexity of retinal circuitry (Masland, 1988; Rodieck, 1998). The AII amacrine cell is small-field and carries rod signals from the rod bipolar to cone bipolars at night (Kolb et al., 1981; Rodieck, 1998). To grasp the function of the AII has been a special challenge because it is coupled by gap junctions to its AII and bipolar cell neighbors, and these two types of electrical coupling are controlled by independently modulated second-messenger systems. The AII also contains voltage-gated Na^+ channels and generates action-potential-like transients. These specialized biophysical properties elegantly solve a signal-processing challenge: in starlight, the AII collects single-photon signals from an array of presynaptic rod bipolars, but synaptic noise is collected even when photons are rare. The AII's strategy, therefore, is to reduce noise by electrical coupling with neighbors, and to nonlinearly amplify the single-photon signal with voltage-gated channels (Smith and Vardi, 1995; Sterling, 1997), removing noise and reshaping the signal before passing it on.

Diversity of Coding

Ganglion Cells

Ganglion cells have exquisite sensitivity to low contrast stimuli over a wide range of light intensity (Kandel et al., 2000). They are specialized into diverse types that code different properties of the visual world (see DIRECTIONAL SELECTIVITY; see also Maturana, Lettvin, and McCulloch, 1960; Kolb et al., 1981; Rodieck, 1998). Some give a tonic response to stationary stimuli (e.g., the X or W cells of cat retina), and others give a more phasic response to signal the presence of flashing or moving stimuli (e.g., the Y cell of cat retina). Many species (lower vertebrates but also mammals) possess ganglion cells with more complex receptive fields; for example, they respond only to small or large moving objects (Maturana et al., 1960; Teeters and Arbib, 1991). In many species color-opponent ganglion cells provide excellent color vision (Dowling, 1987; Rodieck, 1998).

Coding by the Spike Generator

To transmit a signal to the brain, the ganglion cell codes its intracellular voltage (the generator potential) as the firing rate of action potentials along its axon (Kandel et al., 2000). Like synaptic coding, this process is limited by noise and dynamic range, so optimal coding of information is at a premium. The ganglion cell's spike generator, consisting of voltage- and ion-gated channels, traditionally thought to be located in the axon hillock and soma, is responsible for the coding properties. However, ganglion cells have voltage-gated channels in their dendritic membrane, and recently it was shown by simulation that the dendritic tree must contain these channels at sufficient densities to conduct action potentials, for without them the spike rate becomes too high (Fohlmeister and Miller, 1997). Dendritic morphology and slowly activated K^+ channels (Kandel et al., 2000) are also involved in shaping the ganglion cell's response. Simulations have also shown that noise in the spike generator causes variability in the spike rate, and that a significant portion of the information available in the ganglion cells' generator potential is lost in the process.

IPL: Specific Circuits in Sublayers

One problem faced by the spike generator is inherent: it cannot respond well to hyperpolarizations below a certain threshold, and just above threshold, spiking is noisy. To cope with this problem, the retina contains two subclasses of ganglion cell, called *on* and *off*, that respond with opposite polarity to a light stimulus. The on cell increases its firing rate to a flash of light and the off cell reduces its firing rate. Responses of on- and off-ganglion cells in many species are symmetric, which allows the retina to code bright and dark objects without much distortion or noise.

To supply on- and off-ganglion cells with appropriate signals, the IPL is organized into on- and off-layers (sublaminae). Two bipolar cell subclasses, on, and off, respond oppositely to glutamate released by cones. Bipolar and amacrine cell types are divided roughly equally between the two layers, although some arborize in both. The on- and off-layers are in turn organized into specific sublayers defined by microcircuits comprising bipolar, amacrine, and ganglion cells, each generating a specific spatiotemporal code (Sterling, 1997).

On-bipolar dendrites contain *metabotropic* receptors that, when bound by glutamate released by a photoreceptor, signal a cytoplasmic second messenger to turn off the synapse's ionic channels (Dowling, 1987; Sterling, 1997; Rodieck, 1998). Thus, an on-bipolar depolarizes when the photoreceptor decreases its glutamate release (i.e., in response to light). An off-bipolar contains ionotropic glutamate receptors that directly open an ion channel and hyperpolarize to light. Each off-bipolar type contains glutamate receptors with different kinetic parameters, which is the first step in generating a specific temporal code. Some bipolar cells code stimulus velocity, direction, or color (Rodieck, 1998; Haverkamp, Moeckel, and Ammermuller, 1999). These specializations increase

signal fidelity, which is an advantage for a visual signal that is destined to pass through a noisy channel to the brain.

Discussion

There are several explanations for the diversity of retinal circuitry. By discarding part of the information it receives, a neuron specializes in coding specific properties of the signal, e.g., contrast, motion, bright, dark, colored light flashes, and so forth. The exact details of the coding scheme are probably related to the ecological niche occupied by the organism. Rod signals, because of their quantal nature, are qualitatively different from cone signals, so there is an advantage to having a separate rod pathway. Such specialization in coding increases the signal/noise ratio and makes better use of the limited dynamic range of neurons, synapses, and the spike train in the ganglion cell axon (Laughlin, 1994). Specialization in coding also simplifies the task of brain circuitry in visual segmentation, which may imply a function for retinal circuit structure but involves later visual processes as well (see VISUAL SCENE SEGMENTATION).

Local Processing in Retinal Circuits

The receptive fields of many retinal neurons, and particularly of ganglion cells, share important properties, among them a center-surround organization, high sensitivity to contrast, and wide-ranging adaptation. To the extent that each retinal circuit amplifies the signal, it adapts to reduce the signal's dynamic range, which implies that the retina's high sensitivity is achieved at the cost of complexity. For example, the net effect of the OPL circuit is to create for the photoreceptor a receptive field with a broad center region and a wide antagonistic surround (Sterling, 1997; Rodieck 1998; Kandel et al., 2000) that adapts temporally and spatially. By removing information about absolute light intensity, the OPL circuit transmits what is left, i.e., information about contrast. In turn, the IPL circuit removes more information about light intensity and contrast, shaping the signal in time to code transients, and accentuating the spatial center-surround receptive field in bipolar and amacrine cells (Dowling, 1987; Rodieck, 1998). This process further regulates the visual signal's gain to improve discrimination of low-contrast objects from noise and to prevent saturation at high contrast (Shapley and Enroth-Cugell, 1984). The result of these operations is that retinal receptive fields change with background intensity to maximize information transfer (Laughlin, 1994), and the consequence of this processing is the familiar center and surround of the ganglion cell. Thus, it appears that circuits along the retinal pathway all contribute to the ganglion cell's receptive field properties for a similar reason: to prevent noise or saturation from degrading the signal (Laughlin, 1994).

The well-known antagonistic center-surround and adaptation properties of the ganglion cell receptive field, therefore, seem driven by the goal of preserving signal quality. To accomplish this, the circuitry of both OPL and IPL increase the receptive field's lateral extent. But the need for high visual acuity mandates that OPL and IPL circuits not extend laterally too far. Thus, the retina is shaped to compensate for biological limitations by a compromise between spatial acuity and accuracy of coding.

Testing the Theory

Although knowledge of the biophysical components of retinal circuitry and its receptive fields is progressing rapidly, such knowledge does not guarantee a useful theory. For example, whole-cell patch recordings allow the biophysical properties and visual responses of bipolar and amacrine cells presynaptic to a ganglion cell to be measured, and these presynaptic responses contribute to the ganglion cell's receptive field. Yet such knowledge alone cannot answer the question of function in design: what function the individual components add to the circuit, and therefore why they exist. The answer can only be derived from synthetic models that integrate details of the retina's neural circuitry with the noise and dynamic range limitations inherent to neurobiology.

Computational modeling promises to help find the answers (Teeters and Arbib, 1991; Smith, 1995; Smith and Vardi, 1995; Fohlmeister and Miller, 1997; Haverkamp et al., 1999). Once the basic signal flow and function in a retinal circuit have been established, simulations can help determine overall strategies, and with information theory can find what biological limitations are most serious to the circuit (Laughlin, 1994). The effect of noise on the retina's performance can be tested by simulating noise from all the sources in the signal pathway, and comparing the resulting signal/noise ratios as a measure of signal quality.

Road Map: Vision
Related Reading: Color Perception; Directional Selectivity; Motion Perception: Elementary Mechanisms; Visuomotor Coordination in Frog and Toad

References

Dowling, J. E., 1987, *The Retina: An Approachable Part of the Brain*, Cambridge, MA: Harvard University Press. ◆
Fohlmeister, J. F., and Miller, R. F., 1997, Mechanisms by which cell geometry controls repetitive impulse firing in ganglion cells, *J. Neurophysiol.*, 78:1948–1964.
Kolb, H., Nelson, R., and Mariani, A., 1981, Amacrine cells, bipolar cells, and ganglion cells of the cat retina: A Golgi study, *Vision Res.*, 21:1081–1114.
Haverkamp, S., Moeckel, W., and Ammermuller, J., 1999, Different types of synapses with different spectral types of cones underlie color opponency in a bipolar cell of the turtle retina, *Vis. Neurosci.*, 16:801–809, 1999.
Kandel, E. R., Schwartz, J. H., and Jessel, T. M., 2000, *Principles of Neural Science*, 4th ed., New York: McGraw-Hill. ◆
Laughlin, S. B., 1994, Matching coding, circuits, cells, and molecules to signals: General synaptic principles of retinal design in the fly's eye, *Prog. Retinal Eye Res.*, 13:165–196. ◆
Masland, R. H., 1988, Amacrine cells, *Trends Neurosci*, 11:405–410. ◆
Maturana, H. R., Lettvin, J. Y., and McCulloch, W. S., 1960. Anatomy and physiology of vision in the frog (*Rana pipiens*), *J. Gen. Physiol.*, 43:129–175.
Rodieck, R. W., 1998, *The First Steps in Seeing*, Sunderland, MA: Sinauer. ◆
Shapley, R. M., and Enroth-Cugell, C., 1984, Visual adaptation and retinal gain controls, *Progr. Retinal Res.*, 3:263–346. ◆
Smith, R. G., 1995, Simulation of an anatomically defined local circuit: The cone-horizontal cell network in cat retina, *Vis. Neurosci.*, 12:545–561.
Smith, R. G., and van Rossum, M. C. W., 1998, Noise removal at the rod synapse of mammalian retina, *Vis. Neurosci.*, 15:809–821.
Smith, R. G., and Vardi, N., 1995, Simulation of the AII amacrine cell of mammalian retina: Functional consequences of electrical coupling and regenerative membrane properties, *Vis. Neurosci.*, 12:851–860.
Sterling, P., 1997, Retina, in *The Synaptic Organization of the Brain*, 4th ed. (G. M. Shepherd, Ed.), New York: Oxford University Press. ◆
Teeters, J. L., and Arbib, M. A., 1991, A model of anuran retina relating interneurons to ganglion cell responses, *Biol Cybern.*, 64:197–207.

Robot Arm Control

Carme Torras

Introduction

A robot is a multifunctional and reprogrammable mechanism able to move in a given environment. Three broad classes of robots can be distinguished on the basis of their mobility. *Robot arms* have a fixed base, and their mobility comes from their articulated structure; thus, they operate on a bounded three-dimensional (3D) subspace. *Robot vehicles* move on two-dimensional (2D) surfaces by using wheels or other similar continuous traction elements (see Robot Navigation). *Walking robots* are designed to move through rough terrains by using articulated legs. Of course, mixed possibilities also exist, such as robot arms mounted on wheeled vehicles. This article is devoted to robot arms, or manipulators, which we will call simply robots.

Each robot is endowed with a controller that commands its mechanical structure to perform the desired tasks. Controllers are usually *hierarchically* structured from the lowest level of servomotors to the highest levels of trajectory generation and task supervision. The activity taking place at all these levels is conceptually the same: an actual motion (of a single joint, the end-effector, or the entire robot) is made to follow as closely as possible a commanded motion through the use of feedback. The difference lies in the coordinate systems used at each level.

At least four coordinate spaces can be distinguished: the task space (used to specify tasks, possibly in terms of sensor readings), the workspace (six-dimensional Cartesian coordinates defining a position and orientation of the end-effector), the joint space (intrinsic coordinates determining a robot configuration), and the actuator space (in which actual motions are commanded). Because robot control entails transforming a specification in task space into actuator commands, it critically depends on accurate mappings between the various coordinate spaces.

Neural networks have been used to approximate these mappings when they are difficult or impossible to derive analytically (as in the case of flexible or redundant robots, or in tasks entailing sensorimotor coordination) and when, because of environmental changes or robot wear-and-tear, the mappings vary in time and the controller needs to adapt on-line to these variations. This article discusses four such mappings and the neural models used to implement them adaptively.

Neural Adaptivity in Robot Control

A robot, when moving, can be thought of as realizing a mapping from actuator space to joint space, and to the workspace and task space as well. These mappings are referred to as *forward mappings* and are parameterized by the current state of the robot. In the same general terms, a controller can be viewed as implementing *inverse mappings* in that, given the current state and a desired output (sensory pattern or robot pose), the controller has to generate the appropriate commands to attain that output.

Control strategies often rely on models of the various mappings we have delineated. Forward models are used to provide fast internal feedback in order to prevent instabilities in the control loop. Inverse models lie at the core of feedforward control. The learning of such models by means of neural networks is described in Sensorimotor Learning (q.v.), and their use inside robot controllers is discussed in Robot Learning (q.v.).

For the purposes of the present discussion, let us mention that inverse models can be acquired under four schemes, namely *direct inverse modeling, feedback-error learning, distal supervised learning*, and *reinforcement learning* (see SENSORIMOTOR LEARNING for details). These schemes can be applied under both supervised and unsupervised (or self-supervised) training modes and through the use of correlational, reinforcement, or error-minimization adaptation procedures (Torras, 1995). This distinction between adaptation procedures is made on the basis of the type of problem information they use (Figure 1).

Correlational procedures use no problem information, and their goal is to carry out feature discovery or clustering. In a robot control setting, these procedures are often used to represent a given state space in a compact and topology-preserving manner. Two applications to be described later rely on representations of this type for the robot workspace (see discussion under "Inverse Kinematics") and the space of joint positions, velocities, and accelerations (see "Inverse Dynamics"). The correlational procedures most widely used for robot control are SELF-ORGANIZING FEATURE MAPS (q.v.) and ADAPTIVE RESONANCE THEORY (ART) (q.v.).

Error-minimization procedures require complete target information in the form of input-output pairs. The goal of using such procedures is to build a mapping from inputs to outputs that generalizes properly. These procedures are the most widely used in applications. Among others, the LMS rule, backpropagation (see PERCEPTRONS, ADALINES, AND BACKPROPAGATION), locally weighted projection regression, and conjugate gradient optimization have been applied to robot control.

Reinforcement-based procedures lie between both extremes. They make use only of a reward/penalty signal to build a mapping that maximizes reward (see REINFORCEMENT LEARNING). These procedures have been applied for learning sensorimotor maps.

Inverse Kinematics

Inverse kinematics mapping provides joint coordinates as a function of the position and orientation of the robot end-effector, thus relating the workspace to the joint space. The use of neural networks to learn this mapping is of particular interest when a precise model of some joints is lacking or when, because of the conditions of operation of the robot (in space, underwater, etc.), it is hardly possible to recalibrate it.

Feedforward networks using backpropagation have been extensively tested in this context, under both the *direct inverse modeling* and the *distal supervised learning* approaches (Jordan and Rumelhart, 1992), leading to the conclusion that a coarse mapping can be obtained quickly but an accurate representation of the true mapping often is not feasible or is extremely difficult. The reason for this seems to be the *global* effect that every connection weight has on the final approximation obtained (Kröse and van der Smagt, 1993).

A way to avoid this global effect is to use local representations, so that every part of the network is responsible for a small subspace of the total input space. One such representation is the 3D self-organizing feature map (SOM) used by Ritter, Martinetz, and Schulten (1992) to encode the robot workspace. This is combined with the LMS rule to learn the inverse kinematics of a robot arm with 3 degrees of freedom (dof) under a *direct inverse modeling* approach. The inputs to each neuron are the coordinates of the desired end-effector position, and the outputs (after correct learning) are the joint angles and the Jacobian corresponding to that position. Thus, this model provides a discrete encoding of the inverse kinematics mapping augmented by a linear approximation at each sample point that permits interpolating joint angles with higher precision. The network has been shown to self-organize into a reasonable representation of the workspace in about 30,000 learning cycles. This should be taken as an experimental demonstration of the powerful learning capabilities of this model, because the conditions in which it was made to operate are the worst possible ones: no a priori knowledge of the robot kinematics, random weight initialization, and random sampling of the workspace during training.

PROCEDURES	DEGREE OF FEEDBACK	DIAGRAM	KEYWORDS
CORRELATIONAL	none		Unsupervised Classical conditioning Open-loop
REINFORCEMENT	qualitative		Trial-and error Instrumental conditioning Optimal control
ERROR- MINIMIZATION	quantitative		Supervised Reference-model control Closed-loop

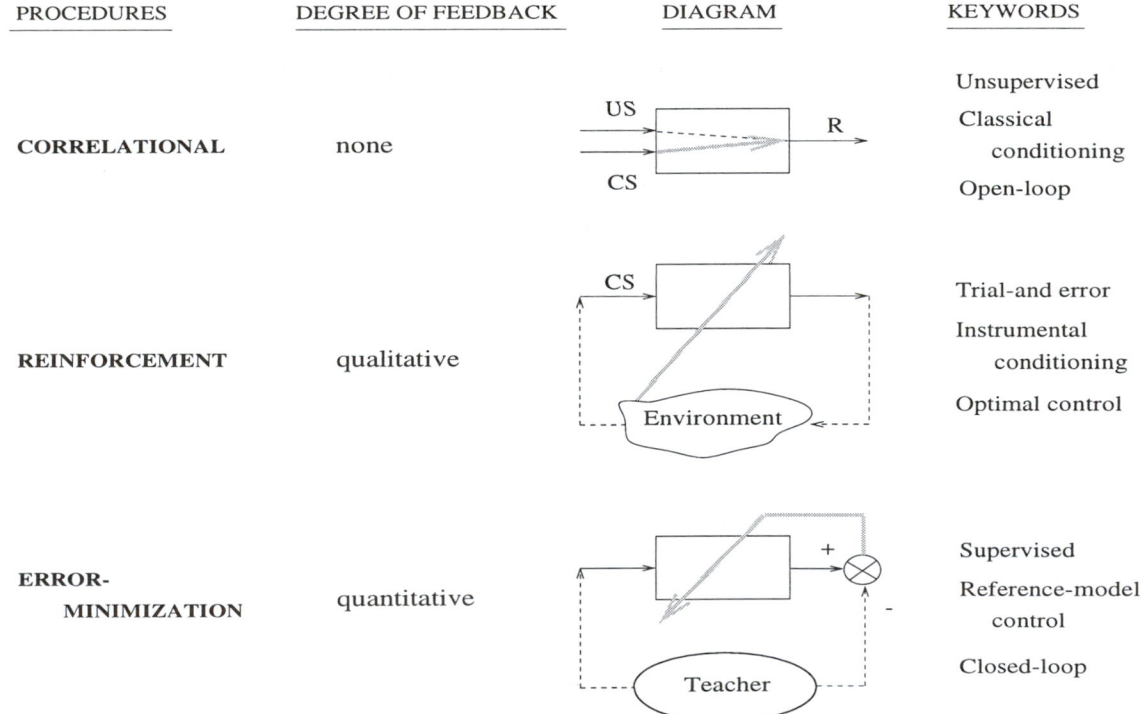

Figure 1. Procedures for neural adaptivity. See Torras (1995) for a detailed explanation.

This basic model has been extended in three directions to cope with higher-dof robots. First, a hierarchical version, consisting of a 3D SOM whose nodes each have associated a 2D SOM, was applied to a 5-dof robot. The 3D net encodes the workspace as before, while each 2D subnet approximates the end-effector orientation space at the corresponding position (Ritter et al., 1992).

Ruiz de Angulo and Torras (1997) have adapted this hierarchical model to suit a practical setting. Thus, instead of learning the kinematics from scratch, only the deviations from the nominal kinematics embedded in the original robot controller are learned. This, together with informed initialization and sampling, as well as several modifications in the learning algorithm aimed at improving the cooperation between neurons, led to a speed-up of two orders of magnitude with respect to the original model. Thus, when applied to the self-calibration of a 6-dof robot installed in a space station mockup, 95% of the decalibration was corrected with the first 25 movements, with the percentage rising to 98% after 100 movements. Moreover, other desirable features in stand-alone applications, such as parameter stability, are guaranteed.

The third extension relies on the generalization of SOMs to parameterized SOMs (PSOMs). The idea is to turn the discrete representation into a continuous one by associating a basis function with each neuron, so that a parameterized mapping manifold is obtained. Moreover, PSOMs make no distinction between inputs and outputs, thus encoding bidirectional mappings. Compared with the SOM, the PSOM considerably reduces the number of training samples required to attain a given precision (Walter and Ritter, 1996), allowing the learning of the full inverse kinematics of a 6-dof robot with less than 800 movements.

Recently, the development of humanoid robots has heightened interest in learning inverse kinematics. Because of the many dofs involved, the aim is no longer learning the mapping for the whole workspace but is focused on a specific trajectory. Following the trend of using localized representations, D'Souza, Vijayakumar, and Schaal (2001) have applied a supervised algorithm, locally weighted projection regression, in this context, with promising results (see Robot Learning).

Inverse Dynamics

When the robot dynamics needs to be taken into account, the control learning problem becomes more involved. An inverse dynamics mapping relating end-effector accelerations to the required joint forces and torques should be considered now.

Because the cerebellum is involved in the production and learning of smooth movements, several cerebellar models have been proposed and applied to control robot arms. The pioneer such model was the Cerebellar Model Articulation Controller (CMAC), developed by Albus in 1975 (see Cerebellum and Motor Control for related material), but today the debate is still open as to what model best captures the functionality of the cerebellum and whether any such model can constitute a practical option to control robots (van der Smagt and Bullock, 1997). A point of agreement is that the cerebellum constructs an inverse dynamics model as it learns. Thus, cerebellar models have been used for this purpose inside robot controllers.

Miller et al. (1990) combined the table look-up facilities provided by CMAC with an error-correction scheme similar to the LMS rule to accomplish the dynamic control of a 5-dof robot. The idea underlying this combination is similar to that of enlarging SOMs with the LMS rule, as described in the preceding section. Here, CMAC is used to represent the state space in a compact and localized manner, as SOMs were used to cover the robot workspace in the preceding section. To teach the robot to follow a given trajectory, successive points along it are supplied to both the neural network and a fixed-gain controller, and then their responses are added up to command the robot. Therefore, the neural network acts as a feedforward component. After each cycle, the actual command given to the robot and its current state are used as an input-output pair to train the neural network, thus following a *direct inverse modeling* approach. As learning progresses, the CMAC network approximates the inverse dynamics mapping, and consequently, the effect of the fixed-gain controller tends to zero. The network converges to a low error (between one and two position encoder units) within ten trials, provided enough weight vectors are used.

The same trajectory learning task as described above was tackled by Miyamoto et al. (1988) using a *feedback-error learning* approach. They used directly as error signal the output of the feedback controller, which can be interpreted as a local linearization of the inverse dynamics mapping if the learning rate is sufficiently small. This error measure is less accurate than that used by Miller et al. (1990) but has the advantage of being directly available in the control loop, thus avoiding the computation of the current state of the robot required in the direct inverse modeling approach. The authors report that, after training the robot to follow a trajectory lasting 6 seconds for 300 trials, the average feedback torque decreased from a few hundred to just a few units, demonstrating that the neural network had taken over control from the fixed-gain controller. Moreover, the mean square error in the joint angles decreased steadily by 1.5 orders of magnitude.

Force-Motor Mapping

For tasks entailing the achievement of a goal using sensory feedback, even programming in task-space coordinates can be very complex. An example is the insertion of components with small clearance, since devising a detailed force-control strategy that performs correctly in all possible situations, and subject to real-world conditions of uncertainty and noise, is extremely difficult. What is needed to accomplish this type of task is an appropriate *sensorimotor mapping* that relates sensory patterns to actuator commands. A relay through the intermediate workspace and joint space representations may or may not be required (see Limb Geometry, Neural Control).

Gullapalli, Barto, and Grupen (1994) have used an associative reinforcement learning system to learn active compliant control for peg-in-hole insertion using a 6-dof robot (see Reinforcement Learning in Motor Control). The system takes the sensed peg positions and forces, as well as the previous position command, as inputs, and produces a new position command as output. Thus, 18 real values are entered into a network with two hidden layers of backpropagation units, and six real values are produced by its output layer of stochastic reinforcement-learning units. The reinforcement signal depends on the discrepancy between the sensed and the desired position of the peg, with a penalty term being activated whenever the sensed forces on the peg exceed a preset maximum. The training runs start with the peg at a random position and orientation with respect to the hole, and end when either the peg is successfully inserted or 100 time steps have elapsed. Experimental results show that after 150 trials, the robot is consistently able to complete the insertion. Moreover, the time to insertion decreases continuously from 100 to 45 time steps over the subsequent 500 training runs.

Visuomotor Mappings

Depending on the task to be performed and the camera-robot arrangement, visuomotor mappings take different forms. Thus, in eye-hand coordination, where cameras external to the robot are used to monitor the pose (position and orientation) of its end-effector, a mapping from the camera coordinates of a desired end-effector pose to the joint angles that permit attaining that pose is

Table 1. Neuroadaptive Procedures Used to Approximate Several Robot Mappings

Mapping	Correlational + Error Minimization	Error Minimization	Reinforcement Learning
Inverse kinematics	SOM + LMS (Ritter et al., 1992; Ruiz de Angulo and Torras, 1997)	BP (Jordan and Rumelhart, 1992; Kröse and van der Smagt, 1993)	
	PSOM + LMS (Walter and Ritter, 1996)	LWPR (D'Souza et al., 2001)	
Inverse dynamics	CMAC + LMS (Miller et al., 1990)	LMS (Miyamoto et al., 1988)	
Force-motor			RL (Gullapalli et al., 1992)
Visuomotor	SOM + LMS (Ritter et al., 1992)	BP (Wells et al., 1996)	
		CG (Schram et al., 1996)	

Abbreviations: SOM, self-organizing feature map; PSOM, parameterized self-organizing feature map; LMS, least-mean-square algorithm; BP, backpropagation; LWPR, locally weighted projection regression; CMAC, Cerebellar Model Articulation Controller; RL, reinforcement learning; CG, conjugate gradient learning algorithm.

sought. This mapping is closely related to the inverse kinematics one, especially if the camera coordinates of selected points in the end-effector uniquely characterize its pose. Therefore, the same models used to learn inverse kinematics have been applied in this context (Ritter et al., 1992).

A camera mounted on a robot arm is used in tasks such as visual positioning and object tracking. The goal of these tasks is to move the camera so that the image captured matches a given reference pattern. The target is thus no longer a position in space but a desired image pattern, and the desired visuomotor mapping needs to relate offsets with respect to that pattern with appropriate movements to cancel them. In visual positioning, the scene is assumed to be static and the main issue is to attain high precision. Applications include inspection and grasping of parts that cannot be precisely placed (e.g., in underwater or space settings). The aim of object tracking is to maintain a moving object within the field of view, speed being the critical parameter here instead of precision.

The classical way of tackling these tasks consists in defining a set of image features and then deriving an interaction matrix relating 2D shifts of these features in the image to 3D movements of the camera (Samson, LeBorgne, and Espiau, 1990). Note that the visuomotor mapping can be implemented with or without a relay through the workspace, depending on how the movements of the camera are commanded.

In the case of visual positioning, Wells, Venaille, and Torras (1996) have used backpropagation to learn the interaction matrix. The training procedure consists in moving the camera from the reference position to random positions and then using the displacement in image features together with the motion performed as input-output pairs. The system thus follows a *direct inverse modeling* approach. In operation, the robot is commanded to execute the inverse of the motion that the network has associated with the given input. The key option in this work is the use of global image descriptors, which permits avoiding the costly matching of local geometric features in the current and reference images. By using a statistical measure of variable interdependence (the mutual information criterion), sets of global descriptors as variant as possible with each robot dof are selected from a battery of features, including geometric moments, eigenvectors, pose-image covariance vectors, and local feature analysis vectors (Wells and Torras, 1998). The results obtained with a 6-dof robot show that after 10.000 learning cycles, translation and rotation errors are less than 2 mm and 0.1 degrees, respectively.

Concerning object tracking, Schram et al. (1996) have used a feedforward network together with a conjugate gradient learning algorithm to make a camera track a cart moving arbitrarily on a table. A visuomotor mapping relating the current and past visual coordinates of the cart with joint displacements is built on-line as the robot moves. Only 2 robot dofs need to be controlled, and thus the network has two outputs, while several numbers of inputs have been tried. The tracking performance improves as more previous

positions of both the cart and the robot are used, attaining an average lag of only 8 mm in the case of seven inputs.

Discussion

After surveying several robot neurocontrol applications entailing the learning of various mappings (Table 1), we have extracted some guidelines.

In the case of *mappings that can be easily sampled*, it seems sufficient to apply a direct inverse modelling approach combined with an error-minimization learning procedure. Some simple inverse kinematics mappings and visuomotor mappings used for visual positioning have been learned in this way. If *the input space is complex*, then many researchers have resorted to a combination of correlational rules for the efficient coding of that space, with error-minimization procedures to build the appropriate association with the outputs. The use of self-organizing feature maps to encode the robot workspace or the sensor space, as well as the application of CMAC to the coding of the robot dynamics state space, fall into this category. When *the task is specified as a goal to be attained* using sensory feedback, without making explicit the movements necessary to attain it, the only possibility is to resort to reinforcement learning procedures, which depend just on the availability of a measure of success rather than on an error measure.

The number of learning cycles required ranges widely in the applications described, depending on the complexity of the mapping to be learned as well as on the accuracy required. Only ten trials are needed to get a useful mapping in the case of inverse dynamics using CMAC. The explanation is that only a very coarse mapping is needed, since the neural controller is used as a feedforward component in combination with a fixed-gain feedback controller. The number of trials rises to a few hundred in the case of force-motor mappings for insertion of components. One hundred learning cycles suffice to correct the distortions in the inverse kinematics mapping resulting from robot wear-and-tear, while this number rises to nearly 1,000 when the full mapping has to be learned from scratch. And the progression continues, to up to 10,000 trials when the inputs are not spatial coordinates but global descriptors extracted from images. Of course, some of these figures might be considerably lower in the future, especially the last one, if more effcient codings of the input space are found.

Road Map: Robotics and Control Theory
Background: Cerebellum and Motor Control
Related Reading: Arm and Hand Movement Control; Identification and Control; Robot Learning; Sensorimotor Learning

References

D'Souza, A., Vijayakumar, S., and Schaal, S., 2001, Learning inverse kinematics, in *Proceedings of the IEEE/RSJ Conference on Intelligent Robots and Systems*, Piscataway, NJ: IEEE Press, pp. 298–303.

Gullapalli, V., Barto, A. G., and Grupen, R., 1994, Learning admittance mappings for force-guided assembly, in *Proceedings of the IEEE International Conference on Robotics and Automation*, Los Alamitos, CA: IEEE Computer Society Press, pp. 2633–2638.

Gullapalli, V., Grupen, R., and Barto, A., 1992, Learning reactive admittance control, in *Proceedings of the IEEE International Conference on Robotics and Automation*, vol. 2, Los Alamitos, CA: IEEE Computer Society Press, pp. 1475–1480.

Jordan, M. I., and Rumelhart, D. E., 1992, Forward models: Supervised learning with a distal teacher, *Cognit. Sci.*, 16:307–354.

Kröse, B. J. A., and van der Smagt, P. P., 1993, Robot control, in *An Introduction to Neural Networks*, 5th ed., Amsterdam: University of Amsterdam, chap. 7. ◆

Miller, W. T., Hewes, R. P., Glanz, F. H., and Kraft, L. G., 1990, Real-time dynamic control of an industrial manipulator using a neural-network-based learning controller, *IEEE Trans. Robot. Automat.*, 6:1–9.

Miyamoto, H., Kawato, M., Setoyama, T., and Suzuki, R., 1988, Feedback-error-learning neural network for trajectory control of a robotic manipulator, *Neural Netw.*, 1:251–265.

Ritter, H., Martinetz, T., and Schulten, K., 1992, *Neural Computation and Self-Organizing Maps*, New York: Addison-Wesley. ◆

Ruiz de Angulo, V., and Torras, C., 1997, Self-calibration of a space robot, *IEEE Trans. Neural Netw.*, 8:951–963.

Samson, C., LeBorgne, M., and Espiau, B., 1990, *Robot Control: The Task Function Approach*, Oxford Engineering Science Series 22, Oxford, Engl.: Oxford Science Publications. ◆

Schram, G., van der Linden, F. X., Kröse, B. J. A., and Groen, F. C. A., 1996, Visual tracking of moving objects using a neural network controller, *Robot. Auton. Syst.*, 18:293–299.

Torras, C., 1995, Robot adaptivity, *Robot. Auton. Syst.*, 15:11–23. ◆

van der Smagt, P., and Bullock, D., Eds., 1997, Can artificial cerebellar models compete to control robots? in *Extended abstracts of the NIPS*97 Workshop*, DLR Technical Report No. 515-97-28, German Aerospace Center (DLR Oberpfaffenhofen).

Walter, J., and Ritter, H., 1996, Rapid learning with parameterized self-organizing maps, *Neurocomputing*, 12:131–153.

Wells, G., Venaille, C., and Torras, C., 1996, Vision-based robot positioning using neural networks, *Image Vision Comput.*, 14:715–732.

Wells, G., and Torras, C., 1998, Selection of image features for robot positioning using mutual information, in *Proceedings of the IEEE Conference on Robotics and Automation*, Los Alamitos, CA: IEEE Computer Society Press, pp. 2819–2826.

Robot Learning

Stefan Schaal

Introduction

Learning robot control, a subclass of the field of learning control, refers to the process of acquiring a sensorimotor control strategy for a particular movement task and movement system by trial and error. Learning control is usually distinguished from adaptive control in that the learning system is permitted to fail during the process of learning, while adaptive control emphasizes single-trial convergence without failure. Thus, learning control resembles the way that humans and animals acquire new movement strategies, while adaptive control is a special case of learning control that fulfills stringent performance constraints, such as may be needed in life-critical systems such as airplanes and industrial robots.

A key question in learning control is what it is that should be learned. In order to address this issue, it is helpful to assume one of the most general frameworks of learning control as originally developed in the middle of the twentieth century in the fields of optimization theory, optimal control, and in particular dynamic programming (Bellman, 1957; Dyer and McReynolds, 1970). Here, the goal of learning control was formalized as the need to acquire a task-dependent control policy π that maps the continuous-valued state vector $\mathbf{x}$ of a control system and its environment, possibly in a time-dependent way, to a continuous-valued control vector $\mathbf{u}$:

$$\mathbf{u} = \pi(\mathbf{x}, \alpha, t) \tag{1}$$

The parameter vector α contains the problem-specific parameters in the policy π that need to be adjusted by the learning system. Figure 1 illustrates the generic control diagram of learning a control policy. Since the controlled system can generally be expressed as a nonlinear function

$$\dot{\mathbf{x}} = f(\mathbf{x}, \mathbf{u}) \tag{2}$$

in accordance with standard dynamical systems theory (Strogatz, 1994), the combined system and controller dynamics result in:

$$\dot{\mathbf{x}} = f(\mathbf{x}, \pi(\mathbf{x}, t, \alpha)) \tag{3}$$

Thus, learning control means finding a (usually nonlinear) function π that is adequate for a given desired behavior and movement system. This formal viewpoint allows discussing robot learning in terms of the different methods that have been suggested for learning control policies.

Methods of Learning Robot Control

Learning the Control Policy Directly

It is possible to learn the control policy π directly, i.e., without splitting it into subcomponents, as explained in later sections. For this purpose, the desired behavior needs to be expressed as an optimization criterion $r(t)$ to be optimized over a certain temporal horizon T, resulting in a cost function

$$J(\mathbf{x}(t)) = \int_{t=0}^{T} r(\mathbf{x}(s), \mathbf{u}(s))ds$$

or

$$J(\mathbf{x}(t)) = \int_{t=0}^{\infty} \frac{1}{\tau} e^{-(s-t/\tau)} r(\mathbf{x}(s), \mathbf{u}(s))ds \tag{4}$$

The second formulation of Equation 4 illustrates the use of an infinite horizon time window by introducing a discount factor that

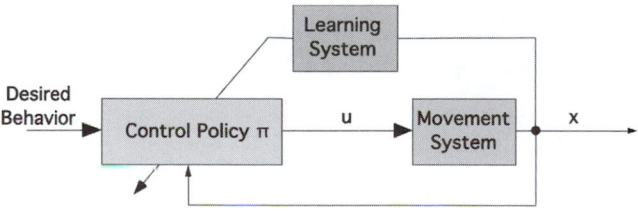

Figure 1. Generic control diagram for learning control.

reduces the influence of values of $r(t)$ in the far future. Note that $r(t)$ is usually a function of the state $\mathbf{x}$ and command $\mathbf{u}$ taken in $\mathbf{x}$; i.e., $r(t) = r(\mathbf{x}(t), \mathbf{u}(t))$. Solving such kinds of optimization problems was developed in the framework of dynamic programming (Dyer and McReynolds, 1970) and its recent derivative, reinforcement learning (Sutton and Barto, 1998; see also REINFORCEMENT LEARNING). For reinforcement learning, $r(t)$ corresponds to the "immediate reward" and $J(\mathbf{x}(t))$ to the "long-term reward." For instance, in the classical task of balancing a pole on a finger, the immediate reward could be $+1$ at every time step at which balancing was successful, and -1000 if the pole was dropped; the task goal would be to accumulate maximal long-term reward, equivalent to balancing without dropping.

The policy π is acquired with reinforcement learning by, first, learning the optimal function $J(\mathbf{x}(t))$ for every state $\mathbf{x}$, usually by a technique called temporal difference learning (see REINFORCEMENT LEARNING), and then deducing the policy π as the command $\mathbf{u}$ in every state $\mathbf{x}$ that leads to the best future payoff, i.e.,

$$\mathbf{u} = \max_{u'} (r(\mathbf{x}(t), \mathbf{u}'(t)) + J(\mathbf{x}(t + 1)))$$

where

$$\mathbf{x}(t + 1) = \mathbf{x}(t) + f(\mathbf{x}(t), \mathbf{u}'(t))\Delta t \tag{5}$$

where Δt is an arbitrarily chosen constant time step for sampling the system's behavior. Many variations of reinforcement learning exist, including methods that avoid estimating the optimization function $J(\mathbf{x}(t))$ (see REINFORCEMENT LEARNING).

Learning the Control Policy in a Modular Way

Theoretically, the techniques of reinforcement learning and dynamic programming would be able to solve any robot learning problem that can be formulated as sketched in the previous section. Practically, however, this is not true, since reinforcement learning requires a large amount of exploration of all actions and states for proper convergence of learning as well as appropriate representations for the function $J(\mathbf{x}(t))$. Traditionally, $J(\mathbf{x}(t))$ needs to be represented as a lookup table; that is, for every state $\mathbf{x}$ a specific table cell holds the appropriate value, $J(\mathbf{x}(t))$. For continuous-valued states, discretization of the individual dimensions is needed. For high-dimensional systems, this strategy leads to an explosion of lookup table cells. For example, for a 30-dimensional movement system where each dimension is split into just two cells, an astronomical number of 2^{30} cells would be required. Exploring all these cells with a real robot would take forever, and even in computer simulations such problems are not tractable. Newer approaches employ special neural networks for learning and representing $J(\mathbf{x}(t))$ (e.g., Sutton and Barto, 1998), but problems with high-dimensional movement systems remain daunting.

A possible way to reduce the computational complexity of learning a control policy comes from modularizing the policy (Figure 2). Instead of learning the entire policy in one big representation, one could try to learn subpolicies that have reduced complexity and

subsequently build the complete policy out of such subpolicies. This approach is also appealing from the viewpoint of learning multiple tasks: some of the subpolicies may be reused in another task, which should strongly facilitate learning new tasks.

Motor control with subpolicies has been explored in various fields under the names of, e.g., schema theory (see SCHEMA THEORY), behavior-based robotics (see REACTIVE ROBOTIC SYSTEMS), pattern generators (see MOTOR PATTERN GENERATION), and movement primitives (Schaal, 1999). Robot learning with such modular control systems, however, is still in its infancy. Reinforcement learning has recently begun to formulate a principled approach to this problem (Sutton, Precup, and Singh, 1999). Another route of investigating modular robot learning comes from formulating subpolicies as nonlinear dynamical systems (Mussa-Ivaldi and Bizzi, 1997; Schaal and Sternad, 1998). However, all this research is still of a preliminary nature and not yet applicable to complex robot learning problems.

Indirect Learning of Control Policies

The previous sections assumed that motor commands are directly generated based on the information of the state of the world $\mathbf{x}$, i.e., from the policy function π. For many movement systems, however, such a *direct* control strategy is not advantageous because it fails to reuse modules in the policy that are common across multiple tasks. This view suggests that, in addition to a modularization of motor control and learning in form of a mixture of simpler policies (Figure 2), modularization can also be achieved in terms of a functional structuring within each control policy. A typical example is to organize the control policy into several processing stages, as illustrated in Figure 3 and also discussed as *indirect* control in MOTOR CONTROL, BIOLOGICAL AND THEORETICAL (q.v.). Most commonly, the policy is decomposed into a planning stage and an execution stage, a strategy that is typical for most robot controllers but also likely to be used in motor control of primates. Planning generates a desired *kinematic* trajectory, i.e., a prescribed way in which the state of the movement system is supposed to change in order to achieve the task goal. Execution transforms the plan into appropriate motor commands.

Separating planning and execution is highly advantageous. For instance, in reaching movements located toward a target, a *direct* approach to robot learning would require learning a new policy for every target location: the desired behavior is to minimize the distance between the hand and the target, and because of the complex dynamics of an arm, different target locations require very different motor commands for reaching. In contrast, an indirect control approach requires learning only the movement execution module, usually in the form of an inverse model (see below). The execution module is valid for any target location. For simplicity, movement plans can be kept the same for every target location, such as a straight line between the target and the starting position of the arm, with a bell-shaped velocity profile. Planning such movement kinematics requires only one-time learning of the robot kinematics model and using standard kinematic planning algorithms (Sciavicco and Siciliano, 1996) that can easily cope with any reachable target location. Thus, after the execution module has been acquired, the problem of reaching is a largely solved, no matter where the target is.

Depending on the task, planning can take place in external kinematic variables (e.g., Cartesian or end-effector space) or in internal kinematic variables (e.g., joint space for a human-like arm). If the planning space does not coincide with the space where motor commands are issued, coordinate transformations are required to map the external motor plan into intrinsic coordinates. This problem is commonly discussed as the inverse kinematics problem of

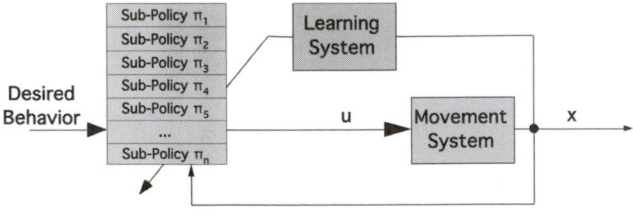

Figure 2. Learning control with subpolicies.

Figure 3. Learning control with functional decomposition.

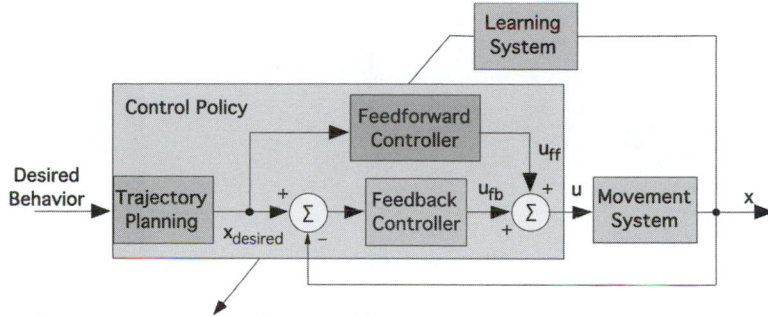

ROBOT ARM CONTROL (q.v.), a problem that equally needs to be addressed by biological movement systems.

To transform kinematic plans into motor commands, standard methods from control theory can be employed (e.g., Sciavicco and Siciliano, 1996). Figure 3 illustrates a typical example that uses a feedforward/feedback mechanism, called a *computed torque controller*, that enjoys popularity in both robotic systems and models of biological motor control (Jordan, 1996). The feedback controller is of classical proportional derivative (PD) type, while the feedforward controller contains an inverse dynamics model of the movement system (see CEREBELLUM AND MOTOR CONTROL).

From the point of robot learning, functional modularity also decomposes the learning problem into several independent learning problems. The modules of the execution stage can be learned with supervised learning techniques (discussed later; see also CEREBELLUM AND MOTOR CONTROL). For various types of movements, kinematic movement plans can be highly stereotyped, as was described for the reaching example, such that no learning is required for planning. For complex movements such as a tennis serve, planning requires more sophistication, and the same reinforcement learning methods of *direct* control can be applied, the only difference being that the motor commands **u** are replaced with a desired change in trajectory $\dot{\mathbf{x}}_d$. Applying reinforcement learning to kinematic planning is less complex than solving the complete *direct* control problem since the highly nonlinear transformation from kinematic plans to motor commands does not need to be acquired anymore, but how to perform reinforcement learning for high-dimensional movement systems still remains an open research problem.

Imitation Learning

A topic in robot learning that is of increasing interest is *imitation learning*. The idea of imitation learning is intuitively simple: a student watches the performance of a teacher and subsequently uses the demonstrated movement as a seed to start his or her own movement. The ability to learn from imitation has a profound impact on how quickly new skills can be acquired (Schaal, 1999). From the viewpoint of learning theory, imitation can be understood as a method to bias learning toward a particular solution, the teacher's. Motor learning proceeds afterward, as described in the other sections of this article. However, not every representation for motor learning is equally suited to be biased by imitation (Schaal, 1997). For instance, a robot using direct control can hardly profit from a demonstration, as motor commands are not perceivable, but a robot using indirect control could first extract a kinematic plan from the demonstration and then use it for starting its own learning. Imitation thus imposes interesting constraints on the structure of a learning system for motor learning.

Learning of Motor Control Components

Whether direct or indirect control is employed in a motor learning problem, the core of the learning system usually requires methods of supervised learning of regression problems, called function approximation in the neural network and statistical learning literature. *Function approximation* is concerned with approximating a nonlinear function $\mathbf{y} = f(\mathbf{x})$ from noisy data, drawn according to the data-generating model:

$$\mathbf{y} = f(\mathbf{x}) + \varepsilon \quad \text{where } \mathbf{x} \in \Re^n, \mathbf{y} \in \Re^m, E\{\varepsilon\} = 0 \quad (6)$$

i.e., **x** is an n-dimensional continuous-valued vector, **y** is an m-dimensional continuous-valued vector, and ε a zero-mean random "noise" variable. By comparing the generic form of a policy in Equation 1 or a dynamics model in Equation 2 with Equation 6, it is apparent that learning such functions falls into the framework of function approximation.

Neural Network Approaches to Function Approximation

Many different methods of function approximation exist in the literature (see LEARNING AND STATISTICAL INFERENCE). For present purposes, it is sufficient to classify all these algorithms into two categories, spatially localized (*local*) algorithms and spatially nonlocalized (*global*) algorithms. The power of learning in neural networks comes from the nonlinear activation functions that are employed in the hidden units of the neural network. *Global* algorithms use nonlinear activation functions that are not limited to a finite domain in the input space (**x**-space) of the function. The prototypical example is the sigmoid function in Figure 4A that outputs a value of roughly one for any input greater than about one. In contrast, *local* algorithms make use of nonlinear activation functions that are different from zero only in a restricted input domain. The Gaussian function in Figure 4B exemplifies this class of functions. Even though both local and global algorithms are theoretically capable of approximating arbitrarily complex nonlinear functions, learning speed, convergence, and applicability to high-dimensional learning problems differ significantly between the two (Schaal and Atkeson, 1998).

To understand how global algorithms approximate nonlinear functions, it is helpful to think of them as an octopus whose tentacles stretch out and span the complex surface described by $\mathbf{y} = f(\mathbf{x})$, except that the tentacles exist in an n-dimensional space. Global algorithms can work quite well for problems with many input dimensions, since their nonlocal activation function (i.e., their tentacles) can span even huge spaces quite efficiently. But global algorithms usually require very careful training procedures so that the tentacles learn how to stretch appropriately into all directions. In particular, if at some point in training, data are only provided for a restricted area in input space, the tentacles may focus too much on approximating this area and, while doing so, forget maintaining the "tentacle posture" in previously learned areas—a phe-

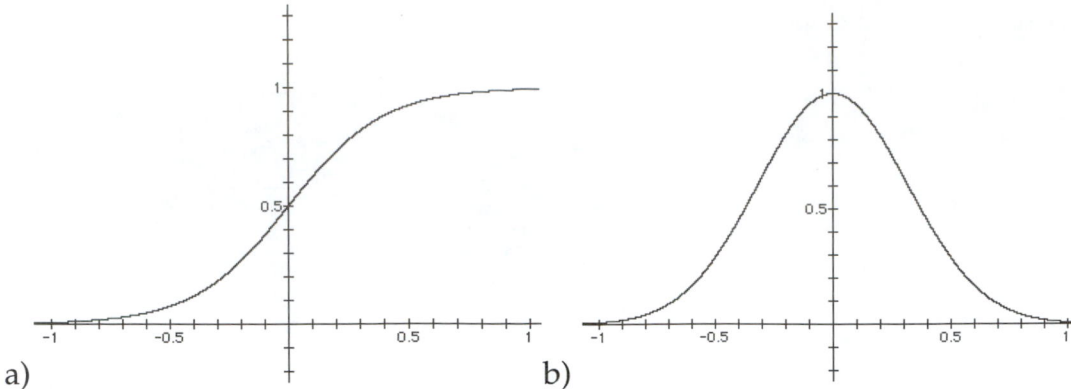

Figure 4. Nonlinear activation functions used in neural networks. *A*, The sigmoid function, a spatially global function. *B*, The Gaussian function, a spatially localized function.

nomenon called catastrophic interference (Schaal and Atkeson, 1998). Catastrophic interference is particularly pronounced in incremental learning problems, where training data come point after point and can only be used once for updating the algorithm. Unfortunately, this is the typical scenario in robot learning. Together with the problem of how to select the right number of hidden units (i.e., the right number of tentacles), it becomes quite complicated to train global algorithms for high-dimensional robot learning problems.

In contrast, local learning algorithms have quite different characteristics. The metaphor for local learning is simply that they approximate the complex regression surface with the help of small local patches, for instance locally constant or locally linear functions (Atkeson, Moore, and Schaal, 1997). Problems of how many patches need to be allocated, where to place them, how large they should be in input space, and how to learn them incrementally have largely been solved (Schaal and Atkeson, 1998). The biggest problem of local algorithms is the curse of dimensionality, i.e., the exponential explosion in the number of patches that are needed in high-dimensional input spaces. For instance, assume that we want to divide every input dimension of a function approximation problem into ten local regions. For two input dimensions, this strategy would result in 10^2 local regions, for three inputs in 10^3 regions, and for n inputs in 10^n regions. Even for only 12 input dimensions, this number reaches the number of neurons in the human brain. The only way to avoid this problem is to make the patches larger, but then the quality of function approximation becomes unacceptably inaccurate. There is theoretically no way out of the curse of dimensionality—but empirically, it turns out not to be a problem. The example demonstrating the curse of dimensionality can be turned around in our favor: How long would it take a robot system to generate all the data points to fill these big spaces? As an example, collecting 10^{12} data points at 100 Hz sampling frequency would take more than 300 years of uninterrupted movement! Thus, no actual robot will ever be able to generate enough data to fill these huge spaces. This argument triggers a most important question: What kind of data distributions are actually realized by robotic (or biological) movement systems? Vijayakumar et al. (2002) found that distribution had only about four to six dimensions locally in a robot learning problem that had 21 input dimensions, a finding that was also duplicated in other robot learning domains (Vlassis, Motomura, and Krose, 2002). Local learning can exploit this property by using techniques of local dimensionality reduction and can thus learn efficiently even in very high-dimensional spaces (Vijayakumar et al., 2002). Thus, for the time being, local learning algorithms seem to be better suited for robot learning.

Specific Function Approximation Problems in Robot Learning

Applying function approximation to problems of robot learning requires a few more considerations. The easiest applications are those of straightforward supervised learning, i.e., where a teacher signal **y** is directly available for every training point **x**. For example, learning a dynamics model of the form of Equation 2 usually falls into this category if the inputs **x** and **u** and the output **ẋ** can be measured directly from sensors. Many other problems of ROBOT ARM CONTROL (q.v.) are of a similar nature.

Learning becomes more challenging when instead of the teacher signal only an error signal is provided, and the error signal is just approximate. Assume we have such an error signal **e** when the network predicted a particular **ŷ** for a given input **x**. From this information, we can create a teacher signal **y** = **ŷ** + **e** and train the network with this target. However, if **e** was only approximate, **y** is not the true target, and later on during learning another (hopefully more accurate) teacher signal may be formed for training the network. Thus, learning proceeds with "moving targets," which is called a nonstationary learning problem. For such learning tasks, neural networks need to have an appropriate amount of plasticity in order to keep on changing until the targets become correct. On the other hand, it is also important that the network converge at some point and average out the noise in the data, i.e., that the network not have too much plasticity. Finding appropriate neural networks that have the right amount of plasticity-stability trade-off is a nontrivial problem, and so far, heuristic solutions dominate the literature.

Nonstationary learning problems are unfortunately quite common in robot learning. Learning the optimization function $J(\mathbf{x}(t))$ in reinforcement learning is one typical example since the temporal difference algorithm (Sutton and Barto, 1998) can only provide approximate errors. Other examples include feedback error learning and learning with distal teachers (Jordan, 1996). Both of these methods address the problem that in learning control, we usually receive errors in only sensory variables, such as positions and velocities, but what is needed to train a control policy is an error in motor commands. Thus, feedback error learning creates an approximate motor command error by using the output of a linear feedback controller as the error signal. Learning with distal teachers accomplishes essentially the same goal, except that it employs a learned forward model to map an error in sensory space to an approximate motor error.

Applications

While the theoretical development of learning control has progressed significantly in recent years, applications in actual robots have remained rather sparse because of the significant computational burden of most learning algorithms and the real-time constraints of actual robots. Reinforcement learning in actual robots remains largely infeasible, and only few examples exist in simplified setups (e.g., see references in Atkeson et al., 1997; Sutton and Barto, 1998; Schaal, 1999). Learning of internal models for robot control has found increasingly more widespread application owing to significant advances in the computational efficiency of supervised learning algorithms (e.g., see references in Atkeson et al., 1997; Vijayakumar et al., 2002; Vlassis et al., 2002).

Discussion

Robot learning is a surprisingly complex problem. It needs to address how to learn from (possibly delayed) rewards, how to deal with very high-dimensional learning problems, how to use efficient function approximators, and how to embed all the elements in a control system with real-time and robust performance. A further difference from many other learning tasks is that in robot learning, the training data are generated by the movement system itself. Efficient data generation, i.e., exploration of the world, will result in fast learning, while inefficient exploration can prevent successful learning altogether (see REINFORCEMENT LEARNING). Insofar as very few robots in the world are equipped with learning capabilities, research on robot learning is still in an early stage of development.

Road Map: Robotics and Control Theory
Related Reading: Imitation; Q-Learning for Robots; Reinforcement Learning in Motor Control; Robot Arm Control; Sensorimotor Learning

References

Atkeson, C. G., Moore, A. W., and Schaal, S., 1997, Locally weighted learning for control, *Artif. Intell. Rev.*, 11:75–113. ◆

Bellman, R., 1957, *Dynamic Programming*, Princeton, NJ: Princeton University Press.
Dyer, P., and McReynolds, S. R., 1970, *The Computation and Theory of Optimal Control*, New York: Academic Press.
Jordan, M. I., 1996, Computational aspects of motor control and motor learning, in *Handbook of Perception and Action* (H. Hever and S. W. Keele, Eds.), New York: Academic Press. ◆
Mussa-Ivaldi, F. A., and Bizzi, E., 1997, Learning Newtonian mechanics, in *Self-Organization, Computational Maps, and Motor Control* (P. Morasso and V. Sanguineh, Eds.), Amsterdam: Elsevier, pp. 491–501.
Schaal, S., 1997, Learning from demonstration, in *Advances in Neural Information Processing Systems 9* (M. C. Mozer, M. Jordan, and T. Petsche, Eds.), Cambridge, MA: MIT Press, pp. 1040–1046.
Schaal, S., 1999, Is imitation learning the route to humanoid robots? *Trends Cogn. Sci.*, 3:233–242. ◆
Schaal, S., and Atkeson, C. G., 1998, Constructive incremental learning from only local information, *Neural Comput.*, 10:2047–2084.
Schaal, S., and Sternad, D., 1998, Programmable pattern generators, in *Proceedings of the 3rd International Conference on Computational Intelligence in Neuroscience*, Research Triangle Park, NC: New York: Association for Computing Machinery, pp. 48–51.
Sciavicco, L., and Siciliano, B., 1996, *Modeling and Control of Robot Manipulators*, New York: McGraw-Hill.
Strogatz, S. H., 1994, *Nonlinear Dynamics and Chaos: With Applications to Physics, Biology, Chemistry, and Engineering*, Reading, MA: Addison-Wesley.
Sutton, R. S., and Barto, A. G., 1998, *Reinforcement Learning: An Introduction*, Cambridge, MA: MIT Press. ◆
Sutton, R. S., Precup, D., and Singh, S., 1999, Between MDPs and semi-MDPs: A framework for temporal abstraction in reinforcement learning, *Artif. Intell.*, 112:181–211.
Vijayakumar, S., D'Souza, A., Shibata, T., Conradt, J., and Schaal, S., 2002, Statistical learning for humanoid robots, *Auton. Robots*, 12:59–72.
Vlassis, N., Motomura, Y., and Krose, B., 2002, Supervised dimension reduction of intrinsically low-dimensional data, *Neural Computat.*, 14:191–215.

Robot Navigation

José del R. Millán

Introduction

Mobile robots are gradually leaving the laboratories to undertake service tasks ranging from providing surveillance of buildings and supervision of plants, to transporting patients and delivery items, to cleaning houses and guiding people. Independently of the assigned task, the basic capability of a mobile robot is to move to its destination—or sequence of targets—efficiently (e.g., along short trajectories) and safely (i.e., without collisions). *Navigation* refers to the capability of selecting and performing a path from a current position to a desired location. Implicit in this definition is the ability to adapt the goal-oriented behavior to the complexity of the task. If a target location is either visible or identified by a landmark (or sequence of landmarks), a simple stimulus-response strategy can be adopted (REACTIVE ROBOTIC SYSTEMS). However, targets are often neither visible nor identified by any sequence of cues. In this case, for a robot to navigate it must first determine its position with respect to the target. This is the *localization* problem. Finally, to perform more flexible and sophisticated navigation (e.g., planning short cuts), the robot needs a model of the environment encoding the spatial relationships between locations. Acquiring such a model is the *map-building* problem.

Like any other robotic system (ROBOT ARM CONTROL), mobile robots must rely on on-line sensory information to take actions. But, unlike most arm robots, sensory information cannot only be proprioceptive (i.e., an odometry process that gives the robot's coordinates based on internal encoders); it must also provide exteroperception (i.e., information about the external environment). Indeed, odometry alone accumulates errors due to slippage, which will make the robot get lost and crash sooner or later. Mobile robots mainly use three types of sensors to perceive their surroundings, namely tactile sensors that inform about contacts, range sensors (lasers, ultrasounds, or infrareds) that return distances after appropriate transformations, and vision. Given the opposite strengths and weaknesses of the different sensors, an orthogonal issue not covered by this article is that of sensor fusion (SENSOR FUSION).

A common property shared by all types of sensors is their noisy responses. This sensor uncertainty, together with the inaccuracy of the robot's actuators and the unpredictability of real environments, makes the design of mobile robot controllers a difficult task. The complexity of the sensorimotor mapping underlying robot navigation yields two main consequences. First, simulations, though useful, are not enough to reproduce the actual agent-environment interaction. Second, robots must build their control strategies based on their own sensory perceptions of the real world (i.e., *embodiment*). Human-made controllers are, except for simple tasks and environments, inadequate because the designer must anticipate every possible situation the robot might face and must tune the controller's parameters to achieve efficient performance. An alternative is to endow robots with *learning capabilities* in order to acquire autonomously their control system and to adapt their behavior to never-experienced situations (i.e., *generalization*).

Artificial neural networks (ANN) offer a suitable learning framework to model the basis of adaptive behavior. Indeed, their noise robustness and generalization capabilities allow robots to cope with the nature of their interaction with the world and to build appropriate sensorimotor mappings. The next three sections discuss ANN approaches to localization, map building, and navigation.

Localization

To solve complex navigation tasks, mobile robots must self-localize in the environment by relying on their exteroceptive and proprioceptive sensory inputs. In general, localization calls on *place recognition*. To localize itself, the robot can either simply memorize the sensory perceptions observed during exploration or can learn a more complex representation (map) encoding spatial relationships between experienced local perceptions. How the robot acquires a map is discussed in the next section.

Strictly speaking, only Thrun (1998a,b) uses an ANN for localization. In the remaining approaches, the robot's perception is matched against the model, which has an ANN organization, and its location is derived from that associated to the winning unit. Actually, the robot's perception can be the current sensory reading plus odometry information (Zimmer, 1996), sensory data averaged as the robot moves (Matarić, 1992), or egocentric views obtained from the sensory perceptions (Recce and Harris, 1996).

An alternative is to transform raw sensory data into a more reliable representation through ANN (Thrun, 1998a). In particular, a feedforward ANN is trained through *backpropagation* to generate a local *occupancy grid* from the current sensory perception. Such a grid is a discrete representation of the space around the robot, where each cell has a value that estimates the occupancy probability of the corresponding area of the world. After exploration, the localization algorithm searches for the previously stored grid that best matches the current local map. There are two advantages of using a neural sensor interpretation to build local occupancy grids: the ANN does not assume any noise distribution, and it interprets sensor readings simultaneously. On the other hand, the shortcoming of this approach is its computational cost, as building an $n*n$ grid requires $n*n$ calls to the ANN.

A totally different approach is to learn what environmental features are the most relevant landmarks for localization. Thrun (1998b) trained a feedforward ANN to optimize a Bayesian measure of probabilistic localization. Training was done on samples collected during an exploration phase in which each sample consisted of a sensory perception and its location. During operation, the robot averaged the ANN response for the k nearest neighbor samples to its estimated location. This approach demonstrated its superiority to hand-coded localization methods based on using doors and ceiling lights as landmarks.

Building

The representations a robot may learn are of two main types, namely *metric* and *topological*. In the former, maps quantitatively reproduce the geometric and spatial features of the environment. This is computationally expensive and vulnerable to errors that affect the metric information. Topological maps are more qualitative and consist of a graph, on which nodes represent perceptually distinct places (landmarks) and arcs indicate spatial relations between them. They are less vulnerable to sensory errors, and enable fast planning since the latter reduces to a simple search process in

a graph. However, topological representations rely on the existence of ever-recognizable landmarks.

One of the most popular approaches to building metric maps is based on the use of occupancy grids. Thrun (1998a) trained a feedforward ANN to create a local occupancy grid modeling the space surrounding the robot. Successive local grids generated as the robot explored its environment were then combined to produce an accurate global metric map. Once the global metric map was available, a topological graph could be abstracted off-line. This greatly reduces the cost of planning paths between different locations in the environment. This approach (in conjunction with the localization process discussed before) is implemented in museum tour-guided robots. An alternative is to use the same neural sensor interpretation but only for deriving coarse geometrical features from which to build up on-line a variable-resolution partitioning of the environment (Arleo, Millán, and Floreano, 1999). The environment is discretized in cells of different sizes, with a high resolution only on critical areas (i.e., around obstacles). The resulting map combines geometrical and topological aspects that are learned simultaneously.

Among topological approaches, Matarić's model (1992) builds a sparse graph in which each node represents a unique predefined landmark. Spatial relationships between landmarks are encoded by neighbor links in the graph, which produces a structure isomorphic to the topology of the environment. Disambiguation between similar sensory patterns is done by spreading expectations from the currently active unit to its neighbors (contextual discrimination) or by attaching metric information to the units. Self-organizing feature maps or Kohonen maps (SELF-ORGANIZING FEATURE MAPS) provide an alternative way of acquiring topological maps (Kurz, 1996; Zimmer, 1996). A self-organizing, or *Kohonen,* map clusters the sensory perceptions gathered during the exploration phase of the robot (Kurz, 1996). The dimensionality of the Kohonen map matches the robot's degrees of freedom, either two or three depending on whether or not the robot moves with a constant orientation. As a result, neighboring units in the learned Kohonen map correspond to neighboring areas in the sensory space. The problem is that there is no guarantee that neighbor areas in sensory space are also close in metric space. Still worse, due to the limitations of its sensors a robot may have similar sensory perceptions from two different metric locations. A possible solution is to include odometry information in the self-organizing process (Zimmer, 1996), which presumes a reliable localization process. Another solution is to use the temporal sequence of sensory perceptions and not just the current one. This can be achieved by means of a recurrent Kohonen map. Finally, instead of using a self-organizing map with a fixed structure (dimensionality and number of units), it is also possible to learn the topological map of the environment by means of a *dynamic self-organizing map*. This method adds a new unit whenever the current sensory perception is sufficiently different from any existing unit (Millán, 1997; Zimmer, 1996), or is using statistical measures (Zimmer, 1996). In this kind of network the topology of the environment is kept in the links between units. It is worth noting that the ADAPTIVE RESONANCE THEORY (q.v.) can yield quantizations of the environment similar to a dynamic self-organizing map, but the resulting map does not exhibit topological relationships between the units.

Map learning systems engineered so far are not as robust, flexible, and adaptable as biological spatial learning solutions. Neurophysiological findings suggest that the spatial memory of mammals is supported by location-sensitive neurons (*place cells*) in the *Hippocampus* (see HIPPOCAMPUS: SPATIAL MODELS). Recent research in robot navigation has moved toward biologically inspired approaches to developing autonomous systems that mimic mammalian spatial learning capabilities. For example, Recce and Harris (1996) put forward a map-building model that ascribes the spatial memory function to the hippocampus. The authors assume that a place cell in the robot's hippocampus memorizes a complete egocentric map of the environment. This is a strong requirement for both robots and animals, especially if operating in middle- and large-scale environments. Arleo and Gerstner (2000) propose a hippocampal model in which unsupervised *Hebbian* learning is applied to acquire a spatial map incrementally and on-line. The representation consists of a population of localized overlapping place fields that provide a stable coarse space code. The robot establishes place fields by extracting spatiotemporal properties of the environment from visual inputs and solves visual ambiguities by taking into account proprioceptive self-motion signals.

Navigation

If the robot has acquired (or is given) a topological map, then whenever it is requested to navigate to a given destination it simply searches for an optimal route in the graph and uses elemental *behaviors* to move from one node to the next along that route. However, building and maintaining consistent global maps of the environment is far from being a trivial problem, since noisy sensory data may introduce errors into the maps. Also, unless the robot is equipped with good exploration strategies, it may fail to model the whole environment and topological relationships. For example, most map building approaches rely on a wall-following (and obstacle avoidance) behavior that prevents the robot from visiting open or cluttered areas. Thus, while in operation, the robot will never take shortcuts. Alternatively, the robot can directly use behaviors to reach its destination without resorting to any map. In this section we discuss how the necessary behaviors can be learned by means of ANN.

A behavior is a set of perception-action rules that provide the robot with a given functionality such as obstacle avoidance (REACTIVE ROBOTIC SYSTEMS). Perception-action mappings can be learned off-line from representative training sets, mainly through *supervised* techniques (Pomerleau, 1993; Sharkey, 1998). Pomerleau's system (1993) is a paradigmatic example of the potentiality of the supervised approach. He trained a feedforward ANN to drive a car in a variety of roads. Training data were gathered by observing a human expert driving the vehicle. In particular, inputs corresponded to images of the road in front of the car and desired outputs corresponded to the driver's steering direction. After learning, the ANN controller made the vehicle follow the road by keeping it in the center of the lane.

Instead of requiring a human for data collection, an alternative is to use a preprogrammed controller as an initial teacher. Sharkey (1998) made feedforward ANN learn from an initial behavior-based controller to approach a target while avoiding obstacles. The final neural controller, obtained through a bootstrapping process, performed better than the original controller did. Nevertheless, the resulting network also inherited limitations of the initial controller. This illustrates one of the fundamental limitations of supervised learning and leads to the necessity of *autonomous* robot learning.

Autonomous robots must train themselves on-line in order to cope with weak and incomplete training examples. REINFORCEMENT LEARNING (q.v.) is an appropriate paradigm to achieve this. A reinforcement-based robot can improve its performance over time without needing extensive previous knowledge about the task. This is quite appealing but, on the other hand, makes the learning process very slow. The following section will describe several extensions to the basic reinforcement learning framework that considerably speed up the convergence to suitable sensorimotor mappings (or policies, as they are customarily called in the control and reinforcement learning fields), thus making it possible to build practical learning mobile robots.

Lin (1991) combined *Q-learning* (a widely studied reinforcement learning technique) and teaching. The controller had one feedforward network for each discrete action the robot can perform. The input to each ANN was the current sensory perception and the output was a prediction of the *Q-value* of that perception-action pair. The robot normally took the action with the highest Q-value (Q-LEARNING FOR ROBOTS). In Lin's experiment, a human teacher brought the robot to its goal several times along efficient paths. Then, the robot learned the appropriate Q-values, and hence good policies, from these examples. The taught navigation sequences helped reinforcement learning by biasing the search for suitable actions toward promising parts of the action space.

Thrun (1995) also used Q-learning, but integrated it with explanation-based learning (EBL). EBL requires a domain theory that is previously learned by a set of feedforward ANN (action models) in a supervised manner, one network for each discrete action the robot can perform. Each network receives the current sensory perception and predicts the next perception and Q-value. In addition to action models, the robot has also a Q network per action similar to that of Lin (1991). As before, the Q networks encode the control policies. Finally, for each actual sequence of actions taking the robot either to the goal or to a failure, the robot explains the observed example in terms of its domain theory by computing the derivatives of the policy with respect to the action model networks. These derivatives are used to bias the supervised learning of the policy (i.e., the Q networks). It is worth noting that since the action models are task independent, they are learned once and can be used across the different tasks faced by the robot.

The previously discussed reinforcement-based robots perform discrete actions, while for smooth operation they should take continuous actions. Millán (1996, 1997) has implemented *Actor-Critic* architectures instead of Q-learning for this purpose. Key components of his learning architecture are the use of *local networks* and the incorporation of *bias* into the network. Local networks make the robot learn incrementally new sensorimotor rules (or tune existing ones) without degrading the performance of other rules. The robots use built-in reflexes (basic domain knowledge) as bias. There are two benefits of bias. First, it accelerates the learning process since it focuses the search process on promising parts of the action space immediately. Second, it makes the robot operational from the very beginning and increments the safety of the learning process. The ANN is trained on-line by means of a combination of reinforcement learning and self-organizing rules. Every time the robot fails to generalize its previous experience to the current sensory perception, it uses the reflexes and adds a new unit to the network. The robot may also add a new unit whenever it receives an advice from humans. This unit is integrated into a dynamic self-organizing map and associates a region around the current perception to either the computed reflex or the advice. The resulting sensorimotor rule is then tuned by means of reinforcement learning and self-organizing rules. Experimental results show that a few minutes suffice for the robot to navigate efficiently in office environments of moderate complexity, in which the robot can easily get trapped inside concave areas.

Recently, reinforcement learning has been shown to be a suitable framework to model reward-based navigation in animals. For example, Arleo and Gerstner (2000) employed Q-learning in continuous space to drive action units one synapse downstream from their hippocampal place cells. Due to the coarse space code provided by the localized overlapping place fields, Q-learning converges in few trials, which is consistent with the rapid acquisition of goal-oriented behavior of animals. Several action modules share the same space representation and guide the robot to multiple targets.

Discussion

For mobile robots to undertake real-world tasks with unreliable sensors and actuators, whose responses greatly depend on the specific working environment, they must exhibit adaptive capabilities. Neural networks naturally cope with the learning task of analyzing the perception-action interactions for navigation, localization, and map building. Even though different ANN approaches have solved some instances of these three aspects of robot navigation, there does not exist a complete navigation system that is purely made of neural components. From an engineering standpoint, such a complete mobile robot must incorporate other types of learning techniques to generate more abstract models of its perceptions, actions, and sensorimotor rules (Kaiser et al., 1995). In addition, the engineering perspective calls for combining learning capabilities with alternative techniques to build successful mobile robots such as those of Thrun and co-workers (Thrun, 1998a). On the other hand, a different perspective looks at animals for inspiration to develop the necessary neural components of a complete robot navigation system. There are numerous efforts along this *bio-inspired* direction (BIOLOGICALLY INSPIRED ROBOTICS and NEUROETHOLOGY, COMPUTATIONAL) in which reinforcement-based learning (REINFORCEMENT LEARNING and Q-LEARNING FOR ROBOTS) and hippocampal models (COGNITIVE MAPS and HIPPOCAMPUS: SPATIAL MODELS) are keystones of this type of future intelligent (because adaptive) mobile robots.

Road Map: Robotics and Control Theory
Related Reading: Cognitive Maps; Embodied Cognition; Hippocampus: Spatial Models; Motion Perception: Navigation; Potential Fields and Neural Networks

References

Arleo, A., Millán, J. del R., and Floreano, D., 1999, Efficient learning of variable-resolution cognitive maps for autonomous indoor navigation, *IEEE Trans. Robot. Automat.,* 15:990–1000.

Arleo, A., and Gerstner, W., 2000, Spatial cognition and neuro-mimetic navigation: A model of hippocampal place cell activity, *Biol. Cyb.,* 83:287–299.

Kaiser, M., Klingspor, V., Millán, J. del R., Accame, M., Wallner, F., and Dillman, R., 1995, Using machine learning techniques in real-world mobile robots, *IEEE Expert,* 10:37–45. ◆

Kurz, A., 1996, Constructing maps for mobile robot navigation based on ultrasonic range data, *IEEE Trans. Syst. Man Cybern.—Part B,* 26:233–242.

Lin, L.-J., 1991, Programming robots using reinforcement learning and teaching, in *Proceedings of the Ninth National Conference on Artificial Intelligence,* Menlo Park, CA: AAAI Press/MIT Press, pp. 781–786.

Matarić, M. J., 1992, Integration of representation into goal-driven behavior-based robots, *IEEE Trans. Robot. Automat.,* 8:304–312.

Millán, J. del R., 1996, Rapid, safe, and incremental learning of navigation strategies, *IEEE Trans. Syst. Man Cybern.—Part B,* 26:408–420.

Millán, J. del R., 1997, Incremental acquisition of local networks for the control of autonomous robots, in *Proceedings of the Seventh International Conference on Artificial Neural Networks,* Heidelberg, Germany: Springer-Verlag, pp. 739–744.

Pomerleau, D. A., 1993, *Neural Network Perception for Mobile Robot Guidance,* Boston: Kluwer.

Recce, M., and Harris, K. D., 1996, Memory for places: A navigational model in support of Marr's theory of hippocampal function, *Hippocampus,* 6:735–148.

Sharkey, N. E., 1998, Learning from innate behaviors: A quantitative evaluation of neural network controllers, *Auton. Robots,* 5:317–334.

Thrun, S., 1995, An approach to learning mobile robot navigation, *Robot. Auton. Syst.,* 15:301–319.

Thrun, S., 1998a, Learning maps for indoor mobile robot navigation, *Artif. Intell.,* 99:21–71. ◆

Thrun, S., 1998b, Bayesian landmark learning for mobile robot localization, *Machine Learn.,* 33:41–76.

Zimmer, U. W., 1996, Robust world-modelling and navigation in a real world, *Neurocomputing,* 13:247–260.

Rodent Head Direction System

David S. Touretzky and William E. Skaggs

Introduction

The brain of the rat contains an inertial compass distributed across a collection of anatomical areas (Figure 1). Head direction (HD) cells in these areas fire maximally when the rat's head is pointed in a specific *preferred direction*, with a gradual falloff in firing as the heading departs from that direction. This directional specificity is independent of the rat's location or behavior. Within a population of HD cells, preferred directions are uniformly distributed around the circle. Although there is no topographic ordering of the cells in any known HD area, it is convenient to refer to a population of HD cells as if they were arranged around a ring according to their preferred directions. Thus, given a population of HD cells, for any direction the rat is facing, a "bump" of activity will be observed over the population, and the bump location will shift around the ring as the animal's heading changes.

Head direction is an internal, cognitive representation, not a simple reflection of sensory stimuli or motor activities. Maintenance of the HD activity bump is thought to be evidence for attractor networks operating in the rodent brain. Because of the HD system's interesting functional properties, it has been the focus of a very productive interaction between neurophysiologists and computational modelers.

Sensory Cues and Head Direction

In order to maintain an accurate heading estimate in the dark or in an unfamiliar environment, the rat must integrate its head angular velocity, which is sensed by the vestibular system. Other possible sources of angular velocity information include motor efference copy and optic flow, but lesions of the vestibular nuclei suffice to abolish stable HD responses (Blair, Cho, and Sharp, 1998). Experiments have shown that even passive rotations, if rapid, are compensated for by the HD system (i.e., the animal's heading estimate changes accordingly), probably because they are above the threshold of the vestibular system. Slow passive rotations are not compensated.

While the bump representation is maintained even in the absence of visual input, when rats forage in the dark in a radially symmetric environment such as a cylinder, the HD system drifts out of alignment after a few minutes, owing to cumulative integration error. Normally the HD system utilizes a correction mechanism based on visual landmarks—and perhaps other perceptual cues—to keep itself aligned with the environment.

In an often repeated experimental paradigm, HD cells are recorded while a rat forages for scattered food pellets in a gray cylindrical arena with a white card on the wall serving as a prominent

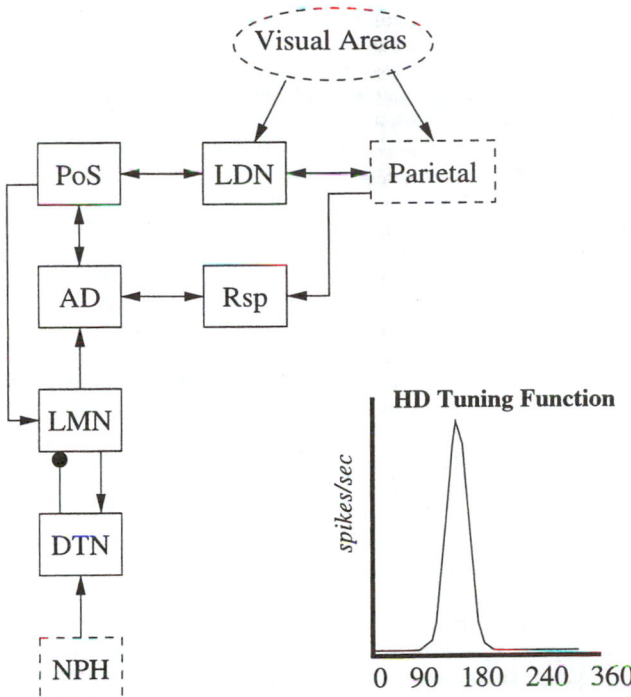

Figure 1. Organization of the rodent head direction system. AD, anterior dorsal nucleus of the thalamus; DTN, dorsal tegmental nucleus; LDN, lateral dorsal nucleus of the thalamus; LMN, lateral mammillary nucleus; NPH, nucleus prepositus hypoglossi; PoS, postsubiculum; Rsp, retrosplenial cortex. Graph at lower right shows the tuning curve of a typical head direction cell.

directional cue. When the cue card is rotated to a different location, the tuning curves of HD cells typically rotate by the same angle as the cue card was rotated, indicating that the cue card is exerting "control" over the HD system. The realignment is a gradual process and may require 1 to 2 minutes to complete (Knierim, Kudrimoti, and McNaughton, 1998).

The influence of visual cues on the HD system is a function of experience. After 1 minute of exposure to a novel environment, little or no control is exerted over the HD system by a cue card, but 8 minutes of exposure is enough for control to develop (Goodridge et al., 1998). The influence of visual landmarks also depends on their being perceived as stable. If rats are repeatedly disoriented before being placed in the cylinder, so that their HD system is randomly oriented, the cue card will appear at a different bearing on each trial, and its influence on the HD system will be substantially diminished (Knierim, Kudrimoti, and McNaughton, 1995).

Conflicts can be introduced between vestibular and visual cues by placing the rat in a cylinder whose floor and wall rotate independently. Under these conditions either the vestibular or the visual cues can win out, depending on circumstances.

The Head Direction Circuit

Head direction cells were first discovered in the postsubiculum (PoS, also called dorsal presubiculum) by Ranck, and studied in depth by Taube, Muller, and Ranck (1990a, 1990b). They were subsequently found in the lateral dorsal nucleus of the thalamus (LDN: Mizumori and Williams, 1993), anterior dorsal thalamic

nucleus (AD: Blair and Sharp, 1995; Taube, 1995), lateral mammillary nucleus (LMN: Blair et al., 1998; Stackman and Taube, 1998), dorsal tegmental nucleus (DTN: Sharp, Tinkelman, and Cho, 2001; Bassett and Taube, 2001), and several other areas. The firing properties of HD cells differ somewhat in the different areas. For example, PoS HD cells are best correlated with the rat's present heading, and their tuning curves are Gaussian shaped and independent of angular velocity. The tuning curves of AD HD cells distort at higher angular velocities, and the activity of these cells is best correlated with the rat's heading roughly 25 ms in the future. This quantity, the *anticipatory time interval* (ATI), was determined by plotting separate tuning curves for left versus right turns. PoS HD cells have an ATI of around zero, but when firing rate is plotted against present heading for an AD HD cell, the peaks of the two curves do not coincide. When firing rate is plotted against future heading, strong overlap of the two tuning curves is obtained for headings around 25 ms in the future. For example, an AD cell whose preferred direction is 120° when the rat is motionless will appear to have a different preferred direction when the rat is turning. During a turn at 320°/s, the cell will fire at its peak rate when the rat's head passes through 112° for a clockwise turn, or 128° for a counterclockwise turn. This can be interpreted as the cell having a fixed preferred direction of 120° but anticipating the rat's heading by 25 ms. The peak firing rates of AD HD cells, but not PoS HD cells, increase with angular velocity.

LMN HD cells have roughly Gaussian tuning curves modulated by angular velocity, but with a preferred turning direction. Cells that prefer clockwise turns increase their firing rate as angular velocity increases in the clockwise direction and decrease their firing rate as angular velocity increases in the counterclockwise direction, relative to the rate observed when the animal's head is not turning at all. Stackman and Taube (1998) observed an ATI of approximately 95 ms for LMN HD cells. But Blair et al. (1998) reported that LMN HD cells have an ATI of only 40 ms, and whereas their peak firing rate changes only slightly with velocity, the width of the tuning curve contracts as angular velocity increases in the preferred turning direction. The tuning curve width does not contract for turns in the opposite direction.

DTN HD cells have much broader tuning curves than PoS, AD, or LMN HD cells. Their firing rate is velocity modulated, and they have a preferred turning direction, as do LMN cells, but their tuning curve widths do not change with velocity (Sharp et al., 2001; Bassett and Taube, 2001). DTN also contains angular velocity cells that are not directionally tuned. These cells fire at a baseline rate when the rat is still, and increase their firing with increasing angular velocity for turns in the preferred direction, or decrease it for turns in the nonpreferred direction. DTN receives projections from the nucleus prepositus hypoglossi (one of the vestibular nuclei), and may be the place where angular velocity information first enters the HD system.

LDN HD cells have tuning curves similar to PoS cells, but they are dependent on visual input (Mizumori and Williams, 1993). If the rat is brought into the recording area in the dark, its LDN HD cells are quiescent. When the lights are turned on, LDN activity increases, resulting in normal HD responses in about 2 minutes. Since LDN projects to PoS, this may be a route by which visual information enters the HD system.

Lesions of AD disrupt the head direction signal in PoS, but lesions in PoS leave the AD HD signal largely intact, although the tuning curve broadens somewhat, and the control of visual landmarks over the HD system is impaired. The persistence of the HD signal may be because AD receives a projection from LMN, and from retrosplenial cortex, which also contains some HD cells. Bilateral but not unilateral LMN lesions abolish the AD HD signal (Blair et al., 1998).

Attractor Models of the Head Direction System

An attractor network is a recurrent neural network whose dynamics generate stable states (attractors) to which the system returns when perturbed. Skaggs et al. (1995) proposed that attractor dynamics could explain the shape of HD cell tuning curves, the stability of HD activity in the face of fluctuating sensory input, the control of the HD system by vestibular and visual cues, and the requirement for landmark stability. Zhang (1996) offered the first mathematical formulation of an attractor network as a model of an HD area. Goodridge and Touretzky (2000) modeled the interactions among PoS, AD, and LMN, including reproducing the distortions of AD tuning curve shapes with angular velocity. Sharp, Blair, and Cho (2001) proposed that the reciprocal connectivity between DTN and LMN could constitute an attractor network at the earliest stage of the HD system. This agrees with the observation that LMN cells have the largest ATI, AD cells anticipate less, and PoS cells, which are even further downstream, are hardly anticipatory at all.

The common mechanism in all bump attractor models is local excitation combined with global inhibition. Assuming for convenience that cells are arranged by preferred direction, each cell excites its nearby neighbors, as in Figure 2, with the strength of the excitatory connection falling off as a Gaussian function of the difference in their preferred directions. To prevent runaway excitation, HD cells also excite global inhibitory units (not shown), which provide uniform negative feedback onto the excitatory population. The stable states of this network consist of a bump of activation located somewhere on the ring. Noise in the network tends to be suppressed by the attractor dynamics, so the shape of the bump persists, and in the absence of external input, its location remains fixed. In addition to accounting for the stability of HD tuning curves, this model also explains the observation of Knierim et al. (1995) that when the HD system drifts, all cells drift in unison: the difference in preferred directions of any two simultaneously recorded cells remains constant.

Applying an external input to a spot on the ring underlying one flank of an attractor bump causes the bump to shift until it is centered over the external input. This is the mechanism Skaggs et al. (1995) proposed to explain how visual landmarks exert control over the HD system. In their model, landmark feature detectors looking at specific egocentric bearings would learn excitatory connections onto the appropriate HD cells as the animal became familiar with its environment. For example, if while facing north the animal saw landmark X ahead and to its right, via Hebbian learning, a feature detector that responds to "X ahead and to the right" would develop excitatory connections onto active HD cells, whose preferred directions would be close to 360°. If the HD system later drifted as a result of accumulated integration error, when the animal attended to the scene, external input from feature detectors would pull the bump back into alignment with the environment.

The greater the magnitude of the external input applied to the flank of a bump, the faster the bump moves. This property can be used to integrate angular velocity if the magnitude of the external input scales with velocity. But if the external input is applied far from the peak, so that it does not lie on the flank of the bump, its effect will be suppressed by the attractor dynamics. If it is applied in equal amounts to both flanks of the bump, the bump will stay put.

Angular velocity integration in an attractor network therefore requires input from a population of velocity-sensitive cells that

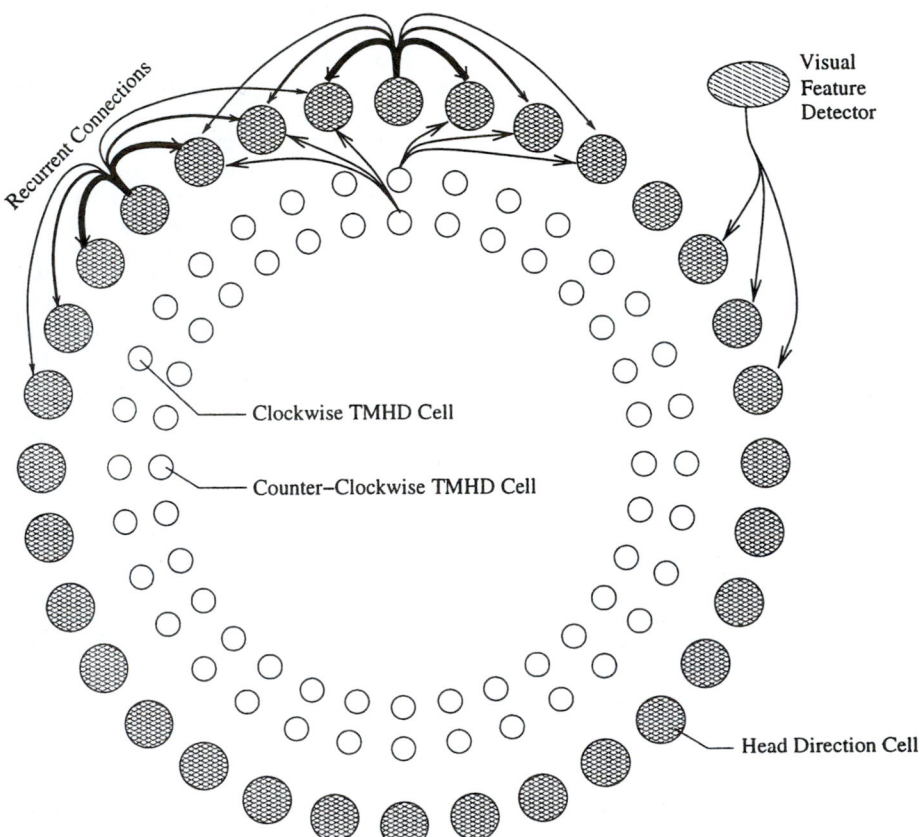

Figure 2. Architecture of an attractor-based head direction system model (after Skaggs et al., 1995).

exhibit HD tuning (so the input is focused on the correct flank of the attractor bump) and a turning preference. Blair and Sharp (1995) called these turn-modulated head direction (TMHD) cells. TMHD cells with a clockwise turning preference should make excitatory projections onto attractor HD cells with preferred directions slightly to the right of their own; TMHD cells with a counterclockwise turning preference should project to attractor HD cells slightly to the left. When the animal is still, both populations of TMHD cells should fire at the same rate, supplying identical input to both flanks of the attractor bump. When the animal is in a clockwise turn, the clockwise TMHD population should increase its firing rate, while the counterclockwise population should decrease its rate, in proportion to the angular velocity. Hence the bump would receive more input on its right flank, and begin shifting to the right. The opposite would occur for counterclockwise turns.

Cells in LMN seem to meet all the requirements for the hypothesized TMHD population: they show normal HD tuning, velocity modulation, and a turning preference. In the Goodridge and Touretzky (2000) model, the clockwise and counterclockwise LMN populations both project to AD. Since AD does not appear to have recurrent connections, it cannot function as an attractor network, and thus cannot exhibit all the stability properties of such a network. But AD HD cells integrate information from LMN, PoS, and perhaps retrosplenial HD cells, and AD projects to PoS. The attractor network is located in PoS, which does have recurrent connections. This model explains why the firing of PoS HD cells is independent of angular velocity, while AD HD cells are influenced by velocity.

In a complementary attractor model by Sharp et al. (2001), DTN cells make inhibitory projections onto LMN cells, which in turn make excitatory projections back onto the DTN population. DTN cells also receive angular velocity information from vestibular nuclei. HD cells in LMN and DTN have different tuning properties, but their interaction is hypothesized to produce the attractor dynamics required to integrate angular velocity.

HD cells in other areas, such as retrosplenial cortex and caudate nucleus, could also contribute to the functioning of the "core" HD system. Further work may explain why there are so many HD areas, and why the difference in ATI values for PoS, AD, and LMN cells is so much greater than can be accounted for by synaptic delays alone.

Road Map: Mammalian Motor Control
Related Reading: Dynamic Remapping; Hippocampus: Spatial Models; Vestibulo-Ocular Reflex

References

Bassett, J. P., and Taube, J. S., 2001, Neural correlates for angular head velocity in the rat dorsal tegmental nucleus, *J. Neurosci.*, 21:5741–5751.

Blair, H. T., Cho, J., and Sharp, P. E., 1998, Role of the lateral mammillary nucleus in the rat head-direction circuit: A combined single-unit recording and lesion study, *Neuron*, 21:1387–1397.

Blair, H. T., and Sharp, P. E., 1995, Anticipatory head direction signals in anterior thalamus: Evidence for a thalamocortical circuit that integrates angular head motion to compute head direction, *J. Neurosci.*, 15:6260–6270.

Goodridge, J. P., Dudchenko, P. A., Worboys, K. A., Golob, E. J., and Taube, J. S., 1998, Cue control and head direction cells, *Behav. Neurosci.*, 112(4):1–13.

Goodridge, J. P., and Touretzky, D. S., 2000, Modeling attractor deformation in the rodent head-direction system, *J. Neurophys.*, 83:3402–3410. ◆

Knierim, J. J., Kudrimoti, H. S., and McNaughton, B. L., 1995, Place cells, head direction cells, and the learning of landmark stability, *J. Neurosci.*, 15:1649–1659.

Knierim, J. J., Kudrimoti, H. S., and McNaughton, B. L., 1998, Interactions between idiothetic cues and external landmarks in the control of place cells and head direction cells, *J. Neurophys.*, 80:425–446.

Mizumori, S. J. Y., and Williams, J. D., 1993, Directionally selective mnemonic properties of neurons in the lateral dorsal nucleus of the thalamus of rats, *J. Neurosci.*, 13:4015–4028.

Sharp, P. E., Blair, H. T., and Cho, J., 2001, The anatomical and computational basis of the rat head-direction cell signal. *Trends Neurosci.*, 24:289–294. ◆

Sharp. P. E., Tinkelman, A., and Cho, J., 2001, Angular velocity and head direction cells recorded from the dorsal tegmental nucleus of Gudden in the rat: Implications for path integration in the head direction cell circuit. *Behav. Neurosci.*, 115:571–588.

Skaggs, W. E., Knierim, J. J., Kudrimoti, H. S., and McNaughton, B. L., 1995, A model of the neural basis of the rat's sense of direction in *Advances in Neural Information Processing Systems 7* (G. Tesauro, D. S. Touretzky, and T. K. Leen, Eds.), Cambridge, MA: MIT Press, pp 173–180.

Stackman, R. U., and Taube, J. S., 1998, Firing properties of rat lateral mammillary single units: Head direction, head pitch, and angular head velocity, *J. Neurosci.*, 18:9020–9037.

Taube, J. S., 1995, Head direction cells recorded in the anterior thalamic nuclei of freely moving rats. *J. Neurosci.*, 15:1953–1971.

Taube, J. S., Muller, R. U., and Ranck, J. B., Jr., 1990a, Head direction cells recorded from the postsubiculum in freely moving rats: I. Description and quantitative analysis, *J. Neurosci.*, 10:420–435.

Taube, J. S., Muller, R. U., and Ranck, J. B., Jr., 1990b, Head direction cells recorded from the postsubiculum in freely moving rats: II. Effects of environmental manipulations, *J. Neurosci.*, 10:436–447.

Zhang, K., 1996, Representation of spatial orientation by the intrinsic dynamics of the head-direction cell ensemble: A theory, *J. Neurosci.*, 16:2112–2126. ◆

Schema Theory

Michael A. Arbib

Introduction

Schema theory complements neuroscience's well-established terminology for levels of *structural* analysis (brain region, neuron, synapse) with a *functional* vocabulary, a framework for analysis of behavior with no necessary commitment to hypotheses on the localization of each *schema* (unit of functional analysis), but which can be linked to a structural analysis whenever appropriate. Schemas provide a high-level vocabulary that can be shared by brain theorists, cognitive scientists, connectionists, ethologists, and even kinesiologists, even though the implementation of the schemas may differ from domain to domain. This article presents a general perspective, notes but does not emphasize learning models for schemas, and focuses on two issues: structuring perceptual and motor schemas to provide an action-oriented account of behavior and cognition (as relevant to the roboticist as the ethologist); and how schemas describing animal behavior may be mapped to interacting regions of the brain. Schema-based modeling becomes part of neuroscience when constrained by data provided by, for example, human brain mapping, studies of the effects of brain lesions, or neurophysiology. The resulting model may constitute an adequate explanation in itself or may provide the framework for modeling at the level of neural networks or below. Such a *neural schema theory* provides a functional/structural decomposition, in strong contrast with models that employ learning rules to train a single, otherwise undifferentiated, neural network to respond as specified by some training set.

Schemas: History and Comparisons

Central to our approach is the notion of the "active organism," which seeks from the world the information it needs to pursue its chosen course of action. In *action-oriented perception*, current sensory input is itself a function of the subject's active exploration of the world, which is directed by *anticipatory schemas*, which Neisser (1976) defines as plans for perceptual action as well as readiness for particular kinds of sensory structure. This view has resonances with that of Piaget (1971, pp. 6–7): "Any piece of knowledge is connected with an action . . . [T]o know an object or a happening is to make use of it by assimilation into an action schema . . . [namely] whatever there is in common between various repetitions or superpositions of the same action." Acting on the basis of an action schema usually entails the *expectation* of certain consequences. Piaget talks of *assimilation*, the ability to make sense of a situation in terms of a stock of schemas, and *accommodation*, whereby the stock of schemas may change over time as the expectations based on assimilation to current schemas are not met. Piaget traces the cognitive development of the child from reflexive schemas through eye-hand coordination and object permanence all the way to schemas for language and abstract thought.

Head and Holmes introduced the term schema to neurology in 1911, speaking of the *body schema* (Frederiks, 1969, reviews relevant literature): "Anything which participates in the conscious movement of our bodies is added to the model of ourselves and becomes part of those schemata: a woman's power of localization may extend to the feather of her hat." A woman with unilateral damage to the parietal lobe may lose awareness that the body on the opposite side actually belongs to her—not only ignoring painful stimuli but even neglecting to dress that half of the body. Damage to the thalamus and the somatosensory system may also produce disorders of the body schema.

Bartlett (1932) carried the schema idea into cognitive psychology, with a schema being "an active organization of past reactions [or] experiences, which must always be supposed to be operating in any well-adapted organic response." He stressed the constructive character of remembering. When people try to recall a story, they reconstitute it in their own terms—relating what they experience to a familiar set of schemas—rather than by rote memorization of details. Instead of thinking of ideas as impressions of sense data, schema theory posits an active and selective process of schema formation (cf. Piaget's notion of assimilation), which in some sense constructs reality as much as it embodies it. More generally, cognitive psychology views schemas as cognitive structures built up in the course of interaction with the environment to organize experience. Not only is sensory input coded by instantiating certain schemas (we say a schema is instantiated when active copies are running, and refer to these copies as "schema instances"), as seeing a chair instantiates an instance of the "chair schema," but the current stock of schema instances may also instantiate related action schemas such as "sitting" and general schemas such as "furniture" while inhibiting other competing schemas. Shallice (1988, p. 308n) stresses that the schema "not only has the function of being an efficient description of a state of affairs—as in, say, Bartlett's usage—but also is held to produce an output that provides the immediate control of the mechanisms required

in one cognitive or action operation. The usage is thus more analogous to Piaget's view than to Bartlett's original concept." In a connectionist vein, Rumelhart et al. (1986) suggest how schemas may be seen as emergent properties of adaptive, connectionist networks, but they neither relate schemas to action nor show how schemas may be combined to form assemblages (see discussion later in this article).

Schmidt (1976) offered a schema theory of discrete motor skill learning. Through experience, the subject builds up a *recall schema* that pairs the response specifications of a movement with the actual outcome. Later, this recall schema can be consulted to infer, from a desired outcome, the response specification that will produce it. Similarly, a *recognition schema* pairs the desired outcome with the expected sensory consequences of each movement. The recall schema is what is now known in the literature of motor control as an "inverse model" (SENSORIMOTOR LEARNING)—it goes from a desired response to a pattern of commands that achieves it, rather than the "direct" causal path from commands to action; while the recognition schema corresponds to Neisser's anticipatory schema.

Arbib (1981; Arbib, Érdi, and Szentágothai, 1998, Chapter 3 for an exposition) offered a schema theory more tightly constrained by the need to explain the neural basis of behavior, stressing that a schema expresses a function that need not be co-extensive with the activity of a single neuronal circuit. (This view was foreshadowed in the work of Kilmer, McCulloch, and Blum (1969) who posed the general question of how the nervous system could set the organism's "overall mode of behavior" through the cooperative computation [no executive control] of modules, each of which aggregates the activity of many neurons.) A *schema* is what is learned about some aspect of the world, combining knowledge with the processes for applying it; a *schema instance* is an active deployment of these processes. A *perceptual schema* not only determines whether a given "domain of interaction" (an action-oriented generalization of the notion of object) is present in the environment, but can also provide parameters concerning the current relationship of the organism with that domain. Each schema instance has an *activity level* that indicates its current salience for the ongoing computation. The activity level of a perceptual schema signals the credibility of the hypothesis that what the schema represents is indeed present, whereas other schema parameters represent other salient properties such as size, location, and motion of the perceived object. Given a perceptual schema, we may need several schema instances, each suitably tuned, to subserve our perception of several instances of its domain. *Motor schemas* provide the control systems that can be coordinated to effect a wide variety of actions. The *activity level* of a motor schema instance may signal its "degree of readiness" to control some course of action (thus enriching somewhat the related notion of motor pattern generators; see MOTOR PATTERN GENERATION).

Schema instances may be combined (possibly with those of more abstract schemas, including coordinating schemas) to form *schema assemblages*. For example, an assemblage of perceptual schema instances may combine an estimate of environmental state with a representation of goals and needs. A *coordinated control program* is a schema assemblage that processes input via perceptual schemas and delivers its output via motor schemas, interweaving the activations of these schemas in accordance with the current task and sensory environment to mediate more complex behaviors. Figure 1 shows the original coordinated control program. As the hand moves to grasp an object, it is *preshaped* so that when it has almost reached the ball, it is of the right shape and orientation to enclose some part of the object prior to gripping it firmly. Moreover (to a first approximation), the movement can be broken into a fast initial movement and a slow approach movement, with the transition from the fast to the slow phase of trans-

Figure 1. Hypothetical coordinated control program for reaching and grasping. Note that different perceptual schemas (at the top) are required to provide parameters for the motor schemas (at the bottom) for the control of "reaching" (arm transport ≈ hand reaching) and "grasping" (controlling the hand to conform to the object). Note too the timing relations posited here within the "Hand Reaching" motor schema and between the motor schemas for "Reaching" and "Grasping." Dashed lines—activation signals; solid lines—transfer of data. (Adapted from Arbib, 1981.)

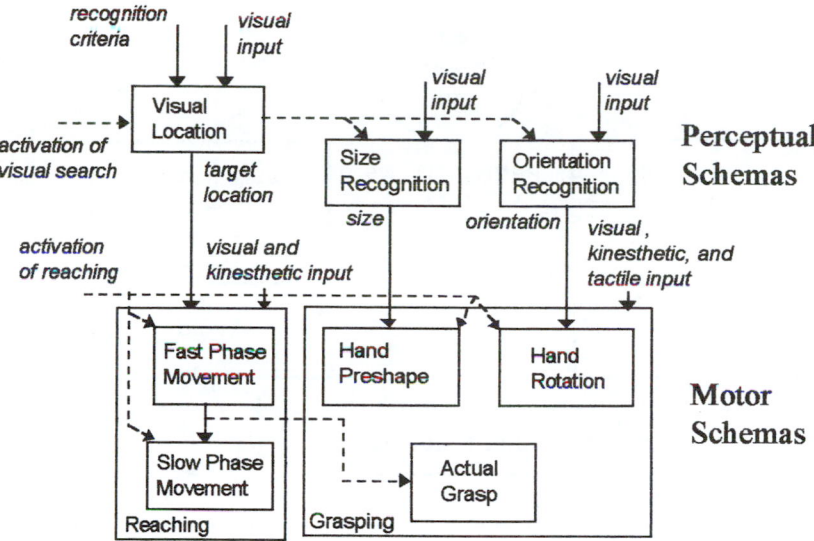

port coming just before closing of the fingers from the preshape so that touch may take over in controlling the final grasp. The top half of Figure 1 shows three perceptual schemas: successful location of the object activates the schemas for recognizing the size and orientation of the object. The outputs of these perceptual schemas are available for the control of the hand movement by concurrent activation of two motor schemas, one controlling the arm to transport the hand toward the object and the other preshaping the hand, with finger separation and orientation guided by the output of the appropriate perceptual schemas. Once the hand is preshaped, it is only the completion of the fast phase of hand transport that "wakes up" the final stage of the grasping schema to shape the fingers under control of tactile feedback. (This model anticipates the much later discovery of perceptual schemas for grasping in a localized area [AIP] of parietal cortex and motor schemas for grasping in a localized area [F5] of premotor cortex. See Grasping Movements: Visuomotor Transformations.)

Neuroscience and cognitive psychology often view working memory as storing a single item (e.g., the location of a target, or a single phone number) for a short delay period between observation of the item and its use in some action, after which it is discarded. Here, we extend the notion to insist that working memory may hold a range of items relevant to upcoming actions, and these items may remain accessible for extended periods so long as they remain relevant. Schema-based modeling of action-oriented perception (Visual Scene Perception) then views the *short-term memory* (STM) of an organism as a working memory that combines the schema instances encoding relevant aspects of, and plans for interaction with, the current environment. This assemblage is dynamic, as certain schema instances are discarded from memory ("de-instantiated") while others are added ("instantiated"). *Long-term memory* (LTM) is provided by the stock of schemas from which STM may be assembled. New sensory input as well as internal processes can update STM. The internal state is also updated by knowledge of the state of execution of current *plans* that specify a variety of coordinated control programs for possible execution. Jeannerod (1997) surveys the role of schemas and other constructs in the cognitive neuroscience of action.

Schemas for *Rana Computatrix*

A schema model becomes a neural model, as distinct from a purely functional model, when explicit hypotheses are offered as

to how the constituent schemas are played over particular regions of the brain. To exemplify this, consider approach and avoidance in the frog (Visuomotor Coordination in Frog and Toad; and see Arkin et al., 2000, for a related discussion of behavioral models of the praying mantis as a basis for robotic behavior). A frog surrounded by dead flies will starve to death, but the frog will snap with equal "enthusiasm" at a moving fly or a pencil tip wiggled in a fly-like way. On the other hand, a larger moving object can trigger an escape reaction. Thus, a highly simplified model of the functioning of the brain of the frog has signals from the eye routed to two basic perceptual schemas, one for recognizing small moving objects (foodlike stimuli) and one for recognizing large moving objects (enemylike stimuli). If the small-moving-object schema is activated, it will in turn trigger the motor schema that gets the animal to approach what is apparently its prey. If the perceptual schema for large-moving-object is activated, it will trigger the motor schema for avoidance, causing the animal to escape an apparent enemy.

The biological model relates these schemas to anatomy. Each eye of the frog projects to regions on the opposite side of the brain, including the important visual midbrain regions called the *tectum* and the *pretectum* (in front of the tectum). If we hypothesize that the small-moving-object schema is in the tectum, while the large-moving-object schema is in the pretectum, the model (Figure 2A) predicts that animals with a pretectal lesion would approach small moving objects, but would not respond at all to large moving objects. However, Peter Ewert in Kassell studied toads with the pretectum removed and found that they responded with approach behavior to both large and small moving objects. This observation leads to the new schema-level model shown in Figure 2B. We replace the perceptual schema for *small* moving objects of Figure 2A by a perceptual schema for *all* moving objects and leave the right-hand column the way it was. The inhibitory pathway from the large-moving-object perceptual schema (in the pretectum) to the all-moving-object schema ensures that the model yields the normal animal's response to small moving objects with approach but not avoidance. This model explains our small database on the behavior of both normal animals and those with a lesion of the pretectum.

We have thus shown how hypotheses about neural localization of subschemas may be tested and refined by lesion experiments. The important point is that models expressed at the level of a network of interacting schemas can really be testable biological

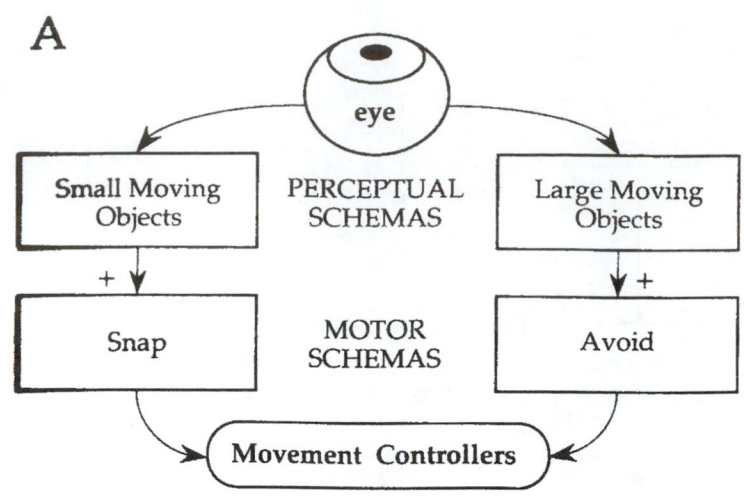

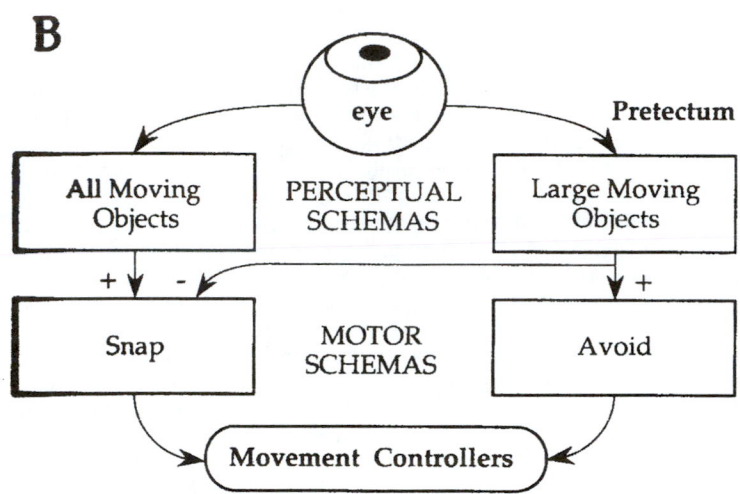

Figure 2. *A*, A "naive" schema program that represents the perceptual and motor schemas for frog approach behavior (snap at small moving objects) as completely separated from those for avoidance. *B*, A schema program for approach and avoidance that takes into account data on the effect of lesioning the pretectum. In particular, the "approach schema" is *not* localized in the tectum alone since it depends on pretectal inhibition for its integrity.

models. Subsequent work has extended work on *Rana computatrix* ("the frog that computes"; Arbib et al., 1998, for a partial review) at the level of both schemas and neural networks for phenomena such as detours and path planning, avoidance behavior sensitive to the trajectories of predators, and details of snapping behavior that link neural control to biomechanics. The work constitutes a grounding example of work in modeling neural mechanisms in overall animal behavior (NEUROETHOLOGY, COMPUTATIONAL).

Coordinated Control Programs and Motor Schemas

We have seen that schemas can be combined to form *coordinated control programs* that control the phasing in and out of patterns of schema co-activation and the passing of control parameters from perceptual to motor schemas. The notion of schema is thus *recursive*—a schema defined functionally may later be analyzed as a coordinated control program of finer schemas, and so on until such time as a secure foundation of neural localization is attained. The model of Figure 1 distinguished two phases of arm movement—a fast phase controlled by a ballistic schema (i.e., one that moves rapidly to completion, unaffected by feedback), followed by a slow phase controlled by a schema that does admit error-correction by use of sensory feedback. However, Jeannerod et al.

(1992) showed that reaching is subject to modification by sensory input even during the fast phase. If the target of a pointing task was perturbed at movement onset, the subject did not complete a ballistic movement toward the initial target before moving on to the new target. Rather, a smooth adjustment was made about 100 msec after target perturbation to a new trajectory terminating at the new target, without loss of accuracy. To address such data (and more), Hoff and Arbib (1993) extended the use of OPTIMIZATION PRINCIPLES IN MOTOR CONTROL (q.v.) by showing how to embed an optimality principle for arm trajectories into a controller that can use feedback to resist noise and compensate for target perturbations, and a predictor element to compensate for delays from the periphery. The result is a feedback system that can *act like* a feedforward system described by the optimality principle in "familiar" situations, where the conditions of the desired behavior are not perturbed and accuracy requirements are such that "normal" errors in execution may be ignored. However, when perturbations must be corrected for or when great precision is required, feedback plays a crucial role in keeping the behavior close to that desired, taking account of delays in putting feedback into effect.

Another claim embodied in Figure 1 is that the transition from preshaping to enclosing is controlled by, but does not influence, the transition in the transport phase. However, data show that when the hand has unexpectedly to open wider (if object size is increased during reach) transport slows by about 200 msec, but if target location is perturbed, the hand temporarily closes so that maximum aperture is delayed as transport takes longer to reach the new target. Hoff & Arbib (1993) designed a controller for the preshape schema to tradeoff an optimality criterion needed to prevent discontinuous "jumps" in the preshape and a "cost" for having the hand open more than a certain amount. The latter yields the partial reclosing of the hand during prolonged movement caused by location perturbation. Their strategy for coordinating the motor schemas is set forth in Figure 3. Here, the Enclose schema is a replica of the Preshape schema with the only exception that its starting point is the maximum aperture achieved by the preshape schema (there seems to be a linear relation between the actual object size and the maximum aperture achieved). The coordinating schema receives from each of the constituent schemas—Transport, Preshape, Enclose—an estimate of the time that it needs to move for execution. Then, whichever schema is going to take longer, Transport or Grasp (Preshape + Enclose), is given the full time it needs, while the other schema will be slowed down to apply its optimality criterion over the longer time base. This yields a satisfactory match between data and simulation.

The implication (a truth better known in motor control than in other areas of neurophysiology) is that much is to be learned at the level of schema analysis prior to, or in concert with, the "lower level" analysis of neural circuitry. Although the hypotheses developed in this section allow us to gain insight into the interaction of a number of different processes, they also pose major challenges for further neurophysiological investigation.

Discussion

Perceptual and Motor Schemas

We have suggested that schemas provide some sort of action-oriented memory, yet have made a distinction between perceptual schemas and motor schemas. Why not combine these two con-

structs into a single notion of schema that integrates sensory analysis with motor control, as suggested in the earlier quote from Shallice? Indeed, there are cases in which such a combination makes sense. However, recognizing an object (an apple, say) may be linked to many different courses of action (to place the apple in one's shopping basket; to place the apple in the bowl at home; to pick up the apple; to peel the apple; to cook with the apple; to eat the apple; to discard a rotten apple, etc.). Of course, once one has decided on a particular course of action, then specific perceptual and motor subschemas may be invoked. But note that, in the list just given, some items are apple-specific whereas other invoke generic schemas for reaching and grasping. It was considerations like this that led me to separate perceptual and motor schemas— a given action may be invoked in a wide variety of circumstances; a given perception may, as part of a larger assemblage, precede many courses of action. Putting it another way, there is no one "grand apple schema" that links all "apple perception strategies" to "every act that involves an apple." At the same time, however, note that, in the schema-theoretic approach, "apple perception" is not mere categorization—"this is an apple"—but may provide access to a range of parameters relevant to interaction with the apple at hand. The *Rana* example shows this in simplest form. In Figure 2A, the two schemas at left may be combined into a single unitary prey schema and the two at right into a single unitary predator schema. However, the lesion study suggested splitting perception from action since it is recognition of the large moving object that inhibits the prey-catching schema—based on the view that tectum and pretectum are "more perceptual" and the brainstem to which they project is "more motor."

A detailed example of how schema theory extends to more "cognitive" realms than basic patterns of sensorimotor coordination is offered by the schema-based interpretation in the VISIONS computer vision system (see VISUAL SCENE PERCEPTION for references). This system shows the importance of schema theory within artificial intelligence (i.e., even when there is no claim to model the brain). Similarly, schemas have played an important role in the development of behavior-based robots (REACTIVE ROBOTIC SYSTEMS).

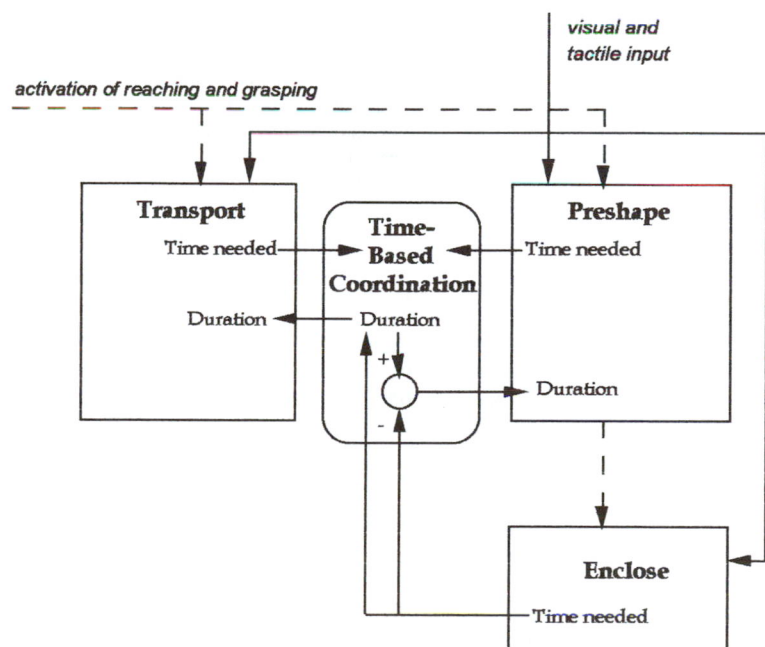

Figure 3. Feedback controllers for transport and preshape. "Cooperative computation" between subprograms is mediated by a coordinating schema ensuring that both reaching and grasping have adequate movement time (Hoff and Arbib, 1993).

Schemas and Their Assemblages Are Adaptable

Head himself considered schemas as plastic entities, which are subject to constant change, and adaptation is at the heart of Piaget's account of assimilation and accommodation. Although the examples of schemas given in the three figures above are fairly stable—as we explored the way in which schemas could be combined into coordinated control programs, and ways in which the psychological or neural correlates of such schema assemblages could be tested—it must be emphasized that schemas, and their connections with each other, change through the processes of accommodation. These processes adjust the network of schemas so that over time they may well be able to better handle a wide range of situations.

Work on HYBRID CONNECTIONIST/SYMBOLIC SYSTEMS (q.v.; see also Sun, 1995) has somewhat similar motivations to schema theory: In decomposing a cognitive model into a network of interacting processes, one may find at a given state of knowledge that quite different models will be appropriate for different components: some cognitive processes are best captured by symbolic models, some by connectionist models, and some by biologically realistic neural models. This leads to the development of hybrid systems. Schema theory is consistent with this in that it allows the schemas in an "assemblage" to be implemented in different ways so long as the input and output codes are compatible on any connection. However, it adds that what may appear to be disjoint schemas when implemented at one level may turn out to involve overlapping networks of subschemas when involved at a more detailed level (a simple example is given in Figure 2B). On the other hand, if we agree to the schema decomposition offered by high-level analysis, we may apply connectionist training procedures to adapt the initial schema structures if these are encoded by (artificial) neural networks.

Beyond Action and Perception

Through learning, a complex schema network arises that can mediate first the child's, and then the adult's, reality. Through being rooted in such a network, schemas are interdependent, so that each finds meaning only in relation to others. For example, a house is defined in terms of parts such as a roof, yet a roof may be recognized because it is part of a house that is recognized on the basis of other criteria such as "people live there." Each schema enriches and is defined by the others (and may change when a formal linguistic system allows explicit, though partial, definition). Though processes of schema change may affect only a few schemas at any time, such changes may "cohere" to yield dramatic changes in the overall pattern of mental organization. There is change yet continuity, with many schemas held in common, yet changed because they must now be used in the context of the new network. Arbib and Hesse (1986) offer an epistemology rooted in this view of schema theory, and show how it may be expanded to link "schemas in the head" with the "social schemas" that form the collective representations (to use Durkheim's phrase) shared by a community. Schemas have also been used in a "computational, neo-Piagetian" approach to language acquisition and may also be used in modeling language processing with special attention to the links between action, action and object recognition, and language (see LANGUAGE EVOLUTION: THE MIRROR SYSTEM HYPOTHESIS) and in relating these processes to neural schemas.

Road Maps: Artificial Intelligence; Psychology
Related Reading: Artificial Intelligence and Neural Networks; Compositionality in Neural Systems; Hybrid Connectionist/Symbolic Systems; Multiagent Systems

References

Arbib, M. A., 1981, Perceptual structures and distributed motor control, in *Handbook of Physiology—The Nervous System II. Motor Control* (V. B. Brooks, Ed.), Bethesda, MD: American Physiological Society, pp. 1449–1480.

Arbib, M. A., Érdi, P. and Szentágothai, J., 1998, *Neural Organization: Structure, Function, and Dynamics*, Cambridge, MA: MIT Press (see Chapter 3). ◆

Arbib, M. A., and Hesse, M. B., 1986, *The Construction of Reality*, Cambridge University Press.

Arkin, R. C., Ali, K., Weitzenfeld, A., and Cervantes-Pérez, F., 2000, Behavioral models of the praying mantis as a basis for robotic behavior, *Robotics and Autonomous Systems*, 32:39–60. ◆

Bartlett, F. C., 1932, *Remembering*, Cambridge University Press.

Frederiks, J. A. M., 1969, Disorders of the body schema, in *Handbook of Clinical Neurology*, 4, *Disorders of Speech Perception and Symbolic Behavior*, (P.J. Vinken and G.W. Bruyn, Eds.), North Holland, pp. 207–240. ◆

Hoff, B., and Arbib, M. A., 1993, Simulation of interaction of hand transport and preshape during visually guided reaching to perturbed targets, *J .Motor Behav.*, 25:175–192.

Jeannerod, M., 1997, *The Cognitive Neuroscience of Action*, Oxford, UK: Blackwell Publishers.

Jeannerod, M., Paulignan, Y., MacKenzie, C., and Marteniuk, R., 1992, Parallel visuomotor processing in human prehension movements, in *Control of Arm Movement in Space* (R. Caminiti, P. B. Johnson, and Y. Burnod, Eds), *Exp. Brain. Res. Ser.*, 22:27–44.

Kilmer, W. L., McCulloch, W. S., and Blum, J., 1969, A model of the vertebrate central command system, *Int. J. Man-Machine Stud.*, 1:279–309.

Neisser, U., 1976, *Cognition and Reality: Principles and Implications of Cognitive Psychology*, San Francisco: W.H. Freeman.

Piaget, J., 1971, *Biology and Knowledge*, Edinburgh University Press, Edinburgh.

Rumelhart, D. E., Smolensky, P., McClelland, J. L., and Hinton, G. E., 1986, Schemata and sequential thought processes in PDP models, in *Parallel Distributed Processing: Explorations in the Microstructure of Cognition* vol. 2 (J. L. McClelland and D. E. Rumelhart, Eds.), Cambridge, MA: MIT Press, Chapter 14.

Schmidt, R. A., 1976, The schema as a solution to some persistent problems in motor learning theory, in *Motor Control: Issues and Trends* (G. E. Stelmach, Ed.), New York: Academic Press, pp. 41–65.

Shallice, T., 1988, *From Neuropsychology to Mental Structure*, Cambridge, MA: Cambridge University Press.

Sun, R., 1995, On schemas, logics, and neural assemblies, *Applied Intelligence*, 5(2):83–102.

Scratch Reflex

Paul S. G. Stein

Introduction

An organism can scratch itself in response to a stimulus at a site on the body surface (Stein, 1983). Mechanical force is the stimulus that has been used in many studies of scratching. In frogs, chemical irritation has also been used to activate scratching. During successful scratching, a nearby limb moves toward and rubs against the site. If a different site is stimulated, different limb movements are required for a successful scratch. The stimulated site may be on a part of the body such as the shell of a turtle (Stein, 1989) or the back of a frog (Berkinblit, Feldman, and Fukson, 1989), or it may be on a part that can move with respect to the body such as the ear of a cat (Kuhta and Smith, 1990) or the elbow of a frog (see Stein, 1983). In each case, the organism can generate a successful scratch. (Since space in the reference list is limited, the reader is referred to the articles by Stein, 1989, Stein and Smith 1997, and other papers by the author for fuller references to the literature.)

Some organisms do not require the entire central nervous system to produce a successful scratch reflex. Some vertebrates with a complete spinal cord transection at the level of the neck or upper back, termed *spinal vertebrates*, can perform a successful hindlimb scratch in response to a stimulus delivered to a site on the body surface posterior to the complete transection. This stimulus excites neural networks in the spinal cord posterior to the complete transection (Stein, 1983, 1989). Scratching has been demonstrated in several spinal vertebrates: dog (Sherrington, 1906), cat (Arshavsky, Gelfand, and Orlovsky, 1986; Orlovsky, Deliagina, and Grillner, 1999), turtle (Stein, Mortin, and Robertson, 1986; Stein, 1989; Earhart and Stein, 2000), and frog. In frog, scratch reflex is also termed *wiping reflex* (Berkinblit et al., 1989; see also MOTOR PRIMITIVES).

Site specificity of scratch reflex in spinal vertebrates is impressive. The spinal frog's hindlimb can wipe off an acid-soaked piece of paper from its elbow. Successful wipes of the elbow by the hindlimb occur when the elbow is close to the neck as well as when the elbow is close to the midbody (see Stein, 1983). Spinal cord neuronal networks can generate complex sensorimotor transformations even when disconnected from supraspinal structures.

Strategies of Scratching: The Forms of a Scratch

The set of all successful scratches is constrained by the physical construction of the organism's limbs and body, i.e., its biomechanics. For some organisms, there may be a set of sites on the body surface, e.g., sites on the middle of the back of a turtle or a human, that cannot be rubbed directly by a limb of that organism. There may be some sites that can be scratched by using only one strategy of movement; for example, a human can scratch some sites on the upper back using only a strategy in which the elbow is placed over the shoulder. These sites belong to a set termed a *pure-form domain*. While the same motor strategy is used to rub against each site within a pure-form domain, parametric adjustment of limb movement is required to reach each specific site. There may be other sites that can be scratched by using either of several strategies; for example, a human can scratch a site on the side of the thorax using either the hand or the elbow. These sites belong to a set termed a *transition zone*. Each scratch movement strategy is termed a *form* of the scratch (Stein, Mortin, and Robertson, 1986). The concept of movement form can be applied to other motor acts. There are several forms of locomotion in mammals, e.g., walk, trot, and gallop (Stein and Smith, 1997; see also GAIT TRANSITIONS). Forward stepping and backward stepping are among the forms of stepping that humans produce.

The spinal turtle produces several scratch strategies. In each strategy, a distinct portion of the hindlimb is used to exert force against the stimulated site (Stein, Mortin, and Robertson, 1986). The turtle uses the dorsum of the foot for *rostral scratching*, the side of the knee for *pocket scratching*, and the side of the foot or heel for *caudal scratching*. Biomechanical constraints play a key role for each of these movement strategies. The rostral scratch is the only strategy that can be used to place a portion of the hindlimb against a site on the region that connects the upper shell and the lower shell in the middle of the body. The foot cannot reach sites in the pocket region just anterior to the turtle's hip; only the side of the knee can be used to generate force against a site in the pocket region. Thus, the spinal turtle can select the biomechanically appropriate form that produces successful scratches; selection of the proper scratch strategy does not require supraspinal structures, i.e., the brainstem and the brain. Experiments described in a later section establish form selection as an intrinsic property of spinal cord neural networks.

Coordinate System Transformations in the Scratch Reflex

Several transformations occur during scratching. First, a stimulus-to-sensory transformation takes place on the body surface when the stimulus activates primary afferent neurons. Second, a sensory-to-motor transformation takes place within the central nervous system (CNS). Third, a motor-to-mechanical transformation takes place in the limb. It is possible to examine all three transformations at the same time during actual scratching. For neuronal network studies, it is useful to examine the first and second transformations in the absence of the third transformation, i.e., in the absence of movement. Experiments that examine the response to a tactile stimulus that elicits scratch motor output while neuromuscular synapses are blocked are described in later sections.

Several coordinate systems help to describe the different transformations. First, the rectilinear orthogonal Cartesian coordinate system is useful in a scientist's description of the site on the body surface that receives the sensory stimulus as well as the position in space of the limb that rubs against the site. Second, the muscle/motor-pool coordinate system is useful for describing the output of the CNS. The set of motor neurons that synaptically activate a given muscle is termed a motor pool. Each muscle of the body and/or its motor pool can be viewed as a dimension of a coordinate system. Each dimension's amplitude is determined by the intensity of activation of each muscle/motor-pool (see MOTONEURON RECRUITMENT). During each movement, there is a distinct *motor pattern* of muscle/motor-pool activation that occupies a region of an abstract space whose dimensions are time and muscles/motor-pools. Third, the body degree-of-freedom, also termed joint-angle, coordinate system is useful for describing multijointed limb movements. Some body joints, e.g., the knee, have a single degree of freedom and involve only a single dimension. Other body joints, e.g., the hip, have several degrees of freedom and therefore require several dimensions. Each movement form has a distinct trajectory in time and degree-of-freedom space.

Coordinate System Analyses of the Turtle Scratch Reflex

Data obtained from studies of the scratch reflex in the spinal turtle (Stein, 1989) allow application of the concepts outlined in the previous section. These data are described in this section. Other data obtained from frog (Berkinblit et al., 1989; see also MOTOR PRIMITIVES) and from cat (Arshavsky et al., 1986) are also consistent with these concepts.

Cartesian Coordinate Description of Receptive Fields

If a stimulus applied to a site on the body surface elicits a specific form of scratch reflex in which a nearby limb reaches toward and rubs against the stimulated site, then that site is within the receptive field for that form of scratch. In the spinal turtle, there is a receptive field for rostral scratch, a receptive field for pocket scratch, and a receptive field for caudal scratch. There is also a rostral-pocket transition zone and a pocket-caudal transition zone (Stein et al., 1986).

Stimulation of most sites in one form's receptive field elicits only scratches of that form; these sites constitute the pure-form domain of that form's receptive field. The *pure-form domain* for each scratch form is the set of sites in which only one scratch form is biomechanically possible. There is also a set of transition-zone sites located between the pure-form domain for one form and the pure-form domain for another form. The *transition zone* is the set of sites in which more than one scratch form is biomechanically possible. Stimulation of a site in this transition zone can elicit either one scratch form, the other scratch form, or a blended response of both scratch forms. There are two types of blends: the switch response and the hybrid response. In a *switch response*, several cycles of one form are followed smoothly by several cycles of the other form. In a *hybrid response*, each of several successive cycles has two rubs per cycle; one rub utilizes one scratch form, and the other rub utilizes the other scratch form.

The occurrence of blends supports the notion that there is shared neural circuitry between the neural network that generates one form of scratch and the neural network that generates another form of scratch. In particular, analyses of blends support the concept that interneurons controlling the rhythm of hip movements are shared among the networks responsible for each of several forms of scratching (Berkowitz and Stein, 1994; Stein et al., 1995; Stein, McCullough, and Currie, 1998; Berkowitz, 2001).

Muscle/Motor-Pool Coordinate Description of Motor Patterns

The electromyographic (EMG) activity of individual muscles that play critical roles for each scratch form may be recorded during scratching in the spinal turtle (Earhart and Stein, 2000). The monoarticular knee extensor muscle is active during the rub against the stimulated site for all three forms of scratch. Scratching in the turtle is rhythmic; all three forms of scratching display rhythmic alternation between hip flexor muscle activity and hip extensor muscle activity. Timing of the monoarticular knee extensor muscle is distinct for each scratch form. The monoarticular knee extensor muscle is active (1) during the latter part of hip flexor muscle activity in a rostral scratch, (2) during hip extensor muscle activity in a pocket scratch, and (3) after the burst of hip extensor muscle activity in a caudal scratch. The motor pattern of muscle/motor-pool activation is distinct for each scratch form.

Body Degree-of-Freedom Coordinate Description of Movement

The time course of hip angle (angle of hip flexion/extension) and knee angle (angle of knee flexion/extension) has been studied during each of the three forms of turtle scratch reflex (see discussion in Earhart and Stein, 2000). Rhythmic alternation between hip flexion and hip extension occurs for all three scratch forms. Timing of

knee extension in the cycle of hip flexion and extension is distinct for each scratch form. The knee extends during the latter part of hip flexion in a rostral scratch; the knee extends during hip extension in a pocket scratch; the knee extends after hip extension is completed in a caudal scratch. A specific *movement pattern* in the joint-angle coordinate system is distinct for each form; that is, there is regulated timing of knee extension in the cycle of hip movement.

The movement pattern for each form in time and joint-angle space is similar to the motor pattern for each form measured in time and muscle/motor-pool space. In both spaces for each form of the scratch, there is a regulated timing of the knee with respect to the cycle of the hip. Similar changes of timing of a distal joint in the cycle of a proximal joint have been observed for other behaviors, e.g., forward versus backward stepping in humans.

Spinal Cord Networks for Scratch Reflex

Spinal cord networks responsible for producing the scratch reflex in the cat (Arshavsky et al., 1986) and in the turtle (Stein, 1989; Currie and Stein, 1992; Berkowitz and Stein, 1994; Berkowitz, 2001; Stein and Daniels-McQueen, 2002) are partially understood. This understanding relies upon the demonstration that the spinal cord can produce a motor pattern in the absence of actual movements. Movements are prevented by muscle acetylcholine receptor blockade with a specific antagonist, e.g., curare. The motor pattern is measured as the electroneurographic (ENG) activities of specific motor pools in response to a stimulation of a site in a scratch receptive field. The ENG motor patterns recorded in the absence of movements are termed *fictive* motor patterns.

The ENG motor pattern for each scratch form in the spinal immobilized turtle is generated in response to stimulation of a site in the receptive field for that scratch form. Each motor pool monitored in the immobilized turtle using ENG recording techniques innervates a muscle that was previously monitored using EMG recording techniques during actual movements. The ENG motor pattern is an excellent replica of the EMG motor pattern recorded during actual movements. These results establish that spinal cord neuronal networks select the appropriate scratch motor pattern in response to stimulation of a specific site on the body surface; thus, motor strategy selection is a property of spinal cord neuronal networks. These rhythmic motor patterns are produced in an open-loop condition without benefit of timing cues from movement-related sensory feedback; thus, rhythmic motor pattern generation is an intrinsic property of spinal cord neuronal networks.

Motor patterns produced in the absence of movement-related feedback are termed *central motor patterns*. The neuronal network responsible for generating a central motor pattern for a behavior is termed a *central pattern generator* (CPG) for that behavior (Stein et al., 1997). A goal of current research is to reveal the properties of the CPG for each scratch form. It is possible that the CPG for one scratch form shares no neural circuitry with the CPG for another scratch form; such a lack of overlap in circuitry is not likely to occur, however. Single-neuron recordings in the turtle support the hypothesis that the CPG for the rostral scratch may share neural elements with the CPG for the pocket scratch (Berkowitz and Stein, 1994; Berkowitz, 2001).

The scratch motor pattern is not independent of movement-related sensory input, however. Motor patterns are subject to important modulations due to sensory input (see MOTOR PATTERN GENERATION). For example, EMG recordings during actual scratching in the cat demonstrate amplitude and phase modulations of the motor pattern due to sensory feedback during paw contact with the stimulated site (Kuhta and Smith, 1990); similar modulations of the EMG motor pattern are also seen in the spinal turtle when the foot catches against the rod that is used to deliver the mechanical stimulus (Stein, 1983).

Localization and Distribution of Spinal Cord Neuronal Networks

The spinal cord is a segmental structure. Each segment receives sensory input from a specific region of the body surface termed the *dermatome* of that spinal segment. Each segment contains the cell bodies of motor neurons that innervate a specific set of muscles. The hindlimb enlargement is the set of spinal segments that contain the cell bodies of motor neurons that innervate hindlimb muscles.

Anterior segments of the hindlimb enlargement play an important role in scratch rhythm generation in the cat (Arshavsky et al., 1986) and in the turtle (Stein, 1989). In all limbed vertebrates, the anterior portion of the hindlimb enlargement contains hip flexor motor neurons and knee extensor motor neurons. A scratch motor rhythm is produced by the most anterior segment of the turtle hindlimb enlargement in response to stimulation of a site in that segment's dermatome. A rhythmic pocket scratch motor pattern is produced by the three most anterior segments of the turtle hindlimb enlargement in response to stimulation of a site in the dermatome of the most anterior segment. The spinal segment just anterior to the hindlimb enlargement also contributes to rhythmogenesis. Thus neuronal networks for scratching are contained in and distributed among a set of spinal segments.

Multisecond Excitability Changes in Scratch Neuronal Networks

The turtle scratch motor response can continue for several seconds after the termination of sensory stimulation (Currie and Stein, 1992). For an additional several seconds after the cessation of motor neuron activity, there is an increased excitability of spinal cord neuronal networks. This afterexcitability is form specific and is a physiological measure of spinal cord selection processes. NMDA receptors contribute to this afterexcitability (Currie and Stein, 1992; see also NMDA RECEPTORS: SYNAPTIC, CELLULAR, AND NETWORK MODELS). The long time constant of NMDA receptor activation is well suited for multisecond excitability changes.

Spinal cord neurons, termed long-afterdischarge interneurons, are activated by stimulation in a region of a scratch receptive field and are active for many seconds after the cessation of stimulation. Long-afterdischarge interneurons may play a role in motor pattern selection in scratch neuronal networks. NMDA receptors contribute to the excitability of long-afterdischarge interneurons (Currie and Stein, 1992).

Broad Tuning of Interneurons in Neuronal Networks for Scratching

There is broad tuning in the responses of individual turtle interneurons activated by stimulation of sites in the receptive fields for the rostral scratch and for the pocket scratch (Berkowitz and Stein, 1994; Berkowitz, 2001). Some of these interneurons are activated throughout the entire region of the scratch receptive fields for each of several forms. Many of these interneurons may be members of both the rostral scratch CPG and the pocket scratch CPG. For each interneuron, there is usually a site whose stimulation results in the highest frequency of action potentials; stimulation of other sites usually results in interneuron firing frequencies that decrease as the distance from the site that evokes the greatest response increases. These data are consistent with the hypothesis that motor pattern selection results from the summed activities of a population of broadly tuned interneurons that are shared by several CPGs.

Scratch CPG Rhythmogenesis

Reciprocal inhibition between hip flexor and hip extensor interneurons plays a major role in spinal cord scratch rhythmogenesis; additional mechanisms for rhythmogenesis must exist, however, since hip flexor motor rhythms are generated in the absence of hip extensor motor activity (Stein et al., 1995; Stein, McCullough, and Currie, 1998). During quiescence of hip extensor motor neuron activity, there is also quiescence of hip extensor interneuron activity (Stein and Daniels-McQueen, 2002). This supports the concept that interneurons that are active during hip flexor motor output are rhythmogenic. Left-right interactions also play a key role in rhythmogenesis (Stein et al., 1995; Stein, McCullough, and Currie, 1998).

Discussion

Scratching can be used to uncover important characteristics of neuronal networks that perform sensory-to-motor transformations. Future experiments are required for a more complete understanding of the properties of these neuronal networks.

Road Maps: Motor Pattern Generators; Neuroethology and Evolution
Related Reading: Gait Transitions; Locomotion, Vertebrate; Motor Primitives

References

Arshavsky, Y. I., Gelfand, I. M., and Orlovsky, G. N., 1986, *Cerebellum and Rhythmical Movements*, Berlin: Springer-Verlag. ◆

Berkinblit, M. B., Feldman, A. G., and Fukson, O. I., 1989, Wiping reflex in the frog: Movement patterns, receptive fields, and blends, in *Visuomotor Coordination* (J.-P. Ewert and M. A. Arbib, Eds.), New York: Plenum Press, pp. 615–629.

Berkowitz, A., 2001, Broadly tuned spinal neurons for each form of fictive scratching in spinal turtles, *J. Neurophysiol.*, 86:1017–1025.

Berkowitz, A. and Stein, P. S. G., 1994, Activity of descending propriospinal axons in the turtle hindlimb enlargement during two forms of fictive scratching: phase analyses, *J. Neurosci.*, 14:5105–5119.

Currie, S. N., and Stein, P. S. G., 1992, Glutamate antagonists applied to midbody spinal cord segments reduce the excitability of the fictive rostral scratch reflex in the turtle, *Brain Res.*, 581:91–100.

Earhart, G. M., and Stein, P. S. G., 2000, Step, swim, and scratch motor patterns in the turtle, *J. Neurophysiol.*, 84:2181–2190.

Kuhta, P. C. and Smith, J. L., 1990, Scratch responses in normal cats: hindlimb kinetics and muscle synergies, *J. Neurophys.*, 64:1653–1667.

Orlovsky, G. N., Deliagina, T. G., and Grillner, S., 1999, *Neuronal Control of Locomotion from Mollusc to Man*, New York: Oxford University Press. ◆

Sherrington, C. S., 1906, *The Integrative Action of the Nervous System*, New Haven, CT: Yale University Press.

Stein, P. S. G., 1983, The vertebrate scratch reflex, *Symp. Soc. Exp. Biol.*, 37:383–403. ◆

Stein, P. S. G., 1989, Spinal cord circuits for motor pattern selection in the turtle, *Ann. NY Acad. Sci.*, 563:1–10. ◆

Stein, P. S. G., and Daniels-McQueen, S., 2002, Modular organization of turtle spinal interneurons during normal and deletion fictive rostral scratching, *J. Neurosci.*, 22:6800–6809.

Stein, P. S. G., Grillner, S., Selverston, A. I., and Stuart, D. G., Eds., 1997, *Neurons, Networks, and Motor Behavior*, Cambridge, MA: MIT Press. ◆

Stein, P. S. G., McCullough, M. L., and Currie, S. N., 1998, Reconstruction of flexor/extensor alternation during fictive rostral scratching by two-site stimulation in the spinal turtle with a transverse spinal hemisection, *J. Neurosci.*, 18:467–479.

Stein, P. S. G., Mortin, L. I., and Robertson, G. A., 1986, The forms of a task and their blends, in *Neurobiology of Vertebrate Locomotion* (S. Grillner, P. S. G. Stein, D. G. Stuart, H. Forssberg, and R. M. Herman, Eds.), London: Macmillan, pp. 201–216. ◆

Stein, P. S. G., and Smith, J. L., 1997, Neural and biomechanical control strategies for different forms of vertebrate hindlimb motor tasks, in *Neurons, Networks, and Motor Behavior* (P. S. G. Stein, S. Grillner, A. I. Selverston, and D. G. Stuart, Eds.), Cambridge, MA: MIT Press, pp. 61–73. ◆

Stein, P. S. G., Victor, J. C., Field, E. C., and Currie, S. N., 1995, Bilateral control of hindlimb scratching in the spinal turtle: Contralateral spinal circuitry contributes to the normal ipsilateral motor pattern of fictive rostral scratching, *J. Neurosci.*, 15:4343–4355.

Self-Organization and the Brain

Christoph von der Malsburg

Introduction

There is a fundamental difference between brain and computer. The computer is based on the algorithmic division of labor. It relies on the separate existence of minds that program and interpret. The brain is a physical, dynamical system to which the algorithmic scheme cannot be applied except in a metaphorical sense. The brain is not digital, not deterministic in any operational sense, and in its inner workings it never gets help from a separate interpreting and planning mind. Instead, the brain is organized on the basis of physical interactions between its elements and of the nested processes of evolution, ontogenesis, and state organization. Unfortunately, our thinking about brain and mind is still very much in the grips of the algorithmic scheme, and we are always in danger of seeing in evolution a programmer and in the genome a program, of taking perception as a mere preparation of material for a "higher level" always just outside our field of view, or of subscribing to a model of learning that relies on the presence of an experimenter to select and prepare the learning patterns and their encoding.

Self-organization is the process by which ordered structures arise in dynamical systems (see PATTERN FORMATION, BIOLOGICAL; COOPERATIVE PHENOMENA; Haken, 1978; Ball, 1999). The theory of evolution has always been a theory of self-organization (EVOLUTION OF THE ANCESTRAL VERTEBRATE BRAIN; EVOLUTION OF GENETIC NETWORKS; EVOLUTION OF ARTIFICIAL NEURAL NETWORKS), and the perspective of self-organization is gaining growing acceptance as well at the level of morphogenesis (not treated here) and the organization of neural connectivity (see DEVELOPMENT OF RETINOTECTAL MAPS; OCULAR DOMINANCE AND ORIENTATION COLUMNS) and brain state (see DYNAMIC LINK ARCHITECTURE). But our ideas about self-organization will have to be developed much further before they can get algorithmic thinking totally out of the way.

Self-Organization in General

Self-organization is the phenomenon by which simple mechanisms of growth and interaction lead to the establishment of complex structures of global order. The phenomenon dominates our world, from the crystalline structure of minute snowflakes to the flow patterns in our coffee cup, atmosphere, and oceans to the formation of stars, planetary systems, and galaxies. Its most awesome expression, however, is found in the structures of the living world. Elementary arrangements cooperate and compete to form more complex patterns, these in turn conspiring to create structures of higher and higher order. What distinguishes winning patterns is the degree of harmony of their elementary arrangements within their smaller and larger contexts. The most interesting aspect of the phenomenon is the tremendous contrast between the simplicity of elementary interactions and the complexity and beauty of the structural order they create. Although a silent revolution in favor of self-organization as a fundamental principle has swept the intellectual world within the past two or three decades, we are still far from realizing the full impact of the phenomenon on our comprehension of things.

Self-organized structures are characterized by inherent order—symmetries, self-similarity, repetition, and many other kinds of regularity: the mechanisms of self-organization are not free to create arbitrary arrangements and can only select from a relatively narrow universe of ordered patterns. For example, although no two snowflakes are ever alike, they realize a vanishing subset of all arbitrary arrangements of water molecules. The amount of information needed to specify a self-organized pattern is therefore very modest, tremendously smaller than the (logarithm of) number of all random arrangements of elements. In consequence, describing phenomena in terms of self-organized structures is a very powerful tool, and focusing attention on those structures is of great scientific importance.

Although science still has to struggle to find and formulate much of the universe of structured patterns that can be realized by self-organization, this universe is preexisting in the mathematical sense. (To give a specific example, the set of all possible periodic crystal lattices can be completely specified mathematically.) It is impressive to see to what extent the structure of this universe is determined by laws and relationships operating at higher levels and independent of the detail of elementary mechanisms and interactions. Structure is determined to a large extent from the top down, supporting the hope that even systems as complex as the brain can ultimately be understood in relatively simple terms.

In an elementary process of self-organization, a system makes the transition from a simple, relatively unstructured initial state that is in the process of becoming unstable to a more structured final state in which the dynamic forces reach equilibrium again. The transition starts with random *fluctuations*, which are small deviations from the initial state. The process is governed by three types of interactions: fluctuations self-amplify, fluctuations cooperate, and fluctuations compete. In the interplay between these interactions, certain constellations of fluctuations collude to form patterns on a larger scale.

A simple and well-understood example of self-organization, originally proposed by Bénard, is a flat pan filled with liquid and heated from below. (Other examples of self-organizing systems are discussed in COOPERATIVE PHENOMENA.) In an initial state, the liquid is at rest. When the temperature gradient is strong enough, the initial state becomes unstable, and fluctuations in the form of small regions of upwelling or downwelling liquid start to grow in amplitude. These fluctuations are self-amplifying, as upward motion draws more hot liquid from the bottom, creating a column of fluid that is hotter and lighter than the surrounding fluid, and similarly for downward motion. Fluctuations cooperate, with vertical movement in one small column dragging along movement in neighboring columns. And they compete, as upward movement in one place must be made up by downward movement in other places. These interactions establish convection cells, regions of coherent motion, which typically take the shape of hexagons or rolls (the latter being akin to the parallel bands of clouds sometimes seen in the sky), often of impressively regular arrangement. In a given system, fluctuations can be defined on several levels. In the Bénard system, for instance, "fluctuations" may be identified with droplets of moving liquid, as I just did, but also with whole coordinated patterns of mutually consistent up-and-down movement, which may have the form of sinusoidal waves fluctuating in amplitude.

The dynamic properties of interacting fluctuations, and consequently the selection of particular final structures, usually is subject to so-called control parameters (among the control parameters of the Bénard system are the temperature gradient, the viscosity, and the depth of the liquid). Moreover, a pattern resulting from self-organization may set the stage for more self-organization, sometimes making a final result dependent on the detailed history of a long chain of processes. This aspect is especially important in biology, whose structures are the result of phylogenetic and ontogenetic history.

Mathematical Methods

There are three types of theoretical tools to describe and understand self-organizing systems: computer simulation, statistical mechanics, and dynamical differential equations and the attendant fields of catastrophe theory and stability analysis. Statistical mechanics is a method to derive relations between global properties of physical systems from the statistics of the constituent atoms or molecules. Typical global parameters are temperature, energy, volume, and pressure. From a very simple basic idea ("all detailed configurations of the system compatible with global parameters are attained with equal probability") all interesting quantities can be derived mathematically (see STATISTICAL MECHANICS OF NEURAL NETWORKS and Hertz, Krogh, and Palmer, 1991). Important applications of statistical physics are phase transition systems. They fall into "universality classes." It is remarkable to what extent the qualitative behavior of systems in a given universality class is independent of detailed material properties. What above was called "harmony" materializes in statistical physics as a quantity called free energy (great harmony is low free energy).

Many self-organizing systems can be completely characterized by continuous variables and their deterministic interactions (in Bénard's system these are the local velocity of the flowing liquid and the forces acting on it). Such systems are conveniently described as systems of coupled differential equations (see Haken, 1978; see also COOPERATIVE PHENOMENA). These are always of nonlinear type and can be solved analytically (that is, with pencil and paper) only in the rarest cases. Computer simulation is a convenient way to explore the behavior of such systems. However, since the behavior of a system can depend in unexpected ways on the precise settings of parameters, it is profitable to analyze this behavior using stability analysis (see DYNAMICS AND BIFURCATION IN NEURAL NETS; COOPERATIVE PHENOMENA; Haken, 1978). As a result, a simpler description of the system is derived in the form of a small number of superimposable patterns ("linear modes") and differential equations describing the behavior of their amplitudes. Stability analysis is thus a powerful conceptual tool to make the transition from a description at the level of microscopic building elements to macroscopic modes of behavior.

Self-Organization in the Brain

The brain is often cited as the most complex entity in the universe. And indeed it is an awesome array of structure that spans many orders of magnitude. Although this can also be said of a simple rock, what distinguishes the brain is the purposeful arrangement of its detail. Pathological alteration at any level—molecular, synaptic, cellular, or macroscopic—easily leads to serious functional deficit. On the other hand, much of the variation from individual to individual, or even from second to second in a given individual, seems to be fully compatible with physiological function. This raises the great puzzle of how the myriad important functional relationships are created and maintained in the brain. According to an old mode of thinking, a Creator, or Mother Nature, or a genetic program is in control of every molecular reaction with exquisite algorithmic foresight. Although this thought pattern of "hetero-organization" under control of a preexisting detailed plan still governs many a thought subconsciously, it is quickly losing dominance, giving way to models of self-organization at all levels—evolution, ontogenesis, learning, and functional organization. As a result, instead of blindly accepting any arbitrary brain structure as of equal a priori likelihood, the explicit examination of mechanisms of organization in evolution and ontogenesis yields powerful constraints on what to expect, reducing the search space of experimental science by many orders of magnitude.

A potent argument against the brain as irreducible heap of structure is the gross mismatch between the amount of information contained in its detail as measured naively and the amount of available genetic information. The direct specification of an arbitrary wiring pattern of the 10^{14} connections between the 10^{10} neurons in the human cerebral cortex would, for instance, take more than 10^{15} bits of information. By comparison, there are little more than 10^9 bits in the human genome. This mismatch of more than six orders of magnitude vanishes if the genes are required only to specify the rules of the game and some control parameters for ontogenetic self-organization. As a consequence, the resulting connectivity patterns, far from random, have to be highly regular. Some of this regularity is known to us and has, for instance, the form of topographic organization. The bulk of the connective architecture of the brain, however, is unknown and very difficult to determine experimentally. The most parsimonious way to describe the brain (including individual variations) would be in terms of generative rules and appropriate theoretical tools to retrace ontogeny. Intimate knowledge of the laws of organization is also a prerequisite for analysis and cure of many ailments of the brain, much more than mere knowledge of static structure (even if it could be had).

The evolution of the brain cannot possibly be imagined as a progression of mutation and selection at the level of individual cells or synapses ("evolution by rote"). This search space would just be too large, even on the time scale of hundreds of millions of years, and the resulting information could not be transmitted from generation to generation through the limited genome. In reality, however, as the genes determine the laws of self-organization and its control parameters, the search space is much smaller. Evolution restricts itself to finding fruitful architectures and tuning them to the particular biological needs of the species by alterations at the control parameter level.

The neurosciences are making extensive use of inductive generalization from a few strategic observations. This is possible only on the basis of the regularities that are the hallmark of self-organization. Progress could be accelerated and many a false start and expensive investigation avoided if we had a clearer picture of the control structures and regularities of the brain as a self-organizing entity. So far the surface has hardly been scratched.

An immense amount of experimental and theoretical work will have to be done. The perspective of self-organization is not a magic bullet that reduces the brain problem to armchair theorizing and a few simple equations. Our nervous system is made up of a bewildering variety of cell types of different anatomy, molecular makeup, and behavioral repertoire, and our brain has an immensely convoluted gross anatomy of interconnected nuclei and areas. Even if the details of neural connectivity could be derived from general laws, these general laws are conditioned from below and above by the underlying behavioral repertoire of the constituent elements and the gross boundary conditions. The amount of information in our genome may be much smaller than any naively calculated information content of the brain, but it is still a very large quantity.

In order for the brain to guide the animal safely through life, it must be in tune with the environment. How can it be so? One important answer evidently is that the brain learns through examples. Unfortunately, this process is far from being fully understood. Each situation with which a brain has to cope is unique. Only appropriate analysis and coding makes information from one scene applicable to others. These mechanisms of analysis and proper representation are unlikely to be learned themselves from example. They exist prior to experience (as postulated by Immanuel Kant) and rely to a large extent on self-organization. Although this sounds like a daring proposition, requiring the universe of self-organized brain structures to be generally in tune with the structure of the environment by "preestablished harmony," no other solution to the epistemology riddle is in sight. The self-organized ontogenesis of brain structures constitutes a natural language, and all evolution had to do was use this language to write the particular text that defines us.

Activity Self-Organization

In the formulation of McCulloch and Pitts (1943), neural networks have binary signals and synchronized switching and are thus equivalent to digital machines. Just as in digital machines, these networks and their activity have no inherent tendency to fall into organized patterns. McCulloch and Pitts do not discuss any mechanism for the generation of networks or the underlying logical functions to be realized. These are based entirely on the algorithmic schema and must be structured on the basis of a separate programmer's insight. With appropriate changes, however, neural networks can be made to self-organize. For this, some combination of giving up synchrony of switching, introducing graded instead of binary signals, and specializing connectivity patterns to near symmetry (between the forward and backward connection between two neurons) seems to be important. Essential for self-organization is a tendency to iteratively approach stationary states (or nearly stationary states).

The self-organization of activity patterns is most simply discussed and modeled in homogeneous two-dimensional sheets of neurons with short-range excitation and longer-range inhibition, assumptions that are consistent with what is known about cortical anatomy. A homogeneous activity distribution in a sheet of neurons becomes unstable when the slope of the input-output function of the tissue grows beyond a critical value (see DYNAMICS AND BIFURCATION IN NEURAL NETS). Small fluctuations in signal strength then start to grow and self-amplify. Due to short-range excitation, they cooperate locally; through longer-range inhibition they compete. As a consequence, organized patterns grow.

Under idealized conditions these patterns may have the form of regular arrays of blobs or of parallel stripes. Under more realistic conditions one observes more or less regular waves or arrays of blobs, closely corresponding in character to ripples in sand under irregularly moving water, and many other systems.

Such activity patterns are found in the visual cortex of cat and monkey with optical or other recording techniques. These patterns may play a role in the generation and expression of the regular columnar arrangement of cellular properties such as OCULAR DOMINANCE AND ORIENTATION COLUMNS (q.v.). They have also been proposed as an explanation for visual hallucinations during migraines or states of intoxication (see PATTERN FORMATION, BIOLOGICAL).

If, as is the reigning opinion, neural connections are the repository of knowledge in the brain, activity self-organization is the mechanism by which elementary knowledge (in the form of connections) is combined into useful thought patterns. An admittedly very simple first model of this process is associative memory (Hertz et al., 1991; see also COMPUTING WITH ATTRACTORS). Activity states are stored by HEBBIAN SYNAPTIC PLASTICITY (q.v.), that is, by strengthening connections between neurons that are simultaneously active in a state. Later, the state can be dynamically recreated by self-organization, starting from an incomplete version of it. The model thus treats self-organization at two levels, the formation of connections and the formation of activity states. The model has been fully analyzed by the methods of statistical physics, which helped to identify important parameters and gave useful information on memory capacity. It may be hoped that the obvious weaknesses of the associative memory model—it only recreates states established previously and cannot generalize to new scenes—can be overcome to create a more realistic model of brain state organization.

The main reason for associative memory's weakness is the monolithic character of its activity states. Lately, much experimental and theoretical study has been devoted to spatiotemporal patterns as a means to segregate the mass of neurons simultaneously active in a given brain state into separate chunks (corresponding to separate objects in a scene) by synchronizing the signals of neurons within chunks and desynchronizing them between chunks (see SYNCHRONIZATION, BINDING AND EXPECTANCY).

Network Self-Organization in Ontogenesis

Network self-organization conforms to a simple scheme (von der Malsburg, 1995). A network and its inputs create activity patterns. These are characterized by statistical correlations between pairs of neural signals. In response to these correlations, individual synapses are changed by HEBBIAN SYNAPTIC PLASTICITY (q.v.). In terms of the general scheme of self-organization discussed above, elementary fluctuations are deviations of synaptic strengths from their initial state. Fluctuations self-amplify as result of the positive feedback between excitatory synapses and the correlations they create. Cooperation rules between synapses that converge on the same neuron if their activity is correlated, as a consequence of which they help each other establish favorable postsynaptic activity. Competition rules between synapses if the activity states they favor are not compatible with each other. The altered network creates modified patterns of signal correlations, which in turn modify synaptic strengths. This feedback loop may create a runaway situation that drives the network state away from the initial, unstructured state. Because of their elementary interactions, natural alliances exist between synapses, and the network that finally wins is a constellation of connections that is optimal in terms of cooperation and competition.

The ontogenesis of fiber projection systems has been studied in great detail in the example of the retinotectal system (see DEVELOPMENT OF RETINOTECTAL MAPS; von der Malsburg, 1995). There seems to be a consensus that three major mechanisms are guiding fibers: gross routing, fiber positioning, and fiber sorting. Apparently, the first two mechanisms are based on gradients of morphogens that guide fibers first to the target structure and then to their target position within that structure. These mechanisms are simple extensions of general themes of morphogenesis (see the chapter on bodies in Ball, 1999). The retinotectal system shows considerable flexibility in dealing with unexpected variations imposed experimentally or by anomalous development. The projection can, for instance, adjust to changed relative size of retina and tectum. The adaptability of the retinotectal system is explained by the third mechanism, fiber sorting. This mechanism has been shown to be dependent on neural activity. It has been modeled with great success and is now a prime paradigm for neural network self-organization. Other instances of network self-organization deal with the ontogenesis of OCULAR DOMINANCE AND ORIENTATION COLUMNS (q.v.; see also von der Malsburg, 1995) and of structures in the barrel field of the rodent cortex.

According to recent evidence, synapses can change their weight on a very rapid time scale (for a review see Hempel et al., 2000). It might be surmised that these changes are controlled by network-created short-term signal fluctuations in a rapid version of HEBBIAN SYNAPTIC PLASTICITY (q.v.). If that is the case, a process of network self-organization may be active, adapting the connectivity pattern of the brain to the current context in which it is operating on time scales of fractions of seconds to minutes (see DYNAMIC LINK ARCHITECTURE).

Conclusion

The theme of self-organization currently receives surprisingly little attention in the brain theory community. And yet there is a tremendous, largely uncharted territory to be explored. The easily accessible geometrical patterns of activity and connectivity have been modeled in hundreds of publications. However, the material with which neural self-organization plays has the form of a *net-*

work, in which neighborhood is defined in terms of neural connectivity and not (or at least not directly) in terms of two- or three-dimensional geometry. We therefore must prepare ourselves for a totally new universe of network and activity patterns in which order is defined in terms of abstract relationships and quantities, and not in terms of pretty pictures. Second, the theory of self-organization has hitherto focused on the establishment of static structures. The nervous system, however, is about the generation of purposeful, nested processes evolving in time. Third, getting the simulation of a self-organizing system to work, that is, to create the intended type of patterns, is still an art. There are usually quite a few control parameters in a system, and they must all be put in the right ballpark. Blind search is usually out of the question for quantitative reasons. In view of the variability of the physiological state of the nervous system, evolution cannot simply have developed fixed values for these parameters. Nature must have developed general mechanisms to actively and autonomously regulate its systems, such as to produce interesting self-organized processes and states.

Finally, it will be important to understand the process of brain organization as a cascade of steps, each one taking place within the boundary conditions established by the previous one, and the theory of such cascades is as yet nonexistent. The tremendous creativity inherent in our brain's state organization cannot be well understood without knowing the arena set up by ontogenesis and learning, and ontogenesis cannot well be understood without understanding the genetic control structure set up by evolution. The perspective of self-organization is more of a program for future work than an accomplished success. There is a new continent to be discovered. It is the continent where our mind lives. It is time to set sail.

Road Map: Dynamic Systems
Related Reading: Cooperative Phenomena; Development of Retinotectal Maps; Ocular Dominance and Orientation Columns; Self-Organizing Feature Maps

References

Ball, P., 1999, *The Self-Made Tapestry: Pattern Formation in Nature*, New York: Oxford University Press. ◆

Haken, H., 1978, *Synergetics: An Introduction. Nonequilibrium Phase Transitions and Self-Organization in Physics, Chemistry and Biology*, 2nd enlarged ed., New York: Springer-Verlag. ◆

Hempel, C. M., Hartman, K. H., Wang, X.-J., Turrigiano, G. G., and Nelson, S. B., 2000, Multiple forms of short-term plasticity at excitatory synapses in rat medial prefrontal cortex, *J. Neurophysiol.*, 83:3031–3041.

Hertz, J., Krogh, A., and Palmer, R. G., 1991, *Introduction to the Theory of Neural Computation*, Redwood City, CA: Addison-Wesley.

McCulloch, W. S., and Pitts, W. H., 1943, A logical calculus of the ideas immanent in nervous activity, *Bull. Math. Biophys*, 5:115–133.

von der Malsburg, C., 1995, Network self-organization in the ontogenesis of the mammalian visual system, in *An Introduction to Neural and Electronic Networks*, 2nd ed. (S. F. Zornetzer, J. Davis, and C. Lau, Eds.), New York: Academic Press, pp. 447–463. ◆

Self-Organizing Feature Maps

Helge Ritter

Introduction

A first and very important step in many pattern recognition and information processing tasks is the identification or construction of a reasonably small set of important features in which the essential information for the task is concentrated.

The *self-organizing feature map* (SOFM) is a nonlinear method by which such features can be obtained with an unsupervised learning process. It is based on a layer of adaptive units ("neurons," Figure 1) that gradually develops into an array of feature detectors that is spatially organized in such a way that the location of the excited units becomes indicative of statistically important features of the input signals.

The linking of input signals to response locations in the map can be viewed as a nonlinear projection from a signal or input space to the (usually) two-dimensional (2D) map layer. The resulting "compressed image" of the (usually higher-dimensional) input space has the property of a topographic map that reflects important metric and statistical properties of the input signal distribution: distance relationships in the input space (expressing, e.g., pattern similarities) are approximately preserved as distance relationships between corresponding excitation sites in the map, and clusters of similar input patterns tend to become mapped to coherent areas whose size varies in proportion to the frequency of the occurrence of their patterns.

This resembles in many ways the structure of topographic feature maps found in many brain areas, for which the SOFM offers a neural model that bridges the gap between microscopic adaptation rules postulated at the single neuron or synapse level and the formation of experimentally better accessible, macroscopic patterns of feature selectivity in neural layers. From a statistical point of view, the SOFM provides a nonlinear generalization of principal component analysis and has proved valuable in many application contexts, ranging from pattern recognition and optimization to robotics (Ritter, Martinetz, and Schulten, 1992; Kohonen, 1995).

The Basic Feature Map Algorithm

The SOFM algorithm provides an unsupervised learning rule by which the adaptive units (neurons) can tune their response prop-

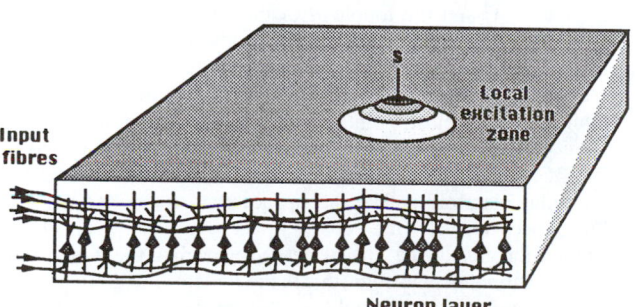

Figure 1. Schematic representation of a feature map. Nerve fibers providing the input signal excite the neurons via synaptic connections. Lateral interactions restrict the neural responses and the synaptic adaptation to a local excitation zone. Each possible position *s* of the excitation zone can be viewed as a compressed image in a two-dimensional space of the original stimulus features.

erties in such a way that the described, topographic map structure arises. The process is iterative and is driven by a sequence of activity patterns on some shared set of (afferent) input lines (Figure 1), at each step activating and adapting some local group of neurons.

Successful self-organization of the map requires the following: (1) the neurons must be exposed to a sufficient number of different inputs; (2) for each input, only the synaptic input connections to the excited group are affected; (3) similar updating is imposed on many adjacent neurons; and (4) the resulting adjustment is such that it enhances the same responses to a subsequent, sufficiently similar input (Kohonen, 1982).

A standard formulation of this process models the input patterns as vectors $\mathbf{x}$ from some pattern space V (whose dimensionality n is given by the number of input lines) and the neural layer as a set of formal neurons occupying discretes sites r in a (e.g., planar) grid A. The response of a neuron at site r is determined by the dot product $\mathbf{x} \cdot \mathbf{w}_r$, where $\mathbf{w}_r$ is the vector of the neuron's synaptic connection strengths with the n afferents carrying the input pattern $\mathbf{x}$.

For each input $\mathbf{x}$, the adaptive changes in the layer are confined to a local group of neurons centered at the site s for which $\mathbf{x} \cdot \mathbf{w}_s$ is maximal. This is achieved by modulating the adaptive changes for other sites r with an activity profile h_{rs} that has its peak at $r = s$ and that decays to smaller values with increasing distance $\|r - s\|$ from s ("neighborhood cooperation"); it is essential that $\|r - s\|$ be taken in the space of the lattice A, not in the original signal space V):

$$\mathbf{w}_r^{(new)} = (1 - \epsilon \cdot h_{rs})\mathbf{w}_r^{(old)} + \epsilon \cdot h_{rs} \cdot \mathbf{x} \quad (1)$$

Equation 1 can be justified by assuming the traditional Hebbian law for synaptic modification together with an additional nonlinear, "active" forgetting process for the synaptic strengths (Kohonen, 1995).

A rather realistic modeling choice for h_{rs} is, e.g., a Gaussian

$$h_{rs} = \exp\left(-\frac{\|r - s\|^2}{\sigma^2}\right) \quad (2)$$

whose variance $\sigma^2/2$ will control the radius of the group.

Consequently, neurons that are close neighbors in A will tend to specialize on similar patterns. After learning, this specialization is used to define the mapping from the space V of patterns onto the (discretized) space A: each pattern vector $\mathbf{x} \in V$ is mapped to one of the discretized neuron sites of A. The image of $\mathbf{x}$ under this mapping is defined to be the location $s = s(\mathbf{x})$ associated with the neuron for which $\mathbf{x} \cdot \mathbf{w}_s$ is largest ("winner neuron").

A frequently useful modification of this basic algorithm is to replace the winner criterion for the site $s(\mathbf{x})$ by a different one. A frequent choice is minimizing the Euclidean difference $\|\mathbf{x} - \mathbf{w}_s\|$ (which is equivalent to maximizing $\mathbf{w}_s \cdot \mathbf{x}$ when the vectors are normalized), but many other similarity measures can also be used to obtain SOFMs.

Visualization of Feature Maps

There are two main ways to visualize a feature map. The first approach labels each neuron in A by the test pattern that excites this neuron maximally (best stimulus). It yields a partitioning of a map into coherent regions of similarly specialized neurons and resembles the experimental procedure by which sites in a brain area are labeled by those stimulus features that are most effective in exciting neurons at this site. In the example in Figure 2, each training and test pattern consisted of 13 simple binary-valued features describing one of 16 animals (Ritter and Kohonen, 1989) whose similarity relationships are reflected in the resulting partitioning of the SOFM.

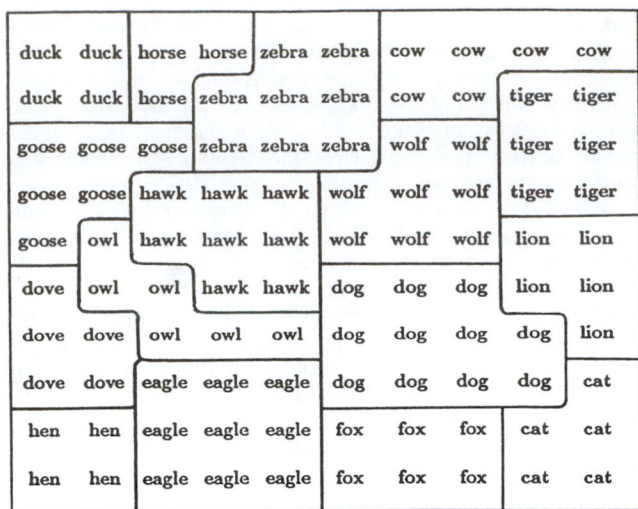

Figure 2. Visualization of a 10×10 feature map for a set of pattern vectors describing binary features of 16 animal species. The spatial arrangement of the labeled map regions reflects the similarity relationships between the animals.

In the second approach, the feature map is visualized as a "virtual net" in the original pattern space V. The virtual net is the set of weight vectors $\mathbf{w}_r$ displayed as points in the pattern space V and connected by lines between those pairs $(\mathbf{w}_r, \mathbf{w}_s)$, whose neuron sites (r, s) are nearest neighbors in the lattice A. While the virtual net is very well suited to display the topological ordering of the map, its use is limited to continuous and at most three-dimensional (3D) spaces. Figures 3A and 3B show the development of the virtual net of a 2D 20×20 lattice A from a disordered initial state (Figure 3A) into an ordered final state (Figure 3B) when the stimulus density is concentrated along the surface $z = x \cdot y$ in the cube V given by $-1 < x, y, z < 1$.

Discussion

The main characteristics of the feature map algorithm. Geometrically, the adaptive process (Equation 1) can be viewed as a sequence of local deformations of the virtual net in the space of input patterns so that it *approximates the shape of the stimulus density $P(\mathbf{x})$ in the space V.* A good approximation is possible if the topology of the virtual net (which is the same as the topology of the lattice A) and the topology of the stimulus density are the same (as, e.g., in Figures 3A and 3B). Otherwise, e.g., if the dimensionalities of the stimulus manifold and the virtual net differ, the resulting approximation can only partially fulfill the goal of matching spatially close points of the stimulus manifold to points that are neighbors in the virtual net. An example is depicted in Figure 3C, where the map manifold is 1D (a chain of 400 units), the stimulus manifold is 2D (the surface $z = x \cdot y$), and the embedding space V is 3D (the cube $-1 < x, y, z < 1$). In this case, the dimensionality of the virtual net is lower than the dimensionality of the stimulus manifold (this is the typical situation), and the resulting approximation resembles a "space-filling" fractal curve.

Properties of the features that are represented in a feature map. The geometric interpretation of the previous section suggests that a good approximation of the stimulus density by the virtual net requires that the virtual net be oriented tangentially at each point of the stimulus manifold. Therefore, a d-dimensional

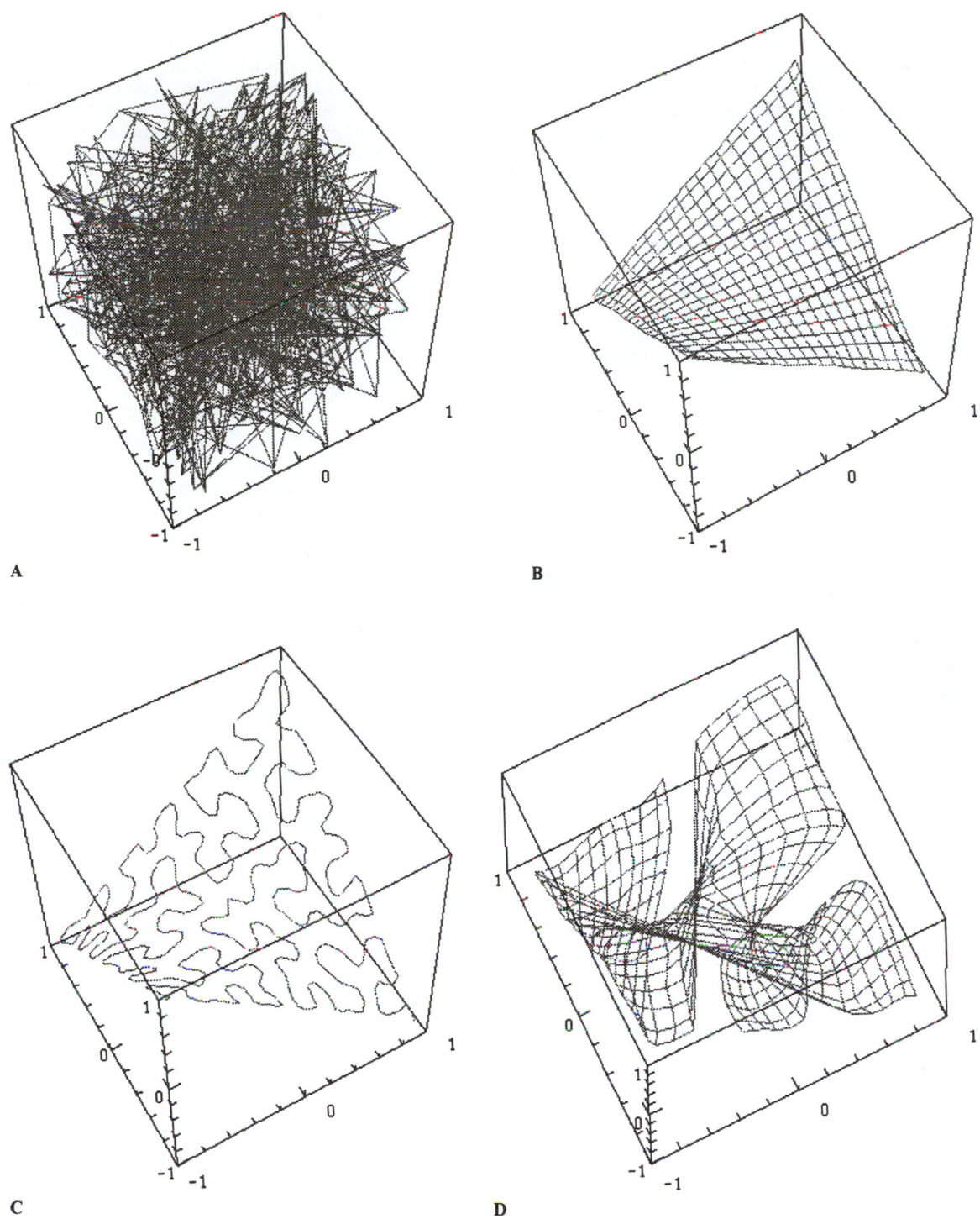

A

B

C

D

Figure 3. Top: Initial, disordered (*A*) and final, ordered (*B*) configuration of the "virtual net" for a two-dimensional feature map, developing under the influence of a two-dimensional stimulus density that is embedded in a three-dimensional signal space. *C, Dimension conflict:* when replacing the two-dimensional feature map of parts *A* and *B* with a one-dimensional chain, a space-filling fractal curve results. *D,* A *topological defect* is characterized by several patches of globally conflicting local orderings.

feature map will select a (possibly locally varying) subset of *d* independent features that capture as much of the variation of the stimulus distribution as possible. This is an important property that is also shared by the method of PRINCIPAL COMPONENT ANALYSIS (PCA) (q.v.). An important difference, however, is that the selection of the "best" features can vary smoothly across the feature map and can be optimized locally. Therefore, the SOFM can be viewed as a nonlinear extension of PCA.

Relationship of the feature map to more traditional approaches. The SOFM shares with a number of other approaches the goal of forming lower-dimensional, distance-preserving mappings of data, which is a general task in data analysis known as *multidimensional scaling* (see DATA CLUSTERING AND LEARNING). Usually, these methods are based on a direct minimization of some *projection index* that quantifies, e.g., the degree of distance distortion, or some measure of "interestingness" (e.g., non-Gaussianity of the resulting image distribution). An example of the first type is the nonlinear *Sammon mapping*, while examples of the latter type are the *projection pursuit methods* that lead to various linear projections (of which PCA can be viewed as a special case when the interestingness measure is just the data variance).

There is also the following relationship with *vector quantization*, which considers the task of finding discrete encodings for continuous signals satisfying certain optimality requirements, such as minimal reconstruction error. The determination of the site $s(\mathbf{x})$ of the winner neuron in a SOFM can be considered as assignment of a code s to a data vector $\mathbf{x}$. From this code, $\mathbf{x}$ can be reconstructed (decoded) approximately by taking $\mathbf{w}_s(\mathbf{x})$ as its reconstruction, with an average (mean square) reconstruction error

$$E = \int P(\mathbf{x})(\mathbf{x} - \mathbf{w}_{s(\mathbf{x})})^2 d^d\mathbf{x} \qquad (3)$$

It can be seen that in the special case $h_{rs} = \delta_{rs}$ (absence of neighborhood cooperation), the adaptation rule (Equation 1) is a stochastic minimization procedure for E, and becomes equivalent to a standard algorithm for finding an optimized set of codebook vectors $\mathbf{w}_s$, in vector quantization terminology. However, a further source of reconstruction errors may be the *confusion* of two codes s', s'' with some probability $p(s', s'')$. This situation requires the minimization of a more general error measure, now given by

$$E = \sum_{s',s''} p(s', s'') \int_{s(\mathbf{x}) = s'} P(\mathbf{x})(\mathbf{x} - \mathbf{w}_{s''})^2 d^d\mathbf{x} \qquad (4)$$

It can be shown that the (approximate) minimization of this error measure, and therefore the construction of an optimal code for this more general situation, is closely related to the feature map formation, provided one takes $h_{ss'} = p(s, s')$; i.e., the neighborhood cooperation in the map is derived from the "confusion matrix" $p(s, s')$ (Luttrell, 1994).

The stationary states of the feature map algorithm. A *stationary state* is a configuration for which the average change of weights per adaptation step vanishes. A stationary state is stable if all sufficiently small perturbations from it decay on the average. However, for a given stable stationary state, this still leaves the possibility that there may exist "very unlikely" sequences of adaptation steps that lead to a different stationary state. If such sequences exist, a stable stationary state is called *metastable*; otherwise it is called *absorbing*. Only the absorbing states are the "true" final states of the time evolution of a feature map. However, if the system is driven into a metastable state, it may become "trapped" for such a long time that the state cannot be distinguished from a true absorbing state within realistic observation times. Usually, the metastable states are those that occur as only partially ordered, while those states that intuitively appear as fully ordered seem to have the property of being absorbing (Erwin, Obermeyer, and Schulten, 1992a, 1992b).

Speed and reliability of the ordering process in relation to the various parameters of the model. The convergence process of a feature map can be roughly subdivided into a first ordering phase, in which the correct topological order is produced, and a subsequent fine-tuning phase. So far, rigorous convergence proofs for the full process have only been obtained for the 1D case, and for the 2D case when the correct topological order is specified along the border of A. Since for many geometrically intuitive definitions of order in dimensions greater than 1 one can show that they do not lead to absorbing states for the SOFM process, a very general ordering proof for higher dimensions is unlikely to exist. For a good overview on these and other theoretical aspects of the SOFM, see Cottrell, Fort, and Pagès (1998).

A very important role for the ordering phase is played by the neighborhood kernel h_{rs}. Usually, h_{rs} is chosen as a function of the distance $\|r - s\|$; i.e., h_{rs} is translation invariant. The algorithm will work for a wide range of different choices (locally constant, Gaussian, exponential decay) for h_{rs}, but for fast ordering the function h_{rs} should be convex over most of its support. Otherwise, the system may get trapped in partially ordered, metastable states and the resulting map will exhibit "topological defects," or conflicts between several locally ordered patches (Figure 3D shows a typical example) (Erwin et al., 1992a, 1992b).

Another important parameter is the distance up to which h_{rs} is significantly different from zero. This range sets the radius of the adaptation zone and the length scale over which the response properties of the neurons are kept correlated. The smaller this range, the larger the effective number of degrees of freedom of the network and, correspondingly, the harder the ordering task from a completely disordered state. Conversely, if this range is large, ordering is easy, but finer details are averaged out in the map. In addition, for Gaussian neighborhood kernels, a sufficiently large range also makes the function h_{rs} convex over the entire network. Therefore, formation of an ordered map from a very disordered initial state is favored by a large initial range (a sizable fraction of the linear dimensions of the map) of h_{rs}, which then should decay slowly to a small final value (on the order of a single lattice spacing or less). Although statistical considerations seem to dictate a $1/t$ decay law, the faster exponential decay is suitable in many cases.

It should be noted that the absence of a general ordering proof is mainly of theoretical concern. In practical applications, one usually will start with an already ordered configuration (oriented, e.g., along the major principal axes of the data distribution) and apply the SOFM process for the fine-tuning phase.

Quantitative characterizion of the ordering achieved with a feature map. The difficulty of characterizing the achieved ordering is partly due to the difficulty of defining order for embeddings of higher-dimensional lattices in higher-dimensional spaces. A more modest goal is the construction of some cost or energy function that is minimized by the algorithm and that then can serve as a measure of "progress" toward a converged state (without, however, necessarily telling much about the geometric ordering properties of such a state). A good candidate is the function E in Equation 4; however, it has been rigorously shown that the SOFM algorithm does not admit an exact energy function, rendering Equation 4 only an approximation. Remarkably, the approximation can be made exact by changing the SOFM winner criterion for the determination of $s(\mathbf{x})$ (Heskes and Kappen, 1993; Luttrell, 1994):

$$s(\mathbf{x}) = \arg \min_r \sum_{r'} h_{rr'} \|\mathbf{x} - \mathbf{w}_{r'}\| \qquad (5)$$

This winner criterion is more costly to compute, and the modified process seems to resemble the SOFM sufficiently closely to warrant the substitution of Equation 5 with the simpler but theoretically less satisfying original winner criterion in practical applications.

In applications, the data topology often is unknown, and the use of a SOFM can only be considered in an attempt to find out how well the (usually) 2D map can approximate the unknown data topology. Various measures of the faithfulness of the resulting maps have been suggested, but their practical usefulness has been limited by their complexity, which usually far exceeds that of the SOFM algorithm itself.

Relationship between stimulus density and weight vector density. During the second, fine-tuning phase of the map formation process the density of the weight vectors becomes matched to the signal distribution. Regions with high stimulus density in *V* lead to the specialization of more neurons than regions with lower stimulus density. As a consequence, such regions appear magnified on the map; that is, the map exhibits a locally varying *magnification factor*. In the limit of no neighborhood, the asymptotic density of the weight vectors is proportional to a power $P(\mathbf{x})^\alpha$ of the signal density $P(\mathbf{x})$ with exponent $\alpha = d/(d + 2)$. For a nonvanishing neighborhood, the power law remains valid in the 1D case, but the original SOFM algorithm leads to a different exponent α that now depends on the neighborhood function (Ritter, 1991). For higher dimensions, the relation between signal and weight vector distribution is more complicated, but the monotonic relationship between local magnification factor and stimulus density seems to hold in all cases investigated so far. Here, too, the modified winner criterion (Equation 5) leads to a simplification and yields a density exponent $\alpha = d/(d + 2)$, independent of the neighborhood function.

The effect of a "dimension conflict." In many cases of interest, the stimulus manifold in the space *V* is of higher dimensionality than the map manifold *A*, and as a consequence, the feature map will display those features that have the largest variance in the stimulus manifold. These features have also been termed *primary*. However, under suitable conditions, further, *secondary* features may become expressed in the map. The representation of these features is in the form of repeated patches, each representing a full "miniature map" of the secondary feature set. The spatial organization of these patches is correlated with the variation of the primary features over the map: the gradient of the primary features has larger values at the boundaries separating adjacent patches, while it tends to be small within each patch. The conditions for the occurrence of secondary features have been analyzed for simplified situations (Ritter et al., 1992; Obermayer, Blasdel and Schulten, 1992). These results show that the stability of a 2D map with only two primary features requires that the ratio of the variance of the primary features across the range of the neighborhood function and of the variance of the signal manifold perpendicular to the directions of the primary features be below a certain threshold. If the signal distribution is such that no such map configuration exists, additional features will become expressed in the map, with the role of the secondary features assigned to the features with the lower variance.

Modeling the properties of observed brain maps. Many regions in the brain are known to be topographic representations of sensory surfaces. It has been shown that the qualitative structure, including, e.g., the spatially varying magnification factor, and certain experimentally induced reorganization phenomena can be reproduced with the Kohonen feature map algorithm (Ritter et al., 1992). A more stringent test is provided by the more complex maps that are found in the visual cortex. In V1, there is a hierarchical representation of the features: retinal position, orientation, and ocular dominance, with retinal position acting as the primary feature. The secondary features, orientation and ocular dominance, form two correlated spatial structures: (1) a system of alternating bands of binocular preference and (2) a system of regions of orientation-selective neurons arranged in parallel iso-orientation stripes such that orientation angle changes monotonically in the perpendicular direction. The iso-orientation stripes are correlated with the binocular bands such that both band systems tend to intersect perpen-

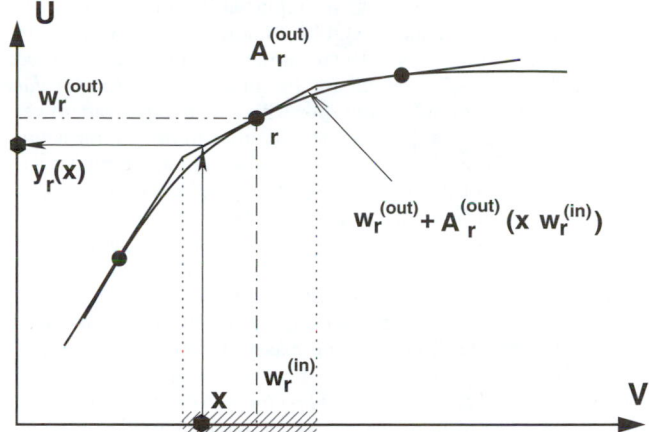

Figure 4. Extended feature map for learning nonlinear input-output mappings. The input-output mapping $V \to U$ is defined by a collection of locally valid linear mappings, one for the vicinity (shaded subregion in *V*) of the (input) weight vector $\mathbf{w}_s^{(in)}$ of each neuron. Defining these mappings requires an additional weight vector $\mathbf{w}_s^{(out)}$ and a matrix $\mathbf{A}_s$ (not shown) per neuron. These additional parameters are adapted with a perceptron error correction rule.

dicularly. In addition, the orientation map exhibits several types of singularities that tend to cluster along the monocular regions between adjacent stripes of opposite binocularity. It turns out that all these features, including even many quantitative aspects, can be remarkably well reproduced by the Kohonen feature map algorithm (Erwin, Obermayer, and Schulten, 1995). One may conclude that despite its computational simplicity, the Kohonen feature map algorithm can successfully model a striking range of features of observed brain maps.

Variants of the basic SOFM algorithm. The basic SOFM algorithm is an on-line learning method that admits the formulation of an analogous batch variant (batch SOFM; Kohonen, 1995) in which adaptation steps occur only after entire epochs, during which all (or a larger number of) patterns have been presented. When T_s denotes the subset of patterns for which neuron *s* was selected as winner in the current epoch, the batch SOFM adaptation step at the end of the epoch is given by

$$\mathbf{w}_r^{(new)} = \frac{\sum_{\mathbf{x} \in T_s} h_{rs} \cdot \mathbf{x}}{\sum_{\mathbf{x} \in T_s} h_{rs}} \tag{6}$$

The advantages of the batch algorithm are the absence of any learning rate and its enlarged possibilities for various optimizations to allow the training also of very large maps and for very large data sets (for details, see Kohonen, 1995).

One major possibility for reducing the number of nodes, as required, e.g., for higher dimensional maps, is the use of *linear interpolation*. In particular, the extension of the basic feature map to produce a vectorial output value from a *locally valid linear map*

$$\mathbf{y}_r(\mathbf{x}) = \mathbf{w}_r^{(out)} + \mathbf{A}_r(\mathbf{x} - \mathbf{w}_r^{(in)}) \tag{7}$$

(Ritter et al., 1992) has proved useful in many contexts. Here, the additional quantities are *output weights* $\mathbf{w}_r^{(out)}$ and matrices $\mathbf{A}_r$. Selection of a winner neuron *s* and adaptation of the input weights $\mathbf{w}_r^{(in)}$ proceed as in the original SOFM algorithm, while the output weights $\mathbf{w}_r^{(out)}$ and $\mathbf{A}$ can be trained with a perceptron rule.

A Bayesian generalization of the SOFM has been proposed and analyzed by Luttrell (1994). Here, both the winner selection $\mathbf{x} \to$

$s(\mathbf{x})$ and the decoding $s \to \mathbf{w}_s$ are replaced by probabilistic mappings, leading to generalized SOFM versions that can be connected with channel coding theory. The resulting formalism has been used to formulate a SOFM variant for the mapping of *distance data* (Graepel and Obermayer, 1999), for which no explicit pattern vectors but only pairwise distances are given as training information. Another idea from statistics, the use of a generative model as a departure point for the generation of topographic maps, has led to the GTM method (Bishop, Svensén, and Williams, 1997). Here the map is derived from a probability density that is concentrated along a low-dimensional, parametrized manifold whose parameters are estimated by the maximum likelihood approach.

A good collection of articles on major recent developments on the SOFM is contained in Oja and Kaski (1999).

Applications of the feature map algorithm. Artificial feature maps have proved useful in many pattern recognition applications. The classic example is the *Neural Typewriter* of Kohonen, where a feature map is used to create a map of phoneme space for subsequent speech recognition. Subsequent work has demonstrated the possibility of creating feature maps of language data that are ordered according to higher-level, semantic categories (Ritter and Kohonen, 1989) and of deriving very large-scale maps to support navigation in very large databases, such as the Internet. Other applications of the feature map include process control, image compression, time series prediction, optimization, generation of noise-resistant codes, synthesis of digital systems, and robot learning. Kohonen's *Self-Organizing Maps* (1995) contains a good survey of SOFM applications, with additional comments on SOFM uses in an Internet database.

Road Maps: Grounding Models of Networks; Learning in Artificial Networks
Related Reading: Competitive Learning; Data Clustering and Learning; Hebbian Synaptic Plasticity; Learning Vector Quantization; Principal Component Analysis

References

Bishop, C. M., Svensén, M., and Williams, C. K. I., 1997, GTM: The generative topographic mapping, *Neural Computat.*, 10:215–234.
Cottrell, M., Fort, J., and Pagès, G., 1998, Theoretical aspects of the SOM algorithm, *Neurocomputing*, 21:119–138.
Erwin, E., Obermayer, K., and Schulten, K., 1992a, Self-organizing maps: Stationary states, metastability and convergence rate, *Biol. Cybern.*, 67:35–45.
Erwin, E., Obermayer, K., and Schulten, K., 1992b, Self-organizing maps: Ordering, convergence properties and energy functions, *Biol. Cybern.*, 67:47–55.
Erwin, E., Obermayer, K., and Schulten, K., 1995, Models of orientation and ocular dominance columns in the visual cortex: A critical comparison, *Neural Computat.*, 7:425–468.
Graepel, T., and Obermayer, K., 1999, A stochastic self-organizing map for proximity data, *Neural Computat.*, 11:139–155.
Heskes, T., and Kappen, B., 1993, Error potentials for self-organization, in *Proceedings of an International Conference on Neural Networks*, vol. 3, New York: IEEE, pp. 1219–1223.
Kohonen, T., 1982, Self-organized formation of topologically correct feature maps, *Biol. Cybern.*, 43:59–69.
Kohonen, T., 1990, The self-organizing map, *Proc. IEEE*, 78:1464–1480. ◆
Kohonen, T., 1995, *Self-Organizing Maps*, 2nd ed., Berlin: Springer-Verlag. ◆
Luttrell, S. P., 1994, A Bayesian analysis of self-organizing maps, *Neural Computat.*, 6:767–794.
Obermayer, K., Blasdel, G., and Schulten, K., 1992, A statistical mechanical analysis of self-organization and pattern formation during the development of visual maps, *Phys. Rev. A*, 45:7568–7589.
Oja, E., and Kaski, S., Eds., 1999, *Kohonen Maps*, Amsterdam: Elsevier.
Ritter, H., 1991, Asymptotic level density for a class of vector quantization processes, *IEEE Trans. Neural Netw.*, 2:173–175.
Ritter, H., and Kohonen, T., 1989, Self-organizing semantic maps, *Biol. Cybern.*, 61:241–254.
Ritter, H., Martinetz, T., and Schulten, K., 1992, *Neural Computation and Self-Organizing Maps*, Reading, MA: Addison-Wesley. ◆

Semantic Networks

John A. Barnden, Mark G. Lee, and Manuela Viezzer

Introduction

Semantic networks (SNs) are a way of representing information abstractly by means of a graphical notation that makes use of interconnected nodes and arcs. They are commonly used in symbolic cognitive science. There are interesting similarities and differences between SNs and neural networks (NNs). Some attempts have been made to implement or emulate SNs in NNs and to form hybrid SN-NN systems.

SNs were originally developed for couching "semantic" information, either in the psychologist's sense of static information about concepts or in the semanticist's sense of the meanings of natural language sentences. However, they are also used as a general knowledge representation tool. The more elaborate types of SNs are similar in their representational abilities to sophisticated forms of symbolic logic. (For more information on SNs, see Sowa, 1984; Rich and Knight, 1991, chaps 4, 9–11; Lehmann, 1992.)

The Nature of Semantic Networks

As with NNs, there are many different styles of SNs. However, all SNs share the following general features:

- The nodes are to be interpreted (by us) as standing for physical or nonphysical entities in the world, classes or kinds of entities, relationships, or concepts.
- The links, which are almost always directed, encode specific relationships between entities, concepts, etc., where the type of the relationship is specified by a symbolic label on the link.

We roughly characterize SNs as being either *restricted* or *general*, although there are cases in between. The restricted class is typified by the small fragment shown in Figure 1. Nodes represent kinds, activities, or individuals (all named in the diagram by lowercase labels). IS-A links and INST links are the characteristic links of restricted SNs. Other links, like MAIN-LOCOMOTION in the fragment, are usually called roles and used to represent properties of the kinds. IS-A is the subkind relationship, whereas INST is the instance (i.e., individual-to-kind) relationship. IS-A links are often labeled as A-KIND-OF or AKO links. The individuals in the fragment are Canny and Osten, whereas the kinds are canary, ostrich, bird, and animal.

The central purpose of a restricted network is to organize concepts, kinds, or classes into a taxonomy, which may or may not be

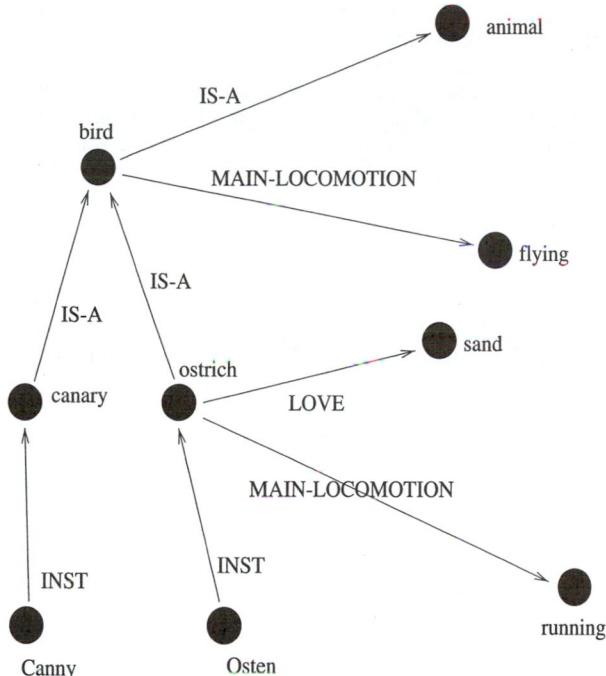

Figure 1. Fragment of a semantic network, restricted class (see text).

strictly hierarchical, and to state properties of the included entities. A general principle is the following:

- Information general to a class, kind, or concept should be held at the node representing it, and not repeated at nodes for subclasses, subkinds, or subconcepts (or particular instances of them); instead, these subentities implicitly *inherit* the information at the former node (inheritance principle).

An allied fundamental principle is the following:

- Information attached to a node can contradict information attached to an ancestor node; in that case the former information overrides the latter (default-overriding principle).

Here, an ancestor node of a node N is a node that can be reached from N by a succession of IS-A links, or by an INST link and then possibly some IS-A links. Thus, the fragment in Figure 1 says that birds (in general) have flying as their main method of locomotion, but that for ostriches (in general), the main method of locomotion is running. On the other hand, canaries in general, and Canny in particular, implicitly inherit the flying because no node between those nodes and the bird node has a MAIN-LOCOMOTION link contradicting the flying. Osten inherits the running of ostriches in general, and their love of sand.

The general type of SN is typified by the fragment shown in Figure 2. The q node represents the proposition that every pig loves rain. Alternatively, it represents the situation of every pig loving rain. The fragment shown is a direct analogue of the logic formula

$$(\forall x)\ \text{is-pig}\ (x) \Rightarrow \text{loves}\ (x, \text{rain})$$

Although general SNs often contain taxonomic information, this information is less important to the overall purpose of the network.

Rather, the focus is on representing entire sentences, propositions, or situations using a network format instead of an algebraic one. The idea goes back to Frege's *Begriffsschrift* and Peirce's relational graphs, and has been exploited to express the semantics of natural language, as, for example, in discourse representation theory (Kamp and Reyle, 1993).

In contrast to restricted networks, general networks usually have only a small selection of link labels, typified by those in Figure 2. Often, labels have a close connection to deep case relationships in natural language semantic theories (see the AGENT and OBJECT links in Figure 2). Relationships such as loving are now represented by nodes (see the *loves* node in Figure 2) rather than by link labels (see the LOVE link in Figure 1). Also, the more elaborate general SNs have facilities analogous to the connectives and quantifiers of formal logic (see the *implication* and *forall* nodes in Figure 2). The QUANT link to the *forall* node says that the q node represents a universally quantified proposition. The VAR link points to the x node, playing the role of the variable x in the formula above. The BODY link points to the body of the proposition, which has the form of an implication proposition (i node). ANTE stands for antecedent, and CONSE represents consequent. PRED links point from nodes representing simple propositions to the nodes for the predicates in the propositions. ARG stands for argument.

One of the problems to be handled when SNs are used to represent propositions is to express correctly the scope of logical operators. This can be achieved by including explicit nodes to represent propositions, like node q in Figure 2, thus turning the SN into what is often called a *propositional semantic network*. The first propositional semantic network to be implemented was the MIND system, by Stuart Shapiro, which then evolved into the SNePS system (see Shapiro and Rapaport, 1992).

Thus, formal logic expressions can be recast as SNs. However, the two forms of representation are not equivalent, partly because SNs implicitly involve implementational assumptions that facilitate some particularly important operations (see below), whereas formal

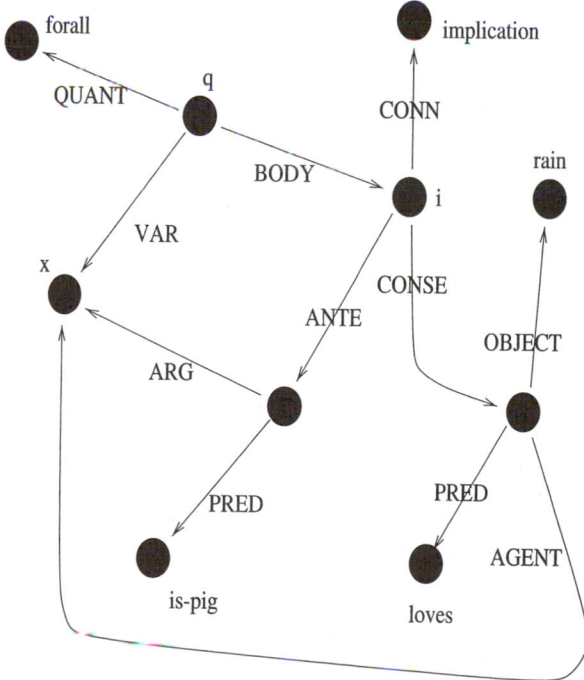

Figure 2. Fragment of a semantic network, general class (see text).

logic is devoid of implementational assumptions. Also, to parallel the inheritance-blocking features of SNs in logic, one has to turn to special, advanced forms of logic (for an introduction, see Rich and Knight, 1991, chap. 7; see also Brachman et al., 1991). Moreover, several SN approaches have made radical claims as to what should and what should not be represented. For example, the SNePS family of SNs argues for a totally intensional representation of knowledge (Shapiro and Rapaport, 1992).

Among current logical systems, description logics capture the features of restricted SNs and are used to reason about taxonomic information. Some versions of description logic support nonmonotonic reasoning and belief revision to cope with the conflicting information that may result from applications of the overriding defaults principle (see Brachman et al., 1991).

Processing in Semantic Networks

Sometimes SNs are used as static data structures that change only when external programs manipulate them. However, it is possible to embed some processing mechanisms in the networks themselves, thus giving SNs a self-modifying ability similar to that of NNs.

One common and basic type of processing in SNs is *spreading activation*. During the course of spreading activation, if one node is active at some moment, then the nodes directly connected to it can become activated. A given episode of activation spreading might only pass activation across links of specific types. Activation here is often a yes-no matter, as opposed to the graded activation typically used in NNs. However, graded activation can be used in SNs.

A common variant of activation spreading is *marker passing*. Markers are symbolic objects, usually of several different types. The markers that a node send out depend in some possibly complex way on the markers it receives from other nodes. Markers are often simple symbolic objects, bearing no information except their type. However, more complex markers are used in some SNs; for instance, a marker can contain information on its node of origin or the nodes or links it has passed through. Complex markers are used in the system of Charniak (1986), for example. A marker can have a graded energy level that affects its ability to cause a receiving node to produce a marker in response (see the system of Hendler in Barnden and Pollack, 1991).

The main motivation for activation spread or marker passing is to allow *intersection search*. For instance, consider an SN system used in understanding natural language text. Marker passing might start with nodes representing the word senses of various words in the text. The collisions of markers at nodes means that paths have been found between word senses. This information can be used to help disambiguate the words (see Yu and Simmons, 1990). Marker passing can also be used to manage simple inheritance reasoning. For instance, in Figure 1, Osten's main locomotion method could be found by sending out a marker from the Osten node and constraining it to travel only along a chain of IS-A links, possibly preceded by a single INST link, and followed by one MAIN-LOCOMOTION link. If the system prefers answers found first to answers found later, the *running* answer is preferred over the *flying* answer, thereby effecting the desired handling of exceptions (blocking of inheritance).

Marker passing is important, but is generally used only for restricted purposes. In general networks that handle more elaborate reasoning, the brunt of the inferencing is typically done by subnetwork matching and construction processes (see Cravo and Martins, 1993, for an advanced implemented system).

In any SN with INST and IS-A links, inheritance reasoning is simpler and quicker than it would otherwise be. In SNs without the special links, or in ordinary logical frameworks, traversal of taxonomic relationships is a more elaborate process. These observations rely on certain strong implementational assumptions that are generally made about SNs, though usually only tacitly. The assumptions apply both to computer implementations of SNs and to hypothesized realizations of SNs in the brain. One of the assumptions is that, if a processing mechanism is attending to a given node N, then it can efficiently transfer attention to nodes connected by single links to N.

Inheritance reasoning can also be given a probabilistic interpretation where every arc between nodes in the SN is given a probability from 1.0 to 0.0 of being traversed. Such networks are termed Bayesian. Bayesian networks are used in reasoning with uncertainty. The probabilities associated with individual arcs can be automatically learned from data. Pearl (2000) gives an extensive overview of such networks.

Finally, SNs can have *attached procedures or rules*. These are algorithms, expressed in some symbolic format, that are attached to nodes or links, and they typically have localized effects supporting particular inference functions. (For a brief introduction to this topic, see Rich and Knight, 1991, chap. 4 and section 10.3.2.)

Marker passing and attached procedures can also be combined, as in Petri nets, where there are passive nodes, called places, active nodes, called transitions, and sets of rules for marking places with tokens and for executing, or firing, transitions.

Contrasts to Neural Networks

In NNs, in contrast to the case of general SNs, activation spread is almost always the only mechanism for short-term computation (as opposed to long-term computation, such as slow adaptation). Moreover, the types of activation spread and marker passing in SNs are typically more complex than activation spread in NNs, especially when complex markers are used. In strong contrast to almost all NNs, the topology of an SN, especially a general SN, can be changed by processing mechanisms in arbitrarily extensive and complex ways in the short term.

NN links do not have type labels. As a result, NNs do not treat different input links differently for the most part. Instead, a weighted sum of the input values is formed, submerging the identities of different links. The most salient exception to this is the differentiation of input links into excitatory and inhibitory links, but this distinction is crude compared with the link differentiation by labels in SNs. Nevertheless, NN links that impinge on other links and modulate them (see NEUROMODULATION IN INVERTEBRATE NERVOUS SYSTEMS) can be used to obtain many of the effects of link typing in SNs.

When an NN link is directed, activation can spread in only one direction across the link. It is less common to impose this constraint in SNs. It is therefore easier in SNs to express asymmetric relationships between nodes without consequently constraining the accessibility of the nodes from each other. As an example of the problem raised for NNs, consider the use of symmetric links in some artificial NNs, notably Hopfield nets (see STATISTICAL MECHANICS OF NEURAL NETWORKS). These allow activation spread in both directions, but do not directly support conceptually asymmetric relationships. More indirect methods are needed to handle such relationships (see Barnden and Srinivas, 1991).

As a result of all these differences, SNs cope much more readily with many of the representational and processing needs that arise in high-level cognitive activities such as commonsense reasoning and natural language understanding. The needs in question are listed in ARTIFICIAL INTELLIGENCE AND NEURAL NETWORKS (q.v.). NNs have difficulty in rapidly creating new, complex bodies of information, and in structurally matching complex, and possibly highly temporary, bodies of information. Certainly, any direct parallel of subnetwork matching and subnetwork creation in SNs is difficult to achieve in typical NNs (but see DYNAMIC LINK ARCHITECTURE). However, some NN systems have been developed that can directly implement SNs (see the next section). They depart from mainstream NNs in that they have more elaborate and specialized structure.

On the other hand, NNs appear to have advantages with respect to other needs posed by high-level cognition (see ARTIFICIAL INTELLIGENCE AND NEURAL NETWORKS). These other needs include context sensitivity, graceful degradation, and automatic adaptation. A contrastive factor here is that link weights are fundamental in NNs but relatively uncommon in SNs. This difference confers a graded associativity quality on NNs that has no direct parallel in most SNs, although the length of a path between two SN nodes has often been assumed to encode the strength of association between them: the shorter the path, the stronger the association.

Bringing Semantic and Neural Networks Together

Several researchers have overtly used NNs to implement or approximately emulate SNs. Other work has aimed at mixed systems that combine NNs with SNs or are compromises between the two. Major examples of the implementation/emulation type of work can be found in Hinton (1989) and in the chapters by Barnden, by Bookman and Alterman, and by Diederich, Dyer, and Shastri in Barnden and Pollack (1991). Touretzky (1990) describes a framework that is not aimed specifically at semantic networks but that could readily implement them. Because of the complexity of the systems that implement or emulate SNs, we omit description of them here.

For examples of combined SN-NN systems, see the chapters by Hendler and Lehnert in Barnden and Pollack (1991). In the Hendler case, nodes in the SN can also serve as input-output nodes in an NN. Markers passed to such SN nodes cause them to inject neural activation into the NN, and vice versa. The symbolic markers have a numeric strength, and this affects the level of neural activation instigated by a marker. The NN acts as an intermediary between SN nodes, allowing an SN node representing one concept to stimulate an SN node encoding a similar concept. The NN is trained by backpropagation to associate concepts with sets of low-level features. Concepts are thereby viewed as similar according to the extent to which they share features. Hendler's system makes symbolic reasoning less rigid by enriching it with similarity-based reasoning.

For compromises between SNs and NNs, see the chapters by Eskridge and Kokinov in Holyoak and Barnden (1994). Unlike Hendler's system, these systems are not divided into separate neural and semantic parts. In Eskridge's system, nodes communicate by means of numerical activation signals, much as in NNs, but symbolic markers travel along with the numerical activation, the links have labels, activation can be constrained to spread only over links with specified labels, links can be dynamically created, and specialized SN processing rules can be invoked. The system performs complex analogical processing, with the symbolic aspects coping with complex structure manipulation and the neural aspects helping with retrieval of source analogues and with weighing of alternatives.

Discussion

NNs and SNs have much in common and should be regarded as two points in a rich, quasi-continuous space of computational architectures rather than as radically different types of network. There are important differences in the nature and usage of links and in the degree to which computation can be thought of as local to individual nodes (although in restricted SNs the computation can be as local as it is in NNs). There are various ways of implementing or emulating SNs in NNs, and of forming hybrid SN-NN systems.

Road Map: Artificial Intelligence
Related Reading: Artificial Intelligence and Neural Networks; Bayesian Networks; Competitive Queuing for Planning and Serial Performance; Connectionist and Symbolic Representations; Graphical Models: Probabilistic Inference; Structured Connectionist Models

References

Barnden, J. A., and Pollack, J. B., Eds., 1991, *Advances in Connectionist and Neural Computation Theory*, Vol. 1: *High Level Connectionist Models*, Norwood, NJ: Ablex.

Barnden, J. A., and Srinivas, K., 1991, Encoding techniques for complex information structures in connectionist systems, *Connect. Sci.*, 3:263–309.

Brachman, R. J., McGuinness, D. L., Patel-Schneider, P. F., Resnik, A. L., and Borgida, A., 1991, Living with Classic: When and how to use a KL-ONE-like language, in *Principles of Semantic Networks: Explorations in the Representation of Knowledge* (J. F. Sowa, Ed.), San Mateo, CA: Morgan Kaufmann, pp. 401–456.

Charniak, E., 1986, A neat theory of marker passing, in *Proceedings of the Fifth National Conference on Artificial Intelligence (AAAI–86)*, Los Altos, CA: Morgan Kaufmann, pp. 584–588.

Cravo, M. R., and Martins, J. P., 1993, SNePSwD: A newcomer to the SNePS family, *J. Exp. Theoret. Artif. Intell.*, 5:135–148.

Hinton, G. E., 1989, Implementing semantic networks in parallel hardware, in *Parallel Models of Associative Memory*, updated edition (G. E. Hinton and J. A. Anderson, Eds), Hillsdale, NJ: Erlbaum, pp. 191–221.

Holyoak, K. J., and Barnden, J. A., Eds., 1994, *Advances in Connectionist and Neural Computation Theory*, Vol. 2: *Analogical Connections*, Norwood, NJ: Ablex.

Kamp, H., and Reyle, U., 1993, *From Discourse to Logic*, Dordrecht: Kluwer.

Lehmann, F. W., Ed., 1992, *Semantic Networks in Artificial Intelligence*, New York: Pergamon Press.

Pearl, J., 2000, *Causality: Models, Reasoning and Inference*, Cambridge, Engl.: Cambridge University Press.

Rich, E., and Knight, K., 1991, *Artificial Intelligence*, 2nd ed., New York: McGraw-Hill. ◆

Shapiro, S. C., and Rapaport, W. J., 1992, The SNePS family, in Lehmann, F. W., 1992, *Semantic Networks in Artificial Intelligence*, New York: Pergamon Press.

Sowa, J. F., 1984, *Principles of Conceptual Structures: Information Processing in Mind and Machine*, Reading, MA: Addison-Wesley.

Touretzky, D. S., 1990, BoltzCONS: Dynamic symbol structures in a connectionist network, *Artif. Intell.*, 46:5–46.

Yu, Y.-H., and Simmons, R. F., 1990, Truly parallel understanding of text, in *Proceedings of the Eighth National Conference on Artificial Intelligence (AAAI–90)*, Menlo Park, CA: AAAI Press, pp. 996–1001.

Sensor Fusion

Allen M. Waxman

Introduction

Sensor fusion is not the sole purview of the modern brain but rather an old and common strategy in nature, and of great relevance to a variety of applications. It is a means by which multiple sensing modalities and interacting modality-specific processing streams can cue one another, enhance or depress cross-modality responses to stimuli, generate cross-modality expectations, and provide complementary evidence supporting or negating a decision (e.g., the detection of prey, or the recognition of an object). Studies of sensory interactions in flatworms, crustaceans, insects, and fishes (see references in Stein and Meredith, 1993), snakes (Newman and Hartline, 1982), cats and monkeys (Stein and Meredith, 1993; Stein, Wallace, and Stanford, 1999), and humans (Stein and Meredith, 1993; Giard and Peronnet, 1999; Shimojo and Shams, 2001) point to multiple levels of sensory integration in brain. From multimodal sensory receptors to midbrain organs (i.e., tectum or superior colliculus) to corticotectal feedback pathways and temporal-prefrontal lobe activation, it is clear that sensor fusion impacts an animal's ability to detect and track objects (i.e., its attentive and orienting behaviors) as well as its decision-making abilities (i.e., to recognize an object from its multimodal signature). Thus, the many sensory pathways that have developed in living systems to process chemical, mechanical, thermal, visual, and auditory stimuli have generally formed two classes of pathways that also project to one another, one that is modality specific and one that is integrated across sensory modalities.

Sensor fusion is of direct relevance to the military defense (Hall and Llinas, 1997), intelligence, remote sensing (Pohl and van Genderen, 1998), medical, robotics, and manufacturing communities. Multiple specialized sensors have been developed to provide the data necessary for decision making in each of these application areas. Yet it is often acknowledged that today's information shortcomings can be overcome, not necessarily with still more and better sensors, but rather with tomorrow's sensor fusion systems. Witness the multitude of methods, systems, and applications for sensor fusion that are reported annually at conferences such as the MSS (formerly IRIS) National Symposium on Sensor and Data Fusion 1988–2002, the International Conference on Information Fusion 1998–2002, and the SPIE conference on Sensor Fusion: Architectures, Algorithms, and Applications 1997–2002. However, approaches motivated by or derived from biological sensor fusion strategies have been embraced by relatively few (Toet, van Ruyven, and Valeton, 1989; Anastasio, Patton, and Belkacem-Boussaid, 2000; Fay et al., 2000; Fisher et al., 2001; Waxman et al., 1995, 1997, 2001).

Biological Insights

There is an extensive and growing literature on sensor fusion in biological systems. Methods of observation in the living animal include electrophysiological recording from single cells, event-related potential (ERP) monitoring from arrays of scalp electrodes, functional magnetic resonance imaging (fMRI) and position emission tomography (PET) of the living brain, and direct psychophysical experiments on humans. Some of the most significant studies lead to the following insights.

Snakes

Newman and Hartline (1982) have studied the integration of visual and thermal infrared signals in the optic tectum of the rattlesnake and python. Both visual signals from the retina and infrared signals from the pit organs project onto the tectum in orderly maps of sensory space (i.e., retinotopically) that are in register with one another. Newman and Hartline identified six classes of bimodal neurons that display highly nonlinear multimodal interactions, including AND cells, OR cells, response-enhanced cells (e.g., cells in which the response to a visual stimulus is enhanced in the presence of an infrared stimulus), and response-depressed cells (e.g., cells in which the response to an infrared stimulus is depressed in the presence of a visual stimulus). These single-cell responses indicate that both cooperative and competitive nonlinear processes are at play, all in the service of orienting the snake toward its potential prey. They are, in fact, reminiscent of opponent-color multispectral interactions observed in primate retinal ganglion cells (Waxman et al., 1997).

Cats and Monkeys

In mammals, the tectum has evolved into the superior colliculus (SC). A midbrain organ involved in attentive and orienting behavior, it aims to *keep your eye on the ball*. The definitive works of Stein and Meredith (1993) and Stein et al. (1999) make clear that the seven-layered SC receives direct sensory input to its deep layers from visual, auditory, and somatosensory neurons, as well as significant feedback from single-modality cortical areas, and that it projects up to higher centers via thalamus and down to brainstem and spinal cord motor pathways in order to control the pointing of sensory organs (see Stein and Meredith, 1993, for anatomical drawings of the SC). These sensory and cortical inputs all form topographically registered maps in the deep layers, in a coordinate system tied to the moving retina (requiring the existence of learned transformations between retinal, head, and body coordinates). Moreover, one also finds motor maps (of vector displacement) in registration as well, providing all sensory modalities common access to the machinery that turns the eyes, ears, and head in order to find and track that target object. More than 50% of deep-layer neurons are multisensory (bimodal and trimodal), exhibiting both cross-modal response enhancement and response depression. These neurons have receptive fields, often with center-surround spatial profiles and noncoincident but overlapping temporal profiles. These cells are well designed (in fact, they develop postnatally, from experience) to detect complementary evidence supporting or negating the detection and localization of targets from their multimodal signatures.

An interesting and significant phenomenon observed among multisensory neurons in SC is that of *inverse effectiveness* in cross-modal response enhancement. Multisensory neurons that respond weakly to unimodal stimuli can be greatly enhanced in their response to multimodal stimuli, in contrast to the modest enhancement observed among multisensory neurons that respond strongly to unimodal stimuli. This effect has been shown to be consistent with the interpretation that multisensory neurons in SC compute the conditional probability (in the sense of Bayesian estimation theory) that a target is present, given the unimodal or multimodal stimulus (Anastasio et al., 2000). However, it is clear from electrophysiological studies that response enhancement in multisensory neurons is due to cortical feedback to the SC that develops after birth (Stein et al., 1999).

Humans

It thus seems likely that the human SC is responsible for our being fooled by both the ventriloquist and the television set. Interactions between visual and auditory activations on registered maps in SC convince us that the sound is actually coming from the mouths of those dummies! Even our perception of human articulated sounds is strongly influenced by the visual shape of moving lips (i.e., the McGurk effect). And what we think we see is easily altered by the sounds we hear, even for very simple stimuli such as flashes and beeps. Shimojo and Shams (2001) review this and many other cross-modality target detection and tracking experiments in which cortical activation is monitored via fMRI and ERP measurements. They note the significance of transient/discontinuous stimuli, regardless of modality, and the apparent ability of these stimuli to influence multimodal perceptions.

Beyond orienting behaviors devised to detect, localize, and track objects, when it comes to the task of object recognition from multimodal signatures, we humans also employ a good deal of cortex while preserving old successful strategies. Observations of ERPs (Giard and Peronnet, 1999) reveal signs of cross-modality response enhancement and response depression as well as new neural activity (not seen with single-modality stimuli derived from the object) in the right frontotemporal area, generally considered an associative area of brain.

Technological Implementations

A great deal of work has been done on the military problem of tracking multiple targets from multiple sensors using Bayesian statistical inference methods, and cast in the context of higher levels of information fusion (Hall and Llinas, 1997). The information-theoretic concept of mutual information, in conjunction with perceptron neural networks, has recently been applied to audiovisual fusion and speaker localization (Fisher et al., 2001).

With application to remote sensing and environmental monitoring, it is commonplace to utilize imagery derived from multiple airborne and space-based sensors (Pohl and van Genderen, 1998). However, most image fusion methods employed are based on global statistical methods (e.g., PRINCIPAL COMPONENT ANALYSIS, q.v.) and false color overlay of separate modalities. These approaches do not derive or benefit from biological approaches to sensor fusion. Early methods for fusion of two complementary imaging modalities, in particular visible (reflected) and thermal (emitted) infrared imagery, also did not utilize biological fusion strategies, but did build on known multiresolution representations in visual processing (Toet et al., 1989). A successful approach to visible-infrared image fusion based on single-opponent color processing in the retina was developed by Waxman et al. (1997) and enabled a color night vision technology. This approach was extended to accommodate three and four imaging modalities by means of double-opponent color processing (as in primary visual cortex), and a target learning and recognition capability based on the fused sensor signature was incorporated (Fay et al., 2000). Biological architectures for visual 3D object learning and recognition, which fuse evidence over multiple views in an *aspect network* and apply to multiple imaging modalities, are summarized in Waxman et al. (1995).

Real-Time Night Vision Enhancement

Figure 1 illustrates an opponent-color architecture for fusing multiple images in real time. It requires that the imagery be collected in an optically registered manner, or separately registered to a common reference frame. Shown here are three modalities of wide dynamic range imagery, low-light visible (VIS), short-wave infrared (SWIR), and thermally emitted long-wave infrared (LWIR), that provide different views into the night. These distinct modalities are fused into a single natural color image (shown here in gray scale,

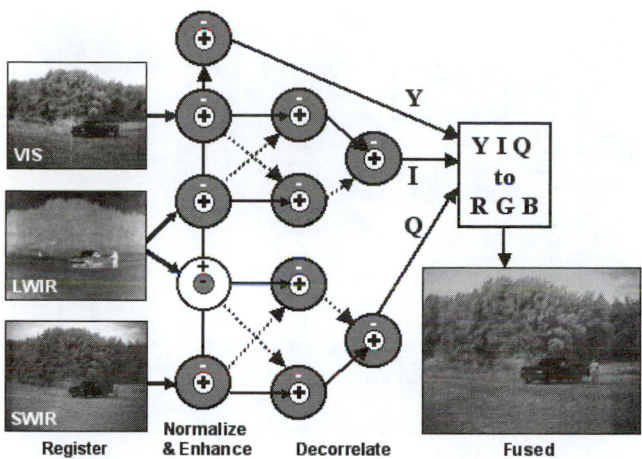

Figure 1. Color night vision through the real-time fusion of multiple imaging sensors (visible, short-wave, and long-wave infrared). Contrast enhancing *on-* and *off-channel* and *opponent-color* receptive fields are built from center-surround shunting neural networks. (See Fay et al., 2000, for color rendering of the fused output image.)

but see Fay et al., 2000, for several color renderings). Multiple center-surround shunting neural networks are used to create enhanced *on-* and *off-center* (e.g., hot and cold LWIR) responses, as well as *single-* and *double-opponent* cross-modality contrasts that serve to decorrelate the input imagery. The outputs of the network are mapped to the human opponent-color YIQ representation and converted to RGB color for display. Similar networks comprised of a variety of such opponent-color fields have been used to fuse two, three, and four imaging modalities, and have been further combined with 3D imagery obtained from a ladar in real-time. Using fuzzy ARTMAP neural networks (Carpenter et al., 1992) in conjunction with a target designation interface, we incorporated field-adaptive target learning and recognition based on fused image data.

Multisensor Fusion and Exploitation

Imagery and signals collected by multiple platforms over a common geospatial area can be brought into registration by means of a 3D site model (i.e., terrain data and building models), as indicated in Figure 2 (Waxman et al., 2001). Forming a layered database of multiple registered modalities, opponent-sensor image fusion (see Figure 1) and spatial feature extraction (oriented edges, extended boundary contours, texture measures, and 3D slopes and curvatures) support interactive 3D visualization and also augment the database. The layered data are well organized for interactive pattern learning and search, for each pixel now corresponds to a complete feature vector. With the aid of a graphical user interface, an analyst selects example and counterexample (context) pixels of the object of interest, and, treating these as training data, a *search agent* is created using fuzzy ARTMAP neural networks. Additionally, the agent sorts the many elements of the feature vector and identifies those features that are salient to the target in context. The agent then conducts a first-pass search for the object of interest (e.g., roads, buildings, vehicles) in the fused imagery. Subsequent searches will use these detections as context in guided search. A separate search agent is trained for each object of interest in the fused data set. These same methods for image fusion and mining have been successfully applied to spectral MRI and MRI/SPECT in medical imaging.

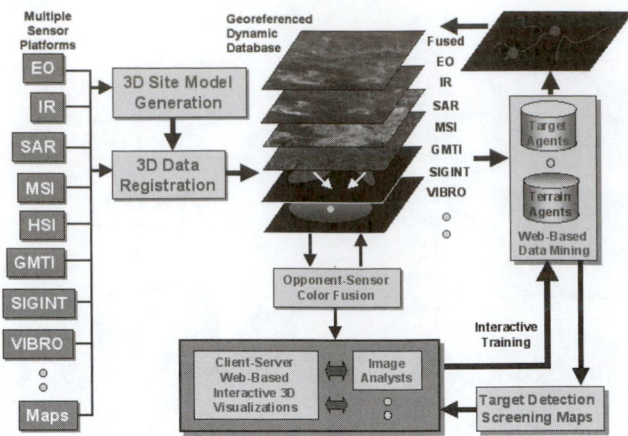

Figure 2. Architecture for fusion and exploitation (i.e., data mining) of multisensor data in a geospatial context. (A prototype fusion system is described in Waxman et al., 2001.)

Discussion

Biological systems, from simple to complex, all demonstrate the capacity for fusing multiple sensing modalities. In humans, auditory-visual fused localization underlies the daily experience of watching television, in which speech seems to emanate from the visual image of the actor on the screen and not from the speakers beside the TV. Lessons learned from the rattlesnake visible-infrared fusion pathway and its similarity to opponent-color processing in the mammalian retina have led to real-time architectures for color-fused night vision. The existence of registered multimodal maps and bimodal neurons in mammalian SC, as well as the cortical feedback pathways to the SC, has led to an architecture and proto-type system for fusion and exploitation of multisensor surveillance data in a geospatial context. Observed interactions in human fronto-temporal cortices reflect associative processes underlying multi-sensor object recognition.

Statistical, information-theoretic, and neural network methods of sensor fusion provide complementary tools for turning data into decisions in the context of knowledge. It remains to be seen if neural methods can rise to the challenge of higher levels of sensor and information fusion, for which knowledge-based systems are required. However, in our experience the unique insights obtained from biological system design yield distinct advantages in the de-velopment of adaptive sensor fusion systems for real-world problems.

Road Maps: Other Sensory Systems; Vision
Related Reading: Collicular Visuomotor Transformations for Gaze Control

References

Anastasio, T. J., Patton, P. E., and Belkacem-Boussaid, K., 2000, Using Bayes' rule to model multisensory enhancement in the superior collic-ulus, *Neural Computat.*, 12:1165–1187.

Carpenter, G. A., Grossberg, S., Markuzon, N., Reynolds, J. H., and Rosen, D. B., 1992, Fuzzy ARTMAP: A neural network architecture for incre-mental supervised learning of analog multidimensional maps, *IEEE Trans. Neural Netw.*, 3:698–713.

Fay, D. A., Waxman, A. M., Aguilar, M., Ireland, D. B., Racamato, J. P., Ross, W. D., Streilein, W. W., and Braun, M. I., 2000, Fusion of 2-/3-/4-sensor imagery for visualization, target learning and search, *Enhanced Synthet. Vision 2000*, SPIE-4023:106–115.

Fisher, J. W. III, Darrell, T., Freeman, W. T., and Viola, P., 2001, Learning joint statistical models for audio-visual fusion and segregation, in *Ad-vances in Neural Information Processing Systems 13* (T. K. Leen, T. G. Dietterich, and V. Tresp, Eds.), Cambridge, MA: MIT Press, pp. 772–778.

Giard, M. H., and Peronnet, F., 1999, Auditory-visual integration during multimodal object recognition in humans: A behavioral and electro-physiological study, *J. Cognit. Neurosci.*, 11:473–490.

Hall, D. L., and Llinas, J., 1997, An introduction to multisensor data fusion, *Proc. IEEE*, 85:6–23. ◆

Newman, E. A., and Hartline, P. H., 1982, The infrared vision of snakes, *Sci. Am.*, 246:116–127.

Pohl, C., and van Genderen, J. L., 1998, Multisensor image fusion in remote sensing: Concepts, methods and applications, *Int. J. Remote Sens.*, 19:823–854. ◆

Shimojo, S., and Shams, L., 2001, Sensory modalities are not separate modalities: Plasticity and interactions, *Curr. Opin. Neurobiol.*, 11:505–509. ◆

Stein, B. E., and Meredith, M. A., 1993, *The Merging of the Senses*, Cam-bridge, MA: MIT Press. ◆

Stein, B. E., Wallace, M. T., and Stanford, T. R., 1999, Merging sensory signals in the brain: The development of multisensory integration in the superior colliculus, in *The New Cognitive Neurosciences*, 2nd ed. (M. S. Gazzaniga, Ed.), Cambridge, MA: MIT Press, pp. 55–71. ◆

Toet, A., van Ruyven, L. J., and Valeton, J. M., 1989, Merging thermal and visual images by a contrast pyramid, *Opt. Engn.*, 28:789–792.

Waxman, A. M., Gove, A. N., Fay, D. A., Racamato, J. P., Carrick, J. E., Seibert, M. C., and Savoye, E. D., 1997, Color night vision: Opponent processing in the fusion of visible and IR imagery, *Neural Netw.*, 10:1–6.

Waxman, A. M., Seibert, M., Gove, A. N., Fay, D. A., Bernardon, A. M., Lazott, C., Steele, W. R., and Cunningham, R. K., 1995, Neural pro-cessing of targets in visible, multispectral IR and SAR imagery, *Neural Netw.*, 8:1029–1051.

Waxman, A. M., Verly, J., Fay, D. A., Liu, F., Braun, M. I., Pugliese, B., Ross, W. D., and Streilein, W. W., 2001, A prototype system for 3D color fusion and mining of multisensor/spectral imagery, in *Proceeds. of the Fourth International Conference on Information Fusion*, I-WeC1, pp. 3–10.

Sensorimotor Interactions and Central Pattern Generators

Avis H. Cohen and David L. Boothe

Introduction

Movement through the world requires that the environment be in-tegrated and understood. An organism must navigate obstacles, seek sustenance, and avoid predators. Movement requires further that the organism integrate the visual, auditory, and other environ-mental information within its machinery for locomotion. Each of us in our daily interactions with the world is familiar with the seamless way in which our nervous system combines sensory and motor information. Thus, we know in a simplistic sense that sen-sory and motor systems are integrated. How this integration is per-formed by a nervous system is currently poorly understood. Much work has been done on motor and sensory systems in isolation. Less work has been done on how these systems interact. In this article we offer an interpretation of currently existing empirical evidence and argue from this evidence for some very basic properties of the biological systems performing sensorimotor integration.

A considerable amount of the experimentation on sensorimotor integration has focused on how sensory information modulates motor system activity. The flow of information commonly explored is from sensory to motor. Two main types of experiment have been performed to elucidate this relationship: reflex-type experiments, and studies of how sensory inputs modulate central pattern generators (CPGs). Peripheral feedback, including that from tactile receptors, muscle afferents, and other proprioceptive feedback, passes up to the somatosensory cortex, but first synapses within the spinal cord, where there are reflex circuits that respond to such inputs. Additionally and perhaps more functionally relevant, sensory input is filtered and processed locally, where the spinal pattern generator circuitry fits its response into the ongoing locomotion as appropriate. Thus, although the brain receives much of the sensory input, the responses to spinal inputs are first the responsibility of the local spinal circuitry. The first section of this article discusses the impact of sensory information on CPGs.

The influence of motor systems on sensory activity is less well characterized. Recent evidence shows that vertebrate motor systems can strongly influence sensory input. In the second section we show that the interplay between sensory feedback and motor output is more complex than is often suggested, and that behavior is strongly affected by movement and movement-related activity.

Studying motor and sensory systems in isolation, one can easily miss the massive interaction between these systems. An understanding of this interaction is crucial for explaining the simplest behaviors of an organism in its environment. What is most surprising about this interaction is not that it exists, but its pervasiveness. Interaction between motor and sensory systems exists from the first steps of sensory detection to the highest levels of processing. In the third section of this article we show that this type of two-way interaction also exists between the cortex and spinal cord.

The older and more usual view is that the spinal cord performs rhythmic and rapid reflexive-type behaviors that require the spinal circuitry and its speed locally, whereas more complex activities are the province of cortex or at least supraspinal centers. In this view, the descending systems send commands to lower-level systems, which respond appropriately. However, this distinction may not be so marked (Jankowska and Lundberg, 1981). Cortical commands now are viewed as integrated with CPG circuitry to produce volitional movements. We present evidence that the integration is considerably richer than the old view or even than the new view would suggest.

There is no doubt that cortical systems contribute to sensorimotor integration. What is in doubt is that motor cortex sends commands to a passively responsive spinal cord. Motor commands are acted on only as spinal circuits independently and thoroughly process all incoming information. In the view that we present, spinal cord and cortex are highly integrated. Movements result from an ongoing interactive process. The actual form that movements take is largely a product of spinal circuitry and its synergies, while the cortex is expected to perform other, more complex tasks that integrate somatosensory and motor systems with other inputs to which the cortex has unique access, such as vision, audition, and olfaction.

In such a limited review, it is inevitable that the material be selective. This review is not intended to be complete but rather to suggest the different types of evidence available.

Sensory to Motor Flow of Information

The most common view of sensory feedback is that it provides information regarding the position of the organism as it moves through space. Appropriate to this role, the feedback can correct a CPG on a cycle-by-cycle basis to maintain the organism in proper relationship to its environment (Rossignol, Lund, and Drew, 1988). For example, the hip joint angle of the cat can trigger a new step cycle as the body is propelled over its respective limb on the ground. Whelan and Pearson (1997) have also found that stretch of muscle spindles can trigger a new step cycle through contractions of appropriate muscles. In these ways, the cycle periods are able to accommodate changes in the velocity of the animal. Similarly, the bending of the tailfin in dogfish or lamprey entrains the swimming so that swim cycles are appropriate lengths for the environmental conditions. Thus, if the body is not able to adequately bend against a strong current, this will be compensated for by a longer cycle. This type of sensory regulation is accomplished at the level of the spinal cord and requires no descending input, although descending input will influence and weaken the responses if present (Whelan and Pearson, 1997). All CPGs must have some stimulus that can trigger or prolong a new cycle as necessary in order to guarantee that the CPG's movements are adaptive.

Another well-documented role for sensory feedback is to elicit reflexive responses to environmental perturbations. This is also accomplished at the spinal level, where sensory inputs are gated through the CPG during ongoing activity (Rossignol et al., 1988). A sensory stimulus can elicit phase-dependent responses that are quite unlike the reflex responses that such stimuli would induce in the absence of CPG activity. For example, an obstacle encountered by the paw dorsum will produce an enhanced flexion during the flexion phase of the step cycle, but it will produce an enhanced extension during the extension phase. This guarantees that the limb is properly supported at the moment it is raised to avoid the obstacle. The contralateral limb is also integrated with such responses. That is, the limb opposite the stimulus must be positioned to support the responsive limb before it will flex over such an obstacle (Hiebert et al., 1994). Such phase-dependent responses to perturbations are very common across CPGs. For each rhythmic movement there are classes of stimuli that elicit such responses (Rossignol et al., 1988). In the case of locomotion, the response requires no input from descending systems and is seen in spinal animals as well as intact animals.

Motor to Sensory Flow of Information

More recently, new evidence has accumulated to indicate that the relationship between the CPG and its sensory feedback is not unidirectional. Dubuc and his colleagues (Nussbaum et al., 1996) first found that there is a feedforward signal coming from the CPG that can be recorded as a dorsal root potential. This is a phasic presynaptic modulation of the sensory terminals in the spinal cord. The modulation is sufficient in some cases to trigger action potentials in the sensory fibers even during fictive locomotion, that is, locomotor pattern generator activity in the absence of movement (reviewed in Nussbaum et al., 1996). Thus, the signals cannot be coming from any source other than the CPG. A similar phenomenon has been found in cockroach flight, in locust walking, and in lamprey swimming. This phenomenon thus seems to be quite general, occurring across a wide range of animals from invertebrates and vertebrates and from cats to lampreys (reviewed in Cohen, 1992).

In the cockroach, the role of phasic modulation seems quite straightforward to interpret. It apparently provides the circal fibers with activity that is phase locked to the flight as a kind of preemptive sensory input during the movement. The situation in cat is more problematic, and the role of presynaptic modulation remains somewhat uncertain. Nussbaum et al. (1996) postulate three possible mechanisms by which the presynaptic modulation, acting as presynaptic inhibition, could influence the activity of primary sensory afferents. First, presynaptic inhibition could reduce the amount of transmitter being released presynaptically. This presynaptic inhibition would reduce the strength of the postsynaptic signal. Second, presynaptic activity could elicit antidromic action potentials in the primary sensory afferent axon. These antidromic action potentials could interfere with orthodromic discharges directly in the axon, or they could desensitize the axon at the first node of Ranvier. This anitidromic stimulation would therefore also reduce the influence of primary sensory afferents on postsynaptic cells. Third, presynaptic inhibition could conceivably cause orthodormic action potentials in other axonal collaterals. These orthodromic action potentials could then cause postsynaptic response elsewhere in the spinal cord. The existence of this third possibility is not well confirmed, nor is the overall functional impact of these effects clear.

Evidence has been accumulating for additional roles that sensory feedback may play. We and others have found that movement and the sensory feedback generated by that movement can change the state of the CPG and significantly alter the pattern of the behavior. In some cases the changes are on a time scale that outlasts a single cycle and have effects that are not predicted by any of the above examples. Two examples will be presented, one invertebrate and one vertebrate.

In the case of locust flight, removal of the hindwing tegulae results in an immediate change in the motor pattern. The wingbeat frequency decreases, and the interval between the activity of depressor and elevator muscles increases. Over a period of 2 weeks, the motor pattern can return to normal even without regeneration of the tegulae (Buschges, Ramirez, and Pearson, 1991). These changes indicate that the intact frequency and phase structure of the movement is normally a function of the CPG as well as the input from the wing sensors.

In the lamprey, slow changes evoked by sensory stimuli can continue over a time period that outlasts the sensory stimulation by varying numbers of cycles (Kiemel and Cohen, 2001). A small-amplitude bending movement of the isolated spinal cord is known to entrain the rhythm of fictive swimming, but more recently it has been found that the bending also leads to a speeding of the bursting that outlasts the bending for one or more cycles. The bending required for this effect can be very low amplitude and can last for as little as one cycle. Consequently, the longer-lasting, slowly decaying excitatory effect of the movement is apt to be seen during intact locomotion. In the latter, the sensory feedback would be a direct consequence of the muscle activation pattern generated by the CPG during its normal activity.

This type of slowly decaying excitation seen in lamprey could be interpreted as an example of positive feedback. That is, the CPG generates movement that in turn causes the CPG to go faster. However, the relationship between the frequency of the bending and the increase in the frequency is weak. If this is indeed positive feedback, then the gain is apparently less than 1, as the effects are limited (Prochazka, Gillard, and Bennett, 1997). The role for this type of excitation is unclear. A modeling study of the slowly decaying excitation (Verschure and Cohen, unpublished) offers some insights into possible roles the excitation might play. The model consists of the six-element neural network model for the lamprey segmental oscillator coupled to a reticulospinal element and receiving tonic drive to initiate bursting. This model was first proposed by Buchanan and Grillner (Grillner, Wallén, and Brodin, 1991). To it was added slowly decaying positive feedback from stretch receptors connected to the motor neuron output. The bursting remained controlled and stable over a wide range of parameter values. Rather than being destabilizing, this type of slowly decay-

ing excitation seemed to offer a new potential control mechanism. Interestingly, the system became autonomous, with no need for tonic drive and with the frequency of bursting highly sensitive to the gain and the duration of the stretch receptor feedback. This type of response may well depend on the balance of excitation and inhibition in a particular network. There was no attempt to test the effect of input with fewer or weaker inhibitory connections. However, it seems apparent that the well-studied lamprey CPG has no shortage of inhibitory neurons (Grillner et al., 1991). While such control mechanisms remain conjectural, the model does suggest that such types of excitation might perhaps be examined in new ways. One fairly definite role that this excitation could play is to change the gain on the system. That is, it seems likely that the excitation could increase the responsiveness of the CPG to other inputs.

In the lamprey (Guan, Kiemel, and Cohen, 2001) the changes induced by the movement have now additionally been implicated in altering the intersegmental coupling of the CPG. In the lamprey, the phase delays among the segments as well as the frequency of the movement are also altered by the movement. This was found in lamprey spinal cords induced to swim with the muscle present. There was no brain or tail, with the spinal cord kept as it is normally during the generation of fictive swimming; the spinal cord was exposed to the bath by removal of the dorsal musculature. The other muscle was left intact, and the preparation was pinned with a single pin at either the rostral or caudal end of the body to provide lateral stability (Figure 1). The burst pattern of the muscle was monitored with electromyography.

The cycle frequencies in such a preparation were consistently faster than the bursting of the respective isolated spinal cord. The phase delays were also consistently shorter. Thus, there is an alteration in the basic parameters of the movement in the presence of the muscle and movement. Using methods developed by Kiemel and Cohen (1998), the characteristics of the intersegmental coupling were measured in spinal cords with the long-range coupling reduced by lesions. Reducing the coupling was necessary since without the reduction, the values for the total coupling are all too near the asymptotic limit to be differentiated. In the presence of movement, the total coupling strength was found to be greatly enhanced in all spinal cords tested in this way. There were also changes in the ratio of ascending to descending short-range coupling. It has been shown in the isolated spinal cord of the lamprey

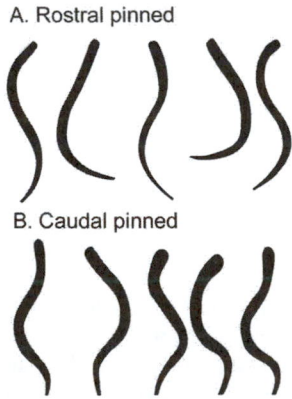

A. Rostral pinned

B. Caudal pinned

Figure 1. Reduced lamprey preparation, with body and muscle largely intact, swimming in response to bath applied D-glutamate (see Guan et al., 2001, for details of the preparation). Shown are the movements during one cycle of swimming when the body was pinned at the rostral end (*A*) and at the caudal end (*B*). Aside from the pinning, there was no difference in treatment between the two episodes of movement.

that after long-range coupling has been almost eliminated through lesions, the ascending short-range coupling is stronger than the descending short-range coupling (Guan et al., 2001). However, in the presence of movement and movement-related feedback, short-range coupling is found to be predominantly descending. Thus, movement and movement-related feedback can alter not only the movement parameters but also the underlying functional properties of the spinal circuitry. The movement could also be strikingly different, depending on which end of the body was allowed to be free (Cohen et al., unpublished) (Figure 1). It is important to note that this complexity is seen in the absence of the brain, and thus depends solely on the spinal cord–body interface.

Spinal Cord-Cortical Interactions

As discussed elsewhere in this *Handbook* (see CHAINS OF OSCILLATORS IN MOTOR AND SENSORY SYSTEMS), many studies of spinal cord treat it as a series of bidirectionally coupled oscillators. The coupling between the segmental oscillators in lamprey has been found to be very strong and is likely to be strong in other vertebrates as well. As such, the removal of one such oscillator or input to any oscillator, will alter the behavior of the other oscillators, regardless of their location within the informational stream. One can conclude from this that as sensory input travels up the spinal cord, it is shared with local circuits before it reaches the cortex. However, additional evidence is needed to truly make the case that motor and sensory systems are integrated across all levels, and not just across the spinal cord.

Interactions between cortex and spinal cord appear to be highly integrated. Indeed, there is evidence that there are neurons in the primary motor cortex of cats that are phasically active during locomotion of the animal. Thus, the strongest descending cortical outputs are most likely to be influenced by preexisting motor activity. This could mean that as the cortical neurons send motor commands to the limbs, the signals are apt to be properly timed to fit within the context of the ongoing locomotion. This is reasonable, as descending neurons must act in the proper context of the animal's movement or the commands will be inappropriate and maladaptive.

Neurons in the posterior parietal cortex of awake, unrestrained rats have also recently been found to exhibit activity linked to motor activity (McNaughton et al., 1994). Many of these cells responded strongly to specific types of locomotion. However, often these same cells would not respond to locomotor movements such as left turns or right turns. If the cells were responding to somatosensory or environmental information alone, one would expect them to respond in either the left turn or right turn case or to some specific position in space. In some animals a specific motion such as turning was compared with an attendant somatosensory state, such as passive bending of the animal. Less than 20% of the movement-related activity seemed to be explained by possible somatosensory or environmental inputs. Thus, the majority seemed to be predominantly motor in their responses.

Recently, it has been shown that the presence of cortical systems can speed up and enhance the responses over that of spinal animals (Hiebert et al., 1994). In some ways, this observation is counterintuitive, as the spinal cord should be faster alone. There are a number of possible explanations for this phenomenon. One is that cortical neurons can alter the response properties of the spinal neurons, making them more excitable, or perhaps the cortex is more adept at responding to unexpected events. Whatever the explanation, while the spinal cord has the capacity to respond by itself, in intact animals the descending systems participate to make the responses more adaptive. This more rapid response in intact animals to certain types of stimuli is still consistent with integration taking place locally, as spinalized animals do respond to the stimuli, but

much more slowly. What the cortex could be providing is some expectation or change in gain such that it picks up that something is novel more quickly than the spinal cord alone.

In conjunction with the discussion in the previous section, the three cases discussed in this section show that sensorimotor interactions across all levels are bidirectional, and that CPG-generated activity has influences on cortical areas thought only to be influenced by or involved in the processing of sensory activity.

Conclusion

Sensory and motor systems are integrated across all levels of the nervous system, from the spinal cord to the cortex. When one considers CPGs and their interactions with sensory input, one sees a remarkable range of phenomena. The simple stimulus-response reflex is a minimal component. At the spinal cord level, responses to sensory stimuli are modulated by the CPG to produce adaptively altered responses, and sensory stimuli adjust the length and amplitude of the CPG cycle. However, sensory input is also filtered by the CPG itself, while sensory input can also alter the state of the spinal activity on a slower time scale and in more ways than is often described. Although sensory input performs the traditionally considered corrective and monitoring functions, in interaction with the CPG it can also change the overall frequency and relative timing of the muscles, as well as altering intersegmental coordination. At the cortical level, CPG input modulates the activity of pyramidal cells, most likely so that their descending signals will occur at appropriate times in the cycle.

The goal is for the organism to produce adaptive behavior. This can only occur if all levels of the nervous system are aware of and responsive to activity at other levels. The cortex is privy to information from all sensory modalities, several of which do not reach the spinal pattern generator. The cortex is responsible for integrating all of this rich sensory input and generating desired responses. However, cortical neurons, while integrating all of this sensory information, must be aware of the state and activity of the limbs and trunk musculature if cortical activity is to move the organism properly through the environment. The spinal pattern generator is the first line of proprioceptive sensory integration, but the spinal cord and the other levels of the nervous system mutually interact to meet the needs of the organism.

Road Maps: Motor Pattern Generators; Neuroethology and Evolution
Related Reading: Chains of Oscillators in Motor and Sensory Systems; Command Neurons and Command Systems; Gait Transitions; Locomotion, Invertebrate; Locomotion, Vertebrate; Spinal Cord of Lamprey: Generation of Locomotor Patterns

References

Buschges, A., Ramirez, J.-M., and Pearson, K., 1991, Reorganization of sensory regulation of locust flight after partial deafferentation, *J. Neurobiol.*, 23:31–43.

Cohen, A. H., 1992, The role of heterarchical control in the evolution of the central pattern generator for locomotion, *Brain Behav. Evol.*, 40:112–124. ◆

Grillner, S., Wallén, P., and Brodin, L., 1991, Neuronal network generating locomotor behavior in lamprey: Circuitry, transmitters, membrane properties and simulation, *Annu. Rev. Neurosci.*, 14:169–199.

Guan, L., Kiemel, T., and Cohen, A. H., 2001, Impact of movement and movement-related feedback on the lamprey central pattern generator for locomotion, *J. Exp. Biol.*, 204:2361–2370.

Hiebert, G., Gorassini, M., Jiang, W., Prochazka, A., and Pearson, K., 1994, Corrective responses to loss of ground support during walking: II. Comparison of intact and chronic spinal cats, *J. Neurophysiol.*, 71:611–622.

Jankowska, E., and Lundberg, A., 1981, Interneurones in the spinal cord, *TINS*, 4:230–233.

Kiemel, T., and Cohen, A., 1998, Estimation of coupling strength in regenerated lamprey spinal cords based on a stochastic phase model, *J. Comput. Neurosci.*, 5:267–284.

Kiemel, T., and Cohen, A., 2001, Bending the lamprey spinal cord causes a slowly-decaying increase in the frequency of fictive swimming, *Brain Res.*, 900:57–64.

McNaughton, B., Mizumori, C., Barnes, C., Leonard, B., Marquis, M., and Green, E., 1994, Cortical representation of motion during unrestrained spatial navigation in the rat, *Cerebral Cortex*, 4:27–39.

Nussbaum, M., El Manira, A., Gossard, J.-P., and Rossignol, S., 1996, Presynaptic mechanisms during rhythmic activity in vertebrates and invertebrates, in *Neurons, Networks, and Motor Behavior* (P. S. G. Stein, S. Grillner, A. I. Selverston, and D. G. Stuart, Eds.), Cambridge, MA: MIT Press, pp. 237–251. ◆

Prochazka, A., Gillard, D., and Bennett, D. J., 1997, Implications of positive feedback in the control of movement, *J. Neurophysiol.*, 77:3237–3251.

Rossignol, S., Lund, J. P., and Drew, T., 1988, The role of sensory inputs in regulating patterns of rhythmical movements in higher vertebrates: A comparison between locomotion, respiration and mastication, in *Neural Control of Rhythmic Movement in Vertebrates* (A. H. Cohen, S. Rossignol, and S. Grillner, Eds.), New York: Wiley, pp. 201–284. ◆

Whelan, P. J., and Pearson, K. G., 1997, Comparison of the effects of stimulating extensor group I afferents on cycle period during walking in conscious and decerebrate cats, *Exp. Brain Res.*, 117:444–452.

Sensorimotor Learning

Daniel M. Wolpert and J. Randall Flanagan

Introduction

Skilled motor behavior is neither the result of rapid sensorimotor processes nor of fast or powerful effector mechanisms. Rather, the secret lies in the way tasks are organized and controlled by the nervous system. What sets humans apart from many robots that are far stronger and faster is our ability to select motor commands—both predictive and reactive—that are tailored to the task at hand and the physical properties of the environment. At the heart of our ability to deal with different tasks and contexts is sensorimotor learning.

Whereas some simple species show no motor learning, the need for motor learning arises in species in which the organism's environment, body, or task change. Specifically, when such changes are unpredictable, they cannot be prespecified in a control system, and therefore flexibility in the control process is required. Skills such as running on complex terrain or manipulating novel tools place a premium on motor learning. Similarly, as body size and proportions change with development, significant changes in the controller are required. Finally, learning is the only mechanism fast enough to allow us to master new tasks that are specified by social conventions, such as writing or dancing.

This article focuses on one perspective of motor learning, that is using internal models to learn transformations between sensory and motor variables. Both experimental and computational approaches to the study of internal model learning are reviewed.

Internal Models

The study of motor control is fundamentally concerned with the relationship between sensory signals and motor commands. Mapping between motor commands and sensory signals is bi-directional, and to specify the direction under consideration, a definition is adopted in which *forward* indicates the causal direction from motor commands into their sensory consequences, and *inverse* indicates the opposite direction; for example, transforming a desired sensory consequence into the motor commands that would achieve it.

The transformations from motor commands to their sensory consequences and vice versa are determined by the physics of the environment, musculoskeletal system, neural conduction and processing, and the sensory receptors. However, these physical transformations may also be represented internally within the central nervous system, and the phrase *internal model* is used to distinguish the actual transformation and it representation in the nervous system. Thus, the internal forward dynamic model is a model within the brain that can predict how our arm will move—and the sensations that will arise—given a specific motor command.

Forward internal models capture the causal relationship between actions and their outcomes. Based on the efference copy produced in parallel with motor commands, the forward model predicts the sensory consequences of the ensuing movement. The central nervous system can use this prediction in several ways (Miall and Wolpert, 1996; ACTION MONITORING AND FORWARD CONTROL OF MOVEMENTS). One use of a forward model is to provide a fast internal loop that helps stabilize feedback control systems. Feedback control in biological systems is subject to potential difficulties with stability, because the sensory feedback through the periphery is delayed by a significant amount. Such delays can result in instability when trying to make rapid movements under feedback control. In predictive control, a forward model is used to provide internal feedback of the predicted outcome of an action. This internal feedback can be used before sensory feedback is available, thereby preventing instability.

Inverse models also play an important role in motor control. A particularly clear example of an inverse dynamic model arises in the vestibulo-ocular reflex (VOR). The VOR couples the movement of the eyes to the motion of the head, thereby allowing an organism to keep its gaze fixed in space (VESTIBULO-OCULAR REFLEX). This is achieved by causing the motion of the eyes to be equal and opposite to the motion of the head. In effect, the VOR control system must compute the motor command that is predicted to yield a particular eye velocity. This computation is an internal inverse model of the physical relationship between muscle contraction and eye motion.

We need to learn an inverse model in order to accurately estimate the motor commands required to achieve a desired sensory response. The feedforward control this allows is essential for most natural movements in which feedback is available too late to guide movement. There have been many control systems proposed in the literature that use direct control; that is, control architectures that do not explicitly use internal models. However, any good controller can be thought of as implicitly implementing an inverse model of the system being controlled. In order words, knowledge about the physical behavior of the system being controlled is employed by the controller.

Internal Model Learning

Skilled motor behavior requires both inverse and forward internal models. These models capture information about the properties of the sensorimotor system. These properties are not static but change throughout life, both on a short time scale, as a result of interactions with the environment, and on a longer time scale, as a result of growth. Internal models must therefore be adaptable to changes in the properties of the sensorimotor system. A major aspect of motor learning can be viewed as the acquisition of forward and inverse internal models appropriate for different tasks and environments (Wolpert and Ghahramani, 2000; Wolpert, Ghahramani, and Flanagan, 2001).

Forward Model Learning

In supervised learning the target output can be provided by an external teacher, for example during imitation learning. However, the target output can also be specified internally based on sensory signals and higher-level goals. Such *self-supervised* learning is involved in the acquisition of a forward model that tries to predict the sensory consequence of an outgoing motor command (Figure 1, top). Here, the desired output of the model is readily available; it is the actual sensory consequence. The environment, therefore, readily provides an appropriate training signal to learn predictors of sensory feedback. The difference between the predicted and actual sensory feedback can be used as an error signal to update a predictive model. The neural mechanisms that lead to such predictive learning in the cerebellum-like structure of electric fishes have recently been partially elucidated (Bell, 2001; ELECTROLOCATION).

Inverse Model Learning: Supervised

An inverse model must learn to convert desired consequences into motor commands. One possible way to do this is with direct inverse modeling in which the inverse model observes the motor system during a "motor babbling" stage in which random motor commands are applied. The inverse model then observes the consequences of the motor commands and learns to associate these consequences (as its input) with the motor command that caused them (as its output). After learning, the inverse model's input is the desired sensory consequence and its output should be the appropriate motor commands. This direct inverse modeling approach is well behaved for linear systems. For nonlinear systems, however, a difficulty arises that is related to the general "degrees-of-freedom problem" in motor control. In many motor systems different motor commands can lead to the same consequence. Therefore, during learning the inverse model will try to associate one outcome with many different motor commands, each of which will lead to this outcome. The inverse model will therefore learn to associate this outcome with the average of all motor commands that can cause it. However, in general, the average of all the motor commands, each of which individually lead to a common outcome, will not lead to the same outcome and therefore, in practice, direct inverse modeling fails.

Two learning mechanisms have been developed to deal with the problem associated with direct inverse model learning, These rely on transforming the outcome error back into a motor error that can be used to train the inverse model. For example, when we throw a dart, the error we receive is coded in visual coordinates. This sensory error must be converted into motor command errors suitable to update the inverse model. The two principal methods proposed in the motor control literature for solving this problem are "feedback error learning" and "distal supervised learning."

Kawato, Furukawa, and Suzuki (1987) developed the feedback error learning approach to inverse model learning, which avoids the problem of direct inverse modeling (Figure 1, bottom). Feedback error learning makes use of a feedback controller to guide the learning of the inverse (feedforward) model. The total motor command acting on the motor system is the sum of the feedback control signal and the output from the inverse model. The feedback controller transforms the trajectory error, in sensory coordinates, into

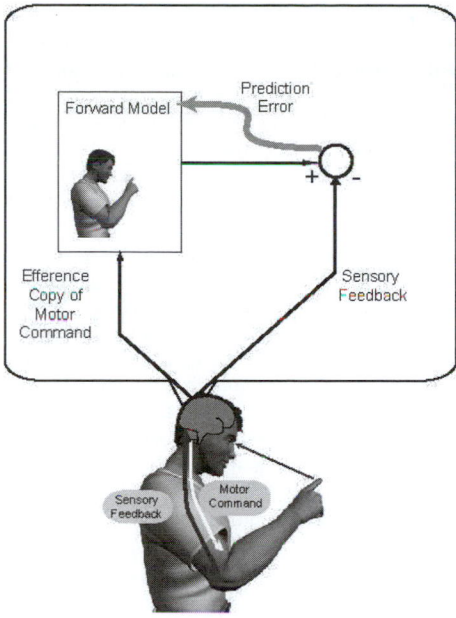

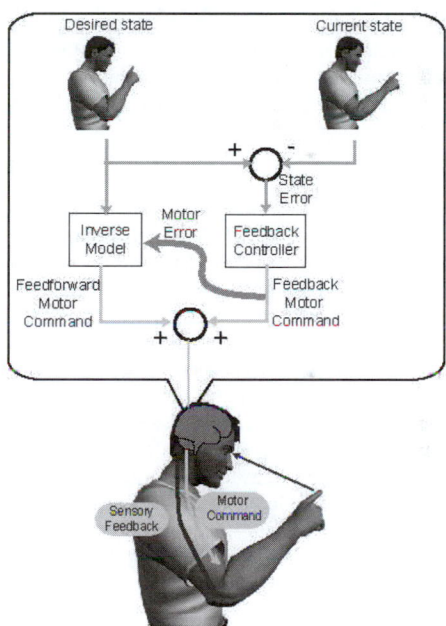

Figure 1. Schematics of forward model and inverse model learning. Top panel shows the forward model using a copy of the descending motor command, known as efference copy, to predict the sensory consequences of action. This prediction can be compared to the actual sensory feedback to generate a prediction error, which can be used (thick arrow) to update the forward model. The bottom panel shows a schematic of feedback-error learning. The aim is to learn an inverse model that can generate motor commands given a series of desired states. A hard-wired and low gain feedback controller is used to correct for errors between desired and estimated states. This generates a feedback motor command that is added to the feedforward motor command generated by the inverse model. If the feedback motor command goes to zero, then the state error will, in general, also be zero. Therefore the feedback motor command is a measure of the error of the inverse model and is used as the error signal to train it.

a feedback motor command, and this forms the error signal used to train the inverse model. This training signal therefore represents the sensory error converted into motor command coordinates. If the feedback motor command can be driven, through learning, to zero, then the inverse model is providing the appropriate motor command (because the outcome error must be zero) and the inverse model has been learned. Even for nonlinear systems, the feedback-error-learning method is generally successful.

In distal supervised learning, a forward model is used to convert outcome errors into errors in the motor command (Jordan and Rumelhart, 1996). The forward model must itself be learned from observations of the motor commands and their consequences on the motor system. The distal supervised learning approach is therefore composed of two interacting processes, one process in which the forward model is learned and another process in which the forward model is used in the learning of the inverse model. For the learning of the inverse model, the inverse model and the forward model are joined together and are treated as a single composite learning system. During this training process, the parameters in the forward model are held fixed and the errors in outcome propagated through the network to update the parameters of the inverse model only. In this way, the forward model is used to convert the outcome errors into motor errors.

Inverse Model Learning: Reinforcement

In *reinforcement learning* (REINFORCEMENT LEARNING IN MOTOR CONTROL), for each input to and output from the learning system, the environment provides feedback in the form of either reward or punishment. The overall performance measure that the system tries to maximize is the sum of total future rewards that may be weighted to favor immediate gain over longer-term gain. The concept of an overall punishment signal, or cost, from reinforcement learning has been very influential in motor control (OPTIMIZATION PRINCIPLES IN MOTOR CONTROL). Because of kinematic redundancy, almost any task can, in principle, be achieved in infinitely many ways. Consider, for example, the number of ways in which you could press an elevator button. Given all these possibilities, it is surprising that almost every study of the way the motor system solves a given task shows highly stereotyped movement patterns, both between repetitions of a task and between individuals on the same task. Such stereotypy is predicted when we consider tasks within the optimal control framework, in which a dynamic system (e.g., the arm) must be controlled so as to minimize a cost function (e.g., error reaching to a target). Mathematically, optimal control theory and reinforcement learning theory are equivalent. The difference is in emphasis: the former usually focuses on continuous state systems with known dynamics and known cost function, while the latter focuses on discrete state systems with unknown dynamics and cost functions that must be learned through experience. An important idea in motor learning has been to try to reverse-engineer the cost function the CNS uses, i.e., what is being optimized, from observed movement patterns and perturbation studies. For example, it has been proposed that there is noise in the motor command and that the amount of noise scales with the magnitude of the motor command. In the presence of such noise the same sequence of intended motor commands, if repeated many times, will lead to a probability distribution over movements. Aspects of this distribution, such as the spread of positions or velocities of the hand at the end of the movement, can be controlled by modifying the sequence of motor commands. In a simple aiming movement, the cost is the final error, as measured by the variance about the target. Assuming the presence of signal-dependent noise, a model that minimizes this cost accurately predicts the trajectories of both saccadic eye movements and arm movements

Different neural structures may be particularly adapted for different computational forms of learning (Doya, 2000). For example, the dopaminergic systems in the basal ganglia have been tied to signals that one would expect in reinforcement learning, such as expected reward, and dysfunctions of these systems are related to movement disorders, addiction, and other problems that could be related to reinforcement signals. Similarly, signals in the cerebellum have been linked to supervised errors. It has been shown that climbing fibres, which may act as a training signal to the cerebellum, can be used to train an inverse dynamic model of the eye (Kawato, 1999).

Novel Dynamic Learning

Recent work on motor learning has focused on the representation of the inverse dynamic model. When subjects make point-to-point movements in which the dynamics of their arm are altered, for example by using a robot or rotating room to generate a force field acting on the arm, they initially exhibit trajectories that deviate from their normal paths and velocity profiles (for reviews see Mussa-Ivaldi, 1999; Lackner and DiZio, 2000). However, over time, subjects adapt and move naturally in the presence of the force field. This can be interpreted as adaptation of the inverse model or the incorporation of an auxiliary control system with a new internal model to counteract the novel forces experienced during movement. Several theoretical questions have been addressed using this motor learning paradigm. The first explored the representation of the controller and in particular whether it was best represented in joint or Cartesian space. This was investigated by examining the generalization of motor learning at locations in the workspace remote from where subjects had adapted to the force field (Shadmehr and Mussa-Ivaldi, 1994). By assessing in which coordinate system the transfer occurred, evidence was provided for joint-based control. Another important advance was made in a study designed to answer whether the order in which states (positions and velocities) were visited was important for learning or whether having learned a force field for a set of states subjects would be able to make natural movements when visiting the states in a novel order. The findings showed that the order was unimportant and argued strongly against a rote learning of individual trajectories. In addition it has been shown that state-dependent fields are learned more efficiently than temporally changing fields, and that during learning both forward and inverse models are simultaneously adapted with the forward model leading.

Modular Learning

Recently, research has begun to shift away from examining learning of a single internal model to considering how we are able to learn a variety of tasks. Many situations that we encounter are derived from a combination of previously experienced situations, such as novel conjoints of manipulated objects and environments. Internal models can be regarded conceptually as motor primitives, which are the building blocks used to construct intricate motor behaviors with an enormous vocabulary. By modulating the contribution to the final motor command of the outputs of a set of internal models, an enormous repertoire of behavior can be generated. One architecture that is capable of learning to act in multiple situations is the MOSAIC model (for review see Wolpert, Miall, and Kawato, 1998). In this architecture a set of forward models (predictors) are used as a set of hypothesis testers to assess which predictor best models the current task. This information is then used to weigh the outputs of a set of corresponding inverse models (controllers). This system can simultaneously learn multiple predictors and controllers as well as how to select the controller appropriate for a given task.

Recent studies have shown that after learning two different contexts, the CNS can appropriately mix the outputs both within the visuomotor domain and across the visuomotor and dynamic domains. Our understanding of the mechanisms of motor learning has gained from examining how learning one task can interfere with learning others. When trying to learn two opposing dynamic or visuomotor rearrangements interference occurs when they are presented in quick succession, but not when they are separated by several hours (Brashers-Krug, Shadmehr, and Bizzi, 1996). This suggests that motor learning undergoes a period of consolidation during which time the motor memory is susceptible to being disrupted. However, if the sensorimotor context is different, then opposite internal models can be simultaneously maintained in motor working memory and subsequently consolidated. For example, subjects can learn and consolidate two opposing force fields if the configuration of the wrist is different for the two fields. In contrast, arbitrary changes in context, such as color cues, are not sufficient for learning of two opposing fields. This suggests that the internal model captures a mapping between motor commands and sensory consequences that is determined by the force field but does not represent the force field per se. Recent studies have suggested that subjects are able to independently learn visuomotor and dynamic transformations presented in close temporal proximity. However, it appears that such independence is only observed when the two transformations depends on different kinematic variables (e.g., a position-dependent visuomotor rotation and a velocity-dependent force field).

Recent evidence indicates that the cerebellum plays a central role in the long-term storage of internal models (for a review see Wolpert, Miall, and Kawato, 1998). In addition it has been suggested that the spinal cord may store a small set of MOTOR PRIMITIVES (q.v.) or basis functions (Bizzi et al., 2000). The idea is to simplify control by combining a small number of primitives, for example patterns of muscle activations (synergies), in different proportions rather than individually controlling each muscle (Mussa-Ivaldi, 1999).

Road Map: Mammalian Motor Control
Background: Motor Control, Biological and Theoretical
Related Reading: Action Monitoring and Forward Control of Movements; Cerebellum and Motor Control; Motor Primitives; Robot Arm Control; Robot Learning

References

Bell, C. C., 2001, Memory-based expectations in electrosensory systems, *Curr. Opin. Neurobiol.*, 11(4):481–487. ◆

Bizzi, E., Tresch, M. C., Saltiel, P., and d'Avella, A., 2000, New perspectives on spinal motor systems, *Nat. Rev. Neurosci*, 1(2):101–108. ◆

Brashers-Krug, T., Shadmehr, R., and Bizzi, E., 1996, Consolidation in human motor memory, *Nature*, 18:252–255.

Doya, K., 2000, Complementary roles of basal ganglia and cerebellum in learning and motor control, *Curr. Opin. Neurobiol.*, 10(6):732–739. ◆

Jordan, M. I., and Rumelhart, D. E, 1996, Forward models: Supervised learning with a distal teacher, *Cognit. Sci.*, 16:307–354

Kawato, M., 1999, Internal models for motor control and trajectory planning, *Curr. Opin. Neurobiol.*, 9(6):718–727. ◆

Kawato, M., Furuwaka, K., and Suzuki, R., 1987, A hierarchical neural network model for the control and learning of voluntary movements, *Biol. Cybernetics*, 56:1–17

Lackner, J. R., and DiZio, P. A., 2000, Aspects of body self-calibration, *Trends. Cogn. Sci.*, 4(7):279–288. ◆

Miall, R. C., and Wolpert, D. M., 1996, Forward models for physiological motor control, *Neural Networks*, 9(8):1265–1279. ◆

Mussa-Ivaldi, F. A., 1999, Modular features of motor control and learning, *Curr. Opin. Neurobiol.*, 9(6):713–717. ◆

Shadmehr, R., and Mussa-Ivaldi, F. A., 1994, Adaptive representation of dynamics during learning of a motor task, *J. Neurosci.*, 14:3208–3224.

Wolpert, D. M., Ghahramani, Z., and Flanagan, J. R., 2001, Perspectives and problems in motor learning, *Trends Cogn. Sci.*, 5(11):487–494. ◆

Wolpert, D. M., and Ghahramani, Z., 2000, Computational principles of movement neuroscience, *Nature Neurosci.*, 3:1212–1217. ◆

Wolpert, D. M., Miall, R. C., and Kawato, M., 1998, Internal models in the cerebellum, *Trends. Cogn. Sci.*, 2:338–347. ◆

Sensory Coding and Information Transmission

John Hertz and Stefano Panzeri

Introduction

The brain is an information-processing machine. Although this statement is commonplace, for a long time most neurobiologists understood the word "information" in it only in the informal, qualitative sense. However, in recent years, quantitative studies based on Shannon's information theory (Shannon, 1948; Cover and Thomas, 1991) have markedly sharpened our understanding of neuronal coding.

Only a few years after Shannon's invention of information theory, MacKay and McCulloch (1952) attempted to estimate the information transmission capacity of single spiking neurons. Assuming that it is limited only by the refractory time (1 ms) and the discriminability of successive spikes, one easily obtains an upper bound on the transmission rate of the order of 1,000 bits/s. A more restrictive bound is obtained by computing the actual entropy of spike trains. This is less than the above limit, because neurons spike less than half the time and different 1 ms intervals are not independent. Still, numbers on the order of 500 bits/s are found.

Now, if neurons are intrinsically very noisy devices, reliable transmission will require a high degree of redundancy, and the actual rate at which they convey information will be correspondingly lower. It has been commonplace to suppose that this is the case, but neural firing may appear noisy to us only because we do not understand it. To achieve even the beginning of an understanding of how the brain works, it is necessary to measure the rate at which neurons actually carry information.

Of course, we do not know how much of the measured information is actually used by downstream neurons. However, measurements of information transmission can usefully identify features of the neural code and thereby help us understand how the brain computes.

An alternative approach to the problem of neural coding is to try to do decoding: optimally estimating the stimulus, given the neuronal response (see, e.g., POPULATION CODES and the review by Borst and Theunissen, 1999).

In the 1970s, Eckhorn and Pöpel (1974, 1975) laid the foundation for much subsequent work on measuring transmitted information by calculating the rate at which neurons in the cat lateral geniculate nucleus carried information about a random train of visual flashes, independent of a priori assumptions about how it was coded. They found rates from about 10 bits/s to as high as 60 bits/s, depending on how fast the stimulus was flashed.

In the 1980s and 1990s, several groups extended this approach. Among them were William Bialek, Rob de Ruyter, and their collaborators (de Ruyter van Steveninck and Bialek, 1988; Bialek and Rieke, 1992), who studied information transmission by single neurons involved in vision in flies, hearing in frogs, and mechanoreception in crickets; and Barry Richmond and co-workers (Optican and Richmond, 1987; Heller et al., 1995), who made similar analyses for spatial pattern vision in monkeys. By now, the quantitative characterization of neurons in terms of information transmission rates has become a standard tool.

Here we review two recent approaches to measuring transmitted information. The first, employed by Bialek and his collaborators, is based on direct estimation of the spike train entropies in terms of which transmitted information is defined. The second, developed by Panzeri and Schultz, is based on an expansion to second order in the length of the spike trains.

Entropy and Information

Whatever system we are interested in, the formal characterization of the problem is the same. The animal is presented a stimulus s from some set S, and the response of a neuron (or several neurons) is measured. For spiking neurons, the response can be represented completely generally in the following way. Time is divided into intervals (typically 1 ms) small enough that there is never more than one spike per interval. The response can then be described by a binary vector with one component per interval, equal to a 1 or 0 according to whether or not the neuron fired a spike in that interval. We denote this vector simply by r and the whole set of responses by R.

To get a grasp of what "transmitted information" means, consider an experiment in which many spike trains are recorded for many stimuli. There is generally intrinsic variability in the system or the measurement process, so we formulate our description of the problem in terms of distributions of stimuli and responses. The fact that the responses depend to some extent on the stimuli means that the stimulus-conditional response probabilities $P(r|s)$ are not in general equal to the unconditional or stimulus-averaged probabilities $P(r) = \Sigma_s P(r|s)P(s)$. We expect that the variability of the responses evoked by a given stimulus will generally be less than that of the entire response set. The transmitted information is a simple measure of this variability difference.

A general way of characterizing variability is as an entropy. Thus, the total or unconditional response entropy $H(R) = -\Sigma_r P(r) \log_2 P(r)$ describes the variability of the entire response ensemble. Analogously, the response entropy conditional on a given stimulus s is $H(R|s) = -\Sigma_r P(r|s) \log_2 P(r|s)$. Its average over s, denoted $H(R|S)$—the average response variability for a fixed stimulus—is termed the *noise entropy*. The transmitted information $I(R; S)$, also called the mutual information between stimuli and responses, is simply the difference between the total and noise entropies: $I(R; S) = H(R) - H(R|S)$. Although the corresponding difference for a single s, $H(R) - H(R|s)$, is not necessarily positive (a single stimulus might evoke highly variable responses), $I(R; S)$ can be proved to be non-negative. It is zero only when the stimulus-response relationship is completely random, and it takes its maximum possible value $H(R)$ only when the response is deterministic (for a given stimulus, every response is identical).

Therefore, the calculation of the transmitted information requires simply the accurate estimation of the conditional probabilities $P(r|s)$ and, from them, the total and averaged conditional entropies, as described above. If one has sufficient data, one can just estimate response probabilities as the fraction of all responses with a particular value of r. This can be difficult because the full response space

has such a high dimensionality: 2^T bins for spike trains T time units long.

The difficulty can be circumvented by employing specific models for the encoding, i.e., for the relevant conditional probabilities. Almost all the work mentioned above was done this way. This reduces the dimensionality of the response space, but at a cost: particular features of the results might be artifacts of the model used. Recent investigations have concentrated instead on model-independent methods, and here we review two sets of studies along these lines.

Direct Calculations

In the approach taken by Bialek's group (Strong et al., 1998), one tries to estimate the probabilities $P(\{t_i\})$ and $P(\{t_i\}|s)$ directly from histograms of the data. (We use the notation $\{t_i\}$ for the response r to emphasize that we mean the entire set of spike times, not just a spike count or some other low-dimensional measure.) These estimated probabilities are then used to calculate the total and noise entropies $H(R)$ and $H(R|S)$ and thereby the transmitted information, as described above.

In the experimental paradigm used, the fly views the moving pattern for very long periods, and we are interested in the information transmission rate. To estimate this, one considers time windows of length T and tries to extrapolate to the limit of very long windows. For small T, it is easy to make reliable entropy estimates directly (consider a 1 ms window in which only two responses are possible, spike or no spike), but these estimates ignore possible correlations between spikes at different times. For very large T, on the other hand, the exponentially growing dimensionality of the space of responses prevents one from estimating their probabilities reliably from histograms based on the data.

The solution is to start with small T, then go to larger and larger windows, trying to identify the large-T trend while the estimates are still reliable. The estimated entropy rates (entropies divided by T) at lower values of T fit a nice straight line as a function of $1/T$, so it is simple to extrapolate to $1/T = 0$ to estimate the asymptotic rates.

The difference between the resulting total and noise entropy rates (Figure 1) gave an estimate of 78 ± 5 bits/s (1.8 bits/spike) for a time-discretization window $\Delta t = 3$ ms. Reassuringly, this number is consistent with those found by other methods (de Ruyter van Steveninck and Bialek, 1988; Bialek and Rieke, 1992).

The noise entropy was just about half of the total entropy; that is, half of the total observed variability in the neuronal firing is signal and half is noise.

Varying Δt, one can explore how much information is encoded in spike timing at different degrees of precision. The transmission rate was found to vary roughly logarithmically with Δt, with a maximum value of 90 bits/s found for a resolution of 0.7 ms.

T-Expansion

Panzeri and Schultz (2001) and Schultz and Panzeri (2001) observed that it was possible to make a formal expansion of both the total and noise entropies in powers of T, the length of the time interval over which the response is measured. The computational advantage of using this expansion is that, working, say, to second order in T, one only need estimate the quantities $P(t^a|s)$ (the probability, given stimulus s, of a spike from unit a at time t^a, conditional on stimulus s) and $P(t_1^a, t_2^b; S)$ (the joint probability of a spike from unit a at time t_1^a and one from unit b at time t_2^b, also conditional on s), not the full conditional response probabilities $P(\{t_i^a\}|s)$. Thus, fewer data are required to make a robust estimation.

Beyond second order in T, the expansion becomes very cumbersome, but the second-order expansion proves quite accurate for

Figure 1. Procedure for estimating total and noise entropy rates. Entropies are estimated for finite-time window width T, plotted functions of $1/T$, and extrapolated to $T = \infty$. Here the bin width $\Delta t = 3$ ms. The upper sets of points are for the total entropy and the lower sets are for the noise entropy. Also shown (open symbols) are the Ma bounds. The dashed lines show the extrapolations $T \to \infty$. (From Strong et al., 1998. Reprinted with permission.)

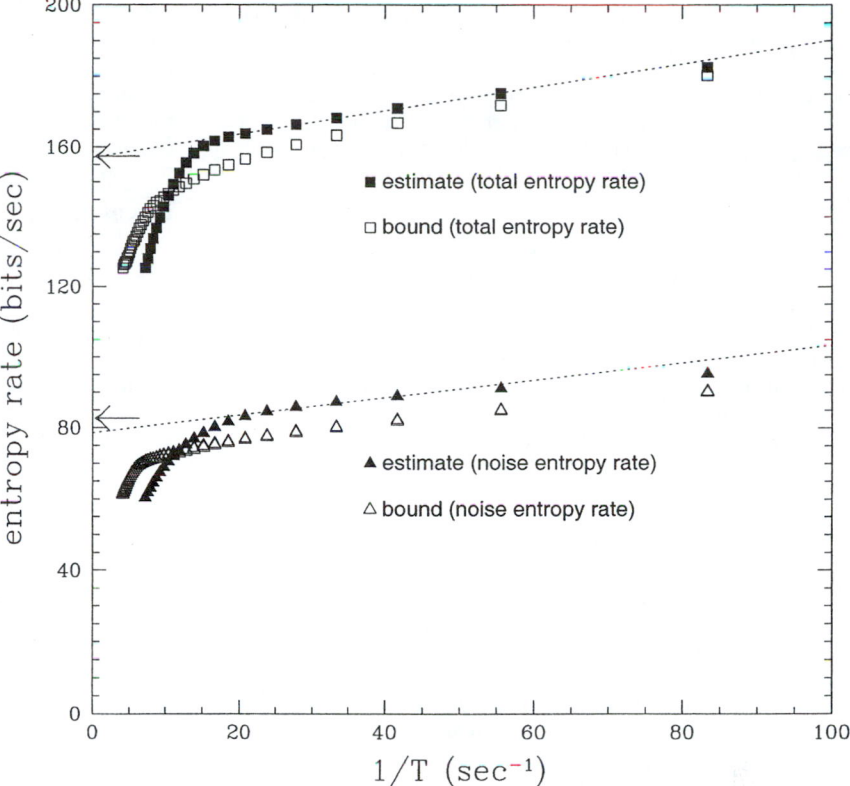

experimentally relevant response times (20–100 ms). Furthermore, the first- and second-order terms can be written in a way that isolates the potential effects of spike timing and of correlation in both signal and noise, permitting direct insight into the nature of the neuronal code.

We now examine these terms. For generality, we consider the case of multiple neurons, labeled by an index a running from 1 to C. The response r is the full set of spike times t_i^a of all the neurons. The expansion takes the form

$$I(\{t_i^a\}; S) = TI_t(\{t_i^a\}; S) + \frac{T^2}{2} I_{tt}(\{t_i^a\}; S) + O(T^3) \quad (1)$$

The first-order term has a very simple form:

$$TI_t(\{t_i^a\}; S) = \sum_{a=1}^{C} \int dt^a \left\langle \bar{r}_a(t^a|s) \log_2 \frac{\bar{r}_a(t^a|s)}{\bar{r}_a(t^a)} \right\rangle_s \quad (2)$$

Here $\bar{r}_a(t^a|s)$ is the average firing rate at time t^a, conditional on stimulus s, and $\bar{r}_a(t^a) = \langle \bar{r}_a(t^a|s) \rangle_s$ is the rate averaged over all stimuli. Since Equation 2 is a linear sum over each time t and cell a, it gives the information gained about the stimulus (i.e., the entropy reduction) from knowing the spike train, if each response time bin and cell were to convey independent information. Deviations from independent information transmission (i.e., synergy or redundancy effects) are expressed by the second-order term, considered next. Correlations between cells or between spikes for a given cell do not enter at first order in T.

At order T^2, correlations between pairs of spikes affect the result. We can describe these correlations by some auxiliary quantities $\gamma_{ab}(t_1^a, t_2^b|s)$ and $v_{ab}(t_1^a, t_2^b)$, defined as follows. Consider, for stimulus s, the joint probability rate of a spike at time t_1^a by neuron a and one by neuron b at t_2^b, which we write in the form

$$P(t_1^a, t_2^a; s) = \bar{r}_a(t_1^a|s)\bar{r}_b(t_2^b|s)[1 + \gamma(t_1^a, t_2^b|s)] \quad (3)$$

If different spikes were independent, the joint probability rate would just be the product of the separate single-spike rates, i.e., $\gamma(t_1^a, t_2^b|s) = 0$. The quantity $v_{ab}(t_1^a, t_2^b)$ measures correlations in the rates across stimuli in an analogous way:

$$v_{ab}(t_1^a, t_2^b) = \frac{\langle \bar{r}_a(t_1^a)\bar{r}_b(t_2^b) \rangle_s}{\bar{r}_a(t_1^a)\bar{r}_b(t_2^b)} - 1 \quad (4)$$

In terms of these quantites, the second-order transmitted information can be written

$$\frac{T^2}{2} I_{tt}(\{t_i^a\};S) = \frac{1}{2 \ln 2} \sum_{ab} \int dt_1^a dt_2^b \bar{r}_a(t_1^a)\bar{r}_b(t_2^b) \Big\{ v_{ab}(t_1^a, t_2^b)$$
$$+ [1 + v_{ab}(t_1^a, t_2^b)] \ln \frac{1}{1 + v_{ab}(t_1^a, t_2^b)} \Big\}$$
$$+ \frac{1}{2} \sum_{ab} \int dt_1^a dt_2^b \langle \bar{r}_a(t_1^a|s)\bar{r}_b(t_2^b|s)\gamma(t_1^a, t_2^b|s) \rangle_s$$
$$\times \log_2 \frac{1}{1 + v_{ab}(t_1^a, t_2^b)} + \frac{1}{2} \sum_{ab}$$
$$\times \int dt_1^a dt_2^b \langle \bar{r}_a(t_1^a|s)\bar{r}_b(t_2^b|s)[1 + \gamma(t_1^a, t_2^b|s)]$$
$$\times \log_2 \Big\{ \frac{\langle \bar{r}_a(t_1^a|s')\bar{r}_b(t_2^b|s') \rangle_{s'}[1 + \gamma(t_1^a, t_2^b|s)]}{\langle \bar{r}_a(t_1^a|s')\bar{r}_b(t_2^b|s')[1 + \gamma(t_1^a, t_2^b|s')] \rangle_{s'}} \Big\} \Big\rangle_s$$
$$(5)$$

We consider the three terms on the right-hand side of Equation 5 separately. The first one is the only one that would be there if there were no correlations between spikes. It is always negative. Since the first-order term (Equation 2) grows linearly with time but the total information is bounded, the rate of information accumulation has to slow down with time, and this term is the first place where we see that effect. The second term reflects the effect of spike correlations, through $\gamma(t_1^a, t_2^b|s)$, but these correlations are averaged over stimuli (weighted in proportion to the rates $\bar{r}_a(t_1^a|s)$ and $\bar{r}_b(t_2^b|s)$ they evoke). Thus, this term describes the effects of *stimulus-independent* firing correlations. The final term, which cannot be negative, is the part of the information due to stimulus-dependent correlations.

This treatment was for the complete neuronal response, i.e., r is the set of firing times t_i^a for all the neurons. Often, one is interested in how much information is carried by the spike count alone, independent of the firing times. This information can be expanded in the same way, and the result is analogous to Equations 2 and 5. The differences are, first, there are no time integrals; second, the conditional and unconditional spike counts replace the full response rates $\bar{r}_a(t^a|s)$ and $\bar{r}_a(t^a)$; and third, there is no longer any time dependence in the correlation coefficients $\gamma_{ab}(s)$ and v_{ab}.

To see what one can learn from this kind of analysis, we review its application to data from rat barrel cortex (Panzeri et al., 2001). In the experiment, single whiskers were stimulated and the responses of 106 neurons were collected and analyzed.

The first significant finding was that a substantial fraction of the total information carried by these neurons about which whisker was being stimulated was encoded temporally. That is, there was considerable information carried by the full response (the complete sets of spike times) that was not carried by the spike counts alone. The size of this effect varied a lot from neuron to neuron, but, on average, including spike timing added about 50% to the information contained in the spike count.

The nature of the temporal code employed by these neurons can be explored further by examining the contributions from the separate terms in Equations 2 and 5. Figure 2 shows the principal findings. Most of the information (83%) could be accounted for without taking any spike correlations into account. More specifically, different stimuli evoke responses with different PSTHs $\bar{r}_a(t^a|s)$, and these differences account for most of the discriminability of the stimuli. For example, $\bar{r}_a(t^a|s_1)$ might rise a lot faster than $\bar{r}_a(t^a|s_2)$. In this case an early spike would be a good indication that it was evoked by s_1 rather than s_2. Indeed, in the present case, the first-

spike time alone conveyed (on average) as much information as could be gained from all spikes, ignoring correlations. Almost all of the remaining 17% of the information (13.5%) was coded in stimulus-independent correlations (i.e., the second term on the right-hand side of Equation 5), with only 3.5% in stimulus-dependent correlations (the final term).

Discussion

These examples illustrate how, given sufficient data, neural information transmission can be measured systematically and accurately, and how one can begin to sort out details of the neural code employed by the brain in specific cases. The computational technology is by now rather well developed, and we can expect that in the future it will be applied to more and more data, in different animals, in different brain regions, and in the context of different brain functions. One can then hope that, integrating this knowledge with the insight gained from exploring the implications of particular coding strategies (see SPARSE CODING IN THE PRIMATE CORTEX and FEATURE ANALYSIS), a coherent general picture of the encoding and computational strategies employed in neural processing will begin to emerge. An extensive and readable treatment of these and related issues can be found in the book by Rieke et al. (1997).

Road Map: Neural Coding
Related Reading: Adaptive Spike Coding; Optimal Sensory Encoding; Rate Coding and Signal Processing

References

Bialek, W., and Rieke, F., 1992, Reliability and information transmission in spiking neurons, *Trends Neurosci.*, 15:428–434.
Borst, A., and Theunissen, F. E., 1999, Information theory and neural coding, *Nature Neurosci.*, 2:947–957. ◆
Cover, T. M., and Thomas, J. A., 1991, *Elements of Information Theory*, New York: Wiley. ◆
de Ruyter van Steveninck, R. R., and Bialek, W., 1988, Real-time performance of a movement-sensitive neuron in the blowfly visual system: Coding and information transfer in short spike sequences, *Proc. R. Soc. Lond. B*, 212:1–34.
Eckhorn, R., and Pöpel, B., 1974, Rigorous and extended application of information theory to the afferent visual system of the cat: I. Basic concepts, *Kybernetik*, 16:191–200.
Eckhorn, R., and Pöpel, B., 1975, Rigorous and extended application of information theory to the afferent visual system of the cat: II. Experimental results, *Biol. Cybern.*, 17:7–17.
Heller, J., Hertz, J. A., Kjær, T. W., and Richmond, B. J., 1995, Information flow and temporal coding in primate pattern vision, *J. Computat. Neurosci.*, 2:175–193.
MacKay, D. M., and McCulloch, W. S., 1952, The limiting information capacity of a neuronal link, *Bull. Math. Biophys.*, 14:127–135.
Optican, L. M., and Richmond, B. J., 1987, Temporal encoding of two-dimensional patterns by single units in primate inferior temporal cortex: III. Information-theoretic analysis, *J. Neurophysiol.*, 57:162–178.
Panzeri, S., Petersen, R., Schultz, S. R., Lebedev, M., and Diamond, M., 2001, The role of spike timing in the coding of stimulus location in rat somatosensory cortex, *Neuron*, 29:769–777.
Panzeri, S., and Schultz, S. R., 2001, A unified approach to the study of temporal, correlational and rate coding, *Neural Comp.*, 13:1311–1349.
Rieke, F., Warland, D., de Ruyter van Steveninck, R., and Bialek, B., 1997, *Spikes: Exploring the Neural Code*, Cambridge, MA: MIT Press. ◆
Schultz, S. R., and Panzeri, S., 2001, Temporal correlation and neural spike train entropy, *Phys. Rev. Lett.*, 86:5823–5826.
Shannon, C. E., 1948, A mathematical theory of communication, *Bell Syst. Tech. J.*, 27:379–423, 623–653. Available: http://cm.bell-labs.com/cm/ms/what/shannonday/paper.htm.
Strong, S. P., Koberle, R., de Ruyter van Steveninck, R. R., and Bialek, W., 1998, Entropy and information in neural spike trains, *Phys. Rev. Lett.*, 80:197–200.

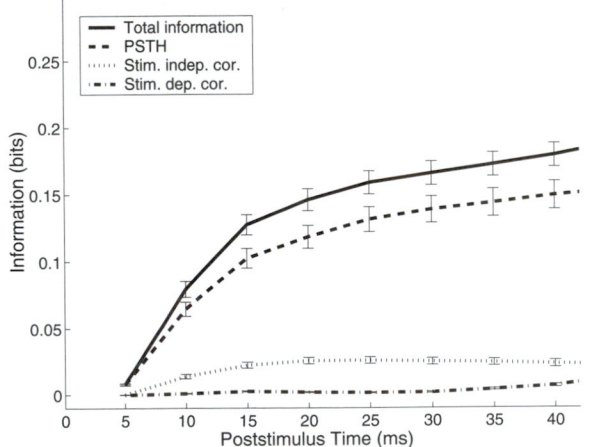

Figure 2. Autocorrelations carry little information about stimulus position in rat somatosensory cortex: Contributions to the transmitted information from PSTHs (dashed line; Equation 2 and the first term on the right-hand side of Equation 5), stimulus-independent correlations (dotted line; second term on the right-hand side of Equation 5), and stimulus-dependent correlations (dashed-dotted line; third term on the right-hand side of Equation 5). Bars denote SEM. (Redrawn from Panzeri et al., 1998.)

Sequence Learning

Peter Ford Dominey

Introduction

The forward linear progression of time imposes a fundamental sequential structure on all behavior, and thus the capacity to store and manipulate sequential information is of central importance for adaptive systems. Sequential structure is not unidimensional, however, and the potentially dissociable aspects of sequence processing are likely to be associated with distinct neural systems. From this perspective, the current article will characterize behavioral sequences in terms of their serial, temporal, and abstract structure, and aspects of the associated neural processing systems.

Serial structure or order is defined by the relation between an element or set of elements, and its successor. This dimension can be characterized in terms of length and complexity. *Length* is the number of elements in the sequence. *Complexity* refers to the maximum number of elements that must be remembered in order to know the correct successor. Temporal structure is defined in terms of the durations of elements (and the possible pauses that separate them), and intuitively corresponds to the familiar notion of rhythm. Thus, two sequences may have identical serial structure and different temporal structure, or the opposite. Abstract structure is defined in terms of generative rules that describe relations between repeating elements within a sequence. Thus, the two sequences A-B-C-B-A-C and D-E-F-E-D-F have different serial structure, but are both generated from the same abstract structure 123-213, and are thus said to be isomorphic. While perhaps not exhaustive, these three dimensions at least partially span the space of possible behavioral sequence structure. This article focuses on how these different dimensions of sequence structure can be encoded in neural systems based on behavioral studies in different patient and control groups, and related simulation studies. Related issues in temporal sequence learning are found in the articles TEMPORAL SEQUENCES: LEARNING AND GLOBAL ANALYSIS; TEMPORAL PATTERN PROCESSING; and RECURRENT NETWORKS: LEARNING ALGORITHMS (q.v.).

Learning Serial and Temporal Structure

Aspects of Recurrent Networks

A fundamental property of a sequence processing system is that the state of the system should contain information about the current sequence element, but should also be influenced by the succession of previous elements. This is the case for recurrent networks in which context units receive inputs from units encoding internal state and feed back into these state units. These recurrent connections between the state and context units allow information from previous time steps to influence the current network activity, thus providing a representation of sequence context. Learning that requires modification of recurrent connections, however, introduces significant technical challenges. Specifically, after an input is presented, multiple network cycles can occur before an output is generated and the error is evaluated and corrected. A given connection weight in the recurrent network has contributed to the error, but in a different way on each successive cycle of information passing through this weight. The technical problem thus arises in unraveling this weight's contribution to the error over these successive time steps in order to implement the error-reducing learning. A number of methods have been developed to deal with the complexity of applying learning algorithms to recurrent connections (Pearlmutter, 1995, and RECURRENT NETWORKS: LEARNING ALGORITHMS). In general, many of these methods of resolving the

problem of learning in recurrent networks over multiple time steps are biologically implausible, because they are not consistent with forward running time, and/or because they have excessive computational and memory storage requirements.

The method used by Elman (1990) in the simple recurrent network (SRN) is to cut off the temporal history at one or two time steps, yielding a simplified learning method but still quite efficient sequence learning capability. The SRN has been demonstrated to be sensitive to serial structure in a number of different domains including representing regularities in the serial structure of language (Elman, 1990), modeling finite-state automata (Cleeremans, Servan-Schreiber, and McClelland, 1989), speech segmentation (Christiansen, Allen, and Seidenberg, 1998), and simulating human performance in sensorimotor sequence learning (Cleeremans, 1993) in serial reaction time (SRT) tasks.

Sequence Learning in the Serial Reaction Time Task (SRT)

The serial reaction time task (SRT) developed by Nissen and Bullemer (1987) has been quite extensively used in the study of human sequence learning, and is thus an interesting object for simulation studies. In the SRT task, reaction times (RTs) for visual stimuli that are presented in a repeating sequence are reduced with respect to RTs for stimuli in randomly presented series (see Figure 1B). This RT difference is the measure of sequence learning. One of the principal manipulations in the SRT paradigm has been the performance of a concurrent or "dual" task that typically impairs the sensorimotor learning (Nissen and Bullemer, 1987). Curran and Keele (1993) proposed the existence of dissociable attentional and nonattentional forms of sequence learning, and that the dual task disrupts attentional sequence learning, while leaving the less efficient nonattentional learning intact. Cleeremans (1993) suggested alternatively that the dual task impairs the processing of successive sequence elements, and he thus introduced random noise to the activity of a subset of units in a simple recurrent network (SRN) during SRT learning, resulting in perturbed performance quite similar to that observed in human subjects in dual task conditions (Cleeremans, 1993). This, however, leaves open the question of how the dual task conditions introduced processing noise to produce such a perturbation in sequence learning.

Stadler (1995) suggested that the dual task condition disrupts sequence learning by preventing consistent temporal organization of the sequence due to the delays introduced during the response-stimulus interval (RSI) by the dual task processing. He thus demonstrated experimentally that the introduction of random delays during the RSI perturbs sequence learning in a manner quite similar to that of the dual task condition, while introducing a purely attentional load with no temporal disorganization does not. This suggested that dual task results could be explained without resorting to dissociable learning mechanisms. Testing this temporal disorganization hypothesis directly in a simulation study would require the presentation of successive elements with realistic RSI delays.

A Temporal Recurrent Network

Temporal structure in sequences can be encoded by systems that employ mechanisms including distributions of delay lines (TEMPORAL SEQUENCES: LEARNING AND GLOBAL ANALYSIS) between units, time-dependant short-term memory elements (TEMPORAL PATTERN PROCESSING), and the temporal dynamics of recurrent networks, though this is not the case for the standard implemen-

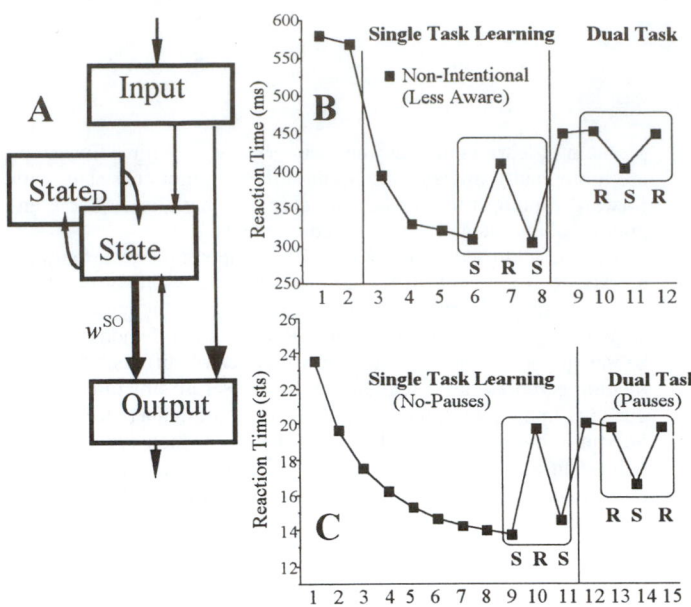

Figure 1. *A*, TRN architecture. Each structure is a 5 × 5 matrix of leaky integrator neurons with sigmoid firing thresholds. Reinforcement learning in w^{SO} synapses binds activation patterns in State to output activations in Output. *B*, SRT learning. Mean RTs for successive blocks of 120 sequence elements. RTs for sequentially presented stimuli in blocks 3–6 are reduced, and then increase in random block 7, revealing learning. Learning expression reduced in dual task as revealed by reduced difference in random (block 11) vs. sequence (blocks 10 and 12) RTs. (Data from Experiment 1 of Curran and Keele, 1993.) *C*, Simulation of SRT learning by the TRN. RTs are reduced as w^{SO} synapses associate sequence-specific State activity with corresponding predictable sequence elements, yielding stronger activation and faster rise to threshold for sequence (S) vs. random (R). Dual task conditions achieved by introduction of random pauses as suggested by Stadler (1995), simulating human data in *B*. (Data from Dominey, 1998.)

tations of the SRN where the next element is expected on the next network cycle as discussed previously. Dominey, Arbib, and Joseph (reviewed in Dominey et al., 1998) introduced an alternative sequence learning model that takes full advantage of the temporal dynamics of a recurrent network, while eliminating the complexity of learning in recurrent connections (see Figure 1*A*). Recurrent connections in the State network of leaky integrator neurons—considered to represent cortico-cortical connections in prefrontal cortex (PFC)—are preset with random values that vary between −0.55 and +0.45, and do not change during learning. Associative learning takes place in modifiable connections between the recurrent state layer and the output layer, corresponding to dopamine-related plasticity in corticostriatal synapses. Neurons in the simulated PFC (State in Figure 1) demonstrated receptive fields sensitive both to the spatial location of sequence elements, and their serial order, as observed in electrophysiological recordings in PFC of the non-human primate (Dominey, Arbib, Joseph in Dominey et al., 1998).

With respect to the SRT task (Figure 1*B*), as a sequence is successively repeated and learned, reaction times for predictable elements in the sequence become progressively reduced due to increased State-Output connection strengths that yield more rapid activation of the leaky integrator neurons in Output for elements in the repeating sequence. Thus the model naturally displays reduced RTs for predictable sequence elements (Figure 1*C*).

Processing of Serial and Temporal Structure

Given its fixed recurrent connections, the TRN exploits the temporal coding capabilities of a recurrent system while avoiding the complexity of recurrent learning, and is thus well adapted to examining the effects of serial and temporal structure in SRT learning. During SRT learning, we introduced random delays during the RSI interval between the model response and the next sequence elements, to simulate the effects of dual task learning as in Stadler's (1995) experiment. This temporally distorted input produced a degraded representation of the sequence in the recurrent network, resulting in weaker activation of the learned State-Output associations, and a corresponding increase in reaction times. This argues for the temporal structure disruption hypothesis of Stadler (1995)

and explains human sensitivity to perturbations in temporal structure of such sequences (Dominey, 1998). In contrast, if temporal structure is introduced in a systematic (rather than random) way that is coherent with the serial structure then these regularities can be represented in a systematic way in the recurrent network and can be learned (Dominey in Dominey and Ramus, 2000).

Indeed, serial and temporal structure are often correlated in behavioral sequences, a condition that likely plays an important role in behavioral sequence learning. In particular, in the earliest phases of language acquisition it is likely that sensitivity to correlations in serial and temporal structure provides the foundation for the construction of more complex linguistic representations. Christiansen et al. (1998) thus demonstrated how the SRN can exploit multiple cues, each of which alone is insufficient, in learning to segment words in a continuous stream. Because of the temporal processing constraints of the SRN, temporal structure is coded symbolically in these simulations, rather than in real time.

In this context the TRN was confronted with human performance in which newborns discriminate between languages in different rhythm classes based on their temporal structure (Dominey and Ramus, 2000). Simulating these results with the TRN, sentences from five different languages were recoded as consonant-verb (C-V) sequences, where the only defining information was the rhythmic structure. Like children, the TRN was able to discriminate between languages from different rhythm classes (e.g., English and Spanish) but not between languages from the same rhythm class (e.g., Dutch and English).

Learning Abstract Structure

Although it has been demonstrated that the serial and temporal structure of sequences can be processed by a common architecture, it is not clear that this generalization extends to abstract structure. In an elegant presentation of abstract structure processing in the infant, Marcus et al. (1999) demonstrated that after only 2 minutes' total exposure to 16 sound sequences such as "le-di-di, ji-we-we . . ." 7-month old infants can extract the common abstract structure (in this case ABB), and can transfer this knowledge in order to recognize new sequences as isomorphic (matching) or not with the learned pattern.

Marcus et al. concluded that infants can learn rules such as ABB, in which A and B represent variables that can be instantiated with new values during generalization and transfer to new sequences, and that such rule representations cannot be realized by statistical methods or standard sequencing models including the SRN. In a series of comments in *Science* and *Trends in Cognitive Science*, opponents argued that if training and transfer domains shared overlapping representations, then statistical learning methods and the SRN would work. Marcus et al. countered that transfer can still be observed even when there is no overlap in the representation, and that systems that require this overlap will fail in these cases.

Addressing this transfer issue, Dienes, Altmann, and Gao (1999) modified the SRN by adding additional units and connections for representing the transfer domain, and for learning the mapping from training to transfer domains. This model has been able to explain a significant set of results from the artificial grammar learning domain, in which this issue of transfer is a central question. Thus the "overlap" problem is solved by learning, but in a manner that avoids representation of the common rule. One behavioral result of this mapping strategy is that transfer is not immediate, but requires significant exposure to the new material for the mapping to be learned.

It remains likely, however, that the "rule" vs. "instance" distinction is behaviorally and neurophysiologically valid (reviewed in Dominey et al., 1998). In this context, we observed in human adults that the serial and abstract structure of sequences, such as ABCBAC and DEFEDF, can be learned independently (Dominey et al., 1998). In implicit (naive) conditions, subjects learned serial structure, but were unable to exploit knowledge of the underlying abstract structure 123-213 when exposed to a new "isomorphic" sequence based on this abstract structure. Indeed, only when subjects were explicitly aware of a possible underlying abstract structure were they able to learn both the serial and abstract structure and rapidly transfer the abstract knowledge to new isomorphic sequences. When exposed to this task, the TRN learned only the serial structure, independant of the abstract structure. This is because the network lacks a representation of the internal relations that characterize abstract structure. To address this representational deficit, we modified the TRN to contain a set of short-term memory (STM) components, that store the 7 ± 2 previous sequence elements, and a recognition function applied to this STM to detect repetition relations, with the recurrent network operating on these relations. In this context, ABCBAC is represented as "u,u,u, n-2, n-4, n-3" where "u" corresponds to unique or nonrepeating, and "n-2" corresponds to repetition of the element 2 positions behind (Dominey et al., 1998). The thus modified abstract recurrent network (ARN) operates on these abstract sequence representations rather than their serial structure. This is consistent with the idea that, to the extent that the training and transfer domain do not overlap, a recurrent network is not enough, and additional hardware is required. For Dienes et al. (1999) the additional hardware was used to construct the mapping between training and transfer domains. In Dominey et al. (1998) it allowed representation of the internal or "abstract" structure of the rule that describes the general mapping itself.

Neuropsychological Evidence for the Serial/Abstract Dissociation

If the hypothesis that serial and abstract structure are treated by dissociable neurophysiological processes is correct, then we should be able to isolate patient groups that display this dissociation. In this context, Parkinson's disease is characterized by motor disorders of akinesia, tremor, and rigidity that result from a massive destruction of midbrain dopamine-producing neurons. This deterioration has significant impact on the functional organization of

the frontostriatal system that is the neuroanatomical correlate of the TRN sequence learning model. Thus, numerous studies indicate that the implicit learning of the serial structure of sensorimotor sequences is impaired in these patients. Interestingly, we demonstrated that these patients retained a significant capability to acquire and transfer knowledge of abstract sequential structure to new isomorphic sequences in a serial reaction time task, suggesting that while implicit sequence learning relies on an intact frontostriatal system, explicit learning of abstract structure does not (or less so). In contrast, it is known that schizophrenic patients tend to perform well on automated, implicit processing, with more difficulty on explicit attentional processing, functionally associated with a hypofrontality. Accordingly, we observed that schizophrenic patients displayed an intact capability to learn serial structure, but failed to learn abstract structure. These results from simulation and neuropsychological studies support the hypothesis that processing of serial and abstract structure rely on dissociable neural mechanisms. These and related studies are reviewed in Dominey et al. (1998).

Relation to Language Processing

Although language clearly requires task specific capacities, it is likely that more generalized capabilities to process serial, temporal, and abstract sequential structure could also come into play. This applies both for learning to segment speech into words (Christiansen et al., 1998), and in the use of abstract generative rules for structural transformations.

Syntactic comprehension is the process of determining "who did what to whom" from a purely syntactic analysis. Considering the sentences "Sally[1] was introduced to Bill[2] by John[3]" vs. "John[3] introduced Sally[1] to Bill[2]," we see that ordering of the agent (John), object (Sally), and recipient (Bill) vary in these active and passive sentences. In a simplified manner, if we consider syntactic comprehension as a recovery of the canonical (active) structure, then the passive to active transformation can be characterized by the abstract rule 123-312. In this context we can predict that if syntactic comprehension shares a common neurophysiological basis with abstract structure manipulation, then performance deficits in the two tasks should be correlated.

In order to test this prediction, we compared performance in syntactic comprehension and in abstract sequential structure processing in a population of aphasic patients with syntactic comprehension deficits. Linear regression revealed that performance in the two tasks was highly correlated, suggesting a common underlying neurophysiological basis. This observation was likewise replicated in a population of schizophrenic patients that displayed correlated deficits in their processing of syntactic and abstract structure (Lelekov et al., 2000).

While such correlation results argue for shared neurophysiological processing, they do not rule out explanations based on a more global cognitive deficit. In order to examine this issue more directly one can exploit brain imagery techniques during the performance of these abstract and syntactic tasks. In this context, we note that the on-line identification of syntactic structures (e.g., active, passive, relative, etc.) is largely guided by closed class function words (e.g., to, by, the) that thus play a crucial role in allowing a parser to apply syntactic knowledge. ERP studies have demonstrated that grammatical function words evoke a left anterior negativity (LAN) between 400–600 ms (reviewed in Hoen and Dominey, 2000). In a related study, Hoen and Dominey (2000) examined brain potentials associated with the processing of special "function" symbols that trigger one of two possible abstract rules that will apply in a cognitive sequencing task. The objective was to determine if these nonlinguistic function symbols would be processed in the same neural networks as grammatical function words in natural language. In order to examine this process in a nonlinguistic sequencing context, two abstract structure conditions were studied (1) ABC*X*BCA and (2) ABC*Y*DEF. In condition (1) the function symbol "X" indicates that the second triplet will be a systematically transformed version of the first triplet. In condition (2) the function symbol "Y" indicates that the second triplet will have no relation to the first. When brain responses to the function symbols X and Y were compared, a relative left anterior negativity was observed for X vs. Y, with a temporal and topographic scalp localization quite similar to the LAN observed for function word processing (Hoen and Dominey, 2000).

These patient and ERP studies suggest a framework in which grammatical markers, either in the form of distinct function words, or as morphological markers, would indicate the appropriate syntactic frames (abstract structure), while these syntactic frames would be applied to open class words for syntactic comprehension. Interestingly, this framework maps quite naturally onto the dual-process TRN/ARN model for the treatment of serial/temporal and abstract structure. Function words (or their morphological equivalents) are processed in the recurrent network of the TRN, thus defining the syntactic context. Open class nouns are stored in the STM components of the abstract network ARN, and based on the syntactic context, these STM components (and thus the contained nouns) are then linked with their corresponding thematic role and retrieved appropriately. In this configuration, the model is able to learn the mapping between syntactic structure and the corresponding conceptual or thematic structure in order to successfully complete a standard syntactic comprehension task. Although this represents an interesting extension of sequential cognition toward language processing, it is clearly a preliminary first step that leaves much work ahead.

Discussion

At the outset of this article, it was suggested that behavioral sequences can be considered in terms of their serial, temporal, and abstract structure. A behavioral sequence learning framework was thus established in which serial and temporal structure are represented in a temporal recurrent network (TRN) with recurrent connections implemented in corticocortical connections of the frontal cortex. State activity in the recurrent network is then functionally associated with behavioral responses via modifiable corticostriatal projections. A dissociated abstract recurrent network (ARN) that is required for manipulating abstract structural relations is potentially implemented in a distributed network that includes the perisylvian cortex in and around Broca's area. The proposal that transfer of sequence knowledge to a new domain requires additional, dissociable, processes remains an open debate. Though the approaches are somewhat different, both Dienes et al. (1999) and Dominey et al. (1998) argued that recurrent networks alone could not address this transfer, which requires additional representational capabilities. Indeed, it is likely that both approaches of between-domain mapping and abstract rule representation are neurophysiological realities.

Road Map: Cognitive Neuroscience
Related Reading: Prefrontal Cortex in Temporal Organization of Action; Speech Processing: Psycholinguistics; Temporal Pattern Processing

References

Christiansen, M. H., Allen, J., Seidenberg, M. S., 1998, Learning to segment speech using multiple cues: A connectionist model, *Lang. Cognit. Proc.*, 13:221–268.
Cleeremans, A., Servan-Schreiber, D., and McClelland, J. L., 1989, Finite state automata and simple recurrent networks, *Neural Comp.*, 1:372–381.
Cleeremans, A., 1993, *Mechanisms of Implicit Learning: Connectionist Models of Sequence Processing*, Cambridge, MA: MIT Press. ◆
Curran, T., and Keele, S. W., 1993, Attentional and nonattentional forms of sequence learning, *J. Exp. Psych.: Learning, Mem. Cog.*, 19(1):189–202.
Dienes, Z., Altmann, G., and Gao, S.-J., 1999, Mapping across domains without feedback: A neural network model of transfer of implicit knowledge, *Cognit. Sci.*, 23:53–82.
Dominey, P. F., Lelekov, T., Ventre-Dominey, J., Jeannerod, M., 1998, Dissociable processes for learning the surface and abstract structure of sensorimotor sequences, *J. Cognit. Neurosci.*, 10(6):734–751. ◆
Dominey, P. F., 1998, Influences of temporal organization on transfer in sequence learning: Comments on Stadler (1995) and Curran and Keele (1993), *J. Exp. Psychol.: Learning, Mem. Cog.*, 24(1):234–248.
Dominey, P. F., and Ramus, F., 2000, Neural network processing of natural language: I. Sensitivity to serial, temporal and abstract structure of language in the infant, *Lang. Cognit. Proc.*, 15(1):87–127.
Elman, J. L., 1990, Finding structure in time, *Cognit. Sci.*, 14:179–211. ◆
Hoen, M., and Dominey, P. F., 2000, ERP analysis of cognitive sequencing: A left anterior negativity related to structural transformation processing, *Neuroreport*, 28;11(14):3187–3191.
Lelekov, T., Franck, N., Dominey, P. F., and Georgieff, N., 2000, Cognitive sequence processing and syntactic comprehension in schizophrenia, *Neuroreport*, 14;11(10):2145–2149.
Marcus, G. F., Vijayan, S., Bandi Rao, S., and Vishton, P. M., 1999, Rule learning by seven-month-old infants, *Science*, 283(5398):77–80.
Nissen, M. J., and Bullemer, P., 1987, Attentional requirement of learning: Evidence from performance measures, *Cognit. Psychol.*, 19:1–32. ◆
Pearlmutter, B. A., 1995, Gradient calculation for dynamic recurrent neural networks: A survey, *IEEE Transactions on Neural Networks*, 6(5):1212–1228. ◆
Stadler, M. A., 1995, The role of attention in implicit learning, *J. Exp. Psychol.: Learning, Mem. Cog.*, 21:674–685. ◆

Short-Term Memory

Emmanuel Guigon, Etienne Koechlin, and Yves Burnod

Introduction

It is generally agreed that two temporally distinct neural processes contribute to the acquisition and expression of brain functions. Transient variations in membrane potential (neuronal activity), on a time scale of milliseconds, reflect the flow of information from neuron to neuron and define the function of neuronal networks. These variations can result in long-lasting (and possibly permanent) alterations in neuronal operations, for instance through activity-dependent changes in synaptic transmission.

There is now strong evidence for a complementary process acting over an intermediate time scale. A wide variety of temporal patterns of activity are actively generated by neurons and local circuits of neurons; an example is the transformation of transient inputs into long-lasting sustained or oscillatory activity. Experimental studies in invertebrates have demonstrated that such temporal patterns produce motor programs and are generated both by the molecular properties of each neuron and by the connectivity of the local network (Harris-Warrick and Marder, 1991; Marder et al., 1996). In vertebrates, long-lasting activities are neural correlates of transient memory processes. These patterns of activity allow past events to be represented and behavioral reactions to future, predictable events to be prepared (see PREFRONTAL CORTEX IN TEMPORAL ORGANIZATION OF ACTION). That these patterns also result from both the intrinsic properties of single neurons and the synaptic interactions between neurons is now well recognized (Llinás, 1988; Marder et al., 1996; Durstewitz, Seamans, and Sejnowski, 2000).

In this article, we discuss cellular and neural network mechanisms that could be involved in the formation of short-term memory (STM) traces in the vertebrate brain. We address three issues: (1) What are the different types of STM traces? (2) How do intrinsic and synaptic mechanisms contribute to the formation of STM traces? (3) How do STM traces translate into long-term memory representations of temporal sequences? We note that we are concerned here neither with exact definitions and properties of psychological concepts nor with detailed biophysical or biochemical mechanisms involved in the characterization of short-term memory processes, but only with computational mechanisms underlying these processes. We also note that these mechanisms may well underlie a wide variety of seemingly different biological processes (e.g., emergence of orientation selectivity in visual cortex, dynamics of head-direction cells in the limbic system, directional tuning in motor cortex) and so may be relevant to understanding brain functions.

Types of Neural Short-Term Memory Traces

As shown in Figure 1, two broad types of STM traces exist. In the first type (Figure 1A), transient inputs are transformed into long-lasting activity patterns. The output traces could represent a membrane potential, a discharge frequency, or any biophysical or biochemical variable (e.g., intracellular calcium concentration). Ideally, the level of maintained activity would be proportional to the intensity of the input stimulus (intensity memory; Figure 1A_1), or tuned about a preferred (spatial) stimulus (spatial memory or

memory field; Figure 1A_2). Spatial and intensity memory mechanisms are relevant to working memory, or the ability to hold relevant information in memory for future utilization in the guidance of behavior. Neural correlates of working memory are found mainly in the anterior regions of the cerebral cortex (e.g., prefrontal cortex) as stimulus-selective sustained neuronal discharges (see PREFRONTAL CORTEX IN TEMPORAL ORGANIZATION OF ACTION). Complete references on the issue of working memory models can be found in Durstewitz et al. (2000).

In the second type of STM trace (Figure 1B), constant inputs are transformed into time-varying outputs, such as ramps with different slopes (Figure 1B_1) or oscillations at different frequencies (Figure 1B_2) or of different amplitudes (not shown). Again, characteristics of the output patterns (slope, frequency, amplitude) should be related to the intensity of the input. Activity ramps are found as correlates of preparatory and anticipatory processes in sensorimotor and cognitive behaviors. They are ubiquitous in cortical parietal and frontal region, and could participate in muscular recruitment, preparation for response, and decision-making processes (Hanes and Schall, 1996). Little attention has been paid to the formation of ramps. Oscillatory activities are mentioned here because they are typical STM traces to which a central role in many behavioral processes has been attributed (see SLEEP OSCILLATIONS). Cellular and network mechanisms of oscillations are dealt with in the literature (see OSCILLATORY AND BURSTING PROPERTIES OF NEURONS) and are not addressed here.

Many other STM traces could be built by combining these two types. Furthermore, in physiological recordings, additional time-varying components would be found in inputs and outputs corresponding to different types of variability in neural processing.

Cellular and Network Mechanisms of STM Traces

Sustained Activity

The basic mechanism for the formation of maintained activities is a neuron with a recurrent excitatory connection

$$\tau \frac{dI}{dt} = -I + wf(I) + I_{in} \tag{1}$$

where I is a variable that could represent the total synaptic current, $f(I) = 1/[1 + \exp(s(0.5 - I))]$, the firing rate of the neuron, w is the weight of the recurrent connection, and I_{in} is the input current. The bifurcation diagram of this equation was plotted with I_{in} as a parameter (Figure 2A). For $I_{in} < I_1$ and $I_{in} > I_2$, the equation has a single, stable, fixed point. Elsewhere there are three fixed points: two are close to the minimum and maximum firing rate, respectively, and are stable (lower and upper branches in Figure 2A). The third one is unstable (dashed middle branch). Transient inputs elicit transition between the stable states (Figure 2B).

This model is illustrative of a general class of neural networks in which persistent states arise from reverberating activity through recurrent excitatory loops (see COMPUTING WITH ATTRACTORS). The main drawback of these models is that the level of maintained activities is close to the neural saturation level, and the resting level is silent (Figure 2A), in contradistinction to physiological observations. More realistic persistent activities are found when excitation and inhibition are represented by different neuronal populations (Durstewitz et al., 2000). Furthermore, low- and high-frequency persistent states can coexist when inhibition slightly dominates excitation.

The models just discussed describe neural processing in terms of firing rate or synaptic current, whereas a physiologically realistic representation is defined by equations governing membrane potential (i.e., Hodgkin-Huxley equations and equations for synaptic inputs; see SYNAPTIC INTERACTIONS). Thus, an open question is

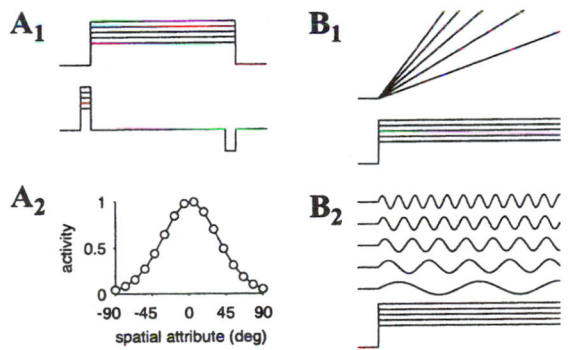

Figure 1. Types of STM traces. A_1, Intensity memory. Intensity of a transient input (lower trace) is translated into a long-lasting activity (upper trace) of equal (or proportional) amplitude. Five activity traces are shown, corresponding to five input intensities (in the same order). Horizontal time scale and vertical intensity scale are not specified (same as for B_1 and B_2). A_2, Spatial memory. The memorized value of a spatial attribute (here 0°) is represented by a tuned activity distribution in a population of neurons selective to this attribute. B_1, Activity ramp. A constant input (lower trace) is translated into a time-varying linearly increasing activity (upper trace). The slope of output activity is proportional to input intensity. B_2, A constant input is translated into oscillations (the output traces are shown separately for clarity). Oscillatory frequency is proportional to input intensity.

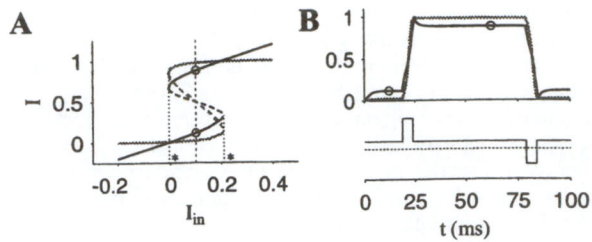

Figure 2. *A*, Bifurcation diagram of Equation 1. The plot depicts the value of equilibrium state synaptic currents (black curve) and corresponding firing rates (gray curve). States belonging to plain (dashed) lines are stable (unstable). Vertical dotted lines delimit a region with three equilibrium states and define input currents I_1 and I_2 (asterisks). *B*, Activity profile (same conventions as in *A*) for $I_{in} = 0.1$ (vertical dashed line in *A*) and transient excitatory and inhibitory inputs (lower trace). Steady states are indicated by ○. Parameters were $\tau = 2$, $s = 10$, $w = 0.8$.

whether similar properties would be found in a biophysically realistic model of a spiking neuron. Simulations show that the ability of a neural network to maintain robust delay activity at physiological rates (e.g., 15–20 Hz) depends on the nature of synaptic transmission. In fact, the largest component of the synaptic transmission, mediated by AMPA receptors, has a fast decay, which leads to persistent discharges at frequencies above 50 Hz (Wang, 1999). The contribution of slow synaptic transmission through NMDA receptors could help bypass this effect and reduce the frequency of persistent activity to the required level (Wang, 1999). However, it is unknown whether the density of NMDA receptors is large enough to play such a role.

We discussed how maintained activity can result from recurrent interactions within neuronal populations. Alternatively, maintained activity could correspond to the depolarized state of an intrinsically *bistable* neuron (Marder et al., 1996). Intrinsic bistability is characterized by the existence of two or more stable states (e.g., a hyperpolarized state and a more depolarized state in which the neuron discharges), with the transition from one state to the other effected by transient synaptic events (Marder et al., 1996). Numerous examples of bistability have been described in the literature, both in invertebrates (e.g., *Aplysia*, crab stomatogastric ganglion) and in vertebrates (spinal cord, cerebellum, thalamus). The cellular bases of bistability generally involve a low-threshold persistent inward conductance, i.e., a depolarizing conductance that activates in the subthreshold range and does not inactivate (see ION CHANNELS: KEYS TO NEURONAL SPECIALIZATION). If the neuron is endowed with a spiking mechanism, the depolarized state corresponds to the discharge of action potentials; otherwise it is a plateau potential.

The models described so far maintained persistent activities in an all-or-none fashion, at a level prescribed by their structure. These observations support the concept of a subset of strongly and uniformly connected neurons representing a discrete attractor (see CORTICAL HEBBIAN MODULES). In the following paragraphs we show that adequate choice of recurrent synaptic interactions allows memory encoding of continuously valued variables (intensity or spatial memory; see Figure 1*A*).

Intensity memory (Figure 1*A*₁) can be addressed in the framework of linear recurrent neural networks, i.e.,

$$\tau \frac{dI}{dt} = -I + WI + I_{in} \qquad (2)$$

where I is the N-dimensional vector of output activities and W is a symmetric synaptic matrix. This equation, which is a multidimensional linear generalization of Equation 1, can be solved explicitly for I,

$$I(t) = \sum_{i=1}^{N} a_i(t)\mathbf{e_i}$$

where $\{e_i\}$ are the eigenvectors of W. Persistent activity appears in the case where one eigenvalue (index k) of W is equal to 1 and all the other eigenvalues are smaller than 1. The solution becomes

$$I(t) \approx \frac{\mathbf{e_k}}{\tau} \int_0^t I_{in}(t') \cdot \mathbf{e_k} \, dt' \qquad (3)$$

This equation shows that the network can hold a faithful memory of the amplitude of a transient input. However, this property is lost when the synaptic matrix is even slightly perturbed. This would also be the case in a nonlinear version of this model.

This principle was used in the framework of conductance-based spiking models by Seung et al. (2000) to explore brainstem networks involved in the control of eye position. In this model, brainstem neurons are integrators that convert transient signals driving changes in eye position into a persistent memory of eye position (Figure 3*A*).

The linear recurrent network described by Equation 2 can also generate *spatial memory* profiles. This occurs when (1) each neuron i is identified by a periodic parameter θ_i (e.g., a preferred direction in $[0; 2\pi]$), (2) the $\{\theta_i\}$ are uniformly distributed in $[0; 2\pi]$, and (3) the synaptic weight between neurons i and j is $W_{ij} = \cos(\theta_i - \theta_j)$. In this case, W has only two non-zero eigenvalues equal to 1, and acts as a filter that suppresses all harmonics ≥ 2 in the input signal. Thus, the network generates and maintains a cosine distribution of activity from any nonuniform transient input. The constraint on the eigenvalues of W can be relieved in a nonlinear version of Equation 2:

$$\tau \frac{dI}{dt} = -I + W[I]_+ + I_{in} \qquad (4)$$

where $[\ ]_+ ([u]_+ = u$ if $u \geq 0$, otherwise $[u]_+ = 0)$ translates current into firing rate. In this case, a spatially selective activity profile can persist in the presence of a constant background (Figure 3*B*). This behavior appears in the case of strong, spatially modulated excitatory connections and corresponds to the existence of a continuous line of stable states (Hansel and Sompolinsky, 1998).

A realistic implementation of spatial memory was described by Compte et al. (2000). Their network involved (1) excitatory and inhibitory neurons modeled as leaky integrate and fire units (see

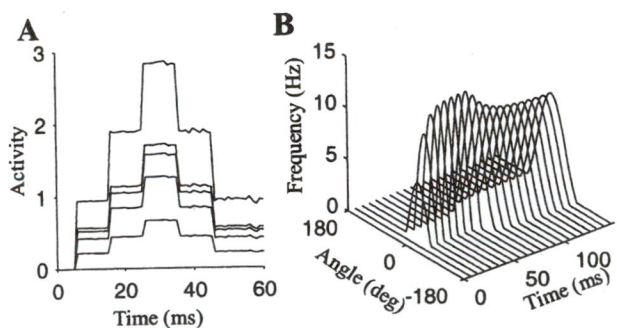

Figure 3. *A*, Intensity memory. Simulation of Equation 3 for five neurons. The eigenvector $\mathbf{e_k}$ was [0 0.25 0.5 0.75 1]. Transient inputs (duration 2 ms) were delivered at times 5, 15, 25 (excitatory), and 35, 45 (inhibitory). *B*, Spatial memory. Simulation of Equation 4. Matrix W was made of local Gaussian excitation and global inhibition. A tuned activity profile (width 40°) was presented at time 10 and replaced at time 50 by an untuned profile of the same amplitude.

SINGLE-CELL MODELS), (2) spatially structured connections between the excitatory neurons, and (3) slow (NMDA) synaptic transmission (Wang, 1999). The model displayed both low spontaneous activity and robust stimulus-evoked selective persistent discharges at physiological frequencies (~20–30 Hz). In the preceding model (Equation 4), spatial pattern formation resulted from a continuous bifurcation. On the other hand, there is genuine network bistability in the present model, which authorizes transition between resting and activated states by transient excitatory inputs. Compte et al. (2000) observed a drift in time of persistent activity patterns in the presence of noise, which resulted in a degraded memory of encoded stimuli. In fact, in all models, the spatial patterns are only marginally stable (Hansel and Sompolinsky, 1998).

An attractive hypothesis would be that both synaptic and intrinsic properties contribute to the formation of persistent activity. Lisman, Fellous, and Wang (1998) proposed that NMDA receptor–mediated bistability could participate in the maintenance of selective working memory activity. Camperi and Wang (1998) used conditional bistability in a continuous attractor network (Equation 4) and showed that it can contribute to the stability of maintained activities against perturbations, although it was not involved in their maintenance per se.

On the whole, these mechanisms provide reasonable clues to how sustained activities can be maintained in neuronal populations. However, several questions remain open: (1) All of the models have built-in instability and require finely tuned synaptic weights to work appropriately. Is this instability a characteristic feature of sustained discharges in the nervous system? How could this instability be removed? Which mechanisms allow the development and maintenance of exact synaptic structures? (2) The models have many features in common and apply to the emergence of orientation selectivity in visual cortex, dynamics of head-direction cells in the limbic system, directional tuning in motor cortex, and persistent activities in prefrontal cortex. Are there definite differences in the neural substrate of these functions? For instance, is the putative role of slow synaptic transmission identified by some models a characteristic feature of prefrontal cortical circuits?

Activity Ramp

When a constant current is injected in a neuron, a time-varying pattern of activity is observed that depends on passive properties of the neuron (membrane time constant) and active membrane characteristics (voltage-gated ionic conductances). The former effect is illustrated by the voltage response of a passive membrane

$$\frac{dV}{dt} = -\frac{V}{\tau} + I$$

for different values of τ and different I. The time to reach a threshold V_θ is given by

$$T_\theta = -\tau \ln\left(1 - \frac{V_\theta}{\tau I}\right)$$

This relation is strongly nonlinear and shows that neither I nor τ can efficiently be used to specify a duration. At best it could be used for durations below 50 ms.

The same is approximately true in a Hodgkin-Huxley model (see AXONAL MODELING) because the sodium and potassium conductances of the action potential are weakly activated in the subthreshold range. The time to reach a given frequency is not yet an appropriate timing mechanism, because steady-state discharge settles within a few time constants.

At the single neuron level, robust STM properties arise from the presence of a slowly inactivating potassium (Ks) conductance (Marder et al., 1996; Delord et al., 2000). The functioning principle of the Ks conductance is the following. It creates a slowly decaying hyperpolarizing current whose initial level can be specified by prior conditioning of the neuron. For instance, prior hyperpolarization sets a large persistent outward current that slows down the rate of membrane potential changes in the subthreshold range during a subsequent depolarization. Figure 4A shows that the latency-to-the-first-spike can be up to 10 s in the presence of a Ks conductance with an inactivation time constant of 2 s, and the relationship between the injected current and the latency is close to linear for a latency of up to approximately 7 s.

The Ks conductance also influences the suprathreshold behavior of the neuron. The discharge frequency gradually increases toward its steady-state level as the Ks current decays (Figure 4B). Both the initial and final frequency increase with the level of injected current, which results in a modest change in the slope of the time–frequency curve with the injected current (Figure 4C). Recruitment at variable rates, as described in Figure 1B₁, can be approached by combining the effect of Ks conductance and synaptic interactions in a population of uniformly connected neurons (Figure 4B) (Delord et al., 2000). In this case, because of recurrent excitation, a smaller amount of injected current is required to obtain a given steady-state frequency. Thus the initial frequencies are lower and vary in a smaller range. Accordingly, the slope is more strongly modulated by the injected current than in the absence of synaptic interactions (Figure 4C). The strength of this modulation is directly controlled by the strength of synaptic weights (Figure 4D). Thus, adaptive recruitment at variable rates is made possible by the simultaneous action of synaptic and intrinsic properties in a neural network. Interestingly, slowly inactivating potassium conductances are found in neurons of most regions of the central nervous system with a time constant ranging from hundreds of milliseconds to several tens of seconds (Llinás, 1988).

Could a similar property be obtained by purely synaptic effects? In fact, the linear recurrent network described by Equation 2 has the required property (Figure 3A). The formation of persistent activities begins by a linear ramp with a slope proportional to the amplitude of the input current (Equation 3). However, as mentioned

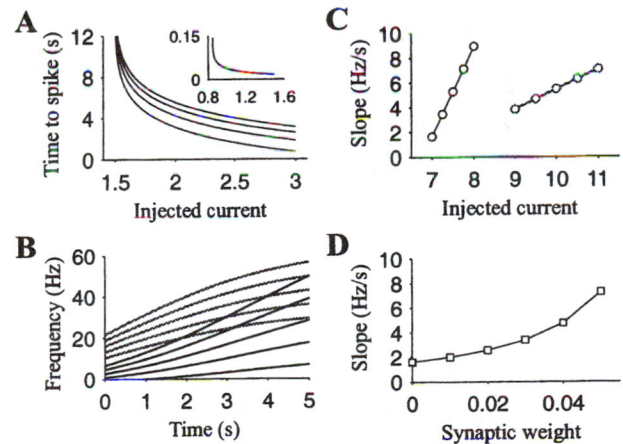

Figure 4. *A,* Time to the first spike as a function of the injected current in the presence of a Ks conductance in a Hodgkin-Huxley model. The curves correspond to different initial level of availability of the Ks conductance (maximal for the upper curve). The result in the absence of Ks conductance is shown at upper right. *B,* Time course of frequency increase for different levels of injected current in a recurrent (dark lines) and nonrecurrent (gray lines) network. *C,* Slope of the frequency increase as a function of the injected current (linear regression on the results of *B*). *D,* Slope of the frequency increase as a function of the synaptic weight in the recurrent network. Details on the methods can be found in Delord et al. (2000).

earlier, exactly tuned synaptic weights are necessary to the proper functioning of the network. It is unclear whether the nervous system can reach the required degree of accuracy in the adjustment of synaptic weights (Seung et al., 2000).

From Short-Term to Long-Term Memory Traces

Synaptic plasticity is a central mechanism in models of learning and memory (see HEBBIAN SYNAPTIC PLASTICITY). The most popular approach involves shaping functions of neural networks by activity-dependent modification of synapses based on Hebbian learning rules. Accordingly, information stored in long-term memory reflects correlation (i.e., temporal contiguity) between transient neuronal activities on a time scale of 0–100 ms. Sutton and Barto (1981) recognized that learning rules based on temporal contiguity are inappropriate to represent temporal dependencies in, for example, the framework of classical conditioning. They proposed that STM traces (synapse-specific and output traces) are involved in the acquisition of new conditioned behaviors. This principle has led to the development of the temporal difference algorithm, which provides a powerful way to learn predictions of future events (see REINFORCEMENT LEARNING). In this framework, STM traces are translated into a long-term representation of the temporal structure of behavior. A related approach applied to the prefrontal cortex is described in Guigon et al. (1995).

Discussion

STM traces become essential as soon as the time scale of behavior extends beyond the duration of phasic signaling (e.g., ~0–500 ms)—in other words, in almost any behavioral situation. We discussed cellular and network mechanisms involved in the formation of STM traces. We described simplified network models that provide mathematical conditions for the formation and stability of STM traces, and more detailed realistic models with which to assess the biophysical basis of these phenomena.

Despite impressive results, our understanding of these mechanisms is far from complete. First, each neuron is endowed with a wealth of intrinsic properties (Llinás, 1988), very few of which have been considered in models. The respective contribution of synaptic and intrinsic factors is unknown. Second, persistent discharges and ramps constitute a small subset of the rich dynamic repertoire of neural populations observed in vivo, and it is unclear how they can be combined to form more complex memory traces. Third, the great majority of models fail to be robust facing noise and inexact tuning of parameters (e.g., synaptic weights). A future

challenge is to relate these pieces of memory to cognitive functions that are very demanding of temporary storage and manipulation of information, such as planning, reasoning, and language use.

Road Map: Dynamic Systems
Background: I.3 Dynamics and Adaptation in Neural Networks
Related Reading: Amplification, Attenuation, and Integration

References

Camperi, M., and Wang, X.-J., 1998, A model of visuospatial working memory in prefrontal cortex: Recurrent network and cellular bistability, *J. Comput. Neurosci.*, 5:383–405.

Compte, A., Brunel, N., Goldman-Rakic, P., and Wang, X.-J., 2000, Synaptic mechanisms and network dynamics underlying spatial working memory in a cortical network model, *Cereb. Cortex*, 10:910–923.

Delord, B., Baraduc, P., Costalat, R., Burnod, Y., and Guigon, E., 2000, A model study of cellular short-term memory produced by slowly inactivating potassium conductances, *J. Comput. Neurosci.*, 8:251–273.

Durstewitz, D., Seamans, J., and Sejnowski, T., 2000, Neurocomputational models of working memory, *Nature Neurosci. Suppl.*, 3:1184–1191.

Guigon, E., Dorizzi, B., Burnod, Y., and Schultz, W., 1995, Neural correlates of learning in the prefrontal cortex of the monkey: A predictive model, *Cereb. Cortex*, 5:135–147.

Hanes, D., and Schall, J., 1996, Neural control of voluntary movement initiation, *Science*, 274:427–430.

Hansel, D., and Sompolinsky, H., 1998, Modeling feature selectivity in local cortical circuits, in *Methods in Neuronal Modeling: From Ions to Networks*, 2nd ed. (C. Koch and I. Segev, Eds.), Cambridge, MA: MIT Press, pp. 499–567.

Harris-Warrick, R., and Marder, E., 1991, Modulation of neural networks for behavior, *Annu. Rev. Neurosci.*, 14:39–57.

Lisman, J., Fellous, J.-M., and Wang, X.-J., 1998, A role for NMDA-receptor channels in working memory, *Nature Neurosci.*, 1:273–275.

Llinás, R., 1988, The intrinsic electrophysiological properties of mammalian neurons: Insights into central nervous system function, *Science*, 242:1654–1663.

Marder, E., Abbott, L., Turrigiano, G., Liu, Z., and Golowasch, J., 1996, Memory from the dynamics of intrinsic membrane currents, *Proc. Natl. Acad. Sci. USA*, 93:13481–13486.

Seung, H., Lee, D., Reis, B., and Tank, D., 2000, Stability of the memory of eye position in a recurrent network of conductance-based model neurons, *Neuron*, 26:259–271.

Sutton, R., and Barto, A., 1981, Toward a modern theory of adaptive networks: Expectation and prediction, *Psychol. Rev.*, 88:135–170.

Wang, X.-J., 1999, Synaptic basis of cortical persistent activity: The importance of NMDA receptors to working memory, *J. Neurosci.*, 19:9587–9603.

Silicon Neurons

Rodney Douglas and Christof Rasche

Introduction

Silicon neurons are analog electronic circuits fabricated in complementary metal-oxide-silicon (CMOS) using very large-scale integration (VLSI) methods. CMOS is a medium for manufacturing transistors whose conductivity can be altered by an applied electric field. This technology is commonly used to construct the digital circuits found in general-purpose computers, but the silicon neurons discussed in this article are not a kind of digital computer. Instead, the same CMOS VLSI technology is used to construct

analog circuits whose physics is analogous to the physics of membrane conductivity. This analogy permits the circuits to emulate the electrophysiological behavior of biological neurons in real time, while the high component density offered by VLSI technology provides a means of fabricating large networks of silicon neurons.

Neuronal systems are difficult to model because they are composed of large numbers of nonlinear elements and have a wide range of time constants. Consequently, their mathematical behavior can rarely be solved analytically. The usual approach is to simulate these problems on a general-purpose digital computer (Koch and Segev, 1998). But for any given computer, the speed of these simulations is limited by the shortest time constant in the problem. Furthermore, the simulation time slows dramatically as the number and coupling of elements increase. By contrast, silicon neurons operate in real time, and the speed of the network is independent of the number of neurons or their coupling. Thus, networks of silicon neurons are especially suited to the investigation of questions that arise from the real-time interaction of the system with its environment. Nevertheless, the design of special-purpose hardware is a significant investment, particularly if it is analog hardware, since analog VLSI (aVLSI) design is still very much an art form.

Analog VLSI has a controversial role in the study of neural computation. This controversy arises out of a debate over the role of precision in computation. Digital computation is guaranteed precise to the number of bits used in the computation. However, the most compact analog circuits have low precision as a result of uncertain calibration between transistors. Some proponents of neuromorphic aVLSI design claim that these circuits provide a natural route for exploring the principles of biological computing, which must also make do with low precision (Mead, 1989). Unlike the ideal components used in conventional computers, real neurons are not homogeneous. Even within a morphological class such as the pyramidal cells of the cerebral cortex, they show a wide range of behavior. They are poorly insulated conductors; they have a variety of nonlinear conductance elements and large amounts of stray capacitance; they are sensitive to environmental changes; and a significant fraction of them malfunction or stop during the operational life of the system. Nevertheless, the smallest vertebrate brain is vastly more competent at interaction with the real world than are our most elaborate supercomputers. From the level of conductances, through synapses to neurons and networks, the nervous system elements obtain precision, speed, and computational power using imperfect elements. Understanding the architectures and adaptive processes that allow the nervous system to extract precise information from a noisy and ambiguous environment with uncalibrated components is a central problem of computational neuroscience (see SYNAPSE TRANSMISSION). Analog VLSI circuits have similar intrinsic variability, and so synthesis of silicon neurons is a method of exploring the principles of computations that must use unreliable components. The philosophy of neuromorphic engineering is that the medium of computation is an intrinsic part of the computation itself.

Mapping Neurons into CMOS

The strategy for mapping neurons into CMOS varies between research groups, and this article will not review the full range of options that are being explored. Instead, we will focus on a few examples that are representative of the various types. The feature that distinguishes a silicon neuron from an ANN neuron is that it includes a large number of time constants. The silicon neuron's dynamical complexity implies that the input-output relationship of silicon neurons cannot be encapsulated by a single sigmoidal function; instead, a given synaptic input will have a different effect on the output, depending on where and when it is applied.

Conceptually, the neuron can be divided into four parts: the dendrite, which receives inputs; the soma, which translates the inputs to an output; the axon, which distributes the output; and the synapses, which transmit the output to the target neurons. At a more physical level, traditional modelers of biological neurons have divided the continuous neuronal membrane of the dendrites and soma into a series of compartments to facilitate numerical computation (Koch and Segev, 1998) (see DENDRITIC PROCESSING). Each compartment is considered to be isopotential and spatially uniform in

its properties. The connectivity of the compartments mirrors the spatial morphology of the modeled cell.

Elias has constructed neuromorphic VLSI neurons with 112 passive compartments that model the leakiness of the cellular membrane and the axial resistance of the intracellular medium using space-efficient switched capacitors to implement resistances (Elias and Northmore, 1999). Each compartment provides passive temporal filtering of the inputs. More recently, we have incorporated circuits that model voltage-dependent conductances into the dendritic compartments (Figure 1D). The resolution of the segmentation is a compromise between the questions that must be addressed by the model, the resources required by each compartment, and error tolerance. For example, neurons with between 5 and 30 compartments are a common compromise for digital simulations of cortical and hippocampal circuits (Koch and Segev, 1998).

The simplest electronic somatic model is a single passive compartment that produces a digital spike event when it is charged to a threshold voltage. This integrate-and-fire neuron (see SINGLE-CELL MODELS) has been used for various purposes ranging from sensors to general network simulations. For example, Elias uses an integrate-and-fire model for his dendrites (Elias and Northmore, 1999). Boahen extended a silicon integrate-and-fire neuron to include a spike-frequency adaptation mechanism. This version is used in a neuromorphic retina.

The oscillatory character of neurons is compactly expressed in mathematical models such as the FitzHugh-Nagumo or Morris-Lecar model (see OSCILLATORY AND BURSTING PROPERTIES OF NEURONS). Both models have been implemented (Linares-Barranco et al., 1991; Patel and DeWeerth, 1997) (Figure 1F). The latter is used to model the intersegmental coordination of the lamprey.

In addition to the passive properties of the lipid membrane, the biological neuronal membrane contains active ionic channels. In the silicon neurons of Douglas and Mahowald (Mahowald and Douglas, 1991), the compartments are populated by modular subcircuits, each of which emulates a particular ionic conductance (see ION CHANNELS: KEYS TO NEURONAL SPECIALIZATION). The dynamics of these circuits is qualitatively similar to the Hodgkin-Huxley mechanism without implementing their specific equations. The various modules that have been designed and tested so far emulate, for example, the sodium and potassium spike currents, persistent sodium current, various calcium currents, calcium-dependent potassium current, potassium A current, nonspecific leak current, and an exogenous (electrode) current source. The prototypical circuits are modified in various ways to emulate the particular properties of a desired ion conductance. For example, some conductances are sensitive to calcium concentration rather than membrane voltage and require a separate voltage variable representing free calcium concentration. Synaptic conductances (see below) are sensitive to ligand concentrations, and these circuits require a voltage variable representing neurotransmitter concentration. This array of ionic conductances, with their different time constants, gives rise to state-dependent dynamics within the compartments. These circuits can be composed to approximate the electrophysiological behavior of various neurons, for example pyramidal cells (Figure 1E). The somatic conductances have been extended to permit the neuron to adapt its discharge sensitivity curve to the statistics of its input current (Shin and Koch, 1999) (Figure 1G; see also ACTIVITY-DEPENDENT REGULATION OF NEURONAL CONDUCTANCES).

Even more detailed models have been fabricated by Dupeyron and colleagues. They used Bi-CMOS technology to implement the detailed differential equations of the Hodgkin-Huxley formalism. Their goal is to build a silicon nerve cell that can interact directly and exactly with real neurons investigated during experiments (Dupeyron et al., 1996)

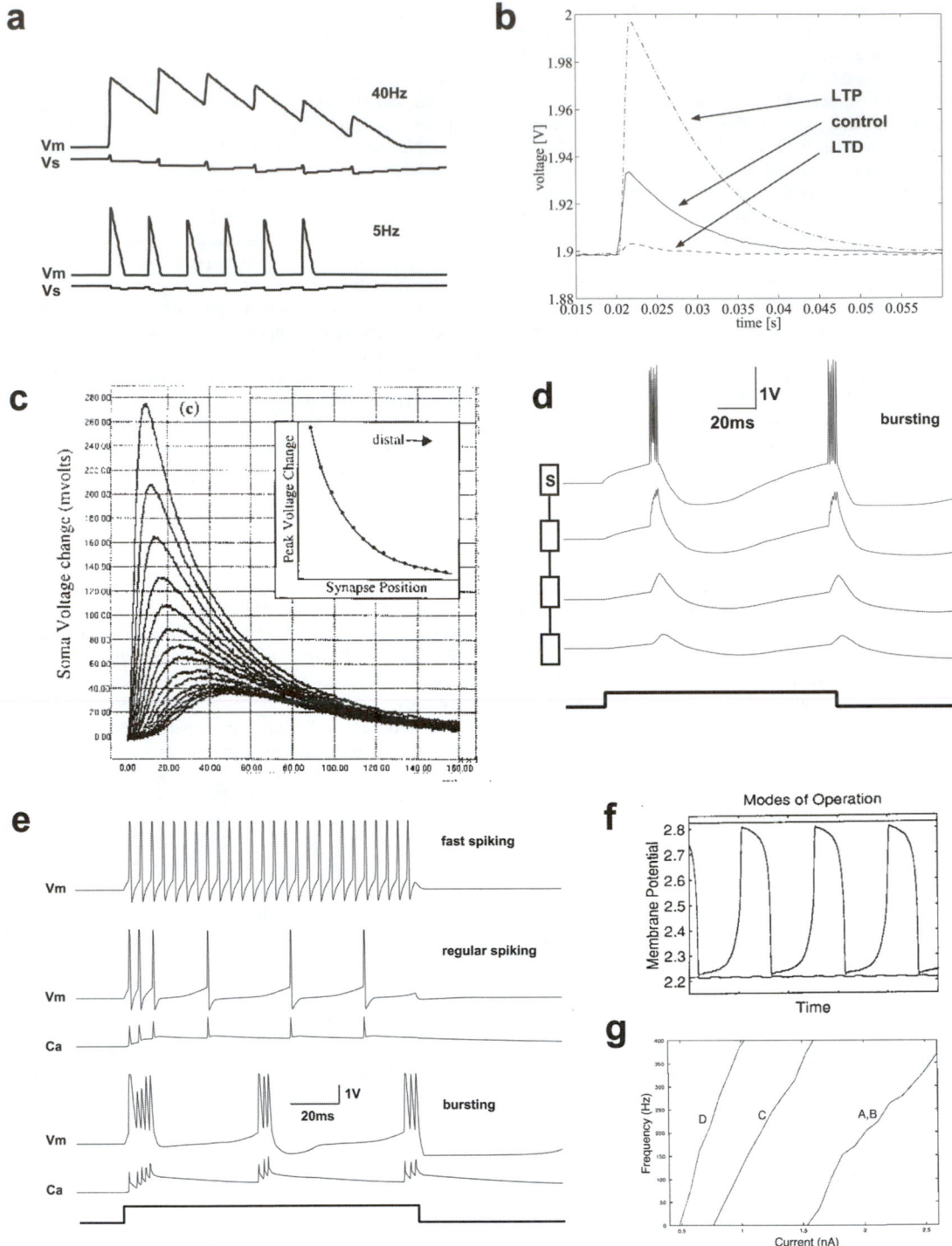

Figure 1. Recording from various silicon synapses, dendrites, and somas. *A*, Short-term depression synapse stimulated at 40 Hz and 5 Hz. *B*, Long-term potentiation (LTP) and depression (LTD). *C*, Excitatory postsynaptic potentials at the soma after spreading along a dendrite. *D*, Backpropagation of somatic bursts into a dendrite containing active conductances (s, soma). *E*, Different spiking modes of a pyramidal cell (Vm, membrane potential; Ca, calcium concentration). *F*, Different spiking modes of a Morris-Lecar neuron. *G*, Modulation of the frequency-current curve of a neuron according to its own input. See text for more details.

Biological neurons communicate with one another through axons that ramify widely to make connections with many target neurons. It is impractical to hardwire every network configuration that one might wish to emulate. Instead, the connectivity of an emulator can be made reconfigurable. One approach is to provide direct connections between neurons that can be configured by sets of switches that are under digital control (Van der Spiegel et al., 1994). This approach requires a large silicon area for the switches, but it has the advantage of continuous communication between neurons. It is appropriate when the neuron output is encoded as a continuous analog variable. An alternative approach is to use the high speed of electrical signals in metal wires to multiplex slow neuronal signals.

Action potential representations of neuronal output are compatible with multiplexing because the output of the neuron is active only during the action potential. Furthermore, the action potential is a digital amplitude signal that can be robustly transmitted between chips. Digital amplitude signals are robust to noise and interchip variability and have been used to advantage in VLSI neural networks (Murray and Tarassenko, 1994). Event-based digital data-encoding methods, such as the address-event representation (AER) (Mahowald, 1994), virtual wires (Elias and Northmore, 1999), and that used by Vittoz et al. (Mortara, Vittoz, and Venier, 1995), broadcast action potential events occurring in neurons onto a common data bus. Many silicon neurons can share the same bus because switching times in CMOS and on the bus are much faster than the switching times of neurons. Events generated by silicon neurons can be broadcast and removed from a data bus at frequen-

cies of more than a megahertz. Therefore, more than 1,000 address-events could be transmitted in the time it takes one neuron to complete a single action potential. Multiplexing strategies are most effective if, as in their biological counterparts, only a small fraction of the silicon neurons embedded in a network are active at any time.

Event-based digital encoding methods facilitate network reconfigurability. These digital multiplexing schemes work by placing on the common communications bus the identity (a digital address) of the neuron generating an action potential. In some implementations, the bus broadcasts this source address to all synapses, which decode the addresses (Figure 2A). In this way those synapses that should be "connected" to the source neuron detect that it has generated an action potential, and they initiate a synaptic input on the dendrite to which they are attached. In other implementations (Deiss, Douglas, and Whatley, 1999), the so-called address-event is translated from a postsynaptic bus to a presynaptic bus through a programmable lookup table that maps the addresses of source neurons to (lists of) destination synapse addresses. The topology of the network is defined by the mapping of source neurons to

a.

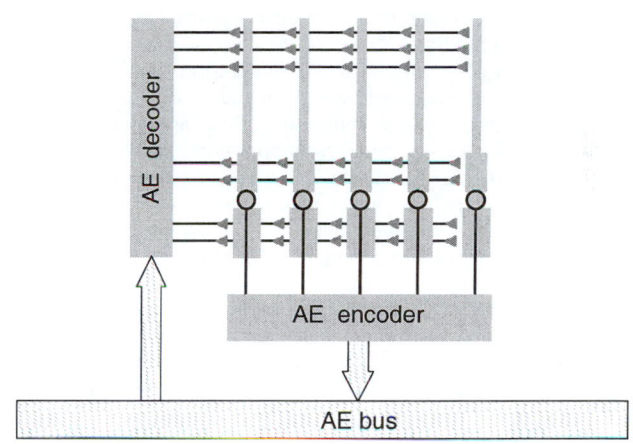

b.   silicon 'cortex'

Figure 2. Connections between silicon neurons based on address-event representation. This figure shows an implementation in which source addresses are broadcast to all synapses, and the synapses decode the addresses. *A*, Multineuron chip attached to an address-event (AE) bus. Action potentials generated by neurons (gray broomsticks) are detected by an on-chip AE encoder that broadcasts the binary addresses of the source neurons on the AE bus. AE decoders activate the destination synapses "connected" to the source neurons. *B*, A silicon retina sends address-events to a number of multineuron chips communicating over a common AE bus in a manner similar to that implemented in the system described in Deiss, Douglas, and Whatley (1999).

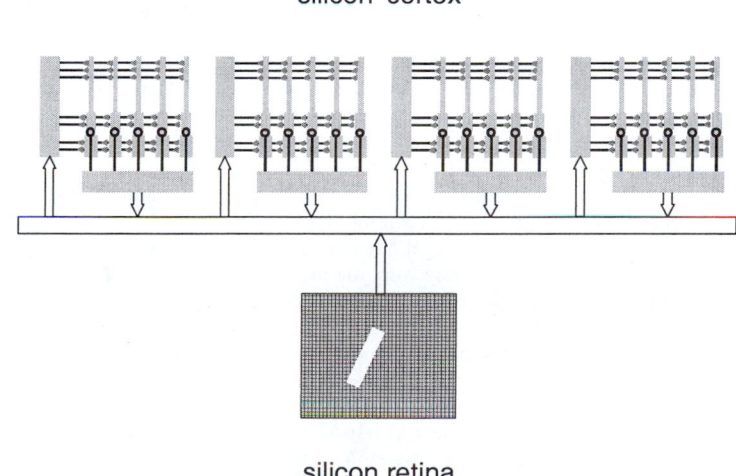

silicon retina

destination synapses as defined by the content of the lookup table.

Synaptic circuits have been developed that approximate AMPA and NMDA (see NMDA RECEPTORS: SYNAPTIC, CELLULAR, AND NETWORK MODELS) excitatory synapses; and also the potassium-mediated and chloride-mediated (shunting) inhibitory synapses (Douglas and Mahowald, 1995). Synaptic response often depends on the history of its own presynaptic input, on a wide range of time scales. We have developed circuits that emulate the short-time-scale synaptic depression (Figure 1A). On longer scales, a spike-based learning synapse has been implemented that modifies its synaptic weight according to the correlation of pre- and postsynaptic spikes (Häfliger and Mahowald, 1999) (Figure 1B).

Working with Analog Silicon

Custom CMOS circuits are created by an iterative process of design, fabrication, and experiment. In the design phase, the correspondence between elements of the analog circuit and those of the neural system are established, and the variable parameters identified. Computer simulations and mathematical analyses of the proposed circuit subunits are useful at this stage. The electronic circuit design is then transposed into a layout design that expresses the circuit as a sandwich of layers in the silicon chip. The layout is drawn with specialized computer-aided design (CAD) software on a workstation or personal computer. The final layout instructions are used by the silicon foundry to fabricate the chip. The MOSIS service at the University of Southern California's Information Sciences Institute (http://www.mosis.org/) accepts layout by electronic mail and returns a fabricated chip in about 10 weeks. Through the MOSIS service, fabrication costs range from approximately $600 for four pieces of a small 2.2×2.2 mm 2.0-μm feature size chip suitable for prototyping a few neurons to $15,000 for 20 pieces of a large 9.4×9.7 mm 1.2-μm feature size chip suitable for fabricating a retina or a network of silicon neurons. The European Union's Europractice initiative offers a similar IC prototyping service (http://www.imec.be/europractice).

It is important to consider the range of desired behaviors when designing the circuits. Within certain limits, the dynamics of the model neurons can be varied parametrically when the neuron is in use. Often, the behavior of analog circuits can be controlled by the voltages applied to the gates of their various transistors. In the Douglas and Mahowald compartmental model neurons, these parameters determine, for example, the temporal dynamics of activation and inactivation, the voltages at which they occur, and the maximum conductance that can be obtained when fully activated. The effect of changing these parameters is immediate. Thus, the electrophysiological "personality" of the silicon neuron can be switched rapidly, for example, from a regular adapting to a bursting pyramidal cell, as in Figure 1E. Of course, only the parameters that were incorporated into the design at the time of fabrication are available for reconfiguring the performance of the neuron. If additional properties are required, another silicon neuron with different morphology or different types of channels can be fabricated using variations of the basic circuit modules.

To produce compact circuits, it may be necessary to make approximations in the design of the circuit modules. For example, the analog conductances may saturate, and hence these neurons would not perform as real neurons if they were clamped at voltages very far away from the resting potential. These errors are insignificant when the cell is operating in the physiological range because the linear regions of the circuits are arranged in such a way that the deviation from true neuronal behavior is minimized within that range.

The circuits constituting the neuron must be arranged spatially on the surface of the chips. One possibility is to distribute the dendritic compartments of individual neurons across multiple chips (Van der Spiegel et al., 1994). This approach is useful because the number of compartments, and hence the number of synaptic inputs to a particular neuron, is not limited by the chip boundaries. However, this division requires a method of transmitting accurately between multiple chips the analog voltages and currents at the compartment boundaries. Even if such analog values are accurately conveyed between chips, the values may be misinterpreted because of the interchip variability, the so-called mismatches, inherent in the technology. The alternative approach of Elias is to fabricate entire silicon neurons, and networks of neurons on the same chip. The single-chip solution is appropriate for networks of simple neurons that have only local connectivity mediated by graded synapses, such as the outer layers of the retina (Mahowald, 1994). It is also appropriate for networks of spiking neurons distributed across multiple chips, where only robust, action potential events need be transmitted between chips. However, the number of neurons that can be fabricated on a single chip is limited and depends on the complexity of the neuron. A large development chip has an area of roughly 100 mm^2. Using 1.2-μm fabrication technology, a retinal chip can accommodate a roughly 100×100 array of simplified photoreceptors together with horizontal cells, bipolar cells, amacrine cells, and retinal ganglion cells (Boahen, 1999). For more comprehensive neurons and more general connectivity, a reasonable target would be a linear array on the order of 100 neurons, each having up to about 10 dendritic compartments. The number of synapses (on the order of 10 to 100) that can be incorporated depends on the size of the synaptic circuits, which in turn depends on their degree of biological realism. There are ways to improve the number of synaptic inputs. One possibility is to map multiple presynaptic inputs into a single postsynaptic circuit. This strategy can raise the effective number of inputs by an order of magnitude. An additional consideration is that as the technology used to implement aVLSI designs continues to evolve toward smaller feature sizes, further improvements in scale can be expected. Nevertheless, an important focus of work must be the development of more compact synapses. Learning synapses that autonomously modify their stored connection strengths in a Hebbian way are another important element of current work (see, e.g., Häfliger and Mahowald, 1999).

Once the chip has been fabricated, its performance is explored using experimental methods similar to those used in a real neurophysiological preparation, except that many more variables can be observed. For example, the response of the analog chip to stimulation is measured in real time with an oscilloscope. Except for the variable parameters included in the design, the circuits cannot be altered after fabrication, and so errors in the specification of the neuron cannot be corrected as easily as in software simulations. Also, care must be taken to plan experiments before the chip is fabricated so that instrumentation circuitry can be included to observe the state of interesting analog variables. The designs of circuits evolve with understanding gained by experiment.

Discussion

A number of groups are currently investigating the properties of analog silicon neurons in networks. At the time of this writing, the scale of these networks ranges from tens of neurons to several thousands of neurons. The next 5 years should see increases in the number of neurons implemented in a single system, owing both to an improvement in the basic fabrication technology and to improved implementations. The optimal degree of biological realism is an open question and is likely to be task dependent. Furthermore, the cost of a computational element ultimately depends on the device physics of the computational primitives, so that more effective methods for performing a computation may eventually become available. The most promising path for the development of these networks is interfacing them to sensors and effectors that can interact dynamically with the real world. Analog VLSI is not the only way to build such systems, but it does have some striking advantages. Analog emulation is inherently parallel, the circuits are extremely compact by comparison with a digital circuit performing an equivalent computation, and the power consumption is often a few orders of magnitude less than their digital equivalents. These properties lend themselves to the construction of small, autonomous neuromorphic systems that can interact directly with the world and so provide a platform for studying animal behaviors by emulation.

In Memoriam. We dedicate this article to our late colleague and co-author, Misha Mahowald.

Road Map: Implementation and Analysis
Background: Single-Cell Models
Related Reading: Analog VLSI Implementations of Neural Networks; Biophysical Mechanisms in Neuronal Modeling; Digital VLSI for Neural Networks; Neuromorphic VLSI Circuits and Systems

References

Boahen, K. A., 1999, Retinomorphic chips that see quadruple images, in *Proceedings of the 7th International Conference on Microelectronics for Neural, Fuzzy and Bio-inspired Systems (MicroNeuro '99)*, Los Alamitos, CA: IEEE Computer Society Press, pp. 12–20.

Deiss, S. R., Douglas, R. J., and Whatley, A. M., 1999, A pulse-coded communications infrastructure for neuromorphic systems, in *Pulsed Neural Networks* (W. Maass and C. M. Bishop, Eds.), Cambridge, MA: MIT Press, chap. 6, pp. 157–178.

Douglas, R., and Mahowald, M., 1995, A construction set for silicon neurons, in *An Introduction to Neural and Electronic Networks*, 2nd ed. (S. F. Zornetzer, J. L. Davis, C. Lau, and T. McKenna, Eds.), San Diego, CA: Academic Press, chap. 14, pp. 277–296. ◆

Dupeyron, D., Le Masson, S., Deval, Y., Le Masson, G., and Dom, J.-P., 1996, A BiCMOS implementation of the Hodgkin-Huxley formalism, in *Proceedings of the Fifth International Conference on Microelectronics for Neural Networks and Fuzzy Systems*, Los Alamitos, CA: IEEE Computer Society Press, pp. 311–316.

Elias, J. G., and Northmore, D. P. M., 1999, Building silicon nervous systems with dendritic tree neuromorphs, in *Pulsed Neural Networks* (W. Maass and C. M. Bishop, Eds.), Cambridge, MA: MIT Press, chap. 5, pp. 135–156.

Häfliger, P., and Mahowald, M., 1999, Spike based normalizing Hebbian learning in an analog VLSI artificial neuron, *Analog Integrated Circuits and Signal Processing 18*, Special issue: *Learning on Silicon*, 2/3:133–139.

Koch, C., and Segev, I., Eds., 1998, *Methods in Neuronal Modelling: From Ions to Networks*, 2nd ed., Cambridge, MA: MIT Press.

Linares-Barranco, B., Sanchez-Sinencio, E., Rodriguez-Vazquez, A., and Huertas, J. L., 1991, A CMOS implementation of FitzHugh-Nagumo neuron model, *IEEE J. Solid-State Circuits*, 26:956–965.

Mahowald, M., 1994, *An Analog VLSI System for Stereoscopic Vision*, Boston, MA: Kluwer Academic. ◆

Mahowald, M. A., and Douglas, R. J., 1991, A silicon neuron, *Nature*, 354:515–518.

Mead, C., 1989, *Analog VLSI and Neural Systems*, Reading, MA: Addison-Wesley. ◆

Mortara, A., Vittoz, E. A., and Venier, P., 1995, A communication scheme for analog VLSI perceptive systems, *IEEE J. Solid-State Circuits*, 30:660–669.

Murray, A., and Tarassenko, L., 1994, *Analogue Neural VLSI*, London: Chapman and Hall.

Patel, G. N., and DeWeerth, S. P., 1997, An analogue VLSI Morris-Lecar neuron, *Electron. Lett. IEEE*, 33:997–998.

Shin, J., and Koch, C., 1999, Dynamic range and sensitivity adaptation in a silicon spiking neuron, *IEEE Trans. Neural Netw.*, 10:1232–1238.

Van der Spiegel, J., Donham, C., Etienne-Cummings, R., Fernando, S., Mueller, P., and Blackman, D., 1994, Large scale analog neural computer with programmable architecture and programmable time constants for temporal pattern analysis, in *Proceedings of the International Conference on Neural Networks*, vol. III, Orlando, FL: IEEE, pp. 1830–1835.

Simulated Annealing and Boltzmann Machines

Emile H. L. Aarts and Jan H. M. Korst

Introduction

Simulated annealing was introduced in the 1980s by Kirkpatrick, Gelatt, and Vecchi (1983) and Černý (1985) as a local search approach to handle hard combinatorial optimization problems. The approach is based on randomized techniques that are quite similar to the Monte Carlo methods used in statistical physics. The origin of the method lies in the physical annealing process, which is used to find low-energy states of solids. Since its introduction, simulated annealing has been extensively used in a remarkably broad range of applications, including computer engineering, molecular physics, biology, chemistry, and cognitive engineering. Meanwhile, the approach has established a strong position as a successful optimization tool. In this article, we concentrate on what is known as *basic simulated annealing*, thus discarding the wealth of generalized approaches that have been developed. (The interested reader is referred to Aarts and Korst, 1989, 2001.)

Boltzmann machines were introduced by Hinton and Sejnowski (1983) as a class of artificial neural networks that can be viewed as an extension of discrete Hopfield networks (Hopfield, 1982) in two ways. First, they replace the greedy local search dynamics of Hopfield networks with a randomized local search dynamics. Second, they replace the relatively simple Hebbian learning rule with a more powerful stochastic learning algorithm. Boltzmann machines are randomized neural networks that implement computational features similar to those used in simulated annealing. The resulting neural networks can perform optimization, classification, and learning tasks. Boltzmann machines apply massive parallelism and adaptive adjustment of neural states and interneural connection weights through the self-organization of stochastic computing elements. This class of neural networks is interesting for three reasons. First, it offers a generalized approach to the three basic connectionist issues, i.e., search, representation, and learning (Hinton, 1989). Second, it is supported by a mathematical formalism that facilitates analysis of the network's dynamics and learning properties. Third, it is relatively easy to implement in hardware. Again, we restrict ourselves in this article to a presentation of the basic properties. For a more elaborate treatment we refer to Zwietering and Aarts (1991).

There is a close relation between simulated annealing and Boltzmann machines. Boltzmann machines can be viewed as a massively parallel implementation of simulated annealing, thus offering a means to speed up considerably the slow convergence of sequential simulated annealing implementations. Moreover, simulated annealing is the built-in self-organization technique of a Boltzmann machine, thus providing this class of neural networks with a powerful stochastic learning and retrieval mechanism.

Simulated Annealing

The use of simulated annealing presupposes the definition of a combinatorial optimization problem and a neighborhood. A *combinatorial optimization problem* is a set of problem instances where each *instance* is a pair $(\mathcal{S}, f)$ with $\mathcal{S}$ the set of feasible solutions and $f : \mathcal{S} \to \mathbb{Z}$ a cost function that assigns a cost value to each solution. The problem is to find a *globally optimal solution*, i.e., an $i^* \in \mathcal{S}$ such that $f(i^*) \leq f(i)$, for all $i \in \mathcal{S}$. Furthermore, $f^* = f(i^*)$ denotes the optimal cost value, and $\mathcal{S}^* = \{i \in \mathcal{S} | f(i) = f^*\}$ denotes the set of optimal solutions. A *neighborhood function* is a mapping $\mathcal{N} : \mathcal{S} \to 2^{\mathcal{S}}$, which defines for each solution $i \in \mathcal{S}$ a set $\mathcal{N}(i) \subseteq \mathcal{S}$ of solutions that are in some sense close to i. The set $\mathcal{N}(i)$ is called the *neighborhood* of solution i, and each $j \in \mathcal{N}(i)$ is called a *neighbor* of i. We shall assume that $i \in \mathcal{N}(i)$ for all $i \in \mathcal{S}$. A solution $\hat{i} \in \mathcal{S}$ is *locally optimal (minimal)* with respect to $\mathcal{N}$ if

$$f(\hat{i}) \leq f(j) \quad \text{for all } j \in \mathcal{N}(\hat{i})$$

The set of locally optimal solutions is denoted by $\hat{\mathcal{S}}$.

Roughly speaking, simulated annealing starts with an initial solution in $\mathcal{S}$ and then continually tries to find better solutions by searching neighborhoods and applying a stochastic acceptance criterion. This is laid out schematically in Figure 1. The procedure INITIALIZE selects a start solution from $\mathcal{S}$, GENERATE selects a solution from the neighborhood of the current solution, and STOP evaluates a stop criterion that determines termination of the algorithm.

Simulated annealing continually selects a neighbor of a current solution and compares the difference in cost between these solutions to a threshold. If the cost difference is within the threshold, the neighbor replaces the current solution. Otherwise, the search continues with the current solution. The sequence $(t_k | k = 0, 1, 2, \ldots)$ denotes the thresholds where t_k is used at iteration k of the algorithm and is given by a random variable with expected value $\mathbb{E}(t_k) = c_k \in \mathbb{R}^+$, $k = 0, 1, 2, \ldots$. The thresholds t_k follow a probability distribution function F_{c_k} over $\mathbb{R}^+$. Simulated annealing uses randomized thresholds with values between zero and infinity, and the probability of a threshold t_k being at most $y \in \mathbb{R}^+$ is given by $\mathbb{P}_{c_k}\{t_k \leq y\} = F_{c_k}(y)$. This implies that each neighboring solution can be chosen with a finite probability to replace the current solution.

The basic simulated annealing version of Kirkpatrick et al. (1983) and Černý (1985) takes for F_{c_k} the negative exponential distribution with parameter $1/c_k$. This choice is identical to the following *acceptance criterion*. For any two solutions $i, j \in \mathcal{S}$, the probability of accepting j from i at the kth iteration is given by

$$\mathbb{P}_{c_k}\{\text{accept } j\} = \begin{cases} 1 & \text{if } f(j) \leq f(i) \\ \exp\left(\dfrac{f(i) - f(j)}{c_k}\right) & \text{if } f(j) > f(i) \end{cases} \quad (1)$$

The parameter c_k is used in the simulated annealing algorithm as a *control parameter*, and it plays an important role in the conver-

gence of the algorithm. A characteristic feature of simulated annealing is that, besides accepting improvements in cost, it also accepts, to a limited extent, deteriorations in cost. Initially, at large values of c, large deteriorations are accepted; as c decreases, only smaller deteriorations are accepted, and finally, as the value of c approaches 0, no deteriorations at all are accepted. Arbitrarily large deteriorations are accepted with positive probability; for these deteriorations, however, the acceptance probability is small.

The Relation with Physics

The origin of simulated annealing and the choice of the acceptance criterion can be found in the physical annealing process. In *condensed matter physics*, annealing is a thermal process for obtaining low-energy states of a solid in a *heat bath*. It consists of the following two steps: first, the temperature of the heat bath is increased to a high value, at which the solid melts; second, the temperature is carefully decreased until the particles of the melted solid arrange themselves in the ground state of the solid. In the liquid phase, all particles of the solid arrange themselves randomly. In the ground state, the particles are arranged in a highly structured lattice, and the energy of the system is minimal.

The physical annealing process can be modeled successfully by computer simulation methods based on *Monte Carlo techniques* such as first proposed by Metropolis et al. (1953), who gave a simple algorithm for simulating the evolution of a solid in a heat bath to *thermal equilibrium*. The analogy between the annealing of a physical many-particle system and the application of simulated annealing to a combinatorial optimization problem is obvious: solutions in a combinatorial optimization problem are equivalent to states of the physical system; the cost of a solution is equivalent to the energy of a state, and transitions to neighbors are equivalent to state changes. The control parameter plays the role of the temperature.

Asymptotic Convergence

Simulated annealing can be viewed as a sampling process whose outcomes are neighboring solutions. This class of processes can be mathematically modeled using finite Markov chains. Let $\mathbb{O}$ denote a set of possible outcomes of a sampling process. A *Markov chain* is a sequence of *trials* satisfying the *Markov property*, which states that the probability of the outcome of a given trial depends only on the outcome of the previous trial. In the case of simulated annealing, a trial corresponds to a transition, and the set of outcomes is given by the finite set of solutions.

The convergence of simulated annealing follows from the *stationarity* property of Markov chains and can be formulated as follows. Let $(\mathcal{S}, f)$ be an instance of a combinatorial optimization problem and $\mathcal{N}$ a neighborhood function that is defined in such a way that any two solutions in $\mathcal{S}$ can be reached from each other in a finite number of steps. Then the Markov chain associated with basic simulated annealing has a stationary distribution $q(c)$, whose components denote the probability of finding a solution $i \in \mathcal{S}$ after a large number of trials at control parameter value c. The components are given by

$$q_i(c) = \frac{|\mathcal{N}(i)| \exp(-f(i)/c)}{\sum_{j \in \mathcal{S}} |\mathcal{N}(j)| \exp(-f(j)/c)} \quad \text{for all } i \in \mathcal{S} \quad (2)$$

Furthermore,

$$q_i^* \overset{def}{=} \lim_{c \downarrow 0} q_i(c) = \begin{cases} \dfrac{1}{|\mathcal{S}^*|} & \text{if } i \in \mathcal{S}^* \\ 0 & \text{otherwise} \end{cases} \quad (3)$$

where $\mathcal{S}^*$ denotes the set of optimal solutions.

```
procedure SIMULATED_ANNEALING;
begin
    INITIALIZE (i_start);
    i := i_start;
    k := 0;
    repeat
        GENERATE ( j from N(i));
        if f(j) − f(i) < t_k then i := j;
        k := k + 1;
    until STOP;
end
```

Figure 1. Pseudocode of the basic simulated annealing algorithm.

Cooling Schedules

The theoretical results just presented imply convergence to optimality after an infinite number of trials. A finite-time implementation of the algorithm, which, as a consequence of the above, can no longer guarantee finding an optimal solution, may result in a much faster execution of the algorithm without giving in too much on the solution quality. A *finite-time* implementation of simulated annealing is obtained by generating a sequence of homogeneous Markov chains of finite length at descending values of the control parameter (Aarts and Korst, 1989). For this, a set of parameters must be specified that governs the convergence of the algorithm. This set of parameters is referred to as a *cooling schedule*. It specifies

- an *initial value* of the control parameter,
- a *decrement function* for lowering the value of the control parameter,
- a *final value* of the control parameter (implicitly), specified by a *stop criterion*, and
- a finite *length* of each homogeneous Markov chain.

Typical cooling schedules in simulated annealing start at sufficiently large initial values of the control parameter, thus allowing acceptance of virtually all proposed transitions. Next, the decrement function and the Markov chain lengths are chosen such that at the end of each individual Markov chain, the probability distribution of the solutions is close to the stationary distribution, which is referred to as *quasi-equilibrium*. Since at large values of c, the probability distribution of the solutions equals the stationary distribution by definition (cf. Equation 2), one may expect that the cooling schedule enables the probability distribution to "closely follow" the stationary distributions, so that, as $c \downarrow 0$, the probability distribution is close to q^*, the uniform distribution on the set of optimal solutions given by Equation 3. It is intuitively clear that large decrements in c require longer Markov chains in order to restore quasi-equilibrium at the next value of the control parameter. Thus, there is a trade-off between large decrements of the control parameter and small Markov chain lengths. Usually, one chooses small decrements in c to avoid extremely long chains, but alternatively, one could use large values for the Markov chain length in order to be able to make large decrements in c.

The search for adequate cooling schedules has been the subject of many studies over the past years. The interested reader is referred to Aarts and Korst (2001).

Issues from Practice

During its 20 years of existence, simulated annealing has been applied to a large variety of problems, ranging from practical, real-life problems to theoretical test problems. VLSI design, atomic and molecular physics, and picture processing are the three problem areas in which simulated annealing is probably most frequently applied. The set of theoretical test problems includes almost all of the well-known problems in discrete mathematics and operations research, such as coding, graph coloring, graph partitioning, and sequencing and scheduling problems (see Aarts and Lenstra, 1997). General overviews of applications of simulated annealing are given by Aarts and Korst (1989) and Collins, Eglese, and Golden (1988).

Broadly speaking, after 20 years of practical experience, it is widely accepted that simulated annealing can find good solutions for a wide variety of problems, but often at the cost of substantial running times. As a result, the true merits of the algorithm become obvious in industrial problem settings, where running times are of

little or no concern. As an example, we mention design problems, since in those cases one is primarily interested in finding high-quality solutions, whereas design time often plays only a minor role. A well-known successful simulated annealing area in this respect is VLSI design.

Boltzmann Machines

A Boltzmann machine is a neural network consisting of a set $\mathcal{U}$ of two-state neurons that are interconnected by a set $\mathcal{C}$ of weighted symmetric connections. A neuron $u \in \mathcal{U}$ can be in one of two states: either it is firing, corresponding to state 1, or it is not firing, corresponding to state -0. A *configuration* k is a $|\mathcal{U}|$-dimensional vector that describes the global state of the neural network. The state of an individual neuron u in configuration k is given by $k(u)$. The set of all configurations is denoted by $\mathcal{R}$. A connection $\{u, v\} \in \mathcal{C}$ is *activated* in a given configuration k if both u and v have state 1, i.e., if $k(u) \cdot k(v) = 1$. The set of connections may contain self-connections whose role is similar to that of thresholds in classical neural networks, i.e., $\{\{u, u\} \mid u \in \mathcal{U}\} \subset \mathcal{C}$. A weight $w_{u,v} \in \mathbb{R}$ is associated with the connection between neurons u and v. By definition, $w_{u,v} = w_{v,u}$ for each pair $u, v \in \mathcal{U}$. The weight is a quantitative measure of the *desirability* that $\{u, v\}$ be activated. If $w_{u,v} > 0$, it is desirable that $\{u, v\}$ be activated; if $w_{u,v} < 0$, it is undesirable. Connections with a positive (negative) weight are called *excitatory* (*inhibitory*). The *energy function* $E : \mathcal{R} \to \mathbb{R}$ assigns to each configuration k a real number, called the *energy*, which equals the negated sum of the weights of the activated connections, i.e.,

$$E(k) = - \sum_{\{u,v\} \in \mathcal{C}} w_{u,v} k(u) k(v) \qquad (4)$$

Generally speaking, the energy is low if many excitatory connections are activated and is high if many inhibitory connections are activated. The energy is a global measure indicating to what extent the neurons in the network have reached a consensus about their individual states, subject to the individual weights. Since the weights impose local constraints, these networks are also often called *constraint satisfaction networks* (Hinton and Sejnowski, 1983). The basic idea of implementing local constraints as connection weights in networks dates back to the work of Moussouris (1974).

Network Dynamics

Self-organization in a Boltzmann machine is achieved by allowing neurons to change their states from 0 to 1 or the reverse. Let the network be in configuration k. Then a *state change* of neuron u results in a configuration l, with $l(u) = 1 - k(u)$ and $l(v) = k(v)$ for each $v \neq u$. Furthermore, let $\mathcal{C}_u$ denote the set of connections incident with neuron u, excluding $\{u, u\}$. Then the *difference in energy* $\Delta E_k(u) = E(l) - E(k)$ induced by a state change of neuron u in configuration k is given by

$$\Delta E_k(u) = (2k(u) - 1)\left(w_{u,u} + \sum_{\{u,v\} \in \mathcal{C}_u} w_{u,v} k(v)\right) \qquad (5)$$

The effect on the energy, resulting from a state change of neuron u, is completely determined by the states of its adjacent neurons and the corresponding connection weights. Consequently, each neuron can locally evaluate its state change, since no global calculations are required.

In a Boltzmann machine, the response of an individual state change of neuron u to its adjacent neurons in a configuration k is a stochastic function that is given by

$\mathbb{P}_c\{$accept a state change of neuron $u \mid k\}$

$$= \frac{1}{1 + \exp\left(-\Delta E_k(u)/c\right)} \quad (6)$$

where $\Delta E_k(u)$ is given by Equation 5 and $c \in \mathbb{R}^+$ again denotes the control parameter.

State changes in a Boltzmann machine are governed by simulated annealing. For the sake of presentation, we distinguish between two models, *sequential Boltzmann machines* and *parallel Boltzmann machines*.

Sequential Boltzmann machines. In a sequential Boltzmann machine, neurons may change their states only one at a time. The resulting iterative procedure can be described as a sequence of Markov chains where each chain consists of a sequence of trials and the outcome of a given trial depends probabilistically only on the outcome of the previous trial. A *trial* consists of two steps: given a configuration k, first a neighboring configuration k_u is generated, determined by a neuron $u \in \mathcal{U}$ that proposes a state change. Second, whether or not k_u is accepted is evaluated. If it is accepted, the outcome of the trial is k_u; otherwise it is k. If the probability of accepting a state change is given by the response function of Equation 6, we obtain the following result, which is analogous to the results of Equations 2 and 3. Given a sequential Boltzmann machine with a response function given by Equation 6, then the following two statements hold:

1. The probability $q(c)$ of obtaining a configuration k after a sufficiently large number of trails carried out at a fixed value of c is given by

$$q_k(c) = \frac{\exp\left(C_k/c\right)}{\sum_{l \in \mathcal{R}} \exp\left(C_l/c\right)} \quad (7)$$

2. For $c \downarrow 0$, Equation 7 reduces to a uniform distribution over the set of configurations with minimum energy.

Parallel Boltzmann machines. To model parallelism in a Boltzmann machine, we distinguish between synchronous and asynchronous parallelism. In *synchronous parallelism*, sets of state changes are scheduled in successive trials, where each trial consists of a number of individual state changes. During each trial, a neuron is allowed to propose a state change exactly once. Synchronous parallelism requires a global clocking scheme to control the synchronization. For an extensive treatment of synchronously parallel Boltzmann machines and related work, see Little and Shaw (1978), Peretto (1984), and Zwietering and Aarts (1991). Here, we briefly summarize the most important results. The main result is a conjecture, which states that under certain mild conditions a stationary distribution different from Equation 7 is attained, which converges as c approaches 0 to a distribution over the set of configurations for which the so-called *extended consensus* is maximal, where the extended consensus is a modified energy function. A proof of this conjecture is an open problem. However, for two special cases, correctness can be proved. These are the cases of *limited parallelism*, where neurons may change their states simultaneously only if they are not adjacent, and *full parallelism*, where in each trial all neurons may change their states simultaneously.

In *asynchronous parallelism*, state changes are evaluated concurrently and independently. Units generate state changes and accept or reject them on the basis of information that is not necessarily up to date, since the states of adjacent neurons may have changed in the meantime. Asynchronous parallelism does not require a global clocking scheme, which is of advantage in hardware implementations. However, this type of parallelism cannot be mod-

eled by Markov chains but requires a completely different approach, and so far little progress has been made in this direction. A brief discussion on the subject can be found in Aarts and Korst (1989).

Combinatorial Optimization and Classification

The ability of a Boltzmann machine to obtain low-energy configurations can be used to handle combinatorial optimization (CO) and classification problems.

Combinatorial optimization. A Boltzmann machine can be used to solve CO problems by defining a correspondence between the configurations of the Boltzmann machine and the solutions of the CO problem in such a way that the cost function of the CO problem is transformed into the energy function associated with the Boltzmann machine. In general, this can be done by formulating the CO problem as a 0–1 integer programming problem. The values of the 0–1 variables correspond to the states of the neurons. The cost function and the constraints that go with the CO problem are implemented by choosing the appropriate connections and their weights. In this way, minimizing the energy in the Boltzmann machine is equivalent to solving the corresponding CO problem. More specifically, it is often possible to construct a Boltzmann machine such that the following properties hold:

1. Each locally minimal configuration of the Boltzmann machine corresponds to a feasible solution.
2. The lower the energy of the corresponding configuration, the better the cost of the corresponding feasible solution.

These properties imply that a feasible solution can be obtained and that configurations with near-minimal values of the energy function correspond to near-optimal solutions of the CO problem. This feature enables Boltzmann machines to be used for approximation purposes, as we have demonstrated for several well-known problems, including the traveling salesman problem, graph coloring, and independent set (Aarts and Korst, 1989).

Classification. A classification problem can be formalized as a pair $(\mathbb{O}, \mathcal{S})$, where $\mathbb{O}$ denotes a set of *objects* and $\mathcal{S}$ a collection of disjoint subsets $\mathcal{S}_1, \ldots, \mathcal{S}_l$ that partition $\mathbb{O}$. The problem is to determine for a given object $o \in \mathbb{O}$ the subset $\mathcal{S}_j \subset \mathcal{S}$ to which it belongs. In practice, the set of objects is usually very large, and providing an explicit description of each subset is impracticable. The subsets are therefore often implicitly described by specifying a number of "typical" examples for each subset. To use a Boltzmann machine for solving classification problems, the set of neurons is subdivided into three disjoint subsets, $\mathcal{U}_i$, $\mathcal{U}_h$, and $\mathcal{U}_o$, denoting the sets of *input, hidden,* and *output neurons*, respectively. The states of the input neurons are fixed by some *input pattern*. This pattern is a coded representation of an object $o \in \mathbb{O}$ that is to be classified. The remaining neurons then adjust their states to minimize the energy, subject to the fixed states of the input neurons. After minimization of the energy, the states of the output neurons represent the subset $\mathcal{S}_j$ to which o is thought to belong. In this way, a Boltzmann machine can implement a given input-output function.

To implement a given input-output function on the input and output neurons, hidden neurons are usually required in addition. The minimum number of hidden neurons required to solve a given classification problem strongly depends on the intrinsic complexity of the input-output function that is to be implemented (Aarts and Korst, 1989). For classification problems, choosing appropriate connection weights is often difficult, since different items may give rise to conflicting connection weights. However, a Boltzmann machine can often acquire a given input-output function by learning from examples, as shown in the next section.

Learning

Learning in a Boltzmann machine takes place by examples that fix the states of the *environmental neurons*, i.e., the input and output neurons. The hidden neurons are used to construct an internal representation that captures the regularities of the examples fixing the states of the environmental neurons. The learning algorithm we discuss starts by setting all connection weights equal to zero. Next, a sequence of learning cycles is completed, each consisting of two phases. In the first phase, or the *fixed phase*, examples of a given input-output function successively fix the states of the environmental neurons, and for each example the Boltzmann machine is equilibrated using the current set of connection weights. In the second phase, the *free-running phase*, all neurons are free to adjust their state, and again the Boltzmann machine is equilibrated. In both phases, we assume the Boltzmann machine to use limited parallelism. At the end of each learning cycle the connection weights are modified using statistical information obtained from the two phases. This process is continued until the average change, over a number of learning cycles, of the connection weights approaches zero. If the learning is successfully completed, then the Boltzmann machine is able to complete a partial example, i.e., a situation where only a subset of the environmental neurons is fixed, by minimizing the energy. In this way a Boltzmann machine not only can reproduce given examples but also is often capable of classifying correctly objects that in some sense resemble the objects that are used during learning.

Extension of the network structure.   The set of environmental neurons is denoted by $\mathcal{U}_{io} = \mathcal{U}_i \cup \mathcal{U}_o$. An *environmental configuration* l is determined by the states of the neurons $u \in \mathcal{U}_{io}$. The state of an environmental neuron u in an environmental configuration l is denoted by $q_l(u)$. $\mathcal{Q}$ denotes the set of all environmental configurations. With each environmental configuration l, a subspace $\mathcal{Q}_l$ can be associated given by

$$\mathcal{Q}_l = \{k \in \mathcal{R} \mid \forall u \in \mathcal{U}_{io} : r_k(u) = q_l(u)\}$$

which consists of all configurations for which the states of the environmental neurons are given by l.

The *learning set* $\mathcal{T}$ consists of the environmental configurations that can be used to fix the environmental neurons during learning. Clearly, $\mathcal{T} \subseteq \mathcal{Q}$.

Toward a learning algorithm.   Here we discuss the basic elements of the Boltzmann machine learning algorithm proposed by Ackley, Hinton, and Sejnowski (1985). The objective of the learning algorithm is to modify the connection weights such that a Boltzmann machine in a free-running phase tends, with a large probability, to be in those environmental configurations that belong to the learning set. To this end we introduce two probability distributions, d and d', defined over the set of environmental configurations. d_l is the probability of obtaining an environmental configuration l in a fixed phase. d'_l is the probability of obtaining an environmental configuration l in a free-running phase. The probability distribution d is determined by the environmental configurations in the learning set and by the frequency at which they are used to fix the environmental neurons. d_l is large if l belongs to the learning set, and l is frequently used to fix the environmental neurons. The probability distribution d' depends on the connection weights and, as is pointed out below, d' can be defined by using the stationary distribution of Equation 7. The objective of the learning algorithm can be formulated as follows: *modify the connection weights of the Boltzmann machine such that d' is close to d. If $d \approx d'$, then the Boltz-*

mann machine can determine for a given input the corresponding output. More generally, if a subset of the environmental neurons is fixed, then the Boltzmann machine can determine the most probable corresponding environmental configuration.

An information-theoretic measure of the distance between the two probability distributions d and d' is the divergence G (Kullback, 1959), given by

$$G = \sum_{l \in \mathcal{Q}} d_l \ln \frac{d_l}{d'_l} \tag{8}$$

It can be shown that $G = 0$ if and only if $d_l = d'_l$ for all $l \in \mathcal{Q}$, and $G > 0$ otherwise. For further properties of G, we refer to Aarts and Korst (1989). The objective of the learning algorithm can be rephrased as: *minimize G by modifying the connection weights.*

Before we describe how G is minimized, we re-address the network dynamics. Using Equation 7, we know that after equilibration in a free-running phase, the Boltzmann machine tends to be in low-energy configurations. If equilibrium is achieved, d'_l is given by

$$d'_l(c) = \sum_{k \in \mathcal{Q}_l} q_k(c)$$

where $q_k(c)$ are the components of the stationary distribution given by Equation 7. The partial derivative of G with respect to $w_{u,v}$ can be written as

$$\frac{\partial G}{\partial w_{u,v}} = \frac{p'_{u,v} - p_{u,v}}{c} \tag{9}$$

where $p_{u,v}$ and $p'_{u,v}$ denote the probabilities of connection $\{u, v\}$ being activated at equilibrium in the fixed and the free-running phases, respectively (see, e.g., Aarts and Korst, 1989). To minimize G, it suffices to collect statistics on $p_{u,v}$ and $p'_{u,v}$, and to iteratively change the connection weight proportionally to the difference between the probabilities, i.e.,

$$w_{u,v} := w_{u,v} + \eta(p'_{u,v} - p_{u,v}) \tag{10}$$

where $\eta \in \mathbb{R}^+$ is called the *learning parameter*.

Informally speaking, the learning algorithm consists of the following steps:

1. Set all connection weights to zero.
2. Complete a number of learning cycles, until $d \approx d'$, where each learning cycle consists of the following steps:
   a. Fixed phase: use a number of examples to fix the environmental neurons, equilibrate for each example, and collect statistics on $p_{u,v}$.
   b. Free-running phase: equilibrate and collect statistics on $p'_{u,v}$.
   c. Modify connection weights.

By definition, environmental configurations l not included in the learning set $\mathcal{T}$ have a corresponding probability $d_l = 0$. Consequently, G is not properly defined for these environmental configurations unless $d'_l = 0$, which can only be realized by infinitely large connection weights, owing to the stochastic nature of the Boltzmann machine optimization. To avoid this problem, a *noise ratio* is introduced that allows the environmental neurons in the fixed phase to change their states with a certain probability. Furthermore, the use of noise suppresses the unlimited growth of connection weights. This was found to be essential for obtaining good results.

The average case performance and time complexity of the learning algorithm depend on the following issues:

1. The parameters of the learning algorithm, viz., the cooling schedule, the learning parameter, noise ratio, and the number of examples per cycle.

2. The ratio between the environmental and the hidden neurons.
3. The way the neurons are connected.
4. The intrinsic difficulty of a given classification problem.

Many studies in the literature have considered the influence of these issues on the performance of the learning algorithm. Most of these studies were based on experimental evaluations. The overall conclusion is that learning in a Boltzmann machine is rather slow. This is essentially due to the time needed to equilibrate and collect statistics. Several approaches that might speed up the learning algorithm have been proposed, including hardware acceleration, multivalued neurons, and higher-order choices for the energy function. For further reading refer to Aarts and Korst (1989).

Road Map: Learning in Artificial Networks
Background: Computing with Attractors
Related Reading: Statistical Mechanics of Neural Networks

References

Aarts, E. H. L., and Korst, J. H. M., 1989, *Simulated Annealing and Boltzmann Machines*, New York: Wiley. ◆
Aarts, E. H. L., and Korst, J. H. M., 2001, Selected topics in simulated annealing, in *Essays and Surveys in Metaheuristics* (C. Ribeiro and P. Hansen, Eds.), Boston: Kluwer, pp. 1–37.
Aarts, E. H. L., and Lenstra, J. K., Eds., 1997, *Local Search in Combinatorial Optimization*, New York: Wiley.

Ackley, D. H., Hinton, G. E., and Sejnowski, T. J., 1985, A learning algorithm for Boltzmann machines, *Cognit. Sci.*, 9:147–169. ◆
Černý, V., 1985, Thermodynamical approach to the traveling salesman problem: An efficient simulation algorithm, *J. Optimiz. Theory Appl.*, 45:41–51.
Collins, N. E., Eglese, R. W., and Golden, B. L., 1988, Simulated annealing: An annotated bibliography, *Am. J. Math. Manag. Sci.*, 8:209–307.
Hinton, G. E., 1989, Connectionist learning procedures, *Artif. Intell.*, 40:185–234.
Hinton, G. E., and Sejnowski, T. J., 1983, Optimal perceptual inference, in *Proceedings of the IEEE Conference on Computer Vision and Pattern Recognition*, pp. 448–453.
Hopfield, J. J., 1982, Neural networks and physical systems with emergent collective computational abilities, *Proc. Natl. Acad. Sci. USA*, 79:2554–2558. ◆
Kirkpatrick, S., Gelatt, C. D., Jr., and Vecchi, M. P., 1983, Optimization by simulated annealing, *Science*, 220:671–680.
Kullback, S., 1959, *Information Theory and Statistics*, New York: Wiley. ◆
Little, W. A., and Shaw, G. L., 1978, Analytic study of the memory storage capability of a neural network, *Math. Biosci.*, 39:281–290.
Metropolis, M., Rosenbluth, A., Rosenbluth, M., Teller, A., and Teller, E., 1953, Equation of state calculations by fast computing machines, *J. Chem. Phys.*, 21:1087–1092. ◆
Moussouris, J., 1974, Gibbs and Markov random systems with constraints, *J. Statis. Phys.*, 10:11–33.
Peretto, P., 1984, Collective properties of neural networks: A statistical physics approach, *Biol. Cybern.*, 50:51–62.
Zwietering, P. J., and Aarts, E. H. L., 1991, Parallel Boltzmann machines: A mathematical model, *J. Parallel Distrib. Comput.*, 13:65–75. ◆

Single-Cell Models

Christof Koch, Chun-Hui Mo, and William Softky

Most of the roughly ten billion neurons in the human cerebral cortex are tiny, membrane-bound bags of saltwater, shaped like trees (including roots). Each is surrounded by more salt water and by other neurons, many of which it is connected to. The vast majority of them communicate by means of brief, all-or-none pulses (called spikes, or action potentials), each lasting a bit less than a millisecond.

Researchers often want to distill the complex shape and behavior of a real neuron into a simpler model, either to guide a neurobiological experiment or to construct a functional network. But choosing which neuronal properties to keep and which to ignore is heavily influenced by how one interprets the pulses. In particular, it is common to reduce the train of action potentials issued by a neuron with an equivalent point process, but beyond that much is in dispute.

Most theories assume that information is carried in the average rate of pulses over a time much longer than a typical pulse-width, so that the occurrence times of particular pulses simply represent jitter in an averaged analog signal. A neural model in such a theory might be a mathematical function that produces a real-valued output from its many real-valued inputs; that function could be linear or nonlinear, static or adaptive, and might be instantiated in analog silicon circuits or in digital software.

However, a few theories assume that each single neural pulse carries reliable, precisely timed information. A neural model in such a theory fires only on the exact coincidence of several input pulses, and quickly "forgets" when it last fired, so that it is always ready to fire on another coincidence. Whether real neurons operate in this regime or in the slower average-rate regime awaits further neurobiological experiment. Both types of codes and single-neuron models have special features and advantages; understanding the models touches issues of bandwidth, nonlinearity, and the fundamental precision and function of single nerve cells. Of course, it is well possible that the nervous system uses both, depending on place, time, and circumstance.

Formal Models

It is easiest to understand and analyze the models that are the least like real neurons. Virtually all such models share two features in common. First, each model neuron combines many inputs, both "excitatory" and "inhibitory," into a single output. And each neuron has at least one internal state variable (conceptually corresponding to the cell's average membrane potential), which increases monotonically with the total amount of excitatory input and decreases with inhibitory input. Thus, the neuron is constrained to "adding up" (in a rough sense) its positive and negative inputs, and *cannot* independently assign an arbitrary value to each of its possible input combinations.

McCulloch-Pitts Model

The McCulloch-Pitts model neuron (see Koch, 1999, for details), more than fifty years old, has many progeny present in digital circuits, in the form of logic gates. The explicit assumptions of this model are that each binary "pulse" represents a logical statement (i.e., *true* or *false*), and that each neuron performs an exact, noise-free, synchronous computation on its input pulses.

If any one of the model neuron's inhibitory inputs is active, the output is shut off, or inactive. Otherwise, all the active excitatory inputs x_i are multiplied by their *synaptic weights* w_i and then added up. However, only if this activity level exceeds a preset *threshold* θ is the output active:

$$Y = \begin{cases} 1 & \text{if } \sum_i w_i x_i > \theta \text{ and no inhibition} \\ 0 & \text{otherwise} \end{cases} \quad (1)$$

McCulloch and Pitts showed that a large enough number of such units, with weights and connections set properly and operating synchronously, could in principle perform any possible computation (Arbib, 1987).

An even simpler model is the *linear* neuron, which simply adds up its inputs and delivers the sum as output, with no thresholds or other nonlinearities. The neuron's real-valued output is the sum of its inputs x_i, weighted by real-valued coefficients w_i:

$$Y = \sum_i w_i x_i \quad (2)$$

Networks of linear neurons can be treated analytically, using well-established matrix methods. Unlike the spikes and rates from real neurons, outputs from the linear model can become negative or arbitrarily large.

Perceptron Model

Rosenblatt's Perceptron model (see Koch, 1999, for details) is formally similar to the McCulloch-Pitts model, having synchronous inputs and producing outputs between zero and one. But the perceptron creates a real-valued (not binary) output, representing the *average firing rate* of the cell. As with the linear model, the internal variable V of a perceptron is the weighted sum of its inputs:

$$V = \sum_i w_i x_i \quad (3)$$

A *threshold* or *bias* θ is subtracted from V and is then passed through a continuous and monotonically increasing function g:

$$Y = g(V - \theta) \quad (4)$$

The nonlinear function g is *sigmoidal*: it asymptotes zero as $V \ll \theta$ and saturates at 1 for $V \gg \theta$ (Figure 1C). This function mimics the empirical relationship between the cell's input current and its firing rate in several ways: the output is non-negative, it is very small below θ, it monotonically increases with input, and the firing rate has an upper bound.

Hopfield Neurons

In Hopfield's binary model (see Koch, 1999, for details), the output of neuron i is the step function of V_i and the threshold θ,

$$Y_i = \begin{cases} 0 & \text{if } V_i < \theta \\ 1 & \text{if } V_i > \theta \end{cases} \quad (5)$$

Unlike the McCulloch-Pitts or the Perceptron model, each Hopfield neuron updates its state at a *random* time, independently of any other neurons.

Both Hopfield's binary and continuous-valued models (Figure 1C) are similar to perceptrons in isolation, but can act as associative memories in highly interconnected networks.

Polynomial Neurons

The appeal of models like those discussed previously is that only a very simple function of the inputs—a weighted sum—is neces-

Figure 1. Simple neuronal models expressed in the commonly used electrical circuit idiom. In (A–C), the entire neuron is reduced to a single spatial compartment (point-model). The summed synaptic input is described by a net current $I(t)$. A, An integrate-and-fire unit. If the voltage V exceeds a fixed threshold, a unit pulse is generated, and all charge on the capacitance is removed by resetting V to zero. The output of this and the leaky integrate-and-fire model (B, in which charge leaks away with a time constant given by the product of the capacitance C and resistance R) is a series of asynchronous spikes (C). In a rate neuron, these discrete pulses are replaced by a continuous output rate whose amplitude is proportional to the inverse of the average interspike interval. The monotonically increasing relationship between V and the output rate $f = g(v)$ can be thought of as the discharge function of a population of spiking cells. D, Nonlinear, saturating interactions can be mediated in a passive dendritic tree by synapses that increase the postsynaptic conductance. The interaction between excitation (circles) and inhibition of the shunting type (elongated boxes) is of the AND-NOT type and is specific in space and time. For instance, the inhibitory synapse i_7 vetos excitation e_3 or e_6 but has only a negligible effect on e_1. (Modified from Koch and Segev, 2000).

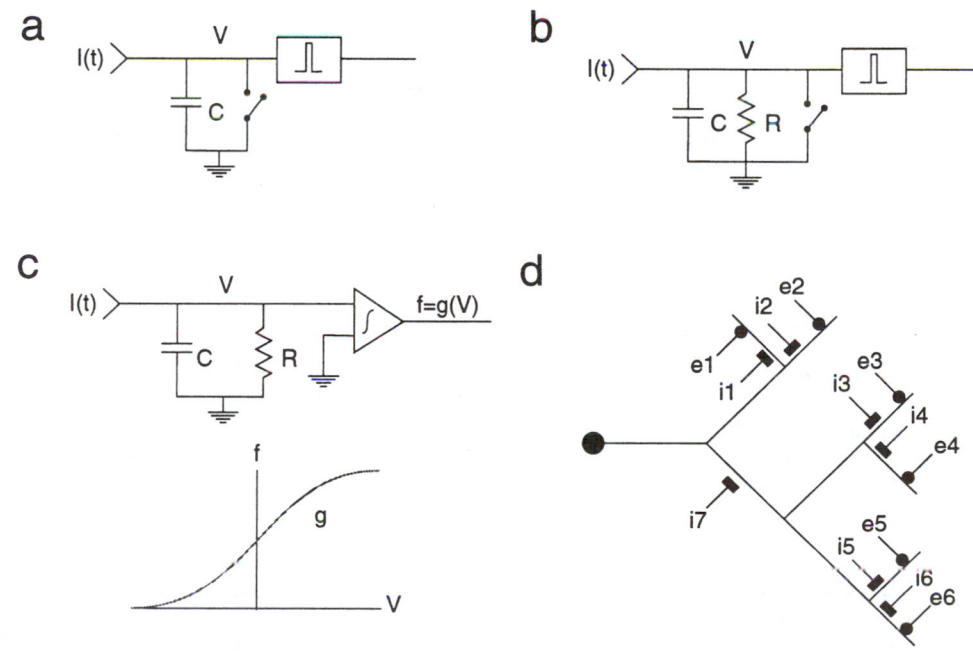

sary for them to work. However, such a sum cannot distinguish among the individual contributions to it. For the neuron to respond strongly to correlations among particular input pairs or groups, one must include multiplicative terms, and then sum over the products. Such a *sigma-pi* (Σ = sum, Π = product) neuron computes its internal state as the sum of contributions from a set of monomials

$$V = a_1 + b_1 x_1 + b_2 x_2 + c_1 x_1^2 + c_2 x_1 x_2 + \cdots \quad (6)$$

This state variable can then be passed through the usual nonlinear function g. It is clear that such "neurons" are computationally richer than linear or threshold units—just one can implement parity, exclusive-or, or *lookup table* functions. Furthermore, such models also better represent the operations of real neurons containing highly branched dendrites with voltage-dependent membrane conductances (Mel, 1994).

Biophysical Models

Although many crucial properties of real neurons remain unknown, biophysical models incorporate some known properties of neural tissue. Like real, spiking neurons, these models produce spikes rather than continuous-valued outputs.

Integrate-and-Fire Models

This family of single-cell models, about a century old, divides the membrane behavior conceptually into two distinct and discontinuous regimes: a prolonged period of linear "integration" (adding up of inputs), and a sudden "firing" (Figure 1A and B). The "integrate-and-fire" model relaxes the requirement that a single set of continuous differential equations describe the cell's two very different regimes. The cell voltage starts from zero, rising or lowering according to the synaptic input. When the voltage reaches a certain threshold θ, the cell instantly fires an output pulse and resets the voltage. After a refractory period—a brief "dead time" during which the cell cannot fire at all—the unit is ready to fire again.

The simplest type of integrator model is a leak-free capacitance (Figure 1A). With steady, DC input current, it acts like a relaxation oscillator or a current-to-frequency converter, producing regular output pulses at a rate depending on the input current.

If the input instead arrives in brief excitatory pulses (e.g., spikes from other cells), so that N pulses are necessary to reach threshold, then this model acts like a divide-by-N counter, firing on every Nth input pulse. Its output rate depends on the *average* of the overall firing rate of the inputs. For small, random input pulses, the output firing will be fairly regular as the input randomness is averaged out. The fact that such a neuron can smooth out input noise is one of its great advantages.

The addition of a leak resistance in parallel to the capacitance makes a *leaky integrate-and-fire neuron,* which will only fire if the excitatory input is strong enough to overcome the leak (Figure 1B). The time constant $\tau = RC$ divides the model's operation into two qualitatively distinct regimes: temporal integration and fluctuation-detection. When τ is larger than the mean time between output spikes, the leak is insignificant and the model temporally integrates its input (Figure 2). When τ is much smaller than the average output interval, then production of a spike depends not on the *average* input but on input *fluctuations*: only a rare fluctuation will bring the voltage above threshold. Here, the output represents a precisely timed threshold-crossing computation with a binary output—in this regime the neuron is neither linear nor analog.

Integrate-and-fire models can account for remarkably many aspects of the behavior of real neurons (Koch, 1999).

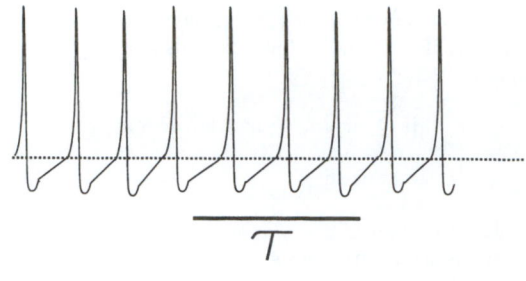

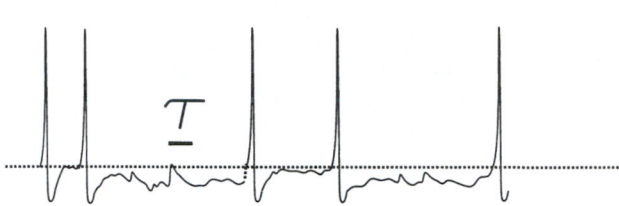

Figure 2. A schematic of the two distinct operating regimes of an integrate-and-fire model. The top trace shows how current input ramps up the neuron's internal "voltage" to produce regular spikes. The input current determines the *average slope* of the voltage between spikes. This can only occur if the interval between spikes is less than the neuron's time constant, so that the spiking frequency reliably reflects the average input current. A strikingly different situation is shown in the lower trace, where a relatively shorter time constant causes the neuron to *forget* when its last spike occurred. Now the input current determines the *average voltage* between spikes, which is nearly constant and below spiking threshold. Here a spike is only generated by a brief fluctuation so that each spike can be interpreted as the distinct binary output of a fast, multiplicative computation, reporting the precise coincidence of several contributing inputs.

The Hodgkin-Huxley Model of Squid Axon

Biophysically much more accurate single-cell models that can account for the very complex, nonstationary behavior of real neurons are lumped under the catch-all name of Hodgkin-Huxley models, since they use a mathematical formalism little different from that set out fifty years ago in the ground-breaking work of Hodgkin and Huxley (1952) on the electrodynamics of the squid axon. The dynamics are modeled by numerous coupled, nonlinear differential equations that describe the behavior of continuous membrane currents that depend in a nonlinear manner on the membrane potential.

In its quiescent state, the inside of a typical neuron has a negative voltage (relative to the extracellular fluid). The cell membrane acts like a capacitor. The electrical charge carriers (various species of ions such as Na^+, K^+, Cl^-, and Ca^{2+}) pass through special pores or *ionic channels* embedded in the membrane (Hille, 1992). Although each individual channel is either open or closed (in a partially stochastic manner), the current through many channels in parallel is well approximated by continuous, deterministic equations, much as the laws of electrical current describe averages over many electrons. That is, the continuous, macroscopic, and deterministic membrane currents derive from binary, microscopic, and stochastic ionic channels.

In the simplest case, the channels' collective behavior resembles an ohmic (or passive) resistor across the membrane. The combination of the resistance and the capacitance creates a membrane time-constant τ, which is typically between 5 and 50 ms.

Other ion channels are nonlinear: their conductance *depends on* voltage. For instance, an action potential occurs when the membrane potential becomes depolarized enough that voltage-controlled sodium channels open, initiating the fast positive-feedback event of a spike. One spike lasts between one-half and one milliseconds, and is followed by a few milliseconds of *refractory period* during which it is difficult or impossible to fire another spike.

This process was described by Hodgkin and Huxley in 1952 in one of the most successful of all models in neurobiology: a four-dimensional set of coupled, nonlinear, partial differential equations. Those equations describe the initiation and propagation of action potentials in axons well enough that they are often treated as "gospel truth," although they are technically imperfect phenomenological fits rather than expressions derived from first principles.

Simplified versions—the so-called *FitzHugh-Nagumo* and van der Pol oscillator equations (see Koch, 1999, for details)—yield qualitatively the same kind of subthreshold behavior and limit-cycle oscillations as the original Hodgkin-Huxley equations, but their reduced parameters are more difficult to be interpreted biophysically.

Although the Hodgkin-Huxley methodology is powerful, it suffers from the drawback that it requires detailed knowledge of a myriad of parameters. It is frequently difficult to properly constrain all of these degrees of freedom.

Modified Single-Point Models

More realistic neural models must account for Nature's rich array of nonlinear currents and additional internal variables, only some of which are understood.

Internal Variables. Most of the simple models outlined previously have only a single internal variable: the membrane potential. An additional variable, such as the concentration of free, intracellular calcium, can give a wider array of functions. Calcium concentration roughly represents a running average of the cell's recent activity. This temporal averaging—along with the ability of calcium ions to remain trapped near synapses—makes it a candidate for modulating synaptic strength. Calcium also participates in "adaptation," a hysteresis effect in which the calcium accumulated from past spikes makes it more difficult to fire new ones.

Additional Ionic Currents. Most neurons typically contain a dozen or more *nonlinear* ion channels, whose conductance depend on the cell voltage. There are slow positive feedback currents, such as calcium and persistent sodium currents, which tend to amplify large voltage excursions. There are also negative-feedback currents like those found for potassium, which tend to hyperpolarize the cell, acting like a kind of active inhibition or adaptation. These "active" currents can strongly influence a cell's response to input, its input, but their strengths in real cells are often unknown. For a discussion of the computational significance of all of these, see Koch (1999).

Compartmental Models

The *single-point* models discussed previously assume that neurons do not have any significant spatial extent. However, most real neurons have intricate dendritic trees (where the synaptic input arrives), as well as an axon and its branches (where the output spike is carried away). The unique shapes of those dendrites and axons can distinguish between various cell classes.

Axons are usually thought of as delay lines without any significant information processing ability (see AXONAL MODELING). Dendrites, however, display a much richer repertoire of information processing operations. The simplest "passive" dendrite model, pioneered by Rall (1989), is a single capacitive, resistive cable. Its voltage is characterized by the *cable equation,* which has two main parameters: τ is the membrane time constant, and λ the electronic space constant, is a characteristic distance over which a steady-state voltage attenuates. Signals always attenuate and temporally

smooth as they spread from their sources in such a dendritic cable (Rall, 1989). For a review of compartmental methods, see the handbook by Koch and Segev (1998).

Because dendrites with branches are not as easily analyzed, modelers resort to discretizing the cable equation (like decomposing the dendritic tree into hundreds of simple electrical compartments connected by Ohmic resistors, as in Figure 3. Note the right branches of the dendritic tree contain arbitrary active membrane component.).

Computation with Passive Dendrites

Low-pass filtering. As predicted by linear cable theory, one important computational function that passive dendrites can perform is low-pass filtering. This operation removes high temporal frequencies from voltage response to input signal and generates voltage attenuation and temporal delay.

Synaptic Saturation. Real synapses—whether slow or fast, inhibitory or excitatory, passive or voltage gated—are best modeled as *conductance* in the cell membrane in series with driving potentials. Synaptic input is not a constant current or voltage source, but rather changes the electronic properties of postsynaptic membrane. Postsynaptic potential (PSP) saturates when synaptic input becomes stronger. As a result, the PSP for two synaptic inputs arriving together is usually smaller than the sum of PSPs of two independent input. When many synapses are simultaneously active, their increased conductance further attenuates distant input (by reducing λ) and makes the cell sensitive to fluctuations at a faster timescale (by reducing τ).

Shunting Inhibition. If the driving potential of the inhibitory synapse is close to the resting potential of the cell, it is called *shunting inhibition.* Such an inhibition can veto excitation locally *only* if the inhibition lies on the path between the location of the excitatory synapse and the cell body. Shunting inhibition enables local non-linear computation at the dendrite level and endows single neurons with more powerful computational abilities (Figure 1*D*).

Computation with Active Dendrites

Experiments have revealed that dendrites contain not only passive membranes but also nonlinear "active" ones (Stuart, Spruston, and Häusser, 1999). These active membranes have voltage-dependent sodium, calcium, or potassium channels that readily perform local nonlinear computation (Figure 3). Given these active channels, action potential can backpropagate to remote dendrites from soma, providing a communication mechanism between soma and dendrites. Such a mechanism can be critical to the Hebbian learning rule-based synaptic plasticity.

Synaptic Input Amplification. Input impedances at distal arbors are usually higher than those of proximal large dendrites. Therefore, distal inputs generate higher local excitatory postsynaptic potential (EPSP), which will be amplified more by local active channels. This amplification can offset the attenuation along the cable so that synapses near and far from the cell body are equally effective. Recent evidence (Magee and Cook, 2000) shows synaptic conductance changes increasing as one moves along the apical dendrite away from the soma in CA1 pyramidal neurons. Such a progressive increase in conductance seems to be the mechanism rendering EPSP size insensitive to input location.

Coincidence Detection. Biophysically plausible proposals for coincidence detection exploit fast sodium action potential generation in spines and distal basal dendrites to achieve sub-millisecond res-

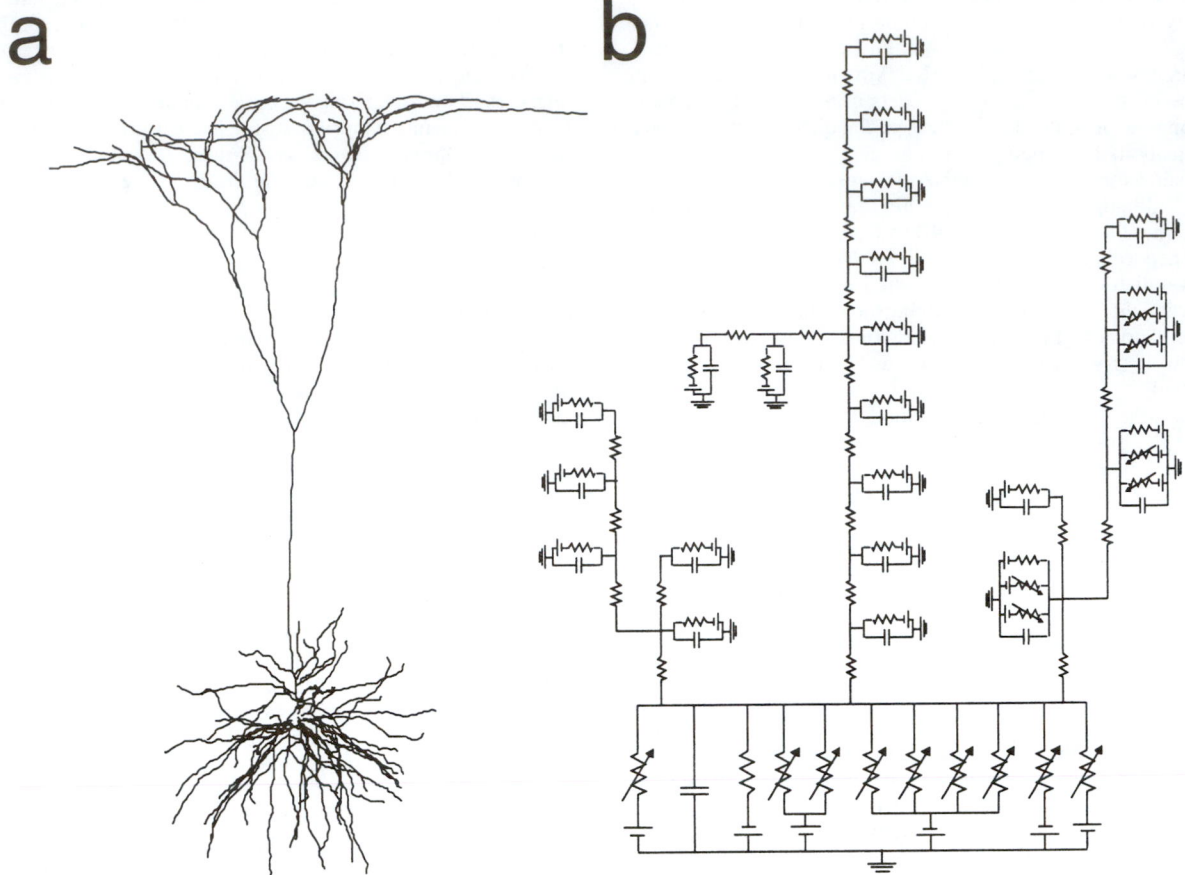

Figure 3. The most realistic form of single-neuron model numerically simulates the electrical properties of a branched cell membrane. First, the observed shape of the cell (*A*) is approximated by a collection of connected cylinders of the appropriate length and diameter. Then, each cylinder is simulated as a single electrical unit composed of an axial resistance and

membrane capacitances and resistances (*B*). Although it is computationally intensive, this numerical approach can treat the whole variety of cell shapes and nonlinear electrical properties, which are ignored by the traditional single-compartment models. Here the right branches of the dendritic tree contains voltage-dependent membrane conductance.

olution (Softky, 1994). Sakmann's group (Larkum, Zhu, and Sakmann, 1999) demonstrated dendritic coincidence detection at the 10 ms level in layer V pyramidal neurons. If an excitatory input at dendrites coincides with somatic-triggered backpropagation action potential, a powerful calcium spike may be triggered at the dendrite level. This long-lasting (10 ms or longer) calcium spike in turn triggers a burst of sodium potential at the soma.

Multiplication Operation. Multiplication is one of the simplest but most important nonlinear operations that serve as the basis for many computation models, such as those for optomotor response of insects and motion perception in primates. Nonlinear interaction by voltage-dependent channels at dendrites might provide a mechanism to implement multiplication.

Synaptic Clustering. The distribution of synapse on active dendrites can be very important because spatially close, simultaneous synaptic inputs will be amplified more by active channels. The difference in amplification is large enough to generate orientation selectivity in V1 cell models (Mel, Ruderman, and Archie, 1998).

Discussion

After several decades of research, we understand only some of the most fundamental functions of nerve cells.

Learning

The most remarkable feature of the nervous system is its ability to change its internal structure in response to previous input—that is, to learn. Theoretical aspects of learning are covered elsewhere (see the three road maps on learning in Part II of the *Handbook*). However, at the single-cell level, there are many issues left to resolve.

Strengthening or weakening a single synapse weight, w_{ij}, seems to involve complex events, including calcium accumulation on both sides of the connection. However, there are several different types of increase and decrease, occurring under different circumstances and lasting from seconds to days. These mechanisms are not yet well understood, especially in the cerebral cortex. Markram and colleagues (1997) controlled the relative timing of presynaptic and postsynaptic action potentials in a pair of excitatory-coupled neurons, measuring its effect on the strength of synaptic coupling between the two cells. If the presynaptic spike preceded the postsynaptic one by as little as 10 ms, synaptic strength increased (long-term potentiation, LTP). Conversely, if the postsynaptic spike preceded the presynaptic one, synaptic coupling decreased (long-term depression, LTD). This gives rise to powerful, temporally asymmetric Hebbian learning rules.

A potent (but poorly understood) type of learning could occur as axonal branches and connections "die off," while other branches form elsewhere and connect to other cells. If such structural plasticity participates in learning, then at least as much information could be stored in the existence/nonexistence of the synaptic connections as in their current-pulse amplitudes or "strengths."

The Dendrites

Although most input to cortical cells arrives on an intricately branched dendritic tree, we do not understand how the tree processes the input. Whether those tiny dendrites smooth out brief, localized input fluctuations—or instead amplify them—depends on the type of nonlinear membrane properties to be found there. Nonlinear dendrites can make a single "neuron" function as a large collection of distinct, multiplicative subunits.

Slow Analog versus Fast Digital

There are two distinct, self-consistent interpretations of single-neuron function, which are diametrically opposed, but there is evidence for both (Figure 2).

In the most popular interpretation, the fundamental computation is like that of a Perceptron or a Hopfield neuron: a slow real-valued output resulting from slowly varying real-valued inputs, in which the timing of single spikes is inconsequential. Indeed, decades of experiments on most parts of the brain have found that only average rates—and not individual spike times—correlate with simple stimuli.

This corresponds to an integrate-and-fire neuron gathering many small inputs, smoothing out their irregularities in the dendritic tree, summing the results in the cell body, and producing a firing rate as output. Here the internal variable is the *average current* into the cell body, and the output firing rate can be interpreted as current into the *next* cell (the cell voltage is just a repeating ramp whose phase has no significance). This form of computation is most effective when the fluctuations in current are small, so that the cell fires in response to the mean current.

An alternative is McCulloch and Pitts' original interpretation of their binary neuron: the "active" state corresponds to a *single spike* rather than to an prolonged firing rate, so that every spike carries some kind of independent message. Although such a model can in principle transmit information much faster than an analog neuron, there are four fundamental criticisms of it: Are binary computations more appropriate than analog ones? Is there any need for such a high bandwidth? Can that high bandwidth be implemented in a realistic cell? And how sensitive is such a cell to the noise that exists in the cortex?

Other neural systems—such as the fly's visual system—can indeed carry significant information by single spikes. And there is a need for *some* improved neural bandwidth to solve problems of segmentation and binding. But there is so far no solid evidence that most cortical areas need such fast temporal resolution.

This single-spike regime corresponds to an integrate-and-fire type of cell that fires according to its instantaneous (rather than average) voltage, so it is sensitive to input fluctuations. However, in order for the cell to respond reliably to fluctuations, the average current must not dominate them—otherwise the mean current will ramp up the voltage and fire the cell, fluctuations or not.

Road Maps: Biological Neurons and Synapses; Grounding Models of Neurons
Related Reading: Axonal Modeling; Biophysical Mechanisms in Neuronal Modeling; Ion Channels: Keys to Neuronal Specialization; Perspective on Neuron Model Complexiy

References

Arbib, M., 1987, *Brains, Machines, and Mathematics,* 2nd ed., New York: Springer-Verlag. ◆
Hille, B., 1992, *Ionic Channels of Excitable Membranes,* 2nd ed., New York: Sinauer. ◆
Hodgkin, A. L., and Huxley, A. F., 1952, A quantitative description of membrane current and its application to conduction and excitation in nerve, *J. Physiol. (Lond.),* 117:500–544.
Koch, C., 1999, *Biophysics of Computation: Information Processing in Single Neurons,* New York: Oxford University Press. ◆
Koch, C. and Segev, I., Eds., 1998, *Methods in Neuronal Modeling: From Ions to Networks,* 2nd ed., Cambridge, MA: MIT Press.
Koch, C., and Segev, I., 2000, Single neurons and their role in information processing, *Nat. Neurosci.,* 3:1171–1177.
Larkum, M. E., Zhu, J. J., and Sakmann, B., 1999, A new cellular mechanism for coupling inputs arriving at different cortical layers, *Nature,* 398:338–341.
Magee, J. C., and Cook, E. P., 2000, Somatic EPSP amplitude is independent of synapse location in hippocampal pyramidal neurons, *Nat. Neurosci,* 3:895–903.
Markram, H., Lubke, J., Frotscher, M., and Sakmann, B., 1997, Regulation of synaptic efficacy by coincidence of postsynaptic Aps and EPSPs, *Science,* 275:213–215.
Mel, B., 1994, Information processing in dendritic trees, *Neural Computat.,* 6:1031–1085.
Mel, B., Ruderman, D., and Archie, K., 1998, Translation-invariant orientation tuning in visual "complex" cells could derive from intradendritic computations, *J. Neurosci,* 18:4325–4334.
Rall, W., 1989, Cable theory for dendritic neurons, in *Methods in Neuronal Modelling* (C. Koch and I. Segev, Eds), Cambridge, MA: MIT Press, pp. 9–62.
Softky, W., 1994, Sub-millisecond coincidence detection in active dendritic trees, *Neuroscience,* 58:15–41.
Stuart, G., Spruston, N., and Häusser, M., Eds., 1999, *Dendrites,* New York: Oxford University Press.

Sleep Oscillations

Alain Destexhe and Terrence J. Sejnowski

Introduction

The brain spontaneously generates complex patterns of neural activity. As the brain falls asleep, the rapid patterns characteristic of aroused states are replaced by low-frequency, synchronized rhythms of neuronal activity. At the same time, electroencephalographic (EEG) recordings shift from low-amplitude, high-frequency rhythms to large-amplitude, slow oscillations. In what follows, we focus primarily on this slow-wave sleep, rather than

rapid eye movement (REM) sleep, whose oscillatory properties resemble those of wakefulness.

The thalamus and cerebral cortex are intimately linked by means of reciprocal projections. The thalamus is the major gateway for the flow of information toward the cerebral cortex and is the first station at which incoming signals can be blocked by synaptic inhibition during sleep. This shift contributes to the transition that the brain undergoes from an aroused state, open to influence from the outside world, to the closed state of sleep. The early stage of quiescent sleep is associated with EEG spindle waves, which occur at a frequency of 7–14 Hz. As sleep deepens, waves with slower frequencies (0.1–4 Hz) appear on the EEG. This article summarizes what is known about the biophysical mechanisms underlying spindle oscillations.

The dramatic reduction in forebrain responsiveness during sleep, the pervasiveness of these changes, and the discovery of the underlying specific cellular mechanisms, suggest that sleep oscillations are highly orchestrated and highly regulated. Experimental and modeling studies have shown how sleep rhythms emerge from an interaction between the intrinsic firing properties of thalamic and cortical neurons and the networks through which they interact (Steriade, McCormick, and Sejnowski, 1993; Destexhe and Sejnowski, 2001). These advances have raised interesting possibilities regarding the function of sleep.

Biophysical Basis of Sleep Spindle Oscillations

Sleep spindles are characteristic of brain electrical synchronization at sleep onset, an electrographic landmark for the transition from

waking to sleep that is associated with loss of perceptual awareness. Spindle oscillations consist of 7–14 Hz waxing-and-waning field potentials, grouped in sequences that last for 1–3 s and recur once every 3–10 s. Spindle oscillations constitute an interesting and well-constrained problem to investigate by computational models for several reasons. First, these oscillations are generated in the thalamus, which is a well-known structure anatomically, with well-defined connectivity between the different cell types. Second, spindles are remarkably well documented experimentally and have been extensively characterized both in vivo and in vitro (reviewed in Steriade et al., 1993; Destexhe and Sejnowski, 2001). Third, this oscillation is generated by an interplay of complex cellular properties, such as burst firing, and synaptic interactions via multiple types of postsynaptic receptors (reviewed in Destexhe and Sejnowski, 2001). Computational models are needed to understand this complex interplay, as we summarize here.

The typical electrophysiological features of spindle oscillations are shown in Figure 1A. The two cell types involved, thalamocortical (TC) and thalamic reticular (RE) neurons, oscillate synchronously and display burst discharges according to a mirror

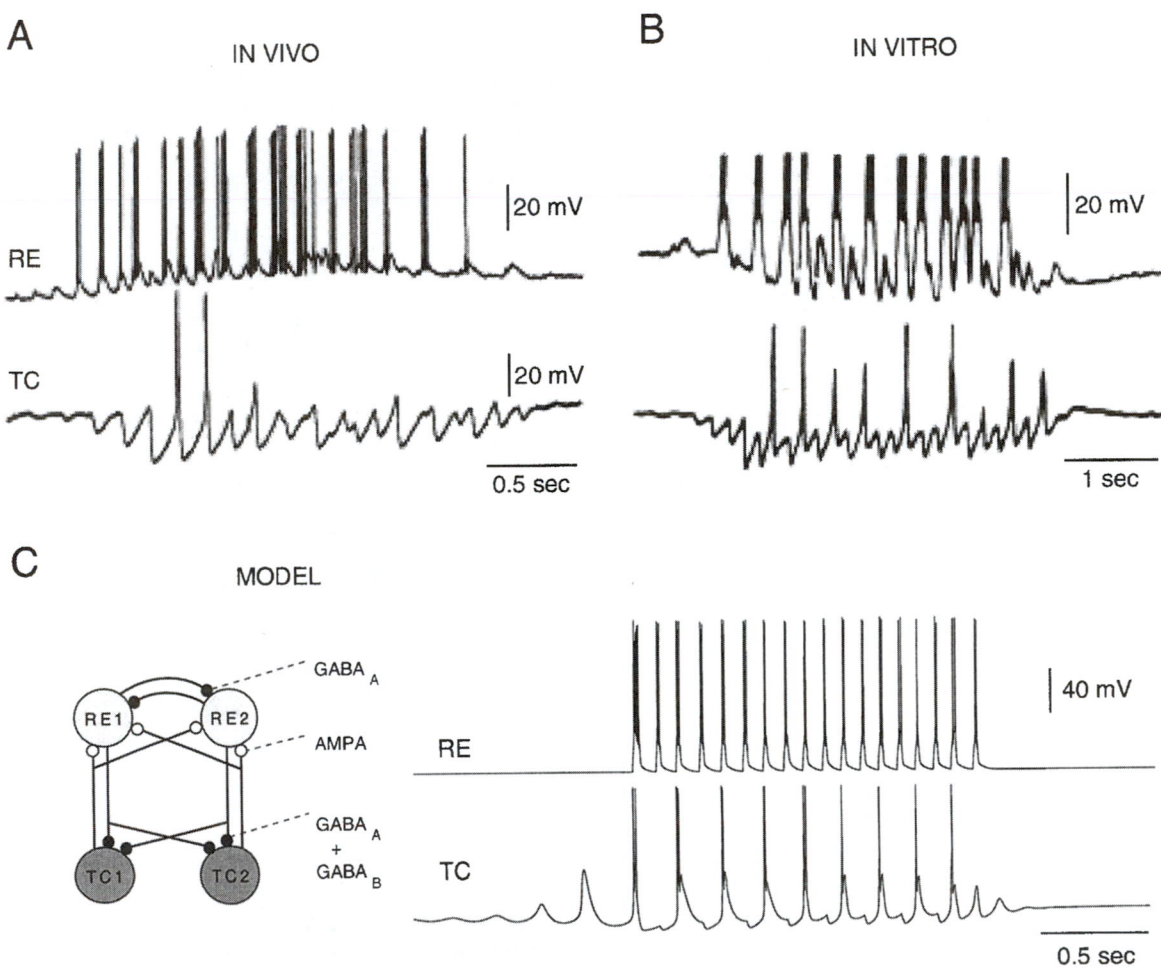

Figure 1. Spindle oscillations in thalamic circuits. *A*, Intracellular recordings of thalamic neurons during spindle oscillations in vivo (cats, barbiturate anesthesia; modified from Steriade et al., 1993). *B*, Intracellular features of spindle oscillations in ferret thalamic slices (spikes truncated; modified from Steriade et al., 1993). *C*, Model of spindle oscillations by interacting TC and RE cells. The intrinsic firing properties of each cell type was simulated by Hodgkin-Huxley type models for Na⁺, K⁺ and Ca²⁺ currents, and kinetic models of postsynaptic receptors (AMPA, GABA_A, and GABA_B; see scheme) were used to represent synaptic interactions (modified from Destexhe et al., 1996; see also Destexhe, Mainen, and Sejnowski, this volume). In all three examples, RE cells generated bursts following EPSPs while TC cells generated bursts following IPSPs once every few cycles.

image: RE cells display bursts following excitatory synaptic potentials (EPSPs) while TC cells burst following inhibitory postsynaptic potentials (IPSPs). Although RE cells tend to burst at every cycle of the oscillation, TC cells only produce bursts once every few cycles. These features are typical of spindles recorded in thalamic neurons in different mammals.

Several hypotheses for the genesis of oscillations by thalamic circuits have been proposed (reviewed in Destexhe and Sejnowski, 2001). These involve reciprocal synaptic interactions between TC neurons and local inhibitory interneurons, loops between TC and RE neurons, or loops within the RE nucleus. The involvement of the RE nucleus was firmly demonstrated in a series of experiments by Steriade's group (reviewed in Steriade et al., 1993; Destexhe and Sejnowski, 2001). In particular, the deafferented RE nucleus in vivo can exhibit spindle rhythmicity in extracellular recordings. In contrast, the RE nucleus does not display autonomous oscillations in vitro, but spindles have been observed in thalamic slices based on TC-RE interactions (see Steriade et al., 1993, for a review of these issues). These in vitro spindles display the same intracellular features as in vivo (Figure 1B).

The genesis of spindle oscillations was investigated with computational models. First, in models of the isolated RE nucleus, RE neurons with sufficiently high connectivity interacting through GABAergic synapses generated spindle rhythmicity (Wang and Rinzel, 1993; Destexhe et al., 1994; Bazhenov et al., 1999; reviewed in Destexhe and Sejnowski, 2001). These models supported the RE pacemaker hypothesis based on in vivo recordings. Second, models including TC and RE cells showed that spindle oscillations can be obtained from TC-RE loops (Destexhe et al., 1996; Golomb, Wang, and Rinzel, 1996). The latter models supported the TC-RE mechanism suggested by thalamic slice experiments. Finally, it remained to explain why the RE nucleus oscillates autonomously in vivo but not in vitro. This apparent inconsistency was addressed by a computational model of the RE nucleus, in which oscillations depended on the level of neuromodulators (Destexhe et al., 1994). The difference between in vivo and in vitro preparations may therefore be explained by the limited connectivity between the RE neurons in the slice, and/or by the fact that slices lack the necessary level of neuromodulation to maintain isolated RE oscillations (Destexhe et al., 1994). The main prediction from this model is that applying neuromodulators to slices of the RE nucleus should induce oscillations similar to those observed in vivo.

The model for the TC-RE loop is shown in Figure 1C. Neurons were modeled using Hodgkin-Huxley type representations of Na$^+$, K$^+$, and Ca^{2+} voltage-dependent currents (see AXONAL MODELING), which were based on voltage-clamp data on thalamic neurons (see details in Destexhe et al., 1996). These models reproduced the most salient intrinsic properties of thalamic neurons, such as the production of bursts of action potentials. Synaptic interactions were modeled using conductance-based kinetic models (see Destexhe, Mainen, and Sejnowski, this volume). Several of the main receptor types (AMPA, NMDA, GABA$_A$, and GABA$_B$) identified in thalamic circuits were incorporated into the model. Under these conditions, the circuit generated 7–14-Hz spindle oscillations with the typical features identified intracellularly in the different thalamic neuron types. The model reproduced the typical mirror image between TC and RE cells during spindles, as well as the phase relations between cells. In particular, TC cells produced bursts once every two cycles, a feature consistently observed experimentally (compare with Figure 1A–B). More irregular behavior, similar to the experiments, was obtained in larger networks or in the presence of the cortex (see the following discussion). The oscillations also showed the typical waxing-and-waning envelope of spindles; this property was due in the model to Ca^{2+}-mediated slow regulation of the I$_h$ current, a prediction that was verified experimentally (Lüthi and McCormick, 1998).

Network Properties of Spindle Oscillations

Network properties were investigated using multiple recordings in vivo (Contreras et al., 1996) and in vitro (Kim, Bal, and McCormick, 1995). Spindle oscillations in vitro showed traveling wave patterns (Figure 2A). The oscillation started on one side of the slice and propagated to the other side, at a constant propagation velocity. Traveling spindle waves were simulated by computational models of networks of interconnected TC and RE cells (one-dimensional extensions of the circuit shown in Figure 1C), in two independent modeling studies (Destexhe et al., 1996; Golomb et al., 1996). These models were similar in spirit to the circuit shown in Figure 1C, but assumed that there was a topographic connectivity between TC and RE layers, consistent with anatomical data. Under these conditions, the models generated traveling waves consistent with in vitro data (Figure 2B).

In contrast to the thalamic slice, in recordings from the intact thalamocortical system in cats in vivo, the oscillations were remarkably synchronized over extended thalamic regions and showed little signs for traveling wave activity (Figure 2C). To simulate the in vivo conditions, a thalamocortical network model was developed by combining the previous model of thalamic slices with a model of deep cortical layers (see details in Destexhe, Contreras, and Steriade, 1998). The principal prediction of this model was that, in order to generate large-scale coherent oscillations, the cortex had to recruit the thalamus primarily through the RE nucleus. Because of the powerful inhibitory action of RE cells, the action of corticothalamic feedback is "inhibitory dominant" on TC cells, which property is essential to maintain large-scale synchrony (Destexhe et al., 1998). In these conditions, the same model was capable of generating large-scale synchrony in the presence of the cortex, and traveling waves in the isolated thalamus (Figure 2D). Consistent with these models, propagating activity has indeed been observed in the thalamus of decorticated cats in vivo (Contreras et al., 1996).

The cortical control of thalamic relay cells in the model through dominant inhibitory mechanisms has important consequences for the function of thalamocortical assemblies (see details in Destexhe and Sejnowski, 2001) and pathological situations such as absence seizures (Destexhe, 1998). As a result of inhibitory dominance, a too strong feedback can activate GABA$_B$ receptors and can entrain the *physiologically intact* thalamus into hypersynchronous rhythms at ~3 Hz. This scheme may explain the genesis of absence seizures, which are hypersynchronous ~3 Hz rhythms that appear suddenly in the thalamocortical system. These seizures can be provoked experimentally by altering the cortex, but a physiologically intact thalamus is required (Gloor and Fariello, 1988). The thalamocortical model accounts for these experiments and could simulate seizures based on inhibitory-dominant corticothalamic feedback (Destexhe, 1998). This model directly predicted that manipulating corticothalamic feedback should entrain the physiologically intact thalamus to generate hypersynchronous rhythms at ~3 Hz, a prediction that has been recently verified by two independent studies (Blumenfeld and McCormick, 2000; Bal, Debay, and Destexhe, 2000).

Finally, computational models have suggested a physiological role for spindle oscillations. The synchronized high-frequency bursts of action potentials in the thalamus provide a powerful input to the cortex, which is ideal for evoking massive calcium entry into pyramidal cells. Massive calcium entry may activate a series of biochemical cascades, leading to permanent changes of previously tagged synapses (Destexhe and Sejnowski, 2001). This scenario provides a biophysical mechanism consistent with the growing evidence that sleep serves to consolidate memories (see Destexhe and Sejnowski, 2001, for further details).

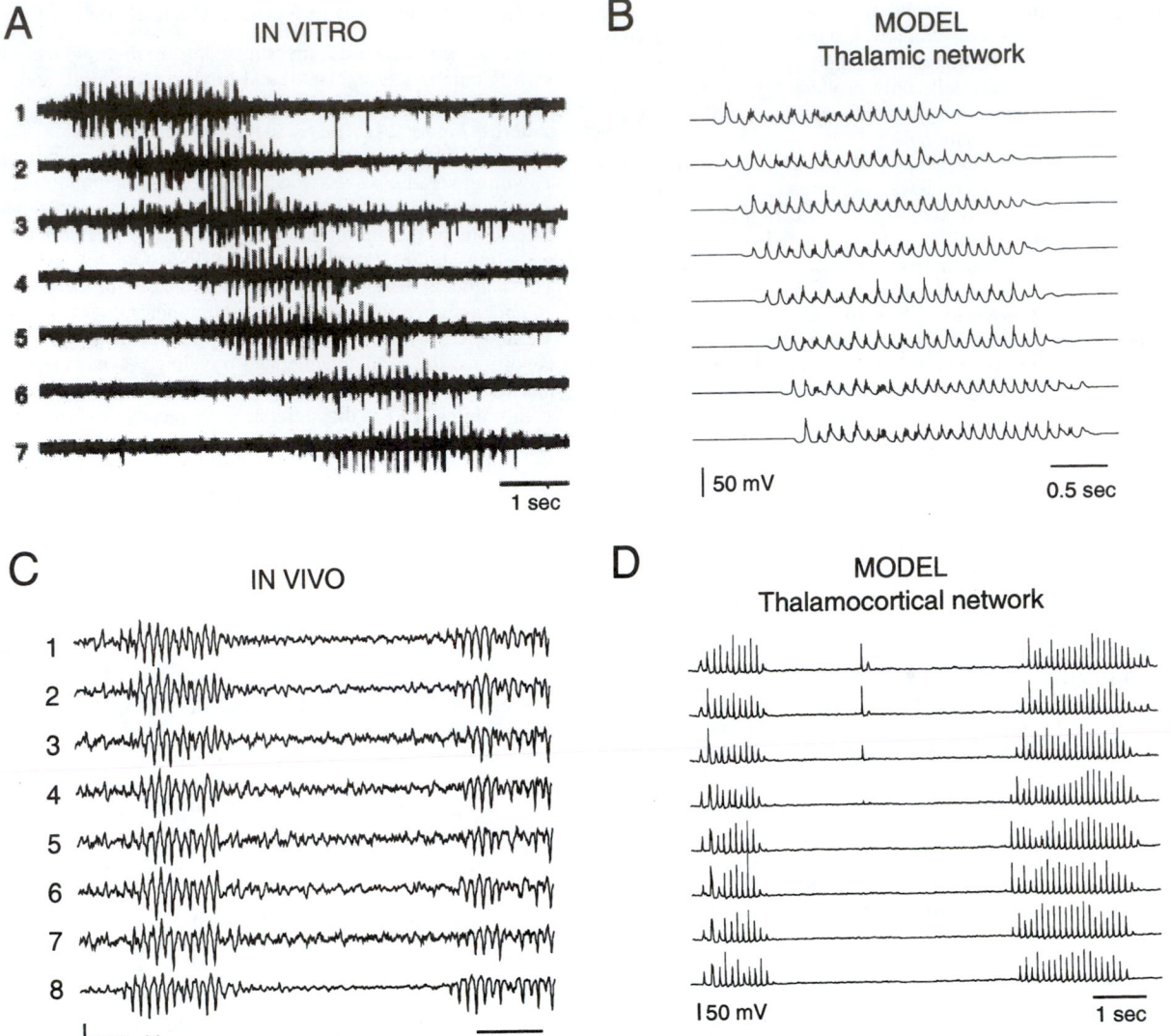

Figure 2. Sleep spindles in thalamic and thalamocortical networks. *A*, Propagating spindles in vitro. Spindle oscillations in an array of seven extracellular electrodes aligned along the dorsoventral axis of the slice (electrodes were separated by 250–400 μm, extending over 2–3 mm in the slice; modified from Kim et al., 1995). *B*, Propagating oscillations in a model thalamic network with reciprocal and topographic connections between TC and RE layers (100 cells total; modified from Destexhe et al., 1996). Each trace shows the averaged membrane potential (computed from ten neighboring TC cells) taken at eight equally spaced sites in the network. *C*, Large-scale synchrony of spindles in vivo. Eight extracellular electrodes were inserted along the dorsoventral axis of the thalamus in cats under barbiturate anesthesia (interelectrode distance of 1 mm; modified from Contreras et al., 1996). *D*, Large-scale synchrony in a thalamocortical network model consisting of four layers of thalamic and cortical neurons interconnected in a topographic fashion (400 cells total; averaged membrane potentials shown at ten equidistant locations; modified from Destexhe et al., 1998). While the oscillation was generated in the thalamus (see Figure 1), the large-scale synchrony depended on the cortex and was generated by corticothalamic interactions (see text for details).

We have shown here that computational models can simulate a large body of experimental data, ranging from isolated thalamic circuits to large-scale thalamocortical assemblies, also including the genesis of pathological behavior such as seizures. The challenge for future studies will be to investigate the physiological role of these slow-wave oscillations. Our present working hypothesis is that the high level of synchrony of these oscillations is ideal to recruit specific calcium-dependent biochemical cascades leading to memory consolidation, which may be one of the principal roles of sleep.

Summary and Conclusions

Computational models of neurons using conductance-based mechanisms integrate electrophysiological data from both in vitro and in vivo preparations. This approach reconciles apparently conflicting experimental data and has generated experimental predictions (some of which have been tested and verified). In particular, a coherent framework has been proposed to explain the genesis of sleep spindles and pathological behavior, such as absence seizures, based on data from the level of ion channels to large-scale network in-

Destexhe, A., Bal, T., McCormick, D. A., and Sejnowski, T. J., 1996, Ionic mechanisms underlying synchronized oscillations and propagating waves in a model of ferret thalamic slices, *J. Neurophysiol.*, 76:2049–2070.

Destexhe, A., Contreras, D., Sejnowski, T. J., and Steriade, M., 1994, Modeling the control of reticular thalamic oscillations by neuromodulators, *NeuroReport*, 5:2217–2220.

Destexhe, A., Contreras, D., and Steriade, M., 1998, Mechanisms underlying the synchronizing action of corticothalamic feedback through inhibition of thalamic relay cells, *J. Neurophysiol.*, 79:999–1016.

Destexhe, A., and Sejnowski, T. J., 2001, *Thalamocortical Assemblies*, Oxford, UK: Oxford University Press. ◆

Hines, M. L., and Carnevale, N. T., 1997, The NEURON simulation environment, *Neural Computation*, 9:1179–1209.

Gloor, P., and Fariello, R. G., 1988, Generalized epilepsy: Some of its cellular mechanisms differ from those of focal epilepsy, *Trends Neurosci.*, 11:63–68.

Golomb, D., Wang, X. J., and Rinzel, J., 1996, Propagation of spindle waves in a thalamic slice model, *J. Neurophysiol.*, 75:750–769.

Lüthi, A., and McCormick, D. A., 1998, Periodicity of thalamic synchronized oscillations: The role of Ca^{2+}-mediated upregulation of I_h, *Neuron*, 20:553–563.

Kim, U., Bal, T., and McCormick, D. A., 1995, Spindle waves are propagating synchronized oscillations in the ferret LGNd in vitro, *J. Neurophysiol.*, 74:1301–1323.

Steriade, M., McCormick, D. A., and Sejnowski, T. J., 1993, Thalamocortical oscillations in the sleeping and aroused brain, *Science*, 262:679–685. ◆

Wang, X. J., and Rinzel, J., 1993, Spindle rhythmicity in the reticularis thalami nucleus—synchronization among inhibitory neurons, *Neurosci*, 53:899–904.

References

Bal, T., Debay, D., and Destexhe, A., 2000, Cortical feedback controls the frequency and synchrony of oscillations in the visual thalamus, *J. Neurosci.*, 20:7478–7488.

Bazhenov, M., Timofeev, I., Steriade, M., and Sejnowski, T. J., 1999, Self-sustained rhythmic activity in the thalamic reticular nucleus mediated by depolarizing GABA$_A$ receptor potentials, *Nature Neurosci.*, 2:168–174.

Blumenfeld, H., and McCormick, D. A., 2000, Corticothalamic inputs control the pattern of activity generated in thalamocortical networks, *J. Neurosci.*, 20:5153–5162.

Contreras, D., Destexhe, A., Sejnowski, T. J., and Steriade, M., 1996, Control of spatiotemporal coherence of a thalamic oscillation by corticothalamic feedback, *Science*, 274:771–774.

Destexhe, A., 1998, Spike-and-wave oscillations based on the properties of GABA$_B$ receptors, *J. Neurosci.*, 18:9099–9111.

Somatosensory System

Oleg V. Favorov and Douglas G. Kelly

Introduction

The somatosensory system provides the central nervous system (CNS) with information about the state of the body and about objects contacted by the body. This information contributes both to perception of the proximal surroundings and to execution of skilled movements. The somatosensory system is unique in the large number of receptor types it employs, which are responsible for qualitatively distinct types of somatic sensations. Several different types of receptors in the skin mediate sensations of contact pressure, texture, movement across the skin, flutter, vibration, pain, and temperature. Receptors located in the muscles, tendons, joints, and the skin overlying the joints mediate proprioceptive sensations of position and movement of the joints and forces acting on them.

Each class of receptors has a separate pathway through the CNS. A typical pathway starts with primary afferent neurons in the dorsal root ganglia outside the spinal cord. These neurons synapse on neurons in the spinal cord (in the case of poorly localized sensations of pain and temperature) or in the dorsal column nuclei in the medulla (in the case of finely discriminative touch and limb proprioception). These second-order neurons in turn project to the ventrobasal complex of the thalamus. The VPL nucleus of this complex receives information from the trunk and limbs, whereas the VPM nucleus receives information from the head. The ventrobasal complex relays the sensory information it receives to the cerebral cortex.

Two areas of the cerebral cortex receive direct inputs from the ventrobasal complex: the primary somatosensory area (SI) in the postcentral gyrus and the secondary somatosensory area (SII) in the lateral fissure. In addition to thalamic inputs, SI and SII also receive dense reciprocal inputs from each other. Although the idea is still controversial, it appears that SI and SII occupy hierarchically parallel, rather than serial, positions in tactile information processing (Zhang et al., 2001).

SI is subdivided into four distinct cytoarchitectonic regions, Brodmann's areas 3a, 3b, 1, and 2. Area 3a is dominated by afferent inputs from muscles, area 3b by afferent inputs from the skin. Skin information is further processed in area 1 and is combined with information from muscles and joints in area 2. SI and SII send their outputs to areas adjacent to them in the insula (for object recognition) and in the parietal lobe (for forming body image and for planning movements in the extrapersonal space), as well as to motor cortical areas (for fine motor control).

A more detailed description of the somatosensory system can be found in Hendry, Hsiao, and Bushnell (1999). The somatosensory system has been studied extensively, and a wealth of information is available about its anatomy and physiology. As a result of pioneering work by Vernon Mountcastle, special emphasis has been placed on quantifying the relationships of various attributes of tactile stimuli (e.g., the frequency and amplitude of stimulus vibration, the direction of stimulus motion along the skin, texture roughness) with the sensations these stimuli evoke in humans or monkeys. To identify the neural mechanisms underlying tactile perception, such psychophysical studies are combined with neurophysiological experiments that compare reports from the subjects with responses from peripheral receptors and from subcortical and cortical neurons. An example of this approach, focusing on the neural mechanisms of stimulus vibration frequency discrimination, is offered by Mountcastle, Steinmetz, and Romo (1990).

While experimental studies have provided many important insights, our theoretical understanding of cortical operations involved in processing somatosensory information is still very limited. Nevertheless, diverse theoretical and modeling studies of the somatosensory system, primarily at the level of the cerebral cortex, have contributed to a progressively more comprehensive understanding of somatosensory information processing. The overall view of this processing is that tactile stimulus representation in the nervous system is changed from an original form (more or less isomorphic to the stimulus itself) to a completely distributed form (underlying perception) in a series of partial transformations in successive subcortical and cortical networks. As demonstrated, for example, by Johnson et al. (1991), at the level of peripheral afferents the representation of a scanned tactile form, such as a letter of the alphabet embossed on a rotating drum, is an isomorphic neural image of that form, because of the topography of the receptor sheet and the small receptive fields (RFs) of those afferents. In contrast, at the level of SI the neural image of the stimulus already has become much more complex, as evidenced by the complexity and heterogeneity of the responses of cortical neurons, which are already sensitive to shape and temporal features of peripheral stimuli, rather than simply reflecting the overall intensity of stimulation of their RFs.

Development of Cortical Topographic Maps

In each somatosensory cortical area the inputs from different body regions are organized topographically into detailed somatotopic maps. This topographic organization of thalamocortical connections is one of the principal determinants of how representations of peripheral stimuli are transformed in the cortex. How the topography is developed and maintained in SI has been the subject of a number of theoretical and modeling studies (see SOMATOTOPY: PLASTICITY OF SENSORY MAPS), which have identified Hebbian plasticity of thalamocortical synapses and Mexican-hat distribution of lateral connections (in which each cortical site excites its closest neighbors but inhibits more distant ones) as two necessary conditions for the development of somatotopy.

In particular, Grajski and Merzenich (1990) demonstrated that these conditions are sufficient to account for the inverse relationship that exists in the cortex between RF size and cortical magnification (i.e., the size of the cortical area representing a unit area of skin). Using a three-layer network (skin, subcortical, and cortical layers) with a Mexican-hat pattern of intrinsic connections and Hebbian plasticity of afferent and intrinsic connectivity, they successfully simulated two experimental studies. In one study, preferential stimulation of a particular restricted skin region resulted in an increase in its cortical representation, coupled with a decrease in RF size. In the second study, cortical magnification was reduced by lesioning a restricted cortical region, which led to an increase in RF size in cortical territories around the lesion.

Modeling studies of Pearson, Finkel, and Edelman (1987), Montague, Gally, and Edelman (1991), and Xing and Gerstein (1996b) offer a mechanistic explanation for the presence of discrete place-defined columns in SI. Cortical columnar organization was first discovered in SI by Mountcastle in 1950s (Hendry et al., 1999). More recently, Favorov and colleagues (Favorov and Kelly, 1996) identified a class of discrete cortical columns (*segregates*) in the SI of cats and monkeys distinguished by the relative RF locations of their constituent neurons. These columns, 0.3–0.6 mm in diameter, are separated from each other by sharp boundaries and compartmentalize SI into a honeycomb-like mosaic. The defining characteristic of segregates is that the *strongest* afferent input to local clusters of neurons *throughout* a given column comes from the *same* focal skin site (the *segregate RF center*). At the borders between segregates, the site of the strongest input shifts abruptly to a new, prominently displaced skin locus.

Although they differ in the details of their models, Pearson et al. (1987), Montague et al. (1991), and Xing and Gerstein (1996b) all identify two characteristic properties of the cortical network as responsible for the emergence of segregates during the perinatal development of SI. These properties are (1) a Mexican-hat distribution of lateral connections and (2) Hebbian-like plasticity of both afferent and lateral excitatory connections. Even though a network with two such properties may initially have somatotopically distributed afferent connections and homogeneously organized intrinsic connections, under repeated sensory stimulation it will nevertheless reorganize and spontaneously resolve into a mosaic of small, discrete regions. The excitatory intrinsic connections among neurons within each such region will strengthen greatly, whereas connections among different regions will weaken profoundly. Afferent connections will reorganize also, and neurons within each region will acquire identical or similar focal RFs, whereas neurons in adjacent regions will acquire nonoverlapping RFs. As a result, across the network, RFs will shift not continuously but in abrupt steps at the borders between these regions.

Minicolumnar Organization of SI

Segregates in SI are composed of smaller, 0.05-mm-diameter columns called *minicolumns*. Neurons located in the same minicolumn have similar RFs, but neurons located in different, even adjacent, minicolumns typically have RFs that differ significantly in size and shape and frequently overlap only minimally on the skin, having in common only the segregate RF center (reviewed in Favorov and Kelly, 1996). Favorov and Kelly (1996) developed a model of a typical SI segregate, made up of 61 minicolumns, to evaluate a hypothesis that the prominent diversity in the RFs among minicolumns in a segregate is an outcome of cortical network self-organization during perinatal development. In the model, each minicolumn consists of three cells representative of different cell types in the cortex: an input *spiny-stellate* cell (which receives thalamic input and distributes it to all other cells of the same minicolumn and, to a lesser degree, to other nearby minicolumns), an intrinsic *double-bouquet* cell (which inhibits adjacent minicolumns), and an output *pyramidal* cell. Connections from thalamus to minicolumns were plastic; they were allowed to self-organize in accordance with a Hebbian rule during a developmental period in which the network was driven by punctate skin stimuli.

During the network's self-organization, each minicolumn is driven by its inhibitory interactions with adjacent minicolumns (mediated by double-bouquet cells) to acquire a set of afferent connections that is different from those of its immediate neighbors. On the other hand, each minicolumn is also driven by the excitatory interactions with a larger circle of its neighbors (mediated by spiny-stellate cells) to make its set of afferent connections similar to theirs. To satisfy these opposing pressures, minicolumns in the segregate arrange their afferent connections in permuted patterns, with shuffled RFs, since such shuffling satisfies the opposing pressures by moving RFs of adjacent minicolumns farther apart, while preventing RFs of the entire segregate from diverging too widely. Thus the model generates complex patterns of RFs across the segregate that are similar to those observed experimentally in microelectrode penetrations through SI segregates (Favorov and Kelly, 1996).

Cortical Cell Tuning

Pinto et al. (1996, based on an earlier model of Kyriazi and Simons) developed a model of the first cortical stage of cell tuning in SI. They modeled the organization of a single cortical *barrel*, a discrete neuronal aggregate in layer 4 of rodent SI that receives its principal input from one of the facial whiskers. Spike trains recorded from real thalamic neurons were used as input to the model network and responses of the model neurons were compared with those recorded from real neurons in cortical layer 4. The crucial features of the model are the following: (1) cortical cells have nonlinear activation properties, (2) inhibitory cells are more responsive than excitatory cells, (3) each excitatory and inhibitory cell receives connections from multiple thalamic cells, and (4) all cortical cells are strongly interconnected. Under these conditions, the model accurately simulates the cortical response to three types of whisker stimulations (brief or prolonged deflection of a single whisker, or a sequential deflection of two whiskers in a condition-test paradigm), and it reproduces the known differences between the response properties of thalamic and cortical neurons. Specifically, excitatory cortical cells share a greater signal-to-noise ratio than thalamic cells, and they have RFs with more tightly focused excitatory centers and stronger inhibitory surrounds than do thalamic cells. Traditionally, focusing of RF properties has been assumed to be achieved by lateral inhibitory interactions among neighboring cortical columns. Pinto et al. (1996) demonstrated a different mechanism of RF focusing, based on the greater responsiveness of inhibitory neurons in a cortical column to weak stimuli applied at the RF margins, and the resulting suppression of the responses of excitatory neurons within the *same* column.

DiCarlo and Johnson (2000) studied the tuning properties of cells in the earliest somatosensory cortical area, area 3b, using scanned, random-dot stimuli and regression analysis to estimate the cells' RF structure. This analysis revealed that area 3b neurons (especially those in the upper layers) are sensitive to the orientation of elongated stimuli and the direction of their motion. The responses of the cells were well described by a spatiotemporal RF model containing three components: (1) a single elongated excitatory region; (2) one or more inhibitory regions, adjacent to and nearly synchronous with the excitatory region and responsible for orientation sensitivity; and (3) a temporally delayed inhibitory region that overlaps partially or totally the excitatory region and is responsible for directional sensitivity. The insightfulness of this model was demonstrated by its ability to accurately predict cells' responses to stimuli (moving bars) that were not used to generate the RFs of the model.

Concerning the nature of cortical cell tuning, Ryder and Favorov (2001) proposed that cortical pyramidal cells tune to causal factors operating in the environment—in the case of the somatosensory cortex, causal factors involved in the physical interactions of the body with objects around it. Causal factors manifest themselves in statistical dependencies—*suspicious coincidences*—among environmental events. Environmental events are reflected only indirectly in the spatiotemporal activity patterns of sensory receptors; in mathematical terms, they can be considered functions over the states of sensory receptors. One way to discover causal factors is to look among various functions over various subsets of sensory receptors, searching for such pairs of functions over nonoverlapping subsets of receptors that will show correlated behaviors. Such *different but correlated* functions will identify a causal factor operating in the environment that is responsible for their correlation.

Ryder and Favorov (2001) proposed that such a search for different but correlated functions is performed by the dendrites of neocortical pyramidal cells. A pyramidal cell has several basal dendrites that extend horizontally in different directions away from the soma, passing through different groups of minicolumns. These different groups of minicolumns provide different basal dendrites of the same cell with different combinations of sensory inputs, over which dendrites can implement a wide variety of nonlinear functions. Which functions? Pyramidal cells seem well set to find *correlated* functions through the plasticity of their synaptic connec-

tions. Synaptic learning in dendrites is controlled both by presynaptic activity and by the output activity of the postsynaptic cell; the latter is signaled to each synapse by spikes that are back-propagated from the soma up through each dendrite. Thus, through its contribution to the cell's output, the output of each basal dendrite can influence the strengths of synaptic connections on the cell's other dendrites, teaching them to behave the way it does, while also learning from them. Through such mutual teaching and learning, different dendrites in a cell can learn to produce correlated outputs in response to their different inputs. That is, the dendrites can discover correlated functions over their different subsets of sensory variables, thereby tuning the cell to the causal factor responsible for this correlation. Ryder and Favorov named this concept of the pyramidal cell SINBAD (a Set of INteracting BAck-propagating Dendrites).

Cortical Dynamics

The cortical network is a complex dynamical system. Xing and Gerstein (1996a) used a model of the cortical network with spiking neurons, topographic projections between skin, thalamic, and cortical layers, and a Mexican-hat pattern of lateral connections in the cortical layer to investigate the contributions of lateral connections to the network's dynamics. They found the balance between lateral excitation and inhibition to be a key network parameter that controls the dynamical stability of the network, the sizes of RFs of cortical neurons, their temporal response patterns, and their spontaneous activity. Xing and Gerstein simulated a number of experimental manipulations of the SI network (such as cortical blockade of the inhibitory GABAergic transmission, cortical microinjections of the excitatory transmitter glutamate, local skin denervation, and local cortical lesions) and were able to account for all current observations of experimentally induced dynamic RF changes in SI, when the cortical layer operated in an inhibition-dominant mode.

Whitsel et al. (1991) proposed a model of cortical dynamics that explains why an initial cortical response to a stimulus undergoes substantial modifications with a continuous or repetitive exposure to that stimulus. According to their model, such modifications could result from activity-dependent increases in extracellular concentrations of potassium and their modulating effects on the state of NMDA receptors and neuromodulators, such as acetylcholine, and on the development of long-lasting afterhyperpolarization in active neurons. These changes in the network state translate into changes in pericolumnar inhibition, leading to progressive changes in the spatial pattern of cortical response. These changes make this pattern progressively more stimulus specific.

Favorov et al. (2002) investigated the nature of cortical dynamics in their model of the SI network, which was an extension of the earlier model of Favorov and Kelly (1996). The model was expanded to a local group of segregates (each made up of 61 minicolumns); it was also expanded to represent both the middle and the upper cortical layers, including their extensive lateral connectivity. The modeled network possesses the full range of dynamics (it exhibits a quasiperiodic route to chaos, capable of generating stable states, periodic and quasiperiodic oscillations, and chaotic fluctuations), depending on particular choices of network parameters. The complexity of the network's dynamics is limited, however, by several factors: (1) Even in the chaotic regime, it can produce only low-dimensional (less than eight) attractors, regardless of increases in the network's structural complexity. (2) Stronger stimuli, as well as moderate levels of random noise, reduce the complexity of dynamics. (3) Stimulus-evoked transients, while complex, are nevertheless to a large degree stereotypical, adhering to particular waveforms that are very stimulus specific.

Based on their model performance, Favorov et al. (2002) argue that, in addition to intended dynamical behaviors, the sheer complexity of a cortical network's structure should promote *spurious* dynamical behaviors. Dynamics observed in the model and in the somatosensory cortex suggest that such unintended dynamical behaviors are likely to be pervasive but relatively simple, contributing to rather than dominating the cortical network's response to stimuli. Many intriguing features of cortical stimulus-evoked behaviors might be attributable to spurious dynamics. We tend to expect specific mechanisms for specific dynamical behaviors, but the presence of spurious dynamics should warn us that a clearly identifiable dynamical feature does not necessarily imply a clearly identifiable cause: the cause might be distributed, everywhere and nowhere. Favorov et al. describe some of the spurious dynamical phenomena associated with the somatosensory cortical response to a brushing stimulation, illustrating how spurious dynamics can affect neurons' functional properties, cortical stimulus representation, and, ultimately, perception.

Discussion

What picture of sensory information transformation in somatosensory cortex emerges from these studies? The first transformation takes place in the input cortical layer, layer 4. The studies of Pearson et al. (1987), Montague et al. (1991), and Xing and Gerstein (1996b) suggest that discrete *macrocolumns* (such as rodent barrels or monkey segregates) are small, sharply delineated cortical regions that, during perinatal development, come to be innervated by a selected group of thalamic neurons, sharing similar RFs, whose axons all terminate extensively *throughout* the territory of that macrocolumn. According to Favorov and Kelly (1996), within a macrocolumn, thalamocortical axons connect to the minicolumns selectively, not uniformly, so that each minicolumn receives afferent connections from a unique subset of the thalamic neurons that project to that macrocolumn. The differences in afferent inputs to neighboring minicolumns are further amplified by their lateral inhibitory interactions, decorrelating almost completely the stimulus-evoked behaviors of neighboring minicolumns. Thus, it appears that local groups of minicolumns together represent a variety of different, but related sensory information concerning a local region of the stimulus space, with adjacent minicolumns tuned to extract only minimally redundant information about what takes place in that stimulus space. Such local cortical environments are exactly the right informational environments for pyramidal cells, to be mined by them in their search for causal factors.

The next transformation of sensory information takes place in the upper and deep cortical layers. Spiny-stellate cells of layer 4 provide their outputs to pyramidal cells lying above and below them in the same and nearby minicolumns. According to Ryder and Favorov (2001), pyramidal cells learn to respond to particular functions over these inputs, functions that identify prominent causal factors operating in the environment. Pyramidal cells then send their outputs to the next cortical area, where the same two-step process of (1) enriching local layer 4 neighborhoods with related sensory information and (2) tuning pyramidal cells of the upper and deep layers to higher-order causal factors is repeated, and so on in all somatosensory cortical areas.

With the prominent causal factors involved in body/object interactions represented explicitly by their pyramidal cells, the somatosensory cortical areas can capture the functional relations among the educed causal factors in the patterns of their ascending, lateral, and feedback connections and can develop an internal working model of mechanical interactions of the body with the outside world. Such an internal model can endow the somatosensory cortex with powerful interpretive and predictive capabilities, crucial for haptic perception of proximal surroundings and for control of object manipulation.

Road Maps: Mammalian Brain Regions; Other Sensory Systems
Related Reading: Cortical Hebbian Modules; Dendritic Learning; Somatotopy: Plasticity of Sensory Maps

References

DiCarlo, J. J., and Johnson, K. O., 2000, Spatial and temporal structure of receptive fields in primate somatosensory area 3b: Effects of stimulus scanning direction and orientation, *J. Neurosci.*, 20:495–510.

Favorov, O. V., Hester, J. T., Lao, R., and Tommerdahl, M., 2002, Spurious dynamics in somatosensory cortex, *Behav. Brain Res.*, in press. ◆

Favorov, O. V., and Kelly, D. G., 1996, Local receptive field diversity within cortical neuronal populations, in *Somesthesis and the Neurobiology of the Somatosensory Cortex* (O. Franzen, R. Johansson, and L. Terenius, Eds.), Basel: Birkhauser, pp. 395–408. ◆

Grajski, K. A., and Merzenich, M. M., 1990, Hebb-type dynamics is sufficient to account for the inverse magnification rule in cortical somatotopy, *Neural Computat.*, 2:77–84.

Hendry, S. H. C., Hsiao, S. S., and Bushnell, M. C., 1999, Somatic sensation, in *Fundamental Neuroscience* (M. J. Zigmond et al., Eds.), San Diego: Academic Press, pp. 761–790. ◆

Johnson, K. O., Phillips, J. R., Hsiao, S. S., and Bankman, I. N., 1991, Tactile pattern recognition, in *Information Processing in the Somatosensory System* (O. Franzen and J. Westman, Eds.), New York: Stockton, pp. 305–318. ◆

Montague, P. R., Gally, J. A., and Edelman, G. M., 1991, Spatial signaling in the development and function of neural connections, *Cereb. Cortex*, 1:199–220.

Mountcastle, V. B., Steinmetz, M. A., and Romo, R., 1990, Frequency discrimination in the sense of flutter: Psychophysical measurements correlated with postcentral events in behaving monkeys, *J. Neurosci.*, 10:3032–3044.

Pearson, J. C., Finkel, L. M., and Edelman, G. M., 1987, Plasticity in the organization of adult cerebral cortical maps: A computer simulation based on neuronal group selection, *J. Neurosci.*, 7:4209–4223.

Pinto, D. J., Brumberg, J. C., Simons, D. J., Ermentrout, G. B., 1996, A quantitative population model of whisker barrels: Re-examining the Wilson-Cowan equations, *J. Comput. Neurosci.*, 3:247–264.

Ryder, D., and Favorov, O. V., 2001, The new associationism: A neural explanation for the predictive powers of cerebral cortex, *Brain Mind*, 2:161–194.

Whitsel, B. L., Favorov, O. V., Kelly, D. G., and Tommerdahl, M., 1991, Mechanisms of dynamic peri- and intra-columnar interactions in somatosensory cortex: Stimulus-specific contrast enhancement by NMDA receptor activation, in *Information Processing in the Somatosensory System* (O. Franzen and J. Westman, Eds.), New York: Stockton, pp. 353–369.

Xing, J., and Gerstein, G. L., 1996a, Networks with lateral connectivity: I. Dynamic properties mediated by the balance of intrinsic excitation and inhibition, *J. Neurophysiol.*, 75:184–199.

Xing, J., and Gerstein, G. L., 1996b, Networks with lateral connectivity: II. Development of neuronal grouping and corresponding receptive field changes, *J. Neurophysiol.*, 75:200–216.

Zhang, H. Q., Zachariah, M. K., Coleman, G. T., and Rowe, M. J., 2001, Hierarchical equivalence of somatosensory areas I and II for tactile processing in the cerebral cortex of the marmoset monkey, *J. Neurophysiol.*, 85:1823–1835.

Somatotopy: Plasticity of Sensory Maps

Sherre L. Florence and Jon H. Kaas

Introduction

Somatotopy, a dominant feature of subdivisions of the somatosensory system, is defined by a topographic representation, or map, in the brain of sensory receptors on the body surface (see SOMATOSENSORY SYSTEM for a review of cortical somatosensory receptive fields and their development). In the mammalian brain, there are orderly representations of cutaneous receptors at various levels: in the spinal cord, lower brainstem, thalamus, and neocortex. In the past, these sensory maps were considered relatively permanent point-to-point representations, with little or no changes in internal organization once the mature patterns had developed. Over the past two decades, however, evidence for plastic changes at all levels of the adult somatosensory system accumulated in a wide range of mammalian species. It is now clear that the somatotopic organization of sensory maps represents both the peripheral distribution of receptors and the dynamic aspects of brain function. Most of the evidence for somatosensory plasticity has accrued from studies of cortical reorganization after peripheral injury; however, changes in the relative levels of sensory stimulation as a result of training can also produce reorganization. Additionally, modifications can occur in sensory maps at all levels of the pathway, including subcortical and cortical somatosensory stations. This article emphasizes work on plasticity in the primate somatosensory system. The following issues are discussed: What features of somatotopic maps change, and under what conditions are the changes produced? How do subcortical changes contribute to cortical plasticity? What mechanisms account for these changes? What are the functional consequences of sensory map changes?

Somatotopic Plasticity in Cortex

The large representation of the hand in the somatosensory cortex of primates is particularly suitable for studies of cortical plasticity, since some of the plastic changes involve small topographic shifts that are harder to detect in the compact representations that exist subcortically. The approach typically is to eliminate the relay of sensory information from a certain portion of the skin surface to the brain. A wide range of denervation procedures has been used, including nerve crush or cut, lidocaine injection, and amputation. The effects of the deprivation on the somatosensory pathway can be studied minutes, weeks, or even years later using microelectrode recording techniques that allow large regions of the nervous system to be sampled in each animal in a relatively limited span of time. In one of the first clear demonstrations of adult plasticity, Merzenich and colleagues (for a review, see Buonomano and Merzenich, 1998; Kaas and Florence, 2000) cut the median nerve that innervates the glabrous (palmar) surface of the thumb, index, and long fingers and the adjacent palmar pads in monkeys. Immediately after the nerve was cut, the majority of neurons in the large cortical zone where median nerve skin is represented were unresponsive. However, at a small number of recording sites, neurons had rapidly acquired new receptive fields on the dorsal rather than the glabrous surfaces of the digits. The immediate appearance of new receptive fields was detected at only a limited number of recording sites; the newly reactivated neurons were located in narrow zones along borders with adjacent intact representations. Thus the somatotopic extent of the change was quite small in scale.

The full potential for reorganization became apparent over an extended time course that required weeks and months after peripheral denervation. In some cases, much longer epochs, such as a year or more, seemed to be needed for all changes to emerge. In their initial studies of the effects of median nerve transection, Merzenich et al. (reviewed by Buonomano and Merzenich, 1998; Kaas and Florence, 2000) noted that more extensive map reorganization occurred in the weeks following denervation. They also determined that the source of the new activating inputs was somatotopically consistent. Neurons throughout much of the deprived median nerve territory had acquired new receptive fields on the hairy (dorsal) surfaces of the denervated digits or on the adjacent ulnar nerve–innervated hand, representations that are spatially adjacent to the deprived cortex. Subsequent investigations, involving a wide variety of sensory denervations, confirmed that alternative sources of activation to deprived representations typically were near neighbors in the sensory map (Figure 1). Thus, after amputation of only a portion of the index finger (digit 2, D2), neurons in the deprived zone closest to the border with D1 were reactivated by D1, and those closest to the intact representation of proximal D2 acquired new receptive fields on D2 (Figure 1B). If all the digits were lost, neurons in the deprived zone were reactivated by inputs from the palm (Figure 1C). If the hand was amputated, the deprived cortical representation was reactivated by inputs predominantly from the forearm (Figure 1D), although there may also have been some expansion of the face representation. Injuries that led to the loss or denervation of even larger extents of the arm resulted in progressively more takeover by inputs from the face (Figure 1E; see also Kaas and Florence, 2000).

Although few studies in primates have looked at the detailed time course of the slowly developing plasticity, it is assumed that reactivations of more than a few millimeters of cortical territory require many months before the full complement of changes could be expressed. For example, 3 weeks after complete cervical dorsal column section to eliminate all tactile inputs from the forelimb, cortical reorganization was still incomplete (reviewed in Jain and Kaas, 1998); however, by 6–8 months, hand cortex was fully reactivated by inputs from the face.

An important caveat of the studies that employ sensory deprivation to induce somatotopic plasticity is that outcomes may differ depending on the integrity of the denervation. For example, if even a few of the dominant inputs are spared, their influence is dramatically amplified and the skin surface that they innervate can take over considerable extents of deprived cortex. This was demonstrated compellingly by Jain and colleagues (see Jain and Kaas, 1998) in a study of the effects of dorsal column transection. In some cases the transection was incomplete and some of the sensory afferents from the hand that ascend in the dorsal columns were spared. At the level of cortex, these spared inputs activated only a small portion of the hand representation initially after the injury. However, over the course of about 5 weeks subsequent to the deprivation, the skin surface represented by the spared inputs expanded markedly and came to occupy the full extent of deprived cortex. Thus, the originally dominant sensory inputs appeared to have much more potency in denervated cortex than other, nondominant inputs.

Changes in cortical somatotopy have also been observed in intact individuals involved in behaviors that alter sensory stimulation patterns. For example, in monkeys trained in behavioral discrimination tasks, the cortical representation of the portion of the hand used to make the discrimination increased in representational area and the neurons in this representation had decreased receptive field sizes (for review, see Buonomano and Merzenich, 1998). Thus, more cortical space was devoted to the behaviorally important skin,

A. Normal area 3b hand representation

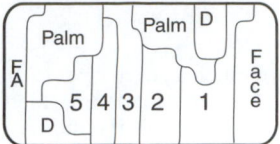

Hand Representation

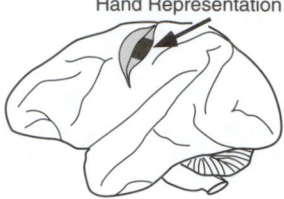

B. Partial amputation of D2

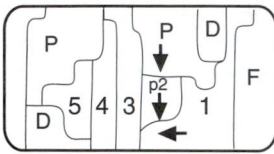

C. Amputation of all digits

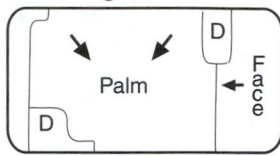

D. Hand amputation

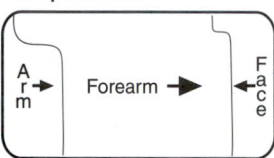

E. Forelimb amputation

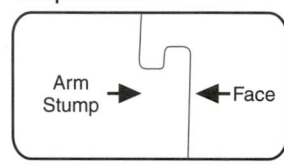

Figure 1. Patterns of topographic organization in area 3b of macaque monkeys after amputation of part or all of the forelimb. The location of cortical area 3b on the posterior bank of the central sulcus is shown in the figurine to the top right. The central sulcus (gray shading) has been opened to show the approximate location of the hand representation (dark gray shading). *A*, Topographic organization of the hand representation in area 3b in normal macaque monkeys. Large numerals 1–5 refer to the representations of digits 1–5, and thin lines indicate borders between representations. *B*, The pattern of reorganization that emerged in the hand representation of a monkey that lost the middle and distal phalanges of digit 2. Arrows indicate that adjacent representations expanded into the deprived zone (reviewed in Jones, 2000). *C*, After loss of all digits on one hand, the region of area 3b where the digits are normally represented is taken over by a large representation of the palm (reviewed in Kaas and Florence, 2000). *D*, After amputation at the level of the wrist, the hand representation is taken over by representations of the forearm (reviewed in Kaas and Florence, 2000). *E*, After amputation at the mid-humeral level of the arm, the deprived region is taken over by an expanded representation of the stump of the arm medially and the face laterally (reviewed in Kaas and Florence, 2000). D, Dors, dorsum of the hand; F, face; FA, forearm; P, palm; p2, proximal phalanx of digit 2.

and at the same time the "grain" of the representation became more refined. The impact of sensory training on cortical somatotopy was similar in humans. Recordings of somatosensory-evoked potentials in hand cortex of blind subjects who learned to read using the Braille method demonstrated that the area of activation for the reading (right index) finger was larger than that for other fingers (Pascual-Leone and Torres, 1993).

Subcortical Contributions to Plasticity

Cortex typically is considered to have more adaptive potential than the subcortical relays; however, there is ample evidence for subcortical plasticity (reviewed by Kaas, Florence, and Jain, 1999; Jones, 2000; Kaas and Florence, 2000). Moreover, subcortical remodeling may be a substrate for some of the plasticity observed in cortex. Immediately after median nerve transection in monkeys,

deprived neurons in the cuneate nucleus of the brainstem acquire new receptive fields on the dorsal skin of the hand, the same types of receptive fields shifts as described in cortex (Xu and Wall, 1999). This suggests that the reorganization observed in cortex is initiated by plasticity mechanisms in the cuneate nucleus.

Also, in monkeys that had undergone forelimb amputation, the pattern of reorganization observed in somatosensory cortex, reactivation of deprived cortex by expanded representations of the stump of the arm and the face, was consistent with changes observed at the level of the brainstem and thalamus. In the cuneate nucleus, the primary sensory afferents from the skin of the forearm adjacent to the amputation, which normally terminate dorsally in the cuneate nucleus, sprouted ventrally to occupy the region where hand inputs normally prevail (Figure 2). Similarly, inputs from the chin of the face, which normally project to the trigeminal nucleus, sprouted into the cuneate nucleus and infiltrated the deprived hand representation (Figure 2; see also Jain et al., 2000). Assuming that the new inputs were functionally potent, their impact would be even more evident at the next levels in the processing sequence, in the ventroposterior nucleus (VP) and consequently in somatosensory cortex (Figure 2), as a result of diverging projections. Indeed, recent studies of the functional organization of VP in monkeys that had sustained forelimb loss demonstrated new patterns of organization in the hand representation of VP (Florence, Hackett, and Strata, 2000) that were consistent with the interpretation that reorganization in the cuneate nucleus leads to map changes at higher-order stations. Other studies in monkeys as well as in humans documented somatotopic changes in the thalamus that mirror those reported in cortex (reviewed in Kaas and Florence, 2000).

Mechanisms Underlying Map Plasticity

Multiple mechanisms contribute to somatotopic plasticity (reviewed in Buonomano and Merzenich, 1998; Kaas and Florence, 2000). Immediate changes have been attributed to an unmasking of existing excitatory connections through a reduction of afferent-driven activation of GABAergic inhibitory neurons (called *disinhibition*). The extent of this immediate reorganization is limited by the amount of overlap of the central projections from different skin regions. Thus, the spatial extent of changes mediated by disinhibition is small in scale. Nonetheless, the accumulation of small changes across subcortical levels of processing could yield a larger cortical reorganization. Changes that take place over a longer time course likely result from a combination of events, with disinhibition accounting for only a proportion of the reorganization. Some of the more slowly developing changes are presumed to involve Hebbian-type mechanisms. A model of cortical plasticity based on Hebbian-like synaptic modifications replicates most of the more limited somatotopic map changes (Sklar, 1991). For example, the model can account for changes in cortical organization after peripheral nerve injury and regeneration, the expansion of representations after the removal of competing inputs (such as after digit amputation), and expansions after overstimulation of a digit. This model is based on the theory that a neuron possesses a synaptic modification threshold that dictates whether the efficacy of synapses impinging on the neuron is strengthened or weakened. The threshold changes in relation to the neuron's recent average postsynaptic activity, so that synapses potentiate when postsynaptic activity is greater than the synaptic modification threshold and weaken when activity is less than the threshold.

Currently, the strongest candidate for the neural mechanism that underlies the Hebbian-type modification is the *N*-methyl-D-aspartate (NMDA) receptor mechanism (see NMDA RECEPTORS: SYNAPTIC, CELLULAR, AND NETWORK MODELS). The NMDA receptor is thought to coexist with other receptors for excitatory amino acids and to mediate synaptic transmission jointly. To test the role of the NMDA receptor mechanism in the reorganization

Normal

Forelimb Amputation

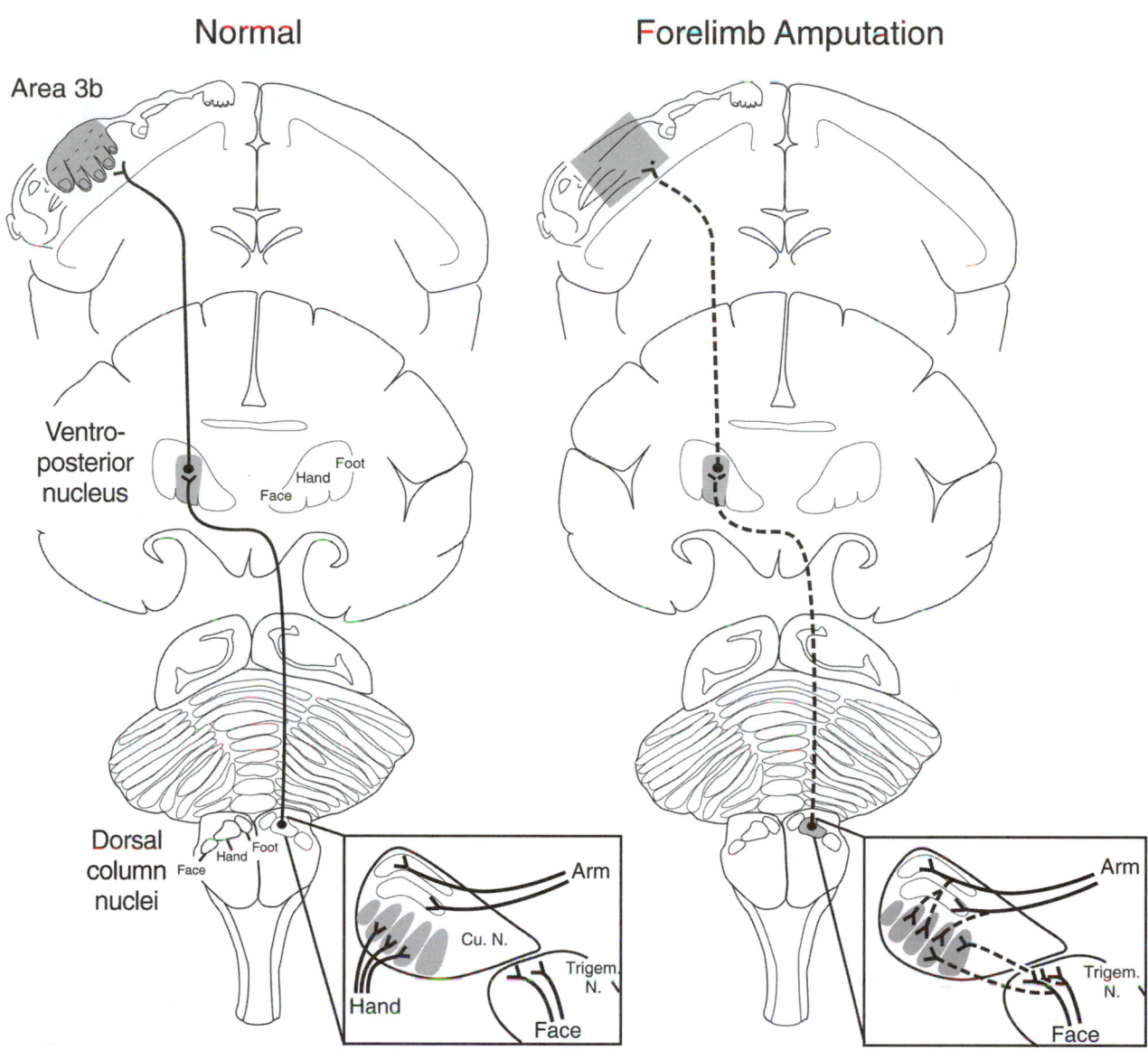

Figure 2. Schematic showing that changes in the dorsal column nuclei produced by longstanding forelimb amputation can lead to reactivations of the hand representations in the ventroposterior nucleus (VP) of the thalamus and cortical area 3b. In normal macaque monkeys (series of cross-sections on the left), only projections from the skin of the hand target the ventralmost cell clusters in the cuneate nucleus (gray shading). These inputs initiate a relay of activation to the hand representations (gray shading) in VP and in area 3b. In monkeys that lost part or all of the forelimb (series of cross-sections on the right), new connections from the arm and from the face (dashed lines in the enlarged image of the cuneate nucleus) sprout into the region of the cuneate nucleus where the hand is normally represented. These new activating inputs alter the maps projected to VP and area 3b (dashed lines), where neurons that normally respond to the hand (gray shading) come to respond to stimulation of the remaining stump of the arm or to the face (see Florence et al., 2000, for a discussion).

of hand cortex after median nerve transection in monkeys, NMDA antagonists were delivered systemically for weeks after the injury (reviewed in Myers et al., 2000). The reactivation of denervated cortex that typically emerged during that time course was blocked, indicating that the NMDA receptor mechanism was essential for the plasticity.

An important distinction of NMDA receptor–mediated plasticity is that it is *not* responsible for the reorganization that occurs immediately after sensory deprivation. As mentioned above, the rapid release of GABA inhibition was thought to be responsible for the plastic changes that appear immediately after a sensory denerva-

tion. To confirm that two mechanisms explain the distinct epochs in the time course of somatosensory plasticity, Myers and colleagues (2000) examined the immediate effects of median nerve transection in monkeys that had undergone systemic blockade of NMDA receptors. If NMDA receptors were required for the rapid appearance of new cortical receptive fields after nerve transection, then NMDA receptor blockade would prevent immediate plastic changes from occurring. However, this was not the case; immediate reorganization was observed in treated monkeys, just as in the control group. Thus, the NMDA receptor mechanism apparently played no role in the rapid phase of the somatotopic plasticity.

Over very long time courses, map reorganizations probably involve additional plasticity mechanisms. The growth of new connections probably accounts for some of the slowly developing changes. New growth, or *sprouting*, was thought to be limited in the mature brain so that the stability of brain function could be preserved. However, over the last decade, sprouting in the adult nervous system has been documented repeatedly. For example, in the spinal cord and lower brainstem, the central processes of both injured and uninjured peripheral nerve axons sprout when nearby synaptic territories are vacated by the removal of other peripheral nerve inputs (reviewed in Mendell and Lewin, 1992). Other evidence for sprouting is the finding of new inputs to the hand representation in the cuneate nucleus of monkeys that had forelimb amputation (described above). Finally, local-circuit neurons in primary somatosensory cortex have the potential for considerable new growth. In monkeys with longstanding forelimb injuries, injections of anatomical tracers into the deprived hand representation resulted in much more extensive zones of label than in normal monkeys (reviewed in Kaas and Florence, 2000). The data suggested that neurons in the deprived region of cortex had extended new connections to nondeprived portions of the sensory representation. The functional impact of the new connections was unclear; however, they may have provided an additional source of activation for the deprived neurons.

Functional Consequences of Sensory Map Changes

It has been commonly assumed that large sensory representations relate to superior sensory abilities, since skin zones with good tactile acuity, such as the hands and lips, have large representations in the somatosensory pathway. To some extent, these large representations reflect a high density of peripheral receptors; however, it also appears that adding neurons to a processing circuit enhances the performance of that circuit. For example, after monkeys were trained in a tactile discrimination task using a specific finger, the cortical representation of that finger expanded and performance improved. Also, human amputees often demonstrated increased tactile acuity for skin zones adjacent to the site of amputation, the same skin whose cortical representation was expanded. In contrast, no improvement in the sensory performance of the reading finger was detected in Braille readers, even though the cortical representation of that finger was expanded (Pascual-Leone and Torres, 1993). Thus, the consequence of the expansion of the sensory representations in cortex remains unclear.

Some cortical reorganization may contribute to sensory mislocalizations. For example, some patients with forelimb amputations reported that tactile stimuli applied to the face produced sensations of touch on both the face and on the missing forelimb (Ramachandran and Hirstein, 1998). These mislocalizations have been attributed to reactivation of the denervated forelimb representation by face inputs, observed using noninvasive imaging techniques (see Elbert and Flor, 1999). The clinical findings suggest that, at least for the case of limb amputation, expanded representations do not lead to better performance. Thus, there must be limits to the extent to which processing circuits can benefit from increasing neuron number. Beyond that limit, additional neurons appear to be a detriment to sensory abilities.

For such profound changes in the topographic organization of the somatosensory cortex to affect the behavior of the individual, the use-driven alterations almost certainly must be relayed through higher-order sensory cortical areas into the motor pathway. Motor cortex appears to be equally as plastic as somatosensory cortex (reviewed by Sanes and Donoghue, 2000), and the interrelationship between the two has been shown in monkeys that develop a task-specific dystonia (abnormal and often painful muscular contrac-

tions) after intensive sensory training. The dystonia has been attributed to alterations in the sensory representations of skin surfaces that are overstimulated during training (Byl, Merzenich, and Jenkins, 1996). Sensory maps appear to be important for sensory control of fine motor skills; thus, it is argued that when the sensory maps are disrupted, sensorimotor feedback is affected and abnormal motor behaviors can emerge. A model of the relationship between the sensory and motor systems predicts that certain plastic changes in somatosensory cortex may exacerbate abnormal motor behaviors, such as dystonias (Sanger and Merzenich, 2000).

Discussion

The reviewed findings show that both peripheral injury and altered sensory experience result in modifications of the body representation in the somatosensory cortex of primates. Current models of cortical function can account for many of the observed changes in somatotopic organization, but no models exist to account for the extensive reorganizations that occur long after massive sensory deprivation. This is largely because such massive reorganizations depend on the growth of new connections, and not only on changing synaptic weights. To successfully explain the types of topographic changes that have been found with large-scale reorganizations, models may need to estimate the role of new growth, and the accumulation of reorganizations relayed from subcortical levels of the somatosensory system.

Acknowledgments. This work was supported by NIH grants NS16446 (to JHK) and NS36469 (to SLF), and by the John F. Kennedy Center for Research on Education and Human Development.

Road Maps: Neural Plasticity; Other Sensory Systems
Background: Somatosensory System
Related Reading: Axonal Path Finding; Development of Retinotectal Maps; Ocular Dominance and Orientation Columns

References

Buonomano, D. V., and Merzenich, M. M., 1998, Cortical plasticity: From synapses to maps, *Ann. Rev. Neurosci.*, 21:149–186. ◆

Byl, N., Merzenich, M. M., and Jenkins, W. M., 1996, A primate genesis model of focal dystonia and repetitive strain injury: I. Learning-induced dedifferentiation of the representation of the hand in the primary somatosensory cortex in adult monkeys, *Neurology*, 47:508–520.

Elbert, T., and Flor, H., 1999, Magnetoencephalographic investigations of cortical reorganization in humans, *Electroencephalogr. Clin. Neurophysiol. Suppl.*, 49:284–291.

Florence, S. L., Hackett, T. A., and Strata, F., 2000, Thalamic and cortical contributions to neural plasticity after limb amputation, *J. Neurophysiol.*, 83:3154–3159.

Jain, N., Florence, S. L., Qi, H-.X., and Kaas, J. H., 2000, Growth of new brainstem connections in adult monkeys with massive sensory loss, *Proc. Natl. Acad. Sci. USA*, 97:5546–5550.

Jain, N., and Kaas, J. H., 1998, The reorganization of the somatosensory system in primates after spinal cord injury, *Adv. Clin. Neurosci.*, 8:437–450.

Jones, E. G., 2000, Cortical and subcortical contributions to activity-dependent plasticity in primate somatosensory cortex, *Annu. Rev. Neurosci.*, 23:1–37.

Kaas, J. H., and Florence, S. L., 2000, Reorganization of sensory and motor systems in adult mammals after injury, in *The Mutable Brain* (J. H. Kaas, Ed.), London: Gordon and Breach, pp. 165–242.

Kaas, J. H., Florence, S. L., and Jain, N., 1999, Subcortical contributions to massive cortical reorganizations, *Neuron*, 22:657–660. ◆

Mendell, L. M., and Lewin, G. R., 1992, Removing constraints on neural sprouting, *Curr. Biol.*, 2:259–261.

Myers, W. A., Churchill, J. D., Muja, N., and Garraghty, P. E., 2000, Role of NMDA receptors in adult primate cortical somatosensory plasticity, *J. Comp. Neurol.*, 418:373–382.

Pascual-Leone, A., and Torres, F., 1993, Plasticity of sensorimotor cortex representation of the reading finger in Braille readers, *Brain*, 116:39–52.

Ramachandran, V. S., and Hirstein, W., 1998, The perception of phantom limbs: The D. O. Hebb Lecture, *Brain*, 121:1603–1630. ◆

Sanes, J. N., and Donoghue, J. P., 2000, Plasticity and primary motor cortex, *Annu. Rev. Neurosci.*, 23:393–415. ◆

Sanger, T. D., and Merzenich, M. M., 2000, Computational model of the role of sensory disorganization in focal task-specific dystonia, *J. Neurophysiol.*, 84:2458–2464.

Sklar, E., 1991, A simulation of somatosensory cortical map plasticity, in *Proceedings of the International Joint Conference on Neural Networks*, vol. 3, New York: IEEE, pp. 727–732.

Xu, J., and Wall, J. T., 1999, Evidence for brainstem and supra-brainstem contributions to rapid cortical plasticity in adult monkeys, *J. Neurosci.*, 19:7578–7590.

Sound Localization and Binaural Processing

Yehuda Albeck

Introduction

In the most general sense, the term *sound localization* means the vivid perception of the location of an object that emits sound. In the more restricted context of psychophysics and neurophysiology, the term denotes the precision with which a subject can point at a sound source and the computational algorithm that the brain uses to complete such tasks. Psychologists can infer the characteristics of the human sound localization system by tuning their models to describe the performance of human subjects. These models emphasize performance: how well people localize sounds and what parameters affect this ability.

Neurobiologists study the underlying neural processing, focusing on neural characteristics and patterns of connectivity such as tuning curves, axonal conduction latencies, and inhibitory or excitatory projections. They use behavioral studies in normal and lesioned animals to study the role and significance of different groups of neurons for sound localization. The two disciplines produce similar but distinct models.

In this article, I concentrate on one aspect of sound localization: the use of the interaural time difference (ITD) to estimate the azimuthal angle of a sound source. I describe one biological model—the ITD detection in the barn owl's brainstem—and two psychological models—the cross-correlation (CRC) model extended by inhibition and monaural processors and the straightness model. These models have much in common. The biological model is well understood in terms of information processing. The psychological models are defined in realistic biological terms, and both contain elements that are present in the biological system. The binaural time pathway in the cat is also well understood (for reviews and references to more biological models, see Yin and Chan, 1988; Casseday and Covey, 1987).

More specifically, these models have a common theoretical foundation, the CRC model. This model suggests that the brain attempts to match the sounds in the two ears by shifting one sound relative to the other. To estimate the match, the brain averages the multiplication of the instantaneous amplitudes. This operation is similar to computing the CRC function of the sounds in the two ears. The shift that produces the best match is assumed to be the one that just balances the *real ITD*. However, the models differ in the detailed composition of the binaural cross-correlator and the way it is interpreted by higher systems. By comparing the models, I intend to highlight the merits of each approach and advocate the need for a unified theory that can satisfy the requirements of both fields.

Models of binaural interaction are founded on a simple logic. The mathematical description, however, is tedious. Thus, the description is only a qualitative introduction. Detailed mathematical formulation, simulation procedures, and experimental paradigms can be found in the original articles (for review, see Yin and Chan, 1988; Yost and Hafter, 1987; and other chapters in these books).

The Cross-Correlation Model

Figure 1 shows a possible implementation of the CRC model (Jeffress, 1948). The ears decompose the sounds to their spectral components using a bank of bandpass filters. Each output line conveys the waveform in a specific spectral channel. Each spectral channel interacts with the corresponding channel from the other ear. The representation of information in distinct spectral channels is called *tonotopic organization*. Each binaural neuron multiplies the signals

Figure 1. Schematic diagram of the cross-correlation model. The binaural processor has two dimensions, frequency and interaural time difference. In this example, each of the four spectral channels, f_1–f_4, has four coincidence detectors. The signals from each ear pass along delay lines on the way along the nucleus toward the contralateral side. Each detector provides an estimate of the cross-correlation of the signals at a specific band f_i for a specific time shift τ_i.

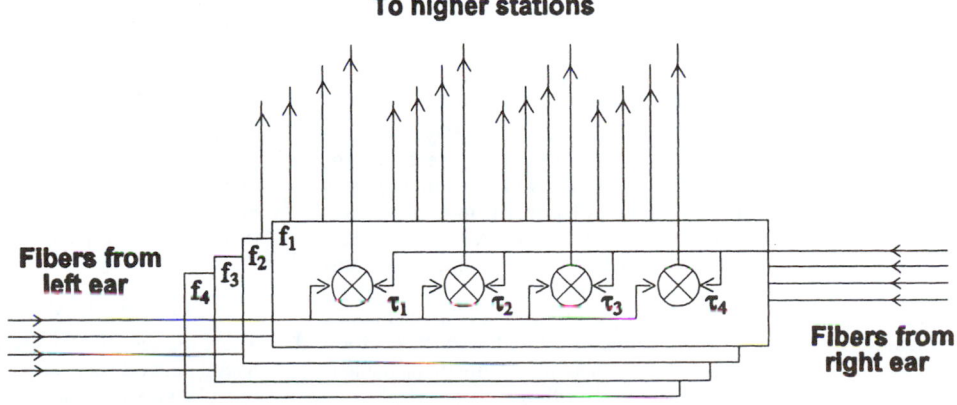

from both sides and averages the signal over the recent past. The inputs from the ears to each binaural neuron are identical; only the relative time shift is different. The signal from the left side reaches the leftmost unit before the signal from the right side does. The opposite is true for the neuron in the right border of the processor. Between these two extremes, the signals are shifted relative to each other by many intermediate values.

The model uses three important features. First, the input signal must represent the temporal structure of the sound. This representation is achieved by phase locking the spikes in the auditory nerve to the signal. In other words, the instantaneous likelihood of observing a spike in the auditory nerve is approximately proportional to the amplitude of the half-wave rectified sound at that time. The barn owl's auditory nerve phase locks to frequencies as high as 9 kHz. Second, the signal has to be accurately delayed to each binaural neuron by selecting the length of the axons from each side to provide the exact amount of conduction delay. The relevant range of ITDs for barn owls is $\pm170\,\mu s$ (the size of the head divided by the speed of sound). Finally, neurons in the binaural processor must effectively multiply the signals. The neural system employs coincidence detectors to mimic the multiplication. These neurons respond only when spikes from the two sides arrive simultaneously, or at least within a fraction of a millisecond. Mathematically, this operation is equivalent to multiplication because the likelihood of a coincidence is the product of the likelihoods of the single independent events (see review in Yin and Chan, 1988). The biophysics of the coincidence detection are not clear (see discussion in Yin and Chan, 1993).

This binaural processor contains a map that *place codes* the azimuth of the target. The neuron for which the axonal interaural delay balances the acoustic interaural delay becomes most active. Its place along the array codes the real ITD. The ITD response of a single cell is usually wider than the behavioral acuity; thus, the brain must use global coding to read the map. The nature of this mechanism is not known.

The Time Pathway in Barn Owls

Barn owls use hearing to locate their prey. When an owl hears a sound, it quickly turns its head to gaze directly at the sound source. The head-turning behavior involves auditory, visual, and motor systems. The auditory system's role is to provide a two-dimensional map of the space. In this map, the location of the target is coded by the firing of a group of neurons. The neurons in the map are organized in a two-dimensional array that resides in the external nucleus of the inferior colliculus. The location of the activity along one axis codes the azimuthal angle of the target. Along the perpendicular axis, the *interaural intensity difference* is represented, which codes the elevation of the target. This map projects to a motor map that controls the owl's neck muscles.

The creation of the ITD map occurs in four computational steps. The brain divides this task among at least eight structures on each side of the brain. A block diagram of the network is shown in Figure 2. The sound is bandpass filtered and transduced to a series of phase-locked spikes in the ears. These series are relayed through the auditory nerve to the nucleus magnocellularis, one of the cochlear nuclei. Each nucleus magnocellularis projects to a nucleus laminaris on both sides. Each nucleus laminaris, in turn, projects to the core of the contralateral inferior colliculus. All of these nuclei are tonotopically organized. The contralateral inferior colliculus projects to the lateral shell of the inferior colliculus on the contralateral side, and the lateral shell projects to the homolateral inferior colliculus. Note that the pathway crosses the midline back and forth three times, but binaural interactions take place only in the nucleus laminaris (see review in Konishi et al., 1988).

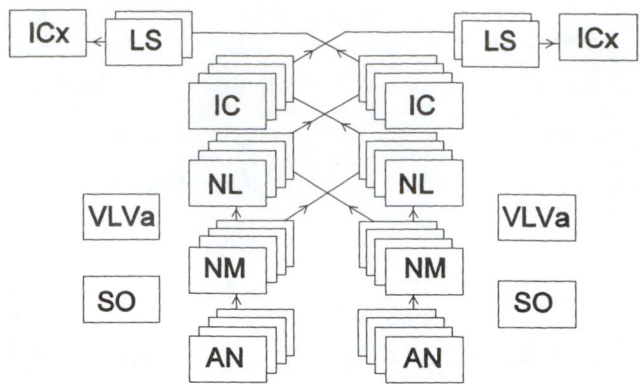

Figure 2. Block diagram of the barn owl's binaural time pathway. The nucleus magnocellularis (NM) relays the auditory nerve (AN) spikes to the nucleus laminaris (NL) on both sides. The NL projects to the core of the inferior colliculus (IC) on the contralateral side. The IC innervates the lateral shell (LS) of the IC, and the LS in turn projects to the inferior colliculus (ICx). Other nuclei, such as the superior olive (SO) and ventral lateral anterior lemniscus (VLVa), also participate, but are not discussed here. Tonotopic organized nuclei are shown in a cascade.

Typical ITD response curves of neurons from the nucleus laminaris, lateral shell, and inferior colliculus are plotted in Figure 3. Recordings in the nucleus laminaris confirm the predictions of the CRC model. The nucleus contains a systematic map of frequencies and ITDs (Carr and Konishi, 1990). In the nucleus laminaris and the contralateral inferior colliculus, the curve is periodic; this phenomenon is called *phase ambiguity*. A typical ITD response in the lateral shell shows a central dominant peak and smaller secondary peaks. In many inferior colliculus neurons, the secondary peaks disappear. This type of neuron is called *space specific*. Note also that the width of the ITD response decreases from approximately 70 μs in the nucleus laminaris to less than 30 μs in the inferior colliculus.

How does the phase-ambiguous curve transform into a space-specific response? It takes a combination of two processes, which are illustrated in Figure 4. The tonotopically organized nucleus laminaris is depicted as a matrix of binaural neurons. Each neuron has its own characteristic frequency and ITD. All neurons that have the same ITD, from all frequency channels, converge in the lateral shell. The convergence creates a composed ITD response curve, with partial suppression of secondary peaks. The real ITD appears in the same location across all of the spectral channels. The secondary peaks are separated from the primary peak by one period of the characteristic frequency; therefore, they have different locations for different frequencies. Thus, the contribution of the secondary peaks is spread out and cannot create a sharp, distinct peak in the composed ITD curve. Consequently, space-specific neurons cannot localize pure-tone stimuli (Takahashi and Konishi, 1986).

The second step involves inhibition (Fujita and Konishi, 1991). Neurons in the lateral shell project to inferior colliculus neurons with the same ITD. Simultaneously, they inhibit other inferior colliculus neurons with different ITDs. The inhibition, along with a high threshold, suppresses the activity in all neurons except those that receive a projection from the central ITD peak.

Psychophysical Models

The CRC model provides a basic mechanism that explains how a neural network can extract the ITD of a binaural signal. Early theoretical approaches used this mechanism to calculate the theoretical

Figure 3. Normalized interaural time difference (ITD) response curves from the barn owl's brainstem. The nucleus laminaris (NL) response is phase ambiguous and has a high baseline. In the lateral shell (LS), the secondary peaks are suppressed. In the external nucleus of the inferior colliculus (ICx), only a narrow range of ITD evokes some response.

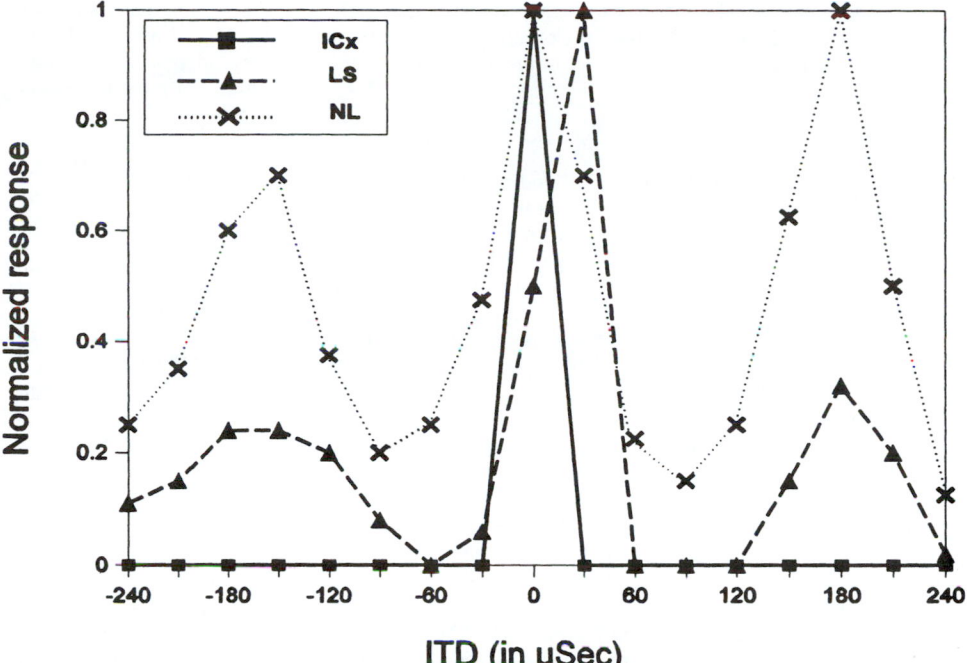

limits on the network's performance derived from the amount of noise in the system (see review in Colburn and Durlach, 1978).

More recent studies focused on how the binaural processor is used to estimate sound locations and enhance detection in a noisy

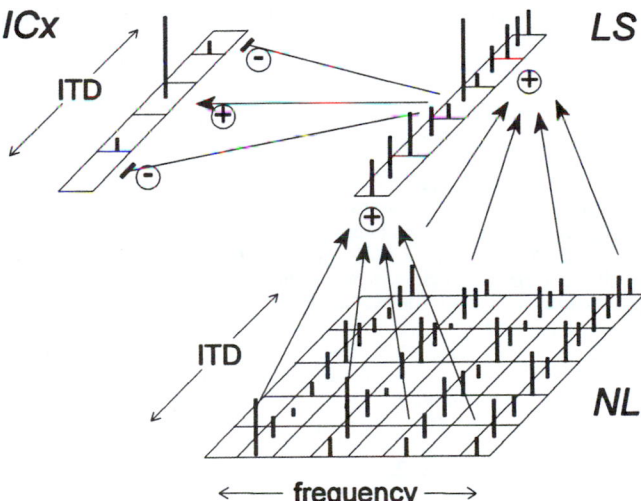

Figure 4. The nucleus laminaris (NL) can be viewed as a matrix of neurons. Each row in this matrix represents a group of neurons with the same characteristic frequency and different ITDs. Columns represent neurons with the same ITD and different characteristic frequency. All the neurons in a specific row excite a single neuron in the lateral shell (LS). The excitation is denoted by an arrow and a plus sign. This projection transforms the NL matrix into a one-dimensional array of ITD-sensitive neurons and destroys the frequency tuning. LS neurons supply excitation to interior colliculus (ICx) neurons with the same ITD and inhibition to other ICx neurons with ITDs larger or smaller than their own. The inhibition is denoted by an arrow with a minus sign. These ICx neurons show a sharp tuning to the sound location and a broad tuning to frequency.

environment (see review in Stern and Trahiotis, 1995). The basic CRC mechanism explains the lateralization experiments. *Lateralization* refers to the perception of an image inside the head that occurs in earphone experiments. *Localization* refers to external perception. The model does not explain how and why the interaural intensity difference can affect lateralization (see, e.g., Yost and Hafter, 1987). This effect is called *time-intensity trading*. The interaural intensity difference cannot change the CRC predictions because the signals from both sides are simply multiplied. Lindemann (1986) suggested that the signal traveling along the binaural processor has two components. The sound-evoked signal attenuates as it travels along the delay line, and it is replaced by a second independent signal. If the sound in the right ear is faint, the binaural units on the right of the processor will multiply it by the left signal and produce a small response. On the other hand, the units on the left multiply the strong signal from the left ear by the independent signal and produce a higher response. The peak of the response is then shifted leftward, and a time-intensity trade results. In addition, Lindemann suggested that each unit in the binaural processor inhibits the input to the other units (for more details, including the distinction between static and dynamic inhibition, see Lindemann, 1986). This inhibition sharpens the ITD peaks and enhances the stronger peak when another peak appears.

These extensions to the CRC model elegantly explain the time-intensity interaction. The model does not explain the interaction between different spectral channels. A pure 500-Hz tone with an ITD of −1.5 ms sounds as if it has an ITD of +0.5 ms. Both solutions are identical for a pure CRC model, but human subjects always perceive the ITD that is smaller in absolute value. As the spectrum of the signal broadens, the perception crosses the midline and moves toward the location that corresponds to an ITD of −1.5 ms. To explain this finding and similar experiments, Stern, Zeiberg, and Trahiotis (1988) stated the *straightness principle*. They suggested that an intermediate mechanism assigns greater weight to units that are active in coincidence with units of different spectral channels but of the same ITD. The weighted image is further processed to lateralize the sound. Neither model provides a perfect fit for every psychophysical experiment (see the review on lateralization in Yost and Hafter, 1987). Each model captures some aspects and probably reflects some characteristics of the biological system.

Discussion

It is instructive to compare the biological and psychophysical approaches. The most striking characteristic of the biological system is its modular structure. Each nucleus performs a limited task. For example, the nucleus laminaris seems to pay little attention to the interaural intensity difference. This feature is taken care of by another nucleus. Also, there is no evidence of monaural processing in the nucleus laminaris. A special pathway is devoted to the preservation of monaural characteristics. The separate pathways converge only in the inferior colliculus. Similar mechanisms exist in other animals (Casseday and Covey, 1987).

The models differ in a more subtle way in across-frequency interaction. The owl employs a two-step process involving excitation and inhibition over the coincidence mechanism suggested in the straightness model. From a computational point of view, the owl's process is a realization of the straightness principle. Lateral inhibition in the inferior colliculus is probable, but in a different context than that suggested by Lindemann.

An important distinction between the models is the purpose of the network. The owl's network is responsible for head turning toward a sound source. Psychophysical models deal with perception, which may involve different brain structures (see DISSOCIATIONS BETWEEN VISUAL PROCESSING MODES for a distinction between *what* and *where* systems in vision). I suggest that models of perception should integrate several modalities and abandon the effort to construct a single, super-binaural processor that accounts for all of the psychophysical data in a single step. A more realistic model should have two separate modules for the processing of ITD and interaural intensity difference as well as a third decision mechanism that weighs both. The decision mechanism should be able to change its strategy based on monaural information, such as spectral composition and envelope structure.

The CRC model is sufficiently detailed to allow a successful silicon implementation of sound localization (Lazzaro and Mead, 1989) that captures the essential features of the biological system. On the other hand, the details of ITD detection at the cellular level are still not known. Intracellular recording in the nucleus laminaris and in analog mammalian structures is difficult; therefore, little is known about its biophysics and pharmacology.

Other biological systems possess some similarity to the owl's time pathway. The jamming-avoiding behavior of the weak electric fish and the echolocation of the bat are well documented (see review in Carr, 1993). However, these models provide little information about the internal representation of the external environment in the brain. Usually, more information is extracted by studying neural pathways that lead to a motor response, such as head turning in owls or frequency adjustments in electric fishes and bats. A more holistic theory of sound localization should unify the biological and psychological models. Such a theory may explain psychophysical phenomena in terms of realistic biological structures and provide testable predictions for experimentalists in both fields.

[Reprinted from the First Edition]

Road Maps: Neuroethology and Evolution; Other Sensory Systems
Related Reading: Collicular Visuomotor Transformations for Gaze Control; Echolocation: Cochleotopic and Computational Maps; Electrolocation

References

Carr, C. E., 1993, Processing of temporal information in the brain, *Annu. Rev. Neurosci.*, 16:223–243. ◆

Carr, C. E., and Konishi, M., 1990, A circuit for detection of interaural time differences in the brain stem of the barn owl, *J. Neurosci.*, 10:3227–3246.

Casseday, J. H., and Covey, E., 1987, Central auditory pathways in directional hearing, in *Directional Hearing* (W. A. Yost and G. Gourevitch, Eds.), New York: Springer-Verlag, pp. 109–145. ◆

Colburn, H. S., and Durlach, N. I., 1978, Models of binaural interaction, in *Handbook of Perception*, vol. 4 (E. C. Carterette and M. P. Friedman, Eds.), New York: Academic Press, pp. 467–518. ◆

Fujita, I., and Konishi, M., 1991, The role of GABAergic inhibition in processing of interaural time difference in the owl's auditory system, *J. Neurosci.*, 11:722–739.

Jeffress, L. A., 1948, A place theory of sound localization, *J. Comp. Physiol. Psychol.*, 41:35–39.

Konishi, M., Takahashi, T. T., Wagner, H., and Carr, C. E., 1988, Neurophysiological and anatomical substrates of sound localization in the owl, in *Auditory Function* (G. M. Edelman, W. E. Gall, and W. M. Cowan, Eds.), New York: Wiley, pp. 721–745. ◆

Lazzaro, J., and Mead, C., 1989, A silicon model of auditory localization, *Neural Computat.*, 1:47–57.

Lindemann, W., 1986, Extension of a binaural cross-correlation model by contralateral inhibition: I. Simulation of lateralization for stationary signals, *J. Acoust. Soc. Am.*, 80:1608–1622.

Stern, R. M., Zeiberg, A. S., and Trahiotis, C., 1988, Lateralization of complex binaural stimuli: A weighted-image model, *J. Acoust. Soc. Am.*, 84:156–165.

Stern, R. M., and Trahiotis, C., 1995, Models of binaural interaction, in *Handbook of Perception and Cognition*, vol. 6: *Hearing* (B. C. J. Moore, Ed.), San Diego: Academic Press, pp. 347–386.

Takahashi, T. T., and Konishi, M., 1986, Selectivity for interaural time difference in the owl's midbrain, *J. Neurosci.*, 6:3413–3422.

Yin, T. C. T., and Chan, J. C. K., 1988, Neural mechanism underlying interaural time sensitivity to tones and noise, in *Auditory Function* (G. M. Edelman, W. E. Gall, and W. M. Cowan, Eds.), New York: Wiley, pp. 385–430. ◆

Yin, T. C. T., and Chan, J. C. K., 1993, Interaural time sensitivity in medial superior olive of cat, *J. Neurophysiol.*, 64:465–488.

Yost, W. E., and Hafter, E. R., 1987, Lateralization, in *Directional Hearing* (W. A. Yost and G. Gourevitch, Eds.), New York: Springer-Verlag, pp. 49–84. ◆

Sparse Coding in the Primate Cortex

Peter Földiák

Introduction

Brain function can be seen as computation, i.e., the manipulation of information necessary for survival. While computation itself is an abstract process, it must be performed in a physical system. Any physical computing system, be it an electronic computer or a biological system consisting of neurons, must use some form of physical representation for the pieces of information that it processes.

Computations are implemented by the transformations of these physical representations of information. The brain receives information via the sensory channels and must eventually generate an appropriate motor output. But before we can even study the transformations that are involved, we need at least some fundamental understanding of the internal representation that these transformations operate on. Neurons represent and communicate information mainly by generating (or "firing") a sequence of electrical impulses. Electrophysiological techniques exist for the recording of these impulses from isolated single neurons in the living brain. Single-cell recording has revealed a remarkably close and highly specific relationship between sensory stimuli, neural activity, and behavioral reports of perceptual states. However, the encoding of events and states into a sequence of neural impulses in a large number of neurons can be highly complex, especially in the cerebral cortex, which contains an elaborate working model of the world. One of the basic questions about this neural code is whether an information item (e.g., a specific sensory stimulus caused by an object) is represented by the activity of a single, individually meaningful cell or is only the global activity pattern across a whole cell population that corresponds to interpretable states. There are now strong theoretical reasons and experimental evidence suggesting that the brain adopts a compromise between these extremes, using a relatively small (though in absolute number still substantial) subset of neurons to represent each item. This is often referred to as sparse coding (Dayan and Abbott, 2001).

Sparse Coding

The brain must encode the state of the environment and its own internal states by the firing pattern of a large but fixed set of neurons. For simplicity, consider coding by units that are either "active" or "passive" where the code assigns states to the subsets of active units. An important characteristic of such a code is the *activity ratio*, the fraction of active neurons at any one time. At its lowest value is *local representation*, where each state is represented by a single active unit from a pool in which all other units are silent. For instance, letters on a computer keyboard (ignoring the Shift and Control keys) are locally encoded. In *dense distributed representations*, each state is represented on average by about half of the units being active. Examples of this are the binary (ASCII) encoding of characters used in computers or the coding of visual images by the retinal photoreceptor array. Codes with low activity ratios are called *sparse codes*.

The activity ratio affects several aspects of information processing, such as the architecture and robustness of networks, the number of distinct states that can be represented and stored, generalization properties, and the speed and rules of learning (Table 1).

The representational capacity of local codes is small: they can represent only as many states as the number of units in the population, which is insufficient for any but the most trivial tasks. Even when the number of units is as high as that in the primate cortex, the number of discriminable states of the environment well exceeds this number. Making associations between a locally encoded item and an output, however, is easy and fast. Single-layer networks can learn any output association in a single trial by local, Hebbian strengthening of connections between active representation units and output units, and the linear separability problem does not even arise. In such a *lookup table*, there is no interference between associations to other discriminable states, and learning information about new states does not interfere with old associations. This, however, also means that there will be no generalization to other discriminable states, which presents a serious problem. If the discrimination is poor, that is a problem in itself. Alternatively, if the discrimination is fine enough to make all the necessary distinctions, we can expect a system never to experience precisely the same pattern of stimulation twice, and so no past experience will ever be used in a new situation.

Dense distributed, or "holographic," codes, on the other hand, can represent a very high number (e.g., in binary codes, 2^N) of different states by combinatorial use of (N) units. In fact, this power is largely superfluous, as the number of patterns ever experienced by the system will never approach this capacity, and therefore dense codes usually have high statistical redundancy. The price to pay for the potential (but unused) high information content of each pattern is that the number of such patterns that an associative memory can store is unnecessarily low. The mapping between a dense representation and an output can be complex (a linearly nonseparable function), therefore requiring multilayer networks and learning algorithms that are hard or impossible to implement biologically. Even efficient supervised algorithms are prohibitively slow, requiring many training trials and large amounts of the kind of training data that is labeled with either an appropriate output or reinforcement. Such data is often too risky, time consuming, or expensive to obtain in a real system. Distributed representations in intermediate layers of such networks ensure a kind of automatic generalization; however, this often manifests as unwanted interference between patterns. A further serious problem is that new associations usually cannot be added without retraining the network with the complete training set.

Sparse codes combine the advantages of local and dense codes while avoiding most of their drawbacks. Codes with small activity ratios can still have sufficiently high representational capacity, while the number of input-output pairs that can be stored in an associative memory is far greater for sparse than for dense patterns. This is achieved by decreasing the amount of information in the representation of any individual stored pattern. As a much larger fraction of all input-output functions are linearly separable using sparse coding, a single supervised layer trained by simple supervised or reinforcement learning methods, following perhaps several unsupervised layers, is more likely to be sufficient for learning target outputs, avoiding problems associated with supervised training in multilayer networks. As generalization takes place only between overlapping patterns, new associations will not interfere with previous associations to nonoverlapping patterns.

Distributed representations are tolerant to damage to the units or noise. However, redundancy far smaller than that in dense codes is sufficient to produce robust behavior. For instance, by simply duplicating units with 99% reliability (assuming independent failures), reliability increases to 99.99%. Sparse representations can be even more tolerant to damage than dense ones if high accuracy is required for a representation to be recognized or if the units are highly unreliable.

Table 1. Properties of Coding Schemes

	Representational Capacity	Memory Capacity	Speed of Learning	Generalization	Interference	Fault Tolerance	Simultaneous Items
Local	Very low	Limited	Very fast	None	None	None	Unlimited
Sparse	High	High	Fast	Good	Controlled	High	Several
Dense	Very high	Low	Slow	Good	Strong	Very high	One

Sparseness can also be defined with respect to components. A busy scene may be encoded in a distributed representation while, at the same time, object features may be represented locally. The number of simultaneously presented items decreases as the activity ratio increases because the addition of active units eventually results in the activation of so many units that the representation of unrelated items ("ghost" items) will be apparent in the set of active units.

To utilize the favorable properties of sparse representations, densely coded inputs must be transformed into sparse form. As the representational capacity of sparse codes is smaller, this cannot be achieved perfectly for all possible patterns on the same number of units. Information loss can be minimized by increasing the number of representation units or by losing resolution—but only in parts of pattern space that are usually not used. Both measures seem to be taken in the cortex. First, the number of neurons in the primary visual cortex is about two orders of magnitude higher than the number of optic nerve fibers that indirectly provide its input. Second, the natural sensory environment consists of patterns that occupy only a small fraction of pattern space; that is, it has large statistical redundancy. Barlow (1972) suggested that it is the nonaccidental conjunctions, "suspicious coincidences" of features, or "sensory clichés" that must be extracted that give good discrimination in populated regions of pattern space. By making explicit, local representations for commonly occurring features of the natural environment, such as facial features, our visual system is much better at discriminating natural images than, for instance, random dot patterns. As events are linked to the causes of sensory stimuli in the environment, such as objects, rather than arbitrary combinations of receptor signals, associations can be made more efficiently, based on such direct representations (Barlow, 1991). There is substantial evidence that the visual system is well adapted to the special statistical properties of the natural visual environment by utilizing sparse coding (Baddeley et al., 1997; Vinje and Gallant, 2000, Simoncelli and Olshausen, 2001).

A simple unsupervised algorithm for learning such representations in a nonlinear network using local learning rules has been proposed (Földiák, 1990) that uses Hebbian forward connections to detect nonaccidental features, an adaptive threshold to keep the activity ratio low, and anti-Hebbian, decorrelating lateral connections to keep redundancy low. Simulations suggest that these three constraints force the network to implement a sparse code with only little information loss. Another interesting effect can be observed: high probability (i.e., known or expected) patterns are represented on fewer active units, while new or low probability patterns get encoded by combinations of larger numbers of features. This algorithm is not limited to detecting only second-order correlations, so it seems suitable for multilayer applications. Other algorithms adjust connection weight by explicitly maximizing measures of sparseness, successfully producing V1 simple-cell-like receptive fields (e.g., Olshausen and Field, 1997), although the biological implementation here is less direct.

Sparse Coding in the Cortex

It is easy to measure sparseness in network models, where the responses of all units can be observed. An idealized "wavelet" filter model of simple cell responses in primary visual cortex has shown that wavelet coefficients of natural images show high kurtosis; that is, for natural images, most wavelet units have outputs near zero and only a small subset of units gives large responses, there being a different subset for each image (Field, 1999). Evaluating the sparseness of coding in brains, however, is difficult: it is hard to record a set of neurons simultaneously across which sparseness could be measured. Techniques such as optical recording and mul-

tiple electrode recording may eventually yield data on the sparseness of coding, but there are presently formidable technical difficulties to overcome. We have more information about individual neurons' breadth of tuning across various stimulus sets than about sparseness per se. Coding across stimuli and coding across cells are, however, closely related (Table 2). For instance, the activity ratio (related to sparseness) averaged across stimuli and breadth of tuning (expressed as a ratio) averaged across units must be equal.

What evidence is there for sparse coding from single unit recordings in sensory cortex? The most immediate observation during physiological experiments is the difficulty of finding effective stimuli for neurons in most cortical areas. Each neuron appears to have specific response properties, typically being tuned to several stimulus parameters. In primary visual cortex, many neurons respond strongly only when an elongated stimulus, such as a line, edge, or grating, is presented within a small part of the visual field, and then only if other parameters, including orientation, spatial frequency (width), stereoscopic disparity, and perhaps color or length fall within a fairly narrow range. This suggests that at any moment during the animal's life, only a small fraction of these neurons will be strongly activated by natural stimuli. The problem of finding the preferences of cells becomes severe in higher visual areas, such as area V4, and especially in inferotemporal cortex (IT). Cells' preferences in IT are often difficult to account for by reference to simple stimulus features, such as orientation, motion, position, or color, and they appear to lie in the domain of shape (Perrett, Rolls, and Caan, 1982; Tanaka, 1996). Cells here show selectivity for complex visual patterns and objects, such as faces, hands, complex geometrical shapes, and fractal patterns, and the responses are usually not predictable from responses to simple stimuli. Cells responding to faces but not to a large collection of control stimuli could be considered, on the one hand, to be very tightly tuned cells in the space of all possible stimuli. On the other hand, they may have quite broad tuning and show graded responses to stimuli within the carefully selected specific categories for which they show selectivity. To estimate, therefore, how often these cells are activated in behaving animals would require much more accurate knowledge of the animals' natural visual environment and behavior, or access to the cell's response during normal behavior.

Cells with apparent selectivity for faces might be selective for the full configural and textural information present in a preferred face stimulus, or may be triggered simply by the presence of two roughly collinear bars (most faces have eyebrows) or by a colored ovoid. One of the possible approaches to explore IT cells' preferences has been employed as systematically as possible by Tanaka and colleagues (Tanaka et al., 1991). Using this approach, they try to determine preferred features of cells by simplifying the stimuli that excite them. This method begins by presenting many objects to the monkey while recording from a neuron to find objects that excite it. Component features of effective stimuli, as judged by the experimenters, are then presented singly or in combination. By assessing the cell's firing rate during the presentation of each sim-

Table 2. Sparseness Versus Breadth of Tuning

		Cell								
		1	2	3	4	5	6	7	8	9
Stimulus	1			0						
	2			0						
	3	1	0	1	0	0	1	0	1	1
	4			0					Sparseness	
	5			1						
	6			0						
	7			0	Breadth of tuning					

plified stimulus, the protocol attempts to find the simplest feature combination that maximally excites the cell. This approach suffers from the problem that even simple objects contain a rich combination of color, orientation, depth, curvature, texture, specular reflections, shading, shape, and other features that may not be obvious to the experimenters. As any feature combination may be close enough to the preferences of a cell for it to become excited, the simplified stimuli that are actually presented are only a small subset of all possible combinations, selected according to the experimenter's intuitions. Hence, it is not possible to conclude that the best simplified stimulus found using this method is optimal for the cell, only that it was the best of those presented. A possible improvement in this area may come from automated neurophysiological experimental stimulus optimization procedures, which use more objective on-line search algorithms in a closed-loop experimental design to find peaks of neural tuning curves in high-dimensional (e.g., image) spaces (Földiák, 2001). However, it may not always be safe to assume that cells code only one optimal set of features, since it is possible that they could exhibit two or more maxima, corresponding to quite different feature combinations (Young, 1993). Recent results from intermediate stages of visual processing, area V4, however, suggest that cells at these stages encode well-localized individual contour components independently of global shape configuration (Pasupathy and Connor, 2001). Even at higher stages, e.g., in IT, cells can show preferences for patterns that are simpler than real visual objects. One interpretation of these results is that IT might consist of a large number of detectors of pattern "partials," which together might constitute an "alphabet." The detection of such partials would seem to suggest that these cells will have broader tuning than cells with selectivity for the full configuration. The idea that an IT cell reliably signals the presence of the particular pattern "partial" seems not to be supported by the results of Tanaka et al. (1991), who showed that the presence of other visual features can disrupt the cell's response to its "partial," a result that is inconsistent with the visual alphabet concept. Hence, the simplification approach captures neither necessary nor sufficient descriptions of the behavior of IT cells, and does not yet present a clear message on the sparseness of representation.

Finally, we note a difficulty in all attempts to measure sparseness in the cortex. In the extreme case, a cell with tuning so precise that it responds only to a single object will sustain its firing near its background rate when shown anything else. Researchers have only limited time and stimuli available to explore the cell's preferences during an experiment, and invariably go on to the next unit if they cannot determine what it is that the cell prefers, which strongly biases estimates of the specificity distribution. So, if there are any cells with extremely high specificity (approaching the specificity of "grandmother cells"), we cannot expect to find them experimentally using current methods. On the other hand, a cell that appears to respond only to a very limited number of a set of stimuli, as, for example, some human medial temporal lobe cells shown in Heit, Smith, and Halgren (1988), cannot be interpreted as conclusive evidence for extremely narrow tuning because of uncertainty about their responses to untested stimuli.

Beyond Sparseness

While breadth of tuning and sparseness are interesting issues both experimentally and theoretically, these issues cover only a minor aspect of neural representation. A much more significant question is what the components of a representation stand for. Imagine a sparse code, where each information item is represented by a randomly selected subset of n units from a pool of N units (e.g., the ASCII code). Alternatively, each unit could represent some meaningful aspect or feature of the item, and each item would be en-

coded by the combination of meaningful properties or features that are applicable to the item (Barlow, 1972). This scheme could have the same sparseness as the random scheme, but the random scheme would only allow us to identify whether the item is present in the representation. The alternative scheme, however, allows much more than that. It allows us to attribute meaning to it. It allows us not only to determine the degree of similarity between items, but the representation of the items also implicitly contain the description of the kind of similarity present between the items. It also allows the system to deal with unknown or new items by generalizing along the relevant dimensions.

Much of the neurophysiological data from high-level visual cortex support Barlow's hypothesis that the neural code is not only sparse, but that the elements of the code stand for meaningful features of the world, such as complex shapes, object-components, and faces (Perrett et al., 1982; Tanaka, 1996), and that even intermediate stages of the ventral visual pathway show selective responses to interpretable shape primitives and contour features, such as angles and curves (Pasupathy and Connor, 2001).

Discussion

The theoretical reasons and experimental evidence discussed here support the hypothesis that sparse coding is used in cortical computations, while the degree of sparseness is still a subject for future research. Even more important may be exploration of the relationship between the responses of single neurons and significant, meaningful features and aspects of the sensory world. The full description of high-level cells will require far more detailed knowledge of their anatomical connectivity and better understanding of the lower-level sensory neurons out of which their responses are constructed.

Road Map: Neural Coding
Related Reading: Localized Versus Distributed Representations; Population Codes; Rate Coding and Signal Processing

References

Baddeley, R., Abbott, L. F., Booth, M. J. A., Sengpiel, F., Freeman, T., Wakeman, E. A., and Rolls, E. T., 1997, Responses of neurons in primary and inferior temporal visual cortices to natural scenes, *Proc. R. Soc. Lond. B*, 264:1775–1783.

Barlow, H. B., 1972, Single units and sensation, *Perception*, 1:371–394.

Barlow, H. B., 1991, Vision tells you more than "what is where," in *Representations of Vision* (A. Gorea, Ed.), Cambridge, Engl.: Cambridge University Press, pp. 319–329.

Dayan, P., and Abbott, L. F., 2001, Sparse coding, in *Theoretical Neuroscience: Computational and Mathematical Modeling of Neural Systems*, Cambridge, MA: MIT Press, pp. 378–383. ◆

Field, D. J., 1999, Wavelets, vision and the statistics of natural scenes, *Philosoph. Trans. R. Soc. Lond. A*, 357(1760):2527–2542.

Földiák, P., 1990, Forming sparse representations by local anti-Hebbian learning, *Biol. Cybern.*, 64:165–170.

Földiák, P., 2001, Stimulus optimisation in primary visual cortex, *Neurocomputing*, 38–40:1217–1222.

Heit, G., Smith, M., and Halgren, E., 1988, Neural encoding of individual words and faces by the human hippocampus and amygdala, *Nature*, 333:773–775.

Olshausen, B. A., and Field, D. J., 1997, Sparse coding with an overcomplete basis set: A strategy employed by V1? *Vision Res.*, 37:3311–3325.

Pasupathy, A., and Connor, C. E., 2001, Shape representation in area V4: Position-specific tuning for boundary conformation, *J. Neurophysiol.*, 86:2505–2519.

Perrett, D. I., Rolls, E. T., and Caan, W., 1982, Visual neurons responsive to faces in the monkey temporal cortex, *Exp. Brain Res.*, 47:329–342.

Simoncelli, E. P., and Olshausen, B. A., 2001, Natural image statistics and neural representation, *Annu. Rev. Neurosci.*, 24:1193–1216. ◆

Tanaka, K., 1996, Inferotemporal cortex and object vision, *Annu. Rev. Neu-rosci.*, 19:109–139. ◆

Tanaka, K., Saito, H., Fukada, Y., and Moriya, M., 1991, Coding visual images of objects in the inferotemporal cortex of the macaque monkey, *J. Neurosci.*, 6:134–144.

Vinje, W. E., and Gallant, J. L., 2000, Sparse coding and decorrelation in primary visual cortex during natural vision, *Science*, 287:1273–1276. ◆

Young, M. P., 1993, Visual cortex: Modules for pattern recognition, *Curr. Biol.*, 3:44–46.

Speech Processing: Psycholinguistics

Nick Chater and Morten H. Christiansen

Introduction

Psycholinguistics refers to the empirical study of the human language processing system, typically using behavioral experiments. This article considers attempts to capture psycholinguistic data using connectionist models (Christiansen and Chater, 2001). We primarily focus on relatively "early" aspects of speech processing—speech segmentation and word recognition.

The article is in three sections. "Connectionist Modeling: A Bridge from Psycholinguistics and Brain Theory?" outlines the gulf between theories of brain function and traditional accounts of language processing. Connectionist modeling promises to help span this gulf, by attempting to ground speech processing in a connectionist processing architecture, a type of architecture initially inspired by attempts to model the computational properties of the brain. The section titled "Segmentation and Recognition: Two Processes or One?" asks how far the problem of segmenting speech into words occurs independently of word recognition—a critical question for computational modeling. The section "Competition and Interaction in Word Recognition" considers connectionist models of word recognition, and their interplay with empirical research and theory.

Connectionist Modeling:
A Bridge from Psycholinguistics to Brain Theory?

Both theoretical and empirical aspects of the psycholinguistics of speech processing seem, at first sight, rather distant from brain theory.

Theoretically, the starting point in psycholinguistics has been to take ideas from linguistics, the study of the abstract structure of language. But a theoretical vocabulary of "phonemes," or "nouns," to say nothing of the subtle notions of modern linguistic theory, seems difficult to relate to neural mechanisms. We shall see, though, that neural network models of aspects of speech processing may be viewed as building a bridge between the abstract domain of linguistic representation and processing and the computational architectures that may capture some general properties of neural machinery.

Empirically, data on psycholinguistics also seem distant from brain theory at an experimental level, because relatively little is known about the detailed structure and function of the rather diverse brain areas involved in processing speech. Partly this is because, in contrast to the study of perception or motor control, it is not possible to gather relevant information from detailed neurobiological studies of nonhuman animals, because natural language appears to be unique to humans. Perhaps more important, it seems unlikely that brain structures underlying speech processing will have a neurophysiological basis as readily interpretable as the topographic maps in the visual and motor cortex. This is because the computational problems of speech processing have no apparent spatial structure that might be expected to map onto cortex in a spatially coherent way. In any case, at present, neurobiological considerations impose relatively coarse constraints on computational models of speech processing. Although data from neuropsychology and functional imaging are becoming increasingly important, the main empirical constraints on psycholinguistic models are derived from the vast body of sophisticated, but often highly equivocal, laboratory studies of human language processing.

Perhaps the strongest constraint on such models is that language processing must somehow be implemented in neural hardware, rather than on a conventional symbolic machine. Conventional symbolic models of language processing in cognitive science and artificial intelligence have typically ignored this constraint, often on the assumption that the brain must be as powerful as a universal Turing machine, and hence able to implement any computable procedure. But this argument ignores the fact that language-processing operations must operate extremely rapidly, using large numbers of slow and simple neural components, and thus require a highly parallel, cooperative style of computation. This style of computation is not easy to reconcile with the very complex chains of sequential symbolic operations involved in most conventional language-processing models.

Connectionist modeling attempts to bridge the gulf between psycholinguistics and neuroscience by capturing detailed psycholinguistic data using computational models that embody at least some of the computational principles of the brain. It also has more general significance as a crucial test case for the viability of neural network models of cognition. Because conventional linguistic theory describes the structure of language in terms of a highly complex set of symbolic rules, language processing appears to represent a very difficult challenge for neural network modeling (see CONSTITUENCY AND RECURSION IN LANGUAGE). At present, connectionist models of speech processing are only partially developed, but prospects are encouraging in a number of areas (Christiansen and Chater, 2001).

The problem of speech processing is, of course, extremely broad, ranging from acoustic processing to semantic analysis. Our discussion focuses on the middle-ground problem of understanding how the brain segments and recognizes individual words in continuous, fluent speech.

Segmentation and Recognition: Two Processes or One?

In speech processing, as in perception, a fundamental question concerns the relationship between the segmentation of sensory input (e.g., the speech signal) into chunks and the recognition of those chunks. Segmentation and recognition appear to stand in a chicken-and-egg relation: it is simply not clear how one could precede the other. Unless the input is segmented, how do we know what chunks of speech we should even attempt identify as specific words (or other linguistic units)? Conversely, unless we know what linguistic unit has been said, how can we know where the boundaries between units lie?

One approach to resolving the paradox is to assume that segmentation and recognition are two aspects of a single process—that tentative hypotheses about each issue are developed and tested simultaneously, and mutually consistent hypotheses are reinforced. A second approach is to suppose that there are segmentation cues in the input that are used to give at least better-than-chance indications of what segments may correspond to identifiable words. So the question is: Does speech processing involve dedicated segmentation strategies prior to word recognition?

Developmental considerations suggest that there may be specialized segmentation methods. The infant, initially knowing no words, seems constrained to segment speech input using some method not requiring word recognition. Moreover, studies have shown that prelinguistic infants may use such methods and are sensitive to a variety of information that is available in the speech stream and potentially useful for segmentation, such as phonotactics and lexical stress—probably before cues based on the possible meaning of what is being said can be used by the child (Jusczyk, 1997).

How can children learn to segment speech? Cairns et al. (1997) note that language is less predictable across, rather than between, words. They trained a recurrent network on a large corpus of phonologically transcribed conversational speech, represented as a sequence of bundles of binary phonetic features. The network was trained to predict the next bundle of features along with the previous and current feature bundles, based on the current input material. Where prediction error was large, it was assumed that a word boundary had been encountered. This model captured some aspects of human segmentation performance. For example, it spontaneously learned to pay attention to patterns of strong and weak syllables as a segmentation cue. However, it was able to reliably predict only a relatively small proportion of word boundaries, indicating that other cues also need to be exploited. Christiansen, Allen, and Seidenberg (1998) showed how multiple, partial constraints on segmentation could yield much better segmentation performance. They trained a simple recurrent network to integrate sets of phonetic features with information about lexical stress (strong or weak) and utterance boundary information (encoded as a binary unit) derived from a corpus of child-directed speech. The network was trained to predict the appropriate values of these three cues for the next segment. After training, the network was able to integrate the input such that it would activate the boundary unit not only at utterance boundaries, but also at word boundaries inside utterances. The network was thus able to generalize patterns of cue information that occurred at the end of utterances to when the same patterns occurred *inside* an utterance. This model performed well on the word segmentation task while capturing additional aspects of infant segmentation, such as the bias toward the dominant trochaic (strong-weak) stress pattern in English, the ability to distinguish between phonotactically legal and illegal novel words, and having segmentation errors being constrained by English phonotactics.

Although it seems likely that segmentation cues are exploited to guide the process of word recognition, this can achieve only limited results. A definitive segmentation of speech can only occur after word recognition has occurred. Empirical evidence strongly indicates that, during word recognition in adulthood, multiple candidate words are activated, even if these correspond to different segmentation of the input. For example, Gow and Gordon (1995) found that adult listeners hearing sentences involving a sequence (e.g., *two lips*) that could also be a single word (*tulips*, in U.S. pronunciation) showed speeded processing of an associate of the second word (*kiss*) and an associate of the longer word (*flower*), indicating that the two conflicting segmentations were simultaneously entertained. This would not occur if a complete segmen-

tation of the input happened before word recognition was attempted. On the other hand, it is not clear how these data generalize to word segmentation and recognition in infancy before any comprehensive vocabulary has been established. How the segmentation and recognition develop into the kind of integrated system evidenced by the Gow and Gordon data remains a matter for future research.

Competition and Interaction in Word Recognition

Gow and Gordon's (1995) result also suggests that word recognition itself may be a matter of competition among multiple activated word representations, in which the activation of the word depends on the degree of match between the word and the speech input. Indeed, many studies, representing a range of experimental paradigms, point toward this conclusion. Such competition is typically implemented in neural networks by a localist code for words (the activation of a single unit represents the strength of evidence for that word, see LOCALIZED VERSUS DISTRIBUTED REPRESENTATIONS), with inhibitory connections between word units. Thus, when an isolated word is identified, a "cohort" of words consistent with that input is activated. As more of the word is heard, this cohort is rapidly reduced, perhaps to a single item.

Although competition at the word level has been widely assumed, considerable theoretical dispute has occurred over the nature of the interaction between different levels of mental representation. *Bottom-up* (or data-driven) models are those in which less abstract levels of linguistic representation feed into, but are not modified by, more abstract levels (e.g., the phoneme level feeds into the word level, but not the reverse). We note, however, that this does not prevent these models from taking advantage of suprasegmental information (an example is the inclusion of lexical stress in the Christiansen et al. segmentation model, described above), provided that this information is available in a purely bottom-up fashion (i.e., no lexical-level feedback). *Interactive* (also *conceptually driven* or *top-down*) models allow a two-way flow of information between levels of representation. Figure 1 shows in abstract form the differences in information flow between the two types of models of word recognition. Note that bottom-up models allow information to flow through the network in one direction only, whereas an interactive model allows information to flow in both directions.

The bottom-up versus interactive debate rages in all areas of language processing, and also in perception and motor control. Here we focus on putative interactions between information at the phonemic and the lexical levels in word recognition (i.e., between phonemes and words), where experimental work and neural network modeling have been intense.

The most obvious rationale for presuming that there are top-down information flows from the lexical to the phoneme levels stems from the effects of lexical context on phoneme identification. For example, Ganong (1980) showed that the identification of a syllable-initial speech sound that was constructed to be between /g/ and /k/ was influenced by lexical knowledge. This intermediate sound was predominantly heard as /k/ if the rest of the word was -*iss* (*kiss* was favored over *giss*), but it was heard as /g/ if the rest of the word was -*ift* (*gift* was favored over *kift*).

The TRACE model (McClelland and Elman, 1986) has an *interactive activation* architecture, with a sequence of layers of units. First-layer units correspond to phonetic features, second-layer units correspond to phonemes, and third-layer units correspond to words. Within and between layers there are fixed inhibitory bidirectional connections between units, which stand for incompatible states, and fixed bidirectional excitatory connections between units, which stand for mutually compatible states. TRACE also deals with the temporal dimension of speech: there are many copies of the entire

Bottom-Up Model

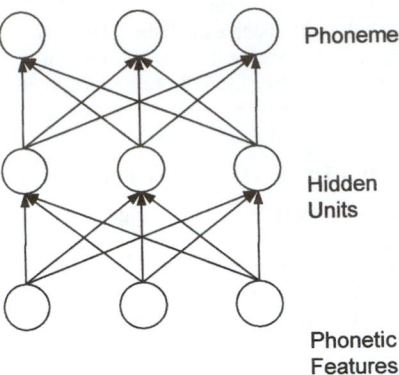

Phonemes

Hidden Units

Phonetic Features

Interactive Activation Model

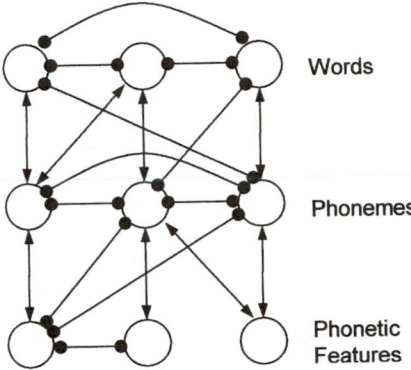

Words

Phonemes

Phonetic Features

Figure 1. A bottom-up model of word recognition and an interactive model. The links in the bottom-up model can be either excitatory or inhibitory, and only allow information to flow upward from the phonetic features through the hidden units to the phonemes on the output. In the interactive activation model, the links are bidirectional and allow information to flow both bottom-up, from the phonetic features through the letter units to the word units, and top-down. Arrows denote excitatory links; solid circles denote inhibitory links.

network, standing for different points in time, with appropriate connections between the units in each copy. TRACE captures effects of lexical context because lexical units influence phonemic input. McClelland and Elman modeled a wide range of data, and their model has proved remarkably robust.

But "context" effects on phoneme recognition can also be explained in purely bottom-up terms. If a person's decisions about phoneme identity depend on both the phonemic and lexical levels, then phoneme identification will be lexically influenced, even though there need be no feedback from the lexical to the phoneme level. For example, the Ganong effect might be explained by assuming that the phoneme identification of an initial consonant that is ambiguous between /g/ and /k/ is directly influenced by the lexical level. Thus, if *gift* is recognized at the lexical level, this will influence the participant to respond that the initial phoneme was /g/; but if *kiss* is recognized, this will influence the participant to respond that the initial phoneme was /k/.

A substantial experimental literature has attempted to distinguish TRACE from bottom-up models, indicating the importance of connectionist modeling in inspiring experimental research. One experimental result (Elman and McClelland, 1988), derived as a novel prediction TRACE, appeared to be particularly persuasive evidence against bottom-up connectionist models. In natural speech, the pronunciation of a phoneme will to some extent be altered by the phonemes that surround it, in part for articulatory reasons. This phenomenon is known as *coarticulation*. Listeners should therefore adjust their category boundaries depending on the phonemic context. Experiments confirm that people do indeed exhibit this "compensation for coarticulation" (CFC; Mann and Repp, 1981). For example, given a series of synthetically produced tokens between /t/ and /k/, listeners move the category boundary toward the /t/ following an /s/ and toward the /k/ following a /sh/.

This phenomenon suggests a way of detecting whether lexical information really does feed back to the phoneme level. Elman and McClelland considered the case in which compensation for coarticulation occurs across word boundaries. For example, a word-final /s/ influences a word-initial phoneme ambiguous between /t/ and /k/ to be heard as a /k/ (as in *Christmas capes*). If lexical-level representations feeds back into phoneme-level representations, the compensation of the /c/ should still occur when the /s/ relies on lexically driven phoneme restoration for its identity (i.e., in an experimental condition in which the identity of /s/ in *Christmas* is obscured, the /s/ should be restored, and thus compensation for coarticulation should proceed as normal). Elman and McClelland confirmed TRACE's prediction experimentally. Recognition of the phoneme at the start of the second word was apparently influenced by CFC, as if the word-final phoneme in the first word had been "restored" by lexical influence.

Surprisingly, bottom-up connectionist models can also capture these results. Norris (1993) provided a small-scale demonstration, training a simple recurrent network to map phonetic input onto phoneme output, for a small (12-word vocabulary) artificial language. When the net received phonetic input with an ambiguous first word-final phoneme and ambiguous initial segments of the second word, an analogue of CFC was observed. The percentages of /t/ and /k/ responses to the first phoneme of the second word depended on the identity of the first word, as in Elman and McClelland (1998). But the explanation for this pattern of results cannot be top-down influence from word units, because there *are* no word units. Moreover, Cairns et al. (1995) scaled up these results using a similar network trained on phonologically transcribed conversational English.

How can an autonomous computational model, where there is no lexical influence on phoneme processing, mimic the apparent influence of word recognition on coarticulation? Cairns et al. (1995) argued that sequential dependencies between the phoneme sequences in spoken English can often "mimic" lexical influence. The idea is that the identification of the word-final ambiguous phoneme favored by the word level is also, typically, favored by transitional probability statistics across phonemes. Analyzing statistical regularities in the phoneme sequences in a large corpus of conversational English, Cairns et al. showed that this explanation applies to Elman and McClelland's (1988) experimental stimuli. If these transitional probabilities have been learned by the speech processor, then previous *phonemic* context might support the "restoration" of the ambiguous word final phoneme, with no reference to the word in which it is contained.

Pitt and McQueen (1998) tested between these two explanations experimentally. They carefully controlled for transitional probabilities across phonemes, and reran a version of Elman and McClelland's experiment: compensation for coarticulation was eliminated. Moreover, when transitional probabilities are manipulated in nonword contexts, compensation for coarticulation effects are observed. This pattern of results suggests that compensation for coarticulation is driven not by top-down lexical influence but by phoneme-level statistical regularities.

Against this, Samuel (1996) argues that the precise pattern of phoneme restoration does indicate the existence of small but discernible top-down effects. He conducted a statistical analysis of people's ability to discriminate whether a phoneme has been replaced by a noise in a word or nonword context, from the case where the phoneme and noise are both present. The logic is that to the extent that top-down factors restore the missing phoneme, it should be difficult to tell whether or not the phoneme is actually present, and hence people's discrimination between the two cases should be poorer. Hence, phoneme present/absent discrimination should be poorer in word contexts than in nonword contexts, because top-down factors should be stronger. This prediction was confirmed experimentally (Samuel, 1996). Predictably, however, purely bottom-up explanations of this finding have since been proposed (Norris, McQueen and Cutler, 2000).

The theoretical debate concerning segmentation and word recognition has been profoundly influenced by connectionism. Connectionist models are now the dominant style of computational account, even for advocates of very different positions (as we have seen in relation to the bottom-up/interactive debate). Attempts to test between the predictions of competing models have generated experimental advances, which in turn have informed how models develop.

Discussion

Connectionist models can provide a rich framework for modeling important aspects of human speech recognition, and are now central to the theoretical and empirical literature in the psychology of language. Moreover, connectionist methods can also be applied both to early processes in speech recognition, concerned with the early analysis of what is a highly complex and variable acoustic stimulus (see READING), and to later aspects of language processing, where the main issues are syntactic and semantic (see CONSTITUENCY AND RECURSION IN LANGUAGE). A critical issue for connectionist modeling is how or whether accounts of different aspects of the speech processing problem might ultimately be integrated into an overall model of speech processing. Presently, such an integration is a long way off. Indeed, although progress has been substantial, connectionist and other models of speech perception are still some way from being able to identify words reliably in fluent continuous speech (and are not used, for example, in state-of-the-art automatic speech recognition), and work on syntactic and semantic analysis is still extremely preliminary.

Connectionist models do appear to provide a promising research direction, for a number of reasons. First, they provide a natural framework for modeling empirical psycholinguistic data. Second, learning is intrinsic to most connectionist networks, and hence the approach provides a natural source of developmental models (see COGNITIVE DEVELOPMENT). Third, connectionist models have provided a means of theoretical integration across different language-processing domains. For example, interactive and bottom-up models of speech recognition as described here are closely analogous to interactive and bottom-up models of single word reading. Fourth, it is widely argued that connectionist networks capture some as-

pects of the computational "style" of the brain, going at least some way to bridge between psycholinguistics and brain theory.

The potential implications of the connectionist approach to language processing are enormous, raising the possibility of a radical rethinking not just of language processing but of language structure itself. Perhaps the ultimate description of language resides in the structure of complex networks and can only approximately be expressed in terms of rigid, grammatical rules. Or perhaps connectionist models can only succeed to by building in standard linguistic constructs; or perhaps connectionist learning methods do not scale up at all (see Seidenberg's and Smolensky's contributions in Christiansen, Chater, and Seidenberg, 1999, for opposing perspectives). The future of connectionist models of language processing may therefore have important implications for the theory of language processing and language structure, and the neural machinery underlying speech processing.

Road Map: Linguistics and Speech Processing
Related Reading: Constituency and Recursion in Language; Motor Theories of Perception; Reading; Recurrent Networks: Learning Algorithms

References

Cairns, P., Shillcock, R., Chater, N., and Levy, J., 1995, Bottom-up connectionist modelling of speech, in *Connectionist Models of Memory and Language* (J. P. Levy, D. Bairaktaris, J. A. Bullinaria, and P. Cairns, Eds.), London: UCL Press, pp. 289–310.

Cairns, P., Shillcock, R., Chater, N., and Levy, J., 1997, Bootstrapping word boundaries: A bottom-up corpus-based approach to speech segmentation, *Cognit. Psychol.*, 33:111–153.

Christiansen, M. H., Allen, J., and Seidenberg, M. S., 1998, Learning to segment speech using multiple cues: A connectionist model, *Lang. Cognit. Proc.*, 13:221–268.

Christiansen, M. H., and Chater, N., 2001, Connectionist psycholinguistics, *Trends Cognit. Sci.*, 5:82–88.

Christiansen, M. H., Chater, N., and Seidenberg, M. S., Eds., 1999, *Connectionist Models of Human Language Processing: Progress and Prospects*, Cognit. Sci., 23:415–634 (special issue).

Elman, J. L., and McClelland, J. L., 1988, Cognitive penetration of the mechanisms of perception: Compensation for coarticulation of lexically restored phonemes, *J. Mem. Lang.*, 27:143–165.

Ganong, W. F., 1980, Phonetic categorization in auditory word perception, *J. Exp. Psychol. HPP*, 6:110–125.

Gow, D. W., and Gordon, P. C., 1995, Lexical and pre-lexical influences on word segmentation: Evidence from priming, *J. Exp. Psychol. HPP*, 21:344–359.

Jusczyk, P. W., 1997, *The Discovery of Spoken Language*, Cambridge, MA: MIT Press. ◆

Mann, V. A., and Repp, B. H., 1981, Influence of preceding fricative on stop consonant perception, *J. Acoust. Soc. Am.*, 69:548–558.

McClelland, J. L., and Elman, J. L., 1986, The TRACE model of speech perception, *Cognit. Psychol.*, 18:1–86.

Norris, D., 1993, Bottom-up connectionist models of "interaction," in *Cognitive Models of Speech Processing* (G. T. M. Altmann and R. Shillcock, Eds.), Hillsdale, NJ: Erlbaum, pp. 211–234.

Norris, D., McQueen, J. M., and Cutler, A., 2000, Merging information in speech recognition: Feedback is never necessary, *Behav. Brain Sci.*, 23:299–370.

Pitt, M. A., and McQueen, J. M., 1998, Is compensation for coarticulation mediated by the lexicon? *J. Mem. Lang.*, 39:347–370.

Samuel, A. C., 1996, Does lexical information influence the perceptual restoration of phonemes? *J. Exp. Psychol. Gen.*, 125:28–51.

Speech Production

Dani Byrd and Elliot Saltzman

Introduction

Understanding speech production requires a synthesis of perspectives found in physiology, motor control, cognitive science, and linguistics. This article presents work in the areas of motor control, dynamical systems and neural networks, and linguistics that is critical to understanding the functional architecture and characteristics of the speech production system.

Centuries of research in linguistics have provided considerable evidence that there are fundamental cognitive units that structure language. Spoken word forms are not unstructured wholes but rather are composed from a limited inventory of *phonological units* that have no independent meaning but can be (relatively freely) combined and organized in the construction of word forms. While languages differ in their selection of phonological units, within a given language there is a relatively small fixed set. Unlike certain other domains of human movement, in which the existence of component action units remains controversial (see MOTOR PRIMITIVES; ARM AND HAND MOVEMENT CONTROL), the production of speech by the lips, tongue, vocal folds, velum (the port to the nasal passages), and respiratory system can be understood as arising from choreographed linguistic action units.

A variety of micro- to macro-level units have been suggested as phonological units, among them features, gestures, phonemes (roughly, segments), moras, syllables, subsyllabic constituents (such as the syllable onset, nucleus, rime, and coda), gestural structures, and metrical feet (see Ladefoged, 2001). Some of these hypothesized units are mutually exclusive by definition (e.g., features and gestures); others have been assumed to coexist or to be hierarchically structured (e.g., feet and syllables and moras). For example, the word "phone" has three phonemes forming one syllable and could be transcribed /fon/, while the word "bone" (/bon/) contrasts in its initial unit and thereby in its meaning. (Two sounds are *contrastive* in a language if a change from one to the other can potentially change the meaning of a word.) Such pairs in a language are called minimal pairs and are appealed to as evidence for certain phonological units. Other types of evidence for phonological units can be gleaned from languages' word formation processes, language games, speech errors, diachronic language changes, and language acquisition. (And certain of these units, for example phonemes and syllables, form the basis of some orthographic systems.)

However, linguists and speech scientists have recognized that when phonological units are made manifest in word and sentence production, their spatiotemporal realization by the articulatory system, and consequent acoustic character presented to the auditory system, is highly variable and context dependent. In fact, the articulatory movements specific to adjacent units are not sequential in nature but are highly overlapped (i.g., co-articulated) and interactive. This has consequences that make the physical speech signal quite different from its familiar orthographic symbolic representation. In the acoustic domain, there is no invariant realization for a particular phonological unit across different contexts, an observation that has been termed *lack of invariance*. Additionally, the edges or boundaries between units are not implicit in the speech signal, a feature we can refer to as *lack of segmentability*. There are no pauses or "blank spaces" systematically demarcating phonological units—neither gestures, nor segments, nor words. (While there are amplitude and spectral discontinuities in the acoustic signal, they do not always indicate edges, although they may be indicative of certain important information regarding segment identity.) This *parallel transmission* of information in the acoustic signal due to co-articulated articulatory movements results in a highly efficient yet complex perceptual event that encodes and transmits information at high rates (see MOTOR THEORIES OF PERCEPTION).

Efforts to understand the relationship between phonological units that structure words and their variable physical realization in fluent speech are an important component of speech production research. A common view is that certain linguistic information seems to be lexically specified (i.e., encoded in our stable knowledge of a particular word), whereas other aspects of word and phrase production seem best understood as resulting from principled modulations of phonological units in the performance of speaking and by peripheral properties of the physical speech production system. For this reason, the speech production system is sometimes viewed as having two components, one, traditionally referred to as *phonology*, concerned with categorical and linguistically contrastive information, and the other, traditionally referred to as *phonetics*, concerned with gradient, noncontrastive information. However, current work in connectionist and dynamical systems models blurs this dichotomy. Speech scientists' views on the cognitive organization of the speech production process are shaped by their hypotheses regarding:

- the coordinate systems in which controlled variables are defined,
- the dynamic versus symbolic nature of phonological units (i.e., primitives),
- the higher-level organization of these units,
- the role of the speaker-listener relationship in shaping speech behavior,
- child language acquisition yielding adult phonology.

We discuss some of the hallmarks of this research in the following sections.

The Speech Production Apparatus

Speaking involves the orchestrated creation and release of constrictions in the supralaryngeal vocal tract (Figure 1). These constrictions are made by the lips and tongue (tip, body, and root) and serve to shape the resonance frequencies of the vocal tract tube. Many speech sounds are differentiated by the location and degree of these constrictions, and most speech sounds (though not all) are *pulmonic*; that is, they are generated using airflow from the lungs.

The sound excitation sources can be several but are primarily the vibratory airstream generated by rapid opening and closing of the vocal folds (*voicing*) and turbulence noise generated at narrow constrictions (*frication*). Vowels, which are voiced and produced with a relatively less constricted vocal tract than consonants, are differentiated in large measure by their first three resonance frequencies or *formants*, determined by the vocal tract shape. Consonants are differentiated largely by movement of the formant frequencies as constrictions at specific locations along the vocal tract are formed and released, by characteristic noise created at the constrictions themselves, and by the presence, absence, and timing of vocal fold vibration. Additionally, the vocal tract tube has a side branch to the nasal passageways that is opened for certain speech sounds by lowering the velum (soft palate). During speech, air may exit the vocal tract from the mouth (velum closed/raised) or from the nose (velum lowered and an anterior closure in the mouth), or from both (velum lowered and no oral closure). (Further information on the articulation and acoustics of speech can be found in

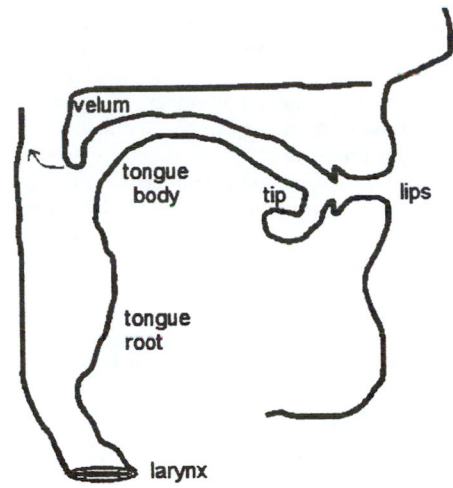

Figure 1. Schematic anatomy of the vocal tract showing the supralaryngeal constrictors (the upper and lower lips, the tongue tip, tongue body, and tongue root); the velum, which rises or lowers to prevent or allow airflow into the nasal passages; and the larynx, which houses the vocal folds that vibrate when adducted under appropriate aerodynamic conditions.

Ladefoged's [2001] *A Course in Phonetics*; for a more sophisticated account of the mapping between vocal tract shape and acoustics, see Stevens' [1998] *Acoustic Phonetics*.) A satisfactory account of human speech production abilities must encompass the great variety of speech sounds used contrastively in the world's languages, including those that contrast in aerodynamic mechanisms, tone, length, and phonation type (see Ladefoged, 2001, and citations therein, e.g., Ladefoged and Maddieson, 1996).

Modeling the Speech Production Process

Linguists have generally adopted a symbolic representation of spoken language. This has proved to be useful in investigating the structure of words and higher-level grammatical processes. Scientists whose primary interest is speech motor control, however, have generally adopted the nonsymbolic formulations provided by dynamical systems and connectionist approaches. The research community interested in spoken language has begun to synthesize these approaches.

Many issues faced in the control and coordination of the speech articulators are the same as those faced in understanding nonspeech skilled actions. In both cases, the multilevel geometry of the system must be specified in terms of a set of appropriate reference frames (coordinate systems) and the set of mappings that is defined among them (see GEOMETRICAL PRINCIPLES IN MOTOR CONTROL; LIMB GEOMETRY, NEURAL CONTROL). Additionally, the appropriate dynamics must be specified within this set of coordinate systems. For speech production, at least four types of coordinate systems and associated dynamics are posited generically in many current models (Figure 2). At the most concrete peripheral level, the *plant* is defined by the actual articulators (e.g., jaw, upper lip) with their neuromuscular (reflexive and muscle activation) and biomechanical dynamics, and may be represented in a coordinate space defined, for example, according to muscle forces and/or equilibrium lengths (see, e.g., Sanguineti, Laboissière, and Ostry, 1998). Commands to this most peripheral level can be shaped with reference to the motions of an internal model of the plant (*model articulators*) (see SENSORIMOTOR LEARNING), whose simulated neuromuscular

and biomechanical behavior can provide significant constraints on the spatial patterning and relative timing (e.g., co-articulation) of movement commands. In turn, model articulator trajectories are shaped with reference to a set of task-space coordinates in which the goals of the language's phonological primitives are represented. Although there are differences in the exact nature of these coordinates among models—e.g., acoustic/auditory goals (Bailly, Laboissière, and Schwartz, 1991; Guenther, 1995) versus vocal tract constriction goals (Browman and Goldstein, 1995; Saltzman and Munhall, 1989)—models generally invoke static attractor dynamics to implement these goals. Thus, in all such models, when a particular phonological primitive is activated, the articulators will move in a coordinated manner to create a task-space *gesture* that attains the acoustic, auditory, or constriction targets and remains there until another primitive is activated or the current primitive is deactivated. In this sense, an *articulatory gesture* is a goal-directed movement of the vocal tract represented in a constriction task space and with an intrinsic duration reflecting the time constant of the attractor.

In order for this arrangement to work, a forward model must represent the mapping from current (model) articulator state to task-space state. A task-space dynamics must define the corresponding set of task-space state velocities ("forces"), and an inverse model must map these task-space state velocities to a corresponding set of (model) articulator state velocities. Finally, a set of activation (or "GO-signal"; e.g., Guenther, 1995) coordinates is required to orchestrate the patterning of these gestural units over time and vocal tract space.

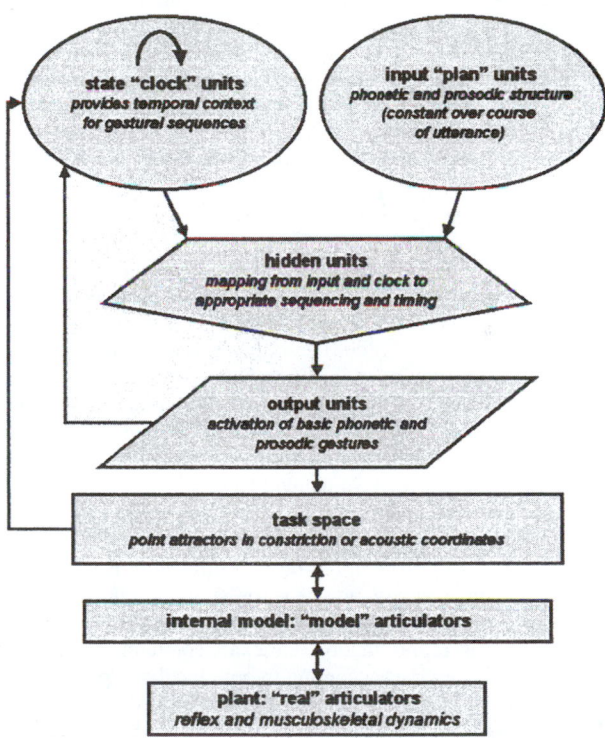

Figure 2. Schematic architecture of the speech production process. Gestural activations are viewed as outputs of a simple recurrent network that drive the articulatory plant through reference signal (model articulator) trajectories generated by task-space dynamics. Feedback connections from the task space and output units to the state unit "clock" modulate clock time flow, owing to the evolving state of the plant and gestural activations, respectively.

Although models generally have adopted connectionist dynamics to shape these activation trajectories, models can be distinguished on the basis of which of two approaches to intergestural timing is adopted. In *chain* models, gestural onsets are triggered whenever an associated preceding gesture either achieves near-zero velocity as it attains its target or passes through another kinematically defined critical point in its trajectory, such as peak tangential velocity (e.g., Guenther, 1995; see also Browman and Goldstein, 1995). In contrast, *clock* models have adopted architectures that are based on or similar to simple recurrent, sequential networks. In these models (e.g., Bailly et al., 1991; Saltzman and Munhall, 1989; see also SEQUENCE LEARNING and references therein), a network's *state unit* activity defines a dynamical flow with a time scale that is intrinsic to the intended sequence and that creates a temporal context within which gestural activations can be shaped by the network's output units. The resultant activation trajectories are determined by the manner in which a static input and the evolving state unit trajectories are mapped nonlinearly onto the output units (see Figure 2). Furthermore, it is noteworthy that many higher-level linguistic properties of both lexical and grammatical encoding can be captured using similar simple recurrent architectures (Dell, Chang, and Griffin, 1999).

Dynamical Units (Gestures) as Phonological Primitives

In our own work we have adopted *articulatory phonology* as a formal account of phonological units and their organization (Browman and Goldstein, 1995, and references to Browman and Goldstein's work therein), and *task dynamics* (Saltzman and Munhall, 1989) as a quantitative model that implements these phonological units in the speech production system in a multilevel dynamical system defined across activation, task-space, and model articulator coordinates. Articulatory phonology views lexical representations as being composed of gestural primitives that act as combinatorial units. Gestures have two functions: they function as units of information (i.e., linguistic contrast) and as units of action (i.e., speech production) (Browman and Goldstein, 1995). The activation waveforms of the gestures in a given utterance are coordinated, or phased, with respect to one another in a highly temporally overlapped pattern that yields the coarticulatory effects that are ubiquitous in speech (Browman and Goldstein, 1995).

To this point, we have mainly discussed the dynamic gesture as the primitive unit of organization in speech production. But gestures can additionally cohere in macro-level structures. Studdert-Kennedy and Goldstein (2002) describe this using the metaphor of gestures as atoms that combine in regular patterns of coordination with one another to form molecules corresponding to larger phonological units such as segments and syllables. Segment-sized units can be viewed as coherent ions—combinations of gestural atoms (one or several) that recur in many different molecules (Studdert-Kennedy and Goldstein, 2002; see also Saltzman and Munhall, 1989). In this way, macro-level phonological structure can be viewed as emerging from micro-level gestural primitives.

Although underlyingly invariant (or at least relatively stable) control units have been postulated in speech production, and certainly for lexical representation, the exact spatiotemporal realization of these units varies according to both local and prosodic context. By way of example, consider the three /o/'s in the sentence "He said *phone* not *folk* on the telephone": the [o] in "phone" will differ from the [o] in "folk" because of the different following consonantal context (e.g., there will be nasal airflow during the [o] in "phone," yielding different formant patterns). It will also differ from the [o] in "telephone" because of the emphatic stress placed on it in its first occurrence in the sentence. These are examples of co-articulatory variability and prosodic variability, respectively. Variation due to neighboring articulation (local context) is straight-

forwardly accounted for by the overlap of gestural units of action (e.g., Saltzman and Munhall, 1989; Browman and Goldstein, 1995, and references therein). However, variation due to prosody (e.g., phrasal position or informational prominence) requires the expression of the underlying primitives to be modulated for communicative ends in the production of a particular utterance. One approach we have pursued to implementing this modulation is via prosodic gestures that have no independent realization in vocal tract space but act vicariously to shape the time course of constriction (or auditory) gestures (Byrd et al., 2000). For example, a prosodic gesture at a phrase edge might slow the central clock (whose rate of time flow determines the local utterance rate), thereby time-stretching the gestural activations and inducing the articulatory slowing and acoustic lengthening that have been observed at phrase edges.

Although we and many in the speech production community adopt the general approach of articulatory phonology to linguistic representation, it is not without competition. A sense of this debate can be gleaned from a 1992 theme issue of the journal *Phonetica* on articulatory phonology (see Browman and Goldstein, 1992, cited in Browman and Goldstein, 1995). This view stands in contrast to a more traditional view among linguists that sees phonological primitives as symbolic (atemporal) elements such as features and segments rather than dynamic gestures. In the symbolic approach, the smallest units are typically binary features, such as [−continuant], [+aspirated], [+labial] (which could jointly describe the segment /p/ in /pat/), that are hierarchically incorporated into larger phonological units such as the syllable, (phonological) word, and phrase. These phonological units are then realized according to various and sundry phonetic implementation rules that mediate between lexical representation and physical realization.

The Role of the Speaker-Listener Relationship in Performance

Speech behavior is adaptive to communicative and situational demands (Lindblom, 1990), and for this reason, listeners can play an important role in shaping the production of the speech signal. The speaker-listener interaction might affect word forms diachronically in the form of language change (see, e.g., Ohala, 1993; see also LANGUAGE EVOLUTION AND CHANGE) or synchronically as a function of the listener's abilities, the opaqueness of the signal, and the environment in which the communication task is taking place. Lindblom (1990) credits the speaker with a "tacit awareness of the listener's access to sources of information independent of the signal and his judgement of the short-term demands for explicit signal information" (p. 403). In Lindblom's view, it is crucial to characterize what constitutes sufficient discriminability in the signal for the listener and how speakers operate to balance the benefits of providing this discriminability against the costs of articulatory precision and effort. This viewpoint diverges from theories of speech production in which the listener plays little or no role in shaping on-line speaker behavior.

The Organization of Speech: Adult Phonology

Whether the units of spoken language are symbolic or dynamic, they must be acquired in learning and utilized in behavior. The acquisition of the units of speech production and the organization of those units in the developing and adult lexicon into patterns appropriate to the language being acquired are broad topics that have just begun to be explored computationally.

While languages vary not only in their inventories of contrastive units but also in the structures (sequential, syllabic, rhythmic) into which those units are marshaled, they also show a large degree of agreement regarding the factors affecting the linguistic acceptability of word forms. A theoretical account of the bases for these cross-linguistic differences and similarities is provided by Prince and Smolensky's Optimality Theory (see, e.g., Prince and Smolensky, 1997; see also OPTIMALITY THEORY IN LINGUISTICS). This approach to phonology (and, by extension, grammar in general) capitalizes on the idea that constraints determining well-formedness of linguistic structure are many but finite, universal (i.e., shared by all human languages), and in conflict within any particular language. The individual constraints are ranked differently from language to language and thereby yield observed cross-language typology. Constraints are thought to concern structural complexity (*markedness* constraints) (where complexity might be conceived, for example, in terms of production, perception [especially distinctiveness], and/or processing) and the relationship of a produced form to some underlying, analogous, or related form (*faithfulness* constraints). All constraints are violable (and indeed many constraints will be violated by any particular word form); however, the optimal candidate word form will be the one that avoids *any* violation of a higher-ranked constraint, regardless of the number of violations of lower-ranked constraints; that is, evaluation is via *strict domination* (Prince and Smolensky, 1997). Prince and Smolensky (1997) have described how the process of selecting optimal word forms might be modeled using connectionist networks in which (1) constraints are embodied in the network connection weights, and (2) optimality is defined according to Lyapunov function ("harmony") values corresponding to activation patterns of the network. Given a particular input, held fixed across a given set of network elements, the network will settle to a pattern that maximizes harmony and that corresponds to the most well-formed linguistic structure. The universality of constraints and the adequacy of particular evaluatory mechanisms for constraint satisfaction are topics of debate. For example, see OPTIMALITY THEORY IN LINGUISTICS for a discussion of probabilistic and variable constraint ranking.

The Organization of Speech: Child Language Acquisition

Finally, we wish to briefly mention the difficult problem of how phonological units emerge in child language production from a signal that clearly cannot be characterized as a sequence of discrete units but is best viewed as an intricately overlapping pattern of vocal tract or auditory goals. The child learner is thus faced with the challenges of *lack of invariance* and *lack of segmentability* in the continuous audiovisual signals with which she is confronted. (Of course, the adult perceiver is in a similar circumstance but brings a much richer semantic and syntactic knowledge, gained through years of experience, to the task.) Further, the child learner faces the additional difficulty of an immature vocal tract apparatus. The acoustics resulting from linguistically significant vocal tract actions of the child are, in certain respects, vastly different from the acoustic properties resulting from articulatorily parallel gestures of the adult (e.g., formant frequencies and fundamental [voicing] frequency are much higher), though their spectral and temporal *patterning* may, importantly, be similar. Further, the child's vocal tract is growing over time, resulting in ongoing changes in the relationship between the child's own articulatory gestures and their acoustic consequences, changes that must be reflected in adjustment to the production system's internal model during development. A recent special issue of the journal *Phonetica* on emergence and adaptation (2000) includes many illuminating articles relevant to the acquisition and development of linguistic systems. In one, Michael Studdert-Kennedy (2000) discusses the emergence of the gestural unit in the process of child language acquisition as occurring via an engagement of the child's own vocal apparatus and its behavioral consequences. He speculates that exemplar models of

learning, facial imitation, and mirror neuron systems might have roles to play in elucidating how children form gestural units defined in terms of vocal tract constrictions in the language acquisition process (Studdert-Kennedy, 2000; see also Studdert-Kennedy and Goldstein, 2002).

Although computational modeling on the acquisition of speech production (i.e., articulation) is still in its infancy (but see Guenther, 1995, and several follow-up articles on his DIVA model for an illuminating treatment of the development of the production system), it is clear that there is an interdependent relationship between the codeveloping perceptual and production systems that relies on a perceptuomotor link (see MOTOR THEORIES OF PERCEPTION), whether learned or innate, and on experience with the phonological and lexical patterning within the child's language. Marilyn Vihman's 1996 book, *Phonological Development*, is an ideal starting point for exploring this relationship, and Beckman and Edwards (2000) specifically address the importance of experience and lexical patterning in the acquisition of spoken language.

Discussion

In order for an individual to articulate a language, she must know words of that language, know how to combine words into phrases, and be able to instantiate those phrases in the physical world through the use of body effectors. Furthermore, this act generally takes place socially in a communicative context involving a perceiver. All of these aspects of producing language shape the research agenda in the field of speech production. In this article we reviewed hypotheses regarding the nature of the units that serve to form words and the architecture of the production system that executes those units. We briefly touched on how the child learner might accomplish this, how the perceiver might play a role in shaping production, and how patterns of word forms within and among languages might be characterized. Although many challenges remain, not the least of which is connecting these insights to theories of brain, it is clear that an interdisciplinary approach involving motor control, cognitive and brain science, and linguistics is essential.

Road Map: Linguistics and Speech Processing
Related Reading: Motor Theories of Perception; Speech Processing: Psycholinguistics

References

Bailly, G., Laboissière, R. L., and Schwartz, J. L., 1991, Formant trajectories as audible gestures: An alternative for speech synthesis, *J. Phonet.*, 19:9–23.

Beckman, M., and Edwards, J., 2000, The ontogeny of phonological categories and the primacy of lexical learning in linguistic development, *Child Dev.*, 71:240–249.

Browman, C., and Goldstein, L., 1995, Dynamics and articulatory phonology, in *Mind as Motion* (R. F. Port and T. van Gelder, Eds.), Cambridge, MA: MIT Press, pp. 175–194. ◆

Byrd, D., Kaun, A., Narayanan, S., and Saltzman, E., 2000, Phrasal signatures in articulation, in *Papers in Laboratory Phonology V* (M. B. Broe and J. B. Pierrehumbert, Eds.), Cambridge, Engl.: Cambridge University Press, pp. 70–87.

Dell, G., Chang, S. F., and Griffin, Z. M., 1999, Connectionist models of language production: Lexical access and grammatical encoding, *Cognit. Sci.*, 23:517–542.

Guenther, F. H., 1995, Speech sound acquisition, coarticulation, and rate effects in a neural network model of speech production, *Psychol. Rev.*, 102:594–621.

Ladefoged, P., 2001, *A Course in Phonetics*, 4th ed., Orlando, FL: Harcourt. ◆

Lindblom, B., 1990, Explaining phonetic variation: A sketch of the H&H theory, in *Speech Production and Speech Modeling* (W. Hardcastle and A. Marchal, Eds.), Dordrecht: Kluwer, pp. 403–439.

Ohala, J. J., 1993, Sound change as nature's speech perception experiment, *Speech Commun.*, 13:155–161.

Prince, A., and Smolensky, P., 1997, Optimality: From neural networks to universal grammar, *Science*, 275:1604–1610. ◆

Saltzman, E. L., and Munhall, K. G., 1989, A dynamical approach to gestural patterning in speech production, *Ecol. Psychol.*, 1:333–382.

Sanguineti, V., Laboissière, R., and Ostry, D. J., 1998, A dynamic biomechanical model for neural control of speech production, *J. Acoust. Soc. Am.*, 103:1615–1627.

Stevens, K., 1998, *Acoustic Phonetics*, Cambridge, MA: MIT Press.

Studdert-Kennedy, M., 2000, Imitation and the emergence of segments, *Phonetica*, 57:275–283.

Studdert-Kennedy, M., and Goldstein, L., 2002, Launching language: The gestural origin of discrete infinity, in *Language Evolution: The States of the Art* (M. Christiansen and S. Kirby, Eds.), Oxford, Engl.: Oxford University Press. ◆

Vihman, M., 1996, *Phonological Development*, Cambridge, Engl.: Blackwell. ◆

Speech Recognition Technology

Françoise Beaufays, Hervé Bourlard, Horacio Franco, and Nelson Morgan

Introduction

Automatic speech recognition, the technology that allows computer systems to transcribe speech waveforms into words, relies on digital signal processing and statistical modeling methods to analyze and model the speech signal. The core technology typically is not based on connectionist methods, even though neural network processing is commonly seen as a promising alternative to some of the current algorithms. Because of the maturity of the current technology, neural networks have to compete with high-performance algorithms to gain acceptance in the field, and it is only recently that researchers have obtained significant performance improvements by using neural networks in specific subsystems of the speech recognizer.

In this article, we review the main neural network approaches to speech recognition. To limit the scope of this review, we will focus on speech recognizers intended to process large-vocabulary continuous speech (as opposed to small-scale systems intended to be integrated into portable electronic devices and which recognize only a few command words), and we will limit the discussion to systems based on multilayer feedforward neural networks or multilayer perceptrons (MLPs).

Automatic Speech Recognition

Traditional speech recognition systems follow a hierarchical architecture. A grammar specifies the sentences allowed by the application. (Alternatively, for very large vocabulary systems, a statistical language model may be used to define the probabilities of various word sequences in the domain of application.) Each word allowed by the grammar is listed in a dictionary that specifies its possible pronunciations in terms of sequences of phones (e.g., k O l for the word *call*). Phones are further decomposed into smaller units whose acoustic realizations are represented by statistical acoustic models.

When a speech waveform is input to a recognizer, it is first processed by a front-end unit that extracts a sequence of observations, or "features," from the raw signal. This sequence of observations is then decoded into the sequence of speech units whose acoustic models best fit the observations and respect the constraints imposed by the dictionary and language model (Figure 1).

Front-End Processing

The purpose of the front end is to extract from the speech signal a set of features that are representative of the lexical content of the signal and invariant to acoustic variations such as those due to ambient noise. Typically, the waveform is divided in overlapping windows or "frames" of approximately 25 ms, over which the signal is assumed to be stationary. Each such frame then undergoes a spectral analysis, from which a feature vector is derived. Many variants of spectral analysis have been used, among them cepstral coefficients (which are the Fourier transform of the log spectrum) computed from a spectrum of the data integrated in a filterbank whose design emulates the auditory system. To model the time dynamics of the signal, the feature vector is augmented with the first and second time derivatives of its components.

Acoustic Modeling

The models used to represent the acoustic realizations of the speech units are based on the underlying assumption that words consist of sequences of units that have varying length, and that each unit has constant spectral properties. The nonstationary characteristics of speech arise as the sequence of units is traversed in time. Although this is not an accurate model for many speech sounds, it is a simplifying assumption that allows powerful statistical techniques to be applied.

The tool most commonly used to model speech units is the hidden Markov model (HMM) (see HIDDEN MARKOV MODELS). HMMs assume that the sequence of feature vectors is a piecewise stationary process. Accordingly, an utterance is modeled as a succession of stationary states, with instantaneous transitions between these states (modeling the temporal structure of speech), and a set of state output processes, one output process associated with each state, that model the actual observed feature vectors (modeling the locally stationary character of the speech signal). This output process is typically represented by a Gaussian mixture model over the feature vectors.

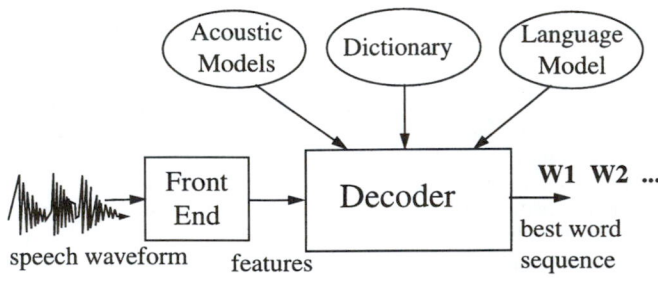

Figure 1. Basic architecture of large-vocabulary speech recognition system.

Although it is theoretically conceivable to have an HMM for every possible utterance, this is clearly unfeasible for all but extremely constrained tasks. Instead, a hierarchical scheme is typically adopted in which a sentence is modeled as a sequence of words and each word is modeled as a sequence of subword units. The units most commonly used are the phones, i.e., the acoustic realizations of phonemes.

A further refinement is the use of context-dependent phone units, usually referred to as triphones, which are the acoustic realizations of phonemes in the specific context defined by the previous and following phonemes. Typically, the phone or triphone HMMs have three states, with a left-to-right structure.

The simplest and most efficient algorithm to train the parameters of the HMMs (the parameters of the Gaussian mixture models as well as the interstate transition probabilities) is based on maximum likelihood techniques, that is, on finding the model parameters that maximize the likelihood of the training data. The most common of these is the forward-backward algorithm, a form of the well-known estimation maximization algorithm (see HIDDEN MARKOV MODELS).

Discriminative Training

Some of the efforts aimed at improving speech recognition have focused on extending the model training paradigm beyond that of maximum likelihood, and on optimizing training criteria more closely related to the actual recognition metric, the recognition error rate.

It has been argued that maximum likelihood training has the potential for poor discrimination between phonetic units because it maximizes the likelihoods of individual models independently of the likelihoods of other (possibly competing) models. Discriminative training instead emphasizes contrasts between phonetic classes. Neural network classifiers based on MLPs provide the simplest architecture for discriminative training: feature vectors extracted from the data frame can be input to an MLP and classified into N classes corresponding to the speech units to be modeled, phones or triphones. When appropriately trained, such an MLP classifier can be shown to minimize the classification error rate over the training data. This form of training explicitly maximizes the discrimination between the correct output class and its competitors. This approach underlies the hybrid MLP/HMM models (Bourlard and Morgan, 1993), which will be described in a later section.

This type of discrimination is local in the sense that it makes the models compete over a single frame of data at a time. Speech recognition, however, is not so much concerned with correctly recognizing individual frames of data as it is with correctly recognizing entire word sequences composed of many data frames. This observation calls for what is referred to as global discrimination, where the training algorithm attempts to increase the likelihood of the correct word string while decreasing the likelihoods of all other competing word strings.

A number of approaches to "global" discriminative training have been proposed. The first approach is that of maximum mutual information, which maximizes the mutual information between the spoken word sequence and its acoustic observations. As a consequence of this formulation, the training procedure maximizes the probability of the correct word sequence while minimizing the probability of all the other possible word sequences (Bahl et al., 1986).

Another popular training criterion is minimum classification error, where an approximation to the number of classification errors in the training data is computed and minimized. The approximation is based on computing the difference between a discriminant function for the correct class and a geometric average of the discriminants for the competing classes, and passing this difference through a nonlinearity that outputs 1 when any of the competing classes

has a higher discriminant value than the correct class, and 0 otherwise (Juang and Katagiri, 1992). This method has been used initially to train neural network classifiers and later to train hybrid HMM/MLP hybrid systems.

Even though discriminative training was introduced early in the speech area, under the form of maximum mutual information, it is really the advent of neural networks that spurred the interest in discriminative approaches.

Acoustic Modeling with MLPs

The idea of combining HMMs and MLPs for the acoustic modeling of speech signals was motivated by the observation that HMMs and MLPs have complementary properties: (1) HMMs are clearly dynamic and very well suited to temporal data, but several assumptions limit their generality; (2) MLPs can approximate any kind of nonlinear discriminant functions, are very flexible, and do not need strong assumptions about the distribution of the input data, but they cannot properly handle time sequences. However, HMMs are based on strict formalisms, making them difficult to interface with other modules in a heterogeneous system. The first such implementations were the so-called hybrid HMM/MLP models.

Context-Independent Hybrid HMM/MLP Models

In hybrid models (Bourlard and Morgan, 1993), an MLP is used to evaluate the likelihoods of the observations given the phones, $p(\mathbf{x}_t|q_j)$, where $\mathbf{x}_t$ denotes the observation vector at time t, and q_j denotes the jth phone state. The MLP is trained as a classifier that estimates phone-class posterior probabilities, $P(q_j|\mathbf{x}_t)$. The posteriors are then inverted with the Bayes rule, according to $p(\mathbf{x}_t|q_j) = P(q_j|\mathbf{x}_t)p(\mathbf{x}_t)/P(q_j)$. The resulting likelihoods are used in lieu of the Gaussian mixture model probabilities computed in a conventional HMM-based system. The rest of the HMM structure (transition probabilities, decoding procedure, etc.) is kept unchanged. Because the MLP learns the boundaries between the phone classes, the hybrid models show better phone discrimination characteristics than traditional ASR systems.

In order to provide the MLP with more contextual information, the phone posterior probabilities can advantageously be conditioned on a window of several consecutive observations (typically nine frames: $\mathbf{x}_{t-4}, \mathbf{x}_{t-3}, \ldots \mathbf{x}_t, \ldots \mathbf{x}_{t+4}$) rather than on a single frame of data.

Extension to Context-Dependent Hybrid Models

In early implementations of hybrid models, the context of a phone, which is known to influence its acoustic realizations because of co-articulation effects, was ignored. This context, denoted here by c_i, can take the form of one or several phones to the right and/or to the left of the current phone, q_j. With context modeling, the likelihood of an observation $\mathbf{x}_t$ can be expressed as $p(\mathbf{x}_t|q_j, c_i) = P(q_j, c_i|\mathbf{x}_t) \cdot p(\mathbf{x}_t)/P(q_j, c_i)$, and, in the context of hybrid models, the posterior probability $P(q_j, c_i|\mathbf{x}_t)$ needs to be estimated by an MLP. Simply extending the context-independent approach to estimate biphone or triphone posteriors would greatly increase the number of outputs of the MLP, and thus the number of parameters to estimate. Because this is undesirable, factorization approaches were proposed in which the posterior probability of a phone and of its context, $P(q_j, c_i|\mathbf{x}_t)$, is decomposed into products of probabilities that can be estimated with smaller MLP classifiers. In Bourlard and Morgan (1993), this posterior is expressed as $P(q_j, c_i|\mathbf{x}_t) = P(c_i|q_j, \mathbf{x}_t)P(q_j|\mathbf{x}_t)$, where both terms on the right-hand side of the equation can be estimated by separate MLPs (further context factorization is possible in the case of left and right context modeling). In Franco et al. (1994), the phone and context posterior is factored as $P(q_j, c_i|\mathbf{x}_t) = P(q_j|c_i, \mathbf{x}_t)P(c_i|\mathbf{x}_t)$, where $p(q_j|c_i, \mathbf{x}_t)$ is estimated by a context-dependent MLP whose training data set contains only tokens whose context is c_i, and which is initialized as the context-independent MLP estimating $P(q_j|\mathbf{x}_t)$. $P(c_i|\mathbf{x}_t)$ is estimated by an MLP classifier similar to that estimating $P(q_j|\mathbf{x}_t)$.

Hierarchical Connectionist Acoustic Models

In very large systems (tens of hours of training data, thousands of HMM states), context classifiers are difficult to train because of the nonuniform distribution of context classes for different phones, and because of the large amount of training data. To overcome this problem, Fritsch (1997) proposed clustering the HMM states in a tree-structured hierarchy and estimating the posterior probability of a given state as a product of the posteriors of the parent nodes in the tree. This approach is very modular and allows as many small MLPs as necessary to be trained for a given task. This was the first connectionist approach to outperform state-of-the-art standard HMM systems on the notoriously difficult Switchboard corpus, a large database of conversational telephone speech.

Recurrent Neural Networks

Recurrent MLPs have been used to incorporate time dependencies in the computation of the HMM's state probabilities (Robinson, 1994). In recurrent MLP implementations of hybrid HMM/MLP recognizers, posterior phone probabilities are estimated based not only on the current observations but also on a set of state variables that are themselves functions of the observations and state variables at previous times. The recurrence built into the state variables allows the network to capture the dynamic evolution of the speech signal in a more principled and efficient way than by increasing the number of data frames in the input window, as in nonrecurrent hybrid systems. The weights of the recurrent MLP are typically trained with the backpropagation-through-time algorithm, a method for "unfolding" the recurrence and treating the time-expanded structure as a long multilayer feedforward MLP (see PERCEPTRONS, ADALINES, AND BACKPROPAGATION).

This approach proved to be competitive with state-of-the-art HMM-based recognizers on large-vocabulary continuous speech recognition tasks (Hochberg et al., 1994).

Multiband Recognition

Hybrid MLP/HMM systems were recently used in multiband recognition, a technique by which the speech frequency band is divided in several subbands that are recognized in parallel. The subband segments can be recombined at the frame, phone, or word level, either with an MLP combiner or with a simpler (nonadaptive) mechanism. This approach has shown great potential for speech environments with band-limited noise (by weighting the clean frequency bands more than the noisy bands) (Bourlard and Dupont, 1996).

MLP Front-End Processing

The front-end unit, which is responsible for extracting feature vectors from the waveform, is probably the most critical component of a speech recognition system in that, ultimately, the performance of the system is limited by the amount of information contained in the speech features.

Although most of the early attempts at incorporating MLPs in recognition systems focused on the acoustic models rather than the front end, MLP-based feature extractors have progressively gained more interest in the speech community. There are several reasons for this.

First, traditional front-end units are designed based on classical signal processing principles, guided to some extent by our knowl-

edge of the human hearing system. They have few parameters, and offer little room for optimization from observed data. The introduction of trainable elements in the front end opens the door to more data-driven designs. Second, MLP-based front ends can be jointly optimized with the acoustic models, thereby allowing a closer integration of the two modules. This is especially relevant in the context of discriminative training. Finally, MLPs are powerful tools for introducing new knowledge sources into the front-end unit, without having to make specific modeling assumptions. The following sections will give a few examples of these points.

Speaker Normalization and Adaptation

Speaker recognition systems are typically trained from utterances spoken by different speakers. These are speaker-independent recognizers. Speaker-dependent recognizers, trained from a single speaker's data, typically outperform speaker-independent systems but are understandably harder to build, because of the difficulty of collecting massive amounts of speech from each user of the system. Part of the performance gap between speaker-dependent and speaker-independent recognizers can be regained with techniques such as speaker adaptation, or adjusting the speaker-independent models to fit a specific voice, and speaker normalization, or factoring out interspeaker differences.

There is a vast body of literature on this topic, most of which does not make use of MLPs. Model adaptation algorithms differ in terms of which parameters are adapted (e.g., Gaussian means only or means and variances), what criterion is used (maximum likelihood or maximum a posteriori), how the transformations are constrained, and so on. Similarly, feature transformations come in different flavors. A few examples of adaptation/normalization implementations using MLPs are given below.

In Neto et al. (1995), a single-layer MLP was inserted between the front end and a speaker-independent connectionist recognizer. It was trained from a small amount of data for each test speaker to normalize out speaker-specific characteristics from the feature stream. This layer was trained by freezing the parameters of the speaker-independent system after it had been trained and backpropagating errors through the recognizer, down to the MLP layer.

To improve the acoustic resolution of the feature transformation Abrash (1997) followed a mixture-of-experts approach. Instead of transforming the speech features with a global transformation according to $\mathbf{x}' = T(\mathbf{x})$, he considered a stack of transformation networks, $T_i(.)$, each specializing at a specific region of the acoustic space, r_i. The overall feature transformation is then expressed as a weighted sum of local transformations, $\mathbf{x}' = \Sigma_i P(r_i|\mathbf{x})T_i(\mathbf{x})$, where the posterior probabilities $P(r_i|\mathbf{x})$ are estimated by a so-called gating network. In particular, the acoustic regions can be defined to correspond to the different phonemes or groups of phonemes.

As mentioned previously, speaker adaptation can also be performed in the model domain by transforming the parameters of the speaker-independent acoustic models. In Abrash et al. (1996), a nonlinear model transformation was proposed to adapt the means of a standard Gaussian mixture–based HMM system. The MLP transformations were trained with a generalization of the Expectation-Maximization algorithm, but with the maximization step performed with a series of steepest ascent iterations, a technique inspired from backpropagation training.

Joint Feature Extraction and Model Training

Steepest descent/ascent training and the concept of backpropagating error gradients throughout a given structure, as is commonly done in the field of MLPs, find applications in various aspects of speech recognition. For example, in Bengio et al. (1992), an MLP feature transformation was trained along with the HMM-based acoustic models to maximize the maximum mutual information criterion for a plosive consonant classification task. Here the feature transformation is speaker independent and is meant to increase acoustic discrimination rather than focusing on speaker variability. Jointly optimizing both sets of parameters gave higher recognition rates than optimizing the two modules separately.

Similarly, in Rahim, Bengio, and LeCun (1997), a feature transformation and a set of acoustic models were jointly trained to minimize the classification errors between subword units. The transformation and the acoustic models were iteratively trained by freezing one of the two modules, training the other one, and vice versa. The authors showed that multiple parallel transformations (one for each word class) gave better recognition results than a single transformation, and that a nonlinear MLP transformation performed better than an affine transformation.

Noise Robustness

Speech recognition systems typically show lower performances when operated in noisy environments (e.g., speech transmitted through a hands-free telephone in a moving car). Noise corrupts the speech waveform and is often difficult to model because of the changing nature of the environment that produces it (speed of the car, quality of the road, etc.).

To help solve this problem, MLPs have been trained to extract clean speech from noisy input signals. In Sorensen (1991), a mapping was performed by presenting noisy speech feature vectors to an MLP and using the corresponding clean feature vectors as target outputs. Experiments were performed with cepstral and auditory features on an isolated word recognition task.

MLPs have also been used to combine knowledge sources, such as instantaneous and sentence-level measures of the signal-to-noise ratio, sentence-level estimates of the noise level, and noise-corrupted speech amplitude to compute an estimate of the noise, and subtract it from the noisy feature vector (Weintraub and Beaufays, 1999). This approach was tested on a large-vocabulary conversational speech database corrupted by additive car noise.

Such approaches resulted in impressive recognition improvement. Nonetheless, noise reduction remains an active research topic awaiting more developments, especially in applications where the noise is nonstationary or is correlated with the speech signal (e.g., speech reverberation in cars).

MLP Front Ends for Speaker Verification

Speaker verification, the task of recognizing a person's identity from his/her voice, is similar in essence to speech recognition: a front-end unit extracts features from the test waveform, and a subsequent classifier uses statistical models of the users's voices to identify the speaker's identity. In Heck et al. (2000), an MLP was trained to perform frame-level classification of speakers. The inputs to the MLP are nine adjacent frames of cepstral features, and the outputs are speaker posterior probabilities. The MLP has four hidden layers, with a bottleneck in the middle. The first two layers can be seen as performing discriminative feature compression, whereas the last two layers perform speaker classification. After training of the MLP, the last two layers are chopped off, and the features computed by the remaining layers are fed into a traditional Gaussian mixture–based speaker classifier.

Confidence in Recognition Results

Although speech recognition has made tremendous progress in the last decade, the technology is not faultless, and error correction mechanisms must be available for a deployed application to be successful. In particular, it is important to assess how confident the recognizer is in its understanding of the user's request before processing it. One way of implementing such a feature is to estimate the posterior probability that each word in the utterance was correctly recognized, and to decide, based on the word posteriors, whether to execute the request or reprompt the user.

MLPs have been used to implement such a mechanism (Weintraub et al., 1997). During recognition, the system collects a set of cues relative to the current word and to its decoding by the recognizer, e.g., how well the acoustic models match the data, whether there are other likely decodings of the spoken segment, how the durations of the subword segments fit their expected distributions, and so forth. These cues act as knowledge sources that are input to an MLP classifier. The MLP is trained with a target output equal to 1 (if the word was correctly recognized) or 0 (misrecognition). At run time, the MLP classifier will output the posterior probability that the word is correctly recognized, given the measured knowledge sources.

Discussion

Speech recognition was already a very mature field by the time multilayer MLPs and the backpropagation algorithm gained general acceptance from the research community. As a consequence, MLPs were experimented with to replace specific components of a well-defined architecture, rather than as a way to solve a brand-new problem. A posteriori, the question is thus where and how MLPs have helped improve recognition systems.

Virtually every possible functionality of multilayer MLPs has been exploited: MLP classifiers were used for phone and triphone classification, MLP estimators proved to be useful in feature transformation and noise estimation, and MLP combiners helped in merging different knowledge sources to estimate confidence measures.

In all these applications, the main advantages of MLPs over other statistical modeling methods are (1) MLP implementations typically require fewer assumptions and can be optimized in a data-driven fashion, (2) backpropagation training can be generalized to any optimization criterion, including maximum likelihood and all forms of discriminative training, and (3) MLP modules can easily be integrated in nonadaptive architectures.

However, most industrial speech recognizers to date count very few MLP components. This can be attributed in part to historical reasons, but more fundamentally, MLPs have some limitations that still hamper their integration in recognition systems. In particular, their training time is typically much greater than that of nonconnectionist models for which closed-form or fast iterative solutions can be derived. This is problematic with a very large data sets, where weeks of training may be necessary to achieve the desired performance. It is even more critical when one considers that, somewhat disconcertingly, increasing the amount of training data and the number of parameters remains to date the best way to improve recognition performance! Nonetheless, MLPs have made great progress in the speech recognition field since the first edition of the *Handbook*: scalable implementations have started to appear in the literature, and MLP-based models have outperformed state-of-the-art traditional recognition systems on some of the most challenging recognition tasks.

Road Map: Linguistics and Speech Processing
Related Reading: Hidden Markov Models; Perception, Adalines, and Backpropagation

References

Abrash, V., 1997, Mixture input transformations for adaptation of hybrid connectionist speech recognizers, *Proceedings of Eurospeech 97, Eu-*

ropean Speech Communication Association, vol. 1, Grenoble, France, pp. 299–302.

Abrash, V., Shankar, A., Franco, H., and Cohen, M., 1996, Acoustic adaptation using nonlinear transformations of HMM parameters, *Proceedings of the IEEE International Conference on Acoustics, Speech, and Signal Processing*, vol. 2, IEEE, Piscataway, NJ, pp. 729–732.

Bahl, L., Brown, P., de Souza, P., and Mercer, R., 1986, Maximum mutual information estimation of hidden Markov models: Parameters for speech recognition, *Proceedings of the IEEE International Conference on Acoustics, Speech, and Signal Processing*, IEEE, Piscataway, NJ, pp. 49–52.

Bengio, Y., De Mori, R., Flammia, G., and Kompe, R., 1992, Global optimization of a neural network-hidden Markov model hybrid, *IEEE Trans. Neural Netw.*, 3:252–259.

Bourlard, H., and Dupont, S., 1996, A new approach based on independent processing and recombination of partial frequency bands, *Proceedings of the International Conference on Spoken Language Processing, Applied Science and Engineering Laboratories*, vol. 1, Wilmington, DE, pp. 426–429.

Bourlard, H., and Morgan, N., 1993, *Connectionist Speech Recognition: A Hybrid Approach*, Boston: Kluwer Academic Publishers.

Franco, H., Cohen, M., Morgan, N., Rumelhart, D., and Abrash, V., 1994, Context-dependent connectionist probability estimation in a hybrid hidden Markov model-neural net speech recognition system, *Comput. Speech Lang.*, 8:211–222.

Fritsch, J., 1997, ACID/HNN: A framework for hierarchical connectionist acoustic modeling, in *Proceedings of the 1997 Workshop on Automatic Speech Recognition and Understanding* (S. Furui, B.-H. Juang, W. Chou, Eds.), IEEE Piscataway, NJ.

Heck, L., Konig, Y., Sönmez, M. K., and Weintraub, M., 2000, Robustness to telephone handset distortion in speaker recognition by discriminative feature design, *Speech Commun.*, 31:181–192.

Hochberg, M., Renals, S., Robinson, A., and Kershaw, D., 1994, Large vocabulary continuous speech recognition using a hybrid connectionist-HMM system, *Proceedings of the International Conference on Spoken Language Processing*, vol. 3, pp. 1499–1502.

Juang, B., and Katagiri, S., 1992, Discriminative learning for minimum error classification, *IEEE Trans. Signal Proc.*, 40:3043–3054.

Neto, J., Alameida, L., Hochberg, M., Martins, C., Nunes, L., Renals, S., and Robinson, T., 1995, Speaker-adaptation for hybrid HMM-ANN continuous speech recognition system, *Proceedings of Eurospeech 95, European Speech Communication Association*, Grenoble, France, pp. 2171–2174.

Rahim, M., Bengio, Y., and LeCun, Y., 1997, Discriminative feature and model design for automatic speech recognition, *Proceedings of Eurospeech 97, European Speech Communication Association, Grenoble, France*, vol. 1, pp. 75–78.

Robinson, T., 1994, An application of recurrent nets to phone probability estimation, *IEEE Trans. Neural Netw.*, 5:298–305.

Sorensen, H., 1991, A cepstral noise reduction multi-layer neural network, *Proceedings of the IEEE International Conference on Acoustics, Speech, and Signal Processing*, IEEE, Piscataway, NJ, pp. 933–936.

Weintraub, M., and Beaufays, F., 1999, Increased robustness of noisy speech features using neural networks, in *Proceedings of a Workshop on Robust Methods for Speech Recognition in Adverse Conditions*, Tampere, Finland, pp. 207–210.

Weintraub, M., Beaufays, F., Rivlin, Z., Konig, Y., and Stolcke, A., 1997, Neural-network based measures of confidence for word recognition, *Proceedings of the IEEE International Conference on Acoustics, Speech, and Signal Processing*, vol. 2, IEEE, Piscataway, NJ, Munich, pp. 887–890.

Spiking Neurons, Computation with

Wolfgang Maass

Introduction

Most artificial neural network models are based on a neuron model (called perceptron or threshold gate) that McCulloch and Pitts proposed in 1943 as an abstraction of the computational function of a biological neuron. Today we know that there exist a number of fundamental differences between computations in such artificial neural networks and computations in circuits of biological neurons. One difference becomes obvious when one considers the output of a neuron. The output of a neuron in an artificial neural network is a bit (in the case of a perceptron) or a real-valued number (in the case of a sigmoidal gate). The output of a biological neuron consists of sharp potential increases (called action potentials, or *spikes*) that are initiated at the initial segment of its axons. These spikes, which last for 1–2 ms, are propagated through its axonal tree, with intermediate restoration of the shape of the spike at the nodes of Ranvier. Since this shape is rather stereotypical (there are no "half-spikes"), one may argue that it corresponds to the binary output of a perceptron: spike = 1, no spike = 0. But in contrast to artificial neural networks, which are usually driven in a synchronous mode, a generic biological neural circuit has no central clock. The times when a neuron fires depend on its current and preceding input. Hence, although at any instance in time the decision whether a neuron fires resembles the computational operation of a perceptron, and although the average number of spikes (with an average taken over time or space) emitted by neurons resembles the real-valued output of a sigmoidal neuron, the resource time plays a completely different role in the computation in a biological neural circuit. Whereas it is trivialized as a computational resource in most digital computers and artificial neural networks, because one takes care that the times at which a gate emits an output adhere to a rigid schedule that is largely input independent, a biological neuron can encode essential information about the input in the times when it fires. This facility can, for example, be used to transmit information very fast through small temporal differences between the spikes sent out by different neurons (see FAST VISUAL PROCESSING), and it can potentially be used to transmit information about relations between neurons through relations between their firing times (e.g., transient correlations between the firing times of a subset of neurons; see SYNCHRONIZATION, BINDING AND EXPECTANCY). Methods from information theory can be used to quantify how much more information about a stimulus can be extracted from spike trains if the precise spike times are taken into account (see SENSORY CODING AND INFORMATION TRANSMISSION). Finally, computing with an input-driven and flexible temporal organization of computational units is potentially beneficial for computing in an on-line manner on a continuous-input stream, since the computation speed can be instantly adjusted to the current input activity, and no energy is wasted by transmitting a central clock signal to all units even if there is nothing to compute. Apparently all of these aspects are essential for understanding biological neural computation. But they also present new ideas for the design of artificial computing machinery that can respond in real time to a complex input stream while spending just a fraction of the energy of a digital processor (see SILICON NEURONS; NEUROMORPHIC VLSI CIRCUITS AND SYSTEMS). Formal models for spiking neural networks are useful for investigating this strange new world of computing with spikes, both in order to formulate reasonable hypotheses about the organization of biological neural computation and to provide an abstract platform for exploring the possible use of spikes and temporal coding in novel artificial computing machinery. These networks of spiking neurons may be viewed as a third generation of neural network models, after perceptrons and sigmoidal neural networks.

A Formal Spiking Neural Network Model

A biological neuron j fires at certain time points $t_j^{(1)}$, $t_j^{(2)}$, . . . , each time sending a stereotyped spike down its axonal tree. At the synapses that connect these axonal branches with other neurons, the spike triggers the emission of neurotransmitter, thereby causing positive pulses (excitatory postsynaptic potentials, EPSPs) or negative pulses (inhibitory postsynaptic potentials, IPSPs) on the membrane potential of the postsynaptic neurons i (Figure 1). The time course of these EPSPs and IPSPs resulting from a firing of neuron j at time $t_j^{(f)}$ can be described by terms of the form $w_{ij}(t) \cdot \varepsilon(t - t_j^{(f)})$, where the function $\varepsilon(t - t_j^{(f)})$ describes a potential hill that has value 0 if $t - t_j^{(f)}$ is less than the transmission time Δ_{ij} from the soma of neuron j to the soma of neuron i, then increases almost linearly and finally decays exponentially back to 0 (typically within 20–80 ms). The factor $w_{ij}(t)$, which describes the efficacy of the synaptic connection from neuron j to neuron i at time t, is positive in the case of an EPSP and negative in the case of an IPSP.

There exist various mathematical models that predict the firing times $t_i^{(1)}$, $t_i^{(2)}$, . . . of a biological neuron i in dependence on the firing times $t_j^{(f)}$ of "presynaptic" neurons j. Because of its mathematical simplicity, the most useful model for a computational analysis is the *spike response model* (see INTEGRATE-AND-FIRE NEURONS AND NETWORKS). Here the membrane potential $u_i(t)$ at time t at the trigger zone of neuron i—i.e., that location on the soma of neuron i where its spikes are initiated—is represented by a sum $\sum_{j,f} w_{ij}(t) \cdot \varepsilon(t - t_j^{(f)})$ consisting of EPSPs and IPSPs that were caused by firings of presynaptic neurons j at preceding times $t_j^{(f)}$, and a refractory term $\eta(t - \hat{t}_i)$ that depends on the last time $\hat{t}_i$ when neuron i has fired before time t. If $t - \hat{t}_i$ is positive but very small (less than 2 ms) then $\eta(t - \hat{t}_i)$ is strongly negative, whereas for larger values of $t - \hat{t}_i$, its value returns back to 0. According to the spike response model the neuron i fires whenever the resulting term for its membrane potential $u_i(t) = \eta(t - \hat{t}_i) + \sum_{j,f} w_{ij}(t) \cdot \varepsilon(t - t_j^{(f)})$ reaches a certain firing threshold ϑ from below.

In comparison with the Hodgkin-Huxley model and the standard equations for integrate-and-fire neurons, this spike response model is much easier to handle for the purpose of analyzing computations, since its formulation does not involve differential equations. On the other hand, with suitable choices of the response functions η and ϵ (which may depend on the neurons i and j) and the functions $w_{ij}(t)$ (which may depend on the specific temporal dynamics of the synaptic connection between neurons i and j), this model is able to capture quite well the dynamics of a biological neural circuit.

Computing with One Spike per Neuron

In order to analyze the computational power of this formal spiking neural network model, one needs in an addition a convention for translating between their inputs and outputs, which are vectors of sequences of spikes ("spike trains") in continuous time, and the types of inputs and outputs of other computational models (which typically are vectors of binary or real-valued numbers). Of particular interest are translations between binary and analog numbers and spike trains that are biologically realistic in the sense that they match translation schemes employed by sensory neurons to encode external stimuli. Several such potential "neural codes" are discussed in INTEGRATE-AND-FIRE NEURONS AND NETWORKS. One of the most intriguing one, which has no analogon in artificial neural network models, is the time-to-first-spike code (also called delay code), where one assumes that the times of the first spikes in each of n incoming spike trains encode n real-valued numbers. Since stronger stimuli tend to produce shorter latencies, one might assign the largest value 1 to the input channel with the earliest first spike, the smallest value 0 to the input channel with the latest first spike, and to the other input channels real values between 0 and 1, corresponding to the position of their first spike relative to the others.

The first interesting observation is that for such code, a spiking neuron can carry out computational operations that have no counterpart in the computational units of traditional neural network models: a spiking neuron can act as *coincidence detector* for incoming pulses by firing only if a certain number of EPSPs arrive almost simultaneously at its soma (Abeles, 1982). Hence if the arrival times of the incoming pulses (EPSPs) encode *analog numbers* x_j, a spiking neuron can detect whether some of these numbers x_j have (almost) equal value. Thus, a spiking neuron can also decide whether the numbers x_j in a vector $\langle x_1, \ldots, x_n \rangle$ are all different, which happens to be a well-known benchmark problem in computer science. It is usually referred to as the element distinctness problem (ED). Since the formal version of this problem requires hair-trigger decisions, one can expect from a physical implementation of a spiking neuron only that it computes a closely related partial function $ED_n : \mathbb{R}^n \to \{0, 1\}$, where for some parameter $c > 0$ (that is related to the amount of imprecision or noise) the output $ED_n(x_1, \ldots, x_n)$ satisfies the equation

$$ED_n(x_1, \ldots, x_n) = \begin{cases} 1, & \text{if there are } j \neq j' \text{ so that } x_j = x_j' \\ 0, & \text{if } |x_j - x_j'| \geq c \text{ for all } j \neq j' \end{cases}$$

A single spiking neuron, modeled according to our formal model, can compute this function ED_n (Figure 2). This is remarkable, since artificial neural networks need a substantial amount of hardware for computing ED_n (even if the network is allowed to give any output it wants if neither of the two cases in the definition of ED_n apply). It was shown in Maass (1997b) that any threshold circuit (i.e., any layered feedforward circuit consisting of McCulloch-Pitts neurons) that computes ED_n needs to have at least $n/2 \log n$ perceptrons on its first hidden layer, and that any feedforward analog neural net (i.e., any multilayer perceptron consisting of sigmoidal neurons) that computes ED_n needs to have at least $n - 6/2$ sigmoidal gates as hidden units.

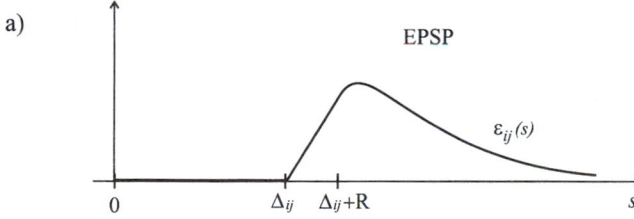

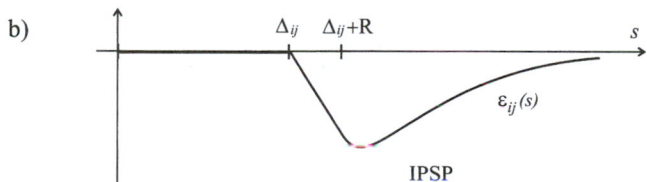

Figure 1. A, Typical shape of an excitatory postsynaptic potential (EPSP). B, Typical shape of an inhibitory postsynaptic potential (IPSP).

a)

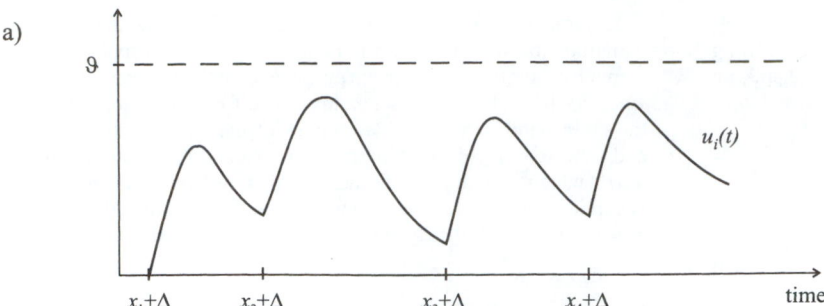

b)

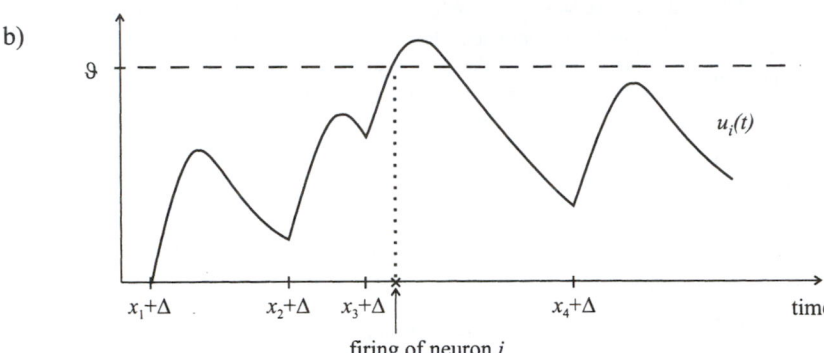

firing of neuron i

Figure 2. *A*, Typical time course of the state variable $u_i(t)$ if $ED_4(x_1, x_2, x_3, x_4) = 0$. *B*, Time course of $u_i(t)$ in the case where $ED_4(x_1, x_2, x_3, x_4) = 1$ because $|x_3 - x_2| \leq c$.

One can exploit the coincidence detection capability of a spiking neuron i even further and raise its firing threshold ϑ so high that EPSPs caused by firings of *all* presynaptic neurons have to arrive nearly simultaneously at the soma of i to make it fire. In this case the spiking neuron implements a variation of an RBF unit (radial basis function unit) in the temporal domain (Hopfield, 1995). If the transmission delays Δ_{ij} from the trigger zone of neuron j to the trigger zone of neuron i all have the same value, then such a neuron with a high threshold ϑ fires if and only if the firing times t_j of all presynaptic neurons j have almost the same value. If these transmission delays Δ_{ij} vary for different j, then the same neuron i will fire if and only if the firing times $\langle t_j \rangle_j$ of the presynaptic neurons j form a specific temporal pattern: $t_j \approx T - \Delta_{ij}$ for all j, where T is some number that is independent of j. In Natschläger and Ruf (1998), the previous construction has been extended to self-organizing RBF networks with the help of lateral inhibition between RBF units.

In the approach for computing with spiking neurons that we have sketched so far, the input consisted of a vector of analog numbers, encoded through temporal delays between the first spikes, but the output of the spiking neuron was binary, encoded through firing or nonfiring of that neuron. Obviously, for multilayer or recurrent computations with spiking neurons, it is desirable to *output* a vector of analog numbers that is encoded in the same way as the input. For that purpose one needs a mechanism for *shifting* the firing time of a spiking neuron i in dependence on the firing times t_j of presynaptic neurons. Such mechanism is provided by the fact that advancing t_j in time tends to advance the firing time of neuron i, and it advances it even more if the intermediate synaptic weight w_{ij} has a large value. This can be used to compute a weighted sum for analog values in such a way that the same temporal code is used for inputs and outputs. Since it is straightforward to simulate the nonlinear activation function of a sigmoidal neuron through the firing mechanism of a spiking neuron, one can simulate in this way any sigmoidal neuron by a spiking neuron where each analog input or output is encoded by the temporal position of a spike. Hence,

one can rigorously prove (Maass, 1997a) that any continuous function $F : [0, 1]^n \rightarrow [0, 1]^m$ can be approximated arbitrarily closely by a network of spiking neurons with inputs and outputs encoded by temporal delays.

As an alternative, Thorpe and co-workers have proposed viewing the *order* of the firing times t_j of different neurons j as the relevant signal conveyed by these neurons, and have explored mechanisms for computing in terms of such code (see Thorpe and Gautrais, 1997, and FAST VISUAL PROCESSING). One may view this firing order code as a digitalized version of the previously discussed delay code.

An interesting general question concerns the theoretical limits of the computational power of spiking neurons, regardless of specific assumption about neural coding. It turns out that if the firing times of spiking neurons were not affected by noise, one could theoretically simulate any Turing machine by some finite network of spiking neurons (Maass, 1996); hence any digital computation could be carried out by such a network. This implies that in order to evaluate the actual computational power of a concrete biological or artificial spiking neural network, one needs to know something about the noise that affects it.

Computing on Spike Trains

In the preceding section we focused on computations where inputs and outputs consisted of a single spike per channel. In this section we will look at the case where inputs and outputs consist of *spike trains*. This can be used for computations on analog variables that are represented in a highly noise-robust manner, or for computations on time series. A simple scheme for converting spike trains into time series of numbers and vice versa is the well-known *firing rate code*, where one interprets the number of times that a neuron i fires (during some sliding time window of a certain length) as the current output of neuron i. Another scheme, this one for interpreting spike trains as codes for analog time series, which requires many fewer spikes but greater precision in the timing of the spikes, results from convolving each spike with a suitable smooth kernel function (see Rieke et al., 1997). In this way each spike train can be viewed as a code for a smooth time-varying function. Possible methods for computing on input functions that are represented in this way by spike trains are discussed in TEMPORAL INTEGRATION IN RECURRENT MICROCIRCUITS (q.v.). A third option for neural coding is the *space-rate code* or *population code*, where the fraction of neurons within a certain pool that fire during a specific short time interval (say, 5 ms) encodes an analog number. It is shown in Maass and Natschläger (2000) that networks of spiking neurons can approximate any given continuous multivariable function if the network inputs and outputs are assumed to encode analog numbers through such a space-rate code. It turns out that the unreliability of synaptic transmission in biological systems (see SYNAPTIC TRANSMISSION) is quite useful for such analog computing in terms of a space-rate code. Furthermore, one can prove that networks of spiking neurons can in principle carry out with regard to a space-rate code more complex operations, where the current output depends not just on the current input but also on previous inputs. One usually refers to such computations as operators or filters, since they map functions of time onto functions of time, rather than mapping numbers on numbers. In this context one can utilize the tails of EPSPs and IPSPs (i.e., their exponentially decaying segments) to implement linear filters via networks of spiking neurons (Maass and Natschläger, 2000). All computations in formal models of spiking neural networks that we have discussed so far can be implemented with static synapses, i.e., with synapses where each synaptic weight $w_{ij}(t)$ has a time-invariant fixed value. In reality, the efficacy of a biological synapse changes on a fast time scale, depending on the frequency and temporal pattern of previous spike arrivals at the synapse (see TEMPORAL DYNAMICS OF BIOLOGICAL SYNAPSES). If one takes this into account, then a feedforward network of spiking neurons can approximate with regard to space-rate coding of time-varying analog inputs and outputs a very large class of nonlinear filters: any nonlinear filter that is time invariant and has fading memory (Maass and Sontag, 2000).

Because of their coincidence-detection capabilities, spiking neurons are quite sensitive to statistical correlations in the firing times of presynaptic neurons (often referred to as *synchronization*). Furthermore, computer simulations suggest that biologically supported learning rules enhance this capability. Since the number of possible relations among presynaptic neurons that can be encoded in this way is exponential, a coding mechanism that involves correlations in firing times may substantially enlarge the expressive capabilities of neural networks. The precise computational operations that can be carried by spiking neurons in the presence of a larger number of competing "relations" encoded through firing correlations of presynaptic neurons has remained elusive (see Milner, 1974; von der Malsburg, 1981; Eckhorn et al., 1988; Maass, 1998).

SYNFIRE CHAINS (q.v.) represent yet another approach for information processing in networks of spiking neurons (Abeles, 1991). Each synfire chain consists of a layered feedforward circuit of spiking neurons, where a wavefront of firing activity is propagated from layer to layer. From the point of view of computation, a single synfire chain just implements a binary register (through its two states, active/nonactive), and hence is not a computational model in a strict sense. But if several synfire chains are superimposed on a spiking neural network, the activity of one or several synfire chains may ignite activity in yet another synfire chain. In this fashion one can, for example, implement an AND gate via a (fairly large) network of spiking neurons. Analog versions of such computations are discussed in Maass and Natschläger (2000).

Discussion

Networks of spiking neurons represent a third generation of neural network models that are biologically more realistic, since they allow that the timing of individual computation steps may transfer salient information. Rigorous proofs imply that formal models for spiking neural networks can carry out all computations that standard neural network models can handle, some of them with substantially fewer gates. In addition, networks of spiking neurons are particularly well suited for carrying out computations on analog time series (see TEMPORAL INTEGRATION IN RECURRENT MICROCIRCUITS). Since spiking neural networks can compute in an input-driven mode without any central synchronization, hardware implementations of such networks offer new ways for real-time sensory processing at the microwatt level (see ANALOG VLSI IMPLEMENTATIONS OF NEURAL NETWORKS). Surveys on biology-oriented models for computations with spiking neurons can be found in Abeles (1991), Rieke et al. (1997), and Cariani (2001). More detailed survey articles on the theory and hardware for implementing computing with spiking neurons are contained in Maass and Bishop (1999). Research papers on the current state of the art can be found in Grossberg, Maass, and Markram (2001).

Road Maps: Grounding Models of Networks; Grounding Models of Neurons
Background: Single-Cell Models
Related Reading: Integrate-and-Fire Neurons and Networks; Synfire Chains

References

Abeles, M., 1982, Role of the cortical neuron: Integrator or coincidence detector? *Israel J. Med. Sci.*, 18:83–92.
Abeles, M., 1991, *Corticonics*, Cambridge, Engl.: Cambridge University Press. (See especially Chapter 3.) ◆
Cariani, P. A., 2001, Neural timing nets, *Neural Netw.*, 14:737–753.
Grossberg, S., Maass, W., and Markram, H., Eds., 2001, *Spiking Neurons in Neuroscience and Technology*, *Neural Netw.*, 14:(6–7) (special issue).
Eckhorn, R., Bauer, R., Jordan, W., Brosch, M., Kruse, W., Munk, M., and Reitboeck, H. J., 1988, Coherent oscillations: A mechanism of feature linking in the visual cortex? Multiple electrode and correlation analysis in the cat, *Biol. Cybern.*, 60:121–130.
Hopfield, J. J., 1995, Pattern recognition computation using action potential timing for stimulus representation, *Nature*, 376:33–36. ◆
Maass, W., 1996, Lower bounds for the computational power of networks of spiking neurons, *Neural Computat.*, 8:1–40.
Maass, W., 1997a, Fast sigmoidal networks via spiking neurons, *Neural Computat.*, 9:279–304.
Maass, W., 1997b, Networks of spiking neurons: The third generation of neural network models, *Neural Netw.*, 10:1659–1671. ◆
Maass, W., 1998, A simple model for neural computation with firing rates and firing correlations, *Netw. Computat. Neural Syst.*, 9:1–17.
Maass, W., and Bishop, C., Eds., 1999, *Pulsed Neural Networks*, Cambridge, MA: MIT Press. (See especially Chapters 1 to 4.) ◆
Maass, W., and Natschläger, T., 2000, A model for fast analog computation based on unreliable synapses, *Neural Computat.*, 12:1679–1704.
Maass, W., and Sontag, E. D., 2000, Neural systems as nonlinear filters, *Neural Computat.*, 2:1743–1772.
Milner, P. M., 1974, A model for visual shape recognition, *Psychol. Rev.*, 81:521–535.
Natschläger, T., and Ruf, B., 1998, Spatial and temporal pattern analysis via spiking neurons, *Netw. Computat. Neural Syst.*, 9:319–332.
Rieke, F., Warland, D., de Ruyter van Steveninck, R. R., and Bialek, W., 1997, *Spikes: Exploring the Neural Code*, Cambridge, MA: MIT Press. (See especially Chapters 1 and 2.) ◆
Thorpe, S. J., and Gautrais, J., 1997, Rapid visual processing using spike asynchrony, *Advances in Neural Information Processing Systems*, vol. 9, Cambridge, MA: MIT Press, pp. 901–907.
von der Malsburg, C., 1981, The correlation theory of brain function, *Internal Report 81-2 of the Department of Neurobiology of the Max Planck Institute for Biophysical Chemistry in Göttingen*, Göttingen, Germany. Reprinted in *Models of Neural Networks II* (Domany et al., Eds.), New York: Springer-Verlag, 1994, pp. 95–119.

Spinal Cord of Lamprey: Generation of Locomotor Patterns

James T. Buchanan

Introduction

The successes in revealing the structure and function of rhythm-generating networks in invertebrates led to the insight that although there are recurring "building blocks" in the evolution of neuronal networks, there is also a great deal of variation in the details of network construction between different classes of organisms (Getting, 1989). Thus, to understand vertebrate neuronal networks, one must study vertebrate nervous systems, and this realization has led to a proliferation of vertebrate models for investigating the cellular and synaptic mechanisms of locomotor rhythm generation (Pearson and Gordon, 2000) (see LOCOMOTION, VERTEBRATE). One of the most favorable adult vertebrate preparations is the lamprey, a jawless fish with close ties to the earliest vertebrates of the fossil record. Significant progress has been made toward revealing features of the lamprey locomotor network, and this preparation has been the focus of numerous modeling studies.

The Lamprey Spinal Cord

The adult lamprey spinal cord has numerous advantages for neurophysiological studies aimed at understanding the cellular and synaptic mechanisms of rhythmic locomotor activity. In overall structure and organization, the lamprey spinal cord resembles the spinal cords of higher vertebrates. For example, the spinal cord consists of a core of nerve cell bodies surrounded by axon tracts, and there are dorsal and ventral roots of sensory and motor functions, respectively. However, when compared with other adult vertebrates, the lamprey spinal cord contains relatively few nerve cells (ca. 1,000 per segment), and the cell bodies of many of these neurons are clearly visible in the thin (ca. 0.3 mm), transparent spinal cord. In addition, the lamprey spinal cord survives and functions well when isolated and can be readily manipulated by adding pharmacological agents to the bathing fluid. This is particularly important in the study of locomotor activity because one can activate the spinal swimming network by adding the excitatory neurotransmitter, glutamate, to the bathing fluid. One disadvantage to using the lamprey nervous system is the lack of uniquely identifiable cells in the spinal cord, a feature that made invertebrate preparations, such as the crustacean stomatogastric ganglion, so successful in the study of network structure and function (see CRUSTACEAN STOMATOGASTRIC SYSTEM). In the lamprey spinal cord we must characterize classes of nerve cells rather than unique individuals, and thus we face the uncertainties associated with defining cell classes.

Fictive Swimming

Like most fish, lampreys swim with lateral body undulations that propagate from head to tail (Figure 1A). These body waves are created by contractions of muscles that alternate between the two sides and propagate down the body. The speed of wave propagation is scaled to the swim frequency so that as the animal swims faster, the propagation speed of the waves increases. In this way, the lamprey maintains about one full wave of body curvature over the length of its body for a wide range of swimming speeds. When the spinal cord is isolated and exposed to glutamate, similar rhythmic activity can be recorded from the ventral roots, the nerves that contain the axons of the motor neurons innervating the body muscles (Figure 1B). As the motor neurons fire action potentials, their

spikes are recorded as rhythmic bursts (ca. 0.5–4 bursts/s) that alternate with ventral roots on the opposite side of the spinal cord (Figure 1B). Ventral roots located more distant from the head show a progressive delay in burst onset. Again, this delay is scaled to the swim frequency, so that there is a constant phase lag in the head-to-tail propagation of the ventral root bursts. This phase lag is about 1% of a cycle period per segment (ca. 100 spinal segments total). Thus, there is a close match between the pattern of muscle electrical activity in the swimming lamprey and the pattern of ventral root bursting in the isolated spinal cord, indicating that the latter represents the neuronal correlate of swimming and is therefore referred to as fictive swimming.

The Lamprey Locomotor Network

The presence of swimming activity in the isolated spinal cord demonstrates that, like other vertebrate and invertebrate preparations, the lamprey spinal cord contains a central pattern generator for locomotion. That is, the neuronal machinery required to produce the detailed locomotor pattern is an emergent property of spinal nerve cells and their synaptic interactions.

One goal of locomotor studies is to understand the structure and function of the locomotor central pattern generator. What do we know about the cells comprising this network and their synaptic interactions? Although uniquely identifiable neurons have not been found in the lamprey spinal cord, several classes of spinal neurons have been characterized on the basis of physiological and anatomical criteria (Figure 1C) (Buchanan, 2001). The alternating pattern of rhythmic activity between the two sides of the spinal cord and the disruption of rhythmic activity by midline cuts suggest that cells with midline-crossing axons (commissural interneurons) are important for locomotor activity (Buchanan, 1999). Therefore, commissural interneurons (CCINs) have been a focus of intracellular studies. One class of CCINs has been shown to make inhibitory glycinergic synapses on motor neurons and interneurons on the opposite side of the spinal cord. These inhibitory CCINs are thought to provide a mechanism for alternation between the two sides and for basic rhythm generation via their reciprocal inhibitory interactions (see HALF-CENTER OSCILLATORS UNDERLYING RHYTHMIC MOVEMENTS). In addition to the inhibitory CCINs, there is a class of small excitatory interneurons (EINs) with short axons confined to the same side of the spinal cord. The EINs provide rhythmic excitation of nearby motor neurons and interneurons via glutamatergic excitatory synapses. Finally, there is a third class of interneurons that are active during fictive swimming, the lateral interneurons (LINs). The LINs inhibit CCINs on the same side of the spinal cord via glycinergic synapses. The LINs have been proposed to provide the early inhibition that is observed in the CCINs and thus to terminate the firing of the CCINs on one side of the cord, allowing the inhibitory CCINs on the opposite side to begin firing.

Modeling Lamprey Locomotion

The lamprey locomotor network has been simulated with a variety of models, from connectionist-style to more detailed biophysical models. These simulations have demonstrated the feasibility of the proposed circuit (Figure 1C), have helped to assess the importance of various electrophysiological parameters in the function of the

Figure 1. Lamprey swimming and the locomotor network. *A*, Images of a swimming lamprey showing the lateral undulations of the body that propagate from head to tail. Images are separated by 67 msec. *B*, Fictive swimming in a 32-segment length of isolated spinal cord exposed to 0.5 mM of D-glutamate. Ventral roots (VR) were recorded with extracellular electrodes. *C*, The proposed lamprey locomotor network consists of three types of interneurons. Each cell represents many neurons. Open triangles indicate excitatory synapses, circles indicate inhibitory synapses, and the dashed line indicates the midline. MN, motor neuron; CC, commissural interneuron; EIN, excitatory interneuron; LIN, lateral interneuron.

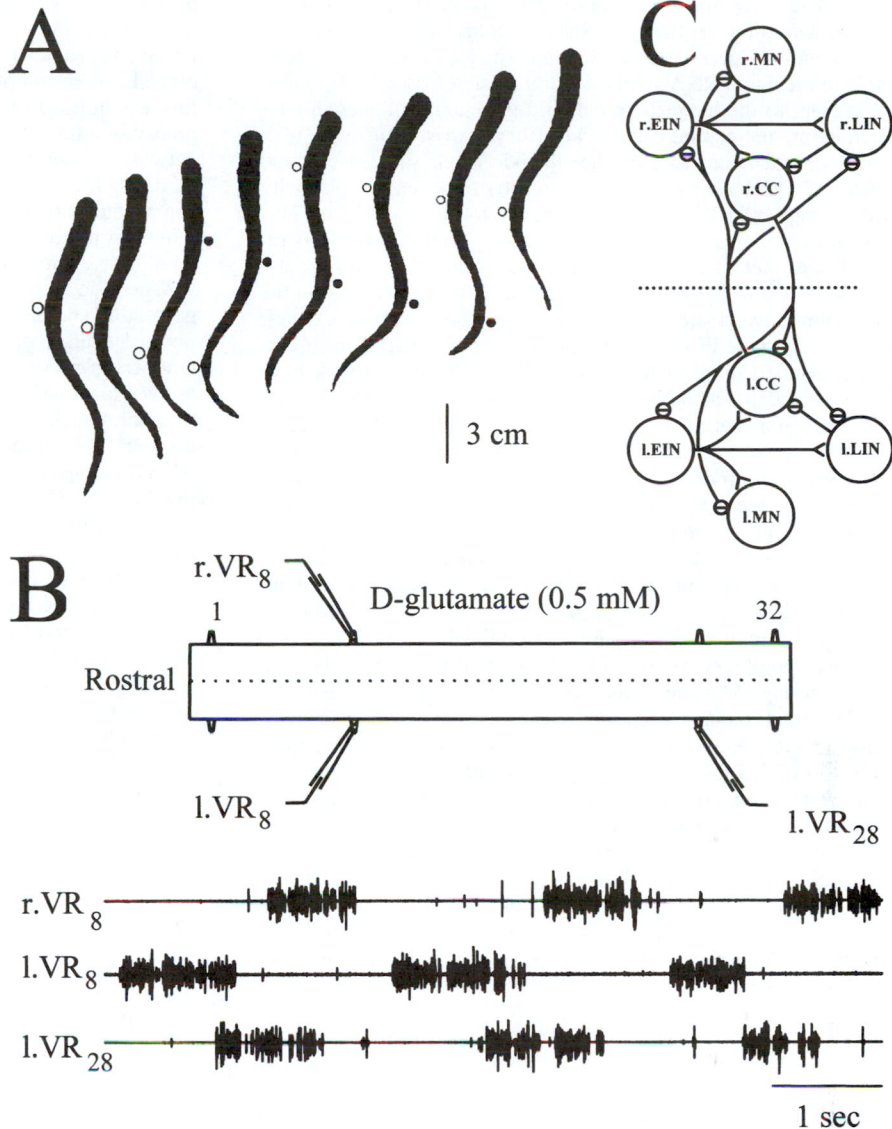

network, and have provided insights into various network issues.

Detailed biophysical models typically use Hodgkin-Huxley (HH)-style kinetic modeling of ion channels that are incorporated into compartmental models of neuronal electrotonic structure. Such models of the lamprey locomotor network suffer from the problem of an overabundance of unspecified and unconstrained parameters because we do not have good voltage-clamp characterizations of the HH parameters for lamprey neurons. An alternative to detailed voltage-clamp analysis has been to use white noise analysis (Murphey, Moore, and Buchanan, 1995). The magnitude and phase responses of lamprey neurons to small-amplitude, subthreshold white noise current or voltage signals have been used to fit model neurons containing voltage-dependent conductances and electrotonic structure. This approach provides a stronger data-based modeling of the nonlinear voltage dependencies and the contributions of dendritic electrotonic structure, but a systematic characterization of the various lamprey spinal neuron classes using this technique has not yet been done.

Although detailed HH-style modeling currently has limitations when applied to lamprey neurons, these or similar detailed bio-

physical models are essential for a full understanding of any neuronal network. For example, neuromodulators often act by subtly altering the activity of voltage-gated or ligand-gated channels, and detailed biophysical models are required to explore the consequences of these ion channel changes on network activity (see NEUROMODULATION IN INVERTEBRATE NERVOUS SYSTEMS). There are a number of neuromodulators present in the lamprey spinal cord that alter the output of the locomotor network, with serotonin, dopamine, and the tachykinins being among the best studied. These substances offer good opportunities to test our knowledge of the locomotor system by combining the cellular and synaptic actions of the modulators into detailed network models.

Interesting new work involving neuromodulators in the lamprey has come from Parker and Grillner (2000). They have been investigating the effects of substance P, a tachykinin neuropeptide. The tachykinins have been well studied in the mammalian spinal cord, where they are involved in pain processing. In the lamprey, application of substance P to the isolated spinal cord has an extremely powerful effect on fictive swimming, increasing the swim burst frequency by three to five times. What is most remarkable is that after only a 10-minute exposure to substance P, the increase in the fictive swimming frequency persists for at least the next 24 hours. This essentially permanent alteration in the locomotor network requires protein and RNA synthesis for its maintenance. Tachykinins are present in the lamprey spinal cord in ventral midline cells located below the central canal, where they coexist in neurons with serotonin and dopamine. At the synaptic level, substance P and serotonin both have strong effects on activity-dependent plasticity at the synapses involved in generating the locomotor rhythm. This type of modulation of activity-dependent synaptic plasticity is referred to as metaplasticity. Not only are serotonin, dopamine, and substance P colocalized in spinal neurons, but their actions on the locomotor network are interdependent. Serotonin can block the effects of substance P on swim frequency and on synaptic metaplasticity. Detailed biophysical models of the lamprey network have demonstrated that metaplasticity can have significant effects on network behavior that are consistent with those observed experimentally (Kozlov et al., 2001). A major challenge for lamprey neurobiology will be to determine when these various neuromodulators are released. Are they coreleased or differentially released in a context-dependent manner?

Given the lack of detailed biophysical information about lamprey locomotor neurons, models that do not depend on details of individual cells have proved useful in advancing our understanding of lamprey locomotion. For example, simplified rhythm generators have been employed to look at larger-scale issues, such as the control of turning (McClellan and Hagevik, 1997). Techniques of bifurcation analysis have been used to examine the dynamic behavior of the network (Figure 1C), especially with regard to its interactions with the brain (Jung, Kiemel, and Cohen, 1996). Efforts have also been made using simpler locomotor networks to expand the levels of modeling to take into account the properties of the muscles, movement through water, and sensory feedback during movement (Ekeberg and Grillner, 1999).

Another application of models with less neuronal detail has been in investigations aimed at understanding the nature of the coupling among the rhythm generators. This is an interesting problem because the speed of the head-to-tail propagation of the rhythmic activity down the spinal cord varies with the speed of swimming, yet conduction delays in axons are fixed. Experimental tests of a model of coupled oscillators (Cohen et al., 1992) (see CHAINS OF OSCILLATORS IN MOTOR AND SENSORY SYSTEMS) led to the conclusion that ascending intersegmental coupling signals have a stronger influence over oscillator coupling in the lamprey spinal cord than do descending signals (Sigvardt and Williams, 1996). Williams (1992) explored coupling using connectionist-style modeling to link chains of unit locomotor networks using the same neurons that generate the rhythmic activity. By adjusting the synaptic strengths of the coupling signals, it was possible to achieve constant phase lags with values similar to that of fictive swimming. While these studies demonstrated the feasibility of this mechanism, we do not yet know sufficient details of the intersegmental connectivity to verify the mechanism experimentally.

Discussion

An underlying motivation for studying the lamprey locomotor network is to learn about vertebrate locomotor networks in general. Does the lamprey tell us anything about higher vertebrates? There is certainly reason for hope that the lamprey network shares some fundamental properties with the locomotor networks of higher vertebrates because of the striking similarities between the lamprey network and that of the frog tadpole spinal cord (Roberts et al., 1998). These two animals swim with similar patterns, so it may not be unexpected that the networks are similar, yet the organisms are evolutionarily quite distant. We would like to believe that the lamprey locomotor network has been conserved to some extent in higher vertebrates as a core rhythm-generating network, and evolution has provided coupling among these core oscillators to generate the more complex sequences of muscle activation required in fins and limbs. In this regard, the salamander offers a promising preparation for studying the interaction of swimming and walking networks because this animal performs both. Connectionist-style modeling has recently been used to explore how a neural circuitry can produce and modulate the two locomotor programs of swimming and walking (Ijspeert, 2001), and several laboratories are beginning to explore these issues experimentally.

Where do we go from here in our attempts to understand the generation and control of vertebrate locomotion? A major limitation to understanding the lamprey locomotor network is the large numbers of nerve cells and the inability to uniquely identify them or even to classify them with confidence. Experimentally, we need to employ techniques that will allow characterization of populations and the synaptic interactions of many cells. Optical imaging of calcium signals or of voltage-sensitive dyes offers some hope in this direction. Further exploration of neuromodulators of the locomotor network will continue to provide opportunities to test our models as we try to account for the network effects of modulators on the basis of their demonstrated cellular and synaptic actions. Modeling of the locomotor network must proceed in parallel with the experimental data; and ultimately, large-scale and detailed biophysical modeling will be necessary. However, given the current limitations in our knowledge about the lamprey locomotor network, modeling that relies less on the details of individual cells will continue to be useful in understanding how locomotion is organized within the lamprey nervous system. Finally, comparisons with other vertebrates will be important for determining what aspects of the locomotor network have been conserved and how the core rhythm-generating network of swimming was modified for walking with limbs.

Road Maps: Motor Pattern Generators; Neuroethology and Evolution
Background: Motor Pattern Generation
Related Reading: Chains of Oscillators in Motor and Sensory Systems; Locomotion, Vertebrate; Sensorimotor Interactions and Central Pattern Generators

References

Buchanan, J. T., 1999, Commissural interneurons in rhythm generation and intersegmental coupling in the lamprey spinal cord, *J. Neurophysiol.*, 81:2037–2045.

Buchanan, J. T., 2001, Contributions of identifiable neurons and neuron classes to lamprey vertebrate neurobiology, *Prog. Neurobiol.*, 63:441–466. ◆

Cohen, A. H., Ermentrout, G. B., Kiemel, T., Kopell, N., Sigvardt, K. A., and Williams, T. L., 1992, Modelling of intersegmental coordination in the lamprey central pattern generator for locomotion, *Trends Neurosci.*, 15:434–438. ◆

Ekeberg, O., and Grillner, S., 1999, Simulations of neuromuscular control in lamprey swimming, *Philos. Trans. R. Soc. Lond. B*, 354:895–902.

Getting, P. A., 1989, Emerging principles governing the operation of neural networks, *Annu. Rev. Neurosci.*, 12:185–204. ◆

Ijspeert, A. J., 2001, A connectionist central pattern generator for the aquatic and terrestrial gaits of a simulated salamander, *Biol. Cybern.*, 84:331–348.

Jung, R., Kiemel, T., and Cohen, A. H., 1996, Dynamic behavior of a neural network model of locomotor control in the lamprey, *J. Neurophysiol.*, 75:1074–1086.

Kozlov, A., Kotaleski, J. H., Aurell, E., Grillner, S., and Lansner, A., 2001, Modeling of substance P and 5-HT induced synaptic plasticity in the lamprey spinal CPG: Consequences for network pattern generation, *J. Comp. Neurosci.*, 11:183–200.

McClellan, A. D., and Hagevik, A., 1997, Descending control of turning locomotor activity in larval lamprey: Neurophysiology and computer modeling, *J. Neurophysiol.*, 78:214–228.

Murphey, C. R., Moore, L. E., and Buchanan, J. T., 1995, Quantitative analysis of electrotonic structure and membrane properties of NMDA-activated lamprey spinal neurons, *Neural Computat.*, 7:486–506.

Parker, D., and Grillner, S., 2000, Neuronal mechanisms of synaptic and network plasticity in the lamprey spinal cord, *Prog. Brain Res.*, 125:381–398.

Pearson, K., and Gordon, J., 2000, Locomotion, in *Principles of Neural Science*, 4th ed. (E. R. Kandel, J. H. Schwartz, and T. M. Jessell, Eds.), New York: McGraw-Hill, pp. 737–755. ◆

Roberts, A., Soffe, S. R., Wolf, S., Yoshida, M., and Zhao, F.-Y., 1998, Central circuits controlling locomotion in young frog tadpoles, *Ann. NY Acad. Sci.*, 860:19–34. ◆

Sigvardt, K. A., and Williams, T. L., 1996, Effects of local oscillator frequency on intersegmental coordination in the lamprey locomotor CPG: Theory and experiment, *J. Neurophysiol.*, 76:4094–4103.

Williams, T. L., 1992, Phase coupling by synaptic spread in chains of coupled neuronal oscillators, *Science*, 258:662–665.

Statistical Mechanics of Generalization

Manfred Opper

Introduction

The theory of learning in artificial neural networks has benefited from various different fields of research. Among these, statistical physics has become an important tool for understanding a neural network's ability to generalize from examples. This article explains some of the basic principles and ideas of this approach.

In the following, we assume a feedforward network of N input nodes, receiving real-valued inputs, summarized by the vector $\mathbf{x} = (x(1), \ldots, x(N))$. The configuration of the network is described by its weights and will be abbreviated by a vector of parameters $\mathbf{w}$. Using $\mathbf{w}$, the network computes a function $F_{\mathbf{w}}$ of the inputs x and returns $\sigma = F_{\mathbf{w}}(\mathbf{x})$ as its output.

In the simplest case, a neural network should learn a binary classification task. That is, it should decide whether a given input $\mathbf{x}$ belongs to a certain class of objects and respond with the output: $F_{\mathbf{w}}(\mathbf{x}) = +1$, or, if the input does not belong, it should answer with $\sigma = -1$ (the choice $\sigma = \pm 1$, rather than, for example, 0, 1, is arbitrary and has no consequence for the learning curves). To learn the underlying classification rule, the network is trained on a set of m inputs $\mathbf{x}^m = \{\mathbf{x}_1, \ldots, \mathbf{x}_m\}$ together with the classification labels $\sigma^m = \{\sigma_1, \ldots, \sigma_m\}$, which are provided by a trainer or *teacher*. Using a *learning algorithm*, the network is adapted to this *training set* $D_m = (\sigma^m, \mathbf{x}^m)$ by adjusting its parameters $\mathbf{w}$ such that it responds correctly on the m examples.

How well will the trained network be able to classify an input that it has not seen before? In order to give a quantitative answer to this question, a common model assumes that all inputs, those from the training set and the new one, are produced independently at *random* with the same probability density from the network's environment. Fixing the training set for a moment, the *probability* that the network will make a mistake on the new input defines the generalization error $\varepsilon(D_m)$. Its *average*, ε, over many realizations of the training set, as a function of the number of examples gives the so-called *learning curve*. This will be the main quantity of interest in the following.

Clearly, ε also depends on the specific algorithm that was used during the training. Thus, the calculation of ε requires knowledge of the network weights generated by the learning process. In general, these weights will be complicated functions of the examples, and an explicit form will not be available in most cases.

The methods of statistical mechanics provide an approach to this problem, which often enables an *exact* calculation of learning curves in the limit of a very large network, i.e., for $N \to \infty$. It may seem surprising that a problem will simplify when the number of its parameters is increased. However, this phenomenon is well known for physical systems like gases or liquids which consist of a huge number of molecules. Clearly, there is no chance of esti-

mating the complete *microscopic* state of the system, which is described by the rapidly fluctuating positions and velocities of all particles. On the other hand, the description of the *macroscopic* state of a gas requires only a few parameters, like density, temperature, and pressure. Such quantities can be calculated by suitably *averaging* over a whole ensemble of microscopic states that are compatible with macroscopic constraints.

Applying similar ideas to neural network learning, the problems that arise from specifying the details of a concrete learning algorithm can be avoided. In the statistical mechanics approach, one studies the ensemble of *all* networks that implement the same set of input/output examples to a given accuracy. In this way the typical generalization behavior of a neural network (in contrast to the worst or optimal behavior) can be described.

The Perceptron

In this section I will explain this approach for one of the simplest types of networks, the *single-layer perceptron* (see PERCEPTRONS, ADALINES, AND BACKPROPAGATION). A study of this network is not of purely academic interest, because the single-layer architecture is a substructure of multilayer networks, and many of the steps in the subsequent calculations also appear in the analysis of more complex networks. Furthermore, by replacing the input vector $\mathbf{x}$ with a suitable vector of nonlinear features, the perceptron (equipped with a specific learning algorithm) becomes a *support vector machine*, an extremely powerful learning device introduced by V. Vapnik and his collaborators (see SUPPORT VECTOR MACHINES).

The adjustable parameters of the perceptron are the N weights $\mathbf{w} = (w(1), \ldots, w(N))$. The output is a weighted sum

$$\sigma = F_{\mathbf{w}}(\mathbf{x}) = \text{sign}\left(\sum_{i=1}^{N} w(i)x(i)\right) = \text{sign}(\mathbf{w} \cdot \mathbf{x}) \quad (1)$$

of the input values. Since the length of $\mathbf{w}$ can be normalized without changing the performance, we choose $\|\mathbf{w}\|^2 = N$.

The input/output relation in Equation 1 has a simple geometric interpretation. Consider the *hyperplane* $\mathbf{w} \cdot \mathbf{x} = 0$ in the N-dimensional space of inputs. All inputs that are on the same side as $\mathbf{w}$ are mapped onto $+1$, those on the other side onto -1. Perceptrons realize *linearly separable* classification problems. In the following, we assume that the classification labels σ_k are generated by some other perceptron with weights $\mathbf{w}_t$, the "teacher" perceptron. (A simple case of a student/teacher mismatch is discussed later.)

The geometric picture immediately gives us an expression for the generalization error. A misclassification of a new input $\mathbf{x}$ by a "student" perceptron $\mathbf{w}_s$ occurs only if $\mathbf{x}$ is between the separating planes defined by $\mathbf{w}_s$ and $\mathbf{w}_t$. If the inputs are drawn randomly from a spherical distribution, the generalization error is proportional to the angle between $\mathbf{w}_s$ and $\mathbf{w}_t$. We obtain

$$\varepsilon(D_m) = \frac{1}{\pi} \arccos (R) \qquad (2)$$

where the "overlap" $R \doteq N^{-1}\mathbf{w}_s \cdot \mathbf{w}_t$ measures the similarity between student and teacher.

Following the pioneering work of Elizabeth Gardner (1988), we assume that $\mathbf{w}_s$ was chosen *at random* with equal probability from all student perceptrons that are consistent with the training set, thereby avoiding the introduction of a concrete learning algorithm. In computational learning theory, the space of consistent vectors has been termed the *version space*. The corresponding probability density is $p(\mathbf{w}_s|D_m) = 1/V(D_m)$ if $\mathbf{w}_s$ is *in* the version space, and $p(\mathbf{w}_s|D_m) = 0$ if it is outside. $V(D_m)$ is the volume of the version space given by

$$V(D_m) = \int d\mathbf{w} \prod_{k=1}^{m} \Theta(\sigma_k \mathbf{w} \cdot \mathbf{x}_k) \qquad (3)$$

Here, the Heaviside step function $\Theta(x)$ equals 1 if x is positive and 0 otherwise. Thus, only coupling vectors for which the outputs σ_k are correct, i.e., $\sigma_k \mathbf{w}_s \cdot \mathbf{x}_k > 0$, contribute.

$V(D_m)$ is related to *Shannon's entropy* $\mathscr{S}$ of the distribution $p(\mathbf{w}|D_m)$ by $\mathscr{S} = -\int d\mathbf{w}\, p(\mathbf{w}|D_m) \ln p(\mathbf{w}|D_m) = \ln V(D_m)$. Similarly, in statistical mechanics the entropy measures the logarithm of the volume of microscopic states that are compatible with given values of macroscopic constraints, such as the total energy of a system. In fact, the constraint of perfect learning of all examples is equivalent to the condition of a minimal "training energy." The learning of an increasing number of examples reduces the set of consistent vectors $\mathbf{w}_s$ and leads to a decrease of the entropy $\mathscr{S}$, i.e., of our uncertainty about the unknown teacher $\mathbf{w}_t$. As we will see, by calculating the entropy one will get the generalization error ε for free.

Entropy and Replica Method

Although $V(D_m)$ fluctuates with the random training set, for large N, the quantity $N^{-1}\mathscr{S}$ will be, with high probability, close to its *average* value $\mathscr{S}_{av}$. This results from the fact that the entropy is roughly additive in the degrees of freedom (which would be exactly true if the components of the weight vector $\mathbf{w}$ were statistically independent). Hence, the fluctuations of $N^{-1}\mathscr{S}$ will be averaged out by the many additive random contributions. A similar argument applies to $R = N^{-1}\mathbf{w}_s \cdot \mathbf{w}_t$.

The calculation of $\mathscr{S}_{av}$ requires another tool of statistical physics, the *replica method*. It is based on the identity

$$\mathscr{S}_{av} = \langle\langle \ln V(D_m) \rangle\rangle = \lim_{n \to 0} n^{-1}(\langle\langle V^n(D_m) \rangle\rangle - 1) \qquad (4)$$

The brackets denote the average over the examples. Often, the average of $V^n(D_m)$, which is the volume of the version space of n perceptrons (replicas) $\mathbf{w}_a$, $a = 1, \ldots, n$, being trained on the same examples, can be calculated for *integers* n. At the end, an analytical continuation to real n is necessary. The calculation of the high-dimensional integral over weight vectors is enabled by two ideas: Since the labels are produced by the teacher perceptron $\mathbf{w}_t$, and the input distribution is *spherical*, the integrand will depend *only* on the angles between the vectors $\mathbf{w}_a$, $a = 1, \ldots, n$, and $\mathbf{w}_t$, i.e., on the overlaps

$$q_{ab} = N^{-1}\mathbf{w}_a \cdot \mathbf{w}_b, a < b$$
$$R_a = N^{-1}\mathbf{w}_a \cdot \mathbf{w}_t \qquad (5)$$

The result can be written in the form

$$\langle\langle V^n(D_m) \rangle\rangle = \int \prod_a dR_a \prod_{a<b} dq_{ab} \exp[N\mathscr{G}(n, \{q_{ab}, R_a\})] \qquad (6)$$

The explicit form of $\mathscr{G}$ has been given in Györgyi and Tishby (1990); see also Engel and Van den Broeck (2001).

The limit $N \to \infty$ (to get a nontrivial result, the number of examples is scaled like $m = \alpha N$, with α fixed) provides a second simplification: The integrals in Equation 6 are dominated by values $R_a(n)$ and $q_{ab}(n)$, for which the exponent $\mathscr{G}(n, \{q_{ab}, R_a\})$ is maximal. Other values have an (in N) exponentially smaller weight. The continuation of these most probable values to noninteger $n \simeq 0$ is by far nontrivial: The symmetry of $\mathscr{G}(n, \{q_{ba}, R_a\})$ under permutation of indices a, b, suggests the *replica symmetric* ansatz $q_{ab}(n) = q(n)$ and $R_a(n) = R(n)$, which is correct for the present perceptron problem. A more complicated scheme called *replica symmetry breaking* (Mézard, Parisi, and Virasoro, 1987) for continuing the matrices q_{ab} to noninteger dimensions can be necessary if the version space of the learning problem is, for example, disconnected or not convex (Monasson and Zecchina, 1995).

Within replica symmetry, the analytic continuation $R = R(n = 0)$ coincides with the average teacher-student overlap needed for the generalization error (Equation 2), and $q = q(n = 0)$ gives the average overlap between two random student vectors in the version space. The resulting learning curve ε as a function of the relative number of examples α is shown as the solid line in Figure 1. For a small size of the training set ($\alpha \to 0$), q and R are close to zero and $\varepsilon \approx 1/2$, which is not better than random guessing. To ensure good generalization, m, the size of the training set must significantly exceed N, the number of couplings. Finally, when the ratio $\alpha = m/N$ grows large, q and R approach 1, and the error decreases slowly to 0 as $\varepsilon \approx 0.62\alpha^{-1}$.

The shrinking of the space of network couplings resembles a similar result obtained for the learning in attractor neural networks,

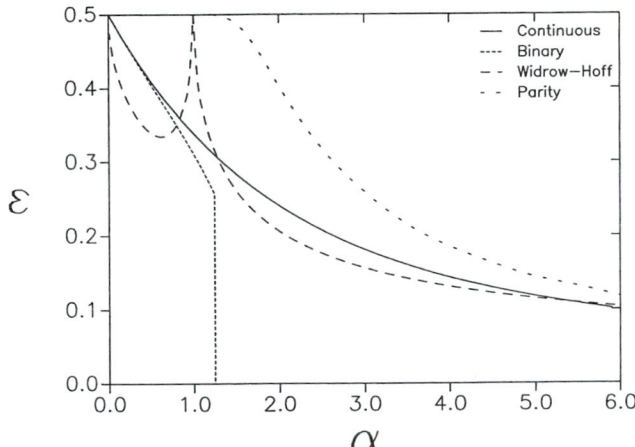

Figure 1. Generalization errors ε for a typical continuous (solid curve) and a typical binary perceptron (dotted curve) as a function of the relative size $\alpha = m/N$ of the training set. For $\alpha = 1.24$, the generalization error drops discontinuously to zero. The dashed curve refers to the linear network formulated in Equation 9. For $\alpha \approx 1$, the mismatch between the nonlinear teacher and the linear student becomes apparent: although all examples are perfectly learned, generalization becomes impossible ($\varepsilon \approx 1/2$). This overfitting phenomenon diappears for $\alpha > 1$, when the algorithm learns with training errors. The curve with small dashes shows the learning curve for a parity tree machine with two hidden units. Nontrivial generalization ($\varepsilon < 1/2$) is impossible for $\alpha < 1.2337$.

as presented in STATISTICAL MECHANICS OF GENERALIZATION (q.v.). For the latter case, however, the output bits of the corresponding perceptron are completely random (given by the random patterns to be stored), instead of being defined by a teacher network. As the number of patterns grows, the volume of couplings decreases to zero already at a non-zero critical capacity $\alpha = 2$.

So far we have discussed the *typical* generalization ability of a perceptron learning a linear separable rule. Is it possible to generalize faster, by using more sophisticated learning strategies? The answer is, not much, if we are restricted to random training examples. Studies of the asymptotics for optimal Bayes classifiers (Opper and Haussler, 1995) yield a generic α^{-1} decay for broad classes of learning models. For linear separable rules and spherical input distribution, the optimal decay is $\varepsilon \simeq 0.44 \, \alpha^{-1}$, only slightly better than the typical error (Watkin, Rau, and Biehl, 1993; Opper and Kinzel, 1995).

The situation changes if the learner is free to ask the teacher questions (Watkin et al., 1993), because she can choose highly informative inputs. Then the decrease in the generalization error ε can be exponentially fast in α.

The approach of statistical mechanics is able to provide information about generalization abilities even in situations where, at present, no efficient learning algorithms are known. Assume, for example, that the perceptron weights are constrained to binary values $w(j) \varepsilon \{+1, -1\}$. This may give a crude model for the effects of a finite weight precision in digital network implementations. For this binary perceptron, perfect learning is equivalent to a hard combinatorial optimization problem, which in the worst case is believed to require a learning time that grows exponentially with N. Using the replica method, the dotted learning curve in Figure 1 is obtained. For sufficiently small α, the discreteness of the version space has only minor effects. However, since there is a minimal volume of the version space when only one coupling vector is left, the generalization error ε drops to zero at a finite value $\alpha_c = 1.24$. Remarkably, this transition is discontinuous. This means that for α slightly below α_c, the few coupling vectors $\mathbf{w}$ that are consistent with all examples typically differ in a finite fraction of bits from the teacher (and from each other).

Phase Transitions and Symmetry Breaking

In statistical mechanics, the overlaps q and R are examples of *order parameters*, which measure the degree of ordering of a system toward an external influence. In our case, the labels, which are provided by the teacher, make the typical student vector more and more aligned with the teacher. This is reflected by the increase in q and R from the minimal values 0 (when there are no examples) to their maximal values 1, when student and teacher align perfectly.

In statistical physics, a variety of systems show *phase transitions*, i.e., ordering sets in *spontaneously* when a control parameter exceeds a critical value. Surprisingly, such phase transitions can also be observed for *multilayer networks*. I will illustrate such a behavior for a simple toy multilayer network with a drastically simplified architecture, the *parity tree*. Here, the set of N input nodes is equally divided into K nonoverlapping groups, each of which is connected to one of K hidden units by N/K adjustable weights, as in a perceptron. The output node computes the parity of the hidden outputs; i.e., a -1 output results from an odd number of negative hidden units and a $+1$ output results from an even number. For $K = 2$, we obtain the learning curve (Hansel, Mato, and Meunier, 1992) with the small dashes shown in Figure 1. Below $\alpha = 1.2337$, the network perfectly memorizes the training examples without being able to generalize at all ($\varepsilon = 1/2$). Above this critical value, generalization sets in, and the generalization error decays smoothly. For $K > 2$, the transition is discontinuous (Engel and Van den Broeck, 2001).

This and similar phase transitions are related to *spontaneous symmetry breaking*. Although a statistical ensemble is invariant under a symmetry transformation, the typical, macroscopically observed state of the system may not show this symmetry. For the parity machine, the symmetry transformation is the inversion of the signs of the couplings corresponding to a pair of different hidden units. For example, for $K = 2$, a network with couplings all equal to, say, $+1$ implements exactly the same classification task as a network with all couplings equal to -1. For small α, the typical student networks trained by a "$+1$" teacher will reflect this $\pm$ symmetry. Their coupling vectors consist of an equal fraction of positive and negative weights without any preference for the teacher (or the reversed teacher), and generalization is impossible. If α exceeds the critical value, the symmetry is broken, and we have *two* possible types of typical students, one with a majority of positive couplings, the other one with a majority of negative couplings. Both types of typical students now display some similarity with the teacher or its negative image, and generalization sets in. A related type of *retarded generalization* can be found in models of *unsupervised learning*, where the learner has to infer an unknown symmetry axis of a high-dimensional probability distribution (Engel and Van den Broeck, 2001). When the number of data is less than a critical value, the estimated direction of the axis will typically be orthogonal to the true one.

Phase transitions for multilayer networks with fully connected architectures are related to the breaking of the permutation symmetry between hidden units (Schwarze and Hertz, 1993; Engel and Van den Broeck, 2001). They can already be observed for *on-line learning* algorithms. Since the change in weights depends on the most recently presented example only, and since each example is seen only once, a detailed study of the dynamics of learning is possible (see STATISTICAL MECHANICS OF ON-LINE LEARNING AND GENERALIZATION).

Algorithms and Overfitting

The statistical mechanics approach can also be applied to the performance of concrete algorithms, if the algorithm minimizes a *training energy*, such as the quadratic deviation

$$E(\mathbf{w}_s | \sigma^m, \mathbf{x}^m) = \sum_{k=1}^{m} (\sigma_k - F_{\mathbf{w}_s}(\mathbf{x}_k))^2 \qquad (7)$$

between the network's and the teacher's outputs (see PERCEPTRONS, ADALINES, AND BACKPROPAGATION).

The ensemble of students is now defined by all vectors $\mathbf{w}_s$ that achieve a certain accuracy in learning, i.e., that have a fixed training energy. We may as well fix the *average* energy, allowing for small fluctuations. Such fluctuations also occur for physical systems in thermal equilibrium, which can exchange energy with their environment. The *Gibbs distribution*

$$p(\mathbf{w}_s | D_m) \propto e^{-\beta E(\mathbf{w}_s | D_m)} \qquad (8)$$

provides the proper probability density for such a case, where the parameter β has to be adjusted such that the average energy achieves the desired value. In physics, $T = 1/\beta$ plays the role of the temperature. For the relation of this concept to the stochastic dynamics of networks, see STATISTICAL MECHANICS OF GENERALIZATION.

For $\beta = \infty$, the distribution p is concentrated at the vector $\mathbf{w}_s$, for which E is minimal, corresponding to a learning algorithm that achieves the total minimum of the training energy. An application to the generalization performance of *support vector machines* can be found in Dietrich, Opper, and Sompolinsky (1999).

Let me briefly illustrate the results of this method for a single-layer perceptron where, during the training phase, the student is replaced by a simple *linear* function

$$F_{\mathbf{w}_s}(\mathbf{x}) = \mathbf{w}_s \cdot \mathbf{x} \qquad (9)$$

in Equation 7. For a teacher of the same linear type, the classification rule is learned completely with $m = N$ examples. A different behavior occurs if the teacher is the *nonlinear* rule (Equation 1), and, for generalization, the student's output is also given by Equation 1. Although all examples are still perfectly learned up to $\alpha = m/N = 1$, the generalization error increases to the random guessing value $\varepsilon = 1/2$ (Figure 1, dashed line), a phenomenon termed *overfitting*.

If $m > N$, the minimal training error E is *greater than zero*. Nevertheless, ε decreases again and approaches 0 asymptotically for $\alpha \to \infty$. This shows that one can achieve good generalization with algorithms that allow for learning errors.

The introduction of a temperature is not merely a formal trick. Stochastic learning with a non-zero temperature may be useful to escape from local minima of the training energy, enabling a better learning of the training set. Surprisingly, it can lead to *better generalization abilities* if the classification rule is not completely learnable by the net. In the simplest case, that happens when the rule contains a degree of noise (Györgyi and Tishby, 1990; Opper and Kinzel, 1995; see also SIMULATED ANNEALING AND BOLTZMANN MACHINES).

The replica method enables us to study the properties of networks at their minimal training energy. However, a real learning algorithm may not reach such a state when local minima are present.

Discussion

The statistical mechanics approach to learning and generalization allows us to understand the typical generalization behavior of large neural networks. Its major tool, the replica method, has been illustrated in this article for simple neural networks like the perceptron. Even for simple models, interesting and unexpected phenomena, such as discontinuous and retarded generalization, can be observed.

The statistical mechanics approach allows us to perform controlled analytical experiments on very large networks. In contrast to real experiments, which will produce an enormous amount of microscopic data that must be evaluated, this analytical method provides us with a small set of order parameters that are directly interpretable in terms of the network's macroscopic performance. Concentrating on typical behavior, the statistical mechanics analysis can complement other theoretical approaches to generalization, such as the worst case PAC bounds (see Engel and Van den Broeck, 2001; Urbanczik, 1996; see also LEARNING AND GENERALIZATION: THEORETICAL BOUNDS).

Presently, the approach is being applied to both novel learning concepts in neural computing, such as support vector machines,

and to a variety of other problems in information science, such as error-correcting codes and hard combinatorial optimization problems (see, e.g., Nishimori, 2001). Siginificant progress has also been made in understanding the *dynamical* properties of concrete algorithms (see Heimel and Coolen, 2001, and STATISTICAL MECHANICS OF ON-LINE LEARNING AND GENERALIZATION).

New and challenging applications are also found in other fields where learning and adaptation in large populations of entities play a role. These fields include ecological systems and economical markets.

Road Map: Learning in Artificial Networks
Background: Perceptrons, Adalines, and Backpropagation
Related Reading: Learning and Statistical Inference; Statistical Mechanics of Neural Networks; Statistical Mechanics of On-Line Learning and Generalization

References

Dietrich, R., Opper, M., and Sompolinsky, H., 1999, Statistical mechanics of support vector networks, *Phys. Rev. Lett.*, 82:2975.
Engel, A., and Van den Broeck, C., 2001, *Statistical Mechanics of Learning*, Cambridge, Engl.: Cambridge University Press. ◆
Gardner, E., 1988, The space of interactions in neural network models, *J. Phys. A. Math. Gen.*, 21:257–270.
Györgyi, G., and Tishby, N., 1990, Statistical theory of learning a rule, in *Neural Networks and Spin Glasses* (W. K. Theumann and R. Koeberle, Eds.), Singapore: World Scientific, pp. 3–36.
Hansel, D., Mato, G., and Meunier, C., 1992, Memorization without generalization in a multilayered neural network, *Europhys. Lett.*, 20:471–476.
Heimel, J. A. F., and Coolen, A. C. C., 2001, Supervised learning with restricted training sets: A generating functional analysis, *J. Phys. A*, 34:9009–9026.
Mézard, M., Parisi, G., and Virasoro, M. A., 1987, *Spin Glass Theory and Beyond*, Singapore: World Scientific.
Monasson, R., and Zecchina, R., 1995, Weight space structure and internal representations: A direct approach to learning and generalization in multilayer neural networks, *Phys. Rev. Lett.*, 75:2432.
Nishimori, H., 2001, *Statistical Physics of Spin Glasses and Information Processing*, New York: Oxford University Press. ◆
Opper, M., and Haussler, D., 1995, Bounds for predictive errors in the statistical mechanics of supervised learning, *Phys. Rev. Lett.*, 75:3772.
Opper, M., and Kinzel, W., 1995, Statistical mechanics of generalization, in *Physics of Neural Networks III* (J. L. van Hemmen, E. Domany, and K. Schulten, Eds.), New York: Springer-Verlag.
Schwarze, H., and Hertz, J., 1993, Generalization in fully connected committee machines, *Europhys. Lett.*, 21:785.
Seung, H. S., Sompolinsky, H., and Tishby, N., 1992, Statistical mechanics of learning from examples, *Phys. Rev. A*, 45:6056–6091.
Watkin, T. L. H., Rau, A., and Biehl, M., 1993, The statistical mechanics of learning a rule, *Rev. Mod. Physics*, 65:499–556.
Urbanczik, R., 1996, Learning in a large Committee Machine: Worst case and average case, *Europhys. Lett.*, 35:553.

Statistical Mechanics of Neural Networks

Annette Zippelius and Andreas Engel

Introduction

Statistical mechanics describes the collective properties of systems composed of many interacting elements on the basis of the individual behavior and mutual interaction of these elements. The term "collective" refers here to properties that result substantially from

the interaction of the constituents and which show up only if the whole system contains a sufficient number of elements. In physics, statistical mechanics bridges the gap between microscopic structure and macroscopic properties of matter. A basic example is the calculation of the equation of state for a gas—i.e., the law according to which pressure changes with temperature—from the equation of motion governing the dynamics of the molecules. Numerous detailed investigations of physical systems have revealed two remarkable features of this approach:

1. The collective properties of a system can be more complex than the simplicity of its constituents seems to allow. This feature is a consequence of the phenomenon of spontaneous *symmetry breaking*, which means that a macroscopic system can be in a state of lesser symmetry (i.e., higher complexity) than the underlying microscopic dynamics. For example, the statistical distribution of atomic *spins* in an unmagnetized bar of iron is symmetrical, but once the iron is magnetized the mean direction of the spins is constrained to lie in a specific direction—the symmetry has been broken. Such symmetry breaking is often the sign of a *phase transition* during which matter changes from one state of organization to another.

2. Very few of the details characterizing the elements of a macroscopic system are essential for the qualitative collective properties. In the example of the gas, an attractive interaction between the molecules results in a condensation point, such that for temperatures below this point there is a phase transition from gas to liquid. Practically any law of mutual attraction would give qualitatively the same transition, just changing the specific value for the transition temperature. The same is true for the characterization of spins in models of magnetization. Consequently, extremely simplified models for the microscopic elements can be used. To find out which microscopic properties are *relevant* is, of course, the first step of the program, usually a nontrivial and decisive one.

Biological as well as technical neural networks are, in many, but not all, cases, made up of a large number of elements (neurons or electronic circuits) strongly interacting through connections (synapses or wires). They can perform information processing of amazing complexity. Although the elements are themselves already rather complicated systems which, at least in the case of biological neurons, are still far from being completely understood, it is generally believed that these abilities for information processing are far beyond the possibilities of a single or a few units and are therefore in some sense collective properties. It is then tempting to assume that, as in complex physical systems, these collective properties are again fairly independent of many of the microscopic details. The aim of a statistical mechanics of neural network models is hence to investigate to what extent the models of physics can be applied to show how, in a large system of simple interacting units reminiscent of biological neurons, there can emerge collective properties for complex information processing comparable to those found in real neural networks.

Within the approach of statistical mechanics, we define a neural network as an ensemble of N neurons of activity S_i, $i = 1, \ldots, N$, which interact via synaptic couplings J_{ij}, $i, j = 1, \ldots, N$. Both the activity and the couplings can be real valued or restricted to a discrete set, and in general evolve dynamically. However, most studies assume a separation of time scales, such that either

- the neurons evolve dynamically, $S_i = S_i(t)$, for a fixed set of couplings J_{ij}, or
- the couplings evolve dynamically, $J_{ij} = J_{ij}(t)$, for a given activity state $\{S_i\}$ or a set of p such states $\{\xi_i^\nu\}$, numbered by $\nu = 1, \ldots, p$.

In the first case the focus is on processing of information. Problems of this kind will be discussed in this article. In the second case the important question is how to adapt the couplings to a particular processing task. Questions concerning this type of learning dynam-

ics are dealt with in other articles in this book (see STATISTICAL MECHANICS OF ON-LINE LEARNING AND GENERALIZATION).

Statistical mechanics provides a quantitative analysis of the properties of a very large network (mathematically in the limit $N \to \infty$). A large class of models can be solved exactly. Examples such as the Hopfield model and strongly diluted networks are discussed below.

Many of the information processing tasks that a neural network can perform involve a set of special configurations $\{\xi_i^\nu\}$ of neuron activity, called *patterns*. Generally, the performance depends on the detailed realization of this pattern set. The focus of statistical mechanics is then on the *typical* behavior of the network, i.e., one wants to know how it performs typically for a given problem rather than to pinpoint the properties specific to one particular pattern set $\{\xi_i^\nu\}$. An effective way to mathematically describe such a typical performance is to generate the pattern set at random according to a given probability distribution (e.g., $\xi_i^\mu = \pm 1$ with equal probability) and to determine averages of the quantities of interest. As it turns out, many interesting quantities are self-averaging, which means that for $N \to \infty$ the performance on a special random pattern set is identical to the average performance. Calculating the average of the relevant quantities, one can hence make reliable predictions for the results of a real or numerical experiment involving just one realization of the pattern set. This approach has been very successful in the theory of disordered physical systems as noncrystalline solids or random magnets, and many of the mathematical techniques developed there have been proven to be adequate for the statistical mechanics of neural networks.

Neuron Dynamics

An extremely simplified model of the individual neurons suitable for a statistical mechanics analysis was introduced in 1943 by Warren McCulloch and Walter Pitts. They devised a neuron as a bistable threshold unit, which is either active (firing) or passive (quiescent). The state of neuron i can therefore be described by a binary variable $S_i = 0, 1$ or equivalently, $S_i = \pm 1$. The former choice was used by McCulloch and Pitts, whereas the latter became standard in statistical mechanics due to its formal similarity with magnetic ("spin") systems, many of which have been studied by physicists under the general heading of *spin glasses*. The interaction between N such neurons takes place via real-valued couplings J_{ij}. More precisely, a neuron S_j contributes to the (postsynaptic) potential of neuron S_i with the value $J_{ij}S_j$ depending on its own activity state. Neuron S_i in turn sums up all these contributions and compares the sum with a neuron-specific threshold θ_i. If the accumulated potential $\sum_j J_{ij}S_j$ exceeds this threshold, neuron S_i becomes (or remains) active, otherwise it remains (or becomes) passive. The discrete-time dynamics of the whole network is therefore given by

$$S_i(t + 1) = \text{sign}(h_i(t)) = \text{sign}\left(\sum_j J_{ij}S_j(t) - \theta_i\right) \quad (1)$$

where $\text{sign}(x) = +1$ for $x > 0$ and $\text{sign}(x) = -1$ otherwise, and where $t = 0, 1, 2, 3, \ldots$ denotes the discrete-time steps.

The collective behavior of an ensemble of such neurons is often understood in the context of associative memory, i.e., the recall of information on the basis of partial knowledge of its content. The use of neural networks as associative memories is built on three main principles (see COMPUTING WITH ATTRACTORS):

- The information, which is to be stored and retrieved in the system, is represented as one or many configurations of neuronal activity, called patterns $\{\xi_i^\nu\}$ ($i = 1, \ldots, N; \nu = 1, \ldots, p$).

- The couplings are designed to make the patterns attractors of the neuron dynamics.
- Association is the dynamic evolution of an arbitrary initial state into one of these attractors.

In this section we discuss the performance of the network for a given set of couplings that we assume to be adapted to a set of patterns $\{\xi_i^\nu\}$. Some of the relevant questions are:

- What are the attractors of the neuron dynamics and how well are they correlated with the patterns?
- What is the capacity, i.e., what is the maximal number of patterns that can be stored and retrieved?
- What are the basins of attraction, i.e., what is the maximal amount of noise permissible in the initial stimulus?
- How long does it take the network to reach an attractor?

Of particular interest are the stationary states of the dynamics, for which $S_i h_i > 0$ for all $i = 1, \ldots, N$ (see Equation 1). If the coupling constants are symmetric, i.e., $J_{ij} = J_{ji}$, and if there are no self-interactions, i.e., $J_{ii} = 0$, then an *energy function*

$$E(\{S_i\}) = -\frac{1}{2} \sum_{i \neq j} J_{ij} S_i S_j + \sum_i \theta_i S_i \qquad (2)$$

exists and is monotonically decreasing for the *asynchronous* dynamics of Equation 1. The stationary states of the dynamics must then coincide with the minima of this energy, which in turn can be analyzed with the methods of equilibrium statistical mechanics.

Before embarking on that analysis, however, it is useful to slightly generalize this approach. By describing the neurons in terms of binary activity variables, we ignored almost all microscopic details of the network. The influence of the neglected microscopic degrees of freedom on the dynamics of the activity states can be modeled by a random noise term changing the deterministic updating process (Equation 1) into a probabilistic one:

$$S_i(t + 1) = \text{sign}(h_i(t) + \varphi_i(t)) \qquad (3)$$

The probability distribution $P(\varphi)$ of the noise is not very critical. A simple choice would be a Gaussian $P(\varphi) = 1/\sqrt{\pi T}$ $\exp(-\varphi^2/T)$, which would imply that neuron i will be firing (quiescent) at time $(t + 1)$ with probability

$$p_\pm = \frac{1}{2}\left(1 \pm \frac{2}{\sqrt{\pi}} \int_0^{h_i(t)/T} dx\, e^{-x^2}\right) \qquad (4)$$

The strength of the noise is denoted by T, such that for $T = 0$ we recover the deterministic dynamics of Equation 1. By analogy with physical systems we will often refer to the noise strength T as the temperature, keeping in mind, however, that it is usually different from the (thermodynamic) temperature of the neural network under consideration. The stochastic process (Equation 3) is also the basic dynamics of Monte Carlo Simulations, which can be used efficiently to *simulate* the dynamics of artificial neural nets. In that context a different choice,

$$P(\varphi) = \frac{1}{2T}\left[\cosh\left(\frac{\varphi}{T}\right)\right]^{-2} \qquad (5)$$

is quite common. It gives rise to a firing probability $p_\pm = (1/2)(1 \pm \tanh(h_i(t)/T)$, which differs only slightly (at most 1%) from Equation 4. Both firing probabilities are such that the system will ultimately converge to a steady-state probability distribution. The macroscopic properties of the system are then given as averages with this distribution. (see Reif, 1982, for a textbook account of relevant results from "ordinary" statistical mechanics).

In deterministic neural networks (see COMPUTING WITH ATTRACTORS), the state of the neural networks will tend toward a single attractor. Once noise is included, no such determinism is possible. Instead, statistical mechanics provides tools to find an *equilibrium distribution* in which each state has a probability of occurrence for which the probability of leaving a state is exactly balanced by the probability of entering it. If we choose the noise statistics of Equation 5, we end up in the equilibrium distribution in which states are distributed according to the Boltzmann distribution in which the probability of a state is given by

$$P(\{S_i\}) = \exp(-\beta E(\{S_i\}))/Z \qquad (6)$$

where $\beta = 1/T$ and Z is a normalization factor, $Z = \Sigma_{\{S_i\}}$ $\exp(-\beta E(\{S_i\}))$. All equilibrium expectation values can then be calculated by summing over all configurations, weighted with their Boltzmann factor. For example, the mean activity of neuron k is given by

$$\langle S_k \rangle_{th} = \frac{\sum_{\{S_i\}} S_k \exp(-\beta E(\{S_i\}))}{\sum_{\{S_i\}} \exp(-\beta E(\{S_i\}))} \qquad (7)$$

where the notation $\langle \cdot \rangle_{th}$ means "average over all states at thermal equilibrium." Note that equivalently we could write

$$\langle S_k \rangle_{th} = \frac{1}{\beta}\frac{\partial F}{\partial \theta_k} \qquad (8)$$

with the free energy $F(\beta, \theta_i)$ defined by

$$F(\beta, \theta_i) = -\frac{1}{\beta} \log \sum_{\{S_i\}} \exp(-\beta E(\{S_i\})) \qquad (9)$$

It is a standard result of statistical mechanics that all averages with the Boltzmann distribution, i.e., all macroscopic quantities, can be calculated similarly by appropriate derivatives of the free energy. The main task within a statistical mechanics analysis is hence the calculation of the free energy.

The inclusion of noise has the effect that many configurations—and not just the minima of E—contribute to the expectation values. In other words, a much larger part of configuration space can be explored. A similar approach has been put forward in optimization theory to include nearly optimal solutions (see SIMULATED ANNEALING AND BOLTZMANN MACHINES and OPTIMIZATION, NEURAL).

In statistical mechanics, powerful methods have been developed to calculate the free energy Equation 9. Most of them, however, only apply in the thermodynamic limit $N \to \infty$. In physics we have abundant experimental evidence that this limit exists. Quantities such as the energy (Equation 2) and the free energy (Equation 9) are expected to be *extensive* variables, increasing linearly with N. Hence the corresponding *intensive* quantities, e.g., the free energy per neuron $f = F/N$ have a well-defined limit as $N \to \infty$. Furthermore, fluctuations of extensive quantities are generally negligible in the thermodynamic limit. Typically the variance relative to the mean decreases like $N^{-1/2}$. Therefore the results obtained theoretically employing the limit $N \to \infty$ very accurately describe real systems with finite but large N. This is a characteristic feature of statistical distributions involving very many degrees of freedom. In a typical neural network application the $N \to \infty$ results of statistical mechanics characterize systems with $N = 100 - 1000$ with an accuracy of a few percent.

Statics of the Hopfield Model

The following choice of couplings was used in early studies of ASSOCIATIVE NETWORKS (q.v.) by Hopfield (1982) and extensively thereafter (see Amit, 1989)

$$J_{ij} = \frac{1}{N} \sum_{\nu=1}^{p} \xi_i^\nu \xi_j^\nu \qquad (10)$$

The patterns are random variables and the synaptic couplings of Equation 10 correspond to one realization of the random process. In the simplest case all ξ_i^ν are statistically independent, identically distributed and equally likely to be ± 1. To further simplify the analysis we set $\theta_i = 0$.

There is no limit on the range of interaction for the coupling matrix of Equation 10, instead each neuron interacts with every other neuron. Hence the *local field*, i.e., the "force" exerted on a single neuron by the activity of all other neurons

$$h_i = \sum_{j=1}^{N} J_{ij} S_j = \frac{1}{N} \sum_{j=1}^{N} \sum_{\nu=1}^{p} \xi_i^\nu \xi_j^\nu S_j \qquad (11)$$

is a large sum of many random numbers, which are only weakly correlated. As long as the number p of patterns remains finite as $N \to \infty$ we can neglect these correlations and replace h_i by its thermal average:

$$h_i \cong \sum_{\nu=1}^{p} \xi_i^\nu \frac{1}{N} \sum_{j=1}^{N} \xi_j^\nu \langle S_j \rangle_{th} \qquad (12)$$

The most important characteristic of an associative memory is the overlap

$$m^\nu = \frac{1}{N} \sum_{j=1}^{N} \xi_j^\nu \langle S_j \rangle_{th} \qquad (13)$$

It describes the average alignment of the stationary states with the patterns. The overlap (as well as the free energy) is self-averaging, i.e., its fluctuations from pattern set to pattern set go to zero in the thermodynamic limit. It is hence equal to its average over the pattern statistics with probability 1: $m^\nu = \langle\langle \xi_i^\nu \langle S_j \rangle_{th} \rangle\rangle_\xi$. In terms of the local field h_i (Equation 12) the activity is given by $\langle S_i \rangle_{th} = \tanh(\beta h_i)$ so that the overlap vector $\boldsymbol{m} = (m^1, m^2, \ldots, m^p)$ is the solution of

$$\boldsymbol{m} = \langle\langle \boldsymbol{\xi}^\mu \tanh \beta \boldsymbol{m} \cdot \boldsymbol{\xi}^\mu \rangle\rangle_\xi \qquad (14)$$

In the context of associative memory we are interested in states $\{S_i\}$, which are correlated with one pattern only, i.e., $m^\nu = m\delta_{\nu\nu_0}$. Such states are called *Mattis* or *retrieval states* and are indeed solutions of Equation 14 below a critical noise level $T_c = 1$. These retrieval states are the global minima of E for $T \simeq T_c$ and for $T \to 0$ and presumably for all T in between. The failure of this property for $T > T_c$ is an example of a *phase transition* in neural networks. Equation 14 also has solutions with several non-zero components of $\boldsymbol{m}$. They correspond to network configurations that resemble mixtures of stored patterns. Such states clearly disturb the retrieval process. One of the surprising results of the statistical analysis is the fact that noise actually improves the efficiency of the network as a an associative memory by eliminating these *spurious states* for $T \geq .5$.

It is also possible to store an extensive number of patterns, i.e., $p \to \infty$ with $N \to \infty$ such that $\alpha = p/N$ finite (Amit, Gutfreund, and Sompolinsky, 1987). This approach gives rise to a *static* random contribution z in the local field h:

$$\langle S_i \rangle_{th} = \tanh \beta h(z)$$
$$h(z) = \boldsymbol{m} \cdot \boldsymbol{\xi}^\mu + \sqrt{\alpha r} z \qquad (15)$$

The overlap $\boldsymbol{m}$ and the variance r of the new noise term have to be calculated from the coupled equations

$$m = \int \frac{dz}{\sqrt{2\pi}} e^{-z^2/2} \langle\langle \xi_i \langle S_i \rangle_{th} \rangle\rangle_\xi$$
$$q = \int \frac{dz}{\sqrt{2\pi}} e^{-z^2/2} \langle\langle \langle S_i \rangle_{th}^2 \rangle\rangle_\xi$$
$$r = \frac{1}{1 - \beta(1 - q))^2} \qquad (16)$$

Thermal noise (T) as well as the static noise (cross-talk, z) resulting from many other stored patterns destroy the retrieval states above a critical line in the (T, α) plane. In the absence of thermal noise ($T = 0$), retrieval states can only exist up to $\alpha_c \simeq 0.14$. This result is in very good agreement with extensive computer simulations of the model. The transition is discontinuous with a sudden jump of the overlap from $m(\alpha \to \alpha_c) \simeq .97$ to $m = 0$ for $\alpha > \alpha_c$. Hence when overloading the network the retrieval quality abruptly changes.

For $\alpha < \alpha_c$ retrieval states coexist with so-called spin glass states. In the latter the neurons build up static random configurations almost uncorrelated with the stored patterns. They can be understood as descendents of the mixture states encountered for finite p now mixing very many patterns. The retrieval states are global minima of the energy E for $\alpha \leq .05$ only.

Numerous extensions and generalizations of the Hopfield model have been discussed. They include the following:

- *Robustness.* It has been shown that the Hopfield model is surprisingly robust with respect to various perturbations, such as synaptic noise or synaptic dilution. Even synaptic clipping, i.e., retaining only the sign of J_{ij}, just reduces the capacity from $\alpha_c \sim 0.14$ to $\alpha_c \sim 0.1$.
- *Forgetting and unlearning.* In the Hopfield model, all memories are destroyed completely upon overloading the network. This distruction can be avoided by using special learning rules that weigh patterns differently thereby forgetting older items in favor of newer ones. It has also been suggested that "unlearning," a procedure to weaken bonds in a specific way, can improve the performance of the network (Hopfield, Feinstein, and Palmer, 1983).
- *Other pattern statistics.* The assumption of uncorrelated patterns in the Hopfield model does not apply to many situations of practical interest. An explicit construction of the coupling matrix for patterns with arbitrary correlations is provided by the pseudo-inverse rule. If the patterns are linearly independent, it is given by

$$J_{ij} = \frac{1}{N} \sum_{\nu,\mu}^{p} \xi_i^\nu (C^{-1})_{\nu\mu} \xi_j^\mu \quad \text{with} \quad C_{\nu\mu} = \frac{1}{N} \sum_{i=1}^{N} \xi_i^\nu \xi_i^\mu \qquad (17)$$

This coupling matrix is nothing but a projector $\sum_j J_{ij} \xi_j^\nu = \xi_j^\nu$, which implies that the patterns are stationary states because

$$h_i \xi_i^\nu = \xi_i^\nu \sum_j J_{ij} \xi_j^\nu = 1 \qquad (18)$$

It has been widely used in the context of self-organizing maps (Kohonen, 1984) as well as attractor neural networks. The storage capacity is $\alpha_c = 1$ and a local learning rule was given to construct the couplings in an iterative scheme. Special cases of correlated patterns include hierarchical correlations, which may be important for the organization of human memory, and biased patterns, which have non-zero average mean activity.

Dynamic Properties

Several interesting questions concern the dynamic behavior of neural networks during retrieval, as, for example:

- How long does it take the system to retrieve a pattern?
- Which initial conditions are iterated into a particular attractor?

If the couplings are asymmetric $J_{ij} \neq J_{ji}$, as in the majority of biological systems, then a neural network is only defined as a dynamic process (Equation 1). Such models have in general no energy function, and complex, time-dependent attractors may occur. Even if one is only interested in stationary states or distributions, these can in general only be obtained as the long time limit of the dynamics. Since the methods of nonequilibrium dynamics are much less developed than those of equilibrium statistical mechanics, it is no surprise that genuine dynamic problems, like the basins of attraction, are much less understood than the stationary properties of neural networks. Nevertheless, nontrivial dynamic behavior is of great importance in biological as well as technical neural networks.

One motivation to study cyclic attractors is the abundant appearance of temporal sequences in cognition and of rhythmic motion in motor control tasks. Hopfield suggested a network, which was designed to store and retrieve a sequence $\xi^1, \xi^2, \ldots, \xi^q$, such that the system, if initialized in pattern ξ^1, makes a collective transition to ξ^2, then from ξ^2 to ξ^3 and so on.

The following set of couplings

$$J_{ij} = \frac{1}{N} \sum_{v=1}^{q} \xi_i^v \xi_j^v + \frac{\lambda}{N} \sum_{v=1}^{q-1} \xi_i^{v+1} \xi_j^v, \quad \lambda > 1 \qquad (19)$$

generate such a temporal sequence of states, provided the neurons are updated synchronously and without any noise, either in the dynamics or in the initial state. Noise tolerance or recall of sequences with asynchronous dynamics can be achieved with delayed synapses, which induce transitions only after the system has been stabilized for a time τ in one of the patterns. The synaptic delay does not have to match the period of the sequence exactly. In fact a broad distribution of synaptic delays is well suited for learning of sequences, whose relevant time scale is represented in the spectrum (see SEQUENCE LEARNING). Connections that match the timescale of the sequence approximately will be enforced, a process which can be seen as learning by selection.

Complex dynamical behaviour naturally occurs in asymmetrically *diluted networks*. The assumption of complete connectivity in the Hopfield model is implausible for biological systems and unacceptable for technical implementations. Hence we are led to consider diluted networks, e.g., a diluted Hopfield model

$$J_{ij} = \frac{c_{ij}}{K} \sum_{v=1}^{p} \xi_i^v \xi_j^v \qquad (20)$$

The $c_{ij} \in \{0, 1\}$ are independent random variables and $c_{ij} = 1$ with probability K/N. In the limit of strong dilution $\log K \ll \log N$ the dynamic model defined by Equations 1 and 20 is exactly solvable (Derrida, Gardner, and Zippelius, 1987). Specializing to retrieval states with overlap $m(t)$ with, e.g., pattern ξ^1 one finds for synchronous updating

$$m(t + 1) = f(m(t)) = \int \frac{dy}{\sqrt{2\pi}} e^{-y^2/2} \tanh \beta(m(t) - \sqrt{\alpha}\, y) \qquad (21)$$

Here we have taken the limit $K \to \infty$ (after $N \to \infty$) and anticipated a finite capacity $\alpha = P/K$ per synapse. Retrieval states correspond to stable fixed points $m_s^* = f(m_s^*) \neq 0$. They exist up to $\alpha \leq \alpha_c = 2/\pi$. As $\alpha \to \alpha_c$, m_s^* decreases continuously to zero, in marked contrast to the discontinuous behavior of m at α_c found in the last

section for the fully connected Hopfield model. Note also that the retrieval states $m_s^* \neq 0$ do not correspond to fixed points in phase space. Although the overlap m is constant in time, there is substantial dynamic activity on the microscopic level. This can be seen from the fact that two states with the same overlap have in general a Hamming distance different from zero and the time delayed autocorrelation function exhibits dynamic noise even at zero temperature.

The size of the basins of attraction is determined by an *unstable* fixed point m_u^* of Equation 21 with $0 \leq m_u^* < m_s^*$. If the system is started in a configuration with initial overlap $m(t = 0)$ larger than m_u^* it will be iterated into m_s^*. If $m(t = 0) < m_u^*$ the dynamics will evolve the state toward $m^* = 0$. The basins of attraction have been calculated in this way for a variety of learning rules in the limit of strong dilution.

Discussion

This article attempts to elucidate how the concepts and methods of statistical mechanics can be successfully applied to understand certain aspects of large neural networks. It has emphasized the goals of statistical mechanics more than the abundance of results. A specific example, namely the Hopfield model for associative memory, has been discussed in detail to show what kind of quantitative result can be expected from a statistical mechanical analysis. To put this model in a more general context, this article has indicated how it can be extended to more complex tasks, and has focused on the dynamics of neurons in the presence of fixed synaptic couplings. The inverse problem—the adaptation of the couplings to given neuronal activity states—has also been analyzed very sucessfully with the methods of statistical mechanics (see STATISTICAL MECHANICS OF ON-LINE LEARNING AND GENERALIZATION). Statistical mechanics of neural networks is a rapidly developing field with widespread research activity. For more information the interested reader is referred to textbooks (Amit, 1989; Domany, van Hemmen, and Schulten, 1991; Hertz, Krogh, and Palmer, 1991; Engel and Van den Broeck, 2001) and the contributions in this *Handbook*.

Road Map: Dynamic Systems
Related Reading: Bayesian Methods and Neural Networks; Dynamics of Association and Recall; Statistical Mechanics of Generalization; Statistical Mechanics of On-Line Learning and Generalization

References

Amit, D. J., 1989, *Modeling Brain Function: The World of Attractor Neural Networks*, Cambrigde: Cambrigde University Press
Amit, D. J., Gutfreund, H., and Sompolinsky, H., 1987, Statistical mechanics of neural networks near saturation, *Ann. Phys.*, 173:30–67.
Derrida, B., Gardner, E., and Zippelius, A., 1987, An exactly solvable asymmetric neural network model, *Europhys. Lett.*, 4:167–173.
Domany, E., van Hemmen, J. L., and Schulten, K. (Eds.), 1991, *Physics of Neural Networks*, Berlin: Springer-Verlag.
Engel, A., and Van den Broeck, C., 2001, *Statistical Mechanics of Learning*, Cambridge: Cambridge University Press ◆
Hertz, J. A., Krogh, A., and Palmer, R. G., 1991, *Introduction to the theory of Neural Computation*, Redwood City, CA: Addison-Wesley. ◆
Hopfield, J. J., 1982, Neural networks and physical systems with emergent collective computational abilities, *Proc. Natl. Acad. Sci. USA*, 79:2554–2558.
Hopfield, J. J., Feinstein, D. I., and Palmer, R. G., 1983, "Unlearning" has a stabilizing effect in collective memories, *Nature* 304:158.
Kohonen, T., 1984, *Self Organization and Associative Memory*, Berlin: Springer-Verlag.
McCulloch, W. S., and Pitts, W., 1943, A logical calculus of ideas imminent in nervous activity, *Bull. Math. Biophys.*, 5:115–133.
Reif, F., 1982, *Fundamentals of Statistical and Thermal Physics*, New York: McGraw-Hill.

Statistical Mechanics of On-Line Learning and Generalization

Michael Biehl and Nestor Caticha

Introduction

In trying to understand how artificial neural networks (ANNs) learn from examples, researchers ask a variety of questions whose answers may require very different approaches. For questions about the typical properties of large ANNs, statistical mechanics (SM) provides a set of tools which was first developed to discern macroscopic properties emerging from microscopic interactions among a large number of units.

The aim of this article is to introduce the reader to the SM theory of on-line training of feedforward neural networks and their generalization ability. The main characteristic of on-line learning is that training examples are dealt with one at a time, as opposed to off-line or memory-based methods, where learning is guided by the minimization of a cost function that incorporates possibly all of the data. In the language of statistical physics, the distinction is between systems that can be thought of as in a state of thermal equilibrium, and off-equilibrium situations in which the network is not allowed to extract all possible information from a set of examples. The equilibrium SM of off-line learning and generalization is reviewed in STATISTICAL MECHANICS OF GENERALIZATION and STATISTICAL MECHANICS OF NEURAL NETWORKS (q.v.).

Although on-line learning is an intrinsically stochastic process, the restriction to large networks, togther with assumptions that are made about the statistical properties of the inputs, permits a concise description of the dynamics in terms of coupled ordinary differential equations. These deterministic equations govern the average evolution of quantities that completely define the macroscopic state of the ANN. The average is taken with respect to the data—an operation that is straightforward if the presented examples are statistically independent.

This off-equilibrium situation can be analyzed for a variety of network architectures and environments. The types of problems that can be investigated in this framework include (1) determining the learning curves for a large class of models, (2) deriving the upper bounds of the typical performance and determining how these bounds might be approached, (3) dynamical symmetry breaking in hidden-layer neurons, which can model rapid transitions to new levels of generalization ability, and (4) analyzing the effects of different types of noise, or changes in the environment. The last issue in particular arises in real-world applications and is an area in which on-line learning is to be preferred. The performance of on-line algorithms compares well with that of sophisticated off-line prescriptions. However, the computational cost and memory requirements of on-line algorithms are significantly lower. Off-line training is not capable of dealing with environmental drift or sudden changes, because no distinction is made between old, possibly irrelevant data and more recent data. This is treated most naturally by on-line methods (see Vicente, Kinouchi, and Caticha, 1998, and references therein).

The Dynamics of On-Line Learning

For illustrative purposes, we will show the theoretical treatment of on-line learning in terms of a specific class of neural networks. It should be noted that many of the restrictions introduced in the discussion can be relaxed without complicating the analysis very much.

We consider student networks with N real-valued inputs, K units in a hidden layer, and one single output. Denote by $\mathbb{J} = (\mathbf{J}_1, \mathbf{J}_2,$ $\ldots, \mathbf{J}_K)$ the set of adaptive student weights that connect the input layer to the hidden units. Here and in the following, boldface vectors are in $\mathbb{R}^N$. The state of a hidden unit is taken to be a function $\sigma_J^k = f_{\mathrm{hid}}(x_k)$ of the projection $x_k = \mathbf{J}_k \cdot \xi$, and the total output is given as $\Sigma_J(\xi) = f_{\mathrm{out}}(\sigma_J^1, \sigma_J^2, \ldots, \sigma_J^K)$. All units may have Boolean (± 1) or continuous (e.g., linear or sigmoidal) transfer functions.

In general, the functions $f_{\mathrm{hid}}, f_{\mathrm{out}}$ can be specified through a set of additional adaptive parameters. For simplicity we will concentrate here on cases where only $\mathbb{J}$ is to be determined in the course of learning and f_{out} is fixed a priori. Learning a finite number of second-layer weights or thresholds is easier and faster than adaptating the $K N$ first-layer weights $\mathbb{J}$ (Riegler and Endres, 1999).

The student network is to learn a rule from examples. For the purpose of modeling it is convenient to parameterize the unknown rule in terms of a teacher network. Let $\mathbb{B} = (\mathbf{B}_1, \mathbf{B}_2, \ldots, \mathbf{B}_M)$ denote its M hidden-unit weight vectors with $y_m = \mathbf{B}_m \cdot \xi$. This teacher net implements the mapping $\Sigma_B(\xi) = f_{\mathrm{out}}(\sigma_B^1, \sigma_B^2, \ldots, \sigma_B^M)$, where $\sigma_B^m = f_{\mathrm{hid}}(y_m)$. For simplicity we will assume that the activation functions are the same in student and teacher. We also restrict our attention to the thermodynamic limit, where $N \to \infty$, but K and M remain finite. Note that in this simplified scheme it is still possible to model a variety of scenarios, including the case of matching complexity ($K = M$), where the rule is perfectly learnable. Obviously, the student can only approximate the rule for $K < M$, whereas the network is *oversophisticated* if $K > M$.

The learning of a linearly separable rule with a so-called single-layer perceptron has served as a prototype model in the development of the entire field (see STATISTICAL MECHANICS OF GENERALIZATION). This scenario is recovered for $K = M = 1$ with threshold hidden activation $f_{\mathrm{hid}}( ) = \mathrm{sign}( )$ and with the output transfer function f_{out} being the identity.

A set of weights $\mathbb{J}^\mu$ is chosen after presentation of $\mu - 1$ examples of the form (ξ_ν, Σ_ν). Here ξ_ν is the input vector drawn at discrete-time ν from a distribution $P(\xi_\nu)$, and Σ_ν is the corresponding training label. The latter can coincide with the true rule output $\Sigma_B(\xi_\nu)$ if reliable example data are available, or it is a noisy version thereof in the presence of stochastic corruption. The aim of learning is to determine $\mathbb{J}^\mu$ such that the teacher and student outputs are close in some respect for a novel, random input ξ. A quite natural choice of an error measure is the quadratic deviation from the correct rule output $e(\xi) = (\Sigma_J(\xi) - \Sigma_B(\xi))^2/2$. The expected value of this quantity with respect to $P(\xi)$ is termed the generalization error $e_G = \langle e(\xi) \rangle_\xi$. Achieving small values of e_G is aimed at by making small changes in $\mathbb{J}^\mu$ at each time step.

Although there is considerable liberty in the choice of a training prescription, some common features are shared by all reasonable algorithms. Here we will consider updates of the student vectors that can be written in the form

$$\mathbf{J}_k^\mu = \mathbf{J}_k^{\mu-1} + \frac{1}{N} F_k \cdot \xi_\mu \tag{1}$$

on presentation of example (ξ_μ, Σ_μ). The central quantities in defining the algorithm are the *modulation functions* F_k, which determine the amount of correction in the direction of the latest example. Often, the update term $F_k \xi_\mu$ can be written as the gradient with respect to $\mathbf{J}_k$ of an instantaneous cost function defined for the latest example. Because of the similarity to pioneering ideas about learning in biological neural networks, algorithms of the type shown in Equation 1 have been termed (generalized) *Hebbian learning*. Modulation functions that vary between different components of the student vectors (*matrix update*) can also be considered (see, e.g., Murata in Saad, 1998; Bös and Amari in Saad, 1998).

The modulation F_k can be a function of several quantities. It utilizes information about the current example and actual student weights. More sophisticated algorithms may depend on several other variables that play the role of hyperparameters. In general, they reflect the fact that the amount of information contained in an example depends strongly on the state of the student network. Learning can introduce so-called hyperparameters to the algorithm that estimate, among other things, the performance of the network, noise levels affecting the data, or parameters that describe the input distribution. Learning will then be efficient, in some cases even as fast as optimal off-line training.

In order to obtain a macroscopic description of the dynamics, we can project the iteration equation (Equation 1) onto $\mathbb{J}$ and $\mathbb{B}$, which immediately yields a set of equations for the overlaps

$$Q_{ij} = \mathbf{J}_i \cdot \mathbf{J}_j \quad \text{and} \quad R_{in} = \mathbf{J}_i \cdot \mathbf{B}_n \qquad (2)$$

The set of (usually) nondynamical parameters $T_{mn} = \mathbf{B}_m \cdot \mathbf{B}_n$ is also introduced here for future reference. In the simplest models, all considered inputs are independent random vectors with uniform density on the sphere $\xi^2 = N$ (referred to as isotropic data in the following discussion). Then, no further directions in $\mathbb{R}^N$ and therefore no other projections are relevant.

Performing the projections brings up great simplifications. First, the number of equations drops from $N K$ to only $(K^2 + K)/2 + K M$. Second, by the law of large numbers, the overlaps in Equation 2, but not their changes, become *self-averaging* quantities in the thermodynamic limit for a large class of algorithms and input distribution. Mean values, as observed in a computer simulation, for instance, will approach the theoretical prediction with increasing N. In many example scenarios, the deviation is found to be on the order $1/N$, yielding excellent results for fairly small systems with, say, $N \sim 100$ already. At the same time, the width of the distribution of quantities in Equation 2, emerging from the randomness in the data, tends to zero with $N \to \infty$. This property is a common feature of so-called order parameters describing disordered systems in SM. A more detailed discussion of self-averaging in on-line learning is given in Reents and Urbanczik (1998).

Finally, the iteration equations for the overlaps reduce to first-order ODE, where the continuous parameter $\alpha = \mu/N$ measures the learning time. Averaging over the last example input ξ_μ and the possibly noisy label Σ_μ leads to the set (indices μ omitted)

$$\dot{R}_{in} = \langle y_n F_i \rangle, \quad \dot{Q}_{ij} = \langle x_i F_j + x_j F_i + F_i F_j \rangle \qquad (3)$$

where the dot denotes a derivative with respect to α. The right-hand side reduces to multidimensional Gaussian integrals if the dependence of F_k on ξ_μ is only through the projections $x_k^\mu = \mathbf{J}_k^{\mu-1} \cdot \xi_\mu$ and $y_m^\mu = \mathbf{B}_m \cdot \xi_\mu$. By means of the central limit theorem, these quantities become correlated Gaussian random numbers in the thermodynamic limit. Hence, their statistics are completely determined by first and second moments, which in the case of isotropic data read

$$\langle x_i \rangle = \langle y_m \rangle = 0, \quad \langle x_i x_j \rangle = Q_{ij},$$
$$\langle y_m y_n \rangle = T_{mn}, \quad \text{and} \quad \langle x_i y_n \rangle = R_{in} \qquad (4)$$

The set of differential equations (Equation 3) can now be integrated, at least numerically, and yields the evolution of R_{ij}, Q_{mn} from arbitrary initial conditions at $\alpha = 0$. Another advantage of the projection is that the generalization error $e_G = \langle e(\xi) \rangle_\xi$ can be written as a function of the overlaps in Equation 2. The particular form depends on the transfer functions, distribution of examples, and the architectures considered.

The formalism outlined here allows one to address a variety of problems: What is the typical behavior of standard algorithms, such as Rosenblatt's perceptron prescription or backpropagation in the soft committee? Which is the best possible decrease of the generalization error, and by what choice of F is it achieved?

In the next section we discuss a few selected results. The following section addresses the learning of classification schemes. Then, regression by means of on-line gradient descent and related methods is discussed, and in closing we summarize some of the many other topics that have been investigated.

Learning of Classification Schemes

The study of binary classifiers presents one of the simplest approaches to categorization. On-line learning of classifications has been investigated for several architectures, ranging from the single-layer perceptron learning a linearly separable rule to fully connected feedforward machines with $(K, M > 1)$, but also for density estimation and unsupervised learning. We will restrict ourselves to the case of supervised learning of a Boolean rule in student-teacher scenarios.

For binary outputs $\Sigma_{J,B} = \pm 1$, it is natural to choose the measure $e(\xi) = (\Sigma_J - \Sigma_B)^2/4 \in \{0, 1\}$, which differs from that introduced above by only a factor $\frac{1}{2}$. Its expected value e_G is the probability of disagreement between student and teacher with respect to a novel random input. As an example, for the single-layer perceptron ($K = M = 1$), one obtains $e_G = \arccos(R/\sqrt{Q})/\pi$ for isotropic inputs.

Instead of a detailed review of results for each particular network architecture and learning scenario, we will describe the properties that are common to successful learning algorithms in terms of the single-layer perceptron. The modulation function F, the central quantities in this analysis, serves as an estimate of the value of the information carried by the example. Different algorithms make different attributions to this value, which leads to differences in performance.

The simplest choice is pure *Hebbian learning*, where $F = \Sigma$ is given by the training label, independent of the actual student weights. This recipe seems to work in the sense that for isotropic inputs, the generalization error decreases as $e_G \propto \alpha^{-1/2}$ if the rule is linearly separable. This hides the fact that it will fail to learn completely for nonuniform distributions. The reason can be tracked to the equal treatment of correctly and incorrectly predicted examples. Rosenblatt's perceptron rule, by paying attention only to errors and disregarding correctly predicted examples, goes further. The resulting algorithm, $F \Sigma_B(\xi) = \Theta(-x \Sigma(\xi))$, i.e., 1 (if wrong) or 0 (if correct), is able to deal with nonuniform distributions, although in the singular isotropic case it is not as fast—$e_G \propto \alpha^{-1/3}$ for large α—as the pure Hebbian prescription (Biehl and Riegler, 1994).

The perceptron rule can be improved by noting two facts. First, not all errors are equally important. Those made on examples far from the decision border should be penalized more than those made on examples near it. The on-line relaxation algorithm with $F = -x\Theta(-x\Sigma(\xi))$ leads to a dramatic improvement with $e_G \propto \alpha^{-1}$ (Biehl and Riegler, 1994). Second, correctly predicted examples may also contain useful information. Their inclusion, however, is not always desired. At the beginning of a learning session, they carry useful information and lead to improved performance; however, their importance decreases as the student net starts to approach the rule. The lesson is that successful algorithms F should be performance dependent.

The effect of noise in the data has been intensely investigated (see Copelli and Caticha in Saad, 1998, for references). The foregoing analysis suggests that algorithms work by constructing a modulation function from information about the *surprise* carried by an incorrectly predicted example and by deciding whether that surprise is expected or not, given the state of the learning process. This strategy is most useful if determined by an estimate of the performance. In the presence of noise, a new ingredient enters: the suspicion that a misclassification is due to noise in the data should suppress large modulations. There is, therefore, the need for a crossover from a regime of surprise to one of *student confidence*, where blame attribution for prediction errors shifts to the data. This idea is implemented, for example, in the on-line Gibbs algorithm (Kim and Sompolinsky, 1996) through a cutoff of the function F at large absolute values of x.

For those cases where learning conditions permit the use of queries, Kinzel and Rujan (1990) have shown that improved performance is achieved by selecting examples at the very edge of the student decision border. To our knowledge, their work constitutes the first description of on-line learning and generalization by means of ODE. Appropriate choices of the actual algorithm F lead their query method to an exponential decay of e_G.

All of these ingredients have been used in building algorithms. They can also be obtained from first principles for a set of model problems by the variational optimization of e_G with respect to the modulation function. The variational method was introduced in Kinouchi and Caticha (1992) with an application to the pure perceptron problem, where $|de_G/d\alpha|$ is to be maximized. It has been extended by several authors but is restricted to working in the limit $N \to \infty$. The obtained optimal modulation function depends typically on the actual performance e_G of the student. Further, it may require knowledge of other unavailable quantities describing the noise or the input distribution, for instance. Obviously, this limits the direct applicability of the prescription in practice. However, the procedure does suggest which are the relevant features of a successful algorithm, and enables establishing lower bounds to $e_G(\alpha)$ in model situations.

The key result in this context is that on-line learning of classifications can be as efficient as the much more involved memory-based training (Kinouchi and Caticha, 1992; Opper, 1996; Van den Broeck and Reimann, 1996). For the single-layer perceptron, e.g., the asymptotic decay of $e_G \propto 1/\alpha$ with $\alpha \to \infty$ differs only by a factor of 2 from the result for optimal off-line learning if examples are noiseless or corrupted by random inversion of the labels. In the case of continuous corruption, such as through additive noise in the inputs, the optimal performances of off-line and on-line training coincide exactly, and $e_G \propto \alpha^{-1/2}$ (see STATISTICAL MECHANICS OF GENERALIZATION). Recently the relation of the variational approach with Bayesian analysis was clarified (Opper, 1996; Opper in Saad, 1998; Solla and Winther in Saad, 1998).

Learning in Continuous Networks

In applications, ANNs with continuous activation are frequently used to solve regression problems. But it is also common practice in classification to approximate the rule with a *soft* or *probabilistic* version thereof. One reason for doing so is that appealing, simple training schemes are available for multilayered architectures. In networks with differentiable activations, the error measure itself is a differentiable function of the network parameters. Therefore, off-line training can be based on gradient descent or similar minimization procedures. The most popular prescription of this kind has been termed *backpropagation of error*, and its success has boosted interest in ANN applications.

As an example architecture, the so-called soft-committee machine has been considered (Saad and Solla, 1995), with sigmoidal $f_{hid}(x) = \mathrm{erf}(x/\sqrt{2})$ and a single linear output with weights fixed to 1. Training is based on the quadratic error for the latest example, i.e.,

$$F_k \xi_\mu = -\eta \Delta_{J_k} e(\xi_\mu)|_{(\mu-1)}$$

in Equation 1, where the gradient is evaluated with the weights at time $\mu - 1$. The dynamics (Equation 3) as well as the generalization error can be worked out analytically for arbitrary K and M (but with $K, M \ll N$).

The learning rate η appears quadratically in the equations of motion (Equation 3); hence its nontrivial influence on the behavior of the system. For example, a critical value η_c exists in matching scenarios, above which the perfect solution $\mathbb{J} = \mathbb{B}$ becomes unstable and even very small deviations from the perfect solution would increase in the training process. For $K < M$ the asymptotic value $e_G(\alpha \to \infty)$ depends explicitly on η, and only in the limit $\eta \to 0$ is the optimal approximation of the rule achieved.

One of the most interesting phenomena in on-line gradient descent is the breaking of permutation symmetry during learning. It can be observed for $K = M = 2$ already: Figure 1 shows a typical learning curve obtained in this scenario when training is based on reliable examples with isotropic inputs. Obviously, the learning process is dominated by a pronounced plateau state in which very little progress is made while the number of examples increases. Only after an extended period of time does the system leave the plateau and approach its asymptotic state exponentially fast.

The occurrence of plateaus can be related to fixed points of the ODE (Equation 3). In the case displayed in Figure 1, the system is very close to a perfectly symmetric configuration with $\mathbf{J}_1 = \mathbf{J}_2$, i.e., $R_{ij} = R$ and $Q_{ij} = Q$ for all i,j. The existence of such a stationary state reflects an underlying symmetry of the problem: the student output and hence the error measure is invariant under permutations of hidden units. Whereas this property leads to phase transitions in equilibrium off-line training (see STATISTICAL MECHANICS OF GENERALIZATION), the effect here is that the system approaches a symmetric state from generic initial conditions.

Properties of such plateaus can be investigated in detail by linearizing the dynamics close to the fixed point. The configuration is unstable, that is, weakly repulsive in a few directions in overlap space. Consequently, the system stays in its vicinity for a long time before eventually leaving the plateau. The observed plateau length depends on the corresponding eigensystem and, in a subtle way, on the initial state. If the student weights are uncorrelated with the teacher before training, one expects random $R_{ij}(0) = \mathbb{O}(N^{-1/2})$ in a finite system. As a consequence, the plateau length and hence the

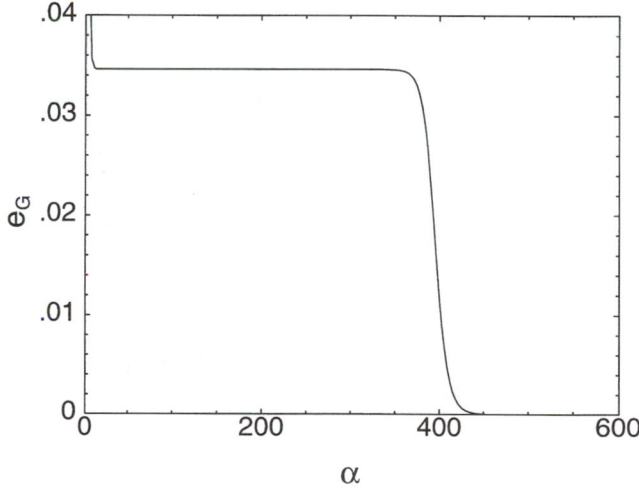

Figure 1. The learning curve of the $K = M = 2$ soft-committee scenario (as described in the text) with $T_{mn} = \delta_{mn}$, $\eta = 1.5$, and initial values $Q_{ii}(0) = 0.5$. All $R_{in}(0)$ as well as $Q_{12}(0)$ were different numbers of order $\mathbb{O}(10^{-12})$.

characteristic learning time will be $\alpha \propto \ln N$, demonstrating the relevance of the phenomenon to the practical treatment of high-dimensional data (Biehl, Riegler, and Wöhler, 1996).

The occurrence of plateaus in learning curves is by no means a feature of the particular scenario considered here. Weakly repulsive fixed points are found for any $K \geq 2$, independent of M. They exist also in systems where the invariance with respect to permutations is replaced by more complicated symmetries. Further, the number of fixed points increases with both K and M, while only the most symmetric states seem to dominate the dynamics from generic initial conditions (Saad and Solla, 1995; Biehl et al., 1996). An interesting observation is the possible existence of attractive fixed points with $e_G > 0$ when $K > M$. Successful training can be impossible if the student is highly oversophisticated for the task to learn.

The deeper reason for the occurence of plateaus is the fact that learning requires the specialization of hidden units. After presentation of only a few examples, it is only reasonable that the student's hypothesis about the rule be as simple as possible. In this sense, unspecialized plateaus can be considered a necessary phase of learning and should be expected quite generally. However, from a practical point of view the question arises as to how the length of this phase can be reduced, potentially to its minimum. To this end, variational methods have been applied to the soft-committee machine as well. Note that the situation is more complicated here than it is in the perceptron or nonoverlapping architectures: e_G is a function of many order parameters and it is not a priori clear that the local maximization of $|de_G/d\alpha|$ yields a successful strategy. Alternatively, the global optimization of e_G achieved after presentation of a certain number of examples has been considered. Both approaches predict that an efficient decrease in plateau length should be possible (Saad and Rattray, 1997; Vicente and Caticha, 1997). The latter is also true for methods that explicitly incorporate curvature information into the learning algorithm. The so-called natural gradient method of Amari deserves particular attention in this context (see Amari, 1967; Rattray and Saad in Saad, 1998; Bös and Amari in Saad, 1998). Its main idea is to base learning on a distance measure that is invariant under reparameterization of the student output.

Discussion

The statistical mechanics approach to on-line learning has allowed for a theoretical understanding of the dynamics of various adaptive systems. In this article we considered selected examples of the success of this method. For a more complete overview of the field and recent developments, see Saad (1998).

The question of on-line learning in systems with discrete degrees of freedom was recently addressed (Solla and Winther in Saad, 1998). A treatment of network parameters that can be trained on different time scales is provided in Riegler and Endres (1999).

The framework of on-line learning and many of the phenomena discussed here carry over immediately to unsupervised learning in high-dimensional spaces (see Biehl et al. in Saad, 1998, for further references).

In a related, alternative approach to on-line learning one preserves the stochastic nature of the Markov process and refrains from taking $N \rightarrow \infty$ beforehand (see, e.g., Heskes and Wiegerinck in Saad, 1998; Leen in Saad, 1998). By means of appropriate expansions and approximations one can then, for example, investigate the dynamics of finite systems. The convergence of on-line algorithms is discussed in the framework of stochastic approximation theory by Bottou (in Saad, 1998).

A question of great importance is that of correlations among the training examples and their influence on the learning dynamics. In this context, training from a limited pool of fixed examples (see chapters by Barber and Sollich, Coolen and Saad, and Heskes and Wiegerinck in Saad, 1998) remains one of the theoretical challenges with great practical relevance.

Road Map: Learning in Artificial Networks
Background: Statistical Mechanics of Neural Networks
Related Reading: Statistical Mechanics of Generalization

References

Amari, S., 1967, A theory of adaptive pattern classifiers, *IEEE Trans. Elect. Comput.*, EC-16:299.
Biehl, M., and Riegler, P., 1994, On-line learning with a perceptron, *Europhys. Lett.*, 28:525.
Biehl, M., Riegler, P., and Wöhler, C., 1996, Transient dynamics of online learning in two-layered neural networks, *J. Phys. A*, 29:4769.
Kim, J. W., and Sompolinsky, H., 1996, On-line Gibbs learning, *Phys. Rev. Lett.*, 76:3021.
Kinouchi, O., and Caticha, N., 1992, Optimal generalization in perceptrons, *J. Phys. A*, 25:6243.
Kinzel, W., and Rujan, P., 1990, Improving a network generalization ability by selecting examples, *Europhys. Lett.*, 13:2878.
Opper, M., 1996, On-line versus off-line learning from random examples: General results, *Phys. Rev. Lett.*, 76:4671.
Reents, G., and Urbanczik, R., 1998, Self-averaging and on-line learning, *Phys. Rev. Lett.*, 80:5445.
Riegler, P., and Endres, D., 1999, Learning dynamics on different timescales, *J. Phys. A*, 32:8655.
Saad, D., Ed., 1998, *On-line Learning in Neural Networks*, Cambridge, Engl.: Cambridge University Press. ◆
Saad, D., and Rattray, M., 1997, Globally optimal parameters for on-line learning in multilayer neural networks, *Phys. Rev. Lett.*, 79:2578.
Saad, D., and Solla, S. A., 1995, On-line learning in soft committee machines, *Phys. Rev. E*, E-52:4225.
Van den Broeck, C., and Reimann, P., 1996, Unsupervised learning by examples: On-line vs. off-line, *Phys. Rev. Lett.*, 76:2188.
Vicente, R., and Caticha, N., 1997, Functional optimization of online algorithms in multilayer neural networks, *J. Phys. A*, 30:L599.
Vicente, R., Kinouchi, O., and Caticha, N., 1998, Statistical mechanics of on-line learning of drifting concepts: A variational approach, *Machine Learn.*, 32:179.

Statistical Parametric Mapping of Cortical Activity Patterns

Karl J. Friston

Introduction

This article addresses the experimental design and analysis of functional brain imaging studies. It considers the neurobiological mo-

tivations for different designs and describes some standard approaches that have been developed to analyze the ensuing data. Functional neuroimaging (positron emission tomography, or PET, and functional magnetic resonance imaging, or fMRI) is generally used to make inferences about functional anatomy on the basis of evoked patterns of cortical activity. Functional anatomy refers to the anatomical organization of the brain as it relates to function. It involves an understanding of what each part of the brain does and how different brain systems interact to support various sensorimotor and cognitive functions. Large-scale organization can be inferred using techniques that image the hemodynamic and metabolic sequelae of evoked neuronal responses. PET measures regional cerebral blood flow (rCBF), and fMRI measures oxygenation changes. Their spatial resolution is on the order of a few millimeters. Because PET uses radiotracers, its temporal resolution is limited by the half-life of the tracers employed (usually a minute or so). However, fMRI is limited only by the biophysical time constants of hemodynamic responses themselves (a few seconds).

An important issue in the design and analysis of functional anatomical experiments is the relationship between conceptual models of brain organization and neurophysiological responses, and how this relationship is realized in the statistical models used in analysis. This article begins by reviewing the distinction between *functional specialization* and *integration* and how these principles serve as the motivation for most analyses.

Statistical parametric mapping (SPM) is used to identify functionally specialized brain regions. Specialized regions respond selectively to experimental cognitive or sensorimotor changes. SPM is used to detect these responses anywhere they occur, irrespective of changes elsewhere. The alternative perspective, that provided by functional integration, requires a different set of (multivariate) approaches that examine the relationship between changes in one area and changes in another. SPM is a voxel-based approach (a voxel is a volume element of an image) that employs standard inferential statistics to make some comment about regionally specific responses to experimental factors at each voxel. In contradistinction to the alternative approach, based on prespecified regions of interest (ROI), SPM examines every part of the brain at the highest resolution afforded by the data. SPM has now almost universally superseded ROI approaches because it avoids preconceptions about evoked responses and avoids many forms of bias. Technically, SPM is a *mass-univariate* approach, in the sense that each data sequence from every voxel is treated as a univariate response. The massive number of voxels is analyzed in parallel, and dependencies among them are dealt with using random field theory at the point of inference. The alternative to a mass-univariate approach is a *multivariate* analysis that considers images as a multidimensional observation with as many components as there are voxels. The general ideas behind statistical parametric mapping are described and illustrated with the different sorts of inferences that can be made with different experimental designs. The article concludes by reviewing multivariate analyses and effective connectivity.

Functional Specialization and Integration

The brain appears to adhere to two fundamental principles of functional organization, functional integration and functional specialization, with the integration within and among specialized areas mediated by *effective connectivity*. This distinction relates to that between *localizationism* and *(dis)connectionism* that dominated thinking about cortical function in the nineteenth century. Since the early anatomical theories of Gall, the identification of a particular brain region with a specific function has become a central theme in neuroscience. However, functional localization per se was not easy to demonstrate. For example, a meeting that took place on August 4, 1881, addressed the difficulties of attributing function to a cortical area, given the dependence of cerebral activity on underlying connections (Phillips, Zeki, and Barlow, 1984). The topic of the meeting was "Localization of function in the cortex cerebri."

Goltz, although accepting the results of electrical cortical stimulation, considered that the excitation method was inconclusive, in that movements elicited might have originated in related pathways, or current could have spread to distant centers. In short, the excitation method could not be used to infer functional localization because localizationism discounted interactions, or functional integration, among different brain areas. It was proposed that lesion studies could supplement excitation experiments; ironically, it was observations on patients with brain lesions some years later that led to the concept of *disconnection syndromes* and the refutation of localizationism as a complete or sufficient explanation of cortical organization. Functional localization implies that a function can be localized in a cortical area, whereas specialization suggests that a cortical area is specialized for some aspect of perceptual, motor, or cognitive processing, and that this specialization is anatomically segregated within the brain. The neuronal infrastructure supporting a single function may then involve many specialized areas whose union is mediated by the functional integration among them. In this view, functional specialization is only meaningful in the context of functional integration, and vice versa. Certain patterns of cortical projections are so common that they could amount to rules of cortical connectivity. "These rules revolve around one, apparently, overriding strategy that the cerebral cortex uses—that of functional segregation" (Zeki, 1990). This is the model upon which the search for regionally specific effects is based.

The analysis of functional neuroimaging data involves many steps, which can be broadly divided into (1) spatial preprocessing, (2) estimating the parameters of a statistical model, and (3) making inferences about modeled effects using the parameter estimates and their associated statistics (Figure 1). We will focus on model estimation and inference.

Statistical Parametric Mapping

Functional mapping studies are usually analyzed with some form of *statistical parametric mapping*, or SPM. SPM refers to the construction of statistical maps to test hypotheses about regionally specific effects like "activations" (Friston et al., 1995). The maps are image processes with voxel values that, under the null hypothesis, are distributed according to a known probability density function (usually Student's T or F distributions). The success of SPM is largely due to the simplicity of the idea. Namely, one analyzes each and every voxel using any standard (univariate) statistical test. The resulting statistical parameters are assembled into an image, the SPM map. SPM$\{T\}$ refers to a map comprising T statistics; similarly, SPM$\{F\}$ denotes a map of F statistics. SPMs are interpreted as spatially extended statistical processes by referring to the probabilistic behavior of stationary Gaussian fields (Friston et al., 1995; Worsley et al., 1996). Stationary fields model both the univariate probabilistic characteristics of an SPM and any spatial covariance structure. "Unlikely" excursions of the SPM are interpreted as regionally specific effects, attributable to the sensorimotor or cognitive process that has been manipulated experimentally. Statistical analysis corresponds to modeling the data in order to partition observed neurophysiological responses into components of interest, confounds, and error. Almost universally, the models employed are general linear models.

The General Linear Model

The general linear model is an equation, $y = X\beta + \varepsilon$, that expresses the observed *response variable* y in terms of a linear combination of explanatory variables X plus a well-behaved error term (see Friston et al., 1995). The general linear model is variously known as

Data transformations

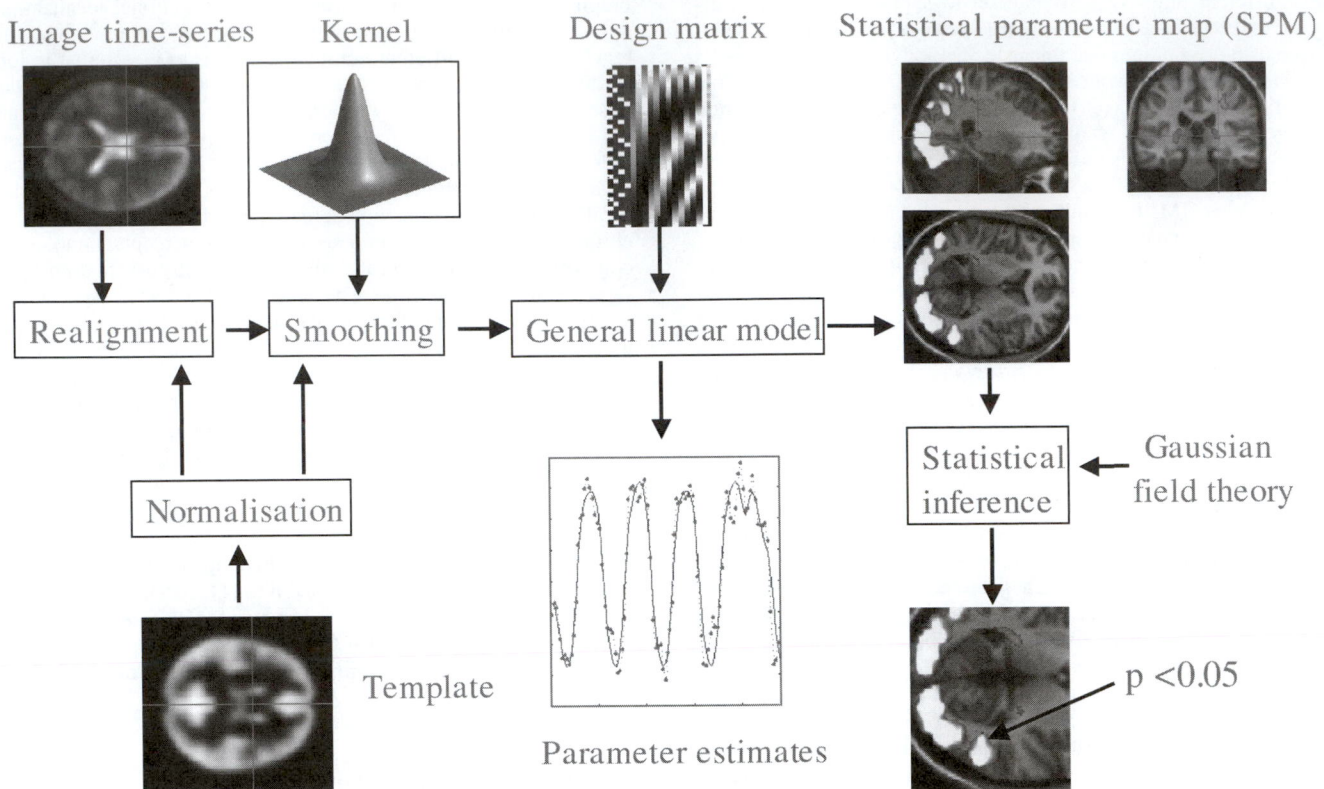

Image time-series   Kernel   Design matrix   Statistical parametric map (SPM)

Realignment → Smoothing → General linear model →

Normalisation

Template

Parameter estimates

Statistical inference ← Gaussian field theory

p <0.05

Figure 1. Schematic depicting the transformations that start with the imaging time series and end with a statistical parametric map (SPM). SPMs can be thought of as x-rays of the significance of an effect. Voxel-based analyses require the data to be in the same anatomical space: realigning the data to remove the effects of subject movement effects this. After realignment the images are subject to nonlinear warping so that they match a template that already conforms to a standard anatomical space. After smoothing, the general linear model is employed to (1) estimate the parameters of the model and (2) derive the appropriate univariate test statistic at each voxel. The test statistics that ensue (usually, T or F statistics) constitute the SPM. The final stage is to make statistical inferences on the basis of the SPM and characterize the responses observed using the fitted responses or parameter estimates. The display format is sometimes a maximum intensity projection (MIP) of the SPM{T} from three views of the brain. The anatomical space conforms to that of the Talairach and Tournoux atlas. This MIP display format in this figure is a thresholded SPM, superimposed on slices through the brain depicting anatomical structures. Such a display format is sometimes preferred when the structure-function relationship is important and can be summarized by reporting a single slice of the SPM.

analysis of covariance or multiple regression analysis, and subsumes simpler variants, like the two-sample T test for a difference in means, to more elaborate linear convolution models such as finite impulse response models for time series. The matrix X that contains the explanatory variables (e.g., designed effects or confounds) is called the design matrix. Each column of the design matrix corresponds to some effect the investigator has built into the experiment or that may confound the results. These are variously referred to as *explanatory variables*, covariates, regressors, or, in fMRI, stimulus functions. The example in Figure 1 relates to an fMRI study of visual stimulation under four conditions. The effects on the response variable are modeled in terms of functions of the presence of these conditions (i.e., boxcars smoothed with a hemodynamic response function) and constitute the first four columns of the design matrix. There follows a series of terms designed to remove or model low-frequency variations in signal due to artifacts such as aliased biorhythms. The final column is whole-brain activity. The relative contribution of each of these columns is assessed using generalized least-squares estimates. These are the estimates of β,

the parameters of the model. Inferences about parameter estimates are made using T or F statistics, depending on whether one is looking at a particular linear combination or several.

The error or noise in neuroimaging has a number of sources and is generally about the same size as the evoked responses themselves. Scan-to-scan error is due to technical measurement noise and neurophysiological noise, inherent in ongoing brain activity. In multisubject designs, between-subject variability in responses is another important error variance component and can sometimes be greater than within-subject or scan-to-scan variability. In fMRI, aliased biorhythms and drifts in the measurement device induce correlations among the errors. This is known as *nonsphericity* and is accommodated in generalized linear models (e.g., Worsley and Friston, 1995). The nonsphericity corrections used to deal with temporal correlations in fMRI are the same as those adopted in conventional analysis of variance.

Generalized linear models can be used to implement a vast range of statistical analyses. The issue is therefore not so much the mathematics but the formulation of a design matrix X appropriate to the study design and inferences that are sought. The design matrix can contain both covariates and indicator variables. Each column of X has an associated unknown parameter. Some of these parameters will be of interest (e.g., the effect of a particular sensorimotor or cognitive condition, or the regression coefficient of hemodynamic responses on reaction time). The remaining parameters will be of no interest and pertain to nuisance or confounding effects (e.g., the effect of being a particular subject, or the regression slope of voxel activity on global activity). Inferences about the parameter estimates are made using their estimated variance. This allows one to test the null hypothesis that all the estimates are zero, using the F statistic to give an SPM{F}, or that some particular linear combination (e.g., a subtraction) of the estimates is zero, using an SPM{T}. The T statistic obtains by dividing a *contrast* or linear combination (specified by contrast weights) of the ensuing parameter estimates by its standard error. The latter is estimated using the variance of the residuals about the least-squares fit. An example of contrast weights would be $[-1\ 1\ 0\ 0\ \ldots]$ to compare the differential responses evoked by the two conditions, modeled by the first two condition-specific regressors in the design matrix. In summary, the T statistic can be regarded as the size of a response, or activation estimate, divided by its variability or standard error. The square of this statistic is the ratio of the sum of squares or variance of interest divided by error variance. This is the F statistic, which can be computed for several linear combinations or *contrasts* of estimated responses at once. This is useful when several parameter estimates are potentially interesting (e.g., using polynomial expansions [Büchel et al., 1996] or basis functions of some parameter of interest).

Statistical Inference and the Theory of Gaussian Fields

Inferences using SPMs can be of two sorts, depending on whether one knows where to look in advance. With an anatomically constrained hypothesis about effects in a particular brain region, the *uncorrected P* value associated with the height or extent of that region in the SPM can be used to test the hypothesis. With an anatomically open hypothesis (i.e., a null hypothesis that there is no effect anywhere in the brain), a correction for multiple dependent comparisons is necessary. The theory of Gaussian fields provides a way of computing this *corrected P* value that takes into account the fact that neighboring voxels are not independent by virtue of smoothness in the original data. This *Gaussian field correction* (GFC) plays the same role for continuous, multidimensional statistical processes like SPM{T} as the *Bonferroni correction* plays in multiple discrete T tests. Provided the data are sufficiently smooth, the correction based on Gaussian field theory is much less severe (i.e., is more sensitive) than a Bonferroni correction for the number of voxels. This is simply because the GFC ensures that the rate of false positive "clusters" is maintained as a nominal level (usually 0.05). The rate of false positive voxels can therefore be much larger, e.g., 0.05 times the expected number of voxels per cluster. The difference between a Gaussian field and a Bonferroni correction increases with smoothness, or expected voxels per cluster.

Experimental Design

Categorical Designs, Cognitive Subtraction, and Conjunctions

The tenet of cognitive subtraction is that the difference between two tasks can be formulated as a separable cognitive or sensorimotor component and that regionally specific differences in hemodynamic responses identify the corresponding functionally specialized area. Early applications of subtraction range from the

functional anatomy of word processing (Petersen et al., 1989) to functional specialization in extrastriate cortex (Lueck et al., 1989). The latter studies involved presenting visual stimuli with and without some sensory attribute (e.g., color, motion). The areas highlighted by subtraction were identified with homologous areas in monkeys that showed selective electrophysiological responses to equivalent visual stimuli.

Cognitive conjunctions (Price and Friston, 1997) can be thought of as an extension of the subtraction technique, in the sense that they combine a series of subtractions. In subtraction, one tests a hypothesis pertaining to the activation in one task relative to another. In conjunction analyses several hypotheses are tested conjointly, with the investigator asking whether all the activations, in a series of task pairs, are jointly significant. Conjunction analyses allow one to demonstrate any context-insensitive component of regional responses.

Parametric Designs

The premise behind parametric designs is that regional physiology will vary systematically with the degree of cognitive or sensorimotor processing or deficits thereof. Examples of this approach include the PET experiments of Grafton et al. (1992), which demonstrated significant correlations between hemodynamic responses and the performance of a visually guided motor tracking task. These relationships, or "neurometric functions," may be linear or nonlinear. Using polynomial regression, in the context of the general linear model, one can identify nonlinear relationships between stimulus parameters (e.g., stimulus duration or presentation rate) and evoked responses. To do this one usually uses an SPM{F} (Büchel et al., 1996).

The example provided in Figure 2 illustrates subtraction, conjunction, and parametric approaches to design and analysis. These data were obtained from an fMRI study of visual motion processing using radially moving dots. The stimuli were presented over a range of speeds using isoluminant and isochromatic stimuli. To identify areas involved in visual motion, a stationary dots condition was subtracted from the moving dots conditions (see contrast weights on the upper right). To ensure significant motion-sensitive responses using both color and luminance cues, a conjunction of the equivalent subtractions was assessed under both viewing contexts. Areas V5 and V3a are seen in the SPM{T}. The responses in left V5 (lower panel) speak to a compelling inverted-U relationship between speed and evoked response that peaks at around 8°/s. It is this sort of relationship that parametric designs try to characterize. Interestingly, the form of these speed-dependent responses was similar using both stimulus types, although luminance cues elicited a greater response. From the point of view of a factorial design, there is a *main effect* of cue (isoluminant *vs.* isochromatic) and a main (nonlinear) effect of speed, but no speed by cue *interaction*.

Factorial Designs

At its simplest, an interaction represents a change in a change. Interactions are associated with factorial designs where two or more factors are combined in the same experiment. The effect of one factor on the effect of the other is assessed by the interaction term. Factorial designs have a wide range of applications (e.g., assessing physiological adaptation with time by condition interactions). Psychopharmacological activation studies are examples of factorial designs. In these studies, cognitively evoked responses are assessed before and after the subject is given a drug. The interaction term reflects the modulatory drug effect on the task-dependent activation. Factorial designs have an important role in the context of cognitive subtraction and additive factors logic by testing for context-sensitive activations, to demonstrate the fallacy of pure in-

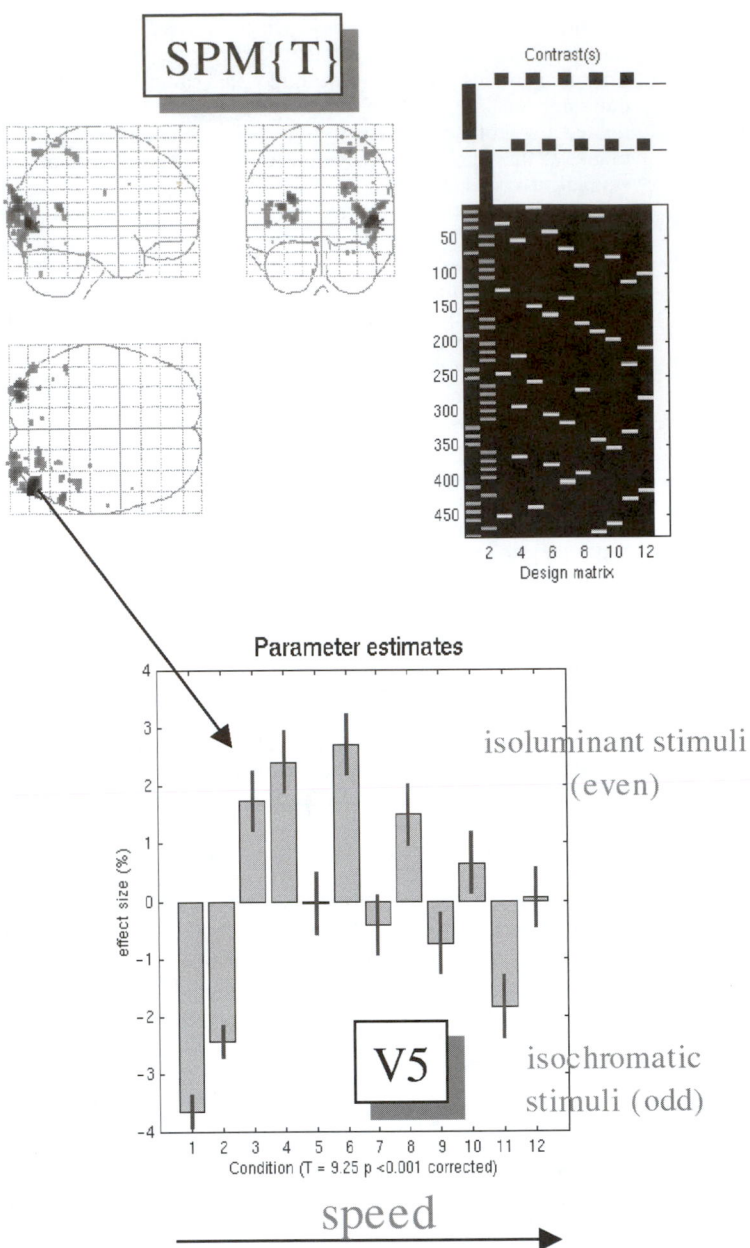

Figure 2. Shown at upper right is an image representation of the design matrix. Contrasts are the vectors of contrast weights defining the linear compounds of the parameters tested. The contrast weights are displayed over the column of the design matrix that corresponds to the effects in question. The design matrix here includes condition-specific effects (boxcars convolved with a hemodynamic response function). Odd columns correspond to stimuli shown under isochromatic conditions, and even columns model responses to isoluminant stimuli. The first two columns are for stationary stimuli and the remaining columns are for conditions of increasing speed. The final column is a constant term. At upper left is a maximum-intensity projection of the SPM{T} conforming to the standard anatomical space of Talairach and Tournoux. The T values here are the minimum T values from both contrasts, thresholded at $P = 0.001$ (uncorrected). The most significant conjunction is seen in left V5. In the lower panel is a plot of the condition-specific parameter estimates for this voxel. The T value was 9.25 ($P < 0.001$ corrected).

sertion. Pure insertion refers to the assumption that the difference between one task and another is completely specified by the difference in task demands. In other words, the difference is inserted without *interacting* with the context established by the extant task components (see Friston et al., 1996). These interaction effects can sometimes be interpreted as (1) the integration of the two or more (cognitive) processes or (2) the modulation of one process by another.

Effective Connectivity and Functional Integration

There is a necessary relationship between functional integration and multivariate analyses because the latter models interactions among brain regions. Multivariate approaches can be divided into those that are inferential in nature and those that are data led or exploratory. Most are based on the singular value or eigen decom-

position of the between-voxel covariances in a neuroimaging time series.

Eigenimage Analysis and Related Approaches

Friston et al. (1993) introduced voxel-based principal component analysis (PCA) of neuroimaging time series to characterize distributed brain systems implicated in sensorimotor, perceptual, or cognitive processes. These distributed systems are identified with principal components or eigenimages that correspond to spatial modes of coherent brain activity. This approach represents one of the simplest multivariate characterizations of functional neuroimaging time series and falls into the class of exploratory analyses. Eigenimage analysis generally uses singular value decomposition (SVD) to identify a set of orthogonal spatial modes that capture the greatest amount of variance, expressed over time. As such, the ensuing

Changes in V5 response to V2 inputs that depend on PPC activity
i.e. a modulatory component of V5 responses

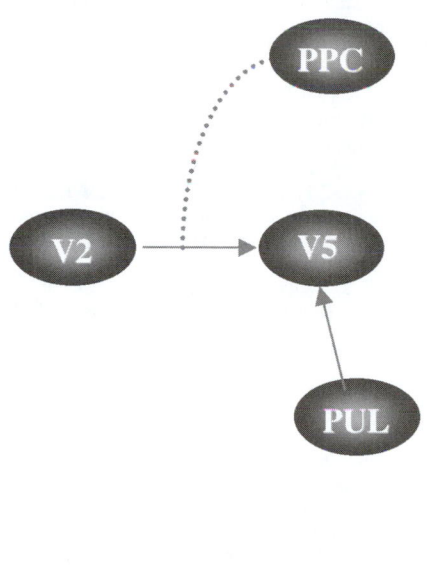

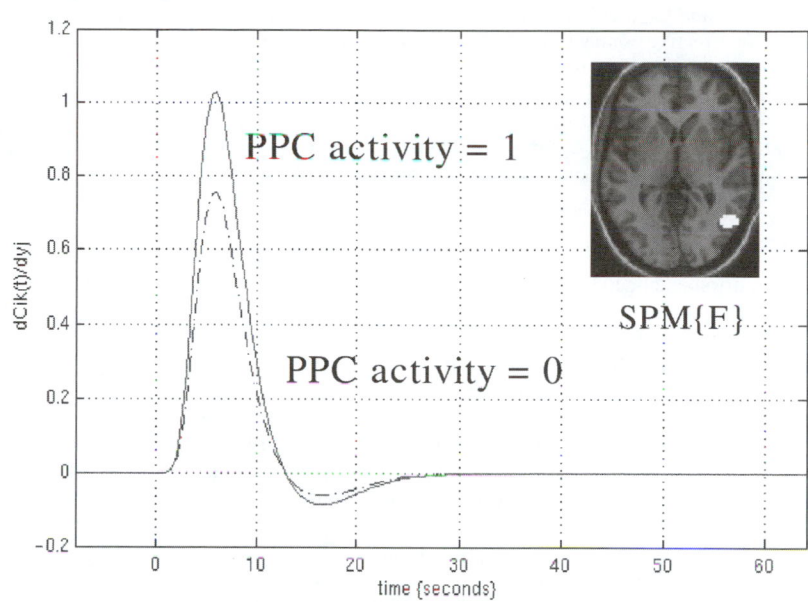

Figure 3. Characterization of effects of V2 inputs on V5 and the modulation of these effects by posterior parietal cortex (PPC). The broken lines represent estimates of V5 responses when PPC activity = 0 according to a second-order Volterra model with inputs based on the activity in V2, PPC, and the pulvinar (all normalized to zero mean and unit standard deviation). The input from V2 corresponded to a square wave of 500 ms duration convolved with a hemodynamic response function. The solid curves represent the same response when PPC activity = 1. It is evident that V2 has an activating effect on V5 and that PPC increases the responsiveness of V5 to these inputs. The insert shows all the voxels in V5 that evidenced a modulatory effect ($P < 0.05$ uncorrected). These voxels were identified by thresholding SPMs of the F statistic testing for the contribution of second-order effects involving V2 and PPC while treating all other components as confounds. Results for one subject are shown. Subjects were studied with fMRI under identical stimulus conditions (visual motion subtended by radially moving dots) while the attentional component of the task (the detection of velocity changes) was manipulated.

modes embody the most prominent aspects of the variance-covariance structure of a given time series. Noting that the covariances among brain regions are equivalent to functional connectivity (see below) renders eigenimage analysis particularly interesting, because it was among the first ways of addressing functional integration in the human brain.

Functional and Effective Connectivity

Imaging neuroscience has firmly established functional specialization as a principle of brain organization in humans. The functional integration of specialized areas has proved more difficult to assess. Functional integration is usually inferred on the basis of correlations among measurements of neuronal activity. Functional connectivity has been defined as *correlations between remote neurophysiological events.* However, correlations can arise in a variety of ways. For example, in multiunit electrode recordings they can result from stimulus-locked transients evoked by a common input, or they may reflect stimulus-induced oscillations mediated by synaptic connections (Gerstein and Perkel, 1969). Integration within a distributed system is usually better understood in terms of effective connectivity. Effective connectivity refers explicitly to *the influence that one neural system exerts over another,* either at a synaptic (i.e., synaptic efficacy) or at a population level. Effective connectivity is dynamic, i.e., activity and time dependent, and it depends

on a model of the interactions. Key here is that effective connectivity may vary from task to task (see next section), even though anatomical connections remain the same. The models employed in functional neuroimaging can be classified as (1) those based on regression models (see next section) or (2) structural equation modeling (McIntosh and Gonzalez-Lima, 1994; see also COVARIANCE STRUCTURAL EQUATION MODELING).

Characterizing Nonlinear Coupling among Brain Areas

Linear models of effective connectivity assume that the multiple inputs to a region are linearly separable. This precludes activity-dependent connections that are expressed in one sensorimotor or cognitive context and not in another. The resolution of this problem lies in adopting nonlinear models that include interactions among inputs. These interactions can be construed as a context- or activity-dependent modulation of the influence that one region exerts over another, where that context is instantiated by activity in other brain regions exerting modulatory effects. These nonlinearities are important in modeling and understanding task-specific changes in effective connectivity. From the point of view of regression models, modulatory effects can be modeled with nonlinear input-output models and in particular a Volterra series formulation (this formulation can be thought of as a polynomial regression on the activity of areas providing inputs, both now and in the recent past).

Because the kernels are high-order, they embody interactions over time and among inputs. The influence of one region j on another i can therefore be divided into two components: (1) the direct influence of j on i, irrespective of activity elsewhere, and (2) an activity-dependent component that represents an interaction with inputs from the remaining regions. The example provided in Figure 3 addresses the modulation of visual cortical responses by attentional mechanisms and the mediating role of activity- or context-sensitive changes in effective connectivity. Figure 3 shows a characterization of this modulatory effect in terms of the increase in V5 responses to V2 input when posterior parietal activity is zero (broken line) and when it is high (solid lines). This sort of result suggests that parietal activity may be a sufficient explanation for attentional modulation of visually evoked extrastriate responses.

Discussion

Functionally specialized brain areas can be identified by some form of statistical parametric mapping. The nature of the specialization and the interactions between various cognitive or sensorimotor factors in engendering a brain response can be established using simple subtraction, parametric, or multifactorial designs. Functional integration is usually assessed using some form of multivariate analysis framed in terms of effective connectivity. Recent advances in modeling effective connectivity emphasize nonlinear interactions among inputs to an area in "causing" its response.

Road Maps: Cognitive Neuroscience; Implementation and Analysis
Related Reading: Brain Signal Analysis; Covariance Structural Equation Modeling; Markov Random Field Models in Image Processing; Synthetic Functional Brain Mapping

References

Büchel, C., Wise, R. J. S., Mummery, C. J., Poline, J.-B., and Friston, K. J., 1996, Nonlinear regression in parametric activation studies, *Neuro-Image*, 4:60–66.

Frackowiak, R. S. J., Friston, K. J., Frith, C. D., Dolan, R. J., and Mazziotta, J. C., 1997, *Human Brain Function*, San Diego, CA: Academic Press.

Friston, K. J., Frith, C., Liddle, P., and Frackowiak, R. S. J., 1993, Functional connectivity: The principal component analysis of large data sets, *J. Cereb. Blood Flow Metab.*, 13:5–14.

Friston, K. J., Holmes, A. P., Worsley, K. J., Poline, J.-B., Frith, C. D., and Frackowiak, R. S. J., 1995, Statistical parametric maps in functional imaging: A general linear approach, *Hum. Brain Mapp.*, 2:189–210. ◆

Friston, K. J., Price, C. J., Fletcher, P., Moore, C., Frackowiak, R. S. J., and Dolan, R. J., 1996, The trouble with cognitive subtraction, *NeuroImage*, 4:97–104.

Gerstein, G. L., and Perkel, D. H., 1969, Simultaneously recorded trains of action potentials: Analysis and functional interpretation, *Science*, 164:828–830.

Grafton, S., Mazziotta, J., Presty, S., Friston, K. J., Frackowiak, R. S. J., and Phelps, M., 1992, Functional anatomy of human procedural learning determined with regional cerebral blood flow and PET, *J. Neurosci.*, 12:2542–2548.

Lueck, C. J., Zeki, S., Friston, K. J., Deiber, M. P., Cope, N. O., Cunningham, V. J., Lammertsma, A. A., Kennard, C., and Frackowiak, R. S. J., 1989, The colour centre in the cerebral cortex of man, *Nature*, 340:386–389.

McIntosh, A. R., and Gonzalez-Lima, F., 1994, Structural equation modelling and its application to network analysis in functional brain imaging, *Hum. Brain Mapp.*, 2:2–22. ◆

Petersen, S. E., Fox, P. T., Posner, M. I., Mintun, M., and Raichle, M. E., 1989, Positron emission tomographic studies of the processing of single words, *J. Cognit. Neurosci.*, 1:153–170.

Phillips, C. G., Zeki, S., and Barlow, H. B., 1984, Localisation of function in the cerebral cortex: Past, present and future, *Brain*, 107:327–361. ◆

Price, C. J., and Friston, K. J., 1997, Cognitive conjunction: A new approach to brain activation experiments, *NeuroImage*, 5:261–270.

Worsley, K. J., and Friston, K. J., 1995, Analysis of fMRI time-series revisited—again, *NeuroImage*, 2:173–181.

Worsley, K. J., Marrett, S., Neelin, P., Vandal, A. C., Friston, K. J., and Evans, A. C., 1996, A unified statistical approach or determining significant signals in images of cerebral activation, *Hum. Brain Mapp.*, 4:58–73. ◆

Zeki, S., 1990, The motion pathways of the visual cortex, in *Vision: Coding and Efficiency* (C. Blakemore, Ed.), Cambridge, Engl.: Cambridge University Press, pp. 321–345.

Stereo Correspondence

John P. Frisby

Introduction

Stereoscopic vision exploits the fact that points in a three-dimensional (3D) scene will in general project to different positions in the images formed in the left and right eyes. These differences are termed *retinal disparities*. They can be analyzed as vectors with horizontal and vertical components. Horizontal retinal disparities are determined both by 3D scene structure and by the positions of eyes in the head, whereas vertical retinal disparities, to first order, contain only information on eye positions (i.e., the prevailing gaze, elevation, and vergence angles of the eyes; Mayhew and Longuet-Higgins, 1982). This geometrical fact allows data from vertical disparities on eye positions to be used for disambiguating the information in horizontal disparities by way of recovering 3D scene structure.

The stereo correspondence problem is, how can a pair of stereo images be mapped into a single representation, called a *disparity map*, that makes explicit the disparities of all points common to both images? A great deal of computer vision research has addressed this problem because a disparity map is a useful first step toward building a representation of 3D scene structure. The problem is illustrated in Figure 1, which shows that the image locations of both correct and false matches fall on geometrical constructs called epipolar lines. The importance of this geometrical constraint is that it makes the stereo matching problem a one-dimensional (1D) search. Without it, the stereo problem becomes formally identical to the two-dimensional (2D) optic flow motion correspondence problem.

Most claims made in this article that are not accompanied by explicit citations are supported by references in Frisby and Pollard (1991) and Howard and Rogers (2002).

Matching Primitives

The first issue in designing any stereo algorithm is deciding what image features should serve as the points to be matched. Edge points are the most common choice because they usually stand in reasonably close correspondence to scene entities and hence they seem a sensible choice, as the ultimate goal is to deliver 3D information about scene structures (Marr, 1982). That property is not

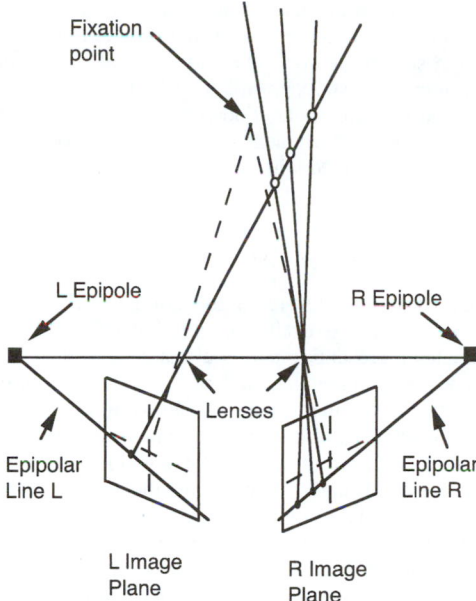

Figure 1. Epipolar geometry and the stereo correspondence problem. A line of sight is shown extending from a left (L) image point through the optic center of the lens out into the world. A sample of the possible locations in the world that could have given rise to that point are shown as unfilled circles. These are imaged in the right (R) image on a geometrical construct known as an epipolar line, thereby reducing to a single dimension the stereo correspondence problem, which is the task of deciding which points in the L and R images are to be matched.

possessed by image point intensities because a given scene entity often produces different pixel/receptor values in the left and right images. Other possible matching primitives that have been tried include image regions, for example in stereo algorithms relying on area cross-correlation (sometimes implemented with coarse-to-fine Fourier filter pyramids), and "corner points," usually defined as image features possessing a sharply peaked autocorrelation function.

Edge and corner points produce sparse disparity maps. It is possible to interpolate a dense disparity surface using processes that lend themselves readily to implementations in neural nets (Blake and Zisserman, 1987). Texture boundary cues help shape such interpolation processes in human vision.

Human stereo vision uses a diverse set of matching primitives, including dots, edges, regions, lines, and texture boundaries. It is clear that stereo matching can be achieved without recourse to matching primitives at the level of objects (chairs, faces, etc.), because human stereo vision can find correctly matching points even when no high-level objects are discernible in each stereo half-image. This is demonstrated by random-dot stereograms, made by taking two copies of a noise field, one for each stereo half-image, and then shifting chosen regions to create disparate zones, but hiding these shifts monocularly by filling in the gaps so generated with new random noise texture, a technique first richly exploited by Julesz.

Exploiting the Epipolar Constraint

Taking advantage of the 1D search characteristic of the stereo correspondence problem requires knowing the location of the right image epipolar line for a given left image primitive, or vice versa. This in turn requires a solution to the nontrivial problem of know-

ing the spatial relationships between the two cameras/eyes, as well as facts about focal length, image aspect ratios, etc. This is the business of camera calibration, as it is termed in the computational literature. Before it has been solved, images are said to be "uncalibrated." For a stereo camera rig it typically involves solving at least 12 free parameters. To find these using image data requires knowledge of at least some matching points, which sets up a vicious circle: matched points are needed to find epipolar lines, so that epipolar lines can be used to find matching points. The circle can be broken using unambiguous corner features as the inputs for an optimal least-squares fit of the various camera parameters.

The calibration problem for human stereovision is usually discussed in the psychophysical literature as a problem in stereoscopic depth constancy. Somehow human vision manages to support a stable or "constant" 3D percept (if the scene itself is unchanging), despite eye movements that radically alter retinal disparities. Therefore, it must have some way of allowing for the effects of changes in fixation position on the disparity vector field. One way to do this is to use vertical disparities to compute eye positions (see the Introduction). Another is to use oculomotor information (inflow and/or outflow) about eye positions. The relative weights given to these two cues, a topical cue integration research issue, may depend on the size of the field of view, the task, the nature of the vertical disparity cues present, and so on.

The stereo calibration problem is less severe if relief rather than metric 3D scene properties are to be recovered. The regional disparity correction theory of Gårding, Porrill, Mayhew, and Frisby (see Frisby et al., 1999) uses vertical disparities to recover 3D surface relief properties (such as planarity, collinearity, etc.) from horizontal disparities by fitting a three-parameter polynomial to regions of the vertical disparity field and then using the coefficients so obtained to correct horizontal disparities to values from which relief properties are easily obtained. Frisby et al. (1999) reported evidence that human vision implements a theory of this type even for small fields of view. Porrill et al. (1999) have shown, using robust Bayesian statistics, that the coefficients used by the regional disparity correction theory have attractive computational properties for pooling vertical disparity measurements to obtain estimates of eye positions. Their scheme is suitable for a simple Hough parameter estimation algorithm that lends itself readily to implementation in a biologically plausible neural network. This pooling scheme is remarkably robust to noise from outliers: using even ten times more incorrect than correct matches still yielded good eye position estimates. It thus allows the epipolar geometry to be recovered without having matched points (see also Zhang et al., 1995). Once epipolar geometry is recovered, it can be exploited in solving the stereo correspondence problem. However, Schreiber et al. (2001) have created stereograms suggesting that human vision does not in fact exploit the epipolar constraint. They conclude that it uses retina-fixed search zones whose size is large enough to cover all locations of the epipolar lines for the usual range of fixation positions. The size of these zones, they suggest, is minimized by the eyes twisting around their lines of sight in a way that reduces the motion of the epipolar lines as the fixation position is changed.

The fact that we can adjust, given time, to perturbations imposed by various distorting lenses shows that the "eye/head calibration" mechanisms in human vision are adaptive in character, suggesting that processes of continual recalibration are at work. These are of obvious benefit in coping with head growth during maturation, as head growth alters the important calibration parameter of interocular separation.

Constraints for Resolving the Matching Problem

Even if used, the epipolar constraint is not sufficient for solving the stereo correspondence problem because several potentially correct matching primitives will often fall on any given epipolar line. Hence other constraints are required, and these must be derived from aspects of the viewed world and its projection into stereo images. From these constraints can be inferred binocular matching rules capable of eliminating false matches while preserving correct ones.

The Constraint of Compatibility of Matching Primitives

The size of the ambiguity problem can be substantially reduced, although not altogether eliminated, by matching features of similar shape and contrast. Marr's (1982) way of expressing this constraint, which he dubbed the compatibility constraint, was to match only left and right features that could have arisen from the same scene entity. To implement this constraint requires careful attention to how scene features appear in stereo projections. This is necessary to determine bounds on the ranges of, for example, size (spatial frequency) and orientation differences allowed between left and right image features if they are to form potential matches.

The Cohesivity Constraint

Marr and Poggio argued that it is reasonable to assume the visual world is made up of matter separated into objects whose surfaces are generally smooth compared with their overall distances from the viewer (see Marr, 1982). In other words, the visual world is not usually made up only of clouds of dust particles or snowflakes. They termed this the cohesivity constraint, and they used it to underpin their continuity binocular matching rule: prefer possible matches that could have arisen from smooth surfaces. This is an example of a smoothness constraint being used as a "regularizer" for solving ill-posed vision problems, so termed because they are either under- or overdetermined (see PROBABILISTIC REGULARIZATION METHODS FOR LOW-LEVEL VISION).

The Uniqueness Constraint

Marr and Poggio also noted that a scene entity cannot be in two places at the same time, from which they derived the binocular matching rule: each matching primitive from each image may be assigned at most one disparity value.

The Figural Continuity Constraint

Mayhew and Frisby in 1981 used the cohesivity constraint to justify a different matching rule: cohesive objects generate surface edges and surface markings that are spatially continuous and therefore prefer matches which preserve figural continuity. That is, give preference to point-for-point matches that are part of an edge whose other component points also have matches, such that the whole forms a figurally continuous structure of matched points. Mayhew and Frisby found psychophysical evidence suggesting that human stereovision exploits this constraint and developed a correspondence algorithm, STEREOEDGE, based on it.

The Ordering Constraint

If opaque surfaces can be assumed, then it is possible to exploit the fact that the order of primitives along an epipolar line in one image is preserved in the other.

Neural Network Stereo Correspondence Algorithms

Much research has attempted to solve the stereo correspondence problem by implementing one or more of the above constraints with processes of excitation and inhibition in networks of elements that represent competing (usually edge-based) matches. Few network modelers have taken seriously the problem of camera calibration, often seeking to solve the (often trivially easy) problems posed by random-dot stereograms, for which rasters are assumed to be the appropriate epipolar lines. Networks differ both in the constraints they try to implement and in the details of how they do so. They will be described with reference to the diagram shown in Figure 2.

Dev's Stereo Neural Network

In 1975, Dev described a stereo algorithm using a neural network in which excitation was exchanged (giving mutual support) between elements representing potential matches with the same disparity (hence lying on the diagonals of Figure 2). The support window was in fact two-dimensional (not shown in Figure 2) because excitation was exchanged between potential matches of the same disparity lying on different epipolar lines within a local neighborhood. This use of excitation implements the cohesivity constraint because it favors matches with roughly the same depth. Inhibition was passed between elements lying on lines orthogonal to the diagonals (lines not shown in Figure 2). Marr (1982) severely criticized that way of using inhibition, arguing that it amounts to the unjustifiable constraint of forbidding double matches along radial lines extending from the viewer.

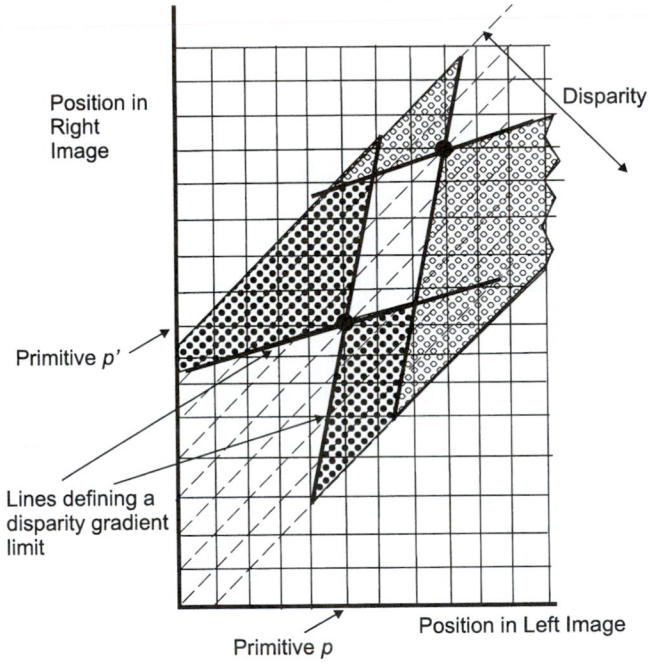

Figure 2. The axes represent the locations of matching primitives on a corresponding pair of left and right epipolar lines. The lines perpendicular to each axis represent lines of sight extending from each primitive, and their intersections represent potential matches. Primitives with zero disparity would fall on the diagonal passing through the origin. Other isodisparity planes lie parallel to that diagonal. The potential match pp' formed from the primitives p and p' and lying in a non-zero disparity plane is shown at the intersection of two bold lines whose slope reflects a particular disparity gradient. The shaded areas on one side of these lines depict, for the region of disparity space shown, zones in which neighbours of pp' would have too steep a disparity gradient with pp' to be allowed to support that match in the PMF stereo algorithm. Gradient limit lines extending from a second match are also shown to emphasize that all matches have their own region of support in disparity space.

Marr and Poggio's Stereo Neural Network

Marr and Poggio's 1976 algorithm was similar to Dev's. The difference lay in the inhibitory connections. These were between elements lying on the same line of sight, shown as the vertical and horizontal lines passing through each potential match in Figure 2. This scheme implements the uniqueness constraint properly. Mathematical analyses showed that states satisfying the cohesivity and uniqueness constraints were stable states of the network, and that the network converges for a wide range of parameter values (Marr, 1982).

PMF and the Disparity Gradient Limit Constraint

A limitation of the Dev and Marr/Poggio algorithms is that they impose a very restricted version of the cohesivity constraint, one that favors isodisparity surfaces. Yet it is evident from inspection of table tops, floors, etc., that human stereo vision copes readily with scenes with a variety of slants. Even locally isodisparity surface patches are far from being a universal characteristic of our visual world. The key idea in Pollard, Mayhew, and Frisby's stereo algorithm, called PMF (Frisby and Pollard, 1991), is that neighboring potential matches exchange support (mutual excitation) if their disparities are similar, not just if they are the same. Similarity is defined in terms of the disparity between potential matches not exceeding a disparity gradient (DG) limit. The butterfly shapes in Figure 2 illustrate the bounds on neighboring matches falling within and outside this limit. DG is defined in PMF as the difference in disparities divided by feature separation.

The use of a disparity gradient limit in PMF was prompted by human psychophysical experiments by Burt and Julesz which showed that if two disparate dots are brought closer and closer together while their disparity is kept unaltered, there comes a point (DG about 1.0) at which binocular fusion breaks down into diplopia.

The Dev and Marr/Poggio algorithms essentially imposed a DG limit of zero, by allowing only matches with the same disparity to exchange support. Using a DG limit greater than zero is much less restrictive: DGs of 1.0 arise from a planar surface with a slant of 84° for a viewing distance of 65 cm and interocular separation of 6.5 cm. One way to view the use of a DG limit is as a means of parameterizing the binocular matching rule of seeking matches that preserve surface smoothness. Perhaps it is better to say parameterizing surface jaggedness, because potential matches falling within the DG limit do not need to arise from smooth surfaces, if by that is meant adopting a selection procedure equivalent to fitting locally planar or curved surfaces. If the DG limit is set close to zero, then the disambiguating power is great, but the range of surfaces that can be dealt with is correspondingly small. This power reduces as the DG limit is increased toward the theoretical limit of 2.0 for opaque surfaces, the value obtained when the viewing direction from one eye to an opaque surface lies in that surface.

The matching strength of each potential match in PMF is computed as the sum of the strengths of all potential matches in a local image neighborhood that satisfy a moderate DG limit with respect to it. The limit used varies as the algorithm proceeds, from an initially prudent 0.5 to a finally generous 1.5. Because the probability of a neighboring match's falling within the DG limit by chance increases (almost linearly) with its distance away from the match under consideration, the contribution of each match in the neighborhood is weighted inversely by its distance away. PMF exploits the uniqueness constraint by selecting the best supported matches using winner-take-all discrete relaxation. To the basic PMF algorithm was added procedures implementing the figural continuity constraint, the use on startup of a set of strong "seed point" matches to speed up selection of subsequent matches, and

an explicit use of the ordering constraint at a late stage to resolve remaining ambiguities. This blend of good ideas, each based solidly on a good constraint, may be in keeping with the style of computation evolved by robust biological vision systems.

Surface Discontinuities and Uncorrelated Points

Even if the cohesivity constraint is utilized in a form that treats the world as "locally not very jagged," it is nevertheless true that many common scenes contain surface discontinuities that are very jagged indeed. For example, tufts of grass or hair are full of discontinuities in depth that exceed a DG limit of 1.0 in almost all directions, yet they give excellent stereo percepts. Any algorithm modeling human stereovision must be able to cope with such objects.

Within the framework of the neural net models being reviewed here, one means for doing this is to compute only the quantity of *support* that exists for a particular match, and not to exact a penalty for neighboring matches that do not satisfy the particular definition of smooth surface being implemented. For example, the extent to which the DG limit is offended by other potential matches in the neighborhood of a candidate match does not directly affect the selection procedure of PMF. The advantage of this design feature can be appreciated by considering a large step between two planar surfaces. This will create steep DGs across it but not necessarily along it. Within-DG-limit support exchanged between neighboring matches will pick out matches lying on one or the other side of the step. This will help their correct selection without introducing inappropriate evidence from the other surface, as would happen if penalties were imposed from neighbors lying outside the DG limit.

Discontinuities from opaque surfaces will usually create features in one image that do not appear in the other image because they are hidden from view. Human vision is remarkably fast at detecting uncorrelated image regions. This suggests they are utilized in some way, not just treated as noise left over after stereo matching has been completed.

The Problem of Transparency

Human stereo vision can deal successfully with points arising from overlapping transparent surfaces. The difficulty they pose is avoiding computations associated with points from one surface becoming entangled with those from other surfaces. Neural network algorithms can solve this problem in the way just described for dealing with discontinuities, namely, by computing the support for any given potential match without imposing a penalty for neighbors that do not satisfy the support rule. For a recent review, experiments, and a neural model, see Gephstein and Cooperman (1998).

Neurophysiological Studies of Disparity Mechanisms

G. F. Poggio's classification scheme for disparity-tuned V1 neurons places them into three broad types, defined in terms of whether they are tuned to disparities close to the fixation point, or to "far," or to "near" disparities. It is controversial whether these are distinct classes or whether they are better regarded as points on a continuum. Cumming and DeAngelis (2001) consider this question in a wide-ranging review of the disparity neuron literature. They note that the signals of V1 neurons differ in many ways from the perception of depth; e.g., they respond to false matches in their receptive fields. They conclude that V1 neurons probably measure binocular correlation over a range of vertical and horizontal disparities, with their outputs exploited in extrastriate cortex for a number of different tasks: stereopsis, vergence control, scene segmentation, and 3D heading judgments. Jannssen, Vogels, and Orban (2000) found that more than one-third of inferior temporal lobe neurons in rhesus monkey were selective for complex surfaces portrayed in random-dot stereograms. This implies that they must be at or after the level at which the stereo correspondence problem is solved. Backus et al. (2001) provide an example of fMRI being used to find brain regions mediating stereopsis in humans. An interesting question stimulated by neurophysiology is whether human vision relies on oriented channels for its matching primitives. Mayhew and Frisby drew a negative conclusion in 1978, based on both psychophysical and logical considerations. Farell (1998), however, reports evidence from an adaptation study suggesting that 2D (non-oriented) matches are derived from 1D (oriented) stimulus components in human stereopsis. To sum up this section, despite much progress in studying neurons linked to stereopsis, an understanding of brain mechanisms that solve the stereo correspondence problem is not yet available.

Learning Algorithms

The neural networks described in this article were hand-crafted by their originators. A topic of considerable interest is how to create networks able to learn their own constraints. O'Toole has described a stereo network model that developed connection weights implementing the smoothness constraint following associative learning of a large number of example mappings from disparity data to surface depth data. Becker and Hinton described a network that replaces an external teacher with internally derived teaching signals generated by the assumption that neighboring parts of the input have common causes in the external world. Small modules look at separate but related parts of the input and discover these common causes by striving to produce outputs that agree with each other, thereby learning to exploit the smoothness constraint. Stone (1996) has devised a learning scheme based on the general principle that perceptually salient visual invariances, such as surface depth, vary smoothly over time. His algorithm uses a learning rule that maximizes the long-term variance of the state of a model neuron and simultaneously minimizes its short-term variance. This approach proved sufficient for estimating subpixel stereo disparities from random-dot stereograms.

Discussion

The main point emphasized throughout has been that neural network approaches to the stereo correspondence problem (as indeed any others) need to be firmly grounded in an analysis of the task to be solved by way of discovering constraints to be implemented in the network. It is also worth emphasizing that solving the stereo correspondence problem as it has been posed here produces a disparity map that is simply another iconic (image-like) representation that itself needs to be interpreted if the information it contains is to be used, for example, for controlling visually guided behavior.

Thus there is much more to stereo vision than solving the stereo correspondence problem. A further limitation of the models described here is that they do not meet the challenges posed by eye movements. In this connection, it is worth noting the potential importance of seeking to establish stereo correspondence in the context of binocular image flows over time.

Road Map: Vision
Related Reading: Motion Perception: Elementary Mechanisms; Perception of Three-Dimensional Structure; Tensor Voting and Visual Segmentation

References

Backus, B. T., Fleet, D. J, Parker, A. J., and Heeger, D. J., 2001, Human cortical activity correlates with stereoscopic depth perception, *J. Neurophysiol.*, 86:2054–2068.
Blake, A., and Zisserman, A., 1987, *Visual Reconstruction*, Cambridge, MA: MIT Press.
Cumming, B. G., and DeAngelis, G. C., 2001, The physiology of stereopsis, *Annu. Rev. Neurosci.*, 24:203–238. ◆
Farell, B., 1998, Two-dimensional matches from one-dimensional stimulus components in human stereopsis, *Nature*, 395:689–692.
Frisby, J. P., Buckley, D., Grant, H., Gårding, J., Horsman, J., Hippisley-Cox, S. D., and Porrill, J., 1999, An orientation anisotropy in the effects of scaling vertical disparities, *Vision Res.*, 39:481–492. ◆
Frisby, J. P., and Pollard, S. B., 1991, Computational issues in solving the stereo correspondence problem, in *Computational Models of Visual Processing* (M. Landy and J. A. Movshon, Eds.), Cambridge, MA: MIT Press, pp. 331–358. ◆
Gephstein, S., and Cooperman, A., 1998, Stereoscopic transparency: A test for binocular vision's disambiguating power, *Vision Res.*, 38:2913–2932.
Howard, I. P., and Rogers, B. J., 2002, *Seeing in Depth, Vol. 1: Basic Mechanisms*, Howard, I. P.; *Vol. 2: Depth Perception*, Howard, I. P., and Rogers, B. J., Published by I. Porteous, 49 Dove Lane, Thornhill, Ontario, L3T 1W1 Canada, iporteous@hpl.crestech.ca.
Jannsen, P., Vogels, R., and Orban, G. A., 2000, Selectivity for 3D shape that reveals distinct areas within Macaque inferior temporal cortex, *Science*, 288:2054–2056.
Marr, D., 1982, *Vision*, San Francisco: Freeman. ◆
Mayhew, J. E. W., and Longuet-Higgins, H. C., 1982, A computational model of binocular depth perception, *Nature*, 297:376–379.
Porrill, J. P., Frisby, J. P., Adams, W., and Buckley, D., 1999, A robust ideal observer model of vertical disparity pooling by the human visual system, *Nature*, 397:63–66.
Schreiber, K., Crawford, J. D., Fetter, M., and Tweed, D., 2001, The motor side of depth vision, *Nature*, 410:819–822.
Stone, J., 1996, Learning perceptually salient visual parameters using spatiotemporal smoothness constraints, *Neural Computat.*, 8:1463–1492.
Zhang, Z. X., Deriche, R., Faugeras, O., and Luong, Q. T., 1995, A robust technique for matching two uncalibrated images through the recovery of the unknown epipolar geometry, *Artif. Intell.*, 78:87–119.

Stochastic Approximations and Efficient Learning

Léon Bottou and Noboru Murata

Introduction

Many learning algorithms work by repeatedly picking one example and updating the learning system parameters on the basis of this example only. The evolving state of the parameters is the only trace of the previously seen examples. These algorithms, called *stochastic algorithms* or *on-line algorithms*, date back to early work on recursive identification and learning systems (Robbins and Monro, 1951; Widrow and Hoff, 1960; Amari, 1967; Tsypkin, 1971). This was the dawn of the computer age. Algorithmic simplicity was a practical requirement.

The analysis of on-line algorithms is much more difficult than that of ordinary optimization algorithms. Practical successes in signal processing (Widrow and Stearns, 1985) motivated the creation of sophisticated mathematical tools known as *stochastic approximations* (Ljung and Söderström, 1983; Benveniste, Metivier, and Priouret, 1990).

On-line algorithms are still extremely useful because they enjoy significant performance advantages for large-scale learning problems (Le Cun et al., 1998). This article describes their properties using the stochastic approximation theory as a very broad framework, and provides a brief overview of newer insights obtained using information geometry (see NEUROMANIFOLDS AND INFORMATION GEOMETRY) and replica calculations (see STATISTICAL MECHANICS OF ON-LINE LEARNING AND GENERALIZATION).

The first section describes and illustrates a general framework for neural network learning algorithms based on stochastic gradient descent. The second section presents stochastic approximation results describing the *final phase*. The third section discusses the conceptual aspects of the *search phase* and comments on some of the latest results.

Stochastic Gradient

This section presents a simplified version of the general framework for stochastic gradient learning algorithms introduced in Tsypkin (1971). Several examples of neural network learning algorithms are discussed in this context.

Stochastic Gradient and Backpropagation

Let us introduce the necessary concepts using the well-known example of multilayer networks (see PERCEPTRONS, ADALINES, AND BACKPROPAGATION). Each example z is a pair composed of an input pattern x and a desired output y. The output of a multilayer network is a differentiable function $f(x, w)$ of the input pattern x and the network weight vector w. The performance of the network on a particular example $z = (x, y)$ is measured by a *loss function* $Q(z, w)$. In the multilayer network case, the loss function usually is the square of the distance between the desired output y and the network output $f(z, w)$:

$$Q_{\text{mse}}(z, w) \overset{\Delta}{=} \tfrac{1}{2} (y - f(x, w))^2 \qquad (1)$$

One seeks a weight vector w that minimizes the loss function averaged over the examples. There is, however, a subtlety in how we define this average. Do we average over the few examples available in the training set, or over all the examples that nature cares to produce? The first average is named *empirical risk* and measures only the training set performance. The second average is called the *expected risk* and measures the much more interesting generalization performance (Vapnik, 1998).

Both empirical and expected risk can be written as:

$$C(w) \overset{\Delta}{=} \mathbf{E}_z Q(z, w) \overset{\Delta}{=} \int Q(z, w)dP(z) \qquad (2)$$

where $dP(z)$ represents a probability distribution of examples and $\mathbf{E}_z$ represents the expectation with respect to this distribution. In the case of the expected risk, $dP(z)$ is an unknown *ground truth distribution* representing the laws of nature. In the case of the empirical risk, $dP(z)$ is a discrete distribution defined by the training set examples $z_{(1)} \ldots z_{(L)}$. The expectation in Equation 2 then reduces to a simple average, $1/L \Sigma_i Q(z_{(i)}, w)$.

It has often been suggested (e.g., Rumelhart, Hinton, and Williams, 1986) to minimize the risk in Equation 2 by using a gradient descent algorithm. Each iteration of the algorithms moves the weights along the steepest descent direction,

$$w_{t+1} = w_t - \gamma_t \int \nabla_w Q(z, w_t)dP(z) \qquad (3)$$

where γ_t is an adequately chosen positive learning rate and $\nabla_w Q$ denotes the gradient of the loss function Q with respect to the

weight vector w. This optimization algorithm cannot be used to optimize the expected risk case because the ground truth distribution is unknown. One must optimize the empirical risk instead and hope that the training set performance is a good predictor of the generalization performance. Each iteration of this *batch gradient descent* involves visiting all of the training examples in order to compute the average gradient.

The *stochastic gradient descent* algorithm is a drastic simplification of the above algorithm. Each iteration consists of picking a single random example z_t, and updating the weight vector w according to the following rule:

$$w_{t+1} = w_t - \gamma_t \nabla_w Q(z_t, w_t) \qquad (4)$$

This algorithm illustrates the concept of *stochastic approximation*. It is hoped that iterating Equation 4 behaves like iterating its mean (Equation 3), despite the noise introduced by this simplified procedure.

The stochastic gradient descent does not need to remember which examples were visited during the previous iterations. This makes this algorithm suitable for the on-line adaptation of deployed systems. In such a situation, the stochastic gradient descent directly optimizes the expected risk, since the examples are randomly drawn from the ground truth distribution.

The stochastic gradient descent can also pick examples from a finite training set. This procedure optimizes the empirical risk. The number of iterations is usually larger than the size of the training set. The examples are therefore presented multiple times to the network.

General Stochastic Gradient Descent

The preceding example suggests a more general framework:

Let us consider a learning system whose goal consists in minimizing a cost function (Equation 2) that can be expressed as the expectation of a loss function, $Q(z, w)$. Each iteration of the *generalized stochastic gradient descent algorithm* consists in picking a random example z_t and updating the parameter vector w using the update rule in Equation 4.

A number of well-known learning algorithms can be viewed as particular cases of the generalized stochastic gradient descent algorithm. A few examples are presented in the following discussion. Additional examples can be found in Bottou (1998). Most results discussed in this contribution are based on the general framework and therefore apply to all of these learning systems alike.

Adaline. The early neural network learning algorithms adapt the parameters of a single threshold unit. Input patterns x are recognized as members of class $y = \pm 1$ according to the sign of dot product $w'x$. Each iteration of the adaline learning algorithm (Widrow and Hoff, 1960) takes one training example $z_t = (x_t, y_t)$ and applies the *delta rule*:

$$w_{t+1} = w_t + \gamma_t(y_t - w'_t x_t)x_t \qquad (5)$$

This is nothing more than an iteration of the stochastic gradient descent algorithm in Equation 4 with the following loss function:

$$Q_{\text{adaline}}(z, w) \overset{\Delta}{=} \tfrac{1}{2} (y - w'x)^2 \qquad (6)$$

The adaline loss function does not take the discontinuity of the threshold unit into account. It is much more difficult to optimize the apparently more natural loss function $(y - \text{sign}(w'x))^2$ because its gradient is null almost everywhere.

Perceptron. The perceptron algorithm provides a slightly different solution. The weights are updated according to the following rule if and only if the current example, $z_t = (x_t, y_t)$, is misclassified:

$$w_{t+1} = w_t + \gamma_t y_t x_t \qquad (7)$$

This learning algorithm can be derived as an on-line gradient descent applied to the following loss function:

$$Q_{\text{perceptron}}(z, w) \triangleq \tfrac{1}{2}(\text{sign}(w'x) - y)w'x \qquad (8)$$

The loss function is not differentiable when $w'x$ is null. It has been shown that the average behavior of the stochastic gradient algorithm is not affected by such mild nondifferentiabilities (Bottou, 1998).

Unsupervised clustering. The k-means algorithm is a popular clustering method that dispatches K centroids $w(k)$ in order to find clusters in a set of points $x_1, \ldots, x_L$. This algorithm can be derived by performing the on-line gradient descent with the following loss function:

$$Q_{\text{kmeans}}(x, w) \triangleq \tfrac{1}{2} \min_k (x - w(k))^2 \qquad (9)$$

This loss function measures the average error achieved when each point x is replaced by the nearest centroid $k^*(x)$. The mild nondifferentiability of this loss function on the cluster region boundaries are handled as in the perceptron case. Equation 4 then yields the k-means algorithm:

$$w_{t+1}(k) = w_t(k) + \gamma_t \begin{cases} x_t - w_t(k) & \text{if } k = k^*(x_t) \\ 0 & \text{otherwise} \end{cases} \qquad (10)$$

Stochastic Gradient Dynamics

Given a suitable choice of the learning rates γ_t, the ordinary gradient descent algorithm (Equation 3) is known to converge to a local minimum of the cost function. This local minimum is a function of the initial parameters w_0. The parameter trajectory follows the meanders of the local attraction basin and eventually reaches the corresponding minimum.

The random noise introduced by stochastic gradient descent (Equation 4) disrupts this deterministic picture. The parameter trajectory can jump from basin to basin. One usually distinguishes a *search phase*, which explores the parameter space, and a *final phase*, which takes place in the vicinity of a minimum.

Final Phase

Convergence

The final convergence phase takes place in the vicinity of a single minimum w^*. The following results rely on the *general convexity* hypothesis:

$$\forall \varepsilon > 0, \quad \inf_{(w - w^*)^2 > \varepsilon} (w - w^*) \nabla_w C(w) > 0 \qquad (11)$$

This hypothesis simply states that the opposite of the gradient always points toward the minimum w^*. This hypothesis usually holds within the final convergence region because the cost function is locally convex.

In order to obtain convergence, the parameter updates $\gamma_t \nabla_w Q(z, w)$ must become smaller and smaller when the parameter vector approaches the optimum w^*. This implies that either the gradients or the learning rates must vanish in the vicinity of the optimum.

The size of the gradients can be described with a first-order expansion of $\nabla_w Q$ in w^*. There usually are constants $A, B \geq 0$ such that the following bound holds within the final convergence region:

$$\mathbf{E}_z(\nabla_w Q(z, w)^2)) \approx \mathbf{E}_z(\nabla_w Q(z, w^*)^2) + \mathbf{E}_z((w - w^*) \ldots)$$
$$< A + B(w - w^*)^2 \qquad (12)$$

The constant A must be greater than the residual variance of the gradients at the optimum $\mathbf{E}_z(\nabla_w Q(z, w^*)^2)$. This residual variance can be zero for certain rare noiseless problems where w^* simultaneously optimizes the loss for every example. It is strictly positive in most practical cases. The average norm of the gradients then does not vanish when the parameter vector w approaches the optimum. Therefore, one must use *decreasing learning rates*, e.g.:

$$\sum \gamma_t^2 < \infty \qquad (13)$$

The presence of constant A in Equation 12 marks a critical difference between stochastic gradient descent and ordinary gradient descent. There is no such constant in the case of the ordinary gradient descent. A simple analysis then yields an expression for the maximal constant learning rate (Le Cun et al., 1998). In the stochastic gradient case, this analysis suggests that the parameter vector eventually hovers around the minimum w^* at a distance roughly proportional to γ_t. Quickly decreasing the learning rate is therefore tempting. Suppose, however, that the learning rates decrease so fast that $\Sigma \gamma_t = R < \infty$. This would effectively maintain the parameters within a certain radius of their initial value. It is therefore necessary to enforce the following condition:

$$\sum \gamma_t = \infty \qquad (14)$$

The general convexity hypothesis (Equation 11) and the three conditions given in Equations 12, 13, and 14 are sufficient conditions for the almost sure convergence of the stochastic gradient descent (Equation 4) to the optimum w^* (Bottou, 1998).

Second-Order Methods

Significant speed-ups of the final phase can be achieved using second-order methods (Le Cun et al., 1998). The simplest second-order method rescales the gradient vector using the inverse of the Hessian matrix $H(w_t)$ in a manner analogous to Newton's algorithm:

$$w_{t+1} = w_t - \gamma_t H(w_t)^{-1} \nabla_w Q(z_t, w_t) \qquad (15)$$

It is, however, preferable to use instead the Gauss-Newton matrix (Le Cun et al., 1998) or the Fisher information matrix (described later under Natural Gradient). These matrices asymptotically behave like the Hessian matrix and also provide superior performance during the search phase.

State-of-the-art batch optimization algorithms (Dennis and Schnabel, 1983) reach so-called superlinear convergence speed *on the training set* using such second-order methods. Such speeds are not possible with stochastic gradient because the convergence speed is determined by the learning rate schedule, which is limited by the condition in Equation 14. This speed limit has often been presented as a severe drawback. However, training algorithms are about the generalization of performance. Well-designed second-order stochastic algorithm have been shown to saturate the Crámer-Rao bound (Murata, 1998). This result means that batch algorithms that converge faster on the training set are merely overtraining.

Search Phase

Although our understanding of the search phase is still very incomplete, empirical and theoretical evidences indicate that stochastic gradient algorithms enjoy significant advantages over batch algorithms.

Stochastic gradient descent can take advantage of the redundancies of the training set. Consider the extreme case, where a training set of size 1,000 is inadvertently composed of 10 identical copies of a set with 100 samples. Averaging the gradient over all 1,000 patterns gives exactly the same result as computing the gradient based on just the first 100. Batch gradient descent is wasteful because it recomputes the same quantity 10 times before one parameter update occurs. On the other hand, stochastic gradient descent will see a full epoch as 10 iterations through a 100-long training set.

The stochastic approximation tools provide only weak results on the search phase (e.g., Bottou, 1998). Stronger results have been obtained using information geometry (see NEUROMANIFOLDS AND INFORMATION GEOMETRY) and statistical mechanics (see STATISTICAL MECHANICS OF ON-LINE LEARNING AND GENERALIZATION). This section reviews what new information has been brought by these new approaches.

Information Geometry

Describing the geometry of the cost function is paramount to understanding the convergence of a training algorithm. The final phase results, for instance, are built on two hypotheses (Equations 11 and 12) that adequately summarize the geometry of the cost function in the final convergence region. This is much more difficult to achieve for the search phase because the parameter vector can explore every aspect of the cost function.

Information geometry provides an elegant description of the global geometry of the cost function. It is best introduced by casting the learning problem as a density estimation problem. A multilayer perceptron $f(x, w)$, for instance, can be regarded as a parametric regression model $y = f(x, w) + \varepsilon$, where ε represents an additive Gaussian noise. The network function $f(x, w)$ then becomes part of the Gaussian location model:

$$p(z, w) = C \exp\left(-\frac{(y - f(x, w))^2}{2\sigma^2}\right) \quad (16)$$

The optimal parameters are found by minimizing the Kullback-Leibler divergence between $p(z, w)$ and the ground truth $P(z)$. This is equivalent to the familiar optimization of the mean square loss in Equation 1:

$$\mathbf{E}_z \log \frac{P(z)}{p(z, w)} = \frac{1}{\sigma^2} \mathbf{E}_z Q_{mse}(z, w) + \text{Constant} \quad (17)$$

The essential idea consists of endowing the space of the parameters w with a distance that reflects the proximity of the distributions $p(z, w)$ instead of the proximity of the parameters w. Multilayer networks, for instance, can implement the same function with very different weight vectors. The new distance distorts the geometry of the parameter space in order to represent the closeness of these weight vectors.

The infinitesimal distance between distributions $p(z, w)$ and $p(z, w + dw)$ can be written as follows:

$$D(w \| w + dw) \approx dw' J(w) dw \quad (18)$$

where $J(w)$ is the Fisher information matrix:

$$J(w) \overset{\Delta}{=} \int (\nabla_w \log p(z, w) \nabla_w \log p(z, w')) p(z, w) dz \quad (19)$$

The determinant $|J(w)|$ of the Fisher information matrix usually is a smooth function of the parameter w. The parameter space is therefore composed of *Riemannian domains* where $|J(w)| \neq 0$, separated by *critical subspaces* where $|J(w)| = 0$.

Natural Gradient

Natural gradient (see NEUROMANIFOLDS AND INFORMATION GEOMETRY) provides an almost ideal way to search a Riemannian domain. The gradient $\nabla_w C(w)$ defines the steepest descent direction in the Euclidian space. The steepest descent direction in a Riemannian domain differs from the Euclidian one. It is defined as the

vector dw that maximizes $C(w) - C(w + dw)$ in the δ-neighborhood:

$$D(w \| w + dw) \approx dw' J(w) dw \leq \delta \quad (20)$$

A simple derivation then shows that multiplying the gradient by the inverse of the Fisher information matrix yields the steepest Riemannian direction. The natural gradient algorithm applies the same correction to the stochastic gradient descent algorithm in Equation 4:

$$w_{t+1} = w_t - \gamma_t J^{-1}(w_t) \nabla_w Q(z, w_t) \quad (21)$$

The similarity between the update rules in Equations 15 and 21 is obvious. This link becomes clearer when the Fisher information matrix is written in Hessian form:

$$J(w) \overset{\Delta}{=} \int -(\nabla_w^2 \log p(z, w)) p(z, w) dz \quad (22)$$

where ∇_w^2 denotes a second derivative. When the parameter approaches the optimum, distribution $p(z, w)$ becomes closer to the ground truth $dP(z)$, and the Fisher information matrix aligns with the Hessian matrix $\nabla_w^2 \mathbf{E}_z Q(z, w)$. The natural gradient asymptotically behaves like the Newtonian algorithm.

Critical Subspaces and Symmetries

Consider a neural network with two fully connected layers and n hidden units. The weight space contains at least $n!$ symmetric Riemannian domains corresponding to all permutations of the hidden units and delimited by critical subspaces. The cost landscape in the vicinity of a critical subspace contains multiple directions along which no first-order change of the cost can be detected. Such critical subspaces create considerable problems for gradient descent algorithms. Batch gradient descent often remains trapped in these extremely flat regions of the cost landscape, because the gradient $\nabla_w C(w)$ is zero along those directions that would allow the algorithm to escape the critical subspace.

These problems arise because the gradient vector no longer carries enough information to describe the local cost geometry. Unlike their batch counterpart, stochastic gradient algorithms have a random component and therefore can resort to luck in picking each training example z_t. A lucky pick sometimes transports the parameter vector into a more interesting area of the cost landscape.

Critical subspaces have both a hierarchical and a symmetric structure (Fukumizu and Amari, 2000). Replica calculations (see STATISTICAL MECHANICS OF ON-LINE LEARNING AND GENERALIZATION) have brought new insights into the symmetry-breaking properties of on-line algorithms. The natural gradient algorithm in Equation 21 seems to perform remarkably well (Rattray and Saad, 1999) in this context too.

Discussion

On-line learning algorithms were introduced early in the computer age because of their low computational requirements. Today, on-line learning algorithms enjoy significant performance advantages for large-scale learning problems (large dimension, millions of examples). On-line algorithms are also mandatory when a system must continuously adapt while being used.

A large number of common learning algorithms can be understood as instances of the general stochastic gradient descent algorithm. The stochastic approximation theory provides a general analysis of the convergence of these algorithms. This analysis describes very accurately the behavior of on-line algorithms in the vicinity of a local solution. Second-order on-line algorithms provide asymptotically optimal convergence speed.

The behavior of on-line algorithms during the search phase is much less understood. Information geometry pictures the search space as an ensemble of Riemannian manifolds separated by critical subspaces. Critical subspaces cause considerable problems to all gradient algorithms. On-line gradient algorithms can overcome these problems, thanks to noise introduced by the random example selection process. Methods from statistical mechanics have recently brought new insights to this topic. These results might be the precursors of vastly more efficient on-line learning algorithms.

Road Map: Learning in Artificial Networks
Related Reading: Neuromanifolds and Information Geometry; Perceptrons, Adalines, and Backpropagation; Statistical Mechanics of On-Line Learning and Generalization

References

Amari, S., 1967, A theory of adaptive pattern classifiers, *IEEE Trans. Electr. Comput.*, EC-16:299–307.
Benveniste, A., Metivier, M., and Priouret, P., 1990, *Adaptive Algorithms and Stochastic Approximations*, Berlin and New York: Springer-Verlag. ◆
Bottou, L., 1998, Online algorithms and stochastic approximations, in *Online Learning and Neural Networks* (D. Saad, Ed.), Cambridge, Engl.: Cambridge University Press, pp. 9–42.
Dennis, J., and Schnabel, R. B., 1983, *Numerical Methods For Unconstrained Optimization and Nonlinear Equations*, Englewood Cliffs, NJ: Prentice Hall. ◆
Fukumizu, K., and Amari, S., 2000, Local minima and plateaus in hierarchical structures of multilayer perceptrons, *Neural Netw.*, 13:317–320.
Le Cun, Y., Bottou, L., Orr, G. B., and Müller, K.-R., 1998, Efficient backprop, in *Neural Networks: Tricks of the Trade*, Lecture Notes in Computer Science 1524, New York: Springer-Verlag. ◆
Ljung, L., and Söderström, T., 1983, *Theory and Practice of Recursive Identification*, Cambridge, MA: MIT Press. ◆
Murata, N., 1998, A statistical study of on-line learning, in *Online Learning and Neural Networks* (D. Saad, Ed.), Cambridge, Engl.: Cambridge University Press. pp. 63–92.
Rattray, M., and Saad, D., 1999, Analysis of natural gradient descent for multilayer neural networks, *Phys. Rev. E*, 59:4523–4532.
Robbins, H., and Monro, S., 1951, A stochastic approximation model, *Ann. Math. Stat.*, 22:400–407.
Rumelhart, D. E., Hinton, G. E., and Williams, R. J. 1986, Learning internal representations by error propagation, in *Parallel Distributed Processing: Explorations in the Microstructure of Cognition*, vol. 1, Cambridge, MA: Bradford Books/MIT Press, pp. 318–362.
Tsypkin, Y., 1971, *Adaptation and Learning in Automatic Systems*, New York: Academic Press. ◆
Vapnik, V. N., 1998, *Statistical Learning Theory*, New York: Wiley. ◆
Widrow, B., and Hoff, M. E., 1960, Adaptive switching circuits, in *IRE WESCON Convention Record*, Part 4, Institute of Radio Engineers, pp. 96–104.
Widrow, B., and Stearns, S. D., 1985, *Adaptive Signal Processing*, Englewood Cliffs, NJ: Prentice Hall. ◆

Stochastic Resonance

Frank Moss

Introduction

Definition of Stochastic Resonance

Stochastic resonance (SR) is an essentially nonlinear phenomenon whereby the addition of a random process, or noise, to a weak incoming signal can enhance the probability that it will be detected by a system. Information about the signal transmitted through the system is also enhanced. An optimal intensity of noise results in maximal enhancements. The information content or detectability of the signal is degraded for noise intensities that are either smaller or larger than the optimal value. The phenomenon is exhibited in Figure 1A where the system can be thought of as a "black box."

Only three ingredients are necessary. The actions within our black box are diagrammed in Figure 1A. The threshold is shown by the dashed line and the subthreshold signal, $A \sin(\omega t)$, by the heavy solid line. The magnitude of the threshold, measured from the mean of the subthreshold signal, is designated Δ_0. A noise (random process), as shown by the gray, irregular line, has been added to the subthreshold signal. Positive-going threshold crossings of the combined signal plus noise are marked above by the train of standard-shaped (narrow) pulses. The noise can be external, for example, environmental noise (perhaps including thermal fluctuations) that adds to the signal to be detected by a sensory neural modality; or it could be internal, for example, deterministic noise generated by dynamical processes within the sensory neurons or even in the brain where the sensory signal is interpreted.

As we can see, it is noise that causes the threshold crossings and hence the output marker pulses above. In the absence of noise there would be no threshold crossings and consequently no output. Thus it is the noise that makes the subthreshold signal detectable in our paradigm. Although the marker pulses, analogous to neural action potentials, seem randomly spaced in time, they carry a surprising amount of information about the subthreshold signal. This is because the probability of threshold crossing is much larger at the locations of the maxima of the signal than at the minima. In sensory neuroscience this is called "rate coding," the mean rate of firings being determined by how close the membrane potential is to the threshold. We can see that the noise serves as a sampling function of the signal, but each sample carries only one bit of information—the time of the threshold crossing. Signal amplitude information is encoded only in the mean rate of threshold crossings.

Thus, only three ingredients are necessary for SR: a threshold, a subthreshold signal, and noise. These three ingredients are ubiquitous in both natural and in manmade systems, so it is not surprising that SR has been found in many of them (Moss, Pierson, and O'Gorman, 1994; Anishchenko et al., 1999).

The threshold: A fundamentally simple nonlinear system. Stochastic resonance appears only in a class of *nonlinear* systems, the simplest examples of which are those systems characterized by a "hard" threshold. Let us consider the input-output characteristic of such a system. If the amplitude of the input is smaller than (or equal to) the threshold, the output is zero. If the amplitude of the input is larger than the threshold, the output equals the input multiplied by some gain factor. Thus, no signal (input) can be detected or transmitted through the system to the output unless the threshold is exceeded.

Thresholds and noise are ubiquitous in both manmade and natural systems; indeed, SR is found in diverse areas. But here we focus on SR as it appears in several biological settings (Moss and Wiesenfeld, 1995): the mechanosensory system of the crayfish, the

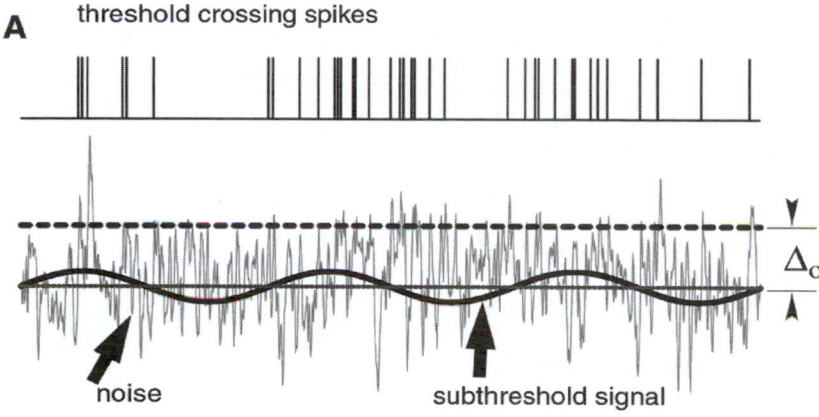

A threshold crossing spikes

noise   subthreshold signal

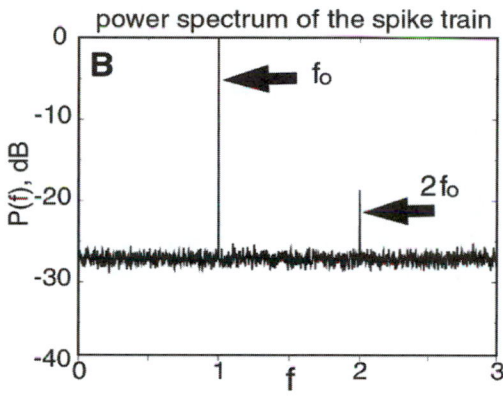

B power spectrum of the spike train

f_0

$2f_0$

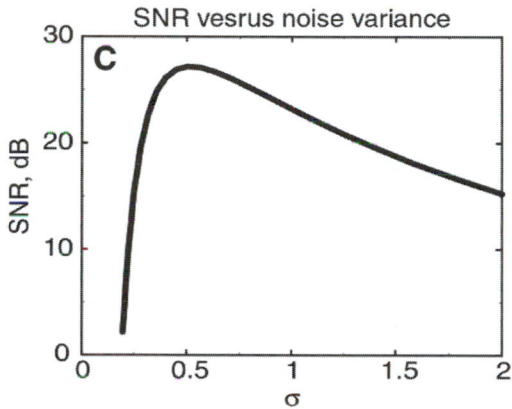

C SNR vesrus noise variance

Figure 1. *A*, The three ingredients necessary for stochastic resonance (SR): a threshold (dashed line), a subthreshold signal (solid sinusoidal line), and noise (irregular shaded line). Threshold crossings of the combined (sinusoid + noise) induce standard responses, or outputs, shown by the train of spikes above. *B*, The power spectrum of the spike train, showing strong evidence of the subthreshold signal as the sharp peaks at f_0 and $2f_0$ riding on a broadband noise background (horizontal irregular line). *C*, The signal-to-noise ratio versus the standard deviation of the noise added to the subthreshold signal in Figure 1*A*. The presence of a maximum at an optimal noise intensity is the signature of SR.

electrosensory system of the paddlefish, human cognition and perception, and the human baroreflexive system. And for simplicity we consider only hard thresholds, though soft thresholds (typically sigmoidal), which abound in neuroscience, also show SR. We consider a simple paradigm: a black box containing the threshold, with an input and output. If the threshold is crossed in the positive-going direction under the influence of an input signal (of sufficient amplitude), the black box outputs a single pulse of standard shape, for example, a narrow pulse of unit amplitude. Otherwise it outputs nothing. This seems somewhat abstract, but it was the earliest model to account for the generation of action potentials by sensory neurons. When a threshold (typically around -50 mV for mammals) is crossed from below by the membrane potential, the neuron "fires," or generates an action potential of standard amplitude and shape that propagates along the axon.

The Signature of Stochastic Resonance

The signature of SR is that some measure of the information content of the marker pulse train shown in Figure 1*A* passes through a maximum at some optimal value of the noise intensity. Considering the noise as a sampling function, we can see that if the noise intensity is too small, the signal is undersampled and information

about it is lost. If the noise intensity is too large, the samples become randomized and information about the signal is masked by the large noise. Thus the information is a maximum at an optimal noise intensity.

One measure, commonly used by communications engineers, is the signal-to-noise ratio (SNR) based on measures of the power spectrum. The power spectrum shows the amount of power contained in the signal on a scale of frequency. Figure 1*B* depicts the power spectrum of the marker pulse train shown in Figure 1*A*. We note sharp peaks (indicating large power) at the signal frequency, f_0, and its second harmonic, $2f_0$. The horizontal irregular line marks the background randomness of the marker train induced by the noise added to the signal. The SNR is the ratio of the power contained within the peak to the power (in a unit bandwidth) of the noise background at the signal frequency. Figure 1*C* shows a graph of the SNR versus the noise intensity, σ. (In this simulation the noise is Gaussian distributed with standard deviation σ.) The graph shows that the SNR passes through a maximum at optimal noise intensity.

Sensory biologists are more familiar with the probability distributions of the time intervals between spikes. A related topic is called "skipping." Skipping occurs when no, one, or just a few spikes are generated near the signal maxima. As can be seen from

Figure 1*A*, the time between spikes at every maximum should be close to the period *T* of the signal. Skipping is represented by time intervals of 2*T*, 3*T*, etc. Thus we expect to see a sequence of maxima in the probability distribution of interspike intervals; indeed, such distributions have been observed in sensory biology for a very long time. Only recently have we achieved a quantitative understanding that such multimodal distributions with exponentially decreasing peak amplitudes are the result of our three ingredients (Longtin, Bulsara, and Moss, 1991). Skipping is related to SR in the sense that there is a maximum of information about the subthreshold signal contained in the multimodal distribution at optimal noise intensity.

Stochastic Resonance in Cell Membrane Ion Channels

Our outline of the development of SR in biology is not chronological; rather, it commences with the application of smallest physical size—a single protein molecule—and proceeds up the scale of size and complexity to whole-animal behavior and human psychophysics.

A few years ago, Bezrukov and Vodyanoy (1995) published the results of a remarkable experiment. They measured the current through an array of artificial, voltage-dependent ion channels, each a single alamethicin molecule embedded in a lipid bilayer. The individual ion channels may open to allow a through-flow of positive ions or close to terminate the current. The probability of opening or closing is determined by the potential. The array is characterized by a sigmoidal threshold curve that is essentially a measure of the mean opening probability of the ion channels as a function of the potential across the bilayer. The key is to modulate the bilayer potential with a weak signal that is a near-subthreshold, periodic potential plus noise, precisely as shown in Figure 1*A*. Then the current through the array, though noisy, carries information about the subthreshold signal. Figure 2*A* shows a power spectrum of the current transmitted through the array. The signal feature shows as a sharp spike at $f_0 = 0.5$ Hz, and its second harmonic at $2f_0 = 1$ Hz is also visible, much like the threshold simulation shown in Figure 1*B*. Figure 2*B* shows that although the amplitude of the signal transduction through the array as a function of the bilayer noise voltage (triangles) increases by about four orders of magnitude, the SNR (circles) passes through but a modest maximum at an optimal noise voltage of approximately 10 mV. The SNR effect is small; nevertheless, this experiment was the first to demonstrate SR at the molecular level.

Stochastic Resonance in Sensory Biology

The Crayfish Mechanoreceptor

In biology, stochastic resonance was first observed in the mechanoreceptor system located on the tailfan of the crayfish (Douglass et al., 1993). This system is adapted for predator avoidance. An array of hydrodynamically sensitive hairs on the crayfish tailfan senses a weak, nearly periodic water motion (8 to 12 Hz) that signals the approach of a predatory fish. Each hair is innervated by an afferent sensory neuron that converges on a ganglion (the sixth, or caudal, ganglion) located just anterior to the tailfan. In their experiment, Douglass and colleagues applied periodic and random hydrodynamic motions simultaneously to the tailfan while recording the spike train from a single afferent sensory neuron identified with its individual hair. The afferents studied were chosen to have low internal noise, allowing the researchers to perform a clean experiment with a single noise source. Power spectra assembled from the spike trains revealed the familiar signature of the three ingredients—a sharp signal feature and its smaller amplitude second harmonic riding on a broadband noise background. The SNRs com-

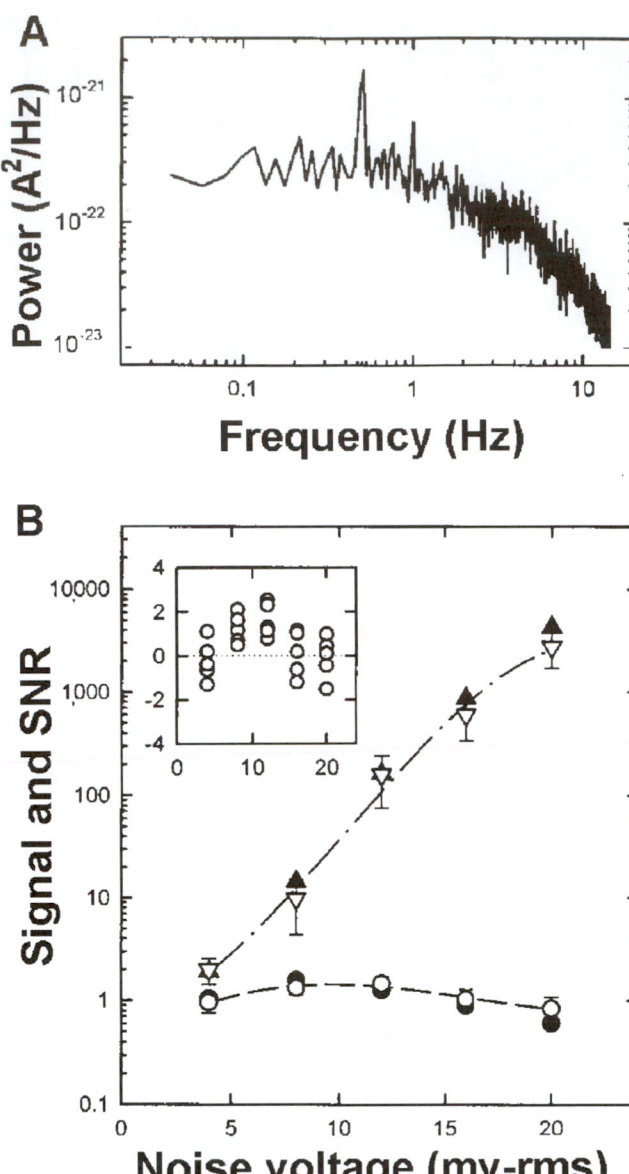

Figure 2. *A*, An experimentally obtained power spectrum from the current transmitted by an array of ion channels through a lipid bilayer (membrane). Note the sharp peak, evidence of the subthreshold periodic signal applied to the bilayer. *B*, The signal amplitude and the signal-to-noise ratio measured as functions of the applied noise intensity. The inset shows a magnified view of the SNR data plotted below with the closed and open circles. The data show a maximum at the optimal noise voltage of approximately 10 mV (rms), thus demonstrating SR. The dashed and dash-dot curves are a guide to the eye. (Reproduced with permission from Bezrukov, S. M., and Vodyanoy, I., 1995, Noise-induced enhancement of signal transduction across voltage-dependent ion channels, *Nature*, 378:362–364.)

puted from these power spectra indicated a clear maximum at an optimal noise intensity. The data are shown in Figure 3*A*. They demonstrate SR at the level of single sensory neurons.

The Cricket Cercal System

Levin and Miller (1996) reported a remarkable experiment—similar to that described above but with many improvements and

A

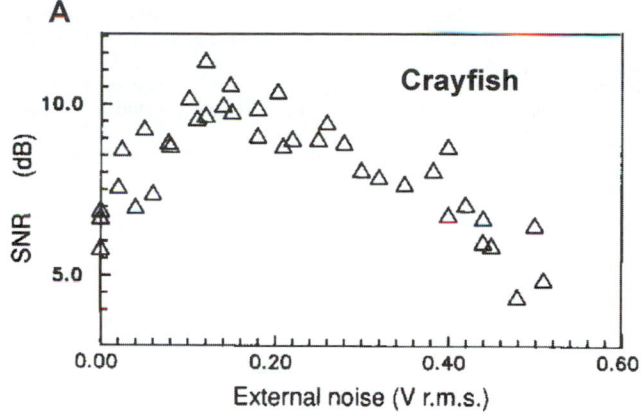

B

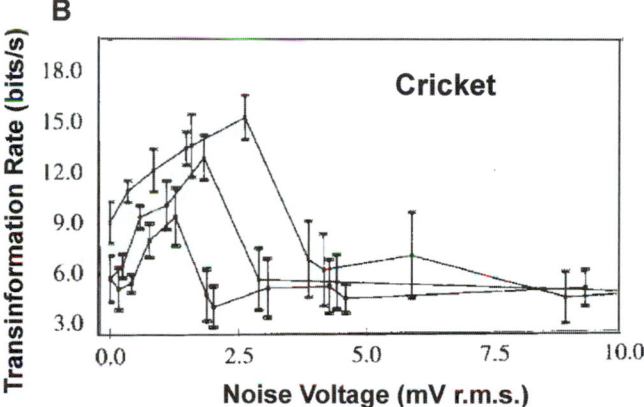

Figure 3. Stochastic resonance in the crayfish and cricket. *A*, signal-to-noise ratio versus noise intensity for the crayfish. (Reproduced with permission from Douglass, J. K., et al., 1993, Noise enhancement of information transfer in crayfish mechanoreceptors by stochastic resonance, *Nature*, 365:337–340.) *B*, Transinformation rate versus noise intensity for the cricket. The curves correspond to three different signal amplitudes increasing from left to right. (Reproduced with permission from Levin, J. E., and Miller, J. P., 1996, Broadband neural encoding in the cricket cercal sensory system enhanced by stochastic resonance, *Nature*, 380:165–168.)

one level up in complexity—using a different animal: the cricket. Their experiment is especially interesting because both the cricket and the crayfish are arthropods and have very similar sensory neural architectures for predator avoidance. The cricket is, however, a land animal; its medium is the air, and its main predator is a specific type of wasp. The flight of the approaching wasp causes perturbations of the air similar to the hydrodynamic perturbations generated by the swimming fish, but the frequency is higher (125 to 150 Hz). The tail of the cricket has two appendages that are covered with hairs adapted to sense nearly periodic weak air motions. As in the crayfish system, each hair is innervated by an afferent sensory neuron, and the neurons converge on a ganglion, collectively called the cercal system. The experiment was performed by applying periodic plus random air motions to the appendages while recording spike trains from within the ganglion. In addition to other improvements, Levin and Miller computed the Shannon transinformation between the stimulating air currents and the neural spike trains instead of the SNR of the spike trains alone. This information measure clearly demonstrates SR at the level of the ganglion in the cricket cercal system as shown by the data in Figure 3*B*.

Stochastic Resonance in Human Psychophysics and Animal Behavior

SR in Human Psychophysics

Stochastic resonance has made its way into human psychophysics. Can the addition of a random process to an applied stimulus enhance the ability of a human subject to perceive the stimulus accurately? An excellent tutorial on protocol design, statistical accuracy, and theoretical interpretations of psychophysics experiments has been provided by Norwich (1993). An early numerical experiment with a neural network model examined the role of the internal noise characteristic of the human brain. The model considered an energy potential with two minima (i.e., stable states) representing the two human perceptions of Necker's famous cube (Riani and Simonotto, 1994). The human percept of the perspective of the cube alternates randomly, and experiments with this percept provided the first quantitative measurements of noise within the brain.

But can noise added to an external stimulus enhance perception? For human hearing, this question has been addressed and answered affirmatively by two experimental groups (Zeng, Fu, and Morse, 2000; Ward et al., 2001). The effect is small (only about 3 dB), and the experiments are difficult owing to the extreme sensitivity of the human ear. It is hard to devise a reliably subthreshold stimulus—one of the three essential ingredients. Nevertheless, both groups have obtained positive results with statistical significance. In their experiment, Zeng and colleagues simply added auditory noise to a weak periodic stimulus; Ward and co-workers, however, made use of the higher perceptive threshold for a beat note from two periodic stimuli of slightly different frequencies, again with added noise.

A suitable protocol has also been devised using noise added to visual stimuli (Ward et al., 2001). In this experiment a well-known visual contrast threshold was exploited. The addition of noise distributed over all pixels in a computer-generated scene displayed on a fast monitor was found to enhance the subject's perceptive ability.

But even earlier, SR had been demonstrated in human tactile sensation (Collins, Imhoff, and Grigg, 1996). In this experiment, an indenter applied a subthreshold "touch" to the skin of a finger. In separate experiments, both mechanical noise and electrical noise were added to the stimulus, and both yielded positive results.

Usher and Feingold (2000) have recently reported an interesting and suggestive experiment on SR in human cognitive ability. They found that the addition of auditory noise can enhance the speed of memory retrieval for arithmetic multiplication rules. This is the first, and to date the only experiment showing SR in a human cognitive function (in contrast to sensory perception).

In a somewhat different approach, the human baroreflexive system was used to demonstrate "functional" SR (Hidaka, Nozaki, and Yamamoto, 2000). This application made use of the coupling between the cardiac and blood pressure regulatory functions. A weak periodic signal was applied to the venous blood pressure and noise to the arterial blood pressure receptor. The noise-enhanced signal was observed in cardiac response, which in turn could compensate for changes (drops) in blood pressure. Stochastic resonance in this application thus mediates an essential physiological function.

Finally, it is worth noting that, in parallel to the human psychophysics experiments, animal behavior experiments (with an electrosensitive fish) have also demonstrated SR as a behavioral perceptive phenomenon (Russell, Wilkens, and Moss, 1999).

Discussion

Stochastic resonance has been demonstrated at several levels in biology: from ion channels in cell membranes to animal and human cognition, perception, and ultimately behavior. The behavioral effects are small, since SR lurks at the edge of human and animal perceptive thresholds. Nevertheless, over evolutionary time scales, SR may have endowed its beneficiaries with a selective advantage. Thus, today we can see its effects in widely diverse living creatures. Such speculations are stimulating and will undoubtedly lead to further study.

Road Map: Dynamic Systems
Related Reading: Amplification, Attenuation, and Integration; Chaos in Biological Systems; Chaos in Neural Systems; Collective Behavior of Coupled Oscillators; Cooperative Phenomena

References

Anishchenko, V., Moss, F., Neiman, A., and Schimansky-Geier, L., 1999, Stochastic resonance: Noise induced order, *Usp. Fiz. Nauk*, 169:7–38; translation in *Sov. Phys. Usp.*, 42(1):7–36.

Bezrukov, S. M., and Vodyanoy, I., 1995, Noise-induced enhancement of signal transduction across voltage-dependent ion channels, *Nature*, 378:362–364.

Collins, J. J., Imhoff, T. T., and Grigg, P., 1996, Noise-enhanced tactile sensation, *Nature*, 383:770–773.

Douglass, J. K., Wilkens, L., Pantazelou, E., and Moss, F., 1993, Noise enhancement of information transfer in crayfish mechanoreceptors by stochastic resonance, *Nature*, 365:337–340.

Hidaka, I., Nozaki, D., and Yamamoto, Y., 2000, Functional stochastic resonance in the human brain: Noise induced sensitization of baroreflex system. *Phys. Rev. Lett.*, 85:3740–3743.

Levin, J. E., and Miller, J. P., 1996, Broadband neural encoding in the cricket cercal sensory system enhanced by stochastic resonance, *Nature*, 380:165–168.

Longtin, A., Bulsara, A., and Moss, F., 1991, Time-interval sequences in bistable systems and the noise-induced transmission of information by sensory neurons, *Phys. Rev. Lett.*, 67:656–659.

Moss, F., Pierson, D., and O'Gorman, D., 1994, Stochastic resonance: Tutorial and update, *Intern. J. Bifurc. Chaos*, 6:1383–1397. ◆

Moss, F., and Wiesenfeld, K., 1995, The benefits of background noise, *Scientific American*, August 273:66–69. ◆

Norwich, K. H., 1993, *Information, Sensation, and Perception*, New York: Academic Press. ◆

Riani, M., and Simonotto, E., 1994, Stochastic resonance in the perceptual interpretation of ambiguous figures: A neural network model, *Phys. Rev. Lett.*, 72:3120–3123.

Russell, D., Wilkens, L., and Moss, F., 1999, Use of behavioral stochastic resonance by paddlefish for feeding, *Nature*, 402:219–223.

Usher, M., and Feingold, M., 2000, Stochastic resonance in the speed of memory retrieval, *Biol. Cybern.*, 83:L11–L16.

Ward, L. M., Desai, S., Rootman, D., Tata, M., and Moss, F., 2001, Noise Can Help as well as Hinder Seeing and Hearing, *Bull. Am. Phys. Soc.*, 46 no.1; paper N23.002 at http://www.aps.org/meet/MAR01/baps/vpr/layn23-002.html

Zeng, F.-G., Fu, Q.-J., and Morse, R., 2000, Human hearing enhanced by noise, *Brain Res.*, 869:251–255.

Structured Connectionist Models

Lokendra Shastri

Introduction

Research in *structured connectionism* is motivated by the twin beliefs that understanding the computational properties of the brain is essential for understanding human cognition, and that insights acquired by disciplines such as computer science, artificial intelligence (AI), psychology, linguistics, and learning theory are crucial for understanding the neural basis of cognition.

Structured connectionist models are networks of nodes and links that are intended to be computational abstractions of neurons and synapses, respectively. Although the structured connectionist approach shares many features with the *distributed* connectionist approach, it differs from the latter in significant ways. The fully distributed approach assumes that each "item" (a concept or mental object) is represented as a pattern of activity distributed over a *common* pool of nodes (van Gelder, 1992). This notion of representation suffers from several fundamental limitations. Consider the representation of *John and Mary*. If *John* and *Mary* are each represented as patterns of activity over the entire network such that each node in the network has a specific value in the patterns for *John* and *Mary*, respectively, then how can the network represent *John* and *Mary* at the same time? The situation gets even more complex if the system has to represent relations such as *John loves Mary* or *John loves Mary but Tom loves Susan*. In contrast to the distributed approach, the structured approach holds that small clusters of nodes can have distinct representational status (for simplicity, structured connectionist models often equate a small cluster of nodes with a single *idealized* node). In particular, there exist small clusters of nodes that act as *focal nodes* or *focal clusters* of learned concepts and provide access to more elaborate structures that make up the detailed encoding of concepts. Such a detailed encoding might include various features of the concept as well as its rela-

tionship to other concepts (see Shastri in Barnden and Pollack, 1991; Shastri, 2001b). The nodes comprising the focal cluster of a concept may be physically distributed, and the focal clusters of two concepts may overlap, although the extent of this overlap is expected to be small.

Another difference between the structured and the fully distributed approaches concerns learning. The latter underplays the importance of prior structure and assumes that the required structure emerges as a result of general purpose learning processes operating on relatively unstructured hidden layers. The structured approach holds that such a tabula rasa view is untenable on the grounds of computational complexity; training unstructured networks using general purpose-learning techniques is not a feasible way to obtain scalable solutions to complex problems. The structured approach emphasizes the importance of prior structure for effective learning and requires that the initial network architecture—for example, the number of layers and the interconnections within and between layers—reflect the structure of the problem.

The structured connectionist approach is sometimes wrongly equated with a narrow interpretation of the grandmother cell approach in which each concept is assumed to be represented by a single neuron. This misunderstanding stems from an incorrect interpretation of the representational role of focal nodes (Page, 2000; see also LOCALIZED VERSUS DISTRIBUTED REPRESENTATIONS).

Some Neural Constraints on Cognitive Models

Representational Constraints

With more than 10^{11} computing elements and 10^{15} interconnections, the human brain's capacity for encoding, communicating, and processing information seems awesome. But if the brain is extremely powerful, it is also extremely limited. First, neurons are slow computing devices. Second, although the spatiotemporal integration of inputs performed by neurons is quite complex, it is unlikely that this integration can encode and decode symbolic structures. Third, neurons communicate via "messages" that encode only a few bits of information. Hence, a neuron's output cannot be expected to encode complex structures.

A specific limitation of neurally plausible systems is that they have difficulty representing composite structures in a dynamic fashion (see COMPOSITIONALITY IN NEURAL SYSTEMS). Consider the representation of the event, *John gave Mary a book*. This event cannot be represented dynamically by activating the conceptual roles *giver, recipient*, and *given-object* and the entities *John, Mary,* and *a book*. Such a representation would be indistinguishable from that of *Mary gave John a book*. The problem is that an unambiguous representation of an event requires the representation of *bindings* between the roles of an event (e.g., *giver*) and the entities that fill these roles in the event (e.g., John). It is easy to represent long-term bindings using dedicated "binder" nodes (such a binder node can be viewed as a conjunction of a bound role and filler pair). But whereas it is feasible to use binder nodes for encoding long-term knowledge, it is implausible to assume that binder nodes can be recruited for representing numerous dynamic bindings arising rapidly during language understanding and visual processing. Binding techniques based on von Neumann architecture cannot be used, since the storage capacity of nodes and the resolution of their outputs are insufficient for storage and communication of names and pointers.

Scalability in Time and Space

We can visually recognize commonplace items in about 100 ms, and we can understand language at the rate of several hundred words per minute, even though doing so involves perceptual processing and the integration of syntactic, semantic, contextual, and pragmatic knowledge. This indicates that the brain can perform a wide range of complex visual, linguistic, and inferential tasks within a few hundred milliseconds. This observation provides a powerful constraint that can inform our search for cognitive models (Feldman and Ballard, 1982; Shastri and Ajjanagadde, 1993).

Although the number of neurons in the brain is large, it is not too large, given the types of problems it must solve. Consider vision. The retinal output consists of a million signals, and hence the "size" of the input processed by the visual system is about a million. Consequently, any model of vision whose node requirement is quadratic (or higher) in the number of inputs cannot be neurally plausible. A similar argument can be made for commonsense reasoning, which occurs with respect to a very large knowledge base.

Examples of Structured Connectionist Models

Early Work

An early structured connectionist model was the interactive activation model for letter perception proposed by McClelland and Rumelhart (1981). The model consisted of three layers of nodes corresponding to visual letter features, letters, and words. Nodes representing mutually exclusive hypotheses within the letter and word layers inhibited each other. For example, all nodes representing letters in the same position inhibited each other. A node in the feature layer was connected via excitatory connections to nodes in the letter layer representing letters containing that feature. Similarly, a node in the letter layer was connected via excitatory connections to nodes in the word layer representing words containing that letter in the appropriate position. Additionally, there were reciprocal connections from the word layer to the letter layer. The

interconnection pattern allowed bottom-up perceptual processing to be guided by top-down expectations. The model could explain a number of psychological findings about the preference of words and pronounceable nonwords over other nonwords and isolated letters.

Other examples of early structured connectionist models were word sense disambiguation models developed by Cottrell and Small (1983) and Waltz and Pollack (1985). Most words have multiple senses, but we are able to exploit contextual and syntactic information to rapidly disambiguate their meanings. These models demonstrated how such disambiguation might occur. Cottrell and Small's model consisted of a three-level network consisting of the word level, the word sense level, and the case level. There were inhibitory links between mutually exclusive senses of a word. A node at the lexical level was connected via excitatory links to all its senses at the word sense level. Connections between the word sense level and the case level expressed all feasible bindings between case roles and objects. As a sentence was input by activating the appropriate lexical items in a sequence, the combination of lexical items, word senses, and case assignments that best fit the input formed a stable coalition.

Another example of an early structured connectionist model was Shastri's (1988) connectionist semantic network (CSN) model. CSN viewed semantic memory (see SEMANTIC NETWORKS) as concepts organized in an IS-A hierarchy (e.g., "Bird IS-A Animal"). Moreover, each concept was assumed to be a collection of property-value pairs. The property-value information consisted of distributional information, such as how many apples are red, green, and yellow, respectively. CSN could infer the most likely value of a specified property for any concept. Furthermore, given a partial description of a concept, CSN could find the concept that best matched the description. CSN found answers by combining available distributional information using the principle of maximum entropy. CSN could deal with partial, exceptional, and conflicting information and disambiguate "multiple inheritance" situations that could not be handled by extant AI models. CSN encoded concepts, properties, and values using focal nodes and IS-A relations as links. Property values were attached to concepts via binder nodes, with link weights capturing distributional information.

Solution to the Binding Problem

A crucial limitation of the structured connectionist models mentioned above was that they could not express dynamic bindings. For example, the McClelland and Rumelhart model could not dynamically bind a letter to a position in a word and required an *n*-fold repetition of letter and feature layers to deal with words of length *n*. Subsequent structured connectionist models have made significant progress in solving the binding problem. These models include CONPOSIT (see Barnden and Srinivas in Barnden and Pollack, 1991), ROBIN (see Dyer in Barnden and Pollack, 1991), SHRUTI (Shastri and Ajjanagadde, 1993), CONSYDERR (Sun, 1992), and LISA (Hummel and Holyoak, 1997). ROBIN and CONSYDERR assign a unique pattern of activity (i.e., a signature) to each concept and propagate signatures to establish bindings. CONPOSIT creates bindings by virtue of the relative position of active nodes and the similarity of patterns. In contrast, SHRUTI and LISA use synchronous firing of nodes to represent and propagate dynamic bindings.

The possible role of synchronous activity in neural representations and feature binding had been suggested by several researchers (see DYNAMIC LINK ARCHITECTURE; SYNCHRONIZATION, BINDING AND EXPECTANCY; SYNFIRE CHAINS; SPIKING NEURONS, COMPUTATION WITH), but SHRUTI was the first model to offer a detailed computational account of how such activity could be harnessed to solve problems in the representation and processing of high-level conceptual knowledge and to support inference.

SHRUTI can encode a large body of semantic and causal knowledge, and yet perform inferences required to establish referential and causal coherence within several hundred milliseconds (Shastri and Ajjanagadde, 1993). For example, given the story fragment "John fell in the hallway. Tom had cleaned it," SHRUTI can rapidly infer that *it* refers to the hallway, the hallway floor was wet because Tom had cleaned it, and John probably fell because he slipped on the wet floor.

SHRUTI encodes relational knowledge (e.g., event frames and action schemas) using neural circuits composed of focal clusters. The focal cluster of a relation P consists of a node $+:P$ whose activity indicates that the system is making an assertion about an instance of P, a node $?:P$ whose activity indicates that the system is seeking an explanation about an instance of P, and role nodes, one for each role associated with P. A dynamic binding between a role and an entity filling that role in a given situation is represented by the synchronous firing of the role and entity nodes. For example, the event "John fell in the hallway" is represented by a *rhythmic* pattern of activity wherein the node $+:fall$ fires, the node $+:John$ fires in synchrony with the role node *fall-patient*, and the node $+:hallway$ fires in synchrony with the role node *fall-location*. A systematic mapping between relations (and other rule-like knowledge) is encoded by high-efficacy links between focal clusters. For example, the knowledge "falling can lead to getting hurt" is encoded by directed links from $+:fall$ to $+:hurt$ and $?:hurt$ to $?:fall$, and by two-way links between *fall-patient* and *hurt-patient* and between *fall-location* and *hurt-location*. Given the above connectivity, the state of activation encoding "John fell in the hallway" evolves so that the role *hurt-patient* starts firing in synchrony with the role *fall-patient* (and hence, with $+:John$), and the role *hurt-location* starts firing in synchrony with the role *fall-location* (and hence, with $+:hallway$). The resulting firing pattern represents not only the event "John fell in the hallway," but also the *inferred* event "John got hurt in the hallway." Thus SHRUTI is able to infer that John got hurt in the hallway, given that John fell in the hallway.

As illustrated by this simple example, inference in SHRUTI results from the propagation of rhythmic activity across interconnected focal clusters. In general, SHRUTI combines predictive inferences with explanatory (or abductive) inferences, exhibits priming, instantiates new entities during inference (if John ran, there must be a path along which he ran), and unifies multiple entities by merging their phases of firing (if John got hurt and if there is a man who got hurt, then the man is likely to be John). These features of SHRUTI allow it to rapidly draw a wide range of inferences within a few hundred milliseconds. The time taken to generate an inference is simply $l * \alpha$, where l is the length of the chain of inference and α is the time required for connected nodes to synchronize.

The use of temporal synchrony for encoding dynamic bindings leads to the prediction that a large number of items may be active at the same time, and a large number of rules may fire simultaneously, provided the number of distinct entities occurring as role fillers in these items remains small (ca. 7). This constraint is motivated by biological considerations; each entity participating in dynamic bindings occupies a distinct phase, and hence the number of distinct entities that can occur as role fillers in dynamic facts cannot exceed $\lfloor \pi_{max}/\omega \rfloor$. Here π_{max} is the maximum delay between consecutive firings of synchronous cell clusters (about 25 ms, assuming that γ band activity underlies the encoding of dynamic bindings), and ω equals the allowable jitter in synchrony (ca. ± 2 ms).

Henderson (1994) has developed an on-line parser for English using a SHRUTI-like architecture. The parser shows that constraints on working memory help explain several properties of human parsing pertaining to long-distance dependencies, garden path effects, and our limited ability to deal with center embedding.

Learning in Structured Networks

Regier's (1996) model for learning the lexical semantics of spatial terms provides an early example of learning within structured connectionist models. The model observes movies of simple two-dimensional objects moving relative to one another, in which each movie is labeled as an example of some spatial term, and learns the association between the label (word) and the event/relation it describes. The model successfully learned several spatial terms for natural languages. The model includes structured network components that reflect prior constraints about the task as well as the usual hidden layers, and demonstrates how structured connectionist models can incorporate flexible learning ability and at the same time leverage prior structure to achieve tractability.

In addition to incremental learning driven by repeated exposure to training data, structured connectionist models have also made use of one-shot learning using *recruitment* learning (see Feldman, 1982; Shastri, 1988, 2001b; Page, 2000). Recruitment learning can be described as follows. Learning occurs within a partially structured network containing a large number of randomly interconnected nodes. Recruited nodes are nodes that have acquired a distinct "meaning" (or functionality) by virtue of their strong interconnections to other recruited nodes and/or sensorimotor (i.e., input/output) nodes. Nodes that are not yet recruited can be viewed as "free" nodes. Such nodes are connected via weak links to a large number of nodes. Free nodes form a primordial network from which suitably connected nodes may be recruited for representing new items. Consider a novel concept y that can be expressed as a conjunct of existing concepts x_1 and x_2. This concept can be learned by (1) identifying free nodes that receive links from nodes representing x_1 and nodes representing x_2 and (2) recruiting one or more such free nodes by strengthening the weights of links incident on these nodes from x_1 and x_2 nodes. Shastri (2001a) has shown that recruitment learning algorithms can be grounded in the biological phenomena of *long-term potentiation* (LTP) and *long-term depression* (LTD), which involve rapid, long-lasting, and highly specific changes in synaptic strength.

The crucial role of structure in neural systems is highlighted by SMRITI, a computational model of episodic memory formation via corticohippocampal interactions (Shastri, 2001a, 2001b). Episodic memory refers to our ability to remember events in our daily lives. A wide array of neuropsychological and imaging data suggests that the hippocampal system, consisting of the entorhinal cortex, the dentate gyrus, the hippocampus proper, and the subicular complex, serves an essential role in the formation of episodic memories. The hippocampal system is known to have a complex and idiosyncratic architecture, and this raises the following question: Does the idiosyncratic architecture of the hippocampal system reflect the functional requirements of the task it is known to subserve? SMRITI suggests that the answer to this question is yes.

Several models have been proposed to explain how the hippocampal system supports episodic memory function, but several key representational problems associated with the encoding of episodic memory remain unsolved. In particular, most existing models view an item in episodic memory as a feature vector or a conjunction of features. But as discussed in Shastri (2001b), a functionally adequate memory trace of an event must be capable of viewing an event as a collection of bindings. Furthermore, the memory trace of an event should be responsive to partial cues, and at the same time, it should be capable of distinguishing between the memorized event and other highly similar events. These requirements suggest that an event's memory trace should be a complex circuit incorporating functional units that serve as binding detectors, binding-error detectors, binding-error integrators, relational-match indicators, and binding reinstators.

SMRITI demonstrates that the idiosyncratic architecture and local circuitry of the hippocampal system is ideally suited for the recruitment of the functional units enumerated above. Specifically, it shows that the propagation of rhythmic activity representing an event can automatically lead to the rapid recruitment of a functionally adequate memory trace within the hippocampal system as a result of LTP. The fine-grained mapping between form and function provided by SMRITI offers the potential for detailed modeling of memory function in normal and patient populations.

Advantages of Structured Connectionism

The structured connectionist approach promotes the development of network models containing different types of nodes, involving different forms of learning, and incorporating anatomical and physiological constraints—although at an abstract computational level. This has led to the development of sophisticated and large-scale models of cognitive function such as memory, reasoning, and language understanding. The representational and expressive power of these models usually exceeds that of parallel distributed networks developed for modeling similar cognitive phenomena. Moreover, instead of viewing networks as black boxes that serve as function approximators for modeling highly circumscribed data sets, the structured connectionist approach attempts to develop networks that model broadly defined cognitive functions (e.g., episodic memory). Finally, the structured connectionist approach explicates the correspondence between structure and function, and this can lead to a better understanding of the neural basis of cognition.

Discussion

Structured connectionism offers a rich framework for developing models of cognition guided by biological, behavioral, and computational constraints. The approach has been productive and has resulted in a number of models informed by insights from such diverse disciplines as computer science, AI, psychology, linguistics, and neuroscience. With some difficult representational problems resolved, the focus of work is shifting toward the study of structured adaptive networks that are grounded in perception and action (Feldman and Bailey, 2000; see SCHEMA THEORY) and tightly constrained by biology (Shastri, 2001b).

Road Map: Artificial Intelligence
Background: Artificial Intelligence and Neural Networks
Related Reading: Cognitive Modeling: Psychology and Connectionism; Connectionist and Symbolic Representations; Dynamic Link Architecture

References

Barnden, J., and Pollack, L., Eds., 1991, *Advances in Connectionist and Neural Computation Theory*, vol. 1, Norwood, NJ: Ablex. ◆

Cottrell, G. W., and Small, S. L., 1983, A connectionist scheme for modeling word sense disambiguation, *Cognit. Brain Theory*, 6:89–120.

Feldman, J. A., 1982, Dynamic connections in neural networks, *Biol. Cybern.*, 46:27–39.

Feldman, J. A., and Bailey, D., 2000, Layered hybrid connectionist models for cognitive science, in *Hybrid Neural Systems* (S. Wermter and R. Sun, Eds.), Heidelberg: Springer-Verlag, pp. 14–27.

Feldman, J. A., and Ballard, D. H., 1982, Connectionist models and their properties, *Cognit. Sci.*, 6:205–254. ◆

Henderson, J., 1994, Connectionist syntactic parsing using temporal variable binding, *J. Psycholinguist. Res.*, 23:353–379.

Hummel, J. E., and Holyoak, K. J., 1997, Distributed representations of structure: A theory of analogical access and mapping, *Psychol. Rev.*, 104:427–466.

McClelland, J. L., and Rumelhart, D. E., 1981, An interactive activation model of context effects in letter perception: Part 1. An account of basic findings, *Psychol. Rev.*, 88:375–407.

Page, M., 2000, Connectionist modeling in psychology: A localist manifesto, *Behav. Brain Sci.*, 23:443–467.

Regier, T., 1996, *The Human Semantic Potential: Spatial Language and Constrained Connectionism*, Cambridge, MA: MIT Press.

Shastri, L., 1988, *Semantic Networks: An Evidential Formalization and Its Connectionist Realization*, Los Altos, CA: Morgan Kaufman. ◆

Shastri, L., 2001a, Biological grounding of recruitment learning and vicinal algorithms in long-term potentiation, in *Emergent Neural Computational Architectures Based on Neuroscience* (J. Austin, S. Wermter, and D. Wilshaw, Eds.), Berlin: Springer-Verlag, pp. 348–367.

Shastri, L., 2001b, Episodic memory and cortico-hippocampal interactions, *Trends Cogn. Sci.*, 6:162–168.

Shastri, L., and Ajjanagadde, A., 1993, From simple associations to systematic reasoning: A connectionist encoding of rules, variables and dynamic bindings using temporal synchrony, *Behav. Brain Sci.*, 16:417–494. ◆

Sun, R., 1992, On variable binding in connectionist networks, *Connect. Sci.*, 4:93–124.

van Gelder, T., 1992, Defining "distributed representation," *Connect. Sci.*, 4:175–191.

Waltz, D. L., and Pollack, J. B., 1985, Massively parallel parsing: A strongly interactive model of natural language interpretation, *Cognit. Sci.*, 9:51–74.

Support Vector Machines

Bernhard Schölkopf and Alexander J. Smola

Introduction

One of the fundamental problems of learning theory is the following: suppose we are given two classes of objects. We are then faced with a new object, and we have to assign it to one of the two classes. This problem, referred to as (*binary*) *pattern recognition*, can be formalized as follows: we are given empirical data

$$(x_1, y_1), \ldots, (x_m, y_m) \in \mathscr{X} \times \{\pm 1\} \tag{1}$$

and we want to estimate a *decision function* $f : \mathscr{X} \rightarrow \{\pm 1\}$. Here, $\mathscr{X}$ is some nonempty set from which the *patterns* x_i are taken, usually referred to as the *domain*; the y_i are called *labels* or *targets*.

A good decision function will have the property that it *generalizes* to unseen data points, achieving a small value of the *risk*

$$R[f] = \int \frac{1}{2} |f(x) - y| \, dP(x, y) \tag{2}$$

In other words, on average over an unknown distribution P which is assumed to generate both training and test data, we would like to have a small error. Here, the error is measured by means of the *zero-one loss function* $c(x, y, f(x)) := (\frac{1}{2}) |f(x) - y|$. The loss is 0 if (x, y) is classified correctly, and 1 otherwise.

It should be emphasized that so far, the patterns could be just about anything, and we have made no assumptions on $\mathscr{X}$ other than it being a set endowed with a probability measure P (note that the labels y may, but need not, depend on x in a deterministic fashion). Moreover, Equation 2 does not tell us how to *find* a function with a small risk. In fact, it does not even tell us how to *evaluate* the risk of a given function, since the probability measure P is assumed to be unknown.

We therefore introduce an additional type of structure, pertaining to what we are actually given—the training data. Loosely speaking, to generalize, we want to choose y such that (x, y) is in some sense similar to the training examples (Equation 1). To this end, we need notions of *similarity* in $\mathscr{X}$ and in $\{\pm 1\}$.

Characterizing the similarity of the outputs $\{\pm 1\}$ is easy. In binary classification, only two situations can occur: two labels can be either identical or different. The choice of the similarity measure for the inputs, on the other hand, is a deep question that lies at the core of the problem of machine learning.

One of the advantages of kernel methods is that the learning algorithms developed are quite independent of the choice of the similarity measure. This allows us to adapt the latter to the specific problems at hand without the need to reformulate the learning algorithm itself.

Kernels as Similarity Measures

Let us consider a symmetric similarity measure of the form

$$k : \mathscr{X} \times \mathscr{X} \to \mathbb{R}$$
$$(x, x') \mapsto k(x, x') \qquad (3)$$

that is, a function that, given two patterns x and x', returns a real number characterizing their similarity. The function k is often called a *kernel*.

General similarity measures of this form are rather difficult to study. Let us therefore start from a particularly simple case and generalize it subsequently. A simple type of similarity measure that is of particular mathematical appeal is a *dot product*. For instance, given two vectors $\mathbf{x}, \mathbf{x}' \in \mathbb{R}^N$, the *canonical dot product* is defined as

$$\langle \mathbf{x}, \mathbf{x}' \rangle := \sum_{i=1}^{N} [\mathbf{x}]_i [\mathbf{x}']_i \qquad (4)$$

Here, $[\mathbf{x}]_i$ denotes the ith entry of $\mathbf{x}$.

The geometric interpretation of the canonical dot product is that it computes the cosine of the angle between the vectors $\mathbf{x}$ and $\mathbf{x}'$, provided they are normalized to length 1. Moreover, it allows computation of the *length* (or *norm*) of a vector $\mathbf{x}$ as

$$\|\mathbf{x}\| = \sqrt{\langle \mathbf{x}, \mathbf{x} \rangle} \qquad (5)$$

Being able to compute dot products amounts to being able to carry out all geometric constructions that can be formulated in terms of angles, lengths, and distances.

Note, however, that the dot product approach is not really sufficiently general to deal with many interesting problems.

- First, we have deliberately not made the assumption that the patterns actually exist in a dot product space. So far, they could be any kind of object. In order to be able to use a dot product as a similarity measure, we therefore first need to represent the patterns as vectors in some dot product space $\mathscr{H}$, called the *feature space*. To this end, we use a map

$$\Phi : ; \mathscr{X} \to \mathscr{H}$$
$$x \mapsto \mathbf{x} := \Phi(x) \qquad (6)$$

Note that we use a boldface $\mathbf{x}$ to denote the vectorial representation of x in the feature space.

- Second, even if the original patterns lie in a dot product space, we may still want to consider more general similarity measures

obtained by applying a nonlinear map (Equation 6). An example that we will consider below is a map that computes products of entries of the input patterns.

Embedding the data into $\mathscr{H}$ via Φ has two main benefits. First, it allows us to deal with the patterns geometrically, and thus lets us study learning algorithms using linear algebra and analytic geometry. Second, it lets us define a similarity measure from the dot product in $\mathscr{H}$,

$$k(x, x') := \langle \mathbf{x}, \mathbf{x}' \rangle = \langle \Phi(x), \Phi(x') \rangle \qquad (7)$$

The freedom to choose the mapping Φ enables us to design a large variety of similarity measures and learning algorithms.

A Simple Pattern Recognition Algorithm

We now design a simple pattern recognizer. We make use of the structure introduced in the previous section; that is, we assume that our data are embedded in a dot product space $\mathscr{H}$. The basic idea of the algorithm is to assign a previously unseen pattern to the class with closer mean. We thus begin by computing the means of the two classes in feature space:

$$\mathbf{c}_+ = \frac{1}{m_+} \sum_{\{i | y_i = +1\}} \mathbf{x}_i \qquad (8)$$

$$\mathbf{c}_- = \frac{1}{m_-} \sum_{\{i | y_i = -1\}} \mathbf{x}_i \qquad (9)$$

where m_+ and m_- are the number of examples with positive and negative labels, respectively, with $m_+, m_- > 0$. We assign a new point $\mathbf{x}$ to the class whose mean is closest (Figure 1). This geometric construction can be formulated in terms of the dot product $\langle \cdot, \cdot \rangle$, leading to

$$\begin{aligned} y &= \text{sgn} \langle (\mathbf{x} - \mathbf{c}), \mathbf{w} \rangle \\ &= \text{sgn} \langle (\mathbf{x} - (\mathbf{c}_+ + \mathbf{c}_-)/2), (\mathbf{c}_+ - \mathbf{c}_-) \rangle \\ &= \text{sgn} (\langle \mathbf{x}, \mathbf{c}_+ \rangle - \langle \mathbf{x}, \mathbf{c}_- \rangle + b) \qquad (10) \end{aligned}$$

Here, we have defined the offset

$$b := \tfrac{1}{2} (\|\mathbf{c}_-\|^2 - \|\mathbf{c}_+\|^2) \qquad (11)$$

which vanishes if the class means have the same distance to the origin.

It is instructive to rewrite Equation 10 in terms of the input patterns x_i, using the kernel k to compute the dot products. To this

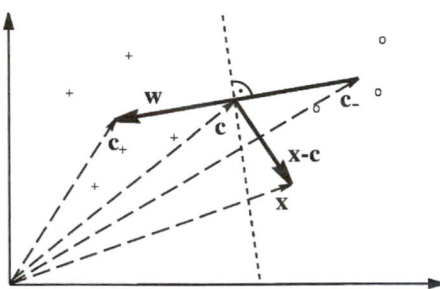

Figure 1. A simple geometric classification algorithm: given two classes of points (depicted by o and +), compute their means $\mathbf{c}_+$, $\mathbf{c}_-$ and assign a test pattern $\mathbf{x}$ to the one whose mean is closer. This can be done by looking at the dot product between $\mathbf{x} - \mathbf{c}$ (where $\mathbf{c} = (\mathbf{c}_+ + \mathbf{c}_-)/2$) and $\mathbf{w} := \mathbf{c}_+ - \mathbf{c}_-$, which changes sign as the enclosed angle passes through $\pi/2$ (From Schölkopf, B., and Smola, A. J., 2002, *Learning with Kernels*, Cambridge, MA: MIT Press. Reprinted with permission.)

end, substitute Equations 8 and 9 into Equation 10 to get the *decision function*

$$y = \text{sgn} \left(\frac{1}{m_+} \sum_{\{i|y_i = +1\}} \langle \mathbf{x}, \mathbf{x}_i \rangle - \frac{1}{m_-} \sum_{\{i|y_i = -1\}} \langle \mathbf{x}, \mathbf{x}_i \rangle + b \right)$$

$$= \text{sgn} \left(\frac{1}{m_+} \sum_{\{i|y_i = +1\}} k(x, x_i) - \frac{1}{m_-} \sum_{\{i|y_i = -1\}} k(x, x_i) + b \right)$$

(12)

Similarly, the offset can be expressed in terms of the kernel. Surprisingly, it turns out that this rather simple-minded approach contains a well-known statistical classification method as a special case. Assume that the class means have the same distance to the origin (hence $b = 0$, cf. Equation 11), and that k can be viewed as a probability density when one of its arguments is fixed.

In this case, Equation 12 takes the form of the so-called Bayes classifier separating the two classes, subject to the assumption that the two classes of patterns were generated by sampling from two probability distributions that are correctly estimated by the *Parzen windows* estimators of the two class densities,

$$p_+(x) := \frac{1}{m_+} \sum_{\{i|y_i = +1\}} k(x, x_i)$$

and   (13)

$$p_-(x) := \frac{1}{m_-} \sum_{\{i|y_i = -1\}} k(x, x_i)$$

where $x \in \mathcal{X}$.

The classifier in Equation 12 is quite close to support vector machines (SVMs). In both cases, the decision function is a kernel expansion corresponding to a separating hyperplane in a feature space.

SVMs deviate from Equation 12 in the selection of the patterns on which the kernels are centered and in the choice of weights that are placed on the individual kernels in the decision function. It will no longer be the case that *all* training patterns appear in the kernel expansion, and the weights of the kernels in the expansion will no longer be uniform within the classes.

Examples of Kernels

So far, we have used the kernel notation as an abstract similarity measure. We now give some concrete examples of kernels, mainly for the case where the inputs x_i are already taken from a dot product space. The role of the kernel then is to implicitly change the representation of the data into another (usually higher-dimensional) feature space. One of the most common kernels used is the polynomial one,

$$k(x, x') = \langle x, x' \rangle^d, \quad \text{where } d \in \mathbb{N}$$

(14)

It can be shown to correspond to a feature space spanned by *all* products of order d of input variables, i.e., all products of the form $[x]_{i_1} \cdot \ldots \cdot [x]_{i_d}$. The dimension of this space is of the order N^d, but, using the kernel to evaluate dot products, this does not affect us. Another popular choice is the Gaussian

$$k(x, x') = \exp\left(-\frac{\|x - x'\|^2}{2\sigma^2} \right)$$

(15)

with a suitable width $\sigma > 0$. Likewise the function

$$k(x, x') = \mathbf{E}[f(x)f(x')] - \int f(x)f(x')d\mathbf{P}(x, x')$$

(16)

is a kernel. Such functions are typically used in Gaussian process estimation (see Williams, 1998, for further details). Examples of more sophisticated kernels, defined not on dot product spaces but on discrete objects such as strings, are the string matching kernels proposed by Watkins (2000) and Haussler (1999).

In general, there are several ways of deciding whether a given function k qualifies as a valid kernel. One way is to appeal to *Mercer's theorem*. This classical result of functional analysis states that the kernel of a positive definite integral operator can be diagonalized in terms of an eigenvector expansion with nonnegative eigenvalues. From the expansion, the feature map Φ can explicitly be constructed. Another approach exploits the fact that the class of admissible kernels coincides with the class of *positive definite* kernels, i.e., functions k such that $\sum_{ij} a_i a_j k(x_i, x_j) \geq 0$ for all $a_i, x_i (i = 1, \ldots, m)$. For positive definite kernels, the feature space can be constructed as the associated *reproducing kernel Hilbert space*.

Hyperplane Classifiers

Statistical learning theory, or Vapnik-Chervonenkis (VC) theory, shows that it is imperative to restrict the set of functions from which f is chosen to one that has a *capacity* suitable for the amount of available training data. VC theory provides *bounds* on the test error, depending on both the empirical risk and the capacity of the function class. The minimization of these bounds leads to the principle of *structural risk minimization* (Vapnik, 1995).

SVMs can be considered an approximate implementation of this principle, by trying to minimize a combination of the *training error* (or *empirical risk*),

$$R_{\text{emp}}[f] = \frac{1}{m} \sum_{i=1}^{m} \frac{1}{2} |f(x_i) - y_i|$$

(17)

and a capacity term derived for the class of hyperplanes in a dot product space $\mathcal{H}$ (Vapnik, 1995),

$$\langle \mathbf{w}, \mathbf{x} \rangle + b = 0 \quad \text{where } \mathbf{w} \in \mathcal{H}, b \in \mathbb{R}$$

(18)

corresponding to decision functions

$$f(\mathbf{x}) = \text{sgn} \left(\langle \mathbf{w}, \mathbf{x} \rangle + b \right)$$

(19)

Consider first problems that are separable by hyperplanes. Among all hyperplanes separating the data, there exists a unique *optimal hyperplane* (Vapnik, 1995), distinguished by the maximum margin of separation between any training point and the hyperplane. It is the solution of

$$\underset{\mathbf{w} \in \mathcal{H}, b \in \mathbb{R}}{\text{maximize}} \min \{ \|\mathbf{x} - \mathbf{x}_i\| \mid \mathbf{x} \in \mathcal{H}, \langle \mathbf{w}, \mathbf{x} \rangle + b = 0, i = 1, \ldots, m \}$$

(20)

Moreover, the capacity of the class of separating hyperplanes can be shown to decrease with increasing margin. The latter is the basis of the *statistical* justification of the approach; in addition, it is *computationally* attractive, since we will show below that it can be constructed by solving a quadratic programming problem for which efficient algorithms exist.

Note that although the form of the decision function (Equation 19) is similar to our earlier example (Equation 10), the training is different. In the earlier example, the normal vector of the hyperplane was trivially computed from the class means as $\mathbf{w} = \mathbf{c}_+ - \mathbf{c}_-$. In the present case, we need to do some additional work. To construct the optimal hyperplane, we have to solve

$$\underset{\mathbf{w} \in \mathcal{H}, b \in \mathbb{R}}{\text{minimize}} \ \tau(\mathbf{w}) = \frac{1}{2} \|\mathbf{w}\|^2$$

(21)

$$\text{subject to } y_i(\langle \mathbf{w}, \mathbf{x}_i \rangle + b) \geq 1 \text{ for all } i = 1, \ldots, m$$

(22)

Note that the constraints in Equation 22 ensure that $f(\mathbf{x}_i)$ will be $+1$ for $y_i = +1$, and -1 for $y_i = -1$. Now, one might argue that for this to be the case, we don't actually need the "≥ 1" on the right-hand side of Equation 22. However, without it, it would not be meaningful to minimize the length of $\mathbf{w}$: to see this, imagine we wrote ">0" instead of "≥1." Now assume that the solution is $(\mathbf{w}, b)$. Let us rescale this solution by multiplication with some $0 < \lambda < 1$. Since $\lambda > 0$, the constraints are still satisfied. Since $\lambda < 1$, however, the length of $\mathbf{w}$ has decreased. Hence $(\mathbf{w}, b)$ cannot be the minimizer of $\tau(\mathbf{w})$.

Let us now try to get an intuition for why we should be minimizing the length of $\mathbf{w}$, as in Equation 21. If $\|\mathbf{w}\|$ were 1, then the left-hand side of Equation 22 would equal the distance from $\mathbf{x}_i$ to the hyperplane (cf. Equation 20). In general, we have to divide $y_i(\langle \mathbf{w}, \mathbf{x}_i \rangle + b)$ by $\|\mathbf{w}\|$ to transform it into this distance. Hence, if we can satisfy Equation 22 for all $i = 1, \ldots, m$ with a $\mathbf{w}$ of minimal length, then the overall margin will be maximized (Figure 2).

The constrained optimization problem (Equation 21) is dealt with by introducing *Lagrange multipliers* $\alpha_i \geq 0$ and a *Lagrangian*

$$L(\mathbf{w}, b, \boldsymbol{\alpha}) = \frac{1}{2} \|\mathbf{w}\|^2 - \sum_{i=1}^{m} \alpha_i(y_i(\langle \mathbf{x}_i, \mathbf{w} \rangle + b) - 1) \quad (23)$$

We use boldface Greek letters as a shorthand for corresponding vectors $\boldsymbol{\alpha} = (\alpha_1, \ldots, \alpha_m)$. The Lagrangian L has a *saddle point* in $\mathbf{w}$, b and $\boldsymbol{\alpha}$ at the optimal solution of the primal optimization problem. This means that it should be minimized with respect to the *primal variables* $\mathbf{w}$ and b and maximized with respect to the *dual variables* α_i. Note that the constraints appear in the second term of the Lagrangian.

Let us try to get some intuition for this way of dealing with constrained optimization problems. If a constraint (Equation 22) is violated, then $y_i(\langle \mathbf{w}, \mathbf{x}_i \rangle + b) - 1 < 0$, in which case L can be increased by increasing the corresponding α_i. At the same time, $\mathbf{w}$ and b will have to change such that L decreases. To prevent $\alpha_i(y_i(\langle \mathbf{w}, \mathbf{x}_i \rangle + b) - 1)$ from becoming an arbitrarily large negative number, the change in $\mathbf{w}$ and b will ensure that, provided the problem is separable, the constraint will eventually be satisfied. Similarly, one can understand that for all constraints that are not precisely met as equalities (that is, for which $y_i(\langle \mathbf{w}, \mathbf{x}_i \rangle + b) - 1 > 0$), the corresponding α_i must be 0: this is the value of α_i that maximizes L. The latter is the statement of the *Karush-Kuhn-Tucker (KKT) complementarity conditions* of optimization theory.

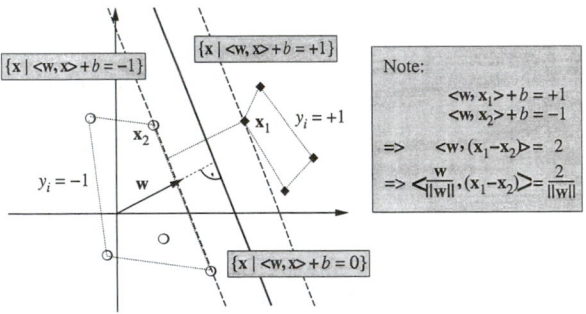

Figure 2. A binary classification toy problem: separate balls from diamonds. The *optimal hyperplane* (Equation 20) is shown as a solid line. The problem being separable, there exists a weight vector $\mathbf{w}$ and a threshold b such that $y_i(\langle \mathbf{w}, \mathbf{x}_i \rangle + b) > 0$ $(i = 1, \ldots, m)$. Rescaling $\mathbf{w}$ and b such that the point(s) closest to the hyperplane satisfy $|\langle \mathbf{w}, \mathbf{x}_i \rangle + b| = 1$, we obtain a *canonical* form $(\mathbf{w}, b)$ of the hyperplane, satisfying $y_i(\langle \mathbf{w}, \mathbf{x}_i \rangle + b) \geq 1$. Note that in this case, the *margin* (the distance of the closest point to the hyperplane) equals $1/\|\mathbf{w}\|$. This can be seen by considering two points $\mathbf{x}_1$, $\mathbf{x}_2$ on opposite sides of the margin, that is, $\langle \mathbf{w}, \mathbf{x}_1 \rangle + b = 1$, $\langle \mathbf{w}, \mathbf{x}_2 \rangle + b = -1$, and projecting them onto the hyperplane normal vector $\mathbf{w}/\|\mathbf{w}\|$. (From Schölkopf, B., and Smola, A. J., 2002, *Learning with Kernels*, Cambridge, MA: MIT Press. Reprinted with permission.)

To minimize with respect to the primal variables, we require

$$\frac{\partial}{\partial b} L(\mathbf{w}, b, \boldsymbol{\alpha}) = 0 \quad \text{and} \quad \frac{\partial}{\partial \mathbf{w}} L(\mathbf{w}, b, \boldsymbol{\alpha}) = 0 \quad (24)$$

leading to

$$\sum_{i=1}^{m} \alpha_i y_i = 0 \quad (25)$$

and

$$\mathbf{w} = \sum_{i=1}^{m} \alpha_i y_i \mathbf{x}_i \quad (26)$$

The solution thus has an expansion (Equation 26) in terms of a subset of the training patterns, namely, those patterns with non-zero α_i, called *support vectors* (SVs). Often, only few of the training examples actually end up being SVs. By the KKT conditions,

$$\alpha_i[y_i(\langle \mathbf{x}_i, \mathbf{w} \rangle + b) - 1] = 0 \text{ for all } i = 1, \ldots, m \quad (27)$$

the SVs lie on the margin (see Figure 2), and this can be exploited to compute b once the α_i have been found. All remaining training examples $(\mathbf{x}_j, y_j)$ are irrelevant: their constraint $y_j(\langle \mathbf{w}, \mathbf{x}_j \rangle + b) \geq 1$ (cf. Equation 22) could just as well be left out, and they do not appear in the expansion in Equation 26. This nicely captures our intuition of the problem: as the hyperplane (see Figure 2) is completely determined by the patterns closest to it, the solution should not depend on the other examples.

By substituting Equations 25 and 26 into the Lagrangian Equation 23, one eliminates the primal variables $\mathbf{w}$ and b, arriving at the so-called *dual optimization problem*, which is the problem that one usually solves in practice:

$$\underset{\boldsymbol{\alpha} \in \mathbb{R}^m}{\text{maximize}} \ W(\boldsymbol{\alpha}) = \sum_{i=1}^{m} \alpha_i - \frac{1}{2} \sum_{i,j=1}^{m} \alpha_i \alpha_j y_i y_j \langle \mathbf{x}_i, \mathbf{x}_j \rangle \quad (28)$$

subject to

$$\alpha_i \geq 0 \text{ for all } i = 1, \ldots, m \text{ and } \sum_{i=1}^{m} \alpha_i y_i = 0 \quad (29)$$

Using Equation 26, the hyperplane decision function (Equation 19) can thus be written as

$$f(\mathbf{x}) = \text{sgn}\left(\sum_{i=1}^{m} y_i \alpha_i \langle \mathbf{x}, \mathbf{x}_i \rangle + b\right) \quad (30)$$

where b is computed by exploiting Equation 27. For details, see Vapnik (1995), Burges (1998), Cristianini and Shawe-Taylor (2000), Schölkopf and Smola (2002), and Herbrich (2002).

Support Vector Classification

We now have all the tools to describe SVMs (Figure 3). Everything in the last section was formulated in a dot product space, which we think of as the feature space $\mathcal{H}$ (see Equation 6). To express the formulas in terms of the input patterns in $\mathcal{X}$, we employ Equation 7. This substitution, which is sometimes referred to as the *kernel trick*, was used by Boser, Guyon, and Vapnik (1992) to develop nonlinear SVMs. It can be applied since all feature vectors only occurred in dot products (see Equations 28 and 30). We obtain decision functions of the form (cf. Equation 30)

$$f(x) = \text{sgn}\left(\sum_{i=1}^{m} y_i \alpha_i \langle \Phi(x), \Phi(x_i) \rangle + b\right)$$

$$= \text{sgn}\left(\sum_{i=1}^{m} y_i \alpha_i k(x, x_i) + b\right) \quad (31)$$

and the following quadratic program (cf. Equation 28):

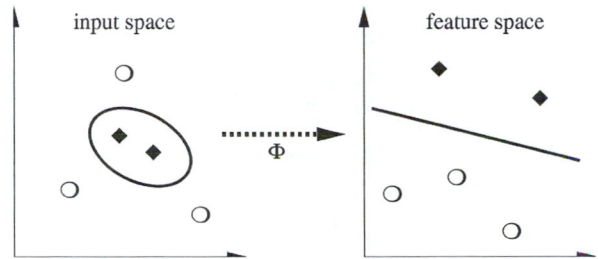

Figure 3. The idea of SVMs: map the training data into a higher-dimensional feature space via Φ, and construct a separating hyperplane with maximum margin there. This yields a nonlinear decision boundary in input space. By the use of a kernel (Equation 3), it is possible to compute the separating hyperplane without explicitly carrying out the map into the feature space. (From Schölkopf, B., and Smola, A. J., 2002, *Learning with Kernels*, Cambridge, MA: MIT Press. Reprinted with permission.)

$$\underset{\alpha \in \mathbb{R}^m}{\text{maximize}} \ W(\alpha) = \sum_{i=1}^{m} \alpha_i - \frac{1}{2} \sum_{i,j=1}^{m} \alpha_i \alpha_j y_i y_j k(x_i, x_j) \qquad (32)$$

subject to

$$\alpha_i \geq 0 \text{ for all } i = 1, \ldots, m, \text{ and } \sum_{i=1}^{m} \alpha_i y_i = 0 \qquad (33)$$

Figure 4 shows a toy example.

In practice, a separating hyperplane may not exist, e.g., if a high noise level causes a large overlap of the classes. To accommodate this case, one introduces slack variables

$$\xi_i \geq 0 \text{ for all } i = 1, \ldots, m \qquad (34)$$

in order to relax the constraints of Equation 22 to

$$y_i(\langle \mathbf{w}, \mathbf{x}_i \rangle + b) \geq 1 - \xi_i \text{ for all } i = 1, \ldots, m \qquad (35)$$

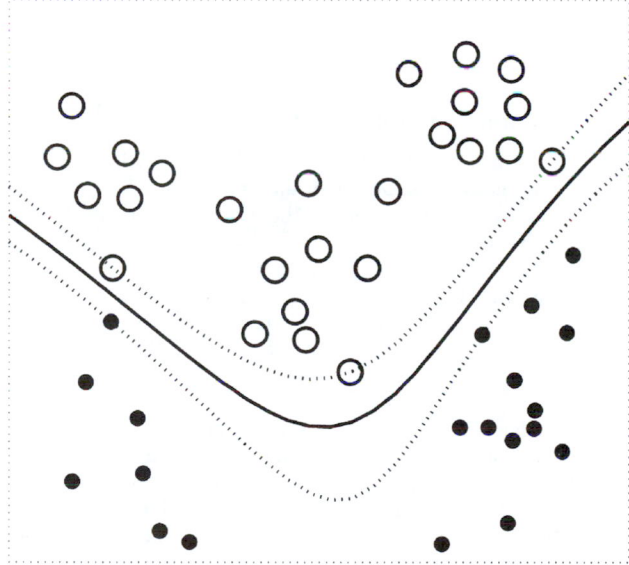

Figure 4. Example of an SV classifier found using a radial basis function kernel $k(x, x') = \exp(-\|x - x'\|^2)$. Circles and points are two classes of training examples; the middle line is the decision surface; the outer lines precisely meet the constraint formulated in Equation 22. Note that the SVs found by the algorithm (sitting on the constraint lines) are not centers of clusters but examples that are critical for the given classification task.

A classifier that generalizes well is then found by controlling both the classifier capacity (via $\|\mathbf{w}\|$) and the sum of the slacks $\Sigma_i \xi_i$. The latter can be shown to provide an upper bound on the number of training errors.

One possible realization of such a *soft margin* classifier is obtained by minimizing the objective function

$$\tau(\mathbf{w}, \xi) = \frac{1}{2} \|\mathbf{w}\|^2 + C \sum_{i=1}^{m} \xi_i \qquad (36)$$

subject to the constraints in Equations 34 and 35, where the constant $C > 0$ determines the trade-off between margin maximization and training error minimization. This again leads to the problem of maximizing Equation 32, subject to modified constraint where the only difference from the separable case is an upper bound C on the Lagrange multipliers α_i.

Another realization uses the more natural v-parametrization. In it, the parameter C is replaced by a parameter $v \in (0, 1)$, which can be shown to provide lower and upper bounds for the fraction of examples that will be SVs and those that will have non-zero slack variables, respectively. Its dual can be shown to consist in maximizing the quadratic part of Equation 32, subject to $0 \leq \alpha_i \leq 1/(vm)$, $\Sigma_i \alpha_i y_i = 0$ and the additional constraint $\Sigma_i \alpha_i = 1$.

Support Vector Regression

Rather than dealing with outputs $y \in \{\pm 1\}$, *regression estimation* is concerned with estimating real-valued functions using $y \in \mathbb{R}$.

To generalize the SV algorithm to the regression case, Vapnik (1995) proposed the *ε-insensitive loss function* (Figure 5),

$$c(x, y, f(x)) := |y - f(\mathbf{x})|_\varepsilon := \max\{0, |y - f(\mathbf{x})| - \varepsilon\} \qquad (37)$$

To estimate a linear regression

$$f(\mathbf{x}) = \langle \mathbf{w}, x \rangle + b \qquad (38)$$

one minimizes

$$\frac{1}{2} \|\mathbf{w}\|^2 + C \sum_{i=1}^{m} |y_i - f(\mathbf{x}_i)|_\varepsilon \qquad (39)$$

Here, the term $\|\mathbf{w}\|^2$ is the same as in pattern recognition (cf. Equation 36). We can transform this into a constrained optimization problem by introducing slack variables, akin to the soft margin case.

An analysis similar to the one above leads to the dual (for $C, \varepsilon \geq 0$ chosen a priori):

$$\underset{\alpha, \alpha^* \in \mathbb{R}^m}{\text{maximize}} \ W(\alpha, \alpha^*) = -\varepsilon \sum_{i=1}^{m} (\alpha_i^* + \alpha_i) + \sum_{i=1}^{m} (\alpha_i^* - \alpha_i) y_i$$

$$- \frac{1}{2} \sum_{i,j=1}^{m} (\alpha_i^* - \alpha_i)(\alpha_j^* - \alpha_j) k(x_i, x_j)$$

$$(40)$$

subject to

$$0 \leq \alpha_i, \alpha_i^* \leq C \text{ for all } i = 1, \ldots, m, \text{ and } \sum_{i=1}^{m} (\alpha_i - \alpha_i^*) = 0 \qquad (41)$$

The regression estimate takes the form

$$f(x) = \sum_{i=1}^{m} (\alpha_i^* - \alpha_i) k(x_i, x) + b, \qquad (42)$$

where $\alpha_i^* - \alpha_i$ is zero for all points that lie inside the ε-tube (Figure 5). Note the similarity to the pattern recognition case (cf. Equation 31 and Figure 6).

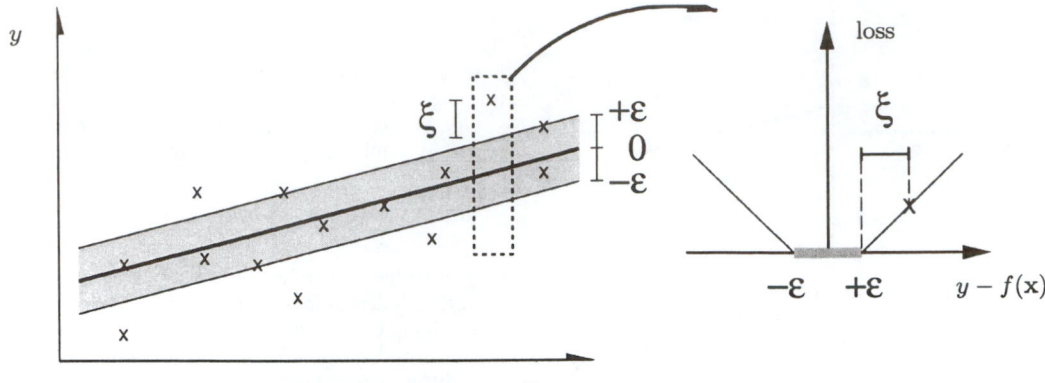

Figure 5. In support vector regression, a tube with radius ε is fitted to the data. The trade-off between model complexity and points lying outside of the tube (with positive slack variables ζ) is determined by minimizing Equa-

tion 39. (From Schölkopf, B., and Smola, A. J., 2002, *Learning with Kernels*, Cambridge, MA: MIT Press. Reprinted with permission.):

Kernel Principal Component Analysis

The kernel trick can be used to develop nonlinear generalizations of any algorithm that can be cast in terms of dot products, such as PRINCIPAL COMPONENT ANALYSIS (PCA) (q.v.).

PCA in feature space leads to an algorithm called *kernel PCA*. It is derived as follows. We wish to find eigenvectors **v** and eigenvalues λ of the so-called *covariance matrix* **C** in the feature space, where

$$\mathbf{C} := \frac{1}{m} \sum_{i=1}^{m} \Phi(x_i)\Phi(x_i)^\top \qquad (43)$$

In the case when $\mathcal{H}$ is very high-dimensional, the computational costs of doing this directly are prohibitive. Fortunately, one can show that all solutions to

$$\mathbf{Cv} = \lambda\mathbf{v} \qquad (44)$$

with $\lambda \neq 0$ must lie in the span of Φ-images of the training data. Thus, we may expand the solution **v** as

$$\mathbf{v} = \sum_{i=1}^{m} \alpha_i \Phi(x_i) \qquad (45)$$

thereby reducing the problem to that of finding the α_i. It turns out that this leads to a dual eigenvalue problem for the expansion coefficients,

$$m\lambda\boldsymbol{\alpha} = K\boldsymbol{\alpha} \qquad (46)$$

where $\boldsymbol{\alpha} = (\alpha_1, \ldots, \alpha_m)^\top$ is normalized to satisfy $\|\boldsymbol{\alpha}\|^2 = 1/\lambda$.

To extract nonlinear features from a test point x, we compute the dot product between $\Phi(x)$ and the nth normalized eigenvector in feature space,

$$\langle \mathbf{v}^n, \Phi(x)\rangle = \sum_{i=1}^{m} \alpha_i^n k(x_i, x) \qquad (47)$$

A toy example is given in Figure 7. As in the case of SVMs, the architecture can be visualized by Figure 6.

Implementation and Empirical Results

An initial weakness of SVMs was that the size of the quadratic programming problem scaled with the number of SVs. This was due to the fact that in Equation 32, the quadratic part contained at least all SVs—the common practice was to extract the SVs by going through the training data in chunks while regularly testing for the possibility that patterns initially not identified as SVs become SVs at a later stage. This procedure is referred to as *chunking*. Note that without chunking, the size of the matrix in the quadratic part of the objective function would be $m \times m$, where m is the number of all training examples.

What happens if we have a high-noise problem? In this case, many of the slack variables ξ_i become non-zero, and all the corresponding examples become SVs. For this case, decomposition algorithms were proposed, based on the observation that not only can we leave out the non-SV examples (the x_i with $\alpha_i = 0$) from the current chunk, but also some of the SVs, especially those that hit the upper boundary ($\alpha_i = C$). The chunks are usually dealt with using quadratic optimizers. Several public domain SV packages and optimizers are listed on the web page http://www.kernel-machines.org.

Modern SVM implementations made it possible to train on some rather large problems. Success stories include the 60,000 example

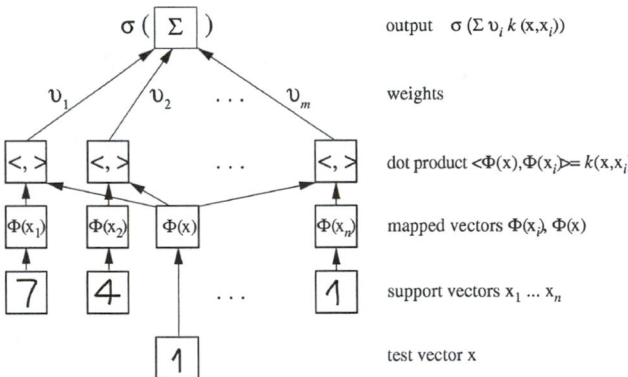

Figure 6. Architecture of SVMs and related kernel methods. The input x and the expansion patterns (SVs) x_i (we assume that we are dealing with handwritten digits) are nonlinearly mapped (by Φ) into a feature space $\mathcal{H}$ where dot products are computed. Through the use of the kernel k, these two layers are in practice computed in one step. The results are linearly combined using weights v_i, found by solving a quadratic program (in pattern recognition, $v_i = y_i\alpha_i$; in regression estimation, $v_i = \alpha_i^* - \alpha_i$) or an eigenvalue problem (kernel PCA). The linear combination is fed into the function σ (in pattern recognition, $\sigma(x) = \text{sgn}\,(x + b)$; in regression estimation, $\sigma(x) = x + b$; in kernel PCA, $\sigma(x) = x$). (From Schölkopf, B., and Smola, A. J., 2002, *Learning with Kernels*, Cambridge, MA: MIT Press. Reprinted with permission.)

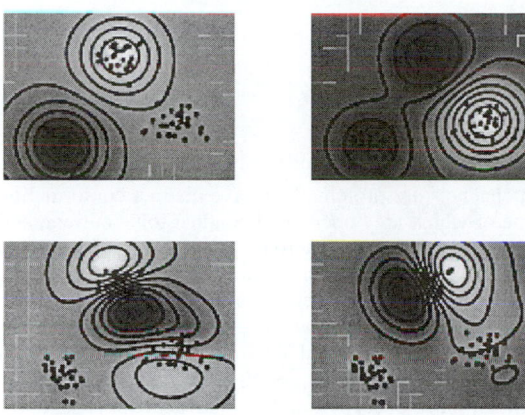
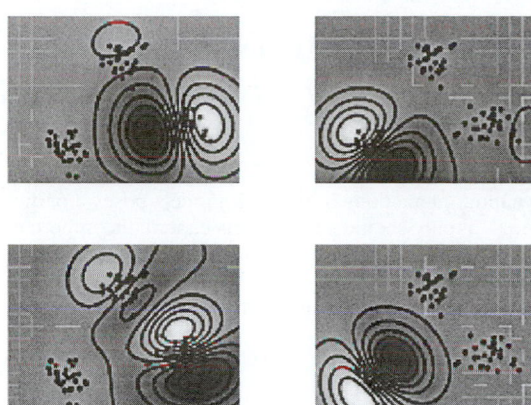

Figure 7. Contour plots of the first eight nonlinear features of kernel PCA using a radial basis function kernel on a toy data set consisting of three Gaussian clusters. In the upper left panel, the first and second component's split the data into three clusters. Note that kernel PCA is not deliberately designed to perform clustering; it tries to find a PCA description of the data in feature space by looking for directions of large variance. In input space, this reveals the cluster structure. The following three components depicted split each cluster in halves (components 3–5), while the last three achieve splits to the earlier ones.

MNIST digit recognition benchmark (with record results, see DeCoste and Schölkopf, 2002), as well as problems in text categorization (e.g., Joachims, 1999) and bioinformatics. For overviews of further applications as well as extensions of the approach to problems such as multiclass classification, density estimation, and novelty detection, the interested reader is referred to Burges (1998), Vapnik (1998), Schölkopf, Burges, and Smola (1999), Smola et al. (2000), Cristianini and Shawe-Taylor (2000), and Schölkopf and Smola (2002).

Discussion

During the last few years, SVMs and other kernel methods have rapidly advanced into the standard toolkit of techniques for machine learning and high-dimensional data analysis. This was probably due to a number of advantages compared to neural networks, such as the absence of spurious local minima in the optimization procedure, the fact that there are only few parameters to tune, enabling fast deployment in applications, the modularity in the design, where various kernels can be combined with a number of different learning algorithms, and the excellent performance on high-dimensional data.

Of particular interest for the cognitive science community are the way in which kernel methods connect similarity measures, nonlinearities, and data representations in linear spaces where simple geometric algorithms are performed. Moreover, it is worthwhile to note that as approaches based on a mathematical analysis of the problem of learning (in the formulation given by Vapnik and Chervonenkis), they are in principle not bound to any particular implementation.

Along with the observation that SV sets contain all the information required to solve a given classification task, this has led to speculation whether they could be related to prototypes believed to be used by the brain for categorization (cf. Poggio, 1990). This question, along with the one of whether SVMs might help explain some aspects of how the brain works, is as yet unanswered.

Road Map: Learning in Artificial Networks
Background: Pattern Recognition

Related Reading: Learning and Generalization: Theoretical Bounds; Principal Component Analysis

References

Boser, B. E., Guyon, I. M., and Vapnik, V., 1992, A training algorithm for optimal margin classifiers, in *Proceedings of the 5th Annual ACM Workshop on Computational Learning Theory* (D. Haussle, Ed.), ACM Press, pp. 144–152.

Burges, C. J. C., 1998, A tutorial on support vector machines for pattern recognition, *Data Mining Knowledge Discov.*, 2:121–167. ◆

Cristianini, N., and Shawe-Taylor, J., 2000, *An Introduction to Support Vector Machines*, Cambridge, Engl.: Cambridge University Press. ◆

DeCoste, D., and Schölkopf, B., 2002, Training invariant support vector machines, *Machine Learn.*, 46:161–190.

Haussler, D., 1999, *Convolutional Kernels on Discrete Structures*, Technical Report UCSC-CRL-99-10, Computer Science Department, University of California at Santa Cruz.

Herbrich, R., 2002, *Learning Kernel Classifiers: Theory and Algorithms*, Cambridge, MA: MIT Press. ◆

Joachims, T., 1999, Making large-scale SVM learning practical, in *Advances in Kernel Methods: Support Vector Learning* (B. Schölkopf, C. J. C. Burges, and A. J. Smola, Eds.), Cambridge, MA: MIT Press, pp. 169–184.

Poggio, T., 1990, *A Theory of How the Brain Might Work*, A.I. Memo No. 1253, Cambridge, HA: Massachusetts Institute of Technology, Artificial Intelligence Laboratory.

Schölkopf, B., Burges, C. J. C., and Smola, A. J., Eds., 1999, *Advances in Kernel Methods: Support Vector Learning*, Cambridge, MA: MIT Press.

Schölkopf, B., and Smola, A. J., 2002, *Learning with Kernels*, Cambridge, MA: MIT Press. ◆

Smola, A. J., Bartlett, P. L., Schölkopf, B., and Schuurmans, D., 2000, *Advances in Large Margin Classifiers*, Cambridge, MA: MIT Press.

Vapnik, V., 1995, *The Nature of Statistical Learning Theory*, New York: Springer-Verlag. ◆

Vapnik, V., 1998, *Statistical Learning Theory*, New York: Wiley.

Watkins, C., 2000, Dynamic alignment kernels, in *Advances in Large Margin Classifiers* (B. Schölkopf, C. J. C. Burges, and A. J. Smola, Eds.), Cambridge, MA: MIT Press, pp. 39–50.

Williams, C. K. I., 1998, Prediction with Gaussian processes: From linear regression to linear prediction and beyond, in *Learning and Inference in Graphical Models* (M. I. Jordan, Ed.), Boston: Kluwer. ◆

Synaptic Interactions

Alain Destexhe, Zachary F. Mainen, and Terrence J. Sejnowski

Introduction

Modeling synaptic interactions in network models poses a particular challenge. Not only should such models capture the important physiological properties of synaptic interactions, but they must do so in a computationally efficient manner in order to facilitate simulations of large networks. This article reviews several types of models that address these goals.

Synaptic currents are mediated by ion channels activated by neurotransmitter released from presynaptic terminals. Kinetic models are expressive enough to describe the behavior of ion channels underlying synaptic currents. Although full representation of the molecular details of the synapse generally requires highly complex kinetic models, we focus here on simpler kinetic models that are more computationally efficient. We show that these models can capture the time course and dynamics of several types of synaptic responses, allowing them to be useful tools for modeling synaptic interactions in large networks.

Models of Synaptic Currents

For neural models that do not include action potentials, synaptic currents are typically modeled as a direct function of the some presynaptic activity measure. In the simplest case, synaptic interactions are described by a sigmoid function, and presynaptic activity is interpreted as the average firing rate of the afferent neuron. Alternatively, the postsynaptic currents can be described by a first-order differential equation in which one term depends on the presynaptic membrane potential through a sigmoid function. Another possibility is to interpret the activity level as the fraction of neurons active per unit of time, thus representing the interaction between neural populations rather than single neurons (Wilson and Cowan, 1973).

A different approach is needed to model synaptic interactions between spiking neurons. It is usually assumed that a presynaptic spike triggers a conductance waveform postsynaptically. A popular model of postsynaptic conductance increase is the alpha function introduced by Rall (1967):

$$r(t - t_0) = \frac{(t - t_0)}{\tau_1} \exp\left[-(t - t_0)/\tau_1\right] \quad (1)$$

where $r(t)$ resembles the time course of experimentally recorded postsynaptic potentials (PSPs) with a time constant τ_1. The alpha function and its double-exponential generalization can be used to approximate most synaptic currents with a small number of parameters that require, implemented properly, low computation and memory requirements (Srinivasan and Chiel, 1993). The disadvantages of the alpha function, or related approaches, include the lack of direct biophysical interpretation and the absence of a natural method for handling successive temporally overlapping postsynaptic currents (PSCs) from a train of presynaptic impulses.

A natural way to model synaptic currents is based on the kinetic properties of the underlying synaptic ion channels. The kinetic approach is closely related to the well-known model of Hodgkin and Huxley (1952) for voltage-dependent ion channels (reviewed in Hille, 2001). Kinetic models can describe in great detail the properties of synaptic ion channels and can be integrated coherently with chemical kinetic models for enzymatic cascades underlying signal transduction and neuromodulation (Destexhe, Mainen, and Sejnowski, 1994). In the next section, we show how to model various types of ion channels with the kinetic formalism.

The Kinetic Description

Ion channels are proteins that have distinct conformational states, some of which are "open" and conduct ionic current, and some of which are "closed," "inactivated," or "desensitized" and do not conduct. Single-channel recording techniques have demonstrated that the transitions between conformational states occurs rapidly and stochastically (reviewed in Sakmann and Neher, 1995). It has furthermore been shown that the behavior of single ion channels is well-described by *Markov models*, in which stochastic transitions between states occur with a time-independent probability.

It is straightforward to move from a microscopic description of single channel behavior to a macroscopic description of a population of similar channels. In the limit of large numbers, the stochastic behavior of individual channels can be described by a set of continuous differential equations analogous to ordinary chemical reaction kinetics. The kinetic analogue of Markov models posits the existence of a group of conformational states $S_1 \ldots S_n$ linked by a set of transitions

$$S_1 \rightleftarrows S_2 \rightleftarrows S_4 \rightleftarrows \cdots$$
$$\Updownarrow \qquad \Updownarrow \qquad\qquad (2)$$
$$S_3 \rightleftarrows \cdots$$

Define s_i as the fraction of channels in state S_i and r_{ij} as the rate constant of the transition

$$S_i \underset{r_{ji}}{\overset{r_{ij}}{\rightleftarrows}} S_j \quad (3)$$

which obeys the kinetic equation

$$\frac{ds_i}{dt} = \sum_{j=1}^{n} s_j r_{ji} - \sum_{j=1}^{n} s_i r_{ij} \quad (4)$$

The wide range of interesting behavior exhibited by channels arises from the dependence of certain transitions on factors extrinsic to the channel, such as the binding of another molecule to the protein or the electric field across the cell membrane. These influences are referred to as *ligand-gating* and *voltage-gating* respectively.

For voltage-dependent ion channels, the transition between two states S_i and S_j occurs with rate constants that are dependent on voltage, such as

$$S_i \underset{r_{ji}(V)}{\overset{r_{ij}(V)}{\rightleftarrows}} S_j \quad (5)$$

The functional form of the voltage-dependence can be obtained from single-channel recordings (see Sakmann and Neher, 1995). The kinetics-based description of the voltage-dependence of channels is quite general. In particular, the well-known model of Hodgkin and Huxley (1952) for the fast sodium channel and the delayed-rectifier potassium channel can be written in the form of a Markov model that is equivalent to the original Hodgkin-Huxley equations.

For ligand-gated ion channels, the transition between two states S_i and S_j can depend on the binding of n molecules of a ligand L:

$$S_i + nL \underset{r_{ji}}{\overset{r_{ij}}{\rightleftarrows}} S_j \quad (6)$$

which can be rewritten as

$$S_i + nL \underset{r_{ji}}{\overset{r_{ij}([L])}{\rightleftarrows}} S_j \quad (7)$$

where $[L]$ is the concentration of ligand and $r_{ij}([L]) = r_{ij}[L]^n$. In this model, there is a simple functional dependence of the rate constants on ligand concentration. For some receptor types, rate constants may also depend on the voltage.

Ligand-gating is typified by *ionotropic synaptic receptors*, which are ion channels that are directly gated by neurotransmitter molecules. By contrast, *metabotropic synaptic receptors* do not have an ion channel and neurotransmitter binding to the receptor induces the formation of an intracellular messenger (calcium or G proteins, for example) that controls the gating of an ion channel independent of the receptor. These two types of synaptic receptors will be considered in the next two sections.

Kinetic Models of Ionotropic Receptors: AMPA, NMDA, and GABA_A

The most common types of ligand-gated synaptic channels are the excitatory AMPA and NMDA types of glutamate receptor and the inhibitory $GABA_A$ receptor. Many kinetic models have been proposed for these receptors (reviewed in Sakmann and Neher, 1995; Destexhe, Mainen, and Sejnowski, 1998). For example, a multistate Markov scheme for AMPA-Kainate receptors (Standley, Ramsey, and Usherwood, 1993) is:

$$D_2 \underset{r_9([L])}{\overset{r_{10}}{\rightleftarrows}} D_1 \underset{r_7([L])}{\overset{r_8}{\rightleftarrows}} C \underset{r_2}{\overset{r_1([L])}{\rightleftarrows}} C_1 \underset{r_4}{\overset{r_3([L])}{\rightleftarrows}} C_2 \underset{r_6}{\overset{r_5}{\rightleftarrows}} O \tag{8}$$

where C is the unbound closed state, C_1 and C_2 are respectively the singly and doubly bound closed states, O is the open state, and D_1 and D_2 are respectively the desensitized singly and doubly bound states. r_1 through r_{10} are the associated rate constants and $[L]$ is the concentration of neurotransmitter in the synaptic cleft.

The six states of this AMPA model are required to account for the electrophysiological properties of these receptors as determined by single-channel recordings (Standley et al., 1993). However, simplified kinetic schemes with fewer states and transitions can constitute fairly good approximations for the time courses and the dynamic behavior of synaptic currents (Destexhe et al., 1994, 1998). In particular, consider the simplest kinetic schemes involving two states

$$C \underset{r_2}{\overset{r_1([L])}{\rightleftarrows}} O \tag{9}$$

or three states

$$\begin{array}{ccc} & r_1([L]) & \\ C & \rightleftarrows & O \\ & r_2 & \\ r_6([L]) \searrow & & \nearrow r_4 \\ r_5 & & r_3 \\ & D & \end{array} \tag{10}$$

In these two schemes, C and O represent the closed and open states of the channel, D represents the desensitized state, and $r_1 \ldots r_6$ are the associated rate constants. Not only are these simple schemes easier to compute than more complex schemes, but the time course of the current can be obtained analytically under some approximations (Destexhe et al., 1994).

Another way to simplify the model is suggested by experiments using artificial application of neurotransmitter, where it has been shown that synaptic currents with a time course very similar to that of intact synapses can be produced using very brief pulses of agonist (reviewed in Sakmann and Neher, 1995). These data suggest that the response time course is dominated by the postsynaptic kinetics rather than the time course of the neurotransmitter concentration. Hence, one can assume that the neurotransmitter is de-

livered as a brief (≈ 1 ms) pulse triggered at the time of each presynaptic spike.

Simplified kinetic schemes for the AMPA response can be compared to detailed kinetic models to judge the quality of the approximation (Figure 1A–D). Both simple and detailed synaptic responses first require a trigger event, corresponding to the release of neurotransmitter in the synaptic cleft. In simulations of the Markov kinetic model, the time course of neurotransmitter was derived using a model that included presynaptic action potentials, calcium-dependent fusion of presynaptic vesicles, and clearance of neurotransmitter. Figure 1A–C shows the AMPA response resulting from a high-frequency train of presynaptic spikes. The amplitude of successive PSCs decreased progressively due to an increasing fraction of receptors in desensitized states. A simplified kinetic scheme using transmitter pulses gave a good fit, both to the time course of the AMPA current (shown in Figure 2A) and to the response desensitization that occurs during multiple successive events (Figure

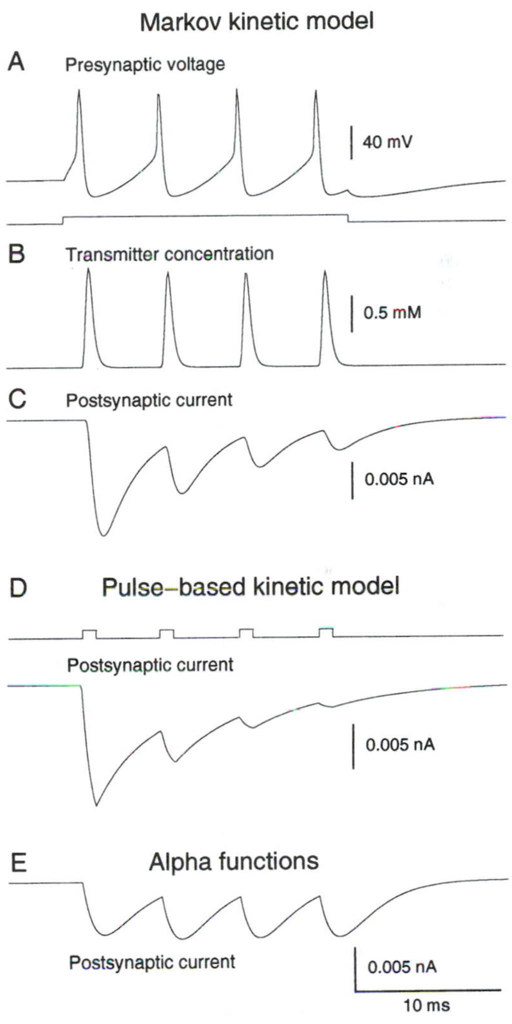

Figure 1. Comparison of three models for AMPA receptors. *A–C,* Markov model of AMPA receptors. *A,* Presynaptic train of action potentials elicited by current injection. *B,* Corresponding glutamate release in the synaptic cleft obtained using a kinetic model for transmitter release. *C,* Postsynaptic current from AMPA receptors modeled by a six-state Markov model. *D,* Same simulation with AMPA receptors modeled by a simpler three-state kinetic scheme and transmitter time course approximated by spike-triggered pulses (trace above). *E,* Postsynaptic current modeled by summed alpha functions. (Modified from Destexhe et al., 1994.)

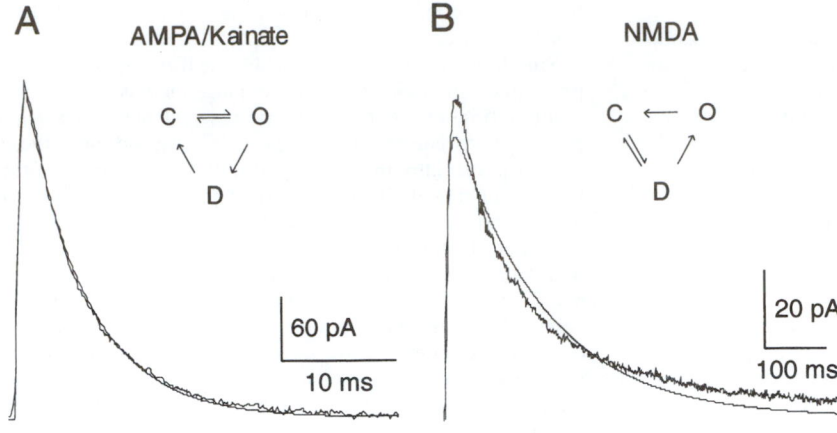

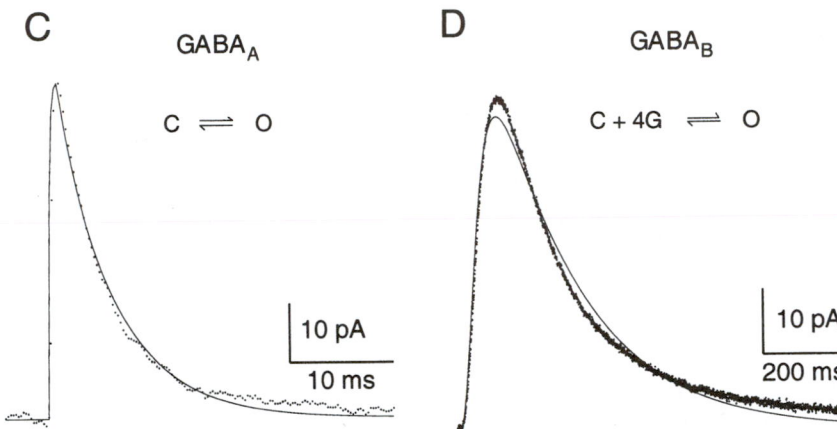

Figure 2. Elementary kinetic schemes provide good models of postsynaptic currents. *A*, AMPA-mediated currents (courtesy of Z. Xiang, A. C. Greenwood, and T. Brown). *B*, NMDA-mediated currents (courtesy of N. A. Hessler and R. Malinow). *C*, GABA$_A$-mediated currents (courtesy of T. S. Otis and I. Mody). *D*, GABA$_B$-mediated currents (courtesy of T. S. Otis, Y. Dekoninck, and I. Mody). The averaged recording of the synaptic current (negative currents upwards for *A* and *B*) is shown with the best fit obtained using simple kinetics (continuous trace— 1 *ms* pulse of agonist for *A*, *B*, *C*). (*A* modified from Destexhe et al., 1994, *B*–*D*, modified from Destexhe et al., 1998. Values of rate constants and other parameters can be found in Destexhe et al., 1998.)

1*D*). Alpha functions, in contrast, did not match the summation behavior of the synaptic current (Figure 1*E*).

Procedures similar to those applied to the AMPA response can be used to obtain simple kinetic models for other types of ligand-gated synaptic channels, including the NMDA and GABA$_A$ receptors. Two-state and three-state models provide good fits of averaged whole-cell recordings of the corresponding PSCs (Figure 2*B*–*C*; for more details see Destexhe et al., 1994, 1998).

Kinetic Models of Metabotropic Receptors: GABA$_B$ and Neuromodulation

Some neurotransmitters do not bind directly to the ion channel, but act through an intracellular second messenger, which links the activated receptor to the opening or closing of an ion channel. This type of synaptic interaction, called *neuromodulation*, occurs at a slower time scale than ligand-gated channels. Neuromodulators such as GABA (GABA$_B$), acetylcholine (M2), noradrenaline (alpha-2), serotonin (5HT-1), dopamine (D2), and others gate a K$^+$ channel through the action of G-proteins (reviewed in Brown, 1990). We have developed a kinetic model of the G protein-mediated slow intracellular response mediated by GABA$_B$ receptors (Destexhe and Sejnowski, 1995) that can be applied to any of these transmitters.

Unlike GABA$_A$ receptors which respond to weak stimuli, GABA$_B$ responses require high levels of presynaptic activity

(Mody et al., 1994). This property might be due to extrasynaptic localization of GABA$_B$ receptors, but it can also be accounted solely from the kinetics of the G-protein cascade underlying GABA$_B$ responses (Destexhe and Sejnowski, 1995). The high level of activity needed to activate GABA$_B$ responses could be reproduced by the following kinetic scheme:

$$R_0 + T \rightleftarrows R \rightleftarrows D \qquad (11)$$

$$R + G_0 \rightleftarrows RG \rightarrow R + G \qquad (12)$$

$$G \rightarrow G_0 \qquad (13)$$

$$C_1 + nG \rightleftarrows O \qquad (14)$$

where the transmitter, T, binds to the receptor, R_0, leading to its activated form, R, and desensitized form, D. The G-protein is transformed from an inactive (GDP-bound) form, G_0, to an activated form, G, catalyzed by R. Finally, G binds to open the K$^+$ channel, with n independent binding sites. A simplified model with very similar behavior can be obtained by assuming quasi-stationarity in Equations 12 and 14, neglecting desensitization, and considering G_0 in excess, leading to:

$$\frac{dr}{dt} = K_1[T](1 - r) - K_2 r \qquad (15)$$

$$\frac{ds}{dt} = K_3 r - K_4 s \qquad (16)$$

Figure 3. Kinetic models of synaptic currents used to simulate a small network of thalamic reticular (RE) and thalamocortical (TC) neurons. These neurones have complex intrinsic firing properties and generate bursts of action potentials following depolarization or hyperpolarization (insets). They are connected with different receptor types (scheme on top: AMPA from TC to RE, GABA$_A$ within RE and a mixture of GABA$_A$ and GABA$_B$ from RE to TC). The simulations exhibit oscillatory behavior in which the exact frequency and cellular phase relationships are dependent on intrinsic calcium- and voltage-dependent currents as well as synaptic currents. Modeling synaptic currents with the correct kinetics was needed to match experimental observations (modified from Destexhe et al., 1996; see also SLEEP OSCILLATIONS).

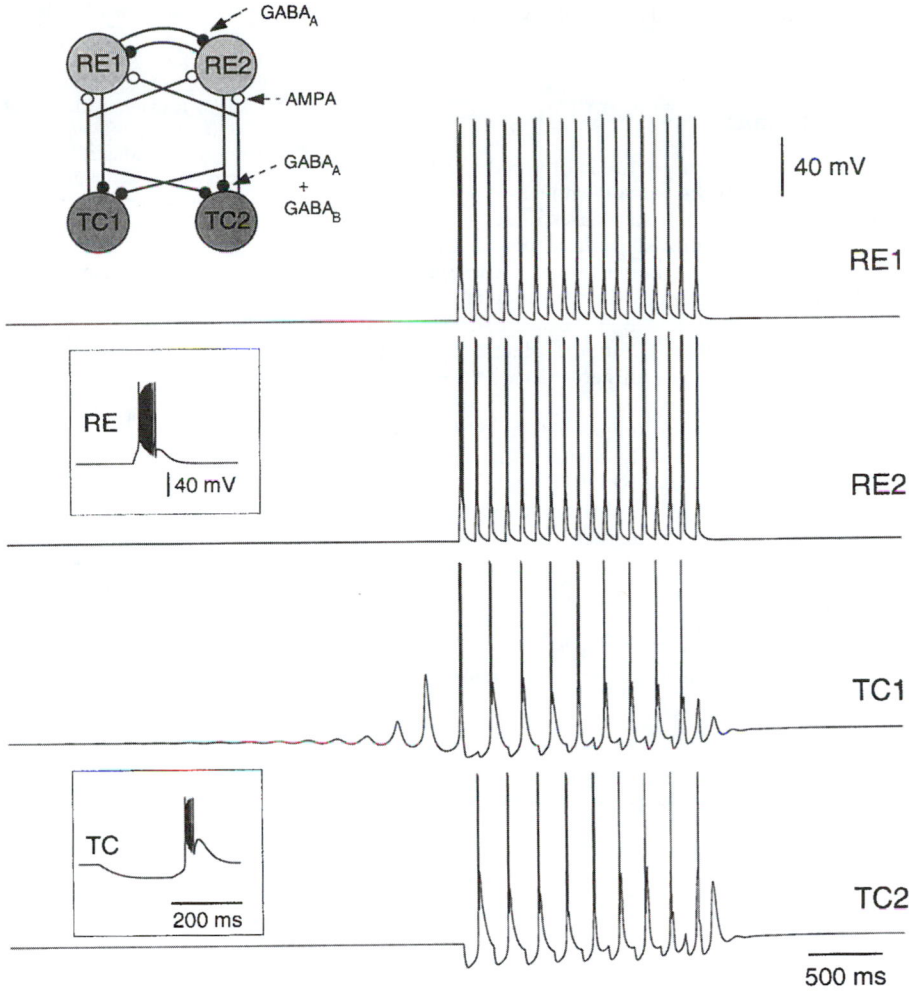

where r is the fraction of receptors in the activated form, g is the normalized concentration of activated G-proteins, and $K_1 \ldots K_4$ are rate constants. The fraction of K$^+$ channels in the open form is then given by:

$$[O] = \frac{s^n}{s^n + K_d} \qquad (17)$$

where K_d is the dissociation constant of the binding of G on K$^+$ channels. This computationally efficient model can fit single GABA$_B$ IPSCs (Figure 2D) and account for the typical stimulus dependence of GABA$_B$ responses (Destexhe and Sejnowski, 1995; Destexhe et al., 1998). Models have shown that this property has drastic consequences for the genesis of epileptic discharges (reviewed in Destexhe and Sejnowski, 2001).

Other neuromodulators listed previously have a G protein-mediated intracellular response similar to that of GABA$_B$ receptors. Details of the rate constants obtained from fitting different kinetic schemes to GABA$_B$ PSC are given in Destexhe et al. (1998).

Simulating Networks of Neurons

Simplified kinetic models of synaptic receptors can be used to model complex cellular interactions that depend on the kinetics of synaptic currents. For example, several types of oscillations are generated by thalamic circuits. Thalamic neurons have complex intrinsic firing properties and can generate bursts of action potentials in rebound to inhibition due to low-threshold calcium currents (see insets in Figure 3). Thalamic neurons are also characterized by different types of synaptic receptors, such as AMPA, GABA$_A$ and GABA$_B$ (see scheme in Figure 3). Modeling this system using Hodgkin and Huxley's (1952) type of models for intrinsic currents and simple kinetics models of synaptic currents led to oscillations in the ~10 Hz frequency range (Figure 3). These simulations have been used to explore the cellular mechanisms for the different types of oscillations in these circuits (Destexhe et al., 1996), which depend on the kinetics of intrinsic and synaptic currents. For example, the ~10 Hz frequency depends on the decay of GABA$_A$-mediated currents and the transformation of these oscillations into more synchronized ~3 Hz oscillations depends critically on the activation properties of GABA$_B$ responses (Destexhe et al., 1996).

This example shows that simplified kinetic models consisting of only a few states can capture the essential properties necessary to explain complex cellular interactions. They are useful for investigating network interactions involving multiple types of synaptic receptors. In addition, kinetic models can be used to model both synaptic currents and voltage-dependent currents, providing a single formalism to describe all currents in a neuron (Destexhe et al., 1994). This approach has been used to model different types of oscillations and pathological behavior in networks of the cerebral cortex, the thalamus, and the thalamocortical system (Destexhe and Sejnowski, 2001).

Summary and Conclusions

Simple and fast mechanisms are needed to model synaptic interactions in biophysically based network simulations involving thousands of synapses. A class of models based directly on the kinetics of the ion channels mediating synaptic responses can be implemented with minimal computational expense. These models capture both the time course of individual synaptic and neuromodulatory events and also the interactions between successive events (summation, saturation, desensitization), which may be critical when investigating the behavior of networks where neurons have complex intrinsic firing properties.

All models shown here were simulated using NEURON (Hines and Carnevale, 1997; see NEURON SIMULATION ENVIRONMENT). Computer generated movies and NEURON programs to simulate these models are available at http://cns.iaf.cnrs-gif.fr and http://www.cnl.salk.edu/~alain/ or on request.

Road Map: Biological Neurons and Synapses
Background: Axonal Modeling
Related Reading: Biophysical Mosaic of the Neuron; Ion Channels: Keys to Neuronal Specialization; Temporal Dynamics of Biological Synapses

References

Brown, D. A., 1990, G-proteins and potassium currents in neurons, *Annu. Rev. Physiol.*, 52:215–242.
Destexhe, A., Bal, T., McCormick, D. A., and Sejnowski, T. J., 1996, Ionic mechanisms underlying synchronized oscillations and propagating waves in a model of ferret thalamic slices, *J. Neurophysiol.*, 76:2049–2070.
Destexhe, A., Mainen, Z. F., and Sejnowski, T. J., 1994, Synthesis of models for excitable membranes, synaptic transmission and neuromodulation using a common kinetic formalism, *J. Computational Neurosci.*, 1:195–230. ◆
Destexhe, A., Mainen, Z. F., and Sejnowski, T. J., 1998, Kinetic models of synaptic transmission in *Methods in Neuronal Modeling*, 2nd ed. (C. Koch and I. Segev, Eds.), Cambridge, MA: MIT Press, pp. 1–26. ◆
Destexhe, A., and Sejnowski, T. J., 1995, G-protein activation kinetics and spill-over of GABA may account for differences between inhibitory responses in the hippocampus and thalamus, *Proc. Natl. Acad. Sci. USA*, 92:9515–9519.
Destexhe, A., and Sejnowski, T. J., 2001, *Thalamocortical Assemblies*, Oxford, UK: Oxford University Press.
Hille, B., 2001, *Ionic Channels of Excitable Membranes*, 3rd ed., Sunderland, MA: Sinauer.
Hines, M. L., and Carnevale, N. T., 1997, The NEURON simulation environment, *Neural Computation*, 9:1179–1209.
Hodgkin, A. L., and Huxley, A. F., 1952, A quantitative description of membrane current and its application to conduction and excitation in nerve, *J. Physiol. (Lond.)*, 117:500–544.
Mody, I., De Koninck, Y., Otis, T. S., and Soltesz, I., 1994, Bridging the cleft at GABA synapses in the brain, *Trends Neurosci.*, 17:517–525.
Rall, W., 1967, Distinguishing theoretical synaptic potentials computed for different some-dendritic distributions of synaptic inputs, *J. Neurophysiol.*, 30:1138–1168.
Sakmann, B., and Neher, E., Eds., 1995, *Single-Channel Recording*, 2nd ed., New York: Plenum Press.
Srinivasan, R., and Chiel, H. J., 1993, Fast calculation of synaptic conductances, *Neural Computation*, 5:200–204.
Standley, C., Ramsey, R. L., and Usherwood, P. N. R., 1993, Gating kinetics of the quisqualate-sensitive glutamate receptor of locust muscle studied using agonist concentration jumps and computer simulations, *Biophys. J.*, 65:1379–1386.
Wilson, H. R., and Cowan, J. D., 1973, A mathematical theory of the functional dynamics of nervous tissue, *Kybernetik*, 13:55–80.

Synaptic Noise and Chaos in Vertebrate Neurons

Philippe Faure and Henri Korn

Introduction

The membrane potential of central neurons undergoes continuous fluctuations called synaptic noise (SN), which is a mixture of ongoing and overlapping inhibitory and/or excitatory postsynaptic potentials. Synaptic noise depends on both the summed firing of action potentials by neurons presynaptic to the investigated cell and the spontaneous release of transmitter, analogous to that producing miniature end-plate potentials. Classical methods such as interevent interval histograms led to the conclusion that SN is stochastic (see references in Faure and Korn, 2000), and in the absence of further understanding it has generally been modeled as such. However, despite its random appearance, SN may be a true signal associated with neural coding, often believed to involve well-defined firing patterns (Perkel and Bullock, 1968; Fujii et al., 1996) including chaotic ones (Skarda and Freeman, 1990; see also CHAOS IN NEURAL SYSTEMS). Tools derived from nonlinear dynamics can be used to address this issue.

The Basic Material

Mauthner (M-) cells are a pair of identified neurons in the hindbrain of teleosts. When the animal is subjected to an unexpected stimulus, one of the cells triggers an escape reaction by activating contralateral motor neurons via a complex reticulospinal network (Figure 1A). Their excitability is controlled by powerful inhibitory presynaptic interneurons that continuously generate an intense SN consisting of successive inhibitory postsynaptic potentials (IPSPs), which can be recorded with intracellular electrodes (Figure 1B, top).

Analysis of Synaptic Noise with Tools Derived from Nonlinear Dynamics

To eliminate nonlinearities due to the asymmetric waveform of synaptic potentials, reliable time series require SN to be converted into time intervals by differentiating the initial signal (Figure 1B, bottom). Thus, the time of occurrence and the peak amplitude of the resulting upstroke "spikes" constitute the raw events train to be used for further analysis. In addition, dynamic parameters can be extracted from these time series with a number of nonlinear methods. Note that the use of these methods requires particular care when dealing with nonstationary and noisy data (see CHAOS IN BIOLOGICAL SYSTEMS).

Figure 1. *A*, M-cell inhibitory ($-$) networks with their excitatory ($+$) inputs. *B*, In upper tier, inhibitory synaptic noise with inverted IPSPs. In lower tier, time derivative of this sample and illustration of the threshold (θ) method. *C*, RP analysis. C_1, At left are trains of three spikes starting at times i and j, with the difference between their intervals $I_1 - I_1'$ and $I_2 - I_2'$ less than and more than ε, respectively. On the right are recurrence plots (RPs) of two almost identical sequences of five intervals each. C_2, RPs of chaotic (left), periodic (right top), and stochastic (right bottom) systems. *D*, Histogram of the number N_L of line segments of length L from a "chaotic" RP. The parameter $\mu(\varepsilon)$ corresponds to the power law of this histogram. Inset: Evolution of $\mu(\varepsilon)$ versus ε (see text). Abbreviations: C, chaotic; P, periodic; S, stochastic. KS indicates the Kolmogorov-Sinai entropy. (C_2 left and *D* adapted from Faure and Korn, 1998.)

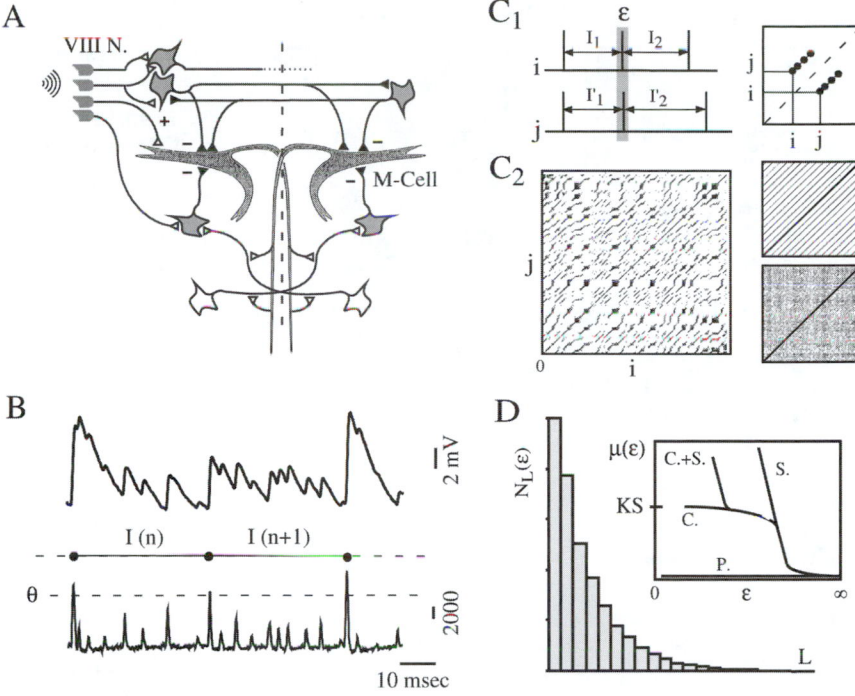

Recurrence Plots

Recurrence plots (RPs) portray the dynamics of a d-dimensional signal in the form of dots interspersed in a square matrix (Eckmann, Kamphorst, and Ruelle, 1985). The plot is an $N*N$ array where a dot is placed at (i, j) whenever the embedded vectors (x_i, x_j) are within a predetermined cutoff distance ε. In a two-dimensional space, the embedded vectors are defined by $x_i = (I_i, I_{i+1})$, where $I_1, I_2, \ldots, I_{N+1}$ is the time interval series and, using a maximum norm, x_i and x_j are close if $\max_{n=0,1}\{|I_{i+n} - I_{j+n}| \leq \varepsilon\}$ (Figure $1C_1$, left). Thus, a diagonal segment of length L indicates the number of recurrent points in the phase space that remain close for L successive time steps. For example, two almost identical trains of six spikes starting at time i and j appear as two diagonal segments of length L = 4 each (Figure $1C_1$, right).

This procedure identifies several dynamics, independent of whether the studied signal is discrete or continuous and embedded in a phase space with appropriate techniques (Schreiber, 1999). The RPs take the form of small-scale discontinuous segments, or of parallel lines, or are homogenous, in the cases of chaotic, periodic, or stochastic systems, respectively (Figure $1C_2$). This approach is useful for detecting periodic and apparently chaotic patterns hidden in SN (Faure and Korn, 1998).

Several sequence-sensitive parameters can be estimated to quantify the degree of determinism using histograms of length L of the upward diagonal segments (Figure 1D). Two are particularly convenient for studies of SN. The first, called percent of determinism (%det), is the ratio of the number of dots in diagonal line segments divided by the total number of dots in the RP (Webber and Zbilut, 1994). The second is defined by the slope $\mu(\varepsilon)$ of the power law of the histogram. It is related to a classical invariant of dynamic systems, i.e., the Kolmogorov-Sinai entropy (Faure and Korn, 1998) and its variations as a function of ε can be used to characterize the dynamics of a time series (Figure 1D, inset).

Return Maps

In the case of time interval series between successive events, one way to look for deterministic relationships between one interval

and the next is simply to plot each interval, I_N, against the next I_{N+1}. The result is a return map (RM), sometimes called a Poincaré map (see DYNAMICS AND BIFURCATION IN NEURAL NETS), that allows the dynamics to be visualized as a sequence of pairs of points. These points are grouped in clusters, in the case of periodic motion, or as an extended structure that is not space filling, in the case of chaotic motion. For studies of M-cell SN, RMs were constructed with subsets of events selected, according to their amplitudes, by varying a threshold θ. As θ was progressively lowered, RMs disclosed three distinct superimposed patterns. The first is periodic and indicates a dominant frequency of the involved IPSPs, denoted fp (Figure $2A_1$). The second and most striking configuration is a triangular motif with its apex at fp (Figure $2A_2$). For the lowest θ's, this pattern is replaced by an undefined partial filling of the map (Figure $2A_3$).

A more refined analysis can be used to determine if temporal processes other than the dominant frequency are hidden in SN. This involves subtracting events associated with fp from the initial time series. RMs reconstructed in this manner revealed at least three populations of IPSPs occurring with distinct and unexpected periodicities, all in the so-called gamma range (Faure, Kaplan, and Korn, 2000).

Unstable Periodic Orbits and Determinism in SN

In a phase space, periodic orbits are the equilibrium state of a dynamic system (see DYNAMICS AND BIFURCATION IN NEURAL NETS). If these orbits are not stable, any trajectory will wander endlessly in a sequence of close approaches followed by rapid divergences, thereby defining unstable periodic orbits (UPOs), which have recently been used as indicators of chaos. In RMs they can be identified by detecting rare sequences of events that approach and depart from a fixed point on the identity line according to strict geometrical rules (So et al., 1998). UPOs were found in SN at the level of the triangular patterns (Figure 2B). In addition, M-cells' SN contains other forms of recurrence defined by repeated sequences of identical intervals.

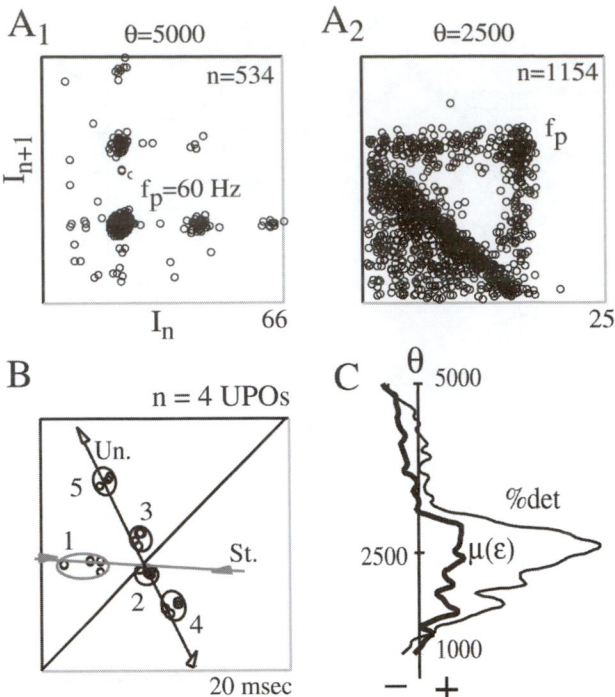

Figure 2. PM analysis. A_1 and A_2, Experimental maps obtained with a 10-s sample of SN for two levels of detection θ. B, four UPOs extracted from the map in A_2, with their stable (St.) and unstable (Un.) manifolds crossing at a period-1 orbit (labeled 2). C, Variation of the significance level of the %det and $\mu(\varepsilon)$ parameters in the same sample, as a function of θ. The vertical line indicates a confidence level at $2e^{-5}$% after comparison with surrogates. (A and B_1 modified from Faure et al., 2000.)

The degree of recurrence, i.e., of determinism, can be quantified to ascertain the nonrandom distribution of the time intervals between events. Both the %det and $\mu(\varepsilon)$ were significantly increased (Faure and Korn, 1998) when SN was studied at intermediate values of θ, in regions of well-defined triangular patterns (Figure 2D). The statistical significance of these results was assessed using surrogate strategies (see CHAOS IN BIOLOGICAL SYSTEMS).

Taken together, results from the M-cell system support the notion that a form of determinism compatible with chaos may be embedded in SN.

Determinism in Presynaptic Networks

Periodic and chaotic processes can be generated by coupled oscillators (Borisyuck et al., 1995), and studies of SN can reveal the presence of such a mechanism in the nervous system. The triangular structures in experimental RMs are consistent with the periodic events varying at random. However, another explanation is possible, namely, that sets of interneurons in the presynaptic networks behave as coupled "oscillators." Two arguments favor this interpretation (Faure et al., 2000). First, analysis of the phase relationships between the identified frequencies indicates a weak coupling between them. The second argument relies on the confrontation of a formal model with observed data. A model of neurons was built that incorporated the fact that M-cells' presynaptic inhibitory interneurons are coupled by chemical and electrical junctions (Figure 1A), with each "neuron" firing action potentials at one of the observed frequency. The coupling between the parent modeled neurons produces fluctuations between action potentials with UPOs

and intermittent locking (not shown). Thus, the diversity of temporal patterns contained in SN may already be present in presynaptic networks.

Transmission of Temporal Patterns; Effects of Learning

If nerve inputs converge from a population of independent channels on an integrating neuron, any information coded temporally in a single one is lost, so that this population can in principle be replaced by a single random channel. But this is only true if these parallel channels induce similar postsynaptic effects (Perkel and Bullock, 1968).

The various, almost periodic components of SN are manifest in the same train if, and only if, some types of events are sometimes above and sometimes below θ. The distribution of the amplitudes of events then allows for gradual transitions between the types of patterns observed (Figures $2A_1$ to $2A_3$) as θ is lowered (Figure 3A). Such properties of RMs are consistent with an involvement of synaptic junctions.

Indeed, the principal feature of evoked transmitter release is its probabilistic nature. That is, chemical transmission is governed by two binomial parameters, n and p (Figure 3B, left), where n represents the population of basic "quantal units," q, capable of responding to a nerve impulse, and p represents their average probability of responding. The product np is the mean quantal content that is equal to the average number of quanta released by a given junction during successive trials (Figure 3B, right). The product npq, where q is the size of a quantum, determines the synaptic efficacy (Korn and Faber, 1991).

Implementing the model in Figure 3C with terminal "synapses" at each oscillator indicates that if np is the same at all of them, the postsynaptic events fluctuate in the same range, and therefore no frequency emerges for a given θ (Figure $3D_1$). In contrast, if the synapses have different synaptic efficacies, the RMs exhibit the hierarchical features of those observed experimentally (Figure $3D_2$). Thus, synaptic heterogeneity confers a "separating power" on the terminals and allows SN to contain precise information about the dynamics of the presynaptic networks. This prediction has been verified experimentally by taking advantage of long-term tetanic potentiation, which increases p in the M-cell inhibitory system. This paradigm of learning sharpens the shape of triangular patterns in PMs and increases the determinism in SN (Faure et al., 2000).

Discussion

Nonrandom patterns compatible with chaos can be detected in SN, and more generally in neural networks (Rabinovich and Abarbanel, 1998; see also CHAOS IN NEURAL SYSTEMS), but it should be stressed that nonlinear dynamics tend now to focus on global modifications of the nervous system rather than on demonstrating chaos per se (see EEG AND MEG ANALYSIS). This aproach can provide unexpected information about the functional organization of neural networks (such as the synchronization of presynaptic cells in the form of coupled oscillators that generate SN) and about their state of activity (such as the enhancement of determinism in SN by learning).

Exept for its influence on the input-output function of neurons (see STOCHASTIC RESONANCE), the role of SN remains uncertain. In the M cells, either one of which triggers a vital escape reaction, the magnitude of inhibitory SN is a critical factor for selecting which of the two cells fires for an appropriate response (Hatta and Korn, 1999). Furthermore, the variability of SN at relay stations of the output pathways introduces uncertainty into the expression of the reflex, and therefore enhances its success in evading predators.

Figure 3. *A,* Schematic time series with three classes of periodic IPSPs, labeled ○, □, and △ according to their parent frequency. Events above and below θ are indicated by filled and empty symbols, respectively. *B,* Transmitter release at a central synapse. At left is an axon with $n = 6$ terminals. Following an action potential, some of them release a quantum, q, whereas the others do not, with probabilities p and $1 - p$, respectively. At right, as a result of successive impulses, the amplitude of postsynaptic events fluctuates in discrete steps, from 0 to n and around the mean quantal content, np (arrow). C', Modeled neurons with their terminal synapses (Syn.) and a sample of their respective spike trains. *D,* Contribution of synaptic properties to the transmission of the presynaptic patterns illustrated in *C.* Return maps constructed with the simulated SN when all the synapses have identical (D_1) or distinct (D_2) quantal contents. (B modified from Faure et al., 2000.)

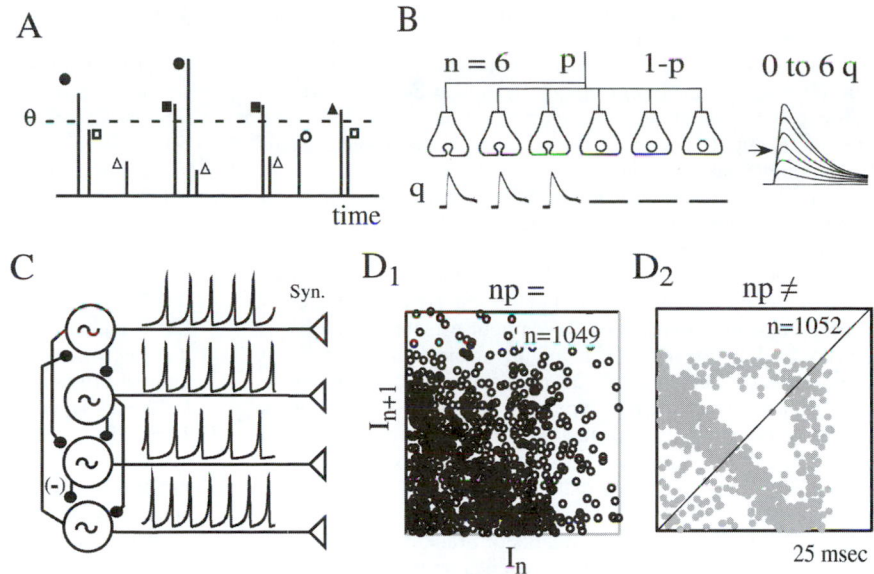

Experimental data are still necessary to assess the possible behavioral advantages of deterministic patterns over truly random ones and to determine how chaotic dynamics affect neural function.

Particularly relevant here are the possible relationships between nonlinear dynamics and higher brain functions. There is growing evidence that the apparent variability of neuronal spike trains, which plays a major role in perception, is mostly the consequence of precise dynamics rather than of a random "noise." That is, the brain would be continuously browsing through various possible internal states until new information induces transitions to a more specific one (Skarda and Freeman, 1990; Tsodyks et al., 1999). Chaos, and possibly SN, may play a role in such adaptive processes (Tsuda, 2001).

Road Map: Biological Neurons and Synapses
Background: Chaos in Biological Systems
Related Reading: Chaos in Neural Systems; Synaptic Transmission

References

Borisyuk, G. N., Borisyuk, R. M., Khibnik, A. I., and Roose, D., 1995, Dynamics and bifurcations of two coupled neural oscillators with different connection types, *Bull. Math. Biol.,* 57:809–840.

Eckmann, J.-P., Kamphorst, S. O., and Ruelle, D., 1987, Recurrence plots of dynamical systems, *Europhys. Lett.,* 4:973–977.

Faure, P., and Korn, H., 1998, A new method to estimate the Kolmogorov entropy from recurrence plots: Its application to neuronal signals, *Physica D,* 122:265–279.

Faure, P., Kaplan, D., and Korn, H., 2000, Synaptic efficacy and the transmission of complex firing patterns between neurons, *J. Neurophysiol.,* 84:3010–3025.

Fujii, H., Ito, H., Aihara, K., Ichinose, N., and Tsukada, M., 1996, Dynamical cell assembly hypothesis: Theoretical possibility of spatiotemporal coding in the cortex, *Neural Netw.,* 9:1303–1350. ◆

Hatta, K., and Korn, H., 1999, Tonic inhibition alternates in paired neurons that set direction of the fish escape reaction, *Proc. Natl. Acad. Sci. USA,* 96:12090–12095.

Korn, H., and Faber, D. S., 1991, Quantal analysis and synaptic efficacy in the CNS, *Trends Neurosci.,* 14:439–445.

Perkel, D. H., and Bullock, T. H., 1968, Neural coding, *Neurosci. Res. Progr. Bull.,* 6(3):221–348.

Rabinovich, M. I., and Abarbanel, H. D. I., 1998, The role of chaos in neural systems, *Neuroscience,* 87(1):5–14. ◆

Schreiber, T., 1999, Interdisciplinary application of non-linear time series methods, *Phys. Rep.,* 308:1–64. ◆

Skarda, C. A., and Freeman, W. J., 1990, Chaos and the new science of the brain, *Concepts Neurosci.,* 1(2):275–285. ◆

So, P., Francis, J. T., Netoff, T. I., Gluckman, B. J., and Schiff, S. J., 1998, Periodic orbits: A new language for neuronal dynamics, *Biophys. J.,* 74:2776–2785.

Tsodyks, M., Kenet, T., Grinvald, A., and Arieli, A., 1999, Linking spontaneous activity of single cortical neurons and the underlying functional architecture, *Science,* 286:1943–1946.

Tsuda, I., 2001, Towards an interpretation of dynamic neural activity in terms of chaotic dynamical systems, *Behav. Brain Sci.,* 24:575–628. ◆

Webber, C. L., and Zbilut, J. P., 1994, Dynamical assessment of physiological systems and states using recurrence plot strategies, *Am. J. Physiol.,* 76:965–973.

Synaptic Transmission

Charles F. Stevens and Yongling Zhu

Introduction

Information flows from one neuron to the next at specialized points of contact known as *synapses*. Because brain function depends essentially on such information flow, synapses play a central role in neural computations. This article reviews the structure and function of synapses, and describes the ways that *synaptic strength*—the magnitude of the effects that synapses produce, often termed the *synaptic weight*—is regulated through the probabilistic nature of synapse function.

Each neuron typically makes synaptic contact with about ten thousand other neurons, and receives synapses from approximately the same number. As a microliter of mammalian neocortex contains about 10^5 neurons, each with about 10^4 synapses, the density of synapses in cortex is about a billion per microliter; the human neocortex has about 10^{10} neurons, so the entire cortex would transmit information between neurons at about 10^{14} synapses.

Synapses provide a unidirectional flow of information, from the *sending* (presynaptic) to the *receiving* (postsynaptic) neuron, but not in the reverse direction. Two distinct types of synapses are present in brain, *excitatory* and *inhibitory*; the excitatory synapses—about 80% of all synapses fall in this category—tend to cause the receiving neuron to produce nerve impulses, whereas inhibitory synapses tend to prevent the receiving neuron from generating nerve impulses. The actual output of a neuron depends, of course, on the joint action of the two types of synaptic inputs. All of the synapses made by a particular neuron are of the same type, so one can divide neurons in the brain into those that are excitatory (make excitatory synapses) and those that are inhibitory (make inhibitory synapses).

Modifiability is one of the hallmarks of brain, and the principle way the function of neural circuits is adapted to the computational needs of the organism is through changes in the average size of the signal generated in the receiving neuron by synaptic action. This synaptic efficacy is usually referred to a *synaptic strength* or *weight*, and the modifications of synaptic strength are key both for the study of artificial and actual neural networks. To understand how synapses function, and how their strength is modified, it is necessary to consider synaptic structure.

Synapse Structure

Three main parts of a synapse can be identified: the *bouton* (the part of the synapse contributed by the sending cell), *postsynaptic structures* (the parts of the synapses contributed by the receiving cell), and the *synaptic cleft* (a 20-nm space that separates the sending and receiving neurons). The bouton contains a cluster of 35-nm diameter spherical structures, the *synaptic vesicles*, a few of which appear to be touching the presynaptic membrane, and the remainder of which fill the regions of the bouton not immediately adjacent to the membrane. The population of vesicles that appear to touch the membrane constitute the *docked vesicle pool*, and the non-docked vesicles are called the *reserve* vesicles (Harris and Sultan, 1995; Schikorski and Stevens, 1997). Vesicles are docked to a specialized region of membrane, called the *active zone*, positioned immediately opposite the postsynaptic structures. Most synapses have only a single active zone, but some large ones have dozens or even hundreds.

The postsynaptic structure of most excitatory synapses is organized around a thorn-like protuberance from the *dendrite* (dendrites constitute another kind of brain "wire" for carrying information) of the receiving neuron, the synaptic *spine* (Harris and Kater, 1994). The spine has a thin neck and a bulb-like head just opposite the bouton. Aligned with the active zone, and having exactly the same size and shape, is a specialized postsynaptic membrane called the *postsynaptic density* (PSD). The synaptic cleft is the extracellular region bounded by the active zone on the sending neuron side and by the PSD on the receiving neuron side.

Outline of Synaptic Transmission

Information flows from the sending to the receiving neuron by the bizarre process known as *synaptic transmission*. The sequence of steps that constitute synaptic transmission are as follows: when a nerve impulse arrives at a bouton, it causes a brief increase in the calcium ion concentration in the bouton that is sensed by a special protein that initiates a process known as *exocytosis* of a synaptic vesicle. The vesicle then releases the fixed amount of *neurotransmitter* it contains.

The postsynaptic density contains *receptors* that bind the neurotransmitter and produce a current known as the *postsynaptic current* (PSC). This current, in turn, produces a voltage change, the *postsynaptic potential* (PSP), that constitutes the postsynaptic signal. The result, then, of a nerve impulse in the sending neuron is an electrical signal in the receiving cell.

Probabilistic Nature of Synaptic Transmission

Early studies, from the middle of the twentieth century, revealed that neurotransmitter release is *quantal* (that is, only an integral number of vesicles can undergo exocytosis) and *probabilistic* (that is, the exocytic event occurs in a probabilistic fashion) (Katz, 1969). The probability that an individual docked vesicle will undergo exocytosis when a nerve impulse arrives is about 0.05, and the number of docked vesicles (although very variable from synapse to synapse) is on the order of 10, so the probability that no neurotransmitter release will occur at a synapse is $(0.95)^{10} = 0.6$; this calculation assumes that the vesicles are independent and identical (neither is likely not to be exactly true). Instances for which a presynaptic nerve impulse fails to cause neurotransmitter release are termed *failures*, and occasions on which release does occur are called *successes*, a terminology taken from the coin-flipping theory that is the mathematical model for the release process. The probability of a success (1 minus the probability of a failure) is commonly called the synapse's *release probability*.

Because the study of individual synapses is difficult, the first evidence that individual synapses are unreliable—in the sense that the probability of a failure is high—was indirect, but more direct methods revealed, at about the same time, that the failure rate is around 0.7 for many synapses (Allen and Stevens, 1994; Bolshakov and Siegelbaum, 1995; Raastad, Storm, and Anderson, 1992). More recently, imaging methods have shown that the release probability for synapses made by a single neuron has a broad distribution, well fitted by a gamma function, with a mean near 0.3 (Murthy, Sejnowski, and Stevens, 1997). Furthermore, this release probability distribution is, as might be expected, produced by a range in synapse sizes and numbers of docked vesicles.

Changes in Synaptic Strength

One of the main insights provided by study of artificial neural networks is that proper adjustment of *synaptic weights* is a key to determining function a neural circuit performs. The physiological analog of the synaptic weight in an artificial network is *synapse strength*, the average size of the postsynaptic response (PSC or PSP) produced by a nerve impulse that occurs on the sending side of the synapse. Synaptic strength is constantly being altered in the functioning brain on many time scales, from a few milliseconds to days or, perhaps, years through many different mechanisms. Some of these mechanisms have been assigned names like *facilitation, augmentation, depression, long-term potentiation*, and *long-term depression*. The very long-term changes are believed to arise from structural modifications in synapse size or number, but the short-term dynamic modification of synaptic strength occurs primarily through alterations in release probability (Dobrunz and Stevens, 1999).

The dynamic regulation of synaptic strength depends on a complicated set of mechanisms that record the history of synaptic use over many time scales, and serve to filter in incoming spike train in a way that reflects the past use of the synapse. Although many of these mechanisms are reasonably well understood at the descriptive level as presented in later sections of this article, the molecular basis and computation significance of the filter is the subject of current study.

The fundamental relation that determines release probability is

$$p = 1 - (1 - \alpha)^n \qquad (1)$$

where p is the probability that a vesicle will be released from an active zone, n is the number of docked vesicles, and α is the average release probability for an individual vesicle to be released (Dobrunz and Stevens, 1997). This equation assumes that vesicles are identical and independent—not quite true—and that at most one vesicle can be released by a nerve impulse at an active zone. Although this and the other equations presented here have a long history, only the more recent references, in which experiments were carried out with modern techniques, are provided; see these references for citations of earlier literature. Release probability is modified both by changes in n, the size of the docked vesicle pool, and α, the probability that an individual vesicle will be released.

The size of the docked vesicle pool (also called the readily releasable pool) varies because of releases (which decrease the size of the pool) and refilling (which tends to restore the pool size to its current capacity N). The difference-differential equation that governs the pool size n during intervals between action potentials is

$$\frac{dP(n, t)}{dt} = -(\rho(N - n) + \lambda n)P(n, t)$$
$$+ \lambda(n + 1)P(n + 1, t)$$
$$+ \rho(N - n + 1)P(n - 1, t) \qquad (2)$$

where $P(n, t)$ is the probability of having n docked vesicles at time t, ρ is the rate constant per vesicle for spontaneous release, and λ is the rate of refilling empty docking sites. Both N and λ in this equation depend on the history of synapse use as described later in this article.

The refilling rate constant λ is increased, through a mechanism that involves intrabouton calcium concentration, by activity according to the equation

$$\frac{d\lambda}{dt} = A \frac{r(t)}{1 + \frac{r(t)}{r_0}} - B(\lambda(t) + \lambda_0) \qquad (3)$$

where A, r_0, B, and λ_0 are all constants and $r(t)$ is the rate at which action potentials enter the terminal (Stevens and Wesseling, 1998).

The maximum size of the docked vesicle pool (N), known as the *pool capacity*, also depends on the history of use according to the pair of equations

$$N = N_0 - \theta(u - u_0) \qquad (4)$$

and

$$\frac{du}{dt} = R(t) - \mu u(t) \qquad (5)$$

where N_0 is the maximum possible capacity, u is the number of vesicles that have been released but not yet recovered by endocytosis, μ is a rate constant (value about .1/s), $R(t)$ is the rate at which vesicles are undergoing exocytosis, and θ is a function whose value is its argument if the argument is non-negative and zero otherwise. These equations describe the process through which unrecovered vesicles start to occlude docking sites once a threshold number (u_0) is reached (Stevens and Wesseling, 1999b).

The equations above describe how synaptic use determines the number of vesicles available for release, and this quantity in turn is a key factor in setting the release probability according to the fundamental equation set out at the start of this discussion. As the number of vesicles in the readily releasable pool declines with use, the release probability also tends to decrease, and synaptic strength

is diminished; this process is generally termed "depression," and it is a prominent mechanism at all synapses.

Several sets of mechanisms also modify synaptic strength through the parameter $\alpha = \alpha_0(1 + \phi(t))$, where α_0 is the resting average release probability per vesicle and $\phi(t)$ is a function of time t that depends on the history of synapse use. The best-studied and most familiar of these mechanisms is known as *facilitation*, a process that remembers synaptic use for about half a second and increases release probability during that period. The function $\phi(t)$ reflects concentration of calcium ions in the bouton but the mechanistic basis is still unclear. Whatever the detailed mechanism, $\phi(t)$ is incremented by an approximately constant amount with each nerve impulse arrival, and it decays exponentially between nerve impulses. Facilitation f is usually defined for a pair of stimuli—this is the way it is studied in the laboratory—and is given by the ratio of the release probability on the second impulse to that on the first. As a consequence of the fundamental relation between number of docked vesicles and release probability, facilitation is given by

$$f = \frac{1 - (1 - p)^{\alpha(t)}}{p} \qquad (6)$$

where p is the release probability in the resting state (the first stimulus of the pair) and $\alpha(t)$ depends on α_0 and $\varphi(t)$ as set out above. A typical value for f at interstimulus intervals of 50 ms would be 2 (Dobrunz and Stevens, 1997).

Another process that increases synaptic strength is called *augmentation*. This phenomenon follows the same equation as facilitation (above), but the increment in $\phi(t)$ per impulse is much smaller than for facilitation, and the decay is much slower (about half a minute). Note that $\phi(t)$ is really the sum of two exponentials, one for facilitation and the other for augmentation. Because augmentation increments a constant amount with each nerve impulse arrival at the synapse and decays exponentially in the time between stimuli, the steady-state augmentation is linearly related to the stimulation frequency. The effect of augmentation can be a large one: with reasonable stimulation rates, augmentation can increase the synaptic strength sixfold or more (Stevens and Wesseling, 1999a).

As noted previously, the processes just described combine to specify synaptic strength in a rather complicated way that defines a type of history dependent filter. Thus, the synapse does not simply relay information from one cell to the next, but rather plays an essential computational role. A major challenge is to define this role and explain how such a filter is related to the other computational mechanisms used by neural circuits.

Road Map: Biological Neurons and Synapses
Related Reading: Single-Cell Models; Synaptic Interactions

References

Allen, C., and Stevens, C. F., 1994, An evaluation of causes for unreliability of synaptic transmission, *Proc. Natl. Acad. Sci. USA*, 91:10380–10383. ◆
Bolshakov, V. Y., and Siegelbaum, S. A., 1995, Regulation of hippocampal transmitter release during development and long-term potentiation, *Science*, 269:1730–1734.
Dobrunz, L. E., and Stevens, C. F., 1997, Heterogeneity of release probability, facilitation, and depletion at central synapses, *Neuron*, 18:995–1008.
Dobrunz, L. E., and Stevens, C. F., 1999, Response of hippocampal synapses to natural stimulation patterns, *Neuron*, 22:157–166.
Harris, K., and Kater, S., 1994, Dendritic spines: Cellular specializations imparting both stability and flexibility to synaptic function, *Ann. Rev. Neurosci.*, 17:341–371.
Harris, K. M., and Sultan, P., 1995, Variation in the number, location and size of synaptic vesicles provides an anatomical basis for the nonuniform probability of release at hippocampal CA1 synapses, *Neuropharmacology*, 34:1387–1395.

Katz, B., 1969, *The Release of Neural Transmitter Substances*, The Sherrington Lectures, Liverpool, UK: Liverpool University Press.

Murthy, V. N., Sejnowski, T. J., and Stevens, C. F., 1997, Heterogeneous release properties of visualized individual hippocampal synapses, *Neuron*, 18:599–612. ◆

Raastad, M., Storm, J. F., and Anderson, P., 1992, Putative single quantum and single fibre excitatory postsynaptic currents show similar amplitude range and variability in rate hippocampal slices, *Euro. J. Neurosci.*, 4:113–117.

Schikorski, T., and Stevens, C. F., 1997, Quantitative ultrastructural analysis of hippocampal excitatory synapses, *J. Neurosci.*, 17:5858–5867.

Stevens, C. F., and Wesseling, J. F., 1998, Activity-dependent modulation of the rate at which synaptic vesicles become available to undergo exocytosis, *Neuron*, 21:415–424.

Stevens, C. F., and Wesseling, J. F., 1999a, Augmentation is a potentiation of the exocytotic process, *Neuron*, 22:139–146. ◆

Stevens, C. F., and Wesseling, J. F., 1999b, Identification of a novel process limiting the rate of synaptic vesicle cycling at hippocampal synapses, *Neuron*, 24:1017–1028.

Synchronization, Binding and Expectancy

Wolf Singer

Introduction

Neuronal systems have to cope with combinatorial complexity. In the context of cognitive functions, combinatorial problems arise because perceptual objects consist of unique constellations of features. Although nervous systems exploit only a limited set of basic features to classify perceptual objects, the diversity of possible constellations of such elementary features is, for all practical purposes, virtually unlimited. Thus, cognitive systems have to explore a huge combinatorial space when searching for the consistent relations among features that define a perceptual object. Combinatorial problems of similar nature have to be solved for the programming and execution of movements. Although the elementary components of motor acts—the movements of individual muscle fibers—are limited in number, the diversity of movements that can be composed by combining the elementary components is, again, virtually infinite. Thus, mechanisms are required that permit rapid analysis and representation of relations between the responses of neurons whose activity signals the presence of particular features.

A common and well-documented strategy for the binding of distributed responses is the implementation of conjunction specific neurons. In the primary visual cortex of mammals, for example, relations are established between the responses of collinearly aligned retinal ganglion cells by having their output converge onto individual cortical neurons. Because of this convergence, cortical cells come to respond preferentially to elongated contours, thereby extracting and encoding the feature "orientation." This strategy of representing relations by selective combination of feedforward connections is common in all sensory systems and at all levels of processing. Its iteration in hierarchically structured processing architectures leads to conjunction-specific neurons that encode increasingly complex relations among elementary features. Representing features and their relations by conjunction units is rapid because it can be realized by feedforward processing, and it is reliable because the response of a particular cell always signals the same content (labeled line coding). However, this coding strategy, if not complemented by additional binding mechanisms, meets with a number of problems. First, large numbers of conjunction units are required for the exhaustive representation of the manifold intra- and cross-modal feature constellations of real world objects. Second, it is hard to see how novel objects and hence entirely new relations among features can be recognized and represented, as this would require rapid reconfiguration of input connections to previously uncommitted cells. Third, unresolved problems arise with the representation of the nested relations among the components of composite objects, such as visual scenes or sentences (for review of the arguments, see Singer, 1999).

A complementary strategy is needed, therefore—one that permits a more flexible definition of relations than can be achieved with hardwired conjunction units. As proposed by Hebb and subsequently elaborated by numerous authors, assembly coding is such a complementary strategy. The assumption is that individual cells represent only components of objects, which may consist of rather complex conjunctions of elementary features but may be common to different objects. Presumably, then, the presence of the whole object is signaled by the simultaneous responses of the ensemble of cells responding to the respective components. In this way, individual neurons can contribute at different times to the representation of different objects by forming ensembles with varying partners. Thus, a neuron tuned to a particular component can contribute to the representation of all objects containing this particular component, and neurons representing elementary features can be recombined in ever-changing constellations to represent novel objects. The requirements for the generation and read out of assembly codes are as follows: (1) Component coding neurons can become bound in variable constellations into different assemblies when input configurations change; (2) assemblies can be stabilized by learning so that a familiar object always activates its corresponding assembly; (3) the responses of cells constituting an assembly can be distinguished as related by subsequent processing stages and do not become confounded with responses of cells participating in other assemblies; (4) assemblies can be read out by triggering the formation of corresponding assemblies at other processing stages rather than by conjunction-specific units.

How to Tag Responses as Related

Numerous theoretical studies have addressed the question how assemblies can self-organize on the basis of cooperative interactions within associative neuronal networks. Here, we focus on the problem of how responses of cells that have been grouped into an assembly can be tagged as related. An unambiguous signature of relatedness is critical for assembly codes because, unlike in labeled line codes, the meaning of responses changes with the context in which they are interpreted; hence, false conjunctions are deleterious. Assembly coding requires a mechanism that assures that the responses of the neurons constituting an assembly are processed and evaluated together at subsequent processing stages and are not confounded with other, unrelated responses. In principle, this can be achieved by raising, jointly and selectively, the saliency of the responses belonging to an assembly. There are essentially three options to achieve this goal. First, unrelated responses can be inhibited and excluded from further processing. Second, the discharge frequency of the selected responses can be enhanced. Third, the selected cells can be made to discharge in precise temporal synchrony. All three mechanisms enhance the relative impact of the selected responses and can therefore be used to tag them as related. Single-cell studies have provided robust evidence that the first two mechanisms play a crucial role in the selection and grouping of responses. However, if joint increases in discharge rate are used for response selection and grouping, certain additional requirements must be fulfilled to comply with processing speed. Estimates based on reaction times, evoked potentials, and latencies of single-cell responses suggest that it takes maximally a few tens of milliseconds per processing stage to perform the computations necessary for the analysis and recognition of patterns of average complexity (Thorpe, Fize, and Marlot, 1996). Given the relatively low discharge rates of cortical neurons, with interspike intervals ranging typically from 20 to many hundreds of milliseconds, decisions on response selection and grouping can only be based on a small number of spikes per neuron. This precludes selection and read out mechanisms that analyze rate changes of individual neurons. It has been proposed that this problem can be overcome by population coding. The idea is that a particular feature is signaled in parallel by a large number of neurons (on average about a hundred) and that downstream neurons average across these population responses. Owing to spatial summation, increases in discharge rate become detectable with sufficiently high temporal resolution, provided that spike density increases significantly across channels within the relevant integration interval. Such changes in the spike density of population responses can result from two, in principle independent, mechanisms. They can result from simultaneous increases in discharge rate if these are sufficiently coherent across channels; or they can result from a coordinated redistribution of individual discharges without this leading to major changes in average discharge frequency of individual channels. What is required in this case is temporal regrouping of discharges across channels, advancing some and delaying others, so that more spikes than predicted by average discharge rates co-occur within the integration interval set by downstream neurons. Evidence suggests that both strategies are used by the nervous system to increase the saliency of responses and to permit rapid read out. In bottom-up feedforward processing, covarying increases in discharge frequency across channels are common because of stimulus locking. In top-down selection of responses, rate increases are made coherent by the coordinating action of attentional mechanisms (reviewed in Engel, Fries, and Singer, 2001). Evidence for rate-independent regrouping of spike timing is more difficult to obtain because it requires correlation analysis between the responses of different but simultaneously recorded neurons. However, such data are now available and reveal the existence of synchronizing mechanisms that can transiently augment cross-channel spike densities above the level predicted by average discharge rate. Frequently, this grouping of discharges occurs on the basis of an oscillatory patterning of the discharge sequences so that there are also periodically reoccurring intervals in which the cross-channel spike density drops below the level predicted by average discharge rate (see below).

Rate Covariation and Synchrony

Because the distinction between rate covariation and synchronization has led to fierce controversies and numerous misinterpretations, a brief comment is warranted here. According to classical conventions, discharge rates of individual neurons are measured over time spans long enough to count at least three or four spikes, i.e., 100 ms to several 100 ms, depending on discharge rate. Over the past few years, however, the duration of the intervals of effective synaptic integration had to be revised toward shorter values. Neurons are now considered capable of discriminating between synchronous and temporally dispersed inputs with a resolution in the millisecond range (Mainen and Sejnowski, 1995). This implies that neurons are sensitive to fluctuations of cross-channel spike densities at time scales at least one order of magnitude shorter than

those relevant for the assessment of rate changes of individual neurons. However, once the relevant integration windows become considerably shorter than the average interspike interval of individual responses, it begins to matter whether the spikes in parallel channels are distributed randomly or clustered in time. Thus, with conventional rate definitions, two variables need to be determined to describe a population response: the changes of discharge rate of the individual cells and the amount of synchrony/asynchrony of spikes across channels. As these measures are defined at different time scales, they can obviously vary independently. An alternative description would be time-resolved counts of cross-channel spike densities. If the time slices are sufficiently short (<10 ms), this measure captures coincident events of putative functional significance that may be independent of rate fluctuations. These cross-channel measurements of spike density are equivalent to a time-resolved assessment of "instantaneous" firing rates of the population; and if the windows for assessment of coincidences and for estimation of population firing rates are of the same duration, fluctuations in the number of coincidences can also be described in terms of ultrarapid fluctuations of population rate. However, by simply counting events across channels, one loses potentially important information—which cells contributed at which time to the population vector. Conditions can be imagined where the population rate is constant but the entries in each successive time slice are provided by different subsets of neurons. Thus, measures of synchrony and measures of cross-channel spike density may dissociate. Because which subset of neurons undergoes an enhancement of response saliency is relevant for the definition of relations, one should expect that it matters which subset of neurons contributes spikes within time slices of 10 ms or less.

Response Selection

While jointly increasing tonic firing is a common strategy of response selection and binding in feedforward processing and labeled line coding, it has several disadvantages if applied to encode relations in assemblies. The reason is that tonic increases in firing lead to sustained enhancement of saliency of the activated channels by augmenting both the frequency of EPSPs in individual channels and the number of coincidences across channels. Thus, sustained increases in rate, if used as the only tag of relations, preclude rapid changes in the assignment of relations. However, a rapid and time-resolved definition of relations is important to comply with fast processing. Assemblies sharing common subsets of neurons cannot be organized strictly simultaneously because it would be unclear which of the shared neurons belong to which assembly. Hence, if assemblies overlap, which is frequently the case, they need to be segregated in time by a multiplexing operation. Processing speed is limited by the rate with which different assemblies can follow one another or, in other terms, by the temporal resolution of the mechanism that labels responses as related. Modulating the saliency of responses by synchronization, i.e., by temporal regrouping of spikes rather than by tonic changes in firing rate, permits definition of relations at very short time scales. As synchronization exploits exclusively spatial summation, with no additional temporal summation, this tagging mechanism can operate, in principle, with a temporal resolution at the level of individual spikes. Using synchronization as a complementary mechanism for the definition of relations has the additional advantage that it permits specification of relations independently of firing rate. The discharge rates of neurons depend on numerous variables such as the physical energy of stimuli or the match between stimulus and receptive field properties, and it may not always be obvious how these modulations of response amplitude can be distinguished from those signaling the relatedness of responses. Not all strong responses are necessarily related. Because synchrony can be modulated independently of rates by temporal regrouping of discharges, it can be used as a tag of relatedness that is orthogonal to rate fluctuations. This can contribute to resolving the ambiguities resulting from stimulus-dependent rate fluctuations. Response amplitudes could thus be reserved to signal the presence and saliency of features, and synchronicity could be used in parallel to signal whether these features are related.

Another advantage of selecting responses by synchronization is that the timing of synchronized input events is preserved with high precision in the output activity of cells because synchronized input is transmitted with minimal latency jitter (Abeles, 1991; Diesmann, Gewaltig, and Aertsen, 1999). This, in turn, could be exploited to preserve the signature of relatedness across processing stages, thus further reducing the risk of getting false conjunctions. Finally, synchronization enhances processing speed also by accelerating synaptic transmission per se because synchronized EPSPs trigger action potentials with minimal delay.

In conclusion, response synchronization appears to be an attractive strategy to encode relations with high temporal resolution and within limits independently of rate fluctuations. However, response synchronization can only be used as a mechanism of response selection and grouping if neuronal networks are able to distinguish synchronous from temporally dispersed activity with a precision in the millisecond range.

Evidence for a Functional Role of Precise Timing

There is increasing evidence that neuronal networks can encode, transmit, and evaluate the temporal structure of stimuli with astounding precision. Temporal resolution is probably highest in the specialized circuits of the auditory system that can exploit latency differences in the submillisecond range for sound localization. Although signal transduction in the retina is slower than that in the ear, the visual system, too, is capable of resolving temporal patterns with a precision in the millisecond range. Thus, timing differences in the millisecond range suffice for the identification of depth cues in rapidly moving patterns, and stimulus onset asynchronies of less than 10 ms seem to support perceptual grouping. The visual system binds simultaneously appearing pattern elements and segregates them from elements presented with temporal offset (for review, see Singer, 1999).

Electrophysiological evidence confirms the ability of neuronal networks to transmit temporally modulated responses with a precision in the millisecond range over several processing stages. Cross-correlations between simultaneously recorded responses of retinal ganglion cells, relay neurons in the lateral geniculate, and cortical cells show that the oscillatory patterning of retinal responses is reliably transmitted to the cortex. Given the high frequency of the retinal oscillations (up to 100 Hz), this implies that the timing of discharges can be transmitted over several synaptic stages with a resolution in the millisecond range, at least when the discharges in parallel channels are precisely synchronized. The well-synchronized cortical responses to flicker stimuli point in the same direction. This temporal fidelity of synaptic transmission is not confined to primary sensory pathways, but holds as well for intracortical transmission. Cortical neurons can engage in oscillatory firing patterns in the γ-frequency range and synchronize their responses with millisecond precision over surprisingly large distances, indicating that cortical networks can handle temporally structured activity with low temporal dispersion (reviewed in Singer, 1999).

Simulation studies indicate that such precision is readily obtained with neurons that operate with conventional time constants if transmission occurs in reciprocally coupled parallel channels, i.e., if a population coding strategy is used (Diesmann et al., 1999). In this case, neurons at the same processing level synchronize their

discharges and these highly coherent pulse packets are then conveyed with minimal dispersion across several synaptic stages as postulated for synfire chains (Abeles, 1991).

Other indications for the high temporal resolution of cortical computations come from recent studies on use-dependent synaptic plasticity. Varying the temporal relations between presynaptic EPSPs and postsynaptic spike responses in simultaneously recorded coupled cortical cells revealed that long-term potentiation (LTP) results when the EPSP precedes the postsynaptic spike within intervals of 10 ms or less while the polarity of the modification reverses to long-term depression (LTD) as soon as the EPSP follows the spike (Markram et al., 1997). Thus, shifts of a few milliseconds in the timing relations between pre- and postsynaptic discharges suffice to invert the polarity of use-dependent synaptic modifications. The mechanism permitting such precise evaluation of the temporal contiguity of pre- and postsynaptic responses is the active dendritic response associated with the backpropagating spike. Recent results from visual cortex slices point in the same direction. In addition, they suggest that the temporal windows for Hebbian coincidence matching are sharpened further if neurons engage in oscillatory responses.

Pyramidal cells of rat visual cortex slices were made to discharge tonically at 20 or 40 Hz by injecting sinusoidally modulated current through a patch pipette. Simultaneously, EPSPs were evoked at 20 Hz by electrical stimulation of excitatory afferents. Changing the phase relations between pre- and postsynaptic activity revealed that the stimulated input tended to undergo LTP when the EPSPs were coincident with the spikes, while afferents consistently underwent LTD when the EPSPs fell in the troughs of the membrane potential oscillations. Thus, although high-frequency pre- and postsynaptic activation overlapped completely on a coarse time scale, phase shifts of about 12 ms between individual EPSPs and spikes reversed the polarity of the synaptic modifications (Wespatat, Tennigkeit, and Singer, in preparation). The temporal windows within which synaptic events or spikes are treated as contingent and related in signal processing must have the same duration as those relevant for Hebbian modifications in order to avoid learning of false conjunctions. Thus, the kinetics of neuronal plasticity imply that precise temporal relations between neuronal discharges matter not only for synaptic modifications but also in signal processing.

In conclusion, the experimental evidence and theoretical arguments indicate that neuronal networks can handle temporal patterns with high precision and that precise timing relations among the discharges of distributed neurons are computationally relevant.

Synchrony as a Code for the Definition of Relations

Following the discoveries that (1) cortical neurons often engage in synchronous oscillatory activity which is not stimulus locked but caused by internal interactions (Gray and Singer, 1989), (2) neurons distributed both within and across cortical areas can synchronize their discharges with a precision in the millisecond range, and (3) synchronization probability reflects common gestalt criteria of perceptual grouping, it had been proposed that the cerebral cortex imposes a temporal microstructure on otherwise sustained responses and uses this temporal patterning to express, through synchronization, the degree of relatedness of the responses (for a review of pertinent literature see Singer, 1999; Engel et al., 2001).

Synchronization of activity is defined operationally as a transient increase of coincident firing of two or more units that exceeds the level of coincidences predicted from estimations of actual discharge rates. Therefore, synchronization must be assessed by correlation analysis and cannot be deduced from comparisons of rate fluctuations alone. When synchronization is caused by internal interactions—as is the case for context-dependent response selection and binding—the time of occurrence of synchronized discharges is locked only loosely or not at all to external events. This intertrial variability precludes detection of synchronized response segments in histograms averaged over successive trials even in cases where synchronization is caused by a transient increase in discharge rate. In the numerous other cases where synchronization is achieved without any noticeable rate changes (e.g., by coordinated latency shifting of individual spikes or by phase locking of oscillatory response patterns), measurements of rate fluctuation cannot in principle disclose the presence of synchronized events even if responses are recorded simultaneously. Thus, internally generated synchrony is detectable only if responses are subjected to a trial-by-trial correlation analysis.

The results of such analyses indicate that synchronization by internal neuronal interactions is a frequent phenomenon that occurs in many cerebral structures (for recent reviews, see Singer, 1999; Engel et al., 2001). It has also been noticed that responses often exhibit an oscillatory patterning that is best revealed by recording jointly the activity of several adjacent cells. The reason for the better detectability of oscillations in population responses is twofold. First, individual cells tend to skip oscillation cycles in an irregular manner; second, oscillatory epochs are usually short and oscillation frequencies are variable. Therefore, the periodicity of oscillatory population responses is often not apparent in the firing patterns of individual cells, even if their discharges are precisely phase locked to the oscillatory activity of the population. For this reason, the search for synchronized oscillatory activity requires methods that assess population responses, such as recordings of multiunit activity, local field potentials (LFPs), or the electroencephalogram (EEG). These global signals can then be correlated with the activity of individual cells to determine whether the discharges of the recorded cells are correlated with the synchronized activity of surrounding cell populations. Such measurements of spike-field coherence have proved highly efficient in detecting changes in the synchronization of neurons and the frequency of oscillatory patterning (see below).

If internally generated synchronization is to serve as a signature of relatedness, it must meet several criteria. First, its precision should be in the millisecond range to match the temporal windows for effective spatial summation and Hebbian modifications. Second, it must be possible to generate and dissolve episodes of synchronous firing at a rate fast enough to be compatible with known processing speed. Third, synchronized activity must be more effective than nonsynchronized activity in driving cells in target structures because it can serve as a tag of relatedness only if it enhances the saliency of the synchronized responses. Fourth, there should be correlations between the occurrence of synchronization patterns and perceptual or motor processes. Fifth, disruption or artificial enhancement of synchrony should lead to changes in cognitive or motor functions.

The postulate that the precision of internally generated synchronization should match the windows for effective synaptic summation and Hebbian contingency matching is supported by cross-correlation data. The widths of the correlation peaks at half-height are typically in the range of less than 10 ms, particularly when the global EEG is in a desynchronized state. In this case, internally generated synchronization is often associated with an oscillatory patterning of the respective responses in the high β- or γ-frequency range (from 20 to 60 Hz). This limits the duration of the episodes of joint firing to the peaks of the oscillations and causes a sharp temporal demarcation of synchronous events because the oscillation troughs tend to be free of spikes.

The second postulate that internally generated synchronization must be established and dissolved very rapidly (within maximally a few tens of milliseconds) has received theoretical and experimental support only recently. Simulations with spiking neurons revealed that networks of appropriately coupled units can indeed undergo very rapid transitions from uncorrelated to synchronized states and vice versa. In physiological recordings, it is not uncommon that neurons engage in synchronous activity, often with additional oscillatory patterning, at the very same time they increase their discharge rate in response to the light stimulus (for review, see Singer, 1999).

Experimental support is also available for the third postulate that synchronized activity should have a stronger impact in target structures than temporally dispersed firing. Simultaneous recordings from coupled neuron triplets along thalamocortical and intracortical pathways in the visual system by Reid and colleagues (Usrey and Reid, 1999) have revealed that EPSPs synchronized within intervals below 2 ms are much more effective than EPSPs dispersed over longer intervals. Simulation studies, *in vitro* experiments, and *in vivo* recordings suggest similar conclusions. Multielectrode recordings from several sites of the cat visual cortex and retinotopically corresponding loci in the superior colliculus indicated that the impact of a particular group of cortical cells on target cells in the colliculus increases substantially whenever the cortical cells synchronize their discharges with other cortical cell groups projecting to the same site in the tectum. Finally, enhanced saliency of synchronized responses can also be inferred from the tight correlation between the strength of neuronal response synchronization and perception observed in experiments on binocular rivalry in cats and human subjects (reviewed in Singer, 1999).

Several mechanisms, some of which have been identified only recently, make synchronously arriving EPSPs more efficient than temporally dispersed EPSPs. First, because of their exponential decay, simultaneous EPSPs summate more effectively than temporally dispersed EPSPs, and there is some evidence for supralinear summation due to voltage-gated dendritic conductances. Second, firing threshold is sensitive to the rising slope of the depolarization and lowers for fast rising depolarizations (C. M. Gray, personal communication). Third, the effect of EPSPs is dramatically enhanced when these coincide with a backpropagating dendritic spike and hence with the input that generated this spike (Larkum, Zhu, and Sakmann, 1999). All three mechanisms are sensitive to dispersions of EPSPs in the range of a few milliseconds.

Putative Functions of Response Synchronization

Attention and Response Selection

A functional role of spike synchronization and the often concomitant oscillatory patterning of responses in the β- and γ-frequency range is suggested by the evidence that both phenomena are particularly well expressed when the brain is in an activated state, i.e., when the EEG is desynchronized and exhibits high power in the β- and γ-frequency range. Such EEG patterns are characteristic for the aroused and attentive brain as well as the dreaming brain, and hence for states in which sensory representations can be activated. Numerous observations in animal and human subjects point in the same direction. Synchronous oscillations in the γ-frequency range and their synchronization become more prominent during states of focused attention or when subjects are engaged in cognitive tasks that put strong demands on feature binding or short-term memory functions (reviewed in Tallon-Baudry and Bertrand, 1999; Engel et al., 2001). Multielectrode recordings from awake cats and monkeys trained to perform discrimination tasks indicate that attentional mechanisms enhance neuronal synchrony in anticipation of the expected task. One observes an increase in oscillatory activity in the γ-frequency range; this is associated with increased coherence between the spontaneous discharges of cells and the oscillations of the local field potential. These attentional effects appear to be selective and are confined to cortical areas and sites that must be engaged for the execution of the anticipated tasks. This priming has the effect that responses to attended stimuli synchronize faster and with greater precision than do responses to nonattended stimuli. These results support the hypothesis that response synchronization is one of the mechanisms by which responses are made more salient and selected for further processing. Recent evidence suggests in addition that the spontaneous γ-oscillations exhibit distinct patterns of coherence that reflect the functional architecture of intracortical association fibers. It has been proposed, therefore, that the spatiotemporal patterns of self-generated oscillatory activity are dynamic correlates of the system's inherent processing rules. The hypothesis is that the a priori knowledge of the system that resides in its functional architecture is permanently translated into dynamic states and that signal processing consists of a matching operation in which afferent sensory activity is compared with these "states of expectancy." This anticipatory nature of cortical computations is probably one reason why processing of sensory signals is so fast (for review, see Engel et al., 2001).

A close correlation between response synchronization and stimulus selection has been found in experiments on binocular rivalry that were performed in strabismic animals (Fries et al., 2002). Owing to experience-dependent modifications of processing circuitry, perception in nonamblyopic strabismic subjects always alternates between the two eyes. We have exploited this phenomenon of rivalry to investigate how neuronal responses that are selected and perceived differ from those that are suppressed and excluded from supporting perception (Figure 1). The outcome of these experiments was surprising because the responses of neurons in areas 17 and 18 were not attenuated during epochs in which they were excluded from controlling eye movements and supporting perception. A close and highly significant correlation existed, however, between changes in the strength of response synchronization and the outcome of rivalry. Cells mediating responses of the eye that won in interocular competition increased the synchronicity of their responses on presentation of the rivalrous stimulus to the other, los-

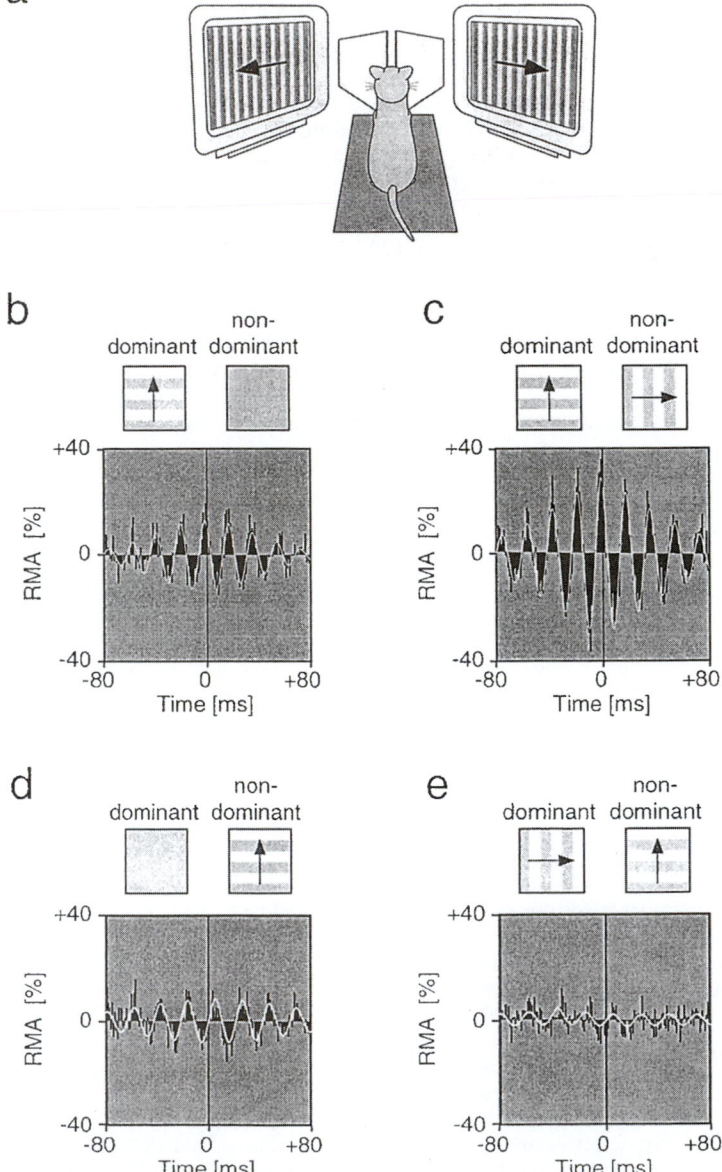

Figure 1. Neuronal synchronization under conditions of binocular rivalry. *A*, Using two mirrors, different patterns were presented to the two eyes of strabismic cats. Panels *B–E* show normalized cross-correlograms for two pairs of recording sites activated by the eye that won (*B, C*) and lost (*D, E*) in interocular competition. Insets above the correlograms indicate stimulation conditions. Under monocular stimulation (*B*), cells driven by the winning eye show a significant correlation, which is enhanced after introduction of the rivalrous stimulus to the other eye (*C*). For cells driven by the losing eye, the reverse is the case (compare conditions *D* and *E*). The white continuous line superimposed on the correlograms represents a damped cosine function fitted to the data. RMA is the relative modulation amplitude of the center peak in the correlogram, computed as the ratio of peak amplitude over offset of correlogram modulation; this measure reflects the strength of synchrony. (Modified from Fries et al., 2002.)

ing eye, while the reverse was true for cells driven by the eye that became suppressed. The synchronized responses exhibited an oscillatory modulation in the γ-frequency range, and differential changes of synchrony were particularly pronounced in measurements of spike-field coherence. Thus, in early visual areas selection of responses for further processing appeared to be achieved by modulating the degree of synchronization among large populations of neurons rather than by modifying the amplitude of responses. It is only at later processing stages that the poorly synchronized responses to the suppressed stimuli fail to elicit suprathreshold responses and that cells respond only to the selected stimulus (Leopold and Logothetis, 1996).

Synchronization and Feature Binding

The hypothesis that internal synchronization of discharges serves to group responses for joint processing predicts that synchronization probability should reflect some of the basic gestalt criteria according to which the visual system groups related features during scene segmentation. In agreement with this prediction, a series of studies provided evidence that neurons distributed across different columns within the same or different visual areas and even across hemispheres synchronize their responses with close to zero phase lag when activated with a single contour, but fire independently when stimulated simultaneously with two different contours. This suggests that synchronization was the result of a context-dependent selection and grouping process. Indeed, the probability and strength of response synchronization reflect some of the elementary gestalt criteria that underlie perceptual grouping. Stimulus configurations that comply with criteria such as continuity, proximity, similarity in the orientation domain, collinearity, and common fate evoke synchronized responses with higher probability than do configurations devoid of groupable features (for review, see Singer, 1999). Early experiments were performed in anesthetized animals, but more recent multielectrode recordings from awake cats and monkeys indicate that these synchronization phenomena are readily observed and even more pronounced when the animals are awake and attentive.

A particularly close correlation between neuronal synchrony and perceptual grouping has been observed in recent experiments with plaid stimuli. These stimuli are well suited for the study of dynamic binding mechanisms because minor changes of the stimulus cause a binary switch in perceptual grouping. Two superimposed gratings moving in different directions (plaid stimuli) may be perceived either as two surfaces, one being transparent and sliding on top of the other (component motion), or as a single surface, consisting of crossed bars, that moves in a direction intermediate to the component vectors (pattern motion). Which percept dominates depends on the luminance of grating intersections because this variable defines the degree of transparency. Component (pattern) motion is perceived when luminance conditions are compatible (incompatible) with transparency (Figure 2A). Here is a case where local changes in stimulus properties cause global changes in perceptual grouping. In the case of component motion, responses evoked by the two gratings must be segregated, and only responses evoked by the contours of the same grating must be grouped to represent the two surfaces. In the case of pattern motion, responses to all contours must be bound together to represent a single surface. If this grouping of responses is initiated by selective synchronization, three predictions must hold (Figure 2B). (1) Neurons that prefer the direction of motion of one of the two gratings and have collinearly aligned receptive fields should always synchronize their responses because they always respond to contours that belong to the same surface. (2) Neurons that are tuned to the respective motion directions of the two gratings should synchronize their responses

in the case of pattern motion because they then respond to contours of the same surface, but they should not synchronize in the case of component motion because their responses are then evoked by contours belonging to different surfaces. (3) Neurons preferring the direction of pattern motion should also synchronize only in the pattern and not the component motion condition.

Cross-correlation analysis of responses from cell pairs distributed either within or across area 18 and the posterior mediolateral suprasylvian sulcus (PMLS) of the cat visual cortex confirmed all three predictions. Cells synchronized their activity if they responded to contours that are perceived as belonging to the same surface (Castelo-Branco et al., 2000; Figure 2C). Interestingly, in contrast to synchrony, variations in response amplitude failed to reflect the transition from component to pattern motion induced by transparency manipulation. Dynamic changes in synchronization could therefore serve to encode, in a context-dependent way, the relations among the simultaneous responses to spatially superimposed contours, biasing their association with distinct surfaces.

Close relations between response synchronization and perception have also been found in animals suffering from developmental disturbances of their visual functions. Strabismic subjects, animals as well as humans, avoid double vision by selecting signals from one eye at a time and suppressing the signals from the other eye. If subjects always select the same eye, the cortical circuits receiving input from the suppressed eye cannot develop normally, and the result is an irreversible perturbation of vision in the suppressed eye—a syndrome known as strabismic amblyopia. Deficits comprise reduced visual acuity, spatial distortions, and problems with perceptual grouping of crowded scenes. Quite unexpectedly, in amblyopic cats, the responses of individual neurons appear normal in the primary visual cortex. Deficits become apparent only in measures that assess the temporal relations among simultaneously recorded responses of distributed neurons. Neurons driven by the amblyopic eye had a drastically reduced ability to synchronize their responses, and this deficit accounts well for some of the perceptual disturbances. Poorly synchronized responses are less salient than well-synchronized discharges; this can explain why the signals from the amblyopic eye always lose the competition with signals from the normal eye and are not perceived when this eye is open. Likewise, if deficiencies in the synchronizing mechanism are equivalent to impaired response selection and grouping, this would account for the reduced visual acuity and the difficulties in scene segmentation that frequently accompany amblyopia.

The interpretation that poorly synchronized activity fails to support perception because of reduced impact on cells at subsequent processing stages agrees with the finding that neurons at higher processing levels fail to respond to the temporally disorganized signals arriving from the primary visual cortex (Schröder et al., 2002).

Further indications for a functional role of precise timing relations between the discharges of distributed neurons have recently been obtained with multielectrode recordings from the motor and prefrontal cortex of monkeys performing a visually cued reaching task (Riehle et al., 1997) and from studies of the insect olfactory system. In insect antennal lobes, as in mammalian olfactory bulbs, odors evoke oscillatory population responses that are synchronized across parallel channels. Interestingly, information about the composition of a particular odor is encoded both in the pattern of rate fluctuations in parallel channels and in the distribution of coincident spikes. When the oscillatory patterning and the resulting synchronization are disrupted by pharmacological manipulations without modification of the spatiotemporal pattern of rate fluctuations, simple, noncomposite odors could still be discriminated while complex, composite odors were confounded (Stopfer et al., 1997).

A

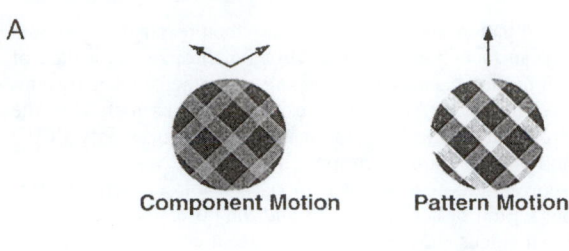

Component Motion   **Pattern Motion**

B

Predictions on Synchronization

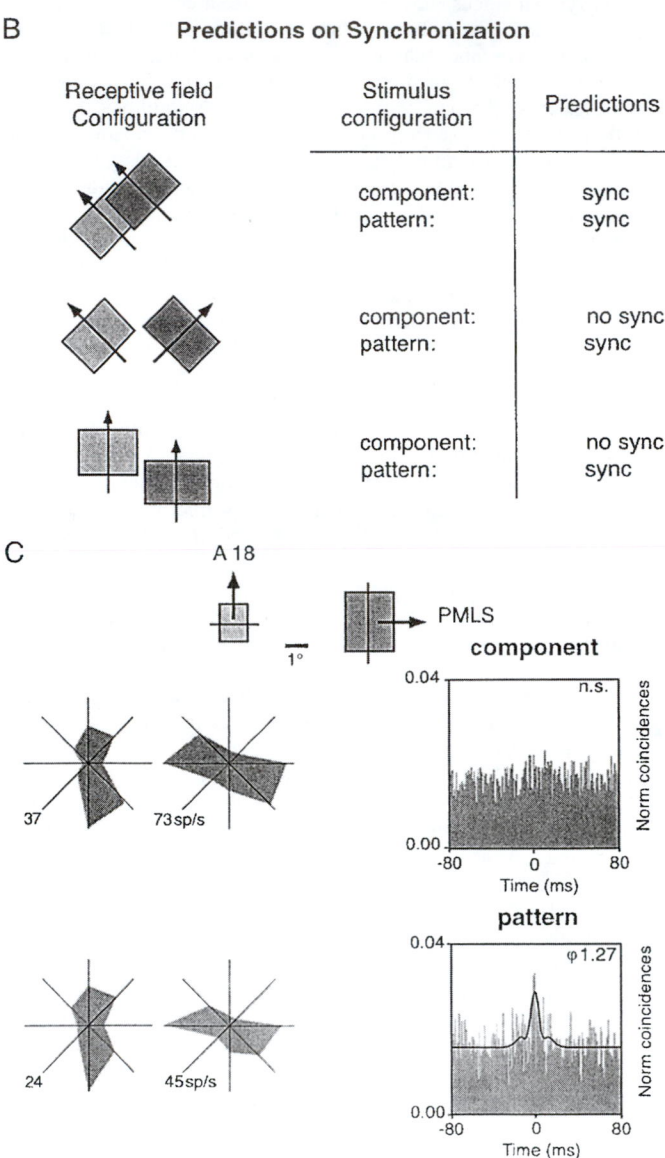

Figure 2. *A*, Two superimposed gratings that differ in orientation and directional drift directions are perceived either as two independently moving gratings (component motion) or as a single pattern drifting in the intermediate direction (pattern motion), depending on whether the luminance conditions at the intersections are compatible with transparency. *B*, Predictions on the synchronization behavior of neurons as a function of their receptive field configuration (left) and stimulation conditions (right). *C*, Changes in synchronization behavior of two neurons recorded simultaneously from area 18 and PMLS that were activated with a plaid stimulus under component (upper graph) and pattern motion conditions (lower graph). The two neurons preferred gratings with orthogonal orientation (see receptive field configuration, top, and tuning curves obtained with component and pattern, respectively) and synchronized their responses only when activated with the pattern stimulus (compare cross-correlograms on the right). (Adapted from Castelo-Branco et al., 2000.)

Conclusions

Taken together, the data and arguments described in this chapter support the notion that neuronal networks are capable of evaluating, with a precision in the millisecond range, the temporal relations among the discharges of neuronal populations and that they exploit this ability for at least three purposes: (1) for the precise signaling of temporal features across processing stages, (2) for the selection of responses, and (3) for the definition of relations among distributed responses with high temporal resolution. It is proposed that this selection and binding mechanism is used in ensemble coding because it meets the requirement for flexible and rapid binding of distributed responses in ever-changing constellations. Assembly coding, in turn, appears necessary in order to cope with the representation of the astronomical number of possible relations among features describing real world objects. It appears, then, that cerebral cortex applies two complementary coding strategies: (1) an explicit representation of features and their conjunctions in the tuned responses of individual, specialized neurons or populations of such neurons; (2) an implicit representation of conjunctions of such explicitly coded contents in dynamically associated assemblies. The first strategy seems to be applied for the representation of a limited set of features and some of their conjunctions and is, in all likelihood, reserved for items that occur very frequently and/or are of particular behavioral importance. The second strategy seems to be reserved for the representation of novel objects and of all those items for which no explicit representation can be realized, either because the explicit representation would require too many neurons or because the contents to be represented are too infrequent to warrant the implementation of specialized neurons.

Road Maps: Neural Coding; Vision
Related Reading: Dynamic Link Architecture; Fast Visual Processing; Laminar Cortical Architecture in Visual Perception; Probabilistic Regularization Methods for Low-Level Vision; Synfire Chains; Tensor Voting and Visual Segmentation; Visual Attention; Visual Scene Perception

References

Abeles, M., 1991, *Corticonics. Neural Circuits of Cerebral Cortex*, Cambridge: UK, Cambridge University Press.

Castelo-Branco, M., Goebel, R., Neuenschwander, S., and Singer, W., 2000, Neural synchrony correlates with surface segregation rules, *Nature*, 405:685–689. ◆

Diesmann, M., Gewaltig, M.-O., and Aertsen, A., 1999, Stable propagation of synchronous spiking in cortical neural networks, *Nature*, 402:529–533. ◆

Engel, A. K., Fries, P., and Singer, W., 2001, Dynamic predictions: Oscillations and synchrony in top-down processing, *Nat. Rev. Neurosci.*, 2:704–716.

Fries, P., Schröder, J.-H., Singer, W., and Engel, A. K., 2002, Oscillatory neuronal synchronization in primary visual cortex as a correlate of perceptual stimulus selection, *J. Neurosci.*, 722:3739–3754.

Gray, C. M., and Singer, W., 1989, Stimulus-specific neuronal oscillations in orientation columns of cat visual cortex, *Proc. Natl. Acad. Sci. USA*, 86:1698–1702.

Larkum, M. E., Zhu, J. J., and Sakmann, B., 1999, A new cellular mechanism for coupling inputs arriving at different cortical layers, *Nature*, 398:338–341.

Leopold, D. A., and Logothetis, N. K., 1996, Activity changes in early visual cortex reflect monkeys' percepts during binocular rivalry, *Nature*, 379:549–553.

Mainen, Z. F., and Sejnowski, T. J., 1995, Reliability of spike timing in neocortical neurons, *Science*, 268:1503–1505.

Markram, H., Lübke, J., Frotscher, M., and Sakmann, B., 1997, Regulation of synaptic efficacy by coincidence of postsynaptic APs and EPSPs, *Science*, 275:213–215.

Riehle, A., Grün, S., Diesmann, M., and Aertsen, A., 1997, Spike synchronization and rate modulation differentially involved in motor cortical function, *Science*, 278:1950–1953.

Schröder, J.-H., Fries, P., Roelfsema, P. R., Singer, W., and Engel, A. K., 2002, Ocular dominance in extrastriate cortex of strabismic amblyopic cats, *Vision Res.*, 72:29–39.

Singer, W., 1999, Neuronal synchrony: A versatile code for the definition of relations? *Neuron*, 24:49–65. ◆

Stopfer, M., Bhagavan, S., Smith, B. H., and Laurent, G., 1997, Impaired odour discrimination on desynchronization of odour-encoding neural assemblies, *Nature*, 390:70–74.

Tallon-Baudry, C., and Bertrand, O., 1999, Oscillatory gamma activity in humans and its role in object representation, *Trends Cogn. Sci.*, 3:151–162.

Thorpe, S., Fize, D., and Marlot, C., 1996, Speed of processing in the human visual system, *Nature*, 38:520–522.

Usrey, W. M., and Reid, R. C., 1999, Synchronous activity in the visual system, *Annu. Rev. Physiol.*, 61:435–456.

Wespatat, V., Tennigkeit, F., and Singer, W., in preparation, Phase sensitivity of Hebbian modifications in oscillating cells of rat visual cortex, *Nature*.

Synfire Chains

Moshe Abeles

Introduction

A synfire chain is a feedforward network with many layers. The term *synfire chain* was coined by Abeles (1982) to account for the appearance of precise firing sequences with long interspike delays that resisted explanation in terms of the known properties of cortical physiology. Figure 1 illustrates such a sequence. Subsequently, a number of studies have considered how such chains might be generated, activity propagation along the chain, how synfire chains can be used to compute, and how they might be detected in electrophysiological recordings. Several critical views of these features have also been published. This article discusses the structure and function of synfire chains and differing views on synfire chain properties.

Structure

A synfire chain is composed of many pools (or layers) of neurons connected in a feedforward fashion. Each neuron in pool i forms about m excitatory connections to neurons in pool $i + 1$, and each neuron in pool $i + 1$ receives about m excitatory connections from neurons in pool i. Each pool is assumed to contain w neurons. The number of such pools in a chain is the *length* of the chain, w is the *width* of the chain, and m is the *multiplicity* of the connections. Typically, the width and multiplicity are assumed to be constant

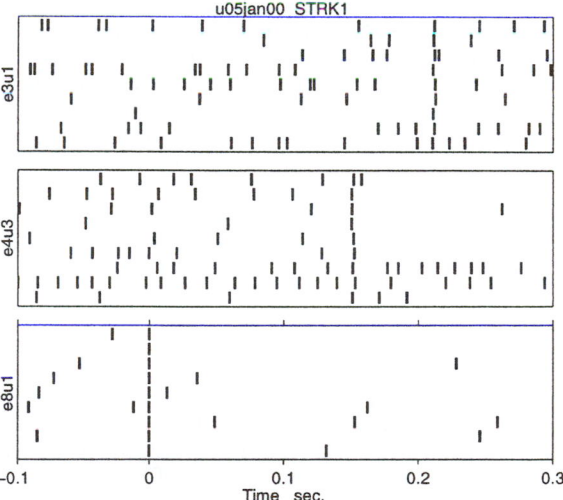

Figure 1. A precise firing sequence. Nine repetitions of the structure unit e8u1 (unit 1 from electrode 8) fired, then within 151.5 ± 1.5 ms, unit e4u3 fired, and also within 211.5 ± 1.5 ms, unit e3u1 fired. This sequence repeated 9 times within 519 seconds. Considering the firing rate fluctuations and the rate correlations among these units, the probability of observing this by chance is less then 4 in 10 million.

along the chain, and the connections between two successive pools are random.

This structure, with $m = w$, was first suggested by Griffith in 1963 as a structure that can ensure a fixed level of activity in a network of excitatory neurons. Griffith called this structure a "complete transmission line." He did not study its properties in any detail. Similar structures were presumably used by Grossberg in 1969 to learn and reproduce complicated space-time patterns.

In a random network with moderate connectivity, many synfire chains can be found by chance (Abeles, 1991). For example, let us examine a random network that might mimic a cortical hypercolumn with 20,000 pyramidal neurons and a connectivity of 25%. If one selects a pool of 100 neurons by chance, there will almost always be another pool of 100 neurons in which every neuron is connected to at least 30 neurons from the first pool. Such random synfire chains may not function reproducibly unless the synaptic connections are strengthened by some appropriate learning rule.

A given neuron can participate in more than one synfire chain. The extent to which such repeated membership can occur without compromising reproducibility is known as the *memory capacity* of synfire chains and is addressed in the next section.

Function

A synfire chain can presumably operate in two modes: asynchronous and synchronous. In the asynchronous mode, each neuron in a pool fires at some elevated firing rate, but the activities are uncorrelated (or only weakly correlated). The activities of one pool are summed by the neurons of the next pool, and each of them fires in an elevated random fashion as well. Shadlen and Newsome (1998) argued that this is the preferential mode of activation.

In the synchronous mode, each pool fires a synchronized volley that induces a large depolarizing wave in the neurons of the next pool, which would then also fire a synchronized volley, and so on. For a synfire chain composed solely of excitatory neurons, this is the preferred mode of activity (Abeles, 1991; Herrmann, Hertz, and Prugel-Bennett, 1995; Diesmann, Gewaltig, and Aertsen, 1999), because each neuron in a pool is subject to approximately the same compound EPSP. Typically, neurons fire during the rising phase of a compound EPSP. The distribution of the times to threshold will be more peaked than the distribution of the firing times of the presynaptic pool.

Diesmann et al. (1999) used EPSP shapes, time constants, thresholds, and so on derived from recordings in cortex and analyzed the transmission between pools numerically. They found that when $m = w = 100$, activity will either propagate as a stable wave with jitter of less than 0.5 ms and saturation of over 90%, or not at all (depending on the initial activation of the chain).

The term *synfire chains* was given to these feedforward structures because of their tendency to transmit activity in this synchronous fashion. The volley of synchronous firing that propagates along a synfire chain is referred to as a *synfire wave*.

Because the effect of a pool resides in the combined synchronous firing of most of its members, the same neuron can participate in a number of pools. This multiple participation is, however, limited. If all neurons participate in every pool, then the network is a fully connected one, and no reproducible synfire waves may be expected.

Bienenstock (1995) and Herrmann et al. (1995) examined how many synfire pools can be embedded in a network of N neurons without interfering with the reproducibility of the activation. Although they used two very different approaches, both came to similar conclusions, namely, the number of pools (P) is proportional to the network size (N), it decreases when the average firing rate in the network increases, and it depends on the width (w) of the pools. A cortical network with an average firing rate of 5 per second and with $w = 100$ may sustain N synfire pools ($P = N$). This means that each neuron can participate in 100 synfire pools.

These pools can be concatenated into one huge synfire chain or into many shorter chains. As pointed out by Maass, any structure that can be wired from individual neurons could just as easily be composed of synfire pools. The advantages would be more reliable operation, shorter input-output delays, and immunity to fallout.

Thus, an average cortical hypercolumn of 20,000 pyramidal neurons may contain 200 synfire chains, each 100 pools long and 100 neurons wide. At 5 spikes per second per neuron, this column will have 300 neurons firing every 3 ms. If the average transmission time between two pools is 3 ms, there could be three synfire waves active concomitantly. These waves may be distributed over three synfire chains or confined to repeated activation of one chain.

Usage

There have only been a few applications using synfire chains. Arnoldi used them to find invariances in a picture, Jacquemin used them to parse and classify French sentences, and Wrigley used synfire chains to parse an auditory scene. However, the main application seems to lie in Bienenstock's (1996) suggestion to use synfire chains for implementing "compositional" systems. He posits that only a few cross-links between two synfire chains that obey appropriate timing constraints are necessary to assure that both synfire chains will act as a wider and more stable synfire chain. This in turn could lock in to activities of other synfire chains, and so on. Thus a large structure of synfire chains can be dynamically generated to represent binding of many simple components into a meaningful composite mental representation. This type of binding is dynamic, so that a single synfire chain may, under different conditions, lock in to a number of other chains and therefore be part of numerous distinct composite representations. In Bienenstock's view, the most important aspect of such dynamic binding is vertical binding, in which a higher-level concept binds to the lower-level elements that compose it.

Abeles et al. (1993) have shown, by way of simulations, that two synfire chains with random connections may learn to lock in to each other if activated synchronously several times and if the synaptic modifications follow a time-asymmetric rule (i.e., synapses are strengthened if the presynaptic spike precedes the postsynaptic spike and weakened if the time order is reversed). Such learning rules were experimentally reported (e.g., Zhang et al., 1998). Hayon has shown by way of simulation that hierarchical systems of synfire chains could be used to separate figure from ground, to implement a minimal description length (MDL) principle, and to exhibit the property of compositionality. However, these demonstrations were for toy problems. It remains to be shown that synfire chains can efficiently solve such problems in real-world situations.

Experimental Evidence

Direct experimental support for the existence of synfire chains requires simultaneous recording of several neurons from one pool and several from the next pool under conditions in which the synfire chain is repeatedly activated. Using current techniques, one can simultaneously record from 10 to 30 neurons in the same hypercolumn. This is far too diluted a sampling. Thus, the most one can hope for is to record a few neurons from the same chain simultaneously. In this case, whenever this chain is activated, one expects to see a precise firing sequence of these neurons. With the numbers given above, each neuron may take part in up to 100 chains within a hypercolumn that contains 200 chains. Thus, the chance that a given neuron will participate in a given chain is approximately 0.5. The chance that three neurons will participate in this chain is 0.125. Because there are many different synfire chains and because one can record from more than three neurons simultaneously, there could be numerous different precise firing sequences in any recording site. This was reported to be the case in behaving monkeys

(Prut et al., 1998). Although the method needed for detecting such excessively repeating firing sequences is still under debate (see the next section), there are examples in which the association of such patterns with behavior demonstrates their functional significance. Such a case is illustrated in Figure 2. Clearly, the time of appearance of the sequence $\langle 1, 4, 1; 116 \pm 1, 198 \pm 1\rangle$ is associated with the monkey's expectation and not with the firing rates of the neurons involved.

Discussion

Synfire chains may be considered a special case of the "cell assembly" suggested by Hebb. A synchronous volley traversing such a chain is equivalent to the concept of "phase sequences." However, Hebb conceived the cell assembly as a network with multiple feedback connections, whereas the synfire chain is a feedforward net. This results in a basic functional difference. Whereas activity in Hebb's cell assembly is characterized by elevated firing rates of all its members for an extended period, a single volley in a prescribed group is enough to characterize the activity in a synfire chain. This allows for much faster computations by synfire chains.

The succession of synchronous volleys generated by a synfire chain can be thought of as a general case of synchrony. Zero-lag synchrony and phase-locked oscillations may be considered special cases. However, the activity wave in a synfire chain is an all-or-none phenomenon. Thus, synfire chains are more suitable for representing categorical mental entities and less suitable for gradual feature representations as required, for instance, by the population vector model.

Several aspects of synfire chain properties have been criticized. These criticisms question the feasibility of their function in cortical environment, self-organization of synfire chains, the existence of precise firing sequences, and their explanatory power.

Shadlen and Newsome (1998) simulated a multilayered feedforward network where in each layer exactly half of the neurons were excitatory and half were inhibitory. They claimed that when two neurons shared fewer than 40% inputs, activity would propagate in the uncorrelated mode through the layers. Their architecture was thoroughly examined by Litvak et al. (submitted), who found that even with 10% of shared inputs, synchrony builds up and renders information transmission by rate codes useless. Furthermore, if the inhibition balances the excitation but is not synchronized with it, synfire waves will develop within two layers.

Bienenstock and Doursat found that in a random network of excitatory neurons, with simple learning rules, if one seeds synchrony by exciting w neurons synchronously from time to time, a synfire chain will spontaneously form. Herz and Prugel-Bennett (1996) tried to replicate these results and found that parameters had to be carefully trimmed in order to grow synfire chains; even then, the chains tended to be short and to form closed loops. Similar results were obtained by Levy et al. (2001), who employed time-

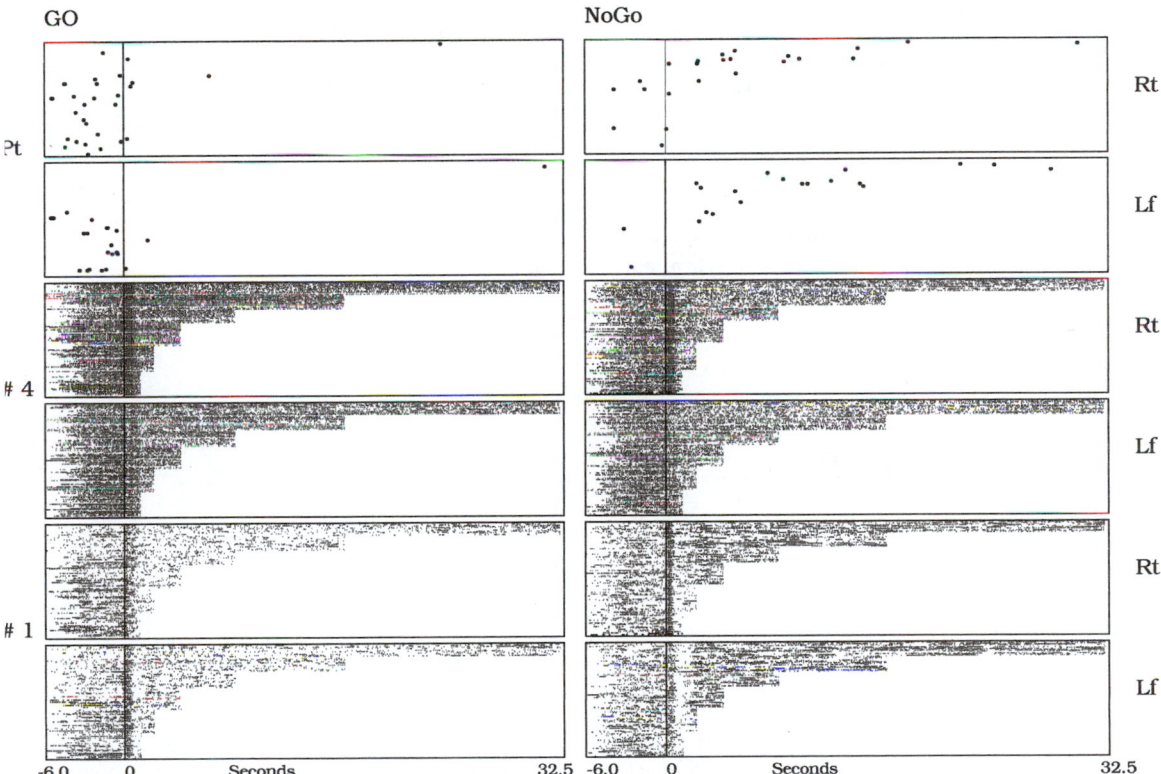

Figure 2. Relations between a precise firing sequence and behavior. A monkey was trained to switch between two modes. In one mode it had to memorize a location of a target for 1–32 seconds and touch it when instructed. In the second mode it had to refrain from moving its hand after the instruction to touch the target. Single-unit activity was recorded from frontal cortex through six microelectrodes. See Prut et al. (1998) for more details. GO, trials in which the monkey behaved in the first mode; NoGo, trials in which the monkey behaved according to the second mode. 1, activity of unit number 1. Each line corresponds to one trial, each dot to one spike. Only the activity from the start of a trial until the instruction to move is shown. Throughout this period the monkey did not move its hand. 4, activity of unit 4; same convention as for unit 1. Pt, times of appearance of the sequence unit 1 fired. After 116 ± 1 ms unit 4 fired, and after 198 ± 1 ms unit 1 fired again. Rt, the target was 15° to the right. Lf, the target was 15° to the left. Time 0 is the time at which a short light blink marked the target to be recalled. Trials were presented at random, but they were sorted and displayed here according to category (Go/NoGo and Rt/Lf) and the delay from marking the target until the instruction to go.

asymmetric learning rules. The network would typically become organized into short cyclical synfire chains, which caused the network to generate cyclical activation of groups of neurons. They called this activity mode *distributed synchrony*. The reasons for these differences are not clear and should be studied further.

Recently, Oram et al. argued that for lateral geniculate nucleus and V1, precise firing sequences carry no specific information on the visual stimuli, nor is there any excess of such sequences beyond what would be expected by chance. However, neither their definition of what constitutes a precise firing sequence nor their analysis of information content fits with what one would expect from the synfire chain model. Baker and Lemon (2000) did treat these sequences as coming from synfire chains but found that their actual number was significantly *smaller* than expected by chance. The main differences between these two last works and earlier works on precise sequences seem to lie in the way the chance level is computed from surrogate spike trains. This and other statistical issues were solved by Abeles and Gat (2001) in a study that confirmed once again the existence of a significant excess of precise firing sequences in data from cortex of behaving monkeys.

A synfire chain is a very simplified structure. There might be other structures with less specific connections that can generate precise firing sequences. Indeed, any network that can produce and recognize precise firing sequences would have all the advantages of a synfire chain. However, to the best of my knowledge, nobody has proposed such a network. Earlier in this article we argued that in a random diluted network, if one chooses w and m appropriately, one can find an almost infinite number of synfire chains by chance. However, the activity in such a network is not reproducible. If we start the activity by activating the same w neurons twice, then even a very small amount of noise will cause the activity patterns to diverge very fast. Van Vreeswijk and Sompolinsky (1996) showed that a random network with balanced excitation and inhibition behaves in this "chaotic" manner.

In summary, classical anatomy and physiology of the cortex sustain the idea that activity may be organized in synfire chains. Synfire chains generate and can recognize sequences of coactivated neurons. Therefore, one can create compositional systems from synfire chains. It remains for future work to show if, when, and where cortical activity is organized in synfire-like modes, and whether real-world problems can be solved by synfire chains.

Road Map: Neural Coding
Related Reading: Hebbian Synaptic Plasticity; Rate Coding and Signal Processing; Sparse Coding in the Primate Cortex; Synchronization, Binding and Expectancy

References

Abeles, M., 1982, *Local Cortical Circuits*, Berlin: Springer-Verlag.
Abeles, M., 1991, *Corticonics: Neural Circuits of the Cerebral Cortex*, Cambridge, Engl.: Cambridge University Press. ◆
Abeles, M., and Gat, I., 2001, Detecting precise firing sequences in experimental data, *J. Neurosci. Methods*, 107:141–154.
Abeles, M., Vaadia, E., Bergman, H., Prut, Y., Haalman, I., and Slovin, H., 1993, Dynamics of neuronal interactions in the frontal cortex of behaving monkeys, *Concepts Neurosci.*, 4:131–158.
Baker, S., and Lemon, R. N., 2000, Precise spatiotemporal repeating patterns in monkey primary and supplementary motor areas occur at chance level, *J. Neurophysiol.*, 84:1770–1780.
Bienenstock, E., 1995, A model of neocortex, *Network*, 6:179–224.
Bienenstock, E., 1996, Composition, in *Brain Theory: Biological Basis and Computational Properties* (A. Aertsen and V. Braitenberg, Eds.), Amsterdam: Elsevier, pp. 269–300. ◆
Diesmann, M., Gewaltig, M.-O., and Aertsen, A., 1999, Stable propagation of synchronous spiking in cortical neural networks, *Nature*, 402:529–533. ◆
Herrmann, M., Hertz, J., and Prügel-Bennett, A., 1995, Analysis of synfire chains, *Network*, 6:403–414.
Hertz, J., and Prügel-Bennett, A., 1996, Learning short synfire chains by self-organization, *Network*, 7:357–363.
Levy, N., Horn, D., Meilijson, I., and Ruppin, E., 2001, Distributed synchrony in a cell assembly of spiking neurons, *Network*, 14:815–824.
Prut, Y., Vaadia, E., Bergman, H., Haalman, I., Slovin, H., and Abeles, M., 1998, Spatiotemporal structure of cortical activity: Properties and behavioral relevance, *J. Neurophysiol.*, 79:2857–2874.
Shadlen, M. N., and Newsome, W. T., 1998, The variable discharge of cortical neurons: Implications for connectivity, computation and information coding, *J. Neurosci.*, 18:3870–3896.
van Vreeswijk, C. A., and Sompolinsky, H., 1996, Chaos in neuronal networks with balanced excitatory and inhibitory activity, *Science*, 274:1724–1726.
Zhang, L. I., Tao, H. W., Holt, C. E., Harris, W. A., and Poo, M., 1998, A critical window for cooperation and competition among developing retinotectal synapses, *Nature*, 395:37–44.

Synthetic Functional Brain Mapping

Barry Horwitz and M.-A. Tagamets

Introduction

The last decade witnessed a conceptual revolution in our understanding of the neural basis of human cognition, emotion, and sensorimotor behavior. This change was driven mainly by the development of functional brain imaging techniques such as positron emission tomography (PET) and functional magnetic resonance imaging (fMRI), and to a lesser degree electric and magnetic encephalography (Horwitz, Tagamets, and McIntosh, 1999). Prior to the use of these methods, the neural correlates of human behavior were inferred primarily by examining the effects of brain lesions on cognitive function, along with extrapolating the results obtained from recordings of neuronal activity in particular brain regions in nonhuman primates while they performed specific sensorimotor and cognitive tasks. Electrical recording and stimulation studies in humans undergoing neurosurgery provided additional important information. These techniques, however, focus on one brain area at

a time. PET and fMRI afford a way to see functional activity in most of the brain simultaneously in awake, normal human subjects as they perform specific cognitive, emotional, and sensorimotor tasks. With these techniques, researchers can determine not only which brain areas are active during one task compared to another, but also how different brain areas interact during a task.

Functional neuroimaging data are rich and complex. However, only recently have neural modeling methods been applied to these kinds of data (for overviews, see Horwitz, Tagamets, and McIntosh, 1999; Horwitz, Friston, and Taylor, 2000). These modeling techniques fall into essentially two distinct categories. One, called *systems-level neural modeling*, aims at determining the network of brain regions mediating a specific cognitive task. This means finding the nodes of the network (i.e., the brain regions) and determining the task-dependent functional strengths of their interregional anatomical linkages (McIntosh et al., 1994). This method uses techniques such as covariance structural equation modeling applied to the correlations (functional connectivities) between (PET- or fMRI-determined) regional brain activities. Examples of questions that can be answered using this approach are: (1) As one learns a task, do the functional links between specific brain regions change their values? (2) Despite similar performance, are the same brain networks being used by healthy subjects and those with illnesses? A discussion of covariance structural equation modeling can be found in COVARIANCE STRUCTURAL EQUATION MODELING (q.v.).

The second category of neural modeling, and one that is the focus of this article, has alternatively been referred to as *synthetic functional brain imaging* (Arbib et al., 1995) or as *large-scale neural modeling* (Tagamets and Horwitz, 1998). The goal is to relate neural electrical activity to functional neuroimaging data. This kind of neural modeling is more ambitious and less (PET/fMRI) data-driven than the first category, but it is crucial for furthering our understanding of the neural basis of behavior. Large-scale modeling entails determining both the neural basis for local brain activations and the neurobiological correlates for the PET/fMRI-determined functional connections.

From a practical point of view, the two methods are connected. Systems-level modeling helps identify the nodes of the network corresponding to the cognitive tasks of interest, especially when little or no nonhuman data are available (e.g., most language tasks). Large-scale modeling enables one to hypothesize about the neural underpinnings for how these tasks are implemented in humans, with PET and fMRI data providing constraints on the possible ways by which these neural systems function.

Functional Brain Imaging Data

PET and fMRI are hemodynamic/metabolic methods that provide indirect measures of neuronal activity (Friston, 1997; Horwitz et al., 2000). Increased blood flow and oxidative metabolism are thought to be needed to restore neuronal ionic concentrations following neural activation, with the largest effects occurring in the vicinity of synapses (for an overview, see Horwitz and Sporns, 1994). In PET, the distribution of brain radioactivity is determined by detecting the coincident gamma rays that are produced by positron-electron pair annihilation. A common method for measuring regional cerebral blood flow (rCBF) involves the bolus injection of $H_2^{15}O$. The half-life of ^{15}O is 123 s, thus permitting multiple scans (e.g., 6–20, each corresponding to a separate injection of tracer) to be performed in an individual subject during a single scanning session. The time interval needed to obtain a single scan is about 1 minute, and the spatial resolution of PET is about 5–6 mm. The most common method for measuring brain functional activity with fMRI is called blood oxygenation level–dependent contrast, or BOLD. Changes in neural activity lead to changes in blood oxygenation and blood volume, and deoxygenated blood acts as an endogenous paramagnetic contrast agent. The spatial resolution of fMRI images can be about 2 mm within plane. The temporal resolution for fMRI seems limited by the slowness of the hemodynamic response to changes in neural activity (about 5–10 s). In a typical scanning session, a time series of activity (e.g., one scan every few seconds) is obtained in a single subject.

There are two primary data analysis techniques used with PET and fMRI data (Friston, 1997; Horwitz et al., 2000). One, called the *subtraction paradigm*, assumes that different brain regions are engaged in different functions (i.e., computations). This technique is implemented by comparing the functional signals between two (in the simplest case) scans, each representing a different experimental condition. The locations of the large differences in signal between the two scans presumably delineate the brain regions differentially involved in the two conditions. The second method, termed the *covariance paradigm*, assumes that the task represented by an experimental condition is mediated by a network of inter-

acting brain regions, and that different tasks correspond to different, but possibly overlapping, functional networks. By examining the covariances in brain activity between different brain areas, one infers something about which areas are important nodes in the networks under study, and how these nodes are functionally connected. Because functional neuroimaging methods obtain data simultaneously from multiple brain regions, they are ideal for use with the covariance paradigm. The subtraction and covariance paradigms complement one another, and both are necessary to get a clear picture of how the brain works.

Large-Scale Modeling of Functional Brain Imaging Data

The subtraction and covariance paradigms use statistical tests to discover important features of the data under examination. Inferences about how the results so obtained are related to other functional brain imaging data, and to other kinds of data (e.g., neuroanatomy, neurophysiology) are generally made post hoc and in a qualitative manner. In this sense, these methods are descriptive. In contrast, neural modeling explicitly chooses from the data what is hypothesized to be important, combines neuroimaging data with results obtained by other methods, makes its hypotheses prior to analysis, and does so quantitatively. As stated before, two major modeling methods have been used for analysis of functional imaging data. The first, covariance structural equation modeling (see COVARIANCE STRUCTURAL EQUATION MODELING), is the natural extension of the covariance paradigm's focus on the functional connectivity between brain regions (McIntosh et al., 1994; Horwitz et al., 1999).

However, several problems make it difficult to directly interpret PET or fMRI imaging data in terms of the underlying neuronal activity (Horwitz and Sporns, 1994; Tagamets and Horwitz, 1998; Horwitz et al., 1999). First, the spatial resolution of human brain imaging devices is large compared with the size of neurons or cortical columns, which means that multiple and diverse neuronal populations are lumped together in any resolvable PET or fMRI region of interest (even a single voxel). Second, whereas the temporal resolution of neuronal events is on the order of milliseconds, the appropriate temporal dimension for the hemodynamic methods is on the order of a few seconds, implying that important transient components of activity can be missed by PET and fMRI. Third, electrical recordings of activity measured in nonhuman animal studies generally reflect the firing of action potentials, whereas hemodynamic measurements most likely reflect synaptic activity to a larger extent than neuronal activity (Logothetis et al., 2001). Furthermore, it is likely that inhibitory synaptic activity, which can lead to decreased neuronal spiking, may result in increased PET or fMRI activity (Horwitz and Sporns, 1994).

Because computational neuroscience provides a framework for integrating data from various methods into an explanatory model, it can address a number of issues related to human brain imaging (Arbib et al., 1995; Tagamets and Horwitz, 1998). For example, because of the large difference between the time scale of neuronal events and the temporal resolution of PET and fMRI data, several different cognitive operations usually contribute to the data from a single scan. Modeling can explicitly examine how each component can alter the results, and thus aid interpretation. Another issue is the effect of synaptic inhibition on imaging data (Tagamets and Horwitz, 2001). As mentioned earlier, an inhibition-induced decrease in neural activity in a region will be reflected as a rise in the PET or fMRI measure, as has been found experimentally in some animal studies (see Horwitz and Sporns, 1994, for details). This issue is closely allied to the question of the relative importance of local versus global connectivity in generating the observed imaging data in a specific region. Several neural modeling efforts have been undertaken to address these questions.

Arbib et al. (1995) used a large-scale model of saccade generation (Dominey and Arbib, 1992) and adapted it to generate simulated PET data, a technique they called *synthetic PET*. The model includes a number of brain structures, such as posterior parietal and visual cortex, superior colliculus, the frontal eye field, the mediodorsal and lateral geniculate nuclei of the thalamus, and the caudate and substantia nigra of the basal ganglia (Figure 1A). Because some of the pathways involving the basal ganglia are inhibitory, the model is a good testing ground for examining the effects of inhibitory synapses on simulated blood flow. The main hypothesis tested in the synthetic PET simulation was that rCBF, as measured by PET, correlates with local synaptic activity in a region. PET activation in the model was computed by summing the absolute values of both excitatory and inhibitory synaptic weights times firing rates of presynaptic neurons and integrating these values over a time period that corresponded to the time scale of PET while the model performed a specific task. To simulate the subtraction paradigm typically used in PET experiments, computed PET activity was calculated during two different tasks (generating simple saccades and memory-driven saccades) and the differences in PET activity between the two conditions were evaluated in all regions of the model. In the simple saccade condition, disinhibition of the superior colliculus allows a saccade to be generated to a target present in the field of view. Memory-driven saccades, however, are driven by activation of a memory loop between the frontal eye field and mediodorsal nucleus (MD) of the thalamus, which is disinhibited by the substantia nigra, generating a saccade (via the superior colliculus) to a remembered target when there is no stimulus present. When compared to the simple saccade task, spiking activity in the modeled MD region increased as a result of the disinhibition, while simulated PET activation decreased in MD (Figure 1B). This result showed how modeling can illuminate a counterintuitive effect: during the simple saccade, synaptic activity from the tonic inhibition of the MD contributes more synaptic activity to the PET measure than the increase in excitation that results from disinhibition.

Tagamets and Horwitz (1998, 2001) developed a large-scale model of working memory that was designed specifically for simulating the quantitative aspects of imaging data. Three types of factors that can influence imaging data were identified and implemented in the model. Emphasis was on using biological constraints for (1) setting local proportions of excitatory and inhibitory connections (Figure 2A), (2) determining interregional connection strengths and patterns (Figure 2B), and (3) determining activation rule parameters that yield appropriate electrical activity behaviors in the local circuits. Because most corticocortical connections are local and excitatory, a basic local circuit that reflects this connectivity pattern was used to construct the model. Local connections account for about 80%–90% of all corticocortical synapses in the model, with the remaining 10%–20% being interregional (Figure 2A). The activation rule (Equation 1) determines the electrical activity of the local circuits:

$$da_{m,i}(t)/dt$$
$$= \Delta\left[1 + \exp\left(-K_m\left(\sum_{q,j} w_{ji}a_{qj} - \tau_m + N_m(t)\right)\right)\right]^{-1} - \delta a_{m,i}(t)$$

where m and q denote the unit type (either E or I, for excitatory and inhibitory, respectively), $a_{m,i}$ is the activity of the ith unit of type m, τ_m is a threshold, and $N_m(t)$ is a noise term for units of type m; w_{ji} is the synaptic weight from unit j to i. Parameters were chosen so that the behavior of a single circuit has maximal flexibility in response to various types of stimuli. For example, for the parameter K (the steepness of the sigmoid, which determines responsiveness of the unit), it was found that a ratio of approximately 2:1 for inhibitory and excitatory units, respectively, yields maximal reactivity to both excitatory and inhibitory inputs.

Simulations with the model suggest that effects such as the interaction between afferent and local connections, interaction between task type and inhibitory input, and effects of feedback con-

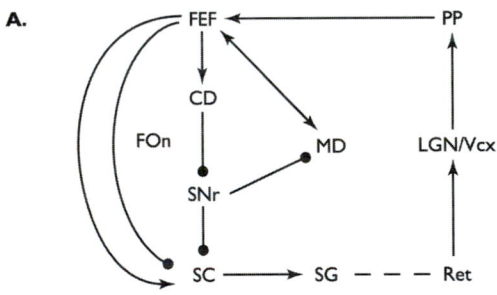

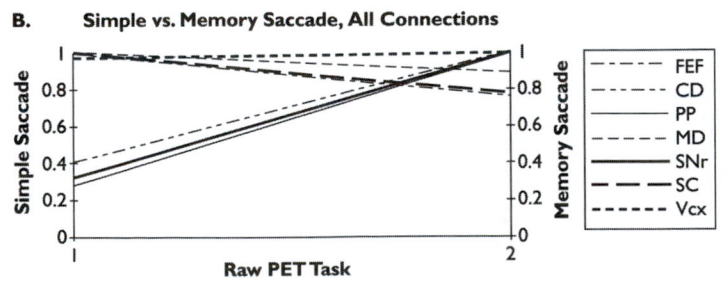

Figure 1. *A*, Simplified schematic model for saccade generation (Dominey and Arbib, 1992). Arrows denote excitatory connections; solid circles, inhibitory connections. CD, caudate; FEF, frontal eye fields; FOn, foveal-on cells; LGN, lateral geniculate nucleus; MD, mediodorsal thalamus; PP, posterior parietal cortex; Ret, retina; SC, superior colliculus; SG, brainstem saccade burst generator; SNr, substantia nigra pars reticulata; Vcx, visual cortex. *B*, Simulated PET activity for each brain area in the neural model of *A* for saccade generation. Simple saccades are given by the values on the left, memory saccades by those on the right. (From Arbib et al., 1995. Reprinted with permission.)

A.

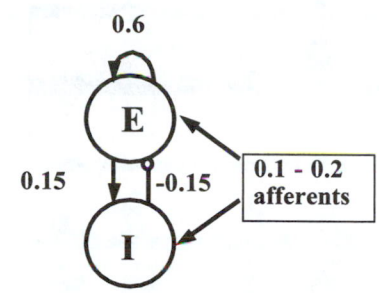

B.

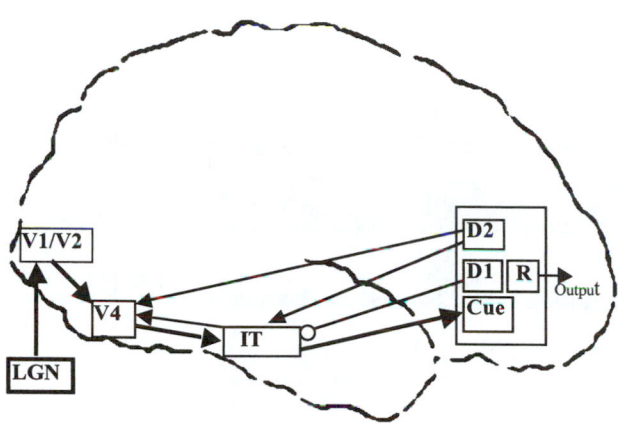

Figure 2. *A,* The basic unit of the Tagamets-Horwitz (1998) model. This local assembly, representing a cortical column, consists of an excitatory group (E) and an inhibitory group (I). Local synaptic activity is dominated by local excitation and inhibition, while afferents from other cortical regions account for the smallest proportion, as indicated by the values of the synaptic weights. *B,* The anatomical regions comprising the Tagamets-Horwitz network. Shown are the regions and the anatomical connections between them. Arrows denote excitatory connections, open circles inhibitory connections. (Modified from Tagamets and Horwitz, 1998.)

nections are likely to play major roles in imaging results (Tagamets and Horwitz, 1998, 2001). The full model is composed of a number of regions along the ventral visual pathway, including V1/V2, V4, inferotemporal cortex (IT), and a prefrontal region (Figure 2*B*). A working memory circuit in the frontal region of the model (Figure *3*) implements a delayed match-to-sample task similar to those used in both electrophysiological experiments in monkeys and human neuroimaging studies. The memory is modulated by a continuous-valued parameter that projects diffusely into all members of a sub-population (D2) of the frontal working memory circuit. When this parameter is set to a low value, the model performs a passive viewing task, stimuli are not kept in memory, and there is little activity in the frontal units during the delay period (Figure 4*A*). At a higher value, this parameter causes two subpopulations of the working memory circuit (D1 and D2) to act as a feedback loop that maintains the memory during the delay interval (Figure 4*B*). Similar to Arbib et al. (1995), simulated PET/fMRI activity is taken to be the absolute value of the local synaptic activity over the time course of the scan. Using this model, it was shown that subtracting a passive viewing task from a match-to-sample task yielded electrical ("spiking") activities that matched those found in monkeys (e.g., Funahashi, Bruce, and Goldman-Rakic, 1990), and simulated PET data that were quantitatively similar to those obtained in human imaging studies of the same tasks, with increases in V4, IT, and frontal regions and little change in early visual cortex (V1/V2) (Haxby et al., 1995). The increases seen in V4 and IT are the result of feedback connections from the frontal working memory circuit.

Although single-cell recordings have been used for years, they have tended to focus on individual neurons that are especially responsive to a particular type of stimulus. Neuroimaging, on the other hand, blends the activity of large ensembles of neurons into a single measure. This leads to the question, to what extent do such "special neurons" contribute to overall activity in a local patch of cortex? Scannell and Young (1999) explored this relationship and discussed the implications for neuroimaging results. They showed that a rise in a population activation can be caused by changes in spontaneous background activity (e.g., via attention) at least as much as by changes in spiking of single stimulus-specific neurons.

The modeling examined in this section focused primarily on relating neural activity to PET signals. Recently, emphasis has shifted toward fMRI studies (Horwitz and Tagamets, 1999; Arbib et al., 2000). For example, the Tagamets-Horwitz model was extended so that fMRI studies could be simulated (Horwitz and Tagamets,

Figure 3. The working memory module in pre-frontal cortex is composed of four types of units, whose electrical activities are similar to the types identified by Funahashi et al. (1990). Each element of the circuit is a basic unit of the type shown in Figure 2*A*. Inhibitory connections are implemented as excitatory connections onto inhibitory units. The attentional modulation is modeled as a diffuse, weak activity directed at the D2 units. For details concerning the connection weights, see Tagamets and Horwitz (1998).

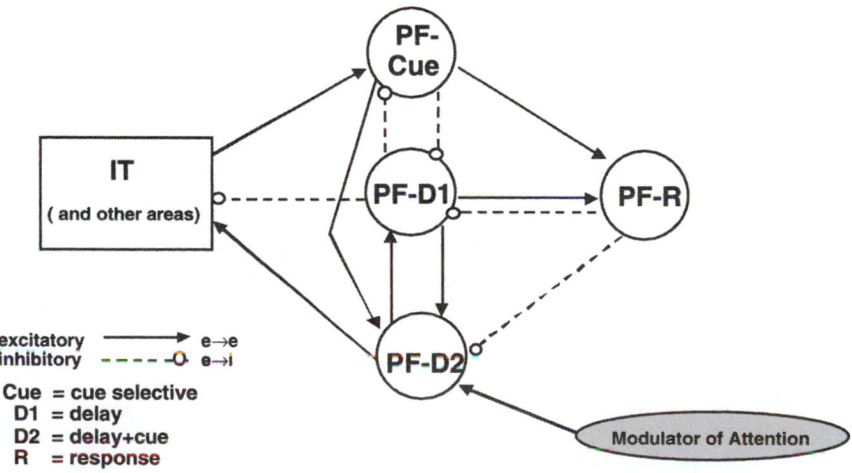

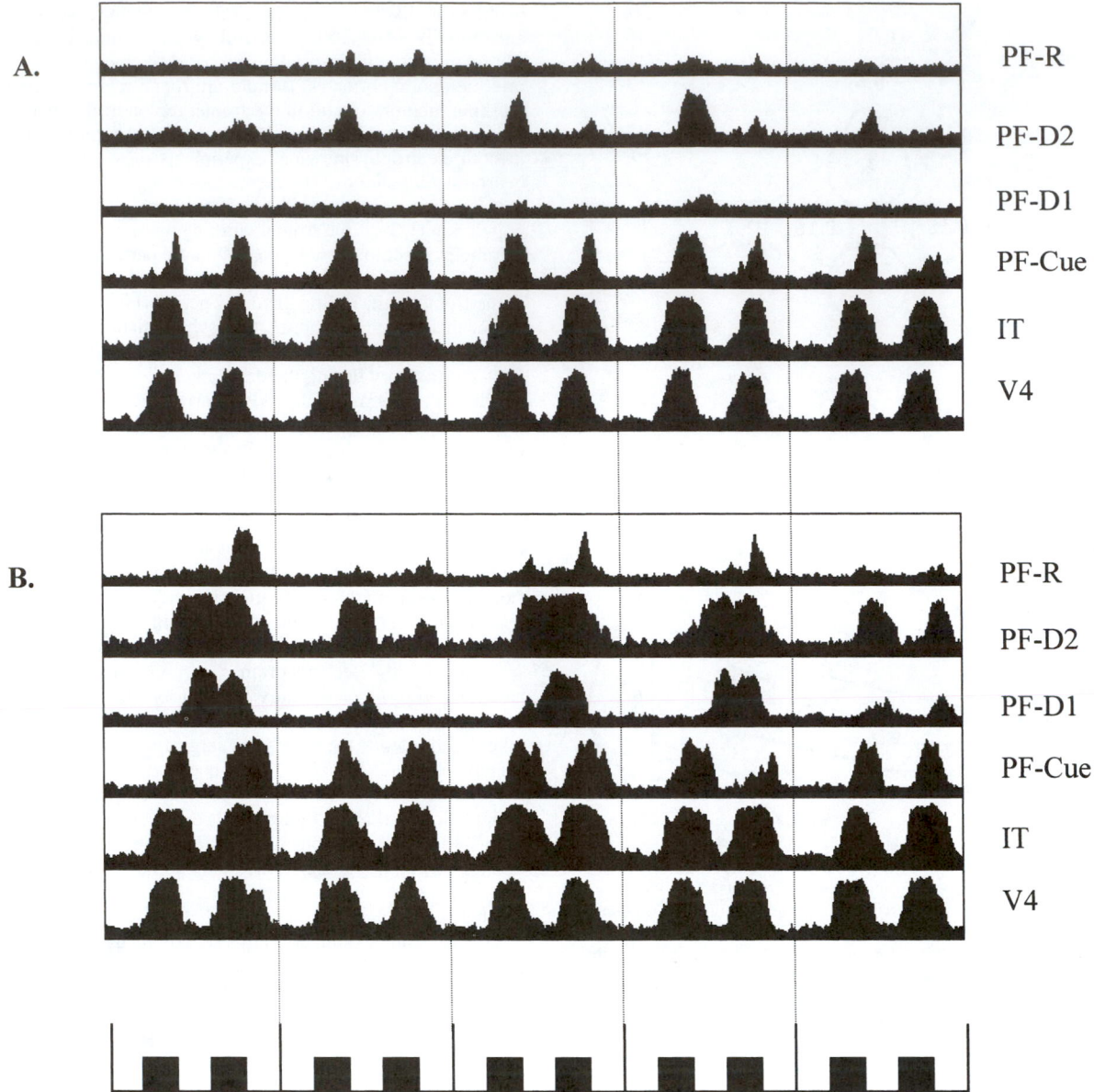

Figure 4. Time course of electrical activities of sample units from the different cortical areas of the Tagamets-Horwitz model during five trials of a task, including each type of frontal unit in the memory circuit. *A*, Low-attention level; *B*, high-attention level. Stimuli are represented by filled blocks in the time line at the bottom of the figure, with each block corresponding to 1 s of simulated time. Trials are separated by dotted lines. (Modified from Tagamets and Horwitz, 1998.)

1999). Rather than integrating the absolute value of the summed synaptic activities in each brain region over the entire experiment, as would be done to simulate a PET study, the integration time was reduced to 50 ms, which compares favorably to the slice acquisition time for many fMRI scanners. The problem of hemodynamic delay must also be dealt with: the brain's vascular response to a transient change in neural activity is delayed and dispersed in time (estimated to be about 5–8 s). A Poisson function was used to represent the hemodynamic delay. One simulation then focused on examining event-related fMRI designs, which use the relatively high temporal resolution of fMRI to capture different components of the cognitive tasks under study. The studies that have been employed to validate these designs generally have been simple sensory or motor tasks. The problem is that in higher cognitive tasks, there can be extensive neural activity in multiple brain regions in the absence of external stimuli, or when no overt motor responses are employed. Moreover, much of this neural activity is not directly under experimental control. Simulations examined these issues and found that fMRI signals often can be misleading, owing to the fact that the hemodynamic delay results in the convolving of neural signals associated with the presence of stimuli and those related to internal processing. These results demonstrated the need for care in interpreting the results of event-related fMRI experiments.

In preliminary work from our laboratories, the neural basis for PET-determined measures of functional connectivity has also been addressed using neural modeling. Because in PET, interregional correlations are evaluated across subjects, to generate subject-to-subject variability we added a "left" hemisphere whose regions are randomly connected (different for each subject) to regions in the right hemisphere that implemented the Tagamets-Horwitz model of visual processing (Tagamets and Horwitz, 1998). Random noise patterns were presented to the left hemisphere, whereas shapes were presented to the right during the simulated PET studies. We found that interregional correlations (i.e., functional connectivity) were smaller during the control task using noise patterns than during the delayed-match-to-sample task for shape. Moreover, for the shape task, the functional connectivity was reduced in value if the strength of an interregional anatomical connection was reduced. Thus, our analysis showed that for two anatomically linked brain regions, the strength of the PET functional connectivity between them depends on the strength of their anatomical connectivity (as embodied in the synaptic weights), and also on the extent to which the circuit in which the two regions are nodes is being utilized.

Another area of research is represented by efforts to relate cognitive models to functional brain imaging data. For example, Just, Carpenter, and Varma (1999) used a computational model of sentence comprehension called 4CAPS (which is a production model) to account for how fMRI activation levels varied as a function of sentence complexity in three brain areas (Broca's, Wernicke's, and dorsolateral prefrontal cortex). In their computational model, resource utilization in a given unit of time in each component of the system is assumed to correspond to the amount of activation observed with the neuroimaging measure in the corresponding component during that time interval. They found good agreement between the experimental number of activated voxels in Broca's and Wernicke's areas and the prediction of their model for three sentence types of different complexity.

Discussion

In this article, we focused primarily on large-scale neural modeling (synthetic brain imaging), which is used to help elucidate the relation between neural activity and functional brain imaging data. Much still needs to be done to effectively utilize neural modeling methods with functional neuroimaging data. Issues to be addressed in the near future include developing a better understanding of the connection between neuronal activity and the concomitant alterations in blood flow and metabolism. Because so many factors regulate blood flow and metabolism, this topic itself will require neurocomputational techniques, perhaps at the level of cortical columns. Researchers will also need to be able to simulate electric and magnetic encephalographic data, because these studies are the best sources of temporal information on high-level cognitive tasks in humans, such as those associated with language processing. Nonetheless, functional brain imaging has become central to cognitive neuroscience and, because the data it generates are so multidimensional and complex, only neurocomputational approaches

such as those discussed here can provide a framework for its integration into a cohesive account of the neural basis of behavior.

Road Map: Cognitive Neuroscience
Related Reading: Covariance Structural Equation Modeling; Statistical Parametric Mapping of Cortical Activity Patterns

References

Arbib, M. A., Billard, A., Iacoboni, M., and Oztop, E., 2000, Synthetic brain imaging: Grasping, mirror neurons and imitation, *Neural Netw.*, 13:975–997.

Arbib, M. A., Bischoff, A., Fagg, A. H., and Grafton, S. T., 1995, Synthetic PET: Analyzing large-scale properties of neural networks, *Human Brain Mapp.*, 2:225–233. ◆

Dominey, P. F., and Arbib, M. A., 1992, A cortico-subcortical model for generation of spatially accurate sequential saccades, *Cereb. Cortex*, 2:153–175.

Friston, K. J., 1997, Imaging cognitive anatomy, *Trends Cogn. Sci.*, 1:21–27.

Funahashi, S., Bruce, C., and Goldman-Rakic, P. S., 1990, Visuospatial coding in primate prefrontal neurons revealed by oculomotor paradigms, *J. Neurophysiol.*, 63:814–831.

Haxby, J. V., Ungerleider, L. G., Horwitz, B., Rapoport, S. I., and Grady, C. L., 1995, Hemispheric differences in neural systems for face working memory: A PET-rCBF study, *Human Brain Mapp.*, 3:68–82.

Horwitz, B., Friston, K. J., and Taylor, J. G., 2000, Neural modeling and functional brain imaging: An overview, *Neural Netw.*, 13:829–846. ◆

Horwitz, B., and Sporns, O., 1994, Neural modeling and functional neuroimaging, *Human Brain Mapp.*, 1:269–283. ◆

Horwitz, B., and Tagamets, M.-A., 1999, Predicting human functional maps with neural net modeling, *Human Brain Mapp.*, 8:137–142.

Horwitz, B., Tagamets, M.-A., and McIntosh, A. R., 1999, Neural modeling, functional brain imaging, and cognition, *Trends Cogn. Sci.*, 3:91–98. ◆

Just, M. A., Carpenter, P. A., and Varma, S., 1999, Computational modeling of high-level cognition and brain function, *Human Brain Mapp.*, 8:128–136.

Logothetis, N. K., Pauls, J., Augath, M., Trinath, T., and Oeltermann, A., 2001, Neurophysiological investigation of the basis of the fMRI signal, *Nature*, 412:150–157.

McIntosh, A. R., Grady, C. L., Ungerleider, L. G., Haxby, J. V., Rapoport, S. I., and Horwitz, B., 1994, Network analysis of cortical visual pathways mapped with PET, *J. Neurosci.*, 14:655–666.

Scannell, J. W., and Young, M. P., 1999, Neuronal population activity and functional imaging, *Proc. R. Soc. Lond. B*, 266:875–881.

Tagamets, M.-A., and Horwitz, B., 1998, Integrating electrophysiological and anatomical experimental data to create a large-scale model that simulates a delayed match-to-sample human brain imaging study, *Cereb. Cortex*, 8:310–320.

Tagamets, M.-A., and Horwitz, B., 2001, Interpreting PET and fMRI measures of functional neural activity: The effects of synaptic inhibition on cortical activation in human imaging studies, *Brain Res. Bull.*, 54:267–273.

Systematicity of Generalizations in Connectionist Networks

Robert F. Hadley

Introduction

The use of the term *systematicity* in relation to connectionist networks originated with Fodor and Pylyshyn's (1988) critique of con-

nectionist architecture. Fodor and Pylyshyn sought to demonstrate that insofar as connectionism offers a novel *architectural* paradigm (as distinct from neurally inspired implementations of symbolic artificial intelligence), it will fail to explain certain fundamental aspects of human cognition. One such aspect, identified by Fodor and Pylyshyn as *systematicity*, consists in the fact that human thought and language comprehension are manifestations of a coherent, underlying system; our ability to entertain certain thoughts (and to understand certain sentences) is *caused* by the very mechanisms that ensure our ability to think (or understand) systematically related variants of the original thoughts and sentences. Thus, humans who can understand sentences of the form *x Relation y* (e.g., *John loves Mary*) can also, as a matter of causal necessity, understand sentences of the form *y Relation x* (*Mary loves John*). Fodor and Pylyshyn provide other, more complex examples of cognitive abilities that "come in clumps" (i.e., the abilities are systematically related). Specifically, they maintain that humans display *systematicity of inference*. Anyone who can perform elementary logical inferences of a given form can perform other elementary inferences of the same logical form.

Even as Fodor and Pylyshyn's 1988 critique went to press, connectionists were preparing rebuttals and counterexamples. Some have argued (see Chalmers, 1990; Smolensky, 1990) that Fodor and Pylyshyn underestimated the manner in which distributed representations can encode compositional structure (see COMPOSITIONALITY IN NEURAL SYSTEMS). Others have argued that Fodor and Pylyshyn's initial conception of systematicity was vague and unworkable (cf. Niklasson and van Gelder, 1994). Nevertheless, the Fodor-Pylyshyn critique spurred a flurry of connectionist research, some of which is described below.

It is important to realize that Fodor and Pylyshyn's conception of systematicity made no reference to learning-based generalization. Rather, they offered indications that causal mechanisms supporting systematicity were innate. At the very least, they viewed systematicity as a *nomologically necessary* feature of human cognition (i.e., it was necessary by virtue of natural law). While acknowledging that connectionist networks might achieve isolated instances of systematicity by means of ad hoc, arbitrary "wiring" configurations, they dismissed such arbitrary devices as scientifically uninteresting.

In 1990, Chalmers offered a refutation of Fodor and Pylyshyn's thesis, based on a simple backpropagation network that transformed distributed representations of active-voice sentences into representations of passive-voice sentences (and vice versa). Significantly, Chalmers demonstrated that *novel* distributed activation patterns can possess structure that bears a systematic relationship to previously encountered, distributed patterns (see CONNECTIONIST AND SYMBOLIC REPRESENTATIONS). This systematic relationship becomes apparent in the presence of trained, weighted link configurations within his three-layer network. Although Fodor and Pylyshyn regard such weighted link configurations as "nomologically arbitrary," it has been argued (Hadley, 1994) that even classical architectures can engender systematicity only when background computational mechanisms are present. The existence of these background mechanisms appears arbitrary from a nomological standpoint.

Independently, Smolensky (1990) described a mathematically sound method, based on tensor products, which ensured that systematically related sentences could all be represented within a single layer of connectionist units. Ignoring for the present the issue of how tensor products can be decomposed, the basic method of representation is straightforward. If a given sentence contains a series of symbols (called fillers), $s_1, s_2, \ldots s_n$, each playing the respective role $r_1, r_2, \ldots r_n$, then the tensor representation is simply the Cartesian product of the numerical activation levels which respectively represent the individual fillers and roles. Viewed mathematically, Smolensky's approach is unproblematic. However, Smolensky did not initially address the issue of whether his tensor product representations could be acquired via training. Thus, their role in generalization was not readily apparent.

Fodor and his colleague McLaughlin soon disputed Smolensky's "solution" to the systematicity challenge (Fodor and McLaughlin, 1990). Among other things, they maintained that Smolensky's tensor product representations constituted "implementations" of classical symbolic structures. Smolensky, however, vigorously stressed the nonclassical aspects of tensor product representations. For example, one may activate the tensor product representation of a compound expression (e.g., the representation of *John loves Mary*) without simultaneously activating the atomic constituents of that expression. Moreover, tensor product representations permit some degree of graceful degradation.

Before we proceed to more complex considerations, a brief explanation of two widely used network architectures may be helpful. Readers already familiar with simple recurrent networks (SRNs) and Recursive Auto-Associative Memory (RAAM) may pass over this digression.

SRNs (Elman, 1990) resemble the familar three-layer backpropagation network except that, in addition to the standard hidden layer, the architecture includes a supplementary *context layer* whose dimensions match the hidden layer's. Links flow from the hidden layer to this context layer, enabling any activation pattern currently present on the hidden layer to be merged with whatever activation pattern happens to be present in the context layer during the current input cycle. Moreover, another set of links flow from the context layer back into the standard hidden layer; hence the adjective *recurrent*. On each input cycle, the hidden layer receives input both from the normal input layer and from the context layer.

RAAM networks (Pollack, 1990) are simple three-layer backpropagation networks whose input and output layers are each divided into regions (*N* regions, let us say). The network is trained to autoassociate, i.e., to reproduce a given pattern of input on the output layer. The purpose of this training is to permit condensed, distributed encodings of those *n*-tuples (or *n*-sequences) of information (which are presented to the *N* regions of the input layer) to be developed on the hidden layer. Once such a distributed encoding has been developed for a given *n*-tuple of information, that encoding may later be presented as input to a single region of the input layer, while the remaining input regions receive similarly derived distributed encodings. The network may then be trained to autoassociate on this more complex set of input information. By following this general iterative pattern, condensed distributed encodings for entire tree structures (such as binary parse trees) can be generated and extracted from the RAAM's hidden layer.

Learning-Based Definitions of Systematicity

As previously noted, Fodor and Pylyshyn's conception of systematicity does not involve a process of learning. It does, however, require that agents extend their understanding of symbolic structures to novel instances. Many of the "novel instances" cited by Fodor and Pylyshyn involved *re-ordered constituents*. For example, any agent who has understood *mice fear cats* will, by virtue of the same mechanisms of understanding, comprehend *cats fear mice*. On their view, these mechanisms involve processes of *semantic compositionality*. Now, although it had been established by 1990 that both SRNs and RAAMs could successfully process sentences in which novel combinations of words were present, it remained unclear whether networks could be trained to accommodate novel orderings of constituents. Indeed, to all appearances, an important form of systematic generalization remained untested. This fact was noted in Hadley (1992), where a hierarchy of degrees of learning-based systematicity was first introduced.

For purposes of the following discussion, it will be helpful to have in mind a brief paraphrase of a portion of this hierarchy. (A somewhat similar though less hierarchical set of distinctions can be found in Niklasson and van Gelder, 1994.)

A cognitive agent, or a connectionist network, might exhibit any of the following degrees of systematicity (or systematic generalization). In the following, *novel* is measured relative to a known training corpus.

1. *Weak systematicity*. An agent is at most weakly systematic if, after training, it can process "test" sentences (or symbol sequences) containing novel combinations of words (symbols) but cannot process sentences containing familiar words in positions that are novel for those words.
2. *Strong systematicity* requires that an agent *learn* to generalize the use of a *significant fraction* of its vocabulary to novel syntactic positions, in both simple and embedded sentences. In this context, a word or symbol is considered to occupy a novel position (e.g., grammatical subject) only if the agent has not encountered that word in that syntactic position at any level of sentential embedding.

The forms of systematicity just listed do not require that an agent be capable of semantically interpreting the sentences in question. Recall, however, that Fodor and Pylyshyn's examples of systematicity included cases where an agent assigns meaning to the sentences involved (e.g., whoever understands *John loves Mary* can also understand *Mary loves John*). Any learning-based conception of systematicity that approaches the depth of Fodor and Pylyshyn's initial challenge must therefore include the ability to assign correct semantic interpretations. For this reason, a more demanding criterion (given below) of systematicity was employed by Hadley and Hayward (1997).

3. *Strong semantic systematicity* (henceforth Semantic-Sys) is displayed when agents not only manifest strong systematicity (i.e., level 2 above), but they are also able to assign appropriate meanings to all words occurring in novel test sentences that could be used to establish a mastery of level 2.

(It is here intended that when an agent assigns an appropriate meaning to a word, the agent can at least map the word onto an internal conceptual representation.)

It is noteworthy that Semantic-Sys presents connectionist networks with an especially demanding challenge. In order to achieve this level of systematicity, networks must not only generalize to novel positions, but simultaneously *retain precision* in the assignment of meanings to each symbol involved. Symbols belonging to the same category (e.g., nouns) must not be conflated. Very few connectionists working on systematic generalization have taken up this challenge, yet it is clear that humans do display Semantic-Sys (see Hadley, 1994).

We have now seen a reasonable sampling of various levels of systematic generalization that connectionist networks might attain (though finer-grained distinctions can be made). The question naturally arises, how have artificial neural networks fared against the challenges posed by these levels? In what follows, we consider connectionist systems belonging to two broad categories: (1) networks that, via training, develop some degree of combinatorial structure in their distributed representations, and (2) networks that possess, a priori, at least one representational layer whose combinatorial structure is prearranged by virtue of the number of nodes present and the configuration of links entering those nodes.

Fundamentally Empirical Approaches

Much connectionist research on systematic generalization has employed network architectures that develop strongly distributed, internal representations, whose topological properties derive both from the statistical nature of input sequences and from the fully connected (and largely general-purpose) link configurations. As in most fully connected networks, the resultant generalization capacities derive largely from the tendency of overlapping activation vectors to be assimilated to one another. Indeed, the very factors that account for "graceful degradation" also play a role in the systematic generalizations formed by these networks. However, in each case, the network possesses additional characteristics that contribute to the systematicity effect. Here we shall consider just two general classes, those that employ a recurrent context layer and those that rely strongly on the distributed nature of input patterns.

Context Layer Effects

By 1990, several connectionist networks had exhibited the capacity to successfully "process," in one sense or another, sentences in which novel combinations of words were present (relative to the training corpus). Six such systems (respectively due to Chalmers, Elman, McClelland and Kawamoto, Pollack, Smolensky, and St. John and McClelland) were examined in Hadley (1994), and of these, five were shown to exhibit at least weak systematicity. Unfortunately, none of the six systems had been subjected to the training and testing regimens necessary to establish strong systematicity. However, Christiansen and Chater (1994) subjected Elman's SRN architecture to appropriate training and testing in an effort to establish its potential for what they dubbed "strong generalization." As in Elman's earlier (1990) work, Christiansen and Chater focused on a syntactic prediction task.

During training, a large corpus of sentences was fed, word by word, through the network's input layer, and backpropagation was employed to train the network to predict (on its output layer) the *next* word to appear in the input stream. As it happened, given the complexity of the training corpus involved, the network eventually learned to predict not just a single word, but a range of possible next words. Throughout the training process, the network's recurrent *context layer* retained a composite (or blended) memory of the main hidden layer's contents during the previous N iterations.

Crucially, during the testing phase, Christiansen and Chater ensured that some sentences presented specific nouns in two grammatical positions they had not occupied during training. The results obtained for these chosen sentences were encouraging in one respect and disappointing in another. Christiansen and Chater emphasized that within one of the selected grammatical positions, their network's predictive capacity was not derailed by the unexpected appearance of hitherto contextually restricted nouns. Importantly, the pervasive effect of the network's context layer explained this ability to "carry on." (Note that the context layer's activation patterns blended with any contextually novel noun's activation. In consequence, the resultant blended activations were only partially novel. Thus, graceful degradation played an essential role in this success.) On the other hand, the network displayed almost no capacity to predict the occurrence of the previously restricted nouns within the critical contexts. (The assigned activation levels were minimal.)

In contrast, Elman (1998) conducted experiments basically similar to Christiansen and Chater's, though with a much smaller grammar and training corpus. Elman examined the behavior of a particular noun (*boy*) that had not appeared as the direct object of any verb during training. However, the noun had appeared as grammatical subject, as had other human nouns. The effects of the SRN's context layer were such that, after 10,000 passes through training corpora of various sizes, the network was able to predict the possible occurrence of *boy* in the position of direct object with nearly the same probability as predicted for the unrestricted human nouns.

Whether Elman has produced a convincing example of positional generalization as opposed to a chance result is not straightforward. In light of the Christiansen-Chater network's failure to make predictions comparable to Elman's successful but solitary example, the robustness of Elman's result is in doubt. Moreover, rigorously extensive experiments, conducted by Hadley with J. Hsiao, failed to reproduce Elman's success when the vocabulary of Elman's simple (noun-verb-noun) grammar was expanded to include roughly twice the initial number of nouns and verbs, and a total of four nouns were positionally restricted during training (as opposed to Elman's single noun).

In any case, it should be borne in mind that the experiments of neither Christiansen and Chater nor Elman addressed the problem of generalizing *while retaining specificity* in assigning semantic interpretations to complete sentences, as would be required to satisfy either the spirit of Fodor and Pylyshyn's initial challenge or the criteria of Semantic-Sys.

Distributed Input Patterns

Working in a different domain, Niklasson and van Gelder (1994) described a backpropagation-trained network that successfully transformed simple logic formulas (in which a single level of embedding is permitted) into expressions of related form. Niklasson and van Gelder explicitly addressed both strong systematicity and the related issue of permitting entirely novel atomic symbols to appear within test sentences. They forthrightly claimed that their network attained 100% accuracy in both kinds of systematic generalization.

The architecture employed by Niklasson and van Gelder involves a hybrid of two standard methods. They train a three-layer RAAM network to develop distributed encodings of the structured logic formulas that comprise the input and output of the transformation task. While this training occurs, the central (hidden) layer of the RAAM is used as the input layer of a separate, three-layer formula-transformation network. The latter network is trained, via backpropagation, concurrently with the RAAM.

Now, although the Niklasson and van Gelder model unquestionably yields intriguing results, some concerns have been voiced (see Phillips, 1994). Among other issues, distributed encodings are assigned a priori to all atomic symbols (including the sole symbol presented, during testing, in a novel context). Crucially, these encodings already include substantial information about the syntactic category of each atomic symbol. Moreover, the featural encoding of these atomic propositional symbols ensures that at least half the features assigned to the lone novel symbol have already been presented, within the crucial context, during the training phase. Thus, the *transformation network* may, in the main, be exhibiting a form of graceful degradation. This agrees with the fact that Niklasson and van Gelder employ a lenient criterion of correctness. Other reservations concern the fact that just one symbol is ever presented in a novel context. Recall that strong systematicity requires that a significant fraction of terms be tested in novel contexts.

In more recent work, Bodén and Niklasson (2000) present a RAAM-based connectionist model that, in their view, displays a form of Semantic-Sys. Fundamental to Bodén and Niklasson's approach is their construal of semantic content. On their construal, any network that develops distributed, *contextually influenced*, internal representations for words in its training corpus will thereby have assigned semantic content to those words. In essence, Bodén and Niklasson equate a word's semantic content with activation patterns that reflect statistical information concerning the word's typical syntactic context.

A problematic aspect of Bodén and Niklasson's construal of semantic content is that this precise kind of statistical information can be extracted when the training and test corpora consist entirely of artificial sentences containing only words that have *no* prior associations with any concept or meaning representation. Thus, their approach would entail that each sentence in such a case has semantic content, although the sentences possess no descriptive (or expressive) relationship to any world situation, state of affairs, or proposition. (It is well known among mathematical logicians that purely syntactic constraints cannot, in general, suffice to uniquely determine the standard semantic interpretation of a set of sentences, including axiom sets.) For these reasons, measured in terms of the definition of semantic systematicity given earlier in this article, the connectionist model of Bodén and Niklasson does not satisfy the Semantic-Sys challenge that has concerned us here.

Apart from the above difficulties, Bodén and Niklasson's case for Semantic-Sys rests on the similarity of an internal activation pattern (which was assigned to a purportedly novel word—call it W—by their network) to activation patterns assigned to certain known words. Yet the activation pattern assigned to W was developed by *training* the network to perform the *same* association task, on a sentence containing W, as the network had (earlier) been trained to perform on sentences containing the aforementioned "known" words. The latter appear in exactly the same syntactic position as W. Given this, it is doubtful whether W should be viewed as novel in the relevant sense.

Combinatorially Endowed Networks

We turn now to network models that, in part, incorporate *preconfigured* node and link structures that intrinsically possess combinatorial properties.

Phillips (1994) employs an intricate architecture that devotes special layers to the calculation and addition of tensor product representations. (See the foregoing discussion of Smolensky, 1990.) The network is trained, via backpropagation, both to autoassociate on simple (noun-verb-noun) sentences and to answer simple queries about roles that words play in those sentences. Five nouns and three verbs were employed in the initial studies. Phillips reported an impressive degree of positional generalization (92% accuracy) even when all five nouns were restricted to a single syntactic position (either agent or patient) during training. However, since embedded sentences were not employed in training or testing, the criteria for *strong systematicity* were not strictly satisfied. It remains to be determined whether the underlying strategy will eventually yield either strong (syntactic) systematicity or Semantic-Sys.

A detailed examination of Phillip's model is not possible here. However, of special significance for the challenge initially posed by Fodor and Pylyshyn (1988) is the structure of layers Phillips employs for creating and storing tensor product representations. The dimensions of these layers are carefully chosen, and wiring leading into each of their units is carefully handcrafted. For example, each unit in the tensor product layer receives just one link from a carefully chosen unit in a special "role vector" layer, and similarly, one link from the network's first hidden layer. Activation functions are also designed to ensure, in the case of the tensor product layer, that addition of tensor products will occur. As a result, the overall appearance and behavior of these crucial layers is strongly reminiscent of conventional hardware networks. Moreover, the layers arguably perform classical structure-sensitive processing, as defined by Fodor and Pylyshyn. Links feeding into these crucial layers are crafted in a manner that is highly sensitive to the structure of the other vectors involved. A plausible case could be made, therefore, that Fodor and Pylyshyn would regard Phillip's model as a connectionist implementation of a classical architecture.

Thus far, the authors we have considered either have addressed only syntactic generalization or have employed a contentious sense of "novel." We now consider a model, due to Hadley and Hayward

(1997), that is designed to achieve the most stringent criterion of systematicity defined above, Semantic-Sys. In contrast to the previous models, training of the Hadley-Hayward network employs no error feedback; all learning arises from Hebbian-inspired processes (Figure 1). During the training regime, two-thirds of all nouns are restricted to a single syntactic position. Nevertheless, the network successfully generalizes and assigns entirely accurate semantic interpretations even when novel levels of clausal embedding are present.

Arguably, the model employs, within its output layer, semantic representations that possess a fundamental classical property, viz., the activation (tokening) of complex representations requires the activation (tokening) of its semantic constituents. Also, Hadley and Hayward employ explicit binding nodes (as in Smolensky, 1990) to ensure that concept and role nodes have the *potential* to bind in novel combinations. This potential is only realized, however, once the model learns to activate role nodes in an appropriate fashion. Such learning arises as a *by-product* of (1) unsupervised spreading activation within the semantic layer and (2) Hebbian learning of associations between words (locally represented in the input layer) and concepts (represented in the semantic layer).

Training involves the presentation of a corpus of sentences, word by word, to the input layer. As each sentence is presented, a target (presumably "guessed") meaning representation for the entire sentence is active within the semantic layer. Hebbian-based incrementing of weights, between simultaneously active nodes, both between layers and within the semantic layer, accounts for all learning. Once learning is complete, the various role nodes become active in an appropriate sequence and bind with appropriate concept nodes. Activation decay plays a crucial role in the binding process, and supports correct attachment of embedded sentence meanings.

Discussion

In light of the preceding, it would appear that the most robust forms of systematicity attained by connectionist networks thus far are found in systems that incorporate at least some classical features, whether in link preconfigurations or in modes of representation. However, we have also seen that, in the cases of Christiansen and Chater (1994) and Niklasson and van Gelder (1994), interesting forms of syntactic generalization have emerged even when little or no classical dispositions are present. These researchers and others continue to explore the potential of radically distributed representations to display stronger forms of systematicity. In this regard, at least two principle challenges now engender further research. First, can networks employing radically nonclassical architectures meet the simultaneous requirements of generalization and specificity imposed by Semantic-Sys? Second, will any of the architectures con-

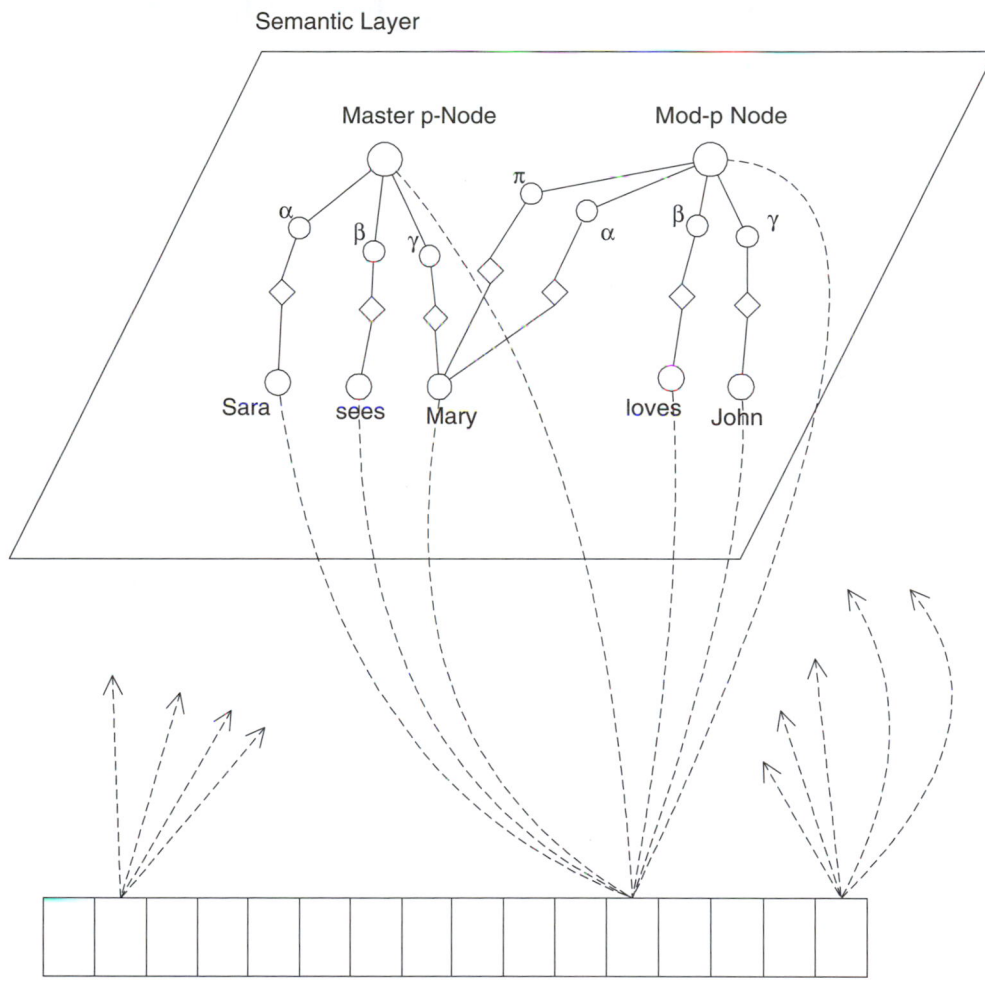

Figure 1. In this illustration, α, β, and γ denote role nodes. Other labeled nodes represent concepts. Diamonds represent binding nodes.

sidered here lead to neurologically plausible solutions to the challenges of systematicity? Arguments offered by Marcus (2001) suggest that the first of these challenges may be theoretically insuperable.

Road Maps: Artificial Intelligence; Psychology
Related Reading: Cognitive Modeling: Psychology and Connectionism; Compositionality in Neural Systems; Constituency and Recursion in Language; Structured Connectionist Models

References

Bodén, M., and Niklasson, L., 2000, Semantic systematicity and context in connectionist networks, *Connect. Sci.*, 12:111–142.
Chalmers, D., 1990, Why Fodor and Pylyshyn were wrong: The simplest refutation, in *Proceedings of the Twelfth Annual Conference of the Cognitive Science Society*, Cambridge, MA.
Christiansen, M. H., and Chater, N., 1994, Generalization and connectionist language learning, *Mind and Language*, 9:273–287.
Elman, J. L., 1990, Finding structure in time, *Cognit. Sci.*, 14:179–212. ◆
Elman, J. L., 1998, Generalization, simple recurrent networks, and the emergence of structure, presented at the Twentieth Annual Conference of the Cognitive Science Society, Madison, WI; available: http://crl.ucsd.edu/elman/Papers/cogsci98.pdf.
Fodor, J. A., and McLaughlin, B. P., 1990, Connectionism and the problem of systematicity: Why Smolensky's solution doesn't work, *Cognition*, 35:183–204.
Fodor, J. A., and Pylyshyn, Z. W., 1988, Connectionism and cognitive architecture: A critical analysis, *Cognition*, 28:3–71.
Hadley, R. F., 1992, Compositionality and systematicity in connectionist language learning, in *Proceedings of the Fourteenth Annual Conference of the Cognitive Science Society*, Mahwah, NJ: Erlbaum, pp. 659–664.
Hadley, R. F., 1994, Systematicity in connectionist language learning, *Mind and Language*, 9:247–272. ◆
Hadley, R. F., and Hayward, M. B., 1997, Strong semantic systematicity from Hebbian connectionist learning, *Minds and Machines*, 7:1–37.
Marcus, G., 2001, *The Algebraic Mind: Integrating Connectionism and Cognitive Science*, Cambridge, MA: MIT Press. ◆
Niklasson, L. F., and van Gelder, T., 1994, On being systematically connectionist, *Mind and Language*, 9:288–302.
Pollack, J. B., 1990, Recursive distributed representations, *Artif. Intell.*, 46:77–105.
Phillips, S., 1994, Strong systematicity within connectionism: The tensor-recurrent network, in *Proceedings of the Sixteenth Annual Conference of the Cognitive Science Society*, pp. 723–727.
Smolensky, P., 1990, Tensor product variable binding and the representation of symbolic structures in connectionist systems, *Artif. Intell.*, 46:159–216. ◆

Temporal Dynamics of Biological Synapses

Larry F. Abbott and Sacha B. Nelson

Introduction

Most experimental and theoretical work on synaptic plasticity in the brain has focused on long-term changes in synaptic strength. However, synaptic function is also profoundly influenced by activity over time scales of milliseconds to seconds. Synapses that exhibit such short-term plasticity are powerful computational elements that can have a profound impact on cortical circuits (Grossberg, 1984; Abbott et al., 1997; Tsodyks and Markram, 1997).

Short-term plasticity was first characterized in studies of the neuromuscular junction that revealed the richness of synaptic dynamics (Magleby, 1987; Zucker, 1989). Both synaptic depression and a number of components of short-term enhancement (facilitation, augmentation, and post-tetanic potentiation) acting over increasingly longer periods of time were observed. Synaptic facilitation appears to result from enhanced transmitter release due to elevated presynaptic calcium levels. Like facilitation, depression can occur with multiple time constants of onset and recovery, and depression and facilitation can coexist at the same synapse. Depression is believed to result, at least in part, from depletion of a readily releasable pool of vesicles. The terminology used to characterize different types of short-term synaptic plasticity is somewhat variable. The following table provides definitions:

Type of Short-Term Plasticity	Onset	Decay
Fast facilitation	1–5 spikes	10–100 ms
Fast depression	1–10 spikes	100 ms–1 s
Slow depression	>10 spikes	>1 s
Augmentation	1–10 spikes	1–5 s
Post-tetanic potentiation	>10 spikes	>5 s

Cortical synapses exhibit short-term plasticity in a variety of forms. Studies of cat visual cortex (Stratford et al., 1996) and rodent somatosensory and motor cortices (Thomson and Deuchars, 1994; Castro-Alamancos and Connors, 1996) indicate that different classes of synapses may exhibit different forms of short-term plasticity. Depression appears to be a particularly prominent feature of transmission at excitatory synapses onto pyramidal cells (Deisz and Prince, 1989; Thomson and Deuchars, 1994; Markram and Tsodyks, 1996; Tsodyks and Markram, 1997; Abbott et al., 1997; Varela et al., 1997).

In addition to having complex short-term dynamics, synapses are stochastic. Indeed, synaptic transmission in the cortex and hippocampus appears to be quite unreliable (Stevens and Wang, 1995). If synaptic transmission occurs with a fixed probability, it is hard to imagine a functional role for this degree of unreliability, since it would act as a significant source of noise. Constructive roles for unreliable transmission become apparent when short-term plasticity is considered in connection with stochastic transmission. The probability that a given presynaptic action potential induces transmitter release at a synapse displaying short-term plasticity is not constant; it depends on the temporal pattern of action potentials that preceded it. Such synapses can act as selective filters, preferentially transmitting particular presynaptic spikes that appear within certain sequences. If the probability of synaptic transmission at cortical synapses is low, synapses are highly selective.

Models

Mathematical models of short-term synaptic transmission were originally developed to describe the neuromuscular junction and other synapses (Krausz and Friesen, 1977; Magleby, 1987) and then extended to deal with cortical synapses (Abbott et al., 1997; Tsodyks and Markram, 1997; Varela et al., 1997). Let A denote the amplitude of the postsynaptic response to a presynaptic action potential. We will discuss a model with one form of facilitation and one form of depression. The same basic model can be extended to more complex cases. We write the postsynaptic amplitude as the product of three factors, $A = A_0FD$. A_0 is a constant equal to the amplitude of the response to a single isolated presynaptic stimulation. F and D are dynamic factors that reflect the effects of facilitation and depression, respectively. In the absence of presynaptic action potentials, F and D both tend toward the value one exponentially,

$$\tau_F \frac{dF}{dt} = 1 - F \quad \text{and} \quad \tau_D \frac{dD}{dt} = 1 - D$$

The time constants τ_F and τ_D reflect the recovery rates of the facilitation and depression processes. When a presynaptic spike occurs, A increases in the case of facilitation and decreases for depression. This is done by making an additive change in F and by modifying D in a multiplicative manner. In other words, whenever a presynaptic spike occurs, we make the replacements

$$F \rightarrow F + (f - 1) \quad \text{and} \quad D \rightarrow dD$$

The parameters f and d, which satisfy $f > 1$ and $d < 1$, determine the onset rate for facilitation and depression, respectively. Facilitation is modeled additively, not multiplicatively, to prevent it from growing without bound. Conversely, depression is modeled multiplicatively to prevent the depression factor from becoming negative. This formalism successfully describes data on cortical short-term plasticity (Varela et al., 1997) and, at the same time, is compact enough to be incorporated easily into network models.

Results

One of the most striking features of the data on cortical short-term plasticity is the dependence of the steady-state amplitude on stimulation frequency. There are strong indications that the synaptic depression seen in cortical slices is the result of a frequency-dependent decrease in the probability of vesicle release. Interpreted in this way, the amplitude of the postsynaptic response is proportional to the probability that a synapse transmits a given presynaptic spike. Experimental results indicate that the synaptic transmission probability for a presynaptic spike train of frequency r is approximately proportional to $1/r$ for $r > 10$–20 Hz (Abbott et al., 1997; Tsodyks and Markram, 1997; Varela et al., 1997). The number of transmitted spikes per unit time is equal to the rate r that presynaptic spikes arrive at the synapse times the probability of transmission, which is proportional to $1/r$. The net result is that the rate at which presynaptic spikes are transmitted is proportional to $r(1/r)$, which is independent of r. Figure 1 illustrates this cancellation of rate dependence. In this example, Poisson spike trains were used as the presynaptic input to a model stochastic synapse with de-

pression. The probability of transmitter release was computed, and the presynaptic spike was transmitted with this probability. Figure 1 shows presynaptic spike trains at two different frequencies, along with the subset of presynaptic spikes actually transmitted by the synapse. Doubling the presynaptic firing rate has only a small effect on the number of successful transmissions. Synaptic depression thus appears to challenge some of our most basic ideas about neuronal coding and signaling.

Synapses that depress transmit action potentials that follow a silent period with a higher probability than action potentials within high-frequency trains. This results in a dramatic enhancement in the response to transient as opposed to static stimuli. Analysis of the response to transients reveals an interesting feature of the $1/r$ dependence of the steady-state depression for these synapses. Suppose that a presynaptic neuron has fired steadily at a rate r long enough to allow the level of depression to reach its steady-state value proportional to $1/r$. Now imagine that the presynaptic firing rate suddenly changes by an amount Δr. Initially, before the level of depression has had time to adjust to its new steady-state level, the first few spikes at the new rate will be transmitted with an amplitude proportional to the previous level of depression. The transient change in the synaptic input to the postsynaptic neuron will be proportional to the change in the presynaptic firing rate, Δr, times the level of synaptic depression, $1/r$. This means that the magnitude of the postsynaptic transient is not proportional to the absolute magnitude of the presynaptic change, Δr, but rather to the fractional or percentage change, $\Delta r/r$.

In psychophysics, the Weber-Fechner law states that the subjective measure of a change ΔI in the magnitude I of a stimulus is proportional to the fraction $\Delta I/I$. Synaptic depression realizes a similar Weber-Fechner relation at the level of individual synapses (Grossberg, 1984; Abbott et al., 1997). The fact that the steady-state postsynaptic response is independent of r, and that the transient response is proportional to $\Delta r/r$, means that a type of firing-rate scale invariance applies to these synapses. This is illustrated in Figure 2. The two spike trains shown are the postsynaptic responses of the same model neuron to 100 synaptic inputs firing asynchronous Poisson spike trains at the rates indicated. The two postsynaptic spike trains are virtually identical despite the fact that the presynaptic firing rates for the two cases are completely different. In one case the firing rate changed by 75 Hz (from 25 Hz to 100 Hz) and in the other by 150 Hz (from 50 Hz to 200 Hz), but the two postsynaptic responses are similar because these change both have $\Delta r/r = 75/25 = 150/50 = 3$.

There are a number of indications that the short-term plasticity of cortical synapses has a significant effect on the dynamics of neural responses. The time course of synaptic depression in slices

input 50 Hz, 14 transmissions

input 100 Hz, 17 transmissions

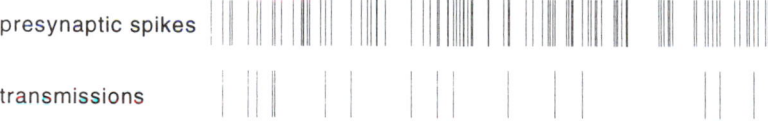

Figure 1. Relative independence of the rate of successful synaptic transmission on the presynaptic firing rate. Poisson spike trains with two different average frequencies were fed into a stochastic synapse model with synaptic depression. Doubling the presynaptic rate increased the number of successful transmissions by only 20%. Note that the spikes shown in the lower rows in this figure represent transmission events, not postsynaptic action potentials.

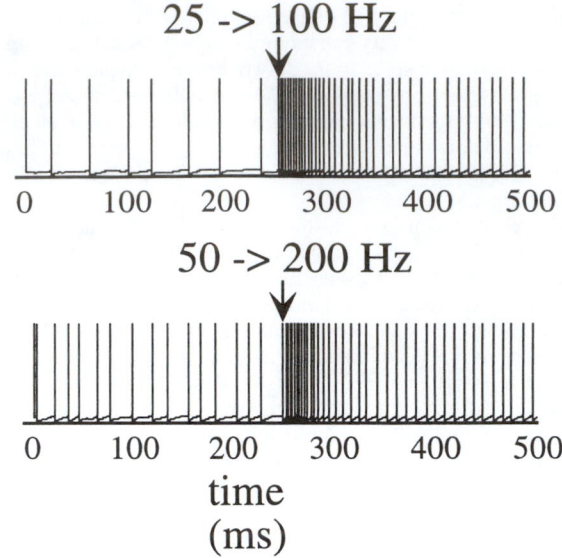

25 -> 100 Hz

0   100   200   300   400   500

50 -> 200 Hz

0   100   200   300   400   500

time
(ms)

Figure 2. Response of a model neuron to a transient increase in the presynaptic firing rate. The spiking pattern shown is that of an integrate-and-fire model neuron driven by 100 presynaptic afferents firing Poisson spike trains through synapses modeled after those measure in cortical slices. In the top panel, the 100 presynaptic afferents all fired at 25 Hz initially, and then this was increased (at the time denoted by the arrow) to 100 Hz. In the bottom panel, the same procedure was followed, but an initial presynaptic rate of 50 Hz was raised to 200 Hz. Despite the difference in presynaptic firing rate, the spike trains are virtually identical, a result of the scale-invariant property of synapses with the type of depression we observed.

of visual cortex (Abbott et al., 1997; Varela et al., 1997) closely parallels the temporal characteristics of cortical responses to visual stimuli (Chance, Nelson, and Abbott, 1998). Neurons in primary visual cortex have relatively low temporal frequency cutoffs, but, paradoxically, they respond briskly to transients containing high-frequency components. The depression measured in cortical slices, when studied in model simulations, reproduces these apparently contradictory effects, enhancing transient and suppressing steady-state responses to high-frequency stimulation. This can account for a number response properties of simple cells, including directional selectivity, response phase, contrast saturation, nonlinear temporal summation, and contrast adaptation (Chance et al., 1998).

Discussion

Because of their probabilistic nature and their dynamics, synapses act as stochastic temporal filters of their presynaptic spike trains. Both facilitation and depression can have important filtering effects. Synapses that exhibit a high degree of facilitation are selective for spikes that appear in groups or bursts (Lisman, 1997). Synapses that depress are selective for transients; they transmit action potentials that follow a period of silence more reliably than those appearing within high-frequency trains.

Synaptic reliability and short-term plasticity are related. At many synapses, changes in release probability are accompanied by changes in short-term plasticity. Synapses with a high probability of transmitter release are more likely to depress, while those with low release probability tend to facilitate (Zucker, 1989). Modula-

tions that affect release probability consequently modify short-term plasticity. Markram and Tsodyks (1996) have found that a form of cortical long-term potentiation can modify the short-term plasticity of synapses between layer 5 pyramidal neurons. This is consistent with the idea that this form of long-term potentiation is acting presynaptically to increase the probability of transmitter release.

Short-term depression has a profound impact on the nature of information transmission between cortical neurons. Synapses showing the degree of synaptic depression seen in cortical slice experiments are relatively ineffective at transmitting information about the rate of presynaptic firing if it is greater than about 10–20 Hz (Abbott et al., 1997; Tsodyks and Markram, 1997). This result challenges a basic assumption, used in virtually all network modeling studies, that synapses transmit signals proportional to their presynaptic firing rates. On the other hand, these synapses transmit information about transient changes in presynaptic firing rates in an extremely efficient, logarithmically compressed, scale-invariant manner.

Road Maps: Biological Neurons and Synapses; Neural Plasticity
Related Reading: Dynamic Link Architecture; Habituation; Synaptic Transmission

References

Abbott, L. F., Sen, K., Varela, J. A., and Nelson, S. B., 1997, Synaptic depression and cortical gain control, *Science*, 275:220–222.
Castro-Alamancos, M., and Connors, B., 1996, Spatiotemporal properties of short-term plasticity in sensorimotor thalamocortical pathways of the rat, *J. Neurosci.*, 16:2767–2779.
Chance, F. S., Nelson, S. B., and Abbott, L. F., 1998, Synaptic depression and the temporal response characteristics of V1 simple cells, *J. Neurosci.*, 18:4785–4799.
Deisz, R., and Prince, D., 1989, Frequency-dependent depression of inhibition in guinea-pig neocortex *in vitro* by GABAb receptor feedback on GABA release, *J. Physiol. (Lond.)*, 412:513.
Grossberg, S., 1984, Some psychophysiological and pharmacological correlates of a developmental, cognitive, and motivational theory, in *Brain and Information: Event-Related Potentials* (R. Karrer, J. Cohen, and P. Tueting, Eds.), New York: New York Academy of Science, pp. 58–142.
Krausz, H. I., and Friesen, W. O., 1977, The analysis of nonlinear synaptic transmission, *J. Gen. Physiol.*, 70:243–265.
Lisman, J. E., 1997, Bursts as a unit of neural information: Making unreliable synapses reliable, *Trends Neurosci.*, 20:38–43.
Magleby, K. L., 1987, Short-term changes in synaptic efficacy, in *Synaptic Function* (G. Edelman, W. Gall, and W. Cowan, Eds.), New York: Wiley, pp. 21–56. ◆
Markram, H., and Tsodyks, M. V., 1996, Redistribution of synaptic efficacy between neocortical pyramidal neurones, *Nature*, 382:807.
Stevens, C. F., and Wang, Y., 1995, Facilitation and depression at single central synapses, *Neuron*, 14:795–802.
Stratford, K. J., Tarczy-Hornuch, K., Martin, K. A. C., Bannister, N. J., and Jack, J. J. B., 1996, Excitatory synaptic inputs to spiny stellate cells in cat visual cortex, *Nature*, 382:258–261.
Thomson, A. M., and Deuchars, J., 1994, Temporal and spatial properties of local circuits in neocortex, *Trends Neurosci.*, 17:119–126. ◆
Tsodyks, M. V., and Markram, H., 1997, The neural code between neocortical pyramidal neurons depends on neurotransmitter release probability, *Proc. Natl. Acad. Sci. USA*, 94:719–723.
Varela, J., Sen, K., Gibson, J., Fost, J., Abbott, L. F., and Nelson, S. B., 1997, A quantitative description of short-term plasticity at excitatory synapses in layer 2/3 of rat primary visual cortex, *J. Neurosci.*, 17:7926–7940. ◆
Zucker, R. S., 1989, Short-term synaptic plasticity, *Annu. Rev. Neurosci.*, 12:13–31. ◆

Temporal Integration in Recurrent Microcircuits

Wolfgang Maass and Henry Markram

Introduction

An essential feature of neural computation in behaving organisms is the capability to produce at any time t a response $y(t)$ that depends on sensory and internal inputs $u(s)$ that the system received at various times $s < t$ back in the past. Such anytime intelligent response to temporally integrated input, which does not have to wait until some algorithm has completed its computation, is also desirable for artificial computing machinery. It would therefore be helpful to understand how neural systems solve this task. Because of the stereotypical features of cortical microcircuits (see Shepherd, 1988; De Felipe, 1997; Douglas and Martin, 1998; von Melchner, Pallas, and Sur, 2000; Thomson et al., 2002), one may hypothesize that there exists a common principle by which neural microcircuits in different cortical areas and species solve the task of adaptive real-time response to temporally integrated information. We survey in this article the primary models that have been proposed for temporal integration in neural microcircuits of the cortex.

Tapped Delay Lines

The most straightforward approach to make past inputs $u(s)$ available for the current output response $y(t)$ is to maintain a finite sliding memory window for inputs $u(t - \Delta)$, $u(t - 2\Delta)$, . . . , $u(t - k\Delta)$ that arrived at a fixed number k of discrete-time points in the past. This memory window has to be updated after every time interval Δ. In a digital computer, such tapped delay line can easily be implemented by a shift operation applied to k registers. An obvious disadvantage of this strategy is the rigid prescribed sampling of inputs u at a discrete set of time points and the rigid prescribed length $k\Delta$ of the memory window, since they may be adequate for some computational tasks but not for others. Neural systems use delay lines for special tasks such as auditory processing or echolocation, but there is no evidence that they use tapped delay lines as the primary tool for temporal integration tasks that require temporal integration over a few hundred milliseconds (ms) and longer. Even for long-range projections such as those across hemispheres or posterior anterior projections, transmission delays between neurons rarely exceed 10–20 ms. Implementing tapped delay lines in the nervous system as a universal solution for temporal integration would also imply a rigid temporal relationship between spatially segregated and specialized brain areas. Furthermore, the largest fraction of synapses in the nervous system (as much as 80%) are those forming local microcircuits, which are characterized by diverse components with highly recurrent connectivity "loops within loops," as shown, for example, in White (1989) and Gupta, Wang, and Markram (2000), rather than uniform units arranged in regular feedforward architectures. The spectrum of delays in information transmission between different neurons of such recurrent microcircuits is in the sub-millisecond to millisecond range, indicating that even the membrane time constant of neurons can perform more temporal integration than delay lines could in recurrent neural microcircuits.

Finite-State Machines and Attractor Neural Networks

Another strategy for making information from past inputs $u(s)$ available for a subsequent response $y(t)$ is to condense all information from earlier inputs that might be needed for a decision at some future time t into the current internal state $x(t)$ of the system. (Such states that contain all information on which future actions of the systems depend are commonly referred to as Markovian states because this property is characteristic for the states in a Markov chain, a well-known model for stochastic systems.) This strategy has the advantage that temporal integration is not restricted to a fixed sampling interval Δ for past inputs nor a fixed memory time window $k\Delta$. The problem of task-specific temporal integration of past inputs is moved here to the definition and implementation of a suitable set X of states $x(t)$ that the system is allowed to assume and a transition function δ that updates the internal state in regular time intervals Δ' in light of new input $u(t)$ arriving at time t:

$$x(t + \Delta') = \delta(x(t), u(t))$$

The transition function δ can be deterministic or stochastic (similar to the stochastic transition function in a Markov chain). This framework for temporal integration is commonly used in formal models for REINFORCEMENT LEARNING (q.v.). In the case in which the state set X is a finite set, one refers to such system as a finite automaton or finite-state machine. To facilitate learning of a transition function δ, the underlying state set X should be fairly small. Popular soft versions of this model that do not require a fixed time interval Δ' for state updates are the attractor neural networks (see COMPUTING WITH ATTRACTORS). The state set X is replaced here by a finite or infinite set of attractors in combination with an infinite set of transient intermediate states. Because of the iterative character of the state update function δ, all these models are in principle compatible with the recurrent connectivity pattern of generic neural microcircuits.

A somewhat problematic aspect of this approach, which constrains its applicability to artificial behaving systems and also its appeal as a model for temporal integration in behaving organisms, is its need for an a priori definition of a suitable set X of internal states or attractors (whereas the transition function δ can in principle be learned through reinforcement learning once the set X has been defined). Attractor neural networks have to cope with the additional difficulty that for the dynamical system defined by a recurrent analog circuit, no general and stable mechanisms are known for controlling the landscape of its attractors and fast online transition between its attractors (except for simulating a discrete finite-state machine). An attractor neural network is in general also not able to produce at any time t a meaningful response $y(t)$ to an ongoing input stream because it is likely to spend most of its time in transient states between attractors. The mathematical theory that underlies attractor neural networks and dynamical systems theory has focused on the case of autonomous dynamical systems (i.e., systems whose input can be encoded in the initial state of the system), usually of a very low dimension. Consequently, there exists a lack of analytical tools for understanding temporal integration of a continuous input stream in the high-dimensional dynamic systems formed by neural circuits.

Using Perturbations of Recurrent Circuits for Temporal Integration

Since the transient dynamics of a recurrent circuit is in general even harder to control than its attractor structure, it might seem hopeless to use it for purposeful computations. However, it turns out that it is not necessary to take control of or manipulate the transient dynamics of a recurrent circuit in order to use it for complex computations requiring temporal integration. If the recurrent circuit is sufficiently complex, its inherent dynamics automatically absorbs and stores information from the incoming input stream (Buonomano and Merzenich, 1995). More precisely, the current state $x(t)$ of a recurrent circuit automatically contains information about preceding inputs $u(s)$. It only remains to read out this information, but this is a standard spatial pattern recognition task requiring no temporal integration. Readout neurons can easily be trained by supervised (Maass, Natschlaeger, and Markram, 2001) or unsupervised (Legenstein, Maass, and Markram, 2002) learning to perform this task, provided that the recurrent circuit—and hence the dimension of its transient states $x(t)$—is sufficiently large. An important class of methods in machine learning (see SUPPORT VECTOR MACHINES) relies on a closely related principle. In fact, one might compare the computational role of a neural microcircuit with a kernel for support vector machines that implements a nonlinear projection of time series (the input stream that has reached the neural microcircuit up to time t) onto points $x(t)$ in a very high dimensional space. If the dimension of this space is sufficiently high, then most complex nonlinear classification problems for time series $u(\cdot)$ are transformed through this nonlinear projection into linearly separable classification tasks for the subsequent state $x(t)$. Hence, in principle, even a single (memoryless) readout neuron can be trained to perform such a task, thereby classifying at time t the input stream $u(\cdot)$ that had reached the recurrent neural circuit up to time t.

From this point of view, a recurrent neural circuit accomplishes more than a tapped delay line, since it not only stores information about the past, but also preprocesses it (in a general-purpose manner, like a kernel, without specialization for a specific task) by projecting it nonlinearly into a very high dimensional space to boost the power of diverse linear readouts for specific tasks.

The abstract computational model on which this view of computation in neural microcircuits is based is the liquid-state machine (see Figure 1; see also Maass et al., 2001, Markram et al., 2002) that is quite different from a Turing machine, the traditional paradigm for universal neural computation. In this new model, a recurrent neural circuit is represented by a generic nonlinear filter L that transforms time-varying input $u(\cdot)$ into a trajectory of internal states $x(t)$ and a task-specific readout of information from $x(t)$ by memoryless readout functions f (see Figure 1). Since in contrast to a finite-state machine the internal state $x(t)$ may change in this new computational model in a "liquid" manner, continuously in time and space, the model is called a *liquid-state machine*. Like Turing machines, the liquid-state machine provides theoretically unlimited computational power if the recurrent microcircuit is sufficiently large but for real-time computing (with fading memory) on continuous input streams, instead of off-line computation on discrete batch inputs, for which Turing machines are universal. The recurrent microcircuit serves in this model as a general-purpose analog fading memory (represented mathematically by a nonlinear filter L). Its current state, $x(t)$, contains, for example, information about the temporal pattern of spike trains that had previously entered the circuit but with lower reliability for spike trains that had arrived farther back in the past (fading memory) (see Figure 2).

So far, we have discussed only the situation in which the readout neuron has to extract information from the current state $x(t)$ of a circuit at one specific time t. But the same mechanisms and principles also apply to the more realistic case in which a target output $y(t)$, requiring integration of information from inputs $u(s)$ at various numbers and combinations of preceding time points $s < t$, has to be provided in real time *at any time t*. From the point of view of a readout neuron, this means that it has to be able to classify states $x(t)$ that occur at different time points t. Hence it has to solve a more complex spatial classification task. But the same principle as before applies: This task can still be solved by simple time-invariant linear readouts if the dimension of the current circuit states $x(t)$ is sufficiently high.

In the context of time-varying outputs $y(t)$, it is biologically more realistic to consider functions $y(t)$ that assume analog values in some interval [0, 1] rather than just discrete values {0, 1}. The target values for such time-varying analog readouts $y(t)$ from recurrent microcircuits could, for example, be predictions of future values of specific inputs, which can be learned in an unsupervised manner (Legenstein et al., 2002). Such time-varying analog readouts could be implemented in a neural system, for example, by a pool P of integrate-and-fire neurons that all receive the same circuit state $x(t)$ as input (but may apply different synaptic efficacies to this common input $x(t)$), where the fraction of neurons in this pool P that fire around time t may be viewed as the time-varying analog readout $y(t)$. It has been shown that any continuous readout map f (see Figure 1) can be approximated by such pool P and that a simple local learning rule suffices for training such pool P of integrate-and-fire neurons to approximate a given function f (Maass et al., 2001). Consider, for example, the case in which a readout neuron has to give the same constant target response $y(t) = y_0$ for all t from some interval $[T, T']$ even if the internal state $x(t)$ (and possibly also the circuit input) keeps changing during this time period. Some of the readouts shown in Figure 3 face exactly this task during those intervals in which their target output, plotted as a dashed line, is constant or almost constant, whereas the circuit input (four spike trains in parallel shown at the top) varies during these time intervals and the internal circuit activity $x(t)$ also varies (this is in fact necessary because other readouts have at the same time quickly varying target outputs $y(t)$, but their weights are assumed to remain fixed after learning). Such diverse readouts are possible because each readout (implemented in this case by a pool P of neurons whose current firing activity represents its current analog output $y(t)$, plotted as a solid line in Figure 3) is trained by the task to define its own notion of equivalence on circuit states $x(t)$ (and thereby implicitly its own neural code). In particular, a readout neuron can give a stable output even if the underlying circuit never reaches a fixpoint attractor, showing that attractors are not necessary for producing stable system outputs. Hence, stable perception is possible even if the internal state of the nervous system may never repeat.

The fact that the previously sketched model for temporal integration of information in a neural circuit does not require to force the internal dynamics $x(t)$ of the circuit to respond to specific time-varying inputs $u(\cdot)$ with specific trajectories $x(\cdot)$ (which is in general very difficult, if not impossible, to achieve for a noisy recurrent circuit) has an additional side benefit. Since the circuit responses $x(t)$ have not been modified to optimally support a particular readout task, different readout neurons can simultaneously extract from

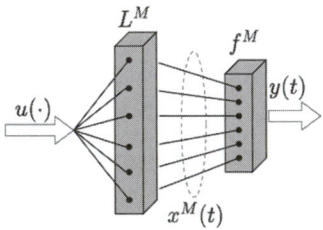

Figure 1. Schema of a liquid-state machine M, consisting of a (in general nonlinear) filter L^M and a memoryless readout map f^M (the latter is applied to the liquid state $x(t)$ defined as the output of the filter at time t for input function $u(\cdot)$). Provided that the available pools of filters L and readout functions f satisfy some rather basic necessary properties (pointwise separation property for filters L—which is approximately met by recurrent neural circuits—and approximation property for readout functions f; see Maass et al., 2001, for details), the resulting liquid-state machines M can in principle approximate any time-invariant fading memory filter. Hence, it can arguably perform any real-time computational task involving temporal integration that a behaving organism might need.

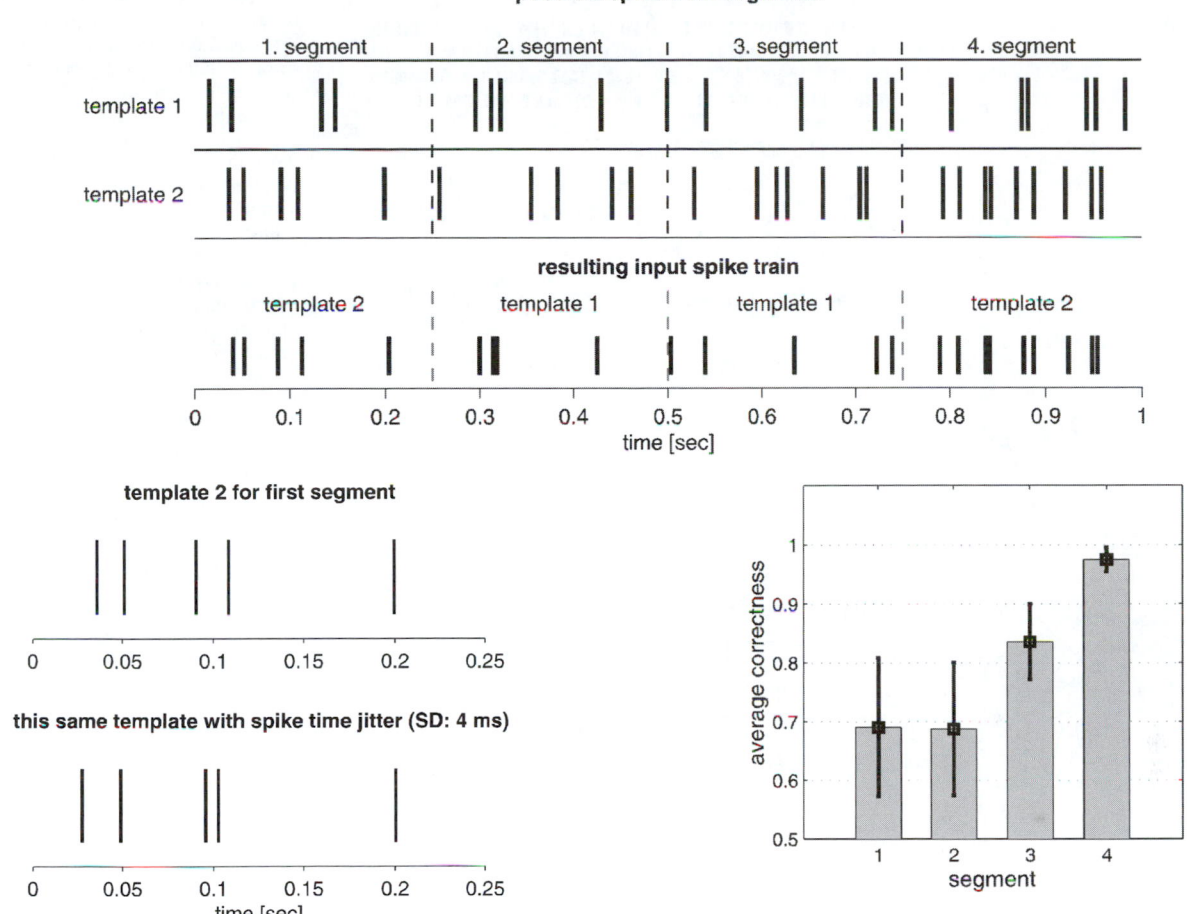

Figure 2. Performance of a recurrent neural microcircuit as analog fading memory. Results shown are from computer simulations of a recurrent (randomly connected) generic circuit of 135 integrate-and-fire neurons. Circuit inputs were spike trains over 1 s. Sixteen temporal patterns of such spike trains had been fixed, each a concatenation of four shorter templates (which were randomly chosen fixed Poisson spike trains over 250 ms, shown at the top of Figure 2A). Two templates were available for each of the 250 ms segments of the spike train, yielding $2^4 = 16$ temporal patterns for spike trains over 1 s. Inputs $u(\cdot)$ to the circuit were noisy variations of these 16 temporal patterns, in which each spike was independently moved by an amount chosen from a Gaussian distribution with SD 4 ms (see Figure 2B for an example). Figure 2C shows the average correctness (for novel test examples of jittered spike trains) of four readout neurons that had been trained to extract from the spatial pattern $x(t)$ of the circuit activity at time $t = 1$ s (i.e., after the spike train $u(\cdot)$ had been sent to the circuit) the information that templates had been chosen for each of the four segments of this input spike train. Error bars shown represent the standard deviation over nine trials with different randomly drawn recurrent circuits and dif-

ferent randomly drawn Poisson spike trains as templates. The ith readout neuron had been trained to fire at time $t = 1$ s if and only if the first one of the two templates had been chosen as template for the ith segment of the preceding spike train. Obviously, this task requires substantial temporal integration of information, since one has to recover information about input segments that had arrived several hundred milliseconds ago. This task is in addition a rather difficult computational task, since the desired information is not contained in any specific interspike interval of the preceding input spike train (owing to the randomly chosen dislocation of spikes). Obviously, the readout neuron that has to recover the identity of the template for the last 250 ms could solve its task with the highest accuracy. However, substantial amounts of information about earlier segments were also recovered, in spite of the fact that all this information had been overwritten in an uncontrollable nonlinear manner by later spikes entering the recurrent circuit. The circuit had not been optimized for this task, and performance can easily be improved by using a larger recurrent circuit or readout units consisting of several neurons. Results shown are from a computer simulation by Maass et al. (2001).

the same trajectory $x(\cdot)$ different temporally integrated information needed for diverse tasks (see Figure 3). The trajectory of internal states of the dynamical system may therefore be viewed as a universal source of information about past inputs, from which different readout neurons can extract different components. Hence this approach not only provides a framework in which purposeful anytime responses to temporally integrated information can be explained, but it also provides a model for parallel real-time computing on temporally integrated information.

We have made two conceptual simplifications in the preceding account. The first one is that synaptic plasticity was assumed to be restricted to readout neurons, while synapses within the recurrent microcircuit itself could remain unmodified. Although this may in principle suffice, the performance of the system could be optimized by adjusting also synapses within the recurrent microcircuit. For example, the dynamic responses $x(t)$ could be optimized by unsupervised learning (for example, nonlinear ICA) for the statistics of actually occurring external stimuli $u(\cdot)$ to provide optimal support

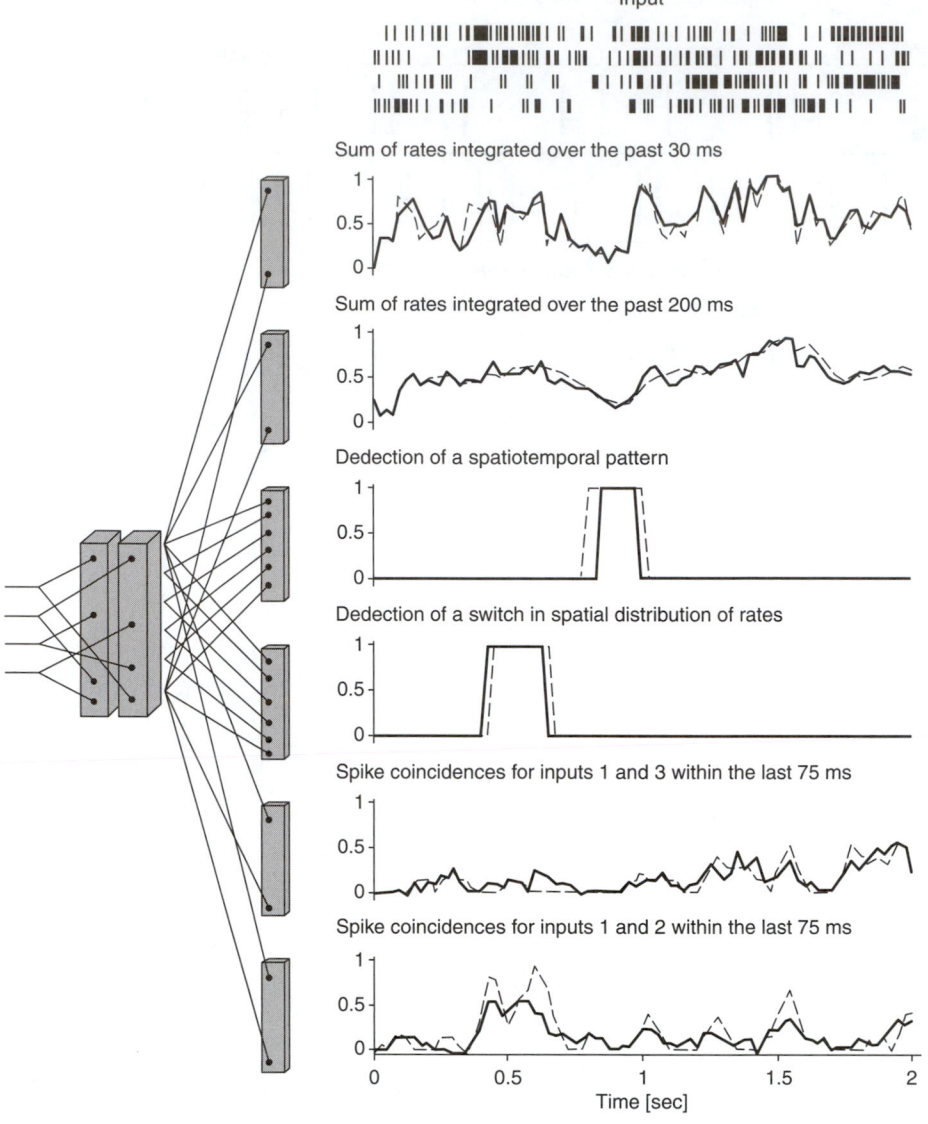

Input

Sum of rates integrated over the past 30 ms

Sum of rates integrated over the past 200 ms

Dedection of a spatiotemporal pattern

Dedection of a switch in spatial distribution of rates

Spike coincidences for inputs 1 and 3 within the last 75 ms

Spike coincidences for inputs 1 and 2 within the last 75 ms

Time [sec]

Figure 3. Six readout units were trained to extract completely different temporally integrated information from the current firing activity of two recurrent circuits (columns) consisting of 135 integrate-and-fire neurons each and both receiving the same four input spike trains over 2,000 ms, shown at the top. The tasks for the readout units were to represent the sum of firing rates of the four input spike trains integrated over the last 30 ms, to represent the sum of firing rates of the four input spike trains integrated over 200 ms, to output a high value only if a specific spatiotemporal pattern occurs, to output a high value only if the firing rates go up in spike train 1 and 2 and simultaneously go down in spike trains 3 and 4, to report the number of spike coincidence (i.e., spikes within a 5 ms window) of spike trains 1 and 3 during the last 75 ms, and to report the corresponding number of spike coincidence for spike trains 1 and 2. Results shown are for novel input spike trains, generated from the same distribution as the spike trains used for training.

for a variety of different readouts (rather than for just one specific readout or task). This may be seen as analogy to a common procedure for support vector machines in machine learning, in which specific kernels are chosen to optimally support a specific family of classification and regression tasks. The other simplification we made was the assumed partition of neurons into neurons that belong to a recurrent microcircuit ("liquid") and neurons that read out information from such recurrent circuit. Of course, in a more sophisticated model of cortical circuitry, one would arrive at a network of many liquid-state machines, in which a neuron that reads out information from one recurrent circuit is embedded into the "liquid" recurrent circuit of another liquid-state machine and also sends backprojections into the recurrent circuit from which it reads out information. In fact, benefits of backprojections from the readout into the recurrent circuit have already been demonstrated by Jaeger (2001), who had independently discovered a closely related computational model (echo-state networks) in the context of artificial neural networks with sigmoidal neurons. Wyss, König, and Verschure (2002) exhibit a complementary mechanism: Static batch inputs are transformed by recurrent circuits into a trajectory

of transient states, from which the identity of the batch input can be recovered.

Summary

We have surveyed the main approaches toward modeling temporal integration in neural microcircuits. Approaches based on tapped delay lines, finite-state machines, and attractor neural networks are suitable for modeling specific tasks. But as models for universal real-time computations in neural microcircuits, they appear to be incompatible with results from neuroanatomy (such as highly recurrent diverse circuitry) and neurophysiology (fast transient dynamics of firing activity with few attractor states). A more recent approach views the transient dynamics of neural microcircuits as the main carrier of information about past inputs, from which specific information, needed for a variety of different tasks, can be read out in parallel and at any time by different readout neurons. This model promises to solve four fundamental problems neural systems face in a real-world situation: (1) how to process continuously changing input, (2) how to respond in real time, (3) how to combine information across a large number and combination of time points (universal temporal integration), and (4) unrestricted parallel processing that allows neuronal activity to partake simultaneously in the perception of multiple features and objects. In other words, this approach supports the solution of binding problems (see Singer and Gray, 1995) by avoiding to scatter information into isolated features at the first level of processing.

This approach has provided so far the only method for using computer models of generic recurrent circuits of integrate-and-fire neurons for complex information processing tasks, in particular for tasks that require temporal integration of inputs. This yields a novel tool for exploring through computer simulations of more and more realistic models for neural microcircuits the specific computational role of the experimentally observed diversity of neurons and synapses with regard to their dynamic behavior and connection preferences (see NEOCORTEX: BASIC NEURON TYPES and Gupta et al., 2000). As a first step in this program, Maass et al. (2001) showed that a recurrent neural circuit serves best as analog fading memory if its statistics of connection lengths is biologically realistic, with primary local connections but also a few long-range connections (whereas preceding theoretical approaches had focused either on recurrent circuits with full connectivity, such as Hopfield nets, or on circuits with strictly local connectivity, such as cellular automata). Furthermore, in contrast to virtually all other theory-based modeling approaches, the liquid-state machine model is enhanced, rather than hampered, by the given biological diversity of circuit components. It also provides a new conceptual framework for the experimental investigation of neural microcircuits and larger neural systems, especially for a possible understanding of the ubiquitous trial-to-trial variations that are traditionally washed out through averaging of data over many trials. It also suggests that beyond neural codes that are clearly understandable for a human observer, there may exist substantially more complex internal neural codes represented through high-dimensional activation states of neural circuits, which are easy to classify for a readout neuron but cannot be adequately characterized in terms of commonly considered special cases of neural codes.

Road Map: Biological Networks

Related Reading: Integrate-and-Fire Neurons and Networks; Recurrent Networks: Learning Algorithms; Recurrent Networks: Neurophysiological Modeling; Spiking Neurons, Computation with

References

Buonomano, D. V., and Merzenich, M. M., 1995, Temporal information transformed into a spatial code by a neural network with realistic properties, *Science*, 267:1028–1030. ◆

De Felipe, J., 1997, Microcircuits in the brain, *Biological and Artificial Computation: From Neuroscience to Technology, Springer Lecture Notes in Computer Science*, 1240:1–14.

Douglas, R., and Martin, K., 1998, Neocortex, in *The Synaptic Organization of the Brain* (G. M. Shepherd, Ed.), Oxford, Engl.: Oxford University Press, pp. 459–509.

Gupta, A., Wang, Y., and Markram, H., 2000, Organizing principles for a diversity of GABAergic interneurons and synapses in the neocortex, *Science*, 287:273–278.

Jaeger, H., 2001, The "echo state" approach to analyzing and training recurrent neural networks, GMD Report 148, German National Research Center for Information Technology.

Legenstein, R. A., Maass, W., and Markram, H., 2002, Input prediction and autonomous movement analysis in recurrent circuits of spiking neurons, submitted for publication.

Maass, W., Natschlaeger, T., and Markram, H., 2001, Real-time computing without stable states: A new framework for neural computation based on perturbations, *Neural Computation*, (in press). ◆

Markram, H., Ofer, M., Natschlaeger, T., and Maass, W., 2002, Temporal integration in recurrent microcircuits, *Cerebral Cortex*, in press.

Shepherd, G. M., 1988, A basic circuit for cortical organization, in *Perspectives in Memory Research* (M. Gazzaniga, Ed.), Cambridge, MA: MIT Press, pp. 93–134.

Singer, W., and Gray, C. M., 1995, Visual feature integration and the temporal correlation hypothesis, *Ann. Rev. Neurosci.*, 18:555–586.

Thomson, A. M., West, D. C., Wang, Y., and Bannister, A. P., 2002, Synaptic connections and small circuits involving excitatory and inhibitory neurons in layers 2 to 5 of adult rat and cat neocortex: Triple intracellular recordings and biocytin-labelling in vitro, *Cerebral Cortex*, in press.

von Melchner, L., Pallas, S. L., and Sur, M., 2000, Visual behaviour mediated by retinal projection directed to the auditory pathway, *Nature*, 404:871–876.

White, E. L., 1989, *Cortical Circuits*, Boston: Birkhaeuser.

Wyss, R., König, P., and Verschure, P. F. M. J., 2002, Invariant representations of visual patterns in a temporal population code, *Proc. Nat. Acad. of Sci.*, in press.

Temporal Pattern Processing

DeLiang Wang

Introduction

Temporal pattern processing is important for various intelligent behaviors, including hearing, vision, speech, music, and motor control. Because we live in an ever-changing environment, an intelligent system—human or robot—must encode patterns over time, recognizing and generating temporal patterns. Time is embodied in a temporal pattern in two ways.

- *Temporal order.* This refers to the ordering among the components of a sequence. For example, the sequence *N-E-T* is different from *T-E-N*. Temporal order may also refer to a syntactic structure, such as subject-verb object, where each component may be any of a category of possible symbols.
- *Time duration.* Duration can play a critical role for temporal processing. In speech recognition, for example, we want rate invariance while distinguishing relative durations of the vowel /i:/ (as in beet) and /i/ (as in bit).

Following Wang and Arbib (1990), a sequence is defined as *complex* if it contains repetitions of the same subsequence, as in *C-O-N-F-R-O-N-T*; otherwise, it is defined as *simple*. For generation of complex sequences, the correct successor can be determined only by knowing components prior to the current one. We refer to the prior subsequence required to determine the current component as the *context* of the component, and the length of this context as the *degree* of the component. The *degree of a sequence* is defined as the maximum degree of its components. Thus, a simple sequence is a degree 1 sequence.

Temporal pattern processing is a challenging topic because the information is embedded in time (thus inherently dynamic), not simultaneously available. Nevertheless, this topic has been studied by a number of investigators; see Sun and Giles (2001) for a recent collection of articles on this topic.

Fundamentally different from static pattern processing, temporal processing requires that a neural network have a capacity for short-term memory (STM) in order to maintain a component for some time. This is because a temporal pattern extends over a time period. How to encode STM thus becomes one of the criteria for classifying neural networks for temporal processing. In this article, I provide an outline of temporal pattern processing, discussing the topics of recognition and generation separately. In the end, I point out several outstanding issues, including time warping and chunking, that require future investigation.

STM Models

Delay Lines

The simplest form of STM uses a fixed-length buffer of N units to maintain the N most recent input items. This can be implemented either by a shift register with a fixed delay between consecutive units or by an array of systematic delay lines. The delay line STM transforms a temporal pattern into a spatial one where time forms another dimension. This idea forms the basis of many recognition models (Waibel et al., 1989).

Decay Traces

Here, an item in STM decays in time, corresponding to the decay theory of forgetting in human STM. The decay usually takes an exponential form. Theoretically, time information can be precisely recovered from the current value. But owing to rapid decay and noise, only a limited number of the most recent items can be reliably discerned from STM. This form has been used by Jordan (1986) and Wang and Arbib (1990), among others. Figure 1A shows a typical decay trace.

Exponential Kernels

Tank and Hopfield (1987) proposed a set of normalized exponential kernels to sample the history, described as

$$f_k(t) = \left(\frac{t}{k}\right)^\alpha e^{\alpha(1 - t/k)} \quad \text{for } k = 1, \ldots, K \quad (1)$$

where α regulates the width of each kernel. Notice that $f_k(t) = 1$ if $t = k$. Figure 1B shows a set of four kernels. There are K units

to represent each symbol. Unlike delay line STM, each unit here samples a symbol within a certain period peaked at a specific time step ($t = k$).

Along similar lines, de Vries and Principe (1992) proposed the *gamma model*, which uses a set of gamma kernels (integrands of Γ-functions, hence the name)

$$g_k(t) = \frac{\mu^k}{(k - 1)!} t^{k-1} e^{-\mu t} \quad \text{for } k = 1, \ldots, K \quad (2)$$

where μ is a parameter between 0 and 1. K is called the order of the memory, and there are K units for storing a symbol S in STM. Figure 1C shows a set of four kernels. Since g_k has a maximum value at $t = (k - 1)/\mu$, μ determines the depth of the peak of each kernel in STM. Thus, unlike normalized exponential kernels, an N-step history may be sampled by less than N gamma kernels. Note that gamma kernels can be computed recursively.

STORE Model

The STM models examined so far are autonomous, for the trace of each item is fully independent of other items in STM. A basic property of human STM is that it has a limited capacity (7 ± 2), so that whether and how long an item is held in STM depends on other inputs entering STM. In addition, the study of human retention of sequences shows a recency factor, where more recent items tend to be better retained, and a primacy factor, whereby the beginning items of a sequence are less prone to forgetting. These two factors together give rise to the bowing effect, which motivated the STORE model (Bradski, Carpenter, and Grossberg, 1992) using a pair of units

$$x_i(t + 1) = x_i(t) + [\beta I_i(t) + y_i(t) - x_i(t)x(t)]I(t) \quad (3a)$$

$$y_i(t + 1) = y_i(t) + [x_i(t) - y_i(t)][1 - I(t)] \quad (3b)$$

where $x(t) = \Sigma_j x_j(t)$ is the sum of STM item values, and $I(t) = \Sigma_j I_j(t)$ is the sum of external inputs. The behavior of STORE has two aspects. The first is the global inhibition term in Equation 3a, which reduces the value of x_i in favor of new items. The second is the excitatory loop between x_i and y_i, which favors old items in STM. Combined, they are able to produce the bowing shape for a

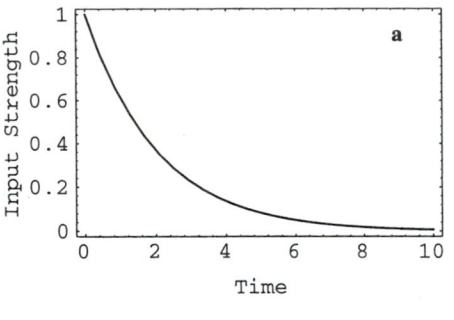

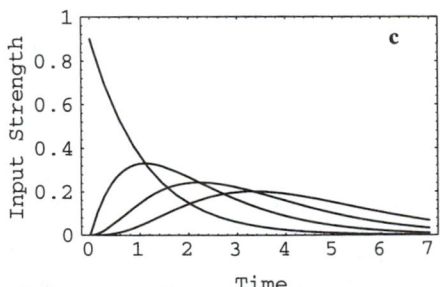

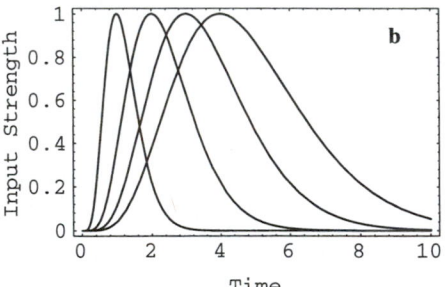

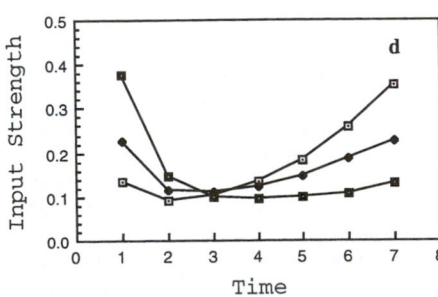

Figure 1. STM traces. *a*, Exponential decay. *b*, Normalized exponential kernels. $\alpha = 5.0$, and $k = 1, \ldots, 4$ for the curves from left to right, respectively. *c*, Gamma kernels. $\mu = 0.9$, and $k = 1, \ldots, 4$ for the curves from left to right, respectively. *d*, The STORE model. $\beta = 0.5$ for the empty square bow, 0.3 for the diamond bow, and 0.15 for the filled square bow. Seven items are kept in STM.

sequence of items. Figure 1D shows three bows generated with different values of β.

Temporal Pattern Recognition

The shared goal of all STM models is to make input history available simultaneously when recognition takes place. With an STM model in place, recognition is not much different from the recognition of static patterns.

Template Matching Using Hebbian Learning

The architecture for this type of recognition is simply a two-layer network: the input layer that incorporates STM, and the sequence recognition layer where each unit encodes an individual sequence. The recognition scheme is essentially template matching, where templates are formed by following Hebbian learning

$$W_{ij}(t) = W_{ij}(t - 1) + Cs_i(t)[x_j(t) - W_{ij}(t - 1)] \quad (4)$$

where W_{ij} is the connection weight from unit x_j in the input layer to sequence recognizer s_i in the recognition layer. Parameter C controls learning rate. Hebbian learning is applied after the presentation of the entire sequence is completed. The templates thus formed can be used to recognize specific input sequences. The recognition layer typically includes recurrent connections for selecting a winner by self-organization (e.g., winner-take-all) during training or recognition.

Kohonen (1990) proposed an architecture, called the *phonetic typewriter* for phoneme recognition. The phonetic typewriter extracts a vector of frequency components using FFT (fast Fourier transform). After this step, his algorithm of feature mapping is applied for recognition, where winner-take-all is applied in both training and recognition. The phonetic typewriter has been applied to recognize Finnish and Japanese phonemes (Kohonen, 1990). Wang and colleagues (Wang and Arbib, 1990; Wang and Yuwono, 1995) adopted a learning method similar to Equation 4, and showed that a recognition algorithm plus either decay trace or shift register can recognize complex sequences.

Associative Memory Approach

The dynamics of the Hopfield associative memory model can be characterized as evolving toward the memory state most similar to the current input pattern. If one views each memory state as a category, the Hopfield net performs pattern recognition: The recalled category is the recognized pattern. This process of dynamic evolution can also be viewed as an optimization process, which minimizes a cost function until equilibrium is reached.

With normalized exponential kernel STM, Tank and Hopfield (1987) described a recognition network based on associative memory dynamics. A layer of sequence recognizers receives inputs from the STM model. Each recognizer encodes a different template sequence by its unique weight vector acting on the inputs in STM. In addition, recognizers form a competitive network. The recognition process uses the current input sequence (evidence) to bias a minimization process so that the most similar template wins the competition, thus activating its corresponding recognizer. Due to the exponential kernels, they demonstrated that recognition is fairly robust to *time warping*, distortions in duration. A similar architecture is later applied to speaker-independent spoken digit recognition.

Multilayer Perceptrons

Multilayer perceptrons (MLP) offer a popular approach to temporal pattern learning. MLPs have been demonstrated to be effective for static pattern recognition. It is natural to combine MLP with an STM model to do temporal pattern recognition. For example, using delay line STM, Waibel et al. (1989) reported an architecture called Time Delay Neural Networks (TDNN) for spoken phoneme recognition. Besides the input layer, TDNN uses two hidden layers and an output layer where each unit encodes one phoneme. The feedforward connections converge from the input layer to each successive layer so that each unit in a specific layer receives inputs within a limited time window from the previous layer. They demonstrated good recognition performance: For the three stop consonants /b/, /d/, and /g/, the accuracy of speaker-dependent recognition reached 98.5%.

Temporal Pattern Generation

In 1969, S. Grossberg introduced an early model of sequence generation, the *outstar avalanche*, which is composed of n sequential outstars. Each outstar $\mathbf{M}_i$ stores a static pattern and is activated by a signal in the vertex v_i. These vertices are connected as: $v_1 \rightarrow v_2 \rightarrow \cdots \rightarrow v_n$. So an initial signal at v_1 can generate sequentially the spatial patterns stored in $\mathbf{M}_1, \mathbf{M}_2, \ldots, \mathbf{M}_n$. See Grossberg (1982) for a more detailed description as well as some of the later extensions. In recent years, a number of more sophisticated solutions have been proposed for temporal pattern generation.

Associative Memory Approach

Since associative memory studies how to associate one pattern with another, its mechanism can be extended to generating a sequence. A sequence is treated as a set of pairs between consecutive components, and these pairs are stored into an associative memory. Hence, after the first component of the sequence is presented, the next component will be activated after some delay, which further activates the third one, and so on. This basic idea, however, leads to ambiguity when generating a complex sequence, where one pattern may be followed by different ones. Several investigators have proposed to use high-order networks to deal with the problem. In a kth-order network, the input to each unit is the weighted sum of k-tuples, instead of individual units, and each k-tuple is a product of k units. In such a network, one component in a sequence is associated by a prior subsequence of length k. Thus, a sequence of degree k can be generated without ambiguity by a kth-order associative memory (Guyon et al., 1988). A major problem with high-order networks is the required number of connections, which grows exponentially with the order of the network.

Multilayer Perceptron Approach

Jordan (1986) described the first MLP architecture with recurrent connections for sequence generation. The input layer has two parts: plan units representing external input and the identity of the sequence and state units that receive one-to-one projections from the output layer, forming decay trace STM. After a sequence is stored into the network by backpropagation training, it can be generated by an external input representing the identity of the sequence. This input activates the first component of the sequence in the output layer. This component feeds back to the input layer and, together with the external input, activates the second component, and so on. A particular component of a sequence is generated by the part of the sequence prior to the component, earlier components having lesser roles due to exponential decay. Elman (1990) later modified Jordan's architecture by having the hidden layer connect to a part of the input layer, called the context layer. The context layer simply duplicates the activation of the hidden layer in the previous time step. Elman used this architecture to learn a set of individual sequences satisfying a syntactic description, and found that the network exhibits a kind of syntax recognition. This result suggests a way of learning high-level structures, such as natural language grammar.

Anticipation Model and Multi-Associative Networks

Generation of complex sequences has been a major issue. The approaches described so far rely either on fixed degree contexts or on a composite vector recording the history. The latter is prone to ambiguity. The former entails high system overhead, because, in order to avoid ambiguity, such a method must use a degree no smaller than the degree of the sequence, which is usually much greater than the degrees of most components. This analysis calls for a mechanism of self-organization, where each component in a sequence can learn the degree of its own context.

By extending basic ideas for complex sequence processing reported in Wang and Arbib (1990), Wang and Yuwono (1995) introduced such a mechanism of self-organization for generating complex patterns. This so-called *anticipation model* is based on the following two ideas. First, the system actively anticipates the next component in sequence learning, and a mismatch between the anticipated component and the actual component triggers context ad-

justment through competitive learning. Second, generation of a sequence component hinges on recognition of the component's context. Figure 2A shows the architecture of the anticipation model, using a shift-register STM model. Each unit in the detector layer recognizes a specific context, and a winner-take-all mechanism is implemented within the detector layer. There is a modulator layer that corresponds to the detector layer, and each modulator receives a downward connection from its respective detector as well as upward connections from every input terminal. The modulators perform a comparison between anticipation from a winning detector and the next input component. Wang and Yuwono (1995) showed that the anticipation model can learn to generate an arbitrary temporal sequence.

Wang and Yuwono (1996) later applied the anticipation model to learn multiple complex sequences sequentially; i.e., new training does not take place until existing sequences are acquired. Using a set of 97 highly correlated complex sequences, they demonstrated that learning a new sequence can interfere with already acquired ones. However, the number of intact sequences increases linearly with the size of the existing memory, while the amount of retraining needed to eliminate interference is independent of the size of the memory, as illustrated in Figure 2B. Such characteristics are largely

a

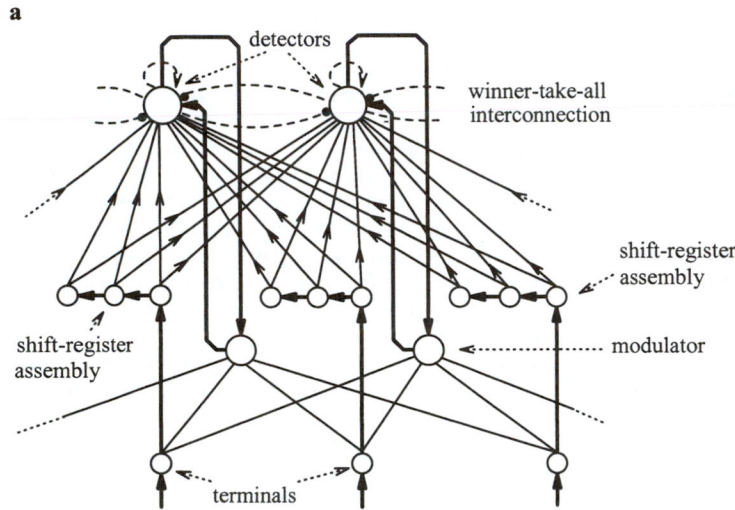

b

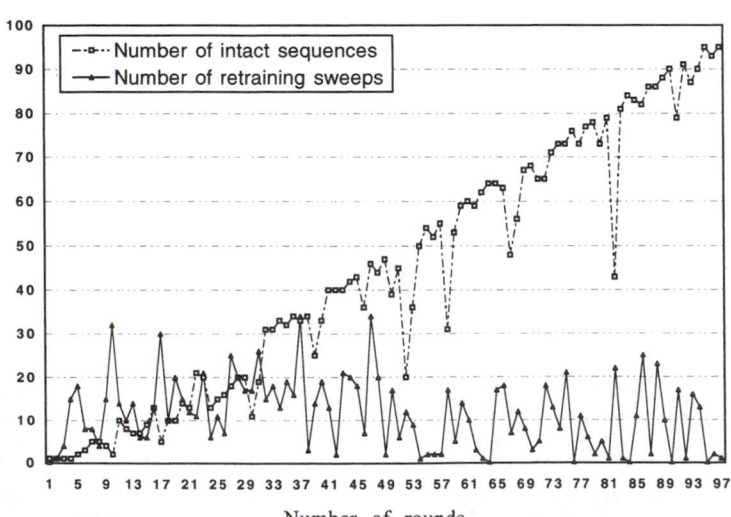

Figure 2. Anticipation model. *a*, Architecture (adapted from Wang and Yuwono, 1995). Thin solid lines denote modifiable connections, thick dashed lines denote fixed connections, and undirected lines denote bidirectional connections. *b*, The number of intact sequences and the number of retraining sweeps with respect to the number of training rounds for individual sequences (adapted from Wang and Yuwono, 1996). The 97 sequences denote all the session titles of the 1994 IEEE International Conference on Neural Networks.

derived from the fact that each sequence is represented in a distributed manner, and different sequences and subsequences within a sequence may share context detectors. The interference properties of the anticipation model are consistent with human retroactive interference, which is well documented in psychology, while contrasting with MLP that shows catastrophic interference in sequential learning.

A limitation of the anticipation model is that it deals with symbol sequences rather than sequences of spatial patterns. Recently, Wang (1999) proposed using multi-associative neural networks for learning and retrieving spatiotemporal patterns. STM is coded as systematic delay lines. The basic idea is that, when dealing with complex sequences, one pattern is allowed to be associated with a set of multiple subsequent patterns, and ambiguity can be eliminated by intersecting multiple sets associated by the previous pattern, the pattern prior to the previous pattern, and so on. A complex sequence of degree k can thus be unambiguously generated with k systematic delay lines. Associations between spatial patterns are established through individual units in a competitive layer. A drawback of this model is that many network operations are algorithmically described, rather than arising from a network autonomously.

Discussion

This brief tour of neural network processing of temporal patterns shows that effective models and techniques exist for both recognition and generation (see SEQUENCE LEARNING for a more biologically oriented review). There are, however, many questions yet to be answered. In my view, the following two problems are particularly interesting and challenging for future research:

1. *Rate invariance and time warp.* Humans show rate invariance to a certain extent in recognizing a temporal pattern. *Rate invariance* is different from what I call *interval invariance*; the former is invariance only to global scaling of durations and the latter is invariance to all changes of durations. Interval invariance is exhibited in several models, but not rate invariance (see Wang, Liu, and Ahalt, 1996, for a comprehensive discussion). One must be careful about time warping. We would like to have invariance over limited warping, but dramatic change in relative duration must be recognized differently.
2. *Chunking.* A fundamental ability of human information processing is chunking, which, in the context of temporal processing, means that frequently encountered and meaningful subsequences organize into chunks that form basic units for further chunking at a higher level. Chunking and STM are closely related. A chunk often corresponds to a meaningful subsequence (such as a melody), but it may be just a convenient way of

breaking a long sequence into shorter parts to cope with limited capacity of STM. One aspect of chunking is studied by Wang and Yuwono (1996), but the general problem of unsupervised chunking has been little addressed and will be increasingly important for future research into temporal pattern processing.

Road Map: Learning in Artificial Networks
Related Reading: Convolutional Networks for Images, Speech, and Time Series; Dynamics of Association and Recall; Helmholtz Machines and Sleep-Wake Learning; Hidden Markov Models; Temporal Sequences: Learning and Global Analysis

References

Bradski, G., Carpenter, G. A., and Grossberg, S., 1992, Working memory networks for learning temporal order with application to three-dimensional visual object recognition, *Neural Comp.*, 4:270–286.
de Vries, B. D., and Principe, J. C., 1992, The gamma model—A new neural model for temporal processing, *Neural Net.*, 5:565–576.
Elman, J. L., 1990, Finding structure in time, *Cogn. Sci.*, 14:179–211.
Grossberg, S., 1982, Associative and competitive principles of learning and development: The temporal unfolding and stability of STM and LTM patterns, in *Competition and Cooperation in Neural Networks* (S. Amari and M. A. Arbib, Eds.), New York: Springer-Verlag, pp. 295–341. ◆
Guyon, I., Personnaz, L., Nadal, J. P., and Dreyfus, G., 1988, Storage and retrieval of complex sequences in neural networks, *Phys. Rev. A*, 38:6365–6372.
Jordan, M. I., 1986, Attractor dynamics and parallelism in a connectionist sequential machine, in *Proceedings of the Eighth Annual Conference of the Cognitive Science Society*, Hillsdale, NJ: Erlbaum, pp. 531–546.
Kohonen, T., 1990, The self-organizing map, *Proc. IEEE*, 78:1464–1480. ◆
Sun, R., and Giles, C. L. (Eds.), 2001, *Sequence Learning*, Berlin: Springer. ◆
Tank, D. W., and Hopfield, J. J., 1987, Neural computation by concentrating information in time, *Proc. Natl. Acad. Sci. USA*, 84:1896–1900.
Waibel, A., Hanazawa, T., Hinton, G. E., Shikano, K., and Lang, K. J., 1989, Phoneme recognition using time-delay neural networks, *IEEE Trans. Acoust. Speech Signal Process.*, 37:328–339.
Wang, D. L., and Arbib, M. A., 1990, Complex temporal sequence learning based on short-term memory, *Proc. IEEE*, 78:1536–1543.
Wang, D. L., Liu, X. M., and Ahalt, S. C., 1996, On temporal generalization of simple recurrent networks, *Neural Net.*, 9:1099–1118.
Wang, D. L., and Yuwono, B., 1995, Anticipation-based temporal pattern generation, *IEEE Trans. Syst. Man Cybern.*, 25:615–628.
Wang, D. L., and Yuwono, B., 1996, Incremental learning of complex temporal patterns, *IEEE Trans. Neural Net.*, 7:1465–1481.
Wang, L., 1999, Multi-associative neural networks and their applications to learning and retrieving complex spatio-temporal sequences, *IEEE Trans. Syst. Man Cybern.—Pt. B: Cybern.*, 29:73–82.

Temporal Sequences: Learning and Global Analysis

Andreas V. M. Herz

Introduction

The capability to process spatiotemporal information is a prerequisite for any action in or reaction to a natural, that is, time-varying, environment. This simple fact explains why biological organisms have developed highly sophisticated mechanisms to recognize, generate, and learn pattern sequences (see SEQUENCE LEARNING; TEMPORAL PATTERN PROCESSING).

A comprehensive theory of the neural processes underlying temporal associations is far beyond the present knowledge (see Herz, 2002, for a review). However, even complicated pattern sequences consist in general of simpler building blocks with a duration of up to a few hundred milliseconds. Hard-wired or learned in a reliable manner, those building blocks are stored in dedicated brain regions such as the cerebellum (see CEREBELLUM AND MOTOR CONTROL) or the hippocampus (see HIPPOCAMPUS: SPATIAL MODELS) and facilitate a faithful replay or recognition of the entire spatiotemporal object.

How could elementary pattern sequences be represented in neural structures at a low architectural and computational cost? What are possible mechanisms to memorize spatiotemporal associations in a robust fashion within model neural networks? Is it possible to understand their global computation on a theoretical level? What is the relevance of these models for biological systems?

This article presents some qualitative and quantitative answers to these questions. It focuses on formal neural networks whose dynamics can be analyzed using methods from nonlinear dynamics and statistical mechanics. Such simplified systems are necessarily caricatures of biological structures. Still, they may capture aspects that are important for more elaborate approaches and real neural systems.

Signal Delays

Signal delays are omnipresent in the brain. Time lags of a few milliseconds are characteristic for axonal propagation of action potentials, synaptic transmission, and dendritic transport processes. The delay times are of the same order of magnitude or slightly smaller than the typical time scale of various important neurobiological phenomena, for example, mean interspike intervals or periods of neural oscillations. The incorporation of signal delays into theoretical models of neural dynamics is thus mandatory, especially if one allows for a distribution of time lags.

Kleinfeld (1986) and Sompolinsky and Kanter (1986) proposed models for temporal associations, using a single delay line between each pair of neurons. Tank and Hopfield (1987) presented a feedforward architecture for sequence recognition based on multiple delays, encoding information relative to the very end of a given sequence. Elements of both approaches have been combined to construct a class of feedback networks with a *broad* distribution of transmission lines (Coolen and Gielen, 1988; Herz et al., 1989). For concreteness, the present contribution focuses on networks with discrete-time dynamics and synchronous updating. Systems with (random) sequential dynamics and other extensions are discussed in Amit (1989); Hertz, Krogh, and Palmer (1991); and Kühn and van Hemmen (1991).

Neural Dynamics

Throughout what follows, a neural network will be described as a collection of N two-state neurons with activities $S_i = 1$ for a firing cell and $S_i = -1$ for a quiescent one. The neurons are connected by synapses with modifiable efficacies $J_{ij}(\tau)$ where τ denotes the delay for the information transport from j to i. For simplicity, a model will be considered in which each pair of neurons is linked by *several* delay lines with time lags $0 \leq \tau \leq \tau_{max}$, which are integer multiples of a small unit time step $\Delta t = 1$ (see Herz et al., 1989, for other network architectures). External stimuli are fed into the system through receptor neurons $\sigma_i = \pm 1$ with normalized input sensitivity γ, $0 \leq \gamma \leq 1$. The postsynaptic potentials h_i are then given by

$$h_i(t) = (1 - \gamma) \sum_{j=1}^{N} \sum_{\tau=0}^{\tau_{max}} J_{ij}(\tau) S_j(t - \tau) + \gamma \sigma_i(t) \quad (1)$$

The network dynamics are assumed to be synchronous, that is, all neurons are updated in parallel. A spike is generated if the postsynaptic potential exceeds the firing threshold. In what follows, this threshold is set to zero for simplicity so that

$$S_i(t + 1) = \text{sign}[h_i(t)] \quad (2)$$

If one takes synaptic noise into account, the postsynaptic potential becomes a fluctuating quantity $h_i + v_i$ where v_i denotes stochastic

contributions due to the probabilistic nature of neurotransmitter release. A careful analysis of synaptic transmission reveals that under the assumption of linear dendritic processing, the variable v_i is distributed according to a Gaussian probability distribution (Amit, 1989). The probability for spike generation may then be approximated by the stochastic dynamics

$$\text{Prob}[S_i(t + 1) = \pm 1] = \tfrac{1}{2} \{1 \pm \tanh[T^{-1} h_i(t)]\} \quad (3)$$

where Prob denotes probability and T represents the noise level. Within the physics literature, the update rule (Equation 3) is known as Glauber dynamics. In the limit $T \to 0$, one recovers the deterministic description (Equation 2). See also DYNAMICS OF ASSOCIATION AND RECALL.

Hebbian Learning

According to Hebb's neurophysiological postulate for learning, information presented to a neural network is physically embedded through an alteration of the network structure: "When an axon of cell A is near enough to excite cell B and *repeatedly* or *persistently* takes part in firing it, some growth process or metabolic change takes place in one or both cells such that A's efficiency, as one of the cells firing B is increased." (Hebb, 1949; see also HEBBIAN SYNAPTIC PLASTICITY). How should this postulate be implemented in a formal neural network with transmission delays?

Let us focus on a connection with delay τ between neurons j and i. According to Hebb's postulate, the corresponding synaptic strength $J_{ij}(\tau)$ should be increased if cell j takes part in *firing* cell i. (In its physiological context, the postulate was formulated for excitatory synapses only, but for simplicity, it will be applied to all model synapses.) Due to the delay τ and the parallel dynamics, it takes $\tau + 1$ time steps until neuron j actually influences the *state* S_i of neuron i: τ time steps for the signal propagation (Equation 1) and one further time step to determine the cell's new firing state given the postsynaptic potential (Equation 2). Following Hebb's rule, $J_{ij}(\tau)$ should therefore be altered at time $t + 1$ by some function of $S_j(t - \tau)$ and $S_i(t + 1)$—most simply by their product. Note that for more general neural dynamics, the term $S_i(t + 1)$ has to be replaced by a properly time-shifted short-term average of the postsynaptic activity. It is worthwhile to compare this theoretical result with recent experimental findings concerning the temporal requirements for synaptic plasticity (Bi and Poo, 1998).

Starting with a *tabula rasa*, $J_{ij}(\tau) = 0$, one obtains after P learning sessions, labeled by μ and each of duration D_μ,

$$J_{ij}(\tau) = \varepsilon(\tau) N^{-1} \sum_{\mu=1}^{P} \sum_{t_\mu=1}^{D_\mu} S_i(t_\mu + 1) S_j(t_\mu - \tau) \equiv \varepsilon(\tau) \tilde{J}_{ij}(\tau) \quad (4)$$

The parameters $\varepsilon(\tau)$ model morphological characteristics of the delay lines; N^{-1} is a scaling factor useful for the theoretical analysis. By Equation 4, synapses act as microscopic feature detectors during the learning sessions: they measure and store correlations of the taught sequences in both space (i, j) and time (τ). This leads to a resonance phenomenon: connections with delays that approximately match the time course of the external input receive maximum strength. Note that these connections are also the ones that would support a stable sequence of the same duration. Thus, due to a subtle interplay between external stimulus and internal architecture (distribution of τs), the Hebb rule (Equation 4), which *prima facie* appears to be instructive in character, exhibits in fact also pronounced selective aspects.

Encoded in a network with a *broad* distribution of transmission delays, an external stimulus enjoys a rather multifaceted representation. According to Equation 4, synaptic couplings with delays that are short compared to the typical time scale of single patterns within the taught sequence are almost symmetric in the sense that $J_{ij}(\tau) \approx J_{ji}(\tau)$. They encode the individual patterns of the sequence as *unrelated static objects*. On the other hand, synapses with transmission delays that approximately match the duration of single patterns of the sequence are able to detect the transitions between patterns. The corresponding synaptic efficacies are asymmetric and establish various temporal relations between the patterns, thereby representing the complete sequence as *one dynamic object*.

Once the learning sessions are over the $J_{ij}(\tau)$ are kept fixed. The retrieval process (Equations 1–3), operating with the very same delays as the synaptic dynamics (Equation 4), is then able to extract the spatiotemporal information encoded in the $J_{ij}(\tau)$. Retrieval is therefore extremely robust as shown in numerous simulations (Herz et al., 1989).

It should be noted that the above mechanism requires delay times that are of the same order as the duration of *single* quasi-static elements of a temporal sequence. The length of the *entire* sequence, however, remains unconstrained. A number of authors have discussed the interplay between neural and synaptic dynamics and, in particular, the role of transmission delays (e.g. Hebb, 1949, and Caianiello, 1961). However, the full consequences, discussed in the present article, have only been explored recently.

Global Analysis

Equations 1–4 describe a "double dynamics" where both neurons and synapses change in time. In general, such a scenario cannot be analyzed mathematically if teaching is performed in a "clamped" fashion where the system evolves according to the external stimuli, $S_i(t_\mu) = \sigma_i(t_\mu - 1)$, so that the synapses measure the true correlations of external stimuli without any interference by the internal dynamics. Clamped learning is achieved by setting $T = 0$ in (3) and $\gamma = 1$ in Equation 1 during learning sessions. Numerical experiments demonstrate that this condition can be relaxed without significant changes in the emergent network behavior.

One may derive approximate equations of motion for the macroscopic network dynamics (for a detailed discussion see Kühn and van Hemmen, 1991). These equations are nonlinear due to the nonlinear signal processing of single neurons (Equations 2 and 3) and contain previous activities due to the memory effects modeled by Equation 1. The solutions agree well with numerical simulations, but an exact analysis is in general not possible.

The mathematics become tractable in the special case where all input sequences $\sigma_i(t_\mu)$ are cyclic with equal periods $D_\mu = D$. If one defines patterns $\xi_{ia}^{\mu 0}$ by $\xi_{ia}^{\mu 0} \equiv \sigma_i(t_\mu = a)$ for $0 \le a < D$, one obtains

$$\tilde{J}_{ij}(\tau) = N^{-1} \sum_{\mu=1}^{P} \sum_{a=0}^{D-1} \xi_{i,a+1}^{\mu 0} \xi_{j,a-\tau}^{\mu 0} \qquad (5)$$

Note that the synaptic strengths are in general still asymmetric in the sense that $\tilde{J}_{ij}(\tau) \ne \tilde{J}_{ji}(\tau)$. They do, however, obey the symmetry $\tilde{J}_{ij}(\tau) = \tilde{J}_{ji}(D - (2 + \tau))$ for $\tau < D - 1$ and $\tilde{J}_{ij}(D - 1) = \tilde{J}_{ji}(D - 1)$. For all networks whose *a priori* weights $\varepsilon(\tau)$ satisfy $\varepsilon(\tau) = \varepsilon(D - (2 + \tau))$ for $\tau < D - 1$ one has thus found an "extended synaptic symmetry,"

$$J_{ij}(\tau) = J_{ji}((D - (2 + \tau))(\text{modulo } D)) \qquad (6)$$

generalizing the symmetry assumption $J_{ij} = J_{ji}$ of Hopfield Networks in a natural way to the temporal domain. The symmetry (Equation 6) suggests that one may be able to find a Lyapunov (or "energy") function for the noiseless retrieval dynamics (Equation 2) (see ENERGY FUNCTIONALS FOR NEURAL NETWORKS). This is indeed the case if $\varepsilon(D - 1) = 0$ (Herz, Li, and van Hemmen, 1991). One takes $\gamma = 0$ in Equation 1 and defines

$$H(t) \equiv -\frac{1}{2} \sum_{i,j=1}^{N} \sum_{a,\tau=0}^{D-1} J_{ij}(\tau) S_i(t - a)$$
$$\times S_j(t - (a + \tau + 1)(\text{modulo } D)) \qquad (7)$$

By Equation 1, Equation 2, and Equation 6 the difference $\Delta H(t) \equiv H(t) - H(t - 1)$ is

$$\Delta H(t) = -\sum_{i=1}^{N} [S_i(t) - S_i(t - D)]h_i(t - 1) \qquad (8)$$

As a finite sum of finite terms, H is bounded. $H(t)$ is nonincreasing because the right-hand side of Equation 8 is nonpositive: the term $S_i(t)h_i(t - 1)$ equals $|h_i(t - 1)|$ due to the dynamics (Equation 2) and is therefore larger than or at least equal to the product $S_i(t - D)h_i(t - 1)$, which is $\pm h_i(t - 1)$. Consequently, $\Delta H(t)$ has to vanish as $t \to \infty$. This is only possible if the system settles into a state with $S_i(t) = S_i(t - D)$ for all i.

The analysis has exposed two important facts: (1) the retrieval process of certain delay networks is governed by a Lyapunov function. The time evolution during retrieval sessions can thus be understood as a downhill march in an abstract energy landscape. (2) The networks relax to a static state or a limit cycle with $S_i(t) = S_i(t - D)$—oscillatory solutions with the *same* period as that of the taught cycles or a period which is equal to an integer fraction of D.

Stepping back for an overview, one notices that H is a Lyapunov function for all networks that exhibit an "extended synaptic symmetry" (Equation 6) and for which the matrix $\mathbf{J}(D - 1)$ vanishes. The Hebbian synapses (Equation 4) are one important special case and will be the main subject of the further discussion.

Statistical Mechanics

The last section shows that certain delay networks relax to fixed points or oscillatory solutions with well-determined periods. Are there limit cycles that resemble the taught sequences? How many sequences can be stored in a given network?

The answers are obtained in a two-step process. First, it is demonstrated that networks with cyclic temporal associations and deterministic dynamics can be mapped onto symmetric Hopfield-like systems without delays. In a second step, one shows that this correspondence holds for the stochastic Glauber dynamics (Equation 3) as well. One may then apply equilibrium statistical mechanics to derive quantitative results. A detailed discussion of the technical issues involved can be found in (Herz et al., 1991). Let me briefly sketch the main ideas.

D-periodic oscillatory solutions of the retrieval dynamics can be interpreted as static states in a fictitious "D-plicated" system with N rows and D columns of cells with activities S_{ia} where $1 \le i \le N$ and $0 \le a < D$. The parallel dynamics of the original system are reproduced by the update rule

$$S_{ia}(t + 1) = \begin{cases} \text{sign}\left[\sum_{j=1}^{N} \sum_{b=0}^{D-1} J_{ij}^{ab} S_{jb}(t)\right] & \text{if } a = t \, (\text{modulo } D) \\ S_{ia}(t) & \text{otherwise} \end{cases} \qquad (9)$$

In terms of the original synaptic efficacies $J_{ij}(\tau)$, the couplings J_{ij}^{ab} are given by $J_{ij}^{ab} = J_{ij}((b - a - 1) \, (\text{modulo } D))$. Due to Equation 6, they are symmetric, that is, $J_{ij}^{ab} = J_{ji}^{ba}$.

The time evolution of the new network has a pseudo-sequential characteristic: synchronous within single columns and sequentially ordered with respect to these columns. The interpretation of the retrieval process is changed significantly: a *limit cycle* of period D in the original network corresponds to a *fixed-point* of the new system of size ND. Storing one cycle $\sigma_i(t_\mu) = \xi_{ia}^{\mu 0}$ in the delay network thus corresponds to memorizing D shifted duplicates $\xi_{ia}^{\mu v}$, $0 \le v < D$, in the equivalent system. This reflects the fact that a cycle with period D can be retrieved in D different time-shifted versions in the original network.

Let me now turn to quantitative results. They were obtained within a replica-symmetric theory (see STATISTICAL MECHANICS OF NEURAL NETWORKS) for the case where each of the P learning sessions corresponds to teaching a (different) cycle of D unbiased random patterns $\xi_{ia}^{\mu 0}$, each lasting for one time step.

The retrieval quality for a given cycle μ is best described in terms of the generalized "overlap" $m^\mu = \max_\nu \{N^{-1}D^{-1}\Sigma_{i,a}\xi_{ia}^{\mu\nu}S_{ia}\}$: this order parameter equals one for perfect recall and zero if the network state is uncorrelated with the μth cycle. Retrieval is possible as long as the network dynamics admit solutions with one large m^μ. Due to interference between different memories, this is only possible if the number P of stored sequences remains below a critical number P_c. The analysis shows that P_c scales linearly with N for large N, $P_c = \alpha_c N$. The factor α_c is called the storage capacity of the network. As in the Hopfield model, the retrieval quality m^μ drops suddenly as P is increased beyond $\alpha_c N$—a first-order phase transition (see COOPERATIVE PHENOMENA and STATISTICAL MECHANICS OF NEURAL NETWORKS).

It should be noted that each cycle consists of D patterns so that the storage capacity for *single* patterns is $\bar{\alpha}_c = D\alpha_c$. During the recognition process, however, each of them will trigger the cycle it belongs to and cannot be retrieved as a static pattern. For systems with a delay distribution that vanishes for $\tau = D - 1$ and is uniform for $\tau < D - 1$, that is, $\varepsilon(\tau) = (D - 1)^{-1}(1 - \delta_{\tau,D-1})$, one obtains

$$
\begin{array}{cccccc}
D & 2 & 3 & 4 & 5 & \infty \\
\alpha_c & 0.100 & 0.110 & 0.116 & 0.120 & 0.138
\end{array}
\tag{10}
$$

The findings agree well with estimates from numerical simulations. The results demonstrate that the storage capacity for temporal associations is comparable to that for static memories. As an example, take $D = 2$. In the limit of large N, $0.100 \cdot N$ two-cycles of the form $\xi_{i0}^{\mu 0} \rightleftarrows \xi_{i1}^{\mu 0}$ may be recalled as compared to $0.138 \cdot N$ static patterns (Amit, 1989); since $2 \times 1.00/1.38 \approx 1.45$, this amounts to a 1.45-fold increase of the information content per synapse.

The influence of the weight distribution on the network behavior is demonstrated by some choices of $\varepsilon(\tau)$ for $D = 4$:

$$
\begin{array}{ccccccc}
\tau = & 0 & 1 & 2 & 3 & \alpha_c & m_c \\
\varepsilon(\tau) = & 1/3 & 1/3 & 1/3 & 0 & 0.116 & 0.96 \\
\varepsilon(\tau) = & 1/2 & 0 & 1/2 & 0 & 0.100 & 0.93 \\
\varepsilon(\tau) = & 0 & 1 & 0 & 0 & 0.050 & 0.93
\end{array}
\tag{11}
$$

The storage capacity decreases with decreasing number of delay lines, but measured *per synapse*, it does increase. However, networks with only a few number of delays are less fault-tolerant as shown by numerical simulations.

Discussion

Learning schemes can only be successful if the structure of the learning task is compatible with both the network architecture and the learning algorithm. In the present context, the task is to store simple temporal associations. It can be accomplished in neural networks with a broad distribution of signal delays and Hebbian synapses which, during learning periods, operate as microscopic feature detectors for spatiotemporal correlations within the external stimuli. The retrieval process utilizes the very same delays and synapses, and is therefore rather robust.

Let me emphasize that the Hebbian mechanism discussed here does *not* limit the overall length of a pattern sequence stored in a neural network with transmission delays. It is the duration of a single pattern within a temporal association that is constrained and cannot exceed the time lags provided by transmission delays.

Quantitative results for the storage capacity and retrieval quality can be obtained for a certain class of delay networks using a global Lyapunov function and techniques from statistical mechanics. Unlike in the general case, the total length of a pattern sequence has to approximately match the maximum time lag to allow for the extended synaptic symmetry (Equation 6). The analytical findings prove that an extensive number of temporal associations can be stored as spatiotemporal attractors for the retrieval dynamics. Numerical simulations with pattern sequences that are long with respect to the available signal delays show a qualitatively similar picture. Both results indicate that dynamic systems with delayed interactions can be programmed in an efficient manner to perform associative computations in the space-time domain.

The approach sketched in this article has also been extended to neural networks with continuous units that store cycles of correlated real-valued pattern sequences (Herz, 1995). Numerical studies have been performed for low-dimensional trajectories (small N) with high numbers of data points (large D). For many examples, good retrieval could be obtained without any need for highly time-consuming supervised learning schemes. However, algorithms of the latter kind are eventually necessary to solve more sophisticated real-world associations. Here, once again, the existence of Lyapunov functions is of great help since it allows for the application of powerful techniques from STATISTICAL MECHANICS OF ON-LINE LEARNING AND GENERALIZATION (q.v.) to a wide class of supervised learning strategies such as spatiotemporal extensions of the Boltzmann Machine (see SIMULATED ANNEALING AND BOLTZMANN MACHINES).

Delays add a new dimension—time—to *any* learning mechanism based on correlation measurements of pre- and postsynaptic events. This extra dimension naturally extends the structure of objects representable in the synaptic code generated by such a learning mechanism, thereby considerably increasing its potential power. Transmission delays do therefore not induce a loss of the associative capabilities of neural networks as one might have feared. On the contrary, if properly included in the learning process, they provide a physical structure to perform spatiotemporal computations at low architectural cost. Nature may have opted to make constructive use of them, as is also indicated by the success of more elaborate models with delayed interactions (see, for example, Gerstner et al., 1996).

Road Map: Learning in Artificial Networks
Related Reading: Dynamics of Association and Recall; Sequence Learning; Statistical Mechanics of Neural Networks; Temporal Integration in Recurrent Microcircuits; Temporal Pattern Processing

References

Amit, D. J., 1989, *Modeling Brain Function—The World of Attractor Neural Networks*, Cambridge, UK: Cambridge University Press. ◆

Bi, G. Q., and Poo, M. M., 1998, Synaptic modifications in cultured hippocampal neurons: Dependence on spike timing, synaptic strength, and postsynaptic cell type, *J. Neurosci.*, 18:10464–10472.

Caianiello, E., 1961, Outline of a theory of thought processes and thinking machines, *J. Theor. Biol.*, 1:204–235.

Coolen, A. C. C., and Gielen, C. C. A. M., 1988, Delays in neural networks, *Europh. Lett.*, 7:281–285.

Hebb, D. O., 1949, *The Organization of Behavior*, New York: Wiley.

Gerstner, W., Kempter, R., van Hemmen, J. L., and Wagner, H., 1996, A neuronal learning rule for sub-millisecond temporal coding, *Nature*, 386:76–78.

Hertz, J., Krogh, A., and Palmer, R. G., 1991, *Introduction to the Theory of Neural Computation*, Redwood City, CA: Addison-Wesley. ◆

Herz, A. V. M., 1995, Global analysis of recurrent neural networks, in *Models of Neural Networks* (E. Domany, J. L. van Hemmen, and K. Schulten, Eds.), Berlin: Springer.

Herz, A. V. M., 2002, How is time represented in the brain? in *Problems in Systems Neuroscience* (J. L. van Hemmen and T. J. Sejnowski, Eds.), Cambridge, UK: Cambridge University Press.

Herz, A. V. M., Li, Z., and van Hemmen, J. L., 1991, Statistical mechanics of temporal association in neural networks with transmission delays, *Phys. Rev. Lett.*, 66:1370–1373.

Herz, A. V. M., Sulzer, B., Kühn, R., and van Hemmen, J. L., 1989, Hebbian learning reconsidered: Representation of static and dynamic objects in associative neural nets, *Biol. Cybern.*, 60:457–467.

Kleinfeld, D., 1986, Sequential state generation by model neural networks, *Proc. Natl. Acad. Sci. USA*, 83:9469–9473.

Kühn, R., and van Hemmen, J. L., 1991, Temporal association, in *Models of Neural Networks* (E. Domany, J. L. van Hemmen, and K. Schulten, Eds.), Berlin: Springer. ◆

Sompolinsky, H., and Kanter, I., 1986, Temporal association in asymmetric neural networks, *Phys. Rev. Lett.*, 57:2861–2864.

Tank, D., and Hopfield, J. J., 1987, Neural computation by concentrating information in time, *Proc. Natl. Acad. Sci. USA*, 84:1896–1900.

Tensor Voting and Visual Segmentation

Chi-Keung Tang and Gérard Medioni

Introduction

In computer vision, we often face the problem of identifying salient and structured information in a noisy data set. In three-dimensional (3D) data sets, constructed from binocular images, surfaces are inferred by obtaining depth hypotheses for points and/or edges using local correlation measures, and then selecting and interpolating appropriate values for all points in the images. In image sequence analysis, the estimation of motion and shape starts with local measurements of feature correspondences, which yields noisy data for the subsequence computation of scene information. Hence, any salient structure estimator must be able to handle the presence of multiple structures and their interaction in the presence of noisy data.

In this article, we analyze representative approaches to early to midlevel vision problems and present our *tensor voting* method for the robust inference of multiple salient structures such as junctions, curves, regions, and surfaces from any combination of point, curve element, and surface patch element inputs in 2D and 3D.

The problem formulation dominates the design of any algorithms, and computer vision is no exception. We can roughly classify major approaches found in computer vision literature into the following five categories, which may not be mutually exclusive:

- *Artificial neural network*—Inspired by biological visual systems, the artificial neural network (ANN) approach devises solutions that mimic operations found in biological neural systems.
- *Regularization*—Because early vision problems are ill-posed inverse problems, extra constraints are introduced to limit the search space of the solution.
- *Consistent labeling*—Computer vision problems are cast as a problem of finding the set of consistent labels for all the image pixels.
- *Statistical methods*—Vision problems are formulated as clustering or parametric model fitting in order to infer relevant visual information.
- *Perceptual saliency approach*—Salient properties emerge from the input data and are detected by a non-maximal-suppression process.

Artificial Neural Network

In the ANN approach, it is suggested that vision problems might be solved computationally if biological vision structures discovered by neurologists can be simulated. An ANN is characterized by a large number of weighted connections among a large number of very simple processing elements. One emphasis is to learn the weighting and internal structure, in either a supervised or an unsupervised way. The absence of explicit models, however, makes the assessment somewhat difficult.

The work by Grossberg and Mingolla (1987) describes a theory and a implementation of surface perception based on the neural network approach. It consists of two interacting systems, the boundary contour system and the feature contour system. Excellent results are obtained on some examples. The use of scalar values can be a limitation.

Regularization

Because of the projective nature of imaging, a single image can correspond to different scene configurations. Because of this ambiguity in image formation, the inverse problem, namely, the inference of structures from images, is ill posed. Below we describe two regularization formalisms. *Regularization theories* entail imposing certain physical constraints, so that the search space can be constrained and algorithmically tractable. *Stochastic regularization* uses a Bayesian formalism to transform the ill-posed problem into one of functional optimization.

Regularization Theory

The underlying spirit of regularization theory is to restrict the solution space by choosing the function that minimizes an appropriate function. For solving the ill-posed problem of finding x from data y, where $y = F(x)$, regularization theories provide the mathematical foundation for choosing the norms and a stabilizing function that characterizes the global constraints of the problem.

In the case of early vision, the problem is transformed into the nonlinear, scalar functional optimization framework, which can then be solved using standard numerical techniques, namely the calculus of variations (Terzopoulos, 1986).

Stochastic Regularization

A Bayesian formalism can also be used to transform ill-posed inverse problem into the functional optimization framework. In Bayesian terms, the task can be described as the maximization problem of a posterior probability density function.

Other modeling approaches, such as minimum description language (Leclerc, 1989), are allowed in describing the model constraints. Various stochastic or probabilistic optimization methods such as simulated annealing (Kirkpatrick, Gelatt, and Vecchi, 1983), genetic algorithm, or evolutionary strategy (Koza, 1992), or the Expectation-Maximization (EM) algorithm are also employed in the search for a solution.

Level Set Approach

Recently, a new implicit representation has been proposed under the name of level set method (Zhao et al., 1988). The main idea is to describe a curve (or a surface) as the zero-level set of a higher-dimension function Φ. Then, instead of evolving the curve, we consider the evolution of the function Φ, and extract the zero levels. This method permits topological changes to be made easily and has proved to be a powerful tool for many applications in physics, geometry, and computer vision (see Sethian, 1996, for a review).

Some interesting results have been reported that also reveal some limitations to this approach. First, the method is based on the computation of a distance function, which may be inaccurate if a large amount of noise is present. It may be difficult to distinguish whether points are relevant or not for the reconstruction.

More generally, concerning the level set formulation itself, even if we do not have any parameters, we are still restricted to consider special shapes. In the 3D case, the formulation can only recover surfaces, not curves. As for the geometrical properties, curves or surfaces can only be enclosed sets, and we cannot represent multiple junctions. Note that in this last problem, solutions have been derived for multiphase problems (Zhao et al., 1988) involving several Φ functions, but the knowledge that such a junction exists must be available beforehand.

In conclusion, level sets (or other implicit representations) rely on shape hypotheses and have a number of inherent limitations. Also, they are representations, and not descriptions, as they do not make explicit edges, crossings, or singularities. This information has to be inferred at a postprocessing stage.

Clustering and Robust Methods

Another major formulation approach is to cast vision problems as a problem in data analysis or classification. *Clustering* methods employ the statistical approach to infer compact groups of points in multidimensional space. *Robust techniques* employ data analysis formalism to perform parametric model fitting.

Consistent Labeling

As pointed out in Medioni, Lee, and Tang (2000), the major issues in computer vision are to infer salient smooth features, detect discontinuities, and identify outliers. Since these roles are mutually exclusive, it seems reasonable to pose early vision problems as problems in *consistent labeling*. A labeling problem is defined by a set of objects, a set of possible labels for each object, a neighbor relation over the objects, and a compatibility relation over labels as *n*-tuples of neighboring objects.

The goal is to assign labels to each object that respect the compatibility relationship. A labeling problem can be formulated as a *relaxation* operation because its formulation is similar to that of a system of linear equations. Three main types of relaxation methods exist: *discrete relaxation labeling, continuous relaxation labeling,* and *stochastic relaxation labeling.*

Discrete relaxation labeling. The labeling problem can be described as one of assigning labels to nodes in the graph defined above. *Discrete relaxation labeling* is an algorithmic approach to tackling this graph-labeling problem. The constraints are required to be expressed by logical assertions. The relaxation is governed by the label-discarding rule: discard a label at a node if there exists a neighbor such that every label currently assigned to the neighbor is incompatible with the label. The discrete relaxation labeling process is defined by the iterative application of the label-discarding rule, applied in parallel at each node, until limiting label sets are obtained.

Continuous relaxation labeling. Continuous relaxation labeling attempts to allow greater flexibility in the constraints by replacing the logical assertions about compatibilities with weighted values representing relative preferences. In addition, by allowing weights to be used for label assignment, the labeling problem is transformed into the functional optimization framework, which can then be solved by numerical relaxation techniques. Because of the mathematical context in which continuous relaxation labeling has come to exist, a number of attempts have been made to develop an underlying theory for the process. We refer readers to articles by Faugeras and Berthod discussed in Faugeras (1993) and Hummel and Zucker (1983) for two different formulations of the continuous relaxation labeling process.

Stochastic relaxation labeling. Stochastic relaxation labeling is similar to continuous relaxation labeling except that the labeling weights and the constraint preferences weights are replaced by probability distributions. Stochastic relaxation labeling makes use of a model of physical phenomena known as Markov random field (MRF) modeling (see Geman and Geman, 1984, for a definition of MRF in the context of computer vision). The MRF model is often combined with the Bayesian estimation technique known as maximum a posteriori (MAP) estimation, forming an MRF-MAP framework for solving computer vision problems. The MRF-MAP approach also requires solving an energy minimization problem. Typically, one uses a global minimum–seeking algorithm such as simulated annealing (Kirkpatrick et al., 1983), evolutionary algorithms (Koza, 1992), or the EM algorithm to minimize the energy functions, which are often nonconvex.

Properties of Consistent Labeling

Regardless of the formulation of the problem, all solutions for consistent labeling entail the intrinsically iterative process of relaxation. As for all iterative processes, the main issues in defining a relaxation process are initialization, updating, and stopping condition. The different formulations just provide different justifications for setting the functions and parameters. Nevertheless, the labeling framework makes it relatively easy to incorporate terms to account for discontinuities.

Clustering

The common use of clustering in solving early vision problems is to create a partition of points such that points in each cluster share similar properties. Partitional clustering methods can be divided into error-square clustering, density estimation clustering, and clustering by graph theory.

Error-square clustering minimizes the squared error for a fixed number of clusters. Density estimation clustering make use of histograms to find clusters. Clustering by graph theory uses geometric structures such as the minimum spanning tree, relative neighborhood graph, and mutual nearest neighborhood to obtain the desired partitions. Methods that use these geometric structures construct the graph first, then remove inconsistent edges of the graph. Inconsistent edges and their elimination are specified for each method. Recently, Shi and Malik (1998) devised a clustering by graph technique called normalized cuts and applied it to image segmentation, motion segmentation, and tracking.

Most of the clustering techniques are iterative and sensitive to the a priori choice of the number of clusters in the feature space. If this choice is poor, the final partition of the space may be incorrect as well. This sensitivity is an important limitation in computer vision, where the number of significant feature properties is rarely known a priori.

Robust Techniques

Another aspect of data analysis is to robustly recover the parameters of a given model from noisy observations.

There are essentially two major issues that needed to be addressed: parameter estimation and inlier/outlier identification (data error correction). Robust estimators often make use of the algebraic properties of the carrier functions and the constraint equation to handle parameter estimation, and apply statistical tools to tackle data error correction. Although techniques such as the Hough transform can be very robust to noise, the parametric formalism of these techniques make it hard to deliver the same robustness in solving early vision problems. In computer vision, usually the models employed are only approximations, and that real data can only be represented by multiple models. Worst, the outliers are often structured, and they obey the same model with a different parameter.

Perceptual Saliency Approach

In 1988, Sha'ashua and Ullman suggested use of a *saliency map* to guide the perceptual grouping process. A saliency map, derived from the input 2D image, is a dense map in which the value of each pixel corresponds to the degree of "perceptual importance," such as smoothness, length, and constancy of curvature. Their method uses an incremental optimization scheme to avoid the exponential complexity involved in picking subsets from a large set of data. A local operator chooses the *optimal continuation* from a given segment. However, this method cannot handle large gaps, and can be fooled by erroneous segments along a correct curve. Moreover, the method is iterative, running on a locally connected network.

Recently, Medioni et al. (2000) combined the representational power of a tensor (introduced by Knutsson, 1989, in the context of signal processing for computer vision) and the computational efficiency of linear voting for salient structure inference. The result is a unified framework for dealing with various input types that retains all the desirable properties of vector voting. The novelty of this approach is that tensor voting avoids searching through the solution space, by formulating the computation as a voting process. Although deriving the best scene description is an optimization problem, the *optimal solution* emerges from the data set.

Unlike regularization and labeling approaches, this formulation avoids all the inherent problems in iterative optimization: no initialization is needed. Thus the choice of size and search direction for each iteration is no longer an issue. The method is noniterative, parameter-free, depends on no critical thresholds, and allows any number of objects in the scene, each of any genus. The only free parameter is the scale of analysis. Also, tensor voting does not need to estimate a large number of parameters, which is common in other statistical approaches. Tensor voting uses dense voting fields, whose designs are based on the good continuity constraint (one of the *Gestalt* principles). When compared with the absence of explicit models in the ANN approach, the analysis of tensor voting is more approachable.

Tensor Voting

We use *tensor* for data representation and *voting* for data communication. A point in the 3D space can assume one of the following configurations: a surface patch, a discontinuity, or an outlier. A point on a smooth surface is very certain about its surface normal orientation (or stick tensor), whereas a point at a junction where surfaces intersect has absolute orientation uncertainty (indicated by a ball tensor). A second-order symmetric tensor in 3D is used to represent this continuum. This tensor representation can be visualized as an ellipsoid.

Overview of the Salient Structure Inference Engine

Figure 1 shows the overall approach in this methodology. Each input token is first encoded as a second-order symmetric tensor.

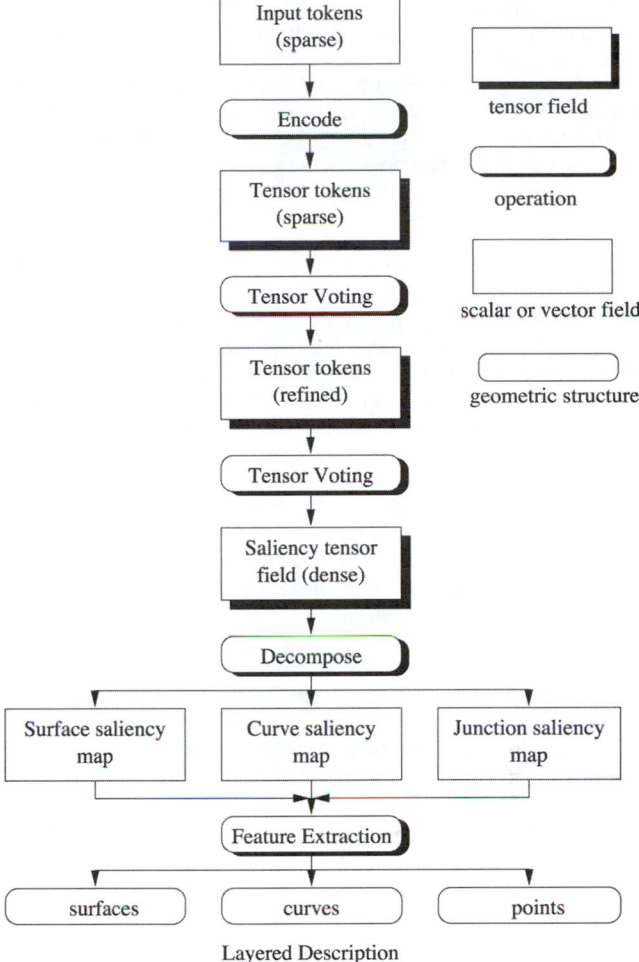

Figure 1. Overview of the essential components of tensor voting.

For instance, if the input token has only position information, it is transformed into an isotropic tensor (a ball) of unit radius.

In the first voting stage, tokens communicate their information to each other in a neighborhood, and refine the information they carry. After this process, each token is now a generic second-order symmetric tensor that encodes confidence of this knowledge (given by the tensor size) and curve and surface orientation information (given by the tensor orientations).

In the second stage, these generic tensor tokens propagate their information in their neighborhood, leading to a dense tensor map that encodes feature saliency at every point in the domain. In practice, the domain space is digitized into a uniform array of cells. In each cell the tensor can be decomposed into elementary components that express different aspects of the information captured.

The resulting dense tensor map is then decomposed. Surface, curve, and junction features are then obtained by extracting, with subvoxel precision, local extrema of the corresponding saliency values along a direction. The final output is the aggregate of the outputs for each of the components.

Tensor Representation

The goal is to extract geometrical features such as regions, curves, surfaces, and the intersections between them. We will first summarize the various differential properties of these entities and their behavior at singularities. Then we discuss using tensors as a representation scheme.

Points can be represented by their coordinates. For curve inference, a first-order local description of a curve is given by the point coordinates and its associated tangent. A second-order description would also include the associated curvature.

For surface inference, a first-order local description of a surface patch is given by the point coordinates and its associated normal information. A second-order description would also include the principal curvatures and their directions.

However, we do not know in advance what type of entity—point, curve, or surface—a token may belong to. Furthermore, singularities occur when these entities intersect each other. For example, when two smooth surfaces intersect, there is no associated normal information at the point of intersection. However, if we consider a small finite neighborhood around a curve junction, it has an associated tangent corresponding to the intersection curves.

Second order symmetric tensor.   To capture first-order differential geometry information and its singularities, a second-order symmetric tensor is proposed that captures both the information and its confidence, or *saliency*. Such a tensor can be visualized as an ellipse in 2D or as an ellipsoid in 3D.

Intuitively, the shape of the tensor defines the type of information captured (point, curve, or surface element), and the associated size represents the saliency. For instance, in 2D, a very salient curve element is represented by a thin ellipse whose major axis represents the estimated tangent direction and whose length reflects the saliency of the estimation. Therefore, it encapsulates both orientation and certainty information at the same time.

In 3D, the second-order symmetric tensor is an ellipsoid that is fully described by its associated eigensystem, with three eigenvectors $\hat{e}_1$, $\hat{e}_2$, and $\hat{e}_3$ and the three corresponding eigenvalues $\lambda_1 \geq \lambda_2 \geq \lambda_3 \geq 0$.

Rearranging the eigensystem, the 3D ellipsoid is given by $(\lambda_1 - \lambda_2)\mathbf{S} + (\lambda_2 - \lambda_3)\mathbf{P} + \lambda_3\mathbf{B}$, $\mathbf{S} = \hat{e}_1\hat{e}_1^T$, $\mathbf{P} = \hat{e}_1\hat{e}_1^T + \hat{e}_2\hat{e}_2^T$, and $\mathbf{B} = \hat{e}_1\hat{e}_1^T + \hat{e}_2\hat{e}_2^T + \hat{e}_3\hat{e}_3^T$, where $\mathbf{S}$ defines a *stick tensor*, $\mathbf{P}$ defines a *plate tensor*, and $\mathbf{B}$ defines a *ball tensor*.

These tensors define the three basis tensors for any general 3D ellipsoid. A linear combination of these basis tensors defines any second-order symmetric tensor.

Tensor Decomposition

The *eigenvectors* encode *orientation (un)certainties*. Surface orientation (normal) is described by the stick tensor, which indicates certainty along a single direction. *Orientation uncertainty* is abstracted by two other tensors. *Curve* junction results from two intersecting surfaces, where the uncertainty in orientation only spans a single plane perpendicular to the tangent of the junction curve, and thus is described by a plate tensor. At *point* junctions, where more than two intersecting surfaces are present, a ball tensor is used, since all orientations are equally probable.

The *eigenvalues*, on the other hand, effectively encode the *magnitude* of orientation (un)certainties, since they indicate the size of the corresponding 3D ellipsoid.

Therefore, we can decompose a tensor token into the following 2-tuples $(s, \hat{v})$, where s is a scalar indicating feature saliency and $\hat{v}$ is a unit vector indicating direction:

- *Surfaceness*: $s = \lambda_1 - \lambda_2$, and $\hat{v} = \hat{e}_1$ indicates the normal direction.
- *Curveness*: $s = \lambda_2 - \lambda_3$, and $\hat{v} = \hat{e}_3$ indicates the tangent direction.
- *Junctionness*: $s = \lambda_3$, $\hat{v}$ is arbitrary.

Token Refinement and Dense Extrapolation

We now turn to our communication and computation scheme, which allows a site to exchange information with its neighbors and infer new information. The input tokens are first encoded as tensors. These initial tensors communicate with each other in order to (1) derive the most preferred orientation information, or refine the initial orientation if given, for each of the input tokens (token refinement); and (2) extrapolate the inferred information at every location in the domain for the purpose of subsequent coherent feature extraction (dense extrapolation).

These two tasks can be implemented by a *voting* process, which involves having each input token aligned with predefined, dense *voting kernels* (or voting fields). This alignment is simply a translation followed by rotation. The dense voting kernels encode the basis tensors (i.e., stick, plate, and ball tensors in the 3D case). This voting process is similar to a convolution, except that the output of this process is a tensor (instead of a scalar).

In the token refinement case, each token collects all the tensor values cast at its location by all the other tokens. The resulting tensor value is the tensor sum of all the tensor votes cast at the token location.

In the dense extrapolation case, each token is first decomposed into its independent elements. By using an appropriate voting kernel, each token broadcasts the information in a neighborhood. The size of the neighborhood is given by the size of the voting kernel used. As a result, a tensor value is put at every location in the neighborhood.

While they may be implemented differently for efficiency, these two operations are equivalent, which can be regarded as tensor convolution.

Results

In this section, we describe inference of junctions, curves, and surfaces from noisy and sparse data in 2D and 3D. Applications of

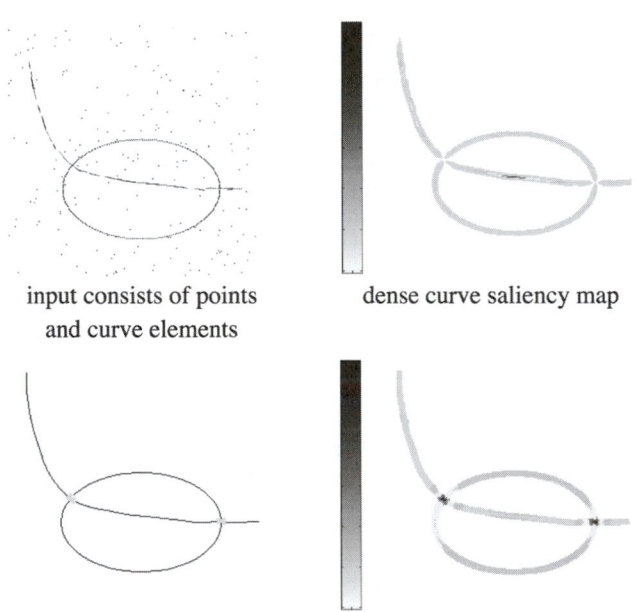

input consists of points and curve elements

dense curve saliency map

extracted curves and junctions

dense junction saliency map

Figure 2. Curve and junction inference from mixed input. The gray levels indicate *curveness* (top) and *junctionness* (bottom). Dark gray indicates a higher value.

Figure 3. Surface and junctions inferred from noisy data sets. *A* and *B* are results on two noisy data sets, the curves and surfaces extracted automatically by tensor voting. (Data courtesy of USC dental school.)

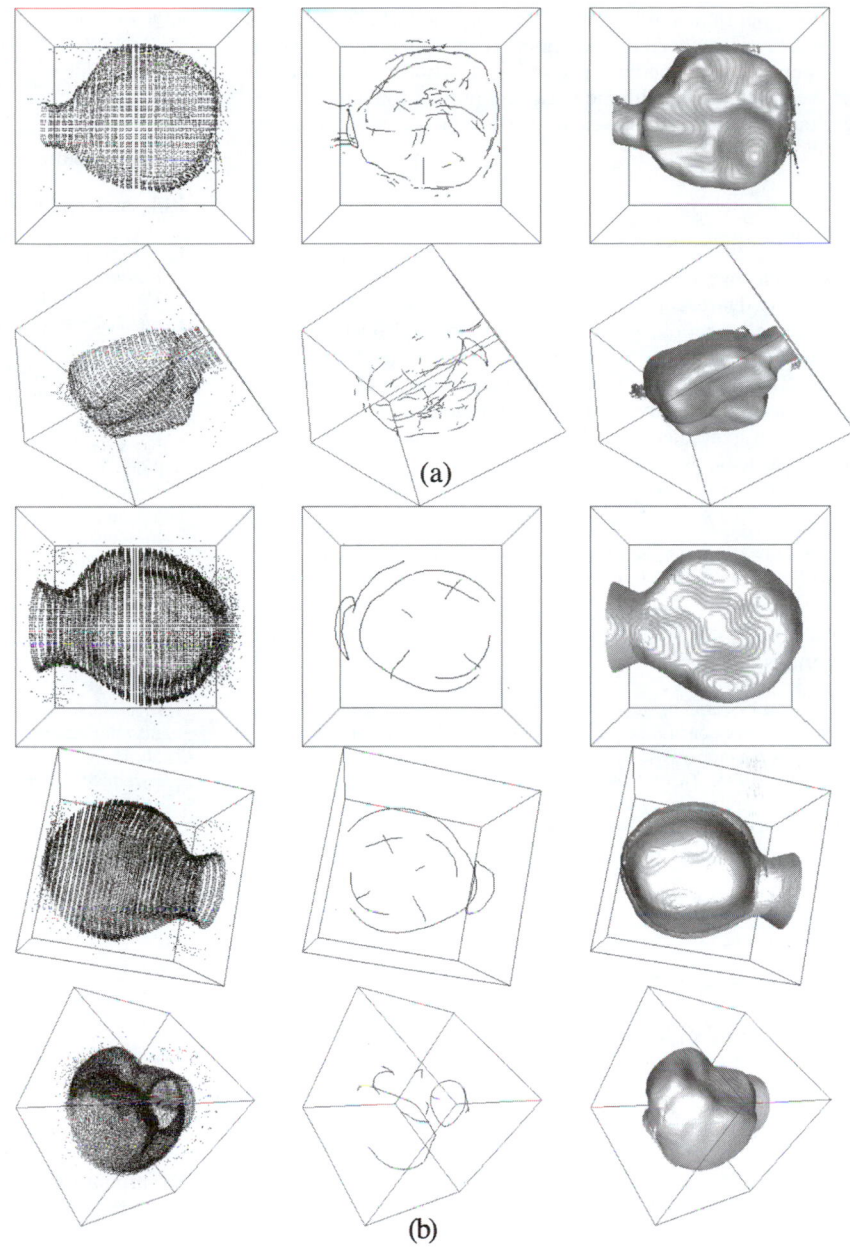

(a)

(b)

tensor voting to midlevel computer vision problems, such as stereo and motion, can be found in Medioni et al. (2000).

2D

In 2D, the second-order symmetric tensor is an ellipse, described by the eigensystem $\lambda_1 \geq \lambda_2$ with corresponding eigenvectors $\hat{e}_1$, $\hat{e}_2$. We have only curveness and junctionness. Also, the number of voting fields is reduced to two: the stick and ball voting fields.

We consider that the input consists of both oriented and nonoriented data as the general case. We first apply tensor voting. Oriented tokens vote with the stick voting field, and nonoriented tokens vote with a ball voting field. Only locations where tokens are present receive votes. A second round of voting is then performed in which we discard the ball component of the tensor. A dense tensor map is produced, which is then decomposed into a junction map and a curve map. Figure 2 shows an example of curve and junction inference from a mixed input consisting of an ellipse made up of curve elements and a curve made up of dots.

Even more generically, we can process input in which the tokens are already in tensor form, simply by decomposing the tokens into ball and stick components and having them vote initially with the corresponding ball and stick fields, only at token locations. The second voting pass is identical.

3D

Figure 3 shows the data (courtesy of USC dental school) and inferred features. The input points are first encoded into perfect balls. The ball voting field is placed at each point, propagating ball votes in each neighborhood. After the preliminary step of ball field voting, a tensor is produced at each point. The stick components (or $\hat{e}_1$) of these tensors denote the normal direction. These inferred sticks then vote again, with the stick voting field for surface inference, exactly as in the basic case for surface inference from surface elements.

Discussion

In this article, we compared representative approaches to visual segmentation. These approaches can be classified as artificial neural network, regularization, consistent labeling, statistical methods, and perceptual grouping. Tensor voting can be placed in the last category. Tensor voting makes use of tensors for data representation and a voting procedure for data communication. Unlike other approaches, it is noniterative, does not have genus limitation, and has only one scale as parameter.

Road Map: Vision
Related Reading: Motion Perception: Navigation; Probabilistic Regularization Methods for Low-Level Vision; Stereo Correspondence

References

Blake, A., and Zisserman, A., 1986, Invariant surface reconstruction using weak continuity constraints, in *Proc. IEEE Comput. Vision Pattern Recogn.*, Los Alamitos, CA: IEEE 62–67. ◆
Faugeras, O., 1993, *Three-Dimensional Computer Vision: A Geometric Viewpoint*, Cambridge, MA: MIT Press.
Geman, S., and Geman, D., 1984, Stochastic relaxation, Gibbs distributions, and the Bayesian restoration of images, *IEEE Trans. Pattern Anal. Machine Intell.*, 6:721–741.
Grossberg, S., and Mingolla, E., 1987, Neural dynamics of surface perception: Boundary webs, illuminants and shape-from-shading, *Computer Vision, Graphics and Image Processing*, 37:116–165. ◆
Hummel, R. A., and Zucker, S. W., 1983, On the foundations of relaxation labeling processes, *IEEE Trans. Pattern Anal. Machine Intell.*, 5:267–287.
Kirkpatrick, S., Gelatt, C. D., and Vecchi, M. P., 1983, Optimization by simulated annealing, *Science*, 220:671–680.
Knutsson, H., 1989, Representing local structure using tensors, in *Proceedings of the 6th Scandinavian Conference on Image Analysis*, Survey UK,: International Association for Pattern Recognition, pp. 244–251.
Koza, J. R., 1992, *Genetic Programming: On the Programming of Computers by Means of Natural Selection*, Cambridge, MA: MIT Press.
Leclerc, Y. G., 1989, Constructing simple stable descriptions for image partitioning, *Int. J. Comput. Vision*, 3:73–102.
Medioni, G., Lee, M. S., and Tang, C. K., 2000, *A Computational Framework for Feature Extraction and Segmentation*, New York: Elsevier.
Sethian, J. A., 1996, *Level Sets Methods*, Cambridge, Engl.: Cambridge University Press.
Sha'ashua, A., and Ullman, S., 1988, Structural saliency: The detection of globally salient structures using a locally connected network, in *Proceedings of an International Conference Computer Vision*, pp. 321–327. ◆
Shi, J., and Malik, J., 1998, Motion segmentation and tracking using normalized cuts, in *Proceedings of an International Conference on Computer Vision*, Los Alamitos, CA: IEEE Computer Society, pp. 1154–1160. ◆
Terzopoulos, D., 1986, Regularization of inverse visual problems involving discontinuities, *IEEE Trans. Pattern Anal. Machine Intell.*, 8:413–424.
Zhao, H. K., Osher, S., Merriman, B., and Kang, M., 1998, Implicit, nonparametric shape reconstruction from unorganized points using a variational level set method, *UCLA Computational and Applied Mathematics Reports 98-7*, Los Angeles: UCLA, Department of *Mathematics*.

Thalamus

Sean Hill and Giulio Tononi

Introduction

The thalamus is the gateway through which all sensory inputs, except olfaction, are relayed to the cortex. The thalamus can effectively control the flow of information to the cortex: during waking, it may subserve attention, selectively enhancing certain inputs to the cortex and attenuating others; during slow-wave sleep, the firing mode of thalamic cells changes, effectively closing the gateway and diminishing the influence of external stimuli on the cortex. Massive feedback from the cortex to the thalamus suggests that the entire thalamo-cortico-thalamic loop plays a role in sustaining and synchronizing cortical activity. Furthermore, certain thalamic nuclei appear to constitute an integral part of the signal flow between different cortical areas. The organization of the projections to and from the thalamus, and the anatomy and physiology of its nuclei are essential to understanding thalamic function from a neurocomputational perspective.

Thalamic Organization and Connectivity

The Thalamus is Organized into Well-Defined Nuclei

The dorsal portion of the thalamus can be subdivided into nuclei based on the source of subcortical afferents (visual, auditory, and somatosensory pathways, the cerebellum, the basal ganglia, etc.). Each thalamic nucleus is anatomically segregated from all the oth-

ers but tightly linked to a specific cortical area. For example, visual input arrives from the retina, via the optic tract, at the lateral geniculate nucleus (LGN) of the thalamus, before being relayed to the primary visual cortex. Auditory input is transmitted to the medial geniculate nucleus, which projects to the primary auditory cortex. The ventral posterior nucleus receives somatosensory inputs such as tactile and kinesthetic information, and projects to the somatosensory cortex. The basal ganglia have direct projections to the ventral anterior nucleus of the thalamus, which projects to motor cortex. The ventral lateral nucleus relays input from cerebellar nuclei to motor cortex. The anterior nuclei receive ascending projections from the subiculum and mammillary body and project densely to olfactory cortex. The intralaminar nuclei, central medial nucleus, and midline nuclei have projections to and from the basal ganglia as well as to the cerebral cortex. Circuits linking other thalamic nuclei with specific cortical areas are less well understood. In some cases, the type of information relayed by these nuclei is not known at all. However, the general principle seems to be that no cortical area is devoid of thalamic afferents.

The dorsal thalamus is surrounded for much of its extent by a thin sheet of cells constituting the ventral thalamus, which includes the thalamic reticular nucleus (TRN) and the perigeniculate nucleus—the visual region of the TRN. These nuclei are pierced by millions of fibers projecting both from thalamus to cortex and from cortex to thalamus, from which they receive collaterals. Unlike nuclei in the dorsal thalamus, the TRN and the perigeniculate nucleus do not send any connections to the cerebral cortex and will be discussed separately.

Sensory Afferents Drive Thalamic Cells and Determine Their Response Properties

The circuit involving the LGN and primary visual cortex is the best understood and will serve as the model for thalamic organization (Figure 1). It is likely that other thalamic nuclei, though subserving other sensory modalities, perform similar operations as the LGN. In the LGN, approximately 75% of the cells are glutamatergic relay cells that receive from the retina and project to primary visual cortex. The remaining 25% of LGN cells are interneurons that form local inhibitory GABAergic contacts. In some mammals, such as rats, interneurons are present in the LGN but are few or missing in other nuclei.

Retinal inputs to the LGN are retinotopically mapped, maintaining the spatial arrangement of the sensory input. The response properties of thalamic neurons are also remarkably similar to those of their retinal afferents. Such afferents make synaptic contacts with both relay neurons and interneurons and provide approximately 10% of the synaptic terminals in the thalamus (Van Horn, Erisir, and Sherman, 2000). They can have strong postsynaptic effects, due to large terminal endings that synapse close to the cell body of target cells (Sherman and Guillery, 2001). They use glutamate as a neurotransmitter by which they activate fast ionotropic receptors. Because they determine the firing properties of thalamic relay cells, these projections are considered the "driving" input to their

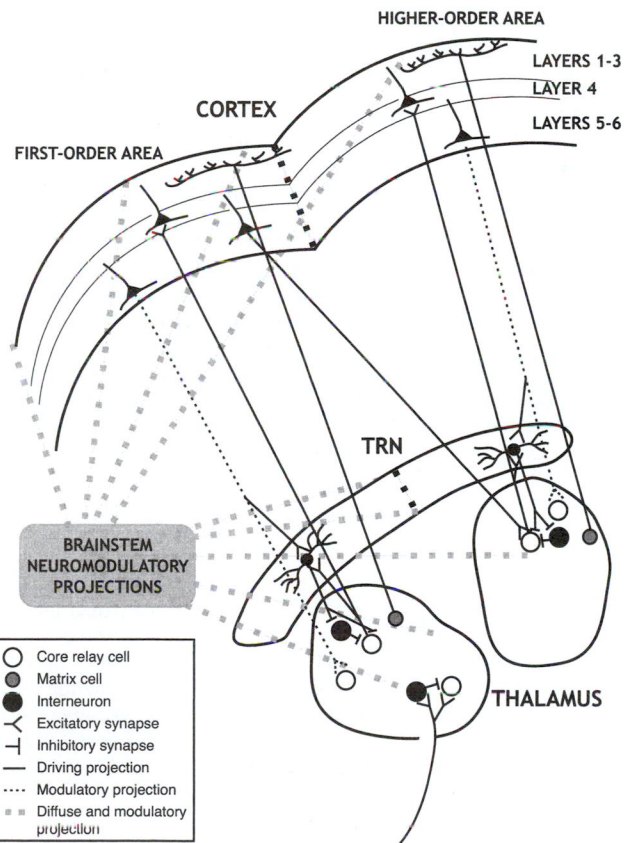

HIGHER-ORDER AREA

LAYERS 1-3
LAYER 4
LAYERS 5-6

CORTEX

FIRST-ORDER AREA

TRN

BRAINSTEM NEUROMODULATORY PROJECTIONS

THALAMUS

○ Core relay cell
◐ Matrix cell
● Interneuron
⊰ Excitatory synapse
⊣ Inhibitory synapse
— Driving projection
···· Modulatory projection
▪ ▪ Diffuse and modulatory projection

Figure 1. Schematic of the primary projections involved in thalamocortical circuitry.

target cells. In thalamic nuclei containing interneurons, one often finds a complex synaptic structure called a glomerulus, in which afferent terminals interact with the dendritic spines of relay cells and interneurons in synaptic triads. Glomeruli and synaptic triads are believed to implement a form of activity-dependent feedforward inhibition.

There is substantial evidence for functional segregation within the LGN that reflects features of the input. Inputs from the left and right retina terminate in different LGN layers. These layers are further segregated into parvocellular and magnocellular cell populations. Parvocellular neurons are more sensitive to color contrast and to stimuli of high spatial frequency; magnocellular neurons are sensitive to luminance contrast and to high temporal frequencies. Such segregation is established in part through activity-dependent processes that take place during early development. It remains to be seen whether functional segregation is at work elsewhere in the thalamus.

Thalamic Cells Relay Sensory Input to Specific Cortical Areas

Relay cells in the thalamus project dense topographic connections to the middle layers of the cerebral cortex—typically layer IV. These cells also form less dense projections to cortical layer VI. The majority of thalamocortical relay projections send collaterals to the TRN and provide excitatory input to the inhibitory population of cells in that nucleus (see discussion later in this article).

Thalamic input represents less than 10% of the synapses in cortical layer IV. Thalamocortical input is fast, strong, and excitatory and is mediated by glutamatergic synapses acting primarily through AMPA receptors. Single spikes in the thalamus can elicit spikes in layer IV cells. These projections are divergent and may synapse with patches of cortex up to 1.5 mm apart. The extent of these axonal arborizations in primary visual cortex corresponds to the size of a visual hypercolumn—representing a small region in the visual field. Projections from a given thalamic cell overlap as much as 600 μm with projections from a neighboring thalamic cell, producing a continuous mapping from thalamus to cortex (Steriade, Jones, and McCormick, 1997). The thalamus also relays afferent input from the basal ganglia and cerebellum to the cortex. However, the degree of organization and precision of these relay projections is not as well understood.

There Are Also Diffuse "Matrix" Projections from the Thalamus to the Cortex

The traditional view of thalamocortical connections is that the focused, highly organized projections to the cortex arise from specific relay nuclei, while broad, diffusely organized projections originate in nonspecific thalamic nuclei, largely identified with the intralaminar nuclei (Jones, 1985). However, recent work has revealed that the key distinction is not between anatomically defined nuclei, but between kinds of cells—core and matrix cells—that can be identified using molecular markers (Steriade et al., 1997). Core cells, which provide the specific, topographically ordered inputs to the cortex, are identified by immunoreactivity to parvalbumin, a calcium-binding protein. Core cells are embedded in a matrix of cells that send diffuse cortical projections and that are immunoreactive for a different calcium-binding protein—D28K calbindin. Matrix cells have been found throughout the thalamus, although they are present in higher numbers in the intralaminar nuclei. The projections of these cells appear to cross the boundaries of cortical areas and to target predominantly the most superficial layers of the cerebral cortex. These connections may play a role in dynamically modulated short-term plasticity such as the augmenting response, in which repetitive stimulation of the thalamus gives rise to an enhancement of thalamic and cortical responses to stimuli (Castro-Alamancos and Connors, 1996).

The Cortex Sends Massive Modulatory Projections Back to the Thalamus

It is customary to describe the flow of signals as going from the thalamus to the cortex. However, there are several times more descending corticothalamic fibers than ascending thalamocortical fibers (Van Horn et al., 2000). It is perhaps to be expected, then, that many corticothalamic projections—those originating from layer VI—modulate, rather than drive, the activity of their thalamic targets. Unlike driving inputs from the sensory periphery, modulatory inputs from layer VI cortical neurons have more subtle postsynaptic effects. Indeed, such inputs are preferentially localized on distal dendrites of thalamocortical cells, have smaller terminal sizes, and may act on both fast ionotropic and slow metabotropic receptors (Sherman and Guillery, 2001).

Connections between the thalamus and cortex are highly reciprocal. Axons originating in layer VI of a specific cortical area project to the same thalamic area that innervates that region of cortex. The arborizations of these axons diverge considerably, extending over an area as wide as 1.5 mm. These arborizations appear to be tightly linked to the hypercolumnar organization of the cortex (Sherman and Koch, 1998). Corticothalamic projections from the cortex form approximately 30% of the synaptic terminals on thalamic cells (Van Horn et al., 2000).

Corticothalamic projections from layer VI also send en passant fibers to the TRN, thus exciting the GABAergic population of thalamic cells in the TRN with the same input that modulates thalamic activity. Corticothalamic and corticoreticular projections have different effective strengths. Recent work has shown that, because of the increased number of glutamate receptor subunits GluR4 at corticothalamic synapses, the effective amplitude of excitatory postsynaptic potentials from synapses in the TRN is more than twice that of corticothalamic synapses in the thalamus (Golshani, Liu, and Jones, 2001). Thus, the influence of the cortex appears to be much greater on the TRN than on the dorsal thalamus.

Cortical deactivation and stimulation experiments have revealed a considerable range of influences of corticothalamic projections on thalamic activity. Initial experiments aimed at determining whether corticothalamic inputs provide excitation or inhibition to thalamic cells produced contradictory results, partly because they necessarily hinged on the combined effect of the corticothalamic projections (excitatory) and cortico-reticulo-thalamic projections (inhibitory). In line with the modulatory nature of these projections, the effect of layer VI cortical inputs appears to be more subtle. Although LGN cells are not orientation-selective, descending input from the cortex renders thalamic cells more sensitive to objects aligned with similar orientation in the visual field. Furthermore, corticothalamic feedback enhances the synchronization of cells responding to a single stimulus (Murphy, Duckett, and Sillito, 1999). Corticothalamic feedback is also essential to maintain the coherence of sleep spindles across the thalamocortical system. After decortication these oscillations continue to be generated by thalamic circuits at their normal frequency of about 7–14 Hz, but they become desynchronized (Contreras et al., 1996). Finally, lesioning the corticothalamic projections can prevent the development of binocular organization in the visual system (Weliky and Katz, 1999).

There Are First and Higher-Order Thalamic Nuclei

The notion that the thalamus merely relays peripheral signals to the cortex is further challenged by another anatomical observation. Several large thalamic nuclei, such as the pulvinar, the mediodorsal nucleus, and the dorsal division of the medial geniculate nucleus do not seem to receive any subcortical afferents capable of providing driving inputs. Instead, these nuclei receive driving input from the cortex itself, specifically from pyramidal cells in layer V. Thus, thalamic nuclei can be placed in two categories: first-order—those that receive driving input from subcortical afferents; and higher-order—those that receive driving input from cortex (Sherman and Guillery, 2001).

Although both classes of nuclei receive modulatory feedback projections from layer VI cortical cells, only higher-order nuclei receive corticothalamic inputs from layer V cells, which share many of the morphological traits of primary afferent inputs. Like retinal inputs, and unlike corticothalamic inputs from layer VI, inputs from layer V terminate in richly branched axons, end with large synapses, mostly on proximal dendrites, and often in triadic arrangements within glomeruli. Moreover, they do not send off collaterals to the TRN, but send branches to various brainstem nuclei. Axons from layer V thus appear to provide strong, driving inputs to higher-order thalamic nuclei. Indeed, the effect of cortical deactivation on the activity of higher-order thalamic nuclei is dramatic. For example, although lesions in the striate cortex alter the response of neurons in the LGN, they eliminate all activity in the pulvinar. Thus, higher-order thalamic nuclei receive driving inputs from one cortical area and relay it further to another cortical area to which they project. From this perspective, the thalamus can be considered an integral part of cortical circuitry, virtually serving as another layer of cerebral cortex that is essential for corticocortical communication (Sherman and Guillery, 2001). It remains to be seen whether any thalamic nucleus receives driving input from more than one cortical area, opening the possibility that the thalamus may be a site for the integration of information from multiple cortical sources.

The Reticular Nucleus Is Interposed Between the Dorsal Thalamus and the Cortex

As mentioned previously, the dorsal thalamus is surrounded by a thin sheet of cells—the thalamic reticular nucleus (TRN) and the associated perigeniculate nucleus. The TRN and associated nuclei receive collaterals from both thalamocortical fibers and corticothalamic fibers originating in layer VI cells, but do not send any projections to the cortex. Since thalamocortical and corticothalamic collaterals are topographically mapped, and they appear to largely overlap, the TRN is organized into functional sectors responsive to different modalities and submodalities (e.g., visual, auditory, somatosensory, and motor).

The TRN contains exclusively GABAergic cells, which project to the dorsal thalamus in a topographically organized manner. GABA released by reticulothalamic cells affects its targets via $GABA_A$ and $GABA_B$ receptors. $GABA_A$ receptors have fast ionotropic responses (tens of milliseconds) acting on the conductance of Cl channels. The kinetics of $GABA_B$ receptors are much slower (hundreds of milliseconds) and influence the conductance of K^+ channels. Since the reversal potential of K^+ is more negative than that of Cl^- (-100 mV vs. -70 mV), the hyperpolarizing effect of the activation of $GABA_B$ receptors is substantially larger than that of $GABA_A$ receptors.

Lesioning the TRN reveals the impact of its inhibitory projections on the thalamus. When the TRN is inactivated, thalamic cells tend to respond more readily to inputs and their receptive field generally becomes broader (Lee, Friedberg, and Ebner, 1994). However, these effects can be complicated by the fact that the TRN also projects to inhibitory interneurons in the thalamus and can thus have an excitatory effect on some thalamic neurons. During sleep, reticulothalamic projections are essential for the generation of spindle oscillations (Steriade et al., 1997)

The different nuclei in the dorsal thalamus are not linked by any direct connections. By contrast, throughout the TRN cells are highly interconnected in a dense meshwork of dendrodendritic connections and axonal arborizations. It is possible that the intrareticular connectivity serves to indirectly link the activities of thalamic nuclei that would otherwise be functionally segregated. As a rule, these reticuloreticular interactions, which are mediated largely by $GABA_A$ receptors, have an inhibitory action. However, due to the relatively high reversal potential of the Cl^- current, if reticular cells become hyperpolarized below -70 mV, as can occur during slow wave sleep, the influence of $GABA_A$ receptors may become excitatory. Recent work suggests that recurrent inhibition in the TRN plays a significant role in desynchronizing thalamic activity. Knockout mice lacking $GABA_A$-mediated inhibition exhibit highly synchronized intrathalamic oscillations that are not normally observed, suggesting that the TRN has a role in reducing synchrony in thalamic circuitry and preventing epileptic seizures (Huntsman et al., 1999).

Brainstem Afferents Modulate the Firing Mode of Thalamic Neurons by Acting on Intrinsic Conductances

A large proportion of the synaptic terminals in the thalamus—estimated to be around 30%—originates from neuromodulatory systems in the brainstem (Van Horn et al., 2000). These include the cholinergic neurons of the pedunculopontine tegmental nucleus, noradrenergic neurons of the locus coerulus, serotonergic neurons of the dorsal raphé, histaminergic neurons of the tuberomammillary nucleus, and glutamatergic cells acting through metabotropic receptors that are distributed throughout the reticular formation. These neuromodulatory projections can have differential effects on thalamic and reticular cells. For example, cholinergic projections excite thalamocortical relay cells but inhibit thalamic interneurons and TRN cells, while noradrenergic projections tend to be excitatory and depolarize TRN cells. Unlike other thalamic inputs, these brainstem inputs are not mapped and have a very broad pattern of termination. Most significantly, the neuromodulators released by these diffuse projections can activate or inactivate intrinsic conductances in thalamic cells and contribute to changes in behavioral state. At the beginning of sleep, for example, decreased activity in these neuromodulatory systems contributes to the hyperpolarization of thalamic neurons and triggers a set of intrinsic conductances leading to a change from tonic firing to burst firing. Bursts of action potentials followed by sustained periods of hyperpolarization effectively interrupt the normal relay functions of the thalamus, thereby closing the gateway and helping to entrain the thalamocortical circuit in repetitive, rhythmic firing.

The switch from tonic to burst firing mode results from the interactions of several conductances and is discussed in detail in SLEEP OSCILLATIONS (q.v.). Key players in burst generation are the conductance responsible for the low-threshold calcium current I_t and the hyperpolarization-activated cation conductance responsible for the depolarizing current I_h. In a minority of thalamic cells, burst firing may also occur during waking. Strong inhibition from the TRN may serve to prime some thalamic relay cells for bursts, which may then be triggered by any small depolarizing input. Such bursting, which occurs with greater frequency during visual stimulation, may serve as a "wake-up call" to the cortex. It has been hypothesized that corticothalamic feedback may then depolarize the bursting cells and lead to a more efficient processing of the stimuli (Sherman and Guillery, 2001).

Discussion

For many years, neurophysiologists have studied the receptive field properties of thalamic cells in the visual thalamus and, to a lesser extent, in the auditory thalamus. Undeniably, the principal finding emerging from these investigations is that the receptive fields of thalamic cells are remarkably similar to those of the primary afferents, retinal or otherwise. From these results, it would appear that the primary function of the thalamus is that of reliably relaying afferent inputs to the cortex.

As mentioned previously, several recent experiments have demonstrated the subtle role played by corticothalamic inputs in shaping the response of thalamic neurons in ways that are not captured by traditional receptive field analysis, such as by facilitating synchronization and contributing contextual influences to orientation selective processing in the LGN. Moreover, the role of the thalamus in gating inputs to the cortex as a function of behavioral state has become clearly established. Corticothalamic feedback is necessary for the synchronization of spindle oscillations throughout the thalamocortical circuit during sleep. The thalamic mode of firing may also influence the way inputs are relayed to the cortex during waking. Most significantly, higher-order thalamic nuclei may play an integral role in the flow of signals between different cortical areas. Finally, it is possible that, under certain circumstances, the thalamus may not only gate but also integrate its inputs.

However, many questions remain about the role of corticothalamic pathways and the function of the thalamus in general. This uncertainty is reflected in the wide array of models designed to address various proposed functions of the thalamus. A number of proposals have suggested that the reticulothalamic circuit is involved in selective attention based on mechanisms for dynamic filtering. It has been suggested that the thalamocortical loop works to complete noisy input patterns based on feedback from the cortex (Harth, Unnikriohnan, and Pandya, 1987). ADAPTIVE RESONANCE THEORY (ART) (q.v.) is an artificial neural network model of these ideas. Active blackboard models combine these ideas with an attention-like mechanism in which a variety of patterns may be selectively enhanced or suppressed (Mumford, 1991). Finally, detailed models of the thalamocortical system have suggested that its dynamic behavior changes considerably when thalamocortical and corticothalamic connections become a functionally closed loop (Lumer, Edelman, and Tononi, 1997). Perhaps the entire thalamocortical loop is the appropriate unit at which to consider the functional role of the thalamus. As with neurocomputational approaches to other brain regions, the principle that function follows form—that is, neuroanatomy—may be most useful in understanding what the thalamus does.

Road Map: Mammalian Brain Regions
Related Reading: Adaptive Resonance Theory; Neuromodulation in Mammalian Nervous Systems; Sleep Oscillations; Visual Attention

References

Castro-Alamancos, M. A., and Connors, B. W., 1996, Short-term plasticity of a thalamocortical pathway dynamically modulated by behavioral state, *Science*, 272(5259):274–277.

Contreras, D., Destexhe, A., Sejnowski, T. J., and Steride, M., 1996, Control of spatiotemporal coherence of a thalamic oscillation by corticothalamic feedback, *Science*, 274(5288):771–774.

Golshani, P., Liu, X. B., and Jones, E. G., 2001, Differences in quantal amplitude reflect GluR4-subunit number at corticothalamic synapses on two populations of thalamic neurons, *Proc. Natl. Acad. Sci. USA*, 98(7):4172–4177.

Harth, E., Unnikriohnan, K. P., and Pandya, A. S., 1987, The inversion of sensory processing by feedback pathways, *Science*, 237:184–187

Huntsman, M. M., Porcello, D. M., Homanics, G. E., DeLorey, T. M., and Hvguenard, J. R., 1999, Reciprocal inhibitory connections and network synchrony in the mammalian thalamus, *Science*, 283:541–543.

Jones, E. G., 1985, *The Thalamus*, New York: Plenum.

Koch, C., 1985, Understanding the intrinsic circuitry of the cat's lateral geniculate nucleus: Electrical properties of the spine-triad arrangement, *Proc. R. Soc. Lond. B. Biol. Sci.*, 225:365–390.

Lee, S. M., Friedberg, M. H., and Ebner, F. F., 1994, The role of GABA-mediated inhibition in the rat ventral posterior medial thalamus. I. Assessment of receptive field changes following thalamic reticular nucleus lesions, *J. Neurophysiol.*, 71(5):1702–1715.

Lumer, E. D., Edelman, G. M., and Tononi, G., 1997, Neural dynamics in a model of the thalamocortical system. I. Layers, loops and the emergence of fast synchronous rhythms, *Cereb. Cortex*, 7(3):207–227. ◆

Mumford, D., 1991, On the computational architecture of the neocortex. I. The role of the thalamo-cortical loop, *Biol. Cybern.*, 65(2):135–145. ◆

Murphy, P. C., Duckett, S. G., and Sillito, A. M., 1999, Feedback connections to the lateral geniculate nucleus and cortical response properties, *Science*, 286(5444):1552–1554.

Sherman, S. M., and Guillery, R. W., 2001, *Exploring the Thalamus*, New York: Academic Press. ◆

Sherman, S. M., and Koch, C., 1998, Thalamus, Chapter in *The Synaptic Organization of the Brain* (G. M. Shepherd, Ed.), New York: Oxford University Press. ◆

Steriade, M., Jones, E. G., and McCormick, D. A., Eds., 1997, *Thalamus: Organization and Function*, New York: Elsevier.

Van Horn, S. C., Erisir, A., and Sherman, S. M., 2000, Relative distribution of synapses in the A-laminae of the lateral geniculate nucleus of the cat, *J. Comp. Neurol.*, 416(4):509–520.

Weliky, M., and Katz, L. C., 1999, Correlational structure of spontaneous neuronal activity in the developing lateral geniculate nucleus in vivo, *Science*, 285(5427):599–604.

Universal Approximators

Věra Kůrková

Universality Versus Complexity

Many classification or pattern recognition tasks can be formulated as mappings between subsets of multidimensional vector spaces by using a suitable coding of inputs and outputs. The goal of a computer scientist in modeling such tasks is to find a computationally feasible procedure capable of recognizing a great variety of patterns by merely changing procedural parameters.

Such versatility in a computational model is often called *universality* with respect to computations to be performed. A classical example of a universal computational model is the Turing machine, which is capable of realizing any algorithm. Within the last decade, it has been shown that many types of feedforward networks, including all standard types that are popular in applications as well as many others that may not have been considered by experimentalists, form a universal computational model with respect to *approximation of mappings between subsets of Euclidean spaces.*

But universality has a price: it cannot be proven within reasonable bounds on *complexity*. Currently, feedforward networks are mostly simulated on classical computers and for such implementations, the limiting factors are number of network units, size, and resolution of their parameters. For most tasks, implementation of theoretically optimal approximation procedures becomes infeasible because of the unmanageably large number of parameters. In particular, high-dimensional tasks are limited by the "curse of dimensionality," i.e., an exponentially fast scaling of the number of parameters with the number of variables.

However, some mappings between high-dimensional representations have been successfully implemented using neural networks of moderate complexity (e.g., NETtalk; see Sejnowski and Rosenberg, 1987). Approximation theory offers some explanation for the feasibility of such implementations by deriving various upper bounds on the complexity, which depend on the number of variables of functions to be approximated together with their other characteristics. Inspection of such bounds shows that we can cope with the "curse of dimensionality" by suitable constraints on characteristics such as smoothness.

This article surveys recent developments in the mathematical theory of feedforward networks and includes proofs of the universal approximation capabilities of perceptron and RBF networks with general activation and radial fnctions, estimates of rates of approximation and description of sets of multivariable functions that can be approximated without the "curse of dimensionality."

Perceptron and RBF Networks

Tasks representable as mappings can be performed by devices computing functions depending on two vector variables: an input vector (corresponding to a coded pattern to be recognized or transformed) and a parameter vector (to be adjusted during learning mode). Due to error-correcting afterprocessing (such as best guess) it is sufficient when such devices compute mappings that perform the tasks only approximately.

Feedforward neural networks compute parametrized sets of functions depending both on the type of computational units and the type of their interconnections. A *computational unit* can be formally described as a function $\phi : \mathcal{R}^q \times \mathcal{R}^d \to \mathcal{R}$, where $\mathcal{R}$ denotes the set of real numbers, and p and d, respectively, are the dimensions of a *parameter* and an *input space*. Since in practical applications all inputs are bounded, it is sufficient to study networks with inputs in some compact (closed and bounded) subset of $\mathcal{R}$; usually, results are formulated for inputs in the interval [0, 1]. By $G_\phi = \{\phi(a, .) : [0, 1]^d \to \mathcal{R} : a \in \mathcal{R}^q\}$ is denoted the set of functions on $[0, 1]^d$ computable by a computational unit ϕ with all possible choices of parameters $a \in \mathcal{R}^q$.

The simplest model of a feedforward network has a single linear output and one hidden layer with n units computing ϕ. Such network can compute all functions from the set $span_n G_\phi$ of all linear combinations of at most n elements of G_ϕ. If an arbitrarily large number of hidden units is allowed, such networks can compute functions from $span\ G_\phi = \bigcup_{n \in \mathcal{N}_+} span_n G_\phi$, where $\mathcal{N}_+$ denotes the set of all positive integers.

As approximation by sets of the form $span_n G_\phi$ exploits flexible choice of n-tuples of inner parameters of computational units, it belongs to *variable-basis approximation* class. Besides neural networks, this class contains free-node splines, rational functions with free poles, and trigonometric sums with free frequencies. In contrast, classical linear approximation can be called *fixed basis approximation*, as it only allows linear combinations of first n elements of a basis with a fixed ordering.

Standard types of hidden units are perceptrons and radial-basis-function units. A *perceptron* with an activation function $\psi : \mathcal{R} \to \mathcal{R}$ computes functions of the form $\phi((v, b), x) = \psi(v \cdot x + b) : \mathcal{R}^{d+1} \times \mathcal{R}^d \to \mathcal{R}$, where $v \in \mathcal{R}^d$ is an *input weight* vector and $b \in \mathcal{R}$ is a *bias*. By $P_d(\psi) = \{\psi(v \cdot x + b) : v \in \mathcal{R}^d, b \in \mathcal{R}\}$ is denoted the set of functions on $[0, 1]^d$ computable by ψ-perceptrons. The most common activation functions are *sigmo-*

idals, i.e., functions $\sigma : \mathcal{R} \to [0, 1]$ such that $\lim_{t \to -\infty} \sigma(t) = 0$ and $\lim_{t \to \infty} \sigma(t) = 1$. Both continuous sigmoidals (like the logistic sigmoid $1/(1 + e^{-1})$ or the hyperbolic tangent) and the discontinuous Heaviside function ϑ defined by $\vartheta(t) = 0$ for $t < 0$ and $\vartheta(t) = 1$ for t $\geq$ 0 are used.

A *radial-basis-function* (RBF) unit with a radial (even) function $\psi : \mathcal{R} \to \mathcal{R}_+$ ($\mathcal{R}_+$ denotes the set of positive real numbers) computes $\phi((v, b), x) = \psi(b\|x - v\|)$, where $v \in \mathcal{R}^d$ is a *centroid*, $b \in \mathcal{R}_+$ is a *width* and $\|.\|$ is a norm on $\mathcal{R}^d$. By $F_d(\psi) = \{\psi(b\|x - v\|) : v \in \mathcal{R}^d, b \in \mathcal{R}\}$ is denoted the set of functions on $[0, 1]^d$ computable by ψ-RBF units networks with distance from centroids measured by the l_2-norm $\|.\|$. Standard choice of a radial function is the Gaussian function $\gamma(t) = e^{-t^2}$.

Note that sigmoidal perceptrons and RBF units are geometrically opposite: perceptrons apply a sigmoidal function to a weighted sum of inputs plus a bias, and so they respond to *nonlocalized* regions of the input space by partitioning it with fuzzy hyperplanes (or sharp ones if the sigmoid is Heaviside's step function. The functions computed by perceptrons belong to the class of *plane waves*. In contrast, RBF units calculate the distance to a centroid, multiply it by a width factor, and finally apply a radial function—hence they respond to *localized* regions. The functions computed by radial units belong to the class of *spherical waves*. Although perceptrons were inspired biologically, plane waves (sometimes also called ridge functions) have been studied for a long time by mathematiciens motivated by various problems from physics. In contrast to integration theory, where functions are approximated by linear combinations of characteristic functions of boxes (called simple functions), the theory of perceptron networks studies approximation by linear combinations of characteristic functions of half-spaces. Expressions in terms of such functions exhibit the strength and weakness of plane waves methods described by Courant and Hilbert (1962): "But always the use of plane waves fails to exhibit clearly the domains of dependence and the role of characteristics. This shortcoming, however, is compensated by the elegance of explicit results."

The Universal Approximation Property

The first theoretical question concerning a given type of a feedforward network architecture is whether a sufficiently elaborate network of this type can approximate all reasonable functions encountered in applications. This capability of a class of neural networks is called the *universal approximation property*. Mathematically, it can be formalized as density in some of standard normed linear spaces. Recall that a subset F of a normed linear space $(X, \|.\|)$ is *dense* in X if $cl F = X$, where $cl F = \{f \in X : (\forall_\epsilon > 0)(\exists_g \in F)(\|f - g\| < \epsilon)\}$. Depending on whether the same quality of performance is required for all input vectors or whether a likelihood or importance of various inputs can be specified, density is studied either in the space $(\mathcal{C}([0, 1]^d), \|.\|_\mathcal{C})$ of all continuous functions on $[0, 1]^d$ with the supremum norm, or in $(\mathcal{L}_p([0, 1]^d, \|.\|_p)$ with the $\mathcal{L}_p$-norm for some $p \in [1, \infty]$. As spaces of continuous functions are dense in $\mathcal{L}_p$-spaces, it is sufficient to investigate the universal approximation property for $\mathcal{C}([0, 1]^d)$.

For RBF networks, the universal approximation capability is intuitively quite clear—one can imagine an approximation of a surface by a combination of Gaussian hills of various widths and heights. The classical method of approximation by convolutions with a suitable sequence of kernels enables one to prove this property for many types of radial functions. The following theorem by Park and Sandberg (1993) is based on the classical method of approximation of continuous functions by convolutions with a sequence of kernels.

Theorem 1. For every positive integer d and for every function $\psi : \mathcal{R} \to \mathcal{R}_+$ with finite non-zero integral and for every norm $\|.\|$ on $\mathcal{R}^d$, span $F_d(\psi, \|.\|)$ is dense in $(\mathcal{C}(\mathcal{R}^d), \|.\|_\mathcal{C})$.

When $\int_\mathcal{R} \psi(t)dt = c \neq 0$, then by properly scaling the function $\psi_0 = (\psi/c)$ we can construct a sequence of kernels $\{\psi_n(t) : n \in \mathcal{N}_+\}$, defined as $\psi_n(t) = n^d \psi_0(nt)$, converging to the Dirac delta function δ. Convolutions $f * \psi_n$ of such kernels with any continuous function on $[0, 1]^d$ converge to f uniformly. Approximating the integrals $\int f(x)(n^d/c)\psi(n(x - v))dv$ by Riemann sums we get a sequence of functions of the form of RBF networks with ψ as a radial function.

In contrast to localized Gaussian radial units, for nonlocalized perceptrons the universal approximation property is far from being intuitively clear. Mathematics extends the range of our visualization and offers tools that enable us to prove this capability for perceptrons with almost any type of activations (it is sufficient that the perceptron is locally integrable and bounded.)

Many ingenious proof techniques have been used to derive the universal approximation property for perceptron networks. They include integral representations of the form of a "neural network with a continuum of hidden units" based either on Fourier or Radon transform, Kolmogorov's representation of continuous functions of several variables by means of superpositions of continuous one-variable functions, arguments by contradiction based on the Hahn-Banach theorem, and several others utilizing Stone-Weiersreass' theorem (for a survey see Pinkus, 1998, and Kůrková, 2002a). Here we illustrate methods of verification of universality of perceptron networks by two theorems with quite elegant proofs.

The following input dimension reduction theorem by Stinchcombe and White (1990) shows that for perceptron networks, it is sufficient to check the universal approximation property only for networks with a single input.

Theorem 2. Let $\psi : \mathcal{R} \to \mathcal{R}$ be any function. Then span $P_1(\psi)$ is dense in $(\mathcal{C}([0, 1]), \|.\|_\mathcal{C})$. if and only if for every positive integer d, span $P_d(\psi)$ is dense in $(\mathcal{C}([0, 1]^d), \|.\|_\mathcal{C})$.

The proof is based on the Stone-Weierstrass theorem, which is Stone's extension of the classical Weierstrass theorem about density of polynomials. It states two conditions on a set of functions $\mathcal{A}$ on a compact (closed and bounded) subset K of $\mathcal{R}^d$ that imply density in $(\mathcal{C}(K), \|.\|_\mathcal{C})$: (1) $\mathcal{A}$ is an algebra (i.e., it is closed under both addition and multiplication of functions), (2) $\mathcal{A}$ separates points (i.e., for each pair of distinct points $x, y \in K$, there exists $f \in \mathcal{A}$ such that $f(x) \neq f(y)$).

The argument takes advantage of existence of an activation function with special properties that allow us to apply the Stone-Weierstrass theorem. This function is $\exp(t) = e^t$. Sets *span* $P_d(\psi)$ are always closed under addition and for reasonable ψ, they also separate points, but they usually fail to be closed under multiplication. Due to special properties of exp, *span* $P_d(\exp)$ is closed under multiplication for all d and hence by the Stone-Weierstrass theorem, it is dense in $(\mathcal{C}([0, 1]^d), \|.\|_\mathcal{C})$. When *span* $P_1(\psi$ is dense in $(\mathcal{C}([0, 1]), \|.\|_\mathcal{C})$, then it can approximate with any accuracy all continuous functions on $[0, 1]$; in particular the function exp. Using composition of two approximations, the first one approximating $f \in \mathcal{C}([0, 1]^d)$ by an element of *span* $P_d(\exp)$, and the second one approximating exp by an element of *span* $P_1(\psi)$, one gets density of *span* $P_d(\psi)$ in $(\mathcal{C}([0, 1]^d), \|.\|_\mathcal{C})$.

Leshno et al. (1993) have shown that the universal approximation property is not restricted to biologically motivated sigmoidals but, with the exception of polynomials, it is satisfied by any reasonable activation function.

Theorem 3. Let $\psi : \mathcal{R} \to \mathcal{R}$ be a locally bounded piecewise continuous function and d be any positive integer. Then span $P_d(\psi)$ is dense in $(\mathcal{C}([0,\ 1]^d),\ \|.\|_e)$ if and only if ψ is not an algebraic polynomial.

The trick of Leshno et al.'s proof is in expressing all powers as limits of higher-order partial derivatives with respect to the weight parameter v of the function $\psi(vx + b)$ (ψ being analytic guarantees that all the derivatives exist). It follows directly from the definition of iterated partial derivative that $(\delta^k(vx + b))/(\delta v^k)$ can be expressed as a limit of functions computable by perceptron networks with activation ψ. More precisely, $(\delta\psi(vx + b))/(\delta v) = \lim_{\eta\to 0}(\psi((v + \eta)x + b) - \psi(vx + b))/(\eta)$, and similarly for $k > 1$. As $(\delta^k\psi(vx + b))/(\delta v^k) = x^k\psi^{(k)}(vx + b)$ and for ψ nonpolynomial, $\psi^{(k)}$ is not identically equal to zero for all k, by setting $v = 0$ and choosing some b_k, for which $\psi^{(k)}(b_k) = c_k \neq 0$, we get a sequence of functions from *span* $P_d(\psi)$ converging to c_kx^k. As polynomials are linear combinations of powers, they can be obtained as limits of sequences of functions from *span* $P_d(\psi)$. So by Weierstrass's theorem and by the previously mentioned input dimension reduction theorem, *span* $P_d(\psi)$ is dense in $(\mathcal{C}([0,\ 1]^d), \|.\|_e)$ for any ψ that is analytic and nonpolynomial. For nonanalytic functions satisfying the assumptions of the theorem, the result can be obtained using suitable convolutions with analytic functions.

Inspection of Leshno et al.'s (1993) proof shows that the theorem is valid even when all network parameters are bounded by an arbitrarily small upper bound. However, to achieve density, the set of hidden unit parameters must have either a finite or an infinite accumulation point.

In practical applications, neural networks are trained to fit to a given set of input/output pairs of data. Hence the domain of the function to be computed by a network is finite, and we can apply results from interpolation theory. They show that for finite domain functions, we can replace *arbitrary close approximation* by *exact representation*. One of the main results of interpolation theory, Miccchelli's (1986) theorem, shows that any function on a finite subset of $\mathcal{R}^d$ can be exactly represented as a network with Gaussian RBF units. An analogous result for sigmoidal perceptron networks has been proven by Ito (1992). However, development of interpolation theory has been motivated by needs to construct surfaces with certain characteristics fitted to a small number of points. Although its results are valid for any number of pairs of data, its application to neurocomputing leads to networks with the same number of hidden units as the number of input/output pairs. For large sets of data, this requirement may prevent implementation. In such cases, estimates of accuracy achievable using networks with fewer hidden units are needed. They can be derived from estimates of rates of approximation that apply to both finite and infinite domains.

Rates of Approximation

Although density guarantees arbitrarily close approximation of all functions from $\mathcal{C}([0,\ 1]^d)$, $\mathcal{L}_p([0,\ 1]^d)$, respectively, for practical purposes, its implications are limited to functions for which a sufficient accuracy can be achieved by networks with n hidden units where n is small enough to allow implementation.

Approximation theory investigates the trade-off between accuracy of approximation and complexity of approximating functions. It has derived various upper bounds on complexity of approximating systems depending on the number of variables of functions to be approximated together with their other characteristics. Inspection of such bounds offers some explanation of feasibility of implementations of high-dimensional tasks, as it shows that we can cope with the "curse of dimensionality" by constraining the characteristics involved.

For example, upper bounds on worst-case errors in linear approximation are of the form $\mathcal{O}(n^{-s/d})$, where d is the number of variables, s degree of smoothness of the functions to be approximated, and n is the number of parameters of the linear approximating family. Thus, in linear approximation, the "curse of dimensionality" can be avoided by increasing smoothness together with the number of variables.

For neural networks, the role of such characteristics is played by norms tailored to computational units. Their definition is fitted to the following Maurey-Jones-Barron's upper bound (see Jones, 1992; Barron, 1993) on rates of approximation by $span_nG$, the set of all convex combinations of at most n elements of G. For a subset M of a normed linear space $(X, \|.\|)$ and $f \in X$, the distance of f from M is denoted by $\|f - M\|$. For simplicity, we present here only the version for Hilbert spaces; however, similar upper bounds hold also for $\mathcal{L}_p$-spaces with $p \in [1, \infty]$ (for a survey see Kůrková 2002b).

Theorem 4. Let G be a bounded subset of a Hilbert space $(X, \|.\|)$ and $s_G = \sup_{g\in G}\|g\|$. Then for every $f \in cl$ conv G and for every positive integer n, $\|f - conv_n G\| \leq \sqrt{(s_G^2 - \|f\|^2)/(n)}$.

As $conv_nG \subseteq span_nG$, the upper bound from Theorem 4 also applies to rates of approximation by $span_nG$. Replacing the set G by $G(c) = \{wg : g \in G, |w| \leq c\}$, we can apply Theorem 4 to all elements of $\bigcup_{c\in\mathcal{N}_+} cl$ conv $G(c)$ (as $conv_nG(c) \subset span_nG(c) = span_nG$ for any $c \in \mathcal{R}$). This approach can be mathematically formulated in terms of a norm tailored to a set G. Let $(X, \|.\|)$ be a normed linear space and G be its subset, then G-*variation* (variation with respect to G) is defined as the Minkowski functional of the set cl $conv(G \cup -G)$, i.e.,

$$\|f\|_G = \inf\{c > 0 : f/c \in cl\ conv(G \cup -G)\}$$

When a set of functions has to be approximated, it is useful to estimate worst-case error, which is mathematically formalized by the concept of *deviation* $\delta(B, Y) = \sup_{f\in B}\|f - Y\|$. The following is a corollary of Theorem 4 formulated in terms of G-variation. If $(X, \|.\|)$ is a normed linear space and $b > 0$, then $B_b(\|.\|)$ and $S_b(\|.\|)$ denote the ball and sphere, respectively, of radius b centered at zero, i.e., $B_b(\|.\|) = \{f \in X : \|f\| \leq b\}$ and $S_b(\|.\|) = \{f \in X : \|f\| = b\}$.

Corollary 5. Let G be a bounded subset of a Hilbert space $(X, \|.\|)$, $s_G = \sup_{g\in G}\|g\|$, $b > 0$, $0 \leq r \leq s_Gb$ and n be a positive integer. Then
(i) for every $f \in X$, $\|f - span_nG\| \leq \sqrt{((s_G\|f\|_G)^2 - \|f\|^2)/(n)}$;
(ii) $\delta(\{f \in B_b(\|.\|_G) : \|f\| \geq r\}, span_nG \leq \sqrt{((s_Gb)^2 - r^2)/(n)}$;
(iii) $\delta(B_b(\|.\|_G), span_nG) \leq (s_Gb)/(\sqrt{n})$.

Corollary 5 shows how to cope with the curse of dimensionality in neural network approximation We can keep rate of approximation by $span_nP_d(\psi)$ or $span_nF_d(\psi)$ within $1/\sqrt{n}$ for all d by restricting approximation to functions from balls in $P_d(\psi)$ variation and $F_d(\psi)$ variation, respectively.

Thus $P_d(\psi)$ and $F_d(\psi)$ variations play a similar role in neural network approximation as the Sobolev norm of the order d does in linear approximation. However in contrast to linear approximation, in neural network approximation sets with worst-case errors bounded by $\mathcal{O}(n^{-1/2})$ are not shrinking with d increasing, as the balls in $P_d(\psi)$, $F_d(\psi)$-variation can be embedded into balls in $P_{d+1}(\psi)$, $F_d(\psi)$-variation, respectively (see Kůrková, 2002b). It was shown by Barron (1993) that balls in Sobolev norms of the order $s > d/2 + 1$ can be embedded into balls in $P_d(\sigma)$-variation. Barron (1993) also described sets of multivariable functions for which neural networks outperform linear approximation methods (see also Kůrková and Sanguineti, 2002.

As Heaviside perceptrons compute characteristic functions of half-spaces restricted to $[0, 1]^d$, $P_d(\vartheta)$-variation is called *variation with respect to half-spaces*. For functions of one variable, variation with respect to half-spaces coincides, up to a constant, with the notion of total variation studied in the integration theory. In $\mathscr{L}_p$-spaces, $P_d(\vartheta)$-variation is equal to $P_d(\sigma)$-variation for any sigmoidal activation function σ (see Kůrková, Kainen, and Kreinovich, 1997). Thus to describe the set of functions that do not exhibit the "curse of dimensionality" in approximation by sigmoidal perceptron networks, it is sufficient to study balls in variation with respect to half-spaces.

Upper bounds on variation with respect to half-spaces can be derived from integral representations of the form of a neural network with a continuum of Heavidise perceptrons (see Kůrková et al., 1997). Lower bounds can be obtained from geometrical considerations (angular relationships to hidden unit functions).

For discussion of the strength and weakness of the method of estimation of rates of approximation by neural networks using Maurey-Jones-Barron's bound see Kůrková, Savicky, and Hlaváĉková, 1998. They have described functions with variations depending on the number of variables exponentially. It is an open question, related to difficult problems of complexity of Boolean functions, whether such functions can be approximated within a small error by one-hidden-layer Heaviside perceptron networks with the number of hidden units depending on the number of variables only polynomially.

Discussion

Within the last decade, it has been shown that many types of feedforward networks are universal approximators. Provided that they contain sufficiently many computational units, their parameters can be adjusted to obtain as an input/output function a good approximation to almost any mapping between subsets of multidimensional spaces.

Each universal computational model determines a hierarchy of complexity on computational tasks with respect to a given type of implementation. Complexity measured by the number of hidden units can be estimated using upper bounds on rates of approximation. Inspection of such bounds shows that it is possible to cope with the "curse of dimensionality" when approximation is restricted to functions with certain norms bounded by a fixed constant independent of the number of variables. For linear approximation, such norms are Sobolev norms of order increasing with the dimension, while for neural networks, such norms are variations with respect to computational units. For sigmoidal perceptrons, they are all equal to variation with respect to half-spaces and for RBF units, they are variations with respect to spherical waves of the shape corresponding to radial functions.

However, examples of functions with variations depending exponentially on the number of variables show that interpretations of upper bounds on rates of neural network approximation of the order of $\mathbb{O}(n^{-1/2})$ as proofs of "dimension-independent" approximation capabilities of neural networks are misleading. It is not possible to

approximate all d-variable functions by neural networks with rates of the order $\mathbb{O}(n^{-1/2})$. To achieve such rates, approximation has to be restricted to functions from balls in variation with respect to the type of computational units.

This work was partially supported by GA ČR grants 201/99/0092 and 201/02/0428.

Road Map: Computability and Complexity
Background: Perceptrons, Adalines, and Backpropagation
Related Reading: Analog Neural Nets: Computational Power; Learning and Generalization: Theoretical Bounds; Radial Basis Function Networks

References

Courant, R., and Hilbert, D., 1962, *Methods of Mathematical Physics*, Vol. 2, New York: Wiley.

Barron, A. R., 1993, Universal approximation bounds for superposition of a sigmoidal function, *IEEE Transactions on Information Theory*, 39:930–945.

Ito, Y., 1992, Finite mapping by neural networks and truth functions, *Mathematical Scientist*, 17:69–77.

Jones, L. K., 1992, A simple lemma on greedy approximation in Hilbert space and convergence rates for projection pursuit regression and neural network training, *Annals of Statistics*, 20:608–613.

Kůrková, V., 2002a, Universality and complexity of approximation of multivariable functions by feedforward networks, in *Softcomputing in Industrial Applications—Recent Advances* (R. Roy, M. Koeppen, S. Ovaska, T. Furuhashi, and F. Hoffmann, Eds.), London: Springer-Verlag. ◆

Kůrková, V., 2002b, Mappings between high-dimensional representations in connectionistic systems, in *Quo vadis Machine Intelligence* (P. Sinĉák, K. Hirota, Eds.), Heidelberg: Physica-Verlag. ◆

Kůrková, V., Kainen, P. C., and Kreinovich, V., 1997, Estimates of the number of hidden units and variation with respect to half-spaces, *Neural Networks*, 10:1061–1068.

Kůrková, V., Savicky, P., and Hlaváĉková, K., 1998, Representations and rates of approximation of real-valued Boolean functions by neural networks, *Neural Networks*, 11:651–659.

Kůrková, V., and Sanguineti, M., 2002, Comparison of worst-case errors in linear and neural network approximation, *IEEE Trans. on Information Theory*, 48:264–275.

Leshno, M., Lin, V. Y., Pinkus, A., and Schocken, S., 1993, Multilayer feedforward networks with a non-polynomial activation can approximate any function, *Neural Networks*, 6:861–867.

Micchelli, C. A., 1986, Interpolation of scattered data: Distance matrices and conditionally positive definite functions, *Constructive Approximation*, 2:11–22.

Park, J., and Sandberg, I. W., 1993, Approximation and radial-basis-function networks, *Neural Computation*, 5:305–316.

Pinkus, A., 1998, Approximation theory of the MLP model in neural networks, *Acta Numerica*, 8:277–283. ◆

Sejnowski, T. J., and Rosenberg, C., 1987, Parallel networks that learn to pronounce English text, *Complex Systems*, 1:145–168.

Stinchcombe, M., and White, H., 1990, Approximating and learning unknown mappings using multilayer networks with bounded weights, in *Proceedings of IJCNN'90*, New York: IEEE Press, pp. III.7–16

Unsupervised Learning with Global Objective Functions

Suzanna Becker and Richard S. Zemel

Introduction

Unsupervised learning algorithms can be distinguished by the absence of any supervisory feedback from the external environment.

Often, however, there is an implicit *internally derived* training signal. This training signal is based on some measure of the quality of the network's internal representation. The main problem in unsupervised learning research is to formulate a performance measure or cost function for the learning, to generate this internal supervisory signal. The cost function is also known as an objective function, since it sets the objective for the learning process. In this article, we review the most promising algorithms for unsupervised learning. We particularly focus on two types of learning procedures: those based on information-theoretic performance measures, and those employing maximum-likelihood density estimation. Another important class of biologically motivated learning algorithms, based on the idea of reinforcement—whether externally provided or internally generated—is covered elsewhere in this *Handbook* (see REINFORCEMENT LEARNING and REINFORCEMENT LEARNING IN MOTOR CONTROL).

Global Objective Functions or Synaptic Learning Rules?

Since our concern is with unsupervised learning in *networks* and their global behavior, we will focus on algorithms based on globally defined objective functions, rather than synaptic learning rules. By viewing the learning process as the optimization of a global objective function, we can reduce a global algorithm to synaptic-level steps (weight changes), but the converse is not necessarily true: a given synaptic learning rule may not correspond to the derivative of any global objective function. Further, a well-defined objective function for the learning allows us to make global predictions about its behavior, which is typically not possible in a bottom-up approach. Finally, the global objective function provides a quantitative measure of the success, or at least convergence, of the learning procedure.

In contrast to this top-down approach, many computational models of learning have been based on synaptic or cellular constraints, such as Hebb's postulate, and more recently, conditions for LTP induction. Hebb postulated that a synapse's efficacy should increase whenever the pre- and postsynaptic neurons are co-active. Hebb's postulate has gained popularity among neurobiologists as a plausible candidate for a cortical synaptic learning mechanism. A typical instantiation of Hebb's rule relates the evolution of the synaptic weight, w_{ij}, to the product of the pre- and postsynaptic activities, y_i, and y_j, as follows:

$$\Delta w_{ij} = \varepsilon y_i \, y_j$$

where ε is a learning rate constant. Although this rule and its variants (see POST-HEBBIAN LEARNING ALGORITHMS) provide a useful way to model cellular- and synaptic-level phenomena, they do not give us much insight into systems-level phenomena arising from neural plasticity. A large multilayered network of neurons all of which follow the same Hebbian rule does not generate particularly useful pattern-processing abilities. Each neuron would tend to behave in a greedy fashion. If we hope to understand large-scale networks of the brain, such as the visual system, we must find more global or network-level constraints on the learning, such as predicting the sensory input over time, that would cause the entire network of neurons to evolve cooperatively toward this common goal. By the same token, once a systems-level goal for the learning has been identified and synaptic-level weight updates have been derived, it is of interest to computational modelers to try to translate their global learning procedures into local, biologically plausible learning rules such as Hebbian learning.

Self-Organization in Perceptual Systems

One of the major motivations for studying unsupervised learning is to discover the general computational principles underlying brain self-organization. Evidence of experience-dependent plasticity has been reported in a wide variety of brain areas. Perhaps the most startling evidence comes from a series of studies by Sur and colleagues (reviewed in Sur, 1989) in which artificially rerouting of the primary visual cortical input pathways to the auditory cortex in ferrets was followed by the "auditory" cortical cells developing responses to visual stimuli and exhibiting characteristics of typical visual cortical receptive fields. These and other experiments have led to the characterization of a plastic brain capable of dynamical restructuring. Thus, the goal of biologically motivated learning research may be stated as the search for the objective function(s) employed by the brain.

Information-Preserving Algorithms

Since there is no external teaching signal for unsupervised learning, the goal of the learning must be stated solely in terms of some transformation on the input that will preserve the interesting structure. The first task, then, is to define what constitutes interesting structure. Perhaps the simplest possible goal is to try to preserve *all* of the information, by, for example, simply memorizing the input patterns. Pattern-associators (see ASSOCIATIVE NETWORKS) operating in auto-associative mode can be used as such by storing each input pattern associated with itself. However, models that perform exact memorization tend to have very poor capacity and are unable to generalize their knowledge to new inputs.

Minimizing Reconstruction Error

Given the limited ability of networks to store a set of patterns exactly, a better strategy might be to try to find a *compressed* representation of the patterns. This may be helpful for preprocessing noisy data, and for modeling early stages of perceptual processing. Later stages of processing may impose additional constraints on the data reduction process, such as the need to map inputs to actions and their consequences. A standard data compression technique is PRINCIPAL COMPONENT ANALYSIS (PCA) (q.v.). Several learning procedures (reviewed in Becker and Plumbley, 1996) have been developed that converge to the first N principal directions of the input distribution. These methods are optimal with respect to minimizing the mean squared reconstruction error for linear networks. However, PCA will often fail to capture interesting structure such as clustering in the data.

A more general method for finding a compressed representation that minimizes reconstruction error is to use a nonlinear backpropagation network as an auto-encoder (Hinton, 1989), by making the desired states of the N output units identical to the states of the N input units in each case. Data compression can be achieved by making the number of hidden units $M < N$. Further, the features discovered by the hidden units may be useful for subsequent stages of processing such as classification. However, with complicated input patterns containing multiple features, it may not be possible to relate the activities of individual hidden units to specific features. One way to constrain the hidden unit representation is to add extra penalty terms to the objective function (see BACKPROPAGATION: GENERAL PRINCIPLES). For example, Zemel (1994) imposed a penalty term on hidden unit activations that caused these units to represent high-dimensional data as localized bumps of activity in a lower-dimensional constraint surface. This encouraged the hidden units to form a map-like representation that best characterized the input. Other penalty terms led to other forms of hidden representations, such as sparse, or combinatorial, representations (see MINIMUM DESCRIPTION LENGTH ANALYSIS).

Direct Minimization of Information Loss

Another approach to ensuring that the important information in the input is preserved in the output is to use concepts from information theory. This use of the term information is in a purely statistical sense, rather than the perhaps more intuitive notion that a sentence is more or less informative based on its semantic content. Viewing a neuron or neural network as a communication channel, one can calculate the rate of information loss through the channel. Atick (1992) provides an excellent review of this and related approaches, as well as a good introduction to information theory. Several learning procedures have been proposed that minimize the information loss in a network, subject to processing constraints (reviewed in Becker and Plumbley, 1996). The common feature of these methods is the preservation of mutual information between input vector $\mathbf{x}$ and output vector $\mathbf{y}$:

$$I_{x;y} = H(\mathbf{x}) + H(\mathbf{y}) - H(\mathbf{x}, \mathbf{y}) \tag{1}$$

where $H(\mathbf{x}) = -\int_{\mathbf{x}} p(\mathbf{x}) \log p(\mathbf{x}) d\mathbf{x}$ is the entropy of random variable $\mathbf{x}$ with probability distribution $p(\mathbf{x})$, and $H(\mathbf{x}, \mathbf{y}) = -\int_{\mathbf{x}, \mathbf{y}} p(\mathbf{x}, \mathbf{y}) \log p(\mathbf{x}, \mathbf{y}) d\mathbf{x} d\mathbf{y}$ is the entropy of the joint distribution of $\mathbf{x}$ and $\mathbf{y}$. The mutual information between two variables is highest when the variables have high entropies individually, but their joint distribution has low entropy. For example, a variable x with a highly peaked probability distribution $p(x)$ has very low entropy, $H(x)$; it is highly predictable a priori, and therefore a given observation of the value of x provides very little information. In contrast, a variable with a uniform distribution has maximum entropy; it is completely unpredictable a priori, and therefore one gains maximal information by having observed its value. Thus, $I_{x;y}$ is high when $\mathbf{x}$ and $\mathbf{y}$ are difficult to predict a priori, but $\mathbf{x}$ becomes predictable after the value of $\mathbf{y}$ is known (and vice versa).

If the network is free of processing noise and has enough units, its output layer can convey all the information contained in the input simply by copying the input. In 1988, Linsker first proposed applying the *Infomax principle* in the presence of Gaussian processing noise at the output layer for linear networks (Linsker, 1997). When the input distribution is Gaussian, the entropy greatly simplifies from the expected value of a log of a Gaussian to a function of the log of the variance (or the log determinant of the covariance matrix, for a multivariate Gaussian) (see, e.g., Atick, 1992). Hence, the information is:

$$I = 0.5 \log \left(\frac{|\mathbf{Q}^y|}{V(n)} \right)$$

where $|\mathbf{Q}^y|$ is the determinant of the covariance matrix of the output vector $\mathbf{y}$ (the signal plus noise) and $V(n)$ is the noise variance. Maximizing this quantity results in a trade-off between maximizing the variances of the outputs and decorrelating them, depending on the noise level. For a single output unit, this is equivalent to maximizing the output variance of a unit, and leads to a simple Hebblike learning rule. In Linsker's more recent work, he has extended this idea to networks with multiple units, nonlinearities, and sparse coding (cited in Linsker, 1997).

A related optimality criterion proposed by Barlow (1989) is to find a minimally *redundant* encoding of the sensory input vector into an n-element feature vector, which should facilitate subsequent learning. If the n features are statistically independent, then the formation of new associations with some event V (assuming the features are also approximately independent conditioned on V) only requires knowledge of the conditional probabilities of V given each feature y_i, rather than complete knowledge of the probabilities of events given each of the 2^m possible sensory inputs. Barlow proposes that one could achieve featural independence by finding a *minimum entropy encoding*: an invertible code that minimizes the sum of the feature entropies (see FEATURE ANALYSIS).

A number of algorithms for Independent Component Analysis (ICA) (for a review, see Lee et al., 2000) instantiate Barlow's principle by direct maximization of entropy. For example, in Bell and Sejnowski's algorithm (reviewed in Lee et al., 2000), a one-layer network of units with sigmoidal activation functions is able to solve the blind source separation problem: given a linear combination of N independent sources such as a mixture of acoustic signals, find a transformation to a set of N statistically independent outputs. Although this algorithm is limited in its applicability to dimensionality-preserving mappings of linear mixtures, it has been applied successfully in a number of domains, including EEG analysis, and thus has gained widespread interest in the signal processing community. More recently, Linsker (1997) has proposed a more biologically plausible version of ICA, also based on entropy maximization. It permits fewer than N output components and employs information locally available to each neural unit.

Our brains may engage in something like blind source separation, for example, when performing auditory streaming. However, unlike many ICA algorithms, which are limited in finding at most N features in an N-dimensional input, the brain has many more neurons than sensory inputs, and employs a sparse, overcomplete representation. Olshausen and Field (1996) proposed an alternative instantiation of Barlow's principle of redundancy reduction that results in such representations. Rather than directly manipulating the entropy of the coding, they minimized the following energy function:

$$E = -\sum_{x,y} \left[I(x, y) - \sum_i a_i \phi_i(x, y) \right]^2 - \lambda \sum_i S\left(\frac{a_i}{\sigma} \right) \tag{2}$$

where the leftmost term is the squared reconstruction error as a function of the image $I(x, y)$ and the weighted unit activations $\phi_i a_i$, and the rightmost term is a nonlinear function (e.g., a zero-mean Gaussian) of the unit activations chosen to enforce sparseness. The sparseness constraint favors a small number of feature detectors being active at a given moment while permitting some redundancy in the representation. The reconstruction term ensures the preservation of as much information in the input as possible. Thus, when exposed to visual images, the model tends to form local, partially overlapping receptive fields at a variety of spatial scales closely resembling those seen in early stages of the mammalian visual system (see FEATURE ANALYSIS).

Preserving Information Within Extracted Features

The methods discussed so far try to extract useful structure from data while assuming minimal prior knowledge, and are good for modeling early sensory processing. But can unsupervised learning be applied beyond these preprocessing stages, to extract higher-order features and build more abstract representations? One approach is to make constraining assumptions about the structure of interest, and build these constraints into the network's architecture or objective function.

Spatiotemporal coherence is a ubiquitous feature of sensory signals. Becker and Hinton's Imax learning procedure (reviewed in Becker, 1996) discovers coherent properties of the input by maximizing the mutual information between the *outputs*, y_a and y_b, of network modules that receive input from different parts of the sensory input (e.g., different modalities, or different spatial or temporal samples). Note how this objective function differs from the Infomax principle: the latter tries to retain *all* of the information in the input by maximizing the mutual information between inputs and outputs, whereas Imax tries to extract only those features common to two or more distinct parts of the input.

Under Gaussian assumptions about the signal and noise, Becker and Hinton simplified the mutual information I down to a log ratio of two variances, that of the signal plus noise and the noise, to derive the following objective function for the learning:

$$I = 0.5 \log \frac{V(y_a + y_b)}{V(y_a - y_b)}$$

This measure tells how much information the average of y_a and y_b conveys about the common underlying signal, i.e., the feature that is coherent across the two input samples. When applied to networks composed of multilayer modules that receive input from adjacent, nonoverlapping regions of the input, Imax discovered higher-order image features (i.e., features not learnable by single-layer or linear networks), such as stereo disparity in random dot stereograms. This illustrates how one part of the brain might self-organize within the visual modality to learn spatially predictive features. The idea could also be applied to the outputs of two different modalities to learn about their common causes (for a review of related work, see Becker, 1996). For example, when we see an object and hear a sound, the two are often correlated and probably help us to learn object categories.

Density Estimation Techniques

So far we have focused on algorithms that try to manipulate the information preserved by the network by imposing various processing constraints or representational assumptions. An alternative approach is to model directly the probability distribution over the input patterns. Many unsupervised learning procedures can be viewed in this way. The general approach is to assume a priori a class of models that constrains the general form of the probability density function, then search for the particular model parameters defining the density function most likely to have generated the observed data. This approach of developing *generative models* of data can be cast as an unsupervised learning problem by treating the network weights as the model parameters θ, and the overall function computed by the network as being directly related to the density function. The goal is to find model parameters that maximize the log likelihood that the model generated the data, x:

$$\log(L) = \sum_x \log (p(\mathbf{x}|\theta)) \qquad (3)$$

Many of the information-maximization algorithms described earlier can also be derived from this generative approach. For example, the reconstruction error in auto-encoder learning can be derived as a data-likelihood term, and the additional penalty terms in the different algorithms can be derived as particular priors over the hidden states (Zemel, 1994). And the Bell-Sejnowski ICA algorithm can be obtained by a particular choice of prior over the sources and a noise model over the input (Pearlmutter and Parra, 1997).

Mixture Models and Competitive Learning

One convenient and popular choice of prior model is a mixture of Gaussians. This model performs a type of cluster analysis, and is the basis for deriving two more biologically plausible models that we will consider afterwards. The prior assumption in this case is that each data point was actually generated by one of n Gaussians having different means μ_i, variances σ_i^2, and prior probabilities π_i. Fixing the model parameters μ_i, σ_i, and π_i, we can compute the probability of a given data point $\mathbf{x}$ under a mixture-of-Gaussians model as follows:

$$p(\mathbf{x}|\{\mu_i\}, \{\sigma_i\}, \{\pi_i\}) = \sum_{i=1}^{n} \pi_i P_i(\mathbf{x}, \mu_i, \sigma_i) \qquad (4)$$

where $P_i(\mathbf{x}, \mu_i, \sigma_i)$ is the probability of $\mathbf{x}$ under the ith Gaussian. Applying Bayes's rule, we can also compute the probability that any one of the Gaussians generated the data point $\mathbf{x}$:

$$p(i|\mathbf{x}, \{\mu_j\}, \{\sigma_j\}, \{\pi_j\}) = \frac{\pi_i P_i(\mathbf{x}, \mu_i, \sigma_i)}{\sum_{j=1}^{n} \pi_j P_j(\mathbf{x}, \mu_j, \sigma_j)} \qquad (5)$$

Given these probabilities, we can now use as a cost function the log likelihood of the data given the model:

$$\log(L) = \sum_x \log (p(\mathbf{x}|\{\mu_i\}, \{\sigma_i\}, \{\pi_i\}))$$

By maximizing this function, we can approximate the true probability distribution of the data, given our prior model assumptions. Note that by taking the log of L, we obtain a cost function that is a sum of log probabilities, rather than a product of probabilities, for each input pattern. The model parameters can then be adapted by performing gradient ascent in $\log(L)$. The Expectation-Maximization (EM) algorithm alternatingly applies Equation 4 (the expectation step) and adapts the model parameters (the maximization step) to converge on the maximum likelihood mixture model of the data.

Competitive learning procedures (see COMPETITIVE LEARNING) can be viewed as performing a discrete approximation to the density estimation algorithm just described, but it can be implemented in a more biologically realistic neural circuit. The general idea is that units compete to respond (e.g., by a winner-take-all activation function or lateral inhibition), so that only the winning unit in each competitive cluster is active. The winning unit learns by moving its weight vector closer to the current input pattern. Hence, each unit minimizes the squared distance between its weight vector and the patterns nearest to it, as in standard k-means clustering. This version of competitive learning is closely related to fitting a mixture-of-Gaussians model with equal priors π_i and equal fixed variances σ_i^2. Using the EM algorithm, every unit (not just the winner) moves its mean closer to the current input vector, in proportion to the probability that its Gaussian model accounts for the current input (Equation 5). Competitive learning approximates this step by making a binary decision as to which unit accounts for the input. Thus, the same learning rule applies, except that the proportional weighting is replaced by an all-or-none decision.

Nowlan (1990) proposed a maximum likelihood competitive learning (MLCL) model for neural networks. Rather than allowing only the winner to adapt, each unit adapts its weights for every input case, in proportion to how strongly it responds on a given case. This is an on-line version of the EM algorithm for Gaussian densities with equal priors, and adaptive means and variances. Nowlan found this method to be superior to traditional competitive learning models on several classification tasks. Becker (1999) extended MLCL to a network that computes the priors using spatio-temporal contextual cues, allowing hierarchical clustering of features based on common contexts. The architecture of Becker's model was motivated by the laminar and columnar organization seen throughout the neocortex. It was shown to learn local views of an object in the first layer, and to group nearby views together into more view-tolerant representations in the second layer.

Combinatorial Representations

A major limitation of mixture models and competitive learning is that they employ a 1-of-n encoding, in which a single unit or feature is assumed to explain each datum. A *multiple causes* model is more appropriate when the most compact data description consists of several independent parameters (e.g., color, shape, size). Some pioneering connectionist work in this area was done by Neal (1992). Neal's multilayer "sigmoid belief networks" (SBNs) resemble stochastic Boltzmann machines (see SIMULATED ANNEALING AND BOLTZMANN MACHINES), but they are strictly feedforward. Output states are held fixed on training patterns selected from the environment, while the hidden unit states are freely but noisily updated. The weights are adjusted so as to increase the probability of the hidden units generating the training patterns. The network thereby learns to represent features in the hidden layer that explain correlations in the pattern set. Unfortunately, Monte Carlo sampling is a prohibitively time-consuming way to search for good hidden layer features. Saul, Jaakkola, and Jordan (1996) proposed a way around this employing a mean field approximation for SBNs.

A major challenge in this area of research is to develop multiple-cause models for multilayered networks with top-down feedback. Perhaps the most noteworthy attempts in this direction are the Helmholtz machine, developed by Hinton et al. (see HELMHOLTZ MACHINES AND SLEEP-WAKE LEARNING), and Rao and Ballard's (1997) model. In the Helmholtz machine, the bottom-up weights embody a "recognition model"; that is, they are used to produce the most probable set of hidden states given the data. At the same time, the top-down weights constitute a "generative model"; that is, they produce a set of hidden states most likely to have generated the data. The "wake-sleep algorithm" maximizes the log likelihood of this model and results in a simple and elegant delta rule for updating either set of weights:

$$\Delta w_{kj} = \varepsilon s_k^\alpha (s_j^\alpha - p_j^\alpha) \tag{6}$$

where p_j^α is the target state for unit j on pattern α, and s_j^α is the corresponding network state, a stochastic sample based on the logistic function of the unit's net input. Target states for the generative weight updates are derived from top-down expectations based on samples using the recognition model, whereas for the recognition weights, the targets are derived by making bottom-up predictions based on samples from the generative model. The Helmholtz machine is restricted in training either the generative or the recognition connections at a given time. In contrast, Rao and Ballard's (1997) model interleaves the training of these connections. This model is based on the extended Kalman filter. At each level, representational nodes combine top-down predictions with bottom-up information to produce two sources of prediction error: (1) a predicted internal state at the next time instant that is sent to the preceding layer for predicting the bottom-up input, and (2) a prediction of the top-down input that is sent to the subsequent layer. Training is cast within a maximum likelihood framework: the model fit depends on the two sources of error mentioned above, as well as model cost terms for each of the model parameters. The model is presented as an account of learning and real-time processing in the visual cortex, and is shown to develop realistic local receptive fields as well as object-level representations when trained on natural image sequences.

Discussion

We have argued in favor of the global objective function approach to modeling unsupervised learning processes and have explored several powerful learning procedures based on this approach. These methods have had success in modeling early perceptual processing. With the incorporation of highly constraining prior models, unsupervised learning procedures can form even more abstract representations of data, and extract higher-order features. A major direction of ongoing research is aimed at finding tractable instantiations of these learning procedures and applying them in multiple learning stages to form a diversity of representational levels. Recent work by Hinton and colleagues on tractable versions of the Boltzmann machine is a promising example of such efforts.

Acknowledgments. The authors acknowledge support from the Natural Sciences and Engineering Research Council of Canada (S. B.) and the Office of Naval Research (R. Z.).

Road Map: Learning in Artificial Networks
Background: Perceptrons, Adalines, and Backpropagation
Related Reading: Competitive Learning; Hebbian Synaptic Plasticity

References

Atick, J. J., 1992, Could information theory provide an ecological theory of sensory processing? *Network*, 3:213–251.

Barlow, H. B., 1989. Unsupervised learning, *Neural Computat.*, 1:295–311. ◆

Becker, S., 1996, Mutual information maximization: Models of cortical self-organization, *Netw. Computat. Neural Syst.*, 7:7–31.

Becker, S., 1999, Implicit learning in 3d object recognition: The importance of temporal context, *Neural Computat.*, 11:347–374.

Becker, S., and Plumbley, M., 1996, Unsupervised neural network learning procedures for feature extraction and classification, *Int. J. App. Intell.*, 6(3):185–205. ◆

Hinton, G. E., 1989, Connectionist learning procedures, *Artif. Intell.*, 40:185–234. ◆

Lee, T., Girolami, M., Bell, A., and Sejnowski, T., 2000, A unifying information-theoretic framework for independent component analysis, *Comput. Math. Appl.*, 39:1–21.

Linsker, R., 1997, Local synaptic learning rules suffice to maximize mutual information, *Neural Computat.*, 9:1661–1665.

Neal, R. M., 1992, Connectionist learning of belief networks, *Artif. Intell.*, 56:71–113.

Nowlan, S. J., 1990, Maximum likelihood competitive learning, in *Neural Information Processing Systems*, vol. 2 (D. S. Touretzky, Ed.), San Mateo, CA: Morgan Kaufmann, pp. 574–582.

Olshausen, B. A., and Field, D. J., 1996, Emergence of simple-cell receptive field properties by learning a sparse code for natural images, *Nature*, 381:607–609.

Pearlmutter, B. A., and Parra, L. C., 1997, Maximum likelihood blind source separation: A context-sensitive generalization of ICA, in *Neural Information Processing Systems*, vol. 9 (M. Mozer, M. Jordan, and T. Petsche, Eds.), Cambridge, MA: MIT Press, pp. 613–619.

Rao, R. P. N., and Ballard, D. H., 1997, Dynamic model of visual recognition predicts neural response properties in the visual cortex, *Neural Computat.*, 9:721–763.

Saul, L. K., Jaakkola, T., and Jordan, M. I., 1996, Mean field theory for sigmoid belief networks, *J. Artif. Intell. Res.*, 4:61–76.

Sur, M., 1989, Visual plasticity in the auditory pathway: Visual inputs induced into auditory thalamus and cortex illustrate principles of adaptive organization in sensory systems, in *Dynamic Interactions in Neural Networks: Models and Data* (M. Arbib and S. Amari, Eds.), New York: Springer-Verlag, pp. 35–51.

Zemel, R. S., 1994, A minimum description length framework for unsupervised learning, PhD diss., University of Toronto.

Vapnik-Chervonenkis Dimension of Neural Nets

Peter L. Bartlett and Wolfgang Maass

Introduction

For any assignment of values to its internal parameters θ (weights, thresholds, etc.) a neural network $\mathcal{N}$ with binary outputs computes a function $x \mapsto \mathcal{N}(\theta, x)$ from D into $\{0, 1\}$, where D is the domain of the network inputs x (e.g., $D = \mathbb{R}^n$). The Vapnik-Chervonenkis dimension (VC-dimension) of $\mathcal{N}$ is a number that may be viewed as a measure of the richness (or diversity) of the collection of all functions $x \mapsto \mathcal{N}(\theta, x)$ that can be computed by $\mathcal{N}$ for different values of its internal parameters θ. Not surprisingly, the VC-dimension of a neural network is related to the number of training examples that are needed in order to train $\mathcal{N}$ to compute—or approximate—a specific target function $h : D \to \{0, 1\}$. We shall discuss a number of different types of neural networks, but typically the VC-dimension grows polynomially (in many cases, between linearly and quadratically) with the number of adjustable parameters of the neural network. In particular, if the number of training examples is large compared to the VC-dimension, the network's performance on training data is a reliable indication of its future performance on subsequent data.

The concept of the VC-dimension, which was introduced by Vapnik and Chervonenkis in 1971, is not specific to neural networks. It applies to any parameterized class F of functions $x \mapsto f(\theta, x)$ from some domain D into $\{0, 1\}$, where θ ranges over some given parameter space, for example, $\mathbb{R}^w$. Related notions for the case of real-valued outputs will be discussed later. The largest possible richness of this class F of functions from D into $\{0, 1\}$ is achieved if *every* function $h : D \to \{0, 1\}$ can be computed by a function $x \mapsto f(\theta, x)$ in F. In this case one says that D is *shattered* by F, and the VC-dimension of F is equal to $|D|$, the number of elements of the domain D. In the general case one defines the VC-dimension of F (VCdim (F)) as the size of the largest subset D' of its domain D so that D' is shattered by F (or, more precisely, by the restrictions of the functions $x \mapsto f(\theta, x)$ in F to inputs $x \in D'$). In other words, the VC-dimension of F is the size of the largest subset D' of its domain D for which every dichotomy h over D' (i.e., each of the $2^{|D'|}$ many functions $h : D' \mapsto \{0, 1\}$) can be computed by some function in F, or in mathematical notation:

$$\forall h : D' \to \{0, 1\} \; \exists \; \theta \forall x \in D'(f(\theta, x) = h(x))$$

Although the definition of the VC-dimension focuses on the shattering effect, it yields a remarkable bound that holds for *all* finite subsets X of the domain D: If d is the VC-dimension of F, then at most $\Sigma_{i=0}^{d} \binom{|X|}{i} \le |X|^d + 1$ functions from X into $\{0, 1\}$ can be computed by (restrictions of) functions in F. This estimate, which is commonly referred to as Sauer's lemma, was independently discovered by several authors, including Vapnik and Chervonenkis in 1971 (see Anthony and Bartlett, 1999, chap. 3, for a review). Results of this form provide the mathematical basis for bounding the number of training examples that are needed for learning functions in F in terms of the VC-dimension of F, as in the following theorem. (This theorem is a consequence of a slightly improved version, due to Talagrand, of a result from Vapnik and Chervonenkis, 1971; see Anthony and Bartlett, 1999, chap. 4, for related references.)

Theorem 1. Suppose that F is a class of functions mapping from a domain X into $\{0, 1\}$, and suppose also that F has VC-dimension $d < \infty$. Let $((x_1, y_1), \ldots, (x_m, y_m))$ be a sequence of m randomly chosen labeled training examples from $X \times \{0, 1\}$. Then, with probability at least $1 - \delta$ over this sequence, any function $f \in F$ has

$$\Pr(f(x) \ne y) \le \frac{1}{m} |\{1 \le i \le m : f(x_i) \ne y_i\}| + \varepsilon$$

provided that $m \ge c(d + \log(1/\delta))/\varepsilon^2$, where c is a universal constant.

In particular, if the sample size is large compared to the VC-dimension of the function class, the function from the class that minimizes the number of errors on a training sample will have near-minimal probability of misclassifying subsequent patterns (see PAC LEARNING AND NEURAL NETWORKS).

The definition of the VC-dimension of a function class F immediately implies that VCdim$(F) \le \log_2 |F|$ if F is finite. Thus, in particular if F is parameterized by w k-bit parameters, VCdim$(F) \le kw$. However, many infinite classes F also have a finite VC-dimension. Consider, for example, the class F_{T2} of functions from $\mathbb{R}^2$ into $\{0, 1\}$ that can be computed by linear threshold gates (McCulloch-Pitts neurons) with two inputs:

$$F_{T2} = \{\langle x_1, x_2 \rangle \mapsto \mathcal{H}(\theta_1 x_1 + \theta_2 x_2 - \theta_3) :$$
$$\theta = \langle \theta_1, \theta_2, \theta_3 \rangle \in \mathbb{R}^3\}$$

where $\mathcal{H}(x) = 1$ if $x \ge 0$, otherwise $\mathcal{H}(x) = 0$. (See Figure 1; the shaded region in each box corresponds to $h(x) = 1$.) Obviously, the set $D' := \{\langle 0, 0 \rangle, \langle 0, 1 \rangle, \langle 1, 0 \rangle\}$ can be shattered by F_{T2} (as illustrated by the eight dichotomies shown in Figure 1). On the other hand it is easy to see that the set $D' \cup \{\langle 1, 1 \rangle\}$ *cannot* be shattered by F (since the dichotomy h that assumes the value 1 on the points $\langle 0, 0 \rangle$ and $\langle 1, 1 \rangle$ and the value 0 on the points $\langle 0, 1 \rangle$ and $\langle 1, 0 \rangle$ cannot be computed by any linear threshold gate). Somewhat less obvious to see is that there exists *no* set $D' \subseteq \mathbb{R}^2$ consisting of four or more points that is shattered by F_{T2}, i.e., that 3 is in fact the VC-dimension of F_{T2}. This follows immediately from the following theorem.

Theorem 2. (Wenocur and Dudley) Let F_{Tn} be the class of functions from $\mathbb{R}^n$ into $\{0, 1\}$ that can be computed by a linear threshold gate, for any $n \in \mathbb{N}$. Then F_{Tn} has VC-dimension $n + 1$.

Sketch of the proof. One can easily verify that the set $S := \{\underline{0}\} \cup \{e_i : i \in \{1, \ldots, n\}\}$ is shattered by $\mathcal{N}$ (where $e_i \in \{0, 1\}^n$ denotes the ith unit vector). Hence VCdim$(\mathcal{N}) \ge n + 1$. The upper bound follows from Radon's theorem, which states that any set S of $\ge n + 2$ points in $\mathbb{R}^n$ can be partitioned into sets S_0 and S_1 such that the convex hulls of S_0 and S_1 intersect. Obviously, such sets S_0 and S_1 cannot be separated by any hyperplane, and hence not by any linear threshold gate. □

Feedforward Neural Nets with Binary Output

Theorem 3. (Cover, 1968; Baum and Haussler, 1989) Let $\mathcal{N}$ be an arbitrary feedforward neural net with w weights that consists of linear threshold gates. Then VCdim$(\mathcal{N}) = O(w \cdot \log w)$.

Sketch of the proof. Let S be some arbitrary set of m input vectors for $\mathcal{N}$. By Theorem 2 and Sauer's lemma, a gate g in $\mathcal{N}$ can compute at most $|X|^{\text{fan-in}(g)+1} + 1$ different functions from any finite set $X \subseteq \mathbb{R}^{\text{fan-in}(g)}$ into $\{0, 1\}$, where fan-in(g) denotes the number of inputs of gate g. Hence $\mathcal{N}$ can compute at most $\Pi_{g \text{ gate in } \mathcal{N}}(m^{\text{fan-in}(g)+1} + 1) \le m^{2w}$ different functions from S into $\{0, 1\}$. If S is shattered by $\mathcal{N}$, then $\mathcal{N}$ can compute all 2^m functions from S into $\{0, 1\}$, which implies that $2^m \le m^{2w}$, and hence

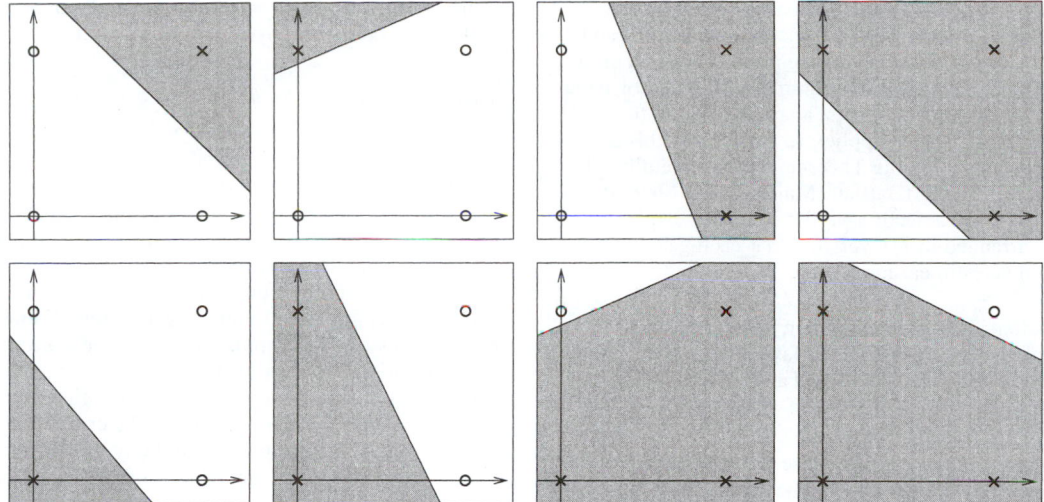

Figure 1. Eight dichotomies of four points in $\mathbb{R}^2$ computed by the class F_{T2} of linear threshold functions. For each of the eight functions $h \in F_{T2}$ illustrated, the shaded region represents the half-space where $h(x) = 1$. When a point x satisfies $h(x) = 1$, it is marked as a cross; when it satisfies $h(x) = 0$, it is marked as a circle. The functions illustrated show that the set $\{\langle 0, 0 \rangle, \langle 0, 1 \rangle, \langle 1, 0 \rangle\}$ is shattered by F_{T2}.

$m \leq 2w \cdot \log m$. It follows that $\log m = O(\log w)$; thus $m = O(w \cdot \log w)$. □

It is tempting to conjecture that the VC-dimension of a neural net $\mathcal{N}$ cannot be larger than the total number of parameters in $\mathcal{N}$, which, in view of Theorem 2, is equal to the sum of the VC-dimensions of the individual gates in $\mathcal{N}$. This conjecture would imply that the $O(w \log w)$ upper bound of Theorem 3 can be improved to $O(w)$. However, the following result (whose proof uses techniques from circuit complexity theory) shows that the superlinear upper bound of Theorem 3 is in fact asymptotically optimal. Hence, with regard to the VC-dimension it is fair to say that a neural net can be "more than the sum of its parts."

Theorem 4. (Maass, 1993) There exist neural networks $\mathcal{N}$ consisting of linear threshold gates whose VC-dimension scales proportional to $w \cdot \log w$, where w is the number of parameters of $\mathcal{N}$.

This superlinear growth of the VC-dimension occurs already for feedforward neural nets with two hidden layers in the case of discrete network inputs. Sakurai (1993) showed that for the case of continuous network inputs it may even occur with a single hidden layer.

Proving upper bounds for sigmoidal neural nets, whose computational units employ some smooth activation function instead of the Heaviside function $\mathcal{H}$, turns out to be quite challenging. For instance, there exists a feedforward neural net consisting of a linear threshold gate as output unit and two hidden units that employ as activation function a very smooth (real analytic) strictly increasing squashing function, which has an infinite VC-dimension. (See, for example, Anthony and Bartlett, 1999; the first result of this form was due to Sontag, 1998.) This shows that it is necessary to exploit more specific properties of a particular activation function, for example, of the logistic sigmoid, in order to achieve a finite upper bound for the VC-dimension of a sigmoidal neural net. The following theorem (Goldberg and Jerrum, 1995) provides the key step in this direction.

Theorem 5. (Goldberg and Jerrum, 1995) Consider the parameterized class

$$F = \{x \mapsto f(\theta, x) : \theta \in \mathbb{R}^d\}$$

for some $\{\pm 1\}$-valued function f. Suppose that, for each input $x \in \mathbb{R}^n$, there is an algorithm that computes $f(\theta, x)$, and this computation takes no more than t operations of the following types:

- the arithmetic operations $+$, $-$, $\times$, and $/$ on real numbers,
- jumps conditioned on $>$, $\geq$, $<$, $\leq$, $=$, and $\neq$ comparisons of real numbers, and
- output 0 or 1.

Then $\mathrm{VCdim}(H) \leq 4d(t + 2)$.

The proof involves counting cells in parameter space. Consider a single thresholded real-valued function, such as a neural network with a single real output that is thresholded at 0. Fix a set of n input patterns. To estimate the VC-dimension, we can estimate the number of distinct dichotomies of those patterns. Suppose two parameter values give distinct output labels for one of these patterns. Then, in moving between these distinct values in parameter space, we must pass through a parameter value where the real output is zero in response to the pattern. Such values form the boundaries of cells in parameter space, and within a cell all classifications are identical. Under appropriate conditions, counting the number of dichotomies reduces to counting the number of these cells. For well-behaved parameterizations, the number of cells defined by these zero sets is closely related to the number of distinct solutions of generic systems of equations. If the output of the network is polynomial in the parameters, classical results give bounds on the number of such solutions, and hence on the number of dichotomies. (Ben-David and Lindenbaum independently obtained this proof and result in a paper that appeared at the same conference as Goldberg and Jerrum's paper.) The argument is essentially unchanged if the parameterized function class is a fixed Boolean function of a number of thresholded functions that are each polynomial in the parameters. If the computation of $f(\theta, x)$ involves few operations, this implies that f can be represented as a fixed Boolean function of a small number of thresholded, low-degree polynomials.

Piecewise Polynomial Activation Functions

As an example of the application of Theorem 5, the output of a linear threshold net can be computed using $O(w)$ of the operations listed in the theorem, where w is the number of parameters, so the VC-dimension is $O(w^2)$. Theorem 3 shows that this bound can be improved to $O(w \cdot \log w)$. Similarly, if the nonlinearity is a piecewise polynomial function with a fixed number of pieces of fixed degree, the number of operations is again $O(w)$, so the VC-dimension bound of $O(w^2)$ again applies. In some cases, this bound also can be improved, by applying Theorem 5 more carefully. This leads to the following bound (Bartlett, Maiorov, and Meir, 1998) on the VC-dimension of a feedforward neural net of piecewise polynomial gates arranged in L layers (so that each gate has connections only from gates in earlier layers).

Theorem 6. (Bartlett, Maiorov, and Meir, 1998)   Suppose $\mathcal{N}$ is a feedforward network with w weights, l layers, and all nonoutput gates having a fixed piecewise-polynomial activation function with a fixed number of pieces. Then $\mathrm{VCdim}(\mathcal{N}) = O(wl \log w + wl^2)$.

Linear threshold gates have a piecewise polynomial activation function. Thus, Theorem 6, together with the lower bound for linear threshold nets (Theorem 4), shows that the VC-dimension of piecewise polynomial networks with a fixed number of layers is also $\Theta(w \log w)$. Perhaps surprisingly, the transition from linear threshold gates to piecewise polynomial gates does not increase the rate of growth of the VC-dimension for networks with a fixed number of layers.

In contrast, if the number of layers is unbounded, the rate of growth of the VC-dimension can be faster for piecewise polynomial networks than for linear threshold networks. The following lower bound applies to networks of gates with an activation function satisfying two conditions: it has distinct left and right limits, and it has non-zero slope somewhere. This result is due to Koiran and Sontag (1997) the refinement to give the dependence on the depth was shown by Bartlett, Maiorov, and Meir, and also by Sakurai.

Theorem 7.   Suppose the activation function $s : \mathbb{R} \to \mathbb{R}$ has the following properties:

1. $\lim_{\alpha \to \infty} s(\alpha) \neq \lim_{\alpha \to -\infty} s(\alpha)$, and
2. s is differentiable at some point $\alpha_0 \in \mathbb{R}$, with $s'(\alpha_0) \neq 0$.

Then for any l and $w \le 10l$, there is a neural network $\mathcal{N}$ with l layers and w parameters, where every gate but the output gate has activation function s, the output gate being a linear threshold gate, and for which the VC-dimension scales as lw. In particular, for $l = \Theta(w)$, there are such networks with $\mathrm{VCdim}(\mathcal{N}) = \Omega(w^2)$.

Sigmoidal Activation Functions

While the VC-dimension of networks with piecewise polynomial activation functions is well understood, most applications of neural networks use the logistic sigmoid function, or gaussian radial basis function. Unfortunately, it is not possible to compute such functions using a finite number of the arithmetic operations listed in Theorem 5. However, Karpinski and Macintyre (1997) extended Theorem 5 to allow the computation of exponentials. The proof uses the same ideas, but the bound on the number of solutions of a system of equations is substantially more difficult.

Theorem 8.   Consider the parameterized class

$$F = \{x \mapsto f(\theta, x) : \theta \in \mathbb{R}^d\}$$

for some $\{\pm 1\}$-valued function f. Suppose that, for each input $x \in \mathbb{R}^n$, there is an algorithm that computes $f(\theta, x)$, and this computation takes no more than t operations of the following types:

- the exponential function $\alpha \mapsto e^\alpha$ on real numbers, and
- all of the operations listed in Theorem 5.

Then $\mathrm{VCdim}(F) = O(t^2 d^2)$.

We immediately obtain bounds for the VC-dimension of sigmoid networks and radial basis networks of the form $O(w^4)$, where w is the number of parameters. This upper bound is considerably larger than the $\Theta(w \log w)$ bound achieved for linear threshold networks or fixed-depth piecewise polynomial networks. It remains open whether it is optimal. For fixed-depth sigmoid networks, the best lower bounds are those implied by Theorems 4 and 7: $\Omega(w \log w)$ for networks of fixed depth, and $\Omega(w^2)$ for arbitrary depth.

If the inputs are restricted to a finite set of integers, a simple parameter transformation allows the machinery of the piecewise polynomial case to be applied to two-layer sigmoid networks, giving the following result. (See Anthony and Bartlett, 1999, for a proof.) A related result applies to Gaussian radial basis networks.

Theorem 9.   Consider a two-layer feedforward network $\mathcal{N}$ with input domain $X = \{-k, \ldots, k\}^n$ (for $k \in \mathbb{N}$) and first-layer computation gates with the standard sigmoid activation function (the output gate being a linear threshold gate). Let w be the total number of parameters in the network. Then $\mathrm{VCdim}(\mathcal{N}) = O(w \log(wk))$.

Feedforward Neural Nets with Real Outputs

All of the results presented so far apply to nets with binary-valued outputs. Neural networks with real outputs are also commonly used, for instance in regression problems. In such cases, the appropriate measure of complexity of the network is a scale-sensitive version of the VC-dimension called the *fat-shattering dimension*.

Suppose that F is a set of functions mapping from a domain X to $\mathbb{R}$, $D = \{x_1, x_2, \ldots, x_m\}$ is a subset of the domain X, and γ is a positive real number. Then we say that D is γ-shattered by F if there are real numbers $r_1, r_2, \ldots, r_m$ such that for all $b \in \{0, 1\}^m$ there is a function f_b in F with

$$f_b(x_i) \ge r_i + \gamma \quad \text{if } b_i = 1$$
$$f_b(x_i) \le r_i - \gamma \quad \text{if } b_i = 0$$

for $1 \le i \le m$. The *fat-shattering dimension* of F at scale γ, denoted $\mathrm{fat}_F(\gamma)$, is the size of the largest subset D of the domain X that is γ-shattered by F.

It is significant that this notion of complexity depends on a scale parameter γ. In a sense, the fat-shattering dimension ignores complex behavior of the function class below a certain scale. If we are concerned with predicting a real value to some accuracy ε then it seems that the behavior of the function class on a scale much smaller than ε should not be relevant. The following result formalizes this intuition by showing that the fat-shattering dimension is related to the number of training examples that are needed to solve a regression problem. Although the result is stated in terms of the squared prediction error, similar results apply to a broad class of loss functions. (The result relies on a generalization of Sauer's lemma to the fat-shattering dimension, from Alon et al., 1997.) See, for example, Anthony and Bartlett, 1999, for a proof.)

Theorem 10.   Suppose that F is a class of functions mapping from a domain X into the real interval $[0, 1]$, and suppose also that F has finite fat-shattering dimension. Let $((x_1, y_1), \ldots, (x_m, y_m))$ be a sequence of m randomly chosen labeled training examples from $X \times [0, 1]$. Then there are constants c_1, c_2 such that, with probability at least $1 - \delta$, any function $f*$ that has the average over the sample of $(f*(x) - y)^2$ within $1/\sqrt{m}$ of the infimum over F satisfies

$$E(f*(x) - y)^2 \le \inf_{g \in F} E(g(x) - y)^2 + \varepsilon \qquad (1)$$

provided that $m \ge c_1(\text{fat}_F(c_2\varepsilon) \log^2(1/\varepsilon) + \log(1/\delta))/\varepsilon^2$.

It is also known that for any learning algorithm to return a function $f*$ that satisfies Equation 1 requires the amount of training data to grow at least as $\text{fat}_F(\varepsilon)$. This shows that the fat-shattering dimension is the right measure of complexity of a function class that is used for regression.

The fat-shattering dimension is also useful for pattern classification using thresholded real-valued functions, like neural networks. Many practical algorithms for such functions typically lead to solutions that have large *margins* on the training data, where the margin of a thresholded real-valued function is the amount by which the function is to the correct side of the threshold. The following result, from Bartlett (1998), shows that in these cases the fat-shattering dimension gives an upper bound on the error.

Theorem 11. Consider a class F of real-valued functions. With probability at least $1 - \delta$ over m independently generated examples $(x_1, y_1), \ldots, (x_m, y_m)$, for every function f in F, the classifier $\mathcal{H}(f)$ has misclassification probability no more than

$$\frac{b}{m} + O\left(\sqrt{\frac{1}{m}\left(\text{fat}_F(\gamma/16)\ \log^2 m\ +\ \log(1/\delta)\right)}\right)$$

where b is the number of labeled training examples with margin no more than γ.

The easiest way to obtain bounds on the fat-shattering dimension for neural networks is via VC-dimension bounds. The following theorem shows that the fat-shattering dimension of a network is no bigger than the VC-dimension of a slightly larger network with one additional input variable. The theorem is a trivial observation involving another combinatorial dimension, called the *pseudo-dimension*; see Chapters 11 and 14 of Anthony and Bartlett (1999) for details.

Theorem 12. Let $\mathcal{N}$ be any neural network with a single real-valued output unit, and form a neural network $\mathcal{N}'$ as follows. The network $\mathcal{N}'$ has one extra real input and one extra computation unit. This additional computation unit is the output unit of $\mathcal{N}'$, and is a linear threshold unit receiving input only from the output unit of $\mathcal{N}$ and from the new input. For any $\gamma > 0$, $\text{fat}_{\mathcal{N}}(\gamma) \le \text{VCdim}(\mathcal{N}')$.

This result and the upper bounds of the previous section immediately imply upper bounds on the fat-shattering dimension of networks with linear threshold gates, with piecewise polynomial activation functions, and with logistic sigmoidal activation functions. These bounds are in terms of the number of parameters in the network, and, significantly, do not depend on the scale parameter γ. In some cases, bounds like this are very loose.

For example, the following theorem (Bartlett, 1998) gives an upper bound on the fat-shattering dimension of a two-layer network with an arbitrary number of computation units (and hence parameters).

Theorem 13. Suppose that $s : R \to [-b, b]$ is a nondecreasing bounded function. For $v \ge 1$, suppose that F is the class of functions from R^n to R computed by two layer neural networks with an arbitrary number of first layer units, each with activation function s, and a linear output unit for which the sum of the magnitudes of the weights is bounded by v. Then

$$\text{fat}_F(\varepsilon) = O\left(\frac{nv^2}{\varepsilon^2} \ln\left(\frac{v}{\varepsilon}\right)\right)$$

It follows that for regression and pattern classification (when the learning algorithm finds a network with large margins on the training data), it is not necessary to restrict the number of parameters in the network, provided the parameters are kept small. Bounds of this kind are also known for deeper networks; see Anthony and Bartlett (1999) for details.

Other Applications to Neural Networks

The VC-dimension of recurrent neural networks was analyzed by DasGupta, Koiran, and Sontag (see Sontag, 1998, for a survey of results for feedforward and recurrent neural nets). In this case it is of interest to consider the case of a time series as the network input. The length k of the time series enters the bounds for the VC-dimension of the neural network as an additional parameter (in most bounds the number w of network parameters is multiplied by a factor of the form $\log k$ or k).

In models for biological neural circuits the transmission delays between neurons enter as additional parameters, which influence the VC-dimension of such circuits even more than the synaptic weights: the VC-dimension of a very simple mathematical model for a single spiking neuron grows superlinearly in the number d of adjustable delays, and the VC-dimension of a feedforward network of such neurons grows quadratically in d (Maass and Schmitt, 1999).

In Koiran (1996), a technique was introduced for using *upper* bounds on the VC-dimension of neural networks for proving *lower* bounds on the size of any sigmoidal neural net (with thresholded output) that is able to compute some concrete function. No other method for proving lower bounds on the size of sigmoidal neural nets is known at present. This technique can, for example, be used to show that there exist functions that can be computed with few spiking neurons, but if they are computed by a sigmoidal neural net, the number of neurons must grow linearly in the number of inputs (see SPIKING NEURONS, COMPUTING WITH).

Discussion

The VC-dimension of a neural net with a binary output measures its "expressiveness." The related notion of the fat-shattering dimension provides a similar tool for the analysis of a neural net with a real-valued output. The derivation of bounds for the VC-dimension and the fat-shattering dimension of neural nets has turned out to be a rather challenging but quite interesting chapter in the mathematical investigation of neural nets. This work has brought a number of sophisticated mathematical tools into this research area, which have subsequently turned out to be also useful for the solution of a variety of other problems regarding the complexity of computing and learning on neural nets. More detailed information about the results presented in this article can be found in Anthony and Bartlett (1999).

Bounds for the VC-dimension (respectively fat-shattering dimension) of a neural net $\mathcal{N}$ provide estimates for the number of random examples that are needed to train $\mathcal{N}$ so that it has good generalization properties (i.e., so that the error of $\mathcal{N}$ on new examples from the same distribution is at most ε, with probability $\ge 1 - \delta$). From the point of view of a single application, these bounds tend to be too large, since they provide such a generalization guarantee for *any* probability distribution on the examples and for *any* training algorithm that minimizes disagreement on the training examples. For some special distributions and specific training algorithms, tighter bounds can be obtained, for instance with the help of heuristic arguments (replica techniques) from statistical physics.

Road Map: Computability and Complexity
Related Reading: Learning and Generalization: Theoretical Bounds; PAC Learning and Neural Networks

References

Alon, N., Ben-David, S., Cesa-Bianchi, N., and Haussler, D., 1997, Scale-sensitive dimensions, uniform convergence, and learnability, *J. ACM,* 44:616–631.

Anthony, M., and Bartlett, P. L., 1999, *Neural Network Learning: Theoretical Foundations,* Cambridge, Engl.: Cambridge University Press. ◆

Bartlett, P. L., 1998, The sample complexity of pattern classification with neural networks: The size of the weights is more important than the size of the network, *IEEE Trans. Inform. Theory,* 44:525–536.

Bartlett, P. L., Maiorov, V., and Meir, R., 1998, Almost linear VC-dimension bounds for piecewise polynomial networks, *Neural Comput.,* 10:2159–2173.

Baum, E. B., and Haussler, D., 1989, What size net gives valid generalization? *Neural Comput.,* 1:151–160.

Cover, T. M., 1968, Capacity problems for linear machines, in *Pattern Recognition* (L. Kanal, Ed.), Washington, DC: Thompson Book Co., pp. 283–289.

Goldberg, P. W., and Jerrum, M. R., 1995, Bounding the Vapnik-Chervonenkis dimension of concept classes parametrized by real numbers, *Machine Learn.,* 18:131–148.

Karpinski, M., and Macintyre, A. J., 1997, Polynomial bounds for VC dimension of sigmoidal and general Pfaffian neural networks, *J. Comput. Syst. Sci.,* 54:169–176.

Koiran, P., 1996, VC-dimension in circuit complexity, in *Proceedings of the 11th IEEE Conference on Computational Complexity,* pp. 81–85.

Koiran, P., and Sontag, E. D., 1997, Neural networks with quadratic VC dimension, *J. Comput. Syst. Sci.,* 54:190–198.

Maass, W., 1993, Bounds for the computational power and learning complexity of analog neural nets, *Neural Computat.,* 6:875–882.

Maass, W., and Schmitt, M., 1999, On the complexity of learning for spiking neurons with temporal coding, *Inform. Computat.,* 153:26–46.

Sakurai, A., 1993, Tighter bounds of the VC-dimension of three-layer networks, *Proc. WCNN 93,* 3:540–543; 45:20–48.

Sontag, E. D., 1998, VC-dimension of neural networks, in *Neural Networks and Machine Learning* (C. M. Bishop, Ed.), Berlin: Springer-Verlag, pp. 69–95. ◆

Vapnik, V. N., and Chervonenkis, A. Y., 1971, On the uniform convergence of relative frequencies of events to their probabilities, *Theory Prob. Appl.,* 16:264–280.

Vestibulo-Ocular Reflex

Thomas J. Anastasio

Introduction

The function of the vestibulo-ocular reflex (VOR) is to stabilize the retinal image by producing eye rotations that compensate for head rotations (Wilson and Melvill Jones, 1979). The VOR forms an integral part of the oculomotor system, which includes the saccadic and pursuit systems (Robinson, 1989). Although it is considered a simple reflex, the neural circuits that mediate the VOR perform diverse computations that include oculomotor command integration, temporal signal processing, temporal pattern generation, and experience-dependent plasticity. Theory and neural network modeling have played an important role in understanding all of these processes.

Classical Analysis and Linear Systems Modeling of the VOR

The VOR works in three dimensions. While modelers have recently turned their attention to the three-dimensional VOR (e.g., Schnabolk and Raphan, 1994), most analysis and modeling has focused on the horizontal VOR. A simplified schematic of the horizontal VOR is shown in Figure 1. The bilateral structure of the real VOR is suppressed in the schematic for clarity.

Eye movements elicited by the VOR describe a temporal pattern called nystagmus, in which compensatory slow-phase eye rotations are interrupted by fast-phase eye rotations that reset the orbital position of the eye. The VOR slow phase is produced in large part by the basic three-neuron arc, which consists of semicircular canal afferent neurons (CAs), vestibular nucleus interneurons (VNs), and eye muscle motoneurons (MNs). The slow-phase signal is transformed by two processes, velocity storage (VS) and neural integration (NI), both of which are essentially leaky temporal integrators (VS is much leakier than NI). The fast phase occurs after reticular burst neurons (BNs) are brought to threshold by VNs.

The cerebellum mediates experience-dependent adaptation of the VOR, and is represented in the schematic by a Purknje cell (PC). The VOR interfaces with other oculomotor subsystems at the VN

level. For example, pursuit signals modulate VNs through the cerebellum (PURSUIT EYE MOVEMENTS).

Semicircular Canals and Canal Afferents

The semicircular canals (SCs) are fluid-filled tori, imbedded in the skull, with a membrane spanning the lumen at one end. Head rotation causes deflection of the membrane against the fluid. Classical analysis of SC dynamics considers the balance of forces associated with head rotational acceleration, fluid inertia and viscosity, and membrane elasticity (Wilson and Melvill Jones, 1979). Due to the dynamic lag introduced by fluid viscosity, membrane deflection is mostly proportional to head rotational velocity. The SC response to an impulse head rotational acceleration would be a deflection of the membrane, followed by an exponential decay back to baseline with a time constant of about five seconds.

Hair cells (HCs) that are sensitive to canal membrane deflection make synaptic contact with CAs, which transmit head rotation in-

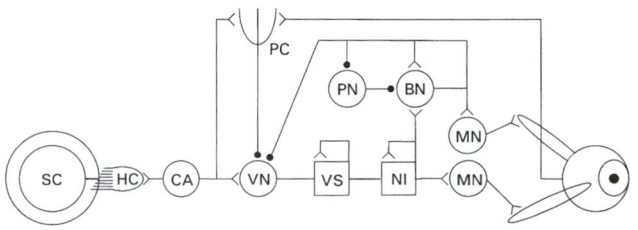

Figure 1. Highly simplified schematic diagram of the neural circuitry that mediates the slow- and fast-phases of the vestibulo-ocular reflex, and adaptive modification of the slow-phase by the cerebellum. SC, semicircular canal; HC, hair cell; CA, canal afferent; VN, vestibular nucleus neuron; VS, velocity storage element; NI, neural integrator; MN, motoneuron; BN, burst neuron; PN, pause neuron; PC, Purkinje cell; bifurcations, excitatory synapses; filled circles, inhibitory synapses.

formation to VNs. The CAs have a baseline firing rate that is modulated up and down for on- and off-direction head rotations, respectively. As expected from SC dynamic analysis, the CA response to an impulse head rotational acceleration decays exponentially with a time constant of about 5 s.

Vestibular Nucleus Neurons and Motor neurons

MNs combine the commands they receive from premotor neurons (such as VNs and BNs) and relay them to the eye muscles (Robinson, 1989). Except for differences in baseline rate and sensitivity, MNs form a homogeneous group. In contrast, VNs receive various oculomotor signals, such as vestibular and pursuit, and combine them in a diverse, seemingly random way (Scudder and Fuchs, 1992). The VNs also form part of the circuits that mediate VS and NI.

The function of VS is to lengthen the CA time constant from about five to about twenty seconds. This prolongs the period during which the VOR can produce compensatory eye movements. Production of the VOR command essentially involves adding the VS and CA signals. Two mechanisms have been proposed whereby this may occur. Raphan, Matsuo, and Cohen (1979) proposed two parallel pathways from VNs to MNs, one carrying the CA and the other the VS signal. Robinson (1981) proposed that VNs feed the CA signal back to themselves through the VS element. Raphan's model predicted that VNs should carry either the CA or the VS signal, while Robinson's model predicted that VNs should carry the VOR signal fully formed. Neither model accounted for the response diversity actually observed for VNs, or for the high sensitivity and low baseline of VNs in comparison to CAs (Baker, Evinger, and McCrea, 1981).

The function of NI is to transform eye velocity commands, such as the VOR signal, into eye position commands. Both velocity and position components are needed to control eye movements (Robinson, 1981). The mechanisms that underlie NI and VS probably involve positive feedback, which is indicated only schematically in Figure 1 using excitatory self-connections. The probable substrate for VS and NI in the nervous system is mutual inhibition between VNs on opposite sides of the VOR pathway, mediated by the inhibitory commissural fibers that interconnect the VNs bilaterally (Wilson and Melvill Jones, 1979). Mutual inhibition allows VNs to integrate push-pull signals in the bilateral pathway without integrating the VN baseline rate. Control systems modeling has demonstrated how commissural connections could produce temporal signal processing in the bilateral VOR and also account for the dynamic properties of VN neurons (Galiana and Outerbridge, 1984).

Burst Neurons and Pause Neurons

Fast-phase eye movements are driven by BNs located in the reticular formation (Shimazu, 1983). BNs are spontaneously silent, due to inhibition from pause neurons (PNs) and perhaps also to intrinsic inhibitory bias. PNs have a constant baseline rate but pause just before and during fast phases. BNs are brought to threshold by VNs and, as a group, inhibit both VNs and PNs. It was widely assumed that the role of PNs is to keep BNs from bursting (Leigh and Zee, 1983). Models of bursting needed a special "trigger" to shut off the PNs before the BNs could burst. No direct evidence for the hypothetical trigger has been provided.

VOR Plasticity and the Cerebellum

The VOR is well known for its ability to undergo experience-dependent adaptation. It can be adapted by altering the normal relationship between head rotation and apparent visual surround rotation. The VOR can also be habituated by prolonged rotation at a low frequency (<0.1 Hz). Analysis of bilateral VOR circuits reveals that commissural connections, in addition to their likely role in temporal signal processing, could provide a powerful site for effecting plastic modification of the VOR (Galiana, 1985). VOR plasticity involves cerebellar processing (Wilson and Melvill Jones, 1979; Robinson, 1989). Models of VOR modification by the cerebellum are based on adaptive linear filters and other concepts from control theory (CEREBELLUM AND MOTOR CONTROL). These models illustrate how VOR adaptation might be guided by error signals. Because they are continuous, they fail to capture the discontinuous phenomena that can be observed during VOR modification.

Neural Network Models of VOR

Previous models of the VOR were based largely on linear control theory (Robinson, 1981; Galiana and Outerbridge, 1984). The introduction of neural networks that allow nonlinear, distributed, and discontinuous processing have contributed new insights and have expanded the range of explicable phenomena. A generic architecture for VOR neural network models is shown in Figure 2. The bilateral model networks have three layers in which the input, hidden, and output units represent CAs, VNs, and MNs, respectively. Inputs can also represent commands from other oculomotor subsystems such as pursuit (not shown). The recurrent connections between hidden units are used to simulate VOR dynamics. Although this generic architecture is a greatly simplified version of the actual VOR pathway, it can be used to understand general principles that should pertain to the real system.

Static Neural Network Models of VOR

Static neural networks have been used to study how vestibular and other oculomotor commands could be distributed over relatively large numbers of VNs (Anastasio and Robinson, 1989). The networks have several pairs of input units, one pair of output units, and forty hidden units. All units compute the weighted sum of their inputs and bound the result sigmoidally between zero and one. The network is trained using backpropagation (BACKPROPAGATION:

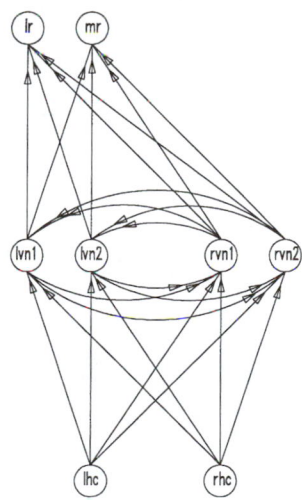

Figure 2. Architecture of adaptive, nonlinear neural network models of the VOR. lhc, rhc, left and right horizontal canal afferents; lvn, rvn, left and right vestibular nucleus neurons; lr, mr, lateral and medial rectus motoneurons on the left side. Figure redrawn from Anastasio (1991).

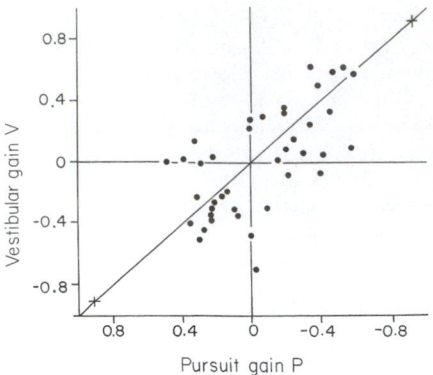

Figure 3. Variability in vestibular and pursuit related activity of forty model vestibular nucleus neurons from an adaptive, static neural network model of the VOR. Figure redrawn from Anastasio and Robinson (1989).

GENERAL PRINCIPLES and PERCEPTRONS, ADALINES, AND BACK-PROPAGATION) to produce push-pull output activations appropriate to the input patterns. The gains of the hidden and output units after training on vestibular (V) and pursuit (P) commands are shown in Figure 3. The MNs (plus signs in Figure 3) have V and P gains that are equal and opposite, as demanded by training. In contrast, the VNs (dots) vary greatly in their relative proportions of V and P gain. They encode the oculomotor commands in a nonuniform, distributed manner. This accords well with the variability in vestibulo-oculomotor behaviors actually observed for VNs.

Dynamic Neural Network Models of VOR

The NI has been modeled as a dynamic neural network (RECURRENT NETWORKS: NEUROPHYSIOLOGICAL MODELING). Dynamic neural networks have also been used to study how a distributed, nonlinear set of model VNs would compute the transformation required for VS (Anastasio, 1991). The dynamic VOR neural network models have recurrent connections and sigmoidal units. They are trained using recurrent backpropagation (RECURRENT NETWORKS: LEARNING ALGORITHMS) to simulate the VOR with VS. The time-varying inputs (Figure 4A and 4B) (dotted line) and outputs (not shown) are exponential decays. Output amplitude is equal

and opposite to input amplitude, but the time constant is four times longer for the output than for the input.

The responses of model VNs in a four-hidden-unit dynamic network after training are shown in Figure 4A and 4B (right side, solid; left side, dashed). The bilateral pair in Figure 4A has developed strong, mutually inhibitory connections. It produces the VS integration in the network. In contrast, the bilateral pair in Figure 4B has almost zero mutual inhibition and produces no VS. It appears that the network has developed parallel pathways to the MNs, one that carries the VS and the other the CA signal. However, the weakly coupled pair projects to and receives from the strongly coupled pair over moderately strong connections. This endows the weakly coupled pair with slowly decaying response tails (Figure 4B). It appears that the weakly coupled pair feeds the CA signal back to itself through the VS element formed by the strongly coupled pair. Thus, the dynamic neural network effectively combines the parallel pathway and feedback mechanisms suggested by Raphan et al. (1979) and Robinson (1981), respectively.

The dynamic network also learns to make use of neural nonlinearly. Hidden units in the trained network have high sensitivity but low baseline. This causes their off-responses to approach zero at the peak of the CA signal. This reduction in the response of one member of the strongly coupled pair leads to a reduction in the amount of lateral interaction and a reduction in VS at the peak of the CA response. Thus, even the strongly coupled pair of model VNs tends to pass the CA signal at its peak. The dynamic neural network model has adaptively found a solution to the VS problem that reproduces the high sensitivity, low baseline, and dynamic diversity of real VNs.

Dynamic and Nonlinear Models of Burst Production

A dynamic, nonlinear model of fast-phase burst generation was studied to gain insight into how an intense, temporally circumscribed burst could be produced by known brainstem circuitry (Anastasio, 1997). BNs excite themselves directly through excitatory collaterals (Shimazu, 1983). BN self-excitation could cause a burst, once inhibition from PNs and other sources is overcome and BNs start firing. But a burst produced by direct self-excitation, once initiated, could not easily be terminated. A transient burst could be produced through a mechanism involving the PNs. The BNs disinhibit themselves by inhibiting the PNs. Thus, the BN-PN loop constitutes another positive feedback pathway onto BNs in addition

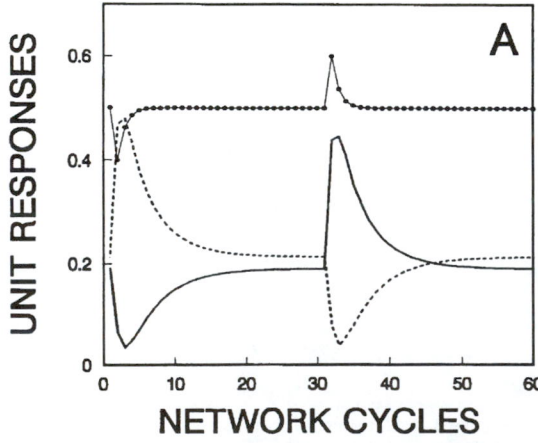
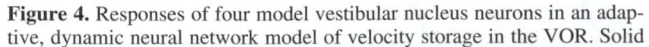
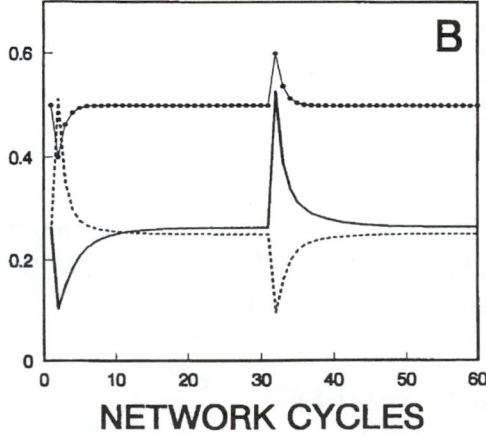

Figure 4. Responses of four model vestibular nucleus neurons in an adaptive, dynamic neural network model of velocity storage in the VOR. Solid and dashed curves, vestibular nucleus neuron responses; dotted curves, canal afferent response. Figure redrawn from Anastasio (1991).

to BN self-excitation. The advantage of the BN-PN loop is that it contributes to BN positive feedback at burst onset, but disengages when the PN pauses and breaks open the BN-PN loop. The BN response could then decay back to zero under the influence of its weaker self-excitation and inhibitory bias.

This idea was explored using a distributed network having ten each of units representing BNs, PNs, and VNs. Each unit computes the weighted sum of its inputs and bounds the result between zero and fifty. Connection polarity is as indicated in Figure 1 but the weights are randomly perturbed about previously defined values. The model produces an intense, temporally circumscribed burst that is synchronized over the population of BNs (not shown). It reproduces the diversity in response characteristics observed for real neurons, particularly the variability in BN response lead (Shimazu, 1983). Thus, PNs in the model function to enhance BN positive feedback at burst onset, and then to reduce BN positive feedback when they pause, allowing the burst to terminate. The hypothetical trigger required for previous models is not needed.

Pattern Correlation Model of VOR Habituation

Discontinuous and nonlinear behavior associated with VOR plasticity was studied using a model based on pattern correlation (Anastasio, 2001). It simulates the performance of the VOR as it undergoes habituation, which is a reduction in VOR gain brought about by prolonged exposure to low-frequency input. The patterns, stored by model PCs, are temporal fragments of the input. The PC whose pattern is most highly correlated with the input at any time reduces the VOR response by the amount of that correlation, multiplied by a preassigned weight. This simple model reproduces the discontinuous and nonlinear behavior of the habituating VOR, including superposition violation (Figure 5). The pattern correlation model suggests that the cerebellum works discontinuously in producing VOR adaptive plasticity.

Discussion

Although many open questions remain concerning VOR performance, the study of the neural mechanisms mediating the VOR has reached maturity and is moving from the laboratory to the clinic (Leigh and Zee, 1983). In contrast, the study of VOR plasticity is still a vibrant area that should continue to provide new results.

Road Map: Mammalian Motor Control
Related Reading: Action Monitoring and Forward Control of Movements; Collicular Visuomotor Transformations for Gaze Control; Pursuit Eye Movements

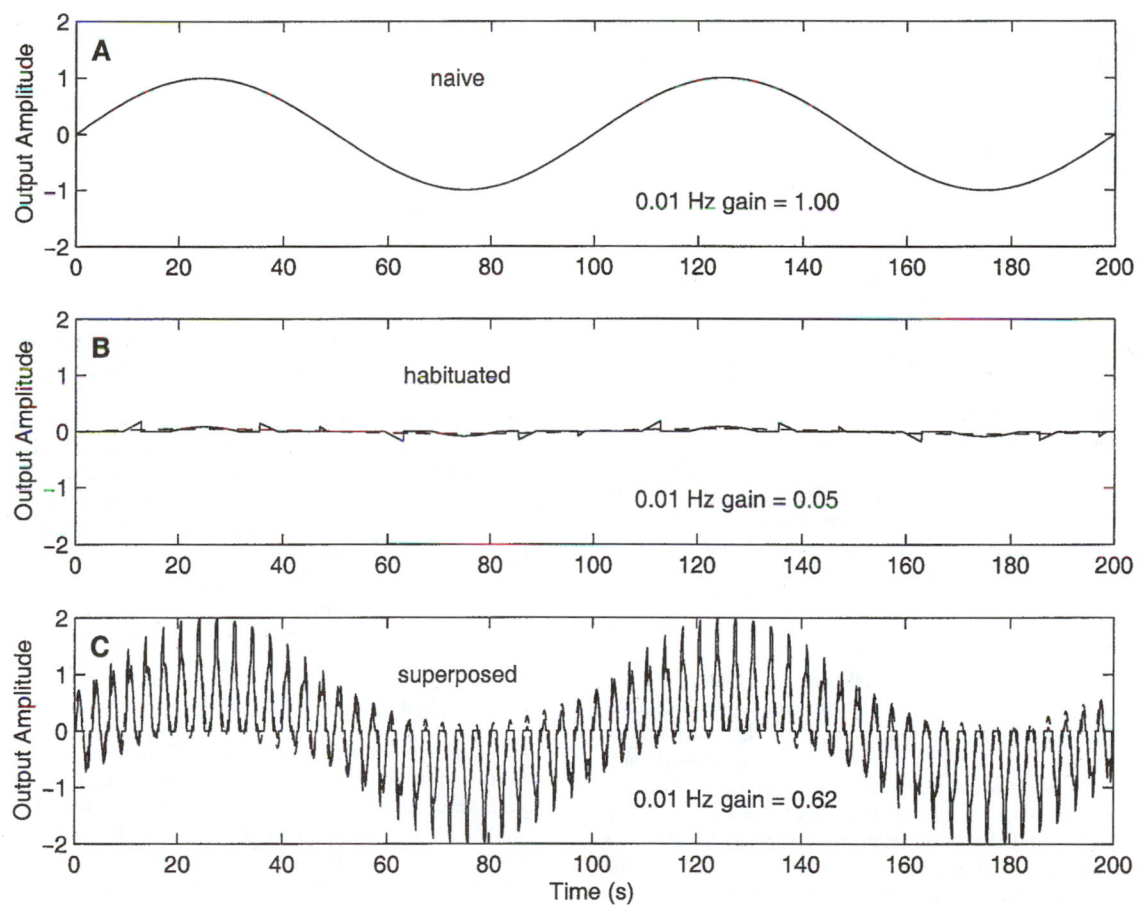

Figure 5. Using the pattern correlation model to simulate superposition violation following VOR habituation. Patterns are taken from an input sinusoid at 0.01 Hz to produce habituation at that frequency. Habituated VOR gain at 0.01 Hz (*B*) increases to more than half the naive level (*A*) when the 0.01 Hz input is combined with a second input component at 0.3 Hz (*C*). Combining the input at the habituating frequency with a second component at a different frequency degrades correlations with patterns taken from the habituating sinusoid, and reduces the amount of habituation. For a system that obeys the superposition principle, gain at a particular frequency should not be affected by the superposition of input components at other frequencies. The pattern correlation model, like the habituated VOR, violates superposition. Figure redrawn from Anastasio (2001).

References

Anastasio, T. J., 1991, Neural network models of velocity storage in the horizontal vestibulo-ocular reflex, *Biol. Cybern.*, 64:187–196.

Anastasio, T. J., 1997, A burst-feedback model of fast-phase burst generation during nystagmus, *Biol. Cybern.*, 76:139–152.

Anastasio, T. J., 2001, A pattern correlation model of vestibulo-ocular reflex habituation, *Neural Networks*, 14:1–22.

Anastasio, T. J., and Robinson, D. A., 1989, The distributed representation of vestibulo-oculomotor signals by brain-stem neurons, *Biol. Cybern.*, 61:79–88.

Baker, R., Evinger, C., and McCrea, R. A., 1981, Some thoughts about the three neurons in the vestibular ocular reflex, in *Vestibular and Oculomotor Physiology* Part IV (B. Cohen, Ed.), New York: The New York Academy of Sciences, pp. 171–188. ◆

Galiana, H. L., and Outerbridge, J. S., 1984, A bilateral model for central neural pathways in vestibuloocular reflex, *J. Neurophysiol.*, 51:210–241.

Galiana, H. L., 1985, Commissural vestibular nuclear coupling, a powerful putative site for producing adaptive change, *Rev. Oculomot. Res.*, 1:327–339. ◆

Leigh, R. J., and Zee, D. S., 1983, *The Neurology of Eye Movements*, Philadelphia: F.A. Davis Company. ◆

Raphan, T., Matsuo, V., and Cohen, B., 1979, Velocity storage in the vestibulo-ocular reflex arc (VOR), *Exp. Brain Res.*, 35:229–248.

Robinson, D. A., 1981, The use of control systems analysis in the neurophysiology of eye movements, *Ann. Rev. Neurosci.*, 4:463–503. ◆

Robinson, D. A., 1989, Control of eye movements, in *Handbook of Physiology, Section 1: The Nervous System, Vol. II, Part 2* (V. B. Brooks, Ed.), Bethesda, MD: American Physiological Society, pp. 1275–1320. ◆

Schnabolk, C., and Raphan, T., 1994, Modeling three-dimensional velocity-to-position transformation in oculomotor control, *J. Neurophysiol.*, 71:623–638.

Scudder, C. A., and Fuchs, A. F., 1992, Physiology and behavioral identification of vestibular nucleus neurons mediating the horizontal vestibuloocular reflex in trained rhesus monkeys, *J. Neurophysiol.*, 68:244–268.

Shimazu, H., 1983, Neuronal organization of the premotor system controlling horizontal conjugate eye movements and vestibular nystagmus, in *Motor Control Mechanisms in Health and Disease* (J. E. Desmedt, Ed.), New York: Raven Press, pp. 565–588.

Wilson, V. J., and Melvill Jones, G., 1979, *Mammalian Vestibular Physiology*, New York: Plenum Press. ◆

Visual Attention

Laurent Itti

Introduction

Selective visual attention is the mechanism by which we can rapidly direct our gaze toward objects of interest in our visual environment. It can be bottom-up (image based) or top-down (task dependent). Attention allows only a small part of the incoming sensory information to reach short-term memory and visual awareness, allowing us to break down the problem of scene understanding into rapid series of computationally less demanding, localized visual analysis problems. Moreover, attention mechanisms can provide feedback modulation of neural activity at the location and for the visual attributes of the desired or selected targets. This feedback may be essential for binding the different visual attributes of an object, such as color and form, into a unitary percept. As such, focal visual attention is often compared to a rapidly shiftable *spotlight* that scans our visual environment overtly (with accompanying eye movements) or covertly (with the eyes fixed). Of course, not all of vision is attentional, as we can derive a coarse understanding from presentations of visual scenes that are so brief they do not leave time for attention to explore the scene. Vision thus appears to rely on sophisticated interactions between coarse, massively parallel, full-field preattentive analysis systems and the more detailed, circumscribed, and sequential attentional analysis system.

In what follows, we focus first on the brain areas involved in the control and deployment of attention; second, on the mechanisms by which attention is attracted in a bottom-up or image-based manner toward salient locations in our visual environment; third, on the mechanisms by which attention modulates the early sensory representation of attended stimuli; fourth, on the mechanisms for top-down or voluntary deployment of attention; and fifth, on the interaction between attention, object recognition, and scene understanding.

Brain Areas

To a first approximation, selecting *where* to attend next is carried out by distinct brain structures from those that recognize *what* is being attended to. This suggests that a cooperation between "two visual systems" is used by normal vision (Didday and Arbib, 1975): selecting where to attend next is primarily controlled by the *dorsal visual processing stream* (or the "where/how" stream), which comprises cortical areas in posterior parietal cortex, whereas the *ventral visual processing stream* (or the "what" stream), comprising cortical areas in inferotemporal cortex, is primarily concerned with localized object recognition (Ungerleider and Mishkin, 1982). It is important to note, however, that object recognition in the ventral stream can bias the next attentional shift by suggesting where the next interesting object may be located. Similarly, attention strongly modulates activity in the object recognition system.

Brain regions participating in the deployment of visual attention (Figure 1) include the lateral geniculate nucleus (LGN) of the thalamus and cortical areas V1 (primary visual cortex) through the parietal cortex along the dorsal stream, as well as subcortical structures instrumental in producing directed eye movements. These include the deeper parts of the superior colliculus, parts of the pulvinar, the frontal eye fields, the precentral gyrus, and areas in the intraparietal sulcus in the macaque and around the intraparietal and postcentral sulci and adjacent gyri in humans.

Bottom-Up Control

One important mode of operation of attention is largely unconscious and driven by the specific attributes of the stimuli present in our visual environment. This so-called *bottom-up control of visual attention* may be studied using simple *visual search* tasks. Based on these experiments, computational models have been developed for how attention is attracted toward salient scene locations.

Visual Search and Pop-Out

One of the most effective demonstrations of bottom-up attentional guidance uses simple visual search experiments in which an odd

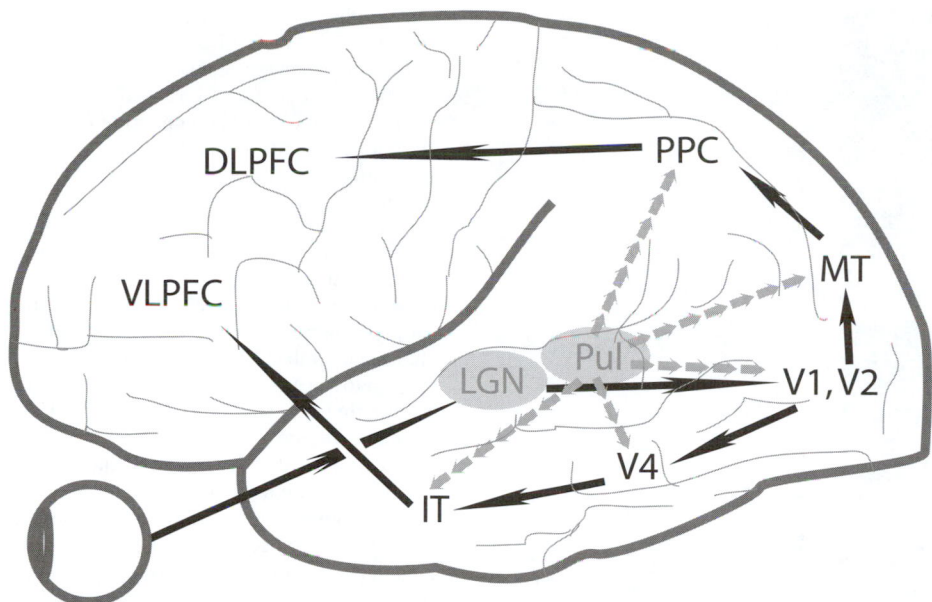

Figure 1. Major brain areas involved in the deployment of selective visual attention. Although single-ended arrows are shown to suggest global information flow (from the eyes to prefrontal cortex), anatomical studies suggest reciprocal connections, with the number of feedback fibers often exceeding the number of feedforward fibers (except between retina and LGN). Cortical areas may be grouped into two main visual pathways: the dorsal "where/how" pathway (from V1 to DLPFC via PPC) is mostly concerned with spatial deployment of attention and localization of attended stimuli, while the ventral "what" pathway (from V1 to VLPFC via IT) is mostly concerned with pattern recognition and identification of the attended stimuli. In addition to these cortical areas, several subcortical areas, including LGN and Pul, play important roles in controlling where attention is to be deployed. LGN, lateral geniculate nucleus; Pul, pulvinar nucleus; V1, V2, V4, early cortical visual areas; MT, medial temporal area; PPC, posterior parietal cortex; DLPFC, dorsolateral prefrontal cortex; IT, inferotemporal cortex; VLPFC, ventrolateral prefrontal cortex.

target stimulus to be located by the observer is embedded within an array of distracting visual stimuli (Treisman and Gelade, 1980). Originally, these experiments suggested a dichotomy between situations in which the target stimulus would visually pop out from the array and be found immediately and situations in which locating the target would require extensive scanning of the array (Figure 2). The pop-out cases suggest that the target can be effortlessly located by relying on preattentive visual processing over the entire visual scene. In contrast, the conjunctive search cases suggest that attending to the target is a necessary precondition to being able to identify it as the unique target, thus requiring that the search array be scanned until the target becomes the object of attentional selection.

Further experimentation has revealed that the fast, parallel pop-out search and the slower, serial search, originally conceived as a dichotomy, represent two extremes on a continuum of search difficulty (Wolfe, 1996). Nevertheless, these experiments clearly demonstrate that if a target differs significantly from its surround (in ways that can be characterized in terms of visual attributes of the target and distractors), it will immediately draw attention to itself. Thus, these experiments are evidence of how the composition of the visual scene alone is a strong component of attentional control.

Computational Models and the Saliency Map

The *feature integration theory* of Treisman and colleagues (Treisman and Gelade, 1980), which was derived from visual search experiments, has served as a basis for many computational models of bottom-up attentional deployment. This theory proposed that only fairly simple visual features are computed in a massively parallel manner over the entire visual scene, in early visual processing areas, including primary visual cortex. Attention is then necessary to bind those early features into more sophisticated object represen-

tations, and the selected bound representations are (to a first approximation) the only part of the visual world that passes through the *attentional bottleneck* for further processing.

The first explicit neurally plausible bottom-up computational architecture was proposed by Koch and Ullman (1985) and is closely related to the feature integration theory. The model is centered on a *saliency map*, that is, an explicit two-dimensional topographic map that encodes for stimulus conspicuity, or *salience*, at every location in the visual scene. The saliency map receives inputs from early visual processing and provides an efficient control strategy by which the focus of attention simply scans the saliency map in order of decreasing saliency.

This general architecture has been further developed and implemented, yielding the computational model depicted in Figure 3 (Itti and Koch, 2001). In this model, the early stages of visual processing decompose the incoming visual input through an ensemble of feature-selective filtering processes endowed with contextual modulatory effects. To control a single attentional focus based on this multiplicity of features, all feature maps provide input to the saliency map, which encodes visual salience irrespective of feature dimensions. Biasing attention to focus on the most salient location is then reduced to drawing attention toward the locus of highest activity in the saliency map. This is achieved using a *winner-take-all* neural network, which implements a neurally distributed maximum detector. To allow attention to shift to the next most salient location, each attended location is transiently inhibited in the saliency map by an *inhibition-of-return* mechanism, such that the winner-take-all network naturally converges on the next most salient location (Koch and Ullman, 1985; Itti and Koch, 2001; see also WINNER-TAKE-ALL NETWORKS).

Many successful models for the bottom-up control of attention are architectured around a saliency map. What differentiates the

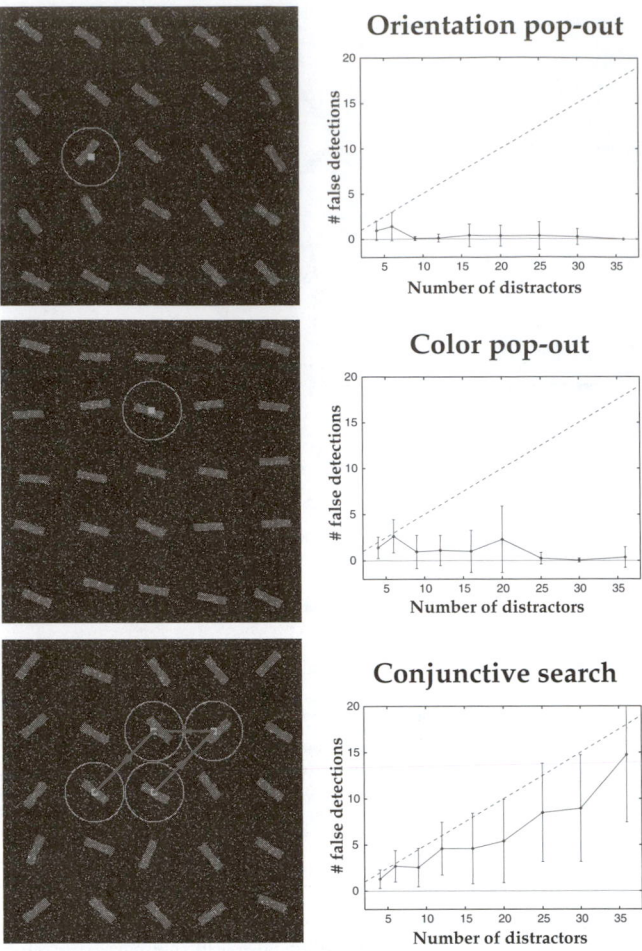

Orientation pop-out

Color pop-out

Conjunctive search

Figure 2. Search array experiments of the type pioneered by Treisman and colleagues. The top two panels are examples of pop-out cases where search time (here shown as the number of locations fixated before the target is found) is small and independent of the number of elements in the display. The bottom panel demonstrates a conjunctive search (the target is the only element that is bright *and* oriented like the darker elements); in this case, a serial search is initiated, which will require more time as the number of elements in the display is increased.

models, then, is the strategy employed to prune the incoming sensory input and extract salience. In an influential model mostly aimed at explaining visual search experiments, Wolfe (1996) hypothesized that the selection of relevant features for a given search task could be performed top down, through spatially defined and feature-dependent weighting of the various feature maps. Although limited to cases where attributes of the target are known in advance, this view has recently received experimental support from studies of top-down attentional modulation (see below).

Tsotsos and colleagues (1995) implemented attentional selection using a combination of a feedforward bottom-up feature extraction hierarchy and a feedback selective tuning of these feature extraction mechanisms. The target of attention is selected at the top level of the processing hierarchy (the equivalent of a saliency map), based on feedforward activation and on possible additional top-down biasing for certain locations or features. That location is then propagated back through the feature extraction hierarchy, through the activation of a cascade of winner-take-all networks embedded within the bottom-up processing pyramid. Spatial competition for salience is thus refined at each level of processing, as the feedfor-

ward paths not contributing to the winning location are pruned (resulting in the fed-back propagation of an "inhibitory beam" around the selected target).

Itti and Koch (2001) recently proposed a purely bottom-up model in which spatial competition for salience is directly modeled after nonclassical surround modulation effects. The model employs an iterative scheme with early termination. At each iteration, a feature map receives additional inputs from the convolution of itself by a large difference-of-Gaussians filter. The result is half-wave rectified, with a net effect similar to a winner-take-all network with limited inhibitory spread, which allows only a sparse population of locations to remain active. After competition, all feature maps are simply summed to yield the scalar saliency map. Because it includes a complete biological front end, this model has been widely applied to the analysis of natural color scenes (Itti and Koch, 2001). The nonlinear interactions implemented in this model strongly illustrate how, perceptually, whether a given stimulus is salient or not cannot be decided without knowledge of the context within which the stimulus is presented.

Many other models have been proposed, which typically share some of the components of the three models just described. It is thus important to note that postulating centralized control based on such a map is not the only computational alternative. In particular, Desimone and Duncan (1995) argued that salience is not explicitly represented by specific neurons but instead is implicitly coded in a distributed modulatory manner across the various feature maps. Attentional selection is then performed based on top-down weighting of the bottom-up feature maps that are relevant to a target of interest. This top-down biasing (also used in Wolfe's (1996) guided search model) requires that a specific search task be performed for the model to yield useful predictions.

Top-Down Modulation of Early Vision

The general architecture for the bottom-up control of attention presented in the previous section opens two important questions about the nature of the attentional bottleneck. First, is it the only means through which incoming visual information can reach higher levels of processing? Second, does it involve only one-way processing of information, from the bottom up, or is attention a two-way process, also feeding back from higher centers to early processing stages?

Are We Blind Outside of the Focus of Attention?

Recent experiments have shown how fairly dramatic changes applied to a visual scene being inspected may go unnoticed by human observers unless those changes occur at the location currently being attended to. These *change blindness* experiments (O'Regan, Rensink, and Clark, 1999) can take several forms, yielding essentially the same conclusions. One implementation consists of alternatively flashing two versions of a same scene separated by a blank screen, with the two versions differing very obviously at one location (for example, a scene containing a jet airplane, with one of its reactors erased from one of the photographs). Although the alteration is obvious when directly attended to, naive observers typically require several tens of seconds to locate it. Not unexpectedly, the most difficult instances of this experiment involve a change at a location of little interest in terms of scene understanding (for example, the aforementioned scene with an airplane also contains many people, who tend to be inspected in priority).

These experiments demonstrate the crucial role of attention in conscious vision: unless we attend to an object, we are unlikely to consciously perceive it in any detail and detect when it is altered. However, as we will see, this does necessarily mean that there is no vision other than through the attention bottleneck.

Figure 3. Typical architecture for a model of bottom-up visual attention based on a saliency map. The input image is analyzed by a number of early visual filters sensitive to stimulus properties such as color, intensity, and orientation, at several spatial scales. After spatial competition for salience within each of the resulting feature maps, input is provided to a single saliency map from all of the feature maps. The maximum activity in the saliency map (detected by a winner-take-all network) is the next attended location. Transient inhibition of return at this location in the saliency map allows the system to shift toward the next most salient location.

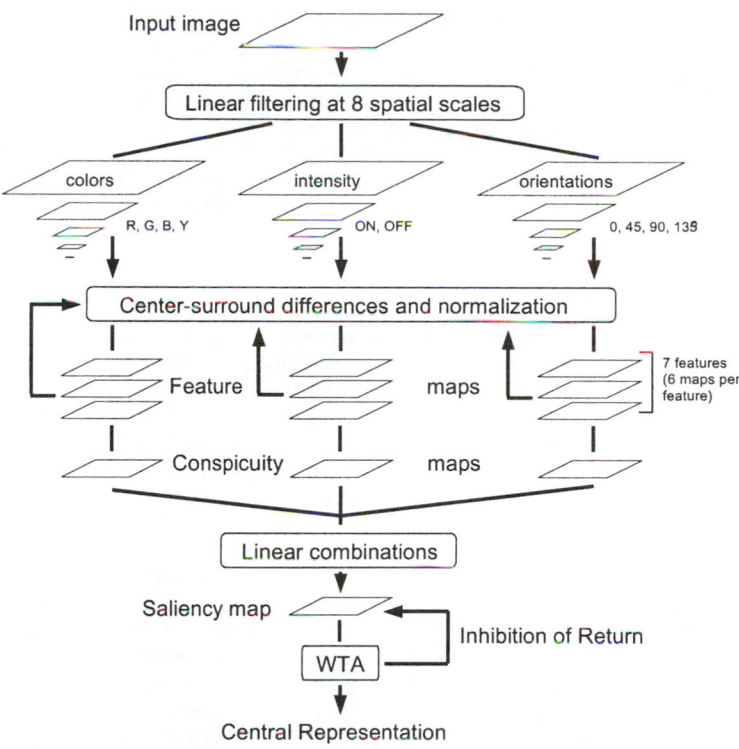

Attentional Modulation of Early Vision

A number of psychophysical and electrophysiological studies indicate that we are not entirely blind outside the focus of attention. At the early stages of processing, responses are still observed even if the animal is attending away from the receptive field at the site of recording or is anesthetized. Behaviorally, we can also make fairly specific spatial judgments about objects not being attended to, though those judgments are less accurate than in the presence of attention. This is particularly demonstrated by *dual-task psychophysical experiments* in which observers are able to simultaneously discriminate two visual stimuli presented at two distant locations in the visual field (Lee, Koch, and Braun, 1999).

Thus, although attention appears not to be mandatory for early vision, it has recently become clear that it can vigorously modulate, top down, early visual processing, both in a spatially defined and in a nonspatial but feature-specific manner (Treue and Martinez Trujillo, 1999). This modulatory effect of attention has been described as enhanced gain, biased or intensified competition, enhanced spatial resolution, modulated background activity, effective stimulus strength, or noise (Itti and Koch, 2001).

Of particular interest from a computational perspective, a recent study by Lee et al. (1999) measured psychophysical thresholds for five pattern discrimination tasks (contrast, orientation, and spatial frequency discriminations, and two spatial masking tasks). They employed a dual-task paradigm to measure thresholds either with attention fully available to the task of interest or with attention poorly available because engaged elsewhere by a concurrent attention-demanding task. The mixed pattern of attentional modulation observed in the thresholds (up to a threefold improvement with attention in orientation discrimination, but only a 20% improvement in contrast discrimination) was quantitatively accounted for by a computational model. It predicted that attention strengthens winner-take-all competition among neurons tuned to different orientations and spatial frequencies within one cortical hypercol-

umn (Lee et al., 1999), a proposition that has recently received additional experimental support.

These results indicate that attention does not implement a feedforward, bottom-up information processing bottleneck. Rather, attention also enhances, through feedback, early visual processing for both the location and visual features being attended to.

Top-Down Deployment

The precise mechanisms by which voluntary shifts of attention are elicited remain elusive, although several studies have narrowed down the brain areas primarily involved (see Itti and Koch, 2001, for a review). Here we focus on two types of experiments that clearly demonstrate how, first, attention may be deployed on a purely voluntary basis one of several identical stimuli, and second, how eye movements over a scene may dramatically differ, depending on task demands.

Attentional Facilitation and Cueing

Introspection easily reveals that we are able to voluntarily shift attention toward any location in our visual field, no matter how inconspicuous that location may be. More formally, psychophysical experiments may be used to demonstrate top-down shifts of attention. A typical experiment involves cueing an observer toward one of several possible identical stimuli, but only at a high cognitive level (e.g., with a verbal cue), so that nothing in the visual display distinguishes the target from distractors. Detection or discrimination of the stimulus at the cued (and presumably attended) location are significantly better (e.g., faster reaction time or lower psychophysical thresholds) than at uncued locations. These experiments suggest that voluntarily shifting attention toward a stimulus improves the perception of that stimulus.

Similarly, experiments involving decision uncertainty demonstrate that if a stimulus is to be discriminated by a specific attribute known in advance (e.g., discriminate the spatial frequency of a grating), performance is significantly improved compared to situations where one randomly chosen of several possible stimulus attributes is to be discriminated (e.g., discriminate the spatial frequency, contrast, or orientation of a grating). Thus, we also appear able to voluntarily select the specific features of a stimulus. These results are closely related to and consistent with the spatial and featural nature of attentional modulation mentioned in the previous section.

Influence of Task

Recording eye movements from human observers while they inspect a visual scene has revealed a profound influence of task demands on eye movements (Yarbus, 1967). In a typical experiment, different observers examine the same photograph while their eye movements are being tracked, but they are asked to answer different questions about the scene (for example, estimate the age of the people in the scene, or determine the country in which the photograph was taken). Although all observers are presented with the same visual stimulus, the patterns of eye movements recorded differ dramatically, depending on the question being addressed by each observer.

Building in part on eye-tracking experiments, Stark and colleagues (e.g., Noton and Stark, 1971) have proposed the *scanpath theory* of attention, according to which eye movements are generated almost exclusively under top-down control. The theory proposes that what we see is only remotely related to the patterns of activation of our retinas; rather, a cognitive model of what we expect to see is at the basis of our percepts. The sequence of eye movements that we make to analyze a scene, then, is mostly controlled top down by our cognitive model, and serves the goal of obtaining specific details about the particular scene instance being observed, to embellish the more generic internal model. This theory has had a number of successful applications to robotics control, in which an internal model of a robot's working environment was used to restrict the analysis of incoming video to a small number of task-dependent circumscribed regions.

Attention and Scene Understanding

We have seen how attention is deployed onto our visual environment through a cooperation between bottom-up and top-down driving influences. One difficulty that arises is the generation of proper top-down biasing signals when exploring a novel scene; indeed, if the scene has not yet been analyzed and understood by means of thorough attentional scanning, how can it be used to direct attention top down? Below we explore two dimensions of this problem. First we describe how merely from a very brief presentation of a scene we are able to extract its gist, basic layout, and other characteristics. This suggests that another part of our visual system, operating much faster than attention, might be responsible for this coarse analysis. The results of this analysis may then be used to guide attention top down. Second, we explore how several computer vision models have used a collaboration between the where and what subsystems to yield sophisticated scene recognition algorithms. Finally, we cast these results into a more global view of our visual system and the function of attention in vision.

Is Scene Understanding Purely Attentional?

Psychophysical experiments pioneered by Biederman and colleagues (Biederman, 1972) have demonstrated how we can derive coarse understanding of a visual scene from a single presentation that is so brief (80 ms or less) that it precludes any attentional scanning or eye movement. A particularly striking example of such

experiments consists of presenting to an observer a rapid succession of unrelated photographs of natural scenes at a high frame rate (over 10 scenes/s). After stimuli have been presented for several tens of seconds, observers are asked whether a particular scene, for example an outdoors market scene, was present among the several hundred photographs shown. Although the observers are not made aware in advance of the question, they are able to provide a correct answer, with an overall performance well above chance (I. Biederman, personal communication). Furthermore, observers are able to recall a number of coarse details about the scene of interest, such as whether it contained humans, or whether it was highly colorful or rather dull.

These and many related experiments demonstrate that scene understanding does not exclusively rely on attentional analysis. Rather, a very fast visual subsystem that operates in parallel with attention allows us to rapidly derive the gist and coarse layout of a novel visual scene. This rapid subsystem certainly is one of the key components by which attention may be guided top down toward specific visual locations.

Cooperation Between Where and What

Several computer vision models have been proposed for extended object and scene analysis that rely on cooperation between an attentional (where) and localized recognition (what) subsystems.

A very interesting instance was recently provided by Schill et al. (2001). Their model aims at performing object recognition, using eye movements to focus on those parts of the scene that are most informative in disambiguating its identity. A hierarchical knowledge tree is trained into the model in which leaves represent identified objects, intermediary nodes represent more general object classes, and links between nodes contain sensorimotor information used for discriminating between possible objects (i.e., bottom-up feature responses to be expected for particular points in the object, and eye movement vectors targeted at those points). During the iterative recognition of an object, the system programs its next fixation toward the location that will maximally increase information gain about the object being recognized, and thus will best allow the model to discriminate between the various candidate object classes.

Several related models have been proposed (see Itti and Koch, 2001) in which scanpaths (containing motor control directives stored in a "where" memory and locally expected bottom-up features stored in a "what" memory) are learned for each scene or object to be recognized. The difference between the various models comes from the algorithm used to match the sequences of where/ what information to the visual scene. These include using a deterministic matching algorithm (i.e., focus next on the next location stored in the sequence being tested against the new scene), hidden Markov models (in which sequences are stored as transition probabilities between locations, augmented by the visual features expected at those locations), or evidential reasoning (similar to the model of Schill and colleagues). These models typically demonstrate strong ability to recognize complex gray-scale scenes and faces, in a translation-, rotation-, and scale-independent manner, but cannot account for nonlinear image transformations (e.g., 3D viewpoint change).

Attention as a Component of Vision

Thus, vision relies not only on the attentional subsystem but also, and more broadly, on cooperation between crude preattentive subsystems for the computation of gist and layout and for bottom-up attentional control, and the attentive subsystem coupled with the localized object recognition subsystem to obtain fine details at various locations in the scene.

This perspective on the visual system raises a number of questions that remain fairly controversial. These are issues of the internal representation of scenes and objects (e.g., view-based versus 3D models, or a cooperation between both) and of the level of detail with which scenes are stored in memory for later recall and comparison with new scenes (e.g., snapshots versus crude structural models). Such issues are beyond the scope of the present discussion. Nevertheless, it is important to think of attention within the broader framework of vision and scene understanding, as this allows us to delegate some of the visual functions to nonattentional subsystems.

Discussion

We have reviewed some of the key aspects of selective visual attention, and how these contribute more broadly to our visual experience and unique ability to rapidly comprehend complex visual scenes.

Looking at the evidence on the brain areas involved in the control of attention has revealed a complex interconnected network, shared with other subsystems, that includes the guidance of eye movements, the computation of early visual features, the recognition of objects, and the planning of actions.

Attention is guided toward particular locations in our visual world under a combination of competing constraints, including bottom up from the visual input and top down from task priorities and scene understanding. Bottom-up control is evidenced by visual search experiments, in which attention is automatically drawn toward targets that pop out from surrounding distractors. It is the best understood component of attention, and computational models exist that replicate some of the human search performance. Most models have embraced the idea that a single topographic saliency map efficiently guides attention. An important theoretical result is the critical role of cortical interactions in pruning the massive sensory input, to isolate conspicuous elements from the scene.

Attention implements an information processing bottleneck, which allows only select elements in the scene to reach higher levels of processing. But not all vision is attentional, and even though we may easily appear blind to unattended image details, there is still substantial residual vision outside the focus of attention. That is, the attentional bottleneck is not strict. In addition, it is a two-way process, such that not only are selected stimuli propagated up the visual hierarchy, they are also enhanced through top-down feedback. Computationally, a proposed unifying mechanism is the activation by attention of a winner-take-all competition among visual neurons representing different aspects of stimulus, making its dominant characteristics more explicit. Top-down attentional modulation appears both location and feature specific.

Introspection evidences how attention is not exclusively controlled bottom up. Improved performance when subjects know in advance where or what to look for provides further support for top-down attentional guidance. The exact mechanisms by which volitional attention shifts remain rather elusive. Nevertheless, high-level task specifications, e.g., a question asked about a visual scene, dramatically influence the deployment of attention and gaze.

Finally, it is important to consider attention not as an autonomous visual subsystem concerned only with stimulus selection. Indeed, it is highly unlikely, or impossible under conditions of very brief presentation, to analyze complex scenes only through attention. Rather, attention, object recognition, and rapid evaluation of scene gist and layout cooperate in a remarkable multithreaded analysis that exploits multiple time scales and levels of details within interacting processing streams. Despite tremendous recent progress, many of the key components of this complex interacting system remain poorly understood and elusive, thus renewing the challenges for future neuroscience research.

Road Map: Vision
Related Reading: Action Monitoring and Forward Control of Movements; Collicular Visuomotor Transformations for Gaze Control; Laminar Cortical Architecture in Visual Perception; Visual Scene Perception; Visual Scene Segmentation

References

Biederman, I., 1972, Perceiving real-world scenes, *Science*, 177:77–80.

Desimone, R., and Duncan, J., 1995, Neural mechanisms of selective visual attention, *Annu. Rev. Neurosci.*, 18:193–222.

Didday, R. L., and Arbib, M. A., 1975, Eye movements and visual perception: A "two visual system" model, *Int. J. Man-Machine Studies*, 7:547–569.

Itti, L., and Koch, C., 2001, Computational modeling of visual attention, *Nature Rev. Neurosci.*, 2:194–203. ◆

Koch, C., and Ullman, S., 1985, Shifts in selective visual attention: Towards the underlying neural circuitry, *Hum. Neurobiol.*, 4:219–227.

Lee, D. K., Koch, C., and Braun, J., 1999, Attentional capacity is undifferentiated: Concurrent discrimination of form, color, and motion, *Percept. Psychophys.*, 61:1241–1255.

Noton, D., and Stark, L., 1971, Scanpaths in eye movements during pattern perception, *Science*, 171:308–311.

O'Regan, J. K., Rensink, R. A., and Clark, J. J., 1999, Change-blindness as a result of "mudsplashes," *Nature*, 398:34.

Schill, K., Umkehrer, E., Beinlich, S., Krieger, G., and Zetzsche, C., 2001, Scene analysis with saccadic eye movements: Top-down and bottom-up modeling, *J. Electron. Imaging*, 10:152–160.

Treisman, A. M., and Gelade, G., 1980, A feature-integration theory of attention, *Cognit. Psychol.*, 12:97–136. ◆

Treue, S., and Martinez Trujillo, J. C., 1999, Feature-based attention influences motion processing gain in macaque visual cortex, *Nature*, 399:575–579.

Tsotsos, J. K., Culhane, S. M., Wai, W. Y. K., Lai, Y. H., Davis, N., and Nuflo, F., 1995, Modeling visual-attention via selective tuning, *Artif. Intell.*, 78(1–2):507–545.

Ungerleider, L. G., and Mishkin, M., 1982, Two cortical visual systems, in *Analysis of Visual Behavior* (D. G. Ingle, M. A. A. Goodale, and R. J. Mansfield, Eds.), Cambridge, MA: MIT Press, pp. 549–586.

Wolfe, J., 1996, Visual search: A review, in *Attention* (H. Pashler, Ed.), London: University College London Press. ◆

Yarbus, A., 1967, *Eye Movements and Vision*, New York: Plenum Press.

Visual Cortex: Anatomical Structure and Models of Function

Jennifer S. Lund and Klaus Obermayer

Introduction

Given a wealth of descriptive detail concerning the anatomical and physiological organization of the mammalian visual cortex, computational approaches have become an important tool with which to explore how its elements of organization interact in analyzing the visual world. Computational approaches are essential to our understanding of cortical function, since it is not easily apparent how anatomical circuitry and functional attributes of single neurons combine to determine activity patterns in large populations of neurons. Also, the anatomist needs indicators as to what connectional features are important for certain visual cortex functions, in order to guide further studies in this most complex of neuropils.

Overview of the Anatomy of Area V1

The anatomy of the mammalian visual cortex has been studied extensively in a variety of species, but here we will discuss primarily the visual cortex of the macaque monkey as a model for the primate including humans (Levitt, Lund, and Yoshioka, 1996). It might be asked to what degree the primate visual cortex is particularly specialized in comparison with other areas of its cortex or in comparison with visual cortex of other mammals. In fact, it appears that most of its cellular components are common to other nonvisual cortical areas in its own brain as well as to the visual cortex of different mammalian species, some of which are long separated from primates in evolutionary history. Moreover, the elaborate patterning of intrinsic intra-areal connections within the primate visual cortex occurs across other cortical areas and across cortex of many other mammalian groups (Tyler et al., 1998; Lund, Yoshioka, and Levitt, 1993). These anatomical commonalities suggests that the mammalian cerebral cortex is a highly conserved neuropil in its evolution. Hence, it is likely that we will find common modes of function in areas of cortex devoted to very different sensory or motor skills within the same brain and in cortical areas of many different species.

Approximately 80% of the neurons in cerebral cortex are excitatory in their influence on other cells and are characterized morphologically by having small spines on their dendrites that act as specialized sites for synaptic contact. These spiny neurons either have dendritic processes that are all of much the same length and are called spiny stellate neurons or have one dendrite on the pial aspect of the cell that is greatly extended compared to the others and are called pyramidal neurons. The extended apical dendrite of the pyramidal neuron allows it to sample different inputs than those to the neuron's soma and basal dendrites. The other 20% of cortical neurons largely lack dendritic spines, are generally stellate in morphology, and usually contain gamma aminobutyric acid (GABA) as their principal neurotransmitter substance. These neurons are called local circuit neurons or interneurons, and they are viewed as being generally inhibitory. A variety of these inhibitory neurons exists and each variety is highly specialized in terms of their choice of postsynaptic cell and the region of the cell on which their axon terminates (see, for example, Tamas, Buhl, and Somogyi, 1997). This leads to marked anatomical specificities in their axon morphologies that serve as key features in their classification (Lund and Wu, 1997; Lund et al., 1993). The excitatory cells have longer axon relays than the inhibitory neurons in terms of lateral projections across the cortical sheet within a cortical area. They terminate on both excitatory and inhibitory neurons, and their axons also make the majority of connections between cortical areas and to subcortical regions.

The cerebral cortex is a sheetlike structure, and in the primate visual area V1, information from the thalamus is first presented across the sheet in a maplike representation of the retina. Relays coming from the right and left eyes do not mix and terminate in interleaved, segregated stripes. In addition, the macaque primary visual cortex receives a unique combination of thalamic inputs, each of which relays a different type, or channel, of visual information from the retina (reviewed by Levitt et al., 1996) and terminates in a different cortical layer. However, the postsynaptic cells' intrinsic lateral connections begin to restructure this information as well as linking different types of information (owing to differential convergence of the different streams onto common postsynaptic cells). Because of this cross-talk, new functional ("receptive field") properties are generated in cortex, and the postsynaptic neuron's properties depend on where the neuron is spatially located. Outputs from area V1 to a variety of surrounding cortical areas, emphasizing different properties, originate from V1 cell groups segregated in depth and laterally from one another, as if they express a high degree of functional specificity, akin to cortical "modules." It seems important that models should reflect this high degree of anatomical order in attempting to determine what is accomplished by the visual cortical neuropil.

There are three major channels of information entering the primate visual thalamus from the retina, and they relay on to primary visual cortex. The best-explored of these pathways are referred to as P and M channels, which originate at the β- and α-retinal ganglion cells and project via the lateral geniculate nucleus (LGN) P and M divisions, respectively, to area V1. The channels differ in chromatic and achromatic sensitivity as well as in spatial and temporal frequency tuning. In area V1 of macaque, thalamic axons from the P and M divisions of the LGN terminate mainly in the lower half (β division) and upper half (α division), respectively, of layer 4C. The third (I) channel of information relays through the LGN, via interlaminar territories inserted between its M and P layers, and terminates primarily in regularly spaced blob-shaped regions in layers 2–3 of area V1 (Yoshioka, Levitt, and Lund, 1994).

In layer 4C of area V1, the excitatory neurons postsynaptic to M and P input are almost all spiny stellate neurons rather than pyramids. These cells have staggered dendritic overlap through the depth of the layer. They send short, rising intrinsic axon projections to three different regions of the overlying layers, the target depending on their depth in layer 4C. Cells in lower 4Cβ project to layer 4A, cells in mid 4C project to the interblob regions of layers 2 and 3, and cells in upper 4Cα project to layer 4B. Their axons also contribute lateral projections to layer 4C, and the extent of these lateral projections is widest at the pial side of the layer. The interneurons within layer 4C can also receive thalamic input, but little is known of their specific relationships with the spiny cells except that one class (the so-called clutch cells) provides input to the spiny stellate cell bodies. The patterns of the inhibitory neuron axon projections relate in part to the projection patterns of the excitatory cells, but they also provide unique patterns of projections between the divisions of layer 4C. Given that the population of GABA cells is about 20% of the total cell population in all layers, any one variety of interneuron is likely to have a fairly economical distribution. This sparse distribution is interesting in that the geometry of the mosaic of inhibitory neuron dendritic surface and axon distribution may itself determine specific response characteristics in the larger population of excitatory spiny neurons with heavily overlapped dendrites. The different patterns of axon projections made by each of the interneuron classes within layer 4C suggest that a different function is fulfilled by each type in the context of processing thalamic inputs to the layer (Lund, 1987).

Anatomical Substrates for Cortical Cell Contrast Sensitivity and Receptive Field Size

Since layer 4C of area V1 receives the bulk of the thalamic input and is the major substrate for the first stage of cortical processing of visual input, it seems very important in terms of understanding cortical function to try to model how the anatomical circuitry of layer 4C and biophysical properties of single neurons might determine the output of the layer. This output must form the substrate for models of further stages of information processing within cortical depth. We know from physiological recording experiments that very important new response properties appear in the depth of layer 4C compared to properties of the LGN neurons. These properties include orientation specificity, binocularity, and direction specificity, and the substrates for determining these properties must lie within layer 4C.

To try to simplify the first stages of modeling, we first considered (Bauer et al., 1999) what might be called basic properties: receptive field size and contrast sensitivity. These properties must be derived by the neurons of layer 4C from input from heavily overlapped thalamic axons synapsing on their surfaces. As was mentioned above, layer 4C can be considered as tripartite in output while only bipartite in input. It would seem very important to determine why this should be and what properties the three outward projections might carry. Physiological measurements of field size and contrast sensitivity are distinctly different in the M and P inputs from the LGN, but in the thalamic input zone of layer 4C, these measures show a continuum of change as cells are recorded sequentially down through the depth of layer 4C, despite the fact that the M and P inputs are segregated into upper and lower halves of the layer, respectively. The answer to how this functional gradient is achieved may lie in the way in which the spiny stellate neurons sample the M and P inputs. As the position of spiny stellate neurons in layer 4C shifts from top to bottom of the layer, the relative degree to which their dendritic fields intrude into M and P termination zones changes. Since the mature synaptic loading of each spiny stellate neuron is a constant, the cells may compute a response characteristic based on the simple weight of M versus P inputs, and their position in depth may be the sole determinant of the ratio of synapses they receive and perhaps the region to which they project.

A connectionist-type neural network model (Bauer et al., 1999) using realistic input properties to a model of layer 4C comprising eight layers in depth demonstrated that the gradient of change in properties could indeed be replicated by using dendritic overlap through the lower two thirds of the 4C layer. However, it was insufficient to explain the continuous and sharply increasing field size and contrast sensitivity observable near the top of the layer. This led us back to consider the anatomy and physiology of the region. There have been reports of very large incoming axons layering along the top half of layer 4Cα and that input conduction velocity is at its highest at the top of layer 4C. There is then the possibility that the M input may have two subpopulations of fibers that terminate at different depths in layer 4Cα. We explored this in our model, giving the inputs properties in the range reported for M LGN cells but giving the largest reported field size and greatest contrast sensitivity to M axons terminating only in the upper half of layer 4Cα. This resulted in a good replication of the actual physiological data and required only feedforward excitation.

However, there is another feature of the anatomy of upper layer 4Cα that could generate the observed increase in field size and contrast sensitivity at that depth. The spiny stellate neurons in upper 4Cα make long lateral connections within the layer that might act to pool the properties of the thalamic recipient neurons and lead to the observed change in properties compared to the deeper neurons. However, in modeling the contributions of lateral connectivity providing recurrent excitation (Bauer et al., 1998), inhibition was necessary to stop runaway excitation. In exploring the parameters for inhibition, it became apparent that inhibition must have higher threshold and gain in upper 4Cα compared to other depths in the layer to replicate the observed change in properties with depth. Returning to our anatomy, we had much earlier reported that there is a change in inhibitory cell type in upper layer 4C compared to deeper regions (the so-called clutch cell provides somatic inhibition to the spiny stellate cells in the lower two thirds of the layer, and this is replaced in the upper one third by the basket neuron type α-6 with long, laterally spreading axon trunks). This anatomical change in the source of inhibition might provide a substrate for a change in the inhibitory properties with depth.

These modeling efforts have greatly helped to crystallize our ideas about the types of anatomical features that are of importance to the issues we have addressed. Further, the modeling has suggested which features are important to address in the next generation of physiological and anatomical studies.

Anatomical Substrates for Orientation Specificity

In the course of physiological explorations of layer 4C, it became apparent that some cells have clear orientation specificity, even though they may not be as sharply tuned as cells in other layers. It is also apparent that the proportion of cells with preferential response to particular orientations of external visual stimuli rises as the recording position rises toward the pial side of the layer. For those cells without orientation specificity, at all levels in layer 4C but most evident in layer 4Cβ, where the majority of cells are not orientation selective, it is clear that with lateral movement of the recording electrode, there is a perfect retinotopic map, interrupted only by the repeat of retinotopy for the segregated interleaved territories of right and left eye inputs. This precise retinotopic mapping in the macaque thalamic input layer appears to argue against Hubel and Wiesel's (1977) model for generation of orientation specificity where direct convergence of thalamic axons arising from spatially offset rows of LGN cells would provide an elongated combined receptive field (though there is some evidence for it in the cat).

Anatomically, the clearest change in structure with depth of primate V1 layer 4C that might accompany the emergence of orientation specificity is the scale and patterning of lateral connections. In the bottom third of layer 4C, lateral connections are very limited in spread; in the middle depth, the spiny stellate cell axons make single sidesteps to terminate in local offset territories; and in the top third of the layer, the excitatory cells make extensive laterally spreading projections with discontinuously distributed stripelike terminal fields. While inhibitory neuron axons are very local in the lower two thirds of the layer, in the upper third, basket neurons provide laterally spreading axons. We have used a computational model (Adorján et al., 1999) to demonstrate that realistic orientation-selective responses can emerge as a result of anisotropic excitatory lateral intracortical projections, with no bias in connectivity of inhibitory connections, even when their spread is limited to the size of one hypercolumn (where both eyes and all orientations are represented for one small region of space). This model study demonstrates that orientation bias and tuning can occur in the same cortical circuits. The model predicts that the first part of the neuron's response will not be orientation specific, since it will be determined by the retinotopic thalamic input, but that orientation specificity appears in the later part of the response as a consequence of the lateral recurrent connections. Recent physiological studies of layer 4C neurons have shown this dual-response characteristic to be a feature of orientation-tuned neurons of that layer. In both model and real life, the orientation tuning is independent of stimulus contrast. The model shows that iso-orientation inhibition is important for controlling runaway excitation, while cross-orientation inhibition, which may be weaker, is involved in obtaining sharply tuned orientation selective cells.

Anatomical Substrates for Surround Modulation of Visual Responses

It is not only the neurons of upper layer 4C that make extensive lateral connections with discontinuously distributed terminal fields; the same pattern of lateral connections, with stripelike terminal fields, continues into the overlying layer 4B, which receives its main input from upper layer 4C (Asi et al., 1996). Here, orientation specificity, binocularity, and direction specificity, which began in layer 4Cα, are fully expressed. In layers 2–3, which receives input from midlayer 4C, the patterning of connections changes. Axons of pyramidal neurons make long-range intra-areal lateral connections with regularly spaced clusters of terminals along their length in a polka-dot pattern. All these lateral connections are reciprocal, with retrogradely labeled neurons clustering at the same locations as the orthograde terminals when appropriate tracers are used. Clusters include the blob zones with direct thalamic input.

Regularly patterned lateral connections, usually stripelike or patchlike, are a striking general feature of superficial layer cortical organization in all areas of mammalian cortex. The connections appear to arise from neurons at every point across the cortex, rather than being a single fixed place system, and are biased to link together cells of common function. Using optical imaging, it has been shown that functions of the same kind repeat across the cortex at a center-to-center distance similar to that between adjacent patches when labeled with small injections of anatomical tracer substances, and in macaque V1, correlations between mutual connections and similar functions have been demonstrated directly (Yoshioka et al., 1996).

Since excitatory connections in the superficial layers of primate V1 spread laterally across the representation of the visual field, it has been suggested that they may form a substrate for long-distance interactions across the cortical map. The physiologically recorded response of single neurons to stimuli in the external world can be modulated by surrounding stimuli that do not enter the region of space that forms the neuron's receptive field; that is, the surround stimuli cannot directly drive activity of the neuron. The monosynaptic reciprocal lateral connections might provide a basis for this modulation (see Stetter, Bartsch, and Obermayer, 2000, for a corresponding modeling study). However, as tested by small deposits of extracellularly deposited tracer substances (such as biocytin or cholera toxin), the range of the lateral connections in area V1 made by any small region appears to cover only the territory that contains neurons whose classical receptive fields share some part of the retinotopic cumulative classical visual field map of the group of neurons taking up the tracer; these connections are not broad enough to allow directly for the often much larger extent of the modulatory surround, unless it is by a multisynaptic pathway. If polysynaptic pathways are in use, there must be a set of active interneurons that mediate the signal transmission. This, however, has not yet been observed.

Another route suggested for surround modulation is via reciprocal connections with extrastriate cortex. In our ongoing anatomical studies (Angelucci et al., 1998) examining interrelations between the early visual cortical areas, we find that any small region of V1, as well as making intrinsic connections to neurons sharing any small part of the injection region's neurons' cumulative classical receptive field, also maps that same retinotopic field onto the visual areas surrounding it. In turn, these extrastriate areas make intrinsic connections with similar rules such that lateral connections from a small injected region reach as far as all neurons sharing a portion of the aggregate classical receptive field of the injected region as well as sending back to single points on V1 a representation of that field. The neurons in the extrastriate areas all have larger classical receptive fields than the V1 neurons at the same retinotopic eccentricity, and the feedback could well provide surround modulation of the right scale to V1. Despite the apparently longer route out to these visual association areas, there need be no more synaptic steps than in the reciprocal monosynaptic connections of the V1 intrinsic lateral connection field, since the V1 afferents can engage at least the basal dendritic fields of neurons feeding back to V1. The feedback pathways to V1 are parceled into distinct clusters of terminals superimposed on the retrogradely labeled cells projecting out to that same visual association area. This suggests that an exquisite match in property must exist between the intrinsic connections patterns of V1 and the extrinsic sources of feedback such that the feedback matches precisely those points of most kinship across the V1 cortical sheet.

Origins of Patterned Anatomical Connections

In our anatomical investigations of these patterned connections across a number of cortical areas in the primate and in the visual cortex of other species, we noted that the size of the clusters of terminals and the intervening uninnervated gaps between them are of equal width. Moreover, this dimension is closely matched to the particular width of the dendritic tree of single pyramidal neurons, making the lattice connections in each area. Since the axons of single basket neurons in the superficial layers of cortex spread three times the diameter of the local pyramidal neuron dendritic fields and contact the cell bodies of the pyramidal neurons, their inhibition will prevent axons of colocalized, coactivated pyramidal neurons from terminating on other pyramidal neurons in the range of the local basket neuron axons (using a Hebbian learning rule). This inhibitory constraint could produce the patchlike connectional fields, even with nonspecific activity patterns. This is particularly important because there is evidence that these connections form in utero in the monkey visual cortex, and indeed the basket neuron axons are visible prenatally. Yet the patterns of connections remain malleable in the early postnatal period and can be shifted in functional allegiance under the influence of afferent drive (e.g., becoming monocular by rearing with alternating monocular input), but the repetitive geometry of the connections remains the same.

Road Maps: Mammalian Brain Regions; Vision
Related Reading: Color Perception; Directional Selectivity; Gabor Wavelets and Statistical Pattern Recognition; Ocular Dominance and Orientation Columns; Orientation Selectivity

References

Adorján, P., Levitt, J. B., Lund, J. S., and Obermayer, K., 1999, A model of the intracortical origin of orientation preference and tuning in macaque striate cortex, *Vis. Neurosci.*, 76:303–318.

Angelucci, A., Lund, J. S., Walton, E., and Levitt, J. B., 1998, Retinotopy of connections within and between areas V1 to V5 of macaque visual cortex, *Soc. Neurosci. Abstr.*, 24:897.

Asi, H., Lund, J. S., Blasdel, G. G., Angelucci, A., and Levitt, J. B., 1996, In macaque V1 lateral connections in layer 4B have a different topography than in layers 2/3, *Soc. Neurosci. Abstr.*, 22:1608.

Bauer, U., Scholz, M., Levitt, J. B., Lund, J. S., and Obermayer, K., 1998, Influence of recurrent excitation and inhibition on receptive field size and contrast sensitivity in layer 4C of macaque striate cortex, in *Artificial Neural Networks—ICANN 98*, vol. 2, pp. 949–954.

Bauer, U., Scholz, M., Levitt, J. B., Obermayer, K., and Lund, J. S., 1999, A model for the depth dependence of receptive field size and contrast sensitivity of cells in layer 4C of macaque striate cortex, *Vision Res.*, 39:613–629.

Hubel, D., and Wiesel, T., 1977, Functional architecture of monkey striate cortex, *Proc. R. Soc. Lond. B Biol. Sci.*, 198:1–59.

Levitt, J. B., Lund, J. S., and Yoshioka, T., 1996, Anatomical substrates for early stages in cortical processing of visual information in the macaque monkey, *Behav. Brain. Res.*, 76:5–19. ◆

Lund, J. S., 1987, Local circuit neurons of macaque monkey striate cortex: I. Neurons of laminae 4C and 5A, *J. Comp. Neurol.*, 257:60–92.

Lund, J. S., and Wu, C. Q., 1997, Local circuit neurons of macaque monkey striate cortex: IV. Neurons of laminae 1–3A, *J. Comp. Neurol.*, 384:109–126.

Lund, J. S., Yoshioka, T., and Levitt, J. B., 1993, Comparison of intrinsic connectivity in different areas of macaque monkey cerebral cortex, *Cereb. Cortex*, 3:148–162. ◆

Stetter, M., Bartsch, H., and Obermayer, K., 2000, A mean field model for

orientation tuning, contrast saturation and contextual effects in area 17, *Biol. Cybern.*, 82:291–304.

Tamas, G., Buhl, E. H., and Somogyi, P., 1997, Fast IPSPs elicited via multiple synaptic release sites by different types of GABAergic neurones in the cat visual cortex, *J. Physiol. (Lond.)*, 500:715–738.

Tyler, C. J., Dunlop, S., Lund, R. D., Harman, A., Dann, J. F., Beazley, L., and Lund, J. S., 1998, Evolutionary conserved features of intrinsic neocortical anatomical organisation: A comparison of the eutherian and marsupial visual cortex, *J. Comp. Neurol.*, 400:449–468.

Yoshioka, T., Blasdel, G. G., Levitt, J. B., and Lund, J. S., 1996, Relation between patterns of intrinsic lateral connectivity, ocular dominance and cytochrome oxidase reactive regions in macaque monkey striate cortex, *Cereb. Cortex*, 6:297–310.

Yoshioka, T., Levitt, J. B., and Lund, J. S., 1994, Independence and merger of thalamocortical channels within macaque monkey primary visual cortex: Anatomy of interlaminar connections, *Vis. Neurosci.*, 11:467–489.

Visual Course Control in Flies

Alexander Borst and Michael Dickinson

Introduction

Motion information plays a prominent role in the visual orientation of many animals. Self-motion displaces retinal images, resulting in an optical flow that depends in a characteristic way on the trajectory described by the animal and the three-dimensional structure of the visual environment. If these are evaluated appropriately, an animal can use different types of motion patterns to initiate and control appropriate behavioral responses. For example, a large-field rotation of the visual world could signal an unintended deviation from its course and initiate a compensatory turn. Just such optomotor reflexes are quite robust in flies and are thought to play an integral role in the animal's autopilot. In contrast, an expansion of a retinal image could signal the imminent approach to an obstacle and initiate a landing or avoidance response. Commensurate with its importance in flight behavior, the fly's nervous system is highly specialized with respect to motor behaviors influenced by visual motion. Since many of the cells that are responsible for motion extraction are large and individually identifiable, the fly is quite amenable to an analysis of sensory processing. Similarly, the small number of muscles and motor neurons used to generate flight maneuvers facilitates studies of motor output. This review provides a summary of recent studies that have begun to elucidate the neural mechanisms underlying the extraction of retinal motion patterns and their transformation into the appropriate motor patterns during flight.

The Organization of the Visual Motion Detecting System

In flies, retinal images are transformed by a cascade of three retinotopically organized layers of nerve cells: the lamina, the medulla, and the lobula complex. The latter is divided into the lobula and the lobula plate, both receiving in parallel input from the medulla. The layers consist of repetitive elements called columns, each column corresponding to one facet in the eye. Owing to their large size and easy access, the neurons within the lamina have been investigated quite extensively. The lamina cells appear to act as high-pass filters of their incoming retinal input and are slightly inhibited by neighboring retinal positions (Laughlin, 1987). Unfortunately, because of their small size, only a few studies have succeeded in recording from the subsequent columnar elements in the medulla

and the lobula; however, the results show that at least some of the neurons in these ganglia display a selective sensitivity to moving stimuli (Douglass and Strausfeld, 1995). In contrast, the large size and external position of cells within the lobula plate have made this ganglion the best characterized region of the visual system (Hausen, 1984).

Each lobula plate contains 60 giant tangential cells (LPTCs) that integrate the output signals of presynaptic columnar inputs. The LPTCs connect either to other regions within the brain or via descending interneurons to motor control centers within the thorax. Most of the LPTCs respond to motion in a directionally selective manner and play an important role in extracting different patterns of retinal motion. Owing to their extraordinary structural constancy and invariant physiological properties, the LPTCs can be identified individually from animal to animal. Three major cell families have been studied in particular detail: the CH-cells, the HS-cells and the VS-cells. HS- and VS-cells synapse onto descending neurons and thus represent output elements of the lobula plate. In contrast, CH-cells are involved in internal signal processing within and between the lobula plates of both hemispheres (Haag and Borst, 2001). HS- and CH-cells respond preferentially to horizontal image motion, whereas VS-cells are most sensitive to vertical motion. However, local directional selectivity is not constant throughout the receptive field of the LPTCs. Rather, it changes systematically in a way that matches the optic flow that would be produced by rotation and translation during flight (Krapp and Hengstenberg, 1996). Both HS- and VS-cells typically respond to visual motion with a graded shift of membrane potential and do not appear to generate full-blown action potentials. Nevertheless, they house a variety of different voltage-activated ion channels that serve, in part, to amplify high-frequency components of their synaptic inputs (Haag and Borst, 1996).

The Flight Motor and Mechanosensory Input

The muscles that control wing motion in flies are segregated into two functionally, morphologically, and physiologically distinct groups—the power muscles and the control muscles (for review, see Dickinson and Tu, 1997). Most of the fly's thorax is filled with two antagonistic sets of power muscles that provide the high levels of mechanical energy required for flight. Contractions in the dorsoventral muscles (DVMs) drive the wings up, while contractions in the antagonistic dorsolongitudinal muscles (DLMs) move the wings down. The power muscles are not attached directly to the wing; rather, they transmit their forces via strains within the thorax and a complex lever system within the wing hinge. In addition, contractions of the power muscles are activated by stretch rather than action potentials in presynaptic motor neurons. The entire thorax functions as a complex resonator whereby contractions in the DLMs initiate contractions in the DVMs and vice versa. Stretch activation relieves these high-frequency muscles from the necessity of maintaining an extensive sarcoplasmic reticulum, thereby freeing the space for contractile filaments and mitochondria, while increasing the output of mechanical power. However, the very properties that make the DLMs and DVMs effective in generating power make them unsuitable for controlling the precision changes in wing kinematics required for sophisticated flight maneuvers. This task falls on a set of 17 small control muscles that insert directly onto the sclerites of the wing hinge. Unlike the power muscles, the control muscles possess extensive sarcoplasmic reticulum and contract in response to motor neuron spikes in the conventional one-to-one fashion. The motor neurons innervating the control muscles possess large-diameter axons and extensive terminal arborizations within their targets. These characteristics are consistent with a design for rapid, neurally controlled reconfigurations of the wing hinge. With one exception, the control muscles are innervated by a single motor neuron each. Thus, understanding

the motor control of flight behavior in flies reduces, in large part, to an understanding of how the nervous system regulates the firing activity of a very small population of cells.

In contrast to the motor neurons of the power muscles, the control muscle motor neurons tend to fire within specific phase bands within the stroke cycle. Important sources of the phasic input to the control muscles include a variety of mechanoreceptors at the base of the wing and haltere (Fayyazuddin and Dickinson, 1996). In flies the halteres are tiny club-shaped organs that are evolutionarily derived from hind wings. They beat in antiphase to the wings during flight and act as gyroscopes to detect angular rotations of the body during flight (Nalbach, 1993). Because they are essential organs for flight control, ablation of the halteres renders a fly catastrophically unstable. Dense fields of mechanosensory cells at the base of the haltere encode both the up and down motions as well as Coriolis force–induced deflections that act on the haltere as the body rotates during flight.

Mechanisms for Computation of Visual Motion

The only information available to the visual system comes from the temporal and spatial variations in brightness values of the retinal images sensed by the photoreceptors. A single photoreceptor, however, cannot detect motion. To do so, the fly's nervous system must process the signals from at least two spatially displaced photoreceptors in an appropriate way. Many years ago, Reichardt and colleagues formulated the "correlation" model to explain motion

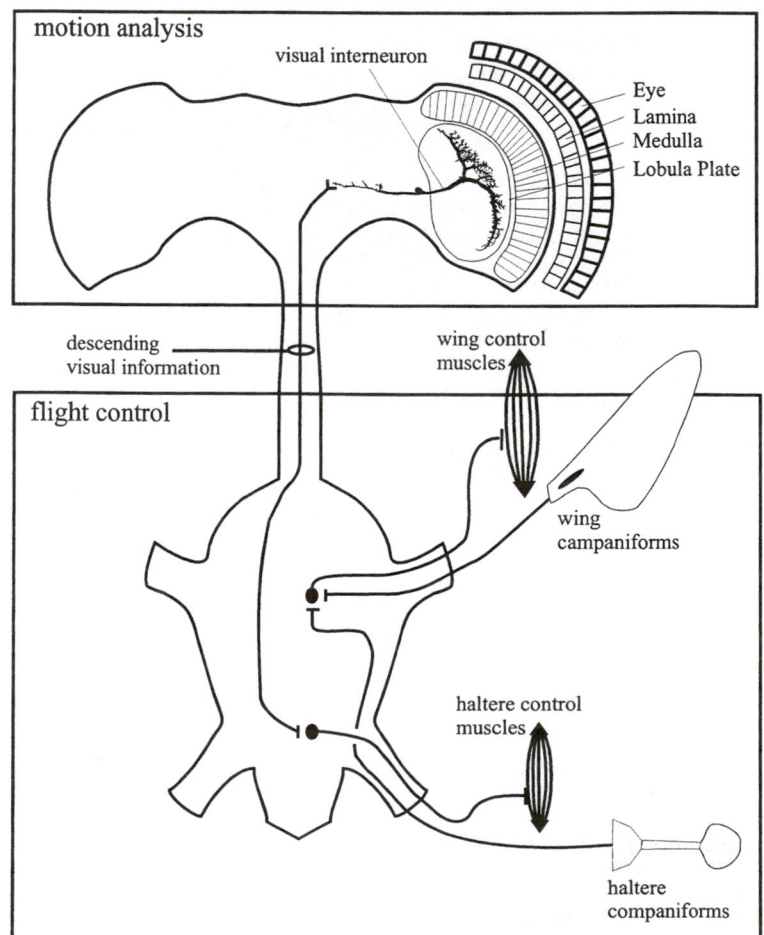

Figure 1. Schematic representation of the fly nervous system with the brain containing the visual ganglia (*top*) and the thoracic ganglion containing the motor control centers (*bottom*). One of the large motion-sensitive tangential cells is shown to contact a descending neuron which runs through the cervical connective. In the thorax, such descending neurons are thought to contact motor neurons controlling the wings and halteres. Haltere mechanosensory sensillae synapse on wing control muscles, thus providing a means by which visual information can directly influence mechanosensory feedback to steering muscles.

detection in the insect visual system (Reichardt, 1961). The original model, based solely on behavioral analysis, posits the existence of two mirror-symmetrical subunits, the outputs of which are subtracted from one another. Each subunit has two input channels that are multiplied after one of the signals has been delayed. Motion measurement comparable to the fly's would require two arrays of such elementary detectors, each encoding a different direction. Output signals suitable for orchestrating motor commands are generated by spatially integrating appropriately tuned movement detectors across the visual field. Unlike a speedometer, the output of a correlation detector is not proportional to image velocity throughout its dynamic range. Rather, a correlation detector has an optimal velocity at which it responds most strongly, and this optimal velocity is a function of the delay unit's time constant. In addition, its response depends on properties of the stimulus pattern such as its spatial frequency and contrast.

Since it was first proposed, Reichardt's model has been subjected to much experimental scrutiny. The first processing step consists of a nonlinear interaction between the neighboring photoreceptor inputs. In the original model, this interaction was realized mathematically as a multiplication of the two adjacent channels. A characteristic of multiplication is its sign rule: signals with the same polarity, either positive or negative, yield positive outputs, whereas input signals of opposite polarity always lead to negative output. This prediction has been tested experimentally in the blowfly using extracellular recordings from the spiking H1-cell. Flies were stimulated with step changes in luminance values in two adjacent parts of the receptive field, an experimental paradigm that creates apparent motion. The apparent motion stimulus elicited a depolarizing response in the H1-cell only when luminance changes had the same sign, i.e., both turning dark or both turning bright. In the other two possible cases, the response of the H1-cell was negative (Egelhaaf and Borst, 1992). These results are taken as confirmation that the first stage of motion detection does indeed involve a functional multiplication, although the underlying physiological mechanisms responsible for this arithmetic operation are not yet known.

Additional experiments support the second step in the Reichardt model, subtraction of adjacent channels. In this case the underlying biophysical mechanisms are better understood. In vitro pharmacological studies indicate that excitatory inputs to LPTCs are mediated by nicotinic acetylcholine receptors, while inhibitory inputs are mediated by GABA (Brotz and Borst, 1996). Blocking GABA receptors with picrotoxin leads to a strong reduction of direction selectivity in postsynaptic LPTCs. In particular, responses to motion in the preferred direction increase, while responses to motion in the null direction reverse sign (Single, Haag, and Borst, 1997). In addition, the motion-induced change of input resistance before and after picrotoxin indicates that picrotoxin application decreases the number of postsynaptic channels that open in response to visual motion, both in the preferred and the null direction. Together, these results suggest that the directional sensitivity of cells providing input to the LPTCs is not particularly strong. Thus, these input cells are activated not only by their preferred direction, but also, though to a smaller extent, by motion in the opposite direction. This antagonistic influence of adjacent inputs with opposite preferred direction appears to sharpen the directional response of the postsynaptic LPTCs.

The final processing step consists of the spatial integration of the local motion signals (Figure 2). As with the subtraction stage, this process takes place in the large dendrites of the LPTCs. Spatial integration appears to serve two quite distinct functions. First, if the optimal flow field required to elicit certain behavioral outputs has different motion vectors in different parts of the visual field, spatial integration must occur over appropriately oriented local motion detectors (Krapp and Hengstenberg, 1996). Second, even if the motion vectors have the same orientation, spatial integration is still

necessary to yield reliable motion measurements because the local signals are corrupted by modulations reflecting variation in local luminance. Such local modulations could indeed be measured in the dendritic tips of LPTCs by optical recordings of cytosolic calcium (Single and Borst, 1998).

Integrating Visual and Mechanosensory Inputs to Tune Motor Output

In order to perform complex flight maneuvers, flies must integrate visual and mechanosensory information. This integration is difficult because these two modalities operate on different time scales. Although the visual system of flies displays a temporal resolution that is unmatched in other animals, it is still sluggish compared to that of the mechanosensory neurons. For visual information to drive steering motor neurons at mechanically phases of the stroke

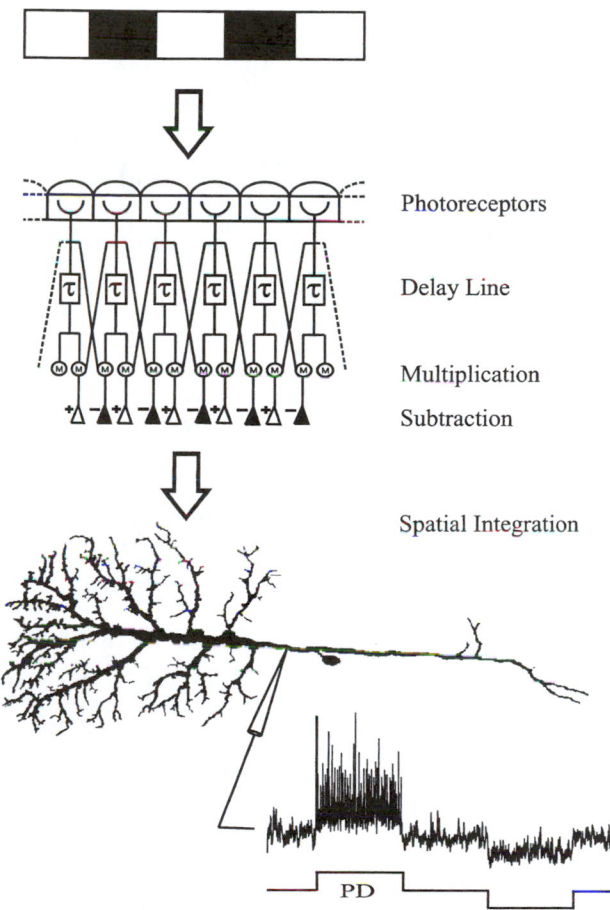

Figure 2. In the first step of motion analysis, motion in different parts of the visual field is computed in parallel by two-dimensional arrays of local movement detectors. A vertically striped pattern moving in the horizontal axis is shown at the top. A one-dimensional array of motion detectors, consisting of two different types, is displayed: One type, tuned to detect rightward motion, makes excitatory synapses onto the dendrite of an HS cell; the other, tuned to the opposite direction of motion, makes inhibitory synapses. In its simplest form, each motion detector measures the light intensities at two points in space. The detector input signals are multiplied by each other after one has been delayed by some sort of temporal filter. Subtraction of opponent signals and spatial integration occurs within the dendrite of the HS cell. Its directional selective response to motion in the preferred (PD) and null direction (ND) is shown at the bottom.

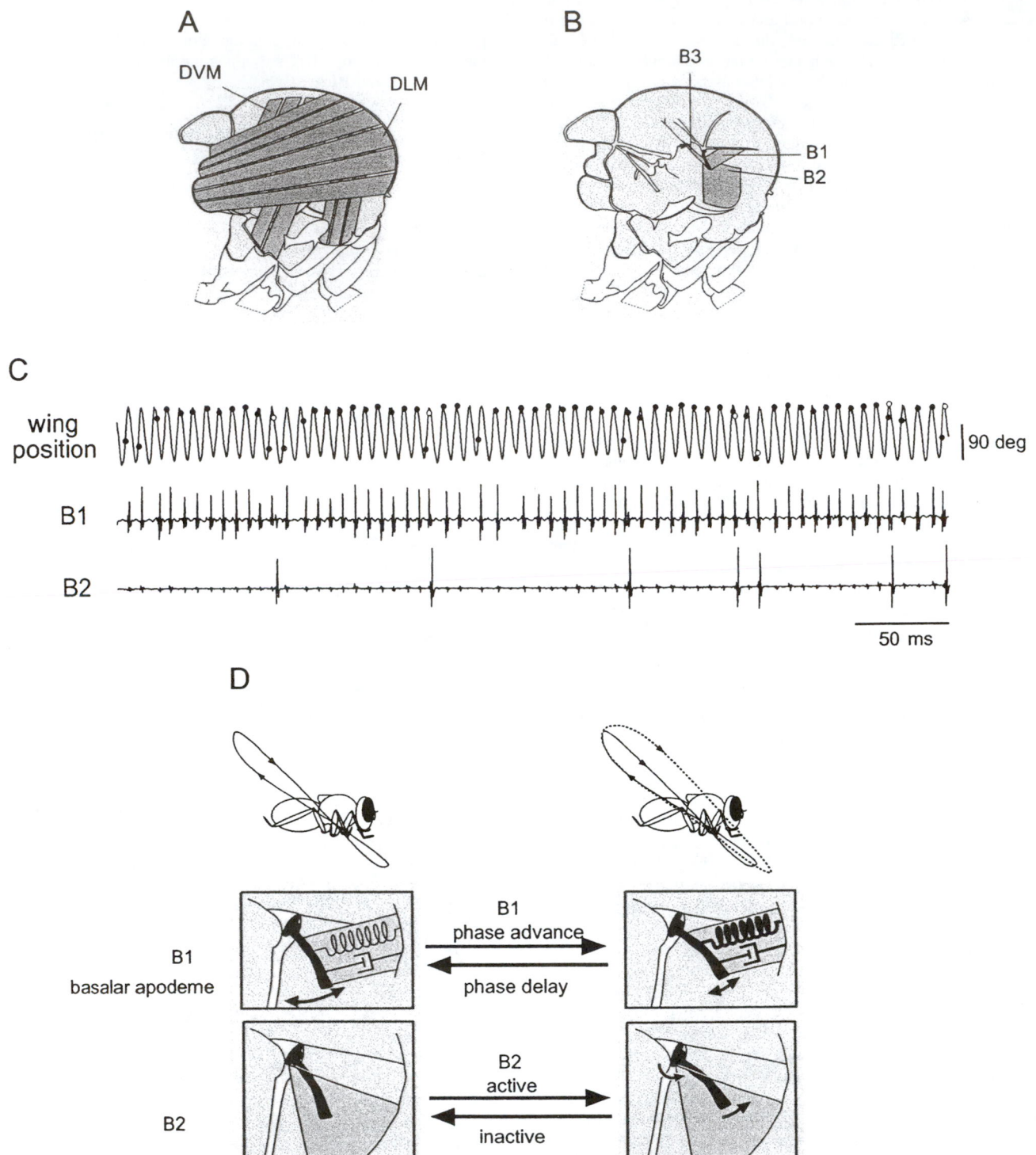

Figure 3. Current model for how two of the steering muscles (B1 and B2) influence wing stroke kinematics. *A*, Most of the thorax is filled with the large indirect asynchronous power muscles (DVMs and DLMs), which provide the mechanical power for flight. *B*, The position of the basalare steering muscles (B1, B2, and B3). The wing hinge contains about a dozen other control muscles, which are not shown. *C*, The firing patterns of B1 and B2 during sequence of tethered flight. The top trace shows the angular motion of the wing within the stroke plane superimposed with the firing times of B1 (solid circles) and B2 (open circles). Note the occasional phase advances of B1, which are often correlated with the presence of B2 spikes. *D*, During flight the basalar apodeme is oscillated back and forth through the action of the other flight muscles. Phase advances in the activation of B1 increase its dynamic stiffness. The increased stiffness damps the oscillation of the adodeme and pulls it forward, resulting in an increase in stroke amplitude and a rostral trajectory during the downstroke. Through its insertion on the head of the basalare, single spikes in B2 can similarly affect phase advances in B1.

cycle, it must be gated by wing beat synchronous feedback. As described below, recent experiments offer a glimpse into the mechanisms by which this integration occurs.

The importance of firing phase in the function of the steering muscles is illustrated by studies on the large basalar muscles, B1 and B2 (Figure 3; for review, see Dickinson and Tu, 1997). The basalare is a nail-shaped sclerite just anterior to the wing that acts like a clutch to reconfigure the wing hinge. Tonic firing of B1 pulls the basalar apodeme anteriorly, causing a gross configurational change in the wing hinge that greatly increases wing stroke amplitude. More subtle alterations in stroke kinematics, however, are associated with changes in firing phase. In the absence of visual input, B1 fires near the upstroke-to-downstroke transition. In response to visual motion toward the contralateral side, the muscle fires 1 to 2 ms earlier in the stroke cycle. As the phase of B1 advances, stroke amplitude increases further and the wing follows a more anterior trajectory during the downstroke. During visually induced turns, B2 is typically recruited within tonic bursts of B1 activity. Single spikes in B2 evoke large transient increases in stroke amplitude, and may underlie the rapid body saccades that some flies display in free flight. Like B1, the magnitude of B2's effect on stroke kinematics depends on the phase at which it is activated within the stroke cycle. Simply by adjusting the activation of the B1 and B2 muscles and the phase at which they fire, the fly can achieve quite complex control over stroke kinematics.

The results discussed above suggest that activation phase is an important control parameter in the flight system of flies. In the case of a tonically active B1, phase is the only variable with which the nervous system can modulate the mechanical properties of the muscle (Dickinson and Tu, 1997). When oscillated and stimulated at 150 Hz, the normal wing beat frequency of *Calliphora*, B1 does not generate positive work, but rather absorbs mechanical energy from the other muscles within the flight system. However, the work required to extend the muscle (i.e., the dynamic stiffness) varies as a function of activation phase. Thus, the flight control system can use B1 as an active spring by varying the firing phase on a cycle-by-cycle basis. From a neural perspective, the important feature of the B1 is that these biomechanical effects are controlled by precise changes in firing phase and not by firing frequency per se.

Visual motion influences stroke kinematics in two ways: by recruiting appropriate steering motor neurons and by adjusting their firing phase. In both cases, the visual input must incorporate mechanosensory feedback in some way, because the visual system does not encode wing motion and thus could not tune muscles to fire at mechanically appropriate phases of the stroke cycle. One mechanism that could explain this fusion of mechanosensory and visual channels signals is the possibility that the two modalities converge directly, either on steering motor neurons or on their premotor interneurons. In this scheme, the wing and haltere would provide phasic synaptic drive to steering motor neurons, but tonic visual input would determine whether or not the motor neurons reach threshold in any given stroke. Such simple convergence could explain how visual motion could recruit steering motor neurons to fire in phase-locked patterns. Although no clear electrophysiological evidence for such direct convergence is currently available, such negative evidence must be viewed with caution, as the appropriate connections might be physiologically gated and thus difficult to identify in the dissected preparations.

A second model of multimodal convergence is that descending visual interneurons alter firing phase and recruitment of steering motor neurons indirectly through their influence on efferent pathways controlling mechanosensory afferents. Like the wing, the haltere is equipped with a set of tiny control muscles that insert upon sclerites at its base. Motor neurons of at least two of these muscles receive input from motion-selective descending visual interneurons (Chan, Prete, and Dickinson, 1998) (Figure 4). It is not yet known what effects these steering muscles have on haltere kinematics, but one possibility is that they might influence the recruitment or firing phase of haltere mechanosensory neurons. These afferents could then relay these temporal changes to wing muscles via their strong connections with steering motor neurons, providing a means by which the visual system could manipulate mechanosensory equilibrium reflexes to cause temporally precise changes in motor output.

In addition to the haltere system, visual input may reverberate through several other sensory motor reflexes en route to the wing steering muscles. For example, descending visual interneurons provide input to muscles that control head position, while mechanoreceptors that encode head motion project to motor neurons of the wing and haltere. Changes in wing motion may alter the firing of wing mechanoreceptors, which themselves project to muscles of the neck, wings, and halteres. Far from a simple reflex arch, descending input from the targets of LPTCs thus might reverberate through this web of overlapping mechanosensory reflexes, integrating essential phasic mechanosensory information with visually controlled motor commands.

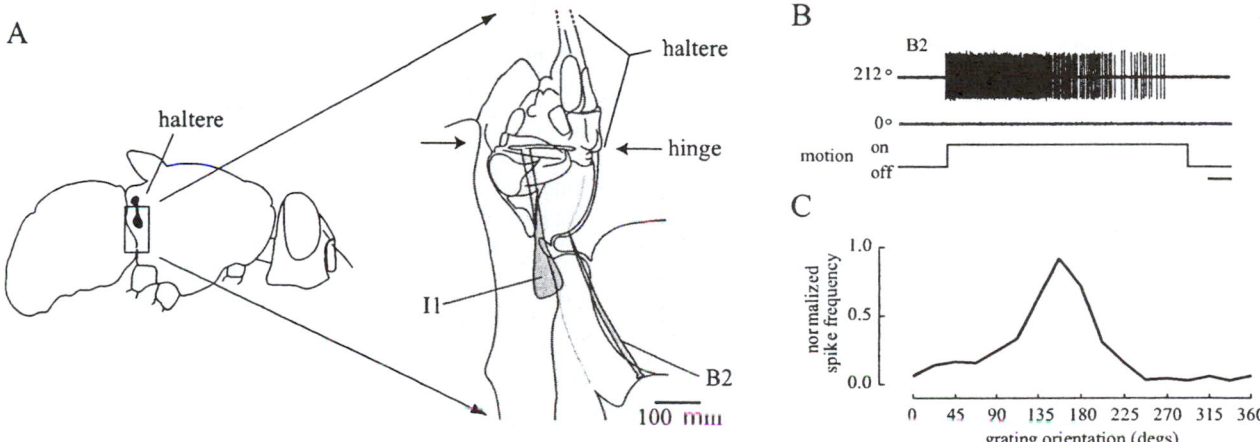

Figure 4. Control muscles of the haltere receive directionally sensitive input from visual interneurons. *A*, Cartoon indicating the position of the haltere and the location of two of its control muscles (I1 and B2). *B*, The motor neuron of the haltere B2 muscle is excited by downward visual motion (212°), but not by upward motion (0°). *C*, Directional tuning curve for the haltere B2 muscle. This tuning is similar to that of lobula plate VS cells.

Conclusions

We have reviewed here our current understanding of visual course control in flies, from the changing retinal images on the fly's eyes all through the nervous system onto the control muscles of the wings. The emerging picture suggests that visual information is first processed in the visual ganglia in order to extract reliable motion information, then sent down to the thoracic ganglion for subsequent integration with mechanosensory inputs. Current research focuses on the physiological implementation of the various processing steps involved in the computation of motion information as well as its translation into precisely timed motor commands that match the biophysics of the effectors.

Road Map: Neuroethology and Evolution
Related Reading: Locust Flight: Components and Mechanisms in the Motor; Motion Perception, Navigation; Visuomotor Coordination in Frog and Toad; Visuomotor Coordination in Salamander

References

Brotz, T. M., and Borst, A., 1996, Cholinergic and GABAergic receptors on fly tangential cells and their role in visual motion detection, *J. Neurophysiol.*, 76:1786–1799.

Chan, W. P., Prete, F., and Dickinson, M. H., 1998, Visual input to the efferent control system of a fly's "gyroscope," *Science*, 280:289–292. ◆

Dickinson, M. H., and Tu, M. S., 1997, The function of dipteran flight muscle, *Comp. Biochem. Physiol.*, 116A:223–238. ◆

Douglass, J. K., and Strausfeld, N. J., 1995, Visual motion detection circuits in flies: Peripheral motion computation by identified small-field retinotopic neurons, *J. Neurosci.*, 15:5596–5611.

Egelhaaf, M., and Borst, A., 1992, Are there separate ON and OFF channels in fly motion vision? *Vis. Neurosci.*, 8:151–164.

Fayyazuddin, A., and Dickinson, M. H., 1996, Haltere afferents provide direct, electrotonic input to a steering motor neuron of the blowfly, *Calliphora, J. Neurosci.*, 16:5225–5232.

Haag, J., and Borst, A., 1996, Amplification of high-frequency synaptic inputs by active dendritic membrane processes, *Nature*, 379:639–641.

Haag, J., and Borst, A., 2001, Recurrent network interactions underlying flow-field selectivity of visual interneurons, *J. Neurosci.*, 21:5685–5692.

Hausen, K., 1984, The lobula-complex of the fly: Structure, function and significance in visual behaviour, in *Photoreception and Vision in Invertebrates* (M. A. Ali, Ed.), New York: Plenum Press, pp. 523–559.

Krapp, H. G., and Hengstenberg, R., 1996, Estimation of self-motion by optic flow processing in single visual interneurons, *Nature*, 384:463–466. ◆

Laughlin, S. B., 1987, Form and function in retinal processing, *Trends Neurosci.*, 10:478–483. ◆

Nalbach, G., 1993, The halteres of the blowfly, *Calliphora.* I. Kinematics and dynamics, *J. Comp. Physiol.*, A173:293–300.

Reichardt, W., 1961, Autocorrelation, a principle for the evaluation of sensory information by the central nervous system, in *Sensory Communication* (W. A. Rosenblith, Ed.), New York, London: MIT Press and John Wiley & Sons, pp. 303–317.

Single, S., Haag, J., and Borst, A., 1997, Dendritic computation of direction selectivity and gain control in visual interneurons, *J. Neurosci.*, 17:6023–6030.

Single, S., and Borst, A., 1998, Dendritic integration and its role in computing image velocity, *Science*, 281:1848–1850. ◆

Visual Scene Perception, Neurophysiology

Edmund T. Rolls and Michael A. Arbib

Introduction

The task of vision is often reduced to the task of recognizing objects, but two further tasks are crucial: (1) finding the spatial disposition of objects and (2) observing features of relevance to planning our actions in the world (consider avoiding collisions when walking down a busy street). *Visual scene perception* includes visual perception of the spatial layout of objects, with properties and relationships relevant to behavior. The article FEATURE ANALYSIS explores the idea that natural images can be decomposed into *objects* composed of *features* and that visual perception can thus benefit from seeing which, among all possible visual features, best reflect the statistics of natural scenes. OBJECT STRUCTURE, VISUAL PROCESSING then suggests how objects may be recognized from approximate spatial relations between fragments. Nonetheless, remarkably little recent modeling or neurophysiology has been done on raising the level from feature, fragment, and object up to scenes. This article, then, is designed to stimulate further work on visual scene perception by juxtaposing two approaches: using as a basis for action a (rather old) theoretical framework for recognizing the layout of objects in a scene and recent neurophysiology suggesting how the context of a natural scene may modify the response properties of neurons responsive to visual features.

What, Where, and How

The vertebrate midbrain can exhibit subtle patterns of visual scene analysis; cortical mechanisms can enrich these basic capabilities. For example, the brain of a frog has basic pattern recognition rou-

tines (*perceptual schemas*; see SCHEMA THEORY) for recognizing small moving objects (prey schema) and large moving objects (predator schema). When activated, these will in turn trigger the motor schema (a control system producing action) for approach or escape, respectively. These basic perceptual schemas in the frog may be localized in the interactions of the tectum and pretectum of the midbrain, while the motor schemas rest on tectum-brainstem interactions driving motor pattern generators in the brainstem for jaw and tongue movements and in the spinal cord for limb movements. Moreover, perceptual schemas provide a parametric description that can be used to tune and calibrate behavior. Recognizing prey, the frog turns and snaps to where the prey is located; similarly, the frog will tend to jump out of the path of the predator. In addition, the frog's behavior can depend on the layout of objects in a scene. If a barrier is present, the frog may detour around it to get to prey or bias its escape from a predator to avoid bumping into the barrier. In short, multiple schemas may be coactivated to control appropriate spatially directed behaviors (Arbib and Liaw, 1995).

The role of tectum in directing whole-body movements in the frog is analogous to that of superior colliculus in directing orienting movements in mammals (see COLLICULAR VISUOMOTOR TRANSFORMATIONS FOR GAZE CONTROL). Moreover, a monkey (or human) without visual cortex appears blind. Humphrey (1970) argued, however, that a monkey without visual cortex should have at least as much visual ability as a frog but that such monkeys had not learned to pay attention to available visual cues. To demonstrate this, he gave two years of attention training to a monkey from which primary visual cortex had been removed. Eventually, the monkey was able to use visual cues to navigate and to grab at moving objects, but no subtlety of pattern recognition was regained. Moreover, it was discovered that humans without primary visual cortex could also "see" in this sense: They could point accurately toward small lights even though they were not aware of seeing the stimuli to which they pointed (they have *blindsight*).

Thus, midbrain visual mechanisms can determine the spatial layout relevant to basic behaviors. Our concern now is with the "added value" provided by cortex. Ungerleider and Mishkin (1982) noted that monkeys with lesions of inferotemporal cortex (IT) were profoundly impaired in visual pattern discrimination but less impaired in solving spatial tasks; the opposite results were observed in monkeys with lesions to posterior parietal cortex (PP). They thus distinguished two cortical systems in primate visual processing: a ventral "what" stream projecting from primary visual cortex, V1, to IT and a dorsal "where" stream projecting from V1 to PP. A variety of data on humans led Goodale and Milner (1992) to suggest that the dorsal system is better seen as a "how" system comprising a number of sensorimotor networks for different actions (including the "where" of object location relevant to a specific task). The "what" and "how" streams usually work together in producing useful actions, with the ventral stream serving for object identification as a precursor to planning, whereas the dorsal stream provides precise motor parameters (see DISSOCIATIONS BETWEEN VISUAL PROCESSING MODES). Indeed, it may have been the utility of object identification invariantly with respect to the size, position, and view of the object on the retina in identifying goals for action that provided the prime pressure for evolution of the ventral ("what") system.

Visual Scene Perception Based on Schemas

The VISIONS system (Draper et al., 1989) is a computer vision system for recognizing outdoor visual scenes. Low-level processes take an image and extract an *intermediate representation*—an up-

datable set of partial representations including regions, lines, surfaces, and vertices, tagged with features such as color, texture, shape, size, and location. Perceptual schemas process different features of the intermediate representation to form confidence values for the presence of objects like houses, walls, and trees. The knowledge required for interpretation is stored in long-term memory (LTM) as a network of schemas, while the state of interpretation of the particular scene unfolds in short-term (STM) or working memory as a network of schema instances (Figure 1). The notion of STM here descends from Didday and Arbib's (1971) slide box metaphor, in which an array of "slides" were placed in retinotopic correspondence with the visual input, each slide providing data related to a given class of objects, both for object recognition and for object-related actions. This anticipates the notion of visuospatial scratchpad presented below.

When a schema instance is activated, it is linked with an associated area of the image and an associated set of local variables. Each schema instance in STM has an associated confidence level which changes on the basis of interactions with other units in STM. The STM network makes context explicit: each object represents a context for further processing. For example, activation of an instance of the roof schema might invoke an instance of the wall schema to check the region beneath the one to which it is linked in the image. If both schema instances achieve a high enough confidence level, they could jointly activate an instance of the house schema.

Miikkulainen and Leow (1995) describe VISOR, a simple schema-based neural network vision system. It has three main modules. The low-level visual module focuses attention on one component of an object at a time, extracts its shape (what) and relative position (where), and sends this information to the schema module. The schema that best matches the input suggests shifting attention to a location where another component of the object it represents is expected. The low-level visual module then shifts attention to

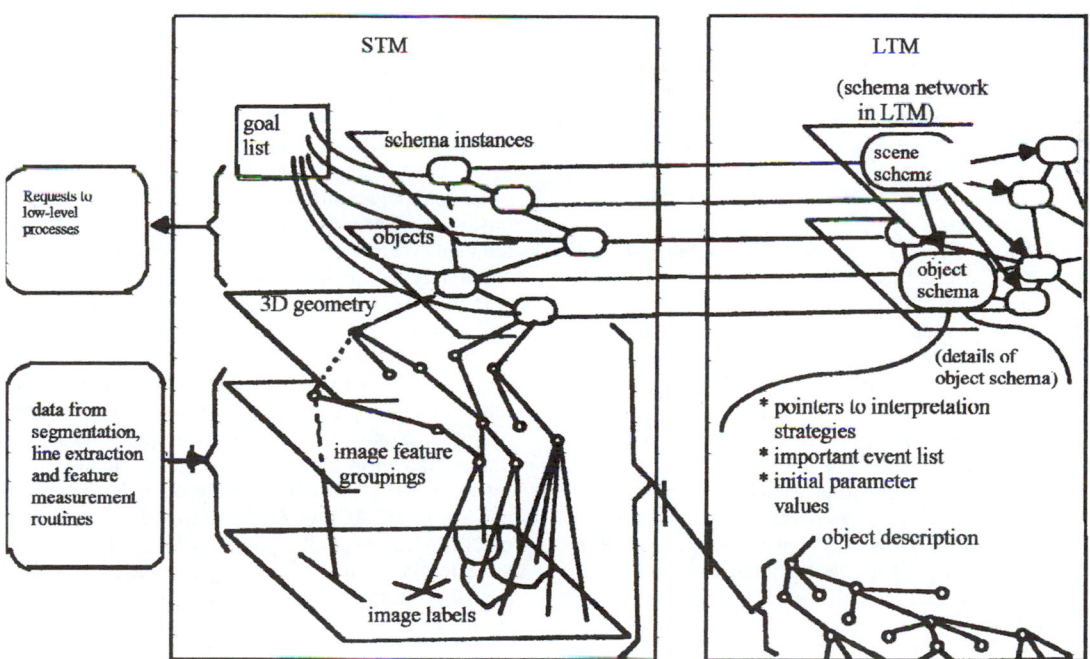

Figure 1. The VISIONS paradigm for cooperative computation in visual scene analysis. Interpretation strategies are stored in schemas that are linked in a schema network in long-term memory (LTM). Under the guidance of these schemas, the intermediate representation is modified and in-

terpreted by a network of schema instances that label regions of the image and link them to a 3D geometry in short-term memory (STM). (From Weymouth, 1986.)

the new position, and the process repeats until VISOR has looked at all the components in the scene. Turning this model into a psychophysical model would require an attempt to analyze the trade-off between the role of different saccadic scanpaths in answering questions about a scene and evidence that much information can be extracted in a single fixation (see FAST VISUAL PROCESSING). Note that an object itself can be viewed as a small scene (see OBJECT STRUCTURE, VISUAL PROCESSING), showing that although PP may be custodian of spatial relations between distinct objects in the large, IT must track, but probably with metric imprecision, the spatial relations of fragments that constitute a familiar object or overlearned scene.

Operation of the Temporal Cortical Visual Areas in Natural Scenes

We now turn toward a neurophysiological approach to how the visual system operates in complex natural scenes and to models at the neuronal network (rather than schema) level. IT contains a representation of objects and faces that has considerable invariance with respect to size, position, and even, for some neurons, view. The neural code (1) is sparse and distributed, with each neuron showing high firing rates to a few stimuli, the rates produced by other stimuli tailing off approximately exponentially; (2) can be read in a short time window from the spike counts of a population of neurons; and (3) has very high capacity in terms of the number of stimuli that can be represented (Rolls, 2000; Rolls and Deco, 2002—henceforth *R&D*).

Until recently, research on translation invariance considered the case in which there is only one object in the visual field. What happens in a cluttered, natural, environment? Rolls, Aggelopoulos, and Zheng (see *R&D*) analyzed the responses of IT neurons to stimuli presented in complex natural backgrounds in which the monkey had to search for one of two objects on a screen. It was found that the response magnitude and selectivity were little affected in natural scenes but that the receptive field sizes of the neurons typically became much smaller in the real scene. It is proposed that this reduced translation invariance in natural scenes helps an unambiguous representation of an object that may be the target for action to be passed to the brain regions that receive input from primate IT. It helps with the *binding problem* (linking distributed patterns of neural firing that together encode one object rather than another) by reducing in natural scenes the effective receptive field of at least some IT neurons to approximately the size of an object in the scene.

It is also found that in natural scenes, the effect of object-based attention on the response properties of IT neurons is relatively small (see *R&D*). Whereas the receptive fields were larger (51° versus 24°) for the attended object versus the nonattended stimulus with a blank background, when tested in a complex background the receptive field sizes were 26.6° (for the attended object) versus 22.8°. Trappenberg, Rolls, and Stringer (2002, see *R&D*) produced a model for this with an attractor network representing IT and a neural input layer with several retinotopically organized modules representing the visual scene in an earlier visual cortical area such as V4. The network has large receptive fields in blank scenes because a weak input in the periphery of the visual field can act as a retrieval cue for the object attractor. On the other hand, in a complex background, the object closest to the fovea acts as the retrieval cue, because the fovea is given increased weight due to the higher magnification factor of the fovea. This results in smaller receptive fields of IT neurons in complex scenes.

Attentional top-down object-based inputs can bias the competition implemented in this attractor model but have relatively minor effects (for example, in increasing receptive field size) when they are applied in a complex natural scene, as then the necessarily

stronger forward inputs dominate the states reached. The results of the investigation thus suggest that object-based attention may be a much more limited phenomenon in complex, natural, scenes than in reduced displays with one or two objects present. The results also suggest that providing strong weight to whatever is close to the fovea is an important principle governing the operation of IT. This principle of operation is important in interfacing the visual system to action systems, because the effective stimulus in making IT neurons fire is in natural scenes usually on or close to the fovea. This means that the spatial coordinates of where the object is in the scene do not have to be represented in IT, nor passed from it to the action selection system, as the latter can assume that the object making IT neurons fire is close to the fovea.

Invariant Visual Object Recognition

Such neurophysiological findings lead to the hypothesis that cortical visual processing for object (including face) recognition is organized as a set of hierarchically connected cortical regions (Figure 2; this also appears as Figure 1 in OBJECT RECOGNITION, NEUROPHYSIOLOGY). There is convergence from each small part of a region to the succeeding region (or layer or stage in the hierarchy) in such a way that the receptive field sizes of neurons (e.g., 0.5° to 1° near the fovea in V1) become larger by a factor of approximately 2.5 with each succeeding stage. This connectivity would be part of the architecture by which translation-invariant representations are computed. Each stage in the hierarchy is considered to act partly as a set of local self-organizing competitive neuronal networks with overlapping inputs. Increasing complexity of representations could also be built in such a multiple-layer hierarchy by similar competitive learning mechanisms. To avoid a combinatorial explosion, low-order combinations of inputs would be learned by each neuron. (See OBJECT RECOGNITION for further data and models on invariant object recognition.)

Although hierarchical processing schemes have been investigated before (see NEOCOGNITRON: A MODEL FOR VISUAL PATTERN RECOGNITION), Rolls (1992, see *R&D*) suggested that translation, size, and view invariance could be computed in such a system by utilizing competitive learning that operates across short time scales to detect regularities in inputs when real objects are transforming in the physical world. The idea is that because objects have continuous properties in space and time in the world, an object at one place on the retina might activate feature analyzers at the next stage of cortical processing, and when the object is translated to a nearby position, because this would occur in a short period (e.g., 0.5 s), the membrane of the postsynaptic neuron would still be in its associatively modifiable state, and the presynaptic afferents activated with the object in its new position would thus become strengthened on the still-activated postsynaptic neuron.

The VisNet model was developed to test and clarify these hypotheses. The network can perform object (including face) recognition in a biologically plausible way and after training shows, for example, translation and view invariance. The network can identify objects shown in a cluttered environment (for example, a natural scene) and can identify partially occluded objects. Elliffe, Rolls, and Stringer (2002, see *R&D*) showed how, by forming high spatial precision feature combination neurons early in processing, it is possible for later layers to maintain high precision for the relative spatial position of features within an object yet achieve invariance for the spatial position of the whole object.

To incorporate top-down processing effects such as attention, associatively modifiable backprojections (*not* backpropagation!) have recently been introduced into the model. They enable the VisNet architecture to show in addition the biased competition effects that characterize attentional modulation of processing in sensory systems. By introducing into the model a dorsal visual stream

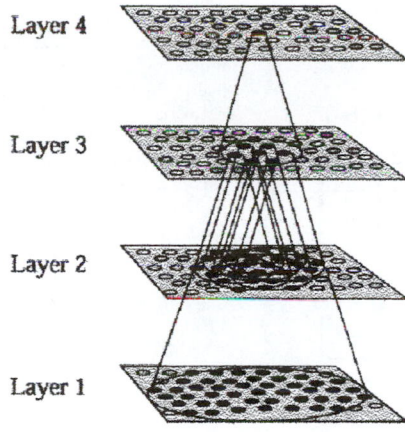

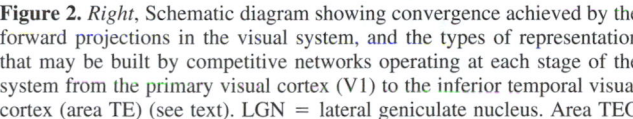

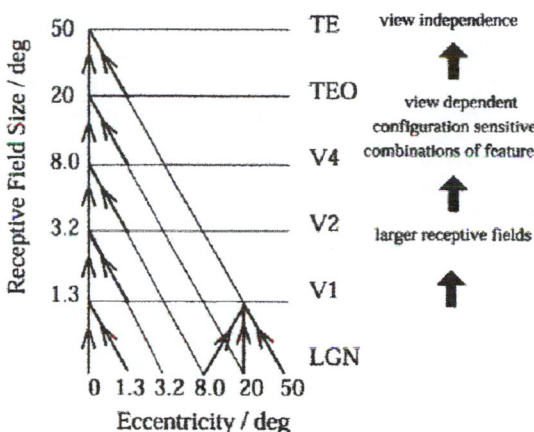

Figure 2. *Right,* Schematic diagram showing convergence achieved by the forward projections in the visual system, and the types of representation that may be built by competitive networks operating at each stage of the system from the primary visual cortex (V1) to the inferior temporal visual cortex (area TE) (see text). LGN = lateral geniculate nucleus. Area TEO forms the posterior inferior temporal cortex. The receptive fields in the inferior temporal visual cortex (e.g., in the TE areas) cross the vertical midline (not shown). *Left,* As implemented in VisNet, Rolls's hierarchical model of invariant visual object recognition (see *R&D*).

module (parietal cortex) that can interact with the ventral stream modules through the topologically mapped V1 and V2 modules, it is possible in a full dynamical model implemented with mean field equations to account quantitatively for many aspects of object search and spatial search in complex scenes.

The Visuospatial Scratchpad and Change Blindness

Given the fact that the responses of IT neurons are quite locked to the stimulus being foveated, it is unlikely that IT provides the representation of the visual world that we think we see, with objects at their correct places in a visual scene. In fact, we do not really see the whole visual scene, as most of it is a memory reflecting what was seen when the eyes were last looking at a particular part of the scene. The evidence for this statement comes from change blindness experiments, which show that humans rather remarkably do not notice if, while they are moving their eyes and cannot respond to changes in the visual scene, a part of the scene changes (Rensink, 2000). Given then that much of the apparent richness of our visual world is actually based on what was seen at previously fixated positions in the scene (this being what IT represents), we may ask where this "visuospatial scratchpad"—another name for the short-term spatial scene memory modeled in terms of schema instances in the VISIONS system—is located in the brain. One possibility is in the right parieto-occipital area, since patients with lesions in this region have (dorsal) *simultanagnosia,* in which they can recognize objects but cannot see more than one object at a time (Farah, 1990).

The neural basis of this is not yet known, but Rolls has suggested that it might consist of a number of separate—that is, local—attractors, each representing part of the space and capable of being loaded by inputs from the IT (see *R&D*). The attractors would be local because they are implemented by the predominantly short-range associatively modifiable excitatory collaterals between cortical pyramidal cells (see Rolls and Treves, 1998, chap. 10). Each attractor network in the visuospatial scratchpad memory would be addressed by information based on the position of the eyes, of covert attention, and probably of the head (see Figure 3). Every module receives the same inputs that represent objects (O) and shapes from the inferior temporal visual cortex and a different position (P) input representing the current place in the environment, probably in egocentric visual field-of-view coordinates and based on the current eye position, covert attention, and perhaps head direction. The network state is cued into a new attractor, which represents the currently foveated object in a scene as indicated by the IT neurons that are firing, when it receives a position input that corresponds to the location of that attractor in the map of the visual scene. The position input must be sufficiently strong that when it is applied to a particular module in combination with the IT input, it forces the attractor to go from a state in which the recurrent collaterals dominate the activity in a stable memory mode to the new state represented by the IT input (see Renart et al., 2001; *R&D,* chap. 12). Each attractor network would be capable of holding active in its short-term memory one of something in the order of 10,000 objects stored in the recurrent collaterals (given the large number of recurrent collaterals on each neuron and the storage capacity equation of attractors storing sparse patterns; see *R&D*).

This schematic architecture would enable the objects present at different locations in a viewed spatial scene to be maintained in a set of spatially separate attractors. Information could be read out from the system from a point in space not currently being foveated by moving a weak, covert, attentional position (P) input to increase the gain in a particular module so that the firing of that module dominates a network receiving from all the attractor modules. If idiothetic (self-motion) inputs reflecting, for example, head direction need to be postulated to dynamically update the position of the object information in the different attractors, then this might be performed in the ways described by Stringer et al. (2002) for performing path integration in spatial continuous attractor neural networks (see also RODENT HEAD DIRECTION SYSTEM and DYNAMIC REMAPPING).

Scene Perception and the Emergence of Planning

Moving beyond visual STM for objects in retinotopic location, note that in action-oriented perception, current sensory stimulation is always interpreted within the ongoing state of the organism; the representation is dynamic and task oriented, linking instances of perceptual schemas to motor schemas, providing parameters, and changing confidence levels. As their activity levels reach threshold, certain motor schemas create patterns of overt behavior. To see this, consider a driver instructed to "turn right at the red barn." At

Local attractor networks for a visuo-spatial scratchpad

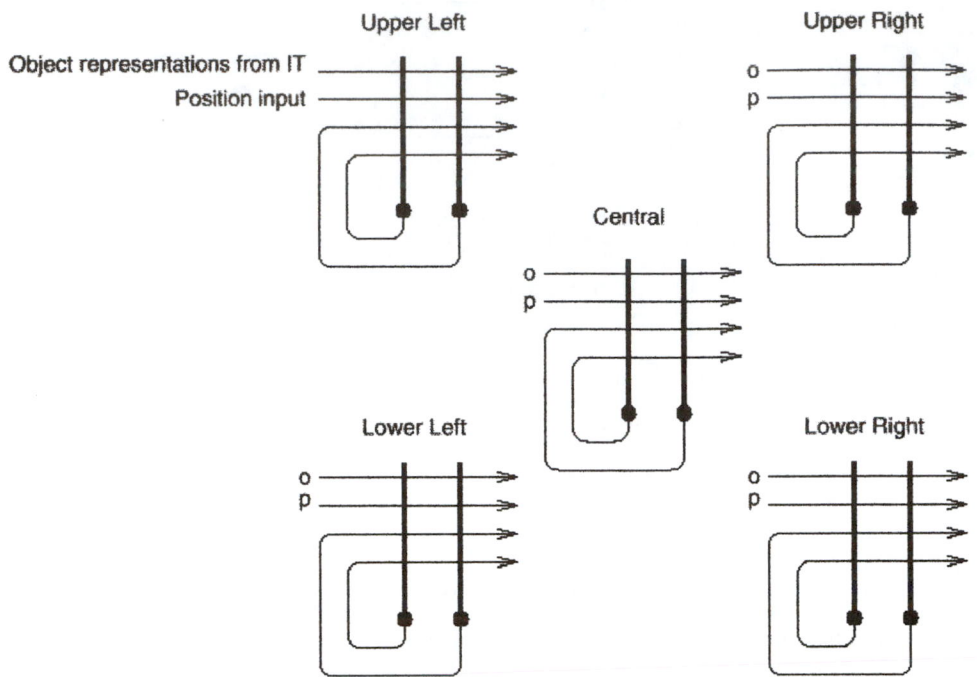

Figure 3. Schematic diagram of a set of attractor networks that it is hypothesized might implement a visuospatial scratchpad in the brain (see text). Each attractor network receives the same input from the IT that represents the object (O) that is being foveated. Each network also receives a position (P) input that enables the attractor currently active in the network to be replaced with a new attractor corresponding to the object at the fovea. The number of attractor networks in the diagram is for illustration only.

first, the person drives along looking for something large and red, after which the perceptual schema for barns is brought to bear. Once a barn is identified, the emphasis shifts to recognition of spatial relations appropriate to executing a right turn "at" the barn but determined rather by the placement of the roadway, and so on. All this is "planning" in a flexible representation strongly conditioned by current goals.

Arbib and Liaw (1995) therefore suggested extending VISIONS by the inclusion of motor as well as perceptual schemas and the dynamic interaction of working memory with changing sensory input. The data reviewed above suggest that activity in IT accentuates perceptual schemas for the current focus of attention. In this case, only a few intermediate schemas may be active, with STM being updated as new results come in from this focal processing. This leads us to reverse the view of activity/passivity of schemas and instances in the VISIONS system. There, the schema in LTM is the passive code for processes (the program for deciding whether a region is a roof, for example), while the schema instance is an active copy of that process (the execution of that program to test a particular region for "roofness"). By contrast, it may be that in the brain, the active circuitry is the *schema*, so that only one or a few instances can apply data-driven updating at a time. This is somewhat reminiscent of the visuospatial scratchpad described above, which stores an object code at each location, while IT processing determines the appropriate schema for the foveal region. However, a possible weakness of that model, demanding further research, is that it requires the IT code for each object to be learned by the attractor network at each position of the scratchpad, rather than dynamically binding, let us say, IT and PP representations of the object to its current location (see DYNAMIC LINK ARCHITECTURE), which would obviate having to repeatedly determine action-relevant properties of the object as it moves. In any case, the post-

VISIONS architecture integrates the "what" system (IT) and the various "how" systems (PP) (see, e.g., GRASPING MOVEMENTS: VISUOMOTOR TRANSFORMATIONS) as follows:

1. In a complex situation, we must recognize which object it is appropriate to interact with, and for what purpose, before the "how" system (PP) can generate appropriate motor parameters. If, then, object recognition is mediated by the ventral system, the question of how to act must be mediated through information from the ventral stream influencing the dorsal stream. For example, if one sees two plums on a plate, the dorsal stream can guide arm and hand in picking up one of the plums, but it may be the task of the ventral stream (and its links to orbitofrontal cortex) to recognize which plum is the riper and thus help to determine the "focus of attention" of the dorsal system.

2. We postulate that PP can be influenced by STM information about goals, etc., maintained in prefrontal cortex. Action is often determined by goals and prior input as much as, if not more than, by current sensory input. Indeed, Fuster (see CORTICAL MEMORY) has reviewed the role of the prefrontal cortex in processes that elaborate, store, and—during the course of behavior—update a plan of action. We hypothesize that at each stage of action, prefrontal cortex, through its extensive system of reciprocal interconnections with parietal cortex, "focuses the attention" of the dorsal stream so that it may elaborate visually based parameters for action. (This raises a question for further research: Is the "visuospatial scratchpad" in the right parieto-occipital area as suggested earlier, or is it part of a larger prefrontal system?) Again, through these reciprocal connections, parietal cortex can apprise the prefrontal system of the progress of motor execution as controlled by premotor cortex, as well as reporting any obstacles to execution of the current plan. This allows the prefrontal system to update the plan, through a mixture of off-line and reactive planning, as the task unfolds.

Discussion

We have sought to show the promise for both theory and experiment of broadening the study of object recognition to encompass visual scene perception. The slide box metaphor, STM in the VISIONS system, and the visuospatial scratchpad provide three perspectives for creating a theory of how the visual perception of objects may be integrated with the perception of spatial layout. The first two stress a schema-theoretic approach, while the latter is strongly tied to visual neurophysiology and modeling in terms of quasi-neural attractor networks. In particular, we have seen that neurophysiological findings made on visual stimuli presented in isolation fail to illuminate crucial aspects of the neural processing of the view of objects embedded in natural scenes. By sandwiching our discussion of neurophysiology between a discussion the "what" and "how" systems and a prospectus for extending the VISIONS methodology to model the dynamic role of vision in the control of action, we have opened the way to future research that will embed the study of visual scene perception in an action-oriented integration of inferotemporal and parietal visual systems.

Road Map: Vision
Related Reading: Dissociations Between Visual Processing Modes; Global Visual Pattern Extraction; Object Recognition, Neurophysiology; Visual Scene Segmentation

References

Arbib, M. A., and Liaw, J.-S., 1995, Sensorimotor transformations in the worlds of frogs and robots, *Artificial Intelligence*, 72:53–79. ◆
Didday, R. L., and Arbib, M. A., 1971, The organization of action-oriented memory for a perceiving system: I. The basic model, *J. Cybernetics*, 1:3–18.
Draper, B. A., Collins, R. T., Brolio, J., Hanson, A. R., and Riseman, E. M., 1989, The VISIONS schema system, *Int. J. Computer Vision*, 2:209–250.
Farah, M. J., 1990, *Visual Agnosia*, Cambridge, MA: MIT Press.
Goodale, M. A., and Milner, A. D., 1992, Separate visual pathways for perception and action, *Trends Neurosci.*, 15:20–25.
Humphrey, N. K., 1970, What the frog's eye tells the monkey's brain, *Brain Behav. Evol.*, 3:324–337.
Miikkulainen, R., and Leow, W. K., 1995, Visual schemas in object recognition and scene analysis, in *The Handbook of Brain Theory and Neural Networks* (M. A. Arbib, Ed.), Cambridge, MA: Bradford Books/MIT Press.
Renart, A., Moreno, R., de la Rocha, J., Parga, N., and Rolls, E. T., 2001, A model of the IT-PF network in object working memory which includes balanced persistent activity and tuned inhibition, *Neurocomputing*, 38–40:1525–1531.
Rensink, R. A., 2000, Seeing, sensing, and scrutinizing, *Vision Res.*, 40:1469–1487.
Rolls, E. T., 2000, Functions of the primate temporal lobe cortical visual areas in invariant visual object and face recognition, *Neuron*, 27:205–218. ◆
Rolls, E. T., and Deco, G., 2002, *Computational Neuroscience of Vision*, Oxford, Engl.: Oxford University Press. ◆
Rolls, E. T., and Treves, A., 1998, *Neural Networks and Brain Function*, Oxford, Engl.: Oxford University Press.
Stringer, S. M., Trappenberg, T. P., Rolls, E. T., and Araujo, I. E. T., 2002, Self-organising continuous attractor networks and path integration: One-dimensional models of head direction cells, *Network: Computation in Neural Systems*, 13:217–242.
Ungerleider, L. G., and Mishkin, M., 1982, Two cortical visual systems, in *Analysis of Visual Behavior* (D. J. Ingle, M. A. Goodale, and R. J. W. Mansfield, Eds.), Cambridge, MA: MIT Press.
Weymouth, T. E., 1986, Using object descriptions in a schema network for machine vision, Ph.D. Thesis and COINS Technical Report 86-24, Department of Computer and Information Science, University of Massachusetts at Amherst.

Visual Scene Segmentation

DeLiang Wang

Introduction

Visual scene analysis, a remarkable achievement of the visual system, involves two basic perceptual processes: segmentation of a visual scene into a set of coherent patterns (objects) and recognition of memorized patterns. In this article, I focus on scene segmentation, which is closely related to figure-ground segregation, whereby one object is segmented from the rest of the scene (background), and perceptual organization.

Humans perform scene segmentation with apparent ease. However, the study of automatic scene segmentation remains a challenging problem, despite dozens of years of intensive research in computer vision and image processing, where *image segmentation* is the commonly used term.

In a natural scene, objects appear as the grouping of similar sensory features and the segregation of dissimilar ones. Studies in visual perception, particularly in gestalt psychology, have uncovered a number of principles for perceptual organization, including the following important principles (see Palmer, 1999, chap. 6):

- *Proximity*: Features nearby in space and time tend to group into the same segment.
- *Similarity*: Features having similar attributes (e.g., brightness) tend to group.
- *Connnectedness*: A uniform, connected region (e.g., a blackboard) tends to form a single segment.
- *Memory*: Features that belong to the same memory pattern tend to group.

Compared to recognition, scene segmentation in neural networks is the subject of far fewer papers. The problem is particularly challenging for neural networks because the binding problem must also be addressed. The binding problem refers to how the coherence of a pattern, generally a large collection of features, is represented in a neural network. One proposal, the grandmother-cell representation, suggests that individual neurons can become so selective as to represent individual objects. Multiple objects in a visual scene would be represented by the coactivation of multiple cells. Another proposal, known as temporal correlation (von der Malsburg, 1981), encodes the binding by the correlation of temporal activities of feature-detecting cells. A special form of temporal correlation is *oscillatory correlation*, where the basic units are neural oscillators (Terman and Wang, 1995). Oscillatory correlation is the underlying representation for a number of recent studies that have substantially advanced the capability of neural networks in scene segmentation.

I first review nonoscillatory approaches, then turn to oscillatory approaches.

Nonoscillatory Approaches

Boltzmann Machine

In an early study, Sejnowski and Hinton (1987) introduced the use of a Boltzmann machine for figure-ground segregation (see SIMULATED ANNEALING AND BOLTZMANN MACHINES). Their network consists of two types of binary units: figure units and edge units. Units in the network are locally and symmetrically connected with fixed excitatory and inhibitory weights. Such connections reflect local cooperation within a connected region and local competition between figure and background. There are two kinds of input to the network: bottom-up input, which contains the location and orientation of edges (or line segments), and top-down input, which corresponds to visual attention and provides a necessary bias for selecting a figure in an image. The desired output of the system is that the units corresponding to a figural object and its boundary be active while the rest of the network units remain silent. Their simulation results on small synthetic images produced the desired results; but, as the authors point out, the applicability of the Boltzmann machine approach to segmenting real images is uncertain.

FBF Model

Grossberg and Wyse (1991) proposed the FBF model for scene segmentation, which iterates between two subsystems—a feature contour system and a boundary contour system—in the order feature-boundary-feature (hence the acronym). The feature contour system detects local features using on-center/off-surround and off-center/on-surround filters, then performs diffusion within an image region; the boundary contour system detects local edges and performs contour completion. Subsequently, a filling-in process spreads a region label until there is a boundary signal. The model has been tested using simple images, but its performance on real images is unclear given the recognized difficulty of contour completion in real images. Labeling by filling-in is rather cumbersome: too few labels may miss significant regions and too many may generate duplicate segments. This labeling process, however, can be significantly improved by introducing top-down attention for selecting one region, as described by Sejnowski and Hinton (1987), and shift of attention for selecting multiple regions sequentially.

Classification-Based Approach

Neural networks are well established as pattern classifiers. Because scene segmentation may be viewed, in some sense, as a classification problem, neural networks have been used in many studies to do image segmentation as classification. A training stage precedes actual classification; in the training stage, multiple classes are formed, corresponding to multiple labels for the regions of interest. After training, the classifier is used to label each individual pixel in the image. Koh, Suk, and Bhandarkar (1995) proposed a hierarchical Kohonen map (see SELF-ORGANIZING FEATURE MAPS) for range image segmentation. At each level of the hierarchy, a Kohonen map is used to segment an image into a given number of regions. A hierarchy is used for two purposes. First, the hierarchy alleviates the requirement to know the number of segments a priori. Second, the hierarchy embodies multiple scales of the input feature space. More recently, Alirezaie, Jernigan, and Nahmias (1997) used both the Kohonen map and a multilayer perceptron for segmenting two-dimensional (2D) magnetic resonance imaging (MRI) images of the human brain. Both networks are trained to classify three kinds of tissue: white matter, gray matter, and cerebrospinal fluid. After training, the two networks are used to segment the same images. Good performance is reported for Kohonen maps and poorer performance for multilayer perceptrons.

A fundamental limitation of all classification-based approaches to segmentation, neural networks or not, is that classification is based on local information only, whereas proper segmentation of a location depends on the image context of that location. This limitation is illustrated in Figure 1, where 12 line segments are arranged in two different ways in Figure 1A and 1B. Because the same set of line segments occurs in both images, local classification produces the same segmentation result, while the two images are perceptually organized very differently. Of course, one can train a system to classify a pixel together with its neighborhood. But fixed neighborhoods cannot capture the variability of image contexts.

Oscillatory Approaches

Early Simulations

Theoretical considerations and the discovery of coherent oscillations in the visual cortex in the late 1980s (see SYNCHRONIZATION, BINDING AND EXPECTANCY) triggered interest in exploring oscillatory correlation as a means to address scene segmentation and figure-ground segregation. Most of the early models employ harmonic oscillators and all-to-all connections to reach synchronization. These models are fundamentally limited in addressing the scene segmentation problem because critical information about the topology of sensory features is lost.

Recognizing the limitation of all-to-all connectivity, Sporns, Tononi, and Edelman (1991) constructed a locally connected network for modeling perceptual organization. To achieve proper synchronization, they used reentrant connections and dynamic weights, which quickly adapt to presynaptic and postsynaptic stimulation. Schillen and König (1994) proposed a network that performs synchronization and desynchronization in multiple feature domains. Their network uses Wilson-Cowan oscillators, which model oscillations from an interacting population of excitatory and inhibitory neurons, and time delays between elements of neighboring oscillators to achieve both synchronization and desynchronization. To deal with multiple-feature domains, the network is extended to include multiple modules and cross-module connections. Both of these studies have been tested using only synthetic stimuli.

LEGION Networks

Terman and Wang (1995) proposed and analyzed a class of locally excitatory globally inhibitory oscillator networks, called LEGION. Each oscillator i in a LEGION network is a relaxation oscillator:

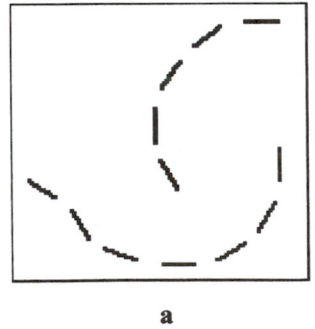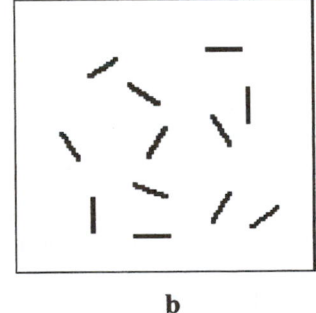

| a | b |

Figure 1. Perceptual organization of line segments. *a*, A spatial arrangement of 12 line segments. *b*, A different arrangement.

$$x_i' = f(x_i) - y_i + I_i + S_i + \rho \qquad \text{(1a)}$$

$$y_i' = \varepsilon(g(x_i) - y_i) \qquad \text{(1b)}$$

Here, $f(x) = 3x - x^3 + 2$ is a cubic and $g(x) = \alpha[1 + \tanh(x/\beta)]$ is a sigmoid (α and β are parameters). I_i denotes external input, and ρ is intrinsic noise. The parameter ε is a small positive number, which yields two time scales that are the defining property of relaxation oscillations. When $I_i > 0$, (1) gives rise to a stable limit cycle, which alternates between a silent phase (small x values) and an active phrase (large x values). Due to ε, the oscillator activity changes slowly within either of the two phases, but the alternation between the two phases takes place rapidly; this phenomenon is known as jumping. S_i denotes the overall input from the network; it contains a local excitatory term and a global inhibitory term. The excitatory term represents the excitatory input from a set of adjacent oscillators that connect to i. In a 2D LEGION network, the set in the simplest case contains four immediate neighbors. This architecture is shown in Figure 2A. The inhibitory term specifies the inhibition from a global inhibitor.

Terman and Wang (1995) conducted an extensive analysis on LEGION networks based on an earlier analysis by Somers and Kopell (1993) on two coupled relaxation oscillators. They showed that LEGION exhibits the mechanism of *selective gating* as follows. When an oscillator jumps to the active phase, its activity spreads to its neighboring oscillators, which further spread the activity to their neighbors, and so on. This leads to synchronization in LEGION. In addition, oscillating groups inhibit each other through global inhibition so that at most one group can be in the active phase at a time. This leads to desynchronization. They proved the following theorem: LEGION networks achieve both synchronization and desynchronization in no greater than m cycles of oscillations, where m is the number of patterns in an input scene, so long as m does not exceed the segmentation capacity. The segmentation capacity refers to the maximum number of patterns that can be segmented by LEGION, corresponding to the ratio of the oscillation period to the duration of the active phase. The capacity is about 5 to 7 for typical parameter values.

The following simulation illustrates the selective gating mechanism. An input image with three caricature patterns—a rabbit, a duck, and a flower—is simultaneously presented to a 30×30 LEGION network, as shown in Figure 2B. The oscillators under stimulation become oscillatory, while those without stimulation

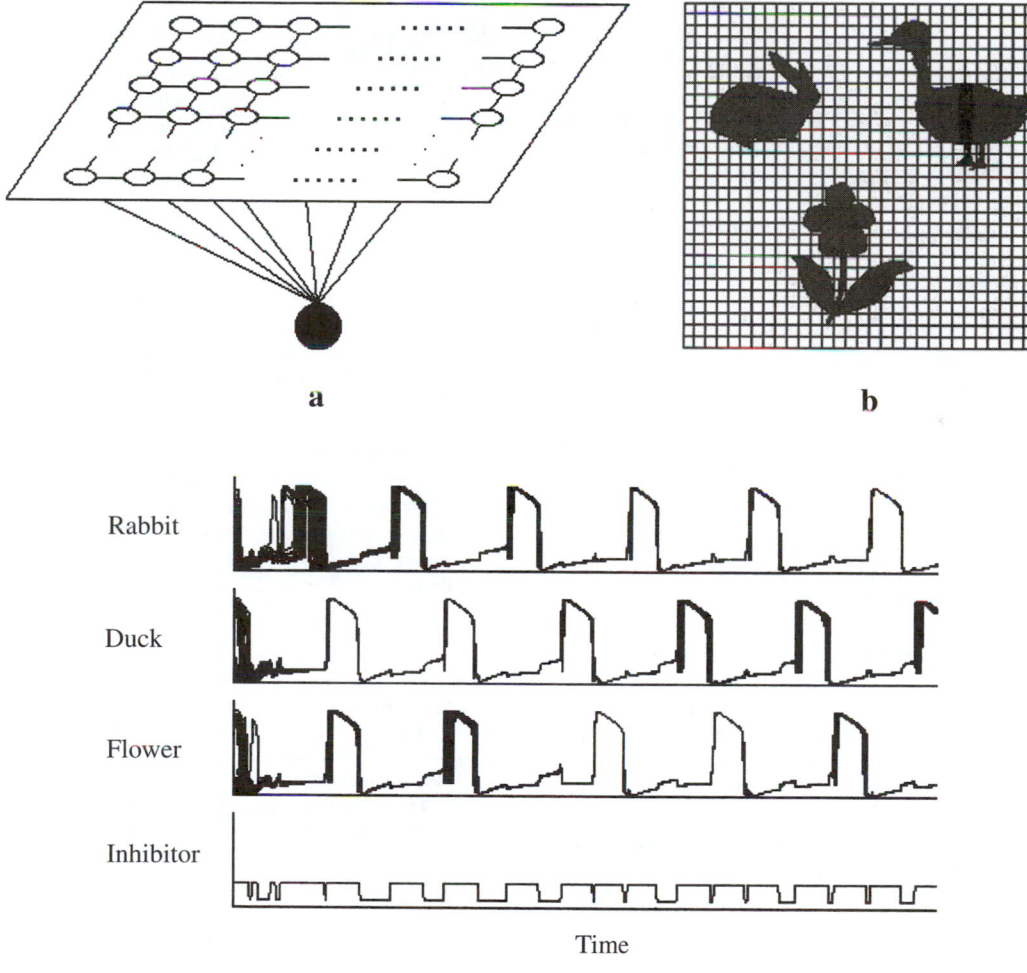

Figure 2. LEGION network. *a*, Architecture of 2D LEGION, where white circles indicate oscillators and the black circle indicates the global inhibitor. *b*, An input image as sampled by a 30×30 LEGION network. *c*, Temporal activity of the network (adapted from D. L. Wang, *Cognitive Science*, vol. 20, p. 425, 1996), where the upper three traces show the combined temporal activities of the oscillator groups corresponding to the indicated patterns. The bottom trace shows the activity of the global inhibitor.

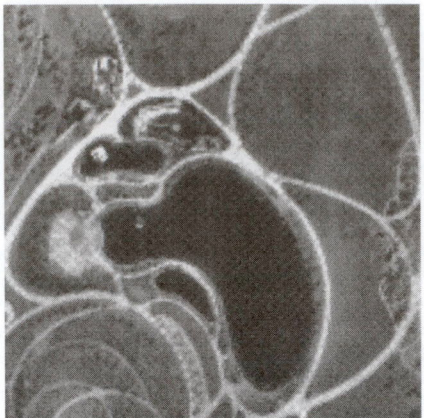 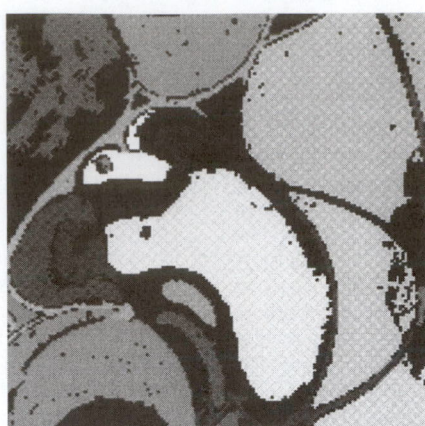

Figure 3. Image segmentation (from Wang and Terman, 1997). *A*, A gray-level image with 160 × 160 pixels. *B*, Segmentation result for panel *A*, where each segment is indicated by a distinct gray level.

cannot oscillate. Figure 2*C* shows the temporal evolution of every stimulated oscillator. The activities of the oscillators representing each object are combined in Figure 2*C*. Although the oscillators in the network start with random phases, the synchronization within each pattern and the desynchronization between different patterns are clearly attained in just two oscillation periods.

Image Segmentation Using LEGION

Wang and Terman (1997) extended LEGION to distinguish between major image regions and noisy fragments; the latter are collected into the background. For gray-level images, each oscillator corresponds to one pixel, and two neighboring oscillators are connected with a weight proportional to pixel similarity. To speed up simulation with the large number of oscillators needed for processing real images, Wang and Terman also abstracted an algorithm that follows LEGION dynamics. To illustrate typical segmentation results, Figure 3*A* shows a gray-level aerial image. Figure 3*B* shows the result of segmentation by the algorithm. The image is segmented into 23 regions, each of which corresponds to a different intensity level in Figure 3*B*, which indicates a distinct phase of oscillators. Note that the segmentation capacity is removed in the algorithm for computational efficiency. In the simulation, different segments pop out from the network sequentially, as similarly shown in Figure 2*C*. As displayed in Figure 3*B*, almost all major regions are successfully segmented. The black scattered areas in the figure represent the background.

A variety of real imagery has been successfully segmented by LEGION networks and their variants, including intensity images such as medical (Shareef, Wang, and Yagel, 1999) and satellite images, texture images, and image sequences (motion). Oscillatory correlation provides a unique way to scene labeling. As illustrated in Figure 2*C*, segmentation is performed in *time*; each segment pops out at a distinct time from the network and different segments alternate in time. Once a segment is in the active phase, all of its features, but none of the ones from competing segments, are simultaneously available for later visual processing such as attention and recognition (Wang and Liu, 2002).

Contour Extraction

Yen and Finkel (1998) used laterally coupled phase oscillators to extract salient contours. Excitatory and inhibitory connections in their network encode orientation relations between edge filters. The salience of a contour is embodied by the total activity of a synchronized oscillator group that corresponds to the contour. Using integrate-and-fire oscillators, Horn and Opher (1999) studied the detection of borders between regions. Their network uses difference-of-Gaussian coupling, and their simulations suggest that, at local minima of total network activity, firing oscillators tend to correspond to edges that separate different regions.

Discussion

The field of neural networks has seen major advances in visual scene segmentation in recent years. The temporal correlation hypothesis is a biologically plausible representation to deal with the binding problem. The selective gating mechanism provides a computational foundation for oscillatory correlation. These advances have finally enabled neural networks to analyze real scenes. I conclude with two issues for future research.

1. *Multi-cue interaction*. There are many grouping cues responsible for perceptual organization. It is important to build systems capable of synergistically integrating multiple cues, not just breaking them into independent modules. Is there, or should there be, a common segmentation mechanism at a deeper level?
2. *Top-down analysis*. Studies in human visual psychophysics demonstrate strong top-down influence on scene analysis. Sources of top-down information include recognition, goal and expectation, short-term memory, and attention. Few studies have seriously addressed these issues in the context of analyzing real scenes. Given their importance, they deserve much more attention.

Road Map: Vision
Background: Phase-Plane Analysis of Neural Nets
Related Reading: Dynamic Link Architecture; Global Visual Pattern Extraction; Markov Random Field Models in Image Processing; Probabilistic Regularization Methods for Low-Level Vision; Synchronization, Binding and Expectancy; Tensor Voting and Visual Segmentation; Visual Scene Perception

References

Alirezaie, J., Jernigan, M. E., and Nahmias, C., 1997, Neural network-based segmentation of magnetic resonance images of the brain, *IEEE Trans. Nuclear Sci.*, 44:194–198.
Grossberg, S., and Wyse, L., 1991, A neural network architecture for figure-ground separation of connected scenic figures, *Neural Net.*, 4:723–742.
Horn, D., and Opher, I., 1999, Collective excitation phenomena and their applications, in *Pulsed Neural Networks* (W. Maass and C. M. Bishop, Eds.), Cambridge MA: MIT Press, pp. 297–320. ◆

Koh, J., Suk, M., and Bhandarkar, S. M., 1995, A multilayer self-organizing feature map for range image segmentation, *Neural Net.*, 8:67–86.

Palmer, S. E., 1999, *Visual Science*, Cambridge, MA: MIT Press. ◆

Schillen, T. B., and König, P., 1994, Binding by temporal structure in multiple feature domains of an oscillatory neuronal network, *Biol. Cybern.*, 70:397–405.

Sejnowski, T. J., and Hinton, G. E., 1987, Separating figure from ground with a Boltzmann machine, in *Vision, Brain, and Cooperative Computation* (M. A. Arbib and A. R. Hanson, Eds.), Cambridge, MA: MIT Press, pp. 703–724.

Shareef, N., Wang, D. L., and Yagel, R., 1999, Segmentation of medical images using LEGION, *IEEE Trans. Med. Imaging*, 18:74–91.

Somers, D., and Kopell, N., 1993, Rapid synchrony through fast threshold modulation, *Biol. Cybern.*, 68:393–407.

Sporns, O., Tononi, G., and Edelman, G. M., 1991, Modeling perceptual grouping and figure-ground segregation by means of active re-entrant connections, *Proc. Natl. Acad. Sci. USA*, 88:129–133.

Terman, D., and Wang, D. L., 1995, Global competition and local cooperation in a network of neural oscillators, *Physica D*, 81:148–176.

von der Malsburg, C., 1981, The correlation theory of brain function, Internal Report 81-2, Max-Planck-Institute for Biophysical Chemistry.

Wang, D. L., and Liu, X., 2002, Scene analysis by integrating primitive segmentation and associative memory, *IEEE Trans. Syst. Man Cybern.*—Part B: Cybern., 32:254–268.

Wang, D. L., and Terman, D., 1997, Image segmentation based on oscillatory correlation, *Neural Comp.*, 9:805–836 (for errata see *Neural Comp.*, 9:1623–1626, 1997).

Yen, S.-C., and Finkel, L. H., 1998, Extraction of perceptually salient contours by striate cortical networks, *Vis. Res.*, 38:719–741.

Visuomotor Coordination in Frog and Toad

Francisco Cervantes-Pérez

Introduction

Frogs and toads (anurans) live within complex, and uncertain, three-dimensional (3D) environments rich in multiple modes of sensory signals (e.g., visual, tactile, olfactory). However, their behavior is guided primarily by visual information. Therefore, they have been widely studied under visuomotor coordination paradigms, where the integration of visual signals with the animal's motor response implies a complex transformation of sensory data. The same locus of retinal activation might release different types of behavior, some directed toward the stimulus (e.g., prey catching) and others directed toward an opposite part of the visual field (e.g., predator avoidance). Furthermore, the efficacy of visual stimuli to release an animal's response is determined by a variety of factors: (1) the stimulus characteristics (e.g., form, size, velocity, geometric configuration with respect to the direction of motion, its location in space, its own current behavior); (2) the current state of internal variables of the anuran's organism, especially those related to motivational changes (e.g., season of the year, time of day, food deprivation); (3) the animal's previous experience with the stimulus (e.g., learning, conditioning, habituation); and (4) the physical condition of the animal's central nervous system (CNS) (e.g., brain lesions). In addition, other types of sensory signals can modulate frogs' and toads' responses to certain moving visual stimuli. For example, the efficacy of a prey-like dummy may be greatly enhanced by the presence of prey odor.

In this article we emphasize how the study of visually guided behaviors in anurans has become significant for scientists working in a variety of fields. In neuroscience (Llinás and Precht, 1976; Vanegas, 1984; Ewert et al., 2001) and in computational neuroscience (see articles by Arbib, Betts, Cervantes-Pérez, an der Heiden, and Lara in Ewert and Arbib, 1989; Corbacho and Weitzenfeld, 2001), people have tried to understand how these animals' CNS integrates sensory information to control motor behavior; whereas in robotics and distributed artificial intelligence, behavioral models generated from the study of amphibians have inspired the development of computer-based action selection algorithms embedded in robots displaying complex sensorimotor behaviors (Arkin in Ewert and Arbib, 1989; Arkin et al., 2000; see also NEUROETHOLOGY, COMPUTATIONAL and REACTIVE ROBOTIC SYSTEMS).

Visually Guided Behaviors in Amphibians

Ethological experiments have shown that frogs and toads are capable of interacting with a wide variety of moving and nonmoving visual stimuli. Even though they have a limited behavioral repertoire, they may display motor actions belonging to different behavioral patterns, and their survival chances depend on their ability to produce the most appropriate action to cope with diverse environmental situations.

Response to Nonmoving Stimuli

A variety of stationary objects may influence the animal's next action. In general, when exploring their surroundings, frogs move toward zones in the visual field where blue is preponderant, probably because this situation might be associated to a pond (a proper habitat) location and to other stimuli whose presence is important for their survival, such as prey to eat, water to maintain their body humidity, and so on (Grüsser and Grüsser-Cornhels in Llinás and Precht, 1976). On the other hand, schema-theoretic models have been used to study those neuronal processes that occur when an obstacle (e.g., a barrier or a chasm) appears between an amphibian and a potential prey. These processes underlie an action selection mechanism that allows the animal to display a *detour behavior*, following predictable routes to avoid the obstacle in order to catch the prey (Arbib in Ewert and Arbib, 1989). Furthermore, these animals *learn to detour* a novel barrier to which they have not been yet exposed. Initially they approach the barrier, trying to go through the gaps of the fence in order to get to the prey. Then they back up and reorient toward one of the neighboring gaps; eventually, they reach the barrier edge and are able to approach the prey. After two or three trials, the dynamical changes in the processing of information allow the *trained frog* to detour without the initial bumping into the barrier (Corbacho and Weitzenfeld, 2001).

Predator Avoidance

Large stimuli at close distances may yield one of several avoidance behaviors, depending on its parametric composition. When a frog is confronted with a large flying stimulus at a close distance, it exhibits a *ducking* behavior, but when the stimulus is far afield, it *orients* toward the opposite direction and *jumps* or *runs away*. In the presence of a ground predator, toads display a *stiff-legged* posture, *puffing up*, orienting toward the predator, and *tilting* the body; then they *sidestep* or *jump away* from the predator's location (see articles by Ingle and Ewert in Llinás and Precht, 1976; Ewert in Vanegas, 1984; Cobas and Arbib in Arbib and Ewert, 1991; Liaw and Arbib, 1993; Roche King and Comer, 1996).

Prey Acquisition

When hunting, amphibians explore the immediate surroundings until a potential prey appears in the visual field; then they might present an action from their prey-catching repertoire: (1) Amphibians *orient* the head and body toward the prey if it appears in the peripheral part of the visual field, aiming to bring the stimulus into the binocular zone. (2) They *stalk* (toad) or *jump toward* (frog) potential prey located far afield in the frontal part of the visual field, *approaching* the prey to bring it closer. (3) Once the prey is within reaching distance, *binocular fixation* occurs to estimate its location in space. (4) If the prey is within the snapping zone, then amphibians *flick* their tongue to catch it. (5) The mechanical stimulation produced by the prey inside the mouth triggers a *gulping reflex*, and amphibians *wipe* the snout with their forelimbs (Ewert in Vanegas, 1984). This ethogram, like the ones described earlier, does not represent a fixed sequence of actions. Rather, all prey-catching responses are episodic and occur on a time scale of hundreds of milliseconds, and their outcome generates new situations with a high probability of activating one of the other prey-catching motor actions. That is, they comprise a sequence of temporally extended actions that leads toward the completion of overall goals (e.g., being fed, avoiding a dangerous situation).

Multisensory Guided Behaviors

Visual information is important not only for releasing well-known visually guided behaviors, it also plays a prominent role in eliciting behaviors requiring the integration of multiple modes of sensory signals. Innate prey recognition processes can be modified when visual prey stimuli are associated with olfactory and gustatory cues. After having a negative experience with distasteful preys (e.g., the red earthworm *Eisenia foetida*, hive bees), frogs and toads avoid attacking these types of prey in future situations (for details see Ewert et al., 2001). In the case of dart-poison male frogs, vocalizations serve, among other things, to regulate male distribution within a given territory. In the field, these animals display fighting behavior against other males, producing the aggression call when in the same territory. However, with the use of dummies and a speaker to play back the call, male frogs hopped toward the sound source but did not attack. That is, acoustic cues alone are not enough to yield frog's fighting behavior. Narins, Holdl, and Grabul (2001) built what they call Roborana, an electromechanical dummy frog sitting on something that looks like a plain old log housing a loudspeaker and an air pump connected to a rubber sac, simulating the dummy's throat sac. By inflating and deflating Roborana's throat sac in synchrony with the playback of the call, these authors showed that, in territorial male frogs, agonistic behavior could be evoked only when both acoustic and visual signals were presented simultaneously.

Neural Basis for Visuomotor Integration

Structural Organization

Neuroanatomical and lesion studies have been used to delineate the structural organization of the visuomotor system in anuran amphibia, which involves both serial and highly parallel interconnections. A direct visuomotor pathway mediating between visual stimulus presentation and the elicitation of prey-catching or predator avoidance behaviors has been identified. Visual signals impinge on visual receptors, producing electrical changes that modify the level of activity displayed by the retina's neuronal elements (i.e., bipolar, amacrine, horizontal, and ganglion cells). The efferent fibers of retinal ganglion cells distribute neural signals, encoding the presence of moving and nonmoving stimuli, to different structures in the animal's CNS. These structures include the optic tectum, the pretectum, the anterior thalamus, and the basal optic nucleus, all of which receive retinotopic mappings. Various types of ganglion cells (i.e., R2, with small receptive fields, and R3 and R4, with larger receptive fields) project to the optic tectum, which in turn projects to the mesencephalic tegmentum and to the reticular formation. These latter structures are reciprocally connected and have been postulated to be involved in generating motor patterns, which are subsequently sent to motor neuron nuclei in the medulla oblongata and the spinal cord. Elements of these motor neuron nuclei exert spatiotemporal control over the activation of specific sets of muscles during the elicitation of a given motor action.

This direct pathway has many modulatory connections with forebrain structures. Pretectal thalamus receives retinotopic projections from retinal ganglion cells with large receptive fields (i.e., R3 and R4) and has reciprocal topographic connections with tectum. These retino-tectal-pretectal interactions have been posited as the basis for prey-predator discrimination, through a dynamical pretectal inhibitory effect on tectum (Cervantes-Pérez, Lara, and Arbib, 1985). Other neural loops involving neuronal elements from the direct processing pathway and from forebrain structures have been identified. Some have been postulated as the basis for motivational effects on prey-catching behaviors (tectum—lateral thalamus—striatum—pretectum—tectum) or for stimulus-specific habituation of visually elicited prey-catching orienting (tectum—anterior thalamus—ventral medial pallium—preoptic/hypothalamus—tectum). For a detailed review of all morphological connections found through anatomical techniques between 1969 and 1999, see Ewert et al. (2001) (see also articles by Grusser-Cornehls and Lázár in Vanegas, 1984, and by Lázár and Weerasuriya in Ewert and Arbib, 1989).

Functional Complexity

Neurophysiological studies reinforce the anatomical hypothesis that visuomotor integration is subserved by a parallel distributed neural information processing system (for a review, see Ewert in Ewert and Arbib, 1989). The retina distributes visual information to different structures and has a great deal of parallelism within itself. Retinal ganglion cells are organized into different classes according to the size of their receptive field; that is, each class extracts information from the complete animal's visual field, but with different resolution. Class R2 cells have an excitatory receptive field (ERF) of $4°$, whereas class R3 cells have an ERF of $8°$ and the ERF of class R4 cells ranges between $12°$ and $16°$. In the same fashion, tectal and pretectal neurons have been grouped into different classes, according to various physiological criteria. Ewert and co-workers offered a classification of ten pretectal cell types (named TH1 to TH10) and nine types in tectum (named T1 to T9). In addition, taking into account their different sensitivities to changes in stimulus configural features, Ewert and colleagues identified several subclasses in some of these tectal cells. T5 cells were divided into four subclasses, T5.1 to T5.4, depending on the way they are activated by visual dummies: *wormlike* objects (i.e., a black rectangle moving against a white background, with its longest axis parallel to the direction of motion), *anti-wormlike* objects (the same object, but with its longest axis moving perpendicular to the direction of movement), and *square* moving objects. It has been postulated that these different types of tectal and pretectal neurons form a *command-releasing system* (see COMMAND NEURONS AND COMMAND SYSTEMS); that is, the activation of a motor pattern generator requires the simultaneous activation of appropriate combinations of specialized neurons. For example, a prey-catching orienting response is elicited only when both T5.2 (prey-feature-selecting unit) and T4 (arousal unit) cells are activated.

In addition, neuroethological data on fixed action patterns point to retino-tectal-pretectal interconnections as the basis for an amphibian's ability to interact with a variety of moving visual stimuli. First, it was suggested that in frogs, retinal ganglion cells with small receptive fields (class R2) were tuned as *bug detectors* (Lettvin et al., 1959). Then, in a more distributed view, the *integrative properties* found in the optic tectum were emphasized as the basis for detecting prey (Grüsser and Grüsser-Cornehls in Llinás and Precht, 1976). Later, prey-predator discrimination was described as the outcome of an *interactive process* among the projection of retinal ganglion cells to tectum (classes R2, R3, and R4) and pretectum (classes R3 and R4), in combination with an inhibitory pretectal effect on tectum (see articles by Arbib, Ewert, Betts, and Cervantes-Pérez in Ewert and Arbib, 1989; Cobas and Arbib in Arbib and Ewert, 1991).

A Tricyclic Approach

The study of anurans' visuomotor coordination has followed a tricyclic approach in which interconnected cycles have been developed to generate scientific and technological contributions. The aim of the theory-experiment cycle between neuroscience and brain theory is to develop an in-depth understanding of the neurobiological basis of behavior through the interplay between experimental and theoretical studies. Theoretical models are used to integrate hypotheses generated by different experimental disciplines (e.g., anatomy, ethology, physiology, pharmacology). By means of computer simulations, theoretical models serve as test bed for studying how these hypotheses yield the appropriate behaviors, and what the critical parametric combinations may be under which these behaviors are displayed (see articles by Arbib, Ewert, and Cervantes-Pérez in Ewert and Arbib, 1989). Formal models of animal behavior, in turn, can provide effective methods for generating biologically inspired *robotic intelligence* (Arkin et al., 2000; see also the article by Arkin in Ewert and Arbib, 1989). Physical experimentation with computer-based machines can also serve to test those hypotheses embedded in the models, which may lead to new ideas, new hypotheses, or the identification of gaps in our current understanding of how these animals' brain works. Thus, a new cycle has been established between the theory-experiment cycle and the fields of robotics and artificial intelligence. Within the reach of this cycle, models can be refined to better represent the phenomenon under study, the next generation of *intelligent* machines may be designed, and future stages in animal experimentation are stimulated.

Within this experimental-theoretical framework, the study of retino-tectal-pretectal interactions as the neural basis for frogs' and toads' visuomotor coordination has been useful in identifying neurobiological operational (computational) principles. Some examples are discussed in the following subsections.

Cooperation and Competition in Neuronal Networks

Ingle (1968) studied a *prey-selection phenomenon*: the snapping behavior of frogs confronted with two fly-like stimuli, each with enough prey-like characteristics (i.e., size, form, type of motion, and distance at which the fly is located in the frontal visual field) to elicit a snapping response. Frogs exhibited one of three reactions: (1) they snapped at one of the flies, (2) they did not snap at all, or (3) they snapped at the *average* fly. Didday (1976) developed a distributed network model of the optic tectum that explains this choice behavior in terms of a cooperation-competition process between two or more input signals. This model permits the network to act as a dynamic filter whose outcome is to transmit only the information encoded in the strongest signal. This process is one of the earliest examples of the *winner-take-all* algorithm (see WINNER-TAKE-ALL NETWORKS). Didday's model offered an architecture whereby different layers in tectum, organized in retino-

topic correspondence, compete in such a way that the most active region in the *foodness and newness* cell layers, receiving direct retinal input, eventually suppresses all other inputs and yields an above-threshold response in the *relative foodness* layer. This process is accomplished through the integration of foodness and newness cell layer activity with a lateral inhibition effect provided by the *sameness* cell layer. It was hypothesized that the level of activation in the foodness layer represented the input to the motor circuitry and encoded information to elicit a snapping response at the corresponding point in space. That is, tectal circuitry has the structural and functional properties to process information about multiple prey-like objects, and to direct animal's actions toward one of them. Amari and Arbib (1977) placed this model in a general theoretical perspective that has been widely used in the field of computer science.

Pattern Representation in the Spatiotemporal Dynamics of Neuronal Networks

Some hypotheses raised by experimental data in frogs and toads address the questions of what information may be stored in the retino-tectal-pretectal interactions, how it is retrieved, and what dynamic processes are activated by the presence of specific stimuli. These questions have also been analyzed by using different kinds of theoretical models.

Ewert and von Seelen (1974) analyzed prey-predator discrimination by considering the retina, the optic tectum, and the pretectum as *filters* working in a serial-parallel configuration (Figure 1). They postulated that within tectum there is a first filter sensitive to wormlike objects, whereas pretectum is modeled as a filter sensitive to anti-wormlike objects. Both filters receive excitatory inputs from the retina and project in turn to a second filter in tectum, which integrates an excitatory effect from the first tectal filter, with an inhibition effect coming from the pretectal filter. The signal processing built into this filter-type model allowed the authors to reproduce Ewert's physiological data: a wormlike object produced a stronger tectal response than a square object, while the antiworm-like object produced little or no response. However, this model is lumped in both space and time, and it describes neither the locus to which the toad directs its response nor the time at which the response is activated.

An der Heiden and Roth (in Ewert and Arbib, 1989) studied the same phenomenon by proposing an alternative model with no pretectal influence. Here, the activation dynamics of tectal cells (i.e., T5.1 and T5.2) are explained as the result of the spatiotemporal summation of retinal signals (i.e., ganglion cells R2 and R3), integrated with recurrent lateral inhibition among tectal elements. This model allowed the authors to reproduce important properties of the worm-antiworm discrimination, but it does not work well for bigger stimuli and does not address the issues of tectal response facilitation after a pretectal lesion or of the intrinsic tectal geometry.

Our group has developed a family of models *(Rana computatrix)* to analyze issues of the possible role played by retino-tectal-pretectal interactions in the processing of sensory signals and their translation into commands for controlling prey-catching and predator-avoidance behaviors. Cervantes-Pérez and Arbib (1990) conducted stability and parameter dependency analyses of the retino-tectal-pretectal neural circuits as organized by functional units (i.e., a layered neural network model), defined as *facilitation tectal columns* (FTCs). It was postulated that short-term memory processes underlying prey-catching facilitation are encoded in the reverberatory activity of tectal self-exciting neural loops rather than in synaptic strengthening. Cervantes-Pérez et al. (1985) presented an extended model consisting of an array of 8 × 8 FTC units, in which the effects of pretectal cell TH3 and ganglion cells R3 and R4 were added (Figure 2). The optic tectum is organized into col-

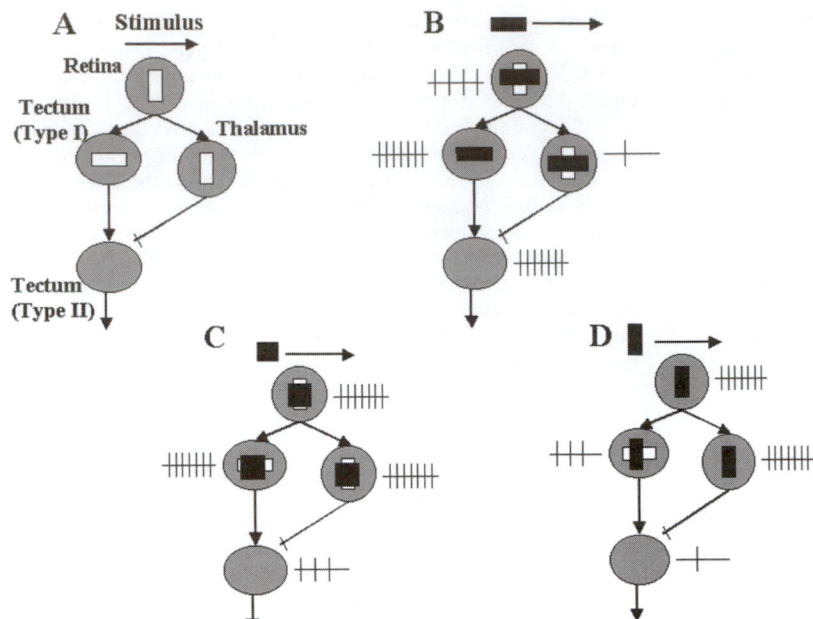

Figure 1. Ewert and von Seelen's filter-type model for prey-predator discrimination. The spike traces show different levels of response intensity. The higher the tectal frequencies, the better the activation of the associated prey-catching response. *A*, The tectal filter is tuned to wormlike stimuli, while the one in the thalamic pretectal area is more sensitive to large and anti-wormlike objects. *B*, During the presentation of a wormlike stimulus, the efferent tectal element presents a strong response, whereas the square produces an intermediate level of activation (part *C*), and the anti-worm elicits little or no response (part *D*). (Adapted with permission from Ewert in Ewert and Arbib, 1989.)

umns composed of different types of processing elements: the large pear-shaped cell (LP), the small pear-shaped cell (SP), the stellate neuron (SN), the pyramidal cell (PY, the only one having projecting axons outside the tectal circuit), and, finally, the glomerulus (GL), representing the convergence in the superficial tectal layers of axon terminals coming from the retina and other brain structures, and dendrite arborizations of tectal cells (see Székely and Lázár in Llinás and Precht, 1976; Lázár in Ewert and Arbib, 1989). GL receives signals from ganglion cells R2 and activates LP and SP cells, which in turn receive inputs from ganglion cells R2 and send axons back to GL, forming positive feedback loops that tend to

recruit tectal activity when a prey-like stimulus is present in the animal's visual field. The LP cell also excites the SN cell, postulated to be the only inhibitory tectal cell, which forms negative feedback loops with LP and SP cells to keep tectal activation in control, especially when the stimulus disappears from the animal's visual field. Finally, the efferent PY cell integrates the overall tectal activity with the inputs it receives from ganglion cells R2, R3, and R4. The PY cell is equivalent to Ewert's T5.2 cells, whose level of activation correlates quite well with the probability of a toad displaying a prey-catching response to a visual stimulus in its visual field.

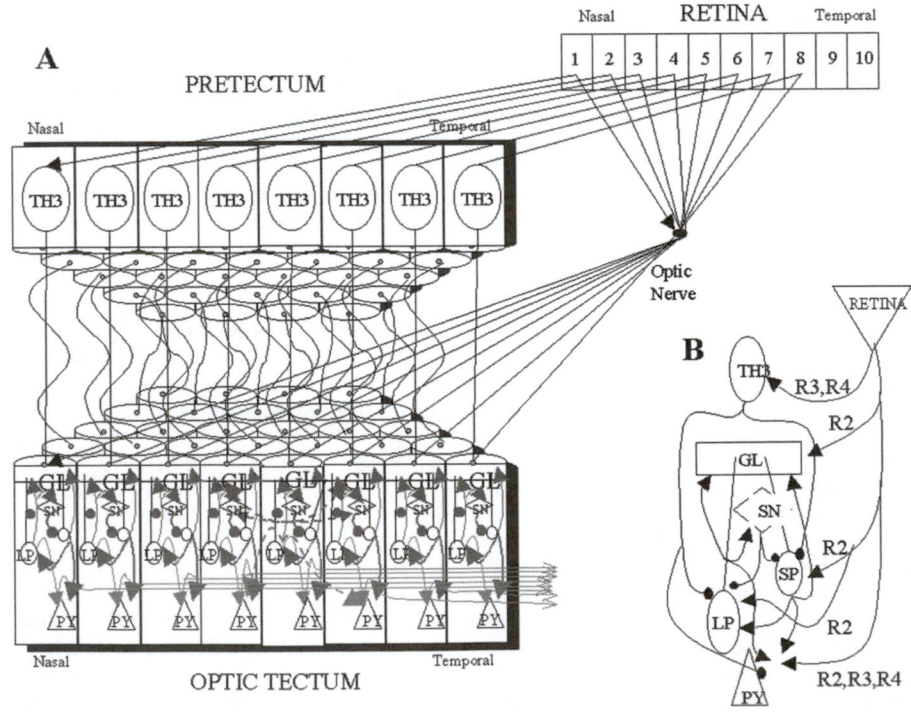

Figure 2. Neuronal network interactions among retina, tectum, and pretectum. *A*, The retina sends efferent fibers retinotopically to both tectum (R2, R3, and R4 ganglion cells) and pretectum (R3 and R4 ganglion cells). There is also a retinotopic projection from pretectal TH3 neurons to different tectal cells. *B*, Structural organization of a facilitation tectal column model; arrows indicate excitatory influences and dark circles inhibitory ones. (From Cervantes-Pérez in Ewert and Arbib, 1989. Reprinted with permission.)

Based on computer simulations, we analyzed how the movement direction invariance of the efficacy of a visual stimulus to elicit prey-catching behavior is a consequence of the tectal architecture. We argued that in the amphibians' visuomotor system, information about prey and predators is distributed among different structures (e.g., retina, tectum, and pretectum), and that its processing is carried out in a serial-parallel fashion. We also posited that the *knowledge* used during prey-predator recognition is *represented* within these neuronal circuits in a *spatiotemporal* way. That is, to signal whether the visual stimulus fits into the prey or the predator categories, it is important not only what neurons get activated, but also their temporal course of activation. In addition, we studied the hypothesis that the pretectal level of activation could be modulated by changes in motivational factors, so that tectum would act as a *dynamic filter* where, depending on the amount of pretectal inhibition, the same stimulus could yield different levels of tectal activation. Although the FTC model was abstracted somewhat crudely from anatomical data (Székely and Lázár in Llinás and Precht, 1976), it has been useful for analyzing how tectal circuitry involving *cooperation-competition* among positive and negative feedback loops works as a dynamic filter. The reverberatory circuits serve as mechanisms for short-term memory processes (prey-catching facilitation) and also as a *content-addressable memory* that stores information related to the probability of a stimulus fitting the prey category. This information is *retrieved* in the presence of a stimulus in the visual field (Cervantes-Pérez et al., 1985; Cervantes-Pérez and Arbib, 1990).

A wide range of those behavioral models (i.e., anurans' prey-catching, predator avoidance, and obstacle avoidance behaviors), in combination with a schema-theoretic model of the behavior of the praying mantis, *Chantlitaxia*, were implemented by Arkin et al. (2000) on a hexapod robot Hermes II equipped with a real-time color vision system. Michael, the robot, was able to properly interact with a 3D environment containing several preys and predators as well as fixed objects. These authors' work demonstrated the feasibility of importing models from the neurosciences community into robotics, and showed that species-specific behaviors can lead to interesting robotic performance.

Command-Releasing System

Experimental and theoretical studies have been conducted to address the question of how are the tectal-pretectal levels of activation used by motor pattern generators to produce the proper behavior. (see articles by Ewert, Grobstein, Matsurnoto, Weerasuriya, and Lázár in Ewert and Arbib, 1989; by Grobstein and by Cobas and Arbib in Arbib and Ewert, 1991; Roche King and Comer, 1996; see also COMMAND NEURONS AND COMMAND SYSTEMS). Tectum and pretectum send efferent fibers to motor pattern–generating networks (i.e., reticular formation, mesencephalic tegmentum) and contain neurons whose level of activation form a *command-releasing system*. The simultaneous activation of appropriate combinations of tectal and pretectal cell populations may be closely correlated with the efficacy of a visual target in producing a given motor response. For example, proper levels of activation in tectal cells T1.3, T3, T4, and T5.2 yield a response to a prey, whereas if tectal cell T5.1 and pretectal cells TH3 and TH4 are activated, then a response to a predator is produced. Additionally, some neuronal elements might participate in releasing behavior toward different types of behavior; for example, in the spring, a response to a *mate* is elicited when tectal cells T4 and T5.1 reach certain levels of activation (see Ewert in Ewert and Arbib, 1989). Furthermore, Cervantes-Pérez et al. (1985) proposed that the locus of activity within tectum and pretectum defines the spatial location of visual stimuli, and that the target location of prey-catching and predator avoidance behaviors is determined by the average of their target loci as weighted by their level of activation. They also assumed a hierarchical relationship between pretectum and tectum; high pretectal activity, closely correlated with the appearance of potential predators in the visual field, should shut off the prey recognition system.

Analyzing experimental data on *direction-selective avoidance behavior*, Liaw and Arbib (1993) offered a neural network model of the retino-tectal-pretectal interactions to account for the anuran's ability to avoid looming objects (potential predators). A visual stimulus activates ganglion cells R3 and R4, which project to tectal cells T3 and T6, which are activated by moving looming objects and also by the presence of a stimulus in the upper part of the corresponding visual field. These authors suggested that the population of T3 neurons gives a spatial map of the stimulus location. The stimulus position is determined by localizing its center, encoded in the peak of activation produced by the stimulus on the T3 neuron population, and the looming stimulus direction of motion is determined by monitoring the shift of the peak of neuronal activity within this population. In addition, the signals generated by these cells are integrated, along with depth information, by pretectal neuron TH6 to indicate whether the stimulus is a looming threat. Their model includes both tectal (T2, postulated to respond to stimuli with temporonasal movement) and pretectal (TH3, sensitive to larger stimuli) neurons. On one hand, the tegmentum integrates and transforms the spatial signals conveyed by T2 and T3 cells to generate a motor heading map that specifies the escape direction. On the other hand, the appropriate motor response selection (e.g., jumping away, ducking) depends on the stimulus size and elevation, which are determined by including TH3 and TH6, and T6 signals, correspondingly.

Different Time-Scale Neuronal Networks as the Basis for Visuomotor Integration

Anurans' prey-catching response can be influenced by changes in motivation (Cervantes-Pérez et al. in Arbib and Ewert, 1991; Merkel-Harff and Ewert in Arbib and Ewert, 1991) or by conditioning or learning processes (see Finkestädt in Ewert and Arbib, 1989; Cervantes-Pérez et al. in Ewert and Arbib, 1989). Through neuroanatomical, neurophysiological, and lesion studies, it has been postulated that those closed loops, formed by tectum and pretectum with telencephalic and diencephalic structures, may be the underlying mechanisms of these modulatory processes (Ewert et al., 2001).

The optic tectum projects to the anterior thalamus, which also receives input from the retina and connects to medial pallium, which in turn sends efferent fibers, directly and through the preoptic area, to dorsal hypothalamus, a structure with direct connection to tectum. This loop has been postulated to subserve *stimulus-specific habituation*, a simple form of learning in which the tendency to respond to a prey-like stimulus declines and eventually disappears when the stimulus remains in the toad's visual field, despite its efforts to catch it. Prey-catching habituation is a stimulus-specific process with almost no analogical generalization, and it shows spontaneous recovery (see Lara in Ewert and Arbib, 1989; Cervantes-Pérez et al. and Wang et al. in Arbib and Ewert, 1991; Ewert et al., 2001). The habituation process does not occur within a single failure trial; rather, it requires that the toad attempt several times to catch the prey without being successful. Thus, we postulated that the *acquisition phase* of habituation is carried out within the telencephalic modulatory path on a much slower time scale (minutes to hours) than that associated to the FTC activation dynamics (hundreds of milliseconds). We also proposed that the build-up of habituation results in an increased inhibition of tectal activity, which reduces the probability of the current stimulus fitting the prey category. That is, the *modulatory path* activity causes a change in the FTC neuronal network *activation dynamics* produced by the visual stimulus rather than changes in the *weight dynamics* related to its structural organization. This phenomenon shows spontaneous recovery, a *forgetting phase*, which may take from minutes to days. Finally, stimulus-specific habituation is a *learning-from-interactions* phenomenon whose characteristics seem to be universal (they appear in studies with different species, e.g., mollusks, rats, and humans).

The complexity of anurans' visuomotor behaviors is also enhanced by changes in factors affecting animal's motivation to display a given behavior. For example, the daytime effect on the efficacy of visual prey like *dummies* to yield prey-catching behavior depends on the time of the day (frogs and toads have a peak of prey-catching activity at dusk). Furthermore, there are also seasonal effects on anurans' prey-catching behavior, which gives the *motivational dynamics* a slow time-varying scale that may go from several hours to several days (Ewert in Ewert and Arbib, 1989).

Discussion

Experimental and theoretical studies have been used to establish how the underlying neural mechanisms of visuomotor integration in amphibians developed into a parallel distributed neural processing system in which tectal circuitry represents more than a visual sensory map. Instead, tectal circuitry can be regarded as the *site of integration* of signals coming from retina and pretectum, as well as from thelencephalic brain regions associated with changes in motivational factors or learning processes that modulate these animals' behavior. There is a wide range of neuronal processes occurring at multiple levels of temporal abstraction. First, on the scale of hundreds of milliseconds, are changes in neuronal activity caused by the stimulus (prey or predator) characteristics and its current spatiotemporal relationship with the toad (or frog); second are signals generated during learning events happening on a temporal scale of minutes to hours; and third are signals generated by changes in motivational factors (e.g., hunger, daily and yearly cycles), which occur on a much slower time scale.

The study of anurans' visuomotor coordination system is an excellent example of how scientists from a range of disciplines (i.e., brain theory, neurosciences, robotics) can work together using theoretical models as an interlingua. This kind of study contributes to neuroscience by analyzing formal models in the quest of testing hypotheses posed by experimental studies and by generating new hypotheses that may stimulate new experimental and theoretical work. In turn, these modeling studies may contribute to building automata that process sensory information "in the manner of the brain" to carry out complex tasks when interacting with a given environmental situation. A good example is provided by the work of Arkin et al. (2000), who implemented a schema-theoretic model of the agent-environment interaction of amphibians and insects in the action-selection control algorithm of a robotic hexapod. This machine is capable of displaying visually guided behaviors equivalent to prey catching, predator avoidance, and obstacle avoidance, and to the praying mantis behavior named "Chantlitaxia" (i.e., in searching for a safe place).

Many mysteries remain to be solved before it can be said that we understand the workings of the anuran brain. However, the results obtained so far are encouraging, and the quest goes on. For the last few years, research attention has focused on the study of behavior modulation, and this trend will likely continue for years to come. People would like to understand how neuronal processes occurring on fast time scales (a few hundreds of milliseconds) can be associated (synchronized) in such a way as to underlie behavioral responses elicited on a time scale of few seconds, or learning processes requiring up to an hour and a half to be consolidated, or motivational changes occurring on a time scale of several hours to days or months.

Road Map: Neuroethology and Evolution
Related Reading: Command Neurons and Command Systems; Habituation; Visual Attention; Visuomotor Coordination in Salamander

References

Amari, S. I., and Arbib, M. A., 1977, Competition and cooperation in neural nets, in *Systems in Neuroscience* (J. Metzler, Ed.), New York: Academic Press, pp. 119–165.

Arbib, M. A., and Ewert, J. P., 1991, *Visual Structures and Integrated Functions*, vol. 3 of *Research Notes in Neural Computing*, New York: Springer-Verlag.

Arkin, R. C., Ali, K., Weitzenfeld, A., and Cervantes-Pérez, F., 2000, Behavioral models of the praying mantis as a basis for robotic behavior, *Robot. Auton. Syst.*, 32:39–60.

Cervantes-Pérez, F., and Arbib, M. A., 1990, Stability and parameter dependency analyses of a facilitation tectal column (FTC) model, *J. Math. Biol.*, 29:1–32.

Cervantes-Pérez, F., Lara, R., and Arbib, M. A., 1985, A neural model of interactions subserving prey-predator discrimination and size preference in anuran amphibia, *J. Theor. Biol.*, 113:117–152.

Corbacho, F., and Weitzenfeld, A., 2001, Learning to detour, in *The Neural Simulation Language NSL: System and Applications*, Cambridge, MA: MIT Press.

Didday, R. L., 1976, A model of visuomotor mechanisms in the frog optic tectum, *Math. Biosci.*, 30:169–180.

Ewert, J. P., and Arbib, M. A., 1989, *Visuomotor Coordination: Amphibians, Comparisons, Models, and Robots*, New York: Plenum Press. ◆

Ewert, J. P., Buxbaum-Conradi, H., Dreisvogt, F., Glagow, M., Merkel-Harff, C., Röttgen, A., Schürg-Pfeiffer, E., and Schwippert, W. W., 2001, Neural modulation of visuomotor functions underlying prey-catching behaviour in anurans: Perception, attention, motor performance, learning, *Comp. Biochem. Physiol. A*, 128:417–461.

Ewert, J. P., and von Seelen, 1974, Neurobiologie and System-Theorio eines Visuellen Muster. Erkennvngs mechanisms bei Kröte, *Kybernetik*, 14:167–183.

Ingle, D., 1968, Visual releasers of prey catching behavior in frogs and toads, *Brain Behav. Evol.*, 1:500–518.

Lettvin, J. Y., Maturana, H., McCulloch, W. S., and Pitts, W. H., 1959, What the frog's eye tells the frog brain, *Proc. IRE*, 47:1940–1951.

Liaw, J. S., and Arbib, M. A., 1993, Neural mechanisms underlying direction-sensitive avoidance behavior, *Adapt. Behav.*, 1:227–261.

Llinás, R., and Precht, W., 1976, *Frog Neurobiology*, Berlin: Springer-Verlag.

Narins, P., Holdl, W., and Grabul, D., 2001, Bimodal signal requisite for agonistic behavior in dart-poison frog, in *Proceedings of the Animal Behavior Society*, 2001, p. 194.

Roche King, J., and Comer, C. M., 1996, Visually elicited turning behavior in *Rana pipiens*: Comparative organization and neural control of escape and prey capture, *J. Comp. Physiol A*, 178:293–305.

Vanegas, H., 1984, *Comparative Neurology of the Optic Tectum*, New York: Plenum Press.

Visuomotor Coordination in Salamander

Richard Woesler and Gerhard Roth

Introduction

For most salamanders, vision is the most important sense (Roth, 1987). To analyze a visual scene, objects have to be segmented from a background. Furthermore, in the context of prey catching, an object has to be selected and identified as prey. Finally, correct motor patterns have to be generated; for example, snapping has to occur only when prey is within reach of the tongue. On the one hand, these computational steps are difficult tasks, especially when self-motion of the salamander is also taken into account. On the other hand, the brains of salamanders are anatomically the simplest among vertebrates, containing only about 1 million neurons (frogs have up to ten times more neurons and humans one million times more). Despite these differences, the salamander (as well as the frog) and the human brain exhibit the same fundamental bauplan, or blueprint, and it is therefore interesting to study the neurobiology and the visually guided behavior of these animals (see VISUOMOTOR COORDINATION IN FROG AND TOAD).

Behavior

Probably the most sophisticated visually guided behavior in salamanders is prey catching (Figure 1). Terrestrial prey catching generally consists of a sequence of the following reactions: First, there is an orienting movement of the head to bring the prey into the binocular visual area. Then, sometimes, differing from species to species, the prey object is approached by walking. Afterwards, an olfactory test may occur. Many salamanders, however, exhibit an "ambush" strategy, that is, they are motionless until a prey object comes within reach of the tongue. A fixation period can usually be observed. Finally, the prey is captured with the tongue and taken into the mouth. These actions may vary in their temporal sequence, depending on the motivation of the animal.

While among frogs there is a larger variety of feeding mechanisms and kinematics (cf. Nishikawa, 1997), salamanders uniformly use their tongues by a forward movement of the hyobranchial apparatus (Roth, 1987). Most species of the large family Plethodontidae have developed projectile tongues that enable them to feed on fast-moving prey such as flying insects. The longest tongue is found in the plethodontid genus *Hydromantes*. This group of salamanders is also capable of catching prey with its tongue up to 45°, or more, laterally.

Neurobiological Results

Retina

The retinal network consists of photoreceptors, a variety of interneurons and retinal ganglion cells (RGCs), which project to further brain areas. In *Hydromantes*, there are about 60,000 photoreceptors and about 50,000 RGCs (Roth, 1987). Most of the RGCs are movement sensitive, that is, they respond with action potentials when a contrast edge moves over receptors within their receptive fields. Three main classes of RGCs can be distinguished: RGC 1 is edge or contrast sensitive, RGC 2 is movement sensitive, and RGC 3 is sensitive for motion of large objects. The RGCs project to the tegmentum, which is thought to provide a self-motion signal to the tectum and to provide various premotor functions (Manteuffel and Naujoks-Manteuffel, 1990), to the thalamus (corpus geniculatum thalamicum, neuropil Bellonci, pars lateralis, and medialis), the pretectum (pretectal neuropil, area uncinata), and the upper layers of the tectum (Roth, Dicke, and Wiggers, 1998). The thalamus is involved in prey/predator distinction and figure/ground separation; for further results concerning thalamic neurons, see Roth and Grunwald (2000). The majority of retinal input runs to the contralateral side. Tongue-projecting salamanders, however, exhibit a substantial proportion of ipsilateral retinal input; this is supposed to be important for catching fast-moving prey with high accuracy in three-dimensional space.

Tectum

The tectum mesencephali (often, but incorrectly, called "optic tectum") is the most important visual brain center regarding prey catching. It receives retinotopic afferents from the retina, ipsilateral lateral amygdala, striatum, thalamus and pretectum, ipsilateral and contralateral nucleus isthmi, and from the medulla oblongata/spinalis (Roth et al., 1998); the latter has premotor functions (see LO-

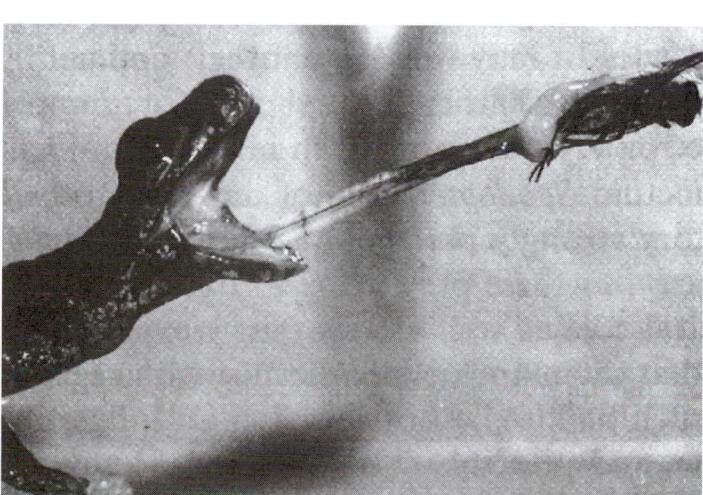

Figure 1. Prey-catching behavior of *Hydromantes italicus*. Protraction and retraction of the tongue takes place within less than 100 ms. (Photo by G. Roth.)

COMOTION, VERTEBRATE). The retinal input originates from RGCs mostly with small excitatory receptive fields in the range of 3°–20°. The tectum of *Hydromantes italicus* contains about 100,000 neurons, about 95% of which are local interneurons (TO-IN); the rest are projection neurons. Five major types of projection neurons can be distinguished (TO1 to TO5). TO1 and TO5 are likely to receive predominantly input from RGC 1, TO2 and TO4 mostly from RGC 2, and TO3 mostly from RGC 3 as well as somatosensory and vestibular input. TO1 to TO3 have large dendritic fields; TO4 and TO5 have smaller ones. Together, these types of neurons constitute a system of parallel ascending (to pretectum, thalamus) and descending (to tegmentum, medulla oblongata/spinalis) pathways mediating information about size, velocity, shape, and movement pattern of prey objects to different brain regions.

Data from freely moving toads demonstrate that certain tectal neurons involved in prey recognition show two different types of reactions (Schürg-Pfeiffer, 1989), which may be called low- and high-firing-rate states. Usually, these neurons show relatively low firing rates depending on the stimulus. Before an action such as an orienting movement takes place, the neurons change to a high-firing-rate state, firing with about 100–150 spikes/s. Further, during this state, the neurons produce double spikes, with interspike intervals of about 6 ms. Possibly, these double spikes are recognized in the motor and premotor areas so that only neurons in the high-firing-rate state can contribute to motor activation. Further, certain tectal neurons respond vigorously only to objects of about prey size (Spreckelsen, Schürg-Pfeiffer, and Ewert, 1995). This differs from the situation found in anesthetized animals in which corresponding tectal neurons do not show absolute size constancy.

Pretectum

The pretectum receives retinal input from ganglion cells with large excitatory receptive fields (30°–90°); it also receives a considerable amount of ipsilateral retinal input (Manteuffel, 1989). Most pretectal cells were found to be sensitive to stimuli moving with about 1°–10°/s in the horizontal plane, and many of them exhibit direction sensitivity, responding best to temporonasal stimulus movement. About half of the neurons studied projected to the tectum; arborization was highly variable, ranging from a single fiber to massive arborization covering almost the entire tectal hemisphere (Luksch et al., 1998). Most neurons (87%) projected to the medulla oblongata and rostral spinal cord. The function of the pretectum is the control of the optokinetic response; it is also assumed to be involved in the prey-enemy distinction (Ewert, 1984).

Models

Compensation of Visual Background Movement

The amphibian nystagmus of the head reaches a maximum gain up to 0.8 at stimulus frequencies of about 0.03 Hz, whereas the gain of the vestibulocollic reflex reaches its maximum at about 0.5 Hz (Manteuffel, 1989). These features can be reproduced in a computer model (Manteuffel, 1989) under both constant velocity and sinusoidal input conditions, taking into account the bell-shaped velocity tuning curves of pretectal neurons and assuming that these signals are fed to the ipsilateral neck motor neurons through a salamander-specific velocity storage system and a linear velocity-to-position integrator. The results suggest that in salamanders, this system is simpler than that found in higher vertebrates and especially that it lacks an effective velocity storage element that serves a more continuous output.

Encoding the Place of a Single Object with High Accuracy

From snapping responses of *Hydromantes*, for example, a high accuracy is known. However, the mean value of the width of receptive fields of recorded tectal neurons was surprisingly large (36°). Within a model called SIMULANDER, Eurich et al. (1995) could show how to encode the place of a single prey with high accuracy using a relatively small number of tectal neurons (100 neurons in the model were sufficient), the fields of which were chosen according to experimental data for tectal neurons. Only one already segmented stimulus was assumed. A neuron was defined to be active in case a part of the object was inside the neuron's receptive field. Binary tectal neurons were sufficient to solve this task. This kind of encoding is called *coarse coding*. The main idea is that a rather small displacement of the object causes it to enter or leave one of the large overlapping fields and therefore yields a change of the neuronal activity pattern. Note that this would not be the case for small fields, because their boundaries are smaller within the snapping region; therefore, the rather large fields in the model are efficient to provide high accuracy.

Segmentation of Objects from Background and Selection of an Object

As has been mentioned, the model of Eurich et al. (1995) does not include segmentation of an object from the background, and no selection of one out of several objects is considered. These questions are addressed in further models (Woesler, 2001). A simplified retinal neural network model is considered, consisting of photoreceptors, interneurons, and RGCs. Anatomical receptor resolution (about 0.2°) and a time constant of the model RGCs (about 0.2 s) are chosen according to data from *Hydromantes*. This network provides segmentation of moving contrast edges from the background. The information is projected to model tectal neurons that integrate the information in a certain binocular receptive field. The center and width distributions of the fields are chosen according to experimental data. A winner-take-all model selects for each tectal hemisphere the neuron with the largest output. Simulation results show that, generally, the winner neurons' fields contain a complete object. For a simplified model (Woesler, 2001), analytical results could be obtained that are in accordance with behavioral findings, for example, concerning optimal prey velocities for prey-catching behavior and "head preference" known from toads. The width distribution of receptive fields in the simplified model arises from a plausible scaling construction within the winner-take-all networks. Comparing the distribution with that found in *Hydromantes* yields a rough correspondence: no or few neurons with small receptive fields, many neurons with relatively small fields, and only very few neurons with very large fields (Figure 2).

The winner-take-all networks exhibit a comparatively low coding accuracy for the place of an object. In the models (Woesler, 2001), the high coding accuracy known from *Hydromantes* is obtained as follows: Roughly speaking, via multiplicative synapses, the winner neurons activate the retinal input within their receptive fields to postsynaptic tectal model neurons, which one may call multiplicative neurons. By this, the multiplicative neurons only "see" the winner object. Via coarse coding, the multiplicative neurons encode the place of the winner object with high accuracy. The multiplicative neurons can be chosen to have binary output values. Note that one may propose that neurons in a state of high firing rate mentioned above correspond to such binary model neurons that are active. Using only 300 neurons in the winner-take-all networks for each hemisphere and 400 multiplicative neurons per hemisphere, the model yields an accuracy of about 1°, which is in good agreement with data from *Hydromantes* (<3°). Note that in *Hydromantes*, there are about 3,000 tectal neurons that project to motor and premotor areas.

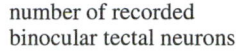
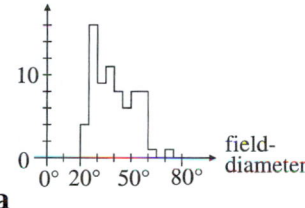
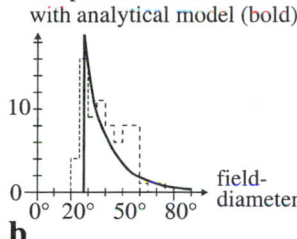

a   b

Figure 2. *A*, Distribution of receptive field diameters of binocular tectal neurons in *Hydromantes italicus*. Data from extracellular recordings of 72 neurons (Roth et al., 1998). *B*, Comparison of the data of part *A* (dashed line) with the corresponding function (curve) of an analytic model (Woesler, 2001). The latter is zero for fields smaller than a threshold value (here fitted to data: 28°), and for larger fields, it is inversely proportional to the field diameter to the third power.

Saccade Generation

As shown in a model of Manteuffel and Roth (1993) based on anatomical and electrophysiological data from tectum and brainstem, the metric properties of salamander saccades are largely the result of visual and motor maps of the tectum. In that model, head movements toward prey were investigated by applying a continuous mapping from the retina to premotor layers of the tectum. Using the coarse coding scheme described above, Eurich et al. (1995) showed that a model with 100 discrete, binary tectal model neurons, 100 interneurons, and 100 motor neurons can exhibit the behavioral accuracy of prey localization.

Approach Behavior, Walking, and Swimming

A corresponding detailed model is described by Ijspeert (see LO-COMOTION, VERTEBRATE).

Snapping

Snapping at prey was modeled for *Hydromantes italicus* (Eurich, Schwegler, and Woesler, 1997). The model was restricted to frontal snapping. It demonstrates that a high distance accuracy of the snapping reaction can be obtained by using 144 tectal neurons, 12 motor neurons, and 12 inhibitory interneurons. Models of the tongue apparatus muscles rectus cervicis profundus and subarcualis rectus 1 were simulated. The snapping distance accuracy was about 0.2 cm, but it was somewhat lower for very close prey. Successful captures of prey usually occurred in more than 90% of the cases.

Discussion

The coarse coding models (Eurich et al., 1995, 1997) have demonstrated how to encode with only a few neurons with large, overlapping receptive fields the place of an object with the high accuracy that is known from the prey-catching behavior of tongue-projecting salamanders. This is in nice relation to the fact mentioned in the introduction that the salamander brain contains so few neurons.

The models have been extended for the case in which several objects are presented to the animal by linking a segmentation network and a winner-take-all-like object selection to a coarse coding network in a biologically plausible way (Woesler, 2001).

Compensation of background movement (Manteuffel, 1989), segmentation of objects, selection of an object, saccade generation,

approaching (see LOCOMOTION, VERTEBRATE), and snapping behavior have been modeled successfully as separate tasks in line with behavioral and neurobiological findings in salamanders. The models remain to be integrated into a more complete model, especially integrating the compensation of background and ego motion with object selection/segmentation (cf. VISUAL ATTENTION).

Models have to be developed for the recent data mentioned concerning thalamus and tegmentum and, finally, for the telencephalon, the largest salamander brain center, for which there are results from lesion studies (Finkenstädt and Ewert, 1983) and detailed findings concerning its connectivity (Roth and Grunwald, unpublished data). It is involved in motivation, learning, and control of "voluntary actions." These functions are challenging with respect to both experiments and modeling, considering that available computer power comes closer to that of a whole salamander brain network, and considering the roughly similar bauplan to that of human brain.

Road Map: Neuroethology and Evolution
Related Reading: Command Neurons and Command Systems; Locomotion, Vertebrate; Neuroethology, Computational; Vestibulo-Ocular Reflex; Visual Attention; Visuomotor Coordination in Frog and Toad

References

Eurich, C. W., Roth, G., Schwegler, H., and Wiggers, W., 1995, Simulander: A neural network for the orientation movement of salamanders, *J. Comp. Physiol. A,* 176:379–389.

Eurich, C. W., Schwegler, H., and Woesler, R., 1997, Coarse coding: Applications to the visual system of salamanders, *Biol. Cybern.,* 77:41–47.

Ewert, J.-P., 1984, Tectal mechanisms that underlie prey-catching and avoidance behaviors in toads, in *Comparative Neurology of the Optic Tectum* (H. Vanegas, Ed.), New York: Plenum Press, pp. 247–416.

Finkenstädt, T., and Ewert, J.-P., 1983, Visual pattern discrimination through interaction of neural networks: A combined electrical brain stimulation, brain lesion, and extracellular recording study in *Salamandra salamandra, J. Comp. Physiol.,* 153:85–98.

Luksch, H., Kahl, H., Wiggers, W., and Roth, G., 1998, Anatomy and connectivity of the salamander pretectum: An in-vitro (whole brain) intracellular recording and staining study, *Cell Tissue Res.,* 292:47–56.

Manteuffel, G., 1989, Compensation of visual background motion in salamanders, in *Visuomotor Coordination: Amphibians, Comparisons, Models, and Robots* (J.-P. Ewert and M. A. Arbib, Eds.), New York: Plenum Press, pp. 311–340. ◆

Manteuffel, G., and Naujoks-Manteuffel, C., 1990, Anatomical connections and electrophysiological properties of toral and dorsal tegmental neurons in the terrestrial urodele *Salamandra salamandra, J. Hirnforsch.,* 31:65–76.

Manteuffel, G., and Roth, G., 1993, A model of saccadic sensorymotor system of salamanders, *Biol. Cybern.,* 68:431–440.

Nishikawa, K. C., 1997, Emergence of novel functions during brain evolution, *BioScience,* 47:341–354. ◆

Roth, G., 1987, Visual behavior in salamanders, *Studies of Brain Function,* vol. 14, Berlin: Springer-Verlag.

Roth, G., Dicke, U., and Wiggers, W., 1998, Vision, in *Amphibian Biology,* vol. 3, *Sensory Perception* (H. Heathwole, Ed.), Chipping Norton, Surrey, Engl.: Beatty & Sons. ◆

Roth, G., and Grunwald, W., 2000, Morphology, axonal projection pattern, and responses to optic nerve stimulation of thalamic neurons in the salamander *Plethodon jordani, J. Comp. Neurol.,* 428:543–557.

Schürg-Pfeiffer, E., 1989, Behavior-correlated properties of tectal neurons in freely moving toads, in *Visuomotor Coordination: Amphibians, Comparisons, Models, and Robots* (J.-P. Ewert and M. A. Arbib, Eds.), New York: Plenum Press.

Spreckelsen, C., Schürg-Pfeiffer, E., and Ewert, J.-P., 1995, Responses of retinal and tectal neurons in non-paralyzed toads *Bufo bufo* and *B. marinus* to the real size versus angular size of objects moved at variable distance, *Neurosci. Lett.,* 184:105–108.

Woesler, R., 2001, Object segmentation model: Analytical results and biological implications, *Biol. Cybern.,* 85:203–210.

Winner-Take-All Networks

Alan L. Yuille and Davi Geiger

Introduction

A winner-take-all mechanism is a device that determines the identity, and sometimes the amplitude, of its largest input. Such mechanisms are necessary in network models for enforcing competition between different possible outputs of the network (Amari and Arbib, 1977). Classic examples include (1) associative memory models (Hertz, Krogh, and Palmer, 1991), where different stored memories compete to explain the input data, (2) cooperative models of binocular stereo, where competition is required to ensure that each feature has a unique match (Dev, 1975; Marr and Poggio, 1977), and (3) Fukushima's neocognitron for feature extraction (see NEO-COGNITRON: A MODEL FOR VISUAL PATTERN RECOGNITION). In addition, such mechanisms are often required for combinatorial optimization problems (see OPTIMIZATION, NEURAL).

There are two important variants of winner-take-all procedures. The first is *k*-winner-take-all, where the *k* largest inputs are identified. The second is a softened version, known as *softmax*, that consists of assigning each input a weight so that all weights sum to one and the largest input receives the biggest weight. In what follows, when "winner-take-all" appears without a noun, it refers to "1-winner-take-all." Winner-take-all can be considered a limiting case of softmax when the biggest weight is set equal to 1. Softmax has been applied to problems in speech recognition (Bridle, 1989) and learning by mixtures of experts (Jordan and Jacobs, 1992). Softmax also appears from a statistical physics analysis of the winner-take-all problem.

It has recently been shown (Maass, 2000) that both these variants are computationally very powerful compared with standard neural network models with threshold gates. The standard models require two layers of nonlinear units in order to represent most functions. By contrast, it can be shown (Maass, 2000) that arbitrary continuous functions can be approximated by circuits employing a single soft winner-take-all gate as their only nonlinear operation. In addition, any boolean function can be computed by a single *k*-winner-take-all unit applied to weighted sums of input variables. Moreover, both approaches require only positive weights. This may be relevant to neuroscience, because positive weights can be implemented by excitatory neural connections but there is no direct way to implement negative weights.

In this article we will concentrate on describing winner-take-all and softmax. We first describe softmax and show how winner-take-all can be derived as a limiting case. We will then describe how they can be both be derived from probabilistic, or energy function, formulations. This leads naturally to several algorithms for calculating them, and their generalization to more complicated systems. Some of these algorithms include the concept of self-annealing (Rangarajan, 2000). We then discuss VLSI and biological mechanisms for implementing these algorithms.

Softmax

The basic idea of softmax is very simple. Suppose we have inputs $I = \{I_a : a = 1, \ldots, N\}$, and let β be a positive parameter. We define a weight $w_a(I; \beta)$ for each input I_a by

$$w_a(I; \beta) = \frac{e^{\beta I_a}}{\sum_b e^{\beta I_b}} \qquad (1)$$

Clearly, because the exponential function is monotically increasing, the largest weight corresponds to the largest input. Moreover,

the size ordering of the weights corresponds to the size ordering of the inputs. The weights sum up to 1, $\sum_a w_a(I; \beta) = 1$. In the limit, as $\beta \to \infty$, the weight of the largest input tends to 1, all other weights tending to 0, and we obtain the classic winner-take-all situation. At the other extreme, as $\beta \to 0$, the weights all tend to $1/N$. Thus the parameter β controls the sharpness of the softmax.

The variables $w_a(I; \beta)$ in Equation 1 will preferentially weigh the largest inputs. They can also be used to calculate a weighted average of the inputs to yield

$$O(I; \beta) = \sum_a w_a(I; \beta) I_a \qquad (2)$$

As $\beta \to \infty$, the output $O(I; \beta)$ will become equal to the largest input value.

We cannot make β arbitrarily large in Equation 1. How large must it be to ensure that we are close to the true winner-take-all solution? If we require that the largest weight differ from 1 by at most ε, then it can be shown that we need to have $\beta \geq (1/|\Delta I|) \log\{(N - 1)(1 - \varepsilon)/\varepsilon)\}$, where $|\Delta I|$ is the difference between the largest and second largest inputs.

Statistical Derivation of Softmax

The winner-take-all problem can be posed as follows: Given a set of N inputs $\{I_a : a = 1, \ldots, N\}$, how can we associate each input I_a with a binary variable V_a, such that $V_{a*} = 1$ for the largest input I_{a*}, and $V_a = 0$ otherwise? We can transform the winner-take-all problem into an optimization problem by introducing the energy function

$$E[V] = -\sum_a V_a I_a \qquad (3)$$

Minimizing Equation 3 with the constraint that $\sum_a V_a = 1$ will select the largest input.

The associated Gibbs distribution (for justification of this distribution, see OPTIMIZATION, NEURAL) is

$$P[V; \beta] = \frac{e^{-\beta E[V]}}{Z} \qquad (4)$$

where the constant $\beta = 1/T$, with T being the "temperature" of the system. Z is a normalization factor, also known as the *partition function*. Hence, $Z = \sum_V e^{-\beta E[V]}$, where we sum over all allowable configurations of V. Because of the global constraint, these configurations are of form $V_a = 1$, $V_b = 0$, for all $b \neq a$. We calculate

$$Z = \sum_b e^{\beta I_b} \qquad (5)$$

We can now directly evaluate the probabilities of the allowable configurations.

These are

$$P[V_a = 1; V_b = 0, b \neq a] = \frac{e^{\beta I_a}}{\sum_b e^{\beta I_b}}, \quad \text{for all } a \qquad (6)$$

This is exactly the softmax formula. So we can interpret the weights given by softmax as the probabilities given by the Gibbs distribution. It is straightforward to design a physical system whose states are specified by the Gibbs distribution so that the probability of unit a firing (i.e., $V_a = 1$) is given by Equation 6.

Alternatively, we can reinterpret the softmax weights as the mean values of the output units (for a binary variable, the means are the same as the probabilities of firing). The means can be calculated by minimizing an effective energy:

$$E_{eff}[w, P; \beta] = -\sum_a w_a I_a + (1/\beta) \sum_a w_a \log w_a$$
$$+ P\left(\sum_a w_a - 1\right) \quad (7)$$

where P is a Lagrange multiplier to impose the constraint $\sum_a w_a = 1$. The second term can be interpreted as an entropy term. It is straightforward to verify that E_{eff} is a convex energy function that is bounded below, and hence has a unique minimum. This minimum can be obtained by extremizing E_{eff} with respect to w and P, yielding

$$\frac{\partial E_{eff}}{\partial w_a} - I_a + (1/\beta)\{\log w_a + 1\} + P = 0$$
$$\frac{\partial E_{eff}}{\partial P_a} = \sum_a w_a = 1 \quad (8)$$

We can solve these equations, eliminating P, to obtain the softmax formula in Equation 1. Moreover, the effective energy can be used (see the next section) to design algorithms for calculating softmax.

Dynamical Systems for Computing Softmax

There are many dynamical systems that converge to the softmax solution. One possibility is to do a variant of steepest descent that is modified to ensure that the constraint $\sum_a w_a = 1$ is satisfied. This corresponds to removing the component of the gradient in the direction that violates the constraints. This yields

$$\frac{dw_a}{dt} = -\frac{\partial E_{eff}}{\partial w_a} + \frac{1}{N} \sum_b \frac{\partial E_{eff}}{\partial w_b} \quad (9)$$

Substituting from Equation 7 gives

$$\frac{dw_a}{dt} = I_a - (1/\beta) \log w_a - (1/N) \sum_b I_b$$
$$+ (1/N\beta) \sum_b \log w_b \quad (10)$$

This update equation ensures that $d/dt(\sum_a w_a) = 0$, so the constraints will always be satisfied (provided the initial conditions are chosen to satisfy them). It can be shown that this equation causes the energy to monotonically increase to the minimum of the effective energy, and hence yield softmax as a solution.

Two other dynamical systems can be adapted from Waugh and Westervelt (1993). Their formulation applies to more general networks such as systems of competitive memories (see the next section). Both systems will converge to the softmax solution. Winner-take-all can be achieved by making β sufficiently large, or by thresholding the softmax solution.

The first is a discrete-time dynamical system:

$$w_a(t + 1) = \exp\{\beta I_a + P(t)\} \quad (11)$$

where $P(t)$ is chosen to ensure that at any time $\sum_a w_a(t + 1) = 1$. This requires that $P(t) = -\log\{\sum_a e^{\beta I_a}\}$. Thus the algorithm converges to the softmax solution $w_a(1) = e^{\beta I_a}/\{\sum_b e^{\beta I_b}\}$ in a single iteration. The simplicity of this algorithm, and its rapid convergence, reflects the simplicity of the winner-take-all/softmax problem. (As discussed later, the algorithm is usually applied to more complex problems.)

The second is a continuous-time dynamical system:

$$\frac{dw_a(t)}{dt} = -w_a(t) + \exp\{\beta I_a + P(t)\} \quad (12)$$

where, as before, $P(t)$ is chosen to ensure that $\sum_a w_a = 1$. It is straightforward to verify that $\lim_{t\to\infty} w_a(t) = e^{\beta I_a}/\sum_k e^{\beta I_k}$, recalling that E_{eff} has a unique minimum and observing that it acts as a *Lyaponov* function for this system (Waugh and Westervelt, 1993). Note that this is only a special case of Waugh and Westervelt's formalism. In the general case, the exponential functions in Equations 11 and 12 could be replaced by other monotonic differentiable functions.

For additional algorithms for this problem and detailed descriptions of the relationship of winner-take-all to effective energies, we recommend Elfadel (1995).

Self-Annealing to Compute Winner-Take-All

A disadvantage of softmax is that it has an unknown parameter β and does not converge to the winner-take-all solution unless we perform annealing on parameter β.

Rangarajan (2000) has suggested an alternative, called "self-annealing." This gives convergence to the winner-take-all solution without requiring a separate annealing schedule.

To perform self-annealing, we rewrite the energy function as

$$E[w] = -\sum_a w_a I_a + \lambda\left(\sum_a w_a - 1\right) \quad (13)$$

The update rule is defined by

$$w_a^{t+1} = \frac{w_a^t e^{-I_a/\alpha}}{\sum_b w_b^t e^{-I_b/\alpha}} \quad (14)$$

It can be proved (Rangarajan, 2000) that this converges to the winner-take-all solution.

Moreover, there is a related continuous-time dynamical system that also converges to the winner-take-all solution:

$$\frac{dw_a}{\partial t} = -w_a + \frac{w_a e^{-I_a/\alpha}}{\sum_b w_b e^{-I_b/\alpha}} \quad (15)$$

Generalizations

Winner-take-all mechanisms are usually part of more complicated systems. In this section we show how they can be generalized to systems of competitive memories. The system converges to the "best" memory rather than to the "best" input. This applies both to softmax and winner-take-all (using self-annealing).

Following Waugh and Westervelt (1993), we now generalize the previous system to more complicated models consisting of neurons grouped into clusters. The variables are $\{w_{ia}\}$, where the index i labels the cluster and a labels the element in the cluster. We impose the constraint $\sum_a w_{ia} = R_i$, for all i to ensure that in the ith cluster, only R_i neurons are firing. The input to the iath neuron is $h_{ia} = \sum_{jb} T_{ijab} w_{jb} + I_{ia}$, where I_{ia} are the external inputs and T_{ijab} are connection strengths. Then the two equations, 11 and 12, are generalized to

$$w_{ia}(t + 1) = \exp\{\beta(h_{ia}(t) + B_i(t))\}, \quad \text{for all } a, i \quad (16)$$

and

$$\frac{dw_{ia}(t)}{dt} - w_{ia}(t) + \exp\{\beta(h_{ia}(t) + B_i(t))\}, \quad \text{for all } a, i \quad (17)$$

where the $B_i(t)$ are chosen to enforce the constraints $\sum_a w_{ia} = R_i$, for all i.

These dynamical systems are guaranteed to converge (Waugh and Westervelt, 1993). Indeed, they will converge (Elfadel, 1995) to a local minimum of an effective energy, generalized from Equation 7, that is given by

$$E_{eff}[w, P; \beta] = -\frac{1}{2} \sum_{ijab} T_{ijab} w_{ia} w_{jb} - \sum_{ia} w_{ia} I_{ia}$$
$$+ (1/\beta) \sum_{ia} w_{ia} \log w_{ia}$$
$$+ \sum_{i} P_{i} \left(\sum_{a} w_{ia} - R_{i} \right) \qquad (18)$$

where the $\{P_i\}$ are Lagrange multipliers.

Waugh and Westervelt's formulation is more general than this. It can be obtained by replacing the exponentials in Equations 16 and 17 with monotonic differential functions F_{ia} and replacing the term $(1/\beta)\Sigma_{ia}w_{ia} \log w_{ia}$ in Equation 18 with $(1/\beta)\Sigma_{ia}\int_{w_0}^{w_{ia}} F_{ia}^{-1}(w)dw$.

Networks with dynamics similar to Equations 16 and 17, and effective energies similar to Equation 18, can also be used to solve optimization problems. They can also be related to the Potts models in statistical physics (see Elfadel, 1995).

The situation is similar for self-annealing (Rangarajan, 2000). We restrict ourselves to $R_i = 1$, $\forall\ i$. Then a discrete iterative algorithm is

$$w_{ia}(t + 1) = \frac{w_{ia}(t)e^{\alpha h_{ia}(t)}}{\sum_{b} w_{ib}(t)e^{\alpha h_{ib}(t)}} \qquad (19)$$

and a continuous-time algorithm is

$$\frac{dw_{ia}}{dt} = -w_{ia} + \frac{w_{ia}e^{\alpha h_{ia}}}{\sum_{b} w_{ib}e^{\alpha h_{ib}}} \qquad (20)$$

VLSI Analog Implementations

There have been several attempts to design analog very large-scale integrated (VLSI) circuits to compute winner-take-all.

Lazzaro et al. (1989) developed a winner-take-all circuit that was used for applications to auditory localization and visual stereopsis. This network was demonstrated to work effectively, and perturbation analysis was performed to demonstrate local stability. Yet, to our knowledge, no global analysis of the network has been performed, and convergence to the optimal solution has not been proved. The circuit takes current as input and outputs voltage.

A second circuit, from Waugh and Westervelt (1993), implements Equation 12. It is guaranteed to converge to the correct solution, provided the components of the circuit correctly implement the equations. In contrast to Lazzaro et al. (1989), the input is gate voltage and the output is current.

More recently, there have been a series of VLSI circuits with biological motivations. These include circuits based on neuronal spikes (Indiveri, 1999) and circuits that emulate visual attention (Horiuchi et al., 1997).

Care must be taken when drawing conclusions from the circuit equations describing these networks. Such equations are idealizations and assume that the networks are built of perfect components. This is unrealistic, and so the design of the network must be robust to imperfections in the components. Analog networks of this type are somewhat fragile and not as robust as simple discrete methods for winner-take-all using analog comparators and digital latches. It seems, however, that latch circuits are only capable of implementing pure winner-take-all and, unlike the analog circuits, cannot perform softmax.

Biological Models

Biological considerations have motivated some winner-take-all models (Elias and Grossberg, 1975). Here we discuss a model pre-

sented by Yuille and Grzywacz (1989). The network is updated by the following equation:

$$\tau \frac{dx_i}{dt} = -x_i + I_i K(x_1, x_2, \ldots, x_{i-1}, x_{i+1}, \ldots, x_N) \qquad (21)$$

where $x_i(t)$ is the state of the ith network element, τ is a constant, and the function K is symmetric in all its variables, decreases (or remains constant) as they increase, and tends to zero when any of them goes to infinity. The initial values of the x_i are set to the inputs I_i, which are constrained to be positive.

The first term on the right-hand side of Equation 21 corresponds to a time decay and the second contains inhibition between the network elements (Figure 1).

Lateral inhibition is a biologically plausible mechanism that is often used in winner-take-all networks to ensure that only one neuron is firing (Amari and Arbib, 1977). An usual aspect of this model is that the output of each element feeds back to inhibit the inputs to other elements (see Figure 1). We consider a special choice of K, which is motivated by a biological mechanism called shunting inhibition (Yuille and Grzywacz, 1989). Let

$$K(x_1, x_2, \ldots, x_{i-1}, x_{i+1}, \ldots, x_N) = e^{-\lambda \Sigma_{j \neq i} x_j} \qquad (22)$$

where λ is a constant that plays a similar role as the parameter β in softmax.

By using the coordinate transformation $z_i = e^{-\lambda x_i}$, Equation 21 can be transformed into

$$\frac{dz_i}{dt} = -\frac{\lambda I_i z_i}{\tau} \frac{\partial E[z]}{\partial z_i} \qquad (23)$$

where

$$E[z] = \frac{1}{\lambda} \sum_{j} \left(\frac{z_j \log z_j - z}{I_j} \right) + \prod_{j} z_j \qquad (24)$$

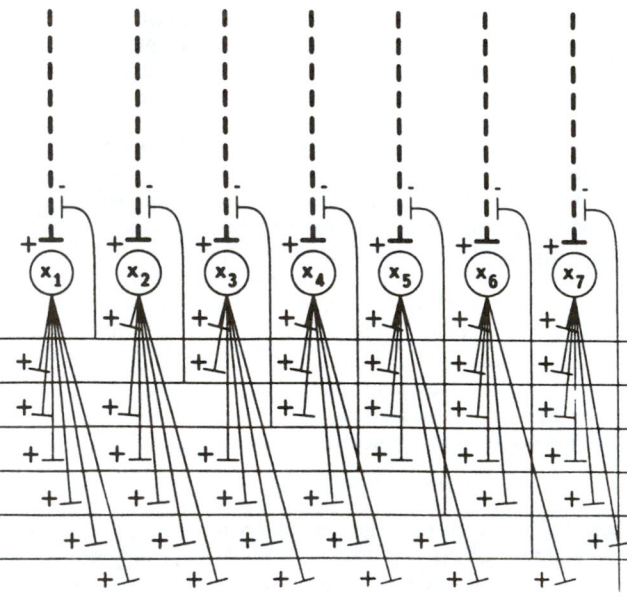

Figure 1. A biologically plausible circuit for winner-take-all. The dashed lines represent the inputs to the individual network elements. Each element excites inhibitory elements (similar to interneurons), which act on the presynaptic inputs of the other elements. Excitatory and inhibitory synapses are labeled with + and − signs, respectively. (From Yuille, A. L., and Grzywacz, N. M., 1989, A winner-take-all mechanism based on presynaptic inhibition, *Neural Computat.*, 1:334–347. © 1989, MIT Press; reprinted with permission.)

satisfies the properties of a Lyaponov function; it is bounded from below and always decreases with time when using the dynamics specified by Equation 23. This can be seen by observing that $dE/dt = -\Sigma_i(\lambda I_{iz_i}/\tau)(\partial E/\partial z_i)^2$ and recalling that the zs are constrained to be positive by definition. Hence the system converges to a minimum of E.

To understand the global convergence of the system, we examine the Hessian of E, the matrix with components $H_{ij} = \partial^2 E/(\partial z_i \partial z_j)$. We see that on the diagonal we have $H_{ii} = 1/(\lambda I_i z_i)$ and off the diagonal $H_{jk} = \prod_{i \neq j,k} z_i$. From Equation 21 we see that the x_i are always positive, and so the z_i lie in the range [0, 1]. Thus the diagonal elements are all greater than $1/(\lambda I_{max})$ and the off-diagonal elements are all less than 1. By making $\lambda \geq (N-1)/I_{max}$ we can ensure that the Hessian is positive definite; hence E is convex, and so there is a single solution that the system converges to. It was shown, in the large λ limit, that this corresponds to the winner-take-all solution (Yuille and Grzywacz, 1989).

Discussion

Winner-take-all is a special case of softmax. Both problems can be formulated in terms of energy minimization, and both can be solved by a number of continuous-time and discrete-time dynamical systems. Some of these systems can be implemented by VLSI circuits or by biologically plausible mechanisms.

These systems can be generalized in a straightforward way to systems of competitive memories or optimization problems. In these cases only convergence to locally optimal solutions is guaranteed.

Finally, recent results on the large computational power of winner-take-all networks, and their need for only positive weights, are very exciting. They ensure that winner-take-all networks will continue to be a major research topic for computation, biology, and VLSI.

Road Map: Dynamic Systems
Background: Computing with Attractors
Related Reading: Modular and Hierarchical Learning Systems; Optimization, Neural

References

Amari, S., and Arbib, M., 1977, Competition and cooperation in neural nets, in *Syst. Neurosci.* (J. Metzler, Ed.), San Diego: Academic Press, pp. 119–165. ◆

Bridle, J., 1989, Probabilistic interpretation of feedforward classification network outputs, with relationships to statistical pattern recognition, in *Neuro-computing: Algorithms, Architectures* (F. Fogelman-Soulie and J. Héfault, Eds.), New-York: Springer-Verlag.

Dev, P., 1975, Perception of depth surfaces in random-dot stereograms, *Int. J. ManMach. Stud.*, 7:511–528.

Elfadel, I. M., 1995, Convex potentials and their conjugates in analog mean-field optimization, *Neural Computat.*, 7:1079–1104.

Elias, S. A., and Grossberg, S., 1975, Pattern formation, contrast control, and oscillations in the short term memory of shunting on-center off-surround networks, *Biol. Cybern.*, 20:69–98.

Hertz, J., Krogh, A., and Palmer, R. G., 1991, *Introduction to the Theory of Neural Computation*, Redwood City, CA: Addison-Wesley. ◆

Horiuchi, T. K., Morris, T. G., Koch, C., and DeWeerth, S. P., 1997, Analog VLSI circuits for attention-based visual tracking, in *Advances in Neural Information Processing Systems 9*, San Mateo, CA: Morgan Kaufmann, pp. 706–712.

Indiveri, G., 1999, Neuromorphic analog VLSI sensor for visual tracking: Circuits and application examples, *IEEE Trans. Circuits and Syst. II Analog Digital Signal Process.*, 46:1337–1347.

Jordan, M. I., and Jacobs, R. A., 1992, Hierarchies of adaptive experts, in *Advances in Neural Information Processing Systems* (J. Moody, S. Hanson, and R. Lippmann, Eds.), San Mateo, CA: Morgan Kaufmann, pp. 985–993.

Lazzaro, J., Ryckebusch, S., Mahowald, M. A., and Mead, C. A., 1989, Winner-take-all networks of O(N) complexity, in *Advances in Neural Information Processing Systems* (D. S. Touretsky, Ed.), San Mateo, CA: Morgan Kaufmann, pp. 703–711.

Maass, W., 2000, On the computational power of winner-take-all, *Neural Computat.*, 12:2519–2535.

Marr, D., and Poggio, T., 1977, Cooperative computation of stereo disparity, *Science*, 195:283–328.

Rangarajan, A., 2000, Self-annealing and self-annihilation: Unifying deterministic annealing and relaxation labeling, *Pattern Recogn.*, 33:635–649.

Waugh, F., and Westervelt, R., 1993, Analog neural networks with local competition: I. Dynamics and stability, *Phys. Rev. E*, 47:4524–4536.

Yuille, A. L., and Grzywacz, N. M., 1989, A winner-take-all mechanism based on presynaptic inhibition, *Neural Computat.*, 1:334–347.

Ying-Yang Learning

Lei Xu

Introduction

This article addresses the issue of simultaneously building (1) a bottom-up pathway for encoding a pattern in the observation space into its representation in a representation space and (2) a top-down pathway for decoding or reconstructing a pattern from an inner representation back to a pattern in the observation space. This approach has been widely adopted in the literature of modeling a perception system for decades. A typical example is the ADAPTIVE RESONANCE THEORY (q.v.), developed by Grossberg and Carpenter starting in the 1970s. In the past decade, this approach has been widely adopted in various studies of brain theory and neural networks. Typical examples include Mumford's integrated theory for the corticothalamic and the corticocortical feedback (see THALAMUS), Kawato's theory on the CEREBELLUM AND MOTOR CONTROL (q.v.), and Hinton and colleagues' HELMHOLTZ MACHINES AND SLEEP-WAKE LEARNING (q.v.). Moreover, the LMSER self-

organizing rule proposed by Xu in 1991 (reference in Xu, 2001a) also uses a bidirectional architecture for statistical unsupervised learning.

The basic spirit of LMSER self-organizing was further developed into the Bayesian ying-yang (BYY) harmony learning in the mid-1990s. BYY harmony learning formulates the two pathways in a general statistical framework. First, a so-called BYY system is proposed for modeling the two pathways in a coordinated fashion via two complementary Bayesian representations of the joint distribution on the observation space and representation space. As a result, a number of existing major learning problems and learning methods are revisited as special cases from a unified perspective. Second, after further developments in the past several years, a harmony learning theory has been developed from which not only new regularization techniques (see GENERALIZATION AND REGULARIZATION IN NONLINEAR LEARNING SYSTEMS) are obtained from a systematic perspective, but also using this theory on the BYY system results in an easily implemented approach for model selection that is made either automatically during parameter learning or sequentially after parameter learning via a new class of criteria. Third, application of the first two achievements to various specific BYY systems with typical structures led to three major learning paradigms, namely unsupervised learning, supervised learning, and temporal modeling, with new insights and a number of new results.

This article provides an introduction to the fundamentals of BYY harmony learning and outlines the major results. Further details are given in Xu (2001a, 2001b, 2002a, 2002b). Moreover, the ability of BYY harmony learning for regularization and model selection is explained from an information-theoretic perspective. A comparative discussion is made to clarify how it differs not only from the minimum message length (MML) and minimum description length (MDL) (Wallace and Dowe, 1999; Rissanen, 1999; also see Minimum Description Length Analysis), as well as Bayesian approach (Mackey, 1992), but also from information geometry theory (Csiszar and Tusnady, 1984; see Neuromanifolds and Information Geometry) and from Helmholtz Machines and Sleep-Wake Learning (q.v.).

The Bayesian Ying-Yang System

We consider a world $\mathbf{X}$ with each object in an observation represented by an $\mathbf{x} \in \mathbf{X}$. Corresponding to each $\mathbf{x}$, there is an inner representation $\mathbf{y} \in \mathbf{Y}$ in the representation domain $\mathbf{Y}$ of a learning system. We consider the joint distribution of $\mathbf{x}$, $\mathbf{y}$, which can be understood from two complementary perspectives.

On the one hand, we can interpret each $\mathbf{x}$ as generated from an invisible inner representation $\mathbf{y}$ via a backward path distribution $q(\mathbf{x}|\mathbf{y})$, called *a generative model* $q(\mathbf{x}) = \int q(\mathbf{x}|\mathbf{y})q(\mathbf{y})d\mathbf{y}$, that maps from an inner distribution $q(\mathbf{y})$. On the other hand, we can interpret each $\mathbf{x}$ as being mapped into an invisible inner representation $\mathbf{y}$ via a forward path distribution $p(\mathbf{y}|\mathbf{x})$, called a *representative model* $p(\mathbf{y}) = \int p(\mathbf{y}|\mathbf{x})p(\mathbf{x})d\mathbf{x}$, that matches the inner density $q(\mathbf{y})$.

The two perspectives reflect the two types of Bayesian decomposition of the joint density $q(\mathbf{x}|\mathbf{y})q(\mathbf{y}) = q(\mathbf{x}, \mathbf{y}) = p(\mathbf{x}, \mathbf{y}) = p(\mathbf{x})p(\mathbf{y}|\mathbf{x})$ on $\mathbf{X} \times \mathbf{Y}$. Without any constraints, the two decompositions should be theoretically identical. However, in a real consideration, the four components $p(\mathbf{y}|\mathbf{x})$, $p(\mathbf{x})$, $q(\mathbf{x}|\mathbf{y})$, $q(\mathbf{y})$ should all be subject to certain structural constraints according to the nature of the learning task. Thus, we usually have two different but complementary Bayesian representations:

$$p(\mathbf{x}, \mathbf{y}) = p(\mathbf{y}|\mathbf{x})p(\mathbf{x}), \quad q(\mathbf{x}, \mathbf{y}) = q(\mathbf{x}|\mathbf{y})q(\mathbf{y}) \qquad (1)$$

where (with compliments to the ancient Chinese ying-yang philosophy) $p(\mathbf{x}, \mathbf{y})$ is called the *yang machine*, which consists of the observation space (*yang space*) $p(\mathbf{x})$ and the forward pathway (*yang pathway*) $p(\mathbf{y}|\mathbf{x})$; and $q(\mathbf{x}, \mathbf{y})$ is called the *ying machine*, which consists of the invisible state space (*ying space*) $q(\mathbf{y})$ and the *ying* (or backward) *pathway* $q(\mathbf{x}|\mathbf{y})$. Such a pair of ying-yang models is called a *Bayesian ying-yang (BYY) system*.

From a set χ of samples from the observed world $\mathbf{X}$, the distribution $p(\mathbf{x})$ is given either by an empirical density $p(\mathbf{x}|\chi)$ or a nonparametric estimate $p(\mathbf{x}|\chi, h^2)$ with a unknown smoothing parameter h, as will be further specified later by Equations 8 and 11. The task of learning on a BYY system consists of specifying all the aspects of $p(\mathbf{y}|\mathbf{x})$, $q(\mathbf{x}|\mathbf{y})$, $q(\mathbf{y})$ as well as h (if any).

First, we need to design the structure of $q(\mathbf{y})$, which depends on learning tasks that are closely related to the complexity of the world $\mathbf{X}$ that we observe. One typical example is a world $\mathbf{X} = \{X, L\}$ that consists of a number of individual objects to observe, with L denoting a set of labels and each $\ell \in L$ denoting an object. In this case, each $\mathbf{x} = \{x, \ell\}$ contains a feature vector $x = [x^{(1)}, \ldots, x^{(d)}]^T$ observed from the object ℓ, subject to a joint underlying dis-

tribution $p(\mathbf{x}) = p(x, \ell)$. Correspondingly, we consider a representation domain $\mathbf{Y} = \{Y, L\}$, subject to a parametric structure of $q(\mathbf{y}) = q(y, \ell)$ that describes the vector $\mathbf{y}$ and the label ℓ jointly. This $q(\mathbf{y})$ is specified by three ingredients. The first consists of a set $\mathbf{k} = \{k, \{m_\ell\}\}$, with k denoting the number of labels in L and m_ℓ being the dimension of either a binary or a real vector $\mathbf{y}$ that corresponds to $\ell \in L$. We call both k, m_ℓ the scales of the representation domain $\mathbf{Y}$. The second ingredient is the functional form of $q(\mathbf{y})$, which is usually prespecified according to the nature of learning task. The third consists of a set θ_y of parameters in this given function form.

Second, we need to design the structures of $p(\mathbf{y}|\mathbf{x})$, $q(\mathbf{x}|\mathbf{y})$ that specify the mapping capacity of $x \rightarrow y$ and $y \rightarrow x$, respectively. Each of the two can be either parametric or structure free. We say $p(u|v)$ is structure free if $p(u|v)$ can be any function that satisfies $\int p(u|v) = 1, p(u|v) \geq 0$. A structure-free distribution is actually specified in learning. Given its functional form, a parametric $p(u|v, \theta_{u|v})$ is structured by a set $\theta_{u|v}$ of unknown parameters.

Putting this all together, the nature of a BYY system depends on the structure of $q(\mathbf{y})$ for describing the representation domain $\mathbf{Y}$, and the architecture of a BYY system is featured by a combination of the specific structures of $p(\mathbf{y}|\mathbf{x})$, $q(\mathbf{x}|\mathbf{y})$. Discarding a useless architecture where both $p(\mathbf{y}|\mathbf{x})$, $q(\mathbf{x}|\mathbf{y})$ are structure free, there remain three choices for a meaningful BYY architecture:

- *Backward architecture (B-architecture):* $p(\mathbf{y}|\mathbf{x})$ is structure-free and $q(\mathbf{x}|\mathbf{y})$ is parametric.
- *Forward architecture (F-architecture):* $q(\mathbf{x}|\mathbf{y})$ is structure-free and $p(\mathbf{y}|\mathbf{x})$ is parametric.
- *Bidirectional architecture (BI-architecture):* Both $p(\mathbf{y}|\mathbf{x})$, $q(\mathbf{x}|\mathbf{y})$ are parametric.

Generally speaking, a learning task includes two subtasks. One is called *parameter learning* and is for determining a value of the set θ that consists of all the unknown parameters in $p(\mathbf{y}|\mathbf{x})$, $q(\mathbf{x}|\mathbf{y})$, $q(\mathbf{y})$ as well as h (if any). The other subtask is called *model selection* and is for selecting the scales of representation, since a collection of specific BYY systems with different scales in $\mathbf{k}$ corresponds to a family of specific models that share the same system configuration but with different scales.

Harmony Learning

We consider learning in a broad sense that starts from two $p(u)$, $q(u)$, with each of them having certain unknown parts, in either or both scales and parameters. The task of learning is to specify all the unknowns from the known parts. Our *fundamental learning principle* is to make $p(u)$, $g(u)$ have the *best harmony in* a twofold sense:

- The difference between the resulting $p(u)$, $g(u)$ should be minimized.
- The resulting $p(u)$, $g(u)$ should be of the least complexity.

Mathematically, we use a functional $H(p\|q)$ to measure the *degree of harmony* between $p(u)$ and $q(u)$. When both $p(u)$, $q(u)$ are discrete densities in the following form:

$$q(u) = \sum_{t=1}^{N} q_t \delta(u - u_t), \quad \sum_{t=1}^{N} q_t = 1 \qquad (2)$$

with $\delta(u)$ being a δ-function, we can simply use the following cross entropy

$$H(p\|q) = \sum_{t=1}^{N} p_t \ln q_t \qquad (3)$$

as a typical example of such a measure. The maximization of $H(p\|q)$ has two interesting natures:

- *Matching nature*: With p fixed, $\max_q H(p\|q)$ pushes q toward

$$q_t = p_t, \text{ for all } t \tag{4}$$

- *Least complexity nature*: $\max_p H(p\|q)$ with q fixed pushes p toward its simplest form

$$p(u) = \delta(u - u_\tau), \text{ with } \tau = \arg \max_t g_t \tag{5}$$

or equivalently $p_\tau = 1$, and $p_t = 0$ for other t, which is of least complexity from the statistical perspective (Xu, 2001a).

Thus, the maximization of this functional indeed implements the above harmony purpose mathematically. As shown by Xu (2001a), we can further represent either a discrete or continuous density $q(u)$ in the form of Equation 2 by considering its sample points $\{u_t\}_{t=1}^N$ via the following normalization:

$$\hat{q}_t = q(u_t)/z_q, \, z_q = \sum_{t=1}^N q(u_t) \tag{6}$$

Putting this into Equation 3, we can get a general form of the harmony measure:

$$H(p\|q) = \int p(u) \ln q(u)du - \ln z_q \tag{7}$$

which reduces to Equation 3 when $q(u)$, $p(u)$ are discrete (as in Equation 2), with u enumerated from $u_1, \ldots, u_N$ deterministically.

Moreover, when $p(u)$ is given by its empirical density (Devroye et al., 1996),

$$p_0(u) = \frac{1}{N} \sum_{t=1}^N \delta(u - u_t) \tag{8}$$

a crude approximation $z_q = 1$ will make $H(p\|q)$ in Equation 7 become the likelihood

$$L(\theta) = \sum_{t=1}^N \ln q(u_t) \tag{9}$$

Thus, finding $\max_q H(p\|q)$ becomes equivalent to conventional maximum likelihood (ML) learning.

Generally, the term $\ln z_q$ imposes a regularization on ML learning. Two typical examples are given as follows:

1. *Normalization learning*: With $p(u)$ given by Equation 8, we approximate either a discrete or continuous $q(u)$ by Equation 6 and get Equation 7 in the form

$$H(p\|q) = L(\theta) - \ln z_q, \, z_q = \sum_{t=1}^N q(u_t) \tag{10}$$

with $\ln z_q$ imposing a de-learning on the ML learning, which avoids $q(u)$ overfitting a finite size data set (Xu, 2001a).
2. *Data smoothing learning*: Consider $p(u)$ given by a Parzen window estimate (Devroye et al., 1996)

$$p(u) = p_h(u) = \frac{1}{N} \sum_{t=1}^N G(u|u_t, h^2 I) \tag{11}$$

where, as hereafter in this article, $G(u|\mu, \Sigma)$ denotes a Gaussian density with mean vector μ and covariance matrix Σ. Under a weak constraint $\Sigma_{t=1}^N p(u_t) \approx \Sigma_{t=1}^N q(u_t) = z_q$, we can approximately get (Xu, 2001a)

$$z_q \approx \frac{z_q^N(h, k)}{N(2\pi h^2)^{k/2}}, \, z_q^N(h, k) = \sum_{\tau=1}^N \sum_{t=1}^N e^{-0.5(\|u_t - u_\tau\|^2/h^2)} \tag{12}$$

where k is the dimension of u. Thus, Equation 7 becomes

$$H(p\|q)$$
$$= \int p_h(u) \ln q(u)du + 0.5k \ln (2\pi h^2) + \ln N - \ln z_q^N(h, k) \tag{13}$$

The first term regularizes ML learning by smoothing each likelihood $\ln q(u_t)$ in the near-neighborhood of u_t, and thus is referred to as *data smoothing*. The role of h^2 is equivalent to the hyperparameter in Tikhonov-type regularization (Bishop, 1995), but with a new feature that the other terms balance the first term such that an appropriate h is learned together with θ (Xu, 2001a).

BYY Harmony Learning

The fact that $\max_\theta \int p_0(u) \ln q(u|\theta)du$ leads to ML learning is well known in the literature. Moreover, $\max_\theta \int p^*(u) \ln q(u|\theta)du$, with $p^*(u)$ being the true distribution of samples, has also been studied in developing the Akaike information criterion (AIC) for model selection (Akaike, 1974). However, the least complexity nature of Equation 5 has rarely been studied because it is regarded as useless in a conventional sense. In contrast, least complexity plays an essential role that enables the harmony learning on a BYY system to implement model selection.

To be specific, we put $p(u) = p(\mathbf{x}, \mathbf{y}) = p(\mathbf{y}|\mathbf{x})p(\mathbf{x})$, $q(u) = q(\mathbf{x}, \mathbf{y}) = q(\mathbf{x}|\mathbf{y})q(\mathbf{y})$ into Equation 7, and get

$$H(p\|q) = \int p(\mathbf{y}|\mathbf{x})p(\mathbf{x}) \ln [q(\mathbf{x}|\mathbf{y})q(\mathbf{y})]d\mathbf{x}d\mathbf{y} - \ln z_q \tag{14}$$

Again, the term $-\ln z_q$ imposes regularization on learning either by normalization similar to Equation 10 or by data smoothing similar to Equation 12. This regularization may be simply ignored by setting $z_q = 1$. The details are given in Xu (2000, 2001a). For example, similar to Equation 10, we can simply get

$$z_q = \sum_{t=1}^N q(\mathbf{x}_t|\mathbf{y}_t)q(\mathbf{y}_t) \tag{15}$$

on a set of samples $\chi = \{\mathbf{x}_t\}_{t=1}^N$, where $\mathbf{y}_t$ is estimated during learning as an inner representation of $\mathbf{x}_t$.

Mathematically, harmony learning is implemented by

$$\max_{\theta, \mathbf{k}} H(\theta, \mathbf{k}), \text{ where } H(\theta, \mathbf{k}) = H(p\|q) \tag{16}$$

Unlike the case of Equation 7, the least complexity nature of a BYY system makes selecting $\mathbf{k}$ possible, because now only $p(\mathbf{x})$ is fixed as a nonparametric estimate, while $p(\mathbf{y}|\mathbf{x})$ is not fixed but able to be pushed into its least complexity form during learning. In a B-architecture, $p(\mathbf{y}|\mathbf{x})$ is free and thus will be determined by $\max_{p(\mathbf{y}|\mathbf{x})} H(p\|q)$, resulting in

$$p(\mathbf{y}|\mathbf{x}) = \delta(\mathbf{y} - \hat{\mathbf{y}}), \, \hat{\mathbf{y}} = \arg \max_{\mathbf{y}} [q(\mathbf{x}|\mathbf{y})q(\mathbf{y})] \tag{17}$$

In turn, the matching nature of harmony learning will further push $q(\mathbf{x}|\mathbf{y})$ and $q(\mathbf{y})$ toward their corresponding least complexity forms. In a BI-architecture, the learning will similarly push $p(\mathbf{y}|\mathbf{x})$ into its least complexity form, e.g., $p(\mathbf{y}|\mathbf{x}) = \delta(\mathbf{y} - f_j(\mathbf{x}, W_{y|x}))$ (Xu, 2001a).

As for $q(\mathbf{y}) = q(y, \ell) = q(y|\ell)q(\ell)$, it is not difficult to observe that letting $p(\ell)$ be zero is equivalent to reducing k by one, and that letting the variance of every $q(y^{(j)}|\ell)$, for all $\ell \in L$, be zero is equivalent to removing the jth dimension (i.e., reducing the dimension m by one). In other words, making θ take a specific value is equivalent to forcing k, m_ℓ to be reduced effectively to appropriate scales. So, model selection may come into effect either in parallel with parameter learning or sequentially after making parameter learning via enumerating k on an appropriate range. That is, we have the following two types of learning implementation:

- *Parameter learning with automated model selection*: We set k, $\{m_\ell\}$ in **k** large enough and then implement harmony learning by

$$\max_\theta H(\theta), \ H(\theta) = H(\theta, \mathbf{k}) \quad (18)$$

The least complexity nature Equation 5 will let θ take a specific value such that $\mathbf{k} = \{k, \{m_\ell\}\}$ are effectively reduced to appropriate scales, i.e., model selection is made automatically in parallel with parameter learning.
- *Parameter learning followed by model selection*: Alternatively, we can make parameter learning and model selection sequentially in two steps. In the first step, we enumerate k, m_ℓ from small values incrementally, and at each specific k, m_ℓ we perform parameter learning Equation 18, to get the best parameter value θ^*. Moreover, to simplify the implementation, we can even assume $q(\ell) = 1/k$ and $q(y|\ell)$ comes from a family that satisfies certain constraint (Xu, 2002a). Then in the second step, we select a best k^*, m_ℓ^* by

$$\min_{k,m_\ell} J(k, m_\ell), \text{ where } J(k, m_\ell) = -H(\theta^*, \mathbf{k}) \quad (19)$$

If there is more than one solution for which $J(k, m_\ell)$ gets the same minimum, we take one with the smallest values on k, $\{m_\ell\}$.

This, two-step implementation can be modified with the first step replaced by alternatives. One is to replace Equation 18 by minimizing the Kullback divergence (see LEARNING AND STATISTICAL INFERENCE)

$$\min_\theta KL(\theta) = \int p(\mathbf{y}|\mathbf{x})p(\mathbf{x}) \ln \frac{p(\mathbf{y}|\mathbf{x})p(\mathbf{x})}{q(\mathbf{x}|\mathbf{y})q(\mathbf{y})} \, d\mathbf{x}d\mathbf{y} \quad (20)$$

as in the initial work of the BYY learning made in 1995 (reference in Xu, 2002a) and other early studies. In this situation, the first step leads us to a number of existing learning models that are based on the maximum likelihood principle or its equivalents. Another alternative is to replace $H(\theta)$ in Equation 18 by $H(\theta) - \lambda KL(\theta)$ with $\lambda > 0$ gradually reducing toward zero from a given value. Both alternatives can reduce the local minimum effect caused by the winner-take-all mechanism of Equation 17, but at the cost of greater difficulty in handling the integral of **y** in Equation 20.

Information-Theoretic Perspective, MML/MDL, and the Bayesian Approach

Alternatively, we can understand harmony learning from an information-theoretic perspective. We consider the transfer of the information in **x** from a sender via a communication line to a receiver. Instead of directly encoding **x** for transmission, **x** is mapped to its inner representation **y**, and then **y** is encoded and sent to the receiver. The receiver then decodes **y** to reconstruct **x**.

Without losing generality, we consider the BYY system with $p(\mathbf{y}|\mathbf{x}) = p(y|x, \theta_{y|x})$, $q(\mathbf{x}|\mathbf{y}) = p(x|y, \theta_{x|y})$, and $q(\mathbf{y}) = q(y|\theta_y)$, as shown in Figure 1. On the sender side, x is mapped into its code y via the yang passage $p(\mathbf{y}|\mathbf{x}) = p(y|x, \theta_{y|x})$ and then y is encoded and sent to the receiver side. On the receiver side, a parametric regression function $\hat{x} = g(y, \theta_g)$ is used to construct x with an error $\varepsilon = x - \hat{x}$. Assuming the functional form of $g(y, \cdot)$ is known at the receiver end, in order to get the original x we need to know not only y but also ε and θ_g, which should be decided at the sender end and then transferred via the communication line, too.

For this purpose, the reconstruction process at the receiver end is simulated by the ying machine at the sender end. First, the yang

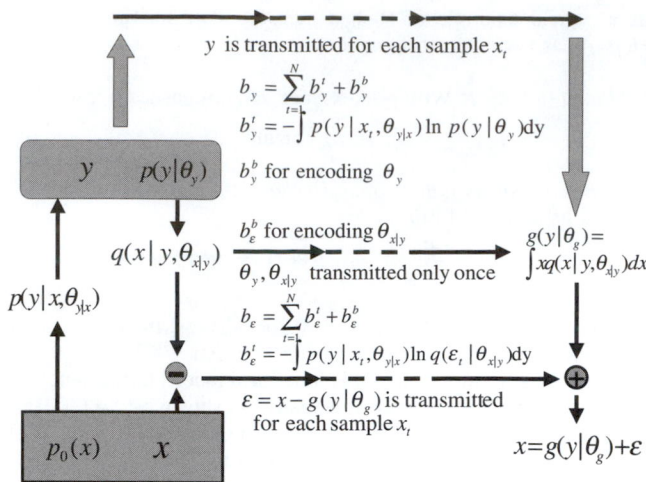

Figure 1. Bayesian ying-yang harmony learning from an information-theoretic perspective.

passage $p(y|x, \theta_{y|x})$ is assumed to come from a known parametric family but with an unknown set of parameters $\theta_{y|x}$. Second, the mapped y is assumed to be exactly described by a distribution of a known parametric family $q(y|\theta_y)$ but with an unknown set of parameters θ_y. Third, we attempt to reconstruct x by the regression $g(y, \theta_g)$ with the residual $\varepsilon = x - g(y, \theta_g)$ that comes from a known parametric family $q(\varepsilon|\theta_\varepsilon)$ but with an unknown set of parameters θ_ε. That is, we have $p(x|y, \theta_{x|y}) = q(x - g(y|\theta_g)|\theta_\varepsilon)$ with $\theta_{x|y} = \{\theta_g, \theta_\varepsilon\}$ and $g(y|\theta_g) = \int xp(x|y, \theta_{x|y})dx$.

We consider the building of the above BYY system from the perspective that the transmission of y, ε, and θ_g is made most efficiently, comparing this approach with the minimum message length (MML) and minimum description length (MDL) approached (Wallace and Dowe, 1999; Rissanen, 1986, 1999), which can be regarded as specific implementations of the more general algorithmic complexity exemplified by the celebrated Kolmogorov complexity (Gammerman and Vovk, 1999).

If we know the true distribution $q(y|\theta_y^*)$ with an exact value of θ_y^*, it follows that the number of bits for encoding y is $b_y^s = \sum_{t=1}^N b_y^t$, with b_y^t being the bits that are needed to encode y for each sample x_t. Since the probability of using a particular y as a code of x_t is $p(y|x_t, \theta_{y|x})dy$, this b_y^t should be the expected number of bits to be used at x_t, i.e., $b_y^t = -\int p(y|x_t, \theta_{y|x}) \ln q(y|\theta_y^*)dy - c_y$, where $c_y = 0$ when $q(y|\theta_y^*)$ is a discrete probability distribution and $c_y = \ln \delta_y$ when $q(y|\theta_y^*)$ is a continuous density, with δ_y being a quantization resolution. Usually c_y is omitted in the MML/MDL literature, since it is regarded as a constant.

However, on a set of finite samples $\{x_t\}_{t=1}^N$, instead of getting exactly θ_y^* we can obtain only an estimate θ_y that is itself a random variable. Thus, the bits for encoding y consist of the above b_y^s plus b_y^b, i.e., $b_y = b_y^s + b_y^b$, where b_y^b is the number of bits for encoding an estimate θ_y, which does not depend on each individual sample but on the entire data set $\{x_t\}_{t=1}^N$, or equivalently the distribution of θ_y.

Similarly, the number of bits for encoding ε also consist of two parts $b_\varepsilon = \sum_{t=1}^N b_\varepsilon^t + b_\varepsilon^b$, where $b_\varepsilon^t = -\int p(y|x_t, \theta_{y|x}) \ln q(\varepsilon|\theta_\varepsilon)dy = -\int p(y|x_t, \theta_{y|x}) \ln q(x_t|y, \theta_{x|y})dy$ for each sample x_t, and b_ε^b for encoding θ_ε. Moreover, we use b_g to count the bits for encoding θ_g, and then use $b_{x|y}^b = b_\varepsilon^b + b_g$ to denote the total bits for encoding $\theta_{x|y} = \{\theta_g, \theta_\varepsilon\}$, which again does not depend on each individual sample but on the entire batch of data.

Summing up, the total description length is $L_T = N b_s + b_\theta$ with $b_s = (1/N)\Sigma_{t=1}^N (b_y^t + b_\varepsilon^t)$ being the average number of bits that is needed for each sample x_t and $b_\theta = b_y^b + b_{x|y}^b = b_y^b + b_\varepsilon^b + b_g$ being the total number of bits for encoding $\theta_{x|y}, \theta_y$. Thus, the average unit length for each sample x_t is $L_U = b_s + (b_\theta/N)$. Since b_θ does not depend on the size N, (b_θ/N) decreases toward zero as N increases.

It further follows that $b_y^t + b_\varepsilon^t = -\int p(y|x_t, \theta_{y|x}) \ln [q(x_t|y, \theta_{x|y}) q(y|\theta_y)] dy$ and thus that

$$b_s = -\int p(y|x_t, \theta_{y|x}) p_0(x) \ln [q(x_t|y, \theta_{x|y}) q(y|\theta_y)] dxdy$$

$$p_0(x) = \frac{1}{N} \sum_{t=1}^N \delta(x - x_t) \tag{21}$$

Comparing this with Equation 14, we have exactly $H(p\|q) = -b_s - \ln z_q^{-1}$, where the second term depends on the specific value of parameters $\theta_{x|y}, \theta_y$ and the complexity of y, but does not depend on each individual sample x_t. Also, it tends to zero as $N \to \infty$, which is consistent with the role of b_θ/N that tends to zero as $N \to \infty$. So, BYY harmony learning relates closely to the MML/MDL spirit in that both have in common minimizing b_s, i.e., the part of the description length for each sample. For this reason, as well as shown experimentally (Xu, 2001a), BYY harmony learning has model selection ability qualitatively similar to that of MML/MDL. This ability can be understood from the interaction between the two parts in $b_y^t + b_\varepsilon^t$. As the representation scale increases, b_y^t increases while b_ε^t decreases. The minimization of the two parts trades off an appropriate scale for representing y.

However, BYY harmony learning differs from MML/MDL on the specific form for encoding θ. One obvious advantage of BYY harmony learning is that using $\ln z_q^{-1}$ instead of b_θ/N is easy in implementation. Usually, b_θ is difficult to compute and has to be replaced by some rough approximation or bound, with consequent poor actual performance. Further studies are warranted to explore the quantitative relation between $\ln z_q^{-1}$ and b_θ/N to see whether the features of the two can be combined.

In the literature on neural networks learning, it has been widely regarded that the Bayesian approach is equivalent to the MDL approach. However, the situation is not so simple, but depends on how the MDL and the Bayesian approaches are implemented.

One typical Bayesian implementation is for parameter regularization, i.e., a priori density on parameters is assumed such that parameters are determined based on the joint distribution of the parameters and the observed sample data. When MDL was first proposed (Rissanen, 1986), it was implemented basically in equivalence to the MML approach (Wallace and Dowe, 1999), which shares the same spirit of Bayesian regularization in that its first part encodes the fitting residuals and its second part corresponds to the a priori density on parameters. According to the original authors of MML, however, MML actually uses an improper prior density if we insist on relating it to the Bayesian perspective.

Another typical Bayesian implementation is the so-called evidence-based Bayesian approach (Mackey, 1992; see also BAYESIAN METHODS AND NEURAL NETWORKS) using what is called the BIC model selection criterion in the literature of statistics. This one has in principle the closet agreement with the MDL principle that considers an average of all the MML code lengths for all distributions in a family instead of a single MML code length (Rissanen, 1999). In various actual implementations, however, it usually degenerates to be identical to MML after selecting a noninformative uniform prior and approximating the integral of the marginal density via considerable simplification. Interestingly, the latest implementation of MDL uses a so-called normalized maximum likelihood model as the universal model (Rissanen, 1999),

which leads to improved code length and becomes different from both MML and the evidence-based Bayesian approach.

BYY harmony learning shares the common spirit of MML as well as Bayesian regularization in the general sense that z_q^{-1} can be regarded as another type of improper prior density on parameters in the BYY system such that the term $-\ln z_q^{-1}$ imposes further regularization on parameter learning, while the interaction between the two parts $b_y^t + b_\varepsilon^t$ in b_s makes model selection implemented either automatically during parameter learning or subsequently after parameter learning via a new class of model selection criteria. It is also possible to further extend BYY harmony learning to share the sprit of MDL and the evidence-based Bayesian approach by normalizing z_q^{-1} into an a priori density $p(\theta)$ and then maximizing an average harmony measure $\int H(\theta) p(\theta) d\theta$. However, this has as extra cost the difficulty in implementing the integral.

Examples of Applications

Applying Equations 18 and 19 to specific BYY systems for various learning tasks, we have obtained not only new insights but also a number of new results. The details are given in Xu (2001a, 2001b, 2002a, 2002b). In the following, we briefly introduce several examples of unsupervised learning.

- *The MSE clustering, number of clusters, and RPCL learning*: Considering a simple B-architecture with $p(\mathbf{y}) = p(y, \ell) = \delta(y - \mu_\ell)/k$ and $p(\mathbf{x}|\mathbf{y}) = p(x|y, \ell) = G(x|y, \sigma^2 I)$, it follows that Equation 18 with the term $-\ln z_q^{-1}$ ignored (i.e., with $z_q = 1$) becomes equivalent to

$$\hat{\ell} = \arg \min_\ell \|x_t - \mu_{\hat{\ell}}\|^2, \min_{all\ \ell} E_2, E_2 = \sum_{t=1}^N \|x_t - \mu_{\hat{\ell}}\|^2 \tag{22}$$

This is exactly conventional least square clustering or vector quantization, which leads to the well-known k-means algorithm and classical COMPETITIVE LEARNING (q.v.). Moreover, we can get several new results. First obtained by Xu in 1997 (reference in Xu, 2002a), it follows that Equation 19 becomes the following criterion for the best number of clusters

$$k^* = \arg \min_k J(k), \text{ with } J(k) = 0.5d \ln E_2 + \ln k \tag{23}$$

Second, with z_q given by the normalization Equation 15 and $p(\mathbf{y}) = p(y, \ell) = \delta(y - m_\ell) p(\ell)$, not only can we get a modified version of Equation 23 from Equation 19, but it also follows that Equation 18 in parallel implementation becomes equivalent to rival penalized competitive learning (RPCL), proposed by Xu, Krzyzak, and Oja in 1993 (reference in Xu, 2002a), that is able to find the correct number of clusters automatically during learning. Third, these results can also be extended to regularized versions (Xu, 2001b).

- *PCA and Gaussian factor analysis (FA)*: For a B-architecture with $p(\mathbf{y}) = G(y|0, I)$ and $p(\mathbf{x}|\mathbf{y}) = G(x|Ay, \sigma^2 I)$, it follows that Equation 18 with $z_q = 1$ becomes equivalent to PRINCIPAL COMPONENT ANALYSIS (PCA) (q.v.) and Equation 19 becomes

$$m^* = \arg \min_m J(m),$$
$$J(m) = 0.5d \ln \sigma^{*2} + 0.5m(\ln 2\pi + 1) \tag{24}$$

for the principal subspace dimension m. Moreover, Equation 18 with $z_q = 1$ becomes equivalent to Gaussian FA when $p(\mathbf{x}|\mathbf{y}) = G(x|Ay, \Sigma)$, with an adaptive EM algorithm developed for its implementation. Also, Equation 18 with z_q given by the normalization Equation 15 will lead to RPCL-type learning that is able to automatically determine the dimension m.

- *Elliptic RPCL, Gaussian mixture, and local PCA*: For a B-architecture with $p(\mathbf{y}) = p(\ell) G(y|\mu_\ell, I)$ and $p(\mathbf{x}|\mathbf{y}) = G(x|A_\ell y,$

$\sigma_\ell^2 I$), from Equation 18 we can obtain (1) both the batch and adaptive EM-type algorithms for either elliptic clustering or ML learning on Gaussian mixtures, (2) an elliptic RPCL algorithm with automated selection on cluster number during learning, (3) extensions to local PCA, and (4) other extensions. Moreover, we can use Equation 19 for selecting both k and the dimensions $\{m_\ell\}$ of local subspaces, which simplifies to

$$[k^*, \{m_\ell^*\}] = \arg \min_{k, \{m_\ell\}} J(k, \{m_\ell\})$$

$$J(k, \{m_\ell\}) = 0.5 \sum_{\ell=1}^{k} p(\ell)[\ln |\Sigma_\ell|$$

$$+ m_\ell(\ln 2\pi + 1)] - \sum_{\ell=1}^{k} p(\ell) \ln p(\ell),$$

$$\Sigma_\ell = A_\ell A_\ell^T + \sigma_\ell^2 I \qquad (25)$$

- *Binary FA, non-Gaussian FA, and local extensions*: For a B-architecture with $p(\mathbf{y}) = \Pi_{j=1}^{m} p(y_j)$ where each $p(y_j)$ is a scalar finite mixture (e.g., Gaussian mixture) and $p(\mathbf{x}|\mathbf{y}) = G(x|Ay, \sigma^2 I)$, from Equation 18 we have obtained both the adaptive EM-type and RPCL-type algorithms for implementing either binary FA when each y_j is binary or non-Gaussian real FA when each y_j is real which was previously studied under the name of Bayesian Ying Yang Kullback dependence reduction in 1998 (reference in Xu, 2000) and further developed with the name changed into the current one. Moreover, from Equation 19 we get criteria for selecting the number m of factors. Furthermore, these results can also be extended to localized versions by considering $p(\mathbf{y}) = p(\ell)\Pi_{j=1}^{m_\ell} p_\ell(y_j)$ and $p(\mathbf{x}|\mathbf{y}) = G(x|A_\ell y, \sigma_\ell^2 I)$.
- *ICA and competitive ICA*: For an F-architecture with $p(\mathbf{y}) = \Pi_{j=1}^{m} p(y_j)$ as above and $p(\mathbf{y}|\mathbf{x}) = \delta(y - Wx)$, from Equation 18 we can revisit (1) the *learned parametric mixture—based ICA* algorithm, first proposed by Xu, Yang, and Amari in 1996 (reference in Xu, 2001a), that works not only on cases where some components of y are super-Gaussian and others are sub-Gaussian, but also on cases where W is not invertible but $|WW^T| \neq 0$. Moreover, it has been further extended to a localized version via competition by considering $p(\mathbf{y}) = p(\ell) \Pi_{j=1}^{m_\ell} p_\ell(y_j)$ and $p(\mathbf{y}|\mathbf{x}) = p(\ell|x)\delta(y - W_\ell x)$ (Xu, 2002a).
- *LMSER learning, principal ICA, and local extensions*: For a BI-architecture with $p(\mathbf{y}) = \Pi_{j=1}^{m} p(y_j)$, $p(\mathbf{x}|\mathbf{y}) = G(x|Ay, \sigma^2 I)$, and $p(\mathbf{y}|\mathbf{x}) = \delta(y - s(Wx))$, Equation 18 leads us not only to revisit LMSER learning that was first proposed by Xu in 1991 and then directly adopted by Karhunen and Joutsensalo (1994) to implement ICA under the name of nonlinear PCA, but also various extensions, including a so-called principal ICA that corresponds to the direct extension of PCA to ICA. Moreover, from Equation 19 we get criteria for selecting the dimension m. Furthermore, these results have also been extended to localized versions (Xu, 2001b, 2002a).

A number of new results have also obtained on supervised learning and temporal modeling.

For supervised learning, new understandings are obtained on three-layer feedforward nets with backpropagation learning, on the popular mixture-of-experts (ME) model with the corresponding EM algorithm (see MODULAR AND HIERARCHICAL LEARNING SYSTEMS), and on the alternative ME model (Xu, Jordan, and Hinton in Xu, 2002a) as well as the normalized radial basis function (NRBF) network and its extensions. Moreover, various adaptive EM-type learning algorithms are developed from both Equation 18 and Equation 20 since 1998. New criteria have been derived from Equation 19 for deciding the number of hidden units, the number of experts, and the number of basis functions. Also, we get an alternative approach for deciding the set of supporting vectors in

SUPPORT VECTOR MACHINES (q.v.). For further details see (Xu, 2001b, 2002b).

Temporal BYY harmony learning has been developed as a general state space approach for modeling data that has temporal relationship among samples, and provides not only a unified point of view on Kalman filter (see KALMAN FILTERING: NEURAL IMPLICATIONS) and HIDDEN MARKOV MODELS (q.v.), but also several new results, such as higher-order HMMs, independent HMMs, temporal ICA, temporal factor analysis, temporal extension of competitive ICA and LMSER learning, and more, with adaptive algorithms for implementation and criteria for selecting the number of states or sources. Further details are supplied in (Xu, 2000, 2001a).

Discussion

Conventional ML learning, as in maximizing $L(\theta)$ in Equation 9, is widely used for estimating θ for a parametric density $q(u|\theta)$ directly on a set $\{u_t\}_{t=1}^{N}$ of samples. For many practical problems, such as perception, u consists of two parts, $u = (x, y)$, with y invisible. What can be observed is a sample set $\{x_t\}_{t=1}^{N}$, and thus ML learning is not directly applicable to $q(u|\theta)$. In such cases, ML learning is usually implemented on the marginal density

$$q(x|\theta) = \int q(u|\theta)dy = \int q(x_t|y, \theta_{x|y})q(y|\theta_y)dy \qquad (26)$$

which is usually called the factor model or latent variable model or *generative model* in the literature.

However, a direct implementation of ML learning on $q(x|\theta)$ is usually not computationally effective. The problem is solved by two closely related approaches. One is the popular EM algorithm, developed under incomplete data theory (IDT) (Dempster, Laird, and Rubin, 1977). The other is the well-known alternative minimization (Csiszar and Tusnady, 1984), also called the *em* algorithm, developed under information geometry theory (IGT) (see NEUROMANIFOLDS AND INFORMATION GEOMETRY). The approaches work on a class of problems where y takes finite discrete values such that either Equation 26 is a finite mixture or the integral in Equation 26 can be analytically solved. However, in the implementation, we have to compute

$$p(y|x) = \frac{q(x|y, \theta_{x|y})q(y|\theta_y)}{\int q(x|y, \theta_{x|y})q(y|\theta_y)dy}, \text{ and } \max_\theta Q(\theta) \text{ } with$$

$$Q(\theta) = \int p(y|x)p_0(x) \ln [q(x|y, \theta_{x|y})q(y|\theta_y)]dxdy \qquad (27)$$

When y is a binary vector of many bits or a non-Gaussian real vector, Equation 27 must be computed either by an exhaustive enumeration or by Monte Carlo approximation, and both those are computationally very expensive. The well-known Helmholtz machine tackles this problem by using a parametric $p(y|x, \theta_{y|x})$ in Equation 20 to avoid the computation on $p(y|x)$, and then minimizes the Helmholtz energy in place of maximizing $Q(\theta)$.

As discussed in the initial work by Xu in 1995 (reference in Xu, 2002a), the BYY system together with implementing Equation 20 provides a unified perspective on understanding not only the above ML learning-related approaches but also a class of information-theoretic approaches. First, $\min_{p(y|x)} KL(\theta)$ in Equation 20 with a free Yang pathway $p(y|x)$ and the empirical density $p_0(x)$ will lead to Equation 27, as well as the equivalence of Equation 20 to ML learning on Equation 26. In other words, the above IDT-and IGT-based approaches are revisited from this new perspective. Second, given a parametric $p(y|x, \theta_{y|x})$, Equation 20 becomes equivalent to minimizing the Helmholtz energy, and a specific design of $p(y|x,$

$\theta_{y|x}$), $q(x|y, \theta_{x|y})$, $q(y|\theta_y)$ will lead us to revisit Helmholtz machine learning. Third, given a parametric $p(y|x, \theta_{y|x})$ but with $q(x|y, \theta_{x|y})$ free, Equation 20 becomes equivalent to minimizing

$$KL_y(\theta_{y|x}, \theta_y) = \int p(y|\theta_{y|x}) \ln \frac{p(y|\theta_{y|x})}{q(y|\theta_y)} dy$$

$$p(y|\theta_{y|x}) = \int p(y|x, \theta_{y|x})p_0(x)dx \qquad (28)$$

which consists of a class of information-theoretic approaches, including both the minimum mutual information approach and the INFOMAX approach for INDEPENDENT COMPONENT ANALYSIS (q.v.).

Moreover, BYY harmony learning goes beyond the approaches discussed above. First, in addition to using Equation 20 for parameter learning, the second step in the two-step implementation of BYY harmony learning provides model selection via a new class of criteria given by Equation 19, sharing a feature similar to the MML/MDL/AC and Bayeisian approaches. Second, the parallel implementation of BYY harmony learning as discussed for Equation 18 provides an easily implementable approach for model selection that is made automatically during parameter learning. Third, the architecture of the BYY system and the term $-\ln z_q^{-1}$ in the harmony function provide new regularization techniques from a systematic perspective. In contrast, learning parameters via minimizing the Kullback divergence is the sole target of the approaches discussed above, while the issues of regularization and model selection are outside the scope of their studies. Even focusing on parameter learning via minimizing Kullback divergence alone, the studies are made from different perspectives with different purposes.

Road Map: Learning in Artificial Networks
Background: Bayesian Methods and Neural Networks; Helmholtz Machines and Sleep-Wake Learning

Related Reading: Adaptive Resonance Theory; Generalization and Regularization in Nonlinear Learning Systems; Learning and Statistical Inference; Model Validation

References

Akaike, H., 1974, A new look at the statistical model identification, *IEEE Trans. Autom. Control*, 19:714–723.

Bishop, C. M., 1995, Training with noise is equivalent to Tikhonov regularization, *Neural Computat.*, 7:108–116.

Csiszar, I., and Tusnady, G., 1984, Information geometry and alternating minimization procedures, *Statist. Decisions*, Suppl. 1, pp. 205–237.

Dempster, A. P., Laird, N. M., and Rubin, D. B., 1977, Maximum likelihood from incomplete data via the EM algorithm, *J. R. Statist. Soc.*, B39:1–38.

Devroye, L., Györfi, L., and Lugosi, G., 1996, *A Probability Theory of Pattern Recognition*, New York: Springer-Verlag.

Gammerman, A., and Vovk, V., Eds. 1999, *Kolmogorov Complexity* (special issue), *Computer J.*, 42(4).

Karhunen, J., and Joutsensalo, J., 1994, Representation and separation of signals using nonlinear PCA type learning, *Neural Netw.*, 7:113–127.

Mackey, D., 1992, A practical Bayesian framework for backpropagation, *Neural Computat.*, 4:448–472.

Rissanen, J., 1999, Hypothesis selection and testing by the MDL principle, *Computer J.*, 42:260–269.

Wallace, C. S., and Dowe, D. R., 1999, Minimum message length and Kolmogorov complexity, *Computer J.*, 42:270–280.

Xu, L., 2000, Temporal BYY learning for state space approach, hidden Markov model and blind source separation, *IEEE Trans. Sign. Process.*, 48:2132–2144.

Xu, L., 2001a, BYY harmony learning, independent state space and generalized APT financial analyses, *IEEE Trans. Neural Netw.*, 12:822–849. ◆

Xu, L., 2001b, Best harmony, unified RPCL and automated model selection for unsupervised and supervised learning on Gaussian mixtures, three-layer nets and ME-RBF-SVM models, *Int. J. Neural Syst.*, 11:43–69. ◆

Xu, L., 2002a, BYY harmony learning, structural RPCL, and topological self-organizing on mixture models, *Neural Netw.*, in press.

Xu, L., 2002b, BYY learning, regularized implementation, and model selection on modular networks with one hidden layer of binary units, *Neurocomputing*, in press.

Editorial Advisory Board

Contributors

Emile H. L. Aarts Media Interaction, Philips Research, Eindhoven, The Netherlands
E-mail: aarts@philips.com
Simulated Annealing and Boltzmann Machines

Larry F. Abbott Volen Center and Department of Biology, Brandeis University, Waltham, Massachusetts
E-mail: abbott@brandeis.edu
Activity-Dependent Regulation of Neuronal Conductances
Temporal Dynamics of Biological Synapses

Moshe Abeles The Interdisciplinary Center for Neural Computation and the Department of Physiology, School of Medicine, Hebrew University, Jerusalem, Israel
E-mail: Abeles@vms.huji.ac.il
Synfire Chains

Kazuyuki Aihara School of Engineering, University of Tokyo, Hongo, Bunkyo-ku, Japan
E-mail: aihara@sat.t.u-tokyo.ac.jp
Chaos in Neural Systems

Yehuda Albeck Bae Systems–Rokar International, Mount Hozvim, Jerusalem, Israel
E-mail: Yehuda.albeck@baesystems.com
Sound Localization and Binaural Processing

Amit Almor Department of Psychology, University of Southern California, Los Angeles, California
E-mail: almor@gizmo.usc.edu
Past Tense Learning

Shun-ichi Amari Laboratory for Mathematical Neuroscience, RIKEN Brain Science Institute, Wako-shi, Hirosawa, Saitam, Japan
Learning and Statistical Inference
Neuromanifolds and Information Geometry

Bagrat Amirikian Brain Sciences Center, Veterans Affairs Medical Center, Minneapolis, Minnesota
E-mail: amiri001@umn.edu
Motor Cortex: Coding and Decoding of Directional Operations

Daniel J. Amit Istituto di Fisica, Universitá di Roma, La Sapienza, Roma, Italia
E-mail: daniel.amit@roma1.infn.it
Cortical Hebbian Modules

Thomas J. Anastasio Beckman Institute for Advanced Science and Technology, University of Illinois at Urbana/Champaign, Urbana, Illinois
E-mail: tja@uiuc.edu
Vestibulo-Ocular Reflex

James A. Anderson Department of Cognitive and Linguistic Sciences, Brown University, Providence, Rhode Island
E-mail: JamesAnderson@brown.edu
Associative Networks

Andreas G. Andreou Department of Electrical and Computer Engineering, Johns Hopkins University, Baltimore, Maryland
E-mail: andreou@jhu.edu
Neuromorphic VLSI Circuits and Systems

Martin Anthony Department of Mathematics and Centre for Discrete and Applicable Mathematics, London School of Economics and Political Science, London, United Kingdom
E-mail: m.anthony@lse.ac.uk
PAC Learning and Neural Networks

Michael A. Arbib USC Brain Project, Computer Science and Neuroscience, University of Southern California, Los Angeles, California
E-mail: arbib@pollux.usc.edu
Backpropagation: General Principles
Language Evolution: The Mirror System Hypothesis
Neuroinformatics
Schema Theory
Visual Scene Perception, Neurophysiology

Ronald C. Arkin College of Computing, Georgia Institute of Technology, Atlanta, Georgia
E-mail: arkin@cc.gatech.edu
Reactive Robotic Systems

Jorge L. Armony Douglas Hospital Research Centre, McGill University, Montreal, Quebec, Canada
Email: jorge.armony@douglas.mcgill.ca
Emotional Circuits

Krste Asanovic MIT Laboratory for Computer Science, Massachusetts Institute of Technology, Cambridge, Massachusetts
E-mail: krste@mit.edu
Programmable Neurocomputing Systems

David Barber Division of Informatics, University of Edinburgh, Edinburgh, United Kingdom
E-mail: dbarber@anc.ed.ac.uk
Bayesian Methods and Neural Networks

José Bargas Biophysics Department, Instituto de Fisiologia Celular, Universidad Nacional Autonoma de Mexico, Mexico D. F., Mexico
E-mail: jbargas@ifcsun1.ifisiol.unam.mx
Ion Channels: Keys to Neuronal Specialization

John A. Barnden School of Computer Science, University of Birmingham, Birmingham, United Kingdom
E-mail: J.A.Barnden@cs.bham.ac.uk
Artificial Intelligence and Neural Networks
Semantic Networks

Peter L. Bartlett Department of Statistics, University of California at Berkeley, Berkeley, California
E-mail: bartlett@stat.berkeley.edu
Vapnik-Chervonenkis Dimension of Neural Nets

Andrew G. Barto Department of Computer Science, University of Massachusetts, Amherst, Massachusetts
E-mail: barto@cs.umass.edu
Reinforcement Learning
Reinforcement Learning in Motor Control

Joseph Bastian Department of Zoology, University of Oklahoma, Norman, Oklahoma
E-mail: jbastian@ou.edu
Electrolocation

Michel Baudry Department of Biological Sciences and Biomedical Engineering, University of Southern California, Los Angeles, California
E-mail: baudry@neuro.usc.edu
NMDA Receptors: Synaptic, Cellular, and Network Models

Douglas A. Baxter Department of Neurobiology and Anatomy, University of Texas Medical School at Houston, Houston, Texas
E-mail: Douglas.Baxter@uth.tmc.edu
Neurosimulation: Tools and Resources

Françoise Beaufays Speech R&D, Nuance Communications, Menlo Park, California
E-mail: francoise@nuance.com
Speech Recognition Technology

Suzanna Becker Department of Psychology, McMaster University, Hamilton, Ontario, Canada
E-mail: becker@mcmaster.ca
Unsupervised Learning with Global Objective Functions

David Beeman Department of Electrical and Computer Engineering, University of Colorado, Boulder, Colorado
E-mail: dbeeman@dogstar.colorado.edu
GENESIS Simulation System

Randall D. Beer Department of Electrical Engineering and Computer Science, Case Western Reserve University, Cleveland, Ohio
E-mail: beer@eecs.cwru.edu
Locomotion, Invertebrate

Kirk W. Beisel Boys Town National Research Hospital, Omaha, Nebraska
E-mail: beisel@boystown.org
Evolution of Genetic Networks

Anthony J. Bell Redwood Neuroscience Institute, Menlo Park, California
E-mail: tony@salk.edu
Independent Component Analysis

Samy Bengio Dalle Molle Institute for Perceptual Artificial Intelligence (IDIAP), Swiss Federal Institute of Technology, Lausanne, Switzerland
E-mail: bengio@idiap.ch
Hidden Markov Models

Yoshua Bengio Departement Informatique et Recherche Opérationnelle, Université de Montréal, Montreal, Quebec, Canada
E-mail: bengioy@iro.umontreal.ca
Convolutional Networks for Images, Speech, and Time Series
Pattern Recognition

Theodore W. Berger Department of Biomedical Engineering and Biological Sciences, University of Southern California, Los Angeles, California
E-mail: berger@bmsrs.usc.edu
NMDA Receptors: Synaptic, Cellular, and Network Models

Öjvind Bernander Division of Biology, California Institute of Technology, Pasadena, California
E-mail: ojvind@klab.caltech.edu
Axonal Modeling

William Bialek Department of Physics, Princeton University, Princeton, New Jersey
E-mail: wbialek@princeton.edu
Adaptive Spike Coding

Michael Biehl Institut für Theoretische Physik, Universität Würzburg, Würzburg, Germany
E-mail: biehl@physik.uni-wuerzburg.de
Statistical Mechanics of On-Line Learning and Generalization

Norman Biggs Department of Mathematics and Centre for Discrete and Applicable Mathematics, London School of Economics and Political Science, London, United Kingdom
E-mail: n.l.biggs@lse.ac.uk
PAC Learning and Neural Networks

Aude G. Billard Autonomous Systems Lab, Ecole Polytechnique Federale de Lausanne, Lausanne, Switzerland
E-mail: aude.billard@epfl.ch, billard@usc.edu
Imitation

David L. Boothe Neuroscience and Cognitive Science, University of Maryland, College Park, Maryland
E-mail: boothe@glue.umd.edu
Sensorimotor Interactions and Central Pattern Generators

Alexander Borst Department of Systems and Computational Neurobiology, Max-Planck-Institute of Neurobiology, Martinsried, Germany
E-mail: borst@neuro.mpg.de
Visual Course Control in Flies

Leon Bottou NEC Research Institute, Princeton, New Jersey
E-mail: leonb@research.nj.nec.com
Stochastic Approximations and Efficient Learning

Hervé Bourlard Dalle Molle Institute for Perceptual Artificial Intelligence (IDIAP), Matigny, Switzerland
E-mail: bourlard@idiap.ch
Hidden Markov Models
Speech Recognition Technology

Jean-Marie Bouteiller Department of Biological Sciences and Biomedical Engineering, University of Southern California, Los Angeles, California
E-mail: bouteiller@java.usc.edu
NMDA Receptors: Synaptic, Cellular, and Network Models

James M. Bower Research Imaging Center, University of Texas Health Science Center, and Cajal Neuroscience Research Center, University of Texas, San Antonio, Texas
E-mail: bower@uthscsa.edu
GENESIS Simulation System

Steven L. Bressler Center for Complex Systems and Brain Sciences, Florida Atlantic University, Boca Raton, Florida
E-mail: bressler@fau.edu
Event-Related Potentials

Paul C. Bressloff Department of Mathematics, University of Utah, Salt Lake City, Utah
E-mail: bressloff@math.utah.edu
Pattern Formation, Neural

Bruce Bridgeman Department of Psychology, University of California at Santa Cruz, Santa Cruz, California
E-mail: bruceb@cats.ucsc.edu
Dissociations Between Visual Processing Modes

Adam S. Bristol Department of Neurobiology and Behavior, University of California at Irvine, Irvine, California
E-mail: abristol@uci.edu
Habituation

Guy J. Brown Department of Computer Science, University of Sheffield, Sheffield, United Kingdom
E-mail: g.brown@dcs.shef.ac.uk
Auditory Scene Analysis

James T. Buchanan Department of Biological Sciences, Marquette University, Milwaukee, Wisconsin
E-mail: james.buchanan@marquette.edu
Spinal Cord of Lamprey: Generation of Locomotor Patterns

Joachim M. Buhmann Institut für Informatik III, Rheinische Friedrich-Wilhelms-Universität Bonn, Bonn, Germany
E-mail: jb@informatik.uni-bonn.de
Data Clustering and Learning
Model Validation

John A. Bullinaria School of Computer Science, University of Birmingham, Birmingham, United Kingdom
E-mail: j.bullinaria@physics.org
Lesioned Networks as Models of Neuropsychological Deficits

Daniel Bullock Cognitive and Neural Systems Department, Boston University, Boston, Massachusetts
E-mail: danb@cns.bu.edu
Competitive Queuing for Planning and Serial Performance
Motoneuron Recruitment

Heinrich H. Bülthoff Max-Planck-Institute for Biological Cybernetics, Tübingen, Germany
E-mail: heinrich.buelthoff@tuebingen.mp.de
Object Recognition, Neurophysiology

Neil Burgess Institute of Cognitive Neuroscience and Department of Anatomy, University College, London, London United Kingdom
E-mail: n.burgess@ucl.ac.uk
Hippocampus: Spatial Models

Yves Burnod INSERM U483, Université Pierre et Marie Curie, Paris, France
E-mail: ybteam@ccr.jussieu.fr
Short-Term Memory

David C. Burr Istituto di Neurofisiologia del CNR, Pisa, Italy
E-mail: dave@in.pi.cnr.it
Motion Perception: Elementary Mechanisms

Dani Byrd Department of Linguistics, University of Southern California, Los Angeles, California
E-mail: dbyrd@usc.edu
Speech Production

John H. Byrne Department of Neurobiology and Anatomy, University of Texas Medical School at Houston, Houston, Texas
E-mail: John.H.Byrne@uth.tmc.edu
Invertebrate Models of Learning: Aplysia and Hermissenda
Neurosimulation: Tools and Resources

Ronald L. Calabrese Department of Biology, Emory University, Atlanta, Georgia
E-mail: rcalabre@Biology.Emory.edu
Half-Center Oscillators Underlying Rhythmic Movements

Thomas J. Carew Department of Neurobiology and Behavior, University of California, Irvine, California
E-mail: tcarew@uci.edu
Habituation

Ted Carnevale Department of Psychology, Yale University, New Haven, Connecticut
E-mail: ted.carnevale@yale.edu
NEURON Simulation Environment

Gail A. Carpenter Department of Cognitive and Neural Systems, Boston University, Boston, Massachusetts
E-mail: gail@cns.bu.edu
Adaptive Resonance Theory

Mauro Carrozzo Human Physiology Section, IRCCS Fondazione Santa Lucia, Roma, Italia
E-mail: carrozzo@caspur.it
Limb Geometry, Neural Control

Nestor Caticha Instituto de Fisica, Universidade de Sao Paulo, Sao Paulo, Brazil
E-mail: nestor@if.usp.br
Statistical Mechanics of On-line Learning and Generalization

Francisco Cervantes-Pérez Departamento Académico de Computación, Instituto Tecnológico Autónomo de México (ITAM), Mexico D. F., Mexico
E-mail: cervante@itam.mx
Visuomotor Coordination in Frog and Toad

Lucía Cervantes Facultad de Ciencias Fisico-Matematicas, Universidad Autonoma de Puebla, Puebla, Mexico
E-mail: lcervant@fismat1.fcfm.buap.mx
Ion Channels: Keys to Neuronal Specialization

Marcin Chady School of Computer Science, University of Birmingham, Birmingham, United Kingdom
E-mail: M.Chady@cs.bham.ac.uk
Artificial Intelligence and Neural Networks

Nick Chater Department of Psychology, Institute for Applied Cognitive Science, University of Warwick, Coventry, United Kingdom
E-mail: nick.chater@warwick.ac.uk
Constituency and Recursion in Language
Speech Processing: Psycholinguistics

Gal Chechik The Interdisciplinary Center for Neural Computation, Hebrew University, Jerusalem, Israel
E-mail: ggal@cs.huji.ac.il
Hebbian Learning and Neuronal Regulation

Rama Chellappa Center for Automation Research, University of Maryland, College Park, Maryland
E-mail: rama@cfar.umd.edu
Markov Random Field Models in Image Processing

Hillel J. Chiel Biology, Neuroscience, and Biomedical Engineering Departments, Case Western Reserve University, Cleveland, Ohio
E-mail: hjc@po.cwru.edu
Locomotion, Invertebrate

Morten H. Christiansen Department of Psychology, Cornell University, Ithaca, New York
E-mail: mhc27@cornell.edu
Constituency and Recursion in Language
Language Evolution and Change
Speech Processing: Psycholinguistics

Paul Cisek Departement de Physiologie, Université de Montreal, Montreal, Quebec, Canada
E-mail: cisekp@magellan.umontreal.ca
Reaching Movements: Implications for Computational Models

Andy Clark Philosophy Department and Cognitive Science Program, Indiana University, Bloomington, Indiana
E-mail: andy@twinearth.wustl.edu
Philosophical Issues in Brain Theory and Connectionism

Dave Cliff Hewlett-Packard Labs Bristol, Bristol, United Kingdom
E-mail: dave_cliff@hp.com
Neuroethology, Computational

Avis H. Cohen Department of Biology and Neuroscience and Cognitive Science and Institute for Systems Research, University of Maryland, College Park, Maryland
E-mail: avis@isrmail.isr.umd.edu
Sensorimotor Interactions and Central Pattern Generators

James J. Collins NeuroMuscular Research Center, Boston University, Boston, Massachusetts
E-mail: jcollins@bu.edu
Gait Transitions

Barry W. Connors Department of Neuroscience, Brown University, Providence, Rhode Island
E-mail: Barry_Connors@Brown.edu
Neocortex: Chemical and Electrical Synapses

Tom Coolen Department of Mathematics, King's College, London, London, United Kingdom
E-mail: tcoolen@mth.kcl.ac.uk
Dynamics of Association and Recall

Jack D. Cowan Department of Mathematics, University of Chicago, Chicago, Illinois
E-mail: cowan@math.uchicago.edu
Pattern Formation, Neural

Francis Crepel Dept. Neurobiol et Pharmacol Synapse, Université Paris VI, Paris, France
E-mail: francis.crepel@snv.jussieu.fr
Cerebellum: Neural Plasticity

Terry Crow   Department of Neurobiology and Anatomy, University of Texas Medical School at Houston, Houston, Texas
E-mail: Terry.Crow@uth.tmc.edu
Invertebrate Models of Learning: Aplysia and Hermissenda

Holk Cruse   Abteilung für Biokybernetik und Theoretische Biologie, Universität Bielefeld, Bielefeld, Germany
E-mail: Holk.Cruse@Biologie.Uni-Bielefeld.DE
Motor Pattern Generation

Rick Dale   Department of Psychology, Cornell University, Ithaca, New York
E-mail: rad28@cornell.edu
Language Evolution and Change

Hervž Daniel   Laboratoire de Neurobiologie et Pharmacologie de la Synapse, Université Pierre et Marie Curie, Paris, France
E-mail: herve.daniel@snv.jussieu.fr
Cerebellum: Neural Plasticity

Bhaskar DasGupta   Department of Computer Science, University of Illinois at Chicago, Chicago, Illinois
E-mail: dasgupta@cs.uic.edu
Analog Neural Networks: Computational Power

John Daugman   Computer Laboratory, University of Cambridge, Cambridge, United Kingdom
E-mail: john.daugman@cl.cam.ac.uk
Gabor Wavelets and Statistical Pattern Recognition

Jules Davidoff   Goldsmiths College, University of London, London, United Kingdom
E-mail: pss01jd@gold.ac.uk
Color Perception

Andrew P. Davison   Department of Neurobiology, Yale University School of Medicine, New Haven, Connecticut
E-mail: andrew.davison@yale.edu
Olfactory Bulb

Peter Dayan   Gatsby Computational Neuroscience Unit, University College, London, London, United Kingdom
E-mail: dayan@gatsby.ucl.ac.uk
Helmholtz Machines and Sleep-Wake Learning

Jeffrey Dean   Department of Biological, Geological, and Environmental Sciences, Cleveland State University, Cleveland, Ohio
E-mail: j.dean@csuohio.edu
Motor Pattern Generation

Michel Desmurget   INSERM 534 Espace et Action, Bron, France
E-mail: desmurget@lyon151.inserm.fr
Eye-Hand Coordination in Reaching Movements

Alain Destexhe   Unite de Neurosciences Integratives et Computationnelles, CNRS, Gif-sur-Yvette, France
E-mail: destexhe@iaf.cnrs-gif.fr
Sleep Oscillations
Synaptic Interactions

Marshall Devor   Department of Cell and Animal Biology, Institute of Life Sciences, Hebrew University, Jerusalem, Israel
E-mail: marshlu@vms.huji.ac.il
Pain Networks

Stephen P. DeWeerth   School of Electrical and Computer Engineering, Georgia Institute of Technology, Atlanta, Georgia
E-mail: steve.deweerth@ece.gatech.edu
Neuromorphic VLSI Circuits and Systems

Michael Dickinson   Department of Integrative Biology, University of California at Berkeley, Berkeley, California
E-mail: flymanmd@socrates.berkeley.edu
Visual Course Control in Flies

Patsy S. Dickinson   Biology Department, Bowdoin College, Brunswick, Maine
E-mail: pdickins@bowdoin.edu
Neuromodulation in Invertebrate Nervous Systems

Thomas G. Dietterich   Department of Computer Science, Oregon State University, Corvallis, Oregon
E-mail: tgd@cs.orst.edu
Ensemble Learning

Peter Ford Dominey   Institut des Sciences Cognitives, Bron, France
E-mail: dominey@isc.cnrs.fr
Sequence Learning

Rodney Douglas   Institute of Neuroinformatics, University/ETH, Zurich, Switzerland
E-mail: rjd@ini.phys.ethz.ch
Silicon Neurons

Kenji Doya   ATR Human Information Science Laboratories, Kyoto, Japan
E-mail: doya@atr.co.jp
Recurrent Networks: Learning Algorithms

Jeng-Ren Duann   Computational Neurobiology Lab, The Salk Institute, La Jolla, California
E-mail: duann@salk.edu
Brain Signal Analysis

Jeff Dugger   Electrical and Computer Engineering, Georgia Institute of Technology, Atlanta, Georgia
E-mail: jeffd@ece.gatech.edu
Analog VLSI Implementations of Neural Networks

Edmund H. Durfee   EECS Department, University of Michigan, Ann Arbor, Michigan
E-mail: durfee@umich.edu
Multiagent Systems

Shimon Edelman   Department of Psychology, Cornell University, Ithaca, New York
E-mail: se37@cornell.edu
Object Structure, Visual Processing

Chris Eliasmith   Departments of Philosophy and Systems Design Engineering, University of Waterloo, Waterloo, Ontario, Canada
E-mail: eliasmith@uwaterloo.ca
Philosophical Issues in Brain Theory and Connectionism

Andreas Engel   Institute for Theoretical Physics, University of Magdeburg, Magdeburg, Germany
E-mail: andreas.engel@physik.uni-magdeburg.de
Statistical Mechanics of Neural Networks

Péter Érdi   Center for Complex System Studies, Kalamazoo College, and Department of Biophysics, KFKI Research Institute for Particle and Nuclear Physics, Hungarian Academy of Sciences, Budapest, Hungary
E-mail: erdi@rmki.kfki.hu; perdi@kzoo.edu
Hippocampal Rhythm Generation
Post-Hebbian Learning Algorithms

Bard Ermentrout   Department of Mathematics, University of Pittsburgh, Pittsburgh, Pennsylvania
E-mail: bard@pitt.edu
Chains of Oscillators in Motor and Sensory Systems
Dynamics and Bifurcation In Neural Nets
Phase-Plane Analysis of Neural Nets

Udo A. Ernst   Institute for Theoretical Neurophysics, University of Bremen, Bremen, Germany
E-mail: uernst@physik.uni-bremen.de
Cortical Population Dynamics and Psychophysics

Christian W. Eurich   Institute for Theoretical Neurophysics, University of Bremen, Bremen, Germany
E-mail: eurich@physik.uni-bremen.de
Cortical Population Dynamics and Psychophysics

Jorg-Peter Ewert   Department of Neurobiology, University of Kassel, Kassel, Germany
E-mail: ewert@uni-kassel.de
Command Neurons and Command Systems

Michèle Fabre-Thorpe   Centre de Recherche Cerveau et Cognition, Université Paul Sabatier, Toulouse, France
E-mail: mft@cerco.ups-tlse.fr
Fast Visual Processing

Adrienne L. Fairhall   Department of Molecular Biology, Princeton University, Princeton, New Jersey
E-mail: fairhall@princeton.edu
Adaptive Spike Coding

Martha J. Farah   Department of Psychology, University of Pennsylvania, Philadelphia, Pennsylvania
E-mail: mfarah@cattell.psych.upenn.edu
Neuropsychological Impairments

Philippe Faure   Biologie Cellulaire et Moléculaire du Neurone, Institut Pasteur, Paris, France
E-mail: phfaure@pasteur.fr
Synaptic Noise and Chaos in Vertebrate Neurons

Oleg V. Favorov   School of Electrical Engineering and Computer Science, University of Central Florida, Orlando, Florida
E-mail: favorov@cs.ucf.edu
Somatosensory System

Jean-Marc Fellous   The Salk Institute for Biological Studies, Computational Neurobiology Laboratory, La Jolla, California
E-mail: fellous@salk.edu
Dopamine, Roles of
Emotional Circuits

Eberhard E. Fetz   Department of Physiology and Biophysics and Washington National Primate Research Center, University of Washington, Seattle, Washington
E-mail: fetz@u.washington.edu
Recurrent Networks: Neurophysiological Modeling

J. Randall Flanagan   Department of Psychology, Queen's University, Kingston, Ontario, Canada
E-mail: flanagan@psyc.queensu.ca
Sensorimotor Learning

Tamar Flash   Department of Computer Science and Applied Mathematics, Weizmann Institute of Science, Rehovot, Israel
E-mail: tamar@wisdom.weizann.ac.il
Optimization Principles in Motor Control

Sherre L. Florence   Department of Psychology, Vanderbilt University, Nashville, Tennessee
E-mail: doc.phillips@comcast.net
Somatotopy: Plasticity of Sensory Maps

Peter Földiák   School of Psychology, University of St Andrews, St Andrews, United Kingdom
E-mail: Peter.Foldiak@st-andrews.ac.uk
Sparse Coding in the Primate Cortex

Carol A. Fowler   Haskins Laboratories, New Haven, Connecticut
E-mail: carol.fowler@haskins.yale.edu
Motor Theories of Perception

Andrés Fraguela   Facultad de Ciencias Físico Matemáticas, Benemérita Universidad Autónoma de Puebla, Puebla, Mexico
E-mail: fraguela@fcfm.buap.mx
Ion Channels: Keys to Neuronal Specialization

Horacio Franco   Speech Technology and Research Laboratory, SRI International, Menlo Park, California
E-mail: hef@speech.sri.com
Speech Recognition Technology

Erik Fransen   Royal Institute of Technology, Stockholm, Sweden
E-mail: erikf@nada.kth.se
Neuromodulation in Mammalian Nervous Systems

Yves Frégnac   Department of Integrative and Computational Neurosciences (UNIC) UPR CNRS, Gif-sur-Yvette, France
E-mail: Yves.Fregnac@iaf.cnrs-gif.fr
Hebbian Synaptic Plasticity

John P. Frisby   Department of Psychology, University of Sheffield, Sheffield, United Kingdom
E-mail: j.p.frisby@sheffield.ac.uk
Stereo Correspondence

Karl J. Friston   Wellcome Department of Cognitive Neurology, Institute of Neurology, London, United Kingdom
E-mail: k.friston@fil.ion.ucl.ac.uk
Statistical Parametric Mapping of Cortical Activity Patterns

Bernd Fritzsch   Department of Biomedical Sciences, Creighton University, Omaha, Nebraska
E-mail: Fritzsch@Creighton.edu
Evolution of Genetic Networks
Evolution of the Ancestral Vertebrate Brain

Kunihiko Fukushima   Katayanagi Advanced Research Laboratories, Tokyo University of Technology, Hachioji, Tokyo, Japan
E-mail: fukushima@karl.teu.ac.jp
Neocognitron: A Model for Visual Pattern Recognition

Joaquín M. Fuster   UCLA Neuropsychiatric Institute, Los Angeles, California
E-mail: joaquinf@ucla.edu
Cortical Memory
Prefrontal Cortex in Temporal Organization of Action

Fabrizio Gabbiani   Division of Neuroscience, Baylor College of Medicine, Houston, Texas
E-mail: gabbiani@bcm.tmc.edu;
Rate Coding and Signal Processing

Bruno Galantucci   Psychology Department, University of Connecticut, Storrs, Connecticut
E-mail: bruno.galantucci@uconn.edu
Motor Theories of Perception

Elvira Galarraga   Departamento de Biofísica, Instituto de Fisiología Celular, Universidad Nacional Autónoma de México, Mexico DF, Mexico
E-mail: egalarra@ifisiol.unam.mx
Ion Channels: Keys to Neuronal Specialization

Valérie Gaveau   INSERM 534 Espace et Action, Bron, France
E-mail: gaveau@lyon151.inserm.fr
Eye-Hand Coordination in Reaching Movements

Davi Geiger   Courant Institute, New York University, New York, New York
E-mail: geiger@cs.nyu.edu
Winner-Take-All Networks

Dedre Gentner   Department of Psychology, Northwestern University, Evanston, Illinois
E-mail: gentner@northwestern.edu
Analogy-Based Reasoning and Metaphor

Apostolos P. Georgopoulos   Brain Sciences Center, Veterans Affairs Medical Center, Minneapolis, Minnesota
E-mail: omega@umn.edu
Motor Cortex: Coding and Decoding of Directional Operations

Wulfram Gerstner   Laboratory of Computational Neuroscience, EPFL, Lausanne, Switzerland
E-mail: wulfram.gerstner@epfl.ch
Integrate-and-Fire Neurons and Networks

Zoubin Ghahramani   Gatsby Computational Neuroscience Unit, University College, London, London, United Kingdom
E-mail: zoubin@gatsby.ucl.ac.uk
Graphical Models: Parameter Learning

Jay R. Gibson   Center for Basic Neuroscience, University of Texas Southwestern Medical Center, Dallas, Texas
E-mail: Jay.Gibson@UTSouthwestern.edu
Neocortex: Chemical and Electrical Synapses

Simon F. Giszter   Neurobiology and Anatomy, MCPHU School of Medicine, Philadelphia, Pennsylvania
E-mail: simon@swampthing.neurobio.mcphu.edu
Motor Primitives

Leon Glass   Department of Physiology, McGill University, Montreal, Quebec, Canada
E-mail: glass@cnd.mcgill.ca
Chaos in Biological Systems

Eric Goles   Departamento de Ingeniería Matemática, Universidad de Chile, Santiago, Chile
E-mail: egoles@uchcecvm.cec.uchile.cl
Energy Functionals for Neural Networks

Geoffrey J. Goodhill   Department of Neuroscience, Georgetown University Medical Center, Washington, D.C.
E-mail: geoff@georgetown.edu
Axonal Path Finding
Development of Retinotectal Maps

Barry Gordon   Cognitive Neurology/Neuropsychology Division, Departments of Neurology and Cognitive Science, Johns Hopkins University, Baltimore, Maryland
E-mail: bgordon@jhmi.edu
Neurolinguistics

Lyle J. Graham   Unité de Neurosciences Intégratives et Computationnelles, CNRS, Gif-sur-Yvette, France
E-mail: lyle@cogni.iaf.cnrs-gif.fr
Biophysical Mechanisms in Neuronal Modeling
Biophysical Mosaic of the Neuron

Jeffrey S. Grethe   Biomedical Informatics Research Network, Department of Neurosciences, University of California, San Diego, La Jolla, California
E-mail: jgrethe@ncmir.ucsd.edu
Cerebellum and Conditioning
Databases for Neuroscience

Yosef Grodzinsky   Department of Linguistics, McGill University, Montreal, Quebec, Canada
E-mail: yosef.grodzinsky@McGill.ca
Imaging the Grammatical Brain

Stephen Grossberg   Department of Cognitive and Neural Systems, Boston University, Boston, Massachusetts
E-mail: steve@bu.edu
Adaptive Resonance Theory
Laminar Cortical Architecture in Visual Perception

Norberto M. Grzywacz   Department of Biomedical Engineering, University of Southern California, Los Angeles, California
E-mail: nmg@bmsr.usc.edu
Directional Selectivity

Emmanuel Guigon   INSERM U483, Université Pierre et Marie Curie, Paris, France
E-mail: guigon@ccr.jussieu.fr
Short-Term Memory

Anirudh Gupta   Brain Mind Institute, Ecole Polytechnique Federale de Lausanne, Lausanne, Switzerland
E-mail: anirudh.gupta@epfl.ch
Neocortex: Basic Neuron Types

Kevin Gurney   Department of Psychology, University of Sheffield, Sheffield, United Kingdom
E-mail: k.gurney@shef.ac.uk
Basal Ganglia

Robert F. Hadley   School of Computing Science, Simon Fraser University, Burnaby, British Columbia, Canada
E-mail: hadley@cs.sfu.ca
Systematicity of Generalizations in Connectionist Networks

Hermann P.J. Haken   Institute of Theoretical Physics, Center for Synergetics, University of Stuttgart, Stuttgart, Germany
E-mail: haken@theo1.physik.uni-stuttgart.de
Cooperative Phenomena

Barbara Hammer   Department of Mathematics/Computer Science, University of Osnabrück, Osnabrück, Germany
E-mail: hammer@informatik.uni-osnabrueck.de
Compositionality in Neural Systems

Dan Hammerstrom   Department of Electrical and Computer Engineering, OGI School of Science and Engineering, Beaverton, Oregon
E-mail: strom@ece.ogi.edu
Digital VLSI for Neural Networks

Paul Hasler   Electrical and Computer Engineering, Georgia Institute of Technology, Atlanta, Georgia
E-mail: phasler@ece.gatech.edu
Analog VLSI Implementations of Neural Networks

Michael E. Hasselmo   Department of Psychology, Program in Neuroscience, and Center for BioDynamics, Boston University, Boston, Massachusetts
E-mail: hasselmo@bu.edu
Neuromodulation in Mammalian Nervous Systems
Olfactory Cortex

Randall D. Hayes   Department of Neurobiology and Anatomy, University of Texas Medical School at Houston, Houston, Texas
E-mail: randall.hayes@uth.tmc.edu
Neurosimulation: Tools and Resources

Simon Haykin   McMaster University, Hamilton, Ontario, Canada
E-mail: haykin@mcmaster.ca
Kalman Filtering: Neural Implications

David Heckerman   Microsoft Research, Redmond, Washington
E-mail: heckerma@microsoft.com
Graphical Models: Structure Learning

Ralf Herbrich   Microsoft Research, Cambridge, United Kingdom
E-mail: rherb@microsoft.com
Learning and Generalization: Theoretical Bounds

John Hertz   Nordita, Copenhagen, Denmark
E-mail: hertz@nordita.dk
Computing with Attractors
Sensory Coding and Information Transmission

Andreas V. M. Herz   Institute of Theoretical Biology, Humboldt University, Berlin, Berlin, Germany
E-mail: a.herz@biologie.hu-berlin.de
Temporal Sequences: Learning and Global Analysis

Charles Heywood   Department of Psychology, University of Durham, Durham, United Kingdom
E-mail: c.a.heywood@durham.ac.uk
Color Perception

Ellen C. Hildreth   Department of Computer Science, Wellesley College, Wellesley, Massachusetts
E-mail: ehildreth@wellesley.edu
Motion Perception: Navigation

Andrew A. V. Hill   Department of Biology, Emory University, Atlanta, Georgia
E-mail: aavhill@yahoo.com
Half-Center Oscillators Underlying Rhythmic Movements

Sean Hill   Department of Psychiatry, University of Wisconsin–Madison, Madison, Wisconsin
E-mail: seanhill@wisc.edu
Thalamus

Michael Hines   Computer Science Department, Yale University, New Haven, Connecticut
E-mail: michael.hines@yale.edu
NEURON Simulation Environment

Neville Hogan   Department of Mechanical Engineering, Department of Brain and Cognitive Sciences, Massachusetts Institute of Technology, Cambridge, Massachusetts
E-mail: neville@mit.edu
Optimization Principles in Motor Control

John G. Holden   Department of Psychology, California State University, Northridge, California
E-mail: jgh62212@csun.edu
Reading

William R. Holmes   Department of Biological Sciences, Ohio University, Athens, Ohio
E-mail: holmes@ohio.edu
Dendritic Spines

Scott L. Hooper   Neuroscience Program, Ohio University, Athens, Ohio
E-mail: hooper@ohio.edu
Crustacean Stomatogastric System

Frank Hoppensteadt   Center for Systems Science and Engineering, Arizona State University, Tempe, Arizona
E-mail: fchoppen@asu.edu
Canonical Neural Models

David Horn   School of Physics and Astronomy, Tel Aviv University, Tel Aviv, Israel
E-mail: horn@neuron.tau.ac.il
Hebbian Learning and Neuronal Regulation

Barry Horwitz   Language Section, Voice, Speech and Language Branch, National Institute on Deafness and Other Communication Disorders, National Institutes of Health, Bethesda, Maryland
E-mail: horwitz@helix.nih.gov
Synthetic Functional Brain Mapping

Michael Hucka   Control and Dynamical Systems, California Institute of Technology, Pasadena, California
Email: mhucka@caltech.edu
GENESIS Simulation System

Auke Jan Ijspeert   School of Computer and Communication Sciences, Swiss Federal Institute of Technology, Lausanne, Switzerland
E-mail: auke.ijspeert@epfl.ch
Locomotion, Vertebrate

Nathan Intrator   School of Computer Science, Tel Aviv University; Institute for Brain and Neural Systems, Brown University, Providence, Rhode Island
E-mail: Nathan_Intrator@brown.edu
Competitive Learning
Information Theory and Visual Plasticity
Object Structure, Visual Processing

Laurent Itti   Computer Science, University of Southern California, Los Angeles, California
E-mail: itti@usc.edu
Visual Attention

Yuri P. Ivanenko   Human Physiology Section, IRCCS Fondazione Santa Lucia, Roma, Italia
E-mail: y.ivanenko@hsantalucia.it
Limb Geometry, Neural Control

Eugene M. Izhikevich   The Neurosciences Institute, San Diego, California
E-mail: Eugene.Izhikevich@nsi.edu
Canonical Neural Models

Robert A. Jacobs   Department of Brain and Cognitive Sciences, University of Rochester, Rochester, New York
E-mail: robbie@bcs.rochester.edu
Modular and Hierarchical Learning Systems

Marc Jeannerod   Institut des Sciences Cognitives, Lyon, France
E-mail: jeannerod@isc.cnrs.fr
Action Monitoring and Forward Control of Movements

B. Keith Jenkins   Signal and Image Processing Institute, University of Southern California, Los Angeles, California
E-mail: jenkins@sipi.usc.edu
Photonic Implementations of Neurobiologically Inspired Networks

Michael I. Jordan   Division of Computer Science and Department of Statistics, University of California at Berkeley, Berkeley, California
E-mail: jordan@cs.berkeley.edu
Graphical Models: Probabilistic Inference
Modular and Hierarchical Learning Systems

Tzyy-Ping Jung   Institute for Neural Computation, University of California, San Diego, La Jolla, California
E-mail: jung@sccn.ucsd.edu
Brain Signal Analysis

Jon H. Kaas   Department of Psychology, Vanderbilt University, Nashville, Tennessee
E-mail: jon.h.kaas@vanderbilt.edu
Somatotopy: Plasticity of Sensory Maps

Raymond T. Kado
(Deceased, May 2002)
Biophysical Mosaic of the Neuron

John F. Kalaska   Departement de Physiologie, Université de Montreal, Montreal, Quebec, Canada
E-mail: kalaskaj@ere.umontreal.ca
Reaching Movements: Implications for Computational Models

Annette Karmiloff-Smith   Neurocognitive Development Unit, Institute of Child Health, London, United Kingdom
E-mail: a.karmiloff-Smith@ich.ucl.ac.uk
Developmental Disorders

Nikola Kasabov   Knowledge Engineering and Discovery Research Institute, Auckland University of Technology, Auckland, New Zealand
E-mail: Nik.Kasabov@aut.ac.nz
Decision Support Systems and Expert Systems

Mitsuo Kawato   ATR Human Information Science Laboratories, Kyoto, Japan
E-mail: kawato@atr.co.jp
Cerebellum and Motor Control

Douglas G. Kelly   Department of Statistics, University of North Carolina, Chapel Hill, North Carolina
E-mail: dgkelly@email.unc.edu
Somatosensory System

Robert Kentridge   University of Durham, Durham, United Kingdom
E-mail: robert.kentridge.@durham.ac.uk
Color Perception

Oussama Khatib   Department of Computer Science, Stanford University, Stanford, California
E-mail: khatib@cs.stanford.edu
Potential Fields and Neural Networks

Christof Koch   Division of Biology and Division of Engineering and Applied Science, California Institute of Technology, Pasadena, California
E-mail: koch@klab.caltech.edu
Axonal Modeling
Single-Cell Models

Etienne Koechlin   INSERM U483, Université Pierre et Marie Curie, Paris, France
E-mail: koechlin@ccr.jussieu.fr
Short-Term Memory

Teuvo K. Kohonen   Neural Networks Research Centre, Helsinki University of Technology, Helsinki, Finland
E-mail: teuvo.kohonen@hut.fi
Learning Vector Quantization

Nancy Kopell   Department of Mathematics and Statistics, Boston University, Boston, Massachusetts
E-mail: nk@bu.edu
Chains of Oscillators in Motor and Sensory Systems

Henri Korn   Biologie Cellulaire et Moléculaire du Neurone, Institut Pasteur, Paris, France
E-mail: hkorn@pasteur.fr
Synaptic Noise and Chaos in Vertebrate Neurons

Jan H. M. Korst   Media Interaction, Philips Research, Eindhoven, The Netherlands
E-mail: jan.korst@philips.com
Simulated Annealing and Boltzmann Machines

Richard J. Krauzlis   The Salk Institute for Biological Studies, San Diego, California
E-mail: rich@salk.edu
Pursuit Eye Movements

Yoshiki Kuramoto   Department of Physics, Kyoto University, Kyoto, Japan
E-mail: kuramoto@scphys.kyoto-u.ac.jp
Collective Behavior of Coupled Phase Oscillators

Věra Kůrková   Institute of Computer Science, Academy of Sciences of the Czech Republic, Prague, Czech Republic
E-mail: vera@cs.cas.cz
Universal Approximators

Francesco Lacquaniti   Human Physiology Section, IRCCS Fondazione Santa Lucia, Roma, Italia
E-mail: lacquaniti@caspur.it
Limb Geometry, Neural Control

Chuck P. Lam   Department of Electrical Engineering, Stanford University, Stanford, California
E-mail: chucklam@stanford.edu
Learning Network Topology

Ning Lan   Department of Biokinesiology and Physical Therapy, University of Southern California, Los Angeles, California
E-mail: ninglan@rcf.usc.edu
Prosthetics, Motor Control

Petr Lánský   Institute of Physiology, Academy of Sciences of the Czech Republic, Prague, Czech Republic
E-mail: lansky@biomed.cas.cz
Diffusion Models of Neuron Activity

Peter E. Latham   Department of Neurobiology, University of Southern California, Los Angeles, California
E-mail: pel@ucla.edu
Population Codes

Yann LeCun   NEC Research Institute, Princeton, New Jersey
E-mail: yann@research.nj.nec.com
Convolutional Networks for Images, Speech, and Time Series Pattern Recognition

Joseph E. LeDoux   Center for Neural Science, New York University, New York, New York
E-mail: ledoux@cns.nyu.edu
Emotional Circuits

Mark G. Lee   School of Computer Science, University of Birmingham, Birmingham, United Kingdom
E-mail: M.G.Lee@cs.bham.ac.uk
Semantic Networks

Michael A. Lehr   SK Communications, Inc., Sunnyvale, California
E-mail: mlehr@skcom.com
Perceptrons, Adalines, and Backpropagation

Svetlana Levitan   SPSS Inc., Chicago, Illinois
E-mail: slevitan@spss.com
Hemispheric Interactions and Specialization

John E. Lewis   Department of Cellular and Molecular Medicine, University of Ottawa, Ottawa, Ontario, Canada
E-mail: jlewis@uottawa.ca
Respiratory Rhythm Generation

Jim-Shih Liaw   Department of Biomedical Engineering, University of Southern California, Los Angeles, California
E-mail: liaw@bmsrs.usc.edu
NMDA Receptors: Synaptic, Cellular, and Network Models

David C. Lin   Department of Biological Systems Engineering, Washington State University, Pulman, Washington
E-mail: davidlin@wsu.edu
Muscle Models

Christiane Linster   Department of Neurobiology and Behavior, Cornell University, Ithaca, New York
E-mail: cl243@cornell.edu
Olfactory Cortex

Jiming Liu   Department of Computer Science, Hong Kong Baptist University, Kowloon Tong, Hong Kong
E-mail: jiming@comp.hkbu.edu.hk
Potential Fields and Neural Networks

Gerald E. Loeb   A. E. Mann Institute for Biomedical Engineering, University of Southern California, Los Angeles, California
E-mail: gloeb@usc.edu
Prosthetics, Motor Control
Prosthetics, Neural
Prosthetics, Sensory Systems

Michael London   Department of Neurobiology, Institute of Life Sciences and the Interdisciplinary Center for Neural Computation, Hebrew University, Jerusalem, Israel
E-mail: mikilon@lobster.ls.huji.ac.il
Dendritic Processing

Fernando H. Lopes da Silva   University of Amsterdam, Kruislaan, Amsterdam, The Netherlands
E-mail: silva@science.uva.nl
EEG and MEG Analysis

David Lowe   Information Engineering, Aston University, Birmingham, United Kingdom
E-mail: d.lowe@aston.ac.uk
Radial Basis Function Networks

Jennifer S. Lund   Moran Eye Center, University of Utah, Salt Lake City, Utah
E-mail: Jennifer.Lund@hsc.utah.edu
Visual Cortex: Anatomical Structure and Models of Function

Giuseppe Luppino   Istituto di Fisiologia Umana, Università di Parma, Parma, Italia
E-mail: luppino@ipruniv.cce.unipr.it
Grasping Movements: Visuomotor Transformations

Wolfgang Maass   Institute for Theoretical Computer Science, Technische Universität Graz, Graz, Germany
E-mail: maass@igi.tu-graz.ac.at
Spiking Neurons, Computation with
Temporal Integration in Recurrent Microcircuits
Vapnik-Chervonenkis Dimension of Neural Nets

Brian MacWhinney   Department of Psychology, Carnegie Mellon University, Pittsburgh, Pennsylvania
E-mail: macw@cmu.edu
Language Acquisition

Zachary F. Mainen   Cold Spring Harbor Laboratory, Cold Spring Harbor, New York
E-mail: zach@cshl.org
Synaptic Interactions

Scott Makeig   Computational Neurobiology Lab, The Salk Institute, La Jolla, California
E-mail: scott@salk.edu
Brain Signal Analysis

Hanspeter A. Mallot   Cognitive Neuroscience, University of Tübingen, Tübingen, Germany
E-mail: hanspeter.mallot@uni-tuebingen.de
Layered Computation in Neural Networks

Eve Marder   Volen Center and Department of Biology, Brandeis University, Waltham, Massachusetts
E-mail: marder@brandeis.edu
Activity-Dependent Regulation of Neuronal Conductances

Arthur B. Markman   Department of Psychology, University of Texas at Austin, Austin, Texas
E-mail: markman@psy.utexas.edu
Analogy-Based Reasoning and Metaphor

Henry Markram   Brain Mind Institute, École Polytechnique Federale de Lausanne, Lausanne, Switzerland
E-mail: Henry.Markram@epfl.ch
Neocortex: Basic Neuron Types
Temporal Integration in Recurrent Microcircuits

Jose L. Marroquin   Center for Research in Mathematics (CIMAT), Guanajuato, Mexico
E-mail: jlm@cimat.mx
Probabilistic Regularization Methods for Low-Level Vision

Anthony Randal McIntosh   Rotman Research Institute, Toronto, Ontario, Canada
E-mail: mcintosh@psych.utoronto.ca
Covariance Structural Equation Modeling for Neurocognitive Networks

David McLaughlin   Courant Institute of Mathematical Sciences and Center for Neural Science, New York University, New York, New York
E-mail: dmac@cims.nyu.edu
Orientation Selectivity

Gérard Medioni   Computer Science Department and Institute for Robotics and Intelligent Systems, University of Southern California, Los Angeles, California
E-mail: medioni@iris.usc.edu
Tensor Voting and Visual Segmentation

Bartlett W. Mel   Biomedical Engineering Department and Neuroscience Graduate Program, University of Southern California, Los Angeles, California
E-mail: mel@usc.edu
Dendritic Learning

David K. Merwine   Department of Biomedical Engineering, University of Southern California, Los Angeles, California
E-mail: dmerwine@bmsr.usc.edu
Directional Selectivity

R. Christopher Miall   University Laboratory of Physiology, Oxford University, Oxford, United Kingdom
E-mail: chris.miall@physiol.ox.ac.uk
Motor Control, Biological and Theoretical

José del R. Millán   IDIAP, Martigny, Switzerland
E-mail: jose.millan@idiap.ch
Brain-Computer Interfaces
Robot Navigation

Kenneth D. Miller   W. M. Keck Center for Integrative Neuroscience, Sloan-Swartz Center for Theoretical Neurobiology, University of California at San Francisco, San Francisco, California
E-mail: ken@phy.ucsf.edu
Ocular Dominance and Orientation Columns

Ennio Mingolla   Department of Cognitive and Neural Systems, Boston University, Boston, Massachusetts
E-mail: ennio@cns.bu.edu
Contour and Surface Perception

Chun-Hui Mo   Division of Biology and Division of Engineering and Applied Science, California Institute of Technology, Pasadena, California
E-mail: mo@klab.caltech.edu
Single-Cell Models

Michael J. Morgan   Applied Vision Research Centre, City University, London, United Kingdom
E-mail: m.morgan@city.ac.uk
Feature Analysis

Nelson Morgan   International Computer Science Institute, Berkeley, California
E-mail: morgan@icsi.berkeley.edu
Speech Recognition Technology

Frank Moss   Center for Neurodynamics, University of Missouri at St. Louis, St. Louis, Missouri
E-mail: mossf@umsl.edu
Stochastic Resonance

David C. Mountain   Department of Biomedical Engineering, Boston University, Boston, Massachusetts
E-mail: dcm@bu.edu
Auditory Periphery and Cochlear Nucleus

Yuko Munakata   Department of Psychology, University of Colorado at Boulder, Boulder, Colorado
E-mail: munakata@psych.colorado.edu
Cognitive Development

Noboru Murata   Waseda University, Tokyo, Japan
E-mail: murata@elec.waseda.ac.jp
Stochastic Approximations and Efficient Learning

James D. Murray   Department of Applied Mathematics, University of Washington, Seattle, Washington
E-mail: murrayjd@amath.washington.edu
Pattern Formation, Biological

Ferdinando A. Mussa-Ivaldi   Department of Physiology, Northwestern University Medical School, Chicago, Illinois
E-mail: sandro@northwestern.edu
Geometrical Principles in Motor Control

Kumpati S. Narendra   Center for Systems Science, Electrical Engineering Department, Yale University, New Haven, Connecticut
E-mail: kumpati.narendra@yale.edu
Identification and Control

Sacha B. Nelson   Department of Biology and Volen Center, Brandeis University, Waltham, Massachusetts
E-mail: nelson@brandeis.edu
Temporal Dynamics of Biological Synapses

Heiko Neumann   Department of Neural Information Processing, Faculty of Computer Science, University of Ulm, Ulm, Germany
E-mail: hneumann@neuro.informatik.uni-ulm.de
Contour and Surface Perception

David C. Noelle   Department of Electrical Engineering and Computer Science, Vanderbilt University, Nashville, Tennessee
E-mail: david.noelle@vanderbilt.edu
Concept Learning

Stefano Nolfi   Institute of Cognitive Sciences and Technologies, CNR, Rome, Italy
E-mail: nolfi@ip.rm.cnr.it
Evolution and Learning in Neural Networks
Evolution of Artificial Neural Networks

Klaus Obermayer   Informatik, Technische Universität, Berlin, Germany
E-mail: oby@cs.tu-berlin.de
Visual Cortex: Anatomical Structure and Models of Function

Erkki Oja   Helsinki University of Technology, Laboratory of Computer and Information Science, Espoo, Finland
E-mail: erkki.oja@hut.fi
Principal Component Analysis

John O'Keefe   Institute of Cognitive Neuroscience and Department of Anatomy, University College, London, London, United Kingdom
E-mail: j.okeefe@ucl.ac.uk
Hippocampus: Spatial Models

Manfred Opper   Neural Computing Research Group, Aston University, Birmingham, United Kingdom
E-mail: opperm@aston.ac.uk
Statistical Mechanics of Generalization

Alice J. O'Toole   Program in Cognition and Neuroscience, University of Texas at Dallas, Richardson, Texas
E-mail: otoole@utdallas.edu
Face Recognition: Psychology and Connectionism

Thomas J. Palmeri   Department of Psychology, Vanderbilt University, Nashville, Tennessee
E-mail: thomas.j.palmeri@vanderbilt.edu
Concept Learning

Stefano Panzeri   University of Newcastle upon Tyne, Newcastle upon Tyne, United Kingdom
E-mail: stefano.panzeri@ncl.ac.uk
Sensory Coding and Information Transmission

Domenico Parisi   Institute of Cognitive Sciences and Technologies, CNR, Rome, Italy
E-mail: parisi@ip.rm.cnr.it
Evolution of Artificial Neural Networks

Judea Pearl   Computer Science Department, University of Southern California, Los Angeles, California
E-mail: judea@cs.ucla.edu
Bayesian Networks

Denis Pélisson   INSERM 534 Espace et Action, Bron, France
E-mail: pelisson@lyon151.inserm.fr
Eye-Hand Coordination in Reaching Movements

Carsten Peterson   Complex Systems Group, Department of Theoretical Physics, Lund University, Lund, Sweden
E-mail: Carsten.Peterson@thep.lu.se
Optimization, Neural

Jan Pieter Pijn
(Deceased, December 1998)
EEG and MEG Analysis

Alexandre Pouget   Department of Brain and Cognitive Sciences, University of Rochester, Rochester, New York
E-mail: alex@bcs.rochester.edu
Dynamic Remapping
Population Codes

Claude Prablanc   INSERM 534 Espace et Action, Bron, France
E-mail: prablanc@lyon151.inserm.fr
Eye-Hand Coordination in Reaching Movements

Tony J. Prescott   Department of Psychology, University of Sheffield, Sheffield, United Kingdom
E-mail: t.j.prescott@shef.ac.uk
Basal Ganglia

Angela L. Purcell   Interdepartmental Neuroscience Program, Yale University, New Haven, Connecticut; and Department of Neurobiology and Behavior, University of California at Irvine, Irvine, California
E-mail: apurcell@uci.edu
Habituation

Wilfrid Rall   NIH Scientist Emeritus, Roseland, Virginia
E-mail: condonrl@ceva.net
Dendritic Spines
Perspective on Neuron Model Complexity

Anand Rangarajan   Department of CISE, University of Florida, Gainesville, Florida
E-mail: anand@cise.ufl.edu
Markov Random Field Models in Image Processing

Christof Rasche   Division of Biology, California Institute of Technology, Pasadena, California
E-mail: rasche@klab.caltech.edu
Silicon Neurons

Peter Redgrave   Department of Psychology, University of Sheffield, Sheffield, United Kingdom
E-mail: p.redgrave@shef.ac.uk
Basal Ganglia

James A. Reggia   University of Maryland, Baltimore, Maryland
E-mail: reggia@cs.umd.edu
Hemispheric Interactions and Specialization
Neurological and Psychiatric Disorders

John E. Remmers   Heritage Medical Research Building, University of Calgary, Calgary, Alberta, Canada
E-mail: jeremmer@ucalgary.ca
Respiratory Rhythm Generation

Bradley J. Rhodes   Cognitive and Neural Systems Department, Boston University, Boston, Massachusetts
E-mail: brhodes@cns.bu.edu
Competitive Queuing for Planning and Serial Performance

Luigi M. Ricciardi   Dept. Matematica e Applicazioni, Università di Napoli Federico II, Napoli, Italia
E-mail: luigi.ricciardi@unina.it
Diffusion Models of Neuron Activity

Magnus J. E. Richardson   Laboratoire de Physique Statistique, Ecole Normale Superieure, Paris, France
E-mail: Magnus.Richardson@lps.ens.fr
Optimization Principles in Motor Control

John Rinzel   Center for Neural Science, New York University, New York, New York
E-mail: rinzel@cns.nyu.edu
Oscillatory and Bursting Properties of Neurons

Helge Ritter Faculty of Technology, Bielefeld University, Bielefeld, Germany
E-mail: helge@techfak.uni-bielefeld.de
Self-Organizing Feature Maps

Mariano Rivera Center for Research in Mathematics (CIMAT), Guanajuato, Mexico
E-mail: mrivera@cimat.mx
Probabilistic Regularization Methods for Low-Level Vision

Giacomo Rizzolatti Istituto di Fisiologia Umana, Università di Parma, Parma, Italia
E-mail: giacomo.rizzolatti@ipruniv.cce.unipr.it
Grasping Movements: Visuomotor Transformations

R. Meldrum Robertson Department of Biology, Queen's University, Kingston, Ontario, Canada
E-mail: robertm@biology.queensu.ca
Locust Flight: Components and Mechanisms in the Motor

Edmund T. Rolls University of Oxford, Oxford, United Kingdom
E-mail: edmund.rolls@psy.ox.ac.uk
Visual Scene Perception, Neurophysiology

Gerhard Roth Brain Research Institute, University of Bremen, Bremen, Germany
E-mail: gerhard.roth@uni-bremen.de
Visuomotor Coordination in Salamander

Constance S. Royden Department of Mathematics and Computer Science, College of the Holy Cross, Worcester, Massachusetts
E-mail: croyden@mathcs.holycross.edu
Motion Perception: Navigation

Eytan Ruppin School of Computer Sciences, Tel Aviv University, Tel Aviv, Israel
E-mail: ruppin@math.tau.ac.il
Hebbian Learning and Neuronal Regulation
Neurological and Psychiatric Disorders

Stuart Russell Computer Science Division, University of California at Berkley, Berkeley, California
E-mail: russell@cs.berkeley.edu
Bayesian Networks

W. Zev Rymer Sensory Motor Performance Program, Rehabilitation Institute of Chicago, Chicago, Illinois
E-mail: w-rymer@northwestern.edu
Muscle Models

Elliot Saltzman Department of Physical Therapy, Boston University, Boston, Massachusetts; and Haskins Laboratories, New Haven, Connecticut
E-mail: esaltz@bu.edu
Motor Theories of Perception
Speech Production

Thomas G. Sandercock Department of Physiology, Northwestern University, Evanston, Illinois
E-mail: sanderco@merle.acns.nwu.edu
Muscle Models

Robert L. Savoy MGH/MIT/HST Athinoula A. Martinos Center for Biomedical Imaging, Charlestown, Massachusetts
E-mail: savoy@nmr.mgh.harvard.edu
Imaging the Visual Brain

Stefan Schaal USC Computer Science and Neuroscience, University of Southern California, Los Angeles, California
E-mail: sschaal@usc.edu
Arm and Hand Movement Control
Robot Learning

Nestor A. Schmajuk Department of Psychological and Brain Sciences, Duke University, Durham, North Carolina
E-mail: nestor@acpub.duke.edu
Cognitive Maps
Conditioning

Georg Schnitger Fachbereich 20, Informatik, Universität Frankfurt, Frankfurt, Germany
E-mail: georg@thi.informatik.uni-frankfurt.de
Analog Neural Networks, Computational Power

Bernhard Schölkopf Max-Planck-Institut für Biologische Kybernetik, Tübingen, Germany
E-mail: bernhard.schoelkopf@tuebingen.mpg.de
Support Vector Machines

Almut Schüz Max-Planck-Institut für Biologische Kybernetik, Tübingen, Germany
E-mail: almut.schuez@tuebingen.mpg.de
Neuroanatomy in a Computational Perspective

Idan Segev Department of Neurobiology, Institute of Life Sciences and the Interdisciplinary Center for Neural Computation, Hebrew University, Jerusalem, Israel
E-mail: idan@lobster.ls.huji.ac.il
Dendritic Processing

Terrence J. Sejnowski The Salk Institute, La Jolla, California
E-mail: terry@salk.edu
Dynamic Remapping
Sleep Oscillations
Synaptic Interactions

H. Sebastian Seung Brain and Cognitive Sciences Department, Massachusetts Institute of Technology, Cambridge, Massachusetts
E-mail: seung@mit.edu
Amplification, Attenuation, and Integration

Reza Shadmehr Department of Biomedical Engineering, Johns Hopkins School of Medicine, Baltimore, Maryland
E-mail: reza@bme.jhu.edu
Equilibrium Point Hypothesis

Shihab A. Shamma Electrical Engineering Department and Institute for Systems Research, University of Maryland, College Park, Maryland
E-mail: sas@glue.umd.edu
Auditory Cortex

Robert Shapley Center for Neural Science, New York University, New York, New York
E-mail: shapley@cns.nyu.edu
Orientation Selectivity

Amanda J. C. Sharkey Department of Computer Science, University of Sheffield, Sheffield, United Kingdom
E-mail: amanda@dcs.shef.ac.uk
Cognitive Modeling: Psychology and Connectionism

Noel E. Sharkey Department of Computer Science, University of Sheffield, Sheffield, United Kingdom
E-mail: noel@dcs.shef.ac.uk
Cognitive Modeling: Psychology and Connectionism
Biologically Inspired Robotics

Lokendra Shastri International Computer Science Institute, Berkeley, California
E-mail: shastri@icsi.berkeley.edu
Structured Connectionist Models

Michael Shelley Courant Institute of Mathematical Sciences and Center for Neural Science, New York University, New York, New York
E-mail: shelley@cims.nyu.edu
Orientation Selectivity

Gordon M. Shepherd   Department of Neurobiology, Yale University School of Medicine, New Haven, Connecticut
E-mail: gordon.shepherd@yale.edu
Olfactory Bulb
Olfactory Cortex

Richard Shillcock   Institute for Adaptive and Neural Computation, University of Edinburgh, Edinburgh, United Kingdom
E-mail: Richard.Shillcock@ed.ac.uk
Language Processing

Larry E. Shupe   Department of Physiology and Biophysics and Washington National Primate Research Center, University of Washington, Seattle, Washington
E-mail: lshupe@u.washington.edu
Recurrent Networks: Neurophysiological Modeling

John J. Shynk   Department of Electrical and Computer Engineering, University of California at Santa Barbara, Santa Barbara, California
E-mail: shynk@ece.ucsb.edu
Filtering, Adaptive

Hava T. Siegelmann   Department of Computer Science, University of Massachusetts, Amherst, Massachusetts
E-mail: hava@cs.umass.edu
Neural Automata and Analog Computational Complexity

Wolf Singer   Max-Planck-Institute for Brain Research, Frankfurt/Main, Germany
E-mail: singer@mpih-frankfurt.mpg.de
Synchronization, Binding and Expectancy

William E. Skaggs   Arizona Research Laboratories, Division of Neural Systems, Memory, and Aging, University of Arizona, Tucson, Arizona
Rodent Head Direction System

Robert G. Smith   Department of Neuroscience, University of Pennsylvania, Philadelphia, Pennsylvania
E-mail: rob@retina.anatomy.upenn.edu
Retina

Alexander J. Smola   Machine Learning Group, Research School of Information Sciences and Engineering, Australian National University, Canberra, Australia
E-mail: Alex.Smola@anu.edu.au
Support Vector Machines

Bo Söderberg   Complex Systems Group, Department of Theoretical Physics, Lund University, Lund, Sweden
E-mail: Bo.Soderberg@thep.lu.se
Optimization, Neural

William Softky   Menlo Park, California
E-mail: bill@softky.com
Single-Cell Models

Zoltán Somogyvári   Department of Biophysics, KFKI Research Institute for Particle and Nuclear Physics, Hungarian Academy of Sciences, Budapest, Hungary
E-mail: soma@sunserv.kfki.hu
Post-Hebbian Learning Algorithms

Olaf Sporns   Department of Psychology, Indiana University, Bloomington, Indiana
E-mail: osporns@indiana.edu
Embodied Cognition

Paul S. G. Stein   Department of Biology, Washington University, St. Louis, Missouri
E-mail: stein@biology.wustl.edu
Scratch Reflex

Charles F. Stevens   The Salk Institute, La Jolla, California
E-mail: stevens@salk.edu
Synaptic Transmission

Leland S. Stone   NASA Ames Research Center, Moffett Field, California
E-mail: lee@vision.arc.nasa.gov
Pursuit Eye Movements

David G. Stork   Ricoh Innovations, Inc., Menlo Park, California
E-mail: stork@rii.ricoh.com
Learning Network Topology

Nobuo Suga   Department of Biology, Washington University, St. Louis, Missouri
E-mail: suga@biodec.wustl.edu
Echolocation: Cochleotopic and Computational Maps

Ron Sun   CECS Department, University of Missouri-Columbia, Columbia, Missouri
E-mail: rsun@cecs.missouri.edu
Hybrid Connectionist/Symbolic Systems

Roland E. Suri   Intelligent Optical Systems (IOS), Torrance, California
E-mail: rsuri@intopsys.com
Dopamine, Roles of

Krisztina Szalisznyó   Department of Biophysics, KFKI Research Institute for Particle and Nuclear Physics, The Hungarian Academy of Sciences, Budapest, Hungary
E-mail: szali@sunserv.kfki.hu
Hippocampal Rhythm Generation

M.-A. Tagamets   Neuroimaging Laboratory, Maryland Psychiatric Research Center, University of Maryland School of Medicine, Baltimore, Maryland
E-mail: mtagamet@mprc.umaryland.edu
Synthetic Functional Brain Mapping

Chi-Keung Tang   Computer Science Department, HKUST, Clear Water Bay, Hong Kong
E-mail: cktang@cs.ust.hk
Tensor Voting and Visual Segmentation

Armand R. Tanguay, Jr.   Departments of Electrical Engineering, Materials Science, and Biomedical Engineering; Neuroscience Graduate Program, University of Southern California, Los Angeles, California
E-mail: atanguay@usc.edu
Photonic Implementations of Neurobiologically Inspired Networks

John G. Taylor   King's College, London, London, United Kingdom
E-mail: john.g.taylor@kcl.ac.uk
Consciousness, Neural Models of

Michael S. C. Thomas   Neurocognitive Development Unit, Institute of Child Health, London, United Kingdom
E-mail: mthomas@ich.ucl.ac.uk
Developmental Disorders

Richard F. Thompson   Department of Psychology and Neuroscience Program, University of Southern California, Los Angeles, California
E-mail: thompson@neuro.usc.edu
Cerebellum and Conditioning

Simon J. Thorpe   Centre de Recherche Cerveau et Cognition, Université Paul Sabatier, Toulouse, France
E-mail: thorpe@cerco.ups-tlse.fr
Fast Visual Processing
Localized Versus Distributed Representations

Bosco S. Tjan   Psychology and Neuroscience Graduate Program, University of Southern California, Los Angeles, California
E-mail: btjan@usc.edu
Object Recognition

James T. Todd Department of Psychology, Ohio State University, Columbus, Ohio
E-mail: Todd.44@osu.edu
Perception of Three-Dimensional Structure

Maria Toledo-Rodriguez Brain Mind Institute, Ecole Polytechnique Federale de Lausanne, Lausanne, Switzerland
E-mail: Maria.Toledo@epfl.ch
Neocortex: Basic Neuron Types

Giulio Tononi Department of Psychiatry, University of Wisconsin–Madison, Madison, Wisconsin
E-mail: gtononi@wisc.edu
Thalamus

Carme Torras Institut de Robotica i Informatica Industrial (CSIC-UPC), Barcelona, Spain
E-mail: ctorras@iri.upc.es
Robot Arm Control

David S. Touretzky Computer Science Department and Center for the Neural Basis of Cognition, Carnegie Mellon University, Pittsburgh, Pennsylvania
E-mail: dst@cs.cmu.edu
Connectionist and Symbolic Representations
Rodent Head Direction System

Claude F. Touzet Laboratoire de Neurobiologie Humaine, University of Provence, Marseille, France
E-mail: touzetc@up.univ-mrs.fr
Q-Learning for Robots

Lyle H. Ungar Department of Computer and Information Science, University of Pennsylvania, Philadelphia, Pennsylvania
E-mail: ungar@cis.upenn.edu
Forecasting

J. A. M. Van Gisbergen Department of Biophysics, University of Nijmegen, Nijmegen, The Netherlands
E-mail: vangisbergen@mbfys.kun.nl
Collicular Visuomotor Transformations for Gaze Control

Stephen D. Van Hooser Department of Biology, Emory University, Atlanta, Georgia
E-mail: vanhoosr@brandeis.edu
Half-Center Oscillators Underlying Rhythmic Movements

John Darrell Van Horn Dartmouth Brain Imaging Center/Center for Cognitive Neuroscience, Dartmouth College, Hanover, New Hampshire
E-mail: John.D.Van.Horn@dartmouth.edu
Imaging the Motor Brain

John Van Opstal Department of Biophysics, University of Nijmegen, Nijmegen, The Netherlands
E-mail: johnvo@mbfys.kun.nl
Collicular Visuomotor Transformations for Gaze Control

Guy C. Van Orden Department of Psychology, Arizona State University, Tempe, Arizona
E-mail: guy.van.orden@asu.edu
Reading

José M. Vidal CSE Department, University of South Carolina, Columbia, South Carolina
E-mail: vidal@sc.edu
Multiagent Systems

Manuela Viezzer School of Computer Science, University of Birmingham, Birmingham, United Kingdom
E-mail: M.Viezzer@cs.bham.ac.uk
Semantic Networks

Philippe Vindras University of Geneva, Geneva, Switzerland
E-mail: vindras@pse.unige.ch
Eye-Hand Coordination in Reaching Movements

Horatiu Voicu Department of Psychological and Brain Sciences, Duke University, Durham, North Carolina
E-mail: hv2@acpub.duke.edu
Cognitive Maps

Christoph von der Malsburg Institut für Neuroinformatik, Ruhr-University Bochum, Bochum, Germany; and Computer Science Department, University of Southern California, Los Angeles, California
E-mail: malsburg@ruhr-uni-bochum.de
Dynamic Link Architecture
Self-Organization in the Brain

Grace Wahba Department of Statistics, University of Wisconsin, Madison, Wisconsin
E-mail: wahba@stat.wisc.edu
Generalization and Regularization in Nonlinear Learning Systems

Guy Wallis Perception and Motor Systems Lab, School of Human Movement Studies, University of Queensland, St. Lucia, Australia
E-mail: gwallis@hms.uq.edu.au
Object Recognition, Neurophysiology

David L. Waltz NEC Research Institute, Princeton, New Jersey
E-mail: waltz@research.nj.nec.com
Memory-Based Reasoning

DeLiang Wang Department of Computer and Information Science, Ohio State University, Columbus, Ohio
E-mail: dwang@cis.ohio-state.edu
Temporal Pattern Processing
Visual Scene Segmentation

Xiao-Jing Wang Center for Complex Systems, Brandeis University, Waltham, Massachusetts
E-mail: xjwang@brandeis.edu
Oscillatory and Bursting Properties of Neurons

Yun Wang Section of Neurobiology, Yale University School of Medicine, New Haven, Connecticut
E-mail: yun.wang@yale.edu
Neocortex: Basic Neuron Types

Alan G. Watts Program in Neuroscience, University of Southern California, Los Angeles, California
E-mail: watts@usc.edu
Motivation

Allen M. Waxman Cognitive and Neural Systems, Boston University, Boston, Massachusetts
E-mail: waxman@cns.bu.edu
Sensor Fusion

Yair Weiss School of Computer Science and Engineering, Hebrew University, Jerusalem, Israel
E-mail: yweiss@cs.huji.ac.il
Graphical Models: Probabilistic Inference

Alfredo Weitzenfeld Departamento Académico de Computación, Instituto Tecnológico Autónomo de México (ITAM), México D.F., México
E-mail: alfredo@itam.mx
NSL Neural Simulation Language

Bernard Widrow Department of Electrical Engineering, Stanford University, Stanford, California
E-mail: widrow@isl.stanford.edu
Perceptrons, Adalines, and Backpropagation

Frances Wilkinson Centre for Vision Research, York University, Toronto, Ontario, Canada
E-mail: franw@yorku.ca
Global Visual Pattern Extraction

Chris K. I. Williams   Division of Informatics, University of Edinburgh, Edinburgh, United Kingdom
E-mail: c.k.i.williams@ed.ac.uk
Gaussian Processes

Robert C. Williamson   Research School of Information Sciences and Engineering, Australian National University, Canberra, Australia
E-mail: Bob.Williamson@anu.edu.au
Learning and Generalization: Theoretical Bounds

Blake Wilson   Research Triangle Institute, Research Triangle Park, North Carolina
E-mail: bsw@rti.org
Prosthetics, Sensory Systems

Hugh R. Wilson   Centre for Vision Research, York University, Toronto, Ontario, Canada
E-mail: hrwilson@yorku.ca
Global Visual Pattern Extraction

Matthew A. Wilson   Department of Brain and Cognitive Science, Massachusetts Institute of Technology, Cambridge, Massachusetts
E-mail: wilson@ai.mit.edu
Olfactory Cortex

Richard J. A. Wilson   Department of Medical Physiology and Biophysics, University of Calgary, Calgary, Alberta, Canada
E-mail: wilsonr@ucalgary.ca
Respiratory Rhythm Generation

Richard Woesler   Institute of Transport Research, German Aerospace Center, Berlin, Germany
E-mail: richard.woesler@dlr.de
Visuomotor Coordination in Salamander

Daniel M. Wolpert   Institute of Neurology, University College, London, London, United Kingdom
E-mail: wolpert@hera.ucl.ac.uk
Sensorimotor Learning

Cai Zhi Wu   Department of Neurobiology, Weizmann Institute for Science, Rehovot, Israel
E-mail: bnczwu@wicc.weizmann.ac.il
Neocortex: Basic Neuron Types

Rolf P. Würtz   Institut für Neuroinformatik, Ruhr-Universität Bochum, Bochum, Germany
E-mail: Rolf.Wuertz@neuroinformatik.ruhr-uni-bochum.de
Face Recognition: Neurophysiology, and Neural Technology

Bradley P. Wyble   Harvard University, Cambridge, Massachusetts
E-mail: wyble@mind.bu.edu
Neuromodulation in Mammalian Nervous Systems

Lei Xu   Department of Computer Science and Engineering, Chinese University of Hong Kong, Shatin, Hong Kong
E-mail: lxu@cse.cuhk.edu.hk
Ying-Yang Learning

Alan L. Yuille   Departments of Psychology and Statistics, University of California at Los Angeles, Los Angeles, California
E-mail: yuille@stat.ucla.edu
Winner-Take-All Networks

Myrka Zago   Human Physiology Section, IRCCS Fondazione Santa Lucia, Roma, Italia
E-mail: m.zago@hsantalucia.it
Limb Geometry, Neural Control

Richard S. Zemel   Department of Computer Science, University of Toronto, Toronto, Ontario, Canada
E-mail: zemel@cs.toronto.edu
Minimum Description Length Analysis
Unsupervised Learning with Global Objective Functions

Li Zhaoping   Department of Psychology, University College, London, London, United Kingdom
E-mail: z.li@ucl.ac.uk
Optimal Sensory Encoding

Yongling Zhu   The Salk Institute, La Jolla, California
E-mail: yzhu@smtp.salk.edu
Synaptic Transmission

Annette Zippelius   Institute for Theoretical Physics, University of Göttingen, Göttingen, Germany
E-mail: annette@theorie.physik.uni-goettingen.de
Statistical Mechanics of Neural Networks

Kie Zuraw   Department of Linguistics, University of Southern California, Los Angeles, California
E-mail: kie@ucla.edu
Optimality Theory in Linguistics

Index